PFENNINGER & FOWLER'S
Procedures *for* Primary Care

FOURTH EDITION

EDITOR IN CHIEF
GRANT C. FOWLER, MD

Professor and Chair
Department of Family and Community Medicine
TCU/UNT Medical School and John Peter Smith Hospital
Fort Worth, Texas

SECTION EDITORS

BETH A. CHOBY, MD, FAAFP
Associate Professor
Department of Medical Education
College of Medicine
University of Tennessee Health Sciences Center
Associate Professor
UT Jackson Medical Residency Program
Jackson, Tennessee

DEEPA IYENGAR, MD, MPH
Professor and Medical Director
Department of Family and Community Medicine
UT Health McGovern Medical School
Houston, Texas

THEODORE X. O'CONNELL, MD
Program Director
Residency Director
Kaiser Permanente
Napa-Solano, California

FRANCIS G. O'CONNOR, MD, MPH
Medical Director
Consortium for Health and Military Performance
Military and Emergency Medicine
Uniformed Services University of the Health Sciences
Bethesda, Maryland

BAL REDDY, MD
Assistant Professor
Predoctoral Director
Department of Family and Community Medicine
UT Health McGovern Medical School
Houston, Texas

GRAHAM V. SEGAL, MD
Assistant Professor
Family Medicine
UT Health McGovern Medical School
Houston, Texas

YU WAH, MD, FAIHM, ABIHM
Assistant Professor
Department of Family and Community Medicine
UT Health McGovern Medical School
Houston, Texas

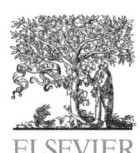

ELSEVIER

PFENNINGER & FOWLER'S PROCEDURES FOR PRIMARY CARE,
FOURTH EDITION

ISBN: 978-0-323-47633-1

Notice

Practitioners and researchers must always rely on their own experience and knowledge in evaluating and using any information, methods, compounds or experiments described herein. Because of rapid advances in the medical sciences, in particular, independent verification of diagnoses and drug dosages should be made. To the fullest extent of the law, no responsibility is assumed by Elsevier, authors, editors or contributors for any injury and/or damage to persons or property as a matter of products liability, negligence or otherwise, or from any use or operation of any methods, products, instructions, or ideas contained in the material herein.

Previous editions copyrighted 2011, 2003, 1994 by Mosby, Inc., an affiliate of Elsevier, Inc.

Library of Congress Control Number: 2018944863

Content Strategist: Sarah Barth
Senior Content Development Specialist: Dee Simpson
Publishing Services Manager: Catherine Jackson
Senior Project Manager/Specialist: Carrie Stetz
Design Direction: Renee Duenow

Printed in Canada

Last digit is the print number: 9   8   7   6   5   4   3

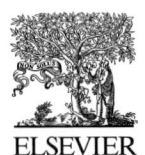

1600 John F. Kennedy Blvd.
Ste. 1600
Philadelphia, PA 19103-2899

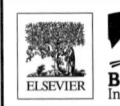

Working together
to grow libraries in
developing countries

www.elsevier.com • www.bookaid.org

As they should have been, the first three editions were dedicated to our families, friends, and colleagues. They both inspired and tolerated us through this process, again and again. Likewise, this edition is dedicated to them.

Special thanks to the faculty, staff, and residents of two different Departments of Family and Community Medicine in Texas for both contributing to and being supportive of this edition.

This book is also dedicated to primary care clinicians who continue to practice "full-scope" family medicine. It is dedicated to those who continue to practice in our current healthcare system as it evolves further, even if we are sometimes just considered a "provider." Many of us now take care of patients in a patient-centered medical home, but our patients still need procedures and appreciate those provided by primary care clinicians. Performing such procedures not only remains a fun part of our practice, but it may also improve our metrics. My prediction persists that patient outcomes and satisfaction as well as healthcare systems will continue to be enhanced when as many procedures as possible are provided by primary care clinicians.

CONTRIBUTORS

Suraj Achar, MD
Associate Clinical Professor, Associate Director of Sports Medicine, University of California–San Diego, San Diego, CA

Christopher F. Adams, MD, MBA
Fellow of Sports Medicine, University of Missouri–Kansas City, Kansas City, MO

Olasunkanmi W. Adeyinka, MD
Assistant Professor, Department of Family and Community Medicine, University of Texas Medical School at Houston; Medical Director, UT Physicians–Family Medicine, Houston, TX

Scott Akin, MD
Medical Staff, Contra Costa Regional Medical Center, Martinez, CA

Haneef Alibhai, MD, CM, CCFP, FCFP
Medical Director, MD Cosmetic & Laser Clinic, Abbotsford, Vancouver, BC, Canada

Philip J. Aliotta, MD, MSHA, FACS, CPI
Chief of Urology, Sisters of Charity Hospitals; Attending, Department of Urology, School of Biomedical Sciences and Medicine, SUNY–Buffalo; Attending and Director of Pelvic Floor Disorders and Neurogenic Bladder, Jacobs Neurologic Institute, Buffalo General Hosptial, Buffalo, NY; Instructor of Urology, New York Osteopathic Medicine, New York, NY; Instructor of Urology Lake Erie College of Osteopathic Medicine, Erie, PA

Michael A. Altman, MD
Associate Professor, Department of Family and Community Medicine, University of Texas Medical School at Houston, Houston, TX

Gerald A. Amundsen, MD
Faculty, Great Plains Family Medicine Residency, Oklahoma City; Physician, Mustang Family Practice, Mustang, OK

John J. Andazola, MD
Program Director, The Southern New Mexico Family Medicine Residency Program, Las Cruces, NM

Fatih Arikan, DDS, PhD
Associate Professor, Department of Periodontology, Ege University School of Dentistry, Bornova, Izmir, Turkey

K.M.R. Arnold, MD
Assistant Clinical Professor, Department of Family Medicine, University of Indiana, Indianapolis, IN

Darrin Ashbrooks, MD
Department of Family Medicine, University of Arkansas for Medical Science AHEC–Southwest, Texarkana, AR; Department of Sports Medicine, University of Kansas City–Missouri School of Medicine, Kansas City, MO

Barry Auster, MD
Clinical Instuctor of Dermatology, Michigan State University, East Lansing; Chair of Dermatology, Sinai-Grace, Detroit; Department of Dermatology, William Beaumont Hospital, Royal Oak, MI

Dennis E. Babel, PhD, HCLD (ABB)
Laboratory Director, Mycology Consultants Laboratory, Holland, MI

Thad J. Barkdull, MD, FAAFP, CAQSM
Clinical Assistant Professor, Department of Family Medicine, John A. Burns School of Medicine, University of Hawaii; Director of Sports Medicine, Family Medicine Residency, Tripler Army Medical Center, Honolulu, HI

Andy S. Barnett, MD
Clinical Instructor, Department of Family Medicine, University of Washington and Madigan Army Medical Center, Tacoma; Staff Physician, Department of Emergency Medicine, Jefferson General Hospital, Port Townsend, WA

Rebecca Beach, MD
Residency Faculty, Mercy Health System Family Medicine Residency; Family Physician, Mercy Clinic South, Janesville, WI; Clinical Assistant Professor, University of Wisconsin–Madison, Madison, WI

Jennifer Bell, MD
Clinical Instructor, Departments of Family and Preventive Medicine, University of Utah, Salt Lake City, UT

J. Michael Berry, MD
Associate Clinical Professor of Medicine, Division of Hematology–Oncology, University of California–San Francisco; Associate Director of HPV–Related Clinical Studies, UCSF Helen Diller Family Comprehensive Cancer Center, San Francisco, CA

Christopher J. Bigelow, MD
Ophthalmologist, MidMichigan Medical Center, Midland, MI

Lee I. Blecher, MD
Assistant Clinical Professor of Family Medicine, Virginia Commonwealth University School of Medicine; Fairfax Family Medicine, Fairfax, VA

David T. Bortel, MD, ABOS
Staff Orthopedic Surgeon–Joint Replacements, MidMichigan Medical Center, Midland, MI

David B. Bosscher, DO, FAAFP
Staff, Allegan General Hospital, Allegan, MI

Jason P. Brewington, MD
Vice Chairman of Academic Family Medicine, John Peter Smith Hospital Family Medicine Residency Program, Forth Worth, TX

Gregory L. Brotzman, MD
Professor of Family and Community Medicine, Medical College of Wisconsin, Milwaukee, WI

Mary Beth Brown, PT, ATC, PhD
Postdoctoral Fellow, Pulmonary and Critical Care, Department of Medicine, Indiana University School of Medicine, Indianapolis, IN

Gregory A. Buford, MD, FACS
Board Certified Plastic Surgeon; Fellowship Trained Cosmetic Surgeon; Founder and Medical Director, Beauty by Buford, Englewood, CO

Christian Burton, MD
Assistant Professor, Department of Family and Community Medicine, Geriatrics, UNT Health Science Center and John Peter Smith Hospital, Fort Worth, TX

Dan F. Casey, MD
Program Director, Family Medicine Residency Program, John Peter Smith Hospital, Fort Worth, TX

Richard Castillo, DO, OD
Clinical Professor, College of Optometry, Northeastern State University; Ophthalmologist, Tahlequah City Hospital, Tahlequah, OK

Jonathan Chan, DO
Associate Physician, Department of Family Medicine, Kaiser Permanente, Southern California Permanente Medical Group, San Diego, CA

C. Mark Chassay, MD, MEd, MBA
Senior Vice Provost, Chief Clinical Officer, University of North Texas Health Science Center, Fort Worth, TX

Marisha Chilcott, MD
Staff Physician, Contra Costa Regional Medical Center, Martinez, CA; Santa Rosa Memorial Hospital, Santa Rosa, CA

Beth A. Choby, MD, FAAFP
Associate Professor, Department of Medical Education, College of Medicine, University of Tennessee Health Sciences Center; Associate Professor, UT Jackson Medical Residency Program, Jackson, Tennessee

Ashley Christiani, MD
Adjunct Clinical Professor, University of California–San Francisco School of Medicine, San Francisco; Adjunct Clinical Professor, College of Osteopathic Medicine, Touro University; Senior Physician, The Permanente Medical Group–Kaiser Vallejo Hospital, Vallejo, CA

Wendy C. Coates, MD
Professor of Medicine and Chair of Acute Care College, UCLA Geffen School of Medicine, Los Angeles; Director of Medical Education, Department of Emergency Medicine, Harbor–UCLA Medical Center, Torrance, CA

Andrew S. Coco, MD, MS
Private Practice, Family Medicine, Lancaster, PA

Nnyekaa Collins, MD
Assistant Professor, Department of Family and Community Medicine, Geriatrics, UNT Health Science Center and John Peter Smith Hospital, Fort Worth, TX

Gregory Costello, MD
Medical Director, RejuviSkin Medical Spa, Verona, NJ

Kevin Crawford, RN, PA, FNP
Owner/Director, Arizona Laser Skin Solutions, Tempe, AZ

Jacob Curtis, DO
Adjunct Assistant Professor of Primary Care, Department of Family Medicine, A.T. Sill University of Health Sciences, Kirksville, MI; Family Physician, Department of Family Medicine, Franklin County Medical Center, Preston, ID; Adjunct Assistant Professor of Primary Care, Department of Family Medicine, Touro University, Nevada College of Osteopathic Medicine, Las Vegas, NV

Paul W. Davis, MD
Associate Clinical Professor of Family Medicine, University of Washington School of Medicine, Seattle, WA; Director of GI Endoscopy, Kanakanak Hospital, Bristol Bay Area Health Corporation, Dillingham, AK

Daniel J. Derksen, MD
Associate Vice President for Health Equity, Outreach and Interprofessional Activities, University of Arizona Health Sciences Center; Professor of Public Health in the Community, Environment and Policy Department, Mel and Enid Zuckerman College of Public Health, Tucson, AZ

Carlos A. Dumas, MD
Assistant Professor, Department of Family and Community Medicine, UT Health McGovern Medical School, Houston, TX

Scott W. Eathorne, MD
Medical Director, Providence Athletic Medicine, Providence Hospital, Southfield, MI

John Eckhold, MD
Staff Physician, Department of Orthopedics, MidMichigan Medical Center, Midland, MI

Steven H. Eisinger, MD, FACOG
Clinical Professor of Family Medicine and Obstetrics and Gynecology, University of Rochester School of Medicine and Dentistry, Rochester, NY

William Ellert, MD, MSN
Clinical Associate Professor, University of Arizona College of Medicine; Chief Medical Officer, Phoenix Baptist Hospital, Phoenix, AZ

Tricia C. Elliott, MD, FAAFP
Vice President, Academic Affairs and Research, Chief Academic Officer and Designated Institutional Official, John Peter Smith Health Network; Professor, Department of Family Medicine, Texas Christian University/University of North Texas Health Science Center School of Medicine, Fort Worth, TX

Mel Elson, AB, MD
Director, Longevity Institute, LLC; CEO, Global Cosmeceutical Innovations, LLC, Nashville, TN

William Jackson Epperson, MD, MBA
Director, Inlet Medical Associates, PA, Murrells Inlet, SC

Joe Esherick, MD, FAAFP
Clinical Associate Professor of Family Medicine, David Geffen UCLA School of Medicine, Los Angeles; Director of Inpatient Medical Services, Ventura County Medical Center, Ventura, CA

Azadeh Esmaeili, MD
Health Science Center, SUNYStony Brook, Stony Brook, NY

Linda Fanelli, RNC, RDMS
Registered Diagnostic Medical Sonographer, Covenant Medical Center, Saginaw, MI

Steven Fettinger, MD, FACOG, FACS
Associate Clinical Professor, College of Human Medicine and Behavioral Sciences, Michigan State University, East Lansing; Attending Physician at Covenant Medical Center and St. Mary's Medical Center, Saginaw, MI

Jeremy Fish, MD
Assistant Clinical Professor, Department of Community and Family Medicine, University of California–Davis; Residency Director, Contra Costa Family Medicine Residency Program, Martinez, CA

David Flinders, MD
Adjunct Assistant Professor, University of Utah College of Medicine, Salt Lake City; Assistant Residency Director, Utah Valley Family Medicine Residency, Provo, UT

Stuart Forman, MD
Attending Physician; Medical Director, Critical Care Unit, Contra Costa Regional Medical Center, Martinez, CA

Grant C. Fowler, MD
Professor and Chair, Department of Family and Community Medicine, TCU/UNT Medical School and John Peter Smith Hospital, Fort Worth, TX

Dan B. French, MD
Cleveland Clinic, Cleveland, OH

Roberta E. Gebhard, DO
Assistant Clinical Professor, SUNY–Buffalo, Buffalo, NY

Jeffrey A. German, MD
Associate Professor of Clinical Family Medicine, Louisiana State University Health Sciences Center, Shreveport, LA

Vincent C. Giampapa, MD, FACS
Assistant Clinical Professor, Department of Plastic and Reconstructive Surgery, University of Medicine and Dentistry of New Jersey, Newark; Attending Physician, Department of Plastic Surgery, Hackensack University Medical Center, Hackensack, NJ

Emily Godfrey, MD, MPH
Assistant Professor of Family Medicine and of Community Health Sciences, University of Illinois–Chicago College of Medicine and School of Public Health; Stroger Hospital of Cook County, Chicago, IL

Mitchel P. Goldman, MD
Volunteer Clinical Professor of Dermatology/Medicine, University of California–San Diego, San Diego, CA

Dolores M. Gomez, MD
Assistant Director, Advanced Hospital Training Fellowship for Family Physicians, Maricopa Integrated Health Systems, Phoenix, AZ

Jennifer L. Good, MD
Associate Director, Altoona Family Physicians Family Medicine Residency, Altoona; Clinical Assistant Professor of Family and Community Medicine, Milton S. Hershey Medical School, Penn State University, Hershey, PA

Ian M. Gralnek, MD, MSHS, FASGE
Associate Professor of Medicine, Rappaport Faculty of Medicine, Technion-Israel Institute of Technology; Chief, Hospital-wide Ambulatory Care Services; Senior Physician, Department of Gastroenterology; Rambam Health Care Campus, Haifa, Israel

Lee A. Green, MD, MPH
Emeritus Professor of Family Medicine, University of Michigan, Ann Arbor, MI

Maury J. Greenberg, MD, CAPT, MC, USPHS
Adjunct Associate Professor of Family Medicine, Uniformed Services University of the Health Sciences, Bethesda, MD; Clinical Associate Professor of Family Medicine, Stony Brook University School of Medicine, Stony Brook, NY

Peter W. Grigg, MD
Colorado Springs, CO

Stephen A. Grochmal, MD
Associate Clinical Professor, Division of Minimally Invasive Surgery; Adjunct Faculty, Department of Obstetrics and Gynecology, Howard University College of Medicine, Washington, DC; Medical Director, Center for Minimally Invasive Gynecologic Surgery and Cosmetic Gynecology, Paramus, NJ

Mark S. Grubb, MD
Associate Clinical Professor of Pediatrics, University of Washington, Seattle; Clinical Staff, Good Samaritan Hospital, Puyallup, WA

Sylvana Guidotti, MD, FACEP
Director of Emergency Department, Ventura County Medical Center, Ventura, CA

Ali Gürkan, DDS, PhD
Assistant Professor, Department of Periodontology, Ege University School of Dentistry, Bornova, Izmir, Turkey

Patrick J. Haddad, JD
Member, Kerr, Russell and Weber, PLC, Detroit, MI

Lesca Hadley, MD
Assistant Professor and Geriatric Fellowship Director, Department of Family and Community Medicine, UNT Health Science Center and John Peter Smith Hospital, Fort Worth, TX

Kim Haglund, MD
Staff Physician, Departments of Family Medicine and Surgery, Contra Costa Regional Medical Center, Martinez, CA

Michael A. Hansen, MD
Clinical Research Fellow, Department of Family and Community Medicine, Baylor College of Medicine, Houston, TX

Basil M. Hantash, MD, PhD
Chair, Elixir Institute for Regenerative Medicine, San Jose, CA

Michael B. Harper, MD
Professor and Chair, Department of Family Medicine, Louisiana State University Health Sciences Center, Shreveport, LA

George D. Harris, MD
Professor of Medicine, Department of Community and Family Medicine; Assistant Dean, Year 1 and 2 Medicine, University of Missouri–Kansas City School of Medicine; Medical Staff, Truman Medical Center–Lakewood, Kansas City, MO

Rebecca H. Hart, MD
Private Practice, League City, TX

Andrew Thomas Haynes, MD
Private practice, Bossier, LA

John Harlan Haynes III, MD, MSc, CPE
Associate Professor, Department of Family and Community Medicine, TCU/UNT Medical School and John Peter Smith Hospital, Fort Worth, TX

Yves Hébert, MD
President, Canadian Association of Aesthetic Medicine, Vancouver, British Columbia, Canada

Harold H. Hedges III, MD
Associate Clinical Professor, Department of Community and Family Medicine, University of Arkansas School of Medicine; Staff, Arkansas Baptist and St. Vincent Hospitals, Little Rock, AR

Scott T. Henderson, MD
Program Director, Mercy Family Medicine Residency, Mercy Medical Center–North Iowa, Mason City, IA

John Hill, DO
Professor of Family Medicine and Sports Medicine; Director of Primary Care Sports Medicine, University of Colorado Health Sciences Center, Denver, CO

John R. Holman, MD, MPH
Officer in Charge, Naval Branch Clinic, Bridgeport, CA

Karl S. Hubach, MD, RVT
Inlet Vein Specialists, PC, Murrells Inlet, SC

Gini Ikwuezunma, MD, MSCR
Department of Obstetrics and Gynecology, University of Tennessee, Memphis, TN

Deepa A. Iyengar, MD
Professor and Medical Director, Department of Family and Community Medicine, UT Health McGovern Medical School, Houston, TX

James L. Jackson, MD, FACS
MidMichigan Medical Center–Midland, Midland, MI

Marjon B. Jahromi, DDS
Assistant Professor, Department of Dental Anesthesiology, Loma Linda University School of Dentistry; Attending Anesthesiologist, Special Care Dentistry Clinic, Loma Linda University, Loma Linda, CA

David James, MD, FCFP(EM)
Clinical Associate Professor, SUNY–Buffalo School of Medicine and Biomedical Sciences; Director, Emergency Department, Millard Fillmore Gates Circle Hospital, Attending Physician, Emergency Department, Valeida Health System, Buffalo, NY; Attending Physician, Emergency Department, Niagara Health System, Welland, Ontario, Canada

Robert E. James, MD
Urologist, Sutter Pacific Medical Foundation; Sutter Medical Group of the Redwoods; Sutter Medical Center of Santa Rosa; Santa Rosa, CA

Raymond F. Jarris Jr, MD
Medical Director, Emergency Department; Assistant Chief, Emergency Medicine, Swedish Medical Center/Ballard, Seattle, WA

Naomi Jay, RN, PhD
Nurse Practioner, Dysplasia Clinic, University of California–San Francisco, San Francisco, CA

Robert L. Kalb, MD
Associate Professor, Medical College of Ohio; St. Anne Hospital, Toledo, OH

Bernard Katz, MD
Co-Chief Executive Officer, Santa Monica Bay Physicians Health Services, Inc., Santa Monica, CA

Barbara F. Kelly, MD
Associate Professor, Department of Family Medicine, University of Colorado–Denver; Medical Director, A.F. Williams Family Medicine Center, Denver, CO

Morteza Khodaee, MD, MPH
Assistant Professor, Department of Family Medicine, University of Colorado–Denver School of Medicine, Denver, CO

Yong Sik Kim, MD, PhD
Assistant Professor, Baylor College of Medicine; Green Health Clinic, Houston, TX

Thomas A. Kintanar, MD
Clinical Associate Professor, Department of Medicine, Indiana University School of Medicine; Director of Medical Education, St. Joseph Hospital, Fort Wayne, IN

Mark A. Koch, MD, FAAFP
Director of Family Medicine Endoscopy, JPS Health Network, Fort Worth, TX

Karyn B. Kolman, MD
Faculty, Maricopa Medical Center, Phoenix, AZ

Donna A. Landen, MD
Assistant Professor, International Family Medicine, University of Virginia School of Medicine, Charlottesville, VA

Dennis LaRavia, MD, FAAFP
Medical Director, Rayburn Correctional Center, Angie, LA; Director, Occupational Health, Temple-Inland Paper Co., Bogalusa, LA

Mark Lavallee, MD, CSCS, FACSM
Assistant Clinical Professor, Indiana University–South Bend School of Medicine; Co-Director, South Bend Sports Medicine Fellowship; Head Team Physician at Indiana University–South Bend and Holy Cross College, South Bend, IN; Co-Chair, Sports Medicine Committee USA Weightlifting, Colorado Springs, CO

Lawrence Leeman, MD, MPH
Associate Professor of Family and Community Medicine and Obstetrics and Gynecology, University of New Mexico School of Medicine; Director of Family Medicine, Maternal and Child Health; Co-Medical Director, Mother-Baby Unit, University of New Mexico Hospital, Albuquerque, NM

Nicholas LeFevre, MD
Assistant Professor and Ultrasound Curriculum Director, Department of Family and Community Medicine, TCU/UNT Medical School and John Peter Smith Hospital, Fort Worth, TX

Whitney LeFevre, MD
Assistant Professor and Clerkship Director, Department of Family and Community Medicine, TCU/UNT Medical School and John Peter Smith Hospital, Fort Worth, TX

Ruth Lesnewki, MD
Medical Director, Department of Family Medicine, East 13th Street Family Practice, New York, NY

Madeline R. Lewis, DO, MS
Private Practice, Family Medicine, East Lansing, MI

Mark Lewis, DO
Private Practice, Obstetrics and Gynecology, East Lansing, MI

Sandy T. Liu, BS
Medical Student, George Washington University School of Medicine, Washington, DC

Benjamin Mailloux, MD
Private practice; Waldo County General Hospital, Belfast, ME

Ashfaq A. Marghoob, MD
Associate Professor, SUNY–Stony Brook, Stony Brook, NY; Associate Member, Memorial Sloan Kettering Cancer Center, Hauppauge, NY

Gregory A. Marolf, MD
Assistant Clinical Director, Sports Medicine Fellowship, Bayfront Medical Center Family Practice Residency; Physician, Bayfront Convenient Care Clinics, St. Petersburg, FL

Reena R. Mathews, MD
Faculty Geriatrician, Medical Director, John Peter Smith Hospital, Fort Worth, TX

Coral D. Matus, MD
Associate Director, The Toledo Hospital Family Medicine Residency Program, Toledo, OH

William L. McDaniel Jr, MD
Retired Clinical Associate Professor of Community Science Program, Department of Family Practice, Mercer University School of Medicine, Macon; Staff Physician, Department of Family Practice, Hamilton Medical Center, Dalton, GA (Whitfield)

Michael McHenry, MA, PA-C
Physician Assistant, Family Medicine Associates, Midland, MI

Greta McLaren, MD
Assistant Professor, University of Colorado Health Sciences Center; Medical Director, RenewSkin Clinic, Denver, CO

James W. McNabb, MD
Adjunct Associate Professor, Department of Family Medicine; Distinguished Teaching Professor of Medical Acupuncture, University of North Carolina School of Medicine, Chapel Hill; Family Physician, Full Circle Family Medicine of Piedmont HealthCare, Mooresville, NC

John M. McShane, MD
Assistant Clinical Professor, Departmet of Family Medicine, Jefferson Medical College, Philadelphia; President, McShane Sports Medicine, Villanova, PA

Thomas H. Mitchell, RRT
Director Cardiorespiratory Services, Truman Medical Center Lakewood, Kansas City, MO

Jason A. Mogonye, MD
Clinical Faculty, JPS Family Medicine Residency Program, Assistant Program Director, JPS Sports Medicine Fellowship Program, JPS Health Network, Forth Worth, TX

Harris Mones, DO
Associate Professor, University of Osteopathic Medicine and Health Sciences, Des Moines, IA; Adjunct Clinical Associate Professor, Lake Erie College of Osteopathic Medicine, Bradenton; Associate Professor, NOVA Southeastern College of Osteopathic Medicine, Ft. Lauderdale; Director of Medicial Education, Westchester General Hospital, Miami, FL

Carlos A. Moreno, MD, MSPH
Professor and Chair, Department of Family and Community Medicine, University of Texas Medical School at Houston; Chief of Family Medicine, Memorial Hermann Hospital–TMC, Houston, TX

Mark Needham, MD
Co-Chief Executive Officer, Santa Monica Bay Physicians Health Services, Inc., Santa Monica, CA

Gary R. Newkirk, MD
Clinical Professor of Family Medicine, University of Washington School of Medicine; Residency Director, Family Medicine Spokane Residencies, Spokane, WA

Mary Jane Newkirk, MS, CCC-SLP
Speech-Language Pathologist, Spokane Public Schools, Spokane, WA

Phuc D. Nguyen, MD
Assistant Professor and Residency Director, Department of Family and Community Medicine, UT Health McGovern Medical School, Houston, TX

Jerry Ninia, MD, RVT, FACOG, FACS
Clinical Associate Professor, SUNY–Stony Brook School of Medicine, Stony Brook, NY; Director of Obstetrics and Gynecology, St. Charles Hosptial, Port Jefferson, NY

Bethany N. Norberg, MD
Assistant Professor and Residency Site Coordinator, Department of Family and Community Medicine, UNT Health Science Center and John Peter Smith Hospital, Houston, TX

John O'Brien, MD
Associate Professor, Department of Family Medicine, Univeristy of Michigan Medical School, Ann Arbor, MI

Theodore X. O'Connell, MD
Program Director, Residency Director, Kaiser Permanente, Napa-Solano, CA

Francis G. O'Connor, MD, MPH
Medical Director, Consortium for Health and Military Performance, Military and Emergency Medicine, Uniformed Services University of the Health Sciences, Bethesda, MD

Kathleen M. O'Hanlon, MD
Professor, Department of Family and Community Health, Marshall University School of Medicine, Huntington, WV

Carol Osborn, MD
Adjunct Professor, Deptartment of Family Practice Medicine, University of Utah Health Sciences Center; Staff Physician, Department of Family Practice Intermountain Healthcare, Salt Lake City, UT

Lori Oswald, PA-C
Physician Assistant, Medical Procedures Center, Midland, MI

Gary Page, MD
Medical Officer, Parker Indian Hospital, Parker, AZ

James R. Palleschi, MD
Urologist, Sutter Medical Network; Sutter Pacific Medical Foundation; Sutter Medical Group of the Redwoods; Sutter Medical Center of Santa Rosa, Santa Rosa, CA

Scott A. Paluska, MD, FACSM
Clinical Associate Professor, University of Illinois–Urbana; Medical Director, OAK Orthopedics, Urbana, IL

Helen A. Pass, MD
Assistant Professor of Clinical Surgery, Columbia University College of Physicians and Surgeons, New York, NY

Dale A. Patterson, MD, FAAFP
Program Director, Memorial Hospital Family Medicine Residency, South Bend, IN

John L. Pfenninger, MD, FAAFP
Clinical Professor, Michigan State University College of Medicine, and retired Private Practice, Midland, MI

Madelyn Pollock, MD
Private Practice, Austin, TX

John Bartels Pope, MD
Professor of Clinical Family Medicine, Louisiana State University Health Sciences Center, Shreveport, LA

Linda Prine, MD
Associate Clinical Professor of Family Medicine, Albert Einstein College of Medicine; Faculty, Beth Israel Residency in Urban Family Practice, New York, NY

Oscar Ramirez, MD, FACS
Clincal Faculty at Cleveland Clinic–Florida; Private practice, Sanctuary Plastic Surgery, Boca Raton, FL

Stephen D. Ratcliffe, MD, MSPH
Program Director, Lancaster General Hospital Family Medicine Residency, Lancaster, PA

Duren Michael Ready, MD
Assistant Professor, Departments of Family and Community Medicine and Medical Humanities, Texas A&M University Health Science Center College of Medicine; Director, Headache Clinic, Department of Neurology, Scott and White Memorial Hospital and Clinic, Temple, TX

Bal Reddy, MD
Assistant Professor and Predoctoral Director, Department of Family and Community Medicine, UT Health McGovern Medical School, Houston, TX

Sumana Reddy, MD, FAAFP
Founder, Acacia Family Medical Group, Salinas; District Director, California Academy of Family Physicians, San Francisco, CA

Peter L. Reynolds, MD
Assistant Professor, Saint Louis University Family Medicine Residency Program, Belleville, IL

Terry Reynolds, BS, RDCS
School of Cardiac Ultrasound, Arizona Heart Foundation, Phoenix, AZ

David Roden, MD
Attending Otolayrngologist, MidMichigan Medical Center, Midland, MI

J.R. MacMillan Rodney, MD
Surgical Resident, Cornell University Medical College, New York, NY

Wm. MacMillan Rodney, MD
Adjunct Professor of Family Medicine, Meharry Medical College, Nashville; Professor and Chair, Medicos para la Familia, Intl., Memphis, TN

Montiel T. Rosenthal, MD
Associate Clinical Professor, Department of Family and Community Medicine, University of Cincinnati College of Medicine; Director, Prenatal Clinic, The Christ Hospital; Director, Family Medicine, Cincinnati Children's Hospital Medical Center; Attending Physcian, Good Samaritan Hospital, Cincinnati, OH

Steven E. Roskos, MD
Associate Professor, Department of Family Medicine, College of Human Medicine, Michigan State University, East Lansing, MI

Scott F. Ross, MD
Family Practicioner, Department of Family Medicine, MidMichigan Medical Center, Midland, MI

Matt D. Roth, MD
Family and Sports Medicine, Promedica Physician Group, Maumee OH

Terry S. Ruhl, MD
Associate Program Director, Altoona Family Physicians Residency, Altoona; Clinical Assistant Professor, Department of Family and Community Medicine, Penn State College of Medicine, Hershey, PA

Edmund S. Sabanegh Jr, MD
Associate Professor and Chair, Department of Urology, The Cleveland Clinic Lerner College of Medicine, Case Western Reserve University; Director, Center for Male Infertility, Cleveland Clinic Foundation, Cleveland, OH

Scott Savage, DO, FACEP, FSCP, FACHE, FAPWCA, CCHP, CHCQM
Associate Professor of Aerospace Medicine, University of Texas Medical Branch, Galveston, TX; Associate Clinical Professor of Emergency Medicine, Boonshaft School of Medicine, Wright State University, Dayton, OH; Space Flight Surgeon, NASA/Wyle/UTMB, Johnson Space Center, Houston, TX

Alon Scope, MD
Visiting Investigator, Dermatology Service, Memorial Sloan-Kettering Cancer Center, New York, NY

Todd M. Sheperd
Clinical Assistant Professor, Department of Family Medicine, Michigan State University College of Human Medicine, East Lansing; Medical Director, Acute Rehabilitation Unit Northern Michigan Regional Hospital; Attending Physician, Bayside Family Medicine, Petoskey, MI

James R. Shepich, MD, FACS
Staff Surgeon, MidMichigan Medical Center, Midland, MI

Julie M. Sicilia, MD
Clinical Assistant Professor, University of Washington, Seattle WA; Clinical Assistant Professor, Providence Alaska Family Medicine Residency, Anchorage, AK

Victor S. Sierpina, MD
W.D. and Laura Nell Nicholson Family Professor of Integrative Medicine; Professor, Family Medicine; Distinguished Teaching Professor of Medical Acupuncture, University of Texas Medical Branch, Galveston, TX

Larry Skoczylas, DDS, MS
Oral and Maxillofacial Surgeon, Midland Oral and Maxillofacial Surgery, PC, Midland, MI

Eric Skye, MD
Associate Professor and Associate Chair for Educational Programs, Department of Family Medicine, University of Michigan, Ann Arbor, MI

Wendy L. Smeltzer, MD, CCFP, FCFP
Medical Director, Medical Esthetics, Sante Wellness Group; President and Medical Director, Medique Skincare Ltd., Calgary, Alberta, Canada

Al Smith, MD
Smith & Robinson Family Medicine; ICAEL Accredited Echocardiography Lab, Raymondville, TX

Eric A. Smith, MD
Associate Staff, Wooster Community Hosptial, Wooster, OH

Farin W. Smith, MD
Clinical Assistant Professor, University of Alabama–Birmingham; Staff, Trauma Surgery and Surgical Critical Care, Huntsville Hospital System, Huntsville, AL

Jeffrey V. Smith, MD, JD
Staff Physician, Departments of Family Medicine and Surgery, Contra Costa Regional Medical Center, Martinez, CA

Gary L. Snyder, MD, RVT, DPM
Medical Director, Apollo International Institute of Medical Sciences, Big Lake, MN

Michael Stampar, DO
Assistant Clinical Professor, Department of Surgery, Michigan State University, East Lansing, MI; Owner, Spago Day Spa, Salon, and Medispa, Punta Gorda, FL

Sandra M. Sulik, MD, MS
Associate Professor Depart of Family Medicine, State University of New York Health Science Center/St. Joseph's Family Medicine Residency, Syracuse, NY

James A. Surrell, MD, FACSm, FASCRS
Associate Clinical Professor of Surgery, College of Human Medicine, Michigan State University, East Lansing; Medical Director, Digestive Health Institute, Marquette General Health System, Marquette, MI

Michelle E. Szczepanik, MD
Resident, Dewitt Army Community Hospital, Ft. Belvoir, VA

Robert S. Tan, MD
Clinical Associate Professor, Department of Family and Community Medicine, University of Texas Medical School at Houston; Associate Professor, Department of Internal Medicine, Baylor College of Medicine; Staff, Michael E. DeBakey VA Medical Center; Extended Care Director, OPAL Medical Clinic, Houston, TX

Sheila Thomas, MD
Primary Care Family Practice Physician, UT Family Practice, University of Tennessee, Memphis, TN

Thomas N. Told, DO, FACOFPdist
Assistant Dean for Clinical Education, and Chief of Division of Rural and Wilderness Medicine, College of Osteopathic Medicine, Rocky Vista University, Parker CO; Kirksville College of Osteopathic Medicine, A.T. Still University, Kirksville, MO

Michael L. Tuggy, MD
Clinical Associate Faculty, University of Washington School of Medicine; Director, Swedish Family Medicine–First Hill Residency, Seattle, WA

Stephen L. Twyman, MD, MPH
Associate Professor, Medical Director, Procedural and Surgical Training Track, John Peter Smith Family Medicine Residency Program, Fort Worth, TX

Cathy Uecker, RN
Registered Nurse, Grand Rapids, MI

Hakan Usal, MD
Surgeon, Department of Plastic Surgery, Usal Cosmetic Surgery Center, Hackensack; Attending Physician, Department of Plastic Surgery, Hackensack University Medical Center, Hackensack; Staff, Department of Plastic Surgery, Valley Hospital, Ridgewood, NJ; Staff, Department of Plastic Surgery, Staten Island University Hospital, Staten Island, NY

Richard P. Usatine, MD
Professor, Departments of Family and Community Medicine and Dermatology and Cutaneous Surgery; Assistant Director, Medical Humanities Education, University of Texas Health Science Center–San Antonio; Medical Director, Skin Clinic, University Health System, San Antonio, TX

Peter Valenzuela, MD, MBA
Chief Medical Officer, Sutter Medical Group of the Redwoods, Santa Rosa, CA

Renier van Aardt, MB, ChB, CCFP
Medical Director, Vitality Medi-Spa, Halifax; Medical Director, Laser Plus Medi-Spa, Truro, Nova Scotia, Canada

Roger K. Waage, MD
Associate Professor, University of Minnesota Medical School–Duluth; Program Director, Duluth Family Medicine Residency, Duluth, MN

M. Amer Wahed, MD
Associate Professor, Department of Pathology and Laboratory Medicine, University of Texas McGovern Medical School, Houston, TX

Matti Waterman, MD
Clinical Lecturer, Rappaport Faculty of Medicine, Technion-Israel Institute of Technology; Senior Physician, Department of Gastroenterology and Department of Medicine, Rambam Health Care Campus, Haifa, Israel; Clinical Fellow, Advanced Fellowship in Inflammatory Bowel Disease, Department of Medicine, Division of Gastroenterology, Mount Sinai Hospital, Toronto, Ontario, Canada

Lydia A. Watson, MD, FACOG
Staff Physician, Department of Obstetrics and Gynecology, MidMichigan Medical Center, Midland, MI

David G. Weismiller, MD, ScM
Professor of Family Medicine, The Brody School of Medicine at East Carolina University; Associate Provost, East Carolina University, Greenville, NC

Stephen J. Wetmore, MD, CCFP, FCFP
Professor, Department of Family Medicine, Schulich School of Medicine and Dentistry, The University of Western Ontario, London, Ontario, Canada

Russell D. White, MD
Emeritus Professor of Medicine, Department of Community and Family Medicine, University of Missouri–Kansas City School of Medicine; Truman Medical Center–Lakewood, Kansas City, MO

Carman H. Whiting, MD
Assistant Professor, Department of Family and Community Medicine, University of Texas Medical School at Houston, Houston, TX

Thad Wilkins, MD
Associate Professor, Department of Family Medicine, Medical College of Georgia, Augusta, GA

Verneeta L. Williams, MD
Associate Director, Riverside Family Medicine Residency, Newport News, VA

Charles L. Wilson, MD
Clinical Associate Professor, Department of Family Medicine, University of Washington School of Medicine; Private Practice, The Vasectomy Clinic, Seattle, WA

Thomas C. Wright Jr, MD
Professor of Pathology, Columbia University, New York, NY

Edward Anthony Yaghmour, MD, FASA
Associate Professor, Northwestern University Feinberg School of Medicine, Chicago, Illinois

Gary Yen, MD
Lecturer, Department of Family Medicine, University of Michigan, Ann Arbor, MI

George G. Zainea, MD
Staff Surgeon, Department of Colon and Rectal Surgery, MidMichigan Physicians Group, Midland, MI

Michael Zeringue, MD
Physician, Sports Medicine and Interventional Pain Management Physician, Ponchartrain Bone and Joint, Metairie, LA

Edward M. Zimmerman, MD, PC
Las Vegas Laser & Lipo, Las Vegas, NV

Edward G. Zurad, MD
Clinical Professor, The Commonwealth Medical College, Scranton; Clinical Associate Professor, Temple University, Philadelphia; Medical Director, Procter & Gamble Paper Products, Mehoophany, PA

The face of medicine has changed dramatically since the first edition of this text was published in 1994, and it continues to change. Electronic medical records (EMRs) have become the framework for most medical practices, especially those that are part of large group practices. And large group practices are becoming the norm, with two-thirds of primary care clinicians now employed. The Affordable Care Act almost succeeded in requiring everyone to have health insurance. But having insurance and being able to afford necessary or important procedures are two different things. Deductibles are higher than ever, so many patients are not able to afford procedures. Therefore, despite all the changes in healthcare, some things have not changed. Patients are still postponing procedures until they can afford them. The performace of procedures by primary care clinicians not only improves access, it also makes it more likely patients will get them and can afford them.

The vision of the primary care clinician "who can provide a breadth and continuity of commonly needed healthcare services for adults and children, who can deliver babies, manage simple fractures, counsel single parents, go to the hospital, maintain an office, and when all else fails, comfort the dying… who provides healthcare from the nursery to the nursing home, without taking the patient to the poorhouse along the way" as defined by Dr. Rodney in the foreword to the first edition still remains. However, attempts to reach this vision are being made in many different ways.

The patient-centered medical home (PCMH) has become mainstream and attempts to provide what is in this vision. PCMHs seem to offer what the primary care clinician aspired to do alone in the past (and still often does in rural settings). In the best PCMHs, the primary care clinician has become both the quarterback and the systems analyst. Levels of PCMH certification are based on measured metrics of quality. In this setting, primary care clinicians performing procedures still makes sense. One of the metrics that PCMHs must follow is the ability to track referrals; what better way to verify patient completion of a referral for a procedure than if a primary care clinician within the group is doing the procedure? Patient satisfaction is another metric; how better to keep the patient satisfied than to have his or her own clinician perform the procedure? What better way to improve your metrics on cancer screening than to be the one who performs this screening?

Direct primary care and concierge medicine are also rapidly evolving as an alternative model of care. The number of providers currently providing this type of care is rapidly increasing. Once again, what a great marketing opportunity: "Your personal care clinician will also perform your procedures"!

The feedback received on the first three editions of this text has been appreciated. New features in this edition include a section on Urgent Care Procedures. Many more primary care clinicians are practicing in this setting. It is also refreshing to note that surveys by the American Board of Family Medicine of recent residency program graduates have shown more interest in performing a wider breadth of procedures than has been seen in the last 20 years.

As an editor of this book over the last 26 years, I have noticed another recent phenomenon. Although the basic steps for many procedures may not have changed, the evidence regarding them has usually become much more robust. Consequently, this is by far the most evidence-based edition. This was the charge and challenge given to section editors: to update chapters where necessary, and if evidence is available regarding a procedure, make every effort to review it. Such evidence is also frequently listed in the Recommended Reading sections.

Another thing that has not changed over the years is the fact that our patients are very busy. They appreciate not having to take the time to go meet another clinician to have a procedure performed. In some cases, that would also mean a higher copayment. It still makes sense for primary care clinicians to perform procedures. A stigma also remains that the primary care clinician performing procedures not only offers one-stop shopping, but they may also perhaps be a better-trained clinician.

Although the problem is not new, public awareness of clinician burnout has been increasing. Part of my personal plan for preventing burnout is to perform and teach procedures. Perhaps other primary care clinicians occasionally need an escape from the mind-numbing process of data entry that EMRs sometimes necessitate. Although the advent of EMRs occurred at about the same time as burnout started being recognized, experts tell us that EMRs are not the cause. Regardless, performing procedures is fun, and procedure notes are usually much more amenable to the use of a template. And my computer monitor never gets between me and the patient when I'm performing a procedure. While I'm not sure of the evidence surrounding whether performing procedures prevents burnout, it seems like an excellent topic for someone to study. So this is a call for more studies!

While there have been many changes in medicine since the first edition, other things have not changed. No matter how complicated our systems become, or how busy we become, or how much technology we adopt, certain aspects of practice should always remain the same. The focus should be entirely upon the patient and family in front of us, especially at the time of the appointment or procedure. As mentioned in the Preface to a previous edition, in our search for the knowledge and expertise to perform the procedures presented in this text, we should never forget that we are first and foremost people who treat patients and their families, not just their symptoms. When it comes to procedures, our goal should always be to perform procedures as a way to prevent disease and to help people feel better and be healthier.

Grant C. Fowler, MD

ACKNOWLEDGMENTS

Thanks to Judith Fletcher for getting this edition started, to Dee Simpson and Carrie Stetz for getting it done, and to Sarah Barth for wrapping it up. Dee and Carrie, thanks for an enormous amount of proofreading and production. You both remained steadfast with the project; Dee throughout the project and Carrie with the page proofs at the end. Clinicians everywhere are grateful for your attention to detail and dedication.

A special acknowledgment goes to Dr. Jack Pfenninger, who has officially retired and sold his practice that was dedicated to office procedures. This book was your idea. We missed you with this edition, the first edition in which you were not an editor, but congratulations! That being said, none of us believes you will give up tilting at windmills.

FOREWORD

The specialty of family medicine in America turned 50 years old in 2019. Much has been accomplished over the past 5 decades. Residencies have been established in more than 450 hospitals, and departments of family medicine exist in most American medical schools. Family medicine has successful ongoing collaborations with general internal medicine, general pediatrics, and with academic programs in nursing, pharmacy, the mental health professions, and physician assistant training. The scholarly work of family medicine faculty members has laid the groundwork for new approaches to clinical care and education in all the primary care disciplines. First published in 1994, *Procedures for Primary Care* is perhaps the best example of such scholarship. It is therefore fitting that a new edition appears as the specialty celebrates its birthday. Through three previous editions, this book has become a staple in the offices of primary care providers around the world. Now in its fourth edition, it includes an encyclopedic catalog of clinical procedures in 235 chapters offering both specific instructions on the best techniques for each procedure and information for patients receiving such care.

Family medicine has undergone major changes since the first edition was published 26 years ago. We have adopted the model of team-based care in the patient-centered medical home. We have worked to fully integrate behavior health into the primary care system. We have adopted electronic health records and can now track population health in new and powerful ways. But the core value of primary care is still based on trusting relationships with patients (continuity of care) and on our ability to deliver a broad scope of services to our communities (comprehensive care). For our care model to work, patients must be able to trust their family physicians to competently care for any problem that is common in the community. Yet there is growing evidence that the very comprehensiveness that makes primary care effective is eroding; referral rates to specialists are rising, and fewer family physicians are delivering the full scope of care intended by our founders. Performing common procedures in the primary care setting lowers the referral rate to specialty care, improves patient confidence and trust in our care, and keeps care located in the community where it can be most efficiently provided. Despite all the changes going on around us, performing common clinical procedures competently and safely remains a critical contributor to both continuity and comprehensiveness. As always, the challenge lies in the very broad scope of services required for successful primary care. This is why an up-to-date and comprehensive reference text for primary care procedures is so important.

Over the course of three previous editions, *Procedures for Primary Care* has also proven useful in emergency medicine and hospital care. The fourth edition now includes a specific section devoted to urgent care procedures. As a result, copies of this book can now be found in settings well beyond primary care offices. Nevertheless, most of the chapter authors continue to be family physicians. Their work stands as a testament to the importance of comprehensiveness in primary care and exemplifies the contributions of family medicine to improving clinical care and medical education in general. Thus, this book is both clinically and historically important. *Procedures for Primary Care* now fills an essential niche in American medicine. Everyone in the primary care community owes a debt of gratitude to the authors, editors, and publisher of this important book.

John W. Saultz, MD
Professor Emeritus
Department of Family Medicine
Oregon Health & Science University
Portland, Oregon

FOREWORD TO THE THIRD EDITION

There are two sides to the complete primary care physician. One side is the compassionate listener, a person who can heal with words. The other side is the talented caregiver who can provide and apply medical science, including necessary or desired procedures for patients. People need people for good health, and those who have a complete primary care physician who knows them and treats them are among the luckiest people in the world. The complete primary care physician is a precious resource that has been endangered but is making a comeback.

Pfenninger and Fowler's Procedures for Primary Care is the bible for the laying on of hands in primary care practice. The first edition in 1994 sold over 40,000 copies and became a fixture in the library of every residency program. It is the one book that is worn and well-used. The second edition in 2003 had 82 new chapters and cemented the book as a must-have in every primary care office. The third edition expands this classic text to an amazing 234 chapters with two new sections, Aesthetic Medicine and Hospitalist Procedures.

The scope of primary care is expanding. After years of decline because of "turf wars" with specialists, health systems are appreciating more than ever that having multitalented primary care physicians is the key to efficient and high-quality healthcare delivery. Comprehensiveness is now back in style for primary care with the Patient-Centered Medical Home as the provider and coordinator of all healthcare services. This is not the "gatekeeping" of managed care but rather a "place" where patients share an information system with their personal physician and have all their services coordinated. The more the primary care physician team can do, the better for everyone.

I am fortunate to be "walking the talk" of the Patient-Centered Medical Home model. In 2009, I was asked to develop a new primary care practice network in a heavily doctored area of southern California. Building off the practice of one physician, we will have 9 offices and 26 physicians in early 2011. We are starting residency programs in family medicine and internal medicine. All practices qualify as advanced medical homes. We have established a variety of "procedure clinics" among our group, performing a wide variety of dermatologic procedures and aesthetics. We have expertise among us in sports medicine. We are developing our own hospitalist service. While no primary care physician will do all the procedures described in this book, among us we will do almost all of them. We will train a new generation of primary care physicians in as many procedures as time and interest allows. *Procedures for Primary Care* is our indispensable guide.

There is a renaissance underway in primary care. The internet and information technology change how we do most everything, and primary care is no exception. Patients now have access to a world of information for free, including healthcare and their medical records.

Primary care physicians have become "information managers" for patients and access to communication online has become continuous. In this new world of information, communication, and continuous care, what patients need and want is shared decision making. For patients, an "I can do that for you" from their primary care physician is usually a welcome relief. The world of specialists is often confusing and usually very expensive. Good primary care exudes value, the combination of quality and efficiency, so needed and welcomed in healthcare today.

Knowledge is power and knowledge is abundantly available in *Procedures for Primary Care*. Jack Pfenninger and Grant Fowler have assembled a phenomenal group of talented authors who all "walk the talk" of their chapters. Need to remove a fishhook? Need to remove a ring from a swollen finger? Remove isolated hairs for good? Apply an Unna boot? Repair an earlobe? This book has procedures for them all, of course, and these examples are only a small slice of what is here. If you want to venture into Botox treatment or provide stress echocardiograms, this book will tell you how. We often go to workshops to learn new procedures, but what is helpful to keep doing them is a handy reference to remind us of all the elements of the procedure.

Patient safety requires that we have a checklist for each procedure and not just rely on what we and our staff remember at the time. This book has all the checklists. I imagine a thousand times a day physicians and office staffs somewhere are reviewing a chapter in this book before going into the treatment room. Copies of these checklists should become part of your office procedure manual.

I am certain that this will not be the last edition of *Procedures for Primary Care*. This resource is simply too valuable not to have, and access to it needs to be in print in every office. With this edition, the patient education sheets have been moved online to make downloading and printing easier and more convenient. I imagine synergy with the internet will grow over time as it has with other classic textbooks. For now, having a readily available copy of *Procedures for Primary Care* will be at the top of your office resources. Use it often to keep your quality of care high and your scope of practice broad for the benefit of your patients.

Joseph E. Scherger, MD, MPH
Vice President, Primary Care
Eisenhower Medical Center
Rancho Mirage, California;
Clinical Professor of Family Medicine
University of California, San Diego
University of Southern California
San Diego, California

FOREWORD TO THE SECOND EDITION

As a comprehensive guide to performing medical and surgical procedures in the office, hospital, or emergency department, *Pfenninger and Fowler's Procedures for Primary Care* might be considered an antidote to the evils that originated from Pandora's box. According to Greek mythology, Pandora (whose name means "rich in gifts") found a buried box and impulsively removed its lid. Out of the box, scattering in every direction, came disease, death, and all the other evils that afflict humankind. Like Eve in the Christian scriptures, Pandora introduced mortality into our world. However, her box also contained an antidote—hope—and she closed the lid just in time to prevent this quality from escaping.

In combating the myriad diseases that Pandora supposedly unleashed, primary care clinicians have long been powerful agents for hope and healing. Because of advances in treatment options, including minimally invasive outpatient surgical techniques, many procedures that previously would have necessitated hospitalization or consultation now can be performed by primary care clinicians in the office, hospital, or emergency room. This arrangement allows continuity of care, hopefully provides excellent patient education, and, by moving some procedures out of the hospital, may offer significant economic advantages. However, as their role expands, these clinicians must continue to use sound judgment and keep the patient's welfare as the uppermost priority. They should avoid procedures beyond their expertise; they should avoid procedures that might necessitate repetition; and they should avoid procedures that might cause them medicolegal problems.

Like Pandora, *Pfenninger and Fowler's Procedures for Primary Care* is rich in gifts, but these are of the life-affirming kind. More than 200 chapters provide up-to-date information for a continually evolving specialty. The book includes practical, step-by-step instructions for performing an extensive array of medical and surgical procedures, as illustrated by line drawings and clear photographs. It also covers indications and contraindications, equipment and suppliers, complications, billing codes, and other practical topics. In the literature for primary care clinicians, few other books cover such a wide range of topics. Indeed, I know of no other volume that is likely to be more useful to its intended audience.

Some readers may wonder why this foreword is being written by a cardiovascular surgeon and not by a primary care clinician. Perhaps they will allow heart disease to serve as an example for many other diseases. Primary care clinicians are at the leading edge of the battle against many diseases—not only in treatment but also in prevention. Regarding heart disease, their advice is often the deciding factor in convincing patients to make positive changes with respect to fat intake, physical activity, cigarette smoking, and other lifestyle factors. An example from the recent literature supports this premise: in a study involving patients with coronary artery disease at Creighton University, recommendations from primary care clinicians concerning the assessment of lipid profiles and use of statin therapy significantly reduced the number of adverse cardiovascular outcomes. As the average age of the population continues to increase and congestive heart failure becomes increasingly prevalent, primary care clinicians can be expected to play an even greater role in diagnosing and treating this disorder. If primary care clinicians can do this with heart disease, it is my hope that they can use their abilities in many other areas of medicine.

The book also contains patient education handouts. When primary care clinicians perform a procedure, they must know the disease well. In so doing, they also have a golden opportunity to teach some prevention principles. I hope that they will never miss the opportunity to treat the whole patient and potentially change the course of the disease by educating the patient before, during, and after performing the procedure.

In conclusion, I congratulate Drs. Pfenninger and Fowler on producing such an excellent volume. It should help improve the quality of care in many aspects of medical practice, and I highly recommend it for every primary care clinician and trainee. There are some who consider me a pioneer in heart disease; I hope that this book encourages medical pioneers everywhere to prevent and treat early the diseases that Pandora supposedly released.

Denton A. Cooley, MD
Surgeon-in-Chief, Texas Heart Institute
Clinical Professor of Surgery
University of Texas Medical School at Houston
Houston, Texas

FOREWORD TO THE FIRST EDITION

In 1930, more than 80% of the physicians in the United States were general family doctors, providing comprehensive health care at a reasonable cost. By 1980, the self-reported percentage of family doctors in the United States was 15%. Along with this trend of dwindling numbers has been a gradual decline of diagnostic and therapeutic skills held by those physicians who do practice general family medicine.

One definition of a generalist physician (formerly a general practitioner) is a family physician who can provide a breadth and continuity of commonly needed healthcare services. These physicians care for children, deliver babies, manage simple fractures, counsel single parents, go to the hospital, maintain an office, and, when all else fails, comfort the dying. Their goal is to provide health care from the nursery to the nursing home, without taking the patient to the poor house along the way

Today, of the 625,000 physicians in the United States, fewer than 10% comprehensively wield the clinical skills needed to provide such care. The headlong rush to subspecialize in medicine has left family physicians in the minority. Still, they are an important minority whose number is now growing in response to the projected needs of the twenty-first century American healthcare system.

Since 1983, a group of family physicians, supported by the American Academy of Family Physicians (AAFP), has constructed a series of demonstration projects to propagate diagnostic and therapeutic skills in family medicine. Many of the procedural pioneers in family practice have quietly and unselfishly contributed their professional energies to the resuscitation of full-service family practice within a medical education system gone far, far astray. This book stands as a contribution to that effort. Although some may view the teaching and learning of clinical skills as "proceduralism," the skills that are depicted in this book represent the desire of physicians to remain clinically excellent. No amount of psychosocial expertise can overcome the credibility lost when a physician cannot perform basic clinical services on behalf of his or her patient.

Recently a prominent dean of a well-known medical school asked me why the residency programs at my institution, the University of Tennessee, persisted in reaching a comprehensive set of procedural clinical skills when, in his opinion, managed care organizations and health maintenance organizations would effectively amputate these skills from the day-to-day practice of family physicians. I disagree with this vision of the future, but it is true that some family physicians voluntarily relinquish many of the clinical skills described in this book. It is my hope that the skills described in its pages will become required curriculum, not only for residents, but, particularly, for faculty. One of the major challenges for the success of this book (and the specialty of family practice) is the development of accountability in a healthcare system that has become overly fragmented, costly, and inaccessible.

Are these skills needed? During the past 20 years, family physicians have been manipulated, exploited, and oppressed in a variety of ways that makes study of their actual needs very complex. For example, a lack of reported interest in obstetrical care cannot be used to justify the tremendous void that exists in women's healthcare as provided by family physicians. Residents are not likely to acquire clinical skills that family physician faculty members cannot themselves demonstrate in their positions as role models. A lack of procedural skill among family practice faculty and practitioners is particularly troubling in rural and underserved communities. These communities cannot afford platoons of various subspecialized physicians.

Although excellent healthcare is available from a combination of obstetricians, pediatricians, and internists, a well-trained, comprehensive-care family physician should be able to deliver continuing healthcare unrestricted by age, sex, organ system, and pregnancy. The physician should be skilled in many of the procedures described here to screen for, prevent, and treat common disease entities. If family practice simply becomes synonymous with "generic primary care," there will be very little need for many of the skills described in this book. My compliments to the editors and the authors for executing a labor of love in an outstanding fashion. They have chosen the road less traveled.

Wm. MacMillian Rodney, MD, FAAFP, FACEP
Meharry/Vanderbilt Professor and Chair
Department of Family and Community Medicine
Professor of Surgery/Emergency Medicine
Meharry Medical College
Nashville, Tennessee

CONTENTS

SECTION 4 Eyes, Ears, Nose, and Throat

Section Editor: GRANT C. FOWLER

SECTION 5 Cardiovascular and Respiratory System Procedures

Section Editor: GRANT C. FOWLER

SECTION 6 Gastrointestinal System Procedures

Section Editor: GRANT C. FOWLER

SECTION 7 Urinary System Procedures
Section Editor: GRANT C. FOWLER

SECTION 8 Male Reproductive System
Section Editor: GRANT C. FOWLER

SECTION 9 Gynecology and Female Reproductive System
Section Editor: DEEPA IYENGAR

SECTION 10   Obstetrics
Section Editor: BETH A. CHOBY

SECTION 11   Pediatrics
Section Editor: BAL REDDY

SECTION 1

Anesthesia

Section Editor: BAL REDDY

CHAPTER 1

PROCEDURAL SEDATION AND ANALGESIA

Sylvana Guidotti

Procedural sedation and analgesia (PSA) is the clinical practice of using pharmacologic agents to achieve a measurable level of sedation while performing typically painful or anxiety-provoking procedures. The term *conscious sedation* is no longer used because it describes neither the intent nor the outcome of the process. PSA allows the nonanesthesiologist to perform selected procedures in a safe and controlled setting.

The Joint Commission (TJC) has produced sedation guidelines to describe and define the spectrum of PSA. More importantly, the American Society of Anesthesiologists (ASA) and the American College of Emergency Physicians (ACEP) have published guidelines for PSA by nonanesthesiologists and emergency physicians, respectively. As defined by the ASA, PSA is a continuum from minimal sedation/analgesia to general anesthesia.

Minimal sedation occurs when the patient continues to respond normally to verbal commands without cardiopulmonary functions being affected. *Moderate sedation* is a state of depressed consciousness where the patient responds appropriately to verbal command with or without light tactile stimuli. *Dissociative sedation* should be considered a form of moderate sedation that occurs when a dissociative pharmacologic agent produces a trancelike state. The result is analgesia and amnesia while protective airway reflexes and cardiovascular stability are maintained. *Deep sedation* causes a depression of consciousness in which the patient is not easily arousable but responds purposefully with repeated or painful stimuli. At this level, the patient may require assistance in maintaining airway and ventilation. *General anesthesia* is at the end of the spectrum; consciousness is lost and the patient is unarousable to any stimuli. The patient requires ventilatory assistance, and cardiovascular function may be affected or impaired.

For coding purposes, the American Medical Association CPT coding manual describes "moderate (conscious) sedation" as a drug-induced depression of consciousness during which patients respond purposefully to verbal commands, either alone or accompanied by light tactile stimulation. No interventions are required to maintain a patent airway, and spontaneous ventilation is adequate. Cardiovascular function is maintained. It does not include minimal sedation (anxiolysis), deep sedation, or monitored anesthesia care (Table 1.1).

PSA is composed of three components. First is the *process of sedation*, which requires a thorough knowledge of the agents being administered. Next is the *intended procedure* to be performed. Finally, there are the *unpredictable side effects* and *untoward reactions* to the sedating medications, which can occur during or in the recovery phase of the procedure.

The clinician should be familiar with all of the appropriate monitoring and rescue equipment. A suitably trained provider should assist with the sedation. All individuals who participate in the care of the patient undergoing PSA must demonstrate ongoing clinical competency and be privileged for the procedure if they will be performing it in a hospital setting.

INDICATIONS

As nonanesthesiologist clinicians become more comfortable with PSA, the roster of appropriate procedures where these agents are beneficial continues to expand. The list includes, but is not limited to, the following:

- Anal procedures
- Biopsy procedures
- Bone marrow aspiration or biopsy
- Bronchoscopy
- Cardioversion (electrical or chemical)
- Dental/oral surgical procedures
- Endometrial biopsy
- Essure contraceptive placement
- Fracture reductions/care
- Gastrointestinal endoscopy
- Hysterosalpingography
- Lumbar puncture
- Magnetic resonance imaging/computed tomography scans/invasive radiographic procedures
- Office dilation and curettage/vacuum aspiration
- Orthopedic procedures
- Phlebectomy
- Plastic/cosmetic/laser procedures
- Wound repair/care, including burns; large excisions

PSA can be used in conjunction with and as a supplement to digital blocks, hematoma blocks, or regional nerve blocks, as well as topical anesthetic agents. These modalities may obviate the need for deeper levels of sedation. Other distractions for the patient such as music or videos are useful adjuncts.

CONTRAINDICATIONS

Elective procedures on pregnant patients should be deferred until after delivery. Patients with severe unstable systemic disease and patients with potentially unstable airways should be directed to a higher level of care. The ASA classification of systemic disease is designed to guide the clinician as to which patients are appropriate candidates for PSA (Table 1.2).

Class II patients include those with well-controlled hypertension, controlled non–insulin-dependent diabetes, and minimal cardiac or respiratory disease. Class III patients include those with insulin-dependent diabetes mellitus, poorly controlled hypertension, significant cardiac or respiratory disease, and significant renal or hepatic disease. Based on individual experience and skill in

TABLE 1.1   Operational Definitions and Characterizations of Levels of Sedation: Analgesia

| Sedation Score | Level of Sedation | Level of Consciousness | Response | | | Ventilation, Oxygenation |
			Verbal	Tactile	Patency	
0	None	Fully aware of self and surroundings	P	P	P	P
1	Minimal	Mostly aware of self and surroundings but sedate	P–L	P	P	P
2	Moderate	Slightly aware of self and surroundings, usually somnolent, arouses easily with stimuli	L–A	P–L	P–L*	P–L*
3	Deep†	Not aware of self or surroundings, little arousal with stimuli	A	L (to pain)	L–A	L
4	General anesthesia	Unconscious, no arousal with painful stimuli	A	A (to pain)	L–A	L–A

A, Absent, inadequate; L, limited, partial, mildly abnormal; P, present, adequate, or normal.
*May need to supplement oxygen to maintain oxygen saturation (SaO$_2$).
†Deep sedation may be indistinguishable from general anesthesia and carries all the same risks.

TABLE 1.2   American Society of Anesthesiologists Physical Status Classification

Classification	Sedation Risk
Class I: normal healthy patient	Minimal
Class II: mild systemic disease without physical limitation	Low
Class III: severe systemic disease with functional limitations	Intermediate
Class IV: severe systemic disease that is a constant threat to life	High
Class V: moribund patient who may not survive without procedure	Extremely high

ASA, American Society of Anesthesiologists.

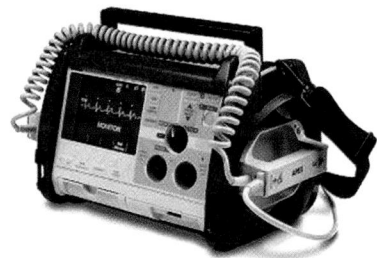

Fig. 1.1   Defibrillator. (Courtesy Zoll Medical Corp., Chelmsford, MA.)

providing sedation, practitioners may decide to limit the amount of patient risk they are willing to accept, using the ASA guidelines.

In general, the nonanesthesiologist clinician who provides PSA in the private office setting should do so on patients with class II status or less. For hospital-based procedures outside the operating room, PSA may be performed on patients up to and including class III status.

The ASA has set forth *preprocedure fasting guidelines* for scheduled elective cases. However, in separate recommendations for PSA, the ASA states, "The literature does not provide sufficient evidence to test the hypothesis that preprocedure fasting results in a decreased incidence of adverse outcomes in patients undergoing either moderate or deep sedation." The current guidelines are the result of consensus, rather than being evidence based, with respect to the risk of aspiration. *The recommendations are 6 hours for solids, cow's milk, and infant formula; 4 hours for breast milk; and 2 hours for clear liquids.* ACEP recognizes that there are certain emergent situations in which the benefits of PSA at any sedation depth outweigh the potential risks. In all other circumstances, it would be best to strictly adhere to the fasting guidelines. Thus, if a patient has not followed the aforementioned fasting guidelines, it would be best to postpone the procedure or to just not use significant PSA.

EQUIPMENT

- A single unit with blood pressure and electrocardiographic measurements, variable-pitch beep pulse oximeter, and recording device is the ideal monitor for PSA. Individual units are acceptable but require repeated manual recordings of the readings on the patient's chart.
- Angiocatheter for intravenous (IV) access (at least 20 gauge), IV solution, and stand.

- Oxygen source.
- Medications for sedation and analgesia.
- Reversal medications.
- Diphenhydramine and epinephrine to be used in the event of severe allergic reactions.
- Crash cart or Banyan kit with equipment and medications for basic and advanced cardiac life support (ACLS; see Chapter 212).
- Suction device.
- Defibrillator (Fig. 1.1).

Although it is not a requirement for class I patients, the *application of oxygen* by nasal cannula should be used for every patient undergoing PSA because each patient has a unique and unpredictable response to the medications. *Capnometry* is another, more sensitive measurement of ventilatory status and is being used frequently as part of PSA monitoring. As a measure of exhaled carbon dioxide, end-tidal CO_2 may detect hypoventilation before the development of oxygen desaturation.

PERSONNEL

At least two providers must be involved in PSA. The clinician who is performing the procedure is also ordering the medications. The assistant is typically a registered nurse who has fulfilled all of the requirements to administer PSA drugs, monitor the patient during the procedure and recovery phase, and participate in any needed resuscitations.

There should be a well-defined response for any cardiopulmonary emergency that results from PSA. Most hospitals have organized a "code team" to respond to such situations. In the nonhospital setting, the clinician should be able to manage the emergency until emergency medical services personnel arrive for transport to a hospital.

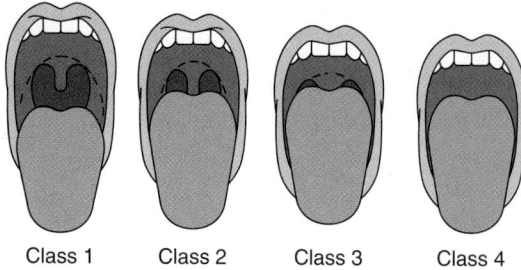

Class 1   Class 2   Class 3   Class 4

Fig. 1.2 Mallampati classification relates tongue size to pharyngeal size. It is based on the pharyngeal structures that are visible. *Class 1*: Visualization of the soft palate, fauces, uvula, anterior and posterior pillars. *Class 2*: Visualization of the soft palate, fauces, and uvula. *Class 3*: Visualization of the soft palate and the base of the uvula. *Class 4*: Soft palate not visible at all. (Modified from Mallampati SR, Gatt SP, Gugino LD, et al. A clinical sign to predict difficult tracheal intubation: a prospective study. *Can J Anaesth.* 1985;32: 429–434.)

TABLE 1.3	Mallampati Classification*
Class I	Full view of soft palate, fauces, uvula, pillars, tonsils
Class II	Visible hard and soft palate, fauces, upper portion of tonsils, and uvula
Class III	Visible hard and soft palate, base of uvula
Class IV	Only hard palate is visible

PREPROCEDURE PATIENT ASSESSMENT

Every patient who undergoes PSA should have a *complete history and physical examination* before the procedure. Included in the documentation are pertinent medical history, current medications, allergies (problems with sedative or analgesics), and review of systems (snoring or obstructive sleep apnea). It should be determined whether there is a history of any past problems with anesthesia or a history of drug or alcohol abuse or dependence. The physical examination should focus on assessment of the airway and cardiovascular system. Anatomic variants (macroglossia, micrognathia) and presence of a beard, dentures, or a short, arthritic neck should be noted. Direct evaluation of the patient's open mouth using the *Mallampati classification* measures how much the tongue obscures the uvula and soft palate (Fig. 1.2 and Table 1.3). Obtain and document an *informed consent* from the patient for both PSA and the procedure. Explain the sedation process, potential for failure, and adverse effects, as well as alternatives to the procedure and the consequences of not providing sedation.

PREPROCEDURE PATIENT PREPARATION

- Reconfirm the initial assessment and the patient's ASA classification.
- Document the fasting time.
- Determine prior history of drug or alcohol abuse or dependence.
- Determine prior history of past problems with anesthesia.
- Check a pregnancy test on age-appropriate women.
- Make certain there is an adult to escort the patient home.
- Ask the patient to void, dress in a gown, and recline on the procedure bed.
- Secure the IV line and ensure it is functioning.
- Apply blood pressure cuff, cardiac monitor, and pulse oximeter and document baseline vitals, including room air oxygen saturation (SaO_2).
- Ensure emergency resuscitation equipment and medications are functional and at the ready.
- Use a PSA monitoring flow sheet to record preprocedure, intraprocedure, and postprocedure data. Document start and completion times and medications and dosages administered, as well as the level of sedation achieved throughout the procedure (see flow sheets available at www.expertconsult.com).
- The practice of premedicating the patient with histamine type 2 blockers or proton pump inhibitors is no longer recommended because of the lack of evidence with regard to the efficacy of these drugs to diminish gastric acid secretion and subsequent risk of aspiration.
- Before sedating the patient, take a "time out" to once again identify the patient, the intended procedure, and the site. Once the procedure has started, encourage the patient to tell the operator about any unusual discomfort, shortness of breath, chest pressure, or itching.

TECHNIQUE

1. Position the patient as comfortably as possible for the procedure, using warm blankets and placing pillows under the head or knees.
2. Use the single dose of medication that will provide a maximum level of sedation required to perform the procedure. Multiple small doses create discomfort for the patient and may culminate in oversedation. For painful procedures, begin IV administrations with a short-acting narcotic. For painless but anxiety-producing procedures, place more emphasis on anxiolysis. Maintain verbal contact with the patient. Observe the patient for slurred speech, droopy eyelids, and calm affect. The patient should stir to verbal commands and be able to follow them. Remember that the effects should start within several minutes but may not peak for up to 7 minutes.
3. Begin the procedure once the patient has achieved the desired depth of sedation.
4. If the patient is not sedated adequately after a modest dose of narcotic, administer a small dose of a short-acting benzodiazepine and continue to observe for effects. Recall the synergistic efforts of these drugs.
5. Record vital signs every 5 minutes. The assistant should remain at the patient's bedside throughout the procedure to observe the response to sedation and to respond to any monitor alarms. Monitor the patient continually for head position, level of consciousness, airway patency, and adequacy of respiration and oxygenation. Observation of ventilation is essential, especially when using supplemental oxygen, which will delay the detection of apnea by pulse oximetry.
6. Naloxone and flumazenil should be at the bedside in the event any reversal is required.
7. The depth of sedation should be assessed at frequent intervals during the procedure. *If the sedation is too light*, the patient may express displeasure or experience discomfort, as well as develop tachycardia or hypertension. *If sedation is too deep*, the patient may develop periods of apnea; the SaO_2 will decrease and trigger the monitor alarm. In addition, if side-stream end-tidal CO_2 is used (capnography), the earliest sign of respiratory compromise would be a steady increase of the end-tidal CO_2 to greater than 40 mm Hg. Finally, the patient's Aldrete score (see flow sheet available at www.expertconsult.com) will decrease if sedation is too deep. If at any time during the procedure there is a change in or deterioration of the patient's condition, either suspend or abort the procedure, assess the patient, and begin any resuscitation.

EDITOR'S NOTE: Although two randomized controlled trials (Deitch, Lightdale) demonstrated the use of capnography during procedural sedation decreased the incidence of hypoxic events, a recent Cochrane systematic review (Wall, 2017) found a lack of convincing evidence that adding capnography to standard monitoring for PSA in the emergency department would reduce the rate of clinically significant adverse events.

TABLE 1.4	Commonly Used Medications for Procedural Sedation and Analgesia					
Medication	**Class**	**Description**	**Initial IV Dose**	**Repeat Dose**	**Minimum Interval**
Etomidate (Amidate)	Sedative-hypnotic	Rapid onset Short duration	0.1 mg/kg	0.1 mg/kg	5 min
Fentanyl (Sublimaze)	Opiate	Short acting	1 μgm/kg, up to 100 μg	25–50 μg	5 min
Flumazenil (Romazicon)	Benzodiazepine antagonist	Reversal agent for benzodiazepine	0.2 mg	0.2 mg, up to 1 mg total	1 min
Midazolam (Versed)	Benzodiazepine	Short acting Sedation/amnesia	1–2 mg	0.5–1 mg, up to 5 mg	5 min
Methohexital (Brevital)	Ultra–short-acting barbiturate	Nonanalgesic amnesia	0.75–1 mg/kg	0.5 mg/kg	2 min
Naloxone (Narcan)	Opiate antagonist	Reversal agent for opiate	0.2–0.4 mg	0.2 mg	2–3 min
Propofol (Diprivan)	Sedative-hypnotic	Rapid onset	1 mg/kg	0.5 mg/kg	3–5 min
Atropine	Anticholinergic Antiarrhythmic	Treatment of symptomatic bradycardia; decrease secretions	0.4 mg	0.4 mg, 3 mg max	3–5 min
Diphenhydramine (Benadryl)	Antihistamine Anticholinergic	Treatment of anaphylaxis; sedative; antiemetic	25 mg	25 mg	5–10 min
Metoclopramide (Reglan)	Central and peripheral dopamine antagonist	Antiemetic	10 mg	—	—
Ondansetron (Zofran)	Serotonin (5-HT$_3$) receptor antagonist	Antiemetic	4 mg	4 mg, 16 mg max	5–10 min

MEDICATIONS

There are several medications in the armamentarium of PSA. The clinician must understand the pharmacology of these drugs and the appropriate settings in which to use them.

A *short-acting analgesic should be used at the onset*. Fentanyl has a very good safety profile with a rapid onset and short duration of action. It does not cause the extent of cardiorespiratory depression that is typical of other opioids. However, its side effects are magnified with benzodiazepines (Table 1.4).

If anxiolysis is the goal of PSA, fentanyl combined with midazolam provides a minimal level of sedation that is ideal for such procedures as cardioversion, endoscopy, lumbar puncture, and certain wound repairs. *When moderate sedation* is desired for particularly painful procedures, fentanyl can be used with etomidate to create relaxation for closed reductions of joint dislocations or fractures. Propofol can be used for moderate or deep sedation. It has no analgesic properties and should be used with fentanyl. It is safest to deliver propofol as a continuous infusion that can be discontinued if any adverse reaction occurs. At low doses, methohexital produces a state of unconsciousness while preserving protective airway reflexes. It is purely an amnestic agent, and careful use with opioids is advised. Hypotension and histamine release are significant side effects.

Ketamine is a dissociative agent that has a long history of use for pediatric PSA. The data supporting the use of ketamine in adults are very few, owing to the increased incidence of hallucinations during emergence from the drug.

COMPLICATIONS

Several factors are associated with adverse outcomes during PSA. In addition to the known effects of the drugs themselves, there are patient factors, inadequate preprocedural evaluation, drug-drug interactions, drug dosing errors, and inconsistent monitoring and observation.

Respiratory depression is the most common and profound adverse effect. All of the drugs used inhibit respiratory drive to some degree. The synergistic effects that occur when the drugs are combined can magnify the inhibition of the respiratory system. If the SaO$_2$ decreases to less than 90%, the procedure should be suspended and the patient evaluated. In addition, *chest wall and glottic rigidity* are catastrophic side effects of fentanyl that can occur when a high dose of the drug is injected rapidly. Under these circumstances the patient may require paralysis and mechanical ventilation until the symptoms resolve.

Sympathetic output from the central nervous system is similarly suppressed by all of the PSA drugs and can result in *bradycardia* and *hypotension*. Furthermore, a preponderance of patients take β-adrenergic blockers and calcium channel blockers, which increase the risk for *dysrhythmias* and cardiovascular collapse during PSA. Atropine *0.4 mg* IV push is used to treat symptomatic bradycardia (i.e., bradycardia associated with hypotension or heart block).

Nausea and vomiting are usually due to opioids. Preventing unwanted gastrointestinal side effects is important when the patient's sensorium is depressed, because emesis could lead to aspiration. Noxious gastrointestinal symptoms also make for an unpleasant experience for the patient. Ondansetron (Zofran) 4 to 8 mg IV is an excellent antiemetic.

Should the patient experience any *itching* or if *urticaria* becomes apparent (allergic reactions), diphenhydramine 25 mg IV should be administered. Auscultate the lungs for wheezing and check vital signs. Inhaled bronchodilators, IV corticosteroids, and subcutaneous epinephrine are appropriate for the management of allergic reactions and anaphylaxis.

In rare instances, *paradoxic reactions* to benzodiazepines can occur. Malignant hyperthermia must also be kept in mind as a potential complication.

POSTPROCEDURE RECOVERY AND PATIENT EDUCATION

Recovery should occur in a place where there is adequate cardiopulmonary monitoring and trained personnel for direct observation because the patient continues to be at risk for development of drug-related complications. If reversal agents are administered, continuous observation is required until sufficient time has elapsed for the last dose to wear off, thus avoiding resedation. The *Aldrete score* uses five criteria to determine a level at which it is safe to discharge the patient. The parameters include a measure of blood pressure and SaO$_2$ and an evaluation of the patient's mental status, airway patency, and motor function. (See flow sheet available at www.expertconsult.com.)

The patient's escort should be given both verbal and written instructions that include postprocedure activities, diet, and medications. Give the patient the following advice:
- Do not drive a car or operate hazardous equipment until the next day.
- Do not make important decisions or sign legal documents for 24 hours.

- Do not take medications, unless your clinician has prescribed them specifically, for the next 24 hours.
- Avoid alcohol, sedatives, and other depressant drugs for 24 hours.
- Notify your health care provider of pain, severe nausea, difficulty breathing, difficulty voiding, bleeding, or other new symptoms.

PATIENT EDUCATION GUIDES

See patient education and consent forms and PSA monitoring flow sheets available at www.expertconsult.com.

CPT/BILLING CODES

See the CPT definition for moderate sedation discussed earlier.

36000	Introduction of needle or intracatheter, vein
96379	IV injection (use in conjunction with J codes for drugs)
94760	Noninvasive ear or pulse oximetry for oxygen saturation
94760	Noninvasive single interpretation
94761	Noninvasive, multiple interpretations
99152	Sedation services provided by the same physician performing the diagnostic or therapeutic service that the sedation supports requiring the presence of an independent observer including monitoring of cardiorespiratory function (pulse oximetry, electrocardiogram, and blood pressure), age 5 years or older, initial 15 minutes. When providing moderate sedation, the following services are included and *not* reported separately:

- Assessment of the patient (not included in intraservice time)
- Establishment of IV access and fluids to maintain patency, when performed
- Administration of agent(s)
- Maintenance of sedation
- Monitoring of SaO_2, heart rate, and blood pressure
- Recovery (not included in intraservice time)

Intraservice time starts with the administration of the sedation agent(s), requires continuous face-to-face attendance, and ends at the conclusion of personal contact by the physician providing the sedation.

99153	Each additional 15 minutes of intraservice time
99156	Moderate sedation services provided by a physician other than professional performing the procedure, first 15 minutes, age 5 years or older
99157	Each additional 15 minutes

SUPPLIERS

(See contact information available at www.expertconsult.com.)

Banyan kits
Banyan International Corp.
Capnometry monitors
Nellcor Coviden Medtronic
Heartstream semiautomatic defibrillator
Philips Medical Systems
Vital signs monitors
Welch Allyn

RECOMMENDED READING

Bahn EL, Holt KR. Procedural sedation and analgesia: a review and new concepts. *Emerg Med Clin North Am.* 2005;23:509–517.

Deitch K, Miner J, Chudnofsky CR, Dominici P, Latta D. Does end tidal CO_2 monitoring during emergency department procedural sedation and analgesia with propofol decrease the incidence of hypoxic events? A randomized, controlled trial. *Ann Emerg.* 2010;55(3):258–264.

Frank LR, Strote J, Hauff SR, et al. Propofol by infusion protocol for ED procedural sedation. *Am J Emerg Med.* 2006;24:599–602.

Goodwin SA, Caro DA, Wolf SJ, et al. Clinical policy: procedural sedation and analgesia in the emergency department. *Ann Emerg Med.* 2005;45:177–196.

Green SM, Roback MG, Miner JR, et al. Fasting and emergency department procedural sedation and analgesia: a consensus-based clinical practice advisory. *Ann Emerg Med.* 2007;49:454–467.

Joint Commission on Accreditation of Healthcare Organizations. *2001 sedation and anesthesia care standards.* www.jointcommission.org.

Krauss B, Green SM. Systemic analgesia and sedation for privileges. In: Roberts JR, Custalow CB, Thomsen TW, eds. *Roberts and Hedges Clinical Procedures in Emergency Medicine.* 6th ed. Philadelphia: Elsevier; 2014:586–610.

Lightdale JR, Goldmann DA, Feldman HA, Newburg AR, Dinardo JA, Fox VL. Microstream capnography improves patient monitoring during moderate sedation: a randomized, controlled trial. *Pediatrics.* 2006;177(6):1170–1178.

Miller MA, Levy P, Patel MM. Procedural sedation and analgesia in the emergency department: what are the risks? *Emerg Med Clin North Am.* 2005;23:551–572.

Practice guidelines for sedation and analgesia by non-anesthesiologists. An updated report by the American Society of Anesthesiologists Task Force on Sedation and Analgesia by Non-anesthesiologists. *Anesthesiology.* 2002;96:1004–1017.

Wall BF, Magee K, Campbell SG, Zed PJ. Use of capnography in emergency department patients being sedated for procedures. *Cochrane Database Syst Rev.* 2017;(3):CD010698.

CHAPTER 2

PEDIATRIC SEDATION AND ANALGESIA

Paul W. Davis

Over the past 2 decades, various professional medical societies and hospital associations have readdressed the challenging issue of sedation and pain control in children, with the goal of developing and updating multidisciplinary guidelines. These societies have included the American Academy of Pediatrics (AAP), the American Society of Anesthesiologists (ASA), and The Joint Commission (TJC). Their recommendations have usually relied on expert opinion and consensus, and some openly advised that all pediatric sedation be performed under the direction of pediatric subspecialists. We and the American College of Emergency Physicians (ACEP) respectfully disagree with the assertion that only pediatricians and anesthesiologists can safely and effectively administer these medications.

The administration of medications for analgesia and moderate or deep sedation was previously termed *conscious sedation*. However, because these medications actually do alter a patient's level of consciousness and perception of pain, the phrase is inaccurate and is now rarely used.

HISTORICAL PERSPECTIVE ON UNDERTREATMENT OF PAIN

Historically, the management of pain and anxiety in the pediatric population outside of the operating room has been inadequate. Indeed, several studies have suggested that inattention to pain may be more prevalent for pediatric procedural care delivered outside of children's hospitals. Nevertheless, any clinician who has performed even minor procedures for infants and children appreciates the value of being able to safely and predictably sedate them. Aside from the psychological shock and trauma imposed on infants and children because of a limited understanding of the purpose for a procedure, developmental responses to pain vary by age and can thwart the most well-meaning clinician's efforts to complete a needed procedure.

At least six factors have been identified as contributing to the undertreatment of pain and anxiety in the pediatric population: (1) lack of familiarity with the use of sedative agents; (2) the erroneous conception that newborns and infants do not feel pain; (3) the incorrect belief that children have a very short-term recollection of painful events; (4) the fear of adverse effects of sedatives and analgesics; (5) the fear of masking the symptoms and signs of progressive injury or complications of treatment; and (6) the overarching underestimation of pediatric pain because of the young patient's inability to describe or quantify it.

DEVELOPMENTAL DIFFERENCES IN THE PERCEPTION OF PAIN

Although the physiologic response to pain is similar in adults and children, studies involving young children and fetuses suggest that they may actually experience a heightened perception of pain. A child's perception and clinical reaction to pain are influenced by several factors, including age, cognitive level, past experiences, extent of control over the situation, parental responses, parental guidance, and perceived cause and expected duration of the painful experience.

The plan for treatment should account for the differences in the pain response at different stages of development:

- *Younger than 6 months*—Anticipatory fear is not present and the infant reflects the level of anxiety of the parent. Withdrawal, facial grimacing, thrashing, and brief crying are typical expressions of pain.
- *6 to 18 months*—Anticipatory reactions begin to appear in response to fear of a suspected painful experience (e.g., withdrawal of a limb at the sight of a needle).
- *18 to 24 months*—Children begin to use words like "boo boo" and "hurt" in response to expected painful stimuli.
- *3 years*—Children are still unable to understand the reason for pain but are able to localize pain and identify its cause. They are more capable of reliably assessing the pain they feel. Their tolerance for a painful procedure is improved by allowing them some sense of control over certain aspects of the situation (e.g., when it will be performed or how they are positioned).
- *5 to 7 years*—Continued improvement in understanding of purpose and necessity of painful stimuli occur at this age with consequent improved cooperation.
- *8 to 12 years*—Comprehension of the whole process continues to grow with improved understanding/localization of internal pain.
- *Adolescence*—Children are adept at qualifying and quantifying pain, and they develop coping strategies similar to those of adults that help to diminish the perception of pain.

This chapter addresses the current breadth of effective pharmacologic and nonpharmacologic methods to alleviate both pain and anxiety in the pediatric patient before surgical operations and other procedures.

NONPHARMACOLOGIC TECHNIQUES

Needlesticks represent the most common source for iatrogenic procedural pain worldwide. From simple immunizations to venipuncture for laboratory studies to anesthetic injection before dermatologic procedures, laceration repair, and orthopedic reductions, needle pain is ubiquitous. In addition, more and more children are undergoing nonmedical procedures such as body piercings and tattooing (or removal of tattoos).

Untreated pain in the pediatric population has been studied extensively and does have long-term emotional and medical outcomes; these may be lifelong. Children now receive more than 20 needlesticks for immunizations before the age of 2 years and many develop needle phobia because only 1 in 9 is done with any kind of pain control. Adolescents may subsequently avoid needed medical treatment, 16% to 75% of adults surveyed refuse to donate blood, patients with human immunodeficiency virus infection may delay needed blood tests and continue to infect sexual partners, and geriatric patients may refuse influenza and pneumococcal vaccines, all owing to lifelong fear of needle pain.

Clinicians who perform neonatal elective circumcisions know first-hand the benefits associated with the oral administration of "sugar water." The analgesic effect and safety of sucrose for procedural pain both with and without the use of a pacifier (nonnutritive sucking) in neonates have been clearly demonstrated. Effectiveness in older patients is less clear, but it is easy to administer and there are no known adverse effects. Aspiration has not been a reported complication. The influence of age, intercurrent illness, type of procedure, and location of procedure is unclear at this time.

The simplest and most common nonpharmacologic method used with children is *voluntary and external distraction*. Giving the child and parent *verbal reassurance* by providing them with information about the procedure before it is started may help to allay anxiety but might also make it worse. *Hypnosis* has been used to help direct children's focus away from the procedure. Young patients can be taught to *repeat positive statements* to themselves for distraction and to relieve anxiety. These behavioral and cognitive approaches represent useful adjuncts that are frequently overlooked because of perceived time constraints in a busy office or emergency department. *Distraction techniques* include counting or saying the "ABCs," listening to music or watching videotapes, blowing bubbles, spinning pinwheels, using party blowers, playing "I Spy" games, and using "medical play" as employed by child-life programs. *Behavioral treatments* include the techniques of desensitization (the gradual, increasing exposure to a procedure over time), positive reinforcement (rewards and positive statements during or after a procedure), and relaxation techniques (the use of breathing, imagery, and self-hypnosis to decrease anxiety). Although all these techniques have been shown to be very effective, they need props, take time, and may require trained personnel.

The dorsal column of the spinal cord forms a common final pathway for several kinds of afferent neurologic stimuli, including pain, position, temperature sensation, and vibration. By applying the gate theory and stimulating nerve fibers with either cold or vibration, the sensation of sharp pain can be decreased or eliminated by interfering with its transmission because of the other impulses. The use of cold water or ice and the application of vibrating massagers represent effective ways of ameliorating pain. Cold sprays (e.g., Pain Ease [ethyl chloride], Gebauer; Frigi-Dent, Ellman International) have been widely used, but the research into their efficacy in children has been equivocal at best. A device that uses vibration (Buzzy; MMJ Labs) has been proven to work as well as topical anesthetics. Pediatric dentists frequently use tactile vibration with their opposite hand in the delivery of oral anesthesia.

TOPICAL ANALGESICS AND ANESTHETICS FOR CHILDREN

Also see Chapter 4.

Ease of administration with minimal trauma for the child and parent would make these the medications of choice for a large variety of procedures. However, the reality has never lived up to the promise.

The topical agent most commonly used for laceration repair in children is LET (a combination of lidocaine, epinephrine, and tetracaine), with an onset of action of 20 minutes. EMLA cream is a eutectic mixture of lidocaine and prilocaine but often requires application approximately 1 hour before the procedure, limiting its usefulness. LMX 4 is a nonprescription 4% liposomal lidocaine preparation that is also effective as a topical anesthetic agent.

Zingo (Powder Pharmaceuticals) has been approved by the U.S. Food and Drug Administration (FDA) for use on intact skin to provide topical local analgesia before venipuncture or peripheral intravenous (IV) cannulation in children ages 3 to 18 years. This needle-free product has a novel delivery system using pressurized gas jets that deliver lidocaine hydrochloride monohydrate directly through the epidermis and into the dermis. Zingo comes as a ready-to-use, sterile, single-use, disposable, needle-free delivery system.

The product consists of a drug reservoir cassette filled with 0.5 mg lidocaine powder (particle size of 40 μm), a pressurized helium gas cylinder, and a safety interlock. The safety interlock prevents premature triggering of the device. Once Zingo is pressed against the skin, the interlock is released, allowing the button to be depressed to deliver the anesthetic. Triggering the device results in a sound not unlike the popping of a balloon. Because the price of this single-use product is between $20 and $25, its use can increase the cost of venipuncture considerably. Although use can be repeated, if necessary, at a different site (a frequent requirement when attempting to place an IV catheter in dehydrated children), repeated use at the same site is not recommended and the clinician needs to pay heed to the total dosage of anesthetic administered to avoid toxicity.

Zingo provides local dermal analgesia within 1 to 3 minutes of application, and analgesia diminishes within 10 minutes of treatment. Most adverse reactions are application site–related and include bruising, burning, pain, contusion, and hemorrhage. These occurred in 4% of pediatric patients. The most common systemic adverse reactions are nausea (2%) and vomiting (1%). Erythema, edema, pruritus, and petechiae occurred in approximately half of all patients and are brief and self-limited.

Hand-held jet injectors (Madajet, Mada Medical) are available that use high pressure to deliver lidocaine or other local anesthetics fairly quietly through a very small orifice and across intact skin (see Fig. 111.5). For whatever reason, they have not seen widespread use in primary care offices or emergency departments, perhaps because of the cost of equipment or the effort needed to clean the equipment after use. However, if multiple uses are anticipated, even with multiple patients, because there are no needles, only the tips need to be changed between patients. Cleaning the equipment can therefore be conveniently done at the end of the shift or the day.

PHARMACOLOGIC AGENTS FOR SEDATION AND ANALGESIA

The ideal pediatric agent for procedural sedation would have certain characteristics. First, it would be both 100% safe and completely effective for the full range of desired properties—amnesia, analgesia, anxiolysis, motor control, and sedation. It would have rapid onset, fast recovery, and a predictable duration of action and would be completely reversible. In addition, it would be easy to titrate and painless to inject, provide choices for administration route, and be easy to administer. Finally, such an ideal agent would be entirely free of adverse effects and complications.

Needless to say, this ideal pediatric sedative agent has yet to be discovered. A wide range of approved short-acting agents is currently available for use as sedative-hypnotics or analgesics in infants and children. Each of these agents offers advantages in select situations and for specific patients. Procedures that are not painful but require patients to cease moving can be performed with sedation alone. However, painful procedures require both sedation and analgesia.

In 1998, ACEP developed an evidence-based clinical policy for the use of pharmacologic agents for sedation and analgesia that included children. This policy was most recently updated in 2013 and focuses on use of ketamine, propofol, and etomidate or combinations of ketamine and propofol in children. Prior guidelines focused on these, as well as use of fentanyl/midazolam, methohexital, and pentobarbital in children. The specific uses, recommendations, and cautions for these and other agents are addressed in the following section. Specific indications and contraindications are addressed individually for each medication. The important characteristics of selected agents are summarized in Table 2.1 for easy reference.

Sedative-Hypnotic Agents

These medications provide anxiolysis, control of movement, sedation, and often amnesia for the painful event but do not provide analgesia.

TABLE 2.1	Summary of Important Characteristics of Selected Agents		
Characteristic	Chloral Hydrate	Fentanyl	Ketamine
Dose and route	Oral: 20–100 mg/kg up to 1 g/dose infants and 2 g/dose older children	IV: 0.5–1.0 μg/kg/dose Titrate q3min to desired effect Suggested max: 2–3 μg/kg	IV: 0.5–1.0 mg/kg; start with 0.25–0.5 mg/kg and titrate to effect q3–5min (suggested max: 1 mg/kg). Combine with atropine 0.01–0.02 mg/kg IV IM: 1–6 mg/kg; usually 2–4 mg/kg, may repeat q5–10 min (suggested max: 6 mg/kg). Combine with atropine 0.02 mg/kg IM Oral: 5–10 mg/kg (suggested max: 6 mg/kg) Combine with atropine 0.02–0.03 mg/kg Rectal: 50 mg/kg
Onset of action/time to peak effect	Onset 15–30 min Peak effect 30–60 min	Onset 1–2 min Peak effect 2–3 min	IV: onset <1 min, peak several minutes IM: Onset 4–10 min, peak 20 min (dose dependent) Oral: Onset >5 min, peak 20 min Rectal: Onset 10–15 min, peak 30 min
Duration of action	60 min; residual sedation may last much longer in neonates and toddlers	20–30 min	IV: 15–45 min IM: 30–60 min Oral: 30–60 min Rectal: 45–75 min
Adverse reactions	Respiratory depression Airway obstruction Paradoxic hyperactivity Delirium Nausea Vomiting Residual sedation (up to 24 hr)	Respiratory depression Bradycardia Dysphoria Delirium Nausea Vomiting Pruritus Urinary retention Smooth muscle spasm Hypotension Allergic reaction Chest wall/glottic rigidity	Laryngospasm Rare respiratory depression Decreased response to hypercarbia Stimulation of salivary and tracheobronchial secretions Mild to moderate increase in blood pressure, heart rate, and cardiac output Emergence phenomena (hallucinations, nightmares, severe agitation) Paradoxic hypotension Skeletal muscle hypertonicity Rigidity Mild disequilibrium Random movements of head or extremities Elevated intracranial and intraocular pressure Nystagmus Vomiting Transient erythematous rash Loss of protective reflexes/aspiration Allergic reaction
Drug Interactions	Coadministration of other sedatives or narcotics increases risk of respiratory complications; can alter warfarin metabolism	Coadministration of other respiratory depressants such as benzodiazepines increases the risk of respiratory depression	Half-life may be prolonged if given with other agents metabolized in the liver Coadministration with benzodiazepines or opiates may decrease the occurrence of hallucinations but may also prolong recovery
Contraindications	Repeated dosing in neonates Patients with significant liver or renal disease Patients with cardiac arrhythmias Patients with porphyria Hypersensitivity	Known allergy or prior serious adverse event	Presence of URI increases risk of laryngospasm to 9% Airway instability (e.g., tracheal stenosis) Presence of potential head injury Known increased intracranial pressure Open globe injury Hypertensive disease Coronary artery disease Psychosis Prior adverse reaction to ketamine Relative contraindications: oral procedures, thyroid disease
Comments	Dose should be decreased in high-risk or debilitated patients Most effective in children <4 years	Slow infusions and lower doses decrease the risk of chest wall rigidity Chest wall and glottic rigidity can be reversed with succinylcholine or naloxone Dose should be decreased in high-risk or debilitated patients Respiratory depressant effects may last longer than opioid effects Use with caution in patients at risk for cholelithiasis Delayed clearance in patients with hepatic disease	Causes dissociative reaction (trancelike state) Provides amnesia, analgesia, immobilization, and sedation All-or-none sedation: no sedation continuum Especially useful for young children (lower incidence of emergence phenomena)
Antagonist	None	Naloxone 10–100 μg/kg IV/IM/SQ Adolescent dose: 0.1–0.8 mg Titrate slowly to patient response waiting 2–3 min between doses	None

BP, Blood pressure; CHF, congestive heart failure; CI, contraindicated; CNS, central nervous system; CO, cardiac output; HR, heart rate; IM, intramuscular; IV, intravenous; SQ, subcutaneous; SVR, systemic vascular resistance; URI, upper respiratory infection.

Lytic Cocktail

This time-honored mixture is addressed briefly here for historical reasons and because many older primary care clinicians have used this regimen extensively in the past with great success. The "lytic cocktail" consists of chlorpromazine (Thorazine), promethazine (Phenergan), and meperidine (Demerol) and is given intramuscularly according to the weight of the child: chlorpromazine, 0.5 mg/kg; promethazine, 0.5 mg/kg; and meperidine, 0.7 to 1.0 mg/kg. It is not recommended because (1) the clinician must deal with the side effects of three medications instead of one (polypharmacy); and (2) its effect can be erratic and unpredictable. Up to one-third of children never obtain moderate to adequate sedation; in the other two-thirds, too deep a level of sedation is reached, and it is difficult to reverse. The mean time to discharge after use is 5 hours; the mean time for the child to return to normal behavior ranges from 4 to 34 hours.

Benzodiazepines (Midazolam)

Benzodiazepines provide sedation, anxiolysis, and amnesia but do not provide analgesia. There are several reasons why midazolam (Versed) is the most commonly used agent in this category and the clear drug of choice for pediatric procedures requiring merely sedation and anxiolysis. Midazolam has a rapid onset of action, short duration of action, and rapid recovery time. Although patients may not appear sedated when it is used as a single agent, they become more relaxed and cooperative, and there is the frequent (but not universal) benefit of a marked amnestic response for the event. Controversy exists as to whether this marked amnestic response actually blocks "intrinsic memory" (i.e., although patients may not consciously recall the painful incident, the traumatic event is still recorded in the brain at the subconscious level). For this reason, it is advisable to coadminister an appropriate analgesic agent for painful procedures.

Midazolam offers great flexibility in route of delivery because it can be administered by the *oral, intranasal, sublingual, rectal, intramuscular (IM), or IV route.* Its efficacy is well established. However, when used as a single agent (i.e., not combined with an opiate, ketamine, or droperidol), it is inferior to other regimens or single agents, and patients may appear to be wide awake.

Recommended dosages vary depending on route of administration. *Oral* midazolam is given at doses of 0.5 to 0.7 mg/kg and results in the onset of mellowness at 10 to 30 minutes. Duration of action is 60 to 90 minutes. *Intranasal* midazolam at recommended dosages of 0.2 to 0.5 mg/kg has a more rapid onset of action at 5 to 15 minutes, duration of action of 45 to 60 minutes, and some effects lingering for up to several hours. The solution is drawn up into a tuberculin syringe, the needle is removed, and the drug is instilled into the child's nares with the child supine or the headed tilted back. Recommended rectal doses of midazolam are 0.25 to 0.5 mg/kg, with efficacy reported variably from 62% to 93% for laceration repair. Agitation (reported in up to 17%) has been the major drawback of this route of administration. The recommended IV dose of midazolam is 0.05 to 0.15 mg/kg, and the IM dose is 0.05 to 0.20 mg/kg; time to peak effect is 2 to 3 minutes for the IV route and 10 to 20 minutes for the IM route. Duration of action is 30 minutes to 2 hours.

Adverse effects are uncommon and include the atypical effects of paradoxic agitation and euphoria after administration or an emergence reaction when given IV (1.4%) or orally (6%). Hypotension and respiratory depression are rare but can occur, especially if a narcotic agent is coadministered. The antagonist flumazenil (Romazicon) at a dose of 0.002 to 0.02 mg/kg IV can be given to reverse the effects of midazolam, but patients will require a longer period of observation in recovery (2 hours is commonly recommended) because this agent may have a shorter duration of action than the benzodiazepine, with consequent recurrence of sedation or respiratory depression after the antagonist has worn off.

Chloral Hydrate

In the recent past, chloral hydrate was considered the mainstay of safe, effective pediatric sedation. Although it has a wide margin of safety, chloral hydrate is primarily used to sedate children younger than 3 years of age for diagnostic imaging because its effects on older children are unreliable. It can be administered orally at a dose of 20 to 100 mg/kg up to 1 g/dose for infants and 2 g/dose for older children. Rectal dosing is no longer recommended due to erratic absorption. Unfortunately, chloral hydrate has an unpleasant smell and taste, making it difficult to entice a child to take much of it orally. Peak action occurs at 30 to 60 minutes, making it much less useful than other agents in the emergency setting. Its duration of action is quite variable, with sedation lasting from 1 to 2 hours after administration.

Adverse effects include prolonged sedation (effects can last up to 24 hours), paradoxic agitation, delirium, and coma, but airway obstruction and respiratory depression can occur and there is no consistent dose below which complications do not occur; deaths have been reported. In one published series, adverse events were reported in 33% of children who received chloral hydrate either alone or in combination with other sedatives. This relatively high rate of complications contrasts markedly with the widespread perception of its safety. There is no reversal agent for chloral hydrate, and its use is contraindicated in patients with cardiac, hepatic, and renal disease as well as those with porphyria. In addition, its sedative effects can be difficult to predict. In the past, this agent was frequently used in unmonitored settings. In light of the difficulty in predicting its sedative effects and the attendant risks with its use, it is imperative that procedural sedation protocols for monitoring patients during and after administration of this agent be strictly followed.

Barbiturates (Thiopental, Methohexital, and Pentobarbital)

Barbiturates are primarily used for sedating children younger than 3 years of age to perform diagnostic imaging. They are relatively safe but are contraindicated in patients with porphyria. Major side effects include respiratory depression with apnea and hypotension, both of which are more common when barbiturates are used in combination with opiates or benzodiazepines.

Thiopental (Pentothal) is a short-acting barbiturate with an onset of action of 30 to 60 seconds when given intravenously and only 5 to 8 minutes when given rectally. It has a duration of effect of 15 minutes when given intravenously but up to 1 hour when given rectally. Given intravenously at doses of 20 to 25 mg/kg, thiopental is generally given rectally to children at a dosage of 5 to 10 mg/kg. Thiopental has the notable side effect of decreasing intracranial pressure; it is therefore particularly useful in patients for whom increased intracranial pressure is a concern.

Methohexital (Brevital) is an ultra-short-acting agent with an onset of action of 30 to 60 seconds and duration of effect of 5 to 10 minutes. It is twice as potent as thiopental and can be administered intravenously at a dose of 0.5 to 1.0 mg/kg to children older than 12 years. It should not be administered in younger children and is contraindicated in children with temporal lobe epilepsy because it can cause seizures in this subgroup. Methohexital is rarely used in the emergency department anymore because of a single study (Zink, 1991) of 102 patients, in which 22 patients developed respiratory depression requiring bag-valve-mask assistance. Five of these 22 patients developed transient apnea. If combined with an analgesic medication, respiratory depression is minimized by first administering the analgesic to control pain and then titrating methohexital to needed effect.

Pentobarbital (Nembutal) is a useful barbiturate sedative for longer radiologic procedures such as magnetic resonance imaging and positron emission tomography scans. It has an onset of action of 3 to 5 minutes when given IV and a duration of effect of 30 to 45 minutes. For children and infants older than 6 months, it can be given intravenously at a dosage of 1 to 3 mg/kg and titrated every 3 to 5 minutes to a maximum dosage of 100 mg or intramuscularly at a dosage of 2 to 6 mg/kg to a maximum dosage of 100 mg.

Etomidate

Etomidate is an ultra-short-acting imidazole (nonbarbiturate) hypnotic agent with no analgesic properties. Although studies have been published supporting its safety and efficacy in children, the FDA does not currently recommend its use in children younger than 10 years.

Its consideration as a potential sedative for children stems from its use in the emergency department for both adults and children as an induction agent in rapid-sequence intubation. After the administration of the recommended dose of 0.3 mg/kg IV, etomidate has a rapid onset of action of 5 to 30 seconds and a duration effect of only 5 to 15 minutes. It has the major advantage of decreasing intracranial pressure, like thiopental, and not adversely affecting hemodynamic stability. Reported adverse effects include myoclonus (22% of children receiving it in one study) and oxygen desaturation. When given with fentanyl for analgesia, its safety and efficacy compare favorably with midazolam and fentanyl. Compared with pentobarbital for pediatric sedation before diagnostic imaging, etomidate provided a shorter duration of sedation, greater overall efficacy, fewer failures, and fewer adverse effects.

Propofol

Propofol is a nonopioid, nonbarbiturate sedative-hypnotic agent that produces deep sedation almost immediately after IV administration (the one arm–brain circulation time is approximately 40 seconds). It has no analgesic properties but does produce a modest amnestic effect (although weaker than that of midazolam) and is affectionately known as "oil of amnesia," although this term would be more aptly applied to midazolam. Propofol has been used extensively by anesthesiologists and pediatric intensivists as either an induction agent for general anesthesia or as a sedative in the pediatric intensive care unit for patients requiring mechanical ventilation or other uncomfortable procedures. It acts as a direct muscle relaxant and has both antiemetic and euphoric properties. It has no adverse effects on hepatic or renal function. Propofol does not increase either the intraocular pressure or intracranial pressure. When given in conjunction with an opioid analgesic agent, it provides very effective analgesia and sedation for painful procedures. It also has the benefit of an extremely short recovery time of 5 to 15 minutes. Even if deep sedation inadvertently drifts into general anesthesia, with the attendant need for assisted ventilation, the patient is likely to awaken within a few minutes after cessation of the IV infusion. Nevertheless, controversy remains intense regarding the use of propofol outside of the operating room or intensive care unit or by nonanesthesiologists.

The recommended induction dosage for children 3 to 16 years of age is 2.5 to 3.5 mg/kg, administered IV over 20 to 30 seconds. A lower dosage should be administered in children with an ASA classification of III or IV. IV infusion should follow using a rate of 200 to 300 µg/kg per minute for children 2 months to 16 years of age, decreasing the dose to 125 to 150 µg/kg per minute after the infusion has been running 30 minutes or longer. Higher infusion rates may be required for children younger than 5 years.

Adverse effects noted with propofol include apnea, hypotension, bacterial contamination of the lipid emulsion, and pain at the site of injection (must be administered with lidocaine). Propofol decreases the systemic vascular resistance by an estimated 15% and cardiac output by more than 10%. Hypotension has been reported to occur between 17% and 92% of the time. Respiratory depression results in decreased tidal volume and unpredictable apnea. Oxygen desaturation has been reported in 5% of cases, and simple airway interventions were required in 3% of patients; increased oxygen concentration sufficed for almost all other patients. The need for endotracheal intubation has been reported in only 0.03% of patients. It is difficult to titrate this drug because of both its potency and its rapid onset of action and time to peak effect. Indeed, this may be the root cause for the frequency with which this agent results in a deeper level of sedation than intended.

In several observational studies, propofol sedation has been reported to be both safe and effective when performed by trained emergency department personnel as long as established practice guidelines and hospital protocols are followed strictly. Because it is considered a general anesthetic agent, a second qualified and credentialed provider (i.e., not the clinician performing the procedure) should be present to administer and monitor the patient throughout the procedure until the patient is fully awake. The patient should be carefully monitored with pulse oximetry, as well as capnography and physical monitoring of spontaneous respiratory effort.

Propofol is relatively contraindicated in patients with a known allergy to eggs or soybeans, because current formulations of propofol contain soybean oil, egg lecithin, and egg yolk phospholipids. The generic form contains sulfites, so the brand name Diprivan must be used for sulfite-allergic patients.

Propofol can be coadministered with ketamine, opioid analgesics, or midazolam, but the initiating and maintenance dosage of propofol will likely need to be decreased. The likelihood of sedation events and complications is increased with the coadministration of narcotics. Adverse events are also more likely when propofol is used for sedation in patients with an ASA classification of III or higher.

Other Agents

Ketamine

Ketamine is a phencyclidine derivative and is unique among the sedative-hypnotic and analgesic agents in that it is a "dissociative sedative." It actually produces a trancelike state and provides amnesia, analgesia, immobilization, and sedation. It is therefore an ideal agent for use in young children, often being used as a single agent, resulting in an enhanced safety profile. Unlike other tranquilizers, there is no "sedation continuum" (i.e., the sedative effect is either present or absent). Ketamine is often used in young children for brief, painful procedures such as fracture reduction and laceration repair.

Not only is ketamine very effective when used according to practice guidelines, it is very safe. Patients almost always retain protective airway reflexes, intact upper airway muscular tone, and spontaneous breathing. It can be administered orally (5 to 10 mg/kg), rectally (50 mg/kg), IM (1 to 6 mg/kg), or IV (0.5 to 1 mg/kg). IV doses can be titrated to effect every 3 to 5 minutes, starting with 0.25 to 0.5 mg/kg. Onset of action is less than 1 minute with IV use, with maximal effect noted at approximately 3 to 4 minutes. Onset of action is 4 to 10 minutes with IM use, with maximal effect noted at 20 minutes. Oral and rectal use results in an even slower onset of action, with peak effect at 20 to 30 minutes. With IV use the duration of effect is short, 15 to 45 minutes, but recovery times are much longer (30 to 75 minutes) and less predictable for oral, IM, and rectal use.

Side effects of ketamine include both vomiting and increased salivation. The latter can be controlled by preadministration of either atropine or glycopyrrolate. Laryngospasm occurs very rarely and can be managed by positive-pressure bag-mask ventilation. Hypertonicity can also occur. Ketamine is most known for the frequent occurrence of unpleasant hallucinations and nightmares, as well as severe agitation during emergence from sedation. These emergence phenomena are much more common in patients older than 15 years and extremely rare in younger children. Coadministration of midazolam has been proposed to minimize this adverse effect, but to date there are no convincing large studies to support this. Although midazolam also decreases the incidence of vomiting with ketamine, it also results in a fourfold to fivefold increase in the incidence of oxygen desaturation. Still, ketamine with midazolam has been associated with fewer adverse events compared with ketamine combined with fentanyl or propofol, especially in children younger than 10 years.

Unfortunately, ketamine has many contraindications, including age younger than 3 months, airway instability, cardiovascular or pulmonary diseases including bronchospasm, glaucoma or eye injury, increased intracranial pressure or head injury, porphyria, thyroid disease, and psychosis.

Nitrous Oxide

Also see Chapter 3.

Inhaled nitrous oxide provides amnesia, mild analgesia, anxiolysis, and sedation when mixed in a 1:1 ratio with oxygen and administered through a demand-valve mask. This system requires patient cooperation, so this method of sedation is generally reserved for children older than 4 years.

At the concentrations usually used for sedation and analgesia, nitrous oxide use preserves protective airway reflexes, normal blood pressure and pulse, and spontaneous respirations. It has an excellent safety profile, and adverse effects are typically mild, including nausea, vomiting, and occasional dysphoria. It can be used alone or in combination with other sedatives and analgesics, and it has a proven track record of efficacy for a variety of painful procedures. Contraindications include pregnancy, vomiting, and the presence of known or presumed "trapped air" (e.g., bowel obstruction, pneumothorax, perforated viscus, or middle ear infection).

Opioid Analgesics (Fentanyl)

Opioids (narcotic agents) are widely used and well-established analgesics. Although morphine is the prototype drug in this class, and meperidine also has been used extensively in the past, fentanyl has rapidly become the opioid agent of choice for children requiring potent analgesia during procedural sedation. Fentanyl is a synthetic opioid that has 75 to 125 times the potency of morphine and a very rapid IV onset of action (1 to 2 minutes) with a relatively short duration of action (20 to 30 minutes). It is administered in an initial IV dose of 0.5 to 1 µg/kg, and its pharmacokinetics permit smooth and safe titration either alone or in combination with midazolam at intervals of approximately 3 minutes until the desired effect is achieved.

Fentanyl has additional *advantages* over the longer-acting narcotic agents. It lacks the histamine release characteristic of morphine and the buildup of very-long-acting metabolites occasionally seen with meperidine (the so-called *serotonin surge syndrome*). It is also effective when administered intranasally or by nebulizer.

Adverse effects of fentanyl include hypoxemia and respiratory depression. Pruritis, bradycardia, nausea, and vomiting can occur. Chest wall and glottic rigidity are uncommon but serious complications and have been reported in neonates receiving a single dose of fentanyl between 3 and 5 µg/kg. In fact, fentanyl has the highest reported complication rate of any agent used for procedural analgesia and sedation. However, fentanyl is rarely used as a single agent so it is likely that much of the excess risk is due to polypharmacy. The practicing clinician needs always to remain vigilant when using opioid-sedative combinations, especially when three or more medications have been administered.

The antagonist naloxone is an effective reversal agent for fentanyl. It is administered IV at a dose of 0.1 mg/kg for children 0 to 5 years of age and 2 mg/kg for children older than 5 years. The dose can be repeated. Its onset of action is 1 to 2 minutes, with a duration of effect of 20 to 40 minutes, resulting in complete reversal as a single dose most of the time when used with fentanyl. Incidentally, when used to reverse the effects of meperidine, naloxone can result in normeperidine-induced seizures. If glottic or chest wall rigidity occurs, a neuromuscular blocking agent such as succinylcholine, rocuronium, or vecuronium may need to be administered to achieve an oral or endotracheal airway, along with bag-mask positive-pressure ventilation.

If any significant sedation and anesthesia is going to be used other than basic anxiolytics (what was formerly called "conscious sedation"), strict adherence to safety and established guidelines is imperative (also see Chapter 1).

EQUIPMENT

The equipment required for pediatric sedation and analgesia comprises everything that is needed to effectively and safely monitor the patient through induction, maintenance, and recovery from the effects of the medications used. In addition, equipment needs to be readily at hand to manage any complication that may arise from the unintended escalation of sedation level to either deep sedation or general anesthesia. A list of basic essential equipment appears in Box 2.1.

BOX 2.1   Equipment Needs and Considerations for Pediatric Procedural Sedation

- Oxygen with a system that is capable of administering at least 90% O_2 at 10 L/min for 60 minutes, nasal cannulas, oxygen mask
- Bag-mask system for positive-pressure ventilation
- Laryngoscope with appropriately sized blades and endotracheal tubes
- Suction catheters and apparatus
- Emergency cart with appropriate medications and Breslow tape
- Defibrillator
- Pulse oximeter, continuous
- Electrocardiograph monitor, continuous
- Noninvasive blood pressure apparatus
- Emergency antagonists, including naloxone and flumazenil
- Succinylcholine if fentanyl is being used
- IV start kit and appropriately sized IV catheters
- 500-mL bags of normal saline and Ringer lactate
- Telephone or radio for summoning assistance in an emergency
- End-tidal CO_2 monitor (when available)
- Equipment for administering blood and blood components need to be readily available if transfusion becomes necessary
- Intraosseous catheter kit should be immediately available if IV access is lost and a standard IV line cannot be started

The majority of this equipment is available in the Banyan kit (a "crash cart in a suitcase"), available commercially.

BOX 2.2   Components of the Children's Hospital of Wisconsin Sedation Model

Monitoring and personnel requirements
Nothing-by-mouth guidelines
Presedation evaluation
Focused present and past history
Focused physical examination
Vital signs
Graded risk assessment documentation
Assignment of ASA physical status score
Generation of sedation plan
Informed parental consent
Equipment and monitoring standards based on actual level of sedation
Quantitative sedation scoring
Time-based recording of vital signs, oxyhemoglobin saturation, and sedation level
Recovery and discharge criteria
Standardized record

Modified from American Society of Anesthesiologists (ASA) and American Academy of Pediatrics (AAP) guidelines. Each of these components is specifically prompted on a uniform sedation documentation record.

PRESEDATION EVALUATION

Box 2.2 summarizes a comprehensive and accepted set of required components for the safe administration of procedural sedation in the pediatric patient. This sedation model was developed at the Children's Hospital of Wisconsin. Pediatric sedation does not relieve the clinician of the need to explain the anticipated procedure to both the child (when their cognitive level warrants) and the parent or

TABLE 2.2	Airway Assessment
Physical Characteristic	**Specific Concerns**
Body habitus	Obese vs. thin
	Size and length of neck
Presence of micrognathia (see Fig. 2.1)	Receding mandible
	Size of mandible in relation to face
Dentition status	Protruding incisors (buck teeth)
	Poor dental condition; caries
	Loose teeth or crowns
	Distance between upper and lower teeth; associated with the presence of high-arched palate
Joint mobility	Mobility of the head at the atlanto-occipital joint (see Fig. 2.2)
	Mobility of the mandible at the temporo-mandibular joint
	Mallampati classification (see Chapter 1, Fig. 1.2)
Thyromental distance (>6 cm, 3 fingerbreadths)	By measuring the thyromental distance, the anatomic proximity of the glottis to the mandible and base of the tongue can be gauged
Intraoral concerns	Status of tonsils, intraoral tissues, torus palatinus, tumors, trauma
	Redundant tissue
	Presence of neonatal teeth
	Intraoral, lingual, or labial body ornaments
Nasal concerns	Body ornaments: studs and rings
	Patient may require a nasal airway rather than oral

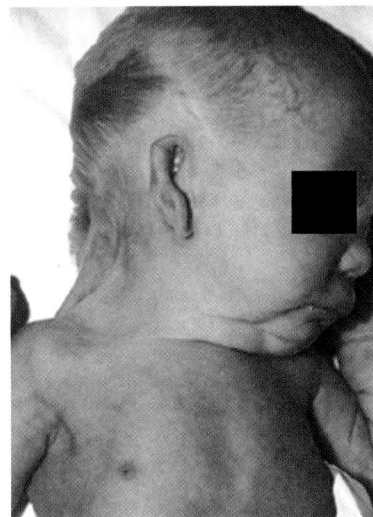

Fig. 2.1   Micrognathia.

guardian. Informed consent for both the sedation and the procedure should be obtained and documented in the medical record. An example of a procedural sedation informed consent form is available at www.expertconsult.com.

A focused history and physical assessment should be performed before administering any sedative or analgesic agent. This evaluation can be performed any time within 30 days of an intended procedure, depending on institutional requirements and standards. However, the patient must be reassessed immediately before initiating procedural sedation to ensure his or her suitability for sedation, as well as to reconfirm the appropriateness of the planned sedation regimen. The sedation plan and choice of sedative/analgesic agent(s) should be clearly documented on the presedation evaluation form.

The history should include allergies, use of medications or illicit drugs, diseases, operations, hospitalizations, previous exposure to sedation or general anesthesia, untoward reactions to anesthetic agents in the past, relevant family history, and the time and content of the last oral intake. The physical examination should include auscultation of the heart and lungs, as well as a careful assessment of the airway (Table 2.2 and Figs. 2.1 and 2.2). Special attention should be given to identifying anatomic or clinical conditions that might interfere with endotracheal intubation and resuscitation should they become necessary. These conditions are summarized in Box 2.3.

Pediatric patients need to be assigned an ASA Physical Status Classification before performing any emergency or elective procedure. This classification is summarized in Table 1.2.

A pediatric patient's suitability for mild, moderate, or deep sedation outside of the operating room can range from excellent to very poor in each of the ASA classes but is generally expected to be good for classes I and II. Formal published recommendations suggest that an anesthesiologist or subspecialist should be consulted for patients with ASA classes of III and IV to assist with airway abnormalities and management, as well as other special needs. At the least, in clinical settings where such assistance is unavailable, a second trained and experienced clinician should be consulted whose entire focus is the management of sedation throughout the procedure. For elective procedures, transfer to a larger facility where such help is available should be seriously considered.

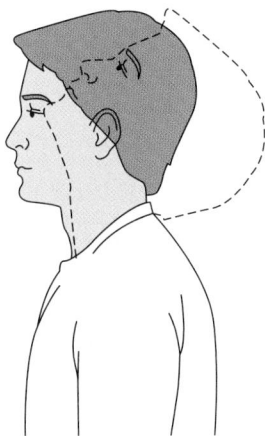

Fig. 2.2   Mobility of the head at the atlanto-occipital joint.

BOX 2.3   Sedation Graded Risk Assessment Tool: Sedation Risk Factors

Snoring, stridor, or sleep apnea
Craniofacial malformation
History of airway difficulty
Vomiting, bowel obstruction
Gastroesophageal reflux
Pneumonia or oxygen requirement
Reactive airways disease
Hypovolemia, cardiac disease
Sepsis
Altered mental status
History of sedation failure
Inadequate nothing-by-mouth time
No identified risk factors

Medical conditions and patient characteristics with known potential for increasing the risk of procedural sedation are specifically prompted on the sedation record.

Fasting Before Sedation

There is limited evidence to support an optimum duration of fasting before sedation to reduce the risk of aspiration. ASA guidelines, which are based on expert opinion and consensus, recommend a minimum fasting period of 2 hours for clear fluids, 4 hours for breast milk, and 6 hours for formula, nonhuman milk, and solids. For children with normal airways and no clinical predisposition to aspiration, a systematic review of randomized trials failed to find any benefit for fasting from fluids for more than 6 hours compared with 2 hours. In addition, no statistically significant differences in intraoperative gastric volumes and pH were noted. It should also be noted that all this research is related to general anesthesia in the operating room; any extrapolation of data to other clinical settings may not apply. According to an expert panel that published their findings in *Annals of Emergency Medicine* in 2007, the following considerations related to the risk of aspiration should dictate the planned depth and length of procedural sedation in the emergency department:

- Possibility of a difficult airway
- Conditions predisposing to esophageal reflux, including elevated intracranial pressure, gastritis, bowel obstruction, or ileus
- Age less than 6 months
- Severe systemic disease with functional limitation (ASA class ≥3)
- Timing and nature of last oral intake
- Urgency of procedure

If the fasting guidelines cannot be followed, the following should be taken into consideration:

- Delay of the procedure.
- Referral to a licensed anesthesia provider to help protect the airway.
- In emergent and urgent situations, the increased risk of aspiration must be weighed against the benefits of the procedure. The lightest effective sedation should be used.

PERSONNEL

Clinicians who administer procedural sedation must fully understand the pharmacology of the medications they use. They must also have the breadth of clinical experience and judgment to select a regimen that is appropriate for both the patient and the intended procedure. Because altered consciousness represents a continuum and not discrete "quantum" levels, clinicians should have the requisite training and current skill to deal effectively with complications arising from the patient drifting to the next deeper level of sedation than that intended.

Two trained and credentialed individuals are required when a patient is significantly sedated for a procedure, one to perform the procedure and the second to administer and monitor the sedation. Ideally, both individuals would be clinicians competent at inducing anesthesia; this choice is probably prudent if deep sedation is planned (at the least, the second individual should be a licensed nurse anesthetist). In practice, the second individual is either a nurse or trained assistant (certified medical assistant, certified nursing assistant, or respiratory therapist). He or she monitors the patient and documents vital signs, level of consciousness, timing and dose of medication administration, and any complications. If the assistant is not a clinician trained in sedation management, the clinician in charge of the procedure must be able to stop the procedure at any time to manage complications arising from sedation and analgesia.

MONITORING

Documentation of any procedure should be scrupulous and complete and include a description of the level of responsiveness of the patient, otherwise known as the sedation score (see Chapter 1, Table 1.1). Document the issues discussed when obtaining informed consent in the patient record. Some medicolegal experts also recommend asking a parent or guardian to sign a form listing each procedure that the clinician might perform. With regard to pediatric sedation, the clinician should document how well the patient tolerated the method used. If side effects are noted or complications encountered, full documentation—including a careful record of all measures and medications used in dealing with them—must be given in the sedation report in the patient's medical record. A time-based record of heart rate (electrocardiographic monitor or pulse oximeter), oxygen saturation (pulse oximeter), and end-tidal CO_2 (if used), as well as nursing assessments and monitoring, must be made until the patient is fully recovered. For patients with an underlying illness or for whom deep sedation is planned, these measurements along with vital signs should be taken and recorded at least every 5 minutes.

The nurse should record all medications given (dose, route of administration, and time given), as well as fluids, blood loss, and any unusual events or complications. Supplemental oxygen should be administered prophylactically in all cases. IV access is strongly encouraged during pediatric sedation and analgesia, although it is not absolutely necessary for lighter levels of sedation or when sedative agents are administered by oral, nasal, rectal, or IM routes. However, in these cases, equipment and skilled personnel capable of immediately establishing vascular access need to be present.

RECOVERY AND DISCHARGE CRITERIA

Monitoring must be continued by trained personnel until the infant or child has met preestablished criteria for safe discharge. These criteria include the following:

- Airway patency and stable cardiovascular function
- Easy arousability with intact protective reflexes
- Ability to talk (if age appropriate)
- Ability to sit up without assistance (if age appropriate)
- Adequate level of hydration

Disabled patients, young children, and infants should be observed until they return to the same level of responsiveness as that noted before sedation. Numerous scoring systems have been published. Table 2.3 outlines the Aldrete Recovery Scale, a common system used at many health care institutions throughout the United States. As most of my residents and nurses have heard me chant, "When they meet the Aldrete, the patient's all ready."

TABLE 2.3	Aldrete Recovery Score	
Measure	**Description**	**Points**
Activity	Voluntary movement of all limbs to command	2
	Voluntary movement of two extremities to command	1
	Unable to move	0
	Apneic	0
Respiration	Breathe deeply and cough	2
	Dyspnea, hypoventilation	1
Circulation	BP ±20 mm Hg of preanesthesia level	2
	BP ±20–50 mm Hg of preanesthesia level	1
	BP >50 mm Hg of preanesthesia level	0
Consciousness	Fully awake	2
	Arousable	1
	Unresponsive	0
Color	Pink	2
	Pale, blotchy	1
	Cyanotic	0

Total score must be >8 at the conclusion of the monitoring.
BP, Blood pressure.

POSTSEDATION CONCERNS

Available evidence suggests that infants and children who have not experienced an adverse event during sedation can be safely discharged after 30 minutes of observation and monitoring.

What about the risk of adverse events occurring after discharge? In a large, well-designed, prospective study of 1341 pediatric sedation events occurring in the emergency department setting, adverse reactions were noted in 14% of patients and potentially life-threatening events occurred in 12%. Only 8% of all adverse events occurred after the procedure. Every child who experienced a postprocedure event had a similar adverse effect earlier in the sedation. All serious, potentially life-threatening events occurred within 25 minutes of the last sedative/analgesic dose. Parents or guardians should nevertheless be advised that minor side effects may occur after discharge from the recovery area and that full recovery after moderate or deep sedation may be prolonged. Discharge instructions should include the telephone number of a trained staff member to field any parental questions or concerns.

PATIENT EDUCATION GUIDES

See the sample patient and parent education handout available at www.expertconsult.com.

CPT/BILLING CODES

99151 Moderate sedation services provided by the same physician performing the diagnostic or therapeutic service that the sedation supports, requiring the presence of an independent trained observer to assist in the monitoring of the patient's level of consciousness and physiologic status in patients younger than 5 years of age, first 15 minutes intraservice time
99152 Patients age 5 years or older, first 15 minutes intraservice time
99153 Each additional 15 minutes intraservice time (List separately in addition to code for primary service)

NOTE: This code list does not include simple or minimal office sedation techniques (anxiolysis).

SUPPLIERS

(See contact information available at www.expertconsult.com.)

Banyan Corporation

RECOMMENDED READING

Afarian HM. Procedural sedation and analgesia. In: Reichman EF, ed. Emergency Medicine Procedures. 2nd ed. New York: McGraw-Hill; 2013:854–868.
American Academy of Pediatrics Committee on Drugs. Guidelines for monitoring and management of pediatric patients during and after sedation for diagnostic and therapeutic procedures. Pediatrics. 1992;89:1110–1115.
Baxter AL. Topical anesthetics in children. MedscapeCME, 2008. http://cme.medscape.com/viewarticle/570327_2.
Blike GT, Cravero JP. Pride, prejudice, and pediatric sedation: a multispecialty evaluation of the state of the art. Report from a Dartmouth summit on pediatric sedation. National Patient Safety Foundation. 2001.
Borland M, Jacobs I, King B, O'Brien D. A randomized controlled trial comparing intranasal fentanyl to intravenous morphine for managing acute pain in children in the emergency department. Ann Emerg Med. 2007;14:335–340.
Brady M, Kinn S, Ness V, O'Rourke K, et al. Preoperative fasting for preventing perioperative complications in children. Cochrane Database Syst Rev. 2009:CD005285.
Chen E, Joseph MH, Zeltzer LK. Behavioral and cognitive interventions in the treatment of pain in children. Pediatr Clin North Am. 2000;47:513–525.
Clinical policy: procedural sedation and analgesia in the emergency department. From the American College of Emergency Physicians Clinical Policies Subcommittee on Procedural Sedation and Analgesia. Ann Emerg Med. 2014;63:247–258.
Cohen LL, MacLaren JE, Fortson BL, et al. Randomized clinical trial of distraction for infant immunization pain. Pain. 2006;125:165–171.
Coté CJ, Wilson S. Guidelines for monitoring and management of pediatric patients during and after sedation for diagnostic and therapeutic procedures: Update 2016. Pediatrics. 2016;138(1):e20161212.
Green SM, Krauss B. Clinical practice guideline for emergency department ketamine dissociative sedation in children. Ann Emerg Med. 2004;44:460–471.
Green SM, Roback MG, Kennedy RM, et al. Clinical practice guideline for emergency department ketamine dissociative sedation: 2011 update. Ann Emerg Med. 2011;57(5):449–461.
Krauss B, Zurakowski D. Sedation patterns in pediatric and general community hospital emergency departments. Pediatr Emerg Care. 1998;14:99–103.
Mace SE, Barata IA, Cravero JP, et al. Clinical policy: evidence-based approach to pharmacologic agents used in pediatric sedation and analgesia in the emergency department. Ann Emerg Med. 2004;44:342–377.
Migita RT, Klein EJ, Garrison MM. Sedation and analgesia for pediatric fracture reduction in the emergency department: a systematic review. Arch Pediatr Adolesc Med. 2006;160:46–51.
Miner JR, Kletti C, Herold M, et al. Randomized clinical trial of nebulized fentanyl citrate versus I.V. Fentanyl citrate in children presenting to the emergency department with acute pain. Acad Emerg Med. 2007;14:895–898.
Newman DH, Azer MM, Pitetti RD, Singh S. When is a patient safe for discharge after procedural sedation? The timing of adverse effect events in 1367 pediatric procedural sedations. Ann Emerg Med. 2003;42:627–635.
Practice guidelines for preoperative fasting and the use of pharmacologic agents to reduce the risk of pulmonary aspiration. Application to healthy patients undergoing elective procedures. An updated report by the American Society of Anesthesiologists Committee on Standards and Practice Parameters. Anesthesiology. 2011;114(3): 895–511.
Press CD. Topical anesthesia. Medscape. http://reference.medscape.com/article/109673; 2015.
Proudfoot J. Analgesia, anesthesia, and conscious sedation. Emerg Med Clin North Am. 1995;13:357–370.
Sacchetti A, Schafermayer R, Geradi M, et al. Pediatric Committee of American College of Emergency Physicians: pediatric analgesia and sedation. Ann Emerg Med. 1994;23:237–250.
Selbst SM, Clark M. Analgesic use in the emergency department. Ann Emerg Med. 1990;19:1010–1013.
Sinha M, Christopher NC, Fenn R, Reeves L. Evaluation of nonpharmacologic methods of pain and anxiety management for laceration repair in the pediatric emergency department. Pediatrics. 2006;117:1162–1168.
Weaver CS, Hauter WE, Brizendine MS, Cordell WH. Emergency department procedural sedation with propofol: is it safe? J Emerg Med. 2007;33:355–361.
Zink BJ, Darfler K, Salluzzo RF, Reilly KM. The efficacy and safety of methohexital in the emergency department. Ann Emerg Med. 1991;20(12):1293–1298.

CHAPTER 3

Nitrous Oxide Sedation

Marjon B. Jahromi

Nitrous oxide (N_2O) sedation was first used as an anesthetic agent in 1844 and can be considered a safe alternative to intravenous (IV) sedation. N_2O sedation has a long history of safety in the medical and dental community. It is now used by approximately 95% of pediatric dentists and is growing in popularity in general dental and medical offices. Most U.S.-trained dentists become proficient in N_2O sedation as part of their undergraduate dental training. It is not necessary to have extensive experience with IV sedation to be able to perform N_2O sedation safely. Gaining experience with N_2O sedation can be achieved by observing an experienced practitioner and performing the sedation under supervision. Alternatively, continuing education courses are available. Practitioners who are not familiar with the technique are encouraged to participate.

N_2O is a relatively insoluble drug and is a rapidly effective sedative with an onset of effects within 2 to 3 minutes of administration and peak effects within 5 minutes. Dosing can be adjusted easily and rapidly to increase or decrease depth of sedation during the procedure. Recovery time is short because elimination through the lungs occurs as rapidly as absorption. N_2O is not metabolized in the body to any significant extent and therefore can be used safely on most patients. Patients remain conscious and protective reflexes are intact, so there is minimal risk of aspiration or oversedation. In addition, N_2O does not cause respiratory depression, making it safer than fentanyl, midazolam, or chloral hydrate. Technically, it is easier to perform than IV sedation because there is no need to gain venous access. N_2O is administered through a face mask or nasal hood that is simply placed on the patient's face.

Indications

- Anxious and apprehensive patients undergoing minor office surgical or dental procedures
- Patients needing increased pain reaction threshold
- Patients who are unable to tolerate other sedatives

Contraindications

- Pregnancy (first trimester)
- Airway obstruction and severe asthmatic conditions
- Severe psychiatric disorders (N_2O can cause dreaming and hallucinations)
- Pulmonary hypertension
- Air embolism
- Pneumothorax
- Severe cardiac disease
- Hyperthyroidism
- Sickle cell anemia
- Chronic bronchitis/emphysema or pulmonary bleb
- Bowel obstruction
- History of stroke (relative)
- Hypotension (relative)

N_2O should *not* be used to replace local anesthesia but rather as an adjunct to local anesthesia. N_2O sedation is not a good option to control defiant or erratic behavior.

Advantages

- Rapid onset; monitoring time during recovery is brief
- Good analgesic and amnestic (limited) properties
- Unlike IV sedation, when N_2O is used alone, a driver is not needed once the patient has recovered. Patients should be monitored for approximately 30 minutes after the use of N_2O to ensure return to baseline functional status before discharge.
- Patients may resume all normal activities after discharge and are not limited in their activities.

Limitations

- Lack of potency
- Expense of equipment
- Training required to become proficient

Equipment

- Inhalation sedation machine (Fig. 3.1)
- Breathing circuit
- Reservoir bag
- Scavenging system
- Nasal hood or facial mask
- Oxygen and N_2O supply (N_2O is stored in compressed form as a liquid in cylinders)
- Pulse oximeter
- Oral pharyngeal airway available
- Emergency cart with appropriate drugs (consider the Banyan kit; see Chapter 212)

Presedation Assessment and Concerns

Fig. 3.2 shows an anesthesia evaluation form that can be used before and after the procedure.

- A complete medical history should be obtained from the patient. Relevant information includes a history of cardiac or respiratory disease, medications, allergies, prior surgeries and complications from anesthesia, history of tobacco use, and history of substance abuse.
- The oropharynx should be thoroughly evaluated for any abnormalities or evidence of obstruction. A history of sleep apnea may indicate airway abnormalities such as narrow airways and tonsillar hypertrophy. Obesity, especially involving the face and neck, may lead to difficulties in spontaneous ventilation under sedation.
- N_2O will potentiate drugs that depress the respiratory system.
- The procedure and all possible sensations should be described to the patient in advance. N_2O can produce a feeling of eupho-

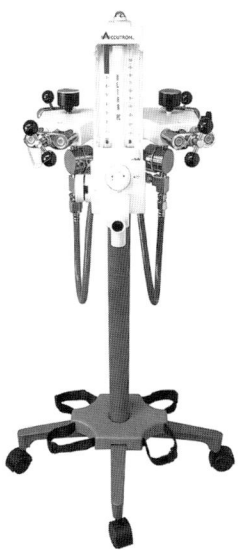

Fig. 3.1 Accutron 4-Cylinder Portable Manifold. (Courtesy Accutron, Inc., Phoenix, AZ.)

ria, dreaminess, and detachment. It can also cause numbness and tingling of the extremities. It may cause nausea, confusion, and sexual hallucinations in higher doses.

PREPROCEDURE PATIENT PREPARATION

- An experienced assistant trained in Basic Life Support should always be present.
- Patients do not need to be fasting if N_2O is the sole anesthetic agent. However, if an oral sedative is to be used in combination with N_2O, confirm that the patient has fasted for at least 6 hours for solid foods and nonclear liquids and at least 6 hours for clear liquids.
- Perform a full check of the inhalation sedation machine to ensure that it is safe to use and that it has an adequate supply of gases for completion of the procedure. N_2O is a compressed liquid at room temperature with a pressure of 745 pounds per square inch. A full E cylinder of N_2O will have 1590 mL of gas. The pressure indicator in a N_2O tank will show a constant pressure until only about 20% (400 mL) of N_2O is left in the cylinder. This is very different from oxygen, which is a nonliquified gas. The pressure indicator in an oxygen tank will indicate a proportional decrease in pressure as the volume of the gas is depleted. Therefore the pressure indicator of a N_2O tank cannot be used to estimate the amount of gas remaining in the cylinder.
- The scavenging system should also be checked for proper functioning. It is below the standard of care to operate a N_2O unit without a scavenging apparatus.
- The health care practitioner should have all the necessary equipment and be prepared to handle all medical emergencies in the event the patient should reach a deeper level of sedation than initially planned. Although not required, a pretracheal stethoscope is an excellent method to monitor the patient's respirations and heart sounds. This may prevent the patient from becoming oversedated and losing consciousness. The conventional or newer wireless pretracheal stethoscope can be easily obtained by any health care practitioner (Figs. 3.3 and 3.4).

DOCUMENTATION

- Informed consent should be obtained for both the planned procedure and the N_2O sedation. All written and verbal instructions, including consent with risks, benefits, alternatives, and contraindications, should be documented.

- The patient's vital signs, including blood pressure, heart rate, and oxygen saturation by pulse oximetry, should be recorded at regular intervals throughout the procedure and during recovery.
- Any standardized anesthesia form can be used for documentation (Fig. 3.5). Alternatively, vitals, level of sedation, and concentration of N_2O being administered can simply be recorded at 5-minute intervals (also see Chapter 1).

TECHNIQUE

1. Always have a Basic Life Support–trained assistant present.
2. Begin the inhalation sedation session with a full check of the inhalation sedation machine to ensure that it is safe to use and that it has an adequate supply of gases to allow the procedure to be completed. Also check the scavenging system for proper functioning.
3. Once the presedation check has been completed, position the patient properly for the procedure to be performed. Obtain and record baseline vital signs, including continuous pulse oximetry. A pretracheal stethoscope may also be placed at the lower end of the trachea and midline to the neck for additional monitoring of respirations.
4. Place a nasal hood or facial mask on the patient's face. The nasal hood should fit snugly around the patient's nose to minimize any leakage of gas. Nasal hoods come in a variety of sizes and may be scented for optimal patient comfort. Most nasal hoods manufactured now are also latex free. It may help to ask the patient to help achieve a snug fit. Also telling them they can adjust the hood or mask as needed gives them a sense of control.
5. Introduce 100% oxygen only. The initial gas flow rate should be set to 6 or 7 L/min for an average-sized adult (4 or 5 L/min for most children). The patient should be instructed to take deep breaths through his or her nose. Adjust the flow rate so that the reservoir bag can be seen moving during each breath. It should not be bulging but rather about two-thirds full before inspiration, and should not empty completely with inspiration. If the reservoir bag empties completely, the flow rate should be increased until about two-thirds of the bag empties with each patient breath. It is best to err with more flow than needed initially to avoid a suffocating feeling. As the patient becomes relaxed, it may be possible to reduce the flow of oxygen.
6. Once the flow rate has been adjusted to the proper level, introduce the N_2O. Patient tolerance and N_2O requirement vary significantly for each person. It is important to titrate the dose slowly to prevent oversedation. Oversedation should be avoided because it can result in unpleasant feelings for the patient. Initially, 10% N_2O is introduced and the patient is allowed to breathe this mixture for 1 minute. The O_2 level should also be adjusted to maintain the constant flow rate that was previously established. Some inhalation sedation machines will also automatically decrease the O_2 flow as the N_2O flow is increased.
7. If this dose provides adequate sedation, the operative or dental procedure can begin. Signs of adequate sedation include a reduction in anxiety, increased relaxation, slowing of the blink reflex, decreased response to painful stimuli, and general decrease in movements.
8. If this level of sedation is not sufficient, provide an additional 10% N_2O and allow the patient to breathe the mixture for 1 minute before reassessment. This cycle can be repeated to a maximum mixture of 70% N_2O to 30% O_2. Document the level and length of N_2O administered in the patient's medical chart. **NOTE:** Minimum dose is 10% N_2O:90% O_2. Maximum concentration is 70% N_2O to 30% O_2. Average maintenance dose is typically between 20% N_2O to 80% O_2 and 40% N_2O to 60% O_2. Almost all ambulatory N_2O/O_2 delivery systems have an oxygen fail-safe mechanism that prevents N_2O from being administered unless there is adequate O_2 flowing to the system. Therefore it is not possible to administer 100% N_2O.

Patient: _____

Operating Surgeon: _____   Procedure: _____

Age: _____   Height: _____   Weight: _____   Pre-Op B/P: _____

MEDICAL HISTORY:

_____

_____

_____

ANESTHETIC HISTORY:

Personal: _____

Family: _____

REVIEW OF SYSTEMS:

Heart:	CP DOE Orthopnea HTN CHF Dysrhythmias	_____
Pulmonary:	COPD Asthma URI Bronchitis Pneumonia	_____
Endocrine:	DM Thyroid Obesity Steroid use	_____
GI:	PUD Reflux HH	_____
Liver:	Hepatitis Cirrhosis	_____
Mus. Skel.:	Fractures MH	_____
CNS:	Seizures CVA Paralysis HA TIA	_____
GU:	CRF Infections Pregnant	_____
Hemo:	Coagulopathy Sickle Cell	_____
Habits:	Smoking EtOH Drugs	_____

MEDICATIONS: _____

ALLERGIES: _____

PHYSICAL EVALUATION:

Heart: _____

Pulmonary: _____

Airway: Classification 1 2 3 4   Head and Neck: _____   FBO: _____   Loose/Missing teeth _____

HOSPITALIZATIONS: _____

_____

ASA CLASSIFICATION: 1 2 3 4 5 E   **NPO:** _____

ANESTHESIA PLAN: General Anesthesia   Monitored Anesthesia Care   Nitrous Oxide

PRE-OPERATIVE MEDICATIONS: _____

CONSENT (Risks/Benefits/Alternatives discussed, Questions answered, Accepts risks) _____

_____

_____   _____

Date / Time   Signature

DISCHARGE SUMMARY: ☐ VSS ☐ Alert/Awake ☐ Ambulatory ☐ IV removed intact ☐ Post-op instructions given to

Post-op transport provided by: Room Air SpO$_2$:   %

POST-DISCHARGE NOTE:

_____

_____

_____

_____

ANESTHESIA EVALUATION

Fig. 3.2   Anesthesia evaluation form used both before and after the procedure to document discharge status.

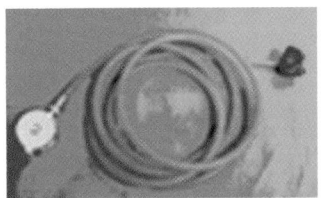

Fig. 3.3 Conventional pretracheal stethoscope. Chest piece from Hull Anesthesia, Inc. Earpiece and cord from Westone.

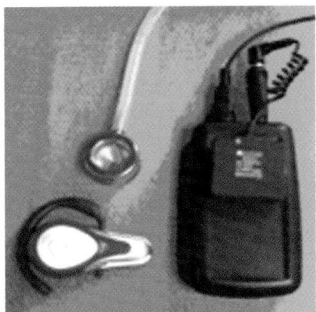

Fig. 3.4 Wireless pretracheal stethoscope. (Courtesy Sedation Resource, Inc., Lone Oak, TX.)

9. Immediately reduce the N_2O concentration with the first sign of oversedation. *Signs of oversedation* include agitation, sweating, nausea, vomiting, lack of cooperation, diaphoresis, inability to keep eyes open, decreased response to questions, and loss of consciousness. The patient is also at risk for silent aspiration if vomit reaches the epiglottis. Patients may also complain of unpleasant feelings such as intense tingling or detachment from reality. It is imperative that the health care provider constantly assess the level of sedation because changes in patient comfort may occur rapidly.

10. With lengthy administration (>30 minutes), reduce the N_2O concentration. The duration of exposure to an anesthetic can have an effect on recovery time. Accumulation of anesthetic in tissues such as muscle, skin, and fat increases with continuous inhalation and can delay recovery time. This is especially true of the more soluble anesthetics, but it can also occur to some degree with low-solubility anesthetics.

11. Once the procedure is complete, the N_2O can be reduced and the patient returned to breathing 100% O_2 for at least 5 minutes. This should be achieved by reducing the inspired concentration of N_2O by 20% per minute until it is reduced to zero. Patients should indicate they are feeling fine and not drowsy, groggy, light-headed, dizzy, or nauseated before removing the 100% O_2.

COMPLICATIONS

- Oversedation or prolonged administration can lead to agitation, sweating, nausea, vomiting, feelings of detachment, confusion, hallucinations, and unconsciousness.
- N_2O can cause myocardial and respiratory depression in high doses (>70%).
- *Chronic* effects of N_2O exposure can include bone marrow suppression, mainly through inhibiting enzymes that depend on vitamin B_{12}. As a result, myelin formation and DNA synthesis may be affected. Megaloblastic anemia, pernicious anemia, peripheral neuropathies, and an increased incidence of miscarriages can also occur as a result of chronic N_2O use. Central nervous system degeneration is common among those who abuse N_2O. Scavenging of waste gases is therefore crucial to protect office staff. The National Institute for Occupational Safety and Health recommends limiting the room concentration of N_2O to 25 ppm.

POSTPROCEDURE MANAGEMENT AND CONCERNS

- Monitoring of vital signs along with pulse oximetry should be continued during recovery.
- The patient should breathe 100% O_2 for 3 to 5 minutes after the procedure to prevent diffusion hypoxia.
- Diffusion hypoxia is a condition caused by the rapid release of N_2O from the blood. Because N_2O is insoluble, it leaves the bloodstream rapidly once the inspired concentration is reduced. If the inspired concentration of N_2O is high, then a large amount of gas will quickly emerge from solution into the alveoli, displacing O_2. This mechanism requires large volumes of N_2O to be released from the alveoli, which usually occurs during the first 5 minutes of recovery. Room air does not have an O_2 concentration high enough to compensate for the high N_2O concentration released from the alveoli after the procedure. Thus, hypoxia can occur if supplemental O_2 is not given and if the patient is not allowed to breathe 100% O_2 for 3 to 15 minutes after the discontinuation of N_2O sedation.
- Symptoms of diffusion hypoxia include disorientation, nausea, and severe headache.
- All written and verbal instructions that were given should be documented.
- Postoperative instructions are more relevant to the actual procedure that was performed; therefore there are no specific postoperative instructions for N_2O sedation.
- The patient should be alert and oriented before discharge. If N_2O was the only sedation used, the patient may drive himself or herself home. However, if an oral sedative was used in combination with N_2O, a driver is required to take the patient home.

CPT/BILLING CODES

01999	Unlisted anesthesia for planned vaginal delivery
99151, 99152, 99155, or 99156	Sedation with or without analgesia (conscious sedation); intravenous, intramuscular or inhalation

NOTE: 99153 or 99157 may be reported for additional intraservice time as necessary.

SUPPLIERS

(Full contact information available at www.expertconsult.com.)

N_2O Machines and Supplies
    Accutron, Inc.
    Henry Schein Dental
Pretracheal Stethoscopes
    Hull Anesthesia, Inc.
    Sedation Resource, Inc.
    Westone

Acknowledgment

The editors recognize the contributions of Jessica Y. Hackman, DMD, and Thomas A. Bzoskie, MD, to this chapter in a previous edition of this text.

M F	Age	Ht	Wt	BP	SpO₂	ASA	1	2	3	4	5	E	NPO

MEDICAL HISTORY:

MEDICATIONS:

ALLERGIES:

PRE-OP MEDICATIONS:

☐ Unable to obtain baseline vital signs, patient is uncooperative

Time:

SpO₂																			
ECG																			
Temperature																			

☐ GA
☐ MAC
☐ Supine
☐

MONITORS
☐ Precordial
☐ Pulse Oximeter
☐ NIBP
☐ ECG
☐ Respirations
☐ Temperature
☐
☐

IV
☐ Hand
☐ Arm
☐ ACF
☐ Foot
☐ R   ☐ L
☐ 20 ☐ 22 ☐ 24

200

150

100

50

Notes   Anes X   Surg O

Oxygen

Total

AIRWAY
☐ Nasal Cannula
☐ Nasopharyngeal
☐ Orotracheal Tube
☐ Nasotracheal Tube
☐ L M A
☐ R   ☐ L
   20   22   24   26

NOTES: ☐ Equipment checked   ☐ Patient examined   ☐ NPO verified   ☐ Consent obtained

ANESTHESIA TIME	Procedure:	Date:	Patient Identification:
Anes end:	Location:		
Anes start:	Surgeon:		
Anes total:			
	Anesthesiologist:		

Fig. 3.5 Anesthesia record.

RECOMMENDED READING

Clark MS, Brunick AL. *Handbook of Nitrous Oxide and Oxygen Sedation*. 4th ed. St. Louis: Mosby; 2014.

Dorsch JA, Dorsch SE. *Understanding Anesthesia Equipment*. 5th ed. Philadelphia: Lippincott Williams & Wilkins; 2008.

Katzung BG. *Basic and Clinical Pharmacology*. 12th ed. New York: Appleton & Lange; 2012.

Meechan JG, Robb ND, Seymour RA. *Pain and Anxiety Control for the Conscious Dental Patient*. Oxford: Oxford University Press; 1998.

Miller RD, Cucchiara RF, Miller ED. *Miller's Anesthesia*. 6th ed. Vols. 2. St. Louis: Elsevier Health Sciences; 2004.

Morgan GE, Mikhail MS. *Morgan and Mikhail's Clinical Anesthesiology*. 5th ed. New York: McGraw Hill: Lange; 2013.

Trojan J, Saunders B, Woloshynowych M, et al. Immediate recovery of psychomotor function after patient administered nitrous oxide/oxygen inhalation for colonoscopy. *Endoscopy*. 1997;29:17–22.

Wiener-Kronish JP, Gropper MA. *Conscious Sedation*. Philadelphia: Hanley & Belfus; 2001.

CHAPTER 4

TOPICAL ANESTHESIA

Suraj Achar • Jonathan Chan

Topical anesthesia offers patients an alternative to local injections. Such an alternative may be very helpful in the anxious patient, especially those in pain from an injury or anticipating pain from a planned procedure. The ideal topical anesthetic would provide 100% anesthesia with a rapid onset, prolonged duration, and no local or systemic side effects. To date, the perfect topical agent has not been developed; however, new formulations have improved efficacy and application options. (Also see Chapters 5, 6, and 183.)

Compared with local injectable anesthetics, there are many benefits and some drawbacks with topical anesthetics. Application of topical anesthetics is painless and does not distort wound margins in laceration repairs. Less sedation may be needed. Drawbacks include the extra time required for topical anesthetics to take effect and, occasionally, inadequate analgesia requiring infiltrative anesthesia.

Although the first topical anesthetic was developed in the latter half of the 19th century (topical cocaine), in recent years, safer and more effective agents have become available. One of the first topical creams developed, TAC (tetracaine, adrenalin, cocaine), also contained cocaine, so it is rarely used any more. Fortunately, LET/LAT (lidocaine, epinephrine/adrenalin, tetracaine) solution-gel has been found to be as effective as TAC. LET eliminates cocaine, thereby lessening the risk for toxicity and seizures, decreasing documentation issues, and lowering the cost.

EMLA (eutectic mixture of local anesthetics), first approved by the U.S. Food and Drug Administration (FDA) in 1992, is now one of the most widely used. A *eutectic mixture* is one in which the melting point of the mixture is lower than that of the individual components; in the case of EMLA, the components (lidocaine and prilocaine) remain liquid at room temperature. LMX 4 (4% liposomal lidocaine) and LMX 5 (5% liposomal lidocaine) are liposomal agents available over the counter. LMX 4 and LMX 5 were formerly called ELA-Max. Liposomes are synthetic biologic membranes composed of an aqueous core surrounded by a lipid layer. This delivery system allows medications to penetrate the stratum corneum more readily because they resemble cell membranes. Consequently, the onset of action is enhanced while, at the same time, the duration of action is lengthened because the lysosomal encapsulation slows metabolism.

More recently, the S-Caine Patch has been developed. This 1:1 eutectic mixture of 70 mg lidocaine and 70 mg tetracaine has a disposable, oxygen-activated heating element incorporated into a patch that enhances anesthetic delivery. This heating element maintains the temperature at 39°C to 41°C for a 2-hour period, excellent for the delivery of topical anesthetic. S-Caine Peel has also been developed which conforms to every surface, hardens, and then can be peeled away prior to a procedure.

Categories of topical anesthetics include those applied to intact skin, to nonintact skin, or alternatively, to mucous membranes. These are important differences; for instance, a topical anesthetic (e.g., lidocaine) applied to the mucous membranes (e.g., nose, mouth, throat, tracheobronchial tree, esophagus, genitourinary tract) may result in significant absorption, resulting in blood levels comparable with those achieved with parenteral administration (Table 4.1). Therefore precautions should be taken against toxicity, especially in children. Available topical anesthetics for intact skin are EMLA/EMLA Disc, LMX 4, LMX 5, S-Caine, S-Caine Peel, and iontophoretic preparations. LMX 5 was designed to be used on rectal mucosa. Lidocaine gel at varying concentrations has also been developed for nonintact skin and mucous membranes. Versions of benzocaine (HurriCaine, Americaine, Cetacaine) at varying concentrations and flavors have been designed for application to mucous membranes. Meanwhile, as more aesthetic procedures have been developed and performed, clinicians have started using various compounded mixtures (see below and Chapter 50).

In addition to creams and ointments, cooling can also be used to provide brief, temporary anesthesia (e.g., ethyl chloride spray or ice cubes). Handheld jet injectors are also available that use high pressure to deliver lidocaine through a very small orifice and across intact skin (see Fig. 111.5 and Chapter 111).

INDICATIONS

Intact Skin

Eutectic Mixture of Local Anesthetics

* FDA: for use on intact skin for local anesthesia and for genital mucous membranes for superficial surgery and pretreatment for infiltrative anesthesia.

LMX 4/LMX 5

* LMX 4: Manufacturer label: temporary relief of pain associated with minor cuts, abrasions, minor burns, skin irritation, and insect bites.
* LMX 5: Manufacturer label: hemorrhoids.
* Literature-supported uses of LMX: venipuncture, venous cannulation, arterial puncture, suture removal, shave biopsy, punch biopsy, chemical peels, curettage of molluscum contagiosum, cryotherapy of venereal warts, intracutaneous allergy testing, epilation, debridement of otitis media with an intact tympanic membrane, removal of an embedded foreign body, circumcision at more than a 37-week gestation, skin grafting, debridement of ulcers, lumbar puncture.
* Adjunct to: vasectomy, dermabrasion, laser resurfacing, postsurgical discomfort.
* Nonsurgical uses: postherpetic neuralgia, meralgia paresthetica.
* When used for intact skin, efficacy is similar to EMLA, but LMX 4 is less expensive. Injected buffered lidocaine appears to provide superior anesthesia to LMX 4 for intravenous catheter insertion.

Lidoderm Patch

FDA: relief of pain associated with postherpetic neuralgia.

BLT Triple Anesthetic Gel (20% Benzocaine, 6% Lidocaine, 4% Tetracaine)

* Used for intact skin.
* Percentages may vary.
* This is usually compounded.

TABLE 4.1 Summary of Topical Anesthetics

Agents	Concentration	Status	Maximum Dose or Area*	Onset of Action	Duration	Pregnancy Category[†]
Intact Skin						
EMLA cream or anesthetic disc	2.5% lidocaine/2.5% prilocaine	Rx	20 g/200 cm² for 7–12 yr of age and >20 kg (A) and (C)	60–120 min	180 min	B
LMX 4/5	4% lidocaine plus vitamin E, propylene glycol, benzyl alcohol, lecithin, cholesterol, carbomer-940, triethanolamine, polysorbate 80	OTC	100 cm² (A)	‡	‡	B
Amethocaine gel	4% tetracaine	Europe	50 mg (A)	40 min	240 min	C
Lidocaine acid mantle (Novartis)	30%–40% lidocaine	Rx		20 min	30–60 min	
Patch (Lidoderm)	5% lidocaine	Rx	420 cm² (three patches)		12 hr max duration of patch time	B (patch not studied in pregnancy)
S-Caine Patch/Peel	Lidocaine 70 mg, tetracaine 70 mg	Rx	One patch	30 min	Patch time	
BLT gel	20% benzocaine, 6% lidocaine, 4% tetracaine			15 min	60 min	C
Ethyl chloride spray	Skin refrigerant	OTC		<1 min	Transient	
Topicaine	4%–5% lidocaine	OTC	600 cm² (A), 100 cm² (C >10 kg)	Rapid	30–60 min	
Nonintact Skin						
LET/LAT	4% lidocaine/1:2000 epinephrine/1% tetracaine	Compounded				
Mucous Membrane						
Xylocaine		Rx	300 mg (A)/100 mg (C)	2–5 min	15–45 min	B
Viscous solution	2% lidocaine			1–2 min	15–20 min	
Liquid	5% lidocaine			2 min		
Ointment	2.5%, 5% lidocaine					
Benzocaine						
Cetacaine						
spray	14% benzocaine	Rx				
liquid	2% tetracaine	Rx				
gel						
ointment						
HurriCaine						
liquid	20% benzocaine	OTC		<5 min	15–45 min	C
gel						
spray						
Cocaine solution	4% and 10%	C-II§	200 mg (A)	1–5 min	30–60 min	C
Ophthalmic						
Alcaine solution	0.5% proparacaine	Rx		20 sec	15–20 min	C
Pontocaine solution	0.5% tetracaine	Rx	50 mg (A)	20 sec	15–20 min	C

*A, Adults; C, children.

†Pregnancy category B: Animal studies have not shown a fetal risk but there are no controlled studies in pregnant women. Pregnancy category C: Animal studies are not available. Safety for use during pregnancy has not been established. Use only when potential benefits outweigh potential hazards to the fetus.

‡No clinical studies.

§C-II: Controlled substances schedule II drug (Controlled Substances Act of 1970). Cocaine must be stored in a locked cabinet; and separate written records must be maintained for a period of 2 years after the drug is dispensed.

EMLA, Eutectic mixture of local anesthetics; LAT, lidocaine, adrenalin, tetracaine; LET, lidocaine, epinephrine, tetracaine; OTC, over the counter; Rx, prescription; TAC, tetracaine, adrenalin, cocaine.

Modified from Huang W, Vidimos A. Topical anesthetics in dermatology. J Am Acad Dermatol. 2000;43:286–298.

S-Caine Patch/S-Caine Peel

- Used for intact skin.
- Approved for children 3 years of age or older.

Nonintact Skin

Topicaine (4% or 5% Lidocaine Gel), Benzocaine Spray

- Minor skin cuts or abrasions.
- Available over the counter.

LET/LAT (Lidocaine, Epinephrine/Adrenalin, Tetracaine)

- Scalp and facial lacerations (LET seems to be less effective on the trunk and extremities).
- Does not work on intact skin.
- Works especially well in young children with wound less than 5 cm in length. In theory, leaving the wound open longer while waiting for anesthesia to take effect may increase the risk of wound infection.
- Some institutions still use cocaine in this mixture (lidocaine, adrenaline, cocaine), but most complications with this technique were associated with mixtures that contain cocaine.

LMX 4

- LMX 4: Manufacturer label: temporary relief of pain associated with minor cuts, abrasions, minor burns, skin irritation, and insect bites.

Mucous Membranes (e.g., nose, mouth, throat, tracheobronchial tree, esophagus, genitourinary tract)

Lidocaine (Xylocaine), Benzocaine, Tetracaine, Cocaine

- Painful, irritated, inflamed mucous membranes; anesthesia before minor surgical procedure and esophagogastroduodenoscopy.
- 2% viscous lidocaine for aphthous ulcers and mucositis in immunosuppressed patients.

Ophthalmic Preparations

- Proparacaine seems to burn less than tetracaine.
- Removal of foreign bodies, short eyelid procedures (e.g., chalazion removal), and placement of eye shields.

Mechanical Methods

Thermal: Ice/Ethyl Chloride Spray

Skin tag clipping, incision and drainage of simple abscess, and injections (blood draws, skin grafting, sports injuries).
Jet injectors: see Fig. 111.5, and Chapter 111.

For Aesthetic Procedures

Many noninvasive aesthetic procedures (e.g., deep skin peels, facial resurfacing) require some type of topical anesthetic. Oral analgesic medications and anxiolytics can also be beneficial. Everyone seems to have his or her own favorite compounded preparation. With the rapid growth of procedures in this field, few studies have been published to compare the various combinations and their efficacy.

BLT (Benzocaine, Lidocaine, Tetracaine) Triple Anesthetic Gel

BLT is a favorite compounded mixture. The percentages may vary (e.g., 20%, 7%, 7%; or 20%, 6%, 4%). With most BLT preparations, it takes 45 to 60 minutes to obtain good effect.

Quadri-Caine

Quadri-Caine (compounding pharmacies listed in "Suppliers" section) is a compounded topical anesthetic that has a more rapid onset (10 to 15 minutes). Standard Quadri-Caine consists of 10% lidocaine, 5% tetracaine, 5% prilocaine, and 1% bupivacaine in an emollient cream plus a penetration enhancer. Quadri-Caine VC contains the vasoconstrictor phenylephrine.

Quadri-Caine, as with most of these potent compounded preparations, should be used only under the direction of clinicians experienced in the use of high-potency topical anesthetics. It is unknown what amounts of the topical anesthetics in Quadri-Caine reach the systemic circulation. The amount to apply must be determined on a case-by-case basis. It is recommended that not more than 3 g of Quadri-Caine be applied in 24 hours.

Quadri-Caine is not for resale. It must be purchased by a medical office or clinic for use during a patient visit or may be ordered by prescription specifically for individual patient use. Quadri-Caine and Quadri-Caine VC are registered trademarks and, as compounded products, have not undergone FDA review.

NOTE: Compounded products are not produced under the same standards as FDA-approved products. The levels of lidocaine may vary dramatically, and toxicity studies using moderate or large amounts of compounded products have not been performed. One of the editors had a patient with delayed (2 hours following procedure) severe headache and significantly elevated systolic blood pressures (up to 260 mm Hg) following a laser procedure. This patient had been premedicated

with topical compounded Quadri-Caine containing phenylephrine. Whether this was an idiosyncratic event or not, this editor no longer uses the Quadri-Caine VC, and in fact, now prefers BLT to Quadri-Caine.

CONTRAINDICATIONS

Most of the preparations are contraindicated in pregnancy and for women who are breast feeding. Many preparations contain preservatives that can cause allergic reactions. If a patient develops an allergic dermatitis while using a topical anesthetic, he or she may not be allergic to the active drug itself, but rather to other components in the cream or ointment. An allergy to lidocaine is extremely rare, if it occurs at all.

LET/LAT

Sensitivity to tetracaine, epinephrine, or lidocaine

Eutectic Mixture of Local Anesthetics

- Advanced liver disease (hepatic metabolism)
- Methemoglobinemia risk

LMX 4/LMX 5

- Sensitivity to lidocaine
- Avoid mucous membranes: absorption increases toxicity risks, especially in children
- Efficacy diminishes as the skin thickness (lack of absorption) and vascularity (rapid clearance) increases. Essentially ineffective on the palms and soles even if occluded for hours.

Lidoderm 5% Patch

- Sensitivity to lidocaine (rare); denuded skin; mucous membranes
- Do not use more than 12 hours out of 24-hour period to avoid toxicity. Do not use with methemoglobinemia-inducing agents on infants younger than 12 months of age (Box 4.1).
- Use with caution in infants younger than 3 months of age (maximum dose of 1 g for 1-hour application if term).

BLT Triple Anesthetic Gel

- Allergy to p-aminobenzoic acid, hair dyes, and sulfonamides
- Sensitivity to benzocaine, lidocaine, or tetracaine

S-Caine Patch/S-Caine Peel

Sensitivity to lidocaine or tetracaine

Topicaine (4% to 5% Lidocaine Gel)

Sensitivity to lidocaine

Thermal: Ice/Ethyl Chloride Spray

- Raynaud phenomenon, cryoglobulinemia
- Not effective for skin biopsy, alters specimen

Lidocaine (Xylocaine), Benzocaine (Mucous Membranes)

- Sensitivity to lidocaine or benzocaine

Ophthalmic Preparations

- Not to be used to control pain over long term
- Inhibits healing and, because no sensation, may lead to inadvertent trauma
- May also eliminate blinking, leading to drying of cornea

TECHNIQUE

NOTE: Precautions must be taken to avoid high blood levels of anesthetics. This is especially true with the use of compounded products or FDA-approved products used under occlusion. Part of the confusion that providers face relates to the need to use occlusion with EMLA because of its poor penetration through the stratum corneum. With LMX 4/LMX 5, occlusion is not needed because the liposomes appear to enhance absorption. However, clinicians may accidently or purposely use these newer agents under occlusion. Small doses of these drugs have been shown to be safe when used with occlusion, but large doses (>60 g) may be toxic.

INTACT SKIN

Eutectic Mixture of Local Anesthetics /Eutectic Mixture of Local Anesthetics Disc

EMLA cream is a eutectic or liquid mixture of 2.5% lidocaine and 2.5% prilocaine. To use, first remove oil from skin with an alcohol or acetone swab. Consider thinning the stratum corneum through tape stripping of superficial cells. Apply the disc or 1 to 2 g per 10 cm² of the cream. Cover with an occlusive dressing (Tegaderm, Opsite, or Band-Aid) for 60 minutes for a 3-mm depth. Every additional 30 minutes provide 1 mm of more depth; a 2-hour maximum time is equivalent to 5 mm. Cream should still be visible when the dressing is removed. If it is not visible, an inadequate amount was used (Table 4.2).

LMX 4/LMX 5

Apply for 15 to 40 minutes without occlusion. A transient erythema may develop, but no serious side effects have been observed. In children weighing less than 20 kg, apply cream to an area no larger than 100 cm² to prevent systemic toxicity.

TABLE 4.2	Recommended Maximum Dose and Application Area of Eutectic Mixture of Local Anesthetics		
Age	Body Weight (kg)	Maximum Total Dose and Time	Maximum Application Area (cm²)
1–3 mo	<5	1 g (1 hr)	10
4–12 mo	>5	2 g (4 hr)	20
1–6 yr	>10	10 g (4 hr)	100
7–12 yr	>20	20 g (4 hr)	200

Modified from Huang W, Vidimos A. Topical anesthetics in dermatology. *J Am Acad Dermatol.* 2000;43:286–298.

Lidoderm 5% Patch

Apply up to three patches at one time to cover the most painful area (e.g., postherpetic neuralgia) for a maximum of 12 hours in a 24-hour period. Patches may be cut to smaller sizes for smaller lesions or impaired elimination (e.g., hepatic disease).

BLT Triple Anesthetic Gel

Apply to intact skin for 10 to 30 minutes. Recent studies note that BLT provides effective analgesia after 15 minutes of application.

S-Caine Patch/S-Caine Peel

Apply S-Caine Patch and use disposable heating element as instructed. Time to effect is 20 to 30 minutes.

Apply S-Caine Peel to area. The cream dries on exposure to air and becomes flexible and is peeled off skin after 20 to 30 minutes. The advantage of this flexible membrane is delivery of topical anesthetic to contoured areas of the body. Do not leave on longer than 30 minutes.

Topicaine

Apply a moderately thick layer (about one-eighth inch) to affected area. Best anesthetic results occur in 20 minutes to 1 hour.

Nonintact Skin

LET/LAT

The facial or scalp laceration should first be placed in a gravity-dependent position. Apply 1.5 to 3.0 mL of LET (or comparable solution) to a soaked gauze and wipe in and over the wound. Alternatively, LET can be poured into the wound and then a LET-soaked gauze or cotton ball applied after 3 minutes. Avoid mucous membranes and end-arteriolar parts of the body such as the digits. Tape or hold the pad in place firmly. Contact with wound should be for a minimum of 15 minutes and a maximum of 30 minutes. Watch for blanching, which correlates with anesthesia. Onset of action is 15 to 30 minutes. LET gel preparations have been found to be as effective as LET solutions, and do not require the gauze or cotton ball pad to be held in place afterward. The gel solutions usually provide more uniform application to tissues, possibly providing better anesthetic effect. Again, it is important to avoid mucous membrane absorption which could result in systemic toxicity, especially in children; fatalities have been reported.

Mucous Membranes

Lidocaine (Xylocaine), Benzocaine, Tetracaine (Mucous Membranes)

Wolfe and colleagues reported in 2000 that atomized lidocaine 4% solution decreased the discomfort of nasogastric tube placement.

The combination of 1.5 mL atomized lidocaine applied intranasally plus 3.0 mL applied oropharyngeally plus 5 mL 2% lidocaine jelly applied intranasally is superior to jelly alone. Caution should be used because of impaired swallowing after use. Patients should expectorate excess anesthetic to avoid systemic absorption and toxicity. Plasma levels are similar to those obtained with intravenous injection. For viscous solution, do not exceed one tablespoon (15 mL) every 3 hours or one teaspoon (5 mL) of 5% liquid in an adult (see Chapters 5 and 6 for maximum doses). Ingestion of food should be avoided for at least 1 hour after oral use to prevent aspiration.

Magic mouthwash contains diphenhydramine elixir, Maalox, and 2% viscous lidocaine and is often used for aphthous ulcers or stomatitis. Anbesol is a popular over-the-counter benzocaine preparation used for dental pain. HurriCaine/Americaine/Cetacaine spray is useful for many oral procedures. It is available in various flavors, requires a prescription, and contains benzocaine. Another compounded formula used for mucous membranes contains lidocaine, prilocaine, and tetracaine (Profound, Steven's Pharmacy).

Thermal: Ice/Ethyl Chloride Spray

For skin-tag clipping hold ice in direct contact for 10 seconds and clip skin tag immediately. For draining an abscess, spray the vaporized coolant for 1 to 2 seconds until the dermis turns white and immediately drain the abscess. Use caution because overapplication causes blistering. Use of thermal cooling may also lessen pain from injections.

Ophthalmic Use

Apply one or two drops in the eye. The effects of the anesthetic are rapid (30 seconds) and persist up to 15 minutes. An additional drop can be placed every 5 to 10 minutes for a total of 7 to 10 drops. Patients should not be discharged with topical ophthalmics unless they are going to be examined daily by the clinician for a worsening condition.

CONCLUSION

Topical anesthetics may offer a painless alternative to painful injectable anesthetics. Since the advent of TAC, there have been numerous advances. EMLA cream and over-the-counter LMX are now available. Moreover, advances in delivery modes, including heat in S-Caine Patch and flexible membranes in S-Caine Peel, allow the provider to tailor topical anesthetics to specific clinical situations. Compounded products (Quadri-Caine, BLT) have further enhanced topical anesthetics.

Acknowledgment

The editors recognize the contributions of William Dery, MD, to this chapter in a previous edition of this text.

SUPPLIERS

(See contact information available at www.expertconsult.com.)

BLT Topical Anesthesia (compounded benzocaine, lidocaine, tetracaine)
Biosense Clinic
Quadri-Caine Topical Anesthesia (compounded bupivacaine, lidocaine, prilocaine, tetracaine)
Keystone Pharmacy (compounding pharmacy)
Portage Pharmacy
Scripts Pharmacy (compounding pharmacy)
Profound (compounded lidocaine, prilocaine, tetracaine)
Steven's Pharmacy

RECOMMENDED READING

Crystal CS, Blankenship RB. Local anesthetics and peripheral nerve blocks in the emergency department. *Emerg Med Clin North Am.* 2005;23:477–502.

Crystal CS, McArthur TJ, Harrison B. Anesthetic and procedural sedation techniques for wound management. *Emerg Med Clin North Am.* 2007;25:41–71.

Eidelman A, Weiss JM, Enu IK, et al. Comparative efficacy and costs of various topical anesthetics for repair of dermal lacerations: a systematic review of randomized, controlled trials. *J Clin Anesth.* 2005;17:106–116.

Eidelman A, Weiss JM, Lau J, Carr DB. Topical anesthetics for dermal instrumentation: a systematic review of randomized, controlled trials. *Ann Emerg Med.* 2005;46:343–351.

Ernst AA, Marvez E, Nick TG, et al. Lidocaine adrenaline tetracaine gel versus tetracaine adrenaline cocaine gel for topical anesthesia in linear scalp and facial lacerations in children aged 5 to 17 years. *Pediatrics.* 1995;95:255–258.

Huang W, Vidimos A. Topical anesthetics in dermatology. *J Am Acad Dermatol.* 2000;43:286–298.

Kundu S, Achar S. Principles of office anesthesia: part II. Topical anesthesia. *Am Fam Physician.* 2002;66:99–102.

Lander J, Brady-Fryer B, Metcalfe JB, et al. Comparison of the ring block, dorsal penile nerve block, and topical anesthesia for neonatal circumcision: a randomized controlled trial. *JAMA.* 1997;278:2157–2162.

Lener EV, Bucalo BD, Kist DA, Moy RL. Topical anesthetic agents in dermatologic surgery: a review. *Dermatol Surg.* 1997;23:673–683.

McGee DL. Local and topical anesthesia. In: Roberts JR, Custalow CB, Thomsen TW, eds. *Roberts and Hedges Clinical Procedures in Emergency Medicine.* 6th ed. Philadelphia: Elsevier; 2014:523–529.

Moy RL, Pfenninger JL. Taking the sting out of local anesthesia. *Pat Care March.* 2000;15:61.

Nestor MS. Safety of occluded 4% liposomal lidocaine cream. *J Drugs Dermatol.* 2006;5:618–620.

Shroeder ED, Taillac P. Topical anesthesia. In: Reichman EF, ed. *Emergency Medicine Procedures.* 2nd ed. New York: McGraw-Hill; 2013:795–799.

Topicaine Topical Anesthetic Gel. http://www.esbalabs.com/top4.htm.

Wolfe TR, Fosnocht DE, Linscott MS. Atomized lidocaine as topical anesthesia for nasogastric tube placement: a randomized, double blind, placebo-controlled trial. *Ann Emerg Med.* 2000;35:421–425.

CHAPTER 5

LOCAL ANESTHESIA

Gerald A. Amundsen

The administration of local anesthesia is important for many clinical settings. Most wounds, traumatic and surgical, require some form of anesthesia before repair to maintain patient comfort and satisfaction. More than 100 million wounds are repaired in the United States each year, so it is important for most clinicians to be comfortable with the medications and techniques used to administer the medications.

The action of local anesthetics at the molecular level is to prevent the generation and conduction of nerve impulses. The overall effect of an anesthetic is to reduce pain associated with trauma or procedures; this effect in turn depends on such factors as blood supply, the size of the area to be anesthetized, and the location of the wound in terms of nerve ending size and density. The fingers, toes, genitals, perianal area, and nose are especially sensitive. Patient factors such as infection, anxiety, and chronic disease (e.g., diabetes, peripheral vascular disease, obesity) also affect the success of the anesthetic. To achieve successful anesthesia, the clinician must be able to make decisions about dose and route of administration while also considering these factors (also see Chapter 4).

INDICATIONS

- To relieve pain from a procedure (incision) or trauma (laceration/fracture)
- Diagnostic nerve blocks to isolate pathology

See Tables 5.1 and 5.2 for a selection of local anesthetics and their characteristics, and Box 5.1 for selection criteria for local anesthetics.

CONTRAINDICATIONS

- "Known" sensitivity to amide anesthetic medications (lidocaine, mepivacaine, bupivacaine) is very rare. The older ester anesthetics (procaine, tetracaine) are more likely to cause true allergic reactions. Fortunately, there is no cross-reactivity between the classes, so the individual with known sensitivity to the ester anesthetics is not likely to experience a reaction with the amide group. The **parabens preservatives** used to prolong shelf life in multidose vials of amide anesthetics may induce sensitivity reactions similar to those of the ester group. Parabens are most likely the cause of any "allergy" ascribed to the amides. However, the incidence of parabens allergy is also quite low. If there is a concern about an allergy, use single-dose vials of the amide anesthetics that lack a preservative and are inexpensive. Other considerations include use of a diphenhydramine (1%) or benzyl alcohol (0.9%) mixture as an alternative injectable anesthetic (see below). Knowing that amide allergy is very rare, one expert has also proposed skin testing by using a 0.1 mL of intradermally administered lidocaine as a skin test. However, other experts suggest that intradermal placement can produce false responses, so they recommend subcutaneous injection of this dose while exercising due caution in the unlikely event that the patient exhibits

a serious reaction. If no reaction occurs in 30 minutes, consider proceeding with the full dose.
- History of central nervous system symptoms (e.g., seizure, tremor, tinnitus) associated with anesthetic toxicity (relative contraindication).
- History of cardiovascular reactions (e.g., hypotension, bradyarrhythmia) associated with previous anesthetic use (relative contraindication).
- Epinephrine, frequently used in local anesthetics to prolong the action as well as to decrease the blood flow, may cause a variety of reactions either directly, in association with other medications the patient uses, or as a result of other existing comorbidities.
- While in the past it was generally recommended that epinephrine be avoided because of vasoconstrictive properties, in the distal extremities (i.e., fingers, toes, penis, nose, earlobes), reports of skin ischemia or sloughing in these situations had generally been observed when concentrations of 1:20,000 were used. Current practice generally uses concentrations in the range of 1:100,000 to 1:200,000. Several experts, supported by studies, suggest that epinephrine at these doses can be safely used in the fingers and toes without adverse sequelae.
- Patients with known peripheral vascular disease may have an exaggerated vasoconstrictor response to epinephrine. Extreme care should be taken if local anesthetics with vasoconstrictors are used in patients with diabetes, hypertension, arteriosclerosis, thyrotoxicosis, heart block, or cerebral vascular disease.
- If a skin flap has marginal viability or if blood flow to a flap is compromised, epinephrine should not be used.
- If a wound is contaminated, epinephrine may increase the likelihood of infection because of the diminished blood flow.
- Do not use epinephrine in patient taking monoamine oxidase inhibitors.

EQUIPMENT

Supplies necessary for the local administration of anesthetic are typically inexpensive and readily accessible.

- Anesthetic agents of choice (see Table 5.1 and Box 5.1)
- 18-gauge needle to draw up solution
- 25- to 30-gauge needles of various lengths
- Syringes (1 to 10 mL)
- Antiseptic (alcohol, povidone-iodine, chlorhexidine) to clean the vial top and the clinical area
- Sodium bicarbonate 7.5% (Neutra-Caine) or sodium bicarbonate 7% to 10% for buffering the anesthetic (e.g., lidocaine or mepivacaine) if desired to reduce the pain of injection (see later discussion; also bupivacaine can be buffered, but to avoid precipitation, lower amounts of sodium bicarbonate should be used)

EDITOR'S NOTES: (1) When equipping the office, it is not necessary to store every type of anesthetic at every concentration, and it is also not necessary to stock the office with every size and length of needle.

TABLE 5.1   Local Anesthetic Agents

Type	Name	Concentration (%)	Onset	Duration*	Maximum Adult Dose
Amino esters	Procaine (Novocain)	2	Slow	15–30 min plain 30–90 min w/epi	500 mg
	Tetracaine (Pontocaine)	0.25	Slow	120–240 min plain 240–480 min w/epi	100 mg plain 200 mg w/epi
	Chloroprocaine (Nesacaine)	2	Fast	15–30 min plain 30–90 min w/epi	800 mg plain 1000 mg w/epi
Amino amides†	Lidocaine (Xylocaine)	0.5–2	Fast	30–120 min plain 60–400 min w/epi	300 mg plain 500 mg w/epi
	Etidocaine (Duranest)	0.5	Fast	120–240 min plain 400 mg w/epi	300 mg plain
	Mepivacaine (Carbocaine)	1	Fast	30–120 min plain 60–400 min w/epi	300 mg plain 500 mg w/epi
	Bupivacaine (Marcaine)	0.25	Moderate	120–240 min plain 240–480 min w/epi	175 mg plain 225 mg w/epi

*Duration of action for adults and older children; prolonged duration of action in neonates and young children possible.
†Allergic reaction to the amides is very rare. If allergic reaction apparent with use, consider parabens preservatives as the cause. Use single-dose vials of anesthetics to avoid parabens.
w/epi, With epinephrine.

TABLE 5.2   Maximum Dosages of Commonly Used Injectable Local Anesthetics

Anesthetic	Concentration (%)	Maximum Adult Dose
Lidocaine (Xylocaine)	1	4.5 mg/kg not to exceed 300 mg (30 mL in adult)
Lidocaine (Xylocaine) with epinephrine	1	7 mg/kg not to exceed 500 mg (50 mL in adult)
Bupivacaine (Marcaine) with epinephrine	0.25	3 mg/kg not to exceed 175 mg (50 mL per average adult)
Bupivacaine (Marcaine)	0.25	3 mg/kg not to exceed 225 mg

From McEvoy GK, ed. *AHFS Drug Information*. Bethesda, MD: American Society of Health-System Pharmacists; 1999.

BOX 5.1   Selection of Local Anesthetics and Effects

Lidocaine (Xylocaine) Without Epinephrine (1%–2%)
Can cause vasodilation
Can last 30–60 minutes depending on site or vascularity
Can use in contaminated wounds
Can use in fingers, nose, penis, toes, earlobes
Can use if vascular disease is present or if patient is immuno-compromised
Can use if there are cerebrovascular or cardiovascular risks
Can use for nerve block

Lidocaine (Xylocaine) With Epinephrine (1%–2%)
Causes vasoconstriction
Has longer duration
Can use in highly vascular areas to improve visualization of field
Can use in clean wounds
In general, use with caution on fingers, nose, penis, toes, and earlobes, especially with patients with vascular disease

Bupivacaine (Marcaine)
For longer duration
For nerve blocks

It is more practical and economical for the clinician to be familiar with the equipment of choice and to stock the office according to preference. Typically, a long- and short-acting anesthetic with and without epinephrine and a few sizes of needles should suffice for most offices. (2) Melman and Siegel (1999) have shown that it is perfectly acceptable **to draw up buffered anesthetic solutions in syringes up to 14 days before use.** When stored at room temperature, there is no increased bacterial contamination or growth, and the anesthetic still functions. We used to pull up our syringes at the beginning of the day and then discard them at the end of the day, but there is no need to do this. We now fill numerous 1-mL syringes, date them, and continue to use them throughout the week. It is much more efficient for the nurse to pull up multiple syringes than to do just one at a time. It is not efficient for the clinician to spend time pulling up anesthetic into the syringe! (3) Advanced Meditech International has designed **a small anesthetic bottle holder that mounts on the wall** (VE-11 Handzfree Anesthetic Bottle Holder; Fig. 5.1). The cost is around $45, but in our office it is indispensable. It holds the anesthetic where it is readily available and makes filling syringes an easy task. It also allows the entire staff to see how much anesthetic is left in the bottle. There is nothing more frustrating than pulling out the drawer with the anesthetic solution and finding that the bottle is empty!

OPTIONS FOR ALLERGIC PATIENTS

- Use a cooling agent (e.g., ice cube, ethyl chloride) instead.
- For small lesions, use no anesthetic.
- Use single-dose vials instead of multidose vials to avoid the parabens preservatives.
- Use bacteriostatic saline alone instead.
- Substitute an amide for an ester (if offending agent can be identified).
- Use a 1% diphenhydramine (Benadryl) or benzyl alcohol (0.9%) mixture as the local injectable anesthetic. Inject 10 to 50 mg (1 to 5 mL of standard 5% [50 mg/mL] parenteral diphenhydramine mixed with 4 mL of normal saline) into the area in manner similar to the other local anesthetics. While it is slightly more painful to inject, and it does not last quite as long, this diphenhydramine mixture has been found to be as effective as 1% lidocaine for pain control. Benzyl alcohol (0.9%) with epinephrine (1:100,000) compares favorably with this diphenhydramine mixture but has a shorter duration than diphenhydramine.

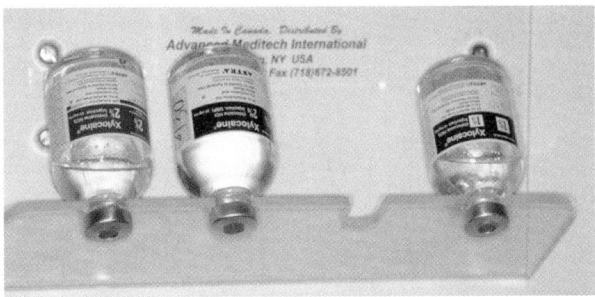

Fig. 5.1 **Anesthetic bottle holder.** (Courtesy Advanced Meditech International, Inc.; VE-11 Handzfree Anesthetic Bottle Holder.)

PREPROCEDURE PATIENT PREPARATION

Patients should be made aware of the anesthesia plan (local, digital block, nerve block, topical) and the potential discomfort they may briefly experience. A standard consent form is used for whatever procedure is to be performed. The risks include allergic reaction to the anesthetic, infection, bleeding, damage to the area resulting in ischemia (if epinephrine or other vasoconstrictors are used), and systematic absorption of the local anesthetic.

GENERAL TECHNIQUES

1. The top of the vial is wiped with alcohol, and the desired volume of anesthetic is withdrawn using an 18-gauge needle. Typically, 5 to 10 mL should suffice for most procedures, although less than 1 mL is usually enough for simple shave or punch biopsy procedures.
2. Discard the 18-gauge needle and replace it with an appropriately sized needle for the location and type of procedure. For most office procedures, a 27- or 30-gauge needle with a length of 1 or 1.5 inches is appropriate.
   EDITOR'S NOTE: To minimize the risk for vasovagal reaction, do not draw up medication in front of the patient. Also, only administer local anesthesia when the patient is in the supine position.
3. The local injection may be intradermal (creating a wheal) or subcutaneous (deep to the skin), depending on the intended procedure. While subcutaneous injections cause less discomfort, and should be preferred, they also require longer for the anesthetic to take effect. Advance the needle to the desired location and draw back on the plunger before injecting to avoid systemic effects associated with injecting directly into a vessel. If there is blood return on aspiration, reposition the needle, aspirate again, and inject if there was no blood return during aspiration.
4. Pain when injecting local anesthesia is primarily a result of skin puncture and subcutaneous injection. Therefore attempt to minimize the number of punctures by redirecting the needle along a different path before entirely withdrawing it. When injecting for laceration repair, inject from the wound edge and advance the needle only in the subdermal layer. This avoids the need for skin puncture. Spread of infection from the wound margin has not been demonstrated clinically with this technique.
5. Before any digital or other block, a review of the related anatomy is recommended. In the case of digital blocks, it is important to remember the location and number of nerves supplying each digit (Fig. 5.2). (See Chapter 7.)

COMMON ERRORS

- Injection while advancing the needle can result in systemic complications from introduction of the anesthetic directly into the vascular system. Inject only while withdrawing the needle.

- Inadequate anesthesia may be the result of failure to wait for the agent to work effectively. Allow time for the drug to diffuse and achieve the desired effect (4 to 5 minutes). If the injection is intradermal (causing a wheal), it will have a more rapid onset. If deeper (subcutaneous), it will take longer to achieve its effect.
- Injection directly into an area of infection will not achieve good anesthesia and may contribute to spread of the infection. Do not inject into an area of infection. Rather, inject around the area in a field block pattern (Fig. 5.3), and do not use epinephrine in areas near infection.
- Although there is no proof that injection directly into a suspected cancer will spread the cancer along the needle track, injection into or through a suspected cancer should be avoided if possible.
- Injection of too much anesthetic may distort a lesion in a way that inhibits the accuracy and completeness of the excision or destruction. It may also mask a lesion and make it difficult to palpate and find if it is below the skin. Use a field block (see Fig. 5.3) to avoid the lesion while achieving anesthesia.
- Inappropriate administration of anesthetic creates increased pain and anxiety for the patient. Methods for reducing the pain of injection are discussed in Box 5.2.
- For adverse reactions and concerns about toxic doses, see Chapter 6.

REDUCTION OF PAIN OF INJECTION

Sodium Bicarbonate

Injection of local anesthetics can cause pain, which is related to the size of the needle, the rapidity of injection, and the temperature of the anesthetic solution. The acidity of the solution (pH 4.05 to 6.49) also causes a significant burning sensation. This short-lived pain can be reduced by using a small needle (30-gauge), pinching up the skin, injecting slowly, warming the solution (room temperature or even body temperature), and adding 1 mL of sodium bicarbonate solution (7% to 10%) to 9 mL of 1% lidocaine or 1% mepivacaine anesthetic. (For bupivacaine, to avoid precipitation, only 0.05 to 0.1 mL of sodium bicarbonate solution [7% to 10%] should be added to 9 mL of 0.5% bupivacaine.) Patients, especially children, will note remarkable improvement in comfort. Infiltration with unbuffered solution has been found to be 2.8 to 5.7 times more painful than infiltration with buffered counterparts. There has been no significant difference detected in the time of onset or duration of anesthesia or in the surface area of skin anesthetized. The addition of bicarbonate will usually make the solution slightly hazy or cloudy, but there are no known adverse effects from this. Other tips to reduce pain with injections are outlined in Box 5.2.

Previously it was indicated that the buffered solution be discarded after 24 hours. Buffered lidocaine is stable for at least 1 week at room temperature. Refrigeration may nearly double that time. Warming the buffered solution to above room temperature may also decrease the discomfort of injection (see Box 5.2).

Topical Anesthetics

Certain clinical situations favor the use of a topical anesthetic (see Chapter 4). Examples include combative children too large for the papoose board and too young to reason with, and patients with nosebleeds, eye injuries, corneal abrasions, or lesions on mucous membranes that need to be treated with painful modalities, such as liquid nitrogen or electrosurgery. Mucous membranes (i.e., nose, mouth, throat, esophagus, anus, and genitourinary tract) can be anesthetized successfully with many of the local anesthetics by direct topical application. Care must be taken to avoid excess systemic absorption of the topical anesthetic near mucous membranes (see Chapter 6). On many occasions, the application of topical anesthetic before injection may allow for more accurate administration of injectable anesthetic.

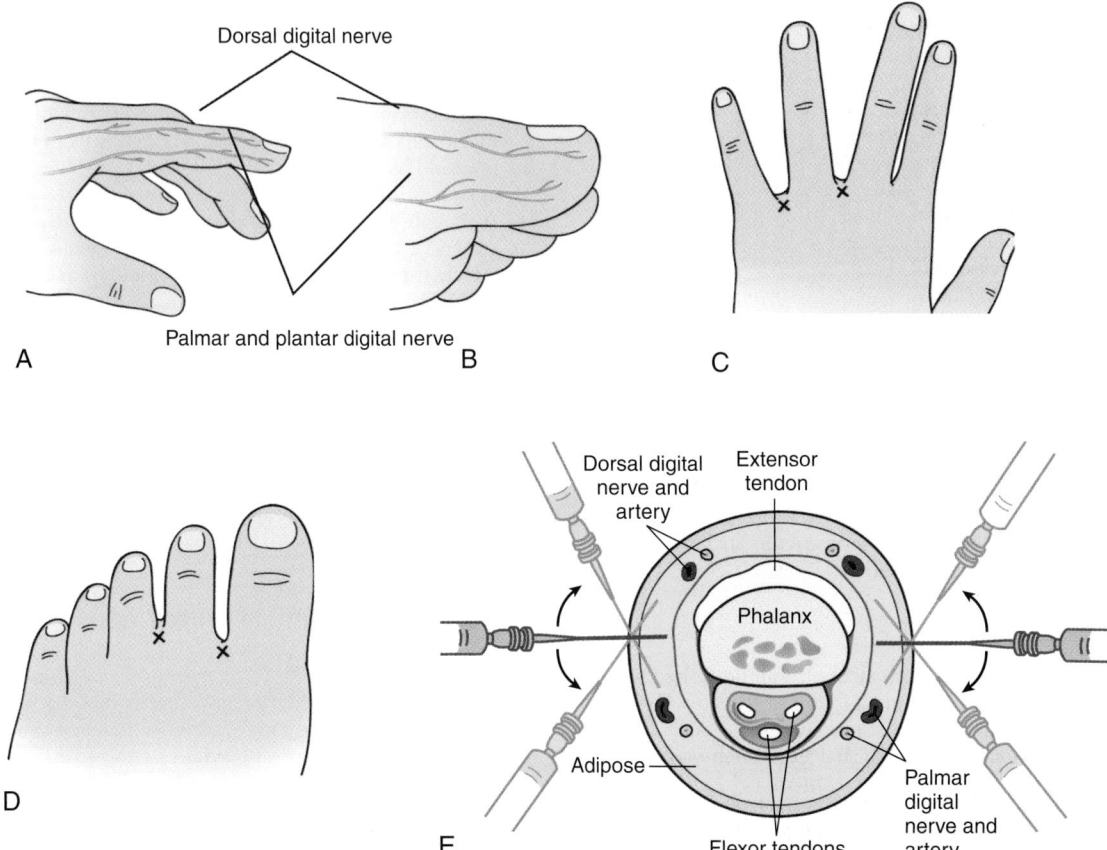

Fig. 5.2 Anatomy of a digital block. In the finger (A) and toe (B), there are four nerves to block in order to obtain a successful digital block. A dorsal and palmar branch on each side of the digit needs to be blocked. If the proper sites of infiltration are chosen (C, finger, or D, toe), the four nerves should be well anesthetized. First, the web space on both sides of each digit is injected. Insert the needle parallel to the digits, directed toward the hand or foot. Insert 1 to 2 cm and inject 1 to 2 mL of anesthetic. Repeat on the other side. After the web space is infiltrated, insert the needle perpendicular to the base of the digit on each side of the digit. Insert until the needle touches bone. Withdraw a few millimeters and inject 1 mL of anesthetic *(red needle and syringe)*. It is also helpful to then perform a "ring block" (E). Inject from the midline on top to the midline on the bottom from both sides to complete a "ring" around the entire digit *(gray needle and syringe)*. A digital block may take several minutes to take effect because there is so much accessory innervation. In the case of a severely inflamed paronychia, or an ingrown toenail in which the nail must be partially or entirely removed, additional local anesthetic may still be necessary just proximal to the site of inflammation to eliminate pain and to allow the removal. It is best to avoid vasoconstrictor agents in local anesthetics for digital blocks. In addition, care should be taken to avoid systemic injection. See Fig. 7.2 for more anatomic details.

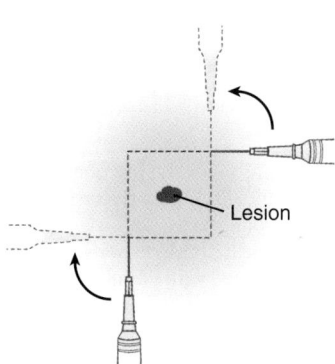

Fig. 5.3 Field block. Inject at 90-degree angles on both sides of the skin lesion to be excised. Usually only two injection sites are necessary. After injecting in one direction, withdraw the needle, rotate it 90 degrees, and inject again. This avoids distortion of the central area around the lesion to be excised.

BOX 5.2   Tips to Reduce Pain With Injections

- Use warm solution (room temperature).
- Use a small needle (30 gauge if possible).
- Inject slowly.
- Inject subcutaneously into the adipose tissue (vs. intradermally, which creates a wheal). It will take longer for subcutaneous injection to take effect but will be less painful.
- Warn the patient that the most sensitive areas are fingers, toes, genitals, nose, and perianal area.
- Use sodium bicarbonate to buffer lidocaine or mepivacaine. (Bupivacaine can be buffered, but a much lower dose of sodium bicarbonate should be used.)
- Pinch up and "shake" the skin while the injection is being given.
- Use a topical anesthetic (see Chapters 4 and 7) before injection.
- Use a topical refrigerant to cool the area before injection (e.g., Frigi-Dent, ethyl chloride, Fluori-Methane [15% dichlorodifluoromethane, 85% trichloromonofluoromethane]).
- Consider distraction techniques in children (see Chapter 2).

COMPLICATIONS

Complications of anesthetic administration are listed here, and adverse effects of the drugs themselves are discussed in detail in Chapter 6. With proper administration, anesthetic complications are quite rare.

- Sensitivity reactions (almost always with esters or multidose vials)
- Central nervous system toxicity: seizure, tinnitus, visual disturbances, altered mental status (if an excess dose is given)
- Cardiovascular toxicity: arrhythmias, bradycardia, hypotension, congestive heart failure exacerbation
- Marked, prolonged vasoconstriction in digit if epinephrine was used (consider rubbing in nitroglycerin ointment for vasodilation)
- Methemoglobinemia
- Infection
- Bleeding
- Tissue/nerve trauma

POSTPROCEDURE MANAGEMENT AND CONCERNS

Patients should be instructed to watch for redness, pus, swelling, streaking, or increased pain, all of which can be indicative of infection or local sensitivity. When a long-acting agent like bupivacaine is used, warn the patient to exercise caution with activity because the long-acting effect will mask pain and allow enough activity to sustain further injury.

CPT/BILLING CODES

Administration of local anesthetic is included in the CPT code for individual procedures, and no extra charge can be generated. When anesthetic is administered as part of a joint injection, the CPT code for the joint injection is used. Injection of an anesthetic for diagnostic purposes or a therapeutic nerve block can be billed under a CPT code.

64400–64489	Introduction/injection of anesthetic (nerve block), diagnostic or therapeutic procedures on the somatic nerves

Acknowledgment

The editors recognize the contributions of Daniel Derksen, MD, to this chapter in a previous edition of this text.

SUPPLIERS

(See contact information available at www.expertconsult.com.)

Ethyl chloride (Gebauer Co)
Frigi-Dent (Ellman Cynosure)
Advanced Meditech International, Inc. (AMI)
Delasco
MD, Inc.

Most medical suppliers can provide syringes and needles as well as anesthetics.

RECOMMENDED READING

Achar S, Kundu S. Principles of office anesthesia. Part 1: infiltrative anesthesia. *Am Fam Physician*. 2002;66:91–94.

Denkler K. A comprehensive review of epinephrine in the finger: to do or not to do. *Plast Reconstr Surg*. 2001;108:114–124.

Denkler K. Dupuytren's fasciectomies in 60 consecutive digits using lidocaine with epinephrine and no tourniquet. *Plast Reconstr Surg*. 2005;115: 802–810.

Ernst AA, Marvez-Valls E, Nick TG, Wahle M. Comparison trial of four injectable anesthetics for laceration repair. *Acad Emerg Med*. 1996;3: 228–233.

Fitzcharles-Bowe C, Denkler K, Lalonde D. Finger injection with high-dose (1:1000) epinephrine: does it cause finger necrosis and should it be treated? *Hand (NY)*. 2007;2:5–11.

Krunic AL, Wang LC, Soltani K, et al. Digital anesthesia with epinephrine: an old myth revisited. *J Am Acad Dermatol*. 2004;51:755–759.

Lalonde D, Bell M, Benoit P, et al. A multicenter prospective study of 3,110 consecutive cases of elective epinephrine use in the fingers and hand: the Dalhousie Project clinical phase. *J Hand Surg Am*. 2005;30:1061–1067.

McGee DL. Local and topical anesthesia. In: Roberts JR, Custalow CB, Thomsen TW, eds. *Roberts and Hedges Clinical Procedures in Emergency Medicine*. 6th ed. Philadelphia: Elsevier; 2014:523–529.

Melman D, Siegel DM. Prefilled syringes: safe and effective. *Dermatol Surg*. 1999;25:492–493.

Moy RL, Pfenninger JL. Taking the sting out of local anesthesia. *Patient Care March*. 2000;15:61–73.

Radovic P, Smith RG, Shumway D. Revisiting epinephrine in foot surgery. *J Am Podiatr Med Assoc*. 2003;93:157–160.

Scarfone RJ, Jasani M, Gracely EJ. Pain of local anesthetics: rate of administration and buffering. *Ann Emerg Med*. 1998;31:36–40.

Schindlbeck MA. Local anesthesia. In: Reichman EF, ed. *Emergency Medicine Procedures*. 2nd ed. New York: McGraw-Hill; 2013:789–795.

Soriano TT, Lask GP, Dinehart SM. Anesthesia and analgesia. In: Robinson JK, Hanke CW, Sengelmann RD, Siegel DM, eds. *Surgery of the Skin: Procedural Dermatology*. Philadelphia: Mosby; 2005:39–58.

Tetzlaff JE. The pharmacology of local anesthetics. *Anesthesiol Clin North Am*. 2000;18:217–233.

Thomson CJ, Lalonde DH, Denkler KA, Feicht AJ. A critical look at the evidence for and against elective epinephrine use in the finger. *Plast Reconstr Surg*. 2007;119:260–266.

Usatine RP, Tobinick EL, Siegel DM. *Skin Surgery: A Practical Guide*. St. Louis: Mosby; 1998.

CHAPTER 6

LOCAL AND TOPICAL ANESTHETIC COMPLICATIONS

William L. McDaniel Jr • Raymond F. Jarris Jr

Many in-office surgical procedures require the use of local or topical anesthetics. Topical anesthetics are used more frequently in children for dermatologic procedures and in persons having oral and dental procedures, nasopharyngoscopy, and esophagogastroduodenoscopy (EGD). Various mixtures of potent topical medications are also being used more frequently, often under occlusion, to cover large surface areas for aesthetic procedures. This markedly increases the risk for reaching toxic levels.

The primary care clinician must have an understanding of the types of complications that may be encountered when using these anesthetics and must be equipped to diagnose and deal with them. For maximum safe dosage, see below.

ALLERGIC REACTIONS

- Low incidence (<1%)
- Older agents such as procaine and tetracaine (esters) are more likely to cause allergic reactions because they are derivatives of para-aminobenzoic acid, a known allergen. However, allergic reactions to ester anesthetics are rare; much more likely is an allergic reaction to the methylparaben preservatives in the solution. Methylparaben preservatives have a structure similar to para-aminobenzoic acid. It should be noted that some patients report a history of an "allergy to Novocaine (procaine) used by a dentist years ago." They frequently attribute any adverse reaction as an allergic reaction. A thorough history may reveal it was not a true allergic reaction. Fortunately, procaine is no longer used in dental practice.
- *Allergic reactions to amide local anesthetics (lidocaine, mepivacaine, bupivacaine) are extremely rare.* Fortunately, there is no cross-reactivity between the ester and amide classes, so the individual with known sensitivity to the ester anesthetics is not likely to experience a similar reaction with the amide group.
- In patients with known or suspected local anesthetic allergy, avoid multidose vials of an amide such as lidocaine. Multidose vials often contain methylparaben preservatives which are much more allergenic than even the ester anesthetics.
- True allergic reactions may vary from mild to life-threatening with anaphylaxis and circulatory collapse. In cases of anaphylaxis:
  - Plasma losses may equal 35% of circulating blood volume within minutes.
  - Rapid replacement of volume with colloid and administration of epinephrine are indicated (see Chapter 212).
  - If epinephrine fails, norepinephrine infusion may be life-saving.

ALTERNATIVES TO OBTAIN PAIN RELIEF IN ALLERGIC PATIENTS

- Use single-dose vials of lidocaine, which lack preservative.
- Substitute an amide anesthetic for an ester.

- A small local anesthetic effect can be obtained by injecting sterile normal saline into tissue.
- Small lesions (e.g., skin tags) may not require an anesthetic for removal/treatment.
- Dilute 50 mg of diphenhydramine (1 mL from a 50 mg/mL vial) with 4 mL sterile normal saline. Inject 1 to 5 mL (10 to 50 mg) of this dilute diphenhydramine locally for anesthetic effect (see Chapter 5).
- Use ice cubes, cold spray (e.g., Pain Ease or ethyl chloride; Frigi-Dent), liquid nitrogen (sparingly) to obtain topical anesthesia.
- Hypnosis

EFFECTS OF EPINEPHRINE IN LOCAL ANESTHETICS

It has long been an admonition to students, residents, and practicing clinicians that epinephrine should never be used in areas of the body supplied by the fine terminal end arterioles such as the fingers and toes, penis, and nose. Theoretically, the epinephrine could cause prolonged spasm leading to ischemia and even necrosis of the tissue. This effect would be potentially magnified if the vessels were already diseased and narrowed, as occurs in smokers and patients with diabetes, peripheral vascular disease, and similar conditions. Hence, in the past, it was literally seen as substandard care to use epinephrine in these areas, especially when there was potential vascular disease or diminished blood supply.

In 2000, a series of articles began appearing in the literature to refute this "theoretical" adverse effect (see Recommended Reading). A paper by Denkler published in 2001 reviewed the literature from 1880 through 2000. The conclusion was: "An extensive literature review failed to provide consistent evidence that our current preparations of local anesthesia with epinephrine cause digital necrosis, although not all complications are necessarily reported. However, as with all techniques, caution is necessary to balance the risks of this technique."

Digits can withstand prolonged periods of ischemia. Successful reimplantations have been reported 42 hours after traumatic amputations.

The usual concentration of epinephrine in local anesthetics is 1:100,000. Studies have been conducted using concentrations of 1:1000 with virtually no adverse consequences.

A multicenter prospective study of 3110 consecutive cases of elective epinephrine use in the fingers and hands (concentration ≤1:100,000) found that "the true incidence of finger infarction in elective low-dose-epinephrine injection into the hand and finger is likely to be remote, particularly with the possible rescue with phentolamine. Phentolamine was not required to reverse the vasoconstriction in any patients" (Lalonde et al., 2005).

"Phentolamine rescue" or reversal of epinephrine (α-adrenergic blockade) is recommended for clinically significant vasoconstrictor-induced tissue ischemia. Phentolamine is usually given by local infiltration of 0.5 to 5 mg diluted 1:1 with saline in the area where the epinephrine has been injected. If local infiltration is ineffective (e.g., area involved is large or there is tension within tissue compartment), then it should be given by intraarterial route. Nitroglycerin ointment has also been suggested to reverse any apparent ischemia, however rare (or even possible) this event is.

It would seem acceptable then to use local anesthetics with epinephrine to control bleeding for optimal wound repair and also to prolong needed anesthesia in areas supplied by end arteries. It would appear that an age-old caveat has been disproven. The prudent clinician would still observe at-risk patients closely and use epinephrine sparingly.

MAXIMUM SAFE DOSAGE

There is no one maximum safe dose of a local anesthetic appropriate for all patients and all conditions. Guidelines for children recommend that plain lidocaine can be used safely in doses up to 4.5 mg/kg, but be cautious and pay special care and attention to dosing in neonates. The addition of epinephrine slows the absorption therefore allowing for a maximum safe dose of 7 mg/kg. In adults, peak blood levels do not correlate well with weight. Hypoxia, acid-base status (acidosis), protein binding, and concomitant drug use all lower a patient's tolerance of local anesthetic agents. Use amide anesthetics with caution in patients with severe liver disease or congestive heart failure. Avoid esters in patients with a known atypical form or a quantitative deficiency of pseudocholinesterase. Understanding a 1% solution means 10 mg/mL, 7.5 mL would only be the usual starting bolus (1 mg/kg for 75 kg adult) for treating an adult cardiac ventricular arrhythmia. While the recommended maximum cumulative dose for a cardiac arrhythmia is 3 mg/kg, it should be kept in mind that this dose would be given intravenously compared to the much slower uptake when injected locally, and even slower when combined with epinephrine.

OVERDOSE REACTIONS

Central Nervous System Toxicity

Local anesthetics reach the central nervous system (CNS) after slow absorption or by direct intravenous (IV) injection. An inadvertent direct IV injection may create a transient high local CNS level of anesthetic, which can cause *seizures*. Most seizures created in this way terminate within minutes, provided the administration of the drug has stopped.

A warning of less serious CNS effects in order of progression include tongue or circumoral numbness, lightheadedness, tinnitus, visual disturbances, muscular twitching, and irrational behavior. Drowsiness, commonly seen with lower doses of lidocaine, is not associated with bupivacaine or etidocaine.

If high serum levels persist, grand mal seizures, apnea, unconsciousness, and death may occur. An alert patient, in most cases, tells the clinician before a seizure develops. This would be absent in the case of rapid inadvertent IV injection.

Acidosis and hypercarbia increase the likelihood of CNS toxicity. Pulse oximetry monitoring during the procedure may be a valuable tool to alert the clinician to some of the effects of toxicity. As mentioned previously, use amide anesthetics with caution in patients with severe liver disease or congestive heart failure. Avoid esters in patients with a known atypical form or a quantitative deficiency of pseudocholinesterase.

With serious CNS toxicity, stop the offending agent and begin oxygen and support ventilation if needed. Alert patients can be asked to hyperventilate, which lowers the $P\text{CO}_2$ level and raises the seizure threshold. This may temporarily alleviate twitching. Seizures can usually be stopped with IV midazolam (Versed), diazepam (Valium), or lorazepam (Ativan). Lorazepam and diazepam are inconsistently absorbed by the intramuscular (IM) route. Midazolam may be used IM if an IV line is not available. Flumazenil (Romazicon) should be available as an antagonist for benzodiazepines in case of respiratory depression from the drugs. Since respiratory depression can occur from either the toxicity or a benzodiazepine, some clinicians prefer an ultrashort-acting barbiturate (e.g., thiopental or sodium methohexital) for the seizures.

Cardiovascular Toxicity

While cardiovascular side effects such as increased cardiac output, heart rate, and arterial pressure can occur at moderate blood concentrations due to CNS stimulation and peripheral vasodilation, cardiovascular toxicity can also occur with any of the local anesthetic drugs. This usually occurs at concentrations well above CNS toxicity levels. Local anesthetics prolong conduction through the Purkinje fibers and heart muscle. *Prolongation of PR interval* and *widening of the QRS* may be observed. Higher concentrations decrease heart muscle contractility. *Hypotension*, *respiratory depression*, and *bradycardia* are observed with lidocaine. In fact, lidocaine is a class Ib antiarrhythmic agent; precaution should be taken with its use in patients taking agents in the same class such as mexiletine and tocainamide. Additive and potentially toxic effects could occur. Tetracaine can produce apnea or cardiovascular toxicity without CNS manifestations.

If cardiovascular toxic effects are suspected, discontinue or remove the agent when possible. Basic cardiopulmonary resuscitation is the cornerstone of immediate management. Advanced cardiac life support protocols should be initiated as necessary for serious rhythm disturbances. Various studies suggest that the cardiotoxicity of bupivacaine is more severe and difficult to treat than that associated with lidocaine. Cardiology and anesthesiology consults should be obtained as soon as available. IV lipid emulsion has been used to resuscitate bupivacaine- and mepivacaine-related cardiac arrest, a situation that is otherwise usually fatal.

CATECHOLAMINE REACTIONS

Catecholamine reactions are rarely associated with administered epinephrine but may be produced as a result of anxiety associated with the administration of a local anesthetic or the initiation of the procedure, or as a result of the initial injury that is being treated. Symptoms may include *tachycardia*, *palpitations*, *hypertension*, *apprehension*, *tremulousness*, *diaphoresis*, *tachypnea*, *pallor*, and, on occasion, *anginal chest pain*. Caution is recommended for patients who have hyperthyroidism, hypertension, or atherosclerotic cardiovascular disease, although these conditions do not contraindicate the judicious use of epinephrine-containing anesthetics. *Patients taking monoamine oxidase inhibitors should not receive epinephrine-containing anesthetics.* The treatment includes stopping further drug administration, observation of the patient, and administration of alpha- or beta-adrenergic antagonists or benzodiazepine agents, if necessary.

NOTE: Compounded products are not produced under the same standards as FDA-approved products. The levels of lidocaine may vary dramatically, and toxicity studies using moderate or large amounts of compounded products have not been performed. One of the editors had a patient with delayed (2 hours following procedure) severe headache and significantly elevated systolic blood pressures (up to 260 mm Hg) following a laser procedure. This patient had been premedicated with topical compounded Quadri-Caine containing phenylephrine. Whether this was an idiosyncratic event or not, we no longer use the Quadri-Caine VC, and now prefer BLT to Quadri-Caine (see Chapter 4).

VASOVAGAL REACTIONS

A marked vasovagal reaction may occur if the patient experiences anxiety when an event, such as the sight or sensation of a needle insertion, causes a loss of sympathetic tone and an increased vagal tone. The resulting hypotension and bradycardia may lead to lightheadedness or syncope. If this occurs, the patient should be placed in the supine position with their legs elevated. Ammonia inhalant ("smelling salts") can be tried initially. A 0.3-mL ampule can be crushed and waved in front of the patient's nose. Should this not be effective, give 0.5 mL of atropine (1 mg/mL) IM. This may also be required for significant bradycardia and may be repeated. Practitioners need to be observant and aware that vasovagal syncope can occur even 10 to 15 minutes after a procedure/injection. This has been reported after immunizations also, and such reactions to the Gardasil vaccine have gained significant press coverage.

EDITOR'S NOTE: I now include the questions, "How well do you tolerate pain?" (choices: well, okay, poorly) and "Do you have a tendency to faint with needles?" (choices: yes, no) on my intake forms and also on specific procedure questionnaires. If patients answer that he or she tolerates pain poorly or has a tendency to faint, I routinely give atropine before the surgery/procedure.

Also, the patient should almost always be supine when getting an anesthetic injection. He or she should almost never observe the needle or syringe prior to the injection nor the anesthetic being drawn up. Injecting more slowly and buffing the anesthetic prior to injection may ease the discomfort and decrease the risk of vasovagal reaction. (See Chapter 5 for these and other techniques to decrease the discomfort associated with injection of local anesthetics.)

METHEMOGLOBINEMIA

Methemoglobinemia is a rare but serious complication of topical and local anesthetic agents. It should be clinically suspected and diagnosed if topical or local anesthetics were given. Early diagnosis and treatment can prevent the serious complications of brain damage and death. One must be especially cautious these days because, as noted, topical anesthesia is being used more frequently for aesthetic procedures.

The best way to illustrate the point is with a case history. A 27-year-old man underwent outpatient EGD and developed unexplained cyanosis. During his recovery phase the nurse noted cyanosis, which did not resolve on high-flow oxygen. Vital signs and arterial blood gases were within the normal range. Diagnoses such as pulmonary thromboembolism or an allergic reaction to meperidine (Demerol) or diazepam (Valium) were considered.

An astute respiratory technician noted that the arterial blood drawn for the arterial blood gases was brown. The diagnosis of methemoglobinemia was suspected and confirmed by discovering a methemoglobin level of 14% (Fig. 6.1).

The patient involved had received Cetacaine spray (a combination of benzocaine, aminobenzoate, and tetracaine) four or five times before the EGD procedure. The endoscopist had requested that the patient swallow the material each time. This spray contains about 14% benzocaine, which was the culprit in this case. The package insert and prescribing information for Cetacaine spray lists methemoglobinemia as a rare adverse effect and cautions that care should be used not to exceed a 2-second spray.

Normal hemoglobin contains iron in the ferrous (+2) state. Methemoglobin contains iron that has been oxidized to the abnormal ferric (+3) state. Normal levels of methemoglobin range up to 3%.

Prevent methemoglobinemia by avoiding overdose of benzocaine, prilocaine, and lidocaine. Prilocaine and lidocaine in a eutectic mixture of 2.5% each (EMLA) is considered safe when used as recommended. EMLA is applied topically and is often used in infants and children. One case of methemoglobinemia has been reported with its use over large areas for a long period of time. It is more likely to occur if used under occlusion for large areas for extended times or if applied to mucous membranes.

The risk for methemoglobinemia is increased in patients with anemia, respiratory or cardiovascular disease, and deficiencies in glucose-6-phosphate or methemoglobin reductase. Other drugs that can cause this side effect include sulfonamides, phenytoin (Dilantin), antimalarials, phenobarbital, amyl nitrate, nitrites, sodium nitroprusside, nitroglycerin dapsone, quinolones, and acetaminophen.

The following signs are noted at the various methemoglobin levels:

- Up to 15%: graying of skin
- 15% to 20%: cyanosis becomes apparent and the blood has a chocolate-brown color
- 20% to 50%: weakness, dizziness
- 50% to 70%: arrhythmias, acidosis, convulsions, and coma may occur
- Over 70%: death and cerebral anoxia may occur

Nitrates, foods, and contaminated well water may predispose to methemoglobinemia and may lower the threshold for such local anesthetic complications.

Treatment varies with the level of methemoglobin present and the condition of the patient. Urgent administration of methylene blue is indicated for symptomatic hypoxia as evidenced by arrhythmias, angina, respiratory distress, seizures, coma, or methemoglobin levels greater than 30%. Methylene blue 1% administered IV slowly over 5 minutes should result in improvement. Adults and children are administered 1 to 2 mg/kg (0.1 to 0.2 mL/kg of 1% solution) or 25 to 50 mg/kg^2. A second dose can be repeated after an hour if the response was inadequate. Do not exceed 7 mg/kg.

Hyperbaric oxygen therapy may help by increasing the amount of dissolved oxygen in the blood. Consider exchange transfusions in the most severely affected patients. This may require a tertiary medical center.

Successful treatment will be unavailable unless the astute clinician considers the diagnosis of methemoglobinemia (Box 6.1).

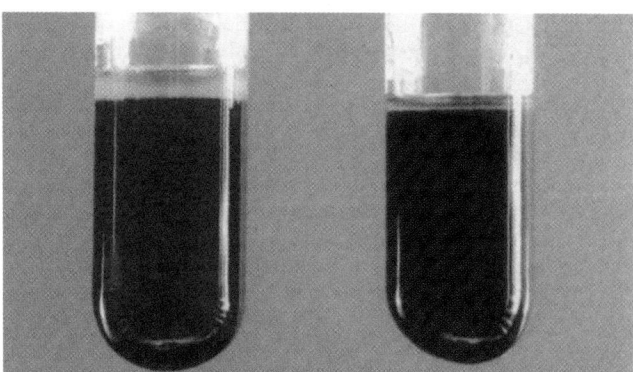

Fig. 6.1 Normal arterial blood versus methemoglobinemia. Compare arterial whole blood with 1% methemoglobin *(left)* with arterial whole blood with 72% methemoglobin *(right)*. Note the characteristic chocolate-brown color of the sample with an elevated methemoglobin level. (From DeBaun MR, Vichinsky E. Hemoglobinopathies. In: Kliegman R, ed. *Nelson Textbook of Pediatrics.* 18th ed. Philadelphia: Saunders; 2007.)

BOX 6.1   Factors Suggesting Acquired Methemoglobinemia

- A local anesthetic agent was used.
- A larger-than-usual dose was needed.
- Environmental predisposition present (nitrates) or other predisposing drugs such as sulfonamides, phenytoin (Dilantin), amyl nitrate, dapsone, sodium nitroprusside, quinolones, nitroglycerin, and methamphetamines.
- Cyanosis does not respond to usual O_2.
- Arterial blood appears chocolate-brown (usually 15%–20% levels of methemoglobin present).
- Infants and the elderly seem more susceptible to development of methemoglobinemia.

OTHER

Gingival mucosa ulcerations have been reported with use of EMLA, so it probably should not be used for mucosal anesthesia.

SUPPLIERS

(See contact information available at www.expertconsult.com.)

Cooling sprays
Gebauer
Ellman Cynosure
Resuscitation equipment
Banyan Corp.
Mukilteo
www.statkit.com

RECOMMENDED READING

Denkler K. A comprehensive review of epinephrine in the finger: to do or not to do. *Plast Reconstr Surg.* 2001;108:114–124.
Denkler K. Dupuytren's fasciectomies in 60 consecutive digits using lidocaine with epinephrine and no tourniquet. *Plast Reconstr Surg.* 2005;115:802–810.

Fitzcharles-Bowe C, Denkler K, Lalonde D. Finger injections with high-dose (1:1000) epinephrine: does it cause finger necrosis and should it be treated? *Hand (NY).* 2007;2:5–11.
Krunic AL, Wang LC, Soltani K, et al. Digital anesthesia with epinephrine: an old myth revisited. *J Am Acad Dermatol.* 2004;51:755–759.
Lalonde D, Bell M, Sparkes G, et al. A multicenter prospective study of 3110 consecutive cases of elective epinephrine use in the fingers and hand: the Dalhousie Project clinical phase. *J Hand Surg Am.* 2005;30:1061–1067.
Lee JJ, Rubin AP. EMLA cream and its current uses. *Br J Hosp Med.* 1993;50:463–466.
Marx JA, Hockberger RS, Walls RM, eds. *Rosen's Emergency Medicine: Concepts and Clinical Practice, 2-Volume Set.* 8th ed. St. Louis: Mosby; 2014.
Radovic P, Smith RG, Shumway D. Revisiting epinephrine in foot surgery. *J Am Podiatr Med Assoc.* 2003;93:157–160.
Reichman EF, ed. *Emergency Medicine Procedures.* 2nd ed. New York: McGraw-Hill; 2013.
Roberts JR, Hedges JR, eds. *Clinical Procedures in Emergency Medicine.* 6th ed. Philadelphia: Saunders; 2014.
Rodriguez LF, Smolik LM, Zbehlik AJ. Benzocaine-induced methemoglobinemia: report of a severe reaction and review of the literature. *Ann Pharmacother.* 1994;28:643–649.
Smith C. Pharmacology of local anaesthetic agents. *Br J Hosp Med.* 1994;52:455–460.
Thomson CJ, Lalonde DH, Denkler KA, Feicht AJ. A critical look at the evidence for and against elective epinephrine use in the finger. *Plast Reconstr Surg.* 2007;119:260–266.

CHAPTER 7

PERIPHERAL NERVE BLOCKS AND FIELD BLOCKS

Morteza Khodaee • Barbara F. Kelly

Many ambulatory procedures lend themselves well to local anesthesia with a field block or a peripheral nerve block. A field block is a method of providing anesthesia to a relatively small area by injecting a "wall" of anesthetic solution across the path of the nerves supplying the operative field (Fig. 7.1). Instead of the injection being made directly into the area of the procedure, it is made into the soft tissue some distance away, where the nerves are situated. Advantages include longer duration of anesthesia and no distortion of the operative field.

A *nerve block* is the infiltration of a local anesthetic near the nerve branch supplying sensation to a particular area. Blocking a nerve provides longer duration of anesthesia than that obtained with local cutaneous infiltration. Knowledge of the anatomy of peripheral nerves and a scrupulous sterile technique are important for successful peripheral nerve blocks. Use of this technique may reduce the amount of anesthetic needed, reduce distortion of tissues, and allow palpation of pathology to be excised.

Using ultrasound to guide nerve blocks may improve the quality and decrease the risk of complications. (See Chapters 171 and 214 for techniques of ultrasound-guided procedures.)

In some sites (e.g., the breast) a nerve block cannot be obtained, and thus the field block is the only reasonable alternative. However, where possible, the nerve block may be the procedure of choice.

Also see Chapter 8.

INDICATIONS

- When local anesthetic at the site of incision may be ineffective (e.g., with infected tissue the pH is lower)
- When the edema from the local anesthetic injection would distort anatomic landmarks and make approximation and repair difficult
- To preserve palpation of the deep tissue to be excised
- When repairs or excisions are quite large and prohibit the use of large amounts of anesthetic
- For burn management, wound exploration, foreign body removal, extensive laceration repair
- For fracture and dislocation care
- For nail removal

CONTRAINDICATIONS

Absolute Contraindications

- If it would require injecting through infected tissue
- Presence of septicemia
- Profound bleeding tendencies
- History of allergy to local anesthetics (True allergy to amide anesthetics such as lidocaine, mepivacaine, and bupivacaine is very rare; see Chapters 5 and 6.)

Relative Contraindications

- Any neurologic damage existing before the procedure. Document findings before injection.
- In the past, it was recommended that epinephrine-containing anesthetic solutions not be used in the fingers, toes, penis, nose, or earlobe. For various reasons, this concept is somewhat outdated (see Editor's note below). However, it is probably still reasonable to avoid use of epinephrine in areas with a poor vascular supply. It should only be used with caution in patients with peripheral vascular disease, or other conditions affecting vascular supply.

EQUIPMENT

- Sterile field and agent for sterile preparation of skin
- 18-gauge needle to draw up solution
- 25- to 30-gauge needle for injection (1 to 10 mL)
- Appropriate-size syringe
- Gloves
- Local anesthetic agent (see Chapter 5), usually 1% or 2% lidocaine

EDITOR'S NOTE: In the past, it was generally recommended that use of epinephrine in local anesthetics be avoided because of its vasoconstrictive properties in the distal extremities (i.e., fingers, toes, penis, nose, earlobes). However, reports of skin ischemia or sloughing in these situations had generally been observed when concentrations of 1:20,000 were used. Current practice generally uses concentrations in the range of 1:100,000 to 1:200,000. Several experts, supported by studies, suggest that epinephrine at these doses can be safely used in the fingers and toes without adverse sequelae.

PREPROCEDURE PATIENT PREPARATION

There are few complications with field and nerve blocks. The benefits of these blocks versus the alternatives (e.g., general anesthesia, no anesthesia, and Bier block) may be explained. Depending on the agent used, the duration of anesthesia may be prolonged, and the patient should be informed of the expected length of action. In rare instances a nerve could be traumatized, but long-term consequences are rare. Any precautionary advice, such as avoidance of heat or cold after the procedure, should be given to the patient. The possibility of paresthesia during the injection should be explained.

TECHNIQUE

Field Block

The technique of administering a field block is similar to the technique discussed for local anesthetics (see Chapter 5). In this instance, however, the area to be incised is spared from the injection. Rather,

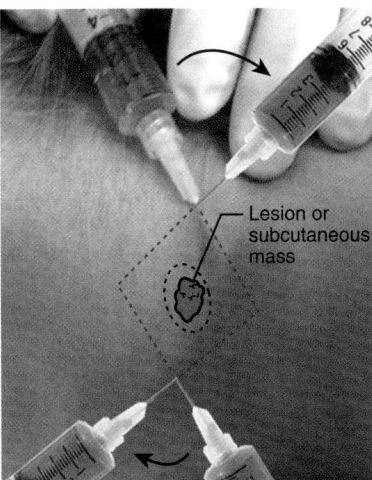

Fig. 7.1 Field block technique. This method of injecting around the lesion prevents distortion of the anatomy and allows any deeper central lesion to remain palpable. The *red lines* indicate the path of the needle (two separate needle insertions, but needle redirected 90 degrees after each insertion). The *black line* indicates the incision line.

the area around the site is injected (see Fig. 7.1). Repeat injections are made until the entire border of the field has been infiltrated. Allowing 5 to 10 minutes for the block to take effect improves the resulting anesthesia.

Nerve Block

1. Before beginning any peripheral nerve block, perform a neurologic examination of the area to be anesthetized and document the results in the medical record. If any neurologic defect is present, include a description of it in the document of informed consent for the procedure, and have the patient sign a statement agreeing that the defect was present before the administration of the anesthetic.
2. Identify the appropriate nerve(s) and anatomic sites to accomplish the block.
3. Carefully clean and prepare the skin over the injection site in a sterile fashion.
4. Draw up the anesthetic. Usually a 25- to 30-gauge needle can be used to inject the anesthetic. The amount of anesthetic used varies depending on the location of the nerve.
5. Insert the needle into the site, withdrawing the plunger slightly to test for intravascular placement of the needle and moving the needle if necessary to avoid intravascular injection. If the patient experiences paresthesia, withdraw the needle slightly because it is probably within the nerve. The goal is to inject perineurally, not into the nerve itself. If no paresthesia is noted at the expected site, confirm that there is no potential for intravascular injection and slowly inject the anesthetic. If the proper site has been identified, often as little as 1 or 2 mL will provide an excellent anesthetic block.
6. Allow 5 to 15 minutes for the block to take effect. Confirm anesthesia to pinprick before making an incision.

Common Nerve Blocks

Also see Chapter 8.

1. **Digital block of finger or toe and nail anesthesia** (Fig. 7.2): Use 4 to 6 mL of 1% to 2% lidocaine without epinephrine for each finger, and 6 to 8 mL of the same for toes. Insert the 25- to 30-gauge, 0.5-inch needle fully into the skin at the base of the finger or toe into the dorsal web space and inject 1 mL (Fig. 7.2B). Repeat this on the other side unless it is the first or fifth digit. Then insert the needle perpendicular to the bone (and parallel to the dorsum

of hand) at the base of the digit, touch the bone, and pull back a little. Inject 1 mL into the lateral aspect, then 1 mL across the dorsal and another 1 mL under the ventral surfaces in the subcutaneous space (Fig. 7.2C). Repeat this on the contralateral side of the digit. The same is done with the thumb (Fig. 7.2D). Alternatively, the needle can initially be inserted dorsally, then ventrally (Fig. 7.2E). The dorsal digital nerves in both instances lie close to bone. As the bone is touched with the needle tip, withdraw 1 or 2 mm and inject the solution.

EDITOR'S NOTE: Having learned to do a ring block for anesthesia for the penis in newborn or adult circumcisions, and noting how effective it is in that situation, many clinicians now use and consider this a ring block of the finger or toe.

If the initial injection is perpendicular to the bone and perpendicular to the dorsum of the hand at the metacarpal head instead of at the level of the digital nerve, it is called a metacarpal block. This will often decrease the discomfort prior to a digital block. Most experts inject these from the dorsal side of the hand or foot as opposed to the palmar/plantar/volar side. Injection of this block through the palmar/plantar/volar side is much more uncomfortable.

Further nail anesthesia can be achieved by a wing block as well (Fig. 7.2F). The injection site is 5 to 8 mm proximal and lateral to the corner of the nail. Direct the needle distally at a 45-degree angle, advance until bone is reached, and pull back slightly to avoid injecting the periosteum. Slowly inject 0.3 to 0.5 mL of anesthetic. This will blanch both the proximal and the lateral nail folds in a "winglike" pattern. To obtain full lateral anesthesia, a second injection of 0.3 to 0.5 mL into the entire length of the lateral nail fold should be performed in addition to the wing block to obtain anesthesia for the lateral half of the nail. A similar procedure can then be carried out on the other side of the toe if full nail anesthesia is needed.

2. **Median nerve block:** The median nerve supplies sensation to the palmar aspect of the thumb, index, and middle fingers as well as the radial half of the palm (Fig. 7.3). A nerve block may be indicated for extensive lacerations and incisions in these areas. The median nerve lies between the flexor carpi radialis and the palmaris longus (Fig. 7.4A). With slight flexion of the wrist and simultaneous flexion of the middle finger only at the metacarpophalangeal joint, the palmaris longus stands out (Fig. 7.4B). The injection should be made at the flexor crease of the wrist just radial to the palmaris longus. Use 3 to 5 mL of 1% lidocaine without epinephrine (Fig. 7.4B–C).

3. **Ulnar nerve block:** The ulnar nerve innervates the dorsal and palmar aspects on the ulnar side of the hand (fifth finger and ulnar side of the fourth finger; see Fig. 7.3). The ulnar nerve divides to dorsal and palmar branches 4 to 5 cm proximal to the wrist. Therefore the easiest way to obtain an ulnar block is to inject the ulnar nerve at the elbow where the nerve lies only 0.5 cm below the skin, between the medial epicondyle and the olecranon (Fig. 7.5A). Each branch can also be blocked separately at the wrist (Fig. 7.5B). The risk of nerve compression and postprocedure paresthesia is higher at the elbow. For all nerve blocks, it is best not to inject directly into the nerve but around it; 2 to 3 mL of 1% lidocaine should be sufficient here.

4. **Radial nerve block:** The radial nerve innervates the dorsum of the thumb, the index and middle fingers, and the radial portion of the dorsum of the hand (see Fig. 7.3). Because of multiple divisions of the radial nerve, 10 mL of anesthetic is often required to obtain good results. Inject 3 mL of solution along the lateral border of the radial artery two fingerbreadths above the wrist. Then lay a superficial ring of solution from this point extending dorsally over the border of the wrist and into the anatomic snuffbox area created by the tendons of the abductor pollicis longus and extensor pollicis brevis muscles. The nerve is in the superficial fascia just deep to the skin (Fig. 7.6).

5. **Wrist block:** Blocking the radial, ulnar and median nerves together, at the wrist, each as described above, provides complete

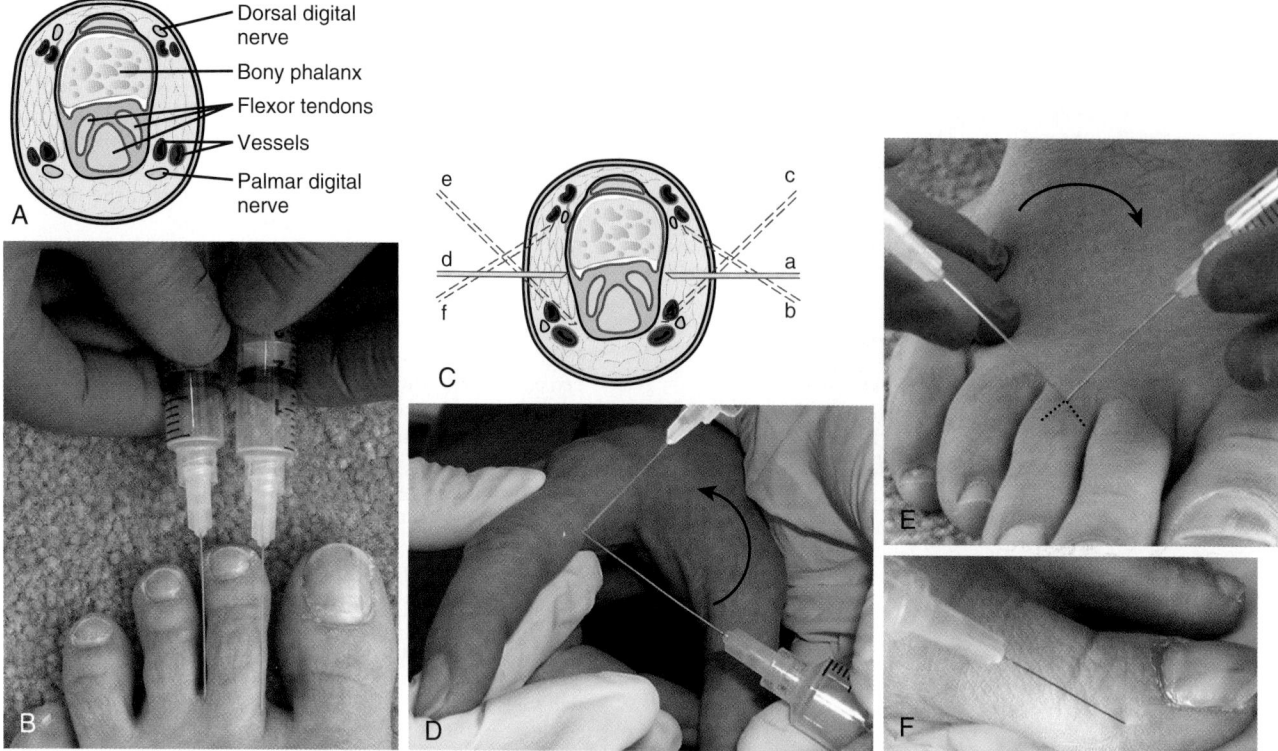

Fig. 7.2 Anatomy and injection technique for digital nerve block. (A) The four digital nerves. The bone is used as a landmark to find the proper plane of the dorsal digital nerve. (B) Site of injection in web space. When removing a toenail, an additional 1 mL of anesthetic can be placed just proximal to the nail. (C–D) Digital nerve block of the finger. The sites of the nerves are injected bilaterally. Insert the needle and, after touching bone, withdraw slightly and then inject 0.5 mL of anesthetic. (E) Digital nerve block of the toe, showing an alternative method of injection from the dorsal aspect. This is followed by a ventral injection in the same manner. (F) Nail wing block.

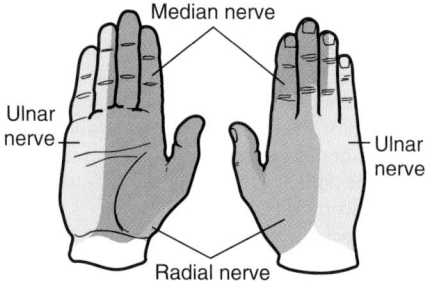

Fig. 7.3 Distribution of cutaneous sensation of the hand by the radial, ulnar, and median nerves.

anesthesia to the hand. This is commonly used for hand surgery. While this block provides reliable anesthesia, it is slow to perform, because it requires the time it takes to block all three nerves.

6. **Facial nerve blocks** (also see Chapter 8):
   - **Supraorbital and supratrochlear nerve blocks (forehead block):** The supraorbital and supratrochlear nerves innervate the forehead and anterior scalp. The nerves exit at the supraorbital ridge. To ensure that both nerves have been injected, infiltrate just above the bone beneath the entire medial two-thirds of the eyebrow (Fig. 7.7A).
   - **Infraorbital nerve block:** Palpate a notch in the infraorbital rim. The infraorbital nerve exits just beneath this small notch. Infiltrate through the skin directly over the infraorbital area, or use an intraoral technique. The latter approach requires a 1.5-inch needle, ideally 27 gauge. Introduce the needle at the gingival–buccal margin over the maxillary canine tooth. Advance it under the skin until the infraorbital foramen is reached. Use approximately 2 mL of anesthetic.

This block is used especially to repair upper lip lacerations so that the vermilion border can be approximated precisely. It can also be used for lacerations of the lower lateral nose and the lower eyelid (Fig. 7.7B–C).
   - **Mental nerve block:** The mental nerve innervates the lower half of the lip. To avoid distortion that is inevitable with local injection around the vermilion border, inject the mental nerve. In adults the nerve exits the mandible just inferior to the second mandibular bicuspid, midway between the upper and lower edges of the mandible, and 2.5 cm from the midline of the jaw. As with the infraorbital nerve injection, introduce the needle at the gingival-buccal margin inferior to the second bicuspid. Another option is a transcutaneous approach 1.5 cm posterior and lateral to the mental foramen, which can be palpated through the skin. After aspiration, inject 2 mL of anesthetic (Fig. 7.7D–E).
   - **Lip block:** The *upper lip* can also be blocked by injection of 5 to 10 mL of anesthetic along two lines in the direction of the nasal alae (Fig. 7.7F). An option for blocking the *lower lip* is to insert the needle at the midpoint of the chin, aiming toward the angle of the mouth (Fig. 7.7G).

7. **Ear block:** Because of complex innervations of the ear, it is impossible to infiltrate a solitary nerve. In addition, it is difficult to infiltrate over the cartilage because the skin here is so thin. A complete block of the auricle can be obtained by infiltrating completely around the ear with approximately 10 mL of 1% lidocaine without epinephrine (Fig. 7.8). This block will not numb the concha or the ear canal.

8. **Foot block:** Foot blocks are indicated not so much to prevent distortion but rather to limit discomfort. The sole of the foot is exquisitely sensitive to injection, and it is often subject to puncture wounds, lacerations, and foreign bodies. Nerve blocks can actually be more comfortable than direct infiltration and are

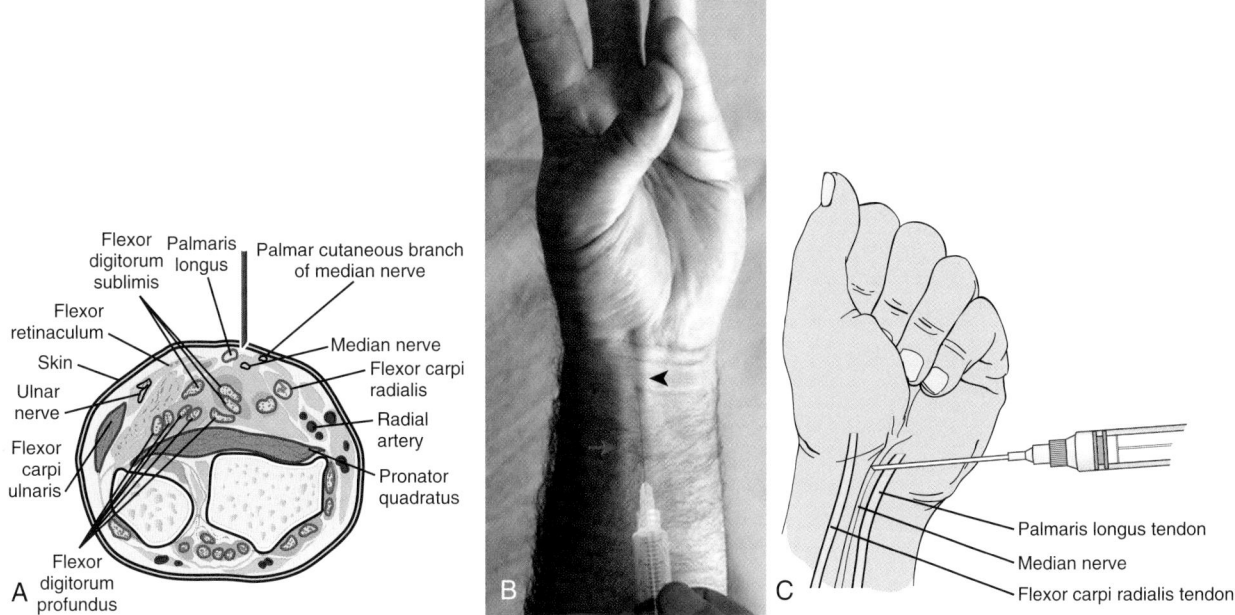

Fig. 7.4 Median nerve block. (A) Cross-sectional anatomy of the wrist (left wrist, palm up). (B) Site of injection between flexor carpi radialis tendon *(arrow)* and palmaris longus tendon *(arrowhead)*. (C) Location of injection. (A and C, Modified from Trott A. *Wounds and Lacerations: Emergency Care and Closure*. 3rd ed. St. Louis: Mosby; 1997.)

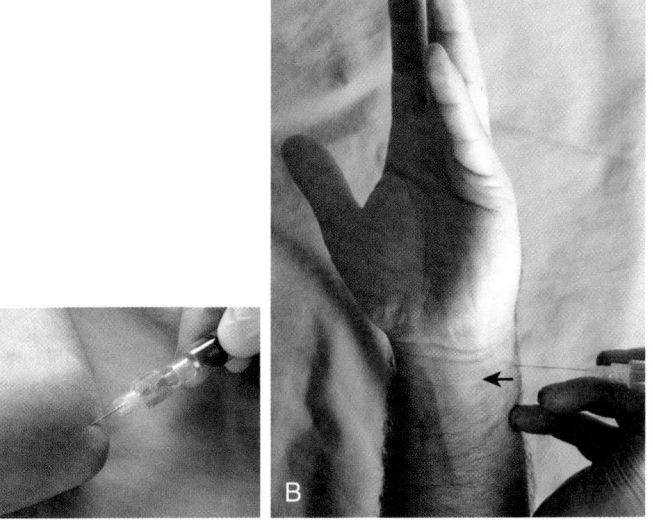

Fig. 7.5 (A) Site of an ulnar nerve block. (B) Site of injection at wrist for palmar branch deep between the flexor carpi ulnaris tendon and ulnar artery *(arrow)*, and for dorsal branch subcutaneously distal to the ulnar styloid process (needle).

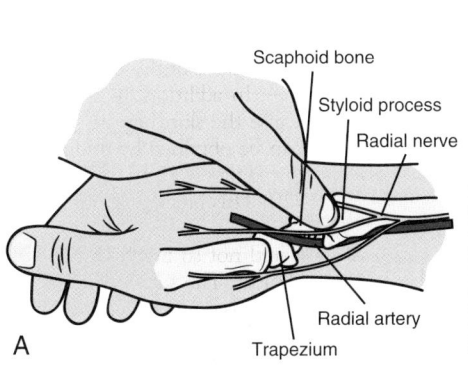
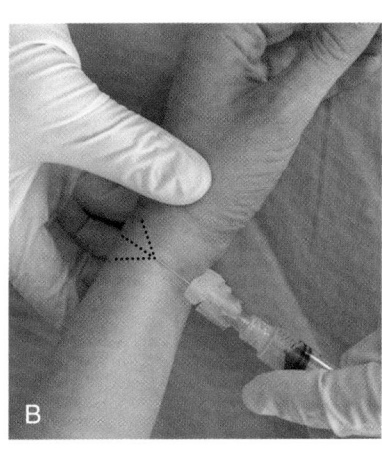

Fig. 7.6 Radial nerve block. (A) Identification of radial artery, the radial styloid, and the anatomic snuffbox. (B) Begin on the ventral surface 2 cm above the wrist, just lateral to the radial artery. Extend over the dorsum of the wrist; *dotted lines* show subcutaneous injection of anesthetic. (A, Modified from Rosen P, Chan TC, Vilke GM, Sternbach G. *Atlas of Emergency Procedures*. St. Louis: Mosby; 2001.)

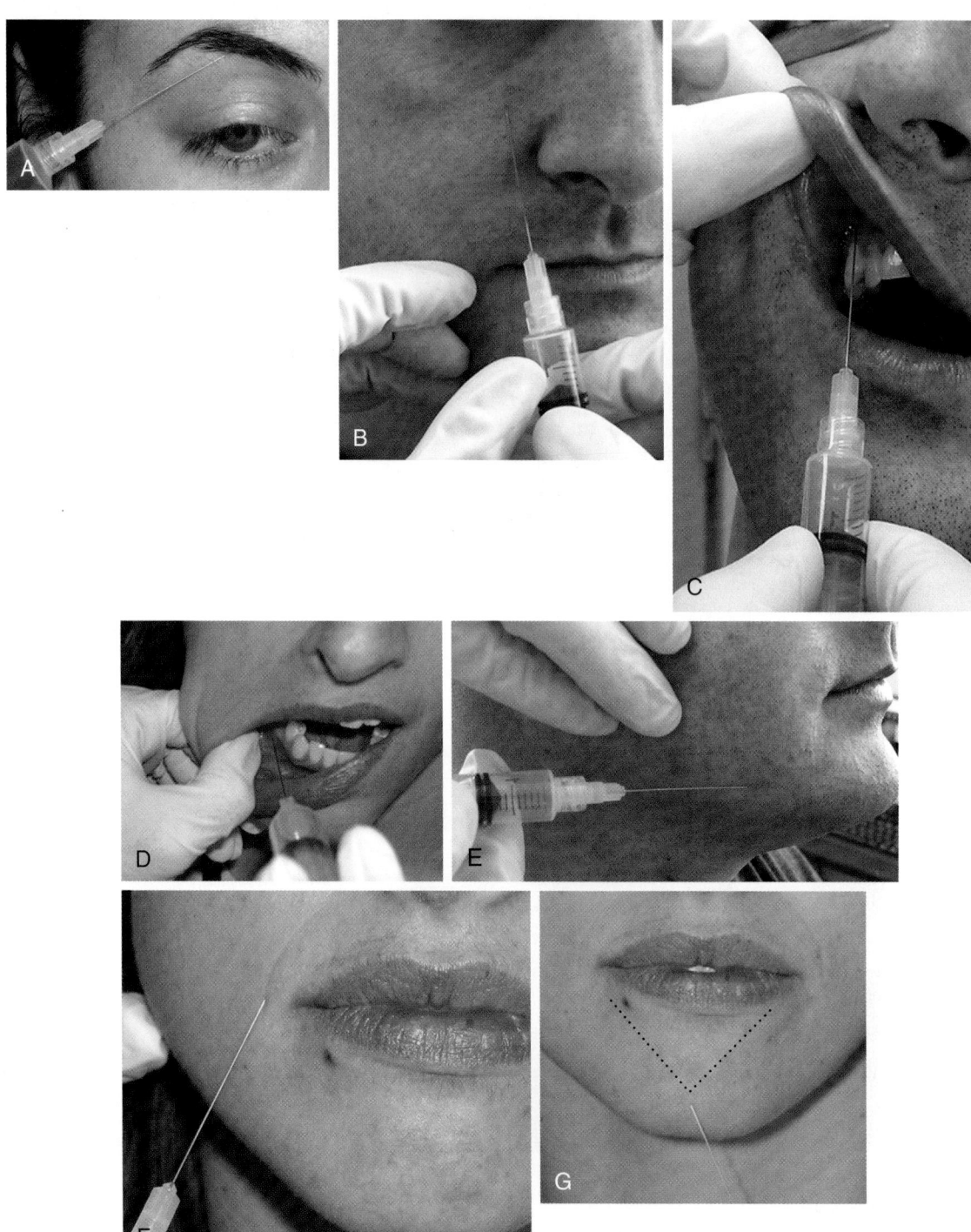

Fig. 7.7 Locations of various nerves of the face and methods to obtain a nerve block. (A) Technique for deposition of anesthetic to accomplish a supratrochlear and su-praorbital (forehead) nerve block. (B) Transcutaneous infraorbital nerve block. (C) Intraoral technique to anesthetize the infraorbital nerve. (D) Intraoral technique to anesthetize the mental nerve. (E) Transcutaneous mental nerve block. (F) Upper lip block. (G) Lower lip block; *dotted lines* show subcutaneous injection of anesthetic. Also see Chapter 8.

discussed in detail in the following. If all four nerves that provide sensation to the foot are blocked, as described below, it will provide complete anesthesia to the foot. However, this takes considerable time to block all four; instead, a single block will often provide adequate anesthesia to work on one area. If all four areas are to be blocked, in order to avoid toxicity, a maximum of 5 mL of 1% lidocaine should be used in each area (1% equals 10 mg/mL, for total of 200 mg for 20 mL).

- **Posterior ankle block:** The sural nerve (Su) runs behind the fibula and lateral malleolus to supply the lateral aspect

of the heel and foot. The tibial nerve (lateral plantar branch of tibial nerve, medial calcaneal branches of tibial nerve, medial plantar branch of tibial nerve) is found between the Achilles tendon and the medial malleolus, and its course is along the posterior tibial artery. The tibial nerve supplies the medial portion of the sole and the medial side of the foot (Fig. 7.9). To block the sural nerve, insert the needle lateral to the Achilles tendon 1 to 2 cm proximal to the level of the distal tip of the lateral malleolus. To ensure that the entire nerve is infiltrated, introduce the needle several times in a fan-shaped

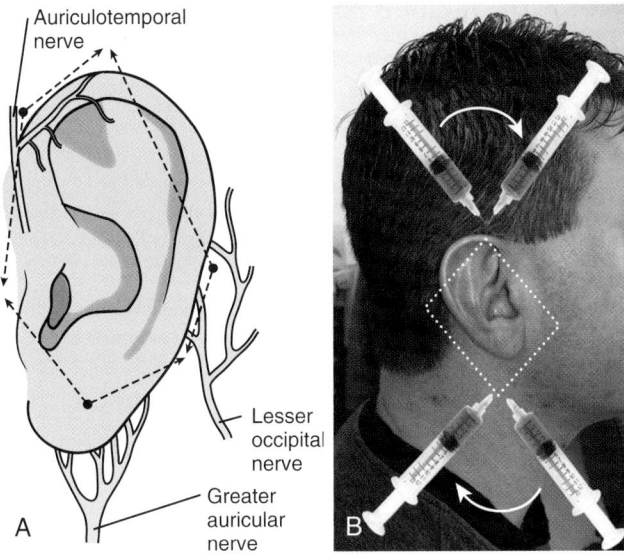

Fig. 7.8 (A) Ear block. *Dots* show insertion sites of needles; *arrows* show direction of needles injecting anesthetic. (B) Alternative technique to achieve field anesthesia of the ear; *dotted lines* show subcutaneous injection of anesthetic. (A, Modified from Robinson JK. *Atlas of Cutaneous Surgery*. Philadelphia: WB Saunders; 1996. B, Modified from Trott A. *Wounds and Lacerations: Emergency Care and Closure*. 3rd ed. St. Louis: Mosby; 1997.)

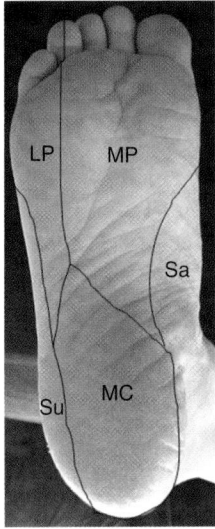

Fig. 7.9 Distribution of sensory innervation to the foot. *LP,* Lateral plantar branch of tibial nerve; *MC,* medial calcaneal branches of tibial nerve; *MP,* medial plantar branch of tibial nerve; *Sa,* saphenous nerve; *Su,* sural nerve.

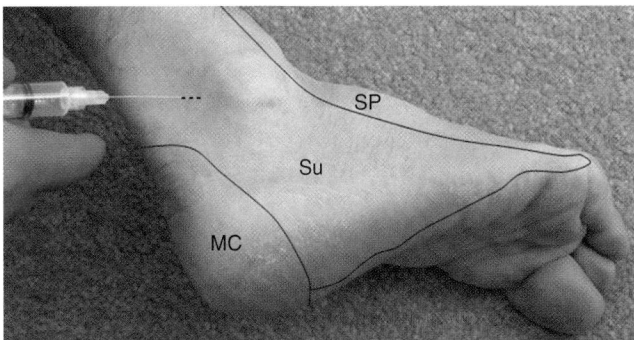

Fig. 7.10 Location of the sural nerve block; *dotted line* shows subcutaneous injection of anesthetic. *MC,* Medial calcaneal branches of tibial nerve; *SP,* superficial peroneal nerve; *Su,* sural nerve.

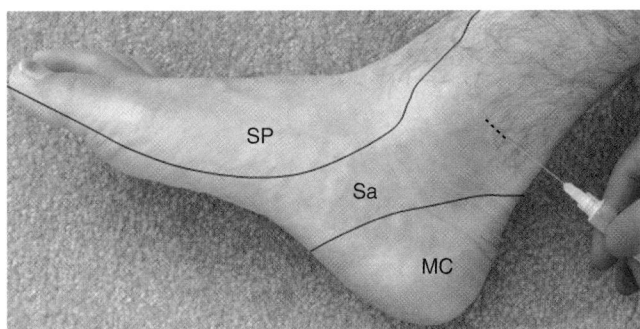

Fig. 7.11 Location of the tibial nerve block; *dotted line* shows subcutaneous injection of anesthetic. *MC,* Medial calcaneal branches of tibial nerve; *SP,* superficial peroneal nerve; *Su,* sural nerve.

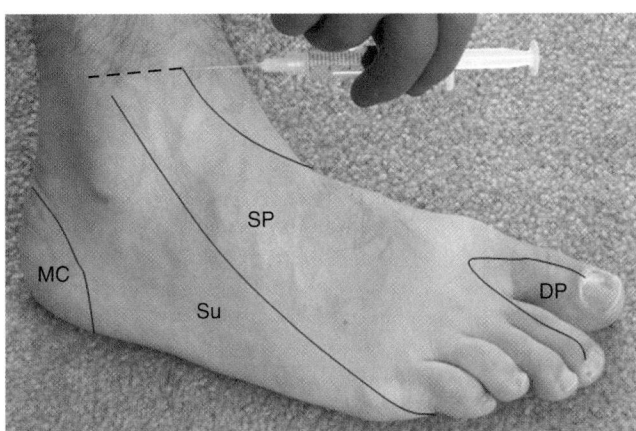

Fig. 7.12 Location of the superficial peroneal nerve block; *dotted line* shows subcutaneous injection of anesthetic. *DP,* Deep peroneal nerve; *MC,* medial calcaneal branches of tibial nerve; *SP,* superficial peroneal nerve; *Su,* sural nerve.

motion, directing it to the posterior medial aspect of the distal fibula (Fig. 7.10). Infiltrate a total of 5 mL of anesthetic.

To obtain a tibial nerve block, identify the posterior tibial pulsation. Pass the needle medial to the Achilles tendon toward the posterior tibial artery behind the medial malleolus. Infiltration is around the artery, and careful aspiration must be carried out to prevent intra-arterial injection (Fig. 7.11). Infiltrate 3 to 5 mL of anesthetic.

- **Anterior ankle block:** The superficial peroneal nerve supplies the majority of the dorsal foot. It can be blocked by inserting the needle subcutaneously at the superior and medial aspect of the medial malleolus (Fig. 7.12). Infiltrate 6 to 10 mL of anesthetic in a transverse line between distal medial and lateral malleoli.
- **Deep peroneal nerve block:** This nerve provides very little sensation to the foot (see Fig. 7.12) and so may not need to be blocked to obtain adequate anesthesia. If a total foot block

is needed, make sure total doses of local anesthetic have not reached near the toxic range. Anatomically, the largest tendon that connects to the dorsal aspect of the great toe is that of the extensor hallucis longus. Identify the anterior tibial artery by its pulse medial to this tendon at the level of the ankle joint. To block the deep peroneal nerve, infiltrate 3 to 5 mL of local anesthetic just medial to the anterior tibial artery and lateral to the extensor hallucis longus at the level of the ankle joint.

9. **Other regional nerve blocks:** Other regional nerve blocks are dealt with in other chapters: oral-facial and nose (Chapter 8), penile (Chapters 102 and 166), paracervical (Chapter 153), pudendal nerve (Chapter 154). Also see Chapters 5 and 6.

CPT/BILLING CODES

64400–64455   Introduction/injection of anesthetic agent (nerve block), diagnostic or therapeutic procedures on the somatic nerves

Be sure to document both the diagnostic and procedural code for the local anesthesia. The CPT system allows separate billing for local anesthetic if it is administered by a physician different than the surgeon, but the CPT code includes local anesthesia for the surgical procedure in most cases. A code for the instrument tray is allowed if the procedure requires more than basic instruments. If the nerve blocks are performed for diagnostic reasons, they can be billed separately.

ICD-10-CM DIAGNOSTIC CODES

ICD-10-CM codes vary depending on the diagnosis.

ADDITIONAL RESOURCES

See the patient education and patient consent forms available at www.expertconsult.com.

Acknowledgment

The editors recognize the contributions of Julie Graves Moy, MD, MPH, to this chapter in previous editions of this text.

ONLINE RESOURCES

American Society of Anesthesiologists: http://www.asahq.org/patientEducation/officebased.htm.
Society for Ambulatory Anesthesia: http://www.sambahq.org.

RECOMMENDED READING

Hadžić A, ed. *Hadzic's Peripheral Nerve Blocks and Anatomy for Ultrasound-Guided Regional Anesthesia.* 2nd ed. New York: McGraw-Hill; 2012.
Hahn MB, McQuillan PM, Sheplock GJ, eds. *Regional Anesthesia: An Atlas of Anatomy and Techniques.* St. Louis: Mosby; 1996.
Krunic AL, Wang LC, Soltani K, et al. Digital anesthesia with epinephrine: an old myth revisited. *J Am Acad Dermatol.* 2004;51:755–759.
Meier G, Buettner J. *Peripheral Regional Anesthesia: An Atlas of Anatomy and Techniques.* Stuttgart: Thieme Medical Publishers; 2007.
Mulroy MF. *Regional Anesthesia: An Illustrated Procedural Guide.* Boston: Little, Brown; 1996.
Reichman EF, ed. *Emergency Medicine Procedures.* 2nd ed. New York: McGraw-Hill; 2013.
Richert B. Basic nail surgery. *Dermatol Clin.* 2006;24:313–322.
Roberts JR, Hedges JR, eds. *Clinical Procedures in Emergency Medicine.* 6th ed. Philadelphia: Saunders; 2014.
Salam GA. Regional anesthesia for office procedures: part I. Head and neck surgeries. *Am Fam Physician.* 2004;69:585–590.
Salam GA. Regional anesthesia for office procedures: part II. Extremity and inguinal area surgeries. *Am Fam Physician.* 2004;69:896–900.
Simon RR, Brenner BE. *Anesthesia and Regional Blocks in Emergency Procedures and Techniques.* 3rd ed. Baltimore: Williams & Wilkins; 1994.
Trott A. *Wounds and Lacerations: Emergency Care and Closure.* 4th ed. St. Louis: Mosby; 2012.

CHAPTER 8

ORAL-FACIAL ANESTHESIA

Larry Skoczylas

The ability to perform site-specific oral and facial regional nerve blocks is an important adjunct to almost any medical practice. Primary care clinicians are often the first to evaluate facial pain. This pain may be due to trauma, localized swelling and infection, or even facial neuralgias and tics. Properly infiltrated local anesthetic can eliminate discomfort when closing wounds, provide pain control to a patient with a tooth abscess until he or she can be treated, or be used as a diagnostic test to see whether a neuralgia is likely due to a peripheral or a central source. If peripheral, pain should be eliminated by the anesthesia. If central, the pain may persist.

This discussion involves both intraoral and extraoral local anesthetic techniques. Therefore an understanding of regional anatomy is crucial to performing these infiltrations and nerve blocks. The sensory innervation of the face and oral cavity is primarily from the trigeminal nerve (fifth cranial nerve). This nerve is divided into ophthalmic (V_1), maxillary (V_2), and mandibular branches (V_3; Figs. 8.1 and 8.2).

The ophthalmic division is purely sensory and supplies the eyeball, conjunctiva, lacrimal gland, parts of the mucous membrane of the nose, the paranasal sinuses, and the skin of the forehead, eyes, and nose. When this nerve is paralyzed, the ocular conjunctiva becomes insensitive to touch. Sensory anesthesia of V_1 is usually obtained by local infiltration with a supraperiosteal extraoral block.

The maxillary division, like the ophthalmic division, is purely sensory. It supplies innervation to the skin of the middle portion of the face, lower eyelid, side of the nose, upper lip, maxillary teeth, and periodontal tissues. In addition, this nerve is sensory to the mucous membranes of the nasopharynx, maxillary sinus, tonsils, and hard and soft palate. This nerve can be blocked by both intraoral and extraoral injection.

The mandibular division has a large sensory as well as a small motor component. Blockage of the motor division can lead to decreased muscle function of the masseter, temporalis, pterygoid, mylohyoid, digastric, and soft palate elevators. Sensory innervation is to the temporal region and ear, cheek, lower lip and chin, parotid gland, temporomandibular joint, and mastoid area. Orally, the mandibular teeth and periosteal tissues, bone of the mandible, anterior two thirds of the tongue, and all intraoral mucosa are affected. The majority of anesthetic given for the mandibular division is intraoral, although some extraoral blocks may be indicated.

INDICATIONS

- Whenever anesthesia is desired in a fairly large anatomic area of the mouth or face
- To limit the amount of medication given
- For laceration repair or lesion removal
- Around infection sites for incision and drainage
- To limit distortion of tissues caused by local anesthetic infiltration and allow a better repair
- To anesthetize periosteum before more painful subperiosteal procedures such as tooth removal

- As a diagnostic block to determine the cause or site of pain
- To control pain

CONTRAINDICATIONS

- History of allergy or reaction to local anesthetics (very rare for amides [lidocaine, mepivacaine, bupivacaine]; more likely, allergy to bisulfite/parabens preservatives [see Chapter 5])
- Risk of hematoma (e.g., in patients with hemophilia or anticoagulant use); trauma to vascular bundles can increase risk of bleeding and hematoma (relative contraindication)
- Uncooperative patients (e.g., pediatric patients or patients with mental retardation may require sedation before local anesthetic; relative contraindication)

COMPLICATIONS

See Chapter 6.

- *Syncope:* Most common untoward reaction to anesthetic injections, often resulting from pain during the injection. A semisupine or supine position and slow injection technique are recommended. Also, do not draw up the medication in front of the patient.
- *Broken needle:* Very rare, but it is best to always leave some needle showing and not to "bury" to the hub when injecting. Also, do not redirect the needle once it has been inserted without withdrawing it to just below the mucosal or epidermal layer.
- *Hematoma:* Rare, often resulting from torn capillaries or vessels that are punctured during injection.
- *Persistent paresthesia:* Occurs after the anesthetic should have worn off. Indicates damage to the nerve from physical or local chemical trauma. Can be temporary or permanent.
- *Ischemic ulcer:* Usually resulting from vasoconstrictor use in relatively avascular tissue (e.g., subperiosteally in the hard palate). Skin is highly vascular, and ischemia is extremely rare when local anesthetic with epinephrine of a low concentration (1:100,000 or 1:200,000) is used.
- *Blanching:* Occurs at the site of injection because of pressure of anesthetic and vasoconstriction. If remote from the injection site, then it is probably due to inadvertent intravascular injection. No treatment is needed.
- *Tachycardia:* Can occur from pain of injection, but it is most likely due to intravascular injection or rapid absorption of local anesthetic with epinephrine.
- *Paralysis:* Results from inadvertent anesthesia of facial nerve (seventh cranial nerve). It is usually temporary. If longer-acting anesthetics such as bupivacaine are used and the patient cannot close the eyelid, the lid can be taped down (to avoid dryness of the eye) until the anesthetic wears off.
- *Visual disturbance:* Rare, probably due to vascular spasm or intraarterial injection. Normal vision usually returns in about 30 minutes.
- *Overdosage:* Seizures and cardiac arrhythmias.

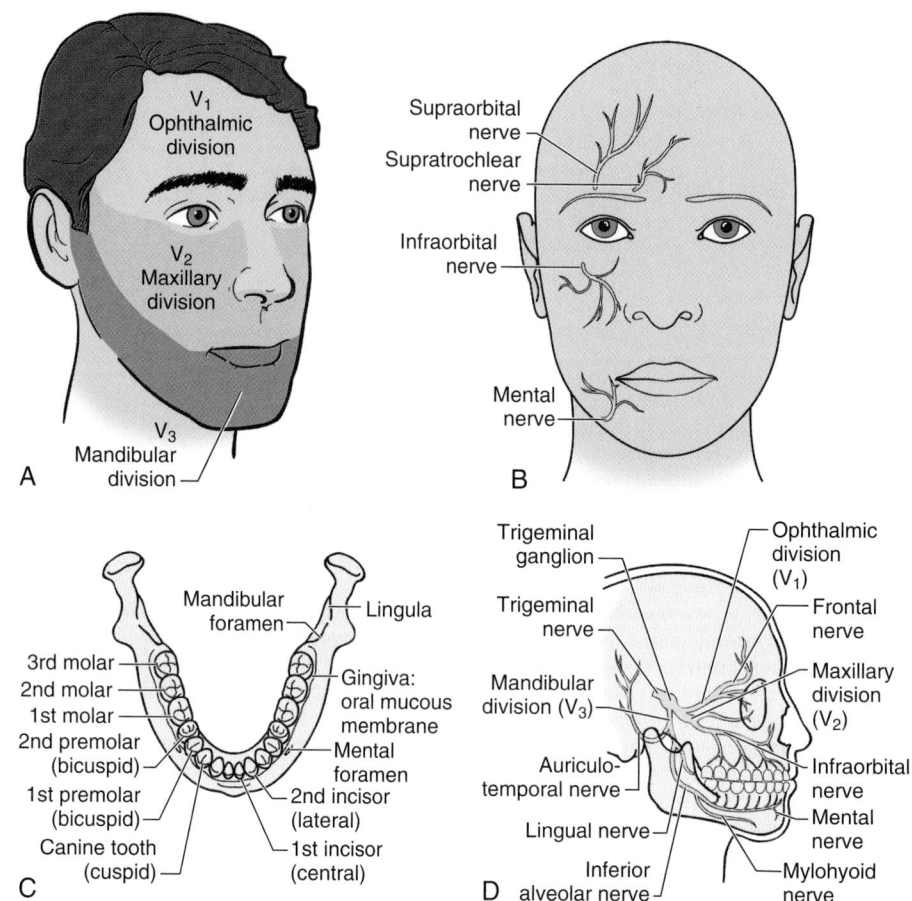

Fig. 8.1 Sensory innervation of the face and oral cavity is primarily from the trigeminal nerve. (A) The trigeminal nerve is divided into three branches: the ophthalmic branch (V_1), the maxillary branch (V_2), and the mandibular branch (V_3). (B) Sensory distribution of the terminal branches of the trigeminal nerve: the supratrochlear nerve, supraorbital nerve, infraorbital nerve, and mental nerve. (C) Anatomy of the mandibular arch and the lower teeth. (D) Distribution of the trigeminal nerve. (D, Modified from Robert RJ. *Roberts & Hedges' Clinical Procedures in Emergency Medicine.* 6th ed. Philadelphia: Elsevier; 2014.)

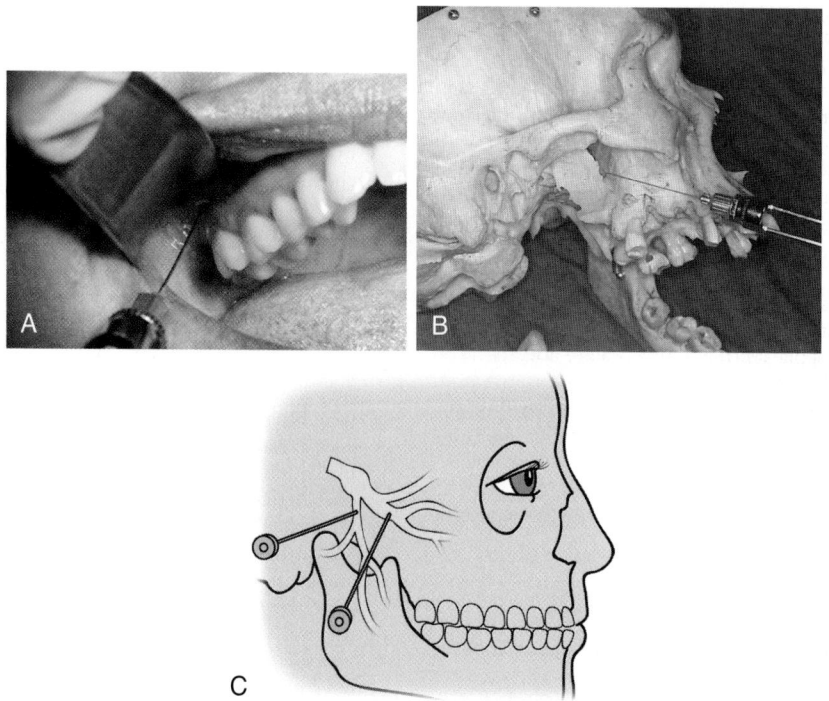

Fig. 8.2 Maxillary nerve block. (A) View with patient. (B) Angle of needle to obtain intraoral maxillary (V_2) block. (C) Location of needles for extraoral block (not described). Note that needle is not placed directly into the nerve.

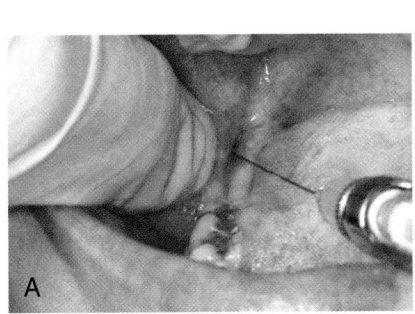
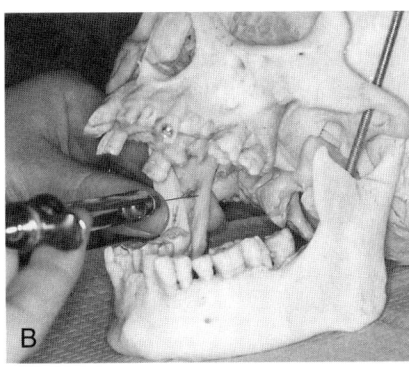

Fig. 8.3 Site of intraoral mandibular (V₃) inferior alveolar block. (A) Patient. (B) Skull.

EQUIPMENT

- 10-mL syringe (preferably with Luer-Lok hub for aspiration)
- 1- or 1.5-inch (25- to 30-gauge) needle
- Local anesthetic, such as 2% lidocaine with or without 1:100,000 epinephrine, or 0.5% bupivacaine with or without 1:200,000 epinephrine.
- Mepivacaine (pK_a 7.6; may give better anesthesia in infected tissue, which usually has an acidic environment [pK_a <7.5])
- Dental aspirating syringe (a good alternative; would need specific anesthetic carpules and needles for this system)
- Topical anesthetic that can be used on mucosal surfaces for intraoral injections (e.g., Benzocaine)

GENERAL TECHNIQUE

1. Anesthetic solution is usually deposited just above the bone around the nerve trunks in the submucosa or subcutaneous tissue, where the nerves exit from the bone itself (e.g., supraorbital, infraorbital, or mental nerves). This technique is known as a *supraperiosteal injection*. It may be approached from either an intraoral or extraoral route, depending on the nerve block desired.
2. If going through facial skin, clean the skin with alcohol. If giving local anesthetic to repair traumatic lacerations, clean thoroughly with normal saline. Tent or support the tissue and slowly infiltrate (for 30 to 60 seconds) into the area to be addressed. Identify landmarks before infiltration; they can become "ballooned" and hard to appreciate after local anesthetic is given.
3. If going through the oral mucosa, tissues are rarely scrubbed before injection. Cleaning any obvious debris in a trauma site with normal saline is indicated before closure. Lift up and tent lips or cheek. The target of the injection should be the procedure site.

INTRAORAL APPROACHES

Most patients dread intraoral injections and appreciate the use of topical anesthesia prior to injection. Make sure to dry the injection site thoroughly with gauze prior to application of topical anesthesia. A cotton-tipped applicator can then be soaked with 20% benzocaine, 5% to 10% lidocaine, 4% cocaine or equivalent and applied to the injection site. The patient can hold the applicator in place for 2 to 3 minutes to allow time for it to take effect. A topical anesthetic spray may also be helpful.

Maxillary (V₂) Intraoral Nerve Block

See Figs. 8.1 and 8.2.

Indications

- Anesthesia of the entire hemimaxilla for trauma repair or pathologic surgery
- For diagnostic blocks of the second division of the trigeminal nerve to evaluate neuralgias and tics
- To aid in anesthetizing infected sites or areas for tooth removal

Advantage

Decreases the amount of anesthetic solution used and the number of injection sites needed for maxillary anesthesia.

Technique

1. Place patient in a semisupine position. Partially open the patient's mouth and pull mandible toward side of injection (mandible to right for upper right injection).
2. Pull taut and retract cheek with index finger to gain visibility.
3. Aim for the area posterior and lateral to back of upper jaw (pterygopalatine fossa area). The area of insertion is the height of the mucobuccal fold above the distal aspect of the upper wisdom tooth area (lateral to the approximate junction of the hard and soft palate). Orient the bevel of the needle toward the bone.
4. Advance the needle slowly in the superomedial direction to a depth of about 30 mm (if necessary, measure the needle beforehand to get an idea of the length).
5. No resistance should be felt. If resistance is noted, the angle of the needle toward the midline is too great.
6. Aspirate and deposit the local anesthetic (2 to 3 mL): continue to aspirate intermittently throughout the course of injection.

Mandibular (V₃) Intraoral Inferior Alveolar Nerve Block

See Figs. 8.1 and 8.3.

Indications

- For anesthesia of entire hemimandible; can be achieved bilaterally if anesthesia of entire mandible or anterior mandible is needed
- For fracture repair, bone biopsy, removal of teeth, or pain control resulting from tooth infection or swelling

Disadvantages

- Not 100% successful (80% to 85%).
- Blind technique (by palpating landmarks). Intraoral swelling can make palpation of landmarks difficult.
- Intraoral landmarks are different in children than in adults. The lingula (a small bony bump) of the inner ramus of the mandible (where the nerve enters the jaw) is at a lower level in children.

Technique

1. Place the patient in a semisupine position and instruct him or her to keep the mouth open.
2. The target site is the lingula, a small bony bump about halfway back on the inner ramus of the mandible, where the inferior alveolar nerve enters the jaw.
3. Place the thumb of the noninjecting hand over the pterygomandibular raphe (the band of tissue in the posterior cheek

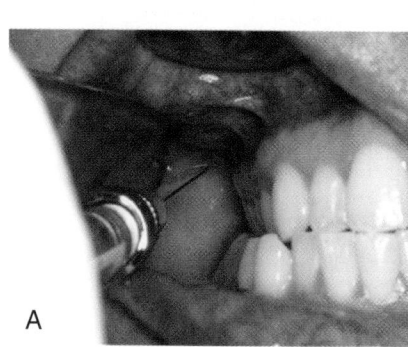
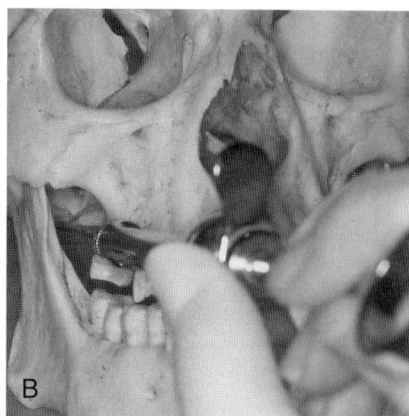

Fig. 8.4   Position of needle for closed-mouth Akinosi intraoral mandibular (V₃) block. (A) Patient. (B) Skull.

between the upper and lower wisdom teeth). Use the thumb to pull the tissue laterally until the deepest depression in the anterior border of the ramus is felt. This creates a tense area for needle penetration.

4. Gently grasp the posterior border of the mandible with the middle finger of the noninjecting hand, as high superiorly as the ear allows. The line between the thumb and finger establishes the vertical height of the target area on the inner aspect of the ramus. The lingula should always be on or just below this line (and will always be below this line in children).

5. The anteroposterior position of the nerve (the target site) is located midway between the thumb and middle finger. The line of needle insertion is an oblique angle estimated by placing the barrel of the syringe over the bicuspid teeth (or mid-mandibular body region) of the opposite side.

6. The needle is inserted to the target site until bone is gently contacted. Depth of penetration is 1 to 2 cm. Always leave part of the needle showing to identify direction. Correct length should be about one-half to three-fourths of a 1.5-inch needle.

7. If bone is contacted before half the length of the needle is inserted, the angle of penetration is usually too anterior. If no bone is contacted, the angle is too parallel to the inner aspect of the ramus of the mandible. In these instances it is best to withdraw the needle and start again.

8. Aspirate and slowly inject over 60 seconds. Continue to aspirate intermittently while injecting.

Akinosi Intraoral Closed Mouth Mandibular (V₃) Block

See Fig. 8.4.

Indications

- For mandibular V₃ anesthesia
- When the patient is unable to open his or her mouth because of pain, swelling, trismus, or infection
- For an uncooperative patient
- When conventional mandibular block has failed

Technique

1. Place the patient in the same position as that for the V₃ block.
2. Place the noninjecting finger (the thumb may be too big) at the greatest depression of the anterior ramus, as previously described for the V₃ block.
3. Identify the maxillary tuberosity—essentially a rounded area of bone just past the upper wisdom tooth area intraorally, which is the end of the maxillary bone.
4. Hold the barrel of the syringe parallel to the plane of the upper teeth, with the bevel of the needle toward the midline of the upper jaw.

5. The needle is inserted at the gingival (gum) level, about 0.5 cm superior to the tooth–gum interface.
6. Advance the needle between your finger and the maxillary tuberosity about 25 mm into the tissue, directing the needle slightly laterally to stay parallel to the plane of the upper teeth.
7. Aspirate and inject 2 to 3 mL of local anesthetic slowly over 60 seconds. Motor nerve paralysis of the masseter and lateral pterygoid muscles often occurs and can help decrease trismus. There can also be a facial nerve palsy if injection is through the sigmoid notch of the mandibular ramus and into the parotid gland. Maintaining the correct depth of penetration will help decrease this complication.

EXTRAORAL (AND SOME INTRAORAL) APPROACHES

Extraoral and Intraoral Block of Infraorbital Nerve

See Figs. 8.1 and 8.5.

Indications

- To anesthetize the upper face, lips, or nose for trauma repair or excision
- To provide local anesthetic effect when infection intraorally causes too much pain to tolerate intraoral injection
- For diagnostic nerve block for neuralgias or tics

This is an easy block to administer, whether the intraoral or extraoral approach is used. It is also frequently used because it avoids the distortion created by direct local injection when lip repair and fine approximation are needed to avoid unsightly scars.

Disadvantage

The technique is performed by blind palpation of infraorbital foramen.

Technique

1. Palpate the infraorbital foramen just below the lowest level of the infraorbital rim, on a line between the pupil and the corner of the mouth.
2. Approach the infraorbital nerve from 1 cm below the bony rim and slightly medial to the palpated foramen. It is *not* necessary to enter the infraorbital foramen. Keep pressure with one finger between the injection site and the lower eyelid while injecting to minimize lid swelling and edema.
3. Slowly deposit 1 to 3 mL of local anesthetic. Paresthesia of the upper lip is sometimes (but not always) noted when the nerve is touched by the needle before injection.
4. For an intraoral approach, use the same anatomic landmarks, and approach the nerve through the mucobuccal fold over the maxillary second bicuspid, aiming at the infraorbital foramen. A long needle will be needed.

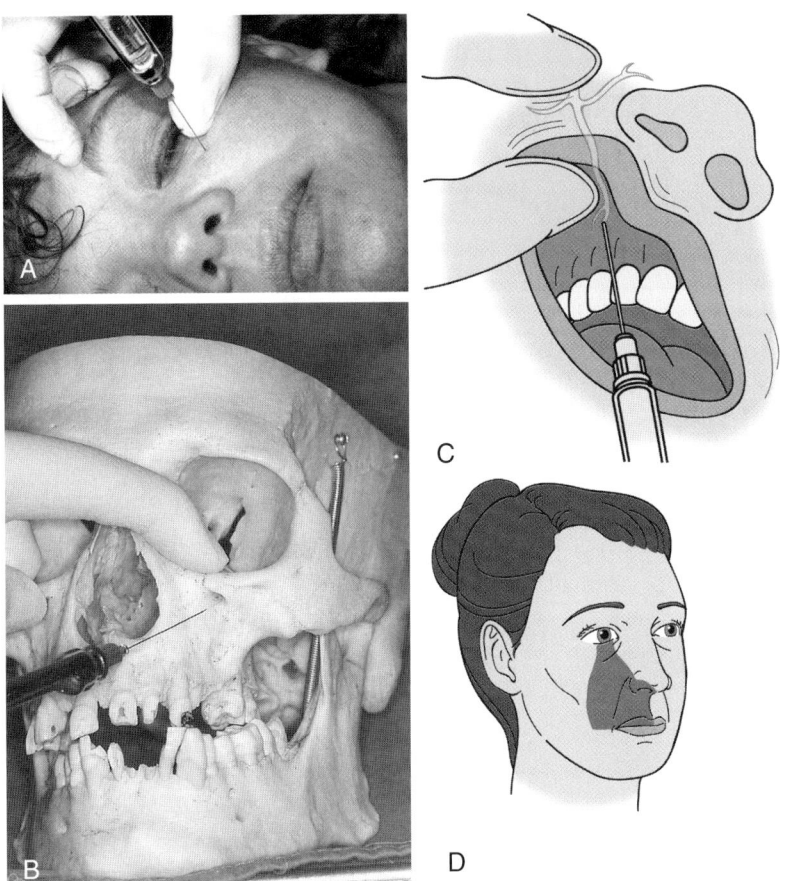

Fig. 8.5 Infraorbital nerve block. (A) View of patient receiving extraoral infraorbital nerve block. (B) Proper location for an extraoral infraorbital nerve block. (C) Intraoral infraorbital nerve block (see text). (D) Area of anesthesia obtained with infraorbital blocks. (C–D, From Rosen P, Chan TC, Vilke GM, Sternbach G, eds. *Atlas of Emergency Procedures*. St. Louis: Mosby; 2001.)

Maxillary Extraoral Block of Supraorbital and Supratrochlear Nerves

See Figs. 8.6 and 8.7.

Indications

- To anesthetize the forehead (supraorbital nerve lateral, supratrochlear nerve medial)
- Use with infraorbital block to anesthetize periorbital tissues

Technique

1. Palpate the supraorbital foramen, which lies just superior to the supraorbital notch. This lies on a vertical line with the pupil when the eye is focused forward.
2. Insert the needle just above the notch and inject 2 to 4 mL of anesthetic. You do *not* need to be injecting directly into the foramen to block the supraorbital nerve.
3. The supratrochlear nerve can be blocked by redirecting the needle to 1 cm below and medial to the supraorbital foramen, staying on the bony rim, and injecting another 2 mL.

Mandibular Extraoral and Intraoral Mental Nerve Block

See Figs. 8.1 and 8.8.

Indications

- To anesthetize the lower lip and chin area for trauma repair or excision
- To provide local anesthetic effect when infection intraorally causes too much pain to tolerate intraoral injection
- For diagnostic nerve blocks for lower face neuralgias and tics

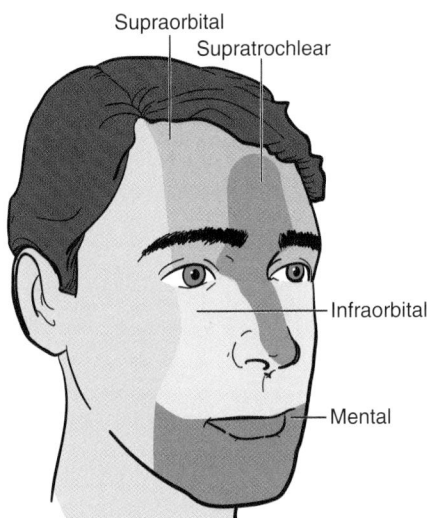

Supraorbital
Supratrochlear
Infraorbital
Mental

Fig. 8.6 Sensory distribution of the terminal branches of the trigeminal nerve.

Disadvantage

The technique is performed by blind approximation of the mental nerve position in the mandible.

Technique

1. Approach the mandible extraorally from a position below the bicuspid teeth. The mental nerve foramen is located in the middle of the lower jaw on a line exactly vertically down from the previously described infraorbital nerve foramen. (This area can also be approached vertically from the inferior border of the mandible.)

Fig. 8.7 (A) Supraorbital nerve block. (B) Supratrochlear nerve block.

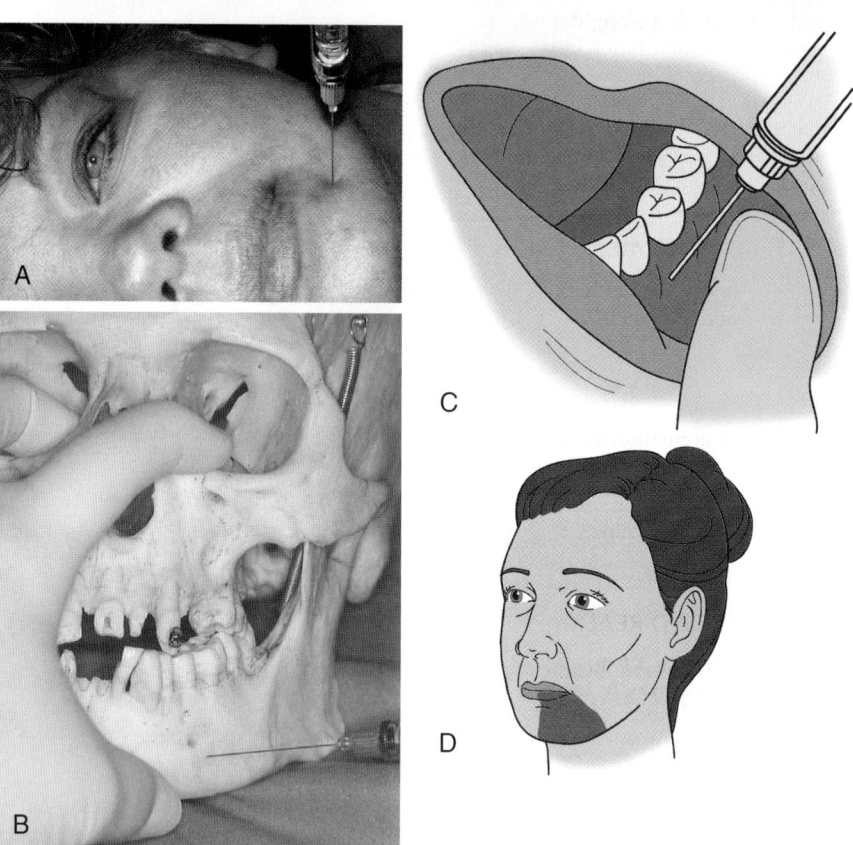

Fig. 8.8 Mental nerve block. (A) View of patient receiving extraoral mental nerve block. (B) Site of extraoral mental nerve block. (C) Intraoral approach. (D) Area of anesthesia obtained with mental nerve block. (C–D, From Rosen P, Chan TC, Vilke GM, Sternbach G, eds. *Atlas of Emergency Procedures.* St. Louis: Mosby; 2001.)

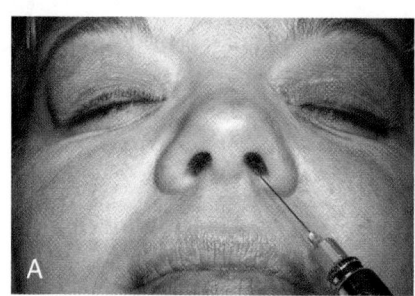
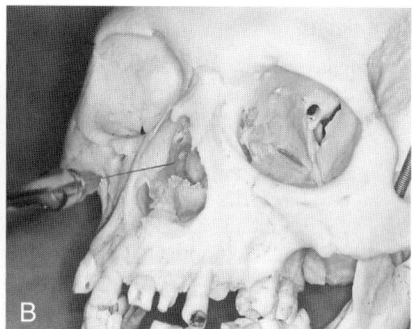

Fig. 8.9 (A) View of patient receiving nasal septal anesthesia. (B) Proper location for administering nasal septal anesthesia.

2. Enter the skin with the needle perpendicular to the bone. Advance the needle until bone is touched, then back off 2 to 3 mm. It is *not* necessary to enter the mental foramen.
3. Deposit 1 to 3 mL of local anesthetic. Paresthesia of the lower lip is sometimes (but not always) noted when the nerve is touched by the needle.
4. The mental nerve can also be approached intraorally. The needle is inserted in front of the teeth at the junction of the gum and lip mucosa at the level of the premolar/molar teeth (fifth tooth from the midline). Direct the needle inferiorly just above bone for approximately 1 cm and inject 2 to 3 mL of anesthetic.

Nose: Skin and Nasal Mucosa

See Fig. 8.9.

Indications

- For paranasal biopsy, or repair of bony or soft tissue nasal trauma (anesthesia for elective rhinoplasty is quite specific and will not be covered)
- Often used in conjunction with extraoral infraorbital nerve block for nasal procedures

Disadvantage

It can be painful to administer in the awake patient.

Technique

1. Apply topical spray anesthetic to each nostril.
2. Cotton-tipped applicators with 20% benzocaine or 4% cocaine solution are then used to paint the nasal mucosa. Leave in place for 5 minutes. Cocaine may be contraindicated in patients with cardiac disease.
3. Perform bilateral infraorbital nerve blocks, extraoral technique (see earlier).
4. Infiltrate the skin along the base of the nares, and continue as subcutaneous infiltration up the nasal-facial crease.
5. Inject the septal mucosa with local anesthetic containing vasoconstrictor to help decrease bleeding, especially in nasal or septal fractures. Use 1.5-inch needle and inject from posterior to anterior. Now inject subperiosteally between the nasal bones and the tissue, and along the lateral nasal region.

CPT/BILLING CODES

64400   Injection anesthetic agent; trigeminal nerve any division or branch

SUPPLIERS

(See contact information available at www.expertconsult.com.)

Benzocaine spray
HurriCaine (20% benzocaine), Beutlich Inc.
Cetacaine (15% benzocaine, 2% butamben, 2% tetracaine), Cetylite Industries

RECOMMENDED READING

Amsterdam JT, Kilgore KP. Regional anesthesia of the head and neck. In: Roberts JR, Custalow CB, Thomsen TW, eds. *Roberts and Hedges Clinical Procedures in Emergency Medicine.* 6th ed. Philadelphia: Elsevier; 2014:541–553.
Bramhall J. Regional anesthesia for aesthetic surgery. In: Kaminer MS, Dover JS, Arndt KA, eds. *Atlas of Cosmetic Surgery.* Philadelphia: WB Saunders; 2002:73–94.
Budac S, Suresh S. Emergent facial lacerations repair in children. *Anesth Analg.* 2006;102:1091–1092.
Eaton JS, Grekin RC. Regional anesthesia of the face. *Dermatol Surg.* 2001;27:1006–1009.
Edlich EF, Rodeheaver GT, Thacker JG. Local and regional anesthesia for wound repair. In: Tintinalli JE, Krome RL, Ruiz E, eds. *Emergency Medicine: A Comprehensive Study Guide.* 8th ed. New York: McGraw-Hill; 2011.
Hahn MB. Distributions of the trigeminal nerve. In: Hahn MB, McQuillan PM, Sheplock GJ, eds. *Regional Anesthesia: An Atlas of Anatomy and Techniques.* St. Louis: Mosby; 1996:45–52.
Hanke CW. The tumescent facial block. *Dermatol Surg.* 2001;27:1003–1005.
Higgenbotham E, Vissers RJ. Local and regional anesthesia. In: Tintinalli JE, Krome RL, eds. *Emergency Medicine: A Comprehensive Study Guide.* 8th ed. New York: McGraw-Hill; 2011.
Kretzschmar JL, Peters JE. Nerve blocks for regional anesthesia of the face. *Am Fam Physician.* 1997;55:1701–1704.
Malamed SF. *Handbook of Local Anesthesia.* 6th ed. St. Louis: Mosby; 2013.
Malamed SF. Nerve injury caused by mandibular block analgesia. *Int J Oral Maxillofac Surg.* 2006;35:876–877.
Mulroy MF. Peripheral nerve blockade. In: Barash PG, Cullen BF, Stoelting RK, eds. *Clinical Anesthesia.* 7th ed. Philadelphia: Lippincott Williams & Wilkins; 2013.
Pascal J, Charier D, Perret D, et al. Peripheral blocks of trigeminal nerve for facial soft-tissue surgery. *Eur J Anaesthesiol.* 2005;22:480–482.
Reichman EF. Dental anesthesia and analgesia. In: Reichman EF, ed. *Emergency Medicine Procedures.* 2nd ed. New York: McGraw-Hill; 2013:1131–1143.
Roberts GJ, Rosenbaum NL. *Color Atlas of Dental Anesthesia and Sedation.* Alesbury, UK: Hazell Books; 1991.
Salam GA. Regional anesthesia for office procedures. *Am Fam Physician.* 2004;69:585–590.
Schimek F, Fahle M. Techniques of facial nerve block. *Br J Ophthalmol.* 1995;79:166–173.
Simpson S. Regional nerve blocks. *Aust Fam Physician.* 2001;30:565–568.
Smith DW, Peterson MR, DeBerard SC. Regional anesthesia. *J Postgrad Med.* 1999;106:69–73. 77–78.
Soriano TT, Lask GP, Dinehart SM. Anesthesia and analgesia. In: Robinson JK, Hanke DW, Sengelmann RD, Siegel DM, eds. *Surgery of the Skin: Procedural Dermatology.* Philadelphia: Mosby; 2005:39–58.

CHAPTER 9

BIER BLOCK

Peter W. Grigg

Intravenous (IV) regional anesthesia, also known as a Bier block, is a useful method of providing operative anesthesia to wide areas of the distal portion of an extremity. When executed with proper technique, the Bier block is a safe alternative to local or hematoma infiltration, and provides anesthesia superior to these other methods. At the same time, it has the advantage of being technically simpler to perform than other regional alternatives (e.g., axillary or brachial plexus block).

INDICATIONS

Although the technique of IV regional anesthesia has been used on the lower extremity, it is most often used in applications involving the upper extremity. Bier blocks are useful for (1) surgery of the wrist, hand, and fingers (e.g., carpal tunnel release, foreign body removal, laceration repair, incision and drainage, and tendon release and repair); and (2) reduction of fractures or dislocation below the elbow. Bier blocks are also used in the treatment of complex regional pain syndromes.

CONTRAINDICATIONS

Documented sensitivity to local anesthesia is an absolute contraindication. Relative contraindications include the following:
- Injuries to the proximal extremity that would be adversely affected by application of a tourniquet (e.g., crush injury)
- Conditions predisposing to arterial thrombosis (e.g., Raynaud phenomenon, homozygous sickle cell disease)
- Fractures about and above the elbow
- Infection at or near the intended IV cannula insertion site
- Preexisting cardiac disorders affected by IV local anesthetic (e.g., untreated third-degree heart block)
- Difficulty in maintaining arterial occlusion with a tourniquet (e.g., inadequate cuff size in a massively obese patient)

EQUIPMENT

- Standard monitoring equipment (cardiac monitor, pulse oximeter, continuous blood pressure monitor)
- Standard Advanced Cardiac Life Support (ACLS) airway supplies and drugs, as well as drugs used for sedation (e.g., midazolam [Versed], fentanyl, and propofol [Diprivan])
- Double-cuff automatic pneumatic tourniquet that can individually or simultaneously inflate or deflate both cuffs to preset pressures (as an alternative, ordinary blood pressure cuffs can be used if the dimensions of the arm can accommodate two appropriately sized cuffs between the axilla and the elbow without overlap)
- Lidocaine (without epinephrine), 1 mL/kg of 0.5% solution for upper extremity blocks, 2 mL/kg of the 0.25% solution for lower extremity blocks
- Two IV catheters, a 22-gauge line for the operative side and a 20-gauge line for the arm on the nonoperative side, which can be used for sedation and administration of emergency drugs if needed

- Sterile skin preparation solution (e.g., povidone-iodine)
- Tape
- Elastic bandage of sufficient size to wrap the entire extremity distal to the tourniquet

Although the risk of serious adverse reaction is very small when the procedure is followed correctly, it should be conducted only in facilities capable of managing serious local anesthetic toxicities (see the Complications section). No reported fatalities directly attributable to use of the Bier block with lidocaine have been reported.

American Society of Anesthesiologists standards require an anesthesiologist (or a similarly qualified practitioner other than the surgeon) to manage the patient during a Bier block. This person should not be the operating surgeon because the surgeon is busy doing the procedure and cannot effectively manage complications of the local anesthetic.

PREPROCEDURE PATIENT PREPARATION

Advise the patient that 95% of patients experience good or complete anesthesia with a Bier block; the remainder require additional analgesics or sedatives. Explain the risks, alternatives, and potential complications to the patient and answer any questions. Note that anesthesia will resolve in 30 minutes or less after tourniquet release. See patient education and patient consent forms available online.

TECHNIQUE

1. Perform a focused history and physical examination to ensure the patient is a candidate for a Bier block. Note NPO status, medical problems, medication allergies, and Mallampati airway classification (see Chapter 1).
2. Attach the cardiac monitor and pulse oximeter. Place the blood pressure cuff on the nonoperative side and note the patient's blood pressure.
3. Place two IV lines—one on the operative side, and one on the nonoperative side. On the operative side, attach the syringe with lidocaine and tape in place. The IV line on the operative side should be as close to the pathologic site as possible.
4. An ACLS-trained practitioner should administer the sedation and monitor the patient as previously noted. An IV tranquilizer such as midazolam (Versed) 2 to 4 mg IV often is given for comfort, although sedation is not required.
5. Test the pneumatic tourniquet or blood pressure cuffs for accuracy and maintenance of pressure and then place them on the proximal portion of the extremity.
6. Have an assistant elevate the extremity above the heart while you wrap the elastic bandage around it, wrapping from distal to proximal (from fingers or toes up to the distal cuff). This will exsanguinate the extremity. Be careful not to dislodge the needle or catheter.
7. Rapidly inflate the proximal cuff to 50 to 100 mm Hg above the systolic blood pressure for upper extremity blocks and twice

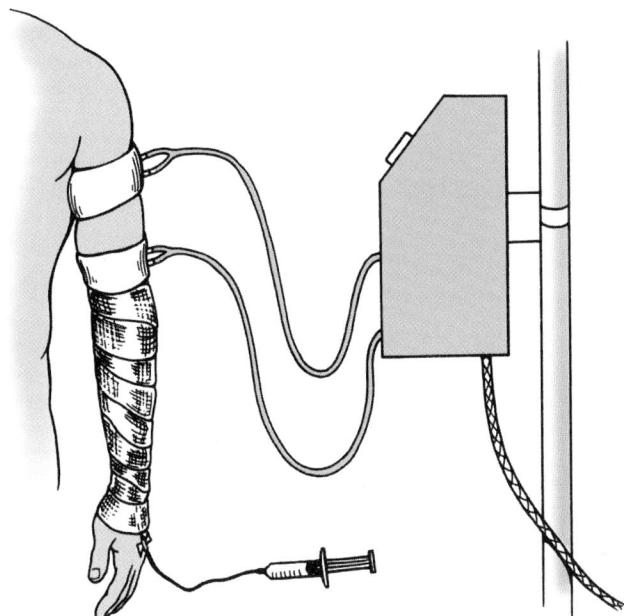

Fig. 9.1 Bier block procedure, before removal of elastic bandage and injection of lidocaine, showing inflation of proximal cuff.

the systolic blood pressure for lower extremity blocks. Assign an assistant to be responsible for continuously monitoring the maintenance of cuff pressure throughout the remainder of the procedure (Fig. 9.1).

8. Lower the extremity, remove the elastic bandage, and check the distal pulses. If no pulse is palpable and the extremity is blanched, inject the appropriate dose of lidocaine.

9. After approximately 10 to 15 minutes, check the adequacy of anesthesia by gently manipulating the operative site. Additional time may be required to achieve full effect.

10. After the initial 10 to 15 minutes, inflate the distal cuff to the same pressure as the proximal cuff, and then deflate the proximal cuff. This use of two cuffs reduces the pain associated with the occlusive tourniquet by allowing infusion of the anesthetic under the proximal cuff before it is inflated.

11. When anesthesia is deemed adequate, the IV line on the operative side may be removed. The limb is then prepared, and the operation may proceed up to a maximum inflation time of 2 hours. Periodically monitor the blood pressure on the contralateral side to ensure proper tourniquet pressure. The tourniquet may remain inflated during the process of taking intraoperative plain films.

12. At the completion of the procedure, but no sooner than 30 minutes after lidocaine injection (to permit diffusion of some of the lidocaine out of the vascular system), deflate and remove the cuffs. Some clinicians recommend cycles of deflation and inflation, but this has no advantage in lowering systemic plasma lidocaine levels.

13. Observe the patient for 10 to 15 minutes for signs of toxicity or adverse reaction.

COMPLICATIONS

See Chapter 6.

* Complications arise from the lidocaine and the equipment used to produce the block. Minor adverse reactions to the lidocaine (e.g., dizziness, tinnitus, bradycardia) occur in fewer than 2% of patients after cuff deflation.
* Allergic reactions are very rare. Anaphylaxis is treated with oxygen therapy, IV fluid, epinephrine, steroids, and antihistamines (see Chapter 212).

* Seizures and cardiovascular collapse occur almost exclusively when the lidocaine is injected with the cuffs deflated—because of operator error or equipment malfunction—and are rare. Seizures may be self-limited and treated with airway management, IV benzodiazepines, barbiturates, or propofol.
* Dysrhythmias are treated according to ACLS algorithms.
* Hypotension may require IV fluids or vasopressors.
* Ecchymosis and subcutaneous hemorrhage can occur underneath the cuff site and can be minimized by placing padding (web roll) on the arm.
* Engorgement of the extremity can occur when arterial inflow of blood continues but venous drainage is restricted by the tourniquet. A fully functional tourniquet and checking for an absent pulse minimize this problem.
* Hematoma formation can occur at sites of unsuccessful IV attempts. Apply pressure for 3 minutes before applying elastic bandage. Apply pressure over the IV site when the functioning catheter is removed.

CPT/BILLING CODES

Anesthesia depends on the procedure performed.

00400 Anesthesia for procedures on integumentary system, upper and lower arm or hand

01810 Anesthesia for all procedures on nerves, muscles, tendons, fascia, and bursae of lower arm, wrist, and hand

01820 Anesthesia for all closed procedures on radius, ulna, wrist, and hand

01830 Anesthesia for open or surgical arthroscopic/endoscopic procedures on distal radius, distal ulna, wrist, or hand

SUPPLIERS

(See contact information available at www.expertconsult.com.)

Double-cuff pneumatic tourniquet
DRE Medical
VBM Medical, Inc.
Zimmer, Inc.

Acknowledgment

The editors recognize the contributions of Robert Williams, MD, MPH, to this chapter in a previous edition of this text.

ONLINE RESOURCES

LipidRescue.org
The New York School of Regional Anesthesia. *World Anesthesia Conference*; 2017. http://www.nysora.com.

RECOMMENDED READING

American Society of Anesthesiologists Task Force on Sedation and Analgesia by Non-Anesthesiologists. Practice guidelines. *Anesthesiology*. 2002;96:1004–1017.
Bannister M. Bier's block. *Anaesthesia*. 1997;52:713.
Blasier RD, White R. Intravenous regional anesthesia for management of children's extremity fractures in the emergency department. *Pediatr Emerg Care*. 1996;12:404.
Bolte RG, Stevens PM, Scott SM, Schunk JE. Mini-dose Bier block intravenous regional anesthesia in the emergency department treatment of upper-extremity injuries. *J Pediatr Orthop*. 1994;14:534.
Brown EM, McGriff JT, Malinowski RW. Intravenous regional anesthesia (Bier block): Review of 20 years' experience. *Can J Anaesth*. 1989; 36:307.

Farrell RG, Swanson SL, Walter JR. Safe and effective IV regional anesthesia for use in the emergency department. *Ann Emerg Med.* 1985;14:288.

Freeman C. Intravenous regional anesthesia. In: Reichman EF, ed. *Emergency Medicine Procedures.* 2nd ed. New York: McGraw-Hill; 2013.

Henderson CL, Warriner CB, McEwen JA, Merrick PM. A North American survey of intravenous regional anesthesia. *Anesth Analg.* 1997;85:858–863.

Lowen R, Taylor J. Bier's block: the experience of Australian emergency departments. *Med J Aust.* 1994;160:108.

Moore N, Kirton C, Bane J. Lipid emulsion to treat overdose of local anesthetic. *Anaethesia.* 2006;61:107–109.

Roberts JR, Carney SK. In: Roberts JR, Hedges JR, eds. *Clinical Procedures in Emergency Medicine.* 6th ed. Philadelphia: WB Saunders; 2014.

Salo M, Kanto J, Jalonen J, Laurikainen E. Plasma lidocaine concentrations after different methods of releasing the tourniquet during intravenous regional anaesthesia. *Ann Clin Res.* 1979;11:164.

Soltesz EG, van Pelt F, Byrne JG. Emergent cardiopulmonary bypass for bupivacaine cardiotoxicity. *J Cardiothorac Vasc Anesth.* 2003;17:357.

Tetzlaff JE. The pharmacology of local anesthetics. *Anesthesiol Clin North Am.* 2000;18:217.

CHAPTER 10

EPIDURAL ANESTHESIA AND ANALGESIA

Peter W. Grigg

Epidural anesthesia (i.e., complete relief of pain and significant motor block) and analgesia (i.e., the relief of pain only, with as little motor block as possible) can be accomplished by injecting opiates, local anesthetics, or a combination of these medications into the epidural space. An epidural is an extremely versatile procedure; it may be used to enhance the birthing experience or to provide anesthesia or analgesia during or after surgical procedures. For prolonged analgesia, a catheter may be left in the epidural space for several days to allow additional medication to be injected by repeated bolus, patient-controlled epidural anesthesia (PCEA) pump, or controlled continuous infusion.

From an anesthetic perspective, the *level* of anesthesia refers to an anatomic level or segment of effect (e.g., up to the level of the umbilicus [T10] or the level of the xiphoid [T8]), whereas *depth* refers to the amount of sensation or motor activity remaining. Depth of blockade is determined by choice of drugs and concentrations. Segmental level of anesthesia or analgesia can be controlled by the level of the injection, the volume of solution injected, as well as other factors (see the note after the "Technique" section), and the depth can be increased or decreased as the clinical situation dictates. Such control is one of the advantages of epidural anesthesia over other forms of regional anesthesia.

Clinicians administering epidural anesthesia or analgesia must have a good understanding of not only the relevant anatomy and needle placement techniques, but the pharmacology and physiology involved. The clinician must be familiar and experienced with the diagnosis and management of possible complications. A review of and familiarity with the updated American Society of Anesthesiologists (ASA) Practice Guidelines for Obstetric Anesthesia (2016) and the ASA Difficult Airway Algorithm are highly recommended for medical professionals providing epidural services to obstetric patients. Epidural anesthesia or analgesia should be performed only in a hospital, surgery center, or facility where equipment and adequately trained personnel are available to manage any and all possible complications. The equipment available should be comparable with that of a hospital operating room.

EDITOR'S NOTE: Although there is general agreement that epidural anesthesia is safe and is the most effective method of pain relief in labor, there has been some controversy regarding possible side effects. Meta-analyses attempting to determine whether epidurals increase the risk for cesarean section are conflicting, but the majority of current evidence suggests they do not. While there seemed to be consensus among studies that epidurals prolonged labor—the first stage of labor by 12 minutes and the second stage of labor by 42 minutes—a recent randomized trial (Shen, 2017) found otherwise. There has also been concern that epidurals increase the need for assisted delivery (Cochrane, 2011) and the likelihood of maternal fever. (The cause of epidural-associated maternal fever is unknown.) Fetal heart rate changes are also common with epidurals during labor. Although the cause of heart rate changes is not known, one theory suggests reduced uterine blood flow from maternal hypotension as the mechanism. Cochrane reviews have found intravenous (IV) fluid preloading (volume expansion) may help reduce the risk of maternal hypotension when traditional high-dose regional anesthetics are used. However, benefit of IV fluid preloading may be reduced if low-dose epidural and combined spinal epidurals are used. Fluid preloading must be performed cautiously or slowly in patients with pregnancy-induced hypertension.

ANATOMIC CONSIDERATIONS

The spinal canal contains the spinal cord, its coverings (i.e., pia mater, arachnoid mater, dura mater), and cerebrospinal fluid. The pia mater is closely attached or adherent to the spinal cord. The dura mater is the separate, toughest, and outermost covering of the spinal cord. The arachnoid membrane is a delicate membrane interposed between the dura mater and the pia mater. It is separated from the pia mater by the subarachnoid space, which contains the cerebrospinal fluid.

The epidural space is a potential space, external to the dura mater and located between the dura mater and the ligamentum flavum (connective tissue covering the vertebrae; Fig. 10.1). Although the epidural space is a potential space, it is filled with spongy connective tissue, fat, and blood vessels. This allows for solutions injected into the space to flow freely in all directions and to bathe the nerve roots as they exit the spinal canal.

PHYSIOLOGIC CONSIDERATIONS

When an epidural is used in labor and delivery, it is important to remember that visceral pain from uterine contractions is partly conducted through the sympathetic nervous system. Impulses travel through the inferior, middle, and superior hypogastric plexuses to the sympathetic chain. This chain then connects to the spinal cord through the 10th, 11th, and 12th thoracic nerves. Any effective analgesic solution must spread cephalad enough to affect these levels.

INDICATIONS

- As an alternative to general or spinal anesthesia for selected surgical procedures
- Requested by patient or suggested by clinician (e.g., to avoid maternal fatigue) for labor and delivery
- Postoperative analgesia

NOTE: Epidural analgesia should not be withheld on the basis of achieving an arbitrary cervical dilation. Consider early placement in patients at high risk (obstetric [e.g., twins, preeclampsia], or maternal [e.g., morbid obesity, difficult airway]) of or with general anesthesia to possibly reduce the need for general anesthesia if an emergent procedure becomes necessary.

NOTE: Continuous epidural analgesia is being used more and more for obstetrics and postoperative analgesia; however, spinal anesthesia is still the most commonly used regional technique for surgical procedures. If labor is anticipated to last beyond a single spinal opioid

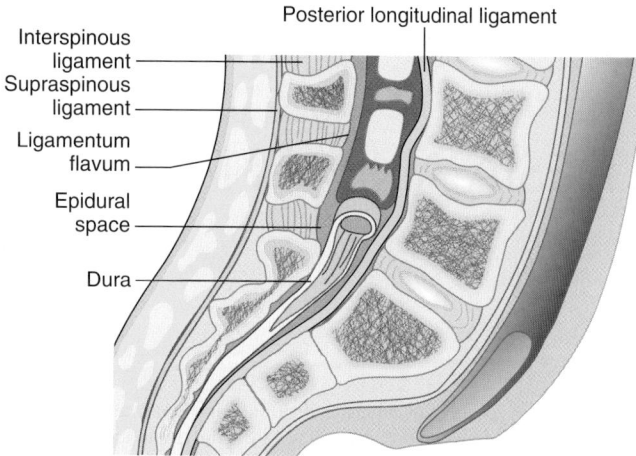

Fig. 10.1   Anatomy of the vertebral column and its contents in the lower lumbar and upper sacral regions.

Labels (clockwise):
Posterior longitudinal ligament
Interspinous ligament
Supraspinous ligament
Ligamentum flavum
Epidural space
Dura

injection, consider placement of an epidural catheter for continuous epidural analgesia. In addition, use of PCEA results in less narcotics usage than continuous epidural analgesia.

CONTRAINDICATIONS

- Patient declines
- Localized infection at the puncture site
- Severe, uncorrected hypovolemia
- Blood dyscrasias; coagulopathy; prolonged international normalized ratio, prothrombin time, or activated partial thromboplastin time; thrombocytopenia
- Anticoagulant therapy (e.g., heparin, warfarin, enoxaparin, clopidogrel, direct thrombin inhibitor [dabigatran], factor Xa inhibitor [fondaparinux, rivaroxaban, apixaban])
- Allergy to specific epidural agents
- Spinal abnormalities, including scoliosis and other structural abnormalities
- Active systemic infection
- Lack of proper resuscitative equipment, skills, or trained staff
- Preexisting neurologic diseases (amyotrophic lateral sclerosis, other degenerative nerve diseases, polio)
- Preoperative headache (relative)
- Aortic stenosis
- Anemia

EQUIPMENT

- Disposable sterile gloves
- Equipment for the clinician to observe universal blood and body fluid precautions
- Disposable epidural tray containing the following:
  1. Appropriate prep solutions, swabs, and sterile 4 × 4 gauze pads
  2. Disposable drapes
  3. Epidural catheter, threading assist guide, and syringe adapter attachment
  4. Syringes
     a. Plastic Luer-Lok (3 mL) for local infiltration of lidocaine 1%
     b. Plastic syringe (20 mL) for administration of epidural agent
     c. Glass Luer-Lok procedural syringe (5 mL) filled with saline for loss-of-resistance technique (Fig. 10.2)
  5. Needles
     a. Skin puncture needle (18 gauge)

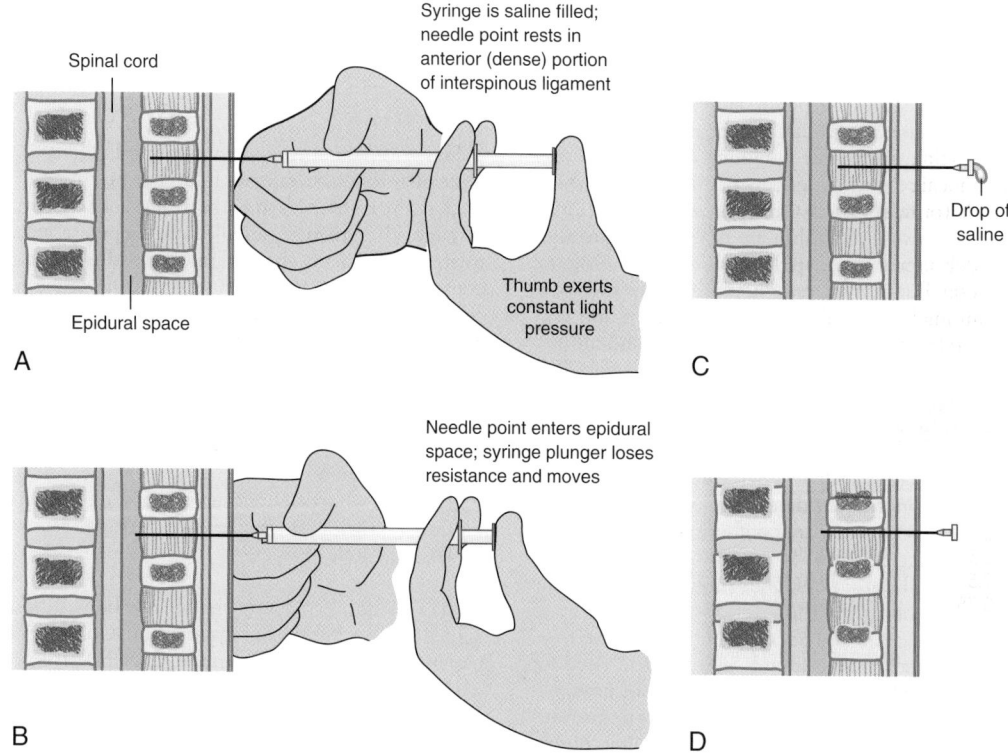

Fig. 10.2   Loss-of-resistance and hanging-drop methods of ascertaining when the point of the needle rests in the epidural space. (A) Needle rests in interspinous ligament. (B) Syringe plunger loses resistance when needle enters epidural space. (C) Saline-filled syringe has been removed, leaving a hanging drop. (D) Hanging drop disappears when needle enters epidural space.

Labels in figure:
Spinal cord
Syringe is saline filled; needle point rests in anterior (dense) portion of interspinous ligament
Drop of saline
Epidural space
Thumb exerts constant light pressure
A
C
Needle point enters epidural space; syringe plunger loses resistance and moves
B
D

   b. Tuohy epidural needle (18 gauge) or other epidural needle; pencil-point needle instead of cutting-bevel needle if combined spinal to be performed
   c. Filter needle (19 gauge) for drawing solutions into the syringes
   d. Skin wheal needle (25 or 27 gauge)
6. Filter (0.2 µm) and filter straw (4 inch)
7. Medications
   a. Lidocaine 1% (5-mL vial) for local infiltration
   b. Sodium chloride 0.9% injectable (10-mL ampule)
   c. Test dose lidocaine 1.5% injectable, with epinephrine 1:200,000 (5-mL vial)
   d. Epinephrine injectable 1:1000 (1-mL vial)
• Epidural medications (Table 10.1)
• Patient-monitoring equipment (e.g., automated blood pressure [BP] device, continuous electrocardiogram monitor, pulse oximeter, fetal monitor [if used for obstetrics])
• Emergency and resuscitative equipment (e.g., suction, Ambubag, oxygen, defibrillator) as well as an anesthesia machine
• Emergency and other drugs not included in the epidural kit:
   1. Ephedrine 5% (1 mL) for use if hypotension develops (usual dose to treat hypotension is 10 mg [0.2 mL] IV) or phenylephrine (Neo-Synephrine). (In the absence of maternal bradycardia, consider phenylephrine.)
   3. Atropine
   4. Diphenhydramine (Benadryl)
   5. Metoclopramide (Reglan), ranitidine (Zantac), and Bicitra (a nonparticulate antacid; the generic is sodium citrate and citric acid solution 3 g/2 g per 30 mL)
   6. Diazepam or midazolam

NOTE: A 1% solution equals 10 mg/mL.

Epidural Agents: Local Anesthetics

The two most commonly used local anesthetics for epidural anesthesia are lidocaine and bupivacaine (see Table 10.1). Lidocaine has a rapid onset (5 to 15 minutes) and lasts 1 to 2 hours, whereas bupivacaine has a slower onset of action (10 to 20 minutes) and a longer duration of action, lasting 2 to 4 hours. In general, increasing the concentration of the drug while maintaining the same volume decreases the latency (time to onset of anesthesia). The addition of epinephrine to lidocaine (available premixed 1:200,000 with lidocaine) or to 0.25% (or less) bupivacaine appears to increase the duration of action.

Bupivacaine is widely used for both obstetric and surgical epidural anesthesia and analgesia. Bupivacaine 0.25% provides adequate sensory analgesia with minimal motor blockade for 1 to 3 hours, and it is well suited for both obstetric and postoperative analgesia (Table 10.2).

When used at 0.5% concentration, bupivacaine produces significant motor blockade. Because of toxicity at higher levels, bupivacaine 0.75% is not recommended for use in obstetrics.

Ropivacaine (Naropin) is a newer agent with less cardiotoxicity than bupivacaine but more than lidocaine. In addition, ropivacaine has a significantly higher threshold for central nervous system toxicity than bupivacaine. In studies, 15 to 30 mL ropivacaine 0.5% provided epidural anesthesia comparable to bupivacaine 0.5% for cesarean section; however, the duration of motor blockade was shorter with ropivacaine.

When lumbar epidural anesthesia is used for surgical procedures, initial volumes of 10 to 20 mL are recommended in adult patients, depending on the concentration of anesthetic and the desired level of anesthesia. Sensory levels are then checked and the dose adjusted accordingly. Additional incremental doses are administered through the epidural catheter as needed. Lower initial volumes (6 to 10 mL) are usually adequate for analgesia in the obstetric patient.

NOTE: The clinician should always use preservative-free local anesthetics and narcotic agents specifically formulated for spinal or epidural anesthesia.

Epidural Agents: Opiates

Anesthetic agents tend to cause motor blockade. Epidural opioids alone are not as effective as dilute concentrations of local anesthetics for anesthesia or analgesia; however, they do not cause motor blockade. When opiates are used in combination with local anesthetic agents, they allow for a reduction in the necessary concentration of the anesthetic agents, thereby minimizing motor blockade. This makes epidural opioids particularly useful in situations where motor blockade is undesirable (e.g., labor, control of postoperative pain). Table 10.3 shows doses and effects of combining bupivacaine and opioids for control of labor pain. Meta-analyses of studies comparing anesthetics combined with opioids versus anesthetics alone found improved analgesic quality with a combination.

PREPROCEDURE PATIENT PREPARATION

A focused history (general maternal health, anesthesia problems, drug allergy, relevant obstetric issues, current medications, and NPO status) and physical examination should be performed with special attention to the airway, BP, heart, lungs, and back for anatomic deformities or skin infection. Expert witnesses in medical liability cases often note a lack of preblock examination by the anesthesiologist. Laboratory studies are obtained on an individualized basis and should include a coagulation profile if indicated.

The patient should be informed of the available anesthesia and analgesia options. A fact sheet can be given to the patient to read before surgery or before the procedure is performed (see the sample

TABLE 10.1	Local Anesthetics Commonly Used for Epidural Anesthesia						
Agent	Concentration (%)	Dose (mL)	Dose (mg)	Onset (min)	Duration (hr)	Sensory Block	Motor Block
Lidocaine	2	10–20	100–400	5–15	1–2	Good	Good
Bupivacaine	0.5	10–20	50–100	10–20	2–4	Good	Good
Ropivacaine	0.5	15–30	75–150	15–30	2–4	Good	Good
Ropivacaine	0.75	15–25	113–188	10–20	3–5	Good	Excellent

TABLE 10.2	Local Anesthetics Commonly Used for Epidural Analgesia						
Agent	Concentration (%)	Dose (mL)	Dose (mg)	Onset (min)	Duration (hr)	Sensory Block	Motor Block
Lidocaine	1	10–20	100–200	5–15	1–2	Good	Good
Bupivacaine	0.125–0.25	10–20	25–50	15–20	1–3	Good	Minimal
Ropivacaine	0.2	10–20	20–40	10–15	0.5–1.5	Good	Minimal

TABLE 10.3	Concentrations of Bupivacaine With or Without Opioids for Labor Analgesia (Bolus Injection) Bupivacaine		
Concentration (%)*	Dose (mL)	Opioid	Result
0.5	5–10	None	Both sensory and motor blockade
0.25	10–15	None	Sensory and partial motor blockade
0.125	10–15	Fentanyl 1–3 µg/mL	Sensory and minimal motor blockade
0.06	10–15	Sufentanil 0.5 µg/mL	Analgesia and no motor blockade

*Higher concentrations are being used less frequently for labor analgesia. The trend is for use of higher-volume lower local concentrations.

patient education form available at www.expertconsult.com) or, for obstetric patients, before the onset of labor. For obstetric care, patients should be informed that any anesthetic procedure is optional and that there are associated risks. Preferably, the fact sheet is given to the patient as a part of the prenatal care. Desired anesthesia or analgesia should be included in the patient's birth plan.

Shortly before performing an epidural, the clinician should answer any questions, review the options again with the patient, including the benefits and specific risks, and obtain signed informed consent. Follow local NPO guidelines (usually nothing to eat 8 hours before the scheduled procedure). ASA guidelines recommend no solid foods in the laboring patient. Patients at high risk of aspiration with surgery (e.g., morbid obesity, diabetes mellitus, difficult airway) may need to be restricted from even clear liquids for more than 2 hours prior to surgery. Early and ongoing communication between the obstetrician or surgeon and the anesthesiologist is vital, particularly when significant anesthetic, obstetric, or surgical risk factors have been identified.

TECHNIQUE

1. Consider giving nonparticulate antacids, H₂ blocker, and metoclopramide 30 minutes before an epidural if a cesarean delivery or postpartum tubal ligation is being performed.
2. Informed consent and permission forms should be signed and in order.
3. Establish IV access with a 20-gauge or larger catheter and give a bolus of 500 to 1000 mL of IV fluids. The patient should be well hydrated before the procedure to minimize the risk of hypotension.
   NOTE: Administer the IV fluids slowly in patients with pregnancy-induced hypertension.
4. Secure the continuous BP, electrocardiogram, and pulse oximetry monitors on the patient and record the initial values. Cycle the BP monitor to observe carefully for hypotension by measuring the BP every 2.5 minutes. Vital signs should be recorded on the anesthesia chart at least every 5 minutes. All medications, doses, routes, and times administered must be noted on the record. For obstetric patients, fetal monitoring should be used.
5. Open the disposable epidural kit and mix the appropriate solutions. Use the filtered needle to draw the solutions that will be administered epidurally. All epidural medications must be preservative free.
6. Place the patient in either the sitting or the lateral position, with the back and neck flexed and the spine straight and not rotated. An assistant should stand in front of the patient during the procedure, helping the patient to remain in that position.
7. Locate the appropriate interspace. Perform the sterile prep and drape the area.
8. A midline approach through the L2–L3, L3–L4, or L4–L5 interspace is most commonly used for epidural anesthesia. Administer local anesthesia (lidocaine 1%) to the interspace area by first making a skin wheal, then injecting into the deeper tissues at the angle the epidural needle will follow. Universal blood and body fluid precautions should be followed.
9. Preliminarily puncture just the skin with an 18-gauge needle to allow for later easy passage of the epidural needle.

10. Pass the Tuohy epidural needle through the skin, angling it appropriately to pass directly toward the spinal canal, until it has firmly passed into the interspinous ligament. Using either the loss-of-resistance technique (with air or saline) or the hanging-drop method (see Fig. 10.2), the needle is now advanced into the epidural space.
    NOTE: The proper angle to direct the tip depends on which interspace is used. The proper angle is almost perpendicular at the L4 to L5 interspace (90 degrees), although it decreases to about 70 degrees at the L2 to L3 interspace. The proper location is usually just below the inferior border of the spinous processes. For epidural anesthesia, insertion angle and location are identical to those used for saddle block anesthesia; however, the depth of insertion is unique to each procedure.
11. Single-shot epidural injections may be used for surgical procedures of short duration. If a longer-duration procedure is anticipated or if postoperative pain relief is desired, place an epidural catheter. Catheter placement must be performed very carefully because improper placement can cause life-threatening complications (e.g., intravascular injection, or total spinal anesthesia if in the subarachnoid space). Rotate the needle so that the catheter will pass either cephalad or caudad as it exits the needle. Note the markings toward the hub of the epidural catheter that are usually 1 cm apart after the first mark. In most cases, the first mark is the same distance from the tip of the catheter as the needle is long. In other words, when inserting the catheter, after the first mark has passed into the needle hub, for every centimeter mark further that the catheter is advanced, the tip advances a centimeter into the spinal canal.
12. Place the tip of the catheter through the hub of the Tuohy epidural needle and advance it slowly through the needle and into the epidural space. A slight resistance is usually encountered as the catheter tip passes through the needle into the epidural space. Advance the catheter 5 cm into the epidural space. The needle is then slowly withdrawn over the catheter, and the catheter secured at the puncture site and along the back with tape. Tape the catheter in place after the patient sits up because the epidural catheter moves when changing from the flexed to straight-up position, and may otherwise come out of the epidural space.
    NOTE: The clinician should never attempt to withdraw the catheter while the needle is in place. The catheter may shear off, leaving the distal segment in the epidural space. Never readvance the needle after the catheter is in place, for the same reason.
13. Secure the catheter hub so that it is easily accessible for injections from the head of the operating table. Fasten the syringe adapter filter to the proximal end of the catheter. Tape the hub to the epidural tubing and to the patient's gown to prevent dislodging with movement.
14. Administer the test dose through the catheter or through the needle hub if not using a catheter. The test dose is performed to detect either intravascular or subdural placement of the catheter or needle. Begin by aspirating to check for the presence of blood or cerebrospinal fluid. If either is present, the needle has been inserted improperly and must be corrected. Next, administer 2 to 4 mL of 1.5% lidocaine with 1:200,000 epinephrine. If the needle is intravascular, a noticeable increase in heart rate, BP, or both will usually be detected within 3 minutes after the injection. The patient may note tinnitus. Sensory and motor function of the lower extremities will be affected after 5 minutes

if the catheter or needle is in the subdural space. If intravascular placement is detected, remove the catheter and repeat the procedure at a different interspace. If the catheter is intrathecal, then options exist: (1) remove and replace the catheter at a different interspace or (2) use as a continuous spinal catheter.

15. After the test dose has confirmed proper placement, the patient is ready for the epidural injection. Aspirate to check for the presence of blood or cerebrospinal fluid before each injection or before placing the patient on an infusion pump or PCEA pump. (Use of infusion pumps or PCEA pumps is beyond the scope of this chapter. Please refer to standard anesthesia textbooks for this information.) Check and record the level of analgesia after the injection. A relatively sharp object (e.g., a toothpick) can be used to do this. Do not use a needle.

16. Some anesthesiologists do a combined spinal/epidural technique, but this is not described here.

NOTE: The factors affecting the level of epidural analgesia include the level of the epidural injection; the volume and concentration of anesthetic solution used; the rate of injection; the addition of a vasoconstrictor; patient age, height, and physical condition; and the position of the patient.

COMPLICATIONS

- Hypotension
  - It is the most common cardiovascular complication of epidural anesthesia.
  - It is caused by widespread sympathetic block.
  - Hypovolemic patients are more susceptible to hypotension.
  - The clinician should treat significant hypotension with positioning, IV fluids, and an IV vasopressor if needed.
  NOTE: Significant bradycardia may be treated with atropine.
- Subarachnoid injection: Injection of large volumes of anesthetic solution into the subdural or subarachnoid space may result in a high or total spinal block, with respiratory arrest, severe hypotension, and possibly cardiac arrest. These conditions must be recognized and treated immediately.
- Postspinal headache: Subdural puncture, always a risk when performing epidural anesthesia, carries a high risk for spinal headache, particularly in younger and pregnant patients. For severe or persistent headache, a blood patch may be necessary (see Chapter 221).
- Toxicity from anesthetic agents
  - See Chapter 6.
  - Accidental injection of local anesthetic into the bloodstream or anesthetic overdose may lead to systemic toxic reactions, including (1) CNS *toxicity* (which begins with numbness of tongue, lightheadedness, dizziness, tinnitus, blurred vision, disorientation, drowsiness, muscle twitching, and tremors, possibly progressing to convulsions); and (2) *cardiovascular toxicity* (initially a mild increase in BP and heart rate is observed, followed by hypotension). The clinician should treat initial hypotension with ephedrine. In severe cases the patient may experience an irreversible state of cardiovascular depression.
  NOTE: For CNS toxicity, treat convulsions by (1) maintaining a patent airway and assisted or controlled ventilation; and (2) administering IV thiopental (sodium pentothal), midazolam, or diazepam. Intubation may be required.
  - Local tissue toxicity is also possible (but it is rare when preservative-free anesthetic solutions are used).
- Respiratory complications, which can be caused by paralysis of intercostal muscles, and hypoxia or hypercarbia can occur, especially in patients with underlying respiratory disease (e.g., chronic obstructive pulmonary disease).
- Neurologic damage: Postepidural neurologic sequelae are due to (1) trauma; (2) anterior spinal artery syndrome (i.e., a syndrome resulting from damage or thrombosis of the anterior spinal artery caused by trauma from the epidural needle), which is almost always avoided by using a midline approach when inserting the needle; and (3) epidural hematoma.

NOTE: Because of decreased peripheral sensation, the patient is at increased risk of lower extremity injury as long as the epidural is in place. Risk of neural injury in the operating room can be kept to a minimum through careful patient positioning. After surgery, patients must be followed closely to detect potentially treatable sources of neurologic injury, including expanding spinal hematoma or epidural abscess, constrictive dressings, improperly applied casts, and increased pressure on neurologically vulnerable sites. A neurologist or a neurosurgeon should evaluate new neurologic deficits promptly to formally document the patient's evolving neurologic status, arrange further testing or intervention, and provide long-term follow-up.

- Catheter complications
  - Epidural catheters may be inadvertently inserted into a blood vessel or into the subarachnoid space. The test dose is used to avoid this possibility and to prevent placing a large dose of anesthetic into either the circulation or the subarachnoid space. Epidural catheters can also migrate into blood vessels and the subarachnoid space, so watch for complications that may occur shortly after insertion.
  - The distal portion of the catheter may break off in the epidural space. This may occur if an attempt is made to withdraw the catheter through the epidural needle. It may also occur if the needle is readvanced after the catheter is deployed. If the catheter will not advance through the needle, remove the needle and catheter together and repeat the procedure at another interspace.

PATIENT EDUCATION GUIDES

See the patient education form available at www.expertconsult.com.

CPT/BILLING CODES

62320	Injection(s) of diagnostic or therapeutic substance(s) (e.g., anesthetic antispasmodic opioid steroid other solution) not including neurolytic substances including needle or catheter placement interlaminar epidural or subarachnoid cervical or thoracic; without imaging guidance
62321	Injection(s) of diagnostic or therapeutic substance(s) (e.g., anesthetic antispasmodic opioid steroid other solution) not including neurolytic substances including needle or catheter placement interlaminar epidural or subarachnoid cervical or thoracic; with imaging guidance (i.e., fluoroscopy or CT)
62322	Injection(s) of diagnostic or therapeutic substance(s) (e.g., anesthetic antispasmodic opioid steroid other solution) not including neurolytic substances including needle or catheter placement interlaminar epidural or subarachnoid lumbar or sacral (caudal); without imaging guidance
62323	Injection(s) of diagnostic or therapeutic substance(s) (e.g., anesthetic antispasmodic opioid steroid other solution) not including neurolytic substances including needle or catheter placement interlaminar epidural or subarachnoid lumbar or sacral (caudal); with imaging guidance (i.e., fluoroscopy or CT)

ICD-10-CM DIAGNOSTIC CODES

For ICD-10-CM codes for other surgical procedures, see the appropriate chapter.

Z33.1	Pregnant state, NOS
O80	Spontaneous vaginal deliveries

Use additional code to indicate outcome of delivery, Z37.0-Z38.8.

Certain conditions have both an underlying etiology and multiple body system manifestations due to the underlying etiology. For such conditions the ICD-10-CM has a coding convention that requires the underlying condition be sequenced first followed by the manifestation. Wherever such a combination exists there is a "use additional code" note at the etiology code, and a "code first" note at the manifestation code. These instructional notes indicate the proper sequencing order of the codes, etiology followed by manifestation. In most cases the manifestation codes will have in the code title, "in diseases classified elsewhere." Codes with this title are a component of the etiology/manifestation convention. The code title indicates that it is a manifestation code. "In diseases classified elsewhere" codes are never permitted to be used as first listed or principle diagnosis codes. They must be used in conjunction with an underlying condition code and they must be listed following the underlying condition.

O60.14XX	Premature labor with delivery (less than 37 weeks)
O321.1XX	Breech presentation
O33.5XXX	Unusually large fetus causing disproportion
O66.0	Shoulder dystocia

The following are codes related to deliveries with forceps or vacuum:

O77.8	Abnormality in fetal heart rate or fetal distress
O63.1	Prolonged second stage of labor

The following are codes related to episiotomy, episiotomy repair, and repair of low vaginal lacerations:

O70.0	First-degree perineal laceration
O70.1	Second-degree perineal laceration
O70.20	Third-degree perineal laceration
O70.3	Fourth-degree perineal laceration
O70.9	Unspecified perineal laceration

The following are codes that relate to pain:

M25.50	Joint pain
M54.5	Back pain
M79.609	Limb or leg pain

NOTE: More specific locations will usually be reimbursed at higher levels.

F45.41	Psychogenic pain, site unspecified
F45.42	Psychogenic pain, other (This code can be used to indicate pain in most areas.)

Acknowledgment

The editors recognize the contributions of Thomas H. Corbett, MD, MPH, to this chapter in previous editions of this text.

SUPPLIERS

(See contact information available at www.expertconsult.com.)

Anesthesia and critical care pharmaceuticals
Baxter Healthcare Corp.
Becton, Dickinson and Co.
Rusch Teleflex
Sims Portex, Smith Medical
Disposable trays, infusion pumps, etc.
B. Braun Medical, Inc.
Epidural and saddle block needles
Kendall Company

RECOMMENDED READING

American College of Obstetricians and Gynecologists Committee on Obstetric Practice. ACOG committee opinion. No. 339: analgesia and cesarean section delivery rates. *Obstet Gynecol.* 2006;107: 1487–1488.

American College of Obstetricians and Gynecologists Committee on Obstetric Practice. ACOG committee opinion. No. 687: approaches to limit intervention during labor and birth. *Obstet Gynecol.* 2017;129: 20–28.

American College of Obstetricians and Gynecologists Committee on Obstetric Practice. ACOG committee opinion. No. 443: optimal goals for anesthesia care in obstetrics. *Obstet Gynecol.* 2009;113: 1197–1199.

American Society of Anesthesiologists Task Force on Management of the Difficult Airway. Practice guidelines for management of the difficult airway: an updated report by the American Society of Anesthesiologists Task Force on Management of the Difficult Airway. *Anesthesiology.* 2013;118:251–270.

American Society of Anesthesiologists Task Force on Obstetric Anesthesia. Practice guidelines for obstetric anesthesia: an updated report by the American Society of Anesthesiologists Task Force on Obstetric Anesthesia and the Society of Obstetric Anesthesia and Perinatology. *Anesthesiology.* 2016;124:270–300.

Anim-Somuah M, Smyth RMD, Jones L. Epidural versus non-epidural or no analgesia in labour. *Cochrane Database Syst Rev.* 2011: CD000331.pub3.

Echt M, Begneaud W, Montgomery D. Effect of epidural analgesia on the primary cesarean section and forceps delivery rates. *J Reprod Med.* 2000;45:557–561.

Hofmeyr GJ, Cyna AM, Middleton P. Prophylactic intravenous preloading for regional analgesia in labour. *Cochrane Database Syst Rev.* 2004: CD000175.pub2.

Horlocker TT. Complications of spinal and epidural anesthesia. *Anesthesiol Clin North America.* 2000;18:461–485.

McClellan KJ, Faulds D. Ropivacaine: an update of its use in regional anesthesia. *Drugs.* 2000; 60:1065–1093.

Shen S, Li Y, Xu S, et al. Epidural analgesia during the second stage of labor: A randomized controlled trial. *Obstet Gynecol.* 2017;130: 1097–1103.

Thorp JA. Epidural analgesia during labor. *Clin Obstet Gynecol.* 1999;42:785–801.

CHAPTER 11

PROCEDURES TO TREAT HEADACHES

Duren Michael Ready

Headaches are an almost universal condition. They are as old as humankind. Headache management evolved beyond "taking two aspirins" with the development of the ergots and migraine-specific triptan medications. However, clinicians still frequently encounter patients who have broken through their prophylaxis, have not responded to acute treatments, and are in need of rescue therapies.

The introduction of sumatriptan and the development of subsequent triptans provided great enhancements to the acute and rescue treatment of migraine and cluster headaches. Triptans are still considered to be underused medications. However, even they have their limits; they work best when used at the onset of mild pain and are of very limited utility 24 hours after onset of the headache. Unfortunately, when we encounter many patients with these difficult headaches, it is too late to use triptans.

Several of the procedures discussed here are older and well established in the medical literature (e.g., greater and lesser occipital nerve block [ONB], sphenopalatine nerve blocks). However, newer techniques (e.g., botulinum toxin, paracervical intramuscular spinal blocks) are under increasing study and are now being used more frequently.

There are multiple benefits to incorporating injection procedures into the management of headaches. They can provide some of the fastest relief (e.g., ONBs, paracervical intramuscular spinal blocks), be the best tolerated (e.g., sphenopalatine ganglion blocks), and provide the most benefit (e.g., botulinum toxin) to patients with refractory headache. They are relatively simple, easy to learn, and provide a great deal of patient satisfaction.

An additional benefit to using injection procedures for acute or rescue management of headaches is the ability to decrease or avoid the use of narcotics. A recent study of acute headache treatments in Canadian emergency departments found that over half of the patients had their first exposure to narcotics in the emergency department as a rescue therapy. There has been a growing consensus among clinicians treating headaches that narcotics should be used only as a last resort, if at all. This is because of their almost universal tendency to sensitize the central nervous system and ultimately make the headaches refractory to treatment.

A history and physical examination are essential before initiating treatment to rule out any red flags for secondary headaches that are caused by treatable conditions. Usually the history will reveal a primary headache disorder that allows for a satisfactory treatment plan. It is also important to discover potential contraindications to these procedures, such as prior cranial surgery. The physical exam primarily excludes secondary causes of headaches. In primary headache disorders, such as migraine or tension-type headache, the physical examination is usually unrevealing (Table 11.1).

Most patients seek help only after they have failed their usual prophylaxis and available acute treatments. Although pharmacologic interventions are still an option, procedural treatments for the most part are simple and safe, and they can be beneficial for the treatment and prevention of many headache disorders. In this chapter, we discuss lower cervical intramuscular blocks, ONBs, sphenopalatine ganglion blocks, and botulinum toxin injections.

Also, see Chapter 7, Peripheral Nerve Blocks and Field Blocks, Chapter 8, Oral/Facial Anesthesia, and Chapter 47, Botulinum Toxin.

LOWER CERVICAL INTRAMUSCULAR INJECTIONS

In 2006, Mellick and colleagues reported a 1-year retrospective review of lower cervical intramuscular injections in over 400 patients treated for headaches in emergency departments. The results were impressive: 65.1% had resolution within 15 minutes and an additional 20.4% had partial relief within 20 minutes. If patients were not pain free 20 minutes after the initial injection, they were reinjected and additional improvement was seen in 59.5% of these patients. The study did not attempt to differentiate between headache subtypes, so the procedure can be tried with most headaches.

Anatomy

Landmarks to identify include the spinous processes of T1, C6, and C7. The injections are then placed 2 to 3 cm lateral to the midline either at the level of C6 or C7; as it turns out, there is some latitude as to their placement. Although there are no major arteries in the area it is always a good practice to aspirate before injecting.

Indications

Although indications have not been well established, generally this procedure is beneficial for *migraine, tension-type, posttraumatic,* and *cervicogenic headaches.*

Relative and Absolute Contraindications

Secondary headache disorders are a relative contraindication (see Table 11.1).

Treatment of the headache should not interfere with treatment of the underlying condition. Although allergy to local anesthetics is very rare, especially allergy to the amides (lidocaine, bupivacaine, and mepivacaine), such an allergy is a contraindication. (See Chapter 5, Local Anesthetics.)

EDITOR'S NOTE: The **parabens preservatives** are used to prolong shelf life in multidose vials of amide anesthetics and may induce sensitivity reactions similar to those seen with the ester group of local anesthetics (procaine, tetracaine). In fact, parabens are the most likely cause of any "allergy" ascribed to the amides. Fortunately, the incidence of parabens allergy is also quite low. There is also no cross-reactivity between the amide and ester anesthetics.

Equipment and Supplies

- Bupivacaine 0.5% 3 mL (1.5 mL injected bilaterally)
- Syringe with 25-gauge, 1.5-inch needle
- Ethyl chloride (Gebauer) or Frigident (Ellman Cynosure) (optional vapocoolant sprays to minimize injection discomfort)

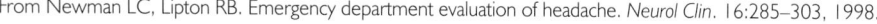

TABLE 11.1   Red Flags for Acute Secondary Headache Disorders

Red Flag	Differential Diagnosis	Possible Workup
Headache beginning after 50 years of age	Temporal arteritis, mass lesion	Erythrocyte sedimentation rate, neuroimaging
Sudden onset of headache	Subarachnoid hemorrhage, pituitary apoplexy, hemorrhage into a mass lesion or vascular malformation, mass lesion (especially posterior mass)	Neuroimaging; lumbar puncture if neuroimaging is negative*
Headaches increasing in frequency and severity	Mass lesion, subdural hematoma, medication overuse	Neuroimaging, drug screen
New-onset headache in a patient with risk factors for human immunodeficiency virus infection or cancer	Meningitis (chronic or carcinomatous), brain abscess (including toxoplasmosis), metastasis	Neuroimaging; lumbar puncture if neuroimaging is negative*
Headache with signs of systemic illness (fever, stiff neck, rash)	Meningitis, encephalitis, Lyme disease, systemic infection, collagen vascular disease	Neuroimaging, lumbar puncture,† serology
Focal neurologic signs or symptoms of disease (other than typical aura)	Mass lesion, vascular malformation, stroke, collagen vascular disease	Neuroimaging, collagen vascular disease evaluation (including antiphospholipid antibodies)
Papilledema	Mass lesion, pseudotumor cerebri, meningitis	Neuroimaging, lumbar puncture†
Headache following head trauma	Intracranial hemorrhage, subdural hematoma, epidural hematoma, posttraumatic headache	Neuroimaging of brain, skull, and (possibly) cervical spine

*Lumbar puncture may follow a negative neuroimaging procedure if suspicion of hemorrhage, infection, or malignancy remains high.
†Suspicion of specific central nervous system infections (e.g., Lyme disease, syphilis) or intracranial hypertension (pseudotumor cerebri) warrants lumbar puncture with cerebrospinal fluid analysis and pressure measurement.
From Newman LC, Lipton RB. Emergency department evaluation of headache. *Neurol Clin.* 16:285–303, 1998.

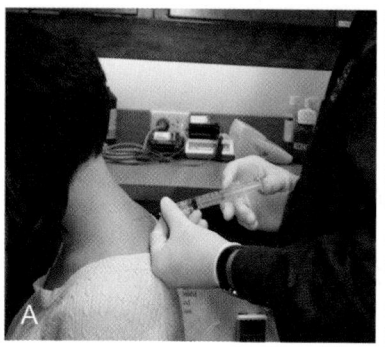
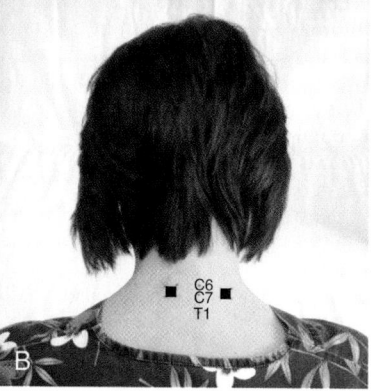

Fig. 11.1 Lower cervical intramuscular injection. (A) A 25-gauge, 1.5-inch needle attached to a 10-mL syringe filled with 3 mL of 0.5% bupivacaine is inserted up to the hub into the paraspinous muscles, 2 to 3 cm lateral to the midline at a level between the C6 and C7 spinous processes and at an angle perpendicular to the cervical spine. The bupivacaine is injected slowly to minimize patient discomfort. After 1.5 mL of bupivacaine has been injected, the needle is withdrawn, the injection site is bandaged, and the procedure is repeated on the other side. (B) Lower cervical intermuscular injection sites. The injections are placed perpendicular to the cervical spine, 2 to 3 cm lateral to the area between the C6 and C7 spinous processes.

Precautions

As with all injections, a sterile technique is essential. Inject slowly to minimize the risk of a vasovagal reaction. It is probably better for the patient to not see the needle nor observe the medication being drawn up into the syringe prior to the injection for the same reason.

Technique

See Fig. 11.1.

1. Have the patient seated with the neck flexed, chin toward chest. The forehead can rest on crossed forearms.
2. Identify the T1 spinous process by finding the superiormost rib. Walk your fingertips medially to the spinous process and move up one or two levels to the C6 or C7 level. Identify the areas for injection bilaterally, 2 to 3 cm lateral to the selected spinous process (two fingerbreadths approximates 3 cm for many people).
3. Insert the needle, all the way to the hub, angled perpendicular to the cervical spine, and toward the anterior neck.
4. Once fully inserted to the needle's hub, aspirate, and if there is no return of blood, inject all of the bupivacaine slowly in one spot. After all of the bupivacaine is injected, withdraw the needle and apply an adhesive strip (Band-Aid) at the site of the injection.
5. Repeat the injection on other side.

6. The injection may be repeated once in 20 to 30 minutes if the headache has not resolved.

It is not known whether relief is a function of resolution of muscle tension, a reflex arc to the spinal trigeminal nucleus, a combination of the two, or some other mechanism of action.

Common Errors

The procedure itself is very simple and does not lend itself to many errors.

Complications

Adverse events are uncommon and limited, but muscle soreness at injection sites, transient weakness of posterior neck muscles, and vasovagal reactions have been reported. If a patient experiences a vasovagal reaction, for the next injection, the patient should be in the supine position with the head flexed off of the table in the position described above.

Postprocedure Management

Typically, placement of a bandage is all that is required after an injection; however, if any complications develop they should be managed before patient discharge.

CPT/BILLING CODES

20552   Injection(s); single or multiple trigger point(s), one or two muscles

This is a common code for cervicalgia, which is frequently associated with headaches.

ICD-10-CM DIAGNOSTIC CODES

Cervicalgia   M54.2

NOTE: Many payers limit the coverage of trigger point injections to specific diagnoses.

GREATER AND LESSER OCCIPITAL NERVE BLOCKS

Greater and lesser ONBs are additional, well-established procedures for the treatment of headaches, and are relatively simple to learn. In a study by Ashkenazi and Young (2005), 89.5% of patients with episodic or transformed migraines responded to greater ONBs (GONB). The GONB has been used as an acute and a preventative treatment for *migraine, cluster, and tension-type headaches*. This block is popular for the treatment of individuals who need quick relief without sedation, although it is slightly more uncomfortable than the lower cervical intramuscular injection. Patients who describe their headaches as "exploding" typically find the greatest relief. The recent discovery of transcranial sensory nerves connecting the scalp and the dura offers an interesting possibility for a mechanism of action, although the exact mechanism has yet to be defined.

Anatomy

The greater occipital nerve (GON) rises out of the dorsal primary rami of cervical spinal nerves 2 and 3. It provides cutaneous sensation to the medial posterior portion of the scalp. The lesser occipital nerve (LON) represents the ventral branches of C2 and C3. These origins suggest a possible mechanism of action: a reflex signal transmitted to the spinal trigeminal nucleus through the C2 nerve.

The GON and LON emerge from underneath the muscles at the level of the nuchal ridge. The GON lies about 2 to 3 cm lateral to the greater occipital protuberance and adjacent to the greater occipital artery. Attempt to palpate the greater occipital artery, which is very near the GON. The GON is frequently tender to palpation during acute headaches.

Indications

The GONB is indicated for prevention and treatment of primary headache conditions and other cephalgias in the back of the neck. Adding steroids to the injection has not been shown in clinical trials to significantly enhance the effectiveness of ONBs, with the noted exception of cluster headaches. When corticosteroids are used, their frequency should typically be no more than one every 3 months, with a continuing assessment of individual risks and benefits. If no steroids are used, the risks (very low) and benefits of repeated injections of local anesthetic should guide decisions about frequency.

Relative and Absolute Contraindications

ONB is relatively contraindicated in the presence of a bony defect. Patients with a prior occipital or mastoid craniotomy should be injected only by a skilled clinician familiar with the patient and his or her anatomic changes to avoid any risk of spinal anesthesia. Caution should also be used in patients with impaired glucose tolerance or diabetes because the steroids may worsen hyperglycemia. In these instances the blocks may be performed with local anesthetic alone.

Equipment and Supplies

Amounts listed here are for unilateral injections. They will need to be doubled for bilateral injections.

- Steroid: typically no more than 1 mL per side
- Intermediate-acting, moderate-potency: triamcinolone acetonide 20 to 40 mg (Kenalog 40 mg/mL)
- Long-acting, high-potency: dexamethasone 4 mg (Decadron 4 mg/mL)
- Local anesthetic: 0.5% bupivacaine 3 mL, *or*
- 1% lidocaine 3 mL with or without epinephrine (*optional*). If lidocaine is used, the patient may report onset of the anesthetic effects of the block while it is still being administered, thereby making the block more tolerable.
- 10-mL syringe with a 25-gauge needle
- The desired quantity of steroid is drawn up into the syringe using a 20-gauge needle and sterile technique, followed by the desired quantities of the bupivacaine or lidocaine. The total volume should be 3 to 4 mL of solution for a unilateral block and 6 to 8 mL of solution for a bilateral block.

Precautions

Always confirm a patient's allergies to medications before any procedure. It is probably better for the patient to not see the needle nor observe the medication being drawn up into the syringe prior to the injection for the same reason.

Procedure

Many techniques have been reported in the literature, but there is no comparison study of the merits of one injection technique over another. It appears best to block the GON and LON by inserting the needle between them and advancing it toward the respective nerves (always aspirating before injection), thereby providing a block that is complete over the superior nuchal ridge. Other clinicians have reported success with blocking the GON and LON using two separate injections.

Greater and Lesser Occipital Nerve Block With One Injection Site

See Fig. 11.2.

1. Have the patient lean forward with the chin flexed forward toward the chest and the head resting on their forearms.
2. Identify the superior nuchal ridge extending from the medial greater occipital protuberance to the lateral mastoid process. Attempt to palpate the greater occipital artery.
3. Introduce the needle between the approximated GON and LON and advance to the skull, withdraw the needle slightly, and administer a small bolus of the solution.
4. Advance the needle medially toward the GON (staying above the nuchal line), aspirate, and inject approximately 2 mL of solution.
5. Withdraw the needle and redirect toward the mastoid process, aspirate, and inject the remaining solution.
6. Repeat the procedure on the contralateral side if the headache is bilateral.

Greater and Lesser Occipital Nerve Blocks as Individual Injections

In this variation, the GON and LON are blocked by two separate injections placed medial and lateral to the anatomic position of the GON and LON.

1. Have the patient lean forward with the chin flexed forward toward the chest and the head resting on their forearms.
2. Identify the greater occipital protuberance at the midline.
3. Inject approximately 2.5 cm lateral to the greater occipital protuberance, just medial to the palpable greater occipital artery. Advance

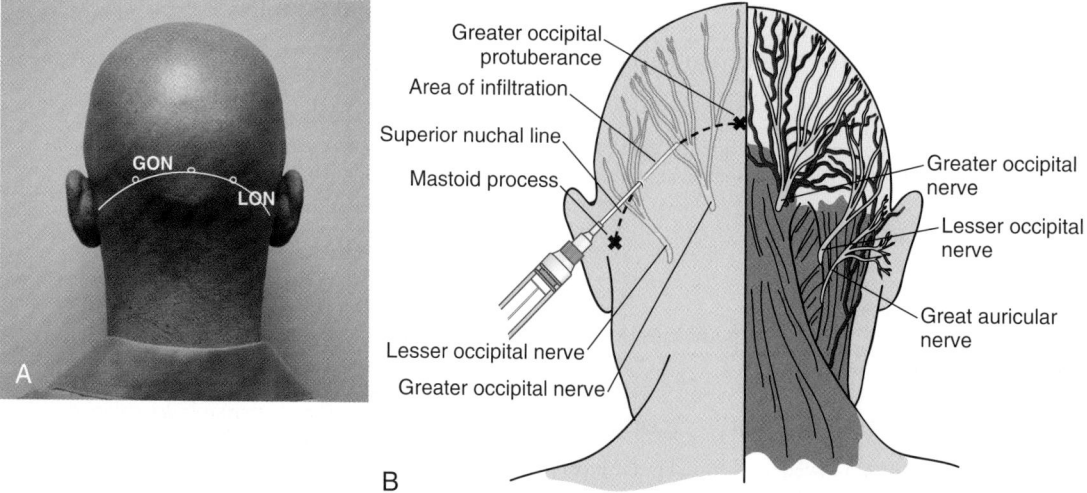

Fig. 11.2 (A) Occipital nerve block. An imaginary curvilinear line is drawn over the superior nuchal line between the greater occipital protuberance and the mastoid process. The line is then divided into thirds. The point of the medial divide (point where medial third meets middle third) represents the approximate position of the greater occipital nerve (GON). The point of the lateral divide (point where lateral third meets middle third) represents the position of the lesser occipital nerve (LON). Injections may be placed over the GON and LON (circles [i.e., nerve sites]), or the injection may be placed between the nerves at the superior nuchal line and directed toward the GON and LON. (B) Occipital nerve block. An imaginary curvilinear line is drawn over the superior nuchal line between then greater occipital protuberance and the mastoid process. The line is then divided into thirds. The point of the medial divide represents the approximate position of the GON. The point of the lateral divide represents the position of the LON. Injections may be placed over the GON and LON (their approximate position [i.e., nerve sites] as labeled on the imaginary curvilinear line), or the injections may be placed between the nerves (marked by the Xs) at the superior nuchal line and directed medially toward the GON and then redirected laterally toward the LON. (B, From Cousins MJ, Carr DB, Horlocker TT, Bridenbough P, editors. *Cousins and Bridenbough's Neural Blockade in Clinical Anesthesia and Pain.* 4th ed. Philadelphia: Lippincott Williams & Wilkins; 2008:421.)

the needle at a slight angle toward the vertex until it strikes the skull. Now withdraw the needle slightly, aspirate, and inject around the target (medially and laterally by approximately 0.5 mm).

4. Place the second injection an additional 2.5 cm lateral to the previous site, approximately two-thirds of the distance along a line drawn from the greater occipital protuberance to the mastoid process. As before, the needle is directed in a slight angle toward the vertex, advanced until contact is made with the skull, and withdrawn slightly; then aspirate and inject in a trigger-point manner.

5. Repeat on the contralateral side if needed.

Common Errors

Intraarterial injection of local anesthetic can usually be prevented by aspirating before injection.

Complications

In addition to the complications reported for lower cervical intramuscular injections, the following may arise:

- As with any repeated steroid injection, it has been suggested that the patient may develop Cushing syndrome or fat atrophy at the injection site (see Chapter 180, Joint and Soft Tissue Aspiration and Injection [Arthrocentesis]).
- It has been suggested that a *seizure* may result from intraarterial injection of the local anesthesia; aspiration before injection will prevent this adverse event.
- Spinal anesthesia has been reported with ONB in a patient with a history of prior cranial surgery. In such patients, it would be best not to perform these procedures unless absolutely necessary, and then only with great caution and appropriate resources. If spinal anesthesia does occur, support the patient until the condition resolves (until the local anesthesia has worn off). The patient may need to be transported to an emergency department or hospital until recovery occurs. The reported cases of spinal anesthesia all occurred in individuals who have bony anomalies or prior craniotomies, and all recovered once the effects of the local anesthesia had resolved.

Postprocedure Management

Postprocedure management is primarily limited to observation of the patient to see if the headache has resolved and to offer additional treatment if needed. If the patient had a vasovagal response, a brief period of observation is appropriate. If a patient experiences a vasovagal reaction, for the next injection the patient should be in the supine position with the head flexed off of the table in the position described above.

CPT/BILLING CODES

64405   Greater occipital nerve blocks

No specific code exists for lesser ONBs. Consider using 64450: Injection, anesthetic agent, other peripheral nerve or branch. You can also charge for the steroid using J-Codes (see Chapter 180, Joint and Soft Tissue Aspiration and Injection [Arthrocentesis]).

Some insurance companies consider ONBs investigational or experimental, so it is important to document the need for the injection in the patient's chart. These reasons could include failure to respond to more conservative therapies, prior positive response, or the acute need for the procedure. Injections with steroids should be limited to no more than four times a year, typically waiting at least 2 months between injections at the earliest. The Michigan Head Pain and Neurological Institute has reported a patient who was self-administering GONBs about four times a day, so any treatment has the potential for abuse. It is hoped that if any clinician encounters these situations, he or she will consult appropriately.

ICD-10-CM DIAGNOSTIC CODES

Headache	R51
Vascular headache	G44.1
Cervicalgia	M54.2

SPHENOPALATINE GANGLION NERVE BLOCK

The sphenopalatine ganglion (SPG) block was first described over 100 years ago by Greenfield Sluder as a treatment for a variety of headaches and facial pain syndromes. The block originally used a cocaine solution. As the medical applications of cocaine came under increasing scrutiny, the procedure became more uncommon. Another likely explanation for the SPG block's fall from favor as a preferred treatment for headaches was the development of ergotamine derivatives, which provided an easier treatment. In the early 1980s, interest in the procedure returned as headache specialists started to report success treating difficult and refractory cephalalgias. Because the SPG represents a crossroad of neurons involved in pain processing, clinicians using SPG blocks have reported its effectiveness in a variety of central pain syndromes, from complex regional pain syndrome to fibromyalgia. A common thread through many of the modern articles about SPG blocks is the question, why is this procedure underused? There are also multiple reports of patients being successfully taught this procedure for self-administration. Although this is a realistic option for some patients, they should be selected carefully on a case-by-case basis.

Anatomy

The SPG (also known as the pterygopalatine or Meckel ganglion) is the largest collection of neuronal cell bodies outside the central nervous system. It is located in the pterygopalatine fossa behind the mid-nasal fossa and in front of the pterygoid canal. Physiologically, there are three major roots: motor, sensory, and sympathetic. It connects the trigeminal and facial nerves and communicates directly with the cervical sympathetic ganglia by the deep petrosal nerve. An SPG block potentially blocks three types of nerve fibers: sensory, sympathetic, and parasympathetic. The zygomatic arch can be an important external landmark because it corresponds to the level of the medial turbinate in the nasopharynx (see also Chapter 8, Oral/Facial Anesthesia).

Indications

The SPG block is indicated for *acute migraine, cluster headaches, and facial neuralgias*. It may be useful for *status migrainosus* and *chronic cluster headaches*. There are reports of varying response to the SPG block for a variety of central pain processes, and given its simplicity and lack of significant adverse events, it is not unreasonable to offer it as a treatment. For central pain conditions (e.g., fibromyalgia, complex regional pain syndrome), it is common to perform several blocks over the space of 1 to 2 weeks.

Relative and Absolute Contraindications

Contraindications are as described for the previously discussed blocks. In addition, a history of nasopharyngeal neoplasms might allow the local anesthetic to cross to the dura and produce spinal anesthesia. History of epistaxis should signal the examiner to proceed with caution; however, this risk is minimized with the use of topical nasal decongestants. Anatomic anomalies in the nasopharynx (e.g., deviated septum, nasal polyps) may also complicate the procedure.

Equipment and Supplies

- Topical, over-the-counter nasal decongestant spray (e.g., Afrin, Neo-Synephrine)
- Sterile cotton swabs (solid wood or hollow plastic)
- 2-inch intravenous catheter (if using the intravenous [IV] catheter technique)
- Local anesthetic: viscous lidocaine 2%, or lidocaine 4% compounded with 1% phenylephrine

Precautions

Nasopharyngeal cancers that communicate with the dura might lead to a spinal block. There has been one reported case of respiratory arrest due to spinal anesthesia. The patient had a complete recovery after the local anesthesia had worn off.

Procedure

The goal is to apply topical anesthesia to the inferior branch of the SPG unilaterally, or bilaterally if needed. Two techniques are commonly described. The traditional technique involves sterile cotton swabs (either wood or hollow plastic—both have advantages that will be discussed). The more recent involves a flexible 1- to 2-inch IV catheter attached to a syringe. A positive response typically occurs in 5 to 10 minutes, although most clinicians keep the applicators in place for 20 to 30 minutes and repeat when necessary.

Sphenopalatine Ganglion Block With Cotton-Tipped Applicators

See Fig. 11.3A–B.

1. With the patient sitting, spray nasal decongestant bilaterally.
2. Apply local anesthetic (viscous lidocaine or lidocaine with phenylephrine) topically to the mucosa of the nasal vestibule and antrum to minimize patient discomfort.
3. Have the patient lie down with a pillow or a towel roll under the shoulders to extend the neck and point the nose toward the ceiling. Allow several minutes for the nasal decongestant and local anesthesia to take effect.
4. Identify the zygomatic arch and use it as a landmark for the middle turbinate.
5. Pass a lidocaine-saturated cotton-tipped applicator into the nasal antrum. Do not force the swab. If you encounter resistance, wait a moment to allow for greater topical anesthesia to occur and then continue advancing the swab gently. Slowly twisting the swab between your fingers as you progress will also ease passage. Continue advancing the swab posteriorly until contact is made with the posterior pharyngeal wall, and then withdraw slightly. At this point, the swab has been inserted to a depth of about 4 inches (10 cm).
6. You may place a second swab unilaterally, posteriorly and superiorly.
7. Repeat insertion if needed on the contralateral side.
8. Leave the swabs in place for 20 to 30 minutes and then withdraw them slowly while rotating them to increase exposure of the ganglion to the topical anesthetic.

PEARLS: Greater exposure to the nasal antrum can be achieved by elevating the nasal apex, thereby opening the nares. Some clinicians have reported additional benefits to rotating the swabs once they are in place, thereby exposing additional anesthetic to the SPG. Some patients are more comfortable having the applicators placed while sitting instead of lying down. One advantage that the hollow plastic swab may have is that once it is in place, small amounts of local anesthesia can be reinstilled through the swab. However, the same process can be accomplished with the wooden swabs by slowly dripping the local anesthetic down the side of the swab. When introducing the additional anesthetic, proceed slowly, using only small amounts to minimize the chance of the patient swallowing the medication. Continued anesthesia can also be accomplished by withdrawing the swabs and replacing them with new ones. Any patient discomfort during the second insertion is greatly diminished because of the preceding anesthesia.

Sphenopalatine Ganglion Block With Flexible Intravenous Catheter

This technique is primarily for unilateral headaches, so treat the affected side (Fig. 11.3C–D).

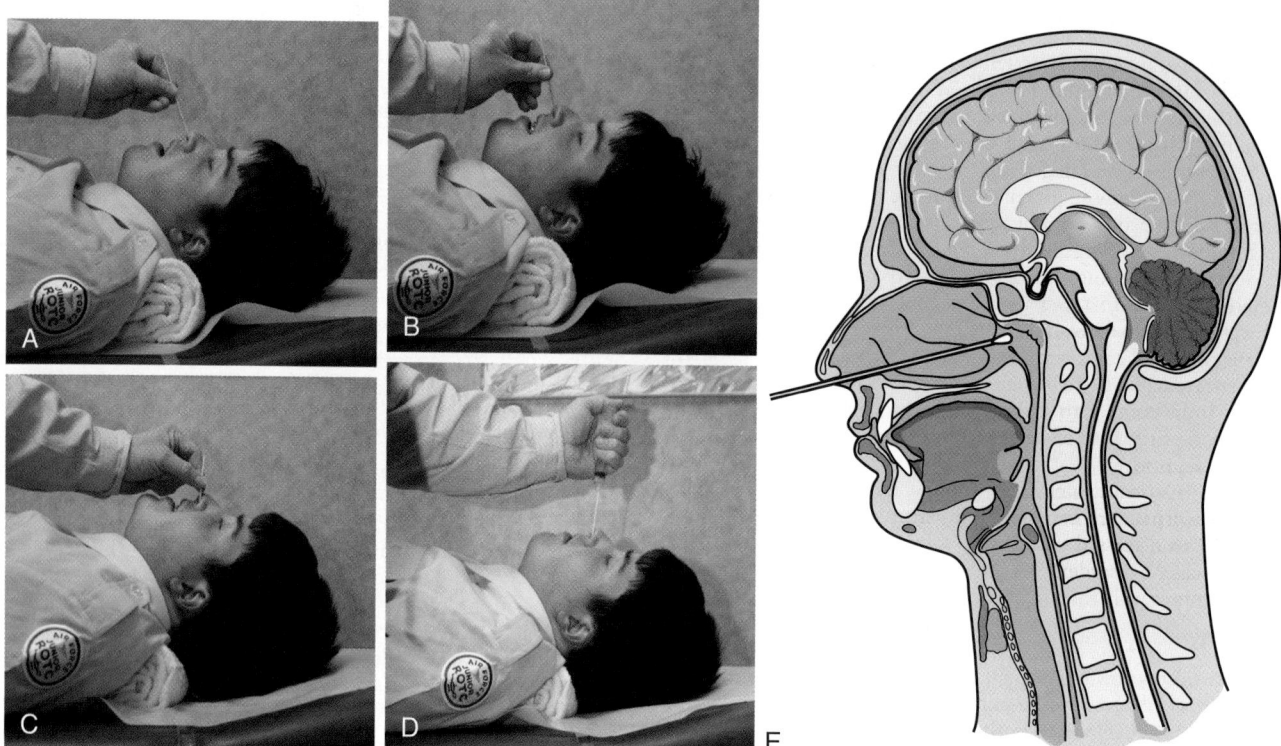

Fig. 11.3   Sphenopalatine ganglion (SPG) block. (A) Step 1: The patient is placed face up with a towel roll under the neck to extend the neck. After applying topical anesthetic to the nasal antrum, the cotton-tipped applicator is introduced into the nostril (targeting the level of the zygomatic arch—the level of the SPG between the first and second turbinates). (B) Step 2: The cotton-tipped applicator is gently advanced, never forced. A twisting motion of the swab between the fingers may ease passage. (C) Step 3: The cotton-tipped applicator is advanced until it touches the posterior pharyngeal wall. It is then withdrawn about 1 cm. It is left in place 15 to 20 minutes and replaced if needed. (D) Step 4: After placement of the applicator, the process may be repeated or additional anesthetic may be applied slowly down the shaft. It will drain down to the cotton tip and replenish the absorbed anesthetic. If a plastic applicator is used, the local anesthetic may be placed inside the hollow shaft. (E) Diagram demonstrating the placement of cotton-tipped applicator in the nasopharynx.

1. Instill 4 mL of 2% viscous lidocaine in a 10-mL syringe, then attach a 2-inch flexible IV catheter from which the needle has been removed.
2. Insert the catheter through the nares toward the posterior nasopharynx, through the middle turbinate.
3. Have the patient turn the head to the side of his or her pain.
4. Slowly administer 2 mL of the viscous lidocaine while having the patient refrain from swallowing or moving the head. Instill the remaining 2 mL after 10 minutes. If the patient is unable to refrain from swallowing, use the cotton swab applicators.

Common Errors

- Incorrect placement of the swab not producing adequate blockade; withdraw and replace the swab or try the IV catheter technique.

Complications

- Epistaxis can occur. It is managed in the usual manner.
- Rarely, toxic effects of the local anesthetic might occur as a result of resorption into a very well-vascularized tumor.
- It has also been suggested that in patients who self-administer the SPG block, mucosal erosions might develop, and that this might lead to some spinal resorption of the local anesthetic. This can be prevented by using a nasal rinse, such as the Sinus Rinse (NeilMed Pharmaceuticals, Inc.), after removal of the cotton-tipped applicator.

Postprocedure Patient Education

- If posterior pharyngeal numbness develops, the patient should not eat or drink until it resolves, typically within 1 hour.

CPT/BILLING CODES

64505   Injection, anesthetic agent; sphenopalatine ganglion

ICD-10-CM DIAGNOSTIC CODES

Migraine	G43.00-G43.99
Cluster headaches	G44.0-G44.02
Neuralgia	G50.0-G51.9

BOTULINUM TOXIN TYPE A

EDITOR'S NOTE: The reader should become totally familiar with the information included in this chapter as well as in Chapter 47, Botulinum Toxin, before injecting Botox for the treatment of headaches. It may be worthwhile testing patients to see if they respond to an injection with a local anesthetic, or even a long-acting local anesthetic (e.g., bupivacaine), in the same location(s) as where the Botox will be injected, to see if they respond. If their headache responds to a local anesthetic, they may be more likely to respond to Botox.

In the early 1980s, Alan Scott was the first clinician to use onabotulinumtoxin A (also known as botulinum toxin type A [BTX-A] or Botox) to treat strabismus in humans. To date, BTX-A is the most widely used and studied form of botulinum toxin. It was during clinical trials using BTX-A for treating brow lines that William Binder, an otolaryngologist, discovered that migraineurs receiving Botox injections for wrinkles experienced fewer headaches. Many of these patients reported fewer migraines or total elimination of migraine pain.

When injected locally, BTX-A binds to acceptor sites on motor or sympathetic nerve terminals and inhibits acetylcholine release by cleaving the SNAP-25 component of the SNARE complex responsible for docking and fusion of the acetylcholine vesicles. BTX-A has also been shown to inhibit release of glutamate, substance P, and calcitonin gene-related peptide from nociceptive neurons, thereby providing a secondary mechanism of action different from neuromuscular junction blockade. The effect is temporary (although it should last several months) and is overcome by regeneration of proximal axons and neuromuscular junctions.

Pooled analyses from the PREEMPT 1 and 2 trials demonstrated that treatment with BTX-A resulted in highly significant improvements in the frequency of headache days versus placebo in patients suffering from chronic migraine. Consequently, the U.S. Food and Drug Administration (FDA) approved BTX-A for headache prophylaxis in patients with chronic migraine, defined as headaches greater than or equal to 15 days per month with headaches lasting 4 hours a day or longer.

Prior to treatment of chronic migraine with BTX-A, it is essential to start with an accurate history, physical, and diagnosis. As with the previously discussed treatments, it is mandatory to rule out secondary headache disorders.

More importantly than for any of the other headache procedures, informed consent with a discussion of costs and expectations must be obtained. Because the level of coverage can vary significantly from one insurance carrier to another, it is essential to determine if the insurance will cover BTX-A injections, and if not, if the patient can afford the treatment course before starting. BTX-A is very expensive, and a treatment can average around $500 or more. Documenting prior treatment failure or adverse events to prior therapies can increase the chance of insurance coverage. Improvement may not be noticed for 1 to 2 weeks after injections; in general, improvements are typically seen in 80% of patients.

BTX-A (Botox) is supplied in single-use vials containing 100 or 200 U of vacuum-dried *Clostridium botulinum* type A neurotoxin complex, 0.5 mg of human albumin, and 0.9 mg of sodium chloride in a sterile, vacuum-dried, preservative-free form. See Chapter 47, Botulinum Toxin, for another description of its use and injection techniques.

Indications

Ninan Mathew, Director of the Houston Headache Clinic, has suggested that the indications for BTX-A include a lack of improvement with preventive pharmacotherapy; severe and intolerable adverse events from preventive therapy; or patient refusal or inability to use daily medications. Contraindications include acute migraine therapy or an elderly patient with chronic migraine. In 2007, Roger Cady and Curtis Schreiber of the Headache Care Center in Springfield, Missouri, suggested BTX-A as an ideal prophylactic agent for patients with frequent disabling headache who have been poorly controlled with previous preventatives secondary to compliance, adherence, or inability to use conventional preventive therapies as a result of adverse events. In a small study of 63 migraineurs, Jakubowski and colleagues (2006) found that 74% of BTX-A responders described their headaches as a pressure from the outside, imploding, or as an "eye-popping" sensation. Conversely, 92% of the nonresponders described their headaches as "exploding," with pressure building up from the inside.

Relative and Absolute Contraindications

* Infection at the injection site
* Known hypersensitivity to any ingredient in the formulation
* Presence of a neuromuscular disorder (e.g., myasthenia gravis, Eaton-Lambert syndrome)
* BTX-A is labeled category C in pregnancy, and its safety in nursing mothers is unknown

Equipment and Supplies

* Botulinum toxin type A
* 1-mL tuberculin syringe

Other gauge needles can be used, but it is generally believed that smaller-gauge needles are less painful.

Precautions

Because the FDA has only approved BTX-A for chronic migraine treatment, for any other headache disorder it may be prudent to limit the amount of BTX-A to 60 U per session until the patient's response to therapy is known.

Preprocedure Patient Education and Forms

* Insurance preauthorization forms. Allergan offers physician and patient assistance through their Botox Reimbursement Solutions website (www.botoxreimbursement.us/Home.apx).
* Checklist visit/encounter form (available at www.expertconsult.com)
* Consent forms

Botulinum Toxin for Headache Treatment and Prevention

Three injection paradigms have been used in clinical trials for patients with chronic daily headache and chronic migraine: (1) fixed-site, fixed-dose; (2) follow the pain; or (3) a combination of the two. A study published in *Headache* also demonstrated a positive response with single bilateral injections of 25 U of BTX-A (Behmand and colleagues, 2003). While the FDA has approved the use of BTX-A injections at 31 sites across seven specific head and muscle groups, what follows is the author's experience with the most successful sites using BTX-A before it was approved by the FDA.

Basic Tenets

1. Preplan the injections using an anatomic drawing for injection sites and units used (see Chapter 47, Botulinum Toxin, for areas of caution).
2. Use a 25-, 27-, 30-, or 31-gauge needle affixed to a tuberculin syringe. Some research has suggested that using a smaller-gauge and slightly longer needle, such as the 31-gauge, 13-mm Steri-Ject needle, minimizes discomfort and allows for injection of the deeper muscles of the head and neck.
3. Inject intramuscularly in a manner that will allow for greater infiltration, avoiding intradermal or periosteal injections.
4. In cosmetically sensitive areas, inject in a symmetric fashion.
5. Injecting at multiple sites in the targeted muscle group allows for a more even dispersal of toxin through the target region.
6. Visualization and avoidance of facial vessels minimizes any subsequent bruising.

Preparation

See Chapter 47, Botulinum Toxin.

1. Reconstitute the BTX-A and draw up into two syringes (one syringe for each side). Dilution with 2 mL of preservative-free normal saline will yield 50 U/syringe, or 5 U/0.01 mL.
2. Return any unused BTX-A to the refrigerator for storage.
3. BTX-A must be used within 24 hours of being reconstituted.

Fixed-Site Protocol

See Fig. 11.4.

* Glabellar region (the area around the smooth prominence between the eyebrows)

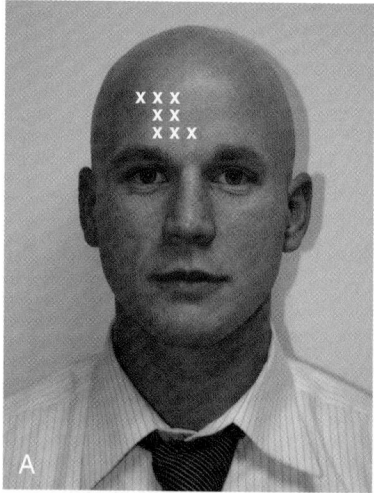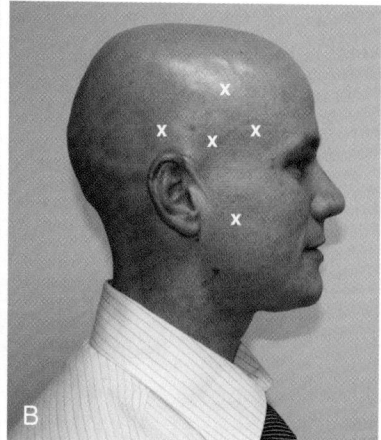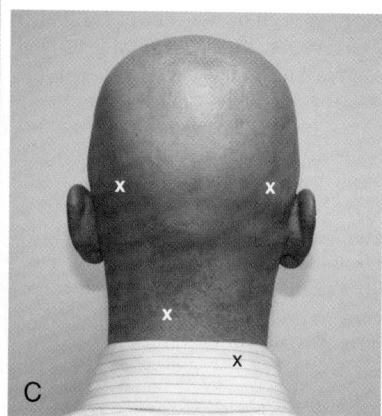

Fig. 11.4 Approximate sites of botulinum toxin injections over the face (A), temple and jaw (B), and occiput and neck (C).

- Smaller fluid volumes minimize spread to adjacent muscles.
- Inject procerus (small muscle that originates at the nasal bone and inserts upward between the eyebrows): Treat as one region, injecting with 2.5 to 4 U.
- Inject corrugators: Inject two sites bilaterally, totaling four sites, 1.5 to 3 cm apart. The corrugators are identified by having the patient frown. Apply pressure at the supraorbital ridge to reduce the potential for inferior extravasation. Grasping the mid-lateral portion of the corrugators between two fingers while injecting the toxin diminishes the risk of eyelid ptosis. See the Precautions section in Chapter 47, Botulinum Toxin.
- Forehead
- Inject the frontalis (forehead muscle, anterior aspect of the occipitofrontalis) with a larger volume (20 to 30 U) over a greater area, typically 8 to 12 sites. Have the patient elevate the eyebrows before injection. Remember to inject symmetrically.
- If the inferolateral frontalis is not painful, do not inject over the lateral third; this will decrease the risk of brow ptosis.
- Lateral injections
- If painful, inject the temporalis (large muscle over the temporal fossa). The temporalis is identified by having the patient clench his or her teeth. Injections are given bilaterally, posterior, superior, and inferior, using 0.2 mL per site in four sites, for a total of 20 U.
- If there is a history of temporomandibular joint syndrome, inject the masseters (large muscle originating from the zygomatic arch and process and inserting into the mandibular ramus and gonial angle) with 5 to 15 U per side.
- Posterior neck muscles
- Inject the trapezius (bilateral large triangular muscle of the upper back that originates at the occipital bone, ligamentum nuchae, and the spinous processes of C7–T12 and inserts into the distal clavicle, acromion, and scapular spine).
- If the trapezius is involved or suspected as a pain generator, inject bilaterally at one to three sites with 5 to 15 U total.
- If posterior neck pain is present, evaluate occipital/cervical paraspinal muscles. Inject one or two sites on each side. The doses vary from 5 to 15 U per side.

"Follow the Pain" Protocol (Most Commonly Treats Tension-Type Headaches)

1. Have the patient identify the areas of origination and radiation of the pain.
2. Inject areas associated with pain and tenderness on palpation.
3. Inject the identified areas with 4 to 12 U, 1.5 to 3 cm apart.

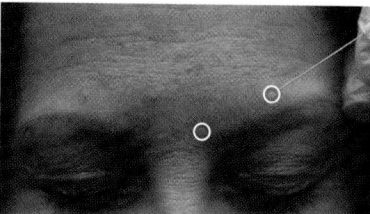

Fig. 11.5 Single-site botulinum toxin type A (BTX-A) injection. Insert the needle at the designated site over the medial brow and advance toward the target on the medial aspect of the procerus. Slowly infiltrate the 25 U of BTX-A while withdrawing the needle to evenly dispense the drug.

Common sites of injection include glabellar and frontal regions, temporalis muscle, occipitalis muscle, and cervical paraspinal region. Inject in similar fashion to the fixed-site injections.

Bilateral Single-Site Protocol

See Fig. 11.5. Significant improvement has been reported with single bilateral injections into the corrugator supercilii muscles with 25 U of BTX-A using a 1-inch, 30-gauge needle. Patients were asked to frown to identify the most lateral attachment of the corrugator supercilii muscle. The needle was then inserted at this most lateral attachment and advanced medially toward the root of the nose. BTX-A was then infiltrated across this path as the needle was withdrawn. Be sure to avoid areas where major nerve branches are present, such as the supraorbital nerve; if injected, significant paralysis may result (see Chapter 47, Botulinum Toxin).

Common Errors

To avoid a ptosis, avoid injecting lateral to the pupil in an area 1 cm superior to the supraorbital rim, out to the lateral eyebrow. Only time will correct this error; typically, ptosis may take upward of 3 months to resolve.

Complications

- Most commonly involve bruising and swelling
- Some patients develop a transient headache that usually resolves within 24 to 48 hours.

- Occasional flulike symptoms may develop and resolve within a day or two.
- A transient ptosis may develop that will resolve over 3 months. This is best avoided by not injecting over the lateral supraorbital muscles. However, if this is an area of pain, this complication may be unavoidable, but it will be essential to warn the patient that a ptosis may result.
- Muscle paralysis at the injection site may occur (although this is a desired effect for the most part).
- There have been reports of antibody formation in patients treated with BTX-A for cervical dystonia or torticollis. These procedures used an older, "less clean" formulation of BTX-A in much higher doses than those used for treating migraines. To prevent antibody formation, current recommendations are to limit BTX-A administration to a minimum of 3-month intervals between injections, with an annual load of 300 to 600 U/year.

Postprocedure Management

Remind patients that improvement is gradual and mostly cumulative over several sessions.

POSTPROCEDURE PATIENT EDUCATION FOR ANY TREATMENT

It is important to maintain a headache diary to provide objective measures for determining the effectiveness of treatment and the direction for future treatments. The goal of most preventive treatments for headache is a 50% reduction in the frequency and severity of the headaches. In the absence of headache diaries, this is very difficult to quantify. If any postinjection wheals or blebs develop, inform the patient that they usually resolve within 2 hours. There may be a reduction in hyperfunctional lines of the face. This should be expected and is not considered an adverse event. It may take several weeks for headache relief, and the greatest benefit is seen with repeated treatments.

ONLINE RESOURCES

Allergan's Botox Reimbursement Solutions website: www.botoxreimbursement. us/. Allergan will help your office preauthorize patients; this is their portal to offer assistance for patients without insurance who are in need.
American Headache Society. Professional Resources: *Headache Journal* toolbox: www.americanheadachesociety.org/resources/
Binder WJ. Beverly Hills Botox treatment: www.doctorbinder.com/proc_botoxmigraines.asp
http://drmiltonreder.com.
The Johns Hopkins Headache Center: www.hopkinsneuro.org/headache/procedure_nerveblock.cfm

SUPPLIERS

See contact information available at www.expertconsult.com.

Botulinum toxin type A
  Allergan, Inc.
Tuberculin syringe 1 mL
  Air-Tite Products Company

RECOMMENDED READING

Ashkenazi A, Young WB. The effects of greater occipital nerve block and trigger point injection on brush allodynia and pain in migraine. *Headache.* 2005;45:350–354.
Behmand RA, Tucker T, Guyron B. Single-site botulinum toxin type A injection for elimination of migraine trigger points. *Headache.* 2003;43:1085–1089.
Blumenfeld AM, Binder W, Silberstein S, Blitzer A. Procedures for administering botulinum toxin type A for migraine and tension-type headache. *Headache.* 2003;43:884–891.
Botox is safe and effective as preventative treatment for chronic migraine. *Clinical Trends and Reviews in Neurology.* 2009;17(10).
Cady R, Schreiber C. Botulinum toxin type A as migraine preventive treatment in patients previously failing oral prophylactic treatment due to compliance issues. *Headache.* 2008;48:900–913.
Jakubowski M, McAllister PJ, Bajwa ZH, et al. Exploding vs. imploding headache in migraine prophylaxis with botulinum toxin A. *Pain.* 2006;125:286–295.
Jankovic D, Wells C. Nasal block of the pterygopalatine ganglion. In: *Regional Nerve Blocks: Textbook and Color Atlas.* 2nd ed. Berlin: Blackwell; 2001:29–30.
Jankovic D, Wells C. Occipital nerve blocks. In: *Regional Nerve Blocks: Textbook and Color Atlas.* 2nd ed. Berlin: Blackwell; 2001:14–16.
Krusz JC. Aggressive interventional treatment of intractable headaches in the clinic setting. *Clin Fam Pract.* 2005;7:545–565.
Lavin PJ, Workman R. Cushing syndrome induced by serial occipital nerve blocks containing corticosteroid. *Headache.* 2001;41:902–904.
Lebovits AH, Lefkowitiz M. Sphenopalatine ganglion block: clinical use in the pain management clinic. *Clin J Pain.* 1990;6:131–136.
Mellick LB, McIlrath ST, Mellick GA. Treatment of headaches in the ED with lower cervical intramuscular bupivacaine injections: a 1-year retrospective review of 417 patients. *Headache.* 2006;46:1441–1449.
Quevedo JP, Purgavie K, Platt H, Strax TE. Complex regional pain syndrome involving the lower extremity: a report of 2 cases of sphenopalatine block as a treatment option. *Arch Phys Med Rehabil.* 2005;86:335–337.
Racz GB, Morton AB, Diede JH. Sphenopalatine ganglion block. In: Waldman SD, Winnie AP, eds. *Interventional Pain Management.* Philadelphia: WB Saunders; 1996:223–225.
Smith KC, Alum P. Botulinum toxin for pain relief and treatment of headache. In: Carruthers A, Carruthers J, eds. *Procedures in Cosmetic Dermatology Series: Botulinum Toxin.* 2nd ed. Oxford: Elsevier; 2007:101–111.
Tobin J, Flitman S. Occipital nerve blocks: when and what to inject? *Headache.* 2009;49:1521–1533.
Waldman SD. Greater and Lesser Occipital Nerve Block. In: *Atlas of Interventional Pain Management.* 4th ed. Philadelphia: Elsevier; 2015:24–27.
Waldman SD. Sphenopalatine Ganglion Block: Transnasal Approach. In: *Atlas of Interventional Pain Management.* 4th ed. Philadelphia: Elsevier; 2015:11–14.
Winner P. Botulinum toxins in the treatment of migraine and tension-type headaches. *Phys Med Rehabil Clin North Am.* 2003;14:885–899.
Yarnitsky D, Goor-Aryeh I, Bajwa ZH, et al. 2003 Wolff Award: possible parasympathetic contributions to peripheral and central sensitization during migraine. *Headache.* 2003;43:704–714.

SECTION 2

Dermatology

Section Editor: THEODORE O'CONNELL

CHAPTER 12

ACNE THERAPY: SURGICAL AND PHYSICAL APPROACHES

Michael A. Altman

Acne is the most common skin disease of childhood and adolescence and is estimated to affect 80% of individuals between 11 and 30 years of age and up to 95% of all adolescents. Acne is a disease of the pilosebaceous unit involving increased sebum production, obstruction of the pilosebaceous glands with keratinization of the canal, bacterial proliferation, and inflammation. Many topical and systemic medications have been developed to treat acne. When these medications fail to control the disease, or when significant lesions develop, several procedures may be used to intervene. This chapter focuses on the procedures a primary care clinician might consider for treatment of acne in their office.

COMEDO REMOVAL

The removal of open comedones (blackheads, noninflamed plugged pores) enhances the patient's appearance while preventing the development of inflamed acne lesions and cysts (with their complications). Instruments, such as the round loop (or oval loop) extractor (Fig. 12.1) or the Schamberg extractor, effectively extract the plug by allowing uniform, smooth pressure to encircle the pore (Fig. 12.2). Downward pressure allows the comedo or pus to exit through the hole in the extractor. Extractors can be obtained from any medical supply provider, and some are even sold over the counter.

Open comedones that offer resistance can be loosened with one of two techniques:

1. Application of tretinoin (Retin-A), a topical keratolytic, for 1 month before comedo extraction.
2. Use of a no. 11 blade scalpel, tip of a needle, or the pointed end of a comedo extractor to stretch the walls or slightly incise the pore opening. The clinician should insert the scalpel point 1 mm into the comedo, following the angle of the follicle opening, and angle the tip to bring the plug upward through the enlarged pore opening.

If there is still resistance, the comedo extractor should be held in the other hand and lateral pressure applied with the blunted end to the base of the lesion as the blade lifts the plug through the center of the extractor. A large amount of sebaceous material may be found beneath the plug and should be removed.

ACNE SURGERY FOR PUSTULES AND CYSTS

The surgical drainage of acne pustules and cysts, when performed correctly, speeds resolution of the lesions, prevents subdermal

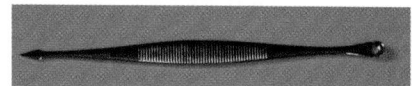

Fig. 12.1   Comedo extractor. Note pointed end and cupped end with central opening.

rupture, and enhances cosmetic appearance. Closed comedones also can be opened to prevent their progression to inflammatory lesions.

Enter the head of a white pustule with a small (25-gauge) needle, with the tip (tiny nick) of a no. 11 blade scalpel, or the pointed end of the comedo extractor. Drain the pustule with lateral pressure or with the assistance of an extractor. Superficial cysts that have thin roofs and easily palpated fluid can be drained by making a small incision less than 4 mm long. Some clinicians advocate that the base of a drained superficial cyst be gently curetted to dislodge any necrotic debris. Nodules and large cysts may best be treated by intralesional corticosteroid injection.

INTRALESIONAL CORTICOSTEROID INJECTION

Individual nodular or cystic acne lesions often dramatically decrease in size after intralesional injection of a corticosteroid. It is reassuring to patients to know that a fast, relatively painless procedure is available when lesions arise. Patients with severe acne often require repeated injections every 2 to 3 weeks. Multiple cysts can be treated in one session.

The steroid preparation triamcinolone acetonide 10 mg/mL (e.g., Kenalog-10) is a preferred agent and should be diluted to about 2.5 mg/mL with saline or local anesthetic (e.g., 1% lidocaine). Saline is the preferred diluent because injections of local anesthetics are painful. Triamcinolone acetonide is particularly useful in that it is insoluble and therefore can remain deposited for months at the injection site, achieving its desired local effect without risk for adrenal suppression.

When preparing for an injection, shake the steroid vial to disperse the suspension. First draw the saline into a tuberculin syringe, followed by an appropriate amount of triamcinolone. (If lidocaine is the diluent, use only single-dose vials to prevent precipitation of the steroid.) An air bubble can be aspirated into the syringe to mix the two. Then insert a 30-gauge needle through the thinnest portion of the cyst roof and deliver 0.05 to 0.2 mL of the resulting 2.5-mg/mL triamcinolone acetonide mixture. Limit the maximum volume to 0.2 mL per lesion to reduce the risk of skin atrophy. The injection usually blanches the cyst.

Inject directly into the cyst, not the skin. Skin atrophy can follow injections if the steroid is deposited into the skin below the cyst or if the steroid concentration is too high. One session of injections should not exceed a total of 10 to 20 mg of triamcinolone, to avoid systemic effects. It may be necessary to repeat intralesional injections at 2-week intervals, not to exceed three total sessions.

Fluctuant lesions can be aspirated first with a large-bore needle attached to a 1- or 3-mL syringe before steroid injection. Skin atrophy remains unlikely, but the patient should be forewarned that atrophy still may occur independent of the injection because of underlying inflammation involving the collagen bed. Secondary bacterial

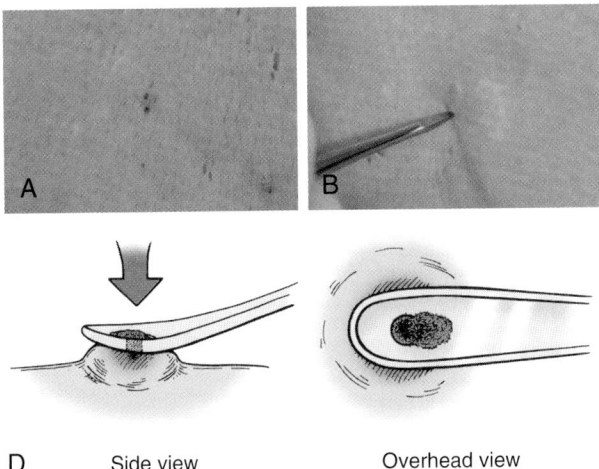

Fig. 12.2 Use of comedo extractor to express cystic contents. (A) Comedo. (B) Incising over comedo to enlarge the opening using the sharp end of extractor. (C) Applying pressure over comedo to express contents through the central opening of the extractor. (D) Graphic representation of extraction.

infections do not occur. Avoid injecting the periorbital and perinasal areas because steroid crystals inadvertently injected into vessels may drain into the cerebral venous sinuses or central retinal artery. Finally, counsel patients that skin depression may occur, but in most cases this is temporary and gradually resolves in 4 to 6 months.

CRYOTHERAPY

Cryotherapy has been found to be effective against pustular acne but not against comedonal or papular acne. It is most effective against superficial cystic lesions and is least effective against deeper lesions. Any softening effect on scars is usually temporary. Application is painful and burning discomfort may last up to 4 hours. In current dermatology, cryotherapy has fallen out of general use for acne management.

OTHER CURRENT APPROACHES

Photodynamic therapy (see Chapter 51, Photodynamic Therapy), microdermabrasion (see Chapter 49, Microdermabrasion and Dermal Infusion), and chemical peels (see Chapter 50, Skin Peels) also can be used to control acne by physical techniques.

SCAR REVISION

NOTE: Scar revisions should not be performed for 6 months to 1 year after use of oral isotretinoin.

1. A variety of procedures can be used to remove or revise acne scars. Deep, "icepick" scars can be excised using a punch biopsy and immediately replacing the scar plug with a full-thickness punch graft of normal skin. This procedure has been relegated to early scar revision now that laser skin resurfacing is available.
2. Another technique, punch-graft elevation, uses a punch just slightly larger than the pitted scar. A cylindrical incision is made into the dermis, allowing the core to "pop out" above the skin surface. A Steri-Strip secures this skin core just above the surrounding skin. Dermabrasion of the remaining treatment site may be required at a later date. Results are unpredictable.
3. Collagen injections can be used to smooth the skin surface, but are a temporary solution (see Chapter 48, Tissue Filler).
4. Dermabrasion involves the use of a high-speed hand drill with a diamond-studded steel sander under local anesthesia to smooth out scars. Microdermabrasion (see Chapter 49, Microdermabrasion and Dermal Infusion) also can be used. It is less aggressive and there is little recovery time, but many (six to eight) visits may be needed. It is best reserved for more superficial scars.

5. Traditional ablative laser resurfacing (using Er:YAG or CO_2 laser) or nonablative fractional laser resurfacing can be used to treat acne scars. Nonablative fractional laser resurfacing is not only less aggressive, less risky, and requires less recovery time, but also is less efficacious and requires multiple treatments.
6. Chemical peels can effectively treat acne scars and are classified as superficial, medium depth, and deep chemical peels. Superficial chemical peels can help improve the appearance of superficial acne scars as well as postinflammatory hyperpigmentation. However, most acne scars require medium depth or deep chemical peels to improve their appearance.

COMPLICATIONS

Complications include adverse pigmentary changes, deeper and longer scars, and increased skin sensitivity to sunlight.

CPT/BILLING CODES

10040	Acne surgery, opening of multiple cysts, comedones, or pustules
10060	Incision and drainage of abscess
11900	Intralesional injection of up to seven lesions
11901	Intralesional injection of more than seven lesions
17360	Chemical exfoliation for acne

ICD-10-CM DIAGNOSTIC CODES

Acne vulgaris	L70.0
Acne conglobate	L70.1
Acne varioliformis	L70.2
Acne tropica	L70.3
Acne excoriee	L70.5
Other acne	L70.8
Acne unspecified	L70.9
Perioral dermatitis	L71.0
Rhinophyma	L71.1
Other rosacea	L71.8
Rosacea unspecified	L71.9
Epidermal cyst	L72.0
Pilar cyst	L72.11
Trichodermal cyst	L72.12
Steatocystoma multiplex	L72.2
Other follicular cysts of skin and subcutaneous tissue	L72.8
Follicular cyst of skin and subcutaneous tissue	L72.9

Acne keloid	L73.0
Pseudofolliculitis barbae	L73.1
Hidradenitis supporativa	L73.2
Other specified follicular disorders	L73.8
Follicular disorder unspecified	L73.9

RECOMMENDED READING

Abdel Hay R, Shalaby K, Zaher H, et al. Interventions for acne scars. *Cochrane Database Syst Rev.* 2016;4:CD011946.

Briden ME. Alpha-hydroxyacid chemical peeling agents: case studies and rationale for safe and effective use. *Cutis.* 2004;73(suppl 2):18–24.

Brody HJ. Complications of chemical resurfacing. *Dermatol Clin.* 2001;19:427–438.

Fife D. Practical evaluation and management of atrophic acne scars: tips for the general dermatologist. *J Clin Aesthet Dermatol.* 2011;4:50.

Garg VK, Sinha S, Sarkar R. Glycolic acid peels versus salicylic-mandelic acid peels in active acne vulgaris and post-acne scarring and hyperpigmentation: a comparative study. *Dermatol Surg.* 2009;25:59.

Goodman GJ. Treatment of acne scarring. *Int J Dermatol.* 2011;50:1179.

Habif TP. *Clinical Dermatology: A Color Guide to Diagnosis and Therapy.* 6th ed. Philadelphia: Elsevier; 2015.

Nguyen QH, Kim YA, Schwartz RA. Management of acne vulgaris. *Am Fam Physician.* 1994;50:89–96.

Ong MW, Bashir SJ. Fractional laser resurfacing for acne scars: a review. *Br J Dermatol.* 2012;166:1160.

Rivera AE. Acne scarring: a review and current treatment modalities. *J Am Acad Dermatol.* 2008;59:659.

Sakamoto FH, Lopes JD, Anderson RR. Photodynamic therapy for acne vulgaris: a critical review from basics to clinical practice: part 1. Acne vulgaris: when and why consider photodynamic therapy? *J Am Acad Dermatol.* 2010;63:183.

Taub AF. Procedural treatments for acne vulgaris. *Dermatol Surg.* 2007;33:1005–1026.

Taylor MN, Gonzalez ML. The practicalities of photodynamic therapy in acne vulgaris. *Br J Dermatol.* 2009;160:1140.

Thiboutot D, Gollnick H, Bettoli V, et al. New insights into the management of acne: an update from the Global Alliance to Improve Outcomes in Acne group. *J Am Acad Dermatol.* 2009;60:S1.

CHAPTER 13

APPROACH TO VARIOUS SKIN LESIONS

John L. Pfenninger

This chapter provides guidelines for the diagnosis and treatment of common skin lesions. Table 13.1 can be used as a guide for proper biopsy and treatment techniques. The specifics of performing the procedures are reviewed elsewhere in this textbook. These guidelines are not intended to be all-inclusive, but they do provide a framework for the approach to common skin lesions.

All excised skin lesions are best sent to the pathologist for definitive diagnosis. With selected lesions, such as skin tags or sebaceous cysts, many clinicians will rely on their clinical judgment and avoid the added laboratory expense. However, in today's litigious society, the clinician must be absolutely certain of the diagnosis when deciding not to send tissue to the pathologist for evaluation. Numerous benign lesions can be placed in a single formalin container (e.g., skin tags, obviously benign nevi) to cover the legal aspects and yet conserve costs. The fee to process each bottle (regardless of the number of samples in it) is approximately $160 to $200 for the routine dermatologic lesion.

EDITOR'S NOTE: finding a good dermatologic pathologist is worth the effort. The pathologist should diagnose just what is seen and not be speculative. For example, if it is an actinic keratosis, that is what should be diagnosed; adding the term "entire extent of lesion not seen, cannot exclude squamous cell carcinoma" is not helpful to the surgeon and might even cause a medicolegal problem many years later.

ANGIOMA (HEMANGIOMA)

If the angiomas are small, use a ball electrode to cauterize them lightly. If larger than 2 mm, local anesthesia may be needed. Tissue should be wiped away and the process repeated until no vessel is seen (Fig. 13.1). Focal cryotherapy or sclerotherapy will also work. If the angiomas are large, a superficial shave excision or curettement followed by light cautery of the base works best.

ACROCHORDON (SKIN TAG)

Although many clinicians prefer to use electrosurgery or cryotherapy to remove acrochordons, the most direct and simple approach is to elevate the tag with pickups and excise it with sharp tissue scissors at the level of the surrounding skin (Fig. 13.2). If it has a broad base, a local anesthetic may be required. Monsel solution (ferric subsulfate) or aluminum chloride may be used for hemostasis. It is essential to have good quality scissors so the lesion is cut, not "pinched." Some clinicians also use a curved small hemostat to very quickly crush the base of the acrochordon before excising it. By crushing the tissue with a hemostat, the sensory nerves are also crushed, effectively providing anesthesia as well as hemostasis.

If the tag is small enough, no cutting is necessary; a ball electrode can be used to lightly and quickly cauterize the tag. It is then simply "wiped away," similar to the treatment of a small angioma (see earlier).

Cryocautery can be effective, but it is difficult to limit the freeze solely to the tag. A unique method with liquid nitrogen is to use the Styrofoam cup method, dipping the flat pickups in the liquid, and then grasping the tag with the cooled metal. The tag usually necrotizes off. The tag should be frozen twice in the same visit. Special thickened metal forceps are available from Brymill Cryogenic Systems (Ellington) that stay colder longer and can be used to treat multiple lesions without having to dip into the liquid nitrogen repeatedly (Fig. 13.3).

ACTINIC KERATOSES

Actinic keratoses (Fig. 13.4) are sun-induced, premalignant lesions. Single lesions can be shaved, cauterized, or, most commonly, treated with *cryotherapy*. When cryotherapy is used, if a 1 mm freeze margin is obtained, there is a 39% complete response rate when the freeze time is less than 5 seconds, a 69% response rate when freeze rates were greater than 5 seconds, and an 83% response rate when freeze times were greater than 20 seconds. However, with 20-second freeze times, there is considerably more hypopigmentation as sequelae. Therefore freeze times should be based upon size and thickness of the lesion as well as location. Multiple lesions can be treated with topical medications (e.g., 5-fluorouracil [5-FU], imiquimod, ingenol mebutate, diclofenac), chemical peels (e.g., trichloroacetic acid), or photodynamic therapy with aminolevulinic acid and red or blue light or methyl aminolevulinate and red light. *Lesions that do not resolve require surgical sampling for histology.* These are frequently squamous cell carcinomas (SCCs; see treatment method, later). The risk that actinic keratoses will progress to SCC is probably less than 1% in early lesions and as high as 10% to 20% for persistent hypertrophic lesions. The patient should be counseled that 5-FU causes significant erythema and tenderness in the areas treated. 5-FU is applied for either 1, 2, or 4 weeks, with the 4-week course demonstrating the greatest benefit. It usually takes 4 to 6 weeks (with half of that being the active treatment) for the skin to progress through erythema, blistering, erosion, and reepithelialization. (See patient education form available at www.expertconsult.com. The manufacturer can also provide a patient education video.) Treatment with imiquimod is twice weekly for 16 weeks. Local adverse events include erythema, scabbing, and flaking. Steroid creams may be used to reduce the inflammatory response. Protection from the sun is essential.

BASAL CELL CARCINOMA

Basal cell carcinomas (BCCs) characteristically have small, centrally ulcerated depressions and raised, pearly borders (*nodular-cystic type*; Fig. 13.5A–B). However, their actual appearance can vary markedly from the classic description. *Sclerosing* (or morpheaform; Fig. 13.5C) BCCs may manifest as flat lesions with nondescript borders. Others are nonhealing ulcerations that never become elevated. Some are *pigmented* (Fig. 13.5D) and may be confused with seborrheic keratoses (SKs), nevi, or even melanomas. They may appear erythematous and bleed easily, mimicking a pyogenic granuloma. *Superficial* (Fig. 13.5E) BCCs commonly occur on the back and are flat and scaly. They may look like an SCC, actinic keratosis, eczema, or even tinea.

TABLE 13.1 Surgical Diagnosis and Management of Common Skin Lesions

Lesion	Punch Biopsy	Shave Biopsy	Shave Removal	Fusiform Excision	Incisional Biopsy	Curettement Alone	Cautery/Curettement (ED&C)	Cryotherapy	Electrosurgery (Radiofrequency)	85% Trichloroacetic Acid	Laser Ablation	Radiation	Fluorouracil 5% (5-FU)	Incision and Drainage	Other
Acrochordon (skin tags)	X^a	X^a	X^a				X^a	X	X						
Actinic keratosis	X	X	X^a	X^l	X	X	X^a	X^a	X^a	X	X		X^{ac}		X^{cok}
Angioma/hemangioma, cherry		X	X			X			X^a		X				
Angioma, spider		X	X					X	X^b		X				X^p
Bowen disease (SCC in situ)	X	X	X	X^{am}	X		X^a if <1 cm	X^a if <1 cm			X				
Cancer, basal cell	X	X		X	X		X^a	X			X	X^n	X^c		
Cancer, squamous cell	X			X^a	X		X	X^a			X	X^n	X^e		
Condylomata acuminata^c	X		X^a	X^d				X		X	X		X^e		X^c
Dermatofibroma	X	X	X^a	X^a	X						X				
Keratoacanthoma	X	X	X	X^a	X	X	X^a	X^a			X		X		
Lentigo	X	X	X	X^a	X			X	X^a	X	X				X^{ap}
Lentigo maligna	X			X^a	X			X^a							X^a
Lipomas	X			X^a											X
Melanoma	X^d	X	X	X^{am}	X	X^a									
Milia	X	X	X			X^a			X					X^a	X^j
Molluscum contagiosum		X	X			X^a		X	X	X					
Mucocele				X				X						X^a	
Neurofibroma	X	X	X^f	X	X		X^g		X^g						
Nevi, acquired	X	X	X^h	X	X				X^g						X
Nevi, atypical	X	X	X^{ai}	X^a	X										
Nevi, giant congenital	X	X		X	X						X^h				X
Paronychia								X						X^a	X
Pyogenic granuloma	X	X	X	X			X^a		X		X				X
Rashes	X	X													X X
Sebaceous cysts	X			X										X^a	
Sebaceous hyperplasia	X	X	X			X	X^a	X	X						X
Seborrheic keratosis	X	X	X^a	X^d	X	X	X	X^a	X^b		X				X^p
Telangiectases					X^d				X	X X	X				X^{ai}
Warts	X	X	X			X	X^a	X^a	X	X	X				X^{ak}
Warts, planar	X	X	X			X^a	X	X	X	X	X				X^{ai}
Warts, plantar	X	X	X					X^a	X		X				X
Xanthelasma	X	X	X	X			X		X		X				

^{a}Procedure of choice.
^{b}Face only; legs require sclerotherapy or laser. Extremely fine veins may require IPL or laser.
^{c}Imiquimod (Aldara), podofilox (Condylox), interferon; see Chapter 138, Treatment of Noncervical Condylomata Acuminata.
^{d}Used only if cancer is a possibility or nature of lesion unknown.
^{e}Not approved by the Food and Drug Administration.
^{f}Followed by cautery and curettement.
^{g}Preceded by shave removal.
^{h}Use only if certain that lesion is not a melanoma.
^{i}If used here, must be sure to use deep, saucer-shaped shave and that entire lesion removed in initial sample (do not use if melanoma is suspected).
^{j}Candida antigen; bleomycin, imiquimod (Aldara): see Chapter 30, Wart (Verruca) Treatment.
^{k}Retin-A.
^{l}Generally not indicated unless large, recurrent, or severely dysplastic.
^{m}See Table 13.2.
^{n}Radiation generally reserved for large, unresectable or recurrent lesions.
^{o}Levulan plus IPL/light therapy.
^{p}IPL, scleropathy.
ED&C, Electrodessication and curettage; IPL, intense pulsed light; SCC, squamous cell carcinoma.

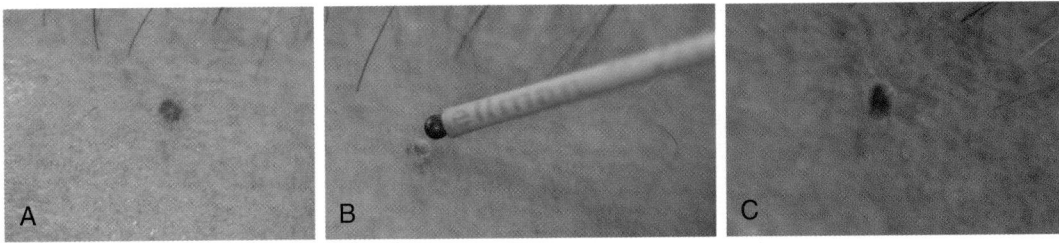

Fig. 13.1   (A) Cherry angioma/hemangioma. (B) Cautery of hemangioma. (C) Hemangioma after cautery.

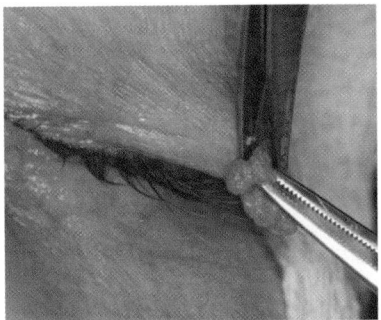

Fig. 13.2   Acrochordon removal with sharp tissue scissors.

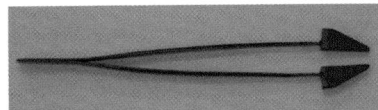

Fig. 13.3   Special cryosurgical forceps (Brymill Cryogenic Systems) with extra mass at tips to allow the freezing of multiple lesions before recooling is needed. No anesthesia is required.

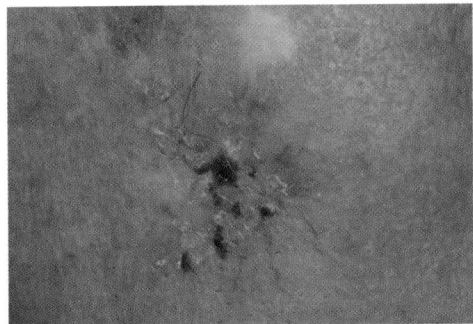

Fig. 13.4   Advanced actinic keratosis of the right cheek.

A biopsy should be taken of all nonhealing, changing, or enlarging skin lesions. Once a diagnosis is made, proper treatment can be planned. Chronic sun exposure, chronic irritation, and human papillomavirus appear to be the most common causative factors.

When a biopsy is taken of a suspected BCC, almost any area of the lesion is appropriate for sampling. If the lesion is ulcerated, it is best to sample the nonulcerated portion because the ulcer may show only necrotic changes if enough depth is not included in the sample. Normal skin from the margin is *not* needed in the specimen.

EDITOR'S NOTE: A pathologist only needs a very small, even miniscule, sample of skin to make the diagnosis of BCC. Therefore, if very sharp iris scissors are used to snip a very small sample of BCC, even without local anesthesia, it may result in less discomfort than an injection of lidocaine.

The treatment of BCCs is rather straightforward. While they are the most common human cancers, as it turns out, they are mostly a cosmetic problem. Mortality from BCC is rare unless there is long-term total neglect. BCC almost never metastasizes, so the failure of treatment will generally lead only to recurrence, which then may need referral or more aggressive treatment. They can be difficult to treat, with higher recurrence rates in the nasolabial folds and the preauricular areas. The inner canthal area can be an especially difficult area to excise and treat because of tear duct involvement. Careful follow-up is needed to detect early recurrence. Any lesion that is less than 5 to 6 mm in any location generally has an excellent response to almost any treatment modality.

There are many approaches to the treatment of BCCs. *Radiation therapy* is rarely used, but it may be necessary when the lesions are located in areas such as the lid margins, and in large lesions found on elderly patients. It is usually not recommended for sclerotic/morpheaform types, around the tear ducts where there can be scarring, or in young people when there can be long-term sequelae from the radiation.

For the majority of lesions that are smaller than 1 cm, treatment with *cautery and curettement (electrodesiccation and curettage [ED&C])* is a rapid and effective solution. Cure rates approach 95% to 98%, and scarring is usually minimal (Figs. 13.6 and 13.7). The technique is as follows:

1. After local anesthesia, scoop out the lesion with a large reusable dermal curette. (The disposable units are usually too sharp for this procedure.) Scrape the base of the lesion until a gritty feeling is encountered. Usually, it is rather easy to determine when all of the soft necrotic tissue is removed. If the lesion has not been previously sampled, send this first curettement to pathology. (Do not include tissue that is obtained after the cautery; see Fig. 13.7B.)
2. Fulgurate or cauterize the entire base with a ball electrode to destroy remaining cells and to control bleeding.
3. After the first cauterization, again vigorously curette the site to remove any of the char. Scrape until "grittiness" is felt once again.
4. Perform fulguration or cauterization a second time, as before.
5. Carry out the third and final curettement with a smaller dermal curette that more easily enters any tiny crevices in the wound site. Be careful not to penetrate too deeply and pass through the entire dermis. If this should happen, a small window of fatty tissue will be visible in the bottom of the wound, and formal excision is indicated because the tumor most likely extends deep into the subcutaneous tissue.
6. After the third curettement, fulgurate or cauterize the lesion for the final time. Place some topical astringent, a small amount of antibiotic ointment, and a dressing. Although the wound appears significantly ulcerated at this point, the long-term cosmetic results of this procedure are excellent if patients follow *moist healing* practices (see the sample patient education form available at www.expertconsult.com).

Encourage the patient to *gently* wash the area three or four times a day with soap and water to prevent an eschar from forming. Immediately after washing, have the patient apply an antibiotic ointment to keep the area moist. The ointment should not contain neomycin

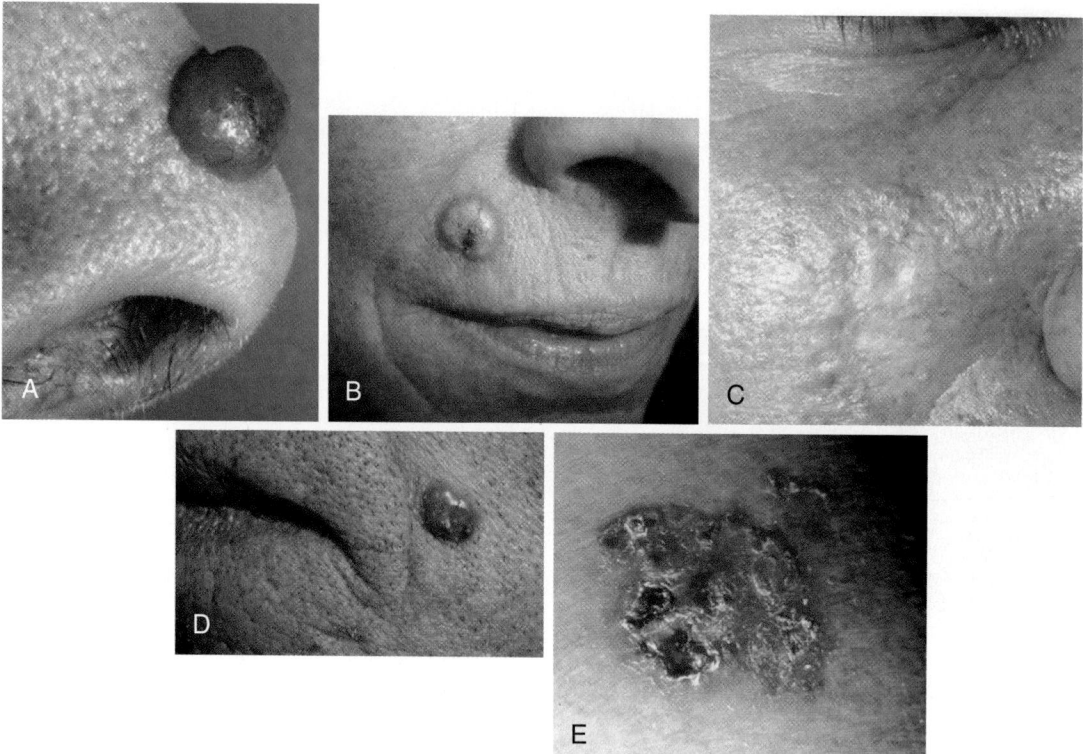

Fig. 13.5 Basal cell carcinoma. (A) Nodular, (B) nodular ulcerative, (C) morpheaform, (D) pigmented, (E) superficial.

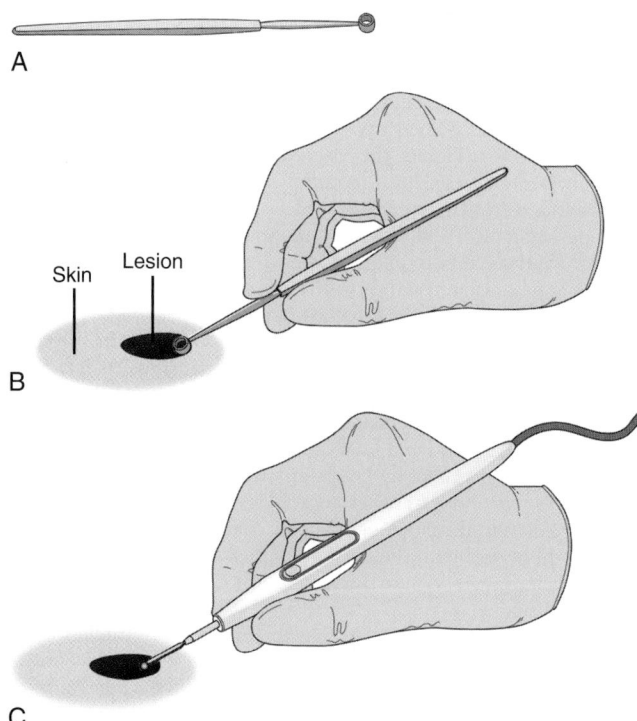

Fig. 13.6 Electrodesiccation and curettage for a basal cell carcinoma. Sequence is repeated a total of three times. (A) Dermal curette (available as disposable and reusable). In general, for cancers, the reusable curettes are used because they are not as sharp and are less likely to penetrate the dermis. (B) Lesion is curetted away. This tissue is sent to pathology for histologic diagnosis. (C) Cautery of curetted area.

(which slows reepithelialization), and it can be applied six or eight times a day, not so much to prevent infection but to aid the reepithelialization of the wound. Petroleum jelly has been found to work just as well. Allow the wound to be open unless it is under clothing. Cover it at night if necessary, to keep it moist.

Lesions in younger patients, larger-sized (>1 cm) lesions, lesions in more aggressive locations (nasolabial folds, preauricular areas, eyelids), sclerosing-type BCC lesions, recurrent lesions, and lesions with ill-defined margins may require *complete excision* to enable the pathologist to examine the margins. Remove 3 to 4 mm of normal skin around all edges (Table 13.2). Margins can be marked to aid in the histologic evaluation. Some clinicians believe that excision is more cosmetically acceptable than ED&C. An advantage of ED&C over cryotherapy is that the necrotic lesion can be "felt" with the curette, so the surgeon knows how far and how deep to proceed with the scraping. If properly cared for, most lesions treated with ED&C will only have some mild depigmentation after 4 to 6 months. They usually heal with a nice flat scar. Although *cryotherapy* reportedly is very successful, the surgeon cannot often "feel" or see the margins of the tumor. All the various clinical factors should be weighed when selecting the method for lesion removal.

Laser therapy can be used to ablate the lesions. *Topical 5-FU* and *imiquimod* have been approved to treat superficial BCCs. *Cryotherapy* has excellent results for lesions less than 1 cm wide. A good freeze 5 mm past the lesion is required, followed by thawing, then a repeat freeze (see Chapter 14, Cryosurgery). It is critical to note the thaw time. Cure rates of 98% are reported (see previous caveat).

Follow-up 3 months after treatment is recommended to ensure success of the treatment. The patient must be followed closely because 30% of patients will develop new BCCs somewhere within 3 years (Table 13.3). Since these often occur in sun-damaged areas, SCCs can also occur.

Mohs surgery is not indicated for the routine treatment of BCCs. Consider it for recurrent, morpheaform-type, or very large lesions. It may also be used for larger lesions in high-risk sites. The cost does not justify routine use because cure rates are so good with the other methods discussed here.

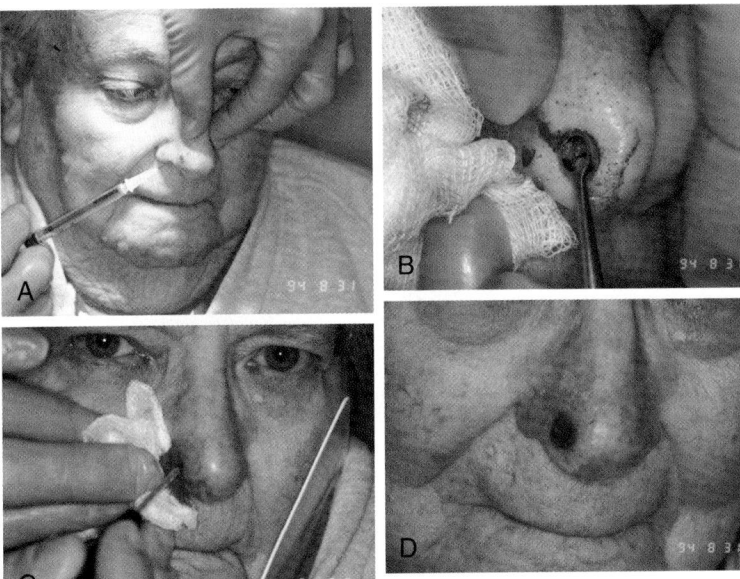

Fig. 13.7 (A) Basal cell carcinoma of right nose. (B) After administration of local anesthetic, the lesion is curetted. (C) Cautery of the base with a ball electrode. Repeat curettement and cautery for a total of three times. (D) Appearance of wound after completion of treatment. (Courtesy The Medical Procedures Center, Midland, Michigan.)

TABLE 13.2	Excisional Margins of Normal Tissue for Various Skin Lesions	
Lesion	**Margins**	
Atypical nevi		
Atypical or mild dysplasia	Be certain margins are clear (shave acceptable)	
Moderate dysplasia	2–3 mm	
Severe dysplasia	3 mm	
Actinic keratosis	2–3 mm	
Bowen disease (squamous cell carcinoma in situ)	3 mm	
Basal cell carcinoma		
Superficial	3 mm	
Nodular/ulcerative	3 mm	
Morpheaform (sclerotic, "aggressive")	5 mm	
Squamous cell carcinoma	5 mm	
Lentigo maligna (Hutchinson's freckle)	3 mm	
Lentigo maligna melanoma	As for melanoma, below	
Melanoma		
In situ	5 mm	
≤2 mm thick	1 cm or consider referral	
2.01–4 mm thick	2 cm; referral advised	
>4 mm thick	2 cm; referral advised	

TABLE 13.3	Follow-up of Various Skin Cancers After Treatment (Nonmetastatic)
Cancer	**Follow-Up**
Basal cell carcinoma	3 mo
Squamous cell carcinoma	3 mo, 6 mo to 1 yr
Melanoma	Every 4–6 mo (2–3 times) first year
	Every 6 mo (2 times) second year
	Every 1 yr lifetime (first-degree family members should be examined and counseled; stress sun avoidance/protection)

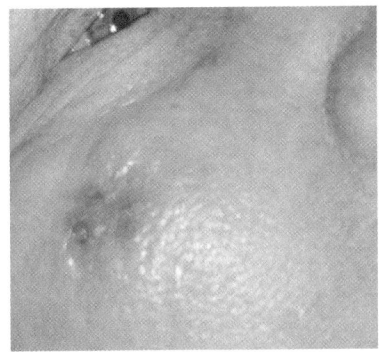

Fig. 13.8 Squamous cell carcinoma.

SQUAMOUS CELL CARCINOMA

SCC (Fig. 13.8) often appears as a diffuse, nonhealing, crusted lesion. It frequently occurs at the base of an actinic keratosis or cutaneous lesion. The lesions may be multifocal in origin and, as with actinic lesions, are due to solar damage. SCCs are more aggressive than BCCs and they can metastasize, although this is rare. Palpation of the lesion can help predict the aggressiveness or the risk of metastasis; the thicker or more indurated the lesion, the higher the risk. Because the margins of these lesions are often not very clear, many clinicians prefer to excise all invasive SCCs. If 5-FU (Efudex) or masoprocol (Actinex) creams or cryotherapy are used to treat diffuse actinic changes, any post-treatment residual lesions (after 6 to 8 weeks) should be removed for biopsy to rule out SCC. When a biopsy is performed on a suspected SCC, try to include portions of the central area. A deep punch biopsy into subcutaneous fat is preferred by many pathologists, but a deep saucer-type shave is adequate, with definitive therapy after pathology results. Early or small lesions can be treated with ED&C (see Figs. 13.6 and 13.7) or with cryotherapy, with excellent results (see earlier). If the lesion is excised, include at least 5 mm margins of normal tissue to be sure the malignancy is removed (see Table 13.2).

SCC in situ (Bowen disease) is a severely dysplastic lesion that has not yet invaded beyond the epidermis. This lesion should be treated similarly to SCC.

Lesions (especially the more invasive ones) should be reevaluated in 3 and 6 months to document cure. Evaluation of the lymph nodes draining the area is also prudent (see Table 13.3).

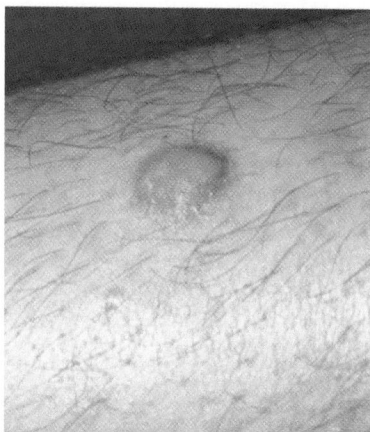

Fig. 13.9   Dermatofibroma.

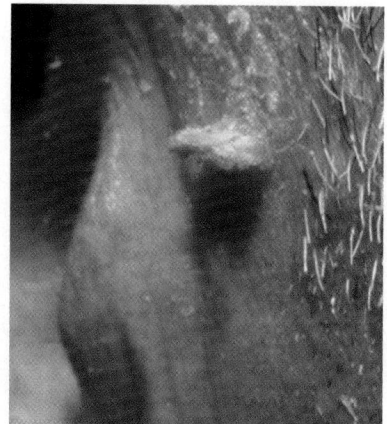

Fig. 13.10   Cutaneous horn.

Coding for skin cancer treatment is complicated. The biller must know the size, location, and method of removal to bill correctly.

CONDYLOMATA ACUMINATA

Many therapeutic interventions are available to treat condylomata acuminata. See Chapter 138, Treatment of Noncervical Condylomata Acuminata.

DERMATOFIBROMA

Dermatofibromas (Fig. 13.9) often occur on the anterior surface of the lower leg, but can frequently be found elsewhere. The etiology is unknown, but dermatofibromas may represent a fibrous reaction to trauma, viral infection, or insect bites. They are often confused with verrucae or nevi. Dermatofibromas do not progress to cancers, and once the diagnosis of dermatofibroma is confirmed, the clinician can merely observe the lesion. However, until the lesion is sampled, only an educated guess is possible. Many BCCs of the lower extremities mimic dermatofibromas. A rapidly growing lesion could also be a dermatofibrosarcoma. Dermatofibromas are generally deep-seated and require excision if complete removal is desired. Cryotherapy can be attempted, but dermatofibromas are generally quite cryoresistant. A punch biopsy is an easy remedy for most dermatofibromas, and provides a pathology specimen, but will leave a small straight-line scar. Because the lesions are often on the legs and are prone to cutting when the patient shaves, the most judicious approach may be for the clinician to shave the lesion flat, which provides tissue for confirmatory diagnosis and reduces the likelihood of further trauma. A pigmented spot may remain, but at least it will be flat. Cryotherapy can be used after the shave. If the final results are not satisfactory, it can still be punched, excised or treated with cryotherapy. The most definitive therapy is punch or excisional biopsy.

CUTANEOUS HORN

A cutaneous horn (Fig. 13.10) is a type of actinic keratosis. Use caution to rule out an early SCC at the base. Usually a deep saucer-type shave is performed, followed by cautery. Tissue should be sent to pathology for verification.

KERATOACANTHOMA

Keratoacanthoma (Fig. 13.11) is a common, benign epithelial tumor found in elderly patients. This lesion may have a viral etiology. Keratoacanthoma often is confused with SCC, but it is a distinct entity and often considered an "SCC variant" because it cannot be differentiated histologically from SCC. In fact, dermatologic pathologists will now often diagnose it as an SCC in situ. (This allows for it to be billed as excision or destruction of a malignant lesion.) The *history of rapid growth* is critical for the pathologist to make the proper diagnosis.

The lesion begins as a dome-shaped papule that continues to enlarge rapidly. It can cause some local aching or tenderness. A fully developed tumor is a round, dome-shaped mass with a central keratin-filled crater often 1 to 2 cm in size. The lesion may stop growing after 6 weeks, and then it may slowly regress over the next 12 months. These lesions often occur on the dorsum of the hands, ears, and neck. Clinically they often appear to be BCCs, but if curettement is attempted they are much more sclerotic and fibrous, unlike the classic BCC.

Because these lesions grow rapidly, most clinicians do not advocate simple observation. Cryotherapy (small lesions only), a deep saucer-type shave, ED&C (×3), or conventional excision with 3- to 5-mm margins provides acceptable treatment. Keratoacanthomas can recur, very rapidly, and patients should be followed closely during and after treatment. The major differential diagnoses for the clinician include BCC and SCC. Because of the rapid growth and high number of mitotic cells, even pathologists experience difficulty and often will report that they "cannot rule out invasive SCC" at the base. Subsequently, the therapeutic approach is essentially the same as for an SCC.

SEBORRHEIC KERATOSES

Seborrheic keratoses (Fig. 13.12) are benign, hyperkeratinized, superficial epidermal lesions that occur commonly with aging. Their size ranges from 2 mm to 3 cm. When magnified, they appear cauliflower-like and merely "stuck on"; patients have been known to call them "barnacles." They have no malignant potential. The typical lesion has the appearance that it can be easily lifted off with a fingernail. Patients often say that they have removed the lesion or rubbed it off with a towel, only to have it recur. SKs are occasionally confused with BCCs, SCCs, nevi, and verrucous lesions. Pigmented lesions can mimic a melanoma. Pathology reports often use the term *verruciform keratosis.*

Most SKs can be easily removed, after local anesthesia, with the *radiofrequency* (electrosurgery) *shave* technique. A curette will also often do the job. Frequently, if performed rapidly, the patient will require no anesthesia. Alternatively, *shave excision with mild curetting* of the base can be performed. This can be done with a single-edge flexible razor, Dermablade, or scalpel followed by curette. Hemostasis can be accomplished with Monsel solution or aluminum chloride. Minimal scarring should result because the lesion is superficial. *Cryotherapy* is the most frequently used method. No anesthesia is needed, but this treatment may cause a little more discomfort. Liquid nitrogen is the quickest approach, especially if multiple lesions are present

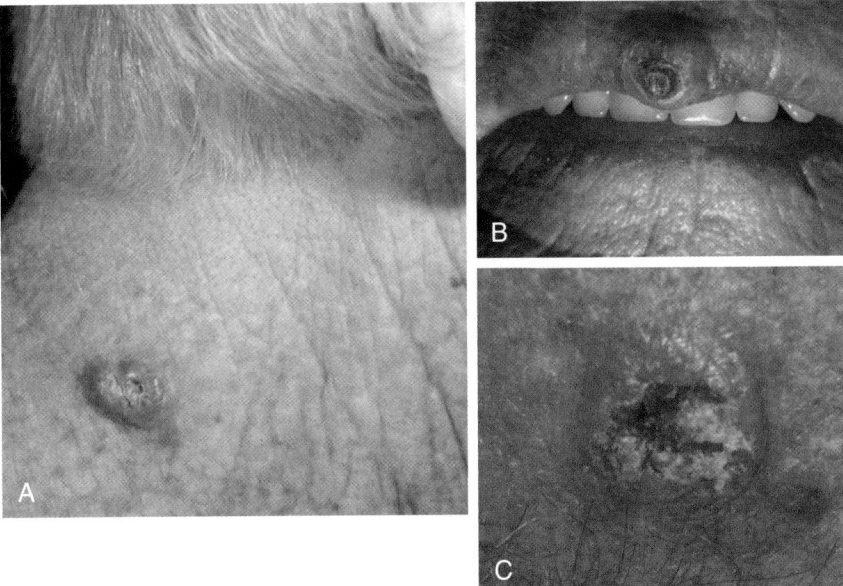

Fig. 13.11   Keratoacanthomas.

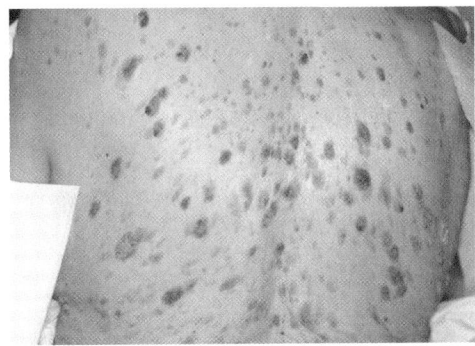

Fig. 13.12   Seborrheic keratoses.

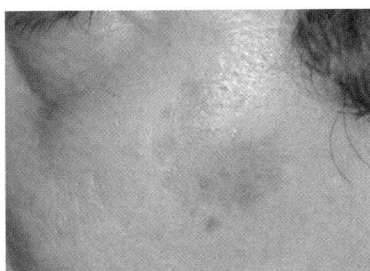

Fig. 13.13   Lentigo.

(use the spray thermos applicators). After treatment, a blister may form or the lesion may just dry up and fall off. It is essential that the clinician be absolutely sure of the diagnosis if cryotherapy is to be used. Any lesions that persist need to be sampled. If many SKs occur all at once, consider an internal malignancy (Leser-Trélat sign).

Medicare does not reimburse for the removal of SKs unless they are inflamed (i.e., markedly irritated or pruritic, bleeding, or rapidly growing), or if the diagnosis is uncertain.

EDITOR'S NOTE: a light pinch ("pinch anesthesia") over a seborrheic keratosis by the clinician before curettement is often briefly numbing and therefore appreciated by patients.

LENTIGO

Lentigos (Fig. 13.13) are common brownish or tan macules that occur on the sun-exposed areas of the face, shoulders, arms, and hands. They are often called "liver spots" or "senior freckles." Lentigos increase in number during childhood and adult life, and occasionally fade spontaneously. Biopsy of lesions with irregular borders or dark pigmentation should be performed to rule out lentigo maligna melanoma. *Cryotherapy* is the treatment of choice of benign lesions. Although bleaching and depigmenting creams may be tried, they will need to be used lifelong. *Superficial ablation techniques* with laser, radiofrequency, or trichloroacetic acid also may work. The latest, most effective approach is to use intense pulsed light (IPL) treatment, but the technology is expensive (see Chapter 44, Fractional Laser Skin Resurfacing).

LENTIGO MALIGNA (MELANOMA IN SITU)

Lentigo maligna is a sun-associated precursor of lentigo maligna melanoma, a type of invasive melanoma. These lesions can grow to be several centimeters in diameter and usually occur on the face. They are slow-growing macules with irregular borders and pigmentation. These lesions often are confused with lentigos, which are smaller, have a homogeneous color, and appear mainly over the dorsa of the hands and forearms. The estimated lifetime risk of transformation from lentigo maligna to melanoma is 4.7%, and some clinicians prefer close observation as the treatment of choice. Unless absolutely sure of the diagnosis, a biopsy should be done. Surgical excision with 5 mm margins is indicated.

LIPOMAS

Lipomas (Fig. 13.14) present as a palpable mass under the skin. Most lesions are nontender, move freely, and have a soft, irregular consistency. The differential includes a sebaceous cyst. Cysts have pores; lipomas do not. Cysts are more tense to palpation. Lipomas usually do not progress to malignancy, but rapidly growing or changing lesions should be removed to rule out liposarcoma. Removal is usually done to alleviate patient concerns or for cosmetic reasons; it may also be necessary when lipomas occur in areas of pressure or when they cause pain or discomfort. Lesions on the lower extremities have a higher likelihood of malignant degeneration. Lesions up to 3 cm are removed by making a 1- to 2-cm incision through the dermis after injecting as little as 1 mL of 2% lidocaine with epinephrine. Sterile preparation and draping are not needed. The clinician should make the incision in line with the skin lines and use hemostats or curved

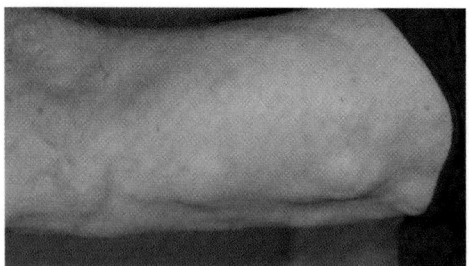

Fig. 13.14 Arm with multiple lipomas.

tissue scissors to dissect the lesion from the surrounding adhering tissue. Pressure on the base of the lesion (lateral pressure, meaning from the lateral aspect) often will extrude the lipoma through the small incision (Fig. 13.15). Some lipomas are encapsulated, but more often the margins are obscure. It may be difficult to determine whether all of the lesion has been removed because the fat involved looks just like normal fat. It is best to remove any loosely adhering fatty tissue in the cavity. Bleeding is minimal. Closure usually can be obtained with Steri-Strips or tissue glue, followed by a pressure dressing. Once the diagnosis of lipoma has been made in one area, other similar lesions do not necessarily require removal unless they are symptomatic. (Lesions that are larger than 3 to 4 cm may require formal excision with a sterile technique and suture closure.)

There are special CPT codes for removal of these lesions under "Excision of Benign Tumors." The code is independent of the method used for removal (see Appendix G, Neoplasms, Skin: ICD-10 Codes).

EDITOR'S NOTE: It is my experience that about 1 in 3 lipomas merely "pop out" with a very small incision, minimal dissection, and application of lateral pressure. Another 1 in 3 require more dissection, and perhaps grasping with a hemostat. The final 1 in 3 require enlarging the incision, grasping with a hemostat, and considerable dissection.

MELANOMA

The major caveat regarding melanomas (Fig. 13.16) is that the *depth of the lesion is very important in determining appropriate definitive treatment.* Primary care clinicians should not feel uncomfortable about performing a biopsy of any lesion with characteristics that may be consistent with a melanoma. A biopsy does not spread the lesion or limit life expectancy in any way. On the contrary, early diagnosis may save the patient's life. The mnemonic A, B, C, D, E, F, G can be used as an aid for remembering the clinical features of malignant melanoma:

Asymmetry
Border irregularity
Color variegation
Diameter more than 6 mm
Elevation above skin surface
Feeling different (including pruritus); "F" also is a reminder to check family history
Growth or change

Because it is so important to determine the depth of the lesion, *never* perform a shave biopsy or shave removal *if melanoma is a consideration* (see Chapter 26, Skin Biopsy). When choosing a site for punch or incisional biopsy within a pigmented lesion, choose the area that is most nodular or atypical (darkest in color, inflamed, or irregular). The majority of pigmented lesions removed are atypical nevi. *Saucer-type shaves are acceptable for biopsy and removal if the clinical impression is that melanoma is unlikely.* All atypical nevi cannot be excised with suture closure. It is too time consuming and costly. If there is a clinical suspicion for melanoma, perform a punch biopsy, which provides depth and the information needed for further

treatment. However, if the working diagnosis is an atypical nevus, a shave biopsy is adequate. To save lives, atypical lesions need to be sampled, and shave excisions are the most expedient. Some unsuspected melanomas may be transected, but at least they will be diagnosed and further care can be initiated.

For lesions that invade less than 2 mm thick, excision with 1-cm clear margins around the lesion is indicated. Excisions margins for thicker lesions is outlined in Table 13.4. It has been difficult to demonstrate survival benefit of wide margin excision over a narrower margin as shown in 2009 systematic Cochrane review (Sladden).

MILIA

Milia are very small (1 to 3 mm) white, keratinized cysts, seen most often on the face and in the genital area. They are frequently seen in the newborn period and may require no treatment because the lesions usually regress spontaneously. However, they can also appear in late childhood or in adults and are often more persistent. Milia can be managed with a punch biopsy, shave biopsy, shave removal, or curettement. The clinician can also manage them similar to molluscum by nicking the surface with a scalpel blade, sterile needle, or sharp end of a comedone extractor and expressing the keratin contents. These small nicks rarely require anesthesia.

MOLLUSCUM CONTAGIOSUM

The lesions of molluscum contagiosum (Fig. 13.17) are small, 2- to 3-mm, papular, wartlike excrescences with central umbilication. They are painless and rarely cause pruritus. They usually appear as a crop of multiple lesions in young children, or later in adolescents and young adults as they become sexually active. Expectant observation is certainly acceptable because the lesions will spontaneously resolve (3 to 18 months), but many patients desire to have these viral lesions removed. Table 13.1 describes the treatments that are possible. Curettement with a small disposable (sharp) dermal curette or cryotherapy is the treatment of choice. Nicking the top of the lesion with a scalpel blade, sterile needle, or sharp end of a comedone extractor may facilitate curettement. Treatment rarely requires anesthesia, but topicals can be tried (see Chapter 4, Topical Anesthesia).

NEUROFIBROMAS

Neurofibromas (Fig. 13.18) are soft, nodular lesions that often appear to be minimally pigmented nevi. However, when a shave excision is performed a soft, jelly-like material is seen at the base. This is the pathognomonic sign of a neurofibroma. The soft tissue is curetted and the base cauterized. A significant cavity may exist, but with moist healing techniques the results are excellent. These lesions do not have to be removed unless they are symptomatic or if a diagnosis is needed. Excision with suture closure is needed for the larger lesions. Free margins of 1 mm are adequate. These lesions may recur, and a local steroid injection may be all that is needed to minimize symptoms. Younger patients (<20 years old) with neurofibromas should be followed because there may be a possibility for conversion to neurofibrosarcoma.

PYOGENIC GRANULOMAS

Pyogenic granulomas (Fig. 13.19) are small, rapidly growing, nodular, friable, vascular lesions that often bleed when touched. They occur at sites of trauma or previous surgery. Because of their vascular nature, pyogenic granulomas are best treated with curettement followed by cautery of the base. These lesions will recur if any tissue remains, and some clinicians advocate complete excision. They are often very easily treated with a punch biopsy, and all attempts should

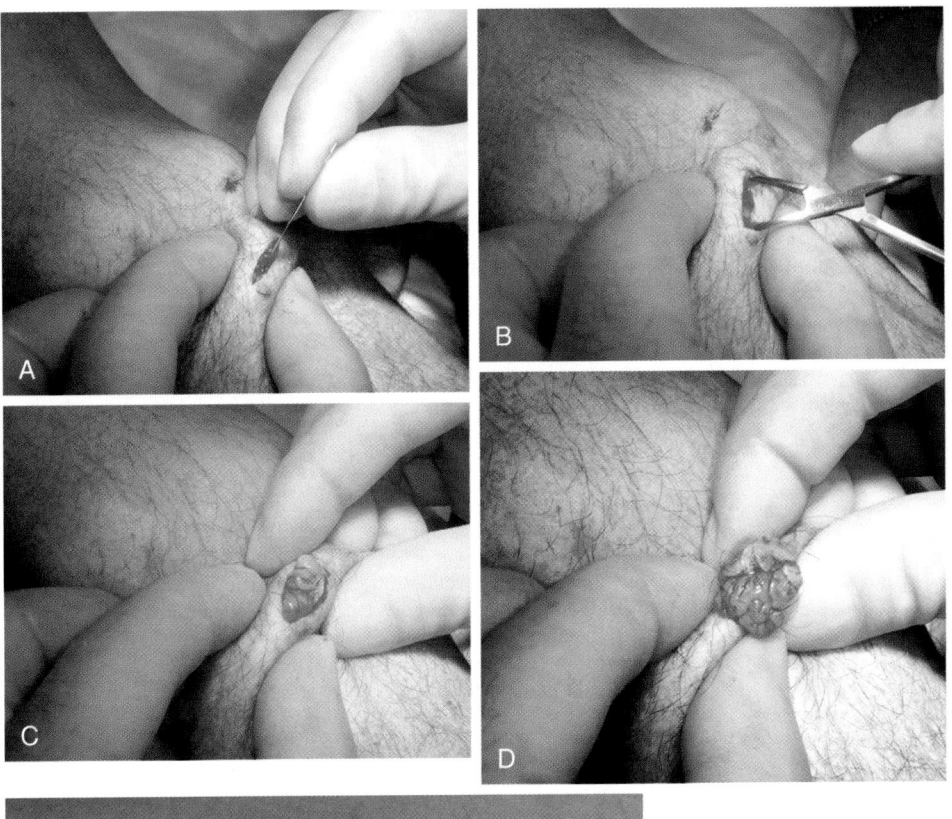

Fig. 13.15 Simple technique for removing lipomas. (A) After local anesthesia is administered, incise and drain the lipoma. (B) Lysing adhesions with hemostat. (C) Expressing the lipoma. (D) Completing removal. Wound is closed with Steri-Strips and a pressure dressing applied. (E) Appearance 1 week after removal of lipoma using this technique.

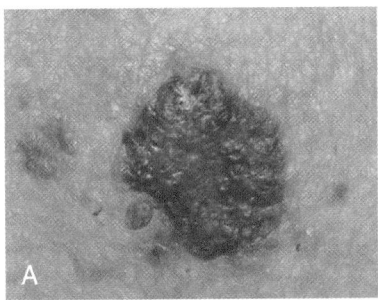
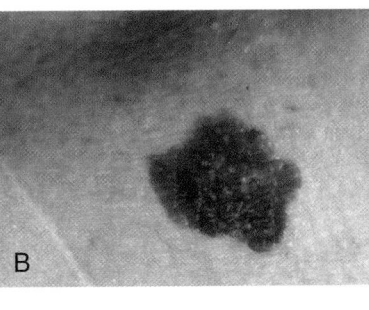
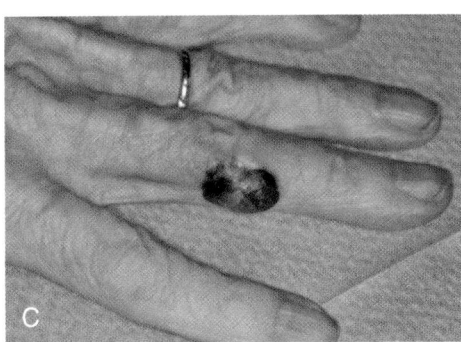

Fig. 13.16 Melanomas.

be made to remove the base to prevent recurrence. Pyogenic granulomas can be confused with BCCs.

ACQUIRED NEVI ("MOLES")

Acquired nevi are benign, melanocytic nevi that are absent at birth and first appear in early childhood. The lesions become more numerous until middle age, and the majority of white adults have several acquired nevi. Lesions are generally found on sun-exposed areas because the sun induces their growth.

Common acquired nevi follow a predictable developmental progression (Fig. 13.20). The earliest lesions are junctional nevi (see Fig. 13.20A), with the nevus cells at the junction between the dermis and epidermis. By late adolescence, the growths develop into compound nevi (see Fig. 13.20B), with nevus cells in both the dermis and epidermis. Compound nevi may develop hairs. By late adulthood, the lesions regress into intradermal nevi and appear nonpigmented (see Fig. 13.20C).

If the lesions lose their pigment, they may turn pink or flesh-colored. At all stages, common benign acquired nevi have smooth,

TABLE 13.4	Treatment of Suspect Pigmented Lesions and Melanomas	
Stage	**Recommended Treatment**	**Survival**
Suspect pigmented lesion	Punch, incisional, or excisional biopsy down to subcutaneous fat	Not affected by biopsy procedure
Suspected positive lymph node with melanoma	Fine-needle aspiration biopsy or excision	Not affected by biopsy procedure
Melanoma in situ (limited to epidermis)	Excision with margin of 5 mm normal skin and layer of subcutaneous tissue No further radiographs or laboratory work indicated	Not affected
Melanoma thickness ≤2 mm	Excision with margin of 1 cm normal skin and subcutaneous tissue down to fascia No further radiographs or laboratory work indicated unless lesion is ulcerated or has high mitotic count	95% (8 yr)
Melanoma thickness 2.01–4 mm	After diagnostic biopsy, wide-margin (2 cm) excision and adjunctive therapy should be considered (refer)	Poor
Melanoma thickness >4 mm	After diagnostic biopsy, wide-margin excision and adjunctive therapy should be considered (refer)	Poor

Modified from NIH Consensus Conference: Diagnosis and treatment of early melanoma. *JAMA.* 1992;268:1314–1319.

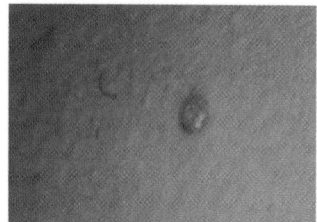

Fig. 13.17   Molluscum contagiosum.

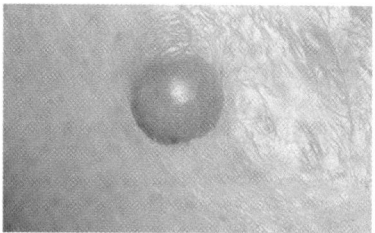

Fig. 13.18   Neurofibroma.

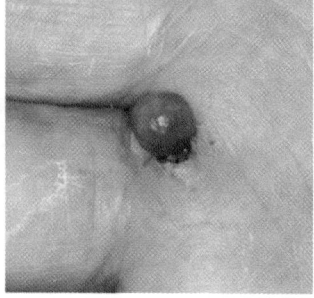

Fig. 13.19   Pyogenic granuloma.

distinct, symmetric borders. Patients with large numbers of acquired nevi should be monitored closely because they are at higher risk for developing melanoma.

Raised or pedunculated benign nevi can best be excised with a shave removal technique (optimized with the radiofrequency technique; see Chapter 25, Radiofrequency Surgery [Modern Electrosurgery]). There should be no suspicion whatsoever of melanoma if a shave technique is used. If malignancy is even a remote possibility, either a full-thickness biopsy of the lesion should be performed before removal, or the lesion should be treated by complete excision rather than shave removal. Treatment of melanomas is based solely on the depth of the lesion (see previous discussion). Superficial nevi usually do not recur, but the deeper compound nevi often do recur unless the full depth of the lesion is excised. It is difficult to determine when the entire lesion has been removed using a shave technique. The deeper dermal lesions are generally flat, whereas the superficial epidermal lesions are raised or pedunculated.

A *halo nevus* (Fig. 13.21) is an acquired nevus that develops a white halo around it. This is a sign that the immune system is activating against the mole, and it will soon disappear. It is the only change in a nevus that does not need a biopsy.

DYSPLASTIC NEVI

Dysplastic nevi (Fig. 13.22; a histologic diagnosis), or atypical moles (a clinical diagnosis but now also used synonymously with "dysplastic" by many pathologists), are acquired nevi that become dysplastic (precancerous) over time. The lesions are usually larger than common acquired nevi (>5 mm) and may have irregular margins, variable pigmentation, and irregular surface contours. They are somewhat common, occurring in approximately 1 in 10 Americans. Because the risk for melanoma is increased in patients with atypical moles and because melanoma can develop from an atypical lesion, some clinicians advocate full excision of suspect lesions. Shave excisions, if done, must be deep and saucer shaped to ensure the entire depth of the lesion is removed. Once the technique of the shave excision is mastered, six to eight nevi can be shaved off in a single 15-minute visit. Using the radiofrequency smoothing technique and moist healing minimizes scarring. Patients can have so many atypical nevi that it precludes excising all of them. These patients need to be followed closely, as do their family members. Sun protection is a must.

Should the pathologist report that the "margins are positive" in an atypical or dysplastic nevus, it may behoove the surgeon to remove more tissue to ensure that the entire lesion has been removed, especially for those lesions with severe atypia. Whether this removal is through another shave or a frank excision with suture closure depends on the exact pathology. In dysplastic nevi with mild to moderate atypia, it may not be as important to reexcise if the margins are positive; close observation may be adequate. Two outcome studies (2009, 2010) demonstrated no development of melanoma in 5-year follow-up (55 dysplastic nevi in one study) whether margins were positive or not in patients with mild to moderate atypia. It should also be kept in mind that there is shrinkage of lesions when placed in formalin, meaning the original margins may have been clear, but the lesion shrank up to the margin in formalin.

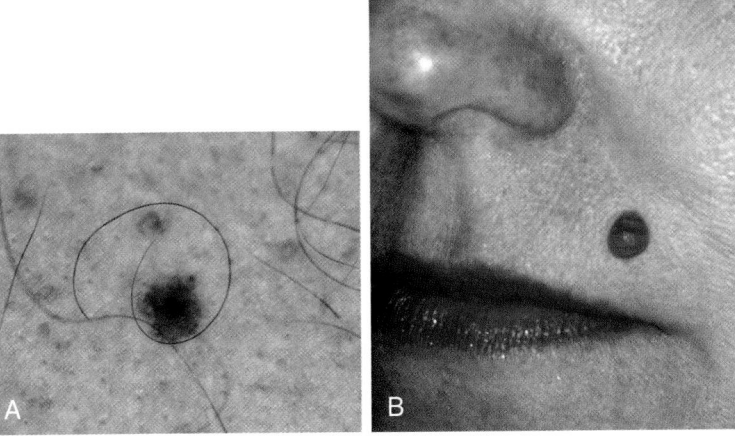
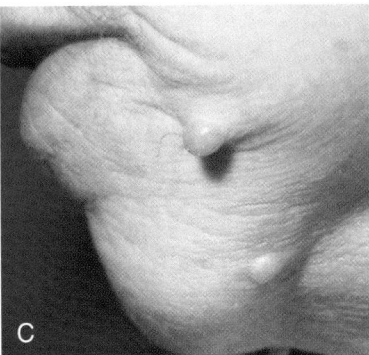

Fig. 13.20   (A) Junctional nevus. (B) Compound nevus. (C) Intradermal nevus.

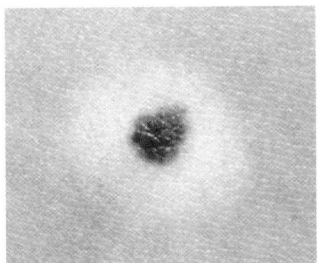

Fig. 13.21   Halo nevus.

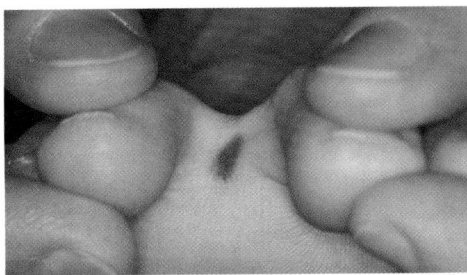

Fig. 13.22   Dysplastic nevus.

CONGENITAL NEVI

The approach to congenital nevi is based on three factors: size, color, and family history. Congenital nevi *larger than 20 cm²* often extend over large portions of the body. The lesions grow proportionally with the anatomic site, their surfaces may be irregular, and they may contain coarse hairs. Their management is controversial because excision is difficult and deforming. The lifetime risk of these nevi developing into melanoma is 5% to 20%; therefore some clinicians advocate early removal and grafting. Others advocate close monitoring. Melanoma can develop at any site in the lesion, and biopsies of the most irregular portions of the lesions may not detect malignant change. Efforts to completely eradicate these lesions must be tempered by the potential for treatment-induced scarring and disfigurement. A 1996 study by De Raeve and colleagues suggests that vigorous curettement in the first weeks of life may be the best alternative.

Lesions between 1.5 and 20 cm² are easier to excise, and this has been generally recommended. Lesions *less than 1.5 cm²* are the easiest to excise but also have the lowest malignant potential. Certainly, those that are located in areas that are difficult to observe (e.g., scalp, buttocks) should be removed. Shave excisions usually are not adequate because congenital nevi are deep lesions.

Another factor to consider is the degree of pigmentation. *Very light moles* are less likely to degenerate into a cancer; when then do, they do so later (after age 20 years), which allows early detection of changes. *Dark, almost black, lesions* are more likely to transform into melanoma; when they do, they do so earlier (teenage years) and are difficult to monitor, making their removal more appropriate.

The most recent recommendations suggest observation for all congenital nevi, as with other nevi, unless changes are observed. The clinician will need to help the patient and the family sort through the various recommendations and decide on a course that is acceptable to all, including the local prevailing medical opinion.

PARONYCHIA

Paronychia (Fig. 13.23) is an infection of the distal phalanx along the proximal and lateral edges of the nail. Paronychia produces signs of local infection, including redness, tenderness, and swelling. Mild paronychia can be treated with soaks and topical antibiotics. More significant infections may develop into abscesses. As with all abscesses, it is best to incise and drain (I&D) them once a loculated area of purulence can be identified. A digital block may be needed, depending on size. The incision technique is illustrated in Fig. 13.24. Occasionally, packing may be used to keep the abscess from reaccumulating, but usually these abscesses are so small that packing cannot be accomplished. Topical antibiotics (e.g., mupirocin [Bactroban]) may be beneficial, but unless there is marked cellulitis or the patient is immunocompromised, systemic antibiotics are rarely indicated. Chronic paronychia may be caused by fungal infection.

RASHES (EXANTHEMS, DERMATOSES)

In many cases, biopsy of a "rash" or ill-defined dermatologic lesion is not very helpful. Unless the clinical diagnosis is fairly clear, the primary care clinician may be wise to obtain a dermatology consultation. Biopsies of these lesions may be indicated for clarification of a fairly discrete differential diagnosis (as with inflammatory dermatoses) or for ruling out a cutaneous neoplasm.

When multiple sites are involved, the following simple guidelines may be followed for selecting a lesion for a biopsy specimen: It is best to *select those areas that have the primary inflammatory changes* but are free from secondary changes such as crusting, fissuring, erosion, ulceration, and infection. *Choose sites where the scar will not be obvious* and where hypertrophic scarring is generally not a problem.

If the primary lesion is a *macule*, select a "fresh" lesion that is more abnormal in color. Generally, perform a punch biopsy, advancing the punch into the subcutaneous fat. *Papules* should be removed completely, if possible. Select a mature lesion without secondary changes. If the lesion is a *plaque*, the biopsy specimen should consist of the thickest area through the full depth into the subcutaneous fat. The same technique is used for *nodular* lesions and *suspected neoplastic* lesions. For *vesicles and bullae*, choose an intact lesion whenever possible. Rupturing a sac makes histologic interpretation more difficult. *Sample these lesions at the margin where the blister roof is attached to the remainder of the specimen, and include normal skin.* This is virtually the only time normal skin is helpful in a biopsy to make a diagnosis (vesicular bullous disease). (See Chapter 26, Skin Biopsy.)

SEBACEOUS HYPERPLASIA (ADENOSUM SEBACEUM)

Adenosum sebaceum, or senile sebaceous gland hyperplasia, is characterized by small growths composed of enlarged sebaceous glands (Fig. 13.25A). These very small, 2- to 5-mm lesions can mimic early BCC. If numerous lesions are present in the temporal and forehead areas, they are very *unlikely* to be cancerous; BCCs usually are solitary. Treatment consists of removal of the elevated portions of the papule with shave, sharp curettement, or electrosurgical techniques. Often the lesion is deeply seated, and, unless curetted, it will not be entirely removed. Unlike a soft necrotic cancer, these lesions are very dense and fibrotic. Biopsy is indicated if the nature of the lesion is uncertain. However, treatment can usually be carried out on the basis of the clinical diagnosis. Cryotherapy also works well for smaller lesions.

SEBACEOUS CYSTS

The *epidermal inclusion cyst*, or *sebaceous cyst*, is a round, tense, keratinizing cyst that is freely mobile and very superficial (see Fig. 13.25B–C).

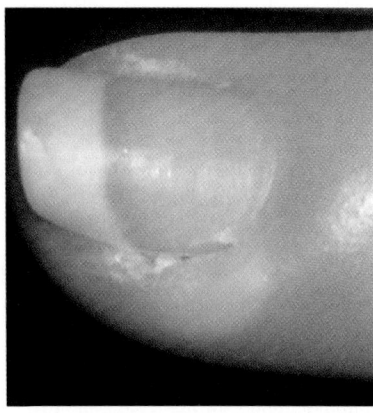

Fig. 13.23   Paronychia.

When located in the scalp, they are called *trichilemmal cysts (wens, pilar cysts).* Most patients present with a slowly growing lesion that on physical examination is subcutaneous, smooth, and nontender. A history of drainage or inflammation with purulent discharge may or may not be present, and this does help solidify the diagnosis. A small central punctum (pore) or opening helps differentiate a sebaceous cyst from a lipoma.

Note the following three precautions:

1. Lesions in the preauricular areas should be examined closely because parotid tumors (both adenomas and adenocarcinomas) can present as apparent "cysts." If there is any question, obtain a needle biopsy or computed tomography scan before attempting removal.
2. "Cysts," especially in infants (but also in children), have a higher likelihood of being dermoids (also known as *fusion plane cysts*), which may have fistulous connections with deeper spaces. Fortunately, cysts in the most common location of the lateral third of the eyebrow can be easily removed. But all others, including on the nasal bridge, the scalp, the neck, and the postauricular areas, may have intracranial connections. Consider magnetic resonance imaging first to exclude a contiguous tract. If present, removal will require a neurosurgical consult. Seventy percent of dermoid cysts will appear by 5 years of age and are more worrisome if they contain hair or capillary changes.
3. "Everything is what it is until it ain't." The majority of sebaceous cysts are easy to differentiate. However, they have been misdiagnosed, with the underlying pathologic process being metastatic melanoma or other cancer. The only way to be sure of the diagnosis is to remove them.

Many clinicians believe asymptomatic lesions can be watched. The down side to this strategy is that the lesion can grow, making removal more difficult. Or, they can become infected. If the patient asks for removal because of irritative symptoms or growth, the lesion should be removed. Once the characteristic sebaceous material and smell are observed, they *do not* need to be sent to pathology.

In the past, a surgeon's adeptness was often judged by whether he or she could remove the lesion intact without rupturing the capsule. This requires a sterile technique and a fairly generous incision over the area with judicious removal of the *entire* sac to decrease the likelihood of any recurrence. The cavity is then irrigated and closed with sutures.

Maintaining an intact sac during removal is no longer thought to be required. A simpler technique may be performed, often described as the minimally invasive technique, especially in areas where the skin is thinner (e.g., face), though it does not work as well with thick skin (e.g., back). When injecting local anesthetic, a minimal amount should be injected into the sac. Most of the anesthetic should be injected superficially so that it spreads immediately under the skin at

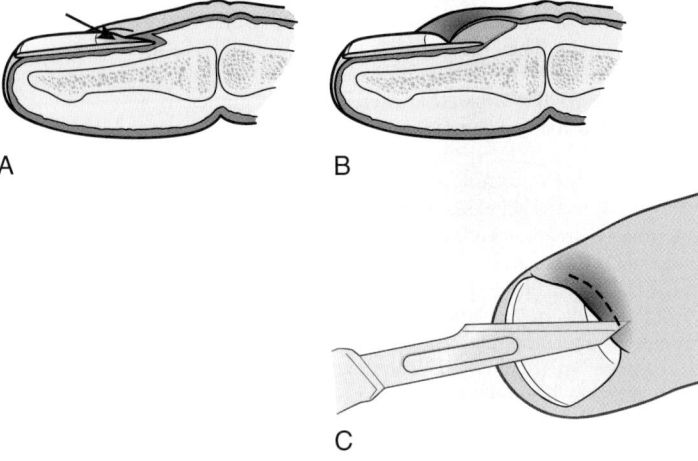

A   B

C

Fig. 13.24   Separation of the cuticle from the nail *(arrow)* (A) can lead to a paronychia (B). In acute paronychia, drain any pus and consider a culture. (C) A simple nick through the most translucent area of the abscess is usually all that is required.

the injection site and over a large portion of the sac. (Avoid inject-ing too near the pore; the anesthetic may shoot straight back at the surgeon.) After local anesthesia is achieved, a small, 5- to 6-mm incision is made directly into the cyst using a No. 11 blade. Some prefer to use a 3- or 4-mm sharp dermal punch, especially in areas where the skin is thick such as the scalp. All contents are expressed using external or lateral pressure. Frequently (especially in scalp cysts, where the sac is thick and firm), this external pressure will not only extrude the sebaceous material of the cyst but the sac itself (Fig. 13.26). (A slightly larger punch biopsy, 4 mm or larger, should be used on the scalp because of the thickness of the skin and sac size.) If the sac is not produced, then curved hemostats are inserted into the wound and repeated attempts are made to grasp the sac and gently tug it out in its entirety. External or lateral pressure should be applied while the sac is grasped and being tugged with a hemostat. A 3- to 4-mm dermal curette can also be inserted into the cavity to curette away any possible residual sac. No suture closure is indi-cated, so a sterile technique (e.g., draping) is not indicated. If blood accumulates or the wound gets infected (both very rare), the patient just expresses it. Should some of the sac be left behind and the cyst reform, then formal excision with suture closure will be required. Usually the recurring cyst is much smaller (pea-sized), and can be removed with a punch biopsy and 1 or 2 interrupted sutures—a much smaller incision than would be necessary if the entire sac had been originally removed intact.

This simple method of cyst treatment is usually successful unless the cyst is quite large (>2 cm), it has been infected previously (should wait at least 2 months after being infected before attempting removal; this allows time for inflammation and induration to resolve), a previ-ous attempt at removal has been made (causing surrounding scarring), or it is deep in the skin tissue. Wens, large and small (0.5 to 4 cm), are almost always treated successfully with the minimal incision tech-nique, even with prior infection. The sacs are much thicker—almost like ping-pong balls. Three to four wens can readily be removed in a 15-minute visit (Fig. 13.27). Most sebaceous cysts can be treated with this simple method with little risk of recurrence.

A variation on the technique just described is to insert two large iodine crystals (iodine crystals USP) into the sac after expres-sion of the contents. The sac contracts around the crystals in 48 to 72 hours; the clinician then easily expresses the entire complex through the incision. This technique also can be used if it appears that the entire sac has not been removed using the simple technique described previously.

For those cysts in which the aforementioned method is not rec-ommended (as noted), excision is necessary. Perform a field block with local anesthesia. Using a scalpel, make a small fusiform inci-sion in the direction of the skin lines over the top of the cyst that includes the punctum. The length should be just less than the size of the cyst. Be careful to incise lightly because the skin is often very thin. Dissect deeply first into the adipose tissue at the two ends of the incision, being careful not to rupture the sac. Curved Metzen-baum scissors work well. Use an Allis clamp to grasp the wedge of skin (still attached) over the cyst. Apply only light pressure because the skin separates easily. However, this traction will lift up the cyst below. Continue dissection until the cyst is free. Should the cyst rupture, one can proceed with the dissection, or express the entire contents, then continue to dissect out the sac. Be sure to remove the entire sac or the cyst is more likely to recur. Irrigate the cav-ity with saline and then close, usually with an intermediate closure technique.

If infected, sebaceous cysts pose a bigger problem. The treatment for an abscess is to I&D it. Formal excision is ill advised because infection is likely to occur if sutures are placed.

Technique

See Chapter 192, Incision and Drainage of an Abscess.
1. Prep with alcohol. Inject 2 mL of 2% lidocaine with epinephrine over the top of the lesion.
2. Use a No. 11 blade to incise the lesion. Be careful because the contents are often under pressure and may come "flying out." All sebaceous material must be removed.
3. Insert hemostats to break up any pockets. Try to remove the sac as noted previously, but it is often too friable. Use a reusable dermal curette and curette the inside, which may remove the sac.
4. Place 0.25-inch iodoform gauze into the wound. Leave a small tail on the outside.
5. Cover with ointment so the dressing does not stick. Change the dressings two to three times per day. Change the gauze in 1 week and replace with clean gauze. Remove the new gauze in 3 weeks and let the wound heal.

Usually the cyst will not recur but rather scar down. If it recurs, formal excision is necessary, but not until the infection has resolved. No antibiotics are necessary after an I&D.

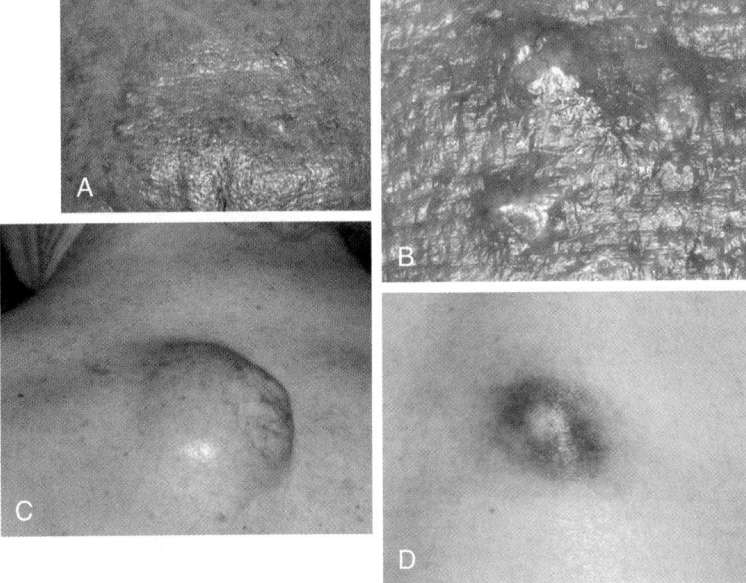

Fig. 13.25   (A) Sebaceous gland hyperplasia on the forehead of a 52-year-old male. Usually lesions are multiple and popular. (B) When larger, or on close inspection, sebaceous gland hyperplasia can resemble basal cell carcinoma (BCC). However, BCCs are rarely multiple like this. (C) Sebaceous cyst. (D) Inflamed sebaceous cyst.

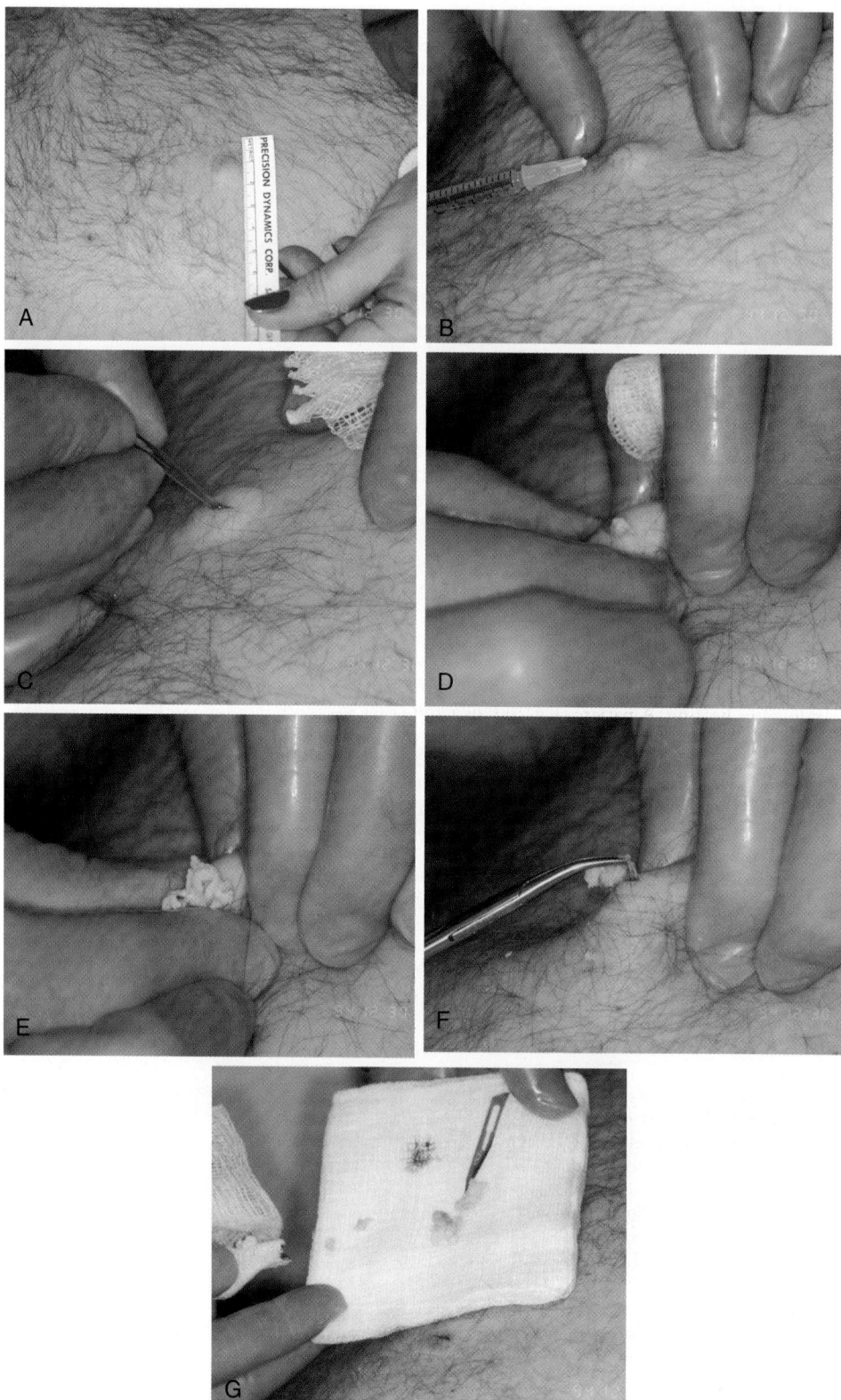

Fig. 13.26 (A) Sebaceous cyst (1.5 to 2 cm). (B) Inject 1 mL of local anesthetic over the top of the cyst to form a wheal. (C) Incise with a No. 11 blade directly into the cyst. (D) Express the contents of the cyst. (E) Sebaceous material. (F) Grasp the sac with hemostats and tease it free with gentle lateral pressure and a rocking motion. (G) Sebaceous material and appearance of wound after removal. No closure is needed for a small incision. (Courtesy The Medical Procedures Center, Midland, Michigan.)

TELANGIECTASES

Small *cherry angiomas* (*hemangiomas*), a type of telangiectasia, are benign, small, red, vascular lesions that do not require treatment. If irritated or bleeding, they can be lightly cauterized and wiped off with a gauze. (See earlier discussion.) Malignancy is not a consideration. *Spider veins*, another type of telangiectasia, are best treated with sclerotherapy if on the legs. Radiosurgery with a 30-gauge needle works extremely well on the face for isolated lesions, but works poorly in the lower extremities (see Chapter 25, Radiofrequency Surgery [Modern Electrosurgery]). Spider veins in the leg can produce significant pain and paresthesias if left untreated (see Chapter 78, Sclerotherapy). When the veins are very fine and dense such as with rosacea, IPL works extremely well.

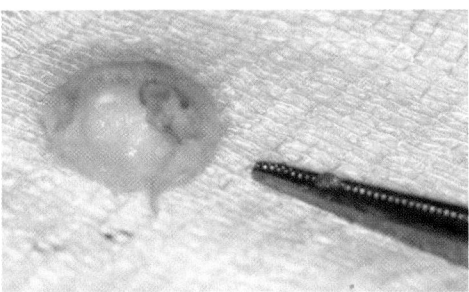

Fig. 13.27 Typical sac from a trichilemmal (pilar) cyst, or wen.

WARTS (VERRUCA VULGARIS AND PLANTARIS)

The recurrence rates associated with all treatments of common warts are 30% or higher. Many over-the-counter and prescription preparations are acidic, caustic solutions. In time, 60% of warts resolve spontaneously. Vitamins enhance the immune system and may aid wart resolution. Numerous treatment methods are used and noted in Table 13.1 (see Chapter 30, Wart [Verruca] Treatment). *Candida* antigen injections are efficacious, cost effective, and the least traumatic of the alternatives, with virtually no residual scarring. Bleomycin injections often work for the most resistant warts.

Plantar warts are treated with methods similar to those used with common warts. Clinicians should avoid surgical excisions on the bottom of the feet because the scar tissue often remains painful after healing. A patient may suffer with the irritated scar, which produces an effect not unlike a pebble in a shoe. Soaking the foot followed by paring of callous tissue will improve the efficacy of any treatment. Cryotherapy is effective and may not result in scarring.

WARTS (CONDYLOMA ACUMINATA)

See Chapter 138, Treatment of Noncervical Condylomata Acuminata.

WENS

See the previous section on sebaceous cysts.

XANTHELASMA

Xanthelasma, the most common form of xanthoma, is a yellow-white plaque on the eyelids. The diagnosis of xanthelasma can be made clinically. The goal of all treatments is to stay very superficial. Light fulguration or cauterization is often sufficient. With radiofrequency loop ablation, it is easier to control depth. Use the large loop at pure cutting level 2 (20 W) and lightly vaporize the lesions until no residual white material exists. Often, if small, an incision can be made with an 18-gauge needle and the lesion can be expressed. Surgically removing the abnormal tissue with a curvilinear elliptical excision provides excellent results when repaired using a 6-0 suture. Because of the nature of the lesion, recurrences are common.

CPT/BILLING CODES

10060   I&D cyst/abscess, simple
10061   I&D cyst/abscess, complex or multiple

NOTE: For a sebaceous cyst, if the sac is removed, gauze is inserted, or a hemostat is inserted to break up adhesions or grasp the sac wall, this is considered "complex."

11200   Skin tag removal by excision or destruction: 1-15
11201   Each additional 10 or portion thereof

Coding and billing of lesion removal and destruction are very complex. There are excision codes with simple and intermediate closures. Shave excisions are another whole section in the CPT code book. Destruction of lesions depends on whether they are benign or malignant, their size, and where they are located. For genital and anal lesions, it also depends on how they are "destroyed." It is of the utmost importance that the clinician differentiates the methods for the treatment of these lesions when coding and billing.

ADDITIONAL RESOURCES

Multiple patient education forms for different diagnoses and conditions are available at www.expertconsult.com.
Multiple DVDs are available from the National Procedures Institute depicting treatment techniques for the methods and approaches discussed in this chapter. www.npinstitute.com (phone 1-866-NPI-CME1).

RECOMMENDED READING

American Cancer Society and National Comprehensive Cancer Network. Melanoma: treatment guidelines for patients (Part 1). *Dermatol Nurs.* 2005;17:119–131.
American Cancer Society and National Comprehensive Cancer Network. Melanoma: treatment guidelines for patients (Part 2). *Dermatol Nurs.* 2005;17:191–198.
American Society of Plastic Surgeons. Evidence-Based Clinical Practice Guidelines. Treatment of Cutaneous Melanoma. *Arlington Heights, IL: American Society of Plastic Surgeons.* 2007.
Bialy TL, Whalen J, Veledar E, et al. Mohs micrographic surgery vs traditional surgical excision: a cost comparison analysis. *Arch Dermatol.* 2004;140:736–742.
Bowen GM, White Jr GL, Gerwels JW. Mohs micrographic surgery. *Am Fam Physician.* 2005;72:845–848.
Cohen PR, Schulze KE, Nelson BR. Cutaneous carcinoma with mixed histology: a potential etiology for skin cancer recurrence and an indication for Mohs microscopically controlled surgical excision. *South Med J.* 2005;98:740–747.
Coit DG, Andtbacka R, Bichakjian CK, et al. Melanoma. *J Natl Compr Canc Netw.* 2009;7:250–275.
Cook J, Salasche S. Mohs surgery: an informed view. *Plast Reconstr Surg.* 2005;115:945–946.
Cook J, Zitelli JA. Mohs micrographic surgery: a cost analysis. *J Am Acad Dermatol.* 1998;39(Pt 1):698–703.
Dandurand M, Petit T, Martel P, Guillot B, for ANAES. Management of basal cell carcinoma in adults: Clinical practice guidelines. *Eur J Dermatol.* 2006;16:394–401.
De Raeve LE, De Coninck AL, Dierickx PR, Roseeuw DI. Neonatal curettage of giant congenital melanocytic nevi. *Arch Dermatol.* 1996;132:20–22.
Dummer R, Hauschild A, Jost L, for the ESMO Guidelines Working Group. Cutaneous malignant melanoma: ESMO clinical recommendations for diagnosis, treatment, and follow-up. *Ann Oncol.* 2008;19(suppl 2):ii86-ii88.
Dummer R, Panizzon R, Bloch PH, Burg G, for the Task Force on Skin Cancer. Updated Swiss guidelines for the treatment and follow-up of cutaneous melanoma. *Dermatology.* 2005;210:39–44.
Essers BA, Dirksen CD, Nieman FH, et al. Cost-effectiveness of Mohs micrographic surgery vs. surgical excision for basal cell carcinoma of the face. *Arch Dermatol.* 2006;142:187–194.
Folberg R, Salomao D, Grossniklaus HE, et al. for the Association of Directors of Anatomic and Surgical Pathology: recommendations for the reporting of tissues removed as part of the surgical treatment of common malignancies of the eye and its adnexa. *Hum Pathol.* 2003;34:114–118.
Fraser MC, Goldstein AM, Tucker MA. Genetic testing for inherited predisposition to melanoma: has the time come? *J Drugs Dermatol.* 2004;3: 93–95.

Gillard M, Wang TS, Johnson TM. Nonmelanoma cutaneous malignancies. In: Chang AE, Ganz PA, Hayes DF, et al., eds. *Oncology: An Evidence-Based Approach*. New York: Springer; 2006.

Guidelines of care for cutaneous squamous cell carcinoma. Committee on Guidelines of Care. Task Force on Cutaneous Squamous Cell Carcinoma. *J Am Acad Dermatol*. 1993;28:628–631.

Guidelines of care for malignant melanomas. Committee on Guidelines of Care. Task Force on Malignant Melanoma. *J Am Acad Dermatol*. 1993;28:638–641.

Habif TP. *Clinical Dermatology: A Color Guide to Diagnosis and Therapy*. 6th ed. Philadelphia: Elsevier; 2016.

Hayes AJ, Maynard L, Coombes G, et al. Wide versus narrow excision margins for high-risk, primary cutaneous melanomas: long-term follow-up of survival in a randomized trial. *Lancet Oncol*. 2016.

Jost LM, Jelic S, Purkalne G, et al. for the ESMO Guidelines Task Force. ESMO minimum clinical recommendations for diagnosis, treatment and follow-up of cutaneous malignant melanoma. *Ann Oncol*. 2005;16(suppl 1):66–68.

Klin B, Ashkenazi M. Sebaceous cyst excision with minimal surgery. *Am Fam Physician*. 1990;41:1746–1748.

Krengel S, Hauschild A, Schäfer T. Melanoma risk in congenital melanocytic nevi: a systematic review. *Br J Dermatol*. 2006;155:1–8.

Kuflik AS, Janniger CK. Basal cell carcinoma. *Am Fam Physician*. 1993;48:1273–1276.

Kunishige JH, Brodland DG, Zitelli JA. Surgical margins for melanoma in situ. *J Am Acad Dermatol*. 2012;66:438.

Kurban RS, Kurban AL. Skin disorders of aging: diagnosis and treatment. *Geriatrics*. 1993;48:30–42.

Lask G, Moyr ED. *Principles and Techniques of Cutaneous Surgery*. New York: McGraw-Hill; 1996.

Leibovitch I, Huilgol SC, Selva D, et al. Basosquamous carcinoma: treatment with Mohs micrographic surgery. *Cancer*. 2005;104:170–175.

Miller SJ. The National Comprehensive Cancer Network (NCCN) guidelines of care for nonmelanoma skin cancers. *Dermatol Surg*. 2000;26:289–292.

Miller SJ, Alam M, Andersen J, et al. for the National Comprehensive Cancer Network: Basal cell and squamous cell skin cancers. *J Natl Compr Canc Netw*. 2007;5:506–529.

Motley R, Kersey P, Lawrence C. Multiprofessional guidelines for the management of the patient with primary cutaneous squamous cell carcinoma. *Br J Dermatol*. 2002;146:18–25.

Nag S, Quivey JM, Earle JD, et al. The American Brachytherapy Society recommendations for brachytherapy of uveal melanomas. *Int J Radiat Oncol Biol Phys*. 2003;56:544–555.

Nguyen TH. Mohs bashing out of hand. *Plast Reconstr Surg*. 2005;115:361–362.

NIH Consensus Conference. Diagnosis and treatment of early melanoma. *JAMA*. 1992;268:1314–1319.

Otley CC. Cost-effectiveness of Mohs micrographic surgery vs. surgical excision for basal cell carcinoma of the face. *Arch Dermatol*. 2006;142:1235. author reply 1235–1236.

Otley CC. Mohs' micrographic surgery for basal-cell carcinoma of the face. *Lancet*. 2005;365:1226–1227; author reply 1227.

Pfenninger JL. *The National Procedures Institute. The NPI Reimbursement Manual for Office Procedures*. Midland: Mich; 2010.

Redondo P, Marquina M, Pretel M, et al. Methyl-ALA-induced fluorescence in photodynamic diagnosis of basal cell carcinoma prior to Mohs micrographic surgery. *Arch Dermatol*. 2008;144:115–117.

Rigopoulos D, Larios G, Gregoriou S, Alevizos A. Acute and chronic paronychia. *Am Fam Physician*. 2008;77:339–346.

Robinson JK, Hanke DW, Siegel DM, eds. *Surgery of the Skin: Procedural Dermatology*. Philadelphia: Saunders; 2015.

Roenigk RK, Roenigk HH. *Dermatologic Surgery: Principles and Practice*. 2nd ed. New York: Marcel Dekker; 1996.

Shindel AW, Mann MW, Lev RY, et al. Mohs micrographic surgery for penile cancer: management and long-term follow-up. J Urol. 2007;178:1980–1985. [See comment in Nat Clin Pract Urol 5:364–365, 2008.]

Shuster S. Mohs' micrographic surgery for basal-cell carcinoma of the face: *Lancet*. 2005;365:1227–1228.

Sladden MJ, Balch C, Barzilai DA, et al. Surgical excision margins for primary cutaneous melanoma. *Cochrane Database Syst Rev*. 2009;(4). CD004835.

Stacano JJ, Juma A, Dhital SK, McGeorge DD. Excision margin for cutaneous squamous cell carcinoma: Is it standardized? *Eur J Plast Surg*. 2004;27:135–139.

Stern RS, Boudreaux C, Arndt K. Diagnostic accuracy and appropriateness of care for seborrheic keratoses. *JAMA*. 1989;265:74–77.

Sterry W, for the European Dermatology Forum Guideline Committee. Guidelines: the management of basal cell carcinoma. *Eur J Dermatol*. 2006;16:467–475.

Stulberg D, Fawcett R, Small R, Usatine RP. Procedures to treat benign conditions. In: Usatine RP, Pfenninger JL, Stulberg DL, Small R, eds. *Dermatologic and Cosmetic Procedures in Office Practice*. Philadelphia: Elsevier; 2012:404–426.

Stulberg DL, Crandell B, Fawcett RS. Diagnosis and treatment of basal cell and squamous cell carcinomas. *Am Fam Physician*. 2004;70:1481–1488.

Stulberg DL, Usatine RP. Diagnosis and treatment of malignant and premalignant lesions. In: Usatine RP, Pfenninger JL, Stulberg DL, Small R, eds. *Dermatologic and Cosmetic Procedures in Office Practice*. Philadelphia: Elsevier; 2012:427–439.

Telfer NR, Colver GB, Morton CA, for the British Association of Dermatologists. Guidelines for the management of basal cell carcinoma. *Br J Dermatol*. 2008;159:35–48.

Tran KT, Wright NA, Cockrell CJ. Biopsy of the pigmented lesion: when and how. *J Am Acad Dermatol*. 2008;59:852–871.

Tromberg J, Bauer B, Benvenuto-Andrade C, Marghoob AA. Congenital melanocytic nevi needing treatment. *Dermatol Ther*. 2005;18:136–150.

Usatine RP, Smith MA, Mayeaux EJ, et al. *The Color Atlas of Family Medicine*. 2nd ed. New York: McGraw-Hill; 2013.

Usatine RP, Pfenninger JL, Stulberg DL, Small R. *Dermatologic and Cosmetic Procedures in Office Practice*. Philadelphia: Elsevier; 2010.

Weiss J, Menter A, Hevia O, et al. Effective treatment of actinic keratosis with 0.5% fluorouracil topical cream in patients with actinic keratosis. *Clin Ther*. 2001;23:908.

Whitaker DK, Sinclair W, for the Melanoma Advisory Board. Guideline on the management of melanoma. *S Afr Med J*. 2004;94(Pt 3):699–708.

CHAPTER 14

CRYOSURGERY

James W. McNabb • John L. Pfenninger

Cryosurgery is the deliberate destruction of diseased tissue by freezing in a controlled manner. It is the most commonly performed dermatologic procedure in the United States; as such, it is important for all primary care clinicians to master the art and technique of cryosurgery. The procedure is often a better alternative than surgical excision, especially when convenience, healing, disability during healing, infectious disease risk (human immunodeficiency virus, hepatitis), discomfort, and scar formation are considered. (See also Chapter 125, Cryotherapy of the Cervix.)

GENERAL CONSIDERATIONS

• Lesions treated with cryosurgery usually heal with minimal or no scar formation. Even if inadvertent excessive freezing is done, scarring is rarely significant.
• Complete healing may take more than 6 to 8 weeks in extreme cases, but the results are usually excellent. Selective destruction of cells occurs during the freeze. However, the collagen and fibroelastic structural framework is preserved, so the epithelial cells grow back in an organized fashion within the preserved matrix.
• The procedure is safe, simple, and easy to learn. It usually takes less time than conventional surgery.
• Patients may prefer to avoid injections of local anesthetic, which is usually possible with cryosurgery.
• A burning sensation is experienced with the initial freeze and again on thawing. Explain to patients that the freezing will feel like an ice cube stuck to the skin. This often reassures them enough to cope with the minimal amount of pain experienced. However, young children often will not accept the procedure without crying. Their fear of the unknown increases when the unpleasant cold sensation starts. They have difficulty trusting that the burning feeling will actually improve in a very short time instead of continually getting worse. In children and in some adults, a local anesthetic will be helpful, especially when freezing multiple or large lesions and when attempting a deep freeze for malignant lesions.
• Other than keeping the lesions clean and protected, patients can essentially ignore the cryotreated lesion between treatments. They appreciate the omission of suture insertion and removal. Patients also welcome being able to bathe and swim while the lesion is healing.
• Secondary infection usually is not a significant problem. Even with overfreezing and with cryosensitive patients who develop with excessive tissue destruction, infection occurs rarely. Excessive freezing may result in wound weeping for longer than 1 to 2 weeks, but infection should not be expected unless the area receives poor skin care.
• Occasionally, a profuse watery discharge may persist more than 3 to 4 days after treatment. Debridement of the wound often alleviates the discharge.
• Two concerns exist regarding cryosurgery and use of the nitrous oxide closed system. The first is the spread of infectious agents by the equipment. Cryoprobes must be cleaned and sterilized

between procedures using Cidex or an autoclave. Second, there can be adverse health effects from prolonged exposure to nitrous oxide at high levels—far higher than will ever be experienced using nitrous oxide closed systems for cryosurgery for mere minutes at a time. Air hunger, dizziness, confusion, headaches, nausea, vomiting, and loss of consciousness or death may occur if nitrous oxide is present in quantities sufficient to dilute the oxygen concentration in the air. This overexposure creates an altered (euphoric or excited) mental state. Long-term exposure to nitrous oxide has been associated with neuropathy, increased rates of spontaneous abortion, and congenital anomalies in offspring. Federal regulations require nitrous oxide gas to be vented outside of the examination/treatment room. This can be accomplished by simply extending the exhaust tube on the unit out a window or by installing vents in an outside wall. The likelihood of a patient receiving enough exposure to do harm is very small and has not yet been reported. In practice, considering the minimal amounts of nitrous oxide used, few practitioners "vent" the rooms. Carbon dioxide (which is an agent nearly as cold) can be substituted for nitrous oxide in a closed system if desired.

ADVANTAGES OF CRYOTHERAPY (CRYOSURGERY)

• Local anesthesia is optional, so needles can usually be avoided.
• Freezing usually produces only minimal pain.
• Final healing is cosmetically excellent, with minimal or no scarring.
• Minimal clinician time is required, and the procedure is easy to learn.
• Preoperative skin preparation is not required.
• Multiple lesions can be treated quickly in one office visit.
• Postoperative infection is rare.
• No complicated postprocedure care is needed.
• No significant disruption of postprocedure activity is required.
• The procedure is ideal for patients with light-complexioned skin.
• The procedure is inexpensive and cost effective.
• A wide variety of lesions can be treated without significant exposure to blood-borne pathogens.
• Units are portable and can be taken to nursing home facilities when needed.
• Units are relatively inexpensive with low start-up costs.
• Units take up little space in the office.

DISADVANTAGES OF CRYOSURGERY

• Use is limited in patients with darker skin because of pigment changes. Even with brief partial-thickness freeze technique, some melanocytes are destroyed and the healed cryolesion may be slightly lighter in color than the surrounding skin, even in fair-skinned individuals.
• Cryosurgery is not recommended in areas of hair growth, such as around the eyebrows and eyelashes, and on scalps with thin hair, because even brief freezing tends to destroy hair follicles.

89

- Healed cryolesions may not tan sufficiently, often are more susceptible to sunburn, and may require added sunscreen protection.
- Tissue is not available for histopathologic diagnosis, so certainty of complete lesion removal is lacking.
- There is the possibility of exposure to nitrous oxide gas if closed units are used (see earlier).

AGENTS USED FOR CRYOSURGERY

There are three basic methods of cryosurgery (Table 14.1).

1. Closed systems (freezing is carried out with a cooled probe as opposed to the application of the agent itself)
   - Nitrous oxide
   - Carbon dioxide
   - CryoPen
2. Liquid nitrogen
   - Thermos bottle/spray unit (Brymill; Wallach)
   - Cotton-tipped applicators and Styrofoam cup
3. Aerosol canister
   - Tetrafluoroethane (Verruca-Freeze, Frigi-Dent)
   - Ether/propane (Histofreezer)

Nitrous oxide is quite unstable, and once it is released into the probe, it immediately breaks down to molecular nitrogen and oxygen. The physical characteristics of the nitrous oxide gas enable the cryotip's temperature to be easily lowered to its boiling point of −89°C. With *carbon dioxide*, the tip is not as cold, and it will take slightly longer to achieve a quality freeze (−78.5°C).

Nitrous oxide comes in a closed gas cylinder (blue tank, versus brown for carbon dioxide and green for oxygen). The hand-held cryogun, which is connected to the tank with tubing, is structured differently from the liquid nitrogen guns. It is designed to allow a controlled, rapid expansion of nitrous oxide gas within the cryoprobe tip, lowering its temperature to −89°C. The storage tanks preserve nitrous oxide virtually "forever" by keeping the gas under pressure with no port for evaporation (except during cryogun activation). The tanks are moved from storage to use on small carts. The cryoprobes (tips) come in numerous shapes and sizes to match the lesion to be treated. The rounded, pointed, and slanted flat tips are popular for dermatologic applications (Fig. 14.1). The hemorrhoid tip is rarely, if ever, used for hemorrhoids, but its shape allows use for multiple dermatologic lesions. The flat and slightly conical 19- and 25-mm tips that are used for cryosurgery of the cervix can also be used for dermatologic applications.

Because nitrous oxide does not achieve a probe temperature as low as liquid nitrogen (−89°C vs. −196°C), it is significantly slower at freezing tissue. This is especially important when treating multiple lesions. Both nitrous oxide and liquid nitrogen are effective for treating malignancies. Overlapping treatment areas for larger lesions using large probes ensures efficacy. Nitrous oxide units have an active defrost mode that rapidly frees the cryotip from frozen tissue.

CryoPen is a closed, self-contained refrigerant system. It uses an internal cryogen that is cooled in a free-standing unit to −95°C. It eliminates the handling of cryogen gases and liquids. CryoPen reusable tips are available in 3-, 5-, 7-, and 10-mm sizes. These are applied directly to the lesion and maintained in place until the clinical end point has been reached.

Liquid nitrogen is the coldest cryogen, effecting a rapid, deep freeze (boiling point −196°C). A large storage container (Dewar) is needed. Newer Dewars can store the liquid nitrogen for up to 1 year. Liquid nitrogen is relatively inexpensive, but if not used it will evaporate. Liquid nitrogen may be applied to the lesion directly using cotton-tipped applicators or sprayed using a thermos-type unit (Brymill CRY-AC and CRY-AC-3 [Brymill Cryogenic Systems], or Wallach UltraFreeze [Wallach Surgical Devices]). The various apertures of the spray tips allow a variable amount of gas to cover a lesion, allowing control over the extent of freezing. A reusable plastic shield is available to limit gas spread. These spray units allow efficient and rapid treatment of multiple lesions in a single office visit. Additional probes are available that allow the thermos to be used as a closed system, but there is no active defrost. Subsequently, the tip may "stick" to the tissue for a significant length of time before it thaws and detaches.

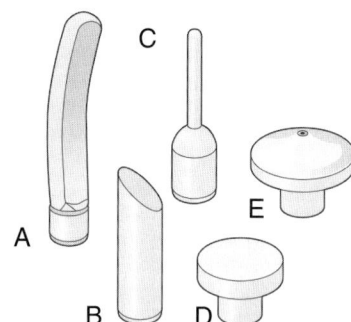

Fig. 14.1 Most cryoprobe tips come in variable sizes. (A) Hemorrhoid tip. (B) Slanted flat tip. (C) Pointed tip. (D) Flat cervical tip. (E) Slight conical cervical tip.

TABLE 14.1	Cryogenic Agents				
	Agents				
	Liquid Nitrogen	**N₂O**	**CO₂**	**Tetrafluoroethane**	**Ether/Propane**
Boiling point	−196°C	−89°C	−78.5°C	−47°C	−25°C
Effective treatment temperature	−196°C	−89°C	−78.5°C	−70°C	−55°C
Use	Thermos-type guns Cotton-tip applicator Stored in large Dewars	Cylinders with applicator gun (cryoprobe)	Cylinders with applicator gun (cryoprobe) Dry ice slush	Aerosol canister	Aerosol canister
Method/system	Open/closed	Closed	Closed/open	Open (spray/cones, buds)	Open (buds)
Shelf life	1 yr max. with best Dewars	Indefinite	Indefinite	5 yr	5 yr+
Flammable	No	No	No	No	Yes
Trade name	Cryogun (Brymill Cryogenic Systems) UltraFreeze (Wallach)	—	—	Verruca-Freeze (CryoSurgery), Frigi-Dent (Ellman Cynosure)	Histofreezer (OraSure Technologies)
Indications	All	All	All	Superficial only (no cancers)	Superficial only (no cancers)

Canister refrigerants are the least expensive agents used for cryosurgery. They come prepackaged in small hand-held canisters the size of a soda can, making them portable for use in nursing homes, satellite clinics, and multiple examination rooms. They have a very long shelf life. Unfortunately, they do not achieve tissue temperatures low enough to treat very many lesions. These agents are not indicated for malignancies, deep lesions, or large lesions. *Trifluoroethane/pentafluoroethane/tetrafluoroethane* (Verruca-Freeze [Cryosurgery, Frigi-Dent [Ellman Cynosure]); (boiling point −47°C). *Dimethyl ether/propane/isobutane* (Histofreezer [OraSure Technologies]) also comes in a canister but is not as cold (−25°C) and is flammable.

Over-the-counter skin refrigerants were approved for use by the US Food and Drug Administration in 2003. Several products are available, including Dr. Scholl's Freeze Away, Wartner Plantar Wart Removal System, and Compound W Freeze Off. The first two products contain dimethyl ether and propane. Wartner's product also adds isobutane to these. Although the manufacturers state that temperatures as low as −57°C are achieved on skin application, such low temperatures were not realized in a clinical study. There is significant concern regarding their ability to create local tissue necrosis because of their inability to reach low temperatures rapidly enough to achieve clinical effect. In contrast to other clinician-applied options, these over-the-counter products are also dangerous because they are extremely flammable.

TISSUE EFFECTS: PRINCIPLES FOR TREATMENT

It is important to recognize that at −2.2°C, cells begin to freeze. At −5°C, cells will supercool, but they usually recover. Large-scale tissue destruction begins only when the temperature is between −10°C and −20°C. A deeper freeze with temperatures between −40°C and −50°C ensures that malignant cells are completely destroyed. Melanocytes are among the most sensitive cells to cryotherapy and can die at temperatures from −4°C to −7°C, hence the risk of hypopigmentation after the procedure. At temperatures less than −20°C, hair follicles and sebaceous glands die. Fibroblasts die at temperatures between −30°C and −35°C. Bone and cartilage are the least sensitive, but temperatures from −50°C to −60°C will also destroy cartilage.

The size of the ice ball that forms around the lesion provides a good estimate of the depth of the freeze. The *lethal zone* (tissue temperature less than −20°C) is 2 to 3 mm *inside* the outer margin of the ice ball (Fig. 14.2). This is especially crucial to remember in cases of premalignant or malignant lesions, which are deeper in the skin. *The size of the ice ball beyond the lesion is the most important criterion in determining how long to freeze.* Factors requiring prolonged freeze time include low tank pressure, increased tissue vascularity, excessive overlying keratin (needs to be removed or moistened), and

poor tip-to-lesion contact. The use of different systems (e.g., nitrous oxide, liquid nitrogen, carbon dioxide, canister gases) dramatically affects the rapidity and depth of freeze. Likewise, the method of applying liquid nitrogen (with the cotton-tipped applicator or in a spray fashion) affects freezing parameters. Once an ice ball of the desired size has been obtained, it is just as important to observe the time it takes for the area to thaw from the outer edge of the ice ball to the lesion edge ("halo thaw time") and the time for all the tissue to thaw (total thaw time; Box 14.1). A brief freeze can turn tissue white, providing the ice ball desired; however, if it remains frozen only momentarily, it will have little effect.

Freeze times should be adjusted according to patient sensitivity, type and size of the lesion, presence of malignancy, and lesion vascularity. Table 14.2 shows the variations with nitrous oxide alone, and Table 14.3 shows those with liquid nitrogen. Age, vascular flow, amount of pigment, depth of lesion, amount of keratin, location on the body, and cell type of the lesion all affect the amount of freezing required to destroy pathologic tissue. Adjust your freeze times accordingly. Applying pressure to the lesion with the fixed probes will increase the depth of freeze. Vascular lesions will require longer freezing times, and pressure from the probe should be applied to squeeze as much blood as possible out of the lesion before freezing. Any active bleeding from a prior shave or curettement will need to be controlled first.

For *benign lesions* (other than warts), a single freeze/thaw cycle is sufficient. The ice ball should extend 2 to 3 mm beyond most lesion margins. Resistant lesions such as warts often require a freeze/thaw/freeze cycle. Complete thaw times should be 2 to 3 minutes for larger lesions.

For *malignant or premalignant lesions*, a freeze/thaw/freeze cycle is recommended. The ice ball should extend 5 mm beyond the lesion margin each time the tissue is frozen. The second freeze is usually quicker and less painful.

Dry, keratinized tissue will not freeze easily and insulates the lesion underneath from freezing. Remove as much keratin as possible before freezing, especially when using nitrous oxide, carbon dioxide, or the canister agents.

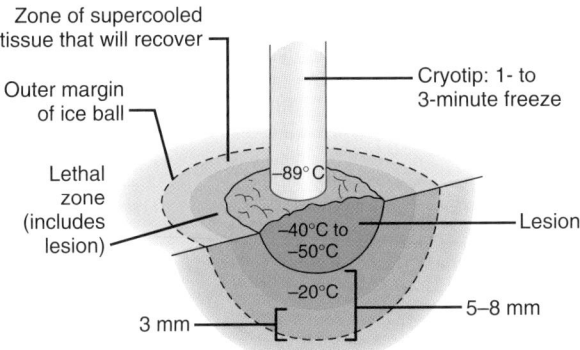

Fig. 14.2 Nitrous oxide full-thickness destruction freeze technique (malignant lesions). Note that the outer supercooled area will recover. Monitoring thaw times for both malignant and benign lesions is extremely important (see Box 14.1).

BOX 14.1 Freezing Guidelines for Skin

Benign Lesions
- Ice ball 2 mm beyond lesion borders
- Correlate with thaw times (see below)
- Consider double freeze for difficult and/or premalignant lesions

Malignant and Most Premalignant Lesions
- Ice ball 5 mm beyond lesion borders
- Double freeze (freeze, thaw, refreeze, using same parameters)

Freeze Time
- Variable, depending on cryogen, pressure applied, size of lesion, type of lesion, size of nozzle/tip, expertise of operator
- Second freeze is faster

Halo Thaw Time
- 1 min (benign)
- 2–4 min (malignant)

Total Thaw Time
- 2–3 min (benign)
- 3–5 min (malignant)

Liquid Nitrogen
- Small swab (small lesions) and large swab (large lesions)
- 10-sec freeze
- Total thaw time: 60 sec (superficial lesions)
- Spray: as noted above for other applications

TABLE 14.2   Freeze Time Guidelines for Nitrous Oxide Technique

Tissue	Lesion	Freeze Time*
Skin	Full-thickness, benign	1–1.5 min
	Full-thickness, malignant	1.5–3 min†
	Plantar warts (after debridement)	40 sec
	Condylomata	20–45 sec
	Verrucae	1–1.5 min
	Vascular lesions (with pressure)	1–1.5 min
	Seborrheic keratoses (2-mm margin)	30 sec†
	Actinic keratoses (3-mm margin)	1–1.5 min†
	Basal cell cancer (3- to 5-mm margin)	1.5 min†
Vascular	Hemorrhoids	
	Cryoligation	2 min
	Cryo without ligation	2–3 min†
Cervix	Cervicitis	3 min
	Cervical intraepithelial neoplasia I, II, III	3 min†
	Cervical intraepithelial neoplasia I, II (alternative method)	5 min

*Freeze times are approximate guidelines and should be adjusted to the size of the ice ball and the thaw time, which are far more important than the freeze time alone. Because nitrous oxide is slower and more controlled, freeze times are more reliable than with liquid nitrogen.
†Freeze-thaw-refreeze.

TABLE 14.3   Freeze Time Guidelines for Liquid Nitrogen Open-Spray Technique

Lesion	Common Freeze Time (Sec)
Actinic keratoses	5–15
Cherry angioma	5–10
Condylomata	5–10
Keloids	20–30
Lentigines	5–10
Molluscum contagiosum	5–10
Mucocele	10–30
Papilloma	5–10
Prurigo nodularis	10–30
Sebaceous hyperplasia	5–10
Seborrheic keratoses	10
Skin tags	5–10
Common warts	10–20

With the nitrous oxide cryotips, once the tip is "frozen" and fixed to the skin, the probe can be pulled back, tenting up the skin, to reduce the depth of freeze, thereby sparing deeper critical structures (such as nerves) from exposure to freezing (Fig. 14.3).

Bandages are not necessary unless the lesion is continually irritated (i.e., by clothing), develops a large blister, or develops a serous discharge.

POSTTREATMENT PHYSIOLOGIC EFFECTS

Erythema and hyperemia are immediate responses to effective freezing. Edema and exudation (blister formation) peak within 24 to 48 hours and usually subside after 72 hours (Fig. 14.4). Blood may accumulate under the blister, making it appear black (Fig. 14.5). The extracellular collagen structures are more resistant to freezing than the cells themselves. Crust formation begins, and this crust will slowly contract over the next several days. Reepithelialization occurs from the outer margin inward. Fibroblasts lay down minimal new collagen along the preserved, well-formed collagen matrix, resulting in a lack of scar formation. However, if the collagen matrix has been destroyed by excessive cryoinjury, fibroblasts will produce collagen randomly, leading to scar formation (Fig. 14.6). Cartilage (e.g., in the ear) is usually preserved.

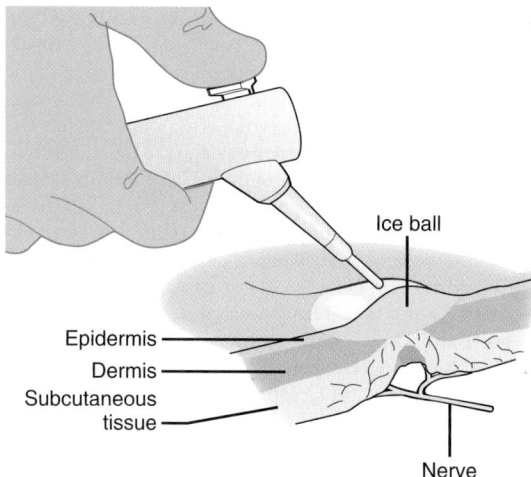

Fig. 14.3 With nitrous oxide, once the cryotip is frozen to the skin, the probe can be retracted to avoid freezing nontarget underlying structures.

If the patient or clinician desires, the treated lesion can be surgically debrided in 24 to 48 hours. During this time, the dermis and epidermis separate, lifting the lesion to the top of the blister. Removal of the prepared lesion with iris or sharp tissue scissors is painless. After 72 hours, however, the lesion may stick like a graft and may bleed on attempts at removal. If completely left alone, the lesion will eventually slough spontaneously. (Surgical debridement 1 or 2 days after freezing effectively removes the lesion and satisfies some patients sooner. However, many patients are quite happy to avoid the early return visit and are willing to wait to see how much of the lesion sloughs before returning for another treatment.) A disadvantage of this technique is that a second office visit is needed for the 24- to 48-hour debridement procedure, and the serous discharge without the intact blister can be quite copious depending on the size of the lesion.

The healed cryolesion is soft, with minimal to no scarring. This allows erections if penile lesions have been frozen. Pigment is often decreased, and hair and sweat glands may be destroyed in the area of freezing. It is best to caution the patient *in advance* that although the area that was frozen is unlikely to develop much of a scar, the skin color may become lighter. The inflammatory response may result in the development of a transient halo of hyperpigmentation. This will usually clear completely over several months.

INDICATIONS

- Actinic keratoses (full-thickness freeze, 83% to 88% cure rate)
- Angiomas or hemangiomas, including congenital strawberry hemangiomas (more difficult)
- Basal cell carcinoma (full-thickness destructive double-freeze)
- Bowen's disease (squamous cell carcinoma in situ)
- Cervical intraepithelial neoplasia (dysplasia), "cryoconization" (see Chapter 125, Cryotherapy of the Cervix)
- Chondrodermatitis nodularis helicis
- Condylomata acuminata
- Dermatofibromas (difficult)
- Digital mucous cyst (ganglion)
- Freckles (lentigines)
- Granulation tissue
- Granuloma annulare
- Hemorrhoids (rarely done)
- Hypertrophic scars (often multiple treatments over time)
- Keloids (as for hypertrophic scars)
- Lentigos
- Lichen planus, hypertrophic

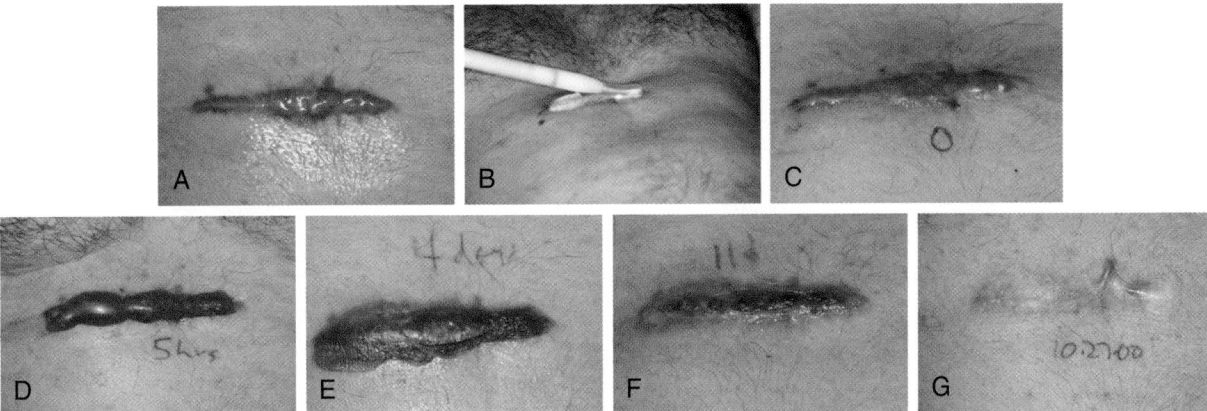

Fig. 14.4 (A) A 10-cm hypertrophic scar over upper abdomen. (B) Application of nitrous oxide probe. (C) Appearance immediately after thawing. (D) Blister formation at 5 hours. (E) Ruptured blister at 4 days. (F) Appearance at 11 days. (G) Final appearance after a second cryotherapy treatment several months later; the small residual scar resolved after the third focal treatment.

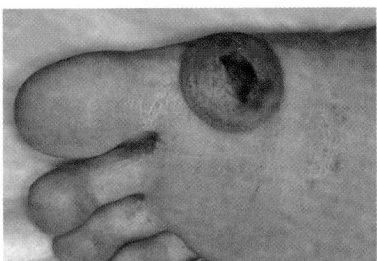

Fig. 14.5 Appearance of a hemorrhagic bulb after cryotherapy of a plantar wart.

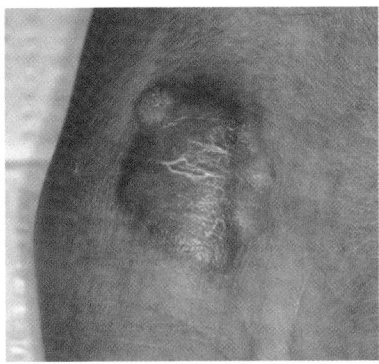

Fig. 14.6 Excessive scarring (rare) after cryosurgery of verrucous lesion over first metatarsophalangeal joint of the large toe on the left foot.

- Molluscum contagiosum
- Mucocele
- Myxoid cysts
- Papular nevi (full-thickness freeze)
- Prurigo nodularis
- Pyogenic granuloma
- Sebaceous hyperplasia
- Squamous cell carcinoma (full-thickness destructive double-freeze)
- Seborrheic keratoses (procedure of choice)
- Skin tags and polyps
- Verrucae (including plantar)
- Xanthoma or xanthelasma

CONTRAINDICATIONS

Absolute Contraindications

- Proven excessive reaction to cryosurgery
- Patient nonacceptance of the possibility of skin pigment changes
- Malignant melanoma
- Areas of end-stage compromised circulation
- Lesions in which identification of tissue pathology is required
- Sclerosing (morpheaform) or recurrent basal cell or squamous cell carcinoma

Relative Contraindications

- Basal cell or squamous cell carcinomas more than 1 cm in diameter
- Any condition with high levels of cryoglobulins (most are noted in this list)
- Immunoproliferative neoplasms (e.g., myeloma, lymphoma)
- Macroglobulinemia
- Active severe collagen vascular diseases
- Severe active ulcerative colitis
- Acute poststreptococcal glomerulonephritis (almost 100% of these patients have high levels of cryoglobulins)
- Active subacute bacterial endocarditis, syphilis, Epstein-Barr virus infection, cytomegalovirus infection
- Chronic severe hepatitis B
- High-dose steroid therapy
- Pigmented nevi should probably not be treated with cryosurgery because if a nevus grows back, it might appear malignant and a biopsy could be suspicious for melanoma (pseudomelanoma)
- Morphea

NOTE: The majority of patients with the preceding conditions are likely to have an exaggerated response to cryosurgery because they have high levels of circulating cryoglobulins. If cryosurgery is appropriate or necessary for any of these patients, be sure to obtain informed consent and perform a pretest in the axilla or thigh area before treating a more prominent or cosmetically sensitive area. Proceed with caution and greatly shorten the freezing times until the response can be predicted. You may be able to freeze lesions effectively and safely with a much shorter freeze time. With overfreezing, the risk of tissue slough and marked hypopigmentation increases. Therefore start slowly and advise patients that extra visits and treatment sessions may be necessary. A conservative approach is best in light of their clinical situation.

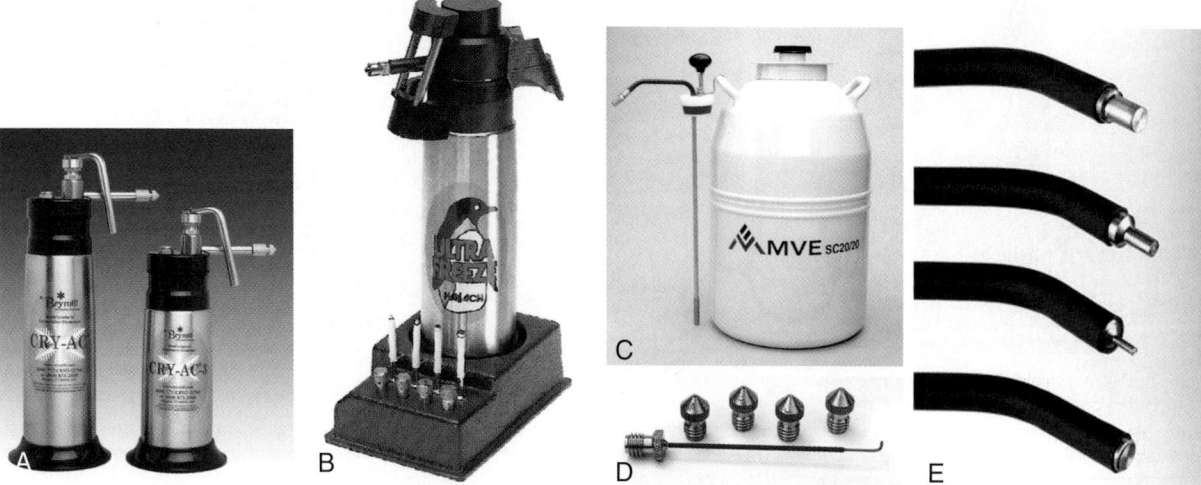

Fig. 14.7 (A) Brymill CRY-AC cryoguns are refillable with liquid nitrogen. (B) Wallach UltraFreeze Cryosurgical System. (C) Liquid nitrogen Dewar. (D) Brymill open-spray aperture tips (openings of tip vary in size, with the A tip the largest). (E) Brymill closed miniprobes. (A and C–E, Courtesy Brymill Cryogenic Systems, Ellington, CT. B, Courtesy Wallach Surgical Devices, Trumbull, CT.)

Lesions Difficult to Treat With Cryosurgery

- Dermatofibroma (these lesions require a longer freeze time)
- Hidradenitis
- Flat nevi (must be absolutely sure the lesion is not a melanoma)
- Squamous cell cancer (usually reserved for practitioners who treat this cancer often)
- Most vascular lesions (especially if extensive, laser or electrosurgery probably preferred), except for venous lake for which cryotherapy is preferred treatment

Areas Not Recommended for Cryosurgery

- Areas where hair loss would be displeasing to the patient
- Areas where pigment changes would be displeasing to the patient
- Feet, ankles, and lower legs when circulation is in question (especially patients with diabetes or peripheral vascular disease)
- Over superficial cutaneous nerves (unless adequate skin traction to pull the skin away from the nerve is possible, usually with nitrous oxide technique)
- Basal cell cancers in the nasolabial fold, in preauricular areas, and on lips (often more extensive and tend to recur)
- Any cancer that has not had histologic confirmation
- Periorbital area (may induce immediate and severe swelling)
- Port wine stain (use laser)

EQUIPMENT

Liquid Nitrogen

- Cryogen spray unit (Fig. 14.7A–B)
- Storage Dewar (Fig. 14.7C)
- Assorted various-sized nozzles (Fig. 14.7D–E)
- Protective plastic shield with assorted opening sizes (Fig. 14.8)
- Styrofoam cups (if thermos canister is not available)
- Cotton-tipped applicators (small and large)
- Metal needle holder, pickups or forceps designed to retain cold (optional; Fig. 14.9)

Nitrous Oxide

- 20-lb tank (the "short, fat, blue one"; Fig. 14.10A)
- Mobile storage cart (Fig. 14.10A)

- Cryoprobe regulator with gun (Fig. 14.10B)
- Cryoprobe tip assortment (Fig. 14.11)
- K-Y Jelly or cryogen gel; do not use anything that is not water soluble (e.g., petrolatum)

Canister Gas Refrigerants

- Can of Verruca-Freeze (Fig. 14.12A) or Frigi-Dent with various sizes of plastic limiting cones and buds (Fig. 14.12A–B)
- Can of Histofreezer with applicators

CryoPen

- CryoPen base unit (Fig. 14.13)
- CryoPen reusable tips (3-, 5-, 7-, and 10-mm sizes)

PREPROCEDURE PATIENT PREPARATION

Before the procedure, the patient should be advised of the basic technique, the expected sensation during treatment, and the possible complications. The advantages of and rationale for using cryosurgery also should be reviewed with the patient.

For all methods listed, consider local anesthesia for patient comfort and the ability to freeze long enough to obtain the desired effect. The need for anesthesia will depend on the size of the lesion, number of lesions, patient age, and other factors.

TECHNIQUE

Liquid Nitrogen

Cup/Cotton-Tipped Applicator, Metal Needle Holder or Pickups Technique

1. Dispense a small amount of liquid nitrogen into a Styrofoam cup to prevent contaminating the primary source of liquid nitrogen.
2. Choose the size of the cotton-tipped applicator to match lesion.
3. Dip a clean cotton-tipped applicator into the cup and then touch the lesion with the applicator.
4. Keep the applicator cold by dipping it into the cup every several seconds and reapplying to the lesion to obtain the desired size of ice ball (Fig. 14.14). Do not place a cotton-tipped applicator that has touched the patient, or the treatment cup supply, into the primary source of liquid nitrogen because contamination can

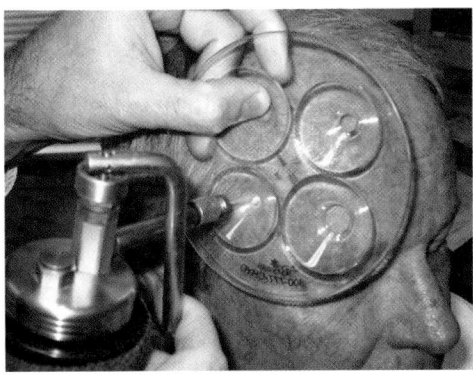

Fig. 14.8 Protective shield (Brymill) with various-sized orifices, which limits the spread of open-spray liquid nitrogen and protects surrounding skin.

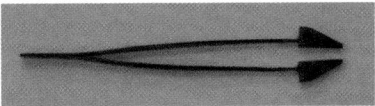

Fig. 14.9 Special cryosurgical forceps (Brymill) with extra mass at tips to allow freezing of multiple lesions before recooling. No anesthesia is needed.

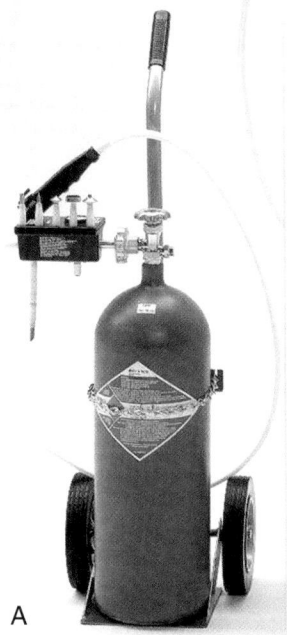

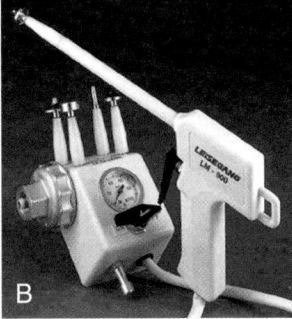

Fig. 14.10 (A) Nitrous oxide cryosurgical unit. Handpiece is placed in holder and connected to a 20-lb tank. (B) CooperSurgical Leisegang cryosurgical hand gun.

occur. Likewise, do not return any unused liquid into the Dewar. Viruses often are not killed by the cold and may be spread to others if contamination of the source occurs.

5. The size of the applicator and amount of pressure applied affect rapidity and depth of freeze.
6. Freezing times are markedly shorter with liquid nitrogen. The cotton-tipped applicator/cup method is not as fast as the cryogun, but it is still significantly faster than nitrous oxide and can be used readily for small lesions, if benign or premalignant (e.g., actinic keratosis).
7. A variant of the foregoing method can be used for pedunculated lesions such as skin tags. Metal needle drivers, metal pickups,

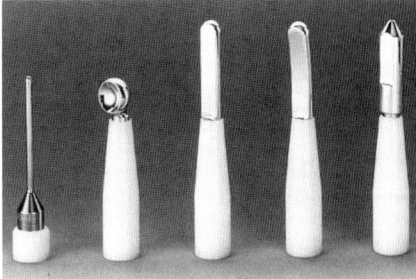

Fig. 14.11 Various cryosurgical tips for treatment of a variety of dermatologic lesions with nitrous oxide. *Left to right:* Fine point, small cup, round tip, hemorrhoid tip, and slightly coned tip.

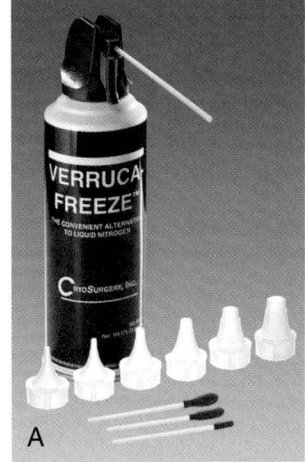

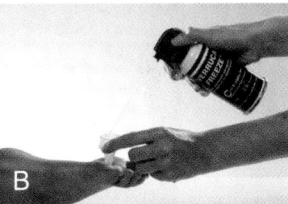

Fig. 14.12 (A) Self-contained Verruca-Freeze unit with various sizes of specula. (B) Application of Verruca-Freeze using a transparent limiting cone.

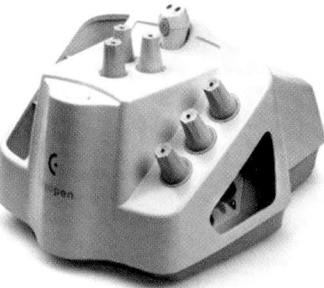

Fig. 14.13 CryoPen base unit.

or specially designed forceps (Brymill) are dipped into the cup of liquid nitrogen. The lesions are then grasped. This technique limits the spread of the freeze and is very effective (Fig. 14.15).

Spray Technique Using a Cryogen Spray Gun: Brymill CRY-AC or Wallach UltraFreeze

The timed-spot freeze technique allows standardization of liquid nitrogen delivery.

1. Select the nozzle size. The C tip is the one chosen most commonly for use with the Brymill; this size is a starting point. The D tip has a smaller opening, the B tip has a larger orifice and can treat large lesions faster. The A tip is larger still (see Fig. 14.7D).
2. Position the nozzle of the spray gun perpendicular to the lesion, 1 to 1.5 cm from the skin surface and aimed at the center of the target lesion (Fig. 14.16A). A tangential spray can be used to create a slower, more controlled freeze.

3. Spray the lesion. The spray gun trigger is depressed and liquid nitrogen is sprayed until an ice ball encompasses the lesion and the desired margin (see Box 14.1). The spray needs to be maintained in either a continuous or intermittent fashion to keep the target field frozen for an adequate time. This time may vary from 5 to 30 seconds. Spraying intermittently will keep the ice ball smaller. If more than one freeze/thaw cycle is required for lesion destruction, complete thawing should be allowed before the next cycle is started (usually 2 to 3 minutes; see Table 14.3).
4. Little movement of the gun is needed unless the lesion is large (>2 cm). Usually it is a direct spray technique as described previously. For large lesions, overlapping direct sprays can be performed, or the lesion can be covered in a paintbrush or enlarging spiral pattern (see Fig. 14.16B).
5. Using a limiting cone or plastic plate shield with variable-sized openings (see Fig. 14.8) is recommended for most smaller lesions because it focuses the spray onto the area desired and limits destruction of normal tissue. It is also helpful around critical areas like the eyes to limit the spread of the spray. Hold it tight against the skin to prevent leakage. Select the cone size to give the desired size of ice ball. The ice

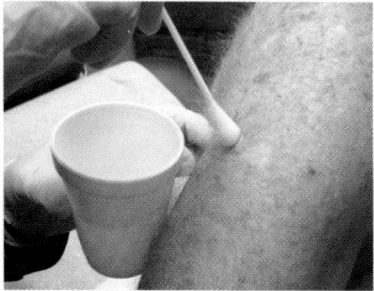

Fig. 14.14 Liquid nitrogen applied directly to a skin lesion using the dipstick technique.

ball will still usually spread 1 to 2 mm beyond the size of the opening. Use freezing guidelines (see Box 14.1) for desired effect.

Liquid nitrogen spray techniques achieve desired freezing levels 8 to 10 times faster than nitrous oxide.

Contact Probes

Small, solid tips much like the nitrous oxide tips also can be used with the thermos guns, but the diameters are only 2 to 4 mm (see Fig. 14.7E).

1. Select the appropriate size and apply the probe tip directly to the skin or lesion (see Fig. 14.16C).
2. Obtain the rim of ice ball size desired.
3. Allow to thaw.

The advantage of these tips is that the ice ball is well-controlled and forms much faster than with nitrous oxide. They can also be used in areas such as around the eyes where it is necessary to avoid a wider spray. The disadvantage of using these probes is that the thawing is passive and can take a long time. Although large tips have been designed to apply to the cervix for dysplasia, studies proving adequacy are not available.

CryoPen Closed System

1. Select the appropriate size reusable tip to match the lesion.
2. Apply the CryoPen tip directly to the lesion.
3. The size of the tip and amount of pressure applied affect rapidity and depth of freeze.
4. Obtain the rim of ice ball size desired.
5. Allow to thaw.
6. Repeat the freeze if indicated.

The advantage of these tips is that the ice ball is well controlled. They can also be used in sensitive areas such as around the eyes where it is necessary to avoid cryogen spray.

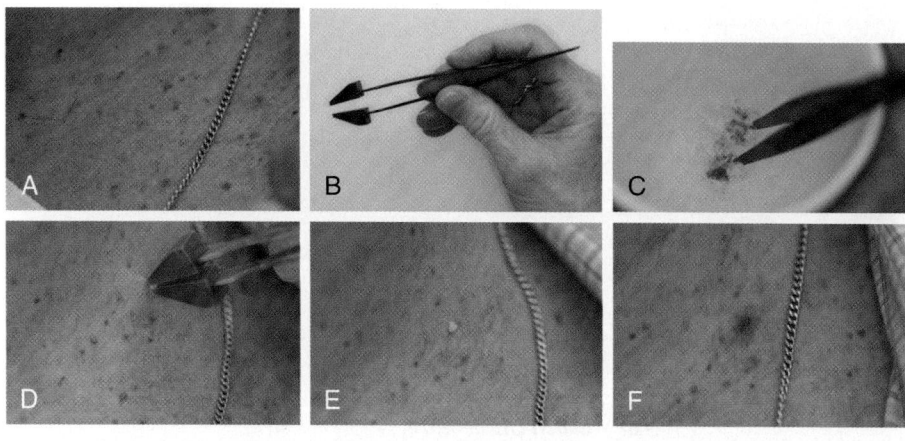

Fig. 14.15 Treatment of a skin tag using cryosurgical forceps (Brymill). (A) Skin tag. (B) Forceps. (C) Forceps in Styrofoam cup with liquid nitrogen. (D) Grasping the skin tag for a few seconds. (E) Frozen tag. (F) Appearance of tag 10 minutes after freezing.

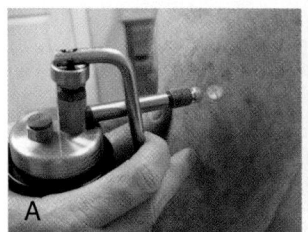
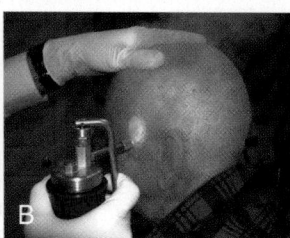
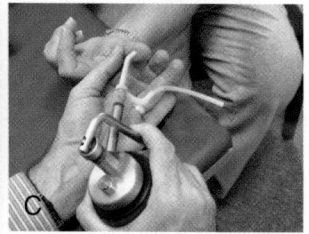

Fig. 14.16 (A) Perpendicular spray technique using liquid nitrogen in a cryogun. (B) Open spray using a spiral pattern to cover a large area. (C) Cryosurgery of a wart using the Brymill CRY-AC with a closed probe.

Nitrous Oxide or Carbon Dioxide Closed System

1. Debride any keratin you can beforehand (e.g., plantar wart). This is usually done using a blade to shave away any callus.
2. Place a thin layer of water-soluble gel on the lesion to hydrate the lesion and to enhance even contact with the cryoprobe. If the lesion is dry, soaking it well with a wet 4 × 4 gauze pad before application of the gel will enhance the effectiveness of the freeze, especially if it is a large lesion.
3. Select a probe with a size and shape that correspond to the lesion size (Fig. 14.17).
4. Hold the handpiece ("gun") with trigger in one hand, and guide the probe tip to a point over the site of freezing (see Fig. 14.17).
5. Place the tip on the lesion and activate the gun. The tip will stick to the skin within 3 to 5 seconds.
6. Freeze until desired ice ball is obtained (Fig. 14.18A).
7. *Thaw.* This will be an active process. Some units will thaw automatically when the freeze trigger or button is released, whereas others require that a second button be pushed. The gas from the tank to the handpiece must be turned on for this to occur. The tip will "release" from the skin within seconds. The frozen skin will then thaw passively (see Fig. 14.18B).

Cryogen Canister: Verruca-Freeze, Frigi-Dent or Histofreezer

See Fig. 14.12.

1. Select a limiting cone size that will completely encompass the lesion (which must be benign) plus 2 mm of normal tissue.
2. Hold the cone securely against the skin to prevent leakage (this is essential; see Fig. 14.12B).
3. Dispense enough liquid from the canister to fill the cone to the line (approximately 0.125- to 0.25-inch). Avoid splattering; use a gentle spray.
4. Allow the fluid to evaporate (30 to 60 seconds).
5. Remove the cone.
6. Repeat, if indicated.

Alternatively, the metal needle driver, forceps, or buds can be frozen and then applied to the lesions much like the cotton-tipped applicators with liquid nitrogen.

TECHNIQUE FOR SPECIFIC LESIONS

Keratin Removal

Lesions with dense keratin coverings (e.g., plantar warts) are very resistant to cryosurgery (especially to nitrous oxide and canister gases). The patient can help prepare a plantar wart with 2 weeks of salicylic acid application. After bathing and cleaning the area, the patient should apply a 17% solution (e.g., Compound W) to the wart(s). A piece of Mediplast (40% salicylic acid) or Trans-Ver-Sal, cut just a little larger than the wart, can also be used. This is left in place 24 hours until the next day's application. (If the pad migrates significantly during the day, it may have to be used at night only.) After 2 weeks, a soft white layer of keratin can be peeled away, revealing the base or root of the plantar wart lesion. Freezing time for the lesion should be shortened once the keratin layer and outer epidermis have been removed.

Alternatively, in lesions with significant keratin, a No. 10 or No. 15 scalpel blade can be used to shave off the keratin in thin layers until the first red punctate vasculature is seen (verruca). Stop debridement at this point (punctate bleeding) to minimize bleeding.

Actinic Keratoses

Usually actinic keratoses are quite superficial. If they are numerous, liquid nitrogen is much quicker to use than nitrous oxide. Anesthesia is rarely needed. Because these lesions are premalignant, however, a full-thickness freeze is suggested. Whichever technique is used, be sure to obtain at least a 3-mm ice ball. It may be best to freeze a second time. Moisten the lesion first (with K-Y Jelly) if nitrous oxide is used.

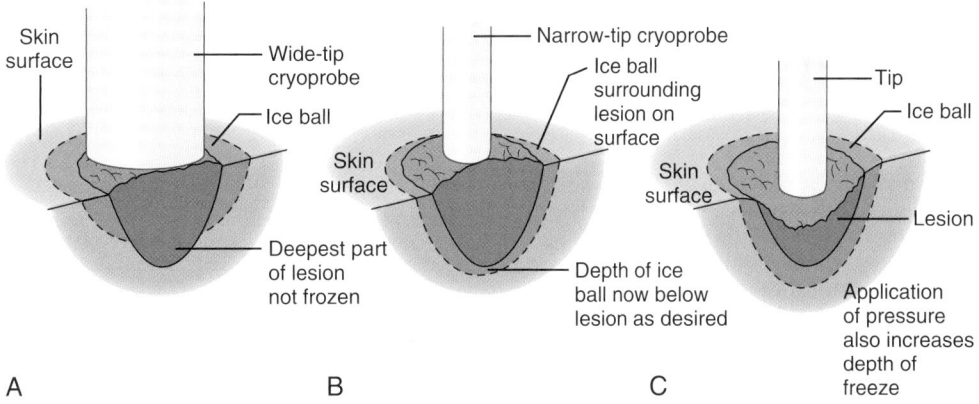

Fig. 14.17 Cryosurgery of a deep but narrow lesion. (A) If a wide cryoprobe tip is used, the deepest part of the lesion will not be frozen even though a 3- to 5-mm margin of ice ball is obtained. (B) To ensure that the entire lesion is frozen, a tip smaller than the lesion may be used, thereby limiting the rapid lateral spread of the ice ball. (C) Alternatively, the cryoprobe tip may be pressed down until the top of the lesion is below the skin surface. The cold will penetrate deeper before too much normal tissue is frozen by lateral spread.

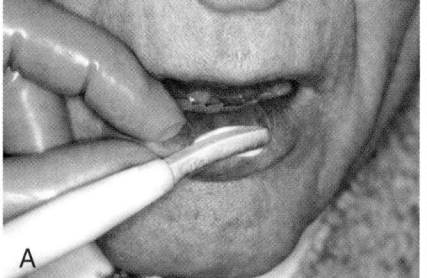
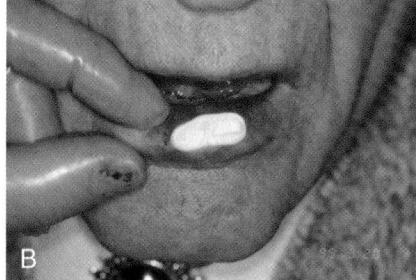

Fig. 14.18 Cryosurgery of a lip lesion using a nitrous oxide closed system with a hemorrhoid tip. (A) Freezing the lesion. (B) Appearance immediately after removing the tip.

Nonmelanoma Skin Cancers

This technique is used for treating malignant lesions such as basal cell carcinomas less than 1 cm. Be sure to confirm the diagnosis by obtaining a biopsy before treatment. Many clinicians do not use cryosurgery on malignancies other than basal cell carcinomas, although studies also would support treating smaller (<1 cm) squamous cell carcinomas. Malignant cells are more cryoresistant, and destruction requires temperatures of −40°C to −50°C. Only liquid nitrogen or nitrous oxide may be used to treat malignancies. The canister cryogens do not achieve low enough tissue temperatures for effective treatment of these lesions. If cryosurgery is the chosen method of destruction for basal cell carcinoma, the probe can be applied directly to the lesion. Alternatively, shave off (debulk) most of the lesion and freeze the now thinned-out residual. Follow the steps outlined previously for the technique used, but continue the freeze until the ice ball is 5 mm beyond the margins of the lesion (see Fig. 14.2). When freezing is complete, allow the lesion to completely thaw and repeat the freezing process a second time. Because a malignancy is being treated, it is wise to document the extent of the freeze and the thaw time. Freeze time will vary depending on the cryogen being used, but the thaw times should be the same—halo thaw time about 2 minutes with complete thaw time 3 to 5 minutes, depending on size (see Box 14.1).

Full-Thickness Freeze Technique for Anatomically Large or Irregular Skin Lesions

Some lesions are too large to be completely frozen by a cryoprobe in a single freeze. Examples include Bowen disease, keloids, vascular lesions, or mosaic warts. In such cases, note the central location of the cryoprobe. This spot will be the lateral margin of the cryoprobe placement (nitrous oxide) for the next adjacent freeze (after thawing occurs). This allows for the 50% overlap that is desired. Freezing of extremely large lesions can begin on one side, and then the opposite side can be frozen while the first is thawing. Progressing from opposite sides to the center will save time and still allow for a 40% to 50% freeze overlap.

Using liquid nitrogen, overlapping direct sprays can be performed or the lesion can be covered in a paintbrush or enlarging spiral pattern. It is important that a good freeze is obtained over the entire lesion.

Hypertrophic Scars and Keloids

Cryosurgery can be used in two different ways to treat scars. It can be used alone or before injection of steroids. The hyperemia and edema that immediately follow freezing and thawing soften the hypertrophic scar or keloid and allow easy penetration by a needle and a more even distribution of intralesional steroid. Cryosurgery alone, without steroids, will reduce the size of large keloids, but numerous treatments may be needed, and more vigorous freezing is needed if steroids are not used (also see Chapter 28, Hypertrophic Scars and Keloids).

Use the following technique for nitrous oxide (see Fig. 14.4):

1. Select a cryotip slightly narrower than the scar. You do not want the ice ball to extend more than 1 mm beyond the scar.
2. Apply a thin coat of water-soluble gel to the scar only. (Do not cover any of the surrounding skin.)
3. Moisten and warm the cryotip in warm water. Freeze until the ice ball progresses just to the edge of the scar, usually for 20 seconds to 1 minute, occasionally longer if necessary.
4. If steroids will be used, wait approximately 10 to 15 minutes for mild tissue swelling, then proceed with intralesional injection using triamcinolone diacetate (Aristocort) or triamcinolone acetonide (Kenalog 10 mg/mL) with a small 30-gauge needle. Use very dilute solutions (0.1 mL diluted with 0.3 mL of a parabens-free

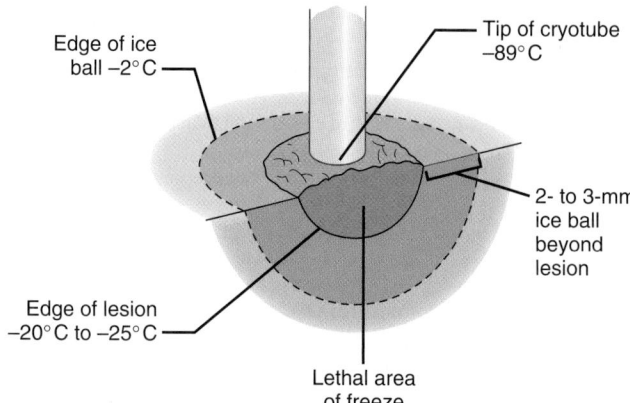

Fig. 14.19 Treatment of benign lesions. To ensure that all of the tissue of the lesion reaches the −20°C to −25°C necessary for destruction, the outer edge of the frozen area (the ice ball) should extend at least 2 to 3 mm in all directions beyond the lesion.

1% lidocaine without epinephrine) and a sufficient volume to infiltrate the entire scar. (Increase the concentration on successive visits as necessary, depending on response.)
5. For large scars, four to five treatments may be necessary at 6- to 8-week intervals to achieve optimal success.

Liquid nitrogen can also be used. It is quicker and very efficacious, but it may be more difficult to limit the size of the freeze with smaller lesions.

Treatment may produce a copious discharge during the first few postoperative days.

Condylomata Acuminata

See also Chapter 138, Treatment of Noncervical Condylomata Acuminata.

1. Penile, perianal, and vulvar areas are sensitive. Individual lesions and small groups of condylomata can be frozen without anesthetic. Topical anesthetics can also be applied before freezing. In some situations, 20% topical benzocaine (HurriCaine), 5% lidocaine, EMLA cream, or ELA-Max may be appropriate. Topical applications may require 30 to 60 minutes to achieve maximum effectiveness. ELA-Max is now available over the counter. Large or multiple lesions may require injections of local anesthetic.
2. Find all the lesions. For women, examine the genitalia and the cervix with a colposcope to look for very small lesions, particularly in the vaginal introitus, on the vaginal side walls, the vulva, and the rectum. Women with external condylomata have a high incidence of cervical dysplasia, and colposcopy may be indicated. (See Chapter 124, Colposcopic Examination, and Chapter 125, Cryotherapy of the Cervix.)
3. If nitrous oxide is used, moisten the skin lesions with a water-soluble gel. Touch the lesion(s) with an appropriately sized probe. Activate the nitrous oxide–powered tip, and effect adherence after 3 to 5 seconds. Then apply gentle traction. Do not pull too hard or you may tear the tissue being treated or the surrounding skin. Freeze for approximately 20 to 45 seconds. Judge actual freezing time by the size of the lesion and the ice ball, which should extend 2 mm beyond the margin of the lesion(s) (Fig. 14.19). Within minutes after freezing, the condylomata darken and then will turn black; they should slough within a few days. If they do not turn dark, refreezing may be necessary.
4. Liquid nitrogen in either form (spray, cotton-tipped applicator, or metal pickups) is quicker for treating multiple lesions. Needle drivers, metal pickups or specially designed forceps (Brymill, Fig. 14.15) dipped into a cup of liquid nitrogen will also work.

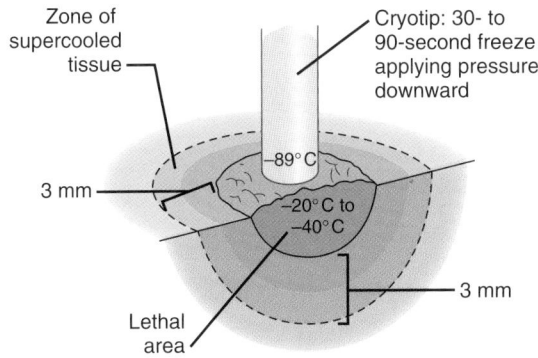

Fig. 14.20 Full-thickness destructive freeze of vascular lesion. Pressure is applied to the tip to express as much blood as possible.

5. A combination of electrosurgery (radiofrequency surgery) and cryosurgery may speed the treatment of extensive perianal, vulvar, or penile lesions. The cryosurgery component will allow preservation of the elastic tissue matrix and expandability of the anal canal, penis, and vulva after healing. The electrosurgery component is used for tissue debridement, making sure not to cut too deep. Then, the base of each lesion is frozen for 20 to 30 seconds. This technique can be used for treatment of large areas of condylomata often seen on the genitalia.

Molluscum Contagiosum

Freezing is often an excellent, nearly painless treatment for molluscum contagiosum. Advise your patients, particularly children, to protect the healing crust to decrease the chance of scar formation.

1. If using nitrous oxide, prepare each lesion with a small amount of water-soluble gel. Freeze each lesion for 30 seconds to 1 minute. Use very fine-tipped probes to avoid freezing normal skin.
2. With liquid nitrogen, only brief freezes of several seconds are necessary.
3. Advise the patient and parent that the lesions should fall completely off within 2 weeks or less. If they do not, the patient should return soon for retreatment to prevent their spread.

Vascular Lesions (Hemangiomas and Strawberry Hemangiomas)

As with malignant lesions, vascular lesions are more cryoresistant, and a freeze/thaw/refreeze technique is recommended (Fig. 14.20). Nitrous oxide may be the preferred method both to control the extent of the freeze and to be able to compress the lesion to remove the blood, although liquid nitrogen can also be used.

1. Moisten and warm the cryotip in warm water, and apply water-soluble gel to the lesion.
2. Make contact with the probe on the hemangioma and exert firm pressure to squeeze the blood out of the vascular channels.
3. Activate the cryogun, and hold pressure against the lesion throughout the freeze. Begin timing when the ice ball becomes visible. For larger lesions, freeze for 1½ minutes or until the ice ball extends out 3 mm. Allow 5 to 7 minutes for thawing, and then repeat the freeze.

Skin Verrucae

Liquid nitrogen spray is the most effective and most rapid treatment option. Use a freeze/thaw/refreeze technique and obtain a 1- to 2-mm margin for each treated wart. Repeat the treatments every 1 to 3 weeks based on response. Debride any necrotic tissue before the next freeze.

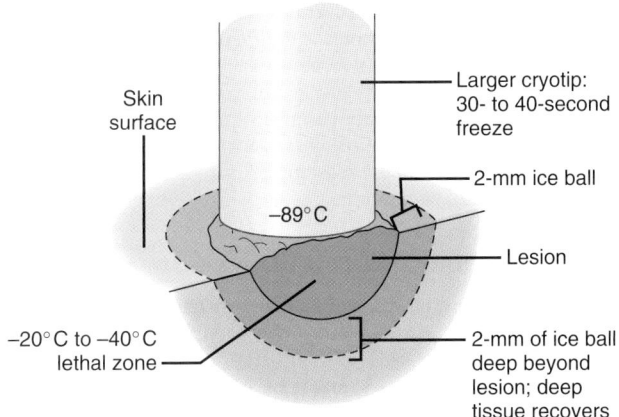

Fig. 14.21 Nitrous oxide partial-thickness freeze used for removal of superficial lesions (e.g., seborrheic keratoses). Cryotip should cover or nearly cover entire lesion to limit depth of freeze. Halo thaw time should be approximately 30 to 45 seconds for all methods.

Seborrheic Keratoses

Seborrheic keratoses are usually quite superficial. However, they frequently demonstrate a thick raised component. They are quickly treated using liquid nitrogen because debridement, anesthesia, and soaking are usually not required. For nitrous oxide, the raised lesions may need to be debrided or hydrated before cryosurgery can be effective. Because the procedure takes longer, anesthesia using 1% lidocaine may be needed with nitrous oxide, especially in larger lesions. A 2-mm ice ball margin is sufficient for treatment (Fig. 14.21).

Cryotherapy for Cervical Intraepithelial Neoplasia

See Chapter 125, Cryotherapy of the Cervix.

COMPLICATIONS AND SHORTCOMINGS

- Pigment cells and hair cells may be destroyed by cryosurgery.
- Hypertrophic scars, verrucae, and vascular lesions are quite resistant to treatment and may recur, requiring several treatments.
- Areas of poor circulation may be susceptible to prolonged ulcer formation, especially in elderly diabetic patients (e.g., anterior tibial compartment).
- Tissue pathology documentation and verification of adequate destruction of malignant lesions is not possible with cryosurgery. Pretreatment biopsy is recommended for all lesions suspicious for malignancy. A presumed "benign" lesion may indeed be malignant and thus insufficiently treated with cryosurgery alone. So, if there is doubt concerning a possible melanoma or squamous cell cancer, biopsy is recommended.
- Cryosurgery in the periorbital area may cause excessive swelling, in which the eyelid may be shut for several hours or days. However, cryosurgery of small, well-localized lesions on the eyelids is usually well tolerated. Be conservative on the freeze time until the individual patient's reaction is documented.
- Peripheral neuropathy (the ulnar nerve at the elbow or peripheral nerves on the lateral aspect of the digits) can result when areas adjacent to nerves are frozen. The nerve sheath is cryoresistant, but the nerve tissue is more susceptible to damage. This side effect can be minimized (if using a closed nitrous oxide or carbon dioxide system) by pulling the skin outward and away from the nerve, once good contact is achieved. If the nerve is affected, recovery occurs within 4 to 6 weeks, although 3 to 6 months may occasionally be required. Sensory nerves are more likely to be affected.
- In general, the skin of infants and the elderly, as well as previously damaged skin, is more susceptible to necrosis and blister-

ing than normal skin. Thin skin can be a result of sun exposure, radiation, and chronic topical steroid application. Reduce freeze times until the reaction of a damaged area is known.

- One of the most common lesions treated with cryosurgery is actinic keratosis. Should any lesion not totally resolve after treatment, especially if it persists after a second cryosurgery session, it should be sampled. These resistant lesions are frequently found to be squamous cell carcinomas.

POSTPROCEDURE PATIENT EDUCATION

The patient should be informed of the anticipated healing time and results, as well as the need to call the office should there be an overreaction to freezing. If the blister enlarges more than 5 to 6 mm beyond the lesion, it might be best to open it. The basic instructions would be the same as those given with a second-degree burn. If the skin from the blister peels off, use moist healing techniques. Document that the patient was told of permanent pigment changes, possible nerve involvement, and hair loss. Placing a copy of the handout that was given to the patient in the chart provides excellent medical-legal documentation as well as an excellent medical reference for staff and physician alike. (See patient education and patient consent forms available at www.expertconsult.com.)

COMMON ERRORS

The most common errors encountered in cryosurgery relate to undertreating the lesion. This usually occurs because of failure to ensure adequate ice ball formation in and around the lesion. Lack of consistent contact of the freezing tip with the lesion or failure to follow proper technique when using the liquid nitrogen spray may lead to clinical failure. Inadequate freeze often occurs in plantar warts because of the insulating effect of keratin. Unless the keratin layer is removed before treatment, cryosurgery is less likely to be effective. Selection of cryogen agent is important, especially when treating malignancy. A canister refrigerant cannot achieve cold enough temperatures to treat malignancy effectively. Conversely, overfreezing lesions may lead to local side effects, especially hypopigmentation.

PATIENT EDUCATION GUIDES

See patient education and patient consent forms available at www.expertconsult.com.

CPT/BILLING CODES

Cryosurgery is billed out as "destruction of lesions." Certain areas require specific codes.

Destruction (Cryocautery, Electrocautery, Laser, Chemical, or Curettement)

Benign Lesions

Site and size not needed, except for locations noted following.

11200	Skin tags, 1–15 lesions
11201	Skin tags, each additional 10 lesions or portion thereof
17000	Destruction of *premalignant* lesion (e.g., actinic keratosis); first lesion
17003	Second through 14 *premalignant* lesions, each (used in conjunction with 17000) (charge for each additional lesion treated)
17004	Destruction of *premalignant* lesions, 15 or more lesions (do not report 17004 in conjunction with 17000–17003)

17106	Destruction cutaneous vascular proliferative lesions, less than 10 cm^2
17110	Destruction of benign other than skin tags or cutaneous vascular proliferative lesions, up to 14 lesions
30117	Destruction of intranasal lesion
45190	Destruction of rectal tumor (e.g., cryosurgery), transanal approach
46615	Anal, ablation of tumor, polyp or other lesion, with anoscopy
46916	Anal (perianal), benign lesion, simple destruction, cryosurgery
46924	Anal (perianal), benign lesion, extensive destruction
54056	Genitals (male), penis, cryotherapy, simple destruction
54065	Genitals (male), penis, cryotherapy, extensive destruction
56501	Genitals (female), vulva/introitus, simple destruction
56515	Genitals (female), vulva/introitus, extensive destruction
57061	Genitals (female), vagina, simple destruction
57065	Genitals (female), vagina, extensive destruction
57511	Cervix
67850	Eyelid, lid margin, up to 1 cm
68135	Eyelid, conjunctiva

Malignant Lesions

See codes 17260 to 17286 as follows.
NOTE: All of these codes have a 10-day global fee surgical period. Destruction by any method, with or without curettement, includes local anesthesia and ablation, and usually does not require closure. Sizes listed describe *lesion* diameter, not the width of the skin area destroyed.

17260	Trunk, arm, or leg (TAL): <0.5 cm
17261	TAL: 0.6–1.0 cm
17262	TAL: 1.1–2.0 cm
17263	TAL: 2.1–3.0 cm
17264	TAL: 3.1–4.0 cm
17266	TAL: >4.0 cm
17270	Scalp, neck, hand, foot, or genitalia (SNHFG): <0.5 cm
17271	SNHFG: 0.6–1.0 cm
17272	SNHFG: 1.1–2.0 cm
17273	SNHFG: 2.1–3.0 cm
17274	SNHFG: 3.1–4.0 cm
17276	SNHFG: >4.0 cm
17280	Face, eyelid, ear, nose, lip, or mucous membrane (FEENLM): <0.5 cm
17281	FEENLM: 0.6–1.0 cm
17282	FEENLM: 1.1–2.0 cm
17283	FEENLM: 2.1–3.0 cm
17284	FEENLM: 3.1–4.0 cm
17286	FEENLM: >4.0 cm

ICD-10-CM DIAGNOSTIC CODES

See under "neoplasm, skin." Then identify anatomic site and whether lesion is benign, malignant (primary or secondary), carcinoma in situ, or uncertain.

Acknowledgment

The editors recognize the contributions of John E. Hocutt Jr, MD, to this chapter in a previous edition of this text.

SUPPLIERS

(See contact information available at www.expertconsult.com.)

Liquid nitrogen
  Brymill Cryogenic Systems
  CryoPen, Inc.
  CryoSurgery, Inc.
  OraSure Technologies
  Wallach Surgical Devices, Inc.
Nitrous oxide units
  CooperSurgical Inc.
  Wallach Surgical Devices, Inc.
  Welch Allyn, Inc.

RECOMMENDED READING

American Academy of Dermatology Committee on Guidelines of Care. Guidelines of care for cryosurgery. *J Am Acad Dermatol.* 1994;31:648–653.

Andrews MD. Cryosurgery for common skin conditions. *Am Fam Physician.* 2004;69:2365–2372.

Bacelieri R, Johnson SM. Cutaneous warts: an evidence-based approach to therapy. *Am Fam Physician.* 2005;72:647–652.

Bowen GM, White Jr GL, Gerwels JW. Mohs micrographic surgery. *Am Fam Physician.* 2005;72:845–848.

Burkhart CG, Pchalek I, Adler M, Burkhart CN. An in vitro study comparing temperatures of over-the-counter wart preparations with liquid nitrogen. *J Am Acad Dermatol.* 2007;57:1019–1020.

Cohen PR, Schulze KE, Nelson BR. Cutaneous carcinoma with mixed histology: A potential etiology for skin cancer recurrence and an indication for Mohs microscopically controlled surgical excision. *South Med J.* 2005;98:740–747.

Dandurand M, Petit T, Martel P, Guillot B, for ANAES. Management of basal cell carcinoma in adults: clinical practice guidelines. *Eur J Dermatol.* 2006;16:394–401.

Essers BA, Dirksen CD, Nieman FH, et al. Cost-effectiveness of Mohs micrographic surgery vs. surgical excision for basal cell carcinoma of the face. *Arch Dermatol.* 2006;142:187–194.

Habif TP. *Clinical Dermatology: A Color Guide to Diagnosis and Therapy.* 6th ed. Philadelphia: Elsevier; 2016.

Jackson A, Colver G, Dawber RPR. *Cutaneous Cryosurgery: Principles and Clinical Practice.* 3rd ed. London: Informa Healthcare; 2005.

Leibovitch I, Huilgol SC, Selva D, et al. Basosquamous carcinoma: treatment with Mohs micrographic surgery. *Cancer.* 2005;104:170–175.

Miller SJ, Alam M, Andersen J, et al. for the National Comprehensive Cancer Network. Basal cell and squamous cell skin cancers. *J Natl Compr Canc Netw.* 2007;5:506–529.

Nguyen TH. Mohs bashing out of hand. *Plast Reconstr Surg.* 2005;115:361–362.

Otley CC. Cost-effectiveness of Mohs micrographic surgery vs. surgical excision for basal cell carcinoma of the face. *Arch Dermatol.* 2006;142:1235; author reply 1235–1236.

Otley CC. Mohs' micrographic surgery for basal-cell carcinoma of the face. *Lancet.* 2005;365:1226–1227; author reply 1227.

Pasquali P. Cryosurgery. In: Robinson JK, Hanke DW, Siegel DM, et al., eds. *Surgery of the Skin: Procedural Dermatology.* 3rd ed. Philadelphia: Saunders; 2015.

Redondo P, Marquina M, Pretel M, et al. Methyl-ALA-induced fluorescence in photodynamic diagnosis of basal cell carcinoma prior to Mohs micrographic surgery. *Arch Dermatol.* 2008;144:115–117.

Shindel AW, Mann MW, Lev RY, et al. Mohs micrographic surgery for penile cancer: management and long-term followup. *J Urol.* 2007;178:1980–1985. [See comment in Nat Clin Pract Urol 5:364–365, 2008.].

Sterry W. for the European Dermatology Forum Guideline Committee: guidelines: the management of basal cell carcinoma. *Eur J Dermatol.* 2006;16:467–475.

Stulberg DL, Crandell B, Fawcett RS. Diagnosis and treatment of basal cell and squamous cell carcinomas. *Am Fam Physician.* 2004;70:1481–1488.

Telfer NR, Colver GB, Morton CA, for the British Association of Dermatologists. Guidelines for the management of basal cell carcinoma. *Br J Dermatol.* 2008;159:35–48.

Usatine RP, Stulberg DL. Cryosurgery. In: Usatine RP, Pfenninger JL, Stulberg DL, Small R, eds. *Dermatologic and Cosmetic Procedures in Office Practice.* Philadelphia: Elsevier Saunders; 2012:182–198.

Usatine RP, Stulberg DL, Colver GB. *Cutaneous Cryosurgery.* 4th ed. New York: CRC Press; 2014.

CHAPTER 15

DERMOSCOPY

Ashfaq A. Marghoob • Azadeh Esmaeili • Alon Scope

Skin cancer, the most common malignancy in the United States, is associated with significant morbidity and mortality. Fortunately, early detection of skin cancer, through visual examination of the entire cutaneous surface, can have a positive impact on patient outcomes. Because dermoscopy can improve their ability to identify cutaneous malignancies, it has been well received by clinicians engaged in skin cancer screening efforts. Dermoscopy can also be used to monitor response to a topical treatment of skin lesions.

Dermoscopy is a technique that requires the use of hand-held magnification devices known as *dermatoscopes*. These instruments illuminate the skin and, by exploiting the optical properties of the skin, allow the clinician to visualize subsurface colors and structures. Dermatoscopes are designed to reduce the amount of light reflected off the skin surface, thereby allowing clinicians to appreciate the appearance of the subsurface anatomic structures of the epidermis and papillary dermis that are otherwise not discernible to the unaided eye. Three types of dermatoscopes are available: one using standard light-emitting diode illumination (i.e., *nonpolarized dermoscopy*) and two using cross-polarized light (contact and non-contact *polarized dermoscopy*; Fig. 15.1). To reduce skin surface light reflection, *nonpolarized dermoscopy* requires direct skin contact in the presence of a liquid interface (e.g., mineral oil, alcohol, clear hand-sanitizing gel) between the dermatoscope and the skin. *Polarized dermoscopy*, however, does not require an immersion liquid. One of the inherent properties of cross-polarized light is to filter out light reflected from the skin surface, allowing only light reflected from deeper layers of the skin to reach the observer's retina. Polarized and nonpolarized dermoscopy provide complementary information. For example, polarized dermoscopy is the preferred method for visualizing blood vessels because it does not require direct skin contact. The ability to see dermoscopic structures without direct skin contact eliminates the effect of contact pressure–induced blanching of the blood vessels. Nonpolarized dermoscopy, on the other hand, is better for visualizing structures within the superficial layers of the epidermis, such as milia cysts, structures important to recognize to correctly identify seborrheic keratoses. With dermascopes, clinicians can appreciate morphologic alterations in skin lesions due to their different shapes and colors (Table 15.1). Because most dermoscopic colors and structures have been correlated with histopathologic findings, dermoscopy can be considered a form of bedside, in vivo, gross tissue inspection that can help predict tissue pathology.

The overall clinical diagnostic accuracy for malignant melanoma (MM), without the added benefit of dermoscopy, for experienced dermatologists is only about 60%. Dermoscopy enhances the diagnostic accuracy for MM and helps triage those lesions requiring a biopsy. In a large meta-analysis of dermoscopy studies, Bafounta and colleagues revealed that dermoscopy increased diagnostic accuracy by 49% compared with unaided examination, with mean sensitivity increasing by 19% and mean specificity by 6%. The increase in specificity with dermoscopy translates into a reduction in the number of excised benign lesions. This is demonstrated in a retrospective analysis that showed a significant reduction in the benign–malignant ratio of excised melanocytic lesions from 18:1 in the predermoscopy era to 4:1 after dermoscopy was implemented by trained clinicians. The benefit of using dermoscopy greatly depends on experience, and reliance on dermoscopy by untrained or less experienced examiners was found to be no better than clinical inspection alone. However, studies indicate that participation in short dermoscopy training courses improves confidence and diagnostic performance of nonexperts when evaluating lesions by dermoscopy. The benefits provided by the use of dermoscopy are presented in Box 15.1.

EVALUATION TECHNIQUE: TWO-STEP DERMOSCOPY ALGORITHM

The two-step dermoscopy algorithm forms the foundation for the dermoscopic evaluation of skin lesions (Fig. 15.2).

The first step in performing dermoscopy requires that the observer classify the lesion as either a growth of melanocytic or nonmelanocytic origin. On nonglabrous skin, the presence of a pigment network, aggregated globules, streaks, or homogeneous blue pigmentation identifies the lesion as melanocytic (Figs. 15.3 through 15.6). In addition, a pseudonetwork pattern can be seen in melanocytic lesions on facial skin (Fig. 15.7). On the other hand, melanocytic

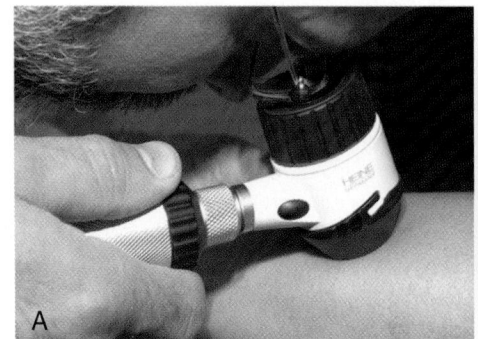
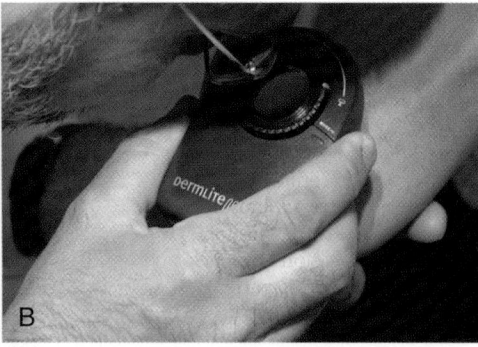

Fig. 15.1 Physician examining a pigmented skin lesion under contact nonpolarized dermoscopy (A) and non-contact polarized dermoscopy (B).

TABLE 15.1 Dermoscopic Structures and Their Histopathologic Correlations

Dermoscopic Structures	Definition	Histopathologic Correlation
Pigment network (reticulation)	Gridlike network consisting of pigmented "lines" and hypopigmented "holes."	Melanin in keratinocytes or melanocytes along the epidermal rete ridges.
Pseudonetwork	In facial lesions, diffuse pigmentation interrupted by nonpigmented follicular openings, appearing similar to a network.	Pigment in the epidermis or dermis interrupted by follicular and adnexal openings of the face.
Structureless (homogeneous) areas	Areas devoid of dermoscopic structures and without regression. These areas can be pigmented or nonpigmented. If the area is uniformly dark, it is referred to as a "blotch" (see below).	Lack of melanin or presence of melanin in all layers of the skin.
Dots	Small, round structures <0.1 mm in diameter that may be black, brown, gray, or bluish.	Aggregates of melanocytes or melanin granules. Black dots represent pigment in the upper epidermis or stratum corneum. Brown dots represent pigment at the dermoepidermal junction. Gray-blue dots represent pigment in the papillary dermis.
Peppering	Tiny, blue-gray granules.	Melanin deposited as intracellular (mostly within melanophages) or extracellular particles in the upper dermis.
Globules	Round to oval structures that may be brown, black, or red with diameters >0.1 mm.	Nests of melanocytes in the dermis and dermal–epidermal junction.
Streaks (pseudopods, radial streaming)	Radially arranged projections of dark pigment (brown to black) at the periphery of the lesion.	Confluent junctional nests of melanocytes.
Blotches	Dark brown to black, usually homogeneous areas of pigment that obscure underlying structures.	Aggregates of melanin in the stratum corneum, epidermis, and upper dermis.
Regression areas	White, scarlike depigmentation (lighter than the surrounding skin, shiny white under polarized dermoscopy) often combined with or adjacent to blue-gray areas or peppering.	Scarlike changes: thickened fibrotic papillary dermis, dilated blood vessels, sparse lymphocytic infiltrates, and variable numbers of melanophages.
Blue-white veil	Irregular, confluent blue pigmentation with an overlying white "ground-glass" haze.	Aggregation of heavily pigmented cells (usually melanoma cells or melanophages) with compact orthokeratosis of the stratum corneum and acanthosis (thickened epidermis).
Vascular pattern	See Table 15.5 for vascular terminology.	Tumor neoangiogenesis and dilated blood vessels in the papillary dermis ("vascular blush").
Milia-like cysts	Round whitish or yellowish structures that shine brightly (like "stars in the sky") under nonpolarized dermoscopy.	Horn pseudocysts.
Comedo-like openings	"Blackhead"-like plugs on the surface of the lesion.	Concave clefts in the surface of the epidermis, often filled with keratin.
Fingerprint-like structures	Thin, light brown, parallel running lines.	Probably represent thin, elongated, pigmented epidermal rete ridges.
Ridges and fissures	Cerebriform surface resulting in gyri (ridges) and sulci (fissures). Confluence of adjacent comedo-like openings will create a fissure.	Wedge-shaped clefts of the surface of the epidermis, often filled with keratin (fissures).
"Moth-eaten" border	Concave invaginations of the lesion border.	Not available.
Leaf-like areas	Brown to gray-blue, discrete bulbous structures resembling a leaf pattern.	Large, complex nodules of pigmented basal cell carcinoma in the upper dermis.
Spoke-wheel–like structures	Well-circumscribed brown to gray-blue-brown radial projections meeting at a darker brown central hub.	Nests of basal cell carcinoma radiating from the follicular epithelium.
Large blue-gray ovoid nests	Large, well-circumscribed areas, larger than globules.	Large nests of basal cell tumor in the dermis.
Multiple blue-gray globules	Round well-circumscribed structures that, in the absence of a pigment network, suggest basal-cell carcinoma.	Small nests of basal cell tumor in the dermis.
Lacunae	Red, maroon, or black lagoons.	Dilated vascular spaces.
Parallel patterns	On acral areas, parallel rows of pigmentation following the furrows (nevi) or ridges (melanoma) of the dermatoglyphics.	Pigmented melanocytes in the furrows (crista limitans) or ridges (crista intermedia) of acral skin.

BOX 15.1 Benefits of Dermoscopy

Allows the observer to formulate a logical differential diagnosis
Differentiates melanocytic from nonmelanocytic skin lesions
Differentiates benign from malignant skin lesions
Provides earlier diagnosis of melanoma
Improves diagnostic accuracy
Increases the confidence in diagnosis
Avoids unnecessary biopsies
Helps isolate suspicious foci within a large lesion
Helps define lesion borders for presurgical margin mapping
Aids in monitoring patients with multiple nevi
Helps reassure patients

lesions on the palms and soles are recognized primarily by the presence of a parallel pigment pattern (Fig. 15.8; see Table 15.1). If, however, the lesion does not manifest any of the aforementioned melanocytic criteria, the observer seeks to identify specific criteria that can identify the lesion as a nonmelanocytic lesion (see Fig. 15.2) such as basal cell carcinoma (Figs. 15.9 through 15.11), squamous cell carcinoma (Fig. 15.12), hemangioma (Fig. 15.13), seborrheic keratosis (Figs. 15.14 and 15.15), or dermatofibroma (Fig. 15.16). In addition, a group of lesions exists that is termed "structureless" in that they do not manifest any melanocytic or nonmelanocytic lesion structures. Because it is not uncommon to encounter amelanotic and hypomelanotic MMs that are structureless, all such lesions should be viewed with extreme suspicion, especially if the lesion manifests linear irregular or dotted blood vessels, both commonly seen in MM (Fig. 15.17).

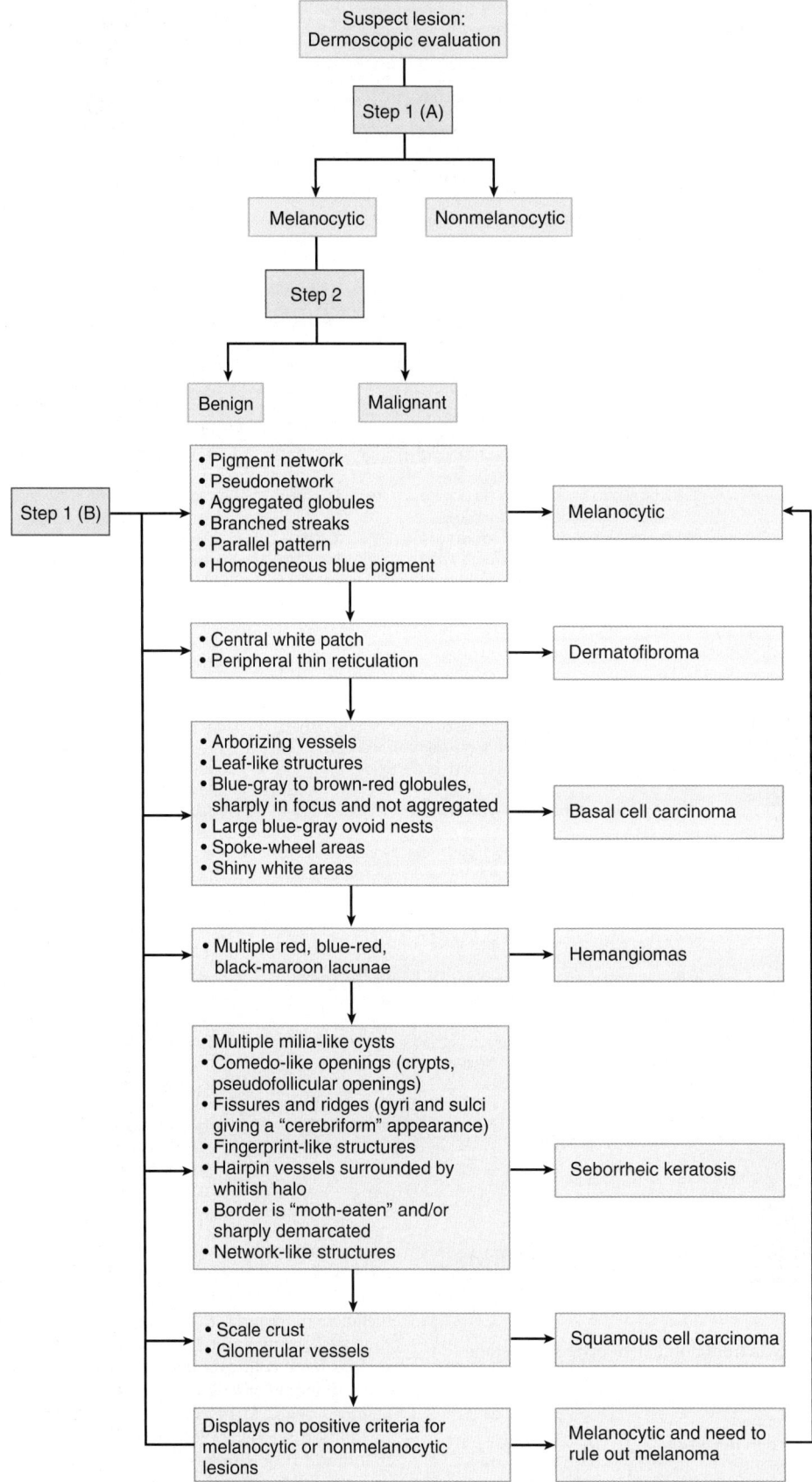

Fig. 15.2 The two-step algorithm for evaluation of a pigmented lesion. In the first step, the observer must decide whether the lesion is of melanocytic or nonmelanocytic origin (Step 1 [A]), using a stepwise evaluation of dermoscopic features (Step 1 [B]). In the second step, the observer differentiates between a benign melanocytic nevus and a melanoma using pattern analysis or one of the score-based algorithms mentioned in the text (e.g., ABCD rule, Menzies method, seven-point checklist).

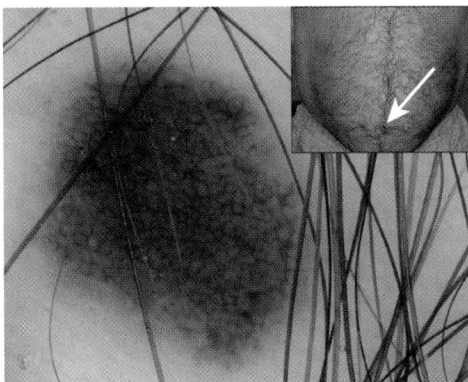

Fig. 15.3 This abdominal pigmented lesion is larger and darker than the patient's other moles *(inset, arrow)* and thus can be considered an "ugly duckling" that requires close-up examination. On dermoscopy, there is a pigmented network, and thus the lesion is melanocytic in origin. The lesion displays a regular network thinning out at the periphery, which is a benign nevus pattern.

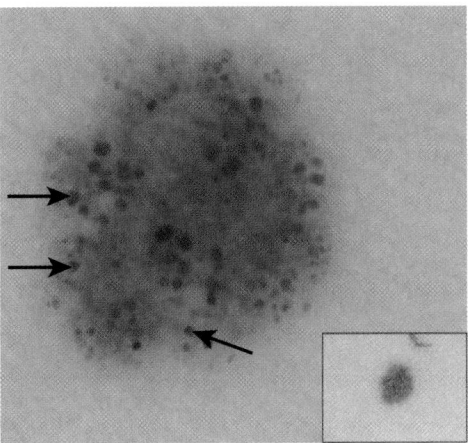

Fig. 15.4 Pigmented lesion featuring aggregated globules *(arrows)* with an overall symmetric distribution, which is a benign nevus pattern.

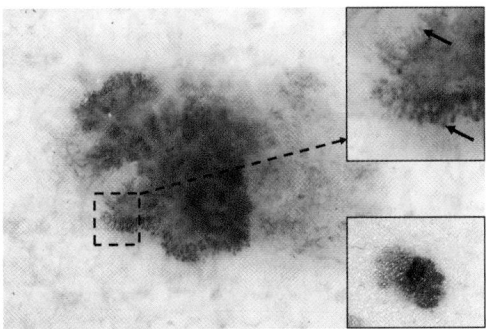

Fig. 15.5 This lesion is clinically suspect by the ABCD criteria for melanoma *(inset)*. On dermoscopy, the lesion does not display any of the benign nevus patterns and has peripheral streaks shaped like pseudopods *(dotted box and corresponding inset)*. The streaks are focally placed; their presence indicates that the lesion is melanocytic and raises concern for melanoma. This was a 0.4 mm thick melanoma.

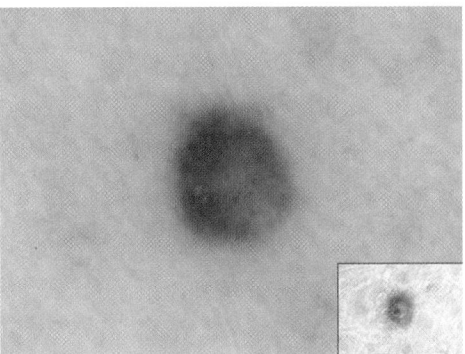

Fig. 15.6 Blue nevus showing homogeneous steel-blue pigmentation (one of the benign nevus patterns: the homogeneous pattern).

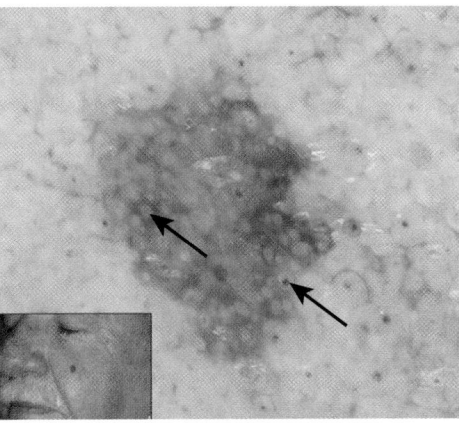

Fig. 15.7 Pigmented lesion on the face featuring a pseudonetwork pattern, produced by pigmentation surrounding adnexal openings such as hair follicles *(arrows)*. This is a benign nevus pattern.

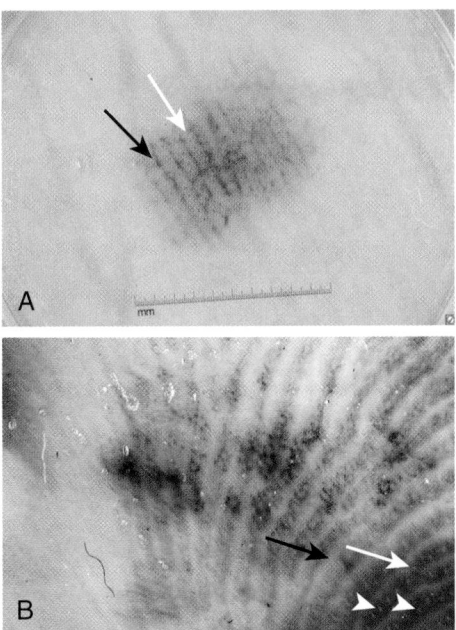

Fig. 15.8 (A) Acral nevus exhibiting a parallel furrow pattern, where pigmentation is seen in the furrows *(black arrow)* but does not involve the ridges *(white arrow)*. (B) Acral melanoma displaying the opposite pattern, with the pigmentation on the ridges *(white arrow)* but not in the furrows *(black arrow)*. To help distinguish ridges from furrows, one can look for the sweat gland openings, which are always located on the ridges *(white arrowheads)*.

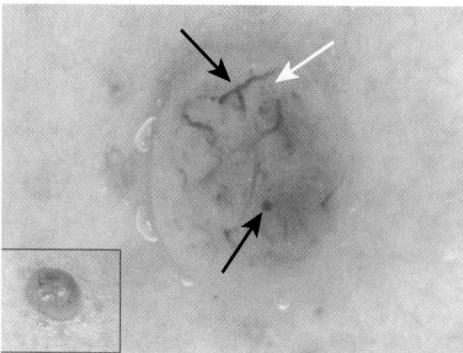

Fig. 15.9 Pigmented nodular basal cell carcinoma featuring arborizing telangiectases *(black arrow, top)*, ovoid nest *(black arrow, bottom)*, and multiple blue-gray globules *(white arrow)*.

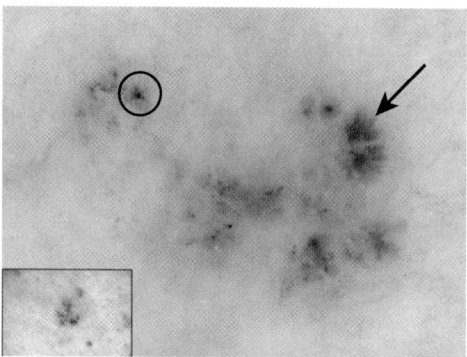

Fig. 15.10 Pigmented basal cell carcinoma showing spoke-wheel–like structures *(circle)* and leaflike areas *(arrow)*. Both of these structures are 100% specific for the diagnosis of basal cell carcinoma.

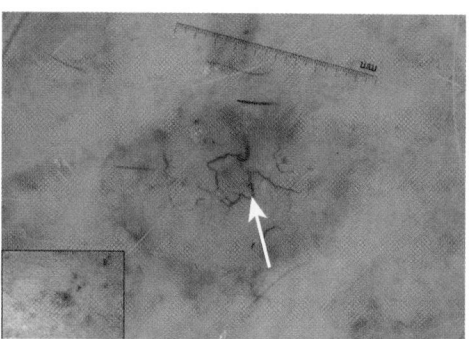

Fig. 15.11 Nonpigmented basal cell carcinoma featuring arborizing telangiectases *(arrow)*.

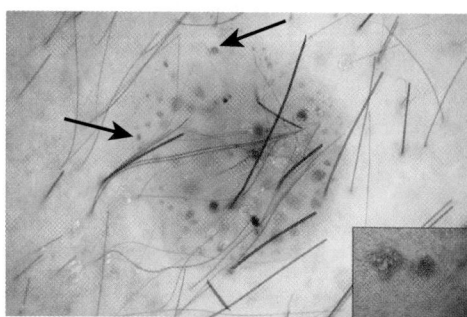

Fig. 15.12 This keratotic lesion *(inset)* reveals clusters of glomeruloid vessels *(arrows)*, suggestive of the diagnosis of squamous cell carcinoma.

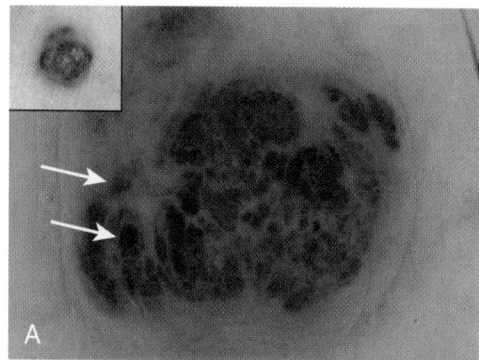

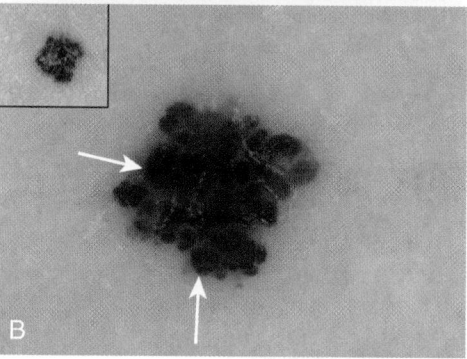

Fig. 15.13 (A) Hemangioma showing multiple lacunae of variable size, with a spectrum of colors from red to blue *(arrows)*. (B) Cherry hemangioma showing multiple bright to dark red lacunae *(arrows)*.

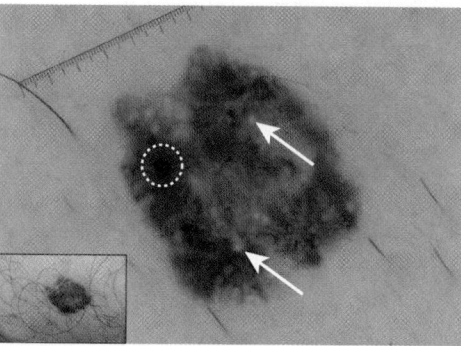

Fig. 15.14 Seborrheic keratosis featuring sharp borders, comedo-like openings *(dotted circle)*, and multiple milia-like cysts *(arrows)*.

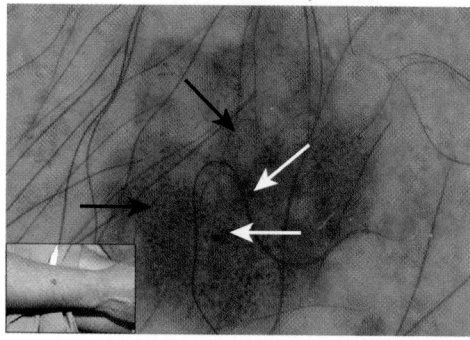

Fig. 15.15 Seborrheic keratosis featuring a cerebriform pattern. The ridges *(gyri, black arrows)* are the raised portion of the lesion, and the fissures *(sulci, white arrows)* are crypts filled with keratin.

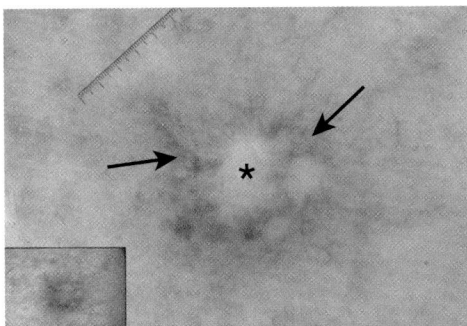

Fig. 15.16 Dermatofibroma featuring a central depigmented scarlike area *(asterisk)* with surrounding peripheral network *(arrows)*.

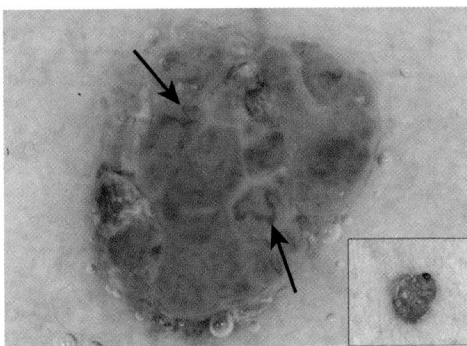

Fig. 15.17 This nodule is amelanotic and lacks specific melanocytic or nonmelanocytic criteria of the two-step algorithm of dermoscopy. Thus, by default, one needs to consider melanoma in the differential diagnosis. Indeed, this lesion features atypical hairpin vessels *(arrows)*, a clue to the correct diagnosis. This proved to be a nodular melanoma.

The second step in the two-step dermoscopy algorithm pertains only to lesions that are deemed to be of melanocytic origin, which include both lesions with melanocytic-specific features (Table 15.2) and those that are structureless. The objective during this second step of the evaluation process is to differentiate benign nevi from MM. Toward this goal, a number of algorithms have been created. Novices in dermoscopy may find one of the score-based algorithms useful in assessing melanocytic lesions (Box 15.2, Tables 15.3 and 15.4, and Figs. 15.18 and 15.19). However, once experience in dermoscopy is attained, most dermoscopists rely on pattern analysis to differentiate between nevi and MM.

Although pattern analysis requires experience, a simplified form of pattern analysis can be taught to novices in dermoscopy (Box 15.3). Fortunately, most benign nevi tend to manifest one of nine benign global patterns, all of which are characterized by symmetry of dermoscopic colors and structures. Hence, knowing these benign global patterns can prevent the excision of many atypical moles, most of which will reveal one of these benign patterns. Any lesion that deviates from one of these global benign patterns needs to be viewed with caution.

The nine benign global dermoscopic patterns include (1) diffuse reticular network, (2) patchy reticular network, (3) peripheral reticular network with central hypopigmentation, (4) peripheral reticular network with central hyperpigmentation, (5) peripheral reticular network with central globules, (6) globular pattern, (7) peripheral globules with central reticular network or starburst, (8) homogeneous pattern, and (9) symmetric multicomponent pattern (Figs. 15.20 and 15.21; see Box 15.3). Based on the aforementioned features common to benign nevi, it stands to reason that most melanocytic nevi will be symmetric, uniform, display less than three colors, and have an organized architecture.

TABLE 15.2	Dermoscopic Criteria for Melanocytic Lesions
Dermoscopic Criterion	**Definition**
Benign Nevi	
Reticular pattern	Pigment network of relative uniform thickness and color with holes of relative uniform size. Small brown or black dots can often be seen overlying the network or within the center of the lesion.
Globular pattern (includes cobblestone pattern)	Numerous, round-to-oval to angulated structures with various shades of brown. The globules are of uniform size, shape, and color and are distributed symmetrically.
Homogeneous pattern	Diffuse brown, gray-blue to blue-white pigmentation.
Starburst pattern	Finger-like projections seen at the edge of the lesion. The pigmented streaks are distributed symmetrically along the entire perimeter of the lesion in a radial arrangement.
Pseudonetwork pattern (face)	Pigmented lesion on facial skin with interruption of the pigment due to the presence of follicular and adnexal openings. This results in a network-like appearance.
Parallel furrow pattern (palms and soles)	Pigment located along the furrows of the palms and soles.
Melanoma	
Multicomponent pattern	Presence of three or more of the aforementioned patterns.
Atypical pigment network	Black, brown, or gray network with irregular-sized holes and thickened network lines. The network is often broken up, creating branched streaklike structures within the lesion.
Irregular dots/globules	Black, brown, round-to-oval structures distributed asymmetrically, not overlying the lines of a network, and often located toward the periphery of the lesion.
Irregular streaks	Finger-like projections seen at the edge of the lesion but distributed asymmetrically and focally along the perimeter of the melanoma.
Blotches	Black, brown, blue, or gray structureless areas distributed asymmetrically and not involving the entire lesion in a homogeneous manner.
Vascular structures	Dotted vessels, linear irregular vessels, thick and tortuous vessels, or erythema.
Annular-granular structures and pseudonetwork (face)	Multiple blue-gray dots surrounding the follicular ostia, creating an annular-granular pattern. Once the pigment becomes confluent, a pseudonetwork-like pattern emerges, which creates rhomboidal-like structures.
Parallel-ridge pattern (palms/soles)	Pigmentation aligned along the ridges on the palms and soles. The openings of the sweat ducts are located on the ridges.

In contrast, MM often exhibits a pattern that deviates from the aforementioned benign patterns, manifests asymmetry of dermoscopic colors and structures, and displays a disordered dermoscopic architecture. For instance, the reticular or globular patterns can look disorganized, there can be nonspecific structureless areas, and they can be multicomponent, meaning several of these findings in the same lesion (Fig. 15.22). *Most MMs also contain at least one of the following nine specific dermoscopic structures:* (1) atypical network, (2) peripheral streaks, (3) atypical dots or globules, (4) negative pigment network, (5) off-center pigmented blotch, (6) blue-white veil overlying flat areas, (7) blue-white veil overlying raised areas, (8) atypical vascular structures, and (9) brown peripheral structureless area (see Figs. 15.22 and 15.23; see Box 15.3).

BOX 15.2   Menzies Method

Negative Features (Neither Feature Found)
Symmetry of pattern (Assess only the colors and structures within the lesion. The symmetry/asymmetry of the contour/silhouette of the lesion is not a factor in this evaluation method.)
Presence of only a single color

Positive Features (At Least One Feature Found)
Blue-white veil
Pseudopods
Scarlike depigmentation
Multiple (5–6) colors
Broadened network
Multiple brown dots
Radial streaming
Peripheral black dots/globules
Multiple blue-gray dots ("peppering")

For melanoma to be diagnosed, the lesion must have neither of the two morphologic negative features and at least one of the nine positive features.

TABLE 15.3   ABCD Rule of Dermoscopy

Components of the ABCD Rule	Description	Score
Asymmetry	In 0, 1, or 2 perpendicular axes; assess not only contour, but also colors and structure	0–2
Border	Abrupt cut-off of pigment pattern at the periphery in 0–8 segments	0–8
Colors	Presence of up to 6 colors (white, red, light brown, dark brown, blue-gray, black)	1–6
Dermoscopic structures	Presence of network, structureless (homogeneous) areas, branched streaks, dots, and globules	1–5

Calculation of Total Dermoscopy Score
A distinction between benign and malignant melanocytic lesions can often be made using the following formula: [(A score × 1.3) + (B score × 0.1) + (C score × 0.5) + (D score × 0.5)].
Interpretation of total score: <4.75, benign nevi; 4.75–5.45, suspicious for melanoma; >5.45, melanoma.

TABLE 15.4   Seven-Point Checklist

Criteria	Score
Major Criteria	
Atypical pigment network	2
Blue-white veil	2
Atypical vascular pattern	2
Minor Criteria	
Irregular streaks	1
Irregular dots/globules	1
Irregular blotches	1
Regression structures	1
Seven-Point Total Score	
Nonmelanoma	<3
Melanoma	≥3

By simple addition of the individual scores, one can differentiate between many benign nevi and melanoma. A minimum total score of 3 is required for the diagnosis of melanoma, whereas a total score of less than 3 is indicative of a benign nevus.

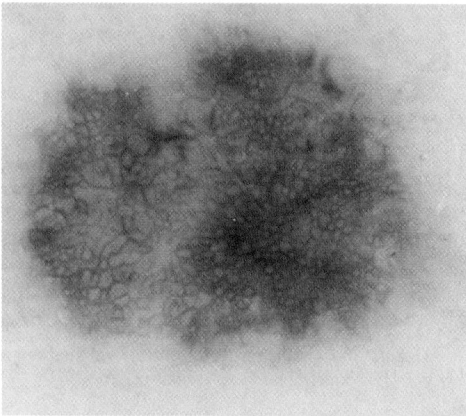

Fig. 15.18 Lesion evaluation using various dermoscopic algorithms. The seven-point checklist of dermoscopy identifies only atypical network (two points). The total score is 2, denoting a benign lesion (i.e., nevus). Evaluation using the Menzies method also leads to the conclusion that this is a nevus because the lesion shows a single color and overall symmetry of structure and pattern. Lesion evaluation using the ABCD rule indicates a total score of 3.3 (A = 1.3 for asymmetry in one axis [comparing right and left halves of the lesion], B = 0 because the lesion gradually fades into the periphery, C = 1 for the color brown, and D = 1 for the presence of network). This score is within the benign range of the ABCD method.

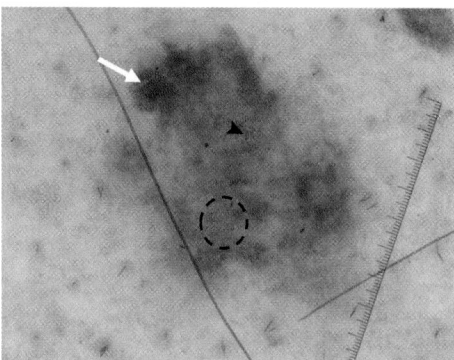

Fig. 15.19 Lesion evaluation using various dermoscopic algorithms. By the seven-point checklist of dermoscopy, the lesion displays an irregular blotch (*arrow*, one point), irregular dots/globules (*arrowhead*, one point), and regression structures with bluish peppering (*dotted circle*, one point). The total score is 3, denoting a melanoma. Evaluating the same lesion by the Menzies method also leads to the same conclusion because the lesion has more than one color and has asymmetry of structure and pattern. It also has blue-gray peppering (*dotted circle*). Thus, this lesion is a melanoma. Lesion evaluation using the ABCD indicates a total score of 6.6 (A = 2.6 for two-axis asymmetry, B = 0 because the lesion fades into the periphery, C = 2 for the presence of four colors [light and dark brown, blue-gray, and red], and D = 2 for the presence of network, structureless areas, and dots and globules). The lesion has dermoscopic features consistent with melanoma.

Although most MMs display at least some degree of asymmetry of pattern, color, and structure, there exists a subset of early MMs that are structureless. Fortunately, most of these early MMs can be correctly identified based on observing their growth dynamics or by visualizing the presence of increased vasculature.

Neoangiogenesis, resulting in an increased blood volume, is required for MM survival and growth. These neoangiogenic blood vessels can often be visualized under dermoscopy, and their presence can help correctly identify many MMs. Studies have shown that the specific morphology of the blood vessels observed under dermoscopy is correlated to specific tumors (Table 15.5). The most common vessel morphologies exhibited by MM are linear-irregular and dotted vessels (Fig. 15.24). Hence, the presence of such vessels in a hypopigmented or amelanotic lesion is an important clue to the diagnosis of MM.

Malignancies, being biologically active, are growing lesions, whereas benign nevi are usually in a state of senescence. This fact can be used by clinicians to help isolate early MMs that have not yet developed any of the MM-specific dermoscopic structures mentioned previously (i.e., structureless MM) from among many benign nevi. The acquisition of sequential dermoscopic images provides clinicians the ability to monitor lesions for change. This ability to compare baseline and follow-up dermoscopic images of the same lesion over time increases the specificity of MM diagnosis while at the same time maintaining a high sensitivity, which results in the appropriate removal of MMs with a concomitant reduction in the unnecessary removal of benign lesions (Figs. 15.25 and 15.26).

Sequential imaging is usually restricted to patients with multiple atypical nevi because it is often more practical to simply remove a single atypical mole on a patient with few to no additional nevi than it is to follow them. For individuals possessing many nevi, the removal of all of their atypical moles would be impractical. In such patients, sequential dermoscopic imaging appears to be a reasonable management strategy. The principle is that if a lesion is found to be stable, the patient can be reassured that the lesion is biologically indolent at that moment in time and thus can be followed routinely.

SHORT-TERM MOLE MONITORING

The most timely method, short of performing a biopsy, for correctly segregating benign lesions from MM is by sequential "short-term" dermoscopic imaging (see Figs. 15.25 and 15.26). Menzies and colleagues (2001) introduced the concept of short-term mole monitoring, which involves sequential reexamination of the same lesion over a 3- to 4-month period. Short-term dermoscopic monitoring is aimed at increasing the specificity of evaluation of equivocal melanocytic lesions. It is used to evaluate melanocytic lesions that lack dermoscopic features of MM, yet appear somewhat atypical to the examiner or have a history of change. In this setting, any morphologic change observed during the 3-month monitoring period warrants an excision. The exceptions to this rule are when one observes an overall increase or decrease in pigmentation without accompanying architectural change or the loss or appearance of milia-like cysts.

The majority (81%) of the lesions followed up in the study by Menzies and colleagues did not change and thus were "spared" from undergoing unnecessary removal. Of the lesions that did reveal change, 11% were found to be MM, all of which proved to be histologically thin tumors, and none revealed any of the MM-specific dermoscopic structures mentioned previously. The specificity for the diagnosis of MM by means of short-term digital monitoring of dermoscopically equivocal lesions was reported to be 83%. In another study, Kittler and associates (2006) followed suspect lesions lacking MM-specific features at baseline for over 8 months. After follow-up of 1.5 to 4.5 months, only 38.2% of the MMs showed specific dermoscopic features for MM. This value increased to 55% after 4.5 to 8.0 months and to 64.9% after more than 8.0 months (Fig. 15.27). The observed changes in MM lesions included asymmetric enlargement, focal changes in pigmentation and structure, regression features, and change in color. Insignificant change observed in lesions after at least 6 months of follow-up included a darker or lighter overall appearance, change in the number or distribution of brown globules, and disappearance of parts of the pigment network. The conclusion of the study was that MM-specific dermoscopic criteria in structureless MMs become readily apparent as the length of follow-up increases. However, MMs that lack any specific features can in fact be detected by the short-term monitoring process. Thus MMs lacking MM-specific dermoscopic features can now be detected based on observing their dynamic evolution over time.

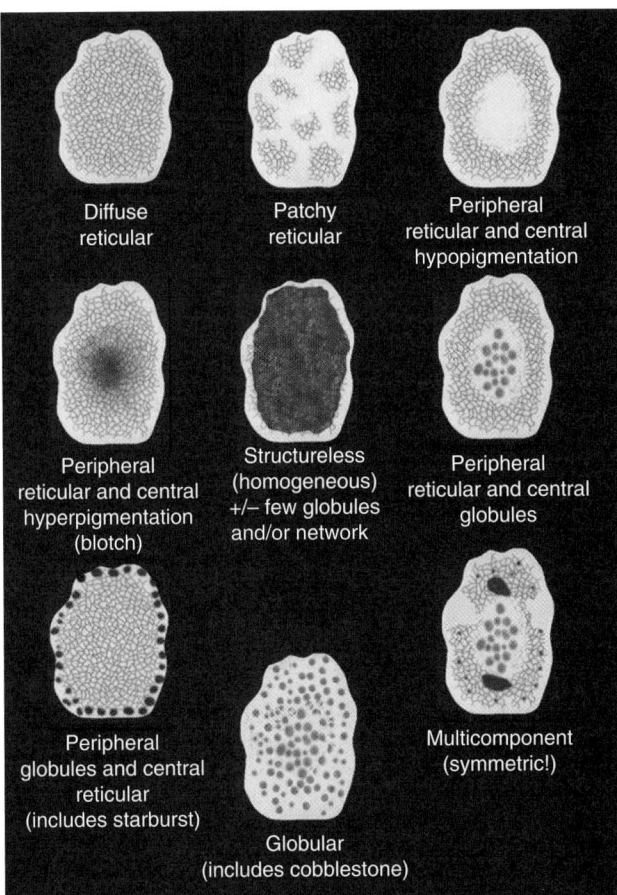

Fig. 15.20 The nine benign global dermoscopic patterns of nevi. "Structureless" refers to a hyperpigmented or hypopigmented blotch.

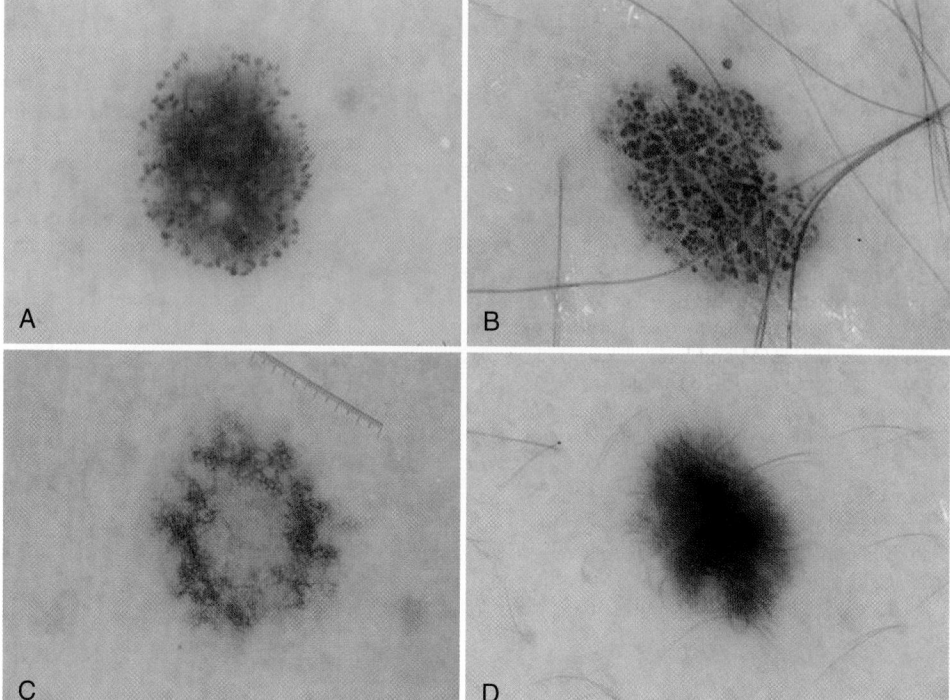

Fig. 15.21 Examples of benign global dermoscopic patterns. (A) Peripheral globules and central reticular. (B) Globular pattern. This variant is called the "cobblestone" pattern because the globules are large and angulated, arranged almost back to back. (C) Peripheral reticular and central hypopigmentation. (D) Peripheral reticular and central hyperpigmentation.

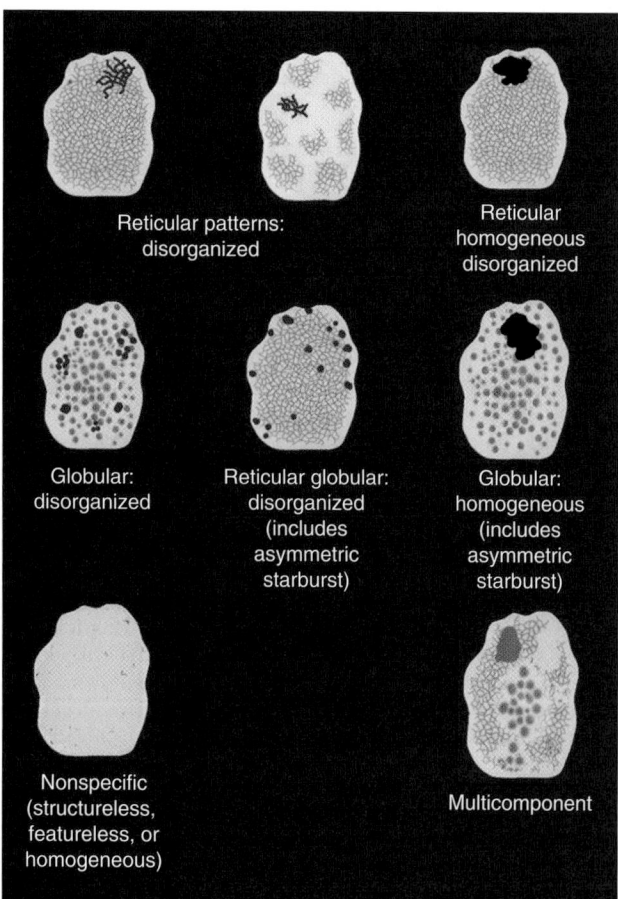

Fig. 15.22 Global dermoscopic patterns commonly seen in melanoma. Specific (local) dermoscopic structures that should raise suspicion for malignancy include atypical network, streaks, atypical dots or globules, negative pigment network, off-center pigmented blotch, blue-white veil overlying flat areas, blue-white veil overlying raised areas, atypical vascular structures, and brown peripheral structureless area.

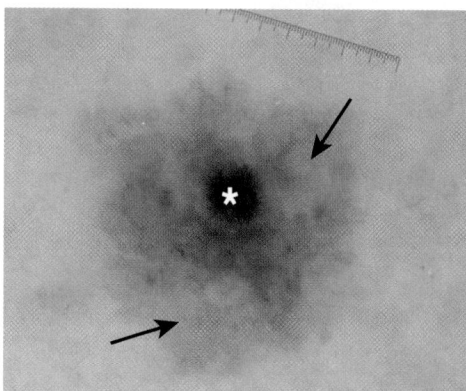

Fig. 15.23 Although this lesion has symmetry of structure and pattern, it does not conform to one of the nine benign patterns. In addition, it has peripheral brown structureless areas (arrows) and an atypical network in the center (asterisk). This was an in situ melanoma.

TABLE 15.5	Vascular Structures With Associated Tumors
Primary Vessel Morphology	**Disease Entity**
Arborizing vessels	Basal cell carcinoma
Comma vessels	Intradermal nevus
	Congenital melanocytic nevus
Corkscrew vessels	Nodular melanoma
	Cutaneous melanoma metastasis
	Desmoplastic melanoma
Dotted and globular vessels	Melanoma
	Spitz nevus
	Dysplastic nevus
	Squamous cell carcinoma
Glomerular vessels	Squamous cell carcinoma
Hairpin vessels	Keratoacanthoma
	Melanoma
	Irritated seborrheic keratosis
	Squamous cell carcinoma
	Spitz nevus
Linear irregular vessels	Melanoma
	Spitz nevus
Milky red area/globule	Melanoma
Polymorphous vessels	Melanoma

DERMOSCOPY IN THE PRIMARY CARE OFFICE

Approximately 40% of office visits to physicians in the United States are to a primary care physician (PCP), and although most patients with MM had at least one primary care visit in the year before diagnosis, only 20% report receiving a skin cancer examination. Compared with MM detection by the patient or family, MM detected by physicians is more likely to be thinner. PCPs, therefore, are in a unique position to perform skin cancer screening. Studies indicate that training PCPs to screen for MM using dermoscopy leads to increased diagnostic sensitivity without a significant decrease in specificity. Argenziano and colleagues (2006) introduced the three-point checklist for the purpose of improving sensitivity in skin cancer (i.e., MM and basal cell carcinoma) screening by PCPs (Table 15.6 and Figs. 15.28 through 15.30). The three-point checklist was meant to serve as a triage tool to help PCPs in deciding on referrals of pigmented lesions to dermatologists. The study indicated that dermoscopy allows PCPs to perform 25.1% better triage of skin lesions suggestive of skin cancer compared with naked-eye examination alone (P = .002).

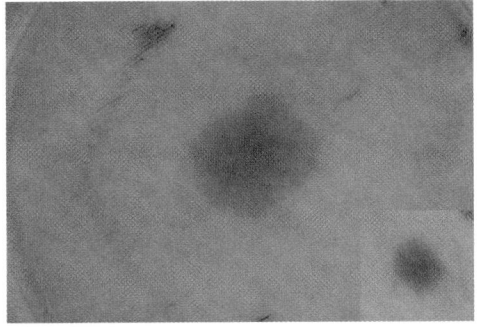

Fig. 15.24 Invasive melanoma (0.45 mm thick) lacking any pigmented dermoscopic features, and showing only dotted vessels throughout the lesion.

In another study among general practitioners, sensitivity for MM diagnosis improved significantly from a clinical baseline pretest of 54% to a post-training dermoscopy diagnosis of 76%. In addition, dermoscopy education created an increased awareness of the clinical appearance of MM among PCPs and improved naked-eye diagnosis of MM. PCPs are encouraged to be formally trained in dermoscopy for the clinical assessment of skin tumors, including MM. Australia and New Zealand have successfully implemented a wide network of skin cancer screening by PCPs. In a study assessing New Zealand general practitioners' diagnosis and management of skin cancer, the participating physicians were shown to have a high level of expertise in making the correct diagnosis and in deciding whether or not to biopsy the lesion.

It is important to acknowledge that dermoscopy constitutes only one portion of a thorough history and physical examination. We caution against *solely* relying on the dermoscopic findings while dismissing other clinical cues. For example, a lesion that appears different (either by clinical or dermoscopic examination) relative to its neighboring lesions, known as the *ugly duckling sign*, should raise suspicion in the observer even in the absence of definitive dermoscopic features of MM. The final decision-making process should always evaluate the dermoscopic findings considering the patient's personal and family history, as well as other clinical parameters of the lesion such as symptoms of pain, bleeding, or itching.

In summary, there is compelling evidence that dermoscopy improves MM diagnosis at an earlier, curable stage while avoiding excessive scarring from removal of benign lesions. As a first-level screening tool, dermoscopy may improve the PCP's ability to detect skin cancer.

CPT/BILLING CODES

There is no CPT billing code for dermoscopy, so use the appropriate evaluation and management code for the visit. If using photography to monitor dysplastic nevus syndrome, can use 99604.

99604   Whole body photography for monitoring of high-risk patients with dysplastic nevus syndrome

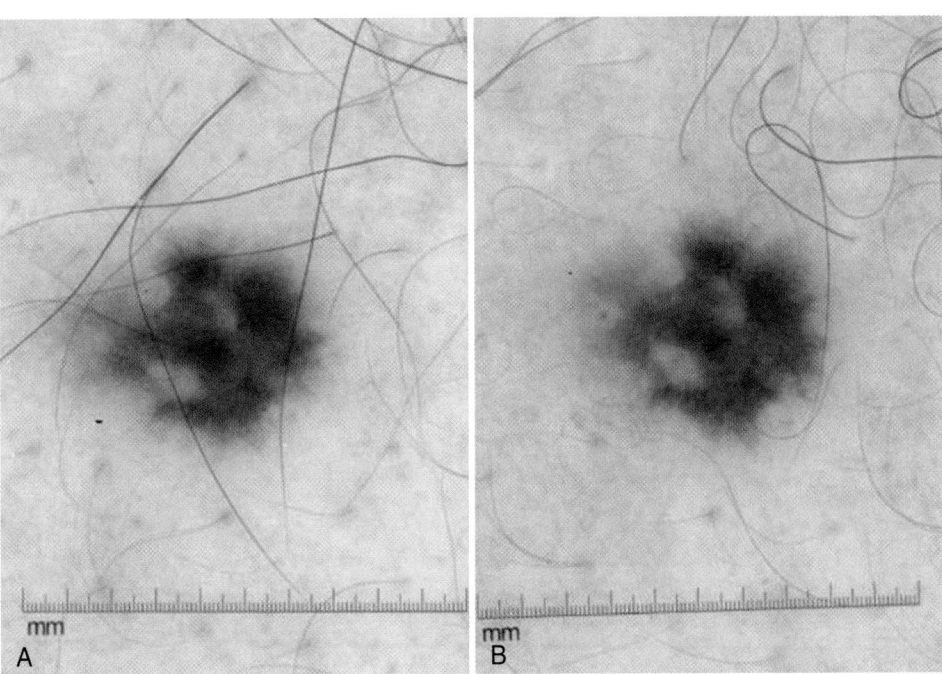

Fig. 15.25 Side-by side comparison of sequential dermoscopic images at baseline (A) and 9-month follow-up (B). No dermoscopic changes are seen on follow-up examination; therefore the lesion is considered biologically benign.

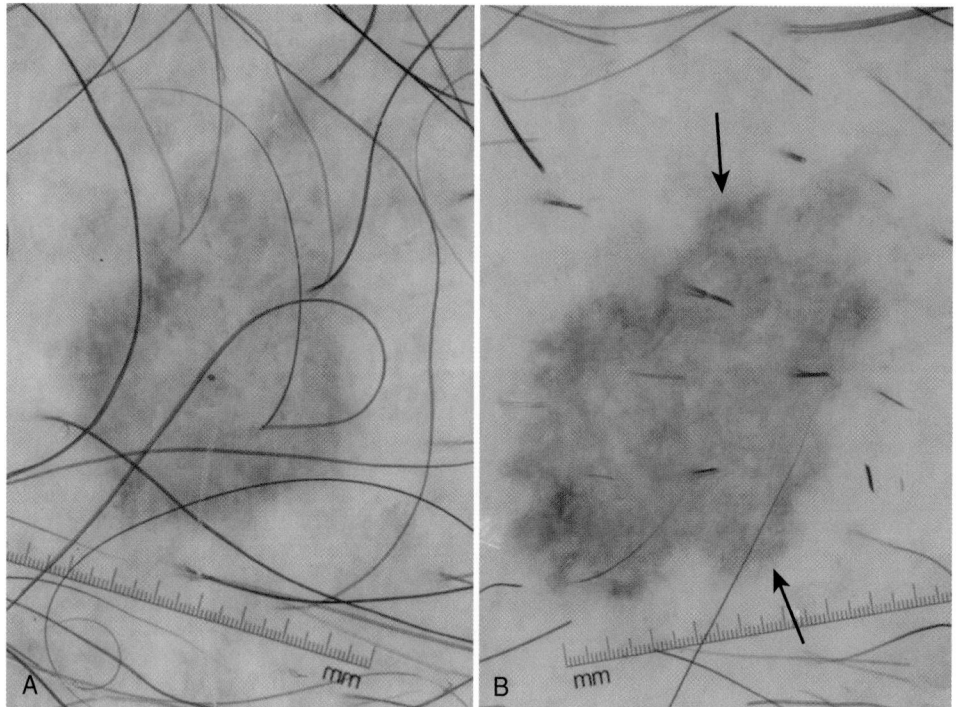

Fig. 15.26 Dermoscopic follow-up using side-by-side comparison of sequential dermoscopic images at baseline (A) and 4-month follow-up (B). At follow-up, radial growth of the lesion can be appreciated (B, *arrows*). This lesion, which otherwise does not display melanoma-specific dermoscopic features, proved to be an invasive melanoma 0.3 mm thick.

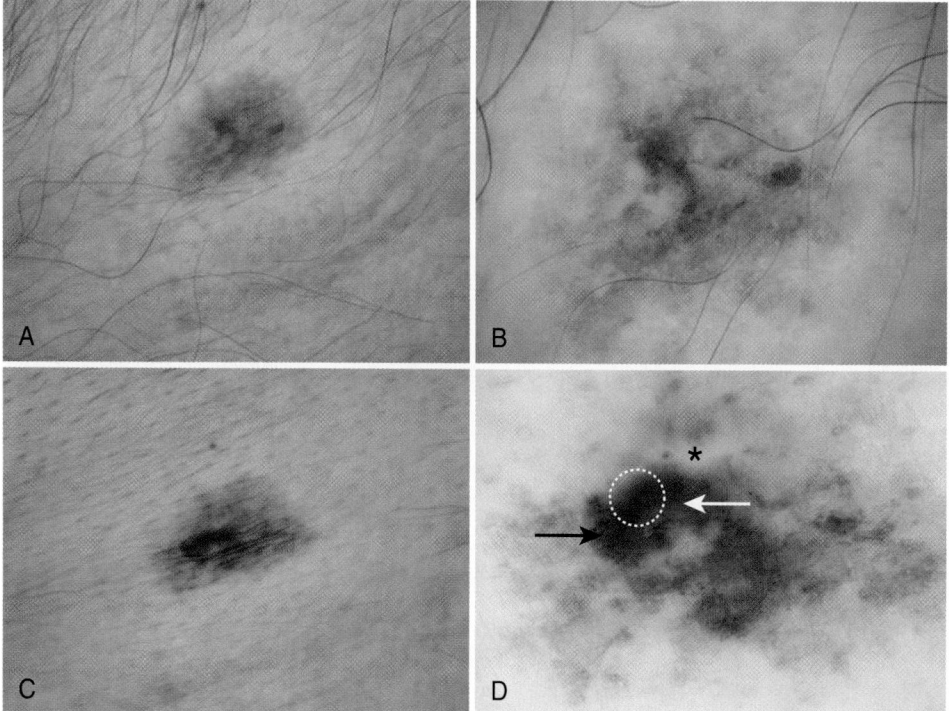

Fig. 15.27 With long-term follow-up, malignant lesions will increasingly show melanoma-specific dermoscopic structures. This lesion was clinically inconspicuous (A) and dermoscopically showed only a reticular homogeneous pattern (B). However, at 2-year follow-up (C), the lesion was clinically more suspect, with asymmetry and multiple colors *(brown, black, and pink)*. On dermoscopy at the 2-year follow-up (D), the lesion showed an atypical network *(black arrow)*, multiple dots *(dotted circle)*, and bluish-gray *(white arrow)* and white scarlike *(asterisk)* areas suggestive of regression. This was a melanoma 1.8 mm thick.

TABLE 15.6	Three-Point Checklist
Three-Point Checklist	**Definition**
Asymmetry	Asymmetrical distribution of colors and dermoscopic structures.
Atypical network	Pigmented network with irregular holes and thick line. Streaks are considered part of an atypical network.
Blue-white structures	Any type of blue or white color, including white scarlike depigmentation, blue-whitish veil, and blue pepper-like granules (regression structures).

The presence of more than one criterion suggests a suspicious lesion.

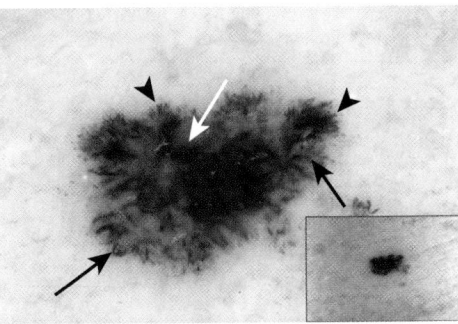

Fig. 15.30 Evaluating this pigmented lesion using the three-point check-list indicates asymmetric distribution of dermoscopic structures, atypical network *(black arrows)*, and blue-white structures *(white arrow)*. The total score is 3. This lesion was a melanoma 0.3 mm in Breslow depth. Of note, the lesion also displays multiple peripheral streaks *(black arrowheads)*, which are considered to be part of the atypical network.

ONLINE RESOURCES

Dermoscopy [educational website]: http://www.dermoscopy.org/; dermoscopy tutorial: http://www.dermoscopy.org/atlas/base.htm. International Society of Dermoscopy: http://www.dermoscopy-ids.org [registration required].
New Zealand Dermatology Society online course: http://www.dermnetnz.org/cme/dermoscopy-course/introduction-to-dermoscopy/.

RECOMMENDED READING

Argenziano G, Puig S, Zalaudek I, et al. Dermoscopy improves accuracy of primary care physicians to triage lesions suggestive of skin cancer. *J Clin Oncol.* 2006;24:1877–1882.

Argenziano G, Soyer HP, Chimenti S, et al. Dermoscopy of pigmented skin lesions: Results of a consensus meeting via the Internet. *J Am Acad Dermatol.* 2003;48:679–693.

Argenziano G, Zalaudek I, Corona R, et al. Vascular structures in skin tumors. *Arch Dermatol.* 2004;140:1485–1489.

Bafounta ML, Beauchet A, Aegerter P, Saiag P. Is dermoscopy useful for the diagnosis of melanoma? Results of a meta-analysis using techniques adapted to the evaluation of diagnostic tests. *Arch Dermatol.* 2001;137:1343–1350.

Benvenuto-Andrade C, Dusza S, Hay J, et al. Level of confidence in diagnosis: clinical examination versus dermoscopy examination. *Dermatol Surg.* 2006;32:738–744.

Benvenuto-Andrade C, Marghoob A. Ten reasons why dermoscopy is beneficial for the evaluation of skin lesions. *Exp Rev Dermatol.* 2006;1:369–374.

Binder M, Kittler H, Steiner A. Reevaluation of the ABCD rule for epiluminescence microscopy. *J Am Acad Dermatol.* 1999;40:171–176.

Bono A, Maurichi A, Moglia D, et al. Clinical and dermatoscopic diagnosis of early amelanotic melanoma. *Melanoma Res.* 2001;11:491–494.

Brochez L, Verhaeghe E, Bleyen L, Naeyaert JM. Diagnostic ability of general practitioners and dermatologists in discriminating pigmented skin lesions. *J Am Acad Dermatol.* 2001;44:979–986.

Carli P, de Giorgi V, Chiarugi A, et al. Addition of dermoscopy to conventional naked-eye examination in melanoma screening: a randomized study. *J Am Acad Dermatol.* 2004;50:683–689.

Carli P, De Giorgi V, Crocetti E, et al. Improvement of malignant/benign ratio in excised melanocytic lesions in the "dermoscopy era": a retrospective study 1997–2001. *Br J Dermatol.* 2004;150:687–692.

Chen SC, Pennie ML, Kolm P, et al. Diagnosing and managing cutaneous pigmented lesions: primary care physicians versus dermatologists. *J Gen Intern Med.* 2006;21:678–682.

Cyr PR. Atypical moles. *Am Fam Physician.* 2008;78:735–740.

Epstein DS, Lange JR, Gruber SB, et al. Is physician detection associated with thinner melanomas? *JAMA.* 1999;281:640–643.

Fox FN. Dermoscopy: an invaluable tool for evaluating skin lesions. *Am Fam Physician.* 2008;78:704–706.

Gachon J, Beaulieu P, Sei JF, et al. First prospective study of the recognition process of melanoma in dermatological practice. *Arch Dermatol.* 2005;141:434–438.

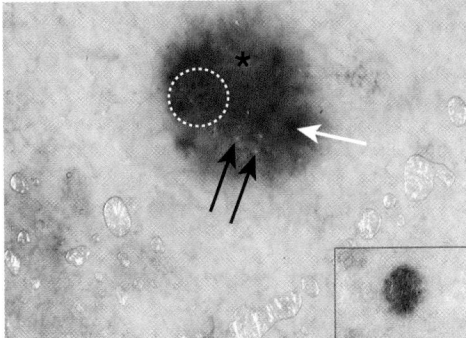

Fig. 15.28 This lesion appears clinically symmetric *(inset)*. However, dermoscopic evaluation reveals asymmetric distribution of the dermoscopic structures: aggregated globules in the top left quadrant *(dotted circle)*, blue-white structures *(asterisk)*, blotches *(white arrow)*, and milia-like cysts *(black arrows)*. By the three-point checklist, the lesion gets a score of 2 for the dermoscopic asymmetry and blue-white structures, denoting a suspect lesion. This lesion was a melanoma 0.5 mm thick.

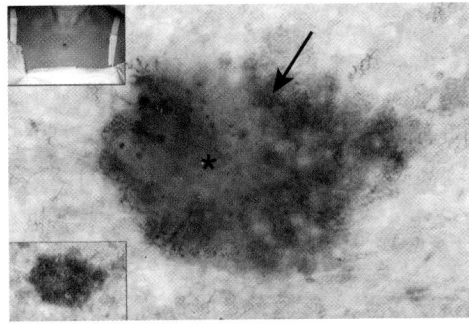

Fig. 15.29 This lesion is an "ugly duckling" that stands out as different on the patient's chest *(top inset)* and shows clinical asymmetry and multiple colors *(bottom inset)*. Evaluating this pigmented lesion using the three-point checklist indicates asymmetric distribution of dermoscopic structures, atypical network *(arrow)*, and blue-white structures *(asterisk)*, for a total score of 3. This lesion was a melanoma 0.5 mm thick.

SUPPLIERS

(See contact information available at www.expertconsult.com.)

Dermatoscope
  Heine USA
DermoGenius
  BIOCAM GmbH
EpiScope
  Welch Allyn
3Gen
  DermLite dermatoscopes

Geller AC, Koh HK, Miller DR, et al. Use of health services before the diagnosis of melanoma: implications for early detection and screening. *J Gen Intern Med.* 1992;7:154–157.

Haenssle HA, Krueger U, Vente C, et al. Results from an observational trial: digital epiluminescence microscopy follow-up of atypical nevi increases the sensitivity and the chance of success of conventional dermoscopy in detecting melanoma. *J Invest Dermatol.* 2006;126:980–985.

Hennings JS, Dusza SW, Wang SQ, et al. The CASH (color, architecture, symmetry, and homogeneity) algorithm for dermoscopy. *J Am Acad Dermatol.* 2007;56:45–52.

Kittler H, Guitera P, Riedl E, et al. Identification of clinically featureless incipient melanoma using sequential dermoscopy imaging. *Arch Dermatol.* 2006;142:1113–1119.

Kittler H, Pehamberger H, Wolff K, Binder M. Follow-up of melanocytic skin lesions with digital epiluminescence microscopy: patterns of modifications observed in early melanoma, atypical nevi, and common nevi. *J Am Acad Dermatol.* 2000;43:467–476.

Kittler H, Pehamberger H, Wolff K, Binder M. Diagnostic accuracy of dermoscopy. *Lancet Oncol.* 2002;3:159–165.

Malvehy J, Puig S, Braun RP, et al. *Handbook of Dermoscopy.* New York: Taylor & Francis; 2006.

Marghoob AA, Malveny P, Braun RP. *Atlas of Dermoscopy.* 2nd ed. Boca Raton, FL: Taylor & Francis; 2013.

Marghoob AA, Korzenko AJ, Changchien L, et al. The beauty and the beast sign in dermoscopy. *Dermatol Surg.* 2007;33:1–4.

McGee R, Elwook M, Adam H, et al. The recognition and management of melanoma and other skin lesions by general practitioners in New Zealand. *N Z Med J.* 1994;107:287–290.

Menzies SW, Gutenev A, Avramidis M, et al. Short-term digital surface microscopic monitoring of atypical or changing melanocytic lesions. *Arch Dermatol.* 2001;137:1583–1589.

Menzies SW, Zalaudek I. Why perform dermoscopy? The evidence for its role in the routine management of pigmented skin lesions. *Arch Dermatol.* 2006;142:1211–1212.

Pagnanelli G, Soyer HP, Argenziano G, et al. Diagnosis of pigmented skin lesions by dermoscopy: web-based training improves diagnostic performance of non-experts. *Br J Dermatol.* 2003;148:698–702.

Scope A, Benvenuto-Andrade C, Agero AC, et al. Correlation of dermoscopic structures of melanocytic lesions to reflectance confocal microscopy. *Arch Dermatol.* 2007;143:176–185.

Soyer HP, Argenziano G, Hoffmann-Wellenhof R, et al. *Dermoscopy: The Essentials.* 2nd ed. Philadelphia: Saunders; 2012.

Usatine RP, (ed). Appendix: Dermoscopy. In Usatine RP, Smith MA, Mayeaux EJ, et al (eds). *The Color Atlas of Family Medicine.* 2nd Ed. New York: McGraw-Hill; 2013.

Wang SQ, Scope A, Marghoob AA. Dermoscopic patterns of melanoma. *G Ital Dermatol Venereol.* 2007;142:99–108.

Westerhoff K, McCarthy WH, Menzies SW. Increase in the sensitivity for melanoma diagnosis by primary care physicians using skin surface microscopy. *Br J Dermatol.* 2000;143:1016–1020.

CHAPTER 16

FLAPS AND PLASTIES

Dennis LaRavia

Appropriate wound closure after excision is essential in achieving a cosmetically pleasing result. Although many elliptical defects can be repaired with a basic side-to-side closure, large or complex defects may require more advanced techniques. Several techniques for wound closure and scar revision are described in this chapter, including advancement and rotation flaps, V-Y plasties, M-plasties, and the management of dog-ears. The specific flaps and plastic surgery closures described are chosen for their utility, reliability, and predictability of aesthetic result.

INDICATIONS

- A soft tissue defect is so large that a simple primary closure is not possible. If an elliptical defect may not be pinched together easily between the fingers with minimal tension, a simple side-to-side closure will likely be insufficient.
- There is excessive skin tension with simple closure techniques, and simple closure would yield a poor cosmetic result.
- Surgical skin remodeling techniques, or "plasties," may be indicated when dealing with dog-ears, complex wounds, or other defects that would cause an undesirable scar.

CONTRAINDICATIONS (ALL RELATIVE)

When performed correctly, the closure techniques described in this chapter generally achieve good results. However, certain risk factors may lead to poor outcomes. Relative contraindications to complex skin closures and flaps include the following:

- Diabetes
- Impaired wound healing history
- Vascular compromise to affected region
- Keloid or hypertrophic scar formation history
- Prior radiation to region
- Coagulopathy (intrinsic or induced through anticoagulants such as warfarin)
- Wound location on lower extremity, especially the feet (due to slow healing)

Good healing can still be accomplished in most cases if the operator carefully engages with the patient to ensure adherence, provides the correct closure technique, and limits platelet aggregation inhibitors (e.g., aspirin, other nonsteroidal antiinflammatory drugs, clopidogrel) for 5 days before surgery, if possible. If the patient cannot stop these agents, the surgery can still be performed, but the patient should expect more intraoperative bleeding and increased likelihood of postoperative oozing and ecchymoses in the operative area. Patients on warfarin or other oral anticoagulants (thrombin or factor Xa inhibitors) can also have extensive plastic procedures with advanced flaps and closures but should expect slower healing and more prolonged bruising in the operative area. The current recommendation is that none of the antiplatelet medications or anticoagulants should be stopped for cutaneous surgery, especially if there is a significant risk of stroke or other cardiovascular event. However, depending on the size of the lesion, the procedures described in this chapter can be quite extensive and involved. Consider "bridge therapy" for those patients who need anticoagulation (see Appendix H).

It is particularly important to ask the patient about any history of abnormal scarring, keloids, or poor healing. Certain areas of the body are especially prone to hypertrophic scar and keloid formation, such as the chest, earlobes, and shoulders (Fig. 16.1). Black skin and children's skin, and the skin of pregnant women, also tend to scar more. Any patient at high risk for keloid formation should receive thorough preoperative counseling before proceeding with any skin surgery. These patients should be followed closely after surgery because early keloid development may be curtailed by the judicious use of steroid injections and silicone gel sheeting. As a general rule, the clinician should avoid the temptation to excise keloids unless special attention is paid to preparation of the area before surgery using intralesional steroids, and the patient agrees to long-term (1 to 2 years) surveillance and follow-up treatment if needed (see Chapter 28, Hypertrophic Scars and Keloids for details). Conservative methods should generally be tried before reexcision, which potentially could lead to more scars.

EQUIPMENT

Most skin excisions and closures can be performed with fairly simple equipment (as shown in the following list). Electrocautery and suction are not always necessary but are strongly recommended for meticulous control of bleeding. Adequate hemostasis is critical in preventing hematomas, wound dehiscence, and infection. Typical equipment should include the following:

- Topical antiseptic wash: povidone-iodine or chlorhexidine gluconate
- 5-mL syringe with needles (16 to 20 gauge to draw up anesthetic and 27 to 30 gauge for tissue injection)
- Injectable local anesthetic: 1% to 2% lidocaine with epinephrine for most areas; previously epinephrine has been avoided in fingers, toes, and genitals. However, newer findings would indicate that it is safe. The lidocaine can be buffered with sodium bicarbonate just prior to injection to take some of the sting out of the injection (see below and Chapter 5, Local Anesthesia).

A 1:1 mixture of 1% lidocaine with 1% lidocaine with epinephrine works well in major revisions or flaps on the nose to minimize the excessive bleeding that often occurs without epinephrine. However, common sense should suggest that epinephrine not be used in an elderly woman with Raynaud disease or poor nasal/facial circulation. It is always helpful to have the vasoconstrictive effect of epinephrine, but if flap viability is going to be a concern, it is best to limit or eliminate its use.

- Sterile drape
- Sterile gloves
- Sterile gauze pads

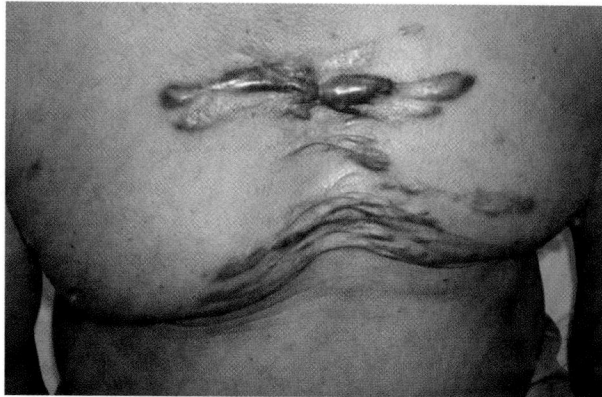

Fig. 16.1 Keloid scars.

- Telfa pad and Tegaderm for wound dressing
- Skin-marking pen (Fine-tipped pens are available and suggested when more cosmetic repairs are important.)
- Nylon suture (4-0, 5-0, or 6-0, depending on location)
- 4-0, 5-0, or 6-0 absorbable suture such as gut, chromic, Vicryl, or Dexon if deep sutures are indicated
- Adson forceps
- Needle holder (smooth)
- No. 15 scalpel
- Suture scissors
- Two skin hooks
- Scissors, Metzenbaum, curved, 5 to 5.5 inches
- Hemostats, curved, mosquito, 2 inches
- Hemostats, straight, small, 2 inches
- Good lighting

Strongly Recommended Equipment

- Electrocautery unit
- Suction device
- Crash cart including defibrillator, oxygen, and intubation equipment on site for emergencies (see Chapter 212, Anaphylaxis)

PREPROCEDURE PATIENT PREPARATION

History and Physical

During the preoperative history, topics of discussion should include the following:

- Medications, including herbal supplements, that the patient has taken in the past 6 weeks
- Allergies or adverse reactions to medications including iodine and local anesthetics, suture material, bandages, and latex
- Past surgical history and any history of keloid formation, hypertrophic scars, or poor wound healing
- Past medical history, including cardiac disease, diabetes, human immunodeficiency virus infection, hepatitis, bleeding disorders, immunosuppression
- Whether the patient has a pacemaker or other implanted electronic device that may preclude the use of electrocautery
- Whether the patient has a history of valvular disease, rheumatic fever, joint replacement, or other indication for antibiotic prophylaxis
- The status of any anticoagulants and when the last dose was taken
- Pregnancy (in reproductive-age women)

Informed Consent

Before the procedure, the patient must give informed consent to undergo surgery. This includes a full description of the risks, benefits, and alternatives to the procedure. The patient must have the opportunity to ask questions regarding the procedure and have the answers provided to his or her satisfaction to constitute informed consent. Informed consent to photography is also recommended to allow a pictorial history. Either still or video recording can be used.

Risks

The risks of the procedure to be discussed with the patient include, but are not limited to, the following:

- Suboptimal result, including the possibility of a worse scar after wound healing
- Infection
- Wound dehiscence
- Hypertrophic scar, keloid formation, or other poor scar result
- Swelling or bruising of the tissue
- Bleeding
- Pain
- Damage to nerves
- An allergic reaction to sutures, dressing, anesthetic, or other medications
- Recurrence of lesion and possible need for further surgery

Benefits

Benefits of the procedure may include, but are not limited to, the following:

- Improved cosmetic result
- Improved wound healing
- Improved overall results compared with conventional side-to-side closure
- Removal of a potentially dangerous lesion such as squamous cell carcinoma, basal cell carcinoma, or melanoma

Alternatives

Alternatives to the cosmetic surgical closures listed previously may include the following:

- Leaving the wound open to heal by secondary intention
- Side-to-side closure
- Performance of a skin graft
- Referral to a plastic surgeon

ANTIBIOTIC PROPHYLAXIS

See Chapter 213, Prevention and Treatment of Wound Infections.
  Surgical antibiotic prophylaxis should be used more liberally when flaps and plasties are performed because the blood supply is often compromised with these closures, increasing the risk of infection. Antibiotic prophylaxis should be strongly considered in the following cases:

- The surgical site involves an extremity or ear, and when it is difficult to keep the area clean such as the axilla, the perineum, genitalia, and other intertriginous areas (e.g., under the breasts)
- Diabetes or immunosuppression
- The wound is dirty, has been open more than 1 hour, or aseptic technique was not ideal
- Patient follow-up is difficult, or the patient is otherwise at increased risk of infection
- History of previously infected wounds for no apparent reason
- Male patients 6 to 16 years of age

PREOPERATIVE MEDICATIONS AND ANESTHESIA

The decision regarding whether to use sedation should be based on personal philosophy, patient desire, and the availability of proper monitoring. When performed correctly, most minor surgical procedures can be completed with minimal discomfort to the patient. However, some sedation may be indicated in anxious patients when the procedure is extensive or if significant discomfort is anticipated (see Chapter 1, Procedural Sedation and Analgesia).

The use of a local anesthetic warrants discussion. Lidocaine with epinephrine is preferable to lidocaine alone for nearly all cutaneous procedures. See the discussion regarding the use of epinephrine in the digits and end artery areas in Chapter 5, Local Anesthesia. In the doses administered in local anesthesia, epinephrine is generally safe and its vasoconstrictive properties are important in controlling bleeding and potentiating analgesia. Because epinephrine takes 7 to 10 minutes to achieve full effect, it is advisable to anesthetize the surgical site before preparing and draping the patient. The addition of 1 mL of sodium bicarbonate to every 9 mL of lidocaine with epinephrine helps neutralize the acidity of the solution and thus decreases the pain with injection. The addition of sodium bicarbonate to plain lidocaine does not benefit to the same extent because plain lidocaine is not as acidified. *Bupivacaine (Marcaine) precipitates at a neutral pH and should never be used with sodium bicarbonate.* When the longer-acting properties of bupivacaine are desired, it may be helpful to anesthetize the region using lidocaine with epinephrine (buffered with sodium bicarbonate) before injecting bupivacaine.

Additional techniques to minimize discomfort include the use of topical anesthetics, cryoanesthesia (e.g., topical ethyl chloride), slow injections, and initiation of the anesthesia injection on the subdermal plane. It is advisable to draw up all injectable medications in advance and to keep scalpels, needles, and syringes out of the patient's view, particularly when working with pediatric patients.

PREPARATION OF SKIN AND HAIR

Hair removal at the surgical site may be accomplished by shaving or by cutting the hair with scissors (to minimize microabrasions that may increase the risk of infection). On the scalp, ointment can be used to spread the hair away from the operative site and to minimize the need to cut the hair. The skin is prepared with a povidone-iodine or chlorhexidine solution with gentle scrubbing. Note that povidone-iodine must be allowed to dry before it is considered effective, and chlorhexidine should be avoided on the face because it is extremely toxic to the eye. Skin markings may be made before or after preparing the patient. An overzealous scrub or an alcohol wipe, however, may remove preoperative markings, and a pen used before the skin preparation is no longer sterile.

DRAPES

Sterile drapes should be used with any skin procedure that requires suturing to protect the suture material from becoming contaminated and introducing bacteria into the tissue. Fenestrated drapes that have adhesive around the opening to affix the hole securely over the surgical site are especially helpful. However, you may need to extend the aperture or design your own by cutting a hole in a sterile surgical drape. Sterile technique is particularly important with flaps and plasties because blood supply may be compromised, predisposing the wound to infection.

TECHNIQUE

Also see Chapters 18 through 22, which cover various types of laceration and incision repair.

Tissue excision should be completed before committing to any particular flap or closure method. It is best to cut the shape of the defect, as well as the flap design, on a cotton towel or drape to practice before cutting the skin. This helps to prevent the common pitfall of creating flaps that are too short. The practitioner need not be limited to the following techniques. Some wounds may even heal best through secondary intention.

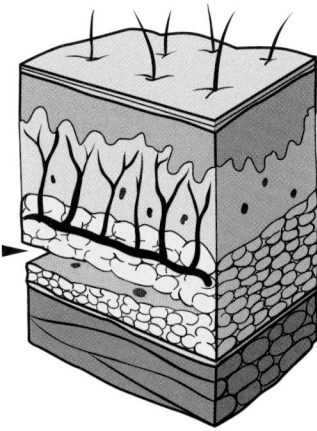

Fig. 16.2 Skin flap (*arrowhead*), with proper level of undermining in subcutaneous adipose layer. This can be performed with a blade or sharp tissue scissors. It is important to maintain integrity of vessels and not create a flap that is too thin.

It is often preferable to convert a nonelliptical defect, such as a large punch biopsy site, to an ellipse along skin tension lines before closure. On occasion, a nonelliptical defect such as a triangle or rectangle may lend itself to a flap closure by advancement or rotation. Regardless of the shape of the defect, the base must be on an even plane in the subcutaneous tissue to allow for a good result.

The key to good wound closure is to provide optimal alignment of the skin edges under minimal tension. High-quality wound closures are best accomplished by adequate *undermining* of tissue, the use of Burow triangles, the appropriate use of corner sutures, and selection of the proper plastic closure for the defect or lesion to be removed. The desired effect is to produce an excellent skin closure with little or no tension. By performing a *layered closure*, tension forces that tend to pull the skin apart can be diverted to the deep structures, limiting scarring on the visible surface area. All *buried sutures*, if necessary, should have the knot inverted (placed away from the skin side). Most skin sutures should be removed within 7 days to prevent the formation of "railroad track" scars. Exceptions are the back and anterior tibial areas, which may require removal of sutures at 14 to 19 days because of slower healing in these areas.

Flaps are composed of skin and subcutaneous tissue cut from the donor site and moved a small distance to a recipient site without removing it from its vascular supply. Local skin flaps consist of rotation flaps that pivot into place and advancement flaps that move laterally. *Rotation flaps* maintain a base of intact skin, whereas some *advancement flaps* are completely incised, with blood being supplied only from the subcutaneous tissues. Because flaps carry their own blood supply, it is important to avoid damaging the subdermal vascular plexus or cutting potential nutrient vessels. Flaps created with parallel incisions are at increased risk for necrosis because of limited blood supply, but they are sometimes unavoidable. Fig. 16.2 illustrates the proper level for undermining the flap tissue.

Tissue handling techniques are important for flap success. It is crucial to handle skin gently with minimal trauma. Lifting the skin with skin hooks is preferable to manipulation with forceps or pickups. Skin forceps should be used primarily for avascular structures and for grasping needles, not for grasping the skin. Skin forceps are capable of exerting forces of greater than 400 pounds per square inch, which will bruise the repaired area and increase the likelihood of skin infection with a poor healing response. If grasping the skin is absolutely necessary, grasp the deep dermis only and avoid the fragile epidermis. Skin forceps without teeth are preferable.

Elliptical Excisions

The elliptical excision technique is appropriate for the vast majority of lesions requiring tissue removal, and it generally facilitates wound

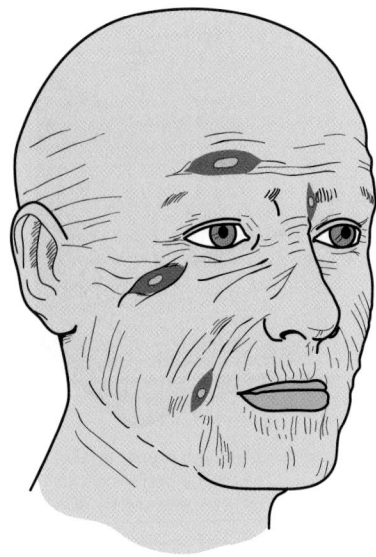

Fig. 16.3 It is essential to place elliptical excisions in relaxed skin tension lines.

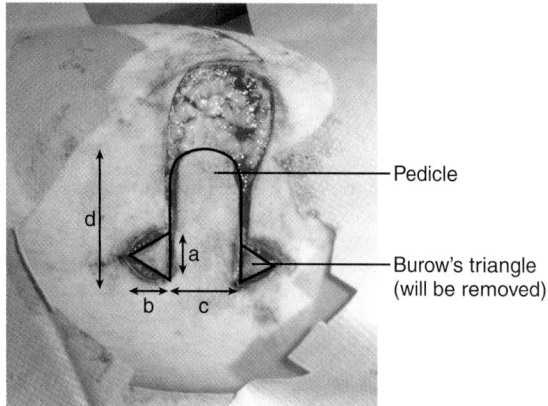

Fig. 16.4 Burow triangle. *a*, Base of Burow triangle; *b*, height of triangle; *c*, base of pedicle; *d*, length of pedicle. In planning Burow triangle, the height (*b*) should equal half the base of its pedicle (*c*). The base of the triangle (*a*) should be one-third the length of the pedicle (*d*).

closure. Length-to-width ratios should be greater than 3:1, and the terminal angles should be less than 30 degrees to avoid dog-ears. The long axis of the ellipse should run along wrinkle lines or, in younger patients, relaxed skin tension lines (Fig. 16.3; see Chapter 18, Incisions: Planning the Direction of the Cut).

If the closure is tight, gentle undermining may create more laxity. With flaps and plasties, some undermining will almost always be necessary. *Undermining* should be performed subdermally (between the skin and subcutaneous adipose tissue) to avoid injury to the vascular plexus (see Fig. 16.2 and Chapter 19, Laceration and Incision Repair). It is critical that the surgeon understands and uses undermining.

Description of Burow Triangle

When side-to-side closure is difficult owing to skin tension, a variety of flaps can be used to close the defect, depending on skin availability and anatomic location. Simple elliptical closures usually have their best results in removal of small defects. Larger defects are almost always closed with a better result and a much lower likelihood of dehiscence with advanced closures and flaps.

In addition to undermining, another concept that must be mastered is the *Burow triangle*. Corner sutures (three-point or half-buried mattress sutures) should be used in closing the Burow triangles and in attaching the free end of the pedicle to the defect site. In most cases, the Burow triangles' height should be approximately half the width of the pedicle, and their base should be approximately one-third the length of the pedicle (Fig. 16.4).

Single Advancement Flap

This flap is a viable consideration for defect closures on the trunk and thighs (Fig. 16.5). Advancement flaps are conceptually simple but have limited application because of the parallel incisions required, as well as the increased skin tension created. The single-pedicle advancement flap, with or without Burow triangles, may be useful in highly vascular, elastic areas. All advancement flaps are moved laterally without any rotation. In planning the flap, remember that *the length of a simple advancement flap should be two to three times the length of the defect to be closed*, depending on skin laxity. On the face, flaps should not exceed a 3:1 length-to-width ratio. As with the planning of all flaps, it may be helpful to cut the defect as well as the planned flap design on a surgical drape or other material, to practice, before cutting the skin.

1. Use a skin-marking pen to draw the desired flap on the patient's skin. In the case of a single advancement flap, it may be preferable cosmetically, although not necessarily, to round the advancing edge, creating a U-shaped closure, depending on the defect

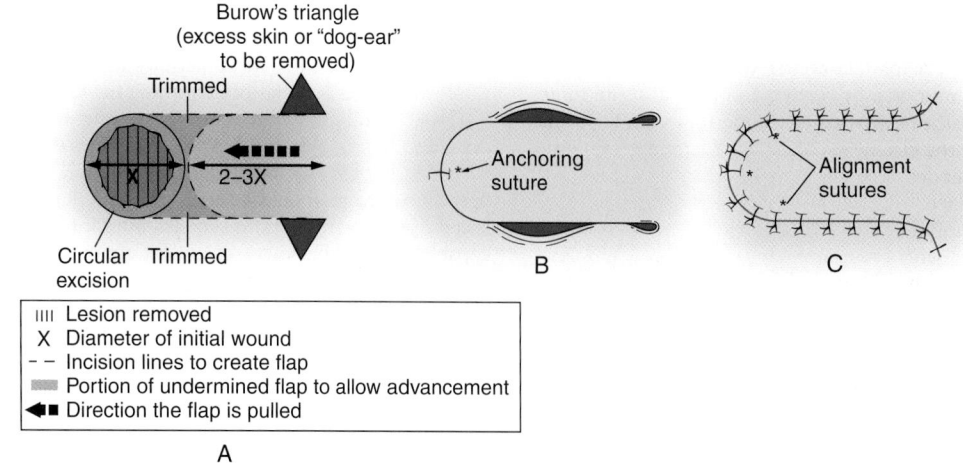

Fig. 16.5 Single advancement flap.

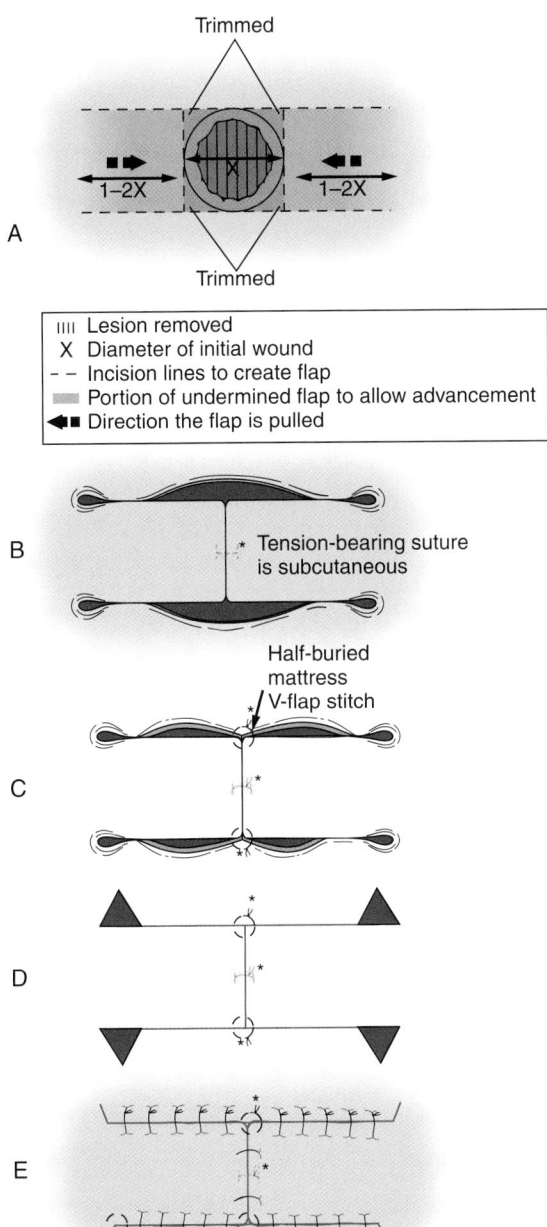

Trimmed

IIII   Lesion removed
X   Diameter of initial wound
- -   Incision lines to create flap
▦   Portion of undermined flap to allow advancement
◄■   Direction the flap is pulled

Fig. 16.6 Double advancement flap. *Asterisk,* Anchoring sutures. For further information, see Chapter 19, Laceration and Incision Repair.

Double Advancement Flap

Consider using double advancement flaps where large defects are encountered on the trunk and the thighs. If a double advancement flap is to be used (advancing a flap from two sides), the length of each flap should generally be one to two times the length of the defect.

1. Excise lesions with appropriate margins.
2. Draw out the anticipated repair with a skin-marking pen and create the incisions as shown. Trim the excess tissue to create a square defect (Fig. 16.6A).
3. Undermine the areas to be advanced.
4. Place a Burow triangle on both sides on both pedicles, similar to the single advancement flap. These Burow triangles should be the following dimensions: the base should be one-third the length of the pedicles, and the height should be one-half the width of the pedicles.
5. Advance the opposing flaps toward each other and place the anchoring (tension-bearing) suture subcutaneously (Fig. 16.6B).
6. Use double corner sutures (three-point/half-buried mattress) at sites where the flaps meet each other and adjacent to normal skin (Fig. 16.6C).
7. Place corner sutures where the Burow triangles were removed (Fig 16.6D).
8. Close the remainder of the wound site with simple interrupted sutures (Fig. 16.6E).

V-Y Plasty or Island Advancement Flap

These closures are satisfactory *for areas with excellent subcutaneous blood supply.* The V-Y plasty or flap is an advancement flap that may be *used in closing a circular defect* (Fig. 16.7). The technique should be limited to skin that is highly mobile. The technique may be useful when a vital structure (e.g., nose in Fig 16.8) prevents the standard elliptical excision or when an elliptical excision is too large to be closed without excessive tension (see Figs. 16.7 and 16.8). There is a reasonable likelihood of loss of part of these flaps if the procedure is not done in a meticulous fashion. For larger lesions, the V-Y flap may be advanced from both sides as a *double V-Y advancement* flap. The *disadvantage* of the V-Y flap is that the entire perimeter of the triangle is incised, which severely reduces the blood supply to only the vessels coming up from beneath the flap and thus limits the distance the flap can travel.

Use of the V-Y flap to close a circular defect is demonstrated as follows (see Fig. 16.7):

1. Excise the defect (see Fig. 16.7A–B).
2. Plan a triangle with a base approximately the diameter of the circular defect and an apical angle of 30 to 45 degrees (see Fig. 16.7C).
3. Incise the triangle and undermine laterally to allow eventual closure of the sides. Do not undermine under the flap itself because the blood supply to the "island" is provided by the subcutaneous vessels (see Fig. 16.7D).
4. Trim the angles at the base of the triangle to fill the defect (see Fig. 16.7E).
5. Using skin hooks, advance the flap into the defect and suture the top together (see Fig. 16.7F).
6. Place a corner stitch at the level of the point of the island, from both sides and under the point of the island. Close the remainder of the incisions with simple interrupted sutures to create a Y-shaped scar (see Fig. 16.7G).

Another method of creating a V-Y repair to close a wound under tension is as follows:

1. Create an elliptical excision large enough to remove the lesion (see Fig. 16.7H).
2. A V-shaped incision is made, then undermined to reduce skin tension (see Fig. 16.7I).

to be closed. At times, a rectangular end may be appropriate. Remember to make the base of the pedicle long and wide enough to avoid tension in the closure of the wound.

2. Undermine the intended flap at the level shown in Fig. 16.2, and pull the flap into place.
3. Burow triangles should be used to facilitate easy tissue movement and a closure with little or no tension. Burow triangles should be placed at the pivot end of the pedicle on either side. This action greatly assists the operator in closing the wound.
4. Using the skin hook, advance the flap and place an anchoring suture. If the pedicle is rectangular rather than rounded, then corner sutures are critical to good position and healing (see Fig. 16.5B).
5. Place the next sutures as shown in Fig. 16.5C to ensure proper alignment of the flap, then complete the closure.

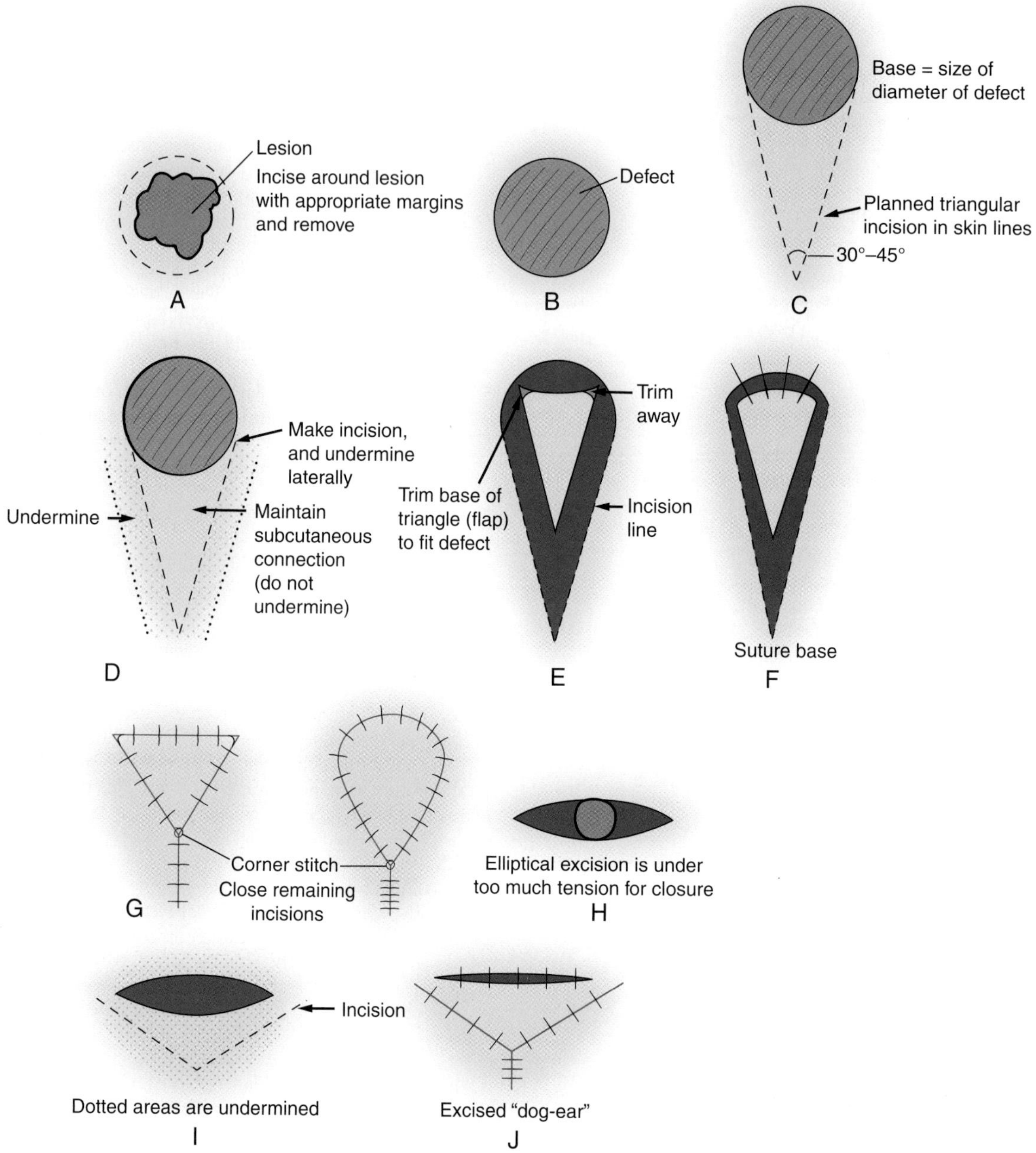

Lesion
Incise around lesion with appropriate margins and remove

A

Defect

B

Base = size of diameter of defect

Planned triangular incision in skin lines

30°–45°

C

Make incision, and undermine laterally

Undermine

Maintain subcutaneous connection (do not undermine)

D

Trim away

Trim base of triangle (flap) to fit defect

Incision line

E

Suture base

F

Corner stitch
Close remaining incisions

G

Elliptical excision is under too much tension for closure

H

Dotted areas are undermined

I

Incision

Excised "dog-ear"

J

Fig. 16.7 V-Y flap.

Fig. 16.8 V-Y plasty or island advancement flap technique. (A) Island advancement repair of perinasal cheek defect. The flap can be advanced a great distance on a nasalis muscular swinging flap, which provides reliable blood supply. (B) Note that although the flap was undersized, the surrounding tissues were undermined, and the flap was inset at the time of repair. (C) There is slight flap elevation, a trapdoor deformity, at 6 months. Philadelphia: Mosby; 2005. (From Robinson JK, Hanke CW, Siegel DM, Sengelmann RD, eds. *Surgery of the Skin: Procedural Dermatology.*)

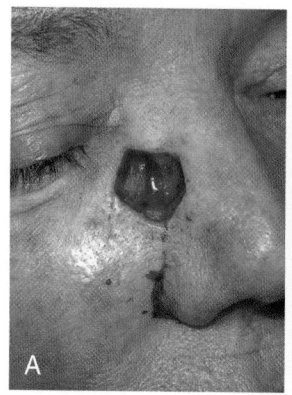
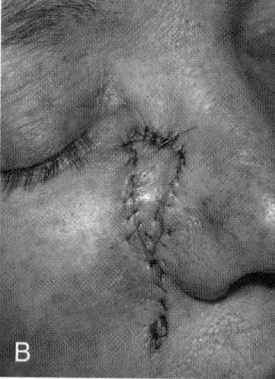
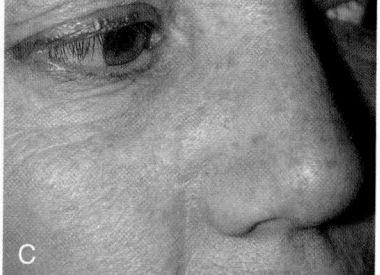

3. Close the ellipse first. When the V is closed, there will be a dog-ear that will need to be excised. Closing this area will form the vertical portion of the Y (see Fig. 16.7J).

The *double V-Y advancement flap* is performed in the same manner but with mirror-image triangular flaps that are advanced toward each other. This technique may be helpful for larger lesions.

1. Mark an elliptical area around the lesion. Excise only the abnormality in a circular fashion (Fig. 16.9A).

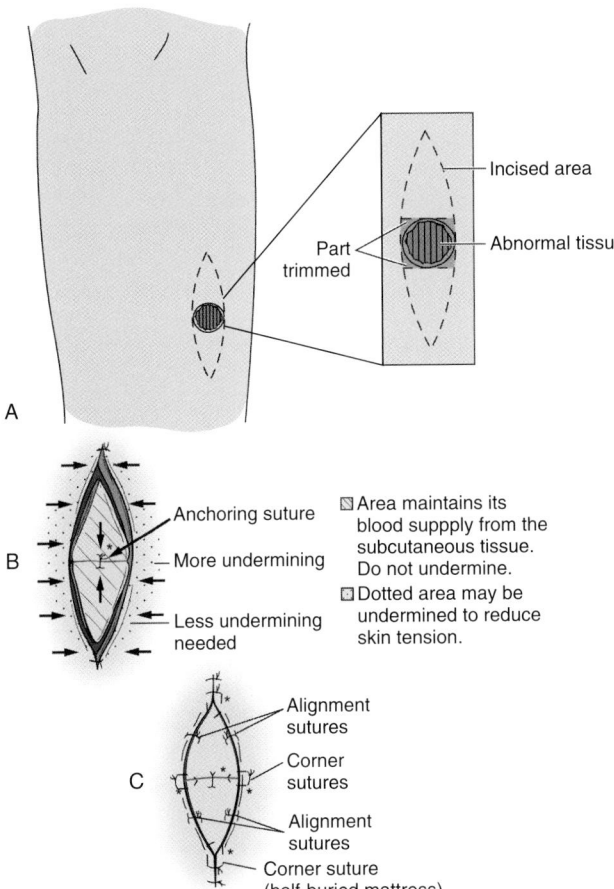

Fig. 16.9 Double V-Y advancement flap. *Asterisk,* Anchoring sutures.

2. *Incise* the triangular flaps that were marked out previously. Undermine laterally only, not under the "triangles." Using skin hooks, gently advance the two flaps toward each other and place the anchoring suture (see Fig. 16.9B).
3. Place the next sutures as shown to provide good alignment, followed by corner sutures. The closure may then be completed with subcutaneous or simple interrupted sutures (see Fig. 16.9C).

Rotation Advancement Flap

The design of a rotation flap should be planned only after the original tissue has been excised completely. The flap length should then be generous (usually an arc length of four to five times the base of the defect to be closed) to allow adequate tissue movement. The advantages of a rotation flap include the provision of good blood supply by avoiding parallel incisions, the ability to undermine the mobilized tissue if needed, and the ability to create a contralateral flap if more tissue is needed. The major disadvantage is that the final result may not blend into natural skin lines. This closure allows the coverage of large defects if used correctly. Some tissues like the face rotate easily. The scalp also closes satisfactorily with this approach. This is an effective closure in the neck region and most other areas where loose skin can be moved to an adjacent area requiring a defect to be closed.

1. The illustrated lesion lends itself to an excision that may be trimmed to create a triangular defect (Fig. 16.10A).
2. Draw the desired arc down to the "pivot point," according to the aforementioned guidelines (i.e., flap edge four to five times the length of the base of the triangular defect). Be sure to allow recruitment of sufficient tissue. As mentioned previously in this chapter, it may be helpful to cut a model of the defect in a surgical towel or drape, first, along with the proposed repair flap design, as practice. One can also practice putting tension over the area to see if the dimensions are correct. This can be done before incising the skin and committing to a particular repair. Then, as always, it is helpful to first carefully draw the arc on the skin, the repair expected, and the Burow triangle before any incisions are made (Fig. 16.10B). Excise the tissue to be removed.
3. Undermine the flap and surrounding tissue with curved Metzenbaum scissors or a blade (Fig. 16.10C). Make the Burow triangle on the opposite side of the arc and at the other end of the arc. The Burow triangle allows you to easily move the tissue of the flap into place (Fig. 16.10D).

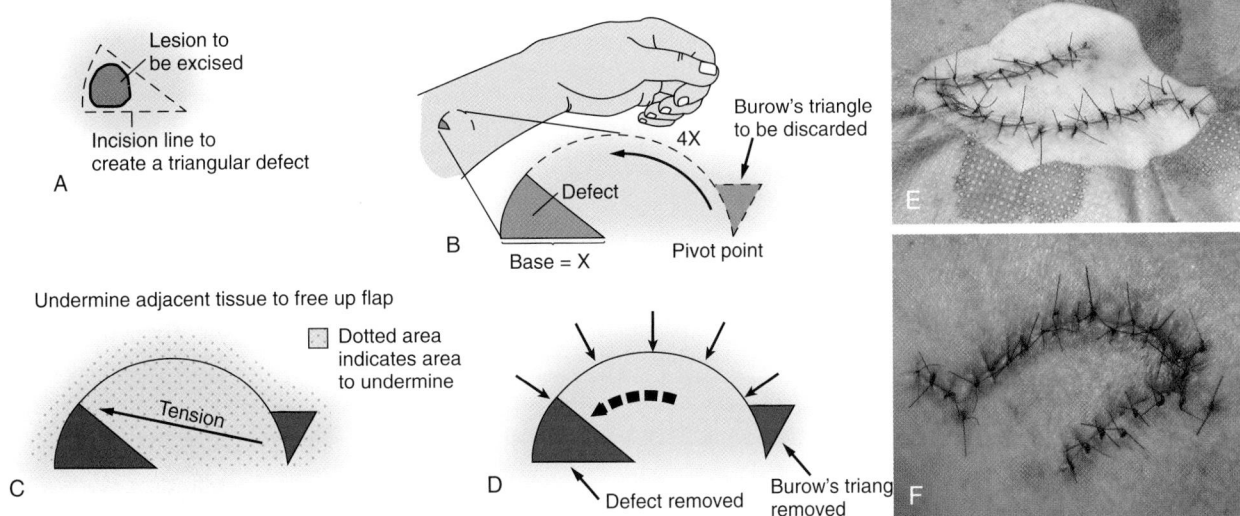

Fig. 16.10 Rotation flap.

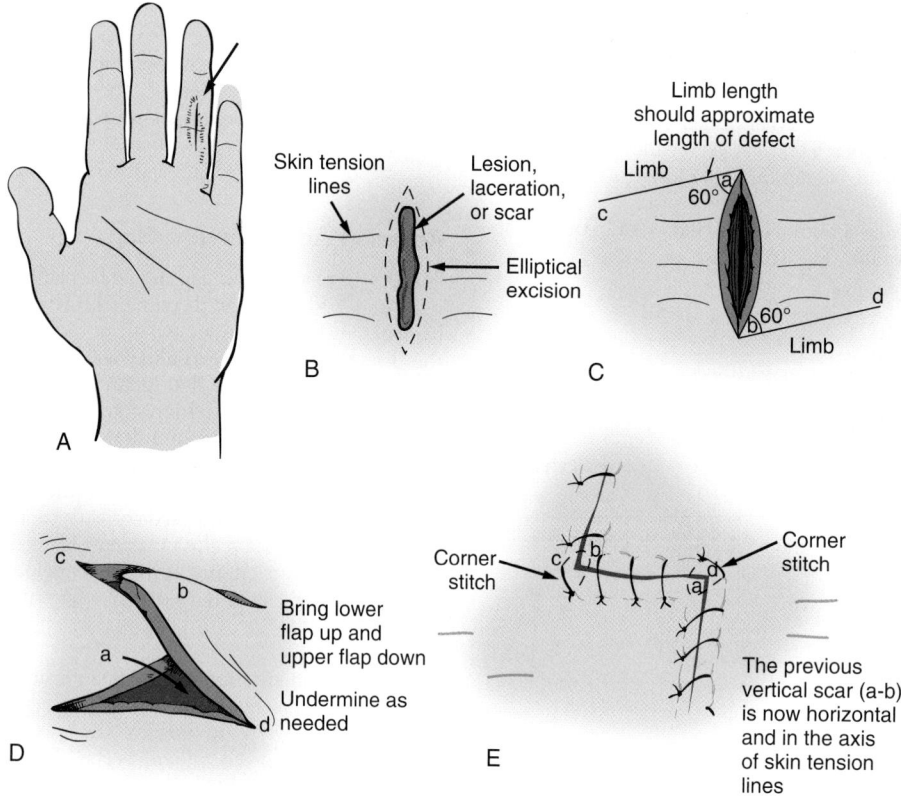

Fig. 16.11   Z-plasty.

4. Rotate the flap into place to fill the defect. The first suture is a corner suture reapproximating the skin at the corner of the Burow triangle, and the second suture is the corner suture to connect the mobile end of the rotation flap to the other corner (Fig. 16.10E).
5. Suture the rest of the skin edges into place with simple interrupted sutures (Fig. 16.10F).

Z-Plasty

The best sites in which to use this closure are over flexor and extensor joints of the hand and the sacral area, where pilonidal cysts occur. The Z-plasty is a particularly useful technique for scar revision to redirect a scar into skin tension lines (making it less visible) or to release scar contractures. Scar contracture is apt to occur when a laceration is perpendicular to skin creases, as in the case of a vertical laceration on the finger (Fig. 16.11A). Healing often contracts the scar, pulling the finger into a flexed position. Redirection of the scar can release skin tension. The major drawback to the technique is that the length of the scar is increased.

1. Excise the linear scar or lesion in a narrow ellipse along its axis (Fig. 16.11B).
2. Create the limbs of the "Z" at 60-degree angles from this axis. The length of each limb should equal the length of the defect (Fig. 16.11C).
3. Using skin hooks, advance the two triangles as shown, by crossing them over one another (Fig. 16.11D). Undermine the flaps as needed.
4. Place a "corner stitch" (half-buried mattress) at each of the flap tips, as shown in Fig. 16.11E. Then complete the wound closure with simple interrupted sutures. The new scar will now lie within the axis of the skin tension lines.

M-Plasty

This is an excellent closure when there is a paucity of skin for rotation or advancement flaps and can be used on the face, scalp, neck, trunk, and

extremities. It is truly a closure suitable for all areas and produces excellent results when the rules are followed. The design of this repair should be based on Langerhans' tension lines so the final closure is parallel with Langerhans' lines. The blood supply following repair is excellent, and it is rare to lose any portion of the flap because of inadequate blood supply. The repair usually blends into the skin lines very well with time.

1. The lesion should lend itself to a linear-type closure. The outline of the lesion to be removed should fit into the center of the M-plasty drawing (Fig. 16.12A). The length/width ratio should be at least 3:1, with the length measured at the internal points of the Burow triangles and the width being the total width of the excision (lesion plus margins). This is an extremely important measurement.
2. The base of each Burow triangle should be approximately the same as the depth (height) to allow ideal closure. There certainly is room for variance while still getting a good closure, but these guidelines are the best.
3. After the M-plasty is drawn on the skin, allowing adequate margins, the entire lesion and excess skin are removed (Fig. 16.12B).
4. The next step is to carefully undermine the surrounding tissue at the same depth as the lesion removed. The area to be undermined is usually about 10 mm, but it needs to be approximately equal to half of the width of the skin excised, with the undermining to be extended around the entire perimeter, including beneath the Burow triangles at each end of the M-plasty.
5. The first suture placed is an anchor suture in the middle of the repair to bring the edges together (Fig. 16.12C). If the wound does not come together easily, then the undermining was inadequate or the 3:1 ratio was not upheld.
6. The second and third sutures to be placed are placed midway between the anchor (middle) suture and either end of the wound to be closed (Fig. 16.12D–E).
7. The fourth and fifth sutures to be placed are modified corner/subcuticular sutures placed near the end of the wound from each side into the subcuticular portion of the skin, then connecting

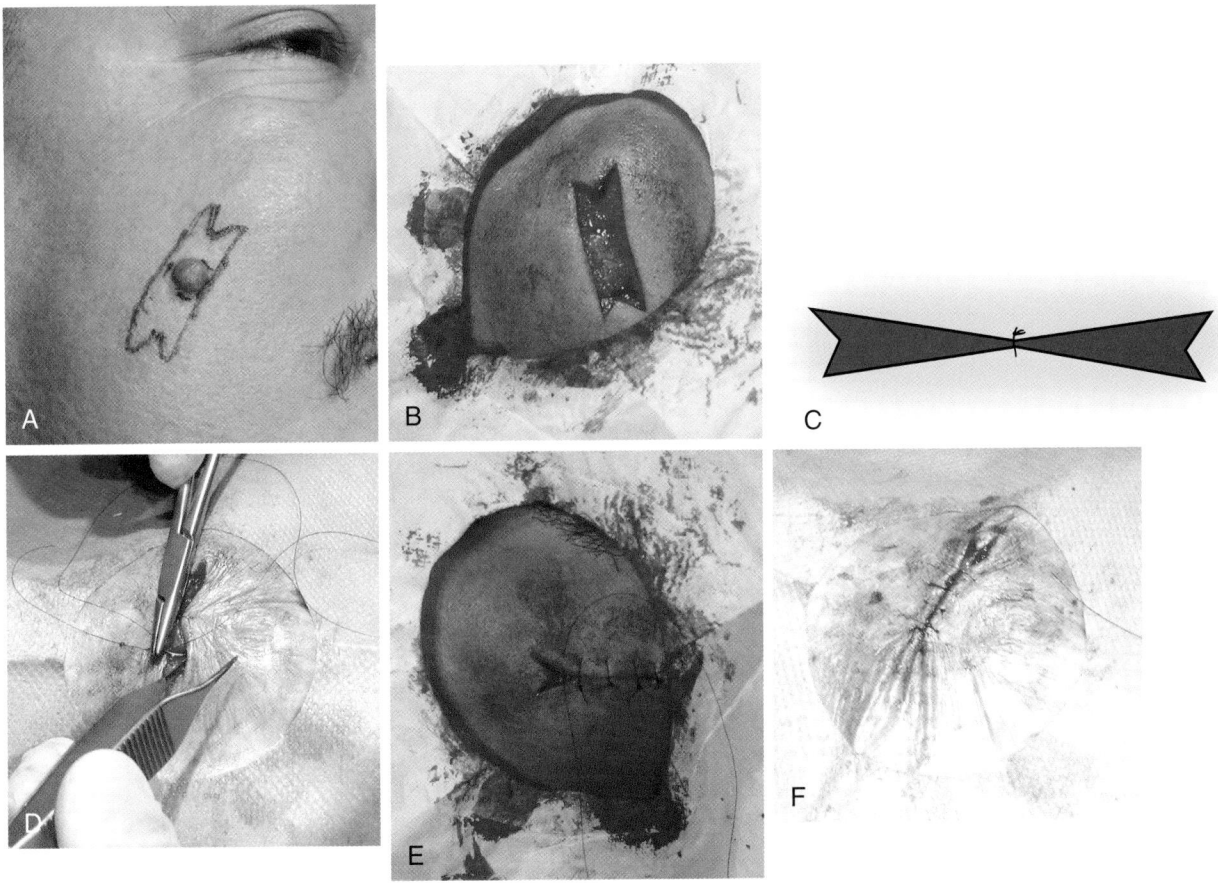

Fig. 16.12   M-Plasty.

the tip of each Burow triangle (through the subcuticular tissue), then out through the subcuticular tissue on the other side and out the skin opposite the entry point on the opposite side of the wound. The suture through the skin should be placed about 2 to 3 mm central to the point of the Burow triangle to allow a gentle pull of the triangle toward the center of the wound (Fig. 16.12F).
8. The other sutures needed are simply interrupted sutures to produce the appropriate closure.
9. When the sutures are removed, it is best to leave the anchor suture as the last one to be removed if the sutures are removed sequentially (not at the same time).

Dog-Ears

Dog-ears are caused by excess skin left at the end of the suture line. They commonly occur when skin edges are rotated or pulled, when interrupted sutures are not placed evenly, or when one side of a wound is longer than the other. Dog-ears can be avoided by (1) closing the ends of an elliptical defect first and distributing the "extra skin" throughout the wound, (2) keeping ellipse incision angles 30 degrees or less, and (3) maintaining 3:1 length-to-width ratios or using advanced closures. The best technique for repair is demonstrated in Fig. 16.13. In this repair, the wound will be lengthened and excess tissue must be removed.

It is easy with this technique to judge the amount of tissue that must be removed.

1. Excess tissue on one side of the wound closure creates a dog-ear (see Fig. 16.13A).
2. At the apex of the wound, incise the tissue at a 150-degree angle to the wound. The length depends on the amount of excess tissue (see Fig. 16.13B). Make the cut on the side of the wound where

the excess tissue exists, making sure that you gently pull the excess tissue toward the wound along the long axis of the wound.
3. Using the skin hook, pull the apex of the dog-ear over the extended incision line and excise the excess tissue with a blade or tissue scissors (see Fig. 16.13C). This action makes the repair close nicely using the Burow triangle approach.
4. Close as shown using a corner suture and then interrupted sutures (see Fig. 16.13D).

POTENTIAL COMPLICATIONS OF ADVANCED CLOSURES AND FLAPS

Acute (Within 2 Weeks)

- Bleeding
- Bruising
- Swelling
- Hematoma
- Pain
- Infection
- Wound dehiscence

Chronic or Permanent

- Scarring/contractures
- "Railroad tracks" from delayed suture removal
- Hypertrophic scars
- Keloid
- Hyperpigmentation
- Hypopigmentation
- Nerve damage
- Ectropion and entropion of eyelid

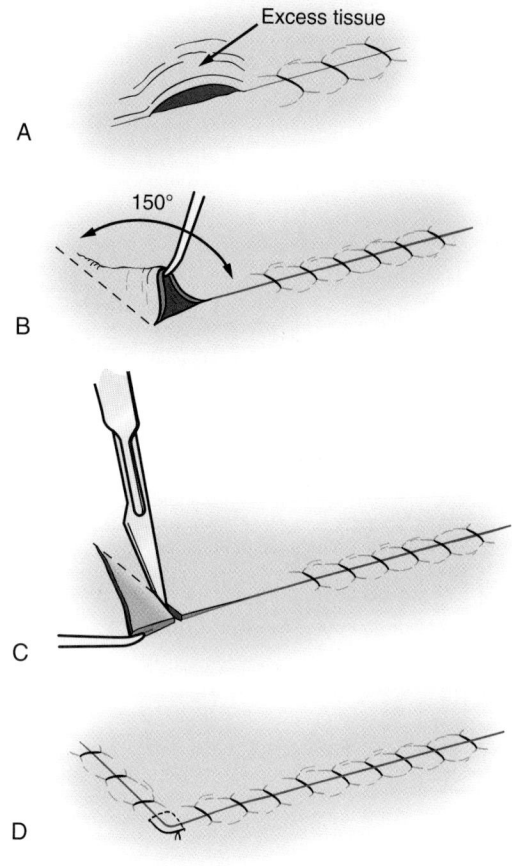

A

150°

B

C

D

Fig. 16.13   Dog-ear repair.

- Disruption of vermilion border of upper lip
- Skin atrophy
- Hair loss
- Recurrence of excised lesion

Additional Considerations

When excising potentially malignant lesions, tumor-free margins must always be obtained before committing to any flap closure. If a later pathology report indicates incomplete excision of a malignant lesion, the appropriate area around the previous closure area will need to be resected. If this involves a flap technique, there may already be significant skin tension, or little skin may be available for further repairs. The patient requiring more extensive repairs or grafting may be left with a large defect. With the correct surgical approach, reexcision to accomplish a cure based on pathology usually is possible.

POSTPROCEDURE PATIENT EDUCATION

Proper postoperative care is more critical with skin flaps and plasties than with simple closures. For the first 24 hours after surgery, the patient must rest and avoid exertion. Instruct the patient to refrain from bending, heavy lifting, and exercising until the sutures are removed. The wound should be kept clean and covered with a thin coat of antibiotic or petrolatum ointment for first 24 hours. The patient should refrain from alcohol and aspirin-containing medicines for at least the first 24 hours after surgery. The wound should be dressed with a small piece of Telfa covered by Tegaderm or roll dressing, depending on the site, so a good seal

develops over the wound. If subcuticular sutures are used, Steri-Strips are placed, followed by the Telfa and Tegaderm dressing. A thick outer dressing of 4 × 4 gauze or other bandage is then placed to provide a pressure dressing that limits bleeding and swelling. Ice on the area for 2 to 4 hours helps relieve pain, swelling, and bleeding.

After 24 hours the thick outer bandage may be removed. Each day the wound should be carefully checked to make sure there is no crust or blood accumulation. If there is blood or crust accumulation, this should be removed with gentle washing using soap and water. The wound should have a very thin layer of antibiotic or petrolatum ointment applied before bedtime. The exceptions to these guidelines are hand and foot wounds in those who will continue to work and play. These selected patients should continue to have a wound covering at least during the daytime after the first 24 hours to keep the wound from getting wet or contaminated. If the wound dressing gets wet or contaminated, it should be replaced with a new dressing of antibiotic or petrolatum ointment and Tegaderm or roll dressing. After 24 hours it is acceptable to shower and wash the wound. The area should not be scrubbed. If the wound bleeds at any time, the patient should apply firm pressure for 15 minutes, and a new dressing should be placed over the wound. Instruct the patient to call the office or go to the emergency department if the wound bleeds significantly despite 15 minutes of firm pressure, if any signs of infection (e.g., purulence, redness, increased pain, swelling, or fever) are noted, or if there is any breakdown in wound or suture integrity.

In the case of surgery on the face, instruct the patient to sleep with his or her head slightly elevated for the first two nights after the procedure and to avoid sleeping on the same side as the wound. The patient should also avoid bending down (head below the heart) for the first 48 hours after the surgery. Arrange for office follow-up based on personal discretion, depending on the complexity of the procedure, the cleanliness of the wound, and patient factors. Sutures on the face are usually removed within 4 to 7 days, depending on the size, position, and tension of the closure. If deep, buried sutures are used, skin sutures may be removed sooner than if no buried sutures are used. Sutures on the neck are generally left in place for 6 to 8 days depending on the size and tension of the closure. On the trunk, groin, and extremities, sutures are left in longer, usually 10 to 21 days, depending on the speed of healing. Usually the slowest areas to heal are the anterior tibial areas and the posterior trunk. Sutures on the scalp are usually removed in 7 to 10 days.

CONCLUSION

Achievement of a durable repair with a good cosmetic result after skin surgery is important. To obtain predictable, good-quality outcomes, focus on simplicity. An ellipse excision with primary closure is best used for small lesions. Larger defects, skin cancers that require wider excision, and any area that is likely to dehisce is usually much better served with a plastic/flap repair if done correctly. When wounds are difficult to close, flaps, skin grafts, and healing by secondary intention are always options, and usually better options for optimal long-term results.

It is prudent to remember the keys to excellent repairs in plastic closures: (1) proper width-to-length ratio of excision, (2) corner sutures placed appropriately, (3) undermining performed carefully with Metzenbaum scissors, and (4) use of Burow triangles to extend and move tissue. Observance of these four parameters will provide optimal outcomes.

PATIENT EDUCATION GUIDES

See the patient education and consent forms available at www.expertconsult.com.

CPT/Billing Codes

Excision or repair by adjacent tissue transfer or rearrangement, including Z-plasty, V-Y plasty, rotation flap, and advancement flaps:

14000 Trunk <10 sq cm
14001 Trunk 10–30 sq cm
14020 Scalp, arms, legs <10 sq cm
14021 Scalp, arms, legs 10–30 sq cm
14040 Forehead, chin, cheek, mouth, neck, axilla, genitalia, hands, feet <10 sq cm
14041 Forehead, chin, cheek, mouth, neck, axilla, genitalia, hands, feet 10–30 sq cm
14060 Eyelids, nose, ears, lips <10 sq cm
14061 Eyelids, nose, ears, lips 10–30 sq cm
14300 Any area, unusual, or complicated repair, more than 30 sq cm
14350 Filleted finger or toe flap, including preparation of recipient site

NOTE: These codes generally apply to full-thickness excision and repair by adjacent tissue mobilization. For reporting laceration repairs, the procedure must be created by the surgeon and not by the incidental shape of the laceration. Refer to the CPT book for further description.

ICD-10-CM Diagnostic Codes

See Appendix G, Neoplasm, Skin: ICD-10 Codes.

Acknowledgment

The editors recognize the contributions of Ashley K. Christiani, MD, and Mats Hagstrom, MD, to this chapter in previous editions of this text.

Suppliers

(See contact information available at www.expertconsult.com.)

Acuderm, Inc.
Delasco Dermatologic Lab and Supply Co.
Integra Life Sciences Corporation
Moore Medical Corp.
SSR Surgical Instruments

Online Resources

Thomsen TW, Barclay DA, Setnick GS. Videos in clinical medicine: Basic laceration repair. *N Engl J Med.* 2006;355:e18–e22.

Recommended Reading

Arndt KA, Dover JS, Alam M. *Procedures in Cosmetic Dermatology Series: scar Revision.* Philadelphia: Saunders; 2006.
Thorne CH, Gurner GC, Chung K, et al., eds. *Grabb and Smith's Plastic Surgery.* 7th ed. Philadelphia: Lippincott Williams and Wilken; 2013.
Botting J, Schofield J. *Brown's Skin and Minor Surgery: A Text and Colour Atlas.* 5th ed. London: CRC Press; 2015.
Denkler K. A comprehensive review of epinephrine in the finger: to do or not to do. *Plast Reconstr Surg.* 2000;108:114–124.
Jackson EA. The V-Y plasty in the treatment of fingertip amputations. *Am Fam Physician.* 2001;64:455–458.
Radovic P, Smith RG, Shumway D. Revisiting epinephrine in foot surgery. *J Am Podiatr Med Assoc.* 2003;93:157–160.
Robinson JK, Arndt KA, LeBoit PE, Wintroub BU. *Atlas of Cutaneous Surgery.* Philadelphia: WB Saunders; 1996.
Robinson JK, Hanke CW, Siegel DM, et al., eds. *Surgery of the Skin: Procedural Dermatology.* 3rd ed. Philadelphia: Saunders; 2014.
Thomson CJ, Lalonde DH, Denkler K, Feicht AJ. A critical look at the evidence for and against elective epinephrine use in the finger. *Plast Reconstr Surg.* 2007;119:260–266.
Usatine RP, Moy RL, eds. *Skin Surgery: A Practical Guide.* 2nd ed. Philadelphia: Elsevier; 2010.
Usatine RP, Pfenninger JL, Stulberg DL, et al., eds. *Dermatologic and Cosmetic Procedures in Office Practice.* Philadelphia: Elsevier; 2012.

CHAPTER 17

FUNGAL STUDIES (AND SCABIES): COLLECTION PROCEDURES AND TESTS

Dennis E. Babel

DIAGNOSTIC METHODS

The three basic methods used to diagnose fungal infections are direct microscopy (e.g., potassium hydroxide [KOH] method), fungal culture, and biopsy with histopathology.

Direct Microscopy

Early diagnosis of cutaneous mycoses can be made in the clinician's office by direct microscopy of infected tissue or lesion exudate. A number of different clearing solutions can be applied to collected material to assist in direct microscopy. These agents help distribute the specimen so fungal structures can be more readily visualized. Included in these solutions are simple saline, potassium, or sodium hydroxide in various formulas and preparations, and various coloring agents.

Fungal Culture

The ultimate identification of fungal pathogens requires their isolation on fungal culture medium. This isolation can take place in the clinician's office using fungal media such as Sabouraud's dextrose agar with cycloheximide (to inhibit fungal contaminants) and chloramphenicol (to inhibit bacterial contaminants). These are commercially available as Mycosel agar (Becton, Dickinson and Company), Mycobiotic agar (Hardy Diagnostics), and Dermatophyte Test Medium (DTM), a presumptive color-change medium (Hardy Diagnostics). Of the three listed, only DTM is a color-change medium. Inoculation of an appropriate patient specimen on these agars should allow the growth only of the true causative fungal organism.

Biopsy and Histopathology

Biopsy specimens obtained from fungal lesions can reveal the in vivo morphology of the infectious agent as well as the host response to this invasive presence. The appropriately stained histopathology section can provide the clinician with proof of the presence of a fungal pathogen, clues to its identity, the extent of infection, and the patient's ability to respond to this invasion. Although this procedure might be considered the gold standard for the diagnosis of human mycoses, it is an invasive procedure, is somewhat costly, and is seldom required for the identification of cutaneous mycoses. A 3-mm punch biopsy is usually sufficient. The pathologist must be alerted if a fungal infection is considered in the differential.

EQUIPMENT

NOTE: Not every item is needed for each collection method.

- Alcohol swabs
- 3 × 3 gauze squares
- Scalpel blade (No. 15)
- Toothbrush
- Cotton-tipped applicator
- Disposable biopsy punch (3 mm)
- Glass microscope slide (1 × 3 in)
- Cover slip (22 × 22 mm)
- 20% KOH (commercial preps are available with dimethyl sulfoxide solution to enhance viewing)
- Chlorazol black E solution (optional, but enhance viewing)
- Microscope with 10× and 40× objectives
- Fungal culture media in tubes, vials, or Petri dishes (see "Fungal Culture" section above)

CUTANEOUS MYCOSES SPECIMEN COLLECTION (FOR KOH PREPARATIONS AND FUNGAL CULTURES)

Hair

The most common mycoses of the hair are tinea capitis and tinea barbae (Fig. 17.1).

- Clean the area of alopecia thoroughly with alcohol to remove foreign debris and minimize bacterial contamination. This will not affect the viability of the fungi in any manner (Fig. 17.2).
- Collect a specimen with a scalpel, glass slide edge, new toothbrush, 3 × 3 gauze square, or cotton-tipped applicator (Fig. 17.3).
- Appropriate specimen could include black dots (hair stubs) or scalp scale from the area of alopecia. (Long hairs and hair clippings are unacceptable because they are seldom actually infected and are frequently contaminated with bacteria.)

Skin

Fungal infections of the skin include tinea corporis, tinea cruris, tinea pedis, tinea manuum, and candidiasis (Fig. 17.4).

- For annular or serpiginous lesions of the skin, clean the advancing lesional edge with alcohol and obtain the scaling epithelium (avoid collecting scale from the center or oldest portion of the lesion because it is unlikely that the fungal pathogen is still present in that "healed" area). Scrape over the area firmly (using the side of a scalpel blade to prevent bleeding). Loosened epithelial debris may be scraped directly onto a glass microscope slide for KOH examination and directly onto the fungal media surface for culture.
- For intertriginous mycoses, once again clean and collect material from the dry scaling edge. (Avoid any central, moist, macerated material because it is usually devoid of any viable fungi and is frequently contaminated with bacteria.)
- For vesicular mycoses of the skin, collect a portion of the vesicle roof by removing with a sterile scissors or scalpel blade. (Vesicular fluid and epithelium from the vesicle base are usually devoid of any fungi.)

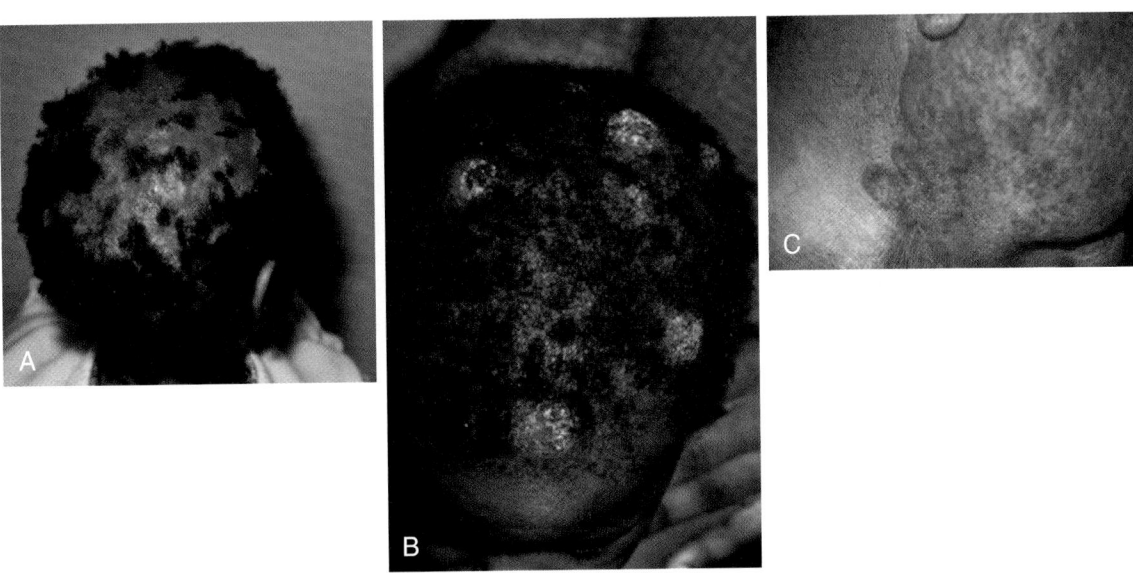

Fig. 17.1   (A) Black dot tinea capitis. (B) Tinea capitis with kerion. (C) Tinea barbae.

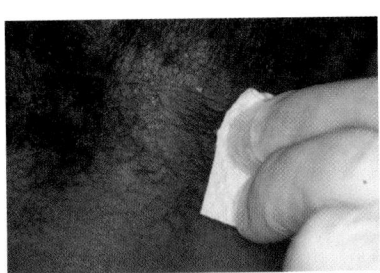

Fig. 17.2   Clean area with alcohol wipe.

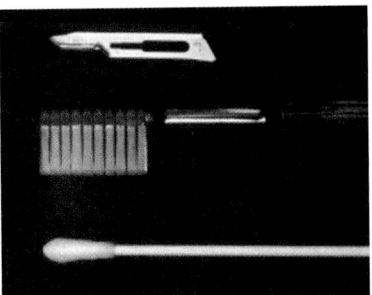

Fig. 17.3   Tinea collection tools.

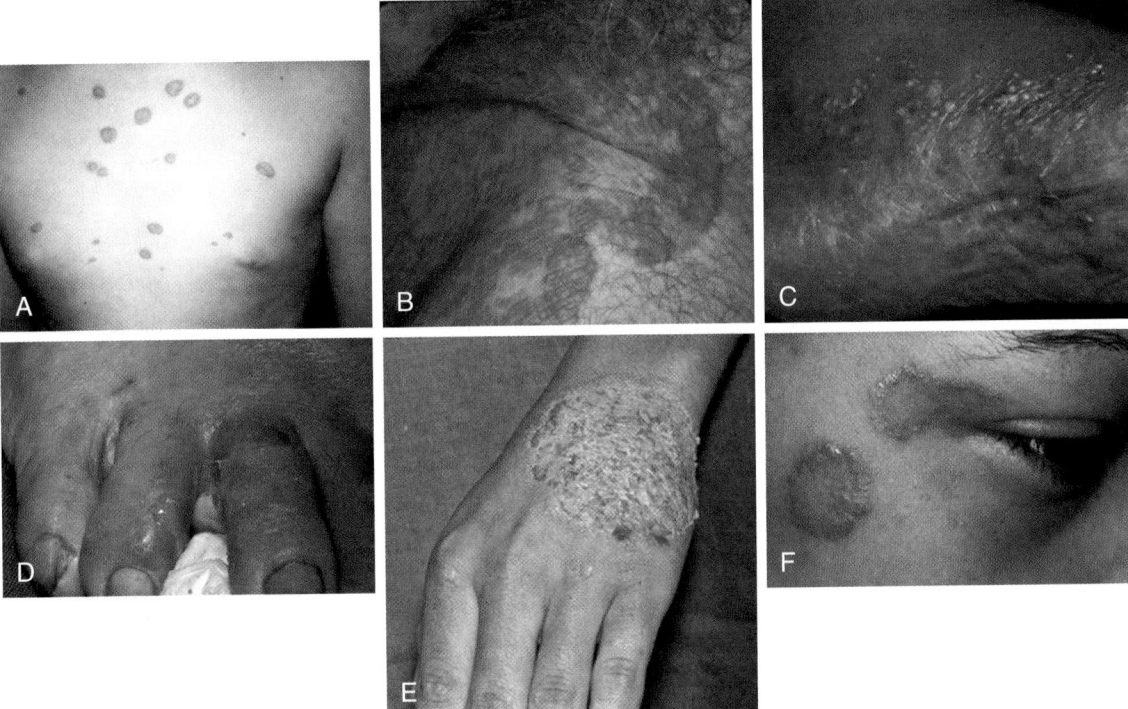

Fig. 17.4   (A) Tinea corporis (annular). (B) Tinea cruris (serpiginous). (C) Tinea pedis (vesicular). (D) Tinea pedis (interdigital). (E) Tinea manuum. (F) Tinea faciei.

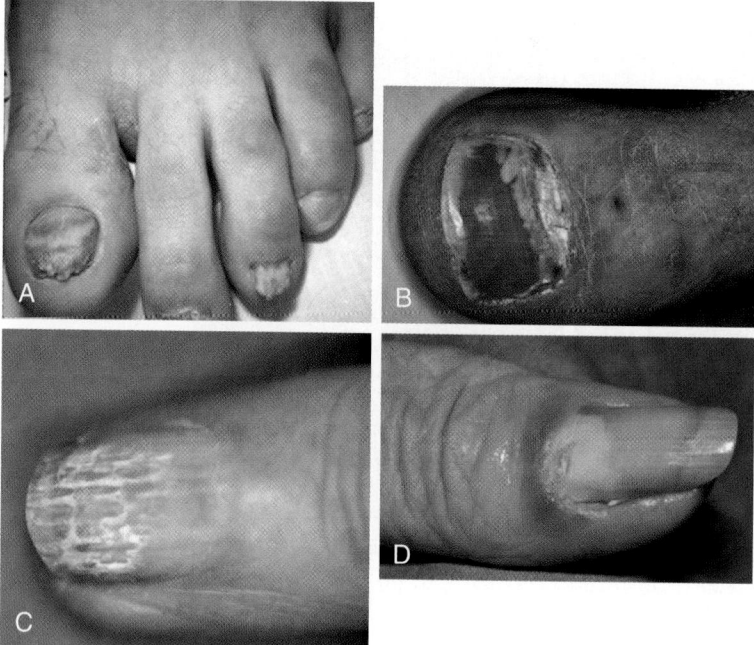

Fig. 17.5 (A) Distal subungual onychomycosis. (B) Proximal subungual onychomycosis. (C) White superficial onychomycosis. (D) Candidal onychomycosis/ paronychia.

Nail

Fungal infection of the nail (onychomycosis) is usually due to dermatophytes (tinea unguium) or *Candida* (Fig. 17.5).

- For *distal* subungual onychomycosis, trim back the nail to the leading edge of infection (edge closest to the proximal nail fold) and discard. Collect keratinaceous debris from beneath the remaining trimmed nail plate edge.
- For *proximal* subungual onychomycosis, reverse this process and collect material from the active edge closest to the distal end.
- For *white superficial onychomycosis*, clean and collect material by simply scraping the surface area of involvement.

NOTE: Less-than-ideal specimens are nail clippings and whole-removed nail plate because the true fungal reservoir is actually the nail bed (the exception being nail plate surface material from white superficial onychomycosis).

TECHNIQUE FOR KOH PREPARATION

See Fig. 17.6A.

1. Place the appropriate specimen (collected as previously described) on a clean glass microscope slide.
2. Add one drop of 20% KOH (enhanced if contains dimethyl sulfoxide solution).
3. If available, add one drop of chlorazol black E solution.
4. Place a cover slip on top of the slide preparation and press down or tap 5 or 6 times to eliminate air bubbles. Tilting one end of the slide up, about 10 degrees, while pressing or tapping may assist in removing bubbles.
5. Blot excess solution from the finished slide preparation.
6. Place the preparation on the microscope stage and examine it with the low-power (10×) objective.
7. To enhance contrast, reduce the microscope illumination by lowering the condenser until epithelial cells are clearly visible.
8. Screen the slide preparation under low power (10×) for the presence of fungal structures, such as hyphae or yeast.
9. Examine suspect structures with the 40× setting (high-power

dry objective) to confirm the presence of fungi (an oil immersion objective is not needed).
10. The observation of hyphae or budding yeast and pseudohyphae constitutes a "positive" KOH preparation for fungus.

EDITOR'S NOTE: The KOH prep can also be used to diagnose scabies. The best location for a sample is a vesicle from between the fingers, on the volar wrist, on the thenar or hypothenar hand, or on the ankles. For infants, lesions on the soles of feet can be helpful. In these areas, vesicles are more common and a better source for diagnosing scabies than burrows. The vesicles should be scraped with more firmness than with fungal studies. The material from 3 or 4 vesicles, if possible, should be wiped onto the slide. The remainder of the procedure follows what is noted above. The test is considered positive when whole mites, parts of mites, whole eggs or parts of eggs, or scybala are noted on the slide. Some clinicians use mineral oil instead of KOH to preserve the specimen. The scabitic elements will dissolve completely 2 to 3 hours after KOH is applied.

Positive Fungal KOH

1. *Dermatophyte (mold) causing tinea.* Look for hyaline, septate filaments with diameters at least four times the diameter of an epithelial cell wall. This diameter should be very consistent (5 to 7 μm). This filament is linear and may course across a number of keratinocytes and occasionally branch (see Fig. 17.6B–F).
2. *Candida (yeast).* Look for round to oval budding cells as well as "stretched out" budding cells (pseudohyphae; see Fig. 17.6G).
3. *Malassezia furfur (pityriasis versicolor).* Look for short, hyaline, septate hyphae as well as round, clustered yeast cells ("spaghetti and meatballs"; see Fig. 17.6F).

Common Errors in KOH Examinations

- Not collecting specimen from the leading edge of infection.
- Not thoroughly cleaning the sample site with alcohol before sampling.
- Not reducing the microscope light by racking down the microscope condenser to maximize contrast.

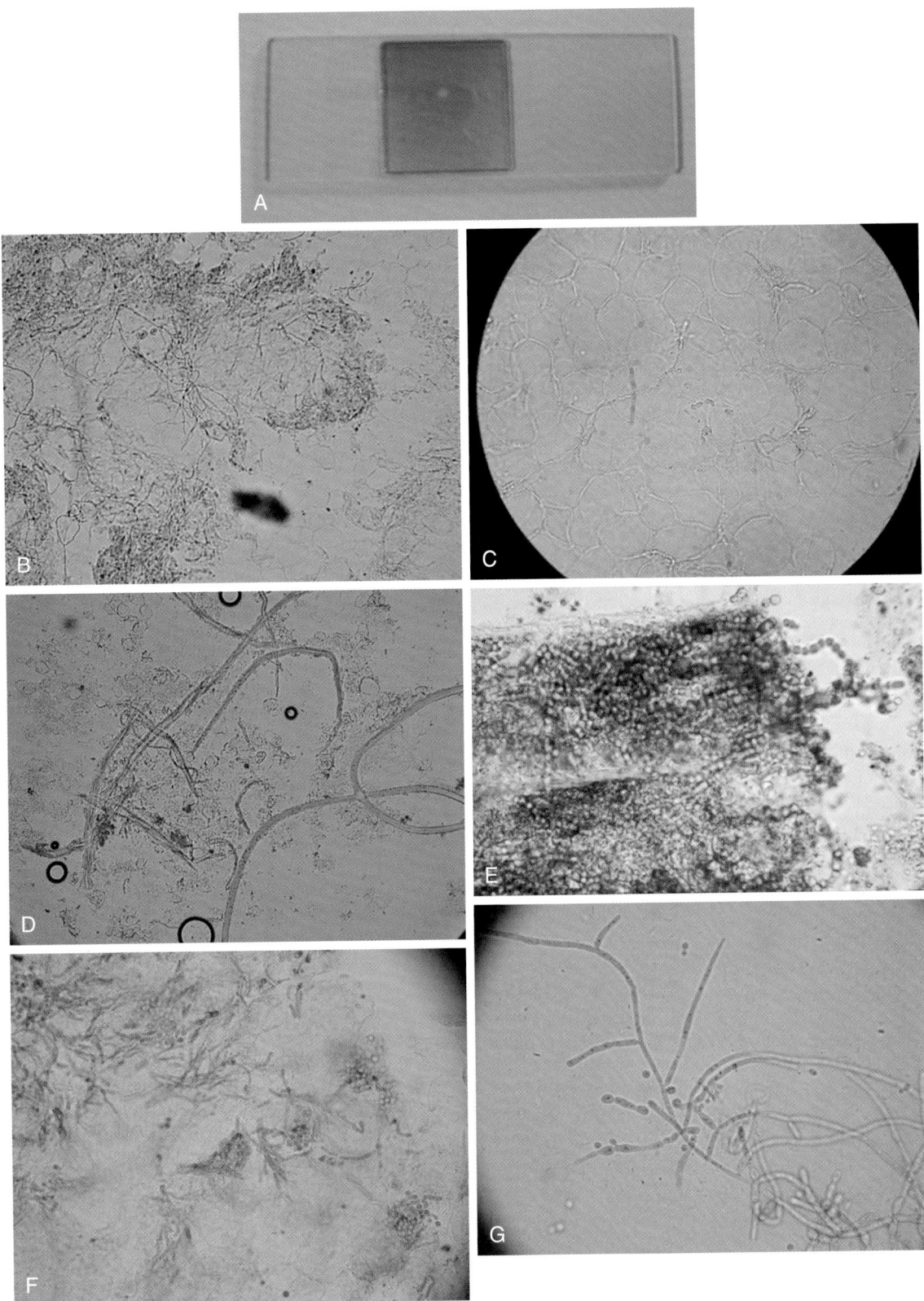

Fig. 17.6 (A) Glass slide potassium hydroxide (KOH) preparation. (B) Positive KOH for hyphae (low power). (C) Positive KOH for hyphae (high power). (D) False-positive KOH preparation with foreign debris. (E) Positive KOH for tinea capitis. (F) Positive KOH for tinea versicolor ("spaghetti and meatballs"). (G) Positive KOH for candidiasis.

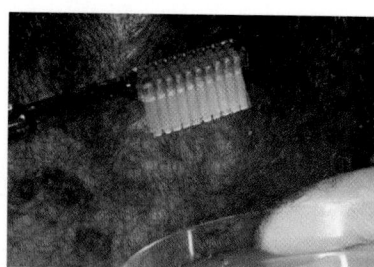

Fig. 17.7   Fungal culture inoculation from tinea capitis with toothbrush.

- Mistaking foreign matter (e.g., sock fibers, dirt, pollen) for fungal structures microscopically.
- Heating a KOH slide preparation to speed up the clearing process to the point where the chemical precipitates out. (Heating a slide preparation should not be necessary if using 20% KOH with dimethyl sulfoxide.)

Technique for a Fungal Culture (Office Procedure)

The greatest recovery of mycotic pathogens by fungal culture is achieved by inoculating lesion material directly onto fungal media (Fig. 17.7). (Alternatively, the patient specimen that will be sent to an outside laboratory for inoculation should be packaged carefully and delivered in a timely fashion.)

1. The patient specimen should be gently pressed onto the agar surface. Minimize "stabbing" and avoid "slashing" the agar because these techniques may lead to a premature drying out of the culture system.
2. Fungal cultures from most cutaneous specimens should be incubated at room temperature (22°C to 27°C) in a draft-free location and out of direct sunlight.
3. Presumptive pathogen media such as DTM, which rely on a color change from orange to red when a fungal pathogen is present, should be observed for the first 10 days. The development of a red agar color after this period should be considered a false-positive result.

Technique for Biopsy

Biopsy specimens can be obtained for both fungal culture and histopathologic confirmation of the organism's presence in vivo.

1. A 3-mm punch biopsy obtained from the lesional edge is usually sufficient for both purposes (see Chapter 26, Skin Biopsy).
2. The biopsy material should be divided longitudinally into two equal parts.

3. One biopsy portion should be placed into *formalin* and sent to the pathology laboratory with a request for "fungal stains."
4. The second biopsy portion should be placed in *sterile saline* and sent to the microbiology laboratory for "fungal culture."

CPT/Billing Codes

87220   Tissue examination for KOH slide of samples from skin, hair, or nails for fungi or ectoparasite ova or mites (e.g., scabies)

Suppliers

(See contact information available at www.expertconsult.com.)

Fungal culture isolation media
  Catalog #X30—Mycobiotic agar, plastic Hardy flask
  Catalog #X15—DTM (Dermatophyte Test Medium), plastic Hardy flask (Hardy Diagnostics)
Instrument for trimming nail plate
  #21-626 Ruskin double action forceps, 6″, straight (Miltex, Inc.)
KOH solutions for micro preps
  20% KOH with DMSO; chlorazol black E fungal stain (Dermatology Lab & Supply, Inc.; Delasco)

Recommended Reading

Babel DE, Fungi. In: Lesher J, ed. *Manual of Cutaneous Microbiology for the Office Laboratory.* Pearl River, NY: Parthenon Publishing; 2000.

Babel DE, Rogers AL. Dermatophytes: their contribution to infectious disease in North America. *Clin Microbiol Rev.* 1983;5:81–85.

Babel DE, Rogers AL, Beneke ES. Dermatophytosis of the scalp: incidence, immune response, and epidemiology. *Mycopathologia.* 1990;109:69–73.

Hall BJ, Hall JC. *Sauer's Manual of Skin Diseases.* 10th ed. Philadelphia: Lippincott-Raven; 2010.

Jung MY, Shim JH, Lee JH, et al. Comparison of diagnostic methods for onychomycosis, and proposal of a diagnostic algorithm. *Clin Exp Dermatol.* 2015;40:479.

Karimzadegan-Nia M, Mir-Amin-Mohammadi A, Bouzari N, Firooz A. Comparison of direct smear, culture and histology for the diagnosis of onychomycosis. *Australa J Dermatol.* 2007;48:18.

Lawry MA, Haneke E, Strobeck K, et al. Methods for diagnosing onychomycosis: a comparative study and review of the literature. *Arch Dermatol* 2000;136.1112.

Usatine RP, Smith MA, Mayeaux EJ, et al. *The Color Atlas of Family Medicine.* 2nd ed. New York: McGraw-Hill; 2013.

Weinberg JM, Koestenblatt EK, Tutrone WD, et al. Comparison of diagnostic methods in the evaluation of onychomycosis. *J Am Acad Dermatol.* 2003;49:193.

CHAPTER 18

INCISIONS: PLANNING THE DIRECTION OF THE INCISION

Julie M. Sicilia

Although generally considered minor procedures, skin incisions are invasive. They cause permanent changes in skin architecture and carry the potential for deleterious patient outcomes in terms of cosmesis and function. Skin incisions must be made with careful, thoughtful consideration and advance planning.

Several general issues should be addressed before deciding to perform an incision:

- Overall health status of the patient, including assessment of risk for:
  - Significant bleeding (bleeding dyscrasias; medications, including herbs)
  - Potential for delayed wound healing (e.g., smoking, collagen vascular disease, diabetes, obesity, immunosuppression, steroid use, malnutrition, peripheral vascular disease)
  - Allergy to any substance being used in conjunction with the procedure, including latex and the parabens preservatives in multiple-dose vials of anesthetics
- Need for antibiotic prophylaxis (e.g., dirty wounds, bites, infection, puncture, immunosuppression, diabetes)
- Ability of the patient or caregivers to properly care for the surgical wound postoperatively
- Expected benefits versus risks of the procedure

The clinician must obtain an informed consent and ensure that the patient knows the basic possible complications of pain, bleeding, infection, recurrence, scarring, damage to nearby structures, and distortion of the anatomy. The clinician must always consider the patient as a whole being and not simply focus on "the lesion." Many pitfalls are avoidable if this is kept in mind.

Technical factors to be considered include the following:

- Avoidance of damage to any underlying vital structures
- Proper orientation of incision lines
- Correct design and size of the excision
- Avoidance of significant anatomic distortion

AVOIDING DAMAGE TO UNDERLYING STRUCTURES

Simple full-thickness skin excisions performed with care usually do not pose a threat to underlying structures. The plane of removal should be at the junction of the adipose tissue and the dermis (Fig. 18.1). Nonetheless, familiarity with the anatomy of the proposed surgical site in regard to underlying nerves, vessels, tendons, bursae, and bony structures is essential. Of special concern are two nerves that lie superficially within the subdermal fat layer: the temporal branch of the facial nerve and the spinal accessory nerve (Figs. 18.2 and 18.3). Injury to the temporal branch of the facial nerve may cause inability to wrinkle the forehead and drooping of the eyebrow on the affected side. Damage to the spinal accessory nerve can lead to loss of use of the trapezius muscle. When performing excisions in these regions,

clinicians should consider less invasive alternative methods for treating the particular lesion, if possible. If an incisional approach must be used, the patient should be advised of the potential complications.

ORIENTATION OF THE INCISION

Skin incisions and excisions must take into account static and dynamic skin tension to minimize scarring and maximize function. Langer lines of minimal skin tension generally lie perpendicular to the long axis of underlying musculature and can usually be demonstrated by pinching together a local area of skin or by having the patient contract the muscles under that area. On the face, wrinkles form along these lines as a result of repeated contraction of the facial musculature. *Linear incisions* (e.g., for removal of underlying lesions such as lipomas or for incision and drainage) should be oriented parallel to wrinkle lines when possible (parallel to the lines of minimal skin tension). With an *elliptical excision*, in which a section of overlying skin is removed, the long axis of the ellipse should lie parallel to the lines of minimal skin tension. Standard depictions of Langer lines (Fig. 18.4) assist in planning incisions, but lines of minimal tension must be evaluated on each patient individually before a procedure. For the face, the patient's simulating various facial expressions will aid in demonstrating natural wrinkle lines. It should also be noted that for certain elliptical excisions (especially on the face), the long axis of the excision may need to curve or angle instead of lying entirely in a straight line (Fig. 18.5). Planning incisions along lines of minimal tension decreases the forces on the wound that tend to pull it apart, thereby reducing scar potential. Certain areas, especially the deltoid and sternum, are invariably prone to experiencing transverse traction, with a subsequent wider scar and a higher propensity for keloid formation. Children also have an increased tendency to develop hypertrophic or keloid scars.

When lines of minimal tension are not apparent, even after the patient performs maneuvers to accentuate them, it may be helpful to first perform a circular excision, undermine the wound circumferentially, and then allow natural skin tension to orient the wound, usually into a more oval shape. At that point the resulting oval can be converted to an ellipse and the wound closed (Fig. 18.6).

Incisions across joint surfaces should be made transversely (or obliquely if necessary). Perpendicular lacerations or incisions across joint space lines have a tendency to contract, thus limiting range of motion. Chapter 16, Flaps and Plasties, includes a review of Z-plasty, an example of a situation in which a laceration extending across a joint is converted to a transverse wound to maximize joint function and minimize contracture.

DESIGN AND SIZE OF THE EXCISION

Surgical marking pens should be used freely in designing incisions. Planning, measuring, and marking are essential steps toward an optimal result. The majority of skin excisions are elliptical in shape.

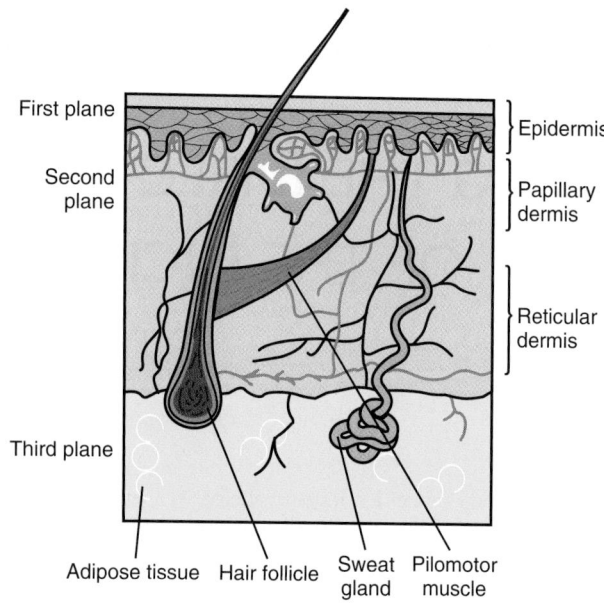

Fig. 18.1   Skin anatomy.

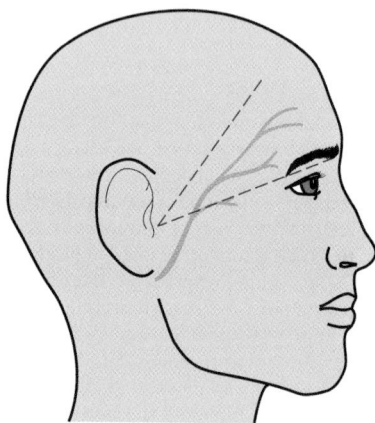

Fig. 18.2   Temporal branch of facial nerve. The nerve lies superficially within a triangle created by a line extending from the tragus to the upper forehead wrinkle area and a line extending from the tragus to the lateral aspect of the eyebrow.

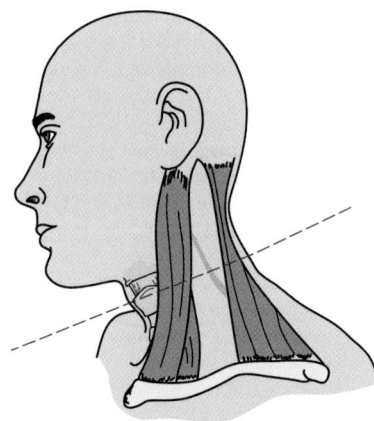

Fig. 18.3   Spinal accessory nerve. The nerve lies superficially within the posterior triangle of the neck at the level of the notch in the superior thyroid cartilage.

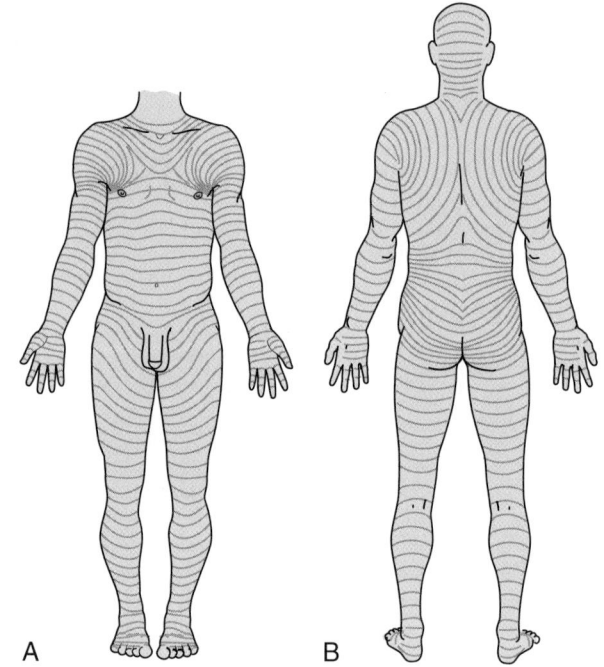

Fig. 18.4   Lines of minimal skin tension. (A) Anterior view. (B) Posterior view.

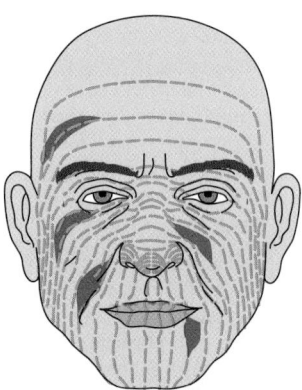

Fig. 18.5   Skin tension lines on the face and proper excision shapes.

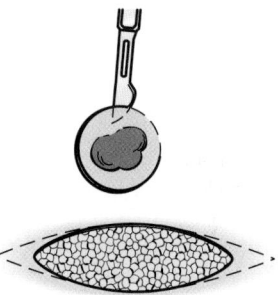

Fig. 18.6   Creating a circular wound, with conversion to an ellipse.

The wound should be three times as long as it is wide (Fig. 18.7). A wound that is not long enough will create dog ears when repaired. Because alcohol will remove most marking pen inks, first use an alcohol wipe and anesthetize the wound, then mark and measure the planned excision, and finally anesthetize the surgical site. Next, prepare the site with povidone-iodine or chlorhexidine gluconate and then drape the patient.

When incising with the scalpel, a no. 15 blade is used and should be held perpendicular to the skin or angled up to 15 degrees with the cutting edge angled away from the lesion (Fig. 18.8A and B). Remember that slight eversion during the repair is desirable (see Fig. 18.8C). Slanting the blade in the opposite direction makes this difficult to accomplish. Remember to "build pyramids, not dig ditches"—when incising, the top of the blade should tilt slightly over the lesion, not away from it (see Fig. 18.8D). Angling the blade more than 15 degrees creates a very thin "slice" of tissue on the remaining skin, which may necrose and lead to more scar formation.

Margins of normal tissue that should be removed vary depending on whether a lesion is benign or malignant, and, if malignant, the margins vary depending on the type of cancer (see Chapter 13 , Approach to Various Skin Lesions). For benign lesions, the incision can be placed close to the lesion with only 1 or 2 mm of normal tissue excised.

The definitive surgical treatment for *primary cutaneous melanoma* is a wide local excision down to the deep fascia. The thickness of the melanoma is a key factor in determining the stage of the lesion and the recommended margin of normal tissue. In situ melanoma can be excised with 5-mm margins, although wider margins may be required for in situ lentigo malignant melanoma, based upon final pathologic evaluation. Melanoma less than 1 mm thick can be resected with a 1-cm margin of normal tissue. If greater than 1 mm deep, consider referral. Melanoma 1 to 2 mm thick should be resected with a 2-cm margin of normal tissue if this is possible without the need for a skin graft (a 1- to 2-cm margin may be adequate if anatomically constrained based upon the location of the melanoma). Melanomas between 2 and 4 mm thick, as well as melanomas greater than 4 mm thickness, generally are excised with a 2-cm margin of normal tissue because clinical trials have not demonstrated a benefit of margins greater than 2 cm.

For *basal cell carcinomas*, remove a 3- to 5-mm rim of normal tissue. Squamous cell carcinomas require at least a 4-mm band of normal tissue around the lesion (with a greater margin for higher risk lesions).

After the ellipse is made down to adipose tissue, the specimen is freed by cutting with the scalpel in the plane between dermis and adipose tissue. Using Adson forceps with teeth, grasp the end of the ellipse and dissect from one end to center. Then grasp the other end and do the same. This technique avoids the tendency to travel too deep within the excision (Fig. 18.9).

AVOIDING DISTORTION OF SURFACE ANATOMY

The clinician should always attempt to estimate the change in surface anatomy that will result from an excision. Pinching together the two sides of a planned ellipse assists in demonstrating whether a defect can be closed in a direct side-to-side fashion and if significant distortion of surrounding tissue will occur. The presternal, scalp, and pretibial regions can be quite difficult to close after a skin excision, as can wider excisions in any location. Excisions necessitating removal of a significant amount of tissue on the forehead, upper lip, and around the eyes often cause distortion of facial appearance (Fig. 18.10). Proper planning creates the best cosmetic results (Fig. 18.11).

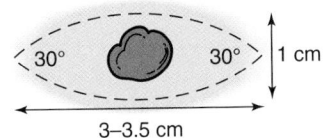

Fig. 18.7 Creating an ellipse (proper dimensions).

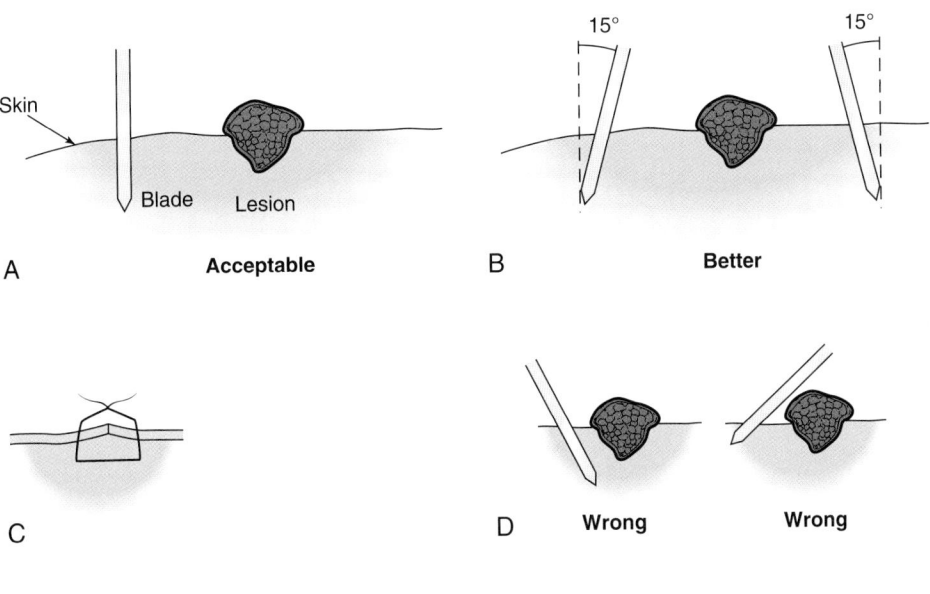

Fig. 18.8 The proper angle of the scalpel when creating an ellipse. (A) Acceptable angle. (B) Better angle. (C) Proper shapes of suture and skin margins on completion of closure. (D) Wrong angles.

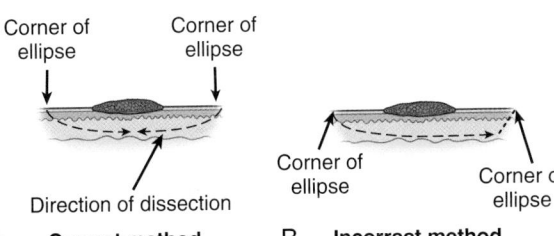

Fig. 18.9 Method of dissecting tissue free after the ellipse is incised. (A) Going from each end to the center. (B) Going from one end to the opposite end (incorrect) leads to too deep of a dissection at the terminal end.

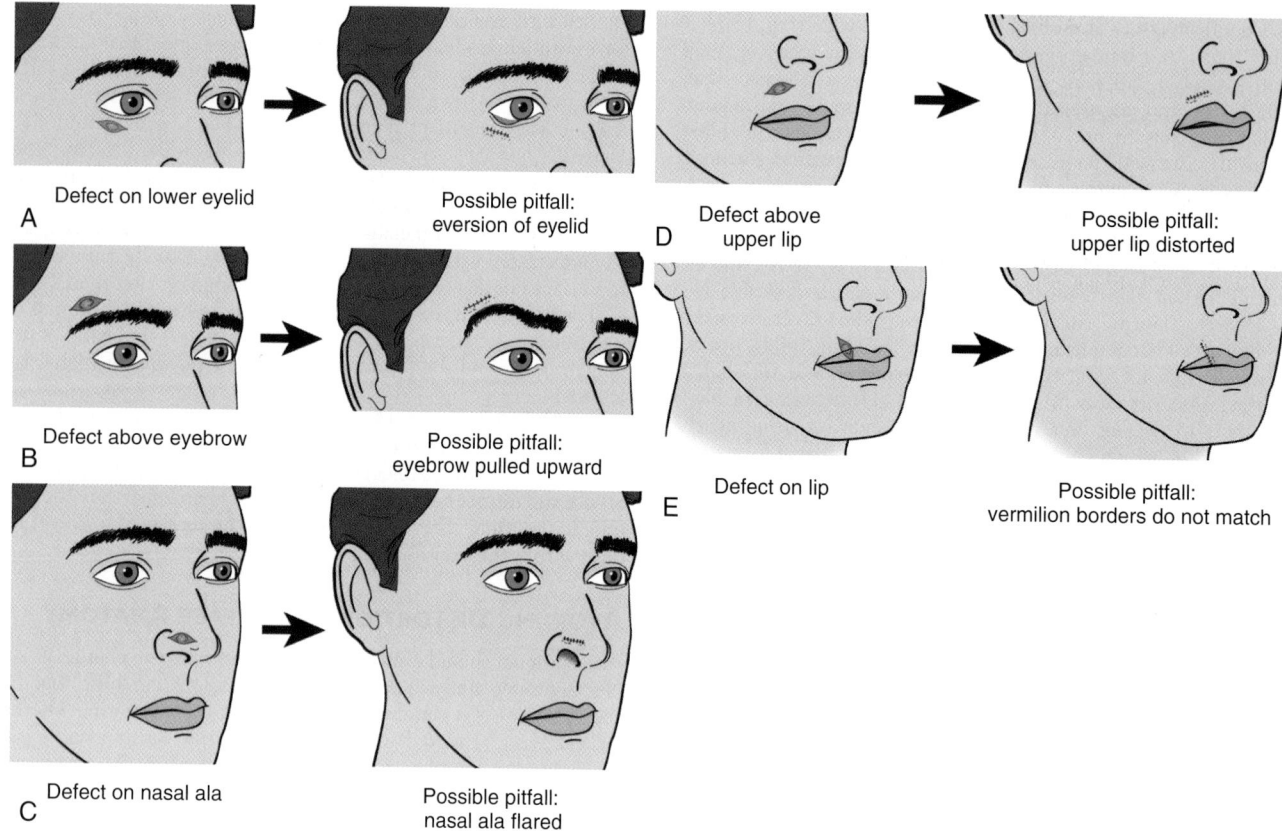

Defect on lower eyelid
A

Possible pitfall:
eversion of eyelid

Defect above eyebrow
B

Possible pitfall:
eyebrow pulled upward

Defect on nasal ala
C

Possible pitfall:
nasal ala flared

Defect above
upper lip
D

Possible pitfall:
upper lip distorted

Defect on lip
E

Possible pitfall:
vermilion borders do not match

Fig. 18.10 Possible pitfalls in closing facial incisions/lacerations. (A) Closing the defect on the lower lid causes an unsightly eversion of the lid. (B) The lateral eyebrow is pulled upward. (C) Nasal ala is flared because of too much tension on the wound. (D) The upper lip is distorted and raised laterally after closure of the excision site. (E) The vermilion borders do not match.

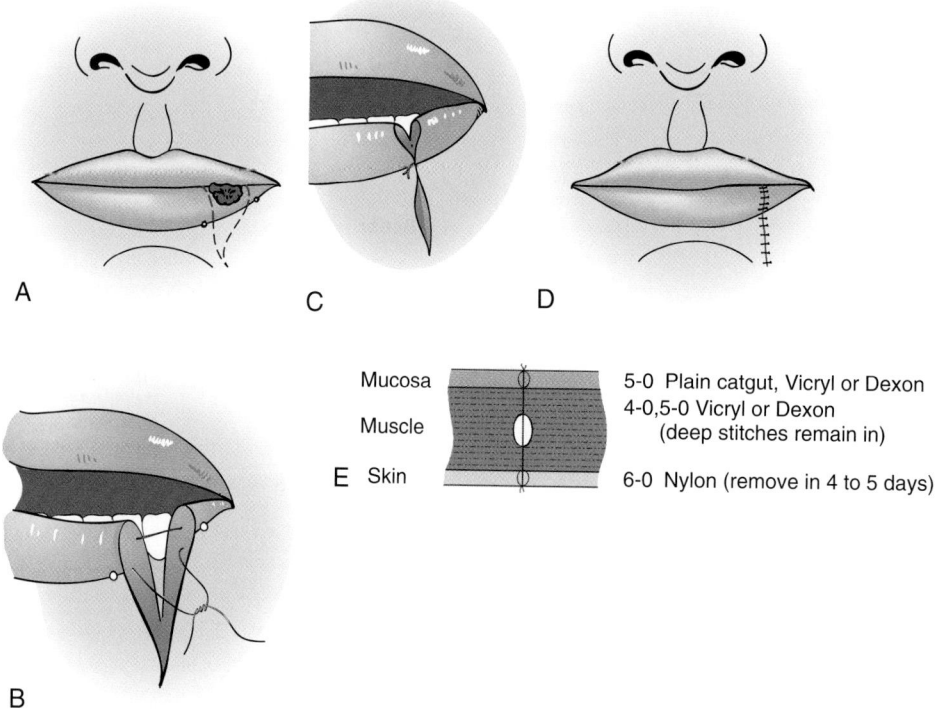

A   C   D

B

Mucosa   5-0 Plain catgut, Vicryl or Dexon
              4-0,5-0 Vicryl or Dexon
Muscle   (deep stitches remain in)

E Skin   6-0 Nylon (remove in 4 to 5 days)

Fig. 18.11 Proper excision and repair of a lip lesion. (A) Dashed lines show planned excision. Mark the vermilion border. (B) Muscle approximation with deep stitch. (C) Vermilion alignment. (D) Final results. (E) Suture material. Vicryl or Dexon inside the mouth will need to be removed. Catgut will absorb in 3 to 4 days.

RECOMMENDED READING

Becker J, Stucchi AF, eds. *Essentials of Surgery*. Philadelphia: Saunders; 2005.

Bratzler DW, Dellinger EP, Olsen KM. Clinical practice guidelines for antimicrobial prophylaxis in surgery. *Am J Health-Syst Pharm.* 2013;70:195–283.

Brodland DG, Zitelli JA. Surgical margins for excision of primary cutaneous squamous cell carcinoma. *J Am Acad Dermatol.* 1992;27:241.

Cascinelli N. Margin of resection in the management of primary melanoma. *Semin Surg Oncol.* 1998;14:272.

Kunishige JH, Brodland DG, Zitelli JA. Surgical margins for melanoma in situ. *J Am Acad Dermatol.* 2012;66:438.

Moy RL, Usatine RP. Elliptical excision. In: Usatine RP, Moy RL, Tobinick EL, Siegel DM, eds. *Skin Surgery: A Practical Guide*. St. Louis: Mosby; 1998:120–136.

Olbricht S. Biopsy techniques and basic excision. In: Bolognia JL, Rapini RP, eds. *Dermatology*. 1st ed. London: Mosby; 2003.

Salasche S, Orengo IF, Siegle RJ. *Dermatologic Surgery Tips and Techniques*. St. Louis: Mosby; 2007.

Salkind AR, Rao KC. Antibiotic prophylaxis to prevent surgical site infections. *Am Fam Physician.* 2011;83(5):585–590.

Trott AT. *Wounds and Lacerations: Emergency Care and Closure*. 4th ed. Philadelphia: Elsevier; 2012.

CHAPTER 19

LACERATION AND INCISION REPAIR

Richard P. Usatine • *Wendy C. Coates*

Lacerations are a commonly seen problem in clinicians' offices, urgent care centers, and hospital emergency departments. Lacerations can be repaired with sutures, wound closure tapes, staples (see Chapter 196, Skin Stapling), or tissue adhesive (see Chapter 198, Tissue Glues).

The goals of laceration and incision repair are as follows:

- Achieve hemostasis
- Prevent infection
- Preserve function
- Restore appearance
- Minimize patient discomfort

In repairing skin, it is helpful to understand the three phases of wound healing, which are listed in Box 19.1. Nonabsorbable skin sutures or staples are used to give the wound strength during the first two phases. After the nonabsorbable skin sutures or staples are removed, wound closure tapes/strips or previously placed deep absorbable sutures play an important role in the final phases of wound healing.

INDICATIONS

- Lacerations that are open and less than 12 hours old (<24 hours old on the face)
- Some bite wounds in cosmetically important areas (close follow-up recommended)
- Repair of sites where a lesion has been surgically removed

CONTRAINDICATIONS

- Wounds more than 12 hours old (>24 hours old on the face)
- Animal and human bite wounds (exceptions: facial or gaping wounds, dog bite wounds)
- Puncture wounds

EQUIPMENT

- Surgical sterile preparation (povidone iodine, chlorhexidine); alcohol swabs (not to be used inside the wound)
- Ruler in centimeters
- Irrigation device for contaminated wounds: 30-mL syringe with 18-gauge angiocatheter or commercially manufactured splash shield device (Fig. 19.1) and sterile saline
- Appropriate anesthetic, usually 1% or 2% lidocaine with or without epinephrine (see Chapter 5, Local Anesthesia)
- 1- to 10-mL syringe
- 27-gauge, 1.25-inch needle (small-gauge needles are preferred to administer anesthesia)
- Sterile drapes; fenestrated drape (applied over the lesion)
- 4 × 4 gauze sponges; sterile cotton applicators are useful for hemostasis
- Sterile pack containing 4.5-inch needle holder; curved or straight iris scissors; one mosquito hemostat; suture scissors; Adson forceps with teeth; skin hook (optional)

BOX 19.1	Three Phases of Wound Healing

Phase 1 (Initial Lag Phase, Days 0–5)
No gain in wound strength

Phase 2 (Fibroplasia Phase, Days 5–14)
Rapid increase in wound strength occurs
At 2 weeks, the wound has achieved only 7% of its final strength

Phase 3 (Final Maturation Phase, Day 14 Until Healing Is Complete)
Further connective tissue remodeling
Up to 80% of normal skin strength

- No. 15 scalpel blade for excisions with blade handle (single disposable unit also available)
- Appropriate suture (see Chapter 21, Laceration and Incision Repair: Suture Selection)
- Allis forceps for removal of deeper masses (optional)
- Skin marking pen (for excision, if wound revision is needed)
- Electrosurgical unit should be available for electrocoagulation
- Specimen jar (when lesions are being excised)
- Sterile or clean gloves (there has been no difference found in infection rates between sterile vs. clean gloves)
- Protective mask with plastic shield for eyes or other types of personal protective equipment

PREPROCEDURE PATIENT PREPARATION

The patient should be informed of the nature of his or her laceration. If the laceration is in a cosmetically important area, consider offering the option of a plastic surgeon for the repair. Advise the patient about the risks of pain, bleeding, dehiscence, infection, and scarring. In the case of lesion removal, warn that it is not always possible to be sure that the entire lesion is removed, so it could recur or require wider/deeper excision. Inform the patient that most repairs cause some permanent scarring, although attempts will be made to optimize the appearance. Patients should apply sunscreen to the area for at least 6 months after repair to minimize scarring. Warn the patient of the risks of hyperpigmentation or hypopigmentation, hypertrophic scars, keloids, nerve damage, alopecia, and distortion of the original anatomy. It is advisable to have the patient sign a consent form (see the consent form available at www.expertconsult.com).

Initial Assessment

The initial evaluation before anesthesia should include a history of how the wound was sustained, factors that might impair healing, tetanus immunization history, and an assessment of peripheral neurovascular status.

For elective excisions, see Chapter 18, Incisions: Planning the Direction of the Incision, to plan the direction of the incision. If a traumatic laceration is to be repaired, see Table 19.1 for essentials of wound

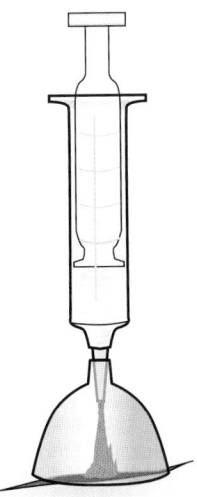

Fig. 19.1 Irrigation of a dirty wound using a syringe and plastic shield.

TABLE 19.1 Essentials of Wound Assessment

Parameters	Factors to Consider
Mechanism of injury	Sharp vs. blunt trauma, bite
Dirty vs. clean	Outdoors vs. kitchen sink
Time since injury	Suture up to 12 hr; 24 hr on face
Foreign body	Explore and obtain radiograph for metal or glass
Functional examination	Neurovascular, muscular, tendons
Need for prophylactic antibiotics	If needed, give as soon as possible and cover *Staphylococcus aureus*; irrigate well

BOX 19.2 Possible Antibiotic Prophylaxis Situations or When to Consider Antibiotic Prophylaxis

Coexisting Conditions
Diabetes mellitus
Peripheral vascular disease
Elderly
Immunocompromised
Previous radiation to the site
Malnutrition (e.g., alcoholism, chemotherapy)
History of previous infection or slow healing
Chronic steroid use
Obesity

Locations
Increased bacteria
Axilla, hand, mouth, anogenital areas
End-arterial locations (fingers, toes) with diseases of vascular compromise
Over joint spaces where there is a possibility of entering joint (e.g., metacarpophalangeal joints)

Contamination
Dirty wounds, especially those sustained at farms, meatpacking plants, etc.
Less than optimal sterile technique (should be rare)
Deep puncture wounds
Bites (especially human and cat bites)
Presence of a retained foreign body

Method of Wound Injury
Crush injury (10-fold increase in infection) with devitalized skin
Penetrating injury

assessment. The clinician should consider the possibility of domestic violence in patients with traumatic wounds, especially if lacerations appear on the face or if multiple injuries of varying ages are noted.

In general, antibiotics are not needed for either wound or subacute bacterial endocarditis prophylaxis for cutaneous procedures. For subacute bacterial endocarditis prophylaxis guidelines, see Chapter 69, Antibiotic Prophylaxis for Prevention of Bacterial Endocarditis. Consideration should be given to coverage for *Staphylococcus aureus* and methicillin-resistant *S. aureus* infection in several situations (Box 19.2).

The following are major goals for prescribing antibiotics before or after skin surgery:

- Prevention of a new wound infection
- Prevention of the spread of an existing local infection
- Treatment of an existing infection
- Prevention of bacterial endocarditis

The clinical decision-making process of whether or not to use antibiotics before or after skin surgery is complex. The clinician must consider host factors, the anatomic location of the surgery, the sources that might contaminate the wound, and method of wound injury. Because this topic concerns wound repair after multiple types of trauma and elective procedures, the full complexity of the decision-making process is beyond the scope of this chapter. Box 19.2 lists the multiple factors to be considered when making a decision about antibiotic prophylaxis for skin procedures. See Chapter 213, Prevention and Treatment of Wound Infections.

The recommendations of the American Heart Association for the *prevention of bacterial endocarditis* were last published in 2007. Endocarditis prophylaxis is not needed for incision or biopsy of surgically scrubbed skin. The 2007 guidelines state that antibiotic prophylaxis is recommended for procedures on infected skin and skin structures for patients with underlying cardiac conditions associated with the highest risk of adverse outcome from infective endocarditis. For individuals at highest risk for endocarditis (see Chapter 69, Antibiotic Prophylaxis for Prevention Bacterial Endocarditis) who undergo a surgical procedure that involves infected skin or skin structures, it is reasonable that the therapeutic regimen administered for treatment of the infection contain an agent active against staphylococci and beta-hemolytic streptococci, such as an antistaphylococcal penicillin or a cephalosporin. Vancomycin or clindamycin may be administered to patients unable to tolerate a β-lactam antibiotic or who are known or suspected to have an infection caused by methicillin-resistant *S. aureus*.

Cummings and Del Beccaro (1995) performed a meta-analysis of randomized studies on the use of antibiotics to prevent infection of simple wounds. They concluded that there is no evidence in published trials that prophylactic antibiotics offer protection against infection of non-bite wounds in patients treated in emergency departments. Cummings (1994) also performed a meta-analysis of randomized trials for antibiotics to prevent infection in patients with dog-bite wounds and found that prophylactic antibiotics reduce the incidence of infection in these patients.

Antibiotics have a role in the treatment of many established skin infections. However, *most skin abscesses are better treated with incision and drainage* than with antibiotics. For skin procedures, there is not a consensus on whether to give an antibiotic nor the appropriate timing for its administration. Recommendations for timing before the procedure vary from 1 hour (which is typical timing for bacterial endocarditis prophylaxis) to within 30 minutes of the procedure. Although a single second dose 6 hours later was the standard in the past, it is no longer currently recommended for bacterial endocarditis prophylaxis but may be advocated for further treatment of the infection.

Controversy exists over which bite injuries should be treated with prophylactic antibiotics. Cat- and dog-bite injuries carry the risk of infection with *Pasteurella multocida,* and human-bite injuries carry the risk of infection with *Eikenella corrodens* and *S. aureus.* Based on the microbiology of these wounds, amoxicillin/clavulanate provides good prophylactic coverage for the bacteria affecting most bite injuries. Alternatives include second-generation cephalosporins or clindamycin with a fluoroquinolone.

The best method for prevention of wound infections is to clean and irrigate traumatic wounds well, rather than relying on prophylactic antibiotics. The clinician needs to weigh the benefits and the risks of antibiotic use based on the individual patient and the circumstances of the wound repair or skin surgery. The factors listed in Box 19.2 and the references at the end of this chapter should provide guidance for the clinician making decisions about antibiotic prophylaxis for skin surgery.

Local Anesthesia

In traumatic wounds, neurovascular integrity should be assessed before administration of anesthesia. The wound should then be fully anesthetized to allow for painless examination of the tissue damage, thorough irrigation, and adequate closure. Many wounds can be adequately anesthetized with 1% or 2% lidocaine. Consider using lidocaine with epinephrine to provide increased hemostasis if there are no contraindications to epinephrine in the patient, the location of the wound, or the wound itself. (See Chapters 5, Local Anesthesia, and 7, Peripheral Nerve Blocks and Field Blocks.) Topical anesthetics are effective for wounds that do not involve mucosal surfaces. A combination of lidocaine, epinephrine, and tetracaine applied with a saturated cotton ball or as a gel formulation directly into the wound provides adequate anesthesia for many wounds.

Perform the following to minimize the pain of injecting local anesthetic:

- Use a small-gauge needle (27 gauge or smaller)
- Inject slowly
- Inject directly into the dermis through the open wound (not through intact skin)
- Warm the anesthetic to body temperature (optional)
- Buffer the anesthetic with sodium bicarbonate (10 to 1 mL) (optional)

Wound Preparation

After the initial assessment and administration of local or regional anesthetic, and antibiotics if indicated, the wound should be inspected thoroughly for foreign bodies, deep tissue layer damage, and injury to the nerve, vessel, or tendon. A radiograph should be obtained to look for retained glass or metal in wounds sustained with broken glass or metal. Complex wounds or those in cosmetically important areas should be closed by a practitioner with the appropriate expertise. Hair removal is rarely necessary prior to closing wounds; shaving should be avoided because it can cause soft tissue trauma and increase the risk of wound infections. Hair can be clipped, but mostly should just be moved or held out of the way. Eyebrows should never be shaved; they can grow back unpredictably or not at all.

Cleansing

After the wound is anesthetized, cleansing of a traumatic wound should be performed by irrigation with normal saline at approximately 15 psi of pressure. This can be accomplished by attaching an 18-gauge angiocatheter or a commercially available splash shield to a 30-mL syringe (see Fig. 19.1). At least 200 mL of irrigation is recommended. Moscati and associates (2007) performed a multicenter comparison of tap water versus sterile saline for wound irrigation,

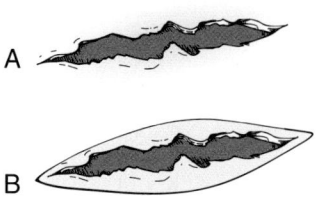

Fig. 19.2 Debridement. (A) Irregular jagged wound. (B) Excise a jagged wound or crush injury to create a more readily reparable wound.

showing equivalent rates of wound infection in immunocompetent patients. The tap water group irrigated their own wounds under the water tap for a minimum of 2 minutes after they had the wound anesthetized. Higher-risk wounds were excluded from the study, suggesting that tap water is a reasonable cleansing alternative only in low-risk lacerations. Chemical compounds such as chlorhexidine gluconate, or povidone-iodine, hydrogen peroxide, or detergents, should not be used inside wounds (these cause tissue toxicity) but may be applied to external, intact skin if desired. Greasy contaminants can be removed with any petroleum-based product, such as bacitracin ointment. To prevent a "road rash" tattoo, wrap petrolatum gauze around the fingers and wipe off the asphalt and other foreign material embedded in the skin after anesthesia.

For elective excisions, irrigation before closure is not generally needed. If there was a ruptured cyst, if the excisional area was open a considerable time, or if there was concern about contamination, irrigation with 10 mL of saline two or three times may be performed.

Debridement

After the cleansing process, wounds should be examined for devitalized tissue that needs removal or debridement. This debridement may convert a jagged, contaminated wound into a clean surgical one and can be accomplished with a scalpel or sharp tissue scissors (Fig. 19.2). Preserve as much tissue as possible in case future scar revision is necessary. After debridement, wound edges should be held together to see if they are under any tension. Wounds under significant tension are best repaired by a two-layer closure. In dirty wounds, however, this may increase the incidence of infection.

EDITOR'S NOTE: Wounds of the face or areas devoid of redundant tissue require conservative debridement to avoid making it difficult to close. Meticulous repair of complex wounds in these areas may have better cosmetic results.

Undermining

Undermining can significantly reduce skin tension when there is a gap to be closed (Fig. 19.3). Undermining may increase the risk of infection and thus should be avoided in dirty wounds. Extreme care is also needed when undermining around vital structures. Approximately one-third to one half of the undermined tissue is freed up to be brought into the defect. Undermine bilaterally as far back as the wound is wide.

TECHNIQUE

Ideally four principles should be incorporated in the process of closing any wound:

1. *Control all bleeding before closure.* This can be accomplished by applying direct pressure for at least 5 minutes, adding epinephrine to the local anesthetic when appropriate, using electrocoagulation, or tying off bleeders with absorbable sutures.
2. *Eliminate "dead space"* where tissue fluid and blood can accumulate (Fig. 19.4).
3. *Accurately approximate tissue layers* to each other. Scars are most visible when shadows are created by depressed or elevated tissue.

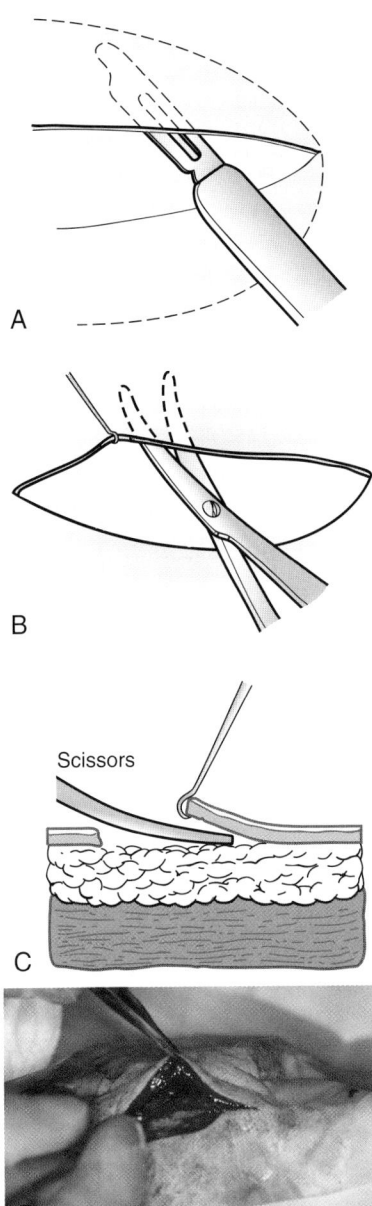

Fig. 19.3 When skin margins approximate with tension, this can be relieved by undermining the margins through the use of a blade (A) or scissors (B and C). Undermine twice as far back as the wound is wide, if possible. The proper level of undermining to mobilize the skin is shown (D). (D, Courtesy The Medical Procedures Center, Midland, Michigan.)

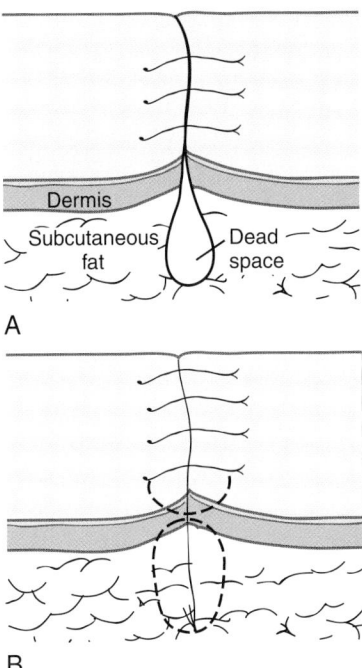

Fig. 19.4 Closing the dead space. (A) Improper closure with dead space not closed, fluid or blood can accumulate. (B) Proper closure with dead space closed by deep sutures.

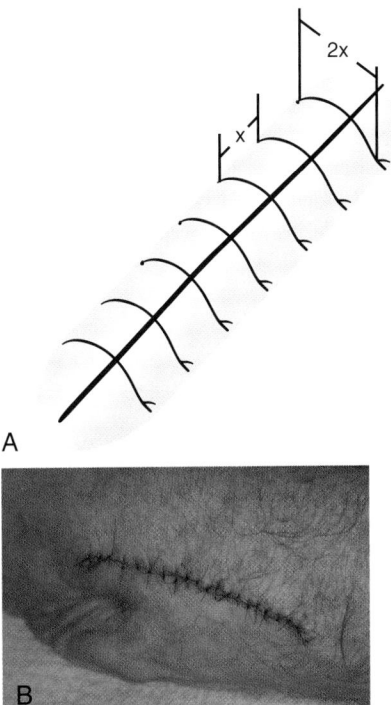

Fig. 19.5 Simple interrupted suture. (A) Proper spacing. (B) Interrupted sutures after excision of a basal cell carcinoma of the elbow. (B, Courtesy The Medical Procedures Center, Midland, Michigan.)

Also be sure that anatomic areas match on each side in critical areas such as the vermilion border of the lip.

4. *Approximate the wound with minimal skin tension.* If there will be significant tension, undermining and deep inverted buried sutures are used to decrease the tension on the skin margin. Ideally, when the repair is completed, the wound will be tented up slightly.

Lacerations and incisions are approximated using a variety of techniques:

- *Simple interrupted suture* (Fig. 19.5). On completion, the skin margins should be slightly everted (Fig. 19.6). The needle should enter the skin surface at a 90-degree angle (Fig. 19.7). The stitch should be as wide as it is deep. The suture on both sides of the wound should be of equal distance from the wound margin and

of equal depth. The final shape should appear like an Erlenmeyer flask (Fig. 19.8). As a general rule, these sutures need to be no closer than 2 mm in a fine plastic closure and can be substantially farther apart in other types of closures. The distance between sutures should equal approximately half the total distance of the sutures across the incision. Avoid tying the knots too tight. The

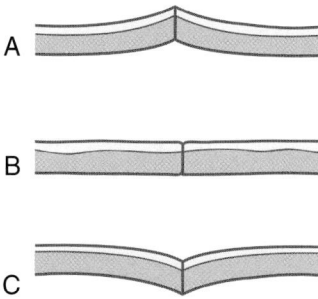

Fig. 19.6 Wound margin appearance after closure. (A) Proper eversion of the skin edges on closure ("build pyramids, not ditches"). (B) Acceptable, but not optimal, closure. (C) Improper closure because healing will lead to further contraction and scar depression.

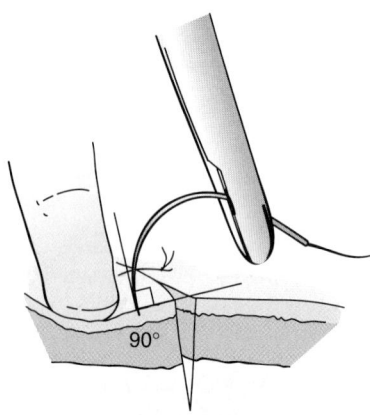

Fig. 19.7 Needle should enter the skin surface at a 90-degree angle. (Revised from Moy R. Suturing techniques. In: Usatine RP, Moy RL, Tobinick EL, Siegel DM, eds. *Skin Surgery: A Practical Guide*. St. Louis: Mosby; 1998:88–100.)

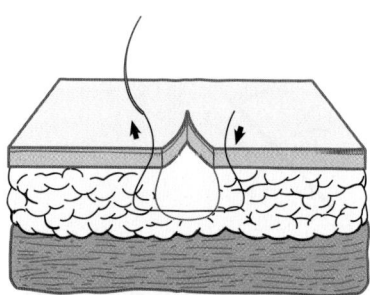

Fig. 19.8 Use the Erlenmeyer flask–shaped pathway to promote eversion of skin edges. (Revised from Moy R. Suturing techniques. In: Usatine RP, Moy RL, Tobinick EL, Siegel DM, eds. *Skin Surgery: A Practical Guide*. St. Louis: Mosby; 1998:88–100.)

knots should be lined up on one side of the wound. The finer the suture, the closer the stitches need to be. See Chapters 20, Laceration and Incision Repair: Needle Selection, and 21, Laceration and Incision Repair: Suture Selection, for needle and suture selection, respectively. See Chapter 22, Laceration and Incision Repair: Suture Tying, for tying techniques.

- *Simple running stitch* (Fig. 19.9). The advantages of the simple running stitch in sterile wounds under little or no tension are that it is quick and distributes tension evenly and provides excellent cosmetic results. Because there is an increased risk of contamination in traumatic lacerations, the simple running stitch is less desirable in these wounds. In case of infection, the entire wound closure would need to be removed. If there is significant

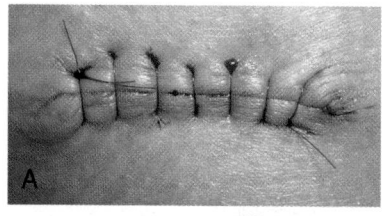

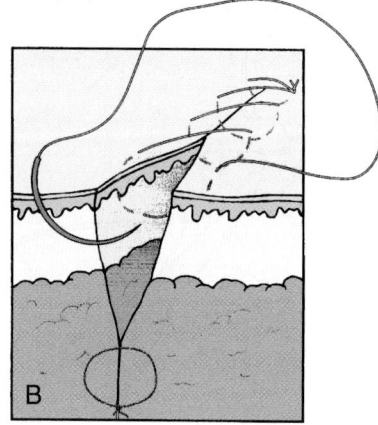

Fig. 19.9 Running stitch. (A) This is a good stitch to use if there is no tension on the wound or after deep stitches have already been placed with good approximation of the wound edges. (B) Always keep the depth of the suture placement the same on each side. (A, Courtesy Richard P. Usatine, MD, San Antonio, Texas. B, From Moy R. Suturing techniques. In: Usatine RP, Moy RL, Tobinick EL, Siegel DM, eds. *Skin Surgery: A Practical Guide*. St. Louis: Mosby; 1998:88–100.)

gaping of the wound, interrupted suture methods should be used. The relative disadvantage is that the entire stitch must be removed at once. With interrupted techniques, some sutures may be removed early for better cosmesis, whereas a few remaining ones can be left for prevention of dehiscence. These can be removed at a later date. This stitch is ideal in the scalp and is the one generally used for episiotomy repairs.

- *Deep suture with inverted knot or "buried stitch"* (Fig. 19.10). Deeper wounds or wounds under tension are best closed by providing structural support and not relying solely on nonabsorbable superficial sutures. Well-placed, deep absorbable sutures can do much to aid in closing a wound, removing tension from the superficial skin sutures, and decreasing scarring by providing increased wound support long after the epidermal sutures have been removed. The inverted knot technique places the bulk of the knot as far below the skin margins as possible to avoid suture spitting (migration of deep sutures to the skin surface). It also keeps the ends of the cut suture from protruding through the wound margin. To start the stitch, begin at the bottom of the wound (in the undermined area if undermining was used) and come up just below the epidermal-dermal junction (remember, "bottoms up!") to start. Go straight across the incision; reenter at the same level at the opposite side; then go down to the base at the same depth as the contralateral side and tie. A skin hook may be used to help gently lift the skin up from the undermined area. Care should be taken to achieve symmetry of depth and width on both sides of the laceration. After the appropriate number of deep inverted sutures are placed to approximate the skin margins, the surface (skin) is then fully closed with the closure of choice (nonabsorbable suture, wound closure tapes, or tissue adhesive).
- *Vertical mattress suture* (Fig. 19.11). This suture promotes eversion of the skin edges. It is useful when the natural tendency of loose skin is to create inversion of the wound margins, which is to be avoided. A good example is the loose skin under the triceps muscle and thin skin in older people. The stitch is also appropriate when the skin is very thin because interrupted sutures have a tendency to pull through.

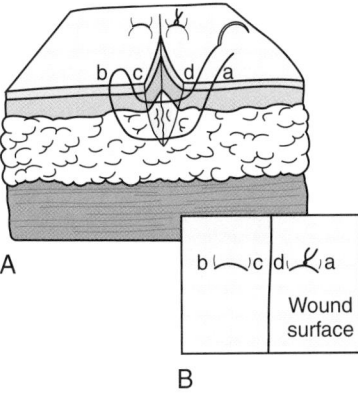

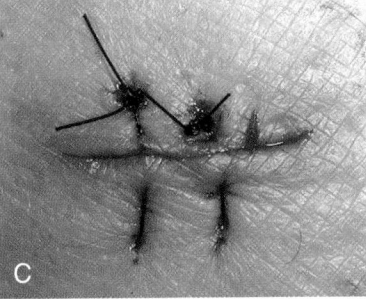

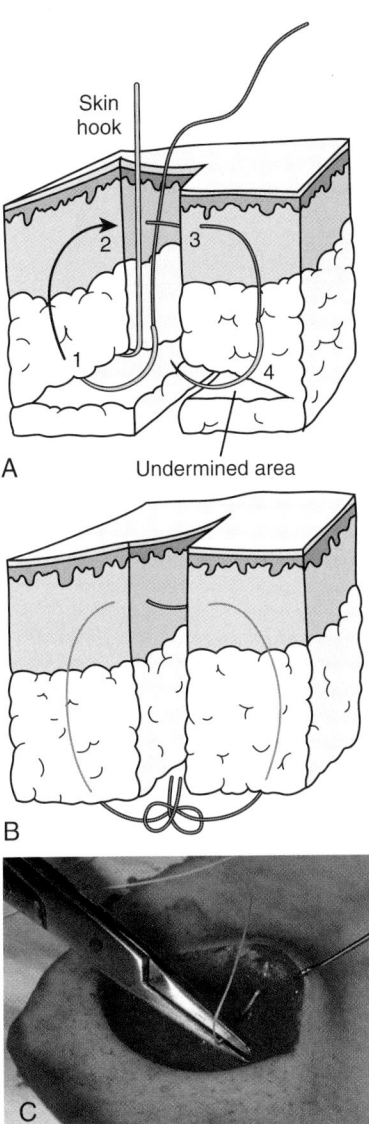

Fig. 19.11 Vertical mattress suture. (A) Cross-section. (B) Overhead view. Begin at *a*, and go deep under skin to *b*. Come out, go in at *c*, and exit at *d*. (C) Two vertical mattress sutures used to obtain wound eversion. (Courtesy Richard P. Usatine, MD, San Antonio, Texas.)

Fig. 19.10 Deep stitch with absorbable suture material. (A) Needle should enter deep in the skin below the dermis where the undermining was accomplished (*1*) and exit in the upper dermis (*2*). The needle re-enters in the upper dermis (*3*) and exits below the dermis where the undermining was accomplished (*4*). A skin hook may help elevate the skin from undermined area. (B) The deep inverted buried stitch is tied at the bottom of the wound to avoid having the knot stick out of the incision. (C) Placing the deep stitch. (C, From Moy R. Suturing techniques. In: Usatine RP, Moy RL, Tobinick EL, and Siegel DM, eds. *Skin Surgery: A Practical Guide.* St Louis: Mosby; 1998:88–100.)

- *Horizontal mattress suture* (Fig. 19.12). This suture is helpful in wounds under a moderate amount of tension; it also promotes wound edge eversion. It is especially useful on palms or soles and in patients who are poor candidates for deep sutures because of susceptibility to wound infection.
- *Subcuticular running suture* (Fig. 19.13). This suture is used to close linear wounds that are not under much tension; it yields an excellent cosmetic result. The two ends can be tied over the wound, or a knot can be placed at each end to prevent slippage. The ends of the suture do not necessarily need to be tied; taping under slight tension preserves approximation. Usually a polypropylene-coated nylon works best. Steri-Strips, tapes, or tissue glue can be used to supplement this type of stitch. Special care must be taken to avoid pressure on the wound because this stitch separates easily. Applying Tegaderm or similar protective sheets provides added protection and strength.

- *Three-point or half-buried mattress suture, also known as the "corner stitch"* (Fig. 19.14). This suture technique is designed to permit closure of the acute corner tip of a laceration or of certain incisional techniques (e.g., Burow triangle) without impairing blood flow to the tip. It is an intradermal stitch in which the needle is inserted initially into the intact skin on the nonflap portion of the wound and passed through the skin at the mid-dermis level; at the same level, the suture is then passed transversely through the tip of the flap, returned on the opposite side of the wound, and brought through the skin, paralleling the point of entrance. The suture is tied by drawing the tip snugly into place in good approximation. Care should be taken not to have the knot tied over the point of the flap (caused by having the needle insertion starting too far laterally). This same approach can be used in closing a stellate laceration, drawing the tips together in a pursestring fashion. Repair of a "T" laceration also uses this technique (Fig. 19.15).
- Repair of a *dog ear* or management of excess tissue can be performed as shown in Fig. 19.16 (see Chapter 16, Flaps and Plasties). Fig. 19.17 reviews the steps in the repair of a *C-flap* laceration.

NOTE: In one study, otherwise healthy children with facial lacerations were randomized to repair using fast-absorbing catgut or nylon suture (Luck and colleagues, 2008). There were no significant differences in the rates of infection, wound dehiscence, keloid formation, and parental satisfaction between the absorbable catgut and the nylon suture. Fast-absorbing catgut suture is not as easy to work with as nylon but does have the advantage of not requiring suture removal in children who may be fearful of the suture removal process.

Wound Closure Tapes or Strips

Wound closure tapes (Fig. 19.18) or strips, sometimes called "butterfly strips," may be used alone for small, superficial wounds (especially in young children). When these tapes suffice to close a wound, they are easily placed without physical or psychological trauma to the patient. Wounds closed with tape are more resistant to infection than are sutured wounds. However, tape cannot

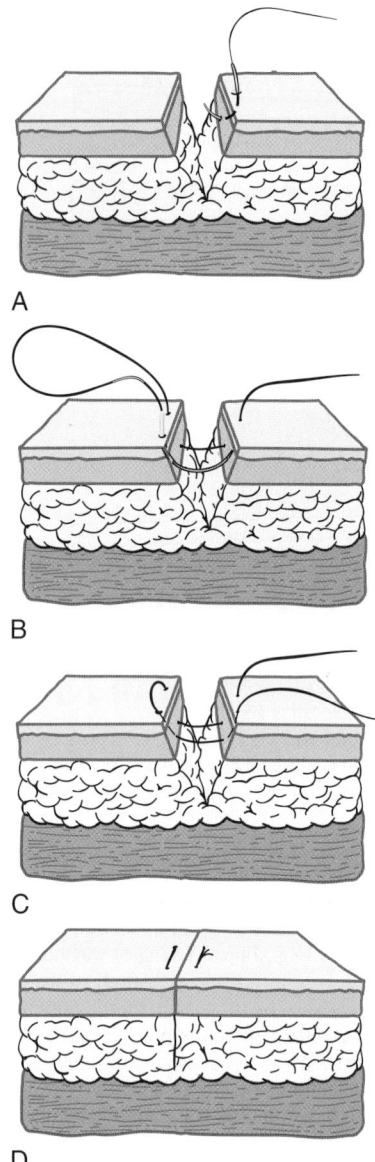

Fig. 19.12 Horizontal mattress suture. (A) Needle is passed 0.5 to 1 cm away from wound edge deeply into the wound. (B) Needle is passed through the opposite side and reenters the wound parallel to the initial suture. (C) Reenter the skin perpendicularly to provide some eversion of the wound edges. Enter and exit both the wound and skin at the same depth; otherwise, "buckling" and irregularities occur in the wound margin. (D) Suture is then tied as shown.

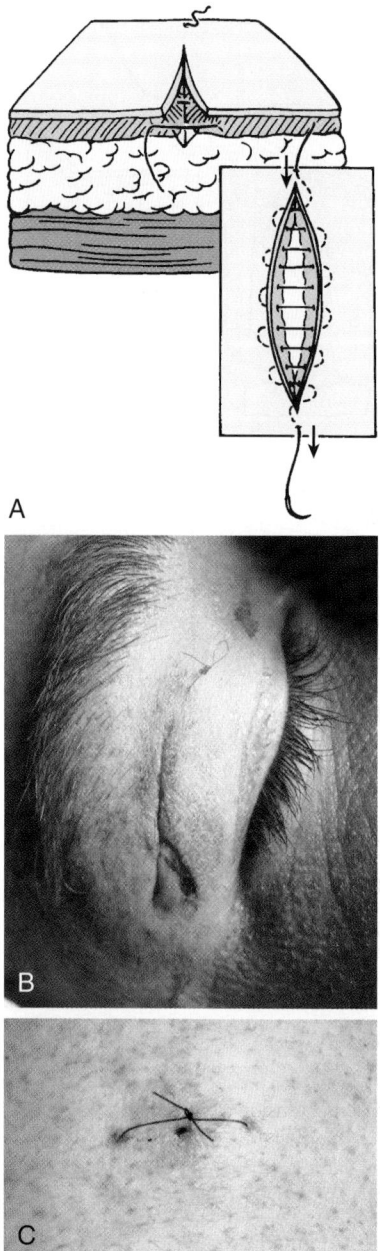

Fig. 19.13 (A) Subcuticular running suture. (B) Prolene was used to repair this eyebrow laceration. The ends are knotted to prevent slippage. (C) Appearance before suture removal after repair of a cheek excision. The ends are tied together to prevent slippage. (B, Courtesy Joe Deng, MD, Loma Linda, California. C, Courtesy The Medical Procedures Center, Midland, Michigan.)

provide adequate skin edge eversion or deep tissue approximation when used alone. Thus tape is most commonly used as an adjunct to sutures or staples. Tape can help reinforce wounds closed subcuticularly or with conventional suturing techniques. Adhesion is enhanced by the application of a sticky substance to the skin surface. Traditionally tincture of benzoin has been used for this purpose, but a preparation containing gum mastic (Mastisol) has been shown to provide stronger adhesion with possibly less risk of contact dermatitis. Wound closure tapes are especially helpful after suture removal to prevent dehiscence and may be left on until they fall off. Patients may shower with them on after the initial 24 hours.

The proper method of applying the tape or strips is to apply benzoin or Mastisol over the entire area, and then place the strips in a parallel fashion without overlapping and without "tacking" strips (see Fig. 19.18).

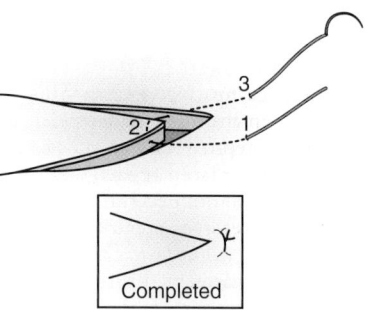

Fig. 19.14 Three-point or half-buried mattress suture to repair a V-flap laceration.

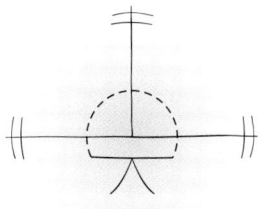

Fig. 19.15   T-laceration repair using half-buried mattress suture technique.

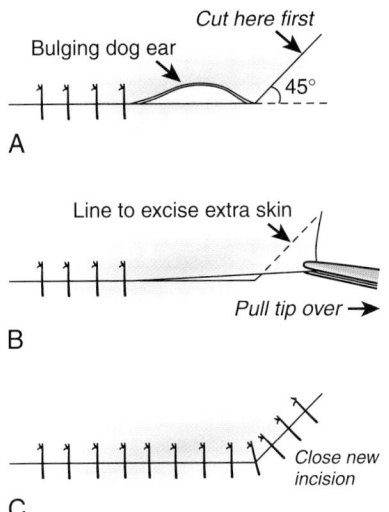

Fig. 19.16   Dog-ear repair. (A) Note site of initial incision of bulging dog ear. (B) Pull the tip over and excise. (C) Close the new incision for skin to lie flat.

Tissue Adhesive

Tissue adhesives may be used to close certain wounds that are not under significant tension and are not at risk for infection (see Chapter 198, Tissue Glues).

Delayed Primary Closure (Tertiary Intention)

Primary closure is defined by the use of sutures, tapes, or adhesives to close the wound at the time of initial surgery or evaluation. Healing by *secondary intention* occurs when no attempt is made to close the wound and the wound granulates in on its own. This method is used after a simple shave biopsy, in grossly contaminated or infected wounds, or in wounds that present far too late to consider closure. Delayed primary closure is healing by *tertiary intention.*

Delayed primary closure is used for wounds that are greater than 12 hours old (24 hours for facial lacerations) but would safely benefit from closure in a few days. Repairing them immediately could increase the chance of infection. After anesthetizing, evaluating, and irrigating the wound, insert a small piece of petrolatum gauze between the wound edges and place the patient on an antibiotic, such as cephalexin, for 5 days. On the third day, the patient should return for definitive repair. The wound is then anesthetized, reirrigated, and closed primarily with nonabsorbable sutures (i.e., no deep sutures because they increase the chance of infection).

See Box 19.3 for a summary of key points for suture repair (also included in Appendix H, Pearls of Practice).

POSSIBLE COMPLICATIONS OF LACERATION REPAIR

The following complications may occur within the first 2 weeks:

- Infection
- Pain
- Bleeding
- Dehiscence
- Hematoma
- Bruising and swelling
- Suture spitting

Prolonged or permanent complications may include the following:

- Scarring
- Hypertrophic scars
- Keloid formation
- Hyperpigmentation
- Hypopigmentation
- Nerve damage
- Imperfect cosmetic alignment (e.g., the vermilion border)
- Suture spitting
- Recurrence of an incompletely excised lesion

POSTPROCEDURE PATIENT EDUCATION

Most wounds are best protected with some sort of dressing during the first 24 to 48 hours after closure. Continued slight oozing of blood might be expected. For hemostasis, a pressure dressing should be applied. This could be folded gauze over a sterile ointment with tape over it or a nonstick type of gauze dressing covered with gauze and tape. Trade names for nonstick dressings include Xeroform, Adaptic, and Telfa. For the extremities, the use of a self-adherent wrap like Coban, CoFlex, and others provides a good pressure dressing to hold things in place. If on the lower extremities, elevation helps for 24 hours. Ice over the area for a few hours will reduce pain, swelling, and bleeding. It is not usually necessary to keep a wound completely dry after 24 hours. Therefore patients may shower after 24 hours and redress the wound after gently drying it. Moist healing (application of some type of ointment after gentle washing twice daily) aids in quicker healing. Although antibiotic ointments traditionally have been used in postsurgical wound dressing, Smack and colleagues (1996) determined that clean wounds heal just as well when white petrolatum is applied. Neomycin and bacitracin are frequent contact allergens. Alternatively, Tegaderm or Opsite (transparent, self-adherent, plastic wrap–type dressings that "breathe out" but do not let anything in) can be applied and left in place until the sutures are removed (Fig. 19.19). If bleeding occurs, the patient can replace the dressing after 24 to 48 hours because it is available over the counter. In addition to providing the optimal moist healing environment, these dressings provide added support to the sutured closure.

Suggestions for the timing for skin suture removal are listed in Table 19.2. See Fig. 19.20 for proper suture removal techniques. Using suture scissors (with a small hook on one of the tips to grasp the suture; see Fig. 19.21) makes removal much easier. Disposable suture removal kits are available with gauze, scissors, and pickups. Because scarring increases the longer the sutures remain in place, consider removing them a few days early and applying a tissue adhesive (see Chapter 198, Tissue Glues) or tape. Early removal is possible only if there is little to no tension on the wound. Even when sutures are removed at the usual times, tape or tissue glues help keep the wound edges opposed. The cost of tissue glues is one barrier to this approach. Adhesive strips or another self-adherent transparent dressing can also be used.

Wounds on the face or scalp may be dressed with a thin layer of antibiotic ointment or petrolatum in lieu of a mechanical dressing. It is best to cover these wounds at night to avoid drying. Instruct patients to return if there are signs of wound infection,

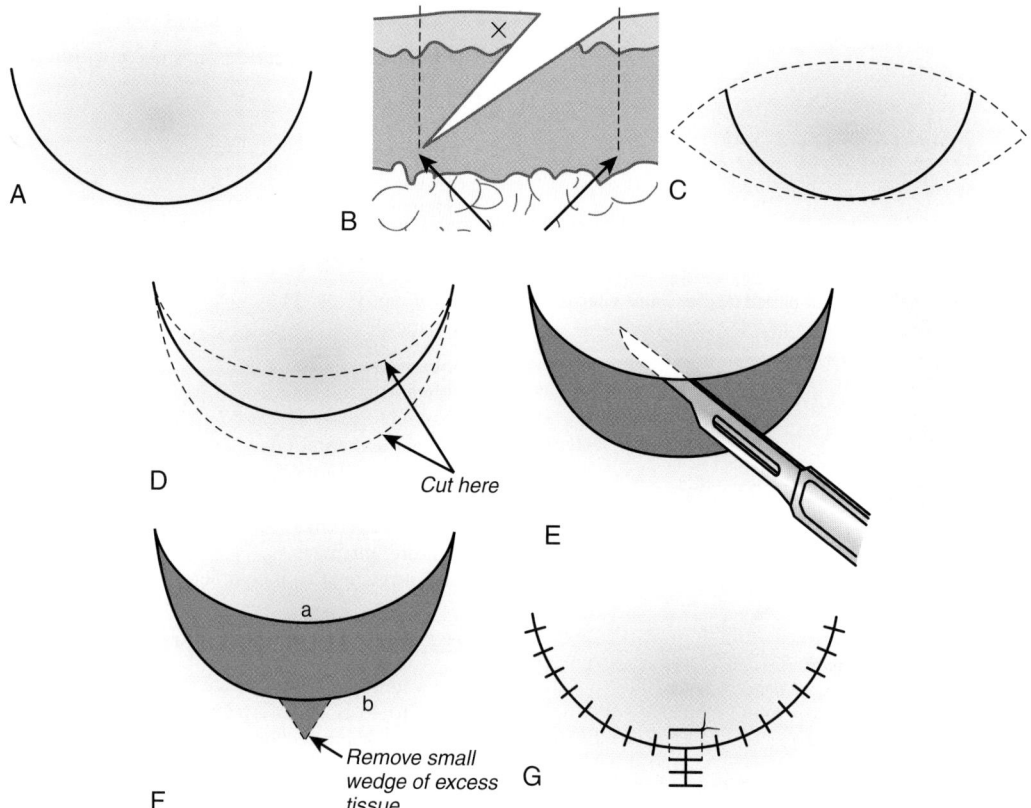

Fig. 19.17   C-flap repair. (A) Laceration. (B) The problem: the point *X* is often very thin and may necrose. Even if it does not, contracture will occur after healing and the slim margin along the *X* will be depressed, causing a more visible scar. (C) If small enough, convert the wound to an ellipse for easier repair. (D) Alternatively, excise the angled margins of skin to obtain "square" borders. (E) Undermine. (F) Close with interrupted sutures. Because side *a* is smaller than side *b*, a small wedge of tissue may need to be removed. (G) Complete closure.

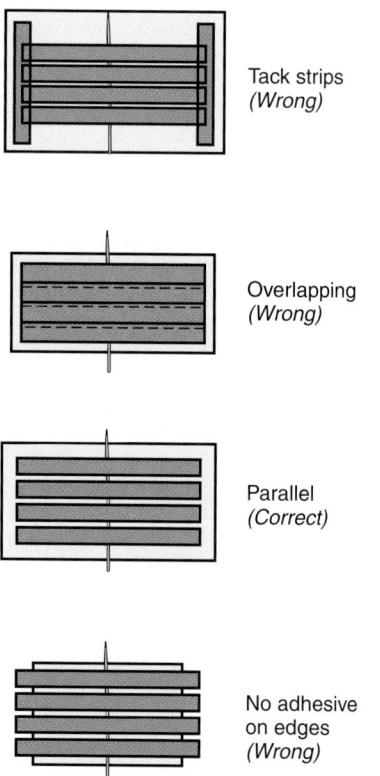

Tack strips
(Wrong)

Overlapping
(Wrong)

Parallel
(Correct)

No adhesive
on edges
(Wrong)

Fig. 19.18   The red strips are the tape; rectangles illustrate where benzoin or Mastisol was applied to the skin.

BOX 19.3   Pearls of Suturing

Use 27- to 30-gauge needle for anesthesia; slow injection; warm solution.

Use 1%–2% lidocaine (epinephrine is helpful to achieve hemostasis). Avoid epinephrine or use with extreme care in fingers, toes, nose, ears, and penis. Do not use epinephrine in digital blocks.

Make elliptical excision at least three times as long as wide.

Follow Langer lines.

Undermine. Undermine. Undermine. Double the width of the wound on each side.

Eliminate all dead space.

Use deep inverted buried absorbable sutures to reduce skin tension ("bottoms up").

Evert skin edges slightly ("build pyramids, not ditches"). Inversion of wound edges results in 300% increase in time for epithelial bridging.

Place interrupted sutures half as far apart as they are across. The more tension, the more sutures needed. Follow the Erlenmeyer flask shape. The finer the suture, the more sutures needed, but the less scarring.

Edema occurs after closure. Only approximate tissues; do not strangulate.

Begin gentle washing of wound after 12–24 hours; if Steri-Strips or tissue glues are not used, apply an ointment to keep the wound moist to speed healing.

Apply Steri-Strips after suture removal.

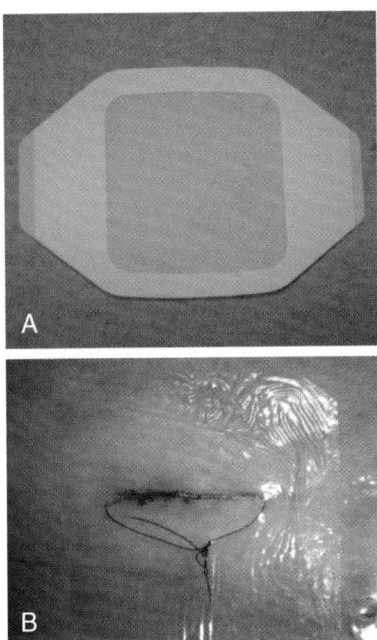

Fig. 19.19 (A) The Tegaderm film patch. (B) The film applied to a newly sutured wound. It is left in place until the subcuticular suture is removed, providing moist healing and support to the wound edges. (Courtesy The Medical Procedures Center, Midland, Michigan.)

TABLE 19.2 Timing for Suture Removal

Anatomic Area	Days Until Removal	External Suture Size	Buried Absorbable Suture Size
Face	4–5	5-0 or 6-0	5-0
Scalp	10–14	4-0, staples	3-0
Upper body	7–10	4-0	4-0
Hand	7–10	4-0 or 5-0	4-0
Lower body	10–14	4-0	3-0
Over joint (splint recommended)	14–21	4-0	3-0

Modified from Coates WC. Face and scalp lacerations. In: Tintinalli JE, Ma OJ, Yealy DM, et al, eds. *Emergency Medicine: A Comprehensive Study Guide*. 8th ed. New York: McGraw-Hill; 2016.

including erythema, pus, lymphangitis, or fever. A routine wound check is unnecessary for patients who understand the importance of monitoring wounds for signs of infection. An instructional handout can be given (see the patient education form available at www.expertconsult.com).

CONCURRENT TREATMENT

Tetanus Prophylaxis

Table 19.3 is based on the current Centers for Disease Control and Prevention recommendations for tetanus prophylaxis in wound management.

Analgesic Medication

Analgesic medication may need to be administered for a few days depending on the extent of the trauma, the pain threshold of the patient, and the concerns of the family. For most patients, over-the-counter medications are sufficient, but in selected patients prescription medication may be indicated. If antibiotics are needed, refer to the earlier discussion under Initial Assessment.

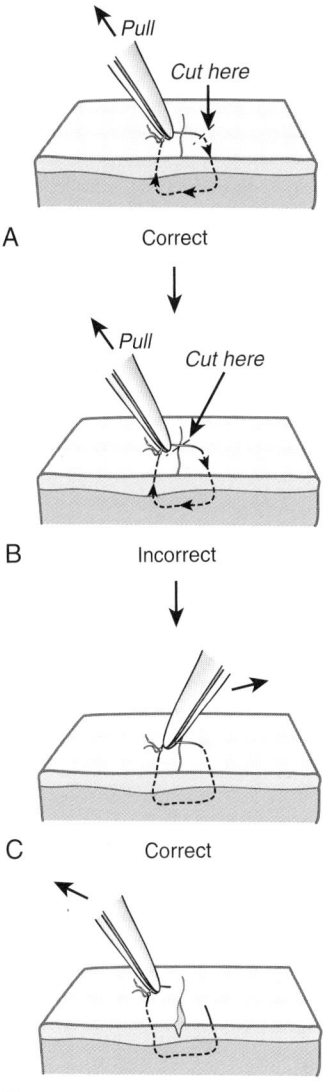

Fig. 19.20 Suture removal. (A) Cut where the suture enters the skin. (B) Cutting suture near knot leaves length of suture that is "dirty" and pulled into the tissue. (C) Pull the forceps over the wound, which approximates wound edges. (D) Pulling suture out this way tends to pull wound edges apart. Also, note dirty length of suture being pulled through wound.

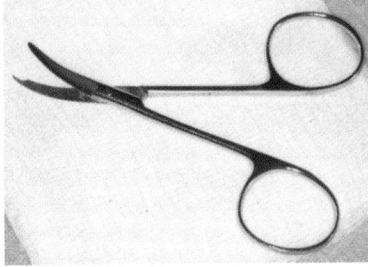

Fig. 19.21 Suture removal scissors. (Courtesy The Medical Procedures Center, Midland, Michigan.)

CONCLUSION

In the treatment of lacerations, careful inspection, adequate irrigation, skilled closure, and appropriate wound care can produce the best functional and cosmetic results. The principles and steps covered in this chapter show how lacerations can be repaired with maximal skill and minimal discomfort to the patient. More advanced

TABLE 19.3   Wound Management and Tetanus Prophylaxis

Previous Doses of Tetanus Toxoid*	Clean and Minor Wound		All Other Wounds†	
	Tetanus Toxoid-Containing vaccine‡	Human Tetanus Immune Globulin	Tetanus Toxoid-Containing Vaccine‡	Human Tetanus Immune Globulin§
<3 doses or unknown	Yes¶	No	Yes¶	Yes
≥3 doses	Only if last dose given ≥10 yr ago	No	Only if last dose given ≥5 yr ago**	No

Appropriate tetanus prophylaxis should be administered as soon as possible following a wound, but should be given even to patients who present late for medical attention. This is because the incubation period is quite variable; most cases occur within 8 days, but the incubation period can be as short as one day or as long as several months.

*Tetanus toxoid may have been administered as diphtheria-tetanus toxoids adsorbed, diphtheria-tetanus-whole cell pertussis (no longer available in the United States), diphtheria-tetanus-acellular pertussis, tetanus-diphtheria toxoids adsorbed (Td), booster tetanus toxoid-reduced diphtheria toxoid-acellular pertussis (Tdap), or tetanus toxoid.

†Such as, but not limited to, wounds contaminated with dirt, feces, soil, or saliva; puncture wounds; avulsions; wounds resulting from missiles, crushing, burns, or frostbite.

‡The preferred vaccine preparation depends upon the age and vaccination history of the patient:
* <7 years: diphtheria-tetanus-acellular pertussis
* Underimmunized children ≥7 and <11 years who have not received Tdap previously: Tdap. Children who receive Tdap between age 7 and 11 years do not require revaccination at age 11 years.
* ≥11 years: a single dose of Tdap is preferred to Td for all individuals in this age group who have not previously received Tdap. Pregnant women should receive Tdap during each pregnancy.
* Td is preferred to TT for those who received Tdap previously and when Tdap is not available.

§250 units intramuscularly at a different site than tetanus toxoid; intravenous immune globulin should be administered if human tetanus immune globulin is not available.
¶The vaccine series should be continued through completion as necessary.
**Booster doses given more frequently than every 5 years are not needed and can increase adverse effects.
Modified from American Academy of Pediatrics. Tetanus (lockjaw). In: Kimberlin DW, Brady MT, Jackson MA, Long SS, eds. *Red Book: 2015 Report of the Committee on Infectious Diseases.* 30th ed. Elk Grove Village, IL: American Academy of Pediatrics; 2015.

skills and knowledge can be developed through experience and by reading Chapter 16, Flaps and Plasties, and the sources listed in the Recommended Reading section.

PATIENT EDUCATION GUIDES

See the patient education and consent forms available at www.expertconsult.com.

CPT/BILLING CODES AND ICD-10-CM DIAGNOSTIC CODES

Coding and billing become very complex for laceration repair and excisions. Important factors to list for billing personnel are as follows:

* Location
* Size of lesion
* Length of closure or excision
* Simple or intermediate repair (intermediate includes either undermining or placement of deep buried sutures)
* Benign or malignant status
* Whether a true skin lesion or subcutaneous tumor or deep tumor (e.g., lipoma) was excised
* Method of removal (shave, excision, destruction)

With an excision, when charging for the size of the lesion, also include the width of the margins. For example, if a basal cell carcinoma that has a diameter of 1 cm is being excised, there should be 0.3-cm free margins. The size charged for the excision would be 1.6 cm. Suture removal is included in the initial charge if the original sutures were placed by the same group of physicians. Suture removal can be billed if performed by an unassociated physician or group.

Anesthetic, materials, and supplies are customarily also included in the reimbursement fees. If a lesion is excised and repaired in a simple fashion (no undermining, deep sutures, flaps, or plasties), the fee for excision then includes local anesthesia, repair, any interval care for 10 days, and suture removal. If an intermediate repair is done with an excision, two codes should be charged (the excision and the repair).

For CPT/billing codes, see Table 19.4. For ICD-10-CM diagnostic codes, see Appendix G, Neoplasm, Skin: ICD-10 Codes. For specific skin lesion sites, and to code out lacerations, go to the ICD-10 manual and look under wounds for the specific site: wound, open (by cutting or piercing instrument) (by firearms) (cut) (dissection) (incised) (laceration) (penetration) (perforating) (puncture) (with initial hemorrhage, not internal). (Laceration ICD codes are too extensive to list in detail here.) For fracture with open wound, see Fracture.

SUPPLIERS

(See contact information at available www.expertconsult.com.)

Zerowet splash shields and Klenzalac wound irrigation systems
Opsite
Smith & Nephew
Tegaderm
3M

ONLINE RESOURCES

Thomsen TW, Barclay DA, Setnick GS: Videos in clinical medicine: Basic laceration repair. N Engl J Med 355:e18–e22, 2006.

TABLE 19.4   CPT/Billing Codes

Benign Skin Excision	
11200	Tags, up to/including 15 lesions
11201	Tags, each additional 10 lesions
11400	TAL <0.6 cm
11401	TAL 0.6–1.0 cm
11402	TAL 1.1–2.0 cm
11403	TAL 2.1–3.0 cm
11404	TAL 3.1–4.0 cm
11406	TAL >4.0 cm
11420	SNHFG <0.6 cm
11421	SNHFG 0.60–1.0 cm
11422	SNHFG 1.1–2.0 cm
11423	SNHFG 2.1–3.0 cm
11424	SNHFG 3.1–4.0 cm
11426	SNHFG >4.0 cm
11440	Face <0.6 cm
11441	Face 0.6–1.0 cm
11442	Face 1.1–2.0 cm
11443	Face 2.1–3.0 cm
11444	Face 3.1–4.0 cm
11446	Face >4.0 cm

Malignant Skin Excision

11600	TAL <0.6 cm
11601	TAL 0.6–1.0 cm
11602	TAL 1.1–2.0 cm
11603	TAL 2.1–3.0 cm
11604	TAL 3.1–4.0 cm
11606	TAL >4.0 cm
11620	SNHFG <0.6 cm
11621	SNHFG 0.6–1.0 cm
11622	SNHFG 1.1–2.0 cm
11623	SNHFG 2.1–3.0 cm
11624	SNHFG 3.1–4.0 cm
11626	SNHFG >4.0 cm
11640	Face <0.6 cm
11641	Face 0.6–1.0 cm
11642	Face 1.1–2.0 cm
11643	Face 2.1–3.0 cm
11644	Face 3.1–4.0 cm
11646	Face >4.0 cm

Simple Skin Repairs

12001	SNAGTE <2.6 cm
12002	SNAGTE 2.6–7.5 cm
12004	SNAGTE 7.6–12.5 cm
12005	SNAGTE 12.6–20.0 cm
12006	SNAGTE 20.1–30.0 cm
12007	SNAGTE >30.0 cm
12011	FEENLMM <2.6 cm
12013	FEENLMM 2.6–5.0 cm
12014	FEENLMM 5.1–7.5 cm
12015	FEENLMM 7.6–12.5 cm
12016	FEENLMM 12.6–20.0 cm
12017	FEENLMM 20.1–30.0 cm
12018	FEENLMM >30.0 cm
12020	Superficial wound dehiscence

Intermediate Skin Repairs

12031	SATAL <2.6 cm
12032	SATAL 2.6–7.5 cm

Benign Skin Excision	
12034	SATAL 7.6–12.5 cm
12035	SATAL 12.6–20.0 cm
12036	SATAL 20.1–30.0 cm
12037	SATAL >30.0 cm
12041	NHFG < 2.6 cm
12042	NHFG 2.6–7.5 cm
12044	NHFG 7.6–12.5 cm
12045	NHFG 12.6–20.0 cm
12046	NHFG 20.1–30.0 cm
12047	NHFG >30.0 cm
12051	FEENLMM <2.6 cm
12052	FEENLMM 2.6–5.0 cm
12053	FEENLMM 5.1–7.5 cm
12054	FEENLMM 7.6–12.5 cm
12055	FEENLMM 12.6–20.0 cm
12056	FEENLMM 20.1–30.0 cm
12057	FEENLMM >30.0 cm

Benign Tumor Excisions (e.g., lipoma)

21550	Biopsy, soft tissue, neck/thorax
21555	Neck/thorax SQ*
21556	Neck/thorax deep* †
21930	Back/flank*
22900	Abdominal wall deep* †
23075	Shoulder SQ
23076	Shoulder deep* †
24075	Upper arm/elbow SQ*
24076	Upper arm/elbow deep* †
25075	Forearm/wrist SQ*
25076	Forearm/wrist deep* †
26115	Hand/finger SQ*
26116	Hand/finger deep* †
27047	Pelvis/hip SQ*
27048	Pelvis/hip deep*
27327	Thigh/knee SQ*
27328	Thigh/knee deep* †
27618	Leg/ankle SQ*
27619	Leg/ankle deep* †
28043	Foot SQ*
28045	Foot deep*
38500	Excision and/or biopsy, lymph node, superficial
41825	Gum/alveolar, no repair
41826	Gum/alveolar, simple rep

Face:	Face, ear, eyelid, nose, lip, or mucous membrane
FEENLMM:	Face, ear, eyelid, nose, lip, or mucous membrane
NHFG:	Neck, hand, foot, or external genitalia
SATAL:	Scalp, axilla, trunk, arm, or leg
SNAGTE:	Scalp, neck, axilla, genitalia, trunk, or extremity
SNHFG:	Scalp, neck, hand, foot, or genitalia
SQ:	Subcutaneous
TAL:	Trunk, arm, or leg

Codes in **bold** have a 10-day global fee surgical period.
The sizes listed in codes 11400 to 11646 describe lesion diameter, not the length of the skin excised.
*90-Day global fee surgical period.
†Deep excision includes subfascial or intramuscular lesions.

RECOMMENDED READING

Coates WC. Face and scalp lacerations. In: Tintinalli J, Ma OJ, Yealy DM, et al., eds. *Emergency Medicine: A Comprehensive Study Guide.* 8th ed. New York: McGraw-Hill; 2016.

Cummings P. Antibiotics to prevent infection in patients with dog bite wounds: a meta-analysis of randomized trials. *Ann Emerg Med.* 1994;23:535–540.

Cummings P, Del Beccaro MA. Antibiotics to prevent infection of simple wounds: a meta-analysis of randomized studies. *Am J Emerg Med.* 1995;13:396–400.

DeBoard RH, Rondeau DF, Kang CS, et al. Principles of basic wound evaluation and management in the emergency department. *Emerg Med Clin North Am.* 2007;25:23–39.

Ellis R, Ellis C. Dog and cat bites. *Am Fam Physician.* 2014;90(4):239–243.

Fincher EF, Gladstone HB, Moy RL. Complex layered facial closures. In: Robinson JK, Hanke CW, Siegel DM, et al., eds. *Surgery of the Skin: Procedural Dermatology.* 3rd ed. Philadelphia: Elsevier; 2015.

Global guidelines for the prevention of surgical site infections. *World Health Organization;* 2016. Available at http://apps.who.int/iris/bitstream/10665/250680/1/9789241549882-eng.pdf?ua=1.

Grossheim LF. General principles of wound management. In: Reichman EF, ed. *Emergency Medicine Procedures.* 2nd ed. New York: McGraw-Hill; 2013.

Haas AF, Grekin RC. Antibiotic prophylaxis in dermatologic surgery. *J Am Acad Dermatol.* 1995;32:155–176.

Houck CS, Sethna NF. Transdermal anesthesia with local anesthetics in children: review, update, and future direction. *Expert Rev Neurother.* 2005;5:625–634.

Jose RM, Vidyadharan J, Bragg TW, et al. Mammalian bite wounds: is primary repair safe? *Plast Reconstr Surg.* 2007;119:1967–1968.

Katz KH, Desciak EB, Maloney ME. The optimal application of surgical adhesive tape strips. *Dermatol Surg.* 1999;25:686–688.

Kundu S, Achar S. Principles of office anesthesia: part II. Topical anesthesia. *Am Fam Physician.* 2002;66:99–102.

Le BT, Dierks EJ, Ueeck BA, et al. Maxillofacial injuries associated with domestic violence. *J Oral Maxillofac Surg.* 2001;59:1277–1283.

Lloyd JD, Marque 3rd MJ, Kacprowicz RF. Closure techniques. *Emerg Med Clin North Am.* 2007;25:73–81.

Luck RP, Flood R, Eyal D, et al. Cosmetic outcomes of absorbable versus nonabsorbable sutures in pediatric facial lacerations. *Pediatr Emerg Care.* 2008;24:137–142.

Moscati RM, Mayrose J, Reardon RF, et al. A multicenter comparison of tap water versus sterile saline for wound irrigation. *Acad Emerg Med.* 2007;14:404–409.

Reichman EF. *Emergency Medicine Procedures.* 2nd ed. New York: McGraw-Hill; 2013.

Robinson JK, Hanke CW, Siegel DM, et al., eds. *Surgery of the Skin: Procedural Dermatology.* 3rd ed. Philadelphia: Elsevier; 2015.

Smack DP, Harrington AC, Dunn C, et al. Infection and allergy incidence in ambulatory surgery patients using white petrolatum vs bacitracin ointment: a randomized controlled trial. *JAMA.* 1996;276:972–977.

Srivastava D, Taylor RS. Suturing technique and other closure materials. In: Robinson JK, Hanke CW, Siegel DM, et al., eds. *Surgery of the Skin: Procedural Dermatology.* 3rd ed. Philadelphia: Elsevier; 2015.

Usatine RP, Moy RL, Tobinick EL, Siegel DM, eds. *Skin Surgery: A Practical Guide.* St. Louis: Mosby; 1998.

Wilson W, Taubert KA, Gewitz M, et al. Prevention of infective endocarditis: guidelines from the American Heart Association. A guideline from the American Heart Association Rheumatic Fever, Endocarditis, and Kawasaki Disease Committee, Council on Cardiovascular Disease in the Young, and the Council on Clinical Cardiology, Council on Cardiovascular Surgery and Anesthesia, and the Quality of Care and Outcomes Research Interdisciplinary Working Group. *Circulation.* 2007;116:1736–1754.

LACERATION AND INCISION REPAIR: NEEDLE SELECTION

William Jackson Epperson

A large variety of needle types have been developed for specific surgical needs. The needle facilitates the appropriate placement of suture. Inappropriate needle selection can damage the tissues, causing poor results and delayed healing. For example, a tapered needle with a round shaft is needed in suturing bowel, where prevention of leakage is imperative. A cutting needle would never be appropriate in the reanastomosis of bowels or blood vessels.

Most needles are made of noncorrosive stainless steel. Through a process of heating the metal, maximum strength and ductility (the ability to bend under pressure without breaking) are achieved. Each needle type is sharpened to a varying degree depending on its use. In addition, to assist with passage through tissues, most needles receive a thin coat of silicone or other lubricant which is preserved as long as they remain in their packaging.

NEEDLE DESIGN

The surgical needle is composed of a swaged eye or shank, a body, and a point (Fig. 20.1). There are three types of needles: the closed eye, the French (split or spring) eye, and the swaged eye. Both closed-eye and French-eye needles must be threaded (Fig. 20.2). Since the 1960s, needles have been almost exclusively swaged because threaded needles have many undesirable characteristics. The swaged portion of the needle is now commonly referred to as the *shank*. Within the shank the metal is molded around the suture, which alleviates most needle-to-suture attachment problems. This also prevents the repeated use of a dull, nonlubricated, or contaminated needle, problems associated with threaded needles.

Many terms have been developed by suture manufacturers to categorize their products for different purposes and to denote their size. Unfortunately, there is no standard nomenclature. On thick skin, "for skin" (FS) needles are acceptable, and most have a reverse

cutting edge. On cosmetic areas, plastic (P), plastic skin (PS), premium (PRE), or precision cosmetic (PC) needles may offer some minor advantages for the surgeon but at a significantly greater cost. These initial designations for the needles are the common nomenclature used by Ethicon as marketing terms for their needles. Ethicon manufactures more than 80% of the needles used in North America. Other manufacturers include Medtronic and Surgical Specialties Corporation; fortunately, they use similar needle description nomenclature.

In general, a larger needle is used for deeply buried sutures, whereas a smaller needle can be used to close a thin layer of skin. Location of closure is also important. For instance, facial closures are often done with a P-3 needle, whereas other areas with thicker skin require an FS-2 or FS-3 needle. It is important to review the descriptions of the needle on the outside of the suture package, and often a picture of the needle will aid in proper needle selection.

Needles should be handled only with needle holders. A proper-sized, high-quality needle holder is needed for suturing; no other instrument is acceptable for this task. This instrument is worth the investment because it can make the suturing experience satisfying, versus totally frustrating with poor instrument selection. In general, gold-handled instruments are of superior quality. The needle should be grasped by the needle holder at a position approximately one needle holder's width past the curved center of the needle. Only one click of needle holder pressure should be applied to hold the needle in place. If the needle slips, it may be that the needle holder is old and no longer will hold the needle, or the suturing attempt being made is not commensurate with the needle size and technique being applied.

A hemostat or other grasping instrument is not an acceptable substitute for a needle holder when suturing. The needle will easily roll out of position because it requires a flat surface to maintain its operative position. Any and all grasping of the needle with any instrument causes a weakening of the metal with risk of breakage. This is less of a concern when a proper-sized needle holder is used with prudent application of force to achieve the desired surgical results.

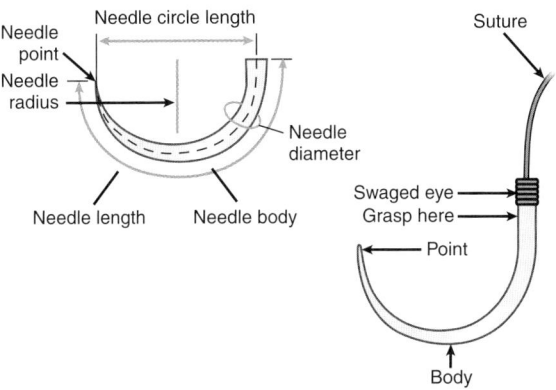

Fig. 20.1 Anatomy of a surgical needle.

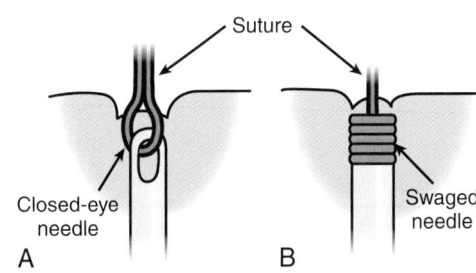

Fig. 20.2 (A) Tissue disruption can be caused by the double-suture strand with a closed-eyed needle. (B) Tissue disruption is minimized by a single-suture strand swaged to needle.

The needle should be grasped below the shank portion but beyond the midbody region (Fig. 20.3). The swaged metal must be sufficiently soft to crimp firmly around the suture and lock it in place. Therefore, if the needle is grasped by the needle holder at the shank, it can easily bend and weaken. The body of the needle is firm, not malleable, and less likely to bend. The tip of the needle holder should just cover the needle, and again, the handle should be closed only to the first click. During needle placement, the force must be advanced in the direction of the curvature of the needle. The wrist must be everted and supinated as the needle goes through tissue to avoid undue pressure and bending.

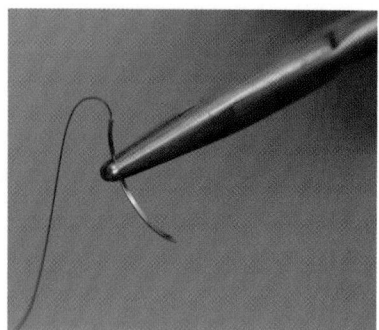

Fig. 20.3 Needle holder with needle in place.

Straight

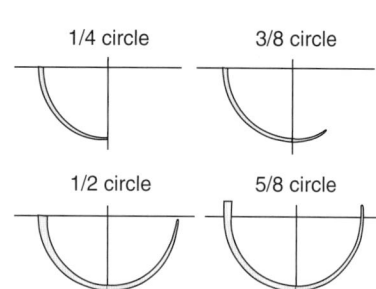

1/4 circle   3/8 circle

1/2 circle   5/8 circle

Fig. 20.4 Needle body shapes.

The body of the needle is important for both strength and grasping by the needle holder. Various shapes of the body are important for added strength, as well as for matching the flow of the needle through the tissues as directed by the point. A flattened body with concave or convex surfaces helps to reduce unwanted needle rotation when suturing. The shape of the body of the needle allows for a variety of uses (Fig. 20.4). In general, a ⅜-inch curvature is adequate for most cutaneous procedures (Fig. 20.5).

Needle points are the most important needle consideration. The basic types of needle points include *cutting*, *tapered*, and *blunt* (Fig. 20.6). The *blunt-point* needle is used for friable parenchymal tissue such as liver and kidney. This point allows for dissection through tissues, avoiding the trauma of a cutting needle.

The two opposing edges of a *cutting needle* allow for easier passage through tough tissues. This makes cutting needles ideal for suturing skin with its dense supporting structures. However, these cutting edges have their drawbacks when it comes to tendons and oral mucous membranes, which are easily damaged by overcutting.

The *conventional cutting* needle has a cutting edge on its inside or concave curvature. The inside cutting in the direction of force is a negative characteristic of this needle. The suture force tends to concentrate at the apex of the triangle, and the tissues outside of the desired suture channel are cut. For this reason, a conventional cutting needle is rarely used compared with the reverse cutting needle (see Fig. 20.6).

The *reverse cutting* needle has its cutting edge on the outer curvature of the needle. This provides a flat surface along the inner edge, thereby reducing the incidence of sutures pulling through tissues into the margin of the wound. Unless specified otherwise, a "cutting needle" now refers to a reverse cutting design.

Tapered cut or *round* needles have an oval body to reduce twisting in the needle holder. These points are useful in less dense tissues that require small holes and minimal tissue injury, such as fascia or bowel.

COMPLICATIONS

When inappropriately small suture needles are chosen, there is a high risk of needle bending or breaking. A lost needle tip can be a serious, time-consuming intraoperative problem. Other causes of needle breakage include an unexpected encounter with bone or scar tissue, inappropriate angle of penetration, or the use of a reshaped needle that was bent during use.

The loss of the whole needle in tissues can be avoided by using good judgment in matching tissue bites to needle length. Avoid

Ethicon
Precision point needles

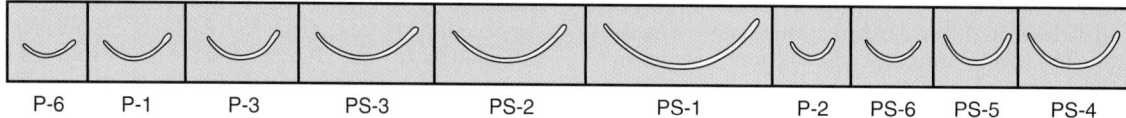

P-6   P-1   P-3   PS-3   PS-2   PS-1   P-2   PS-6   PS-5   PS-4

Precision cosmetic needles

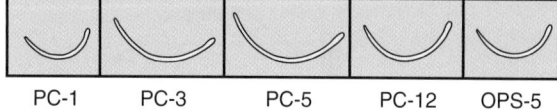

PC-1   PC-3   PC-5   PC-12   OPS-5

Davis & Geck

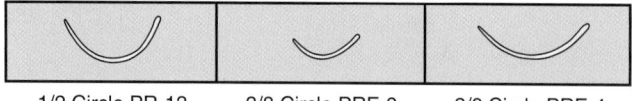

1/2 Circle PR-13   3/8 Circle PRE-2   3/8 Circle PRE-4

Fig. 20.5 Ethicon and Davis & Geck (Kendall) needle nomenclature for facial closures (actual sizes).

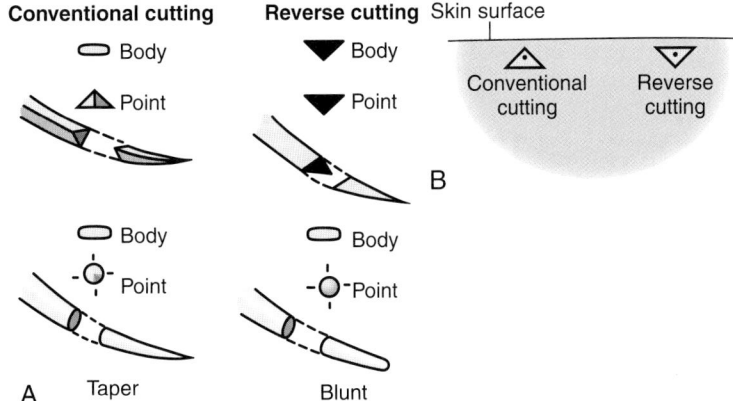

Fig. 20.6 (A) Needle points and body shapes. (B) In conventional cutting needles the pressure is concentrated on the apex of the triangle; the needle therefore has a tendency to tear through tissue. In reverse cutting, the advantage of piercing through tissue still exists, but the pressure from the suture is distributed over the whole base so unwanted tearing is reduced. *Black dot* indicates suture.

firm grasping of the suture material near the shank with the needle holder or forceps because it can weaken or cut the suture material, leaving an unattached needle. This free needle becomes a risk to the surgeon for needlestick injury, as well as an opportunity for complications in the patient.

The shank is the thinnest metal portion of the needle, and this thin metal is therefore the weakest portion of the needle. Care must be taken never to apply force or attempt to use the needle holder on the shank when suturing. When a needle bends during suturing, the act of straightening it further weakens the metal. The surgeon must remain aware of this potential risk for complications.

In addition, multiple needle passes through tissue and associated frequent re-arming of the needle holder wear away the needle lubricant coating, which increases the force required for subsequent needle passes.

CONCLUSION

Often an ordinary suturing procedure becomes more difficult than expected. This difficulty can be ameliorated by reassessing the appropriateness of the instruments being used. Needle selection is often a key factor in facilitating the ease of the operation and ensuring ultimate good surgical results.

SUPPLIERS

(See contact information available at www.expertconsult.com.)

Ethicon, Inc.
Medtronic, Inc.
Surgical Specialties Corporation

Most medical supply firms carry any suture material needed.

RECOMMENDED READING

Brunicardi FC, Andersen DK, Billiar TR, et al. *Schwartz's Principles of Surgery.* 10th ed. New York: McGraw-Hill; 2015.

Ethicon Inc. *Wound Closure Manual.* Somerville, NJ: Ethicon, Inc; 2005. Available online at: http://www.uphs.upenn.edu/surgery/Education/facilities/measey/Wound_Closure_Manual.pdf.

Goldwasser MS, Bailey JS, eds. Diagnosis and management of skin cancer. *Oral Maxillofac Surg Clin.* 2005;17:133–240.

Grossheim LF. Skin and soft tissue procedures. In: Reichman EF, ed. *Emergency Medicine Procedures.* 2nd ed. New York: McGraw-Hill; 2013:619.

Lammers RL, Smith ZE. Methods of wound closure. In: Roberts JR, Custalow CB, Thomsen TW, eds. *Roberts and Hedges Clinical Procedures in Emergency Medicine.* 6th ed. Philadelphia: Elsevier; 2014:654–655.

Moy RL. Suture material. In: Usatine R, Moy R, Tobinick E, Siegel D, eds. *Skin Surgery: A Practical Guide.* St. Louis: Mosby; 1998:77–87.

Rohrer TE, Cook JL, Nguyen TH, et al. *Flaps and Grafts in Dermatologic Surgery.* Philadelphia: Saunders; 2007.

Srivastava D, Taylor RS. Suturing technique and other closure materials. In: Robinson JK, Hanke DW, Siegel DM, et al., eds. *Surgery of the Skin: Procedural Dermatology.* Philadelphia: Elsevier; 2015.

CHAPTER 21

LACERATION AND INCISION REPAIR: SUTURE SELECTION

William Jackson Epperson

Numerous suture types have been developed for specific tissue properties in the body. The qualities most important for suture choice include flexibility, strength, secure knotting, and a low propensity to contribute to inflammation or infection. The goal of suturing is to maintain the approximation of tissue securely until healing allows for tissue strength to recover.

The two main categories of suture are *absorbable* and *nonabsorbable*. All types of suture are foreign to the body; therefore the degree to which the body reacts against the suture is an important consideration in suture choice.

Absorbable suture is a sterile strand of synthetic polymer or mammal-derived collagen. The rate of absorption and duration of tensile strength are important considerations. For example, the suture may lose effective strength long before it has been absorbed. Various coatings and materials have been developed to prolong the retention of tensile strength in absorbable sutures. These coatings also aid in the passage of suture through tissues by decreasing friction.

The natural absorbable suture (mammalian collagen or gut sutures) are derived mainly from the submucosa of sheep intestine, the serosa of cattle intestine, or the flexor tendons of cattle. They are available in plain or chromic (coated with chromic salts to help delay absorption) forms. Tensile strength is determined by the percentage of collagen in the gut suture. Any collagen materials in the gut suture can cause severe tissue reactions, so purity of the protein is very important. Rare true suture allergy can be caused by foreign collagens or chromic salts in "gut" suture.

Common synthetic absorbable suture materials include polyglactic acid (Vicryl), polyglycolic acid (Dexon), and polydioxanone (PDS). These materials have the desirable property of extended duration of tensile strength (Fig. 21.1).

Nonabsorbable suture is used for skin and for long-term internal placement, as in cardiovascular, orthopedic, and plastic surgery. Many raw materials are used, including silk, cotton, stainless steel, nylon, polyester, and polypropylene (Table 21.1). Table 21.2 reviews the various features of each of these sutures. All suture materials except stainless steel will lose at least some tensile strength if left in the body for long enough periods.

Nonabsorbable sutures are removed from the skin when no longer needed. In vascular and orthopedic applications there is often a need for more permanent materials that retain their tensile strength. Tendon repair requires prolonged healing times, so sutures need long-term tensile strength to give adequate time for self-repair. Vascular grafts must have the support of suture for an indefinite period. The anastomosis of a graft and a blood vessel is never secured by the fibroblast and collagen of the body alone.

Braided suture adds strength and helps to secure the knotting but is more likely to leak fluid, which is called *capillarity*. This quality also increases the likelihood of harboring bacteria and subsequent infection. Monofilament is therefore better to use in the presence of infection, but its knots are less dependable. Tissue reaction is important

in delicate tissues where scar and tissue formation may be a problem, which is why gut suture may not be a good choice for use on the face.

Suture size is indicated by the use of a "0," with more "0"s designating smaller sutures (e.g., 4-0 is smaller than 3-0). Suture materials are standardized by specific regulations, which ensure the consistency of tensile strength.

Other suture characteristics are also important. Tensile strength is the force necessary for a suture to break divided by its cross-sectional area. Tensile strength can be altered by twisting, braiding, increased age, heating, and moisture. Suture coatings reduce friction when the suture is passing through tissues. Braided suture has more friction than monofilaments. Coatings used include silicone, Teflon, and wax. Polyglactic suture has also been coated with triclosan, which is an antibacterial agent that may reduce the incidence of staphylococcal infections. *Memory* describes the characteristics of a suture material in returning to its original shape after bending. Increased memory is found in nylon and polypropylene, and the knots of both are more likely to untie spontaneously.

Sutures are foreign to tissues, and all induce inflammatory responses. The larger stranded and multistranded sutures generally cause more tissue reactions than thin or monofilament sutures. Synthetic sutures of nylon and polypropylene cause less reaction than silk or surgical gut. The dissolution of absorbable sutures is accomplished by the homeostatic immune response. In general, less immunogenic suture materials are smaller diameter, synthetic, monofilament, and nonabsorbable. A greater immunologic response comes from suture materials that are larger in diameter, made of natural fiber, multifilament, and absorbable.

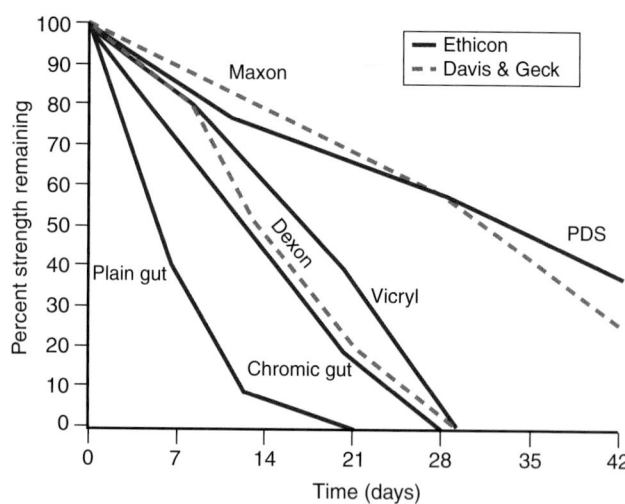

Fig. 21.1 In vivo strength retention of absorbable sutures. *PDS,* Polydioxanone.

Knots are an important consideration in terms of whether they remain tied and do not cause a significant reduction in the tensile strength of the suture material. The knot is the weakest part of the completed suture ligature. Proper knotting technique requires application of the square knot or a double loop followed by a square knot tie. Often knots are accomplished as half hitches that are weak and do not remain secure. The more friction the suture has, the less likely it is to incur slippage and loss of knot integrity. Braided suture knots rarely slip, whereas monofilament often comes untied in the absence of proper knotting technique. For proper tying techniques, see Chapter 22, Laceration and Incision Repair: Suture Tying.

CHOOSING A SUTURE

Each surgeon has his or her own choice of suture based on training and individual preferences. Choosing the appropriate suture characteristics in relation to the various applications will facilitate the operation and lead to an acceptable result. Table 21.3 generalizes some recommendations for sutures commonly used in an office setting. In general, the smaller the suture, the lower the tensile strength; thus more sutures will be needed, but the cosmetic result will be better. Therefore, to help minimize scarring, choose the suture of the smallest possible size that is capable of securely closing the wound. Clinicians vary greatly in their preferences, and no one suture is satisfactory for all situations. Nylon is a good, all-around, inexpensive material for surface skin suturing. It is not quite as strong or slippery as polypropylene, but it ties more easily and requires fewer knots. Polypropylene is stronger and glides through tissue easily, but it requires at least three if not four knots and still may not remain tight. Polypropylene works well for running subcuticular stitches, and, because it is stronger, a smaller size can be used for interrupted closures.

COMPLICATIONS

Suture breakage can be a time-wasting inconvenience for the surgeon and can present significant problems for wound healing. The direct application of inappropriate force to suture material may result in suture breakage, as may irregular surgical angles, rapid suture decomposition by infection, difficult-to-access surgical sites, and postoperative patient mobility. Complications may be reduced

TABLE 21.1   Nonabsorbable Sutures

Material	Type	Tensile Strength	Tissue Reaction	Cost
Silk	Braided	Poor	High	Low
Nylon (Ethilon,* Dermalon†)	Mono	Good	Minimal	Low
Polypropylene (Prolene,* Surgipro†)	Mono	Excellent	Minimal	High
Uncoated braided polyester (Dacron,* Mersilene*)	Braided	Good	Moderate	High
Coated braded polyester (Ti-cron,† Ethibond*)	Braided	Good	Moderate	High
Polybutester (Novafil†)	Mono	Good	Minimal	Moderate

*Ethicon, Inc.
†Covidien/Medtronic, Inc.

TABLE 21.2   Common Suture Materials

Suture	Types	Makeup	Usage	Tissue Reaction	Absorption Time or Rate (Total)	Tensile Strength Retention
Absorbable Sutures						
Gut	Plain multifilament twisted	Mammalian collagen	Superficial vessels and quick-healing subcutaneous tissues	High	70 days	7–10 days
Gut	Chromic multifilament twisted	Mammalian collagen	Versatile; also good in the presence of infection; do not use on skin because of reaction	Moderate	90 days	10–21 days
Polyglycolic acid (Dexon*)†	Mono	Synthetic polymer	Buried sutures; good tensile and knot strength	Mild	40% in 7 days	20% in 15 days, 5% in 28 days
Polydioxanone (PDS‡)	Mono	Polyester polymer	Versatile; body cavity closure; bowel; buried skin suture where more strength and longer retention needed	Mild	210 days	70% in 14 days, 50% in 28 days
Polyglactic acid (Vicryl‡)	Braided	Coated polymer	Subcutaneous skin; buried sutures	Mild	60–90 days	60% in 14 days, 30% in 21 days
Polyglyconate (Maxon*)	Mono	Polyester	Smoother knot and excellent first-throw holding; buried	Mild	180–210 days	80% in 14 days, 60% in 28 days
Nonabsorbable Sutures						
Cotton	Twisted fibers	Cotton fiber	Ligating, some skin but generally too reactive	Minimal	Nearly permanent, encapsulated in the body	50% in 6 mo, 30% in 2 yr
Silk	Braided	Silkworm-spun fiber	Ligating, some skin but rarely used	Moderate	2 yr	Gone in 1 yr
Steel	Mono	Alloy Fe-Ni-Cr	Tendons, sternum, abdominal wall	Low	Never; encapsulated in the body	Indefinite
Nylon (Ethilon,‡ Dermalon*)	Mono	Synthetic polymer	Skin	Very low	20% per yr	Loses 20% per yr
Polyester (Mersilene‡)	Braided	Polyester	Cardiovascular, general, and plastic surgery	Minimal	Nearly permanent; encapsulated in the body	Nearly indefinite
Polypropylene (Prolene,‡ Surgilene*)	Mono	Synthetic polymer	Skin, vascular, plastic surgery—very "slippery" so needs extra knots; "stronger" than nylon	Minimal	Considered permanent; encapsulated in the body	Nearly indefinite

*Covidien/ Medtronic, Inc.
†Dexon Plus has a synthetic coating to facilitate knot tying and passage through tissue.
‡Ethicon, Inc.

TABLE 21.3	Common Sutures for Cutaneous Surgery		
Area of Body	Skin (Interrupted)	Skin (Running Subcuticular)	Buried
Face	5-0 or 6-0 nylon	4-0 or 5-0 polypropylene	4-0, 5-0, or 6-0 synthetic absorbable
Extremities, trunk	4-0 or 5-0 nylon	3-0 or 4-0 polypropylene or 3-0 or 4-0 synthetic absorbable (rarely used on extremities)	3-0 or 4-0 synthetic absorbable; occasionally 4-0 polypropylene if quite deep

by applying an increased number of ligatures and by using suture of a diameter that is commensurate to the forces most likely to be experienced in the surgical situation. Of course almost all applications of suture can reduce tissue blood supply; proper surgical technique reduces the incidence of this complication. Running loops of suture, used in an effort to accomplish quicker wound closure, increase the risk of wound dehiscence in the event of suture breakage. Interrupted suture ligatures greatly reduce this complication but their placement is extremely time-consuming compared with that of running ligatures.

The tensile strength of the suture can be reduced by actions that cause fragmentation or splitting of the suture fibers, also known as *frays*. Common causes of frays include friction caused by tying, especially with tension applied during long knot rundowns. Also, scar tissue, bone, or foreign material may damage suture within tissues, while retractors, forceps, clamps, and needle holders can cause damage to suture within the surgical field.

TIPS

When purchasing a supply of office sutures, consider the following:

1. Nylon is most commonly used and least expensive for interrupted sutures in the skin (3-0 through 6-0).
2. For running subcuticular sutures, nylon will work, but only for shorter lengths. It is not very slippery and may break on removal. Polypropylene (Prolene) is "more slippery" and stronger.

3. For deep inverted sutures, generally use polyglactic acid (Vicryl) or polyglycolic acid (Dexon). Vicryl lasts a little longer.
   - If longer retention and greater strength are desired, consider polydioxanone (PDS II).
   - If a permanent deep suture is preferred, consider clear nylon.

PATIENT EDUCATION GUIDES

See the patient education form on care of sutures available at www.expertconsult.com.

SUPPLIERS

(See contact information available at www.expertconsult.com.)

Ethicon Inc.
Covidien/Medtronic Inc.

Most medical supply firms carry any suture material needed.

RECOMMENDED READING

Brunicardi F, Andersen D, Billiar T, et al., eds. *Schwart's Principles of Surgery.* 10th ed. New York: McGraw-Hill; 2015.

Ethicon Inc. *Wound Closure Manual.* Somerville, NJ: Ethicon, Inc; 2005.: http://www.uphs.upenn.edu/surgery/Education/facilities/measey/Wound_Closure_Manual.pdf.

Forsch RT. Essentials of skin laceration repair. *Am Fam Physician.* 2008;78: 945–951.

Goldwasser MS, Bailey JS, eds. Diagnosis and management of skin cancer. *Oral Maxillofac Surg Clin.* 2005; 17:133–240.

Lammers RL, Smith ZE. Methods of wound closure. In: Roberts JR, Custalow CB, Thomsen TW, eds. *Roberts and Hedges Clinical Procedures in Emergency Medicine.* 6th ed. Philadelphia: Elsevier; 2014:652–654.

Moy RL. Suture material. In: Usatine R, Moy R, Tobinick E, Siegel D, eds. *Skin Surgery: A Practical Guide.* St. Louis: Mosby; 1998:77–87.

Reichman EF, Powell C. Basic wound closure techniques. In: Reichman EF, ed. *Emergency Medicine Procedures.* 2nd ed. New York: McGraw-Hill; 2013.

Robinson JK, Hanke CW, Siegel DM, et al., eds. *Surgery of the Skin: Procedural Dermatology.* 3rd ed. Philadelphia: Elsevier; 2015.

Rohrer TE, Cook JL, Nguyen TH. *Flaps and Grafts in Dermatologic Surgery.* Philadelphia: Saunders; 2007.

Srivastava D, Taylor RS. Suturing technique and other closure materials. In: Robinson JK, Hanke CW, Siegel DM, et al., eds. *Surgery of the Skin: Procedural Dermatology.* 3rd ed. Philadelphia: Elsevier; 2015.

Way LW. *Current Surgical Diagnosis and Treatment.* 9th ed. Norwalk, CT: Appleton & Lange; 1991.

CHAPTER 22

LACERATION AND INCISION REPAIR: SUTURE TYING

Ronald D. Reynolds

The knot is the weakest point of any suture. Even when properly tied, the knot is less than half the strength of the suture material in which it is tied; it will always be the point at which a suture fails. Knots will slip apart if not correctly constructed. If excessive tension is applied, even to a properly tied suture loop, it will break at the knot because of internal shearing forces.

It is incumbent on the clinician to know what suture material and size to use for each type of tissue that is to be approximated (see Chapter 21, Laceration and Incision Repair: Suture Selection). Once a suture is placed, it must be tied in an appropriate manner—not too tight or too loose and with a knot that will not fail before the tissue has healed. The knot must not be excessively large because inflammation and infection correlate directly with knot volume in tissue.

GENERAL PRINCIPLES OF KNOT TYING

A few generalities can be made about all knot tying. The suture material must always be treated with respect. Grasping the suture with an instrument will weaken it, and so this should be avoided except when holding a tail that will be cut away after an instrument tie. Shearing forces created by sawing two strands upon one another will weaken the strands. The first throw of a knot should just approximate the tissue, but subsequent throws must be tied firmly for knot security. Ideally, knots should be tied with equal tension on both strands. Tension should be applied parallel to the loop being closed (and being used to close tissue) and along the axis of the knot being tightened. Excessive throws do not add to knot security; they only add time and bulk.

KNOT MECHANICS

Suture knots are at the mercy of a number of factors. If the knot is tied in a *monofilament* material such as gut, nylon, polypropylene (Prolene), or polydioxanone (PDS), the *coefficient of friction* within the knot will be low, leading to a tendency to slip. These materials also have *memory*, a tendency to maintain the shape in which they were manufactured, giving a straightening tendency that can lead to untying. The *pliability*, or ability to form a tight loop, of nylon is higher than that of the other monofilament materials. Braided *multifilament* suture materials such as silk, polyester (Mersilene, Ethibond), polyglactin (Vicryl), and polyglycolic acid (Dexon) have a higher coefficient of friction and less memory, making them easier to tie and less prone to slippage. The absorbability of a suture does not have a direct influence on its tying characteristics.

When knots are tied, great care must be taken as to the details. The *square knot* (Fig. 22.1A) is the prototype suture knot because it is easy to tie, is strong, and does not loosen easily.

Each twisting layer of the knot is called a *throw*. A square knot is constructed of one helical twist for the first throw followed by one

helical twist in the opposite direction for the second throw. If both helices are in the same direction, a *granny knot* (Fig. 22.1B) results. Granny knots slip much more easily than square knots and therefore should be avoided in tying sutures.

After a helix for a knot throw is made with two suture strands, it must be kept in a helical configuration as the knot is tightened. If too much tension is applied to one strand, that strand will straighten and a *half hitch* (Fig. 22.1C) in the other strand will result. As is obvious from their appearance, half hitches will slip on the straightened member of the suture and therefore are also to be avoided. It is unfortunately common for a clinician who thinks that square knots are being laid down to instead make a series of slipping half hitches (Fig. 22.1D). This occurs because too much tension is being applied to one strand during the tightening phase of tying.

If there is excess tension on wound edges when a square knot is being tied, the first throw of the knot may loosen before the second throw is placed and allow the edges to gape apart. The *surgeon's knot* (Fig. 22.1E) is an adaptation of the square knot with two helical twists in the first throw. This additional twist increases the friction within the first throw and helps to hold it tight while the second throw is made. It is almost always used, but whenever a surgeon's knot seems necessary, the clinician should always be sure that the deep space has been closed with a deep suture, if possible, to approximate wound edges and take tension off the skin closure.

CHOOSING A SUTURE TYING TECHNIQUE

All physicians should learn knot tying skills during medical school and become familiar with one- and two-handed ties as well as instrument ties. There are some important points to consider when you decide which of these tying techniques to use.

Most procedures performed by primary care clinicians are office procedures performed on the skin. Clinicians cannot afford to waste excess suture material just for the sake of knot tying. Studies of the economics of suture tying show that at least two to four times as many sutures can be constructed in a given length of suture material with an *instrument tie* than with a *hand tie*. Although instrument tying is slightly slower than hand tying, it is much more economical and is the preferred technique for all skin procedures.

If a hand tie is to be done, the preferred method is the two-handed tie. Although the one-handed tie may be slightly faster than the two-handed tie, it is difficult to do well. One-handed ties are liable to create a series of half hitches because it is common to keep too much tension on one strand during tying. Also, because most wounds are sutured with the needle movement directed toward the clinician and it is this closest strand (with its needle attached) that is primarily manipulated during a one-handed tie, there is a risk of needlestick injury during a one-handed tie. Therefore one-handed tying is not covered in this chapter.

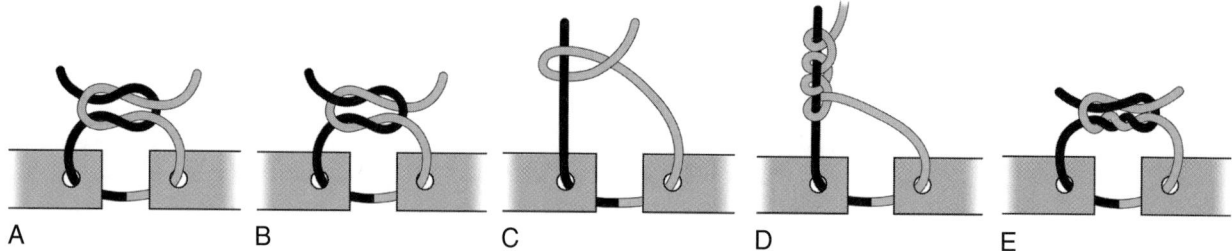

Fig. 22.1   (A) Square knot. (B) Granny knot. (C) Half hitch. (D) Series of "square" half hitches. (E) Surgeon's knot. (Modified from Zimmer CA, Thacker JG, Powell DM, et al. Influence of knot configuration and tying technique on the mechanical performance of sutures. *J Emerg Med.* 1991;9:107–113.)

HOW TIGHT TO TIE THE LOOP

To appropriately approximate tissue, sutures must bring wound edges into apposition, without placing excessive force on the tissues ("approximate but don't strangulate"). If a suture loop is tied too loosely, a gap will persist and the wound will not heal by primary intention; instead, it will have to heal by secondary intention from deeper within the defect. If tied too tightly, a suture loop will strangulate the tissue within, creating ischemia and poor wound healing. A too-tight skin suture will cut into the skin surface across the wound, creating a permanent "railroad track" scar.

Whether incised by accidental laceration or by an intentional surgical wound, all tissue will swell somewhat from the inflammation that is attendant to the healing process. Some allowance must be made for this anticipated swelling in tying each suture. It is the tension of the first throw, and maintenance of this tension while the second throw locks it in place, that is critical. Additional throws beyond these do not change the tension within the original loop.

As tension is applied to the first throw of a knot, the tissue edges should just barely touch. If the edges are bunched together initially, subsequent swelling will make the loop too tight. With skin sutures, two subtle indications of excess loop tension include (1) a puckering effect of each suture that makes the wound mound up slightly between each loop and (2) a pale color of the skin underneath the suture. *It is far better to remove and replace an improperly tied suture than to leave it and hope for the best.*

HOW MANY THROWS TO PLACE

How many additional throws to place on top of the basic square or surgeon's knot for knot security is a slippery question. Suture manufacturers will say only, "additional throws as indicated by the surgical circumstance and the experience of the surgeon" (medicolegal concerns keep them from committing themselves).

For a knot to be secure, additional throws are needed beyond the basic two throws. Without added throws, the knot will slip loose when tension is applied to the loop. Any loosely tied knot will slip, so all throws past the first must be tied quite firmly but without excessive force, which will damage the integrity of the suture material.

Placing more throws than needed will unnecessarily add operative time and increase the bulk of the knot without adding strength to it. Extra throws in a skin suture knot add operative time but have no consequence for the tissue because they are not buried. If the knot is buried, as in a subcuticular suture, additional bulk adds to the tissue reaction and can increase the risk for infection. It is therefore necessary to know the minimum number of throws needed to tie a secure knot in a variety of suture materials.

As a general rule, studies have shown that when 3- to 4-mm tails are left, monofilament materials need a total of four firm square throws to be secure, and braided materials need three. Obviously if the knot is not tied squarely (made of alternating throws with helices in different directions), is tied loosely, or consists of half hitches rather than square throws, even the recommended number of throws will not suffice.

There are two exceptions to this general rule. First, nylon is pliable enough that it holds with three firm square throws. Second, when the suture is cut on the knot and no tails are left, one additional throw is required for knot security.

TECHNIQUES

Instrument Tie

An instrument tie uses the needle holder to form the twists in each throw. Directions are for a right-handed clinician. Left-handed clinicians can reverse the handedness in the directions and look at the figure in a mirror.

1. Place the suture moving toward yourself, and pull it through until just 2 to 3 cm of the tail is left outside the entry hole. Drop the needle beside the wound to minimize needlestick risk. Pick up the long end of the suture with your left thumb and index finger about 8 cm from its exit and hold it above the wound.

2. Create the first throw by making a single twist (for a square knot) or double twist (for a surgeon's knot) around the tip of the needle holder with the long strand. To do this, the needle holder is held closed but not locked, facing toward the left. The instrument tip approaches the long strand moving toward the clinician. Both it and the long strand are moved in a clockwise motion to wrap the strand around the tip (Fig. 22.2A), with care taken not to pull the suture through the wound. Grasp the short end with the very tip of the needle holder. Pull the short end through the loops around the needle holder's tip (Fig. 22.2B). Keep even tension on both strands as you pull the short strand toward you with the needle holder and the long strand away from you with your left hand (Fig. 22.2C). The sutures should maintain a helical configuration all the way down to the wound. Apply enough tension to just appose the wound. Release the short end.

3. The second throw is created by reversing the rotation of the long strand around the needle holder tip. While still holding the long strand in your left hand, bring it toward you while moving the needle holder away from yourself. As the needle holder tip touches the long strand, wrap counterclockwise around it (Fig. 22.2D). Again grasp the short end in the needle holder tip (Fig. 22.2E) and pull the short strand away from yourself while pulling the long strand toward you (Fig. 22.2F). Carefully pull the throw down square to lock the knot. As you tighten this critical second throw, do not pull hard enough to disturb the first throw—this might loosen the careful apposition.

4. Additional throws must be made, with the number depending on the suture material and circumstances. Repeat the cycle of clockwise-counterclockwise throws, being careful to lay each throw down with opposite rotation to the last throw. Tie each throw square (not half-hitched) with firm and even tension on both ends as the knot is snugged tight. When the knot is completed, excess material is cut away, either on the knot if it is to be buried or leaving 3- to 4-mm tails if it is a skin suture.

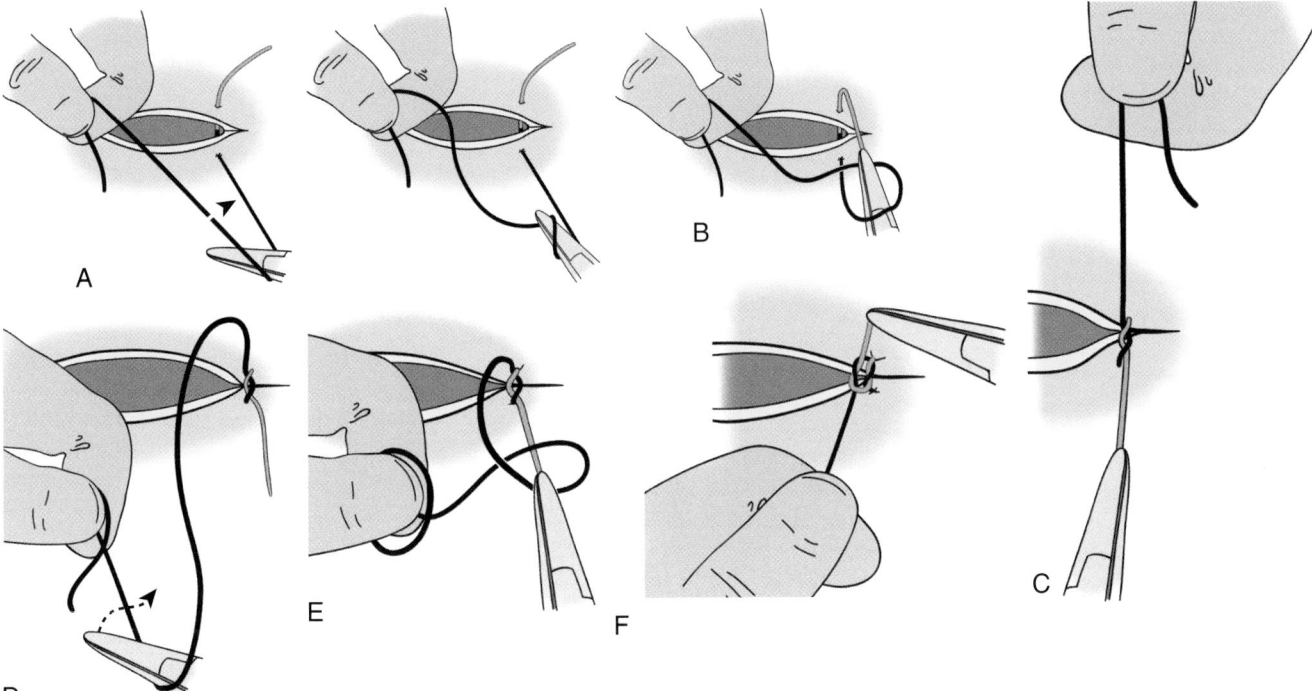

Fig. 22.2 Instrument tie. (A) The first clockwise wrap around the needle holder tip. (B) Grasping the tail. (C) Tensioning the first throw. (D) Counterclockwise wrap for the second throw. (E) Grasping the tail. (F) Tensioning the second throw.

Two-Handed Tie

This version of the two-handed tie presumes that the suture to be tied has been sewn toward you, with the needle on your side of the wound. Following this sequence prevents you from having to cross your hands over the top of the wound, a motion that blocks your vision of the knot being formed.

1. The two-handed tie starts like the instrument tie with the suture being placed in the tissue and being pulled through, but leaving about 10 cm of the tail outside the wound. Grasp the tail in your right hand and the long end in your left hand. Palms are up when initially grasping the strands, which are held between the last three fingers and the palm. To start the knot, grasp the short end between your right index finger and thumb. Use the back of your left thumb to hold the long end as shown. Lay the short end across the side of your left thumb to form a loop (Fig. 22.3A).
2. Drop your left index finger to contact the pad of your left thumb and hold the loop open. Maintaining the pinch, drop the loop off your thumb and move down to pinch the short end (Fig. 22.3B), leaving your left index finger inside the loop. Push the free end up through the loop with our left thumb by extending your left wrist (Fig. 22.3C). Release the free end from your right hand and regrasp it as it is pulled through the loop. This same maneuver can be redone to make the second twist needed for a surgeon's knot. Draw down the first throw and tighten it evenly by bringing your left hand away from and your right hand toward you (Fig. 22.3D).
3. The second square throw is created by reversing these maneuvers. As you draw the long end back toward you with your left hand, use your left index finger to begin to create a loop. Reach under the short end with your left thumb (Fig. 22.3E) and push your thumb up to hold the side of the loop. Bring your left thumb and index finger together inside the loop (Fig. 22.3F). Lift the short end in your right hand and place it in the pinch of your left thumb and index finger. Push the short end down through the loop with your left index finger, release it from the right hand, and then regrasp it. The second throw is then brought down by

bringing the right hand away and the left hand toward you (Fig. 22.3G). Be careful not to disturb the first throw as this critical second throw is tightened.

4. Additional throws are added as needed by alternating the same process of the first and second throws. Alternating the helix of the throws will keep the knot square. When the knot is completed, excess material is cut away, either on the knot if it is to be buried or leaving 3- to 4-mm tails if it is a skin suture.

Half Blood Knot

It is useful to know one additional knot for tying suture—the half blood knot. Fishermen use this slipping knot to tie lures onto the ends of fishing lines. It is a very strong knot, retaining almost all of the strength of the suture material. The half blood knot is the best knot for securing the beginning of a running suture, particularly with monofilament material. General surgeons commonly use it to secure the beginning of a running suture in the linea alba in closing the abdomen, but it also works well to start a running cuticular or subcuticular suture.

After the suture is placed in the tissue, the tail is passed around the working strand of the suture. Four twists of the tail around itself are made. More than four twists do not add to the strength of the knot. The tail is then passed up through the first loop, parallel to the working strand (Fig. 22.4). The knot is tightened by pulling on the tail with a needle holder, which is then slipped down to secure the tissue. The working end continues on to construct a running suture line.

COMMON ERRORS

- If the first throw of a knot slips loose before the second throw can be tied, additional measures are needed:
- A double helix can be used as the first throw, creating the *surgeon's knot*.
- An absorbable deeper suture can be placed to take tension off of the closure.

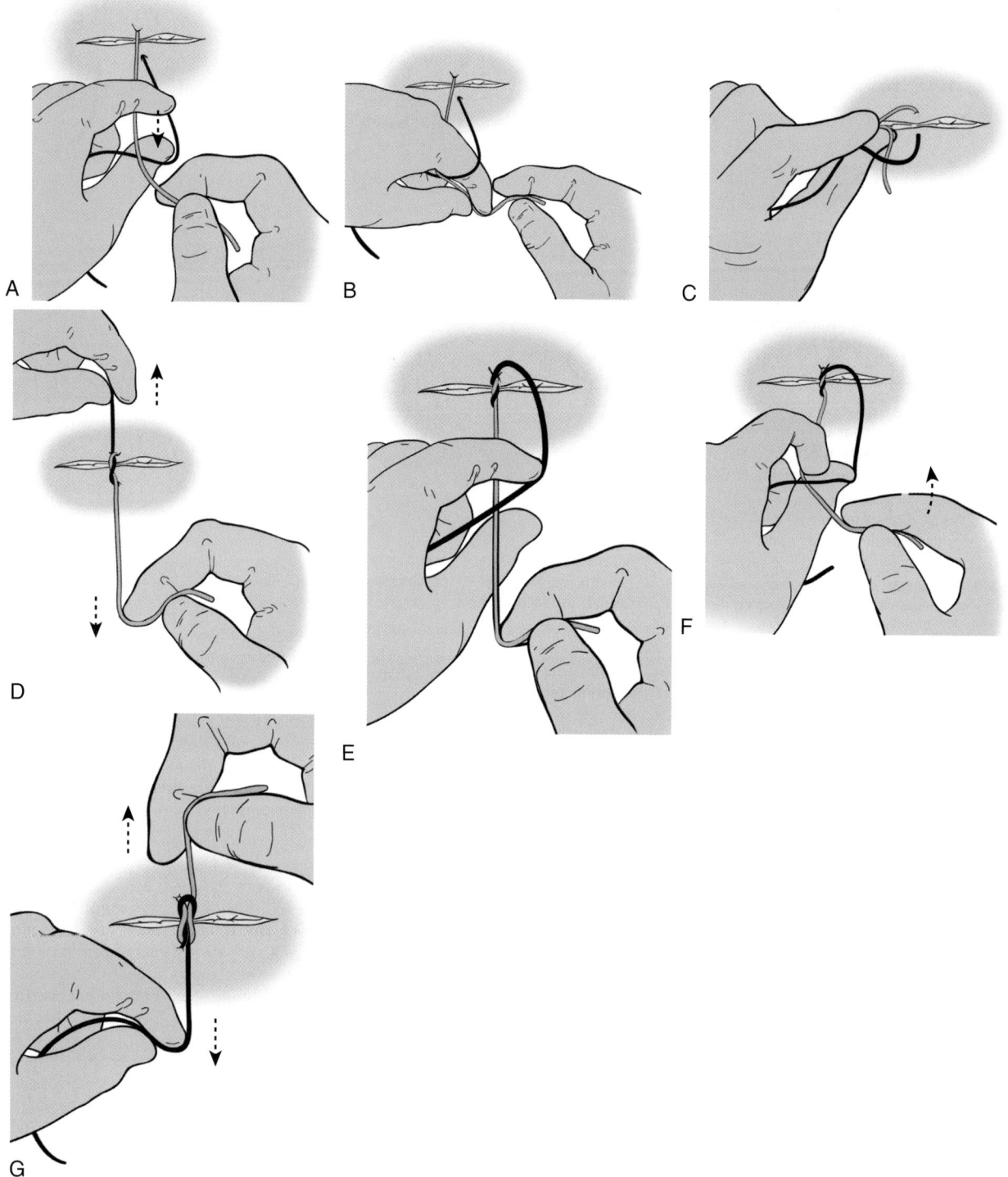

Fig. 22.3   Two-handed tie. (A) Starting position. (B and C) Creating the first throw. (D) Tensioning the first throw. (E and F) Creating the second throw. (G) Tensioning the second throw. (Modified from James JD, Wu MM, Batra EK, et al. Technical considerations in manual and instrument tying techniques. *J Emerg Med*. 1992;10:469–480.)

- The extra hands of an assistant can hold the wound edges together as the suture loop is being tied.
- A "helper" stitch can be placed and later removed. A horizontal mattress suture is placed in the middle of the wound to bring the skin edges partway together. Once the wound has been closed completely, this helper stitch is often loose and can then be removed.
- A series of half hitches is tied rather than locking square knots. To prevent this, the surgeon must apply even tension to both

strands as the knot is tightened rather than holding one strand taut and tightening the other.
- The knot is tied too loosely. This may be caused by two different problems. First, the first throw must be tied tightly enough to just appose the wound edge. Second, the surgeon should not pull tension on either strand as the second throw is tied because this often loosens the first throw.

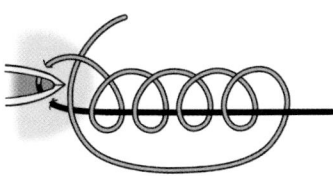

Fig. 22.4 Half blood knot. The tail is passed around the long strand, then it loops four times around itself, and finally the tail is put through the first loop.

- The knot is tied too tightly. As each knot throw is constructed, attention must be given to not strangulating the tissue because this can lead to tissue ischemia and necrosis. The common result of too tight a suture loop is a "railroad track" appearance of the scar when the sutures are removed. It is best to remove and replace an improperly tied suture.

CONCLUSION

Suture tying is an art that develops with experience. Close attention to detail is necessary when one is approximating tissue. The goal is to bring the tissue edges into apposition without causing strangulation inside the loop as postoperative swelling develops. The instrument tie is preferred for skin sutures. If a hand tie is to be done, the two-handed technique is preferred. The clinician must tie firm, square throws by using even tension on each end and must know how many throws to place with each type of suture material to ensure knot security.

PATIENT EDUCATION GUIDE

See the patient education form on suture care available at www.expertconsult.com.

SUPPLIERS

The useful *Knot Tying Manual* and "knot tying board" are available free of charge from Ethicon, Inc. (see contact information available at www.expertconsult.com).

ONLINE RESOURCES

Half Blood Knot
https://www.youtube.com/watch?v=cE5jxbNEVkA.
Instrument Tie
http://www.bumc.bu.edu/surgery/training/technical-training/instrument-tie/.
https://www.youtube.com/watch?v=VmaenFTww9w.
Two-Handed Tie
http://www.bumc.bu.edu/surgery/training/technical-training/two-hand-tie/.
https://www.youtube.com/watch?v=_lvQ2YJ0RjQ.

RECOMMENDED READING

Behm T, Unger JB, Ivy JJ, Mukherjee D. Flat square knots: are 3 throws enough? *Am J Obstet Gynecol.* 2007;197:172.e1–172.e3.

Ethicon Inc. *Wound Closure Manual.* Somerville, NJ: Ethicon, Inc.; 2005. http://www.uphs.upenn.edu/surgery/Education/facilities/measey/Wound_Closure_Manual.pdf

Fong ED, Bartlett AS, Malak S, Anderson IA. Tensile strength of surgical knots in abdominal wound closure. *Aust N Z J Surg.* 2008;78:164–166.

Kim JC, Lee YK, Lim BS, et al. Comparison of tensile and knot security properties of surgical sutures. *J Mater Sci Mater Med.* 2007;18:2363–2369.

Lammers RL, Smith ZE. Methods of wound closure. In: Roberts JR, Custalow CB, Thomsen TW, eds. *Roberts and Hedges Clinical Procedures in Emergency Medicine.* 6th ed. Philadelphia: Elsevier; 2014:655–669.

Reichman EF, Powell C. Basic wound closure techniques. In: Reichman EF, ed. *Emergency Medicine Procedures.* 2nd ed. New York: McGraw-Hill; 2013.

Scott DJ, Goova MT, Tesfay ST. A cost-effective proficiency-based knot-tying and suturing curriculum for residency programs. *J Surg Res.* 2007;141:7–15.

CHAPTER 23

Nail Plate, Nail Bed, and Nail Matrix Biopsy

Steven E. Roskos

Nail biopsy is a simple procedure that can be used to diagnose tumors, inflammatory diseases, and infections of the nail. *Nail plate* biopsy is the simplest of the nail biopsies and is useful for diagnosing proximal subungual onychomycosis, as well as distinguishing melanoma from other types of nail pigmentation. *Nail bed* biopsy is helpful in diagnosing many disorders, including psoriasis, lichen planus, squamous cell carcinoma, melanoma, and subungual epidermoid inclusions. *Nail matrix* biopsy is used to distinguish between benign pigmented streaks (longitudinal melanonychia) and melanoma.

The presence of melanocytes in the germinal tissue of the nail matrix makes this a possible site for development of melanoma. Primary subungual melanomas frequently appear as pigmented bands or streaks in the nail plate, and they account for up to 3.5% of all cutaneous malignant melanomas (15% to 20% in blacks). Distinguishing between the numerous benign causes of pigmented streaks (trauma, malnutrition, and normal occurrence in many blacks and Asians) and malignant lesions is frequently difficult. Biopsy is often recommended to confirm the diagnosis.

ANATOMY

The *nail plate* is the hard, translucent structure composed of keratinized squamous cells, commonly called the "nail" itself. The *nail bed* refers to the softer tissue beneath the nail that provides germinal tissue for the nail plate and to which the nail plate is attached (Fig. 23.1). The nail matrix lies beneath the proximal nail fold and synthesizes 90% of the nail plate (see Chapter 24, Nail Bed Repair, for a more thorough discussion of nail bed anatomy).

INDICATIONS

- Thickened, distorted nail plate with a negative evaluation for fungal infection (potassium hydroxide [KOH] scraping, culture)

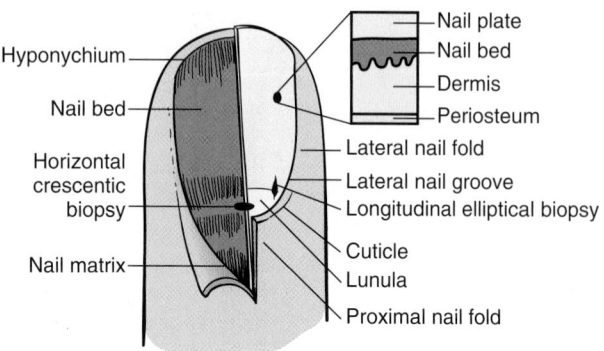

Fig. 23.1   Anatomy of the nail, dorsal view. Also shows possible shapes for obtaining a nail biopsy. For more anatomic details, see Chapter 24, Nail Bed Repair.

- Longitudinal pigmented linear streak in the nail plate suspicious for malignancy
- Tumor of the nail bed
- Subungual hyperkeratosis
- Diagnosis of disorders such as psoriasis and lichen planus

CONTRAINDICATIONS

- Allergy or sensitivity to local anesthetics (see Chapter 5, Local Anesthesia)
- Bleeding diathesis or uncontrolled anticoagulation therapy (there is no routine need to stop anticoagulants [warfarin, factor Xa inhibitors], aspirin, or clopidogrel)

EQUIPMENT

- Antiseptic (chlorhexidine, povidone-iodine, or alcohol)
- Sterile gloves
- 3-mm disposable skin biopsy punch
- Local anesthetic (e.g., 1% or 2% lidocaine) *without* epinephrine
- 27-gauge needle (for toes) or 30-gauge needle (for fingers)
- Sterile scissors with straight blades (or a narrow Locke periosteal elevator)
- Sterile rubber band, small Penrose drain, or Ellman disposable digit tourniquet
- Two sterile, straight hemostats
- 5-0 or 6-0 nylon suture
- Needle driver
- Suture scissors
- Tissue forceps
- No. 15 scalpel
- Periosteal elevator (for nail bed and matrix biopsy)
- Fine sterile scissors with curved blades (for nail bed and matrix biopsy)
- Steri-Strips (for nail matrix biopsy)
- Sterile gauze and tubular gauze dressing
- Antibiotic ointment (Bacitracin or Polysporin)
- Adhesive bandage or an adhesive wrap such as Coban or CoFlex tape
- Sterile specimen container filled with 10% formalin (for histology)
- Sterile specimen container without formalin (for fungal culture)

PRECAUTIONS

When sampling the nail matrix, be careful not to damage the proximal matrix. Most linear melanomas (95%) originate from the distal matrix. Biopsies of the distal nail matrix are very unlikely to produce permanent scarring because this part of the matrix produces the ventral portion of the nail plate. Biopsies of the proximal nail matrix will usually cause a permanent nail plate abnormality in the form of a longitudinal fissure. For pigmented streaks less than 3 mm wide, punch biopsy as described in this chapter is an adequate technique. Larger lesions require more extensive excision and are more likely to cause nail deformity.

PREPROCEDURE PATIENT EDUCATION

It is important to explain to the patient what information you hope to gain from the biopsy and how it will affect treatment decisions. Explain that a biopsy is not guaranteed to produce an accurate diagnosis. Describe the procedure in detail, including the anesthesia. Make sure the patient understands the risks, which include bleeding, distortion of the nail during regrowth, infection, onycholysis (separation of nail from nail bed), permanent nail abnormality, and scarring. The patient should be given an opportunity to read the patient education handout and the consent form before signing it (see patient education and patient consent forms available at www.expertconsult.com).

TECHNIQUE

Nail Plate (Nail) Biopsy

1. Soak the affected digit and nail in warm water for 10 minutes to soften the nail plate.
2. With steady pressure, hold the punch perpendicular to the nail; rotation of the punch will produce a round biopsy specimen without pain. No anesthetic is required.
3. Elevate the biopsy sample, and lyse it from the underlying nail bed tissue with the scissors or scalpel.
4. Place the specimen in a sterile container if it is being sent for fungal culture, or a formalin-filled container if it is being sent for histology or periodic–acid Schiff (PAS) staining.

Nail Bed Biopsy

1. Soak the digit in warm water for 10 minutes to soften the nail plate.
2. Prepare the patient's hand with antiseptic.

3. Perform a digital ring block (Fig. 23.2) or distal wing block (see Chapter 7, Peripheral Nerve Blocks and Field Blocks) using 2% lidocaine without epinephrine.
4. Apply a tourniquet proximally to decrease bleeding at the site and allow easier removal of specimen. The tourniquet can be placed over the ring block and, if placed tightly enough, can provide further anesthesia by placing compression on the digital nerves. Allow time for the anesthetic to take effect.
5. Partially remove the nail plate according to the procedure outlined in Chapter 194, Ingrown Toenails.
6. When the affected nail bed has been exposed, use a 3- or 4-mm punch to obtain the biopsy specimen as close as possible to the proximal origin of the pigmentation. However, there is a higher chance of a deformed nail if the biopsy is obtained from the root portion of the nail under the proximal nail fold. The biopsy specimen should be 2 to 3 mm in thickness. Alternatively, small elliptical excisions can be made (see Fig. 23.1 and Chapter 26, Skin Biopsy).
7. Close the biopsy site with one or two 5-0 or 6-0 nylon sutures oriented along the longitudinal plane.
8. Remove the tourniquet.
9. Apply a dressing of antibiotic ointment and sterile gauze.

Nail Matrix Biopsy

1. Soak the digit in warm water for 10 minutes to soften the nail plate.
2. Prepare the patient's hand with antiseptic.
3. Perform a digital ring block using lidocaine without epinephrine (see Fig. 23.2).
4. Apply a tourniquet proximally to decrease bleeding at the site and allow easier removal of the specimen. The tourniquet can be placed over the ring block and if placed tightly enough, can provide further anesthesia by placing compression on the digital nerves. Allow time for the anesthetic to take effect.
5. Make two lateral incisions in the proximal nail fold at an angle of 45 degrees using a no. 15 scalpel (Fig. 23.3).
6. Use a periosteal elevator to detach the proximal nail fold from the nail plate. This should expose the entire nail plate and allow you to visualize the origin of the pigmented streak (longitudinal melanonychia). The nail plate can be left in place (Fig. 23.4) or reflected (see Fig. 23.3).

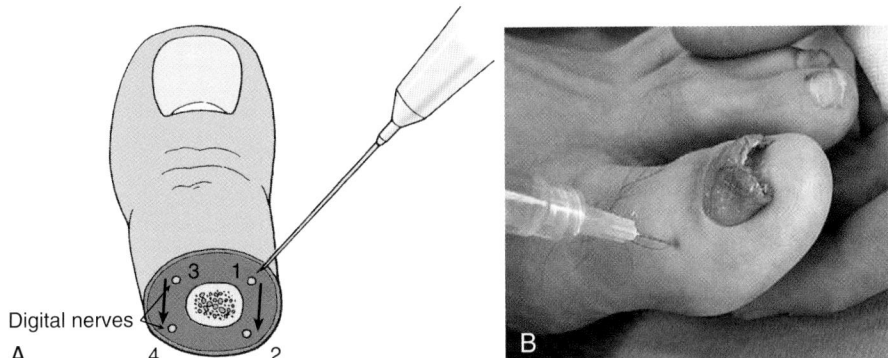

Fig. 23.2 (A) Ring block technique for digital nerve block. *1,* Raise a wheal at the dorsal surface of the base of the digit. *2,* Direct the needle toward the plantar surface, delivering 1 mL of anesthetic to the extensor and 1 mL to the plantar branches of the digital nerve. *3,* Perform a second puncture at the corresponding site of the other side. *4,* Advance the needle in the plantar direction to allow delivery of 1 mL of anesthetic to each branch of the digital nerve. A minimum of 4 mL of anesthetic is used. Also see Chapter 7, Peripheral Nerve Blocks and Field Blocks. (B) Administering a distal wing block. Insert needle 5 to 8 mm proximal and lateral to the junction of the proximal nail fold and lateral nail fold. Inject anesthetic until it progresses as far as possible down the nail fold toward the tip of the digit, distending and blanching the lateral nail fold. This has the appearance of a "wing." Repeat on the other side of the nail. If necessary, inject at other already anesthetized areas around the nail until the entire digital tip is swollen and white.

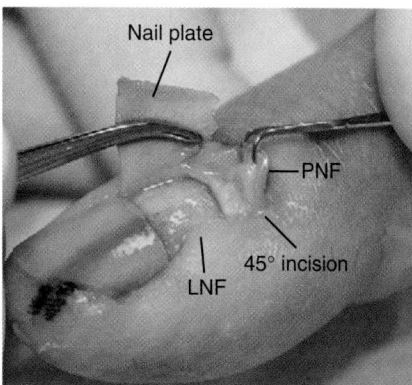

Fig. 23.3 Proximal nail fold (PNF) is reflected (with skin hook) and proximal nail plate is partially avulsed and reflected (with hemostat), exposing the nail matrix. The nail plate can be reattached with nylon sutures to the lateral nail fold (LNF).

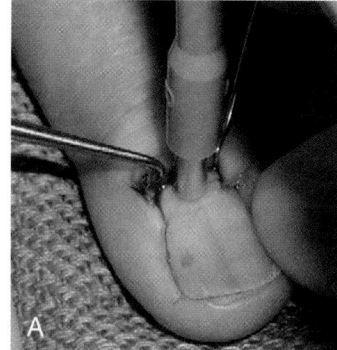 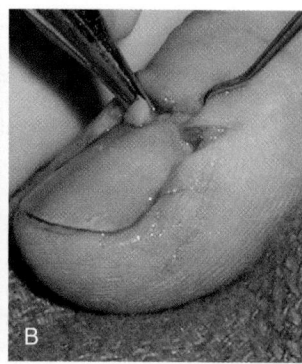

Fig. 23.4 (A) Nail matrix biopsy with nail plate in place. The proximal nail fold is reflected (with skin hooks, optional) while punch is held perpendicular to nail plate over origin of linear pigmentation (nail plate has not been reflected in this figure). Scarring is more likely to occur if the germinal matrix is sampled. (B) Removing punch sample. Gently lyse adhesions to the bone using fine curved scissors, held nearly perpendicular to the nail plate.

7. Place a 3-mm punch against and perpendicular to the nail plate directly over the origin of the pigmented streak (see Fig. 23.4A).
8. Rotate the punch between the thumb and forefinger.
9. After scoring the nail, check to be sure the origin of the band is entirely encompassed by the punch.
10. Reapply the punch and continue to rotate until you contact bone.
11. Gently lyse adhesions to the bone using fine curved scissors (see Fig. 23.4B).
12. Gently remove the specimen using the scissors or tissue forceps, and place the whole specimen, including nail plate (which may be stuck inside the punch), in the formalin-filled specimen container. *Be careful not to crush the specimen.*
13. Apply Steri-Strips to the two lateral incisions and the defect in the nail plate.
14. Remove the tourniquet.
15. Dress the site as described in the next section.

The possible shapes and types of biopsies are summarized in Fig. 23.5.

POSTPROCEDURE MANAGEMENT

1. Apply topical astringent (e.g., Monsel solution) before removing the tourniquet, and control bleeding with pressure, if needed.
2. Place a bulky dressing of gauze over the surgical site (except for nail plate biopsy, where a simple adhesive bandage may be applied over antibiotic ointment). Use multiple 2 × 2 gauze pads, folded in half and wrapped over the nail transversely and longitudinally. Secure these tightly with tape or adhesive dressing to create a pressure dressing.
3. Observe the patient for 10 to 15 minutes. If blood soaks through the bandage, apply pressure to the lateral digital arteries and remove the bandage. Apply a clean, dry gauze pressure dressing while holding pressure on the arteries.

POSTPROCEDURE PATIENT EDUCATION

The patient should keep the limb elevated until the next day to decrease throbbing. Acetaminophen or ibuprofen may be used for pain. If the patient experiences increasing pain several hours after the procedure, the dressing may be acting as a tourniquet and should be removed. Otherwise, the patient should leave the dressing in place for 24 to 48 hours, after which he or she may remove the dressing, wash the wound with a 1:1 mixture of hydrogen peroxide and tap water or simple soap and water, and apply a large adhesive bandage over gauze and antibiotic ointment. After the first 24 hours, wash only with soap and water. The patient should repeat this procedure two to three times daily until the area has healed.

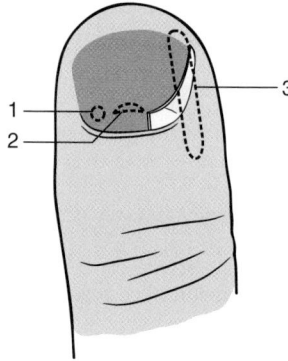

Fig. 23.5 Alternative biopsy techniques. *1,* Punch biopsy of nail matrix; *2,* transverse biopsy of nail matrix, used for longitudinal pigmented streaks between 3 and 6 mm; *3,* longitudinal nail biopsy for lateral nail pigmentation.

NAIL BIOPSY ENCOUNTER FORM

See Encounter Form, Nail Biopsy, available at www.expertconsult.com.

COMPLICATIONS

- Bleeding
- Infection
- Distortion of nail with regrowth and permanent nail abnormality (the greatest concern if the germinal matrix is sampled)
- Onycholysis (separation of the nail plate from the nail bed)
- Scarring

PATIENT EDUCATION FORMS

See patient education and consent forms available at www.expertconsult.com.

CPT/BILLING CODES

11730 Avulsion of nail plate, partial or single
11732 Avulsion, each additional
11755 Biopsy of nail unit (e.g., plate, bed, matrix, hyponychum, proximal and lateral folds)
11765 Wedge excision of skin of nail fold (e.g., for ingrown toenail)

ICD-10 Diagnostic Codes

B35.1	Dermatophytosis nail (tinea unguium)
B48.8	Other specified mycosis
B49	Unspecified mycosis
I60.0	Ingrowing nail
I60.1	Onycholysis
I60.2	Onychogryphosis
I60.3	Nail dystrophy
I60.4	Beaus lines
I60.8	Other nail disorders
I03.011	Cellulitis right finger
I03.012	Cellulitis left finger
I03.019	Cellulitis unspec toe
I03.031	Cellulitis right finger
I03.032	Cellulitis left finger
I03.039	Cellulitis unspec finger

See Appendix G: Neoplasm, Skin: ICD-10 Codes for neoplasm table.

Online Resources

Onumah N, Scher RK. Nail surgery. eMedicine. http://www.emedicine.com/derm/topic818.htm.

Sinni-McKeehen B, Rich P. Fungal nail infections: Treating from head to toe. http://medscape.com/viewarticle/470942_19.

Recommended Reading

André J, Lateur N. Pigmented nail disorders. *Dermatol Clin.* 2006;24:329–339.

Braun RP, Baran R, Le Gal FA, et al. Diagnosis and management of nail pigmentations. *J Am Acad Dermatol.* 2007;56:835–847.

Haneke E, Baran R. Longitudinal melanonychia. *Dermatol Surg.* 2001;27:580.

Jellinek N. Nail matrix biopsy of longitudinal melanonychia: diagnostic algorithm including the matrix shave biopsy. *J Am Acad Dermatol.* 2007;56:803–810.

Jellinek NJ. Nail surgery: practical tips and treatment options. *Dermatol Ther.* 2007;20:68–74.

Rich P. Nail surgery. In: Bolognia JL, Jorizzo JL, Schaffer JV, eds. *Dermatology.* 3rd ed. New York: Elsevier; 2012.

Richert B. Basic nail surgery. *Dermatol Clin.* 2006;24:313–322.

Usatine RP, Smith MA, Mayeaux EJ. *The Color Atlas of Family Medicine.* 2nd ed. New York: McGraw-Hill; 2013.

CHAPTER 24

NAIL BED REPAIR

John Eckhold

The fingernail is a highly evolved structure designed to enhance the functions of the distal finger. The fingernail functions to (1) protect the distal phalanx, (2) enhance fine touch and fine digital movements, (3) facilitate scratching and grooming, and (4) provide aesthetic and cosmetic detailing.

Any disruption of the normal anatomy distal to the tendinous insertions of the extensor and deep flexor tendons on the finger or the thumb may adversely influence the growth, configuration, quality, and function of the nail plate unit. Sometimes a crushing injury with no penetration of the nail may cause more disfigurement than a sharp penetration, which may extend through the nail to the underlying phalanx. A good primary repair of the injured nail bed yields a high percentage of good results. Meanwhile, the results of excessively delayed repairs and revisions of faulty repairs have a much poorer prognosis. A severely deformed fingernail can be a source of embarrassment or functional impairment.

Consideration for repair includes (1) a thorough anatomic knowledge of the structure to be restored; (2) availability of all the sterile equipment required (including excellent lighting and magnification); (3) the ability to counsel the patient on what to expect over the 6 to 12 months of follow-up that will be required to see the final nail growth; and (4) the ability to recognize those injuries that may exceed the clinician's training and experience, requiring referral to a hand surgeon.

Informing the patient *before* any repair effort that the resultant fingernail may be deformed or absent in spite of best efforts spares the clinician and the patient much grief in the end. Preoperative (close-up) photographs provide documentation of the severity of the injury. Patients sometimes forget what the clinician had to start with and instead recall only how wonderful the fingernail looked before the injury, expecting the clinician to replicate the preinjury status.

ANATOMY

The nail unit is composed of four distinct epithelial structures: the *proximal nail fold, germinal matrix, sterile matrix,* and *hyponychium* (Fig. 24.1). The *lateral nail folds* (Fig. 24.2) are adjacent normal epidermal folds that border the nail unit laterally. The proximal nail fits into a groove of tissue, a virtual space, termed the *proximal nail fold.* The skin over the dorsum of the nail fold is the *nail wall.* The *eponychium* is the fold of skin cells that produce the *cuticle,* the thin membrane of dead cells extending from the nail wall onto the dorsum of the nail. The *lunula* is the curved, white opacity in the nail, just distal to the eponychium. It is the indicator of the junction between the germinal and sterile matrix. The *germinal matrix* is the most important component of the nail unit because it is responsible for the formation of the nail plate. A detailed anatomic understanding of the perionychial components of the nail area is required for consideration of nail repairs. The components are as follows:

1. *Nail plate (nail).* Formation begins in the germinal matrix under the proximal nail fold. It is made up of desiccated, keratinized, squamous cells. Note how the nail plate fits into the groove of the proximal nail fold (see Fig. 24.1).

2. *Nail bed.* This lies under the nail plate, beginning at the proximal edge of the nail matrix and continuing until the hyponychium. It is very vascular and thus appears pink. The space between the nail bed and underlying bony structure is very thin (1 to 3 mm) without any subcutaneous tissue. The nail bed consists of the following:
   - The *eponychium,* which includes the dorsal roof of the proximal fold, is adherent to the nail and serves as protection for the underlying germinal matrix and provides a thin layer of cells producing the shiny dorsal nail surface
   - The *germinal matrix,* where nail production begins and which extends distally just beyond the eponychium to end at the distal border of the lunula
   - The *sterile matrix,* described by some observers as the "road bed" for the advancing nail, and which adds squamous cells to thicken the nail and enhance its adherence to the nail bed

NOTE: The sterile matrix is the distal portion of the nail bed, beyond the germinal matrix. The germinal matrix serves as the nail origin; the sterile matrix only adds to the nail thickness.

3. *Hyponychium.* The distal site where the nail separates from the nail matrix. This area allows the nail to become independent of the nail matrix.
4. *Paronychium.* Consists of the lateral nail folds and adjacent cutaneous portions of the lateral nail borders.
5. *Lateral nail folds.* Epithelium bordering the nail laterally.
6. *Cuticle.* The translucent vein of tissue that extends out to the surface of the nail where it emerges from beneath the proximal nail fold. It acts as a barrier or seal to protect the nail unit from external irritants and seals the proximal nail fold to the nail.

PHYSIOLOGY

Nail formation occurs in three layers. The *dorsal* layer arises from the dorsal roof of the nail fold, the *intermediate* layer from the ventral floor and the lateral walls of the proximal nail, and the *ventral* layer from the sterile matrix of the nail bed. The ventral layer provides adherence and enhances the nail thickness to compensate for wearing away on the dorsal surface. The nail grows distally as a result of the force of the pressure placed on the growing cell mass beneath the proximal nail fold. The resultant nail advances distally, hugging the underlying nail bed. Any distortion of these anatomic templates (e.g., proximal nail fold, nail matrix contour and composition) can lead to a deformed and unattractive nail.

Full-length fingernail growth takes 4 to 6 months and is frequently suspended completely for 3 weeks after an acute traumatic event. Fingernails reportedly grow four times as rapidly as toenails. Peak nail growth rate occurs at approximately 30 years of age.

FRACTURES

An x-ray examination must be performed on any crush, impact, or penetrating injury for possible involvement of the distal phalanx.

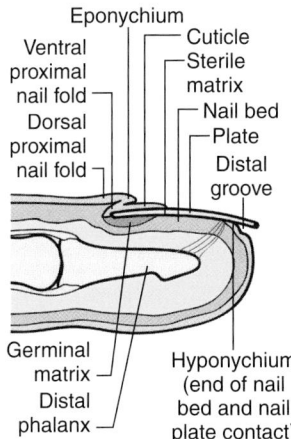

Fig. 24.1 Sagittal view of the nail and distal phalanx.

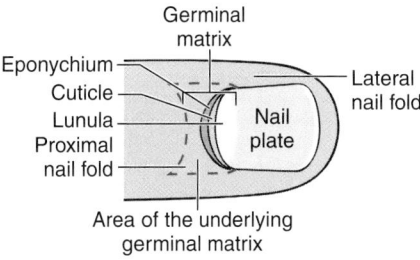

Fig. 24.2 Dorsal view of the nail. The sterile matrix underlies the nail plate distal to the lunula (proximal to the lunula is the germinal matrix) under the nail plate.

This helps to avoid missing a fracture that may deform the nail bed if left unreduced or unstable. Fractures accompanied by bleeding from under or around the nail plate, including a drained subungual hematoma, automatically become open fractures and must be treated with the appropriate caution and care. Fractures may require reduction and internal fixation before nail bed repair. Proximal nail bed injuries or avulsions in children are often open Salter epiphyseal fractures of the distal phalanx and should be treated appropriately.

SUBUNGUAL HEMATOMA

See Chapter 193, Subungual Hematoma Evacuation.

The nail bed is a highly vascular area subject to bleeding with either sharp or nonpenetrating blunt trauma. To release the painful smaller hematoma, first cleanse the finger with povidone-iodine solution for several minutes (no anesthesia is required if the nail plate does not need to be removed). Use of a heated (red-hot) paper clip, drill, or microcautery releases the underlying pressure with minimal discomfort. The heated tip passes through the nail with minimal pressure and is cooled by the hematoma, thus not causing injury to the nail bed. The hole should be at least 2 mm in diameter to allow drainage to continue and not seal up when clot forms. If the nail is to be removed to inspect and possibly repair the nail bed, do not place the hole in the nail until the location of the repair site is known. After nail bed repair, the vent hole should *not* overlay the repair site directly to achieve maximal contouring effect from the replaced nail plate.

If the trauma produces a large hematoma suspected of causing a significant nail bed injury, some experts suggest the nail should be removed to facilitate meticulous magnified inspection and careful repair of the nail bed. The prerequisites for inspection include (1) good anesthesia, (2) good light and magnification, (3) essential sterile equipment, (4) sterile saline for irrigation, and (5) adequate retraction assistance to carefully investigate the area deep to the proximal and lateral nail folds.

EQUIPMENT

- Surgical loupes or appropriate magnification providing 2.5× magnification or greater
- Freer septum elevator, Kutz periosteal elevator or small Key elevator (all three may be needed for significant repairs)
- English nail splitter
- Small bone rongeur
- Single- and double-pronged skin hooks
- No. 11 or 15 surgical blade and handles
- Small cuticle scissors
- Needle holders
- Suture scissors
- 0.375-inch Penrose drain or finger tourniquet
- Small hemostats (2)
- 6-0 and 7-0 absorbable suture (gut, chromic or white Vicryl)
- 5-0 and 6-0 monofilament (nylon) suture
- Silicone sheeting (0.020-inch thick)
- Petrolatum gauze
- Antibiotic ointment (e.g., Neosporin)
- Small syringe and 30-gauge needle
- Lidocaine 1% to 2% plain (generally no epinephrine in the fingers; however, see the discussions in Chapter 5, Local Anesthesia, and Chapter 6, Local and Topical Anesthetic Complications)
- Adson pickups, with and without teeth
- Finger dressing material, small metal splints, and arm sling for postoperative elevation

NAIL PLATE AVULSION (SURGICAL)

EDITOR'S NOTE: Some experts suggest that for a simple subungual hematoma, if the nail is firmly adherent and disruption of the surrounding tissue is minimal, even in the presence of a tuft fracture, there is no indication to remove the nail to search for nail bed laceration. Despite the presence of a nail bed laceration, a good result can be expected as long as the tissue is held in anatomic approximation by the intact fingernail (see Lammers and Smith).

Other experts suggest that the nail must be removed when there is a large subungual hematoma or when the nail bed injury/laceration is directly visualized or strongly suspected (e.g., there is avulsion of the distal nail from the hyponychium or proximally from the eponychium; see also the Editor's Note after the Recommended Readings). Verify at this time if there is (1) displaced, unstable phalangeal fracture (requiring fixation); (2) large nail bed avulsion (with missing tissue requiring nail bed grafts); or (3) significant distal amputation of tissue (requiring some type of graft for closure). Consider early referral of the injury if it exceeds personal training, experience, or comfort level.

Exploration of the nail bed can be completed under general anesthesia, scalene block, axillary block, Bier block, or digital block (see Chapter 9, Bier Block, and Chapter 7, Peripheral Nerve Blocks and Field Blocks). The first four can be used with an arm tourniquet and additional sedation as required for longer procedures in which multiple digits are involved. Uncooperative adults and restless children may be managed better with the use of a more formal type of anesthetic setting. Practitioners prefer to save the patients any additional anesthetic charges, if possible, but their desire to economize should not compromise the examination or repair in any way when the patient is being uncooperative and moving about during a delicate repair under magnification.

After anesthesia is achieved, the surgical field is prepared and draped in the usual manner to ensure sterility of the surgical field. At this time, if no other form of tourniquet is in use, a digital tourniquet can be established by use of a sterile 0.375-inch Penrose drain

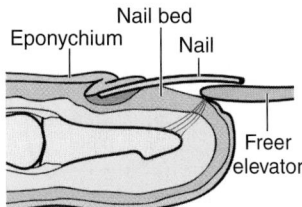

Fig. 24.3 Freer elevator placed under the nail. The nail bed is made up of the germinal matrix proximal to the lunula and the sterile matrix distally.

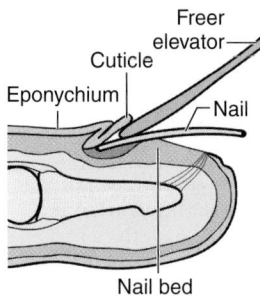

Fig. 24.4 Freer elevator placed under the cuticle.

placed smoothly around the finger and secured with a small hemostat to occlude flow through the digital vessels. Depending on the site of the injury and personal preferences, there are two techniques to remove the nail and visualize the nail bed.

Distal Technique

The Freer elevator is placed under the free edge of the nail (Fig. 24.3) and advanced proximally, following the plane of cleavage between the nail plate and the nail bed. Substantial resistance is encountered along the nail bed until the germinal matrix is reached, where the progress becomes easier. Be careful to avoid advancing the elevator excessively into the proximal nail groove. Now gently work the elevator medially and laterally to free up the last of the soft tissue attachments deep to the nail plate. Place the elevator under the cuticle (on the dorsum of the nail; Fig. 24.4) and dissect under the ventral portion of the proximal nail fold. Continue the dissection laterally on both sides to release any remaining soft tissue attachment while a hemostat is used to apply gentle distal traction, pulling distally. (The goal is to free the nail from any residual soft tissue attachments while not digging too deeply into either the proximal or lateral folds and not worsening any existing trauma.)

Proximal Technique

The proximal approach is often used when a distal cleavage plane cannot be identified because trauma or other pathology (such as onychomycosis) exists. The Freer elevator is placed under the cuticle and advanced to the proximal nail fold and worked to free the proximal and lateral gutters while avoiding damage to the cells in the depth of the folds. Proximal relaxing incisions (Fig. 24.5) facilitate exposure. Advance the elevator to locate the proximal edge of the nail plate. The skin hooks are now used to hold the eponychium folded proximally while the elevator comes over the top, then directed distally just deep to the nail plate as it dissects the plane between the nail plate and the nail bed. Keep the plane of the elevator turned so that the blade conforms as well as possible to the exact curvature of the nail plate in all areas.

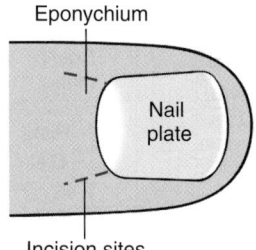

Fig. 24.5 Proximal relaxing incisions are used to facilitate exposure.

GENERAL CONSIDERATIONS FOR REPAIR

When the nail is removed (by the trauma or the surgeon), carefully cleanse the area and examine it with magnification. Make an adequate record of the status of the entire nail bed, the proximal and lateral nail folds, and the hyponychium. Record these findings as part of the operative findings of the distal phalanx.

Carefully scrape any residual nail bed tissue off the nail undersurface, and place the nail in sterile saline to soak while the nail bed is examined. With the tourniquet inflated, cleanse and lavage the nail bed. With excellent light and magnification, the defects can be identified and any gross irregularities trimmed while leaving all the tissue that can be repaired and contoured.

The best sutures for nail bed repair are absorbable 6-0 or 7-0 gut, chromic or Vicryl. Alternatively, the nail bed may be repaired using skin glue (e.g., Dermabond). Strauss and colleagues (2008) studied 40 consecutive patients with acute nail bed lacerations, and there was no statistically significant difference in physician-judged or patient-perceived cosmetic outcome, pain, or functional ability between repairs using skin glue versus 6-0 chromic suture. The skin glue also had a shorter average time of repair.

Either a 4-0 or 5-0 monofilament suture is used to repair lacerations or incisions in the skin.

Sometimes the germinal matrix and nail bed may be avulsed from their proximal origin below the proximal fold. When this occurs, use of a monofilament (5-0 or 6-0) horizontal mattress suture (Fig. 24.6) restores the anatomy.

After repair of the nail bed, replace the nail. The nail serves as a stent to keep the nail folds open and to approximate the edges of the repair. If the germinal matrix has been repaired and the nail used as stent to keep nail folds open (see Fig. 24.6), the nail will already have a proximal horizontal mattress suture attaching it to the finger. The nail is finally stabilized by the placement of a 5-0 or 6-0 monofilament suture through the distal nail into the fingertip area (Fig. 24.7). If the nail was merely avulsed from the distal aspect, anchoring it with a distal monofilament suture to the distal phalanx may prevent further injury to the area. This suture will have to be removed in a few weeks to months as the nail grows out.

If the nail is not available or is damaged too badly to use as a stent, alternative materials may be used to provide contouring and protection to the nail bed. Materials such as medical-grade silicone sheeting (0.020 inch), petrolatum gauze, or Xeroform can be shaped to approximate the original nail (see Figs. 24.6 and 24.7). They must be placed carefully so that they occupy the space of the proximal and lateral nail folds to prevent them from permanently scarring down. These stents must be anchored by a 6-0 monofilament or similar suture through the proximal portion of the nail folds to ensure their position. Placing a distal suture through the distal stent to the fingertip area will further stabilize it. These stents will (1) protect the nail bed while healing, (2) maintain the contour of the nail bed and subsequent nail plate, and (3) prevent adherence of the proximal nail fold to the matrix.

Avoid making the postoperative dressing too tight. Instruct the patient to elevate the hand at all times. If nonadherent gauze is used as a stent on the nail bed to hold open the nail folds, the sutures may

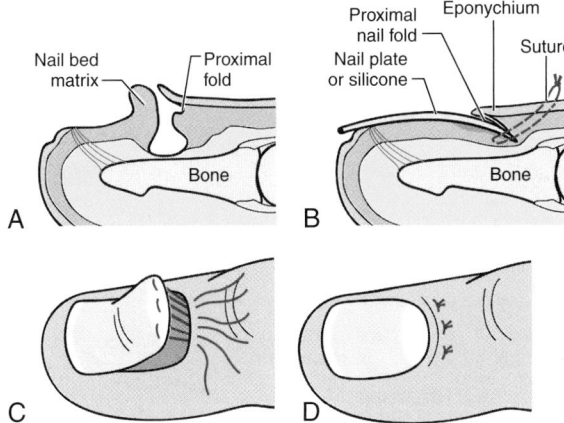

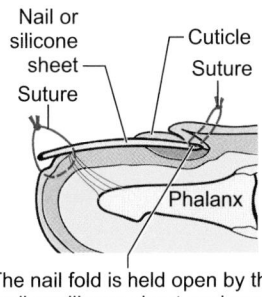

The nail fold is held open by the nail or silicone sheet anchored by the horizontal mattress suture

Fig. 24.7 Replacement of the nail or substitute. The nail fold is held open to prevent it from scarring down when the nail bed has been avulsed or severely damaged. The nail itself or a silicone sheet is anchored by the horizontal mattress suture. A distal suture through the nail and fingertip will prevent the nail or silicon sheet from popping up.

- Avulsed segment available for repair (see Fig. 24.8E)
- Small avulsion (<2 mm width)
- Large avulsion that requires a split- or full-thickness graft from adjacent finger or toe donor site

Treatment Guidelines

Type I injuries often go untreated or may benefit from decompression of the hematoma if throbbing pain occurs when the hematoma is small (see Chapter 193, Subungual Hematoma Evacuation).

According to some experts, *type II* injuries involve nail removal and suture repair of the nail matrix. Replace the nail plate as a template into the proximal and lateral nail folds, and anchor with 5-0 nylon sutures through the distal nail and hyponychium to prevent accidental removal (Fig. 24.9).

A careful search of the nail fragments should be undertaken to find segments of nail bed that can then be removed carefully with a small elevator and reattached to the nail bed as a free graft to reapproximate the original undamaged nail bed. Again, the intact nail plate or the silicone sheet is used to contour and protect the nail bed during the healing stage.

With *type III* injuries, remove the nail. Stabilize unstable or displaced fractures with small C-wires. Repair the viable matrix with absorbable suture, and replace the nail for splinting (Fig. 24.10). If the nail is unavailable or unusable, create a template from sterile silicone sheeting (0.020 inch) and secure in the place of the nail plate.

If the fracture is nondisplaced at the time of the x-ray examination but is so unstable when examined surgically that it cannot be trusted to remain in anatomic position, it must be stabilized with C-wire fixation. Any inadvertent displacement of the dorsal phalangeal cortex during the healing leads to nail bed irregularities and resultant deformed fingernails. The previous principles of repair apply, and serial radiographs are required to verify position of bone fragments and to observe for evidence of osteomyelitis. As in other open fractures, prophylactic antibiotics are required until indication of proper wound healing is demonstrated.

With *type IV* injuries, remove the nail and carefully repair the epithelial fragments. This may involve trimming some severely traumatized fragments with very minimal debridement because the nail plate will hold the fragments down into a vascular bed and contour them to heal with the nail bed.

For *type V* injuries, perform the following:

- With an available avulsed segment, carefully remove it from the nail plate and reattach it to the nail bed with a 6-0 or 7-0 absorbable suture.
- Small avulsions (<2 mm wide) may be closed primarily if the nail bed can be undermined with a small elevator and the tissue closed without tension using a 6-0 or 7-0 absorbable suture.

Fig. 24.6 Proximal nail bed avulsion. The nail plate has been removed. The *nail bed* consists of the germinal and the sterile matrix. The *matrix* extends from a point just distal to the insertion of the extensor tendon to the end of the fingernail attachment. The *germinal matrix*, which produces most of the nail, begins just 3 to 5 mm proximal and deep to the *eponychium* and extends distally to the lunula. The *lunula* is the white portion of the germinal matrix just beyond the *cuticle*. It marks the end of that portion of the germinal matrix that produces the fingernail. The *sterile matrix* begins proximally at the distal edge of the lunula and extends distally to the *hyponychium*. It also plays some role in production of the nail. The *eponychium* is the flap or tuft of skin that covers over the proximal nail. (A) Nail bed has been avulsed from its normal location and displaced dorsally. (B) Side view, horizontal mattress suture through the nail wall is used to anchor the nail bed into proper site for healing. Proximal nail fold must be held open (with fingernail or substitute) to prevent scarring down and closure of nail fold. The nail plate or silicone sheet has been placed and anchored (with suture) to hold the proximal nail fold open. (C) Same as seen from above. (D) Appearance of wound after suturing. Sutures are removed from the nail in 3 weeks. The replaced nail or silicone sheet will dislodge in 1 to 3 months.

be removed at 7 to 10 days, and the gauze will subsequently peel off on its own. If the nail plate has been replaced, it will usually come off in approximately 3 weeks. Explain to the patient that the fingernail will require 6 to 12 months to grow out and to allow its final status to be determined. Trim the advancing rough edges to prevent accidental snags.

Classification of Nail Bed Injuries

A *type I* nail bed injury (Fig. 24.8A) is a small hematoma (<30% of visible nail) with no major matrix injury. Any injury that produces a subungual hematoma can be classified as a type I injury, including superficial lacerations of the nail bed.

A *type II* injury (see Fig. 24.8B) is a large hematoma (>30% of visible nail) with a likely matrix injury (e.g., a severe crushing injury). These injuries have a poor prognosis because the fragments are much more difficult to reassemble anatomically, and the viability of this tissue is severely reduced compared with that of simple or stellate lacerations. The need for radiographs to visualize fracture patterns and stability is increasingly important in these more complex injuries. The same general techniques as described previously are used, but more time is spent informing the patient of the poor prognosis and of the likely need for further surgery and possible partial or complete loss of the nail.

A *type III* nail bed injury (see Fig. 24.8C) with or without a hematoma has a phalangeal fracture (distal phalangeal fracture–nail bed lacerations). These fractures may be nondisplaced or displaced and, more important, stable or unstable.

A *type IV* nail bed injury has extensive matrix fragmentation, but the bone is intact. The proximal nail plate may or may not be avulsed from the proximal nail fold (see Fig. 24.8D).

A *type V* nail bed injury, involving matrix avulsion, can be categorized as follows:

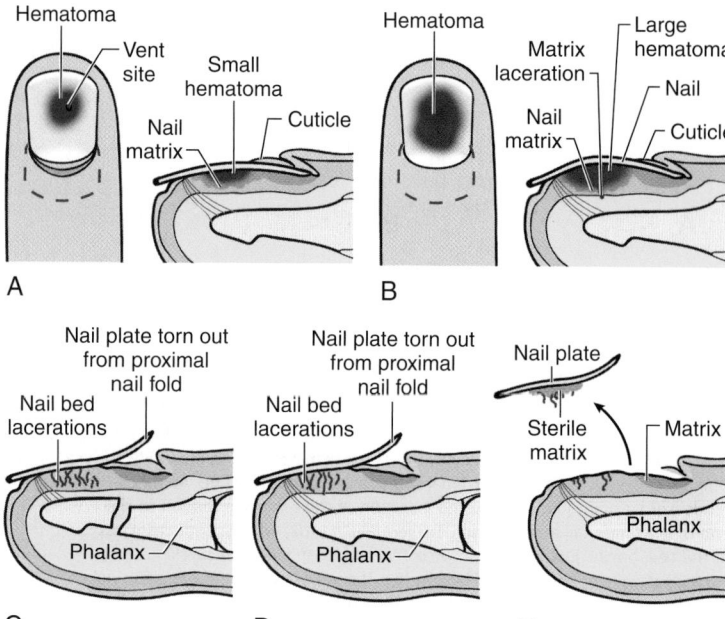

Fig. 24.8 (A) Type I nail bed injury: small hematoma. (B) Type II nail bed injury: large hematoma (>30%) with likely matrix injury. (C) Type III nail bed injury with phalangeal fracture. (D) Type IV nail bed injury: extensive matrix injury with intact phalanx. (E) Type V nail bed injury with matrix avulsion. This particular matrix avulsion shows an avulsed segment available for repair still attached to bottom of nail.

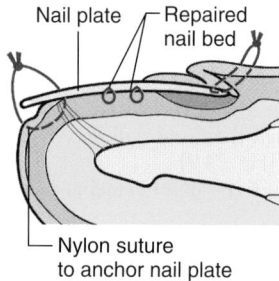

Fig. 24.9 Repair of type II injury with nail reattached. The nail bed is repaired and the nail plate or substitute is anchored proximally and distally.

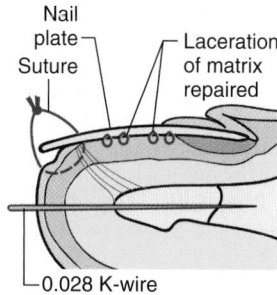

Fig. 24.10 Repair of type III injury. The unstable fracture is stabilized, the matrix repaired, and the nail plate secured by nylon suture.

- Larger avulsions require split- or full-thickness grafts from adjacent fingers or toes (see Shepard, 1990a and 1990b).

As mentioned previously, with an avulsed nail bed, look carefully for remnants of the nail bed on large pieces of the nail plate that may accompany the patient. Ask family members or coworkers to look for any amputated fingertips, which may provide needed tissue for the nail bed reconstruction. Sometimes a fingernail and part of the nail bed may still be inside a glove that was worn at the time of injury. If an adjacent finger was amputated or is otherwise irreparable, it may

serve as a donor for a full- or partial-thickness nail bed graft for the defect in question. A small defect may be repaired with a small split-thickness graft from an undamaged segment of the involved nail. In larger defects, a split-thickness graft from the sterile matrix (do not include the germinal matrix) of the great toe can be used. After removal of the great toenail, use a sterile surgical blade with a thick graft sawing motion to shave approximately 0.014 inch from the nail bed (it is preferable to cut too thin than too thick). Carefully sew the graft in place with fine absorbable sutures, reapply the nail or other template, and secure in place when properly positioned to maintain the proximal and lateral folds in an open position.

In general, consider perioperative antibiotic use for type III, IV, and V injuries, including distal amputations. Verify that tetanus status is up to date, because many of these wounds are grossly contaminated.

LATE RECONSTRUCTION OF THE NAIL MATRIX

Delayed reconstruction efforts are frequently associated with disappointment for the patient and the clinician. Patients must know upfront that odds of a major improvement after surgery are very guarded, and it is possible for the nail to look even worse regardless of best efforts and surgical technique.

- *Nail ridges* can result from either a scar below the nail bed or a fracture healing with a prominence on the dorsal phalangeal surface. Correction requires smoothing of the healed bone surface and removal of the scar tissue. The defect created by the scar removal must be closed either by undermining and direct approximation or by grafting, as mentioned previously.
- *Split nails* can result from a ridge or longitudinal scar in the germinal or sterile matrix. Resection of the scar in the sterile matrix and use of a free graft, if primary closure is impossible, may be helpful. Use of the proximal eponychial incisions to visualize and graft the germinal matrix may provide some improvement. Some authors advocate use of the second toe as a donor rather than the great toe to avoid cosmetic alteration of the larger great toenail. Use a germinal matrix graft of similar size and shape to fill the resected scar site as a free graft.
- *Nonadherence* of the nail is caused from scars in the sterile matrix. Resection of the scar and replacement with a free split- or full-thickness matrix graft provides the best results.

CPT/BILLING CODES

11720   Debridement of nail(s) by any method; 1–5
11721   Debridement of nails by any method; 6 or more
11730   Avulsion of nail plate; partial or complete, simple; single
11732   Avulsion of each additional nail plate
11740   Evacuation of subungual hematoma
11760   Repair of nail bed
11762   Reconstruction of nail bed with graft

ICD-10-CM DIAGNOSTIC CODES

S60.111X–S60.159X	Contusion of finger with damage to nail
S61.101X–S61.109X	Open wound of thumb with damage to nail
S61.111X–S61.119X	Laceration thumb w/o foreign body with damage to nail
S61.121X–S61.129X	Laceration thumb w/foreign body with damage to nail
S61.131X–S61.139X	Puncture wound thumb w/o foreign body with damage to nail
S61.141X–S61.149X	Puncture wound thumb w/foreign body with damage to nail
S61.151X–S61.159X	Open bite thumb with damage to nail
S61.300X–S61.309X	Open wound of finger with damage to nail
S61.310X–S61.319X	Laceration finger w/o foreign body with damage to nail
S61.320X–S61.329X	Laceration finger w/foreign body with damage to nail
S61.330X–S61.339X	Puncture wound finger w/o foreign body with damage to nail
S61.340X–S61.349X	Puncture wound finger w/foreign body with damage to nail
S61.350X–S61.359X	Open bite finger with damage to nail

Add appropriate seventh character: A = initial, D = subsequent, S = sequela.

Acknowledgment

The editors recognize the contributions of Douglas R. Jackson, MD, to this chapter in previous editions of this text.

RECOMMENDED READING

Fleckman P, Christopher A. Surgical anatomy of the nail unit. *Dermatol Surg.* 2001;27:257–260.

Hanke E. Nail surgery. In: Robinson JK, Hanke DW, Siegel DM, et al., eds. *Surgery of the Skin: Procedural Dermatology.* 3rd ed. Philadelphia: Saunders; 2014.

Lee HD, Mignemi ME, Crosby SN. Fingertip injuries: an update on management. *J Am Acad Orthop Surg.* 2013;21:756.

Moossavi M, Scher RK. Complications of nail surgery: a review of the literature. *Dermatol Surg.* 2001;27:225–228.

Reardon CM, McArthur PA, Survana SK, Brotherston TM. The surface anatomy of the germinal matrix of the nail bed in the finger. *J Hand Surg Br.* 1999;24:531–533.

Rich P. Nail biopsy: indications and methods. *Dermatol Surg.* 2001;27:229–234.

Scher RK, Daniel CR III, eds. *Nails: Therapy, Diagnosis, Surgery.* 3rd ed. Philadelphia: Saunders; 2005.

Shepard GH. Management of acute nail bed avulsions. *Hand Clin.* 1990a;6:39–56.

Shepard GH. Nail grafts for reconstruction. *Hand Clin.* 1990b;6:79–102.

Strauss EJ, Weil WM, Jordan C, et al. A prospective, randomized, controlled trial of 2-octylcyanoacrylate versus suture repair for nail bed injuries. *J Hand Surg Am.* 2008;33:250.

Van Beek AL, Kassan MA, Adson MH, Dale V. Management of acute fingernail injuries. *Hand Clin.* 1990;6:23–35.

Zook EG, Van Beek AL, Russell RC, Beatty ME. Anatomy and physiology of the perionychium. a review of the literature and anatomic study. *J Hand Surg.* 1980;5:528–536.

EDITOR'S NOTE: There is some controversy regarding the necessity to remove the nail regardless of the hematoma size. Traditional teaching recommended removal. The study by Roser and Gellman (1999) and others questions this practice. Consult the following sources:

Fieg EL. Letter to the editor. *Am Fam Physician.* 2002;65:1997.

Lammers RL, Smith ZE. Methods of wound closure. In: Roberts JR, Hedges JR, eds. *Clinical Procedures in Emergency Medicine.* 6th ed. Philadelphia: Elsevier; 2014.

Magdy A, Durani Y, Weihmiller SN. Minor trauma. In: Shaw KN, Bachur RG, eds. *Textbook of Pediatric Emergency Medicine.* 7th ed. Philadelphia: Lippincott Williams & Wilkins; 2015.

Roser SE, Gellman H. Comparison of nail bed repair versus nail trephination for subungual hematomas in children. *J Hand Surg Am.* 1999;24:1166–1170.

Wang QC, Johnson BA. Fingertip injuries. *Am Fam Physician.* 2001;63:1961–1966.

CHAPTER 25

RADIOFREQUENCY SURGERY (MODERN ELECTROSURGERY)

John L. Pfenninger

Radiofrequency (RF) surgery—modern electrosurgery—has become a versatile tool for the primary care clinician in dermatologic, surgical, and gynecologic applications. It is both time- and cost-effective, providing efficacious treatment for a multitude of lesions. Appropriate selection of waveform and current intensity allows excision (cutting), cutting and coagulation (blend), pure coagulation (hemostasis), or fulguration. Tissue can either be removed delicately with excellent cosmetic results or totally ablated. The electrosurgical unit (ESU) can be used for the treatment of both benign and malignant lesions.

This chapter is based on the Ellman Surgitron (Ellman Cynosure), a portable generator that creates high-frequency current of 3.8 to 4.0 MHz, which is comparable to the radiowave frequency for broadcasting (Figs. 25.1 and 25.2). ESU wave frequency for different brand models can vary from 500,000 to 4 million cycles (4.0 MHz) per second. All units can be used with a multitude of electrode tips for a large variety of applications. After the advent of the loop electrosurgical excision procedure (LEEP) in the 1990s, many

other companies introduced units into the market. Unless otherwise noted, discussion here is in reference to the Ellman Surgitron because it is widely adapted to many dermatologic procedures. The reader can generalize the discussion to most other units quite readily.

There is a choice of three waveform outputs plus a fulguration current (four modes). By changing waveforms, practitioners obtain different effects. The settings of the Ellman unit are described as *filtered fully rectified, fully rectified,* and *partially rectified.* These correspond with a *pure cutting* effect (90% cutting, 10% coagulation), a *blended* current to allow 50% cut and 50% coagulation, and a 90% *coagulation* (hemostasis) effect, respectively. A separate outlet also provides a spark-gap fulgurating current (referred to as *hyfrecation*) for very superficial cautery (Fig. 25.3).

Advantages of using RF technique include rapidity of treatment, a nearly bloodless field, minimal postoperative pain, and rapid healing. Local anesthetic is used except in rare instances. Because the frequency is so high, the current from this unit passes through the body without causing painful muscle contractions or nerve stimulation

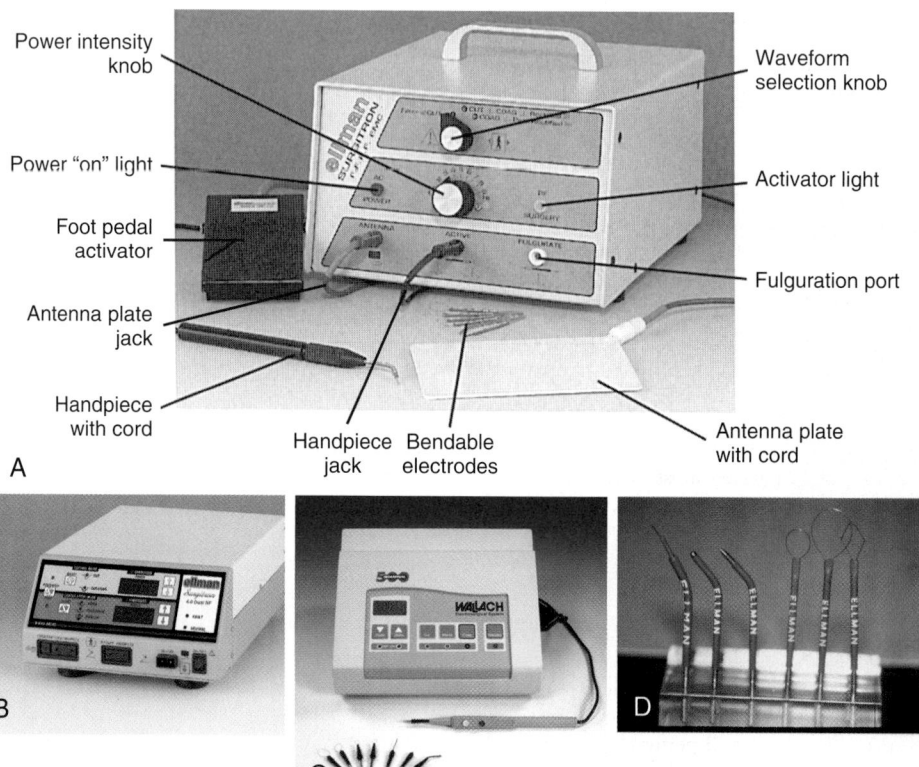

Fig. 25.1 (A) Ellman Surgitron radiofrequency unit with foot pedal, antenna plate, and hand wand tip holder. Various electrode tips are lying above the white antenna plate. (B) Ellman Dual Frequency IEC II. (C) The Wallach Q500 electrosurgical unit with finger control handpiece and a variety of electrodes. (D) Typical electrodes (Ellman) for skin electrosurgery *(left to right):* vari-tip cutting wire, ball electrode and pointed electrode for cautery or fulguration, small and large loops, diamond-shaped electrode. (A, B, and D, Courtesy Ellman Cynosure, Hicksville, New York. C, Courtesy Bruno Ratensberger.)

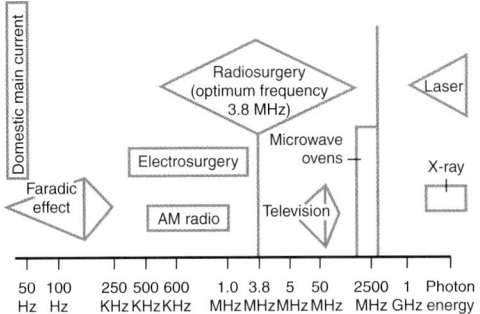

Fig. 25.2 Comparison of uses and effects of various electrical frequencies. (Courtesy Ellman Cynosure, Hicksville, New York.)

Mode or function	Waveform	Configuration
Electrocoagulation Hemostasis Cautery	Partially rectified	
Blend Cut and coag	Fully rectified	
Cutting Electrosection	Fully filtered and fully rectified	
Fulguration Electrodesiccation	Markedly damped	

Fig. 25.3 Common terminology for various modes, waveform characterization, and waveform configurations for the outputs of the radiofrequency unit.

(Faraday effects). Radiosurgery using the *cutting wave* cuts without pressure, needing only a feather-like touch, and thus minimizes tissue damage. The tissue damage that does occur is very superficial and comparable to that of proper laser use. This is in contrast to true cautery, which causes damage similar to third-degree burns. In addition, radiosurgery avoids the risk of electrical burns to the patient. Instead of a ground plate, an antenna is used to focus the "radio waves." In contrast to other electrical units, this antenna does not have to be in contact with a patient's skin; instead, it only needs to be under the patient near the operating field. (Most ESUs with lower-frequency output, however, do require true grounding pads or plates, so the manufacturer's recommendations must be followed.)

The high-frequency energy of this unit is concentrated at the tip of each electrode. During each procedure, the electrode itself remains cold; however, the highly concentrated electrical energy creates molecular energy inside each cell it contacts, thereby creating intracellular heat and actually vaporizing the cell, much as a laser does. The amount of heat generated depends on the amount of time the tip is in contact with the tissue, the size of the electrode, the power setting, the type of waveform selected, and the wave frequency. Higher frequency means less contact time, finer wire, less power, a more "cutting" waveform, and less tissue damage.

High-frequency electrosurgery is now replacing many laser applications because of the minimal tissue damage, low cost of equipment, minimal maintenance, ease of treatment, and excellent long-term results. It has replaced most laser applications for the gynecologic treatment of dysplasia (conization) and condylomata. It is now also being used for blepharoplasties, radio-assisted uvulopalatoplasty for snoring, spinal procedures, skin tightening (dual-frequency unit), and many more applications.

INDICATIONS

RF surgery can be used for a variety of skin and mucosal lesions. It is especially helpful when good cosmetic results are essential. It is also very helpful in well-perfused areas like mucosa and the anal area because the "cut and coag" setting can be used to control bleeding. Common uses and lesions treated are listed in Box 25.1.

BOX 25.1   Common Uses of and Lesions Treated With Radiofrequency Surgery

Actinic keratosis
Basal cell cancers
Blepharoplasties
Cauterization of "bleeders"
Cervical biopsies
Cervical conizations (LLETZ, LEEP)*
Chalazions
Condylomata
Curettement and cautery (e.g., warts)
Electroepilation
Excisions
Hair transplants
Hemangiomas
Hemorrhoid tags
Incisions
Mucosal lesions
Nail plate ablation†
Nevi (benign)
Pyogenic granulomas
Radioassisted uvulopalatoplasties (RAUP)
Rhinophyma
Sebaceous gland hyperplasia
Seborrheic keratosis
Shave removals
Skin tags
Skin tightening (Radiage)
Squamous cell carcinomas
Syringomas
Telangiectases (spider veins) face (not recommended for legs)
Verrucae
Xanthelasma

---

* See Chapter 127, Loop Electrosurgical Excision Procedure for Treating Cervical Intraepithelial Neoplasia.
† See Chapter 194, Ingrown Toenails.

CONTRAINDICATIONS

- *Cardiac pacemakers* (relative contraindication): Do not work near the heart, and place the antenna (or grounding) plate well away from the heart. Use the least power possible. Activate the handpiece intermittently rather than continuously. The cutting mode is the most risky, so avoid it if possible. Use another form of treatment if that is an option. The pacers are purportedly "shielded" and the current in the ESUs should not affect them, but all things are not perfect! Therefore caution is needed. Asystole and tachycardia are potential adverse outcomes.
- Uncooperative patient.

EQUIPMENT

- Alcohol wipe
- Local anesthetic (e.g., 2% lidocaine with or without epinephrine)
- 1-mL syringe with 30-gauge needle
- ESU
- Electrode tips (depending on procedure performed): reusable or disposable
- No. 15 scalpel blade
- Antenna (or grounding) plate
- Handpiece for tips (unit can be finger-activated from this handpiece if desired)
- Foot pedal to activate handpiece (or use handpiece as indicated earlier); foot pedal preferred for delicate surgeries
- Smoke evacuator (human immunodeficiency virus [HIV] and human papillomavirus [HPV] have been found in smoke plume)

- Room air purifier or exhaust fan (removes residual odor)
- Movable cart to hold the ESU, smoker evacuator, tips, and all equipment for the procedures
- Mask
- Nonsterile gloves and equipment to follow universal blood and body fluid precautions
- Aluminum chloride for topical control of bleeders (or Monsel solution if the face is not involved)
- Antibiotic ointment
- Bandage
- Patient education handout on moist healing (which is essential to obtain optimal results). (See the sample patient education handout available at www.expertconsult.com.)
- For LEEP supplies, see Chapter 127, Loop Electrosurgical Excision Procedure for Treating Cervical Intraepithelial Neoplasia.

The *most common tips* used for removal of skin lesions are the large and small loops. The ball electrode is used frequently for coagulation and the ablation of lesions. Special tips are available for matrixectomy (see later discussion and Chapter 194, Ingrown Toenails) and skin tightening (see Chapter 45, Nonablative Radiowave Skin Tightening With the Ellman S5 Surgitron [The Pellevé Procedure]).

Disposable tips are convenient but can be costly. Reusable tips must be shiny and free of carbon buildup to obtain best results. After cleaning and sterilizing and before repeat use, the tip must be examined. If it is not shiny, the carbon can be removed in several ways:

- Use a 2 × 2 inch piece of fine sandpaper and, using the index finger to support the back side of the loop, rub it over the sandpaper. Turn it over and use it on the reverse side. Be sure to clean the entire wire loop.
- Purchase the available cleaning "blocks."
- Place the units in an ultrasonic cleaner.
- Use a moistened piece of 4 × 4 inch gauze, insert the tip into the folded material, and activate it on the cutting setting, level 5.

When complete, the wire should be shiny (like new). One of the most common reasons for poor cutting and "stalls" during RF surgery is "dirty" (carbon-covered) reusable loops, which is avoided if disposable tips are used.

Most ESUs have digital readouts for *wattage* (power intensity). The Ellman simply has an intensity dial labeled 1 to 10. Each unit roughly corresponds to 10 W. For skin surgery a setting of 2 to 4 (20 to 40 W) is usually needed. (As a "default," remember "pure cutting on level 2.")

Use of a *smoke evacuator* is essential. Not only have HPV and HIV been found in smoke plume (no infections have been documented), but the smell of burning flesh is very offensive, and the examination room and office can smell for hours afterward.

The dual-frequency units (Ellman Pellevé S5, Surgitron Dual RF S5, Surgitron Dual RF 120, and Surgitron Dual/EMC 90, and AcuSect; see Fig. 25.1B) are being used with increasing frequency for surgical and esthetic procedures. Their coagulation potential is much better and they can coagulate in a "wet" (bloody) field using the bipolar modality. This is achieved through the dual frequencies of 4 MHz for cutting but 1.7 MHz for bipolar coagulation. Other benefits include a higher frequency (4.0 vs. 3.8 million cycles per second) than the earlier models. There is still minimal thermal damage when cutting. These units are more expensive, so the clinician must determine whether the benefits warrant the extra cost. Only the Pellevé S5 and Surgitron Dual RF S5 energy sources are compatible with their proprietary GlideSafe Wrinkle Treatment Handpieces for skin-tightening procedures. The physician considering offering esthetic procedures in his or her practice may want to consider these units.

TECHNIQUE

Universal blood and body fluid precautions should be followed. Proper technique is accomplished when the loop electrodes pass through the tissue smoothly, like cutting through soft butter. Generally, a motion of 5 to 8 mm/s is appropriate. If there is excess sparking and smoke, the power setting is too high. If the flow is not smooth, the operator is going too fast, the power setting is too low, the skin is too dry or hyperkeratotic, or the electrode is dirty (debris or carbon buildup). It is important to remember that the least tissue damage occurs with the pure cutting setting. Coagulation causes the most tissue destruction. If cosmetic results are desirable, judicious use of the coagulation setting and using as little power (watts) as possible is important.

The most common use for the RF unit in primary care is removal of elevated skin lesions such as nevi and seborrheic lesions. Commonly, when using a blade to shave off a benign nevus, two things result: bleeding and an irregular surface. As the surgeon tries to smooth out the "highs" in the base of the wound, blood obscures the area. Then, as the blade is used to shave off these highs, too much tissue is removed, leaving "dips." The "lows" (too much tissue removed) and the "highs" (too little) result in adverse outcomes with undesirable scarring. Using the RF technique, both bleeding and an uneven wound base can be avoided. In addition, any focal areas of undesirable residual tissue are removed and the edges can be smoothed for a more pleasing cosmetic result. Because the tissue left behind has minimal thermal damage, healing is quick and scarring minimized.

The most successful technique for removing lesions appears to be first to debulk the majority of the lesion with a No. 15 blade in a shave fashion (see Chapter 26, Skin Biopsy). Then, the loop electrode on a pure cutting setting of 2 (20 W) is used to smooth out or vaporize the base of the wound. Pinch the skin around the area to control bleeding, activate the loop, and very superficially pass the tip over/through the tissue, gradually going down until the lesion is smoothed out adequately (Fig. 25.4). This "smoothing out" of the base provides an excellent outcome with rapid healing. The cutting setting has 10% coagulation so bleeding is nicely controlled. The tissue is literally vaporized cell layer by cell layer. Healing results are excellent. Another advantage with the method described is that the tissue sent to pathology has no burn artifact.

Some advocate the removal of lesions primarily with the loop only (as opposed to using the blade). *Extreme caution is needed!* The loop cuts so quickly that it often goes too deep. Even in experienced hands too much tissue may be removed unless the process is very slow and meticulous with only a small amount of tissue removed each time. *Do not try to remove the entire lesion with the first pass!* The only time the "layered" or "feathering" removal technique is recommended is for larger condylomata (Fig. 25.5).

Another advantage of shaving the lesion first with a blade is that a good specimen is available for pathology. If the loop is used, there will always be some coagulation artifact, albeit minimal. If total vaporization or the coagulation technique is used, minimal (if any) tissue can be sent. It is best that all pigmented lesions be sent for histology because this is a very litigious area of medicine, and the less artifact on a specimen the better.

The Ellman unit does have a fulguration port. This setting provides a very intense but superficial burn/coagulation. It can be used in place of the coagulation mode in many instances, but in general it has little benefit over the coagulation setting and is rarely used.

Novices are most concerned about the proper choice of settings when beginning electrosurgery. Following are some pointers:

- For removal of tissue, use pure cutting mode.
- For cutting the skin, or for the shave technique noted previously, usually an intensity of 2 (≤20 W) is sufficient. For removing large areas (e.g., cervical conization) or if the skin is hyperkeratotic, the intensity will have to be increased, but rarely over 4 (40 W) for the skin and 6 for the cervix. Remember the "default" setting: cutting, level 2. The larger and drier the tissue, the higher the power will have to be.
- When tissue destruction (matrixectomy, epilation, telangiectases) or bleeding control is needed, turn to the coagulation

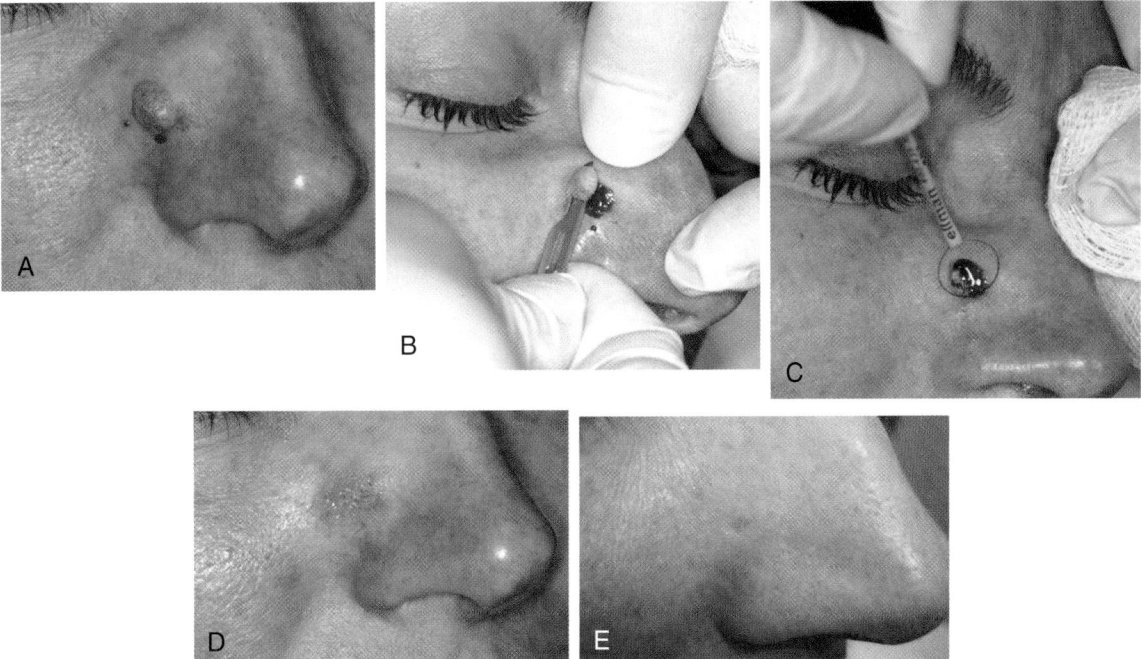

Fig. 25.4 Preferred technique for removal of raised lesions with a broad base. (A) Nasal nevus after infiltration with lidocaine. (B) Shave the lesion with a No. 15 blade. Remove most of the lesion, being careful not to go too deep. (C) Smooth out the base and control bleeding with a large loop electrode (cutting, 2). "Sculpt" the final result. Proceed very superficially and remove a few cell layers at a time to blend the edges. (D) Appearance on completion of removal. (E) Appearance 2 years after removal. (Courtesy The Medical Procedures Center, Midland, Michigan.)

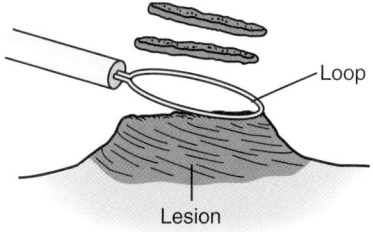

Fig. 25.5 "Feathering" technique for lesion removal. Rather than removing the entire lesion in one pass, it is removed a small amount at a time. This avoids removing too much and going too deep, causing scarring.

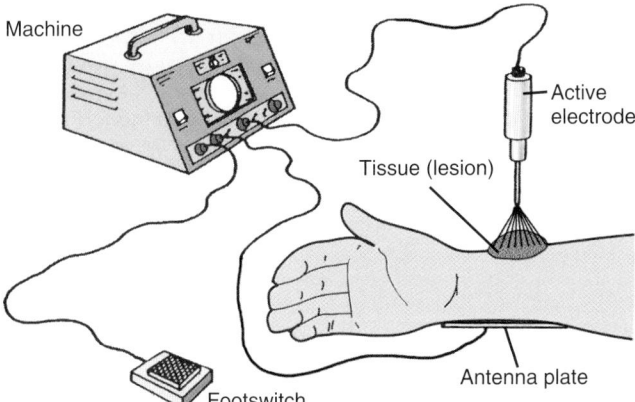

Fig. 25.6 Radiosurgery showing the distribution of energy and the appropriate placement of the antenna plate near the lesion. (Courtesy Ellman Cynosure, Hicksville, New York.)

mode. Most applications will require a level of 3 (30 W). When small areas are treated without anesthesia (epilation, telangiectases of the face), reduce the power level to 1.

- Use the cut/coagulation mode when bleeding is likely (e.g., inner lip, buccal mucosa) or where scarring is not so much of an issue

(external hemorrhoidal tags). The setting will have to be a little higher (3, or 30 W).

- For removal of cervical tissue, the goal is to limit tissue artifact so the pathologist can readily read the specimen and discern if the entire lesion was removed. Use a pure cutting mode; although scarring is not a concern, bleeding still is. Amazingly, however, there is generally very little bleeding, even with pure cutting, and the pathologist will be able to read to the margins of the excision because the cutting mode leaves little burn artifact (see Chapter 127, Loop Electrosurgical Excision Procedure for Treating Cervical Intraepithelial Neoplasia).
- All electrosurgery will be accomplished more easily at lower power (therefore causing less tissue destruction) if the tissue is moist and hyperkeratotic material has been removed. Use a moistened 4 × 4 inch gauze pad and wipe it across the tissue after each pass or two.
- Most lesions will have to be anesthetized before removal with the RF unit.
- In general, place the antenna plate or grounding pad as close to the lesion as possible to limit the spread of the current and increase the intensity at the desired site (Fig. 25.6).
- The proper electrode tips and power settings are summarized in Table 25.1.
- Be sure to hold the handpiece like a pencil, and place the fifth finger on the patient for stabilization. If the patient jumps or moves, your hand moves as well. Otherwise the patient may experience a significant laceration or burn.

Specific Approaches for Various Lesions

There are a multitude of applications possible with the variety of tips available (Fig. 25.7; see Fig. 25.1D). There are loop and straight-wire electrodes for excising, incising, or shaping tissue; ball electrodes for coagulation; and pointed rod electrodes for fulguration and desiccation. More specific electrodes are available for nail matrixectomies and LEEP of the cervix. The tips are changed in the handpiece much like the bits are changed in an ordinary drill. Most treatments are accomplished with simple local anesthesia,

TABLE 25.1	Proper Electrode Tips and Power Settings		
Procedure	**Mode**	**Power (Ellman/Watts)**	**Electrode**
Condylomata	Cutting	2/20	Large or small round loop
Ear piercing	Cutting or cut/coag	2/20	Narrow, pointed tip
Electrodesiccation and curettage	Coag	3/25–30	Ball
Epilation	Coag	1/10	Vari-tip, 33-gauge needle on hub adaptors, or insulated needle
Epistaxis	Coag	3/30	Ball electrode
Hemorrhoid tags	Cut/coag	3/25–30	Large loop or vari-tip
Hemostasis, skin	Coag	2–3/20–30	Ball electrode
Incisions	Cutting	2–3/20–30	Vari-tip, fine needle, blade
LEEP	Cutting	4/35–40	Long, special LEEP electrodes
LEEP	Coag base/hemostasis	6/40–60	Long, special LEEP ball
Matrixectomy	Coag	2–3/20–30	Special insulated matrixectomy electrodes, raise up on the eponychium, do not overcoagulate
Rhinophyma	Cutting	2/20	Large loop or rounded surgical blade (no. 10A)
Shave excision/smoothing	Cutting	2/20	Large or small loop
Skin tags/small condylomata	Coag	3/25–30	Pickups with ball electrode, bipolar pickups
Telangiectases	Coag	1/10	Vari-tip, 33-gauge needle on hub adapters, or insulated needle
Undermining	Cutting or cut/coag	2–3/20–30	Vari-tip, blade
Vasectomy (cauterizing vas ends)	Coag	3/30	Narrow, pointed tip
Verruca	Cutting	3/25–30	Large loop, special cutting curette
Verruca	Coag	3/30	Ball electrode
Xanthelasma	Cutting	2/20–25	Large loop

LEEP, Loop electrosurgical excision procedure.

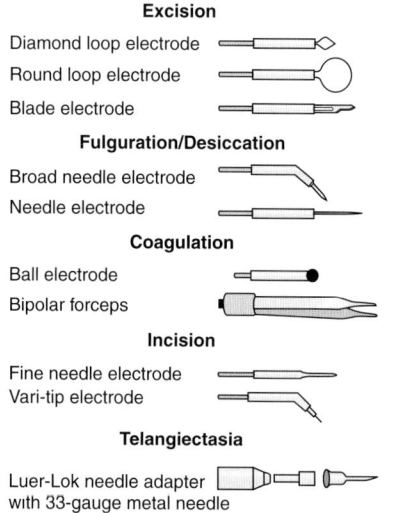

Fig. 25.7 Multiple electrode tips available for the Ellman Surgitron radiofrequency units.

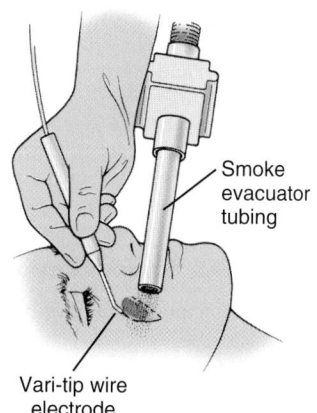

Fig. 25.8 Use of the vari-tip wire electrode to carry out an elliptical excision.

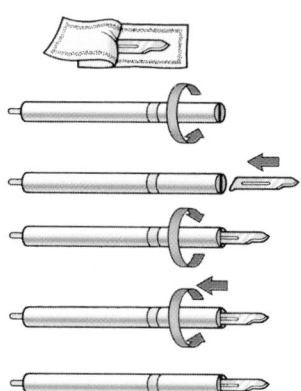

Fig. 25.9 Technique of inserting scalpel blade into handle for radiofrequency surgery. Most surgery is carried out with the loop electrodes or vari-tip wire. The scalpel is used most frequently for "bloodless" undermining.

regional field blocks, or digital blocks. Radiosurgery is relatively atraumatic when correctly applied; consequently the risks of scar tissue formation are minimal compared with those associated with scalpel surgery.

For the majority of cases, the handpiece is inserted into the color-coordinated handpiece port on the unit to enable the selection of various output modes. (If inserted into the fulguration port, that will be the only output.)

Biopsies or excisions of lesions may be accomplished with the standard ellipse technique using the vari-tip electrode (Fig. 25.8) or a scalpel blade inserted into a chuck adapter (Fig. 25.9). The vari-tip has a fine wire that can be pulled out at variable distances to cut from 1 to 2 mm up to 1.5 cm deep. The unit is set at cutting mode. The proper power is usually between 2 and 3. The thickness and dryness of skin may cause some variation in the latter setting. Remove any hyperkeratinized tissue first, and be sure the skin is moist. In addition to incising and excising, these two electrodes are often used to undermine skin because bleeding will be controlled if the cut/coag (blend) mode is used. The cutting is very fast, so be careful not to excise too deeply.

If the lesion to be removed is large and elevated, a biopsy specimen may be obtained by simply using the loop electrodes to remove the sample (Fig. 25.10). (See previously discussed precautions.)

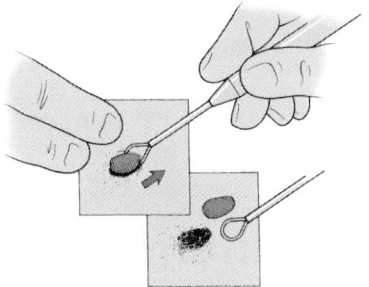

Fig. 25.10 Another technique for removing a raised skin lesion with a broad base. Care must be taken not to excise too much tissue.

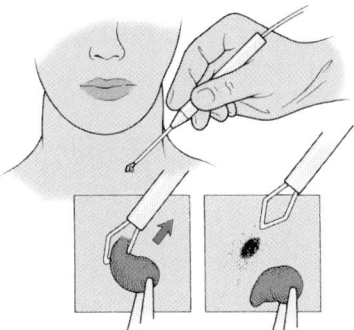

Fig. 25.11 Technique for removing a lesion with a pedunculated base.

However, with smaller, flatter lesions, using the loop to obtain a shave biopsy specimen may cause sufficient artifact in the tissue specimen to obscure pathology. For smaller lesions, then, use a regular scalpel blade (without current) to obtain a shave biopsy specimen. Then use the loop electrode to smooth out the base and control bleeding. Remember, when obtaining a biopsy sample for suspected melanoma, the depth of lesion penetration is *very important*. Do not perform a shave biopsy of a pigmented lesion unless you are certain it is not a melanoma (see Chapter 26, Skin Biopsy).

Basal cell cancers are often best treated using a combination of curettement and cautery (or fulguration). A ball electrode is used in the handpiece with coagulation mode and the power set at approximately 3 to 4. After curetting the lesion, the base of the wound is cauterized. Cautery and curettement are usually carried out three times on the same visit. The tissue from the first curettement is sent for histology to confirm the clinical diagnosis (see Chapter 13, Approach to Various Skin Lesions, and Chapter 26, Skin Biopsy). Lesions less than 1 cm have a cure rate greater than 98%.

Condylomata acuminata may be excised using a loop electrode with the unit set at cutting (most commonly) or at cut/coag and power set at approximately 2 to 3. For larger lesions, debulk them with the initial pass, then successively remove more tissue, and finally feather out the edges with a very light touch. Be very careful not to go too deep and remove too much tissue with the first pass! Using a colposcope for magnification during the removal is very helpful. (Alternatively, any residual after the initial pass may be removed with coagulation of the bases of the wound.) *Small warts* on all parts of the body may be destroyed easily using a ball electrode with the unit set at coagulation and a power setting just strong enough to "cook" the lesions (1 to 2). The smaller lesions can also be grasped with metal pickups and the electrode applied to the pickups while lifting the lesion. Apply enough current so that the lesion can be wiped off with moist gauze after being coagulated.

Xanthelasma may be treated easily using a large loop in the cutting mode set at level 2. Use very superficial passes over the lesion until all white material has been removed. Use ophthalmic ointment to keep the wound moist until it is healed. No suture closure is required.

Fibroepithelial skin tags may be removed simply, usually without anesthesia, with the loop electrode on the cut (or cut/coag) mode and power setting at slightly less than 2 (Fig. 25.11). They can also be treated like small condylomata, as noted previously. Larger lesions will require anesthesia.

Hemorrhoidal tags can be removed similarly to skin tags. Be careful that the local anesthesia does not distort the base of the tag, which can create a false sense that more tissue has to be removed. This could leave a larger wound than needed. The cut/coag mode at level 3 to 4 works best. Usually the wound is left open.

Seborrheic keratoses are successfully treated using the technique described previously for shave excisions. Remember that the lesion is very superficial, so deep removal is not necessary. This will minimize scarring. Use a blade to shave off the bulk of the lesion and follow it with a large loop, cutting mode, and setting of 2, using the feathering technique.

Sebaceous cysts may be uncovered for intact removal or extraction of the capsule by using a small ellipse around the central pore. The cutting mode is selected, and the power dial is set at no more than 2. The length and depth of the ellipse obviously depend on the size of the cyst and thickness of the skin. The vari-tip electrode is set at skin thickness (estimate). With an Allis clamp, put slight traction on the ellipsed area over the cyst wall itself. The lesion is then bluntly dissected from surrounding deep tissue and removed.

Telangiectases (face only) are effectively treated with the electrocoagulation technique. Use the coagulation (hemostasis) mode with the power set at 1, and a fine needle. A hypodermic Luer-Lok needle adaptor is available for the handpiece; a short 33-gauge hypodermic needle with a metal hub is then attached to the adaptor for this procedure (see Fig. 25.7). Insulated needles can also be purchased from the manufacturer (Fig. 25.12). The special needles are insulated and active only at the very tip. Generally, topical anesthetic is used (see Chapter 4, Topical Anesthesia). Treatment lasts a fraction of a second. The unit is activated before touching the telangiectases. Vessels should be penetrated minimally at approximately 1- to 2-mm intervals. Begin distally and work proximally. (Doing the opposite— proximal to distal—causes the vessels to go into spasm, making them hard to locate.) Facial lesions respond the best, whereas spider veins on the lower extremity do not resolve well. There is often prolonged pigmentation and recurrence with leg veins. Sclerotherapy is the procedure of choice for the lower extremities (see Chapter 78, Sclerotherapy). *Spider angiomas* anywhere can be treated with the fine needle. Occasionally all that is needed is coagulation of one central vessel. *Cherry hemangiomas* are best treated using light ball electrode desiccation and then wiped away.

Epilation of isolated hairs deploys a similar technique and needle. Choose the coag setting at level 1, grasp the hair with pickups, and slide the needle down the shaft. Activate the electrode; as the hair follicle is "cooked," the hair comes out easily. Trichiasis is treated in this fashion too. For large areas of unwanted hair, use the modern techniques of removal (see Chapter 38, Laser and Pulsed-Light Devices: Hair Removal).

Actinic keratoses are very dry and, unless small, are best treated with cryosurgery or shave technique. If the electrodesiccation technique is used, however, those lesions that do not respond appropriately should be studied further to rule out neoplastic changes. If there is any doubt, obtain a shave biopsy sample before treatment.

Plantar warts are treated in a multitude of ways (see Chapter 30, Wart [Verruca] Treatment). When other methods fail (e.g., *Candida* antigen injections, topicals, cryotherapy, bleomycin), the wart may have to be removed with curettement and coagulation. Perform this carefully because scarring on the bottom of the feet can cause painful nodules. Some residual scarring is the norm rather than the exception. After anesthesia, curette the lesion and follow with ball electrode coagulation. Curette again to ensure all wart tissue has been removed. Do not penetrate the dermis; warts are epithelial. Alternatively, a loop can be used to excise the lesion, but it frequently

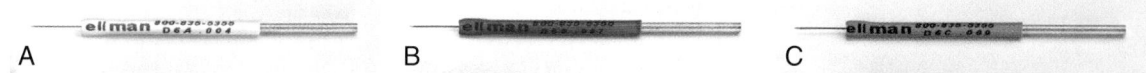

Fig. 25.12   Insulated needles available for the treatment of telangiectasia. (A) #D6-A, 0.004; (B) #D6-B, 0.007; (C) #D6-C, 0.009. (Courtesy Ellman Cynosure, Hicksville, New York.)

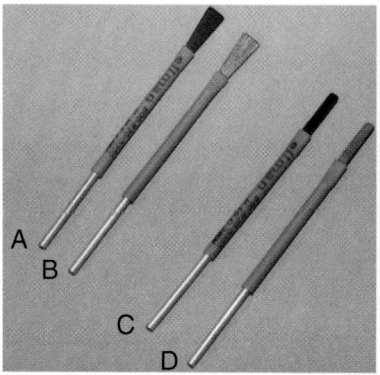
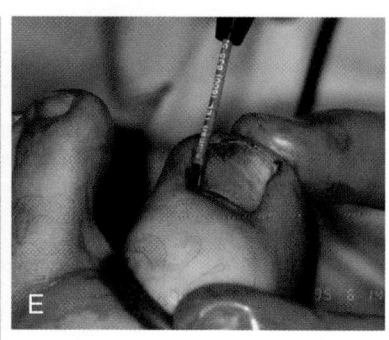

Fig. 25.13   Toenail matrixectomy electrodes. (A) Wide blade, coated Teflon side up. (B) Wide blade, brass uncoated side up. (C) Narrow blade, coated Teflon side up. (D) Narrow blade, brass uncoated side up. The brass (active) side goes down, facing the matrix. The Teflon (coated protective side) faces and lifts up against the eponychium as it is slowly withdrawn. (E) Proper application of the matrixectomy electrode into the nail groove.

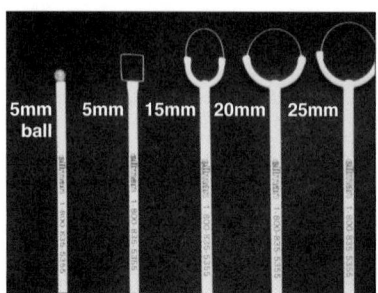

Fig. 25.14   Large loop excision of the transformation zone (LLETZ) electrodes used to perform office cervical conizations. (Courtesy Ellman Cynosure, Hicksville, New York.)

goes too deep (see precautions discussed previously). The electrified curette works very well, but it too can go too deep, too fast, and too easily. Be careful and go slow.

For *ingrown toenail surgery*, where ablation of part or all of the growth center is desired, the matrixectomy electrodes perform superbly (Fig. 25.13; see Chapter 194, Ingrown Toenails).

For *ear piercing*, use the thin, pointed electrode at the cutting or cut/coag settings, 2 to 3, or 25 to 30 W. Identify the sites bilaterally and mark them. Stabilize the earlobe and then advance the tip through the anesthetized tissue. Remove the tip and insert the earring stud.

For *cervical dysplasia:* For those trained in colposcopy and the treatment of cervical intraepithelial neoplasia, this unit can be adapted to the large loop excision of the transformation zone (LLETZ) procedure with a special set of electrodes designed for this purpose (Fig. 25.14). This office procedure allows for a "tailored" cervical conization (see Chapter 127, Loop Electrosurgical Excision Procedure for Treating Cervical Intraepithelial Neoplasia).

For *Rhinophyma*, extra tissue is removed using the large round electrode and sculpting the nose back to the original form (Fig. 25.15). Use pure cutting, level 2. Keep the tissue moist by continually wiping with a moist gauze pad.

For *skin tightening*, the basic concept is to heat collagen, which then contracts during the healing process. No anesthesia is necessary. Special tips are used for this procedure (Fig. 25.16; see Chapter 45, Nonablative Radiowave Skin Tightening with the Ellman S5 Surgitron [The Pellevé Procedure]). The GlideSafe wands range in size from 7.5 to 20 mm, depending on the part of the body that is being treated.

For this procedure, a dual-frequency Ellman unit that is compatible with the GlideSafe wand must be used. Long-term effects remain to be seen. Good immediate improvement can be seen in some patients, but contraction and thus tightening will continue for up to 3 months.

Typical power levels for the face are 16 to 20 W, with less for the neck (14 to 15 W) and much less for the eyelids (4 to 7 W) when done with the 7.5-mm tip.

Circular motions are recommended by the manufacturer, but a sweeping motion also works well. Most patients experience a pleasant sensation of warmth throughout the treatment of a given area until just before it is time to move the tip. At this point, it goes from feeling comfortable to very hot in a matter of 2 to 3 seconds. When the tip becomes too hot, move on to a new area. The excessive heat dissipates and patients are again comfortable in 2 to 3 seconds. Patients do not seem to mind this as long as the reason for it is explained to them at the beginning of the treatment.

Do not lift the wand off the skin with the handpiece activated. It will cause a small electrical shock that is uncomfortable for the patient.

Forty-five minutes is the typical treatment time for the face, including eyelids (use plastic eye shields). This does not include setup or cleanup time.

Ninety days is the expected time for revision and new collagen formation to be complete. Repeat treatment, if needed, may take place any time after that.

When the eye shields are being used, coat the inside with ointment-type eye lubricant to protect the corneal epithelium. Drops are not adequate. Erythromycin ophthalmic ointment works but may cause allergic reactions. Consider overnight eye lubricants, such as GenTeal PM. Most of these seem to contain petrolatum (like LacriLube). The vision may be blurry for 1/2 hour or so after removal. This does not seem to be a problem if one treats the eyes first and then immediately removes the eye shields, giving time for the lubricant to dissipate during the remainder of the treatment (see Chapter 45, Nonablative Radiowave Skin Tightening With the Ellman S5 Surgitron [The Pellevé Procedure]).

For *other lesions*, including tattoos, sebaceous hyperplasia, eccrine hidrocystomas, milia, verrucae plana, verrucae vulgaris, venous lakes, and trichoepitheliomas. For physicians performing laparoscopy, radiosurgical techniques can be used to treat endometriosis, pelvic inflammatory disease, myomectomy, and, in skilled hands, ectopic pregnancy. The vari-tip has also been used to treat blepharoplasties. The larger pointed tips can be used for body piercing. Uvuloplasties are quite simple using excision or ablation techniques.

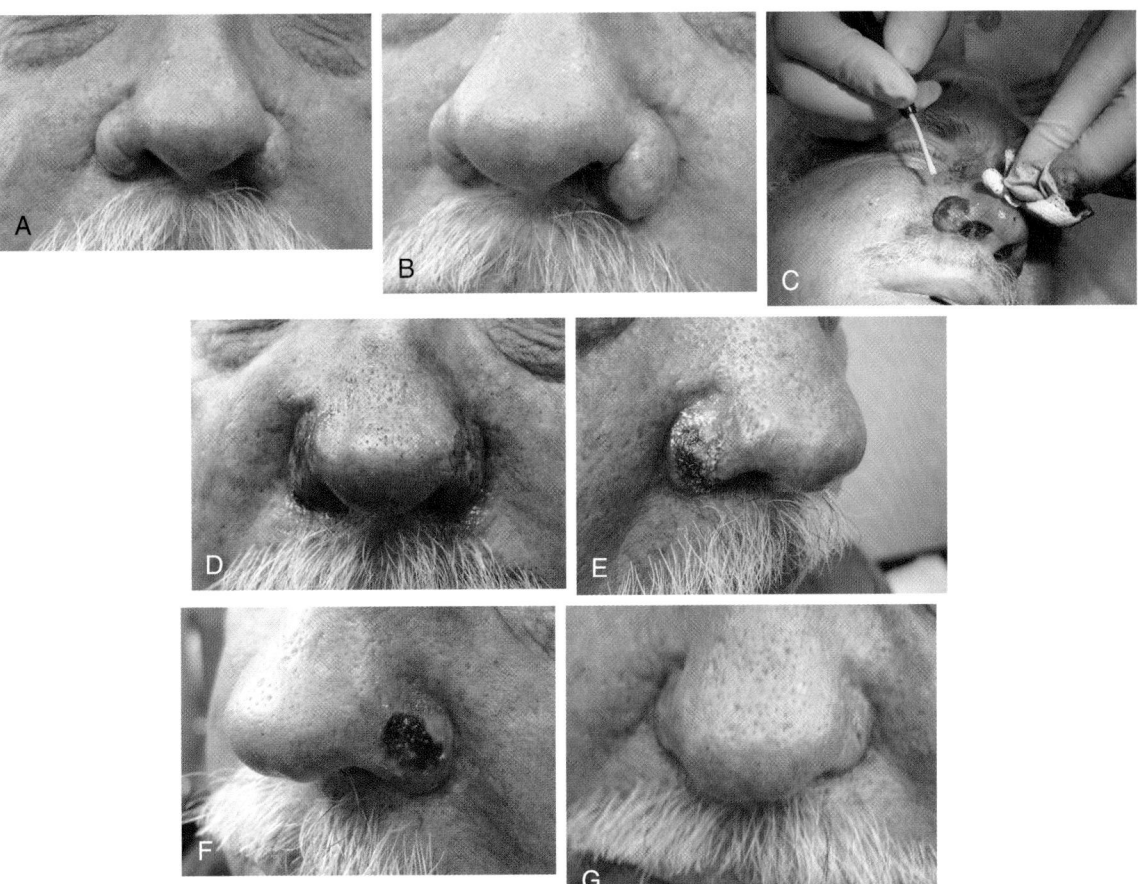

Fig. 25.15 Use of radiofrequency loop to treat rhinophyma. (A) Preoperative appearance. (B) Preoperative appearance of left naris. (C) Using the loop to remove tissue after a nasal block with lidocaine. (D) Immediate postoperative appearance. (E) Two weeks postoperative appearance, right naris. (F) Two weeks postoperative appearance, left naris. (G) One month postoperative appearance.

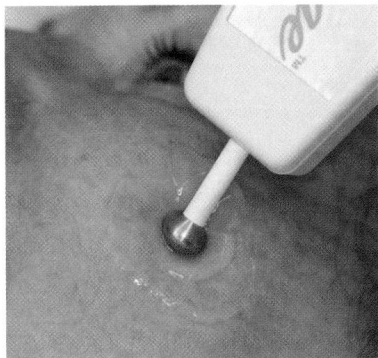

Fig. 25.16 Technique for skin tightening (Radiage) using the special handpiece and tip.

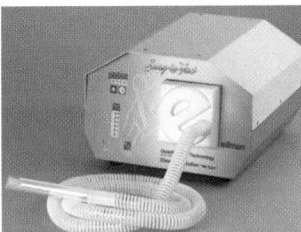

Fig. 25.17 Smoke evacuator with both viral and charcoal filters. (Courtesy Ellman Cynosure, Hicksville, New York.)

Warning: As with laser, vaporization of viral particles (HPV and HIV) in the smoke plume that accompanies destruction or excision of tissues with these techniques has been documented. Those present in the room should wear protective masks, and a smoke evacuation system is mandatory (Fig. 25.17). The suction should be no further than 2 cm from the operative site. Proper vacuums have a viral filter as well as a charcoal filter to limit the offensive odor. Compact portable units are available from the same manufacturers who supply the ESUs.

Some clinicians have created their own vacuum exhaust systems leading to the exterior of the building or installed bathroom-type exhaust fans in the room.

Modern electrosurgery (RF) techniques are easily mastered and are best accomplished by attending a workshop on radiosurgery or by following the instructions given in Pollack's *Electrosurgery of the Skin.* These instructions can be practiced at home on a piece of beefsteak. Simplicity, economy, and versatility are unique to this instrument. The lesions that can be removed are myriad, depending on the practitioner's scope of practice and versatility.

Key Points

- If the ESU is adjusted to the correct settings, the tissue will cut like soft butter.
- If the power is too low, the stroke too fast, the skin too dry, or the electrodes not totally clean, the electrode will stick or catch.
- If the power is too high, there will be excessive sparking and smoke. The principle is to minimize the lateral heat. Less tissue

damage occurs with the finer the tip, the less energy used, the less time the electrode stays in one spot, the more moist the tissue, use of a cutting mode, and use of a higher-frequency unit:

$$H = \frac{T \times I \times W \times S \times R}{F}$$

where heat (H) depends on time (T), intensity of current (I), waveform (W), area of surface contact or electrode size (S), and resistance of tissue (R) divided by frequency (F).

- Once the lesion has been removed, any remaining bleeding can be controlled with topical astringents. Monsel solution or aluminum chloride works best (see Chapter 199, Topical Hemostatic Agents).

COMPLICATIONS

- Broken wire causing laceration (discard worn tips).
- Too deep an excision, causing excessive scarring and trauma to undesired tissue.
- Destruction of tissue for pathologic review, caused by improper technique.
- Handpiece in wrong port or unit in wrong mode to obtain desired effect.
- Pacemaker dysfunction.
- Inadvertent burns, on either the patient or operator, resulting from unintended activation of handpiece.
- Poor healing.
- Pain, bleeding, and infection (extremely rare).
- Scarring (usually very minimal, but could result in a depression, hypopigmentation, or hyperpigmentation).
- Incomplete removal of a lesion.
- Recurrence of the lesion.
- Inadvertent shaving of a pigmented lesion that turns out to be a melanoma.
- Spreading infection between patients.
- Explosion of colonic gas (methane) from exposure to a spark (if the patient is asleep, a moist gauze should be placed in the anus to reduce the chance of a burn if a procedure is being performed in that area).
- Sparks can cause explosions should alcohol or other flammable agents be nearby.

Although some of these complications can be avoided, they still do occur on occasion. Removing a lesion on someone who is taking aspirin or anticoagulant therapy may be accompanied by increased bleeding, necessitating heavier use of the coagulation waveform. But do not discontinue oral anticoagulants, warfarin, aspirin, or clopidogrel. Another complication that may be seen in diabetic or older patients with thin, poorly perfused skin is slow or delayed healing. In this case, patients can be instructed in self-care of the wound, with periodic inspections by the clinician. Performing any procedures with these techniques on the lower extremities of diabetic patients can certainly be fraught with problems related to delayed healing and possibly secondary infection. Scarring must also be considered a complication; however, once proper technique is established, a scar by this method of treatment is often less pronounced than those produced by other surgical and excisional techniques. Excising too deeply increases the likelihood of scars.

POSTPROCEDURE PATIENT CARE

Several approaches are acceptable in the postprocedure care of these lesions. In general, the areas that were treated should be washed lightly four times a day with mild soap and water. The patient can use a washcloth for light debridement to prevent eschar formation. A topical antibiotic ointment is then applied as frequently as necessary to keep the lesion moist (even Vaseline will work). A dressing is not needed except at bedtime (or if under clothing) to ensure that the area stays moist (see the patient education handout at www.expertconsult.com). Moist healing and the prevention of eschar (scab) formation are essential to decrease the likelihood of scarring.

Moist healing can also occur when the lesion is simply covered with a small piece of synthetic material (e.g., Op-Site, Tegaderm; see Chapter 33, Wound Dressings). Leave these coverings in place for 1 week provided that there is no excessive accumulation of serum. If serum does accumulate, the dressing should be changed. Usually, after 7 days, the wound can be left open to continue its healing process without any covering unless it is in an area that may be irritated by clothing. This method is not practical in hair-bearing sites or if multiple lesions are removed.

PATIENT EDUCATION GUIDES

See patient education and consent forms available at (www.expertconsult.com.)

CPT/BILLING CODES

Billing codes for RF surgery are diverse depending on what was done. There is no special reimbursement if RF is used. Codes vary with the lesion size, benign or malignant characteristics, location, and type of removal. Some lesions would be billed as true "excision." Others would be billed as "shave excision," and still others would be termed "destruction" or "biopsy." Consult the most recent CPT coding manuals and other sections of this text.

Acknowledgment

I thank J. Drlik, MD, for his contribution to the section on skin tightening.

SUPPLIERS

(See contact information available at www.expertconsult.com.)

Ellman Cynosure International, Inc.
Wallach Surgical Devices, Inc.

For other suppliers, see Chapter 127, Loop Electrosurgical Excision Procedure for Treating Cervical Intraepithelial Neoplasia.

RECOMMENDED READING

Bolotin D, Alam M. Electrosurgery. In: Robinson JK, Hanke DW, Siegel DM, et al., eds. *Surgery of the Skin: Procedural Dermatology*. 3rd ed. Philadelphia: Elsevier; 2015.

Brown JS. Electrocautery. In: *Minor Surgery: A Text and Atlas*. 4th ed. New York: Oxford University Press; 2000.

Chiarello S. Controlled radio-vaporization of tumor tissue utilizing 4.0 MHz radiofrequency cutting current through a patented radiofrequency blade. *Dermatol Surg*. 2001;27:157.

El-Gamal HM, Dufresne RG, Saddler K. Electrosurgery, pacemakers and ICDs: a survey of precautions and complications experienced by cutaneous surgeons. *Dermatol Surg*. 2001;27:385–390.

Hainer BL. Fundamentals of electrosurgery. *J Fam Pract*. 1991;4:419–426.

Hainer BL, Usatine RB. Electrosurgery for the skin. *Am Fam Physician*. 2002;66:1259–1266.

Kannon GA. Moist wound healing with occlusive dressings: a clinical review. *Dermatol Surg*. 1995;21:583–590.

O'Grady KF, Easty AC. Electrosurgery smoke: hazards and protection. *J Clin Eng*. 1996;21:149–155.

Pfenninger JL. Electrosurgery. In: Usatine RP, Pfenninger JL, Stulberg DL, Small R, eds. *Dermatologic and Cosmetic Procedures in Office Practice*. Philadelphia: Saunders; 2011.

Pollack SV. *Electrosurgery of the Skin*. New York: Churchill Livingstone; 1991.

Rex J, Ribera M, Bielsa I, et al. Surgical management of rhinophyma: report of eight patients treated with electrosection. *Dermatol Surg*. 2002;28:347–349.

Usatine RP. Electrosurgery. In: Usatine RP, Moy RC, eds. *Skin Surgery: A Practical Guide*. St. Louis: Mosby; 1998:165–199.

Wedman J, Miljeteig H. Treatment of simple snoring using radio waves for ablation of uvula and soft palate: a day-case surgery procedure. *Laryngoscope*. 2002;112:1256–1259.

CHAPTER 26

SKIN BIOPSY

John L. Pfenninger

Examination and appropriate history suffice to establish most dermatologic diagnoses. However, at times, biopsies are necessary. A skin biopsy is typically performed to make or confirm a diagnosis and to guide definitive treatment. In many instances a biopsy serves as the means of both diagnosis and treatment if it removes the entire lesion. Needle aspiration biopsy (see Chapter 68, Fine-Needle Aspiration Cytology and Biopsy) is usually reserved for deeper lesions but at times can also be used to diagnose skin lesions.

Skin biopsies are generally quick, simple, and cost effective. Diagnoses obtained by biopsy also serve to build a clinician's experience and skill in dermatologic diagnosis by providing feedback and confirming the clinical diagnosis, perhaps reducing the need for future biopsies of similar lesions.

To enable the pathologist to provide the most information possible, provide a good history with each specimen submitted. Include aspects of the "seven D's":

1. *Demographics* (e.g., patient's age, history of travel, location of lesion)
2. *Diseases* (other diseases the patient has [e.g., lupus])
3. *Duration* (how long it has been present)
4. *Drugs* applied to the lesion or taken by the patient that could be the cause or change the appearance of the lesion (e.g., topical or oral steroids)
5. *Description* (e.g., papular, vesicular, hyperkeratotic)
6. *Diameter*
7. *Diagnosis* suspected

Skin biopsies are either partial or full thickness. Partial-thickness biopsies include shave excision and curettage. Full-thickness biopsies include standard excisional and incisional biopsies and the punch biopsy. Punch biopsies take only 5 to 7 minutes to complete; excisional or incisional types take longer. All of these may readily be incorporated in a primary care setting and can be performed when the patient first presents.

Priorities to be kept in mind when performing skin biopsies are (1) maintaining patient comfort and safety, (2) obtaining an appropriate tissue sample for pathologic diagnosis, and (3) producing the best cosmetic (least scarring) and functional result possible. Although written consent forms are usually not necessary for a skin biopsy, it is still important that patients understand the nature of the procedure, why it is being performed, and the possible complications.

INDICATIONS

- To obtain a tissue sample for diagnosis by histopathology, electron microscopy, or immunofluorescence testing
- To perform an excision for curative or cosmetic purposes
- To obtain a deep culture (bacterial or fungal) while avoiding superficial contamination of wounds (e.g., decubitus ulcers)

NOTE: Lyme disease can be confirmed through cultures of biopsy material.

In general, the main reasons to do a skin biopsy are to rule out cancer and to determine the disease process present. If the clinician's answer to the question, "What is it?" is "I don't know," that may be an indication for biopsy (not necessarily referral). The next question should be, "Could this be a melanoma?" If the answer is "yes," then a full-thickness biopsy (punch, incision, or excision) is indicated.

CONTRAINDICATIONS

- Significant coagulopathy (warfarin, factor Xa, or direct thrombin inhibitors, clopidogrel, and aspirin do not need to be stopped in patients with normal renal function).
- Preparations, anesthetics, preservatives, or other materials to which the patient is allergic.
- Partial-thickness biopsies are discouraged, if not contraindicated, if melanoma is suspected (must "biopsy for depth").

A biopsy does *not* spread or activate the disease, distort a future diagnosis of a melanoma, or compromise future care (unless possibly if a melanoma is shaved and transected). The only potential error that can be made in sampling a lesion is to shave a melanoma and not include the entire depth. If the entire lesion is removed so its depth can be assessed, there is no consequence. However, if when performing a shave biopsy/removal, part of the lesion is left behind, thereby making it impossible to determine prebiopsy thickness, it could compromise appropriate care. Melanoma treatment and prognosis are based on depth of the neoplasm. Thus, if there is a true consideration for melanoma, it is best to perform "biopsy for depth," which means a punch or excision. The fear that any pigmented lesion "could be" a melanoma should not deter a clinician from doing a biopsy. In practice, the majority of atypical nevi are removed using a shave technique. It is impractical to remove every such nevus with a full-thickness frank excision using suture closure. It is far better to shave and transect a melanoma than to ignore a lesion and miss the melanoma. The point is to sample suspect lesions or to refer the patient for biopsy and definitive care.

EQUIPMENT

- Nonsterile gloves (sterile if sutures are to be placed)
- Alcohol wipes
- Local anesthetic (0.5 to 1.0 mL of 1% to 2% lidocaine with or without epinephrine, can be buffered with sodium bicarbonate to decrease "sting" (see Chapter 5, Local Anesthesia)
- Hemostatic agents (see Chapter 199, Topical Hemostatic Agents)
- Antibiotic ointment
- Adhesive bandage
- Specimen container, usually containing formalin

NOTE: Tissue for culture may need to be placed in saline, whereas immunofluorescent studies may require that the tissue be placed in dry ice. Check with the pathologist or lab to determine the proper handling of tissue for the diagnosis of Lyme disease.

For Punch Biopsy

- A 2-, 3-, or 4-mm punch biopsy tool; disposable biopsy punches are convenient and inexpensive, and it is not necessary to clean, sterilize, or sharpen them. The 2-mm punch is used only for areas where scarring is to be avoided, because such a small amount of tissue may lead to a missed diagnosis, or the tissue can become inappropriately crushed. Biopsies greater than 4 mm in size will leave more scarring and, if sutured, may leave a "dog-ear effect."
- Pickups.
- Sharp fine tissue or iris scissors.
- Suture kit or Steri-Strips (only if the biopsy site is 4 mm or larger).

For Curettage

A dermal curette (Fig. 26.1) is used. *Disposable* curettes are recommended for nonmalignant lesions. Disposables are very sharp and will cut into the skin quite readily, so they must be used with caution. They do have a tendency to bend if a lesion is fibrotic (e.g., verruca). *Reusable* curettes do not bend but are not as sharp and often are inadequate for benign lesions where tissue adhesion is good. On the other hand, neoplastic tissue (e.g., basal cell carcinoma, squamous cell carcinoma) is necrotic and easily curetted. When used for this purpose, reusable curettes are also less likely to cut into the normal skin structures. The curette blade (see Fig. 26.1C–D) is interesting and has some excellent features. The curette is disposable, so it is sharp and fits on a scalpel handle. It also does not bend, so when curetting fibrotic tissue, such as verrucae, it maintains its shape and curetting function. Curettes of 2, 3, 4, 5, and 6 mm should be available. The size used depends on the size of the lesion.

For Shave Excisions

A single-edge flexible razor blade, DermaBlade (see Fig. 27.14), or scalpel blade (No. 10 or 15) is used (Fig. 26.2). A scalpel handle is not needed; not only does it take time to insert and remove the blade on the handle, but medical personnel can be injured during the process. The blade itself or a radiofrequency unit may be used to smooth out the surface after the shave excision. (See Chapter 25, Radiofrequency Surgery [Modern Electrosurgery], to review the technique.) Sharp tissue scissors (iris or Metzenbaum) can also be used to perform the "shave" by clipping off elevated lesions.

For Incisions and Excisions

- Minor surgical or laceration tray with scalpel, skin hooks, pickups, tissue scissors, and suture (see Chapter 18, Incisions: Planning the Direction of the Incision; Chapter 19, Laceration and

Incision Repair; and Chapter 21, Laceration and Incision Repair: Suture Selection)
- Radiofrequency unit, if desired (see Chapter 25, Radiofrequency Surgery [Modern Electrosurgery])

TECHNIQUE

Choosing a Biopsy Site

Although any skin area can be sampled, being selective improves final outcome. See Table 26.1 for recommendations specific to particular lesions and Table 26.2 for anatomic sites.

It is *not necessary to include normal tissue* in the sample, except when sampling a vesiculobullous lesion. It is then necessary to sample (usually a punch) right at the margin where the epidermis is being lifted from the underlying tissue (Fig. 26.3). If the lesion is small, a deep shave removing the entire lesion is also acceptable.

When there are multiple lesions that could be sampled, avoid the following areas:

- Cosmetically important areas
- Upper chest and deltoid regions, where hypertrophic scarring is more common
- Fingers, toes, and areas overlying joints
- Regions in which secondary infection (e.g., axillae and groin) or delayed healing (e.g., pretibial) is common
- Areas that compromise underlying structures, including superficial nerves and vessels
- Old lesions (choose well-developed but "fresh" lesions free of excoriation or excessive inflammation)
- Ulcerated lesions (if the only available lesion is ulcerated, include a border of the lesion in the specimen)
- Areas of poor circulation

Punch Biopsy

The punch biopsy instrument is used to obtain a full-thickness cylindrical specimen. Punch biopsy is a good choice for complete removal of small lesions (<5 mm) or whenever there is doubt as to the diagnosis or optimal treatment for a particular lesion. Punch biopsy is strongly recommended when melanoma is a significant consideration because it provides information on the depth of the lesion. The whole lesion does not have to be removed at the time of biopsy, and a biopsy does not change the natural history of the lesion's progression in any way.

1. Prepare the selected site with alcohol. Sterile technique should be followed if sutures are intended; otherwise, nonsterile gloves can be used. Biopsies of 2 or 3 mm do not need to be closed with sutures. A 4-mm biopsy on the face may need to be sutured, and a 5-mm biopsy nearly always requires suturing.

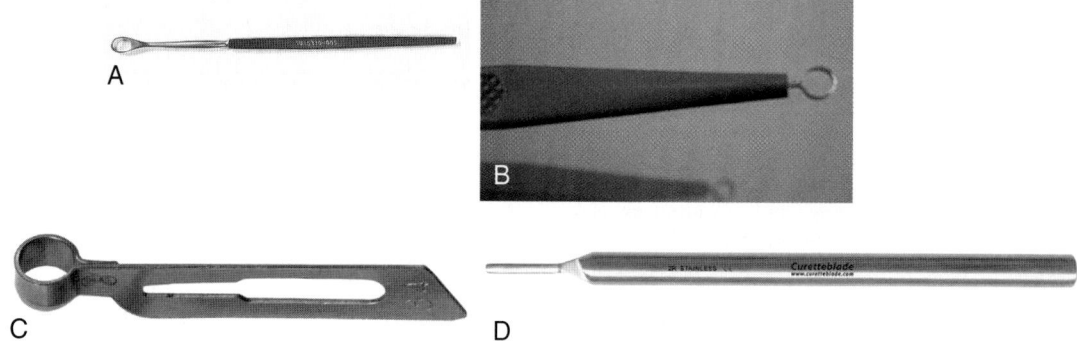

Fig. 26.1 (A) Fox dermal curette (reusable). (B) Acuderm disposable curette. (C) Disposable curette blade. D, Curette blade with smooth handle. (B, Courtesy Acuderm, Inc., Fort Lauderdale, Florida)

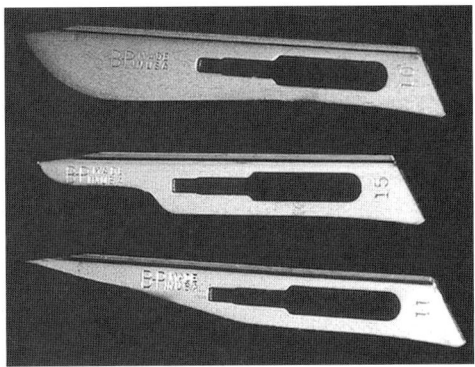

Fig. 26.2 No. 10, 15, and 11 scalpel blades used for shave excisions.

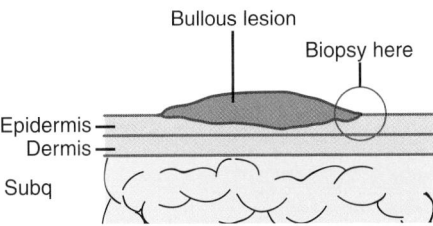

Fig. 26.3 Obtaining a skin biopsy when a vesicle or bulla is present. Normal tissue should be included in the specimen. "Fresh" lesions that have not ruptured and are not crusted should be chosen.

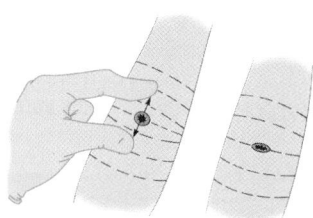

Fig. 26.4 Proper stretching of skin tension lines before punch biopsy (arm). On release, the tendency of the skin is to make the circular biopsy become more elliptical and thus more cosmetically pleasing when healed.

TABLE 26.1	Selection of Biopsy Site Based on Lesion Type
Lesion Suspected	**Where to Biopsy**
Basal cell carcinoma	Raised, nonulcerated area
Squamous cell carcinoma	Central, thickened area
Melanoma	Darkest, raised portion
Vesiculobullous disease	Fresh lesion at the margin; include some normal tissue (see Fig. 26.4)
Rashes	Primary lesion without secondary excoriation or infection

Normal tissue is not needed in most instances (only with vesiculobullous lesions).

A biopsy does not spread cancer.
In sampling a suspected melanoma, go for depth (i.e., a punch instead of a shave).
Most chronic dermatitis is nonspecific on biopsy. A dermatologic consult may be indicated and be more beneficial.

TABLE 26.2	Site-Specific Biopsy Guidelines
Location	**Comments**
Breast	Punch or shave
Cervix	Mini-Townsend or baby Tischler forceps (see Chapter 124, Colposcopic Examination)
Eyelid	Sharp iris or tissue scissors for shave removal
Gingiva	Shave; consider radiofrequency unit to limit bleeding if lesion is elevated
Intra-anal	Cervical biopsy forceps or flexible sigmoidoscopy biopsy forceps
Lip	Punch (bloody; heals quickly) or shave
Muscle	See Chapter 188, Muscle Biopsy
Nail bed	Remove portion of nail; use small punch (see Chapter 24, Nail Bed Repair)
Penis	Thin skin; use shave technique; stay superficial; iris or tissue scissors or sharp curette works best
Perianal	Sharp iris or tissue scissors
Pinna	Shave; superficial punch; curette
Tongue	Punch; bloody; use suture; curette
Trunk	Any method
Vagina	Cervical biopsy forceps
Vulva	Hair-bearing area: use punch for depth Non–hair-bearing area: shave biopsy (see Chapter 139, Vulvar Biopsy)

2. Place a ring of anesthesia around the lesion (field block) or deep to the lesion.

   EDITOR'S NOTE: the clinician should be aware of what is directly beneath what is about to be punched. Although a punch biopsy can be performed over a nerve or artery (e.g., digital nerve, digital artery), the clinician should be a little more cautious and make sure not to advance the instrument very far below the dermis. In addition, inspect the base of the cylinder of skin being removed to make sure nothing else (e.g., nerve, artery) is involved or damaged.

3. Choose the appropriate-sized punch unit (2 to 5 mm). Remember that 2-mm biopsies may not provide adequate tissue for diagnosis and are somewhat difficult to handle (e.g., the specimen is slightly more difficult to remove from the instrument). To minimize scarring, stretch the skin on both sides of the planned biopsy site away from the site, perpendicular to the lines of minimal skin tension, using the thumb and index finger of the nondominant hand (Fig. 26.4). Then push the unit vertically into the skin and rotate it back and forth to cut through the skin to the subcutaneous fat (Fig. 26.5A). A decrease in resistance should be felt at the point where the dermis is completely penetrated (much like doing a lumbar puncture). Again, if there is a vital organ (e.g., nerve, artery) beneath the area being biopsied, make sure not to advance far below the dermis.

4. Withdraw the punch. Push down with the fingers on each side of the biopsy. If the "plug" goes down with the skin, the biopsy has not gone deep enough. If the plug pops up instead of going down, then the adipose tissue has been entered and the tissue has been freed adequately. Gently grasp the specimen with forceps or a skin hook. Lift the specimen, and free it by cutting the subcutaneous base with sharp tissue scissors (see Figs. 26.5B–C and 26.6). Apply pressure for hemostasis. Avoid chemical astringents in punch sites if the wound is to be closed with sutures, Steri-Strips, or glues; otherwise, apply Monsel solution, aluminum chloride, silver nitrate, or Gelfoam to control the bleeding. (Biopsies 3 mm or less rarely, if ever, need closure.) Rarely, electrocautery will be needed to control bleeds. A small pressure dressing with a folded 2 × 2 gauze under a bandage is usually sufficient (Fig. 26.7).

5. Large punch instruments (>5 mm) are available, but closure of these wounds may require conversion of the circular defect into an ellipse because closure would otherwise cause dog ears.

6. Use of absorbable sutures provides the same outcome cosmetically as does the use of nonabsorbable sutures, but they are more costly. With punch biopsies of 4 mm or less, outcomes are the same regardless of whether a suture is placed.

Curettage

Curettage is a partial-thickness technique and is particularly well suited for biopsy removal of basal cell carcinomas and hyperkeratotic epidermal lesions such as warts, molluscum contagiosum, seborrheic keratoses, and actinic keratoses (see Chapter 13, Approach to Various Skin Lesions). A potential disadvantage of curettage in terms of obtaining a laboratory specimen is that, usually, multiple fragments of specimen are produced and the presence of disease-free margins cannot be determined. The clinician performing the procedure decides if the removal is adequate. Many times, the initial curettement will reveal necrotic tissue consistent with a neoplasm such as a basal cell carcinoma. If the decision is made to proceed with treatment at that time, only the first curettement specimen is sent to pathology.

NOTE: With benign lesions, it is clinically apparent when the abnormal tissue has been removed. For treatment (not just biopsy) of malignant lesions, continue curettement until there is a "gritty"

tissue sensation, which is then followed by cautery. This process of curettement followed by cautery is done three times to ensure complete removal of any foci of *neoplastic* tissue (e.g., basal cell carcinoma, advanced actinic keratosis, or squamous cell carcinoma).

1. Prepare the area with alcohol and obtain an anesthetic wheal. Use the curette to scrape away or scoop out the lesion, typically in multiple fragments. Send the curetted tissue to pathology. (Remember to use disposable instruments for more fibrotic lesions and reusable curettes for necrotic tissue; see earlier discussion.)
2. Continue the curettage until only normal tissue remains at the margins. Usually, this is the upper aspect of the dermis, which feels "gritty" or "sandy" under the curette and demonstrates punctate surface bleeding. Use hemostasis as needed with topical hemostatic agents or light ball cautery. Carcinomas and severely dysplastic lesions generally feel soft and scrape out easily. Remember, when using curettage to treat a carcinoma, repeat a process

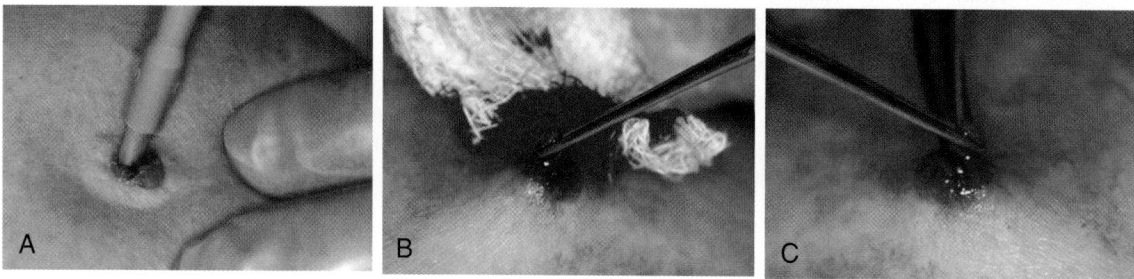

Fig. 26.5   (A) Applying the punch for a skin biopsy. (B) Excising the tissue freed by the punch. (C) Typical cylinder of tissue obtained from a 3-mm punch. (Courtesy The Medical Procedures Center, Midland, Michigan.)

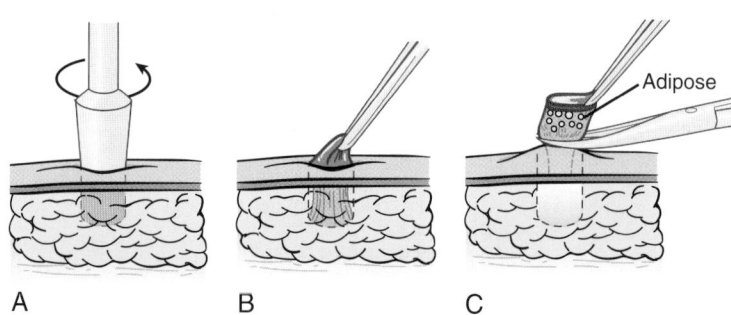

Fig. 26.6   Punch biopsy technique. (A) Twisting the punch with gentle pressure. (B) Picking up the loosened piece. (C) Cutting with scissors or a blade.

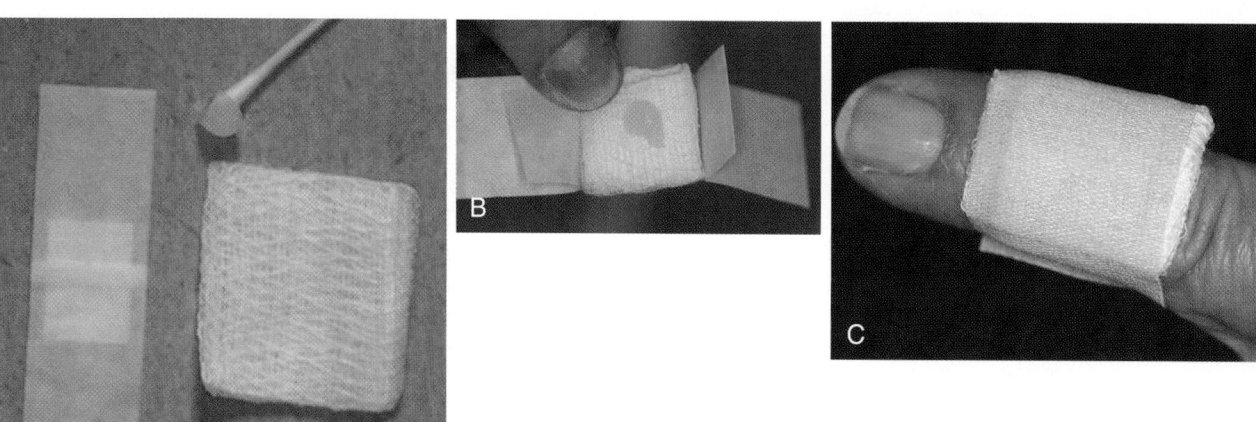

Fig. 26.7   Pressure dressing for a biopsy. (A) Components: gauze pad, antibiotic ointment, and adhesive bandage. (B) Gauze pad with antibiotic ointment. (C) Pressure dressing on finger.

of curettage and cautery three times (Fig. 26.8; see Chapter 13, Approach to Various Skin Lesions).

3. If, in the case of cancer, curettage (or shave excision) produces a full-thickness skin wound and adipose tissue is entered, this indicates that the tumor has probably invaded below the dermis. Set up a sterile field, excise the area, and close the wound with suture.

Shave Biopsy

Shave biopsy is used frequently and is best suited to remove the protruding portion of a raised skin lesion when a full-thickness sample is not required. Flat lesions such as nevi also can be removed/sampled using this technique, but rather than shaving flat across the surface, a saucer-shaped incision is made to go deeper in the center to remove the lesion.

Shave excisions should not be performed if a melanoma is suspected, because they may interfere with the pathologist's ability to grade the depth of invasion. A melanoma is treated based on the depth of invasion, and a difference of 0.1 mm or even 0.01 mm could be the difference between little further treatment and a large resection. Lesions most amenable to shave excision include compound or intradermal nevi, skin tags, seborrheic keratoses, actinic keratoses, lentigines, and small basal cell carcinomas.

Advantages of shave excision include minimal time requirement, simple equipment, lack of need for suturing, and generally excellent cosmetic results. In addition, the pathologist can determine if the entire lesion has been removed.

1. Prepare the area with alcohol and use clean technique; sterile gloves are not necessary. Reserve full sterile setup for full-thickness skin excisions that will be sutured. Instill a local anesthetic within the dermis underneath the lesion to elevate the lesion slightly, facilitating removal.

2. Excise the lesion by shaving with a slightly bowed, flexible, single-edge razor blade, DermaBlade, or with a scalpel blade kept parallel to the skin (Fig. 26.9). The resulting defect should be essentially level, or minimally depressed, in relation to the surrounding skin. The greater the depth of the shave into the dermis, the more likely there will be resultant scarring. Apply simple pressure, pinpoint electrodesiccation, radiofrequency loop smoothing (pure cutting level 2/20 watts), or topical agents such as aluminum chloride or Monsel solution to achieve hemostasis. Topical applications theoretically may inhibit healing. Monsel solution and silver nitrate carry the risk of temporary staining.

3. Shave excision can also be performed using a radiofrequency loop. However, heat artifact may occur at the margins of the excision, hindering histopathologic evaluation, or in the case of a very thin lesion, obliterating the lesion entirely. In addition, because of the ease of cutting with the radiofrequency unit, the novice user may inadvertently go too deep with the loop, causing excessive and unnecessary scarring. Many practitioners perform a shave biopsy with a scalpel blade then use a radiofrequency loop to feather out the edges of the defect created to complete the procedure (see Chapter 25, Radiofrequency Surgery [Modern Electrosurgery]).

4. Sharp iris or tissue scissors can be used, especially for pedunculated lesions, to effectively shave off the abnormality.

5. A variation of the shave biopsy is the *saucer excision.* With this technique, the central aspect of the biopsy, instead of being flat, is more depressed than the periphery. This technique might be used for actinic lesions, nevi, or dermatofibromas. In cases of suspected dysplastic nevi (but not a melanoma), one may cautiously perform a "deep saucer shave" because it allows histopathologic review of the tissue to ensure everything has been removed. However, be sure not to partially transect a melanoma; this is a very fine line. When in doubt, perform a deep punch biopsy first to confirm the nature of the lesion.

EDITOR'S NOTE: A good dermatologic pathologist can make the diagnosis of a basal cell carcinoma with a minute amount of tissue. With experience, some clinicians merely snip a portion of a basal cell carcinoma with very sharp iris or tissue scissors using NO anesthesia (other than "pinch" anesthesia, in which the clinician pinches the area briefly to induce numbness) to confirm the diagnosis. With very

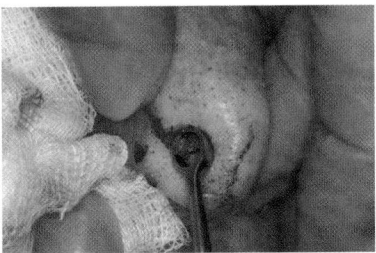

Fig. 26.8 Skin biopsy performed using a reusable curette to obtain a sample. (Courtesy The Medical Procedures Center, Midland, Michigan.)

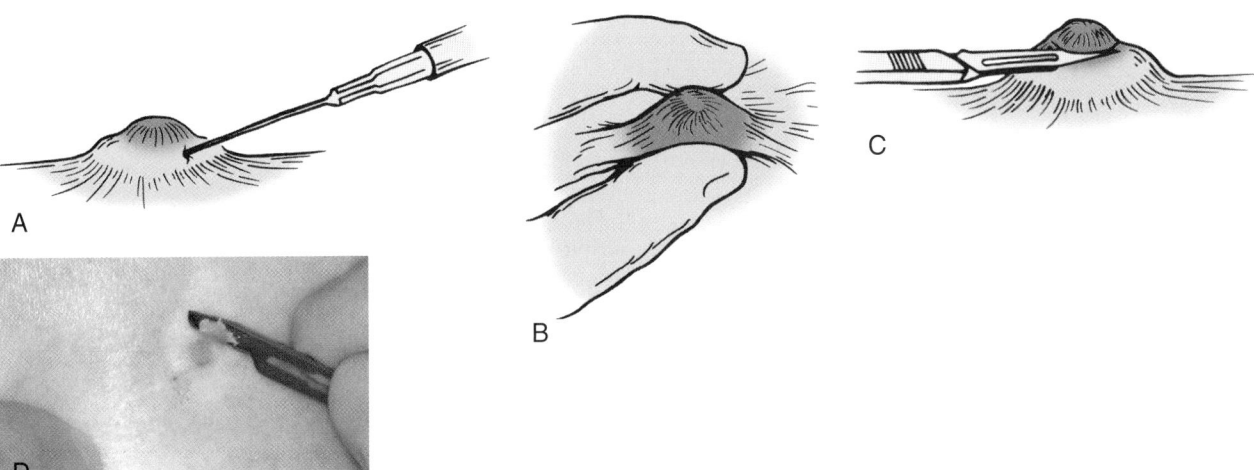

Fig. 26.9 One technique of shave biopsy. (A) Inject a local anesthetic to elevate the lesion. (B) Roll the skin between the thumb and forefinger to create a flat cutting surface and a tamponade effect on the surrounding blood vessels. (C) Holding a No. 15 blade parallel to the skin or at a slight downward angle, shave the lesion flush with or slightly below the surrounding skin. (D) Shave technique using a No. 15 blade. No scalpel handle is necessary. (A–C, Courtesy The Medical Procedures Center, Midland, Michigan.)

sharp scissors, for most people, a few very fast snips are less uncomfortable than a lidocaine injection.

Excisional or Incisional Biopsy

An *excisional biopsy* is used to remove an entire lesion in a manner that obtains a full-thickness specimen of skin. It generally refers to traditional frank excision with suture closure. Diagnosis and treatment can be carried out at the same time. Excisional biopsy can be used for removal of malignant, or suspected malignant, skin lesions where margins can then be assessed. The problem with this approach is that the recommendations for "clear margins" vary depending on the lesion involved (e.g., 1 to 2 mm for benign lesions, 3 mm for a basal cell carcinoma, 5 mm for a squamous cell carcinoma, 10 mm for invasive melanoma <2 mm deep), and this is often unknown until the histology report is obtained. Doing a primary excision for a biopsy may lead to an excessive and unnecessarily large excision or may require repeat surgery so that more tissue can be removed. An *incisional biopsy* removes only a portion of a larger lesion, and residual abnormal tissue remains. In general, a single punch biopsy (or more, if the lesion is very large) would be quicker and more acceptable when the diagnosis is uncertain. Then, once the diagnosis is known, appropriate treatment may be addressed.

1. In performing an excision, use sterile technique. Establish anesthesia, preferably in a field block pattern. Use a surgical marking pen to outline the planned margins of excision, and orient the long axis of the excision parallel to the lines of minimal skin tension (see Chapters 19, Laceration and Incision Repair, through Chapter 22, Laceration and Incision Repair: Suture Tying). Form the planned excision in the shape of an ellipse with a length that measures three times its width. The corners of the ellipse should subtend approximately 30 degrees (Fig. 26.10). See Chapter 13, Approach to Various Skin Lesions, for a discussion of appropriate margins for various lesions.

2. With the scalpel, make the initial incision along the outlined excision, then free up one corner of the ellipse, excising the full thickness of skin. Excise from one end to the center, then from the opposite end to the center, obtaining a specimen of uniform thickness. (A common error is to perform only a partial-thickness excision in the corners or lateral aspects of the wound.)

3. After the specimen is freed, undermine the edges on each side of the wound to a distance measuring the width of the original wound (Fig. 26.11). Undermine between the dermis and subcutaneous tissue with a scalpel blade, tissue scissors, or a radiofrequency unit using a vari-tip or fine needle with the unit set on the cut and coagulation setting.

4. A simple single-layer closure suffices for wounds with minimal tension. Otherwise, absorbable subcutaneous sutures (e.g., Dexon, Vicryl, PDS II) placed with an inverted knot can be used to reduce tension on the skin edges before final closure is completed (Fig. 26.12; see also Chapter 19, Laceration and Incision Repair).

NOTE: The following topics can be found in their respective chapters: planning the excisional site (Chapter 19, Laceration and Incision Repair), choosing and administering the anesthetic (Chapter 5, Local Anesthesia), selecting the suture (Chapter 21, Laceration and Incision Repair: Suture Selection), performing proper closures (Chapter 22, Laceration and Incision Repair: Suture Tying), and choosing dressings (Chapter 33, Wound Dressing).

COMPLICATIONS

- *Pain*: Generally insignificant.
- *Infection*: If the patient washes the area three to four times per day with soap and water and applies ointment (antibiotic or otherwise) to keep it moist, infection rarely develops.
- *Excessive bleeding*: Almost nonexistent.
- *Scarring*: Always a possibility. With punch biopsies, there may be an acne-like pockmark. Obviously, excision and incision leave a line and possibly suture tracks. All methods can leave hypopigmentation. Some topical hemostatic agents (Monsel solution and especially silver nitrate) can leave prolonged staining.
- *Missing the correct diagnosis*: A lesion may be sent for biopsy, but unless it is completely removed, the most significant area could be missed. (Likewise, the practitioner could unknowingly shave and transect through a melanoma; therefore, if there is any doubt, perform the biopsy for depth.)
- *Allergic reactions*: To topical antibiotics, the anesthetic, dressings, and other agents (usually indicated by redness and itching).
- *Recurrence*: Even if it was thought that the entire lesion was removed, both benign and malignant lesions can recur.

POSTPROCEDURE PATIENT EDUCATION

Shave excisions and curettage require moist healing, as described for radiofrequency shave excisions in Chapter 25, Radiofrequency Surgery (Modern Electrosurgery). Care for sutured full-thickness

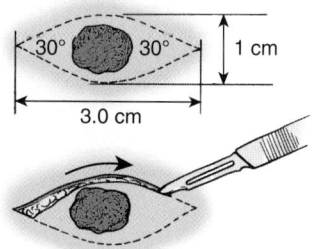

Fig. 26.10 Elliptical excision biopsy technique.

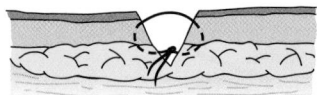

Fig. 26.12 Deep inverted absorbable sutures to close dead space after excision.

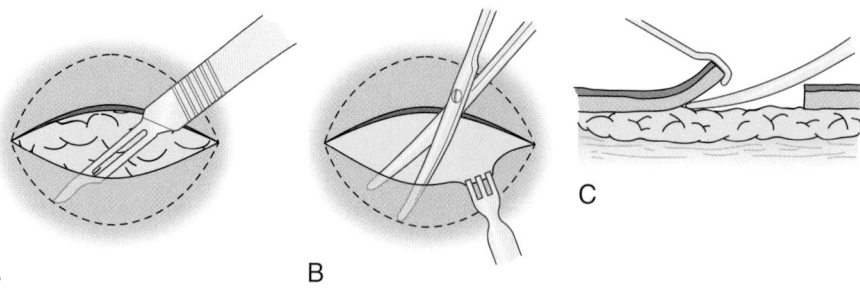

Fig. 26.11 Subcutaneous undermining to release tension on wound margins with scalpel (A) and scissors (B). Proper level for undermining within subcutaneous fat (C).

wounds is like that for primary clean lacerations and incisions described in Chapter 19, Laceration and Incision Repair.

CPT/BILLING CODES

11100	Skin biopsy, one lesion
11101	Biopsy, each additional lesion
11300	Shaving of epidermal or dermal lesion, single lesion, trunk, arms or legs, 0.5 cm or less
11305	Shaving of epidermal or dermal lesion, single lesion, scalp, neck, hands, feet, genitalia, 0.5 cm or less
11310	Shaving of epidermal or dermal lesion, single lesion, face, ears, eyelids, nose, lips, 0.5 cm or less
11755	Biopsy nail unit
30100	Biopsy intranasal
38500	Biopsy/excision lymph node, superficial
38505	Biopsy lymph node, by needle
41100	Tongue, anterior two thirds
41105	Tongue, posterior one third
45100	Biopsy anorectal wall
54100	Biopsy penis, cutaneous
54105	Biopsy penis, deep
56605	Biopsy lesion, vulva or perineum
56606	Vulva, each additional
57100	Biopsy vagina, simple
57105	Biopsy vagina, extensive
57500	Biopsy cervix
68100	Biopsy of conjunctiva
69100	Biopsy external ear or pinna
69105	Biopsy ear canal

ICD-10-CM DIAGNOSTIC CODES

See Appendix G for a listing of ICD-10-CM codes for the skin.

SUPPLIERS

(See contact information available at www.expertconsult.com.)

Disposable and reusable punches, curettes, and DermaBlade
Acuderm, Inc.
American Safety, Inc
Curetteblade, Stoeker and Associates Technology Company
Integra Miltex

Any office medical supplier should be able to supply the basic instruments needed for skin biopsy.

ADDITIONAL RESOURCES

See information on moist healing in Chapter 25, Radiofrequency Surgery (Modern Electrosurgery).
See patient education and patient consent forms available at www.expert consult.com.

RECOMMENDED READING

Achar S. Principles of skin biopsies for the family physician. *Am Fam Physician.* 1996;54:2411–2418.

Bergfield WF, Pfenninger JL, Weinstock MA. Skin biopsy: selecting an optimal technique. *Patient Care.* 2001;30:11.

Boyd AS, Neldner KH. How to submit a specimen for cutaneous pathology analyses: using the "5 D's" to get the most from biopsies. *Arch Fam Med.* 1997;6:64–66.

Coit DG, Andtbacka R, Bichakjian CK, et al. Melanoma. *J Natl Compr Canc Netw.* 2009;7:250–275.

Dummer R, Hauschild A, Jost L, for the ESMO Guidelines Working Group. Cutaneous malignant melanoma: ESMO clinical recommendations for diagnosis, treatment and follow-up. *Ann Oncol.* 2008;19(suppl 2):86–88.

Gabel EA, Jimenez GP, Eaglstein WH, et al. Performance of nylon and an absorbable suture material (Polyglactin 910) in the closure of punch biopsy sites. *Dermatol Surg.* 2000;26:750–752.

Garbe C, Hauschild A, Volkenandt M, et al. Evidence-based and interdisciplinary consensus-based German guidelines: systemic medical treatment of melanoma in the adjuvant and palliative setting. *Melanoma Res.* 2008;18:152–160.

Garbe C, Hauschild A, Volkenandt M, et al. Evidence and interdisciplinary consensus-based German guidelines: surgical treatment and radiotherapy of melanoma. *Melanoma Res.* 2008;18:61–67.

Harvey DT, Fensje NA. The razor blade biopsy technique. *Dermatol Surg.* 1995;21:345–347.

Jost LM, Jelic S, Purkalne G, for the ESMO Guidelines Task Force, et al. ESMO minimum clinical recommendations for diagnosis, treatment and follow-up of cutaneous malignant melanoma. *Ann Oncol.* 2005;16(suppl 1):66–68.

Oppenheim EB. Failure to biopsy skin lesions prompts litigation. *Medical Malpractice Prevention.* 1990.

Pfenninger JL, Usatine RP. Choosing the biopsy type. In: Usatine RP, Pfenninger JL, Stulberg DL, Small R, eds. *Dermatologic and Cosmetic Procedures in Office Practice.* Philadelphia: Elsevier; 2012:70–85.

Saiag P, Bosquet L, Guillot B, et al. Management of adult patients with cutaneous melanoma without distant metastasis. 2005 update of the French standards, options and recommendations guidelines. Summary report. *Eur J Dermatol.* 2007;17:325–331.

Salasche SJ, Grabski WJ. Transverse sectioning of a pigmented lesion. *Dermatol Surg.* 1997;23:578–582.

Schanbacher CF, Bennett RG. Postoperative stroke after stopping warfarin for cutaneous surgery. *Dermatol Surg.* 2000;26:785–789.

Stulberg DL, Kattalanos N, Usatine RP. Elliptical excision. In: Usatine RP, Pfenninger JL, Stulberg DL, Small R, eds. *Dermatologic and Cosmetic Procedures in Office Practice.* Philadelphia: Elsevier; 2012:111–132.

Tran KT, Wright NA, Cockerell CJ. Biopsy of the pigmented lesion: when and how. *J Am Acad Dermatol.* 2008;59:852–871.

Usatine RP. The punch biopsy. In: Usatine RP, Pfenninger JL, Stulberg DL, Small R, eds. *Dermatologic and Cosmetic Procedures in Office Practice.* Philadelphia: Elsevier; 2012:98–110.

Usatine RP. The shave biopsy. In: Usatine RP, Pfenninger JL, Stulberg DL, Small R, eds. *Dermatologic and Cosmetic Procedures in Office Practice.* Philadelphia: Elsevier; 2012:86–97.

CHAPTER 27

Skin Grafting

Thomas N. Told

PINCH (PATCH) GRAFTING

Pinch grafting (also known as *patch grafting*; first described in 1872) is a method of treating leg ulcers by grafting small pieces of full-thickness skin, usually harvested from the patient's medial thigh, to the ulcer site. With pinch grafting, leg ulcer healing rates of 20% to 50% can be anticipated, depending on the cause of the ulcer. Pinch grafting should be considered as an adjunct to conservative therapy and a therapeutic alternative for the inpatient or ambulatory management of leg ulcers. (Chapter 29, Unna Paste Boot: Treatment of Venous Stasis Ulcers and Other Disorders, describes another method for treating lower extremity venous ulcers using the Unna boot.) Pinch grafting requires no special training and no specialized equipment or supplies, but it does require a prolonged period of leg elevation and bed rest after the procedure. Clinicians should consider pinch grafting as an adjunct to conservative therapy for the treatment of leg ulcers, especially when other therapies like the Unna boot have failed.

NOTE: Unna boots do not make a good outer covering dressing for skin grafts because they tend to apply too much compression for optimum vascularization of the new graft.

Indications

Pinch grafting can be used to treat any leg ulcer or any other small, slow-healing ulcer of the trunk or extremities. Success rates for pinch grafting are highest for arterial ulcers (50%) and lowest for venous ulcers (20% to 40%). Compared with patients treated with conservative therapy, patients treated with pinch grafting have a shorter time to healing (reepithelialization) and a longer time until ulcer recurrence.

Contraindications

- Allergy to anesthetic or antiseptic agents
- Skin infection at potential donor sites
- Lack of granulation base in ulcer (relative contraindication)
- Patient unwillingness or inability to comply with postprocedure instructions

Equipment

- Syringe and needle for anesthetic injection
- 1% or 2% lidocaine without epinephrine
- Antiseptic agent for donor site preparation (e.g., povidone-iodine, chlorhexidine)
- Sterile drape for donor site
- Sterile gloves
- Tissue forceps with teeth
- No. 15 scalpel blade (a 3- to 5-mm punch biopsy can be used instead)
- Ruler
- Dressings for grafted ulcer (options include petrolatum-impregnated gauze; saline-soaked fine-mesh gauze, Adaptic [Johnson & Johnson] nonadhering dressing, Biobrane [Smith & Nephew], or Xeroform gauze [Covidien])
- Two layers of dry gauze and a light pressure dressing
- Telfa pad (Covidien) to transport grafts
- Petrolatum gauze, Telfa pad, Adaptic or Xeroform (bismuth tribromophenate) gauze to dress the donor site (there is also a dissolving petrolatum gauze that works well)

Preprocedure Patient Preparation

The patient must be willing and able to comply with postprocedure activity restrictions. The leg ulcer must be clean and must have a granulation base. The ulcer base can be debrided with wet-to-dry saline gauze dressings for 3 to 4 days before the procedure. The relative risks and benefits of pinch grafting should be explained to the patient. All supplies and equipment should be gathered at bedside or in the examination/treatment room. The ulcer should be measured to provide an estimate of the number of grafts needed. The donor site (the proximal medial thigh is preferred) and the skin around the ulcer should be prepared in a sterile manner. Pinch grafting should be performed under sterile conditions.

Technique

1. Prepare and drape both donor site(s) and ulcer(s).
2. Measure the ulcer(s).
3. *Inject local anesthetic* (without epinephrine) into the donor site to form wheals of 5 to 10 mm in diameter (the number of wheals should equal the number of grafts needed; Fig. 27.1).
4. Grasp the anesthetized skin with the tissue forceps and *remove full-thickness skin pieces* 3 to 5 mm in diameter, avoiding subcutaneous fat (Fig. 27.2). Trim off any fat that may be adherent. A 3- to 5-mm punch biopsy can be used in the same manner, punching only down to (avoiding or trimming off) subcutaneous fat.
5. *Store the graft pieces* on a Telfa pad moistened with normal saline.
6. *Place the skin pieces on the leg ulcer.* Leave 2- to 5-mm spaces between grafts as well as between grafts and the ulcer edge to allow drainage of wound secretions (Fig. 27.3).
7. *Dress the ulcer and grafts* with fine-mesh petrolatum-impregnated gauze (e.g., Adaptic or Xeroform) to cover the whole ulcer, followed by an occlusive dressing with 4- by 4-in gauze pads and a compressive dressing.
8. *Dress the donor site* with fine-mesh petrolatum-impregnated gauze (e.g., Adaptic or Xeroform) followed by dry gauze in at least two layers and light compression with an Ace wrap or Coban (3M).
9. See later for postoperative care.

Substitutes for Autographs

The mathematics of skin loss is very precise; the body cannot afford to lose too much skin surface area before it is fatally compromised. In some cases there may not be adequate skin to harvest, or the

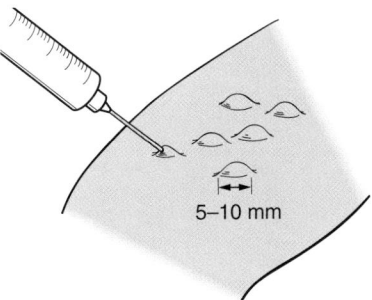

Fig. 27.1 Local anesthetic (without epinephrine) is injected into the donor site, forming wheals 5 to 10 mm in diameter.

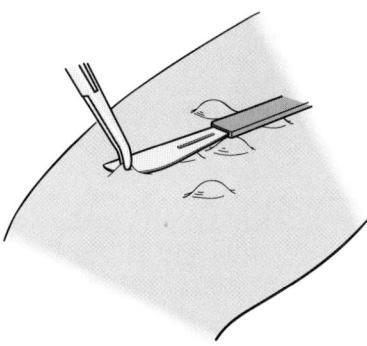

Fig. 27.2 Anesthetized skin is grasped with the tissue forceps. Full-thickness pieces of skin, 3 to 5 mm in diameter, are removed.

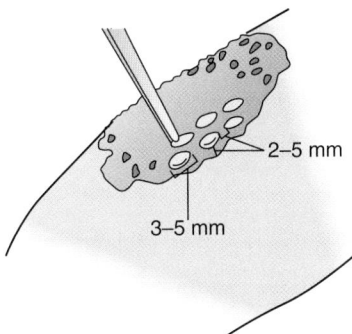

Fig. 27.3 Skin pieces are placed on the leg ulcer, with 2- to 5-mm spaces left between grafts as well as between grafts and the ulcer edge to allow drainage of wound secretions.

condition of the patient's skin may be too poor to supply autografts to cover defects. In these cases substitutes are available to cover defects and allow protection and healing.

Early *skin substitutes*, such as Biobrane, which is a collagen-impregnated fabric that imparts a framework for fibroblasts to adhere to on the wound surface and thus accelerate the healing process, have been available for years. Unlike Telfa dressings, where the slick, shiny side of the dressing touches the wound to prevent adherence, with Biobrane the rough, collagen-bearing fabric side is placed next to the wound and left there until it falls off weeks later. With deep second-degree skin loss, this is all that may be needed to stimulate healing.

Heterografts such as pig skin may be used to temporarily stabilize and debride large areas of skin loss that may need temporary coverage until autografting can take place with the patient's own skin.

Synthetic skin has undergone remarkable development from the early days of culturing fibroblasts from the foreskins of circumcised

infants to today's modern techniques of growing customized skin using stem cell technology. Currently the major problem with these grafts is their lack of durability and short life span.

Allografting with banked cadaver skin is the mainstay of burn centers today. It is used for covering large, full-thickness areas of skin loss. There is a good supply of this material, but the potential to spread serious tissue-borne diseases must always be kept in mind and could limit general use.

Most of these materials are supplied in sheets, as a mesh, and are ready to be applied using the basic techniques for grafting previously discussed. Before using them one must be familiar with all the supplier's recommendations for use.

Complications

- The most common complication is graft failure.
- Infections at the donor site or the ulcer are rarely reported.
- Deep venous thrombosis is a possible complication of this procedure because of immobilization.
- Bleeding at the donor site occurs frequently but is almost always minor and easily controlled with local pressure.
- Cosmetic outcome should be considered because grafts heal with a permanent studded appearance to the wound, so they work best on smaller lesions in less cosmetically sensitive areas such as legs and ankles.

Postprocedure Patient Education and Care

- Give the patient a handout on postoperative care. (See the sample patient education form available at www.expertconsult.com.)
- Patients must be placed on bed rest, with toilet privileges, and the grafted leg elevated for 7 days.
- The donor site dressing can be removed and replaced two to three times a day as needed. Wash gently with soap and water. Cover with petrolatum or antibiotic ointment, followed by the dressing.
- At 7 days after the procedure, the petrolatum gauze covering the ulcer is removed (if wound secretions are profuse, the compresses covering the petrolatum gauze are changed daily). After the petrolatum gauze has been removed, a nonadherent dressing is applied and held in place with an elastic bandage. This dressing may be made by impregnating a stockinette with petrolatum ointment, or a commercially prepared product such as Adaptic or Xeroform gauze may be used.
- At 7 days after the procedure, the patient is allowed to ambulate.
- At 14 days after the procedure, the stockinette is removed and the ulcer dressed with gauze as needed.
- Some authorities recommend that low-molecular-weight heparin or other deep venous thrombosis prophylaxis be given to patients at high risk of venous thrombosis for 7 to 10 days after pinch grafting.
- Prophylactic antibiotics have generally not been used but may be considered in high-risk situations. If topical antibiotics are used, it is best to avoid products containing neomycin owing to the high rate of allergic reactions.

FULL-THICKNESS AND SPLIT-THICKNESS SKIN GRAFTS

Every primary care physician who manages wounds will encounter full-thickness skin loss that cannot be closed by conventional suturing methods. One of the best ways to solve these full-thickness skin loss problems is through the use of skin grafting techniques. The cutaneous surgeon possessing the basic skills of skin closure can easily master this very useful procedure. Donor skin reduces the size of the defect and speeds healing time. A properly selected and applied graft creates a minimal donor site defect and contributes to good function and cosmetic results.

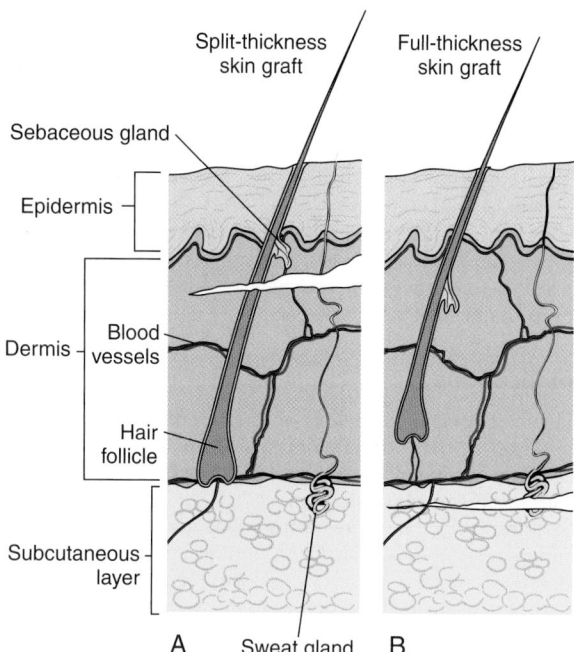

Fig. 27.4   Free skin grafts are divided into two main types: split thickness (A) and full thickness (B).

Indications

- Full-thickness abrasions and burns where skin loss creates defects 1 cm or more in width between viable skin edges
- Full-thickness skin loss on areas that have tight skin that cannot be advanced or undermined (e.g., tip of the nose, fingers, and toes)
- Large areas of skin loss that need to be minimized for better function
- Essential covering for defects that cannot be closed (e.g., large skin excision sites, full-thickness skin flap donor sites, tendons, cartilage, and bone)
- Areas of skin loss where excessive scarring of secondary granulation tissue may impair function or create adverse cosmetic results

Contraindications

- Infection at the donor site
- Infection at the recipient site
- Excessive bleeding at the recipient site
- Contamination of the recipient site with embedded foreign material
- Excessive edema at the recipient site
- Inadequate blood supply to sustain a graft

NOTE: Defects that are smaller than the size of a dime (1 cm in diameter) will heal well on their own with no need for grafting. If wounds are contaminated with foreign material or are infected, a delay of the grafting procedure will allow for the recipient site to establish granulation tissue that will better support the graft.

Skin Graft Types

Skin grafts are divided into two categories: *full thickness* and *split thickness* (Fig. 27.4):

Full-thickness grafts consist of the epidermis and the entire dermis. Full-thickness grafts are harvested by sharp dissection with a scalpel, and the thickness of the graft is determined by the region of the body where the donor skin originates.

Split-thickness grafts consist of the epidermis and a variable depth of dermis. Split-thickness grafts take only a part of the dermis, leaving the rest of the dermis at the donor site to regenerate. There are three grades of a split-thickness graft: thin (0.005 to 0.010 inch), medium, and thick.

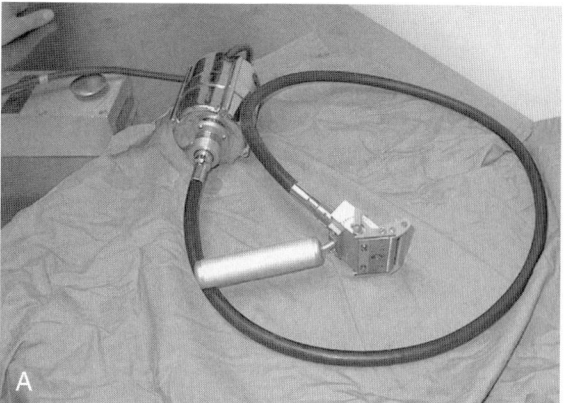

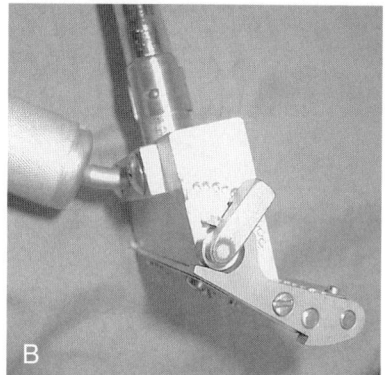

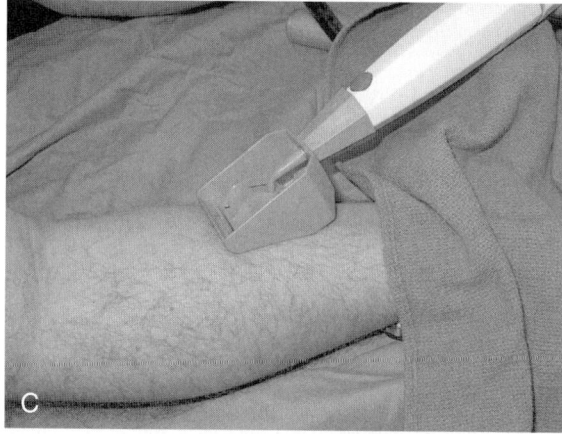

Fig. 27.5   (A) Adjustable-thickness motorized dermatome. (B) Adjustment lever on the motorized dermatome that cams the blade up or down to control the thickness of the skin graft. (C) Battery-powered dermatome with disposable fixed-depth and fixed-width detachable head.

The thickness is varied by the downward pressure the surgeon exerts on the dermatome handle or by a steeper angle applied to the cutting blade. Mechanical dermatomes are available that have an adjustable gate, or a preset thickness setting, that will determine graft thickness (Fig. 27.5).

Whether the surgeon uses a freehand shave technique or a preset dermatome, it takes practice to produce skin grafts of appropriate and uniform thickness.

NOTE: The tendency of the novice operator is to produce thicker split-thickness grafts than intended, even with the mechanical dermatome set on the thinnest settings.

Split-Thickness Grafts

ADVANTAGES:

- Split-thickness grafts can be "meshed" and made to cover large areas of skin loss. In this technique, small slits are cut in the graft similar to the holes in a pie crust, allowing the sides of the graft to be stretched by an expansion ratio of 1 to 1½ times (Fig. 27.6).

- Thicker grafts can be placed in a mechanical mesh maker (Fig. 27.7) to form a uniform mesh pattern that covers large areas of skin loss from full-thickness burns. Extensive meshing promotes drainage of blood and serum from under the graft and improves success of donor skin revascularization.
- Very thin grafts (0.010 to 0.015 inch) vascularize quickly and heal much more rapidly.
- Split-thickness grafts tend to contract as they heal, thus drawing down the size of the original defect.
- Donor sites heal more rapidly.
- Grafts require less blood supply to survive and may be the best choice for sites where vascularization is less than optimal.

Graft thickness can be chosen to satisfy the need for wear, appearance, hair growth, and speed of healing. Thin grafts heal rapidly but are not as cosmetically pleasing. Grafts thicker than 0.015 inch look better and resist wear better but heal more slowly.

DISADVANTAGES:

- Split-thickness skin grafts are not as resistant to trauma and can be injured easily in areas of friction and wear.
- They are less like normal skin in color, texture, suppleness, and hair growth. The mesh pattern is permanent and is not used in cosmetically sensitive areas such as the face or anterior neck.
- Meshing or "pie crusting" causes additional scarring and skin hypertrophy.

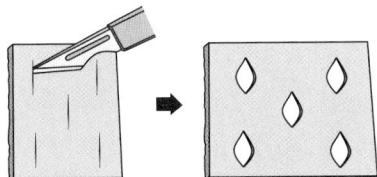

Fig. 27.6   Split-thickness grafts can be expanded by "pie crusting" or cutting small slits in places that need expansion. This can expand a graft by 50% over the original size.

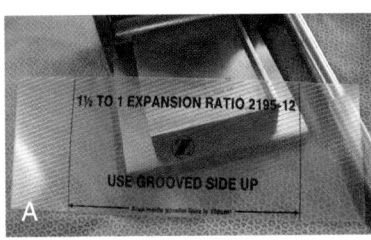
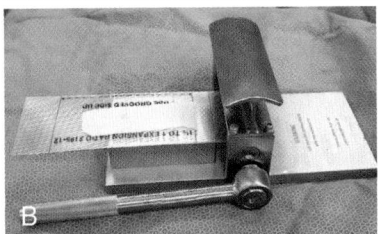

Fig. 27.7   (A) The skin graft is placed on the disposable clear plastic template with the dermis side resting on the grooves of the template. (B) The handle is turned clockwise, rolling the graft through the press. A uniform meshed graft emerges on the opposite side. Meshing allows a 2-inch-wide graft to expand to cover a defect of 3 inches (1:1.5 ratio) and facilitates drainage of blood and fluids that may accumulate under the graft.

- Split-thickness grafts do not germinate over bone without periosteum or cartilage without perichondrium.
- A dermatome must be used; for large grafts, an operating suite is necessary.
- Freehand technique produces only postage stamp–sized grafts.
- These grafts do not work well over joints because they are more likely to cause contracture and restriction of the joint.

Full-Thickness Grafts

ADVANTAGES:

- Full-thickness grafts match normal skin contours, color, and texture better than any other form of graft and are more esthetically pleasing over time.
- They undergo less postoperative contracture and will not influence the size of the defect.
- Thick grafts resist friction and wear better than the thinner grafts.
- Full-thickness grafts can be used to cover bone without periosteum and cartilage without perichondrium.

DISADVANTAGES:

- Full-thickness grafts cannot be used to cover large areas without carrying their own blood supply.
- Large full-thickness donor sites must be covered with split-thickness grafts to heal.
- Full-thickness grafts need a good supply of blood at the recipient site to survive.
- Thick grafts do not contract in total diameter with healing, as split-thickness grafts do.
- Full-thickness grafts take the longest time of any graft to vascularize.
- The size of the donor site is determined by the defect size, and the graft cannot be meshed to expand its surface coverage.

Equipment

- Dermatome
  - Adjustable type with thickness settings, flexible shaft, and external power (see Figs. 27.5A and B)
  - Battery-powered, disposable-head type (see Fig. 27.5C)
- Sterile tongue blade
- 5 to 10 mL sterile mineral oil
- Petrolatum-impregnated gauze, Tegaderm (3M), or fine-mesh gauze
- Minor surgical tray
- 5-0 suture (polyethylene or Vicryl)
- Skin stapler if sutures are not used
- Steri-Strips
- Kerlix roll
- Ace wrap, Coban, or elastic stockinette
- No. 10 or larger scalpel blade or a razor blade
- Two Adson tissue forceps
- 5-inch Halsey needle holder
- 4-inch curved iris scissors
- 6-0 or 5-0 nylon sutures (monofilament, not braided)

Donor Sites

Full-Thickness Grafts

See Fig. 27.8.

- Postauricular area
- Supraclavicular area
- Suprapalpebral area
- Antecubital area
- Volar wrist area
- Lower abdominal area
- Inguinal area

Split-Thickness Grafts

See Fig. 27.9.

- Posterior lateral thigh
- Superior buttocks
- Anterior abdomen
- Anterior thigh
- Inner surface of the upper arm for hairless skin
- Flexor surface of the forearm

NOTE: Facial defects should be repaired with full-thickness grafts because these grafts cause less cosmetic disruption. Never use skin for the face from areas below the clavicle because these grafts do not

match in color or texture and they contain hair follicles, resulting in lifelong deformity.

Techniques

Full-Thickness Grafts

1. Make sure no active folliculitis or cellulitis exists close to the donor site.
2. Prepare the skin for surgery using aseptic technique.
3. Drape the donor site.
4. Infiltrate the skin to be transferred with lidocaine without epinephrine for anesthesia.
5. Remove a fusiform piece of skin large enough to cover the defect without creating tension (Fig. 27.10A and B). Try to stay above the subcutaneous fat layer.
6. Remove as much subcutaneous fat as possible from the graft without button-holing the graft (see Fig. 27.10C and D).
7. Place the graft dermis side down on a saline-soaked gauze pad until ready for transfer.
8. Trim the graft to fit the defect.
9. Suture the graft into the defect, taking care to notice the skin lines and skin edges (Fig. 27.11A).
10. Use polyethylene suture, staples, or Steri-Strips.
11. Care must be taken to use the suture size and technique that will result in the least damage to the edges of the skin graft (small premium needles [size P-3] and suture 5-0 or less). Excessive bleeding at the edges will allow blood to flow under the new graft and prevent adherence of the graft.

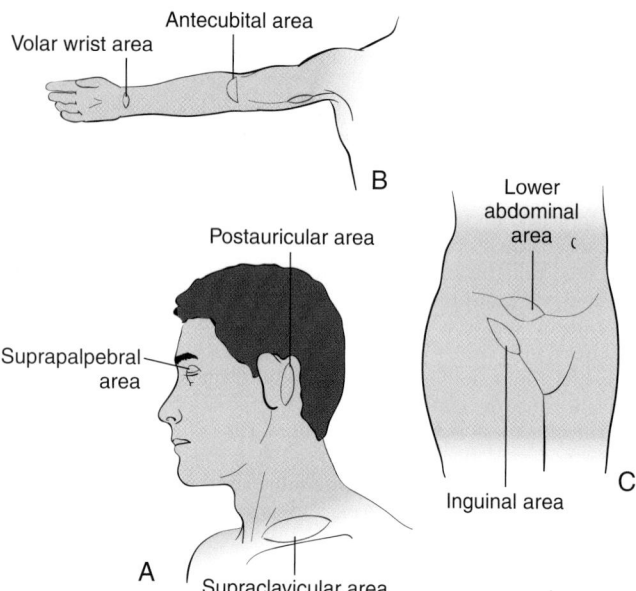

Fig. 27.8 Potential harvest areas for full-thickness grafts. (A) Head. (B) Arm. (C) Lower abdomen and inguinal areas. Do not use grafts from areas shown in (B) and (C) to graft the face, head, and neck (A). The color will not match and a permanent defect will remain.

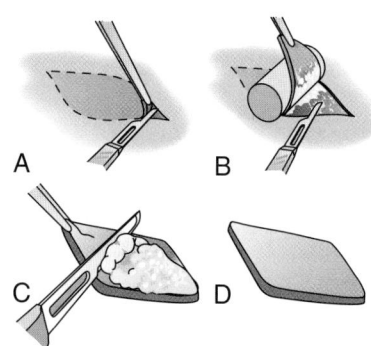

Fig. 27.10 Full-thickness grafts should have all the subcutaneous fat removed before being placed on the graft site. (A) Excising the graft. (B) Using a small cotton roll to aid in keeping the graft flat. (C) Removing the subcutaneous fat from donor skin. (D) Graft skin ready to be applied.

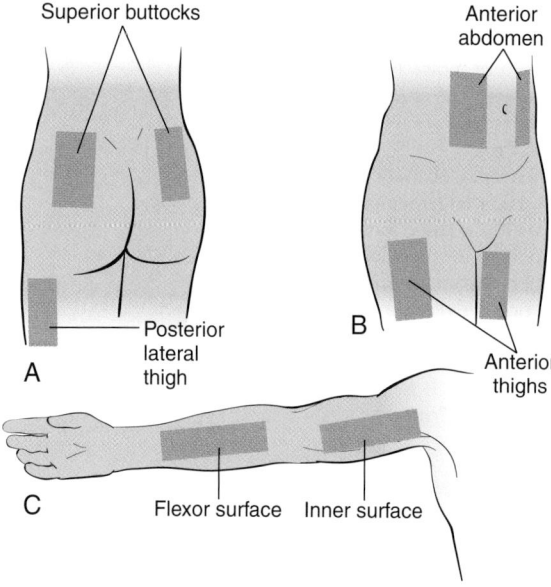

Fig. 27.9 Potential harvest areas for split-thickness grafts. (A) Posterior buttocks and lateral thigh. (B) Anterior abdomen and thighs. (C) Hairless areas of the arm.

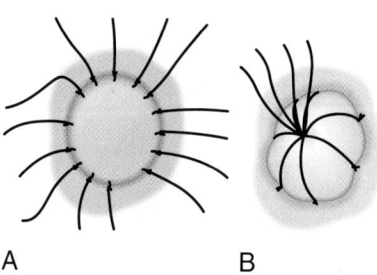

Fig. 27.11 Grafts can be secured best by using a stent. Suture tails are left long at the time of attachment of the graft (A), then tied over the gauze dressing (B) to provide pressure and anchor the graft in place. An initial layer of nonadherent material is applied, or the graft may be lubricated with antibiotic ointment to prevent the gauze stent from sticking.

12. A stent dressing best secures the graft (see Fig. 27.11B). A stent dressing basically holds a piece of gauze in between the sutures and the graft for a week.
13. Close the donor site in the usual fashion with sutures or staples. If the donor site cannot be closed without excess tension, a split-thickness graft can be used to cover it.
14. Place a nonadherent dressing on the donor site and treat as a laceration.

Split-Thickness Grafts

HARVESTING TECHNIQUES: DERMATOME:

1. Make sure no active infection or atrophic skin diseases exist on or near the donor or recipient site.
2. Prepare and drape the area with surgical scrub and drapes.
3. Ready the dermatome by setting the desired thickness on the gauge. Usually the best intermediate setting is the thickness of a scalpel blade. Thin grafts should transmit light, like frosted glass. Disposable dermatome heads will produce thin grafts; the operator simply needs to decide on the blade width, because various heads have various widths.
4. Anesthetize the skin to be harvested with local or regional anesthesia for small grafts. General anesthesia can be used when the areas to be grafted are large.
5. Place a thin film of sterile mineral oil on the skin that will be run through the dermatome. This lubricates the surfaces and helps maintain a uniform thickness.
6. Have an assistant use the sterile tongue blade to depress the skin in front of the dermatome and provide countertraction to straighten out any wrinkles in the skin.
7. Start the dermatome and approach the skin at a fairly steep angle until the blade catches the skin and begins cutting. When this happens, flatten the angle so the undersurface of the dermatome is aligned perfectly parallel with the skin surface. Downward pressure on the handle will place the blade deeper in the dermis and produce a thicker graft (Fig. 27.12).
8. The split-thickness graft will bunch up behind the blade, and an assistant will have to grasp the leading edges of the graft and gently lift them straight up (the way a thin slice of cheese is lifted from a cheese cutter to keep it from bunching up). The total length of the graft can easily be determined as it is lifted off the blade.
9. When the desired graft length is reached, release downward pressure on the dermatome handle and point the blade at a steep upward angle, severing the graft.
10. Spread the graft out carefully, with the dermis side down, on saline-soaked gauze. In the case of extremely thin grafts, the skin can be floated on the surface of sterile saline in a basin before being transferred to the recipient site.

   NOTE: The shiny side is always the dermis side (vs. epidermis) and must go next to the vascular surface of the recipient site; otherwise it would be like laying grass sod upside down.

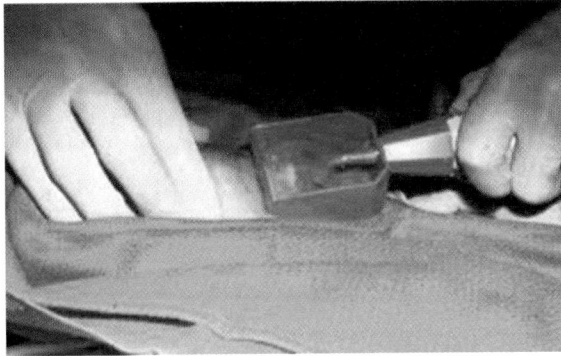

Fig. 27.12 Battery-powered dermatome at the correct cutting angle.

11. The donor site is dressed with Tegaderm, Adaptic, Biobrane, or Xeroform gauze or fine-mess gauze, which is left in place until it falls off in about 2 weeks. A gauze wrap and an Ace bandage can further protect the wound and reduce scar hypertrophy.

HARVESTING TECHNIQUES: FREEHAND: This technique is well-suited to the outpatient setting or emergency department, where small areas of skin loss elude conventional closure and require grafting.

1. A half-dollar–sized (3 × 3 cm) area on the forearm or thigh is infiltrated with 2% plain lidocaine without epinephrine, prepared with antiseptic solution, and draped for surgery (Fig. 27.13A).
2. Using a scalpel blade with a long straight cutting edge, like the no. 20, 21, or 22 in a scalpel handle (Fig. 27.13B), shave the skin at the desired thickness with a gentle slicing motion (Fig. 27.13C). A DermaBlade (Fig. 27.14) or a thin, standard double-edged razor blade can be used. Both blades are straight when not in use and are grasped between the thumb and index finger and gently bent into a U-shaped arc (see Fig. 27.14). The closer the thumb and index finger are drawn together the narrower the strip of skin will become. The DermaBlade is more expensive than a standard double-edged razor blade, but it has the advantage of

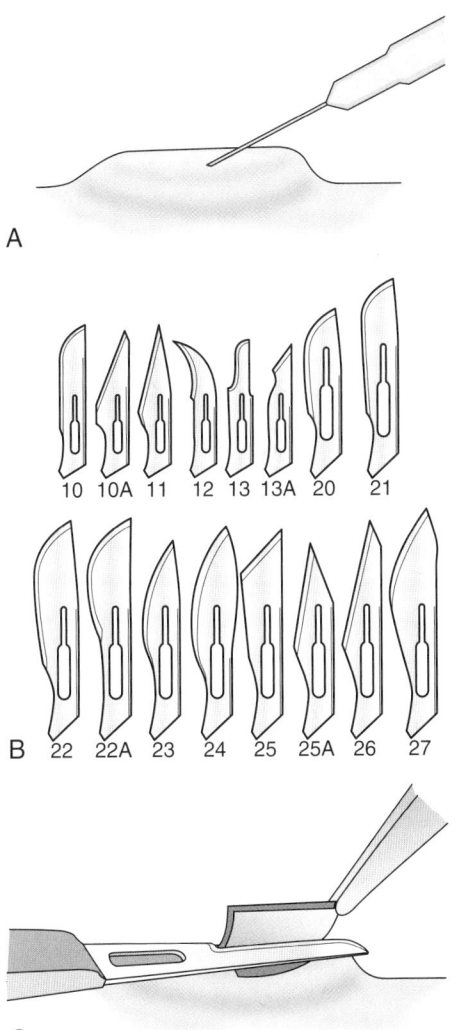

Fig. 27.13 Freehand split-thickness graft. (A) Infiltration with local anesthesia will slightly raise the skin, making cutting easier. (B) Scalpel blades of various sizes. (C) The large scalpel blade is held at a shallow angle to the skin, and the graft is shaved off to a desired length.

being completely sterile and much safer to use. The graft is taken by applying light downward pressure on the blade and moving it side to side in smooth oscillating strokes. The greater the downward pressure on the blade, the thicker the graft.

3. Widths up to 2 cm can be removed up to the length needed.
4. The skin can be transferred directly to the defect and sutured in place like any other split-thickness graft.

Recipient-Site Preparation and Graft Stabilization

1. In the case of full-thickness grafts, meticulous hemostasis is the key to graft survival. Bipolar cautery (as opposed to the monopolar cautery generally used) is the best way to achieve homeostasis with very little thermal damage.
2. The full-thickness graft must be tailored precisely to the defect at the time of placement, whereas split-thickness grafts may overlap the margins.
3. The survival of split-thickness grafts depends on the growth of capillary beds into the raw undersurface of the graft; it may take several weeks for granulation tissue to develop to provide these capillary beds. During this time, try to use natural methods of debridement and capillary bed enhancement; if possible, avoid enzymatic débriding agents, which will attack the graft as well.
4. The graft must not move during the period of revascularization. The graft can be secured with a 6-0 or 5-0 monofilament suture. One tail of the suture is intentionally left twice as long as the diameter of the defect so that a stent dressing can be tied over the graft (see Fig. 27.11). The dressing will stay in place for 7 to 10 days. Avoid the temptation to look under the dressing during the healing process.
5. Use as few sutures as necessary. Simple interrupted suture with monofilament material is the best tolerated. Do not put too much tension on the graft or the sutures. If more stabilization is needed, Steri-Strips can be used. Some surgeons report good success with

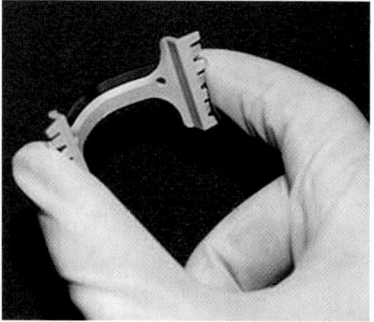

Fig. 27.14 The DermaBlade is bent in a U-shape between the thumb and forefinger in preparation for harvesting a free-hand split-thickness graft. Widening the distance between the thumb and forefinger will widen the strip of skin being harvested. T-shaped gripping bars at each end of the blade improve control. (Courtesy American Safety Razor, Cedar Knolls, New Jersey.)

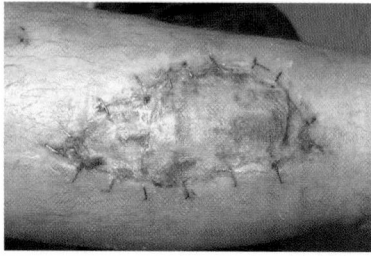

Fig. 27.15 Split-thickness skin graft attached with skin staples 10 days after surgery.

Steri-Strips alone. Dermabond, a commercial dermal adhesive, can stabilize fragile grafts; however, care must be taken not to allow the adhesive to flow between the graft and recipient site, which will prevent adherence.

6. In the case of large split-thickness grafts, skin staples can be used. This is a more rapid method of attachment and is relatively atraumatic (Fig. 27.15).
7. Large skin grafts may require a "pie crust" maneuver to vent bubbles or blood from under the graft itself. Small holes can be cut in the graft with fine scissors or a scalpel to let out the fluid (see Fig. 27.6).
8. Cover the graft with nonadherent material like Adaptic, Biobrane, Xeroform gauze, or Telfa. Make sure the new graft stays moist and out of the ambient air for extended periods. Cover the nonadherent material with saline-moistened gauze and at least two layers of protective gauze wrap and a light compressive dressing of Ace wrap or Coban.

    The dressings are not changed for the first 24 to 48 hours after graft placement unless soiled or bloody; then, for the next two daily outer dressing changes, moistened gauze is replaced over the nonadherent dressing. It is best not to disturb the nonadherent dressing in direct contact with the graft to prevent movement of the new graft.
9. The graft must be protected from trauma and from loss of contact with the vascular bed. Some cutaneous surgeons prefer to roll a cotton-tipped applicator over the surface of the new graft, rolling from the middle of the newly applied skin to the outside. This expresses unwanted blood, fluids, or air bubbles that will lift the healing graft away from the recipient bed.

Common Errors

- Placing the wrong surface of the graft against the donor site. Care must be taken at all times to ensure that the graft is not turned over in transferring it from the donor site to the recipient site. Split-thickness grafts are the most susceptible to this mistake.
- Allowing split-thickness grafts to dry out between harvesting and placement. The graft should be kept in moist gauze or a small basin of saline. Blot, do not rub, the surfaces of the graft.
- Causing excessive bleeding to the donor site before graft placement. Excessive debridement or wiping of the site with antiseptic-saturated gauze may cause bleeding that will lift the graft from the surface after placement and encourage infection.
- Not removing large air bubbles. Air bubbles can become trapped under the graft during the placement process and before application of the dressing. Care must be taken to remove such bubbles or fluid pockets.
- Not removing all the fat and subcutaneous tissue from the dermal side of a full-thickness skin graft. The dermal side of a full-thickness graft should be free of any material that will block the migration of vascular elements into the skin graft.
- Allowing edema or venous stasis to occur in the grafted extremity. Edema and vascular congestion will cause the buildup of fluid under the graft and lift it away from the recipient site.
- Attempting to remove an adherent covering in direct contact with the graft in less than 7 days. Dressing edges can be trimmed when they spontaneously lift away from the surgical site, but the dressing should never be pulled off.
- Loose-fitting dressings. Loose dressings will cause excessive shear forces on the skin graft during the 7- to 14-day healing process. Movement of the graft will impede healing and adherence.

Complications

The major complication of skin grafting is infection at the donor site (causing it to become a full-thickness defect) and loss of the graft at the recipient site (causing another full-thickness defect). The use of prophylactic antibiotics cannot make up for poor planning and bad surgical technique; therefore it is important to approach full-thickness skin loss with proper preparation.

POSTPROCEDURE PATIENT EDUCATION AND GUIDES

See the sample patient education form available at www.expert consult.com.

CPT/BILLING CODES

15100	Split graft, trunk, arms, legs, first 100 cm²
15120	Split graft, face, scalp, eyelids, mouth, neck, ears, orbits, genitalia, hands, feet, first 100 cm²
15200	Full-thickness graft, free, including direct closure of the donor site, trunk, 20 cm² or less
15220	Full-thickness graft, free, including closure of the donor site, including scalp, arms, legs, 20 cm² or less
15240	Full-thickness graft, free, including donor site closure, forehead, cheeks, chin, mouth, neck, axilla, genitalia, hands and feet, 20 cm² or less
15260	Full-thickness, free, including closure of the donor site, nose, ears, eyelids, and/or lips, 20 cm² or less

ICD-10-CM DIAGNOSTIC CODES

Split-Thickness Grafts and Full-Thickness Grafts

L97–L98.49	Ulcers, nonpressure chronic
L89–L89.95	Ulcers, pressure
L90.5	Scar
S01.00X–S01.95X Head	Open wounds
S31.20X–S31.45X Genitalia	
S61.001X–S61.559X Wrist, hand, fingers	
S91.201X–S91.359X Ankle, foot and toes	
S81.000X–S81.859X Knee and lower leg	
T20.000X–T25.799X	Burns

Add appropriate seventh character: A = initial; D = subsequent; S = sequela. See Appendix G for ICD-10 codes for neoplasms.

Acknowledgment

The editors recognize the contributions of Paul M. Paulman, MD, to the chapter on pinch (patch) grafting in a previous edition of this text.

SUPPLIERS

(See contact information available at www.expertconsult.com.)

Adjustable dermatomes
  Zimmer Biomet
  Bard Medical (battery powered)
  Humeca (battery powered)
Medical and surgical supplies
  Bergen Brunswig Medical Corp.
Surgical instruments
  Integra LifeSciences

RECOMMENDED READING

Acota AE, Aasi SZ, MacNeal RJ, et al. Skin grafting. In: Robinson JK, Hanke DW, Siegel DM, et al., eds. *Surgery of the Skin: Procedural Dermatology*. Philadelphia: Elsevier; 2015.

Adams DC, Ramsey ML. Grafts in dermatologic surgery: review and update on full- and split-thickness skin grafts, free cartilage grafts, and composite grafts. *Dermatol Surg.* 2005;31:1055–1067.

Andreassi A, Bilenchi R, Biagioli M, D'Aniello C. Classification and pathophysiology of skin grafts. *Clin Dermatol.* 2005;23:332–337.

Brunicardi FC, Andersen DK, Billiar TR, et al., eds. *Schwart's Principles of Surgery*. 10th ed. New York: McGraw-Hill; 2015.

Collins L, Seraj S. Diagnosis and treatment of venous ulcers. *Am Fam Physician.* 2010;81:989–996.

Doherty GM, ed. *Current Diagnosis & Treatment: Surgery*. 14th ed. New York: McGraw-Hill; 2015.

Haas AF, Glogau RG. Composite graft. In: Robinson JK, Arndt KA, LeBoit PE, Wintroub BU, eds. *Atlas of Cutaneous Surgery*. Philadelphia: WB Saunders; 1996:165–168.

Hjerppe A, Sand M, Huhtala H, Vaalasti A. Pinch grafting of chronic leg ulcers. *J Wound Care.* 2010;119:37–40.

Kontos AP, Qian Z, Urato NS, et al. The use of a flexible razor blade in skin graft harvesting. *Dermatol Surg.* 2009;35:120–123.

Leffell DJ. Split-thickness skin grafts. In: Robinson JK, Arndt KA, LeBoit PE, Wintroub BU, eds. *Atlas of Cutaneous Surgery*. Philadelphia: WB Saunders; 1996:149–156.

Ogawa R, Hyakusoku H, Ono S. Useful tips for successful skin grafting. *J Nippon Med Sch.* 2007;74:386–392.

Oien RF, Hakansson A, Hansen BU. Leg ulcers in patients with rheumatoid arthritis: a prospective study of aetiology, wound healing and pain reduction after pinch grafting. *Rheumatology.* 2001;40:816–820.

Oien RF, Hansen BU, Hakansson A. Pinch graft skin transplantation for leg ulcers in primary care. *J Wound Care.* 2000;9:217–220.

Orgill DP. Excision and skin grafting of thermal burns. *N Engl J Med.* 2009;360:893–901.

Phillips TJ. Current approaches to venous ulcers and compression. *Dermatol Surg.* 2001;27:611–621.

Roenigk RK, Zalla MJ. Full-thickness skin grafts. In: Robinson JK, Arndt KA, LeBoit PE, Wintroub BU, eds. *Atlas of Cutaneous Surgery*. Philadelphia: WB Saunders; 1996:157–164.

CHAPTER 28

HYPERTROPHIC SCARS AND KELOIDS

Harris Mones • Dennis LaRavia

The skin of predisposed individuals may respond to injury or surgery by developing excessive growths known as *hypertrophic scars* or *keloids*. Hypertrophic scars are self-limited growths that enlarge within the boundaries of a wound and then often regress over time. Many hypertrophic scars spontaneously involute within 2 years. Keloids are benign, hard, fibrous proliferations of collagen that expand, either slowly or rapidly, beyond the original size and shape of a wound. They tend to persist and often invade surrounding tissue. They may become painful or pruritic as well as unsightly.

Hypertrophic scars and keloids represent abnormalities in the synthesis and degradation of collagen and extracellular matrix components. Hypertrophic scars have a threefold increase in collagen synthesis enzymes compared with normal scars, whereas keloids may exhibit 20 times the normal levels. Hypertrophic scars can occur at any site of skin injury. Those following surgical incisions usually remain linear. Burns frequently produce unsightly, pink, hypertrophic scars that may contract. The scars may itch, but generally they do not produce the pain and hyperesthesia seen with keloids.

The most important risk factor for keloid formation is a wound healing by secondary intention. This is especially true if wound healing time is greater than 3 weeks. Although most cases of keloids are sporadic, some are familial. In familial cases, the mode of inheritance is unknown.

The incidence of keloids in dark-skinned individuals is 15 to 20 times that found in light-skinned people and is higher in Asians. Overall, there is an equal incidence of lesions in males and females, although young females have a higher incidence than young males. Hypertrophic scars and keloids are found only in humans, occur in 5% to 15% of wounds, and are rarely seen in people older than 65 years of age. Keloids appear frequently in anatomic sites that are subject to motion, that overlie bony prominences, or in areas of increased skin tension or recurrent stretch, such as the shoulders, upper back, and presternal areas. Keloids may develop on the face and scalp after acne or on the earlobe after ear piercing. They are seen more frequently in wounds that cross skin lines. Blood type A may be a risk factor. Children and pregnant women are more likely to experience both hypertrophic scars and keloids.

This chapter focuses on office techniques used in the treatment of hypertrophic scars and keloids. Because of the natural regression of hypertrophic scars, therapy for these lesions is usually limited to topical application or injection of steroids and compression. Keloids are considered by some clinicians to be low-grade, benign, cutaneous tumors, and radiation therapy has been advocated. That therapy is not reviewed here. The malignancy potential of radiation in the treatment of a benign disease as well as its expense makes radiation therapy a last resort. No single therapy for keloids has proven superior. Location, size, and duration are factors in choosing the most appropriate therapy. Cryotherapy, corticosteroid injection, surgical excision, pressure therapy, and irradiation—or a combination of these modalities—may be chosen for the treatment of keloids.

PREVENTION

The most important thing to consider in the management of keloid scar formation is prevention. Before surgical procedures are performed, a thorough history of abnormal scar formation or a family history of keloid scar formation should be obtained from the patient. If a history of keloid formation is obtained, all nonessential surgery should be avoided, especially at sites that are at higher risk. In circumstances where surgery cannot be avoided, all attempts should be made to minimize skin tension and secondary infection. Antibiotics, meticulous sterile technique, and perioperative steroid injections (mixed with lidocaine) are helpful in prevention as well.

CRYOTHERAPY

Tissue destruction techniques used for treating keloids can incite further keloid formation. Cryotherapy, however, has been used with good results in 65% to 75% of cases. Both liquid nitrogen and nitrous oxide methods can be efficacious (see Chapter 14, Cryosurgery, Fig. 14.4). The more recently the keloid developed, the better the response to cryotherapy. A 10- to 15-second freeze with *liquid nitrogen* (−189°C) is usually required for keloids on most sites other than the mid-sternal region (small scars will take less time). Freezing for more than 10 to 15 seconds with liquid nitrogen can produce persistent posttreatment hypopigmentation. A 30- to 45-second freeze is usually adequate for most keloids when *nitrous oxide* (−89°C) is used. A better guide for any modality is to continue the freeze until 1 to 2 mm of normal tissue is involved and the complete thaw time is 1.5 to 2 minutes. During each treatment visit, the entire lesion must be treated with two to three freeze/thaw cycles.

After cryotherapy, tissue edema will develop in 20 to 60 minutes. Within hours, a significant bulla (blister) will appear. A rather copious serous discharge may follow. A moist environment (semiocclusive dressing) will aid healing. In southern and temperate climate areas, particularly during the summer months, occlusive therapy may prolong healing and increases the likelihood of secondary infection. Depending on the size of the lesion, five to eight treatments may be needed at 6-week intervals. Start conservatively and increase the freeze times if there are no adverse effects.

Cryotherapy can also be used to soften hard keloids immediately before injection of steroids. Edema of the skin allows better dispersal of the steroid and minimizes its deposition into the subcutaneous or surrounding normal tissue. Cryotherapy before injection (liquid nitrogen spray for 3- to 5-second bursts) may also improve keloid regression; it allows for lower injection pressures and decreases the pain associated with injections. Allow 20 to 60 minutes for the edema to develop before proceeding with the injection.

CORTICOSTEROID INJECTIONS

Once a scar is palpable, topical corticosteroids, even under occlusion (e.g., flurandrenolide [Cordran] tape), are rarely beneficial. Raised hypertrophic scars and keloids, however, may be softened and flattened by intralesional corticosteroid therapy. Corticosteroids represent effective monotherapy for some hypertrophic scars and small keloids, and they are frequently used as the initial therapy for large keloids.

Early, small, or narrow lesions are initially treated with an intralesional injection every 4 to 6 weeks. Early keloids are softer and more responsive to injection than older, inactive lesions. Avoid injecting into surrounding normal skin to prevent perilesional subcutaneous atrophy and telangiectasia formation. When a lesion flattens to nearly the level of the skin surface, allow more time to pass before injecting again and decrease the concentration of the injections. Overaggressive therapy can lead to hypopigmentation and a depression resulting from subcutaneous atrophy.

Injections are frequently performed with a 27- or 30-gauge needle on a Luer-Lok syringe. Locked syringes help to prevent needle disengagement when injecting under pressure. Consider using cryotherapy immediately beforehand (see the previous section) to ease injection and improve dispersal of the steroid.

Many steroid regimens have been developed, and there is considerable variation in guidelines and recommendations for dosages and drugs. No clear advantage has been shown for any one type of corticosteroid. Triamcinolone acetonide 10 mg/mL (Kenalog-10) is a popular choice because of its 4- to 6-week duration of action. Although undiluted steroid can be used for unresponsive or dense lesions, it is more prudent to dilute the triamcinolone 1:3 with physiologic saline or 1% lidocaine (single-dose vials) to create a 2.5-mg/mL solution. This dilute concentration limits postinjection hypopigmentation and atrophy. Injecting only lidocaine around the lesion using a 27- to 31-gauge needle before steroid injection improves patient comfort. Once the individual patient response is known, the concentration of triamcinolone acetonide can be increased to a dilution of 1:2 or 1:1 with lidocaine for future injections to increase the effect. If little effect is seen even without dilution, triamcinolone 40 mg/kg can be used and diluted as indicated. **A common error is to be too aggressive.** Go slowly to avoid the complication of atrophy. Hyaluronidase can be added to the solution to help disperse the steroid.

Administer the corticosteroid as the needle passes through the lesion. Keep the bevel of the needle pointed down. The scar may blanch temporarily with the injection. Try to keep the injection within the confines of the lesion to prevent side effects in the adjacent tissue. Firm lesions may limit the amount of medication that can be administered. The total amount will vary significantly depending on the size of the lesion. Keloids over 1 to 1.5 cm in diameter generally do not resolve as quickly or completely as smaller keloids. When the lesion is too dense to inject, consider treating with cryotherapy first, as previously discussed.

Another method of injecting steroids is to use the MadaJet Injector (see Pearl no. 8 in Appendix H, Pearls of Practice). The same concentration is used. The spring-loaded "gun" fires (dispenses) the solution, which is under pressure, into the lesion. No needles are involved, and there is less pain. Injections may need to be repeated every 4 to 6 weeks to gain maximum benefit. The same dilutions are used.

Systemic effects from the corticosteroids are rare but are possible with repeated injections of higher concentrations. Local effects include hypopigmentation, hyperpigmentation, perilesional atrophy, perilymphatic linear atrophy, and local telangiectasia. These effects often improve over time. This therapy is generally considered safe and effective.

SURGICAL EXCISION

Therapy of keloids limited to traditional surgical excision with primary closure leads to a recurrence rate of greater than 50%. Mixing corticosteroids with the local anesthetic at the time of surgical removal provides superior results. In treating recalcitrant keloids over 1 to 1.5 cm, the best surgical results have been obtained using intralesional corticosteroid injections of triamcinolone (diluted to 2.5 to 5.0 mg/mL) into the immediate subcutaneous interface of the keloid and normal deep skin structures. The steroid injections can be administered 3 months and 6 weeks before scheduled surgical excision and again on the day of skin surgery immediately before the procedure. Follow-up at 4 and 8 weeks after surgery is important to detect any recurrence, which can be aborted with further injections. For smaller lesions, many clinicians will just inject at the time of surgery.

Proper surgical technique during the excision reduces the recurrence of keloids. Because tissue trauma may incite excessive growth, the wound bed and surrounding tissues must be handled gently. Avoid the use of instruments that crush tissue as well as overly aggressive cautery. Superpulse carbon dioxide lasers allow precise excision and cautery and cause minimal thermal damage to surrounding tissue. This, despite their relative expense, makes them useful in excising some keloids. Radiofrequency surgery has similar results (see Chapter 25, Radiofrequency Surgery [Modern Electrosurgery]).

When an excision is performed, close the skin under minimal tension. Consider gentle undermining to decrease wound tension. Some surgeons avoid subcuticular absorbable sutures, which may increase tissue reaction. Skin closure should be accomplished with a very fine nonabsorbable suture material, such as 6-0 nylon. Topical adhesives ("tissue glues" such as Dermabond, SurgiSeal, Histoacryl Blue, or Periacryl) and wound closure strips help to close the wound with the least possible trauma and reduce tension on wound edges. They may also reduce the total number of sutures needed.

Some surgeons advocate removal of every vestige of a keloid; however, wide excision of normal skin around keloids does not reduce the rate of recurrence. Others advocate leaving a rim of incompletely excised keloid in place to serve as a barrier to further keloid growth. It is unclear whether this technique provides significant benefit over standard excision.

Local advancement flaps can be used to limit the wound tension after excision. Fig. 28.1 shows a low-tension flap created after the removal of a globular earlobe keloid. Although some practitioners advocate skin grafting to provide low-tension skin closure, large donor-site keloids can also develop. Advanced closure techniques such as rotation advancement or M-plasty to cover large areas of keloid removal may be indicated to minimize tension on skin edge closure.

Evidence suggests that the use of Silastic-silicone preparations (e.g., Mederma, ReJuveness, Biodermis, Mepiform, Kelo-cote) immediately after surgery may reduce the occurrence of keloids in those prone to excessive scarring.

A final surgical method of removing keloids is radiofrequency surgery. The large loop is used on a pure cutting setting. After anesthesia (with a dilute steroid included), the keloid is shaved off, followed by radiofrequency surgery/smoothing (Fig. 28.2).

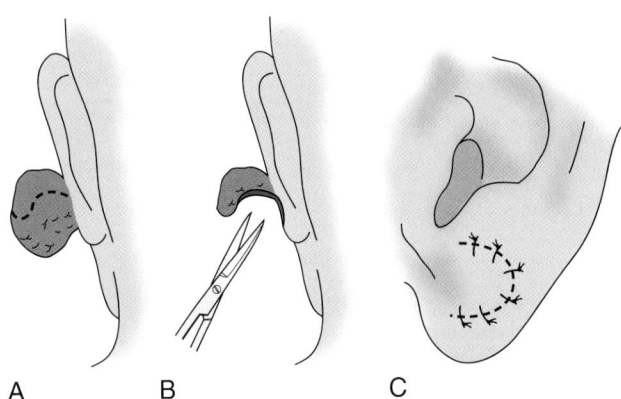

A   B   C

Fig. 28.1 Resection of a keloid on an earlobe. The skin overlying a keloid can be used to create a low-tension wound closure. (A) Half the skin is selected for the flap. (B) The skin is sharply dissected from the underlying keloid and the subcutaneous keloid is totally excised. (C) The wound is closed with simple, interrupted, nonabsorbable 6-0 nylon suture.

Before attempting surgical excision of a keloid, counsel the patient well. Patients with current or previous hypertrophic scars or keloids are more likely to form these types of scars after most surgical procedures, including dermabrasion. However, sculpting hypertrophic scars with traditional dermabrasion or carbon dioxide laser is usually beneficial and generally does not lead to the recurrence of hypertrophic scars. Such recurrence is more common in cases that are complicated by other factors, such as previous isotretinoin therapy, infection, or patient noncompliance with postoperative therapy. A detailed informed consent is useful in creating appropriate patient expectations. Photographs can be helpful before the procedure, immediately after the procedure, 3 months after the procedure, and 1 year after the procedure.

Postoperative results vary widely, and patients must understand that keloids may recur regardless of the treatment methods used. Warn patients that pigment variations may take several months after surgery to resolve. Sunscreens are essential. Patients should be seen at monthly intervals to identify any recurrence, and steroid injections or silicone treatments should be initiated or reintroduced early before the lesion becomes mature and large. It is recommended that patients should agree to surveillance of the wound closure site at least every 3 months for 1 to 2 years to ensure early intervention with postoperative intralesional corticosteroid injection if there is evidence of return of the keloid.

PRESSURE THERAPY

Pressure applied to burn sites can prevent hypertrophic scar formation or induce regression of early hypertrophic scars. Similarly, pressure dressings and garments after keloid surgery reduce their rate of recurrence. Pressure bandaging is used until the scar is no longer red; however, patient compliance may be poor when months or years of therapy are required. Many clinicians prefer to use postoperative injections to ensure adequate therapy. However, when wounds are large or numerous, fitted pressure garments may be the best alternative.

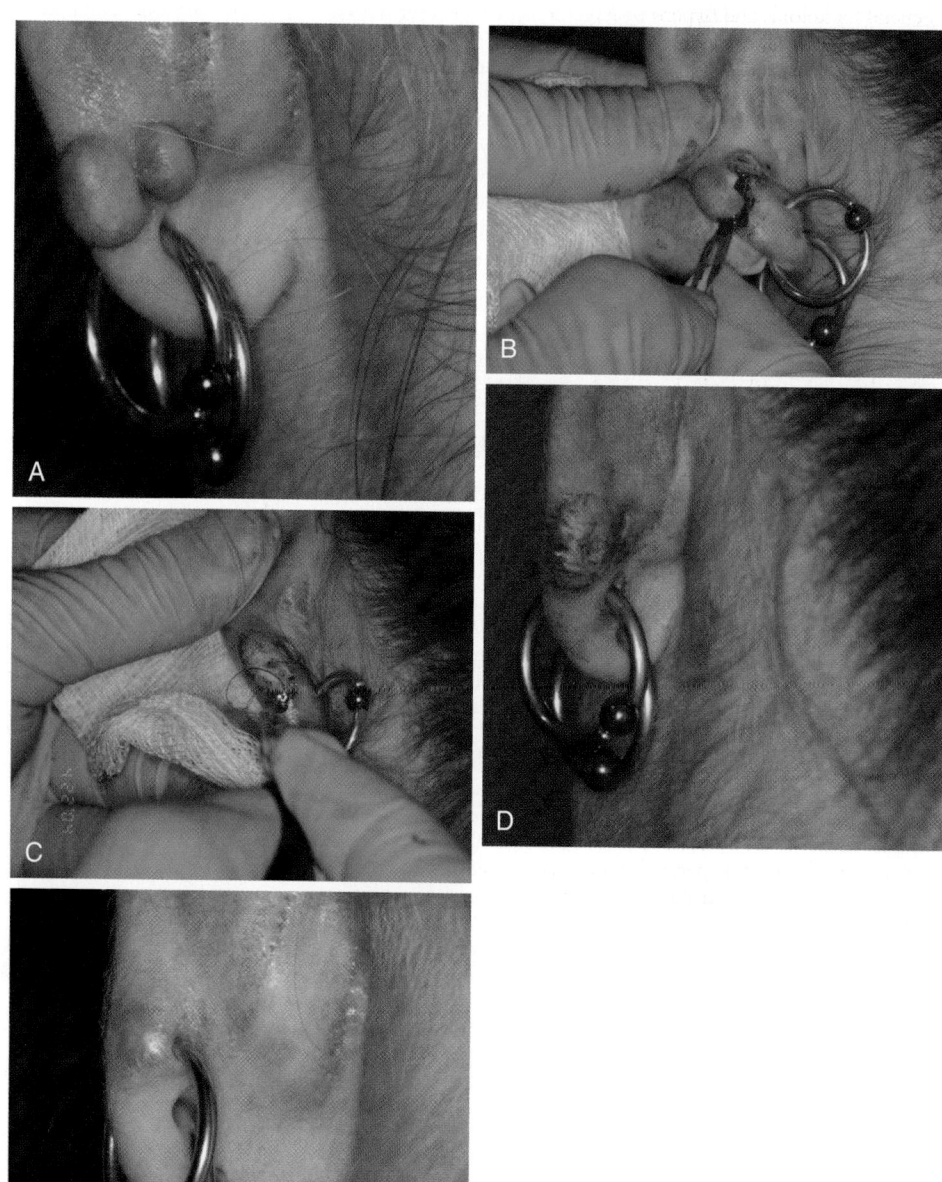

Fig. 28.2 Removal of earlobe keloid using radiofrequency technique. (A) Keloid. (B) Shave removal of lesion after local anesthesia, including low-dose steroid. (C) Radiofrequency smoothing of wound base using pure cutting setting. (D) Appearance of wound on completion of procedure. (E) Appearance 1 month later. Unfortunately, the patient had repierced the area.

After earlobe keloid excision, a pressure earring can be worn as soon as the skin sutures are removed (usually 5 to 7 days). A spring-loaded, light-pressure earring prevents the complication of skin necrosis. Hypoallergenic pressure earrings with a self-adjusting clasp are available from Delasco Dermatologic Lab and Supply (www.delasco.com) and many other medical supply companies. These earrings cost about $25 to $40 a pair and are available in a variety of styles and colors, encouraging prolonged use. A less expensive alternative is to use large, flat, back-clip earrings lined with Silastic sheeting cut to fit. Silastic sheeting alone has been therapeutic in reducing keloids and hypertrophic scars but is best combined with repetitive intralesional steroid injections and compression to hold it in place.

LASER THERAPY

Pulsed dye laser, carbon dioxide laser, and neodymium-yttrium-aluminum-garnet (Nd:YAG) laser therapy has been reported to be beneficial for keloids and hypertrophic scars. Laser therapy works by destroying small blood vessels, followed by hypoxemia and altered collagen production, which leads to improved scar color, height, texture, and pliability. However, evidence from high-quality studies for the treatment of hypertrophic scars and keloids is limited and the efficacy of laser treatment for hypertrophic scars remains uncertain.

ALTERNATIVE METHODS

Some investigators inject *hyaluronidase* with steroids after cryotherapy, with improved results. Others have applied *imiquimod 5%* cream postoperatively to help prevent keloid recurrence after surgical excision. The cream is applied postoperatively on alternate nights for 8 weeks. *Topical silicone gel* and *silicone sheeting* have been used with success, although their mechanism of action is unknown. The gel's impermeability to water is thought to minimize evaporation and provide a semiocclusive dressing that accelerates healing and shortens the inflammatory phase. Topical Silastic gels and Mederma gel (a vegetable oil extract) have proved to be beneficial in reducing both the volume and redness of lesions. The silicone sheets (e.g., Mederma, ReJuveness, Biodermis, Mepiform, Kelocote) must be worn 12 to 24 hours per day for 3 months or more. They are applied under tape or a pressure garment. The sheet is 3.5 mm thick and is applied over the scar only. It is held in place with paper tape and removed and washed daily. Its effect is unrelated to pressure. Perioperative injection with *interferon* has been used. One study of 12 patients showed a recurrence rate of less than 10% after traditional excision, interferon injection, and follow-up of nearly 15 months. Intralesional *bleomycin* and *mitomycin* have been used with some success. *5-Fluorouracil* 50 mg/mL mixed with triamcinolone 1 mg/mL injected one to three times weekly into hypertrophic scars may be efficacious in decreasing scar tissue. Verapamil, botulinum toxin A, cyclosporine, D-penicillamine, relaxin, topical mitomycin C, Cordran tape, and tacrolimus are other options that have been studied.

CONCLUSION

Stepwise treatment as well as a combination of modalities may prove to be the most effective approach to the treatment of keloids. If initial topical (or injected, high-potency) steroids and compression do not resolve the lesion, cryotherapy may soften the lesion and allow improved injectability. Next, excision or careful vaporization of the bulk of the lesion with carbon dioxide superpulse laser may be indicated. If resection is attempted, careful low-tension closure with minimal sutures or healing by secondary intention is recommended. Excision followed by several sessions of 500- to 600-nm pulsed light or laser or low-dose radiation is also an option. Application of topical gels and pressure dressings combined with various modalities seems to produce acceptable results even with difficult lesions.

PATIENT EDUCATION GUIDES

See patient education and consent forms available at www.expertconsult.com.

CPT/BILLING CODES

There are no specific codes for treatment or excision of hypertrophic scars or keloids.

11900   Intralesional injection; up to and including 7 lesions
11901   Intralesional injection; more than 7 lesions

Also include the J code and amount for substance used.

ICD-10-CM DIAGNOSTIC CODES

L91.0   Keloid or scar

Acknowledgment

The editors recognize the contributions of Edward M. Zimmerman, MD, to this chapter in a previous edition of this text.

SUPPLIERS

(See contact information online at www.expertconsult.com.)

MadaJet injector
  Mada Medical
Mederma gel
  Merz Pharmaceuticals
Mepiform (self-adherent silicone dressing)
  Mölnlycke Health Care
PhotoDerm and lasers of all wavelengths
  Lumenis (formerly ESC Medical Systems), Syneron Candela
Pressure earrings
  Delasco Dermatologic Lab and Supply
ReJuveness silicone sheets
  ReJuveness, Inc.
Silastic gel sheeting and topical products
  Biodermis
Silastic topical gel (Kelo-cote)
  Kelocote, Inc.

RECOMMENDED READING

Alster TS, Williams CM. Treatment of keloid sternotomy scars with 585 nm flashlamp-pumped pulsed-dye laser. *Lancet.* 1995;345:1198–1200.

Alster TS. Laser treatment of hypertrophic scars, keloids, and striae. *Dermatol Clin.* 1997;15:419.

Al Arno, Gauglitz GG, Barret JP, et al. Up-to-date approach to manage keloids and hypertrophic scars: a useful guide. *Burns.* 2014;40(7):1255–1266.

Chuangsuwanich A, Gunjittisomram S. The efficacy of 5% imiquinod cream in the prevention of recurrence of excised keloids. *J Med Assoc Thai.* 2007;90:1363–1367.

de Oliveira GV, Nunes TA, Magna LA, et al. Silicone versus nonsilicone gel dressings: a controlled trial. *Dermatol Surg.* 2001;27:721–726.

España A, Solano T, Quintanilla E. Bleomycin in the treatment of keloids and hypertropic scars by multiple needle punctures. *Dermatol Surg.* 2001;27:23–27.

Fitzpatrick RE. Treatment of inflamed hypertrophic scars using intralesional 5-FU. *Dermatol Surg.* 1999;25:224–232.

Gold MH. Topical silicone gel sheeting in the treatment of hypertrophic scars and keloids. *J Dermatol Surg Oncol.* 1993;19:912–916.

Gold MH, Foster TD, Adair MA, et al. Prevention of hypertrophic scars and keloids by the prophylactic use of topical silicone gel sheets following a surgical procedure in an office setting. *Dermatol Surg.* 2001;27:641–644.

Gold MH, Berman B, Clementoni MT, et al. Updated international clinical recommendations on scar management: part 1 evaluating the evidence. *Dermatol Surg.* 2014;40:817.

Habif TP. *Clinical Dermatology.* 6th ed. Philadelphia: Elsevier; 2015.

Juckett G, Hartman-Adams H. Management of keloids and hypertrophic scars. *Am Fam Physician.* 2009;80:253–260.

Kantor GR, Wheeland RG, Bailin PL, et al. Treatment of earlobe keloids with carbon dioxide laser excision: a report of 16 cases. *J Dermatol Surg Oncol.* 1985;11:1063–1067.

Koike S, Akaishi S, Nagashima Y, et al. ND-YAG laser treatment for keloids and hypertrophic scars: an analysis of 102 cases. *Plast Reconstr Surg Glob Open.* 2014;2:3272.

Ledon JA, Savas J, Franca K, et al. Intralesional treatment for keloids and hypertrophic scars: a review. *Dermatol Surg.* 2013;39:1745.

Mahdavian Delavary B, van der Veer WM, Ferreira JA, et al. Formation of hypertrophic scars: evolution and susceptibility. *J Plast Surg Hand Surg.* 2012;46:95.

Marneros A, Noris JEC, Olsen BR, Reichenberger E. Clinical genetics of familial keloids. *Arch Dermatol.* 2001;137:1429–1434.

Rusciani L, Rossi G, Bono R. Use of cryotherapy in the treatment of keloids. *J Dermatol Surg Oncol.* 1993;19:529–534.

Usatine RP, Smith MA, Mayeaux EJ, et al. *The Color Atlas of Family Medicine.* 2nd ed. New York: McGraw-Hill; 2013.

Wolff K, Johnson RA, Saavedra AP. *Fitzpatrick's Color Atlas and Synopsis of Clinical Dermatology.* 7th ed. New York: McGraw-Hill; 2013.

Wolfram D, Tzankov A, Pülzl P, et al. Hypertrophic scars and keloids a review of their pathophysiology, risk factors, and therapeutic management. *Dermatol Surg.* 2009;25:171.

CHAPTER 29

UNNA PASTE BOOT: TREATMENT OF VENOUS STASIS ULCERS AND OTHER DISORDERS

Paul W. Davis

BACKGROUND

Venous stasis leg ulcers are the most common type of ulcers on the lower extremities, accounting for 70% to 90% of ulcers found on the lower leg. They most often occur on the medial aspect of the ankle, and can be either partial or full thickness. Their shape is usually irregular, and there is often associated edema, skin hyperpigmentation, induration, and thickening of the dermis and epidermis. Plaquelike lesions, called *lipodermatosclerosis*, are frequently observed. Erythema may be present, especially when the feet are dependent. This remarkable redness can make it difficult to distinguish between stasis dermatitis and cellulitis. These ulcers are often painful and are accompanied by a significant amount of exudative drainage, again suggesting cellulitis.

Leg ulcers affect an estimated 500,000 to 1 million people annually in the United States. One percent of people in industrialized countries will suffer from a leg ulcer at some point in their lives, and the vast majority of these are secondary to venous problems. Venous leg ulcers are the end result of chronic venous insufficiency (CVI), which leads to venous hypertension, inadequate venous blood return, and increased capillary pressure in the lower extremities. Chronic and recurrent venous obstruction, progressive valvular damage, and impairment of the calf muscle pump are the root causes of CVI.

A variety of hypotheses have been proposed to explain the pathophysiology of venous ulceration. One theory is that sluggish venous flow leads to the *adherence of leukocytes* to the capillary walls, resulting in obstruction of the local capillaries and the migration of additional leukocytes into the surrounding subcutaneous tissue. Proteolytic enzymes and toxic metabolites are released, increasing capillary permeability and destruction. Local ischemia, tissue necrosis, and ulceration are the final result. The *fibrin cuff theory* suggests that increasing venous hypertension causes fibrinogen molecules to leak out of the damaged capillary endothelial cells, polymerizing to fibrin and forming thick deposits around the remaining capillaries. Thus "fibrin cuffs" develop, posing a barrier to diffusion of oxygen and nutrients throughout the tissues of the lower extremities and leading to fibrosis, necrosis, and ulceration.

The *trap hypothesis* incorporates the theories described previously and, in addition, suggests the extravasation of erythrocytes from the capillary bed further contributes to the problem. These "trapped" red blood cells are broken down in the tissues and release hemoglobin, which is metabolized to hemosiderin. This hemosiderin is responsible for the brown hyperpigmentation, often referred to as *brawny edema*, characteristic of the advanced stages of CVI. The associated thin, glistening skin and induration of brawny edema result from the associated fibrin cuffs and fibrosis. Already prone to ischemia and tissue necrosis, the involved areas develop venous stasis dermatitis and

attendant intense pruritus, resulting in scratching, skin breakdown, and ulceration.

Surgical repair is not the standard or first-line treatment for venous stasis ulcers. The application of a firm compression garment to the lower leg has been used for thousands of years for various ailments. For more than 300 years, compression in one form or another has been the mainstay of treatment for venous stasis leg ulcers and CVI. As early as the 1600s, a rigid lace-up stocking was used, but it was not until the mid-1800s that elastic bandages were invented and used for treating this condition. Multiple forms of compression therapy are available today, including hosiery, bandages, boot systems, orthotics, pneumatic pumps, and various combinations of these.

The exact mode of action of compression is not fully understood, but the theory is that pressure applied to the calf muscle raises interstitial pressure, reduces venous insufficiency, lowers superficial venous hypertension, and facilitates venous return by supporting the calf muscle pump. Additional proposed benefits include the softening of lipodermatosclerosis, reduction of venous reflux, increase of arterial flow to the ulcer site, improvement in the microcirculation, increased oxygenation to the wound site, and stimulation of fibrinolysis. In short, continuous compression decreases venous congestion, lowers retained volume in the lower extremities, and facilitates a favorable wound-healing environment.

This chapter considers only one frequently used type of compression therapy—the Unna boot. Although the Unna boot was popular for many years, several factors have led to its decline in popularity in recent years. An Unna boot is messy, makes driving and bathing difficult, and requires training in the appropriate application technique. In addition, an Unna boot may provide suboptimal compression pressure. As a result of these downsides, elastic bandages and compression hosiery are often used as initial therapy for the treatment of venous ulcers. When choosing a treatment modality for venous stasis ulcers, remember that compression is more effective than no compression, high compression is more effective than low compression, and multilayered systems are more effective than single-layer systems. While a recent Cochrane review (O'Meara, 2012) found that elastic compression therapy may be more effective for healing ulcers than inelastic compression therapy such as the Unna boot, there is some controversy in the result. Apparently the level of compression was not adequately measured with the elastic dressings, and in fact, they may have had compression properties similar to those of the Unna boot.

The Unna paste boot is used primarily when a semi-immobilizing, soft-pressure, or gradient-pressure dressing over a joint, extremity, or even the scalp is needed. It is commonly available in a 3- or 4-inch roll or bandage that is impregnated with a calamine–gelatin–zinc oxide compound (Fig. 29.1). Unna paste dressings are soothing and

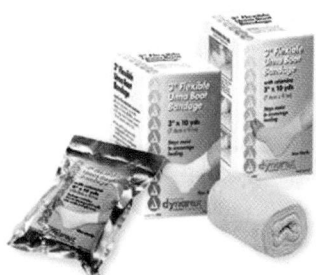

Fig. 29.1 Examples of commercial Unna paste boot materials. (Courtesy Dynarex Corporation, Orangeburg, New York.)

antipruritic and require less frequent dressing changes than conventional dressings. When dressing changes can be scheduled in 3 to 11 days, instead of one to three times per day, both health care cost savings and increased patient convenience can be realized.

INDICATIONS

- Phlebitis and thrombophlebitis of the lower extremity
- Venous stasis ulcers
- Postphlebitic syndrome
- Lymphedema
- Split- and full-thickness skin graft sites
- Split- and full-thickness skin graft donor sites
- Ankle sprains as an alternative to simple elastic compression bandage

Unna paste dressings continue as a treatment option for chronic venous disease with or without venous stasis ulcers. Without some type of dressing, healing-associated pruritus can lead to scratching and subsequent enlargement of the ulcers. The Unna boot can be used as a symmetric gradient-pressure dressing for venous stasis ulcers to help reduce venous hypertension, control edema, and counteract delayed venous return. As such, the Unna boot is a proven, effective part of overall therapy. Debridement, if indicated, should be carried out before application, and then the ulcer should be covered with a permeable dressing, such as Tegaderm (pouched or regular).

Recent studies have advocated Unna paste dressings over split- or full-thickness skin grafting of burns on extremities. The advantages of using the Unna paste dressing compared with conventional dressing changes two to three times per day include earlier hospital discharge, patient comfort (because of fewer painful dressing changes), and higher graft acceptance rate (nearly 100% in some studies, probably because of less graft disturbance during critical microcirculation formation).

Unna paste dressings have been used over skin graft donor sites on the scalp. Use on scalp donor sites led to a significant reduction in a complication called *concrete scalp* (thick exudative crusting over the hair-bearing scalp, which tends to scar).

When pediatric patients excoriated their lower extremity skin grafts because of pruritus, the Unna paste dressings allowed healing and higher percentage skin graft acceptance. Parents spent less time changing the dressings (15 minutes vs. 3.5 hours/week), and children had fewer play- and sleep-time disturbances compared with conventional three-times-per-day dressing changes and use of antihistamines.

When Unna paste dressings were used over skin-grafted, molten metal burns of the lower extremity, the benefits included early ambulation and earlier hospital discharge and return to work (44 vs. 84 days).

CONTRAINDICATIONS

- Sprains with acute fractures (might swell further)
- Significant arterial insufficiency when used with compression covering

- Venous stasis ulcers that are infected and need debridement and cleaning (e.g., ulcers with heavy exudate and crusted ulcers with associated cellulitis)
- Active superficial phlebitis if infection is a major concern
- Sensitivity to any of the dressing components

Acute fractures can continue to swell. Because the gauze in the Unna paste dressing is nondistensible, pressure sores or compartment syndrome may occur if there is marked swelling after application.

Circulatory compromise and necrosis have been reported when a compression dressing is used in the presence of arterial insufficiency. Use a handheld Doppler and blood pressure cuff to compare the ankle and brachial pressures. The ratio of the systolic pressure at the posterior tibial or dorsalis pedis artery divided by the brachial artery pressure should be equal to or greater than 1. If the ratio is 0.7 or less, significant arterial insufficiency is present and compression is contraindicated (see also Chapter 77, Noninvasive Venous and Arterial Studies of the Lower Extremities). If infection is a concern, using a dressing that is not changed for 3 to 11 days may mask progressive infection and postpone appropriate treatment.

TECHNIQUE

1. Cleanse the skin with slightly warm water or saline. If the skin is dry, petroleum jelly can be used as a moisturizer. Avoid topical antibiotics, povidone iodine, and chlorhexidine, which can be topically sensitizing and cause a contact dermatitis. Topical steroids can be applied after washing if dermatitis is present.
2. For venous stasis ulcers, debride the ulcer. Hydrocolloid dressings such as DuoDerm can aid in healing. Some experts recommend extending the DuoDerm 1 inch past the edge of the ulcer. It is normal for these moist dressings to develop an anaerobic odor that does not necessarily indicate an infection. Alternatively, the ulcer can be covered with a permeable dressing like Tegaderm.
3. A smooth, snug layer of Kling or Kerlix can be used as an underwrap if desired. This may prevent chafing of the skin as the Unna paste dries.
4. For the lower extremity, keep the ankle at a right angle. Start wrapping at the metatarsal heads and roll proximally with a 50% overlap. It is important to avoid ridges, which can cause discomfort (Fig. 29.2).
5. Cover the heel completely. Alternate a horizontal wrap to cover the Achilles tendon with an oblique turn to cover the posterior aspect of the heel. Cut the dressing and start another wrap around the heel. Wrap snugly and cut the dressing frequently during the wrap. Avoid applying the edge of the dressing on the joint line; instead, cross the ankle with the full width of the wrap. This helps prevent constriction bands and a tourniquet effect. *Do not reverse directions* as with plaster casting material; wrap only in one direction (clockwise or counterclockwise) to prevent ridges.
6. Wrap the Unna paste dressing in three layers and proceed all the way to the tibial tuberosity.

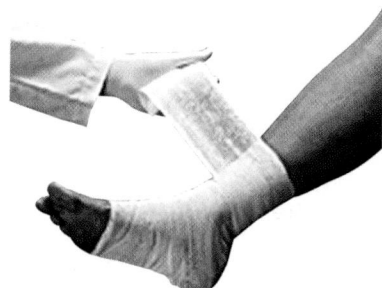

Fig. 29.2 Application of first layer of Unna paste boot with zinc oxide–impregnated gauze. (Courtesy Dynarex Corporation, Orangeburg, New York.)

7. Several options for covering the Unna paste dressing include elastic bandage, Coban, Kling, or stockinette. Both the elastic bandage and Coban dressing help with needed compression (Fig. 29.3).

8. The final boot will consist of two or three distinct layers, in addition to the specialized wound dressing if a venous leg ulcer is present (Fig. 29.4).

9. For wounds that are moist and draining, the dressing may need to be changed more frequently, as often as every 3 days. If moist discharge is minimal, the dressing can be changed about every 7 days (even extended up to 11 days) for patients on protracted therapeutic regimens. For patients with new applications of the Unna boot, it is wise to examine the patient and change the dressings more frequently to ensure that there are no complications.

10. The Unna "cap" for a skin graft donor site on the scalp is applied with an initial layer of Aquaphor gauze followed with an Unna paste dressing. Excellent results with no "concrete scalp" complications were achieved with dressing changes every 3 days in one small study.

11. An Unna boot placed over Webril is an alternative to a simple elastic bandage in an ankle sprain. Apply the Unna boot in a figure-of-eight configuration, similar to how an elastic bandage would be applied. Once in place, wrap the ankle with an elastic bandage or roller gauze. The patient can cut the dressing off at home at the time designated by the clinician, depending on severity of the sprain (see also Chapter 175, Ankle and Foot Splinting, Casting, and Taping.)

COMPLICATIONS

- Occasional contact dermatitis
- Neurovascular compromise if the dressing is applied too tightly or in the presence of arterial insufficiency
- Masking of cellulitis developing in a stasis ulcer under the dressing

POSTPROCEDURE PATIENT EDUCATION

- The dressing must be kept dry.
- Patients should cover the entire dressing with a plastic bag or other impermeable covering to bathe.

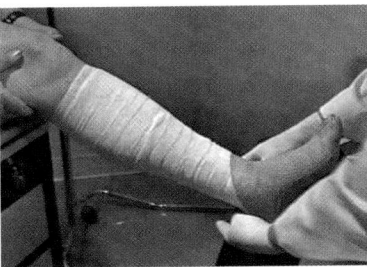

Fig. 29.3 Application of second layer of Unna paste boot with Ace, Coban, Kling, or gauze wrap. (Courtesy Dynarex Corporation, Orangeburg, New York.)

- Remove the boot with a pair of large bandage scissors. Lifting the bandage away from the skin and applying a thin film of petroleum jelly on the scissors can prevent discomfort or inadvertent injury during removal.
- Cleanse and dry the skin thoroughly. When the boot is used for stasis ulcers, inspect the area carefully for the presence of infection and debride again if necessary before applying a new boot. Venous stasis ulcers can take 2 to 3 months or more to heal.
- For best results, the patient must comply with all other aspects of medical therapy.
- As the swelling subsides in sprains, the compression advantage will be lost. Instruct the patient to return in 2 or 3 days or when the Unna paste dressing becomes loose or develops wrinkles, because these can cause pressure sores. A new boot will need to be applied, or more appropriate therapy, such as an inflated splint, may be used.
- Teach the patient to check for signs of impaired circulation and to report any paresthesia, discoloration, or worsening discomfort promptly.

CPT/BILLING CODES

29580   Unna paste boot application

(When the code 29580 is used with the modifier 22, the procedure applies to the application of a multilayered, sustained, graduated high-compression bandage system, *not* to the standard three-layer Unna boot application.)

ICD-10-CM DIAGNOSTIC CODES

I80–I80.9	Phlebitis and thrombophlebitis
I83–I83.93	Varicose veins
I89.9	Noninfectious disorders of lymphatic channels
I89.0	Lymphedema
I87.3–I87.9	Chronic venous hypertension
I87.0–I87.099	Post thrombotic syndrome
L89–L89.95	Ulcer pressure
L97–L97.929	Ulcer nonpressure
R60–R60.9	Edema
S92.301X–S92.356X	Fracture metatarsal

Fracture—use appropriate seventh character; A = initial closed fx, B = initial encounter open fx, D = subsequent with routine healing, G = subsequent fx delaying healing, K = subsequent fx nonunion, P = subsequent encounter malunion, S = sequela.

Some Medicare Carriers (MCs) and Fiscal Intermediaries specify the diagnoses that support medical necessity for CPT 29580. One MC in Arkansas will cover Unna boots only for ulcers of the lower extremity. Other MCs and Fiscal Intermediaries will accept a wider

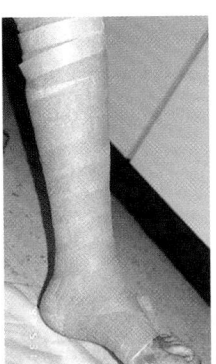

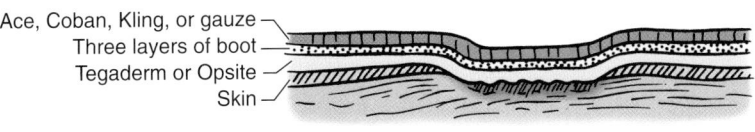

Ace, Coban, Kling, or gauze
Three layers of boot
Tegaderm or Opsite
Skin

Fig. 29.4 (A) Unna paste boot, completed application. (B) The layers of a completed boot application.

A

B

set of ICD-10-CM codes, so it is advisable to consult their written Articles and Local Coverage Decisions to ascertain what codes are covered in a specific locale.

SUPPLIERS

(See contact information available at www.expertconsult.com.)

Unna Paste Boot dressing is a trade name, and more than 25 companies make these dressings. Check with your local medical supply company or contact one of the following:

Unna-Z Bandage
  Medline, Inc.
Flexible Unna Boot Bandage
  Dynarex, Inc.
Medicopaste Bandage
  Graham-Field, Inc.
Unna's Boot Elastic Paste Bandage
  Surgical Supply Service
Unna-FLEX Bandage
  ConvaTec

RECOMMENDED READING

Amsler F, Willenberg T, Blattler W. In search of optimal compression therapy for venous leg ulcers: a meta-analysis of studies comparing diverse [corrected] bandages with specifically designed stockings. *J Vasc Surg.* 2009;50:668.

Barone CM, Mastropieri CJ, Peebles R, Mitra A. Evaluation of the Unna boot for lower-extremity autograft burn wounds excoriated by pruritus in pediatric patients. *J Burn Care Rehabil.* 1993;14:348–349.

Bello Y, Charles CA, Falabella AF, et al. Leg ulcer management. In: Robinson JK, Hanke DW, Sengelmann RD, Siegel DM, eds. *Surgery of the Skin: Procedural Dermatology.* 3rd ed. Philadelphia: Elsevier; 2015.

Carter YM, Summer GJ, Engrav LH, et al. Incidence of the concrete scalp deformity associated with deep scalp donor sites and management with the Unna cap. *J Burn Care Rehabil.* 1999;20:141–144.

Chudnofsky CR. Splinting techniques. In: Roberts JR, Custalow CB, Thomsen TW, eds. *Roberts and Hedges Clinical Procedures in Emergency Medicine.* 6th ed. Philadelphia: Elsevier; 2014:1024.

Collins L, Seraj S. Diagnosis and treatment of venous ulcers. *Am Fam Physician.* 2010;81:989–996.

Cullum N, Nelson EA, Fletcher AW, Sheldon TA. Compression for venous leg ulcers. *Cochrane Database Syst Rev.* 2001:2.

Davis J, Gray M. Is the Unna's boot bandage as effective as a four-layer wrap for managing venous leg ulcers? *J Wound Ostomy Continence Nurs.* 2005;32:152–156.

Grube BJ, Heimbach DM, Engrav LH. Molten metal burns to the lower extremity. *J Burn Care Rehabil.* 1987;8:403–405.

Latz CA, Brown KR, Bush RL. Compression therapies for chronic venous leg ulcers: interventions and adherence. *Chronic Wound Care Manag Res.* 2015;2:11–21.

Mauck KF, Asi N, Elraiyah TA, et al. Comparative systematic review and meta-analysis of compression amodalities for the promotion of venous ulcer healing and reducing ulcer recurrence. *J Vasc Surg.* 2014;60:71S.

O'Donnell Jr TF, Lau J. A systematic review of randomized controlled trials of wound dressings for chronic venous ulcer. *J Vasc Surg.* 2006;44:1118.

O'Donoghue JM, O'Sullivan ST, Beausang ES, et al. Calcium alginate dressings promote healing of split skin graft donor sites. *Acta Chir Plast.* 1997;39:53–55.

O'Meara S, Cullum NA, Nelson EA, Dumville JC. Compression for venous leg ulcers. *Cochrane Database Syst Rev.* 2012;11:CD000265.

Palfreyman SJ, Nelson EA, Lochiel R, Michaels JA. Dressings for healing venous leg ulcers. *Cochrane Database Syst Rev.* 2006:3.

Partsch H. Compression therapy. *Int Angiol.* 2010;29:391.

Partsch H, Mortimer P. Compression for leg wounds. *Br J Dermatol.* 2015;173:359.

Sanford S, Gore D. Unna's boot dressings facilitate outpatient skin grafting of hands. *J Burn Care Rehabil.* 1996;17:323–326.

Schaum KD. Unna boots versus multilayered, sustained, graduated high compression bandage systems. *Ostomy Wound Manage.* 2005;51:28–30.

Summer GJ, Hansen FL, Costa BA, et al. The Unna "cap" as a scalp donor site dressing. *J Burn Care Rehabil.* 1999;20:183–188;discussion 182.

Wells NJ, Boyle JC, Snelling CF, et al. Lower extremity burns and Unna paste: Can we decrease health care costs without compromising patient care? *Can J Surg.* 1995;38:533–536.

Zarchi K, Jemec GB. Delivery of compression therapy for venous leg ulcers. *JAMA Dermatol.* 2014;150:730.

Zenilman J, Valle MF, Malas MB, et al. *Chronic Venous Ulcers: A Comparative Effectiveness Review of Reatment Modalities.* Rockville, MD: Agency for Healthcare Research and Quality; 2013.

CHAPTER 30

WART (VERRUCA) TREATMENT*

Lori Oswald • John L. Pfenninger

Warts are a disease of antiquity. They have no regard for class or social status. They do not discriminate by race or color. There is an equal political distribution between Republicans and Democrats. They are annoying, sometimes disfiguring and painful, and to the angst of patient and clinician, they frequently recur. With ardent attempts to rid the pest by heating, freezing, burning, cutting, and electrifying, treatment has induced as much anxiety as the disease itself. But the clinician persists.

William C. Everts, DO

Verrucae vulgaris (warts) are caused by the human papillomavirus (HPV). There are over 100 individual types and they are identified by numbers. *Common warts* are caused by types 1, 2, 4, 7, 27, 29, and 57; *flat (planar) warts*, by types 3, 10, 28, and 49; and *plantar warts*, by types 1, 2, and 4. Another series of HPVs cause cervical dysplasia and condylomata. Most verruca vulgaris lesions form after a latent period of weeks to several months. The peak incidence occurs in late childhood and adolescence.

HPV also causes numerous epithelial cancers. Cervical dysplasia and cervical cancer are the most commonly recognized types. However, 31% of squamous cell carcinomas and 36% of basal cell carcinomas of the skin contain HPV in nonimmunosuppressed patients. In immunosuppressed patients, 65% of squamous cell carcinomas and 60% of basal cell carcinomas contain HPV. As a result, treatment becomes more than just a cosmetic issue.

Warts have the following various presentations:

- Flat (planar)
- Filiform (small, fine, elongated lesions)
- Mosaic (a cluster of warts that fuse together)
- Verruca vulgaris, including periungual ("common wart")
- Plantar
- Genital/anal wart (condylomata acuminata)
- Laryngeal papillomatosis

DIFFERENTIAL DIAGNOSIS

- Actinic keratosis
- Seborrheic keratosis
- Nevus
- Molluscum contagiosum
- Callus
- Corn
- Nonspecific papule
- Cutaneous dysplasia

It can be difficult to differentiate the true nature of a plantar lesion. Hypertrophic callus buildup makes identification confusing. The telltale sign of a plantar wart is that, as the callus is pared away, the practitioner sees small, punctate sites of bleeding. This is nearly pathognomonic for HPV disease. Biopsies can be obtained if the diagnosis remains unclear.

---

*For the treatment of genital warts (condyloma), see Chapter 138, Treatment of Noncervical Condylomata Acuminata.

INDICATIONS FOR TREATMENT

- Pain
- Bleeding
- Recurrent trauma
- Lack of spontaneous resolution
- Psychosocial sequelae
- Employment repercussions (e.g., waitress)
- Rapid growth or multiplication
- Concerns regarding transmission
- Persistence as a possible cause of malignancy

A large number of verruca do not resolve spontaneously. A longitudinal study concluded that only 40% of patients cleared their warts over a 2-year follow-up. HPV can remain dormant for long periods and then suddenly grow rapidly or multiply. With any treatment, the role of the immune system should not be underestimated. Induced inflammation from whatever treatment modality is used may finally trigger the immune system to recognize and then resolve the wart.

The virus itself is never totally eliminated. Rather, the immune system merely keeps it in remission, much like herpes. The virus can recur with any immunosuppressed state at any time during the patient's life. The goal of treatment is to eradicate active disease, not to eliminate the virus itself.

CONTRAINDICATIONS

- Lack of compliance
- Cellulitis
- Allergy to treatment modality
- Ambiguous diagnosis
- Bleomycin in the very young (relative)

TREATMENT

See Box 30.1 and Fig. 30.1.

General

Transmission of HPV occurs by direct person-to-person contact or, possibly (and rarely), from fomites. The patient may also cause autoinoculation of verruca vulgaris by scratching, shaving, or traumatizing the skin. It is important to *enhance the immune system* as much as possible during the treatment of all wart manifestations. Smoking is known to increase the growth potential and persistence of warts on the cervix. Smoking reduces the cells of Langerhans in the skin in general and subsequently decreases all immunity. The patient must be advised to *stop smoking* (if applicable). *Illicit drugs* have been known to suppress the immune system and they, too, should be avoided. On the other hand, various *vitamins* (e.g., folic acid) have been shown to play a beneficial role in suppressing HPV. Consequently consider using a good multivitamin with minerals to maximize the immune system's capabilities. The patient should also be instructed to eat a *diet* that includes five helpings of fruits and

BOX 30.1   Modalities for Treating Warts (Verruca Vulgaris)

General guidelines (maintaining a healthy immune system)
    Eating a diet high in fruits and vegetables
    Taking vitamins with folic acid (may supplement folic acid up to 1 mg/day)
    Avoiding smoking and secondhand smoke
    Avoiding any immunosuppression when possible
Expectant observation
Hypnosis
Chemicals: topical
    Over-the-counter medication (usually an acid preparation)
    Topical salicylic acid 17%–40%
    Formalin
    Cantharidin (Cantharone) 0.7% collodion solution
    Trichloroacetic acid
    Cidofovir (topical)
    Tretinoin (Retin-A 0.05% solution, or 0.025%, 0.05%, or 0.1% cream)
    5-Fluorouracil (Efudex, Fluoroplex) 5% cream
    Imiquimod (Aldara)
    Podofilox (Condylox)
    Silver nitrate
Chemicals: oral
    Acitretin
    Zinc sulfate 10 mg/kg to maximum of 600 mg/day (three divided doses, 2 mo maximum)
Chemicals: injection
    Candida antigen (Candin) 1:500 solution or generic 1:1000 solution
    Bleomycin (Blenoxane) 15-U vial
    Interferon
    Cidofovir (Vistide)
Mechanical
    Tape occlusion
    Cryotherapy
    Liquid nitrogen (−196°C)
    Nitrous oxide (−89°C)
    Carbon dioxide (−78°C)
    Tetrafluoroethane (−47°C/−70°C): Frigident, Verruca Freeze
    Dimethyl ether/propane (−29°C/−55°C): Histofreezer, Compound-W, Wartner, Dr. Scholl's
Electrodesiccation and curettage
Electrocautery (ball electrode)
Laser (pulsed dye or carbon dioxide)
Photodynamic therapy
Infrared coagulator
Radiofrequency loop removal
Excision (discouraged)

See also Chapter 14, Cryosurgery, and Chapter 138, Treatment of Noncervical Condylomata Acuminata.

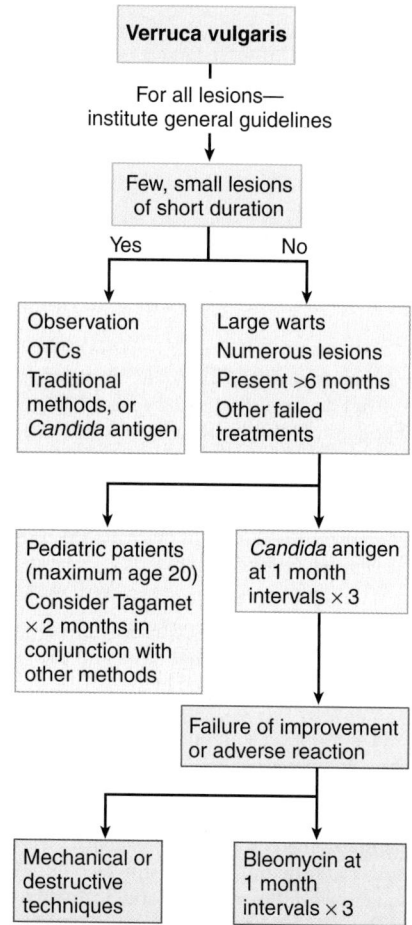

Fig. 30.1   Selected modalities for treating verrucae. At each visit, reinforce general guidelines. At times, especially with extensive lesions, bleomycin and *Candida* antigen can be injected at the same visit (use separate syringes). *Candida* and bleomycin may have to be used more than three times. As long as progress is being made, there is no need to change treatment. *OTC*, Over the counter.

vegetables a day to optimize immune function. Medications such as *steroids* that suppress immunity should be limited if possible.

Treatment of verrucae in patients who are pregnant, have had organ transplants, are immunosuppressed as a result of diseases such as acquired immunodeficiency syndrome, or are taking immunosuppressants of any sort is difficult. Patients should be made aware that the success rate in such cases is poor.

Research into the efficacy of various treatments for warts is difficult. Some studies have shown that even hypnosis can resolve warts. Many folktales carry the belief that banana peel, raw potatoes, cerumen, spiderwebs, and other items can resolve warts. Spontaneous resolution is always possible and often occurs for no apparent reason.

Many clinicians recommend *expectant observation*. An old maxim states that "wart" patients should not be referred to a clinician friend for treatment because it will generally make the clinician look bad! Anyone who has treated warts can become frustrated in dealing with them. Not only can they persist, but they may indeed multiply. Sometimes treatment of a single wart with a modality such as cryotherapy or cautery will result in a ring of warts around the area that was frozen or burned. The simple common wart has indeed humbled the best clinicians. Therefore many again recommend simple observation.

Warts have no "roots" and are completely epidermal lesions. Treatment ideally should not cause scarring. There is no communication between warts—no "mother wart!" However, treatment of a single wart or some of the warts can lead to resolution of all the warts because of immune activation. Obtaining patient compliance for any regimen is often difficult, and home remedies frequently fail owing to lack of consistency in applying the treatment. It is not uncommon for a clinician to have to treat a lesion or lesions four or more times to resolve it.

Chemicals: Over-the-Counter Medications

Numerous over-the-counter (OTC) medications, usually mild acids in liquid form, are available for the treatment of warts. These include Compound-W, Mediplast, Trans-Ver-Sal, Occlusal-HP, Duofilm, Premier, Salactic Film, Sal-Plant gel, Tinamed, Warticide, Wart Off, and Duoplant. Forty percent salicylic acid treatments (Compound-W maximum-strength pads, Mediplast pads, Dr. Scholl's clear-away maximum-strength pads and invisible strips) may also be used and applied every 48 hours. (See also the discussion of Tape Occlusion in the section titled Mechanical Methods.)

Method: Pare away callus after soaking lesions in warm water. Hydrating the keratin allows better penetration of the liquid or agent being applied. Apply medication, patch, or pad as directed by the supplier and occlude the area. Repeat every other day, being sure to remove the dead tissue with paring, a metal nail file, or a pumice stone. Treatment is nonscarring and generally effective but requires extreme persistence with daily treatments, often for 4 to 6 weeks.

Chemicals: Clinician Applied

Trichloroacetic Acid (50% to 85%)

This is a potent chemical and should not be provided for home treatment.

Method: Prepare the lesion as described for OTC medications. Apply the acid, being careful to avoid normal skin. If the lesion is raised and convoluted, work the acid into the lesion with a toothpick. Cover. Repeat weekly until the wart has resolved.

Cantharidin 0.7% (Cantharone, Verr-Canth)

Cantharidin causes blistering at the dermoepidermal junction.

Method: Apply the chemical directly on the wart and cover it with tape for 48 hours. Evaluate the patient weekly and remove any residual blister, then reapply the cantharidin. Repeat until the wart has resolved.

Prescription Creams

Tretinoin Cream (Retin A)

Method: Cream or solution at a concentration of 0.025%, 0.05%, or 0.1% is rubbed in thoroughly at bedtime. This is frequently used with diffuse flat warts on the legs or face, so it is rubbed over the entire area. The application may be repeated daily. The goal is to have a mild erythema with fine scaling. Not uncommonly, it may take months for the warts to resolve. This method can be used in combination with 5-fluorouracil (5-FU) or imiquimod.

5-Fluorouracil (5-FU, Efudex)

5-FU is a second-line treatment for truly resistant warts, and it has not been approved by the US Food and Drug Administration (FDA) for this indication.

Method: A 2% solution or 5% cream is applied similarly to tretinoin cream. It is important to rub it in thoroughly. 5-FU can also be used for condylomata (see Chapter 138, Treatment of Noncervical Condylomata Acuminata). 5-FU can cause significant inflammation in intertriginous areas and in areas with actinic skin change.

Imiquimod (Aldara)

Imiquimod is not a caustic agent but rather an immune enhancer. It is supplied in boxes of 12 or 24 packets. It is not approved by the FDA for verrucae (only for condylomata in those 12 years of age and older) but is frequently used as the sole treatment or as an adjunct in combination with other treatments. It is essential to pare down

the callus (especially on a plantar wart) and to rub in the imiquimod thoroughly. For verrucae, it is applied *daily*, usually in the evening before sleep, and removed after 8 hours. It is not necessary to discard a packet if only a portion has been used.

Podofilox (Condylox) Liquid

Refer to Chapter 138, Treatment of Noncervical Condylomata Acuminata.

Chemicals: Oral

Oral Zinc

Zinc sulfate taken orally at 10 mg/kg per day to a maximum of 600 mg in three divided doses has been reported to result in complete resolution of resistant warts in 60.9% after 1 month and in 86.9% after 2 months. However, patients generally become nauseated, and 20% have experienced vomiting, which limits its overall acceptance.

Chemicals: Injected

Candida Antigen

AUTHOR'S NOTE: After OTC topicals, this method is my absolute first choice to treat all but the simplest verrucae. I have not tried it on condylomata. It can be used on single large warts, on mosaics, or to treat patients with 80 to 100 lesions! I have used it for many years now, and results are excellent, with few adverse reactions and no scarring. Multiple studies confirm its effectiveness.

Candida antigen is used for verruca vulgaris (nongenital HPV; Fig. 30.2). It has not been studied on condylomata acuminata. Although this antigen has been approved for over 40 years as the control for tuberculosis testing, it does not have FDA approval for treating verrucae. Its use is nevertheless covered by malpractice policies even in the treatment of warts. *Candida* antigen can be especially helpful for large, extensive lesions, multiple lesions, and periungual lesions where other modalities would cause too much trauma (Fig. 30.3).

The concept is that nearly everyone has antibodies to *Candida*. When the antigens are injected into an area, there is an immediate immune response (redness, some swelling, occasionally mild pruritus). The increased immune activity in the area leads to recognition of the foreign material of the verruca, and an immune response ensues against that antigen as well. The body is then "sensitized" to the wart and eliminates all such lesions.

Pfenninger Protocol

- *Candida* antigen is available as Candin (1:500) and as a generic (1:1000). *Caution:* Some allergy desensitization extracts may be in concentrations as high as 1:50, which can cause excessive reactions.
- Mix 1:1 Candin and lidocaine 1% or 2% without epinephrine, or 1 part generic antigen with four parts lidocaine. (In spite of its lower concentration, the generic preparation appears to cause more reaction and thus needs greater dilution.)
- Topical anesthetic may be applied 15 minutes before injection.
- Inject 0.1 to 0.3 mL per wart (depending on size), using a 30-gauge needle and 1-mL Luer-Lok syringe. The Luer-Lok (screw-on) connection is important because it often takes con-

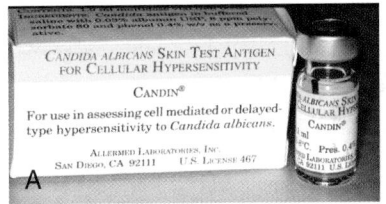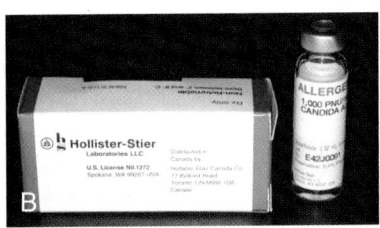

Fig. 30.2 *Candida* antigen preparations: (A) proprietary and (B) generic.

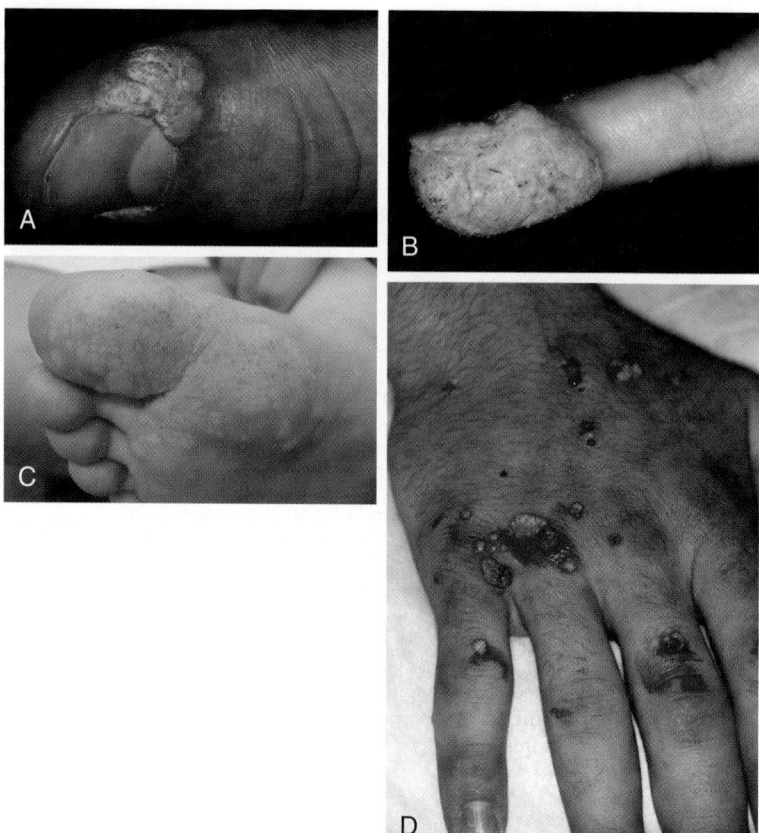

Fig. 30.3 Examples of verrucae that are difficult to treat but are well suited to *Candida* antigen injections: (A) periungual; (B) large finger lesion; (C) mosaic, toe, and plantar aspect of metatarsal head; (D) multiple lesions on the hand of a patient who had both hands affected (postinjection).

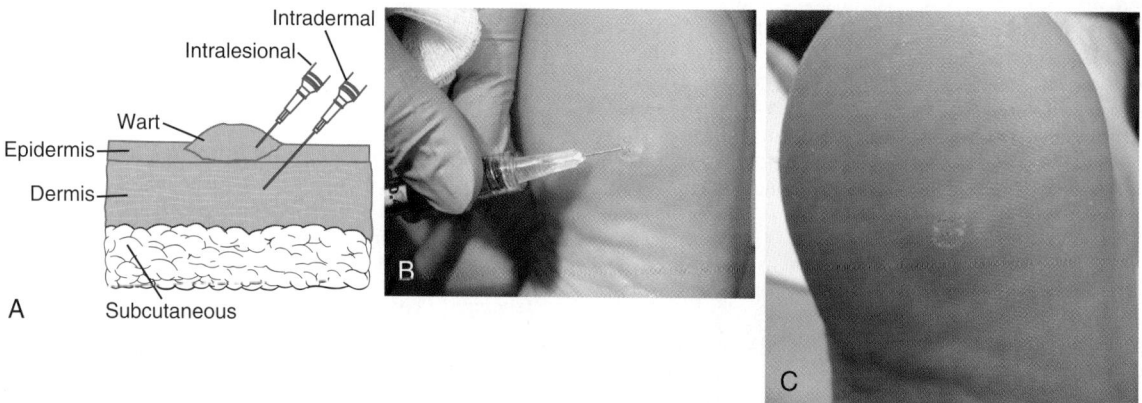

Fig. 30.4 Injecting *Candida* antigen for the treatment of warts. (A) Intralesional injection and intradermal injection. If injected into the subcutaneous tissue, the level is too deep. (B) Injecting a heel lesion. (C) Appearance postinjection.

siderable pressure to inject the solution into the wart/skin. This can cause a needle that is just pressed on to come off, spraying fluid everywhere.

- Try for an *intradermal* or *intralesional* injection to create an immune response. If the solution goes in easily, it is in too deep. Create a bleb if possible. Wear protective glasses because the material often squirts out through a verruca's pore (Fig. 30.4).
- Limit the total amount to 1 mL at any one visit. If there are numerous warts, this may mean injecting only minute amounts into each one. Even if all the warts are not injected individually, the immune response may generalize and all warts may disappear.
- Repeat injection in 1 month if residual tissue remains.
- If the injections have not worked after three attempts 1 month apart, then they probably will not be successful. However, when warts are extensive, there are not many other options. As long as

there is some progress, good results have been obtained even after five or six monthly injection sessions.
- Expect 65% to 75% effectiveness with the first injection. Of the remainder, approximately 50% respond with each succeeding injection.
- Expect pruritus, drying of the lesion, and peeling of dead tissue. The lesion may turn black, regress spontaneously without any outward signs, or become erythematous (localized).
- Adverse reactions include rash (allergy), adenopathy, and persistence of the lesion, all of which are very rare.

The advantages of the *Candida* antigen injection are that if the immune system can be activated to recognize the foreign tissue, all lesions will resolve. Allergic reactions are extremely rare. There is usually none of the scarring, hyperpigmentation, or hypopigmentation that can occur more commonly after some of the other modalities of treatment. There is no "downtime"; patients can exercise, play sports, go back to work, and do whatever they want immediately after treatment. There is minimal pain. The pain at the time of injection can be reduced through the use of the MadaJet to inject the solution (see Appendix H, Pearls of Practice). However, expensive solution is lost just to prime the "gun." The real advantage to using *Candida* antigen is that, unlike many of the other modalities, the immune system is induced into responding and resolving the lesion or lesions. Recurrences are rare, and efficacy is 80% to 85% after three treatments at monthly intervals. This regimen can be used in combination with almost all of the other treatment modalities to effect a synergy between the agents.

Proprietary *Candida* antigen is expensive, but a generic form is available. Practitioners often supply the antigen for the first visit but write a prescription for the patient to bring the antigen in at subsequent visits. Outpatient hospital pharmacies usually carry it, but any pharmacy can order it. This markedly reduces costs for the clinician's office. Insurance companies generally do not reimburse the physician as there is no J code, but they will commonly pay for the patient's prescription. Note on the prescription, "Bring to the next office visit for treatment of warts." Some insurance companies will not pay if the antigen is being used for diagnostic purposes.

The most critical aspect of treatment is to inject the solution into the lesion itself or intradermally just below it. Do not go below the dermis. The injection should be difficult; if the solution goes in easily, the placement is too deep.

Bleomycin

When all other methods have failed, intralesional bleomycin can be considered. Pregnancy must be excluded before a bleomycin injection is given.

Method: A 15-U vial of bleomycin sulfate (Blenoxane) is diluted with 5 mL of bacteriostatic water or 0.9% sodium chloride to form a 3-U/mL solution. When stored at 4°C, the solution can be used for up to 4 months. Mix one part of this solution with five parts of 1% lidocaine without epinephrine (i.e., 0.1 mL of bleomycin with 0.5 mL of lidocaine). This provides 0.6 mL of solution with 0.5 U/mL of bleomycin. Use a 30-gauge needle. Inject directly into the wart as follows:

Amount of Solution (0.5 U/mL Bleomycin) for Size of Wart
Less than 5 mm: 0.1 to 0.2 mL
5 to 10 mm: 0.2 to 0.4 mL
Greater than 10 mm: Up to 1 mL
Multiple warts: Up to 3 mL (1.5 U) per visit

Warts will initially appear hemorrhagic and then clear (48% to 92%; Fig. 30.5). Repeat injection can be performed in 2 to 4 weeks. Three to four treatments may be required for resistant lesions. Alternatively, the drug can be "dropped" onto the wart and pricked into the lesion using a Monolet needle. If tolerated well, the concentration of bleomycin can be gradually increased to 1:3 (bleomycin 0.5 U/mL to lidocaine).

Bleomycin is expensive. One vial will treat many patients. Patients can be given a prescription, which allows them to bring the drug to the office and saves office expense. It is also quite painful. The main mode of action of bleomycin is the inhibition of DNA synthesis, with some evidence of RNA inhibition. When injected locally, it causes vascular microthrombosis; therefore the patient may develop a hemorrhagic blister and may want it drained if the blister becomes uncomfortable. Do not use it near the base of a nail or use it on a very diluted basis because it can cause a distorted nail bed and nail. Rarely (maybe 1 in 200 to 300 cases), it can cause hyperpigmentation (especially in children); if too much is given, it can cause lipodystrophy. There have been very

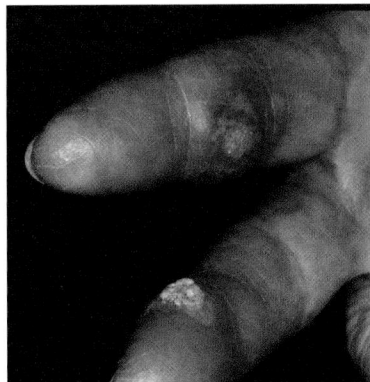

Fig. 30.5   Bleomycin response 3 days after injection.

rare reports of Raynaud phenomenon occurring after intralesional injection of bleomycin.

AUTHOR'S NOTE: We have used bleomycin extensively for 20 years, treating five or six patients per week in a referral clinic. We have never seen Raynaud phenomenon as a complication when using bleomycin as described.

Interferon

Alfa interferon is approved by the FDA for treatment of condylomata in patients older than 18 years of age. Two preparations are available:

- Alferon N injection (interferon alfa-n3): 1-mL vial, 0.05 mL per wart injected two to three times per week for up to 8 weeks
- Intron-A (interferon alfa-2b): 10 million IU per vial, 0.1 mL (reconstituted) per wart three times per week for 3 weeks

Some practitioners use interferon for verrucae as well. It is expensive and can often be followed by flu-like symptoms for 24 hours. Consequently its use is quite limited. For more details on the use of interferon, see Chapter 138, Treatment of Noncervical Condylomata Acuminata.

MECHANICAL METHODS

Tape Occlusion (Patient Applied)

For young children or those who are afraid of needles, tape occlusion can be tried. However, evidence regarding the effectiveness of this technique is conflicting. One trial in children demonstrated superiority of treatment with standard duct tape compared with cryotherapy. A meta-analysis of two placebo-controlled randomized trials failed to find a statistically significant difference between duct tape and placebo. If this technique is to be tried, the wart is simply covered with tape (usually duct tape) for a week. Tape is removed for 12 hours and then reapplied. The patient is seen 1 week later and macerated tissue is removed. The cycle is repeated until the wart or warts resolve, usually in 4 to 6 weeks. Obviously this method is useful only if there are a limited number of lesions and if there is patient compliance. One of the major difficulties is keeping the tape in place. If the tape has been in place for 12 hours, the skin will usually be moist and softened, so some clinicians advise paring with a metal nail file or the use a pumice stone to remove the dead or overlying skin and as much of the wart as possible each time the tape is removed.

Cryotherapy (Over-the-Counter and Clinician-Applied)

Cryotherapy is a destructive treatment of the skin because the cold by itself does not kill HPV. The real advantage to cryotherapy is that it involves little disability and usually no scarring. The patient

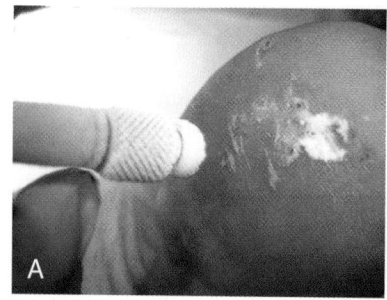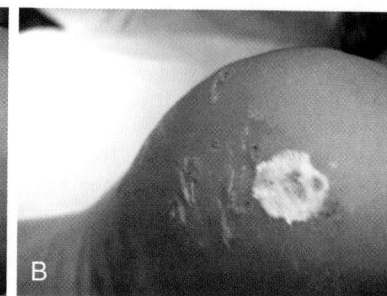

Fig. 30.6   Treating a plantar wart with liquid nitrogen. (A) Freezing the wart. (B) Appearance after cryotherapy.

may initially experience localized erythema and edema, followed by blister formation. Some persistent hypopigmentation may occur. Cryotherapy with liquid nitrogen is usually performed using a thermos bottle spray unit or cotton-tipped applicators (Fig. 30.6). OTC freeze treatments are also available. They contain dimethyl ether and propane but are not as effective because they do not reach as cold a temperature as liquid nitrogen (−196°C). Examples of these products are Compound W-Freeze Off, Wartner-Freezing Wart Remover, and Dr. Scholl's Freeze Away (also makes a combination kit with salicylic acid). See Chapter 14, Cryosurgery, for further details.

Electrodesiccation and Curettage or Electrocautery

Warts can be treated readily with electrocautery. Small ones can be touched with the battery-powered "hot wires" and wiped away. Similarly, electrical units can be placed on fulguration or coagulation settings and the warts coagulated with the ball tips. It helps to have them moistened first. Smaller lesions can be grasped with metal pickups and the current transferred to the wart by touching the cautery tip to the forceps.

All lesions must be anesthetized. Keratin (as in plantar warts) must be pared away because it has little moisture and does not coagulate readily. That is why many practitioners curette the wart first and then coagulate the base. Bleeding from the curettage is controlled with digital pressure.

The major complication from electrodestruction is scarring, which occurs to some degree in all areas treated this way except for very small superficial lesions. The provider must be especially careful not to create a hypertrophic scar on the plantar surface of the feet. This can become a persistently painful area analogous to walking on a stone in a shoe.

The greatest advantage of using curettage before electrocautery is that the abnormal tissue will usually separate from normal skin, defining what is abnormal from the normal tissue. A sharp disposable curette is needed; reusable curettes are often too dull. Unfortunately the disposable curettes frequently bend. The Curetteblade (see Chapter 26, Skin Biopsy) is sharp and strong, so it does not bend. Cautery is then applied, and repeat light curettage is performed. This limits excessive removal of normal tissue and scarring. Alternatively, large warts can be shaved off to debulk them before cautery, but this will leave a significant amount of wart tissue behind and make cautery more difficult. Simply passing electric current through warts will damage them, so the goal of electrocautery is not to cause a full-thickness "burn" but rather to cauterize just enough to raise a blister in a few days (partial thickness).

Primary excision using radiofrequency loop removal (see Chapter 25, Radiofrequency Surgery [Modern Electrosurgery]) is to be discouraged because the loop cuts so rapidly that it is easy to excise too much of the lesion and leave a large pit and subsequent scarring. Tendons, nerves, and periosteal tissue can be injured inadvertently, even by the experienced practitioner. It is critical to be familiar with the relevant anatomy when using any of the electrocautery techniques.

Of all methods, the electrocautery technique is one of the most effective. However, it has the disadvantages of prolonged healing with an open sore, scarring, and pain.

Pulsed-Dye Laser

Pulsed-dye laser has been used to treat warts. Warts should be pared prior to treatment, and a series of treatments is usually required. Treatment intervals of 3 to 4 weeks were associated with higher success rates than longer treatment intervals. Combining pulsed-dye laser with the application of salicylic acid has been shown to decrease the number of laser treatments needed.

Possible side effects of laser therapy include blistering, pain, hyper- or hypopigmentation, and scarring.

Infrared Coagulation (Redfield)

Infrared coagulation is infrequently used to treat warts, but it is quick and effective. Much of the research has been done on condylomata. Local anesthesia is necessary. The probe is placed on the wart for 0.75 to 1 second and the trigger is pulled. Blistering followed by sloughing and then superficial ulceration can be expected. Scarring is possible. See Chapter 87, Office Treatment of Hemorrhoids, for a discussion of the infrared coagulator.

Excision

Many pedunculated and filiform warts can be grasped with pickups and quickly excised with sharp tissue scissors, a curette, or a blade (shave excision). To promote resolution of the wart, consider using Candida antigen with lidocaine mixed per the Pfenninger protocol as the local anesthetic before excision. This means treating the wart with two different modalities. After removal, cauterize the base lightly, not only to control the bleeding but also to destroy any residual wart tissue. It is only in the extremely rare case (as with an isolated wart or two that has resisted everything) that full-thickness skin excision with suture placement is necessary. This is especially discouraged on the plantar surface of the feet because painful scarring can be a significant complication.

Table 30.1 shows the optimal methods of treating various wart presentations. OTC medications are often tried first. Treatments can also be combined to improve outcomes.

COMBINATION THERAPY FOR RESISTANT WARTS

- Candida antigen solution for treatment and anesthesia followed by cryotherapy.
- Imiquimod (Aldara) cream or 5-FU cream can be used in addition to most therapies (especially Candida antigen injection). If mechanical methods are used, it will be necessary to allow some healing before applying the cream. The creams may be used immediately after paring away the hyperkeratotic tissue on plantar warts; however, they will be more efficacious if the callus is removed.
- For extensive lesions (e.g., entire planter surfaces) Candida antigen injections can be used for some lesions along with bleomycin for others.

TABLE 30.1	Treatments of Choice Listed in Order of Preference	
	Primary	**Secondary**
Filiform wart	STS excision	Electrocautery, cryotherapy, curettement
Flat warts (planar)	*Candida* antigen	Tretinoin, 5-FU, cryotherapy
Verruca		
Single or few, small	Cryocautery/*Candida* antigen	Electrocautery
Multiple	*Candida* antigen	Cryocautery
Mosaic	*Candida* antigen	Cryocautery
Plantar	*Candida* antigen	Cryocautery
Periungual	*Candida* antigen	Cryocautery
Resistant to *Candida* × 3	Bleomycin injection (off-label)	Cryocautery, electrocautery, IRC
Condylomata*	85% TCA	Radiofrequency loop excision, IRC, cryotherapy, imiquimod
Urethral meatus*	5-FU	STS excision; electrocautery
Vaginal*		
Few	85% TCA	Electrocautery, nitrous oxide cyrotherapy
Multiple	Imiquimod, 5-FU (both off-label)	Laser
Anal, vulvar*	85% TCA	Imiquimod, radiofrequency excision, cryocautery, IRC
Rectal*	85% TCA	Cryocautery, electrocautery, imiquimod, radiofrequency excision
Laryngeal papillomatosis	Laser	Mumps or *Candida* antigen (injection; off-label)

*See also Chapter 14, Cryosurgery, and Chapter 138, Treatment of Noncervical Condylomata Acuminata.
5-FU, 5-Fluorouracil; *IRC*, infrared coagulator; *STS*, sharp tissue scissor; *TCA*, trichloroacetic acid.

- Always reinforce the importance of a good diet and folic acid supplements with any treatment. Zinc can also be considered alone or in addition to any treatment modality, but it is poorly tolerated.

FURTHER TREATMENT OPTIONS

Because of the quest for the most efficacious treatment, multiple other treatments have been tried, including the following—only limited studies have been done to determine their effectiveness:

- Zinc sulfate orally at 10 mg/kg daily, up to 600 mg/d in three divided doses (61% with complete clearing)
- Garlic extracts topically
- Topical or intralesional cidofovir (Vistide, an antiviral approved for cytomegalovirus treatment)
- Oral acitretin
- Carbon dioxide laser therapy
- Photodynamic therapy

COMPLICATIONS

- Allergic reactions
- Infection
- Blistering
- Scarring
- Persistence of lesion
- Pain
- Bleeding
- Traumatic seeding and increase in number of warts

PATIENT EDUCATION GUIDES

See patient education and patient consent forms available at www.expertconsult.com.

CPT/BILLING CODES

Intralesional Injection

11900	Up to and including 7
11901	Over 7

For injections there is also generally a charge for the medication used, but there is no J code for *Candida* antigen. The provider is advised to provide a prescription to be taken to the pharmacy by the patient.

The J code for bleomycin is J 9040. However, it may be advisable to give the patient a prescription to be filled, as is done with *Candida*.

Destruction (Electrocautery, Cryotherapy, Laser, Chemicals, and Curettement)

17110	Benign lesions (e.g., flat warts) destruction, any method, up to 14
17111	15 or more

ICD-10-CM DIAGNOSTIC CODES

B07.0–B07.9	Viral Warts
A63.0	Anogenital (venereal warts)

SUPPLIERS

(See contact information available at www.expertconsult.com.)

Candida antigen (Candin or generic)
Nielsen BioSciences
Allermed Laboratories (Stallergenes Greer)
Hollister-Stier Allergy Laboratories
Many companies that manufacture antigens for allergy testing
MadaJet
Mada Medical Products
For cryotherapy, radiofrequency, and electrocautery units, see the appropriate chapters mentioned throughout this chapter. For the infrared coagulator, see Chapter 87, Office Treatment of Hemorrhoids.

Acknowledgment

The editors recognize the contributions of William C. Everts, DO, to this chapter in a previous edition of this text.

RECOMMENDED READING

Al-Gurairi FT, Al-Waiz M, Sharquie KE. Oral zinc sulphate in the treatment of recalcitrant viral warts: randomized placebo-controlled clinical trial. *Br J Dermatol*. 2002;146:423–431.

Amer M, Diab N, Ramadan A, et al. Therapeutic evaluation for intralesional injection of bleomycin sulfate in 143 resistant warts. *J Am Acad Dermatol*. 1988;18:1313–1316.

Brodell R, Marchese Johnson S. *Warts, Diagnosis and Management: An Evidence-Based Approach*. London: Martin Dunitz, Taylor and Francis Group; 2003.

Broganelli P, Chiaretta A, Fragnelli B, et al. Intralesional cidofovir for the treatment of multiple recalcitrant cutaneous viral warts. *Dermatol Ther*. 2012;25:468.

Burkhart CG, Pchalek I, Adler M, et al. An in vitro study comparing temperatures of over-the-counter wart preparations with liquid nitrogen. *J Am Acad Dermatol*. 2007;57:1019–1020.

Cha S, Johnson L, Natkunam Y, Brown J. Treatment of verruca vulgaris with topical cidofovir in an immunocompromised patient: a case report and review of the literature. *Transplant Infect Dis*. 2005;7:158–161.

Cordro AA, Guglielmi HA, Woscoff A. The common wart: intralesional treatment with bleomycin sulfate. *Cutis*. 1980;26:319–322.

Davis M, Gostout B, McGovern R, et al. Large plantar wart caused by human papillomavirus-66 and resolution by topical cidofovir therapy. *J Am Acad Dermatol*. 2000;43:340–343.

De Haen M, Spigt MG, van Uden CJ, et al. Efficacy of duct tape vs placebo in the treatment of verruca vulgaris (warts) in primary school children. *Arch Pediatr Adolesc Med*. 2002;156:971.

Epstein E. Immunotherapy of warts with masoprocol cream. *Cutis*. 1997;59:287–289.

Eriksen K. Treatment of the common wart by induced allergic inflammation. *Dermatologica*. 1980;160:161–166.

Field S, Irvine AD, Kirby B. The treatment of viral warts with topical cidofovir 1%: our experience of seven paediatric patients. *Br J Dermatol*. 2009;160:223.

Fleischer Jr AB, Feldman SR, McConnell RC. The most common dermatologic problems identified by family physicians, 1990–1994. *Fam Med*. 1997;29:648–652.

Focht III D, Spicer C, Fairchok M. The efficacy of duct tape vs. cryotherapy in the treatment of verruca vulgaris (the common wart). *Arch Pediatr Adolesc Med*. 2002;156:971–974.

Glass A, Solomon B. Cimetidine therapy for recalcitrant warts in adults. *Arch Dermatol*. 1996;132:680–682.

Habif TF. *Clinical Dermatology*. 6th ed. Philadelphia: Elsevier; 2016.

Haen M, Spigt M, Caro JT, et al. Efficacy of duct tape vs. placebo in the treatment of verruca vulgaris (warts) in primary school children. *Arch Pediatr Adolesc Med*. 2006;160:1126–1129.

Haller KH. *Candida* antigen injection proves effective treatment for warts. *Am Fam Physician*. 2000;61:478.

Johnson SM, Roberson PK, Horn TD. Intralesional injection of mumps or *Candida* skin test antigens: a novel immunotherapy for warts. *Arch Dermatol*. 2001;137:451–455.

Kwok CS, Gibbs S, Bennett C, Holland R, Abbott R. Topical treatments for cutaneous warts. *Cochrane Database Syst Rev*. 2012;(9): CD001781.

Lipke M. An armamentarium of wart treatments. *Clin Med Res*. 2006;4:273–293.

Marchese-Johnson S, Kincannon JM, Horn TD. *A novel treatment for warts: Immunotherapy using mumps and Candida antigen*. San Francisco: Presented at the Scientific Poster Discussion Session. 58th Annual Meeting of the American Academy of Dermatology; 2000.

Marchese-Johnson S, Roberson PK, Horn TD. Intralesional injection of mumps or *Candida* skin test antigens: a novel immunotherapy for warts. *Arch Dermatol*. 2001;137:451–455.

Miller OM, Brodell RT. Human papillomavirus infection: treatment options for warts. *Am Fam Physician*. 1996;53:135–143.

Munn SE, Higgins E, Marshall M, Clement M. A new method of intralesional bleomycin therapy in the treatment of recalcitrant warts. *Br J Dermatol*. 1996;135:969–971.

Muzio G, Massone C, Rebora A. Treatment of non-genital warts with topical imiquimod 5% cream. *Eur J Dermatol*. 2002;12:347–349.

Naylor MF, Neldner KH, Yarbrough GK, et al. Contact immunotherapy of resistant warts. *J Am Acad Dermatol*. 1988;19:679–683.

Phillips RC, Ruhl TS, Pfenninger JL, Garber MR. Treatment of warts with *Candida* antigen injection. *Arch Dermatol*. 2000;136:1274–1275.

Price N. Bleomycin treatment for verrucae. *Skinmed*. 2007;6:166–171.

Robson KJ, Cunningham NM, Kruzan KL, et al. Pulsed-dye laser versus conventional therapy in the treatment of warts: a prospective randomized trial. *J Am Acad Dermatol*. 2000;43:275.

Shamanin V, zur Hausen H, Lavergne D, et al. Human papillomavirus infections in nonmelanoma skin cancers from renal transplant recipients and nonimmunosuppressed patients. *J Natl Cancer Inst*. 1996;88:802–811.

Signore R, Gillis K. *Candida Albicans Intralesional Injection Immunotherapy of Warts: A Novel Therapeutic Approach*. San Francisco: Presented at the Scientific Poster Discussion Session. 58th Annual Meeting of the American Academy of Dermatology; 2000.

Sollitto RJ, Pizzano DM. Bleomycin sulfate in the treatment of mosaic plantar verrucae: a follow-up study. *J Foot Ankle Surg*. 1996;35:169–172.

Sontheimer D, Brown M. Are oral agents effective for the treatment of verruca vulgaris? *J Fam Pract*. 2006;55:353–354.

Sparreboom EE, Luijks HG, Luiting-Welkenhuyzen HA, et al. Pulsed-dye laser treatment for recalcitrant viral warts: a retrospective case series of 227 patients. *Br J Dermatol*. 204(171):1270.

Stulberg D, Hutchison A. Molluscum contagiosum and warts. *Am Fam Physician*. 2003;67:1233–1240.

Thomas K, Koegh-Brown M, Chalmers J, et al. Effectiveness and cost-effectiveness of salicylic acid and cryotherapy for cutaneous warts: an economic decision model. *Health Technol Assess*. 2006;10(iii): ix–87.

Tosti A, Piraccini BM. The nail unit: surgical and non-surgical approaches. *Dermatol Surg*. 2001;27:235–239.

Trozak D, Tennenhouse D, Russell J. *Dermatology Skills for Primary Care: An Illustrated Guide*. Totowa, NJ: Humana Press; 2006.

Usatine RP, Moy RL, Tobinick EL, Siegel DM, eds. *Skin Surgery: A Practical Guide*. St. Louis: Mosby; 1998.

Vanhooteghem O, Richert B, de la Brassinne M. Raynaud phenomenon after treatment of verruca vulgaris of the sole with intralesional injection of bleomycin. *Pediatr Dermatol*. 2001;18:249–251.

Wenner R, Askari S, Cham P, et al. Duct tape for the treatment of common warts in adults. *Arch Dermatol*. 2007;143:309–313.

PILONIDAL CYST AND ABSCESS: CURRENT MANAGEMENT

James A. Surrell

A *pilonidal cyst* or *abscess* is located in the gluteal crease, usually within 5 to 10 cm of the anal verge. This lesion was originally described in the mid-1800s, and there has been considerable debate in the literature over whether it is an acquired or a congenital lesion. Most experts now believe that this is an acquired lesion resulting from penetration of the skin at this level from shafts of hair. Therefore such cysts are more common in hirsute individuals. A pilonidal sinus frequently contains multiple hairs that are microscopically noted to be tapered at both ends, like hairs that have been shed. The existence of hair follicles in the wall of the pilonidal sinus tract has never been demonstrated conclusively, so the hairs are shed from somewhere else. Pilonidal sinus and abscess is a disease of the younger population, and 75% of cases are seen in males. Most patients develop symptoms of pilonidal disease between the ages of 20 and 25 years. A typical patient develops an abscess or experiences recurrent infection and drainage at the base of the spine. The disease is characterized by the development of multiple sinus tracts in this location.

Examination of the patient with suspected pilonidal disease generally reveals an area of inflammation in the midline of the gluteal crease, with one or more sinus openings (Fig. 31.1). The openings may be slightly off the midline. Careful inspection of this site often reveals loose hairs projecting from the sinus openings. Note that these hairs are *not* growing in the pilonidal sinus cavity but rather are shed loose hairs that have migrated to this dependent site in the gluteal crease. If the pilonidal sinus has an associated abscess, the patient will complain of pain, and the examiner may note swelling and erythema at this site. Spontaneous and ongoing drainage is the common indicator, however, and if an abscess is present, it is usually small. As a general guideline, if the patient gives a history of recurrent infection at the base of the spine, this in itself is almost diagnostic of pilonidal sinus disease. Some difficulty in diagnosis may occur if the pilonidal sinus is located in the more caudal position closer to the anal canal. This position raises the possibility of an anal fistula as the cause of the infection. If, however, hairs are found in the lesion, this offers convincing confirmatory evidence that the clinician is dealing with a pilonidal sinus or abscess.

INDICATIONS

Surgical treatment should be performed for the following:

- Acute abscess formation in the superior gluteal crease area (simple incision and drainage [I&D] may be adequate, but recurrences are common).
- Patients with a history of recurrent infections and drainage at the base of the spine are better treated with complete excision of the area. (Antibiotic therapy should be considered only as temporizing and palliative because recurrence will be the rule until adequate I&D or excision is accomplished.)

CONTRAINDICATIONS

- Patient with a paucity of symptoms, such as only minimal drainage with little or no discomfort or inflammation occurring only once or twice per year
- History of bleeding disorder

EQUIPMENT

- Local anesthesia.
- No special equipment is necessary to perform a simple I&D; a No. 11 blade is adequate.
- Only a minor surgical setup tray, a dermal curette, and shaving equipment are required for excision.
- Methylene blue dye (optional).

PREPROCEDURE PATIENT PREPARATION

The procedure of choice is I&D; for recurrent abscesses or persistent draining, excision of the involved area is needed. The wound is left open to heal by secondary intention. With this technique, the patient must be informed of a prolonged healing time. The wounds are not at all disabling and they can be expected to close, but this process takes 8 to 12 weeks. Other options for treatment of pilonidal disease must be reviewed; they include excision with primary closure as well as using a skin flap or other plastic procedures for more extensive and complex involvement.

TECHNIQUE

A simple I&D may be all that is needed for a small abscess or first-time presentation. For recurrent disease, an elliptical incision can be made at the site of the pilonidal disease to include the obvious sinus tract(s) (Fig. 31.2). The lateral and deep margins should extend to noninfected tissue that appears healthy. This procedure can be performed under local anesthesia (with or without intravenous sedation) or under general anesthesia in the operating room. Because of the spine's proximity to the infected site, spinal anesthesia is not recommended. Thoroughly inspect the wound during the procedure, shave any local hair around the wound, and curette all chronically infected granulation tissue so that the remaining wound defect is lined with healthy-appearing tissue with no obvious remaining sinus tracts. Some surgeons inject methylene blue dye into the sinuses and make sure all dyed tissue is removed surgically or with the curette. If the resultant wound defect is not too deep, depending on the extent of the disease and the body habitus of the patient, marsupialization of the wound may be considered; this is done by tacking the skin edges to the base of the wound with an absorbable running simple suture (Fig. 31.3) to help prevent premature secondary wound closure. Total procedure time is generally 30 minutes or less.

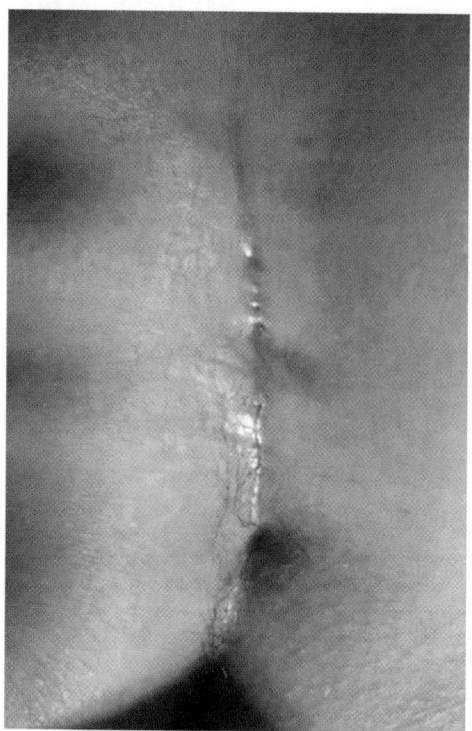

Fig. 31.1 Multiple (six) pilonidal sinus openings in the natal cleft. (From deParedes V, Bouchard D, Janier M, et al. Pilodinal sinus disease. *J Vasc Surg.* 2013;150[4]:237–247.)

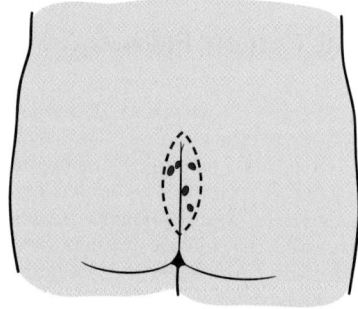

Fig. 31.2 Area of elliptical excision for pilonidal sinus.

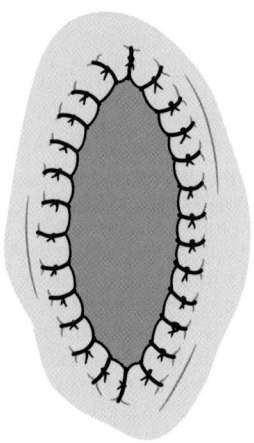

Fig. 31.3 Marsupialization after excision of pilonidal sinus, closed with interrupted absorbable sutures.

COMPLICATIONS

Clearly the most common complication of surgery for pilonidal disease is recurrence. The results are variable, but most clinicians report that the open technique poses less risk of a recurrence than the closed technique. The obvious disadvantage to the open technique is the prolonged healing time, but these wounds generally do not cause significant morbidity during this longer healing process. With the open technique, bleeding, excessive pain, and infection are rare. Two randomized trials have compared a surgical "flap" procedure with primary closure. Both studies found the flap procedure to be superior in terms of pain, healing, complications, and return to work, but these surgical procedures are more extensive and should be performed only by an experienced surgeon. The flap procedure may be the best option for persistently recurrent pilonidal disease.

POSTPROCEDURE PATIENT EDUCATION

If the procedure is performed and the wound left open, instruct the patient on proper wound management. An open wound should be cleansed several times daily with soap and water, either by showering or other irrigation.

During the early stages of wound healing, the wound is packed with moistened gauze sponges that are changed twice daily. During the early phases of postprocedure recovery, the patient should be examined weekly to assess progress. At this time, if hair regrowth is occurring, any hair from around wound edges should be shaved. Every effort to prevent loose hairs from entering the healing wound should be made. Finally, the patient should be instructed on the concept of the wound healing from the inside out, so that premature skin bridging does not occur before the entire cavity is obliterated. Typical time off from work is approximately 1 week. Laser depilation can be used for effective long-term hair removal from the area (see Chapter 38, Lasers and Pulsed Light Devices: Hair Removal).

CPT/BILLING CODES

10080	Incision and drainage of pilonidal cyst, simple
10081	Incision and drainage of pilonidal cyst, complicated
11770	Excision of pilonidal cyst or sinus, simple
11771	Excision of pilonidal cyst or sinus, extensive
11772	Excision of pilonidal cyst or sinus, complicated

ICD-10-CM DIAGNOSTIC CODES

L05	L05.92 Pilonidal cyst and sinus

RECOMMENDED READING

Corman ML, Nichols RJ, Fazio VW, et al. *Colon and Rectal Surgery.* Philadelphia: Lippincott Williams & Wilkins; 2013.

Gordon P, Nivatvongs S. *Principles and Practice of Surgery for the Colon, Rectum, and Anus.* 3rd ed. St. Louis: Informa Healthcare; 2007.

Nelson H. Pilonidal disease. In: Townsend DM, ed. *Sabiston Textbook of Surgery.* 19th ed. Philadelphia: Elsevier; 2012.

CHAPTER 32

WOOD'S LIGHT EXAMINATION

Roberta E. Gebhard

The Wood's lamp (black light) produces ultraviolet rays with a wavelength of 365 nm (or higher) by projecting a beam of light through a filter of glass containing nickel oxide. Invisible light in the long-wave ultraviolet range and visible blue-white light are created. The fluorescence produced as the light hits objects varies in color, depending on the qualities of the surface itself. With magnification, characteristic appearances have been described for several dermatologic conditions; consequently, a Wood's lamp provides a quick, inexpensive, and useful adjunct in their diagnosis (Fig. 32.1).

Diagnostic uses for the examination include the following:

- Tinea capitis
- Erythrasma
- Vitiligo, albinism, tuberous sclerosis, and other pigmentary conditions
- *Pseudomonas* infections
- Tinea versicolor
- Porphyria cutanea tarda
- Detection of some chemicals that are applied to the skin or taken systemically
- Detection of corneal abrasions or herpetic corneal lesions
- Identification of ejaculate in rape/sexual assault

INDICATIONS

- Any dermatitis in body folds such as the inguinal, perianal, interdigital, axillary, or inframammary areas (e.g., erythrasma, *Pseudomonas* infections)
- Patches of scalp scaling and partial hair loss, especially when the hairs are broken or shorter than normal (tinea capitis)
- Pigmentary conditions
- Blisters or punctate erosions on the exposed portions of the hands and forearms, with follow-up urine examination (porphyria cutanea tarda)
- Patches of scaling and altered pigmentation of the skin, "sun spots" (tinea versicolor)
- Suspected corneal abrasion or infection, sexual assault, porphyria, ethylene glycol poisoning
- Evenness of application of salicylic acid–containing (fluoresces green) chemical peels (see Chapter 50, Chemical Peels)

TECHNIQUE

Let the light warm for a few minutes. From a distance of approximately 8 inches, focus the Wood's light on the area of interest. Darken the room to improve visualization of the resultant fluorescence. Observe and record findings carefully. It is crucial to observe the specific color of fluorescence, not simply its presence. Soaps, lotions, cosmetics, urine, other chemicals, and fragments of scaling skin may themselves yield fluorescence. In addition, *patients should not bathe 24 hours before the examination*. Otherwise the examination may show little or no fluorescence.

COMMON FINDINGS

- *Tinea capitis*: The majority of cases in the United States are caused by *Trichophyton tonsurans*, which does not fluoresce. Instead, a "black dot" pattern is noted under magnification, caused by broken hair shafts at the scalp surface. *Trichophyton verrucosum* does not fluoresce either. Hair (but not the skin of the scalp) may fluoresce yellow-green if infected with *Microsporum canis* or *Microsporum audouinii*, or a pale white-green in the rare event of *Trichophyton schoenleinii* infection. In these cases, sensitivity may be relatively low. Sensitivity of approximately 50% has been reported for *M. canis* (Kefalidou and colleagues, 1997). Fluorescence of affected hair should be sought, particularly in the follicular portion of the hair. Potentially infected, broken-off hair may be plucked and the subepidermal portion then viewed under the Wood's lamp (Fig. 32.2).
- *Tinea corpora*: Fungal infections of the skin do not fluoresce, except for tinea versicolor (usually a golden yellow).
- *Erythrasma*: This produces a brilliant coral-red fluorescence. Erythrasma, frequently confused with tinea, is not fungal in origin but is caused by *Corynebacterium minutissimum*. Treatment is with topical clindamycin or erythromycin in most cases (Fig. 32.3). In cases of topical treatment failure, oral erythromycin, single-dose clarithromycin (1 g), or amoxicillin-clavulanate can be chosen for systemic therapy.
- Pseudomonas *infection*: This fluoresces aqua-green or white-green. Wood's light examination can be used to screen burn patients because infection fluoresces before it becomes clinically apparent. *Pseudomonas* can also be found in hot tub folliculitis, ear discharge, intertrigo pedis, and secondary pseudomonal infection of the scrotum.
- *Vitiligo*: Wood's light accentuates hypopigmented areas and is particularly useful for examining patients with fair complexions.
- *Tuberous sclerosis*: Wood's light is helpful in highlighting characteristic hypopigmented skin lesions exhibiting the shape of a mountain ash leaf.
- *Tinea versicolor*: This produces a pale yellow-gold fluorescence. In this case, Wood's light helps differentiate it from skin lesions such as vitiligo.
- *Porphyria cutanea tarda*: Urine fluoresces a bright pink-orange. This may be accentuated by acidifying the urine with 10% HCL or acetic acid (Fig. 32.4).
- *Tetracycline*: In patients taking tetracycline systemically, some inflammatory lesions (including acne papules) may exhibit a yellow fluorescence under the Wood's lamp. This fluorescence may also be observed in dried or concentrated urine containing the drug.
- *Fluorescein*: The dye is used topically by moistening a small strip of impregnated paper (available commercially) and allowing a drop to run off into the eye or the inferior cul-de-sac (see Chapter 200, Corneal Abrasions and Removal of Corneal or Conjunctival Foreign Bodies). Any areas of denudation (e.g., trauma, herpes) on the cornea then fluoresce when viewed through the Wood's lamp (Fig. 32.5).

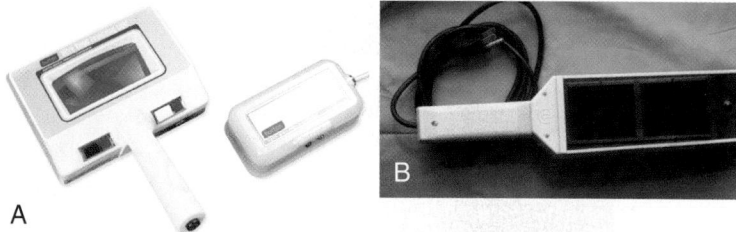

Fig. 32.1 (A) and (B) Examples of Wood's lamps (ultraviolet light). (B, Courtesy Dennis Babel, PhD.)

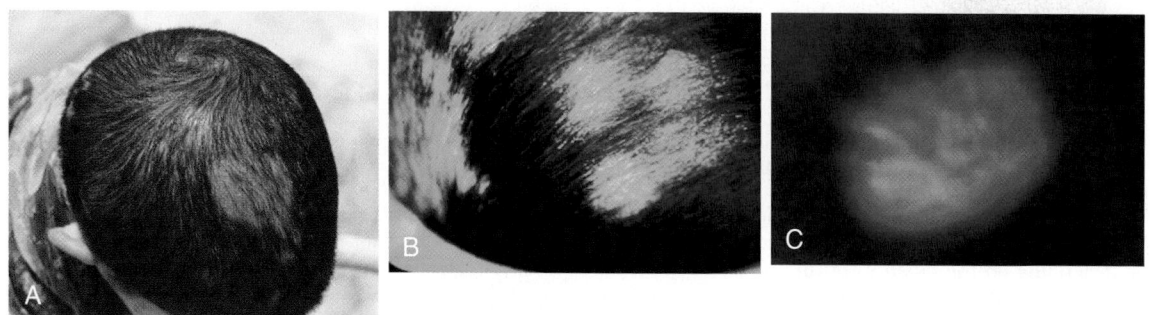

Fig. 32.2 (A) Clinical picture of nonfluorescent "black dot" (hair follicles break at scalp surface, forming black dot pattern) tinea capitis. This is the most common presentation seen in North America. (B–C) Wood's light–positive (fluorescent) tinea capitis. This fluorescence is caused by the fungal metabolite pteridine. (Courtesy Dennis Babel, PhD.)

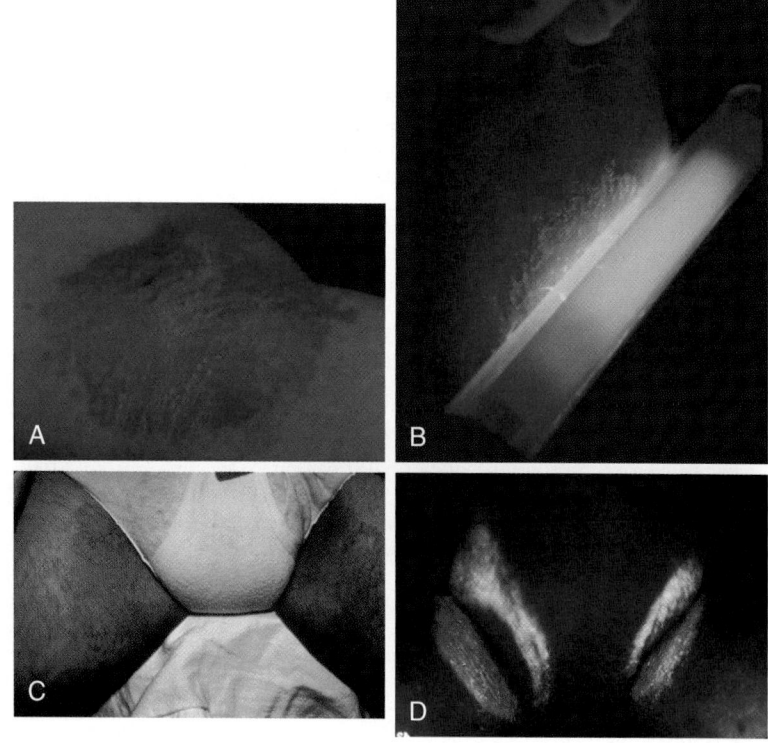

Fig. 32.3 (A–B) Erythrasma under Wood's light. (C) Crural erythrasma caused by the bacterium *Corynebacterium minutissimum*. (D) Wood's light–positive crural erythrasma. (A, From Papadakis MA, McPhee SJ. *Current Medical Diagnosis and Treatment*. New York: McGraw-Hill; 2017. B, Courtesy Richard P. Usatine, MD, Florida State University, Tallahassee. C–D, Courtesy Dennis Babel, PhD.)

- *Ethylene glycol overdose:* Many ethylene glycol–based antifreeze solutions contain fluorescein to allow mechanics to locate leaks with a Wood's light. While lack of fluorescein in urine does not rule out a significant exposure, high levels of fluorescein suggest significant ethylene glycol ingestion. Since certain urine specimen containers can cause false-positive results, comparison with a normal urine specimen may help rule out false positives.
- *Miscellaneous:* Many cosmetics, topical medications, industrial chemicals, and even urine may be detected on the skin by their fluorescence. For this reason, the Wood's lamp is very useful for identifying areas for collection of samples for fo-

rensic study in suspected sexual abuse, rather than as proof of assault.

PRECAUTIONS

- Not all tinea fluoresces.
- Patients washing before the examination may yield a false-negative result.
- Do not confuse a pathologic process with other substances, such as lint, sulfur-laden scales of skin, serum exudate, ointment, deodorants, soaps, or tetracycline.

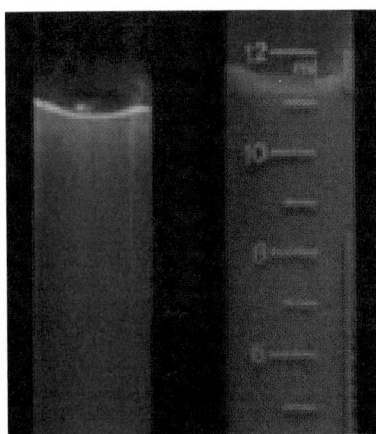

Fig. 32.4   Urine fluoresces a bright pink-orange in porphyria cutanea tarda under Wood's light. (From Wolff K, Johnson RA, Suurmond D. *Fitzpatrick's Color Atlas and Synopsis of Clinical Dermatology*. 7th ed. New York: McGraw-Hill; 2013.)

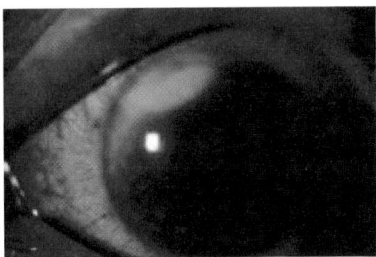

Fig. 32.5   Corneal abrasion with fluorescence under Wood's light. (From Knoop KJ, Stack LB, Storrow AB, Thurman RJ. *Atlas of Emergency Medicine*. 4th ed. New York: McGraw-Hill; 2016.)

CPT/Billing Codes

Use standard "Evaluation and Management" codes.

ICD-10 CM Diagnostic Codes

L08.1	Erythrasma
B35-B36.9	Dermatophytosis

Acknowledgment

The editors recognize the contributions of Stephen K. Toadvine, MD, MPH, to this chapter in a previous edition of this text.

Suppliers

(See contact information available at www.expertconsult.com.)

Burton Medical Products

RECOMMENDED READING

Bechtel K, Bennet BL. Evaluation of sexual abuse in children and adolescents. In: Rose BD, ed. *UpToDate*. 2016. www.uptodate.com.

Chuh AA, Wong WC, Wong SY, Lee A. Procedures in primary care dermatology. *Aust Fam Physician*. 2005;34:347–349.

Dean AJ, Lee DC. Bedside laboratory and microbiologic procedures. In: Roberts JR, Custalow CB, Thomsen TW, eds. *Roberts and Hedges Clinical Procedures in Emergency Medicine*. 6th ed. Philadelphia: Elsevier; 2014:1414–1415.

Habif TP. *Clinical Dermatology: A Color Guide to Diagnosis and Therapy*. 6th ed. Philadelphia: Saunders; 2015.

Kefalidou S, Odia S, Gruseck E, et al. Wood's light in *Microsporum canis* positive patients. *Mycoses*. 1997;40:461–463.

Wolff K, Johnson RA, Suurmond R, Saavedra AP. *Fitzpatrick's Color Atlas and Synopsis of Clinical Dermatology*. 7th ed. New York: McGraw-Hill; 2013.

CHAPTER 33

WOUND DRESSING

Marisha Chilcott

Wound management is an often overlooked and undervalued aspect of patient care. Nonetheless, wounds are a source of significant patient, family, and clinician distress, causing readmission, long-term morbidity, and avoidable mortality. This brief overview of wound care and dressing selection intends to demystify basic wound management and improve patient outcomes.

There are three basic tenets to wound management:

1. To get rid of the "ick" (i.e., slough, pus, and necrotic debris)
2. To promote healthy tissue growth
3. To achieve wound closure

The key steps in attaining these goals are *first to prepare the wound bed and then to manage the progressive development of the healing tissue.* Selection of appropriate dressings is critical to success in these simple endeavors, and there is no single recipe that will work for all wounds. Dressing selection is determined by the wound itself, the available materials, and the psyche and physical health of the patient. For example, a wound in the perineum requires very different considerations than a wound on the scalp or back. A lower extremity wound in the exact same location is very different if the patient is diabetic, has peripheral vascular disease, or is an otherwise well patient with Hansen disease (with neuropathy).

In addition to the general wound types most frequently encountered (e.g., pressure ulcers, venous stasis ulcers, nonhealing infected surgical wounds), the clinician will occasionally have to address the recalcitrant and fungating malignant wound of neoplasia. These wounds may need to be addressed somewhat differently because their management objective may not be actual healing. Rather, the objective may be to maintain quality of life for the patient who must live with the open wound for the remainder of his or her life. Thus management of odor and appearance is of greater import than achieving resolution of the wound site.

Wounds with toxins, such as those produced by brown recluse spider bites or infiltrated chemotherapeutic agents, are also treated differently in that they require aggressive, usually wide surgical debridement to remove the offending agent and limit ongoing damage to tissue.

The range of dressing choices includes a variety of materials, forms, and structures. Their individual characteristics are governed by their principal purpose, be that absorption, bacterial growth inhibition, pain relief, debridement, occlusion, compression, or simple protection. Effective management of the stages of wound healing requires an understanding of the processes and the roles potentially played by the dressings available.

WOUNDS 101

The word *wound* is defined as a break in the epithelial integrity of skin with disruption of possibly deeper tissues, including dermis, fascia, muscle, and bone. Wounds then divide neatly into acute versus chronic, and clean versus infected. The ideal wound, from the standpoint of speed of healing, cosmesis, and function, is clean and

acute. An example is the classic surgical wound created in a sterile environment and approximated to maximize the probability of primary closure. The most challenging wound, from either a patient's point of view or a clinician's management perspective, is infected and chronic. These can be decubitus sacral ulcers exposed to feces, foot injuries on the diabetic patient with severe tinea pedis and onychomycosis, abdominal wounds that have dehisced secondary to infected seromas, or any of a number of unfortunate breakdowns in integumentary integrity.

Clean or sterile acute wounds can heal by either primary or secondary intention and are relatively straightforward to manage. The fundamentals of that process are the basis for all wound care. In fact, the goal of the management of the chronic infected wound is to modify its conditions to approximate a clean acute wound so as to follow the same uneventful healing process.

Healing of acute wounds involves a cascade of overlapping processes that includes first *hemostasis*, then *inflammation*, followed by *proliferation*, and culminating with *remodeling*. Chronic wounds become chronic when they get stuck in the stage of inflammatory processes because of infection, poor circulation, inadequate enervation, repeated trauma, or some combination of those conditions. The role of dressing selection and wound care management comes down to ameliorating those conditions that impair the progression from inflammation to proliferation.

Wound types generally can be categorized by their cause, their depth, and their appearance. Causes are almost always multifactorial, but the underlying pathologic process that predisposes a particular patient toward wound development is relevant in the overall care of the wound and the person who hosts it.

Depth is both a physical measurement (in millimeters to centimeters) and a characterization of penetration through the skin and underlying tissues. It is generally divided into *surface, partial thickness*, and *full thickness*.

A categorization for pressure ulcers was developed in 1975 by J. D. Shea, then refined and promoted as a tool to promote clear communication between clinicians in 1989 by the National Pressure Ulcer Advisory Panel (NPUAP). In 1997 and 2007 the NPUAP updated their pressure ulcer staging system to reflect the growing understanding of the multifactorial nature of wound development. The NPUAP further updated their terminology in 2016, with the term "pressure injury" replacing "pressure ulcer" to more accurately describe pressure injuries to both intact and ulcerated skin. The following NPUAP definitions describe pressure injuries and do not apply to wounds from other causes (e.g., venous insufficiency, diabetic foot wounds):

Stage 1 pressure injury: nonblanchable erythema of intact skin.
Intact skin with a localized area of nonblanchable erythema, which may appear differently in darkly pigmented skin. Presence of blanchable erythema or changes in sensation, temperature, or firmness may precede visual changes. Color changes do not include purple or maroon discoloration; these may indicate deep tissue pressure injury (DTPI).

Stage 2 pressure injury: partial-thickness skin loss with exposed dermis. Partial-thickness loss of skin with exposed dermis. The wound bed is viable, pink or red, and moist and may present as an intact or ruptured serum-filled blister. Adipose (fat) is not visible and deeper tissues are not visible. Granulation tissue, slough, and eschar are not present. These injuries commonly result from adverse microclimate and shear in the skin over the pelvis and shear in the heel. This stage should not be used to describe moisture-associated skin damage (MASD) including incontinence-associated dermatitis (IAD), intertriginous dermatitis (ITD), medical adhesive–related skin injury (MARSI), or traumatic wounds (skin tears, burns, abrasions).

Stage 3 pressure injury: full-thickness skin loss. Full-thickness loss of skin, in which adipose (fat) is visible in the ulcer and granulation tissue and epibole (rolled wound edges) are often present. Slough and/or eschar may be visible. The depth of tissue damage varies by anatomic location; areas of significant adiposity can develop deep wounds. Undermining and tunneling may occur. Fascia, muscle, tendon, ligament, cartilage, and/or bone are not exposed. If slough or eschar obscures the extent of tissue loss, this is an unstageable pressure injury.

Stage 4 pressure injury: full-thickness skin and tissue loss. Full-thickness skin and tissue loss with exposed or directly palpable fascia, muscle, tendon, ligament, cartilage, or bone in the ulcer. Slough and/or eschar may be visible. Epibole (rolled edges), undermining and/or tunneling often occur. Depth varies by anatomic location. If slough or eschar obscures the extent of tissue loss this is an unstageable pressure injury.

Unstageable pressure injury: obscured full-thickness skin and tissue loss. Full-thickness skin and tissue loss in which the extent of tissue damage within the ulcer cannot be confirmed because it is obscured by slough or eschar. If slough or eschar is removed, a stage 3 or 4 pressure injury will be revealed. Stable eschar (i.e., dry, adherent, intact without erythema or fluctuance) on the heel or ischemic limb should not be softened or removed.

DTPI: persistent nonblanchable deep red, maroon, or purple discoloration. Intact or nonintact skin with localized area of persistent nonblanchable deep red, maroon, purple discoloration or epidermal separation revealing a dark wound bed or blood-filled blister. Pain and temperature change often precede skin color changes. Discoloration may appear differently in darkly pigmented skin. This injury results from intense and/or prolonged pressure and shear forces at the bone-muscle interface. The wound may evolve rapidly to reveal the actual extent of tissue injury or may resolve without tissue loss. If necrotic tissue, subcutaneous tissue, granulation tissue, fascia, muscle, or other underlying structures are visible, this indicates a full-thickness pressure injury (unstageable, stage 3, or stage 4). Do not use DTPI to describe vascular, traumatic, neuropathic, or dermatologic conditions.

TYPES OR HEALING STAGES OF WOUNDS

Acute wounds heal in a relatively orderly and well-organized fashion, with "coordinated actions of both resident and migratory cell populations within the extracellular matrix environment leading to repair of injured tissues." In contrast to this, some wounds fail to heal in a timely and orderly manner, resulting in chronic nonhealing wounds. As mentioned earlier, the usual stages of healing are hemostasis, inflammation, proliferation, and epithelialization.

Chronic wounds are those that fail to progress through the normal stages of healing. Although the most common place for a chronic wound to get "stuck" is in the inflammatory stage, a wound that is exposed to repeated trauma (because of a patient who "picks") can also be functionally chronic. The biologic foundations for the variety of reasons a wound becomes chronic are complex, but the facts that wounds have stages of evolution and that clinical interventions

TABLE 33.1	Chronic Wound Characteristics and Descriptions
Wound Characteristic	Features
Necrotic	Devitalized epidermis Blackened in color Dry and retracted
Sloughy	Containing a layer of viscous, adherent slough Yellow in color Wet Potentially malodorous
Granulating	Significant amounts of highly vascularized granulation tissue Beefy red or deep pink in color
Epithelializing	Evidence of pink margin Isolated pink islands on the surface

play a role in their development are the obvious motivations behind wound care and dressing selections (Table 33.1).

WOUND BED PREPARATION

A clean acute wound has, by definition, a prepared wound bed. That is, the injured tissue is disrupted but not necrotic or burdened by foreign bodies or bacterial load. It is ready to start healing and needs dressings that simply protect it and keep it on its natural course by preventing it from becoming infected, necrotic, or otherwise healing impaired. This is described further later.

Whether acute or chronic, a dirty wound has a wound bed that will not heal well because the inflammatory cascade is upregulated and proliferation of the various cell lines that make up the new tissue (basal cells, fibroblasts, myofibroblasts, and epithelial cells) is inhibited. Thus the first step in the care of a dirty wound is to prepare its bed.

Wound bed preparation means creating an optimal environment for healing with a well-vascularized foundation that is stable and has minimal exudate. This preparation requires reducing the bacterial load, removing necrotic tissue, and optimizing host systemic factors. Bacterial load reduction is achieved through both appropriate systemic antibiotics and selection of a dressing that is bactericidal or at least bacteriostatic.

Dakin solution and acetic acid solutions have been used for more than a century to decontaminate wounds. There is now clear clinical evidence that these solutions are toxic to fibroblasts and impair healing. However, this does not mean that they do not have a role. Both are extremely effective at reducing the bacterial burden of a wound infected with gram-negative organisms, particularly Pseudomonas. Although there is an element of toxicity to the polymorphonuclear neutrophils and fibroblasts that slows healing, infection and colonization probably impair healing even more significantly. The judicious course of practice is to make staged use of these solutions as part of 1 to 2 days of wet-to-dry dressing management before converting to a more long-term, tissue-promoting (but less bactericidal) dressing choice.

Virtually all necrotic tissue requires removal to develop a healthy wound bed. The notable exception to this rule is the case of dry necrosis without infection. These cases occur under relatively special circumstances of severe frostbite, ischemic injury, and rare other circumstances. Such completely dry necrotic tissue can be allowed to autoamputate; however, if the dry necrosis is actually an eschar overlying wet necrosis, intervention is necessary. If there is any indication of infection (i.e., wet necrosis), aggressive debridement is a prerequisite to wound bed preparation and healing.

Debridement can be achieved through progressive dressing changes using a hydrogel and mechanical removal with gauze, surgical/sharp debridement, use of a vacuum device, or, if tolerable, larval therapy (see Chapter 34, Maggot Treatment for Chronic Ulcers).

TABLE 33.2	Examples of Antimicrobial Dressings	
Silver-Based Dressings	**Iodine-Based Dressings**	**Other Antimicrobials**
Acticoat (Smith & Nephew)	Iodosorb (Smith & Nephew)	Metronidazole (Metrogel; Galderma, Lausanne, Switzerland)
Silvadene Cream (Monarch Pharmaceuticals)	Iodoflex (Smith & Nephew)	Bacitracin zinc and polymixin B sulfate (Polysporin; Johnson & Johnson)
Actisorb Silver 220 (Acelity)		Neomycin sulfate, polymixin B sulfate, and bacitracin (Neosporin; Johnson & Johnson)
Aquacel Ag (ConvaTec)		Mupirocin (Bactroban; GlaxoSmithKline, London)

Under the appropriate conditions, larval therapy is the safest, fastest, and most efficacious method of wound debridement.

As implied earlier, wound bed preparation involves more than simply the local management of the wound. It also requires a perspective that includes the individual patient who harbors the wound. This means thinking about the patient as a whole person and recognizing that the greater milieu of the patient's health state is hugely influential on the outcome of the healing process. Glycemic optimization and nutritional support are often at the foundation of this multidisciplinary approach. A nutritional consult can aid tight glycemic control and suggest if supplementation of key minerals (e.g., zinc) and vitamins (e.g., vitamins A, C, and E) can benefit. Note that, although supplementation with zinc in patients with deficiency enhances collagen formation, supplementation with zinc in patients who are not deficient can paradoxically cause copper deficiency. Copper deficiency in turn weakens scar tissue through decreased tensile strength. In addition, vitamin stores and intake can vary widely depending on individual patient circumstances. Thus a formal nutrition consult to assess a patient's current and impending status should guide supplementation, rather than wholesale recommendations for general replenishment. Occupational therapy consultation may aid with appropriate bed/chair fitting and selection. In addition, edema should be minimized through compression and elevation, and immunosuppressive drugs such as steroids should be avoided.

DRESSINGS BY DESIGN

The general objective of all dressings is to promote rapid and cosmetically acceptable healing with minimal patient discomfort. However, within this greater expectation, dressing types vary greatly in their material composition and primary application. Absorption, infection prevention, infection amelioration, debridement, pain management, and protection are different dressing purposes.

The following describes various dressing types and their characteristics. Each description is followed by a table that includes brand name dressings in each category (where applicable). This section is by no means meant to be an endorsement of any specific product, nor does it claim to be an exhaustive list of products currently available. Nonetheless, it is often difficult for the clinician to recognize based on name or product labeling just what category a given product might fit into. Many health care organizations do not stock the entire line of a given supplier's products, and how to mix and match what is available at an institution to address the progressive dressing needs of a given wound can be very confusing. The purpose of the tables is to provide a basis for this sort of cross-reference.

Dressing Types and Characteristics

Antimicrobial

Antimicrobial dressings are used for locally infected or colonized wounds to reduce the microbiologic load (Table 33.2). Solutions of acetic acid or dilute bleach (Dakin solution) have been used for years for this purpose but except in specific and judicious applications should be replaced with the less host-toxic options now available. Dressings made with silver, in ionic or nanocrystalline form, have been demonstrated to be very effective antimicrobials with bactericidal rather than just bacteriostatic qualities. Silver dressings include both silver-infused creams and meshes (Figs. 33.1 and 33.2).

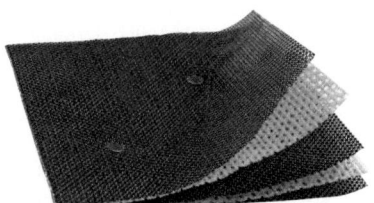

Fig. 33.1 Acticoat, a silver-impregnated antimicrobial barrier dressing. (Courtesy Smith & Nephew, St. Petersburg, Florida.)

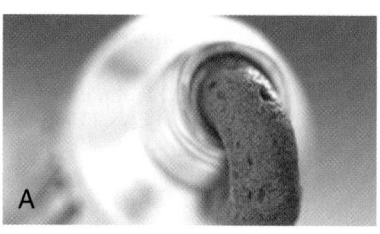

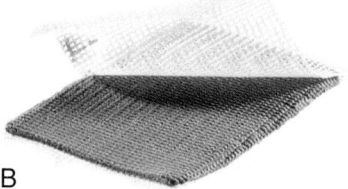

Fig. 33.2 Iodine-containing products. (A) Iodosorb cream. (B) Iodoflex mesh. (Courtesy Smith & Nephew, St. Petersburg, Florida.)

Iodine is an excellent bacteria eradicator, but in some forms it has been clearly demonstrated to delay healing. Povidone-iodine (Betadine) in particular has been implicated as more toxic than others for overall healing in spite of its efficacy against bacterial infection and colonization. It remains an extremely effective preoperative skin preparation agent but should not be used directly in open wounds. However, there are other iodine-based dressings that are indicated for wound care (see Fig. 33.2). For patients with thyroid disease, caution needs to be maintained and thyroid function monitored because it has been demonstrated that there is systemic uptake of iodine through dressings.

Other antibiotic ointments and creams are useful in that they create a barrier to prevent new infection and can reduce the risk of cross-colonization with other wounds or uninfected tissues. Ointments or creams can be used directly on or over a wound and subsequently covered with a dry gauze or bandage to form a basic antibacterial dressing.

Low-Adherent and Nonadherent

Low-adherent and nonadherent dressings are designed to reduce their adherence to the wound bed and either permit (hydrophilic) or prevent (hydrophobic) drainage of fluid from the wound (Table 33.3). The hydrophobic low-adherent and nonadherent dressings thus are also a form of occlusive dressing. The hydrophilic dressings are designed to be used with an overlying absorptive dressing that is in turn usually occlusive (e.g., a foam or gel dressing).

Most of these are in the form of tulles, textiles, or multilayered or perforated plastic films.

Semipermeable

Semipermeable films consist of transparent polyurethane sheets that are coated with hypoallergenic acrylic adhesives. They promote a moist environment by occluding the wound, adhering to the healthy skin (but not wound), and allowing visualization of the wound and

TABLE 33.3 Low-Adherent and Nonadherent Dressings

Hydrophilic	Hydrophobic
Adaptic (Johnson & Johnson)	Vaseline Gauze (Kendall, Ltd.)
Xeroflo (Kendall, Ltd.)	Xeroform (Kendall, Ltd.)
Mepore (Mölnlycke Health Care)	Telfa (Kendall, Ltd.)
Tegapore (3M)	
N-Terface (Winfield Labs)	
Fine-mesh gauze or chiffon (type of cloth)	

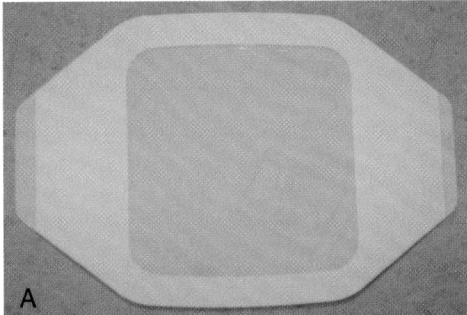

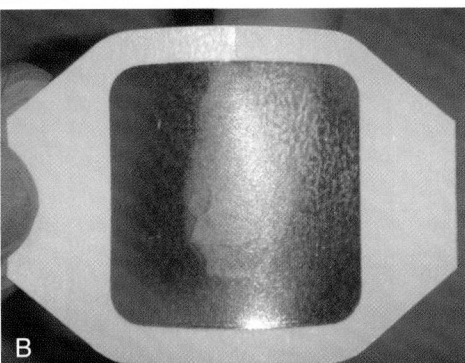

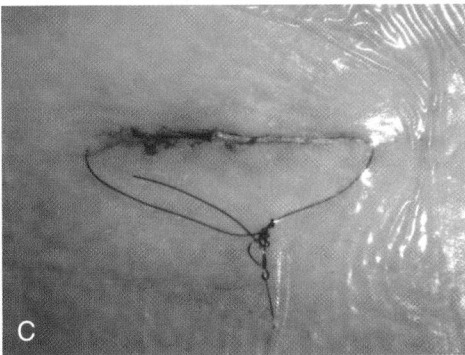

Fig. 33.3 Tegaderm, a hydrophobic low-adherent dressing. (A) The dressing with the protective backing in place. (B) The protective backing has been removed, leaving a transparent window for proper application. (C) Tegaderm placed over a recently closed excision (subcuticular running closure). The dressing provides moist healing/protection and support to the wound margins. (Courtesy The Medical Procedures Center, Midland, Michigan.)

surroundings skin (Fig. 33.3). However, because they are just a film over the wound, they do not provide any padding, nor do they address the amount of exudate an infected wound often produces (Box 33.1). Thus they are most suitable for flat, shallow wounds with low exudates or for use as a secondary dressing (i.e., in lieu of tape covering dry gauze to create an occlusive dressing). These dressings are often used over sutured wounds not only to provide protection and moist healing but to decrease the tension on wound margins. Care is minimal because these covered wounds can become wet (e.g., bathing) without consequence.

Hydrocolloids

Hydrocolloids are a class of nonbiologic occlusive dressings that contain a hydrocolloid matrix composed of carboxymethylcellulose, gelatin, elastomers, and pectin on an adhesive sheet or wafer, or in a paste or powder. Although their forms vary by brand and type, the hydrocolloid dressings have in common that they form a gel on contact with wound exudates (Box 33.2). Although there is little clinical evidence based on randomized, controlled trials to guide dressing choices generally, it has been fairly well established that hydrocolloids are more effective than either paraffin gauze or wet-to-dry gauze dressings.

Hydrogels are a matrix of insoluble polymers, usually sodium carboxymethylcellulose, modified starch, or sodium alginate, that are partially hydrogenated and able to simultaneously donate water molecules to the wound surface (maintaining moistness) and absorb some wound exudates. They are the standard for management of sloughing or necrotic wounds. They promote wound debridement by rehydration of nonviable tissue, thus encouraging autolysis (Fig. 33.4). All hydrogels may be left in place for multiple days but require a secondary dressing overlying them. For very dry wounds, the secondary dressing should be occlusive, such as a semipermeable film (Box 33.3).

Alginates

Alginates are made of the calcium and sodium salts of alginic acid, found in a class of brown seaweed (Phaeophyceae). Commercially produced alginates are either 100% calcium alginate or a combination of calcium with sodium alginate at a ratio of 80:20 (Box 33.4). The alginates, like the hydrocolloids, react on contact with the wound exudate to form a gel. Typically, they can absorb 15 to 20 times their weight of fluid and are excellent choices for highly exudative wounds. They should not be used in wounds with little exudate because they will dry out the wound surface, adhere to it, and cause pain on removal. With respect to removal, alginates need to be changed daily and to have a secondary dressing overlying them (i.e., gauze or film; Fig. 33.5). Those with higher concentrations of mannuronic acid (e.g., Kaltostat) can be washed off with saline, whereas

BOX 33.1 Examples of Semipermeable Film Dressings

Bioclusive (Johnson & Johnson)
CarraFilm (Carrington Laboratories)
Mepore Film (Mölnlycke Health Care)
OpSite Flexigrid (Smith & Nephew)
Tegaderm (3M)

BOX 33.2 Examples of Hydrocolloid Dressings

Comfeel (Coloplast)
Cutinova Hydro (Smith & Nephew)
DuoDerm (ConvaTec)
Hydrocol (Dow Hickam Bertek Mylan)
Nu-Derm (Johnson & Johnson)
Tegasorb (3M)

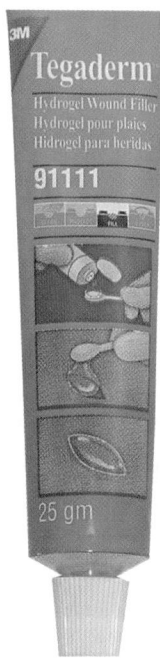

Fig. 33.4   Tegaderm hydrogel. (Courtesy 3M, St. Paul, Minnesota.)

BOX 33.3	Examples of Hydrogel Dressings

GranuGEL (ConvaTec)
Intrasite (Smith & Nephew)
Nu-Gel (Johnson & Johnson)
Purilon (Coloplast)
Tegagel (3M)
Vigilon (Bard)

BOX 33.4	Examples of Alginate Dressings

AlgiDERM (Bard)
Algosteril (Johnson & Johnson)
Kaltostat (ConvaTec)
Seasorb (Coloplast)
Sorbsan (Aspen Medical)
Tegagen (3M)

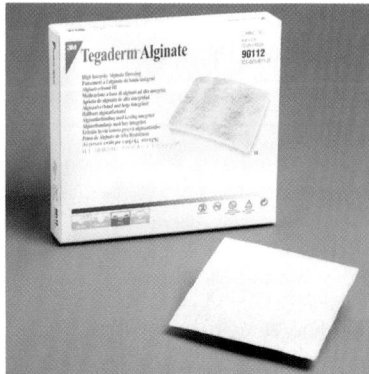

Fig. 33.5   Tegaderm alginate. (Courtesy 3M, St. Paul, Minnesota.)

those higher in guluronic acid (e.g., Sorbsan) will retain their structure and can be removed as a single piece.

Foam Dressings

Foam dressings are manufactured from either a polyurethane or silicone foam and are available as sheets (with and without integrated adhesives) or cavity-filling chips. Foam dressings are excellent for absorbing large amounts of exudates, providing a level of protection in the form of padding, and being generally occlusive, thus not requiring additional overlying dressing. Furthermore, under most circumstances, they may be left in place for 2 to 3 days at a time, reducing the cost and discomfort of frequent dressing changes (Table 33.4 and Fig. 33.6).

Vacuum Dressings

A vacuum dressing is a mechanical device that uses a reticulated foam dressing cut to the shape of the individual wound and then covered by an occlusive drape through which a sealed vacuum tube is placed. The tube is connected to a pump, which provides 50 to 125 mm Hg of negative pressure to the wound environment (see V.A.C., Figs. 33.7 and 33.8). The technology is available through KCI Acelity Medical. The V.A.C. device has been demonstrated to enhance local blood flow, diminish edema, limit bacterial proliferation, and accelerate granulation tissue formation. It has excellent capacity to remove drainage and exudates and acts as an effective debridement tool. Indications for using a V.A.C. include chronic open wounds, dehisced incisions, meshed grafts, and flaps, as well as either chronic or acute traumatic wounds. Contraindications to its use are fistulas to organs or internal cavities, necrotic tissue in eschar, untreated osteomyelitis, and malignancy in the wound.

General Recommendations

Among the review articles and other published works on wound management from the past 15 years, there is a consensus statement by experts published in 2007 (Vaneau and colleagues, 2007). A steering committee selected a panel of 27 experts who had no declared conflicts of interest; they worked first from questionnaires, then discussion, followed by working-group peer review. Their recommendations are given here regarding the application of specific dressing types for specific wound stages:

- Acute wounds, epithelialization stage (i.e., postoperative): low-adherent dressings
- Epithelialization stage: hydrocolloid and low-adherent dressings
- Debridement stage: hydrogels
- Granulation stage: foam and low-adherent dressings
- Hemorrhagic wounds: alginates (effective both for absorption of exudates and hemostasis)
- Malodorous wounds: activated charcoal; metronidazole gel (good for anaerobic bacteria)

However, it should be noted that a paucity of published evidence based on actual trials limits these recommendations. In particular, firm conclusions could be drawn on only three types of dressings (hydrocolloid, alginate, and foam dressings), and the committee made no comment one way or the other on either surgical/sharp debridement techniques or larval therapy (maggots) as methodologies for removal of necrotic tissue from wounds.

Other criteria that were agreed on as useful for individual clinicians' decision making but for which there was insufficient evidence to make specific recommendations included the following:

- Pain or discomfort on application and removal
- Management of exudates
- General dressing tolerance (e.g., ability of caregiver/nursing staff and patient to accept larval therapy)

TABLE 33.4	Foam Dressings	
Foam Adhesive Sheets	**Foam Nonadhesive Sheets**	**Foam Cavity Fillers**
Allevyn Adhesive (available in different shapes and sizes) (Smith and Nephew) Allevyn Gentle (Smith and Nephew) Biatain Adhesive (Coloplast) Lyofoam Extra Adhesive (Mölnlycke Health Care) Tielle and Tielle Lite (Johnson & Johnson)	Allevyn (Smith and Nephew) Allevyn Lite (Smith and Nephew) Lyofoam, Lyofoam Extra, and Lyofoam Max (Mölnlycke Health Care) Mepilex XT (Mölnlycke)	Allevyn Cavity and Allevyn Plus Cavity (Smith and Nephew) Cavi-Care (Smith and Nephew)

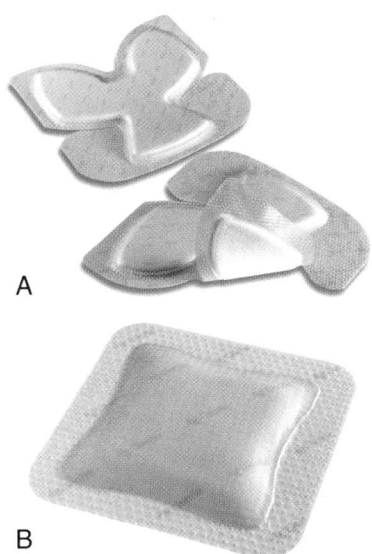

A

B

Fig. 33.6 Allevyn Adhesive foam dressing in two shapes. (Courtesy Smith & Nephew, St. Petersburg, Florida.)

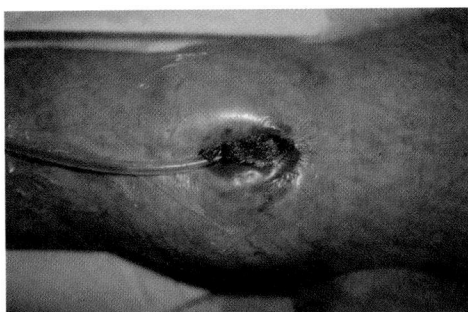

Fig. 33.7 V.A.C. dressing in place in knee wound.

Dressings for Specific Wound Types

Table 33.5 and Box 33.5 present general recommendations for types of dressings based on wound types and the healing objective of the dressing.

OTHER CONSIDERATIONS IN WOUND MANAGEMENT AND DRESSING APPLICATION

One of the most common problems in wound management is failure to protect the surrounding healthy skin or tissue and resultant expansion of the wound area. Although much of this discussion has focused on dressing choices that take the clinician away from traditional wet-to-dry gauze dressings, these outdated techniques nonetheless remain one of the most common choices (familiarity and lack of knowledge about other choices being the most likely reasons for this). A common error made by many nurses, physicians, and other

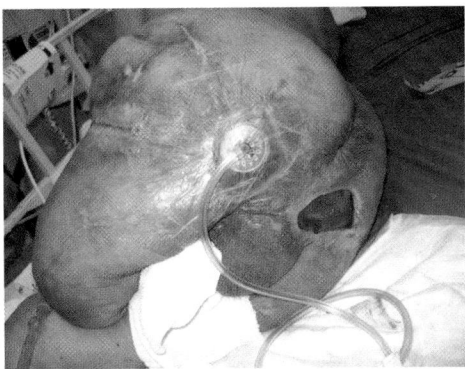

Fig. 33.8 V.A.C. dressing in sacral wound, with adjacent wound before second dressing has been placed.

caregivers who change dressings is that of allowing wet material to macerate dry, intact skin. This can be a problem with any dressing that either does not keep up with absorption of exudates or is oversized and sits on intact skin. For areas that are constantly exposed to moisture, a layer of hydrophobic ointment or thick cream (e.g., zinc oxide, A&E ointment, or Desitin cream) can prevent maceration and further breakdown of the skin.

Of additional concern, the dry, intact skin surrounding a wound is exposed to the adhesives of the binding layer of the dressing (i.e., plastic or paper tapes, Coban, clear occlusive dressing), which can cause skin tears and irritation such as blisters and rash. Care should be taken to protect intact skin by using a skin protectant, either a thin liquid applied and dried or even a thin film dressing (e.g., Tegaderm or OpSite), on areas of intact skin that are repeatedly exposed to adhesives and the mechanical irritation of their repeated removal and reapplication.

In addition to the general wound types most frequently encountered (e.g., pressure ulcers, venous stasis ulcers, nonhealing infected surgical wounds), the clinician will occasionally have to address the recalcitrant and fungating malignant wound of neoplasia. These wounds may need to be addressed somewhat differently because their management objective may not be actual healing. Rather, the objective may be to maintain quality of life for the patient, who must live with the open wound for the remainder of his or her life. Thus management of odor and appearance is of greater import than achieving resolution of the wound site. Activated charcoal can reduce unpleasant odors and is found in dressings such as Actisorb and Lyofoam.

Wounds containing toxins, such as those produced by brown recluse spider bites or infiltrated chemotherapeutic agents, are also treated differently in that they require aggressive, usually wide surgical debridement to remove the offending agent and limit ongoing damage to tissue.

SUMMARY AND RESOURCE REFERENCES

Wound management is a challenging element of patient care that requires a multidisciplinary approach for optimization of the final

TABLE 33.5   Dressing Recommendations Based on Wound Type and Dressing Objectives

Wound Type	Dressing Objective	Dressing Recommendation
Incisional/Surgical wounds	Protect wound from contamination Immobilize wound edges Compression	Benzoin + Steri-Strips Antibacterial ointment Low-adherent dressing Semipermeable film
Skin tears	Protect wound from contamination Immobilize wound edges	Antibacterial ointment Low adherent dressing Semipermeable film
Partial-thickness wounds or donor sites	Facilitate epithelialization Absorb exudate Protect wound from contamination	Low-adherent dressing + overlying absorptive layer (foam or gauze) Antibiotic cream/ointment + gauze or foam Occlusive dressing with absorptive property (hydrocolloid sheets or foam dressing)
Full-thickness wounds (pressure wounds, surgical site dehiscence, third-degree burns)	Maintain moisture Absorb exudate Debridement	Hydrogels Alginates Foam dressings V.A.C. dressing
Any wound with heavy load of necrotic tissue	Absorb exudate Debridement	Larval therapy/dressing V.A.C. dressing
Malignant wound	Maintain moisture Absorb exudate Odor control	Foam dressings for absorption Metronidazole gel Activated charcoal (Actisorb Plus or Lyofoam C)

BOX 33.5   Factors Influencing Dressing Selection

Wound Depth
- Superficial
- Full thickness
- Cavity

Wound Description
- Necrotic
- Sloughing
- Granulating
- Epithelializing

Wound Characteristics
- Dry
- Moist
- Heavily exudative

Bacterial Profile
- Sterile
- Colonized
- Infected
- Infected and potential source of serious cross infection

outcome. It is incumbent on the clinician(s) to be willing to change course as the wound's character evolves. Dressing selection is a vital and dynamic, but not singular, element of the total wound care. No amount of dressing expertise can overcome the deleterious effects of ignoring the patient's condition as a whole—medical, metabolic, social, and emotional states are crucial for healing in the global sense.

CPT/BILLING CODES

Procedures 16000 to 16030 refer to local treatment of burned surface only. Note codes 11045, 11046 are out of numerical sequence.

11000	Debridement eczema/infected skin—first 10% of body surface
11001	Debridement of eczema/infected skin—each additional 10% of body surface
11042	Debridement skin and subcutaneous tissue, first 20 cm^2 or less
11045	Each additional 20 cm^2
11043	Debridement skin, subcutaneous tissue, and muscle, first 20 sq cm or less
11046	Each additional 20 cm^2
11044	Debridement skin, muscle, bone, first 20 sq cm or less
11047	Each additional 20 cm^2
15852	Dressing change (for other than burns) under anesthesia (other than local)
16000	Initial treatment, first-degree burn, when no more than local treatment is required
16010	Dressing/debridement, initial or subsequent, under anesthesia, small
16015	Under anesthesia, medium or large, or with major debridement
16020	Without anesthesia, office or hospital, small
16025	Without anesthesia, medium (e.g., whole face or whole extremity)
16030	Without anesthesia, large (e.g., more than one extremity)

ONLINE RESOURCES

Dressings.org: www.dressings.org.
V.A.C. Therapy: www.acelity.com/wound-management
Monarch Labs: www.monarchlabs.com.
World Wide Wounds: www.worldwidewounds.com.

RECOMMENDED READING

Bluestein D, Javaheri A. Pressure ulcers. *Am Fam Physician.* 2008;78:1186–1196.

Chaby G, Senet P, Vaneau M, et al. Dressings for acute and chronic wounds: a systematic review. *Arch Dermatol.* 2007;143:1297–1304.

Enoch S, Price P. Cellular, molecular and biochemical differences in the pathophysiology of healing between acute wounds, chronic wounds and wounds in the aged. http://www.worldwidewounds.com/2004/august/Enoch/Pathophysiology-Of-Healing.html.

Kramer SA. Effect of povidone-iodine on wound healing: a review. *J Vasc Nurs.* 1999;17:17–23.

Levin Y, Brown KL, Phillips TJ. Wound healing and its impact on dressings and postoperative care. In: Robinson JK, Hanke CW, Siegel DM, et al., eds. *Surgery of the Skin: Procedural Dermatology.* 3rd ed. Philadelphia: Elsevier; 2015.

Morykwas MJ, Argenta LC, Shelton-Brown EI, McGuirt W. Vacuum-assisted closure: method for wound control and treatment: animal studies and basic foundation. *Ann Plast Surg.* 1997;38:553–562.

National Pressure Ulcer Advisory Panel. *NPUAP Pressure Injury Stages, presented at the NPUAP 2016 Staging Consensus Conference.* (Chicago), IL: Rosemont; 2016.

Piacquadio D, Nelson DB. Alginates: a "new" dressing alternative. *J Dermatol Surg Oncol.* 1992;18:990–998.

Reddy M, Gill SS, Kalkar SW, et al. Treatment of pressure ulcers. JAMA. 2008;300:2647–2662.

Sanchez R. Wound dressing. In: Pfenninger JP, Fowler GC, eds. *Procedures for Primary Care*. 2nd ed. Philadelphia: Mosby; 2003:295–304.

Stahl-Bayliss CM, Grandy RP, Fitzmartin RD, et al. The comparative efficacy and safety of 5% povidone-iodine for topical antisepsis. *Ostomy Wound Manage*. 1990;31:40–49.

Thomas S. A structured approach to the selection of dressings. www.worldwidewounds.com/1997/july/Thomas-Guide/Dress-Select.html.

Thomas S. MRSA and the use of silver dressings: Overcoming bacterial resistance. www.worldwidewounds.com/2004/november/Thomas/Introducing-Silver-Dressings.html.

Vaneau M, Chaby G, Guillot B, et al. Consensus panel recommendations for chronic and acute wound dressings. *Arch Dermatol*. 2007;143:1291–1294.

CHAPTER 34

MAGGOT TREATMENT FOR CHRONIC ULCERS

Kim Haglund • Marisha Chilcott

Pressure ulcers and other types of chronic wounds are commonly encountered by primary care providers, especially those who provide care for nursing home residents. Getting such wounds to heal can be a daunting task and requires attention not only to optimal wound dressings but to pressure relief measures, nutrition, and hygiene. The first step toward wound healing is to remove necrotic tissue from the wound and create a clean wound base. Necrotic tissue removal may be accomplished by surgical debridement, either in the operating room or at the bedside; chemical debridement with products that soften or liquefy dry necrotic tissue; or mechanical debridement, such as traditional "wet-to-dry" gauze dressings that pull adherent necrotic tissue from the wound bed when the gauze packing is removed. Although all of these methods have a role in chronic wound management, they all have some disadvantages. Each method can cause damage to adjacent viable tissue and can be uncomfortable for the patient. Surgical debridement in the operating room also exposes the patient, who may have multiple comorbidities, to the risks of anesthesia. Maggot debridement, on the other hand, has the advantages of not harming viable tissue, debriding accurately and completely even in areas of undermining or tunneling, and, in our experience, being very well tolerated in terms of patient comfort.

INDICATIONS

- Debridement of soft tissue wounds with any type of devitalized tissue including dry eschar, densely adherent fibrinous exudates, or purulent exudates
- Pressure ulcers, venous stasis ulcers, neuropathic foot ulcers, and nonhealing traumatic or surgical wounds

RELATIVE AND ABSOLUTE CONTRAINDICATIONS

- Maggot therapy does not work very well for ischemic wounds because the maggots may debride tissue from the wound edges that, although not visibly necrotic, is not really viable owing to very poor perfusion, thereby enlarging the wound area. Such wounds should be revascularized first; once good perfusion is restored, maggots may be used if needed.
- Wounds such as fistulas that communicate with internal organs or body cavities should never be treated with maggots.
- Wounds that are manifestations of an acute life- or limb-threatening infection, the patient should be stabilized first.
- Allergy to brewer's yeast or soy protein (both used to grow the larvae).
- Allergy to the blowfly larvae.
- Bleeding from the wound bed is common during maggot debridement and, in patients on anticoagulation or with a coagulopathy, may be severe enough to require stopping therapy. Caution should be exercised when deciding whether to use maggot therapy for a patient on anticoagulation or with a coagulopathy.

EQUIPMENT AND SUPPLIES

- Medical-grade maggots. Regulated by the FDA and available in the United States from Monarch Labs (Fig. 34.1). Vial cost for 250 to 500 larvae is approximately $190 (2016 pricing), with overnight shipping $52 to $64 additional. They should be used within 24 hours of receipt.
- "Cage" material, either Dacron chiffon (order from Monarch) or other small-pore fabric. We have used cut-up TED (thromboembolic deterrent, or compression) hose with good results when Dacron was unavailable. Monarch will also provide custom-cut pieces of Dacron if you need a bigger piece. The Monarch website states that nylon stockings can be used, but you must select stockings with a weave that is tight enough to prevent the maggots from escaping when they are still small.
- Hydrocolloid dressing to protect skin around the wound (optional)
- Protective skin prep solution
- Adhesive solution (e.g., benzoin)
- Saline solution
- Dry gauze
- Tape or semipermeable transparent dressing to secure cage
- Cotton-tipped applicators
- Two plastic (red, biohazard) trash bags for disposal
- Ethyl chloride
- Gloves

PREPROCEDURE PATIENT EDUCATION

Maggot therapy is not well known to the general public or even to many nurses or physicians. Thus, when instituting maggot treatment, it is important for the provider to demystify the procedure and remove the "yuck" factor as much as possible. Try to stress to patients that maggots work like tiny, flexible, and mobile surgical instruments to remove dead or infected tissue from tight corners or tunnels under the skin where human hands and instruments cannot reach. For patients who may be living in a long-term care facility, let the family know when and why maggot therapy is planned because they may misinterpret maggots in the wound as a sign of neglect. See the patient education form available at www.expertconsult.com.

TECHNIQUE

Application of Maggots

1. Before starting, check the viability of the maggots—you should be able to see them crawling along the walls of the vial. If none are moving, make sure the vial is warm (room temperature at least). If still no movement after warming, contact Monarch Labs for a replacement.

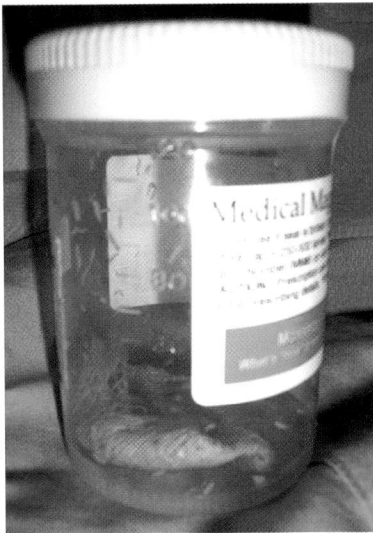

Fig. 34.1   Vial of medical-grade maggots.

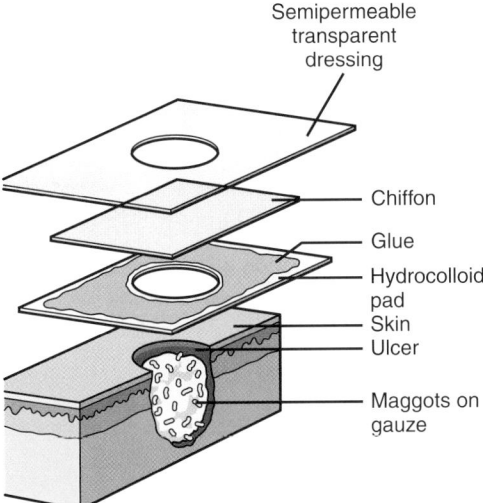

Semipermeable
transparent
dressing

Chiffon
Glue
Hydrocolloid
pad
Skin
Ulcer

Maggots on
gauze

Fig. 34.2   Cut a hole in the dressing to match the size of the wound. Typical layering of materials when using maggot therapy.

2. Wearing gloves, apply protective skin prep solution to intact skin around wound.
3. Cut a donut (or square with hole in it) of hydrocolloid dressing to fit around the wound. (This step is not strictly necessary but does protect vulnerable skin and allows the application of potentially irritating adhesive to the dressing rather than directly to skin.) The hole needs to match the wound in size and shape, leaving 2 to 3 cm of hydrocolloid margin around the wound (Fig. 34.2).
4. Apply the hydrocolloid donut to the skin, making sure it sticks securely and has no wrinkles.
5. Apply a layer of adhesive (benzoin works well) to the top surface of the hydrocolloid. If hydrocolloid is not being used, apply the adhesive to the prepared skin.
6. With an open plastic trash bag tucked under the body part to which the maggots are being applied (to catch "runaways" and make cleanup easy), open the vial of maggots and gently use cotton-tipped applicators to nudge them into the wound bed. The recommended dose of maggots is five to eight maggots per square centimeter of wound area. For wounds larger than 5 × 5 cm, simply use the whole vial. The piece of damp gauze that comes in the vial may be used to gently wipe the maggots from the sides of

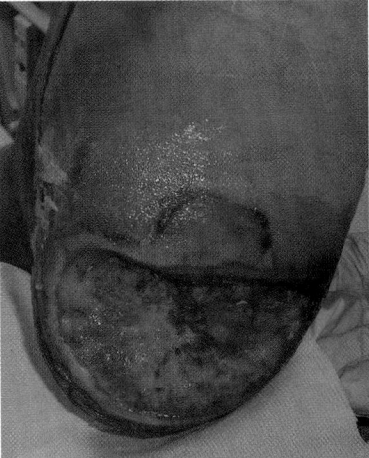

Fig. 34.3   Ulcer prepared for medical maggot treatment.

the vial (many more will already be burrowed into the gauze itself) and then apply them to the wound. The gauze is then placed in the wound bed. The maggots tend to collect on the underside of the vial lid and in the crevice of the vial lid, so bang the vial against a hard surface before beginning to knock them to the bottom of the vial. If you are having trouble getting them out, an easy way is to pour a little saline in the vial, swirl, and pour out onto a gauze pad. Then put the damp gauze and maggots into the wound.
7. Once the maggots are in place, apply a little damp, loosely fluffed gauze to cover them and keep the wound bed moist.
8. Apply the Dacron (chiffon) or other fabric "cage" over the wound, sticking it to the prepared hydrocolloid while being careful to avoid wrinkles. Wrinkles create tunnels through which maggots can escape. The edges of the fabric can be taped to the skin or hydrocolloid for an extra measure of security. Semipermeable transparent dressing cut in similar fashion to the hydrocolloid donut (see Fig. 34.2) can instead be used to secure the cage.
9. Put a few squares of dry gauze on top of the fabric cage to absorb drainage, then secure with tape. Do not use too thick a pad of dry gauze or the maggots will be smothered. This dry dressing should be changed as often as needed, usually a few times a day. Although there may be substantial drainage, avoid the temptation to use an abdominal pad or other occlusive absorbent material, because you will find that the maggots do not tolerate the lack of oxygen (Figs. 34.3 and 34.4).
10. When the maggots are secured in place, the patient may lie on the wound without concern for killing the maggots.
11. Put all maggot-related trash in plastic biohazard bag, double-bag, and dispose. You cannot save maggots for future use if you do not use them all.
12. Remove maggots (see next section) in 2 to 3 days and reapply new maggots in 1 to 2 days with a fresh "cage" and dressings if debridement is incomplete.

Removal of Maggots

1. Place a biohazard plastic bag under the body part to be debrided.
2. Remove the dry gauze, fabric cage, and damp gauze from the wound bed and place in the trash bag. The damp gauze will have lots of maggots crawling in it. They should be much bigger than when applied—at least the size of grains of cooked rice—but there may seem to be many fewer because some may have died.
3. If there is any undermining or tunneling of the skin, maggots likely are in these spaces. Probe into tunnels with cotton-tipped applicators, wipe the wound with gauze, or flood the wound with saline to flush them out.

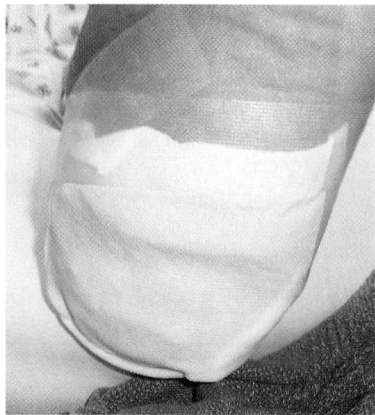

Fig. 34.4   Ulcer dressed with medical maggots in place.

4. If you think there may be maggots left behind, apply a damp gauze dressing to the wound bed, cover with a fabric cage, and secure as for a regular maggot dressing. The maggots will stop eating when they are full and will migrate out of the wound and into the gauze. There is no danger of them eating healthy tissue even if all the necrotic tissue has been removed—they will simply migrate out of the wound and hide in the gauze. Change the gauze three or four times a day for a day or two, and all the maggots should be gone.

5. Even if you are sure all the maggots appear to be gone, damp-to-dry gauze dressing changes should be made three to four times daily for the 1 to 2 days between cycles of maggot therapy. This helps to remove any material that has been liquefied by the maggots but not consumed.

6. Reapply a new vial of maggots 1 to 2 days after removal of the first set. Most wounds require only two or three cycles of maggot treatment. Very large wounds may need up to five or six treatments.

7. The hydrocolloid donut may be left in place for up to 1 week through multiple cycles as long as it is still adhering well and the skin beneath does not appear macerated.

8. If maggots are escaping from the trash bag while you are trying to remove them from the wound bed, they can be sprayed with ethyl chloride to slow them down.

Once the maggots have debrided all of the necrotic tissue and a clean wound bed is present, the wound will heal by secondary intention. The debrided wound may be left open or may be covered with a usual dressing to maintain a clean, moist wound environment.

Once maggots have died, they should be removed. Otherwise, they may trigger an allergic response or become a catalyst for further infection.

COMMON DIFFICULTIES

- Escaped maggots due to wrinkles in cage material or tape.
  Resolution: Make sure the material is flat when laid down on the adhesive and take care with taping. Multiple pieces of flat tape are better than a few pieces with wrinkles or folds.
- Dead maggots when dressing removed.
  Resolution: Make sure the gauze dressing over the maggots is not too occlusive or too dry. Maggots need plenty of oxygen and a moist environment.
- Maggots escaping through the cage despite it being adequately secured around the edges.
  We have only had this problem when using nylon stockings to cover leg wounds, never with the Dacron chiffon pieces supplied by Monarch. Use the Dacron or a tightly woven stretch fabric (TED hose works) rather than ordinary pantyhose.

COMPLICATIONS

The most serious potential complication is bleeding. Although most wounds will have mild oozing from a healthy granulating base once the maggots have debrided off necrotic tissue, rarely will there be such heavy bleeding that maggot therapy will have to be abandoned. If the wound includes necrotic tissue through which blood vessels course, maggot debridement may also cause significant bleeding by débriding away the vessel wall. If this happens, the bleeding vessel will need to be controlled with a figure-of-eight stitch, or cautery if the vessel is very small.

Maggots can also cause pain or discomfort. This usually occurs at 24 to 36 hours into therapy and increases as larvae grow larger. If analgesics do not help, remove the dressing, which generally affords immediate relief. Do not apply local anesthetics.

BILLING AND CODING

Medicare/Medicaid and most insurance companies will cover maggot therapy. If a patient is uninsured or his or her insurance does not cover maggot therapy, the BioTherapeutics Education and Research Foundation (BTER Foundation) provides Patient Assistance Grants to subsidize the cost of maggot therapy. See the BTER Foundation website (www.bterfoundation.org) or the Monarch Labs website for more information.

PATIENT EDUCATION GUIDES

See patient education forms available at www.expertconsult.com.

CPT/BILLING CODES

ABC code for Maggots (EAACT) or HCPCS misc code A9270.

| 97597 | Debridement, for wounds 20 cm^2 or less |
| 97598 | Debridement, for wounds greater than 20 cm^2 |

ICD-10-CM DIAGNOSTIC CODES

| L89–L89.94 | Ulcers Pressure |
| L97–L97.929 | Ulcer nonpressure |

Open wound S00.00X–S99. 359X (by site)

For open wound, use appropriate seventh character: A – initial, D = subsequent encounter, S = sequela.

If reimbursement is denied, appeal. The BTER Foundation will assist with appeals as well as provide Patient Assistance Grants.

SUPPLIERS

BioTherapeutics Education and Research (BTER) Foundation
Monarch Labs

ONLINE RESOURCES

BTER Foundation: http://www.bterfoundation.org.
Monarch Labs: http://www.monarchlabs.com.

RECOMMENDED READING

Andersen AS, Sandvang D, Schnorr KM, et al. A novel approach to the antimicrobial activity of maggot debridement therapy. *J Antimicrob Chemother*. 2010;65:1646.

Courtenay M, Church JC, Ryan TJ. Larva therapy in wound management. *J R Soc Med*. 2000;93:72–74.

Davies CE, Woolfrey G, Hogg N, et al. Maggots as a wound debridement agent for chronic venous leg ulcers under graduated compression bandages: a randomized controlled trial. *Phlebology*. 2015;30:693.

Jukema GN, Menon AG, Bernards AT, et al. Amputation-sparing treatment by nature: "surgical" maggots revisited. *Clin Infect Dis.* 2002;35: 1566–1571.

Margolin L, Gialeanell P. Assessment of the antimicrobial properties of maggots. *Int Wound J.* 2010;7:202.

Nigam Y, Morgan C. Does maggot therapy promoto wound healing? The clinical and cellular evidence. *J Eur Acad Dermatol Venereol.* 2016;30:776.

Opletová K, Blaizot X, Mourgeon B, et al. Maggot therapy for wound debridement: a randomized multicenter trial. *Atch Dermatol.* 2012;148:432.

Sherman RA. Maggot therapy for treating diabetic foot ulcers unresponsive to conventional therapy. *Diabetes Care.* 2003;26:446–451.

Sherman RA, Sherman J, Gilead L, et al. Maggot debridement therapy in outpatients. *Arch Phys Med Rehabil.* 2001;82:1226–1229.

SECTION 3

Aesthetic Medicine

Section Editor: YU WAH

CHAPTER 35

INTRODUCTION TO AESTHETIC MEDICINE

Haneef Alibhai

As our world continues to evolve, investment in health and wellness is now, more than ever, a top priority for people living longer, healthier, and more active lives. With this comes an ever-growing demand for various surgical and nonsurgical cosmetic medical procedures to enhance one's appearance and overall wellness.

In 2015, over 12 million cosmetic medical procedures were performed in the United States. Eighty-five percent of these procedures were nonsurgical (American Society of Aesthetic Plastic Surgeons). Since 2011, surgical procedures increased by 17% and nonsurgical procedures by 44%. Ninety percent of the procedures were performed on women. The top five nonsurgical cosmetic procedures in 2015 were botulinum toxin (Botox) injections (4,267,038 procedures), hyaluronic acid dermal filler treatments (2,148,326 procedures), laser hair removal (1,136,834 procedures), chemical peels (603,305 procedures), and microdermabrasion (557,690 procedures). The most popular procedure among people younger than 35 years of age was laser hair removal, whereas the most popular procedure among people older than 35 years was botulinum toxin injection. In 2015, Americans spent more than $13.5 billion on cosmetic procedures.

POPULATION TREND

Currently people aged 35 to 50 years are the most powerful consumers in the world of aesthetic and cosmetic treatments, accounting for 40% of total procedures and spending $5.1 million in 2015. Although cosmetic procedures remain highly popular among people aged 51 and older (with 30% of total procedures performed in people aged 51 to 64, and 10% in people older than age 65), consumption is also on the rise for the younger population. People aged 34 years and younger accounted for nearly 20% of total procedures performed in 2015.

FACIAL AGING PROCESS

As we age, our skin matures (chronologic aging). This is generally accelerated by a process known as *photoaging*. Photoaging refers to premature aging from sun exposure and can be exacerbated by environmental conditions, smoking, and genetic predisposition. *Healthy skin* is defined as skin that is smooth, firm, glowing, clear of blemishes and vascular lesions, and plump with natural moisture. *Unhealthy skin* is defined as skin that is uneven, blotchy with pigmentation, poor in tone and elasticity (thin), leathery, dull, and covered with age spots, telangiectases, fine lines, and wrinkles. These unwelcome changes are brought about by the pull of gravity and cumulative damage to DNA, collagen, and cell membranes by free radicals produced from normal cellular metabolism, environmental elements, and sun exposure. (Also see the discussion of aging skin in Chapter 50, Skin Peels.)

For centuries we have striven to slow the aging process in an attempt to look and feel younger. The facial rejuvenation process aims to achieve the following goals:

- Reverse sun damage and reduce the signs of aging (vascular and pigmented lesions)
- Renew and retrain skin cells to appear younger and function more effectively to maintain youthful appearance (smooth skin)
- Relax overactive muscles that cause wrinkles
- Replace lost volume
- Tighten sagging and loose skin
- Stimulate dermal collagen production

During the past decade, much progress has been made in the field of noninvasive facial rejuvenation. The list of noninvasive facial rejuvenation techniques has grown considerably in response to the aging baby boomer's demand for procedures that combine safety, efficacy, predictability, and, of course, minimal downtime. The following noninvasive facial rejuvenation techniques are the most widely performed and sought-after procedures:

- Cosmeceutical skin care
- Microdermabrasion and dermal infusion
- Chemical peels
- Photofacial rejuvenation (intense pulsed light [IPL])
- Laser/IPL treatment of hair, veins, pigmented lesions, acne, and tattoos
- Ablative laser resurfacing (carbon dioxide, erbium:yttrium-aluminum garnet)
- Light-based therapies (e.g., radiofrequency [RF], light-emitting diode [LED] photomodulation, infrared [IR] devices, fractional resurfacing)
- Nonablative/fractional skin resurfacing
- Nonablative/fractional skin tightening (RF, IR)
- Ablative/fractional skin resurfacing
- Photodynamic therapy (PDT)
- Sclerotherapy
- Botulinum toxin injections
- Dermal filler treatments

More recently, cosmetic physicians have begun combining rejuvenation techniques in an attempt to provide better and longer-lasting results. Depending on the patient's concerns and goals, most facial rejuvenation procedures can be performed in concert to provide patients with the best results. Indeed, when combined, these procedures offer results far superior to those from any single procedure.

Without question aesthetic medicine is an exciting and rapidly growing field of medicine today. Given this staggering growth, it is more important than ever for providers to constantly seek educational opportunities to keep up to date with recent advances in technology and new procedures. This section of the text provides an overview of the most popular and sought-after cosmetic rejuvenation procedures available today. Those who want to enter the field of aesthetic medicine are strongly encouraged to undergo intensive hands-on clinical training with an experienced aesthetic clinician.

INITIAL COSMETIC AND AESTHETIC ASSESSMENT VISIT

Regardless of the reason for the initial visit, it is essential that a full evaluation be made of the patient's overall health status. The general health history questionnaire can be used for an overview, but specific questions should then be asked about the skin (Fig. 35.1). It is important to determine exactly what it is the patient is concerned about, because another procedure may be more appropriate than what the patient has in mind.

For light-based therapies, it is important to determine the Fitzpatrick skin type (see Chapter 38, Lasers and Pulsed-Light Devices: Hair Removal, section on Fitzpatrick Skin Types and Treatment Implications, and Fig. 38.7) because the amount of energy needed will vary depending on the skin type.

It is also important to determine if there has been recent use (within 6 months) of isotretinoin (Accutane), because it markedly increases the skin's sensitivity to light and many other products.

If the patient has a history of herpes simplex, it may be wise to use antiviral prophylaxis to prevent an outbreak if generalized facial procedures like ablative laser resurfacing or aggressive peels are to be performed (e.g., valacyclovir [Valtrex] 2 g immediately, followed by 2 g 12 hours later).

Knowing what the patient has used for skin care and what is available to improve the appearance of the skin is very helpful (see Chapter 36, Cosmeceuticals and Skin Care).

Effective *topical anesthetics* are beneficial for many procedures. Care must be taken that they be used appropriately, especially if applied under occlusion, because side effects can be significant (see Chapter 6, Local and Topical Anesthetic Complications, and Chapter 4, Topical Anesthesia). In some instances, an *anxiolytic* drug (e.g., diazepam [Valium] 10 mg 30 minutes before the procedure) will make the experience easier (e.g., ablative laser resurfacing).

This initial visit allows not only a comprehensive physical evaluation of the patient but also enables the provider to assess the patient's psychological makeup. An honest discussion of findings is essential. Conditions such as body dysmorphic syndrome should be recognized and dealt with in a straightforward fashion lest the patient be harmed further. The main objective of the initial consultation is to educate the patient on the various nonsurgical cosmetic procedures that are available. The discussion focuses on the procedures deemed to be most appropriate for the particular patient. Based on the patient's concerns, time line, goals, and budget, a customized treatment plan will be developed (Fig. 35.2). It is imperative that realistic expectations be set in discussing outcomes. Experience over the years has proved that it is best to be honest with patients and to "underpromise and overdeliver."

BEFORE AND AFTER PHOTOGRAPHS

Obtaining before and after photographs can be very beneficial in an aesthetic practice and is strongly recommended. Photographs document the appearance before an intervention for both the patient and the provider. Patients frequently "forget" their initial appearance and see only what remains to be done. Having a "before" photograph can document the changes. Clinicians can also use the photographs to gauge which interventions have had the most impact over time.

General Tips

- Ideally, all photographs should be taken in a designated room using a blue background.
  - Lighting, distance, background, and views taken should be duplicated for both the before and the after photographs.
  - Additional background options: dark solid wall color, posterboard, felt, blue window shade mounted on the back of a door.

- Limited or no jewelry for both before and after photographs.
- Hair pulled away from the face.
- Views should be consistent: full face/oblique/profile/close-up of treatment area.

"Before" Tips

- The "before" photograph should be taken during the initial consultation, before any treatment.
- If face has not been cleansed, use a makeup-remover wipe to remove the majority of makeup.

"After" Tips

- "After" photographs should be as similar as possible to the "before" photograph.
  If no makeup is worn in the "before" photo (recommended), the "after" also should be taken without makeup.
- "After" photographs should be taken at predetermined time frames, such as 7 to 10 days postpeel and again at 3, 6, 9, and 12 months.

Preparing for the Photograph

- Take a photograph of the name on the chart before taking a photograph of the patient.
- If the picture is taken with a digital camera, the photograph should not have a yellow hue.
- For dermal filler photographs, turn the flash off. With a digital camera, the flash washes out folds.
- Turn on the date stamp feature for recording the date the photograph is taken.
- The patient should be seated on a stool with no back.
  - The patient should be sitting up straight and not leaning back against anything.
  - Position the stool approximately 1 foot from the wall; check viewfinder for shadows.
  - Pull the patient's hair back away from the face and remove all or large jewelry.

Taking the Photo

- Head position
  - The ala-tragus line should be parallel to the floor (the ala-tragus line is an imaginary line that runs from the nostril to the cartilaginous projection in the middle of the ear).
  - Another way to check head position is to be sure the occlusal (biting) surface of the teeth is parallel to the floor.

FULL-FACE PHOTO

- Have the patient sit up straight.
- Head position should be straight; make sure the ear is not tipped toward either shoulder.
- Pull hair away from jaw line.
- Eyes should be open and focused straight ahead, not looking up or down.
- For "blinkers," ask the patient to keep the eyes closed until you have the view in focus and then to open the eyes.

Additional Checks

- Ala-tragus line or occlusal surface should be parallel to the floor.
- Chin should not be tipped too far up or down.
- Lips should be in a neutral position—not smiling or frowning.
- The head should take up the entire frame—do not crop off hair or chin.

AESTHETIC SERVICES PATIENT PROFILE

Name: _____ DOB: _____ Age: _____ Gender: M/F

Have you completed our medical history form?   Yes_____   No_____
Are you pregnant?   Yes_____   No_____
Do you wear contact lenses?   Yes_____   No_____
Have you had any skin cancers?   Yes_____   No_____   Abnormal moles removed?   Yes_____   No_____
Precancerous skin changes (actinic keratoses)?   Yes_____   No_____
Do you currently have a sunburn/windburn/red face?   Yes_____   Why?_____   No_____
Are you in the habit of going to tanning booths?   Yes_____   No_____   Last visit?_____
Please circle what best describes how your skin reacts to the sun (Fitzpatrick Classification):
   I   Always burns, never tans—light white skin
   II   Always burns, sometimes tans—light white skin
   III Sometimes bums, always tans—medium white skin
   IV   Rarely burns, always tans—dark/olive white and Asian skin
   V   Moderately pigmented—light brown skin
   VI   Black skin—medium to dark brown, African and African-American skin
Do you currently get facial waxing/electrolysis/use depilatories?   Yes_____   No_____
Are you currently using Biore/snore strips?   Yes_____   No_____
Are you currently using Retin-A/Renova/Differin?   Yes_____   No_____   What Strength?_____
          For how long? _____ How frequently? _____ Where applied? _____
Are you now or have you ever used Accutane?   Yes_____   No_____   How long? _____   When? _____
Have you ever had microdermabrasion?   Yes_____   No_____   When? _____   Where? _____
Do you have regular dermal filler injections?   Yes_____   No_____
Do you have regular Botox injections?   Yes_____   No_____
Have you ever had a chemical peel?   Yes_____   No_____   Within the last 14 days?   Yes_____   No_____
   What kind? _____   Describe your reaction: _____
Have you recently had facial surgery?   Yes_____   No_____   Describe: _____   When? _____
Have you recently had laser resurfacing?   Yes_____   No_____   When? _____   What Kind? _____
What type of work do you do? _____   Airline travel?   Yes_____   How often? _____   No_____
Do you participate in vigorous aerobic activity or sports?   Yes_____   No_____   What type? _____
Do you smoke?   Yes_____   No_____
Do you develop cold sores/fever blisters?   Yes_____   No_____   Last breakout? _____
Are you allergic/sensitive to (check all that apply) milk_____   apples_____   citrus_____   grapes_____
   aloe vera_____   aspirin_____   perfumes_____   latex_____   hydroquinone_____
   Other allergies? If so, what? _____
Are you sensitive to alcohol-based products?   Yes_____   No_____
Please list all medications you take especially thyroid supplements, hormone replacement therapy, birth control pills,
Accutane, Coumadin: _____
How would you describe your skin? (check all that apply) Thick_____   Thin_____   Sagging_____   Firm_____
   Normal_____   Dry_____   Oily_____   Acne_____   Blackheads_____   Milia_____   Cysts_____   Breakouts_____
   Acne scarred_____   Large pores_____   Small pores_____   Rosacea_____   Eczema_____   Freckled_____
   Sun-damaged_____   Uneven/blotchy_____   Mature_____   Wrinkled_____   Patchy dryness on_____
   Sallow_____   Melasma_____   Perfume-stained_____   Hypopigmented_____   Hyper-pigmented_____   Psoriasis_____
   Dehydrated (lacking moisture)_____   Telangiectasia (broken surface blood vessels)_____
Do you have a tendency to scar?   Yes_____   No_____   Form keloids?   Yes_____   No_____
Do you consider your skin sensitive_____   resilient_____   not sure_____
Eye color: Blue_____   Green_____   Hazel_____   Gray_____   Lt Brown_____   Med Brown_____   Dk Brown_____
Hair color: Blonde_____   Red_____   Lt Brown_____   Med Brown_____   Dk Brown_____   Black_____   Gray/Silver/White_____
Skin tone: Pale/Whlte_____   Light_____   Medium_____   Reddish_____   Freckled_____   Lt Olive_____   Med Ollve_____
   Dark Olive_____   Lt Brown_____   Med Brown_____   Dk Brown_____   Soft Black_____   Black_____
What is your hereditary makeup (what nationality)? _____
Are you using glycolic/AHA home care products? Yes_____   No_____   If so, which one(s)?_____
How does your skin react to them? _____
Have you ever used any products that caused a bad reaction? Yes_____   No_____   Describe _____
What is your daily home care regimen? _____
What are the cosmetic improvements you would like to see in your skin? _____

Patient/Client Signature: _____   Date: _____
Treatment recommendations: _____
_____
_____
_____

Patch test: _____   Date _____   Solution _____   Test area _____   Result _____
Physician/Aesthetician Signature _____   Date: _____

Fig. 35.1   Aesthetic Services Patient Profile form.

CUSTOMIZED AESTHETIC TREATMENT PLAN

Name of Patient: _____ M _____ F _____ Date of Birth: _____

Date first evaluated: _____ Date photos taken: _____

SUBJECTIVE: Patient's initial concerns:

1. _____
2. _____
3. _____
4. _____

PAST MEDICAL HISTORY: Reviewed. See medical history form. Initial _____
PERTINENT FACTS:

Previous skin cancer:	Y ___ N ___	Previous actinics:	Y ___ N ___	Sun exposure:	Y ___ N ___
Cold sores:	Y ___ N ___	Tanning booth use:	Y ___ N ___	Scar easily:	Y ___ N ___
Heal poorly:	Y ___ N ___				

PREVIOUS TREATMENTS: Y ___ N ___ What _____ When _____ Where _____
AESTHETIC QUESTIONNAIRE FORM: Reviewed. Initial _____
SKIN TYPE: I   II   III   IV   V

OBJECTIVE:

_____
_____
_____

ASSESSMENT:

1. _____
2. _____
3. _____
4. _____

TREATMENT PLAN:

Botox: 1st Area: _____ Price: $ _____ Date Sch'd: _____ Date Tx: _____ Date Tx: _____
             2nd Area: _____ Price: $ _____ Date Sch'd: _____ Date Tx: _____ Date Tx: _____
             3rd Area: _____ Price: $ _____ Date Sch'd: _____ Date Tx: _____ Date Tx: _____

Cosmoderm: Area: _____ Price: $ _____ Date Sch'd: _____ Date Tx: _____ Date Tx: _____
Juvederm: Area: _____ Price: $ _____ Date Sch'd: _____ Date Tx: _____ Date Tx: _____

LIGHT SHEER/HAIR REMOVAL:

             Area: _____ Price: $ _____ Date Sch'd: _____ Date Tx: _____ Date Tx: _____
             Area: _____ Price: $ _____ Date Sch'd: _____ Date Tx: _____ Date Tx: _____
IPL: 1st Area: _____ Price: $ _____ Date Sch'd: _____ Date Tx: _____ Date Tx: _____
             2nd Area: _____ Price: $ _____ Date Sch'd: _____ Date Tx: _____ Date Tx: _____
Radiage: Area: _____ Price: $ _____ Date Sch'd: _____ Date Tx: _____ Date Tx: _____
Active FX: Area: _____ Price: $ _____ Date Sch'd: _____ Date Tx: _____ Date Tx: _____
Microdermabrasion: _____ Price: $ _____ Date Sch'd: _____ Date Tx: _____ Date Tx: _____
Chemical Peel: _____ Price: $ _____ Date Sch'd: _____ Date Tx: _____ Date Tx: _____

Skin Care Products: _____ Price: $ _____
Skin Care Samples: _____

Customized Plan Notes:

_____
_____
_____

PROVIDER SIGNATURE:

_____ Date: _____

Fig. 35.2 Customized Aesthetic Treatment Plan form.

Oblique View and Profile Views

- Repeat aforementioned positioning checks.
- Rotate the stool, not just the person's head.

PATIENT EDUCATION AND CONSENT

Probably more than in any other area of medicine, the time must be taken to evaluate the patient's condition and wishes. A frank discussion of risks, benefits, possible complications, alternative therapies, and expected outcomes is essential. It is important not to "oversell" a procedure (see consent forms available at www.expertconsult.com). Educational handouts explaining the procedure; before, during, and after photographs from previous patients; and written postprocedure instructions can be very helpful. Most of the procedures in this section are elective, and it is essential that patients have realistic expectations of what can be accomplished.

Aesthetic medicine can be a very enjoyable and rewarding area in which to practice. The key to success is combination therapy, because no single procedure will address all the concerns that may bring a patient to a cosmetic clinic. Clinicians must therefore be well trained and seek continuing education as this field goes on growing rapidly. Ultimately, honest communication, patient education, outstanding customer service, and ethical care are the cornerstones of success in aesthetic medicine.

Acknowledgment

We thank Cathy Uecker for her contributions to the section "Before and After Photographs."

RECOMMENDED READING

Alam M, Silapunt S. *Procedures in Cosmetic Dermatology Series: Treatment of Leg Veins.* 2nd ed. Philadelphia: Elsevier Saunders; 2010.

Arndt KA. *Procedures in Cosmetic Dermatology Series: Scar Revision.* Philadelphia: Elsevier Saunders; 2006.

Carruthers A, Carruthers J. *Procedures in Cosmetic Dermatology Series: Botulinum Toxin.* 3rd ed. Philadelphia: Elsevier; 2012.

Carruthers A, Carruthers J. *Procedures in Cosmetic Dermatology Series: Soft Tissue Augmentation.* 3rd ed. Philadelphia: Elsevier; 2012.

Donofrio LM. Evaluation and management of the aging face. In: Robinson JK, Hanke DW, Siegel DM, Fratila A, Bhatia ACohrer TE, eds. *Surgery of the Skin: Procedural Dermatology.* 3rd ed. Philadelphia: Elsevier; 2014.

Draelos ZD. *Procedures in Cosmetic Dermatology Series: Cosmeceuticals.* 2nd ed. Philadelphia: Saunders; 2008.

Glaser DA, Layman J. Psychosocial issues and the cosmetic surgery patient. In: Robinson JK, Hanke DW, Siegel DM, Fratila A, Bhatia ACohrer TE, eds. *Surgery of the Skin: Procedural Dermatology.* 3rd ed. Philadelphia: Elsevier; 2014.

Hruza G, Avram M. *Procedures in Cosmetic Dermatology Series: Lasers and Lights.* 3rd ed. Philadelphia: Elsevier; 2012.

Goldman MP. *Procedures in Cosmetic Dermatology Series: Photodynamic Therapy.* 2nd ed. Philadelphia: Saunders; 2007.

Haber RS, Stough D, Alam M. *Procedures in Cosmetic Dermatology Series: Hair Transplantation.* Philadelphia: Saunders; 2006.

Hanke CW, Sattler G, Dover JS. *Procedures in Cosmetic Dermatology Series: Liposuction.* Philadelphia: Saunders; 2006.

Moy RL, Dover JS. *Procedures in Cosmetic Dermatology Series: Advanced Face Lifting.* Philadelphia: Saunders; 2006.

Moy RL, Fincher EF. *Procedures in Cosmetic Dermatology Series: Blepharoplasty.* Philadelphia: Saunders; 2006.

Tung R, Rubin MG. *Procedures in Cosmetic Dermatology Series: Chemical Peels.* 2nd ed. Philadelphia: Saunders; 2010.

Usatine RP. *The Color Atlas of Family Medicine.* 2nd ed. New York: McGraw-Hill; 2013.

CHAPTER 36

COSMECEUTICALS AND SKIN CARE

Wendy L. Smeltzer

Products applied to the skin can range from purely cosmetic products to prescription drugs, but many fall somewhere in between and are commonly referred to as *cosmeceutical agents*. The term *cosmeceutical* is widely used in the skin care industry but is still not recognized by many regulatory bodies such as the U.S. Food and Drug Administration (FDA). However, cosmeceuticals are a reality, as evidenced by the widespread use of this term and a growing number of textbooks and symposia in the medical aesthetics field on this subject. The share of the skin care market comprising cosmeceuticals continues to grow and is the fastest-growing segment of skin care products in the marketplace.

DEFINITIONS

The term *cosmeceutical* was coined by Dr. Albert M. Kligman in the 1970s to focus on the ill-defined territory that falls between cosmetic products and therapeutic medications (drugs). Historically, topical skin care products have been divided into either cosmetics or drugs as defined by the Food, Drug and Cosmetic Act of 1938. A *cosmetic* is defined as "an article intended to be rubbed, poured, sprinkled, sprayed on, introduced into or otherwise applied to the human body or any part thereof for cleansing, beautifying, promoting attractiveness or altering appearance." The definition of a *drug* is "an article intended to affect the structure or any function of the body or articles intended for use in the diagnosis, cure, mitigation, treatment or prevention of disease in man." At a fundamental level, cosmetics alter the appearance of the skin, whereas drugs alter the structure and function of the skin.

Cosmetics do not require premarketing clearance, and it is up to the manufacturer to ensure that the ingredients and amounts used are not subject to drug regulations and that the product is safe when used as intended. On the other hand, drugs are subject to extensive premarketing research to prove their efficacy and safety. According to regulators, the intended use of a product can also determine its classification. Thus it is not only the ingredients in a skin care product but the claims in labeling and advertising that can affect its classification as a cosmetic or drug. Cosmeceuticals bridge the gap between cosmetics and drugs and comprise products that achieve cosmetic results by means of some degree of physiologic action. Other terms for cosmeceuticals are *performance cosmetics*, *active cosmetics*, *functional cosmetics*, and *dermoceuticals*.

COSMECEUTICAL CLASSES

Categories of cosmeceuticals, some of which overlap, include the following:

* Retinoids
* Exfoliants
* Vitamins
* Antioxidants
* Peptides
* Growth factors
* Skin-lightening agents
* Others

Retinoids

The *retinoids* are compounds that have the basic core structure of vitamin A and its derivatives. *All-trans retinoic acid* is the active form of vitamin A in the skin. It works by interacting with nuclear receptor proteins to form complexes that interact with DNA sequences to affect the transcription and regulation of gene expression for skin keratinocyte growth and differentiation. This causes increased cell turnover in the epidermis. All-trans retinoic acid is quite irritating to the skin and has teratogenic effects. Derivatives such as *retinol* are commonly used in skin care products because they have a lower irritation profile and fewer safety concerns. Once applied to the skin, retinol converts to retinaldehyde and then all-trans retinoic acid. The science and benefits of retinoids are well documented, with proven results in reducing photo damage and fine lines of the skin as well as efficacy against acne and psoriasis.

Exfoliants

The two key exfoliant cosmeceuticals are *alpha hydroxy acids (AHAs)* and *beta hydroxy acids (BHAs)*. The difference in their chemical structures leads to significant differences in their mechanisms of action, although both cause superficial skin cells to desquamate at an increased rate. This results in a smoothing of skin texture and reduction in photo damage.

Alpha Hydroxy Acids

The most widely used AHA in skin care products is *glycolic acid* because of its small molecular size and hence excellent penetration into the epidermis. However, *lactic acid* and other larger AHAs are found increasingly in skin care products. There have been many studies on the science and effectiveness of AHAs since the introduction of these products in 1974 by Van Scott and Yu. The AHAs cause desquamation of skin cells in the epidermis by reducing the cellular cohesion between keratinocytes. It is postulated that AHAs bind calcium, which decreases local calcium ion concentrations from cell adhesion molecules, thus disrupting intercellular adhesion and increasing exfoliation. There are also some stimulating effects on the dermis, including increased synthesis of collagen and glycosaminoglycans, which also results in a moisturizing effect.

AHAs are very effective in the treatment of photo-damaged skin as well as dry skin, seborrheic dermatitis, acne, and keratoses. Concentrations up to 10% are used in home care products, whereas higher concentrations are used in professional treatments.

Beta Hydroxy Acids

Salicylic acid is the only BHA used extensively in skin care products. It has proven keratolytic effects and affects only the stratum corneum. It decreases cohesion between the corneocytes by denaturing glycoproteins and disrupting desmosomal attachments. It has been used to treat hyperkeratotic conditions such as corns, warts, seborrheic dermatitis, psoriasis, and dandruff. Because salicylic acid is lipophilic, it is also very useful in the treatment of acne as well as photoaging and dyschromia. Concentrations of 0.5% to 2% are commonly used in home care products. Higher concentrations are used in patches to treat calluses, corns, and warts. The concentration is usually limited by the amount of irritation it causes.

Amino Acid Filaggrins

These amino acids, found naturally in skin, foster moisture retention. However, they are used topically as mild chemical peels to reduce wrinkles and improve skin texture, although more peer-reviewed research is required to define their optimal use.

Vitamins

Vitamin C

Vitamin C is a valuable topical cosmeceutical in skin care with significant data supporting its biologic activity and benefits to the skin. Vitamin C is useful in treating photoaging because it has an antioxidant effect as well as a skin-lightening effect through the inhibition of tyrosinase. It is also an essential cofactor for collagen production in the skin and has proven effects on wrinkle reduction. In addition, vitamin C is helpful in treating acne because of its antiinflammatory properties, which are due to the deactivation of some factors responsible for the production of proinflammatory cytokines. The active form of vitamin C is L-ascorbic acid, which is difficult to incorporate in topical products because of stability and absorption issues. It oxidizes easily, which leads to loss of potency, and has poor skin penetration. Enhanced delivery systems and the use of more stable derivatives such as magnesium ascorbyl phosphate allow the use of topical vitamin C as a mainstay in skin rejuvenation treatments.

Vitamins B and E

Vitamin B_3 (niacinamide) is used topically in skin care because it is well absorbed and well tolerated. The mechanism of action is not clearly elucidated, but it is a precursor to enzyme cofactors that are important in many cellular metabolic functions. There is some evidence that it improves the skin barrier function, which reduces skin redness and irritation. It may also reduce hyperpigmentation and improve skin texture and wrinkle depth.

Vitamin E (i.e., the tocopherols) is an antioxidant and a well-documented free radical scavenger. In topical application to the skin, there is good evidence that is it photoprotective, helping prevent damage from ultraviolet (UV) radiation. There is some controversy about its use in wound healing and scar prevention, and it may have some benefit in the treatment of photo-damaged skin.

Vitamin K

Vitamin K is a potent agent that increases the coagulation of blood. When applied to the skin topically, there is some evidence that it may reduce bruising. There are studies showing reduced purpura after pulsed-dye laser treatments, but more research is required.

Antioxidants

Antioxidants protect the skin from free radical damage due to oxidant stress generated by sunlight and pollutants. The mechanism of action is the scavenging of singlet oxygen and reactive oxygen species. Many antioxidants have proved effective when taken orally, but not all are effective topically. The challenge is to get sufficient skin absorption of the correct form of the antioxidant agent with enough activity to achieve the desired effect. In addition to the following agents, some of the vitamins reviewed earlier are also antioxidants.

Ubiquinone

Ubiquinone, or coenzyme Q10, has been proven to be absorbed after topical application to skin. There are some studies to support improvement in the photoaging of skin as well as decreased stratum corneum cell size due to a lessening of the slowdown of cell division that occurs with intrinsic aging.

Alpha Lipoic Acid

Alpha lipoic acid is a potent antioxidant that penetrates the dermis. There is some evidence that it may reduce both the intrinsic and extrinsic aging of the skin that has occurred due to free radical damage; it may also decrease UV-B–induced erythema. Further investigation and peer-reviewed studies are still required.

Idebenone

This newer antioxidant is a synthetic version of ubiquinone. Some initial studies indicate that it may be effective in the treatment of photo-damaged skin, but more studies are required.

Peptides

Peptides are short chains of the amino acid sequences that make up larger proteins. There are three key cosmeceutical peptides that are useful topical agents for antiaging skin treatments, all with very different mechanisms of action. The cost and delivery mechanisms for these ingredients are challenging. There are limited peer-reviewed studies on these products, and research is ongoing.

Argireline

Argireline (acetyl hexapeptide-3; Lipotec) is a hexapeptide that inhibits neurotransmitter release. It can therefore theoretically reduce muscle movement. It may decrease skin wrinkles when it is delivered to targeted facial muscles, such as fine lines around the eyes and lips. It does not penetrate deep into facial muscles and is not a substitute for botulinum toxin in the treatment of dynamic wrinkles.

Matrixyl

Matrixyl (palmitoyl pentapeptide-3), a pentapeptide fragment of dermal collagen, acts as a feedback stimulator to increase collagen synthesis. It is nonirritating to skin and preserves the skin's barrier function. It is useful in helping to reduce wrinkle depth in aging skin.

Copper Peptide

Copper is a trace element necessary for wound healing and enzymatic processes that enhance collagen production and antioxidant activities. A tripeptide carrier may help to deliver elements such as copper into the skin. The major effect of this peptide is as a delivery system rather than because of its own biologic activity.

Growth Factors

Growth factors are regulatory proteins that act as chemical messengers between and within cells. Hundreds of growth factors have now been identified, with many acting synergistically in wound healing and tissue regeneration; however, their mechanisms of action are still poorly understood. Growth factors can be extracted from plants, cultured epidermal cells, placental cells, and human fibroblasts for use in cosmeceuticals. Some studies show improvement in photo-damaged skin, which is similar to a chronic wound. There is also controversy about whether these molecules are too large to be absorbed as well as theoretical concerns about their potential to contribute to hypertrophic scarring or cancerous growth. Growth factors used in skin care products include kinetin, a plant growth factor, and human growth factor (HGF).

Skin-Lightening Agents

Unwanted pigmentation in the skin may be treated with a variety of cosmeceutical agents. However, only pigments in the epidermis will respond to topical agents; the deeper dermal pigments will not. Some of the aforementioned cosmeceuticals will decrease pigmentation, such as vitamins C and B_3, retinoids, and the AHAs and BHAs. Other agents are also useful as topical products to lighten pigmentation.

Hydroquinone

Hydroquinone (HQ) has been the standard treatment of hyperpigmentation for many years. Its main mechanism of action is through the inhibition of tyrosinase, an enzyme necessary for the production of melanin, but it may also alter the formation of melanosomes and selectively damage melanosomes and melanocytes. Although very effective, it commonly causes skin irritation and may have a cytotoxic effect on melanocytes. Concern over cytotoxicity has resulted in the banning of HQ from use in skin products in some countries.

Others

Kojic acid is a naturally occurring derivative from a fungus that acts as a tyrosinase inhibitor. At the 2% to 4% concentration used in skin products, it is mildly irritating and a possible allergen.

Azelaic acid, another effective skin-lightening agent, is isolated from *Pityrosporum ovale* and also inhibits tyrosinase. It is safe, although it may require a higher concentration (20%), which can cause contact dermatitis.

Other tyrosinase inhibitors—such as *arbutin* from bearberry fruit, *paper mulberry* extract from mulberry leaves, *aloesin* from aloe vera, and *glabridin* from licorice extract—may also be used as skin-lightening agents.

Other Cosmeceutical Agents

Dehydroepiandrosterone

Dehydroepiandrosterone (DHEA) is an adrenal steroid, levels of which naturally decline with age. There is some evidence that topically applied DHEA may increase collagen synthesis and decrease collagen breakdown, although more studies are needed.

Dimethylaminoethanol

Dimethylaminoethanol (DMAE) is a precursor of choline that increases neurotransmitter release and muscle tone. When applied topically, it may increase muscle tone, which may cause skin tightening for skin rejuvenation. Given that other cosmeceutical peptides designed for skin rejuvenation act by doing the reverse—relaxing muscle tone to smooth out wrinkles—one can see the potential for consumer confusion and the need for more research and clinical studies.

SUNSCREENS

Although sunscreens technically are not cosmeceutical agents, no discussion of skin care products is complete without a review of sunscreens. Sunscreens are regulated by the FDA as over-the-counter (OTC) drugs and require a drug identification number (DIN). The use of a broad-spectrum sunscreen with minimum sun protection factor (SPF) of 30 is important in any skin care regimen to prevent photoaging as well as skin cancers. Although in the past there has been a focus on damage caused by UV-B radiation (290 to 320 nm), we now know that UV-A radiation (320 to 400 nm) is also significant in both carcinogenesis and photo damage. UV-A has been called "the silent killer" because erythema does not occur with exposure, as it does with UV-B radiation. The SPF number indicates the dose of UV radiation required to produce one minimal erythema dose (MED) on protected skin after the application of 2 mg/cm^2 of product divided by the UV radiation needed to produce one MED on unprotected skin. Because erythema is produced by UV-B radiation only, the SPF rating refers to its ability to protect from UV-B and *not* UV-A. There is no standard measure of UV-A protection. It is therefore important to choose a sunscreen that provides broad-spectrum protection and lists both UV-B (an SPF rating) and UV-A radiation (no current rating available) on its label.

Sunscreens can be categorized as either physical or chemical sunscreens. Physical sunscreen agents work by physically blocking the penetration of UV radiation into the skin by reflecting or scattering light. The most common physical sunscreen agents are titanium dioxide and zinc oxide. Both of these block UV-A and UV-B radiation and are well tolerated on the skin, with a low risk of irritation. Chemical sunscreen agents work by absorbing the harmful UV rays and transforming them to harmless longer-wave radiation.

PABA (para-aminobenzoic acid) was one of the first chemical sunscreen agents available. It absorbs UV-B radiation but causes significant skin sensitivities, so it has generally been replaced by newer agents. Table 36.1 lists some of the common chemical sunscreen agents and their primary filtering actions.

Another factor to consider with sunscreens is their water resistance classification. For sunscreens to be labeled "water resistant," they must maintain their SPF level after 40 minutes of water immersion. "Very water resistant" sunscreens (formerly called "waterproof") maintain their SPF level after 80 minutes of water immersion.

COSMETIC SKIN CARE PRODUCTS

In addition to the various cosmeceutical agents and sunscreens, it is important also to understand the use of cosmetic skin care products. Adults use an average of seven skin care products daily and billions of dollars are spent annually in the United States on skin cleansers and moisturizers; thus it behooves the clinician to have some understanding of skin care basics. The stratum corneum plays a key role in the use of cosmetic skin care products. The general appearance of the skin depends on the status of the stratum corneum. When it has adequate moisture, the stratum corneum is soft, pliant, and smooth, and it reflects light. The skin will then have a "radiance" or "glow." When the stratum corneum does not have adequate moisture, the skin will be rough and may have scaling or cracks. This roughness scatters light, and the skin then has a dull appearance. Skin care involves cleansing the skin and ensuring adequate moisture content in the stratum corneum by preserving the integrity of the epidermal barrier. Skin care regimens involve the daily use of cleansers, toners, and moisturizers.

Cleansers

The basic function of a cleanser is to cleanse the skin. There is a hydrolipid film covering the surface of the skin that becomes soiled through contact with dirt and pollutants as well as by secretions from sebaceous and sweat glands. Shed corneocytes, decomposition products from the cornification process, as well as microorganisms may also contaminate this hydrolipid film. The challenge for cleansers is to remove this soil and not strip the hydrolipid film in the process, which would impair the epidermal barrier. There are two major categories of cleansers: *soaps/detergents* and *emulsion cleansing agents*.

TABLE 36.1	Common Chemical Sunscreen Agents (U.S. Food and Drug Administration–Approved in the United States)	
UV-A Filters	**UV-B Filters**	**UV-A + UV-B Filters**
Avobenzone (Parsol 1789)	Para-aminobenzoic acid (PABA)	Dioxybenzone
Encamsule (Mexoryl SX)	Cinoxate	Drometrizole trisiloxane (Mexoryl XL)
Methyl anthranilate	Homosalate	Ensulizole (Eusolex 232)
	Octyl methoxycinnamate (octinoxate; Eusolex 2292)	Helioplex (combo avobenzone/oxybenzone)
		Octocrylene
	Octyl salicylate (octisalate)	
	Oxybenzone (Eusolex 4360)	
	Sulisobenzone	

Soaps and detergents contain surfactant agents that increase the affinity of dissimilar phases for each other. This allows oil and water to mix. These are foaming cleansers and generally remove oil from skin and thus are best as cleansers for oily skin. Soaps are the alkali salt of a fatty acid and leave an alkaline residue on the skin. This raises the pH of the skin, which increases counts of *Propionibacterium acnes* and can exacerbate acne. There are very few true soaps remaining in the marketplace; most have been replaced by synthetic detergents. Common detergent agents found in skin cleansers are sodium and ammonium lauryl sulfate, sodium laureth sulfate, cocamidopropyl betaine, and lauramphocarboxyglycinate.

Emulsion cleansing agents are oil-in-water or water-in-oil emulsions. They are usually cleansing milks or cleansing creams. They are less drying generally than detergents and can leave a residue of oil on the skin. These cleansers are better suited to drier skin types.

Toners

Toners are leave-on products applied to the skin after cleansing. They are designed to freshen and tone the skin and prepare it for the application of a moisturizer. When soaps were commonly used as cleansers, toners also served to remove the alkali residue and restore the acid mantle of the skin. In addition, toners are used to remove surface oil and debris and can serve as a delivery vehicle for other agents applied to the skin. Many toners have astringent agents such as witch hazel, ethanol, citrus extracts, and potassium alum as their key components. These are best for oily skin types. Alternatively, toners may have humectant agents—such as propylene glycol, butylene glycol, and sorbitol—which may increase the moisture content of dry skin.

Moisturizers

Moisturizers are products applied to the skin to promote and restore the epidermal barrier function and thus increase the water content of the stratum corneum. We lose approximately 500 mL of water daily through our skin (i.e., transepidermal water loss). Moisturizers are designed to maintain the water content of skin between 10% and 30%. Skin moisturizers are classified as *occlusive agents*, *humectant agents*, and *emollient agents*. Occlusive agents act as enhanced skin barriers by adding a hydrophobic film to the surface of the skin. This further impairs evaporation and conserves the moisture content of the stratum corneum. Common occlusive agents include petrolatum, mineral oil, paraffin, silicone, fats, and wax. *Humectant agents* attract water into the stratum corneum. This water is usually drawn from the dermis, but humectants can also attract water from the environment if the ambient humidity is over 70%. It is important to note that humectants can increase transepidermal water loss if the epidermal barrier is not intact. Humectant ingredients commonly found in skin moisturizers are glycerin, hyaluronic acid, urea, propylene glycol, gelatin, honey, and sorbitol. *Emollient agents* are substances that fill in the cracks and crevices in the stratum corneum. They are usually also barrier agents and include substances such as mineral oil, lanolin, ceramides, silicone, fatty esters, and fatty alcohols.

Most moisturizers are formulated as *creams*, which are water-in-oil emulsions, or as *lotions*, which are oil-in-water emulsions and are lighter than the cream formulations. The heaviness of the moisturizer depends on this formulation as well as the amount and characteristics of the occlusive agents. Night creams are examples of moisturizers designed as heavier creams, whereas a light, nongreasy moisturizer may be a lotion containing a weaker occlusive agent with the addition of humectant agents.

Choosing a Skin Care Regimen

Proper skin cleansing and moisturizing must work in harmony to maintain the integrity of the epidermal barrier and adequate hydration of the stratum corneum. Before choosing a skin care regimen, it is important to consider the skin's condition. Note the status of the stratum corneum and the epidermal barrier and determine whether the skin is oily or dry and whether it appears dehydrated. Sensitivities should be considered. The presence of acne lesions, dyschromias, and other signs of photo damage should be noted. The environment should also be considered, because humidity, temperature, wind, and pollutants are factors affecting skin care choices.

There are as many individual skin care regimens as there are products to choose from. It is impossible to give a standard skin care regimen or list all brands of skin care products on the market. The following is this author's approach and may provide some general guidance.

For oily skin types, choose a foaming cleanser with an astringent toner and lighter moisturizer with less occlusive and more humectant properties. For drier skin types, a cleansing milk or cream is preferable with a humectant toner and heavier moisturizer with increased occlusive and emollient effect.

The choice then to add cosmeceutical agents to the basic regimen depends on the desired structural changes for the skin conditions present.

For acne-prone skin, the use of lotions for moisturizing is preferable to creams. AHAs and BHAs are very beneficial in exfoliating the skin and unblocking sebaceous glands. Retinols may also be useful, as well as the anti-inflammatory action of vitamin C serums.

For hyperpigmentation, products containing hydroquinone have been the mainstay of treatment. Other lightening agents—such as kojic acid and azelaic acid—are beneficial, as is vitamin C serum. Exfoliating agents such as retinol should be used, and daily use of a sunscreen is important.

The largest demand for skin care advice is in the realm of skin rejuvenation and the treatment of photo damage and aging of the skin. In addition to the basic skin care regimen of appropriate cleansing and moisturizing, products with active cosmeceutical ingredients are beneficial, along with a sunscreen to prevent further damage. The daily use of a medical exfoliant such as retinol and an AHA is an important step in any skin rejuvenation regimen, along with the topical application of vitamin C serum. The use of a peptide cream with Argireline and Matrixyl may also be beneficial. A broad-spectrum sunscreen with a minimal SPF of 30 should be used daily. Although this is one suggested approach to skin rejuvenation, there are many other cosmeceutical ingredients and regimens that may be useful.

CHALLENGE OF COSMECEUTICALS

Cosmeceuticals represent the next new frontier in aesthetic medicine and the fastest-growing segment of the skin care industry. They are the driving force in the field of skin care research. However, there are very few peer-reviewed clinical trials for most of these products and there is little incentive to conduct extensive scientific research and studies. There is the concern that if research proves efficacy, then the product would no longer be considered a cosmeceutical but would be classified as a drug and be subject to the rigorous governmental approval processes. The dilemma for skin care companies is that clinicians require scientific proof of efficacy, yet this proof would then remove the newly developed product from the cosmeceutical market and subject it to scrutiny as a new drug. The current confusion in the marketplace about cosmeceuticals and the issue of hope versus hype versus fact is likely to remain until new regulations are in place.

RECOMMENDED READING

Draelos Z. Cutaneous exfoliation. *Cosmet Dermatol.* 2000;10:51–57.

Draelos Z. *Procedures in Cosmetic Dermatology Series: Cosmeceuticals.* 3rd ed. Philadelphia: Saunders; 2015.

Draelos Z, Thaman L, eds. *Cosmetic Formulation of Skin Care Products.* New York: Taylor & Francis; 2006:167–215.

Farris P. Cosmeceuticals: A review of the science behind the claims. *Cosmet Dermatol.* 2003;16:59–70.

Geffken C. What's in a name? *Global Cosmetic Industry (GCI).* 2004;5:28–30.

Kligman D. Cosmeceuticals. *Dermatol Clin.* 2000;18:609–615.

O'Rourke K. Cosmetic pharmaceuticals in dermatology. *Curr Probl Dermatol.* 2000;12:291–293.

Small R. Skin care products. In: Usatine R, ed. *Dermatologic and Cosmetic Procedures in Office Practice.* Philadelphia: Saunders; 2010.

Talakoub L, Neuhaus IM, Yu SS. Cosmeceuticals. In: Alam M, ed. *Cosmetic Dermatology.* Philadelphia: Saunders; 2009.

CHAPTER 37

GINGIVAL MELANIN HYPERPIGMENTATION

Ali Gürkan • Fatih Arikan

Hyperpigmentation of the gingiva is caused by excessive deposition of melanin. It is more frequently observed in Asian, African, and Mediterranean populations and has also been called *racial* or *physiologic pigmentation*. Pigmentation may vary not only among subjects of the same ethnic background but within different regions of the mouth. This kind of pigmentation presents as a well-demarcated, bilateral, dark-brown asymptomatic coloration in the keratinized gingiva, mostly in the anterior region. It is due to melanocyte overactivity; both dark- and light-skinned subjects have similar numbers of melanocytes in the gingiva. Because toxic agents in tobacco smoke induce melanocytes to produce melanin, smoking can cause hyperpigmentation in subjects with light skin and may aggravate pigmentation in dark-skinned individuals ("smoker's melanosis"). The severity and extent of melanosis are usually correlated with the duration and quantity of smoking, and the condition improves after the cessation of smoking. Environmental tobacco smoke has also been shown to influence the prevalence and the severity of gingival hyperpigmentation.

Gingival melanin hyperpigmentation is an aesthetic problem rather than a medical problem. The appearance of the gingiva while smiling is essential to overall personal aesthetics. Because brown-black melanotic lesions mostly involve the anterior vestibular gingiva, they cause an unaesthetic smile. Therefore depigmentation procedures have attracted much interest, and numerous techniques have been introduced to reverse this change (e.g., surgical debridement, laser treatments, cryotherapy, Table 37.1). A gingival melanin depigmentation method using radiofrequency (RF) surgery offers superior results and many advantages including speed, reliability, lack of postoperative pain, virtually no bleeding, and no discomfort from local anesthetic injection.

DIFFERENTIAL DIAGNOSIS

The patient presenting with pigmented gingiva should be thoroughly evaluated regarding dental and medical history and have an extraoral and intraoral examination as well as laboratory tests when indicated. Addison's disease (adrenal insufficiency) can also cause gingival hyperpigmentation.

Assess the following:

- Smoking habit (duration and number per day)
- Duration of pigmentation
- Skin pigmentation
- Perioral pigmented lesions (lips, face)
- Systemic diseases (e.g., Addison disease)
- Systemic symptoms of malignancy (fatigue, malaise, weight loss)
- Medications
- Lymph nodes
- Characteristics of the pigmented lesions (size, number, distribution, shape, color, surface, and borders)

A biopsy should be performed if a lesion cannot be explained by other factors.

INDICATION

- Removal of gingival melanosis

CONTRAINDICATIONS

- Cardiac pacemakers, cardiac defibrillator implants, cochlear implants (relative contraindication)
- Uncooperative patient

EQUIPMENT

- RF device (see Chapter 25, Radiofrequency Surgery [Modern Electrosurgery]).
- Small ball-tip (No. 135 or D8D; Ellman International Cynosure, Inc.) or, preferably, L-shaped advanced-composition alloy electrode (Ellman no. 136, F1D or 133D); the L-shaped no. 136 electrode has a flat end, making it suitable for a "tapping" action.
- 10% lidocaine spray.
- Mouth retractor.

TABLE 37.1	Comparison of Gingival Depigmentation Methods					
Method	Bleeding	Needle Anesthesia	Postoperative Pain	Periodontal Dressing	Ease of Access to Interdental Papillary Region	Major Disadvantage of Method
Scalpel surgery	+	+	+	+	−	Bleeding
Particle abrasive methods	+	+	+	+	−	Bleeding
Laser	−	+	−	−	+	Expense
Gas cryosurgery	−	−	−	−	−	Safety
Tetrafluoroethane cryosurgery (e.g., Envirotech Freezer Spray, Medi-Frig, and Verruca-Freeze)	−	−	−	−	−	Lack of access to interdental papillary region
Radiofrequency surgery	−	−	−	−	+	None

TECHNIQUE (DUAL FREQUENCY)

- Place the retractor and apply anesthetic spray to the region of interest.
- Adjust the device to the cutting mode (10 to 11) for thick gingiva or to the coag mode (7) for thin gingiva.
- Melanocytes are primarily located in the basal and suprabasal cell layers of the epithelium. Therefore, touch the pigmented areas lightly with the electrode tip. Remove the electrode as soon as the tissue around the electrode turns whitish. A "tapping" type approach covering all the pigmented areas works best (Fig. 37.1).

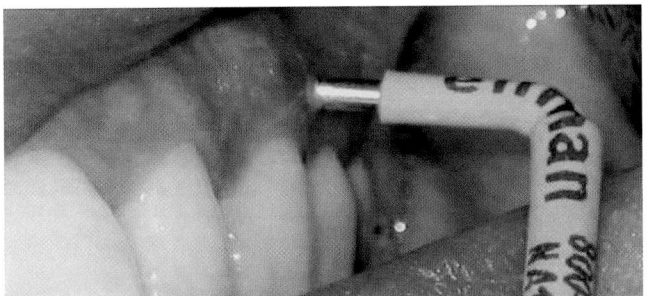
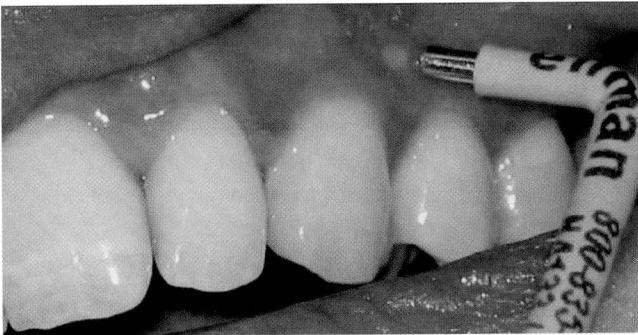

Fig. 37.1 Tapping the electrode on the pigmented gingival tissues. A topical anesthetic has been applied.

- Repeat the procedure for all pigmented areas.
- During the following week, slight redness is observed around the margins of the RF-treated lesions.
- Epithelialization is completed in 10 days, and at 2 weeks after the first treatment, a second procedure can be performed to treat any residual pigmentation.

Figs. 37.2 to 37.5 illustrate the results of RF surgical treatment of gingival hyperpigmentation in a variety of cases.

POSTPROCEDURE CARE

- Gentle brushing
- Antiseptic rinse
- Analgesic drugs the day of surgery (usually not needed)

COMPLICATIONS

- If the electrode is held in place longer than necessary or if too high a setting is used, excessive tissue necrosis can occur, increasing postoperative pain and compromising healing.
- We have never observed hypopigmentation of the pigmented gingiva after treatment. After the healing period at 2 weeks, the brown gingiva becomes pale pink, like the neighboring tissues. We have followed these patients for up to 1 year and observed no recurrence, even when they have not changed their smoking habits. In the event of recurrence, the simple procedure can easily be repeated. All of our patients indicated that they were willing to repeat the procedure if needed, scoring their satisfaction with the results as "excellent."

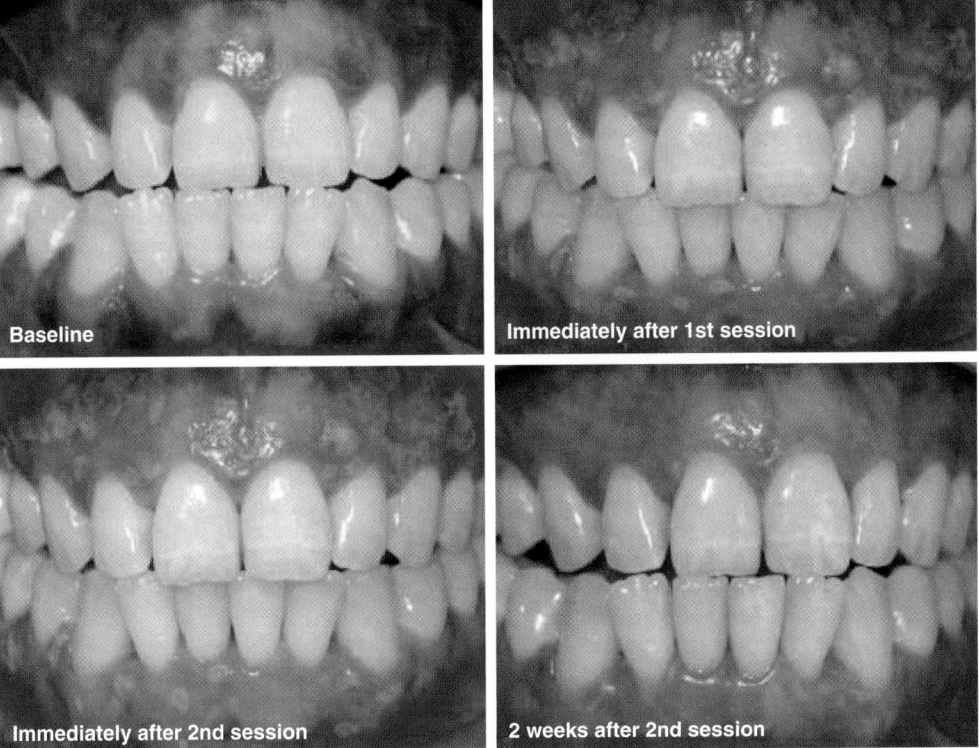

Baseline

Immediately after 1st session

Immediately after 2nd session

2 weeks after 2nd session

Fig. 37.2 Clinical view of a case before and after the procedure.

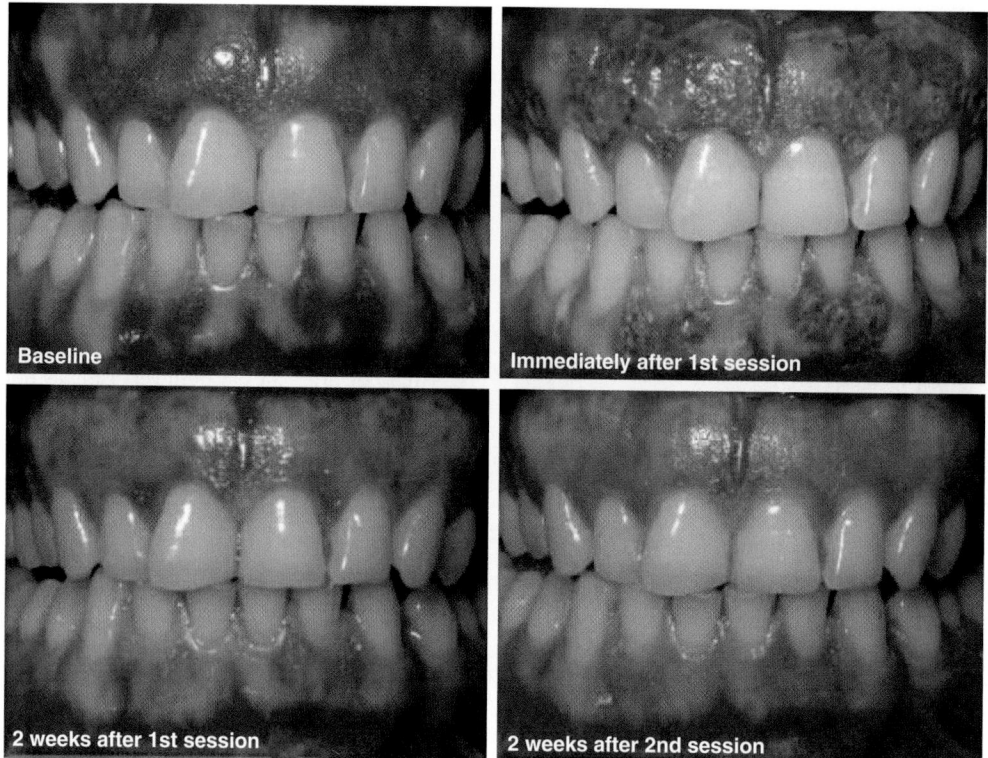

Fig. 37.3   Total removal of heavily pigmented lesions with two radiofrequency sessions over a 4-week period.

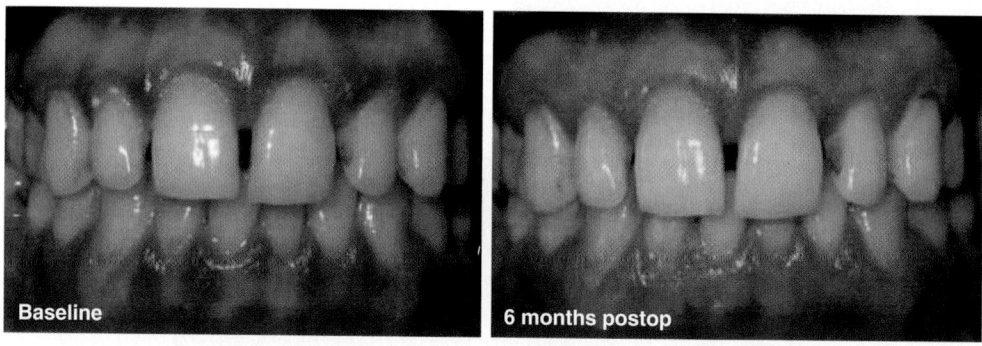

Fig. 37.4   Clinical view of a case before and 6 months after radiofrequency depigmentation treatment.

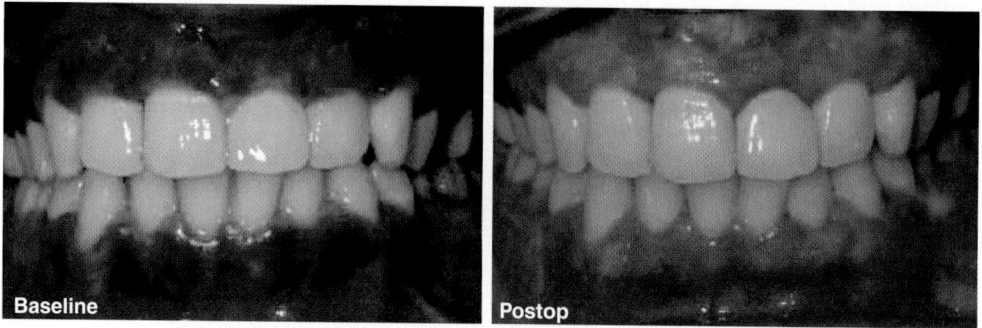

Fig. 37.5   Aesthetic results achieved after crown lengthening (gingivectomy) and depigmentation with radiofrequency surgery.

RECOMMENDED READING

Arikan F, Gürkan A. Cryosurgical treatment of gingival melanin pigmentation with tetrafluoroethane. *Oral Surg Oral Med Oral Pathol Oral Radiol Endod*. 2007;103:452–457.

Axéll T, Hedin CA. Epidemiologic study of excessive oral melanin pigmentation with special reference to the influence of tobacco habits. *Scand J Dent Res*. 1982;90:434–442.

Basha MI, Hegde RV, Sumanth S, Sayyed S, Tiwari A, Muglikar S. Comparison of Nd:YAG Laser and Surgical Stripping for Treatment of Gingival Hyperpigmentation: a clinical trial. *Photomed Laser Surg*. 2015;33(8):424–436.

Hedin CA. Smokers' melanosis: occurrence and localization in the attached gingiva. *Arch Dermatol*. 1977;113:1533–1538.

Kauzman A, Pavone M, Blanas N, Bradley G. Pigmented lesions of the oral cavity: review, differential diagnosis, and case presentations. *J Can Dent Assoc*. 2004;70:682–683.

Kishore A, Kathariya R, Deshmukh V, Vaze S, Khalia N, Dandgaval R. Effectiveness of Er:YAG and CO2 lasers in the management of gingival melanin hyperpigmentation. *Oral Health Dent Manag*. 2014;13(2):486–491.

Lin YH, Tu YK, Lu CT, Chung WC, Huang CF, Huang MS, et al. Systematic review of treatment modalities for gingival depigmentation: a random-effects poisson regression analysis. *J Esthet Restor Dent*. 2014;26(3):162–178.

Sherman JA. *Oral Radiosurgery: An Illustrated Clinical Guide*. 3rd ed. Basingstoke, UK: Taylor & Francis; 2005.

Yadav R, Deo V, Kumar P, Heda A. Influence of environmental tobacco smoke on gingival pigmentation in schoolchildren. *Oral Health Prev Dent*. 2015;13(5):407–410.

CHAPTER 38

LASERS AND PULSED-LIGHT DEVICES: HAIR REMOVAL

Barry Auster • Gary Page

Photoepilation (laser hair removal) is one of a variety of methods for the removal of unwanted hair. Others include electroepilation, mechanical epilation, depilatories, and waxing. Laser hair removal has rapidly evolved over the past 20 years and there are now numerous laser or intense pulsed-light (IPL) devices available for hair removal that are approved by the U.S. Food and Drug Administration (FDA). The current technologies evolved from the clinical observation of hair reduction in laser-treated congenital (pigmented) hairy nevi. The potential market for laser hair removal is tremendous.

PRINCIPLES FOR PHOTOEPILATION WITH LASERS

Light energy emitted from a monochromatic laser (a single wavelength of light) or an IPL source (which produces a broad spectrum of light using filters to block unwanted wavelengths) is absorbed by a pigmented object (in this case, hair) and is converted into heat energy. This heat energy destroys the hair follicle, causing a long-term reduction in hair growth. This process of transforming light to heat energy and destroying targeted pigmented tissue is called *selective photothermolysis*.

The concept of selective photothermolysis was first presented by Anderson and Parrish in 1983. Using this process, based on two important concepts, thermal damage is confined to the particular target tissue. The first concept is that *chromophores* (e.g., hair, blood vessels, melanosomes/pigment) are objects that preferentially absorb light of specific wavelengths (Fig. 38.1). The second concept is the *thermal relaxation time* (TRT), which is defined as the time required for an object to cool to 50% of the temperature resulting from laser exposure. When the target tissue absorbs the laser light, energy is changed to heat, which causes thermal tissue damage and heat transference to the surrounding tissues. For lasers, *pulse width* is the duration (in milliseconds [msec]) that the light energy is applied. A laser with a pulse width less than the TRT of the target conducts very little heat to the surrounding tissues. Consequently it is possible to confine the laser's destructive effect to a specific area of tissue based on the chromophore content and the rapidity with which the light energy is applied (Fig. 38.2).

Lasers are *monochromatic*, which means that the light is of a single wavelength or color. Each type of laser has a different wavelength and each chromophore absorbs the specific light energy in that laser wavelength, converting it to thermal energy. Melanin is the target chromophore for photoepilation. Hemoglobin, another chromophore, is targeted to destroy vascular lesions. Water and collagen are also chromophores. Each chromophore has a spectral absorption pattern that determines the wavelengths of light that are most absorbed and converted to thermal energy. It is important to match the wavelength of the laser with the specific chromophore to target destruction while avoiding damage to adjacent tissues. *The amount of energy needed to destroy the hair follicle is usually close to the energy level at which skin damage occurs. Determining the treatment energy level for a particular patient without causing excessive surrounding tissue damage is the most clinically demanding task for this procedure.* Certain types of lasers or devices are then chosen because they are more effective at destroying hair follicles without causing excessive surrounding damage, which could lead to burns or scarring.

The lasers used for epilation fall into four categories: alexandrite (755 nm), neodymium-doped yttrium aluminum garnet (Nd:YAG; 1064 nm), ruby (694 nm), and diode (810 nm). Ruby lasers were the first to be used for hair removal. However, lasers with this wavelength and short device pulse widths cause very high melanin absorption with a higher risk of complications; therefore they are generally no longer used.

Treatment tips or spot sizes vary from 2 to 15 mm, and pulse widths vary from 10 to 100 msec. In addition, the repetition rate can vary from 1 to 10 or more pulses per second (hertz). Faster repetition rates improve efficiency in treating larger areas, such as the back or legs. The size of the area being affected by each burst of energy (spot size) is variable from machine to machine and from laser tip to laser tip. In general, the larger the spot size, the greater the depth of light penetration at the same energy level. Lasers and IPL machines most often measure the energy level delivered to the skin in joules per square centimeter (J/cm^2), also known as *fluence* (Fig. 38.3A).

IPL (Fig. 38.3B–C) devices are flash-lamp devices that emit light over the entire visual spectrum and hence are not monochromatic, like lasers. Specificity for different hair colors and skin types may be achieved with various cutoff filters and fluence settings. IPL devices have increased in popularity over the years because of their versatility and cost effectiveness. With one device and multiple handpieces/filters, clinicians can treat most conditions. With regard to photoepilation, IPL devices are now as effective as lasers. In addition, a hybrid device (Syneron Candela) uses a combination of IPL followed by radiofrequency. It is based on the principle of electrical impedance, whereby electrical energy flows preferentially to a warmer target. This device reportedly has some beneficial effects for gray and white hairs. One disadvantage of this technique is that radiofrequency tends to be a more painful method of delivering energy to the skin.

The ideal patient for photoepilation is someone with light skin and dark hair, so that all the generated thermal energy is focused on the melanin chromophore of the hair. Light hair is very difficult to treat because it is not differentiated from the surrounding light skin. Similarly, it is very difficult in most instances to treat black hair on black skin. When patients are tanned, care must be taken lest the skin itself be burned during the treatments.

Cooling during treatment is important. IPL devices contact the skin and use a combination of a chilled gel and a chilled sapphire tip. The latter is a vast improvement over glass tips, which frequently cracked from the stress of temperature changes. Some devices (e.g., Light-Sheer Diode Laser; Lumenis) use a cold-water chamber to cool tissue.

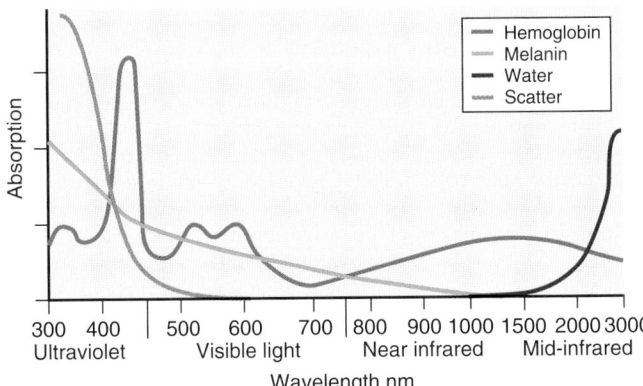

Fig. 38.1 Relative absorption of light by biologic tissues. By selecting specific wavelengths of light, a selective effect on biologic tissue is achieved. Whenever light hits tissue, it can be transmitted, scattered, reflected, or absorbed, depending on the type of tissue and the selected wavelength(s) (color) of the light. However, light absorption and subsequent tissue heating must take place to achieve any biologic effect, and a given wavelength of light may be strongly absorbed by one type of tissue and be transmitted or scattered by another. Different tissues have different absorption characteristics depending on their specific components (i.e., skin is composed of cells, hair follicles, pigment, blood vessels, sweat glands). The main absorbing targets, or chromophores, of tissues are (1) hemoglobin in blood; (2) melanin in skin, hair, and moles; and (3) water (present in all biologic tissue).

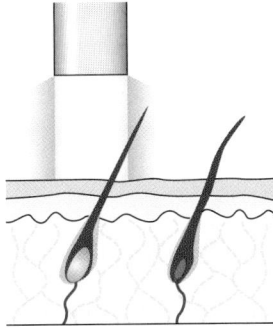

Fig. 38.2 The three principles of selective photothermolysis should be applied to damage target tissue. (1) Penetrating wavelength of light should be absorbed selectively by target tissue; (2) pulse duration should match thermal relaxation time of target tissue; and (3) sufficient fluence (J/cm²) should be used. (Modified from Brian Zelicksen, MD.)

Dynamic cooling devices use a chlorofluorocarbon, a refrigerant spray approved by the U.S. Environmental Protection Agency. This is available only on lasers produced by Candela, which has proprietary rights to the technology. A final alternative chilling method is using cold air blown on the site being treated (Zimmer MedizinSystems Corp.).

The FDA has also approved home-use laser devices for hair removal. Limited evidence suggests that some of these devices may have modest results. The technology, specifications, ease of use, maintenance, and price can differ greatly between different devices.

HAIR GROWTH PHASES AND TREATMENT IMPLICATIONS

Hair follicles have been difficult to treat with lasers. There is a wide variation in depth at different anatomic sites, with the deepest follicular bulbs at 5 mm. This is beyond the range of penetration of most lasers (Figs. 38.4 and 38.5). Whereas upper lip hair follicles range from 1 to 2.5 mm in depth, pubic and axillary hairs may lie as deep as 5 mm. In addition, most authorities agree that *only the anagen phase* of follicular growth is responsive to laser-induced thermal energy damage. The

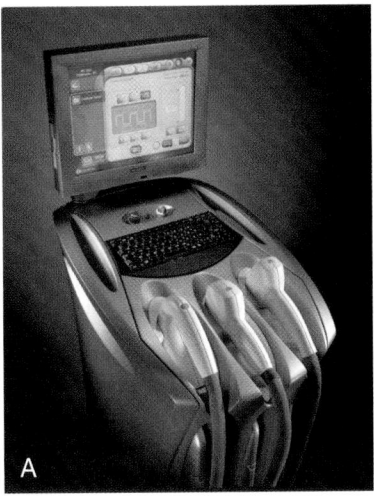

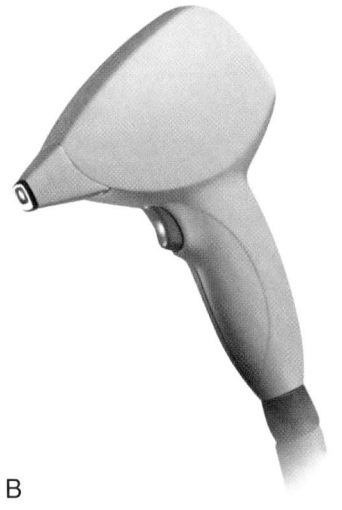

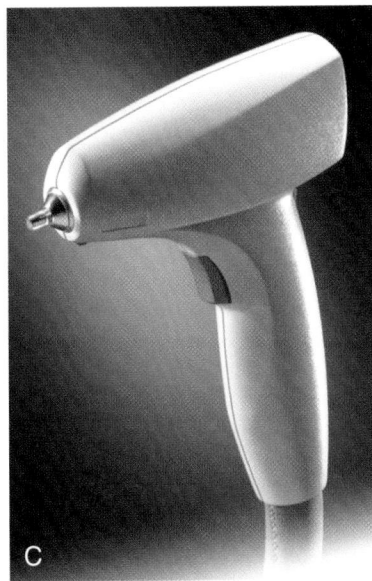

Fig. 38.3 Intense pulsed-light and laser system. (A) Lumenis One. (B) LightSheer handpiece. (C) Multi-Spot Nd:YAG handpiece. (Courtesy Lumenis, Santa Jose, California.)

percentage of follicles in the anagen phase at any one anatomic site varies from 30% on the trunk to as high as 80% on the scalp. Therefore, to understand laser hair removal more fully, a knowledge of the anatomy and development of hair is necessary.

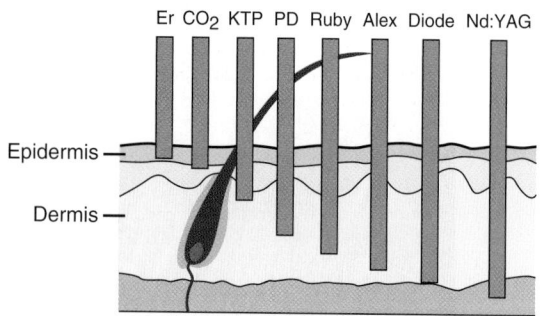

Fig. 38.4 Depth of penetration of various cutaneous lasers. *Alex,* Alexandrite; *Er,* erbium; *KTP,* potassium titanyl phosphate; *PD,* pulsed dye.

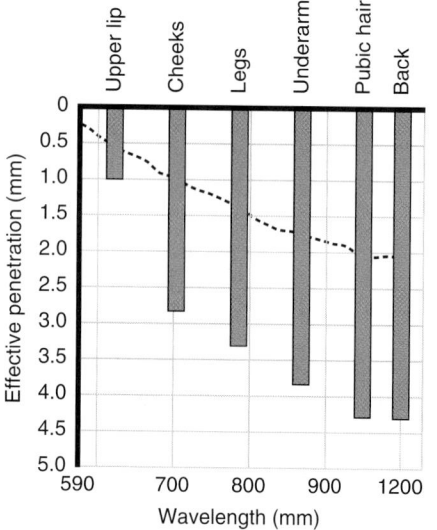

Fig. 38.5 Depth of hair follicles in different body locations. *Dotted line* indicates penetration depth of light frequency.

Hair is composed of keratinous fibers that grow from follicles over the entire body surface except the palms and soles. The number of follicles is finite at birth. Growth involves three stages (Fig. 38.6). *Anagen* is the active growth phase of the hair follicle, during which the hair contains abundant melanin. *Catagen* is a period of regression, when cell division terminates in the long part of the follicle and the lower part of the follicle begins to involute. The final, resting phase is called *telogen,* during which the old hair is emitted and shed before the development of a new hair begins. During telogen there is very little or no melanin in the follicle and hence laser treatments will have very little to no effect. The length of these three individual phases of hair growth varies widely with anatomic site (Table 38.1). Because of this, patients must be advised that 100% hair reduction may be impossible because of the relative unresponsiveness of the telogen follicle to laser photoepilation. Hairs, particularly on the trunk, may remain in telogen for longer than 3 months. Therefore patients must be advised that follow-up treatments may be needed up to 1 year after initiation of therapy to allow for the conversion of telogen hairs to anagen.

Hairs are of two types: *terminal hairs,* which are thick, long, and pigmented with melanin and found throughout the body surface, and *vellus hairs,* which are thin, short, and depigmented.

Fig. 38.6 demonstrates the structure and life cycle of a typical hair. The hair itself grows from the bulb, which consists of the hair matrix and dermal papilla. The *papilla* is an area of highly vascularized connective tissue that provides the nutrients for the rapidly dividing cells of the matrix. During periods of active growth, matrix cells divide every 24 to 72 hours and migrate upward to become keratinized and packed into layers that compose the hair shaft.

The "bulge," which is a protrusion near the attachment of the arrector pili muscle, has recently been determined to consist of stem cells important in hair regeneration. The bulge is generally located 1 to 1.5 mm below the cutaneous surface. As mentioned previously, hairs grow in recurrent cycles (see Table 38.1). Therefore the target of laser thermolysis is twofold: the bulge and the papilla.

FITZPATRICK SKIN TYPES AND TREATMENT IMPLICATIONS

As the thermolytic hair removal technique has developed, it has become clear that proper patient selection is critical for success. The

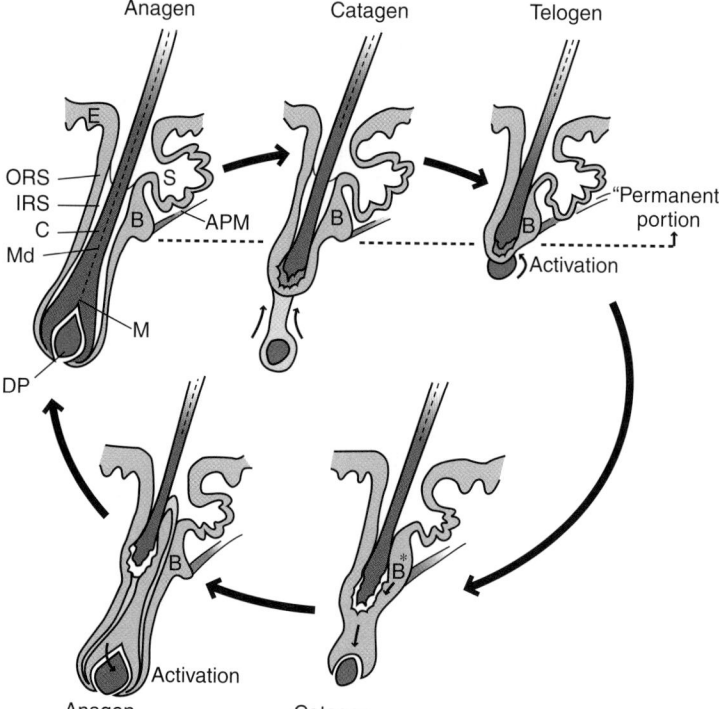

Fig. 38.6 Different phases of the hair cycle: anagen, catagen, and telogen. Labeled structures include arrector pili muscle *(APM),* bulge *(B),* cortex *(C),* dermal papilla *(DP),* epidermis *(E),* inner root sheath *(IRS),* matrix *(M),* medulla *(Md),* outer root sheath *(ORS),* and sebaceous gland *(S).* B and B* denote quiescent and activated bulge cells, respectively. Follicular structures above the *dotted line* form the permanent portion of the follicle; keratinocytes below the bulge degenerate during catagen and telogen. (Modified from Cotsarelis G, Sun TT, Lavker RM. Label-retaining cells reside in the bulge area of pilosebaceous unit: implications for follicular stem cells, hair cycle, and skin carcinogenesis. *Cell.* 1990;61:1329–1337.)

TABLE 38.1 Hair Depth and Hair Cycle

Body Area	Telogen Hair (%)	Anagen Hair (%)	Telogen Duration	Follicles Density (1/cm²)	Follicle Depth (mm)
Scalp	13	85	3–4 mo	350	3–5
Beard	30	70	10 wk	500	2–4
Upper lip	35	65	6 wk	500	1–2.5
Axillae	70	30	3 mo	65	3.5–4.5
Trunk	70	30	12 wk	70	2–4.5
Pubic area	70	30	12 wk	70	3.5–4.5
Arms	80	20	18 wk	80	2.5–4
Legs and thighs	80	20	24 wk	60	2.5–4
Breasts	70	30	12 wk	65	3–4.5

two preeminent factors in patient selection are skin type and hair color (Fig. 38.7). Skin types are based on the Fitzpatrick classification system:

Type I Always burns, never tans
Type II Always burns, sometimes tans
Type III Sometimes burns, always tans
Type IV Rarely burns, always tans
Type V Moderately pigmented
Type VI Black skin

Fitzpatrick grouped patients into the six different skin types based on the amount of pigmentation found in the skin. Skin type I has the least pigment and type VI has the most. The lower skin types are most sensitive to ultraviolet (UV) radiation ("sunburn") and to the development of solar damage such as pigmentation, skin thinning, actinic changes, and skin cancer. More freckles are also found in skin types I and II and fewer in type III and above. The higher the skin type, the more melanin is present in the epidermis and the more resistant the skin is to sunburn. Hair removal treatment is easier in patients who are most sensitive to UV radiation because they have less melanin in their skin to absorb the therapeutic light. More light energy passes through to the hair follicle itself and there is less risk of photothermal damage to the skin.

In general, skin types I and II are most easily treated. Types III, IV, and V are more difficult to treat. Skin type VI may be treated only in rare circumstances. Because of increased epidermal melanin, there is a higher risk of thermal damage to the skin in types V and VI, which may cause scarring or pigmentary alterations such as hypopigmentation or postinflammatory hyperpigmentation. Only a few devices (Nd:YAG and diode lasers) have received FDA approval to treat type VI skin. Extreme care must be taken in treating type V and VI skin types, particularly if the hairs are fine or light. Permanent depigmentation may occur if such patients are overtreated.

INDICATIONS

- Hypertrichosis
- Hirsutism
- Cosmetic reasons (e.g., bikini lines)
- Pseudofolliculitis barbae and pubis

Hypertrichosis, or excessive vellus or lanugo hair, may be localized or generalized and may occur in both men and women. It is not related to excess testosterone.

Hirsutism involves the development of coarse terminal hair (e.g., on the face) in children or women resulting from increased levels of male hormone. In women, the most common clinical causes are congenital adrenal hyperplasia and polycystic ovaries. If a woman has symptoms of these disorders (e.g., irregular menses, infertility,

obesity, acne), appropriate laboratory testing should be performed. These tests should be carried out under fasting conditions and should include insulin level, glucose, luteinizing hormone, follicle-stimulating hormone, prolactin, dehydroepiandrosterone (DHEA), and free testosterone. If a woman does demonstrate androgen excess, either treatment or referral to an endocrinologist will be appropriate. Spironolactone, a competitive inhibitor of DHEA binding, may be used supplementally; it is also effective in women with hypertrichosis without androgen excess.

Pseudofolliculitis barbae and pubis resulting from ingrown hairs is improved dramatically by photoepilation. When the number of hairs is reduced, the severe infection may be significantly diminished and the patient's symptoms markedly improved. Although there may be some pigmentary changes, they may improve over time and the risks may be outweighed by the benefit to the patient's quality of life. Unwanted permanent hair loss may also occur because of treatment.

CONTRAINDICATIONS

Absolute

- History of keloids
- Isotretinoin (Accutane) use in past 6 months

Relative

- Herpes simplex (use antiviral drugs if there is a history; start the day before and continue for 5 days afterward)
- Active infection in the area, such as cellulitis or pustular acne
- Dermatoses such as vitiligo or active psoriasis or eczema in the treatment area
- Photosensitizing medications (e.g., St. John's wort, tetracycline, thiazides)
- Recent plucking, waxing, electrolysis or use of a depilatory cream or bleaching product in last two weeks
- Bleeding disorder (e.g., thrombocytopenia or anticoagulant use)
- Pregnancy or breastfeeding (general precautions; no adverse effects are known)
- Body dysmorphic disorder
- White hair
- Seizures
- Uncontrolled systemic condition
- Photosensitization disorder (e.g., systemic lupus erythematosus)
- Cardiac pacemaker
- Deep chemical peel, dermabrasion or radiation therapy in the area in the last 6 months
- Skin atrophy (chronic oral steroid use or genetic syndromes such as Ehlers-Danlos syndrome)
- Self-tanning product used in last 2 weeks
- Recently tanned skin (relative, because the degree of tan is important and only a change in the parameters for treatment may be required; patients with a tan should know that treatments must be more conservative and therefore may not show the optimal benefit)

Individuals with a history of herpes simplex should be treated prophylactically with antiviral drugs before and during treatment. Individuals who have been on isotretinoin within 6 months tend to have adverse healing and susceptibility to hypertrophic scarring. In addition, patients on photosensitizing medications or supplements may be treated, but treatment settings should be conservative. Because the hair itself is the major chromophore for the laser, patients should be advised to avoid waxing, electrolysis, plucking, depilatories, or shaving immediately before treatment because the resulting inflammatory process generally involves more pigmentary changes, which will absorb the light energy. In female patients who have plucked hair on a daily basis, this last requirement may pose a problem because an effective treatment requires approximately 1 mm of hair protruding above the skin surface. Between treatments,

Skin Typing

For successful hair removal, it is necessary to determine the correct typing of your skin. Your doctor will consider your skin type when planning your treatment program.

Skin type is categorized by the Fitzpatrick skin type scale, which ranges from Type I (fair) to Type VI (black). The main factors that influence skin type are genetic disposition and reaction to sun exposure and tanning habits.

Skin type is determined genetically and is one of the many aspects of overall appearance. Genetics also determines the eye color, hair color, and the way skin pigments react to light. The way your skin reacts to sun exposure is important in correctly assessing your skin type. Sunbathing or artificial tanning (e.g., tanning creams) affects the evaluation of your skin color.

Please take a few minutes and fill out this questionnaire to help us determine your skin type and treat you properly.

Genetic Disposition

	0	1	2	3	4	Score
What color are your eyes?	Light blue, gray, green	Blue, gray, green	Blue	Dark brown	Brownish black	
What is the natural color of your hair?	Sandy red	Blonde	Chestnut/dark blonde	Dark brown	Black	
What color is your skin (unexposed areas)?	Reddish	Very pale	Pale with beige tint	Light brown	Dark brown	
Do you have freckles on unexposed areas?	Many	Several	Few	Incidental	None	
					Genetic Disposition Total	

Reaction to Sun Exposure

	0	1	2	3	4	Score
What happens when you stay too long in the sun?	Painful redness, blistering, peeling	Blistering followed by peeling	Burns sometimes followed by peeling	Rare burns	Never had burns	
To what degree do you turn brown?	Hardly or not at all	Light tan	Reasonable tan	Tan very easy	Turn dark brown quickly	
Do you turn brown with several hours of sun exposure?	Never	Seldom	Sometimes	Often	Always	
How does your face react to the sun?	Very sensitive	Sensitive	Normal	Very resistant	Never had a problem	
					Reaction to Sun Exposure Total	

Fig. 38.7 Sample form to determine skin type. (Courtesy John L. Pfenninger, MD, The Medical Procedures Center, Midland, Michigan.)

Tanning Habits

	1	2	3	4	5	Score
When did you last expose your body to sun (or artificial sunlamp/tanning cream)?	More than 3 months ago	2–3 months ago	1–2 months ago	Less than a month ago	Less than 2 weeks ago	
Did you expose the area to be treated to the sun?	Never	Hardly ever	Sometimes	Often	Always	
					Tanning Habits Total	

Add up the total scores for each of the three sections for your Skin Type Score. This will give you a better evaluation of your skin type.

Summary

Genetic Disposition Total	
Reaction to Sun Exposure Total	
Tanning Habits Total	
Skin Type Score	

Your Fitzpatrick Skin Type

Skin Type Score	Fitzpatrick Skin Type
0–7	I
8–16	II
17–24	III
25–30	IV
Over 30	V–VI

Note: This questionnaire is intended as a guideline for skin typing. Final evaluation of skin type should be determined by your doctor.

Fig. 38.7,cont'd

patients are allowed to continue their own hair removal methods, with shaving being the preferred method.

SAFETY ISSUES

Clinicians who use lasers for hair removal should be acutely aware of the potential for ocular damage. All of the devices may cause blindness. The importance of eye protection for both the practitioner (or technician) and the patient is paramount and cannot be overstressed. Laser goggles should be labeled with the wavelength they block. For working around the orbit, metallic, totally occlusive goggles are preferred (Oculo-Plastik, Inc.); in some cases a corneal shield inserted under the lids is best. The laser or IPL handpiece must be carefully guarded, and those using it must ensure that it is pointed away from the eyes at all times. Some office practices designate one of the clinical personnel as the "laser safety officer" in charge of ensuring that eye protection is worn by all in the treatment rooms and that warning signs are posted outside the door when the laser is in operation. The warning sign should be taken down when the laser is not in use or it will soon be ignored.

FACTORS INFLUENCING TYPE OF EQUIPMENT USED

- Reliability
- Purchase price
- Technical support
- Training provided
- Cost of maintenance contract
- Space needed in office for storage
- Disposable materials cost
- Ease of operation
- Warranty period
- Length of time the particular company representative has been in the business

Purchasing a hair removal device is a challenging task. It is important to determine the reliability of the unit, the available warranty, and exchange and support contracts, including costs, because these units are mechanically complicated and do break down. The cost of a service contract should be considered part of the acquisition cost. Even more important is the educational support and training provided by the company for current and future staff members. All units involve a learning curve, and training seminars with on-site education on an ongoing basis are crucial for safety and efficacy of treatments. Appropriate technical support is also an important consideration, as are anticipated upgrades. Repairs must be guaranteed on a timely basis. Finally, it is prudent to have frank discussions and pose questions to other clinicians who currently use the equipment being considered and have experience with it.

EQUIPMENT

- 4- by 4-in gauze pads.
- Hair clippers.
- Alcohol to cleanse the skin.
- Cooling gel or Zimmer Chiller (depends on device used).
- Topical anesthetic. EMLA (eutectic mixture of local anesthetics) cream is preferable because of its vasoconstrictive

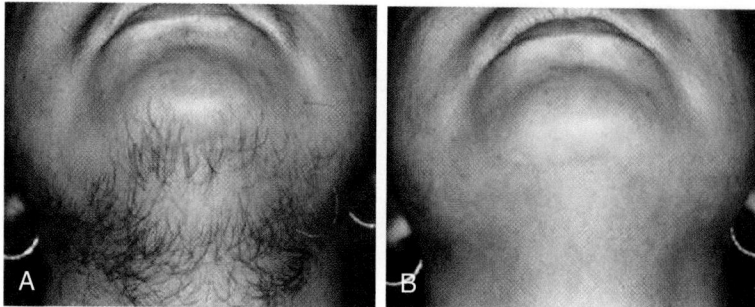

Fig. 38.8 Before (A) and after (B) laser treatment of the neck and face. (Courtesy Nimish Patel, MD, The Laser Center, Ahmedabad, India.)

effect, which reduces the competing chromophore of hemoglobin. Many offices use topical anesthetics prepared by specialty pharmacies that contain much higher concentrations of lidocaine. Many of these have not been tested for safety. Operators should be aware that these agents may be absorbed percutaneously, with resultant neurologic and cardiac effects. Several deaths have been reported from the topical overuse of these agents. Care should be taken to apply limited quantities and avoid occluding them if large areas are involved. (See Chapter 6, Local and Topical Anesthesia Complications, and Chapter 4, Topical Anesthesia.)

- Protective laser eyewear (goggles and metal eyepieces).
- Laser/IPL equipment.
- Cooling pack/ice for posttreatment care.
- Smoke evacuator or a room exhaust fan to remove the smell of burning hair.
- For offices that have not previously used lasers there are certain U.S. Occupational Safety and Health Administration (OSHA) requirements for the treatment room. There should be no mirrors, or any mirror present must be covered with paper. If the room is on the first floor, it should have no windows, or they should be covered with blackout shades. If the door to the room has a window, it should also be covered. The door also should have a sign on the outside that says "Laser in Use." Although uncommon, OSHA inspections may result in fines in the tens of thousands of dollars if infractions are discovered.

PREPROCEDURE PATIENT PREPARATION

The patient should fill out the aesthetics questionnaire form (see Chapter 35, Introduction to Aesthetic Medicine, Fig. 35.1) and be supplied with educational materials before the visit with the clinician (see patient education and consent forms available at www.expertconsult.com). The patient must not tan for 4 weeks prior and should not pluck any hair for at least 5 days prior.

It is extremely important to know the medical history, including use of medications and tanning history, and to determine Fitzpatrick skin type. The power settings for the full treatment are determined at this time and recorded. During the initial visit, many practitioners perform test patches with the settings that will be used. This is particularly important in types V and VI skin. For the darker skin types, adverse reactions such as edema and crusting may become evident up to 2 days after treatment. Some practitioners will treat the ideal patient (Fitzpatrick type I or II with dark brown or black hair) at this initial appointment but will observe the effect of the test spots on other skin types before initiating the full treatment.

A useful adjunct for patients who have a combination of coarse and fine hairs is topical eflornithine (Vaniqa; Allergan SkinMedica, Inc.). This product inhibits hair growth. It is useful for vellus hairs and does not affect the treatment of terminal hairs. It can be used to improve the overall appearance at completion of the treatment process and can be started immediately after the consultation session. However, hair growth tends to recur once the medication is stopped.

PROCEDURE AND TECHNIQUE OF HAIR REMOVAL

1. The patient's skin type is determined on the Fitzpatrick skin type scale (see Fig. 38.7).
2. Proper settings are selected (individualized with each unit). Each company will provide training with its particular unit. The settings are too variable to list individually here.
3. The hair is clipped to a 1-mm length.
4. The skin is wiped with alcohol.
5. Various topical anesthetics may be used before treatment.
6. The cooling gel is applied; most lasers and IPL devices have integrated cooling systems.
7. Eye protection is provided to the practitioner and the patient.
8. Photoepilation is performed.
9. The tissue reaction is observed and evaluated (see later discussion).
10. An ice pack or chilled aloe gel is applied.
11. Follow-up sessions are scheduled.

At the treatment session, hairs are clipped to a 1-mm length; if long hairs are left on the skin surface, there is a risk that they will act as a heat sink and singe the underlying epidermis. Protective goggles are placed on the patient, laser operator, and anyone else present in the room. Proximity of the spot treatments varies from one device to another, but in general they should either be abutted or slightly overlapped (10% to 20%). *Observation of clinical response during the treatment is essential.* If either obvious burning of the skin or no effect to hairs or follicles is noted, energy fluences should be adjusted accordingly. The ideal cutaneous response is discrete perifollicular erythema and edema without coalescence into solid erythema. Observe for shearing or fracture of about 20% to 30% of the hairs during the treatment session and note the sulfur-like smell of thermally damaged hair. Patients should be advised that additional hairs will fall out over the ensuing 2 to 3 weeks (Figs. 38.8 to 38.10).

COMPLICATIONS

- *Anesthesia complications*: Topical anesthetic creams may be used before treatment, but caution should be used because some deaths have been attributed to toxicity of anesthetics applied under occlusion over large areas.
- *Discomfort* associated with photoepilation is generally mild and transient and has been described as similar to a large rubber band snapping against the skin when the light pulse is triggered. *If the patient reports severe pain during the treatment, this should be considered as an indication of excessive energy with the potential for significant thermal injury.* Power should be immediately lowered and ice applied if the treated sites appear bright red or edematous.
- Ocular burns and blindness.
- Second-degree burns.
- *Hypopigmentation* is a difficult problem to treat, but it usually improves on its own over a period of months to years.
- *Postinflammatory hyperpigmentation* may be treated with prescription as well as over-the-counter bleaching creams, light chemical peeling, or even pigment-specific lasers. Over-the-counter

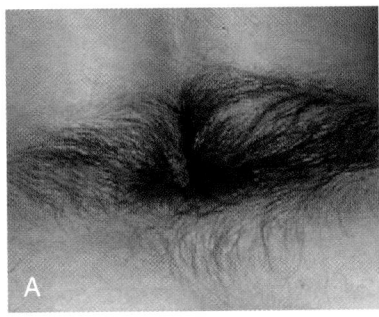

Fig. 38.9 Before (A) and after (B) laser treatment of the lower back. (Courtesy of Nimish Patel, MD, The Laser Center, Ahmedabad, India.)

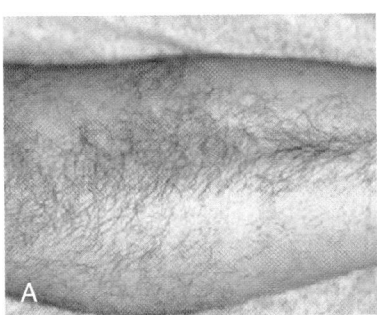
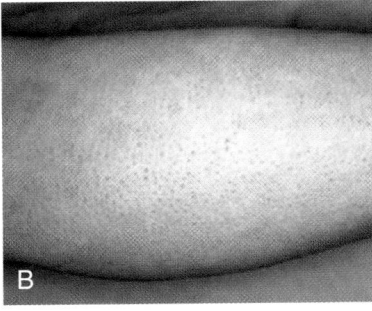

Fig. 38.10 Before (A) and after (B) laser treatment of the arm. (Courtesy of Valeria B. Campos, MD, Christine C. Dierickx, MD, and R. Rox Anderson, MD, Wellman Laboratories of Photomedicine, Harvard Medical School, Boston, Massachusetts.)

bleaching agents contain 2% hydroquinone and are modestly effective for this problem. Prescription agents containing 4% hydroquinone combined with tretinoin and fluocinolone (e.g., Tri-Luma Cream; Galderma Laboratories) are far more effective.

- *Scarring:* Hypertrophic scarring or keloids should be treated with currently acceptable modalities, which include intralesional steroid injections, silicone gel sheathing, and pulsed-dye laser treatments.
- Lack of satisfactory response with regrowth.
- *Stimulation of hair growth (rare):* This is a rare event but does occur more commonly in dark type III or IV skin types. This may be due to a biostimulatory rather than destructive effect. If it occurs, treatment with an alternative, longer-wavelength laser should be attempted.

POSTPROCEDURE PATIENT EDUCATION

The patient should be given the following instructions and advice:

- Do not pick at any skin peeling that may occur.
- Plucking of residual hair after treatment is acceptable.
- Soothing gel, lotion, or cool packs may provide comfort after treatment.
- Makeup can be applied after 2 hours.
- Erythema may last for several hours.
- Sunscreen (sun protection factor [SPF] ≥30) should be used between sessions.
- Multiple treatments will be required at all anatomic sites, but the number varies.
- Treatment intervals will be every 3 to 4 weeks or longer depending on the site for five to six treatment sessions, then every 3 months for a year.

Cool compresses can be applied for 2 to 3 hours after treatment but are usually not needed after this time. On occasion, patients experience blistering, which causes crusting. This usually does not occur until the following day. If it does occur, the patient can apply warm compresses and a topical antibiotic ointment. Future treatments will require that the settings be adjusted.

CONCLUSION

Photoepilation is a well-developed technology in the cosmetic medical field. Compared with electrolysis, treatments are more rapid, comfortable, and effective. The key to a successful laser hair removal practice is correct selection of patients for whom the treatment would be effective. Patients with dark skin types and light hair are poor candidates. Providing appropriate expectations for the patients before the onset of treatment is crucial. As our understanding and experience with this technology improve in the future, improved treatment responses as well as more acceptable home-use devices are likely to be seen.

CPT BILLING CODES

17380   Electrolysis, epilation, each half-hour

ICD-10-CM DIAGNOSTIC CODES

L68.0-L68.9   Hirsutism, hypertrichosis
L73.8   Pseudofolliculitis barbae
L73.9   Disease of hair and follicle, NOS

CHARGES

There is wide variation in the charges for photoepilation between practices and within a practice. Variables that determine pricing include local competition, cost of equipment, size of the area being treated, and the duration of the treatment. Larger treatment areas require more provider or technician time and cause more "wear and tear" on the equipment. Most hair removal is considered to be cosmetic; thus patients must pay out of pocket at the time of service. It is important that they understand this and sign an agreement beforehand stating that the fees are known to them.

SUPPLIERS

(See contact information available at www.expertconsult.com.)

Equipment

Candela Corp.
Cynosure, Inc. (now also owns Palomar Medical Technologies)
Lumenis, Inc.
Zimmer MedizinSystems, Inc.

Patient education materials

MJD Patient Communications

RECOMMENDED READING

Anderson RR, Parrish JA. Selective photothermolysis: precise microsurgery by selective absorption of pulsed radiation. *Science.* 1983;220:524–527.

Babilas P, Schreml S, Szeimies RM, Landthaler M. Intense pulsed light (IPL): a review. *Lasers Surg Med.* 2010;42:93–104.

Draelos ZD. Hair removal techniques. In: Merli GJ, ed. *The Clinics Atlas of Office Procedures: Basic Cosmetic Procedures.* Philadelphia: WB Saunders; 2000:142–149.

Eremia S, Li C, Newman N. Laser hair removal with alexandrite versus diode laser using four treatment sessions: 1-year results. *Dermatol Surg.* 2001;27:925–929.

Eremia S, Li CY, Umar SH, Newman N. Laser hair removal: long-term results with a 755 nm alexandrite laser. *Dermatol Surg.* 2001;27:920–924.

Hession MT, Markova A, Graber EM. A review of hand-held, home-use cosmetic laser and light devices. *Dermatol Surg.* 2015;41(3):307–320.

Hruza G, Avram M. *Procedures in Cosmetic Dermatology Series: Lasers and Lights.* 3rd ed. Philadelphia: Elsevier Saunders; 2012.

Goldberg DJ, Arndt KA. Is a medical degree necessary to perform laser and surgical procedures? *Dermatol Surg.* 2000;26:85–86.

Grossman MC, Dierickx C, Farinelli W, et al. Damage to hair follicles by normal-mode ruby laser pulses. *J Am Acad Dermatol.* 1996;35:889–894.

Orf RJ, Dierickx C. Laser hair removal. In: Kaminer MS, Arndt KA, Dover JS, Rohrer TE, Zachary CB, eds. *Atlas of Cosmetic Surgery.* 2nd ed. Philadelphia: Saunders; 2008.

Page GW. Is there a doctor in the spa? *Bodyworks.* 2006;12:10.

Ross EV, Cooke LM, Timko AL, et al. Treatment of pseudofolliculitis barbae in skin types IV, V, and VI with a long-pulsed neodymium:yttrium aluminum garnet laser. *J Am Acad Dermatol.* 2002;47:263–270.

Sadick NS, Shaoul J. Hair removal using a combination of conducted radiofrequency and optical energies: an 18-month follow up. *J Cosmet Laser Ther.* 2004;6:21–26.

Small R. Hair removal with lasers. In: Usatine RP, Pfenninger JL, Stulberg DL, Small R, eds. *Dermatologic and Cosmetic Procedures in Office Practice.* Philadelphia: Elsevier; 2012:309–326.

Sun TT, Cotsarelis G, Lavker RM. Hair follicular stem cells: the bulge-activation hypothesis. *J Invest Dermatol.* 1991;96(suppl 5):77S–78S.

Tanzi EL, Alster TS. Long-pulsed 1064nm Nd:YAG laser-assisted hair removal in all skin types. *Dermatol Surg.* 2004;30:13–17.

Tope WD, Hordinsky M. A hair's breadth closer [editorial]. *Arch Dermatol.* 1998;134:867.

Wagner RF, Tomich JM, Grande DJ. Electrolysis and thermolysis for permanent hair removal. *J Am Acad Dermatol.* 1985;12:441–449.

Willey A, Torrontegui J, Azpiazu J, Landa N. Hair stimulation following laser and intense pulsed light photo-epilation: review of 543 cases and ways to manage it. *Lasers Surg Med.* 2007;39:297–301.

CHAPTER 39

LASERS AND PULSED-LIGHT DEVICES: PHOTOFACIAL REJUVENATION

Renier van Aardt

In 1983, Anderson and Parrish described the concept of selective *photothermolysis*. Their article stated that the matching of a specific wavelength and pulse duration of light can obtain selected effects on a targeted tissue with minimal changes to surrounding structures.

This was a breakthrough in the application of light and laser technology for the purpose of skin rejuvenation. Patrick Bitter is credited for developing the treatment and for coining the word *photofacial*, referring to the cosmetic improvement of facial skin using nonablative light-based technology.

Lasers have a relatively short history in medical use. In 1964, the Nd:YAG (neodymium-doped yttrium-aluminum garnet) laser and CO_2 (carbon dioxide) laser were developed at Bell Laboratories. Researchers found that a CO_2 laser beam could cut tissue like a scalpel, but with minimal blood loss. The surgical uses of this laser were investigated extensively from 1967 to 1970 by pioneers such as Thomas Polanyi and Geza Jako. By the early 1970s, use of the CO_2 laser in ear/nose/throat and gynecologic surgery had become well established but was limited to academic and teaching hospitals.

The single most significant advance in the use of medical lasers was the concept of "pulsing" the laser beam, which allowed for the aforementioned selective photothermolysis. The first lasers to fully exploit this principle were the pulsed-dye lasers introduced in the late 1980s for the treatment of port wine stains and strawberry birthmarks in children. Soon afterward, the first Q-switched lasers were used for the treatment of tattoos.

Another major advance was the introduction of scanning devices in the early 1990s, enabling precision computerized control of laser beams. Scanned, pulsed lasers revolutionized the practice of plastic and cosmetic dermatologic surgery by making safe, consistent laser resurfacing possible.

In recent years the main focus of dermatologic laser research and development has been on laser hair removal, photo rejuvenation, and the treatment of vascular lesions, including leg veins, using lasers and intense pulsed light (IPL). The thrust of current research is directed toward *nonablative laser resurfacing* (e.g., laser skin toning, photofacial), *fractionated ablative resurfacing, plasma resurfacing,* and *improved photodynamic therapy* (for treatment of sun damage and skin cancer as well as for hair removal).

The treatment known as *photofacial rejuvenation* stems from the inherent human desire to be socially acceptable and to appear young and attractive. Social pressure demands a flawless skin; when obvious blemishes are present, the individual can suffer significant psychologic trauma. Patients seek treatments that will improve facial blemishes such as pigmented lesions, vascular lesions, scars, texture, rhytids, and tone without downtime and preferably without risk.

Skin deterioration is the result of a number of external and internal factors. The most common *external factor* is ultraviolet (UV) light from prolonged sun exposure as well as the popular use of tanning beds. The effects of UV light are cumulative over a person's lifetime and can result in telangiectases, matting, poikiloderma, broken capillaries, actinic keratoses, skin cancer, seborrheic keratoses, solar lentigines, progression of chloasma and melasma, textural deterioration, accelerated skin atrophy, redundant skin, and the formation of rhytids. These findings are more likely in patients with lighter skin types (Fitzpatrick types I, II, and III), who have less natural defense against UV light, resulting in more severe sun damage. Patients with sun-damaged skin are usually good candidates for IPL photo rejuvenation, although expectations should be realistic and focused on the improvement of chromophores (pigmented spots) rather than rhytids. Mild to moderate rhytids can be improved with fractional, plasma, and ablative technologies, as outlined in the next section.

Internal factors that cause the skin to lose its youthful appearance include acne, rosacea, chronic illness, endocrine diseases, skin diseases, drug abuse, smoking, and congenital skin lesions.

It is therefore essential for any person desiring attractive skin in later life to practice healthy lifestyle habits, including sun avoidance and regular use of topical sun protection products, not smoking, and consuming a healthy diet and ample water. The degree of improvement of lesions will vary depending on the origin and characteristics of the lesion and the chosen treatment modality and parameters.

TREATMENT OPTIONS

Photofacial treatment can be categorized into two main types: *ablative* and *nonablative*. Ablative treatment vaporizes tissue at very high temperatures, whereas nonablative treatment uses gentler heat that may denature protein in certain targets but is insufficient to vaporize tissue. Photofacial treatments can be subdivided further into those that need downtime to recover versus those that have little or no downtime. Nonablative technologies typically do not require significant downtime, whereas ablative treatment at a reasonable depth of treatment does. The exception is *fractional ablative therapy*, where tiny islands of tissue known as *microscopic treatment zones* (MTZs) are destroyed. The areas of normal tissue between the treated areas (Fig. 39.1) allow for a much more rapid healing time and needing little, if any, downtime. The treatment causes macroscopic erythema and edema that typically resolves within 24 to 72 hours. The success of both ablative and nonablative laser treatments still depends on the skill of the operator. Fig. 39.2 shows the pattern and depth of various treatments.

Ablative Laser

The two most commonly used ablative lasers are the CO_2 and the erbium lasers. The CO_2 laser was the first to be used for ablative skin resurfacing and tends to create coagulation and significant bulk heating of the skin; therefore it carries a higher risk of complications such as hypopigmentation and permanent scarring. In skilled hands it remains the most effective way to achieve the best results in skin rejuvenation. CO_2 lasers emit light in the near-infrared region at 10,600 nm. They target intracellular water, which heats cells instantly to more than 100°C, resulting in vaporization and removal of a surface layer of cells, coagulation necrosis of cells, denaturing of extracellular proteins in a subjacent residual layer, and nonfatal damage to cells in a still deeper zone. The entire epidermis and a variable thickness of dermis are removed, with a resultant smoother skin due to heat-induced shrinkage of deeper collagen. Patients must accept posttreatment edema, burning, and crusting and an average of 4.5 months of posttreatment erythema. Traditional ablative therapy carries the risk of pigmentary changes, acne flares, herpes simplex virus infection, scars, milia formation, and dermatitis.

Erbium (Er:YAG) lasers are solid-state lasers whose lasing medium is erbium-doped yttrium aluminum garnet (Er:Y$_3$Al$_5$O$_{12}$). The erbium laser has become a more popular resurfacing modality than the CO$_2$ laser because of its precision and lower degree of bulk heating. It also targets intracellular water at 2940 nm, but it is considerably less ablative than the CO$_2$ laser. The ablation is more superficial and wounds heal more quickly, but it is less effective at equal fluence and with a similar number of passes compared with the CO$_2$ laser. To achieve an effective thermal damage effect to improve solar elastosis and rhytids, a longer pulse duration is required when using the erbium laser. A combination of erbium and CO$_2$ lasers may be used as an alternative to the CO$_2$ laser alone.

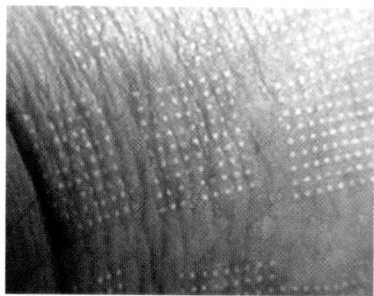

Fig. 39.1 Appearance of the skin after application of the fractional laser, showing the typical areas of ablation (*dots*) and the spared areas in between that allow a much more rapid healing time. The treatment causes macroscopic erythema and edema that typically resolve within 24 hours. The beneficial effects of collagen contraction and skin tightening may continue for 4 to 6 months.

Nonablative Laser

Nonablative lasers can be used to selectively injure the dermis or a target in the skin while protecting the epidermis by cooling during treatment, such as the Nd:YAG laser used for collagen remodeling of the dermis or the treatment of leg, truncal, and facial veins. Like ablative lasers, nonablative lasers emit coherent light at wavelengths absorbed by water. This approach has less predictable efficacy compared with ablative laser techniques.

Fractional Therapies

Fractional photothermolysis using the erbium laser has been developed to overcome the disadvantages of conventional ablative and nonablative laser therapies. It produces columns of thermal damage or ablation called *foci*, or MTZs, ranging between 50 and 150 μm in diameter and located at specific depths from 0 to 550 μm (Fig. 39.3). Treatment time for each pulse (exposure duration) ranges between 3 and 30 ms. The density of treatment corresponds to the inter-MTZ space and is adjustable. Because the MTZs are surrounded by uninjured tissue, keratinocytes have a shorter migration path and healing is much quicker (Fig. 39.4). The technique coagulates both the epidermis and dermis without affecting the stratum corneum, which acts as a natural bandage that protects the tiny wounds as they heal. To improve solar elastosis, scars, and rhytids, a course of treatments, typically three to five, is spaced at least 2 weeks apart. The treatments have fewer and less severe side effects than traditional, nonfractional ablative resurfacing and, with the exception of deep rhytids, the results in terms of skin tone, texture, dyschromia, and scars are essentially equivalent. More aggressive CO$_2$ laser fractional treatment vaporizes tiny columns of tissue entirely and may require fewer treatments than erbium devices, but it causes more downtime because of erythema and even crusting that can last a few days, with a possible higher incidence of postinflammatory hyperpigmentation. The ratio of risk to benefit always must be considered when choosing the appropriate device for the condition to be treated.

Fractional light therapy can be nonablative, using IPL or laser, or ablative with the CO$_2$ and erbium laser, with varying degrees of coagulation. Compared with a chemical peel, dermabrasion, or other forms of laser treatment, fractional laser allows the surgeon to customize the surgery more safely, not only to each patient but to each area of the face.

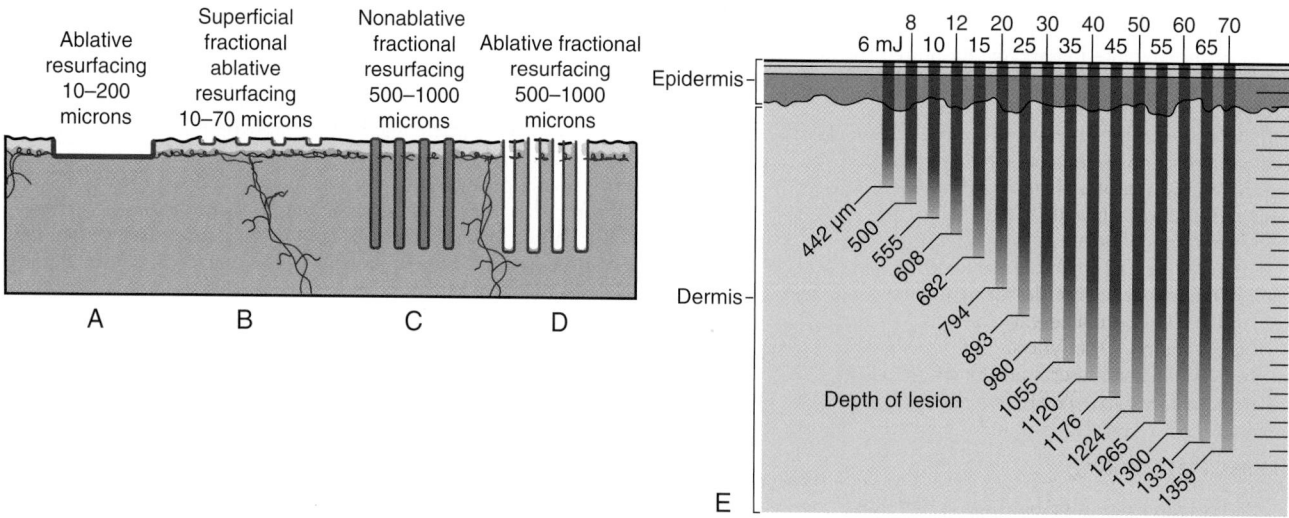

Fig. 39.2 Diagram illustrating the difference between ablative and fractional resurfacing. (A) Superficial layer of tissue is completely vaporized. (B) Columns of tissue have been vaporized, leaving areas of normal tissue in between, which speeds healing. (C) Nonablative fractional resurfacing, showing heated (injured) tissue that remains in the microchannels. (D) Ablative fractional treatment with the tissue in the microchannels vaporized. Ablative and nonablative fractional laser treatments can essentially penetrate to the same depth; however, ablative laser vaporizes tissue, whereas nonablative laser leaves a plug of necrotic debris. (E) Human skin and depth of penetration of the Fraxel laser with corresponding energy settings. (E, Courtesy Solta Valeant, Hayward, California.)

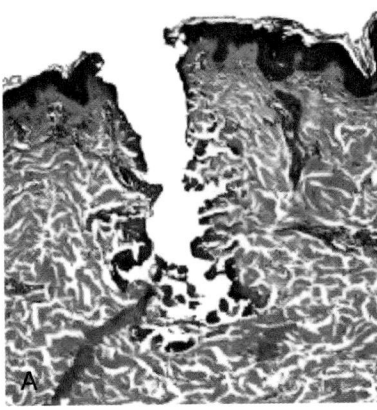 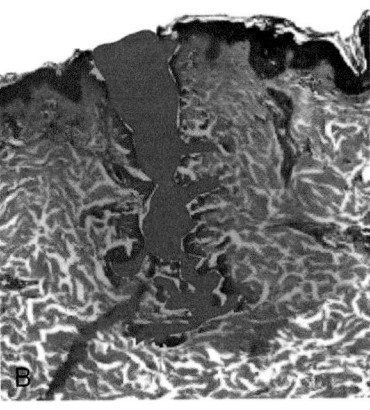

Fig. 39.3 (A) Immediately after ablative fractional laser treatment. Treatment depth up to 1500 μm. With fully ablated microchannels, necrotic tissue is completely vaporized, with the following results: (1) no residual heating, (2) more comfortable procedure, and (3) faster healing time. (B) Immediately after nonablative fractional laser treatment. Treatment depth up to 1500 μm. Necrotic debris stays in the tissue, with the following results: (1) wide, deep zone of thermal necrosis, (2) more painful procedure, and (3) longer recovery time.

Intense Pulsed Light

Intense pulsed-light technology has been increasingly competitive with lasers since the mid-1990s, and owing to enhanced engineering and favorable pricing versus many lasers, IPL devices have proliferated in the skin rejuvenation market. These devices are quickly gaining acceptance in medical offices and spas; although the technology was initially decried as "the poor man's laser" and dismissed as having too many side effects and too little efficacy, the newest generation of devices have proved so popular that even long-established companies are adding IPL to their product offerings.

IPL has both advantages and disadvantages compared with lasers. Lasers are useful because they permit exquisite control of where and how much one heats the skin. Lasers allow for smaller handpieces, whereas IPL treatment heads house the flash lamp, cooling apparatus, and high-voltage wires, resulting in a bulkier and heavier handpiece. Like lasers, IPL devices are becoming smaller, more efficient, more powerful, and less expensive. Lasers are more intricate than IPL and therefore more vulnerable to breakdown, resulting in higher purchase costs and more expensive maintenance. Because laser is collimated light, it is less eye-safe than IPL. Collimated light is light whose rays are nearly parallel; therefore they spread slowly as the light propagates. A laser beam delivers more focused energy to the target than IPL and hence is potentially more harmful to the retina. It is imperative, therefore, to use protective eyewear when operating or undergoing treatment with any light-based device.

Because the *three main chromophores* in skin (hemoglobin, water, and melanin) have broad absorption peaks, monochromacity is not a prerequisite for selective heating, making IPL an adequate substitution for or, in some instances, even preferable to lasers. When treating sun damage, the targets consist of brown pigmentation (solar lentigines), redness (enlarged capillaries), and water and collagen (textural deterioration). Wavelengths between 515 and 600 nm are optimally absorbed by oxyhemoglobin and melanin, making this spectrum ideal for selective photothermolysis in treating the typical patient with sun-damaged skin (i.e., pigmented areas and redness). IPL devices use flash lamps, computer-controlled power supplies, and bandpass filters to generate light pulses of prescribed duration, intensity, and spectral distribution (see Chapter 38,Fig. 38.1). Flash lamps are high-intensity gas-discharge lamps filled with xenon gas that produce bright light when an electrical current passes through the gas. Electrical energy stored in capacitor banks is converted into optical energy, pulsing the lamps and covering the entire spectrum of light between UV and infrared.

To ensure an even flow of energy, most modern IPL systems use partial-discharge technology. Mirrors surround the xenon flash lamp, and the lamp is cooled by water circulating around a quartz envelope, filtering out most of the harmful far-UV output of the lamp. The light output is directed toward the distal end of the handpiece, and a sapphire or quartz block couples the light output to the skin. The normal, unfiltered output of a xenon lamp is between 370 and 1800 nm.

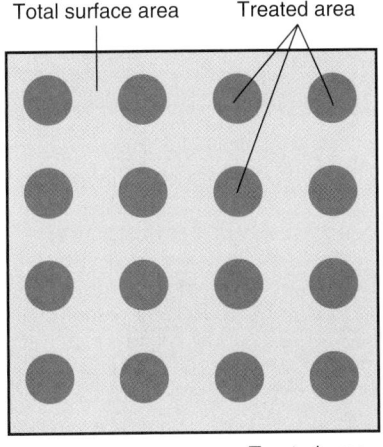

Total surface area   Treated area

Treatment coverage $= \dfrac{\text{Treated area}}{\text{Total surface area}}$

Fig. 39.4 Fractionated columns of light versus the traditional laser. With fractional applications, the treated areas are affected by focal columns of light, leaving "dots" of destroyed tissue within the total surface area. In traditional laser ablation, the entire surface area (i.e., the box) would be orange, denoting the affected/ablated area.

Photofacial resurfacing devices include the following:

- Matrix RF (radiofrequency device; Syneron Candela, Inc.)
- Erbium (Er:YAG) fractional lasers
  - Lux2940 (Palomar Cynosure Medical Technologies, Inc.)
  - Sciton Profractional (Sciton, Inc.; Fig. 39.5)
- CO_2 fractional lasers
  - Smartxide DOT (Deka Laser)
  - Fraxel repair (Solta Medical, Inc.)
  - Pixel CO_2 (Alma Lasers, Ltd.)
  - SmartSkin CO_2 (Cynosure, Inc.)
- Harmony^{XL} (pixel laser; multimodality skin rejuvenation; Alma Lasers, Ltd.; see Fig. 39.5)

Plasma Resurfacing

Skin resurfacing can also be accomplished with a plasma-based device (Rhytec Portrait PSR3; Rhytec, Inc.) instead of a laser, although its superiority to laser-based devices remains an open question. Nitrogen plasma energy is delivered to the skin to stimulate skin remodeling while creating a coagulated barrier from the skin's outer layers to mitigate infection. Studies are lacking to assess its efficacy compared with traditional devices.

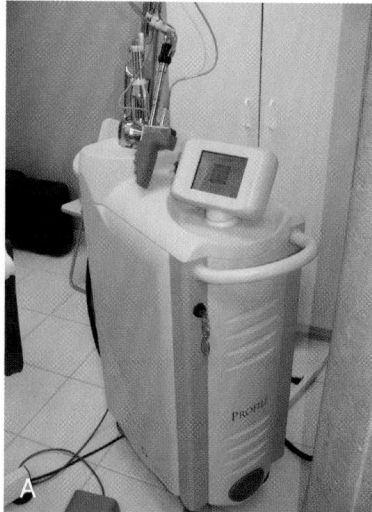
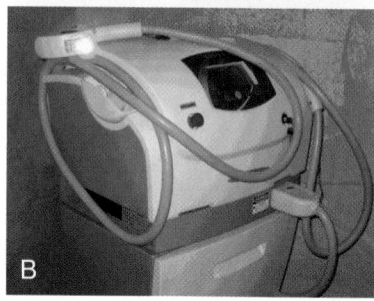

Fig. 39.5   (A) Sciton Profractional laser. (B) Alma Harmony intense pulsed-light device.

Most IPL devices use dichromic filters to transmit a desired range of wavelengths. In other words, they use filters to select the wavelength of light desired to treat the particular entity (e.g., pigment, vessels, collagen). By adjusting the fluence, number of pulses, pulse duration, and the cutoff filter, and considering the patient's particular skin type, various skin targets can be selectively heated to achieve the desired clinical outcome. Most IPL devices have different spot sizes to choose from, facilitating adequate treatment over small or large surface areas.

When using light-based therapy for type I photo rejuvenation (see later), photo rejuvenation is also sometimes known as a photo-facial treatment (Figs. 39.6 through 39.8). The majority of photo-facial treatments are performed with IPL devices, and IPL has become a popular treatment in clinician offices and spas.

INDICATIONS

Type I Photorejuvenation or Photofacial Treatments (Intense Pulsed Light and Fractional Laser)

- Mild to moderately photoaged skin
- Actinic lesions
- Angiomas, both spider and cherry
- Benign vascular lesions (telangiectases, flushing, symptoms of rosacea)
- Broken capillaries
- Chloasma
- Diffuse erythema and poikiloderma
- Dyschromia
- Erythema after laser resurfacing
- Pigmentary sun damage
- Melasma
- Mottled pigmentation
- Hyperpigmentation, including postinflammatory hyperpigmentation
- Rosacea

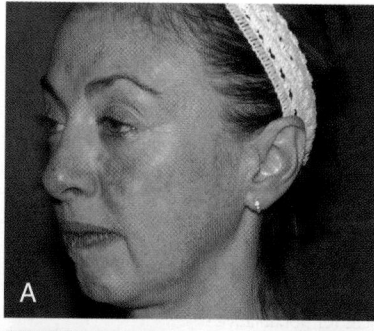
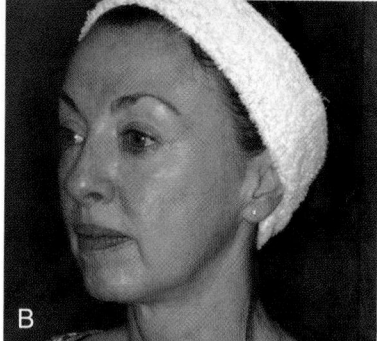

Fig. 39.6   Before (A) and 1 month after (B) a series of five intense pulsed-light treatments with the Vasculight (Lumenis). Improvements in erythema and pigmentation are noted.

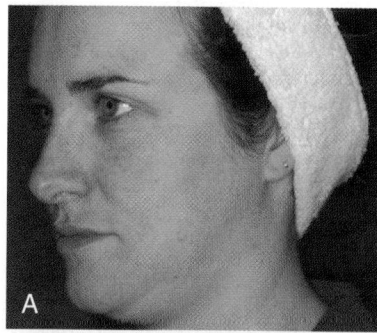
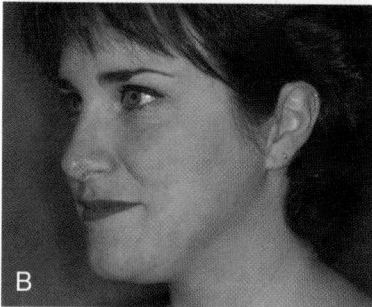

Fig. 39.7   Before (A) and 2 weeks after (B) a single intense pulsed-light treatment with the Vasculight (Lumenis), showing improvement in dyschromia.

- Solar lentigines
- Telangiectases

Skin texture and pore size may also improve from the stimulation of fibroblasts, resulting in collagen production and tightening. The final result of a series of photofacial treatments may be evident only a few months later, because skin remodeling is a gradual process. Collagen may continue to contract for up to 3 months after treatment.

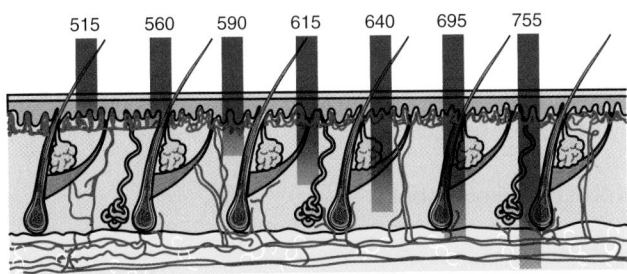

Fig. 39.8 Depth of penetration of various cutoff filters used in intense pulsed-light devices for nonablative selective photothermolysis. A wavelength of 515 to 590 nm targets melanin and vascular structures and is used mainly for skin rejuvenation; 640 to 695 nm is used mainly for hair removal; and 755 nm is used for skin tightening. Besides wavelength, fluence and spot size also determine the depth of penetration.

Type II Photorejuvenation (Fractional and Ablative Lasers)

- Dermal and epidermal structural changes
- Rhytids
- Elastotic changes
- Collagenous and connective tissue changes
- Large pores

Contraindications

- Patients with darker skin types, such as Fitzpatrick types V and VI, are naturally protected from most UV damage and are therefore less likely to need photo rejuvenation. As is turns out, they are also generally not good candidates for this procedure, with the possible exception of mild to moderate fractional laser resurfacing to address scars and melasma. They are also much more likely to suffer side effects from light-based treatments because of the high absorption of light by melanin. Practitioners should exercise particular caution because these patients are also more likely to develop keloid scars and hyperpigmentation or hypopigmentation if they sustain a burn wound from overly aggressive treatment.
- A generalized active inflammatory or infectious process of the skin.
- A history of herpes simplex without receiving antiviral prophylaxis (some procedures).
- Photosensitizing medications: If a patient is on Accutane, at least 6 months should pass after a course is completed before laser or IPL is used in order to avoid irreversible skin discoloration.
- Suntan: Patients should wait for a tan to fade before treatments commence to avoid burning the epidermis and risking hypopigmentation, which may take months or longer to heal.

Preprocedure Patient Education

See patient information and consent form available at www.expertconsult.com. In general, IPL treatments should be performed in a series of three to six treatments 2 to 4 weeks apart.

A medical history and clinical examination are required before treatments can commence. The skin should be carefully examined to rule out skin lesions such as actinic keratoses, basal cell carcinoma, squamous cell carcinoma, and melanoma; such lesions should be treated appropriately before beginning light-based therapies.

Technique

The patient is placed in a comfortable reclined or supine position; good ambient lighting is needed. The skin must be cleansed and all makeup and skin cream removed before the procedure. Eye protection must be supplied for the patient and can consist of snug fitting metal eye shields or disposable stick-on eye protectors specifically designed for IPL use. The technician must wear appropriate IPL eye protection, and the use of gloves is recommended. Most IPL devices require the application of cool or chilled clear ultrasound gel to provide a consistent light path and cooling to the skin. Devices that have handpieces with built-in cooling of the light guide require a thin layer of gel; if built-in cooling is absent, a thicker layer of cold gel serves to cool and protect the epidermis. Each manufacturer has specific recommendations for gel use and application related to its particular device design.

The spot size of IPL light guides varies, but the average size is about 2 × 0.75 inches, whereas laser spot sizes are usually smaller. The handpiece and light guide must be properly cleansed and disinfected between treatments with a medical-grade chemosterilant/high-level disinfectant such as hydrogen peroxide 7%. The starting fluence for the first treatment is generally modest and is usually increased with each consecutive treatment. It is good practice to perform two or three test pulses in the preauricular area and monitor the treated area for 2 minutes or more to ensure that the chosen energy level does not cause excessive redness, swelling, ecchymosis, or blistering. It should be sufficient to cause end-point pigment darkening and capillary contraction or color changes. Manufacturers will provide suggested treatment settings related to their particular device.

The face is treated in sections that typically consist of each cheek area, from preauricular to midface, with the midface consisting of the nose, upper lip, chin area, and forehead. Care must be taken not to pass over the vermillion of the lips and not to treat closer than 0.5 inch from the eyebrows and hairline. Because most IPL wavelengths have a strong affinity for melanin and may cause a permanent reduction in darker hair, patients must be made aware of this fact, especially men, who may not want their beard hair decreased by treatment.

It is important to note that the midface is more sensitive than other areas of the face; the patient should be informed of this and that despite the eye protection, they will see bright flashes of light that will not be harmful to their eyesight. Depending on the device, the parameters, and the protocol, one or more passes may be made of the face or certain areas using the same or different cutoff filters. When the treatment has been completed, the gel must be removed, the skin gently cleansed, and a soothing aloe-based gel or protective moisturizing cream applied. The treatments are repeated every 2 to 3 weeks, with a total of three to six treatments being typical. Herpes simplex prophylaxis should be prescribed when laser or IPL devices are used in treating the perioral region for patients with a past history of herpes simplex type 1 infection. Valacyclovir 2 g 1 hour before the procedure and 2 g 12 hours after the first dose is generally effective.

Maintenance IPL treatments can be performed every 3 to 4 months, choosing parameters based on any skin pigmentary changes in the interim. Other areas of the body can be treated, including the neck, décolleté area, arms, hands, back, and legs. The fee for the procedure is calculated by either area or the number of pulses used.

Postprocedure Patient Education

Patients must be instructed to avoid sun exposure and use a good-quality UV-A/UV-B broad-spectrum sunscreen (sun protection factor [SPF] 15 to 30) daily. If a patient has acquired a tan between treatments, any further treatments should be postponed until the tan has faded. Appropriate skin care is beneficial for patients undergoing a series of photofacial treatments. Exfoliation of the stratum corneum with microdermabrasion or gentle chemical peels can assist in removing surface pigmentation between IPL treatments, and using a daily moisturizer can treat dry skin caused by increased skin turnover after IPL treatment. Patients should also be made aware that maintenance treatments will be required every 3 to 4 months to avoid a gradual return to baseline. Patients should be educated regarding the dangers of UV light exposure and the value of continued use of a sunscreen, because this information will help them prolong the beneficial effects of their photofacial treatments.

Complications

Surface cooling of the skin is extremely important with IPL to avoid side effects such as burns, which can lead to pain, blisters, infection, scars, and hyperpigmentation, especially on darker skin types. Newer IPL devices have built-in contact cooling, allowing the light guide to be placed directly on the skin, thus achieving effective cooling and precisely duplicable results with each pulse. Other cooling methods include cold ultrasound gel, cold air devices, and cryogen spray.

Common Errors

- Single, aggressive treatments can yield impressive results, especially for superficial pigmentation; however, this approach is painful, the risk of short-term side effects is higher, and most patients desire a no-downtime treatment with an acceptable comfort level. Achieving a no-downtime treatment regimen requires starting treatments at a modest fluence and incrementally increasing the energy in subsequent treatments toward a target level.
- Care must be taken not to use too much pressure when treating capillaries because excessive pressure will result in blanching and the target will be lost and not effectively treated.
- Some IPL devices rely on the use of cold ultrasound gel to be placed on the skin for cooling and "drifting" the light guide in the gel just above the skin surface. Although the technique is effective, the skill and experience of the operator are important in achieving consistent results.

Adjunctive Treatments

5-Aminolevulinic Acid (Levulan)

An adjunctive treatment that complements IPL extremely well is the use of the photosensitizing agent 5-aminolevulinic acid (Levulan, DUSA Pharmaceuticals, Inc.) to broaden the overall benefits and improve the end results achieved with photofacial treatments. The treatment is known as *photodynamic therapy* (also see Chapter 51). 5-Aminolevulinic acid is approved for the treatment of actinic keratoses. It is also used in the treatment of nonmelanoma skin cancer and of systemic cancers. It is applied off-label with excellent results for the treatment of acne. Levulan is prepared by breaking chambers in a vial. It is then applied directly to skin that has been prepared with microdermabrasion or by acetone or alcohol scrub to break down the skin's lipid barrier. The material is allowed to be absorbed over time, which increases the effectiveness of light therapy. The interval between application and the start of IPL treatment is referred to as the *incubation time*.

When combined with IPL, short incubation times between 15 minutes and 1 hour can be used with good clinical response. Improved reduction of brown and red pigments, textural improvement, and shrinkage of pores can be expected with this approach. Patients must avoid any sunlight or bright indoor light exposure to the treated skin for 24 hours after treatment to minimize erythema and avoid burns. Some erythema, flaking, swelling, or peeling can be expected with 5-aminolevulinic acid treatment.

Retinoids

Topical retinoids (i.e., tretinoin and isotretinoin) are other adjunctive treatment options that have been shown to improve the outcome of IPL treatments. Patients should be motivated and prepared for possible erythema and dry, flaking skin with the use of topical retinoids. Patients should start using retinoids at least 2 weeks before commencing IPL, discontinue application 2 days before IPL, and resume use a day after treatment. Because retinoids are photosensitizing, increased flushing and some downtime may occur when they are used in conjunction with IPL to treat sun damage. For this reason, retinoids are reserved for more severe sun damage. Microdermabrasion is never employed with the use of retinoids because of increased skin fragility and should be considered only after the

retinoid has been discontinued for at least 1 month. Waxing should also be avoided when retinoids are being used. Retinoids alone have beneficial effects on sun-damaged skin, improving texture and dyschromia with consistent use, and may be used over the long term to reduce the frequency of maintenance IPL treatments.

Nonfacial Treatments

Other body areas can be treated with IPL with equal efficacy, including the neck, chest, arms, and legs. Fluence should be lowered in treating the neck and décolleté areas and always adapted to the particular skin area color. With years of sun damage, more exposed areas may have increased background melanin than less exposed areas and should be treated accordingly.

CONCLUSION

Photofacial treatments have become an accepted method of improving the appearance of the skin, especially photo-damaged and aging skin. Many modalities are available, and it is up to the practitioner to decide on the most appropriate treatment to address the patient's concerns. In some cases combination treatments may be required. The patient's expectations, budget, and clinical concerns must be considered when deciding on the appropriate treatment method. IPL has become the most common and popular treatment option for photo-damaged skin because of its good safety profile, minimal downtime, low cost, and excellent results.

When IPL is used for the appropriate candidate, results can be dramatic and very pleasing for the patient as well as rewarding for the practitioner. The technology has seen significant advances in recent years, overcoming many of the initial barriers and objections to its use to such an extent that in some cases it is now preferred over laser treatment. For the cosmetic dermatology practitioner, IPL is a modality that can be combined with other, traditional laser devices to satisfy the demands of patients and allow for a comprehensive armamentarium of light-based skin treatment devices to be available to address various skin concerns.

PATIENT EDUCATION GUIDES

See the patient information and consent forms available at www.expertconsult.com.

J CODE

J7308 5   Aminolevulinic acid (Levulan)

CPT/BILLING CODES

Insurance providers do not reimburse for cosmetic procedures. However, they will reimburse for some of the following treatments:

17106	Destruction of cutaneous vascular proliferative lesions (e.g., laser) <10 cm^2
17107	Destruction of cutaneous vascular proliferative lesions 10 to 50 cm^2
17108	Destruction of cutaneous vascular proliferative lesions >50 cm^2
17110	Destruction of benign lesions, up to 14
17111	Destruction of benign lesions, >14
96567	Photodynamic therapy by external application of light to destroy malignant and/or nonmalignant lesions of the skin and adjacent mucosa (e.g., lip) by activation of photosensitive drug(s), each phototherapy session

ICD-10-CM DIAGNOSTIC CODES

I78.1	Nevus Nonneoplasm
L57-L57.9	Skin changes nonionizing radiation
L71.0-L71.9	Rosacea
L91.0-L91.9	Hypertrophic disorders
L90.0-L90.9	Atrophic disorders
L82-L82.1	Seborrheic keratosis
L98.5	Mucinosis of skin
L70.0-L70.8	Acne
L81.0-L81.9	Pigmentation disorder

SUPPLIERS

(See contact information available at www.expertconsult.com.)

Selected IPL manufacturers

Alma Lasers, Ltd.
Cynosure, Inc.
Lumenis
Palomar Cynosure
Solta Medical
Sciton, Inc.
Syneron Candela, Inc.

AUTHOR'S NOTE: Many manufacturers produce IPL devices today, some of which are inexpensive and of low power, often purchased by spas and salons. High-quality equipment, supported by reputable clinical studies, ensures high-quality treatment, the best results, and high-quality support by the manufacturer. Proper research, discussion with peers, and attendance at national and international laser conferences, such as that of the American Society of Laser Medicine and Surgery, are strongly recommended before any purchase is made.

ONLINE RESOURCES

American Board of Laser Surgery: www.americanboardoflasersurgery.org.

RECOMMENDED READING

Alster TS, Tanzi EL, Welch EC. Photorejuvenation of a facial skin with topical 20% 5-aminolevulinic acid and intense pulsed light treatment: a split-face comparison study. *J Drugs Dermatol.* 2005;4:35–38.

Anderson RR, Parrish JA. Selective photothermolysis: precise microsurgery by selective absorption of pulsed radiation. *Science.* 1983;220:524–527.

Bjerring P, Christiansen K, Troilius A, Dierickx C. Facial photo rejuvenation using two different intense pulsed light wavelength bands. *Lasers Surg Med.* 2004;34:120–126.

Geronemus R. Fractional photothermolysis: current and future applications. *Lasers Surg Med.* 2006;38:169–176.

Goldman M. Clinical pearl: observations on the use of fractionated CO_2 laser resurfacing. *J Drugs Dermatol.* 2009;8:82–86.

Hruza G, Avram M. *Procedures in Cosmetic Dermatology Series: Lasers and Lights.* 3rd ed. Philadelphia: Elsevier; 2012.

Ross EV. Laser versus intense pulsed light: competing technologies in dermatology. *Lasers Surg Med.* 2006;38:261–272.

Saluja R, Khoury J, Detweiler S, Goldman M. Histologic and clinical response to varying density settings with a fractionality scanned carbon dioxide laser. *J Drugs Dermatol.* 2009;8:17–20.

Small R, Hoang D. Photorejuvenation with lasers. In: Usatine RP, Pfenninger JL, Stulberg DL, Small R, eds. *Dermatologic and Cosmetic Procedures in Office Practice.* Philadelphia: Elsevier; 2012:322–335.

Tan KL, Kurniawati C, Gold M. Low risk of postinflammatory hyperpigmentation in skin types 4 and 5 after treatment with fractional CO_2 laser device. *J Drugs Dermatol.* 2008;7:774–777.

Waibel J, Beer K. Ablative fractional laser resurfacing for the treatment of a third-degree burn. *J Drugs Dermatol.* 2009;8:294–297.

CHAPTER 40

LASERS AND PULSED-LIGHT DEVICES: ACNE

Renier van Aardt

Acne vulgaris is a common chronic disease affecting the pilosebaceous follicles of the face, neck, back, chest, and other areas of the body. It affects 50 million Americans annually. At least 50% of adults admit to having suffered with some degree of acne in their lifetime. In the past, people have treated it in many different ways, with everything from handfuls of vervain (a flowering herb) to bloodletting (India). Even arsenic and x-rays were used with little benefit and considerable risk because people were willing to try anything for even minor improvements. Given the prevalence and number of patients who suffer from refractory acne, alternatives to existing treatments are constantly sought. Acne vulgaris is a disease that not only causes physical blemishes but has major psychologic effects on its sufferers, including social withdrawal, clinical depression, and suicide. In recent years, the use of laser- and light-based devices has had a significant impact on the ability to manage acne.

CLINICAL APPEARANCE AND GRADING

Acne has been classified from grades 1 to 4, depending on its severity. Variations include minor blackheads and whiteheads and clogged pores (grade 1) that can become infected and inflamed (grade 2), leading to large red papules and pustules (grade 3) and cysts and nodules (grade 4). Lesions are often "popped" or picked by the patient. With the larger lesions, scarring is often the result. The usual type of depressed scarring can last throughout a person's life and can become an extremely noticeable facial imperfection. Scars can be erythematous, irregular, textured lesions; enlarged pores; or deep "icepick" and cratered lesions. Treatment is primarily directed at reducing inflammation and preventing scars. However, light-based technologies also make scar reduction and skin remodeling possible, thus improving the patient's appearance.

Internal Causes

There are many contributing factors to the severity of acne, but no clear single cause has been identified. Acne develops as the patient progresses through puberty and the sebaceous glands grow and secrete more sebum. Acne is more prevalent and severe in males because of the increased production of *testosterone* during puberty. Adult-onset acne in women may be attributed to cyclic variations in sex hormones, with an increase in androgenic hormone levels resulting in an increase in sebum production. This increase in sebum, coupled with the keratinization of the hair follicle, causes occlusion of the ducts and in turn the formation of comedones.

There is a correlation between the *depth of the hair follicle* and the size of the lesion. The deeper the follicle, the deeper the occlusion, which in turn results in a larger lesion.

The bacterium *Propionibacterium acnes* causes inflammation either because of an immune system reaction, inflammatory enzymes from the bacteria, or a combination of the two. *P. acnes* is a normal colonizer of the sebaceous follicles; it is a gram-positive microaerophilic bacterium that, as part of its normal metabolic and reproductive processes, produces and accumulates endogenous porphyrins, namely protoporphyrin, uroporphyrin, and coproporphyrin III. Porphyrins can be visualized using a Wood's lamp or digital fluorescence photography because they absorb light energy at the near-ultraviolet and blue-light spectrum. This unique attribute of the bacterium contributes to the therapeutic effects of some light-based treatments.

EXTERNAL CAUSES

External factors vary from patient to patient, but there are several that can affect the severity of acne. *Diet* will affect each patient individually, and although dairy products seem to cause problems in women, no other universal dietary factors have been identified. *Thick makeup, hair spray, greasy hair gels,* and *hats, sweat bands,* or *athletic helmets* are all external factors that contribute to the severity of acne because of the combination of mechanical or chemical irritation, oil gland occlusion, and bacterial colonization. In some work environments, exposure to industrial products like cutting oils may produce acne. In addition, *inadequate cleansing* contributes to the development of acne. In all cases, the external factors aggravate acne but are not the root cause of the disease.

Patients should be advised not to rub, scratch, pick, or squeeze their skin because mechanical irritation can aggravate acne and lead to scarring. Careful and controlled extraction of comedones by a trained aesthetician or nurse after steaming and appropriate skin preparation may be beneficial. Some drugs can cause or worsen acne, including iodides, bromides, and oral or injected steroids. A proper skin care regimen is helpful to minimize the severity of acne by removing impurities and irritants.

TREATMENT OPTIONS

Because the pathogenesis of acne involves four factors (hypercornification of the pilosebaceous duct, increased sebum production, colonization by *P. acnes*, and the development of inflammation), a stepwise and systematic approach to treatment is best. Because acne is a chronic disease, its treatment is an ongoing process that requires educating the patient as well as patience on the part of both patient and clinician. It takes time for each step in the treatment process to take effect. Treatments aimed at the clearance of *P. acnes* alone generally provide short-lived improvement; therefore combination therapy is recommended (Table 40.1).

The first universal step is appropriate skin care. Cleansing the skin seems to help all patients, if only slightly, but acne is not directly caused by dirt. Cleansers have an antibacterial effect and may reduce bacterial colony counts. Toners may be helpful in restoring the pH balance of the skin after cleansing to an acidic state. Using gentle exfoliation such as *microdermabrasion* or *glycolic facials* may be helpful

TABLE 40.1	Treatment Options in Acne Management			
Grade 1	**Grade 2**	**Grade 3**	**Grade 4**	**Rosacea Acne**
Gentle skin care and extraction of comedones	Gentle skin care and extraction of comedones	Gentle skin care	Gentle skin care	Gentle antiinflammatory skin care
Topical retinoids	Blue light	Blue light and red light	Blue light and red light	Topical antibiotics and/or systemic tetracyclines
Exfoliation: peels and/or microdermabrasion	Topical retinoids	Topical retinoids	Systemic antibiotics	Glycolic acid peels
	Benzoyl peroxide	Benzoyl peroxide	Hormonal therapy	
		Systemic and/or topical antibiotics	IPL (not with tretinoin) and photodynamic therapy	
	Topical antibiotics			IPL and photodynamic therapy
	Exfoliation: peels (salicylic/glycolic) and/or microdermabrasion	Hormonal therapy	Systemic isotretinoin	
	Photodynamic therapy	Exfoliation: peels (salicylic/glycolic) and/or microdermabrasion		Avoid triggers
		IPL and photodynamic therapy		

IPL, Intense pulsed light.

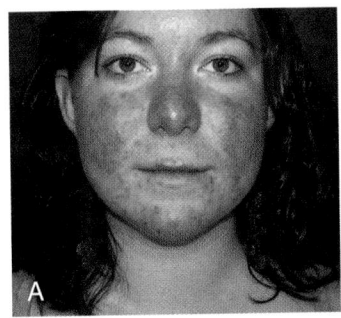 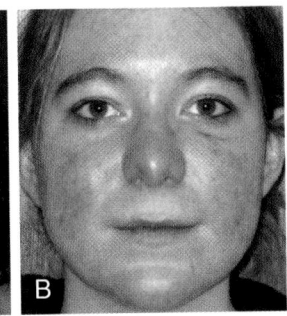

Fig. 40.1 Treatment of inflammatory acne with scars. Five intense pulsed-light treatments were performed with the Vasculight SR handpiece (Lumenis, San Jose, California) combined with three photodynamic therapy treatments with incubation periods lasting 30 to 90 minutes. (A) Before treatment. (B) After treatment.

to remove excessive keratin from the epidermis and open pores, allowing sebum to drain freely. Overscrubbing is not recommended, because the skin becomes dry, damaged, and inflamed; as a result, it can become less receptive to topical products. Abrasive home scrubs are therefore not recommended for acne-prone skin. *A gentle cleanser* is all that is necessary to cleanse the skin properly. *Moisturizers* that are noncomedogenic are helpful to prevent skin dehydration and to counteract the drying effect of many other active ingredients, such as benzoyl peroxide. The most commonly used cleansers are available over the counter and include Clearasil and PHisoderm, but aesthetic clincians' offices and spas also have a variety of excellent brands available.

As with many other cosmetic treatments, combination therapy is the best approach to treating acne, which leads to the *second step of treatment.* Using topical products, such as *topical retinoids*, maximizes the effect that an intense pulsed-light (IPL) treatment will have. Retinoids are comedolytic and act on the keratinization of the hair follicle. They are therefore beneficial for acne grades 1 and 2, where comedones predominate. Adapalene (Differin) is the least irritating, but others, such as tretinoin (Retin-A) or tazarotene (Tazorac), may also be used. There are many over-the-counter retinoid creams on the market, but these do not usually deliver consistent levels of retinoid to the dermis.

Retinoids decrease the occlusion of sebaceous ducts, thus preventing oil from accumulating in the sebaceous glands and creating a favorable environment for bacterial colonization. Inflammatory acne, on the other hand, responds better to *topical antibiotics and photodynamic therapy* (PDT; Fig. 40.1). Preparations that combine antibiotics like clindamycin with benzoyl peroxide are available for better efficacy than could be achieved with single antibiotics alone. In addition, *blue light* (415-nm wavelength) has excellent antibacterial properties against porphyrin-producing bacteria because porphyrins release singlet oxygen when

activated by this wavelength of light. Singlet oxygen is toxic to the bacteria (see Chapter 51, Photodynamic Therapy).

Hormonal therapy is a useful adjunct to the treatment of acne in female patients who have perimenstrual flare-ups or those with acne in combination with other hyperandrogenic features. One important pathogenic factor in acne is increased sensitivity of the pilosebaceous unit to androgens. Combination oral contraceptives (COCs) inhibit ovulation, reduce the production of androgen in the adrenal glands and ovaries, block androgen receptors, and increase the production of sex hormone–binding globulin (hence lowering free circulating androgens). COCs containing progestins with an antiandrogenic potential or no androgenic effect are preferred. The full effect of COCs may take 6 to 9 months to appear and it is important to identify risk factors and contraindications before prescribing them (e.g., clotting disorder, thromboembolism, headache, and migraine, smokers over 35 years of age, history of breast or endometrial malignancy). A Cochrane review of oral contraceptive pills (OCPs) (Arowojolu, 2012 Update) found that ethinyl estradiol combined with any of several progestins (e.g., levonorgestrel [also used in intrauterine devices], cyproterone, desogestrel, dienogest, drospirenone, norethindrone, norgestimate) was effective for the treatment of acne.

Oral antibiotics and isotretinoin (Accutane) constitute the next level of traditional therapy. However, the availability of lasers, IPL devices, and PDT now provides excellent treatment options that avoid possible systemic side effects, leaving oral treatment as an alternative for severe and unusually refractive cases. *Intralesional steroids* are infrequently used and are more appropriate for early nodular lesions; they should not be a standard treatment for acne. Newer *devices that extract comedones* in the course of IPL treatment are excellent for grades 2 and 3 acne. Gently extracting large comedones and draining superficial cysts may be helpful in providing full-face treatments such as IPL and PDT. In order to avoid spreading infection, strong pressure should never be applied. *Oral antibiotics* such as minocycline are very effective in treating acute flare-ups of papulopustular acne. Oral antibiotics also reduce the severity of acne in conjunction with or before the initiation of light-based therapy. Combining tetracyclines with light therapy is a relative contraindication because the skin is more photosensitive, but in my experience the increased posttreatment erythema is worth the benefit. Patients need to be informed of the possible side effects.

Rosacea

Although rosacea differs from acne vulgaris, it warrants discussion here because of the many similarities between the two, including an inflammatory component and small papules and pustules. When treating rosacea, skin care should be restricted to mild, hypoallergenic products. Prescription metronidazole preparations such as Rosasol and Metrogel are effective at controlling the disease activity, and IPL and PDT treatments can be highly effective in reversing erythema, telangiectasia, and the activity of the disease (Fig. 40.2).

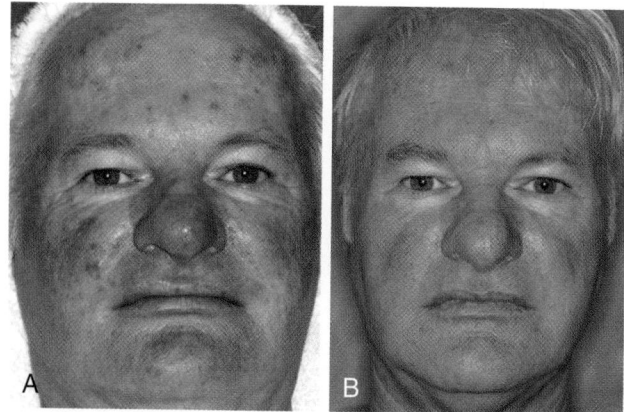

Fig. 40.2 Treatment of refractory rosacea acne with five intense pulsed-light treatments with the Vasculight and three photodynamic therapy treatments with incubation periods of 60 to 120 minutes. (A) Before treatment. (B) After treatment.

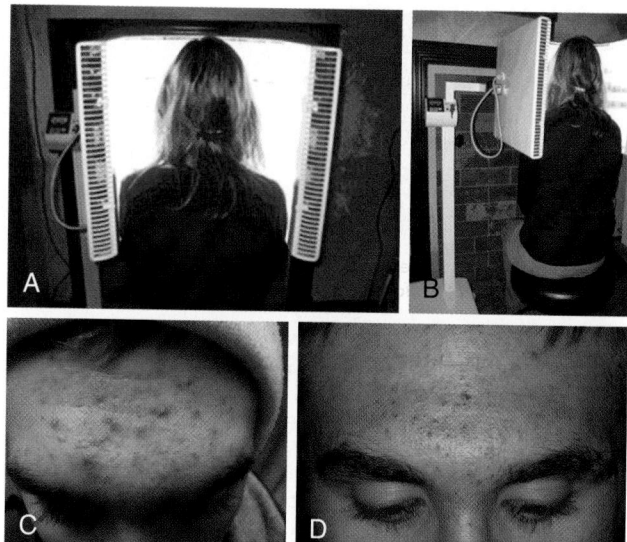

Fig. 40.3 (A–B) Blue light sessions combined with extractions and skin care. Before (C) and after (D) a 6-week course of twice-weekly treatments.

Blue Light and Red Light Therapy

Approximately 70% of patients report improvement of their acne after sunlight exposure. In vivo studies, however, have provided insufficient evidence to justify the use of ultraviolet A and B as antiacne treatment, especially given their potential carcinogenicity. Because the strongest porphyrin photoexcitation band that produces singlet oxygen lies between 407 and 420 nm, irradiation of *P. acnes* with blue light leads to predictable bacterial destruction. Studies have shown a mean acne lesion reduction of 64% for papulopustular acne in a treatment course of two 15-minute sessions per week over 5 weeks. Various devices are available, such as the Clearlight, the Blu-U, and 410-nm IPL devices. The treatments are painless and have no side effects (Fig. 40.3).

Although *blue light* has the strongest porphyrin photoexcitation ability, it is limited by its depth of penetration in skin. *Red light*, although a less effective photoexciting wavelength, has an increased depth of penetration in human skin and may also induce antiinflammatory effects by stimulating cytokine release from macrophages. Improvements as high as 76% have been achieved in combined blue and red light studies, perhaps because of a synergistic effect of these wavelengths.

Photodynamic Therapy

PDT (see also Chapter 51, Photodynamic Therapy) refers to the topical application of D-aminolevulinic acid (ALA; e.g., Levulan) to the skin, which, when preferentially absorbed by pilosebaceous units, is metabolized through the heme synthesis pathway to produce protoporphyrin IX. PDT has been widely used for the treatment of a variety of skin diseases, including nonmelanoma skin cancer, actinic keratoses, warts, psoriasis, cutaneous T-cell lymphoma, and acne vulgaris.

When protoporphyrin IX is photoactivated by the appropriate wavelengths of light (IPL, pulse light, or blue light), singlet oxygen species and free radicals, which have cytotoxic effects, are produced. Not only is *P. acnes* destroyed, but the pilosebaceous unit is damaged or destroyed as well. ALA application time, also referred to as the incubation period, can vary between 15 and 120 minutes. Red light, blue light, IPL, diode laser, pulsed-dye laser, and light-emitting diode sources have all been shown to be effective in activating protoporphyrin IX. Studies have shown a decrease in acne lesion counts, which persists from 10 to 20 months after one to four treatments. Typically three treatments are performed at 2- to 4-week intervals to achieve a remission of this duration. PDT results in a temporary reduction in skin oiliness, improvement in acne severity, and a cosmetic improvement of the skin, with textural improvement and a

reduction in sun damage and pore size. Cosmetic improvement of the skin is maximized when IPL parameters for skin rejuvenation are used at a moderate fluence. Possible side effects include initial burning discomfort, self-limiting crusting, erythema, mild edema, and hyperpigmentation. The side effects are reduced with short incubation periods and are self-limiting. Patients must stay out of the sun and bright rooms for a minimum of 24 hours after ALA is applied.

Intense Pulsed-Light Therapy

Intense pulsed light involves the use of a broadband light source that emits multiple wavelengths, typically produced by a xenon flash lamp, coupled with light filters to select specific bands of wavelengths to treat specific conditions. With acne, the wavelengths used (400 to 600 nm) are highly absorbed by the sebum, the bacteria within the lesions, and the sebaceous glands. IPL systems (available from ClearTouch, Palomar Cynosure, etc.) can be used on all skin types. Lumenis has equipment that may be faster and can be used on all but the darkest skins. Caution must be exercised in treating darker skins because these wavelengths have an extremely high melanin absorption coefficient; without proper settings, effective epidermal cooling, and testing, therefore, the risk of burning is high. The broad range of emitted wavelengths covers the peak absorption of endogenous porphyrins produced by *P. acnes* as well as that of hemoglobin in blood vessels close to the inflamed acne lesions, leading to both antibacterial and antiinflammatory effects (Fig. 40.4).

Patients must be protected from any possible sun exposure before treatment because increased skin pigment (tanning) will increase the risk of epidermal burning from the artificial light sources. A very small amount of sun exposure can alter the pigment of the skin, restricting the technician's ability to treat at optimal settings. Self-tanning creams are also contraindicated, because any darkening of the skin increasing the absorption of light energy where it is not desired will restrict the amount of power that can be safely used. Areas of higher melanin concentration and areas of more sensitive skin should be evaluated and treated accordingly. Pretreatment of the skin with topical hydroquinone 4% twice a day for 2 to 4 weeks for patients with Fitzpatrick skin type 4 or higher will reduce the incidence of hyperpigmentation after laser and IPL treatments.

Treatment with light-based technology incorporates the ability to tailor both the pulse duration and fluence energy used. Contact cooling before, during, and after the light pulse is also important. Tailoring pulse duration means altering the duration of light being emitted from the flash lamp in milliseconds. The delay between

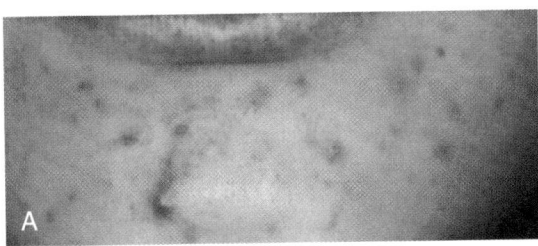
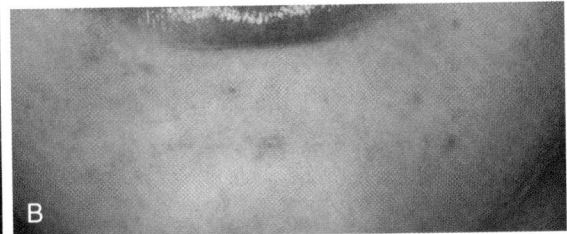

Fig. 40.4   Treatment of recalcitrant acne on the chin. The patient received 2 weeks of twice-weekly treatments with the LuxV handpiece (Palomar Cynosure Medical Technologies, Westford, Massachusetts). (A) Before treatment. (B) After treatment.

pulses allows some cooling of surrounding tissue, while targeted chromophores absorb additional energy with the second, shorter pulse. Cooling of the epidermis allows the user to deliver a larger amount of energy to the target and also to reach deeper into the skin while protecting its superficial layers. Some additional cooling may be necessary after treatment, both for comfort and to prevent blistering (e.g., ice packs). Using these principles, the initial treatment settings are often 100-ms pulse duration with fluences of 10 to 14 J/cm^2, followed by a second pass using a 20-ms pulse with fluences of 8 to 12 J/cm^2. Subsequent treatments will have the same pulse durations, but with increasing fluence. The first pulse penetrates deeper and allows for a longer heating time to affect the cysts and glands, whereas the second pass attacks the more superficial lesions. Most patients notice improvement with five to six treatments. If the fluence is not increased throughout the course of treatment, results may not meet expectations. The treatment will cause some discomfort, and some redness is to be expected, but it typically clears within hours.

Treatments should be conducted at 2- to 3-week intervals for teenagers because their flare-ups seem to occur within this time frame, whereas adults respond better to monthly treatments. When treatment intervals are too short, flare-ups may occur; however, too long an interval between treatments will also diminish their cumulative effect and the ultimate outcome.

With regard to complications, as stated earlier, there is a large amount of melanin absorption at these wavelengths; therefore patients should be advised that permanent hair reduction may occur in the treated areas. Men are required to shave before treatment on the face, and some pain is to be expected in these areas. There can be lateral spread of the effect owing to diffusion of light in the skin, so if the clinician is trying to avoid a hairline or eyebrow, it is important to stay at least 2 cm away from it to make sure that there will be no thermal damage to the hair bulb or stem cells.

"Major" complications include superficial blisters and burns. These are ultimately caused by overtreatment, too much sun exposure, or a patient's failure to follow posttreatment instructions. Most burns and blisters can be treated with a class I steroid (clobetasol cream), and blisters can be treated with antibiotic/healing creams. Most burns resolve spontaneously within 2 months; however, hypopigmentation can still be seen after 8 to 12 months on some darker-skinned patients.

After treatment, in addition to immediate cooling with a cold pack, patients are told to limit sun exposure, use a non-comedogenic moisturizer that includes a sunscreen, and avoid external heating factors that could create an adverse reaction. Most patients are able to continue their combination oral or topical therapies during the treatment course, including tetracycline antibiotics. Combination therapy increases the treatment success rate. Some erythema secondary to the thermal damage is to be expected. This can be treated by short-term use of an over-the-counter hydrocortisone cream, which will not affect the treatment or cause further breakouts. The use of light-emitting diodes has also been proven to aid the body in the thermal healing response.

Laser Therapy

Lasers with wavelengths used to treat vascular lesions and superficial pigmented lesions can also be used to treat acne. These wavelengths also act through photoactivation of bacterial porphyrins as well as potentially causing nonspecific thermal injury to sebaceous glands. Devices such as the Aura (Boston Scientific), a potassium titanyl phosphate laser, and other pulsed-dye lasers (e.g., Energist) have been shown to provide a reduction in acne severity. Studies with a single treatment or biweekly treatments for 2 weeks have been reported to reduce acne by 39% to 50%. Treatment was found to be more effective in combination with topical therapy than when lasers were used alone.

Infrared lasers have recently become one of the most effective available acne treatments because of their depth of penetration into the dermis. Experience with isotretinoin use has shown shrinkage of sebaceous glands and marked reduction of sebum production during treatment. Although sebum production returns to normal after cessation of treatment, many patients remain clear of acne, leading to the hypothesis that a temporary effect on sebaceous glands may be adequate to induce long-term acne clearance. With infrared lasers, the target chromophore is water, which is the dominant chromophore in sebaceous glands. The laser produces an injury zone in the dermal layer, where sebaceous glands are located, and in theory causes enough injury to arrest the overproduction of sebum, thereby eliminating acne.

Both 1450- and 1540-nm lasers have been studied in trials. Initial biopsies confirmed thermal coagulation of the sebaceous gland, but biopsies at 2 and 6 months revealed no long-term alteration of the skin. Studies combining pulsed-dye laser with infrared laser have shown synergistic effects, suggesting that infrared laser may have clinical use as a primary or adjunctive acne treatment in patients requiring an alternative to more traditional methods of treatment. Side effects are transient and local, including erythema and discomfort during treatment, without any delayed adverse effects.

Radiofrequency

Although radiofrequency (RF) is not a light-based technology, it has a similar effect on the sebaceous unit as laser by producing thermal injury to the dermis, including the sebaceous gland. Various frequencies have been studied and show encouraging results in reducing acne and improving acne scarring, although the study sizes have been small with limited follow-up, underscoring the need for larger studies with longer follow-up.

CONCLUSION

A proper history and physical examination with accurate diagnosis is imperative before the treatment of acne commences. A stepwise approach and the establishment of realistic expectations are important. Patients need to understand the chronic nature of the disease and the possibility that their acne will be refractory to treatment. Combination therapy remains the best approach in the treatment of acne.

Comedonal acne is best managed with skin care that includes appropriate exfoliation and topical retinoids. If multiple lesions are inflamed and infected, benzoyl peroxide and topical or oral antibiotics must be prescribed along with skin care to reduce infection. Blue light, IPL, and PDT can be added for more severe cases.

Nodulocystic acne is unlikely to respond to topical therapy and, if the severity warrants, is best treated with oral antibiotics and PDT in combination with IPL and blue light or isotretinoin (Accutane).

The use of light-based technology has greatly increased the treatment success rate for acne. It may be considered after oral and topical therapy have failed in patients with inflammatory acne without scarring or in conjunction with current therapies as part of a first-line of therapy in patients presenting with both active acne and acne scars. However, cost, discomfort, erythema, multiple office visits, and complications are potential downsides to laser and other light-based therapies. Although a systematic review (Hamilton et al., 2009) found some forms of light therapy to be effective, especially in the short term, the authors point out that there are few studies comparing light therapy with conventional acne treatments. Consequently insurance companies still consider it somewhat experimental and many refuse to reimburse for it. They do acknowledge, however, that some patients may find it easier to be compliant with this regimen as opposed to more conventional treatments despite the initial discomfort.

These newer treatments provide an attractive alternative for noncompliant patients and are free of complications such as antibiotic resistance and teratogenic side effects. With continued technologic advances in the ability to selectively target *P. acnes* and sebaceous glands, a new frontier of acne treatment is evolving, providing patients with safer and more effective treatment choices for one of the most prevalent and distressing skin conditions.

CPT/BILLING CODES

10040	Acne surgery
10060	I&D one abscess
10061	I&D multiple abscesses
11900	Intralesional injection, up to and including 7 lesions
11901	Intralesional injection, more than 7 lesions

ICD-10-CM DIAGNOSTIC CODES

L71.0–L71.8	Rosacea
L70.0–L70.8	Acne

SUPPLIERS

(See contact information available at www.expertconsult.com.)

Blue-U (blue light)
Clarion Medical Technologies, Inc.
Candela Smoothbeam diode laser
Candela, Inc.
Intense pulsed-light devices
Clarion Medical Technologies, Inc.
Alma Lasers, Inc.
Palomar Cynosure Medical Technologies, Inc.
Isolaz Deep Pore Laser Therapy
SkinRx Distribution
Levulan
Clarion Medical Technologies, Inc.
Radiofrequency devices
Ellman Cynosure
Solta Medical

RECOMMENDED READING

Ammad S, Gonzales M, Edwards C, Finlay AY, Mills CJ. An assessment of the efficacy of blue light phototherapy in acne vulgaris. *J Cosmet Dermatol.* 2008;7(3):180–188.

Alexiades-Armenakas M. Long-pulsed dye laser-mediated photodynamic therapy combined with topical therapy for mild to severe comedonal, inflammatory, or cystic acne. *J Drugs Dermatol.* 2006;5:45–55.

Arowojolu AO, Gallo MF, Lopez LM, Grimes DA. Effect of birth control pills on acne in women. *Cochrane Database Syst Rev.* 2012;(7):CD004425.

Bettoli V, Zauli S, Virgili A. Is hormonal treatment still an option in acne today? *Br J Dermatol.* 2015;172(suppl 1):37–46.

Calderhead RG. The photobiological basics behind light-emitting diode (LED) phototherapy. *Laser Ther.* 2007;16:97–108.

Gold MH, Bradshaw VL, Boring MM, et al. The use of novel intense pulsed light and heat source and ALA-PDT in the treatment of moderate to severe inflammatory acne vulgaris. *J Drugs Dermatol.* 2004;3(suppl):S15–S19.

Gold MH, Rao J, Goldman MP, et al. A multicenter clinical evaluation of the treatment of mild to moderate inflammatory acne vulgaris of the face with visible blue light in comparison to topical 1% clindamycin antibiotic solution. *J Drugs Dermatol.* 2005;4:64–70.

Goldberg DJ, Russell BA. Combination blue (415 nm) and red (633 nm) LED phototherapy in the treatment of mild to severe acne vulgaris. *J Cosmet Laser Ther.* 2006;8:71–75.

Hamilton FL, Car J, Lyons C, Car M, Layton A, Majeed A. Lasers and other light therapies for the treatment of acne vulgaris: a systematic review. *Br J Dermatol.* 2009;160(6):1273–1285.

Hongcharu W, Taylor CR, Chang Y, et al. Topical ALA-photodynamic therapy for the treatment of acne vulgaris. *J Invest Dermatol.* 2000;115:183–192.

Hruza G, Avram M. *Procedures in Cosmetic Dermatology Series: Lasers and Lights.* 3rd ed. Philadelphia: Elsevier; 2012.

Na JI, Suh DH. Red light phototherapy alone is effective for acne vulgaris: randomized, single-blinded clinical trial. *Dermatol Surg.* 2007;33(10):1228–1233.

Taub AF. Photodynamic therapy for the treatment of acne: a pilot study. *J Drugs Dermatol.* 2004;3(suppl):S10–S14.

Tzung T-Y, Wu K-H, Huang M-L. Blue light phototherapy in the treatment of acne. *Photodermatol Photoimmunol Photomed.* 2004;20:266–269.

Usatine RP. *The Color Atlas of Family Medicine.* 2nd ed. New York: McGraw-Hill; 2013.

CHAPTER 41

LASERS AND PULSED-LIGHT DEVICES: SKIN TIGHTENING

Gregory Costello

Advances in aesthetic and antiaging medicine have led to treatments that were not available just a few decades ago. A multitude of options other than surgical intervention are now available to the patient who wishes to improve his or her appearance. The trend in aesthetic medicine has increasingly shifted from the concept of painful, long surgical recovery to multiple procedures with minimal downtime and little to no pain. This is especially true in the area of skin tightening.

In the past, the concept of skin versus muscle laxity was irrelevant in terms of treatment because in either case the only treatment was surgical. However, with the advent of novel technologies that cause contraction, synthesis, and remodeling of collagen, "loose skin" can be addressed by noninvasive means. Laxity below the eyes, lowering of the brows, prominence of nasolabial folds, and the formation of "jowls," among a multitude of other skin laxity issues, can be easily improved without painful surgery, long recovery times, or the risks of anesthesia.

Some types of sagging were and are still treated with surgery, such as an abdominoplasty (Fig. 41.1). This procedure is painful and requires general anesthesia. In addition, the procedure is costly, requires significant down time for recovery, and often leaves an unsightly scar.

This chapter focuses on the latest technologies developed specifically for tightening lax and sagging skin, which in turn reduces wrinkles and improves surface irregularities of the skin (Fig. 41.2). The latest technologies include intense pulsed light (IPL), radiofrequency (RF), and laser modalities to achieve a similar goal of dermal heating and thus to produce changes in the skin. (Also see Chapter 45, Nonablative Radiowave Skin Tightening With the Ellman S5 Surgitron [Pellevé Procedure].) Most of these modalities show some immediate short-term results owing to temporary protein contraction; however, because of the stimulation of collagen formation, maximum results, which are also longer lasting, require up to 8 months to complete the remodeling process.

SKIN STRUCTURE AND BREAKDOWN

As we age, our skin's structure deteriorates as a result of sun exposure, dietary habits, and natural processes. As the collagen in the skin breaks down, the skin's tightness and general elasticity decreases, causing a sagging or loose appearance. This tissue breakdown occurs at a depth of 3 to 5 mm in the dermis.

TREATMENT EVOLUTION

The new technology that has evolved from older treatments involves passing certain types of light or current through the top layers of the skin, leaving them undamaged but affecting a specific target deeper in the dermis, which in turn stimulates the production of "good" collagen. These treatments are mostly noninvasive and in most cases involve very little pain. They do involve multiple treatments, and the results are most noticeable over time.

LIGHT-BASED TECHNOLOGY

In recent years many systems have been developed using light to target the condition of loose skin. These systems use various wavelengths and different types of technology. In principle, light penetrates deep into the skin, where it is absorbed by water and converted to heat energy. The thermal conversion then stimulates fibroblasts to produce new collagen. Some of the original systems, such as the CoolTouch system, used the 1320-nm neodymium-doped yttrium–aluminum garnet (Nd-YAG) wavelength. The 1440-nm Nd-YAG wavelength has also been used, but the results have been only slightly better than those with the 1320-nm systems. Good results have also been achieved with the use of IPL technology to deliver specified wavelength bands for a more efficient heating process. IPL technology uses several wavelengths banded together by light cutoff filters to specifically target certain chromophores in the skin. In the case of skin tightening, the target chromophore is water. Accordingly, for the treatments to be effective, the system must use wavelengths that are well absorbed by water.

Infrared Light

Infrared laser technology can be used to target water as a chromophore for photothermolysis. There are many examples of infrared technologies, both ablative and nonablative, that can be used to promote collagen growth in the dermis. The Cutera 1064-nm Nd-YAG laser targets the microvasculature to produce subdermal heating using high peak energies delivered through microsecond pulses. This gentle heating of the skin causes the formation of type I collagen, resulting in improvement in skin firmness and texture. Type I collagen is the most abundant type of collagen in the body and is found in blood vessels, multiple organs, tendons, and bone as well as in skin. The proportion of type I collagen increases when tissue repair or healing occurs.

There are other wavelengths in the infrared spectrum that are surface ablative and promote collagen growth by means of deep dermal heating. Use of these lasers improves surface defects in the skin (e.g., roughness, sun damage, rhytids) and also promotes collagen growth. The 2790-nm yttrium-scandium-gallium garnet laser (Cutera) uses water as a chromophore, causing vaporization of approximately 10 to 30 μm of epidermal tissue and coagulation of an additional 20 to 60 μm of tissue. Below this layer of coagulation the tissue is heated. Collagen stimulation occurs in this heated subcoagulation region. The coagulated tissue acts as an occlusive dressing that quickly peels off, leaving behind a layer of skin where collagen remodeling occurs. The most widely used parameters for this treatment are between 1.0 and 3.5 J/cm^2, with a pulse width of 0.3 to 0.5 msec. Maximal dermal heating occurs with a higher pulse width with this procedure.

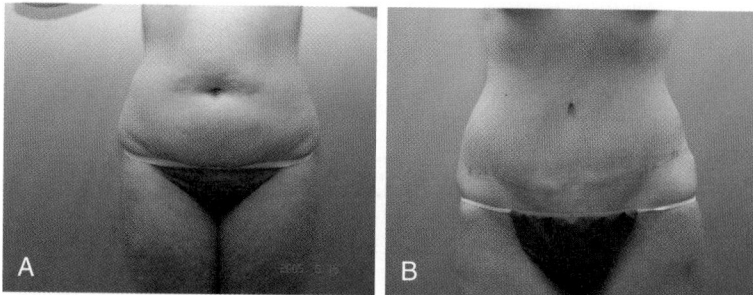

Fig. 41.1 (A) Preoperative photograph showing laxity of the abdominal skin. (B) Same patient after abdominoplasty. (From Hunstad and Repta: Atlas of Abdominoplasty. London: Saunders; 2009.)

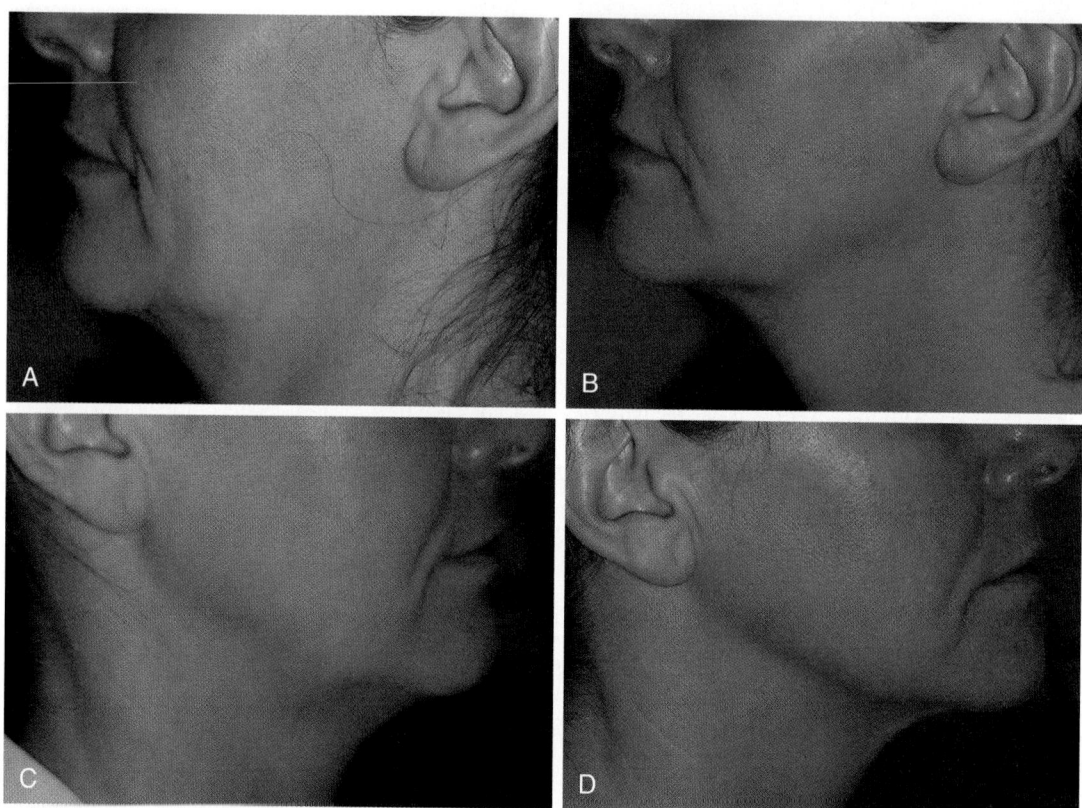

Fig. 41.2 (A, C) Preoperative photograph taken from the side showing laxity of the neck skin. (B, D) Same patient 1 month after treatment. (From Alexiades-Armenakas M. Aging facial skin: infrared broad band light technologies. Facial Plast Surg Clin North Am. 2011;19:361–370.)

Fractionated Infrared Light

The use of *fractional light delivery* with infrared light allows for a higher fluence, resulting in a deeper thermal effect and thus deeper tightening. The idea of fractional energy delivery, which has been made popular recently by the Reliant Fraxel (Solta Medical) and Palomar Lux IR (Palomar Cynosure Medical Technologies) systems, involves controlled thermal damage. The concept centers on the principle of using microlenses for focusing light to create a significant amount of thermal damage in one column while leaving the surrounding tissue relatively undamaged. This stimulates the skin's normal healing response, including fibroblast activity that promotes new collagen production. In the case of the Palomar Cynosure Lux IR fractional system, fractional delivery is combined with optimum wavelength selection to allow for deep thermal injury with minimal pain and risk. Cooling is absolutely necessary because these wavelengths are all very highly absorbed by water, and at the fluencies that are being used, a burn is likely without proper cooling. This system is equipped with contact sensors, which allow the system to fire only if proper contact is achieved. This ensures that the skin is adequately cooled.

Intense Pulsed Light

Intense pulsed-light technology, in the infrared wavelengths, uses a spectrum of wavelengths to achieve collagen production through fibroblast stimulation. The Cutera Titan XL uses flash-lamp technology in the 1100- to 1800-nm wavelengths, where water is the dominant chromophore. The challenge in IPL technology has always been to provide enough energy to the desired target without causing thermal damage to the surface tissue. The Titan XL overcomes this risk through a cycle of cooling before and after the delivery of energy to the desired target. The treatment area is covered with a thin layer of gel and the 3- by 1-cm IPL handpiece crystal is placed directly in contact with the skin. One second of cooling is followed by the delivery of heat at the selected fluence, followed by 2 more seconds of cooling. Both the cooling and delivery of energy take place through the contact crystal and are preprogrammed to occur automatically without having to lift the handpiece from contact with the skin. This automated cycle allows for the delivery of high amounts of energy deep into the skin while protecting the surface from visible damage.

RADIOFREQUENCY

RF, unlike light-based technologies that operate based on absorption coefficients, is based on passing an RF current deep into the skin; it is designed to denature collagen deeper in the skin while leaving the top layer undamaged. This causes immediate tightening and thermal damage, which stimulates new collagen growth. The thermal effect is generated by the tissue's natural resistance to the movement of ions within an RF field.

The ThermaCool TC system from Thermage (Solta Medical) is an example of a monopolar RF technology. This system uses a capacitive coupling membrane to couple the RF to the skin. A grounding plate is attached to the patient to dissipate the current, and the RF generator is then turned on. This type of delivery allows for deep penetration by the RF and, as a result, much better heating than that obtained with RF bipolar electrodes. Monopolar delivery of RF causes excellent volumetric tissue heating. Monopolar RF treatments are moderately painful and do pose a risk for scarring and burns when not administered correctly. (Also see Chapter 45, Nonablative Radiowave Skin Tightening With the Ellman S5 Surgitron [The Pellevé Procedure].)

Another approach to skin tightening using RF technology is the addition of IPL. The ReFirme ST from Syneron Candela uses pulses of infrared light in the 700- to 2000-nm wavelength range simultaneously with bipolar RF. The pulse of infrared light uses melanin and hemoglobin as chromophores, thus heating the dermis. The heating effect creates a path of optimal electrical conductivity or lower impedance. Because electricity prefers the path of lowest impedance, the electrical bipolar RF energy is concentrated at the target site preheated by the optical energy. Contact cooling at the treatment site minimizes electrical conduction to the epidermis and allows most of the energy to penetrate into deeper parts of the dermis.

TIPS AND COMMON ERRORS

- Choose the right patient for best results. These systems are designed only to tighten skin, so muscle laxity and excessive fat will not improve in appearance.
- Be cautious with darker skin types (types 3 to 6) in any system that uses melanin as a chromophore.

CONCLUSION

As with most aesthetic procedures, patient selection is of the highest priority to maximize patient satisfaction. The aforementioned procedures work best in patients with mild to moderate skin laxity. The procedures will produce a subtle tightening of the loose or sagging skin but are not intended for the correction of muscle laxity, severe skin laxity, or excess skin in overweight patients. In order to attain the greatest patient satisfaction from any skin-tightening procedure, physicians must fully explain to patients what they should expect and what not to expect from their treatments.

SUPPLIERS

(See contact information available at www.expertconsult.com.)

Cutera
Palomar Cynosure Medical Technologies, Inc.
Syneron Candela Medical Ltc.
Thermage, Inc. (Solta Medical Valeant)

ONLINE RESOURCES

American Board of Laser Surgery: www.americanboardoflasersurgery.org.

RECOMMENDED READING

Anderson RR, Parrish JA. Selective photothermolysis: precise microsurgery by selective absorption of pulsed radiation. *Science.* 1983;220:524–527.
Dierickx CC. The role of deep heating for noninvasive skin rejuvenation. *Lasers Surg Med.* 2006;38:799–807.
Goldberg D. *Procedures in Cosmetic Dermatology Series: Lasers and Lights, Volume 1: Vascular/Pigmentation/Scars/Medical Applications.* Philadelphia: Saunders; 2005.
Goldberg D. *Procedures in Cosmetic Dermatology Series: Lasers and Lights, Volume 2: Rejuvenation/Resurfacing/Treatment of Ethnic Skin/Treatment of Cellulite.* Philadelphia: Saunders; 2005.
Goldberg DJ. Histologic changes after treatment with intense pulsed light. *J Cutan Laser Ther.* 2000;2:53–56.
Goldman M. Clinical pearl: observations on the use of fractionated CO2 laser resurfacing. *J Drugs Dermatol.* 2009;8:82–86.
Kauvar A, Hruza G, eds. *Principles and Practices in Cutaneous Laser Surgery.* Boca Raton, Fla: Taylor and Francis; 2005.
Moy RL, Dover JS. *Procedures in Cosmetic Dermatology Series: Advanced Face Lifting.* Philadelphia: Saunders; 2006.
Sadick N. Combination radiofrequency and light energies: Electro-optical synergy technology in aesthetic medicine. *Dermatol Surg.* 2005;31:1211–1217.
Saluja R, Khoury J, Detwiler S, Goldman M. Histologic and clinical response to varying density settings with a fractionality scanned carbon dioxide laser. *J Drugs Dermatol.* 2009;8:17–20.
Schmults CD, Phelps R, Goldberg DJ. Nonablative facial remodeling: erythema reduction and histologic evidence of new collagen formation using a 300-microsecond 1064-nm Nd:YAG laser. *Arch Dermatol.* 2004;140:1373–1376.
Small R, Hoang D. Combination cosmetic treatments. In: Usatine RP, Pfenninger JL, Stulberg DL, Small R, eds. *Dermatologic and Cosmetic Procedures in Office Practice.* Philadelphia: Elsevier; 2012:377–381.
Small R. Wrinkle reduction with nonablative lasers. In: Usatine RP, Pfenninger JL, Stulberg DL, Small R, eds. *Dermatologic and Cosmetic Procedures in Office Practice.* Philadelphia: Elsevier; 2012:336–350.
Tan KL, Kurniawati C, Gold M. Low risk of postinflammatory hyperpigmentation in skin types 4 and 5 after treatment with fractional CO2 laser device. *J Drugs Dermatol.* 2008;7:774–777.
Waibel J, Beer K. Ablative fractional laser resurfacing for the treatment of a third degree burn. *J Drugs Dermatol.* 2009;8:294–297.

CHAPTER 42

LASERS AND PULSED-LIGHT DEVICES: LEG TELANGIECTASIA*

Mitchel P. Goldman

Lasers and intense pulsed light (IPL) are used to treat leg telangiectasia for various reasons. *First*, both treatments have a futuristic appeal, not only to the general public but also to physicians. By virtue of their advanced technology, they are perceived as state-of-the-art treatment modalities and are sought by the general public because "high tech" is thought of as safer and better than traditional sclerotherapy. Unfortunately these perceptions have often resulted in unanticipated adverse sequelae (scarring and pain) at an increased cost to the patient (lasers cost considerably more to purchase and maintain than a needle, syringe, and sclerosing solution).

Lasers may also have theoretical advantages compared with sclerotherapy for treating leg telangiectasia. Sclerotherapy treatment of leg veins has been associated with pigmentation in up to 30% of patients, the development of new blood vessels in up to 10% of patients, and, very rarely, allergic reactions. These temporary but bothersome adverse effects are perceived not to occur with laser treatment. This chapter discusses the author's experience in treating leg veins with sclerotherapy, lasers, and IPL since 1983.

MECHANISM OF ACTION FOR LASERS AND INTENSE PULSED LIGHT

Lasers and IPL are pulsed, so that they act within the thermal relaxation times of blood vessels to produce specific destruction of vessels of various diameters based on the pulse duration (Table 42.1). Lasers of various wavelengths and broad-spectrum IPL are used to selectively treat blood vessels by taking advantage of the difference between the light absorption of the components in a blood vessel (oxygenated hemoglobin, deoxygenated hemoglobin, and methemoglobin) and the overlying epidermis and surrounding dermis to selectively thermocoagulate blood vessels. Deoxygenated hemoglobin has distinct optical properties, with two absorption spectrum peaks at approximately 545 and 580 nm and a broader peak beyond 650 nm (Fig. 42.1). The main feature to note in the curve is the strong absorption at wavelengths below 600 nm, with less absorption at longer wavelengths. This is because the absorption coefficient in blood is higher than that of surrounding tissue for wavelengths between 600 and 1064 nm.

The goal is to deliver sufficient energy to thermocoagulate the target vessel while the overlying epidermis and perivascular tissue remain unharmed. To accomplish this selective preservation of tissue, some form of epidermal cooling is also required. A number of different laser and IPL systems have been developed toward this end.

An understanding of the appropriate target vessel for each laser or IPL device is important, so that treatment will be tailored to the appropriate target. As detailed in sclerotherapy textbooks, most telangiectases arise from reticular veins. Therefore the single most important concept to keep in mind is that feeding reticular veins must be treated completely before treating telangiectasia. This minimizes adverse sequelae and enhances therapeutic results. Failure to treat feeding reticular veins and short follow-up periods after the use of lasers may give inflated values to the success rates of laser treatment.

HISTOLOGY OF LEG TELANGIECTASIA

The choice of the proper wavelength, degree of energy fluence, and pulse duration of light exposure are all related to the type and size of target vessel treated. Deeper vessels necessitate a longer wavelength to allow penetration. Large-diameter vessels necessitate a longer pulse duration to effectively thermocoagulate the entire vessel wall, allowing sufficient time for thermal energy to diffuse evenly throughout the vessel lumen. The correct choice of treatment parameters is aided by an understanding of the histology of the target telangiectasia.

Venules in the upper and middle dermis typically maintain a horizontal orientation. The diameter of the postcapillary venule ranges from 12 to 35 μm. Collecting venules range from 40 to 60 μm in the upper and middle dermis and enlarge to 100 to 400 μm in diameter in the deeper tissues. Histologic examination of simple telangiectases demonstrates dilated blood channels in a normal dermal stroma with a single endothelial cell lining, limited muscularis, and adventitial layers. Most leg telangiectases measure from 26 to 225 μm in diameter. They are found 175 to 382 μm below the stratum granulosum. The thickened vessel walls are composed of endothelial cells covered with collagen, elastic, and muscle fibers.

REVIEW OF AVAILABLE LASERS

Patients seek treatment for leg veins mostly for cosmetic reasons. Any effective treatment should be relatively free of adverse sequelae.

Krypton Triphosphate and Frequency-Doubled Nd:YAG (532 nm)

Modulated krypton triphosphate lasers have been reported to be effective at removing leg telangiectases using pulse durations between 1 and 50 ms. The 532-nm wavelength is one of the hemoglobin absorption peaks. Although this wavelength does not penetrate deeply into the dermis (about 0.75 mm), relatively specific damage (compared with argon laser) can occur in the vascular target by selecting an optimal pulse duration, enlarging the spot size, and adding epidermal cooling (Fig. 42.2).

---

* Portions of this chapter are excerpted from Goldman MP, Bergan JB, Guex JJ.: Sclerotherapy: Treatment of Varicose and Telangiectatic Leg Veins, 4th ed. London: Mosby; 2006.

TABLE 42.1	Thermal Relaxation Times of Blood Vessels
Diameter (mm)	**Seconds**
0.1	0.01
0.2	0.04
0.4	0.16
0.8	0.6
2.0	4.0

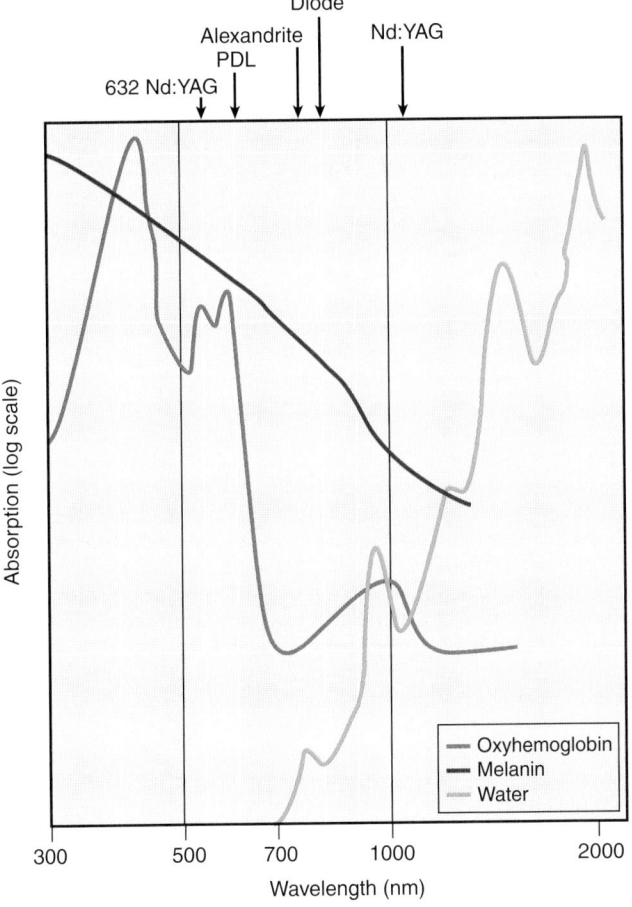

Fig. 42.1 Oxygenated and deoxygenated hemoglobin. Water and melanin absorption curves are given as a function of wavelength. PDL, Pulsed-dye laser. (Modified from Boulnois JL. Photophysical processes in recent medical laser developments: a review. *Lasers Med Sci.* 1986;1:47–66.)

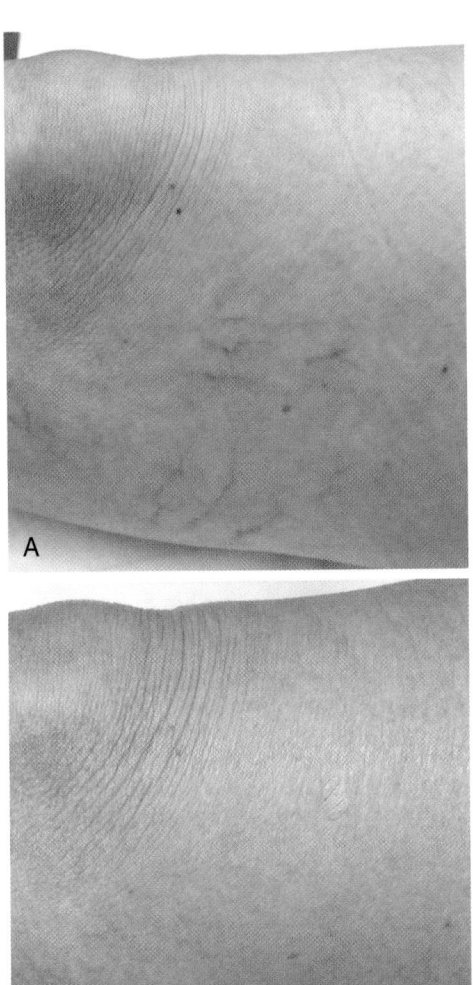

Fig. 42.2 Leg telangiectasia. (A) Before treatment. (B) After treatment. (Courtesy David Vasily, MD, Bethlehem, Pennsylvania.)

Effective results have been achieved by tracing vessels with a 1-mm projected spot. Typically the laser is moved between adjacent 1-mm spots following the vessels at 5 to 10 mm/s. Immediately after laser exposure, the epidermis is blanched. Lengthening of the pulse duration to match the diameter of the vessel is attempted to optimize treatment.

We and others have found the long-pulse 532-nm laser (frequency-doubled Nd:YAG) to be effective in treating leg veins less than 1 mm in diameter that are not directly connected to a feeding reticular vein. When used with a 4°C chilled tip, a fluence of 12 to 15 J/cm² is delivered as a train of pulses in a spot size 3 to 4 mm in diameter to trace the vessel until spasm or thrombosis occurs. Some overlying epidermal scabbing is noted, and hypopigmentation is not uncommon in dark-skinned patients. Although individual physicians report considerable variation in results, usually more than one treatment is necessary for maximum vessel improvement, with only rare reports of 100% resolution of the leg vein. Efficacy is technique dependent, with the potential for achieving excellent results.

Patients must be informed of the possibility of prolonged pigmentation at an incidence similar to that seen with sclerotherapy as well as temporary blistering and hypopigmentation that is predominantly caused by epidermal damage in pigmented skin (type III or above).

Pulsed-Dye Laser (585 or 595 nm)

The pulsed-dye laser (PDL) has proved to be highly effective in treating cutaneous vascular lesions consisting of very small vessels, including port wine stains, hemangiomas, and facial telangiectasia. The depth of vascular damage is estimated to be 1.5 mm at 585 nm and 15 to 20 μm deeper at 595 nm. Consequently penetration to the typical depth of superficial leg telangiectasia may be achieved. However, telangiectases over the lower extremities have not responded as well, with less lightening and more posttreatment hyperpigmentation. This may be due to the larger diameter of leg telangiectases compared with dermal vessels in port wine stains and larger-diameter feeding reticular veins, as described previously.

Vessels that should respond optimally to PDL treatment are red telangiectases less than 0.2 mm in diameter, particularly those vessels arising as a function of telangiectatic matting after sclerotherapy (Fig. 42.3). This is based on the time of thermocoagulation produced by this relatively short-pulse laser system (see Table 42.1).

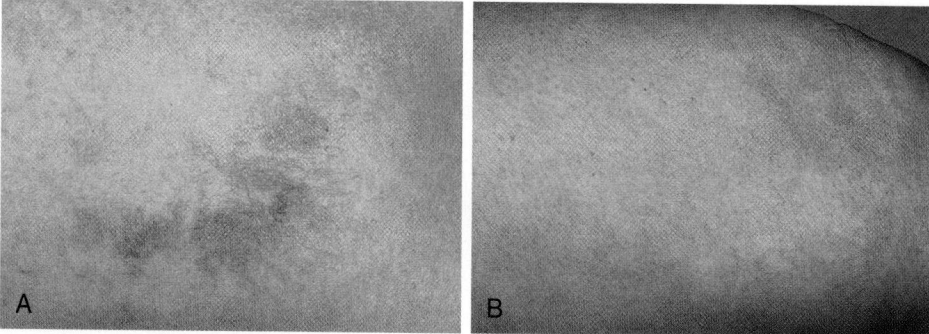

Fig. 42.3   Red telangiectasia. (A) Before treatment. (B) After treatment. (From Goldman: Sclerotherapy: Treatment of Varicose and Telangiectatic Leg Veins, ed 6. Philadelphia: Elsevier; 2017.)

In an effort to thermocoagulate larger-diameter blood vessels, the pulse duration of PDL has been lengthened to 1.5 to 40 ms and the wavelength increased to 595 nm. This theoretically permits more thorough heating of a larger vessel. These longer pulse durations are created by using two separate laser beams each emitting a 2.4-ms pulse. These lasers operate at 595 nm with an adjustable pulse duration from 0.5 to 40 ms delivered through a 5-, 7-, or 10-mm diameter spot size or an elliptical spot 3 by 10mm or 5 by 8 mm in diameter. Dynamic cooling with cryogen spray is also available, with the cooling spray adjustable from 0 to 100 ms given 10 to 40 ms after the laser pulse or as continuous 4°C air cooling at a variable speed. A fluence of 10 to 25 J/cm^2 can be delivered through a spot 3 by 10 mm or 5 by 8 mm in diameter.

We use the PDL at pulse durations matching the thermal relaxation time of the leg veins. The energy fluence used is just enough to produce vessel purpura or spasm. We use stacked pulses to achieve this clinical end point. Because of the need for multiple treatments and the significant occurrence of long-lasting hyperpigmentation, we reserve the use of PDL for sclerotherapy-resistant red telangiectases less than 0.2 mm in diameter.

Diode Lasers

Multiple *diode-pumped lasers* are now available, including 532-, 810-, 915-, and 940-nm lasers (Table 42.2). Diode lasers generate coherent monochromatic light through the excitation of small diodes. As a result, these devices are lightweight and portable with a relatively small desktop footprint. Diode laser therapy is more painful than sclerotherapy in almost all patients, with equal efficacy noted by the patients who had had both sclerotherapy and laser treatment. A combination diode laser at 915 nm with radiofrequency at levels up to 100 J/cm^2 has been used to treat leg telangiectasia.

Treatment with diode lasers is limited by the resultant pain and adverse effects. Of note, unless feeding reticular veins are treated, the distal treated telangiectases recur at 6 to 12 months posttreatment. Some authors appear to be able to achieve better results than others using similar parameters. The addition of RF to the diode appears to offer little advantage.

Intense Pulsed Light

The high-intensity pulsed-light source was developed as an alternative to lasers to maximize efficacy in treating leg veins (PhotoDerm VL; ESC/Sharplan, now Lumenis). This device permits sequential rapid pulsing, longer-duration pulses, and longer penetrating wavelengths than other laser systems. Theoretically, a phototherapy device that produces a noncoherent light as a continuous spectrum longer than 550 nm should have multiple advantages over a single-wavelength laser system. First, both oxygenated and deoxygenated hemoglobins absorb light at these wavelengths. Second, blood vessels located deeper in the dermis are affected. Third, thermal absorption by the exposed blood vessels should occur with less overlying epidermal absorption because the longer wavelengths penetrate deeper and are absorbed less by the epidermis.

With the theoretical considerations just mentioned, IPL emitting in the 515- to 1000-nm range was used at varying energy fluences (5 to 90 J/cm^2) and various pulse durations (2 to 25 ms) to treat venectases 0.4 to 2.0 mm in diameter. Clinical trials using various parameters with the IPL, including multiple pulses of variable duration, have demonstrated efficacy ranging from over 90% to total clearance in vessels less than 0.2 mm in diameter, 80% in vessels 0.2 to 0.5 mm, and 80% in vessels 0.5 to 1 mm in diameter. The incidence of adverse sequelae is minimal, with hypopigmentation occurring in 1% to 3% of patients and resolving within 4 to 6 months. Tanned or darkly pigmented patients with Fitzpatrick type III skin are more likely to develop hypopigmentation and hyperpigmentation in addition to blistering and superficial erosions. The choice of a cutoff filter is based on skin color, with a 550-nm filter used for light-skinned patients and a 570- or 590-nm filter for darker-skinned patients.

The use of IPL to treat leg veins has produced encouraging results, but these are far from being easily reproduced. Optimal use of this technology requires significant experience and surgical ability. Various parameters must be matched to the patient's skin type as well as to the diameter, color, and depth of the leg vein. With older machines that do not have integrated cooling through sapphire crystals, a cold gel must be placed between the IPL crystal and skin surface to provide optimal elimination of epidermal heat. Dozens of IPL units are now available from many manufacturers (see Table 42.2).

Long-Pulse Nd:YAG Laser (1064 nm)

The 1064-nm Nd:YAG laser is probably the most effective laser available to treat leg telangiectasia. In an effort to deliver laser energy to the depths of leg veins (often 1 to 2 mm beneath the epidermis) with thermocoagulation of vessels 1 to 3 mm in diameter, 1064-nm lasers with pulse durations between 1 and 250 ms have been developed. However, because of the poor absorption of deoxygenated and oxygenated hemoglobin with a 1064-nm wavelength, higher fluences must be used. Depending on the amount of energy delivered, the epidermis must be protected to minimize damage to pigment cells and keratinocytes (Fig. 42.4). Three mechanisms are available to minimize epidermal damage through heat absorption. First, the longer the wavelength, the less energy will be absorbed by melanocytes or melanosomes. This will allow darker skin types to be treated with minimum risks to the epidermis because of decreased melanin interaction. Second, delivering the energy with a delay in pulses greater than the thermal relaxation time for the epidermis

TABLE 42.2   Lasers and Light Sources for Leg Veins

Supplier	Product Name	Device Type	Wavelength (nm)	Energy (J)	Pulse Duration (ms)	Spot Diameter (mm)	Cooling
American Bio-Care	OmniLight FPL	Fluorescent pulsed light	480, 515, 535, 550, 580–1200	Up to 90	Up to 500		External continuous
Adept Medical	Ultrawave	Nd:YAG	1064	5–500	5–100	2, 4, 6, 8, 10, 12	None
Alderm	Prolite	IPL	550–900	10–50		10 × 20, 20 × 25	
Asclepion-Meditech	Pro Yellow	Copper bromide	578	55	300	1, 5	None
Candela	Vbeam	Pulsed dye	595	25	0.45–40	5, 7, 10, 12	DCD
	Cbeam	Pulsed dye	585	8–16	0.45	5, 7, 10	DCD
	Gentle YAG	Nd:YAG	1064	Up to 600	0.25–300		DCD
CoolTouch	Varia	Nd:YAG	1064	Up to 500	300–500	3–10	DCD
Cutera	Vantage	Nd:YAG	1064	Up to 300	0.1–300	3, 5, 7, 10	Copper contact
	XEO	Pulsed light	600–850	5–20	Automatic		None
Cynosure	PhotoGenica V	Pulsed dye	585	20	0.45	3, 5, 7, 10	Cold air
	PhotoGenica V-Star	Pulsed dye	585–595	40	0.5–40	5, 7, 10, 12	Cold air
	SmartEpill II	Nd:YAG	1064	1–200	Up to 100	2, 5, 7, 10	Cold air
	Acclaim 7000	Nd:YAG	1064	300	0.4–300	3, 5, 7, 10, 12	Cold air
	PhotoLight	Pulsed light	400–1200	3–30	5–50	46 × 18; 46 × 10	None
	Cynergie	Pulsed light + Nd:YAG	595 + 1064	20 + 160	0.5–40 + 0.3–300	7	Cold air
DDD	Ellipse	IPL	400–950	Up to 21	0.2–50	10 × 48	
DermaMed USA	Quadra Q4	Pulsed light	510–1200	10–20	60–200	33 × 15	None
Fotana	Dualis	Nd:YAG	1064	Up to 600	5–200	2–10	None
Iridex	Apex-800	Diode	800	5–60	5–100	7, 9, 11	Cooling handpiece
Laserscope	Lyra	Nd:YAG	1064	5–900	20–100	1–5 CA	Cooling handpiece
	Aura	KTP	532	1–240	1–50	1–5 CA	Cooling handpiece
	Gemini	KTP	532	Up to 100	1–100	1–5 CA	Cooling handpiece
		Nd:YAG	1064	Up to 990	10–100	1–5 CA	Cooling handpiece
Lumenis	Quantum	Pulsed light	515–1200				Cooled sapphire crystal
	Vasculite Elite	Pulsed light	515–1200	3–90	1–75	35 × 8	
		Nd:YAG	1064	70–150	2–48	6	Cooled sapphire crystal
	Lumenis One	Pulsed light	515–1200	10–40	3–100	15 × 35, 8 × 15	Cooled sapphire crystal
		Nd:YAG	1064	10–225	2–20	2 × 4, 6, 9	Cooled sapphire crystal
Med-Surge	Quantel Viridis	Diode	532	Up to 110	15–150		None
	Prolite II	Pulsed light	550–900	10–50		10 × 20, 20 × 25	
OpusMed	F1	Diode	800	10–40	15–40	5, 7	None
Orion Lasers	Harmony	Fluorescent pulsed light	540–950	5–20	10, 12, 15	40 × 16	None
		Nd:YAG	1064	35–145	40–60	6	None
		Nd:YAG	1064	35–450	10	2	None
Palomar	MediLux	Pulsed light	470–1400	Up to 45	10–100	12 × 12	None
	EsteLux	Pulsed light	470–1400	Up to 45	10–100	16 × 46	None
	StarLux	Pulsed light/Nd:YAG	550–670/870–1400/1064	Up to 700	0.5–500		
Quantel	Athos	Nd:YAG	1064	Up to 80	3.5	4	None
Sciton	Profile	Nd:YAG	1064	4–400	0.1–200		Contact sapphire crystal
	Profile BBL	Pulsed light	400–1400	Up to 30	Up to 200	30 × 30, 13 × 15	
Syneron	Aurora SR	Pulsed light/RF	580–980	10–30/2–25 RF	Up to 200	12 × 25	
	Polaris	Diode/RF	900	Up to 50/up to 100 RF			
	Galaxy	Diode	580–980	Up to 140/up to 100 RF	Up to 200		
WaveLight	Mydon	Nd:YAG	1064	10–450	5–90	11	Contact or cold air

CA, Continuous adjustable; *DCD*, dynamic cooling device; *KTP*, krypton triphosphate; *Nd:YAG*, neodymium-doped yttrium aluminum garnet; *RF*, radiofrequency.
Modified from Goldman MP. *Cosmetic and Cutaneous Laser Surgery*. Philadelphia: Mosby; 2006.

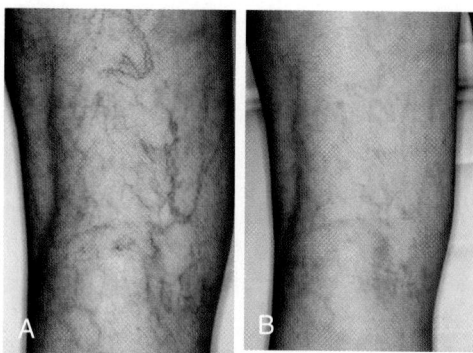

Fig. 42.4 Large leg veins. (A) Before treatment. (B) After treatment.

(1 to 2 ms) allows the epidermis to cool conductively between pulses. This cooling effect is enhanced by the application of cold gel on the skin surface, which conducts epidermal heat away more efficiently than air. Finally, the epidermis can be cooled directly, thus allowing the photons to pass through without generating enough heat to cause damaging effects.

Epidermal cooling can be provided in many different ways. The simplest method is continuous-contact cooling with chilled water, which can be circulated in glass, sapphire, or plastic housings. The laser impulse is given through the transparent housing, which should be constructed to ensure that the laser's effective fluence is not diminished. This method is referred to as *continuous-contact cooling*. Its benefit lies in its simplicity. The disadvantage is that the cooling effect continues throughout the time that the cooling device is in contact with the skin. This results in a variable degree and depth of cooling determined by the length of time the cold housing is in contact with the skin. This nonselective and variable depth and temperature of cooling may necessitate additional treatment energy, so that the cooled vessel will heat up sufficiently to thermocoagulate.

Another method of cooling is *contact precooling*. In this approach, the cooling device contacts the epidermis adjacent to the laser aperture. The epidermis is precooled and then treated as the handpiece glides along the treatment area. Because the cooling surface is not in the beam path, no optical window is required and better thermal contact can be made between the cooling device and the epidermis. The drawback is the nonreproducibility of cooling levels and degrees, which are based on the speed and pressure with which the practitioner uses the contact cooling device.

Yet another method for cooling the skin is to deliver a cold spray of refrigerant to the skin that is timed to precool the skin before laser penetration and also to postcool the skin to minimize thermal backscatter from the laser-generated heat in the target vessel. This method, along with continuous air cooling, reproducibly protects the epidermis and superficial nerve endings. In addition, it acts to decrease the perception of thermal-laser epidermal pain by providing another sensation (cold) to the sensory nerves. Finally, it allows for efficient use of laser energy because of the relative selectivity of the cooling spray, which can be limited to the epidermis.

Because the target vessel poorly absorbs the 1064-nm wavelength, a much higher fluence is necessary to cause thermocoagulation. Whereas a fluence of 10 to 20 J/cm² is sufficient to thermocoagulate blood vessels when delivered at 532 or 585 nm, a fluence of 70 to 150 J/cm² is required to generate sufficient heat absorption at 1064 nm. Various 1064-nm lasers are available that meet the criteria for selectively thermocoagulating blood vessels (see Table 42.2). All long-pulse 1064-nm Nd:YAG lasers are not the same. Variables include the spot size, laser output (in both fluence and how the long laser pulse is generated), pulse duration, and epidermal cooling.

I have found the 1064-nm long-pulse Nd:YAG lasers to be beneficial in the treatment of leg telangiectasia not responsive to sclerotherapy or other lasers. The advantage of using a 1064-nm laser

is that its longer wavelength can penetrate more deeply, allowing effective thermosclerosis of vessels up to 3 to 4 mm in diameter. In addition, the 1064-nm wavelength permits treatment of patients of skin types I to VI with or without a tan because melanin absorption is minimal. The 1064-nm long-pulse laser systems are not entirely without side effects. Cutaneous burns with resulting ulcerations, pigmentation, and telangiectatic matting have been observed with each of these systems as parameters are being tested. The dynamically cooled, 1064-nm Nd:YAG laser appears to produce the best clinical resolution with the least pain and adverse effects.

Combination/Sequential 595-nm Pulsed-Dye Laser and 1064-nm Nd:YAG (Cynergy)

The latest laser to enter the market uses a novel sequential 595-nm PDL pulse followed by a 1064-nm Nd:YAG laser pulse. The rationale for enhanced efficacy is that the 595-nm pulse generates methemoglobin, which is more strongly absorbed by 1064-nm wavelengths. Lower energies from both lasers can therefore be used, with the possibility of less pigmentation and adverse sequelae. Preliminary experience is promising in treating bright red vessels less than 0.1 mm in diameter, which are the most difficult vessels to treat with sclerotherapy.

CONCLUSIONS

Because sclerotherapy is still considered to be more effective than laser vein therapy and is relatively cost-effective compared with laser or IPL treatment, when is it appropriate to use the more advanced therapy? Obviously, needle-phobic patients will tolerate the use of this technology even though the pain from lasers and IPL is more intense than that from sclerotherapy with all but hypertonic solutions. Patients who are prone to telangiectatic matting from injected sclerosants are also appropriate candidates. Vessels below the ankle are particularly appropriate to treat with light because sclerotherapy has a relatively high incidence of ulceration in this area owing to the higher distribution of arteriovenous anastomoses. Finally, patients who have vessels that are resistant to sclerotherapy are excellent candidates. A 75% clearance rate with two to three IPL treatments has been documented in sclerotherapy-resistant vessels.

The optimal treatment plan for common leg telangiectasia includes sclerotherapy to treat the feeding venous system and laser or IPL to seal superficial very tiny vessels to prevent extravasation with resulting pigmentation, recanalization, and telangiectatic matting.

PATENT EDUCATION GUIDES

See patient consent form available at www.expertconsult.com.

ONLINE RESOURCES

The American Board of Laser Surgery. www.americanboardoflasersurgery.org.

RECOMMENDED READING

Adrian RM. Treatment of leg telangiectasias using a long. Pulse frequency. Doubled neodymium:YAG laser at 532 nm. *Dermatol Surg.* 1998;24:19–23.

Alam M, Silapunt S. *Procedures in Cosmetic Dermatology Series: Treatment of Leg Veins.* 2nd ed. Philadelphia: Saunders; 2010.

Bernstein EF. Clinical characteristics of 500 consecutive patients presenting for removal of lower extremity spider veins. *Dermatol Surg.* 2001;27:31–33.

Eremia S, Li CY. Treatment of leg and face veins with a cryogen spray variable pulse width 1064.nm Nd:YAG laser: a prospective study of 47 patients. *J Cosmet Laser Ther.* 2001;3:147–153.

Garden JM, Tan OT, Kerschmann R, et al. Effect of dye laser pulse duration on selective cutaneous vascular injury. *J Invest Dermatol.* 1986;87:653–657.

Goldman MP. Are lasers or non.coherent light sources the treatment of choice for leg veins? A look into the future. *Cosmet Dermatol.* 2001;14:58–59.

Goldman MP. Laser and sclerotherapy treatment of leg veins: my perspective on treatment outcomes. *Dermatol Surg.* 2002;28:969.

Goldman MP, Weiss RA. *Treatment of Varicose and Telangiectatic Leg Veins.* 5th ed. Philadelphia: Saunders; 2011.

Hruza G, Avram M. *Procedures in Cosmetic Dermatology Series: Lasers and Lights.* 3rd ed. Philadelphia: Elsevier; 2012.

Kaudewitz P, Kloverkorn W, Rother W. Treatment of leg vein telangiectasias: 1.year results with a new 940 nm diode laser. *Dermatol Surg.* 2002;28:1031–1034.

Lupton JR, Alster TS, Romero P. Clinical comparison of sclerotherapy versus long.pulsed Nd:YAG laser treatment for lower extremity telangiectases. *Dermatol Surg.* 2002;28:694–697.

Sadick NS. Long.term results with a multiple synchronized. Pulse 1064 nm Nd:YAG laser for the treatment of leg venulectasias and reticular veins. *Dermatol Surg.* 2001;27:365–369.

Sadick NS. Laser treatment with a 1064.nm laser for lower extremity class I.III veins employing variable spots and pulse width parameters. *Dermatol Surg.* 2003;29:916–919.

Sadick NS, Trelles MA. A clinical, histological, and computer. Based assessment of the Polaris LV, combination diode, and radiofrequency system, for leg vein treatment. *Lasers Surg Med.* 2005;36:98–104.

Schroeter CA, Wilder D, Reineke T, et al. Clinical significance of an intense, pulsed light source on leg telangiectasias of up to 1mm diameter. *Eur J Dermatol.* 1997;7:38–42.

Weiss MA, Weiss RA. Three year results with the long pulsed Nd:YAG 1064 laser for leg telangiectasia. *Presented at the Annual Meeting of the American Society for Dermatologic Surgery.* Dallas; 2001.

Weiss RA, Weiss MA. Early clinical results with a multiple synchronized pulse 1064 nm laser for leg telangiectasias and reticular veins. *Dermatol Surg.* 1999;25:399–402.

CHAPTER 43

LASERS: TATTOO REMOVAL

Kevin Crawford

Decorative tattoos have been a part of human history for thousands of years (Fig. 43.1). The recent discovery of a tattooed, frozen, early European more than 5000 years old in a glacier in Italy clearly supports this fact. If tattoos have been placed in the skin for over 5000 years, clinicians have likely been trying to remove them for the same length of time.

Currently 40% of Americans between the ages of 36 and 50 have tattoos. It is estimated that 50% or more of all people with tattoos will eventually want them removed completely. Approximately 40% of all tattoo removal patients do not want to remove all of the tattoo ink. In fact, they want only to change the existing tattoo and have a new tattoo placed over it.

TATTOO TYPES

Amateur tattoos or home tattoos are usually black, based on India ink. The carbon-based India ink dyes are, fortunately, the easiest to remove safely. Amateur tattoos are often placed in the dermis by simply dipping the end of a needle into the ink and then dotting the skin to form a design or pattern. The depth of the ink in the dermis is very irregular. Therefore the density and uniformity of the ink in the design are often very uneven (Fig. 43.2).

Professional tattoos are placed using a repetitively oscillating needle, which in skilled hands will place the ink at a relatively consistent depth in the dermis. Uniform depth can be an advantage for the removal process; therefore one would think that the removal of professional tattoos would have a more consistent success rate. However, with professional tattoos, the various colors and the density of the ink complicate the removal process (Fig. 43.3).

Cosmetic tattoos or permanent cosmetics such as lip liners, eyeliners, and eyebrow color enhancers pose unique challenges for removal because of their location and the variety of mixed colors (Fig. 43.4).

Traumatic tattoos are most often the result of an explosion (gunpowder embedded in the skin) or a bicycle or motorcycle accident (asphalt/tar embedded in the skin). Scar tissue often surrounds the embedded particles. The particles are not very deep and can usually be removed easily with a quality-switching (QS) laser (Fig. 43.5).

Although the mechanism of laser tattoo removal is not fully known, electron microscopy has demonstrated disrupted ink pigment particles in lysosomes after treatment of a tattoo with a QS laser. It is likely that the disrupted particles are then removed by macrophages through the lymphatic system. What is known is that very short bursts of high energy in the nanosecond or shorter wavelength range are needed to destroy tattoos. QS lasers are in this wavelength range and store a large amount of optical energy in the laser cavity through the use of an optical shutter. When a QS laser fires by opening the shutter, it is able to release a high-energy, short-wavelength pulse with an extremely short pulse duration. Lasers with even shorter pulse durations in the picosecond range, than the QS lasers, are now also being used. These are ideally suited for the removal of ink tattoo pigment particles, which all range in size between 40 and 300 nm, even smaller than melanosomes.

CONTRAINDICATIONS

Absolute

- Pregnancy
- Breastfeeding
- Known allergy to pigment
- Uncontrolled systemic disease
- Active untreated bacterial or viral infection in the area of the tattoo
- Use of Accutane in the preceding 6 months (this is controversial and may not be an issue)
- Immunosuppressive disorder

Relative

- Scarring abnormalities
- Bleeding abnormalities
- Hepatitis
- Poorly controlled diabetes mellitus
- Peripheral vascular disease
- Seizure disorder
- Unreasonable client expectations

FORMER TREATMENT METHODS

Until recently, all tattoo removal modalities caused disfiguring scars. In the past, the most popular options included salabrasion (salt-based dermabrasion), mechanical dermabrasion, CO_2 (continuous-wave) laser ablation, and infrared photocoagulation.

LASER TREATMENT AND REMOVAL

Fortunately the majority of tattoos are still predominantly composed of black ink. However, vibrant colors are becoming more popular and are more difficult to remove. There are three common QS lasers that are frequently used for removing tattoos: the *QS ruby laser* (QSRL; 694-nm red), the *QS Nd:YAG laser* (QSYL; both 1064-nm infrared and 532-nm [FD-QSYL] green wavelengths), and the *QS alexandrite* (QSAL; 755-nm red) laser. *QS*, sometimes known as *giant pulse formation*, is a technique by which a laser can be made to produce a pulsed output beam. This allows the production of light pulses with extremely high (gigawatt) peak power, much higher than would be produced by the same laser if it were operating in a continuous-wave (constant output) mode.

All three of these lasers have strong absorption by black ink. The color of the ink will determine the wavelength of laser needed (Fig. 43.6). The amount or density of the ink and the depth of the ink will determine the approximate number of treatments required. The QSYL has been the dominant laser used for removing tattoos. QSYLs, by design, produce shorter, higher-peak-power pulses than either QSRL, and the QSYL can also produce two very useful output wavelengths. HOYA Cynosure makes lasers with handpieces that convert the 532-nm wavelength to either 585 or 650 nm, effectively

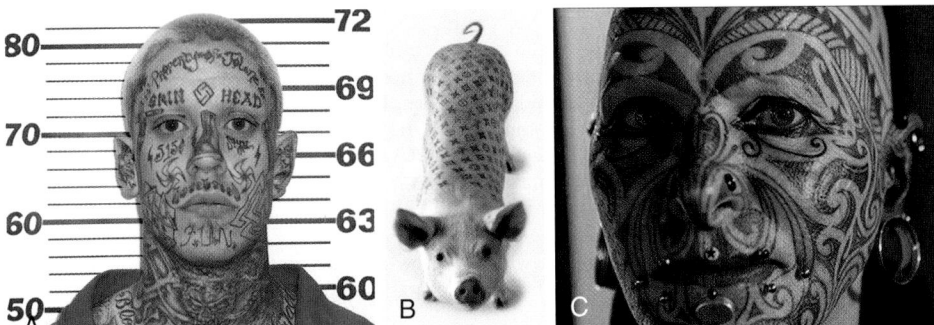

Fig. 43.1   (A) Prison tattoos, Utah State Prison. (B) Tattooed pig. (C) Tattoo convention, Berlin, 2007.

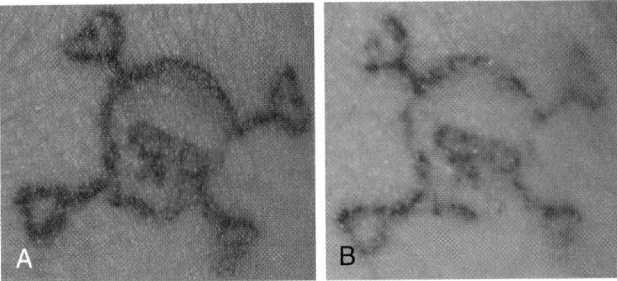

Fig. 43.2   Amateur tattoo. Before (A) and after (B) treatment with HOYA ConBio Revlite, 6.5 J, 6-mm spot size, 1064 nm.

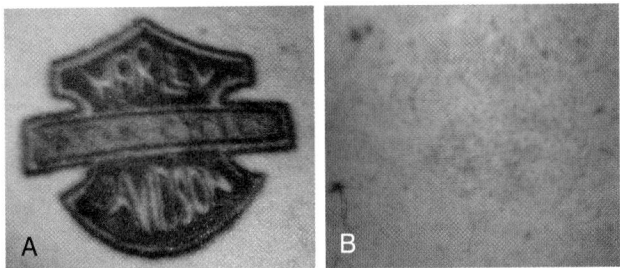

Fig. 43.3   Professional tattoo. Before (A) and after (B) seven treatments over 18 months with VersaPulse-C, 1 to 3 J, 3-mm spot size, 1064 and 532 nm.

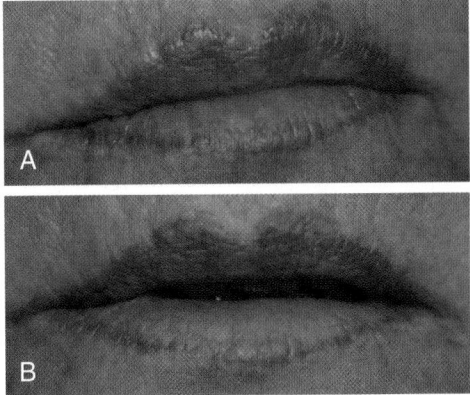

Fig. 43.4   Cosmetic tattoo. Before (A) and immediately after (B) one treatment with HOYA ConBio Revlite, 1.5 J, 4-mm spot size, 1064 nm.

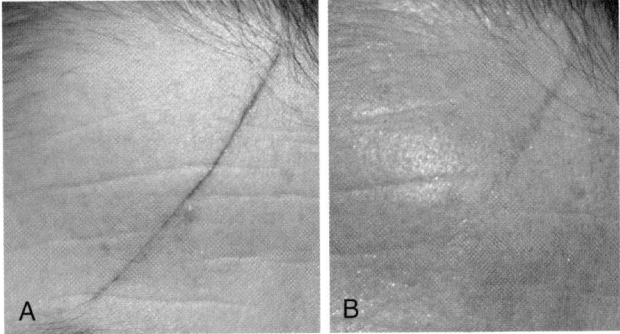

Fig. 43.5   Traumatic tattoo. Before (A) and after (B) 18 treatments over 24 months with VersaPulse-C, 1 to 3 J, 3-mm spot size, 1064 nm. (Courtesy Richard Burmeier, MD, Perfect Skin Laser Center, Tempe, Arizona.)

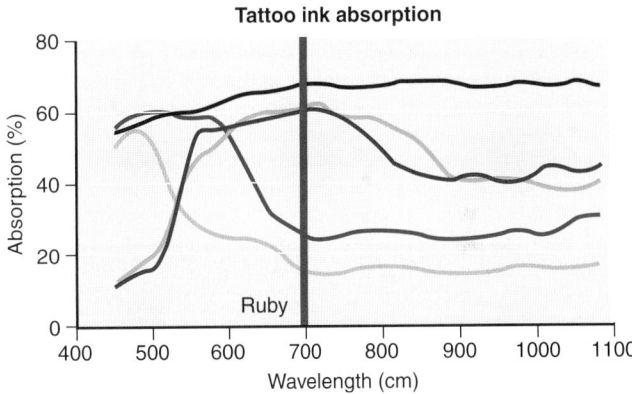

Fig. 43.6   Various wavelengths and absorption of different ink colors.

offering two additional wavelengths. Candela offers lasers with "laser-pumped-laser" technology and handpieces that convert the 755-nm wavelength to 532 or 1064 nm to purportedly improve removal of all tattoo colors. The choice of an appropriate laser may depend on the prevalence of the type/color of the majority of the

tattoos seen in the practice. The QSYL has become popular because of its ability to treat black, red, orange, yellow, and blue inks. The QSYL pulses faster than the ruby- or alexandrite-based laser, so more surface area can be treated in less time.

Predicting success for a particular tattoo is difficult. In general, amateur tattoos require 4 to 8 treatments; professionally placed tattoos call for 9 to 15 treatments for satisfactory removal. Using the QS 1064/532-nm ND:YAG and 755-nm alexandrite laser, prognostic factors for the clearance of professional tattoos were formally examined. Smoking, tattoos larger than 30 cm^2 and older than 36 months, location on the feet or legs, colors other than black or red, high color density, short intervals between treatments (<8 weeks), and darkening of the tattoo during treatment were all associated with reduced clearance. Green- and yellow-ink tattoos seemed to have the worst response. However, overall successful removal of tattoos with these lasers was 47.2% after 10 treatments and 74.8% after 15 treatments, respectively.

Lasers may be used for tattoo removal in patients of all skin types (Fitzpatrick types I through VI). However, patients with darker skin types (Fitzpatrick types IV through VI) are at higher risk for side effects, specifically hyperpigmentation and hypopigmentation.

PREPROCEDURE PATIENT PREPARATION

- Cleanse area of any makeup.
- Laser tattoo removal is painful. Clinicians may decide to apply a topical anesthetic with or without occlusion. If this is the case, the topical anesthetic cream must be applied for approximately 45 minutes to 1 hour before commencing treatment. Infiltrative anesthesia or nerve blocks can be used for larger tattoos (see Chapter 4, Topical Anesthesia; Chapter, 5 Local Anesthesia; and Chapter 7, Peripheral Nerve Blocks and Field Blocks). As an alternative to anesthetic creams or blocks, a flexible gel ice pack may be used. Apply ice packs for approximately 30 to 45 seconds before laser treatment. Use caution not to freeze the skin.

TECHNIQUE

1. For a given color of ink, choose the most appropriate laser based on wavelength and other characteristics (Table 43.1).
2. Limit the treatment area for any given treatment session. Normally the largest area treated at a given time is 24 to 30 square inches. If the tattoo area is larger, the client may come in biweekly to treat additional portions so that the entire tattoo can be treated every 6 to 8 weeks.
3. Start off with a lower power setting. Test a small area first to make sure settings on laser are working correctly. There are no set parameters to use with tattoo removal as to joules/power, just a range. Setting knowledge comes with time and experience (see Table 43.1).
4. Make sure everyone in the room has protective eyewear in place and that the door is closed.
5. Begin your treatment with the 1064-nm wavelength to treat the dark ink in the tattoo. The surface of the skin should turn a mild hazy white color each time the laser pulse strikes the skin. Some slight overlap is acceptable from pulse to pulse, but it is not advisable to repeatedly cover the same area, because once the skin turns white, it reflects subsequent laser pulses. If the tattoo ink

appears yellowish or brown immediately after the laser pulse, increase the fluence to obtain a white spot. **NOTE:** Dark tattoos with high concentrations of ink will require lower starting fluences and larger spot sizes than lighter, faded tattoos.

6. After completion of the pass over the black ink in the tattoo, the red ink can be treated with the 532-nm wavelength of the QSYL. As with the 1064-nm wavelength, the 532-nm pulses are applied evenly to the red areas of the tattoo until there is white color covering the entire treated area (Fig. 43.7). **NOTE:** Treating with 532 nm first will cause the skin to reflect the 1064-nm wavelength, thus minimizing successful treatment of the black ink.

COMMON ERRORS

- Overtreatment does not increase the speed of clearance of the tattoo and only increases the risk of negative side effects. It should be noted that it is very common for red ink to blister after treatment.
- In the mid-1990s, latex-based tattoo ink was introduced. This ink is vibrant from the first day it is placed in the dermis and the bright colors remain glossy. During the initial evaluation, the tattoo appears to have the appearance of high-gloss oil-based paint. This ink cannot be removed by any laser. It "shrinks" when heated with a laser, causing deep ulcerations that take months to heal and almost certainly resulting in deep, depressed scars.
- Cosmetic tattoos pose other problems. In general, cosmetic tattoos are black or dark red and are used to accentuate margins or borders. They include lip liners, eyeliners, and eyebrow enhancers. When treated with a high-powered QS laser, oxidation occurs and the ink turns black. When the red lip liner changes to a black lip liner, the patient becomes very disconcerted. The black ink tattoo can be removed and should be treated in the same way as any other black ink tattoo. In general cosmetic tattoos can be effectively cleared; however, care and a thorough consultation are very important.
- Titanium dioxide is a white ink that, when exposed to a QS pulse of light, can turn black. Gold atoms in some inks can change from gold to purple to black depending on the change in oxidation state. Again, subsequent treatments are usually successful in removing the changed ink color, but it is very disturbing to the patient to note such a dramatic change in color.

POSTPROCEDURAL CARE

- Normally there is erythema and edema immediately after treatment. Provide an ice pack/ice pillow after treatment to remove the heat from the treated area and reduce posttreatment discomfort.
- Ointments such as Aquaphor are applied to the treated area, which is covered if desired. If epidermal damage does occur, use topical ointments for moist healing to prevent scabbing of the wound (see patient education form for Chapter 25, Radiofrequency Surgery [Modern Electrosurgery], available at www.expertconsult.com).

TABLE 43.1	Laser Characteristics for Removal of Different Tattoo Ink Colors	
Ink Color	**Laser Characteristics***
New black or dark blue	1064 nm, 6 mm, 1.0–2.0 J
Faded black or dark blue	1064 nm, 4–6 mm, 3.0–6.4 J
Red/orange/yellow/purple	532 nm, 3 mm, 2.0–3.5 J
Faded red/orange/yellow/purple	532 nm, 3–4 mm, 2.0–4.0 J
Green	650 nm, 2 mm (preset)
Sky blue	585 nm, 2–3 mm (preset)

*Wavelength (nm), spot size (mm), energy level (J).

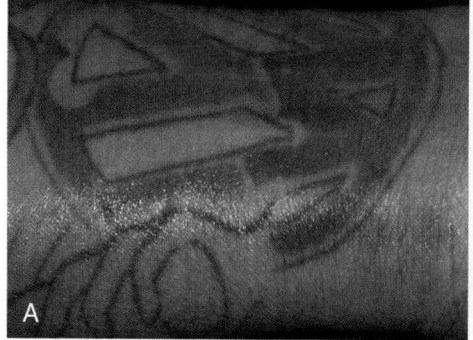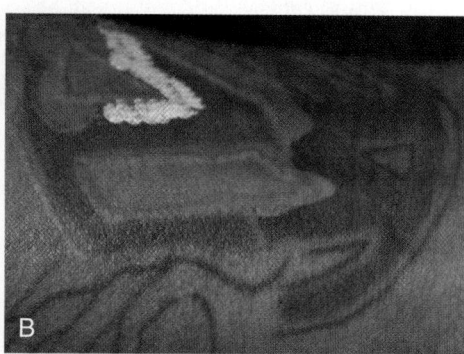

Fig. 43.7 Before (A) and during (B) treatment of red ink tattoo with Palomar Q-YAG 5, 1.5 J, 4-mm spot size, blended 1064/532 nm.

- In addition to the proper wound care, the prevention of sun exposure to the treated area is very important. Because the treated area has been traumatized by the laser pulses, the skin is more sensitive to hyperpigmentation by exposure to the sun. Encourage the use of a sun protection factor (SPF) 45 product during the entire treatment period. The accepted treatment interval is 6 weeks.
- Some clinicians feel that waiting 2 months or even longer between treatment sessions may be advantageous. Common sense says that it takes time for the macrophages to clean up the pigment after each treatment and prior to another treatment.

COMPLICATIONS

Although the treatment and removal of tattoos with QS lasers is considered a very safe procedure, potential side effects and risks do exist, including the following:

- Allergic reactions
- Blistering
- Infection
- Pain
- Swelling
- Scabbing
- Bleeding
- Itching
- Hypertrophic scarring
- Atrophic scarring
- Hyperpigmentation
- Hypopigmentation
- Incomplete tattoo removal
- Color changes in dyes

Allergic reactions to tattoo inks are occasionally seen. Red inks can produce very severe reactions in patients after QS laser treatments. After treatment of a red tattoo, in particular, patients often complain of itching. This is a sign of an allergic reaction to mercuric oxide in the tattoo ink. These patients should not be treated with a QS laser. Other, nondispersive methods of removal, such as surgical excision or erbium laser resurfacing, may be beneficial.

Although rare, hypertrophic and atrophic scarring is the most common complications associated with QS laser tattoo removal. In both cases, the scar formation can be attributed to overly aggressive treatment sessions or poor postoperative wound care by the patient. Keeping the wound clean and covered and preventing the wound from drying out and scabbing are of paramount importance. Conservative posttreatment wound care and strong patient compliance are the keys to preventing hypertrophic scarring.

Because the density of tattoo ink is always an unknown, the number of treatments necessary to remove a tattoo completely can only be estimated. Patients may become frustrated and impatient during the process. It is not uncommon to find tattoos or parts of tattoos that need greater than 10 treatment sessions, and some patients require 20 or more treatment sessions to remove very stubborn inks. As the number of treatment sessions increases, the degree of dermal fibrosis also increases and the texture of the skin changes as well. Patients must be aware of this.

Postinflammatory hyperpigmentation (PIH) should be considered a transient side effect related to the impact of the high-intensity laser pulse. PIH may fade on its own after the initial treatment, but the need to perform 7 to 10 treatments will, on average, increase the risk of developing PIH. Twice-daily treatment with hydroquinone and broad-spectrum sunscreens on fully healed skin usually resolve hyperpigmentation within a few months, although in some patients resolution can be prolonged. Overall, these changes usually resolve in 6 to 12 months. Patients with Fitzgerald skin types IV to VI are more likely to develop PIH and should be advised accordingly.

During treatment, portions of the treated area may completely lose pigmentation. This is a more significant problem in treating colored tattoos on darker skin types. When the tattoo removal treatment is completed and if the melanocytes are permanently disabled, the treated area will exhibit hypopigmentation or depigmentation in the same shape as the tattoo that was removed. If there are still active, nondamaged melanocytes in the treated area, it should slowly repigment after repeated sun exposure.

One of the most difficult problems to resolve is incomplete removal of the tattoo. If the majority of the ink is removed in the first five or six sessions, then extending the intervals between sessions to 12 to 16 weeks will benefit the patient because it will permit more clearance of the ink to take place. At a certain point, further treatments will yield minimal if any improvement and the decision to discontinue treatment can be made.

PATIENT EDUCATION GUIDES

See patient education and patient consent forms available at www.expertconsult.com.

SUPPLIERS

(See contact information available at www.expertconsult.com.)

Lasers for tattoo removal
AlexTriVantage, Candela Lasers
Q YAG 5, Palomar Medical Cynosure
Revlite and C6, HOYA ConBio Cynosure
Versapulse, Lumenis
VRM 3, Lutronic

Dealers offering used lasers
www.hotlasers.com/
www.medproonline.com/
www.thelaseragent.com/

RECOMMENDED READING

Alster TS. Q-switched alexandrite laser treatment (755 nm) of professional and amateur tattoos. *J Am Acad Dermatol.* 1995;33:69–73.

Anderson RR, Parrish JA. Selective photothermolysis: precise microsurgery by selective absorption of pulsed radiation. *Science.* 1983;220:524–527.

Bencini PL, Cazzaniga S, Tourlaki A, et al. Removal of tattoos by Q-switched laser: variables influencing outcome and sequelae in a large cohort of treated patients. *Arch Dermatol.* 2012;148:1364–1369.

Dirks M. Making innovative tattoo ink products with improved safety: possible and impossible ingredients in practical usage. *Curr Probl Dermatol.* 2015;48:118–127.

Greveling K, Prens EP, Liu L, van Doorn MB. Non-invasive anaesthetic methods for dermatological laser procedures: a systematic review. *J Eur Acad Dermatol Venereol epub.* 2017.

Hruza G, Avram M. *Procedures in Cosmetic Dermatology Series: Lasers and Lights.* 3rd ed. Philadelphia: Elsevier; 2012.

Kirby W, Kartono F, Small R. Tattoo removal with lasers. In: Usatine RP, Pfenninger JL, Stulberg DL, Small R, eds. *Dermatologic and Cosmetic Procedures in Office Practice.* Philadelphia: Elsevier; 2012:367–376.

Kauvar A, Hruza G. *Principles and Practices in Cutaneous Laser Surgery.* New York: Taylor and Francis; 2005.

Kilmer SL, Lee MS, Anderson RR. Treatment of multi-colored tattoos with a frequency doubled Q-switched Nd:YAG laser: a dose-response study with comparison to the Q-switched ruby laser. *Lasers Surg Med.* 1993;(suppl 5):54.

Levine V, Geronemus RG. Tattoo removal with the Q-switched ruby laser and the Q-switched ND: YAG laser: a comparative study. *Cutis.* 1995;55:291–296.

Naga LI, Alster TS. Laser Tattoo Removal: an Update. *Am J Clin Dermatol.* 2017;18:59.

Pritzker RN, Iyengar V, Rohrer TE, Arndt KA. Laser treatment of tattoos and pigmented lesions. In: Robinson JK, Hanke CW, Siegel DM, Fratila A, Bhatia AC, Rohrer TE, eds. *Surgery of the Skin.* 3rd ed. Philadelphia: Elsevier; 2015.

Ross V, Naseef G, Lin G, et al. Comparison of responses to picosecond and nanosecond Q-switched ND: YAG lasers. *Arch Dermatol.* 1998;134:167–171.

CHAPTER 44

FRACTIONAL LASER SKIN RESURFACING

Gregory A. Buford

HISTORY OF LASER RESURFACING

Facial aging follows a rather predictable course. As we age, our skin thins and becomes translucent, the collagen fibers in the deep dermis diminish in number and become more randomly organized, and pigmentary changes appear in more superficial layers as a result of years of actinic damage. Some of these changes can be ameliorated or reversed. To do so, the skin must be injured in a predictable manner that stimulates it to reorganize and rejuvenate during the healing process. Chemical peels, microdermabrasion, and laser rejuvenation have been used successfully in the past, but each has its own inherent advantages and disadvantages. In this chapter we focus on laser resurfacing and, most important, fractional laser resurfacing.

Lasers were developed in 1960 on the foundation of Einstein's quantum theory of radiation. Over time, the use of different lasing media allowed for the development of specific lasers and ultimately specific applications. Ablative laser resurfacing was first introduced in the 1990s with the advent of the CO_2 laser; soon thereafter, the erbium-doped yttrium aluminum garnet (Er:YAG) laser was released.

Although these two lasers formed the foundation of ablative resurfacing, they provided slightly different outcomes with respect to treatment efficacy, downtime, and risk for adverse events. The shorter wavelength of the erbium laser (2940 nm) versus the CO_2 laser (10,600 nm) allowed for more effective absorption of laser energy by water and thus a significantly higher absorption coefficient (Er = 12,000 vs. CO_2 = 800). As such, residual thermal damage was significantly less with use of the erbium laser than with the CO_2 laser. In addition, faster reepithelialization was noted with the erbium laser. But were these advantages necessarily decisive? Perhaps not—although the erbium laser has been associated with less downtime and erythema and a faster recovery, its overall results have been less dramatic than those attained with use of the CO_2 laser.

In response to the prolonged downtime associated with traditional ablative resurfacing, which is quite aggressive, a number of nonablative technologies were developed, with the aim to provide noninvasive facial rejuvenation but to do so with minimal to no downtime. Technologies such as intense pulsed light, radiofrequency lasers, and infrared lasers were ultimately developed. While the downtime with these devices was definitely less, the overall results also were less impressive.

The next evolution of laser technology, around 2004, involved reintroduction of the erbium laser but in a "fractional pattern," with the first device to pioneer this technology being the Fraxel Laser (Solta Medical, Inc.). Fractionated resurfacing uses many small, separate columns of light to create microthermal treatment zones with bridges of untreated tissue in between. In the case of the Lumenis Ultrapulse Encore, spot size varies from 0.12 mm (DeepFX) to 1.3 mm (ActiveFX) and can be applied in a square, rectangular, linear, or other shaped configuration. The treated area appears as many small ablated "dots," as opposed to a single large, homogeneous ablated area. By leaving areas untouched, treated areas heal faster because of ingrowth from the surrounding untreated zones. The result is dramatic improvement with significantly less downtime.

Although fractionated erbium laser technology was a significant step ahead of its predecessors, the disadvantages were also clear. Most patients were seeing improvement, but it came at the cost of at least three to five treatment sessions. So although downtime was minimal, the overall duration of therapy was prolonged. Eventually, fractional technology was extended to a CO_2 platform, which then allowed for more effective rejuvenation in as little as one treatment.

BASICS OF LASER THERAPY

Ablative devices such as the CO_2 and erbium laser use water as a target chromophore. As previously noted, the erbium wavelength is nearly 20 times more highly absorbed than the CO_2 wavelength. This difference effectively differentiates the two lasers. The absorbed laser energy then exerts two effects on the treated tissue: ablation and coagulation. *Ablation* involves actual destruction and removal/vaporization of tissue, and can be beneficial in improving the superficial tone, texture, and appearance of the skin. *Coagulation*, on the other hand, is the result of heat transference to the tissue and is thought to encourage collagen remodeling and ultimately tissue tightening.

The amount of ablation and coagulation is controlled by the amount of laser fluence (power) and pulse duration (or pulse width; length of time power is applied). Short pulse durations and high fluence produce greater ablation, whereas longer pulse widths and lower fluencies emphasize coagulation. Settings can therefore be individualized for the desired patient outcome.

The percentage of skin treated is dictated by the density setting. Higher density settings affect a greater area within a specific treatment zone (i.e., the columns of light energy are closer together) and can be especially effective for dyschromias. The downside is that there may be a prolonged healing time, depending on the chosen fluence, because there are fewer untreated skin islands surrounding treated areas.

Although there are basic recommendations for treatment parameters for each device, in reality there is considerable variation among practitioners (Table 44.1). In the beginning stages, it is best to incorporate more conservative settings and accept the potential need for additional treatment, versus using more aggressive settings with the greater potential for complications.

PATIENT SELECTION

Patient education and selection are essential for achieving optimal results with fractional laser resurfacing. Fitzpatrick skin type classification is a basic way to identify patients at higher risk for pigmentary changes associated with laser resurfacing (see Chapter 35). Lighter-skinned patients (Fitzpatrick types I to III) are at lowest risk for postprocedure pigmentary changes, whereas darker-skinned patients (Fitzpatrick types IV and V) are at a much higher risk. Although darker-skinned patients can still be treated, more conservative settings must be chosen, and they must be carefully counseled about the specific risks they may encounter.

Continued

TABLE 44.1   Fractional Technologies Comparison Chart

Supplier Product Name	Device Type	Wavelength	Energy Output	Pulse Length	Price	Accessories
Alma Lasers						
Pixel 2940	Fractional Er:YAG handpiece for Harmony^{XL} system	2940 nm	2500 mJ/p	N/A	Contact manufacturer	Pixel 2940 handpiece
Pixel CO$_2$	Fractional CO$_2$ system	10,600 nm	30 W	N/A	$69,900	7 × 7 and 9 × 9 pixels array handpieces, two surgical handpieces
Pixel Omnifit	Pixelized handpiece for existing CO$_2$ systems	10,600 nm	N/A	N/A	$34,900	7 × 7 and 9 × 9 pixels array configuration
Cutera, Inc.						
Pearl Fractional	Fractional 2,790 nm YSGG	2,790 nm	60–320 mJ per microspot	600 ms	Contact manufacturer	Smoke evacuator connector
Cynosure						
Affirm CO$_2$	CO$_2$ with scanner	10,600 nm	30 W	0.2–20 ms ablative, 0.2–2 ms microablative	Contact manufacturer	Scanner (microablative and full ablative)
Eclipse, Ltd.						
SmartXide Dot	CO$_2$ laser and scanner system	10,600 nm	30 W	0.2–80 ms	Contact Eclipse	Scanner offers standard or dot scanning mode
Ellipse, A/S						
Juvia	Fractional CO$_2$ laser	10,600 nm	0.1–15 W	N/A	Contact manufacturer	Truly flexible fiber delivery Built-in parameter controls on handpiece Adjustable scan dwell times: 2 ms, 3 ms, 4 ms, 5 ms, 6 ms, 7 ms Scan density: 7 × 7; 9 × 9; 11 × 11 MTZ/cm^2 Scan area: 1 cm^2; MTZ (spot) size: 500 μm No consumables
Focus Medical						
NaturaLase Er	Er:YAG	2940 nm	Up to 24 J/cm^2	350 ms	$74,900	Fractional handpiece with system 100–150 μm spots size Up to 8 Hz
Lasering USA						
MiXto SX	CO$_2$ laser	10.6 nm	0.5–30 W	2.5–16 ms	$79,000	Patent pending MiXto SX fractional scanner system 300 μm spot scanner for optimal heat delivery and collagen production 5%–40% density adjustment Optional 180 μm spot scanner for deep ablation and skin tightening
Velure S5 MiXto VX	Diode laser	532 nm	0.1–5 W	10–1000 ms	$53,900	MiXto VX fractional scanner Focusing handpieces with spot sizes of 0.3 mm, 0.5 mm, 1.5 mm

TABLE 44.1   Fractional Technologies Comparison Chart—cont'd

Supplier Product Name	Device Type	Wavelength	Energy Output	Pulse Length	Price	Accessories
Lumenis						
UltraPulse ActiveFX	Fractional CO$_2$ laser	10,600 nm	1–225 mJ	<1 ms	Contact manufacturer	Single, minimal downtime treatment for wrinkle/pigment results
UltraPulse DeepFX	Fractional CO$_2$ laser	10,600 nm	2.5–50 mJ	<1 ms	Contact manufacturer	Fractional CO$_2$ treatment for wrinkles, scars, and deep collagen treatment
UltraPulse TotalFX	Fractional CO$_2$ laser	10,600 nm	1–225 mJ	<1 ms	Contact manufacturer	Blended fractional CO$_2$ treatment for customized patient outcomes
Lutronic						
eCO2	CO$_2$ laser	10.6 mm	240 mJ	10.56 ms	Contact manufacturer	
Palomar Cynosure						
StarLux 500 Platform						
Lux2940 Fractional	2,940 laser	2,940 nm	N/A	N/A	Contact manufacturer	
Lux1540 Fractional Laser handpiece	1540 laser	1540 nm	Up to 70 mJ per microbeam	1–500 ms	Contact manufacturer	
LuxDeepIR Fractional Infrared handpiece	Infrared light	850–1350 nm	Up to 175 J	2.5–10 s	Contact manufacturer	
Sandstone Cynosure Medical Technologies						
Matrix LS.25	CO$_2$ laser	10,600 nm	25 W	Adjustable to 100 ms	$50,000	Ultrafine FS Fractional Scanner, 150 mm focusing handpiece
UltraFine.FS Fractional Scanner	Fractional scanner (adapts to most CO$_2$ lasers)	10,600 nm	N/A	N/A	$19,995	Fractional scanner
Sciton						
ProFractional.XC	Tunable laser 2940 µm	2940 µm	Up to 400 J/cm^2	Variable	Contact manufacturer	Expandable module
ProFractional	Tunable laser 2940 µm	2940 µm	Up to 400 J/cm^2	Variable	Contact manufacturer	Expandable module/density 1.5%–60%
Solta Medical						
Fraxel re:store	Erbium-fiber laser	1550 nm	4–70 mJ/MTZ	N/A	Contact manufacturer.	Intelligent Optical Tracking System (IOTS) / Variable optical spot size using telescope / Maximizes lesion depth for a chosen pulse energy / Ergonomic handpiece and roller tip
Fraxel re:fine	Single mode fiber laser	1410 nm	5–20 mJ/MTZ	N/A	Contact manufacturer	Same as above / Built-in smokeless evacuation system / IOTS
Fraxel re:pair	Fractional CO$_2$ laser	10,600 nm	5–70 mJ/MTZ	N/A	Contact manufacturer	Ergonomic handpiece and roller tip
Syneron Candela						
eMatrix Matrix RF	Radiofrequency electrical energy	N/A	Up to 20 J	N/A	Contact manufacturer	Spot size 12 × 12 mm, 3-year warranty
eMax Matrix RF						
eLight Matrix RF						
eLaser Matrix RF						

Data subject to change; please refer to Suppliers section for supplier contact information. Not all devices are FDA cleared for the application(s) indicated. From The Aesthetic Guides, January–February 2009. www.miinews.com.

MTZ, Microthermal treatment zone.

The most important area of patient education, however, is in the identification of expectations. Although laser resurfacing can achieve some degree of skin tightening and improve tone and texture, it is no replacement for surgical intervention in the patient who really needs a facelift or necklift. Sagging skin and jowling are surgical problems and cannot effectively be addressed with laser resurfacing alone. Using various combinations of procedures, however, these patients can often achieve synergistic results that go far beyond either intervention (surgical or nonsurgical) alone. In addition, realistic healing and recovery time must be discussed with the patient, as well as the need for patience while waiting for final results, which may take 4 to 6 months. Proper patient selection before treatment is essential for achieving optimal results and can generally allow one to avoid many of the pitfalls associated with unrealistic expectations.

INDICATIONS

- Laser resurfacing can be an effective means for treating the following age-related conditions:
  - *Dyschromias (pigment changes)*: Areas of hyperpigmentation can effectively be addressed with fractional resurfacing. Because only light treatment settings are required, the downtime is often as short as 2 to 3 days (Fig. 44.1).
  - *Textural changes*: As aged skin is replaced with new tissue, there is diminishment in the wrinkled, crepey appearance because the collagen matrix is stimulated to regenerate and reorganize (Figs. 44.2 and 44.3).
  - *Fine lines and wrinkles*: Improvement in fine lines and wrinkles has been noted after laser resurfacing, but improvement is known to be enhanced after pretreatment with botulinum toxin type A. With movement stabilized in the

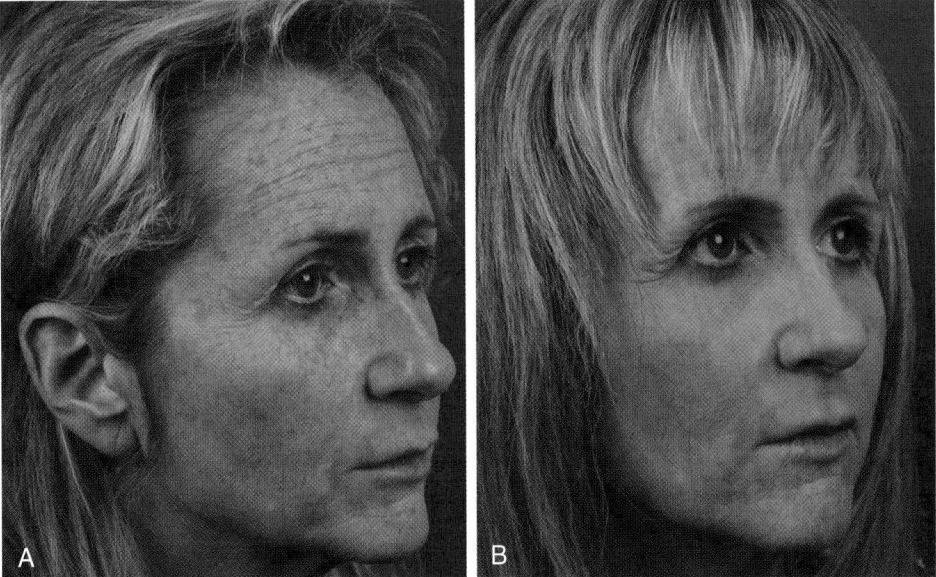

Fig. 44.1 Treatment of dyschromias using a Lumenis Ultrapulse Encore Laser. ActiveFX: 100 mJ, 600 Hz, density 100%, single pass; DeepFX: 12.5 mJ, 300 Hz, density 15%, single pass. (A) Before treatment. (B) Three months after treatment. (Courtesy Gregory A. Buford, MD, FACS, Denver, Colorado.)

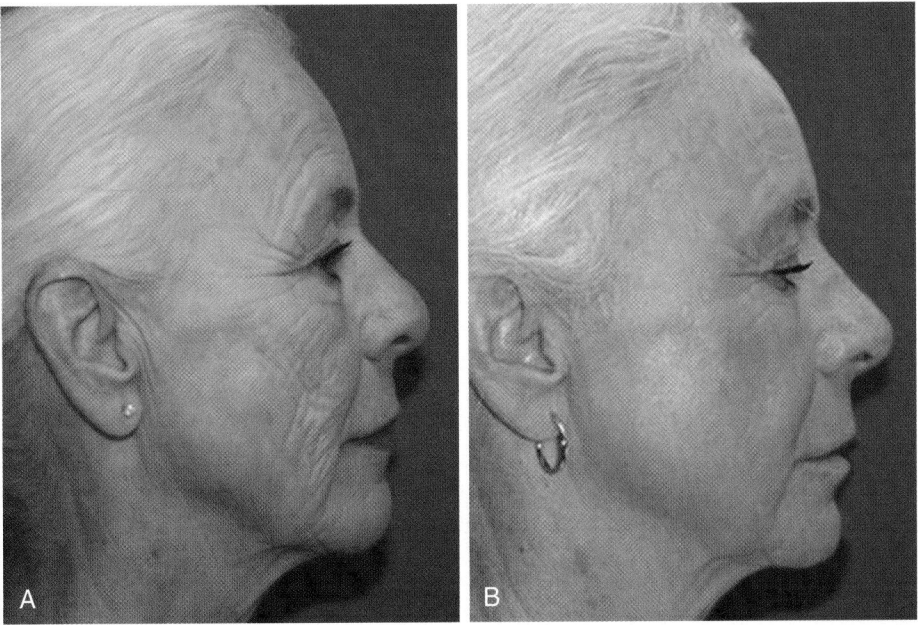

Fig. 44.2 Treatment of coarse lines and wrinkles and crepey skin using a Lumenis Ultrapulse Encore Laser. ActiveFX: 125 mJ, 125 Hz, density 82%, double pass. (A) Before treatment. (B) After treatment. (Courtesy Robert Bushman, MD, La Mesa, California.)

treated areas, the newly regenerated skin is allowed to heal in a more stable environment (Fig. 44.4).

- *Dilated pores*: Many patients notice refinement of pore size, although this effect may take upward of 6 months to fully achieve.
- *Scars (surgical vs. traumatic vs. acne vs. burns)*: By effectively planing down the scar and stimulating collagen remodeling, fractional resurfacing can have a beneficial effect on the appearance of scars from a variety of sources (Figs. 44.5 through 44.9).
- *Stretch marks (questionable efficacy)*: Although results are variable, some practitioners report improvement in the appearance of stretch marks; however, there are very few well-controlled studies in this area.

CONTRAINDICATIONS

Absolute

- Keloid formers
- Active bacterial or viral skin infection
- Use of isotretinoin in the past 12 months
- Scleroderma
- Prior radiation therapy to area
- History of localized poor healing
- Melanoma or identified lesions suspect for skin cancer in area to be treated
- Ectropion

- Vitiligo
- History of noncompliance with previous treatments

Relative

- Impaired immune system or known autoimmune disease
- Collagen vascular disorder
- Lower lid laxity
- Photosensitizing medications
- Fitzpatrick skin type IV or V

PRETREATMENT PATIENT EVALUATION

- *Skin type classification*: Fitzpatrick skin type classification should be determined before treating any patient with fractional or nonfractional laser resurfacing (see Chapter 35). Darker skin types are at a higher risk for long-term pigmentary changes even with fractional technology, so the degree and number of treatments should be adjusted accordingly.
- *Current medications*: Any medications that will delay or impede wound healing should be discontinued before laser resurfacing.
- *Previous treatment with lasers or deep chemical peels*: Prior treatment with either deep chemical peels or lasers in the same area should be considered before retreatment, given the potential for delayed or impaired healing.

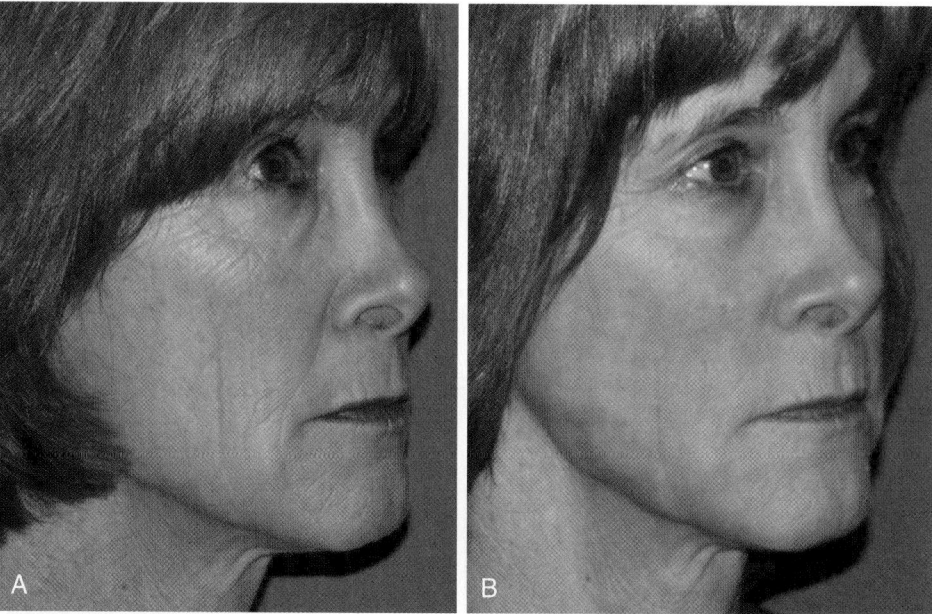

Fig. 44.3   Treatment of coarse lines and wrinkles and crepey skin using a Lumenis Ultrapulse Encore Laser. ActiveFX: 125 mJ, 100 Hz, density 82%, single pass. (A) Before treatment. (B) One month after treatment. (Courtesy Gregory A. Buford, MD, FACS, Denver, Colorado.)

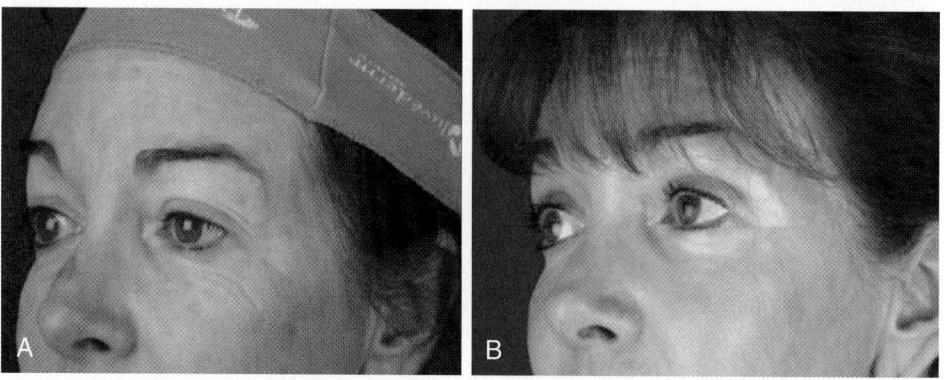

Fig. 44.4   Treatment of fine lines and wrinkles (periorbital area) using a Lumenis Ultrapulse Encore Laser. ActiveFX: 90 mJ, 125 Hz, density 68%, single pass; DeepFX: 12.5 mJ, density 5%, single pass. (A) Before treatment. (B) Three months after treatment. (Courtesy Gregory A. Buford, MD, FACS, and Beryl Reker, PMA, Denver, Colorado.)

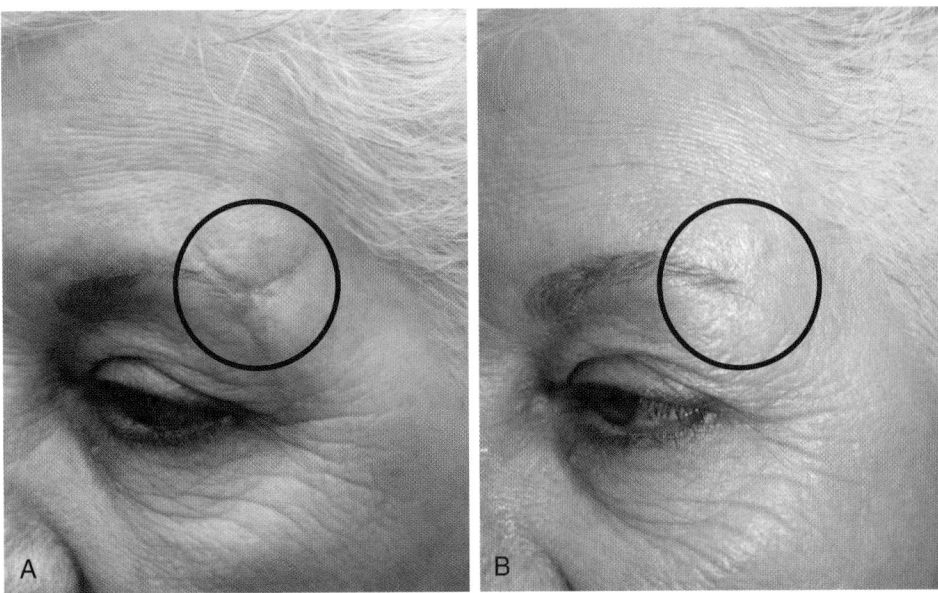

Fig. 44.5 Laser scar revision using a Lumenis Ultrapulse Encore Laser. Treatment settings not available. (A) Before treatment. (B) After treatment. (Courtesy Joseph Niamtu III, DMD, Richmond, Virginia.)

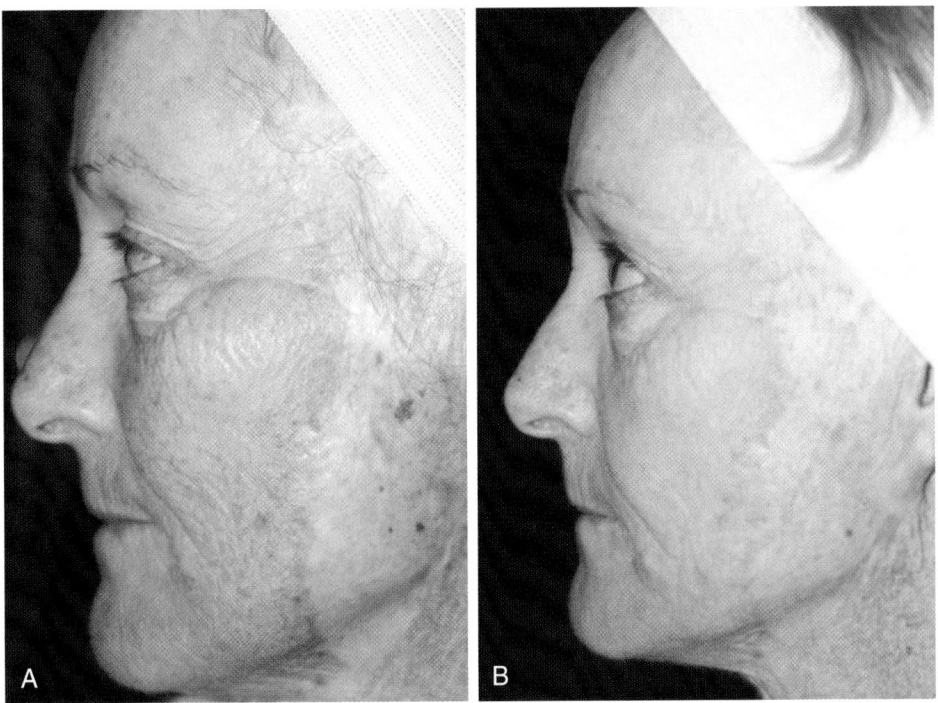

Fig. 44.6 Laser scar revision using a Lumenis Ultrapulse Encore Laser. ActiveFX: 80 mJ, 55% coverage, single pass; DeepFX: 12.5 mJ, 15% coverage, single pass. (A) Before treatment. (B) After treatment. (Courtesy Jill Waibel, MD, West Palm Beach, Florida.)

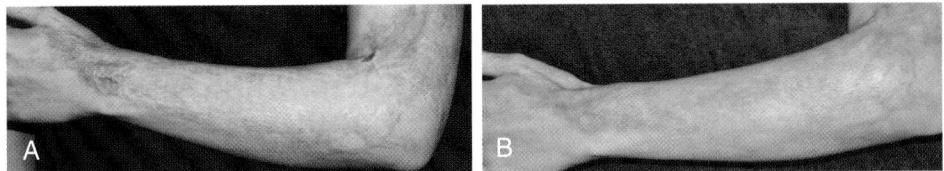

Fig. 44.7 Laser scar revision using a Lumenis Ultrapulse Encore Laser. Treatment settings not available. (A) Patient's arm with 20-year-old burn scar. (B) After treatment. (Courtesy Jill Waibel, MD, West Palm Beach, Florida.)

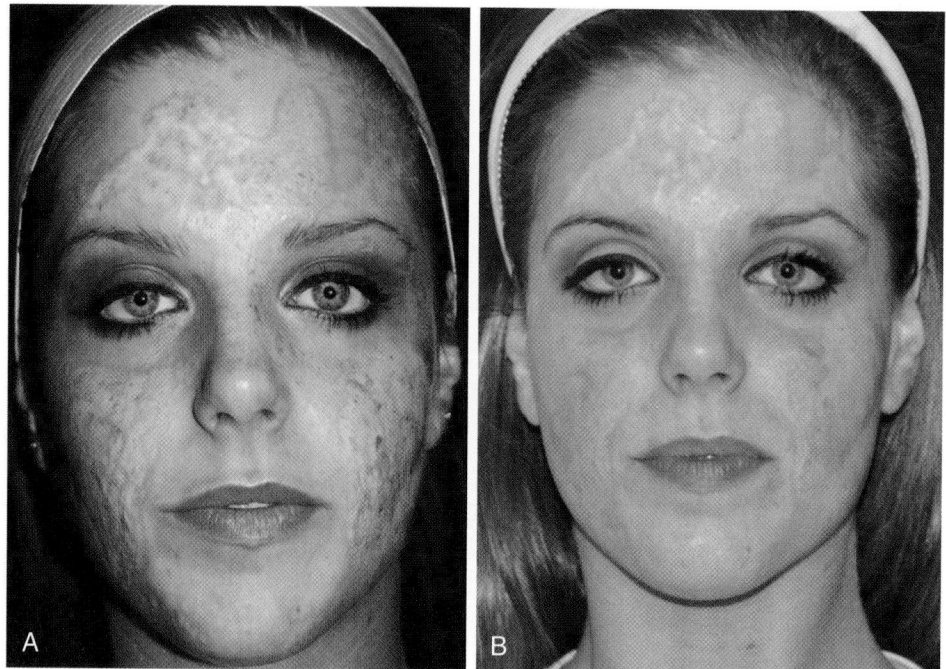

Fig. 44.8 Laser scar revision using a Lumenis Ultrapulse Encore Laser. Treatment settings not available. (A) Before treatment. (B) Seven months after treatment. (Courtesy Jill Waibel, MD, West Palm Beach, Florida.)

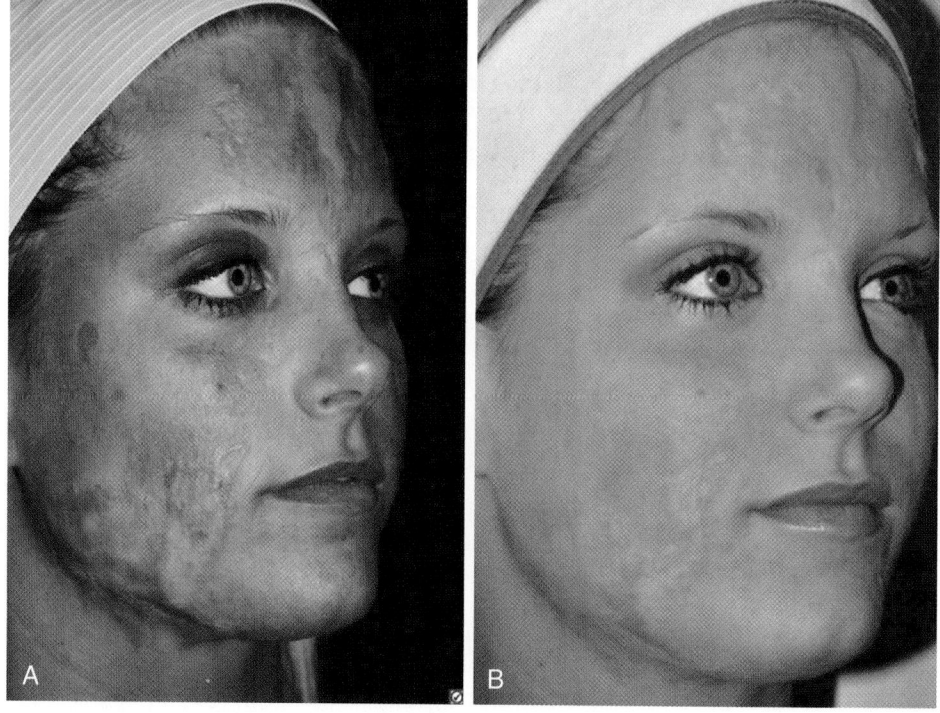

Fig. 44.9 Laser scar revision using a Lumenis Ultrapulse Encore Laser. Treatment settings not available. (A) Before treatment. (B) Seven months after three total treatments using TotalFX. (Courtesy Jill Waibel, MD, West Palm Beach, Florida.)

- *Desired end result*: One of the most critical variables in success is patient expectation, so it is important to have an open and honest discussion with each patient before moving forward with any aesthetic procedure. Managing expectations before treatment will better prepare your patient for outcome in both the short and long term. Speak candidly and honestly about the following:
- Number of treatments
  - Anticipated costs
  - Recovery time
  - Degree of discomfort

- *Pretreatment/posttreatment protocol* (e.g., skin care products, patient instructions): The outcome of any aesthetic procedure is often the result not only of the success of the procedure itself but of the patient's compliance with recommended protocol instructions before and after the treatment. This is especially true with laser resurfacing. Although some experts dispute the importance of an individualized and guided medical skin care regimen before the laser procedure, most agree that it is essential during the healing period.
- *Adjunctive treatment with botulinum toxin type A*: As demonstrated by multiple authors, treatment with botulinum toxin type A

allows for more optimal and potentially sustained results when undertaken before laser resurfacing. As one study supports, the practice effectively prevents dynamic facial muscular action in treated areas and potentially minimizes the reestablishment of expressive wrinkles and folds.

- *Discussion of risks/benefits and informed consent:* As with any procedure, informed consent must be obtained after discussion with the patient of associated risks and benefits. Be realistic in describing downtime and discomfort, with the understanding that there is a degree of variation depending on individual patient characteristics, treatment settings, and the specific device used.
- *Pretreatment photographs:* The importance of pretreatment photographs cannot be overemphasized. Aside from the ability to document degree of improvement from the pretreatment to posttreatment stages, taking photographs of your patients also provides you a means with which to educate other patients on the efficacy of these procedures.

BEFORE THE PROCEDURE

The laser treatment itself must be performed by a trained laser professional under medical supervision. State laws dictate the actual degree of medical supervision and who can actually perform the procedure.

Pain control should be addressed and individualized, and is really a factor of four variables.

1. Patient pain tolerance
2. Specific device
3. Depth of treatment
4. Area of treatment

With other rejuvenative procedures, some patients require very little analgesia, whereas others have less tolerant pain thresholds. The key is to understand the average patient's needs, begin there, and then fine-tune accordingly. It is always better to make your patients more comfortable than less because their experience will largely be shaped not only by the outcome they eventually receive but by the initial experience they perceive.

A variety of methods can be used to manage pain in an office setting:

- *Topical anesthesia:* For all fractional laser treatments, this is the foundation of pain management and may include a wide variety of topical agents. A frequently used compounded combination is a 23% lidocaine/7% tetracaine cream, which is applied 45 to 60 minutes before treatment. As with any treatment, check for potential allergic reactions before proceeding and watch for signs and symptoms of toxicity. Although with facial resurfacing there is less risk than with extended treatment areas (e.g., laser hair removal), the risk is not zero, and so all patients must be observed for evidence of impending toxicity and a resuscitation plan must be in place before any treatment is begun.
- *Nerve blocks* (see Chapters 7 and 8): For more aggressive treatments around the mouth, infraorbital and mental nerve blocks can be used. One milliliter of 2% lidocaine with epinephrine per injection is extremely effective in achieving an acceptable degree of patient comfort. However, warn the patient when transitioning from a blocked to a nonblocked area. Pain control can be so effective using blocks that it can make the transition to an area where only a topical anesthetic was used significantly more sensitive.
- *Oral medications:* Although many practitioners combine some type of either narcotic or nonnarcotic (e.g., nonsteroidal anti-inflammatory drugs) pain medication with an anxiolytic for their pain management program, it does more to manage acute anxiety than pain. As such, a light anxiolytic (diazepam) may be best so that the patient is still aware of her or his surroundings but, at the same time, lightly relaxed.

PREPARING FOR THE TREATMENT (AT LEAST 1 WEEK PRIOR)

- Discuss and obtain informed consent from the patient (see the sample consent form available at www.expertconsult.com).
- Review all written postprocedure wound care instructions with the patient and encourage her or him to call the office for any concerns or suspicion of poor healing associated with the treatment.
- Take pretreatment photographs.
- Schedule postprocedure appointments.
- Make sure that the patient has the necessary skin care products for the immediate postprocedure healing period.
- Give the patient Swiss Therapy Eye Masks (if performing periorbital rejuvenation).
- Give the patient prescriptions for all medications related to the treatment and encourage him or her to fill these before the day of the procedure:
    - Antiviral (regardless of prior history of herpes simplex)
    - Ophthalmic antibacterial ointment (if performing periorbital rejuvenation)
    - Anxiolytic or analgesic
- Patients should discontinue the use of aspirin, nonsteroidal anti-inflammatory drugs, vitamin E, St. John's wort, and other dietary supplements, including ginkgo biloba, evening primrose oil, garlic, feverfew, and ginseng, at least 2 weeks before treatment to reduce the risk of bleeding.
- Remind the patient to bring sun-protective clothing (e.g., wide-brimmed hat and sunglasses) on the day of the procedure.
- Arrange for a driver for the day of the procedure (regardless of whether the patient will be medicated for the actual treatment).

SUPPLIES

Before

- Topical anesthetic (to be applied 45 to 60 minutes before the procedure)
- Metal eye shields (intraocular vs. extraocular) plus ophthalmic ointment and anesthetic drops
- Protective laser goggles for all present during the treatment
- Smoke evacuator
- Gloves
- Surgical mask
- 4 × 4 gauze sponges (for wiping away fluid from treated areas and from periorbital area)
- Moistened towels (to be placed below the neck to protect the chest)
- Zimmer Chiller (or other cooling device)
- Laser

After

- 4 × 4 gauze sponges
- Ice water
- Bowl
- Hand towels*
- Aquaphor
- Swiss Therapy eye masks

SKIN PREPARATION

Before the actual procedure, the skin must be prepared in the following steps:

---

*Before the procedure, the towels are placed in the ice-water slurry to chill. After treatment, the chilled towels are applied to treated areas and left in place for at least 10 minutes. The skin is then gently dried, and a thick coating of Aquaphor is applied.

1. All makeup removed
2. Skin cleansed with mild cleanser
3. Numbing eye drops placed (when using intraocular eye shields)

TREATMENT

- The patient should arrive 45 to 60 minutes before the procedure. At that time, all makeup is removed, the skin is cleansed with a mild cleanser, and topical anesthetic is applied to treatment areas. The anesthetic is left in place a minimum of 45 minutes.
- Immediately before the procedure, topical anesthetic cream is removed and the skin is again cleansed with a mild cleanser.
- Position the patient so that both the clinician and patient are comfortable. Whereas some prefer to treat in a flat, supine position, others find it easier to elevate the head of the bed to approximately 30 degrees and treat from the standing position.
- If using eye shields, instill one or two drops of ophthalmic anesthetic solution into each eye. Lubricate the shield side facing the cornea with an appropriate ophthalmic ointment. If the patient is wearing contact lenses, remove them. Gently place the corneal eye shields onto the patient's eyes.
- Make sure that all staff members present have the appropriate laser-protective eyewear.
- Next, consider the following variables when deciding on specific treatment settings:
  - Specific treatment area
  - Desired depth of treatment
  - Desired effect of treatment
  - Specific skin type
- Choose the appropriate settings (i.e., fluence, density, pulse width, shape, repeat time) for the patient and select them for the device. Each particular laser has certain parameters recommended by the company. It will be important to receive training for the unit purchased. Begin with the suggested parameters and adjust them as needed only after gaining experience (Tables 44.2 through 44.4).
- Perform a test spot on a tongue depressor to ensure that the laser is functioning correctly and that you have chosen appropriate treatment settings.
- Begin treatment, observe reactions of the skin to the laser energy, and make any appropriate adjustments. Most practitioners will treat a specific zone as a whole and then move onto the next zone. This provides for a more coordinated approach and allows for differential treatment settings for each individual zone.
- Inform the patient when you are moving onto a different treatment area and be cognizant of her or his pain tolerance. Application of the laser feels like a rubber-band snap and can be startling to the patient if the area being treated suddenly shifts from the chin to the upper forehead. Remember, pain tolerance is highly subjective, and some patients will need to have their treatment settings adjusted accordingly.
- After standard treatment has been concluded, dial down the settings and "feather" along the jawline and hairline. Feathering blends the treated and untreated areas so there will not be a fine demarcation line between the two when healing is complete. It

TABLE 44.2	Recommended Treatment Settings for Lumenis Ultrapulse Encore Laser ActiveFX (1.3 mm Spot Size)						
Treatment	Energy (mJ)	Scan Size (mm)	Density	Hertz	Repeat Delay (sec)	Cool Scan	No. of Passes
PigmentFX facial	80–125	6–7	2–3	100–150	0.3–1.5	On	1
Moderate photoaging/facial	80–125	6–7	2–3	100–150	0.3–1.5	On	1
Severe photoaging/facial	100–125	6–7	2–3	100–200	0.3–1.5	On	1–2
Skin types V–VI/facial	70	5–6	1–2	75–100	0.3–1.5	On	1
Neck, décolleté	80–100	5–6	1–2	125–150	0.3–1.5	On	1
Hands, forearms	50–60	5–6	1–2	125–150	0.3–1.5	On	1

Courtesy Lumenis, Inc., San Jose, California.

TABLE 44.3	Recommended Treatment Settings for Lumenis Ultrapulse Encore Laser DeepFX (0.12 mm Spot Size)						
Treatment	Energy (mJ)	Scan Size (mm)	Density	Hertz	Repeat Delay (sec)	No. of Pulses	No. of Passes
Deep wrinkles/facial	15–22.5	10	5%–10%	300–400	0.3–1.5	1	2
Periorbital	10–17.5	10	5%–15%	300–400	0.3–1.5	1	1
Perioral	17.5–22.5	10	15%–25%	300–400	0.3–1.5	1	1
Surgical scars	17.5–22.5	10	10%–15%	300–400	0.3–1.5	1–2	1
Hypertrophic scars	15–22.5	10	10%–15%	300–400	0.3–1.5	1–2	1

Courtesy of Lumenis, Inc., Santa Jose, California.

TABLE 44.4	Recommended Treatment Settings for Lumenis Ultrapulse Encore Laser TotalFX (ActiveFX + DeepFX)						
Treatment	Energy (mJ)	Scan Size (mm)	Density	Hertz	Repeat Delay (sec)	No. of Pulses	No. of Passes
ActiveFX							
Acne scars	100	7	3	100–150	0.3–1.5	N/A	1
Rhinophyma	100–125	6	2	125	0.3–1.5	N/A	1
Burn scars*	80–125	7	1	100	0.3–1.5	N/A	1
DeepFX							
Acne scars	15–22.5	10	10%–20%	300–600	0.3–1.5	1	1
Rhinophyma	20	10	15%–20%	300–600	0.3–1.5	1–2	1
Burn scars	12.5–22.5	10	5%–15%	300–600	0.3–1.5	1–2	1

*Settings depend on thickness of scar tissue and body area treated.
Courtesy of Lumenis, Inc., San Jose, California.

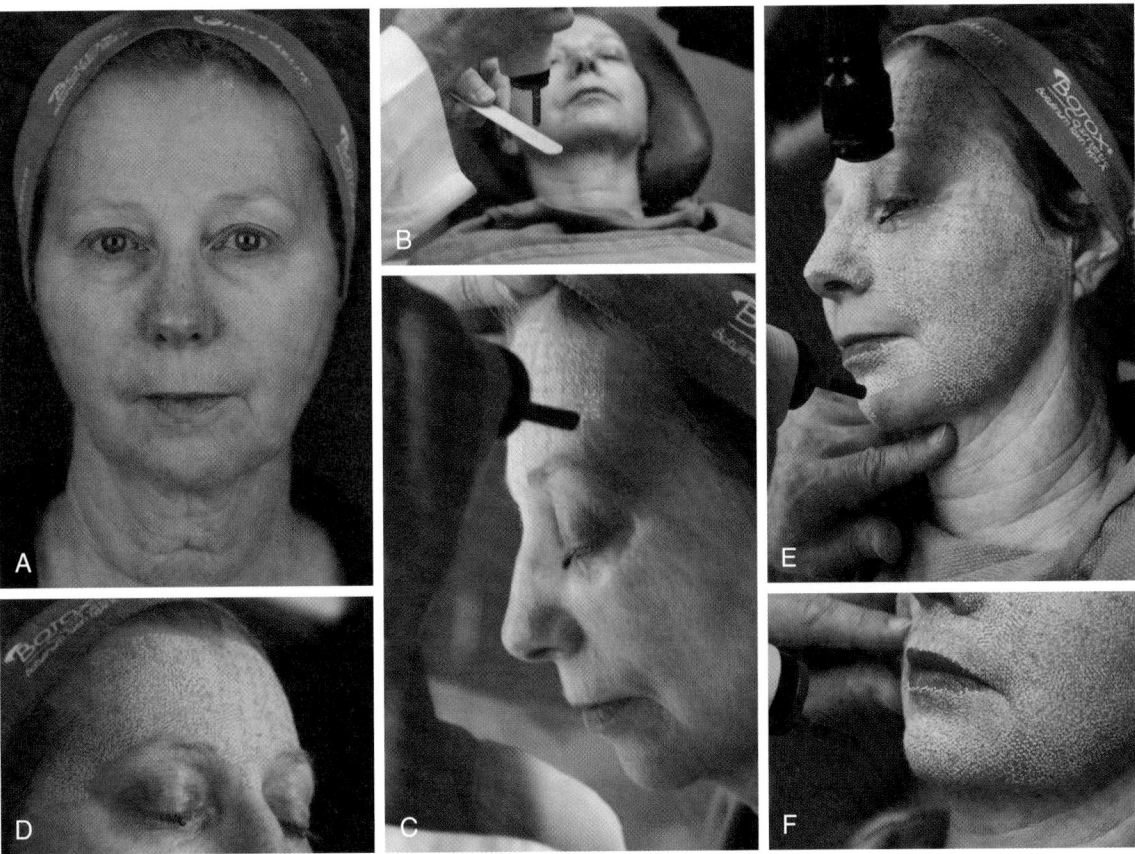

Fig. 44.10 Client treatment using the Lumenis Ultrapulse Encore fractionated CO_2 laser. (A) Preprocedure photograph. (B) Testing settings on a tongue depressor before treatment. (C) Treatment of the forehead aesthetic subunit. (D) Completion of treatment of the forehead aesthetic subunit. (E) Treatment of the perioral subunit with overlapping of pulses with use of the Zimmer cooling unit for intraprocedure pain relief. (F) Treatment of the perioral subunit with two passes at the same setting to address more advanced localized aging.

can be done in several ways: turning the treatment probe at an angle so the penetration is not so deep, or moving the handpiece faster to spread out the density of the columns.

- When treatment is complete, immediately remove the eye shields or protective eyewear and apply cool, damp towels to all treated areas. The towels should remain in place for at least 10 minutes to allow for egress of any residual heat.

- The skin is then dried and an occlusive dressing or ointment applied. This is extremely important, and the patient must understand the importance of keeping the treated tissues moist for the next several days.

- The patient is then discharged and asked to call in the morning for a status report, or earlier if having problems. Encourage plenty of fluids to stay well hydrated because patients tend to lose a significant amount of fluid from their skin during the early healing process. Also suggest avoidance of high-sodium meals, because increased salt intake will merely add to the normal and anticipated degree of postprocedure swelling.

Details of an Actual Patient Treatment

The patient is a 65-year-old white woman with advanced facial aging and significant facial laxity. Although she would have benefited from an aggressive ablative CO_2 laser resurfacing, she did not want the associated downtime. The Lumenis Ultrapulse Encore fractionated CO_2 laser treatment was recommended. She underwent this initial treatment in the office with topical anesthetic cream alone and was very comfortable.

Key areas during her treatment session and a few pearls are as follows:

- The patient is a middle-aged white woman with advanced facial aging (a combination of coarse and fine rhytids, facial laxity, and scattered dyschromias; Fig. 44.10A).

- After 45 minutes of topical anesthetic cream use, her skin is degreased, cleansed, and dried. Instill topical anesthetic drops into her eyes and then place lubricated metal eye shields to provide corneal protection during treatment. Once settings have been chosen, test them on a tongue depressor before actual treatment (Fig. 44.10B).

- While the patient is in a semiupright position, treat the forehead first (Fig. 44.10C–D). This area generally requires moderate treatment settings, and this patient was pretreated 2 weeks earlier with botulinum toxin type A to the upper third of the face to ensure a relaxed posttreatment healing environment.

- Fig. 44.10C–D show the application of outward-directed tension to the treated skin to achieve more even penetration of the laser to this area. The pattern is overlapped by around 10% to 20% on the borders. Fig. 44.10E shows detail of the fractional pattern, which leaves intact interspersed skin bridges.

- Fig. 44.10E also shows treatment of the lower perioral subunit and emphasizes the overlap of treatment zones (which provides for more even treatment).

- Fig. 44.10F shows application of a second pass. The skin is stretched in this area because the patient has a moderate degree of laxity and, if not stretched, her skin would be unevenly affected. This second pass is reflected as a much darker treatment zone.

- When treating around the eyes, the upper lids are usually done first, followed by the lower lids. This area requires extreme caution. Eyelid skin is the thinnest skin on the body, and so great care must be taken to avoid complications. Before treating this area, be sure to assess for lower lid laxity (to minimize the risk for postprocedure ectropion), and always have eye shields in place. Fig. 44.10G shows the treatment lines beginning 1 to 2 mm directly above the upper lash line, followed with another row directly above. The skin is stretched to achieve even penetration.

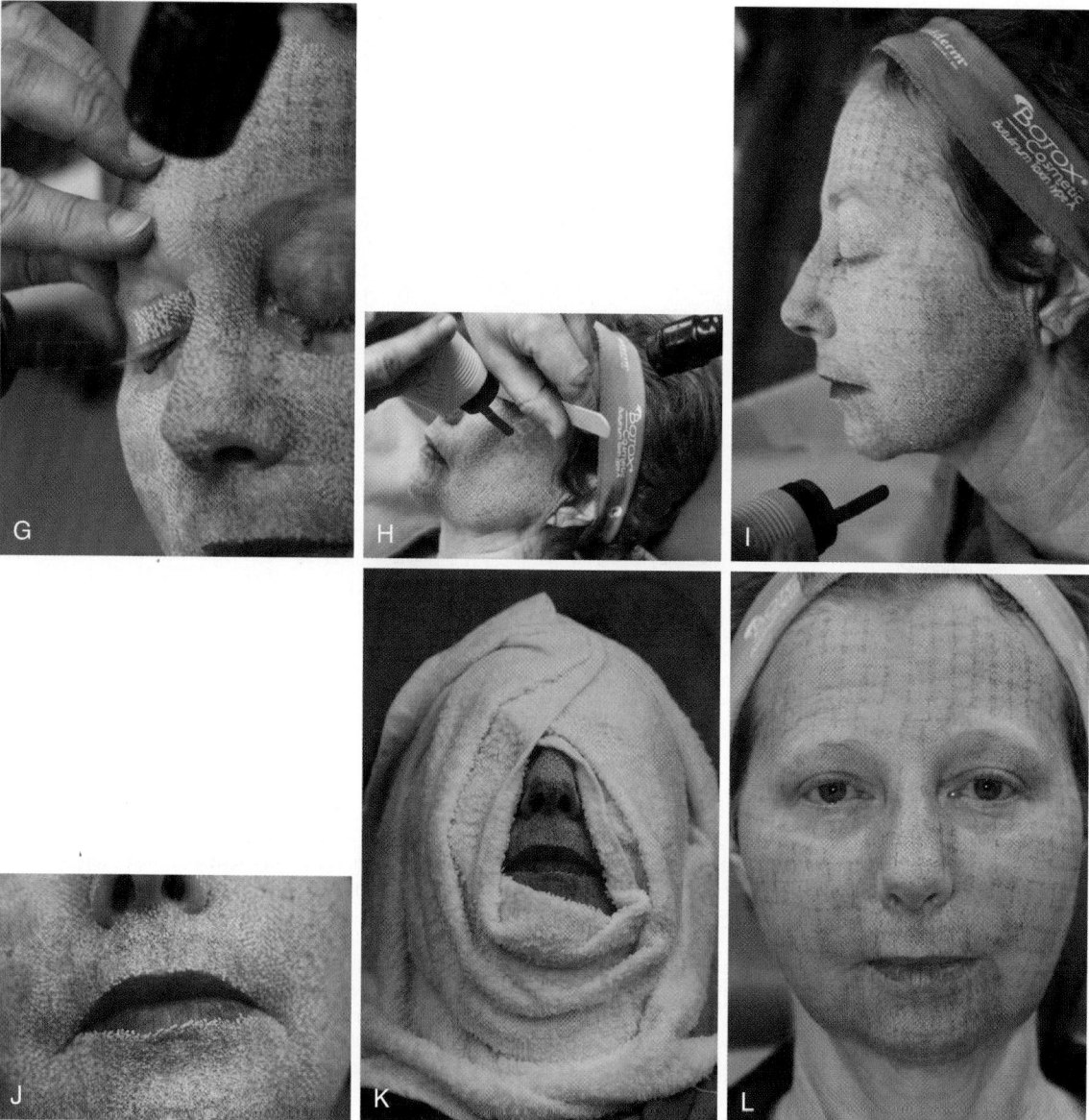

Fig. 44.10, cont'd   (G) Treatment of the upper and lower lids. (H) Treatment of the lower lid skin and use of a tongue depressor to decrease eyelash singeing. (I) Feathering of the junction between treated and nontreated tissue. (J) Close-up of the perioral treatment area to illustrate appearance of a double pass. (K) Placement of moist, cool towels to the face immediately after treatment. (L) Patient appearance after treatment and 15 minutes of cooling. (Courtesy Gregory A. Buford, MD, FACS, Denver, Colorado.)

- For the lower lids (Fig. 44.10H), use a tongue depressor to sweep the eyelashes superiorly to reduce the risk of singeing them. Begin about 1 to 2 mm below the lower lash line and then paint a line across the treatment area, followed by blending with the previously treated upper cheek zone. To complete the periorbital area, change to a smaller pattern and effectively fill in the blanks.
- Once all subunits are treated, feather all the edges (see earlier discussion) by dialing down the energy and turning the handpiece at an angle so that the beam appears elongated. Also, move the wand rather than holding it stationary. Fig. 44.10I demonstrates feathering the lower jawline onto the neck.
- Fig. 44.10J shows the final appearance after a single ActiveFX pass to the face as well as a second pass to the perioral area. The second pass effect around the mouth creates a slightly denser appearance, but was necessary, given the degree of facial aging in this area.
- Remove the patient's eye shields and rinse the eyes with balanced salt solution. Apply cool, moist towels (that have been sitting in an ice-water slurry during the actual treatment) and

leave them on for at least 15 minutes to allow heat to dissipate from the patient's skin (see Fig. 44.10K).
- Reiterate the essentials of the postprocedure care regimen with both the patient and whoever is accompanying her for discharge. There will be an early striping effect (which is natural) and a mild to moderate degree of swelling (see Fig. 44.10L). Emphasize that the swelling will be pronounced for the next 3 days but that it will resolve, how quickly depending on the depth of treatment. During that time, the patient needs to stay upright as much as possible and keep the area cool to facilitate lymphatic drainage and resolution of postprocedure edema.
- Give your office and on-call number and instruct the patient to call for any significant concerns. Complications of laser resurfacing can generally be avoided if the appropriate steps are taken early.

Treatment Caveats

As with any treatment, there are a number of ways to achieve optimal results. There is significant variation among practitioners as to which

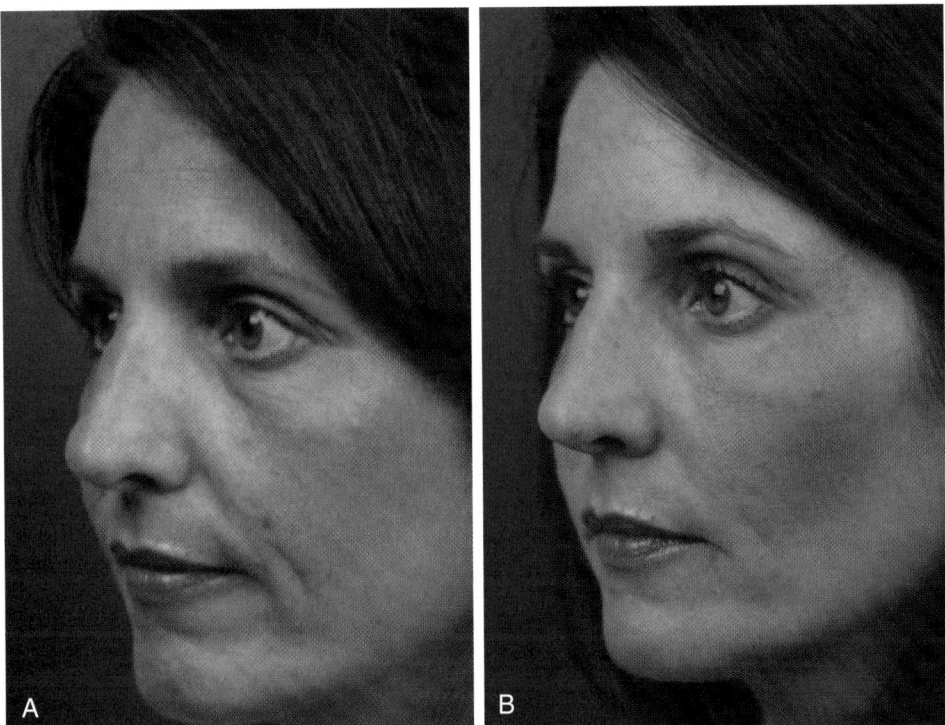

Fig. 44.11 Combination therapy using a Lumenis Ultrapulse Encore Laser. *Periorbital area*: ActiveFX: 80 mJ, 125 Hz, density 82%, single pass; DeepFx: 12.5 mJ, 300 Hz, density 15%, single pass. *Remainder of face*: ActiveFX: 125 mJ, 125 Hz, density 82%, single pass; DeepFx: 17.5 mJ, 300 Hz, density 15%, single pass. *Pretreatment with Juvederm Ultra*: medial cheeks and tear trough area. *Pretreatment with botulinum toxin type A*: forehead, glabella, lateral brow, and crow's feet. **(A) Before treatment. (B) After treatment.** (Courtesy Gregory A. Buford, MD, FACS, Denver, Colorado.)

variables provide the best outcome. Keep in mind that the safest treatment is generally the simplest treatment and that exotic settings, although they may prove successful in highly experienced hands, can be dangerous in the hands of someone in the beginning stages. Use the most basic settings when you start and adapt as you gain experience. Your patients are much more likely to respect an approach where they may need to come back for a second treatment, rather than an overly aggressive approach where they may be at risk for adverse events.

There are a number of controversies in the medical field as to which settings are most important and which should be emphasized when addressing specific needs or end points. With that said, the following are a few suggestions, but they are by no means the only ways to achieve optimal results:

- *Pulse coverage*: Position the coverage area for each pulse so that treatment zones are adjacent with very little (maximum of 10%) to no gapping between them.
- *Density*: Use a density setting right in the middle when treating photo-aged skin. For the patient with dyschromias, dial down the fluence and dial up the density so that there is a more focused treatment directly over the affected area. For generalized dyschromias, treat the entire area this way; for a localized area of pigmentation, focus simply on the specific area.
- *Fluence*: There is a tremendous amount of controversy as to the optimal fluence. Look at the patient to decide. For a patient with mild photoaging, use a light setting; for an older patient with more advanced photoaging, dial up the setting. However, be very careful in the older patient, whose thinner skin may not tolerate a higher setting, leading to delayed healing.
- *Pulse stacking*: Avoid this until comfort is gained with a specific device. Pulse stacking takes a particular fluence and associated depth of penetration, and drives it even deeper. Although there are many advocates of a low fluence doubly stacked, there is still significant controversy as to whether this is more effective than simply increasing the fluence in the first place. There is also the issue of heat dissipation. Keep in mind that double stacking may not allow for adequate

heat dissipation, so there may be more of a coagulative effect. That can be good and bad, as discussed earlier. I would strongly discourage you from incorporating this technique until you have considerable experience with your specific laser, because the results can often be unpredictable even in the hands of a highly experienced practitioner.

- *Hertz rate*: This is another controversial area. When treating scars, a higher hertz rate may be necessary. However, the science behind this approach is still being actively investigated.
- *Treatment of erythema*: More and more patients want less and less downtime but ultimately the same results. The problem, however, is that the treatment injures the tissue and the tissue needs to fully heal to achieve optimal results. It is best not to reduce the erythema for at least 4 to 6 weeks, because this enhanced vascularity is part of the overall healing process. Encourage the patient to be patient, and if the erythema is reasonable, wait for at least 4 weeks before intervening with either steroids or intense pulsed light.
- *Combination therapy*: There are a number of excellent reports documenting enhanced long-term results using pretreatment with botulinum toxin type A 1 to 2 weeks before the actual laser treatment. In addition, deep placement of volumizing fillers in conjunction with laser rejuvenation can also provide for a more comprehensive result, because laser therapy will do nothing to replace lost volume (Figs. 44.11 through 44.13).
- *Treatment of nonfacial areas*: Extension of laser resurfacing to the neck, chest, and hands allows blending of treated with nontreated areas, but it also carries an increased risk for adverse events. These areas lack the abundant adnexal glands present in the face and thus tend to heal less effectively. In addition, tissue of the chest and hands tends to be much thinner, with very little underlying subcutaneous tissue. The close proximity of bone to the skin can create a heat sink and actually prevent effective heat dissipation. Aggressive treatment in these areas can lead to delayed healing and worse. Be conservative. Educate your patients about the differences in these areas, and tell them that it may take several treatments instead of the single treatment that was effective for their face (Fig. 44.14).

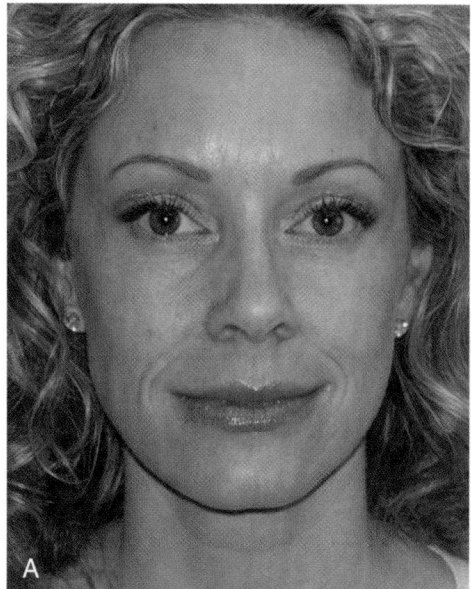
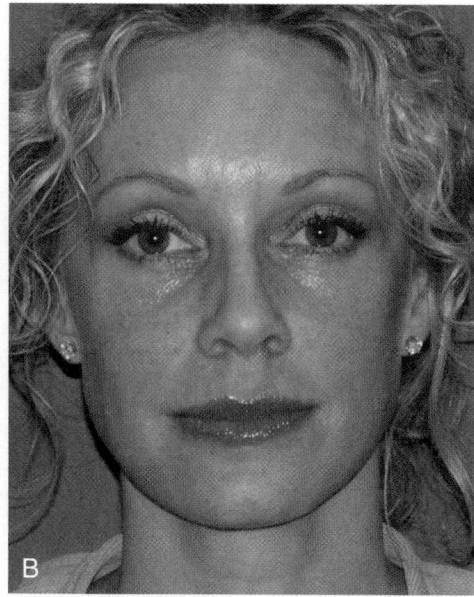

Fig. 44.12 Combination therapy using a Lumenis Ultrapulse Encore Laser. *Periorbital area*: ActiveFX: 80 mJ, 125 Hz, density 82%, single pass; DeepFx: 12.5 mJ, 300 Hz, density 15%, single pass. *Remainder of face*: ActiveFX: 125 mJ, 125 Hz, density 82%, single pass; DeepFx: 15 mJ, 300 Hz, density 15%, single pass. *Pretreatment with Juvederm Ultra*: superficial cheek lines. *Pretreatment with botulinum toxin type A*: forehead, glabella, lateral brow, and crow's feet. (A) Before treatment. (B) After treatment. (Courtesy Gregory A. Buford, MD, FACS, Denver, Colorado.)

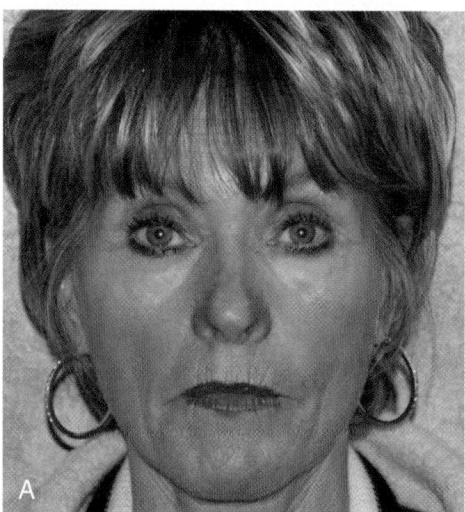
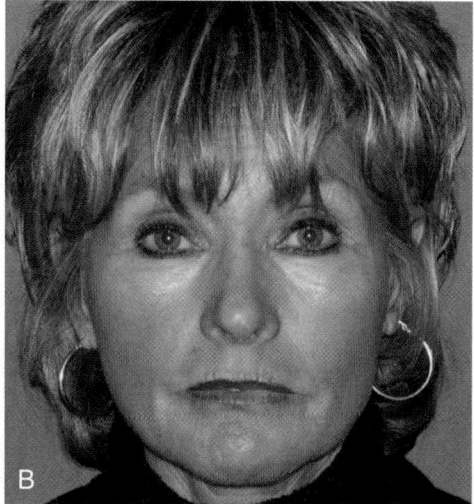

Fig. 44.13 Combination therapy using a Lumenis Ultrapulse Encore Laser. *Periorbital area*: ActiveFX: 80 mJ, 125 Hz, density 82%, single pass; DeepFx: 12.5 mJ, 300 Hz, density 15%, single pass. *Perioral area*: ActiveFX: 125 mJ, 125 Hz, density 100%, single pass; DeepFx: 22.5 mJ, 300 Hz, density 20%, single pass. *Remainder of face*: ActiveFX: 125 mJ, 125 Hz, density 82%, single pass; DeepFx: 17.5 mJ, 300 Hz, density 15%, single pass. *Pretreatment with poly-L-lactic acid*: medial and lateral cheeks. *Pretreatment with botulinum toxin type A*: forehead, glabella, lateral brow, and crow's feet. (A) Before treatment. (B) After treatment. (Courtesy of Gregory A. Buford, MD, FACS, Denver, Colorado.)

POSTPROCEDURE PATIENT CARE AND INSTRUCTIONS

There are a number of ways to optimize results after laser treatment. The following home care guidelines are one example.

Immediately After Treatment

1. Make a 1-week follow-up appointment.
2. Avoid direct sunlight to the face, even when just driving home from the office.
3. When in the car, turn on the air conditioner or roll down a window to aim cool air at the treated area.
4. Place a piece of gauze between the bridge of the nose and eyeglasses to avoid irritation to the treated skin if that area was treated.

First 2 to 4 Hours After Treatment

1. Take an analgesic (acetaminophen or ibuprofen) for discomfort.
2. You will be sent home with a container of Thermal Spring Water. Spray this on your skin as often as needed to cool the skin.
3. Avoid direct application of ice to skin. Apply cooling vinegar compresses with cold, wet washcloths using 1 tablespoon of white vinegar in 1 cup of cold water. This will help draw out heat.
4. Blow air from a fan to help with the cooling process.
5. When intense heat subsides, apply Aquaphor Moisturizer, avoiding the area close to the eyes. Keep treated areas covered (thickly) with Aquaphor Moisturizer up to 3 to 4 days, depending on the depth of treatment. The skin must not dry out! For the area around the eyes, apply the ophthalmic ointment prescribed and

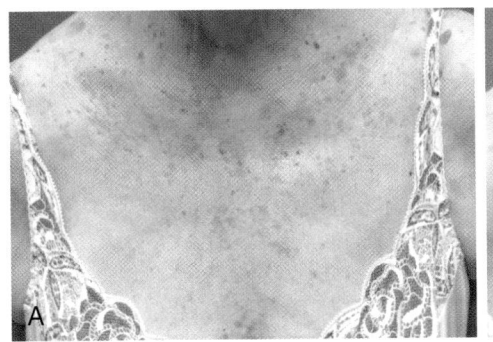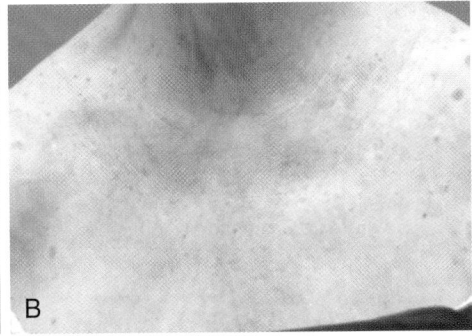

Fig. 44.14 Treatment of nonfacial areas using Lumenis Ultrapulse Encore Laser (décolleté). ActiveFX: 100 mJ, 125 Hz, density 68%, single pass. (A) Pretreatment. (B) Two months after treatment. (Courtesy Gordon H. Sasaki, MD, FACS, Pasadena, California.)

cover with a Swiss Therapy Eye Mask. These will tend to warm and dry out in about 20 to 30 minutes, so always keep an extra one in an ice-water bath and change as necessary.

First Night

1. Sleep on your back and with your head slightly elevated (continue every night until swelling subsides). TIP: Place a towel over your pillow to protect it from the Aquaphor Moisturizer.
2. Avoid environmental irritants (e.g., dust, dirt, sun, hairspray) during the healing process.

Day 1 (First Day After Treatment)

1. Stay indoors and avoid direct sunlight.
2. Begin washing treated areas two to three times a day by gently removing Aquaphor Moisturizer with the vinegar/water combination, and then cleansing with gentle cleanser and tepid water. Do not rub the skin—gently pat it! Tepid showers and washing the hair are permitted. TIP: Stand with your back to the shower.
3. Generously (thickly) reapply occlusive ointment to all treated areas.
4. Hydrate and eat healthy foods. Avoid alcohol because it will tend to dehydrate you. Also avoid exercising until the areas are completely healed.

Day 2

1. Continue to wash the face two to three times a day with gentle cleanser and tepid water.
2. Itching (particularly along the jaw line) begins and is generally an indication that the healing process has started. Mild to moderate itching is normal; if there is severe itching, call the practitioner's office.
3. Clinique Medical Recovery Week Complex works well for the itching areas.
4. Continue to apply extra Aquaphor ointment and cool compresses. An oral antihistamine such as diphenhydramine or loratadine may help.
5. Avoid picking and scratching.

Day 3

1. Continue to wash the face up to two to three times a day with gentle cleanser and tepid water.
2. Itching may persist. Use your Clinique Medical Recovery Week Complex.
3. The central area of the face may begin to exfoliate (peel), leaving behind soft, pink tissue.

Days 4 to 7 (Progress Depends on Depth of Treatment)

1. Itching has usually subsided. If not, continue using an antihistamine, especially at bedtime.

2. Exfoliation begins. Use the NIA 24 Cleansing Scrub if your skin has completely healed.
3. Transition to the Clinique Medical Optimizing Treatment Cream with or without the Recovery Week Complex and spot treat drier areas with Aquaphor Moisturizer.
4. Start your Clinique Medical sunscreen.
5. Most female patients will be able to apply mineral makeup to treated areas. For male patients, solid sun protection factor is available to help camouflage temporary redness. Be sure to use a fresh applicator and cleanse it with antibacterial soap between applications.

Day 7 and Beyond

1. Start your regular skin care program as long as the treated area is healed. Do not use harsh, very active, or strong acids (e.g., Prevage, Retin-A) for 1 month.
2. Continue to apply sunscreen and (female patients) use mineral makeup to protect the treated areas.
3. Avoid exposure to excessive sun for up to 4 weeks. Hat or clothing must be used to protect the treated areas.
4. You may fully return to your normal exercise program.

SIDE EFFECTS

Side effects are common with laser resurfacing, including the following:

- Erythema
  - Generally caused by increased blood flow to the area (which is not necessarily a bad thing)
  - Tends to resolve with the overall healing process but may be prolonged in certain patients
  - Often correlated with depth of treatment and specific type of treatment device
- Inflammation
  - Most people experience moderate swelling after treatment, but individual results vary.
  - The skin may feel tight because of tissue edema in combination with the actual skin-tightening effect of the laser. This effect may wax and wane, depending on multiple variables (e.g., treatment depth, individual patient reaction).
- Allergic reactions: These usually occur in response to a specific medication or cream.
- Milia formation: These are usually the result of use of moisturizers or the injudicious use of irritant cleansers.
- Acne
  - Generally associated with the use of heavy emollients during the recovery period
  - Treated by changing topicals or adding oral antibiotics
  - Helpful to use Aquaphor because it is water-based
- Scarring/keloids: This usually occurs because of some secondary factor (e.g., infection, scratching, poor wound care) that interferes with healing.

- Xerosis (dry skin): This is very common because we are effectively denuding the protective epithelial covering and allowing for greater evaporative water loss from the skin.
- Desquamation: Although most patients tend to have some degree of peeling, this is variable and depends on a number of factors, including depth of treatment, skin quality, and so forth.
- Pruritus: Although many patients experience some degree of itching that reflects the normal healing process, watch for severe or protracted pruritus, because it can herald a more worrisome underlying etiology.

COMPLICATIONS

Complications after laser resurfacing can occur as early as the initial healing phase or as late as several months after the procedure. As such, it is important to educate your patients about signs of an impending complication and ask them to notify the office if they suspect such. The most common complications include the following:

- Infection
  - Bacterial: Usually seen as adherent yellow crusting papules or increased pain/delayed healing.
  - Viral (herpes simplex virus): Watch for clustered vesicles, although herpes simplex virus infection can have an unusual presentation in the denuded epidermis within a few weeks after treatment.
  - Yeast: Symptoms may be subtle and often present simply as increased redness or itching (sometimes confused with contact dermatitis).
- Pigmentary changes
  - Although the incidence of pigmentary changes has dramatically decreased with the use of fractional laser resurfacing, pigmentary changes can still occur, and steps should be taken before, during, and after treatment to prevent such changes, as well as to identify individuals at higher risk for both hypopigmentation and hyperpigmentation.
  - Contributing factors include the following:
    - Fitzpatrick skin types IV to VI
    - Prior history of pigmentary changes
    - More aggressive treatment settings
  - Treatment options
    - Prevention is the key.
    - Identify increased risk before treating higher Fitzpatrick skin types.
    - Pretreatment (e.g., Tri-Luma) is helpful.
    - Posttreatment protocol generally involves a combination of glycolic acid and hydroquinone.
- Delayed wound healing
  - Have high suspicion for potential underlying infection
  - Greater association with more aggressive treatment options
  - Increases potential risk for localized scarring
- Most important ways to minimize or potentially prevent complications
  - Patient education
  - Good pretreatment and posttreatment care
  - Early recognition of future problems during the initial consultation
  - Early recognition of issues during the healing period and prompt intervention

SUPPLIERS

(See contact information available at www.expertconsult.com.)

Alma Lasers, Ltd.
Cutera, Inc.
Cynosure, Inc. (includes Ellman, Palomar, and Sandstone Medical)
Eclipse, Ltd.
Ellipse, A/S
Focus Medical
Lasering USA
Lumenis, Inc.
Lutronic, Inc.
Sciton, Inc.
Solta Medical Valeant
Syneron Candela

ONLINE RESOURCES

American Society for Aesthetic Plastic Surgery: www.surgery.org.
American Society for Laser Medicine and Surgery: www.aslms.org.
American Society of Plastic Surgeons: www.plasticsurgery.org.
eMedicine: www.emedicine.medscape.com.

RECOMMENDED READING

Alexiades. Armenakas M. Fractional laser resurfacing. *J Drugs Dermatol.* 2007;6:750–751.
Alster TS, Tanzi EL. Laser skin resurfacing: ablative and nonablative. In: Robinson JK, Hanke CW, Siegel DM, Sengelmann RD, eds. *Surgery of the Skin: Procedural Dermatology.* Philadelphia: Mosby; 2005:611–624.
Beer K, Waibel J. Botulinum toxin type A enhances the outcome of traditional fractional resurfacing of the cheek. *J Drugs Dermatol.* 2007;6:1151–1152.
Carruthers J, Carruthers A. The adjunctive usage of botulinum toxin. *Dermatol Surg.* 1998;24:1244–1247.
Chen KH, Tam KW, Chen IF, et al. A systematic review of comparative studies of CO2 and erbium:YAG lasers in resurfacing facial rhytides (wrinkles). *J Cosmet Laser Ther.* 2017.
Dierickx C, Khatri K, Alshuler G, et al. Fractionated delivery of Er:YAG laser light to improve efficacy and safety of ablative resurfacing procedure. *Lasers Surg Med.* 2007;(suppl 19):16.
Goldman M. Clinical pearl: observations on the use of fractionated CO2 laser resurfacing. *J Drugs Dermatol.* 2009;8:82–86.
Hruza G, Avram M. *Procedures in Cosmetic Dermatology Series: Lasers and Lights.* 3rd ed. Philadelphia: Elsevier; 2012.
Manstein D, Herron GC, Sink RK, et al. Fractional photothermolysis: a new concept for cutaneous remodeling using microscopic pattern of thermal injury. *Lasers Surg Med.* 2004;34:426–428.
Perkins SW, Balikian R. Treatment of perioral rhytids. *Facial Plast Surg Clin North Am.* 2007;15:409–414.
Perkins SW, Castellano R. Use of combined modality for maximal resurfacing. *Facial Plast Surg Clin North Am.* 2004;12:323–337.
Rahman Z, Tanner H, Tournas J, et al. Ablative fractional resurfacing for the treatment of photodamage and laxity. *Lasers Surg Med.* 2007;(suppl 19):15
Saluja R, Khoury J, Detweiler S, Goldman M. Histologic and clinical response to varying fractionality settings with a fractionality scanned carbon dioxide laser. *J Drugs Dermatol.* 2009;8:17–20.
Small R. Anesthesia for Cosmetic Procedures. In: Usatine RP, Pfenninger JL, Stulberg DL, Small R, eds. *Dermatologic and Cosmetic Procedures in Office Practice.* Philadelphia: Elsevier; 2012:242–247.
Tan KL, Kurniawati C, Gold M. Low risk of postinflammatory hyperpigmentation in skin types 4 and 5 after treatment with fractional CO2 laser device. *J Drugs Dermatol.* 2008;7:774–777.
Waibel J, Beer K. Ablative fractional laser resurfacing for the treatment of a third-degree burn. *J Drugs Dermatol.* 2009;8:294–297.
West TB, Alster TS. Effect of botulinum toxin type A on movement-associated rhytides following CO2 laser resurfacing. *Dermatol Surg.* 1999;25:259–261.
Yamauchi PS, Lask G, Lowe NJ. Botulinum toxin type A gives adjunctive benefit to periorbital laser resurfacing. *J Cosmet Laser Ther.* 2004;6:145–148.
Yu K, Small R, Maas C. Skin resurfacing with ablative lasers. In: Usatine RP, Pfenninger JL, Stulberg DL, Small R, eds. *Dermatologic and Cosmetic Procedures in Office Practice.* Philadelphia: Elsevier; 2012:351–356.
Zimbler MS, Holds JB, Kokoska MS, et al. Effect of botulinum toxin pretreatment on laser resurfacing results: a prospective, randomized, blinded trial. *Arch Facial Plast Surg.* 2001;3:165–169.

NONABLATIVE RADIOWAVE SKIN TIGHTENING WITH THE ELLMAN S5 SURGITRON (PELLEVÉ PROCEDURE)

Michael Stampar

The demand for procedures to rejuvenate aging skin has never been greater, and the baby boomer market demands results without downtime. Nonablative monopolar radiofrequency energy has been shown to contract skin in both a horizontal and vertical axis through "volumetric" heating of the dermis and subdermis. This radiofrequency (RF) energy is conducted/passed through from the dome-shaped active handpiece touching the skin, directly to a passive antenna plate placed behind the body part. Heat is generated at the dermal-subdermal junction, where fat provides the highest resistance to the flow of electrons. This increased impedance causes heating of adjacent deep dermal type 1 and 3 collagen fibrils and causes contraction of skin in a horizontal plane. Further deeper heating, with conduction through vertical connective tissue bands, running through fat from the deep dermis to the underlying fascia, has been shown to be the mechanism responsible for vertical contraction, or a "shrink-wrap" effect with nonablative monopolar radiofrequency energy. Many different RF devices have become available, but primary care providers interested in providing anti-aging procedures require technology that offers reliable results, with little to no risk of true complications, at a reasonable cost, and with a predictable range of efficacy.

The Ellman Dual Frequency S5 Surgitron device (Fig. 45.1) is unique because of the very high frequency (4 MHz, or 4 million cycles per second) it produces as compared with other RF devices. Earlier monopolar versions have been available for more than 20 years as a source of RF energy for office surgery, with diverse applications in many specialties (see Chapter 25, Radiofrequency Surgery [Modern Electrosurgery]). More recently, dome-shaped, handheld, alloy electrode treatment tips have been developed. They are to be used only with the S5 Surgitron device, to allow continuous, gradual, volumetric dermal, and subdermal heating. These smooth-edged domes use low energy levels and allow constant visual, tactile, and patient-generated feedback to ensure safety.

The efficacy of thermally induced skin contraction appears to be temperature dependent and based on the number of repeat passes required to induce collagen denaturation and restructuring in any given patient. This gradually progressive heat-generating technique allows thermal injury to occur in both deep and more superficial levels of the dermis. Controlled thermal injury causes three-dimensional skin contraction with immediate as well as delayed improvement in wrinkles, texture, and pore size. Horizontal dermal contraction provides lift and tightening, whereas vertical contraction firms the skin by making the subdermal fat layer more compact. Patients seeking dermal fillers have had enough dermal thinning to allow collapse and creasing. Volume replacement is aided by firming the subdermal "compartment" where the volumizing products are deposited. By treating not only to the point of visible contraction, but to an end point of no further observable contraction, a demonstrable result can be achieved in almost every case in a single treatment session.

The degree of improvement depends on the "skin age" more than chronologic age. The more reversibly bound collagen fibrils remaining, the better, and more rapid, the immediate result. When properly used, the dome-shaped handpieces allow the physician to deliver each patient's therapeutic dose painlessly, without significant safety concerns. Favorable results have been seen in patients ranging from a 19-year-old fashion model with early fine forehead lines to an 81-year-old with coarse neck creases. Skin in other areas of the body also has responded when heated thoroughly. The safety, reliability, and low treatment cost make skin tightening with the Ellman Dual Frequency unit (Ellman Cynosure International, Inc.) a reasonable treatment modality for the primary care physician providing anti-aging services. At this time, the Pellevé procedure has received FDA clearance for the treatment of moderate-to-fine facial wrinkles and folds in types I to IV skin. Neck and body use mentioned in this chapter represent off-label use, as does treating types V and VI skin in the United States. There are no such restrictions outside the United States.

ANATOMY

The pertinent anatomy for skin tightening includes the location of the collagen bundles and vertical fibrous connective tissue bands. The greatest densities of bundles of collagen fibrils are in the deep dermis just superficial to the dermal–subdermal junction, but they are present throughout the dermis. The decrease in density of these bundles with photodamage and aging leads to dermal softening, allowing lines and creases to form. Thermal denaturation of collagen occurs at a temperature of 65°C, which causes a breakdown of covalent bonds and restructured contraction of the helical fibrils; cooling appears to cause more rapid skin contraction. The inflammatory response and subsequent repair of the thermal injury bring fibroblasts that lay down new collagen, further improving the appearance of the skin by reversing, to some degree, the aging process of the skin. The more superficially the dermis is injured by vertical penetration of the accumulating heat energy, the greater the effect on fine lines and texture.

The vertical fibrous septa provide the path of least resistance for further energy flow to the passive electrode. The energy flows down these bands to their fascial origin, resulting in vertical contraction of the fibrous septa surrounding fat compartments that remain cool (Fig. 45.2).

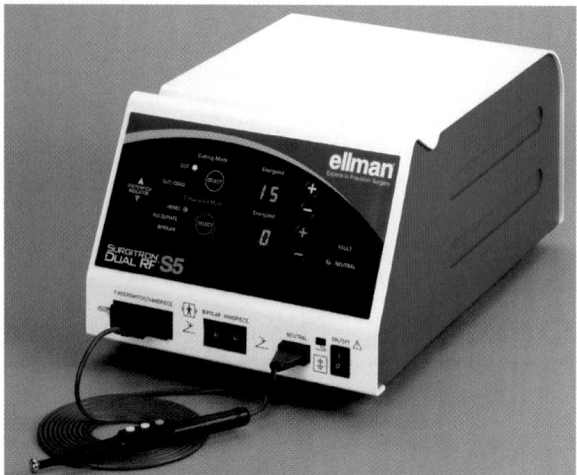

Fig. 45.1   Ellman Cynosure Dual Frequency electrosurgical unit used for the Pellevé skin tightening procedure.

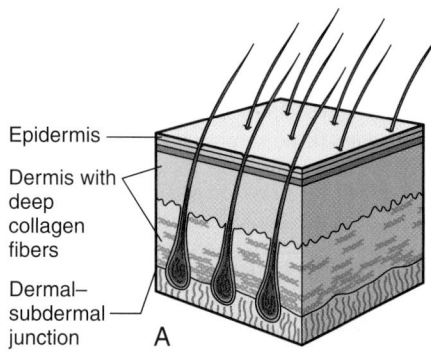

Epidermis

Dermis with deep collagen fibers

Dermal–subdermal junction

A

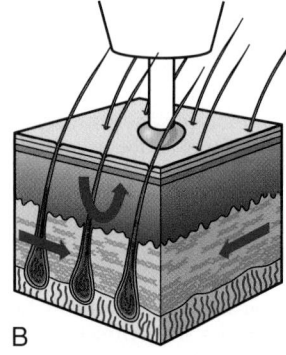

B

Fig. 45.2   (A) Diagram of actinically damaged or aged skin. (B) Application of the S5 Surgitron probe. *Straight arrows* show horizontal saturation of deep collagen. *Curved arrow* shows heat rising more superficially to affect wrinkles.

INDICATIONS

RF-generated thermal skin tightening with the Pellevé procedure is indicated in anyone showing signs of photodamaged or aging skin. Skin laxity—ranging from early softening of contours causing a vague, tired appearance to overt sagging—can benefit from the restoration of dermal collagen integrity. Ptotic brows and jawline, double chins, and an overall "melting" appearance of the skin on the face can be improved.

Significant improvement has been seen in these areas:
- Softened jaw contours (jowling)
- Flattened brow arch with or without forehead creasing
- Nasolabial and melolabial folds
- Crow's feet

- Excess upper lid skin
- Forehead and glabellar creasing and softening
- Double chin
- Neck softening and creasing
- Perioral lip lines
- Large pores and thick skin on the nose and chin
- Aged loose skin in the face, neck, arms, and abdomen (off-label)
- Dermal-filler patients (off-label)

CONTRAINDICATIONS AND RELATIVE CONTRAINDICATIONS

Currently in the United States, the Pellevé procedure is cleared for use in patients with types I to IV skin. Despite the general acceptance that RF energy is "color blind," no patients with type V or VI skin were included in the study population. When combining RF skin tightening with botulinum toxin (Botox) or fillers, tighten first, then inject. Successful skin tightening will alter the amount of filler needed in glabellar and perioral lines and folds, so filling after skin tightening is advised. On the other hand, studies have shown no detrimental effects of heating with RF energy over all commonly used dermal fillers. Avoid heating over areas injected with Botox within 7 days to allow proper tissue penetration.

Contraindications include the following:
- The presence of any topical, local, regional, or general anesthetic that can alter the patient's perception of heat on the skin. Patients need to provide feedback on heat sensation to avoid burns and overheating.
- Pacemakers and implanted defibrillators (The "shielding" built into new devices decreases the risk, but patients should be cleared by a cardiologist familiar with the specific device before proceeding.)
- Open skin lesions in the treatment area
- Any neuropathy that alters pain sensation to the areas being treated

NOTE: The use of anticoagulation is not a contraindication.

EQUIPMENT AND SUPPLIES

- Ellman Cynosure Dual Frequency 4.0 RF generator with antenna plate (Other, lower-frequency units, and coagulation- or hyfrecation-only units will not work safely!)
- Dome-shaped skin tightening handpieces: 5 mm for eyelids, 10 mm for face, 15 mm for face and neck (off-label)
- Pellevé cooling gel (Ultrasound gels also work well, but others may coagulate or allow burns.)
- Reusable soft gel cool packs
- Eye shields for direct eyelid treatment and anesthetic ophthalmic drops
- Nonsterile 4 × 4 gauze pads
- Elastic headband

NOTE: Do not use any topical anesthetic on the skin!

PREPROCEDURE CARE

- Ask patients to arrive with no makeup or to remove makeup on arrival.
- Tell patients not to take pain medications or sedatives and avoid antiinflammatory medicines for 1 week before and 4 weeks after the procedure, if possible, to avoid blunting the inflammatory response to the treatment.

PROCEDURE

Photos are vital and should be taken. Take them with the patient standing in five positions and with appropriately lit close-ups of wrinkles in the forehead, periorbital, cheek, or lip areas. The lighting, positioning, and framing should be standardized for your camera and facility to ensure reliable comparisons of before and after photographs. Asymmetry between the two sides of the face or brow position, orbital height, or cheek volume should be reviewed with the patient in the mirror before starting the procedure. A headband can be used to keep dispersion gel out of the patient's hair, and also adds consistency to photographs.

The Pellevé procedure is performed with the patient placed in the supine position on a treatment table that allows the operator to sit at the head. Adequate lighting should be provided to allow close observation of changes in skin redness and texture as the treatment progresses. The passive electrode pad is placed against the skin of the upper back for face and neck treatments or, when treating other areas, directly under the treatment area. The pure cut waveform is used for the most efficient delivery of the RF energy. For facial applications, the 10-mm tip is used. When treating on or around the eyelids, eye shields provided with the device should be carefully inserted after topical anesthetic drops are instilled (see Chapter 4, Topical Anesthesia). Dispersion gel can be applied directly to the skin, or the dome-shaped electrode can be dipped into a reservoir of the gel, and is spread with the continuous random circular or linear movement of the tip on the treatment area. Failure to cover all areas with a layer of gel can result in rapid excessive heat delivery and burns. The dispersion gel provides smooth gliding over the skin and keeps the epidermis cooler than the dermis, where the therapeutic heating occurs. To provide the treatment safely and painlessly, contact of the treatment electrode with the skin through the dispersion gel must be established before activating the electrode.

Prior to activating the electrode on facial skin, "patient tuning" can be done on the back of the hand to determine the approximate heat threshold for each patient. Because of variability in local and total body impedance between patients, all treatments should be started with continuous movement at a power level of 20 watts on pure cutting mode and increased a few watts at a time to find an effective but comfortable working level. Comfortable treatment levels will vary over the face and neck, with lower levels on the thinner skin of the forehead and periorbital area, and higher levels in the cheek and neck areas.

The power setting should be adjusted based on patient feedback to allow a gradual, progressive warming from a "3 to 4" to a "7 to 8" on a scale, where "10" would cause the patient to pull away. To optimize treatment time and patient comfort, a proper level of energy will require 10 to 15 seconds of continuous random-pattern contact to reach the heat perception level of 7 to 8 over an area of 6 to 10 cm^2.

Treatment level and heat perception can be adjusted by changing the power level of the pure cut mode or by changing the speed of movement or amount of area covered between passes. Initially, the provider may completely depend on the patient's feedback to decide when to move to the next treatment area. But, with experience, observed color and texture changes will indicate that the tissue temperature is near threshold before the patient needs to alert you to increased heat sensation. A dialogue should be maintained between the operator and patient to develop an understanding of the patient's heat tolerance and variations in heat perception in all treatment areas. Handheld infrared temperature guns can be used to spot-monitor the temperature to help avoid undertreating easily reddened skin and to monitor progress.

Slower, more concentrated movements in an area will often result in jumping from a 5 to 9 on the heat perception scale, whereas rapid movements over a large area may seem never to achieve that threshold temperature to allow collagen remodeling. A compromise between these two extremes should be reached.

Passes over sensitive areas such as the orbital rim under the brow are incorporated into other periocular passes over crow's feet and the temple, because all these areas require a lower treatment energy than the thicker cheek and forehead skin. Avoid heating directly over the brow hairs, as this may cause a spark gap or tattooed brows to change color.

So, in addition to patient feedback, control of the treatment level also requires observing the skin for redness, visible smoothing, and contraction. A "pass" is counted each time an area is taken from warm to almost too warm on threshold temperature, when visible contraction is seen or the patient states "that's hot." Circular or linear motions can be made (Fig. 45.3). If the patient repeatedly reports the sensation is too warm too quickly, the power setting should be turned down on the unit. Passes should be repeated until no further contraction or smoothing occurs with continued energy delivery. This end point must be reached for a demonstrable result. In general, when addressing wrinkles directly, the operator will return to the previously treated area for additional passes after going over the next one or two adjacent areas to allow some gel pack cooling between passes. When performed properly at appropriate energy settings, the procedure should be essentially painless.

In contrast to other devices that are limited by pulses to be delivered, continuous confluent energy should be applied to all facial skin, hairline to hairline laterally, and to the clavicle inferiorly when treating the neck (off-label in the United States). By extending the facial treatment to the firm, adherent skin of the scalp and over the sternocleidomastoid muscle in the neck, the contraction achieved after several passes has an anchor point for pulling the skin taut rather than simply contracting concentrically. In the midface, more energy should be delivered laterally and across the jawline, where maximal horizontal contraction and tightening will occur relative to the medial cheek fat pad areas, where vertical contraction will firm and smooth the skin. Excessive malar flattening should be avoided. All forehead and neck areas are treated evenly to the therapeutic end point of definitive visible firming, contraction, or smoothing. It will take several passes over an area to get to a point that the skin can be seen to contract, firm, or smooth with each additional application of heat, followed by a cold pack. In a split-face, 1-month study of four consecutive patients, the author demonstrated greater midface contraction when heating and cooling, versus just heating, was used.

The time it takes to treat adjacent areas to tolerance allows enough cooling time to then return to the initial area for added passes. If discomfort occurs immediately, decrease the energy level or terminate the treatment for that area. The skin will progress to a point of no further contraction in two to five additional passes after seeing contraction after the first pass. Typically, one pass in each area per decade of age is required for maximal contraction and smoothing.

A full face and neck procedure takes approximately 40 to 60 minutes, depending on the skin condition and size of the patient.

At the point of completion for an anatomic area, cold gel packs are applied with gentle pressure in the desired direction of contraction to rapidly chill the freshly denatured collagen bundles, primarily in the midface, where three-dimensional contraction provides lift. The theory behind this is that rapid cooling will force tighter contraction of covalent bonding of the collagen helices, similar to setting a molten mold.

NOTE: Care should be taken not to activate the electrode treatment tip before skin contact is established and not to lose contact while energy is being delivered. Disrupting the contact between the treatment electrode and the dispersion gel while the electrode is active will cause a spark gap to occur, which causes an electric shock–type feeling. This can happen if the patient pulls away, the operator pulls away, a dry area is touched, or thicker hair is crossed. This typically startles the subject but has not been observed to cause any significant epidermal damage. If stretching the skin is desired, hold gauze with a gloved hand on a dry area away from the actual active treatment site to avoid grounding yourself.

With this technique of treating gradually but progressively to the point of apparent maximal skin contraction, every patient should see and feel tightening, smoothing, lifting, or sculpting, depending on the aging characteristics being addressed. The degree of improvement depends on the "skin age" more than

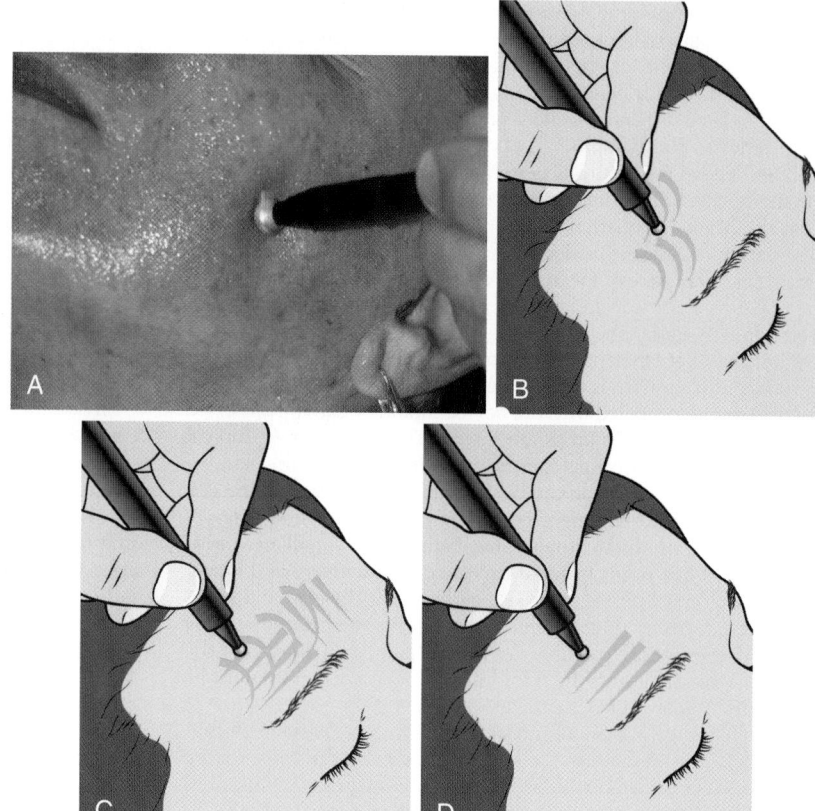

Fig. 45.3 The energy is delivered using random geometric patterns such as swirls and horizontal and vertical strokes. The purpose is to deliver a confluent heating to all treated skin and to avoid any nonrandom movement that could theoretically leave a treatment pattern visible in the soft tissues. (A) Pellevé probe contacting the skin. (B) Circular pattern. (C) Linear and circular patterns (superimposed). (D) Linear pattern.

chronologic age. The more reversibly bound collagen fibrils remaining, the better, and the more rapid the immediate result. Skin in all areas can be tightened. A photograph of the half-treated face can be taken to document the treatment effects compared with the untreated side.

Fig. 45.4 shows a patient before treatment and 2 months after Pellevé treatment. In most patients, a touch-up treatment 4 to 8 weeks after the original treatment typically yields an additional 10% to 20% improvement, possibly addressing posttreatment relaxation or incomplete collagen denaturation. These "touch-ups" typically take only two to four passes and always show more rapid heating than the original treatment. The greater the laxity, the greater the response to a second or third procedure. The patient should be advised that treatment results should continue to improve for up to 4 months based on the physiology of thermal tissue injury, and that they may repeat the procedure every 1 to 2 years as needed after a desired end point is reached.

COMPLICATIONS

- Very limited
- Discomfort if power is set too high
- Rarely, a burn caused by activating the electrode before making contact or after losing contact
- Possible lack of intended tightening because of inadequate residual collagen
- Inadequate effort

POSTTREATMENT CARE

There should be no downtime with the Pellevé skin tightening procedure when performed properly. Transient reddening of the skin should resolve in 1 to 3 hours, and no change in skin care is required. Makeup can be applied immediately. Patients are also advised to take

1000 mg of vitamin C daily in oral form for 6 months to ensure an adequate systemic supply for collagen synthesis. Patients are reevaluated at 6 weeks, 6 months, and 1 year following the procedure. Additional RF treatments are recommended every 6 to 8 weeks for 6 months, or until the patient is satisfied a maximal result has been achieved (for patients with excessively wrinkled or lax areas). Light peels, filler injections, Botox injections, or surgery can be done any time after the treatment.

Ellman Cynosure is the sole supplier of the device worldwide. The most significant observed advantages of this device and treatment relative to other RF-based devices and treatments are the tactile control of the treatment; gradual, progressive, continuous heating rather than pulsing; demonstrable results in a single, essentially painless treatment; and the cost of delivery. A bipolar treatment tip is being evaluated at this time and will be available with the same device if additional efficacy is seen.

PATIENT EDUCATION GUIDES

See patient education and patient consent forms available at www.expertconsult.com.

CODING AND BILLING

This is an aesthetic procedure so there are no CPT/ICD-10 codes.

SUPPLIERS

(Contact information also available at www.expertconsult.com.)
Ellman Cynosure International, Inc.
Westford, Massachusetts
Phone: 800-886-2966, 978-256-4200
www.ellman.com

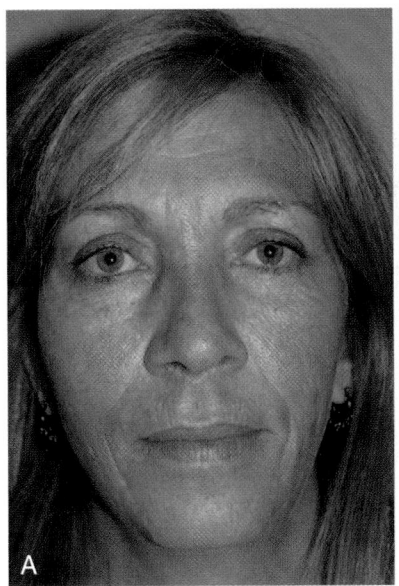 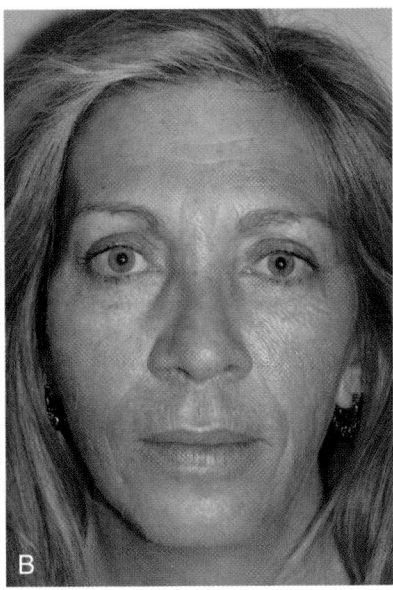

Fig. 45.4 Appearance of the skin before (A) and after (B) Pellevé treatment.

ONLINE RESOURCES

www.www.pelleve.com.
www.www.lookyoungeratanyage.com.

RECOMMENDED READING

Arnoczky SP, Aksan A. Thermal modification of connective tissues: basic science considerations and clinical implications. *J Am Acad Orthop Surg.* 2000;8:305–313.

Beasley KL, Weiss RA. Radiofrequency in cosmetic dermatology. *Dermatol Clin.* 2014;32(1):79–90. https://doi.org/10.1016/j.det.2013.09.010.

Bridenstine JB. Use of ultra-high frequency electrosurgery (radiosurgery) for cosmetic surgical procedures. *Dermatol Surg.* 1998;24:397–400.

el-Domyati M, el-Ammawi TS, Medhat W, et al. Radiofrequency facial rejuvenation: evidence-based effect. *J Am Acad Dermatol.* 2011;64(3): 524–535.

England LJ, Tan M, Shumaker PR, et al. Effects of monopolar radiofrequency treatment over soft tissue fillers in an animal model. *Lasers Surg Med.* 2005;37:356–365.

Rusciani A, Curinga G, Menichini G, et al. Nonsurgical tightening of skin laxity: a new radiofrequency approach. *J Drugs Dermatol.* 2007;6:381–386.

Small R. Wrinkle reduction with nonablative lasers. In: Usatine RP, Pfenninger JL, Stulberg DL, Small R, eds. *Dermatologic and Cosmetic Procedures in Office Practice.* Philadelphia: Elsevier Saunders; 2012:336–350.

Zelickson BD, Kist D, Bernstein E, et al. Histologic and ultrastructural evaluation of the effects of a radiofrequency-based non-ablative dermal remodeling device: a pilot study. *Arch Dermatol.* 2004;140:204–209.

CHAPTER 46

EPILATION OF ISOLATED HAIRS (INCLUDING TRICHIASIS)

Kathleen M. O'Hanlon

The method used to permanently remove problem hairs, such as misdirected eyelashes or ingrown hairs, depends on the anatomic location of the hair and the condition of the surrounding skin. The simplest approach, typically used by electrologists, applies electrical current to cause follicular destruction. In radiofrequency surgery, household current is converted to a frequency of 3.9 MHz, resulting in heating and vaporization of water in the tissue and subsequent destruction of the hair root. This process results in minimal lateral heat transfer, allowing for selective ablation of lash follicles without the side effects on the lid previously experienced with electrocautery (see section "Complications"). In the presence of inflammatory disease with ingrown hairs, a more comprehensive skin care program should be used first to decrease the density of papules and pustules. For removal of large areas of hair, lasers and intense pulsed-light devices are quite effective. The units are expensive but time saving and effective (see Chapter 38, Lasers and Pulsed-Light Devices: Hair Removal).

PHYSIOLOGY

Hair is formed by the replication of cells in hair follicles. The growth phase (anagen) commences with germinal papillae descending into the dermis. This is followed by cellular proliferation (catagen), during which a bulb and a hair are formed. Once growth has ceased, the follicle shrinks and enters into the resting phase (telogen). The duration of each phase of the cycle depends on the type and location of the hair. Short hairs, such as human eyelashes, spend the majority of their time in the telogen phase, during which the germinal cells reside near the base of the follicle. Hair ablative procedures therefore need to apply heat energy (electrolysis or radiosurgery) specifically to the base of these follicles.

Trichiasis

Abnormal eyelashes may be congenital or may result from trauma, infections, diseases such as Stevens-Johnson syndrome, chronic disease, and allergies, medication use, or even the aging process. *Cilia inversum* is a rare finding in which a lash originates in the tarsal conjunctiva instead of anterior to the tarsal plate. *Cilia incarnata*, an anomaly akin to ingrown hair, develops when a lash is trapped beneath the skin near the lid margin. In *distichiasis*, lashes grow from the meibomian gland orifices posterior to the normal lashes. True trichiasis, an acquired condition in which one or more lashes is misdirected posteriorly toward the conjunctiva or cornea, may pose a range of problems, from irritation to corneal abrasion or ulceration. Localized hairs may be suitable for tweezing, followed by permanent ablation if they recur. On the upper lid, the eyelash bulb has been determined to be about 2.4 mm below the surface of the lid margin, and the lower lid follicles are about 1.4 mm deep. Lanugo hairs or widespread trichiasis may require more specialized surgical procedures and should be referred to an ophthalmologist.

Ingrown Hairs

Ingrown hairs, *pili incarnati*, originate from a variety of causes. Razor-shaved hair ends have very sharp tips that may curve back toward the skin surface and reenter the epidermis a short distance from the mouth of the follicle (common in black people or people with curly hair). Double-edged razors, in which the hair is pulled out of the follicle by the first razor and cut by the second razor, leave the resultant hair tip recoiled in the follicle below the surface of the skin. The curved hair may then grow into the follicular wall. As the hair tips pierce the epidermis or penetrate the dermis, a foreign body inflammatory reaction ensues. Usually the ingrown hairs are completely buried, but they may have an identifiable recurving loop. In treating such hairs, the unattached end of the hair must be exposed above the surface of the skin using sharp forceps. Impacted hairs, which cannot be freed, should be left in place until a subsequent visit.

INDICATIONS

- Trichiasis
- Ingrown hairs (e.g., pseudofolliculitis barbae and other related disorders)

RELATIVE CONTRAINDICATIONS

- History of recurrent herpes (premedicate before epilation)
- Inflammatory skin condition (controlled)
- "Demand" cardiac pacemaker (radiofrequency wave can cause pacemaker malfunction, resulting in palpitations or even asystole)

ABSOLUTE CONTRAINDICATION

Active herpetic outbreak

EQUIPMENT

- Radiosurgery unit (Surgitron; Ellman Cynosure)
- Ellman's "insulated needle electrode," fine wire (A2D, A8D or similar), or flexible probes (TA1B or similar, fine wires or 33-gauge needles) may be necessary for the curvaceous ingrown hairs (Fig. 46.1).
- Small tweezers
- Alcohol wipe
- Loupes or magnification lamp (optional but very helpful)
- Topical anesthetic (optional; e.g., EMLA, ELA-Max, Hurricaine Gel; see Chapter 4, Topical Anesthesia)

PRECAUTIONS

- Excess insertion depth of epilation needle can cause unnecessary scarring.

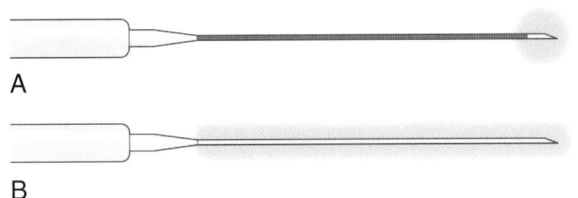

Fig. 46.1 Two common needles used for epilation. (A) Coated with only the tip active. (B) Uncoated with entire needle active. (Courtesy Ellman Cynosure, Hicksville, NY.)

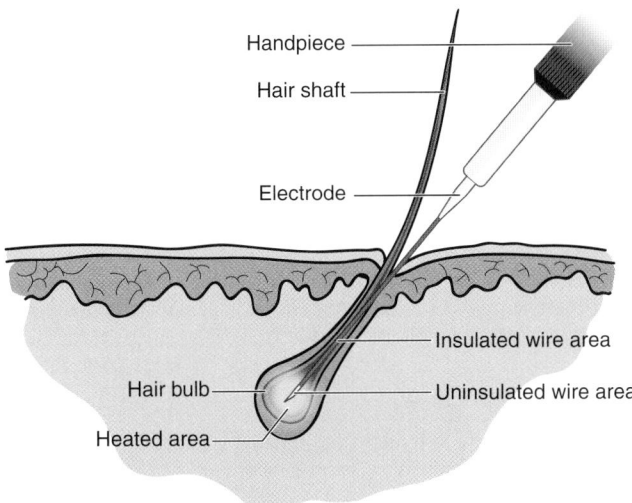

Fig. 46.2 Using a fine needle or wire electrode for epilation. (Courtesy Ellman Cynosure, Hicksville, NY.)

- Power set too high can result in lid or corneal side effects, including scarring.
- In the case of the ingrown hair, the shaft should be pulled gently to indicate the direction of the follicle, and a preferably flexible probe should be inserted for epilation. Probes that do not conform to the curvature of the hair may not reach the hair root. Although rare, incomplete electrolysis may create an ingrown hair if a distorted follicle is sealed off by the current.

PREPROCEDURE PATIENT EDUCATION AND FORMS

See patient education, encounter, and consent forms available at www.expertconsult.com.

PROCEDURE

See Fig. 46.2.

- Prepare area with alcohol.
- Apply topical anesthetic (optional).
- Set the Ellman Surgitron to 10 W or less (level 1) in the coagulation mode.
- Place the insulated needle or fine wire electrode into the handpiece. Alternatively, use the 33-gauge needle and a needle hub adapter.
- Identify the exposed end of the hair and, pulling the shaft gently with tweezers, insert the needle into the follicle until resistance is met, and activate the unit.
- Remove the hair with tweezers. It should come out easily.

SAMPLE OPERATIVE REPORT

See sample operative report available at www.expertconsult.com.

COMMON ERRORS

- Inadequate penetration depth, resulting in unsuccessful permanent ablation
- Excessive cautery to the tissue

COMPLICATIONS

Although extremely rare, the following are potential complications:

- Recurrence of hair growth ("permanent" ablation is not 100% effective)
- Eyelid complications, including cellulitis, hypopigmentation or hyperpigmentation, lid deformities (e.g., notching, scarring—much more likely with *electrocautery*, which is not recommended by the author)
- Cicatricial conjunctival disease due to heat damage (also more likely with *electrocautery*)
- Potential hazard to the globe (due to close proximity)
- Activation of herpes zoster

POSTPROCEDURE MANAGEMENT

Antibiotic (eye) ointment for 3 to 5 days or until localized pits have granulated.

PATIENT EDUCATION GUIDES

See patient education and consent forms and sample operative and encounter forms available at www.expertconsult.com.

CPT/BILLING CODES

17380	Electrolysis epilation; each half-hour
67820	Correction of trichiasis; epilation by forceps only
67825	Correction of trichiasis epilation by electrosurgery, cryosurgery, or laser

ICD-10-CM DIAGNOSTIC CODES

H02.001-H02.009	Entropion
H02.051-H02.059	Trichiasis
H02.861-H02.869	Hypertrichosis eyelid
L68.0-L68.9	Hypertrichosis
L67.0-L67.9	Hair color and shaft abnormalities

RECOMMENDED READING

Bartley GB. An experimental study to compare methods of eyelash ablation. *Ophthalmology.* 1987;94:1286–1289.

Crutchfield CE. The causes and treatment of pseudofolliculitis barbae. *Cutis.* 1998;61:351–356.

Elder MJ. Anatomy and physiology of eyelash follicles: relevance to lash ablation procedures. *Ophthal Plast Reconstr Surg.* 1997;13:21–25.

Ferreira IS, Bernardes TF, Bonfioli AA. Trichiasis. *Semin Ophthalmol.* 2010;23(3):66–71.

Hurwitz JJ. Experimental treatment of eyelashes with high-frequency radio wave electrosurgery. *Can J Ophthalmol.* 1993;28:62–64.

Kezirian GM. Treatment of localized trichiasis with radiosurgery. *Ophthal Plast Reconstr Surg.* 1993;9:260–266.

CHAPTER 47

BOTULINUM TOXIN

Edward M. Zimmerman

In 1978, a San Francisco ophthalmologist, Alan B. Scott, published the first paper on the use of botulinum toxin in humans. He used it to treat strabismus in 1980. The US Food and Drug Administration (FDA) first approved botulinum A exotoxin (BTX-A or BoNT A) in 1989 for the treatment of strabismus and blepharospasm. It has also been approved for treatment of dystonia, spasticity, severe hyperhidrosis of the axillae, chronic migraine headaches, and urinary detrusor instability. In 2002, the FDA approved Botox Cosmetic for temporary alleviation of dynamic wrinkles of the glabellar area, and in 2013 it was approved for the treatment of crow's feet. All other uses are "off-label." This chapter discusses the cosmetic uses of BTX-A, which include the temporary alleviation of dynamic wrinkles of the face and neck; the lifting of nose tips, oral commissures, and brows; the thinning of hypertrophic masseter muscles; and smoothing the pebbly appearance of a "walnut" chin. Botox injections have become the most common cosmetic procedure in the world. In 2015, nearly 7 million cosmetic injections were performed, a continued increase since it was introduced.

BTX-A is available in several forms. Botox, now called onabotulinum toxin A by the FDA, is a purified neurotoxin complex produced by Allergan, Inc. It is available in 100-unit vials. A branch of Ipsen Pharmaceuticals makes Dysport in England in 500-unit vials. It was FDA approved to be distributed in the United States as Dysport, or abobotulinum toxin A, by Ipsen and Galderma. Botox is three to four times as potent per unit as Dysport. Incobotulinum toxin A (Xeomin; Merz Pharmaceuticals) was FDA approved in 2011 for temporary improvement in the appearance of moderate-to-severe glabellar lines in adults. Xeomin may be used in equivalent dose as Botox clinically. Other, non–FDA-approved forms are available outside of the United States, including Relatox in Russia, Botulax in Korea, Neuronox in Korea and South America, and Chinatox in China.

There are seven serotypes of BTX, designated A through G. Type A is the most potent, and it was the first one commercially available. BTX-A and BTX-E work at the level of the neuromuscular junction of striated muscle, where they irreversibly bind, and after cleaving 9 and 25 amino acids, respectively, from the C-terminus of the SNAP 25 protein, they inhibit the release of acetylcholine. This causes paralysis of that muscle until a new neuromuscular junction is sprouted by the nerve ending, a process that can take weeks to months depending on the density of innervation and on the site, amount, and concentration of the solution injected. The onset of muscle paralysis, reduced sweating, or pain control varies from site to site and patient to patient. Most patients notice a gradual increasing response in 3 to 7 days that plateaus and lasts for 2 to 11 months, with a gradual redevelopment of wrinkles, sweating, or pain. The duration of effect on sweating (6 to 9 months) is significantly longer than on wrinkles (3 to 4 months). Some patients respond more quickly and completely to the injections. A small percentage of patients are minimally responsive, even to large amounts of Botox. Some become resistant to injections. Resistance in patients treated with less than 100 U per session for either blepharospasm or aesthetic purposes is rare. Patients who become resistant to BTX-A because of antibody development after repeated, large doses, and laboratory workers, who are specifically immunized, may respond to BTX-B and BTX-F, which are currently undergoing clinical trials. BTX-B (Myobloc, now called rimabotulinum toxin B by the FDA) was approved by the FDA in December 2000 for treatment of patients with cervical dystonia. It is produced by Solstice Neurosciences. It has a rapid onset of action (hours to days), loses effect after about 6 to 12 weeks, and is currently used to treat cervical dystonia. BTX-A is about 50 times as potent as BTX-B. In theory, if a patient has developed an immune reaction to BTX-A, BTX-B might be an alternative. In reality, few clinicians use BTX-B anymore due to its low potency compared with BTX-A and the actual rarity of immunity to BTX-A.

SAFETY OF BTX-A

The LD_{50} of Botox in humans is estimated to be 2500 to 3000 U of toxin for a 70-kg human, or approximately 40 U/kg. For cosmetic purposes, doses of Botox are limited to 100 U; therefore Botox Cosmetic can be considered a safe and useful chemical. No irreversible clinical effects have been reported.

Similarly, the suggested limit for cosmetic uses of Dysport is 300 U, but up to 1000 U may be used to treat cervical dystonia if needed. No formal drug interaction studies have been conducted with Dysport. However, the package insert lists much the same suggested interactions as could occur with other types of BTX-A.

Suggested dose of Xeomin for glabellar lines is 20 units per treatment session, it may be used up to 400 units for upper limb spasticity. Co-administration of XEOMIN and aminoglycoside antibiotics or other agents interfering with neuromuscular transmission is cautioned, as these agents may potentiate the effect of the toxin. Use of anticholinergics after administration of Xeomin may enhance systemic anticholinergic effects.

INDICATIONS

Food and Drug Administration-Approved Indications for Botox

- Strabismus
- Blepharospasm
- Adult focal spasticity
- Adult chronic migraine
- Adult cervical dystonia (spasmodic torticollis)
- Overactive bladder (and associated incontinence) when other medications (anticholinergics) fail or cannot be tolerated
- Primary axillary hyperhidrosis
- Dynamic glabellar and lateral canthal rhytids

Food and Drug Administration-Approved Indications for Dysport

- Adult cervical dystonia and upper limb spasticity
- Pediatric lower limb spasticity
- Dynamic glabellar rhytids

Food and Drug Administration-Approved Indications for Myobloc

* Adult cervical dystonia

Food and Drug Administration-Approved Indications for Xeomin

* Adult upper limb spasticity
* Cervical dystonia
* Blepharospasm
* Dynamic glabellar rhytids

Other Indications for BTX

* Cosmetic reduction of dynamic wrinkles in face, lips, and neck
* Hyperhidrosis of the palms, soles, and forehead
* Anal fissures resulting from an increase in rectal sphincter tone (see Chapter 85, Anal Fissure and Lateral Sphincterotomy and Anal Fistula)
* Headaches, both tension, and migraine
* Asymmetric face, acquired (e.g., Bell's palsy, hemifacial spasm, or after facial trauma, the unaffected side causes reduced movement or unopposed muscle tension)

Anecdotally, it is well accepted to perform superficial skin treatments (microdermabrasion, superficial peels, nonablative laser, and light treatments) first and then administer BTX-A afterward on the same visit. Injections can also be performed after minor surgeries to different parts of the face (e.g., inject the glabella and brow after blepharoplasty) without causing a deficit in onset or duration of action of BTX-A. More invasive chemical peels, deeper laser resurfacing, and facelifts cause enough inflammation to decrease the duration of action of BTX-A. Injections are usually done 4 to 8 weeks after these procedures.

CONTRAINDICATIONS

* Pregnancy or nursing
* Preexisting neuromuscular diseases (This is a relative contraindication; consider obtaining a neurologist's opinion before initiating BTX-A for cosmetic reasons in these patients.)
* Inability to contract muscles in treatment area prior to treatment
* Skin atrophy (e.g., chronic oral steroid use or genetic syndromes such as Ehlers-Danlos syndrome)
* Periocular or ocular surgery within last 6 months
* Bleeding abnormality
* Sensitivity or allergy to any of the constituents of reconstituted Botox (e.g., BTX-A, human albumin)
* Infection (e.g., pustular acne, active herpes, cellulitis) or active dermatosis (e.g., psoriasis, eczema) at proposed injection sites
* Some medications decrease neuromuscular transmission and may potentiate the effect of large doses of BTX-A (usually not a problem for the small doses used for cosmetic procedures). These include aminoglycosides and similar antibiotics, neuromuscular blocking agents (succinylcholine), penicillamine, quinidine, quinine, and calcium channel blockers.
* Sun exposure has been shown to decrease the effect and duration of BTX-A injections.
* Unrealistic expectations
* Body dysmorphic disorder

EQUIPMENT

* One vial of Botox (50 U or 100 U), Dysport (300 U) or Xeomin (50 U, 100 U or 200 U). These are labeled as "single use or single patient use," which some states (e.g., Nevada) are now enforcing—meaning single use on a single patient at a single time. For many years, clinicians have reconstituted these drugs and then used separate, sterile syringes of medication on different patients for enhanced economy to the patient with no side effects or problems.
* Sterile normal saline *without preservatives* (single-dose vials). (Although not recommended by the company, saline *with* the preservative benzyl alcohol is commonly used to reconstitute Botox. This solution stores safely in a refrigerator for several weeks and may be less painful to inject because of the numbing effect of the preservative.)
* 20-gauge needle to reconstitute the vial of BTX-A with saline.
* 1-mL syringes and 30-gauge, ½-inch needles for injection, *or* 0.3-mL insulin syringes with 30- or 31-gauge needles
* Alcohol wipes to cleanse injection sites (*optional*)
* Facial tissues or clean gauze to hold pressure on injection sites
* Nonsterile gloves to wear during injection
* vIce packs or small bags of ice to topically anesthetize the skin and constrict blood vessels at injection sites before injection

PREPROCEDURE PATIENT PREPARATION

Botox and Dysport are delivered by overnight transport in a thick Styrofoam container packed with dry ice to keep the potent toxin stable. Xeomin requires no refrigeration. Allergan and Ipsen recommend storage of the unmixed Botox and Dysport toxins at 5°C or lower (frozen). Potency of the toxin is measured in units (U), where 1 U is the amount of toxin that kills 50% (LD_{50}) of a standardized mouse model when injected intraperitoneally. Each vial of Botox contains either 50 or 100 U of toxin, plus 0.5 mg of human albumin and 0.9 mg of sodium chloride. The toxin is lyophilized and sealed in the vial under negative pressure.

Dysport is supplied in a single-use, sterile vial for reconstitution intended for intramuscular injection. Each vial contains 500 or 300 U of lyophilized abobotulinumtoxinA, 125 µg human serum albumin, and 2.5 mg lactose. Dysport may contain trace amounts of cow's milk proteins.

Xeomin is supplied in 50, 100, or 200 U lyophilized powder in a single-dose vial. Once reconstituted, it needs to be stored in a refrigerator (2°C to 8°C) and used within 24 hours.

The FDA-recommended dose for treatment of dynamic glabellar rhytids with Botox or Xeomin is 20 U, compared with the recommended dose of 50 U for Dysport.

BTX-B (Myobloc) is delivered premixed in several quantities: 2500 U in 0.5 mL, 5000 U in 1 mL, and 10,000 U in 2 mL. (BTX-B may be stored undiluted in the refrigerator at 2°C to 8°C for up to 21 months. If diluted, it should be used promptly because it contains no preservatives.)

An injection site record (Fig. 47.1) should be available before the procedure begins.

RECONSTITUTION AND HANDLING OF BTX-A

Alcohol used to cleanse the rubber stoppers and injection sites can inactivate the toxin. Allow it to evaporate completely before proceeding. Allergan recommends that from 1 to 10 mL of sterile saline *without preservatives* (single-dose vials do not contain preservatives—see previous comment) be mixed in the vial of Botox, using the large needle to reconstitute it. A vial that does not demonstrate a vacuum should not be used and will be replaced by the company. The reconstituted Botox should be mixed by gently rolling or swirling the vial. Shaking the vial (i.e., causing foaming) was thought to denature Botox, leading to decreased potency of the solution, but this has proven not to be an issue. Once reconstituted, the toxin should be kept at 2°C to 8°C (refrigerated) and used as quickly as possible. Practitioners may choose to store the solution in the glass vial and use a larger needle to fill the solution into 1-mL syringes as needed, or remove the rubber stopper and withdraw the fluid with the small needle on insulin syringes to inject the solution. The package insert recommends using this "single-use vial" of toxin within

BOTOX Cosmetic Injection Site Record

Patient Name:_____
Chart#/Ident.:_____

Notes

	Area 1	Area 2	Area 3	Area 4
Location				
Botox Lot Number				
Botox Expiration Date				
Treatment Date				
Dilution (cc)				
Units/0.1 cc				
Total Units/Site				
Site A				
Site B				
Site C				
Site D				
Total Units Used				

Fig. 47.1 Sample record of injection sites.

4 hours when mixed with sterile saline without preservatives. Group consensus and studies have shown minimal loss of potency in either refrigerated or frozen solution made with saline, with or without preservatives, at 30 days. However, most patients agree that injections reconstituted with saline with preservatives are more comfortable.

Botox dilution varies by use and personal preference. More concentrated dilutions seem to cause effects sooner, but may be more difficult for a clinician to inject accurately and last no longer than injections of more dilute solutions. Most clinicians dilute 100 U of lyophilized Botox with 1 to 6 mL of saline. Dilutions of 100 U/1 mL (10 U/0.1 mL), 100 U/2 mL (5 U/0.1 mL), or 100 U/3 mL (3.3 U/0.1 mL) are commonly used for cosmetic procedures, headache treatments, and hyperhidrosis (Table 47.1). The area of effect associated with each injection point can be up to 2 to 3 cm in diameter.

Dysport can be reconstituted with 1 to 3 mL of saline, and Xeomin 0.25 mL to 5 mL of saline depending on required concentration and the clinician's preference, and used in a similar fashion.

TABLE 47.1 Dilutions of Botox (100 U/Bottle as Supplied)

Amount of Saline (mL)	Units/0.1 mL	Units/1 mL
1	10	100
2	5	50
3	3.3	33
4	2.5	25
5	2.0	20

PATIENT EDUCATION

Before injection, the patient should review and sign the informed consent (see the patient consent form online at www.expertconsult.com). The patient should appreciate that the treatment produces temporary results (3 to 4 months) and will take up to 10 days for the full effect. The FDA has recently added a

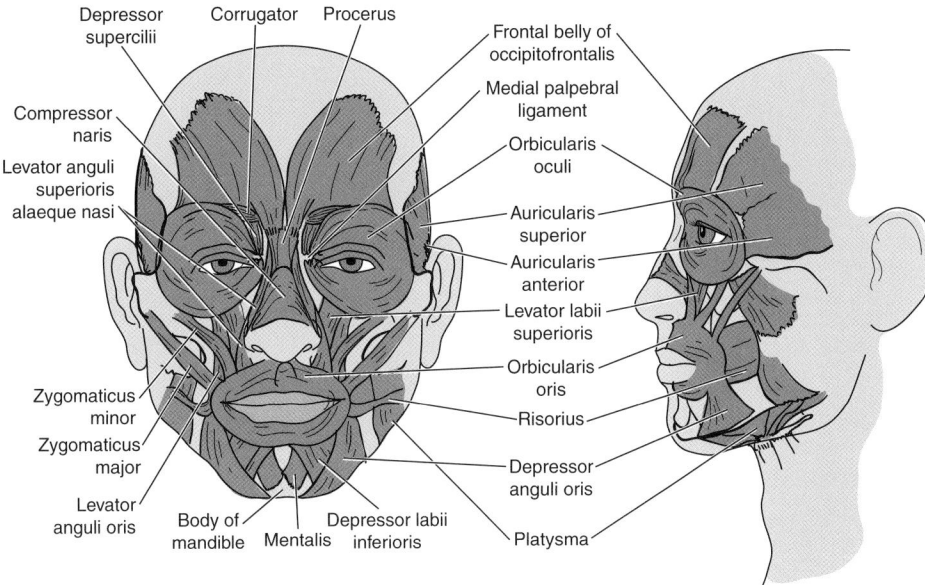

Fig. 47.2 Anatomy of the face with masseter muscles noted.

Labels (clockwise): Depressor supercilii · Corrugator · Procerus · Frontal belly of occipitofrontalis · Medial palpebral ligament · Orbicularis oculi · Auricularis superior · Auricularis anterior · Levator labii superioris · Orbicularis oris · Risorius · Depressor anguli oris · Platysma · Depressor labii inferioris · Mentalis · Body of mandible · Levator anguli oris · Zygomaticus major · Zygomaticus minor · Levator anguli superioris alaeque nasi · Compressor naris

revised form, included with the BTX-A vial, for patient distribution every time BTX-A injections are to be given. It discusses the risk of "potentially life threatening distant spread effects after local injection" because these injections have become so commonplace that some patients may underestimate the associated risk. Conversely, by minimizing the amount of toxin used (to decrease risk of side effects), some wrinkles may not be totally eradicated. However, a "natural" rather than "frozen" face is aesthetically desirable. Efficacy and duration of action vary from patient to patient, but both generally increase with serial injections over time as a result of increasing muscle atrophy. At times, a "touch-up" could be of value 2 to 3 weeks after the initial injections, should there be areas where the muscles have not been affected enough or with bilateral symmetry.

Caution the patient against prior use of aspirin, large doses of vitamin E, garlic, ginger, and diet pills, which increase the risk of bruising. Cosmetics covering treatment areas can be removed just before injection and reapplied immediately after, provided the patient *does not rub the treatment areas afterward*. Rubbing the treatment areas can spread the Botox into areas not intended for treatment, increasing the risk of complications such as ptosis. Conversely, the clinician may massage Botox toward or away from areas intentionally.

TECHNIQUE

Cosmetic uses for Botulinum toxin include the following:

- *Forehead wrinkles* caused by frontalis muscle contraction
- *Glabellar (frown or "11") lines* and *ridges across the bridge of the nose* caused principally by corrugator and procerus contraction
- *"Bunny lines"* formed across the upper nose (the expression of nose scrunching when someone smells something foul) caused by nasalis muscle contraction
- Lateral *crow's feet, inferior eyelid wrinkles, and ptotic eyebrows* from orbicularis oculi tension
- *Lipstick lines* from orbicularis oris contraction; *chin clefting and elevation* from overactive mentalis muscles
- *Depressed lateral commissures* from overactive depressor anguli
- *Ptotic nose tips and "gummy smiles"* caused by depressor septi nasi and levator labii superioris muscle contraction
- Masseter hypertrophy that causes *lower face broadness* and even *neck bands* from overactive platysma (Fig. 47.2)

Treatment of any site starts with appropriate patient selection, education, and consent. Injections are usually performed in the

seated position. It is advisable to take dated, pretreatment photographs of the patient at rest, frowning, smiling, nose scrunching, puckering, and with the brows raised, both front and side views as needed, for later evaluation of treatment efficacy and duration.

1. Cleanse the area to be injected with alcohol, and allow it to dry completely.
2. Topically applied anesthesia (e.g., Betacaine, TripleCaine, or equivalent) may be used at injection sites. It should be applied at least 30 minutes in advance to be beneficial.
3. Apply a cold gel pack or glove with ice or water to the proposed injection site to decrease injection discomfort and to cause vasoconstriction.
4. After injection, apply a dry gauze or tissue and ask the patient to hold pressure for a few minutes to reduce bruising and flatten any tissue elevation. Do not let the patient rub the area, lest the BTX-A be spread to unwanted areas.
5. Injections are most effective and comfortable when made into the subcutaneous tissue, rather than into the muscle or periosteum, or intradermally.

TREATMENT OF FOREHEAD WRINKLES AND FRONTALIS MUSCLE CONTRACTION HEADACHES

Horizontal forehead wrinkles and some "stress" or tension headaches are caused by contraction of the frontalis muscle. This muscle usually runs in two bands from the upper margin of the orbits to the scalp. Midforehead creases are usually "sympathy" wrinkles, but this area occasionally requires injection as well. Be aware and careful that inadvertent frontalis contraction may be masking brow ptosis, which would allow excess upper lid skin to collapse down toward or onto the upper lashes. This will be unmasked when Botox or Dysport is administered. Look for this by pushing the forehead down into a fully relaxed/smooth position, and see if the patient has or complains of the excess skin on the upper lid.

1. Take pretreatment photographs of the patient.
2. Cleanse the injection sites with alcohol and allow them to dry.
3. Have the patient raise the eyebrows to delineate the muscles.
4. Inject a total of 20 to 30 U of Botox or 50 to 100 U of Dysport *subcutaneously* (Fig. 47.3) into the *ridges* between the wrinkles (furrows) at indicated sites (2.5 to 5 U Botox or 5 to 15 U Dys-

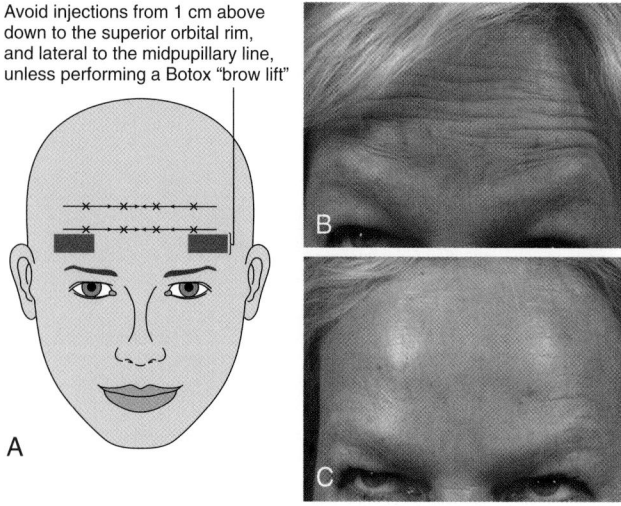

Fig. 47.3 (A) Treatment of frontalis muscle (forehead wrinkles). (B) Before. (C) After.

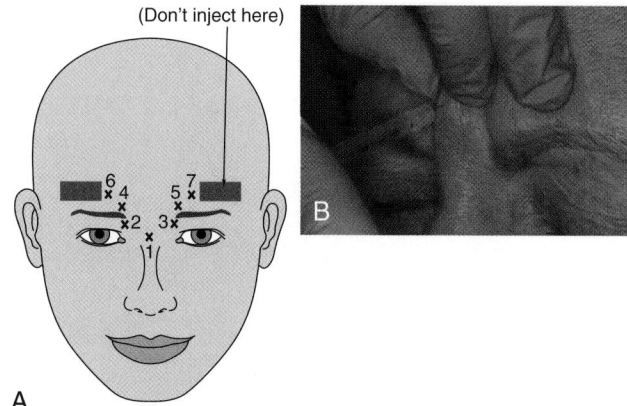

Fig. 47.4 (A) Treatment of frown lines (glabellar muscle). Direct the needle into the bulk of the contracted muscle for corrugator, procerus, and lip injections. All others are directed subcutaneously. (B) Injecting botulinum toxin into the glabellar area for frown lines.

port per site). Injections can be made relatively perpendicularly to the forehead or threaded under the tissue and injected as the needle is withdrawn. Intramuscular injections tend to bleed more, are less comfortable, and do not provide a better response. Avoid the area between the eyebrows and 1 cm above the superior edge of the orbit lateral to the midpupillary line (or the lowest frontal wrinkle) to decrease the risk of iatrogenic ptosis. Always stay above the lowest line. Eyebrow or upper lid ptosis can last weeks before fading. For treatment of lid ptosis, see the "Complications" section.

Treatment of Glabellar Wrinkles (Frown Lines)

Frown lines are caused by the contraction of several muscles; the corrugator runs diagonally from the skin of the medial brow to the bony bridge (root) of the nose. The procerus is a Y-shaped muscle that runs up the bridge of the nose to the forehead. The orbicularis oculi courses around the orbit of the eye. The depressor supercilii muscle is between them. It adds to the depression of the medial brow. Have the patient frown and scrunch his or her nose to identify the dynamic wrinkles, and inject a total of 20 to 40 U of Botox into these areas after each site is cleansed with alcohol, thoroughly dried, and chilled. Toxin is injected into each of the five to seven injection sites proportional to the effect desired. The injection sites are as follows (Fig. 47.4):

- Site 1: The bridge of the nose at the level of the lower margin of the upper lid with the eye normally open (5 to 6 U Botox, 10 to 15 U Dysport)
- Sites 2 and 3: Directly above each medial canthus at or above the level of the medial orbital bone (4 to 5 U Botox, 10 to 15 U Dysport; injecting below the edge of the orbit may cause lid ptosis)
- Sites 4 and 5: About 1 cm above and slightly lateral to sites 2 and 3 following the direction of the corrugator on each side (4 to 5 U Botox, 10 to 15 U Dysport)
- Sites 6 and 7: About 1 cm above the brow at each midpupillary line, if necessary (4 to 5 U Botox, 10 to 15 U Dysport; see Fig. 47.4)

Variations in muscular anatomy should be appreciated and treated accordingly in terms of dose and injection location. Do not inject below the superior edge of the orbit, even if the patient has preexisting brow ptosis; this can result in worsening brow ptosis and new upper lid ptosis.

Treatment of Lateral Orbital or Canthus Wrinkles (Crow's Feet)

Lateral orbital creases are created by contraction of the orbicularis oculi and photoaging. Photoaging and lateral brow ptosis cause static wrinkles, which may not be removed by BTX-A injections alone. Therefore in older patients who have significant photoaging, the objective of treatment is to minimize rather than abolish the wrinkles entirely. A total of 9 to 15 U of Botox or equivalent dose of Dysport (1 U Botox to 2.5 to 4 U Dysport) is injected in a fanlike pattern into two to five sites on each side, 1 cm lateral to the edge of the orbit (Fig. 47.5). Occasionally, anatomy dictates a second row of injections be placed farther out from the lateral canthus to control a wider orbicularis oculi. Injections made too close to the lower lid margin may cause temporary lower eyelid droop or scleral show, or may worsen infraorbital festoons. Laser treatments and conservative filler injections to the static wrinkles complement the use of Botox in this area. If there are hypertrophic orbicularis oculi muscle folds under the eye with smiling or unapposed, dynamic, inferior orbicularis wrinkles are present, an additional 2 to 4 U of Botox or an equivalent dose of Dysport may be injected subcutaneously at the level of the lower lid crease. Reevaluate results in 2 weeks, and re-treat as needed.

Insert the needle from a lateral approach to make a smooth entrance into the subcutaneous tissue. Brace or rest your hand(s) on the patient to have the best control over the needle tip and plunger. Start superiorly and inject 2 to 3 U of Botox into each furrow (two to five wrinkles), following the shape of the lateral orbital margin.

Botox "Brow Lift" and Shaping the Brow

The Botox "brow lift" (Fig. 47.6) relaxes the lateral brow depressors (orbicularis oculi) and medial aspect of the corrugator so that the action of the frontalis muscle is unopposed. To lift the lateral brow, inject 3 to 5 U of Botox at or above the lateral orbit into the brow where you feel the suture line between the frontal and temporal bones on each side. Then inject 3 to 5 U into the corrugator above the medial canthus on each side if the medial brow needs elevation as well. Do not inject the frontalis above these areas, or little lift will be achieved. If there is too much elevation of the medial brow (sad look) or lateral brow ("Spock eyed"), the frontalis muscle may be conservatively injected with a unit or two of Botox at a time until reasonable brow shape and symmetry are restored.

Treatment of Perioral Lines

Contraction of the orbicularis oris can cause vertical lines through and above the vermilion margin, which worsen with smoking and

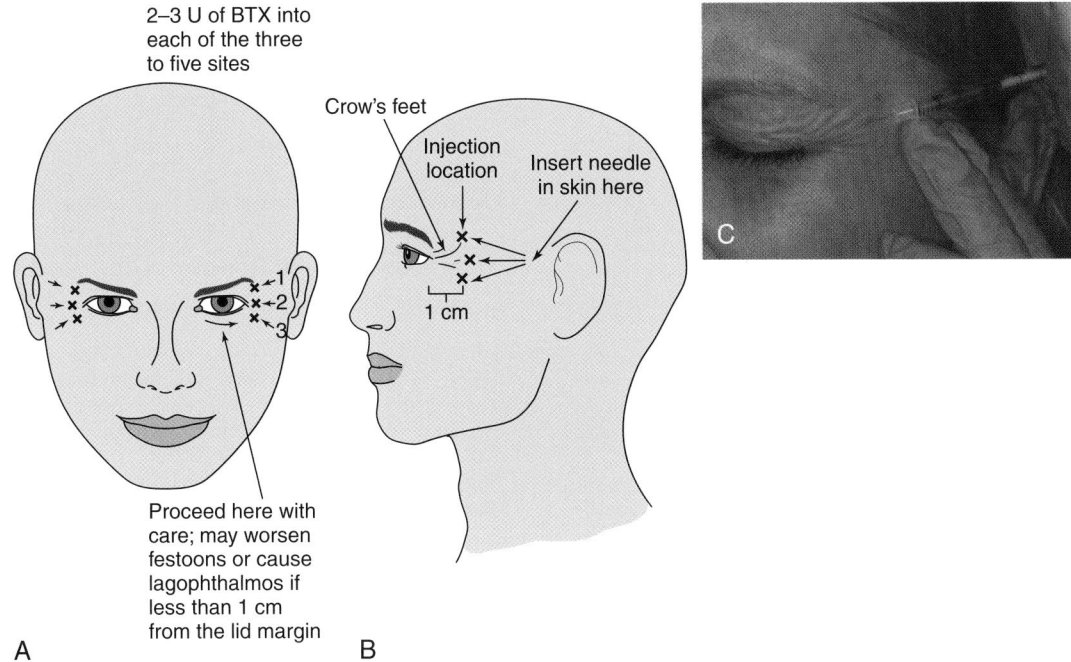

Fig. 47.5 Treatment of lateral orbital wrinkles (crow's feet). In this case, three crow's feet wrinkles are treated with three injections. (A) Frontal view. (B) Lateral view. (C) Injecting botulinum toxin for rhytids of the lateral canthal area.

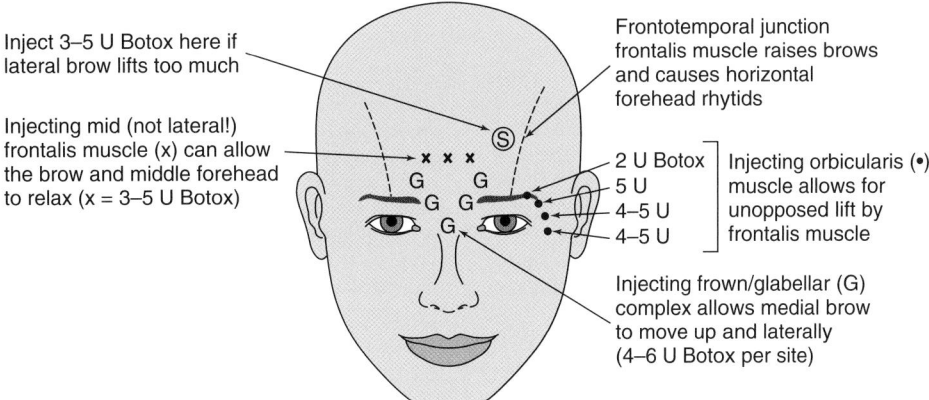

Fig. 47.6 Brow lift injection sites.

photoaging. Careful injection of 1 to 2 U of Botox into the *valley* of the wrinkle at one or two sites per side into the orbicularis oris muscle helps alleviate contraction (Fig. 47.7). This helps decrease a "gummy smile" in select patients, but they must be warned about the risk of temporary lip droop, which leads to drooling, or lessened or asymmetric smiles. If the "gummy smile" persists, 3 to 5 U of Botox can be injected into the levator labii superioris muscle (see Fig. 47.2 for a depiction of the muscle) in the area of the canine fossa bilaterally. Subtle relaxation of orbicularis allows for an increase in vertical height of the lip (outward pout) by everting the dry vermilion.

After these very precise injections, have the patient avoid rubbing the injection sites to decrease the risk of migration of the toxin to adjacent muscles.

Treatment of Depressed Commissures

Inject 3 to 5 U of Botox along the margin of the jaw directly below each corner of the mouth into the depressor anguli oris muscle (see Fig. 47.2), just anterior to the masseter muscle, which can be palpated at the level of the mandible when the patient grits his or her teeth. Check results in 2 weeks. Reinforce with further injections if needed.

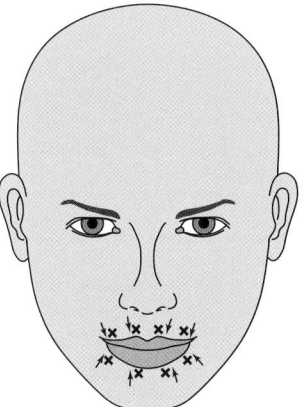

Fig. 47.7 Treatment of perioral lines. Inject up to 2 U of botulinum toxin into each valley caused by orbicularis oris contraction.

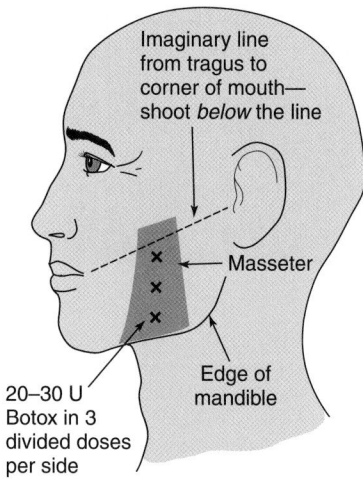

Imaginary line from tragus to corner of mouth— shoot *below* the line

Masseter

Edge of mandible

20–30 U Botox in 3 divided doses per side

Fig. 47.8 Treatment of hypertrophic masseter muscles to narrow lower face.

Treatment of Wrinkled ("Walnut") or Elevated Chin

Inject 5 to 10 U of Botox centrally into the lower part of the chin (mentalis muscle; see Fig. 47.2) or 5 U/side to a clefted chin. Too high an injection in this area can cause lower lip droop. Check results in 2 weeks. Reinforce with further Botox as needed.

Treatment of Hypertrophic Masseter Muscles

Some (usually female) patients have an angular/squared-off jawline that appears bulky and masculine. Reducing the bulk of the lower half of the masseter muscle helps soften and round that area to obtain a more feminine/oval shape to the face or balance the "pear" shape that patients demonstrate with age. This treatment is more requested by patients of Asian descent. It is also useful for helping to treat patients who chronically grind their teeth or have temporo-mandibular joint dysfunction.

Draw an imaginary line between the tragus and the corner of the mouth. Inject 20 to 30 U of Botox per side, in three divided doses, below the level of the line, down to the level of the mandible, into the bulk of the masseter muscle (Fig. 47.8). This preserves upper cheek volume while the lower face subjectively thins (masseter muscle atrophies from lack of use) after several months, and can be maintained indefinitely.

Treatment of Neck Bands

Botox is more effective on vertical platysmal bands than horizontal bands. Grasp each band where it is most prominent and inject 2 to 5 U of Botox or equivalent dose of Dysport *subcutaneously*, every 1 to 2 cm, and reevaluate in 2 weeks. Avoid accidently treating the strap muscles or making deep injections that could cause dysphonia, dysphagia, and neck weakness.

Treatment of Primary Hyperhidrosis

Excessive sweat production of the hands and armpits are common conditions that are often treated with topical applications of aluminum salts, iontophoresis, and local and systemic anticholinergic medications. When such treatments fail or give unacceptable side effects, studies have shown that Botox injections may inhibit sweating for 1 to frequently up to 8 months without muscle weakness or other side effects. A 100-U vial of Botox is diluted with 1 to 2 mL of sterile saline, yielding an effective dose of 10 or 5 U per 0.1 mL, respectively. A starch iodine test may be performed to evaluate the major area(s) of hyperhidrosis by thinly applying a liquid iodine solution to the affected areas, allowing it to dry, and then dusting the

areas with corn starch. The affected areas will turn blue and can be injected. However, most patients will be able to identify where the area of sweating is most prominent. Approximately 20 small, 2.5-U, subcutaneous blebs are injected, spaced every 1 to 2 cm, into an affected axilla or palm. Topical anesthetics, ice, or continual cold air anesthesia make these injections tolerable. Patients may note some increase in apparent sweat production in surrounding untreated areas and need further treatment.

SAMPLE OPERATIVE REPORT AND PROGRESS NOTE

See Fig. 47.1. The following is a sample SOAP (Subjective, Objective, Assessment, Plan) note for Botox treatment of crow's feet:

S—48-year-old woman with no medical problems or contraindications requests Botox chemodenervation of orbicularis oculi muscles to decrease the appearance of dynamic crow's feet.

O—After informed consent and preoperative pictures were obtained, the patient was positioned sitting upright with head supported. Topical anesthetic was applied for 30 minutes and topical ice momentarily applied before three injections of three-plus units of fresh Botox were injected subcutaneously via 30-gauge needle about a centimeter lateral to the lateral orbit on each side. Topical compression was applied to each site. There was no bruising. The injections were tolerated well.

Botox lot no.:_____   Expiration date:_____   Mix date:_____

A—Botox Chemodenervation of Orbicularis Oculi Muscles; Bilateral; 20 U

P—Patient discharged in stable condition with written instructions. Recheck in 2 weeks or as necessary.

USE OF COMMON BTX-A PREPARATIONS AVAILABLE IN UNITED STATES—DYSPORT VERSUS BOTOX VERSUS XEOMIN

Dysport is currently a bit less expensive to effectively treat an area for a similar duration of action as Botox or Xeomin. Dysport is not a household name in the United States, but it has been safely used elsewhere for more than 2 decades. Xeomin is the most recent addition to the U.S. market among the three, and its FDA approval for cosmetic use is limited to glabellar lines. The onset of action of Dysport appears to be slightly sooner than that of Botox. The injection techniques are similar once it is understood that 1 U of Botox is equivalent to 1 U of Xeomin or 2.5 to 4 U of Dysport.

The easiest, least risky place to inject is the glabella. Once you have mastered that area, try the lateral eyes and then the forehead and brow shaping. Lower face injections are mastered once you are comfortable and consistent with upper face treatments and bundling BTX-A treatments with fillers, skin treatments, and skin care programs. Symmetric injection is preferable unless you are trying to correct facial asymmetry. Start with lower doses. Increase the dose to increase the effect and duration. If an area does not respond after 2 weeks, try increasing the dose by 30% to 50%. If it still does not work, you may have one of the few patients who do not respond to these treatments. It is better to inject too high above the brow and leave horizontal forehead rhytids than to drop the brow or upper eyelid. BTX-A is a powerful and forgiving tool for performing minimally invasive, temporary facial shaping. Patients who get the best results are usually working with a clinician who integrates various modalities to address loss of facial and neck volume and proportion, skin texture, tone, color, clarity, and elasticity.

COMPLICATIONS

* Brow ptosis
* Ptosis of the upper eyelid
* Double vision

- Temporary discomfort
- Headache, nausea, or flulike symptoms
- Swelling
- Bruising
- Lip droop and drooling
- Temporary facial asymmetry
- Abnormal or lack of facial expression
- Dry mouth (reported after Myobloc injections)
- Incomplete or poor results
- Possible unknown long-term effects (e.g., muscle atrophy, nerve irritability, production of antibodies with unknown effects to general health)

There have been no long-term adverse effects or health hazards related to the use of Botox. Little if any allergy or hypersensitivity has been documented. Repetitive doses of greater than 300 U may lead to production of antibodies, making the patient resistant to further treatment with that particular serotype of BTX. However, it is rare that more than 100 U of Botox is used at any one time for cosmetic uses, or greater than 200 U used at one sitting for the treatment of hyperhidrosis.

Ptosis of the upper eyelid is infrequent (1% to 2%). This temporary side effect of Botox injection can be treated with apraclonidine 0.5% (Iopidine; Alcon Laboratories) ophthalmic drops (two drops three times daily to affected eyes). Alternatively, a compounding pharmacy can dilute Neo-Synephrine (phenylephrine) 2.5% ophthalmic drops to 1.25%. Neo-Synephrine drops give relief of lid ptosis in over 80% of patients for 3 to 4 hours, but may cause pupillary dilation with associated photophobia and difficulty with near vision temporarily.

Some patients find injections uncomfortable, which can be minimized by the use of topical anesthetic, ice before injection, small-gauge needles, subcutaneous injections, and topical and verbal distraction during injections. Chilling the tissue to be injected briefly with cold air or direct-contact chilling (e.g., devices available from Zimmer MedizinSystems [www.zimmerusa.com] and ThermoTek [www.thermotekusa.com]) can improve comfort and decrease bruising as well. The risk of bruising and swelling at injection sites is minimized by preinjection chilling and postinjection direct pressure, as described previously. Aspirin and other antiplatelet medications should be avoided for 2 weeks before treatment if possible. Keep injection volumes low. Do not inject below or less than 1 cm above the superior orbital margin lateral to the midpupillary line to prevent brow and upper lid ptosis.

POSTPROCEDURE PATIENT EDUCATION

It is important that the patient understands that Botox injections may not entirely alleviate all dynamic wrinkles every time and that the results of the treatment are temporary. Most patients achieve a 60% to 90% improvement 3 to 14 days after their injections. Recheck the patient in about 2 weeks. Review the preinjection photographs, and reinject the areas that have not responded satisfactorily. Remind patients that the objective of treatment is improvement, not perfection, and that some movement is preferred over a frozen face.

It is best if the patient does not lie down or participate in vigorous exercise for at least 4 hours after the injection. Exercising the facial muscles injected by raising the eyebrows, furrowing the brows, and frowning deeply 10 times every 15 minutes for 4 hours will enhance the binding effect of BTX-A.

CONCLUSION

Botulinum toxin has been used safely in humans since the early 1980s. The FDA approved Botox for cosmetic use in 2002. Botox has been demonstrated to be a safe and effective therapy in a number of studies. It is well accepted in the medical community as a valuable adjunct for the treatment of dynamic wrinkles of the face and neck, control of muscle contraction and vascular headaches, and treatment of hyperhidrosis. The effects of the injections generally last from 3 to 5 months and then fade gradually, with the exception of hyperhidrosis, where they are more likely to be effective for 7 to 9 months.

PATIENT EDUCATION GUIDES

See the patient education preinjection and postinjection information and patient consent forms available at www.expertconsult.com.

CPT/BILLING CODES

Note that for cosmetic purposes, there are no CPT codes, nor is there insurance coverage. Insurances vary in their coverage for any Botox injection, and it is best to have the patient clarify this with his or her carrier before doing any injections. The fees are often in the thousands of dollars, and patients need to be aware of their financial responsibilities.

64612	Chemodenervation of muscle(s); muscles innervated by facial nerve, unilateral (e.g., blepharospasm, hemifacial spasm). (Use for migraines, tension headaches.) For bilateral, use modifier 50
64615	Chemodenervation of muscles innervated by facial, trigeminal, cervical spinal and accessory nerves, bilateral (e.g., for chronic migraine)
64616	Chemodenervation of neck muscles, excluding muscles of the larynx, unilateral (e.g., spasmodic torticollis). For bilateral, use modifier 50
64642	Chemodenervation of one extremity, 1–4 muscles (e.g., dystonia, cerebral palsy)
64643	Each additional extremity, 1–4 muscles
64644	Chemodenervation of one extremity, 5 or more muscles
64645	Each additional extremity, 5 or more muscles
64646	Chemodenervation of trunk muscles, 1–5 muscles
64647	Chemodenervation of trunk muscles, 6 or more
64650	Chemodenervation of eccrine glands; both axillae
64653	Chemodenervation of other areas (e.g., scalp, face, neck) per day
64999	For hands or feet (unlisted procedure, nervous system)

ICD-10-CM DIAGNOSTIC CODES

The cost of Botox is about $5.25 per unit (100-U vial) and under $1.50 per unit for Dysport. Charges for injections range from $8 to $15 per Botox unit, depending on additional overhead, amount used, and prevailing charges in the area.

G43-G43.91	Headache Migraine
G44.2-G44.229	Headache Tension
G24.5	Blepharospasm
L74.510-L74.519	Hyperhidrosis

J Codes

J0585	Botulinum Toxin A per unit (e.g., Botox)
J0587	Botulinum Toxin B per 100 units (e.g., Myobloc)

SUPPLIERS

(See contact information available at www.expertconsult.com.)

Anatomic chart stickers for documenting Botox injections
George Tiemann and Co.
Betacaine LA and Betacaine Plus
Custom Scripts Pharmacy
University Compounding Pharmacy

Botox
　Allergan, Inc., sells and distributes the product
Cold Air and Contact Analgesia Units
　ThermoTek, Inc.
　Zimmer Medizin Systems
Customizable patient education brochures
　Contemporary Health Communications
　MJD Patient Communications
Dysport
　Ipsen (Basking Ridge, New Jersey) and Galderma (Fort Worth, Texas)
Xeomin
　Merz Aesthetics North America (Raleigh, North Carolina)
Topical Anesthetics
　See Chapter 6, Local and Topical Anesthetic Complications

ONLINE RESOURCES

DVDs: *Learning to Work with Botox (Botulinum Toxin Type A): A Guide for Clinicians (Paul A. Fox, MD, 2004) and Introduction to Botox (Botulinum Toxin Type A) for the Patient:* http://www.npinstitute.com/product-p/learning-to-work-with-botox.htm.

NOTE: There are numerous didactic and clinical training courses on cosmetic Botox injection for clinicians (e.g., National Procedures Institute [http://www.npinstitute.com]).

RECOMMENDED READING

Allergan, Inc. Botox Cosmetic (botulinum toxin type A) purified neurotoxin complex (Package Insert). Irvine, Calif, Allergan, Inc.

Bartfield JM, May-Wheeling HE, Raccio-Robak N, Lai SY. Benzyl alcohol with epinephrine as an alternative to lidocaine with epinephrine. *J Emerg Med.* 2001;21:375–379.

Botulinum toxin (Botox Cosmetic) for frown lines. *Med Lett Drugs Ther.* 2002;44:47–48.

Carruthers A, Carruthers J. *Procedures in Cosmetic Dermatology Series: Botulinum Toxin.* 3nd ed. Philadelphia: Saunders; 2012.

Carruthers A, Carruthers J, eds. Special issue: update on botulinum toxins. *Dermatol Surg;* 2007;33(suppl 1):S1–S110.

Carruthers J, Fagien S, Matarasso SL. Botox Consensus Group: consensus recommendations on the use of botulinum toxin type A in facial aesthetics. *Plast Reconstr Surg.* 2004;114(suppl 6):S1–S22.

Gart MS, Gutowski KA. Overview of botulinum toxins for aesthetic uses. *Clin Plast Surg.* 2016;43(3):459–471.

Glogau RG. Botulinum A neurotoxin for axillary hyperhidrosis: no sweat Botox. *Dermatol Surg.* 1998;24:817–819.

Kaminer MS, Arndt KS, Dover JS, Rohrer TE, Zachary CB, eds. *Atlas of Cosmetic Surgery with DVD.* 2nd ed. Philadelphia: WB Saunders; 2009.

Kim JH, Yum KW, Lee SS, et al. Effects of botulinum toxin type A on bilateral masseteric hypertrophy evaluated with computed tomographic measurement. *Dermatol Surg.* 2003;29:484–489.

Lowe N, Bradbury E, Flynn T, et al. Proceedings of the facial aesthetics conference and exhibition, royal college of physicians, London, 24–25 June 2006. *J Cosmet Laser Ther.* 2006;8:203–222.

Matarasso SL, Shafer D. Botox cosmetic. In: Nahai F, Nahai F, Codner MA, eds. *Minimally Invasive Facial Rejuvenation. Techniques in Aesthetic Plastic Surgery Series.* Philadelphia: Saunders; 2009:1–20.

Naver H, Aquilonius S-M. The treatment of focal hyperhidrosis with botulinum toxin. *Eur J Neurol.* 1997;4(suppl 2):S75–S79.

Scaglione F. Conversion ratio between Botox, Dysport, and Xeomin in clinical practice. *Toxins.* 2016;8(3):65.

Small R. Botulinum toxin. In: Usatine RP, Pfenninger JL, Stulberg DL, Small R, eds. *Dermatologic and Cosmetic Procedures in Office Practice.* Philadelphia: Elsevier; 2012:248–258.

Sundaram H, Signorini M, Liew S. Global Aesthetics Consensus: botulinum toxin type A: evidence-based review, emerging concepts, and consensus recommendations for aesthetic use, including updates on complications. *Plast Reconstr Surg.* 2016;137(3):518e–529e.

Walker TJ, Dayan SH. Comparison and overview of currently available neurotoxins. *J Clin Aesthet Dermatol.* 2014;7(2):31–39.

Xeomin Important Safety Information, Xeomin Important Safety Information. http://www.xeomin.com/physicians/safety.

CHAPTER 48

TISSUE FILLER

Mel Elson

Soft tissue augmentation has been performed since the 15th century, when physicians transplanted fat en bloc to correct defects, usually facial disfigurements related to wartime injuries. The modern era began in 1981, when the US Food and Drug Administration (FDA) approved Zyderm I, a suspension of 3.5% bovine collagen with 0.3% lidocaine. Although not particularly long-lasting or effective for a great many indications, it was sufficient to treat acne scars and fine lines and wrinkles, such as nasolabial folds, oral commissures, and crow's feet.

Over the past 30 years, products and techniques have evolved so that there are now more than 300 different filling materials. Table 48.1 lists the most common filling of those used around the world. Modern techniques and products are used not only for the classic indications for soft tissue augmentation but also to rebuild and renew faces by replacing lost tissue volume so that they appear much younger.

INDICATIONS

The indications for soft tissue augmentation have evolved over the years. Although they remain in the realm of cosmetic treatment, some, such as the soft-tissue injectables for human immunodeficiency virus (HIV) lipoatrophy, are life-changing. The areas of treatment have also expanded from the injection of nasolabial folds (Fig. 48.1), oral commissures, crow's feet, and glabella to neck lines, hands, cheeks (Fig. 48.2), bridge of the nose, chin (Fig. 48.3), and any area of atrophy.

CONTRAINDICATIONS

There are both absolute and relative contraindications as well as those that are generally applicable to all fillers and those that are specific to certain fillers.

- Allergies: Most filler materials are based on hyaluronic acid (discussed in detail later), which does not elicit a delayed hypersensitivity response. In addition, only rarely do these materials contain lidocaine, so allergy is not a substantive problem. In the past there was much more bovine material in fillers, and any allergy to bovine protein would preclude their use; to avoid reactions, skin testing had to be performed. Only Bellafil (formerly Artefill, Suneva Medical) still uses bovine materials. Interestingly, there is one hyaluronic acid product from avian sources (cock's comb), which is used to treat osteoarthritic joints; this product, however, does not require skin testing.
- Any active infection or skin disease in the area to be injected is a contraindication.
- Location: Injection of robust substances such as Cosmoplast or biphasic fillers into the glabellar complex must be avoided.
- Patients who are pregnant or breastfeeding should not undergo augmentation.

Relative contraindications include the following:

- Unrealistic expectations.

- Body dysmorphic disorder or patients seeking a psychologic boost after a life-changing event such as a divorce, the death of a family member, or loss of a job. Patients should wait and let things settle down before rushing into a procedure that may or may not be right for them and will not solve their emotional issues.
- Coagulopathy or use of anticoagulants. In addition, preparation for the injections to prevent bruising, particularly when biphasic fillers are used, should consist of discontinuing aspirin and vitamin E for at least 72 hours; if the patient is on warfarin or any other oral anticoagulant, the patient should consult his or her primary care clinician regarding the feasibility of discontinuing the drug for a few days. If this cannot be done, the patient should not be injected with biphasic fillers and extreme caution should be taken even with hyaluronic acid fillers. Topical vitamin-K cream twice a day for a week before and after treatment will significantly decrease bruising.

INITIAL EXAMINATION AND PATIENT PREPARATION

A complete history and physical examination should be performed before soft tissue augmentation, and particular emphasis should be placed on any prior injections or botulinum toxin (Botox) treatments, what the patient is using for skin care, and any allergic reactions or difficulties with any cosmetic procedures in the past.

Obtaining good-quality photographs before injection from all patients is strongly encouraged.

Informed consent should include all the pertinent information regarding possible side effects, cost, and alternative treatments as well as a statement at the end that the patient has been asked if he or she has any further concerns or questions. It is also prudent, if at all possible, to schedule another session for injections for the patient 2 to 3 weeks after treatment to see if what both the patient and clinician desired has been accomplished. Do not describe this as a session "for a possible touch-up" but one for possible additional injection if needed. The problem with calling a second injection a "touch-up" is that often the patient will feel that something may have been done incorrectly with the first injection and may therefore be hesitant to pay this additional session.

EQUIPMENT FOR SOFT TISSUE AUGMENTATION

- Injectable material of choice
- Appropriate-gauge needles for the material of choice
- Anesthetic material
- Ice
- Topical vitamin K
- Alcohol swabs for skin preparation

Material for Injection

At this point things become very complicated because there are a myriad materials available. It is not possible to obtain expertise or

TABLE 48.1   Common Filling Materials Worldwide

Manufacturer	Filling Material	Main Ingredient	Needle Gauge	Indication	Status
Alcon	Silkon 1000	Silicone	30	All except fine work	Off-label use
Allergan	CosmoDerm	Human-based collagen	30	Fine work	Worldwide
	CosmoPlast	Human-based collagen	30	Deeper; lips; base	Worldwide
	Juvéderm Ultra	Nonanimal HA	30	All except fine work	Worldwide
	Juvéderm Ultra Plus	Nonanimal HA	27	Deeper; lips; base	Worldwide
	Juvéderm Vollure,	Nonanimal HA	27	Moderate to severe wrinkles/folds	Worldwide
	Juvéderm Volbella,	Nonanimal HA	27		Worldwide
	Juvéderm Voluma	Nonanimal HA	27	Deeper, lips Cheeks	Worldwide
Anika	Elevesse	HA with lidocaine	27	Mid to deep	Worldwide
Contura	Aquamid	Polyacrylamide gel	27		EU; 30 countries
	Aquamid Recon		27 or 30		
Dermik/Sanofi Aventis	Sculptra	Polylactic acid	27	Very deep	Worldwide
Genzyme	Captique	HA	27	Mid to deep	Worldwide
Laboratories ORGéV	MacDermol S	Avian HA, non–cross-linked	30	Moisturizing	CE mark
	MacDermol R	Avian HA, cross-linked	30	Medium depth	CE mark
Medicis Valeant; Qmed; Galderma	Restylane	NASHA	30	Deep; lips	Worldwide
	Restylane touch	NASHA	32	Contour; not for fine or lips	Worldwide
	Perlane	NASHA	27	Contour; lips; not for fine lines	Worldwide
	Restylane Sub Q	NASHA	27	Medium depth	Worldwide
Mentor/Johnson & Johnson	Prevelle	HA, cross-linked	30	Finer	Worldwide
Merz (Anteis)	Belotero (Esthelis)	Non-animal HA	27	Three forms, from fine to deep	Worldwide
	Radiesse	70% acrylic hydrogel with 30% calcium hydroxylapatite	27	Biphasic, very deep	Worldwide
Prollenium	HylaNew	HA, cross-linked	30	Medium	Canada, some Asia
	HylaNew Ultra	Higher concentration	27	Deeper; lips; base	Canada, some Asia
	Hyladex	HA + hypromellose	27	Deeper except lips	Canada, some Asia
	Revanesse Versa	HA	27	Mid to deep	Worldwide
Suneva	Artefill/Bellafill	PMMA and bovine carrier	26	All except fine work	Worldwide
Teoxane SA	Teosyal 27	HA	27	Medium-deep	Worldwide
	Teosyal 30	HA	30	Fine work	Worldwide

*The European Conformity (CE) mark indicates that the product has met EU consumer safety, health, and environmental requirements. It applies to all countries of the EU as well as the four countries of the European Free Trade Area (Iceland, Liechtenstein, Norway, and Switzerland) and Turkey.
EU, European Union; *HA*, hyaluronic acid; *NASHA*, stabilized nonanimal hyaluronic acid; *PMMA*, polymethyl methacrylate.

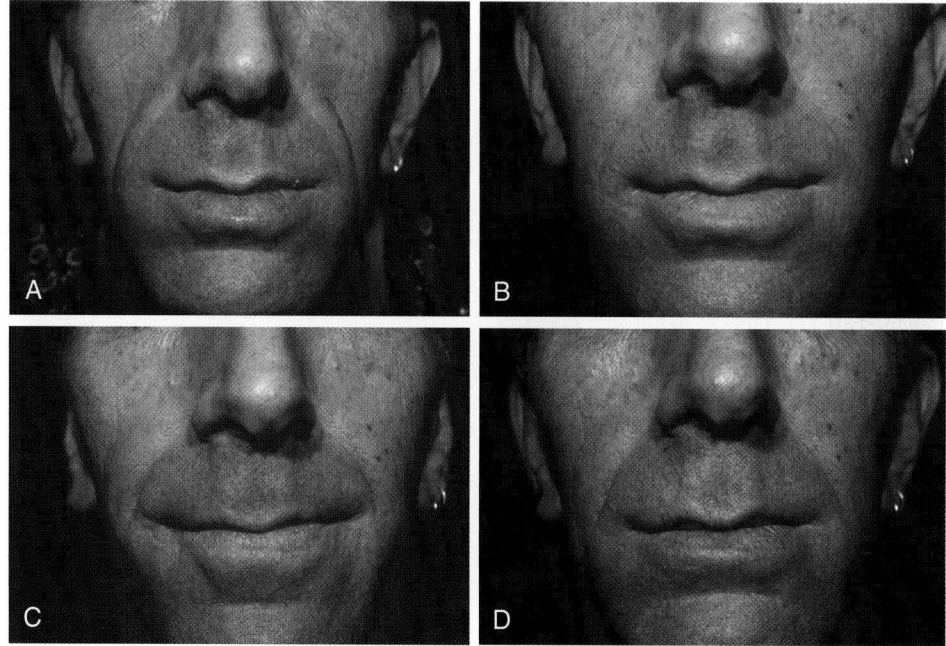

Fig. 48.1   Radiesse injection of the nasolabial folds. Before (A) and 3 months (B), 6 months (C), and 12 months (D) after treatments. Volume injected: baseline, 4 mL; 1 month, 0 mL; 6 months, 2 mL; total, 6 mL.

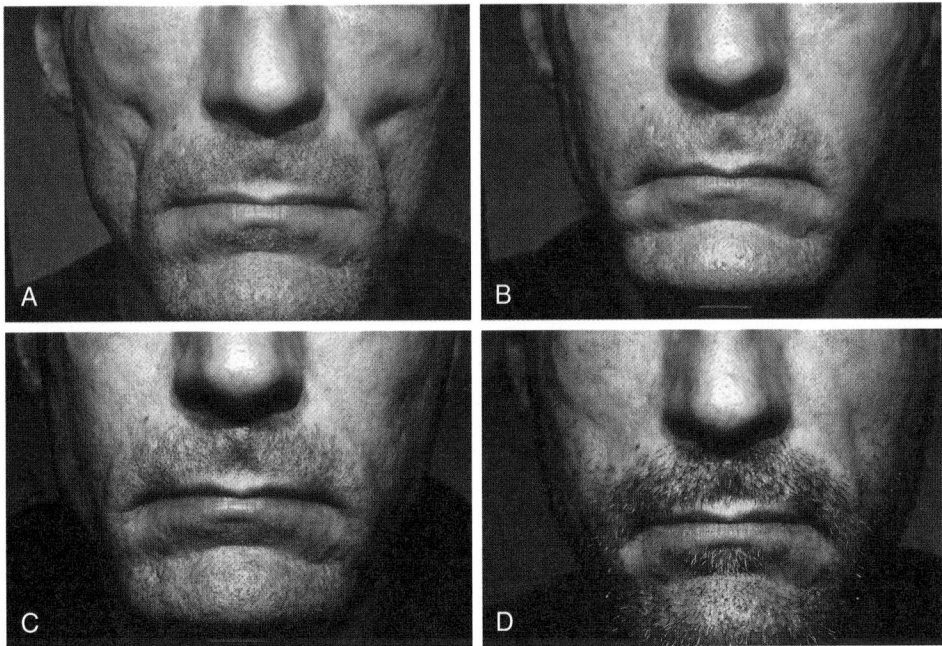

Fig. 48.2 Radiesse injection of the cheeks. Before (A) and 3 months (B), 6 months (C), and 12 months (D) after treatments. Volume injected: baseline, 8 mL; 1 month, 5 mL; 6 months, 5.7 mL; total, 18.7 mL.

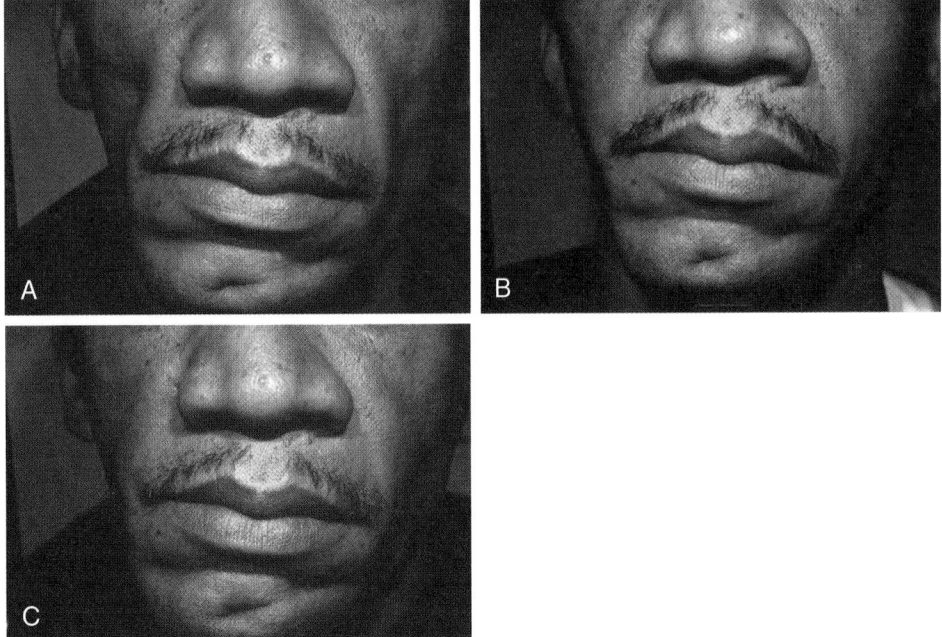

Fig. 48.3 Radiesse injection of the chin. Before (A), 3 months (B), and 12 months (C) after treatments. Volume injected: baseline, 6 mL; 1 month, 0.8 mL; 6 months, 2 mL; total, 8.8 mL.

even experience with all filling materials that are currently on the market; however, familiarity with a few will provide an armamentarium that will suffice for most needs (Table 48.2).

Collagen Products From Human Fibroblasts

CosmoDerm basically replaced Zyderm, which contained bovine collagen, because it is the same material with the same indications but with the collagen derived from human foreskin fibroblasts; therefore it does not require allergy skin testing. CosmoPlast is the same as Zyplast, which also contained bovine collagen but is now also derived from human tissue.

Collagen Products From Bacterial Hyaluronic Acid

Most of the materials currently available are based on hyaluronic acid. Such products have become very popular around the world, and there are indeed many of them, but the most significant in this category are the products from Q-med in Sweden (Restylane, and Perlane Restylane Fine Lines, versions now also marketed by Medicis/Valeant and Galderma) and those from Inamed Allergan (Juvéderm Ultra, Juvéderm Ultra Plus, and Juvéderm Fine Line—also known as Juvéderm 24, Juvéderm 30, and Juvéderm 18). All of these products are manufactured by bacterial fermentation in the laboratory, after which the hyaluronic acid undergoes various degrees of

TABLE 48.2   Common Uses of Major Fillers

Filler	NLF	OC	Glabella	Periocular	Lips
Restylane	1.5 mL	1 mL	0.3 mL	0.1 mL	1–2 mL
Juvéderm	1–2 mL	1 mL	0.2 mL	0.1 mL	1–2 mL
Radiesse	0.8 mL	0.4 mL	—	—	—
Teosyal	1 mL	0.5 mL	0.2 mL	0.1 mL	1–2 mL
Revanesse	1 mL	0.5 mL	0.2 mL	0.1 mL	1–2 mL

NLF, Nasolabial folds; *OC*, oral commissures.
For this table, it is assumed that the clinician understands the following:
- Every patient is different and the volumes given are averages only.
- There are a number of different fillers in each line designated for certain uses that are not interchangeable (e.g., Restylane is for NLF, Perlane is better for lips).
- Teosyal has seven different products in the line, so each product should be used in the appropriate area.
- Never use a biphasic filler in the lips.
- Never use a robust filler around the eyes or in the area of the glabella.
- The volumes refer to each side of treatment.

cross-linking and folding to increase the longevity of the implant. Without any manipulation of the molecule to increase cross-linking and molecular weight, the implant would be very short-lived, because pure hyaluronic acid lasts only hours to a few days when injected into the skin. A product used in Asia, called Hyalan, is actually injected into the skin to act as a moisturizer. Hyaluronic acid traps and attracts water. This is also the reason why, when hyaluronic acid is injected as filler, the end result is a smooth surface—because water is absorbed into the area of injection. Although there is great similarity between different types of hyaluronic acid fillers available, there is much debate as to which is the longest-lasting, which produces the smoothest results, and which is most comfortable for the patient. The higher-molecular-weight products are used for more aggressive augmentation, as for scars, lip augmentation, and some degree of sculpting. The lower-molecular-weight products are used for fine lines such as crow's feet and lip lines. Midrange products are used for the majority of augmentation needs, such as the treatment of nasolabial folds, oral commissures, and the glabellar area.

The most common fillers used in the United States are Restylane and Perlane (Medicis Valeant) and Juvéderm Ultra and Juvéderm Ultra Plus (Allergan), although there are also some others.

Noncollagen, Non–Hyaluronic Acid Products

Some widely used products are not collagen-based and do not contain hyaluronic acid; these include Sculptra (called New-Fill in Europe) and Radiesse. Sculptra (Dermik/Sanofi Aventis) is a polymer of lactic acid that is provided as a powder to be mixed before injection with water or lidocaine. Since it is difficult to force into solution, it is recommended that the product be mixed the day before use if possible. It was initially approved in the United States for HIV lipoatrophy and is used in many areas for soft tissue augmentation, including cheek augmentation and post-rhinoplasty defects. *It induces new collagen formation* as the implant itself degrades to lactic acid and is absorbed completely by the body. There has been a report of this material inducing a correction lasting for 40 months, although probably 12 to 24 months is more likely. It is injected into the lowest part of the dermis at the junction with the subcutaneous tissue using a 26-gauge needle and does require some degree of anesthesia.

Radiesse (Bioform Medical Mertz) is one of the most popular filling materials because it is a biphasic filler that produces long-lasting results (although they are not permanent, because the second phase is biodegradable). With a biphasic filler, phase one corrects the defect and triggers the second phase, which induces the patient to form collagen from fibroblast infiltration. The key point is that any biphasic material should be both biocompatible and biodegradable, so that eventually the only substance that remains is the patient's own collagen producing the correction. Radiesse consists

of 70% acrylic hydrogel with 30% calcium hydroxylapatite beads. Calcium hydroxylapatite has been used as a dental material for more than 20 years. Radiesse has been approved by the FDA for vocal-fold augmentation, as a radiographic marker, and for maxillofacial augmentation. More recently, the FDA approved the material for the treatment of HIV lipoatrophy and nasolabial fold augmentation. It is injected at the junction of the dermis and subcutaneous tissue using a 27-gauge needle. When augmenting cheeks or correcting nasolabial folds, use of a 27-gauge 1.25-inch needle is recommended, rather than the more common half-inch needle, which can be used in shorter areas such as the oral commissures.

The Radiesse injection technique is more specific than those used with other materials. The needle should be inserted through the dermis (where resistance is felt) and then into the subcutaneous space (where there is little resistance). The material is injected in a retrograde fashion with care taken to discontinue injecting before withdrawal to avoid inadvertent injection into the dermis. Although this is difficult to master, it is imperative that the injections be done in this manner to avoid foreign-body reactions. Rather than a single pass, multiple passes are made.

- To correct the nasolabial fold, material is injected under the fold in the manner just described and then closer to the nose, with still a third linear thread just onto the cheek slightly above the fold. Care should also be taken to make the injections in the linear thread smooth, without hesitation during the injection, so that lumps do not occur. This technique will form a "scaffold" under the nasolabial fold to elevate it.
- To augment cheeks the same technique is used, but with an additional triple linear thread at right angles to the first set. This would also apply to the correction of HIV lipoatrophy, rhinoplasty defect, or any other true augmentation.

Also see later under Plane of Injection, in the Technique section.

The gel and the particles are injected into the desired area of correction. The gel dissipates over a 3- to 4-month period; during this time the particles that have been delivered induce fibroblasts to collect, stimulating new collagen formation. As the gel disappears, the new collagen remains, producing correction for approximately 18 months or more. The main advantage to Radiesse is that the calcium hydroxyapatite particles are biodegradable and disappear over time, avoiding the possible problems of permanent fillers.

This filler also contains no anesthetic, so it is advisable to provide the patient with some form of anesthesia. Augmentation of the nasolabial fold, oral commissures, and the like may require only a topical anesthetic such as Ela-Max or Betacaine, but cheek augmentation or treatment of HIV lipoatrophy usually requires a nerve block. Radiesse should not be used for lip augmentation because significant beading may result.

GENERAL GUIDELINES

In using materials for soft tissue augmentation, certain guidelines should be kept in mind:

- The shortest-lasting (low-molecular-weight) materials are the ones that are injected highest in the dermis with the smallest-gauge needle (30, 32, or 33 gauge); they may require overcorrection, can be repeated often, and are forgiving if an error occurs. They will usually last 3 to 4 months.
- Mid-molecular-weight materials should be injected with a 30-gauge needle into the middle dermis and can be expected to last approximately 6 to 12 months.
- The most robust (highest-molecular-weight) materials are injected deeper into the tissues, use larger needles (26 or 27 gauge), must never be overcorrected, cannot be repeated very often (e.g., no more than twice a year), and may be totally unforgiving in the event of an error on the part of the injector. Inexperienced injectors should begin with more forgiving materials such as

CosmoDerm, Restylane, and Juvéderm Ultra and should receive one-on-one instruction from an experienced injector to obtain proper knowledge of soft tissue augmentation.

PREPROCEDURAL PATIENT PREPARATION

Once a history, physical examination, photographs, and informed consent are obtained, the areas to be injected should be cleansed with alcohol. The patient should not be wearing makeup. Ice can be applied both before and after the procedure for patient comfort. If more anesthesia is desired or required, a field block, nerve block, or mixing the filler material with 0.2 mL of 2% lidocaine with epinephrine will provide greater patient comfort.

TECHNIQUE

The patient should be in the upright position for injection. Technique depends on the goal for each individual patient. Provide traction by pulling the skin in the direction of the defect and aligning the needle with the defect to be injected. Use the smallest-gauge needle possible (usually provided by the manufacturer with the material). The plane of injection and degree of correction are critical to achieve complete, smooth, and long-lasting correction of the defect.

Basic Technique

Whenever a dermal filler is being injected—regardless of the material being used, the level of injection, or the defect being corrected—the key technical concept is to inject smoothly. One should consider the material flowing through the needle, and the syringe-needle unit should be seen as a continuation of the injector's hand and arm. The action should be smooth, like laying down icing on a cake. Once movement begins, do not stop until the end point is reached.

Plane of Injection

Collagen should be injected into the superficial dermis with some overcorrection. All hyaluronic acid products should be injected into the dermis with just slight undercorrection, because water will come into the area immediately and continue to do so over time, enhancing the correction. All biphasic (e.g., Artefill and Radiesse) and robust (e.g., Sculptra) fillers must be placed at the dermal-subcutaneous junction with no overcorrection and care taken to avoid placing any material in the dermis.

When biphasic materials are being injected, a fan-like scaffold, also known as the fern technique, should be formed under the defect to hold up the defect (see the earlier discussion in the section titled Noncollagen, Non–Hyaluronic Acid Products). This is performed by entering the subcutaneous space (as soon as resistance gives, one has entered that space) and injecting in the same plane but at varying angles and not exiting through the dermis before discontinuing the injection so that no material is deposited into the dermis, thus avoiding a possible granulomatous response.

COMMON ERRORS IN SOFT TISSUE AUGMENTATION

- Overcorrecting in areas of fine lines (e.g., periorbital and perioral)
- Injecting biphasic fillers into the dermis
- Injecting too robust a filler into the glabellar complex
- Not providing sufficient anesthesia to make the patient comfortable
- Not following up with a second patient visit
- Not taking before and after photographs
- Not obtaining informed consent
- Not taking a complete medical history before injection

- Using a permanent filler of any type
- Not asking patients which type of filler they had injected by a former physician

COMPLICATIONS

- *Bruising:* Some degree of bruising is the most common complication. It can be eliminated or decreased with the application of ice and topical vitamin K before and after the injection session. (See the earlier discussion of relative contraindications.)
- *Erythema:* This is common after injection of any material and is easily addressed with topical vitamin K and ice.
- *Edema:* This is not unusual and is particularly common with hyaluronic acid products; it is temporary and of no consequence.
- *Infection:* Although infection is theoretically possible with dermal fillers, I have never seen this occur in over 25 years of practice.
- *Skin necrosis:* This can occur anywhere on the face from the injection of any material; however, the most common area of occurrence is the glabellar complex, owing to the paucity of collateral circulation in this area. The necrosis is not due to injection into a vessel but to the material crimping a vessel in this area, thus occluding the blood supply. If there is sudden blanching and the patient states the injection has become painful, stop immediately and apply nitroglycerin paste or dimethyl sulfoxide to increase the circulation in the area.
- *Uneven results:* The possibility of this occurrence is the primary reason to schedule a second injection session 2 weeks after the first. This is also one of the primary reasons to take pretreatment photographs of every patient; we are not symmetric to begin with, and some patients do not realize that.

POSTPROCEDURAL PATIENT CARE AND EDUCATION

- Apply ice immediately after injection.
- Apply topical vitamin K twice daily for at least 5 days.
- No warfarin, aspirin, or vitamin E for 48 hours.
- No significant sun exposure for 48 hours.

Patient should be advised to do the following for overall skin health:

- Apply a sun protection factor (SPF) 30 product every morning (ultraviolet A and B block).
- Apply retinoids each evening.
- Do not smoke.
- Avoid tanning beds completely.
- Return for another injection session in 2 weeks and then whenever desired in the future but before all the correction has subsided.

PEARLS

- Use the smallest-gauge needle through which the material can flow.
- Use ice before and during the injection session for more patient comfort.
- When injecting the lips, move slightly onto the lip (about 1 mm) to achieve longer-lasting correction.
- To avoid lumpy results, make sure your movements are smooth.
- Try using a 32- or 33-gauge needle for fine lines.
- Change needles before the syringe is empty because the skin dulls needles.
- Always underestimate how long correction will last—in other words, underpromise and overdeliver.
- Do not attempt to learn technique except from an expert (one on one if possible).
- Never talk patients into procedures they are not certain they really want.
- If you are not sure, then do not do it.

CPT/Billing Codes

11950	Subcutaneous injection of filling material (e.g., collagen), 1 mL or less
11951	1.1 to 5 mL
11952	5.1 to 10 mL
11954	over 10 mL

Suppliers

(See contact information available at www.expertconsult.com.)

Providers of filler material and videos for injection technique
Allergan
BioForm Medical Mertz (Radiesse)
Medicis Valeant Aesthetics

Additional Resources

See the treatment record form available at www.expertconsult.com.

Videotapes and DVDs

Clinician Education

Carruthers J, Carruthers A. *Procedures in Cosmetic Dermatology Series: Soft Tissue Augmentation with DVD.* 3rd ed. Philadelphia: Elsevier; 2012.

Patient Education

U.S. Food and Drug Administration: Dermal Fillers (Soft Tissue Fillers): https://www.fda.gov/MedicalDevices/ProductsandMedicalProcedures/CosmeticDevices/WrinkleFillers/default.htm.

Recommended Reading

Ahn MS. Calcium hydroxylapatite: Radiesse. *Facial Plast Surg Clin North Am.* 2007;15:85–90.

Ballin AC, Brandt FS, Cazzaniga A. Dermal fillers: an update. *Am J Clin Dermatol.* 2015;16(4):271–283.

Bass LS. Injectable filler techniques for facial rejuvenation, volumization, and augmentation. *Facial Plast Surg Clin North Am.* 2015;23(4):479–488.

Busso M, Applebaum D. Hand augmentation with Radiesse (calcium hydroxylapatite). *Dermatol Ther.* 2007;20:385–387.

Busso M, Voigts R. An investigation of changes in physical properties of injectable calcium hydroxylapatite in a carrier gel when mixed with lidocaine and with lidocaine/epinephrine. *Dermatol Surg.* 2008;34(suppl 1):S16–S23.

Duranti F, Salti G, Bovani B, et al. Injectable hyaluronic acid gel for soft tissue augmentation: a clinical and histologic study. *Dermatol Surg.* 1998;24:1317–1325.

Elson ML. Soft tissue augmentation. In: Elson ML, ed. *Evaluation and Treatment of the Aging Face.* New York: Springer-Verlag; 1986:79–96.

Elson ML. The role of skin testing in the use of collagen injectable materials. *J Dermatol Surg Oncol.* 1989;15:301–303.

FDA. Soft Tissue Fillers Approved by the Center for Devices and Radiological Health. https://www.fda.gov/MedicalDevices/ProductsandMedicalProcedures/CosmeticDevices/WrinkleFillers/ucm227749.htm.

Ferneini EM, Beauvais D, Aronin SI. An overview of infections associated with soft tissue facial fillers: identification, prevention, and treatment. *J Oral Maxillofac Surg.* 2017;75(1):160–166.

Hanke CW, Tierney EP, Countryman NB, Rzany B, Sattler G. Soft-tissue augmentation. In: Robinson JK, Hanke CW, Sengelmann RD, Siegel DM, Fratila A, eds. *Surgery of the Skin: Procedural Dermatology.* 2nd ed. Philadelphia: Elsevier; 2014:367–392.

Lowe N, Maxwell CA, Lowe P, et al. Hyaluronic acid skin fillers: adverse reactions and skin testing. *J Am Acad Dermatol.* 2001;45:930–933.

Serra M. Facial implants with polymethylmethacrylate for lipodystrophy correction: 30 months follow-up. *Antiviral Ther.* 2001;6(suppl 4):75.

Sherman RN. Sculptra: the new three-dimensional filler. *Clin Plast Surg.* 2006;33:539–550.

Small R. Dermal fillers. In: Usatine RP, Pfenninger JL, Stulberg DL, Small R, eds. *Dermatologic and Cosmetic Procedures in Office Practice.* Philadelphia: Elsevier; 2012.

Small R. Dermal Fillers for Facial Rejuvenation. In: Mayeaux EJ, ed. *The Essential Guide to Primary Care Procedures.* 2nd ed. Philadelphia: Wolters Kluwer; 2015.

Sundaram H, Liew S, Signorini M, et al. Global Aesthetics Consensus Group. Global aesthetics consensus: hyaluronic acid fillers and botulinum toxin type A-recommendations for combined treatment and optimizing outcomes in diverse patient populations. *Plast Reconstr Surg.* 2016;137(5):1410–1423.

Vedamurthy M, Vedamurthy A, Nischal K. Dermal fillers: do's and dont's. *J Cutan Aesthet Surg.* 2010;3(1):11–15.

Werschler WP. Treating the aging face: a multidisciplinary approach with calcium hydroxylapatite and other fillers. *Cosmet Dermatol.* 2007;20:739–742.

CHAPTER 49

MICRODERMABRASION AND DERMAL INFUSION

Basil M. Hantash • Sandy T. Liu

MICRODERMABRASION: BACKGROUND

The concept of smoothing the skin by removing or abrading the upper layers can be dated back to 1500 BC, when Egyptian physicians used a type of sandpaper to treat scars. Modern dermabrasion was developed in Germany in the early 1900s by Kromayer, who used human-powered rotating wheels and rasps to abrade the epidermis and superficial portions of the dermis. This new technology was mainly used to treat scars, hyperpigmentation, and keratoses; however, acceptance was not forthcoming. It was not until Kurtin, Burks, and others began using motorized wire brushes for dermabrasion in the early to mid-1950s that the power of the technology began to be realized. In spite of possible great benefits with dermabrasion, there are potential negatives: need for anesthesia, scarring, prolonged downtime, wound care, infection, and contaminated operative field with aerosolized particles that endanger the practitioner and staff. Many of these problems are also encountered with other techniques, such as laser resurfacing and deep chemical peels. These factors, as well as economic considerations, pushed for development of a new technology that is less debilitating, safer, and more affordable: microdermabrasion (MDA).

MDA was developed in Italy in 1985, introduced in the United States during the mid-1990s, and has spread at an explosive rate. According to data from the American Society for Aesthetic Plastic Surgery, an estimated 557,690 MDA procedures were performed in the United States in 2015.

MECHANISM OF ACTION

The most superficial layer of the skin is the *stratum corneum*, which is a lifeless accumulation of protein and lipids derived from flattened, dead keratinocytes; this layer forms a barrier to protect the skin from a myriad of invasive insults. From the time a keratinocyte is formed in younger skin it takes approximately 28 days to mature, die, and flake off the skin surface as dander. As humans age, keratinocyte transit times dramatically increase, trapping pigment and debris in the superficial epidermal layers to give the characteristic stained appearance of aging or solar (actinic) damage. Another skin cell of major importance is the dermal fibroblast, which lies within the dermis and synthesizes extracellular matrix components, including proteoglycans (e.g., dermatan sulfate), glycosaminoglycans (e.g., hyaluronic acid), collagen, and elastin. This function also decreases with aging and actinic damage. The process of MDA addresses both the stained, debris-laden epidermis and the sluggish fibroblast production of extracellular matrix, especially collagen.

Epidermal Effects of Microdermabrasion

The micrographs in Fig. 49.1 exhibit the immediate sequential thinning and smoothing of epidermal structures from the abrasive effect of crystals moving rapidly across the skin surface. The gentle planing of the upper layers of skin removes pigmentary impurities and debris held within the stratum corneum and yields a smoother, softer skin surface. Each pass of the MDA handpiece is estimated to ablate approximately 15 μm of skin, roughly equal to one pass of the erbium laser. In addition to immediate smoothing of the skin, the abrasive process seems to stimulate keratinocyte turnover. Shehadi and colleagues have shown 9% increases in epidermal thickness in porcine skin with MDA.

Dermal Effects of Microdermabrasion

Most MDA machines are quite simple in principle, having a reservoir of abrasive crystals to be fed through a flexible tube to a handpiece that is moved across the skin. The skin is "tented up" by the negative pressure generated in the machine, and the abrasive crystals, usually aluminum oxide (corundum), are simultaneously blown and "sucked" across the skin. This removes the upper layers of the epidermis in a fine "sandblasting" technique. Other types of particulate materials are also available such as sodium chloride crystals, sodium bicarbonate (baking soda), and magnesium oxide crystals. However, aluminum oxide seems ideal because it is widely available, inert, very hard, has multiple sharp edges, does not readily absorb liquid, and is nontoxic even if inadvertently inhaled. Used crystals and cutaneous debris are then removed with suction and collected in a separate waste container, thus creating a closed-loop system that avoids the airborne contaminants of open dermabrasion. The handpieces usually can be fitted with either reusable metal tips or disposable plastic tips. The metal tips must be sterilized before each use.

Treatments are superficial enough to not cause bleeding or "serum ooze." Patients with very sensitive skin may experience slight discomfort, but most treatments are considered painless and are well tolerated. No topical anesthetics are needed. After each pass, the bulk of crystals should be removed before continuing. The second pass should be at right angles, or perpendicular, to the direction of the first pass. An optional third pass is performed with a swirling or circular motion, making sure that the skin is taut and the handpiece tip is moving and not stationary over a single skin point. Skilled operators also pay close attention to the direction of lymphatic flow, especially in areas such as the face, to avoid obstructing drainage or causing unnecessary edema.

Skin changes are cumulative and treatment sessions are repeated at 7- to 14-day intervals. Depending on the type and severity of the skin problem(s), usually between 4 and 15 treatments are offered on an as-needed basis over 1 to 4 months. The patient is usually able to return to normal activities immediately unless the skin is extremely sensitive. Mild erythema may be observed and usually resolves within 12 to 24 hours after treatment.

The operator has great flexibility in treating patients and improving outcomes by varying the depth of penetration to match each

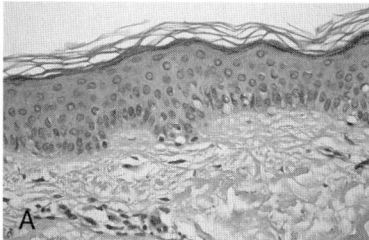
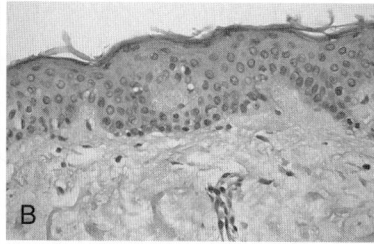
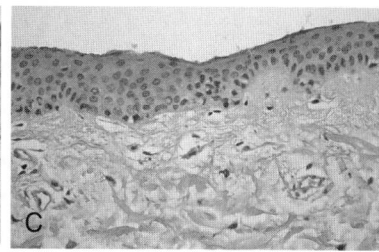

Fig. 49.1 (A) Pretreatment photomicrograph of human skin of the upper back showing fully intact stratum corneum and stratum granulosum. (B) Upper back skin on same patient after two passes. Note that the stratum corneum has been markedly ablated. (C) Upper back skin after four passes, same region of the back as A and B, but separated by 20 minutes, exhibiting total removal of the stratum corneum and most of the stratum granulosum. (Courtesy Rick Wilson, MD, Dallas, TX.)

patient's unique circumstances and requirements. This is accomplished by controlling the following four factors:

1. Density of crystal flow
2. Number of passes completed
3. Vacuum pressure
4. Handpiece speed over the skin surface

In rare instances (e.g., acne scarring), high vacuum settings (≥20 mm Hg) may be required. The operator should expect variability in vacuum settings and crystal flow with different machines.

INDICATIONS

- Minor acne scarring
- Postoperative/traumatic scarring
- Fine lines and wrinkles
- Superficial pigmentation such as lentigines and ephelides
- Melasma and other disorders of pigmentation
- Postinflammatory hyperpigmentation due to acne or eczema, among other causes
- Blending post-laser hyperpigmentation
- Skin texture irregularities
- Actinic keratoses
- Enlarged pores
- Clogged pores and blackheads
- Whiteheads
- Some mild forms of acne
- Keratosis pilaris
- Rosacea (using dermal infusion; see later discussion)
- Striae distensae

MDA is best used in combination with a regimen of topical cosmeceuticals such as a retinoid, a bleaching agent, sunscreen, and antioxidants; the regimen is better absorbed and more effective when applied to thinner skin. Patients with stage I, II, or III acne have done well when MDA is combined with topical retinoid therapy (Fig. 49.2). Although MDA does not entirely eliminate stretch marks, it can be an effective treatment option when combined with topical therapies. In a study by Abdel-Latif and Elbendary (2008), better results were seen when treating striae rubra than for striae alba, suggesting that treatment may be limited to more recent-onset stretch marks. Moreover, molecular studies showed that type I collagen expression was upregulated in the skin of patients with striae post-MDA treatment. This provides a biologic mechanism for the benefits of MDA treatment in patients with striae rubra. More recently, cosmeceutical agents such as vitamin C have been proposed as therapies for striae. In addition, work by Lee and colleagues (2003) demonstrated that treatment of ex vivo skin with MDA significantly increased the uptake of vitamin C. It will be interesting to see whether a combination of MDA and topical vitamin C will improve clinical outcomes for striae treatment.

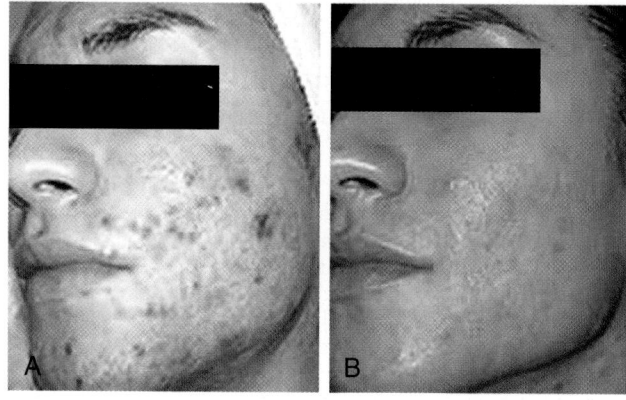

Fig. 49.2 (A) Patient with stage II acne on chronic daily topical retinoids. (B) Same patient after six SilkPeel treatments combined with dermal infusion of an antiacne solution.

DERMAL INFUSION

Background

Dermal infusion is an innovative procedure that uses MDA technology to increase delivery of active ingredients to treat skin conditions such as hyperpigmentation, telangiectasia, papulopustular acne, eczema, photodamage, dehydration, rosacea, and fine lines. It is unique in that it uses a closed-loop vacuum system with a recessed diamond tip, rather than microcrystals, to exfoliate the skin while simultaneously infusing the topical dermaceutical into the deeper dermal layers. The size, coarseness of the diamond tip, vacuum, and flow rates can all be adjusted depending on the patient's treatment. A major advantage of dermal infusion is minimal posttreatment erythema and decreased risk of postinflammatory hyperpigmentation compared with the harsh and abrasive standard MDA treatments. Furthermore, dermal infusion is ideal for treatment of the lips, papulopustular acne, and rosacea, which are all relatively contraindicated with crystal-based MDA. The optimal treatment regimen involves 4 to 6 treatments every 1 to 2 weeks and monthly treatments thereafter.

In a 2007 unpublished histologic study conducted by Moy, patients were pretreated with dermal infusion in the preauricular area 1 to 3 days before undergoing an elective facelift. During the procedure, the marked dermal infusion-treated area was removed, fixed with formalin, processed, and then analyzed. The author found that the dermal infusion treatment created a smooth and uniform abraded surface confined to the granular layer approximately 30 to 35 μm deep. The epidermal layer and the keratinosomes in it that help create the hydrophobic barrier remained intact after treatment. Moreover, addition of a hydrating serum to the abrasive surface showed vacuolization of keratinocytes, displacement of the nucleus, and edema around collagen fibers near the upper papillary dermis.

Furthermore, epidermal thickness was increased by 70% after dermal infusion, consistent with effective absorption and penetration into the papillary dermis. These findings are consistent with rapid hydration of the underlying dermis and help explain the mechanism for the observed clinical improvement in fine wrinkles after MDA plus dermal infusion treatment.

Intense Pulsed Light Therapy

MDA-thinned skin enhances penetration of intense pulse light therapy (see Chapters 38 to 44).

Rosacea Treatment

Current treatments of rosacea include avoiding triggers such as sunlight exposure, administration of topical and oral antibiotics, and use of laser and light therapies. Treatment usually lasts 3 to 6 months and is associated with side effects such as skin irritation and dryness, erythema, bruising, and photosensitivity. Moreover, MDA is not recommended for patients with rosacea because it can further aggravate the skin, causing angiogenesis, inflammation, and reactive oxygen species. Dermal infusion, however, will not exacerbate the deeper epidermal layers and can be considered an alternative monotherapy for rosacea. In a study by Desai and colleagues (2006), 30 patients with erythematotelangiectatic or papulopustular rosacea underwent MDA plus dermal infusion treatment twice a month for 12 weeks. The authors chose to use 2% erythromycin and 2% salicylic acid as their infusion solution to decrease inflammation and induce exfoliation, respectively. Twenty patients completed the study: six patients with erythematotelangiectatic rosacea and 14 patients with papulopustular rosacea. There was a statistically significant reduction in erythema, papules, and pustules in all patients by the 12th week, with a reduction noted as early as week 4. The authors reported a 42% improvement in erythema in the erythematotelangiectatic group and a 69% decrease in papules and 55% decrease in pustules in the papulopustular group. In addition, photographs taken throughout the study documented an overall improvement in the patients' condition, and there was positive patient feedback regarding tolerability, satisfaction, and overall quality of life. The adverse event most commonly reported by the study participants was transient erythema, which resolved in 3 to 6 hours.

Tattoo Treatment

An interesting case report by Wray and colleagues (2005) documented the first successful treatment of traumatic tattoo with SilkPeel (Envy Medical, Inc.) MDA treatment during isotretinoin (Accutane) therapy. The adolescent male patient had suffered a traumatic tattoo around the upper and lower eyelids after an explosive accident. The first treatment was performed 48 hours after the accident, with two other treatments on days 3 and 12 postaccident. Comedonal extractors and Vigilon wound dressing were used as adjunctive therapy. After the first treatment, more than half of the tattoo marks disappeared; further improvement was reported with each ensuing treatment. The patient was extremely satisfied with the cosmetic outcome and no complications were reported.

Hyperpigmentation Treatment

Envy Medical, the manufacturer of the SilkPeel MDA system, introduced a novel approach for the treatment of hyperpigmentation that involves four MDA treatments spaced 1 week apart, in combination with infusion of a skin-lightening solution (Lumixyl) developed by the same company. This approach represents a potential breakthrough in the treatment of hyperpigmentation because the skin-lightening formulation does not include the possibly toxic hydroquinone. It can thus be used safely in women of child-bearing age, even if pregnant or breastfeeding. Fig. 49.3 shows the results for an Asian patient with Fitzpatrick type IV skin before and after 4 weekly treatments using this approach.

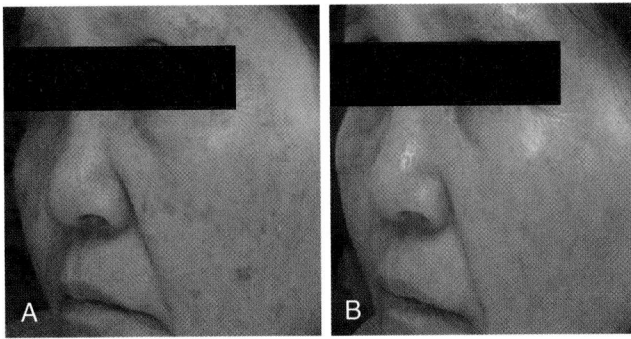

Fig. 49.3   (A) Baseline appearance of patient with Fitzpatrick phototype IV skin and melasma. (B) Same patient after four SilkPeel treatments combined with dermal infusion of Lumixyl, a novel skin-lightening formulation that does not contain retinoids or corticosteroids.

Other Dermal Infusion Systems

HydraFacial, manufactured by Edge Systems, is another dermal infusion unit currently used by dermatologists and aestheticians. Similar to SilkPeel, the HydraFacial device simultaneously resurfaces the stratum corneum and delivers active serum into the treated tissue. The exfoliation is achieved with a patented crystal-free tip, patented disposable HydroPeel tip, or a Spa Aggression tip. Various skin-specific solutions such as glucosamine, lactic acid, salicylic acid, and antioxidants (vitamins A and E and white tea extract) are used for infusion. The Tissue Nutrient Solution serum developed by SkinMedica is exclusively designed for the HydraFacial system. The serum consists of NouriCel-MD, a patented formulation of human growth factors, cytokines, soluble collagen, antioxidants, and matrix proteins that enables greater skin rejuvenation.

In a study by Freedman (2008), two study groups were randomized to either a series of hydradermabrasion treatments with antioxidant dermal infusion or treatments with the same antioxidant applied manually. Histologic and clinical assessments showed improvement in skin quality in the hydradermabrasion group. The treated skin showed a statistically significant increase in antioxidant levels and an increase in epidermal and papillary dermal thickness, collagen hyalinization, and fibroblast density. There was also a decrease in wrinkles, pore size, and hyperpigmentation after hydradermabrasion treatment. The skin with manually applied antioxidant, however, showed no detectable change in structure or antioxidant levels. MDA with antioxidants as an infusion agent may be a reasonable treatment option for those patients who wish to prevent or stop the signs of aging.

In another study by Freedman (2009), 10 patients were treated in split-face fashion with either MDA with infusion of an antioxidant serum or MDA alone. Patients underwent a total of six treatments, each 1 week apart. Histologic assessment of posttreatment biopsies revealed that patients treated with MDA plus antioxidants had a marked increase in epidermal and papillary dermal thickness, as well as an increase in fibroblast density and deposition of collagen. Digital photography indicated that skin quality improved more with the combined treatment than MDA alone. Raman spectroscopy was used to measure skin polyphenolic levels. The dermal infusion-treated skin was found to have a 32% increase in antioxidant levels. Unfortunately, the author did not report the effect of MDA alone on polyphenolic levels, so it remains unclear whether the increase in antioxidant levels is attributable to topical infusion therapy, MDA, or a combination of the two.

A number of other MDA infusion systems have also been commercially developed. The HydraFacial and SilkPeel systems have appropriate patent protection.

CONTRAINDICATIONS

SilkPeel has been safely used in patients with inflammatory disorders such as psoriasis or eczema without complications. This is due to its ability to abrade up to specific depths by altering the grit of the diamond used for abrasion. Other MDA systems have not been reported to share this safety advantage. Similarly, many practitioners are using MDA for the treatment of actinic keratoses. However, frank malignancy is a contraindication because of fear of spread of the lesion after treatment. It should be noted that this concern is theoretical and not based on any published reports.

Absolute contraindications to MDA include the following:

- Accutane use within the past 12 months (except SilkPeel)
- Presence of skin malignancy (excluding actinic keratoses; see earlier discussion)
- Presence of herpetic lesion(s)
- Presence of eczema or psoriasis (except SilkPeel)
- Presence of autoimmune disease

Relative contraindications to MDA include the following:

- Accutane use within the past 12 months (for SilkPeel only)
- Patients with thin skin
- Patients with compromised wound healing (e.g., smokers, diabetic patients)
- Patients with compromised immune systems
- Current use of anticoagulation therapy (excludes diamond-based MDA)

PATIENT SELECTION

MDA is safe and effective; however, proper patient selection is essential. Poor patient selection will cause patient dissatisfaction, staff frustration, and ultimate failure of the MDA program in any given practice.

MDA is an excellent modality for all skin types, even those patients with Fitzpatrick skin types V and VI (see Chapter 35, Introduction to Aesthetic Medicine). These patients are especially vulnerable to hyperpigmentation or hypopigmentation when more aggressive skin resurfacing treatments are administered. MDA is safe in these patients because the depth of penetration is usually limited to the superficial epidermis. Elderly patients with thin skin are not good candidates for MDA unless pretreated with other modalities to improve skin quality. Pregnant women should not undergo MDA because of hormonal changes that cause increased skin sensitivity, delayed wound healing, and increased melanocyte melanin production. Consequently, the risk of postinflammatory hyperpigmentation and scarring can be significant during pregnancy, and any procedure should be avoided until after delivery. Patients on anticoagulant therapy are also not good candidates for crystal-based MDA and should be treated with caution because it can be difficult for the practitioner to adequately control the abrasion depth, potentially injuring blood vessels in the papillary dermis and causing excessive bleeding.

It is recommended that patients who have had a recent chemical peel or other skin procedure such as collagen injections, waxing, tanning, or sun exposure wait at least 2 weeks before undergoing MDA.

INITIAL EVALUATION

Every patient must be seen and evaluated by the clinician before initiation of treatment. Unfortunately, some offices turn the MDA practice over to an aesthetician and the process runs independent of clinician input. This situation is more appropriate for a beauty salon. A clinician has the responsibility of seeing and evaluating every patient who is treated in his or her practice. Anything less than this compromises patient care.

After filling out the usual history form, with special attention to current medications, the clinician should evaluate the patient with particular attention to the following:

- Fitzpatrick skin typing (see Chapter 38, Lasers and Pulsed-Light Devices: Hair Removal)
- Skin thickness
- Skin tone
- Site-specific rhytids
- Depth and severity of rhytids
- Dryness
- Acne
- Acne scarring
- Other scarring
- Vascular anomalies
- Telangiectases
- Ecchymosis
- Nevi
- Pigmentation problems
- Skin malignancies
- General actinic damage
- Actinic keratoses
- Current tanning status
- Poikiloderma
- Open sores
- Herpetic lesions

Once these and other individual factors are considered, a treatment protocol can be determined for the patient. Instructions should be written or checked off on a patient encounter form and treatment plan communicated with the MDA technician (Fig. 49.4; also see Chapter 35, Introduction to Aesthetic Medicine, Fig. 35.1).

Pretreatment and posttreatment photographs are recommended and should become a part of the patient's permanent record. They will also facilitate assessment of clinical outcomes. However, do not expect miracles with every patient. It may be extremely difficult to photographically document improvement in patients whose initial skin quality is good and who just wanted "freshening." Certainly, those patients with major pigment problems, acne scarring, and other extreme conditions yield documentable photographic improvement. Recent advances in digital photographic systems provide improved sensitivity, allowing detection of less dramatic improvements in patients with reasonable baseline skin quality.

COMPLICATIONS

Complications can result from any type of treatment, regardless of how innocuous the technology may seem. Certainly, MDA is no different. However, the very factor that has contributed to MDA's widespread success is that it has very few, if any, long-term complications. The clinician and staff should receive bona fide training before embarking on patient treatments and know the potential complications and treatment options to provide a good outcome.

Erythema is the most common side effect of MDA, and its severity has a nearly linear relationship with the aggressiveness of the treatment. Some patients (e.g., those suffering from dermatographism, rosacea, certain types of urticaria) have very sensitive skin and will exhibit some erythema no matter how mild the treatment settings. Most erythema resolves spontaneously within a few hours. Inform the patient to avoid sun or tanning bed exposure during the time of his or her treatment sessions because this will surely increase skin irritation. All patients must use daily sunscreen (preferably SPF 30 or greater) to protect their skin.

Most patients experience mild tingling, which is very tolerable. However, a few patients complain of burning and skin discomfort for up to 24 hours after the peel. These patients can be treated effectively with moisturizers.

Chemical Peel/Microdermabrasion
New Patient Consultation Checklist

Name: _____   Date: _____

Analyze the Skin: **Initial Photographs:**
_____ Visually
_____ Patient Profile Form
_____ Consent Form signed (copy to patient)
_____ Fee Schedule Form signed (copy to patient)
_____ Photos taken

Discuss Peel Treatments with Patient:
_____ Expectations
_____ Possible Reactions and Side Effects
_____ Sunblock Use

Home Care Program:
_____ Sample Kit
_____ Instructions
_____ Home Care Regimen
_____ Post Peel Tip Sheet

Peel Appointment:
_____ Preparation for Peel Treatment
_____ Date of First Treatment

Fig. 49.4 Sample chemical peel/microdermabrasion new patient consultation checklist. (Courtesy John L. Pfenninger, MD, The Medical Procedures Center, Midland, MI.)

Purpura, ecchymosis, and petechial hemorrhages are all a function of overly aggressive vacuum settings. They are more common with crystal-based MDA treatments and relatively uncommon with diamond-based ones. Also, poor patient selection, such as treating patients with thin skin or those on anticoagulants (gingko, vitamin E, aspirin, and nonsteroidal antiinflammatory drugs, among others), can lead to these side effects. Apply ice to the area when first noticed and decrease the vacuum setting to minimize the problem. If one of these complications should occur, do not return to the affected area for peeling at that same treatment session. Skin should return to normal appearance in most patients younger than 50 years within 10 to 14 days. It may take longer to resolve these problems in older patients.

Scarring is rare with MDA, but can occur in the following unusual situations:

- Patient circumstance demands aggressive therapy (e.g., treatment of mild to moderate acne scarring on the cheeks, which requires deep planing).
- Aggressive treatments administered to patients currently using Accutane or patients who have been on Accutane within 1 year of initiating MDA.
- Mild skin abrasion in patients who are noncompliant, have compromised immune function and subsequent wound contamination, or have active infection.
- Being too aggressive or allowing the handpiece to stop or dwell on specific skin areas for too long.

Minor skin abrasions can occur. Simply having the patient clean these areas and apply petroleum jelly or antibiotic ointment until reepithelialization has occurred should alleviate the situation.

Ocular damage is a potential complication. Protection of the eyes for both the patient and practitioner is absolutely essential. Tsai and associates (1995) discussed development of ocular pain, photophobia, epiphora, and conjunctival congestion with crystal adherence to the cornea and punctate keratopathy resulting from ophthalmologic crystal contamination during MDA. Ocular contamination can be prevented by placing moist, folded 4 × 4 gauze pads over the eyes and holding them in place with suntanning goggles. Alternatively, special eye shields (see next section) can be used alone. After treatment, the technician must meticulously remove crystals from the periorbital region before allowing the patient to get off the treatment table and wash.

EQUIPMENT

- MDA unit with tips (sterile, reusable metal; plastic disposable; Fig. 49.5)
- Power examination table and adjustable stool for the technician
- Alcohol wipes
- Crystals (usually aluminum oxide); approximately one-half of a cup (30 to 35 mL) for the face and more for larger areas
- Nonsterile gloves
- Moist 4 × 4 gauzes
- Surgical cap for patient
- Suntanning goggles for patient (alternatively, Derm-Aid Non-Laser Disposable Eye Shields [Honeywell Uvex] work very well)
- Saline eye wash
- Towel or gown to drape around patient's neck
- Protective glasses with shields for operator
- Mask for operator (to reduce inhalation)
- Postoperative moisturizer (e.g., Theraplex, aloe, Kinerase) and sunscreen (with zinc or titanium)
- Flow sheet to record settings and progress
- Digital camera with macro feature for close-up pictures (ideal but optional)
- Solutions to be used for dermal infusion (contact manufacturers)
- Cleaning solutions (contact manufacturers)

Crystals vary widely in quality and cost. Cheaper materials contain variable-sized particles and may not be pure. Fine, powdery substances are not only less effective but also aerosolize when the containers are emptied. Not only do these substances cause a sediment in the room, they may be irritating to the patient or clinician. The lower limit of particle size should be 20 μm. Crystals should also be prepared in a "medically clean" way to avoid any type of contamination.

The apertures that the crystals traverse eventually wear larger from the passage of crystals. Check to see if the tip needs repair

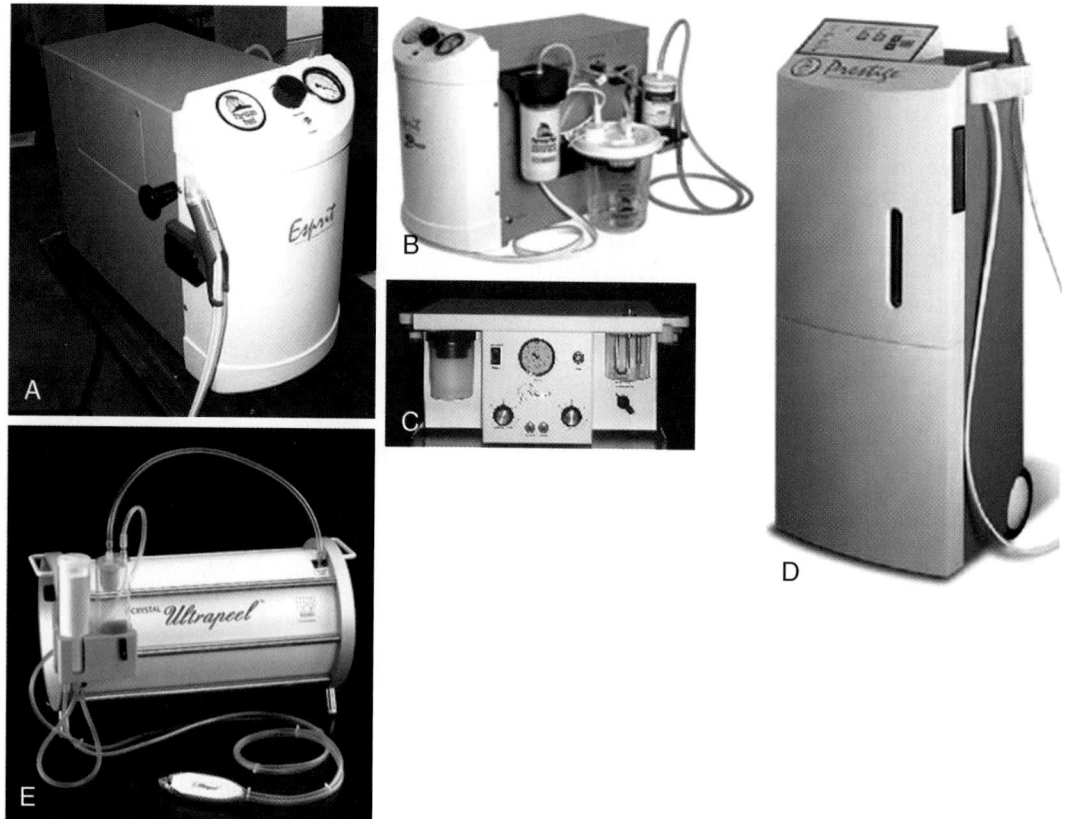

Fig. 49.5   (A) Parisian Peel Esprit. (B) Inside view of Parisian Peel unit showing the crystal container and collection system. (C) BellaMed microdermabrasion machine. (D) Prestige microdermabrasion machine. (E) Ultrapeel Crystal. (A, B, and D, Courtesy Aesthetic Technologies, Broomfield, CO. C, Courtesy Bella Products, Foothill Ranch, CA. E, Courtesy Mattioli Engineering, McLean, VA.)

/replacement before each treatment by observing the crystal flow. A wider crystal flow that lacks uniformity indicates the need for tip replacement.

Handpiece tips must be replaced or sterilized (cold or hot) for each patient. Angled handpieces are somewhat more comfortable for the operator to use.

PREPROCEDURE PATIENT PREPARATION

- Have the patient wash his or her face to remove all makeup and lotions.
- The patient must wear eye protection and a surgical cap to keep crystals from getting into the eyes and hair. Should crystals get into the eye, they can be very irritating and must be washed out with saline.
- The patient is placed in the supine position on the treatment table. The technician is seated at the head with clear three-sided access to the patient.
- Place a towel or gown around the patient's neck to keep crystals from getting on the patient's clothing.
- Cleanse the patient's face with isopropyl alcohol or acetone to remove any lingering skin oils, makeup, and lotions.
- Examine the skin in the areas to be treated. Open sores should be avoided. Also, be attentive for any type of herpetic outbreak. If the patient does exhibit a herpetic lesion, cancel the treatment for at least 2 weeks and make sure the patient is treated with the appropriate antiviral medication (e.g., Valtrex, Zovirax). Prophylaxis for patients with frequent herpetic outbreaks may be required; however, it should be individualized to each patient's circumstance.

TECHNIQUE

See specific manufacturers' guidelines for each particular unit.

1. Select the appropriate grit and size of the diamond-tip treatment head. The heads vary in coarseness from smooth (no diamond chips) to fine (120 grit) and coarse (30 grit). The 6-mm head is recommended for the face and the 9-mm head for larger areas such as the arms and legs. The usual power setting for initial treatment starts at 12 to 14 mm Hg and works up to 18 to 20 mm Hg for most patients (those with special problems such as acne scarring may require 20 to 35 mm Hg). *Tip:* The practitioner can make a good estimate of the correct suction level by applying the handpiece to a colored page from a magazine for 3 to 4 seconds. If all color is removed, the power is too high. If most is removed, it is just right. If most color is left, it is too low.

2. With a nonsterile, gloved hand, spread the skin between the thumb and index or middle finger with a moderate amount of tension. Place the MDA treatment head on the skin and move the handpiece parallel to the direction of tension between the two fingers (Fig. 49.6A). Keep the handpiece head moving, and definitely avoid stopping and holding it in contact with one area of the skin; this could cause deep penetration, serious damage to the skin, and scarring. Hold the handpiece perpendicular (90 degrees) to the skin.

3. For the first pass, strokes should be from the central face to the periphery. After completing a small area of skin with parallel strokes, move the handpiece for a *second pass* perpendicular to the direction of movement of the first pass (see Fig. 49.6B). This crosshatches the area and decreases any streaking or linear erythematous markings. It is recommended to start at the forehead, proceed down the bridge of the nose, and cover the cheeks, chin, and around the mouth.

4. If a third pass is to be made, use a circular or swirling motion. When initiating MDA with a new patient, it may be prudent to see how two passes are tolerated and their effects before making a third.

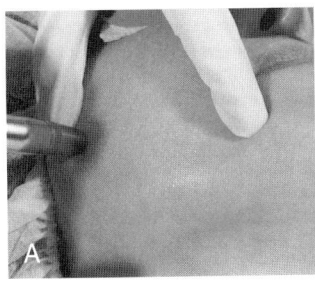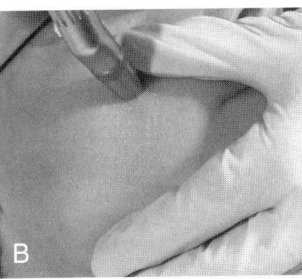

Fig. 49.6 (A) First microdermabrasion pass on the patient's right cheek. The technician's fingers are tensing the skin in a horizontal direction while using parallel movements of the handpiece. (B) A second pass on the right cheek with the skin tensed in a more vertical orientation, perpendicular to the direction of the first pass in A. Note crystal residue on skin.

5. After two or more passes, some patients exhibit a darkened or grayish hue to the skin because of the crystal interaction with skin oils. This is no cause for alarm because it will be removed completely with posttreatment cleansing. (For treatment of the neck, only one pass with vertical strokes is sufficient. For treatment of the chest, use two passes with strokes from the midline to the periphery. For treatment of the hands, have the patient make a fist around a towel and perform two passes with strokes parallel and then perpendicular to the axis of the forearm.)
6. When the treatment is completed, the technician should remove the crystals from the face while the patient is still in the supine position, taking great care to remove all crystal remnants from the periorbital region by suction or gentle removal with a moist cloth.
7. Have the patient cleanse with mild soap and water.
8. A light moisturizer, such as aloe, Theraplex, or Kinerase, will decrease any mild irritation. Also apply sunscreen with SPF 30 or greater (containing zinc or titanium).

After a treatment, it is important to leave the crystal container heater on whenever the machine is not in use to prevent moisturization of the crystals, which would result in poor crystal flow and possible malfunction.

POSTPROCEDURE PATIENT EDUCATION

Instruct the patient to avoid applying makeup, if possible, for the next 12 to 18 hours and to avoid significant sun exposure for 3 to 4 days after each treatment. The patient must wear sunblock whenever going outdoors and avoid applying irritant products such as retinoids, astringents, alpha-hydroxy acids, and depilatories for 1 week. See the sample patient education form available at www.expertconsult.com.

PURCHASING A MICRODERMABRASION SYSTEM

Before purchasing an MDA machine, consider several factors:

- Do you currently have access to a patient base that is appropriate for the use of this technology?
- Can ancillary treatments or therapies be offered to enhance the patient's results and to generate additional income (e.g., skin care products)?
- Do you have the personnel to support these new activities?
- Do you have the office space to dedicate to the MDA unit and a practitioner for the procedure?
- Make sure the local region is not saturated with MDA units. Is there a realistic market potential?
- Evaluate machine functions such as crystal flow, vacuum capacity, and the operator's ability to vary treatment parameters. Machine flexibility is important in treating a variety of skin types, conditions, and problems.
- Evaluate the propensity of the machine to clog, which may occur in a humid, moist environment. Most machines have a crystal heater that maintains dry crystals. The heater is left on continually.

- In today's market, warranty coverage, technical support, and possible shared marketing arrangements have become increasingly important factors in determining purchase decisions.
- Along with designated staff, attend a course that covers the essentials of MDA. These courses are usually sponsored by the equipment manufacturer or clinician experts in the field.

PATIENT EDUCATION GUIDES

See the sample patient education and consent forms available at www.expertconsult.com.

CPT/BILLING CODES

15780	Dermabrasion,* total face (e.g., for acne scarring, fine wrinkling, rhytids, general keratosis)
15781	Dermabrasion,* segmental, face
15782	Dermabrasion,* regional, other than face
15783	Dermabrasion,* superficial, any site (e.g., tattoo removal)
15786†	Abrasion, single lesion (e.g., keratosis, scar)
15787†	Abrasion, each additional 4 lesions or less (list separately in addition to code for primary procedure)

ICD-10-CM DIAGNOSTIC CODES

L71.9	Rosacea unspecified
L90.8	Wrinkling of skin; rhytids facialis
L57.0	Actinic keratosis
L70.0	Acne vulgaris
L81.9	Dyschromia, unspecified
L81.1	Melasma
L90.5	Scar conditions and fibrosis of skin

Acknowledgment

The editors recognize the contributions of Dexter W. Blome, MD, to this chapter in a previous edition of this text.

SUPPLIERS

(See contact information available at www.expertconsult.com.)

BellaMed
Bella Products, Inc.
Bio-Brasion
Bio-Therapeutic
ClairDerm
Medical Aesthetics
Delphia/HydraFacial
Edge Systems
DermaGenesis
Genesis Biosystems
Dermaglide Legacy KS/Microglide
Advanced Laser Centers
DermaPod
Silhouet-Tone USA
DermaSweep
Cosmetic R & D
DermGlow
Aesthetic Solutions
Esprit Pro-xp
MedSurge Advances, Inc.
Facial H20
Syneron, Inc.
ImageDerm
ImageDerm

MegaPeel
   DermaMed, Inc.
NaturaBrador
   Focus Medical, LLC
NewAPeel/DiamondTome
   Altair Instruments
Parisian Peel (Prestige, Esprit, Entrée)
   Aesthetic Technologies, Inc.
PortaPeel
   ImageDerm, Inc.
PowerPeel and Ultrapeel
   Mattioli Engineering
Pristine
   Viora Medical, Inc.
Salt-A-Peel
   Med-Aesthetic Solutions
Sapphire 3 Abrasion
   Raja Medical
SilkPeel
   Envy Medical, Inc.
SmartPeel
   SoundSkin Corp.
Vibraderm
   Vibraderm, Inc.

RECOMMENDED READING

Abdel-Latif AM, Elbendary AS. Treatment of striae distensae with micro-dermabrasion: a clinical and molecular study. *J Egypt Womens Dermatol Soc.* 2008;5:24–30.

Abu Ubeid A, Wang Y, Zhao L, Hantash BM. Short-sequence oligopeptides with inhibitory activity against mushroom and human tyrosinase. *J Invest Dermatol.* 2009;129:2242–2249.

American Society for Aesthetic Plastic Surgery. 2015 Statistics on cosmetic surgery. http://www.surgery.org/sites/default/files/ASAPS-Stats2015.pdf.

Ash K, Lord J, Zukowski M, McDaniel DH. Comparison of topical therapy for striae alba (20% glycolic acid/0.05% tretinoin versus 20% glycolic acid/10% L-ascorbic acid). *Dermatol Surg.* 1998;24:849–856.

Bhatia A, Hsu JTs, Hantash BM. Combined topical delivery and dermal-infusion of decapeptide-12 accelerates resolution of post-inflammatory hyperpigmentation in skin of color. *J Drugs Dermatol.* 2014;13(1):84–85.

Coimbra M, Rohrich RJ, Chao J, Brown SA. A prospective controlled assessment of microdermabrasion for damaged skin and fine rhytides. *Plast Reconstr Surg.* 2004;113:1438–1443.

Desai TD, Moy LS, Kirby W, et al. Evaluation of the SilkPeel system in treating erythematotelangiectatic and papulopustular rosacea. *Cosmet Dermatol.* 2006;19:51–56.

Elsaie ML, Baumann LS, Elsaaiee LT. Striae distensae (stretch marks) and different modalities of therapy: an update. *Dermatol Surg.* 2009;35:563–573.

Fields KA. Skin breakthroughs in the year 2000. *Int J Fertil Womens Med.* 2000;45:175–181.

Freedman BM. Hydradermabrasion: an innovative modality for nonablative facial rejuvenation. *J Cosmet Dermatol.* 2008;7:275–280.

Freedman BM. Topical antioxidant application enhances the effects of facial microdermabrasion. *J Dermatol Treat.* 2009;20:82–87.

Freedman BM, Rueda-Pedraza E, Waddell SP. The epidermal and dermal changes associated with microdermabrasion. *Dermatol Surg.* 2001;27: 1031–1033.

Hantash BM, Jimenez F. Treatment of mild to moderate facial melasma with the Lumixyl topical brightening system. *J Drugs Dermatol.* 2012;11(5):660–662.

Hernandez-Perez E, Ibiett EV. Gross and microscopic findings in patients undergoing microdermabrasion for facial rejuvenation. *Dermatol Surg.* 2001;27:637–640.

Karimipour DJ, Karimipour G, Orringer JS. Microdermabrasion: an evidence-based review. *Plast Reconstr Surg.* 2010;125(1):372–377.

Lawrence N, Mandy S, Yarborough J, Alt T. History of dermabrasion. *Dermatol Surg.* 2000;26:95–101.

Lee WR, Shen SC, Kuo-Hsien W, et al. Lasers and microdermabrasion enhance and control topical delivery of vitamin C. *J Invest Dermatol.* 2003;121:1118–1125.

Mahuzier F. Microdermabrasion of stretch marks. In: Mahuzier F, ed. *Microdermabrasion or Parisian Peel in Practice.* Marseille, France: Solal; 1999:25–65.

Monheit GD, Chastain MA. Chemical and mechanical skin resurfacing. In: Bolognia JL, Schaffer JV, Cerroni L, eds. *Dermatology.* 4th ed. Philadelphia: Elsevier; 2018:2593–2609.

Moy LS, Maley C, Skin management: a practical approach. *Plast Surg Pract.* https://www.slideshare.net/Silkpeel/article-skin-management-a-practical-approach-moy-clinical-study-plastic-surgery-products-magazine.

Shehadi IE, Larson DL, Archer SM, Zhang LL. Evaluation of histologic changes after micordermabrasion in a porcine model. *Aesthet Surg J.* 2004;24:136–141.

Shim E, Barnette D, Hughes K, Greenway H. Microdermabrasion: a clinical and histopathologic study. *Dermatol Surg.* 2001;27:524–530.

Tan MH, Spencer JM, Pires LM, et al. The evaluation of aluminum oxide crystal microdermabrasion for photodamage. *Dermatol Surg.* 2001;27:943–949.

Tsai RY, Wang CN, Chan HL. Aluminum oxide crystal microdermabrasion: a new technique for treating facial scarring. *Dermatol Surg.* 1995;21:539–542.

Wray A, Marshall D, Cleaver L. Effective treatment of traumatic tattoo with SilkPeel microdermabrasion during isotretinoin treatment. http://silkpeelturkiye.com/wp-content/uploads/2013/04/5.-Traumatic-Tattoo.pdf.

CHAPTER 50

SKIN PEELS

Cathy Uecker

With the tremendous increase in numbers of older Americans as the baby-boomer population ages, more and more patients are seeking treatments for photodamage and other conditions commonly seen with aging skin (e.g., uneven color, tone, and texture). In fact, skin rejuvenation has become one of the most common reasons for patients to consult a plastic surgeon, dermatologist, or clinical skin care provider. Oral isotretinoin (Accutane) prevents much of the deep scarring once seen from acne. However, patients routinely request treatment for minor scarring and postinflammatory hyperpigmentation, usually the result of previous acne lesions. Chemical peels and topical medications continue to be reliable methods used to rejuvenate skin damaged by all of these conditions.

Superficial peels are very common and are deemed so safe that nonclinicians now perform them in health spas and salons. However, many patients would prefer to have even superficial peels performed under the trusted supervision of their primary care clinician if the procedure were made available to them.

Although skin aging is both intrinsic (Table 50.1) and extrinsic (Table 50.2), the majority of damage is from extrinsic causes. Intrinsically, chronic use of the muscles of expression and dermal thinning combine with the loss of collagen fibers due to aging to produce wrinkles and skin lines. Most intrinsic aging, such as that associated with hormonal changes, is the result of both chronologic and genetic causes.

Extrinsic aging is caused by environmental hazards, such as ultraviolet radiation, wind, smoking, and chemical exposure. Years of exposure from the sun and tanning booths can produce wrinkles and pigmentary or surface changes. The stratum corneum thickens and the granulosum and spinosum layers become thinner. Atypical cells develop, the skin becomes less translucent, and pigmentation often becomes markedly irregular. Lentigines (freckles) and actinic precancerous lesions may develop (Fig. 50.1), the papillary dermis thins, and the skin loses elasticity while developing a sallow color. Extrinsic aging causes blood vessels to dilate, telangiectases to proliferate, and collagen to become sparse (clumping in bundles). In turn, the reticular dermis fills with abnormal elastin fibers. Eventually, hair follicles and pores dilate and become filled with desquamated debris.

In America, from the early 1900s until the 1950s, chemical peels were popular for skin rejuvenation. When dermabrasion was developed in the 1950s, it soon became the favored skin resurfacing technique. With newer commercial preparations available and the aging population able to afford cosmetic treatments, chemical peels became popular again. Recent developments in cryotherapy and laser have also become available for more complex interventions.

TOPICAL TREATMENTS AND ADJUNCTS TO PEELS

Considerable improvements in sun-damaged skin can be achieved with topical therapy alone if the patient is willing to be consistent and compliant with a skin care program. Topical retinoids, such as tretinoin (Retin-A), have been shown to clinically and histologically reverse sun damage. In fact, the more severely damaged the skin, the better the response. Newer tretinoin products have gained popularity owing to advances in their delivery systems geared toward reducing the common side effects of dryness and irritation. For example, Renova (Ortho Dermatologics Valeant) is delivered in an emollient base. Retin-A-Micro (Ortho Dermatologics Valeant) has a patented microsphere delivery system, and Atralin (Valeant Pharmaceuticals) is delivered in a water-base, alcohol-free vehicle, with added hydrating and moisturizing ingredients. Compliance and consistency with topical therapy are much greater when dryness and skin irritation are decreased. After the use of topical retinoids, biopsies demonstrate deposition of new dermal collagen, formation of new blood vessels, and normalization of epidermal atypia. Accumulated melanin in the basal layer is transported to the surface and shed, improving pigmentation. Epidermal cell turnover is stimulated, producing a proliferation of new cells and improving skin texture. Improved blood supply to the dermis enhances both skin color and the transportation of nutrients to the skin. However, a minimum of 24 weeks is necessary to manifest visible signs of improvement. Unfortunately, topical treatments must continually be used to maintain improvements. When topical treatments are discontinued, the skin gradually returns to its previous condition.

Fortunately, retinoids are now available generically, so their cost has decreased; however, some dermatologists insist that the generic preparations have a higher risk of skin irritation because of their preservatives. Those likely to benefit the most from retinoids are fair-skinned individuals in their 30s and 40s who have blotchy pigmentation, sunspots, or fine lines around their eyes.

Lustra (Medicis Valeant) is an antiaging cream that contains 2% glycolic acid (GA), antioxidants, and 4% hydroquinone. Hydroquinone, a tyrosinase inhibitor, disrupts the synthesis of melanin, thus lightening the skin or pigmented areas. It is also available in a preparation that contains a complete sunblock (Lustra AF). This type of preparation can be used in combination with topical retinoids to treat areas of hyperpigmentation, such as melasma. Use of a combination of topical preparations is likely to be slightly irritating to the skin. To avoid irritation that may cause patients to discontinue their regimen, it is wise to start with every-other-day application for the first 2 weeks, and then daily.

If skin irritation occurs and becomes problematic, a mild steroid cream or ointment (triamcinolone 0.1%), applied sparingly and concomitantly once a day, may reduce the associated erythema and flaking.

α-Hydroxy acids (AHAs) can be applied at low strength (2% to 20%) by patients as part of their daily skin care regimen to improve collagen and elastin synthesis and promote protein regeneration. AHA is a "blanket" term for a variety of fruit acids. Studies have indicated that both the papillary dermis and the epidermis can be thickened, elastic fibers improved, and melanin dispersed with the use of AHAs. Benefits visible to the patient include the reduction of fine lines and wrinkles along with improved skin color, tone, and texture. At low doses these occur without inflammation. Because AHAs do not cause angiogenesis (as opposed to retinoids), they are the preferred treatment for patients with telangiectases from rosacea.

TABLE 50.1	Intrinsic (Chronologic and Genetic) Aging of the Skin
Cause	**Effect**
Decreased vascularity	Yellow skin
Dermal thinning	Atrophy
Decreased dermal cellularity	Irregular texture
Loss of elastic fibers	Fine lines or wrinkles
Decreased mechanical properties with decreased elastic recoil after stretching	Laxity

Modified from Lewis AB, Gendler EC. Resurfacing with topical agents. *Semin Cutan Med Surg.* 1996;15:139–144.

TABLE 50.2	Extrinsic (Solar and Environmental) Aging of the Skin
Cause	**Effect**
Altered cell maturation	Dry, coarse texture, actinic keratoses
Melanocyte alteration (overstimulated or destroyed)	Solar lentigines, mottled pigmentation
Decreased collagen fiber number and strength; elastic fiber curling, branching, and thickening; degeneration into solar elastoses	Fine wrinkling
Loss of collagen support of vessels	Solar (senile) purpura
Alteration of vascular network	Yellow hue, loss of pink color

Modified from Lewis AB, Gendler EC. Resurfacing with topical agents. *Semin Cutan Med Surg.* 1996;15:139–144.

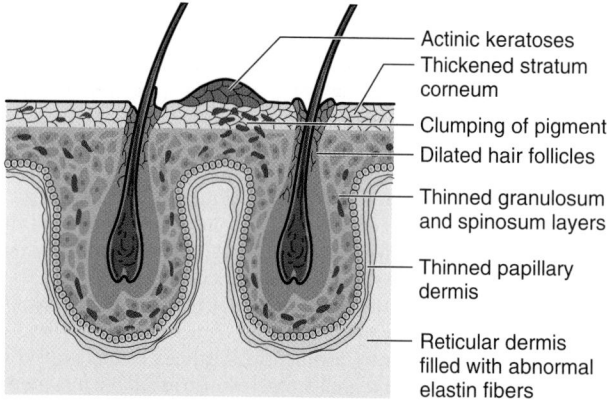

Actinic keratoses
Thickened stratum corneum
Clumping of pigment
Dilated hair follicles
Thinned granulosum and spinosum layers
Thinned papillary dermis
Reticular dermis filled with abnormal elastin fibers

Fig. 50.1 Skin damage from years of sun exposure. (Modified from Edwards L, Maibach HI, Roenigk HH. What can be done for photoaged skin? *Patient Care.* 1996;30:68.)

In addition, because AHAs work by a different mechanism, they can be used concurrently with retinoids.

The following is a list of some of more commonly used AHAs or ones you may see as ingredients in skin care products:

- *Glycolic acid (GA):* Derived from sugar cane, by far the most common and widely used. Because it has the smallest molecular size of all the AHAs, it easily penetrates the skin and is often used as a delivery system in skin care products.
- *Lactic acid:* Comes from sour milk and is used as a skin softener and exfoliator.
- *Citric acid:* Vitamin C is most commonly used as an antioxidant.
- *Malic acid:* Derived from unripe and green grapes.
- *Tartaric acid:* A fermentation byproduct from wine making.
- *Mandelic acid:* Derived from almond extract and has antibacterial properties. It is a larger molecule than GA, making it widely tolerated by almost all skin types.

Because of increased sun sensitivity, retinoids are usually applied at night, whereas AHAs are most often applied during the day, along with the recommendation of a sun protection product with an SPF of 15 or greater. Skin texture, and to some degree skin pigmentation, may benefit at any age from retinoids, AHAs, or both. If irregular or abnormal pigmentation is persistent, consider incorporating hydroquinone, a tyrosinase inhibitor, or kojic acid, a melanin inhibitor, to the patient's treatment program.

There are many AHA preparations available, buffered to various pH levels. It has been theorized that the beneficial or antiaging effects of AHAs are due to activation of transforming growth factor-β, which is increasingly activated at cutaneous pH levels below 5. The prolonged application of "acid" AHAs may reduce the cutaneous pH and thus activate this growth factor. Most unbuffered AHAs have a low pH; however, a low pH also increases the risk of local skin irritation. Buffered preparations with pH levels above 2 are available and may be preferred if skin irritation occurs. In addition, using a low-strength AHA before a chemical peel not only will allow the clinician to judge patient tolerance, but will enhance the penetration of the peel.

ALTERNATIVE PROCEDURES TO CHEMICAL PEELS

Alternatives to chemical peels include the following:

- Cryopeels
- Dermaplaning
- Dermabrasion
- Microdermabrasion/dermalinfusion
- Ablative laser resurfacing
- Fractional ablative laser resurfacing
- Nonablative laser (intense pulsed light [IPL])

Of the alternatives to chemical peels, cryopeels are the most similar in effect (see Chapter 14, Cryosurgery). Many primary care clinicians already use liquid nitrogen for freezing pigmented spots (lentigines), warts, actinic keratoses, seborrheic keratoses, and angiomas. With considerable experience, and often aided by a special attachment, the clinician can treat the entire face with cryotherapy to produce a cryopeel. It is less expensive for the patient than having a deep chemical peel, and with proper patient selection results may last up to 1 to 2 years. Although a cryopeel may result in more swelling initially, results are often comparable with those of a medium-depth chemical peel.

Originally designed to remove acne scars, surgical skin planing, or dermaplaning, was soon found to be useful for scarring from other causes, such as photodamage. After freezing, the skin layers are removed mechanically. Although postoperative healing is slower with dermaplaning and the cost is much higher than for a peel (as much as $4000 for a full-face dermaplane), more severe lesions can be treated, and the results of the skin resurfacing last longer (5 years or more). A more common and less invasive dermaplaning procedure is accomplished by scraping the skin with a no. 12 blade. After cleansing the skin, a light coating of povidone–iodine (Betadine) is applied and allowed to dry. Visualizing the change of color while gently scraping the skin allows the clinician to carefully remove only the most superficial layers of the epidermis. Repeat treatments may be done every 4 to 6 weeks at a cost of $150 to $200 per treatment. Although chemical peels are the procedure of choice for fine wrinkles, dermaplaning has a more prolonged effect and is superior for deep acne scars. Dermabrasion is similar to dermaplaning (e.g., preparations, indications) and is most often used to improve the look of facial scars caused by accidents or previous surgery or to smooth out fine facial wrinkles. The patient should be aware that after dermaplaning or dermabrasion, the immediate postprocedure effects on the face will be quite obvious to friends and colleagues, with an average downtime of at least 10 to 14 days or even longer.

TABLE 50.3 Levels of Chemical Peeling		
Type of Peel	**Chemical Formula**	**Indications**
Superficial, stratum granulosum/papillary dermis (up to 0.06 mm)	AHA (GA 20%–70%) BHA (SA 20%–30%) 5-Fluorouracil TCA (10%–20%) Jessner solution: 14 g resorcinol, 14 g SA, 14 g lactic acid 95% ethanol (quantity sufficient to add up to 100 mL) Unna paste Carbon dioxide (solid)	Fine rhytids (wrinkles) Bad skin texture Acne vulgaris (comedonal/inflammatory, papular-pustular) Acne rosacea (papular-pustular) Pigmentary changes (especially postinflammatory) Superficial actinic keratoses
Superficial to medium (0.06–0.45 mm)	20%–30% TCA Series of AHA (GA 20%–70%) or BHA (SA 20%–30%) peels (see Table 50.4)	Persistent fine rhytids or bad skin texture Persistent acne vulgaris or rosacea Persistent mild pigmentary changes Isolated but deeper actinic keratoses
Medium, upper reticular dermis (0.45–0.6 mm)	50% TCA or 35% TCA plus initial keratolytics Initial keratolytics: Jessner's solution, carbon dioxide (solid), or 70% GA	Moderate rhytids (wrinkles) Chronic photodamage Multiple epidermal/premalignant lesions Pigmentary changes and solar lentigines Multiple actinic keratoses Multiple flat warts
Deep, mid-reticular dermis (0.6–0.8 mm)	Baker-Gordon formula: 3 mL 88% phenol, three drops croton oil, eight drops hexachlorophene, 2 mL distilled water	Severe rhytids (wrinkles) Epidermal lesions Superficial neoplasms Deep pigmentary changes

AHA, α-Hydroxy acid; *BHA,* β-hydroxy acid; *GA,* glycolic acid; *SA,* salicylic acid; *TCA,* trichloroacetic acid.

Microdermabrasion (see Chapter 49, Microdermabrasion and Dermalinfusion) is a technique in which the skin is buffed with aluminum oxide crystals. This method has grown in popularity because there is virtually no downtime. It has been coined "the lunchtime peel" and it is much less expensive than dermabrasion (about $50 to $100 per treatment). Three to six treatments are needed at weekly intervals for significant results. Among aesthetic skin care providers, microdermabrasion is the closest equivalent to superficial facial chemical peels. A potential drawback for primary care clinicians is the initial cost of $3500 to $10,000 for equipment.

Carbon dioxide laser resurfacing is another option. Traditionally, lasers were used to obtain a deep resurfacing that often required general or tumescent anesthesia. The cost was as much as $3500 to $5000 per treatment. Although studies have not been published comparing laser surgery with dermabrasion, anecdotal evidence indicates it to be as effective as dermabrasion for removing deep wrinkles around the mouth. There have been no comparative studies showing advantages of laser resurfacing of the whole face over dermabrasion or chemical peeling.

Long-pulse (i.e., 1000 ms) erbium-YAG lasers and CO_2 lasers are now being used to achieve results similar to superficial and medium-depth chemical peels. Using special techniques (fractional ablation techniques), islands of skin are left unaffected within the treated area. This leads to a more rapid recovery time (5 to 7 days) as opposed to previous laser therapy (6 weeks). These lasers can be used anywhere on the body with only topical anesthesia and some oral sedation (see Chapter 41, Lasers and Pulsed-Light Devices: Skin Tightening, and Chapter 44, Fractional Laser Skin Resurfacing). These units require a considerable investment ($70,000 to $140,000).

With the exception of ethnically darker skin types, IPL therapy works best for pigment reduction, redness, flushing, or dilated capillaries, and can also be used for overall skin rejuvenation. There is no downtime for patients and minimal discomfort during the four to six required treatments. Unfortunately, the cost of equipment ($40,000 to $80,000) again prevents many primary care clinicians from offering this procedure. Certain IPL technologies can also be successful for hair reduction. However, if using IPL therapy for hair reduction, Fitzpatrick skin types IV through VI will present a challenge in both treatment safety and efficacy (see Chapter 46, Epilation of Isolated Hairs [Including Trichiasis]).

CHEMICAL PEELS

If self-applied over-the-counter AHAs alone are unsatisfactory, they can be used at higher strengths (20% to 70%) or with other agents to cause an inflammatory response or a skin peel. Chemical peeling relies on penetration of an irritating exfoliant into the dermal level to produce a controlled-depth wound that results in sloughing of the superficial skin layers of the epidermis. The injury also evokes a nonspecific tissue regeneration that produces a smoother and more youthful-appearing skin. A peel can be used after the skin has been prepared over time with retinoids, AHAs, or both, or it can be used as an alternative to the continuous application of these topicals.

It is not surprising that AHAs improve the skin; fermented food products that contain them have long been used to exfoliate the skin. Ancient Egyptians used the "hemayet" fruit, Greeks used facial masks, and Romans applied various combinations of salts and plants for this purpose.

Four levels of chemical peels are available: (1) superficial, (2) superficial to medium, (3) medium, and (4) deep (Table 50.3). The deeper the peel, the higher the risk of complications, patient inconvenience, and discomfort. A downtime of 1 or 2 weeks is to be expected with medium-depth and deeper peels, and it is usually obvious to the patient's friends and colleagues that a cosmetic procedure has been performed. On the other hand, most superficial peels can be performed on a Thursday with the patient able to return to work the following Monday with little noticeable skin damage.

Because of the potential for postinflammatory hyperpigmentation, scarring, and hypopigmentation, superficial peels are the procedure of choice for individuals with ethnically darker skin. **NOTE:** With the ability to achieve many of the effects of deep peels by repeated superficial peels combined with retinoid preparation, the need for deep peels has diminished. For this and other reasons (including a higher risk of permanent skin damage and scarring with deep peels), deep peels should be performed only by someone formally trained or significantly experienced in advanced peels. For this chapter, deep peels are discussed only for the sake of completeness and to provide the clinician with an understanding of older, alternative techniques.

Although chemical peels are the least complex of the many cosmetic procedures discussed here, they should not be taken lightly or performed without proper training, experience, and knowledge of managing potential adverse events. With chemical peels, there is less control of the depth of skin penetration and damage than with other skin procedures; therefore in unskilled hands it is wise to start with superficial peels. Deeper peels should not be performed until the clinician has significant clinical experience with various peeling agents.

Advantages of chemical peels over dermabrasion and laser include the lower cost of equipment and a shorter learning curve, especially for superficial and medium-depth peels.

Various chemicals have been used for skin peels, also known as chemexfoliation and *chemabrasion*, in addition to AHAs. These include phenol, trichloroacetic acid (TCA), and β-hydroxy acid (BHA; i.e., salicylic acid [SA]). Combinations are also used. For single agents, lactic, glycolic, and salicylic acids are used most frequently. The difference between BHA and AHA is that AHAs are water soluble, whereas SA (the only BHA) is lipid soluble.

Weaker chemicals such as resorcinol have been used and are relatively free of side effects. Resorcinol is rarely used alone; it is most commonly used in Jessner solution (see Table 50.3).

The effects of a single light peel are so subtle that friends, colleagues, and even the patient may not realize that a cosmetic procedure has been performed. For greater patient satisfaction, a series of peels or alternating superficial peels with microdermabrasion treatments is recommended.

GA is often the first choice of experts for skin peels. Among the many benefits of using GA is the fact it is stable and water soluble. In addition, GA is colorless, odorless, and nontoxic if ingested. Disadvantages of GA include the fact that the peels are somewhat variable: some patients have a brisk inflammatory response to only 30% GA, whereas others have only a slight response to as high as 70% GA. There is some dispute concerning the degree of buffering to be used with GA. Even though it is water soluble, some controversy also exists on how best to neutralize it after application.

Salicylic acid is self-limiting and does not require neutralization after application. Another benefit of SA over GA or any of the AHAs is that the end product is a visible precipitate, or "frost," after application. This allows the clinician to verify that the application is even. If a frost is not clearly visible after the application of one coat, and drying time has been allowed, an additional coat can be applied. SA fluoresces under a Wood's light, which can be used to ensure complete application. These characteristics may be important when clinicians are first learning the procedure. Because it penetrates the epidermal lipids of the skin more deeply than GA, SA usually causes more desquamation (allowing patients to see the peeling and note the changes).

In addition, because SA is lipid (oil) soluble it is naturally comedolytic and is able to penetrate into the pore and exfoliate the buildup of sebum and dead skin cells. Therefore it is perhaps the best preparation to use with acne rosacea.

With these differences, it would appear that SA is superior to the AHAs; however, in reality most experts do not use these differences to make their choice, but rather their own personal experience.

TCA, AHAs, and SA (at the listed strengths) are not as deeply absorbed through the skin and do not burn the skin nearly as deeply as phenol. Therefore once the clinician is adequately trained on proper patient selection, the application process, and how to manage potential adverse events, using only these preparations avoids most of the long-term sequelae associated with deep phenol peels (e.g., total loss of pigmentation, irregular pigmentation, hypertrophic scars). Because of these risks and a theoretic risk of toxicity if absorbed, phenol peels are used much less frequently than other modalities.

With safe and effective AHA and SA peels available, there is a question as to whether primary care clinicians should even use TCA or phenol, both of which work by coagulating skin proteins.

Decreasing the concentration of TCA toward 20% decreases the depth of exfoliation, perhaps making it safer. Before the advent of AHAs and BHA (i.e., SA), TCA was found to be safer than phenol for treating transition zones, such as the area between the face and neck. It was also found to be excellent for treating the thin skin of the hands. In both of these areas, a deeper burn might increase the risk of scar formation.

With AHAs, application of a series of superficial peels, especially if the skin has been prepared by the use of topical retinoids for many weeks, may produce the same effects as one medium peel or even some of the effects of a deep peel. With experience, AHAs allow you to customize the treatment to the area of the body.

INDICATIONS

See Table 50.3.

- Skin rejuvenation—freshen and brighten skin
- Minor to moderate photodamage, especially in 25- to 50-year-old patients
- Dissatisfaction with results from home topical therapy program alone
- Irregular skin texture
- Actinic keratoses
- Acne vulgaris (comedonal and inflammatory, papular and pustular)
- Acne rosacea (papular and pustular)
- Irregular pigmentation (e.g., melasma, freckles, hyperpigmentation, lentigines)
- Superficial acne scars
- Fine wrinkles
- Multiple flat warts

NOTE: If peels are used to treat acne or the complications of acne, the acne should be approximately 75% resolved with whatever primary treatment is being used (e.g., oral antibiotics or topical treatments) before using a peel. In addition, SA is probably the chemical of choice for acne rosacea.

CONTRAINDICATIONS

Absolute

- Concurrent or recent (within 6 months) isotretinoin (Accutane) therapy. It is best to obtain a release from the prescribing physician before performing a chemical peel.
- Concurrent radiation therapy.
- Impaired healing (e.g., due to immunosuppression).
- History of keloid or hypertrophic scarring.
- Allergies or hypersensitivities to agents used for chemical peels.
- Presence of melanoma or squamous cell or basal cell carcinoma in the region to be treated (if diagnosis is uncertain, obtain a biopsy first).
- Hemangiomas and nevus flammeus do not respond to chemical peels.
- Alcoholism (heavy alcohol use will impair healing, making it futile to do a peel).
- Body dysmorphic disorder.
- Pregnancy or nursing.
- Skin atrophy (e.g., chronic steroid use or genetic syndrome such as Ehlers-Danlos).

Relative

- Concurrent hormone therapy (increased risk of postinflammatory hyperpigmentation).
- Herpes simplex virus. If there is a history of outbreaks, pretreat with an antiviral medication during the treatment period.
- Inflammatory lesions (e.g., herpes simplex, acute acne papule, cellulitis, severe seborrheic dermatitis) should be avoided during

chemical peels. More peeling occurs in areas of inflammation, and hyperpigmentation can result. Dermatitis, areas of broken skin, and infection should be controlled before peels; otherwise the chemicals will penetrate more deeply.

- Smoking results in impaired healing and a greater risk of infection. Changes induced by peels will not counteract the damage to the skin from heavy smoking.
- Medium and deep chemical peels of the neck should be approached with extreme caution. In this area there is difficulty controlling the depth of the peel, thus increasing the risk of hypertrophic scarring.
- Although peels are not absolutely contraindicated, patients with as little as 1/32 Native American heritage may be at increased risk of persistent erythema and subsequent hyperpigmentation after a peel. This may be due in part to a reaction to chemicals.
- Patients with a history of allergy to parabens or perfumes may be at the same risk of excessive reaction and pigmentation.

Every precaution should be taken to prevent an allergic reaction to any agents, preservatives, or perfumes (see the Technique section). Oral and topical steroids for potential allergies should be considered. For patients with the potential for excessive reactions and subsequent hyperpigmentation, consider using a tyrosinase inhibitor (hydroquinone) early in the process (see the Complications section for a formula or the Suppliers section to order BleachEze from Medical Center Pharmacy).

EQUIPMENT AND SUPPLIES

- Water source in treatment room
- Eye wash or sterile saline
- Headband
- Towels
- Glass beaker for the peel solution
- Gentle facial cleanser
- 4 × 4 gauze pads
- Clock or timer
- Petroleum jelly
- Ultrasound gel
- Cotton-tipped applicators/swabs
- Acetone (for degreasing the skin)
- Hand-held fan for cooling (allows patient to maintain "control" by participating in comfort measure)
- Tepid water or 10% to 15% sodium bicarbonate solution for neutralizing
- Bowls for water
- Nonirritating moisturizer such as Aquaphor (available in drugstores)
- Sunblock to apply immediately after the peel
- Preprocedure photograph
- Postpeel instruction sheet
- Optional topical anesthetic for medium-depth peels (also see Chapter 4, Topical Anesthesia)
  - Lidocaine 2.5% and prilocaine 2.5% (EMLA) mixture
  - Lidocaine 4% (ELA-Max)
  - Lidocaine 7% or tetracaine 7% or benzocaine 20% cream (will need to be compounded)
  - BLT ointment (benzocaine 10%, lidocaine 20%, tetracaine 4%)
  - Quadri-Caine (compounded bupivacaine, lidocaine, prilocaine, tetracaine)*

---

*Quadri-Caine enhanced cream is a combination of four anesthetics formulated in a topical cream base containing a penetration enhancer (n-decyl methyl sulfoxide 0.25%). Each gram contains 100 mg of lidocaine USP, 50 mg of tetracaine USP, 50 mg of prilocaine hydrochloride, and 10 mg of bupivacaine hydrochloride.

TABLE 50.4	**Protocols for Serial Glycolic Acid Peels (Performed 2–4 Wk Apart)**					
	Peel 1		Peel 2		Peel 3	
Indication	Conc. (%)	Time (min)	Conc. (%)	Time (min)	Conc. (%)	Time (min)
Acne	70	2	35	3	50–70	1–3
Melasma	70	3	35	4	50–70	2–4
Actinic keratoses	70	4	50	3	70	5–7
Fine wrinkles	70	5	50	4	70	4–8
Solar lentigines	70	6	70	3	70	4–8
Back or chest (any indication)	70	7	70	4	70	5–10

Conc., Concentration
Modified from Gendler EC. Topical treatment of the aging face. *Dermatol Clin.* 1997;15:561–567.

NOTE: Compounded products are not produced under the same standards as FDA-approved products. The levels of lidocaine may vary dramatically, and toxicity studies using moderate or large amounts of compounded products have not been performed. One of the editors had a patient with delayed (2 hours following procedure) severe headache and significantly elevated systolic blood pressures (up to 260 mm Hg) following a laser procedure. This patient had been premedicated with topical compounded Quadri-Caine which apparently contained phenylephrine (should not have contained phenylephrine, was not the Quadri-Caine VC). Whether this was an idiosyncratic event or not, this editor no longer uses the Quadri-Caine VC, and in fact, now prefers BLT to Quadri-Caine.

Superficial Peels

Kits are available for superficial chemical peels, ranging in price from $4 to $10 per peel. The patient is charged from $65 to $100 per peel. Treatment for photodamage usually obtains optimal benefit after four to six peels, each 1 month apart.

- TCA 10% to 20%
- SA 20% to 30%
- AHAs 20% to 70% (e.g., glycolic, lactic, citric, malic, mandelic, tartaric)

NOTE: Although lower pH (i.e., pH < 2) GA solutions (50% to 70%) create more necrosis, there is no evidence that this leads to a more favorable peel. Additional necrosis produces additional crusting, making it more obvious that the patient has had a procedure performed as well as increasing the risk of complications. Therefore partially buffered or neutralized GA solutions (i.e., pH > 2) are recommended.

Superficial to Medium-Depth Peels

- TCA 20% to 30%
- A series of AHA or BHA peels (Table 50.4)

Medium-Depth Peels

- TCA 50% or TCA 35% plus initial keratolytics

NOTE: For patient safety and standardization, TCA should be compounded by a weight-to-volume method (i.e., 15% TCA is made by diluting 15 g of TCA crystals in distilled water up to a total volume of 100 mL).

PREPROCEDURE PATIENT PREPARATION

Obtain informed consent from the patient before treatment (see sample consent form available at www.expertconsult.com).

In many cases patients will be asked to pretreat the skin with topical retinoids for 3 to 5 weeks before the peel. Benefits of pretreatment include the fact that it accelerates epidermal turnover, which will reduce healing time. If the topical retinoids cause bothersome or severe desquamation, they should be discontinued for several days and then resumed on alternate days.

For superficial and most medium-depth peels, patients can be informed that after the face is cleansed and prepared, applying the chemicals to produce the peel takes very little time, usually less than 1 minute (see Technique section). However, deep peels may require several hours, allowing time to make the patient comfortable, prepare the face, apply the chemical, complete the peel, and permit patient recovery if an antianxiety medication, pain management, or any type of anesthesia was used during the peel.

It is very important to know Fitzpatrick skin types before doing peels (see Chapter 35, Introduction to Aesthetic Medicine). Be aware that anyone of Native American heritage will be much more sensitive. Anyone with allergies to parabens, perfumes, or other skin preparations needs to inform the clinician so that precautions can be used. He or she needs to receive a patient teaching guide and must inform the clinician of any other possible contraindication. (See the sample patient education handouts available at www.expertconsult.com.)

For superficial peels, patients may experience a stinging or burning sensation during application of the peel. This increases for 2 minutes after application, reaches a peak at 3 minutes, then dissipates over the following few minutes, resulting in a feeling similar to a sunburn. The chemicals themselves cause superficial anesthesia, and patients may find this information psychologically reassuring. In addition, patients usually report a slight tightness and smoothness of the skin immediately after superficial peels.

Within several days, some patients experience slight skin crusting, swelling, and possibly purpura in the lower eyelid areas, which generally resolve over the next 24 to 72 hours depending on the chemical used and the patient's skin type. Erythema almost always resolves in a few weeks.

Whenever the skin is peeled or wounded, there is a risk of scarring and infection. Also, pigmentary augmentation is both a short-term risk (it almost always resolves) and a long-term, permanent risk. The deeper the peel, the higher the risk of all of these side effects and complications.

Superficial peels very rarely cause complications; medium and deep peels are higher risks.

Patients should be aware that their postoperative appearance may be frightening, especially after medium or deep peels. This is rare for superficial peels. Patients should use hypoallergenic, nonscented, complete sunblock (SPF 30 or greater).

For superficial peels, the patient can wear makeup the day of the peel. It will be removed in the clinician's office. Topical retinoids should be stopped 3 days before the procedure. For medium and deep peels, the skin should be washed the evening before the procedure to remove all cosmetics and cleansed again in the office before applying the peeling agent.

NOTE: Disappointment with a chemical peel is most often the result of unrealistically high expectations on either the clinician's or patient's part. Patients should be given a patient teaching guide and made aware that superficial peels yield only modest clinical effects. After multiple peels, patients should be able to better appreciate the benefits. Patients should also be reminded that the effect of a medium-depth peel is not comparable to a face lift. Professional-strength peels increase the effectiveness of GA or other AHA solutions that are used later at home by the patient.

TECHNIQUE

For a sample documentation form, see Fig. 50.2.

Superficial Peels

1. Choose the proper mixture or concentration for the patient. AHA 20% to 70%, BHA (i.e., SA) 20% to 30%, or TCA 10% to 20% causes detachment of keratinocytes at the lower concentrations and epidermolysis at the higher concentrations.
2. Cleanse skin of residual debris, makeup, and body surface oils with alcohol or, preferably, acetone.
3. Using cotton-tipped applicators, apply a thin coat of petroleum jelly at the lash line, taking care to protect the medial and lateral canthi of the eyes, the mouth corners, and the edges of the nose (i.e., nasoalar junction; Fig. 50.3A–C). These are typically dry areas of the face and therefore need protection. Any inflamed lesion, such as an active acne lesion, should be avoided. Ask the patient if there are any other dry areas of the face that need protection from the peel. Patients usually know which areas of their nose and face are the driest.
4. After cleansing and applying protectant jelly, eye patches are placed to prevent accidental eye damage (see Fig. 50.3D).
5. Starting on the forehead, apply the acid mixture evenly to the entire face, being careful not to pass your hand directly over the patient's eyes. Gentle stretching of the skin will allow the fluid to coat the depths of wrinkles evenly (see Fig. 50.3E–F). In general, facial peels do not need to go beyond, but should generally be feathered just below, the jaw line and the fluid should not be applied closer than a couple of millimeters to the eyelid margin. Feather the solution into the hairline and along the chin to prevent a line of demarcation between the treated and untreated areas. If desired, the solution can also be used to extend the peel to the chest, neck, arms, and hands.
6. Allow the mixture to remain in place for the appropriate time (usually 3 to 5 minutes; see Fig. 50.3G). Use a timer or a clock, but even more important, assess the patient and skin; do not rely on the timer alone. If there are any areas showing increased penetration, intense redness, or pain ("hot spots"), they can be neutralized with a cotton-tipped applicator dipped in ultrasound gel. The gel does not run like water, so it dilutes the acid effect on the area and decreases discomfort.
7. Neutralize and gently blot the treated areas with either water or sodium bicarbonate solution unless the acid you are using is self-limiting and does not require neutralizing, such as SA or Jessner solution.
8. A hypoallergenic, nonscented moisturizer (e.g., Aquaphor) and complete sunblock should be applied immediately after the peel (see Fig. 50.3H).

Superficial to Medium-Depth Peels

1. As for superficial peels, choose the proper mixture technique to obtain a superficial to medium-depth peel. A single agent can be used (TCA 20% to 30%) or superficial peels may be repeated every 2 to 4 weeks for a deeper peel effect or until the desired results are obtained. For AHAs or TCA, three or four treatments may be adequate (see Table 50.4); however, often six to eight SA peels are performed. In most cases, the best results are obtained if the patient waits 1 month between peels.
2. If TCA 20% to 30% is chosen, the skin to be peeled must first be dekeratinized to ensure uniform TCA penetration. AHA or SA superficial peels applied in the office a few days before the TCA procedure can be used for this purpose. Dekeratinization can also be performed by the patient before arrival by applying topical retinoids to the skin surface daily for 3 to 5 weeks.
3. Although anesthesia is not necessary, intravenous conscious sedation or topical anesthesia (see earlier discussion) may be used.
4. Protect the necessary areas of the face with petroleum jelly in the same manner as for superficial peels.
5. Using a cotton-tipped applicator with the tip wrung out well to avoid dripping or splashing, apply the TCA to the entire face. It should be applied evenly to produce a smooth, white surface.

Chemical Peel Progress Note

Patient Name: _____ M/F ____ D.O.B. _____ Date _____

Allergies: _____

Patient Concern/Goals: _____

Skin Assessment: Fitzpatrick skin type: I   II   III   IV   V   VI

Check all that apply:

- ❏ Normal   ❏ Sensitive   ❏ Telangiectasias   ❏ Hyperpigmentation
- ❏ Oily   ❏ Dehydrated   ❏ Excoriations   ❏ Hypopigmentation
- ❏ Dry   ❏ Rosacea   ❏ Scars   ❏ Other

Home Program:
Skin care products: _____
Current facial mediations: Retin-A (strength)_____ Ranova (strength)_____
Taxorac (strength)_____ Tazorac (strength)_____ Differin (gel or cream)_____
Other: _____

Treatment Plan:
Vitalize Peel   Lot #: _____ Treatment #: _____
Illuminize Peel   Lot #: _____ Treatment #: _____

Treated Area: ❏ Face   ❏ Neck   ❏ Chest

Step 1: Prepping Solution Lot #: _____ Pressure Applied: ❏ Light ❏ Medium ❏ Strong

    Areas of Pressure Applied: _____

Step 2: Prepping Solution Lot #: _____ Pressure Applied: ❏ Light ❏ Medium ❏ Strong

    Number of Passes: 1   2   3

    Areas of Pressure Applied: _____

Optional Step: Retinoic acid (not supplied with this kit).   Number of passes: 1   2

Step 3: Sunscreen

Skin Reaction:
Erythema: ❏ none ❏ mild ❏ moderate ❏ severe   Areas affected: _____
Burning: ❏ none ❏ mild ❏ moderate ❏ severe   Areas affected: _____
Frosting: ❏ none ❏ mild ❏ moderate ❏ severe   Areas affected: _____

Recommendations and Comments: _____
_____
_____

Provider's Signature: _____

Fig. 50.2 Sample skin peel documentation form. (Courtesy John L. Pfenninger, MD, The Medical Procedures Center, PC, Midland, MI.)

Greater penetration in certain areas may be achieved by rubbing the applicator vigorously. Gently stretching the skin will allow the fluid to coat the depths of wrinkles evenly. The peel should not be extended below the jaw line. Desired areas of the hands and arms may also be treated.

6. Treatments may be repeated, if necessary, in 1- to 3-month intervals to achieve the desired effect.

Medium-Depth Peels

Pretreatment with 0.1% tretinoin (Retin-A) daily for at least 2 weeks will enhance wound healing from medium-depth peels.

Using a Combination of 70% Glycolic Acid and 35% Trichloroacetic Acid

1. After protecting areas of the face with petroleum jelly in the same manner as for superficial peels, apply a 70% GA mixture to the entire face.
2. Allow the mixture to remain in place for 2 minutes. A fan in the room may ease patient discomfort from the stinging associated with the peel.
3. Wash with water.

4. Optional but effective: Apply a topical anesthetic for 30 minutes without occlusion.

NOTE: A study comparing two topical anesthetics (EMLA and ELA-Max) with each other and with a placebo found a statistically significant decrease in pain with both topical anesthetics and no difference in efficacy between the two anesthetics. Neither anesthetic affected the depth of penetration of the peel. Other topical anesthetics can be used based on clinician preference.

5. Remove the topical anesthetic and apply 35% TCA to the entire face as previously described.
6. If successful and there are no complications, this technique can be extended to the hands, arms, and chest during the next peel. Depending on the chemical used, be aware of toxicity levels when treating multiple zones and larger surface areas.
7. A cool compress applied to the area after a peel may ease patient discomfort.

Using Trichloroacetic Acid 50%

The technique for a superficial to medium-depth peel with TCA 50% is the same as that noted for the combination 70% GA/35% TCA peel in the previous section.

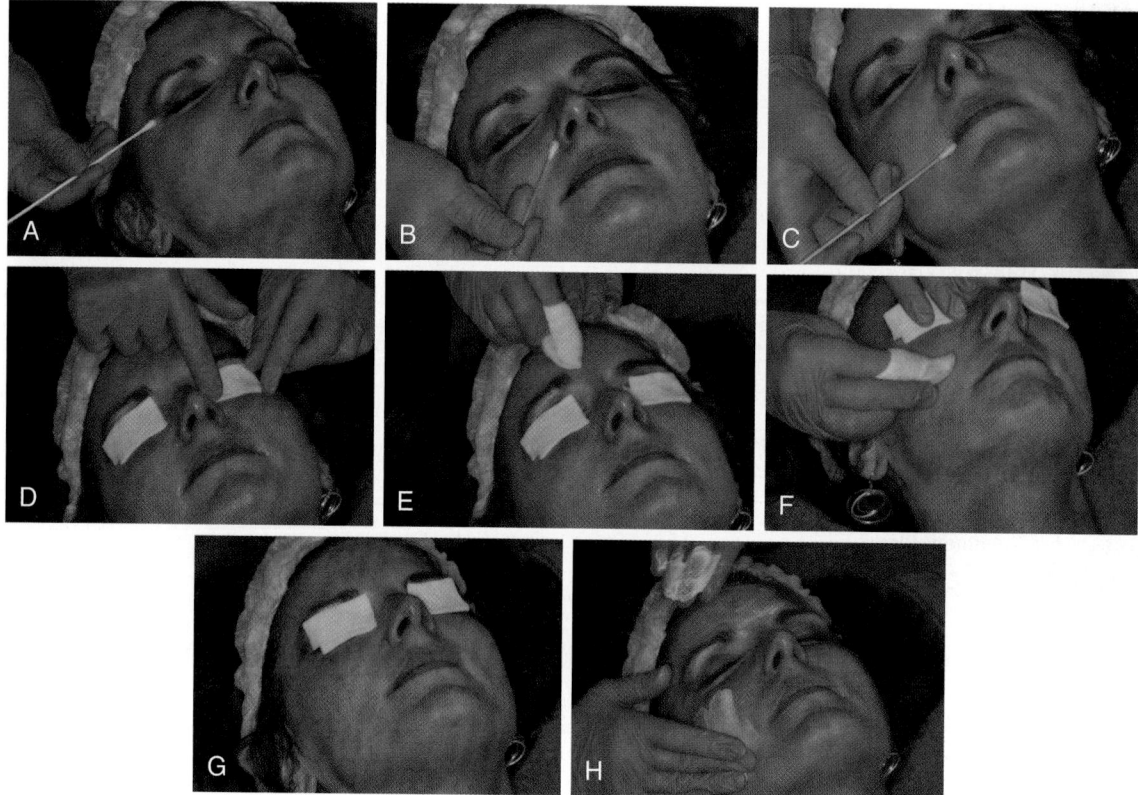

Fig. 50.3 (A–H) Steps in a skin peel procedure. In this case, the Illuminize Peel followed by TNS Ceramide treatment (SkinMedica Allergan, Inc., Carlsbad, CA) were used. (Courtesy John L. Pfenninger, MD, The Medical Procedures Center, PC, Midland, MI.)

COMPLICATIONS

Persistent hyperpigmentation is a slight risk, but it is often adequately treated with a tyrosinase inhibitor (hydroquinone, often combined with steroids). One published formula combines 30 g of parabens-free corticosteroid cream, 15 g of 4% hydroquinone, and 20 g of Retin-A 0.1% into a cream to be applied starting 2 weeks after the procedure if hyperpigmentation is developing. Another option is BleachEze (see the Suppliers section).

The use of oral corticosteroids for 2 weeks after the procedure, followed by a steroid cream, may prevent persistent hyperpigmentation in those at risk or with a history of previous hyperpigmentation.

POSTPROCEDURE PATIENT EDUCATION

For superficial peels, the effect is maximal at 48 hours, so the patient should attempt to avoid the sun completely for at least 3 days. If going outside is unavoidable during this time, the patient must use a sunscreen and wear a broad-brimmed hat and large sunglasses. The skin is most vulnerable to damage during this time and sun exposure can cause many problems, including swelling, a deepening of the peel, postinflammatory hyperpigmentation, and potential scarring.

Actual peeling usually begins 2 days after the treatment and can last for up to 7 days. Most patients peel in the central part of the face more heavily than peripherally, and only lightly on the forehead. Some patients peel in fine sheets, but most peel in flakes.

As stated previously, immediately after a superficial peel patients usually report a slight tightness, much like the feeling of a sunburn. A smoothness to the skin is felt and some patients may experience slight skin crusting. Occasionally, swelling occurs, as well as purpura in the lower eyelid areas. These symptoms resolve within a few days. The deeper the peel, the more likely the patient will have these side effects, and the longer they will last.

The effect of a medium-depth peel is maximal at 48 hours. Crusting and some swelling are to be expected and usually subside within the first week. Use of continuous lubrication and sunblock is

essential to protect the new skin. If a home care skin regimen is not implemented and maintained, the result of the peel will likely wane by the third month after the procedure.

Aspirin and nonsteroidal antiinflammatory drugs work very well for postpeel discomfort. A prescription for a mild pain medication may relieve any tingling or throbbing.

In about 7 to 10 days, new skin will be apparent and the patient should be healed sufficiently to return to normal activities. Patients should continue to protect their skin and avoid being in the sun without protection for several months.

After all peels, sunburn may occur at lower doses of sunlight and lead to hyperpigmentation or hypopigmentation. Preservatives, scents, or the chemicals used may also provoke a sensitivity reaction and cause persistent erythema; therefore a hypoallergenic, unscented, complete sunblock (SPF 20 or greater) for sensitive skin should be used. Even after healing, the postpeel skin is thinner and more susceptible to sun damage and sunburn. The patient should make a habit of wearing a broad-brimmed hat and large sunglasses, as well as using a complete sunblock every day, and should avoid direct sunlight as much as possible.

Thinner or irritated skin is also more susceptible to desiccation. Thus, a moisturizer should be applied daily.

PATIENT EDUCATION GUIDES

See the sample patient education handouts available at www.expertconsult.com.

CPT/BILLING CODES

15788	Chemical peel, facial; epidermal
15789	Chemical peel, facial; dermal
15792	Chemical peel, nonfacial; epidermal
15793	Chemical peel, nonfacial; dermal

ICD-10-CM Diagnostic Codes

Although most insurers consider chemical peels a cosmetic procedure, occasionally they reimburse for treatment of acne, actinic keratoses, or acne rosacea.

L71.0–L71.8	Rosacea
L57.0	Actinic keratosis
L70.0–L70.8	Acne
L81.0–L81.9	Other pigment disorders
L90.5	Scar conditions
L98.8	Other disorder skin and subcutaneous tissue

Acknowledgment

The editors recognize the contributions of Grant C. Fowler, MD, and Stephen F. Ramirez, MD, to this chapter in a previous edition of this text.

Suppliers

(See contact information available at www.expertconsult.com.)

Betacaine and BleachEze
  Custom Scripts Pharmacy
BLT Topical Anesthesia (compounded bupivacaine, lidocaine, tetracaine)
  Biosense Clinic
Cosmeceutical skin care, Jessner solution, salicylic acid, and glycolic peels
  Allergan, Inc.
  Newport Cosmeceuticals, Inc.
  SkinMedica Allergan, Inc.
  Theraplex Company
  Visual Changes Skin Care
Glycolic acid
  Valeant Pharmaceuticals
Quadri-Caine Topical Anesthesia (compounded bupivacaine, lidocaine, prilocaine, tetracaine)
  Keystone Pharmacy (compounding pharmacy)
  Portage Pharmacy
  Scripts Pharmacy (compounding pharmacy)
Trichloroacetic acid, glycolic acid, and other supplies
  Delasco/Dermatologic Lab and Supply, Inc.

Online Resources

American Society of Plastic Surgeons. Chemical peel. https://www.plasticsurgery.org/cosmetic-procedures/chemical-peel.
American Society of Plastic Surgeons. Dermabrasion. https://www.plasticsurgery.org/cosmetic-procedures/dermabrasion.
Plastic Surgery Network. The Art of Deep Chemical peels. http://www.psenetwork.org/lecture.aspx?cid=ced8c722-6ed3-4d83-a6d4-c18b7e4016b4.

Recommended Reading

Arndt KA, Kaminer M, Wheeland RG. The promises and limits of cosmetic dermatology. *Patient Care*. 1999;33:97.

Bernstein EF. Chemical peels. In: Kaminer MS, Dover JS, Arndt KA, eds. *Atlas of Cosmetic Surgery*. 2nd ed. Philadelphia: Saunders; 2009:117–134.

Brody HJ. *Chemical Peeling and Resurfacing*. Emory University: Digital Library Publications; 2009.

Coleman III WP, Coleman KM. Techniques for peeling of the face. In: Merli GJ, ed. *The Clinics Atlas of Office Procedures: Basic Cosmetic Procedures*. Philadelphia: Saunders; 2000.

Cox SE, Soderburg J, Butterwick KJ. Chemical peels. In: Robinson JK, Hanke CW, Siegel DM, Sengelmann RD, Alina Fratila MD, eds. *Surgery of the Skin: Procedural Dermatology*. 2nd ed. Philadelphia: Elsevier; 2010:393–414.

Dayal S, Amrani A, Sahu P, Jain VK. Jessner's solution vs. 30% salicylic acid peels: a comparative study of the efficacy and safety in mild-to-moderate acne vulgaris. *J Cosmet Dermatol*. 2017;16(1):43–51.

Deprez P. *Textbook of Chemical Peels: Superficial, Medium, and Deep Peels in Cosmetic Practice*. 2nd ed. Abingdon, United Kingdom: Informa Healthcare; 2016.

Edwards L, Maibach HI, Roenigk HH. What can be done for photoaged skin? *Patient Care*. 1996;30:68.

Farber GA. Prolonged erythema after chemical peel. *Dermatol Surg*. 1998;24:934–935.

Fulton Jr JE. Acne: its causes and treatments. *Int J Cosmet Surg Aesthet Dermatol*. 2002;4:95–105.

Holzer G, Pinkowicz A, Radakovic S, Schmidt JB, Tanew A. Randomized controlled trial comparing 35% trichloroacetic acid peel and 5-aminolevulinic acid photodynamic therapy for the treatment of multiple actinic keratosis. *Br J Dermatol*. 2016.

Kligman D, Kligman AM. Salicylic acid peels for the treatment of photoaging. *Dermatol Surg*. 1998;24:325–328.

Koppel RA, Coleman KM, Coleman WP. The efficacy of EMLA versus ELA-Max for pain relief in medium-depth chemical peeling: a clinical and histopathologic evaluation. *Dermatol Surg*. 2000;26:61–64.

Lewis AB, Gendler EC. Resurfacing with topical agents. *Semin Cutan Med Surg*. 1996;15:139–144.

Matarasso SL, Hanke CW, Alster TS. Cutaneous resurfacing. *Clin Dermatol*. 1997;15:569–582.

Moy R, Luftman D, Kakita L. *Glycolic Acid Peels. Vol 22: Basic and Clinical Dermatology*. Abingdon, United Kingdom: Informa Healthcare; 2002.

Rees TD. Chemabrasion and dermabrasion. In: Rees TD, LaTrenta GS, eds. *Aesthetic Plastic Surgery*. 2nd ed. Philadelphia: WB Saunders; 1994:757–766.

Small RA. *Practical Guide to Chemical Peels, Microdermabrasion & Topical Products*. New York: Lippincott; 2012.

Small R, O'Hanlon K. Chemical peels. In: Usatine RP, Pfenninger JL, Stulberg DL, Small R, eds. *Dermatologic and Cosmetic Procedures in Office Practice*. Philadelphia: Elsevier; 2012.

Taylor MB, Zaleski-Larsen L, McGraw TA. Single Session Treatment of Rolling Acne Scars Using Tumescent Anesthesia, 20% Trichloracetic Acid Extensive Subcision, and Fractional CO2 Laser. *Dermatol Surg*. 2017;43(suppl 1):S70–S74.

Tosti A, Grimes PE, De Padova MP, eds. *Color Atlas of Chemical Peels*. Berlin: Springer-Verlag; 2005.

Tung R, Rubin MG. *Procedures in Cosmetic Dermatology Series: Chemical Peels*. 2nd ed. Philadelphia: Elsevier; 2010.

Vossen M, Hage JJ, Karim RB. Formulation of trichloroacetic acid peeling solution: a bibliometric analysis. *Plast Reconstr Surg*. 2000;105:1088–1094.

CHAPTER 51

PHOTODYNAMIC THERAPY

Greta McLaren

The history of photodynamic therapy (PDT) dates back to the early 1900s. Various chemicals were found to have cytotoxic effects on specific cells, after absorption, when activated by light. In the presence of oxygen, they became photosensitizers. PDT is currently used to treat various dermatologic conditions, connective tissue disorders, and malignancies. This chapter reviews the various dermatologic conditions, both medical and cosmetic, that can be treated in the office setting using topical PDT. Both U.S. Food and Drug Administration (FDA)–approved applications as well as off-label applications are discussed.

PDT, using the topical photosensitizer 5-aminolevulinic acid (ALA-PDT), has been gaining popularity over the last 2 decades among dermatologists and primary care clinicians alike. The procedure received FDA approval in 1999 for the treatment of minimally to moderately thick actinic keratoses of the face and scalp. However, multiple off-label uses have been investigated and found to be both safe and effective. Some of the more common off-label protocols include the treatment of acne, photodamage, sebaceous gland hyperplasia, and hidradenitis suppurativa. Extensive research regarding the off-label use of ALA-PDT in the treatment of nonmelanoma skin cancers, including basal cell carcinoma and Bowen disease, has been published. However, these topics are not covered in this chapter. Refer to the Recommended Reading for more information on these subjects (e.g., Gilbert, 2007).

The most common form of ALA used by clinicians in the United States is 20% 5-ALA (Levulan Kerastick; Dusa Pharmaceuticals, Inc.). This photosensitizing chemical has the unique property of being absorbed by the outer layer of the skin and being taken up selectively by cells undergoing rapid turnover. As a result, this procedure allows for the targeting of rapidly reproducing, unhealthy, sun-damaged, precancerous, and cancerous skin cells.

Once applied to the skin and allowed to incubate and be absorbed, ALA is converted to a potent photosensitizer (PS), protoporphyrin IX (PpIX). When exposed to oxygen and light of various wavelengths, PpIX reacts and becomes cytotoxic (via singlet oxygen) to the targeted cells. The absorption peaks for PpIX show a maximum peak at 409 nm, with lesser peaks at 509, 544, 584, and 635 nm (Fig. 51.1). Higher fluencies (light energy) are needed for the lesser peaks, although the deeper penetration at the longer wavelengths may have an added benefit.

O_2 + PS + light → singlet oxygen (which destroys the target).

ALA-PDT used off label in the treatment of acne vulgaris works in two ways: (1) by destruction of *Propionibacterium acnes*, the bacterium associated with the disorder; and (2) by shrinkage of the oil glands resulting in less production of oil. This procedure is considered an alternative to isotretinoin (Accutane), with results in some studies lasting for up to 2 years.

In the presence of ALA, *P. acnes* makes a large amount of photosensitive porphyrins, increasing its photosensitivity. The pilosebaceous unit itself selectively accumulates the photosensitizer, PpIX. Light application again produces a chemical reaction that in turn kills the bacteria and also causes involution of the sebaceous gland.

A second PDT photosensitizer, *methyl aminolevulinate* (Metvix, Galderma Laboratories and PhotoCure AS), has been FDA approved as second-line therapy for the treatment of nonhyperkeratotic actinic keratoses of the face and scalp not amenable to conventional therapy.

Lasers and light sources capable of emitting wavelengths of light that correspond to the absorption peaks for PpIX (see Fig. 51.1) are possible sources for activation of ALA. *BLU-U*, a 417-nm wavelength light manufactured by Dusa Pharmaceuticals, is the activating light source used in FDA approved protocol. Multiple other light and laser sources noted in the Equipment section below have also been found to be effective in activating ALA. Devices such as intense pulsed light (IPL) or pulsed-dye laser (PDL) can be synergistic in that not only are they capable of activating ALA, they are also able to target other chromophores such as hemoglobin or melanin. As a result, these devices can simultaneously treat telangiectases and solar lentigines while activating ALA, thereby enhancing the cosmetic result for photodamaged skin. This procedure using a PDL or IPL source is often referred to as photorejuvenation with ALA.

INDICATIONS

U.S. Food and Drug Administration Approved

Actinic keratoses, mild to moderate thickness.

Off-Label Use

- Acne vulgaris
- Acne rosacea
- Cosmetic photorejuvenation
- Sebaceous hyperplasia
- Hidradenitis suppurativa
- Nonmelanoma skin cancers
- Actinic cheilitis
- Warts

CONTRAINDICATIONS

Absolute

- Pregnancy
- Breastfeeding (not studied)
- Planned sun exposure within 48 hours
- Isotretinoin (Accutane) use within the previous 6 months

Relative

- Seizure disorder
- Diabetes
- Photosensitizing drug use
- Tobacco use

EQUIPMENT

- Acetone and 4 × 4 gauze for skin preparation
- Microdermabrasion machine (optional)
- 20% 5-ALA (Levulan Kerastick)
- BLU-U (417 nm), ClearLight (405 to 420 nm; Lumenis, Ltd.), Omnilux Blue Light (415 nm; Photo Therapeutics, Inc.), PDL (585 or 595 nm), broadband light source or IPL (410 to 1200 nm)
- Zimmer chiller (optional)

PATIENT SELECTION AND PRECAUTIONS

- Photodynamic therapy with ALA can be used on all skin types, Fitzpatrick I through VI, if indicated, using one of the previously noted light devices. Photorejuvenation using an IPL or PDL should be reserved for patients with skin types I through IV only. Patients with darker skin types (Fitzpatrick IV and above) are more susceptible to postinflammatory hyperpigmentation after this procedure. These patients should be well informed of the potential risk of postinflammatory hyperpigmentation before undergoing the procedure. For the first PDT treatment in skin types IV and above, a shorter incubation time should be considered. The incubation time for subsequent treatments may be gradually increased in 15-minute increments if tolerated (Table 51.1). It is prudent in these patients to take prophylactic measures by prescribing a skin-lightening agent such as hydroquinone 4% gel or cream 2 weeks before and up to 4 weeks after the procedure when treating skin types IV or higher.
- The side effects and potential downtime with this procedure vary significantly from patient to patient. Some of the more common side effects are erythema, swelling, peeling, crusting, dryness, and discomfort. As a general rule, the amount of target tissue present, such as the prevalence of actinic keratoses or severity of acne, along with the length of the incubation period, will determine the amount of downtime and side effects.
- Retinoid use before the procedure may enhance the results but will also increase the downtime. For better predictability of downtime and side effects, retinoids can be discontinued 1 to 2 weeks before the procedure, unless the enhanced effect, with its potential increased severity of downtime, is desired and discussed with the patient during the consultation.
- ALA-PDT should not be performed on patients who have used isotretinoin (Accutane) within the previous 6 months.
- The use of photosensitizing drugs, including tetracyclines, must be taken into consideration when performing this procedure. It is acceptable to continue the medication during the treatments; however, the incubation time of ALA is decreased by 15 minutes on the initial treatment to determine if increased side effects due to photosensitivity are likely to occur.
- The discomfort and nerve irritation that may occur with ALA-PDT may stimulate a herpes simplex virus recurrence in patients with a history of cold sores. Antivirals should be used prophylactically to prevent this potential side effect in such patients.

PATIENT EDUCATION AND POSTTREATMENT GUIDELINES

Because of the potential severity of side effects and reactions to this procedure, an initial consultation with the patient by a clinician with a full explanation of the potential risks, downtime, and side effects is recommended. Once ALA is applied and absorbed in the skin, it may remain reactive to sunlight for the next 24 to 48 hours, regardless of cleansing after the application. It is therefore imperative that patients understand the need to avoid sunlight, both direct and indirect, for a minimum of 48 hours after the procedure. An educational handout and informed consent should be reviewed with the patient during the initial consultation.

PROCEDURE

1. Baseline photographs are always helpful.
2. Review consent form and posttreatment guidelines with the patient.
3. Review the history to note any contraindications or use of photosensitizing drugs.
4. Note any cold sore risk and prescribe antivirals if indicated.
5. Cleanse and prepare the skin with either a vigorous acetone scrub or microdermabrasion.
6. Crush the Levulan Kerastick according to directions and shake the solution for 3 minutes.
7. Protect the patient's eyes and mouth with petrolatum ointment or gauze, and apply the Levulan solution to the treatment area (face, neck, chest, back, arms, hands, or legs). Areas with more severe disease may be treated with a second coat of Levulan.
8. Incubate to allow for sufficient absorption of the Levulan depending on area, disease severity, and skin type (see Table 51.1).

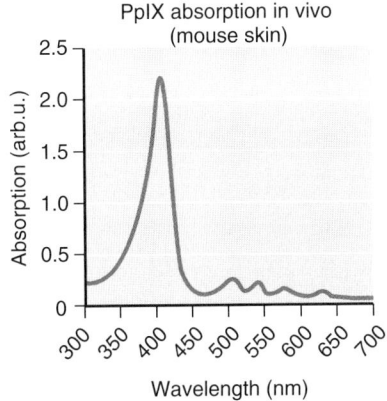

Fig. 51.1 Absorption peaks for protoporphyrin IX (PpIX). (Courtesy Dusa Pharmaceuticals, Inc., Wilmington, MA.)

TABLE 51.1	Levulan Incubation Time for ALA-PDT Treatment				
Area	Treatment Number	Fitzpatrick Skin Type	Disease Severity	Occlusion	Time (min)
Face/scalp	First	I–III	Mild to moderate	No	60
	Second–Fifth	I–III	Same as above	No	60–90*
	First	I–III	Moderate to severe	No	30
	Second–Fifth	I–III	Same as above	No	45–60*
	First–Fifth	IV–VII	All	No	30–45
Chest, back, arms or legs	First–Fifth	I–III	Mild to moderate	Yes	120
	First–Fifth	I–III	Moderate to severe	Yes	90–120
Chest, back	First–Fifth	IV–V	All	Yes	60–90
	First–Fifth	VI	All	Yes	60

*Incubation time may be gradually increased with subsequent treatments if the patient's reaction is well tolerated.

9. Areas other than the face and neck, such as chest, back, hands, arms, and legs, require longer incubation times for sufficient absorption of the Levulan. If treating these areas, occluding the area with cellophane (kitchen plastic wrap) and tape will enhance the absorption and decrease the incubation time required (see Table 51.1).

10. When significant acne and/or photodamage are present, or if the patient has a darker skin type and is at risk for postinflammatory hyperpigmentation, consider a shorter initial incubation time. Gradually increase incubation times with subsequent treatments, depending on tolerance. Do not exceed a 30-minute incubation time in Fitzpatrick skin type VI because of the increased risk of postinflammatory hyperpigmentation (see Table 51.1).

11. Wash the treated area with a gentle cleanser and water after incubation, before starting the light treatment.

12. Activate the Levulan by exposing the treated area to a light source. Narrow-band blue light, IPL, PDL, and light-emitting diode light that falls within the required wavelength absorption spectrum for PpIX (see Fig. 51.1) are all possible activators of Levulan. The operator should use the chosen device in accordance with its operating protocol. If using the BLU-U light alone, the exposure time is approximately 15 minutes. The recommended energy for the Omnilux 415-nm light, according to the manufacturer, is 48 J/cm^2 for 20 minutes. However, this energy setting can cause significant discomfort, so start with a setting of 24 J/cm^2 for 20 minutes. Energy settings can always be increased. For significant photodamage, actinic keratoses, or deep cystic acne, use IPL at 25 to 45 J/cm^2, depending on the skin type and cooling mechanism, followed by additional exposure using blue light (410 to 417 nm) at 10 to 48 J/cm^2 for 3 to 8 minutes, depending on the energy settings used.

13. Apply a gentle moisturizer or Aquaphor.

14. Inform the patient that the redness and swelling will likely intensify over the next 48 hours. The patient should use a hat or umbrella and sunscreen to guard against any sun exposure for the next 48 hours.

15. Patients appreciate a follow-up by phone or office visit in 24 to 72 hours.

16. To help prevent postinflammatory hyperpigmentation, prescribe a lightening agent such as hydroquinone 4% cream for darker skin types (IV to VI) once the skin is fully recovered.

17. When IPL with ALA is used for sebaceous gland hyperplasia, at a 7- to 10-day follow-up, treat the majority of the lesions still present. After two to three treatments with ALA-PDT, there is a significant reduction in the number of newly occurring lesions.

COMPLICATIONS

- Postinflammatory hyperpigmentation is a potential complication of this procedure. If this occurs, prescribe a combination cream of hydroquinone 4%, tretinoin 0.05%, and fluocinolone acetonide 0.01% to be used once or twice daily for up to 8 weeks. Microdermabrasion every 2 weeks may also be added.

- Sun exposure in the first 48 hours may result in blistering, severe discomfort, and peeling. Cold compresses, pain medication, Aquaphor, and frequent follow-up visits to monitor for infection are recommended.

- Infection is rare but can occur. If impetigo occurs, mupirocin topical antibiotic ointment or cephalexin 500 mg twice daily may be prescribed for 7 to 10 days. If herpes simplex virus infection occurs, antivirals such as acyclovir should be prescribed.

- Also see some of the common after-effects noted previously.

POSTPROCEDURE MANAGEMENT

Avoiding sun exposure and keeping the treated area moist are essential. Aquaphor is a preferred healing ointment. To soften any significant crusting, apply wet gauze soaked in a solution of 1 teaspoon of vinegar to 1 cup of water. This may be applied for 10 minutes three times daily.

RESULTS

With three to five photorejuvenation treatments with ALA-PDT (60-minute incubation time) in combination with IPL followed by BLU-U for 3 minutes (Fig. 51.2A–B); or with three to five acne treatments with ALA-PDT (60-minute incubation time) and BLU-U exposure alone for 15 minutes (Figs. 51.3 and 51.4), the patient satisfaction rate is very good.

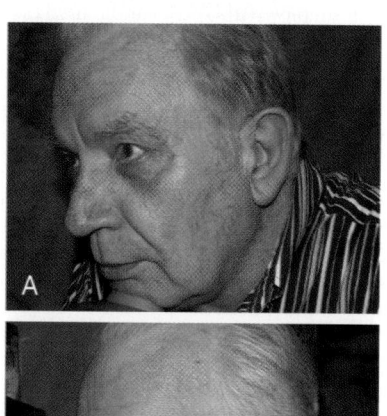

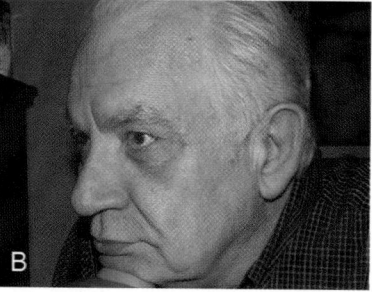

Fig. 51.2 (A) Photodamage before treatment. (B) Photodamage after three photodynamic therapy treatments with intense pulsed light and BLU-U.

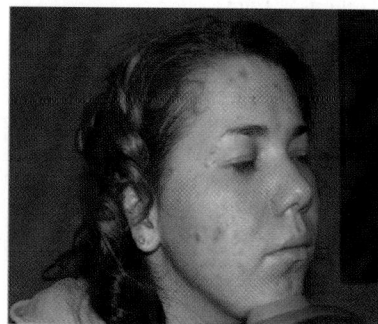

Fig. 51.3 Acne before treatment.

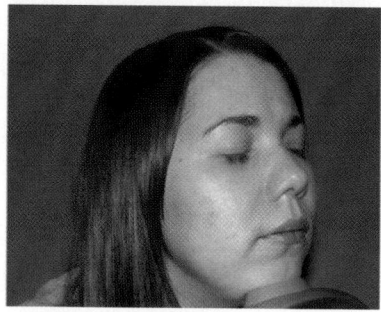

Fig. 51.4 Acne after three photodynamic therapy treatments with BLU-U.

PATIENT EDUCATION GUIDES

See the patient education and patient consent forms available at www.expertconsult.com.

CPT/BILLING CODES

Limited reimbursement for the FDA-approved treatment of actinic keratoses is available through some insurance companies. The majority of the off-label uses of ALA-PDT are considered cosmetic and are unlikely to be covered by insurance.

* For treatment of actinic keratoses, use the CPT code 17004 (destruction premalignant lesions, 15 or more).
* 96567- Photodynamic therapy by external application of light to destroy premalignant and/or malignant lesions of the skin and adjacent mucosa by activation of photosensitive drug(s), each phototherapy exposure session
* Use J code 7308 for amino-levulinic acid.

For support in documentation and billing and current CPT codes, Dusa Pharmaceuticals has a reimbursement and coding support center (http://www.dusapharma.com/levulan-pdt-proce-dures-coding-billing-guide.html; telephone: 822-533-3872 [United States/Canada]).

ICD-10-CM DIAGNOSTIC CODES

| L70.0-L70.8 | Acne |
| L57.0 | Actinic Keratosis |

SUPPLIERS

(See contact information available at www.expertconsult.com.)

20% 5-ALA (Levulan Kerastick) and light sources for activation of ALA
Dusa Pharmaceuticals, Inc.
Broad-band light (BBL)
Sciton
ClearLight and Omnilux Blue
Lumenis
Photo Therapeutics, Inc.
Intense pulsed light
(See Chapters 38 to 44 for other units.)
Cutera
Palomar Cynosure
Pulsed-dye laser
Candela Syneron

ONLINE RESOURCES

American Society for Laser Medicine & Surgery. https://www.aslms.org.

RECOMMENDED READING

Alexiades-Armenakas M. Aminolevulinic acid photodynamic therapy for actinic keratoses/actinic cheilitis/acne: vascular lasers. *Dermatol Clin.* 2007;25:25–37.

Barbaric J, Abbott R, Posadzki P, et al. Light therapies for acne. *Cochrane Database Syst Rev.* 2016;9:CD007917.

Blume JE, Oseroff AR. Aminolevulinic acid photodynamic therapy for skin cancers. *Dermatol Clin.* 2007;25:5–14.

Boen M, Brownell J, Patel P, Tsoukas MM. The role of photodynamic therapy in acne: an evidence-based review. *Am J Clin Dermatol.* 2017.

Gilbert DJ. Incorporating photodynamic therapy into a medical and cosmetic dermatology practice. *Dermatol Clin.* 2007;25:111–120.

Gold MH. Introduction to photodynamic therapy: early experience. *Dermatol Clin.* 2007;25:1–4.

Gold MH. Photodynamic therapy in dermatology: the next five years. *Dermatol Clin.* 2007;25:119–120.

Gold MH, Bradshaw VL, Boring NM, et al. The use of novel intense pulsed light and heat source and ALA-PDT in the treatment of moderate to severe inflammatory acne vulgaris. *J Drugs Dermatol.* 2005;3(suppl 6):S15–S19.

Goldman MP. *Procedures in Cosmetic Dermatology Series: Photodynamic Therapy.* 2nd ed. Philadelphia: Saunders; 2007.

Goldman MP, Massaki ABMN. Photodynamic therapy. In: Goldman MP, Fitzpatrick RE, Ross EV, Kilmer SR, Weiss RA, eds. *Lasers and Energy Devices for the Skin.* 2nd ed. Boca Raton: CRC Press; 2013:222–271.

Maranda EL, Lim VM, Nguyen AH, Nouri K. Laser and light therapy for facial warts: a systematic review. *J Eur Acad Dermatol Venereol.* 2016;30(10):1700–1707.

Nestor MS. Evolving use of 5-aminolevulinic acid (ALA) topical photodynamic therapy clinically and cosmetically: a clinician's perspective. *Cosmetic Dermatol.* 2005;18:2–5.

Nestor MS. The use of photodynamic therapy for the treatment of acne vulgaris. *Dermatol Clin.* 2007;25:47–57.

Nootheti PK, Goldman MP. Aminolevulinic acid-photodynamic therapy for photorejuvenation. *Dermatol Clin.* 2007;25:35–45.

Richey DF. Aminolevulinic acid photodynamic therapy for sebaceous gland hyperplasia. *Dermatol Clin.* 2007;25:59–65.

Taub AF. Photodynamic therapy: other uses. *Dermatol Clin.* 2007;25:101–109.

CHAPTER 52

CELLULITE TREATMENTS

Yves Hébert

Cellulite is a condition that occurs mostly in postpubescent women in which the skin of the lower limbs, abdomen, and pelvic region becomes dimpled. The term was first used in the 1920s in France and began appearing in English-language publications in the late 1960s.

Descriptive names for cellulite include orange-peel syndrome and cottage cheese skin. Synonyms include adiposis edematosa, liposclerosis, dermopanniculosis deformans, sclerotic-fibrous-edematous panniculopathy, and gynoid lipodystrophy.

ANATOMY OF CELLULITE

Fat is stored in fat cells that lie between the skin and the muscle underneath. The fat cells are grouped together into large collections that are separated by fibrous strands, or *septa* (Fig. 52.1). These septa run vertically between the muscle and the skin, especially in women (in men, they tend to run in more of a crisscross pattern, including over the thighs and buttocks). As the fat cells expand with weight gain, the gap between muscle and skin expands, but unfortunately the septa cannot stretch. This results in the dimpling characteristic of cellulite.

The layers of fat are separated into three zones by two planes of connective tissue (Fig. 52.2):

* The *upper zone*, where the fat cell chambers stand vertically separated by radially running septa of connective tissue
* The *middle and lower zones*, where the squat fat chambers and the septa of connective tissue run tangentially to the fascia

CLASSIFICATION

Cellulite is classified using the Nurnberger-Muller scale:

* Stage 0: Skin surface is smooth while standing or lying, but folds or furrows appear when the skin is pinched.
* Stage 1: Skin surface is smooth while standing or lying, but dimples appear when the skin is pinched.
* Stage 2: Cellulite is present when standing, but disappears when lying.
* Stage 3: Cellulite is present regardless of position.

PATHOPHYSIOLOGY

The overlying skin begins to bulge as excess fat is stored in the subcutaneous fat cells. With time, the accumulating fatty deposits compress the circulation and create congestion. As congestion increases, fluid and sugars leak out of the vessels to form complex sugar chains that draw even more fluid out of the vasculature through osmolarity. Fat cells begin to organize within fibrous nets to become fatty lobules. Gradually, these fatty lobules invade the skin's dermis and the fibrous nets become more rigid, finally creating skin dimpling ("peau d'orange").

CAUSES OF CELLULITE

Currently, the causes of cellulite are poorly understood. It is widely accepted that hormonal factors play a dominant role:

* Estrogens seem to initiate and aggravate cellulite.
* Insulin, catecholamines, epinephrine and norepinephrine, thyroid hormones, and prolactin participate in the development of cellulite.

Disorders of water metabolism, abnormal hyperpolymerization of the connective tissue, and chronic venous insufficiency are also involved in the pathogenesis of cellulite.

Many predisposing factors are identifiable:

* Sex
* Race (affects all races, but more common in whites than Asians or African-Americans)
* Phenotype
* Lifestyle
* Smoking status
* Predisposition to circulatory insufficiency
* Abnormal distribution of subcutaneous fat (apple or pear shape)
* Obesity

TREATMENT OF CELLULITE

Detoxification Diet

The detoxification diet has been shown to affect the development and amount of cellulite, but it is not a definite cure for cellulite. This diet recommends less alcohol, caffeine, refined food (salt), saturated fat, refined carbohydrates, smoking, diet pills, sleeping pills, laxatives, and diuretics, and more fresh vegetables and fruits, water, fibers and whole-grain foods, essential nutrients (calcium, potassium, vitamins B and C, glucosamine), and essential fatty acids. All patients wishing to improve the appearance of cellulite should adopt most of the recommendations of this diet but must understand that diet by itself is not a cure for cellulite.

Exercise

Exercise plays an important role and is one of the most effective and inexpensive measures for cellulite reduction. Exercise improves the following:

* Muscle tone
* Circulation
* Lymphatic drainage

Aerobic activity, yoga, Pilates, swimming, walking, biking, and stair climbing are excellent forms of exercise for patients with cellulite. Exercise is a fundamental part of the treatment of cellulite and should be strongly encouraged in all patients.

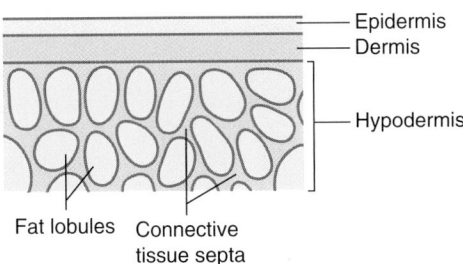

Fig. 52.1   Skin and subcutaneous tissue with fat lobules and septa.

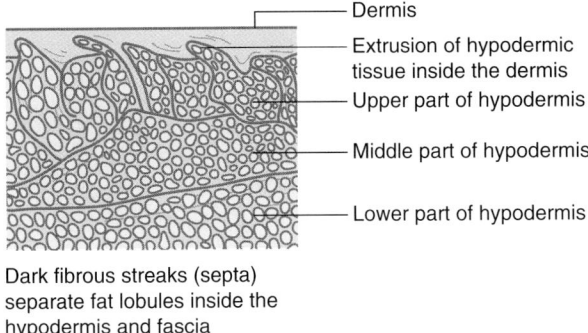

Dark fibrous streaks (septa) separate fat lobules inside the hypodermis and fascia

Fig. 52.2   Zones of connective tissue in the hypodermis.

Physical and Mechanical Methods

Numerous therapies have been attempted:

* Iontophoresis (transdermal transmission of medication using small electrical charges)
* Ultrasound (high-frequency sound waves)
* Thermotherapy (induced localized hyperthermia)
* Pressotherapy (pneumatic massaging in the direction of the circulation)
* Lymphatic drainage (massage technique to stimulate lymphatic flow)
* Electrolipophoresis (application of a low-frequency electric current)

However, no reports in the scientific literature have shown consistent results. They are possibly helpful in selected patients with lymphatic drainage deficiency.

Pharmacologic Agents

Several drugs that act on fatty tissue, connective tissue, and the microcirculation have been tried as therapeutic agents. They can be used topically, systemically, or transdermally:

* Methylxanthines (theobromine, theophylline, aminophylline, caffeine), which act through phosphodiesterase inhibition
* Pentoxifylline, which improves the microcirculation
* β-Adrenergic agonists (isoproterenol and epinephrine)
* α-Adrenergic agonists (yohimbine, piperoxan, phentolamine, dihydroergotamine)
* Methylxanthine enhancers (coenzyme A and the amino acid L-carnitine)
* Drugs with connective tissue activity (silicium and *Centella asiatica*)
* Microcirculation-active drugs (Indian chestnut, gingko biloba, and rutin)

None of these medications has been reported in the scientific literature as having a significant effect on cellulite. Some patients could benefit temporarily from an effect on microcirculation.

Anticellulite Creams

Anticellulite creams provide a temporary reduction in cellulite by plumping up the skin and creating a smoother texture. They do not remove the "orange-peel" cellulite appearance. The key ingredients in the creams have antioxidant and antiinflammatory effects:

* Aminophylline: reduces the bumpy, dimpling effect of cellulite
* Retinol and α-hydroxy acids (AHAs): improve skin texture by exfoliation of dead cells
* Caffeine: reduces fat content in cells by blocking phosphodiesterase, an enzyme that inhibits fat breakdown.

These creams have an indirect effect on cellulite by improving the quality of the skin through skin rejuvenation.

Mesotherapy

Originating in France in the 1950s, mesotherapy is still very controversial in North America. It is practiced extensively in Europe and South America. Small amounts of medications and vitamins are intradermally injected directly into cellulite-affected areas to increase circulation, to decrease fibrosis of the connective tissue, and to decrease fat cells.

Indications

* Spot and cellulite reduction
* Weight loss
* Skin rejuvenation

Side Effects

* Redness and burning that may last for a few days
* Swelling and sensitivity around the treated area for several weeks

Treatment Protocol

Ten to 15 weekly sessions are necessary to achieve visible results. NOTE: While there have been good reports from Europe and South America about the results of this treatment, products are not readily available in North America; hence the procedure is uncommon.

Lipodissolve

Lipodissolve is a nonsurgical medical procedure that involves the injection of phosphatidylcholine (PPC) into the skin to dissolve fat. The treatment is meant to destroy fat cells, which are eliminated from the body through normal waste removal. The desired end result is precise body contouring in localized areas. PPC is a naturally occurring enzyme and is the main component of soy lecithin. Lecithin has been medically proven to have the ability to break down fat and reduce cholesterol. PPC has been used for fat removal and cellulite reduction by clinicians for several years as a safe, noninvasive alternative to surgical procedures such as liposuction.

Treatment Protocol

* Multiple microinjections directly in the subcutaneous tissue
* One to three treatment sessions about 6 weeks apart

The procedure is still very controversial and possibly harmful if done by inexperienced providers because of risk of tissue necrosis. It should be used on selected patients only with localized pockets of fat tissue.

Devices and Technologies

Med Sculpt

See Fig. 52.3A. Through a nonmechanical massage and a powerful ultrasound beam, the Med Sculpt system (Sound Surgical

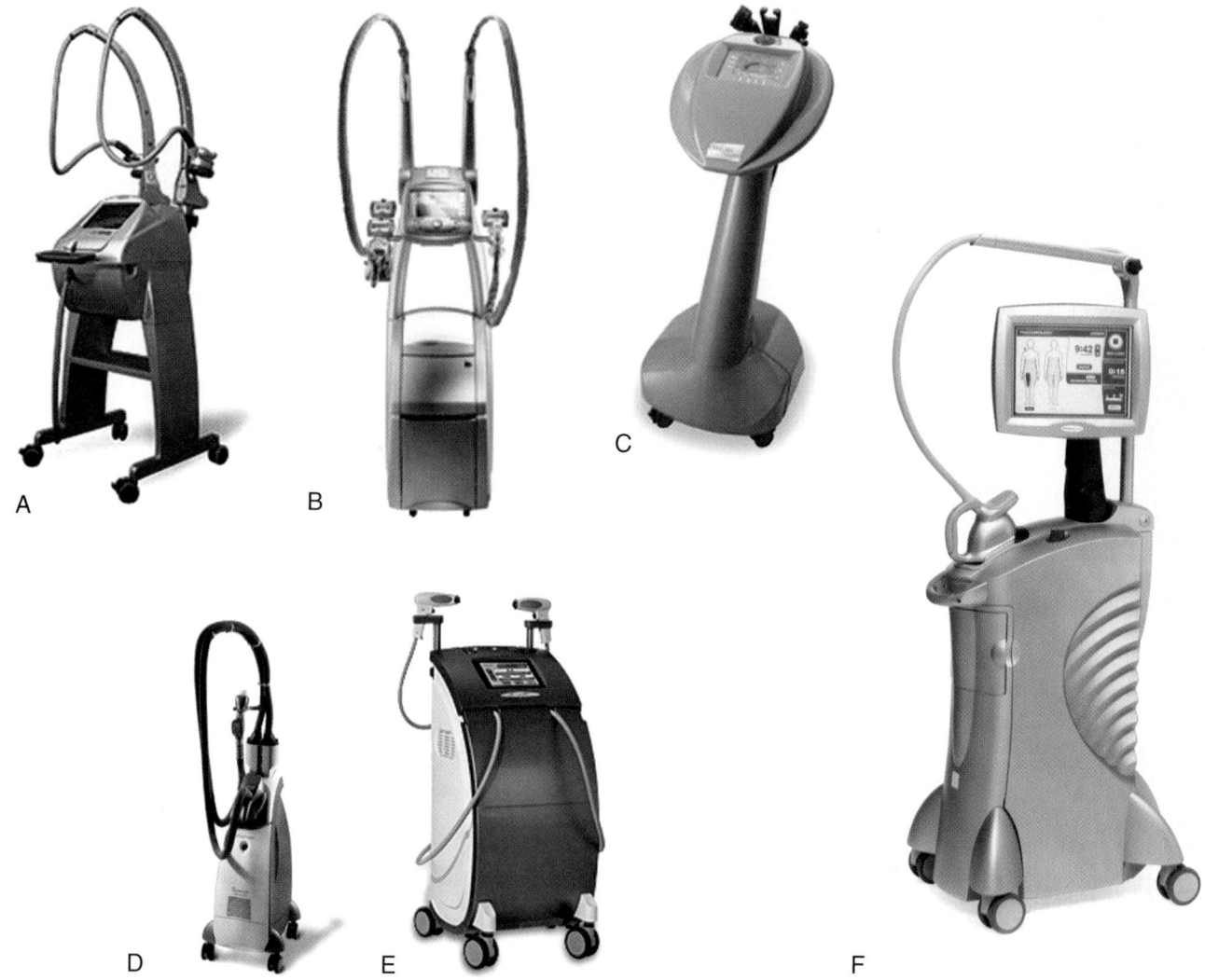

Fig. 52.3   (A) Med Sculpt (Solta Medical Valeant). (B) Endermologie (LPG Systems). (C) TriActive Cellulite Workstation (Cynosure). (D) VelaShape (Syneron Candela). (E) Accent^{XL} (Alma Lasers, Ltd.). (F) SmoothShapes XV system (Elemé Medical Cynosure). (A, Courtesy Solta Medical Valeant.)

Technologies) generates lipoclasis and stimulates the connective layers of the skin for a toned and smoother appearance to the treated areas (mechanical, thermal, and cavitational effects).

PROTOCOL:

- Eight sessions twice a week with the vacuum-operated massage
- Four to six sessions at 3-week intervals with the hydrolipoclasia treatment (infiltration of physiologic solution before applying a strong ultrasound beam)
- Ten sessions twice a week of massage only

CLINICAL BENEFITS:

- Compact loosening of the fatty tissue matrix
- Stimulation of lymphatic and venous circulation
- Redistribution of subcutaneous fat
- Moderate results on mild cases of cellulite

Endermologie

See Fig. 52.3B. Endermologie (LPG Systems) is a temporary cellulite reduction technique. Mechanical rollers and suction provide intense massage to cellulite-affected areas by stimulating circulation to the affected zone. It is said to increase circulation by up to 200%, creating a smoother and toned effect to the cellulite problem areas.

CLASSIC TREATMENT PROTOCOL:

- Thirty to 45 minutes per session, one to two times per week until the desired cellulite reduction has been achieved.
- An average of 15 to 18 treatments is required to achieve visible results, and more treatments are required to maintain the results.

LIPOMASSAGE BY ENDERMOLOGIE. This form of Endermologie delivers more intense treatments for faster results with newly designed rollers. Six treatment sessions are recommended.

ENDERMOLOGIE EXPRESS. Sessions are more vigorous and energetic, requiring subject participation. Soliciting the muscles with contraction–relaxation repetitions, the new protocols isolate fat layers and work them more intensively.

NOTE: Endermologie technology is very operator dependent and patients should inquire about the experience and the training of the technician operating the machine. Results are temporary, as with most of these technologies.

TriActive Cellulite Workstation

See Fig. 52.3C. The TriActive Cellulite Workstation (Cynosure, Inc.) provides a comfortable mechanical massage and rhythmic aspiration to distend the skin in various directions and enhance microcirculation, thereby increasing skin elasticity and improving lymphatic drainage. Six diode lasers penetrate tissues to stimulate fibroblasts for collagen production, yielding smoother, healthier-looking skin. The system can be used in combination with other therapies to enhance the outcomes of surgical and nonsurgical procedures such as liposuction and dermal fillers. This technology provides limited temporary action on superficial cellulite.

VelaShape

See Fig. 52.3D. The VelaShape (Syneron Candela, Inc.) is a U.S. Food and Drug Administration–cleared system for circumferential reduction through four mechanisms of action:

- The vacuum induces vasodilation and allows deeper penetration of bipolar radiofrequency (RF).
- Massage trough roller movements soften tissues and assist in lymphatic drainage.
- Infrared light (IR) combined with vacuum provides strong, nonspecific dermal heating, leading to skin toning and firming through collagen stimulation.
- Optimized, controlled RF delivery results in greater depth of penetration and higher peak temperature in the subcutaneous tissue.

TREATMENT PROTOCOL:

- Four to eight sessions using both applicators
  - Vsmooth for larger areas
  - Vcontour for smaller areas and localized action

CLINICAL INDICATIONS:

- Circumferential reduction
- Cellulite reduction
- Body reshaping through cellulite treatment
- Postliposuction treatment through circumferential reduction
- Postpartum treatment through circumferential reduction

NOTE: The combination of massage, vacuum, and heat (IR and RF) provides interesting results, improving cellulite through skin tightening and circumferential reduction. Patients should be made aware of the short duration of the results and the importance of a maintenance program.

Accent^XL

The Accent^XL (Alma Lasers, Ltd.) is an upgradeable, multiapplication, multitechnology, RF-based platform that performs volumetric thermotherapy for the noninvasive treatment of wrinkles and rhytids (see Fig. 52.3E). A dual-mode RF system tightens and recontours the skin using proprietary unipolar (for deep subcutaneous remodeling) and bipolar (for superficial skin tightening) RF energy, delivered with separate handpieces. Figs. 52.4 and 52.5 show the results of treatment with the Accent^XL.

TREATMENT PROTOCOL. Four to six sessions 3 to 4 weeks apart.

CLINICAL INDICATIONS:

- Skin tightening and rejuvenation
- Cellulite reduction
- Body contouring
- Scar improvement
- Postliposuction touch-ups
- Acne improvement

NOTE: The dual-mode RF system (bipolar and unipolar) improves the appearance of cellulite, but patients should be advised that results are temporary and need maintenance.

SmoothShapes

See Fig. 52.3F. The SmoothShapes XV system (Elemé Cynosure) effectively treats cellulite by improving the overall condition of enlarged fat cells and inflexible fibrous septae through a proprietary

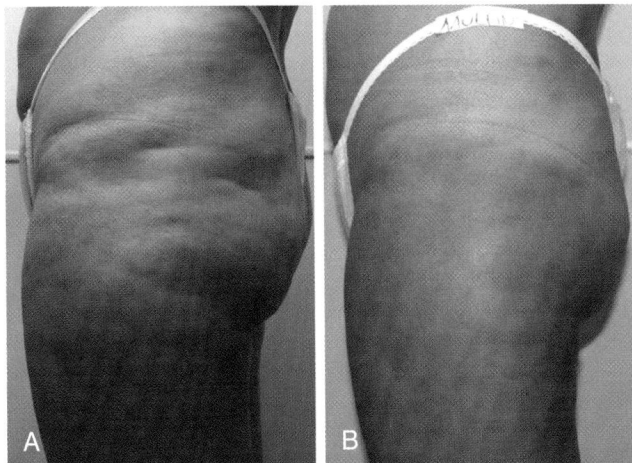

Fig. 52.4 Before (A) and 2 weeks after (B) one Accent^XL treatment using the unipolar handpiece. (Courtesy Emilia del Pino, MD, and Ramon Rosado, MD, Mexico City.)

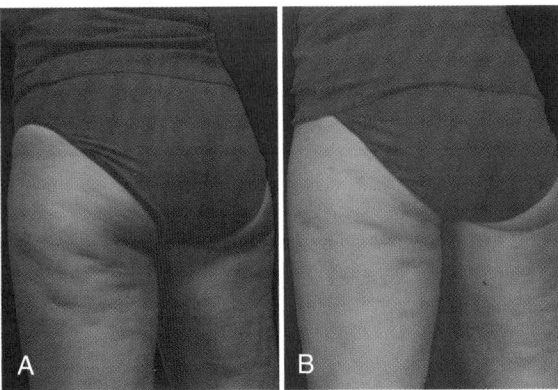

Fig. 52.5 Before (A) and 4 weeks after (B) seven Accent^XL treatments using the unipolar handpiece. (Courtesy David McDaniel, MD, Assistant Professor of Clinical Dermatology and Plastic Surgery, Eastern Virginia Medical School, Norfolk, VA.)

technology called Photomology, which is nondestructive. Photomology restores enlarged cells through a unique mechanism of action that combines dynamic laser and light energy with mechanical manipulation (vacuum and massage) to specifically target problem cellulite resulting in smoother looking skin.

The 915 nm wavelength penetrates well into the tissue and is preferentially absorbed by lipids, causing a thermal effect. The temperature inside the adipocytes is slightly elevated. Contoured rollers move liquefied lipids from the interstitial space to the lymphatic system for dynamic drainage.

TREATMENT PROTOCOL. Eight to 10 sessions on a weekly schedule.

SUPPLIERS

(See contact information available at www.expertconsult.com.)

Alma Lasers, Ltd.
Cynosure, Inc.
Elemé Cynosure
LPG Systems
Solta Medical Valeant
Syneron Candela, Inc.

RECOMMENDED READING

Alizadeh Z, Halabchi F, Mazaheri R, Abolhasani M, Tabesh M. Review of the mechanisms and effects of noninvasive body contouring devices on cellulite and subcutaneous. *Fat Int J Endocrinol Metab.* 2016;14(4):e36727.

Draelos ZD. *Procedures in Cosmetic Dermatology Series: Cosmeceuticals.* 2nd ed. Philadelphia: Saunders; 2008.

Goldman MP, Peterson JD, Fabi SG. Laser, light and energy devices for cellulite and lipodystrophy. In: Goldman MP, Fitzpatrick RE, Ross EV, Kilmer SR, Weiss RA, eds. *Lasers and Energy Devices for the Skin.* 2nd ed. Boca Raton: CRC Press; 2013:339–347.

Goldman MP, Hexsel D, eds. *Cellulite: Pathophysiology and Treatment.* 2nd ed. New York: Taylor & Francis; 2010.

Hruza G, Avram M. *Procedures in Cosmetic Dermatology Series: Lasers and Lights.* 3rd ed. Philadelphia: Elsevier; 2012.

Knobloch K, Kraemer R. Extracorporeal shock wave therapy (ESWT) for the treatment of cellulite-a current meta-analysis. *Int J Surg.* 2015;24(Pt B):210–217.

Luebberding S, Krueger N, Sadick NS. Cellulite: an evidence-based review. *Am J Clin Dermatol.* 2015;16(4):243–256.

Madhere S, ed. *Aesthetic Mesotherapy and Injection Lipolysis in Clinical Practice.* Abingdon, United Kingdom: Informa Healthcare; 2007.

The Aesthetic Guide. http://miinews.com/the-aesthetic-guide.

Turati F, Pelucchi C, Marzatico F. Efficacy of cosmetic products in cellulite reduction: systematic review and meta-analysis. *J Eur Acad Dermatol Venereol.* 2014;28(1):1–15.

CHAPTER 53

THREAD LIFT USING BARBED SUSPENSION SUTURES FOR FACIAL REJUVENATION

Vincent C. Giampapa • Hakan Usal • Oscar Ramirez

Surgeons and patients alike are constantly searching for methods of facial rejuvenation that can be performed with minimal tissue invasion, with the least amount of anesthesia, and with no downtime. This is the holy grail of aesthetic surgery. One of the latest procedures in this field is the *barbed thread lift,* although suture suspension during lifting has been successfully performed for more than 2 decades. The original type of suture suspension for the midface and neck required an open or a semiopen procedure. Suture suspension worked because of the wide undermining and repositioning of the soft tissues in the elevated position, which was held over the long term by the sutures until scar formation allowed tissue reattachment in the new position. However, when suture suspension was applied in a percutaneous fashion, the general complaint was that the suture tended to act like a cheese-cutting wire that would eventually cut through the tissues and diminish the effect over a period of time. The reason this happened was that the sutures were smooth instead of barbed. The advent of the barbed suture represented a new concept in facial lifting because of the ability of barbed sutures to hold and support tissues along their entire length, rather than just at the loop made by the smooth sutures. This mechanical advantage provided by the barbed suture permitted its use without the need for tissue undermining.

The barbed suture also makes it easy to insert in one direction and difficult to move in the opposite direction. Once the suture is introduced in the soft tissues, it can be lifted to a position in one direction, and the barbs will theoretically prevent the tissues from drooping to their former, original position. Although in principle this made a lot of sense, early configuration of the barbed sutures was not effective enough. Over time, the surgical principles evolved and surgeons modified and improved the configuration of the barbed sutures.

HISTORY OF BARBED SUTURES

In 1964, New Jersey physician J.H. Alcamo patented a roughened suture that offered resistance in one direction only. However, there is no reference to its clinical use. In 1984, Fukuda patented the surgical barbed suture.

The next important landmark was the work done by Russian cosmetic surgeon Marlene Sulamanidze, who, working with Georges Sulamanidze and Tatiana Paikidze from 1986 to 1998, studied a series of subdermal thread insertions using threads from 5 to 18 cm long. This is the first clinical report of the concept and technique of barbed sutures. They described the application of barbed sutures in the subcutaneous plane without undermining. They called their suture design *Aptos (antiptosis) threads.* These sutures were introduced in the United States under the name *Featherlift sutures.* However, the

Featherlift design did not gain U.S. Food and Drug Administration approval until June 2004.

In the United States in the late 1990s, Gregory Ruff invented what is now called the Contour Thread. The difference between the Featherlift and Contour Thread sutures is that the latter is a bidirectional, free-floating device that does not require specific anchoring, whereas the former is a unidirectional barbed suture with needles attached to both ends. The Featherlift requires a hollow cannula for insertion and is not anchored to a fixed structure. It is a self-anchoring device with one barbed segment used to "lift" the lower tissues while the upper barbed segment provides support in a higher position. The first-generation Contour Thread had a unidirectional barb configuration and one needle attached to each end. One long, straight needle is used to thread the suture into the tissues to be lifted (e.g., cheek), and the other end is used to anchor the thread in a fixed structure (e.g., temporal fascia). Subsequently, Leung and Ruff patented other variations and configurations of sutures, such as bidirectional barbed sutures with different types of needles and suture lengths.

BIOMECHANICS OF BARBED SUTURES

Not all barbed sutures are the same. The Aptos barbed sutures are made of 3-0 blue polypropylene with cogs that are relatively longer and thinner than the Contour Thread cogs (Fig. 53.1). The Contour Thread sutures are made of 2-0 clear polypropylene.

The Aptos thread is introduced using a hollow cannula of larger diameter than the suture, whereas the Contour Thread has attached needles of slightly larger diameter than the suture. Because the Aptos suture is inserted through a wider channel, this theoretically may make the cog engagement slightly looser. The Contour Thread needle also widens the channel through which the suture is placed. The flexible needle configuration of the Contour Thread allows the suture to be introduced in a zigzag fashion (Fig. 53.2), which in turn allows better anchoring of the barbs in the tissue. Biomechanical studies have also shown that the shorter the length of the barbs, the stronger their grip on tissues. The Aptos thread has longer barbs than the Contour Thread. Needle attachment at both ends, as well as the bidirectional barb configuration, gives the Contour Thread the additional versatility of permitting a change in direction at the end of the path to apply suture knots if needed or to anchor in a loop of the central, nonbarbed segment. The newer sutures feature a helicoidal distribution of cogs, offering an even better grip. A recently developed design uses absorbable suture (NovaThreads, Silhouette InstaLift) that can be used in semiopen or open methods of tissue lifting. Cones are also being used instead of barbs, and the cones theoretically stimulate collagen deposition. Thread lifts are also

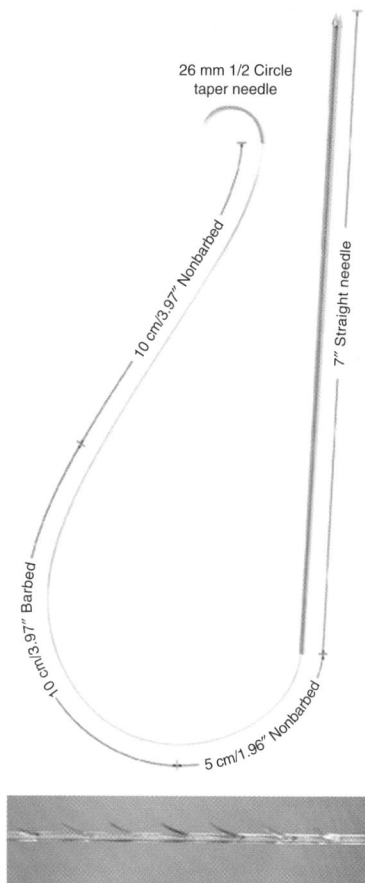

Fig. 53.1   Contour Thread. *Bottom*, Magnified barbed section of thread.

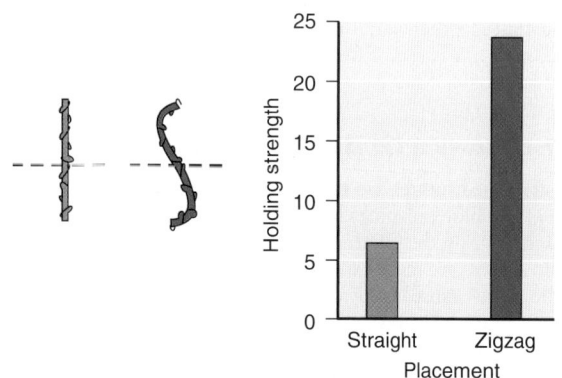

Fig. 53.2   Optimized placement patterns.

being combined with dermal fillers, lasers, and nonsurgical facial treatments for optimal effect.

As with all cosmetic surgery procedures, patient selection is the key initial decision in obtaining optimal results. The Contour Thread procedure fulfills the demands of cosmetic patients because it is a minimally invasive yet effective procedure. It offers significant improvement in facial rejuvenation with minimal downtime and potential complications.

ANATOMY

There are four natural aging changes one needs to consider when seeking to rejuvenate the midface. These were originally described by Hester and colleagues (2000) and include (1) gradual ptosis of

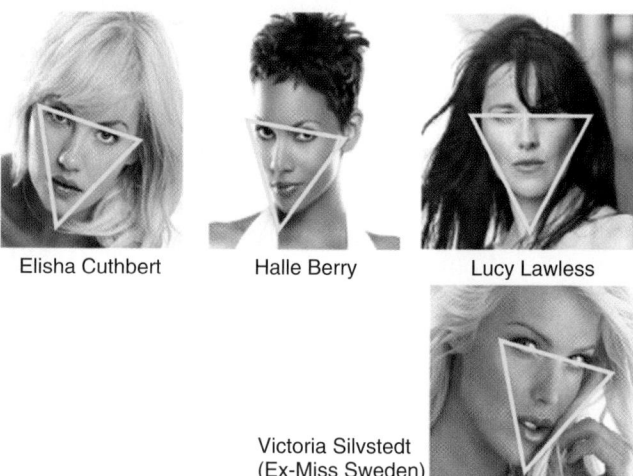

Elisha Cuthbert   Halle Berry   Lucy Lawless

Victoria Silvstedt
(Ex-Miss Sweden)

Fig. 53.3   Triangle of youth.

the cheek skin below the inferior orbital rim with descent of the lax lower eyelid skin (this creates a skeletonized appearance with hollowness around the infraorbital area); (2) descent of the malar fat pads with loss of malar prominence in projection; (3) a prominence and deepening of the tear trough area; and (4) a marked enhancement of the nasolabial fold. These anatomic areas have been called the *triangle of youth* (Fig. 53.3); a youthful facial appearance and contour can be retained by limiting the effects of aging in these areas.

INDICATIONS AND USES

* Mild to moderate facial laxity
* Midface laxity
* Neck laxity

The longevity (anywhere from 2 to 4 years) of the rejuvenation obtained depends on the patient's age and quality of facial anatomy. The best result is obtained in a younger individual who displays early signs of facial aging. Patients with strong skeletal support also have better results and greater longevity with the procedure. The poorest candidate is the older individual with severe sagging, redundant skin, and poor skeletal support.

CONTRAINDICATIONS

* Older individuals with severely sagging, redundant skin and poor skeletal support
* Uninformed patients with exaggerated expectations
* Patients who are unwilling to comply with a proper postoperative care program

The goal of midface rejuvenation centers around restoring the triangle of youth, which consists of the malar eminence, nasolabial fold, corners of the mouth, and labiomandibular area (see Fig. 53.3). With appropriate placement of Contour Threads, specific areas of the midface can be individually targeted for improvement. It is important to inform prospective patients that results using Contour Threads will not equal those obtained with an open facelift, either immediately or in the long term. The ideal patient is one with mild to moderate (class I to III) facial laxity. In particular, patients with laxity in the midface and neck area do very well (Fig. 53.4).

EQUIPMENT AND SUPPLIES

* 0.5% lidocaine with epinephrine
* Sodium bicarbonate to buffer the lidocaine
* 24-gauge, 4-inch spinal needle
* 27-gauge, 1.5-inch needle

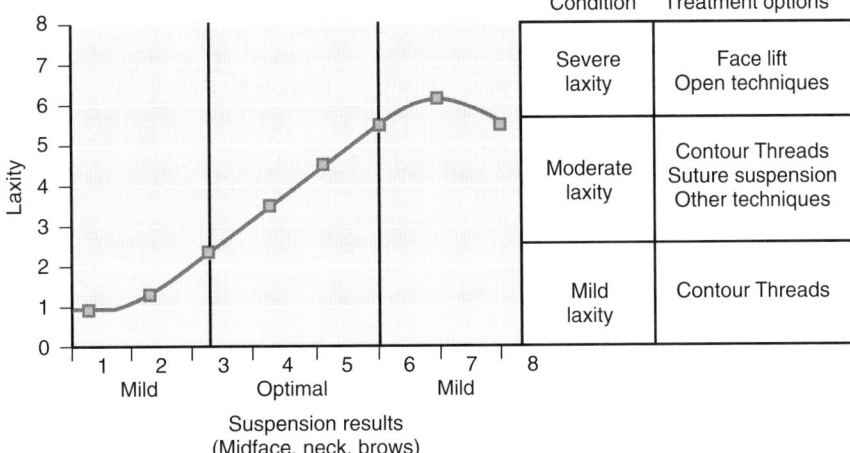

Fig. 53.4 Patient selection factors.

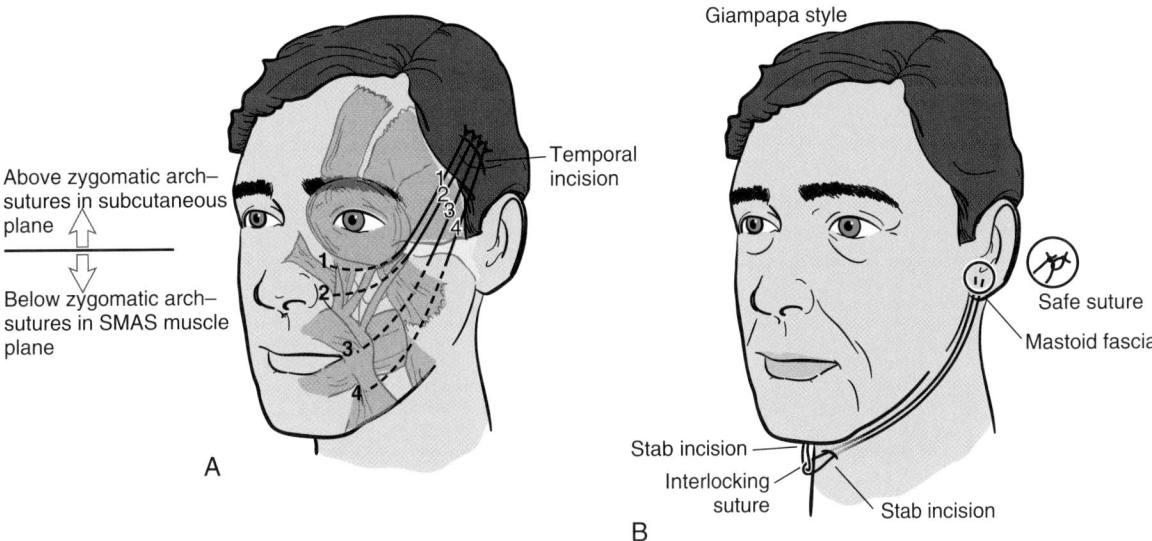

Fig. 53.5 (A) Basic suture placement for midface rejuvenation. *(1)* Infraorbital hollow and orbital rim depression; *(2)* malar eminence descent and superior portion of nasolabial fold; *(3)* ptosis of lateral commissure of mouth and inferior nasolabial fold; *(4)* labiomandibular fold. (B) Neck lift with interlocking suture (Giampapa style). *SMAS,* Superficial muscular aponeurotic system.

- No. 15 scalpel blade and handle
- 4 × 4 gauze pads
- Alcohol wipes
- Lifting thread of choice (e.g., Contour Threads)
- Steri-Strips
- Elastic foam dressing

PREPROCEDURE PATIENT PREPARATION

No special preparation is needed before the patient comes to the office for the procedure. Standard consent forms are used.

TECHNIQUE

Midface Lift

1. The patient is premedicated with oral diazepam (Valium) 5 mg, oxycodone/acetaminophen (Percocet) 5 mg, and Dramamine 25 mg 30 minutes before the procedure.
2. Mark the patient as shown in Fig. 53.5.
3. Lidocaine 0.5% with epinephrine 1:200,000 (up to 100 mL) is mixed 10:1 with sodium bicarbonate (buffering lessens the stinging effect). This is injected into the incision sites on the temporal scalp, as well as the proposed needle pathways with a 27-gauge needle and a 24-gauge, 4-inch spinal needle.
4. A small, 1- to 2-cm incision is made in a temporal hair-bearing area to introduce the Contour Threads (2-0 polypropylene suture) for the midface lift.
5. The Contour Threads are placed through the temporal incision and directed downward. This technique focuses on improving the four key anatomic areas to maximally restore the triangle of youth and provide a more youthful appearance. Each anatomic area is corrected using a specific thread for a specific purpose (see Fig. 53.5).
6. The placement of thread #1 is designed to improve lateral orbital rim and infraorbital rim hollowness, which is a key sign of aging in the triangle of youth. To avoid palpation of the suture, the subcutaneous plane is gently pinched between the thumb and index fingers during suture placement.
7. Thread #2 restores the descent of the malar pad and improves the superior portion of the nasolabial fold. Over the malar eminence and below the zygomatic arch, the suture is placed deeper into the superficial muscular aponeurotic system (SMAS) level and slowly introduced with a weaving action before it exits with a slight curve.

8. #1 and #2 threads are then anchored to the temporal fascia and pulled in a cranial direction. The tension and correction on the tissue will indicate how tight to pull the threads. The barbs are engaged with gentle digital pressure over the entire thread. At the exit points, deeply buried suture knots are tied and kept well below the subcutaneous level to avoid suture palpability.

9. Thread #3 is placed next. This thread corrects descent of the corner of the mouth and improves the lower half of the nasolabial fold and definition of the inframalar area.

10. Thread #4 corrects descent of the labiomandibular area and improves the labiomandibular fold. For the submalar area and corners of the mouth, the same principles are followed, and the sutures are placed deep into the SMAS level in the lower third of the face. Sutures are kept lateral to the nasolabial folds.

11. The remaining sutures (#3 and #4) are now secured and tied as described previously.

12. Steri-Strips are then applied to the face with cranial-directed traction.

13. The patient's face and neck are gently dressed with elastic foam dressing for 48 hours to avoid any initial tension in the wrong direction along the barbed section of the sutures.

POSTPROCEDURE PATIENT CARE

Patients are advised to avoid excessive facial mimicking/movement and laughter for 96 hours. Patients are seen in the office after 48 hours for dressing removal. Facial cleansing should be performed in a cranial direction to avoid disengagement of the barbed segment of the sutures within the first week. Acetaminophen and other standard pain medications are recommended for pain, as well as the use of an ice compress on the evening after surgery.

Patients are not ready to return to work or engage in social activities until at least 7 to 10 days after the procedure.

Proper early postoperative care is important. The face must be protected from pressure to avoid disengagement of the cogs from the lifted tissues. Patients are instructed to sleep on their backs. Talking and chewing are to be minimal and limited as much as possible. This may restrict the patient's function at work or socially. Facial and scalp cleansing and washing have to be performed in a cranial direction. All of these precautions should be observed for 2 weeks after the procedure, at which time the connective tissue around the cogs may be strong enough for the patient to engage in more liberal activity.

KEY POINTS

All threads are placed in the deep subcutaneous plane above the zygomatic arch and then pass into the superficial SMAS plane below the zygomatic arch. It is here that the barbed portion of the suture interacts with the SMAS, so that it is firmly anchored and supports the underlying tissues in a deeper context, similar to a standard facelift technique. This support of the underlying facial musculature and SMAS level creates the initial improvement as well as the long-lasting results desired.

COMMON ERRORS

- Sutures placed too deeply
- Sutures placed too superficially
- Sutures not anchored securely
- Sutures pulled too tight or not tight enough

COMPLICATIONS

- Nerve injury (extremely rare)
- Facial asymmetry
- Ecchymoses
- Skin puckering or dimpling, especially at the suture ends

If any excessive pull or contour deformity is seen after the procedure, the barbs can be released up to 2 weeks after the procedure. This is performed with moderate digital pressure downward over the area that appears to have a "divot" or overtied effect. The bunching effect of skin over the zygoma and postauricular areas and transient tightness and overcorrected look with skin tension improve over the next 1 to 2 weeks, resulting in a very natural appearance.

Furthermore, although it is uncommon, some patients develop significant dimpling at the exit points of the sutures, an uneven contour of facial curvatures with grooving along the cheeks, and waviness and skin folding along the hairline and around the ears. Bruising is rare and resolves within 10 to 14 days. Suture rejection is also rare.

DISCUSSION

The barbed suture technique provides initial marked improvement in the triangle of youth and an extremely high level of patient satisfaction. In our practice we also apply autologous fat injections to the midface as an adjunct procedure to improve midface volume loss. We have noted an initial contraction of the skin in approximately 1 week to 10 days, followed by marked long-term improvement in the patient's overall facial contour. It has been observed that the sutures retain their effect through the formation of a capsule (scarring) around the barbed segments and gradually retract the tissues even more over time. Because the Contour Threads are placed through the SMAS level to ensure final anchoring, it is anticipated that long-term results will be significant, based on the fact that the basic fundamental principles are the same for open face lifting in general.

The closed form of the mid-facelift procedure described here can provide approximately 60% to 70% of the results of a standard open facelift procedure. The patient will lose some of the initial lifting results because the immediately apparent postoperative effect relaxes by approximately 30% in the first 6 to 12 weeks. (Overcorrecting is common because loosening can be performed up to 2 weeks after surgery.) The thread lift is certainly not a replacement for the more enduring and proven facelift procedure, nor is it a lunchtime procedure. It is still a surgical procedure that requires local anesthesia and in some select cases intravenous sedation. The degree of facial edema, ecchymosis, discomfort, and tightness can be significant.

If patients have realistic expectations as to the degree of facial rejuvenation attainable with this procedure and understand the need to allow appropriate time for postoperative recovery, then this procedure can yield very good results (Figs. 53.6 and 53.7).

Barbed suspension sutures for midface rejuvenation are safe and reliable. The technique is relatively easy to perform after a moderate

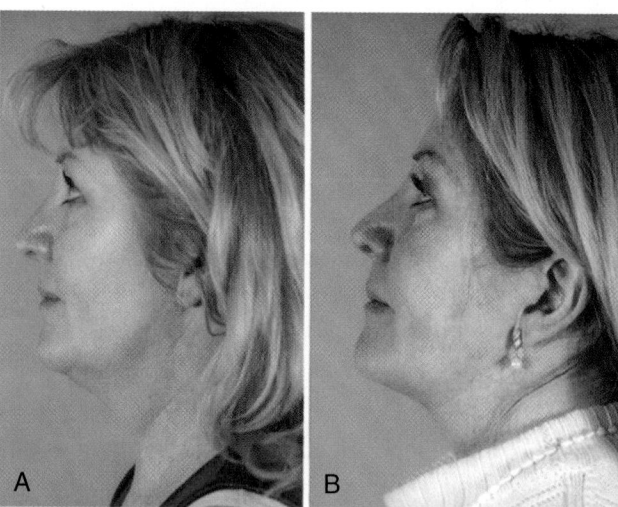

Fig. 53.6   Preoperative (A) and postoperative (B) images of neck lift.

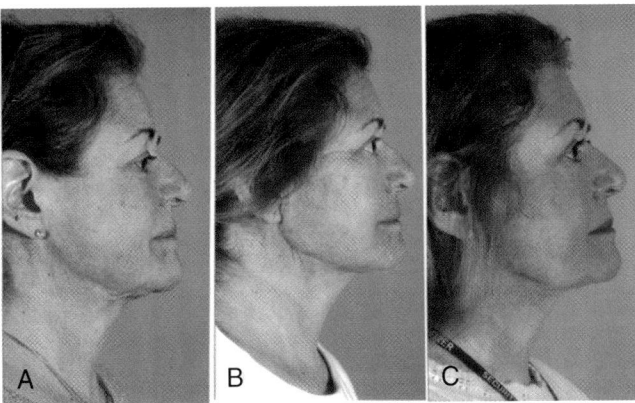

Fig. 53.7 Preoperative (A) 2-month postoperative (B), and 14-month postoperative (C) images of combined midface and neck lift.

learning curve has been traversed. Nerve injury or facial asymmetry is rare. Like most new procedures, the surgical techniques and technology of barbed sutures have evolved and will likely continue to improve. The final chapter on the barbed suture suspension technique has not yet been written. Despite some controversy, this procedure will certainly find a place in the cosmetic physician's armamentarium and gain popularity in years to come.

SUPPLIERS

(See contact information available at www.expertconsult.com.)

Contour threads
    Surgical Specialties Corporation

RECOMMENDED READING

Abraham RF, DeFatta RJ, Williams 3rd EF. Thread-lift for facial rejuvenation: assessment of long-term results. *Arch Facial Plast Surg.* 2009;11(3):178–183.

Atiyeh BS, Dibo SA, Costagliola M, Hayek SN. Barbed sutures "lunch time" lifting: evidence-based efficacy. *J Cosmet Dermatol.* 2010;9(2):132–141.

Badin AZ, Forte MRC, Silva OL. Scarless mid and lower face lift. *Aesthetic Surg J.* 2005;25:340–347.

Garvey PB, Ricciardelli EJ, Gampper T. Outcomes in threadlift for facial rejuvenation. *Ann Plast Surg.* 2009;62(5):482–485.

Hester Jr TR, Codner MA, McCord CD, et al. Evolution of technique of the direct transblepharoplasty approach for the correction of lower lid and midfacial aging: maximizing results and minimizing complications in a 5-year experience. *Plast Reconstr.* 2000;105:393–406.

Sulamanidze MA, Fournier PF, Paikidze TG, Sulamanidze G. Removal of facial soft tissue ptosis with special threads. *Dermatol Surg.* 2000;28:367–371.

Sulamanidze MA, Shifman MA, Paikidze TG, et al. Facial lifting with APTOS threads. *Int J Cosmet Surg Aesthetic Dermatol.* 2001;4:275–281.

Villa MT, White LE, Alam M, Yoo SS, Walton RL. Barbed sutures: a review of the literature. *Plast Reconstr Surg.* 2008;121(3):102e–108e.

Wu WTL. Nonsurgical face-lifting with the Woffles Lift. Presented at the American Society of Aesthetic Plastic Surgeons (ASAPS) Annual Meeting, Hot Topics Symposium, Vancouver, Canada, April 16–21, 2004.

Wu WTL. Barbed sutures in facial rejuvenation. *Aesthetic Surg J.* 2004;24:582–587.

CHAPTER 54

RADIOFREQUENCY-ASSISTED UPPER BLEPHAROPLASTY FOR THE CORRECTION OF DERMATOCHALASIS

Richard Castillo

Lid droop secondary to redundant skin (dermatochalasis) affects nearly all individuals at some point. It is more common on the upper eyelids but also occurs to a lesser extent on the lower lids. It is typically a bilateral condition, most often manifesting in patients older than 50 years. Occasionally, it is observed in younger adults.

Examination of the eyelids reveals redundant, lax skin. An excess fold of skin in the upper lid is characteristic, and the normal upper lid crease may be hidden by the excess tissue. Patients will frequently use the frontalis muscle to augment eyelid opening. This reduces the degree of lid droop but often results in exaggerated wrinkling or furrowing of the forehead and may lead to muscle tension headaches. Dermatochalasis can present both as a cosmetic problem as well as a functional one by interfering with the superior visual field. In this case, surgical correction is considered reconstructive rather than cosmetic.

The introduction of the 4-MHz Dual-Frequency Surgitron (Ellman Cynosure) has made the successful office-based management of dermatochalasis commonplace. The use of the device's unique radiofrequency profile coupled with the proprietary electrode handpieces allow for excellent management of the delicate and highly vascular skin of the eyelid. With proper patient selection, office-based blepharoplasty for the treatment of dermatochalasis is an effective and convenient option (see Chapter 25, Radiofrequency Surgery [Modern Electrosurgery]).

ANATOMY

Successful surgery on the eyelids requires a detailed knowledge of the normal anatomic structures and their functional relationships. Good surgical outcomes depend on correcting anomalies while maintaining or reestablishing normal anatomic relationships. The anatomy relevant to the successful correction of dermatochalasis is reviewed here. The recommended readings at the end of this chapter contain several excellent text references that practitioners may use to supplement the following review.

In the primary position of gaze (i.e., eyes staring straight ahead), the palpebral fissure measures anywhere from 9 to 12 mm vertically. The horizontal dimension is generally 28 to 30 mm. The upper eyelid margin lies 1.5 to 2 mm below the superior corneal limbus in the adult. The upper eyelid's marginal contour reaches its highest point slightly nasal to the midpupillary line. The lower eyelid margin is normally positioned directly at the inferior corneal limbus.

The upper eyelid crease (Fig. 54.1) typically lies 8 to 12 mm above the eyelid margin. It is generally lower in males and higher in females. In non-Asian eyes, the crease must be reformed as part of the blepharoplasty procedure to reestablish a normal cosmetic appearance. In a large percentage of Asian eyes, the crease may be lower in position than 8 to 12 mm above the eyelid margin or absent

altogether. This factor must be taken into account and discussed with the patient before the procedure so that one does not inadvertently "westernize" an Asian eye against the patient's desires.

The skin of the eyelid is the thinnest skin in the body. The epidermis itself may be only three to four cell layers thick. The combined epidermis and dermis of the eyelid may be only 1 mm thick. The underlying dermis is also scant and poorly defined. It lacks the interdigitations (rete ridges and rete pegs) found in overlying epidermis in other areas where skin is thicker. Thus the epidermis is only loosely adherent to the dermis. We exploit this unique characteristic during blepharoplasty by delivering local anesthetic into this space. The skin of the eyelid also lacks the subcutaneous fat present in skin elsewhere. The skin of the eyelid thus lends itself to healing nicely from properly formed incisions. One tends not to see the depressions found in scars in other areas of the body when the collagen fibers and adipose tissue in the dermis are disrupted.

Below the skin of the eyelid lies the orbicularis muscle complex (Fig. 54.2). This is a sheet of striated muscle innervated by branches of the facial nerve, which acts to close the eyelid. The muscle is subdivided into an orbital portion, which overlies the orbital rim, and a palpebral portion overlying the eyelid itself. The palpebral orbicularis is further divided into a superior preseptal portion overlying the orbital septum and a pretarsal portion overlying the tarsus of the lid. The pretarsal portion ends medially and laterally in fibers that form components of the canthal tendons, which hold the lid margins against the globe. The medial portion is well developed and forms a structure known as the *Horner muscle*. Care must be taken in excising redundant skin from these areas so as not to damage these structures; otherwise resultant lid malpositions may develop. The orbicularis functions not only in eyelid closure but also in the proper functioning of the lacrimal system.

Posterior to the orbicularis is an avascular fascial plane composed of loose areolar tissue. Anatomically it separates the orbicularis from the underlying orbital septum or *levator aponeurosis complex*. This is an important surgical reference plane: it marks the posterior limit of dissection during blepharoplasty for the correction of dermatochalasis.

Note the position of the supraorbital nerve in Fig. 54.3 as it emerges from the supraorbital foramen. Care should be taken to avoid this area during administration of anesthesia as well as while making incisions to avoid trauma to this nerve.

INDICATIONS

- Dermatochalasis of the upper eyelids without significant prolapse of orbital fat
- Pseudoptosis of the upper eyelids due to redundant skin folds

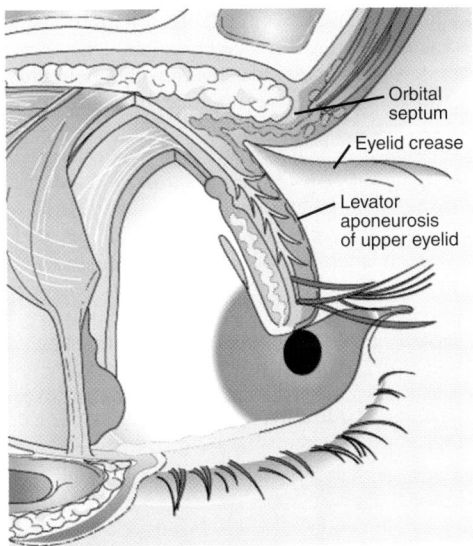

Fig. 54.1   Components of the eyelid and the invagination that forms the visible lid crease.

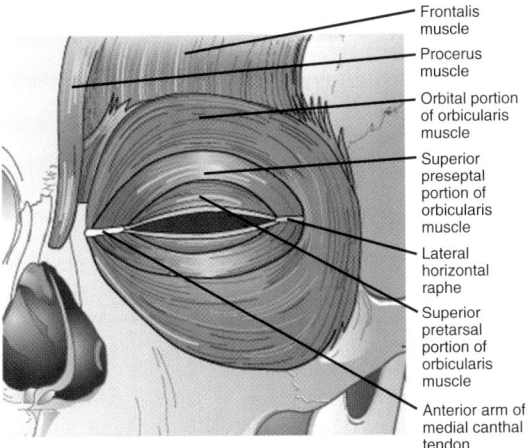

Fig. 54.2   Multiple components of the orbicularis muscle.

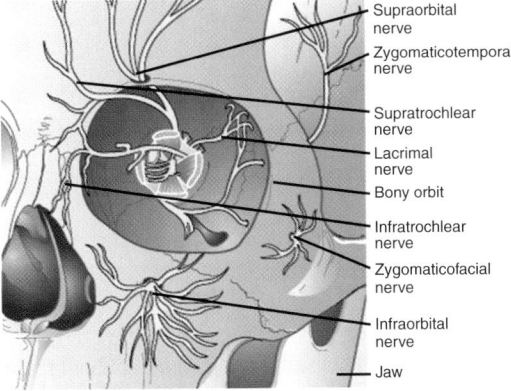

Fig. 54.3   Sensory nerves of the periorbital area. Note the position of the supraorbital nerve.

Good surgical outcomes depend as much on accurate diagnosis and proper patient selection as on good surgical technique. In the case of blepharoplasty, mistaking a case of "true" ptosis for pseudoptosis, or lid droop attributed solely to dermatochalasis, will inevitably yield a poor surgical result. The correction of true ptosis involves more than removal of redundant skin. It almost always

requires dissection posterior to the orbital septum and into the orbit, manipulation of the levator aponeurosis and the levator palpebrae superioris themselves, and dissection of the preseptal fat pads that are contiguous with the orbital adipose tissue. Depending on the etiology of the ptosis, treatment may require fascial slings or tarsectomy. A thorough preoperative evaluation is therefore mandatory to establish a proper diagnosis and determine whether one is dealing strictly with dermatochalasis.

Evaluation of Lid Droop

1. A problem-focused history is essential and should include the following:
   - Systemic conditions possibly associated with ptosis, such as myasthenia gravis, must be ruled out.
   - History, if any, of past ocular disorders (including the lids and surrounding skin).
   - History, if any, of prior ocular surgery.
   - History, if any, of wearing contact lenses (giant papillary conjunctivitis secondary to contact lens wear can present as a droopy lid).
   - Is lid droop congenital or acquired?
   - Was it gradual or sudden onset?
   - Are there symptoms of visual obstruction, ocular irritation, or *dry eyes*?
   - Are there complaints of diplopia (suggestive of myopathy, neuropathy, or a mass lesion effect)?
2. The physical examination should be aimed at determining the etiology of the lid ptosis as well as detecting conditions that could increase the likelihood of surgical complications.
   - Note the position of the eyebrows. The brows should be at or above the level of the superior orbital rim; otherwise the patient has brow ptosis, which must be dealt with separately.
   - Note the amount of dermatochalasis.
   - Note the presence of and measure the height of the eyelid crease. A n absent crease is a sign of levator dehiscence and cannot be corrected simply by addressing the dermatochalasis component (if present). The normal eyelid crease is found anywhere from 8 to 12 mm above the central eyelid margin (in the primary position of gaze).
   - Note the position of the upper and lower lid margins in both up gaze and down gaze. The margins should be flush against the globe with lashes directed out. There should be no inversion (entropion) or eversion (ectropion) of the eyelid margins noted.
   - Measure levator function. The levator palpebrae superioris is the primary elevator of the eyelid. Measuring levator function is an important part of determining the etiology of the ptosis and can be done as follows: use a millimeter ruler to measure the upper eyelid margin excursion from far down gaze to far up gaze while blocking frontalis function (manually fix the brow with your hand). Normal for an adult is between 12 to 16 mm of travel. Less than this usually signifies a problem other than dermatochalasis.
   - Note any preexisting eyelid scars.
   - Are there any palpable masses?
   - Are the eyes proptotic?
   - Perform a thorough cranial nerve examination.
   - Document any degree of preexisting strabismus or diplopia.
   - Obtain photographs to document findings. Photographs are taken with the eyes in primary position of gaze (Fig. 54.4) as well as a lateral view (Fig. 54.5). These are essential for reimbursement purposes.
   - Perform a screening visual field examination (i.e., tangent screen or automated field) bilaterally with the lids in normal position and then again with the lids held or taped up. To qualify for third-party reimbursement, field testing must show a superior defect within 15 degrees of central vision that im-

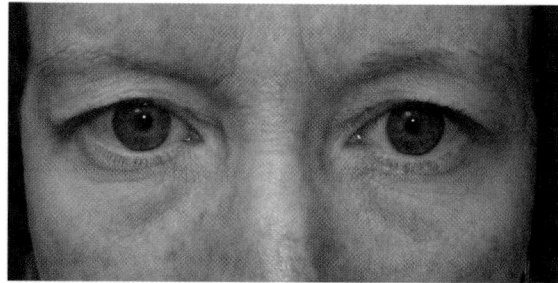

Fig. 54.4 Frontal photograph showing redundant skin of the upper lids typical of dermatochalasis (redundant skin). Note that the lid margins themselves are in normal position and pupils free of obstruction. This particular patient would not be expected to show a significant degree of superior visual field restriction.

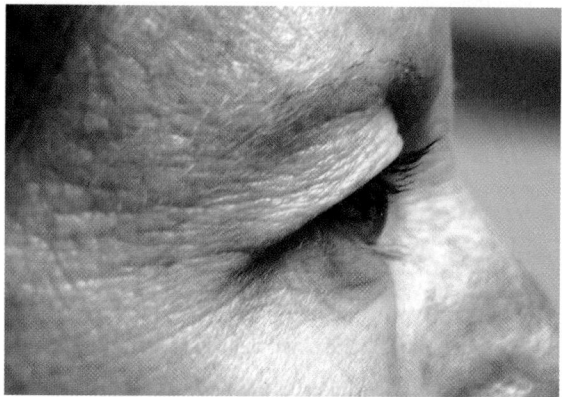

Fig. 54.5 Lateral photograph showing skin overhanging the lid margin to rest on the eyelashes.

proves when the lids are held or taped up. In most cases an inexpensive tangent screen (Wilson Ophthalmic) testing device can be set up in a small room in the office and the field testing performed by an assistant in less than 5 minutes. One need not perform a full 360-degree field test on each eye. All that is required is one superior isopter mapped out for each eye with the lids in normal position and then with the lids taped up.

- Note the condition of the external eye.
- Perform ophthalmoscopy.
- Visual acuities (bilateral) are recorded before performing any procedure on or around the eyes.

Once all other potential causes of ptosis have been excluded, a diagnosis of dermatochalasis without other mitigating factors can be established as the cause of the lid droop. Clinically one should pay close attention to the position of the eyelid margin. Sometimes redundant skin folds must be gently lifted up and out of the way to observe the actual eyelid margin. Normally the lid margin is 1 to 2 mm below the superior limbus. If the lid margin is at or below the superior pupillary border (or within the pupillary zone) with the patient in the primary position of gaze (i.e., staring straight ahead), reconsider the decision to proceed with surgery. In such a case there is likely a secondary cause of the ptosis exclusive of any degree of dermatochalasis.

CONTRAINDICATIONS

Dermatochalasis with associated fat prolapse: Correction requires more extensive resection of prolapsed orbital fat posterior to the orbital septum.

Any type of ptosis not due solely to dermatochalasis (redundant skin):
- May require more complicated reconstruction such as advancement of the levator aponeurosis, repair of aponeurotic dehiscence, or plication of the aponeurosis tendon.

- May further require frontalis suspension techniques, frontalis sling with tarsectomy, supramaximal levator resection, or other steps that require incising the orbital septum and therefore would not be deemed appropriate to attempt in an office setting.

History of previous eyelid surgery: Previous surgical trauma and distorted anatomy may prevent tissues from responding in the expected manner and therefore make outcomes difficult to predict.

History of thyroid orbitopathy (Graves disease): Potential for exacerbating lagophthalmos, dry eye syndrome, and exposure keratitis.

History of dry-eye syndrome: Potential for exacerbating preexisting condition.

History of corneal disease: Potential for exacerbating preexisting condition.

History of keloid scar formation: May make it difficult to predict outcomes based on poor healing response.

Diabetes: May make it difficult to predict outcomes based on poor healing response. Patients may be more susceptible to postoperative infection.

Hypertension: A heightened risk of intraoperative/postoperative hemorrhage.

Anticoagulants: A heightened risk of intraoperative/postoperative hemorrhage.

Pacemakers: Contraindication for certain radiofrequency devices.

History of myasthenia gravis:
- Difficult to predict final lid height/position.
- May inadvertently overcorrect, causing severe lagophthalmos.

Any patient who cannot be properly positioned or would otherwise not be an acceptable risk for office-based surgery.

EQUIPMENT AND SUPPLIES

- Povidone-iodine (Betadine) 10% or similar skin cleanser (chlorhexidine)
- Proparacaine topical ophthalmic anesthetic
- Corneal shields (Ellman Cynosure)
- Skin marking pen (fine point)
- Millimeter ruler (disposable)
- Two suture-tying forceps without teeth
- Sterile plastic drapes
- Large cotton-tipped applicators
- Sterile 4 × 4 inch gauze pads
- Lidocaine 2% with epinephrine 1:100,000
- Sterile saline solution
- 0.12-mm toothed forceps
- Westcott scissors (sharp tips)
- Ellman Surgitron Unit (Ellman Cynosure)
- Empire Micro Needle Electrode for incising the skin (Ellman Cynosure)
- Coagulation forceps (Ellman Cynosure)
- 6-0 silk suture
- Needle driver
- Antibiotic ointment

PRECAUTIONS

- Anticoagulants such as aspirin and warfarin should be discontinued (if possible) at least 7 days before the planned procedure to minimize intraoperative bleeding and postoperative bruising. Vitamin E and fish oil can also increase bleeding tendencies in these lax tissues.
- If signs of blepharitis (lid margin infection) are present (i.e., flaking, crusting, debris between the lashes, erythema of lid margins), surgery should be postponed until lids have been treated and are clear of infection.
- A corneal shield should always be used while making incisions and carrying out dissection with sharp instruments.

- An etiology of "true" ptosis must be ruled out. This would include congenital, myopathic, neurologic, aponeurotic, and posttraumatic causes of lid droop. Prior evaluation by an ophthalmologist or optometrist is important.

PROCEDURE: UPPER EYELID BLEPHAROPLASTY FOR DERMATOCHALASIS (WITHOUT FAT EXCISION)

1. After a diagnosis of pseudoptosis secondary to dermatochalasis, an informed consent form is reviewed with the patient and signed. The patient is given the opportunity to ask questions. Realistic expectations for the surgery are discussed. Patients are informed that the goal of the procedure is to remove the redundant skin obstructing vision along the superior visual field.
2. The patient is then escorted into the operative suite and placed in supine position. Monitoring devices (electrocardiography, pulse oximetry) and oxygen may be used at the physician's discretion.
3. One drop of a topical ophthalmic anesthetic (e.g., proparacaine) is instilled in each eye.
4. The lower incision line is marked.

NOTE: Incision lines are marked before administration of subcutaneous anesthetic because administration of an anesthetic bolus will distort normal anatomy and make accurate measurements impossible.

- The lower incision line is marked with a fine-tipped skin marker and placed within the eyelid crease (if present). Otherwise, a new crease position is planned 9 to 12 mm above the central eyelid margin (slightly higher in women and slightly lower in men).
  - The line is extended and tapered laterally to the lateral canthus (orbital rim), ending approximately 6 mm above the lid margin. It is often helpful to place the lateral incision line in a preexisting rhytid or "crow's foot" wrinkle line.
  - Extend the line medially to the area approximately 5 mm directly above the punctum. Do not extend this line any further medially to avoid trauma to the lacrimal apparatus. The natural contour of the eyelid crease is followed (Fig. 54.6).
5. Mark the upper incision line.
  - With the patient's eyes gently closed (and before administration of subcutaneous anesthetic), determine the upper incision line by grasping the excess skin gently directly above the center of the lid margin with a pair of smooth forceps (Fig. 54.7). Use the forceps to grasp (Fig. 54.8) and bunch up the excess skin until the closed eyelids just begin to open (<1 mm). Mark this point with the skin marker. Repeat this process for additional three or four points medially and three or four points laterally until the outline of the upper incision line is apparent. Again, the normal contour of the lid should be followed (Fig. 54.9).
  - The "dots" are now connected, creating a smooth continuous line from the medial to the lateral canthus (Fig. 54.10).
  - Care should be taken to ensure that the angle formed by the intersection of the upper and lower incision lines at the lateral and medial canthi does not exceed 60 degrees, or webbing may result (i.e., the approach is too steep when the skin margins are sutured together).
6. Recheck the amount of skin to be excised by gently "pinching" the upper and lower incision lines together to confirm that the closed eyelids do not open more than 1 mm (Fig. 54.11). If the latter is the case, the patient may be left with an iatrogenic lagophthalmos that could require subsequent repair.

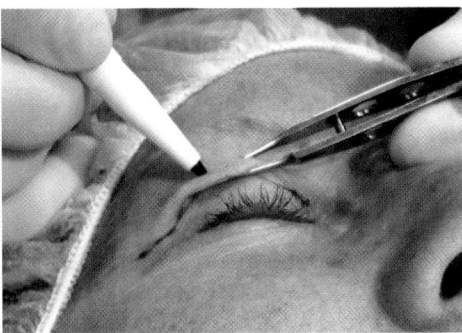

Fig. 54.6 Marking the incision lines. The incision is carried and tapered laterally to the orbital rim and no further medially than the superior punctum.

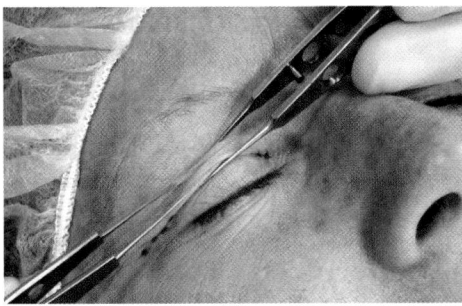

Fig. 54.7 Redundant skin is bunched up using smooth forceps to determine the amount of tissue to be excised.

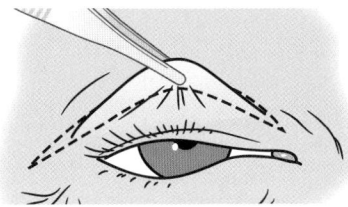

Fig. 54.8 Measuring the amount of skin to be excised using the "pinch" method.

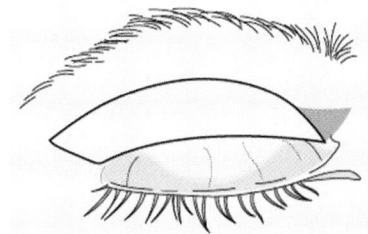

Fig. 54.9 Typical skin incision lines for upper blepharoplasty.

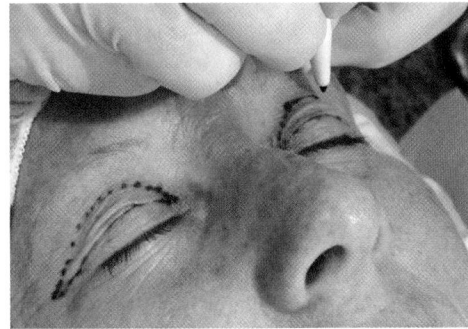

Fig. 54.10 Marking the superior incision line.

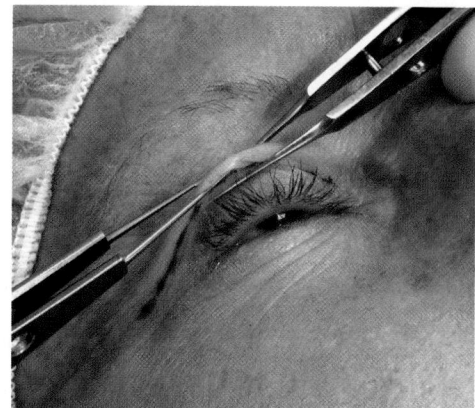

Fig. 54.11 Rechecking the amount of skin to be excised using the "pinch" method. Note the eyelid margins should pull apart no more than 1 mm.

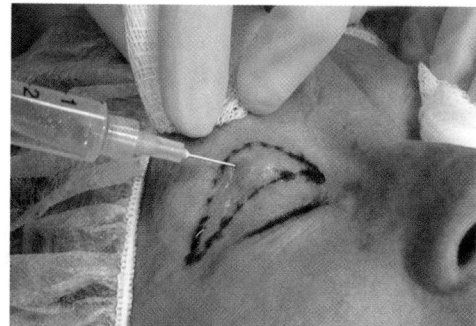

Fig. 54.12 Infiltrative subcutaneous anesthesia using lidocaine 1% with epinephrine 1:100,000. Drapes omitted for visibility.

7. Administer local anesthetic.
   * Inject 1.0 to 1.5 mL of local anesthetic (lidocaine 1% or 2% with epinephrine) subcutaneously beneath the marked area. Care is taken to direct the tip of the needle away from the globe during injection to avoid trauma to the globe itself (Fig. 54.12).
   * Use a piece of 4- by 4-in gauze to massage the area and dissipate the bolus of anesthetic.
   * Allow 5 to 10 minutes for the anesthetic to take effect and for the epinephrine to provide some degree of vasoconstriction and hemostasis.
8. Cleanse the skin with povidone-iodine 10% or a similar surgical preparation formula. This step can be performed while the anesthetic is taking effect. At a minimum, the forehead, periorbital region, eyelids, nose, and upper cheek should be cleansed bilaterally.
9. Isolate the surgical field with sterile drapes. Disposable plastic sheets with adhesive along one edge work well. A Nevyas drape retractor (Wilson Ophthalmic Corp.) can be used to keep the drape off the patient's nose and mouth.
10. Check for adequate anesthesia by pinching along the incision lines with toothed forceps. Administer supplementary anesthetic where needed.
11. Place a corneal shield before incising the skin.
    * A corneal shield (Ellman Cynosure) is placed directly over the cornea and sclera of the eye being worked on to minimize the risk of trauma while the skin incision/dissection is being performed.
    * The shield can be lubricated on the inside with a drop of topical anesthetic and inserted (and removed) with a smooth forceps.
12. The Ellman Surgitron (Fig. 54.13) radiosurgical handpiece with Empire needle electrode tip installed is used to make the skin incisions (Fig. 54.14). The unit is set to the cut/coag blended waveform. Care is taken to keep the power setting to the minimum required to create the skin incision. It is helpful to lightly moisten the skin with a piece of wet 4- by 4-in gauze because this facilitates the cutting action of the radiosurgical electrode. Gentle tension along the incision line also facilitates creating the incision. Remember that the total thickness of the epidermis and dermis combined is about 1 mm. The depth of the incision is no greater than that required to visualize the separation of the skin margins as the Empire needle moves along the surface of the incision line. Always cut along the inside of the inked incision line.
13. Dissect and excise an en bloc skin-muscle flap.
    * Grasp the lateral corner of the skin flap with toothed forceps and tent up the skin in this area. Using the Empire needle electrode and light horizontal strokes, carefully

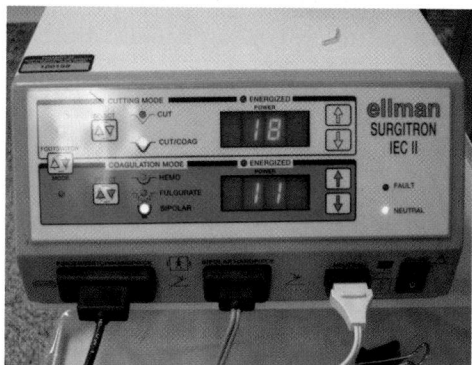

Fig. 54.13 Ellman Dual-Frequency Surgitron II Unit. (Courtesy Ellman Cynosure, Hicksville, NY.)

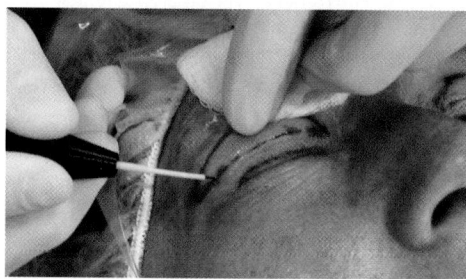

Fig. 54.14 Skin incision created using the Ellman Empire Micro Needle Electrode set to the blended cut/coag waveform.

dissect the skin/orbicularis flap free from the underlying orbital septum along the plane of the suborbicularis fascia (Fig. 54.15). Alternatively, one may remove the skin, leaving the orbicularis intact. Carefully cauterize any bleeders encountered with light cautery using either bipolar coagulation forceps (Fig. 54.16) or the lateral edge of the Empire needle electrode itself.
   * Once the myocutaneous flap has been dissected free of the underlying tissue bed and significant bleeders controlled with cautery, a piece of 4- by 4-in gauze soaked in chilled sterile saline may be placed over the exposed bed to constrict the remaining bleeders and achieve hemostasis. This can be done while the skin flap is being excised from the other eye.
14. Close the incision.
   * With the skin flap excised and proper hemostasis achieved, all that remains is to close the incision. The author's preference is 6-0 silk suture placed in simple interrupted fashion (Fig. 54.17). Alternatively, 6-0 Prolene running sutures may be used.

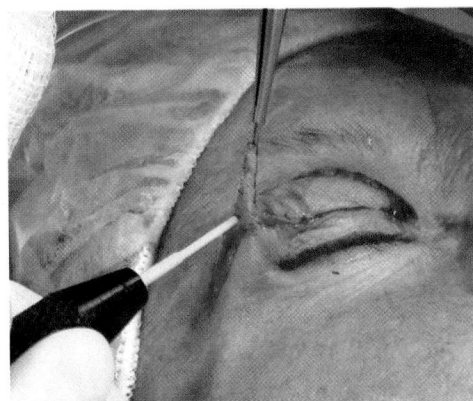

Fig. 54.15 Myocutaneous flap is dissected free with the Ellman Empire Micro Needle Electrode.

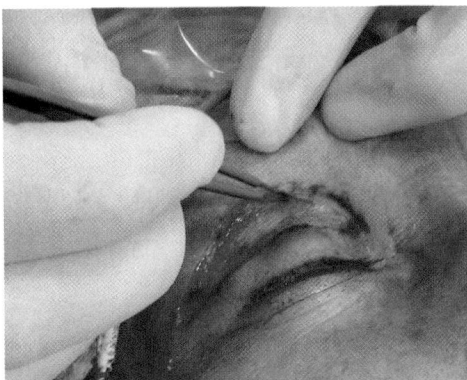

Fig. 54.16 Light bipolar cautery being applied to small bleeders. Note the relatively blood-free field, which is characteristic of radiofrequency dissection.

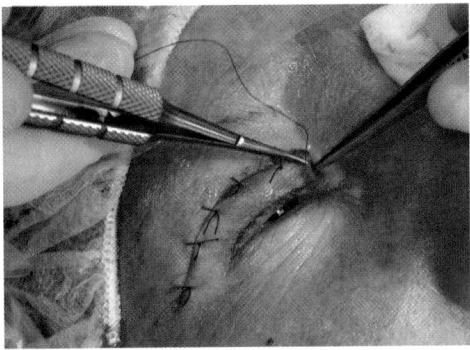

Fig. 54.17 Placement of simple interrupted sutures using 6-0 silk. The lid crease is reformed by taking small bites of the underlying fascia as the skin edges are reapproximated.

- The position of the eyelid crease is fixed or reformed by taking a small bite of the underlying fascia as the suture is passed from wound margin to wound margin before it is tied off. Recall that the eyelid crease is usually lower or completely absent in Asian eyes. Both the patient and physician should have a clear understanding of how the eyelid crease will be managed before the procedure is performed.
- Antibiotic ophthalmic ointment is applied to the incision lines, monitoring equipment is removed, the face is gently cleansed, and the patient is escorted to the recovery area.

SAMPLE OPERATIVE REPORT

See the sample operative report available at www.expertconsult.com.

COMPLICATIONS

Overcorrection (lagophthalmos)
- Usually due to overly aggressive "pinch" estimation while bunching up the excess skin with forceps to establish incision lines.
- A small degree of overcorrection (<2 mm) will usually correct itself with prescribed forced-blink exercises (e.g., blink as hard as you can 10 times then relax. Repeat six to eight times per day for 1 week).
- Overcorrection noticed immediately after surgery may be due to the fact that the orbicularis muscle is still paralyzed from the anesthetic and not functioning fully. This situation is transient and will typically correct itself within a few hours to days.
- If there is any degree of lagophthalmos present, the patient should be given artificial tears to use six to eight times per day to keep the ocular surface (primarily the corneal surface) moist. Antibiotic ointment can be used to protect the ocular surface at night.
- Persistent severe lagophthalmos may require a corrective procedure.

Undercorrection
- Usually due to poor technique or too conservative an estimation of how much skin to remove.
- Postoperative edema can give the false appearance of undercorrection.
- Cold packs should be started as soon as possible after the procedure and continued for at least 48 hours.
  In select cases where edema persists, a short course of oral steroids may be helpful.

Dry-eye syndrome/tear film dysfunction
- Typically affects older women.
- Lagophthalmos (as mentioned previously) may cause exposure keratitis.
- Transient decreased blink frequency after surgery can cause dry-eye symptoms.
- Any dry-eye complaint should be treated first with artificial tears supplementation.
- Persistent dry-eye complaints or frank lagophthalmos should be referred for evaluation.

Contour deformity

Abnormal/asymmetric lid crease height

Hemorrhage
- Some degree of lid ecchymosis is to be expected.
- Subconjunctival hemorrhage may occur and will resolve spontaneously in 7 to 10 days.
- Retrobulbar hemorrhage is rare but potentially organ-threatening. Features of retrobulbar hemorrhage include massive subconjunctival hemorrhage, often accompanied by proptosis of the globe. Ocular motility may be affected. There may be a ring of erythema/ecchymosis along both upper and lower eyelids. Pain and decreased vision often accompany this complication. Intraocular pressure is elevated. Check the optic nerve head with an ophthalmoscope. If the optic nerve head is swollen, the patient must be referred immediately for an emergent lateral canthotomy. Regardless of nerve status, if retrobulbar hemorrhage is suspected, urgent referral is advised.

Infection: Rare; however, the clinician should diligently examine the incisions and the surrounding skin for signs of infection/cellulitis at all follow-up visits and instruct the patient on how to monitor for signs of infection/cellulitis.

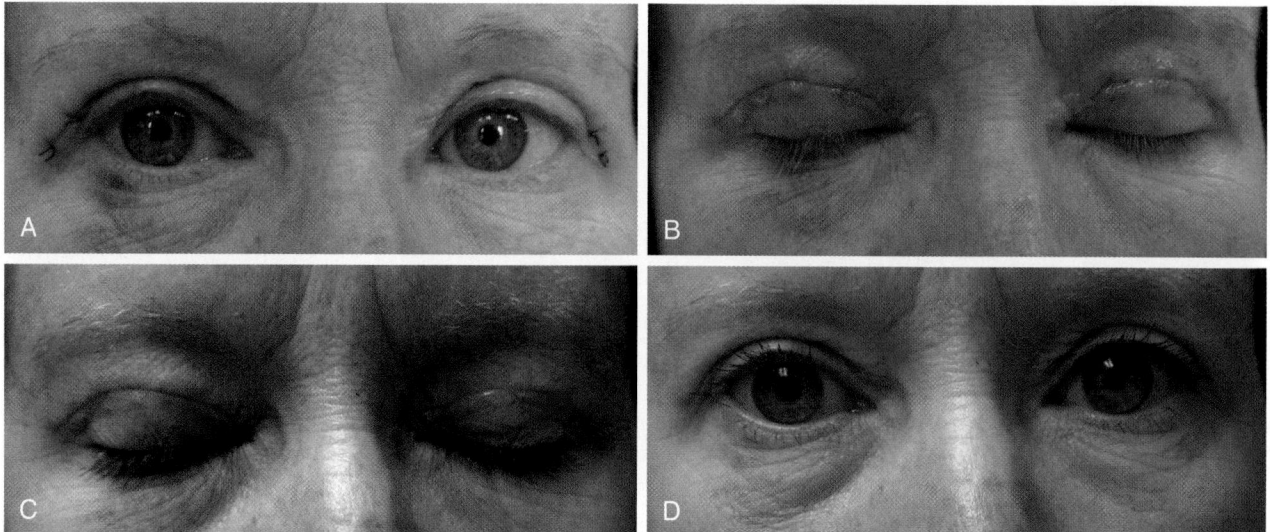

Fig. 54.18   (A) One week after surgery, before suture removal. Mild edema of the lids is evident. This resolves quickly once sutures have been removed. (B) One week after surgery with sutures removed. (C) Appearance of incisions 2 weeks after surgery. (D) Front view, 2 weeks after surgery.

POSTOPERATIVE MANAGEMENT

- Antibiotic ointment is applied sparingly to the incision lines three times per day for 1 week or until the next follow-up visit.
- Cold packs are applied directly to the lids (alternate 15 minutes on with 15 minutes off every hour while awake) for the first 48 hours. If edema persists, this may be extended.
- The area is to be kept clean and dry by gently cleansing with mild soapy solution (e.g., baby shampoo), which is rinsed with clean water and patted dry (do not rub!). Antibiotic ointment is then reapplied during the first week.
- Patient may use his or her usual choice of over-the-counter pain medication (e.g., Tylenol, Motrin) for discomfort if needed. Prescription-strength painkillers are generally not indicated.
- The patient is to return to clinic in 5 to 7 days for suture removal (Fig. 54.18).
- The patient should be advised to try to avoid exposure to direct sunlight for prolonged periods. If the patient is going to be outdoors, he or she should wear sunglasses with ultraviolet protection or a hat with a wide brim.
- After discontinuation of the antibiotic ointment at 1 week, the patient should continue to use a good skin moisturizer (preferably with a sunblock) along the incision lines for up to 8 weeks.
- The patient should be advised that the incisions will continue to heal for a period of 3 to 6 months and that the incision lines will gradually fade over the next 6 months to 1 year.

PATIENT EDUCATION GUIDES

See patient education and sample operative report available at www.expertconsult.com.

CPT/BILLING CODES

15823   Blepharoplasty, upper lid excessive skin weighting down
For bilateral procedures add-50 modifier.
Major surgical follow-up global period of 90 days.
150% total payment (adjustment) for bilateral procedures applies.

ICD-10-CM DIAGNOSTIC CODES

| H02.41-H02.419 | Ptosis mechanical |
| H02.831-H02.839 | Dermatochalasis of eyelid |

SUPPLIERS

(See contact information available at www.expertconsult.com.)

Ellman Cynosure
Wilson Ophthalmic Corp.

RECOMMENDED READING

Chen W. *Oculoplastic Surgery: The Essentials*. New York: Thieme; 2001.
Collin JRO. *A Manual of Systematic Eyelid Surgery*. 3rd ed. London: Butterworth-Heinemann; 2006.
Fagien S. *Putterman's Cosmetic Oculoplastic Surgery*. 4th ed. Philadelphia: WB Saunders; 2007.
Leatherbarrow B. *Oculoplastic Surgery*. London: Martin Dunitz, The Livery House; 2002.
Moy RL, Fincher EF. Blepharoplasty. In: Dover JS, ed. *Procedures in Cosmetic Dermatology*. Philadelphia: Saunders; 2006.
Tse DT. *Color Atlas of Oculoplastic Surgery*. 2nd ed. Philadelphia: Lippincott Williams & Wilkins; 2011.
Tyers AG, Collin JRO. *Colour Atlas of Ophthalmic Plastic Surgery*. 3rd ed. London: Butterworth-Heinemann; 2007.

CHAPTER 55

BODY PIERCING

Peter Valenzuela

Modification of the body in the form of piercing and skin art has been demonstrated in virtually every culture dating back to at least 2000 BC. Egyptian pharaohs pierced their navels and Roman soldiers pierced their nipples. Perhaps better known are the piercings and body art of African and Native American communities. In the United States, female ear piercing has long been accepted, but in the last 25 years male ear piercing and the piercing of other body areas has become widespread. Today navel piercing is one of the most fashionable piercings. More extreme piercings of the eyebrows, nipples, lips, tongue, and genitals have also become common. With this in mind, primary care clinicians may decide to offer body piercing to their patients.

Primary care clinicians have the advantage of being trained in anatomy, physiology, and aseptic technique, which are vital to performing safe piercings. In addition, these clinicians can recognize potential complications and have the capacity to therapeutically intervene early and effectively. Even if primary care clinicians choose not to perform body piercing, they need to be familiar with the techniques and complications that are unique to body piercing.

ANATOMY

Commonly pierced areas of the body include the ears, eyebrows, tongue, nose (i.e., ala, septum, and bridge), umbilicus, nipples, lips, and genitals. Each site carries unique risks. The clinician needs to be cognizant of these risks when evaluating whether to pierce a specific location and must counsel the patient accordingly.

INDICATIONS

- Cosmetic procedure
- No traditional medical indications
- The clitoral hood piercing may improve the sexual experience for women who have lost sensitivity

CONTRAINDICATIONS

- *Skin and systemic disorders:* Medical contraindications to body piercing are related to external factors involving the skin and to systemic conditions. Local skin infection, a cyst, severe eczema, or any other significant skin disorder at the site is a contraindication to piercing. A history of keloid formation (not necessarily hypertrophic scarring) is also a condition that warns against piercing.
- *Steroid use and coagulation disorders:* Chronic steroid use or a coagulation disorder also precludes the procedure. (This may be a relative risk, depending on dose or severity.)
- *Immunodeficiency syndromes:* Patients with an immunodeficiency disorder, such as acquired immunodeficiency syndrome (AIDS), present unique difficulties. For many of these patients, body modification is an important part of life, and the piercing would benefit their overall sense of well-being. Although, theoretically, AIDS might be considered a contraindication to piercing, piercing

can be successfully accomplished in the patient with AIDS unless the his or her T-cell levels are significantly compromised.

- *Pregnancy:* Clinicians should discuss pregnancy intentions with women seeking nipple or navel piercings because healing can take 2 to 4 months. Controversy exists regarding whether a nipple piercing affects lactation. There are 15 to 20 milk ducts in the nipple. Although scar tissue may occlude some ducts, a properly placed piercing with appropriate jewelry should not adversely affect breast function. Excessive scarring may lead to duct occlusion, which could cause decreased or absent milk expression, persistent breast engorgement, and increased risk of infection or abscess formation during lactation. Women interested in nipple piercings should be aware of the unknown and potentially adverse effects on the ability to breastfeed. Also, because the infant may aspirate the jewelry or develop metal allergies, the jewelry must be removed during actual breastfeeding.

Navel piercings can take 6 to 10 months to heal. This should also be taken into consideration if a pregnancy is being considered. Navel piercings also tend to migrate. Tissue distortion that occurs during pregnancy can exacerbate this problem, and it may be necessary to remove the jewelry as gestation progresses.

EQUIPMENT

Jewelry

It is important to use the proper jewelry so as to avoid complications. Patients should wear only jewelry made of surgical-grade stainless steel (316 L [low carbon], 316 LVM [low carbon, volume melt]), titanium, niobium, platinum, solid white or yellow gold (14K or 18K), or Tygon. Gold-plated jewelry contains reactive metals such as nickel and can cause allergic reactions. Silver will tarnish in the moist environment of a new piercing or in contact with any mucosal surface.

The most common types of jewelry are bead rings, captive bead rings, straight barbells, circular barbells, and curved barbells (Fig. 55.1). Size is defined in terms of gauge and either diameter or length. If the jewelry is not provided by the clinician's office, patients should be advised to purchase the jewelry that is appropriate for the piercing they desire and bring it with them. Table 55.1 summarizes the initial jewelry commonly used for each location.

The bead ring and captive bead ring are opened and closed either by hand or with specialized ring-opening/ring-closing pliers. The use of other pliers may distort the shape of the ring. It is important to maintain the integrity and shape of the ring when opening and closing it.

Piercing Equipment

- Appropriate jewelry: sterilize in an autoclave.
- Antiseptic cleanser: use povidone-iodine, chlorhexidine, ethyl alcohol, or equivalent.
- Ring-closing pliers: use with captive or bead rings; usually not

needed if jewelry is annealed. (The annealing process allows jewelry to be manipulated more easily, particularly by hand.)
- Piercing needles: have various sizes available, including 10, 12, 14, 16, and 18 gauge. (For most piercings, the needle size should match the gauge of the jewelry being inserted [Fig. 55.2].)
- Needle-receiving tube: use for piercings involving the nostril, septum, penis, clitoral hood, and some parts of the ear cartilage (Fig. 55.3).
- Rubber bands: use to provide tension for piercing clamps.
- Insertion taper: a solid metal rod that is larger at one end and gradually becomes smaller at the other end; gauge measurement is based on size of larger end; use to help transfer jewelry or for stretching; in a fresh piercing, the taper's gauge will be the same as the jewelry gauge. *Transfer* means to place the tip of the jewelry into the needle or taper and pass it into place in the hole previously made by the needle.
- Needle pusher/acrylic needle holder: helps pass the needle through skin.
- Tissue forceps: use Pennington, mini-Pennington, or ring forceps; slotted style is optional. (The forceps is tensioned with two rubber bands; this helps to avoid clamping skin too tightly.)
- Surgical marking pen: use very fine point. (Sharpie Fine Point pens can be used.)
- Gentian violet: to mark tongue and oral cavity piercings.

- Toothpicks: to apply gentian violet.
- Cotton applicators: use to adjust the size or site of insertion marks at the piercing site; erase or fine-tune the marks with alcohol-soaked applicators.
- Gauze: to cleanse the site after piercing.
- Gauge wheel: to confirm gauge of needle or jewelry.
- Caliper: to confirm size of jewelry.
- Sterile barrier field: to cover instrument tray.
- Cork: to cover needle tip after insertion (protects against needle injury).
- Ethyl alcohol (70%): can be used as a skin cleanser (removes excess ink marks).
- Sterile saline.
- Topical anesthetic for certain locations: topical lidocaine (EMLA) or benzocaine (Hurricaine).

Sterilization

Most piercing equipment can be sterilized in an autoclave (270°F under high-pressure steam for at least 10 minutes). Items that are reusable should be cleansed in an ultrasonic cleaner before sterilization. Those items that are heat-sensitive can be cleansed with a broad-spectrum environmentally safe germicide that kills such organisms as human immunodeficiency virus (HIV), hepatitis (particularly B, C), and tuberculosis. When possible, piercing guns should be avoided because most cannot be properly sterilized. Those patients choosing to have a body piercing done at a piercing salon should be advised to search for members of the Association of Professional Piercers. In addition, the piercer should possess certifications for basic life support/cardiopulmonary resuscitation and blood-borne pathogens training.

PREPROCEDURE PATIENT EDUCATION AND FORMS

Inform the patient of all possible complications of piercing in general and those specific to the location requested. Thorough documentation of the informed consent is mandatory. All patients younger than 18 years of age need legal guardian consent. Patients should anticipate the average healing time depending on the location of the piercing (Table 55.2). (See the sample patient education and consent forms available at www.expertconsult.com.)

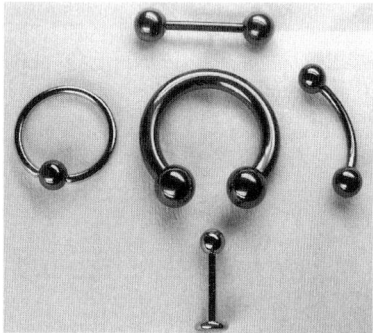

Fig. 55.1 Jewelry styles: straight barbell *(top)*, captive ring *(left)*, circular barbell *(center)*, curved barbell *(right)*, and labret stud *(bottom)*.

TABLE 55.1	Jewelry Selection		
Location	**Type and Size**	**Gauges***	**Comments**
Earlobe	BR, CBR, or LB; ⅜ to ½ in	18–10	Avoid ear studs; occlusive and difficult to clean
Ear cartilage (outer)	BR, CBR, or LB; 5/16 to 7/16 in	18–14	Choose jewelry least likely to be uncomfortable during sleep
Ear cartilage (tragus)	BR, CBR, or BB; 5/16 to ⅜ in	18 or 16	Choose jewelry least likely to be uncomfortable during sleep
Eyebrow	BR, CBR, BB, or LB; ⅜ to 7/16 in	18 or 16	Risk of tearing with smaller gauges; risk of migration with larger gauges
Nostril	Nostril screw; BR, CBR; 5/16 to 7/16 in	20; 18	Nostril screw has small loop at right angle to hold it in place
Nasal septum	BR, CBR, BB or CB; ⅜ to ½ in	16–10	Use a needle-receiving tube
Tongue	BB; ¾ to 1 in	14–10	Length accounts for initial edema; downsize jewelry in 2–3 weeks; minimal ball size is 6 mm
Labret	Labret stud; ⅜ to ½ in	14	Minimal ball size is 5 mm; can downsize later
Nipple (female)	BR, CBR, BB, or CB; ⅝ to ¾ in	14–10	Consider future breastfeeding plans; postpone piercing if pregnancy is in the near future
Nipple (male)	BR, CBR, BB, or CB; 9/16 in	14 or 12	
Navel	BR, CBR, or LB; 7/16 to ⅝ in	14 or 12	Pierce navel fold; avoid small jewelry that can constrict skin
Clitoral hood (vertical)	BR, CBR, or LB; 7/16 to 9/16 in	14 or 12	Position jewelry so that ball rests on the clitoris
Penis (Prince Albert)	BR, CBR, LB, or CB; 9/16 to 1 in	12 or 10	Use a needle-receiving tube

*In using gauge readings, the size actually decreases as the gauge number gets larger.
BB, straight barbell; *BR*, bead ring; *CB*, circular barbell; *CBR*, captive bead ring; *LB*, curved barbell.

TECHNIQUE

Universal precautions should always be followed. Instruments and jewelry must be appropriately sterilized. In rare circumstances, certain jewelry will have to be soaked in an antiseptic solution for 30 minutes. This jewelry is removed from the solution with alcohol before insertion. Anesthesia is usually not indicated for these procedures. However, for sensitive areas such as the genitals and mucosa, topical anesthetics like topical lidocaine (EMLA cream) or benzocaine (Hurricaine) can be applied before the procedures.

Navel Piercing

1. Prepare the sterile instrument tray (Fig. 55.4).
2. Clean the navel and the surrounding abdominal wall with an antiseptic solution (sterile preparation).
3. Mark entry and exit points with the surgical marker (Fig. 55.5). Confirm acceptability of location with the patient before proceeding. Use the crest of the navel fold as a guide. On the abdominal wall, mark the entrance site at a distance half the length of the curved barbell or the diameter of the ring from the edge of the skin fold. On the undersurface of

Fig. 55.2 Piercing needle. This is a hollow, tribeveled needle. Jewelry is held against the nonpointed end of the needle for passage through the skin. After passage, a cork can be placed on the needle tip to prevent needlestick injuries.

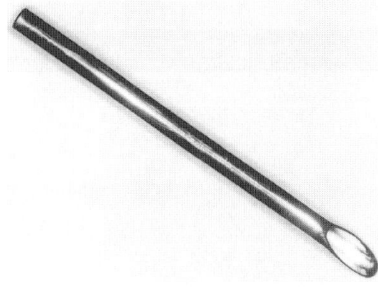

Fig. 55.3 Needle-receiving tube. This is a hollow tube that is used in ear cartilage, nostril, and genital piercings. The needle tip is passed through the area being pierced into the tube. The tube protects adjacent structures from inadvertent injury.

the navel skin fold, mark the exit site at the same distance from the edge of the fold as the entrance site. This is above the deep, flat base of the umbilicus. Have the patient lie, sit, stand, protrude, and retract the abdomen to evaluate placement of the markings, as they vary with each position. Make adjustments in the markings if needed. If an umbilical hernia or other anatomic variants are present, a navel piercing should be avoided.

NOTE: Our preferred method is to start with the patient in a supine position and mark the exit hole within the fold of skin over the navel. Have the patient stand and evaluate tissue above the navel fold for a natural indentation. Mark this site as the entrance hole. Choose the appropriate jewelry size (7⁄16, 1⁄2, 9⁄16, or 5⁄8) to match the navel's anatomy as determined by the placement of the markings.

4. Place rubber bands on the forceps and adjust the tension. Grasp and tent the skin with traction. Avoid actually clamping the forceps because this will crush the skin (Fig. 55.6).
5. Position the piercing needle perpendicular to the tented skin and parallel to the floor and the markings (Fig. 55.7).
6. Pass the needle through the skin. Remove the forceps. Attach the jewelry to the nonpointed end (see Fig. 55.2) of the needle, then pass the jewelry into the piercing. For a captive ring, the ring must be twisted back and forth to allow easy transfer (Fig. 55.8). After the ring is in place, straighten the ring and insert the ball (Fig. 55.9).
7. Remove the antiseptic cleansing agent with sterile saline.

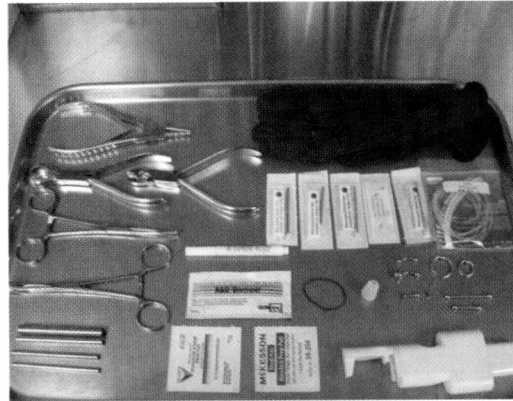

Fig. 55.4 Instrument tray. Items shown: gloves, marking pen, cotton applicators, calipers, gauze, captive bead ring, piercing needle, insertion taper, Pennington forceps, and rubber bands. All items are appropriately sterilized. (Courtesy Armando Escajeda Jr.)

TABLE 55.2	Average Healing Times for Piercing Locations
Location	**Healing Times**
Ear lobe	4–6 wk
Ear cartilage	2–3 mo
Eyebrow	6–8 wk
Nostril	2–3 mo
Nasal septum	4–6 wk
Tongue	4–6 wk
Labret	6–8 wk
Nipple (female)	2–3 mo
Nipple (male)	2–3 mo
Navel	6–10 mo
Clitoral hood	4–6 wk
Penis (Prince Albert)	4–6 wk

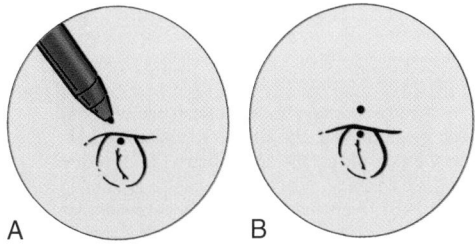

A   B

Fig. 55.5 Skin markings for umbilical piercing. The longitudinal line in the circular area represents the base of the umbilicus. The transverse line represents the navel skin fold. The area between the longitudinal and transverse lines represents the undersurface of the skin fold. The markings are usually equidistant from the edge of the fold.

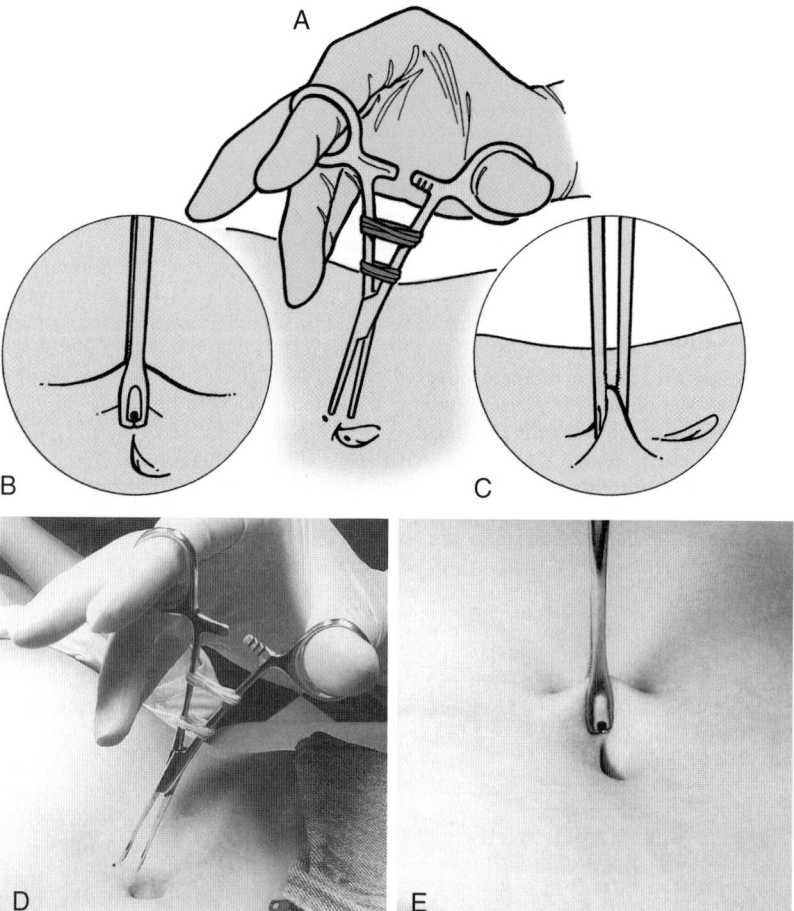

Fig. 55.6 Forceps application for umbilical piercing. The patient is supine. (A) The navel skin fold has been marked *(center)*. (Note markings above and below the marked skin fold.) The forceps have two rubber bands in place for tensioning. The skin fold will be gently held by the forceps. (B) The markings are positioned at the edge of the clamp opening. The skin fold is then gently tented and held perpendicular to the floor. It is important not to engage the clamp's ratchets (not to close the clamp). (C) Forceps application. The skin fold is gently tented and held perpendicular to the floor. Note the deep aspect of the umbilicus is not involved in the piercing. (D) Photograph of step A. (E) Photograph of step B.

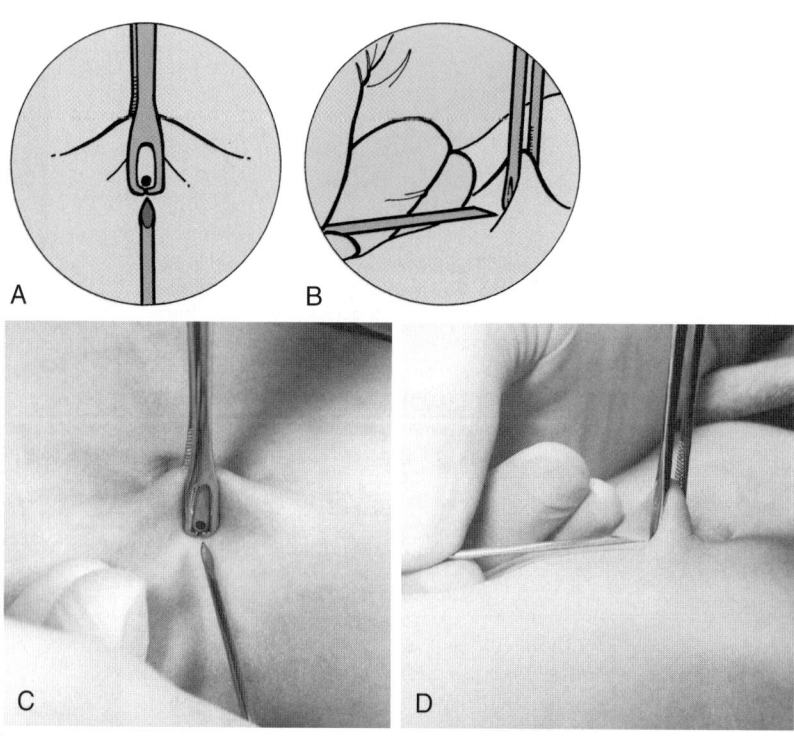

Fig. 55.7 Needle position for umbilical piercing. (A) With the skin gently tented, the needle is positioned perpendicular to the skin and parallel to the floor. The direction of the piercing is cranial to caudal (i.e., the needle is pointing toward the foot). (B) The needle is positioned perpendicular to the skin fold and parallel to the floor. The needle is aligned with the markings and is pointing cranial to caudal (i.e., toward the foot). (C) Photograph of step A. (D) Photograph of step B.

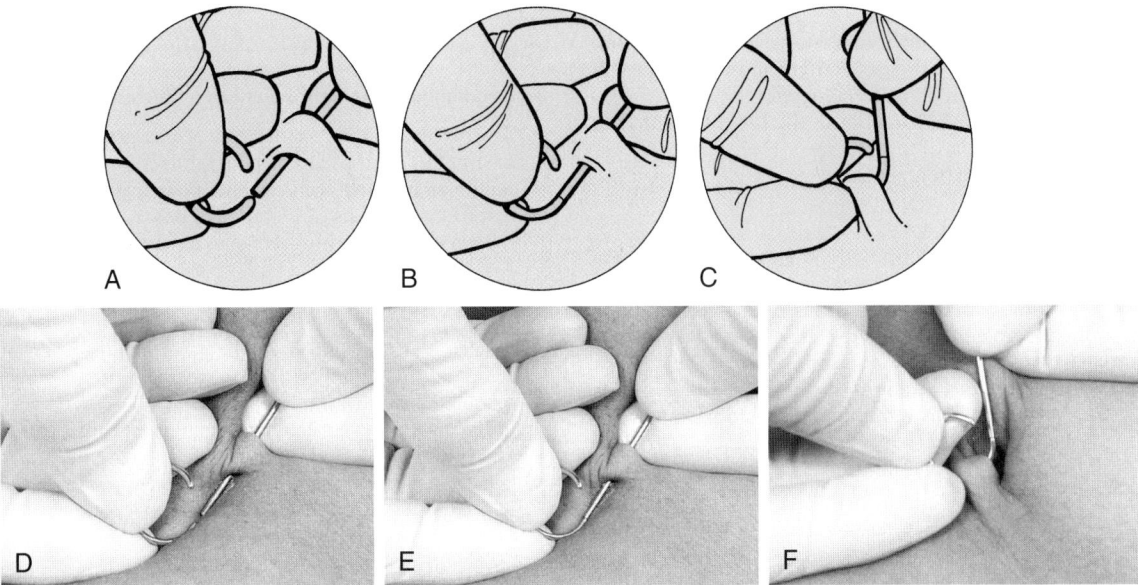

Fig. 55.8 Jewelry transfer for umbilical piercing. (A) The sharp end of the needle is held with the fingers of one hand (hand on right side of images). The point can be protected with a cork while being held. (B) The jewelry is positioned against the nonpointed end. (C) The skin fold is stabilized against the finger during transfer. The jewelry is gently pushed and twisted to help clear the skin fold. (D) Photograph of step A, showing jewelry positioning. The sharp end of the jewelry is held with the fingers of one hand. The jewelry is being placed on the nonpointed end of the needle. The jewelry is gently pushed and twisted to help clear the skin fold. (E) Photograph of step B. The jewelry abuts the nonpointed end of the needle. The skin fold is stabilized against the finger holding the sharp end. (F) Photograph of step C showing jewelry transfer. The jewelry has been transferred through the skin fold. During the transfer, the jewelry is held against the nonpointed end of the needle. The jewelry is gently twisted to help clear the skin fold.

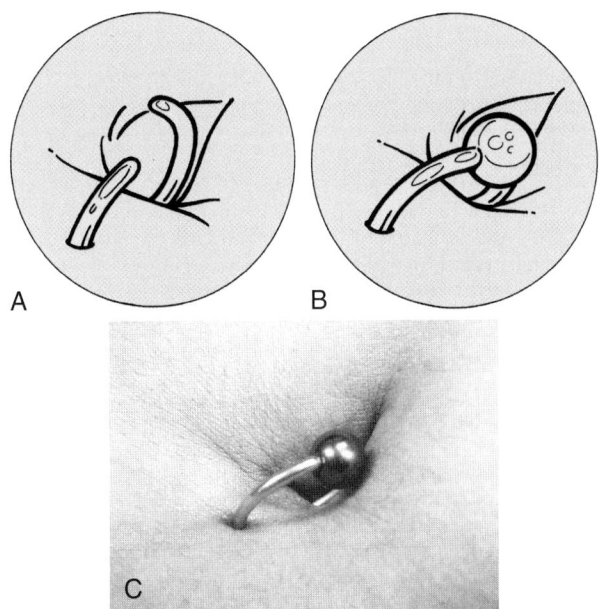

Fig. 55.9 Jewelry for umbilical piercing. (A) The ring has a gentle twist and must be untwisted for bead placement. (B) The bead has indentations, and these are positioned between the ends of the ring. (C) The captive bead ring is positioned in the navel's skin fold.

Other Piercings

Earlobe

1. Cleanse the front and back of the lobe.
2. Mark the front and back in the center of the lobe.
3. Use the Pennington forceps to stabilize the lobe when passing the needle. Do not ratchet down the forceps. (Disposable ear piercing kits are also available.)
4. Pierce perpendicular to the plane of the lobe.

Ear Cartilage

1. Clamping is not recommended for cartilage because of potential crushing and increased risk of complications.
2. Use a freehand technique or a needle-receiving tube.
3. Pierce perpendicular to the plane of the cartilage.

Eyebrow

1. Can be performed similar to the navel technique.
2. The piercing is placed over the lateral third of the eyebrow to avoid the supraorbital nerve.
3. Slant the piercing toward the nose with the lower mark made medial to the upper mark.
4. Avoid a shallow piercing because this can lead to migration.

Nostril

1. The entrance point is at the natural indentation of the alar fold; the direction of the piercing is external to internal.
2. Use a needle-receiving tube placed inside the nostril to avoid tissue damage.
3. Avoid using a clamp on the ala because this will crush the cartilage.

Nasal Septum

1. Piercing is done through the soft membrane inferior to the nasal cartilage.
2. The piercing is located ¾ in from the external tip of the nose and ⅛ in below the cartilaginous edge.
3. Use a needle-receiving tube to stabilize the septum.

Labret or Lip

1. These are unique piercings because they involve two different tissue surfaces, facial skin and the mucosa of the oral cavity.
2. The piercing site in the skin is usually placed below the vermilion border of the lip.
3. On the mucosal surface, the site is positioned so the jewelry does not rest on the gums.
4. Appropriate jewelry for these piercings are rings or labret studs (see Fig. 55.1). Jewelry size is ⅛ to ½ inch.

Cheek

1. Before the piercing, use a penlight to identify vascular structures, particularly the branches of the facial artery and vein. This will help to avoid the branches of the facial nerve.
2. Pierce through the facial skin anterior to the laugh line into the oral cavity.
3. Inside the oral cavity, the hole should avoid the parotid duct.

Tongue

1. Choose a central and midline location in the natural bend of the tongue. Have the patient cup the tongue to find this indentation.
2. The exit site is anterior to the frenulum. Avoid the veins that are easily visualized on the underside of the tongue.
3. Use gentian violet to mark the entrance and exit sites. With the tongue in an extended position, the entrance and exit sites should be perpendicular. This allows for a slightly angulated position when the tongue is retracted.
4. During the piercing, hold the tongue in an extended position with gauze or a sponge forceps.

Nipple

1. The horizontal axis is preferred for women, but they may prefer the piercing to be vertical. The horizontal or vertical axis can be used for men.
2. For women, the piercing is placed through the base of the nipple at or just below the midline. In men, placement is at the junction of the nipple with the areola at or just above the midline.

Clitoral Hood

Actual clitoral piercings are rare, and they depend on the size of the clitoris. Damage to the neural tissue can occur. Most patients who request a clitoral piercing actually want the clitoral hood piercing.

VERTICAL PIERCING

1. Find the apex of the hood at the base of the clitoris.
2. Mark the outer skin of the hood at this site.
3. Measure the distance to the edge of the hood and to the head of the clitoris. Choose a jewelry size that allows the ball to rest on the head. Typically the jewelry will be a half-inch curved barbell.
4. Insert the jewelry; the preferred jewelry is a curved barbell.

HORIZONTAL PIERCING

1. Pierce through the clitoral hood tissue at a similar distance from the clitoris as in the vertical piercing.
2. Avoid the veins that pass down the hood; use a penlight to identify the veins.
3. Use lightweight jewelry because the weight of the jewelry can pull the hood beyond the clitoris, and the desired effect will be lost.

Penis (Prince Albert)

1. This is the most commonly requested penile piercing.
2. Place the piercing in the thin, soft, triangular skin on the ventral side of the penis just below the corona of the glans at the frenulum.
3. Evaluate the penis in both a flaccid and an erect state to locate the entrance site that accommodates an erection.
4. Choose the jewelry size based on the erect state of the penis; the jewelry is generally ⅝ to ¼ inch long.
5. Mark the entrance site at the frenulum.
6. Place a needle-receiving tube through the meatus into the urethra. Position the end of the tube (which is now inside the urethra) at the entrance site.
7. Pass the needle through the skin into the receiving tube.
8. Remove the tube and protect the sharp end of the needle with a cork.
9. Position the jewelry on the needle and transfer.

NOTE: The Prince Albert has a tendency to bleed for several days after the piercing.

COMPLICATIONS

General

Some complications are inherent in all piercing procedures.

- The most common complication is infection from staphylococcal or streptococcal species. Bacterial infections can occur because of improper piercing technique or poor hygiene. Local infections can be cared for using warm compresses, antibacterial soap, and topical mupirocin. In severe skin infections, oral antibiotics such as the first-generation cephalosporins (i.e., cephalexin, cefadroxil) or dicloxacillin may be indicated and are appropriate treatment options for more serious wound infections. If Pseudomonas is suspected, use ciprofloxacin. If methicillin-resistant Staphylococcus aureus is suspected, consider oral trimethoprim/sulfamethoxazole (Bactrim) or clindamycin.
- Other infection: Tuberculosis, tetanus, hepatitis, HIV infection, and toxic shock syndrome have been attributed to contamination at the time of piercing. Genital piercings increase the risk of hepatitis and HIV infections from sexual contact because of the open wounds and associated trauma.
- Pain.
- Bleeding.
- Hypertrophic scarring.
- Keloid formation.
- Granuloma or cyst formation.
- Migration or expulsion of jewelry.
- Contact dermatitis or other skin reaction.
- Possible social stigma.

Specific Complications by Location

Navel

- Migration
- Frictional irritation
- Scar formation

Ear Cartilage

- Associated with poor healing and more serious infection because of the avascular nature of auricular cartilage.
- Auricular perichondritis and perichondral abscess (typically occurring in the first month after piercing, especially during the warm-weather months).
- Infection from Lactobacillus or Pseudomonas more common.
- Toxic shock syndrome (very rare).
- In one study, 34% of ear piercings experienced complications such as mild infection, pain, and allergic reaction.

Earlobe

- Keloids, especially in black individuals
- Enlargement of the opening and traumatic lacerations tearing through the lobe
- Lack of symmetry between the two sides

Eyebrow

- Periorbital infection
- Damage to the supraorbital nerve

Nostril

- Damage to cartilage
- Infection (staphylococcal)

Nasal Septum

- Pressure necrosis of cartilaginous border and alae

Tongue

- Damage to dentition and gums
- Loss of bone supporting the teeth

- Lingual nerve damage
- Hematoma
- Aspiration of jewelry

Labret and Lips

- Damage to dentition and gums

Cheek

- Damage to parotid duct branches of the facial artery, vein, and nerve
- Uncontrolled drooling

Nipple

- Interference with lactation
- Mastitis and abscess formation

POSTPROCEDURE PATIENT EDUCATION

Advise the following:

- Always wash hands thoroughly before touching the piercing.
- Avoid tight clothing, which can cause increased friction at the piercing site.
- Expect serosanguineous fluid to ooze and crust around the entrance and exit sites. This crusting will last until the piercing has healed completely. Only when the crusting has stopped can jewelry be exchanged or a stretching procedure considered. The crusted material harbors bacteria and must be removed. Soak the piercing site with a warm sea salt solution (1/4 teaspoon of sea salt in 8 oz of distilled water) using a soft cloth, gauze, or an inverted glass for 5 to 10 minutes. Then remove the crusted material with a clean damp cloth or cotton-tipped applicators before carefully twisting the jewelry in the moistened area to make sure that it is not trapped.
- Use a mild antibacterial soap that does not contain fragrances. We prefer Provon (GOJO Laboratories, Akron, OH) and Septicare (Sage Laboratories, Hudson, NH). If using soap, lather the area and the jewelry, then rinse well with water. Allow to air-dry. If using Septicare, allow it to dry without rinsing.
- If redness and swelling develop, use warm compresses four times a day for 24 hours. If the redness and swelling do not go away or if a purulent discharge (pus) develops, see a clinician.
- For tongue piercings, use an antibacterial mouthwash that does not contain alcohol or a saline solution after meals and smoking. Gargle for 30 to 60 seconds. It is preferable to avoid smoking. Use a new toothbrush and change it every 30 days. Brush the jewelry with the toothbrush to remove plaque.
- Do not use antibacterial ointments such as bacitracin, Neosporin (polymyxin B sulfate, neomycin and bacitracin) or Polysporin (polymyxin B sulfate and bacitracin). These ointments are petroleum-based and can occlude the piercing. Occlusion will trap serosanguineous fluid and dead cells, delay healing, and promote possible infections. Prolonged use of antibacterial ointments can also irritate the skin. If necessary, use mupirocin (Bactroban) ointment for the first 24 to 48 hours if mild redness or swelling develops. Rub the ointment gently on the jewelry and the surrounding skin until a thin, invisible layer is present.
- Avoid using alcohol, which can dry the skin and the cells involved in healing the piercing.
- Avoid using hydrogen peroxide and povidone-iodine, which are toxic to healing tissues.

CONCLUSION

Body piercing is an elective procedure; patients may be surprised to learn that a primary care clinician can understand and perform it. Anatomic evaluation, aseptic technique, appropriate aftercare, and proper selection of jewelry to fit the location are keys to a successful piercing procedure. In order to obtain an excellent result, it is necessary to understand the patient who requests a piercing.

PATIENT EDUCATION GUIDES

See the sample patient education and consent forms available at www.expertconsult.com.

The following brochures are available from the Association of Professional Piercers (APP) (www.safepiercing.org). The APP has also written the *APP Procedural Manual*.

- Picking Your Piercer
- Aftercare Guidelines for Facial and Body Piercings
- Aftercare Guidelines for Oral Piercings
- Body Piercing Troubleshooting: For You and Your Healthcare Professional

CPT/BILLING CODES

Because this is a cosmetic procedure, providers must collect payment directly from the patient.
However, there is an ICD-10-CM code for ear piercing.

ICD-10-CM DIAGNOSTIC CODES

Z41.3   Encounter for ear piercing

SUPPLIERS

(See contact information available at www.expertconsult.com.)

Anatometal
Body Circle Designs
Body Jewelry Shop
Body Vision
Hinged
Industrial Strength Body Jewelry
Unimax Supply Company

ONLINE RESOURCES

Answers.com:Bodypiercing.https://health.answers.com/Q/What_is_a_body_
   piercing.
Association of Professional Piercers. www.safepiercing.org.
Atomic Tattoos and Body Piercing. www.atomictattoos.com.
Body Jewellery Shop. www.bodyjewelleryshop.com.
Tribalectic Body Piercing Community. www.tribalectic.com.

RECOMMENDED READING

American Academy of Dermatology. Position Statement on Body Piercing. https://www.aad.org/forms/policies/uploads/ps/ps-body%20piercing.pdf; 1998.
American Academy of Dermatology. Caring for Pierced Ear. https://www.aad.org/public/skin-hair-nails/skin-care/caring-for-pierced-ears.
American Academy of Dermatology. Piercings and Tattoos: cool or Dangerous. https://www.aad.org/public/kids/skin/piercings-tattoos.
Angel E. The worst piercing story. *The Point.* 2002;23:15.
Campbell A, Moore A, Williams E, et al. Tongue piercing: impact of time and barbell stem length on lingual gingival recession and tooth chipping. *J Periodontol.* 2002;73:289–287.
Er N, Ozkavaf A, Berberoglu A, Yamalik N. An unusual cause of gingival recession: oral piercing. *J Periodontol.* 2000;71:1767–1769.
Gawkrodger DJ. Nickel dermatitis: how much nickel is safe? *Contact Dermatitis.* 1996;35:267–271.
Landeck A, Newman N, Breadon J, Zahner S. A simple technique for ear piercing. *J Am Acad Dermatol.* 1998;39:795–796.
Liden C, Menne T, Burrows D. Nickel-containing alloys and platings and their ability to cause dermatitis. *Br J Dermatol.* 1996;134:193–198.

Meltzer D. Complications of body piercing. *Am Fam Physician*. 2005;72:2029–2034.

Meyer D. Body piercing. Old traditions creating new challenges. *J Emerg Nurs*. 2000;26:612–614.

More DR, Seidel JS, Bryan PA. Ear-piercing techniques as a cause of auricular chondritis. *Pediatr Emerg Care*. 1999;15:189–192.

Samantha S, Tweeten M, Rickman LS. Infectious complications of body piercing. *Clin Infect Dis*. 1998;26:735–740.

Staley R, Fitzgibbon JJ, Anderson C. Auricular infections caused by high ear piercing in adolescents. *Pediatrics*. 1997;99:610–611.

Stone DB, Scordino DJ. Foreign body removal. In: Roberts JR, Custalow CB, Thomsen TW, eds. *Roberts and Hedges Clinical Procedures in Emergency Medicine*. 6th ed. Philadelphia: Elsevier; 2014:709.

Yang S, Wang D, Zhang Y, et al. Transmission of hepatitis B and C virus infection through body piercing: a systematic review and meta-analysis. *Medicine (Baltimore)*. 2015;94(47):e1893.

SECTION 4

Eyes, Ears, Nose, and Throat

Section Editor: GRANT C. FOWLER

CHAPTER 56

MUCOCELE REMOVAL

Andy S. Barnett

Oral mucous cysts (mucoceles) form as a result of obstruction or trauma involving the ducts of minor salivary glands. Mucoceles are the most common benign soft tissue masses of the oral cavity. Mucoceles occur most frequently in the mucosa of the lower lip. They appear as soft, nontender, compressible lesions with a pink or bluish tinge. Typical sizes range from a few millimeters up to 1 cm, but they can be much larger. Superficial mucoceles may rupture (as when bitten) and not recur, but larger lesions usually remain persistent or recurrent unless treated. Simple aspiration is not usually curative.

ANATOMY

Because most labial mucoceles occur as a result of mild trauma, location adjacent to the lower lip incisors is most common. Lesions on the lower lip can occur in any layer of tissue from the mucosal lining to beneath the submucosa; they usually involve minor salivary glands but not significant neurovascular structures.

INDICATIONS

- Growth, pain
- Lesions refractory to superficial treatment (e.g., simple puncture or topical cryotherapy)
- Uncertain of clinical nature and biopsy is indicated
- Cosmetic concerns

CONTRAINDICATIONS

- Atypical location (e.g., gingival or sublingual)
- Atypical gross appearance when perhaps just a biopsy is indicated
- Pulsating mass (consider an arterial aneurysm) (relative)

EQUIPMENT

- Lidocaine 2% with 1:100,000 epinephrine
- Antiseptic solution (alcohol or povidone-iodine)
- 1- to 3-mL syringe with a 0.5- to 1-inch 27- or 30-gauge needle
- Scalpel with No. 11 blade and possibly a No. 15 blade
- Cryocautery or electrocautery unit
- Antibiotic ointment or petroleum jelly (optional)
- Ferric subsulfate (Monsel) solution (large lesions)
- Absorbable or silk suture (marsupialization or micromarsupialization technique)

PRECAUTIONS

Depending on location, consider a proximal duct stone or tumor occluding the duct. Be sure to include any unusual or palpable/thickened tissue in the specimen. Lesions that are atypical in appearance or location should be sent for pathologic evaluation to exclude carcinoma.

PREPROCEDURE PATIENT PREPARATION

See the patient education handout available at www.expertconsult.com.

PROCEDURE

Small Lesions or Initial Treatment

After applying antiseptic solution, an injection of lidocaine with epinephrine is given under the mucocele to produce anesthesia and minimize bleeding by inducing vasoconstriction. The injection will often elevate the lesion, making it easier to see. Injecting in or above the lesion may have just the opposite effect.

With a No. 11 blade, a small stab wound is made in the cyst laterally, and the seromucinous contents are expressed. A freeze of the lesion (see Chapter 14, Cryosurgery) is performed to produce a 2- to 3-mm rim of ice around the lesion. As an alternative to cryotherapy, electrocautery may be used to lightly desiccate the lesion after incision and drainage. The ball cautery tip can be inserted directly into the cavity. An antibiotic ointment or petroleum jelly can then be applied.

Larger Lesions

Because the tissue is so pliable, it is often difficult to stabilize the lip. Consider using a large chalazion clamp, which also effectively controls bleeding.

Option 1

For larger lesions, recurrence is less likely if the roof is shaved off with a No. 15 blade before proceeding to cryotherapy or electrodesiccation (Fig. 56.1). Compress the area firmly between the fingers to reduce bleeding. If cryotherapy is chosen, hemostasis should be obtained before the freeze. A chemical coagulant, such as Monsel solution, is useful here. The wound is allowed to heal by secondary intention, which takes 5 to 7 days. Caution the patient not to bite on the areas, which is tempting to do.

Option 2

Alternatively, after anesthesia, use a radiofrequency loop (cutting 20 W and coagulate 30 W or, if a single "cut and coag" setting is available, about level 3 or 4) to remove the top of the lesion. Be careful not to go too deeply. Mucinous material appearing much like saliva will often come out of the cyst. A deeper wall of the cyst is usually evident at this point. Generally a ball electrode is used to destroy the base, or cryotherapy can be considered. Cryotherapy can also be used first and then combined with electrosurgery (see Fig. 56.1).

Recurrent Lesions

Recurrent lesions may be retreated as described previously, but with a more aggressive approach. Persistently recurrent lesions or cysts located more deeply in the submucosa may need to be completely excised or marsupialized with interrupted fine absorbable sutures around the margins of the lesion (Fig. 56.2).

A micromarsupialization technique (Fig. 56.3) has recently been described that involves the placement of a 4-0 silk suture through the widest diameter of the dome of the lesion without involvement of the base. A surgical knot is made and the suture is left in place for 7 days. Patients must return to have the suture replaced if it is lost during this 7-day period. The suture should be removed at 7 days.

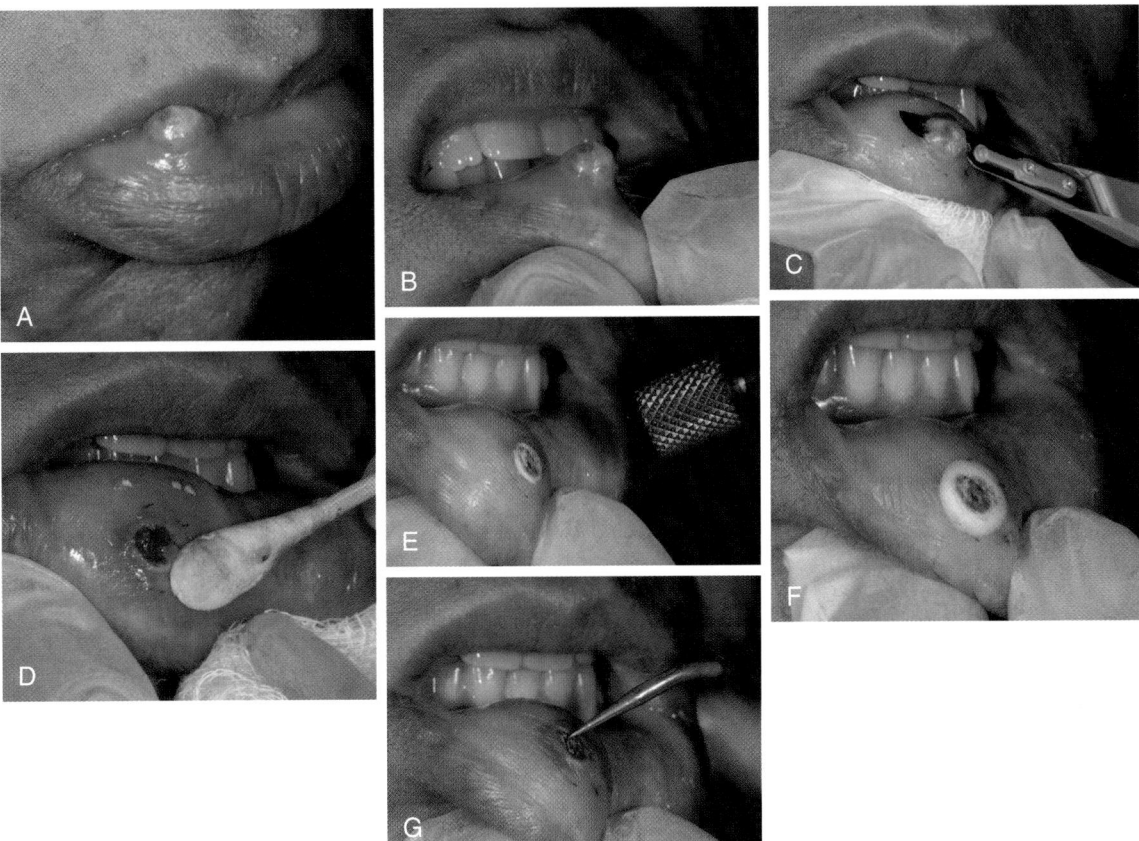

Fig. 56.1 Mucocele removal. (A) Large mucocele on the lip that recurred after previous incision, drainage, and cryosurgery. (B) The lip is stabilized for administration of local anesthesia with lidocaine and epinephrine. (C) The protruding tip of the mucocele is shaved off with a No. 15 blade. (D) Preliminary hemostasis is achieved with Monsel solution. (E) Liquid nitrogen is sprayed to destroy the underlying lesion. (F) Cryospray is continued until a 2-mm halo of normal tissue is frozen around the affected area. (G) Electrosurgery is used to achieve final hemostasis after cryosurgery. (From Usatine RP, Moy RL, Tobinick EL, Siegel DM, eds. *Skin Surgery: A Practical Guide*. St. Louis: Mosby; 1998.)

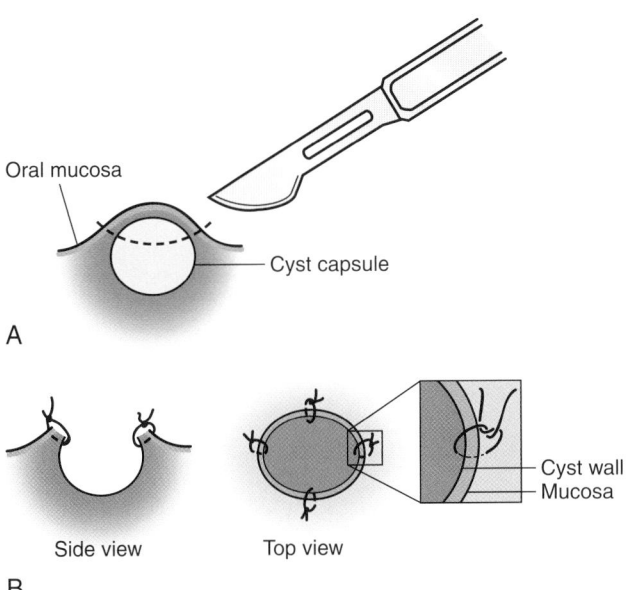

Fig. 56.2 Marsupialization technique to allow continued drainage and promote epithelialization of mucocele cyst. (A) Unroof the cyst with a No. 15 blade. (B) Simple interrupted sutures (4-0 or 5-0 absorbable such as plain or chromic catgut, which dissolves quickly) are placed circumferentially through the cyst and oral mucosa.

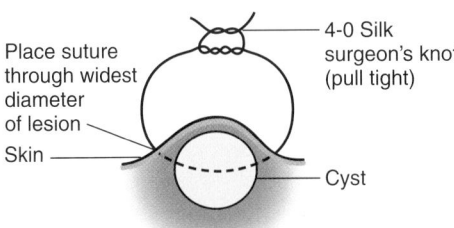

Fig. 56.3 Micromarsupialization technique. Remove suture after 7 days.

SAMPLE OPERATIVE REPORT

Procedure: Mucocele excision (or destruction)

Indication: Lower lip mucocele, refractory to simple cryotherapy

Consent: A consent form was signed and witnessed after a discussion with the patient/guardian of the risks (including but not limited to pain, bleeding, infection, scar formation, slow healing, recurrence of lesion, and failure to diagnose more serious pathology), benefits (treatment of lesion), and alternatives (including but not limited to simple aspiration, topical cryotherapy, and watchful waiting).

Technique: The mucosa surrounding the lesion was cleansed with Betadine and then anesthetized with lidocaine 1% with epinephrine 1:100,000 through a 30-gauge needle, using a total volume of

3 mL. Anesthesia was confirmed and then the lesion was unroofed around the margins of the dome with a sterile No. 15 blade. The removed portion was sent to pathology for histologic evaluation. Hemostasis was achieved with application of Monsel solution. The base of the lesion was frozen, with a 2-mm rim of normal tissue included, for 5 seconds. Final hemostasis was achieved with brief application of electrocautery to any visible areas of bleeding. Antibiotic ointment was applied to the lesion.

Complications: None

Estimated blood loss: Less than 5 mL

Follow-up: If needed for any signs or symptoms of infection or recurrence of lesion and pending the pathology report.

COMPLICATIONS

Postoperative complications are very rare because of the forgiving nature of oral mucosal tissue.

- A minimal amount of postoperative bleeding can be controlled with direct pressure and should resolve within hours.
- Any infection should be treated with antibiotics to cover typical oral pathogens.
- Pain can be treated with over-the-counter medications.
- If the biopsy specimen indicates atypical, dysplastic, or neoplastic tissue, conservative reexcision or referral should be considered based on the findings.
- Recurrence is the most common complication and can be dealt with using a more aggressive approach, as noted previously, or with referral.
- Perforation/"buttonhole" is a rare complication if the excision or treatment (especially with a radiofrequency loop) goes too deep. Often the wound can be left to heal on its own. If it is gaping open, a subcuticular closure may be necessary to limit scarring. Alternatively, an absorbable suture on the mucosal side may close the exterior wound nicely.

POSTPROCEDURE MANAGEMENT

Frequent topical application of antibiotic ointment or petroleum jelly may speed healing and prevent irritation of the healing mucosa by the adjacent teeth. Healing, even in delayed cases, should be complete within 2 weeks. Incomplete mucosal healing is suspect for a more serious underlying pathologic process, which requires excisional biopsy. Swelling is to be expected. Pain can generally be controlled with over-the-counter medications.

PATIENT EDUCATION GUIDES

See the sample patient education forms available at www.expert consult.com.

CPT/BILLING CODES

40490	Biopsy of lip
40808	Biopsy, vestibule of the mouth
40810	Excision/destruction, lesion of mucosa and submucosa (e.g., mucocele), vestibule of mouth, without repair
40812	With simple repair
40814	With complex repair
40820	Destruction of lesion or scar of vestibule of mouth by physical methods (e.g., laser, thermal, cryo, chemical)

ICD-10-CM DIAGNOSTIC CODES

K11.6   Oral mucocele

Lip Lesion (Upper and Lower)

C00.0	Malignant neoplasm skin upper lip, external
C00.1	Malignant neoplasm skin lower lip, external
D23.0	Benign neoplasm skin lip
D10.0	Benign neoplasm mucosa, vermilion border
D00.01	Carcinoma in situ
D49.0	Uncertain behavior

Acknowledgment

The editors recognize the contributions of Stephen K. Toadvine, MD, MPH, to this chapter in a previous edition of this text.

ONLINE RESOURCES

Flaitz CM, Hicks MJ. Mucocele and ranula. www.emedicine.medscape.com.

RECOMMENDED READING

Ata-Ali J, Carrillo C, Bonet C, et al. Oral mucocele: a review of the literature. *J Clin Exp Dent.* 2010;2(1):e18–e21.

Delbem AC, Cunha RF, Vieira AE, Ribeiro LL. Treatment of mucus retention phenomena in children by the micro-marsupialization technique: Case reports. *Pediatr Dent.* 2000;22:155–158.

Gill D. Two simple treatments for lower lip mucocoeles. *Australas J Dermatol.* 1996;37:220.

Usatine RP, Moy RL, Tobinick EL, Siegel DM, eds. *Skin Surgery: A Practical Guide.* St. Louis: Mosby; 1998.

Holtzman LC, Hitti E, Harrow J. Incision and Drainage. In: Roberts JR, Custalow CB, Thomsen TW, eds. *Roberts and Hedges Clinical Procedures in Emergency Medicine.* 6th ed. Philadelphia: Elsevier; 2014:756–757.

CHAPTER 57

CHALAZION AND HORDEOLUM

James L. Jackson

Patients with a chalazion or hordeolum, focal inflammatory conditions of the eyelids, are frequently encountered in primary care. Invariably they complain of a "stye." Both conditions may be treated by the prudent nonophthalmologist, either medically or with a minor surgical procedure in the office. However, care must be taken not to injure the eye, the eyelid, or other delicate components, particularly the lacrimal drainage system (tear ducts) or the eyelid margin.

A *chalazion* (Fig. 57.1) is an acute or chronic granulomatous inflammation of a meibomian gland in the eyelid and is usually painless. A *hordeolum* is an acute, painful abscess of a hair follicle or the meibomian, Zeis, or Moll gland (see Fig. 57.10). An *internal hordeolum* points onto the conjunctival surface of the lid, whereas an *external hordeolum* points onto the external surface of the skin or the margin of the lid.

The meibomian glands are basically sebaceous glands located deep within both eyelids (Fig. 57.2). They produce a lipid material that drains through long ducts and emerges from orifices at the eyelid margin. This lipid material then enters the tear film to help keep the surface of the eye lubricated while also slowing evaporation of the tears.

Meibomian secretions are naturally viscous, but under certain conditions they become thick enough to plug the duct of the gland. Because the gland continues to produce secretions, they must go somewhere (similar to a sebaceous cyst); consequently the secretions eventually leak between the cells of the gland into the surrounding tissue of the eyelid. Here the secretions incite a chronic granulomatous inflammatory reaction (chalazion). As more secretions are produced, the inflammation worsens, and it may smolder chronically, sometimes for a year or longer.

Clinically the inflammation causes localized swelling, edema, or a nodule within the lid, sometimes associated with erythema and mild tenderness. A chalazion may be located at the lid margin or up to a few millimeters away. At times it may be prominent externally, but more commonly a chalazion will be found on the inner surface (palpebral conjunctiva) of the lid. Associated inflammation may cause a soft or even liquid center, and patients may report spontaneous drainage internally, externally, or through the lid margin, which may lead to clinical improvement or resolution. A chalazion may also wax and wane; about 25% will go away on their own without treatment.

Some people experience multiple chalazia over time or even concurrently. Multiple chalazia are more commonly seen in people with acne rosacea, seborrhea, diabetes, or hyperlipidemia and in those who use old or contaminated eye makeup, do not remove their eye makeup completely, or have chronic blepharitis. Chronic blepharitis is characterized by eyelid margin inflammation, thickening, and erythema associated with bacterial colonization and crusting at the base of the eyelashes. Chronic blepharitis usually requires a slit-lamp examination to make the diagnosis (see Chapter 201); even with a slit lamp, the findings are often subtle and not easily detected by the nonophthalmologist.

In contrast to a chalazion, a *hordeolum* is an acute bacterial abscess of a hair follicle or a meibomian, Zeis, or Moll gland (see Fig. 57.2). Hordeola are classified as internal or external based on the primary anatomic focus of the inflammation (which is usually obvious). Typically characterized by an acute tender mass within the eyelid associated with erythema and a collection of pus, hordeola are often accompanied by acute cellulitis of the eyelid. Such cellulitis, in turn, is characterized by erythema, edema, and tenderness of the surrounding skin. (*Eyelid cellulitis* is a different, much more localized entity than the less common *orbital cellulitis*, a systemic vision- and life-threatening condition with which the patient is toxic, with a high fever.) A hordeolum usually drains spontaneously at 5 to 7 days, often relieving the symptoms. Hordeola are frequently associated with staphylococcal infections and acute blepharitis, both of which usually respond to antibiotics.

Differentiating a chalazion from a hordeolum can be a clinical challenge. The same things associated with multiple chalazia can be associated with a hordeolum (acne rosacea, seborrhea, diabetes, hyperlipidemia, use of old or contaminated eye makeup, inadequate removal of eye makeup, chronic blepharitis). Although a hordeolum is usually more tender and tense, with obvious fluctuance, a chalazion may have a liquefied center; however, it is usually not a collection of pus. The presence of significant eyelid cellulitis also usually suggests a hordeolum, but a chalazion may be associated with a degree of surrounding erythema and edema (although usually to a lesser degree). The natural history of a hordeolum is usually more acute, yet a chalazion can also present acutely. It may also be important to differentiate a chalazion or hordeolum from other eyelid disorders. If the swelling is located nasal to the medial canthus (the corner where the upper and lower eyelids meet), the patient likely has *dacryocystitis* rather than a chalazion or hordeolum. In this situation, strongly consider prompt referral to an ophthalmologist, because dacryocystitis can lead to serious sequelae. Because of the facial anatomy, bacterial dacryocystitis can dissect posteriorly to the cavernous sinus and beyond, with grave consequences.

CHALAZION

Medical Management

A chalazion may respond to one or more of the following medical treatments:

- Warm washcloth compresses to the eyelid (four times a day if possible).
- Eyelid scrubs of the lid margins at bedtime each night (at base of eyelashes) with commercially available ocular cleansing pads or diluted baby shampoo (diluted to half strength with water, applied with a cotton swab or washcloth).
- Application of antibiotic ointment (usually erythromycin) to eyelid margin after washing.
- Oral doxycycline.
- Intralesional steroid injection (e.g., triamcinolone acetonide 40 mg/mL, 0.2 to 0.4 mL) using a 30-gauge needle through the conjunctival (inner) surface of the eyelid, after the application of topical anesthesia (e.g., proparacaine or tetracaine drops). However, steroid injection carries the risk of skin hypopigmentation, especially in dark-skinned individuals.

Indications for Excision

- Chalazion unresponsive to medical management
- Substantial size (large enough to palpate)
- Cosmetic deformity
- Visual problems (e.g., astigmatism or blurry vision from pressure on the eye)
- Patient's request

Contraindications to Excision

- Chalazion has recently drained through the skin or with very thin overlying skin (relative contraindication, increases risk of a full-thickness "buttonhole" defect of the eyelid, leading to a visible scar and prolonged healing time).
- Skin crusted or markedly inflamed (excision is usually performed from the inner surface of the eyelid and, again, a buttonhole defect may result).
- Anticoagulated patient (relative contraindication).
- Chalazion near the lacrimal punctum. This punctum is a tiny opening in the nasal aspect of each eyelid margin. Tears drain through the punctum into the canaliculus, which runs just beneath the skin toward the nose. Damage to the punctum or canaliculus may lead to chronic tearing and the need for a complicated surgical repair. If the chalazion is close enough to the punctum that it could have been damaged, the patient should be referred to an ophthalmologist for excision.

Equipment

See Fig. 57.3.

- Equipment needed to follow universal blood and body fluid precautions (e.g., mask and goggles)
- Sterile tray
- Skin marking pen
- Topical ophthalmic anesthetic drops (e.g., proparacaine or tetracaine)
- Alcohol pads
- Local anesthetic for injection (2% lidocaine with epinephrine), 3-mL syringe, 30-gauge needle
- Povidone-iodine swabs
- Sterile gloves
- Sterile drape, fenestrated
- Chalazion clamps (two or three sizes)
- Scalpel (No. 15 blade)

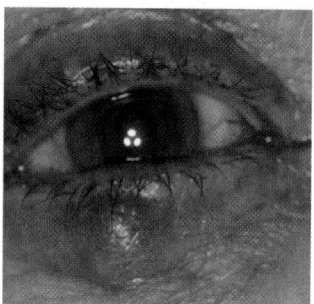

Fig. 57.1 Chalazion, lower lid.

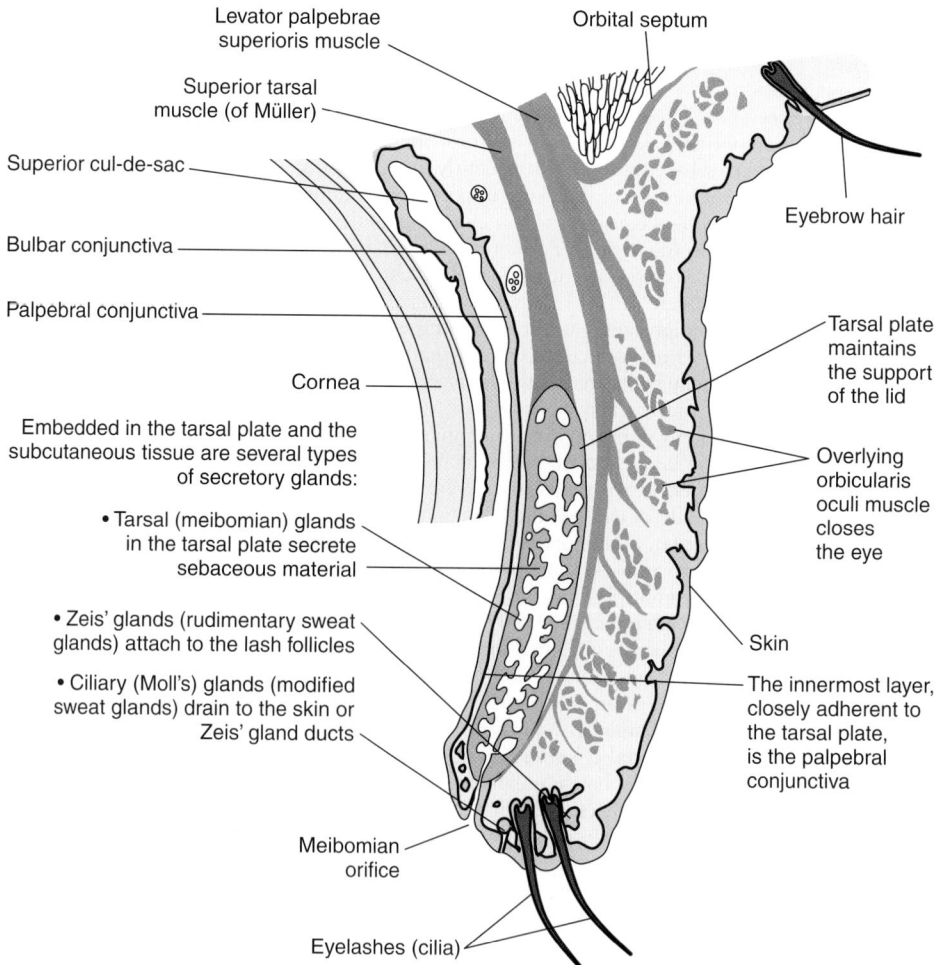

Levator palpebrae superioris muscle

Orbital septum

Superior tarsal muscle (of Müller)

Superior cul-de-sac

Bulbar conjunctiva

Palpebral conjunctiva

Cornea

Eyebrow hair

Tarsal plate maintains the support of the lid

Overlying orbicularis oculi muscle closes the eye

Embedded in the tarsal plate and the subcutaneous tissue are several types of secretory glands:

- Tarsal (meibomian) glands in the tarsal plate secrete sebaceous material

- Zeis' glands (rudimentary sweat glands) attach to the lash follicles

- Ciliary (Moll's) glands (modified sweat glands) drain to the skin or Zeis' gland ducts

Skin

The innermost layer, closely adherent to the tarsal plate, is the palpebral conjunctiva

Meibomian orifice

Eyelashes (cilia)

Fig. 57.2 Anatomy of the eyelid.

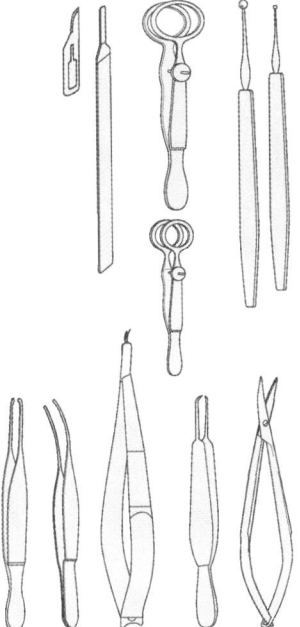

Fig. 57.3 Instruments for chalazion excision. *Top row, left to right:* Scalpel (No. 15 or No. 11 blade), chalazion clamps, chalazion curettes. *Bottom row, left to right:* Ocular tissue forceps, needle holder, suturing forceps, Westcott conjunctival scissors.

- Chalazion curettes (two sizes)
- Cotton swabs
- Ocular tissue forceps, 0.2 tips
- Westcott conjunctival scissors
- 4 × 4 gauze pads
- Antibiotic-steroid combination ophthalmic ointment (e.g., neomycin, polymyxin, dexamethasone or tobramycin, dexamethasone)
- Eye patches (two or three) and medical tape
- Suture (6-0 nylon), needle holder, and suture scissors (only in the event of a full-thickness eyelid defect occurring as a complication)

Preprocedure Patient Preparation

Unless the patient is at high risk for cardiovascular events, he or she should discontinue aspirin or other antiplatelet medications for 1 week and anticoagulants for 4 days before the procedure. The patient should be counseled about the risks of scarring, a possible need for sutures, the risk of recurrence and need for repeat excision, short-term swelling/bruising of the eyelid, excessive bleeding, infection, and, rarely, damage to the lacrimal drainage system resulting in chronic tearing. It will be important for the patient to remain motionless during the procedure. The patient may experience some discomfort and tearing with injection of the anesthetic.

Technique

Universal blood and body fluid precautions should be followed. The clinician can achieve good access to the eye by sitting near the top of the head. The patient should lie supine. Good lighting is essential. Injection of the local anesthetic may make palpation of the chalazion difficult, so it is helpful to use a skin marker before administering the injection.

1. Administer several drops of a topical ophthalmic anesthetic. Then inject 2% lidocaine with epinephrine through the skin, infiltrating the area where the chalazion clamp is to be applied (Fig. 57.4A).
2. Place a chalazion clamp over the chalazion, with the open side inside the eyelid (see Fig. 57.4B). Avoid damaging the eyelid

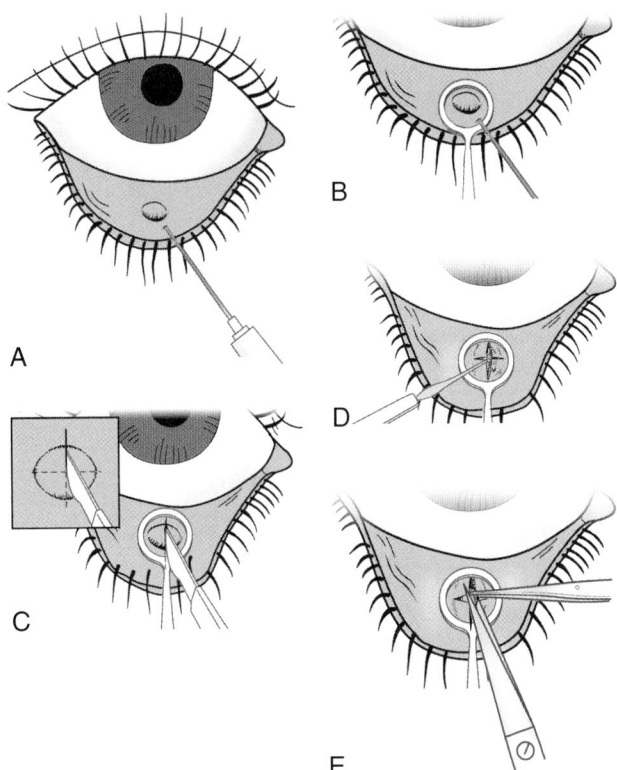

Fig. 57.4 Chalazion excision. (A) Inject anesthetic. (B) Place chalazion clamp. (C) Incise with scalpel, making an "X" over the lesion. (D) Curette interior of chalazion to remove soft, inflamed material. (E) Remove small amount of inflamed tarsus with Westcott conjunctival scissors and tissue forceps.

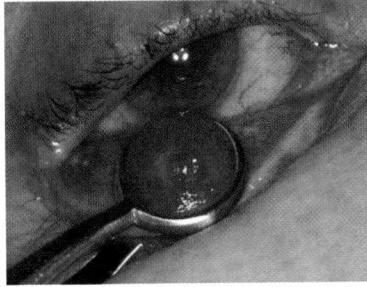

Fig. 57.5 After topical anesthetic drops are instilled, a chalazion clamp is used to stabilize and evert the lid.

margin. Tighten the clamp to achieve a firm grip on the eyelid; this will maintain hemostasis during the procedure. Do not overtighten. Evert the eyelid using the clamp as a lever (Fig. 57.5). The chalazion should now be evident and bulging through the opening of the clamp.
3. With a no. 15 blade, make two incisions in the form of a cross, taking care not to go through the eyelid skin but only into the substance of the chalazion (Figs. 57.6 and Fig. 57.4C). Some soft material may be released, confirming that the incision is in the correct location.
4. Use the curettes and cotton swabs to remove as much soft, inflamed material as possible (Figs. 57.7 and 57.4D). Remove as much granulation tissue as you can with forceps (Fig. 57.8).
5. Using the Westcott conjunctival scissors and tissue forceps, remove a small amount of the inflamed tarsal plate (the cartilage underneath) if necessary (see Fig. 57.4E). Take care not to tent the deeper tissue, which can lead to inadvertent incision of the skin and cause a "buttonhole" defect. Again, avoid damaging the eyelid margin.

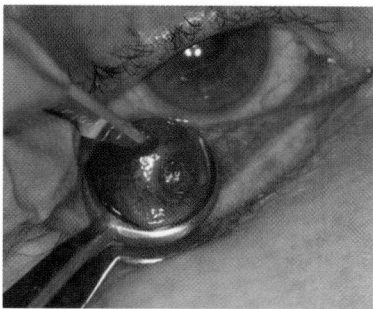

Fig. 57.6 Incising the chalazion using a No. 15 blade. Make an "X" over the lesion.

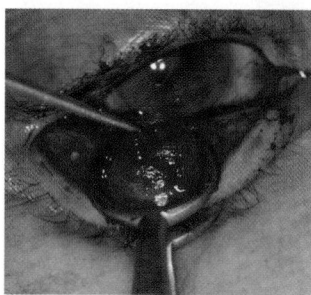

Fig. 57.7 Removing contents with a chalazion curette.

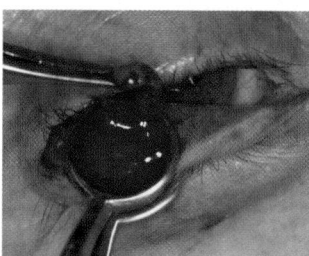

Fig. 57.8 Removing granulation tissue with forceps (pickups).

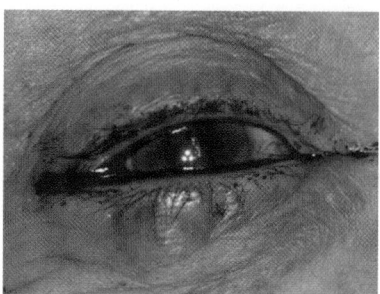

Fig. 57.9 Postoperative appearance after chalazion removal.

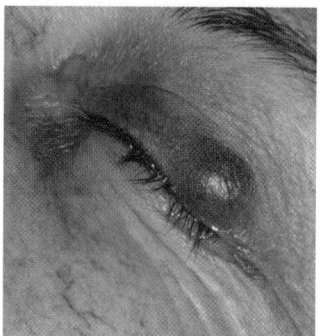

Fig. 57.10 Hordeolum of upper lid.

6. Remove the chalazion clamp, which will likely lead to significant bleeding because of the excellent vascularity of the eyelid. Apply direct pressure with cotton swabs or gauze pads to achieve hemostasis. This may take 5 to 10 minutes (Fig. 57.9). Once hemostasis has definitely been achieved, apply an antibiotic-steroid eye ointment and place a pressure patch on the eye (see Chapter 200 and Fig. 200.5 for a technique of pressure patching).

7. If a full-thickness eyelid defect is present, after external application of povidine-iodine solution, suture the outer skin while taking care that the suture does not include the conjunctival (inner) surface of the eyelid; this would cause a great deal of irritation and possibly a corneal abrasion. If damage to the lacrimal punctum or canaliculus has occurred, promptly refer the patient to an ophthalmologist.

8. Beware of recurrent or multiple chalazia in older patients, especially with associated ocular inflammation. This could represent sebaceous cell carcinoma, which is very aggressive and not always noted on pathologic examination of an excised chalazion. If a presumed chalazion does not behave as expected after excision, particularly in an elderly patient, sebaceous cell carcinoma should be suspected even if the initial pathology report is negative. In that situation, the patient should be referred to an ophthalmologist.

Postprocedure Patient Education

The patient may remove the patch the evening of the procedure. Tell the patient that he or she can expect a large amount of clotted blood and matting of the eyelid. The patient should then begin to apply an antibiotic eye ointment (e.g., erythromycin) to the eye twice a day until it is judged to be "back to normal." If the eyelid begins to bleed again, the patient should apply pressure until it stops and should seek medical attention if the bleeding does not stop. If sutures were placed, they should be removed in 5 days.

HORDEOLUM

Medical Management

If less severe and not yet "pointing," the hordeolum may be treated with frequent warm washcloth compresses and an oral antibiotic directed against *Staphylococcus*. In fact, most hordeola respond to this management, with spontaneous drainage and resolution occurring within 5 to 7 days. However, if the patient is being treated medically, he or she should be watched closely in case the need for incision and drainage develops.

Indications for Incision and Drainage

- Hordeolum that fails medical management (Fig. 57.10)
- Hordeolum causing significant pain
- Hordeolum with significant localized accumulation of pus
- Previous or current eyelid cellulitis associated with hordeolum

Contraindications to Incision and Drainage

If the hordeolum is located near the lacrimal punctum (i.e., nasal to the medial canthus), refer the patient to an ophthalmologist because of the risk of damaging the lacrimal drainage system.

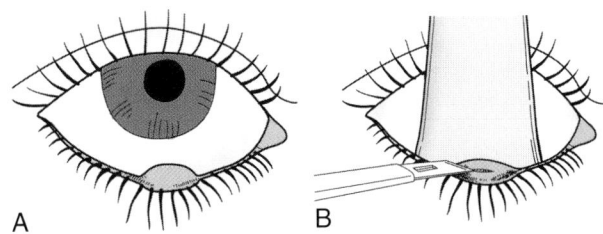

Fig. 57.11 Hordeolum excision. (A) Hordeolum pointing externally. (B) Incision and drainage of external hordeolum, with a tongue blade or metal elevator protecting the eye.

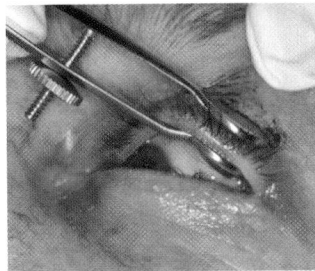

Fig. 57.12 Stabilizing the hordeolum with a chalazion clamp.

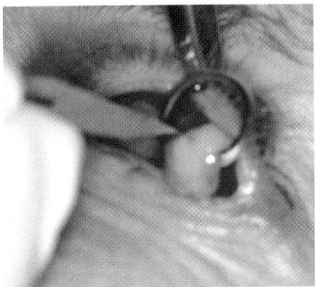

Fig. 57.13 Incising the hordeolum: acute infection and drainage are evident.

Equipment

- Equipment needed to follow universal blood and body fluid precautions (e.g., mask and goggles)
- Topical ophthalmic anesthetic drops (e.g., proparacaine or tetracaine)
- Alcohol pads
- Local anesthetic for injection, 2% lidocaine with epinephrine, 3-mL syringe, 30-gauge needle
- Nonsterile gloves
- Scalpel (No. 11 blade)
- Cotton swabs
- 4 × 4 gauze pads
- Tongue blade or metal elevator

Preprocedure Patient Preparation

Unless the patient is at high risk for cardiovascular events, he or she should discontinue aspirin or other antiplatelet medications for 1 week and anticoagulants for 4 days before the procedure (although it is usually necessary to perform the procedure without much advanced planning). The patient should be counseled about the risks of scarring, recurrence, possible need for repeat incision and drainage, short-term swelling/bruising of the eyelid, excessive bleeding, spread of infection, and, rarely, damage to the lacrimal drainage system resulting in

chronic tearing. It will be important for the patient to remain motionless during the procedure. The patient may experience some discomfort and tearing with the injection of local anesthetic.

Technique

Universal blood and body fluid precautions should be followed. The hordeolum will point either internally or externally and should be incised from whichever surface allows the best access to the collection of pus (Fig. 57.11A).

1. Administer several drops of topical ophthalmic anesthetic. Then inject 2% lidocaine with epinephrine through the skin, infiltrating the area around the hordeolum. (Remember that anesthesia is more difficult to obtain in the presence of inflammation.) A tongue blade or metal elevator can be inserted behind the lid to protect the eye (see Fig. 57.11B). It may be helpful to stabilize the hordeolum and lid with a chalazion clamp (Fig. 57.12).
2. Use a No. 11 scalpel blade to make an incision into the hordeolum until pus is obtained, taking great care to avoid a through-and-through eyelid defect or injury to the eyelid margin or eye. If significant cellulitis is present, it may be prudent to send a sample of the pus for culture and sensitivity testing.
3. After the pus is expressed (Fig. 57.13), apply direct pressure with gauze pads to achieve hemostasis. This may take 5 to 10 minutes. An eye patch is not necessary.
4. If a full-thickness eyelid defect is present, do not suture the skin because of the presence of acute bacterial infection. Consider appropriate systemic antibiotic therapy for significant cellulitis of the eyelid. (Spread of infection can lead to preseptal cellulitis.) If damage to the lacrimal duct has occurred, promptly refer the patient to an ophthalmologist.

Postprocedure Patient Management

If the eyelid begins to bleed again, the patient should apply pressure until it stops and should seek medical attention if he or she is having difficulty controlling the bleeding. The patient will be given an oral antibiotic (with good coverage for *Staphylococcus*), and should be seen the next day. He or she may need to be seen daily for several days after the procedure until it is evident that the cellulitis is resolving and that pus is not reaccumulating. Thereafter the patient should make an appointment in 2 to 3 weeks to further assess healing. It may take several weeks for the swelling and tissue distortion to return to normal.

PATIENT EDUCATION GUIDES

See the patient education and consent forms available at www.expertconsult.com.

SAMPLE OPERATIVE REPORTS

See sample operative reports available at www.expertconsult.com.

CPT/BILLING CODES

For chalazion excision

67800	Excision of chalazion, single
67801	Excision of chalazion, multiple, same lid
67805	Excision of chalazion, multiple, different lids

For incision and drainage of hordeolum

67700	Blepharotomy, drainage of abscess, eyelid

ICD-10-CM DIAGNOSTIC CODES

H00.11–H00.19	Chalazion
H00.01–H00.19	Hordeolum, NOS or external
H00.21–H00.029	Hordeolum, internal

Acknowledgment

The editors recognize the contributions of Lewis E. Mehl, MD, PhD, to this chapter in a previous edition of this text.

SUPPLIERS

(Any medical instrument supplier can provide the necessary equipment. See contact information available at www.expertconsult.com.)

Accutome
Storz (Bausch and Lomb)

ONLINE RESOURCES

For Patients

http://www.aao.org/eye-health/diseases/what-are-chalazia-styes.
http://www.merckmanuals.com/home/eye-disorders/eyelid-and-tearing-disorders/chalazion-and-stye-hordeolum.

For Clinicians

Bessette M. Hordeolum and stye in emergency medicine: www.emedicine.com/EMERG/topic755.htm.
Deschenes J, editor. Chalazion. www.emedicine.com/EMERG/topic94.htm.

RECOMMENDED READING

Jacobs PM, Thaller VT, Wong D. Intralesional corticosteroid therapy of chalazion: a comparison with incision and curettage. *Br J Ophthalmol.* 1984;68:836–837.
Knoop KJ, Dennis WR. Ophthalmologic Procedures. In: Roberts JR, Custalow CB, Thomsen TW, eds. *Roberts and Hedges Clinical Procedures in Emergency Medicine.* 6th ed. Philadelphia: Elsevier; 2014:1292–1294.
Neff AG, Carter KD. Benign eyelid lesions. In: Yanoff M, Duker JS, eds. *Ophthalmology.* 4th ed. St. Louis: Elsevier; 2014:1295–1305.

CHAPTER 58

TONOMETRY

Deepa A. Iyengar • Grant C. Fowler

Tonometry is used to detect increased intraocular pressure, which is common in patients at risk for glaucoma. Glaucoma is actually caused by a group of conditions, all of which can lead to optic nerve damage and a loss of visual function. It is estimated that three million persons in the United States have glaucoma, a leading cause of blindness after age 60 years, and its incidence increases with age. It is the second leading cause of blindness worldwide. Despite the fact that most blindness caused by glaucoma is preventable, or at least able to be delayed, there are estimates that only about half of patients with glaucoma know they have it. Tonometry remains one of the easiest methods of screening for glaucoma; however, patients with glaucoma can have normal intraocular pressures and, vice versa, not all patients with increased intraocular pressures have glaucoma. Researchers are currently pursuing other risk factors associated with glaucomatous changes in the eye to develop additional practical screening techniques. When this succeeds, glaucoma will be more readily diagnosed, even in those with normal intraocular pressure. Until then, tonometry, in combination with funduscopic examination and visual field testing, is the most sensitive and specific method for detection of glaucoma. Patients at high risk should be screened with all three.

There are three basic types of tonometry. *Impression tonometry* measures the depth of the impression produced on the ocular wall by a given force, and the Schiøtz tonometer uses this method. *Noncontact/air-puff tonometry*, originally considered the least accurate and therefore designed for screening (especially for children), has turned out to be fairly accurate even when compared with applanation tonometry, the gold standard. *Applanation (Goldmann) tonometry* measures the force necessary to flatten an area of the cornea. Because applanation tonometry is more accurate than Schiøtz tonometry, most optometrists and ophthalmologists use this technique; however, it requires the ability to use a slit lamp (see Chapter 201, Slit-Lamp Examination). Consequently, the Schiøtz tonometer is still the standard for measuring intraocular pressure in the offices of primary care clinicians, in many urgent care centers, and in some emergency departments. The Schiøtz tonometer is also less expensive (about $250). Many urgent care centers and emergency departments also now have available a hand-held portable device (e.g., Tono-Pen; Reichert, Inc.) that uses applanation technology, although it is somewhat more expensive (about $3000) than the Schiøtz tonometer. Regardless of the method of tonometry, the clinician may recommend other tests or a referral if the initial test result is abnormal. This chapter discusses the techniques used in impression (Schiøtz) and applanation (Tono-Pen, Goldmann) tonometry.

NOTE: If no instruments are available, a relatively unskilled examiner can detect the very high intraocular pressure of acute angle closure glaucoma by merely palpating one eye and comparing it to the other normal eye. With the patient looking down, and without closing their eyes, the examiner rests both hands on the patient's forehead. With an index finger, enough pressure can then be applied to the suspicious eye to indent it slightly. This should be compared to the pressure it takes to indent the opposite eye with the other index finger. With acute angle closure glaucoma, the affected eye will be rock hard compared with the softer, more compliant normal eye.

INDICATIONS

Screening Those With Risk Factors

- Age older than 40 years (older than 35 years in African Americans)
- Age older than 60 (sixfold increased risk)
- Family history of glaucoma (fourfold to ninefold increased risk)
- African Americans (sixfold to eightfold higher risk than Caucasians)
- Hispanics at higher risk than those of European descent, especially if older than 60 years
- Asian Americans (increased risk of angle-closure glaucoma, but this causes <10% of glaucoma)
- Diabetes mellitus
- Hypertension
- Decreased visual acuity (myopia or hyperopia)
- Central corneal thickness less than 0.5 mm
- Prior injury: blunt or penetrating trauma, eye surgery, eye inflammation (e.g., uveitis) can cause glaucoma acutely or years later
- Prior or current medications: use of corticosteroids (including high-dose inhaled corticosteroids), mydriatics, phenothiazines, and sympathomimetics can precipitate glaucoma

Diagnosis

- Ocular pain (usually unilateral, especially if associated with signs or symptoms of angle-closure glaucoma such as acute-onset red eye, cloudy or smoky cornea, fixed mid-position pupil, blurry vision, halos around lights, nausea and vomiting, frontal headache)
  NOTE: Patients with angle-closure glaucoma may complain more about nausea and vomiting than eye symptoms.
- Red eye (usually unilateral, especially if associated with signs or symptoms of angle-closure glaucoma)
- History of visual field loss

Determining Baseline Intraocular Pressure

- Uveitis: patients with iritis or uveitis can develop both open- and closed-angle glaucoma. Corticosteroid treatment of uveitis can also cause glaucoma.
- After blunt ocular trauma: patients with hyphema often have an acute rise in intraocular pressure.
- Orbital fracture: measuring intraocular pressure and comparing with opposite eye can predict risk of ocular injury.

CONTRAINDICATIONS

- Eye infection (although Tono-Pen can be used because it uses disposable tip covers, noncontact tonometry may be preferred)
- Corneal abrasion (although Tono-Pen can be used in another area of the cornea, tonometry is commonly deferred until a subsequent visit)
- Recent eye trauma (Tono-Pen/Schiøtz tonometry should not be performed in patients with suspected penetrating ocular injury or ruptured globe; pressure on the globe can result in extrusion of intraocular contents. Dilated slit-lamp examination should be performed to exclude perforation and posterior scleral rupture which can be very subtle. Scleral rupture should be associated with significant visual loss and prominent swelling of periorbital tissue)
- Patients who cannot keep their eyes still or open (Schiøtz and applanation tonometry cannot be used in patients with severe eyelid swelling or those unable to open their eyes; however, the Tono-Pen can sometimes be used)

EQUIPMENT

- Topical ophthalmic anesthetic drops, such as proparacaine hydrochloride 0.5% or tetracaine 7% (tetracaine causes less burning sensation than proparacaine)
- Gloves, mask, goggles (whatever is needed to follow universal blood and body fluid precautions)
- For Schiøtz: Schiøtz tonometer kit (each kit contains the tonometer, three plunger weights, a concave test block, conversion tables, pipe cleaners, and instructions for care)
- For Tono-Pen: Tono-Pen unit, condom-style disposable tip covers, optical-grade canned air for cleaning
- For applanation: slit lamp with Goldmann applanation device attached, sterile fluorescein strips

PREPROCEDURE PATIENT PREPARATION

Explain the reason for measuring the intraocular pressure with the tonometer (e.g., presence of glaucoma risk factors, symptoms, or positive physical findings). Briefly explain the procedure as well as the fact that this test only detects increased intraocular pressure. Contact lens should be removed prior to instillation of a topical ocular anesthetic or fluorescein. The patient should know that anesthetic ophthalmic drops may sting a little as they are instilled; after that is it not painful. They should know that the instrument will contact their tear films on the eye. The patient should also know that having normal intraocular pressures does not completely exclude glaucoma. If glaucoma is suspected, even with normal intraocular pressures, tonometry should be combined with the other tests mentioned previously. It is not necessary to obtain informed consent because tonometry is part of the routine eye exam.

TECHNIQUE

Schiøtz or Tono-Pen

1. Check and record the patient's visual acuity. Examine the eyes. Immediately after the funduscopic examination, place two drops of topical ophthalmic anesthetic in each eye. (The anesthetic will have time to take effect while you prepare the tonometer.) The clinician should follow universal blood and body fluid precautions.
2. Assemble the Schiøtz tonometer with the 5.5-g weight in place, and test for accuracy on the convex metal test block (Fig. 58.1). The Schiøtz tonometer is precalibrated by the manufacturer and must be returned for repair if it does not read "0" when resting on the test block. This test should also assure smooth motion of the device. The Tono-Pen (Fig. 58.2) should also be calibrated

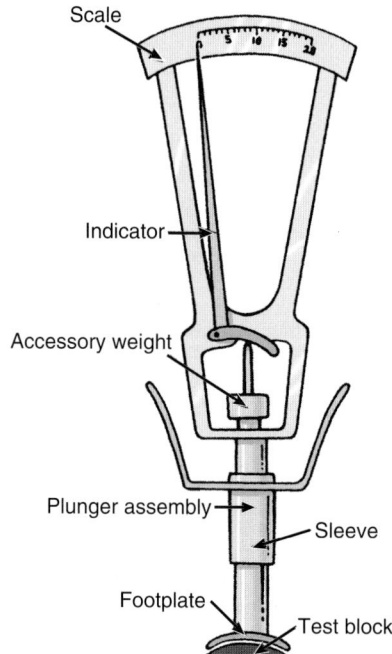

Fig. 58.1   Schiøtz tonometer.

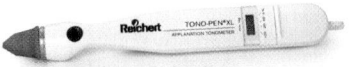

Fig. 58.2   Hand-held tonometer (Tono-Pen XL). (Courtesy Reichert, Inc., Depew, NY.)

before each use. Turn the transducer tip straight down and push the operation button twice within 1.5 seconds. It will beep and the liquid crystal display (LCD) will read "CAL." Although it may take up to 15 seconds, the Tono-Pen will then beep and display "UP." Immediately invert the tip straight upward, and if it is functioning properly, it should beep again and display "Good" in the LCD, which means it is calibrated. It is now ready for use, so the tip should be covered with a disposable cover.

NOTE: Beware of latex allergy in patients if latex Tono-Pen tip covers are being used.

Press the operation button again, and the instrument will display "[8.8.8.8]" followed by a single row of dashes and then a double row of dashes followed by a beep. Proceed with obtaining intraocular pressure readings within 15 seconds.

NOTE: Any time the operation button is depressed twice within 1.5 seconds, the instrument will attempt to calibrate and will display "CAL." While attempting to calibrate, if "Bad" is displayed in the LCD, repeat the process. If further attempts are unsuccessful, press the RESET button and repeat the process. If still unsuccessful, use optical-grade canned air to clean the probe tip for about 2 seconds, wait 3 minutes for the instrument to stabilize thermally, and then repeat the calibration process. If still not working, the batteries should be replaced and the process repeated. ("Lob" on the display also indicates low batteries.) Further unsuccessful attempts to calibrate warrant a call to technical support (1-800-866-6736 [TONO-PEN], www.reichert.com/products.cfm?pcId=474reichert.com/products. cfm?pcId=474).

3. For Schiøtz tonometry, have the patient lie on a table in the supine position and keep both eyes wide open. Ask the patient to relax and fix his or her gaze on a spot on the ceiling, with the line of vision perpendicular to the table. Retract the lids of the eye against the bony margin of the orbit with one hand, being careful to touch only the orbital margin because pressure directed into

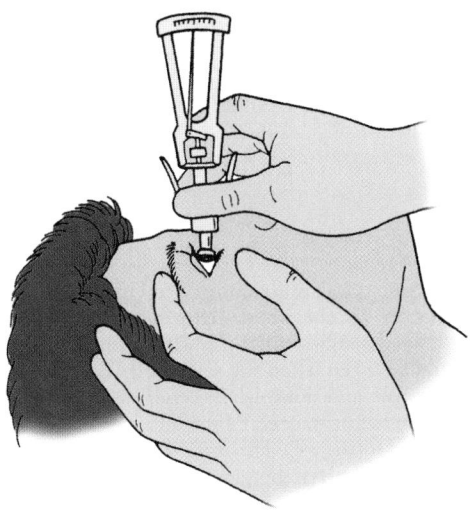

Fig. 58.3 Examination with the Schiøtz tonometer.

TABLE 58.1	Sample Calibration Scale for Schiøtz Tonometer			
	Intraocular Pressure (mm Hg) by Plunger Load			
Scale Reading	**5.5 g**	**7.5 g**	**10.0 g**	**15.0 g**
0	41	59	82	127
0.5	38	54	75	118
1.0	35	50	70	109
1.5	32	46	64	101
2.0	29	42	59	94
2.5	27	39	55	88
3.0	24	36	51	82
3.5	22	33	47	76
4.0	21	30	43	71
4.5	19	28	40	66
5.0	17	26	37	62
5.5	16	24	34	58
6.0	15	22	32	54
6.5	13	20	29	50
7.0	12	19	27	46
7.5	11	17	25	43
8.0	10	16	23	40
8.5	9	14	21	38
9.0	9	13	20	35
9.5	8	12	18	32
10.0	7	11	16	30
10.5	6	10	15	27
11.0	6	9	14	25
11.5	5	8	13	23
12.0		8	11	21
12.5		7	10	20
13.0		6	10	18
13.5		6	9	17
14.0		5	8	15
14.5			7	14
15.0			6	13
15.5			6	11
16.0			5	10
16.5				9
17.0				8
17.5				8
18.0				7

From Schiøtz Tonometer Kit literature, courtesy Gulden Ophthalmics, Elkins Park, PA.

the orbit will cause the tonometer reading to be falsely elevated. Hold the tonometer by its handles with the thumb and middle finger of the other hand. After the patient has relaxed from the involuntary muscle contraction that occurs when the tonometer is first placed in his or her line of sight, center the foot plate of the tonometer over the cornea and gently lower the tonometer until it is resting on the cornea (Fig. 58.3). The indicator will come to rest at a position to the right of 0. The tonometer should be perpendicular to the cornea in a vertical position. Record the scale reading. If it is less than 4, repeat the reading because this indicates an elevated intraocular pressure. Perform another reading after adding the 7.5- or 10-g weight, as necessary, to obtain a scale reading between 4 and 8. Convert the scale reading to millimeters of mercury using the calibration scale included with the kit (Table 58.1). Record the intraocular pressure in the patient's chart. If the intraocular pressure in the other eye is going to be measured, immediately clean the foot plate with an alcohol swab and allow it to air dry for 1 to 2 minutes.

NOTE: Closing the eyelids or blinking or looking toward the nose can increase intraocular pressure by 5 to 10 mm Hg. Repeated or prolonged measurements have been found to lower intraocular pressure by 2 mm Hg and may also lower pressure in the opposite eye. Overhydration (e.g., four large cups of coffee, six cans of beer) can also lower pressure.

4. If the Tono-Pen is used, the patient can be in any position. However, the head should be supported so that the patient cannot pull away when the Tono-Pen is placed in his or her line of vision. Have the patient fix his or her line of vision by looking straight ahead.

NOTE: Regardless of technique used, to assist patients in fixing their gaze, ask them to extend an arm straight upward or out and to stare at their thumbnail placed over a spot on the wall or ceiling.

5. The clinician should consider bracing the heel of his or her hand on the patient's cheek for stability and then touch the tip of the Tono-Pen lightly to the central cornea directly over the pupil (the cornea does not need to be indented; indentation may lead to inaccurate readings). If the cornea is abraded over the pupil, touch the Tono-Pen to the cornea elsewhere. While holding the Tono-Pen perpendicular to the corneal surface, tap the cornea lightly several times. The Tono-Pen will chirp after each valid intraocular pressure reading is obtained. After four valid readings, the Tono-Pen will sound a final beep and display a mean intraocular pressure (mm Hg) with a horizontal line under it on the LCD. The statistical reliability of the measurement is also displayed, and if the reliability measure (standard deviation) is 20% or higher, a repeat measurement is recommended. Likewise,

a single row of dashes in the LCD indicates an insufficient number of valid readings were collected, so after pressing the operation button, additional measurements should be made. When a valid intraocular pressure is displayed, record it in the patient's chart.

NOTE: The tip of the Tono-Pen is a very sensitive probe that can be easily damaged, so it should never be touched by anything except a tip cover and then the cornea or the airflow from the optical-grade canned air when it needs to be cleaned.

6. Carefully clean the Schiøtz tonometer after each use to prevent transmission of disease. It can then be soaked in a special stand that soaks the tip only. A sterilizing solution that can eliminate human immunodeficiency virus should be used. Rinse carefully and allow to dry before using again. Alternatively, set the tonometer in an ultraviolet sterilizer stand. The tonometer should be disassembled at the end of each day and a pipe cleaner soaked with sterilizing solution run through the barrel to remove any debris. Accumulated debris could interfere with the motion of the plunger. Next, a dry pipe cleaner should be used to dry the barrel. The tonometer should not be oiled. If a Tono-Pen is used, it should not be immersed in fluids because the electronics will be damaged. Instead, the tip of the Tono-Pen should be cleaned of accumulated dust with optical-grade canned air; this step should be completed after it has been used for about 30 to 40 patients, or at least once a month. The tip cover should be changed after

Fig. 58.4 (A) Semicircles too wide: excessive moisture. (B) Semicircles too thin: excessive dryness. (C) Intraocular pressure greater than knob setting (semicircles are correct width). (D) Intraocular pressure equals knob setting (applied pressure). (E) Intraocular pressure less than knob setting.

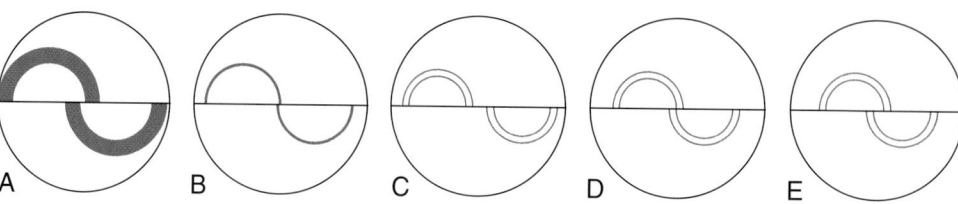

each use. A fresh tip cover should also be in place when the Tono-Pen is stored in the provided storage case. If the Tono-Pen is not going to be used for an extended period of time, the batteries should be removed.

Applanation

1. Check and record the patient's visual acuity. Examine the eyes. Immediately after the funduscopic examination, place two drops of anesthetic in each eye. (The anesthetic will have time to take effect while you prepare the slit lamp and attached Goldmann tonometer tip.) The clinician should follow universal blood and body fluid precautions.
2. Stabilize the patient's head by putting his or her chin on the chin rest and placing the forehead firmly against the headrest of the slit lamp (see Chapter 201, Slit-Lamp Examination). Each eye should be stained with fluorescein and the patient then asked to gaze straight ahead. His or her vision can be further fixated by asking him or her to focus on the clinician's ear on the side opposite the eye being examined.
3. The slit lamp should be on low-power magnification, the light filter switched to cobalt blue, and the slit diaphragm opened completely. Angle the light arm at about 45 to 60 degrees to the clinician's line of observation while shining the light on the plastic tonometer tip.
4. Set the pressure knob on the tonometer to 1 g (10 mm Hg). The patient should hold his or her eyes wide open and try to avoid blinking. The clinician may have to help the patient hold the lids open by applying pressure on the lids (only on the orbital rim).
5. Watching from the side (not through the slit lamp), the joystick should be used to move the tonometer tip up to the center of the patient's cornea, and then gentle contact is made. When contact is made, an immediate bluish glow should be noted all the way to the margin of the cornea. Avoid touching the lid margins with the tonometer tip because it will provoke blinking.
6. Through the slit lamp, the clinician should see two blue semicircles, each bordered by an arc of green light. These semicircles should be of equal extent above and below a horizontal dividing line. If the dividing line is not horizontal, the tonometer tip should be withdrawn and rotated on the holder until it is horizontal and reapplied to the cornea. If the semicircles extend beyond the illuminated field, there is too much pressure on the tonometer tip, so it should be backed away slightly from the eye.
7. The width of the arcs can be used to judge whether enough or excessive moisture is present. The width should be approximately {1/10} the diameter of the flattened surface contained within the arc. If the width is greater than {1/10} the diameter of the flattened area (Fig. 58.4A), too much moisture is present, either because of the tonometer tip being wet before application or because of excessive tears. The tip should be withdrawn from the patient's eye, dried, and reapplied. If the width of the arc is too narrow (see Fig. 58.4B), the tear film has dried excessively. The tip should be withdrawn from the patient's eye and he or she should be asked to blink several times.
8. The blue semicircles and the surrounding green light will pulsate synchronously with the cardiac rate. If the intraocular pressure is greater than 10 mm Hg, the semicircles will not touch (see Fig 58.4C). The clinician should turn the pressure knob up

until the semicircles are touching (see Fig. 58.4D). If the knob is turned up too far, the semicircles will overlap (see Fig. 58.4E). Because the semicircles will move with cardiac pulsations, readings should be taken when the semicircles touch about midway between systole and diastole. In other words, when the knob pressure matches intraocular pressure, the semicircles should glide back and forth past each other through excursions of equal distance. If the width of the semicircles suddenly shrinks, either the patient has withdrawn from the scope or the instrument has been inadvertently backed away from the eye.
9. Record the intraocular pressure reading in the chart. Clean the tip of the tonometer with an alcohol swab immediately after use, and let it air dry for 1 to 2 minutes. Repeat the procedure on the contralateral eye if needed for comparison.

POSTPROCEDURE PATIENT EDUCATION

Routine prophylactic topical antibiotics are no longer prescribed after the procedure. The patient should be instructed to avoid rubbing, touching, or traumatizing the eyes for 1 or 2 hours after the test, when the anesthesia has worn off, to avoid injuring the cornea. A contact lens should not be worn until the eye regains sensation. Patients should be warned that an anesthetized eye is easily traumatized and they should call the clinician's office immediately if symptoms of a corneal abrasion occur. If the result is abnormal (increased intraocular pressure), follow-up care should be discussed. Most clinicians recommend consultation with an ophthalmologist if the pressure in either eye is greater than 21 mm Hg. In the setting of an orbital fracture, a pressure greater than 22 mm Hg or a difference of 3 mm Hg between eyes is a good marker of ocular injury and should be referred. Intraocular pressure less than 9 mm Hg with recent eye surgery or trauma should also be discussed with an ophthalmologist. Reading of 22 to 25 mm Hg should be followed up with an ophthalmologist within 2 to 3 days. Emergent consultation with an ophthalmologist or treatment should be considered if the pressure is greater than 26 mm Hg. Patients need to know the importance of follow-up; however, they should be aware that increased intraocular pressure does not always mean that they have glaucoma and, vice versa, that normal intraocular pressure does not always exclude glaucoma.

COMPLICATIONS

- Trauma to the cornea during tonometry is uncommon; however, a corneal abrasion can occur after the procedure while the cornea is still anesthetized.
- Infection can usually be avoided by properly cleaning the tonometer and using fresh Tono-Pen tip covers or applanation tips.
- Low-pressure glaucoma may be missed; therefore patients with suspiciously cupped disks on ophthalmic examination should be referred.

LIMITATIONS

Falsely elevated intraocular pressure readings can be a normal variant, or they can be the result of an inflamed cornea, a scarred cornea, or pressure placed on the globe during the procedure. They can also occur with a thick or steeply curved cornea (Tono-Pen minimally affected). Falsely low measurements can be a normal variant, or they can result from high-grade myopia or rapidly repeated measurements.

PATIENT EDUCATION GUIDES

See patient education and patient consent forms available at www.expertconsult.com.

CPT/BILLING CODES

Ophthalmologic services constitute integrated services. Itemization of tonometry is not applicable.

92002 Ophthalmologic services: medical examination and evaluation with initiation of diagnostic and treatment program; intermediate, new patient

92012 Ophthalmologic services: medical examination and evaluation with initiation or continuation of diagnostic and treatment program; intermediate, established patient

92100 Serial tonometry (separate procedure) with multiple measurements of intraocular pressure over an extended time period with interpretation and report, same day (e.g., diurnal curve or medical treatment of acute elevation of intraocular pressure)

99173 Screening test of visual acuity, quantitative, bilateral (e.g., Snellen chart) (This cannot be used with 92002 or 92012)

ICD-10-CM DIAGNOSTIC CODES

H57.10–H57.13	Ocular pain
H53.8–H53.9	Other visual disturbances
H40–H42	Glaucoma

SUPPLIERS

(See contact information available at www.expertconsult.com.)

Schiøtz tonometer kit
  Gulden Ophthalmics: https://www.guldenophthalmics.com.
Tono-Pen and applanation (Goldmann) tonometry equipment
  Reichert, Inc: http://www.reichert.com/products.cfm?pcId=474.

ONLINE RESOURCES

Eye Care America, Eye Care America: Foundation of the American Academy of Ophthalmology. www.eyecareamerica.org (offers glaucoma risk assessment, educational materials, and access to care, all available in multiple languages).

Glaucoma Research Foundation, Glaucoma Research Foundation. www.glaucoma.org (has patient information in Spanish).

National Eye Institute, National Eye Institute. www.nei.nih.gov/ (has patient information in Spanish).

The Glaucoma Foundation, The Glaucoma Foundation. www.glaucomafoundation.org.

RECOMMENDED READING

Crouch ER, Crouch ER, Grant TR. Ophthalmology. In: Rakel RE, Rakel DP, eds. *Textbook of Family Medicine*. 9th ed. Philadelphia: Elsevier; 2016:274–304.

Knoop KJ, Dennis WR. Ophthalmologic procedures. In: Roberts JR, Custalow CB, Thomsen TW, eds. *Roberts and Hedges Clinical Procedures in Emergency Medicine*. 6th ed. Philadelphia: Elsevier; 2014:1282–1288.

Verplanck MW, Rolain M, Cohn AD. Intraocular Pressure Measurement (tonometry). In: Reichman EF, ed. *Emergency Medicine Procedures*. 2nd ed. New York: McGraw-Hill; 2013:1032–1038.

Sharma R, Brunette DD. Ophthalmology. In: Marx J, Hockberger R, Walls R, et al., eds. *Rosen's Emergency Medicine e-dition*. 8th ed. Philadelphia: Elsevier; 2014:909–930.

CHAPTER 59

AUDIOMETRY

Gerald A. Amundsen

Hearing is measured according to its two main components: frequency/pitch and intensity/loudness. Audiometry is a procedure used to measure and graph an individual's hearing over a range of frequencies (measured in cycles per second [Hz, for hertz]) at various intensity levels (measured in decibels [dB]). Although it is used frequently to test young children and the elderly (the groups at highest risk for hearing loss), audiometry is also an important component of any successful occupational hearing loss prevention program. In many instances, formal audiometry is performed by an audiologist; however, because screening audiometry is not a complex procedure and only a minimal amount of equipment is required, it is often performed by primary care clinicians. A recent systematic review concluded that adults who report hearing loss (spontaneously or on questioning) should have an audiogram; those who deny hearing loss should be screened with the whispered voice test or audioscopy (Bagai et al., 2006). They found little value to the Weber and Rinne tests. Even if not performing audiometry, primary care clinicians should have a basic understanding of not only the procedure but also the possible results.

An audiometer consists of a variable frequency oscillator that produces electrical impulses across the audible/perceptible frequencies, a transducer to convert the electrical impulses into sound or vibrations, and an attenuator to create variations in intensity. The device may be a stationary part of a designated testing facility or a portable unit with the flexibility to be used in a variety of settings. When sound is transmitted through headphones or an earpiece worn by the patient, and the patient responses are then recorded, an *air conduction audiogram* is produced. Air conduction audiometry evaluates both sensorineural and conductive hearing.

Sensorineural hearing refers to that produced by the cochlea of the inner ear, the auditory nerve, and the cochlear nuclei of the brain. There are both acquired and congenital causes of sensorineural hearing loss (Box 59.1). Age-related hearing loss is the most common cause of acquired sensorineural hearing loss, eventually impacting about 90% of older adults, and half of this is genetically determined. There are also risk factors for age-related hearing loss. Males tend to get the genetically determined versions at a younger age and to a more severe degree. Exposure to certain chemicals (e.g., toluene, styrene) or illicit drugs (e.g., ecstasy) seems to increase the risk for this type hearing loss as well as certain medications (progestin as well as ototoxic drugs). Other medications may be slightly protective (estrogen, aldosterone). If not causing vitamin deficiency, low or moderate alcohol consumption does not seem to increase risk; abuse may increase the risk. There may be slightly reduced risk with high folate intake. Chronic medical problems such as diabetes, renal failure, atherosclerosis, or immunosuppression may increase the risk of age-related hearing loss. Smoking may increase the risk slightly.

To test sensorineural hearing alone, a *bone conduction audiogram* is performed. With this procedure, similar to using a tuning fork when performing a physical examination, a bone conduction oscillator or vibrator is held against the mastoid process or forehead. Usually secured by a headband, the vibrator sets the skull into oscillation, producing a disturbance of the fluid in the cochlea. This disturbance is sensed by the cochlea and transmitted down the auditory nerve to the cochlear nuclei, *all without use of the middle ear system*. Results are graphed as the bone conduction audiogram. With pure sensorineural hearing loss, both air and bone conduction are impaired, and the impairments are about the same.

With air conduction hearing loss (usually due to middle or outer ear problems), air conduction is impaired but bone conduction is preserved. In the normal ear, the differences between the air and bone conduction thresholds, or the air–bone gap, should not exceed 10 dB. A gap larger than this indicates an air conduction problem (again, usually due to a middle or outer ear problem) as the source of hearing loss. Patients with air conduction hearing loss frequently respond to surgery, and cochlear implants are now available for severe or profound sensorineural hearing loss. In many patients, hearing impairment is due to a combination, or a *mixed hearing loss*, and these also usually respond somewhat to surgery.

BOX 59.1 Causes of Sensorineural Hearing Loss

Newborn
- Anoxia, asphyxia, hypoxia
- Bacterial infections
- Birth trauma
- Congenital syphilis
- Genetic causes, expressed at birth
- Hyperbilirubinemia (at levels requiring exchange transfusion)
- Prematurity
- TORCH syndrome (toxoplasmosis, other agents, maternal rubella, cytomegalovirus, herpes simplex)

Acquired
- Age-related hearing loss (about half of which is genetic)
- Autoimmune inner ear disorders
- Bacterial meningitis
- Congenital or acquired syphilis
- Cranial radiation therapy
- Excessive occupational or leisure noise or exposure to loud music (noise trauma)
- Genetic
- Glomus tumors
- Acoustic neuroma
- Head trauma (temporal bone fractures or labyrinthine concussion)
- Herpes zoster
- Human immunodeficiency virus infection/acquired immunodeficiency syndrome
- Labyrinthitis
- Lyme disease
- Measles
- Meniere disease
- Mumps
- Ototoxic medications
- Vascular disorders

	Response*		
Modality	**Ear**		
	Left	**Unspecified**	**Right**
Air conduction: earphones			
Unmasked	X		O
Masked	□		Δ
Bone conduction: mastoid			
Unmasked	>	∧	<
Masked	]		[
Bone conduction: forehead			
Unmasked	L	v	⌐
Masked	Γ		⌐
Air conduction: sound field	X	s	∅

Fig. 59.1 Standardized symbols for recording audiogram results. *For "no response," use a downward 45-degree arrow pointing to the left for the right ear symbols, and to the right for left ear symbols (e.g., ↙ for no response in the right ear unmasked).

The symbols used on an audiogram (Fig. 59.1) have been standardized by the American Speech-Language Hearing Association (ASHA; www.ahsa.org) since 1989. Traditionally, symbols representing the right ear were recorded in red, whereas results from the left ear were recorded in blue. Because color is potentially lost in photocopying, different symbols specific to each ear are now used on most audiograms.

Frequency is represented on the horizontal axis of the graph from low to high, from left to right. Although the normal human ear is capable of hearing a range from 20 to 20,000 Hz, an audiogram usually tests the range most necessary for hearing and the understanding of speech (usually 250 to 8000 Hz). Intensity, the measurement of "loudness," is represented on the vertical or left axis of the graph, and usually ranges from 0 to 100 or 120 dB. Data points plotted on the graph represent the lowest decibel intensity that can be heard by the individual 50% of the time at each frequency, and this is the *auditory threshold* for that particular frequency.

Results are interpreted relative to 0 dB, or *audiometric zero*. *Audiometric zero* was originally defined as "normal" by the American National Standards Institute and is derived from sampling a large population of ear-disease–free young adults. In other words, if a person's threshold at a given frequency is 20 dB, it means that the individual can hear sound at that frequency only when it is 20 dB louder than that needed by an average disease-free young adult. More recently, the American Speech Language Hearing Association has provided their definitions for normal hearing and levels of hearing impairment (Table 59.1).

NOTE: From 1 to 6 of 1000 newborns have severe hearing loss, usually sensorineural in origin. The Joint Committee on Infant Hearing recommends screening all infants for hearing loss at no later than 1 month of age. If the screening test result is abnormal, they should have comprehensive audiologic evaluation at no later than 3 months of age (e.g., behavioral observation audiometry, auditory brain stem response, acoustic immittance, otoacoustic emissions testing, visual reinforcement audiometry, conditioned play audiometry), and an intervention if deaf or hard of hearing. (Such an evaluation and treatment is beyond the scope of this text.) Likewise, one-third of adults from 61 to 70 years of age and 80% of those over 85 years have hearing loss. After hypertension and arthritis, hearing loss is the most common chronic health problem in older adults. The American Academy of Family Physicians recommends screening everyone older than 60 years for hearing loss during the periodic health examinations.

INDICATIONS

- General screening in children at the earliest age possible
- Exposure to one (or more) of the causes for sensorineural hearing loss (see Box 59.1)
- Speech delay in children
- Persistent behavioral problems or changes in children or the elderly
- Screening of adults 60 years or older when performing periodic health examination, and especially when performing geriatric assessment (see Appendix M, Special Considerations in Geriatric Patients)
- Patient complaints of hearing loss
- Persistent serous otitis media, especially bilateral in children
- Anyone undergoing tympanometry with suspected sensorineural hearing loss (an abnormal tympanogram usually implies conductive hearing loss; however, sensorineural hearing loss may also be present)
- Formal audiometric evaluation of a failed screening test
- Patient complaints of tinnitus, dizziness, or vertigo
- After severe head trauma
- After use of ototoxic drugs
- After meningitis, encephalitis, or other serious viral or bacterial infections that could affect hearing
- Occupational screening and follow-up for individuals with noisy work environments

NOTE: Up to 5% of school-age children will have fluctuating hearing loss during the school year because of middle ear effusions. Retesting is imperative.

CONTRAINDICATIONS

- Inexperienced technician
- Acute otitis media
- Local pinna infection that would cause pain from the earphone or earpiece application
- Uncooperative patient
- Uncontrollable background noise in the room when testing
- Occlusion of the canal by cerumen (see Chapter 62, Cerumen Impaction Removal) or a foreign body (see Chapter 204, Removal of Foreign Bodies from the Ear and Nose)

EQUIPMENT

- Audiometer: These range from simple hand-held screening instruments that test one ear at a time with a limited range of frequencies and intensities to more comprehensive devices. Audiometers may test air conduction alone or may be equipped to test both bone and air conduction. The most comprehensive units test frequencies from 125 to 8000 Hz at 0 to 100 or 120 dB. Audiometers are either stationary or portable, and many modern units interface directly with a laptop computer to record, store, and interpret patient evaluations.
- An individual trained in proper techniques for obtaining reliable, reproducible, and valid test results. (For occupational/industrial screening, the individual should be certified by the Council for Accreditation of Occupational Hearing Conservationists [www.caohc.org].)
- Quiet or sound-treated room, preferably tested (by an outside company) for acceptable background/ambient noise levels. If ambient noise levels are too high, thresholds may be artificially elevated, particularly in the lower frequencies.

PREPROCEDURE PATIENT PREPARATION

The indications for the procedure should be explained to patients, and they should be reassured that the process is painless. Patients should know that they will be hearing tones of varying degrees of loudness and pitch, and that they should signal both when they first hear a tone and when the tone disappears. They should also know how to signal (e.g., raising their hand or a finger, pushing a button). Patients should sit in a relaxed and comfortable position and look straight ahead. If they can hear noise from outside the earphones or earpiece, they should inform the clinician. If bone conduction testing will be performed, the source and nature of the vibrations should be explained to the patient.

TECHNIQUE

1. The examination must be administered using a properly calibrated instrument in a room with an acceptable level of background noise. The ear canal should have been checked for patency by the clinician.
2. The patient should be comfortably seated facing neither the monitor nor the examiner. (Usually patients are seated in a position that provides a side profile view to the examiner.)
3. Anything that may interfere with earphone application (or earplug insertion) should be removed (earrings, glasses, hats), and the headphones must be appropriately seated on the patient's head (or the earplugs properly inserted), sealing the ears from environmental noise.
4. Instruct the patient to respond to the faintest detectable sound at each frequency. Responses can consist of raising a hand or finger or pressing a test button when sound is first heard. The patient should continue to signal for the duration of audible sound. Having the patient indicate the entire duration of audible sound allows the examiner to determine if the responses are reproducible. If reproducible, the threshold should be the same at the beginning and at the end for a particular frequency, at least 50% of the time; this can then be recorded. Patients should be tested from low to high decibels and then back to low. This step helps the examiner exclude false-positive responses.
5. Threshold testing is initiated in the better ear (or the right ear if hearing is equal in both) with the following recommended sequence of frequencies: 1000, 2000, 4000, 8000, 1000 (repeated), 500, and 250 Hz. Start with 0 dB hearing levels and produce the tones for 1 to 2 seconds unless the patient responds.
6. Increase the tone by 5 dB, and, if the patient responds, reduce it by 10-dB increments until it is inaudible.
7. Continue repeated ascents in 5-dB increments and descents in 10-dB increments until a 50% reproducible response is obtained. Generally this requires three to four repetitions, with the patient attaining the same response at least half of the time. This result is then entered with the appropriate symbol on the audiogram.
8. Test through the frequencies sequentially as previously noted, starting 15 to 20 dB below the threshold of the previously tested frequency. Continue testing until all frequencies have been tested.
9. If bone conduction testing is planned, this same sequence can be applied and the results recorded with the appropriate symbols.
10. It may be necessary to mask or obscure one sound with another when the difference in hearing loss between the ears is great (e.g., a 40-dB difference for air conduction testing, a 5-dB difference for bone conduction hearing) or there is a 10-dB air–bone gap in the ear being tested. In these situations, if unmasked, crossover

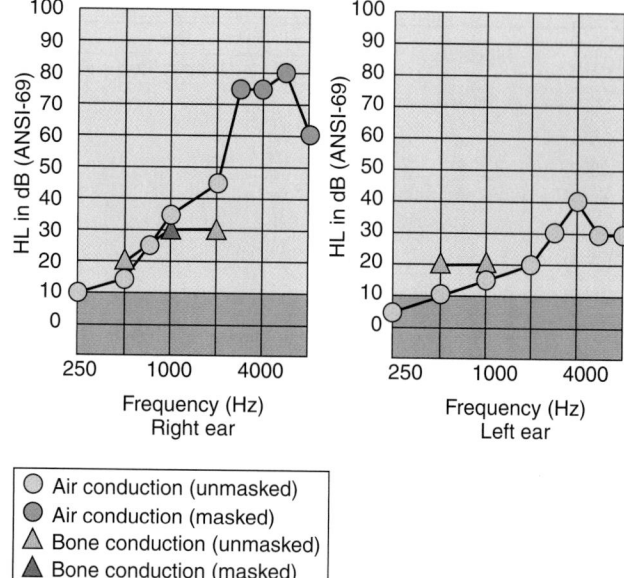

Legend:
- ○ Air conduction (unmasked)
- ● Air conduction (masked)
- △ Bone conduction (unmasked)
- ▲ Bone conduction (masked)

Fig. 59.2 Sixty-year-old man with suspected right acoustic neuroma. Note the unilateral hearing loss. (The corresponding tympanograms would be type A or normal.) *HL,* Hearing loss. (Modified from Jacobsen JT, Northern JL, eds. *Diagnostic Audiology.* Austin, TX: Pro-Ed; 1991.)

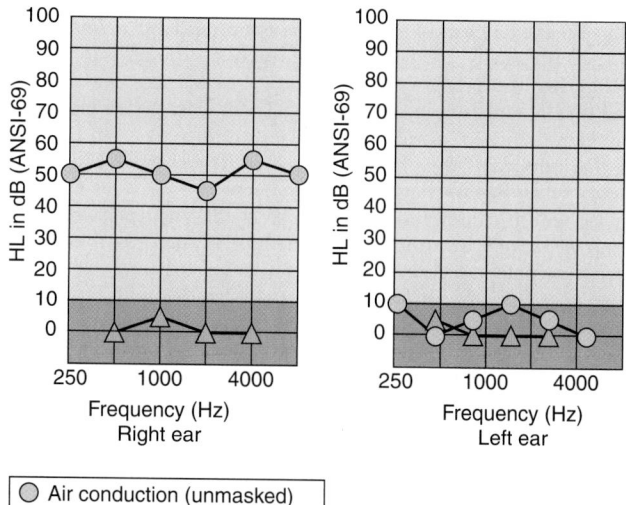

Legend:
- ○ Air conduction (unmasked)
- △ Bone conduction (unmasked)

Fig. 59.3 Nine-year-old boy with right acute otitis media with effusion. Using masking, the curves would probably appear the same; however, there would be slightly more assurance of the accuracy of the study. (The corresponding tympanogram would be type B.) *HL,* Hearing loss. (Modified from Jacobsen JT, Northern JL, eds. *Diagnostic Audiology.* Austin, TX: Pro-Ed; 1991.)

of sound to the better ear may occur and artificially lower the threshold of the impaired ear; therefore masking is applied to the nontest ear. Masking is usually done by providing constant noise to the nontest ear to "keep it busy." Audiometers are calibrated so that a 10-dB masking noise will block a 10-dB pure signal.

INTERPRETATION

Air conduction testing alone can approximate the degree of hearing loss. However, to differentiate between conductive, sensorineural, and mixed hearing loss, it is often best to test both air and bone conduction hearing.

TABLE 59.1	Classification of Severity of Hearing Loss (American Speech Language Hearing Association)
Degree of Hearing Loss (dB)	**Level of Severity**
−10–15	Normal
15–25	Slight
26–40	Mild
41–55	Moderate
56–70	Moderately severe
71–90	Severe
>90	Profound

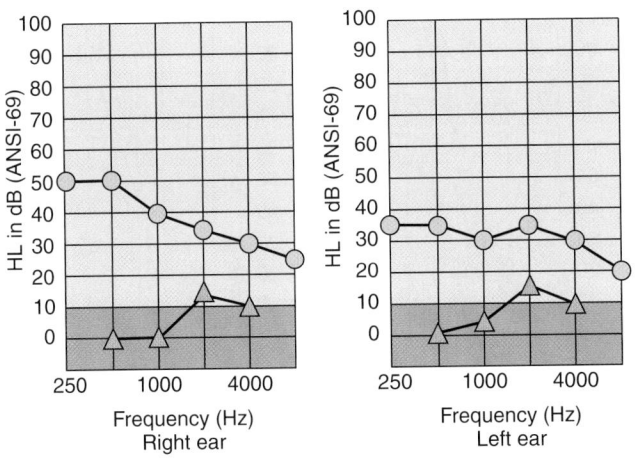

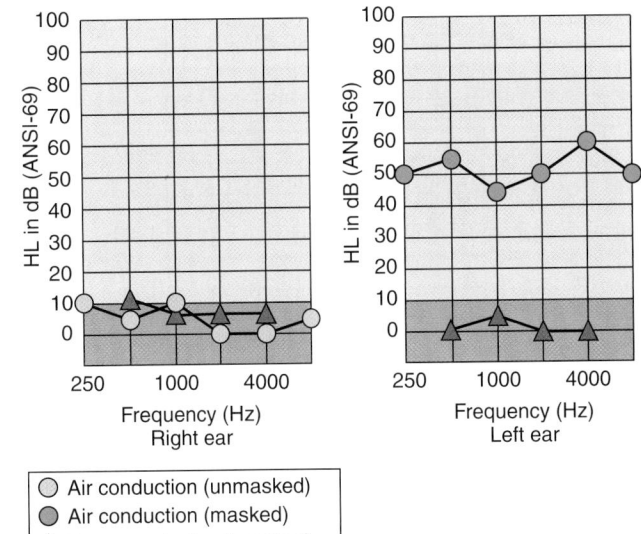

Fig. 59.4 Forty-year-old woman with bilateral otosclerosis. (The corresponding tympanograms would be type A or A_S.) This disorder is autosomal dominantly inherited with about 40% penetrance. *HL*, Hearing loss. (Modified from Jacobsen JT, Northern JL, eds. *Diagnostic Audiology*. Austin, TX: Pro-Ed; 1991.)

Fig. 59.5 Twenty-year-old man with ossicular disruption on the left after mild head trauma. (The corresponding left ear tympanogram would be type A_D.) *HL*, Hearing loss. (Modified from Jacobsen JT, Northern JL, eds. *Diagnostic Audiology*. Austin, TX: Pro-Ed; 1991.)

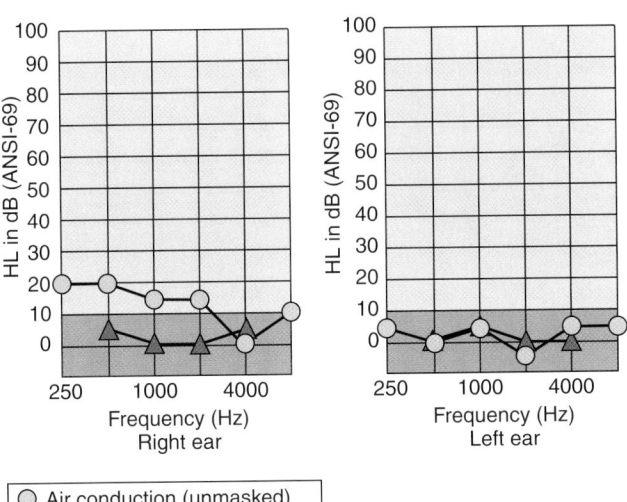

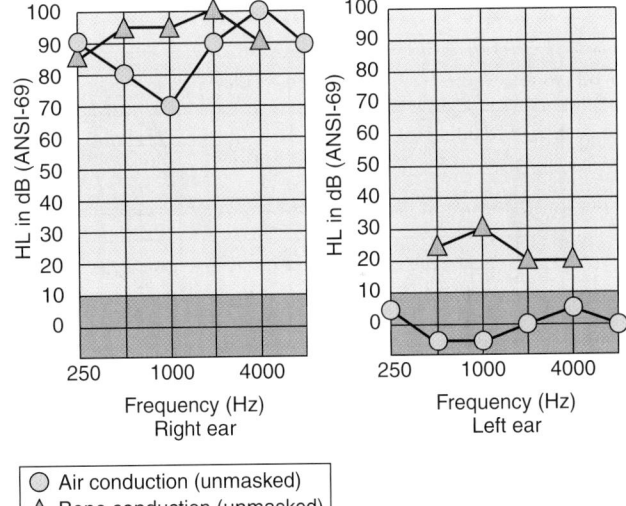

Fig. 59.6 Fifteen-year-old girl with right tympanic membrane perforation. (The corresponding right ear tympanogram would be type B.) *HL*, Hearing loss. (Modified from Jacobsen JT, Northern JL, eds. *Diagnostic Audiology*. Austin, TX: Pro-Ed; 1991.)

Fig. 59.7 Forty-year-old man with suspected functional (factitious) hearing loss *(HL)* after industrial accident with a single exposure to high-intensity noise (e.g., an explosion). Bone conduction should be intact after a single exposure. (The corresponding tympanograms would be type A or normal.) (Modified from Jacobsen JT, Northern JL, eds. *Diagnostic Audiology*. Austin, TX: Pro-Ed; 1991.)

A threshold of up to 15 dB is considered normal. Above that, hearing loss can be divided into degrees of severity (see Table 59.1). Certain patterns of hearing loss, especially unilateral, can indicate specific diseases. Hearing asymmetry of more than 20 dB, especially if it is suspected to be sensorineural in origin, may indicate a retrocochlear lesion or mass (Fig. 59.2). Such patients should be evaluated further with imaging or referred. The tympanometer may be used as an additional tool to assess mobility of the tympanic membrane when conductive hearing loss is

diagnosed by audiometry. Conversely, audiometry is often used as an adjunct to tympanometry when a persistently abnormal tympanogram is present (see Chapter 60, Tympanometry, for more details).

Figs. 59.2 through 59.11 illustrate classic patterns of hearing loss. In the examples, hearing thresholds have been converted to hearing loss. In addition, because each ear was recorded separately, the standardized symbols were not necessary to distinguish left from right.

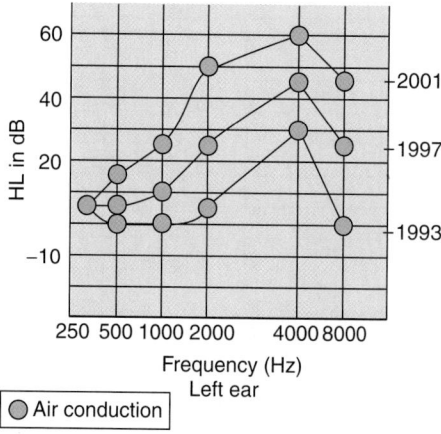

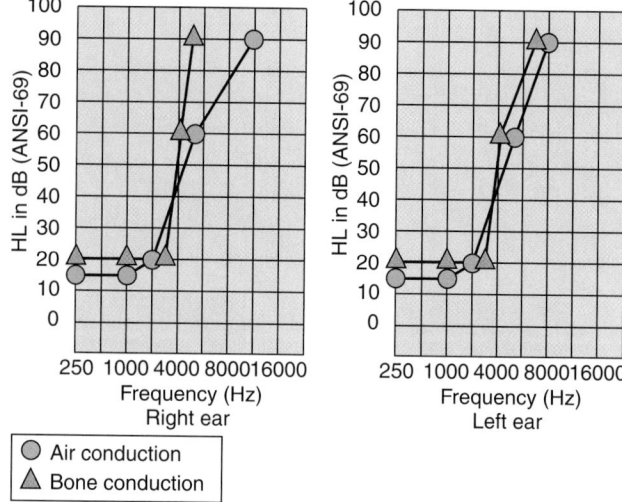

Fig. 59.8 Fifty-five-year-old man with gradually progressive left neurosensory hearing loss *(HL)* over several years. Such a hearing loss can be seen in a person who hunts and shoots left-handed. In most such cases, the audiogram differs from that of presbycusis because it spares the upper frequencies (8000 Hz). (The corresponding tympanogram would be type A or normal.) (Modified from Jacobsen JT, Northern JL, eds. *Diagnostic Audiology*. Austin, TX: Pro-Ed; 1991.)

Fig. 59.9 Eighty-year-old man with presbycusis, or hearing loss *(HL)* caused by advancing age. It is usually bilateral, and in men it often affects the higher frequencies more severely. In women, in addition to symmetric high-frequency loss, there may be hearing loss in the lower frequencies. (The corresponding tympanograms would be type A or normal.) (Modified from Jacobsen JT, Northern JL, eds. *Diagnostic Audiology*. Austin, TX: Pro-Ed; 1991.)

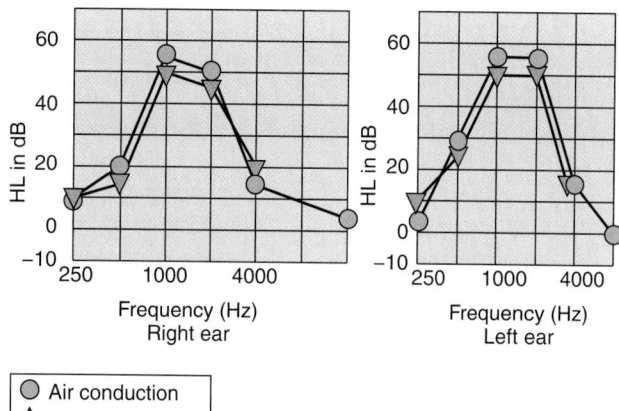

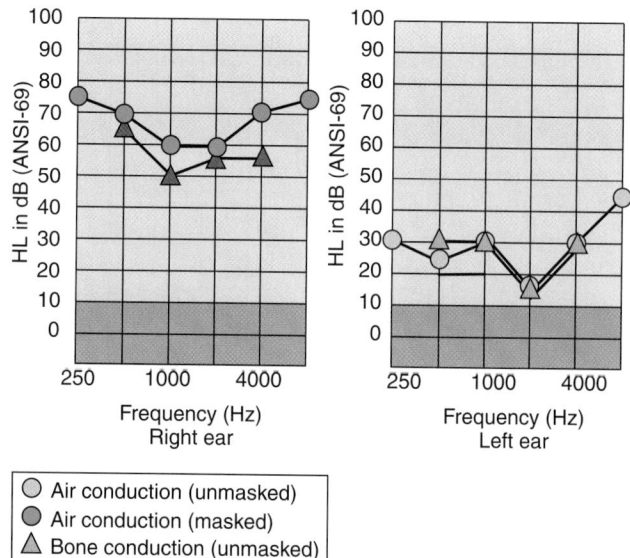

Fig. 59.10 Fifty-year-old woman with long-term exposure to loud occupational noise, which could include loud music. Note the speech frequencies are more affected than the higher frequencies. (The corresponding tympanogram would be type A or normal.) (Modified from Jacobsen JT, Northern JL, eds. *Diagnostic Audiology*. Austin, TX: Pro-Ed; 1991.)

Fig. 59.11 Fifty-two-year-old man with Meniere disease, predominantly affecting right ear. This hearing loss *(HL)* is often associated with episodes of tinnitus and vertigo, frequently at the same time. Remission can occur, as well as exacerbation. Over time, the hearing loss typically progresses to moderate or moderately severe and persistent. (The corresponding tympanograms would be type A or normal.) (Modified from Jacobsen JT, Northern JL, eds. *Diagnostic Audiology*. Austin, TX: Pro-Ed; 1991.)

CPT/Billing Codes

92551   Screening test, pure-tone, air only (e.g., single-decibel-level device with selected frequencies)
92552   Pure-tone audiometry, threshold; air only
92553   Pure-tone audiometry, threshold; air and bone
92555   Speech audiometry, threshold
92556   Speech audiometry, threshold; with speech recognition
92557   Comprehensive audiometry, threshold evaluation and speech recognition (92553 and 92556 combined)

ICD-10-CM Diagnostic Codes

H91.20-H91.23	Hearing loss, sudden, unspecified
H90.0-H90.A32	Hearing loss, conductive and sensorineural hearing loss
H91.0-H91.93	Hearing loss, high or low frequency
H91.90-H91.93	Unspecified hearing loss (deafness NOS)
S04.60-S04.62	Injury acoustic nerve (traumatic deafness)
Z82	Family history of hearing loss
Z01.110-Z01.118	Hearing exam following failed hearing screening
Z01.10	Hearing exam

Acknowledgment

The editors recognize the contributions of Gregory J. Forzley, MD, to this chapter in previous editions of this text.

Suppliers

(See contact information available at www.expertconsult.com.)

Benson Medical Instruments
Castle Group
Gordon Stowe
Grason-Stadler, Inc.
Maico Diagnostics
Micro Audiometrics
Otometrics
Welch Allyn, Inc. (including handheld)

RECOMMENDED READING

American Academy of Family Physicians. American Academy of Otolaryngology-Head and Neck Surgery, American Academy of Pediatrics Subcommittee on Otitis Media with Effusion. Otitis media with effusion [clinical practice guideline]. *Pediatrics.* 2004;113:1412–1429.

American Academy of Pediatrics. Joint Committee on Infant Hearing: year 2007 position statement. Principles and guidelines for early hearing detection and intervention programs. *Pediatrics.* 2007;120:898–921.

American Academy of Pediatrics. Joint Committee on Infant Hearing: supplement to the JCIH 2007 position statement. Principles and guidelines for early intervention after confirmation that a child is deaf or hard of hearing. *Pediatrics.* 2013;131(4):e1324–e1349.

American Speech-Language-Hearing Association. Guidelines for audiometric symbols. *ASHA.* 1990;32(suppl 2):25.

American Speech-Language-Hearing Association. Audiologic Guidelines for the Assessment of Hearing in Infants and Young Children. http://audiologyweb.s3.amazonaws.com/migrated/201208_AudGuideAssessHear_youth.pdf_5399751b249593.36017703.pdf; 2012.

Bagai A, Thavendiranathan P, Detsky AS. Does this patient have hearing impairment? *JAMA.* 2006;295(4):416–428.

Cunningham M, Cox EO. Committee on Practice and Ambulatory Medicine and Section on Otolaryngology and Bronchoesophagology. Hearing assessment in infants and children: recommendations beyond neonatal screening. *Pediatrics.* 2003;111:436–440.

Hall JW, Antonelli PJ. Assessment of peripheral and central auditory function. In: Johnson JT, Rosen CA, eds. *Bailey's Head and Neck Surgery-Otolaryngology.* 5th ed. Philadelphia: Wolters Kluwer Lippincott William & Wilkins; 2014:2275–2290.

Isaacson JE, Vora NM. Differential diagnosis and treatment of hearing loss. *Am Fam Physician.* 2003;68:1125–1132.

Walling AD, Dickson GM. Hearing loss in older adults. *Am Fam Physician.* 2012;85:1150–1156.

CHAPTER 60

TYMPANOMETRY

Gerald A. Amundsen

The tympanometer is a tool that has been used since the 1970s to assist in evaluation of middle ear and eardrum (tympanic membrane) function. Despite the current availability of multiple other tools and measuring instruments, tympanometry, with or without pneumatic otoscopy, continues to be a useful tool in the primary care clinic. Tympanometry has a sensitivity and specificity of 70% to 90% for detection of middle ear fluid in a cooperative patient. The tympanogram, a graphic display of the information obtained from the tympanometer, provides the clinician an ability to objectively evaluate *otitis media with effusion*, *acute otitis media*, suspected or known *perforation of the tympanic membrane*, *patency of pressure equalization tubes* (PE tubes), *ossicular chain function*, and suspected *eustachian tube dysfunction*. When added to the history, clinical signs, and otoscopic findings, a tympanogram usually improves the clinician's diagnostic accuracy as well as his or her ability to monitor treatment.

The tympanometer consists of the probe, which is inserted into the external ear canal, and the associated hardware that produces stimuli (air and sound) to be directed toward the tympanic membrane; it then measures the response, and records the results. The probe has three ports, each of which has an independent function. The speaker port transmits the tone toward the tympanic membrane; the air port transfers air to vary the pressure in the canal. The third port has a microphone to gather sound waves reflected from the tympanic membrane. The remaining components of a tympanometer include the air pump, the oscillator (produces the tone transmitted through the speaker port), a manometer, a recorder, and an impedance bridge to translate information received through the microphone.

Ultimately, the tympanometer evaluates *immittance*, a measurement of the performance of the tympanic membrane and the middle ear. The word *immittance* was coined by combining the words *impedance* and *admittance*. *Admittance* is the term used to describe the flow of energy into the middle ear; *impedance* is the opposition to this flow of energy.

INDICATIONS

- Ear pain, vertigo, or hearing loss
- Evaluate patency of PE tubes
- Abnormalities (e.g., fluid, tympanic membrane retraction) on otoscopic or pneumatic otoscopic examination
- Possible tympanic membrane perforation (or to follow-up previously diagnosed perforation)
- Suspected eustachian tube dysfunction when the tympanic membrane appears normal on examination
- Persistent middle ear effusion or otitis media with effusion

CONTRAINDICATIONS

- Fulminant otitis externa
- Occlusion of the canal by cerumen (see Chapter 62, Cerumen Impaction Removal) or a foreign body (see Chapter 204, Removal of Foreign Bodies from the Ear and Nose)
- Age younger than 7 months (relative contraindication)

NOTE: Age younger than 7 months is a relative contraindication because although a positive result (type B curve) likely indicates an effusion, a negative result may be falsely negative. Even in the presence of a significant effusion, the soft, highly compliant ear canals in infants may result in a normal tympanogram.

EQUIPMENT

- Probe covers of various sizes to create a good seal in ear canals of different sizes (universal to all models).
- A tympanometer with air pressure range of −400 to +100 mm H_2O is preferable. Air pressure is also measured in decapascals (daPa; 1.0 daPa = 1.02 mm H_2O).
- Oscillator in tympanometer that produces a tone of 226 cycles per second (hertz [Hz]; 220 Hz is actually optimal).
- Most units, even the handheld units, have some version of a printer for documentation.
- (*Optional*) Memory (may store data from one or more patients, with one or two tests per patient).
- Units range from handheld models to more expensive models equipped with a graphic acoustic reflex display or the instrumentation to perform audiometry. Although the basic tympanometer is a generally affordable tool for the office, these other features can increase the cost of equipment.

PREPROCEDURE PATIENT PREPARATION

After educating the patient about the indication(s) for the procedure, reassure him or her that the process is painless. Describe the tone that may be heard and the slight bursts of air that will be felt in the canal. Emphasize the importance of remaining still during the test to ensure accuracy and ease of data collection.

TECHNIQUE

1. Check the ear canal for patency and visualize the tympanic membrane with the otoscope. At this point, the use of pneumatic otoscopy may improve diagnostic accuracy.
2. Select the probe tip; choose the size that occludes the canal and creates a seal without entering too deeply.
3. Place the patient upright in the seated position, or in the lap of a parent in the case of a young child.
4. Apply posterior-superior traction to the helix to straighten the ear canal (posterior-inferior traction in the young child), and place the probe into the outer canal (Fig. 60.1).
5. Once a seal has been obtained, the tympanometer will automatically deliver the sound, vary the air pressures, and record the various parameters.

COMMON ERRORS

- Failure to remove cerumen impaction or a foreign body leads to false-positive results (type B curves) or inability to complete the test owing to "occlusion."
- Inappropriate probe tip size leads to "occlusion" or "air leak."

NOTE: Typical devices display results on a graphic screen when a test is successfully completed. Error messages such as "occlusion" or "leak" indicate the need for repositioning the probe or selection of a more appropriate tip size. The test will usually not run to completion unless occlusions in the canal have been removed and an appropriate seal has been achieved and maintained.

INTERPRETATION

The tympanogram is a graph of middle ear compliance on the vertical axis and pressure on the horizontal axis. From this graph, four useful pieces of information can be obtained for interpretation (Fig. 60.2 and Table 60.1):

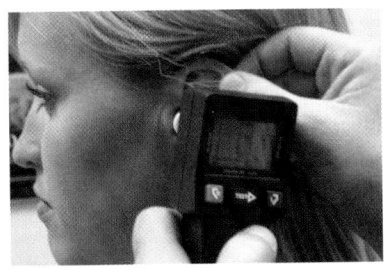

Fig. 60.1 With the patient seated upright, apply traction to the helix and insert the probe.

- **Canal volume** is a measurement of the approximate volume between the probe tip and the tympanic membrane. It is usually 0.2 to 2.0 mL, but varies with age and bony structure. Abnormally high volume is indicative of a patent PE tube or a perforation. Abnormally low volume may indicate obstruction or a bulging tympanic membrane due to effusion.
- **Compliance** of the tympanic membrane when receiving sound at various pressures. The peak of the curve (maximal compliance) typically occurs when the air pressure is equal on both sides of the tympanic membrane (0 mm H_2O or daPa).
- **Pressure** (mm H_2O or daPa) at which the compliance peaks: usually 0 mm H_2O, but may be negative with eustachian tube dysfunction or a retracted tympanic membrane, or greater than 0 mm H_2O or daPa when the membrane is bulging.
- **Width of the curve** is calculated by the device. This may be too wide with early or resolving effusion or tympanosclerosis. This is the least useful portion of the data because the result is quite variable and the diagnostic reliability for middle ear pathology is uncertain.

It should be noted that a localized abnormality (e.g., perforation of the tympanic membrane) may obscure the ability to evaluate the rest of the middle ear system. However, compared with pneumatic otoscopy, the tympanogram is usually more accurate; pneumatic otoscopy may elicit movement of a tympanic membrane despite a pinpoint perforation, whereas a tympanogram will likely make the correct diagnosis. In contrast, middle ear mucosal edema may be sufficient to mask even a large perforation on a tympanogram.

POSTPROCEDURE PATIENT EDUCATION

The tympanogram is used to help direct treatment and monitor progress. The patient should be informed of the result and treatment plan. Appropriate consultation should be requested when indicated.

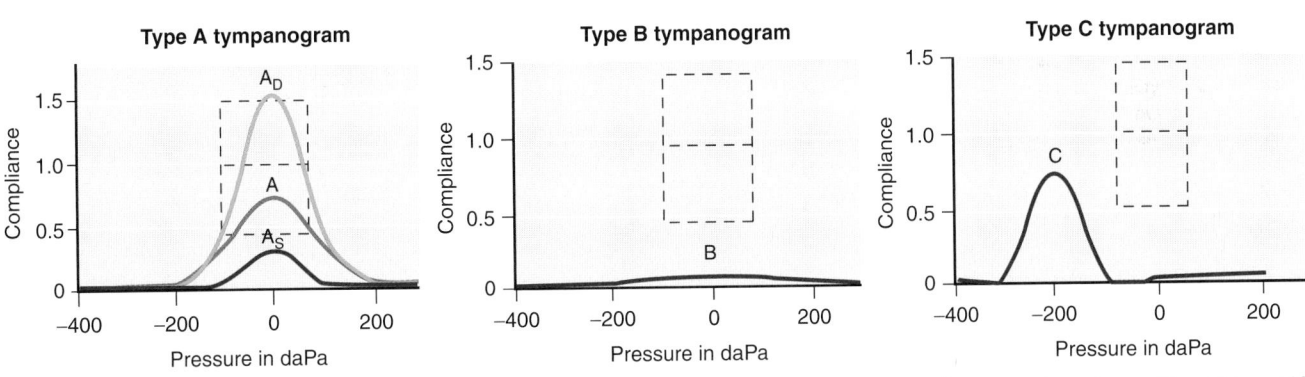

Fig. 60.2 Tympanograms. Compliance and pressure are normal for adults if the curve crosses into the rectangles at any point and normal for children <10 years if the curve crosses into the lower rectangle. See Table 60.1 for interpretation.

TABLE 60.1	Interpretation of the Tympanogram	
Tympanogram Result	**Characteristics**	**Possible Diagnoses**
Type A	The "normal" curve Peak compliance is at 0 mm H_2O or daPa	Normal or negative tympanogram
Type A_D	Tall (deep) peak at 0 mm H_2O or daPa indicating high compliance	Monomeric (one layer) tympanic membrane due to healing perforation, disruption of the ossicular chain
Type A_S	Short (shallow) peak at 0 mm H_2O or daPa indicating low compliance	Thickened tympanic membrane, ossicular fixation, presence of middle ear fluid
Type B	Flat or minimal peak indicating minimal compliance	*With low canal volume:* cerumen impaction, foreign body, wrong probe *With high canal volume:* pressure equalization tubes, perforation *With normal canal volume:* middle ear fluid
Type C	Peak compliance at negative pressure (<−100 mm H_2O or daPa)	Retracted membrane, eustachian tube dysfunction with or without effusion

Adults with new onset unilateral, recurrent (more than 2 episodes per year) acute otitis media or persistent (>6 weeks) otitis media with effusion should be evaluated further or referred to an otolaryngologist to rule out the rare obstruction due to nasopharyngeal carcinoma.

CPT/BILLING CODES

92567   Tympanometry (impedance testing)

ICD-10-CM DIAGNOSTIC CODES

H61.20–H61.23	Cerumen impaction
H65.00–H65.07	Acute serous otitis media
H65.20–H65.23	Chronic serous otitis media ✕
H66.00–H66.009	Acute suppurative otitis media w/o rupture
H66.011–H66.019	Acute suppurative otitis media w/rupture
H65.111–H65.119	Acute and subacute allergic otitis media
H65.191–H65.199	Other acute nonsuppurative otitis media
H72.0–H72.93	Perforation tympanic membrane
H73.811–H73.899	Disorder tympanic membrane
H92.01–H92.09	Otalgia
S09.20XX–S09.22XX	Perforation: traumatic

Use appropriate seventh character: A = initial, D = subsequent encounter, S = sequela.

Acknowledgment

The editors recognize the contributions of Gregory J. Forzley, MD, to this chapter in previous editions of this text.

SUPPLIERS

(See contact information available at www.expertconsult.com.)

Tympanometers
Gordon Stowe (www.gordonstowe.com)
Grason-Stadler, Inc. (www.grason-stadler.com)
Maico Diagnostics (www.maico-diagnostics.com/us/)
Micro Audiometrics (www.microaud.com)
Otometrics (www.otometrics.com)
Welch Allyn, Inc. (www.welchallyn.com)

RECOMMENDED READING

American Academy of Family Physicians. American Academy of Otolaryngology-Head and Neck Surgery; American Academy of Pediatrics Subcommittee on Otitis Media with Effusion. Otitis media with effusion [clinical practice guideline]. *Pediatrics.* 2004;113:1412–1429.

Green LA, Culpepper L, de Melker RA, et al. Tympanometry interpretation by primary care physicians: a report from the International Primary Care Network (IPCN) and the Ambulatory Sentinel Practice Network (ASPN). *J Fam Pract.* 2000;49:932–936.

Hall JW, Antonelli PJ. Assessment of Peripheral and Central Auditory Function. In: Johnson JT, Rosen CA, eds. *Head and Neck Surgery-Otolaryngology.* 5th ed. Philadelphia: Wolters Kluwer Lippincott William & Wilkins; 2014:2275–2290.

Harmes KM, Blackwood RA, Burrows HL, Cooke JM, Van Harrison R, Passamani PP. Otitis media: diagnosis and treatment. *Am Fam Physician.* 2013;88(7):435–440.

Onusko E. Tympanometry. *Am Fam Physician.* 2004;70(9):1713–1720.

CHAPTER 61

TYMPANOCENTESIS AND MYRINGOTOMY

Mark S. Grubb

Tympanocentesis is a puncture of the tympanic membrane performed with a hollow needle to aspirate fluid for diagnostic or therapeutic purposes. A myringotomy is an incision in the tympanic membrane made with a myringotomy knife. Ventilation of the middle ear space by either method instantly relieves pain and pressure associated with acute otitis media. Culture of middle ear aspirate establishes disease etiology and enables precisely targeted antibiotic therapy. Tympanocentesis or myringotomy can also relieve discomfort and hearing loss associated with chronic middle ear effusions.

At this time, myringotomy is performed almost exclusively during tympanostomy tube insertion, for which the patient is under general anesthesia. Tympanocentesis is the more suitable procedure for primary care settings. Needle puncture of the tympanic membrane is easy to accomplish, requires only local anesthesia, poses less risk than a myringotomy incision, and permits drainage for up to 5 days.

The ear that would benefit from tympanocentesis will have fluid behind the tympanic membrane, and the membrane will have either a bulging or retracted appearance resulting from positive or negative pressure in the middle ear space. Despite this distorted appearance, the location of the umbo and the orientation of the manubrium usually remain discernible. Tympanocentesis is performed on the inferior half of the membrane at the location of maximal bulge, usually in the anterior quadrant. The puncture or incision should be performed nearer to the tip of the manubrium than to the fibrous annulus. Do not perform the procedure on the fibrous annulus, over the incus or stapes, or directly over the round window (Fig. 61.1).

INDICATIONS

Tympanocentesis

- Immediate relief of pain and pressure associated with acute otitis media
- Aspiration of middle ear fluid for culture to target antibiotic therapy
- Adjunct to watchful waiting for acute otitis media; tympanocentesis relieves symptoms and promotes therapeutic drainage during the observation period, and enables accurate drug selection for patients who remain symptomatic after 48 hours
- Persistent acute otitis media or in episodes that have failed to respond to antibiotic therapy
- Otitis media in immunocompromised patients or those with multiple antibiotic allergies
- Complicated otitis media such as that associated with unusually severe pain, signs of toxicity, facial nerve palsy, mastoiditis, meningitis, encephalitis, brain abscess, or dural sinus thrombosis
- Alleviation of conductive hearing loss or discomfort associated with chronic serous otitis media
- Alternative therapy for patients who wish to avoid antibiotics

Myringotomy

- Immediate relief of pain and pressure associated with acute otitis media
- Placement of tympanostomy tubes

EDITOR'S NOTE: it should be noted that myringotomy or tympanocentesis may be helpful to relieve pain or to obtain samples for culture; however, there is no advantage in duration of effusion or risk of recurrence of acute otitis media.

CONTRAINDICATIONS

- Known anomalous positioning of the jugular bulb
- Cochlear implant
- Tympanostomy tubes (intact)
- Acute otitis externa (relative contraindication)
- Uncooperative patient (relative contraindication)
- Obscure landmarks (consider referral to otolaryngologist)

EQUIPMENT

- Local anesthesia: 0.5 mL of 8% tetracaine otic solution, eyedropper
- Cotton balls
- Hydrogen peroxide 3%
- Tissue wicks
- Procedural restraint board or other patient restraint (as needed)
- Tympanocentesis
  - CDT (channel directed tympanocentesis) speculum method: A CDT (Walls Precision Instruments) 3- or 5-mm speculum and aspirator bulb, and an otoscope with pneumatic, diagnostic, or operating head. The CDT instrument has a protected needle and other safety features enabling safe completion of the procedure without restraints for most patients (Fig. 61.2).
  - Tympanocentesis collector method: A 3-inch 20- or 21-gauge spinal needle with a tympanocentesis aspirator attached, a second aspirator with flexible tubing, an otoscope with operating head, and a vacuum pump or wall suction (Fig. 61.3). Note the need for positional restraint.
  - Syringe method: A 3-inch 20- or 21-gauge spinal needle bent at the hub to about 60 degrees, a 3-mL syringe, and an otoscope with operating head (Fig. 61.4).
- Myringotomy
  - Myringotomy knife, an otoscope with operating head (Fig. 61.5).
  - Aspiration after myringotomy will require a vacuum pump, and either an aspirator or a Baron suction tube combined with an inline suction trap.

NOTE: In all instances where an operating otoscope head is used, the clinician may elect to move the lens of the otoscope out of the field of view and use a head-mounted portable binocular microscope instead.

PREPROCEDURE PATIENT EDUCATION AND FORMS

Explain the indications, the procedure, risks of the procedure, options for procedural anesthesia, and available alternative therapies. The patient should be warned that working near the tympanic membrane can be noisy. Unless conscious sedation is used, they should also be aware that they will experience some discomfort. Obtain signed informed consent and document it in the patient's chart.

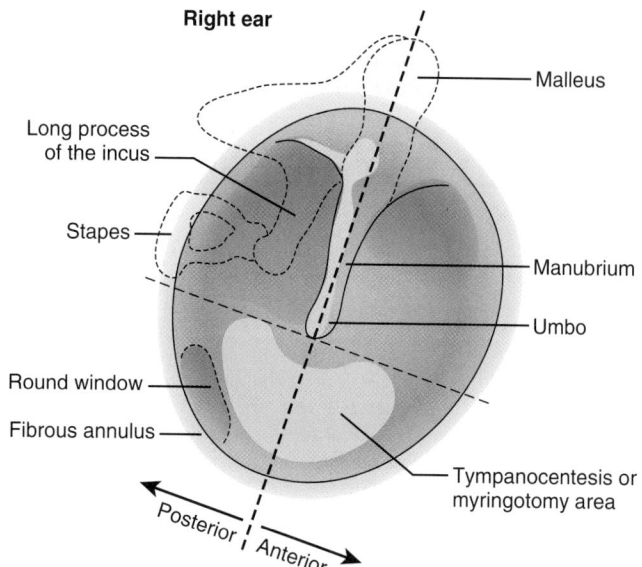

Right ear

Malleus

Long process
of the incus

Stapes

Manubrium

Umbo

Round window

Fibrous annulus

Tympanocentesis or
myringotomy area

Posterior | Anterior

Fig. 61.1 Tympanic membrane of the right ear. (Courtesy David Spaugh.)

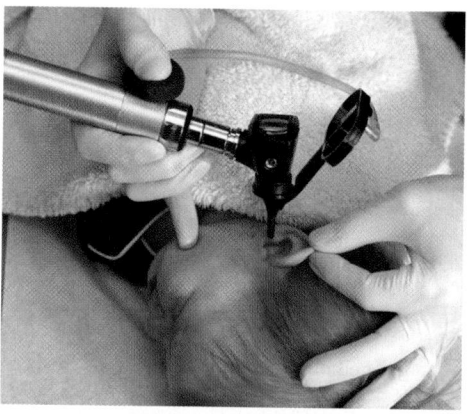

Fig. 61.2 Tympanocentesis with channel directed tympanocentesis (CDT) speculum and CDT aspirator bulb. No procedural positioner is used.

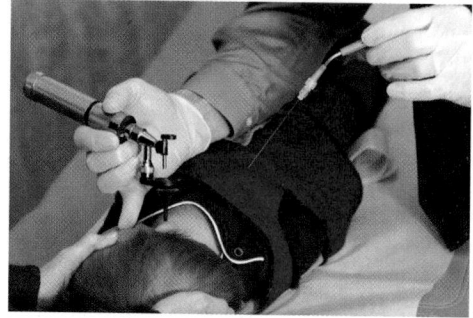

Fig. 61.3 Tympanocentesis with aspirator attached to vacuum pump. Note the procedural restraint.

TECHNIQUE

Tympanocentesis

1. Remove any cerumen from the canal (see Chapter 62, Cerumen Impaction Removal).
2. Initiate the desired preprocedure anesthesia or analgesia. The methods most frequently used are the following:
   - 8% tetracaine otic solution applied topically to the membrane, held in place for 15 minutes with a cotton dam or wick

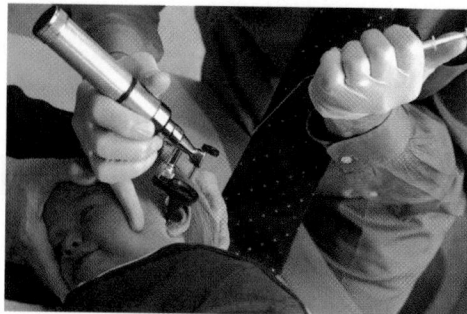

Fig. 61.4 Tympanocentesis with spinal needle attached to 3-mL syringe.

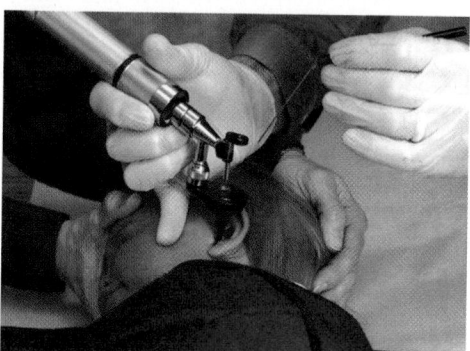

Fig. 61.5 Myringotomy with disposable myringotomy knife.

   - Acetaminophen with codeine, given orally 30 minutes before the procedure
   - Midazolam (requires training in conscious sedation; see Chapter 1, Procedural Sedation and Analgesia) or pediatric sedation (see Chapter 2, Pediatric Sedation)

NOTE: Topical anesthetic solutions are typically bacteriostatic. If the clinician intends to culture aspirated fluid, excess anesthetic solution must be removed from the external auditory canal before the procedure.

3. Lay the patient in the supine position with head turned to one side. A procedural restraint is usually necessary in a child when the procedure is performed with an unprotected sharp. Use a tissue wick to remove excess anesthetic solution from the canal and membrane.
4. Insert the speculum into the ear canal, and visually determine the point of the intended perforation.
5. Extend the needle 2 mm through the tympanic membrane at the point of maximal bulge in the inferior portion of the tympanic membrane.
6. Aspirate fluid while the tip of the needle is in the middle ear space, as follows:
   - CDT method: Release thumb pressure on the aspirator bulb (see Fig. 61.2).
   - Collector method: Occlude the trap opening with a finger (see Fig. 61.3). An assistant can be helpful with this step. As soon as pus appears in the aspirator trap, release the trap opening. This is the fluid to send for culture. Use the other aspirator with flexible tubing to suction the remaining pus, serosanguinous fluid, and debris from the external auditory canal.
   - Syringe method: Retract the syringe plunger with the thumb (see Fig. 61.4).
7. Retract the needle and then the speculum from the patient's ear.
8. Irrigate the canal with 3% hydrogen peroxide solution and remove excess fluid with a tissue wick.
9. Send the aspirated fluid for culture and sensitivity if desired.

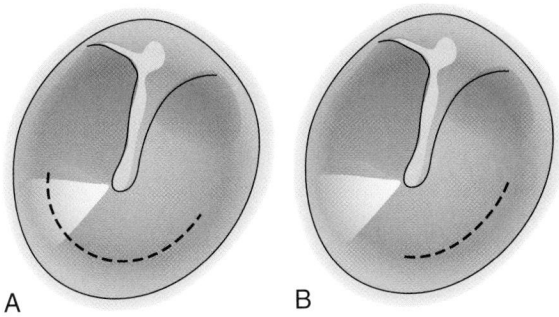

Fig. 61.6 Locations for myringotomy. A tympanocentesis could precede either of these myringotomy incisions in the same location. (A) Wide myringotomy incision through the tympanic membrane might be used in patient with refractory purulent otitis media or for prolonged drainage of pus if necessary. (B) More limited myringotomy incision.

Myringotomy

1. The steps for office myringotomy are essentially the same as for tympanocentesis, except a myringotomy knife is used to make a curved incision in the tympanic membrane (see Fig. 61.5). A myringotomy may be preceded by tympanocentesis in the same location (Fig. 61.6).
2. If aspiration is to accompany myringotomy, it is accomplished by reentering the myringotomy incision with aspiration equipment before removing the speculum from the patient's ear. (If fluid is sent for culture, this would be the method to obtain it. Postprocedure aspiration of exudate directly from the canal is not recommended for culture because the aspirate may be contaminated by canal flora.)
3. Do not irrigate the ear canal or use peroxide-saturated wicks after myringotomy.
4. Other than applying topical antibiotic solutions, the ear canal should be kept dry for 5 days after myringotomy.

COMPLICATIONS

Potential complications include chronic perforation, bleeding, puncture of abnormally positioned bulb of jugular vein, a scar on the tympanic membrane, damage to facial nerve or oval window, disruption of the ossicles, or hearing loss (especially if using a method with unrestricted needle traverse). Authors of the current medical literature and those who use tympanocentesis in clinical settings describe a zero incidence for these complications.

POSTPROCEDURE MANAGEMENT

Tympanocentesis

Purulent or serosanguinous drainage may continue for up to 5 days. Twice-daily cleaning of the external canal with peroxide and tissue wicks will remove residual drainage and prevent external otitis.

Myringotomy

Purulent or serosanguineous drainage may continue for up to 5 days. Peroxide rinse of the external canal is not recommended after myringotomy. Patients should be instructed to keep the ear dry for 5 days after myringotomy, with particular attention to care when bathing or washing hair.

CPT/BILLING CODES

NOTE: Presently, there is no differentiating CPT code for tympanocentesis. The procedure is coded and billed using the myringotomy codes.

69420	Myringotomy including aspiration and/or eustachian tube inflation (also used for tympanocentesis)
69420	LT or 69420.RT (Use LT or RT modifiers for the left or right ear)
69420.50	(Use the .50 modifier for bilateral procedures)
69421	Myringotomy including aspiration and/or eustachian tube inflation requiring general anesthesia

ICD-10-CM DIAGNOSTIC CODES

H61.20–H61.23	Cerumen impaction
H65.00–H65.07	Acute serous otitis media
H65.00–H65.23	Chronic serous otitis media
H66.00–H66.009	Acute suppurative otitis media w/o rupture
H66.011–H66.019	Acute suppurative otitis media w/rupture
H65.111–H65.119	Acute and subacute allergic otitis media
H65.191–H65.199	Other acute nonsuppurative otitis media
H65.41–H65.93	Other chronic nonsuppurative otitis media
H72.0–H72.93	Perforation tympanic membrane
H73.811–H73.899	Disorder tympanic membrane
H92.01–H92.09	Otalgia
T70.0XXX	Otitis media due to barotrauma
T75.89XX	Otitis media due to barotrauma, late effect

Use appropriate seventh character: A = initial, D = subsequent encounter, S = sequela.

SUPPLIERS

CDT (channel directed tympanocentesis) Speculum kits
  Walls Precision Instruments

ONLINE RESOURCES

Treatment of otitis media. www.omew.com/research/tympanocentesis.htm
University of Texas Medical Branch: Acute otitis media. www.utmb.edu/pedi_ed/AOM-Otitis/default.htm
Tympanocentesis in children with acute otitis media. NEJM procedure video, 2011. https://www.nejm.org/doi/full/10.1056/NEJMvcm0706756

RECOMMENDED READING

Brook I. Tympanocentesis in the diagnosis and treatment of otitis media. *Infect Med.* 2001;18:363–366.
Casselbrant ML, Mandel EM. Otitis media in the age of antimicrobial resistance. In: Johnson JT, Rosen CA, eds. *Bailey's Head and Neck Surgery-Otolaryngology.* 5th ed. Philadelphia: Wolters Kluwer Lippincott William & Wilkins; 2014:1479–1506.
Dudley JP. Making tympanocentesis easier. *J Emerg Med.* 1990;8:765–767.
Hoberman A, Paradise JL, Wald ER. Tympanocentesis technique revisited. *Pediatr Infect Dis J.* 1997;16(suppl 2):S25–S26.
Jones PJ. Tympanocentesis. In: Reichman EF, ed. *Emergency Medicine Procedures.* 2nd ed. New York: McGraw-Hill; 2013:1075–1078.
Lieberthal AS, Carroll AE, Chonmaitree T, et al. The diagnosis and management of acute otitis media. *Pediatrics.* 2013;131(3):e964–e999.
Pichichero ME, Wright T. The use of tympanocentesis in the diagnosis and management of acute otitis media. *Curr Infect Dis Rep.* 2006;8:189–195.

CHAPTER 62

CERUMEN IMPACTION REMOVAL

Michael McHenry

Cerumen impaction is one of the most common otologic problems encountered by primary care clinicians (approximately 150,000 ears are irrigated per week in the United States to remove cerumen). Cerumen is produced by ceruminous glands in the lateral two-thirds of the external auditory canal and pilosebaceous glands at the roots of hairs, and is mixed with sloughed squamous epithelial cells. It is a naturally occurring lubricant, is somewhat water repellent, and has antimicrobial activity; therefore it is a protectant of the external auditory canal. The predominant form is a wet, sticky, honey-colored wax that can darken. A dry, scaly form also occurs in some patients. Normally cerumen is carried from inside the canal to outside by tiny cilia, an activity that is enhanced by chewing movements. Accumulation of cerumen can cause symptoms such as decreased hearing, tinnitus, vertigo, infection, or a sensation of increased pressure. The hearing loss is usually quite sudden when the cerumen seals off the canal; it is often described by the patient as a "blocked ear." Accumulation is common in elderly patients, in developmentally delayed individuals, and in patients working in dusty environments. Patients often do a poor job of removing cerumen with cotton-tipped swabs, other instruments, or over-the-counter preparations, leaving the clinician to complete the procedure. In fact, overzealous use of these applicators frequently disrupts the natural ciliary cleaning process. For removal by the clinician, topical anesthesia may be desired; foreign bodies may also need to be removed. (See Chapter 204, Removal of Foreign Bodies from the Ear and Nose, which also describes a technique for injecting anesthetic for external canal field block.) The overall goal of this procedure is to remove cerumen under direct visualization or by irrigation without causing injury. The risk of injury is not to be taken lightly because ear irrigation is one of the more common causes of iatrogenic injuries treated by otolaryngologists. Asymptomatic cerumen buildup does not require removal; in fact, most people do not need a regular schedule for prevention of ear wax. Rather, only patients at risk for impaction (e.g., prior or recurrent impaction) should be taught how to perform his or her own ear irrigation to clean the ears. They can then keep them clean by following a home self-irrigation maintenance schedule, usually several times a year following an overnight application of a ceruminolytic. There is some data that mere use of a ceruminolytic on a regular basis may also prevent cerumen impaction.

While using ceruminolytic drops appears better than no treatment (drops prior to irrigation may improve success rate by as much as 97%), there is a lack of evidence regarding which ceruminolytic is superior. Many studies comparing different agents are surprisingly comparable in their outcomes regarding effectiveness. This may explain why irrigation is so frequently successful; any ceruminolytic may be helpful. Most authors recommend waiting at least 15 minutes after the application of drops before attempting to remove cerumen. Hydrogen peroxide is commonly used, but has not been studied extensively. The liquid stool softener docusate sodium in some studies was more effective than commercially available ceruminolytics. A 5% or 10% solution of sodium bicarbonate was also found to be more effective than commercially prepared ceruminolytics. (The sodium bicarbonate solution can be made at home by dissolving ¼ teaspoon sodium bicarbonate [baking soda] in 10 mL of water.) Triethanolamine is one available commercial preparation. Olive oil has also been used to some effect. If nothing else is available, even water or saline are effective at cerumen softening and disintegration.

NOTE: Hollow ear candles have been found ineffective; in fact, ear candling can cause serious damage to the ear canal or tympanic membrane.

INDICATIONS

Recently the term "impacted" has been defined more clearly as cerumen that causes patient symptoms or prevents a necessary examination.

- Tympanic membrane or ear canal obscured by cerumen with otologic complaint
- Patient complaint of decreased hearing ("blocked ear"), fullness, itching, odor, discharge, otalgia, tinnitus, vertigo, reflex cough, unsteady gait associated with cerumen, or problems with hearing aid (cerumen can damage hearing aids or cause feedback sound)
- External otitis associated with cerumen (the ear should be dried meticulously after the procedure)
- Tympanic membrane or ear canal obscured by cerumen and clinician needs to examine or patient needs hearing tested
- Patient with cerumen buildup who may not be able to complain about symptoms such as young children or cognitively impaired individuals

CONTRAINDICATIONS

- Uncooperative patient or infant who cannot be adequately restrained.
- Clinician unfamiliar with or unable to define anatomy of the external auditory canal.
- Patient with distorted anatomy (e.g., prior or current injury obscuring normal anatomy, neoplasm of ear canal), although this is a relative contraindication.
- Previous ear surgery with resultant scarring, tympanoplasty/myringoplasty, or radiation therapy to the head and neck, both resulting in increased risk of perforation (relative contraindication).
- Known or suspected cholesteatoma.
- The affected ear is the only hearing ear (relative contraindication, but referral should be considered).
- Consideration should be made to refer patients with diabetes, an immunocompromised state, or on anticoagulation therapy or with a coagulopathy who also have any of the other contraindications listed above.
- For irrigation, acute otitis media, known/suspected perforation of the tympanic membrane, or presence of tympanostomy tube is a contraindication. In these situations, the curette or suction catheter should be used under direct visualization.

EQUIPMENT

- Equipment necessary for clinician to observe universal blood and body fluid precautions (gloves, mask, goggles)
- Ear curette
  - Metal: rigid, Buck, Shapleigh, or Yankauer; flexible, Billeau flexible earloop
  - Plastic: Flex-loop ear curette, disposable ear curette, or infant ear scoop
- Otoscope with moveable posterior lens or shield, or ear speculum and light source
- Ear forceps
- Ball-tipped ear hook
- Local anesthetic solution or suspension (e.g., lidocaine solution, viscous lidocaine, antipyrine/benzocaine)
- For suction: Various ear suction catheters with suction source (Fig. 62.1)
- For irrigation
  - Ear syringe (large stainless steel syringe with irrigant deflector), or a commercially available jet irrigator (on "ENT table units," or an oral Waterpik), or a 22-gauge butterfly intravenous catheter tubing (with needle and butterfly removed) and a 20- to 50-mL syringe. An 18-gauge Angiocath type IV catheter can also be used with a syringe.
  - Lukewarm tap water ("lukewarm" is confirmed when a drop placed on the inner forearm of the examiner is comfortable, similar to testing baby formula)
  - Towels, Chux, or plastic drape
  - Cotton gauze strip
  - Emesis or ear basin to collect irrigant
  - Ceruminolytic (see discussion above for choice of ceruminolytic)

PREPROCEDURE PATIENT PREPARATION

- For curette and suction removal, discuss the chance of perforation and minor trauma to the ear canal associated with pain.
- For irrigation removal, discuss the risk of perforation and potential dizziness during the irrigation. Local discomfort may also be experienced, especially when the ear syringe is used.
- Stress the importance of remaining still during the procedure.
- The patient should expect to hear occasional loud noises while the clinician is working in the ear, especially if suction is used.
- Patients should be aware that firmly adherent cerumen frequently tears the skin lining the ear canal when removed, regardless of the technique used. As a result, there may be some bleeding. Slight bleeding does not indicate perforation. There is also a slightly increased risk of external otitis after cerumen removal. For both reasons, antibiotic ear drops are frequently prescribed.

TECHNIQUE

The clinician should follow universal blood and body fluid precautions when performing these procedures.

Curette or Suction Technique

A curette is usually the fastest way to remove cerumen and may be preferred for small amounts of easily visible and reachable wax. It is also usually the easiest method for children, who may find it difficult to remain still for suction or irrigation. In adults, suction can be used for deeper or slightly more adherent impactions. Suction works best for multiple tiny fragments or for soft cerumen; it often fails when there is a single, hard, irregular, and impacted cerumen plug. Young children are often frightened by the noise suction makes. For children and adults, irrigation will be necessary for dense, adherent, or circumferential impactions.

1. Seat the patient on the examination table. If available, a neck rest, such as those on a dental or otolaryngology (ears, nose, throat [ENT]) chair, may help adults remain immobile. Children often tolerate the procedure better if held securely or swaddled with a sheet in a parent's lap or, if supine, with the parent or assistant stabilizing the head. A positional restraint board may be helpful.
2. Using the otoscope, first visualize the opposite canal to become familiar with the patient's anatomy. Next, visualize the cerumen in the affected canal by applying traction on the helix as necessary. In adults, traction is usually applied posteriorly and upward on the pinna while simultaneously pulling it slightly out from the head. In the small child, the pinna is pulled down, back, and slightly out from the head. Five to 10 mL of local anesthetic instilled in the ear will usually result in increased patient comfort for the duration of the procedure; however, it may obscure the canal briefly, so sometimes it is better just to remove the cerumen.
3. Using the selected curette, ear hook, or suction catheter, reach through the partially open magnifying posterior lens of the otoscope and gently remove the impacted cerumen. Take care to avoid traumatizing the bony ear canal. Work either through the scope (Fig. 62.2A) or, after identifying the location of the cerumen, by direct visualization (Fig. 62.2B).

   NOTE: The clinician's hand should be stabilized by remaining firmly in contact with the patient's head at all times. This should minimize the risk of scraping the wall of the external canal or perforating the tympanic membrane. Even the most cooperative patient may move involuntarily because of a stimulated vagal nerve cough reflex.

4. If hard wax is encountered, installation of 8 to 10 drops of ceruminolytic (e.g., 3% hydrogen peroxide, docusate sodium, or 5% to 10% sodium bicarbonate) for at least 15 minutes should facilitate removal. For wax adherent to the tympanic membrane,

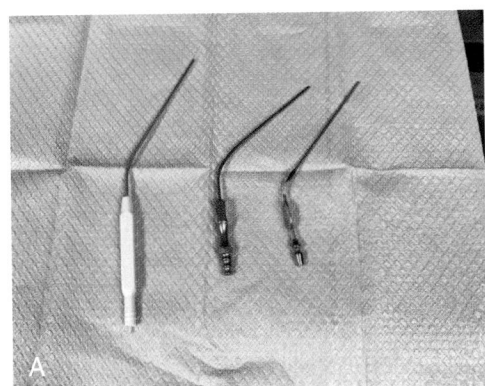 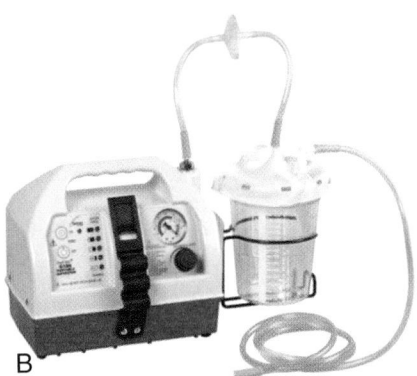

Fig. 62.1 Suction catheters (including Frazier) (A) and basic suction pump (B) can assist in managing ear canal obstruction.

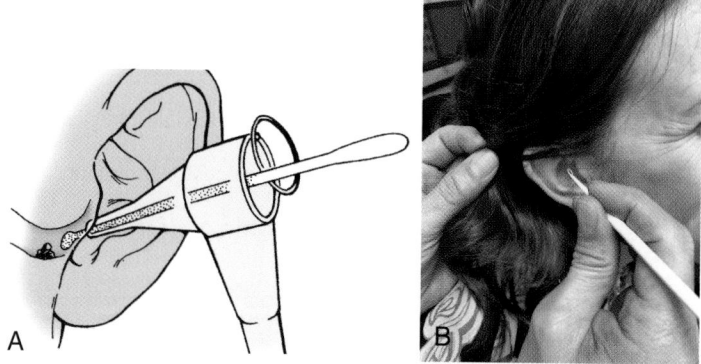

Fig. 62.2 (A) Removal through the otoscope. (B) Foreign bodies or cerumen in the ear canal can often be removed with direct visualization after careful, magnified, otoscopic examination is completed. Notice how the patient's head is supported and the clinician's hand rests on the patient's face.

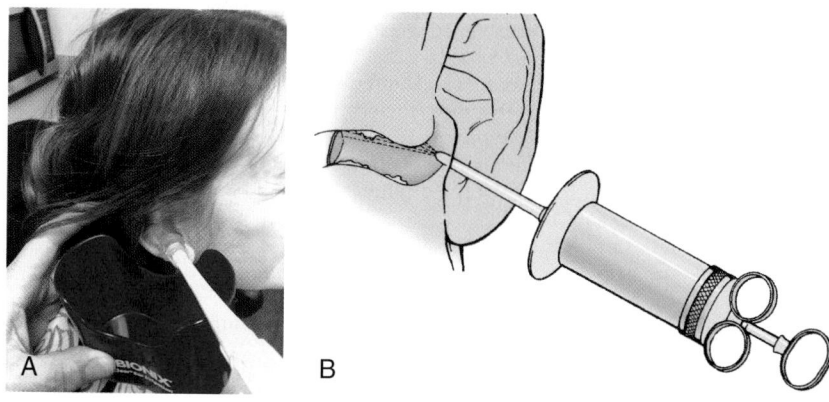

Fig. 62.3 Typical ear canal irrigation setup. The water should be at body temperature. Patients often feel reassured when allowed to help hold the basin (A). The initial stream should be directed toward the superior aspect of the canal (B). Cover the upper torso with a splash bib.

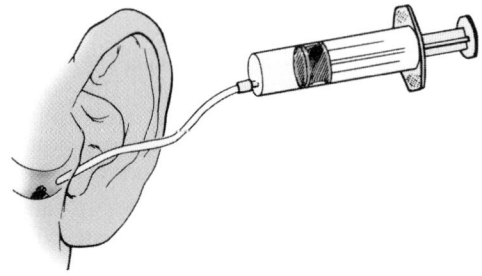

Fig. 62.4 Alternative irrigation setup. Use an 18-gauge plastic intravenous catheter or butterfly tubing with needle and butterfly removed.

irrigation or suction may be necessary. Suction catheters (see Fig. 62.1) are quite loud when used in the external canal, so if suction is used, the patient should be warned and instructed not to pull away from the noise.

5. Firmly adherent cerumen frequently tears epithelium as it is removed. Consider prescribing topical otic antibiotics afterward if epithelium is disrupted.

Irrigation Technique

The irrigation technique (Figs. 62.3 to 62.5) takes longer than the curette or suction technique. However, irrigation rarely fails; it is also the safest technique. While irrigation is the technique used most often by nonotolaryngologists, it is often used when other techniques have failed or caused pain.

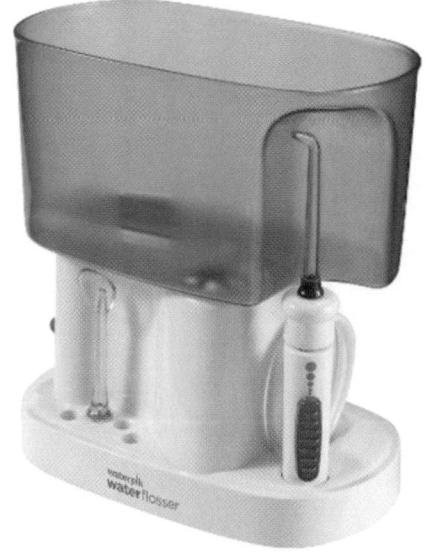

Fig. 62.5 Waterpik oral cleaning system (not marketed by the company for cerumen impaction removal). (Courtesy Waterpik, Inc., Fort Collins, CO.)

1. Fill the irrigator (syringe) with body temperature tap water. Using water at this temperature reduces the chance for stimulation of the vestibular reflex which could cause nystagmus and nausea. Test the water temperature by placing a drop on the inner forearm of the examiner. It should feel neither warm nor cold to touch.

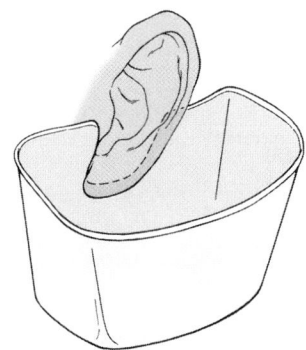

Fig. 62.6 Basin cup that fits under ear.

NOTE: If the jet irrigator (e.g., Waterpik) is used, adjust the pressure to the lowest setting to reduce the risk of perforation or acoustic trauma. Even at low pressures, jet irrigators have been known to rupture the tympanic membrane; therefore some experts no longer recommend use of jet irrigators for cerumen removal. If a jet irrigator is used, the clinician may want to use a "safe" irrigation tip (see Suppliers section).

2. Protect the patient and prepare to collect excess water with a towel, Chux, or plastic sheet.
3. Have the patient tilt his or her head to the side being irrigated, and hold the ear basin (Fig. 62.6) below the patient's earlobe. Patients often feel reassured when allowed to help and hold the basin. Advise the patient not to pull his or her head away from the irrigating tip.
4. Using the selected device, direct the water jet superiorly toward the occiput, allowing space for the return of the water and cerumen. Directed in this manner, water circulates first above and behind the cerumen, and then it pushes the cerumen out of the ear. The irrigation should not be directed onto the tympanic membrane. No irrigation device should be inserted more than 1 cm into the canal.
   - If the ear syringe is used, fairly vigorous force may be needed. The use of large (25- to 50-mL) syringes prevents excessive pressure. Be sure that air bubbles are removed from the syringe before use.
   - If the jet irrigator or catheter–syringe unit is used, after directing the flow superiorly, rotate the tip back and forth to change the direction of spray.
5. Often the cerumen washes out in one or two large pieces in a few seconds, at which point the canal is reexamined. If the canal is clear, stop the irrigation and dry the canal by inserting and removing a small length of cotton gauze. If the patient has otitis externa, the ear canal should be dried meticulously.
6. Occasionally the impacted cerumen will need to be prodded with an ear curette. If irrigation is still unsuccessful after a few moments, terminate the procedure and send the patient home to use a liquid ear wax softener. Have the patient return in a few days for a repeat irrigation.
7. Consider prescribing topical otic antibiotics if the epithelium was disrupted to provide prophylaxis against external otitis.

COMPLICATIONS

- Tympanic membrane perforation and damage to ossicles with possible hearing loss
- Otitis externa
- Vertigo or nausea and vomiting
- Minor canal wall abrasions—as mentioned earlier, some bleeding may occur if hard wax is adherent to the epithelium and causes desquamation with removal (if noted, antibiotic otic drops should be used for a few days)
- Tinnitus

POSTPROCEDURE PATIENT EDUCATION

Instruct the patient to contact the clinician's office for fever or vertigo or for decreased hearing, purulent drainage, or pain in the affected ear. Slight bleeding from the affected ear may be expected if the skin was disrupted. Diabetic and other immunocompromised patients should be especially observant for signs of infection because they are prone to development of malignant otitis externa (often due to *Pseudomonas*), with its resultant high morbidity and mortality rates.

Inform patients with recurring cerumen impactions, unless contraindicated, to perform monthly or bimonthly ear cleansing using hydrogen peroxide, docusate sodium, 5% to 10% sodium bicarbonate (mixed as previously described in Equipment section), a commercial ceruminolytic, or distilled water as an irrigant from a squeeze bulb ear syringe (similar to nasal bulb syringe used in newborns; both are available at local pharmacies). Advise the patient to avoid self-instrumentation of the ear canal with cotton-tipped applicators or any other instrument. It may be helpful to explain that cotton-tipped applicators or other instruments often disrupt the cilia and other natural ear cleansing mechanisms, even *causing* an accumulation of cerumen. Cotton-tipped applicators should be used only on the external ear and never inserted into the canal. Another option is the instillation of two to three drops of mineral oil, pure vegetable oil, or liquid docusate sodium every couple of weeks in the ear canal to soften the wax (these are contraindicated with suspected perforation). Again, there is no consistent evidence that one ceruminolytic is better than another. Patients who use hair spray should cover the ears when spraying to avoid hardening the cerumen.

CPT/BILLING CODES

69210 Removal impacted cerumen requiring instrumentation, unilateral (for bilateral, report with modifier 50)

ICD-10-CM DIAGNOSTIC CODES

H61.20–H61.23 Cerumen impaction
H60.391–H60.399 Otitis externa (secondary diagnosis)

Acknowledgment

The editors recognize the contributions of Gregory J. Forzley, MD, and Gary R. Newkirk, MD, to this chapter in previous editions of this text.

SUPPLIERS

(See contact information available at www.expertconsult.com.)

Metal and plastic disposable curettes
Cardinal Health
Miltex, Inc.
Spectrum Surgical Instruments

Plastic curettes and safe irrigation tips
Bionix Corporation: www.bionix.com/medicaltech/product/otoclear-ear-irrigation
Elephant Ear Washer Bottle System: www.healthykin.com/p-5058-elephant-ear-washer-bottle-system-by-doctor-easy.aspx

RECOMMENDED READING

Burton MJ, Doree C. Ear drops for the removal of ear wax. *Cochrane Database Syst Review.* 2009;(1):CD004326.
Dinsdale RC, Roland PS, Manning SC, Meyerhoff WL. Catastrophic otologic injury from oral jet irrigation of the external auditory canal. *Laryngoscopy.* 1991;101:75–78.

Hand C, Harvey I. The effectiveness of topical preparations for the treatment of earwax: a systematic review. *B J Gen Pract.* 2004;54:862–867.

McCarter DF, Courtney AU, Pollart SM. Cerumen impaction. *Am Fam Physician.* 2007;75(10):1523–1528.

Murtagh J. Ear Wax and Syringing. In: Murtagh J, ed. *Practice Tips.* 6th ed. Sydney, Australia: McGraw-Hill; 2012.

Riviello R. Otolaryngologic procedures. In: Roberts JR, Custalow CB, Thomsen TW, eds. *Roberts and Hedges Clinical Procedures in Emergency Medicine.* 6th ed. Philadelphia: Elsevier; 2014:1311–1313.

Roberts RR. Cerumen Impaction Removal. In: Reichman EF, ed. *Emergency Medicine Procedure.* 2nd ed. New York: McGraw-Hill; 2013:1070–1074.

Robinson AC, Hawke M. The efficacy of ceruminolytics: everything old is new again. *J Otolaryngol.* 1989;18:263–267.

Schwartz SR, Magit AE, Rosenfeld RM, et al. Clinical practice guideline (update): earwax, (cerumen impaction). *Otolaryngol Head Neck Surg.* 2017;156(IS):S1–S29.

Wilson SA, Lopez R. What is the best treatment for impacted cerumen? *J Fam Pract.* 2002;51:117.

CHAPTER 63

EARLOBE REPAIR

Dennis LaRavia

Constant or repetitive traction by jewelry worn in a pierced earlobe may eventually cause a large, elongated hole (Figs. 63.1A and 63.2). Over time, the defect may even extend through the tip of the lobe, creating a bifid lobe that is completely reepithelialized (see Fig. 63.1B). More acutely, an earring can be pulled or ripped through the lobe, resulting in a laceration. This area is also a common site for cysts. Regardless of the cause, the patient often finds the results cosmetically unacceptable; it may also become difficult or impossible for the patient to wear an earring at that site. Although some patients will opt for clip-ons or piercing at an adjacent site and wear large earrings to cover the defect, others will choose to repair the lobe.

Primary care clinicians can repair the earlobe in the office, often bringing great satisfaction to a patient by improving both cosmetic appearance and convenience for wearing jewelry. The usual charge from a plastic surgeon for such a repair is $450 to $650; consequently primary care clinicians can usually work something out that is beneficial to both the patient and the clinician.

EQUIPMENT

- Sterile preparation and setup (alcohol or chlorhexidine, sterile drapes and gloves).
- Lidocaine 1% or 2% without epinephrine if doing field block or with epinephrine if injecting into the actual lobe repair site.
- Laceration repair kit including skin hooks and 6-0 nylon suture.
- Scalpel with a No. 15 or 15c blade, and possibly a No. 11 blade.
- Antibacterial ointment or petroleum jelly.
- Sterile dressing.
- If available, an electrosurgical or radiofrequency unit (e.g., Ellman Surgitron) with a fine cutting needle or wire works well to excise the tissue (see Chapter 25, Radiofrequency Surgery [Modern Electrosurgery]).

PREPROCEDURE PATIENT PREPARATION

Although the patient may desire this procedure, it is often considered a cosmetic procedure by insurance companies and may not be a covered expense. Explain this possibility as well as the possible complications of the procedure, which may include discomfort, bleeding, infection, and a cosmetic defect. The patient should be aware that there will be a scar after the repair and that the repaired earlobe will not be identical to the contralateral one but that every attempt will be made to minimize any additional cosmetic defect. If the patient tends to develop keloids or hypertrophic scars, these may result from the procedure. Obtain informed consent. Also explain the discomfort of injected local anesthetic and the necessity for the patient to remain very still during the procedure.

TECHNIQUE

1. After sterile preparation has been performed, sterile technique is used, and universal blood and body fluid precautions are observed.
2. A wheal of lidocaine without epinephrine placed circumferentially around the entire base of the ear will provide good anesthesia (ear block; see Chapter 7, Peripheral Nerve Blocks and

Field Blocks). The concha and ear canal retain sensation. Use of the circumferential block as opposed to injection directly into the lobe avoids distortion of the local anatomy. Alternatively, if the injection is made into the site on the lobe, using a much smaller amount of lidocaine with epinephrine can help to minimize bleeding. Or, both blocks can be used.

3. Excise the defect with a No. 15 or 15c blade, a No. 11 pointed blade, or with the electrosurgical or radiofrequency unit (e.g., Ellman Surgitron; level 2, pure cut, Varitip or fine needle; Figs. 63.3 through 63.5). If the defect is a large hole, it is often easier just to excise all the way through the lobe to create a "V" (see Fig. 63.3). Various sterilized objects with a flat surface have been used to support the lobe during the excision because it is so flaccid, but with gentle traction by the clinician's nondominant hand, the lobe should remain stable. The radiofrequency unit makes this step easier, especially if the defect is a hole and there is an effort to preserve the lower intact rim of tissue (see Figs. 63.4 and 63.5). Care should be taken to excise

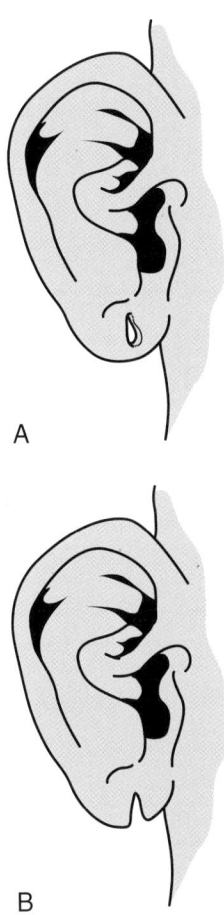

A

B

Fig. 63.1 Torn earlobe defect. (A) Incomplete tear with resulting large hole. (B) Complete tear.

a smooth line and treat the exposed subcutaneous tissue and wound edges extremely gently. If needed, skin hooks may be used. Absolutely avoid grasping the skin edges with forceps; this delivers a crushing force, induces unnecessary trauma, and increases scarring. Earlobe cysts are removed and repaired in the same manner (Fig. 63.6).

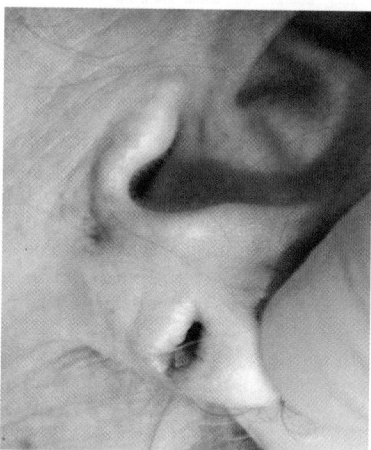

Fig. 63.2   Chronic earlobe laceration.

4. Control bleeding with pressure.

5. Close the skin edges anteriorly to posteriorly with interrupted 6-0 nylon. It is wise to begin suturing anteriorly first so that any malalignment is confined to the posterior aspect. Also, sutures may be placed intermittently at first and then the gaps filled in to conclude the repair. Proper approximation at the tip of the lobe is important (Fig. 63.7; see also Figs. 63.3 and 63.4). The wound edges may try to invert; a vertical mattress stitch may help to prevent this. Z-plasties and sliding flaps have also been described to minimize risk of a cleft in the final scar (see Sokol in the recommended readings).
   EDITOR'S NOTE: Although some clinicians recommend repiercing the ear later, at 6 weeks, others clinicians insert a single small gold stud in the location the patient chooses within the incision just after it is closed. Stitches must be close enough together on either side of the stud to prevent wobble. Make sure the stud is long enough to extend beyond the skin anteriorly and posteriorly to prevent it from becoming embedded. If the patient turns the stud very carefully in place on a daily basis as the incision heals, it may also help to prevent it from becoming embedded. Earrings should not be attached for 6 weeks. For patients with a prior history of keloids or hypertrophic scars, pressure earrings are available, or they may benefit from corticosteroid injections before the repair, at the time of repair, and after the repair (see Chapter 28, Hypertrophic Scars and Keloids).

6. Apply antibacterial ointment or petroleum jelly.

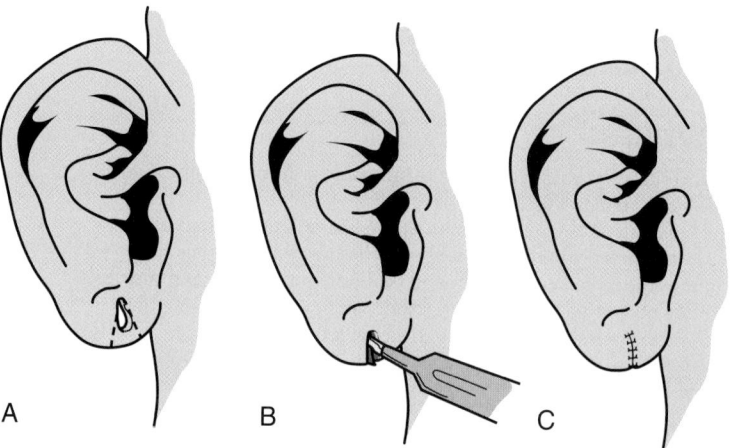

Fig. 63.3   Excising reepithelialized skin within the defect using a No. 11 blade. (A) Area to be excised. In this case, a large opening is being converted into a "V." Alternatively, for a smaller hole, a small elliptical excision could be made around it to preserve the lower margin of the lobe. (B) Making the excision. (C) Appearance after closure.

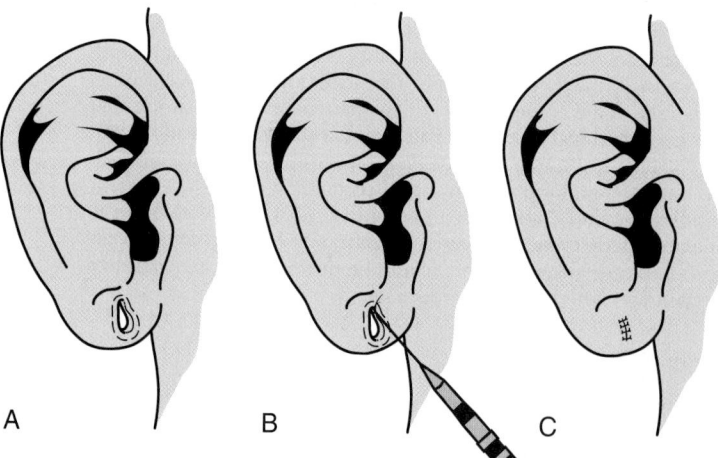

Fig. 63.4   Excising reepithelialized skin within the defect using a radiofrequency unit and a fine needle (this maintains integrity of the lower rim). This procedure can also be carried out with a No. 11 blade but is more difficult. (A) Area to be excised. (B) Making the excision. (C) Appearance after closure.

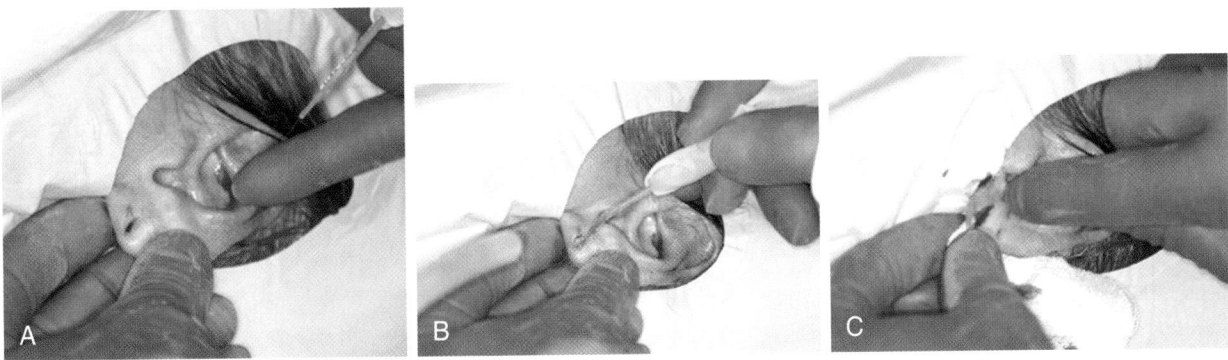

Fig. 63.5 Excising reepithelialized skin with a radiofrequency unit. (A) Chronic earlobe laceration from earring. Anesthetic ear block has been obtained. (B) Using the radiofrequency unit, the healed margins of the wound are excised. (C) Wound margins can now be approximated using fine nylon suture.

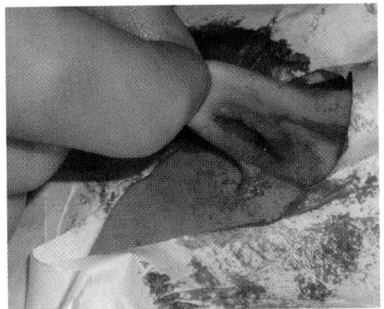

Fig. 63.6 Earlobe cysts are removed and repaired in the same manner.

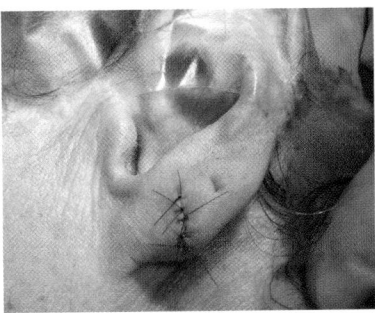

Fig. 63.7 Appearance after suture closure.

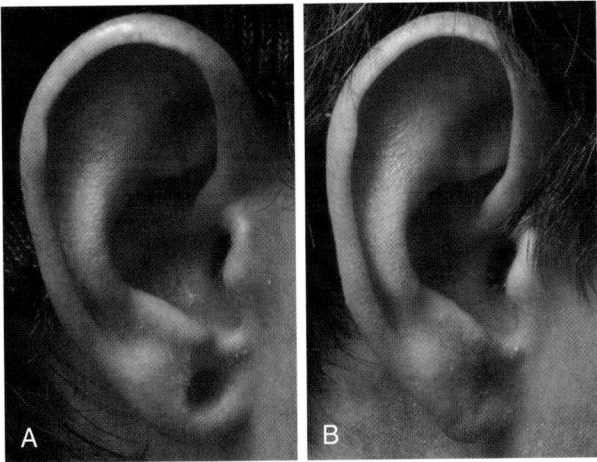

Fig. 63.8 Before (A) and after (B) earlobe repair using radiofrequency unit. (Courtesy Greg Lawrence.)

7. Place a pack behind the earlobe and against the mastoid process to secure the lobe and ensure that it will not suffer trauma or excessive motion. Cover the wound with a sterile pressure dressing. Overall, patients generally appreciate the final result (Fig. 63.8).

POSTPROCEDURE PATIENT EDUCATION

1. For the first few hours, the patient should lie on the side that was repaired to compress the area and reduce bleeding.
2. The patient should remove the dressing in 12 to 24 hours and all blood and crusts should be removed with alcohol or hydrogen peroxide on cotton-tipped applicators to minimize the risk of scarring and infection. Thereafter the area should be washed gently twice a day with soap and water. A small amount of antibacterial ointment (avoid neomycin, which can inhibit reepithelialization) or petroleum jelly should then be applied with a new cotton-tipped applicator.
3. The patient should return for suture removal in 5 days. Some clinicians use Steri-Strips to give additional support for several days.
4. Repiercing of the ear may be performed after 6 to 8 weeks in a location off of the wound line. For patients with a prior history of keloids or hypertrophic scars, pressure earrings are available.

5. The patient should be instructed to avoid heavy, dangling, or large loop earrings in the future to avoid repeated undue traction on the lobe.

PATIENT EDUCATION GUIDES

See the sample patient education form available at www.expertconsult.com.

CPT/BILLING CODES

12011 Repair, simple, of superficial wounds of ear (2.5 cm or less)
12012 Repair, simple, of superficial wounds of ear (2.6 cm to 5.0 cm)
12051 Repair, intermediate, layer closure of ear (2.5 cm or less)
12052 Repair, intermediate, layer closure of ear (2.6 cm to 5.0 cm)

ICD-10-CM DIAGNOSTIC CODES

S01.301X-S01.309X   Laceration, external ear (pins) unspecified
S01.311X-S01.319X   Laceration, external ear (pins) w/o foreign body
S01.321X-S01.329X   Laceration, external ear (pins) w/foreign body
S01.80X   Unspecified wound of other parts of head

Add appropriate seventh character: A = initial, D = subsequent, S = sequela.

Acknowledgment

The editors recognize the contributions of Stephen K. Toadvine, MD, to this chapter in a previous edition of this text.

RECOMMENDED READING

Nikko A, Hsu S, Quan LT, Greenbaum SS. Surgical pearl: repair of partially torn earlobes: punch technique versus conversion to complete tear. *J Am Acad Dermatol.* 2000;43:99–101.

Russo CJ, Desai A. Management of specific soft tissue injuries. In: Reichman EF, ed. *Emergency Medicine Procedures.* 2nd ed. New York: McGraw-Hill; 2013:661–662.

Silapunt S, Goldberg LH. Repair of the split earlobe, ear piercing and ear-lobe reduction. In: Robinson JK, Hanke CW, Siegel DM, Fratila A, eds. *Surgery of the Skin: Procedural Dermatology.* 3rd ed. Philadelphia: Elsevier Saunders; 2015:781–792.

Smith C, Glaser DA. Surgical pearl: repair of split or deformed ear lobe with tongue blade for stabilization during surgery. *J Am Acad Dermatol.* 1998;38:990–991.

Sokol JA, Schwarcz RM. A better way to repair torn earlobes using a modified z-plasty. *Dermatol Surg.* 2011;37:1–3.

CHAPTER 64

NASOLARYNGOSCOPY

Grant C. Fowler • Phuc D. Nguyen

Fortunately, the mortality rates for cancers of the oral cavity, pharynx, and larynx have declined over the last 30 years. That said, cancers of the oropharynx and larynx remain two of the most common cancers in the upper aerodigestive tract, with approximately 16,000 and 13,000 new cases diagnosed, respectively, each year in the United States. Both types of cancer can be diagnosed with nasolaryngoscopy, and the earlier the diagnosis, the better the cure rate. At the same time, the number of nasopharyngeal complaints in the offices of primary care clinicians has increased. Sinusitis is now one of the most common chronic diseases in the United States. These facts—combined with the fact that many primary care clinicians have difficulty visualizing the nasal passages, oropharynx, and larynx—have led many practitioners to seek alternatives to mirror or direct laryngoscopy. Nasolaryngoscopy has now been used for over 35 years. The ease of learning the technique (especially for clinicians already performing endoscopic procedures), its low risk (no need for sedation), the expediency of the procedure (most procedures can be completed in 10 to 20 minutes), and the relatively low cost of equipment ($3500 to $7000) have resulted in increasing numbers of primary care clinicians using this valuable diagnostic tool. In addition, patients appreciate the immediately available results, especially when nasolaryngoscopy is performed in the familiar and comfortable environment of their primary care clinician's office. Recent developments include biopsy ports, smaller-diameter scopes, and distal-chip optical systems (improve visualization and may be less prone to fogging). Narrow-band imaging, an image enhancement system, is now available in some models and increases the contrast in the background when visualizing capillaries and veins. This may allow clinicians to diagnose smaller lesions at an earlier stage. In addition, biopsies, dilations, botulinum toxin (Botox) injections, and in-office laser procedures can now be performed through these small-diameter scopes. Although these scopes may in turn be replaced by those capable of performing transnasal esophagoscopy, at present nasolaryngoscopy remains a popular procedure.

The indications for nasolaryngoscopy by primary care clinicians are chronic upper respiratory complaints, especially in smokers or those with unilateral conditions. Nasolaryngoscopy is also helpful in patients with certain acute disorders (e.g., one study found nasolaryngoscopy more effective than sinus films for diagnosing acute maxillary sinusitis). Nasolaryngoscopy is helpful when there is difficulty examining the larynx with an indirect mirror (see Chapter 65, Indirect Mirror Laryngoscopy), such as when there is unusual anatomy or persistent gagging or if the clinician does not have much experience with this technique. The only other option is per-oral rigid fiberoptic laryngoscopy, and that is beyond the scope of this text.

INDICATIONS

Chronic Conditions

- Chronic hoarseness or voice change (>3 weeks)
- Chronic sinusitis or sinus discomfort, especially unilateral
- Chronic serous otitis media or eustachian tube dysfunction in an adult, especially unilateral
- Recurrent otalgia
- Suspected neoplasm
- Chronic cough
- Chronic nasal obstruction or postnasal drip
- Chronic rhinorrhea
- Chronic pharyngeal pain
- Halitosis
- Previous head and neck cancer
- Previous conservative treatment of laryngeal polyps
- Head or neck mass or adenopathy
- Recurrent epistaxis
- Dysphagia
- Globus hystericus
- Foreign body sensation in pharynx
- Evaluation of snoring
- Vocal cord paralysis
- Further reassurance against serious disease in any chronic upper respiratory condition, especially in smokers
- Chronic acid (reflux) laryngitis

NOTE: More than 60% of patients with reflux laryngitis do not have the classic gastroesophageal symptoms of heartburn and reflux. Instead, they may present with chronic intermittent hoarseness, vocal fatigue, chronic cough, dysphagia, sore throat, stridor, croup, postnasal drip, frequent throat clearing, globus sensation, or a choking sensation. They may also have associated asthma, pulmonary fibrosis, chronic bronchitis, or pneumonia.

Acute Conditions

- Hemoptysis
- Acute sinusitis
- Acute epistaxis (without profuse hemorrhage)
- Suspected nasal foreign body
- Suspected laryngeal foreign body
- Acute onset of hoarseness after straining voice

CONTRAINDICATIONS

- Acute epiglottitis (may precipitate complete airway obstruction)
- Acute epistaxis (bleeding source may be difficult to visualize with profuse hemorrhage)
- Uncooperative patient
- Respiratory distressed patient
- High grade airway obstruction
- Supraglottic hematoma that is expanding
- Facial fractures, especially midface, or basilar skull fractures with possible cribriform plate injuries (relative contraindication, otolaryngoscopy may be a better option, but see text regarding a bite block)
- Recent nasal or oropharyngeal surgery (may be relative contraindication, depending on nature and location of the surgery)

EQUIPMENT

- Flexible nasolaryngoscope with light source. Similar to recently manufactured gastroscopes and colonoscopes, newer nasolaryngoscopes are available with distal-chip digital optical systems (i.e., camera at the tip) where the cameras have basically replaced the fiberoptic technology. However, fiberoptic nasolaryngoscopes are still manufactured and tend to be less expensive. Recently manufactured scopes (both fiberoptic and distal-chip) are also completely immersible, which simplifies cleaning and disinfection. Light sources used for other endoscopes in the office may be adaptable to a nasolaryngoscope. This might be an important consideration when purchasing a flexible sigmoidoscope, gastroscope, or colonoscope.

NOTE: Since there are few things to occlude the scope or block visualization, there is little need to increase the cost by upgrading to distal-chip cameras from fiberoptic technology. A recent study (Plaat et al., 2014) found distal-chip to be no better than fiberoptic regarding diagnostic accuracy. (However, image quality and interrater reliability was slightly better with distal-chip technology.)

- Nasal speculum
- Decongestant*: phenylephrine (0.25% to 2%) spray (Neo-Synephrine, Vicks) or epinephrine 1:50,000 (Adrenalin), ephedrine (3%), or oxymetazoline hydrochloride 0.05% spray (Afrin, Neo-Synephrine 12 hour)
- Anesthetic: lidocaine (2% to 10%) solution in an atomizer spray bottle or benzocaine spray (14% to 20%) (Cetacaine)†
- Goggles, mask, and gloves (equipment necessary to follow universal blood and body fluid precautions)
- Sterilizing solution, such as glutaraldehyde (Cidex)
- Optional supplies include cotton balls or pledgets soaked in either a decongestant or anesthetic. Three ear, nose, and throat spuds with soaked cotton applicators are another option. Cocaine solution (4% to 10%) can be used for both decongestion and anesthesia. At this strength, it does not produce a euphoric effect; however, many clinicians choose not to stock cocaine because of the mandatory record keeping and the risk of burglary. If cocaine is considered for the anesthetic, patients should be informed of the risk of finding its metabolites in their urine in case they have on-the-job drug screening.

PREPROCEDURE PATIENT EDUCATION

After explaining the procedure, inform the patient that he or she may experience an intense tickling sensation on insertion of the scope. Warning the patient beforehand can minimize his or her response. Use of a topical decongestant or an anesthetic may decrease this sensation, and they should be told if this is going to be used. Although nasolaryngoscopy can be performed without these, visualization and patient tolerance are usually improved with their use. This may be especially helpful with inexperienced operators or anxious patients. Next, the objectives of the procedure should be described. Explain that he or she may speak during the procedure, and they should inform the clinician if they are having any significant discomfort other than pressure. The patient will be asked to say certain words or sounds and may be asked to swallow or to avoid swallowing at different stages. The patient should keep his or her eyes open and focused straight ahead to minimize the gag reflex. Breath holding can also trigger the gag reflex, so the patient should be encouraged to breathe through the mouth.

TECHNIQUE

1. Before performing the procedure, a thorough head and neck history and examination, as well as the remainder of a complete history and physical examination, should be performed. The procedure is brief enough to be performed on the initial visit. If nasolaryngoscopy is not performed on the initial visit, when the patient returns, obtain the interval history and again examine the head and neck. Explain the procedure again.

2. Before applying decongestant or anesthetic, the patient should gently blow their nose to clear the nasal passage. Give the patient some tissues to hold in one hand and a plastic emesis basin in the other. The patient should have an absorbent sheet draped over the shoulders that is then tucked inside the collar. The clinician should follow universal blood and body fluid precautions.

3. With the patient sitting up, apply decongestant generously by spraying the atomized solution into both nostrils. If the same spray nozzle is to be used with another patient, it should not touch this patient. One spray should be directed superiorly and a second posteriorly. After spraying, have the patient tilt his or her head back to allow the liquid to drain as far back as possible. The patient should then swallow any residual. Unless both nares need to be intubated, determine by visual inspection which nostril is the least obstructed. After decongestion, this is the nostril that should be anesthetized for scope insertion.

4. After waiting 5 to 10 minutes for the decongestant to take effect, anesthetize the chosen nostril(s). Spray liberal amounts of lidocaine or benzocaine aerosol spray; direct the spray superiorly for 1 second and then posteriorly for about 1 second with the patient tilting his or her head back and again swallowing any residual. The patient should be warned that lidocaine has a sour taste. Swallowing the anesthetic assists with suppression of the gag reflex. For patients with a hyperactive gag reflex, gargling with lidocaine solution or a generous spraying of the pharynx with benzocaine may be helpful. The patient is ready for the procedure when he or she reports no sensation at the back of the throat.

   As an alternative to spraying, soaked cotton balls or pledgets can be inserted with offset or bayonet forceps through the nasal speculum. One cotton ball (or pledget) should be inserted superiorly, another inserted in the middle meatus, and a third posteriorly. They should remain in place for 5 to 10 minutes and then removed before insertion of the scope. Three otolaryngoscopy spuds with cotton applicators can be used in the same manner. If cotton balls, pledgets, or spuds are used, the back of the pharynx should also be sprayed with anesthetic to suppress the gag reflex.

5. Before insertion of the scope and while waiting for the anesthesia to take effect, the clinician may want to get reacquainted with the scope (for those who do not regularly perform endoscopic procedures). Deflect the tip both ways to observe which direction and how far it moves for a given movement of the deflector. The focal length on most scopes is about 5 mm or greater, and viewing an object through the scope (e.g., a penny, a piece of gauze) before insertion may give the clinician a better sense of distance and magnification. In general, as it is advanced, the tip of the scope moves toward whatever structure is directly in the center of the field of view. Note that for these very small scopes, a slight deflection of the tip can cause a marked change in direction of the scope. It should also be noted that the most difficult aspect of nasolaryngoscopy may not be manipulating the scope, but rather maintaining familiarity with the complex anatomy of the nose and throat. Clinicians who do not frequently perform the procedure may benefit from a brief review of the anatomy before each procedure. Atlases and CD-ROMs/ DVDs are available for such reviews (see the Recommended Reading section).

6. Place the patient in either an erect (sitting) or supine position. Both examiner and patient should be in a position that they can maintain comfortably for 20 minutes. The patient is reasonably protected from injury caused by his or her own sudden movements or by jumping away from the scope if in the supine position. Patients who are sitting can be protected by placing their head all the way back against a high, firm headrest. A small child may want to sit in a parent's lap; the parent should then hold the child firmly, especially the head, to help protect from any injury that might be caused by sudden involuntary

---

*Should be used with caution in those who are severely hypertensive or have a history of sensitivity to the agent.

†Should be used with caution in those who have a history of an allergy or sensitivity to the agent..

movements. Most clinicians prefer the sitting position over the supine because gravity will pull the tongue and scope posteriorly, both of which make viewing the anteriorly placed larynx more difficult.

7. Rest the hand you will be using to guide the endoscope on the patient's cheek. Your middle, ring, and little fingers should form a tripod to support the index finger and thumb while handling and guiding the tip of the scope. As you gain more experience, you may wish to rest this tripod on the patient's forehead to sense for tensing of the frontalis muscle, which is often the first sign that the patient is experiencing significant discomfort. Turn on the light source. Tell the patient to close his or her eyes and to expect a bright light and possibly a tickling sensation. Insert the tip through the least-obstructed nostril and past the nasal hairs at the vestibule. If the scope is prone to becoming fogged, rest it against the nasal septum to warm it. Warming the scope usually defogs it.

8. The floor of the nasal cavity, which is in the inferior meatus, usually offers the most open channel and the best passage for intubations (Fig. 64.1). (The meatus is the space below each turbinate.) Advance the scope only toward visualized objects; avoid advancing the scope blindly or against significant resistance. As with other endoscopic procedures, if only white is visible (a "whiteout"), the scope is probably resting against mucosa and should be withdrawn until the actual structure that the mucosa is covering is visualized. A deviated septum or large maxillary ridge may impede advancement of the endoscope along the floor. In this situation, make an attempt to pass the scope through the middle meatus, keeping in mind that the patient usually experiences discomfort whenever the scope is directed or advanced superiorly. If this is unsuccessful, withdraw the scope and intubate the other nostril.

NOTE: If unable to intubate either nostril, after spraying the back of the pharynx with benzocaine to suppress the gag reflex, the scope can be passed through the oropharynx. In this situation, the patient might damage the scope by biting it. To minimize this risk, the barrel of a 10-mL syringe (minus the plunger) can be cut in half (cut crosswise/across the diameter), and the remaining barrel placed between the patient's upper and lower front incisors. If the scope is then inserted through the barrel, it will serve as a bite-block.

If possible, avoid touching the posterior pharynx, the base of the tongue, or the epiglottis which may elicit the gag reflex. In this manner, the scope should be advanced to visualize the pharynx, and then past the epiglottis to visualize the structures below.

9. As the scope is advanced along the floor, the feet of the medial crura (of the lower lateral septal cartilages) can frequently be seen protruding from the medial aspect of the nasal passage. The inferior turbinate is visualized about 1 cm into the passage. Note the texture and size of the inferior turbinate, as well as any

polypoid degeneration or any swelling of the covering mucosal membranes. Flexion of the scope slightly upward often illuminates the middle turbinate in the distance and its meatus. The nasolacrimal duct drains into the inferior meatus and is usually not seen; however, purulent fluid draining from it is evidence of a nasolacrimal gland infection. If the patient has had surgical antral windows placed into the maxillary sinus, the openings are frequently located in the inferior meatus. These openings can often be entered with a scope (Fig. 64.2). Note the condition of the mucosa if the antral windows are entered.

10. Next, pass the scope posteriorly about 4 to 5 cm until the choana comes into view. The choana is the junction between the nasal fossa and the nasopharynx, and it looks just like a posterior "nostril." It should form a halo in front of adenoid tissue. If desired, move the scope laterally and superiorly to allow entry into the middle meatus. However, because superior reflection of the scope may result in discomfort, it may be prudent to examine the middle meatus on the way out after visualizing the larynx. Again, if the nasal floor is obstructed, there may be no choice but to attempt passage of the scope through the middle meatus.

11. Upon entering the choana, the adenoid pad appears on the posterior wall of the pharynx. Star-shaped scarring may be all that is seen if the patient has had an adenoidectomy. Advance the endoscope into the nasopharynx, and when the posterior margin of the septum is passed (when it is no longer seen), slightly flex the tip of the endoscope and rotate 90 degrees laterally to observe the torus tubarius. The torus is the valve at the opening of the eustachian tube (Fig. 64.3). Ask the patient to say "key, key, key" while you observe valve function. The eustachian tube should open and close slightly. Adenoid or lymphoid hyperplasia may be noted in this area or elsewhere throughout the procedure. It may

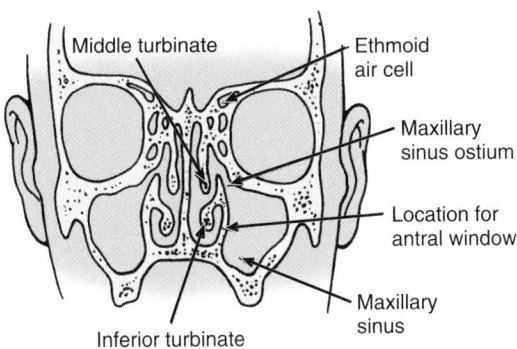

Fig. 64.2 Frontal section of the head. In this section, eight ethmoid air cells (four on each side) are shown in their locations medial to the orbit. A rather large maxillary sinus ostium is demonstrated, as well as the location in the inferior meatus for surgical placement of antral windows.

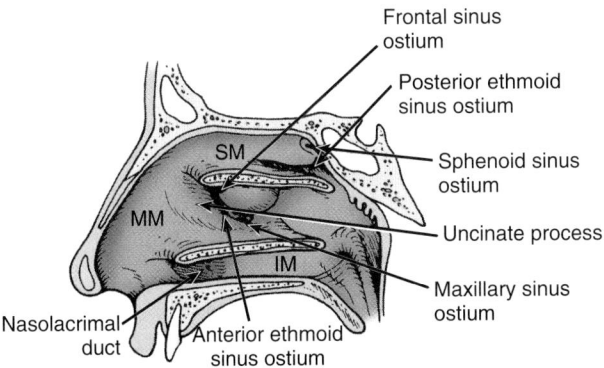

Fig. 64.1 Sagittal section of the head with the turbinates removed to demonstrate ostia of the paranasal sinuses and the nasolacrimal duct. *IM*, Inferior meatus; *MM*, middle meatus; *SM*, superior meatus.

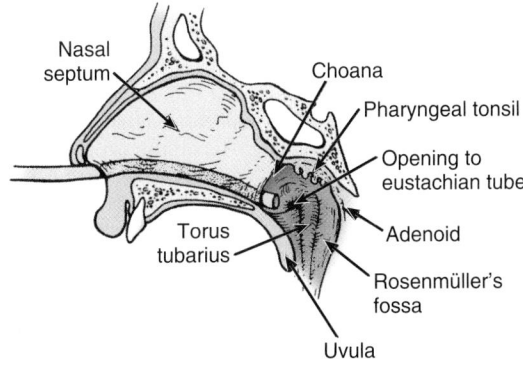

Fig. 64.3 Anatomy of nasopharynx and oropharynx.

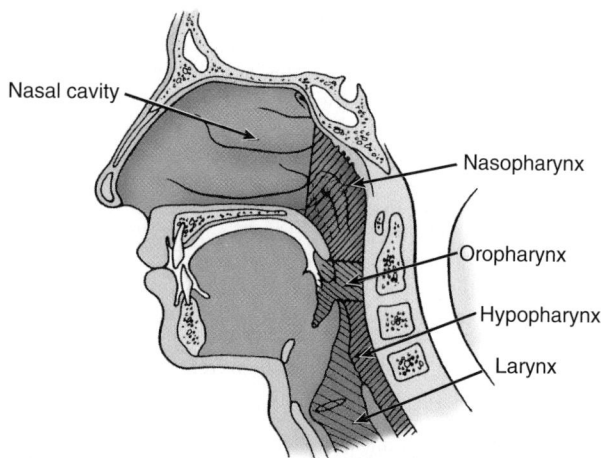

Fig. 64.4 Anatomic divisions of the upper airway. All five divisions may be inspected with a fiberoptic nasolaryngoscope.

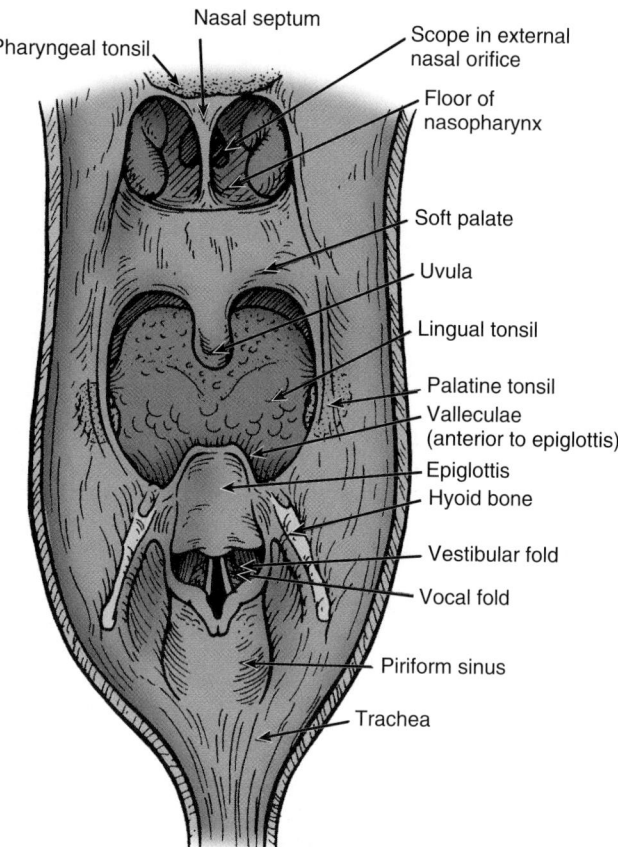

Fig. 64.5 Oropharyngeal and laryngeal areas, viewed from posterior.

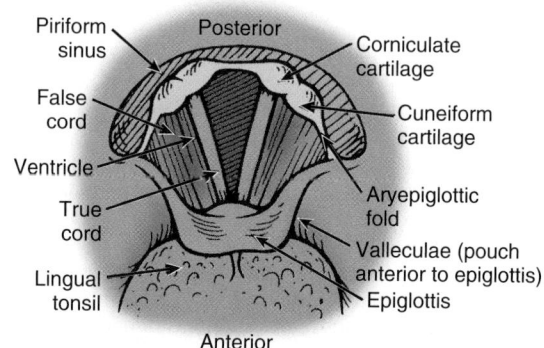

Fig. 64.6 Larynx viewed from above and oriented as it would be seen with a fiberoptic nasolaryngoscope.

actually block the torus tubarius. By advancing the scope slightly and rotating 180 degrees while avoiding the septum (make sure to avoid contact with the septum!), the opposite torus is illuminated. Its function should also be observed. Purulent fluid may be seen draining from a eustachian tube and should be noted. Posterior to both tori and anterior to the adenoid pad lie the clefts of Rosenmüller, each of which should be carefully inspected. Most nasopharyngeal malignancies are found in this area.

12. Next, advance the scope inferiorly and toward the posterior wall of the oropharynx (Fig. 64.4).
    NOTE: If possible, avoid touching the posterior pharynx or the base of the tongue, which may elicit the gag reflex.

    Instruct the patient to breathe through his or her nose to keep the soft palate from obstructing the view. As the patient swallows or talks, the normal movement of the soft palate can be seen. Downward flexion and slight rotation of the scope as it nears the posterior wall will allow for inspection of the uvula, the soft palate, and the lateral and posterior walls of the pharynx. The epiglottis should be seen in the distance. Note the presence of any masses, scarring, inflammation, exudate, mucosal irregularities, or pulsations. In some cases, dysphagia may be explained by lymphoid hyperplasia in this area, especially if the hyperplasia is associated with enlarged palatine tonsils and an exudate.

13. When the scope has passed the soft palate, it enters the oropharynx. Again, for the remainder of the procedure, attempt to avoid touching the posterior pharynx while keeping the scope as close as possible to it. If the scope becomes fogged, tell the patient to swallow; this often clears the scope. With slight flexion and rotation, examine the posterior tongue, lingual tonsils, palatine tonsils, epiglottis, and medial and lateral glossoepiglottic folds. Avoid touching the base of the tongue, which can trigger the gag reflex. Examine the valleculae from above (Figs. 64.5 and 64.6). Ask the patient to stick out his or her tongue to improve visualization of the valleculae.

14. When the scope has passed the epiglottis, it enters the hypopharynx (see Fig. 64.4). Ask the patient to refrain from swallowing; at this level, swallowing can induce an unusual foreign body sensation or provoke coughing. Assure the patient that if it is unavoidable, it is all right to swallow; however, he or she may experience the sensation of swallowing the scope. If this sensation becomes too strong, the scope may be withdrawn until the sensation passes. The arytenoid cartilages, the corniculate and cuneiform cartilages, and the aryepiglottic folds can be visualized at this level. The piriform sinuses posterior to the cords should be at least partially inspected. Closely examine the false and true vocal cords and the ventricles during quiet respiration (see Fig. 64.6). Tell the patient to hold a prolonged high "eee" sound while you

watch for symmetry of cord mobility as well as edema, hemorrhages, erythema, nodules, or masses of the cords or surrounding structures. Record any mucosal or structural abnormalities.

Vocal cord nodules, cysts, and polyps usually occur at the junction of the anterior and middle third of the cord. Nodules are generally caused by vocal abuse and are usually bilateral, small, white, sessile, and firm. Vocal cord cysts are usually unilateral and filled with caseous material, and can be due to vocal abuse (i.e., epidermoid). Mucous retention cysts are also usually unilateral due to an obstructed duct and filled with mucoid material. Polyps are also caused by vocal abuse, are usually unilateral, and can be sessile or pedunculated with a prominent feeding vessel on the superior aspect of the vocal cord. There may be evidence of preceding hemorrhage. Reinke's edema, also known as polypoid degeneration of

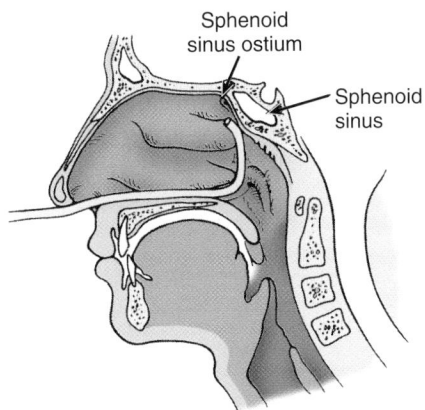

Fig. 64.7 Nasolaryngoscope is withdrawn to a position just anterior to the choana and retroflexed.

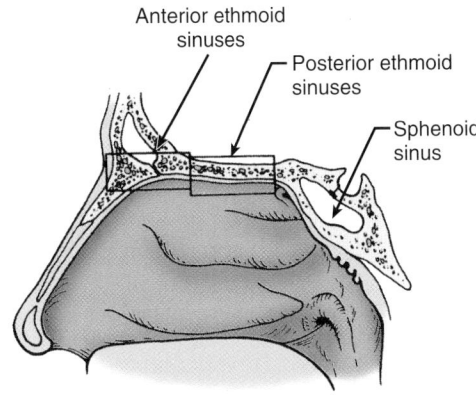

Fig. 64.8 Parasagittal section of the head showing the relationship of the anterior and posterior ethmoid sinuses. The bone in this area is eggshell thin.

the vocal cords, appears as sausage-shaped edematous vocal cords. It is usually due to tobacco abuse, but can also be at least partly due to vocal abuse and gastroesophageal reflux disease. Other findings associated with reflux laryngitis can be diffuse or limited to the vocal cords. The ventricles can be obliterated, the arytenoids thickened, and there may be erythema, edema, or "cobblestoning" of the posterior aspect of the larynx or trachea.

NOTE: The scope should never touch or pass below the cords. When nearing the cords, if the patient accidentally swallows, the operator should be prepared to quickly withdraw the scope enough to avoid touching them. If the cords are touched, severe laryngospasm can occur with resultant patient asphyxia.

15. Next, withdraw the scope to a position just anterior to the choana and direct it very superiorly, almost inverted on itself (Fig. 64.7). With the tip in this position, carefully withdraw the scope slightly again, and the sphenoid bone should appear. (The sphenoid bone will appear in what was previously an inferior position in scope orientation, before inversion.) The superior turbinate may be seen, as might an anatomic variant, the supreme turbinate. The ostia of the sphenoid sinus—medial to the superior turbinate—should be visible. The sphenoid sinus, which can be thought of as a large posterior ethmoid air cell (Fig. 64.8), is usually the only sinus in the posterior ethmoid group with a visible ostium (see Fig. 64.1). Again, care is necessary when directing the scope superiorly. This is an area where anesthesia is frequently incomplete, and this maneuver may cause the patient some discomfort.

16. Straighten the scope and withdraw to the level where the complete choana comes into view. Move the scope in a superior and lateral direction to allow examination of the middle meatus. In most cases it is easier to examine the middle meatus from posterior to anterior. The frontal sinus, anterior ethmoid cells, and maxillary sinus ostia are located in the middle meatus, with the maxillary sinus ostia the most likely to be visualized. Observe for any drainage from ostia.

NOTE: Drainage of pus from an ostium is diagnostic of acute sinusitis, with accuracy possibly greater than radiographs.

Inflammation should be recorded, and attempts should be made to identify the source of any purulent fluid or polyps protruding from or occluding the ostia. The majority of polyps are seen in the middle meatus, originating from the anterior ethmoid cells. Typical polyps are slightly yellow, translucent, and relatively avascular. They can originate from nasal mucosa (most common) or they can result from polypoid degeneration of a turbinate. Polyps can be filled with mucus or fluid. Frequently they have a stalk, or extension of mucosa, that can be traced back to their sinus of origin. Through air drying and subsequent keratinization, polyps can develop benign squamous metaplastic changes, becoming more opacified and whiter or grayer in appearance.

17. On completion of the examination, withdraw the scope and explore the opposite nasal cavity, if indicated.

NOTE: As with any endoscopic procedure, the natural tendency during nasolaryngoscopy is for the examiner to move toward whatever is being visualized. This action may form a tight loop in the scope outside the patient's nose. Such a tight loop may actually break the scope or the fibers in the scope (if a fiberoptic scope). To prevent this tendency, remember to relax and maintain the same distance from the patient throughout the procedure. If you straighten the scope at the end of the procedure before removing it from the patient's nose, the patient is usually grateful.

CARE AND CLEANING OF EQUIPMENT

Although nasolaryngoscopes are fairly indestructible, they are composed of fibers/lenses or cameras that can be broken; hence, avoid bending the scope into tight angles (especially a fiberoptic scope) or traumatizing the tip. Wash the scope with soap and water between procedures, and then soak it for 10 minutes in glutaraldehyde. Make sure the glutaraldehyde is thoroughly rinsed from the scope, before air drying, to prevent chemically irritating the next patient's mucosa. Clean the lens with lens cleaner and paper.

COMPLICATIONS

- An adverse reaction to anesthetic or decongestant (most common)
- Sneezing and gagging severe enough to prevent completion of the procedure
- Laryngospasm with possible asphyxia; prevented by remaining above the level of the vocal cords
- Blood pressure elevation (very rare and usually related to an adverse drug reaction)
- Vasovagal reaction (rare)
- Epistaxis (it is possible to dislodge eschar or to traumatize a tumor)
- Vomiting with possible aspiration

CPT/BILLING CODES

92511   Nasopharyngoscopy with endoscope
99070   Supplies and materials (except spectacles) provided by the clinician over and above those usually included with the office visit or other services rendered (list drugs, trays, supplies, or materials provided)

ICD-10-CM DIAGNOSTIC CODES

Z85.21   Laryngeal cancer, history
C32.9   Laryngeal cancer, NEC
F44.0–F44.9   Globus hystericus

F45.8	Psychogenic dysphonia or cough
H66.3x1–H66.3X9	Otitis media, chronic suppurative, unspecified
H66.001–H66.019	Otitis media, acute suppurative, unspecified
H66.40–H66.93	Otitis media, unspecified, chronic or acute
H92.01–H92.09	Otalgia unspecified
J33.9	Nasal polyp unspecified
J33.8	Sinus polyp
J31.0	Rhinitis, chronic
J31.2	Pharyngitis, chronic
J32.0	Sinusitis, chronic, maxillary
J32.1	Sinusitis, chronic, frontal
J32.2	Sinusitis, chronic, ethmoidal
J38.1	Laryngeal or vocal cord polyp
J38.00–J38.02	Vocal cord paralysis, unspecified
J41.0	Simple chronic bronchitis (cough, smoker's)
R22.1	Localized swelling, mass, and lump, neck
R04.0	Epistaxis
R49.1	Aphonia (loss of voice)
R49.8	Hoarseness
R19.6	Halitosis or choking sensation
R06.00	Dyspnea, chronic
R06.83	Snoring
R06.1	Stridor
R05	Cough, chronic
R04.2	Hemoptysis
R13.10	Dysphagia
T17.200–T17.208	Foreign body in hypopharynx, nasopharynx, or pharynx
T17.300–T17.308	Foreign body, larynx

Acknowledgment

The editors recognize the contributions of Rolf O. Montalvo, MD, to this chapter in a previous edition of this text.

SUPPLIERS

(See contact information available at www.expertconsult.com.)

Flexible nasolaryngoscopes with light source
Olympus America Inc.
Pentax Precision Instruments Corporation
Laborie Cogentix Vision-Sciences, Inc. (manufactures a scope as well as disposable sheath covers for various brands of scopes)

RECOMMENDED READING

American Academy of Family Physicians. *Nasolaryngoscopy for the Family Physician [CD-ROM or DVD]*. Leawood, KS: American Academy of Family Physicians; 1998.

Charous S. Laryngoscopy. In: Reichman EF, ed. *Emergency Medicine Procedures*. 2nd ed. New York: McGraw-Hill; 2013:1113–1120.

Corey GA, Hocutt JE, Rodney WM. Preliminary study of rhinolaryngoscopy by family physicians. *Fam Med*. 1988;20:262–265.

Courey MS, Roediger FC. Laryngoscopy. In: Snow JB, Wackym PA, eds. *Ballenger's Otorhinolaryngology Head and Neck Surgery*. 17th ed. Shelton, CN: Hamilton: Ontario, BC Decker Peoples Medical Publishing House; 2009:955–962.

Hayes JT, Houston R. Flexible nasolaryngoscopy: a low-risk, high-yield procedure. *Postgrad Med*. 1999;106:107–110. 114.

Hocutt JE, Corey GA, Rodney WM. Nasolaryngoscopy for family physicians. *Am Fam Physician*. 1990;42:1257–1268.

Holsinger FC, Kies MS, Weinstock YE, et al. Videos in clinical medicine. Examination of the larynx and pharynx. *N Engl J Med*. 2008;358(3):e2 https://www.nejm.org/doi/full/10.1056/NEJMvcm0706392 or www.youtube.com/watch?v=2ZDC4nQNjRs.

Corporation Olympus. *Fiberoptic Examination of the Pharynx and Larynx [videotape]*. Melville, NY: Olympus Corporation; 1994.

Corporation Olympus. *Nasolaryngoscopy: the Inside View [video]*. Greenville, NC: East Carolina University School of Medicine, Center for Medical Communications; 1988.

Patton D, DeWitt DE. Flexible nasolaryngoscopy: a procedure for primary care. *Prim Care Cancer*. 1992;12:13–21.

Corporation Pentax. *Current Concepts in Examination of the Nasopharynx and Larynx [video]*. New York: Pentax Corporation; 1995.

Plaat BE, van der Laan BF, Wedman J, Halmos GB, Dikkers FG. Distal chip versus fiberoptic laryngoscopy using endoscopic sheaths: diagnostic accuracy and image quality. *Eur Arch Otorhinolaryngol*. 2014;271(8):2227–2232.

Riviello RJ. Otolaryngologic procedures. In: Roberts JR, Custalow CB, Thomsen TW, eds. *Roberts and Hedges Clinical Procedures in Emergency Medicine and Acute Care*. 7th ed. Philadelphia: Elsevier; 2019:1338–1383.

Usatine RP. *The Color Atlas of Family Medicine*. New York: McGraw-Hill; 2009.

CHAPTER 65

INDIRECT MIRROR LARYNGOSCOPY

Grant C. Fowler • Carlos A. Dumas

Although flexible nasolaryngoscopy is often available for visualization of the upper respiratory tract, indirect mirror laryngoscopy remains the simplest, fastest, least expensive, and often most helpful method of examining the upper tracheal rings, vocal cords, epiglottis, larynx, and hypopharynx. In certain cases, mirror laryngoscopy combined with an adequate history will be all that is needed to make the diagnosis. Experienced clinicians appreciate the glare-free lighting of the laryngeal structures provided by mirror laryngoscopy, which allows for observation of subtle color variations. Mirror laryngoscopy requires very little preparation, very little time to perform, and very little effort afterward to care for a few inexpensive instruments. The upper respiratory tract in most adults and children older than 6 or 7 years of age will be easily visualized by experienced clinicians. Examples of when mirror laryngoscopy may be useful include when nasolaryngoscopy is not available, in patients at low risk of malignancy, and during follow-up for a known lesion after complete nasolaryngoscopy has excluded other lesions. It may also be useful as a preliminary examination before nasolaryngoscopy. To keep oriented, clinicians should recall that when using a mirror, everything is seen in reverse. Before performing the procedure, it may be helpful for clinicians to refamiliarize themselves with the anatomy of the oropharynx, hypopharynx, and larynx (see Figs. 64.4 through 64.6 in Chapter 64).

NOTE: When not done on a regular basis, the necessary coordination of patient and instruments to perform mirror laryngoscopy may make it difficult and occasionally impossible to examine the patient's larynx—even for expert laryngologists. This fact was highlighted when a survey in the 1980s found that less than 30% of primary care clinicians practicing in Ohio were able to visualize a larynx, and that less than 4% included inspection of the larynx as part of their complete physical examination. Primary care clinicians in Ohio are probably representative of those elsewhere, and a few commented anonymously that they had never visualized a larynx!

INDICATIONS

- Chronic hoarseness (>3 weeks)
- Suspected or previous neoplasm
- Chronic cough
- Chronic dyspnea
- Halitosis
- Head or neck mass or adenopathy suggestive of malignancy
- Dysphagia
- Phonation disturbance, such as vocal weakness in the elderly or psychogenic dysphonia
- Chronic foreign-body sensation in pharynx
- Hemoptysis
- Suspected laryngeal foreign body
- Acute onset of hoarseness after straining voice
- Stridor, particularly inspiratory stridor
- Posttraumatic evaluation
- Any chronic unilateral upper respiratory complaint in a smoker
- Any clinical situation in which visualization of the oropharynx, hypopharynx, and larynx will aid in diagnosis or therapy

CONTRAINDICATIONS

- Acute epiglottitis. (Patient usually appears toxic (meaning very ill), will be leaning forward, drooling secretions, and may not be able to talk.) Laryngoscopy may precipitate complete airway obstruction.
- Infants and young children who are unable to cooperate.
- Acute inflammation or infection of the throat (relative contraindication).
- Patient who cannot open his or her mouth adequately (relative contraindication).

EQUIPMENT

- Bright headlight or head mirror with external light source
- No. 4 and 5 laryngeal mirrors; smaller sizes for children
- 4 × 4 inch gauze sponges
- Local anesthetic: lidocaine* spray (2% to 4%) or benzocaine* spray (14%)
- Goggles, gloves, and mask (to follow universal blood and body fluid precautions)
- Alcohol lamp or bowl of hot water to warm mirrors (optional); antifogging solutions also available

PREPROCEDURE PATIENT PREPARATION AND EVALUATION

After obtaining and performing a thorough head and neck history and examination as well as the remainder of a complete history and physical examination, explain the indications and alternatives for the procedure as well as what will happen during the procedure. Every effort should be made to relax the patient. The clinician should maintain a gentle, unhurried manner and perhaps show the patient the instruments by touching the patient with them in a nonthreatening area such as the hand or arm. Gently inform the patient that it will be important to relax and that the mirror will be placed in the top of the back of his or her mouth, avoiding the throat and the gag reflex. The patient should know that if the procedure is performed properly and an anesthetic is used, the risk of gagging should be minimized, especially if the patient keeps his or her eyes open and looks straight ahead (which diminishes the gag reflex). Possible complications should be explained, and the patient should remove any dentures.

TECHNIQUE

1. The patient should sit upright and straight, preferably in a high-backed chair with a headrest. Tell the patient to lean slightly forward. The head and jaw should be jutted forward in a "sniffing" position (Fig. 65.1). The chin should be up.

---

*Should be used with caution in those who have a history of an allergy or sensitivity to the agents (see Chapter 5).

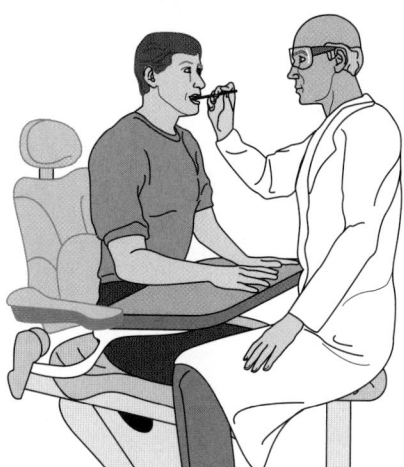

Fig. 65.1 Proper positioning of the patient is essential for successful visualization of the larynx.

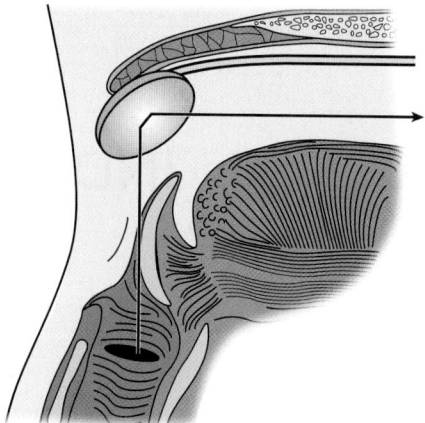

Fig. 65.2 The laryngeal mirror is inserted into the pharynx, lifting the uvula but avoiding contact with the posterior pharyngeal wall.

2. Sit slightly to the side of the patient; sitting slightly higher than the patient will also facilitate visualization of the laryngeal structures. Position the light source so that the light is directed parallel to your visual axis and focused on the patient's posterior pharynx. The clinician should be comfortable and understand that the use of a hurried approach can make this procedure more difficult. The clinician should follow universal blood and body fluid precautions.

3. Spray the patient's pharynx with the anesthetic and have him or her gargle and spit it out.

4. Select the largest mirror that will fit comfortably into the back of the patient's throat and warm it over the alcohol lamp, in the warm water, or inside the patient's cheek. Warming the mirror should prevent fogging. If the mirror is externally warmed, check its temperature on the back of your hand to make sure that it is not too hot before inserting it. In addition, you can touch the warmed mirror to the hand or arm of the patient, not only to reassure the patient that the temperature is acceptable but also to demonstrate that the mirror is nonthreatening.

5. Have the patient protrude his or her tongue. Cover it with gauze and grasp it firmly between the thumb and middle finger of your nondominant hand. In effect, the ventral surface of the tip of the tongue is rolled over your middle finger. Do not pull so hard as to cause discomfort. Use your index finger to retract the patient's upper lip.

6. Ask the patient to breathe in and out through the mouth or to "pant like a puppy." This opens the space between the soft palate and the tongue. Remind the patient to keep his or her eyes open and to perhaps focus on your forehead or headband to serve as a distraction.

7. With the warm mirror in your dominant hand and the glass surface pointing downward, slowly introduce the mirror and visualize the epiglottis. Next, slowly and gently apply the posterior aspect of the mirror to the uvula and a portion of the soft palate. With a smooth, gentle movement, slowly lift them upward and backward out of the way. Avoid touching either the posterior pharyngeal wall or the base of the tongue. Touching these might stimulate the gag reflex (Fig. 65.2).
   NOTE: In certain patients, adequate anesthesia is not attainable for this portion of the procedure. In those cases, flexible nasolaryngoscopy should be performed.

8. With the mirror gently lifting the uvula and soft palate out of the way, tilt it in various directions to visualize the larynx, the hypopharynx, and the anterior oropharynx, including the base of the tongue. Move your head toward and away from the mirror to focus the light source maximally on visualized objects

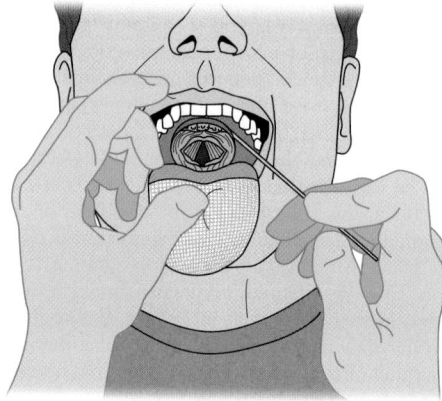

Fig. 65.3 The tongue is pulled forward with gauze and the mirror tilted in various directions to visualize the larynx, hypopharynx, and anterior oropharynx.

(Fig. 65.3). Continue to encourage the patient to breathe gently in and out through the mouth. If the structures are not adequately visualized after lifting the soft palate and uvula out of the way, check the positioning of the patient's chin and neck. Reposition if necessary.

9. With the larynx visualized (see Fig. 64.6 in Chapter 64), observe vocal cord activity during quiet respiration. Next, observe cord activity while the patient makes a prolonged high "eee" sound. This lengthens the vocal cords and moves the larynx upward vertically, which should allow visualization of the anterior commissure. Observe for symmetry of cord mobility and for edema, hemorrhage, erythema, nodules, or a mass on the cords or in the surrounding structures. Note any other mucosal or structural abnormalities.
   NOTE: All structures viewed will be seen in mirror image (upside down and backward).

10. If the mirror fogs during the procedure, it must be reheated. If it is heated externally, it must be tested again on your hand or arm before use. For those patients whose pharynx is not suitably visualized by this technique or those in whom a closer evaluation of an abnormality is indicated, nasolaryngoscopy should be performed or referral to an otolaryngologist considered.

FINDINGS

- Epiglottis: This usually has a slightly curved and regular upper edge but is sometimes acutely curved and conical ("infantile type"). It may hang backward and obscure the view of the cords in the relaxed state or hang forward to hide the valleculae. If the epiglottis is floppy, small lesions on the laryngeal surface of the epiglottis may be difficult to see. The apices of the pyriform sinuses are also not usually visualized. The epiglottis rises upward and forward during phonation. Pooling of secretions in the valleculae (anterior to the epiglottis) indicates tongue weakness; pooling of secretions in the piriform sinus (posterior to the epiglottis) indicates pharyngeal wall weakness.

- Aryepiglottic folds: May have swelling or an ulceration.
- Interarytenoid area: May be thickened or covered with papilla.
- False cords: May show swelling or an ulceration.
- Vocal cords must be examined for the following:
  - Color: Normal color is pearly white.
  - Movement: May be restricted by paresis or by infiltration of tumor. Arthritis of the cricoarytenoid joint may also cause limited movement.
  - Surface: May be intact or ulcerated.
  - Edge: May be irregular.
  - Anterior commissure: Not always seen because of anatomic variations.
- Subglottic space: Difficult to examine, but swellings may be seen below the level of the vocal cords.

COMPLICATIONS

- Possible laceration of the undersurface of the tongue from stretching the tongue over the teeth
- Possible adverse reaction to anesthetic
- Vomiting, with possible aspiration
- Failure to diagnose an abnormality because of inadequate visualization

CPT/BILLING CODES

No separate code is available for this procedure. Consider using a more comprehensive E/M code.

ICD-10-CM DIAGNOSTIC CODES

C32.9	Laryngeal cancer, NEC
F17.200	Nicotine addiction, or addiction in remission
F45.8	Psychogenic dysphonia
R22.1	Localized swelling, mass and lump, neck
R49.1	Aphonia
R49.8	Hoarseness
R19.6	Halitosis
R06.02	Dyspnea, chronic
R06.1	Stridor
R05	Cough, chronic
R04.2	Hemoptysis
R13.10	Dysphagia
T17.200-T17.208	Foreign body in hypopharynx, nasopharynx, oropharynx, or pharynx
T17.300-T17.308	Foreign body, larynx

RECOMMENDED READING

Fink DS, Roediger FC, Courey MS. Laryngoscopy. In: Wackym PA, Snow JB, eds. *Ballenger's Otorhinolaryngology Head and Neck Surgery.* 18th ed. Shelton, CT: Peoples Medical Publishing; 2016.

Riviello RJ. Otolaryngologic Procedures. In: Roberts JR, Custalow CB, Thomsen TW, eds. *Roberts and Hedges Clinical Procedures in Emergency Medicine and Acute Care,* 7th ed. Philadelphia: Elsevier; 2019:1338–1383.

CHAPTER 66

TONSILLECTOMY AND ADENOIDECTOMY

Thomas N. Told

Tonsillectomy is one of the oldest surgeries known. It was first described in 50 AD by Celsus, who used a hook to grasp the tonsil and his finger to excise the bulk of the tonsillar tissue. By the 6th century, hygienic concerns had led to the use of knives and other instruments to complete the surgery. These early surgeons were quick to recognize the importance of following the correct tissue planes to be successful, a fact that holds true today. The pain of doing surgery without anesthesia led to the development of instruments that would remove the tonsils quickly. These methods often failed to remove all the tonsillar tissue and obstruction would recur. Throughout the first half of the 20th century, tonsillectomy was performed under local anesthesia and later general anesthesia without airway protection. The procedure was often performed with very few indications in healthy individuals. Adenotonsillectomy reached its peak when 1.4 million procedures were performed in the United States in 1959.

Over the last 50 years, the frequency of tonsillectomy and adenoidectomy has declined in America; however, it still remains the most common surgery performed on children younger than 15 years of age. With improved antimicrobial therapy, the indications for tonsillectomy and adenoidectomy have also shifted from recurrent infection to obstruction. Currently 75% of tonsillectomies are performed to remove obstruction. There are many techniques and innovations that have been tried through the years, from snares to lasers. Many fell out of favor because of concerns over excessive blood loss, tissue damage, excessive postoperative pain, or extended intraoperative time.

This chapter focuses on three of the most popular techniques used today. These are cold knife and snare with or without electrocautery, harmonic ultrasonic scalpel (Ethicon Endosurgery), and bipolar radiofrequency ablation or Coblation (Arthrocare Smith & Nephew).

Most studies agree that the less heat introduced into the pharyngeal tissue, the less postoperative pain experienced by the patient. A Cochrane review (Pinder, 2011) found more pain if monopolar cautery is used versus the cold knife technique. Cold knife and snare removal puts no heat into the system, but cold steel does nothing to stop the bleeding. Bleeding is the most feared complication of tonsillectomy, and electrocautery or sutures must be used as a supplemental measure to control any brisk bleeding, if it occurs. Electrocautery produces considerable heat at the operative site (400°C; Fig. 66.1A). Electrocautery and figure-of-eight sutures also cause collateral tissue damage for several millimeters around the bleeding site. This heat and tissue damage nullifies any benefits the cold knife procedure may have had with respect to lower pain levels or prompter healing rates. Both the harmonic ultrasonic scalpel and the radiofrequency Coblation wand cut and coagulate at the same time, resulting in very little blood loss. Hemostasis is achieved by the production of a protein plug in the end of the cut vessel from the ultrasonic or plasma energy of the devices. The harmonic scalpel generates operative site temperatures

of only 70°C to 80°C, and the radiofrequency Coblation wand produces a slightly lower temperature of 60°C (see Fig. 66.1B). Less heat should translate into slightly lower postoperative pain scores for the Coblator compared with the harmonic ultrasonic scalpel, especially in the first few days. However, total recovery time is nearly identical, so the temperatures should not be a significant factor when deciding between these two techniques. A recent Cochrane review of Coblation versus standard technique (2017) had this same conclusion, despite much larger differences in temperatures. The investigators also concluded that despite the large number of studies, the current evidence is of very low quality. All studies agree that lower pain scores and decreased recovery time also come from gentle and careful removal of all of the tonsillar tissue. Therefore the best method for tonsillectomy is the technique with which the operating clinician is most comfortable, or has the most experience.

ANATOMY OF THE TONSIL BED

See Fig. 66.2 for an overview of tonsil bed anatomy.
- Superior: soft palate
- Inferior: lingual tonsil
- Deep: superior constrictor muscle
- Anterior: palatoglossus muscle
- Posterior: palatopharyngeus muscle
- Vascular supply to the tonsil (Fig. 66.3)
  - Superior pole
    Ascending pharyngeal artery
    Lesser palatine artery
  - Inferior pole
    Tonsillar branches of facial artery
    Dorsal lingual artery
    Ascending palatine artery

NOTE: The key to controlling brisk tonsillar bed bleeding is to direct efforts toward the superior or inferior poles first before trying to control every bleeder in the tonsillar bed because the poles are the vascular points of entry.

INDICATIONS FOR TONSILLECTOMY

Absolute Indications

- Hypertrophy resulting in obstructive sleep symptoms in adults or children that lead to adverse pulmonary or cardiovascular conditions
- Hypertrophy and airway obstruction leading to malformation of the facial bones or malocclusion of the teeth requiring dental attention
- Hypertrophy resulting in dysphagia and poor weight gain
- Recurrent peritonsillar abscesses requiring drainage that fail to heal with appropriately dosed medications (see Chapter 206, Peritonsillar Abscess Drainage)

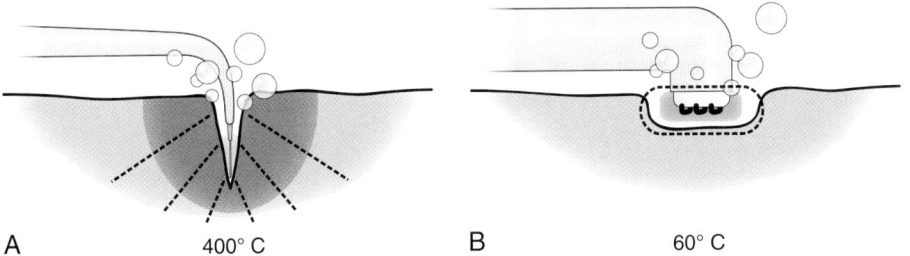

Fig. 66.1 (A) Electrocoagulation produces excessive heat at the operative site and results in a wide area of thermal damage (400°C). (B) The bipolar radiofrequency ablation (Coblation) wand and the ultrasonic cutting and coagulating instrument (harmonic scalpel) produces low heat (60°C) at the tissue interface while achieving good hemostasis. (Courtesy Arthrocare Smith & Nephew ENT.)

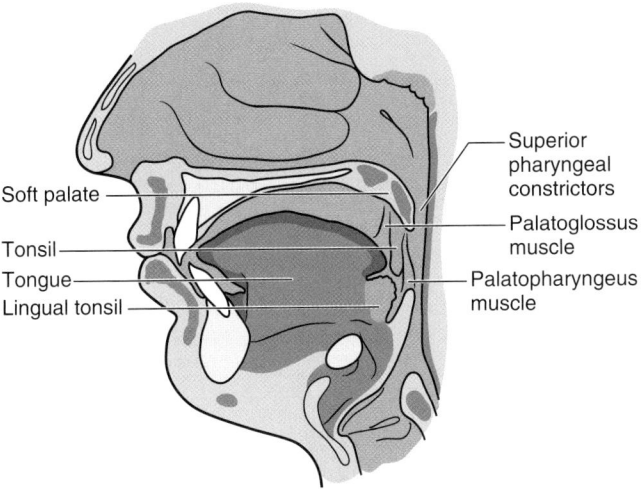

Fig. 66.2 Anatomy of the tonsil bed.

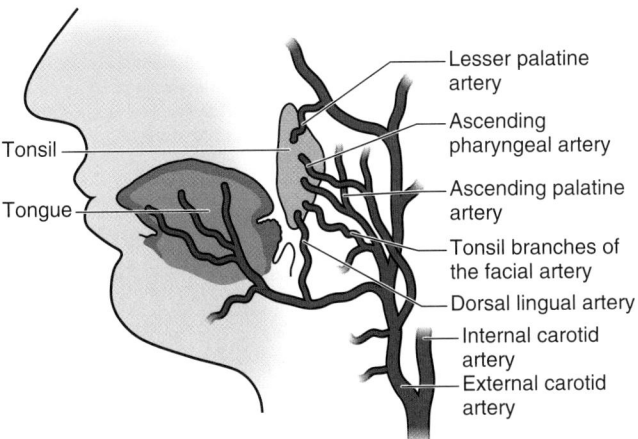

Fig. 66.3 The tonsil is sustained by a rich supply of vessels that enter through the inferior pole. Only two branches enter the superior pole. Directing maximum hemostatic effort to the inferior pole controls most of the potential intraoperative bleeding.

- Tonsillitis that spawns febrile convulsions
- Tonsils with suspicious growth or anatomic characteristics that may require biopsy for the exclusion of malignancy

Relative Indications

- Seven or more clearly documented (sore throat associated with fever >38.2°C, cervical lymphadenopathy, tonsillar exudate or positive strep test) episodes of acute tonsillitis within a year, five or more episodes per year over the last 2 years, or three or more per year over last 3 years. (Some clinicians recommend tonsillectomy in children who miss 2 or more weeks of school annually because of tonsillar infections.)

  NOTE: Children who undergo tonsillectomy for recurrent tonsillitis may have a higher risk of postoperative hemorrhage than those who undergo the procedure for obstructive symptoms.
- Children with multiple antibiotic allergies or intolerance, a history of aphthous stomatitis, pharyngitis and adenitis with fever (PFAPA), or a history of peritonsillar abscess.
- Persistent episodes of a foul taste in the mouth or malodorous breath that do not clear with appropriate medical therapy.
- Chronic bouts of tonsillitis in a streptococcal carrier that do not respond to beta lactamase–resistant antibiotics.
- Nocturnal enuresis where upper airway obstructive sleep disorder also is present from large tonsils and adenoids.
- Attention deficit hyperactivity disorder resistant to treatment with coexistent upper airway obstructive sleep disorder.

CONTRAINDICATIONS TO TONSILLECTOMY AND ADENOIDECTOMY

- Poor anesthetic risk
- Uncontrolled medical illness
- Anemia
- Acute bilateral infections
- Anticoagulated patient or patient with coagulopathy (either the anticoagulation/coagulopathy should be reversed or otolaryngology consulted)

COMPLICATIONS OF TONSILLECTOMY AND ADENOIDECTOMY

- Hemorrhage during surgery, immediately in the postoperative period, or 5 to 7 days after surgery when the scabs slough off the adenotonsillar bed. Intraoperative bleeding around the endotracheal tube may form a clot and lead to airway obstruction after extubation. Swallowed blood can lead to postoperative nausea and vomiting.
- Dehydration
- Temporary weight loss during the postoperative period
- Perforation of the anterior or posterior tonsillar pillars, a benign complication
- Airway obstruction
- Death
- *Specific to adenoidectomy:* nasopharyngeal stenosis and velopharyngeal insufficiency (nasal regurgitation of food and hypernasal speech)

NOTE: Patients with significant airway obstruction due to adenotonsillar hypertrophy may be at risk for postobstructive pulmonary edema syndrome once the obstruction is removed.

PREPROCEDURE PATIENT EVALUATION AND CONSIDERATIONS

- Complete blood count, prothrombin time/international normalized ratio, and bleeding time if there is a suspicion or a history of a bleeding disorder.

- Caution in children younger than 3 years, or with history of prematurity, seizures, neuromuscular conditions, or asthma, and in anyone with a significant history of obstructive sleep apnea or other severe medical conditions or extenuating circumstances.
  NOTE: These patients may have to be monitored more closely in the postoperative period, and some may have to remain overnight to exclude delayed complications.
- Evaluate and possibly remove extremely loose deciduous teeth that could be dislodged during the course of the surgery and threaten the airway.
- Patients should not eat solid foods for 8 hours before surgery.
- A single intraoperative intravenous (IV) dose of dexamethasone (0.5 mg/kg) during tonsillectomy or adenotonsillectomy in children results in less pain after surgery, less vomiting, and a return to eating a normal diet sooner. IV antibiotics may also reduce postoperative fever.
- Injection of local anesthetics into the tonsillar or adenoid beds at the start of surgery may decrease hemorrhage and improve postoperative recovery.
- Universal blood and body fluid precautions should be followed, whichever technique is performed.

TYPES OF TONSILLECTOMY

Fig. 66.4 illustrates the two types of tonsillectomy.

Intracapsular (Tonsillotomy)

This method removes only the body of the tonsil down to the level of the capsular membrane, which remains in contact with the pharyngeal musculature. The tonsillar tissue is removed in small pieces using suction along with some type of tissue ablation such as electrocautery, a harmonic scalpel, or Coblation. The incremental removal is useful when extremely friable tonsillar tissue will not allow grasping or traction with a tonsillar forceps to perform a subcapsular procedure. This procedure also theoretically decreases postoperative pain and recovery time. *All the tonsillar tissue must be removed to reduce the risk of bleeding and recurrence.*

Subcapsular/Extracapsular

This technique is the favored method in use today. It involves the gentle traction and careful dissection of the tonsil and the capsule from the musculature surrounding the tonsillar bed. Using blunt cold dissection, dissection with the aid of a harmonic ultrasonic scalpel, or radiofrequency ablation, the entire tonsil with accompanying capsule is removed from the tonsillar bed. No redundant capsule or tonsillar tissue is left behind, reducing the risk of delayed complications.

COLD KNIFE AND SNARE METHOD

This is the oldest and most widely recognized method of tonsil removal. Bleeding must be controlled by other means such as electrocautery, vasoactive topical agents, packing, or placement of absorbable sutures.

Equipment

See corresponding numbers in Fig. 66.5.
- Self-retaining mouth gag and tongue retractor (1)
- Three sizes of tongue blades
- Operative suction and cautery (2)
- Curved tonsillar tenaculum (3)
- Posterior throat pack with attached retrieval string and small hemostat (4)
- Tonsil dissector and pillar retractor (5)

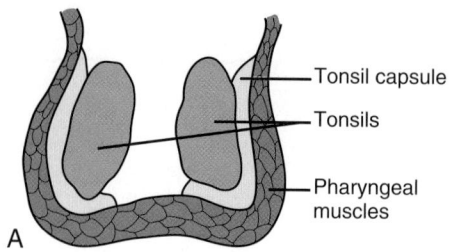
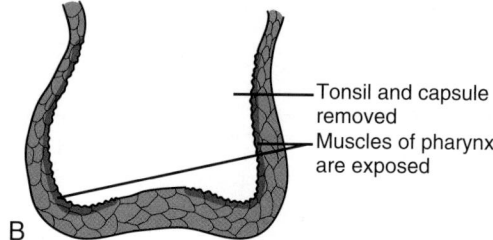
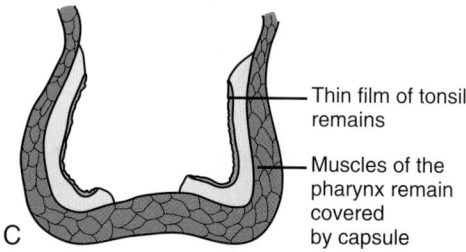

Fig. 66.4 (A) The tonsil is separated from the pharyngeal muscle by a fibrous capsule. (B) Extracapsular (subcapsular) tonsillectomy removes the tonsil and capsule, leaving the pharyngeal muscle to epithelialize in several weeks. (C) Intracapsular tonsillectomy leaves the capsule and some tonsil attached. Tonsil regeneration is greater with this procedure.

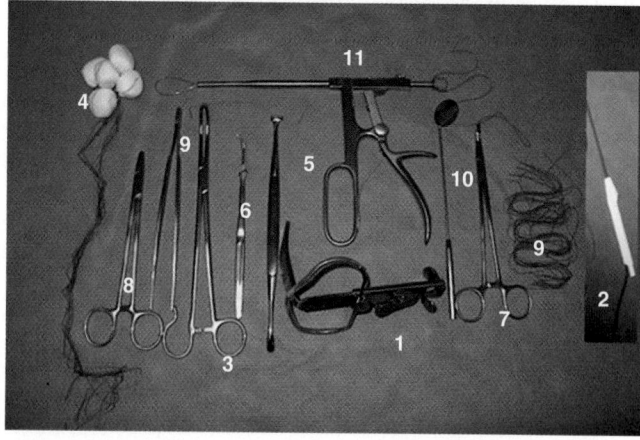

Fig. 66.5 Equipment for tonsil removal. See the "Equipment" section under "Cold Knife and Snare Method" for corresponding numbered parts.

- Curved tonsil knife (6)
- Tonsillar bed hemostat (7)
- Needle holder (8)
- 0 or 2-0 plain gut suture on tonsil needle (9)
- Laryngeal mirror (10)
- Tonsil snare and wire (11)

Technique

1. The patient is placed supine on the operating table, and the head is hyperextended using a dropped headrest or a shoulder roll. The head must be secured on a donut-style headrest or on head pads.
2. The airway is protected by endotracheal intubation. A self-retaining mouth gag and tongue retractor is placed in the mouth to expose the tonsils. Exposure can be increased by suspending the handle of the tongue retractor from the Mayo stand. Some clinicians prefer to retract the soft palate with a small red rubber catheter placed through the nose and out of the mouth. It can then be secured over the mouth gag with a clamp; however, such a catheter is not always necessary for adequate exposure.
   NOTE: The mouth gag and tongue retractor places pressure on the base of the tongue, so it should be released intermittently to restore circulation to the tongue and, it is hoped, reduce postoperative pain.
3. A throat pack is placed in the posterior pharynx. There should be a string or umbilical tape firmly applied to the pack for later retrieval. A hemostat is placed on the tape and left in place to ensure the pack is removed at the end of the procedure.
4. The tonsil is then grasped at its midpoint using a tonsillar tenaculum. Care should be taken not to grasp the anterior (palatoglossus muscle) or posterior pillars (palatopharyngeus muscle) when grasping the body of the tonsil. The tenaculum is used to apply medial traction on the tonsil, thereby tenting the tonsil into the tonsillar fossae and oral cavity.
5. Begin the dissection superiorly. Using a curved tonsil knife, an incision is made down to the palatoglossus muscle along the posterolateral aspect of the muscle in the plane of the muscle fibers.
6. Using a tonsillar dissector, the tonsil is bluntly and gently dissected away from the bed and removed. The dissection should start from the superior portion of the tonsillar bed and work downward toward the lower one-third or inferior portion of the tonsillar bed.
7. Leaving the inferior portion of the tonsil attached to the tonsillar bed, the snare is then applied. (The snare can then be applied over the tonsillar tenaculum's special handle [Fig. 66.6], or the tenaculum removed and then replaced through the loop of the snare.)
8. The snare is now tightened slightly so that it nearly approximates the size of the body of the tonsil, but it is not yet tightened around the tonsil.
9. The tip of the snare is then moved to the back of the pharynx, to a point posterior to the body of the tonsil. The wire loop will be bent slightly inferiorly and medially relative to the body of the tonsil.
10. This snare is then closed briskly and firmly, which bluntly dissects the inferior portion of the tonsil away from the tonsillar bed. Bleeding will be brisk from the superior and inferior aspects of the tonsillar fossae. This can be controlled by placing packs into the bleeding tonsillar bed and waiting for the bleeding to stop. Applying figure-of-eight sutures to the superior and inferior aspects of the tonsillar fossae using 0 or 2-0 plain gut sutures on a tonsil needle may help with hemostasis. (Avoid placing the sutures too deeply, which could damage nearby structures, including blood vessels such as the carotid artery.) Unipolar or bipolar cautery, with or without suction, can also be used to ablate the bleeding areas (Fig. 66.7).
11. The procedure is repeated on the opposite side.

HARMONIC SCALPEL METHOD

This procedure requires the use of an ultrasonic generator that passes energy to a special titanium rod that vibrates at 55,000 times per second (Hz). This generates enough energy to vaporize tissue at the point of contact with the tip, and this can be limited to the width

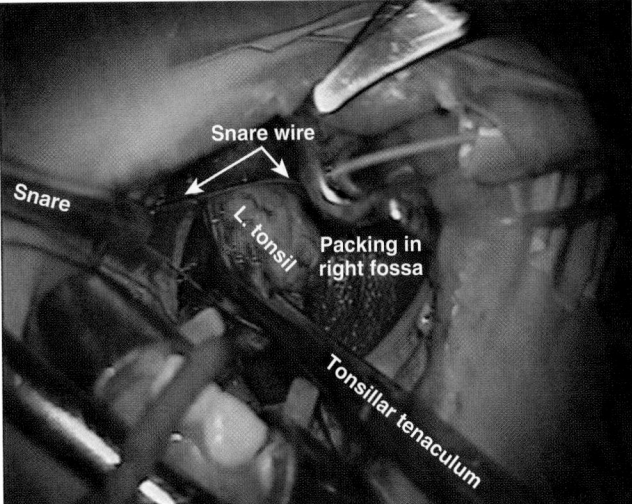

Fig. 66.6 The right tonsil has been removed and is packed. The left tonsil has been bluntly dissected from superior to medial, and the tonsil snare is being applied to clip off the inferior pole. Note the generous amount of bleeding in the throat and mouth. (Courtesy Kevin T. Kavanaugh, MD.)

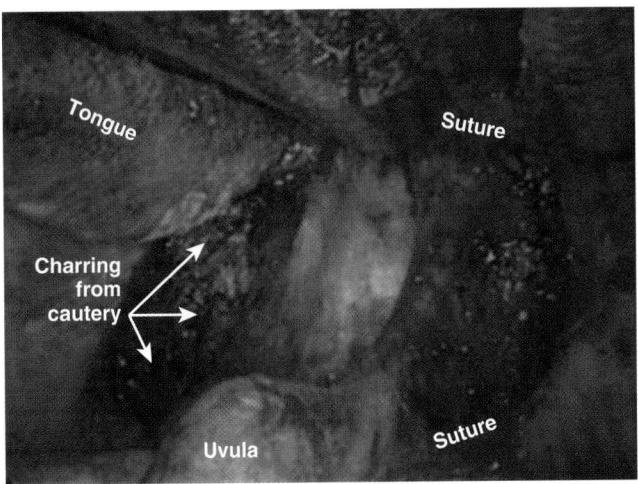

Fig. 66.7 If simple packing fails to control postoperative bleeding, then suture ligatures and suction cautery need to be used. The image shows the charring of conventional cautery on the left and the area on the right for most effective suture placement to control hemorrhage. (Courtesy Thomas N. Told, DO.)

of a knife blade. The ultrasonic energy also generates enough heat (70°C to 80°C) to form protein plugs in the severed ends of blood vessels (Fig. 66.8).

There are two energy settings on the generator, a low setting (level 3) and a high setting (level 6). Unlike conventional electrocautery, where higher settings result in greater cautery power, the ultrasonic harmonic scalpel creates more hemostasis on the lower settings. The best setting for tonsillectomy is level 3.

The vapor that is generated from cell destruction helps undermine the tissue layers as well.

The tip is disposable and contains a blunt, curved back portion, a sharply hooked front, and large flat sides (Fig. 66.9). Most of the surgery is performed with the blunt, curved back part of the tip because it produces better bleeding control than the sharp, hooked front of the tip (see Fig 66.9). The large, flat side surfaces can also be used for hemostasis in areas like the superior and inferior tonsillar poles where the major blood vessels enter. The sharp, hooked portion of the front of the blade can be used to

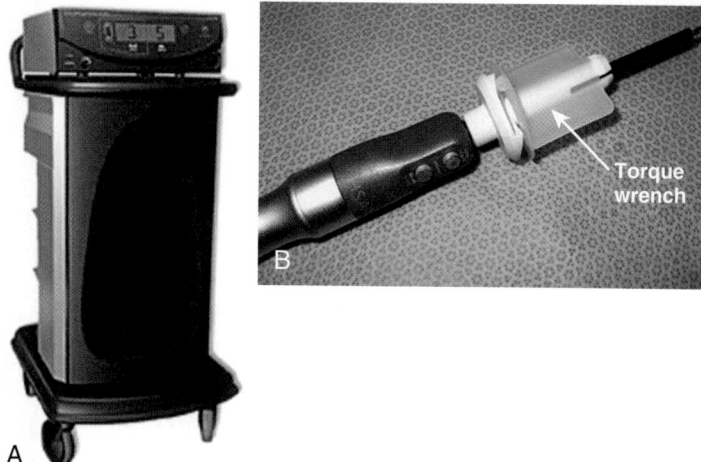

Fig. 66.8 (A) The ultrasonic generator forms a high-frequency sound wave that is transmitted to the handpiece, where it causes a titanium rod to vibrate at 55,500 Hz. (B) A special torque wrench ensures proper fit between handle and titanium rod to prevent loss of energy. (Courtesy of Ethicon Endo-Surgery, Inc.)

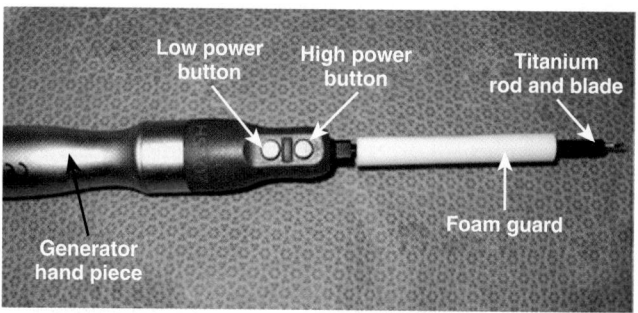

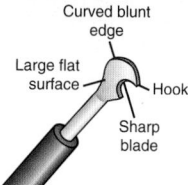

Fig. 66.9 Heat can be generated along the rod, so a foam guard covers the rod where it could touch lip and other mouth parts. High power cuts quickly but gives less hemostasis. Low power controls bleeding the best. *Bottom,* Magnified view of the hooked blade shows the operative surfaces. (Courtesy Ethicon Endo-Surgery, Inc.)

divide the nonvascular membranes or the thick, tough tissue that has been cauterized by the curved back part of the tip. Although the harmonic scalpel can control the usual bleeding that occurs during the course of a normal procedure, other measures such as unipolar cautery or sutures may be required to control larger, more brisk bleeders that cannot be occluded by the harmonic scalpel tip.

Equipment

See the corresponding numbers in Fig. 66.10.
- Harmonic scalpel generator and disposable hooked dissection tip (1)
- Self-retaining mouth gag and tongue retractor (2)
- Three sizes of tongue blades (3)
- Curved tonsillar tenaculum (4)
- Posterior throat pack with attached retrieval string and small hemostat (5)
- Operative suction and cautery (6)
- Laryngeal mirror
- Sucralfate liquid
- 0 or 2-0 plain gut tonsil suture, and curved, long-handled needle holder on standby

Technique

1. Patient preparation and exposure are the same as with the cold knife and snare technique.
2. The body of the tonsil is grasped with the tonsillar tenaculum and retracted medially into the tonsillar fossae/oral cavity. This will tent the palatoglossus muscle and accentuate the boundaries of the tonsillar body.
3. The dissection begins near the boundary of the palatoglossus muscle with the anterior aspect of the body of the tonsil.
4. Using the blunt, curved back portion of the tip as a scalpel (see Fig. 66.9), and extremely light downward pressure, the tip is energized and moved back and forth a few millimeters each way. Proceed slowly and carefully to deliver the tonsil (Fig. 66.11).
5. There will be some vapor and foam released by the tip. This vapor tends to separate the tissue planes and make the dissection easier. The capsular tissue under the tip will turn white to slightly brown; it is important to stay in this plane. The tonsillar capsule will remain a white and glistening membrane, whereas the delivered tonsil will have an egglike appearance. Continue this maneuver in a lateral and inferior or superior direction until the entire anterior portion of the tonsil is released.
6. If the tip of the harmonic scalpel penetrates the body of the tonsil, the tonsillar tissue will bubble up with the appearance of fresh-cooked oatmeal. If this happens, change the direction and pressure of the tip slightly until you again enter the correct plane.
7. The dissection can then proceed inferiorly or superiorly, depending on which direction the tonsil releases easiest from the bed.
8. The tonsillar tenaculum can be manipulated and twisted to more easily expose the different surfaces of the tonsil (Fig. 66.12).
9. The largest vessels enter the tonsil from the inferior aspect of the tonsillar bed near the lingual tonsil. When dissecting this area, most clinicians use the larger, flat side of the harmonic scalpel tip to create a greater area of hemostasis and less bleeding (Fig. 66.13).
10. When the body of the tonsil is completely released from the superior or inferior tonsillar bed, the tenaculum can then be reapplied to facilitate removal of the tonsil from the palatopharyngeus muscle of the posterior pillar.
    NOTE: When removing the tonsil body from the muscle where tissue planes have been destroyed by infection, it is important to confine the dissection to the tonsillar side rather than the muscular side.
11. When the tonsil is completely removed, residual bleeding can be controlled by placing the flat portion of the dissection tip against the bleeding site and gently tamponading the bleeding.

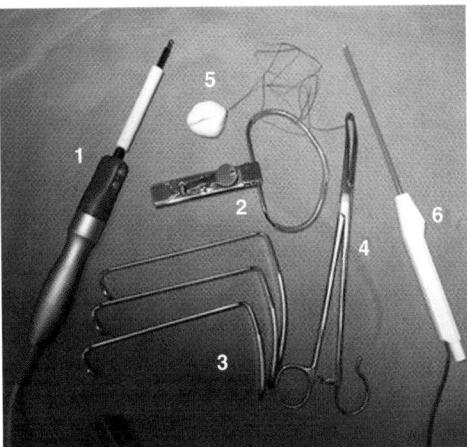

Fig. 66.10 Harmonic scalpel method equipment. See the "Equipment" section under "Harmonic Scalpel Method" for corresponding part numbers. (Courtesy Ethicon Endo-Surgery, Inc.)

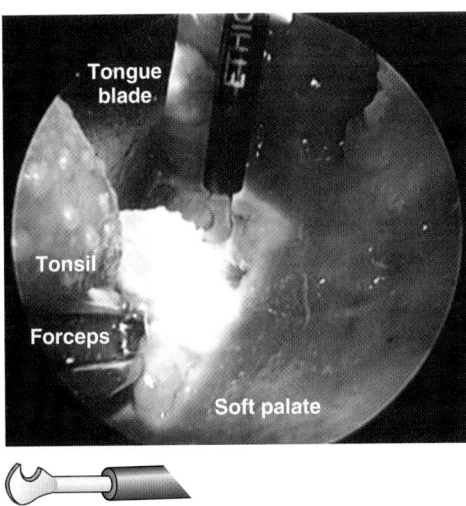

Fig. 66.11 Dissection of the middle and superior portion is done with the blunt, curved side of the hooked blade. The traction on the tonsil clamp is in the direction opposite to the plane being operated. Note the white hemostatic capsular plane under the scalpel. *Bottom,* The curved edge *(arrow)* is the best dissector and is used to do most of the procedure. (Courtesy Thomas N. Told, DO.)

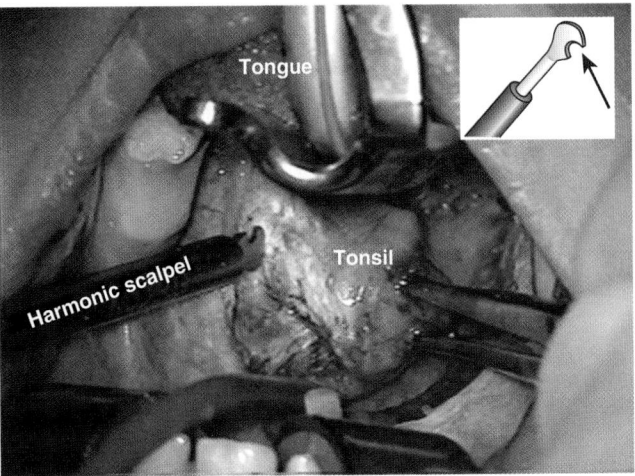

Fig. 66.12 The sharp, hooked portion of the harmonic scalpel is not frequently used because it cuts too rapidly to provide effective hemostasis. It is best used on thin tissue in the superior portion of the tonsil, or to cut tough, thick capsule. *Inset,* The sharp, hooked blade *(arrow)* can be used to do fine dissection or transect large avascular tissue.

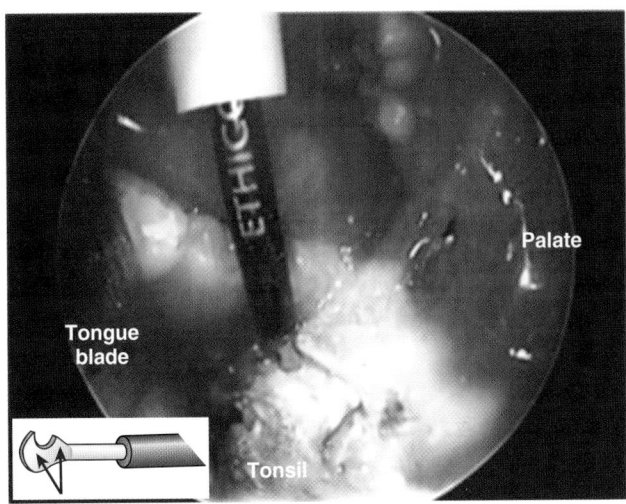

Fig. 66.13 The flat portion of the hooked blade is used on the inferior aspect of the tonsil near the tongue blade, where the major blood vessels enter. This achieves maximum hemostasis. Extremely large vessels are gently compressed with the large, flat surface of the blade and power applied for 5 to 10 seconds. *Inset,* The flat surface of the blade *(arrows)* provides the best hemostasis. (Courtesy Thomas N. Told, DO.)

The tip can be placed on low power for 10 seconds to coagulate the bleeding. Small amounts of capillary bleeding can also be controlled by lightly moving the activated tip over the bleeding site until the bleeding stops or a light char appears.

NOTE: When controlling bleeders, it is important that the clinician be very careful not to apply excessive downward pressure to the tip because it will quickly bury the tip into deeper layers and cause serious bleeding.

12. The procedure is repeated on the opposite tonsil.
13. The tonsillar beds are painted with sucralfate liquid, and the self-retaining retractor released to check for any residual bleeding. The posterior throat pack is removed and the posterior pharynx is then thoroughly suctioned, if necessary.

COBLATION METHOD

This technique is the favorite for many surgeons because it is relatively fast and produces less heat and pain, all leading to shorter initial recovery times. The wand in this unit contains both suction and bipolar cautery. It produces tissue vaporization by passing a bipolar radiofrequency current through normal saline (Fig. 66.14A). This results in the production of a plasma field of sodium ions (see Fig. 66.14B). This plasma field is able to vaporize tissue at low temperatures (60°C) and coagulate blood in any severed vessels. As previously mentioned, the instrument possesses a built-in suction feature that removes excess water and blood. Larger vessels that are not controlled with the plasma field can be cauterized with the built-in electrocautery. Set the electrocautery feature on the lowest settings that will work to avoid collateral tissue damage. The Coblator is the only device that can do both tonsillectomy and adenoidectomy (see Fig. 66.14C). The power of the Coblator's plasma field also can be varied so that the operator can perform either dissection or ablation.

The Coblation wand is more than twice the diameter of the harmonic scalpel, but its curved tip makes it easy to use. Like the harmonic scalpel, the Coblation wand must be used slowly and carefully during dissection

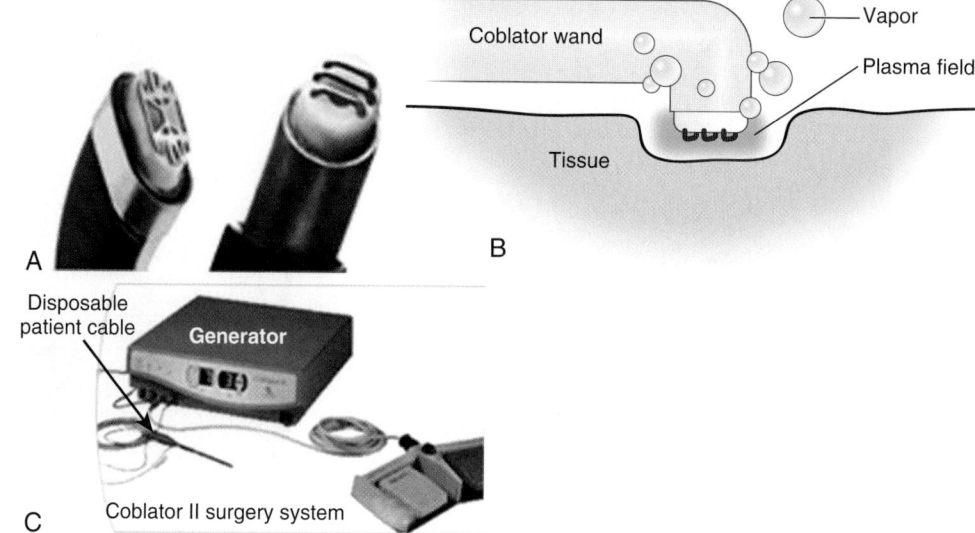

Fig. 66.14 (A) The Coblation wand provides both suction and bipolar cautery. (B) It produces tissue vaporization by passing a bipolar radiofrequency current through normal saline. (C) The Coblator is the only device that can do both tonsillectomy and adenoidectomy. (Courtesy Arthrocare Smith & Nephew ENT.)

for the best results. This device can also perform either an intracapsular or a subcapsular tonsillectomy without requiring extra equipment.

Equipment

See Fig. 66.10 for pieces 2 through 5.
- Bipolar radiofrequency Coblator unit and wand (see Fig. 66.14C)
- Self-retaining mouth gag and tongue retractor (2)
- Three sizes of tongue blades (3)
- Curved tonsillar tenaculum (4)
- Posterior throat pack with attached retrieval string and small hemostat (5)
- Laryngeal mirror
- Sucralfate liquid

Technique

1. Patient preparation and exposure are the same as with the cold knife and snare technique.
2. The tonsil is grasped with a tonsillar tenaculum and retracted medially.
3. The tip of the wand is used to carefully dissect the anterior portion of the tonsil away from the surrounding muscle. The tip of the wand is always pointed toward the tonsillar tissue to prevent injury to underlying tissue (Fig. 66.15). The tonsil is manipulated to expose the lateral and inferior surfaces to the tip of the wand.
4. Larger vessels are point cauterized with the electrocautery feature. Care must be taken to use the lowest setting to avoid excess tissue damage.
5. The procedure is repeated on the opposite tonsil.
6. The tonsillar fossae are painted with sucralfate solution.
7. The mouth gag is released and the beds are inspected for bleeding.
8. The posterior throat pack is removed and the posterior pharynx is suctioned, if necessary.
9. Both fossae are inspected for the presence of any tonsil tissue (Fig. 66.16).

INDICATIONS FOR ADENOIDECTOMY

- Large adenoids causing upper airway obstruction and resulting in obstructive sleep apnea.
- Children with large adenoids, with or without large tonsils, resulting in snoring and mouth breathing.

NOTE: There is no evidence that adenoidectomy improves chronic otitis media; therefore, its use is *discouraged* for this condition.

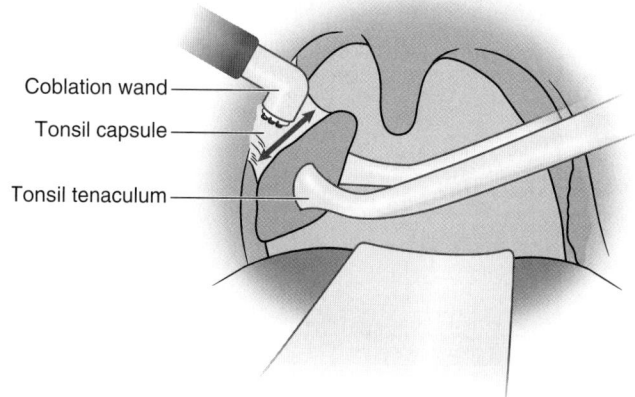

Fig. 66.15 The Coblation wand uses a sodium ion cloud at the tissue interface to cut tissue and coagulate blood vessels. Bipolar cautery is also provided to coagulate large bleeding vessels. The wand also contains a suction tip that removes vapor and blood obscuring the operative field. Traction is maintained in an opposing direction to the wand, which aids in separating the tissue planes. (Courtesy Arthrocare Smith & Nephew ENT.)

CONTRAINDICATIONS TO ADENOIDECTOMY

Only conservative adenoidectomy should be performed in the presence of occult submucous cleft palate; therefore both the hard and soft palates should be examined visually and manually for a cleft palate.

EQUIPMENT

See the corresponding numbers in Fig. 66.17.
- Self-retaining mouth gags and tongue retractor (1)
- Palate retractor (2)
- Adenoid curettes (3)
- Punch adenotome (6)
- Posterior throat pack with attached retrieval string and small hemostats (4)
- Laryngeal mirror (5)
- Suction cautery (optional)
- Nasal suction catheter of appropriate caliber
- Coblation equipment and wand (for Coblation method)

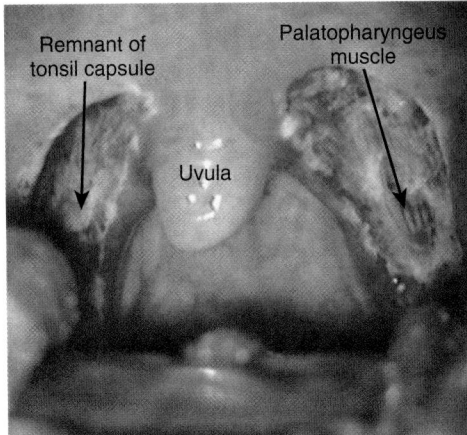

Fig. 66.16 The pharynx with both tonsils ultrasonically removed, exposing the posterior tonsil pillars with a thin film of capsule and exposed palatopharyngeus muscle. Note the absence of the charring usually present with conventional electrocautery. (Courtesy Arthrocare Smith & Nephew ENT.)

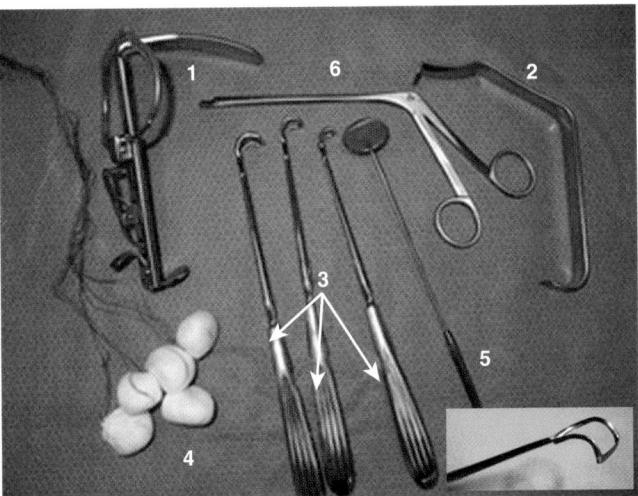

Fig. 66.17 Adenoid curettes come in three widths, and care must be taken to choose one that is not too wide. A curette that is too wide may injure the opening to the eustachian tube adjacent to the adenoid tissue. Adenoid tissue around the eustachian tube can be removed with the punch adenotome. See the "Equipment" section under "Adenoidectomy" for corresponding part numbers. *Inset,* Curette blade. (Courtesy Thomas N. Told, DO.)

TECHNIQUE

Curette Method

1. A self-retaining mouth gag is placed in the mouth and suspended from the Mayo stand.
2. The hard and soft palates are inspected visually and manually for occult submucous cleft palate. If there is no cleft palate, the soft palate is then retracted with a red rubber catheter that is placed through the nose and out the mouth, and clamped over the retractor to expose the adenoid bed.
3. The adenoid bed is inspected with the laryngeal mirror for the presence of adenoid tissue. Adenoid tissue decreases with age and is often gone by the teenage years.
4. An adenoid curette is placed on the adenoid tissue extending superior to the soft palate. It is placed high in the nasopharynx, basically abutting the posterior aspect of the nasal septum.
5. Downward pressure is applied to the curette while the curette is moved along the plane of the posterior pharyngeal muscle (Fig. 66.18). Take care not to penetrate deeply into the prevertebral tissue.

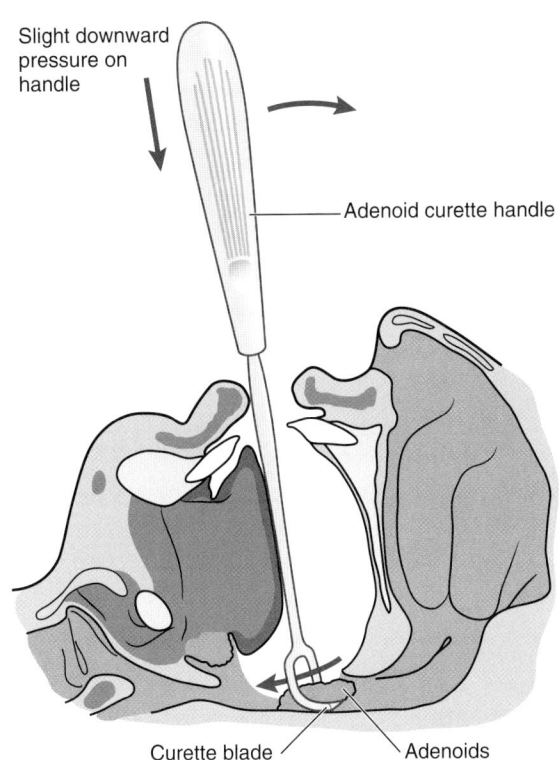

Fig. 66.18 The handle of the adenoid curette moves back slightly as the blade moves forward, curetting the tissue. Slight downward pressure is applied to keep the blade in contact with the posterior pharyngeal wall.

6. The bulk of the adenoid tissue is removed with the first pass.
7. Occasionally a second pass may be needed with grossly enlarged adenoids. Take care not to venture too far laterally to avoid injuring the torus tubarius or eustachian tube opening.
8. Redundant tissue around the opening of the eustachian tube can be carefully removed with a punch adenotome.
9. A nasal suction catheter is inserted, and continuous suction is applied for 2 to 3 more minutes, until bleeding stops. Nasopharyngeal packing may also help.
10. Rarely does this technique produce enough bleeding for cautery to be required. Persistent postoperative oozing may be controlled somewhat by nasal decongestant drops.

Coblation Method

1. Patient preparation and exposure are the same as with the curette method.
2. The soft palate is retracted with a red rubber catheter placed through the nose and out the mouth and then clamped over the retractor to expose the adenoid bed.
3. Using a laryngeal mirror, the area to be ablated is inspected.
4. The Coblator is set on level 6 or 7 and the tip of the wand is energized. The tissue is removed to the level of the pharyngeal muscle (Fig. 66.19). Take care not to venture too far laterally, which increases the risk of injury to the openings of the eustachian tubes on both sides of the pharynx.
5. Bleeding can be controlled with the built-in electrocautery feature.

POSTPROCEDURE EVALUATION AND ORDERS AFTER TONSILLECTOMY AND ADENOIDECTOMY

- Most procedures can be done in same-day surgery.
- Continue IV maintenance fluids until the patient tolerates oral fluids.

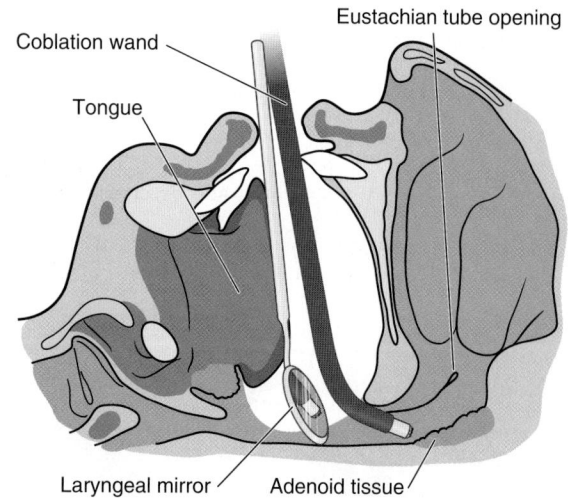

Fig. 66.19 Coblation adenoidectomy. (Courtesy Arthrocare Smith & Nephew ENT.)

- Oral fluids can be started after surgery when the patient is awake enough to protect the airway.
- Some children benefit from postoperative ice collars and cool mist vaporizers.
- Nausea can be controlled with promethazine 12.5 to 25 mg IV every 4 to 6 hours in adults or 0.25 to 1 mg/kg IV every 4 to 6 hours in children. Promethazine should never be given as IV push, only slowly with IV drip. Ondansetron (Zofran) 6 to 8 mg IV every 6 hours in adults and 0.15 mg/kg IV every 4 to 6 hours in children also works well.
- Give IV analgesics such as meperidine 25 to 50 mg IV every 3 hours in adults, and 0.25 to 0.5 mg/kg IV every 3 hours in children for severe pain.
- Morphine sulfate 2.5 to 10 mg every 2 to 4 hours in adults, 0.05 to 0.2 mg/kg every 4 hours in children, also can be given for severe pain.
- Alternatively, if the patient can tolerate oral fluids, give acetaminophen/hydrocodone 500/7.5/15 mL 2.5 to 5 mL orally every 4 hours to children, and 10 to 15 mL orally every 4 hours to adults. **NOTE:** Some clinicians avoid narcotics in the postoperative patient because codeine has not been found to be superior to acetaminophen and it may contribute to nausea, vomiting or constipation.
- Guidelines suggest nonsteroidal antiinflammatory drugs (NSAIDs), with the exception of ketorolac (which may increase risk of postoperative bleeding), can be used safely for the treatment of postoperative pain.
- The role of sucralfate to reduce pain in the postoperative period is still debated, but 1 teaspoon orally four times a day can be of benefit in both children and adults.
- A Cochrane review (Steward, 2011) concluded that children given a single IV dose of dexamethasone during tonsillectomy or adenotonsillectomy have less pain after surgery and return to eating a normal diet sooner. It can also prevent vomiting for one in every five children treated. For those not given an IV dose, dexamethasone elixir 0.03 to 0.3 mg/kg per day can be given to children, 0.75 to 9 mg/day to adults, divided into two doses. This can be used in the postoperative period to reduce swelling and nausea. Given in the immediate postoperative period, dexamethasone is also probably of benefit to those patients at risk of laryngeal edema or airway obstruction. Dexamethasone given in these doses is relatively free of side effects.
- Some experts suggest amoxicillin given orally for 1 week after surgery has been shown to decrease morbidity. However, another Cochrane review (2012) found that antibiotics did not reduce pain,

need for painkillers, or bleeding. But they may reduce fever. That said, the investigators concluded the fever reduction may be due to weaknesses in the studies rather than a direct antibiotic effect.
- Children who cannot tolerate oral opioids usually do very well on regular doses of acetaminophen, but they should avoid all aspirin or NSAID-containing products.
- Adults who can tolerate oral tablets can be sent home on oral analgesics that contain no aspirin or NSAIDs.

PATIENT EDUCATION GUIDES

See patient education form available at www.expertconsult.com.

CPT/BILLING CODES

42825   Tonsillectomy, primary or secondary, younger than age 12
42826   Tonsillectomy, primary or secondary, age 12 or over
42830   Adenoidectomy, primary, younger than age 12
42831   Adenoidectomy, primary, age 12 or over

ICD-10-CM DIAGNOSTIC CODES

J35.01   Tonsillar hypertrophy with chronic tonsillitis
J35.02   Tonsillar enlargement with chronic adenoiditis
J35.03   Tonsillar hypertrophy (hyperplasia) with chronic adenoiditis and tonsillitis
J35.8   Tonsillar remnant or tag
J35.9   Tonsillar disease, chronic
J35.3   Tonsillar hyperplasia with adenoid hyperplasia
J35.1   Tonsillar enlargement or hyperplasia

SUPPLIERS

(See contact information available at www.expertconsult.com.)

Coblator
   ArthroCare Smith & Nephew ENT
Harmonic scalpel
   Ethicon Endo-Surgery, Inc. (Johnson & Johnson)

ONLINE RESOURCES

ENT USA: Tonsillectomy: Tonsil and adenoid surgery (video presentation of tonsillectomy and adenoidectomy using various methods). www.entusa.com.

RECOMMENDED READING

Baugh RF, Archer SM, Mitchell RB, Rosenfeld RM, Burns AR, et al. Clinical practice guideline, tonsillectomy in children. *Otolaryngol Head Neck Surg.* 2011;14(suppl 1):S1–S30.
Dhiwakar M, Clement WA, Supriya M, McKerrow W. Antibiotics to reduce post-tonsillectomy morbidity. *Cochrane Database Syst Rev.* 2012;(12):CD005607.
Mahant S, Keren R, Localio R, Luan X, Song L, et al. Variation in quality of tonsillectomy perioperative care and revisit rates in children's hospitals. *Pediatrics.* 2014;133(2):280–288.
Pinder DK, Wilson H, Hilton MP. Dissection versus diathermy for tonsillectomy. *Cochrane Database Syst Rev.* 2011;(3):CD002211.
Pynnonen M, Brinkmeier JV, Thorne MC, Chong L, Burton MJ. Coblation versus other surgical techniques for tonsillectomy. *Cochrane Database Syst Rev.* 2017;(8):CD004619.
Steward DL, Grisel J, Meinzen-Derr J. Steroids for improving recovery following tonsillectomy in children. *Cochrane Database Syst Rev.* 2011;8:CD003997.
Tonsillectomy and adenoidectomy. In: Flint PW, Haughey BH, Lund V, et al., eds. *Cummings Otolaryngology: Head and Neck Surgery.* 6th ed. Philadelphia: Elsevier; 2015.

CHAPTER 67

ALLERGY TESTING AND IMMUNOTHERAPY

Harold H. Hedges III

The primary methods of allergy skin testing are (1) single skin prick tests (SPTs; pricking the skin at a 45-degree angle through previously placed allergens); (2) skin puncture tests (puncturing the skin at a 90-degree angle through previously placed allergens); and (3) preloaded multiple-allergen testing devices that apply multiple allergens simultaneously. All three of these tests are confined to the epidermis and are considered the in vivo tests. Multiple-allergen applicators have gained popularity because of their safety, ease of use, and test reproducibility and readability. Three tests that are commercially available are the Multi-Test II (Lincoln Diagnostics; Fig. 67.1), Quintest (Hollister-Stier Laboratories; Fig. 67.2), and Omni (Stallergenes Greer Laboratories).

As opposed to the prick and puncture tests, the intradermal (ID) test goes deeper, into the dermis. Older scratch testing methods are not as reproducible or reliable as SPTs and are not recommended.

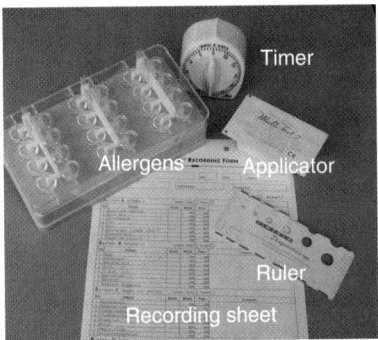

Fig. 67.1 **Lincoln Diagnostics Multi-Test.** (Courtesy Lincoln Diagnostics, Decatur, IL.)

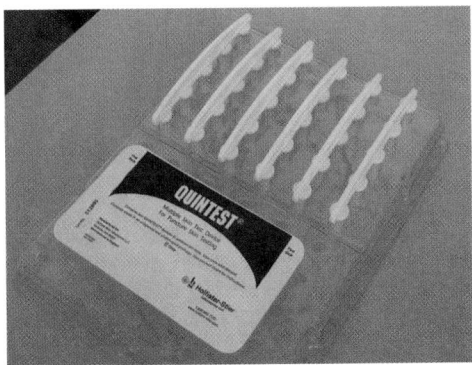

Fig. 67.2 **Hollister-Stier Quintest.** (Courtesy Hollister-Stier Laboratories, Spokane, WA.)

Although considered an SPT, Multi-Test II is comparable to an intradermal (ID) test using a 1:1000 dilution of allergen. Several studies have shown that a positive ID skin test (1:100 dilution) after a negative SPT (using 1:20 concentrates) has little or no clinical significance; thus it is not recommended (see later discussion).

In vitro blood tests (e.g., radioallergosorbent test [RAST]) are performed by a reference laboratory. Kits are not available for office testing because the test involves drawing and sending a blood sample to a reference lab. It is the test of choice for patients exhibiting dermographism, hyporeactive skin, poorly controlled asthma, eczema, or any skin condition limiting the placement of skin tests (i.e., skin testing unable to be performed).

EDITOR'S NOTE: Many insurance companies will not authorize or approve RAST testing unless skin testing is contraindicated or unable to be performed.

The identification of allergens helps direct patient avoidance measures and medical therapy; it also provides the basis for immunotherapy. As an expert stated long ago, "Immunotherapy provides the only potentially curative treatment available because of its unique ability to change the natural history of allergic respiratory disease and Hymenoptera (e.g., bee, wasp) sensitivity. Many suggest that starting immunotherapy is a reasonable option that can provide safe and cost-effective management for a substantial number of patients." Starting immunotherapy earlier in allergic conditions may prevent (rather than just reduce) the inflammatory response, prevent the development of asthma in children with rhinitis, and allow treatment to begin at lower levels of patient sensitivity. It may be the only safe modality for patients whose jobs require alertness and who cannot tolerate antihistamines (e.g., pilots, truck drivers). That said, it is also known and accepted that a positive SPT or in vitro test does not necessarily mean clinical sensitivity, so correlation with the clinical history is essential if immunotherapy is to be successful.

INDICATIONS

Perennial or seasonal rhinitis, rhinosinusitis, rhinoconjunctivitis, rhinitis with otitis media, and anaphylaxis from Hymenoptera stings are the major indications for allergy testing. Patients should be tested for tree, grass, and weed pollens; mold sensitivity; and appropriate insects or animal dander. Latex allergy can now be confirmed with very high sensitivity and specificity (90% to 98%, 100%, respectively) using commercially prepared extracts. Limited food testing may be performed. There is increased risk when testing asthmatic patients and when placing them on immunotherapy, so the risk-benefit ratio must be considered carefully. Many people with asthma have concomitant allergic rhinitis, which, when treated, aids in asthma control.

EDITOR'S NOTE: Although up to 15% of parents believe their children have food allergies, these allergies have only been confirmed in 1% to 3% of Americans. Food intolerance, food dislikes, and other conditions can mimic food allergy and are much more common. The foods that produce allergic symptoms most frequently are milk, eggs, seafood, peanuts, and tree nuts. Fortunately, more than 70% of children will outgrow milk and egg allergies by early adolescence; peanut allergies usually remain throughout life. Unfortunately, sensitivity (20% to 60%) and specificity (30% to 70%) of skin testing using commercially prepared extracts for food allergies is not as high as for inhalant allergies (80% to 97%, 70% to 95%, respectively). Although skin testing and in vitro serum immunoglobulin E (IgE) assays may help in the evaluation of suspected food allergies, they should not be performed unless the clinical history suggests a specific food allergen to which testing can be targeted. Furthermore, these tests do not confirm food allergy. Confirmation requires a positive food challenge or a clear history of an allergic reaction to a food and resolution of symptoms after eliminating that food from the diet.

CONTRAINDICATIONS

- Any condition that compromises the patient's ability to withstand the rare anaphylactic reaction (e.g., patients with uncontrolled hypertension or significant unstable cardiovascular disease).
- Although most allergic patients can be safely tested and treated by the primary care clinician, an allergist should be consulted for the evaluation and treatment of patients with history of anaphylactic reactions (particularly to stinging insects), reactions to anesthetics, and difficult-to-control, moderate to severe, persistent asthma. Great caution must be exercised in these patients.
- Immunotherapy usually is not initiated during pregnancy. However, allergic patients on maintenance therapy who become pregnant may continue the desensitization process throughout the pregnancy.
- Patients taking β-blockers should have alternative medications prescribed before they are tested and placed on immunotherapy because β-blockers interfere with the response to epinephrine, which is needed to treat anaphylaxis should it occur.
- Those with dermographism (which makes skin testing unreliable), those with chronic skin diseases that limit access to normal skin, and those (physically or psychologically) unable to communicate symptoms should be tested by in vitro testing.
- There is no specific age limit (young or old) for allergy testing to check for suspected inhaled allergens, but usually it is not done before the age of 3 years. Allergic food reactions can be detected by limited food testing (SPT or RAST). Other (nonallergic) adverse food reactions require single or multiple food elimination diets.
- Antihistamines and steroids may blunt the response to skin testing and should be eliminated before testing. Older, short-acting antihistamines should be stopped 48 hours before testing. Longer-acting antihistamines require a drug-free period of 7 to 10 days. Steroids may need to be withheld for 2 to 4 weeks. Positive and negative controls are essential, especially when these medications have been used, and help to validate skin test results. The positive control (histamine) usually responds with a 7- to 10-mm wheal (and is always read as a 3+ reaction). If the response is less, it is still being blunted by the antihistamine or other medication. In vitro tests (e.g., RAST) are not affected by antihistamines, steroids, or other medication and thus can be used at any time.

SCREENING FOR ALLERGIES

It is appropriate and cost effective to screen patients for allergies with a limited set of 6 to 10 allergens before applying a complete geographic panel of allergens (Fig. 67.3). A typical screen consists of a positive (histamine) and negative (glycerol-saline) control; house

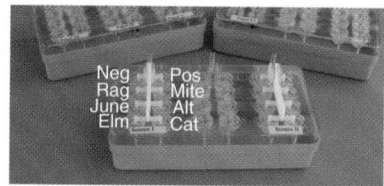

Fig. 67.3   A typical screening panel with six allergens.

dust mite mix; cat; and most tree, grass, weed, and mold allergens of the geographic area. Clinicians and patients reluctant to rely on only six allergens for screening may use a second panel of eight allergens consisting of dog; cockroach; feathers; silk; and secondary tree, grass, weed, and mold preparations.

Always check the positive and negative control sites before interpreting the response to the allergens. When all screening test sites are negative (excluding the positive control; see Fig. 67.3), the probability of allergy is less than 3%. Approximately 50% of patients with rhinitis tested by Multi-Test or an in vitro test will have negative findings. These patients have *nonallergic rhinitis*. Identification of nonallergic triggers is critical for medical care. Decongestants (not antihistamines), nasal steroids, nasal ipratropium, and nasal astemizole are the appropriate medications for nonallergic rhinitis. However, approximately 50% of patients with rhinitis have an allergic basis for their symptoms. Many patients have mixed rhinitis, meaning they have both allergic and nonallergic rhinitis simultaneously.

As noted, allergy screening can be performed using either SPT (in vivo) or in vitro methods. Phadiatop (Thermo Fisher Scientific) and the Multiple Inhalant Allergy screen (MIA; LabCorp) are two RAST screens using 10 allergens. In vitro screens usually have ±10 of the most common allergens, including tree, grass, weed, and molds from a geographic area; house dust mite; and cat. In vitro screens are performed by various laboratories. A blood sample is sent to the company for testing. Again, many insurance companies will not authorize or approve RAST testing unless skin testing is contraindicated or unable to be performed.

When the aforementioned screening tests are negative, no further testing is needed. Screening is very cost effective in selecting out the nonallergic patient. (The Blue Cross/Blue Shield usual and customary reimbursement for SPTs is currently $7.00 per allergen. The negative and positive controls are not reimbursed, hence the $42 payment. The $15 to $25 fee for in vitro testing varies from company to company.)

A history of symptoms in early spring generally correlates with positive skin tests to tree allergens. Summer symptoms usually correlate with grass sensitivity, and fall symptoms often correlate with weed sensitivity. In the warmer climates there is much overlap. Year-round (perennial) symptoms correlate with house dust mite, mold, or insect or animal sensitivity. Perennial symptoms with seasonal exacerbations frequently occur in the same patient.

PREPROCEDURE PATIENT PREPARATION

- Establish that the history is compatible with rhinitis or asthma.
- Explore hereditary factors, allergic and nonallergic triggers, previous and present medications, severity and duration of symptoms, secondary infections, and quality-of-life limitations caused by the symptoms.
- Perform a physical examination to evaluate for signs of atopic disease: rhinorrhea (especially if clear and combined with nasal congestion and pale blue, swollen turbinates), allergic "shiners" under the eyes, conjunctivitis, and evidence of reversible airway disease.
- Spirometry or peak expiratory flow rates are helpful to identify and follow associated asthma (see Chapter 81, Pulmonary Function Testing). Patients with poorly controlled asthma (forced

expiratory volume in 1 second [FEV₁] <70% of their personal best effort) should not be skin tested or receive immunotherapy until treated and stable. In vitro testing, however, is safe and recommended in this situation.

- Inform patients about the nature of testing, the risk of possible reactions, the types of reactions encountered (local and systemic), and the treatment available should a reaction occur. Patients or parents of minors should sign an informed consent. (Refer to Lockey et al., 2014.)
- Instruct patients to avoid older, short-acting antihistamines 48 hours before skin testing. Longer-acting antihistamines should be avoided 7 to 14 days before testing. Remember, the positive histamine control must produce a 7- to 10-mm wheal to validate skin testing.
- Explain the frequency and duration of immunotherapy (weekly or biweekly injections for 3 to 5 years), the expected response, and the criteria for discontinuation (symptom-free control with little or no medication and no increase in symptoms with increasing intervals between injections).

EQUIPMENT

For Skin Testing

- Multiple allergen applicators and loading docks (Multi-Test II, Quintest)
- Individual applicators for the occasional testing of one or two allergens (Duotip [Lincoln Diagnostics], Morrow Brown Needle [Morrow Brown Diagnostics]); or a tip from a multiple-allergen applicator can be broken off and used separately
- Alcohol sponges to clean the testing site
- 30 to 50 standardized or 1:20 weight/volume [w/v] allergen concentrates identified for the specific geographic locale by published data or suggested by providers of allergy diagnostics (house dust mite comes only as a 1:100 dilution as the concentrate)
- Histamine phosphate (2.75 mg/mL) for the positive control and saline for the negative control
- Recording form (Fig. 67.4)
- Black skin-marking pen
- Timer capable of timing at least 20 minutes
- Millimeter ruler
- EpiPen, Ana-Kit, or epinephrine; albuterol
- Resuscitation equipment in the rare event of anaphylactic reaction (the same as that for giving any injections in the office; see Chapter 212, Anaphylaxis)
- Disposable tuberculin syringes fitted with a 26- or 27-gauge needle for the vial test (see the section on Intradermal Testing and the Vial Test)

For Radioallergosorbent Testing or Other in Vitro Tests

- Equipment for drawing blood
- Mailing packages or instructions provided by the RAST laboratory

TECHNIQUE

Skin Prick and Puncture Tests

Skin prick tests are performed by placing a drop of allergen concentrate (usually 1:20 w/v) on the arm or back, then pressing a needle through the drop into the epidermis at a 45-degree angle. The tip of the needle is then lifted up, producing the pricking sensation. If performed correctly, no bleeding should occur (Figs. 67.5 and 67.6A). The skin puncture test is similar, but the skin is punctured at a 90-degree angle (see Fig. 67.6B). Several skin testing devices

were listed previously. The use of Multi-Test II is described in detail here because it has been found to be safe, easily learned, reproducible, and reliable. A DVD/video of the procedure is available from Lincoln Diagnostics.

Multi-Test Applicator Method

Multi-Test II is a sterile, disposable, multiple-test applicator used to apply eight allergens simultaneously. Although considered an SPT, its reliability is comparable to ID techniques using a 1:1000 dilution of allergen. Laboratories that supply the allergen concentrates will help determine the most relevant allergens for the patient's geographic area based on established patterns. The system consists of plastic applicators and the Dipwell tray (Fig. 67.7).

Loading the Dipwell Tray

1. Establish a master list of allergen panels (each containing eight allergens) to be tested and enter them on the recording form. It is crucial to load each allergen in the same test well each time. Make copies of this list for recording test results and refer to it when replenishing allergens.
2. Label (number) each panel A, B, C, D, and so forth.
3. Allergen panels are made by adding 1 mL (enough for 100 applications) of each allergen concentrate (1:20 w/v in 50% glycerin or standardized extract) to each well numbered 1 through 8. Applicator heads are numbered 1 through 8 also and correspond to the numbered wells. Each Dipwell tray accommodates three allergen panels, each with eight testing heads (see Fig. 67.7).
4. Panel A (screening panel) contains the positive control in well A1 and the negative control in well A8. A2 through A7 contain the most common tree, grass, weed, and mold allergens from a geographic area, plus house dust mite mix and cat.
   NOTE: This panel will identify over 95% of those in the allergic population. A negative (except for the positive control) screen indicates a nonallergic cause of rhinitis or asthma. No further allergy testing is indicated. This reduces the cost of total allergy testing. When the screen is positive, additional allergens of the geographic area are tested (usually 30 to 40). An additional panel can also be used to check for allergies to common foods (e.g., milk, corn, wheat, egg, soy, sugar, baker's yeast, and pork).
5. Trays are stored in the refrigerator and stack easily.

Application of Multi-Test

1. Place the Dipwell tray, which has been filled as noted previously, on a flat surface with the "cradle" for the T-handle facing away from you.
2. Remove the sterile applicator from the package (held with the blue dot at the top) by pulling the label at the blue dot. This positions the T-handle away from you for correct placement in the Dipwell tray (Fig. 67.8).
3. Place the applicator in the loaded Dipwell tray (see Fig. 67.7). The applicator now has the allergen on the respective tips.
4. Cleanse the skin with an alcohol wipe and allow it to dry.
5. Mark (number) the test sites on the skin corresponding to the placement of the applicators (A, B, C, D, etc.) with a black skin-marking pen. From this point forward, universal blood and body fluid precautions should be followed.
6. Apply panel A (screening panel) to the volar surface of the forearm (supported with a pillow to keep the arm flat) with the T-handle toward the patient's head (Fig. 67.9). Apply with a rocking motion, to and fro and side to side. When applied with correct pressure, a footprint of each testing head will be visible. No bleeding should occur; if it does, reduce the amount of pressure applied. The correct amount of pressure will be realized after several applications.
7. A positive reaction to any one of the tree, grass, weed, or mold allergen(s) is followed by testing all remaining significant allergens of the area suggested by history. The total number is

Multi-Test Recording Form

Patient Name: _____ Age: _____ Sex: _____ Date: _____

Patient ID: _____ Ordered by: _____ Tested by: _____

❒ Initial Test   ❒ Re-test

Battery A Screen I   Location: ❒ Back   ❒ Forearm

Site	Antigen	Grade	Wheal	Flare	Comments
1	Positive control		mm	mm	
2	Mite mix		mm	mm	
3	Alternaria		mm	mm	
4	Cat		mm	mm	
5	Elm		mm	mm	
6	Bluegrass/June (std.)		mm	mm	
7	Ragweed mix		mm	mm	
8	Negative control		mm	mm	

Battery B Screen II   Location: ❒ Back   ❒ Forearm

Site	Antigen	Grade	Wheal	Flare	Comments
1	Dog		mm	mm	
2	Cockroach		mm	mm	
3	Feather mix		mm	mm	
4	Silk		mm	mm	
5	T.O.E.		mm	mm	
6	Epicoccum		mm	mm	
7	Bermuda		mm	mm	
8	English Plantain		mm	mm	

Battery C Panel III (molds)   Location: ❒ Back   ❒ Forearm

Site	Antigen	Grade	Wheal	Flare	Comments
1	Pullularia		mm	mm	
2	Aspergillus		mm	mm	
3	Cephalosporium		mm	mm	
4	Cladosporium		mm	mm	
5	Fusarium		mm	mm	
6	Mucor		mm	mm	
7	Penicillium		mm	mm	
8	Helminthosporium		mm	mm	

Battery D Panel IV (trees)   Location: ❒ Back   ❒ Forearm

Site	Antigen	Grade	Wheal	Flare	Comments
1	Alder		mm	mm	
2	Birch		mm	mm	
3	E. Cottonwood		mm	mm	
4	Hackberry		mm	mm	
5	Maple/Box Elder		mm	mm	
6	Pine		mm	mm	
7	Sweet Gum		mm	mm	
8	Sycamore		mm	mm	

Fig. 67.4 Sample recording form. (Courtesy Lincoln Diagnostics, Decatur, IL.)

Battery E Panel V (grass)	Location:	❏ Back	❏ Forearm		
Site	Antigen	Grade	Wheal	Flare	Comments
1	Oak		mm	mm	
2	Hickory/Pecan		mm	mm	
3	Mtn. Cedar		mm	mm	
4	Timothy (std.)		mm	mm	
5	Grass Smuts		mm	mm	
6	Bermuda (std.)		mm	mm	
7	Johnson		mm	mm	
8	Bahia		mm	mm	

Battery F Panel VI (weeds)	Location:	❏ Back	❏ Forearm		
Site	Antigen	Grade	Wheal	Flare	Comments
1	Cocklebur		mm	mm	
2	Dock		mm	mm	
3	Lambsquarter		mm	mm	
4	Nettle		mm	mm	
5	Pigweed/Careless		mm	mm	
6	Marshelder, R.		mm	mm	
7	Russian Thistle		mm	mm	
8	W. Water Hemp		mm	mm	

Battery G Foods	Location:	❏ Back	❏ Forearm		
Site	Antigen	Grade	Wheal	Flare	Comments
1	Beef		mm	mm	
2	Corn		mm	mm	
3	Egg		mm	mm	
4	Milk		mm	mm	
5	Pork		mm	mm	
6	Soybean		mm	mm	
7	Wheat		mm	mm	
8	Baker's Yeast		mm	mm	

Battery H	Location:	❏ Back	❏ Forearm		
Site	Antigen	Grade	Wheal	Flare	Comments

Fig. 67.4, Cont'd

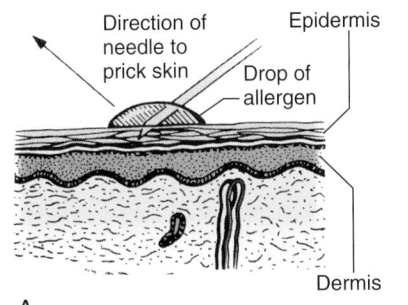
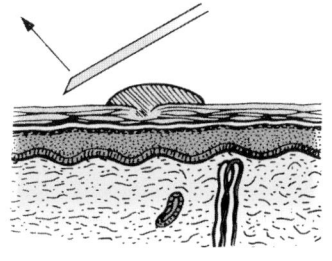

A   B

Fig. 67.5 Method for percutaneous skin prick testing. (A) The drop of allergen is placed on the skin and a 27-gauge needle (bevel up) is placed through the allergen drop into the superficial epidermis. (B) The needle pricks the skin at a 45-degree angle, allowing allergen to come in contact with sensitized mast cells located in the epidermis, and then is lifted up. The dermis is not violated and bleeding at the site is nonexistent or minimal.

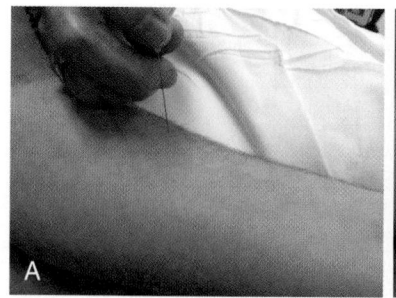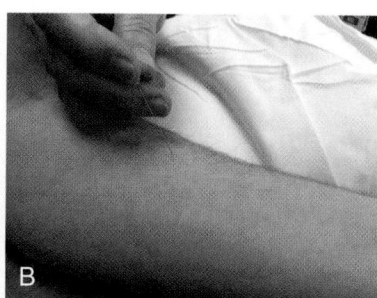

Fig. 67.6 (A) Skin prick test (90-degree angle). (B) Skin puncture test (45-degree angle). In both methods, only the epidermis is penetrated.

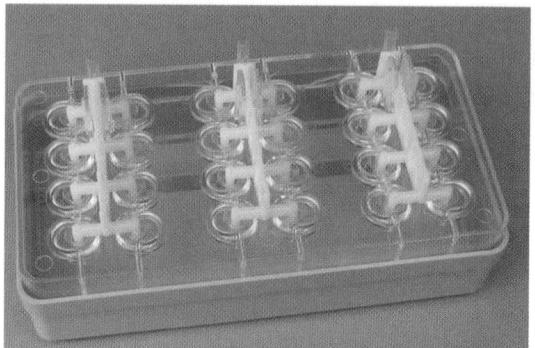

Fig. 67.7 Plastic applicators in the Dipwell tray.

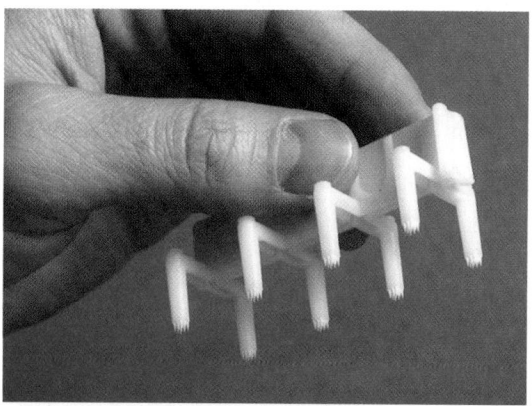

Fig. 67.8 Disposable plastic applicator for Multi-Test II.

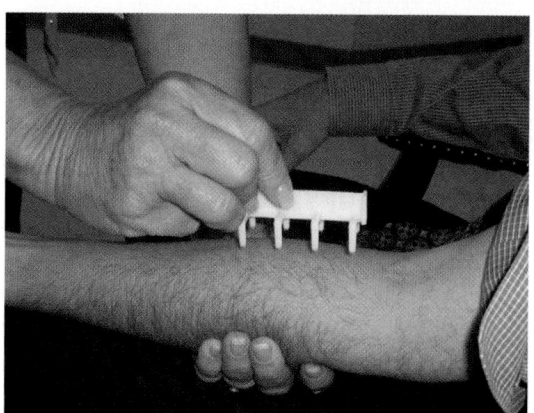

Fig. 67.9 Applying loaded applicator.

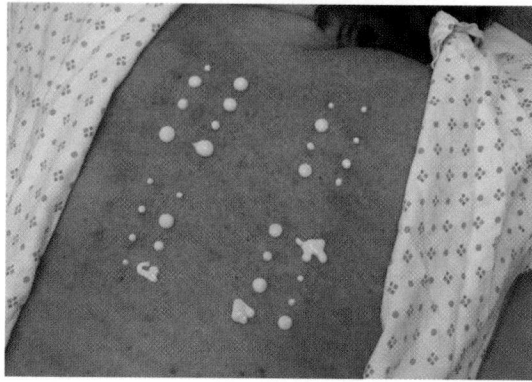

Fig. 67.10 Additional panels on patient's back.

BOX 67.1   Scoring of Multi-Test (Used in Fivefold Dilution Systems)

Multi-Test is scored by comparing the reaction of allergens to the negative (glycerol–saline) and positive (histamine 1 mg/mL) controls applied at the same time and in the same general location.

0   No reaction or a wheal up to 3 mm in size may occur at the negative control site
1+   Wheal larger than the negative control, usually 3–4 mm
2+   Wheal 5–7 mm
3+   Wheal 7–10 mm (size of the positive control)
4+   Any reaction with a wheal larger than the positive control without pseudopods
5+   Any reaction larger than the positive control with pseudopods

---

variable from area to area, usually 20 to 40. These are placed on the patient's back with the patient lying face down and can be applied at this visit (Fig. 67.10). Sites must be kept flat to prevent allergens from running and contaminating other sites. Hairy sites should be avoided because this interferes with readability.

Interpretation of Results

See Box 67.1. Positive responses are noted by wheals. Erythema may be present but is not used in scoring.

- The wheal is the white or gray raised area at the test site. This wheal may be surrounded by an area of erythema called the *flare*. The size and shape of the *wheal* only are used in scoring reactions (see Box 67.1) and are noted on the recording form in the corresponding position.
- The wheal produced at the positive (histamine) control site (Fig. 67.11), usually 7 to 10 mm in an adult and 6 mm in a child, is

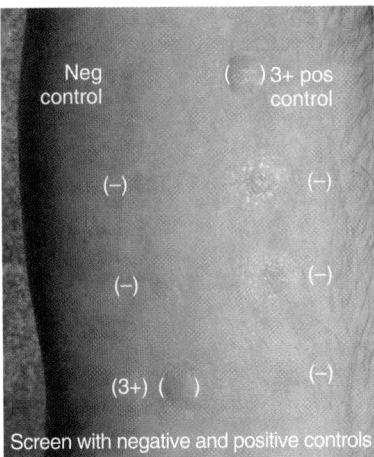

Fig. 67.11 Example of a positive allergy screen (3+ reaction). A positive reaction at the tree, grass, weed, or mold site dictates completing local allergy panels.

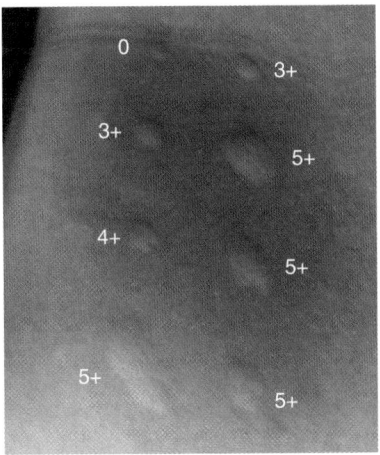

Fig. 67.12 Scoring results. The negative control in the left upper corner shows a 1+ reaction.

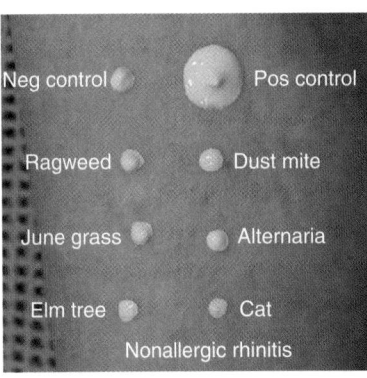

Fig. 67.13 Nonallergic allergy screen. Positive and negative controls are appropriate; all other test sites are negative. The diagnosis is nonallergic rhinitis or asthma.

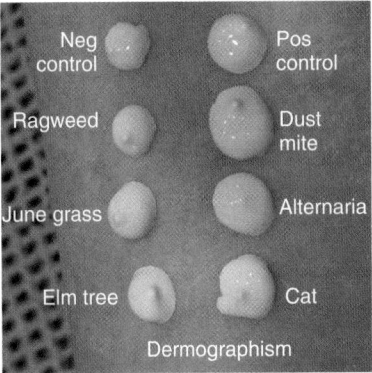

Fig. 67.14 Dermographism. Negative control is positive and all other test sites are positive.

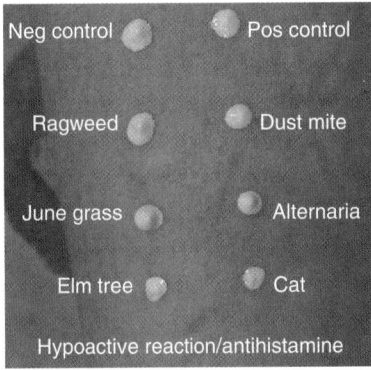

Fig. 67.15 Positive (histamine) control is nonreactive, which invalidates skin response at other test sites. Suspect antihistamine or other medications.

read and recorded as a 3+ reaction. Should the reaction at the positive control site be less than 7 mm or more than 10 mm, it should always be scored as a 3+ reaction, and should be read and recorded at 10 minutes because it will begin to fade. Other sites should be read at 20 minutes.

- Reactions comparable to those at the negative control site (saline or glycerol-saline) are negative. It is not unusual to see a small wheal (1 to 3 mm) at the negative control site (Fig. 67.12). 2+ reactions are generally 5 to 7 mm in size, and 3+ reactions 7 to 10 mm or as large as the positive control. Reactions read as 4+ are greater than the reaction at the positive control site but retain their circular form. Reactions read as 5+ are larger than the positive control site with spreading pseudopods.
- Reactions equal to or greater than the positive (histamine) control site generally correlate best with a history of exposure to allergic triggers. 2+ reactions correlate less, and 1+ reactions even less. Correlation of all test responses to history is important in compounding immunotherapy sets.
- When the positive control is positive and all other tests are negative (Fig. 67.13), nonallergic rhinitis or asthma is present. This result occurs 50% of the time.
- Dermographism (Fig. 67.14) should be suspected when all tests are positive, including the negative control. Such patients must be tested by RAST.

- When reactions at all test sites are negative (Fig. 67.15), including the positive control site, suspect an antihistamine or other medication, which may decrease the skin response.
- Results of tests are recorded (see Fig. 67.4), and a signed copy is the prescription sent to the laboratory for compounding immunotherapy (see later discussion).
- When house dust mite (Fig. 67.16), cat (Fig. 67.17), or both, are the only positive reactions, no further testing need be done at this time. Avoidance measures and immunotherapy are instituted for either or both of these allergens. House dust mite avoidance includes covering pillows and mattresses, dusting regularly, and removing stuffed animals, carpets, and overstuffed furniture. Bedding should be washed weekly with water at 130°F.

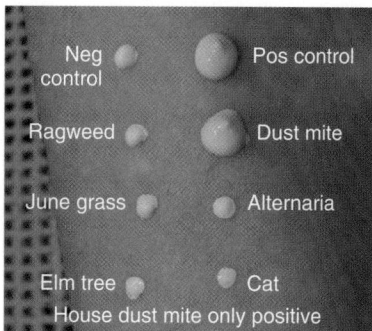

Fig. 67.16   House dust mite is the only positive.

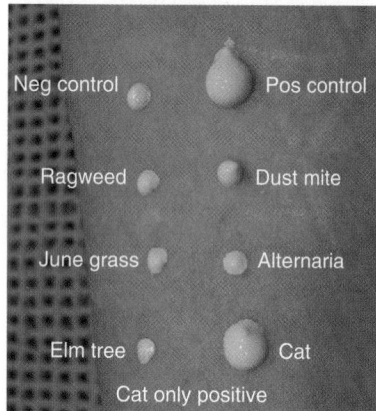

Fig. 67.17   Cat is the only positive.

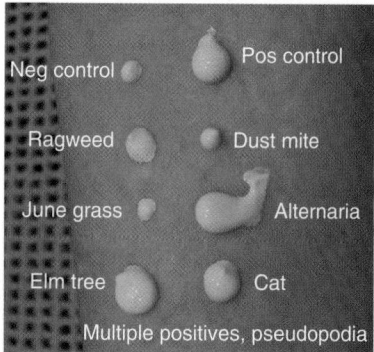

Fig. 67.18   Allergic rhinitis. Pseudopod is best seen with the *Alternaria* allergen.

Lowering humidity to below 50% is helpful. High-efficiency particulate air filtration helps remove small particulate matter. Ideally, cats should be eliminated from the home, but it has been shown that less than 25% of patients or families comply. (At the very least, cats should be kept out of the bedroom and off the bed.) Weekly washing of the cat will decrease the allergen load. Later, additional allergy testing can be done if symptoms do not improve.

- Pseudopods (Fig. 67.18) occur frequently and are recorded as 4+ or 5+ reactions.
- Testing for other nonpollen allergens, such as dog, cockroach, feathers, and laboratory and farm animals, may be suggested by history.

Complications

- Itching at the positive test sites is expected. Highly allergic patients may have rapid and large skin responses and will begin

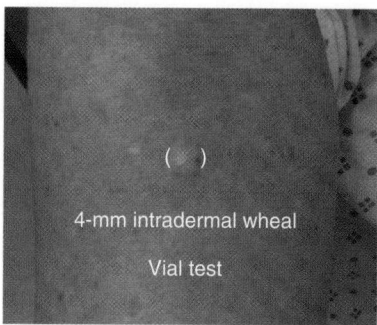

Fig. 67.19   A 4-mm intradermal wheal for the vial test.

to show wheals, erythema, and itching within minutes. These individual reactions should be wiped clean with alcohol, being careful not to contaminate a nearby test site. These will proceed to react despite wiping and can be treated with oral antihistamines or steroid creams if necessary. The reaction will usually resolve in 30 minutes to 1 hour.
- Rarely, systemic symptoms occur that may include hives, urticaria, itching of the roof of the mouth, a sensation of throat closure, shortness of breath, an increase in presenting symptoms (sneezing, rhinorrhea, or wheezing), and anxiety. All allergens should be removed with alcohol. Give 50 to 100 mg of diphenhydramine (Benadryl) orally or intramuscularly and observe closely, monitoring vital signs. Epinephrine, 0.3 mL (1:1000 dilution) for adults and 0.1 to 0.15 mL for children, should be nearby and used as needed if symptoms proceed to anaphylaxis. This occurrence is very rare. In addition to epinephrine, maintenance of the airway, correction of hypotension, and other general measures are used for treatment. Bronchodilation per inhaled albuterol should be given if asthma is precipitated. Monitor the patient's general condition, including blood pressure and respirations using peak flow measurement or spirometry, for several hours as needed. Transfer to an emergency department for more intensive help may be indicated (see Chapter 212, Anaphylaxis).
- False-negative results.
- When there is no reaction whatsoever at the positive control site, hypoactive skin due to antihistamines, steroids, or other medications should be suspected. The clinician should retest after an appropriate time off medication or consider an in vitro test, which is not affected by any medication.
- Delayed reactions (usually at mold sites) may occur up to hours after testing and last for 2 to 7 days. This reaction is an inflammatory response rather than IgE mediated, and it does not respond to immunotherapy. Local steroids may be helpful.

Intradermal Testing and the Vial Test

Historically, ID testing has followed negative or equivocal SPT results when the history strongly indicates a particular allergen. Studies have questioned the presence of clinically significant sensitivity if the SPT is negative but the ID test is positive. The use of positive ID tests after negative SPTs may not be an appropriate basis for selecting patients for immunotherapy. However, an ID test is used for the vial test before starting immunotherapy. The vial test affirms the safety of the immunotherapy set. It is needed only with the initial vial. The clinician should create a 4-mm ID wheal (Fig. 67.19) by injecting about 0.03 mL of the weakest vial (1:100,000 dilution) on the upper outer arm, using an allergy syringe and a 26- or 27-gauge needle. The test is read in 15 minutes. Growth of the ID wheal beyond 15 mm indicates increased sensitivity, and a further 10-fold (1:1,000,000) or fivefold dilution of the vial is necessary. The clinician should take 0.5 mL of the allergen vial and add it to 4.5 mL of phenolated saline (diluting fluid) and repeat the vial test. Rarely, the vial test may cause reproduction of presenting symptoms (e.g., sneezing, rhinorrhea, congestion, asthma). This recurrence indicates increased exposure to an allergen(s) in the mix that may have pollinated since testing and initiation of immunotherapy. Further dilution of the immunotherapy may be indicated.

Radioallergosorbent Blood Test

A reference laboratory processes in vitro tests. The same principles of screening apply as for SPT, and most laboratories will provide a geographic screening panel before completing an extensive specific regional in vitro panel; if not, one can be designed based on the allergens in the clinician's local area. A negative in vitro screen requires no further testing. In vitro testing is not affected by any medication. Box 67.2 shows indications for in vitro testing.

In in vitro testing, an allergen is coupled to a paper disk or placed in a cellulose suspension to which the patient's serum is added. An antigen–antibody complex is formed that, when tagged with radioactive anti-IgE, forms an antigen–antibody–anti-IgE complex scored by a gamma counter. A grading system provides quantifying levels of IgE antibody on which immunotherapy is based. In vitro–based immunotherapy uses either fivefold or 10-fold dilutions. In vitro laboratories usually provide immunotherapy sets or will suggest an immunotherapy-compounding laboratory. As with skin testing, results must be interpreted in light of the clinical history.

In vitro testing is an accepted method of testing for specific allergies and can be used by clinicians who do not want to perform skin testing.

ADVANTAGES OF SKIN TESTING

- The patient can be tested and results known within minutes, whereas in vitro results may not be available for a week or longer, depending on the laboratory.
- The patient sees and experiences the reaction, which reinforces the need for avoidance. This is especially helpful in house dust mite and cat or dog allergy.
- There is much less difficulty with insurance companies over payment for skin allergy testing. As mentioned previously, a significant number of insurance carriers will deny payment for in vitro testing unless skin testing is contraindicated or unable to be performed.
- In vitro testing is more expensive than SPT ($3 to $4 per skin test vs. $8 to $15 per RAST).

POSTPROCEDURE PATIENT EDUCATION

Avoidance procedures and medications are prescribed where appropriate. Brochures describing general allergen avoidance and specific house dust mite and animal dander measures are readily available. Immunotherapy is considered an adjunct to treatment.

IMMUNOTHERAPY

Immunotherapy is indicated based on the demonstration of immediate hypersensitivity by SPT, Multi-Test, or any in vitro test that correlates with the patient's history and physical findings. This correlation is imperative for success. When beginning therapy on a patient for the first time, perform an ID test (the vial test) as noted previously. Increasing amounts of allergen are given subcutaneously until the highest tolerated dose is reached.

Conventional immunotherapy is based on a 10-fold dilution system and is started at 0.1 mL of 1:100,000 dilution of each allergen. Injections are graduated (0.1, 0.2, 0.3, 0.4, 0.5 mL) weekly through dilutions of 1:100,000, 1:10,000, 1:1000, and 1:100 until maintenance is reached. Some laboratories use a fivefold dilution system (1:325,000, 1:62,500, 1:125,000, 1:2500, 1:500, 1:100) for immunotherapy. The maintenance dose in either system is the highest tolerated dose that can be attained without causing a significant local (painful knot or erythema lasting more than 24 hours) or systemic reaction. Some patients may not be able to tolerate injections of the 1:100 dilutions because of local or systemic reactions, but immunotherapy at lower dilutions will usually be effective for them. Using the fivefold dilution system, Multi-Test and in vitro testing allow the starting dose to be tailored based on the degree of sensitivity to the allergen. The higher the sensitivity, the more dilute the starting dose; the lower the sensitivity, the more concentrated the starting dose. Immunotherapy is usually started at a level 5 to 25 times weaker than the test scores, and then graduated until maintenance is reached.

Based on testing, an allergy laboratory will compound an immunotherapy set consisting of four vials each containing increasing concentrations of all the relevant allergens. If more than 12 allergens are to be included, 2 sets are needed. As a clinician's allergy practice grows, compounding immunotherapy in the office can be considered. This requires additional space and personnel. By law, immunotherapy sets made by commercial laboratories are "quarantined" for 2 weeks to ensure sterility. This does not apply in office compounding. Phenolated saline with glycerin or glycerinated saline is used as the diluent in mixing, providing ample sterility and stability.

Escalation of immunotherapy (Table 67.1) proceeds on a weekly schedule with doses adjusted as needed because of local or systemic reactions. Increasing symptoms and skin responses that occur during a pollinating season may require slowing or holding of escalation until pollination ceases. As the season passes, escalation can then proceed with no further problem. Local swelling, wheals, or "knot" formation greater that 2 cm lasting more than 24 hours is considered significant. The subsequent dose should be reduced to one not causing a reaction and escalated at a slower rate for patient comfort. Doses for smaller local reactions of swelling and redness should be repeated or reduced as tolerated. Immunotherapy should be omitted or delayed (1) when a febrile illness is present, (2) when the patient is extremely fatigued, (3) after acute exacerbation of allergic symptoms during a pollinating season, (4) or during or after an asthma attack. The peak expiratory flow rate should be above 70% of the patient's personal best effort. Asthmatic patients should be free of wheezing, cough, or shortness of breath before being tested or receiving an allergy injection. Asthmatic patients should monitor their own status with a peak flow meter.

Actions to prevent untoward reactions and anaphylaxis during immunotherapy include the following:

- Evaluate the patient's condition before injection.
- Minimize the chance of errors in dosing and administration by checking and rechecking the patient's dosing schedule and reactions to previous injections.
- Have the patient identify the vial to be used by name and birthday on the vial.
- Use more dilute allergen in highly sensitive patients (by history or testing).
- Observe patients in the office for 20 to 30 minutes after injection.
- Check the patient and injection site before allowing the patient to leave.

TABLE 67.1 Example of Escalation Schedule for Weekly Immunotherapy*

Vial D

1:100,000 w/v	Green vial
Dose 1	0.05 mL
2	0.10
3	0.20
4	0.30
5	0.40
6	0.50

Vial C

1:10,000 w/v	Blue vial
Dose 7	0.05 mL
8	0.10
9	0.20
10	0.30
11	0.40
12	0.50

Vial B

1:1000 w/v	Gold vial
Dose 13	0.10 mL
14	0.20
15	0.30
16	0.40
17	0.50

Vial A

1:100 w/v	Red vial
Dose 18	0.05 mL
19	0.10
20	0.15
21	0.20
22	0.25
23	0.30
24	0.35
25	0.40
26	0.45
27	0.50

Maintain for 1 year, then go to every 2 weeks for 3–5 years, then try to discontinue.
*The same antigen mixture is used in vials A through D, but with varying concentrations.

TABLE 67.2 Resuming Immunotherapy After Missed Doses During Escalation

3–10 days	Continue escalation
10–14 days	Repeat last dose
14–21 days	Reduce dose 0.1 mL
>21 days	Reduce dose by half and gradually reescalate

TABLE 67.3 Resuming Immunotherapy After Missed Doses During Maintenance

1–4 weeks	Continue maintenance dose
4–12 weeks	One-half maintenance dose, rebuild to maintenance
3–6 months	Drop dilution by full 10-fold (e.g., if maintenance is 0.5 mL of vial A [1:100 dilution], drop back to 0.5 mL of vial B [1:1000 dilution])

Attempts to discontinue immunotherapy can be made after 3–5 years if the patient is symptom free. The interval between injections can be lengthened from every 2 weeks to 3 or 4 weeks. If there is no exacerbation of symptoms after 6 months to 1 year, immunotherapy may be discontinued. Approximately one-third of patients will return within 2 years to restart their immunotherapy program.

chronic asthma patients not only reduced asthma symptoms and use of medications, but the benefit was comparable to that of inhaled steroids. An older review (Calderon, 2007) found significant improvement in symptoms and reduction in medication use when immunotherapy was used for seasonal allergic rhinitis. Maintenance doses should be continued for 3 to 5 years, and the time between doses increased to 2 weeks after the first year, then 2 to 4 weeks after the second year, with symptom return used as the guide. The patient may miss doses in the buildup and maintenance phases of immunotherapy. Guidelines for treatment after missed doses are found in Tables 67.2 and 67.3.

On completion and discontinuance of a program after 5 years of therapy, one-third of patients may return to restart immunotherapy because of return of symptoms. Reasons for allergy treatment failures are given in Box 67.3.

Sublingual Immunotherapy

Sublingual immunotherapy (SLIT), first described in 1934 in the United States, is being increasingly recognized by clinicians as an alternative to allergy shots. It is a common practice in European countries, especially in Italy and France. The safety and efficacy of SLIT are well documented in peer-reviewed journals in the United States and abroad. SLIT is an evidence-based practice and recommended by the World Health Organization and the Cochrane Review. There has never been a death or serious anaphylactic reaction reported in patients using SLIT.

Since 2014, the Food and Drug Administration (FDA) has approved several SLIT tablets for use in immunotherapy. As of 2019, two SLITs have been approved for grass pollen, one for dust mites, and one for ragweed. Allergens used for compounding SLIT are the same as those used for subcutaneous administration and are also approved by the FDA. Low-dose and high-dose treatments have been shown to be effective. Weekly doses are nearly equally effective to those used in subcutaneous immunotherapy (SCIT). SLIT is used for 3 to 5 years before discontinuing it, similar to SCIT. The route of administration is the only significant difference.

In addition to its efficacy and safety profile, advantages of SLIT include the following:

- Sublingual drops or tablets can be given at home daily.
- The cost of preparation of sublingual drops or tablets is similar to that of injections.

BOX 67.3 Reasons for Allergy Treatment Failures

Development of new allergens
Erratic dosage schedule
Inaccurate diagnoses
Inadequate dose of immunotherapy
Incomplete diagnoses (allergic and nonallergic factors)
Immunotherapy dose beyond the optimal dose
Lack of appropriate patient education
Nonallergic food and chemical sensitivities
Noncompliance with avoidance
Noncompliance with medication
Rhinitis medicamentosa

- Reduce the first dose of newly prepared extracts by half.
- Reduce the dose when local or systemic reactions occur.
- Avoid shots to asthmatic patients whose peak flow is less than 70% of their personal best effort.
- Avoid immunotherapy in the presence of a febrile illness.
- Avoid giving immunotherapy to patients on β-blockers.

About 80% of allergic patients respond to immunotherapy, whereas some 20% show little or no response (Box 67.3). A Cochrane review (Abramson, 2010) found that use of immunotherapy in

- The cost of allergen administration decreases because no injection is necessary.
- There is no loss of time or income or inconvenience incurred in driving to and from an office to obtain an allergy injection, wait for the injection, wait after the injection, and return to work.
- There is no loss of time from school or missing after-school activities to get an allergy shot.
- There is no needle fear, as seen in children (and some adults).
- There is no erythema or painful local reaction at the injection site.
- SLIT can be used in children 3 years of age and older.

The disadvantages of SLIT are few:

- Doses have to be given on a daily basis rather than weekly.
- It may be difficult to get children to hold a sublingual dose in the mouth for 30 seconds or longer.
- The immune response may be somewhat slower than with SCIT.

Labeling and Storage of Extracts

- Each vial of extract should be labeled with the patient's name, chart number, birth date, expiration date, and dilution strength.
- Vials are stored in the refrigerator overnight but may be kept out and readily accessible for daily use.
- Dilutions should be discarded and remade after 6 months if not used. Glycerin is added to ensure stability.
- 2.5-mL vials are used in sets for escalation of doses (five doses will be used in 5 weeks [0.1, 0.2, 0.3, 0.4, 0.5 mL = 1.5 mL]). The remainder may be used to repeat doses if necessary, or simply discarded.
- Ten-dose vials (number of milliliters [usually 5 mL] will vary depending on the maintenance dose) are formulated for maintenance therapy.

Summary

Studies have shown beneficial effects on acute allergic disease and long-lasting symptom control after a successful course of immunotherapy. The measurable antiinflammatory influences of immunotherapy do not occur with antihistamines and steroids, suggesting that immunotherapy should be used earlier and more often in the treatment of allergic rhinitis and asthma.

EDUCATIONAL GUIDE

Lincoln Diagnostics provides a video describing the Multi-Test II (http://www.lincolndiagnostics.com/products/multi-test-ii/instructions/).

CPT/BILLING CODES
Testing and Immunotherapy

86003	RAST per test
86005	RAST multiallergen disk (screen)
95004	Multiple puncture test, SPT, per test
95024	Intradermal test, per test; vial test (intradermal)

Allergy Injections

95115	Allergy injection, single (injection only)
95117	Allergy injection, multiple (injection only)
95120	Allergy injection, single antigen (plus antigen if provided)
95125	Allergy injection, multiple antigen (plus antigen if provided)

95165	Allergy extract (specify number of doses) (vial of antigen)

Other Services

99002	Mail out charge
99071	Educational supplies
99080	Medical reports

ICD-10-CM DIAGNOSTIC CODES

R51	Headache
H10.45	Other chronic allergic conjunctivitis
H65.90	Allergic otitis media unspecified ear
J30.2	Allergic rhinitis seasonal
J01.91	Acute recurrent sinusitis
J45.20	Asthma
K52.29	Other allergic and dietetic gastroenteritis
L20.89	Eczema dermatitis
L50.0	Allergic urticaria/hives
R0	Cough
T78.2XXA	Anaphylaxis
T78.3XXA	Angioedema

SUPPLIERS

(See contact information available at www.expertconsult.com.)

Allergen extracts, immunotherapy sets, supplies
Allergy Laboratories
ALK-Abello Laboratory
Greer Laboratories, Inc.

Devices for skin testing (multiple-allergen applicators)
Greer Laboratories, Inc.
Hollister-Stiert Laboratories LLC
Lincoln Diagnostics

Laboratories providing RAST services
Commonwealth Medical Laboratories
LabCorp
MRT Laboratories
Quest Diagnostics
Serolab
SmithKline Beecham Clinical Laboratories

RECOMMENDED READING

Abramson MJ, Puy RM, Weiner JM. Injection allergen immunotherapy for asthma. *Cochrane Database Sys Rev.* 2010;(2):CD001186.

Ahlstedt S, Murray CS. In vitro diagnosis of allergy: how to interpret IgE antibody results in clinical practice. *Prim Care Respir J.* 2006;15:228–236.

Altman CA, Becker WB, Williams PV, eds. *Allergy in Primary Care.* Philadelphia: WB Saunders; 2000.

Bousquet J, van Cauwenberge P, Khaltaev N, World Health Organization. Allergic rhinitis and its impact on asthma: executive summary of the workshop report, 7–10 December 1999, Geneva, Switzerland. *Allergy.* 2002;57:841–855.

Canonica GW, Bousquet J, Casale T, et al. Sub-lingual immunotherapy: World Allergy Organization position paper 2009. *Allergy.* 2009;64(suppl 91):1–59.

Cox LS, Linnemann DL, Nolte H, et al. Sublingual immunotherapy: a comprehensive review. *J Allergy Clin Immunol.* 2006;117:1021–1035.

Craig T, Sawyer AM, Fornadley JA. Use of immunotherapy in a primary care office. *Am Fam Physician.* 1998;57:1888–1894.

Emanuel I. In vitro testing for allergy diagnosis. *Otolaryngol Clin North Am.* 1998;36:879–8931998.

Hedges H, Squillace S. *Asthma, Allergic Rhinitis, and Immunotherapy. AAFP Home Study Monograph 235*. Kansas City: MO: American Academy of Family Physicians; 1998.

Kaliner MA. *Current Review of Allergic Diseases*. Philadelphia: Current Medicine; 2000.

Kniker WT. Multi-Test skin testing in allergy: a review of published findings. *Ann Allergy*. 1993;71:485–491.

Krouse JH, Sadrazodi K, Kerswill K. Sensitivity and specificity of prick and intradermal testing in predicting response to nasal provocation with timothy grass antigen. *Otolaryngol Head Neck Surg*. 2004;131:215–219.

Li JT. Allergy testing. *Am Fam Physician*. 2002;66:621–624.

Lockey RA, Ledford DK, eds. *Allergens and Allergen Immunotherapy*: Subcutaneous, Sublingual and Oral. 5th ed. New York: CRC Press; 2014.

Adkinson NF, Bochner BS, Burks AW, Busse WW, Holgate ST, et al., eds. *Middleton's Allergy: Principles and Practice*. 8th ed. Philadelphia: Saunders Elsevier; 2014.

Nelson HS, Lahr J, Buchmeier A, McCormick D. Evaluation of devices for skin prick testing. *J Allergy Clin Immunol*. 1998;101:153–156.

Normansell R, Kew KM, Bridgman A. Sublingual immunotherapy for asthma. *Cochrane Database of Syst Rev*. 2015;2:CD011293.

Schwindt CD, Dykewicz MS, Hutcheson GA, et al. Role of intradermal skin tests in the evaluation of clinically relevant respiratory allergy assessed using patient history and nasal challenge. *Ann Allergy Asthma Immunol*. 2005;94:627–633.

Yawn BP, Fenton MJ. Summary of the NIAID-sponsored food allergy guidelines. *Am Fam Physician*. 2012;86(1):43–50.

Radulovic S, Calderon MA, Wilson D, Durham S. Sublingual immunotherapy for allergic rhinitis. *Cochrane Database Syst Rev*. 2010;12(2):CD002893.

CHAPTER 68

FINE-NEEDLE ASPIRATION CYTOLOGY AND BIOPSY

Lee A. Green

Fine-needle aspiration (FNA) and biopsy is a rapid, safe, relatively painless method of sampling solid and cystic masses in a variety of anatomic sites for cytologic examination. Both benign and suspected malignant conditions can be diagnosed with FNA.

Although the procedure is used to sample lesions of the prostate, salivary glands, and intra-abdominal and intrathoracic organs, as well as for culturing cellulitis, the primary care clinician will find FNA most useful for masses in the breast and thyroid, and for lymph nodes (especially solitary supraclavicular nodes). For tumors of these sites, positive and negative predictive values for malignancy are typically in the 92% to 98% range, with overall diagnostic accuracy of greater than 70%. However, these rates are highly dependent on the skill of the clinician. It is clear from the literature that FNA should be performed by clinicians who are skilled at technical procedures and well-trained in FNA to obtain adequate diagnostic accuracy. The availability of a cytopathologist skilled in reading FNA specimens is also crucial. Liquid-based cytology (e.g., ThinPrep Non-Gyn or CytoLyt [Hologic Corporation]; SurePath [Becton Dickinson]) is now standard, eliminating the potentially error-prone step of direct slide smear preparation at the time of aspiration. However, slides are still acceptable for the clinician skilled at preparing them.

As implied by the overall diagnostic accuracy rate, as much as one-fourth of specimens will return with nondiagnostic results, necessitating repeat aspiration or open biopsy. However, FNA will provide diagnosis in most cases with a procedure that is safer, more comfortable, less invasive, and less costly than open biopsy. These same advantages allow FNA to be used with less hesitation than with open biopsy. For example, many samples can be drawn over time from breast lesions in a patient with fibrocystic disease, whereas repeated open biopsy with subsequent scarring would be unacceptable.

Although false-negative results are generally more common than false-positive results with FNA, the reverse is true for breast aspirations among young women; more than half of all "suspect" FNAs of palpable breast masses among women younger than 30 years of age prove to be benign on excisional biopsy. Fibroadenomas can show cellular atypia, nuclear overlapping, hyperchromasia, and epithelial clustering, and are thus easily overinterpreted.

Some authors advocate use of FNA of breast lesions as one component of a *triple test*, comprising clinical examination, mammography or ultrasonography, and FNA. When all three elements are concordant for malignancy or nonmalignancy, the negative predictive value of the triple test approaches 100%. The majority of the predictive value of the triple test is the FNA result, but attention to a discordance—suspect abnormal clinical and imaging findings with a negative or nonspecific FNA—may help the clinician identify potential false-negative FNAs for further workup. In the breast, *any palpable mass that is new and clinically suspect must be removed if fluid cannot be aspirated, regardless of other test findings.*

In all breast complaints, FNA provides significant information. If a mass is palpable, FNA is carried out. If thin, nonbloody cystic fluid is retrieved and the mass is gone, the woman can be reassured of the extremely low likelihood of cancer if the mass does not recur within 6 to 8 weeks. If it does recur, repeat aspiration should be performed. If it recurs a third time, it should be excised. Mammograms are usually done for baseline or confirmation a week after the aspiration.

FNA is widely used for evaluation of thyroid masses, where it has similar predictive values. Nondiagnostic thyroid FNAs prove malignant in approximately 7% of cases. Malignancy is more likely in younger (<20 years), older (>40 years) and male patients, in those with a family history of papillary or medullary thyroid cancer, in those with high-normal thyroid-stimulating hormone levels, and in solitary lesions, especially if more than 2 cm diameter. Solitary hyperfunctioning nodules with low-normal thyroid-stimulating hormone or patients with more than two nodules are less likely to harbor malignancy. Two successive nondiagnostic FNAs of a thyroid mass should prompt suspicion. More than two FNAs are not generally useful.

INDICATIONS

- Presence of a palpable, suspect mass in the breast
- Thyroid nodule
- Clinically suspect lymph node or group of nodes
- Any palpable, superficial, nonpulsatile mass

The primary care clinician ordinarily does not perform plain radiography– or computed tomography–guided FNA of nonpalpable lesions, but if an office ultrasound machine is available it can readily be used to guide FNA (see Chapter 214, Emergency Department, Hospitalist, and Office Ultrasound [POCUS]). Endocrinologists now frequently bill for a thyroid or head and neck ultrasound with the initial office visit and an ultrasound-directed FNA during a follow-up visit. Regardless, FNA is the procedure of first choice, even over imaging studies, for evaluating thyroid nodules and detecting the rare parathyroid tumor.

CONTRAINDICATIONS

- Unskilled clinician (relative)
- Absence of a cytopathologist capable of proper interpretation of the slides
- Sites of active pyogenic infection, although suspected granulomatous infection (fungal or mycobacterial) of a node does not contraindicate FNA, and FNA can be used (with sensitivity of approximately 20% to 30%) to obtain culture material from cellulitis
- Masses near the carotid bifurcation (may be a carotid body tumor and should not be biopsied)
- Nonpalpable lesion (unless readily visualized with ultrasound and office ultrasound is available)

FNA may be performed safely in the anticoagulated patient (if international normalized ratio in the therapeutic range for warfarin), with proper attention to compression of the site afterward to avoid hematoma. It may be performed in all but the most severely immunocompromised patients.

EQUIPMENT

One of the following syringe or needle systems:
- The syringe pistol holder shown in Fig. 68.1 is available in various sizes from Belpro or Comeco.
- Cooper Surgical Milex Products (Trumbull, CT) supplies a breast aspiration biopsy needle (Fig. 68.2), which is unique because of its separate cutting port near the tip. A control syringe is also available with finger grips.
  NOTE: A 23-gauge needle was found to be more comfortable than a 21-gauge in the patient without local anesthesia and had equal diagnostic yields (Brennan). A 25-gauge needle was also found to have equal diagnostic yields (Tangpricha).
  - A 21- or 23-gauge butterfly needle can be connected to a syringe. The assistant aspirates the syringe while the clinician manipulates the needle.
  - A 21- or 23-gauge needle can be used on the end of a regular 3-, 5-, or 10-mL syringe.
- Two sterile, plain (nonanticoagulant), evacuated blood tubes.

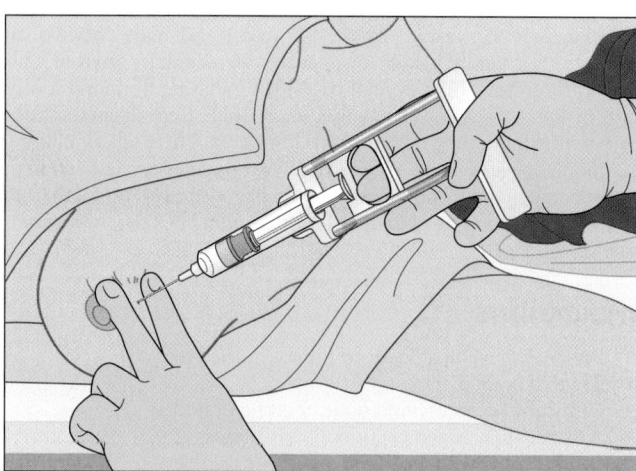

Fig. 68.1 Breast fine-needle aspiration using Cameco syringe holder.

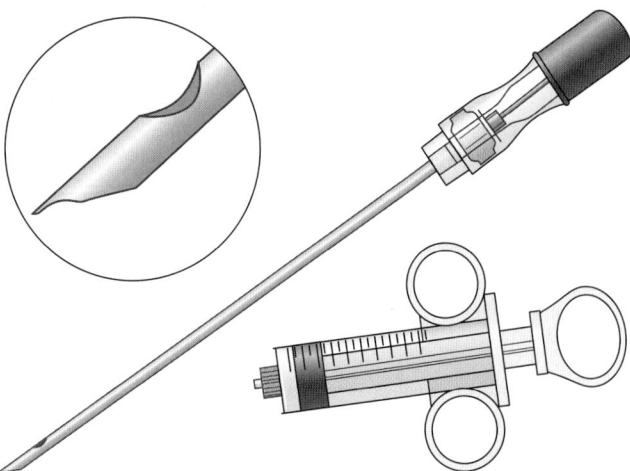

Fig. 68.2 Milex needle used for needle biopsy. Note the special extra side port to sample more tissue. (Courtesy Cooper Surgical Milex Products, Chicago.)

- 21-, 22-, or 23-gauge needle.
- Syringe of appropriate size.
- 120-mL specimen containers with 30 mL ThinPrep, CytoLyt, or SurePath solution in each.
- 4 × 4 gauze pads.
- Sterile gloves.
- Isopropyl alcohol pads or povidone–iodine or chlorhexidine swabs.
- 1-mL syringe with 30-gauge ½-inch needle (or insulin syringe and needle) and 1% or 2% plain lidocaine for anesthesia of skin (optional).

PREPROCEDURE PATIENT PREPARATION

Advise patients of the risks and benefits of the procedure, the indications, the alternatives, and the comparative risks and benefits of the alternatives. (See the sample patient education and consent forms available at www.expertconsult.com.)

Significant complications of FNA are rare. A small hematoma or ecchymosis for a few days (especially from thyroid FNA) and some mild soreness are to be expected. The patient must understand that nondiagnostic results occur commonly and may require repeat FNA or open biopsy, and that false-negative and false-positive results are possible. Patients undergoing FNA of breast lesions should wear a supportive brassiere.

TECHNIQUE

Setup and Preparation

Prepare the skin with 70% isopropyl alcohol. Povidone–iodine or chlorhexidine preparation may be used but is not required for FNA. Sterile draping is not required, although neither the needle nor the skin entry site should be touched, except with a sterile glove after the skin is prepared.

Fig. 68.3 illustrates the typical equipment setup for FNA. The sterile tray contains both a 5-mL syringe for freehand aspiration and a 20-mL syringe for use with the aspirator handle; ordinarily one or the other is used, not both. Both 21- and 23-gauge needles are illustrated; either size may be used, although 23-gauge may be preferred in the thyroid and 21-gauge for dense masses and the breast. The 1-mL syringe with a 30-gauge, ½-inch needle may be used for skin anesthesia, if desired. The specimen containers use the same CytoLyt fluid used for ThinPrep-method Papanicolaou (Pap) smears, but it is best to use a container distinct from that used for Pap smears because the laboratory may mistakenly process the FNA specimen as a Pap, destroying it. The sterile plain (nonanticoagulant) blood specimen tubes are for cyst fluid, if obtained. Alternatively, the fluid can just be placed in the CytoLyt. Again, if breast fluid is nonbloody (thin, urine-colored or green), it does not need to be sent to pathology (for cell block, cytology, or anything else) and should be discarded.

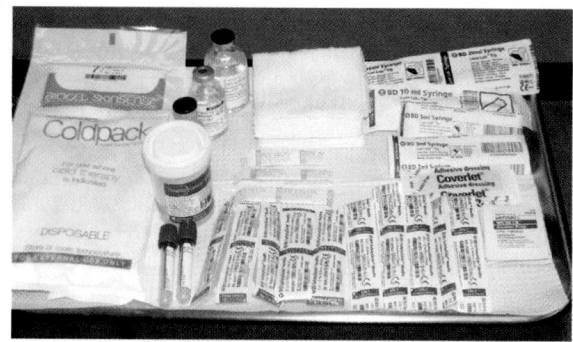

Fig. 68.3 Setup tray for fine-needle aspiration.

Skin anesthesia is often not necessary for FNA because the needles are small and not painful. If desired, however, excellent anesthesia can be obtained with 1% or 2% lidocaine (plain or with epinephrine) by using a 30-gauge needle on a 1-mL syringe. If the lidocaine is injected slowly and in small volume (approximately 0.5 mL) into the subcutaneous tissues without raising a skin wheal, and then allowed to remain for 5 minutes, anesthesia can be achieved painlessly and without obscuring the lesion to be aspirated. Buffering the lidocaine to near-neutral pH just before injection by mixing it in a 9:1 ratio with 1 mEq/mL sodium bicarbonate solution can further reduce injection discomfort.

Sampling

Pneumothorax has been reported with needle aspiration and needle biopsy of the breast. To prevent this, aspirate with the mass positioned over a rib, or keep the needle at a tangential angle as opposed to perpendicular to the body. If the person is thin or the lesion is deep, it may be prudent to have the patient hold her breath while sampling. For thyroid FNA, placing a pillow beneath the patient's shoulders will extend the cervical spine slightly, which thins the soft tissue over the thyroid. The needle should be directed medially toward the thyroid and away from the more lateral carotid artery. Lymph nodes in the neck may be made more prominent by rotating or flexing or extending the neck.

Fig. 68.4 illustrates the aspiration of a thyroid nodule using one-handed manual withdrawal of the syringe plunger to create vacuum. The fingers hold the plunger while the thumb exerts pressure on the syringe top flange. Fig. 68.1 illustrates aspiration of a breast cyst using the syringe holder to withdraw the plunger. Whatever technique is used, the fingers of the nondominant hand stabilize the lesion to be aspirated and provide tactile feedback when the needle has been placed in the lesion.

Before the puncture is made, draw air into the syringe, filling approximately one fifth of its volume. The purpose of this is to have the air to flush out the needle and its contents onto a slide. Without the air, there is no good way to empty the needle. (Do not aspirate air after withdrawing the needle from the mass, because this will spread the sparse contents all over the inside of the syringe, making it hard to retrieve.) Carefully note the position of the plunger against the syringe markings, and then introduce the needle into the lesion. The standard technique is to then withdraw the plunger to create vacuum and sample the lesion, but recent research suggests that suctionless fine-needle sampling may be equally effective.

Fig. 68.5 illustrates the technique of sampling a solid lesion or a cyst that remains palpable after fluid has been drained. Make several (3 to 20) passes into the lesion, filling the needle with cells and sampling all areas of the lesion (Fig. 68.6). Return the plunger to its previously noted resting position before withdrawing the needle from the mass to avoid aspirating the cells into the syringe when the needle is withdrawn. The cytologic specimen is now in the needle or the hub of the needle. Withdraw the needle from the lesion and skin, and use the air that was in the syringe to express the sample from the needle into the specimen container. Aspirate 1 to 2 mL of the liquid cytology solution into the syringe, agitate it gently, and express it gently back into the container. Repeat the procedure if necessary. NOTE: Some experts make only three passes with a needle, and recommend all three passes be in a different direction. Others recommend the same number of passes; however, they suggest all passes be in the same direction to minimize tissue trauma, risk of hemorrhage, and dilution of the specimen with blood. Most clinicians make from 3 to 20 passes with the needle, using short, quick motions.

If a lesion is cystic and fluid is obtained, draw as much as possible into the syringe. Withdraw the needle and empty the syringe; then perform another aspiration if more fluid remains. Alternatively, detach the needle from the syringe and leave the needle in place, empty the syringe and reattach it, and withdraw more fluid. After draining a cyst, any residual mass should be biopsied to rule out cystic carcinoma.

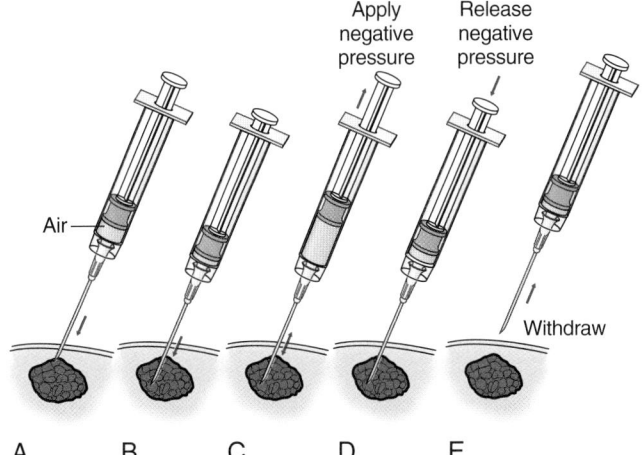

Apply negative pressure   Release negative pressure

Air

Withdraw

A   B   C   D   E

Fig. 68.5 Fine-needle aspiration technique of a solid lesion or cyst (a palpable breast mass, in this case) that remains palpable after fluid has been drained. (A) Aspirate 1 to 2 mL of air into syringe before inserting needle. (B) Insert the needle into the mass and aspirate. If cystic fluid is not obtained or the mass does not resolve, the mass is solid. (C) Maintain negative pressure in the syringe and move the needle back and forth through the tissue from 3 to 20 times to collect cells for analysis (see Fig. 68.6). (D) Release the plunger. (E) Withdraw needle; use the previously aspirated air to expel and spread contents into fixative or onto a slide, which is immediately fixed.

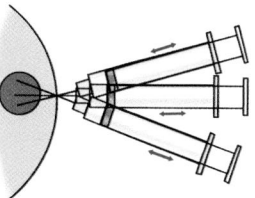

Fig. 68.6 Redirecting the needle to carry out step C in Fig. 68.5. Some experts do not redirect the needle. The needle is passed multiple times into the mass to obtain adequate sampling.

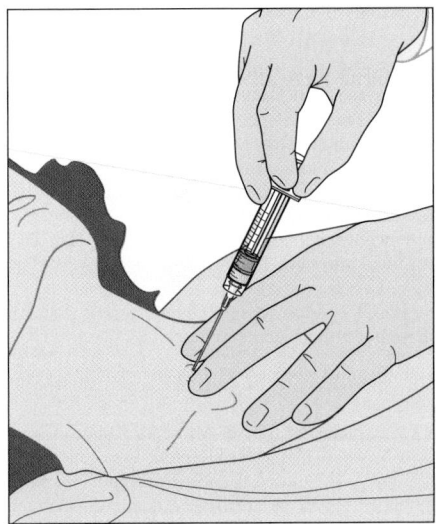

Fig. 68.4 Thyroid fine-needle aspiration using ordinary syringe.

Fluid obtained from cysts other than breast cysts can be placed in liquid cytology solution or submitted in bulk in a sterile tube. (Standard evacuated blood tubes are sterile; use those without anticoagulants.) As previously mentioned, when a breast cyst is aspirated, the fluid should be submitted for pathologic evaluation only if tinged with blood or thick and tenacious. Thin, yellow, or green fluid is diagnostic of benign breast cysts, and cytology is unnecessary. A sterile tube can also be used to submit semisolid material such as that obtained from a lymph node for culture. If infection is suspected, fluid and solid specimens can be submitted in transport media as well.

SLIDE PREPARATION

If a slide is to be prepared, the goal is to leave a thin, monolayer of cells on the slide for microscopic examination. To start, the specimen should be deposited at the labeled end of the specimen slide. The spreading slide is then touched to the specimen slide and drawn down the slide while thinly spreading the specimen. After consultation with the cytopathology lab regarding their preferred method, the slide can be allowed to air dry or sprayed with a fixative, or both. Air drying should be accomplished rapidly; many labs use a hair dryer or handheld air fan to hasten drying. A spray fixative usually contains polyethylene glycol mixed with either isopropyl or ethyl alcohol. Instead of using a spray fixative, the slide can just be immersed in 95% ethyl alcohol.

POSTPROCEDURE CARE

Compression of the site with a gauze pad for 5 to 15 minutes will minimize bruising, especially of the highly vascular thyroid area. A compression dressing of folded gauze pads under Elastoplast tape can be applied on suitable sites. In breast biopsies, placement of a stack of folded gauze pads under a snug brassiere forms an effective compression dressing that may be left in place for several hours to prevent hematoma formation. Some clinicians apply a small ice pack to the FNA site for 15 to 60 minutes after the procedure.

COMPLICATIONS

Complications of FNA are limited primarily to diagnostic failure or to false-negative and false-positive results. The incidence of failure is strongly dependent on the operator. Minor hematoma formation is a frequent occurrence but is seldom of clinical significance. Pneumothorax has been reported in rare instances. Before the widespread use of FNA, concern was often expressed about the possibility of seeding the needle track with malignant cells or releasing malignant cells to spread through lymphatics. Neither of these theoretical complications has been documented to occur, and they should not be considered complications of FNA. Damage to local anatomic structures (e.g., recurrent laryngeal nerve injury with thyroid FNA) is possible but occurs rarely; most large case series have not reported such injuries. The lack of complications is probably due to the small diameter of the needles used for FNA, in contrast to cutting-needle biopsies, which do cause injury with some frequency.

PATIENT EDUCATION GUIDES

See the sample patient education and consent forms available at www.expertconsult.com.

CPT/BILLING CODES

10021	Fine-needle biopsy w/o imaging
19000	Puncture aspiration of a breast cyst
19001	Puncture aspiration of a breast cyst; each additional cyst
19100	Core needle biopsy breast, not using imaging
20206	Muscle biopsy, percutaneous needle
38505	Lymph node biopsy, needle
60100	Biopsy thyroid, percutaneous core needle
60300	Aspiration and/or injection, thyroid cyst
76942	Ultrasonic guidance for needle placement (e.g., biopsy, aspiration, injection, localization device), imaging, supervision and interpretation

ICD-10-CM DIAGNOSTIC CODES

C50.019	Cancer, breast, areola unspecified female breast
C50.119	Cancer, breast, central unspecified female breast
C50.219	Cancer, breast, upper inner quadrant unspecified female breast
C50.319	Cancer, breast, lower inner quadrant unspecified female breast
C50.419	Cancer, breast, upper outer quadrant unspecified female breast
C50.519	Cancer, breast, lower outer quadrant unspecified female breast
C50.619	Cancer, breast, axillary tail unspecified female breast
C73	Malignant neoplasm of thyroid
D24.9	Benign lesion unspecified breast
D34	Benign neoplasm of thyroid
N60.09	Solitary cyst of unspecified breast
N60.19	Fibrocystic breast disease unspecified breast
N60.29	Fibroadenosis of unspecified breast
N63.0	Unspecified lump in unspecified breast
R59.9	Enlarged lymph node

SUPPLIERS

(See contact information available at www.expertconsult.com.)

Cameco syringe
  Belpro Medical, Inc.
CytoLyt solution
  Hologic Corp.
SurePath
  Becton, Dickinson and Company
Special syringe
  Cooper Surgical Milex Products, Inc.

ONLINE RESOURCES

Papanicolaou Society of Cytopathology. www.papsociety.org/fna.html.

RECOMMENDED READING

Abati A, Simsir A. Breast fine needle aspiration biopsy: prevailing recommendations and contemporary practices. *Clin Lab Med.* 2005;25:631–654.

Baloch ZW, LiVolsi VA. Fine-needle aspiration of thyroid nodules: past, present, and future. *Endocr Pract.* 2004;10:234–241.

Brennan PA, Mackenzie N, Oeppen RS, et al. Prospective randomized clinical trial of the effect of needle size on pain, sample adequacy and accuracy in head and neck fine-needle aspiration cytology. *Head Neck.* 2007;29(10):919–922.

Cady B, Steele Jr GD, Morrow M, et al. Evaluation of common breast problems: guidance for primary care providers. *CA Cancer J Clin.* 1998;48:49–63.

Donnegan WL. Evaluation of a palpable breast mass. *N Engl J Med.* 1992;327:937–942.

Florentine BD, Staymates B, Rabadi M, et al. Cancer Committee of the Henry Mayo Newhall Memorial Hospital: the reliability of fine-needle aspiration biopsy as the initial diagnostic procedure for palpable masses: a 4-year experience of 730 patients from a community hospital-based outpatient aspiration biopsy clinic. *Cancer.* 2006;107:406–416.

Gupta RK, Naran S, Lallu S, Fauck R. The diagnostic value of fine needle aspiration cytology (FNAC) in the assessment of palpable supraclavicular lymph nodes: a study of 218 cases. *Cytopathology.* 2003;14:201–207.

Hammond S, Keyhani-Rofagha S, O'Toole RV. Statistical analysis of fine-needle aspiration cytology of the breast. *Acta Cytol.* 1987;3:276–280.

Handa U, Mohan H, Bal A. Role of fine needle aspiration cytology in evaluation of paediatric lymphadenopathy. *Cytopathology.* 2003;14:66–69.

Layfield LJ, Chrischilles EA, Cohen MB, Bottles K. The palpable breast nodule: a cost-effectiveness analysis of alternate diagnostic approaches. *Cancer.* 1993;72:1642–1651.

Layfield LJ, Cibas ES, Gharib H, Mandel SJ. Thyroid aspiration cytology: current status. *CA Cancer J Clin.* 2009;59:99–110.

Lau SK, McKee GT, Weir MM, et al. The negative predicative value of breast fine-needle aspiration biopsy: the Massachusetts General Hospital experience. *Breast J.* 2004;10:487–491.

Ogilvie JB, Piatigorsky EJ, Clark OH. Current status of fine needle aspiration for thyroid nodules. *Adv Surg.* 2006;40:223–238.

Perez-Reyes N, Mulford DK, Rutkowski MA, et al. Breast fine-needle aspiration: a comparison of thin-layer and conventional preparation. *Am J Clin Pathol.* 1994;102:349–353.

Pothier DD, Narula AA. Should we apply suction during fine needle cytology of thyroid lesions? A systematic review and meta-analysis. *Ann R Coll Surg Engl.* 2006;88:643–645.

Salzman B, Fleegle S, Tully AS. Common breast problems. *Am Fam Physician.* 2012;86(4):343–349.

Tangpricha V, Chen BJ, Swan NC, et al. Twenty-one-gauge needles provide more cellular samples than twenty-five-gauge needles in fine needle aspiration biopsy of the thyroid. *Thyroid.* 2001;11(10):971–976.

Cardiovascular and Respiratory System Procedures

Section Editor: GRANT C. FOWLER

CHAPTER 69

ANTIBIOTIC PROPHYLAXIS

Coral D. Matus • Scott F. Ross

ANTIBIOTIC PROPHYLAXIS FOR INFECTIVE ENDOCARDITIS

The publication of American Heart Association (AHA) guidelines for the prevention of infective endocarditis by Wilson and associates in 2007 in *Circulation* represented a major change. The AHA originally published guidelines for infective endocarditis prevention in 1955, and since then there have been multiple updates. Before the 2007 update, the last changes were in 1997. Since these 2007 guidelines were released, several studies have tracked the incidence of viridans group streptococcal infective endocarditis, and it has trended downward, both locally and nationally. The efficacy of antimicrobial prophylaxis to prevent infective endocarditis in patients undergoing dental, gastrointestinal (GI), genitourinary (GU), and respiratory tract procedures has also been questioned by other groups. In the United Kingdom, the National Institute for Health and Care Excellence published guidelines in 2008, updated in 2015, that recommended *against routine* prophylaxis for endocarditis in people undergoing dental and various nondental procedures. These nondental procedures include those involving the upper and lower GI tract, urinary tract (including urologic, gynecologic, and obstetric procedures and childbirth), and upper and lower respiratory tract (including ear nose and throat procedures and bronchoscopy). The European Society of Cardiology also released guidelines in 2015, which recommend prophylaxis for endocarditis only for those patients at highest risk. Those seeking further discussion beyond that presented here are referred to the guidelines from the AHA and other such organizations. It should be kept in mind that there may be other reasons for antibiotic prophylaxis (see the sections on surgical site wound prophylaxis, GI, GU, and gynecologic and obstetric surgeries later in the chapter).

Major changes in the 2007 AHA guidelines included the following:

- Emphasis that most cases of infective endocarditis are caused by random bacteremia related to daily exposures, such as chewing, tooth brushing, flossing, and use of toothpicks.
- Review of the literature showing that prophylaxis prevents a very small number of cases of infective endocarditis.
- The risk of antibiotic-associated adverse events appears to exceed the benefit of prophylactic antibiotic therapy, which seems to be very small.
- Recommendations are based on consideration of those conditions most likely to have an adverse outcome from infective endocarditis, not necessarily those with the highest lifetime risk of acquiring infective endocarditis.
- Although the committee acknowledged that there was no convincing evidence that prophylaxis is effective, prophylaxis is considered reasonable for those with the highest risk of adverse outcomes from infective endocarditis.
- Mitral valve prolapse, which is the most common underlying condition that might predispose to infective endocarditis, is not on the list of recommended conditions for prophylactic antibiotic

use because the absolute incidence of infective endocarditis in this population is very low, and poor outcomes are extremely uncommon.

Box 69.1 lists the conditions that are at highest risk for poor outcomes with infective endocarditis and should therefore be considered for prophylaxis with antibiotics for some procedures. If prophylaxis is used, the chosen antibiotic should cover organisms that can cause endocarditis. As mentioned previously, while there may be other reasons for prophylaxis (see the sections on surgical site wound prophylaxis, GI, GU, and gynecologic and obstetric surgeries later in the chapter), no other cardiac conditions should be considered for prophylaxis for any dental, GI, GU, or respiratory procedures.

Prior recommendations separated *dental procedures* into those for which prophylaxis was or was not recommended, based on risk of bacteremia and subsequent development of infective endocarditis. The 2007 guidelines recommend prophylaxis only for those at high cardiac risk (see Box 69.1) for any dental procedure that might involve manipulation of the gingival tissues or apical region of the teeth or perforation of the oral mucosa, including teeth cleaning. Box 69.2 lists dental procedures for which antibiotic prophylaxis is *not* recommended for anyone.

For those undergoing incision or biopsy of the *respiratory mucosa*, including tonsillectomy or adenoidectomy, prophylaxis for infective endocarditis with antibiotics is only recommended for those with the cardiac conditions at highest risk for poor outcomes (see Box 69.1).

BOX 69.1   Cardiac Conditions with High Risk of Adverse Outcome

Prosthetic cardiac valve
Previous infectious endocarditis
Congenital heart disease including only the following:
- Unrepaired cyanotic congenital heart disease
- Palliative shunts and conduits
- Completely repaired congenital heart defect with prosthetic material or device (placed surgically or by catheter) during first 6 mo after procedure (until endothelialization of prosthetic material occurs)
- Repaired congenital heart disease with residual defects at site of prosthetic patch or device (because endothelialization may be inhibited)

Cardiac transplant recipients with cardiac valvulopathy

Modified from Wilson W, Taubert KA, Gewitz M, et al. Prevention of infective endocarditis: Guidelines from the American Heart Association. A guideline from the American Heart Association Rheumatic Fever, Endocarditis, and Kawasaki Disease Committee, Council on Cardiovascular Disease in the Young, and the Council on Clinical Cardiology, Council on Cardiovascular Surgery and Anesthesia, and the Quality of Care and Outcomes Research Interdisciplinary Working Group. *Circulation.* 2007;116:1736–1754.

This recommendation is in spite of a lack of conclusive data linking respiratory tract procedures to infective endocarditis.

In contrast to prior AHA guidelines, prophylaxis for infective endocarditis is *no longer recommended for GI or GU procedures*, including diagnostic esophagogastroduodenoscopy or colonoscopy with or without biopsy. The only exception to this guideline is for those patients with cardiac conditions at highest risk for poor outcomes who have an enterococcal urinary tract infection or colonization at the time of a GU procedure. The 2007 guidelines reaffirmed that vaginal hysterectomy, vaginal delivery, cesarean section, dilation and curettage, therapeutic abortion, insertion of an intrauterine device, and sterilization procedures do not need prophylactic antibiotics in anyone to prevent endocarditis. (However, as noted in the sections that follow, there may be a benefit in antibiotic prophylaxis in some of these individuals to prevent surgical site infections.)

Antibiotic prophylaxis for infective endocarditis for *routine skin procedures* is not recommended. For surgical procedures involving *infected* skin, skin structures, or musculoskeletal tissue, antibiotic choice should be active against staphylococci and beta-hemolytic streptococci, but again only for those patients listed in Box 69.1.

The 2007 AHA guidelines not only simplified the decision-making process for clinicians regarding who should or should not receive antibiotic prophylaxis for infective endocarditis; they also shifted the emphasis to improved dental care and oral health to decrease routine exposure to bacteremia from oral microflora related to daily activities, which likely cause the vast majority of cases of infective endocarditis.

Fig. 69.1 illustrates an approach to appropriate antibiotic selection for those high-risk individuals undergoing a procedure for which prophylaxis for infective endocarditis is indicated. Table 69.1 indicates appropriate doses for adults and children of selected antibiotics used for prophylaxis.

SURGICAL SITE WOUND PROPHYLAXIS

Also see Chapter 213, Wound Infections.

Surgical site infections account for 14% to 18% of all health care infections. Perioperative antimicrobial surgical prophylaxis is recommended for operative procedures that have a high rate of postoperative wound infection, when foreign material is implanted, or when the wound infection rate is low but the development of a wound infection would be catastrophic.

Several studies have found a moderate correlation between the type of wound and the risk of surgical site infections. A common classification system describes the wound as clean, clean-contaminated, contaminated and dirty. Antibiotic prophylaxis is probably justified for most clean-contaminated wounds. The use of antibiotics for contaminated, dirty, or infected wounds is considered treatment, not prophylaxis.

Wound care is an important part of a busy outpatient and office practice. For dirty, traumatic wounds, copious irrigation is the most important means of decreasing the incidence of wound infection. Smaller, low-risk wounds and those in more vascular areas usually require less volume, but in most cases the best approach is to follow the dictum "The solution to pollution is dilution." Irrigation with normal saline is recommended (and warmed saline offers the additional benefit of increased patient comfort over room-temperature

---

BOX 69.2 Dental Procedures for Which Antibiotic Prophylaxis Is Not Recommended

Adjustment of orthodontic appliances
Bleeding from trauma to the lips or oral mucosa
Dental radiographs
Placement of orthodontic brackets
Placement of removable prosthodontic or orthodontic appliances
Routine anesthetic injection through noninfected tissue
Shedding of deciduous teeth

Modified from Wilson W, Taubert KA, Gewitz M, et al. Prevention of infective endocarditis: Guidelines from the American Heart Association. A guideline from the American Heart Association Rheumatic Fever, Endocarditis, and Kawasaki Disease Committee, Council on Cardiovascular Disease in the Young, and the Council on Clinical Cardiology, Council on Cardiovascular Surgery and Anesthesia, and the Quality of Care and Outcomes Research Interdisciplinary Working Group. *Circulation.* 2007;116:1736–1754.

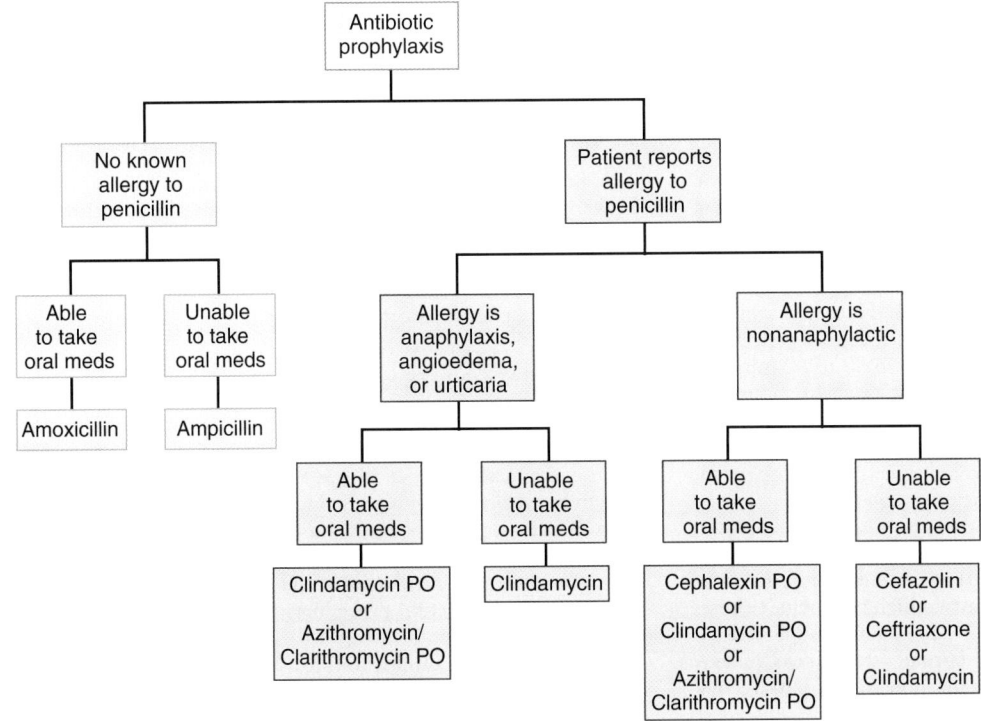

Fig. 69.1 Appropriate antibiotic selection for high-risk individuals undergoing a procedure for which prophylaxis for infective endocarditis is indicated. *PO,* Orally.

TABLE 69.1   Antibiotic Doses for Prophylaxis of Infective Endocarditis

Antibiotic	Adult Oral Dose	Pediatric Oral Dose	Adult IV/IM* Dose	Pediatric IV/IM* Dose
Amoxicillin	2 g	50 mg/kg	N/A	N/A
Ampicillin	N/A	N/A	2 g	50 mg/kg
Cefazolin	N/A	N/A	1 g	50 mg/kg
Ceftriaxone	N/A	N/A	1 g	50 mg/kg
Cephalexin	2 g	50 mg/kg	N/A	N/A
Clindamycin	600 mg	20 mg/kg	600 mg	20 mg/kg
Azithromycin or clarithromycin	500 mg	15 mg/kg	N/A	N/A

*Avoid IM doses in patients who are anticoagulated.

IM, Intramuscular; *IV,* intravenous; *N/A,* not applicable.

Modified from Wilson W, Taubert KA, Gewitz M, et al. Prevention of infective endocarditis: Guidelines from the American Heart Association. A guideline from the American Heart Association Rheumatic Fever, Endocarditis, and Kawasaki Disease Committee, Council on Cardiovascular Disease in the Young, and the Council on Clinical Cardiology, Council on Cardiovascular Surgery and Anesthesia, and the Quality of Care and Outcomes Research Interdisciplinary Working Group. *Circulation.* 2007;116:1736–1754.

solution), but tap water may be an acceptable alternative in nonbite wounds. Povidone–iodine (Betadine) surgical scrub solution, and other antiseptic solutions such as hydrogen peroxide, may be toxic to wound tissue and therefore impede healing. A dilute Betadine solution (1:10), however, may be useful for contaminated wounds. Debridement of the wound plays an equally important role in preventing infection because permanently devitalized tissue impairs the wound's ability to resist infection. In situations in which foreign bodies such as particulate matter or bone fragments may be present, exploration with a metal probe and use of radiographs are indicated. Opening the wound further to permit adequate visualization may be necessary in some cases.

Clean, sterile technique is mandatory in any surgery and with the excision and repair of any wound in the skin. The 11 most common causes of a wound infection may truly be the naso-oral area and the 10 fingers of the operating clinician! Also, see the discussion on wound prophylaxis in Chapter 19, Laceration and Incision Repair.

Optimal antimicrobial agents for surgical site prophylaxis should be bactericidal, nontoxic, inexpensive, and active against the typical pathogens that can cause surgical site infection postoperatively. Although antibiotic prophylaxis can reduce surgical site infections, the benefits must be weighed against the risks of toxic and allergic reactions, selecting for resistant bacteria, drug interactions, and possibly unnecessarily increasing the costs of health care. Consensus panels most often recommend cefazolin (1 or 2 g for most patients, 3 g for patients >120 kg) and other cephalosporins because they meet the aforementioned criteria. However, there are sites where other antibiotics are recommended due to local flora (see the GI, GU, and gynecologic and obstetric sections that follow). To maximize its effectiveness, intravenous perioperative prophylaxis should be administered within 30 to 60 minutes before the surgical incision. Antimicrobial prophylaxis should be of short duration to decrease toxicity and antimicrobial resistance and to reduce cost. However, repeat dosing should be considered for procedures lasting longer than two half-lives of the drug, or in which there is excessive blood loss.

For most elective dermatologic and plastic surgeries, antibiotic prophylaxis for wound infection is not routinely indicated unless the procedure is expected to last more than 3 hours or the patient is at high risk for wound infection. Patients at high risk include those with diabetes mellitus, significant obesity, immunosuppression, vascular insufficiency, malnutrition, chronic steroid use, coexisting infection at a distant site, colonization with a pathogenic

organism, a prolonged preoperative stay, lymphedema, as well as older patients. It is best to give the antibiotic 1 hour before surgery (vancomycin and fluoroquinolones 90 to 120 minutes before surgery), but there are benefits to administration even up to 4 hours later. There is no benefit to extending prophylactic therapy beyond 24 to 48 hours. For most procedures, cefazolin, which is effective against streptococci and staphylococci, is an effective and narrow-spectrum choice. However, any antibiotic effective against streptococci and staphylococci, such as erythromycin, may be used. For office surgeries in which prophylaxis is desired, also consider cephalexin and drugs effective against methicillin-resistant *Staphylococcus*.

GASTROINTESTINAL PROCEDURES

Antibiotic prophylaxis is not required for routine endoscopic procedures associated with a low risk of bacteremia, even in patients with the highest risk cardiac conditions. However, antibiotic prophylaxis is suggested for patients with severe neutropenia (absolute neutrophil count <500 cells/ mm^3), advanced hematologic malignancies, or cirrhosis with ascites undergoing procedures such as esophageal dilation or endoscopic sclerotherapy, though data to support this recommendation are lacking. The antibiotics to be used in this situation should cover for bacteremia, the same as in Box 69.2. Antibiotic prophylaxis is also recommended prior to percutaneous endoscopic gastrostomy and jejunostomy tube placement to minimize the risk of peristomal wound infections. Prophylaxis should be with cephazolin, as discussed previously, unless methicillin resistant *S. aureus* is a possibility; in that situation, vancomycin should be considered. There may be benefit of preprocedure screening for methicillin resistant *S. aureus* if endemic.

GENITOURINARY PROCEDURES

Antibiotic prophylaxis is recommended prior to cystoscopy only in high risk patients. Coverage with ciprofloxin 500 mg orally or 400 mg intravenously should be adequate. An alternative is one oral double strength trimethoprim-sulfamethoxazole tablet. These same antibiotics can be used prior to prostate biopsy. A meta-analysis of nine trials (Yang, 2015) found that prophylactic antibiotics prior to prostate biopsy significantly reduced the risk for bacteriuria, bacteremia, fever, urinary tract infection, and the need for hospitalization.

GYNECOLOGIC AND OBSTETRIC PROCEDURES

Cefazolin (2 g for most patients, 3 g for patients >120 kg) should be given intravenously prior to cesarean section. Doxycycline 100 mg should be given orally an hour prior to an abortion and 200 mg after the procedure. For a hysterosalpingogram, doxycycline 100 mg should be given twice daily for 5 days. Antibiotic prophylaxis is not recommended prior to laparoscopic surgery.

PROSTHETIC JOINTS

Most prosthetic joint infections are due to contamination during the original surgery from colonization of the prosthesis or airborne contamination of the wound. Infection of prostheses through hematogenous spread is much less common. In those situations of hematogenous spread, most are due to S aureus bacteremia, skin infections, or urosepsis. In 2014, the American Dental Association recommended against the routine use of prophylactic antibiotics prior to dental procedures in patients with prosthetic joints. Likewise, patients with prosthetic joints in general do not require antimicrobial prophylaxis for GI, GU, or respiratory tract procedures.

RECOMMENDED READING

American College of Obstetricians and Gynecologists. *Antibiotic Prophylaxis for Gynecologic Procedures. ACOG Practice Bulletin no. 104.* Washington DC: ACOG; 2009.

Bratzler DW, Dellinger EP, Olsen KM, Perl TM, Auwaerter PG, et al. Clinical practice guidelines for antimicrobial prophylaxis in surgery. *Surg Infect.* 2013;14:73.

Enzler MJ, Berbari E, Osmon DR. Antimicrobial prophylaxis in adults. *Mayo Clin Proc.* 2011;86(7):686–701.

Ernst AA, Gershoff L, Miller P, et al. Warmed versus room temperature saline for laceration irrigation: a randomized clinical trial. *South Med J.* 2003;96:436–439.

Graham L. AHA releases updated guidelines on prevention of infective endocarditis. *Am Fam Physician.* 2008;77:538–545.

National Institute for Health and Clinical Excellence. *Prophylaxis Against Infective Endocarditis [NICE Clinical Guideline No. 64];* 2008 , Updated 2016. www.nice.org.uk/CG064.

Sollecito TP, Abt E, Lockhart PB, et al. The use of prophylactic antibiotics prior to dental procedures in patients with prosthetic joints. *J Am Dent Assoc.* 2015;146(1):11–16.

Taubert K. Endocarditis prophylaxis: an evolution of change. *Am Fam Physician.* 2008;77:421–422.

Yang L, Gao L, Chen Y, Tang Z, Liu L, et al. Prophylactic antibiotics in prostate biopsy: a meta-analysis based on randomized controlled trials. *Surg Infect.* 2015;16:733–747.

Wilson W, Taubert KA, Gewitz M, et al. Prevention of infective endocarditis: guidelines from the American Heart Association. A guideline from the American Heart Association rheumatic fever, endocarditis, and kawasaki disease committee, council on cardiovascular disease in the young, and the council on clinical cardiology, council on cardiovascular surgery and anesthesia, and the quality of care and outcomes research interdisciplinary working group. *Circulation.* 2007;116:1736–1754.

CHAPTER 70

OFFICE ELECTROCARDIOGRAMS

Jason A. Mogonye

The electrocardiogram (ECG) is a graphic description of the electrical activity of the heart, recorded from skin surface electrodes positioned to demonstrate this activity from a variety of spatial perspectives. The waves of electrical activity are represented as a sequence of deflections on the ECG (P wave, QRS complex, and T wave). The resting ECG is the most widely used cardiovascular diagnostic test in the United States. Current estimates are that half are performed or interpreted by clinicians without fellowship training in cardiology. The clinician supervising, performing, or interpreting ECGs must be familiar with the proper use of the machine and electrode placement. In addition, guidelines and clinical competency statements are available (see Recommended Reading section).

The validity of using the resting 12-lead ECG as a screening test for cardiovascular disease in asymptomatic individuals has never been demonstrated convincingly. One reason is the relatively low prevalence of ECG abnormalities in the general population (ranges from 1% to 10%). Such a low prevalence limits the ECG's sensitivity for screening, its predictive accuracy, and its usefulness (Fig. 70.1). Likewise, the ECG can appear completely normal in patients experiencing an acute coronary event. Therefore it is important for the clinician to consider each ECG in the context of the clinical situation. Pertinent to each ECG are the patient's age, risk factors, medications, symptoms, physical findings, and laboratory results as well as findings from any previous ECGs (for comparison).

INDICATIONS

In the office, the following situations are the most common to warrant an ECG:

- Chest pain, especially if suspected to be of cardiac origin
- Palpitations
- Acute-onset dyspnea
- Syncope
- Presence of a new cardiac finding on examination (e.g., murmur, gallop, rub)
- Dysrhythmia recognition and management
- Baseline or longitudinal data for patients with hypertension, diabetes, chronic kidney disease (defined as glomerular filtration rate <60 mL/min), or other chronic diseases that might cause ECG changes or increase cardiac risk
- Preoperative screen for patients with known coronary artery disease (CAD), significant arrhythmia, peripheral arterial disease, cerebrovascular disease, or other significant structural heart disease, except those undergoing low-risk surgery. It may also be reasonable to screen any patients undergoing surgery except those undergoing low-risk surgery.
- Electrolyte abnormalities that may cause ECG alterations (e.g., potassium, calcium)
- Before administration of pharmacologic agents that are known to have a high incidence of cardiovascular effects (e.g., medications causing a QT prolongation, cancer chemotherapy) and for monitoring QTc after starting therapy

- Before exercise testing (to evaluate for any contraindications)
- Before beginning an exercise program in those at high risk (e.g., known CAD, first-degree relative with hypertrophic cardiomyopathy)
- Individuals in special occupations that require high cardiovascular performance or who would immediately endanger others if they experienced a cardiovascular event
- Possibly for a baseline during a physical examination of those older than 40 years, especially patients with risk factors for CAD

Patients can be classified into three major groups when undergoing an ECG: (1) patients with known cardiovascular disease or dysfunction, (2) patients who are suspected of having or who are at increased risk of developing cardiovascular disease or dysfunction, and (3) patients with no apparent or suspected heart disease or dysfunction.

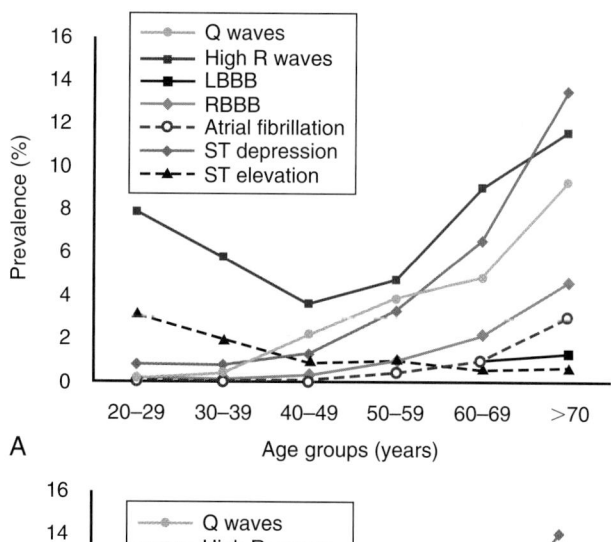

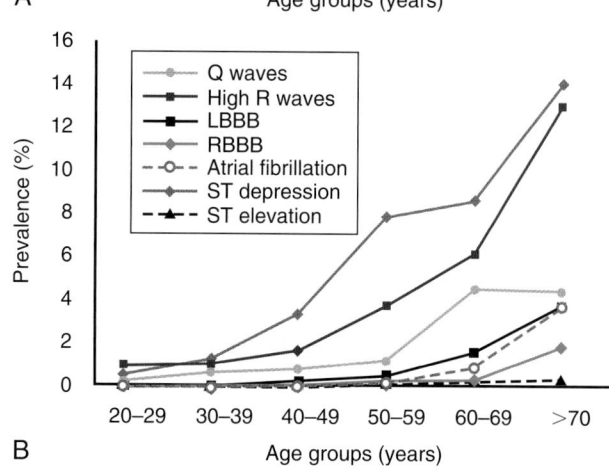

Fig. 70.1 Prevalence of electrocardiogram abnormalities in men (A) and women (B). *LBBB*, Left bundle branch block; *RBBB*, right bundle branch block.

For patients in the first two groups, an ECG is indicated if there has been a change in symptoms or if the therapy may change based on the ECG. The ECG may show changes during symptoms and in response to treatment, which would confirm a cardiac basis for symptoms. It also may demonstrate preexisting structural or ischemic heart disease (e.g., left ventricular hypertrophy, Q waves). However, a normal ECG, or one that remains unchanged from the baseline, does not exclude the possibility that chest pain is ischemic in origin. The last group (those without apparent or suspected cardiac disease) represents a large proportion of the patients treated in the usual office practice.

NOTE: The routine use of a resting ECG to screen for CAD in asymptomatic adults is not recommended by the American College of Physicians or the Canadian Task Force on Preventive Health Care. The American Academy of Family Physicians and the US Preventive Services Task Force recommend against routine screening for CAD with resting ECG in asymptomatic, low-risk adults. They also find insufficient evidence to recommend for or against routine screening with resting ECG in patients at increased risk for events from CAD.

Although the American Heart Association likewise does not recommend routine or repeated ECGs for risk assessment, various ECG abnormalities have been reported to have predictive power. For example, the most common abnormal ECG findings (Q waves, ST segment depression, nonspecific T-wave abnormalities, left ventricular hypertrophy [LVH], and bundle branch blocks) on the resting ECG have been found to have independent predictive power for both coronary mortality and total cardiovascular mortality. In some studies, patients with one or more of these abnormalities were associated with two to four times increased cardiovascular risk (i.e., multivariate-adjusted relative risks between 2.0 and 4.0). These study results indicate that ECG abnormalities might suggest an increased clinical risk in certain patients and therefore warrant further investigation or risk reduction. Persistent abnormalities on the resting ECG on serial tracings are associated with a higher clinical risk than transient findings alone.

Screening for cardiac disease in asymptomatic athletes during the preparticipation examination (sports physical) is becoming more common. Sudden cardiac death is the leading cause of mortality during sports participation, and identification of conditions that may predispose athletes to sudden cardiac death may allow clinicians to exclude those from participation who are at high risk. Criteria have been developed for interpretation of screening ECGs for athletes based on the consensus of an international panel of experts. These criteria are recognized and endorsed by multiple international sports medical societies. Changes on ECGs are thought to be related to the relative increase in vagal tone and cardiac chamber size in those who engage in regular exercise or training for sport and range in age from 12 to 35. Many of those changes are considered normal for athletes, while others are worrisome and require further evaluation. The full consensus statement and an online training module are available for those interested in conducting screening ECGs in athletes (see Recommended Reading and Online Resources).

EDITOR'S NOTE: an endurance athlete is defined as anyone performing an hour a day of aerobic activity most days of the week. This can result in increased vagal tone; consequently, first-degree AV block and Mobitz type I second-degree block can be considered somewhat normal in an endurance athlete.

CONTRAINDICATIONS

- Emergent need for airway maintenance or management of breathing or circulation (these needs should be addressed before attempting to obtain an ECG)
- Patient phobia, refusal, or inability to remain still or in one position (relative contraindication in life-threatening situation)
- Skin conditions (e.g., burns, infections) that would interfere with electrode placement (relative contraindication in life-threatening situation)

EQUIPMENT

- Electrodes.
- ECG machine with appropriate patient cables and paper.
- If computerized storage is expected (e.g., in an electronic medical record [EMR]), an appropriate connection, or having available electronic storage for later transfer to the EMR, should be ensured.

PREPROCEDURE PATIENT PREPARATION

Explain the procedure to the patient and discuss why the patient needs to remain as still as possible, breathe normally, and not talk during the procedure. Occasionally, there is a need to reassure the patient that the procedure is safe and will not cause an electrical shock (e.g., "It reads the electricity your heart produces and does not shock you with electricity"). The patient should be aware that further cardiac workup may be necessary regardless of the outcome of the ECG. The patient should also be aware that a normal ECG does not eliminate the possibility of CAD or significant heart disease. Moreover, abnormal ECGs do not always indicate significant cardiac disease.

TECHNIQUE

Most modern ECG machines are so simple that an operator's manual is not needed. Standardization is accurate with digital machines, which often automatically adjust for excessive voltage. Perform the ECG procedure in a room away from powerful electrical equipment (e.g., electric motors, x-ray equipment), if possible. Electrode placement remains the biggest challenge.

1. Place the patient in the supine position on the table. Generally, the patient has a pillow under his or her head. Arms should rest at the sides of the torso. Legs should be flat, apart, and not touching each other. If the patient is in a position other than supine (e.g., head elevated to relieve orthopnea), the heart's electrical axis is altered, possibly an issue when comparing serial tracings. In such cases, a note should be made on the ECG strip of degree or angle of patient elevation so that future ECGs can be obtained with the patient at the same angle for comparison. Although the patient's chest and distal extremities are exposed during lead placement, keep the rest of the body covered. Once the leads are placed, a sheet or blanket may be used to cover the patient. This not only protects patient dignity but should also help prevent shivering, which can cause a tremor artifact on the ECG tracing.
2. Bring the ECG machine near the table and turn it on. The usual paper speed is 25 mm/sec and the amplitude 1 mV/10 mm.

NOTE: Older equipment, especially analog equipment, occasionally needs to be standardized. If available, review the operator's manual regarding standardization. Standardize the machine when it is tracing at 25 mm/sec by briefly depressing the standardization button. One millivolt should deflect exactly 10 mm, and full standardization should be used if possible. If standardization is not performed or is allowed to vary, evaluation of serial tracings is less accurate.

3. Wipe the areas for electrode placement with an alcohol swab. It may be necessary to shave some areas so that the electrodes stick. We recommend shaving after using the alcohol swab to avoid applying alcohol to any abrasions resulting from shaving. Gentle abrasion with a fine-grit sandpaper or equivalent may also reduce noise and artifact and improve the quality of the ECG. We also recommend using adhesive electrodes with a tab for fastening the clips from the cable lead.
4. Place the limb electrodes. The red electrode is for the left leg and is labeled "left leg." The electrode for the right leg is universally green and is labeled "right leg." The electrode for the right arm is often banded in white and labeled "RA." The electrode for the

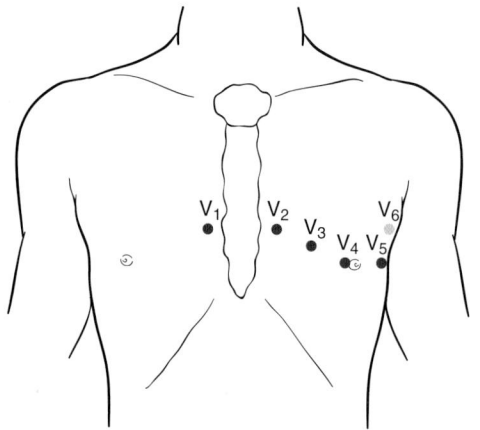

Fig. 70.2 Placement of electrodes. Note that V_6 is in the same horizontal plane as V_4 and V_5, but more lateral, in the midaxillary line.

left arm is banded in black and labeled "LA." Traditionally, limb electrodes were placed on the wrists and ankles. However, with the development of high-quality disposable electrodes, many clinicians have started applying the limb electrodes below the hips and on the upper arms. Applying the electrodes more proximally in this manner may reduce motion artifact.

5. Place the chest electrodes in the following order (Fig. 70.2):
   - V_1 (red): fourth intercostal space at right sternal border
   - V_2 (yellow): fourth intercostal space at left sternal border
   - V_4 (blue): fifth intercostal space at the mid-clavicular line
   - V_3 (green): halfway between V_2 and V_4
   - V_5 (tan): anterior axillary line at the same level as V_4 (directly lateral and in the same transverse plane)
   - V_6 (violet): mid-axillary line at the same level as V_4 and V_5 (again, directly lateral to V_5)

   For a landmark in men, the nipples are usually in the mid-clavicular line and overlie the fourth intercostal space. For consistent placement, use only bony landmarks for precordial electrodes. It may be necessary to ask a female patient to raise her left breast to allow for proper placement of the leads. The electrodes should not be placed on the breast itself to avoid erroneous tracings. Once the leads are placed, the patient may allow her breast to rest naturally with her hands at her side. The sternal angle, between the manubrium and body of the sternum, is immediately above the second intercostal space. The V_4 through V_6 electrodes are placed in the same horizontal plane (not necessarily in the same intercostal space).

6. Perform the ECG procedure with the electrodes in their proper locations. For dysrhythmias, an extended rhythm strip or another attempt at a 12-lead ECG may be indicated for improved technical quality. Multichannel machines are superior to single-channel machines for rhythm strips. When a second channel is available, it is best to display lead II for rhythm and V_5 for ischemia. If three channels are available, it is best to display leads aVF, V_2, and V_5.

   NOTE: For continuous monitoring (telemetry), any lead can be used; however, most coronary care units use a modified bipolar chest lead. The negative electrode is near the left shoulder and the positive is the traditional V_1. A third is placed at a more remote area of the chest and serves as a ground. However, of all leads, V_5 is the most sensitive for the diagnosis of ischemia. Ventricular arrhythmias are more ominous when ischemia is present (see Chapter 73, Ambulatory Electrocardiography: Holter and Event Monitoring). If a single channel is all that is available and ischemia is a concern, V_5 should be used.

7. Remove the electrodes from the patient, dispose of them, and clean the areas on the patient where the electrodes were attached. Modern adhesive electrodes are dry and leave very little residue.

INTERPRETATION

Although computer interpretive programs provide the noncardiologist with a quick and convenient second opinion, they do not provide advice on what to do with an abnormality. The following discussion is aimed at supplementing the available interpretive programs with a suggested course of management, including troubleshooting for errors.

Limb Lead Reversal

Limb lead reversal is the most common noticeable error involving the frontal leads. It usually occurs between the right and left arm electrodes, probably because these leads are usually grouped, bundled, or connected together. Lead reversal has become more common as inexperienced personnel replace ECG technicians. Fortunately, the right and left leg electrodes can be switched without affecting the recorded ECG. The clinician should consider arm lead reversal as a possibility whenever the computer interpretation is marked right axis deviation, especially if it is new compared with a previous tracin. It can also be considered when precordial leads do not exhibit the normal R-wave progression. Also, the precordial leads and aVF will be normal, whereas limb lead I will be inverted. Normally, limb lead I somewhat matches V_6 in terms of morphology of the P-wave and QRS direction; this will not be the case with arm lead reversal. When every tracing from an ECG machine exhibits this pattern, the actual ECG leads may be mislabeled.

The second most common placement error is reversal of V_1 and V_3 (again, frequently in the same group or bundle of leads). This should be considered a possibility when R-wave amplitude does not increase from V_1 to V_3 and there is T-wave inversion in V_3.

Management includes repeating the ECG procedure after checking previous ECGs for the patient, checking the ECG machine, and verifying lead placement. If limb lead reversal is excluded and the finding is still not explained, check the precordial leads for normal R-wave progression. If the R waves do not progress normally, move the precordial leads to the patient's right side and record for the possibility of dextrocardia. If dextrocardia is confirmed, correlation with a chest radiograph is the next step.

Wolff-Parkinson-White

Wolff-Parkinson-White (WPW) is an ECG pattern characterized by a short PR interval followed by a delta wave and a prolonged QRS duration. The QRS duration may be longer than 120 msec, but it may also be shorter, depending on the degree of fusion of conduction. These characteristics are due to aberrant conduction of activation through an accessory pathway. WPW occurs in 1 of 10,000 individuals and can be entirely asymptomatic, or it can be associated with tachycardia and palpitations. When WPW is present, the ST segments cannot be used to identify ischemia. Q waves are actually negative delta waves and are not due to infarction. Individuals who are incidentally found to have this ECG finding are usually otherwise normal. However, they should be questioned about symptoms of palpitations or syncope. Also, a family history of syncope or sudden death could have significance. If either of these symptoms has occurred or the family history is positive, referral to an electrophysiology cardiologist is appropriate.

Right Atrial Abnormality (Not Present on Prior Electrocardiograms)

If the right atrial abnormality or P-pulmonale is new compared with previous ECGs, consider the clinical possibilities of a pulmonary embolus (e.g., tachycardia, pleuritic chest pain, cough, fever, hypoxia, presence of cancer, or immobilization) versus an exacerbation of lung disease.

Right Atrial Abnormality (Present on Prior Electrocardiograms)

If the right atrial abnormality is a consistent finding, examine the patient for chronic lung disease (e.g., prolonged expiration, hyperresonance, rhonchi and distant breath sounds, lowered diaphragms) and consider the overall history, including possible exposure to asbestos, coal dust, or cigarette smoke. Pulmonary function testing may be indicated.

Left Atrial Abnormality (Not Present on Prior Electrocardiograms)

If the left atrial abnormality or P-mitrale is new compared with previous tracings, consider the clinical possibilities of new congestive heart failure (CHF) or mitral valvular insufficiency. Mitral valvular insufficiency is confirmed by a holosystolic murmur radiating into the axilla and, if necessary, by echocardiography.

Left Atrial Abnormality (Present on Prior Electrocardiograms)

If the left atrial abnormality or P-mitrale is consistent compared with previous tracings, evaluate the ECG for additional LVH criteria. LVH plus left atrial abnormality can be an ominous marker for future events such as CHF, stroke, or death. Physical examination and an echocardiogram can confirm the findings.

Right Axis Deviation (Not Present on Prior Electrocardiograms)

When right axis deviation is a new finding, it can be due to an exacerbation of lung disease, a pulmonary embolus, or simply a tachycardia. If right axis deviation is a change from previous ECGs, question the patient for symptoms consistent with an exacerbation of lung disease or a pulmonary embolus. If the patient has findings consistent with embolus, a nuclear ventilation/perfusion ({Vdot}/{Qdot}) scan or computed tomographic angiogram is usually indicated.

Right Axis Deviation (Present on Prior Electrocardiograms)

Chronic right axis deviation is normal in those younger than 21 years and in athletes. It can also be a chronic finding in patients with lung disease, right ventricular hypertrophy, an old lateral wall myocardial infarction, or a left posterior hemiblock.

Left Axis Deviation

Left axis deviation (LAD) is the most common "abnormality" in adults, occurring in over 8% of patients. It can be part of the criteria for LVH, but in isolation it has little significance. Marked LAD (45% or more) is called *left anterior hemiblock* or *left anterior fascicular block*. If LAD is present and the patient is not known to be hypertensive, it may be worth efforts to exclude the diagnosis of hypertension with frequent blood pressure checks or ambulatory blood pressure monitoring (see Chapter 72, Ambulatory Blood Pressure Monitoring). LAD can also be seen after an old inferior wall myocardial infarction.

Right Bundle Branch Block

Right bundle branch block (RBBB) can be normal (occurring without underlying disease) or due to trauma, increased right ventricular pressure, ischemia, or infarction. An incomplete RBBB has a QRS duration of less than 120 msec and an RSR′ pattern in V_1 and V_2 without an R wave greater than the amplitude of the S wave. It sometimes is simply called an *RSR′ pattern* and usually is a normal finding. Very rarely, it can be associated with an atrial septal defect. Incomplete RBBB or right ventricular conduction delay (RVCD) is not necessarily a precursor of RBBB or any conduction abnormality. Such atypical right ventricular conduction patterns are seen more frequently in people younger than 21 years, in athletes, and can also be normal variants. Although wide splitting of the second heart sound (S2) is a very common finding among normal patients, fixed splitting of S2 can also be associated with an atrial septal defect. Remember that the abnormalities of S2 must be heard in the sitting position because splitting is often wide in normal individuals when supine. If present, an echocardiographic air contrast ("bubble") study is indicated. Any pulmonary disease process can be associated with RVCD, and RVCD can occur acutely with exacerbation of lung disease or a pulmonary embolus. Clinical correlation is necessary; either treatment of the lung disease or a {Vdot}/{Qdot} scan/computed tomographic angiogram might be indicated.

Left Bundle Branch Block

Left bundle branch block (LBBB) can result from severe trauma (car accident), ischemia, or infarction. It is often associated with LVH or left ventricular dilation. LBBB can also result from fibrosis of the conduction system. LBBB has a weak predictive power in a young, asymptomatic population (consistent with Bayes' rule), but is quite ominous in an older population as a marker for an increased risk of death, stroke, and CHF. Incomplete LBBB and hemiblocks are usually not associated with cardiac disease. Clinical correlates, including the cardiac examination, should direct any further studies in response to a new LBBB. If the patient has an enlarged heart with signs or symptoms of CHF, an echocardiogram is usually indicated. If a patient with LBBB has prolonged ischemic-type chest pain, the patient is experiencing an ST-elevation myocardial infarction until proven otherwise. Percutaneous coronary intervention, or fibrinolysis is indicated. If the patient is asymptomatic and clearly not having an acute myocardial infarction, unfortunately neither the resting nor the exercise ECG can be used as a diagnostic tool. Instead, a stress echocardiogram or a nuclear perfusion test is required.

Right Ventricular Hypertrophy

Right ventricular hypertrophy can be a normal finding in people younger than 21 years and in athletes. It can also be associated with chronic obstructive pulmonary disease, primary and secondary pulmonary hypertension, some types of congenital heart disease, pulmonary embolus, and CHF. Clinical correlation is indicated. If the right ventricular hypertrophy is new compared with previous tracings, consider the clinical presentation for pulmonary embolus or exacerbation of lung disease. The patient may require hospitalization and treatment with heparin for pulmonary embolism, or bronchodilators, antibiotics, and steroids for chronic obstructive pulmonary disease. If the pulmonary disease ECG criterion is not a new finding, examine the patient for chronic lung disease (e.g., prolonged expiration, hyperresonance, rhonchi and distant breath sounds, lowered diaphragms) and consider the overall medical history, including possible exposure to asbestos, coal dust, or cigarette smoke. Pulmonary function testing and an echocardiogram may be indicated.

Left Ventricular Hypertrophy

LVH requires clinical correlation, beginning with blood pressure measurement and physical examination for cardiac size, murmurs, and morbid obesity. A complete medical history should be obtained with emphasis on symptoms of aortic valve disease (e.g., angina, syncope) and CHF. If CHF or aortic stenosis is suspected after the history or examination, or there is an abnormal cardiac examination, an echocardiogram may be indicated. LVH is one of the most ominous ECG indicators of risk for future cardiovascular events in patients older than 30 years. In isolation, it is not a reliable indicator of cardiac disease in well-trained athletes.

ST Segment Depression

Acute ST segment depression can be associated with ischemia, unstable angina/non–ST segment elevation myocardial infarction (acute coronary syndrome), electrolyte abnormalities, osmolality changes, hyperventilation, standing up, and certain drugs. An ECG should be obtained in any patient with chest pain of uncertain etiology because an acute ST shift can confirm that it is due to ischemia. ST segment depression may also be associated with subendocardial damage, as opposed to Q waves, which are usually associated with transmural damage from infarction. Although chronic ST segment depression is nonspecific as a marker for cardiac disease, it is associated with a poor outcome. It can be due to electrolyte abnormalities and drugs, particularly digoxin. The patient should be questioned about a past or present history of cardiac ischemic pain. Blood chemistries, including electrolytes, glucose, calcium, magnesium, blood urea nitrogen, and creatinine, should be obtained. All medications should be recorded carefully and any nonprescription drugs that the patient may be taking should be noted. Many nonprescription drugs, especially from other countries, contain diuretics and even digoxin.

Prolonged QT Interval

Diagnosis of a prolonged QT interval is complicated by the inherent difficulty in identifying T-wave end and the inaccuracy of Bazett's formula when correcting for heart rate. It may be preferable to judge the QT interval as prolonged when it changes in length or when it exceeds 50% of the R-R interval. QT prolongation can be due to multiple causes, but its importance is its association with premature ventricular contractions, ventricular tachycardia, and ventricular fibrillation; in other words, it is associated with vulnerability to a lethal arrhythmia. The following is a list of some of the conditions that can cause QT prolongation: hereditary syndromes (rare), electrolyte–metabolic abnormalities (hypokalemia, hypomagnesemia, or hypocalcemia), medications (e.g., type Ia antiarrhythmics such as quinidine; tricyclic and other antidepressants, antipsychotics, antihistamines, anticholinergic drugs, antibiotics [e.g., fluoroquinolones and macrolides], and antifungals), central nervous system disorders, systemic illnesses, and myocardial infarction. Obtain blood chemistries, including electrolytes, glucose, calcium, magnesium, blood urea nitrogen, and creatinine. Take a careful medication history, including noncardiac drugs such as decongestants, antigastroesophageal reflux disease medications, and antibiotics. Ask specifically about any family history of syncope, sudden death, or syndromes associated with deafness. (See www.crediblemeds.org for a list of meds that prolong the QT interval and/or have been associated with life-threatening arrhythmia torsades de pointes.)

Troubleshooting

- Arm lead reversal can result in false-negative or false-positive signs of ischemia.
- Older ECG machines use thermal-head printers that automatically adjust for tracing intensity. Most newer machines use laser printers that actually write the grid. They use regular paper rather than the more expensive, heat-sensitive grid papers. Extra paper, styluses, or printer cartridges should always be available.
- For a wandering baseline, there is either poor electrode contact or a bad cable, or the patient is slowly moving or breathing deeply. For older equipment, especially analog equipment, the machine may not be warmed up adequately.
- A jagged baseline is from wall current (AC) interference, a broken wire, improper grounding, or other electrical interference.
- For older equipment with heat-sensitive paper, if the baseline is too light or thin, the stylus is not hot enough. If the baseline is too thick, the stylus is too hot (refer to the operating manual). Improper stylus pressure is detected by using the standardization pulse. With proper pressure, the standardization pulse should produce a tracing with sharp corners. Rounded or exaggerated angles indicate improper pressure.
- Technicians and other medical personnel responsible for obtaining ECGs should have training and periodic retraining in skin preparation, lead placement, and patient positioning.

COMPLICATIONS

- Local skin irritation or allergic reaction to electrode placement or adhesive
- Patient distress over abnormal ECG
- Incorrect interpretation because of improper lead placement, ECG performance, or computer or clinician error
- Unnecessary diagnostic workup or treatment (and the adverse events associated with these additional interventions) because of false-positive results, no prior ECG tracing with which to compare, an inadequate clinical correlation, or a normal ECG variant

POSTPROCEDURE PATIENT EDUCATION

The patient should be scheduled for an appropriate follow-up visit with his or her clinician, regardless of the ECG result (especially those with persistent symptoms). The patient should be given the results of the ECG, as well as instructions for medications, follow-up, or further workup, as necessary. The clinician may wish to give the patient a copy of the ECG or ECG interpretation for his or her personal records.

PATIENT EDUCATION GUIDES

See patient education form available at www.expertconsult.com.

CPT/BILLING CODES

93000 Electrocardiogram, routine, with at least 12 leads; with interpretation and report
93005 Tracing only, without interpretation and report
93010 Interpretation and report only

NOTE: An ECG is usually needed to rule out a contraindication to exercise testing; however, Medicare will not reimburse for an ECG on the same day as an exercise test. For this and other reasons, it is usually better to bring the patient back on another day for an exercise test. Before every exercise test, another comparison ECG is performed; it is just not reimbursable by Medicare.

ICD-10-CM DIAGNOSTIC CODES

I10   Hypertension
I15.0   Hypertension, renovascular
I15.9   Hypertension, secondary, unspecified
I21.09 MI, acute, anterolateral
I21.09 MI, acute, anterior, NOS
I21.19 MI, acute, inferolateral
I21.11 MI, acute, inferoposterior
I21.19 MI, acute, other inferior wall, NOS
I21.29 MI, acute, other lateral wall
I21.29 MI, acute, true posterior
I21.4   Non-ST elevation MI
I21.3   ST elevation MI, unspecified site
I25.2   MI, old
I25.10 Coronary atherosclerosis, native coronary artery, without angina
I25.89 Ischemic heart disease, chronic, other
I25.9   Ischemic heart disease, chronic, unspecified

I25.5	Ischemic cardiomyopathy
I44.2	Atrioventricular block, third degree
I44.7	Bundle branch block, left
I45.10	Bundle branch block, right
I44.0	Atrioventricular block, first degree
I44.1	Atrioventricular block, Mobitz II
I44.1	Atrioventricular block, Wenckebach block
I45.81	Long QT syndrome
I47.1	Tachycardia, paroxysmal SVT
I48.91	Atrial fibrillation
I48.92	Atrial flutter
I49.01	Ventricular fibrillation
R00.1	Sinus bradycardia, NOS
I50.9	Heart failure, congestive, unspecified
I50.20	Heart failure, systolic, unspecified
I50.21	Heart failure, systolic, acute
I50.22	Heart failure, systolic, chronic
I50.30	Heart failure, diastolic, unspecified
I50.32	Heart failure, diastolic, chronic
I50.40	Heart failure, combined, unspecified
I51.7	Cardiomegaly
I70.90	Unspecified atherosclerosis
I70.91	Generalized atherosclerosis
R00.0	Tachycardia, NOS
R00.2	Palpitations
R07.9	Chest pain, unspecified

Acknowledgment

The editors recognize the contributions of Mark Clasen, MD, PhD, Jerry Hizon, MD, Victor Froelicher, MD, Russell D. White, and George D. Harris to this chapter in previous editions of this text.

SUPPLIERS

See Chapter 74, Stress ECG Testing, for a list of suppliers.

ONLINE RESOURCES

American Heart Association: www.americanheart.org.
Canadian Task Force on Preventive Health Care: www.ctfphc.org.
Clinical Exercise Physiology Consortium: examples of ECG abnormalities and what to do about them: www.cardiology.org.
ECG Interpretation in Athletes: training module for interpretation of pre-participation ECGs in athletes: https://www.amssm.org/BMJ_ECGModules.php.
KG-EKG Press (ECG interpretive aids): www.ekgpress.blogspot.com.

RECOMMENDED READING

2014 ACC/AHA guideline on perioperative cardiovascular evaluation and management of patients undergoing noncardiac surgery. *Circulation.* 2014;130:278–333.

Ashley EA, Raxwal VK, Froelicher VF. The prevalence and prognostic significance of electrocardiographic abnormalities. *Curr Probl Cardiol.* 2000;25:1–72.

Drezner JA, Sharma S, Baggish A, et al. International criteria for electrocardiographic interpretation in athletes: consensus statement. *Br J Sports Med.* 2017;51(9):704–731. https://doi.org/10.1136/bjsports-2016-097331.

Fowler-Brown A, Pignone M, Pletcher M, et al. Exercise tolerance testing to screen for coronary artery disease: a systematic review for the technical support for the U.S. Preventive Services Task Force. *Ann Intern Med.* 2004;140:W9–W24.

Froelicher V, Quaglietti S. *Handbook of Ambulatory Cardiology.* Philadelphia: Lippincott-Raven; 1997.

Grauer K. *A 1st Book on ECGs.* Gainesville, FL: KG EKG Press; 2014.

Grauer K. *12-Lead ECGs: A "Pocket Brain" for Easy Interpretation.* 6th ed. Gainesville, FL: KG EKG Press; 2014.

Grauer K. *A Practical Guide to ECG Interpretation.* 2nd ed. St Louis: Mosby; 1998.

Grundy SM, Bazzarre T, Cleeman J, et al. Prevention conference V: beyond secondary prevention: identifying the high-risk patient for primary prevention: medical office assessment: writing group I. *Circulation.* 2000;101:E3–E11.

Kadish AH, Buxton AE, Kennedy HL, et al. ACC/AHA clinical competence statement on electrocardiography and ambulatory electrocardiography: a report of the ACC/AHA/ACP-ASIM task force on clinical competence (ACC/AHA Committee to develop a clinical competence statement on electrocardiography and ambulatory electrocardiography) endorsed by the International Society for Holter and noninvasive electrocardiology. *J Am Coll Cardiol.* 2001;38:2091–2100.

Kligfield P, Gettes LS, Bailey JJ, et al. Recommendations for the standardization and interpretation of the electrocardiogram: part I: the electrocardiogram and its technology. A scientific statement from the American Heart Association Electrocardiography and Arrhythmias Committee, Council on Clinical Cardiology; the American College of Cardiology Foundation; and the Heart Rhythm Society endorsed by the International Society for Computerized Electrocardiology. *J Am Coll Cardiol.* 2007;49:1109–1127.

Mason JW, Hancock EW, Gettes LS, et al. Recommendations for the standardization and interpretation of the electrocardiogram: part II: electrocardiography diagnostic statement list. A scientific statement from the American Heart Association Electrocardiography and Arrhythmias Committee, Council on Clinical Cardiology; the American College of Cardiology Foundation; and the Heart Rhythm Society Endorsed by the International Society for Computerized Electrocardiology. *J Am Coll Cardiol.* 2007;49:1128–1135.

U.S. Preventive Services Task Force. Coronary heart disease. Screening with electrocardiography. https://www.uspreventiveservicestaskforce.org/Page/Document/UpdateSummaryFinal/coronary-heart-disease-screening-with-electrocardiography. 2012.

CHAPTER 71

Preoperative Evaluation*

Whitney LeFevre • Maury J. Greenberg

The preoperative medical consultation may be one of the most misunderstood services provided by primary care clinicians. Often incorrectly referred to as a "clearance," it is more properly a consultation provided by the patient's primary clinician, at the request of the operating surgeon. The goals of this consultation are first is to assess the patient's overall medical condition and then minimize risks of untoward events related to a proposed surgical intervention.

In some instances, the operating surgeon is also the primary care clinician. In this case the preoperative evaluation may be conducted as part of the overall decision-making process surrounding the need for an office- or otherwise-based diagnostic or therapeutic procedure. In others, the consultation may be performed before surgery by another clinician. In either case, it provides an opportunity for the primary care clinician to review the patient's overall health status and to bring up a variety of issues, such as recommended screening tests, medication adjustments, and lifestyle modifications. It may afford an opportunity, separate from the annual wellness exam, to review previous recommendations the patient has failed to pursue, such as screening colonoscopy, smoking cessation, weight loss, vaccination, or, in the case of children, developmental assessments.

As a consultation, the results must be reported to the requesting surgeon in a timely fashion and in a usable format, and must include clear, concise, and specific recommendations related to the proposed surgical procedure. It should be noted that, particularly in the case of procedures performed in hospitals, the preoperative evaluation will become a part of the patient's medical record. As such, should complications arise or unexpected events occur, this evaluation may provide the only comprehensive medical history immediately available. That said, most facilities require a history and physical examination to be performed and documented in the patient's medical record within the week prior to a procedure. It is also recommended by the most current American Society of Anesthesiologists (ASA) guidelines that the patient be reevaluated immediately before the procedure.

Finally, it must be recognized that "standards" change. Ongoing research and evidence result in changes to our understanding of what is best for optimizing a patient's condition and to limit risks. For example, changes to American Heart Association (AHA) guidelines for prevention of bacterial endocarditis (www.americanheart.org) and other preoperative guidelines have altered the use of antibiotic prophylaxis in many patients (see Chapter 69, Antibiotic Prophylaxis). It is thus important for every clinician to be current with guidelines and to seek expert consultation when indicated.

SURGICAL RISK

Determining the relative risk of a given procedure considers the patient's underlying condition, the specific risks of the procedure itself, the risks of anesthesia, and the possibility of postoperative complications. In most cases, "risk" refers to the possibility of cardiovascular complications in adults or respiratory complications in children. However, in the face of underlying conditions such as bleeding disorders, steroid dependence, or renal insufficiency, an otherwise simple procedure can present risks that require careful preoperative preparation. The timing of an elective procedure can also modify the risk, particularly during the postpartum period, or in a patient with a recent myocardial infarction or coronary intervention. Methods of calculating risk specific to a particular procedure will be discussed in a later section.

Urgency of Procedures

By AHA guidelines, an *emergent procedure* is one that is life- or limb-preserving and is usually performed in less than 6 hours, so there is little time for clinical evaluation prior to the procedure. An *urgent procedure* is also life- or limb-preserving and generally performed in 6 to 24 hours; this may allow some time for a limited clinical evaluation. A *time-sensitive procedure* is generally performed in 1 to 6 weeks, a time frame allowing for clinical evaluation and possible changes in management without negatively affecting the outcome. Oncologic procedures often fall into this category. An *elective procedure* is one that can be delayed up to a year.

Risk From Procedures

- *High-risk procedures* (often >5% risk) include cardiac procedures, aortic and other major vessel vascular procedures, peripheral arterial procedures, prolonged procedures, and procedures in which large volumes of fluid are shifted.
- *Intermediate-risk procedures* (1% to 5% risk) include intraperitoneal, intrathoracic, carotid or aortic stent, carotid endarterectomy, orthopedic, head and neck, and prostate procedures. Although each of these types of surgery may entail specific risks such as anticipated blood loss, risk of airway compromise, or risk of intraoperative or postoperative neurologic complications, they are not unanticipated and are addressed by the operating surgeon together with the anesthesiologist as part of the operative plan.
- *Low-risk procedures* (<1% risk) include cataract surgery, plastic surgery, most endoscopic procedures, and breast, superficial skin, and ambulatory noncardiac surgeries. Since intermediate and high-risk procedures are managed in generally the same way, the AHA and others have combined these groups into those of *increased risk* (≥1%). Most office-based procedures such as skin biopsy, colposcopy, vasectomy, and others that require no anesthesia or only topical or local anesthesia do not increase the risk of cardiac or pulmonary events in otherwise healthy individuals and are considered low risk. Such procedures, including dental procedures performed with clinician-administered 50% nitrous

---

*The opinions contained in this chapter are solely those of the author and do not represent the official policy or doctrine of the Department of Defense, the U.S. Public Health Service, or the Uniformed Services University of the Health Sciences.

BOX 71.1 Conditions With Increased Risk of Cardiac Complications

Uncontrolled coronary occlusive disease (e.g., unstable angina, recent [<30 days] myocardial infarction)
Uncontrolled congestive heart failure
Significant valvular disease (especially aortic and mitral stenosis)
Cardiac dysrhythmias associated with hemodynamic instability

TABLE 71.1 American Society of Anesthesiologists Physical Status Classification System

Class	Description
1	Healthy patient with no significant medical problems
2	Patient with mild systemic disease
3	Patient with severe systemic disease that is not incapacitating
4	Patient with severe systemic disease that is a constant threat to life
5	Moribund patient, not expected to live 24 hr regardless of treatment
6	Brain-dead patient who is an organ donor
E	"E" suffix is added to any class to indicate that the surgery is emergent.

oxide or other diagnostic and therapeutic procedures performed without sedation or analgesia, do not usually require a separate or specific preoperative consultation.

Patient Risk Factors

Risk is further determined by considering the patient's medical conditions, including that which resulted in the need for surgery. Clinical predictors of increased risk of cardiac complications associated with surgery are included in Box 71.1.

Concurrent medical conditions such as morbid obesity, uncontrolled hypertension, diabetes, obstructive pulmonary disease (asthma or emphysema), poor nutritional status, bleeding disorders, anticoagulant therapy, hypercoagulable states, ischemic cerebrovascular disease, liver disease, kidney disease, or immune deficiency also require assessment and specific interventions to reduce risk, if possible.

In some cases, the decision to defer an elective procedure should be made until risk factors have been fully evaluated and appropriate interventions performed.

Although it may be intuitive to assign greater risk of a given procedure to patients of advanced age, there is no evidence for age as an independent variable correlating with increased incidence of poor outcomes. The perception of increasing age resulting in increased risk is more likely associated with increased incidence of comorbid conditions (i.e., adults >55 years have a higher incidence of cardiovascular disease, cerebrovascular disease, and diabetes). Simply put, healthy elderly people will have the same risks of surgery as healthy young people. That said, among older people (age >65 years), there is generally a higher risk for acute ischemic stroke, since age greater than 62 years is an independent risk factor for perioperative stroke. More postoperative complications, increased lengths of stay, and inability to return home after hospitalization are seen among "frail" adults older than 70 years (e.g., those with impaired cognition who are dependent on others for their activities of daily living) than in healthy, younger adults. For patients with known cognitive defects undergoing general anesthesia, their caregiver should be counseled regarding increased risk of postoperative delirium and the potential for accelerated change in cognition afterward (see Appendix M, Special Considerations in Geriatric Patients).

Risk From Anesthesia

Selection of type of anesthesia may also affect the overall risk of surgery, but the notion that local, regional, or spinal anesthesia is automatically safer than general anesthesia is not valid. The availability of a tracheal tube in a patient under general anesthesia allows optimal airway control and protection, which may offset the risks of such anesthesia in some patients.

The use of "sedation analgesia," also known as moderate (conscious) sedation, allows the performance of certain procedures while the patient is still able to respond to commands and maintain his or her own airway (see Chapter 1, Procedural Sedation and Analgesia). The selection of this technique, however, mandates strict adherence to monitoring and the availability of resuscitative equipment. Clinicians who use moderate (conscious) sedation for

procedures performed in office settings need to make considerable investments in training, equipment, and personnel. This is because they should provide essentially the same level of care as is provided in a hospital setting.

For procedures performed in hospitals or ambulatory facilities that provide anesthesia team services, in the absence of compelling issues, it is usually best to leave selection of specific anesthetic modalities to the anesthesiologist. Specific concerns should of course be discussed with the surgeon and anesthesia team when indicated. It is helpful, however, for all clinicians to understand the risk classification system used by the ASA (Table 71.1).

PREOPERATIVE HISTORY AND PHYSICAL EXAMINATION

History

A careful and complete history is critical to providing good care and appropriate recommendations. The reasons for the planned procedure should be noted and should include the laterality of the affected organ or body part, if appropriate. Events leading up to the procedure, especially those associated with trauma, should be reviewed for possible indicators of medical causes. For example, a fractured hip may be secondary to a fall, but the fall may be secondary to syncope related to intermittent complete heart block, which in turn may be secondary to Lyme disease. Identification of these underlying medical problems and appropriate interventions prior to surgery can help prevent complications.

The past surgical history, including any reactions to anesthesia as well as any family history of such reactions, must be noted and investigated. Any allergies to medications as well as sensitivity to latex must be prominently included in the report forwarded to the surgeon. Any history of a difficult airway would be good to note, as well as whether there has been frequent or repeated exposure to sedation or analgesic agents.

A complete list of medications being taken by the patient, including dose, route, and frequency, should include not only prescribed medications but vitamins, supplements, and herbal treatments. The common use of aspirin is an obvious concern, but other products such as nonsteroidal antiinflammatory drugs (NSAIDs), omega-3 fatty acids, ginkgo biloba, or high-dose vitamin E can also affect bleeding. St. John's wort interacts with many medications.

Aspirin, which irreversibly interferes with platelet function by inhibiting cyclooxygenase, has effects that last the entire 10-day lifespan of platelets. The decision to stop antiplatelet therapy depends on the patient's cardiac history and risk, along with the type of surgery being performed. The American Academy of Chest Physicians Perioperative Anticoagulation Clinical Guideline from 2012 recommends that patients who have a low risk of cardiovascular events should stop aspirin 7 to 10 days before the procedure. For patients with known coronary or cardiovascular disease, the decision is more complex and discussed later in this chapter.

Other NSAIDs, such as ibuprofen and naproxen, affect cyclo-oxygenase, but in a reversible fashion that lasts until the drug has effectively been cleared. This usually occurs after approximately 5 half-lives, which for ibuprofen takes 10 hours, but for naproxen takes longer, up to 3 to 4 days. There is limited evidence to guide clinicians on when it is ideal to stop NSAIDs preoperatively, but the decision to stop these medicines must consider the surgical bleeding risk versus the indication for the NSAID. Knowing that not all NSAIDs have the same half-life is important to ensure they are appropriately stopped in relation to the time of surgery.

Patients should be questioned about any history of angina, myocardial infarction, and symptoms suggestive of congestive heart failure such as dyspnea, orthopnea, recent rapid weight gain, or edema, as well as any recent cardiac testing. The availability of a recent stress test or echocardiogram might obviate the need for repeat studies. For those with an implanted defibrillator or pacemaker (collectively known as cardiovascular implantable electronic devices), it is helpful to know if they have seen the clinician managing their device for query in the last 6 months (implantable defibrillator) or a year (pacemaker). The preoperative team should also consult this clinician to develop a plan for the surgical procedure (Crossley et al., 2011, Heart Rhythm Society/ASA Expert Consensus Statement).

A history of respiratory or cardiac conditions that might suggest the need for preoperative testing, or interventions such as bronchodilator treatments, should be noted and appropriate recommendations made. Factors such as obesity, likelihood of immobility, or altered coagulation and immunologic states should also prompt appropriate suggestions for both preoperative and postoperative care. Risk of postoperative deep venous thrombosis with secondary pulmonary embolism is increased by immobility and should prompt suggestions for prevention, which may include early ambulation if possible, use of sequential leg compression devices, or postoperative anticoagulation with heparin, enoxaparin, warfarin, or other anticoagulants. In some cases, it may be prudent to discontinue medications that have prothrombotic properties, such as estrogen or oral contraceptives that contain estrogen.

A family history of deep venous thrombosis, early stroke, or other events that might suggest the possibility of an inherited hypercoagulability might prompt testing for such issues as factor V Leiden mutation, prothrombin mutation, lupus anticoagulant, and abnormalities of protein S or protein C, among others.

For children, the history should include the birth history, any prenatal or perinatal complications, growth and developmental milestones, immunization status, any history of asthma or seizures, and any recent illness, particularly respiratory infections.

The last menstrual period for women must be noted, as well as methods of birth control, menstrual history, and date of last Papanicolaou test and mammogram. For patients with planned gynecologic surgery, a pregnancy history should be taken, including types of delivery, obstetric anesthesia, and birth outcomes.

A history of nutritional deficiency for adults as well as children may have profound implications for wound healing and postoperative morbidity, and must be mentioned. It should prompt specific recommendations for preoperative nutritional evaluation and possibly the need for preoperative or postoperative nutritional support.

Smoking status must be reviewed and noted. Discontinuation of smoking 6 to 8 weeks before surgery is clearly beneficial in terms of reduced risk of cardiac and respiratory complications, as well as long-term health if the patient does not resume smoking. The longer the period of smoking cessation before surgery, the better. There is debate, however, about the effects of more proximate smoking cessation, especially if the patient discontinues cigarette use only a few days before surgery, which may lead to increased mucus mobilization as well as nicotine withdrawal symptoms. Alcohol consumption and nonmedical drug use or abuse are also important factors that should be considered in order to avoid unexpected withdrawal.

Elements of the patient's history may affect recommendations for antibiotic prophylaxis, including recent prosthetic joint surgery or other implanted devices, the need for endocarditis prophylaxis or the need for prophylaxis for certain surgeries (see Chapter 69, Antibiotic Prophylaxis), or the need for other specific pharmacologic pretreatment such as stress doses of cortisone for dependent patients (e.g., patients with steroid-dependent asthma or Addison disease).

Physical Examination

The physical examination starts with an accurate recording of the patient's vital signs, including temperature, pulse, respiratory rate, and blood pressure. Orthostatic testing should be performed if there is risk or suspicion of hemodynamic compromise. Document height, weight, and body mass index (BMI). Head circumference should be noted for children younger than 2 years. The temptation simply to ask a patient his or her weight must be avoided, and only values and measurements obtained at the time of the consultation should be considered valid. For example, without an accurate weight, a recent rapid gain due to decompensated heart failure might be missed. There are weight limits for certain types of anesthesia (e.g., BMI > 40 or 45 for moderate [conscious] sedation) in certain facilities and risks associated with morbidly obese patients, which is discussed in the "Bariatric Surgery" section.

A full examination is performed with emphasis on the patient's known medical conditions and the type of surgery anticipated, remembering that the patient's care may not be ultimately limited to the procedures, interventions, and types of anesthesia initially planned.

The report of the physical examination should mention pupil equality and reactivity, especially if the patient exhibits anisocoria (unequal pupils) at baseline. The condition of his or her dentition and the presence of braces, dentures, or other removable dental appliances should be noted, as should the absence of teeth, which should be identified by tooth number. The presence of previously uninvestigated carotid bruits or jugular venous distention indicates the need for further workup.

Recalling that the most serious surgical risk is associated with cardiovascular and pulmonary complications, careful attention should be paid to the examination of the heart and lungs, being alert for murmurs, gallops (especially S_3), wheezes, rales, crackles, or other signs of valvular disease, respiratory conditions, or congestive heart failure. The abdominal examination should include palpation for pulsatile abdominal mass that might prompt an assessment for aortic aneurysm, and for renal bruits. The presence of ascites or a previously undocumented enlarged liver or spleen will prompt the need for additional evaluation.

Assessment of extremity function, including motor strength, is important in patients undergoing joint surgery. Evaluation of peripheral vascular competency, including distal pulses and capillary refill, is essential in all patients because peripheral vascular disease is an important predictor of postoperative cardiac complications. Pedal edema, especially of recent onset, may suggest anemia, hypothyroid, or decompensated heart failure.

The neurologic examination should at minimum include a mental status evaluation that will serve as a baseline against which postoperative neurologic compromise will be measured. In some cases, it may also be important in establishing the patient's ability to give informed consent.

As mentioned previously, the preoperative medical evaluation may be the patient's only opportunity for a complete medical assessment, and it may be appropriate to perform other health care maintenance exams, even if they are not directly related to the planned procedure.

LABORATORY AND RADIOGRAPHIC TESTING

Preoperative laboratory testing should be based on the individual patient's underlying conditions, the potential for surgically related problems that relate to laboratory findings, or the potential that baseline or preoperative laboratory results might be helpful, should complications arise perioperatively. Most laboratory and diagnostic tests are unnecessary in healthy patients undergoing low-risk or even some elevated-risk (intermediate) procedures, and in fact may lead to additional unnecessary testing if insignificant abnormalities are identified.

A baseline electrocardiogram (ECG) is not routinely recommended unless an indication is present. A preoperative ECG is reasonable for patients with known cardiovascular disease (coronary heart disease, arrhythmia, peripheral artery disease, cerebrovascular disease) undergoing elevated-risk surgery. For patients with diabetes, hypertension, chest pain, congestive heart failure, smoking, inability to exercise, or morbid obesity, it is also reasonable to get an ECG if there is none on file in the last year for patients undergoing intermediate to high-risk procedures. An ECG is not useful for asymptomatic patients undergoing low-risk surgical procedures. It is also never indicated for cataract surgery, regardless of age.

The patient with chest pain, new symptoms of congestive heart failure, or arrhythmias including ectopic beats should also be considered for noninvasive cardiac testing (e.g., exercise stress ECG testing, nuclear stress testing, stress echocardiography, pharmacologic stress testing, Holter monitoring). An echocardiogram may also be helpful in assessing risk in patients with murmurs, physical findings suggestive of cardiomegaly, or symptoms that indicate decreased ventricular function. Results of recent testing may obviate the need for repeat studies if the patient's symptoms are chronic and unchanged in the past year or two.

The emergence of medications for treatment of erectile dysfunction has improved awareness of this condition as a marker for peripheral vascular disease and possible concomitant coronary artery disease. Patients taking these medications who have not previously been evaluated might benefit from a careful review of cardiac symptoms, and even possibly preoperative noninvasive cardiac testing.

Hemoglobin measurement should not be routinely done. The risk of complications of asymptomatic, normovolemic anemia prior to surgery is unknown, and the optimal hemoglobin level is related more to the patient's baseline and functional capacity than to a specific value. A hemoglobin can be considered in patients with history of anemia, bleeding or other hematologic disorders, hepatic disorders, or those with a planned surgery in which significant blood loss is anticipated. Preoperative supplementation of iron and vitamin C (or when documented deficiency exists, folic acid or vitamin B_{12}) may help optimize hemoglobin levels. The use of erythropoietin should be avoided in the absence of documented deficiency, usually related to renal or neoplastic disease.

Renal function and serum electrolytes are reasonable studies to obtain for patients undergoing increased risk procedures who have significant systemic disease and are on diuretics, angiotensin-converting enzyme inhibitors, or angiotensin II receptor blockers. Those on digoxin should also have a magnesium level drawn. Liver function tests (aspartate and alanine aminotransferases, alkaline phosphatase, serum bilirubin) may be considered in patients with significant liver disease undergoing increased risk surgery. While several meta-analyses did not find the value of preoperative natriuretic peptide testing in general (Rodseth, 2014), other studies found the natriuretic peptide level to be predictive of events in the 30 days following vascular surgery (Rajagopalan, 2008).

Before ordering any of the above tests, be aware that the ASA's Choosing Wisely Campaign recommends against routine preoperative Complete Blood Count, Basic Metabolic Panel, Comprehensive Metabolic Panel, or coagulation studies in patients without significant systemic disease undergoing low-risk surgery when blood loss is expected to be minimal.

A preoperative chest radiograph should not be routinely performed. Consider ordering a chest radiograph if a patient has known cardiopulmonary disease that is unstable, or has signs or symptoms suggestive of new disease.

Assessment of nutritional status can be helpful in planning the need for nutritional support, especially in patients with signs of malnutrition. Measurement of serum albumin below 3.2 g/dL or prealbumin below 15 mg/dL suggests the need for nutritional evaluation and possible supplementation before and after surgery. In some cases, it may be prudent to postpone nonemergent surgery in nutritionally depleted individuals until this issue has been addressed.

Other preoperative laboratory evaluation should be specific to the patient's comorbid conditions or the specific nature and risks of the planned procedure. This may include a pregnancy test for women of childbearing age, or a thyroid stimulation hormone level in a patient with a history of thyroid disease who has not had recent lab testing.

Patients on warfarin therapy will need to have the international normalized ratio (INR) checked before surgery, to ensure a return to normal levels if treatment was stopped, or to ensure therapeutic values if treatment is to continue uninterrupted. In the past, patients at high risk of a cardiovascular event if warfarin therapy was discontinued were given "bridging" therapy with low-molecular-weight heparin or heparin. This is discussed in the "Anticoagulation" section.

Patients With Cardiac and Pulmonary Disease

Patients with a past history of cardiac disease or at high risk of cardiac disease should be evaluated and managed preoperatively (see the "Further Evaluation" section and Fig. 71.1), if stable. Patients with destabilized conditions, such as those with recent myocardial infarction or unstable angina (acute coronary syndrome), significant valvular disease, hemodynamically significant dysrhythmias, or uncompensated heart failure, should be managed according to disease-specific guidelines. Comorbid conditions such as pulmonary disease, diabetes (especially insulin requiring), kidney disease, and uncontrolled hypertension (diastolic blood pressure >100 mm Hg) require careful consideration for preoperative evaluation and management.

Recent coronary stent placement presents specific issues related to the risk of early stent thrombosis. Dual antiplatelet therapy (aspirin plus an adenosine diphosphate receptor inhibitor such as clopidogrel, prasugrel, or ticagrelor) is recommended in patients who have recently received coronary or carotid stents to prevent early stent occlusion until epithelialization has occurred. Decisions regarding the risk of bleeding in a particular procedure weighed against the risk of stent closure must be made when evaluating a patient preoperatively. It is best that the decision to continue or discontinue dual antiplatelet therapy in stented patients be made in partnership with the surgeon, anesthesiologist, cardiologist, and patient.

AHA guidelines from 2014 suggest delaying elective noncardiac surgery for a month in patients with a bare metal stent, and a year for patients with a drug-eluting stent. However, it may be acceptable to perform elective surgery 180 days after a drug-eluting stent if at that point the risk of delaying surgery further is greater than the risk of stent thrombosis. In an update in 2016, there is some evidence that even shorter durations for drug eluting stents may be acceptable. For nonelective, urgent, or emergent surgery at less than 4 to 6 weeks, they recommend continuing dual antiplatelet therapy unless the risk of bleeding is greater than the risk of stent thrombosis. If dual antiplatelet therapy is discontinued, aspirin should be continued if possible, and dual therapy restarted as soon as safely possible.

Patients with known or suspected valvular disease of moderate of higher severity are at a higher cardiac risk. It is reasonable for patients with known or suspected valvular disease (moderate or higher) to undergo echocardiogram prior to surgery if there is no echocardiogram on file for the last year or they have developed worsening symptoms. There is some evidence to suggest that if a patient qualifies for a valve repair surgery due to severity or symptoms prior to an elective, noncardiac surgery, that valve repair/replacement before surgery may reduce their perioperative risk. If

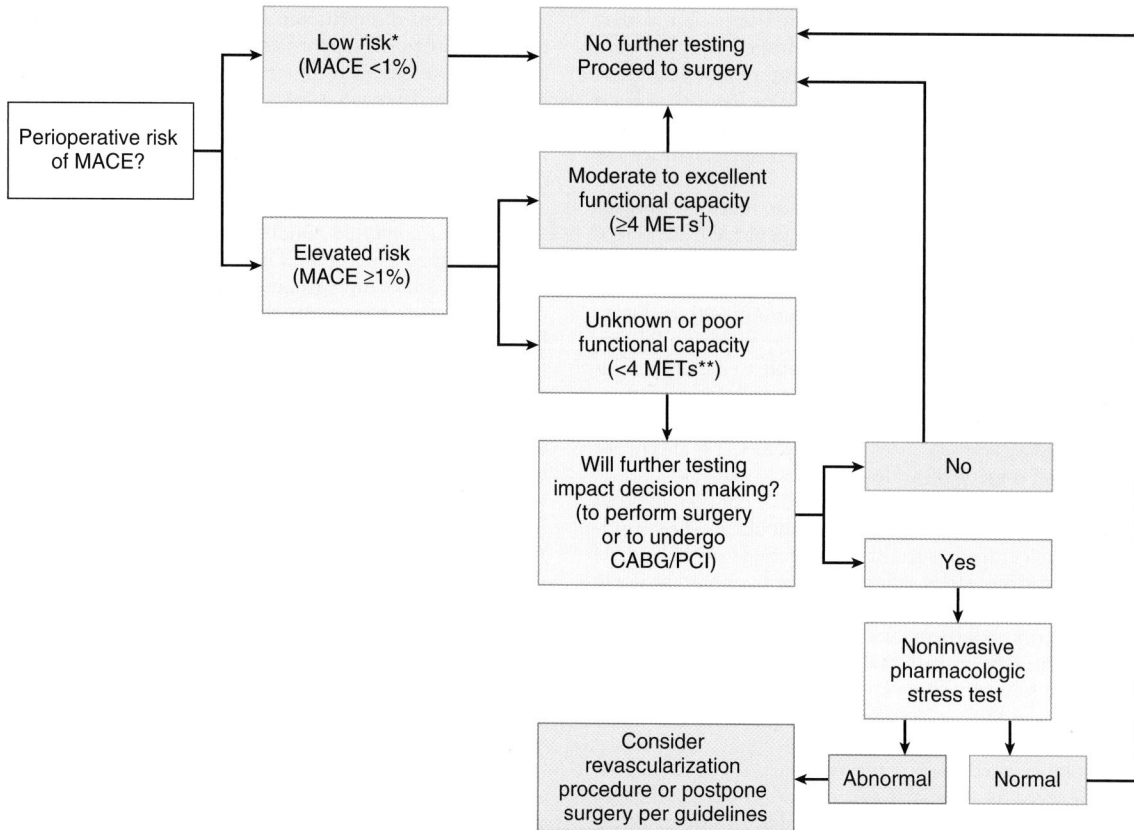

Fig. 71.1   Preoperative assessment for patients with coronary artery disease in the outpatient setting. This tool is used for nonemergent surgery in the clinically stable patient who does not have acute myocardial ischemia. *Some surgeries (e.g., cataract removal, cosmetic surgery) have a low risk of major adverse coronary events even in a high-risk patient and should follow the low-risk algorithm. †Examples of moderate metabolic equivalents (METs) include performing light housework (e.g., cleaning, sweeping, scrubbing floors), climbing a flight of stairs, walking on level ground at 4 mph, running a short distance. Examples of poor functional capacity (1 to 3 METs) include only being able to walk a block or two on level ground at 2 to 3 mph or walking around the house. *CABG,* Coronary artery bypass grafting; *PCI,* percutaneous coronary intervention. (Modified from Fleisher LA, Fleischmann KE, Auerbach AD. 2014 ACC/AHA guideline on perioperative cardiovascular evaluation and management of patients undergoing noncardiac surgery: a report of the American College of Cardiology/American Heart Association Task Force on Practice Guidelines. *Circulation.* 2014;130[24]:278–333.)

valve repair surgery is not done, in patients with severe, asymptomatic aortic or mitral stenosis, it is reasonable to use preoperative and postoperative hemodynamic monitoring. Likewise, it is reasonable to use such monitoring in patients with severe, asymptomatic mitral and aortic regurgitation (if there is a normal ejection fraction).

When considering the value of various cardiac tests as part of a preoperative medical consultation, the clinician must consider the individual patient's risk of progressive disease, as well as the risk of the test itself compared with the risks of the surgery. The concerns of the patient, the anesthesiologist, and the surgeon who will be performing the procedure must be factored into the decision-making process. It is important to maintain an open dialogue with patients, surgeons, and anesthesiologists to achieve trust and confidence among all involved.

Anticoagulation

Long-term anticoagulation with warfarin is common among certain patients with atrial fibrillation, artificial heart valves, or risk factors for thrombotic complications. The safety of discontinuing warfarin before surgery depends on the type of surgery and the underlying condition requiring anticoagulation. In some cases, the patient may require bridging heparin or low-molecular weight heparin therapy while warfarin is discontinued for surgery and until a therapeutic INR is achieved after restarting warfarin. Such patients include those at a high risk of thromboembolism, such as those with older mechanical heart valves or a history of recurrent deep venous thrombosis, especially if associated with

hypercoagulable states. The American Society of Gastrointestinal Endoscopy (ASGE) guidelines recommend bridging when the CHADS2-VASc score is 2 or greater, there is an older mechanical aortic heart valve that is not bileaflet or a mechanical mitral valve, there has been a recent cerebrovascular accident, or there is a thromboembolic risk factor (prior venous thromboembolism while on anticoagulation, recent [last 6 months] transient ischemic attack or cerebrovascular accident). Bridging therapy with low-molecular-weight heparin or heparin may be considered in these patients.

In recent years, more research studies are calling into question the practice of bridging anticoagulation, as there is more evidence of increased bleeding risks without significant reductions in thromboembolic events. Meta-analyses have demonstrated a higher risk of bleeding without differences in thromboembolic events in patients bridged with heparin periprocedurally (Siegal, 2012). A follow-up randomized control trial published in 2015 known as the BRIDGE study (Douketis, 2015) also showed a higher risk of bleeding and no decrease in thromboembolic events when bridging patients with atrial fibrillation (average CHADS2 score of 2.3). Hence the ASGE and the AHA relaxed their guidelines to only bridge those previously discussed. Conversely, the ASGE has also suggested that anticoagulation does not always need to be discontinued if a procedure is at low risk for bleeding (see Chapter 90, Colonoscopy and Chapter 91, Esophagogastroduodenoscopy), which includes many gastrointestinal procedures, including mucosal biopsy. Therefore, the decision about bridging anticoagulation should be made on a case by case basis, depending on the patient and the procedure.

If the decision to bridge warfarin is made, the drug can usually be discontinued 3 days before surgery and restarted at the usual dose on the first postoperative day if the surgeon deems the risk of postoperative bleeding to be low. This would allow the patient's INR to slowly return to normal around the time of surgery, and slowly return to a therapeutic level after surgery without leaving the patient fully untreated for more than 72 hours.

EDITOR'S NOTE: Although no guidelines have been written to support it, certain experts use oral dabigatran (Pradaxa), apixaban (Eliquis), or rivaroxaban (Xarelto) for bridging therapy, and withhold them 2 days prior to major surgery or 1 day for less significant surgery. Since apixaban is taken twice a day due to its shorter half-life, it would seem quicker to reverse by withholding it.

Patients with protein S or C deficiency, factor V Leiden mutation, lupus anticoagulant, or other inherited causes of hypercoagulability may require heparin therapy while warfarin treatment is restarted to avoid thrombosis.

Close communication with the operating clinician, surgeon, or dentist is important to avoid conflicting and confusing instructions to the patient.

Other Medications

β-Blockers should be continued in most patients already taking them, and initiation of such treatment before surgery should be considered in patients with high cardiac risk (ischemia on preoperative testing) who are scheduled for vascular surgery and other procedures that present increased risk of cardiac stress. It may also be reasonable to start perioperative β-blockers in patients with three or more cardiac risk factors (e.g., diabetes, heart failure, renal insufficiency, cerebrovascular accident). β-blockers should not be started the day of surgery. If there would be benefit of initiating them, it is reasonable to start them at least 1 day prior to surgery, which should be long enough to assess safety and tolerability. These patients may be at high risk of perioperative cardiac events, and expert consultation may be of benefit in determining appropriate therapy. AHA guidelines suggest that continuing angiotensin-converting enzyme inhibitors and angiotensin receptor blockers perioperatively is reasonable. If they are stopped, it is reasonable to restart them postoperatively as soon as clinically feasible, especially after euvolemia has been established in order to decrease the risk of perioperative renal dysfunction. Alpha-2 agonists are no longer recommended for prevention of cardiac events in patients undergoing noncardiac surgery.

Statins, widely used for long-term control of serum cholesterol, are also known to have beneficial effects in stabilizing atherosclerotic plaques. They should be continued in patients undergoing noncardiac surgery. Perioperative initiation is reasonable in patients undergoing vascular surgery. Otherwise, initiation of statins should be directed by guidelines.

Pulmonary Disease

Preoperative evaluation of patients with pulmonary disease, including asthma, emphysema, or conditions that may affect oxygen diffusion such as lupus or sarcoidosis, involves assessing their control prior to surgery. Routine spirometry before noncardiothoracic surgery is of minimal benefit, as there is no numerical value at which the risks of surgery are unacceptable (Qaseem, 2006). Spirometry is useful for cardiothoracic surgery and has a role in undiagnosed lung disease prior to surgery. Optimization of therapy with inhaled β-agonists, inhaled steroids, and oral steroids may help reduce postoperative complications such as atelectasis, pneumonia, and exacerbations of obstruction. Intravenous stress doses of steroids (e.g., hydrocortisone sodium succinate [Solu-Cortef] 100 mg) might also be considered in patients who are steroid dependent. This may need to be balanced against considerations of steroid effects on wound healing and fluid balance. A preoperative nebulizer treatment with albuterol or another β-active medication is often helpful. Patients with increased risk of postoperative atelectasis, including those with planned thoracic or abdominal surgery, may also benefit from preoperative lessons on the use of an incentive spirometer.

Sleep apnea, most common in adult men, should be noted in previously diagnosed individuals and considered in patients with typical body habitus (obese, short neck) and history of snoring, fatigue, and observed apneic episodes while sleeping. Sleep studies may be appropriate, and the use of postoperative continuous positive airway pressure might be considered.

According to AHA guidelines, it is reasonable to continue phosphodiesterase type 5 inhibitors, soluble guanylate cyclase stimulators, endothelin receptor antagonists, and prostanoids in patients with pulmonary hypertension unless contraindicated or not tolerated. If time allows, it is also reasonable to consult a pulmonary hypertension specialist prior to surgery.

PATIENTS WITH DIABETES

Control of blood glucose levels as well as recognition of conditions that are frequently associated with diabetes are important concerns in the preoperative evaluation of diabetic patients. If sufficient time is available before surgery, an attempt should be made to bring the patient under good glycemic control through adjustment in their usual oral medications or insulin dosages, or initiation of insulin therapy if necessary. Attempting to maintain normal blood sugars postoperatively, especially after major surgeries, has been proven beneficial for diabetic patients. In addition, undiagnosed patients at risk for metabolic disease, including diabetes, would benefit from screening before surgery.

The stress response to surgery can result in hyperglycemia, and this should be considered in the planning of diabetic therapy. Patients who require insulin prior to surgery will still require insulin even if they are NPO for a procedure, though doses may need to be adjusted. For example, in a type 1 diabetic, holding basal insulin and only covering hyperglycemia with short-acting sliding-scale insulin for a procedure may precipitate diabetic ketoacidosis.

Non-insulin-requiring patients with diabetes who are undergoing a planned minor surgical procedure and expected to resume a normal diet soon after surgery should continue their oral medications up until the morning of surgery. Holding oral diabetic medications the morning of the surgery can decrease complications such as hypoglycemia from sulfonylureas or kidney injury due to metformin. Oral regimens may be resumed when the patient returns to a normal diet.

When deciding what to do in patients with diabetes who require insulin, the decision to adjust their insulin will depend on a number of factors. Patients taking a long-acting insulin (e.g., glargine [Lantus, Toujeo], detemir [Levemir], degludec [Tresiba]) may be instructed to take a reduced dose of their evening or morning insulin before surgery. In general, it is recommended to decrease the basal insulin dose by 20% to 25% the night before and/or the morning of surgery (depending on when the patient routinely injects their basal insulin). For a type 1 diabetic, it is recommended they receive 80% of their usual basal insulin requirements the night before and/or the morning of surgery. For type 2 diabetic patients on intermediate acting insulin (NPH) or premixed preparations (70/30), insulin doses should be decreased by 20% the night before surgery and 50% the morning of surgery. It is also recommended to hold the morning dose of NPH or premixed insulin in type 2 diabetic patients with a fasting blood sugar less than 120 mg/dL. In general, it is wise to hold any regularly scheduled short-acting insulin the morning of surgery while a patient is NPO (Duggan, 2017).

Longer procedures that entail more extensive periods of NPO status require a more detailed approach to preoperative glycemic control. Type 1 and some type 2 insulin-requiring diabetic patients may require continuous insulin infusion preoperatively, along with a separate intravenous glucose infusion. The use of subcutaneous doses of short-acting insulin may yield unpredictable responses in patients with altered peripheral perfusion, and these patients may also benefit from continuous intravenous insulin infusion that can be monitored and adjusted with greater accuracy. Careful attention to fluid balance and serum electrolytes, especially potassium, is also critical to avoiding complications.

Patients with diabetes are at risk for silent ischemia as well as ventricular dysfunction, and may benefit from preoperative cardiac evaluation if not recently performed. Renal status should also be confirmed, understanding that a normal preoperative serum creatinine level, although somewhat comforting, may not reflect the patient's reserve capacity and response to surgical stress.

Communication with the surgeon, anesthesia team, and postoperative nursing staff is important in the management of diabetic patients, and may best be done directly rather than through written means if concerns about the patient's perioperative management exist. The trend toward ambulatory surgery and early discharge also requires careful instructions to the patient about postoperative management and may warrant specific preadmission teaching.

PATIENTS WITH LIVER OR KIDNEY DISEASE

Liver Disease

The presence of known liver disease, including cirrhosis, hepatitis, or obstructive biliary disease, may predispose patients to nutritional deficiency as well as coagulation disorders. Preoperative evaluation should include studies to identify such disorders, including serum albumin or prealbumin, clotting time, prothrombin time (INR), and CBC to assess hemoglobin and platelets. Even though an elevated INR in a cirrhotic patient may not accurately reflect their bleeding risk (in fact, they may be more prothrombotic at an elevated INR due to procoagulant and anticoagulant imbalance), there are no better laboratory tests at this time to determine their status. Thus some patients may require perioperative administration of fresh frozen plasma or other blood products, supplementation of vitamin K to correct elevated INR, or specific clotting factors. Platelet infusions have a very brief benefit and should be used only if counts are critically low. Most patients with platelet counts above 50,000 do not exhibit abnormal bleeding on the basis of thrombocytopenia and can undergo procedures. Some procedures in smaller spaces such as eye surgery or neurologic surgery may require platelet levels greater than 100,000.

Antibiotics that are cleared through the liver should be avoided or dosages adjusted appropriately, and sedatives with hepatic metabolism must be used with caution. Amide anesthetics (e.g., lidocaine, bupivacaine, mepivacaine) commonly used for local and regional anesthesia are cleared through the liver and must be used with caution in patients with known liver disease, as well as elderly patients whose hepatic function may be naturally reduced.

Kidney Disease

Patients with kidney disease may have stable mild chronic renal insufficiency, which, if their reserve is minimal, may progress to acute renal failure perioperatively. Others may already be on dialysis; a third category is those somewhere between these two extremes.

Chronic renal disease predisposes patients to anemia, platelet dysfunction, metabolic acidosis, hyperkalemia, and uremia. They also have higher incidences of peripheral vascular disease, coronary artery disease, and ischemic cerebrovascular disease. Preoperative evaluation therefore must identify individuals at risk of electrolyte imbalance and fluid status abnormalities and increased risk of worsening renal impairment, as well as of cardiac and respiratory disease.

Preoperative testing should include measurement of serum electrolytes, bicarbonate, creatinine, blood urea nitrogen, calcium, CBC with platelet count, coagulation studies (prothrombin time/INR, bleeding time), urinalysis, and arterial blood gas if bicarbonate is decreased (<16 to 18 mEq/L). Unless the patient is undergoing dialysis, results of recent measurement of renal function, including creatinine clearance, should be reviewed. An ECG and chest radiograph should be reviewed for evidence of worsening cardiac disease or fluid overload and repeated if not recent.

Timing of dialysis in enrolled patients should be discussed with the nephrology or dialysis team, and is usually performed on the day before surgery to optimize fluid status and reduce uremic bleeding complications. Serum potassium levels should be checked within 3 to 6 hours before surgery and corrected to less than 5 to 5.5 mEq/L using bicarbonate/dextrose/insulin infusion, unless the patient has responded well to previous use of binding resins. Anemia as low as 7 to 8 g/dL hemoglobin may be well tolerated in patients with chronic renal failure; however, if functional capacity, coronary ischemia, respiratory compromise, or likelihood of significant surgical blood loss are a concern, the patient may benefit from judicious transfusion of packed red cells. If time permits, erythropoietin therapy may be considered.

BARIATRIC SURGERY

The growth of the availability and variety of surgical procedures aimed at treating obesity has offered hope for many patients who have struggled with weight loss. In many cases, these procedures offer life-changing remedies, and the results of surgery are often encouraging to patients, their families, and their clinicians. As this field grows, more research is needed to understand the perioperative risks.

Primary care clinicians are increasingly being asked to provide "clearance" for their patients. The American Society of Metabolic and Bariatric Surgery has a recommended standard preoperative checklist. While many bariatric surgeons will refer patients for subspecialty consultations in cardiology, pulmonary, endocrinology, gastroenterology, psychiatry, as well as for dietary and nutritional counseling, to meet many of the items on the checklist, there is still a role for the primary care clinician. In particular, screening for obesity-related comorbidities, documenting the patient's weight loss history, as well as smoking cessation counseling, ongoing nutrition and weight loss counseling, pregnancy counseling, and appropriate cancer screening should all be done prior to bariatric surgery. Primary care has a central role in all of these matters. Providing surgical clearance, however, can be perceived by some clinicians as medicolegal defensiveness on the part of the surgeon, especially in the setting of many other specialists' consultations. As such, many primary care clinicians may choose to withhold an opinion as to the fitness of their patients for bariatric surgery. Instead, they limit their consultative reports to an accounting of the patient's medical history, including that of their obesity and attempts at weight loss, offering help with smoking cessation, and ensuring patients are up to date on cancer screening. They then leave recommendations about preoperative optimization to the other specialists involved.

It should be noted that due to an increased risk of sleep apnea, possibly an increased risk of difficult airway and aspiration, and due to weight limitations for the equipment, many surgery centers have set a BMI limit less than 40 or 45 for moderate sedation.

PREGNANT PATIENTS

Nonobstetric surgery may be required during the course of nearly 2% of otherwise normal pregnancies. Appendectomy, cholecystectomy, orthopedic procedures after trauma, or other emergent procedures must not be delayed because of concurrent pregnancy. Surgery that is nonobstetric but related to pregnancy, such as urologic interventions or ovarian surgery, may also be required. In these cases, the axiom that a pregnant patient is treated in the same fashion as a nonpregnant patient applies. The safety and well-being of the fetus depend in the greatest degree on the health of the mother.

When possible, elective surgical procedures should be performed during the second trimester, when organogenesis is less affected and the risk of preterm labor is decreased. Advanced pregnancy may affect diaphragmatic excursion and predispose the patient to atelectasis and postoperative risk of pneumonia. Medication selection should avoid drugs with known fetal adversities, such as tetracycline in early pregnancy or NSAIDs near term.

Preoperative medical evaluation of the pregnant patient centers on the same considerations of operative and anesthesia risk, patient risk factors, and the need for perioperative care as with a nonpregnant patient.

CALCULATION OF RISK

Current AHA guidelines give three options for the calculation of risk: the Revised Cardiac Risk Index (RCRI), the American College of Surgeons National Surgical Quality Improvement Program (NSQIP) Risk Calculator (www.riskcalculator.facs.org), or the American College of Surgeons NSQIP Myocardial Infarction and Cardiac Arrest (www.surgicalriskcalculator.com/miorcardiacarrest).

The RCRI is an older, simple, well-validated, and accepted tool that has six predictors of risk for major cardiac complications, such as myocardial infarction, pulmonary edema, primary cardiac arrest, complete heart block, or ventricular fibrillation. The six risk factors are a creatinine level of 2.0 mg/dL or greater, heart failure, insulin-dependent diabetes, suprainguinal vascular surgery, intrathoracic surgery or intraabdominal surgery, history of stroke or TIA, and ischemic heart disease. A patient with 0 or 1 of these risk factors would be considered low risk (<1%) for these cardiac complications; 2 or greater risk factors places the patient at increased risk (≥1%).

The other two options are newer risk predictors created by the American College of Surgeons based on prospectively collected data from more than 1 million surgeries performed in more than 525 hospitals in the United States. The NSQIP Myocardial Infarction and Cardiac Arrest takes into consideration the type of surgery to be performed, using inguinal hernia as the index, and predicts risk of cardiac arrest or MI. Although the data is from one large multicenter study, it was found to be slightly more accurate than RCRI for predicting risk, especially in patients about to undergo vascular surgery. The NSQIP calculator uses the current procedural terminology code to produce a procedurally specific risk assessment. The calculator also uses 21 patient-specific factors, such as age, sex, BMI, previous MI, dyspnea, and functional status, for a patient-specific calculation. The final product is risk of major adverse cardiovascular event, death, and eight other adverse events. One limitation to the calculator is that it has not been validated in a population outside the NSQIP population. Another is the fact that it also uses the ASA classification system (see Table 71.1) for patients, which has poor interrater reliability, even among anesthesiologists. It may also be unfamiliar to clinicians other than anesthesiologists.

Further Evaluation

If the patient is calculated to be in the low-risk (<1%) category, surgery should proceed. If a patient has an elevated risk for a major adverse cardiac event based on their calculated risk (≥1%), further evaluation is deemed appropriate. The next step is to assess functional cardiac capacity based on questions of tolerance of physical activity. The inability of the adult patient to perform activity equaling at least four metabolic equivalents (METs) or unknown functional status (exercise capacity) usually suggests the need for additional preoperative cardiac evaluation. Examples of activities that correspond to four METs or more include playing doubles tennis, climbing a flight of stairs, walking on level ground at 4 miles per hour, running a short distance, or doing moderately heavy gardening or housework such as pushing a mower, raking leaves, sweeping and scrubbing floors, or moving furniture without symptoms. For those with moderate/good (≥4 to 10) to excellent (>10) METs, no further testing is necessary and the surgery can proceed. For patients with poor METs (<4) or unknown functional exercise capacity, if further testing will impact management decisions or

perioperative care, noninvasive testing pharmacologic stress testing is reasonable.

Individuals with moderate symptoms of heart failure or mild valve disease should be considered for preoperative cardiac testing, especially if the planned procedure is high risk, because perioperative stresses may unmask or exacerbate previously controlled or compensated disease. Guidelines specific to these diseases should be followed. Patients whose history and clinical presentation suggest the need for a cardiac evaluation independent of the planned surgery should have such an evaluation regardless of their risk factors or the calculated risk of the specific procedure.

To be more specific regarding the patient with known or risk factors for coronary artery disease, if the procedure is emergent, clinical risk stratification should be performed, and medical management maximized to deal with risk as the surgery is performed. In the presence of acute coronary syndrome, appropriate guidelines should be followed. Otherwise, the risk of the specific surgical procedure should be calculated using one of the three techniques previously described. See Fig. 71.1 for a stepwise guide or algorithm to the preoperative cardiac evaluation.

COMMUNICATING RECOMMENDATIONS

The results and report of the preoperative consultation should be forwarded to the requesting surgeon (or dentist, clinician) promptly. Inpatient consultations will be posted to the patient's chart and reviewed by the surgeon and anesthesia team. Although local protocols may request that reports of outpatient medical evaluations be sent directly to the hospital or ambulatory surgical center, it is the responsibility of the consultant (the primary care provider in this case) to ensure that findings and recommendations are in fact received by the surgeon. For this reason, many clinicians forward the preoperative evaluation to the surgeon and directly communicate the need for him or her to provide the results to the hospital or other surgical facility. The establishment of good communication and relationships helps guarantee effective information sharing for the benefit of the patient.

Many formats, forms, and designs for both printed and electronic transmittal of preoperative medical evaluations are available, but the standard dictated letter that includes the patient history, physical examination, laboratory, and diagnostic findings and recommendations may be most useful and, as previously noted, may constitute the only comprehensive document containing this information in the patient's chart. It should include a statement of the patient's condition relative to his or her fitness for the planned procedure, indicating that no current medical contraindications exist, or, if they do exist, what specific steps need to be taken to reduce the risks compared with the urgency of the surgery. The patient's estimated risk should be included.

CPT/BILLING CODES

99241–99245	Office consultations
99251–99255	Inpatient consultations

NOTE: Determining the level of complexity for consultations is similar to determining use for other office- and hospital-based evaluation and management (E&M) services.

ICD-10 DIAGNOSTIC CODES

Z01.810	Encounter for preprocedural cardiovascular examination
Z01.811	Encounter for preprocedural respiratory examination
Z01.812	Encounter for preprocedural laboratory examination
Z01.818	Encounter for other preprocedural examination

ONLINE RESOURCES

CHADS2-VASc Calculators

https://www.mdcalc.com/chads2-score-atrial-fibrillation-stroke-risk.
https://www.chadsvasc.org.

Apps

CHADS2-VASc calculator: Cardio Calculator by Blue Maple Technologies
Preoperative app: Pre-Op Eval by Joshua Steinberg

RECOMMENDED READING

ACC/AHA Guideline on Perioperative Cardiovascular Evaluation and Management of Patients Undergoing Noncardiac Surgery. *Circulation.* 2014;130:278–333.

American Society for Gastrointestinal Endoscopy (ASGE). Standards of Practice Committee: guideline on the management of antithrombotic agents for patients undergoing GI endoscopy. *Gastrointest Endosc.* 2016;83(1):3–16.

Abbas N, Makker J, Abbas H, Balar B. Perioperative care of patients with liver cirrhosis: a review. *Health Services Insights.* 2017;10.

Crossley GH, Poole JE, Rozner MA, et al. The Heart Rhythm Society (HRS)/American Society of Anesthesiologists (ASA) expert consensus statement on the perioperative management of patients with implantable defibrillators, pacemakers and arrhythmia monitors: facilities and patient management. *Heart Rhythm.* 2011;8:1114–1154.

Douketis JD, Spyropoulos AC, Spencer FA, et al. Perioperative management of antithrombotic therapy: antithrombotic therapy and prevention of thrombosis, 9th ed: American College of Chest Physicians Evidence-Based Clinical Practice Guidelines. *Chest.* 2012;141(suppl 2):e326S–e350S.

Douketis JD, Spyropoulos AC, Katz S, the BRIDGE study group, et al. Perioperative bridging anticoagulation in atrial fibrillation. *N Engl J Med.* 2015;373:823–833.

Duggan EW, Carlson K, Umpierrez GE. Perioperative hyperglycemia management: an update. *Anesthesiology.* 2017;126(3):547–560.

Feely M, Collins CS, et al. Preoperative testing before noncardiac surgery: guidelines and recommendations. *Am Fam Physician.* 2013;87(6):414–418.

Institute for Clinical Systems Improvement (ICSI). *Preoperative evaluation.* 5th ed. Bloomington, MN: ISCI; 2014.

Petty B, Tice J. *Society of General Internal Medicine Choosing Wisely: 5 Things Physicians and Patients Should Question;* April 2016. https://www.sgim.org/File%20Library/JGIM/Web%20Only/Choosing%20Wisely/Pre-Operative-testing.pdf.

Practice Guidelines for Moderate Procedural Sedation and Analgesia 2018. A Report by the American Society of Anesthesiologists Task Force on Moderate Procedural Sedation and Analgesia, the American Association of Oral and Maxillofacial Surgeons, American College of Radiology, American Dental Association, American Society of Dentist Anesthesiologists, and Society of Interventional Radiology. *Anesthesiology.* 2018;128:437–479.

Qaseem A, Snow V, Fitterman N, et al. Risk assessment for and strategies to reduce perioperative pulmonary complications for patients undergoing noncardiothoracic surgery: a guideline from the American College of Physicians. *Ann Intern Med.* 2006;144(8):575–580.

Rajagopalan S, Croal BL, Bachoo P, et al. N-terminal pro B-type natriuretic peptide is an independent predictor of postoperative myocardial injury in patients undergoing major vascular surgery. *J Vasc Surg.* 48:912–917 2008.

Rodseth RN, Biccard BM, Le MY, et al. The prognostic value of preoperative and post-operative B-type natriuretic peptides in patients undergoing noncardiac surgery: B-type natriuretic peptide and N-terminal fragment of pro-B-type natriuretic peptide: a systematic review and individual patient data meta-analysis. *J Am Coll Cardiol.* 63:170–180 2014.

Siegal D, Yudin J, Kaatz S, Douketis JD, Lim W, Spyropoulos AC. Periprocedural heparin bridging in patients receiving vitamin K antagonists: systematic review and meta-analysis of bleeding and thromboembolic rates. *Circulation.* 2012;126:1630–1639.

Wani S, Azar R, Hovis CE, et al. Obesity as a risk factor for sedation-related complications during propofol-mediated sedation for advanced endoscopic procedures. *Gastrointest Endosc.* 2011;74(6):1238–1247.

Wolk MJ, Bailey SR, Doherty JU, et al. American College of Cardiology Foundation Appropriate Use Criteria Task Force. ACCF/AHA/ASE/ASNC/HFSA/HRS/SCAI/SCCT/SCMR/STS 2013 multimodality appropriate use criteria for the detection and risk assessment of stable ischemic heart disease. *J Am Coll Cardiol.* 2014;63(4):380–406.

CHAPTER 72

AMBULATORY BLOOD PRESSURE MONITORING

Russell D. White • Thomas H. Mitchell

Ambulatory blood pressure monitoring (ABPM) is an automated, noninvasive technique for obtaining blood pressure measurements at predetermined intervals over an extended period of time (usually 24 hours or more) while the patient goes about his or her daily activities. The process involves attaching a measuring and recording device to the patient. These devices are lightweight and use either the auscultatory (i.e., microphone and Korotkoff sounds) or the oscillometric method (i.e., senses arterial waves) to determine blood pressure. Although the auscultatory method needs low ambient noise levels to obtain its most accurate results, it tolerates patient movement better than the oscillometric method. While the oscillometric method tolerates high levels of environmental noise, it is most accurate when the patient is less physically active. These days, the majority of equipment uses the oscillometric method. Regardless of technique, the recordings are downloaded for analysis.

Hypertension was redefined in 2014 by the 8th Joint National Committee (JNC8, James, et al) as an office systolic blood pressure of 140 to 150 mm Hg or higher, or diastolic blood pressure of 90 mm Hg or higher; However, the American College of Cardiology (ACC) and the American Heart Association (AHA), collaborating with 13 other groups, defined hypertension in 2017 as an office systolic blood pressure of 130 mm Hg or higher or a diastolic blood pressure of 80 mm Hg or higher. Elevated systolic blood pressure is frequently isolated (i.e., elevated in the absence of elevated diastolic blood pressure), especially in the elderly. More than 100 million Americans are now considered hypertensive, a major risk factor for such common diseases as cardiovascular disease, stroke, aortic aneurysm rupture, renal failure, and retinopathy. Because some patients are hypertensive only during specific hours of the day, documentation of adequate blood pressure control over 24 hours is imperative to prevent sequelae. Studies have shown that hypertension diagnosed with ABPM more often correlates with target organ damage than hypertension noted on sporadic blood pressure measurements in the office setting (especially in patients with albuminuria or echocardiographically determined left ventricular hypertrophy). Patients whose average pressures by 24-hour ABPM are greater than 135/85 mm Hg have twice the risk for a cardiovascular event compared with those with 24-hour mean blood pressures less than 135/85 mm Hg, regardless of the blood pressures measured in the office. In most people, blood pressure decreases by 10% to 20% at night; those without such a reduction (i.e., nondippers) are at increased risk of cardiovascular events. Conversely, overtreatment of hypertension can lead to complications such as transient hypotension, dizziness, myocardial ischemia and falls. In addition, as many as 21% of patients with mild blood pressure elevation in the office are incorrectly diagnosed with and treated for hypertension. Likewise, although having the patient monitor his or her blood pressure at home (i.e., self-monitored blood pressure) can improve blood pressure control, there have been few studies in the United States that correlate such a practice with fewer cardiovascular events. However, both the JNC8 and 2017 ACC/AHA hypertension guidelines recommend increased use of home blood pressure monitoring. In addition, the ACC/AHA guidelines agree with the United States Preventive Services Task Force (USPSTF) in that ABPM is the best method for diagnosing hypertension; it is now considered the reference standard.

INDICATIONS

Routine, properly obtained, sporadic blood pressure measurements in the office setting remain the recommended method to screen for and monitor hypertension. While ABPM should not be used indiscriminately as a screening device, blood pressure measurements in the office can lead to both false-positive and false-negative results, Fig. 72.1 provides a helpful algorithm. Indications may include the following:

- Normal or borderline office hypertension with target organ damage (e.g., left ventricular hypertrophy, heart failure, angina or prior myocardial infarction, prior coronary revascularization, stroke or transient ischemic attack, dementia, chronic kidney disease [glomerular filtration rate <60 mL/min], peripheral arterial disease, retinopathy) or increased overall risk of cardiovascular disease (CVD)
- Persistent office hypertension without target organ damage
- Discrepancy between office and home blood pressure measurements (especially in diabetic and elderly patients)
- Considerable blood pressure variability found during same office visit or over different visits
- Episodic hypertension (e.g., smoking raises blood pressure acutely, and the level returns to baseline about 15 minutes after stopping)
- Episodic angina or pulmonary congestion unrelated to exercise
- Determination of the duration or efficacy of antihypertensive medications during the 24-hour treatment cycle
- Dosage adjustment of antihypertensive medications
- Documented hypertension unresponsive to treatment ("drug resistance")
- Suspected pressor ("white coat") hypertension and no target organ damage
- Office blood pressure elevated during pregnancy and preeclampsia suspected
- Autonomic dysfunction
- Hypotensive symptoms while on antihypertensive medication
- Evaluation of syncope or pacemaker syndromes

CONTRAINDICATIONS AND LIMITATIONS

- Cost: Although covered by Medicare, some insurance companies may not reimburse for ABPM
- Irregular, rapid heart rate: limits ability to obtain blood pressure measurements and limits the accuracy of ABPM
- Severe obesity: limits ability to obtain blood pressure measurements and limits the accuracy of ABPM

Ambulatory blood pressure monitoring

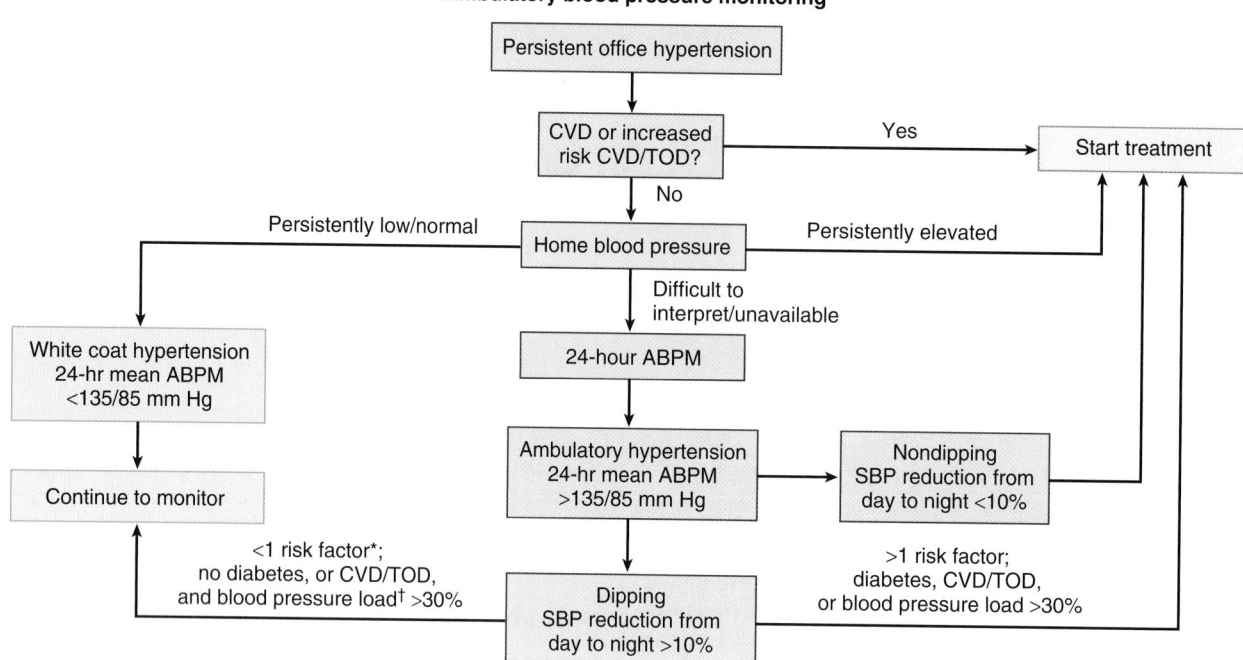

Fig. 72.1   Algorithm for appropriate use of ambulatory blood pressure monitoring (ABPM). *CVD,* cardiovascular disease; *SBP,* systolic blood pressure; *TOD,* target organ damage. *Major cardiovascular risk factors in patients with hypertension include smoking, dyslipidemia, diabetes, age older than 60 years, gender (men and postmenopausal women), family history of early cardiovascular disease chronic kidney disease, physically inactive. †The proportion of blood pressures during the monitoring period that are increased relative to preset thresholds (140/90 mm Hg awake, 120/80 mm Hg asleep). (Modified and updated from Ernst ME, Bergus GR. Ambulatory blood pressure monitoring: technology with a purpose [editorial]. *Am Fam Physician.* 2003;67:2262–2263.)

- Severe patient anxiety regarding instrument

PREPROCEDURE PATIENT PREPARATION

The procedure should be explained to the patient as well as its risks, benefits, and any alternatives. Obtain either verbal or written consent. Patients should be instructed to record any symptoms or events that occur during the monitoring period and any medications they are taking (and when they take them). In most cases, they should be instructed not to speak or move during cuff deflation (recording phase). Patients should also usually avoid strenuous activity (e.g., running or racquet sports) during the study. They should know how long they will be monitored, where to go to have the equipment removed, and when they might expect the results. If not contraindicated, the clinician may choose to offer the patient a sleep medication to minimize the equipment's interference with sleep.

EQUIPMENT

- Monitor (with instructions) for ABPM
- Automatic blood pressure cuff and sphygmomanometer
- Connectors and tubing
- 24-hour diary for events, activities, and medications

TECHNIQUE

1. The clinician should follow the manufacturer's instructions for attaching the equipment and performing the procedure. However, this usually means placing the microphone/sensor over the brachial artery proximal to the elbow of the *nondominant* arm (Fig. 72.2). *Proper positioning of the microphone/sensor is critical.*
2. Select the appropriate cuff size. The bladder inside the cuff should encircle 80% of the upper arm circumference without overlap.
3. Attach and secure the automatic cuff to the upper arm. To prevent shifting of the cuff on the arm, an adhesive-backed strap is usually

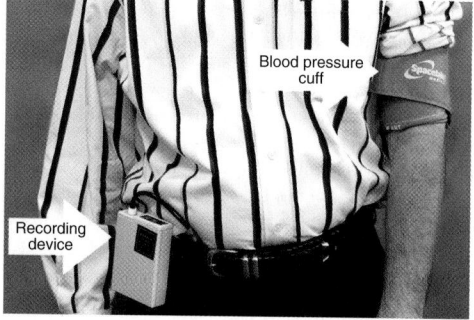

Fig. 72.2   Placement of ambulatory blood pressure monitoring unit.

placed on the arm. The cuff is then placed around the arm and secured to the adhesive-backed strap, often by snapping it in place.
4. Connect the cuff–microphone/sensing unit to the monitor.
5. The connecting tubing is passed under upper body clothing to the monitor worn on the waist in a carrying pouch.
6. Calibrate the monitor for each patient in the lying, sitting, and standing positions. Measure blood pressure simultaneously with a manual cuff and sphygmomanometer or sphygmomanometer attached to the monitor through a T-tube device. (Three consecutive measurements should be within 3 to 5 mm Hg of one another.)
7. Secure the hose and microphone/sensor cable in a manner that will minimize patient discomfort.
8. Set the frequency of recordings (typically three to four times per hour during waking hours and one to two times per hour during sleeping hours).
9. Instruct the patient to record any symptoms or events, his or her activities, and which medications were taken and when they were taken during the monitoring period.
10. Instruct the patient to not speak or move during cuff deflation (i.e., recording phase).

TABLE 72.1	Average Normal Ambulatory Blood Pressure Monitoring Values		
Blood Pressure (mm Hg)	**Day**	**Night**	**24-Hr**
Average	123/76	106/64	118/72
Systolic range	101–146	86–127	97–139
Diastolic range	61–91	48–79	57–87

From Staessen JA, Fagard RH, Lijnen PJ, et al. Mean and range of the ambulatory pressure in normotensive subjects from a meta-analysis of 23 studies. *Am J Cardiol.* 1991;67:723–727.

11. Instruct the patient to avoid strenuous activity (e.g., running or racquet sports) during the study.
12. Remove the monitoring and recording device at the end of the study period, and retrieve the recorded data.

COMPLICATIONS

- Inaccurate or incomplete results
- Interference with normal sleep patterns
- Inconvenience related to device
- Petechiae at measurement site
- Arm edema distal to cuff
- Transient arm discomfort
- Dermatitis
- Ulnar nerve palsy (rare)

INTERPRETATION OF RESULTS

Information acquired from ABPM normally includes (1) average blood pressures (usually average systolic, diastolic, and mean blood pressures); (2) diurnal fluctuations in blood pressure; and (3) short-term variability of blood pressure.

Most normotensive individuals exhibit a circadian pattern of blood pressure, reaching a peak during the daytime hours and a nadir after midnight (however, shift workers may reverse this pattern). Hypertensive patients also usually follow this diurnal pattern, with (as mentioned previously) an average blood pressure greater than 135/85 mm Hg when awake and greater than 120/75 mm Hg during sleep. Blood pressure usually increases after awakening and with increased activity in the early morning. Staessen and colleagues (1991) reviewed several studies and summarized average diurnal blood pressures (Table 72.1). Combining these data with subsequent meta-analyses (Table 72.2), the following diagnostic criteria are suggested:

- *Hypertension* is diagnosed if more than 30% of the 24-hour systolic readings are greater than 140 mm Hg, or greater than 90 mm Hg for diastolic readings (Fig. 72.3). This is an abnormal blood pressure load (percentage of elevated systolic and diastolic pressures during a 24-hour period). In patients with diabetes or target organ damage, hypertension should be diagnosed if more than 30% of the 24-hour systolic readings are greater than 130 mm Hg, or greater than 80 mm Hg for diastolic readings.
- Average systolic arterial pressure greater than 125-130 mm Hg or average diastolic pressure greater than 75-80 mm Hg is considered hypertension. Also, daytime average systolic pressure greater than 130-135 mm Hg or daytime average diastolic pressure greater than 80-85 mm Hg, or nighttime average systolic pressure greater than 110-120 mm Hg or nighttime average diastolic pressure greater than 65-70 mm Hg is considered hypertension (2017 ACC/ AHA and 2018 European Society for Hypertension–European Society for Cardiology guidelines).
- A *nondipper* is diagnosed if the patient's blood pressure does not decrease by at least 10% at night. If the patient is being treated for hypertension, medications may need to be given at bedtime or a medication with a longer half-life chosen.

TABLE 72.2	Definitions of Hypertension According to Office, Ambulatory, and Home Blood Pressure (BP) Levels (mm Hg)		
	SBP		**DBP**
Office BP[a]	≥140	and/or	≥90
Ambulatory BP (mean)			
Daytime (or awake)	≥135	and/or	≥85
Nighttime (or asleep)	≥120	and/or	≥70
24 h	≥130	and/or	≥80
Home	≥135	and/or	≥85

DBP, Diastolic blood pressure; *SBP,* systolic blood pressure.
[a]Conventional office BP rather than unattended office BP.
Data from Whelton PK, Carey RM, Aronow WS, et al. ACC/AHA/AAPA/ABC/ACPM/AGS/APhA/ASH/ASPC/NMA/PCNA guideline for the prevention, detection, evaluation, and management of high blood pressure in adults: a report of the American College of Cardiology/American Heart Association Task Force on Clinical Practice Guidelines. *J Am Coll Cardiol.* 2018;71:e127–e248; and Williams B, Mancia G, Spiering W, et al. 2018 ESC/ESH guidelines for the management of arterial hypertension. *Eur Heart J.* 2018;39:3021–3104.

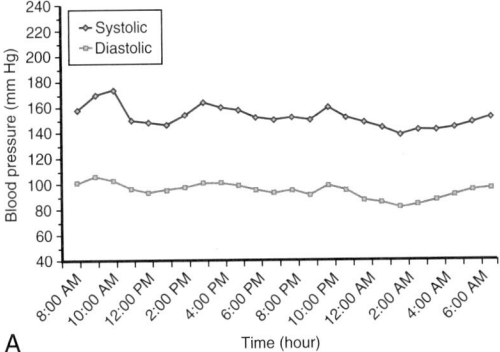

A

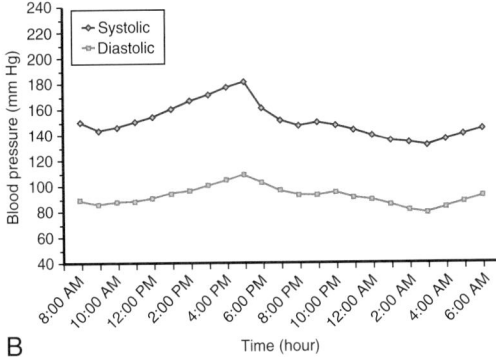

B

Fig. 72.3 Examples of 24-hour ambulatory blood pressure monitoring recordings in hypertensive patients. (A) The first patient is newly diagnosed and needs to be treated. (B) Report for a different patient on a low-dose antihypertensive medication; the dose needs to be increased. If the patient has symptoms, it is unlikely to be due to the medication.

- Finally, patients whose blood pressure recordings vary widely during 24-hour ABPM may require medication changes to provide control during the entire 24 hours.

CPT/BILLING CODES

93784 Ambulatory blood pressure monitoring, utilizing a system such as magnetic tape and/or computer disk, for 24 hours or longer, including recording, scanning analysis, interpretation, and report
93786 Recording only
93788 Scanning analysis with report
93790 Physician review with interpretation and report

ICD-10-CM Diagnostic Codes
Hypertension

I10	Hypertension, essential
I11.0	Hypertensive heart disease with heart failure
I11.9	Hypertensive heart disease without heart failure
I12.0	Hypertensive chronic kidney disease with stage 5 end-stage renal disease
I12.9	Hypertensive chronic kidney disease with stage 1 to 4
I13.0	Hypertensive heart and chronic kidney disease with heart failure stage 1 to 4
I13.10	Hypertensive heart and chronic kidney disease without heart failure stage 1 to 4
I13.11	Hypertensive heart and chronic kidney disease without heart failure stage 5
I15.9	Secondary hypertension unspecified
I15.0	Benign, renovascular
R03.0	Elevated blood pressure reading without diagnosis (incidental without diagnosis)

Hypotension

I95.1	Orthostatic or postural
I95.0	Chronic hypotension, permanent, idiopathic
I95.81	Iatrogenic, abnormally low blood pressure post procedural
I95.89	Other specified hypotension
I95.9	Hypotension, unspecified

Syncope

R55	Syncope, cardiac, vasovagal, fainting, pre- or near-syncope
G90.09	Carotid sinus or idiopathic peripheral autonomic neuropathy
G90.9	Disorder of autonomic nervous system, unspecified

Cardiomyopathy

I42.1	Hypertrophic obstructive cardiomyopathy
I42.4	Endocardial fibroelastosis
I42.9	Cardiomyopathy unspecified (primary)(secondary)
I42.6	Alcohol cardiomyopathy
I42.8	Nutritional/metabolic cardiomyopathy
I43	Cardiomyopathy in other diseases classified elsewhere (e.g., progressive muscular dystrophy, sarcoidosis)
I42.8	Other cardiomyopathy

PATIENT EDUCATION GUIDES

See patient education form available online at www.expertconsult .com.

Acknowledgment

The editors recognize the contributions of Peter Hanson, MD, and Diane Lillis, RN, to this chapter in a previous edition of this text.

SUPPLIERS

(See contact information online at www.expertconsult.com.)

Advanced BioSensor, Inc.
Colin Medical (Omron)
Lifesource Medical (A & D Medical)
SpaceLabs Healthcare
SunTech Medical
Welch Allyn

A list of validated devices for ABPM is available: https://bihsoc. org/bp-monitors/bp-monitors. Accessed January 3, 2019.

RECOMMENDED READING

Chobanian AV, Bakris GL, Black HR, et al. Committee on prevention, detection, evaluation, and treatment of high blood pressure. national heart, lung, and blood institute; national high blood pressure education program coordinating committee: seventh report of the joint national committee on prevention, detection, evaluation, and treatment of high blood pressure: JNC 7. *Hypertension.* 2003;42:1206–1252.

Clement DL, De Buyzere ML, De Bacquer DA, et al. Prognostic value of ambulatory blood-pressure recordings in patients with treated hypertension. *N Engl J Med.* 2003;348:2407–2415.

Ernst ME, Bergus GR. Ambulatory blood pressure monitoring: technology with a purpose [editorial]. *Am Fam Physician.* 2003;67:2262–2263.

Gardner SF, Schneider EF. 24-Hour ambulatory blood pressure monitoring in primary care. *J Am Board Fam Pract.* 2001;14:166–177.

James PA, Oparil S, Carter BL. 2014 evidence-based guidelines for the management of high blood pressure in adults. Report from the panel members appointed by the eighth joint national committee (JNC 8). *JAMA.* 2014; 311:507–520.

Mancia G, De Backer G, Dominiczak A, et al. 2007 Guidelines for the management of arterial hypertension: the Task Force for the Management of Arterial Hypertension of the European Society of Hypertension (ESH) and of the European Society of Cardiology (ESC). *Eur Heart J.* 2007;28:1462–1536.

Mancia G, Facchetti R, Bombelli G, et al. Long-term risk of mortality associated with selective and combined elevation in office, home, and ambulatory blood pressure. *Hypertension.* 2006;47:846–853.

Marchiando RJ, Elston MP. Automated ambulatory blood pressure monitoring: Clinical utility in the family practice setting. *Am Fam Physician.* 2003;67:2262–2270.

Niiranen TJ, Hänninen MR, Johansson J, Reunanen A, Jula AM. Home-measured blood pressure is a stronger predictor of cardiovascular risk than office blood pressure: the Finn-Home study. *Hypertension.* 2010;55:1346–1351.

Ohkubo T, Kikuya M, Metoki H, et al. Prognosis of "masked" hypertension and "white-coat" hypertension detected by 24-h ambulatory blood pressure monitoring: 10-year follow-up from the Ohasama study. *J Am Coll Cardiol.* 2005;46:508–515.

Sheps SG, Clement DL, Pickering TG, et al. Ambulatory blood pressure monitoring: hypertensive diseases committee, american college of cardiology. *J Am Coll Cardiol.* 1994;23:1511–1513.

Staessen JA, Fagard RH, Lijnen PJ, et al. Mean and range of the ambulatory pressure in normotensive subjects from a meta-analysis of 23 studies. *Am J Cardiol.* 1991;67:723–727.

Verdecchia P. Prognostic value of ambulatory blood pressure: current evidence and clinical implications. *Hypertension.* 2000;35:844–851.

Whelton PK, Carey RM, Aronow WS, et al. 2017 guideline for high blood pressure in adults. ACC/AHA/AAPA/ABC/ACPM/AGS/APhA/ASH/ASPC/NMA/PCNA guideline for the prevention, detection, evaluation and management of high blood pressure in adults: a report of the American College of Cardiology/ American Heart Association Task Force on Clinical Practice Guidelines. *H J Am Coll Cardiol.* 2018;71:e127–e248.

Williams B, Mancia G, Spiering W, et al. 2018 ESC/ ESH guidelines for the management of arterial hypertension. *Eur Heart J.* 2018;39:3021–3104.

White WB, Berson AS, Robbins C, et al. National standard for measurement of resting and ambulatory blood pressures with automated sphygmomanometers. *Hypertension.* 1993;21:504–509.

CHAPTER 73

AMBULATORY ELECTROCARDIOGRAPHY: HOLTER AND EVENT MONITORING

David Flinders • Scott Akin

Norman Holter developed ambulatory electrocardiography (AECG) in the form of Holter monitoring in the early 1960s. The first device weighed about 85 pounds and was worn as a backpack. As the technology, availability, size, and convenience of the equipment improved, use of AECG increased. Although in the past, Holter monitoring was primarily requested, provided, and interpreted by cardiologists, this procedure, and other forms of AECG, have become increasingly popular among primary care clinicians. As our population ages, the prevalence of arrhythmias will increase, along with the prevalence of cardiovascular disease. Routine use of AECG generally involves the evaluation of patients who report symptoms possibly related to cardiac arrhythmias, such as unexplained palpitations, unexplained syncope, presyncope, or episodic dizziness. More advanced (and in some cases more controversial) uses of AECG include arrhythmia detection in asymptomatic patients with cardiac risk factors, ST segment monitoring for silent myocardial ischemia in the patient with coronary artery disease (CAD), assessment of antiarrhythmic drug therapy, and assessment of pacemaker/implantable cardioverter-defibrillators (ICD) function.

As primary care clinicians have become more competent using AECG devices, they have often provided increased access to them in their offices. The benefits of this include more readily, and perhaps more rapidly, available data for their patients. These data allow for more complete and definitive care for many patients. AECG is also attractive to clinicians or practices because it requires little clinician time to interpret the results and is therefore a time-efficient, income-generating test. With more widespread use, the cost of equipment has decreased. However, acquisition of an office monitoring system is not a decision to be taken lightly. Although it is relatively easy to interpret the results, it is considerably more difficult to apply them clinically. The clinician must have a clear interest in and understanding of cardiac arrhythmias and be willing to invest the time needed to learn the system. They must also commit to promptly interpreting the results of all tests performed. Realistically, with training and a modicum of practice, clinicians can interpret and dictate the results of most Holter reports within 5 to 15 minutes. Interpretation of event monitoring usually takes less time. That said, despite being more readily available, ambulatory monitoring should not be considered a routine procedure. From the patient's and insurer's perspective, it is expensive and time consuming. It should be reserved for specific indications. This chapter outlines the different types of AECGs, their indications, and the techniques necessary for use; it also provides a foundation for basic AECG interpretation.

OVERVIEW AND COMPARISON OF AVAILABLE METHODS OF EVALUATION AND ARRHYTHMIA MONITORING

12-Lead Electrocardiogram and Rhythm Strip

- Only monitors cardiac rhythm for a short period. Therefore, unless the patient is symptomatic at time of electrocardiogram (ECG), it is difficult to correlate clinically.

- Can diagnose certain conditions associated with worrisome arrhythmias (hypertrophic cardiomyopathy, Brugada syndrome, long QT syndrome, etc.).
- Inexpensive and readily available.

24-Hour Holter Monitor (Often Extended to 48 or 72 Hours)

- Standard monitoring modality for arrhythmias that occur frequently (i.e., several times daily).
- Patient wears two to three electrodes on the chest with leads attached that communicate continuously with a data-collecting device worn on the patient's belt.
- Patient completes a diary that enables a correlation of symptoms with the timing of arrhythmias.
- Because the recording period is short (24 to 72 hours), it only detects arrhythmias that are responsible for symptoms approximately 10% of the time. It may miss infrequent, but potentially dangerous, arrhythmias.
- Can identify subjects with worrisome arrhythmias (as well as quantify the frequency, duration, etc.) and silent ischemia. However, the interpreter must be aware of the tremendous spontaneous variability in frequency not only of ectopy, but also of ST segment changes that may or may not indicate ischemia (see later discussion).
- Moderately expensive ($250 to $500 per test in most institutions).

Postevent Recorders

- The device is kept by the patient at all times for up to several weeks. When experiencing symptoms, the patient places the device on the chest and activates it (the device does not record the ECG until the patient activates it). The patient can then transmit the recording over the telephone or internet.
- The patient keeps the device until several recordings have been made, or for an agreed-upon time frame (usually between 2 and 6 weeks).
- The patient must be aware of arrhythmias when they occur and must maintain consciousness long enough to activate the device.
- Short-lived arrhythmias, and those preceding activation of the device, may be missed.
- Some newer devices are credit card sized—small enough to carry in a wallet or to be worn as a necklace or wristwatch.
- Use is not recommended in the setting of arrhythmias that may cause serious symptoms such as syncope.
- Compliance can be problematic because of waning patient motivation without recurrent symptoms or patient error in correctly activating the device.
- Cost is more expensive than Holter monitoring.

External Preevent Recorders ("Loop Recorders")

- The patient wears a recording device and electrodes (that are changed by the patient every several days and removed for bathing), usually over the period of a month.
- The standard device continuously records 5 to 10 minutes of ECG data. When the device is activated, the preceding data are captured or "frozen." a Aditional data are saved for a few minutes following activation at the time of an event. The data can then be transmitted over the telephone or internet to a center for analysis. If the button is not pushed, the ECG loop continuously replaces the old data. Technicians may be on call 24 hours a day to interpret the data when transmitted. If necessary, they can coordinate a trip to the emergency department.
- The device can be programmed to detect asymptomatic arrhythmias and to then alert the patient to transmit data for evaluation.
- It is the recommended initial monitoring modality for patients with syncope because the activation button can be pressed once consciousness has been regained.
- It is also the recommended initial monitoring modality in the workup of most patients with palpitations for which AECG monitoring is deemed appropriate.
- Compliance can be problematic (similar to postevent recorders), and, in addition, some patients report problems with electrode attachment and skin irritation.
- Cost is more expensive than Holter monitoring.

Implantable Loop Recorders

- For very infrequent arrhythmias, a device the size of a pack of gum is implanted subcutaneously in the chest under local anesthesia and is left in place for up to 24 months.
- Like other loop recorders, it stores ECG data, which can be telephonically or wirelessly transmitted. The device can be programmed to store 1 minute of data prior to and 1 minute of data after automatic activation for a total of approximately 20 events. The device can also be activated externally and programmed to record up to 8 minutes of preactivation data and 2 minutes of postactivation data.
- It can be programmed to detect bradyarrhythmias or tachyarrhythmias on a prespecified basis.
- This device is generally used in the patient who has undergone previous noninvasive testing that was nondiagnostic but who continues to have infrequent symptoms.
- This method is not a good choice for high-risk patients (those with prior myocardial infarction [MI] or conduction abnormalities on ECG) in whom other testing, such as tilt-table or electrophysiologic testing, may make a diagnosis earlier and thus allow for earlier treatment.
- Cost is more expensive than preevent external loop recorders.

Electrophysiology Studies

- Electrophysiology (EP) studies are helpful when Holter or event monitoring results are equivocal, particularly in patients with a low ejection fraction, documented ischemic heart disease, and a history of syncope or near syncope.
- Used in post-MI patients at high risk of a life-threatening arrhythmia.
- Can determine whether an arrhythmia is inducible.
- Very expensive and higher risk (can provoke refractory or life-threatening arrhythmias).

Signal-Averaged Electrocardiogram

- Signal-averaged ECG (SAECG) enables detection of the substrate for potentially dangerous arrhythmias, such as ventricular tachycardia (VT), by using computed filtering and averaging of ECG complexes, which facilitates the detection of very low amplitude cardiac potentials not detectable by routine ECG.
- Generally 200 to 400 QRS complexes with the same morphology are averaged over approximately 3 to 7 minutes to record an adequate SAECG.
- Can be used to stratify risk for ventricular arrhythmias and sudden cardiac death, but only in specific settings, such as post-MI, cardiomyopathies, Brugada syndrome, arrhythmogenic right ventricular dysplasia, mitral valve prolapse, ventricular aneurysms, and idiopathic VT.
- Used more widely in the past, it is now known that the positive predictive value of SAECG is poor. As a result, utility is more for its negative predictive accuracy.
- It does not quantitate the frequency of premature ventricular complexes (PVCs).
- The procedure has limited availability and is moderately expensive.

Exercise Electrocardiogram (Stress) Testing

See also Chapter 74, Stress ECG Testing.

- Commonly used as a screening or diagnostic test for underlying cardiac ischemia or significant CAD.
- May confirm ischemia as the etiology of an arrhythmia or document its association with an arrhythmia.
- Demonstrates the effect of activity on ventricular arrhythmias.
- May detect some forms of complex ventricular ectopy not detected by Holter monitoring.
- ST segment depression in the absence of chest pain may alert the clinician to silent ischemia (but may be falsely positive).
- Not nearly as sensitive as Holter monitoring for the detection of PVCs.
- Systems are now available to check for T-wave alternans, a risk factor for ventricular arrhythmias, particularly in patients with a dilated cardiomyopathy or post-MI with a decreased ejection fraction.

Mobile Cardiac Outpatient Telemetry

- Continuous ECG monitoring from three leads that communicate with a palm-sized monitor. On detection of arrhythmia, real-time data are automatically transmitted via cell phone to a remote monitoring center. The device can generally store data for transmission if the patient is temporarily in an area where cell phone transmission is unavailable.
- Allows up to 2 weeks of continuous monitoring.
- Does not require the patient to activate the device, unlike postevent and loop recorders. Technicians are on call 24 hours a day to interpret the data when transmitted. If necessary, they can coordinate a trip to the emergency department.
- May have a higher yield of arrhythmia detection or exclusion than loop recorders, though validation is still in progress.
- Expensive.

BENEFITS AND DRAWBACKS OF AVAILABLE MONITORING METHODS

Physical examination and cardiac auscultation are unreliable for differentiating supraventricular from ventricular premature beats. The least expensive yet reliable method to document these arrhythmias is a standard 12-lead ECG with a short rhythm strip. Unfortunately, with an ECG, the cardiac rhythm is monitored only for a short period of time. Considering that the commonly accepted definition of "frequent" ventricular ectopy is more than 10 to 30 PVCs an hour, it becomes easy to see how even "frequent" PVCs can be overlooked by this method. On the other hand, if any PVCs are noted on a short rhythm strip, it is likely that the patient has both frequent and complex ventricular ectopy. Both would probably be detected during a longer period of monitoring, such as a Holter monitor study.

In the past, Holter recordings of only a few hours' duration were used for arrhythmia detection. Although practical and economical, such brief recordings do not accurately reflect the severity of cardiac arrhythmias in many individuals. This point is best illustrated by reviewing what is known about the frequency of ventricular arrhythmias over the course of a 24-hour period. Simply stated, even with the same patient, a tremendous amount of spontaneous variability in PVC frequency exists between one Holter recording and another. Similarly, marked variability in PVC frequency also occurs in patients with chronic ventricular arrhythmias. PVC frequency varies greatly from one day to the next, between successive 8-hour monitoring periods, and even from hour to hour within a single day. Certain individuals exhibit PVCs primarily during the day; others manifest them principally at night. As might be expected, PVC frequency often varies with physical activity and emotional state. However, in many individuals, marked spontaneous variability in PVC frequency persists even when monitoring conditions are kept absolutely constant.

Because of such fluctuations in PVC frequency, a monitoring period of at least 24 hours has become the standard for adequate characterization of an arrhythmia, and thus Holter monitors are generally worn for 24 hours, though occasionally the time period is extended to 48 hours. For most individuals, 24 hours of monitoring not only permits recognition of diurnal variations in arrhythmias, but it also allows detection of the maximal grade of ectopy.

The key caveat of 24-hour Holter monitoring is that no conclusions can be reached about whether a symptomatic arrhythmia exists unless symptoms occur during the 24 hours of monitoring. As noted previously, a patient may even have a malignant symptomatic ventricular arrhythmia that occurs only intermittently, sometimes as infrequently as once every few weeks. Event monitors, either in the form of a "postevent" device that necessitates patient activation or more commonly a continuously recording preevent ("loop") device, circumvent the short time limitation of the Holter monitor, as patients use these devices for several weeks at a time.

Although many variations of event monitoring exist, patients are generally issued a device that transmits the patient's rhythm over the telephone or internet. Usually the equipment remains with the patient for a few days or weeks. For cases of extremely infrequent arrhythmias, subcutaneously implanted units may be used for months or years. The principal weakness of the postevent monitor is that patients must be aware of arrhythmias when they occur, and they must maintain consciousness long enough to capture or transmit the rhythm. In the case of preevent (loop) recorders, the patient can activate the device after regaining consciousness, and the preceding data will be saved. Some loop recorders can be programmed to detect asymptomatic arrhythmias and alert the patient to transmit data for evaluation. These automatic detection devices typically have greater data storage capability because they may not reliably discriminate arrhythmias from artifacts, potentially creating a lot of false-positive events.

In the past, most clinicians began with full 24-hour Holter monitoring and then proceeded to event monitoring only for those cases when symptoms persisted despite negative Holter findings. However, because asymptomatic Holter results are often complicated and confusing, and there is a low yield of positive findings on Holter monitoring when arrhythmias are infrequent, event monitoring is now more commonly ordered. Overall, event monitoring is at least as effective as Holter monitoring for detection of symptomatic arrhythmias; event monitoring also has the advantage of less frequently recording asymptomatic background arrhythmias (for which treatment is unnecessary). In the case of syncope and the evaluation of unexplained palpitations, the diagnostic yield of preevent loop recorders over Holter monitors has been validated, and is the preferred initial AECG modality (Kinlay, 1996).

When Holter or event-monitoring results are equivocal, EP studies may be helpful. Although EP is an invasive study, the information obtained may be critical. Patients in whom a clinically relevant arrhythmia can be induced during EP testing usually have a worse prognosis, even if asymptomatic, than patients in whom an arrhythmia cannot be induced. However, EP testing does have a small but significant false-negative rate; results in patients with nonischemic cardiomyopathy are also difficult to interpret.

SAECG is a noninvasive test that has been advocated for risk stratification in potentially lethal ventricular arrhythmias. Although its main initial use was following MI, SAECG use has expanded to include patients with cardiomyopathies, Brugada syndrome, arrhythmogenic right ventricular dysplasia, mitral valve prolapse, ventricular aneurysms, and idiopathic VT. By computer-averaging signals for several hundred recorded beats, background "noise" can be filtered out to allow detection of low-amplitude, high-frequency late potentials after the QRS. These late potentials are suggestive of areas of slower conduction that may facilitate development of ventricular reentry. Unfortunately, the positive predictive accuracy of late potentials on SAECG following MI is less than optimal, around 15% to 20% for prediction of VT or ventricular fibrillation (VF). Therefore, negative findings on this test are more useful. SAECG is of established value in the evaluation of the syncope patient, but only in the setting of ischemic heart disease, and again its value is in its negative predictive accuracy.

Exercise ECG testing (EET; see Chapter 74, Stress ECG Testing) is a common method for evaluating PVCs (especially in older patients or those with coronary risk factors) and other arrhythmias (especially exercise-induced arrhythmias). It serves as a convenient, noninvasive test to screen for or to diagnose underlying CAD. EET may be indicated if ischemia is diagnosed with AECG. If CAD is diagnosed, EET can also evaluate its severity and assist with its management. EET also demonstrates what effect exercise has on arrhythmias. In general, PVCs that diminish with progressively increasing activity are less worrisome and tend to be associated with a better prognosis than those brought on by low levels of exercise. Recent evidence suggests that PVCs occurring during recovery from EET are associated with increased mortality, whereas PVCs during the EET are not (Dewey, 2008). Although not nearly as accurate as Holter monitoring for quantitative or qualitative assessment of PVCs, complex ventricular arrhythmias (including VT) and symptoms are sometimes elicited only by vigorous exercise. Chronotropic incompetence (unable to obtain heart rate >120 beats/min) on EET may suggest sick sinus syndrome, which is best diagnosed with a Holter monitor. Holter monitoring and EET may thus be complementary procedures that provide different information, and both tests should sometimes be considered for the complete evaluation of patients with ventricular arrhythmias.

It should be emphasized that detection of PVCs per se on EET is not indicative of an ischemic response. However, PVCs are cause for more concern when they occur in association with evidence of ischemia, such as ST segment depression or substernal chest pain in patients who are likely to have CAD. Thus, it is inadvisable to allow a middle-aged individual who has coronary risk factors to exercise in an unsupervised manner if EET produces frequent PVCs and ST segment depression or symptoms. Instead, further evaluation for CAD or ischemic or structural heart disease may be warranted.

On the other hand, many clinicians are much more comfortable allowing healthy young adults who have frequent PVCs to exercise vigorously if EET does not produce ST segment depression or if PVCs resolve with exercise. This is especially the case if they have a normal echocardiogram and laboratory tests (e.g., electrolytes, thyroid-stimulating hormone, complete blood count, sed rate). When these younger, asymptomatic, and otherwise healthy adults go out and exercise, their PVCs and symptoms will probably resolve with activity. Moreover, such individuals are much less likely to have underlying ischemic heart disease. Rare, life-threatening complex arrhythmias, seen only at peak exercise, will also be excluded with EET.

Mobile cardiac outpatient telemetry (MCOT) is an emerging technology that allows up to 2 weeks of continuous "real-time" ECG monitoring. Data collected are automatically transmitted via cell phone to a monitoring center. Benefits include less patient error because the device does not require patient activation, unlike postevent and loop recorders. A small industry-sponsored study suggested that MCOT devices may have a higher yield of arrhythmia detection or exclusion than loop recorders, although full validation is still in progress (Rothman, 2007).

An all-too-often-ignored adjunct for monitoring is the patient's history (perception) of symptoms compatible with an arrhythmia. Although many individuals are totally unaware of their arrhythmias, others are able to sense each and every ectopic beat. For individuals with non-life-threatening arrhythmias who have this awareness—and in whom AECG has confirmed a temporal relationship between symptoms and the occurrence of their arrhythmias—the *patient's account of symptoms* may serve as a fairly reliable and cost-effective adjunct for long-term monitoring (i.e., it may greatly reduce the need for [and expense of] repeated Holter recordings for judging the effect of treatment).

Consider the case of a young patient who is markedly symptomatic from extremely frequent ventricular ectopy. Baseline Holter monitoring reveals several thousand PVCs during the day of monitoring but no runs of VT and no evidence of ischemia. The echocardiogram is normal; there is no evidence of pericarditis, cardiomyopathy, or a metabolic cause for the PVCs, and the patient's diary confirms a definite temporal relationship between symptoms and periods of greatest ectopy. If treatment with a β-blocker (or a reduction in stimulants such as caffeine) leads to complete resolution of symptoms, does the Holter recording need to be repeated? The answer to this key question is often found by asking two additional questions: Would repeating the Holter recording alter treatment? Will the patient's account of symptoms (i.e., the "poor person's Holter") be adequate for guiding management? In many instances, such as in this particular case, experts would consider that monitoring the patient's symptoms alone to be adequate.

INDICATIONS

- Palpitations
- Chest pain
- Syncope or near syncope
- Vertigo
- Arrhythmias and response to antiarrhythmic therapy or post ablation therapy
- Transient ischemic episodes
- Dyspnea
- Evaluation of MI survivors with ejection fraction of 40% or less
- In patients with CAD to correlate symptoms (e.g., chest pain) with ST depression

Evaluation of Patients With Symptoms Possibly Related to Rhythm Disturbances

Symptoms of patients with VT or VF include palpitations (i.e., a sensation in the chest of a rapid or irregular cardiac rhythm), dizziness, and unexplained syncope. These symptoms may suggest a hemodynamically compromising arrhythmia.

However, not all patients with symptoms of palpitations, dizziness, and syncope need Holter monitoring. An occasional episode of skipped, dropped, or racing beats is not suggestive of VT or VF. Symptom duration and severity, the likelihood of underlying cardiac disease based on a history of risk factors or echocardiogram results, the existence and effect of potentially reversible extracardiac factors (e.g., caffeine, alcohol, sleep deprivation, viral illness, electrolyte abnormalities, hyperthyroidism, nonessential medications, normal sedimentation rate), the patient's or clinician's "need to know," and cost concerns should all be considered. Therefore, on a patient's first visit, do *not* routinely order Holter monitoring for patients who lack underlying heart disease or risk factors, especially if symptoms are of recent onset and are not particularly bothersome to the patient. On the other hand, you probably should consider some form of AECG monitoring for a patient with activity-limiting symptoms, especially when the symptoms are persistent, and especially when the patient has possible underlying structural heart disease or multiple risk factors for CAD.

AECG can also be of use in evaluating the patient with unexplained syncope, presyncope, or episodic dizziness. The American College of Cardiology/American Heart Association (ACC/AHA) guidelines give a class I recommendation for an AECG in such patients "in whom the cause is not obvious" (Crawford, 1999). Although syncope is a prevalent disorder, it is only infrequently secondary to a cardiac cause. However, the mortality rate is quite high in patients with a cardiac cause of syncope, and it is an independent predictor of sudden death. (One pearl: The older the patient is with the first episode of syncope, the more likely the syncope is due to a cardiac cause and the worse the prognosis.) Unfortunately, the yield of AECG monitoring in the patient with syncope is low because most patients do not have symptoms during the time they are being monitored. In fact, it is estimated that AECG establishes a diagnosis in only 2% to 3% of syncope patients. Because syncope can be a symptom of a potentially serious underlying problem, an AECG is prudent to pursue in the high-risk patient. In the evaluation of syncope, the most appropriate type of AECG monitoring is usually the loop recorder, which can be activated by the patient once he or she regains consciousness. The higher yield of loop recorders over Holter monitors was demonstrated in a prospective randomized trial (Sivakumaran, 2003). Sometimes results of the AECG can determine whether the patient with syncope would benefit from being evaluated in the electrophysiology laboratory. For example, the syncope patient with structural heart disease noted to have nonsustained VT (NSVT) on AECG has a high likelihood of having a serious underlying ventricular tachyarrhythmia induced in the EP laboratory.

Evaluation of unexplained recurrent palpitations, a widely accepted indication for AECG monitoring, was also given a class I recommendation by the ACC/AHA. Unexplained palpitations may be secondary to a potentially dangerous underlying arrhythmia, and it is prudent to identify high-risk patients. Although the diagnostic yield of identifying the cause of frequent palpitations from a 24-hour Holter monitor is approximately 35%, the percentage is doubled if one uses a loop recorder. Therefore it is considered more cost-effective to start the AECG evaluation of palpitations with a loop recorder rather than a Holter monitor. Often (perhaps in one-third of patients) a symptom is reported in the patient's symptom diary that does not correlate with any abnormality on the ECG, a scenario that is helpful to exclude a cardiac cause, reassure the patient, and consider pursuing other noncardiac causes of the patient's symptoms.

Evaluation of palpitations with AECG is a special case, with insight provided in a study (Weber, 1996) showing that one-third of patients coming to an emergency facility with palpitations as their chief complaint had a psychological cause for this symptom (either generalized anxiety or panic disorders). Four factors were found in this study to be independently predictive of a cardiac (arrhythmia) cause: male gender, a history of heart disease, subjective sensation of an irregular heartbeat, and symptom duration (palpitations) of more than 5 minutes. Awareness of these findings may help in the decision of when to order an objective form of arrhythmia detection.

Evaluation of Antiarrhythmic Drug Therapy

In the past, AECG was commonly used to evaluate the efficacy of an antiarrhythmic drug; however, it is now used less frequently for this indication because interpretation is limited by a high spontaneous variability in the frequency and type of arrhythmia within each individual and a lack of correlation between suppressing an arrhythmia and patient outcome. This limitation was particularly evident in the cardiac arrhythmia suppression trial (CAST; Echt, 1991), in which attempted arrhythmia suppression with flecainide, encainide, and moricizine resulted in an increased mortality rate. This study outcome led to class I antiarrhythmics no longer being recommended as long-term therapy for arrhythmia suppression, resulting in less AECG monitoring. Furthermore, approximately 25% of patients with ventricular arrhythmias have spontaneous resolution within 12 to 17 months, making it difficult to establish benefit (or causality) after antiarrhythmics are started. When AECG is chosen for monitoring drug response, it is done so under three specific circumstances: (1) to document drug response in a patient with known baseline of arrhythmias that are reproducible; (2) to detect proarrhythmic response to an antiarrhythmic drug; or most commonly, (3) to assess rate control in chronic atrial fibrillation.

A review of the statistics behind spontaneous variability in PVC frequency is essential if the practitioner is to use Holter recordings to evaluate the effectiveness of antiarrhythmic therapy, especially now that nonrepetitive ventricular ectopy is treated much less often than it was in the past. To *statistically* exclude a spontaneous variation in response following antiarrhythmic therapy, a reduction in PVC frequency of at least 70% to 90% between Holter recordings is required.

Evaluation of Rate Control for Atrial Fibrillation

In general, adequate rate control can be documented in older or sedentary individuals by checking their heart rate after a brisk walk around the office or upstairs. For younger or active individuals, either a Holter monitor or exercise ECG test can be used to evaluate adequacy of control. In the patient where strict rate control is the goal (heart rate <80 beats/min), which has not been found to have better outcomes than lenient rate control (heart rate <110 beats/min, Van Gelder, 2010), Holter monitoring may need to be done on a regular basis until rate control is achieved and then periodically thereafter to assure rate control. In this group, Holter monitoring is frequently performed after each change of medication or dose to evaluate control and to exclude bradycardia.

Evaluation for Silent Myocardial Ischemia

Silent myocardial ischemia, defined as objective evidence of ischemia without chest discomfort or any anginal equivalent, is the most common manifestation of CAD. It is estimated that more than 75% of ischemic episodes occur without symptoms while patients go about their activities of daily living, and since episodes of silent myocardial ischemia are not alarming to the patient, they frequently go undetected and untreated. AECG monitoring to detect ST segment changes was first investigated in the mid-1970s, but there was much skepticism, particularly regarding a high number of false-positive results. In monitoring for silent ischemia, the Holter monitor continuously records ST segments, which can be assessed for flat or downsloping ST depression of 1 to 2 mm or more (see discussion of Equipment Settings). However, because of large day-to-day variability of ST segment changes, ST segment depression as detected by Holter monitors may not be indicative of ischemia. In recent years, technologic improvements have resulted in increased specificity for ischemia particularly in certain population subgroups. We now know that ischemia detected by Holter monitoring is associated with increased coronary events and increased mortality risk, but this applies only to patients with known CAD, particularly those who

have had an MI. At this point, there is no role for monitoring for silent myocardial ischemia in patients without CAD. For this reason, the ACC/AHA do not strongly support the routine use of AECG to assess for silent myocardial ischemia (with one exception being the patient with suspected variant [Prinzmetal] angina). Furthermore, Holter monitoring should not be used as an alternative to EET to diagnose ischemia. It has been suggested that Holter monitoring may allow for further risk stratification in patients who have had a positive EET, by assessing for ischemia while patients perform their routine activities. Such detection of ischemia by Holter monitoring may help to identify groups of patients who would benefit most from more aggressive antiplatelet and antiischemic therapy.

Risk Assessment in High-Risk Asymptomatic Patients

There are approximately 450,000 sudden cardiac deaths per year in the United States; most are due to ventricular tachyarrhythmias such as VF or VT. One key role of AECG is, in certain high-risk patient populations, to detect arrhythmias that are precursors to sudden death so that there is time to consider an intervention that may reduce the patient's chance of sudden death. Patients who survive VF or sustained VT are likely to have recurrences (particularly if they have CAD or structural heart disease), and, unfortunately, many such recurrences are fatal. Much attention has been given to the prevention of sudden cardiac death, particularly with the development of ICDs, which have shown a mortality risk benefit in select patient populations. Antiarrhythmic drugs, although less effective in certain subgroups for primary and secondary prevention of sudden cardiac death, are often used in conjunction with ICDs to reduce the frequency of shocks.

Conditions associated with ventricular arrhythmias and sudden cardiac death include CAD, dilated or hypertrophic cardiomyopathy, right ventricular dysplasia, long QT syndrome, electrolyte abnormalities, use of antiarrhythmic drugs, and valvular heart disease. As noted earlier, AECG can be used to identify high-risk patients who may be at risk for sudden cardiac death. Currently there are only three conditions for which the ACC/AHA support (albeit weakly with class IIb recommendations) risk assessment in the absence of symptoms: post-MI patients with left ventricular ejection fraction (LV EF) less than 40%, patients with congestive heart failure, and patients with hypertrophic cardiomyopathy.

In general, patients with ischemic heart disease, especially those with a history of MI, have a very high risk for a serious or fatal arrhythmic event. Frequent and complex PVCs are an independent risk factor associated with a two- to fivefold increased risk of death after an MI. AECG (particularly Holter monitoring) is sometimes performed in post-MI patients with a low EF (<40%) as a risk assessment tool.

It is well established that patients with congestive heart failure and underlying cardiomyopathy have an increased risk of sudden death. Much attention has been paid to the possible role of AECG as a way to further identify those patients who may or may not benefit from ICDs. However, the data are contradictory, and the role for using AECG in this population is not well established.

Patients with hypertrophic cardiomyopathy have an increased risk of sudden death. AECG monitoring for NSVT has been proposed in this patient population, with the idea that NSVT may be a marker for sudden death. However, this has not been clearly established, and arrhythmia treatment has not been shown to improve mortality risk. Therefore AECG for risk assessment in this population remains unclear.

Evaluation of Pacemaker or Implantable Cardioverter-Defibrillator Function

In the past, Holter monitors were commonly used to assess the function of a pacemaker or an ICD, and the data were used to guide programming, for example, by changing pacing thresholds. This practice is becoming less frequent because newer generation devices generally have the ability to store ECG data that can be retrieved and analyzed. However, AECG is still recommended in several situations, such as to evaluate for device failure or malfunction (e.g., pacemaker-induced tachycardia in the setting of frequent palpitations, syncope, or near syncope) or to assess the response to adjunctive pharmacologic therapy in patients receiving frequent ICD discharges.

CONTRAINDICATIONS

As with other office-based procedures, AECG monitoring can be overutilized. More information is not necessarily better, particularly when the information could be misleading, such as may be the case with a false-positive result in a low pretest probability setting (e.g., a low-risk patient with a constellation of vague symptoms). AECG should not be used as a screening tool in the low-risk asymptomatic patient or for the evaluation of chest pain in low-risk patients who can exercise. Similarly, the ACC/AHA discourages AECG for patients with syncope or palpitations in whom another etiology has been identified or in the assessment of a patient who has had a cerebrovascular accident but has no evidence of arrhythmia.

PREPROCEDURE PATIENT EDUCATION AND PREPARATION

- Explain to the patient why Holter or event monitoring is necessary.
- Explain to the patient the need for a symptom diary.

An essential part of the Holter recording is the patient's symptom diary. Consider how often supraventricular and ventricular ectopy are found in the general population and how frequently patients come to a clinician with symptoms suggestive of cardiac arrhythmias; the importance of establishing a cause-and-effect relationship between the two should be evident. For example, if symptoms are noted at 10 AM, 2 PM, 5 PM, and 11 PM, but no cardiac arrhythmias are seen at these times, it is unlikely that the symptoms are cardiac related. Therefore a lot of useful information may be obtained from Holter recordings even in the absence of arrhythmias—provided the diary is carefully completed.

In symptomatic individuals who actually demonstrate cardiac arrhythmias during Holter monitoring, one can determine whether the arrhythmias are likely to be the cause of their symptoms by the temporal relationship in the diary. For example, if long runs of ventricular bigeminy occur while the patient is relaxed and totally unaware of the arrhythmia—and palpitations or chest discomfort are noted only during periods of sinus rhythm—ventricular bigeminy is probably not related to the patient's symptoms.

Unfortunately, in clinical practice, completion of the diary is all too often neglected. As a result, consider the following:

- Emphasize the importance of filling out the diary to your patient.
- Be sure that the patient can read and write before providing the diary. If the patient is illiterate, see if someone can help the patient fill out the diary.
- For hospitalized patients, consider actively involving the nursing staff to ensure accurate completion of the patient diary.

NOTE: Use of event monitoring is much more conducive to correlating symptoms with arrhythmias than Holter monitoring because the occurrence of symptoms is what prompts the patient to initiate the event monitor recording.

EQUIPMENT

- Holter, event, or other AECG monitor with desired capabilities (check for cracked or broken wires and for damage to the carrying case)
- Fresh, alkaline batteries
- Printer paper, ink, extra cassettes (for the Holter report to be printed out for interpretation)
- Razor
- Rubbing alcohol
- Electrodes
- Lead attachment kit

Most of the time, hospitals and commercial Holter or event laboratories employ trained technicians to scan Holter recordings for the interpreting clinician. This is a tremendous time-saving feature because the technician can highlight the principal findings, thus sparing the clinician the need to meticulously scan each of the full-disclosure printouts.

On the other hand, the luxury of having a trained technician to scan tracings is not available to many clinicians who have purchased their own Holter monitoring system. In this case, options include the following:

- Having the hard copy of the Holter recording processed and scanned by a commercial laboratory—an expensive and rarely used option.
- Hiring or training a technician to scan, which may be the most cost-effective solution for the busy practitioner who has a nurse or technician with the interest and expertise in arrhythmia interpretation.
- Not printing 24 hours of full disclosure. (Full disclosure means that the Holter device prints out a miniaturized strip of each hour of the 24 hours tracing.) Depending on the area's third-party payment regulations, the practitioner may not receive full reimbursement unless 24 hours of full disclosure is printed out.
- Printing out, but ignoring the 24-hours full disclosure, or looking only at those portions of the printout that seem relevant to the clinical problem (i.e., looking at full disclosure only at times when symptoms are noted in the diary or at times of densest ectopy as suggested on the hourly summary). This saves time, but if something is missed, it will be documented.
- Printing 24 hours of full disclosure and scanning the printout yourself. Although this takes a greater amount of time to accomplish, it may be time well spent.
- Purchasing a Holter system that does not provide full disclosure. If reimbursement for this modality in your area is comparable to that for full-disclosure systems, this alternative may be both cost and time effective, especially if the practitioner does not have great interest or expertise in arrhythmia interpretation. However, such systems are more likely to yield equivocal findings, and they may overlook potentially important arrhythmias. Personal interpretation of Holter data recorded on such systems is only as good as the system's computer software.

NOTE: The authors feel that a full 24 hours of disclosure is indispensable for optimal Holter interpretation. Many experts suggest that it is essential for the interpreter to scan the entire recording, even when trend analyses, hourly summaries, and selected rhythm strips are normal.

Systems that offer data compression do not provide full disclosure. Using signal averaging to evaluate compressed data, and then re-expanding it, does not allow every QRS complex to be reproduced.

TECHNIQUE

1. The patient's report form (see Fig. 73.14) should be completed with relevant patient information, such as date of birth and indications for procedure. Recorded data such as cardiac risk factors, medications, activity level, and other medical problems that may affect the management following interpretation would also be helpful.
2. Monitoring parameters on the equipment should be set.

TABLE 73.1	Equipment Settings
Automatic high rate	120 beats/min
Automatic low rate	40 beats/min
Automatic pause	2.00 sec
Automatic supraventricular ectopic	25%
Automatic ST level	2 mm
Automatic abnormal	3/hr
Periodic storage	2 hr
Strips per hour	5

3. Attach the ECG electrodes in the locations indicated for the particular model of Holter or event monitor (see the operating instructions or illustrations provided by the monitor manufacturer). In general, limb leads are placed more centrally than with an office ECG.

Equipment Settings

Most Holter systems provide the operator some flexibility in selecting the parameters used to scan for abnormalities. Some routine settings are shown in Table 73.1. In this example, the computer will record a full-size rhythm strip for those tachycardias that are faster than 120 beats/min (automatic high rate); for bradycardias slower than 40 beats/min (automatic low rate); and for pauses longer than 2 seconds (automatic pause). Since automatic abnormal is set at three events, the machine should record the first three incidents of tachycardia that occur during any given hour, to a maximum of five strips per hour for any reason—which may potentially yield a total of 120 rhythm strips to review (up to 5 strips per hour × 24 hours = 120 strips).

Because periodic storage is set at 2 hours, the computer should record at least one rhythm strip every 2 hours, even if no abnormalities occur. This guarantees that the interpreter will have at least 12 rhythm strips to view, even if the Holter result is completely normal. NOTE: We are generally uncomfortable accepting the computer's reading of normal unless a minimal number of normal full-size rhythm strips are displayed.

One reason for favoring 120 beats/min as the upper rate limit is that lower numbers (e.g., 100 or 110 beats/min) are more likely to produce an excessive number of benign sinus tachycardia strips, whereas higher numbers (e.g., 130 or 140 beats/min) might prevent the detection of significant tachycardias with relatively slow rates, such as VT at 125 beats/min. NOTE: Selection of equipment settings always involves a compromise, and the setting of 120 beats/min may occasionally yield a monotonous deluge of sinus tachycardia strips at 120 to 125 beats/min.

For similar reasons, a lower rate limit of 40 beats/min is favored. For example, selecting a lower rate limit of 50 beats/min might result in a deluge of benign sinus bradycardia strips if the Holter examination was performed on an otherwise healthy individual who happened to have a slow resting heart rate.

Pauses of up to 2 seconds are common, especially in the elderly, and are usually benign. Longer pauses, especially those accompanied by frequent episodes of bradycardia with rates of fewer than 40 beats/min, suggest the possibility of sick sinus syndrome, particularly in the setting of structural heart disease.

The automatic supraventricular ectopic (SVE) setting of 25% should record rhythm strips demonstrating a greater than 25% variation in R-R interval. This record is how atrial fibrillation or premature atrial contractions (PACs) are detected. Setting the SVE lower (e.g., at 10%) would detect many more PACs but would also pick up sinus arrhythmia. Higher settings might miss too many PACs. Even with a setting of 25%, imagine the number of strips that would result when the underlying rhythm is atrial fibrillation!

The most controversial parameter is the automatic ST segment level, which is usually set at 2 mm, unless the reason for performing

the Holter monitoring is to "seek and search for" silent ischemia (which is only recommended in the known CAD patient). Resolution of ST segment images may be less than ideal, and because of marked day-to-day variability of ST segment changes, in an otherwise unselected population, the majority of episodes of ST segment depression between 1 and 2 mm will demonstrate false-positive results; that is, they will not represent true silent ischemia. Setting the ST segment parameter at 2 mm greatly increases the specificity for true silent ischemia. The tradeoff is that some patients with CAD may have frequent episodes of silent ischemia with lesser degrees of ST segment depression. Although the ST segment trend analysis (see Fig. 73.4) should reflect this, it is important to document the phenomenon by recording at least a few full-size strips that demonstrate definite ST segment depression. This is one benefit of lowering the ST segment parameter to 1 mm when the principal reason for performing the Holter test is to evaluate the patient with known CAD for silent ischemia.

NOTE: The technique and equipment settings for event monitors are usually similar to those for Holter monitors.

INTERPRETATION OF RESULTS

Appreciation of the wide range of normal is essential for meaningful interpretation of ambulatory ECG recordings. Premature supraventricular and ventricular contractions and certain other cardiac arrhythmias are common in otherwise healthy, asymptomatic individuals without underlying structural heart disease or CAD. Additional evaluation of such individuals is potentially expensive and may be harmful.

Although a detailed description of all of the variants of "normal" is beyond the scope of this chapter, a brief discussion of the prevalence of ventricular arrhythmias and then an overview of the clinical perspective of the process may be helpful.

Prevalence of Premature Ventricular Contractions in the General Population

Premature ventricular contractions are common. They are found in up to 50% of otherwise healthy, asymptomatic young adults. Their frequency increases with age; thus, most adults over 60 have some ventricular ectopy during a 24-hour period of monitoring. Less well appreciated is the fact that in the absence of underlying heart disease, complex forms of ventricular ectopy (e.g., ventricular couplets, salvos, or longer runs of VT) are uncommon and when present in this population are generally associated with a low risk of sustained VT or sudden death. The excellent prognosis for such patients has been documented in patients with primary electrical disease (Kennedy et al., 1985) and competitive athletes. In contrast, both frequent and complex ventricular ectopy are common when underlying heart disease is present.

The term *frequent* when used to quantify ventricular ectopy is subject to interpretation. In a population of middle-aged individuals with underlying heart disease, frequent ventricular ectopy is most often defined as an average of more than 10 to 30 PVCs per hour during a 24-hour period of monitoring (i.e., at least 240 PVCs per day). In contrast, among otherwise healthy, asymptomatic young adults, a much lower number should probably be used to define *frequent*. As noted earlier, although up to half of these individuals have some PVCs during 24 hours of monitoring, it is unusual for them to have as many as 100 PVCs per day.

Clinical Significance of Premature Ventricular Contractions

The significance of ventricular ectopy depends on the clinical setting in which it occurs. Patients with PVCs who do not have underlying heart disease tend to have a benign prognosis. Even among individuals with primary electrical disease and frequent, complex

PVCs (as noted previously), treatment may not be indicated in the absence of both symptoms and underlying heart disease, as This was demonstrated in the cardiac arrhythmia suppression trials (CAST I and II), which found that antiarrhythmic treatment was associated with an increased mortality rate.

In a study of 355 athletes aged 14 to 35 years who underwent a 24-hour Holter study due to palpitations or frequent PVCs noted on routine ECG (Biffi et al., 2002), there were no deaths during a mean 8-year follow-up in the group (284 athletes) noted to have fewer than 2000 PVCs in 24 hours. The 71 athletes who had 2000 or more PVCs per day were excluded from competitive athletics. There was only one sudden death in this excluded group in an individual with arrhythmogenic right ventricular cardiomyopathy; it occurred while playing field hockey against medical advice.

In contrast, in the setting of acute ischemia, especially if associated with angina, any ventricular ectopy at all must be viewed as significant and as a potential trigger of VF. Data suggest that this is particularly true of PVCs that occur in recovery following exercise. This was seen in a study following exercise ECG (stress) testing (Dewey, 2008).

Although left ventricular function is the most important predictor of death during the year following acute MI, PVCs are also an independent risk factor. Death in this year is related to the frequency of ventricular ectopy, as detected by Holter monitoring before discharge from the hospital. Patients with less than one PVC per hour tend to have a low (<10%) mortality rate. This figure rises sharply as a function of PVC frequency. About half of the total PVC-associated deaths happen at PVC frequencies as low as three per hour. A mortality rate plateau (20% to 30% for the ensuing year) is reached above PVC frequencies of 10 per hour. Thus a predischarge Holter monitor recording obtained for a post-MI patient needs to be interpreted in a different light than that of one obtained on a patient with chronic ventricular ectopy. The definition of frequent ventricular ectopy should probably be adjusted downward in post-MI patients.

The frequency of ventricular arrhythmias detected in the postinfarction period is time dependent. PVCs are infrequent for 3 to 5 days following infarction. They tend to increase in frequency over the next 6 to 12 weeks, and then the frequency levels off. Despite the tendency of PVC frequency to increase after discharge from the hospital, it may be more practical to obtain a baseline Holter monitor in selected patients *before* they go home.

Repetitive forms of ventricular ectopy (e.g., ventricular couplets, and especially salvos and longer runs of VT) are additional cause for concern. Their presence more than doubles the first-year mortality risk after MI over that of patients who do not demonstrate repetitive forms. In contrast to previous thinking, multiform PVCs and R-on-T complexes are considered much less worrisome than repetitive forms.

Much less can be said about the clinical benefit of drug treatment for PVCs in postinfarction patients. β-Blockers are generally favored as a first-line therapy because they are well tolerated, have a low proarrhythmia effect, and reduce both postinfarction mortality *and* ventricular ectopy rates. As mentioned, the CAST studies demonstrated a two- to threefold *increase* in mortality rate when postinfarction patients with ventricular arrhythmias were routinely treated with flecainide or encainide. Treatment of such patients with a class Ia, Ib, or Ic antiarrhythmic agent when β-blockers cannot be used is not recommended. Because these antiarrhythmic drugs may produce significant side effects, increase mortality risk, or be proarrhythmic or ineffective, the decision to use them should never be taken lightly.

Fortunately, there are alternatives to pharmacologic therapy. ICDs are often lifesaving, but expensive, and may be associated with morbidity from repetitive shocks. That said, ICDs are often recommended in patients with prior MI who have an EF less than 30%, and in survivors of sudden cardiac arrest. Most patients with VT and normal LV function may not require or be candidates for ICDs. Catheter ablation of the ectopic focus or reentry circuit is another potential alternative for some of these patients.

SAMPLE HOLTER MONITOR

Many types of Holter monitor systems are on the market. Each has its own advantages and disadvantages. The field continues to evolve at an amazingly rapid pace, so that current drawbacks of a particular system may be corrected by the next version of that system. It behooves the interested clinician to become familiar, at least in general terms, with the pros and cons of several types of Holter systems. This familiarity will assist the clinician in selecting those operative features that are likely to be most applicable for a particular practice setting.

In the following section, the information provided by one particular full-disclosure Holter system is illustrated. Although resolution quality of P wave and ST segment morphology is admittedly less than optimal with this system, it should still be adequate for office monitoring. The general principles illustrated by this Holter system are applicable to other systems and to many of the principles involved in event monitoring. The main difference with event monitoring is that 24-hour full disclosure is not included.

CASE STUDY

A 60-year-old man has dyspnea on exertion, which has been increasing for 1 month. He had an MI in the distant past, but he has been active for years and is otherwise doing well and is not on cardiac medications. He has not complained of chest pain or palpitations but recently described frequent episodes of intense dyspnea, weakness, and dizziness, most often associated with activity. Physical examination is unremarkable, and a resting ECG reveals normal sinus rhythm without any acute changes. Because of the frequent occurrence of symptoms with activities of daily living, the practitioner has decided to obtain a Holter monitor before exercise testing.

Patient Diary

It is important for patients to keep a diary to aid in interpreting the results of Holter monitoring. As mentioned earlier, symptoms of potential cardiac etiology and arrhythmias are common in the general population. The only way to prove that symptoms are cardiac related is to document a temporal correlation between their occurrence and the occurrence of arrhythmias on a Holter monitor.

As emphasized earlier, completion of a diary can provide the clinician with very useful information, even if the Holter result is entirely normal. Thus, if multiple symptoms are noted on the day of monitoring and no arrhythmias are detected on the Holter, the patient can be reassured that symptoms are unlikely to be cardiac in origin. The diary (Fig. 73.1) is especially helpful in this case because it indicates eight symptomatic episodes of weakness, dizziness, or shortness of breath.

Time	Activity	Symptoms
1PM	Lunch, relax	
2PM	Rake leaves	Weak, dizziness
4PM	Sitting, resting	Weak, dizziness
6PM	Resting	Weak
7PM	Watching TV	Dizziness
9PM	Went to bed	Dizziness
7AM	Breakfast	Short of breath
8AM	Resting	Short of breath, dizzy
9AM	Drove to doctor's office	Weak, dizziness

Fig. 73.1 Patient diary for Holter monitoring.

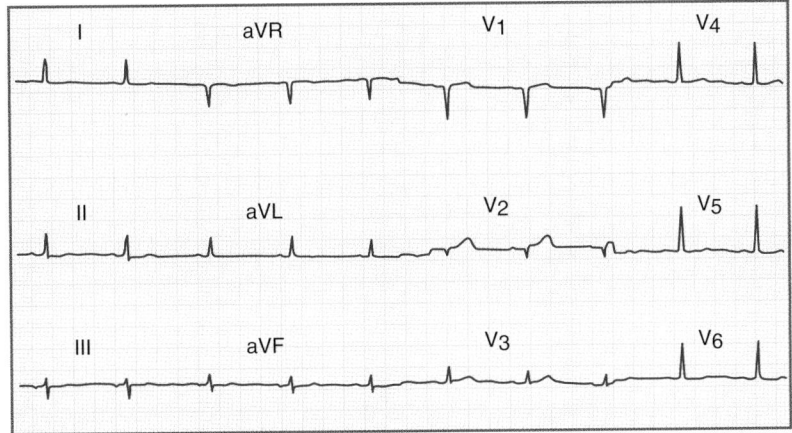

Fig. 73.2 Baseline 12-lead electrocardiogram.

12-Lead Electrocardiogram

Many clinicians obtain a preprocedure 12-lead ECG on all patients scheduled for Holter monitoring to screen for baseline artifact. If there is a significant artifact on the 12-lead ECG, such artifact will likely be seen on the Holter recording and might preclude accurate assessment of the rhythm strip. However, this additional step may be considered unnecessary and time consuming by technicians because the patient has usually undergone a 12-lead ECG at a recent clinical visit. In most cases, proper attention to lead placement precludes baseline artifact.

If there has been a frequent problem with the quality of Holter results, certain systems offer the ability to test the three or five leads of a Holter recording through a 12-lead ECG at the time of lead attachment. Others require the use of a "block," a conversion device available from the manufacturer, to connect the Holter monitor to a 12-lead ECG for testing.

In this case example, despite the fact that the P wave amplitude is small on the patient's 12-lead ECG (Fig. 73.2), the underlying rhythm fortunately turns out to be clearly identified as sinus on the eventual Holter (since the P wave is upright in lead II). Although this overall Holter study is interpretable, on many of the selected rhythm strips, as predicted by the 12-lead, a sinus rhythm is harder to identify with certainty.

Other benefits of obtaining a baseline 12-lead ECG include accurate determination of intervals (PR, QRS, and QT) and a much better appreciation of the baseline ST segment (many patients have baseline ST depression, which is not indicative of ischemia). As a result, determination of ST segment shifts (i.e., possible silent ischemia) is greatly facilitated. In this Holter study example, all intervals are normal. There is some nonspecific ST-T wave flattening in the inferolateral leads, but no significant ST segment depression and no acute changes.

Narrative Summary

Some Holter monitors produce a narrative summary (Box 73.1) that consolidates the principal findings detected by the computer. Practically speaking, the main task of the interpreter is to verify that this computed summary of pertinent findings is accurate.

In this case example, the narrative summary indicates a number of abnormal findings. The interpreter will certainly want to see representative samples of the following:

- Episodes of tachycardia (with a heart rate of up to 160 beats/min)
- Episodes of bradycardia (with a heart rate between 36 and 39 beats/min)
- Pauses (between 2.14 and 3.29 seconds in duration)
- Rhythm strips at the time the patient activated the event button (which occurred on two occasions)

BOX 73.1   Narrative Summary of Holter Recording*

- During this period the average heart rate was 75 beats/min with a maximum heart rate of 160 beats/min at 16:45 and a minimum heart rate of 36 beats/min at 03:38.
- There were 29 tachycardic episodes detected during the monitoring period.
- These episodes ranged in rate from 120 to 160 beats/min.
- There were 7 bradycardic episodes detected during the monitoring period.
- These episodes ranged in rate from 36 to 39 beats/min.
- There were 57 pause episodes detected during the monitoring period.
- These episodes ranged in duration from 2.14 to 3.29 sec.
- There were 25 SVE episodes detected during the monitoring period.
- The patient pressed the event button two times during the monitoring period.
- There were no ST segment episodes detected during the monitoring period.
- During the monitoring period there were 1144 abnormal beats detected.
- There were two successive abnormal episodes detected during the monitoring period.

---

*The patient was monitored for a period of 23:36 (hours and minutes).
SVE, Supraventricular ectopy.

- Abnormal beats (1151 were detected), including the two episodes of successive abnormal episodes

The clinician-interpreter does not need to find each of the 1144 abnormal beats. Nevertheless, he or she should verify that the beats are truly abnormal (not artifactual), whether the "abnormal" beats are truly PVCs, and whether these PVCs seem to be occurring frequently enough to explain the computer count. Practically speaking, it matters little if there are 1144 abnormal beats or 1100 abnormal beats—or 800 or 500, for that matter—since the difference between 1151 and 800, or 500, is still well within the range for spontaneous variability. Clinically, it is unlikely that treatment would differ for a patient who has 1151 PVCs or 500 PVCs. In both situations, it is probably sufficient to say that there are frequent PVCs.

REMEMBER: Evaluate any intervention; a reduction of at least 70% to 90% of the PVCs from one Holter to the next must be demonstrated to rule out the possibility of spontaneous variation. Therefore, in this particular case, the number of PVCs would have to be reduced from 1144 to less than 350 to eliminate this possibility.

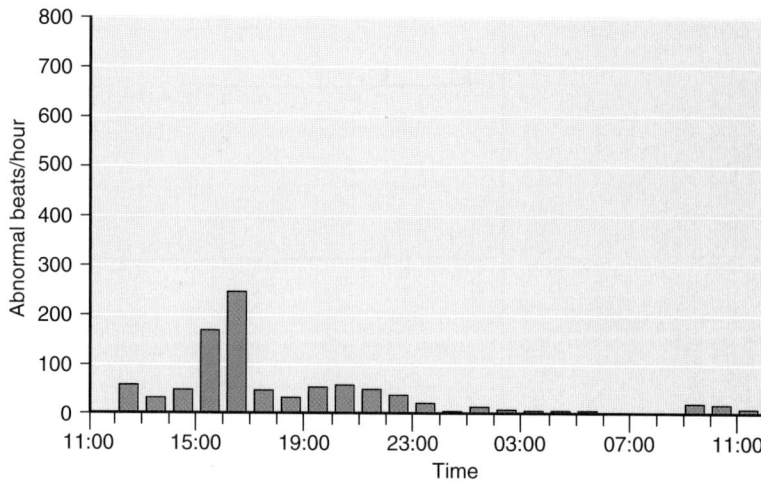

Fig. 73.3 Trend analysis of abnormal heartbeats during 24-hour Holter monitoring.

Finally, this particular Holter system does not indicate whether the PVCs are uniform or multiform; it simply gives the sum of all abnormal beats. Once again, practically speaking, this really does not matter in view of the following facts:

- The prognostic implications of multiformity are not nearly as ominous as previously thought. Much more important than the multiform PVCs are *repetitive* PVCs (e.g., couplets, salvos, and longer runs of VT).
- Almost all individuals with frequent ventricular ectopy over a 24-hour period demonstrate at least some degree of multiformity.

Trend Analysis of Abnormal Beats

The trend analysis of abnormal beats allows the interpreter, at a glance, to see what time of day PVC frequency peaks. In this case, minimal ventricular ectopy occurs at night, and maximal ectopy occurs during the daytime and evening hours (e.g., between noon and midnight) when the patient is active (Fig. 73.3).

Identifiable periods of peak ventricular ectopic activity may suggest a specific approach to treatment. For example, patients who manifest diurnal variation or increased ectopic activity during the hours of maximal daily activity often have an increase in sympathetic tone as part of their etiology. Therefore, these patients are optimal candidates for β-blocker therapy. Patients on antiarrhythmic therapy who demonstrate a peak in ectopic activity 6 to 10 hours after the last dose of their medication may benefit from an increased dosing frequency or by use of a sustained-release product.

Trend Analysis of Heart Rate and ST Segment Level

The heart rate trend analysis demonstrates, at a glance, heart rate variations throughout the day. In this case, it is easy to see that a tachycardia of approximately 150 beats/min was sustained for most of the period between 16:00 and 17:00 (Fig. 73.4). The ST segment level trend analysis shows that 1 mm of ST segment depression was sustained throughout much of this same period (*arrow*), suggesting that the ST segment depression is likely to be at least partially rate related.

The ST segment level trend analysis may facilitate quantitative assessment of the type and duration of ST segment depression in patients with silent ischemia.

Hourly Summary

Most Holter systems produce an hourly summary in some type of tabular format. Although it usually takes some time and practice to become familiar with this type of format, doing so tremendously facilitates interpretation. The hourly summary shows exactly where to look on the full-disclosure tracings to verify abnormal findings.

The hourly summary in this case (Fig. 73.5) indicates the following:

- The lowest heart rate (36 beats/min) was recorded between 03:00 and 04:00. The fastest heart rate (160 beats/min) was recorded between 16:00 and 17:00. The greatest hourly frequency of PVCs, or isolated abnormalities, (235) occurred between 16:00 and 17:00.
- The event button was activated twice (once between 15:00 and 16:00, and once between 09:00 and 10:00).
- All 57 pause episodes (38 + 19) occurred between 19:00 and 21:00.

Selected (Full-Size) Rhythm Strips

Inspection of selected representative full-size rhythm strips is essential for verifying pertinent computer findings and is generally performed next. These strips have usually been selected by the reviewing technician as discussed previously. The rhythm strips should include portions of the tracings that were patient activated (i.e., the patient was symptomatic at the time the device recorded the strip) and any abnormalities noted by the technician. Thus, in this case, the patient had a 10-beat run of paroxysmal atrial fibrillation at 13:03:20 (Fig. 73.6). He was in a regular, presumably, sinus rhythm of 80 beats/min at 15:03:20 (Fig. 73.7). An ever-so-slightly irregular supraventricular tachycardia (rapid atrial fibrillation) is evident at 15:51:09 (Fig. 73.8).

Another rhythm strip was automatically recorded at 15:55:53 (Fig. 73.9), presumably because of the rapid, irregular rhythm and associated ectopic activity. Finally, a rhythm strip is shown at 21:56:13 (Fig. 73.10) when the computer probably interpreted the tracing, mistakenly, as representing ventricular ectopic beats. Close inspection suggests that the baseline irregularity is in fact due to artifact.

Full-Disclosure Strips

Many insurance carriers now require full disclosure as a prerequisite for maximal financial compensation. The obvious benefit of full disclosure is that it enables the interpreter to review any or all events of the day. The interpreter can also print out a full-size rhythm strip of any abnormality not initially recognized by the computer or technician. Interpretation of full-disclosure tracings probably seems like an overwhelming task to the uninitiated; however, this need not be the case.

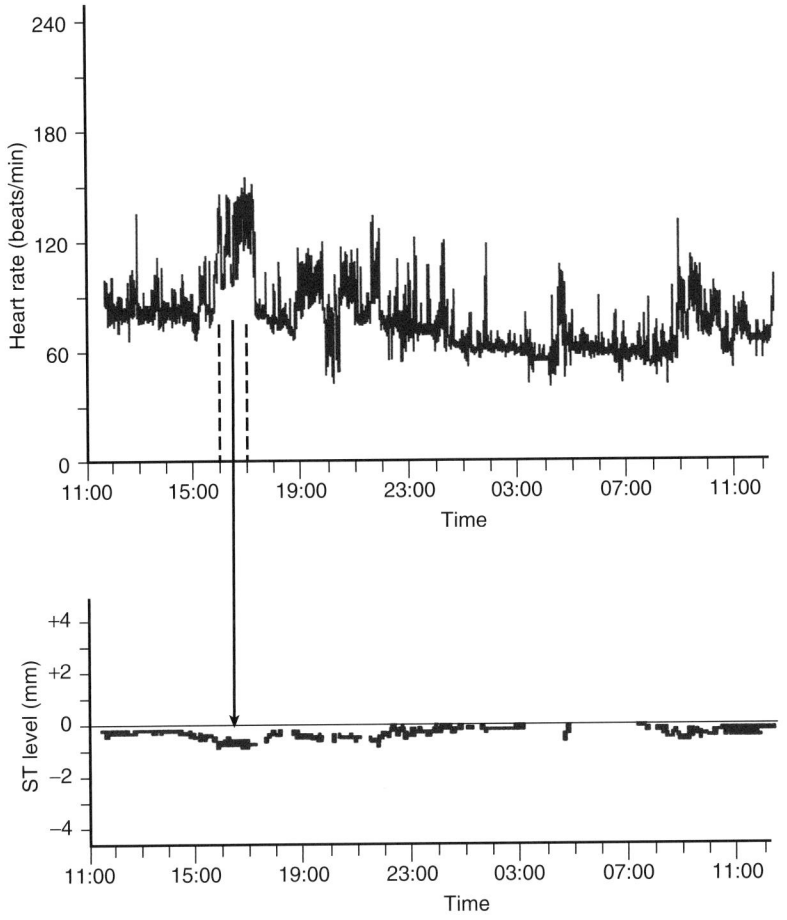

Fig. 73.4 Heart rate and ST segment trend analysis during Holter monitoring.

Time	Heart Rate			S/T		Tachy EPS	Brady EPS	Pause EPS	SVE	Iso. abn.	Coup.	Succ. abn.	Pat. event
	Avg	Max	Min	LEV	SLP								
11:00	87	105	70	−0.4	−02	0	0	0	0	5	0	0	0
12:00	82	105	62	−0.4	−02	0	0	0	0	64	0	0	0
13:00	80	139	63	−0.4	−01	0	0	0	1	40	0	0	0
14:00	81	114	68	−0.4	−02	0	0	0	0	67	0	0	0
15:00	94	153	63	−0.8	−09	3	0	0	2	176	0	0	1
16:00	129	160	89	−1.0	−17	8	0	0	10	235	0	0	0
17:00	83	159	67	−0.4	−04	4	0	0	3	71	0	0	0
18:00	82	136	63	−0.2	−01	2	0	0	0	57	0	0	0
19:00	85	141	37	−0.4	−01	4	3	38	1	79	0	0	0
20:00	87	129	44	−0.4	−02	4	0	19	0	86	0	0	0
21:00	84	144	50	−0.4	−06	4	0	0	1	62	0	0	0
22:00	73	126	51	−0.2	−03	0	0	0	1	51	0	0	0
23:00	73	124	56	−0.2	−03	0	0	0	0	32	0	0	0
00:00	62	94	43	0.0	−04	0	0	0	0	9	0	0	0
01:00	61	122	53	0.0	−05	0	0	0	0	16	0	0	0
02:00	58	81	39	0.0	−04	0	1	0	2	9	0	0	0
03:00	58	110	36	0.0	−05	0	1	0	0	6	0	1	0
04:00	63	105	42	0.0	−03	0	0	0	0	7	0	1	0
05:00	58	91	50	0.0	−03	0	0	0	1	4	0	0	0
06:00	56	91	39	0.0	−03	0	1	0	0	3	0	0	0
07:00	56	99	38	0.0	−03	0	1	0	1	4	0	0	0
08:00	87	137	53	−0.4	−01	0	0	0	1	23	0	0	0
09:00	72	101	55	−0.2	−01	0	0	0	0	20	0	0	1
10:00	70	93	48	−0.2	−01	0	0	0	1	13	0	0	0
11:00	70	105	55	−0.2	−03	0	0	0	0	5	0	0	0
Avg	75			−0.2	−04	1	0	2	1	48	0	0	0
TOTAL						29	7	57	25	1144	0	2	2

Fig. 73.5 Hourly summary for 24 hours Holter study. *Abn.*, Abnormality (i.e., primarily premature ventricular contractions); *Avg*, average; *Brady*, bradycardia; *Coup.*, couplets; *EPS*, events per section; *Iso.*, isolated; *LEV*, level above (+) or below (−) baseline in mV; *max*, maximum; *min*, minimum; *pat.*, patient; *S/T*, ST segment; *SLP*, slope; *Succ.*, successive; *SVE*, supraventricular ectopy; *Tachy*, tachycardia. Boxed values are maximum or minimum for 24 hours.

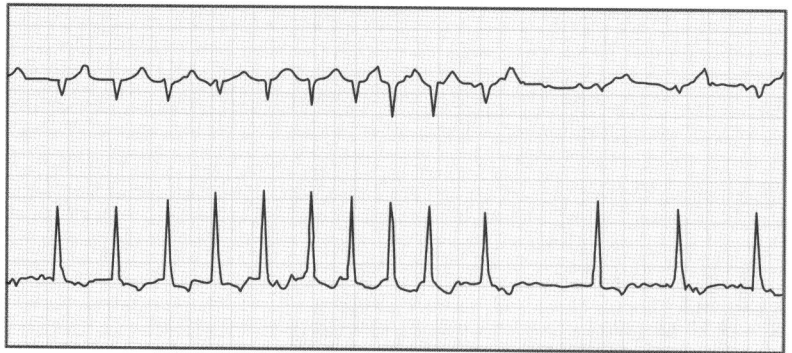

Fig. 73.6   Selected rhythm strip at 13:03:20.

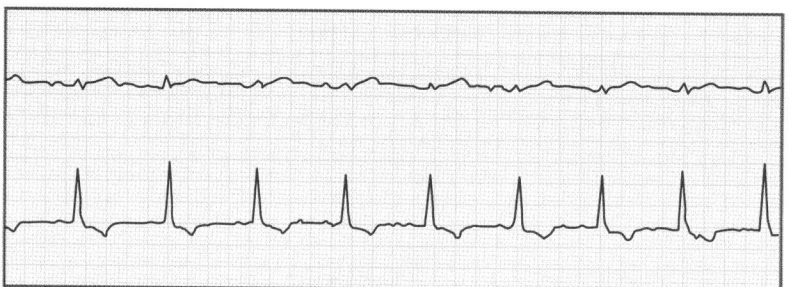

Fig. 73.7   Selected rhythm strip at 15:03:20.

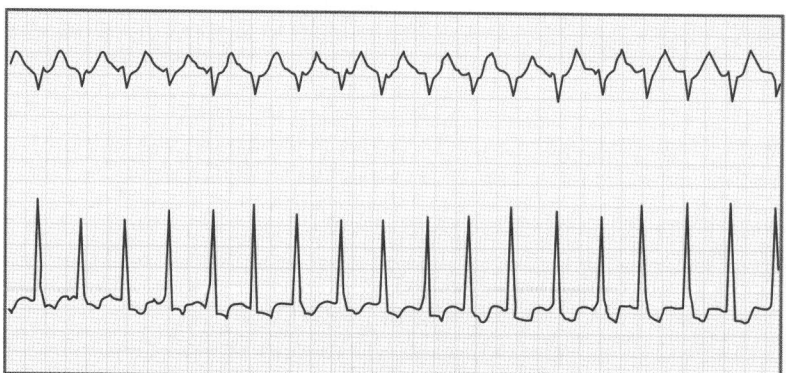

Fig. 73.8   Selected rhythm strip at 15:51:09.

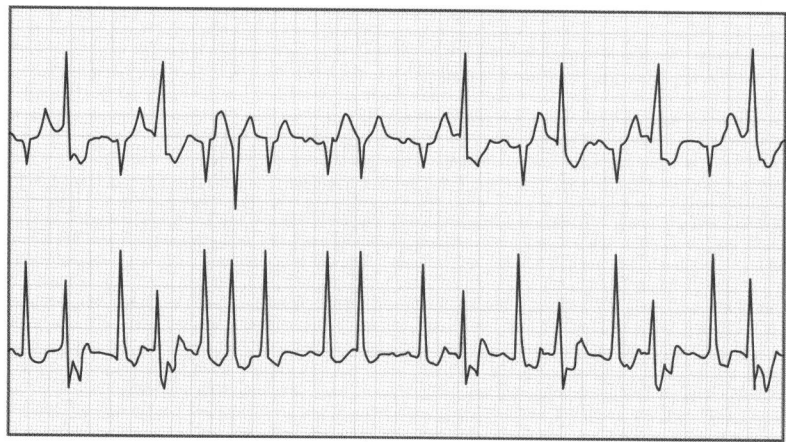

Fig. 73.9   Selected rhythm strip at 15:55:53.

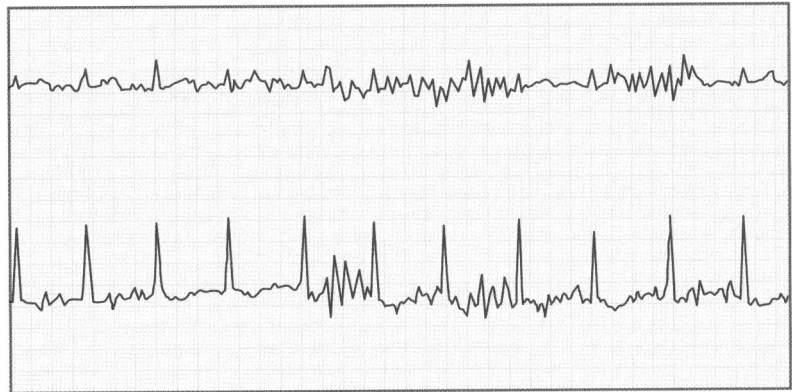

Fig. 73.10   Selected rhythm strip at 21:56:13.

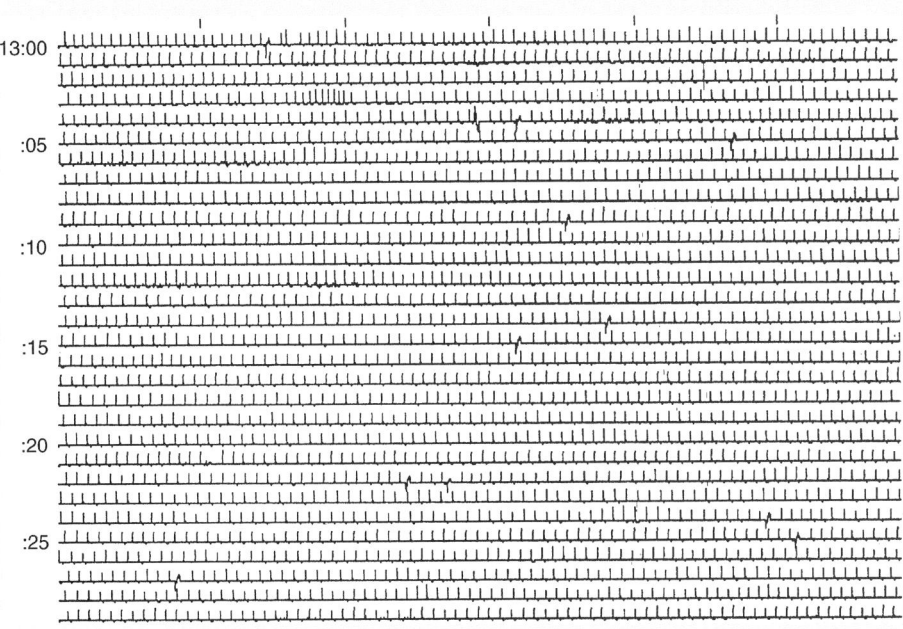

Fig. 73.11   Full-disclosure strip between 13:00 and 13:29.

For orientation to full-disclosure tracings, portions of three pages from the case example Holter study are displayed. Normally, each page contains a miniaturized account of a full hour of Holter recording from a single monitoring lead. One minute of recording is represented by each of the 60 lines on the page. Due to the space constraints of this chapter, only half of a page (30 minutes) is used for each demonstration. Thus the period from 13:00 to 13:29 is shown in Fig. 73.11; from 15:30 to 15:59 in Fig. 73.12; and from 16:00 to 16:29 in Fig. 73.13.

A scan of the first few lines of Fig. 73.11 shows how relatively easy it is to identify the short run of supraventricular tachycardia that occurs between 13:03:10 and 13:03:20. (See Fig. 73.6 for the full-size recording of this short burst of tachycardia.) Also note how easy it is both to spot the "different looking" (i.e., abnormal) beats, which are PVCs, and to see that the baseline undulation on the 13:06 and 13:12 lines is likely due to artifact.

With practice, self-discipline, and diligent concentration, the interpreter should be able to scan each page (i.e., each hour of recording) rapidly (in <10 seconds) and still be able to identify most major abnormalities on the page.

Now look at Fig. 73.12. The selected full-size rhythm strips previously reviewed demonstrated rapid atrial fibrillation at 15:51:09 (see Fig. 73.8) and rapid atrial fibrillation with frequent ventricular ectopy at 15:55:53 (see Fig. 73.9). Find these arrhythmias on the full-disclosure tracing.

Once a particular abnormality has been seen on the miniaturized full-disclosure tracing, it becomes relatively easy to spot other episodes of that abnormality. Thus, other short runs of frequent ventricular ectopy on lines 15:52, 15:53, 15:54, and 15:56 are easily noticed. Finally, look at Fig. 73.13. Note how the patient has a sustained tachycardia for a substantial portion of this monitoring period. Actual-size rhythm strips reveal persistence of rapid atrial fibrillation during much of the hour.

INTERPRETATION OF CASE STUDY

This case study is an excellent example of how to use a Holter system to determine the cause of a patient's symptoms. In this case, the patient's symptoms were not well defined; they included increasing dyspnea, weakness, and dizziness over the previous month. There were no palpitations, and apart from some non-specific ST-T wave changes, the patient's baseline ECG was unremarkable. With this history, although most clinicians would include a cardiac arrhythmia in the differential diagnosis, other

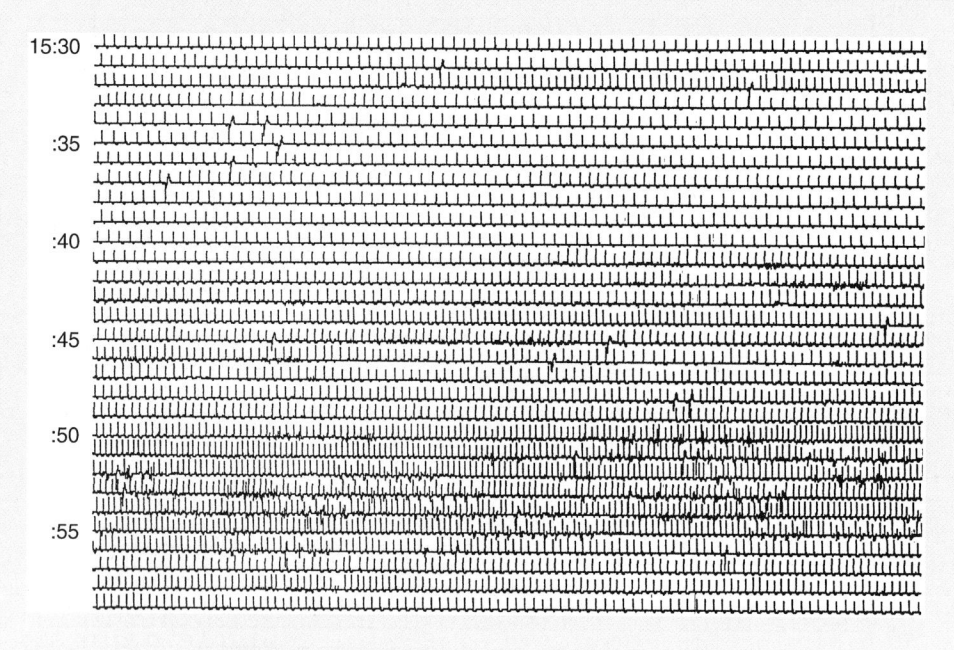

Fig. 73.12 Full-disclosure strip between 15:30 and 15:59.

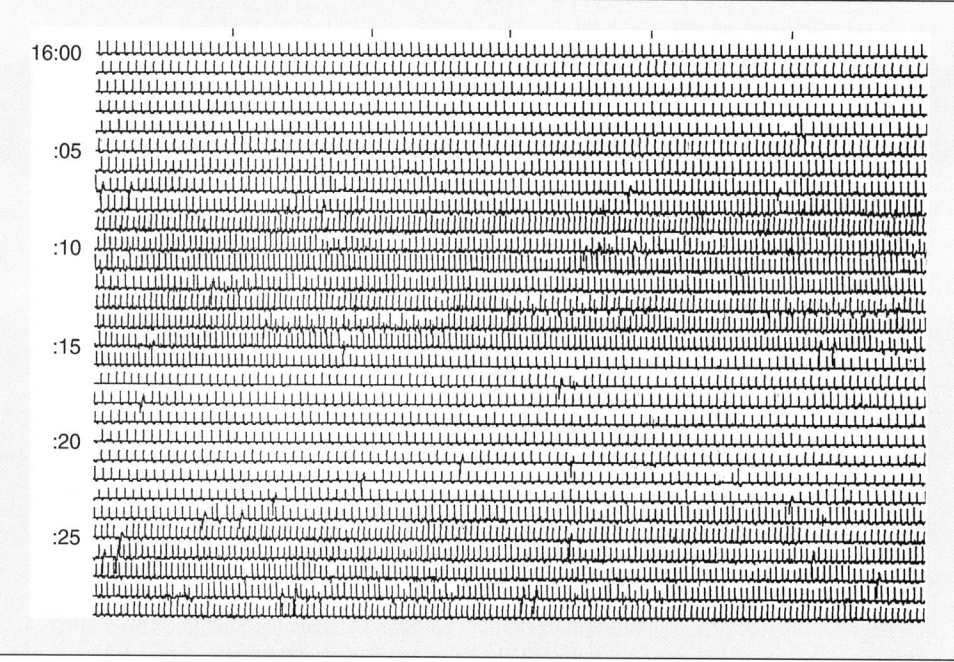

Fig. 73.13 Full-disclosure strip between 16:00 and 16:29.

possibilities would merit equal attention. However, after combining the results of this Holter data with the diary, there is little doubt as to the final diagnosis.

Final Interpretation

- Sinus rhythm with periods of sinus bradycardia down to 36 to 40 beats/min.
- Several episodes of rapid, paroxysmal atrial fibrillation lasting minutes, with heart rate up to 160 beats/min.
- Normal intervals.
- No significant ST segment shifts.

- Frequent PVCs (1144 recorded), especially during the waking hours—but virtually no repetitive forms.
- Diary indicates eight symptomatic episodes of weakness, dizziness, and dyspnea that correlate precisely with episodes of rapid, paroxysmal atrial fibrillation. These findings strongly suggest that the patient's symptoms are cardiac related (and should be treated).

Despite notation on the narrative summary of 57 pause episodes of up to 3.29 seconds, close inspection of full-disclosure tracings did not reveal any sustained pauses, suggesting that this count may reflect computer error.

Standard Interpretation Form

Use of a standardized form greatly facilitates the task of Holter interpretation. The two-sided form (Fig. 73.14) organizes the key components of an ambulatory ECG study. In so doing, it not only saves time, but also ensures consistency in interpretation, provides clear documentation of findings, and facilitates the reporting of information in an easily understood, clinically relevant manner.

Several components of this form deserve special mention. Because artifact is often misread by the computer as ventricular ectopy, a boxed commentary (under "Arrhythmias") is included on the form to reflect the interpreter's assessment of the computer's PVC count. The interpreter should indicate whether the count is likely to be accurate or a distortion produced by artifact. Rather than focusing exclusively on the number of ectopic beats, a greater emphasis is placed on whether the occurrence of premature atrial, junctional, and ventricular contractions (including couplets and runs of VT) is "common," "occasional," or "rare/absent."

Finally, it is occasionally difficult to convey the clinical relevance of a patient's diary, especially when attempting to correlate it with the ambulatory ECG recording. The relative scales on the back of the interpretation form can help to resolve this problem. They attempt to clarify the interpreter's assessment of the validity of the patient's diary and the correlation (if any) between patient symptoms and the arrhythmias that are noted.

Holter Interpretation Form

Name of patient _____ Name of clinician _____ Date _____

Indications for testing _____

Baseline ECG interpretation _____

_____

PR interval _____ QRS duration _____ QTc: Normal ☐ Borderline ☐ Long ☐

Trend analysis:

    The heart rate varies from ____ to ____, with an average rate of ____ /min .

    ST segment shifts? ☐ Yes   ☐ *No significant ST segment shifts*

    ST elevation? ☐ ST depression? ☐ with Sx? ☐ without Sx? ☐

    Estimated duration of ST segment depression over 24 hours _____.

Rhythm:

    Selected strips show the rhythm to be _____.

Arrhythmias:

Number of **PVCs** *counted* by computer _____.

    Probable *accuracy* of computer **PVCs count**

    Poor   Moderate   Excellent

    (PVCs are rare;   (Computer count

    much artifact present)   is probably accurate)

True **PVCs appear to be:** Common ☐ Occ ☐ Rare/absent ☐   Multiform? ☐

    Number of ventricular couplets _____. Couplets are: Common ☐ Occ ☐ Rare/absent ☐

    Number of runs of VT (≥ 3 PVCs) _____. VT runs are: Common ☐   Occ ☐ Rare/absent ☐

Number of **PACs/PJCs** counted by computer _____.

PACs/PJCs are: Common ☐ Occ ☐ Rare/absent ☐

Longest tachyarrhythmia (type) _____. *No significant tachyarrhythmias* ☐

    Duration of run _____. Time _____ with Sx? ☐ without Sx? ☐

Longest bradyarrhythmia (type) _____. *No significant bradyarrhythmias* ☐

    Duration of run _____. Time _____ with Sx? ☐ without Sx? ☐

Longest pause (type) _____. *No significant pauses* ☐

    Number of pauses >2.0 sec _____ at _____. with Sx? ☐ without Sx? ☐

Fig. 73.14 Standardized interpretation form. *PAC,* Premature atrial contraction; *PJC,* premature junctional contraction; *PVC,* premature ventricular complex. (Modified from Grauer K, Leytem B. A systematic approach to Holter monitor interpretation. *Am Fam Physician.* 1992;45:1641.)

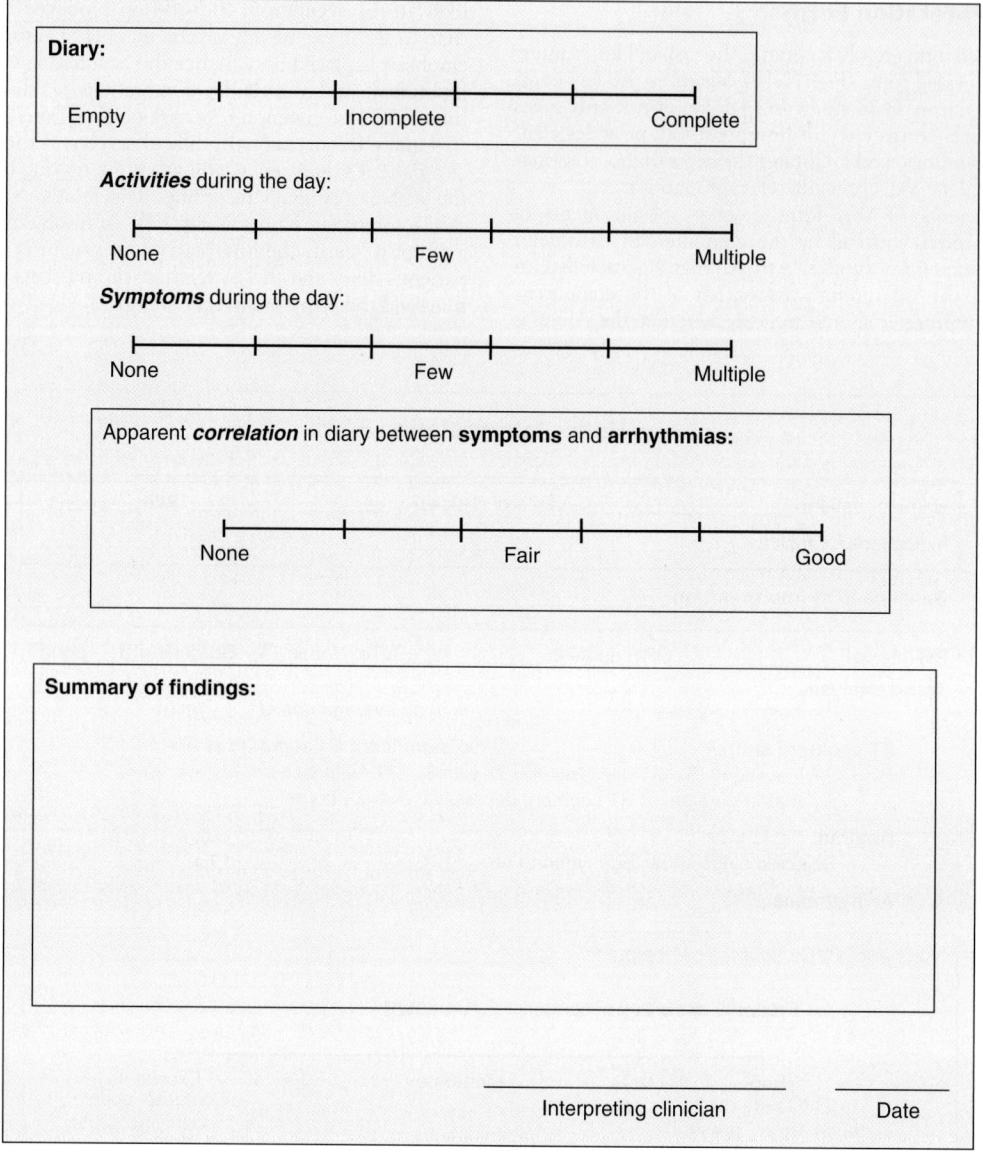

Fig. 73.14, Cont'd

CPT/BILLING CODES

93224   External electrocardiographic recording up to 48 hours by continuous rhythm recording and storage; includes recording, scanning analysis with report, review and interpretation by physician or other qualified health care professional

93225   Recording (which includes connection, recording, and disconnection)

93226   Scanning analysis with report

93227   Review and interpretation by a physician or other qualified health care professional

99228   External mobile cardiovascular telemetry with electrocardiographic recording, concurrent computerized real time data analysis and greater than 24 hours of accessible ECG data storage (retrievable with query) with ECG triggered and patient selected events transmitted to a remote attended surveillance center for up to 30 days; review and interpretation with report by a physician or other qualified health care professional

99229   technical support for connection and patient instructions for use, attended surveillance, analysis and transmission of daily and emergent data reports as prescribed by a physician or other qualified health care professional

93268   External patient and, when performed, auto activated electrocardiographic rhythm derived event recording with symptom-related memory loop with remote download capability up to 30 days, 24 hours attended monitoring; includes transmission, review and interpretation by a physician or other qualified health care professional

93270   Recording (includes connection, recording and disconnection)

93271   Transmission and analysis

93272   Review and interpretation by a physician or other qualified health care professional

93278   Signal-averaged electrocardiography (SAEG), with or without ECG

ICD-10-CM Diagnostic Codes

I25.2	Old MI (healed; past MI diagnosed on ECG, but currently no symptoms)
I25.812	Coronary atherosclerosis, of native coronary artery w/o angina
I25.719	Coronary atherosclerosis, of autologous vein bypass graft unspecified angina
I25.709	Coronary atherosclerosis, of artery bypass graft unspecified angina
I25.89	Chronic coronary insufficiency
I44.7	Left bundle branch block, complete
I45.10	Right bundle branch block
I45.6	Anomalous atrioventricular excitation (Wolff-Parkinson-White syndrome)
I45.9	Conduction disorder, unspecified
I44.0	Atrioventricular block, first degree
I44.1	Atrioventricular block, Mobitz type II
I44.1	Atrioventricular block, Mobitz type I (Wenckebach's)
I45.81	Long QT syndrome
I47.1	Paroxysmal supraventricular tachycardia
I47.2	Paroxysmal ventricular tachycardia
I46.9	Cardiac arrest
I48.91	Atrial fibrillation
I48.92	Atrial flutter
I49.01	Ventricular fibrillation
I49.40	Premature beats, unspecified
I49.1	Supraventricular premature beats
I49.49	Ventricular premature beats, contractions, or systoles
I49.5	Sinoatrial node dysfunction, sick sinus syndrome, sinus bradycardia
I49.8	Other rhythm disorder, including bradycardia
I50.1	Dyspnea, cardiac, also includes left-sided heart failure
R55	Syncope, presyncope and collapse, including vasovagal and cardiac syncope
R42	Dizziness
R00.2	Palpitations

Acknowledgment

The editors recognize the contributions of David Feller, MD, and Ken Grauer, MD, to this chapter in a previous edition of this text.

Suppliers

Holter systems

Mortara (Cardiac Science Diagnostics): www.mortara.com

GE Healthcare: www2.gehealthcare.com/portal/site/usen/menuitem.d9d1e5260a507013d6354a1074c84130/?vgnextoid=15466f6bba930210VgnVCM10000024dd1403RCRD&plCode=205&pcChannelObj=Diagnostic+ECG&pcChannelId=e9fda52fcea2d110VgnVCM100000258c1403

Philips Medical Systems: www.healthcare.philips.com/main/products/cardiography/products/holter/holter.wpd

Preevent recorders ("loop recorders")

Lifewatch (Instromedix): http://www.lifewatch.com

NOTE: The authors recommend a system from a company with a proven track record. Many companies have come and gone over the years. Often, the companies with a proven track record also produce equipment for other procedures, such as ECG stress testing. Choosing such a company may simplify service contracts.

Recommended Reading

Abbott AV. Diagnostic approach to palpitations. *Am Fam Physician.* 2005;71:743.

Biffi A, Pelliccia A, Verdile L, et al. Long-term clinical significance of frequent and complex ventricular tachyarrhythmias in trained athletes. *J Am Coll Cardiol.* 2002;40:446.

Cain ME, Anderson JL, Arnsdorf MF, et al. Signal averaged electrocardiography: ACC expert consensus document. *J Am Coll Cardiol.* 1996;27:238.

Crawford MH, Bernstein SJ, Deedwania PC, et al. ACC/AHA guidelines for ambulatory electrocardiography: executive summary and recommendations. A report of the american college of cardiology/american heart association task force on practice guidelines (Committee to revise the guidelines for ambulatory electrocardiography) developed in collaboration with the north american society for pacing and electrophysiology. *Circulation.* 1999;100:886.

Dewey FE, Kapoor JR, Williams RS, et al. Ventricular arrhythmias during clinical treadmill testing and prognosis. *Arch Intern Med.* 2008;168:225.

Echt DS, Liebson PR, Mitchell LB, et al. Mortality and morbidity in patients receiving encainide, flecainide, or placebo. The Cardiac Arrhythmia Suppression Trial. *N Engl J Med.* 1991;323:781.

Enseleit R, Duru R. Long-term continuous external electrocardiographic recording: a review. *Europace.* 2006;8:225.

Gibson CM, Ciaglo LN, Southard MC, et al. Diagnostic and prognostic value of ambulatory ECG (Holter) monitoring in patients with coronary heart disease. *J Thromb Thrombolysis.* 2007;23:135.

Issa ZF, Miller JM, Zipes DP. Sinus node dysfunction. In: Issa ZF, Miller JM, Zipes DP, eds. *Clinical Arrhythmology and Electrophysiology: A Companion to Braunwald's Heart Disease.* 2nd ed. Philadelphia: Elsevier; 2012:164–174.

January CT, Wann LS, Alpert JS, et al. 2014 AHA/ACC/HRS guideline for the management of patients with atrial fibrillation: a report of the american college of cardiology/american heart association task Force on practice guidelines and the heart rhythm society. *Circulation.* 2014;130:e199–e267.

Kennedy HL, Whitlock JA, Sprague MK, et al. Long-term follow-up of asymptomatic healthy subjects with frequent and complex ventricular ectopy. *N Engl J Med.* 1985;312:193.

Kinlay S, Leitch JW, Neil A, et al. Cardiac event recorders yield more diagnoses and are more cost-effective than 48-hour Holter monitoring in patients with palpitations: a controlled clinical trial. *Ann Intern Med.* 1996;124:16.

Rothman SA, Laughlin JC, Seltzer J, et al. The diagnosis of cardiac arrhythmias: a prospective multi-center randomized study comparing mobile cardiac outpatient telemetry versus standard loop event monitoring. *J Cardiovasc Electrophysiol.* 2007;18:241.

Runser LA, Gauer RL, Houser A. Syncope: evaluation and differential diagnosis. *Am Fam Physician.* 2017;95(5):303–312B.

Semelka M, Gera J, Usman S. Sick sinus syndrome: a review. *Am Fam Physician.* 2013;87(10):691–696.

Sivakumaran S, Krahn AD, Klein GJ, et al. A prospective randomized comparison of loop recorders versus Holter monitors in patients with syncope or presyncope. *Am J Med.* 2003;115:1.

Solomon H, DeBusk RF. Contemporary management of silent ischemia: the role of ambulatory monitoring. *Int J Cardiol.* 2004;96:311.

Spragg DD, Tomaselli GF. Principles of electrophysiology. In: Kasper D, Fauci A, Hauser S, et al., eds. *Harrison's Principles of Internal Medicine.* 19th ed. New York: McGraw-Hill; 2014.

Van Gelder IC, Groenveld HF, Crijns HJ, et al. Lenient versus strict rate control in patients with atrial fibrillation. *N Engl J Med.* 2010;362:1363–73.

Weber B, Kapoor W. Evaluation and outcomes of patients with palpitations. *Am J Med.* 1996;100:138.

ECG Interpretation And Cardiac Arrythmias

Dubin D. *Rapid Interpretation of EKGs.* 6th ed. Tampa, FL: Cover Publishing; 2000.

Grauer K. *A Practical Guide to ECG Interpretation.* St Louis: Mosby; 1998.

Huff J. *ECG Workout: Exercises in Arrhythmia Interpretation.* 7th ed. Philadelphia: Lippincott Williams & Wilkins; 2016.

Thaler M. *The Only EKG Book You'll Ever Need.* 9th ed. Philadelphia: Lippincott Williams & Wilkins; 2019.

Van Gelder IC, Groenveld HF, Crijns HJ, et al. Lenient versus strict rate control in patients with atrial fibrillation. *N Engl J Med.* 2010;362: 1363–1373.

CHAPTER 74

STRESS ECG TESTING

Grant C. Fowler • Michael A. Altman • John H. Haynes

Seventeen million Americans have known coronary artery disease (CAD); however, in more than half of those diagnosed with CAD, the diagnosis will follow a bad outcome—namely, a myocardial infarction (MI) or sudden cardiac death. Approximately one-fourth of all deaths in the United States are due to heart disease, and almost 400,000 deaths per year are caused by CAD, the leading cause of death in both sexes. Stress electrocardiography testing (ET) is a safe (<1 event per 10,000 properly selected patients) and cost-effective method for diagnosing CAD, and it is probably the most cost-effective method to screen for and manage CAD. ET can also be used to reassure patients about the safety of exercise and to customize their exercise prescription.

For the diagnosis of CAD, although much money, time, and effort have been spent designing and applying other tests with greater sensitivity, the sensitivity of ET exceeds 90% (perhaps 95%) for significant CAD—meaning patients with CAD who develop left ventricular (LV) dysfunction at a low level of exertion. This is usually due to left main CAD or multivessel disease with resultant left main equivalent CAD. These are patients where an intervention has often been proven beneficial. Supporting this, several studies have examined the incremental value of exercise myocardial perfusion imaging compared with ET for diagnosis and risk stratification of CAD. In an analysis of these studies, the modest incremental benefit of imaging did not appear to justify its cost (which has been estimated at $20,550 per additional patient correctly classified). Consequently, the American College of Cardiology (ACC) and the American Heart Association (AHA) continue to recommend a stepwise strategy for diagnosing CAD in patients with an intermediate pretest likelihood, using an ET as the initial test, and not an imaging procedure. If the patient is able to exercise, has a normal resting ECG, and is not taking digoxin ET is recommended as the first test* (ACC/AHA/ASNC [American Society of Nuclear Cardiology] guidelines and multiple others). (See Chapter 76, Stress Echocardiography, for testing patients with an abnormal resting ECG or who are taking digoxin, and for a dobutamine echo protocol for patients unable to exercise.) Recent data (Duvall, 2015) also suggest that there is no value added with imaging (no improvement in mortality) if a patient has an exercise capacity of 10 metabolic equivalents (METs, which will be explained later) or achieves their predicted maximal heart rate (MHR) during the stress test. A randomized controlled trial (Shaw, 2011) also found no event-free survival benefit over 2 years from use of myocardial perfusion imaging versus stress testing in symptomatic women at intermediate risk of CAD.

With medical management of CAD more successful than ever, primary care clinicians' skills in managing it have become more important. Performing ET is one method of maximizing these skills. In fact, using the Duke Treadmill Score (DTS) or nomogram for positive tests, primary care clinicians can now risk-stratify and provide prognoses for CAD as well as their cardiologist colleagues. It should be noted that in the latest guidelines (Wolk et al, 2014)

from AHA/ACC for management of stable CAD, an ET is a reasonable test for risk stratification in patients with a normal resting ECG and who are able to exercise. In part, these guidelines are based on "the simplicity, lower cost, and widespread familiarity with the performance and interpretation of the standard ET." Also, when patients divided into risk groups using ET have been studied with imaging (Gibbons, 1999), few patients (<5%) who have a low-risk DTS (≤1% annual cardiac mortality rate) are identified as high risk after imaging, and thus the cost of identifying these patients again argues against routine imaging. Those patients identified as high risk (≥3% per year annual cardiac mortality) should probably be referred directly for cardiac catheterization and a possible intervention (again, see Chapter 76, Stress Echocardiography). *Only those patients with an intermediate DTS (>1% and <3%) seem to benefit from an imaging study to further differentiate low-risk patients from those who might benefit from an intervention.*

Performing a maximal ET provides additional information for predicting prognosis, such as exercise capacity and heart rate in recovery (HRR, explained later), even if the ECG cannot be used for interpretation or predicting prognosis (as might be the case with ECGs with baseline ST segment abnormalities by themselves or as associated with right or left bundle branch block). From a study of 7163 patients (Diaz, 2001) with known or suspected CAD undergoing myocardial perfusion imaging at the Cleveland Clinic and for whom a DTS could not be calculated (e.g., patient taking digoxin, resting ECG abnormalities), the independent prognostic values of exercise capacity and HRR were determined. Patients were followed for an average of 6.7 years. When compared with results of myocardial perfusion imaging, exercise capacity and HRR provided additional prognostic information, and abnormal exercise capacity and HRR portended a higher risk of mortality than the results of the myocardial perfusion test in nonrevascularized patients. Since these studies were published, the reproducibility and durability of HRR as a risk factor have been challenged, but additional studies such as the St. James Women Take Heart study (Gulati, 2003) have demonstrated that the exercise capacity alone is a potent predictor of prognosis, perhaps independent of the DTS, in women.

Primary care clinicians can also use ET to screen certain asymptomatic individuals. Such screening may be especially helpful for diabetic patients, firefighters, many individuals about to undergo noncardiac surgery, high-risk patients after revascularization, patients about to undergo cardiac rehabilitation, and older individuals with risk factors about to embark on a vigorous exercise program. Although the ACC/AHA are not currently recommending ET to screen all asymptomatic individuals, there is emerging evidence that this will be a future growth area for the procedure. A negative ET demonstrating good exercise capacity combined with a negative multidetector (>32-slice) computed tomography (CT) angiogram, which has a false negative rate of less than 2% for CAD, will likely be our ultimate screening test for CAD. In the meantime, with estimates that 12% of deaths in the United States are due to a lack of exercise, any method to motivate patients to exercise should be beneficial. ET can be used not only to reassure individuals of the

---

*ET has a higher specificity in the absence of 1 mm ST segment depression due to resting ST segment changes, LV hypertrophy, and digoxin use.

safety of exercise, but also to customize their exercise prescription. After almost every ET, patients should receive some type of customized exercise prescription based on their true MHR, their exercise (aerobic) capacity, and the test results. We now know that almost every patient benefits from an exercise program, even cardiac transplant recipients. In fact, of all the options available, exercise may be the single best method for lowering risk, and may be superior to any single medication.

Benefits of performing ET in the primary care clinician's office include having test results immediately available, improving communication and referral patterns to cardiologists, and improving primary care clinicians' ECG reading skills. Clinicians performing ET also naturally improve their understanding of CAD pathophysiology and exercise physiology. With results immediately available, patient satisfaction usually improves and liability from failure to diagnose should decrease. Using the DTS when there is a positive study, the patient can immediately be counseled from an outcomes or prognosis perspective. Such data allow a patient to make a truly informed decision before undergoing a major procedure, such as coronary artery bypass graft (CABG) surgery. With personalized data, the patient can weigh his or her known risks of forgoing surgery against available known risks of an intervention, with interventions reserved for those who choose to accept the risks.

For primary care clinicians covering emergency departments or urgent care centers, or those working as hospitalists, knowledge of a patient's recent ET results may be helpful for perioperative evaluation. Management of patients with an acute chest pain syndrome is also greatly facilitated when ET is available. For many patients, after myocardial damage has been excluded by serial blood tests, resolution of the symptoms, and stabilized ECG findings, an ET may be useful for triage or early discharge. National guidelines with algorithms are available, and they have been demonstrated to be both safe and useful. For hospitalists, the diagnostic cardiac test is often what is preventing hospital discharge for a patient; many hospitalists now supervise ETs or cardiac imaging tests, which are then interpreted by cardiologists (often via digital transmission). This process often hastens hospital discharge.

PHYSIOLOGY OF EXERCISE ECG TESTING

Performing exercise increases total oxygen demand and consumption, with the amount of increase depending on the size of the muscles used and the exercise intensity. In other words, the larger the muscles used, the more oxygen is consumed; oxygen consumption also increases as the intensity of exercise increases. In response to increased exercise and oxygen demand, the body increases ventilation, oxygenation, cardiac output, and oxygen extraction by tissues. Unless there is moderate to severe lung disease (e.g., chronic obstructive pulmonary disease) or a process severely limiting oxygen transport or extraction (e.g., severe anemia), cardiac output is usually the factor limiting an individual's maximal exercise capacity. In turn, the limiting factor for cardiac output in those with obstructive CAD is usually coronary blood flow. Maximal exercise capacity can therefore be limited by coronary blood flow. Maximal exercise capacity is usually quantified by measuring or estimating an individual's maximal oxygen uptake (VO_2 max). In other words, maximal exercise with large muscles can be used both to estimate VO_2 max and to evaluate limitations in coronary blood flow.

Cardiac output is calculated by multiplying the stroke volume by the heart rate; therefore, increases in either the stroke volume or the heart rate will increase the cardiac output. Increasing the stroke volume is generally a more efficient method of increasing cardiac output (i.e., requires less oxygen). However, unless the patient is taking a β-blocker, the initial physiologic response to increased demand for cardiac output is usually an increase in heart rate. (In part, this is why β-blockers work in treating angina; they block the increase in heart rate when there is a need for increased cardiac output, thereby forcing an increase in stroke volume and keeping the increased myocardial

oxygen demand to a minimum). Therefore, as intensity of exercise increases, heart rate increases up to a maximum (MHR), usually when the patient has reached maximal voluntary effort or exertion.

In normal patients there is a linear relationship between myocardial oxygen demand and heart rate. In other words, the faster the heart rate, the more oxygen the heart requires. Because the heart rate continues to increase as exercise intensity increases, so does the myocardial oxygen demand. MHR can be crudely estimated based on age (i.e., 220 − age in years ≅ MHR) or by using graphs; however, true MHR is best determined with a maximal ET. MHR is the heart rate noted when the patient is at maximal voluntary effort (voluntarily fatigued), and this number should be recorded and given to the patient at the completion of each ET when the clinician is customizing an exercise prescription.

There is also a linear relationship between myocardial oxygen demand and systolic blood pressure (SBP). In other words, the higher the SBP, the harder the heart is working (and consequently the higher the myocardial oxygen demand). Therefore, one method of quantifying the overall myocardial oxygen demand is to multiply the SBP by the heart rate; the product obtained is the *double product*, also known as the *rate-pressure product* (RPP). At any given moment, the RPP is an estimate of total myocardial oxygen demand. As long as the demand has not exceeded the supply, it is also a measure of total myocardial oxygen uptake or consumption. In other words, the higher the RPP, the more oxygen the heart is demanding; if supply matches demand, the higher the capacity of the heart to deliver its own oxygen.

When the myocardium demands more oxygen, there are two options for supplying it: the coronary arterial flow increases or the extraction of oxygen from the flow increases. As it turns out, increased myocardial oxygen demand during exercise is met primarily through an increase in coronary arterial flow rather than through increased oxygen extraction. This is because myocardial tissue is very efficient at extracting almost all of the available oxygen from the coronary arterial flow, even in the resting state. Therefore, coronary arterial flow is usually the limiting factor for cardiac oxygenation. This is especially true in patients with obstructive CAD.

With gradually increasing levels of exertion in the patient with obstructive CAD, a threshold is eventually reached where the heart's supply of oxygen cannot meet the demand. At this threshold, the heart becomes ischemic, initially at the subendocardial layer. With subendocardial ischemia, the patient usually demonstrates ECG changes in the form of ST segment depression. Usually, and eventually, this is followed by chest discomfort (i.e., angina). Because in most cases the ischemia is due to a fixed lesion, patients develop these ECG changes at about the same threshold or RPP every time. Granted, this can vary according to other factors such as inotropic state, but by and large it remains the same. If symptoms occur, they also usually occur at the same RPP and follow the same pattern every time. In other words, angina caused by a fixed lesion does not radiate only into the left arm one day and into the right arm another day. Sure, it can extend to additional areas (e.g., up into the neck, further down the arm) as the RPP increases, but it does not move from side to side. If ST segment depression occurs (due to ischemia) and angina is not experienced, the diagnosis is silent ischemia.

Large muscles, such as leg muscles, rapidly increase the oxygen demand with increased exertion (i.e., using a treadmill or bicycle). VO_2 max is the greatest amount (i.e., volume) of oxygen that a person can extract from inspired air while performing dynamic exercise. It is usually reached when the patient is in the anaerobic range. Measuring VO_2 max is a method of quantifying maximal exercise capacity, and VO_2 max varies with body weight, heredity, sex, and exercise habits. It often decreases progressively with age, but this decrease may be purely due to inadequate exercise habits. Performing aerobic exercise on a regular basis may maintain a constant VO_2 max for life. There is a nearly linear relationship between VO_2 max and the maximum cardiac output; therefore the VO_2 max is a measure of the functional capacity of the cardiovascular system. It can be measured directly with inspired/expired gas analysis or more easily estimated from a maximal ET. As mentioned previously, in those with CAD, VO_2 max may be limited by coronary blood flow. With prognosis data discussed later in this chapter, estimating VO_2 max is very important for predicting outcomes from a cardiovascular perspective.

Basal oxygen consumption, or 1 MET, defines the amount of oxygen an average individual consumes sitting at rest, which is approximately 3.5 mL/kg per minute (i.e., 1 MET = 3.5 mL/kg per minute O_2). VO_2 max is often quantified as a multiple of the basal oxygen consumption in METs. For instance, walking 2 miles per hour (mph) on level ground requires approximately 2 METs. Walking 4 mph on level ground requires approximately 4 METs. Moderately active young men usually have a VO_2 max of at least 42 mL/kg per minute, or 12 METs. This means they are able to consume 12 times the amount of oxygen that they consume at rest. Obviously, METs can also be used as a conversion factor between types of exercise. Charts are available (Fig. 74.1) to estimate a patient's exercise capacity or maximal METs by cross-referencing MET levels with different daily activities. This estimate may then be used to predict performance before placing a patient on a treadmill. Performing a maximal ET remains one of the more accurate and available methods of estimating maximal METs. An individual's maximal METs, whether determined on a bicycle or a treadmill, have significant management and prognosis implications if the person has CAD. Even if the test is positive for CAD, achieving certain MET thresholds can be very reassuring for prognosis.

During a maximal ET, a perceived exertion scale (PES) may be helpful for monitoring the patient. The PES is similar to a pain scale; however, the patient quantifies "effort" or "exertion" instead of "pain" during the test. Originally studied and published with a scale from 5 to 20 (with 20 being the subjective maximum that an individual could work and 5 being minimal or no work at all), it has now been modified. Most clinicians in the United States use a range from 1 to 10 (Box 74.1) for the PES. Although it is a subjective measurement, in most patients the PES level is very reproducible; in other words, if they were asked to repeat the ET in 2 weeks, they would report the same PES level at the same workload and duration for both ETs. Interestingly, their heart rate is also usually very similar at a given PES. As a result, a PES target can be given to most patients to use as part of their exercise prescription. This replaces the patient's need to check the heart rate during exercise, and anything that simplifies an exercise prescription will, it is hoped, increase the chance of adherence/compliance.

A positive test result occurs when subendocardial ischemia causes *ST segment depression* on the ECG tracing. Because this is a "global" phenomenon, meaning much of the subendocardial layer is affected, it is almost always seen in more than one lead; if suspected, it should be confirmed in an area of the ECG tracing where the baseline is relatively flat. True ischemia will cause ST segment depression for at least three beats in a row, and the ischemia (ST changes) usually persists or worsens during the recovery period. ST segment depression occurs because ischemia impairs the sodium/potassium adenosine triphosphatase (Na^+/K^+ ATPase) pump at the cellular level. Such an ST segment change can also be noted in patients taking digitalis, whose site of action is the Na^+/K^+ ATPase pump. When the pump is affected, there is a resultant change in the Na^+/K^+ intracellular gradient and a subsequent small shift in polarity. This shift in polarity is what is noted on the ECG tracing as ST segment depression.

With exercise-induced ischemia, ST segment depression becomes a global phenomenon, meaning it involves the entire subendocardium. When one area of the subendocardium becomes ischemic, there is a "failsafe" mechanism that responds, meaning this subendocardial segment reduces its workload or shuts down before becoming permanently damaged. As a result, the remaining and surrounding subendocardium must work harder to compensate. This surrounding area subsequently becomes ischemic, and a domino effect occurs, cascading around the entire subendocardium. Consequently, ST segment depression is usually seen in multiple leads. In fact, this is such a global phenomenon that the coronary vessels involved cannot be predicted based on the leads that demonstrate ST segment depression. (If knowledge of the coronary vessels involved or the total burden of ischemia is needed, an imaging test [myocardial perfusion or echocardiogram, see Chapter 76, Stress Echocardiography] should be added to the stress test.)

If the entire wall of the myocardium (full thickness) becomes ischemic, such as from severe CAD, ST segment elevation may be noted. It may appear very similar to that seen with a transmural/ST-elevation infarct or a ventricular aneurysm. In this situation, unless the clinician is certain that the finding is due to a ventricular aneurysm (e.g., associated with Q waves, the clinician previously diagnosed/managed the infarct, an aneurysm was noted on an echocardiogram or during cardiac catheterization), the ET should be stopped. If either transmural ischemia or a new infarction is

---

VETERANS' ADMINISTRATION SPECIFIC ACTIVITY QUESTIONNAIRE

Instructions to patient: Draw a line below the activities done routinely with minimal or no symptoms, such as shortness of breath, chest discomfort, and fatigue.

1 MET:	Eating, getting dressed, working at desk
2 METs:	Taking a shower
3 METs:	Walking slowly on a flat surface for one or two blocks
	Doing a moderate amount of work around the house, such as vacuuming, sweeping the floors, or carrying groceries
4 METs:	Doing light yard work (e.g., raking leaves, weeding, light carpentry, or painting)
5 METs:	Walking briskly (5 mph), dancing
6 METs:	Playing nine holes of golf carrying own clubs, performing heavy carpentry or mowing lawn with a push mower
7 METs:	Playing tennis (singles), carrying 60 lbs
8 METs:	Moving heavy furniture
	Jogging slowly, climbing stairs quickly, carrying 20 lbs upstairs
9 METs:	Bicycling at a moderate pace, sawing wood, jumping rope (slowly)
10 METs:	Swimming briskly, bicycling up a hill, walking briskly uphill, jogging 6 mph
11 METs	Skiing cross-country
	Playing basketball (full court)
12 METs:	Running briskly and continuously (level ground, 8-minute miles)
13 METs:	Rowing, backpacking, any competitive activity, including those that involve intermittent sprinting, running competitively

Fig. 74.1 Veterans Administration Specific Activity Questionnaire MET, Metabolic equivalents.

BOX 74.1 Perceived Exertion Scale
0: Nothing at all
0.5: Very, very weak
1: Very weak
2: Weak
3: Moderate
4: Somewhat strong
5–6: Strong
7–9: Very strong
10: Very, very strong

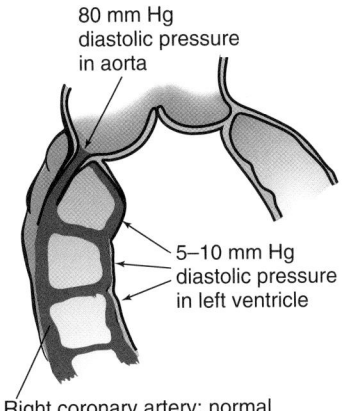

80 mm Hg
diastolic pressure
in aorta

5–10 mm Hg
diastolic pressure
in left ventricle

Right coronary artery: normal

Fig. 74.2 Normal myocardial perfusion. Note perfusion gradient is from 80 mm Hg to 5 to 10 mm Hg. (Modified from Ellestad MH. *Stress Testing: Principles and Practice*. 4th ed. Philadelphia: FA Davis, 1996.)

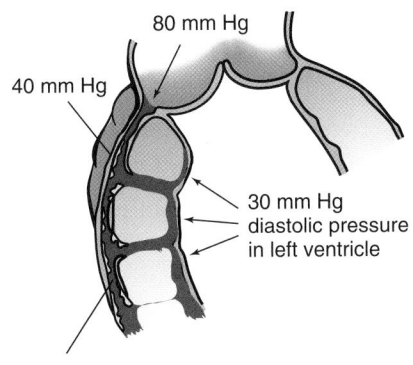

80 mm Hg

40 mm Hg

30 mm Hg
diastolic pressure
in left ventricle

Right coronary artery: CAD

Fig. 74.3 Myocardial perfusion in coronary artery disease (CAD). Note perfusion gradient is only from 40 to 30 mm Hg. (Modified from Ellestad MH. *Stress Testing: Principles and Practice*. 4th ed. Philadelphia: FA Davis; 1996.)

occurring, the potential for an arrhythmia is very high. However, transmural ischemia is rare in a community setting. In almost all positive ETs, ST segment depression is what is noted, the same as with what used to be called a *subendocardial infarct*. The subendocardial layer is usually the first to become ischemic because it is the "watershed" area of the heart, or the farthest from the arteries that are located in the epicardium (Figs. 74.2 and 74.3).

Certain other conditions may also make it difficult to perfuse the subendocardial layer, even in the absence of CAD. Normally, the subendocardial layer is perfused during diastole and relies on perfusing "downhill" from 80 to 90 mm Hg of diastolic blood pressure (DBP) to an area where there is only 5 to 10 mm Hg pressure (i.e., end-diastolic pressure [EDP]). Thus, the pressure gradient, or the difference between "uphill" DBP and "downhill" EDP, is 80 or 90 minus 5 or 10, which is a 75 to 85 mm Hg difference (DBP − EDP = 75 to 85). If hypertension is poorly controlled, EDP may be elevated, reaching as high as 30 to 40 mm Hg, with the resultant drop in this pressure gradient (DBP − EDP = 40 to 60). In other words, there is much less "pressure" for blood to flow "downhill." Anything causing diastolic dysfunction, such as profound hypothyroidism or severe valvular disease, can also result in an elevated EDP, a decreased pressure gradient, and a false-positive ET result. A thickened myocardial wall, as seen in LV hypertrophy, can make it physically difficult to perfuse through the wall, thereby causing subendocardial ischemia and ST segment depression, even without CAD. In addition to

physical causes, other situations that can cause false-positive results include hypokalemia and other electrolyte imbalances. Inadequate potassium prevents the Na$^+$/K$^+$ ATPase pump from functioning correctly, resulting in ST segment changes. As mentioned previously, digitalis may also result in ST segment depression, even at physiologic doses.

Normal and Abnormal Clinical Responses to Exercise ECG Testing

1. A gradual increase in heart rate to MHR where MHR is estimated by the formula 220 − age (i.e., 220 − age ≅ MHR). If a heart rate of 120 beats/min cannot be achieved, the diagnosis of *chronotropic incompetence* is possible (see the Interpretation section).
2. Return of the heart rate to resting values within the first few minutes after exercise. The rate of return of the heart rate to its resting value depends partly on the exercise conditioning effect on vagal tone (i.e., frequent exercise or "being fit" increases vagal tone). An abnormal HRR is declared when the heart rate does not decrease by at least 12 beats/min in the first minute of recovery (see the Interpretation section).
3. A gradual rise in SBP. SBP is usually the highest at maximal workload. A drop in SBP during the exercise phase of ET, especially if it drops below the resting standing SBP, may indicate severe CAD. It is an indication to stop the test. An SBP greater than 214 mm Hg is designated a *systolic hypertensive response to exercise* (see the Interpretation section).
4. A return of SBP and DPB to resting values by approximately 3 minutes after exercise. Failure of return of either blood pressure (BP) to normal by 3 minutes of recovery is also a *hypertensive response to exercise* (see the Interpretation section).
5. Minimal change or a decrease in DBP during exercise. During exercise, the legs produce lactic acid, one of the most potent vasodilators known. As a result, a significant amount of blood volume flows into the legs. Because of this vasodilation, and the effects of exercise on Korotkoff sounds, diastolic pressure by auscultation can decrease all the way to zero in normal individuals. An increase in DBP of more than 10 mm Hg is also designated a *diastolic hypertensive response to exercise* (see the Interpretation section).
6. Most patients perceive an increase by 1 to 3 points on the PES per stage of exercise. Few ever admit to reaching a full 10 points on the scale. For many patients, PES level increases rapidly from 7 to 9 when they are near maximal effort.

INDICATIONS

Comprehensive, national guidelines are available regarding the appropriate use of ET, including special cases and situations (e.g., diabetic patients, patients in the emergency department, firefighters, before noncardiac surgery, before and after revascularization). There are three general indications for ET: *diagnosing CAD* (especially helpful when evaluating atypical chest pain and screening asymptomatic patients at significant risk), *managing CAD*, and *providing data for an exercise prescription* while determining exercise capacity and safety. In certain cases, several of these indications are evaluated during the same procedure. An example would be a patient who has an intermediate pretest likelihood and is found to have CAD when performing the ET. Because the diagnosis has now been made, if it is considered safe to continue the procedure, prognosis may also be determined. Exercise capacity (i.e., aerobic capacity) could be determined if the patient were allowed to complete a maximal ET; this is helpful for determining prognosis. Based on the results, an exercise prescription along with cardiac rehabilitation might be initiated. In this manner, the diagnosis, management (e.g., prognosis, cardiac rehabilitation), and exercise prescription could all be determined during the same test.

General Indications

Diagnosing CAD

- Patients with an intermediate (20% to 70%) pretest probability of CAD based on sex, age, and symptoms (see Determination of Pretest Likelihood, later; Fig. 74.4 and Table 74.1).
- Asymptomatic patients with multiple risk factors, possible myocardial ischemia on ambulatory ECG monitoring, or a high-risk coronary calcium score from electron-beam computed tomography (EBCT) scan. It should be noted that asymptomatic patients are included in the graphs and tables (see Fig. 74.4 and Table 74.1) used to determine pretest probability.

    NOTE: For diagnosing CAD, determining pretest likelihood is important. This is explained for patients with symptoms by examples in the section Determination of Pretest Likelihood.

Managing CAD*

- Patients with known or highly probable CAD, for initial assessment or for a change in symptoms.
- For risk assessment, to evaluate medical management, prior to revascularization or possibly prior to noncardiac surgery.
- After MI or revascularization (especially those at high risk), for prognostic assessment, activity prescription, evaluation of medical therapy, or cardiac rehabilitation.
- Demonstrating proof of ischemia before revascularization.
- Consider for perioperative evaluation of patients with CAD *only* if results would change management.

Determining Exercise Prescription Data, Exercise Capacity, and Safety

- Evaluation of exercise-related symptoms, including possible exercise-induced arrhythmias* (also see Chapter 73, Ambulatory Electrocardiography: Holter and Event Monitoring).
- Graded treadmill ET is one of the best methods for determining an individual's MHR. The exception is the elite athlete, for whom a sport-specific ET should be used.
- True MHR must be known to calculate a training heart rate range, which can be used as a guideline for aerobic training.
- An ET can also be used to estimate an individual's VO_2 max, which is helpful in determining the current level of fitness or conditioning.

Specific American College of Cardiology/American Heart Association Indications

For the sake of completeness of this chapter, most of the indications for ET in adults from the ACC/AHA guidelines will be listed. Guidelines for special cases (e.g., children, ET with expired ventilatory gas analysis) may be found in the ACC/AHA reference or on the AHA website (www.americanheart.org), under "Science and Professional, Scientific Publications, Scientific Statements." The ACC/AHA guidelines use the following classification system for indications:

Class I: Conditions for which there is evidence and/or general agreement that a given procedure or treatment is useful and effective.
Class II: Conditions for which there is conflicting evidence and/or a divergence of opinion about the usefulness/efficacy of a procedure or treatment.
Class IIa: Weight of evidence/opinion is in favor of usefulness/efficacy.

Class IIb: Usefulness/efficacy is less well established by evidence/opinion.
Class III: Conditions for which there is evidence and/or general agreement that the procedure or treatment is not useful/effective and in some cases may be harmful.

Exercise ECG Testing in Diagnosis of Obstructive Coronary Artery Disease

Class I: Adult patients (including those with complete right bundle branch block [RBBB] or less than 1 mm of resting ST segment depression) with an intermediate pretest probability of CAD based on sex, age, and symptoms (see Determination of Pretest Likelihood, Fig. 74.4, and Table 74.1).
Class IIa: Patients with vasospastic angina.
Class IIb: Patients with a high or low pretest probability of CAD by age, symptoms, and sex; patients with less than 1 mm of baseline ST segment depression and taking digoxin; patients with ECG criteria for LV hypertrophy (LVH) and less than 1 mm of baseline ST segment depression.
Class III: Patients with the following baseline ECG abnormalities: preexcitation syndrome (i.e., Wolff-Parkinson-White [WPW] syndrome), electronically paced ventricular rhythm, greater than 1 mm of resting ST segment depression, complete left bundle branch block (LBBB); patients with a documented MI or prior coronary angiography demonstrating significant disease and who have an established diagnosis of CAD. (Note that for diagnostic purposes, ET may not be useful. However, overall risk for individuals can be determined from obtaining VO_2 max if it is deemed safe to test [see following sections Risk Assessment and Prognosis in Patients with Symptoms or a History of CAD, Exercise ECG Testing after Myocardial Infarction, and Exercise ECG Testing before and after Revascularization].)

Risk Assessment and Prognosis in Patients With Symptoms or a History of Coronary Artery Disease

Class I: Patients undergoing initial evaluation with suspected or known CAD. Patients with suspected or known CAD previously evaluated but now with a significant change in clinical status (specific exceptions noted in Class IIb). Low-risk patients with unstable angina (moderate or high likelihood of CAD with new-onset or progressive angina with walking) 8 to 12 hours after presentation or intermediate-risk unstable angina (prolonged [>20 minutes] or at-rest angina; patients with prior MI, CABG, atherosclerotic cerebrovascular disease [ASCVD], or peripheral artery disease; aspirin use; age older than 70 years; or troponins negative or slightly elevated [<0.1 mg/mL]) 2 to 3 days after presentation; both groups of patients with unstable angina should have been free of active ischemic or heart failure symptoms.
Class IIa: Intermediate-risk patients with unstable angina who have initial cardiac markers that are normal, a repeat ECG without significant change, cardiac markers that are normal 6 to 12 hours after the onset of symptoms, and no evidence of ischemia during observation.
Class IIb: Patients with the following resting ECG abnormalities: preexcitation (i.e., WPW syndrome), electronically paced ventricular rhythm, greater than 1 mm of resting ST segment depression, complete LBBB. Patients with a stable clinical course who undergo periodic monitoring to guide treatment.
Class III: Patients with severe comorbidity likely to limit life expectancy or candidacy for revascularization. Patients with high-risk unstable angina (prolonged, ongoing >20 minutes pain at rest; pulmonary edema; new or worsening mitral regurgitant murmur; new/worsening rales; hypotension; bradycardia; tachycardia; age older than 75 years; transient ST segment changes; or elevated troponin [>0.1 mg/mL]).

---

*Patients with LV dysfunction, history of recent (within 7 to 10 days) acute coronary syndrome, severe valvular (aortic) stenosis, or complex or life-threatening arrhythmias are considered a higher-risk group. Exercise testing for them should be performed in the hospital by a clinician with significant experience treating patients with CAD or with consultation by a cardiologist.

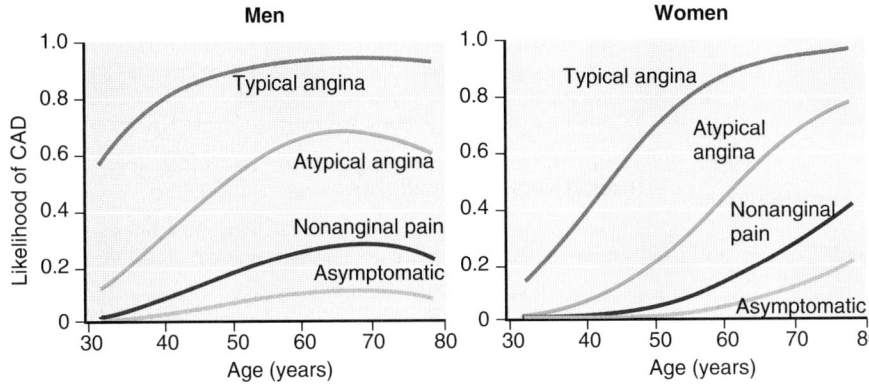

Fig. 74.4 Pretest likelihood of coronary artery disease (CAD). (Modified from Diamond GA, Forrester JS. Analysis of probability as an aid in the clinical diagnosis of coronary-artery disease. *N Engl J Med.* 1979;300:1350–1358.)

TABLE 74.1   Pretest Likelihood of Coronary Artery Disease Based on Symptoms

Age (yr)	Asymptomatic	Nonanginal Chest Pain	Atypical Angina	Typical Angina
Women				
35	0.3	1	4	26
45	1	3	13	55
55	3	8	32	79
65	8	19	54	91
Men				
35	2	5	22	70
45	6	14	46	87
55	10	22	59	92
65	12	28	67	94

Modified from Diamond GA, Forrester JS. Analysis of probability as an aid in the clinical diagnosis of coronary artery disease. *N Engl J Med.* 1979;300:1350–1358; and Fowler GC, Evans CH, Altman MA. Office procedures: exercise testing. *Prim Care* 1997;24:375–406.

Exercise ECG Testing After Myocardial Infarction

Class I: Before discharge for prognostic assessment, activity prescription, or evaluation of medical therapy (submaximal at about 4 to 7 days). Early after discharge for prognostic assessment, activity prescription, evaluation of medical therapy, and cardiac rehabilitation if the predischarge ET was not done (do a symptom-limited ET at about 14 to 21 days). Late after discharge for prognostic assessment, activity prescription, evaluation of medical therapy, and cardiac rehabilitation if the early ET was submaximal (do a symptom-limited ET at about 3 to 6 weeks).

Class IIa: After discharge for activity counseling or exercise training as part of cardiac rehabilitation in patients who have undergone coronary revascularization.

Class IIb: Patients with preexcitation syndrome (i.e., WPW syndrome), electronically paced ventricular rhythm, greater than 1 mm of resting ST segment depression, complete LBBB, digoxin therapy, LVH. Periodic monitoring in patients who continue to participate in exercise training or cardiac rehabilitation.

Class III: Patients with severe comorbidity likely to limit life expectancy or candidacy for revascularization. At any time after MI if there is uncompensated congestive heart failure (CHF), cardiac arrhythmia, or noncardiac conditions that limit the patient's ability to exercise.

Exercise ECG Testing in Asymptomatic Patients Without Known Coronary Artery Disease

Class I: None.

Class IIa: Evaluation of asymptomatic persons with diabetes mellitus who plan to start vigorous exercise (this indication has somewhat been superseded by evidence suggesting it is safe for a diabetic to begin a gradual exercise program if they remain asymptomatic and do not meet other indications for an ET).

Class IIb: Evaluation of patients with multiple risk factors as a guide to risk reduction therapy. Evaluation of asymptomatic men older than 45 years and women older than 55 years (or with two or more risk factors for CAD) planning to start vigorous exercise (especially if physically inactive), or involved in occupations in which impairment might affect public safety, or at high risk for CAD because of other diseases (e.g., peripheral vascular disease, chronic renal failure).

EDITOR'S NOTE: there are no outcome trials comparing preexercise stress test screening versus encouraging light exercise with gradual increases in exertion.

Class III: Routine screening of asymptomatic men or women.

NOTE: The class IIb indication evokes controversy because of the increased risk of false-positive results. However, with good clinical judgment or consultation of a table (see, e.g., Fig. 74.4, Table 74.1), the clinician may determine that the patient has a pretest likelihood as high as 15% to 20%, making the patient a reasonable candidate for ET.

Exercise ECG Testing for Valvular Heart Disease

Class I: In chronic aortic regurgitation, assessment of functional capacity and symptomatic responses in patients with a history of equivocal symptoms.

Class IIa: In chronic aortic regurgitation, evaluation of symptoms and functional capacity before participation in athletic activities. For prognostic assessment before aortic valve replacement in asymptomatic or minimally symptomatic patients with LV dysfunction.

Class IIb: Evaluation of exercise capacity in patients with valvular heart disease.

Class III: Diagnosis of CAD in patients with moderate to severe valvular disease or with baseline ECG abnormalities (preexcitation, electronically paced ventricular rhythm, >1 mm ST segment depression, complete LBBB).

Exercise ECG Testing Before and After Revascularization

Class I: Demonstration of proof of ischemia before revascularization. Evaluation of patients with recurrent symptoms suggesting ischemia after revascularization.

Class IIa: After discharge for activity counseling or exercise training as part of cardiac rehabilitation in patients who have undergone coronary revascularization.

Class IIb: Detection of restenosis in selected, high-risk (multivessel CAD, proximal left anterior descending CAD, family history of sudden cardiac death, diabetes, hazardous occupations, suboptimal results from the revascularization, saphenous vein graft,* CHF [congestive heart failure]*) asymptomatic patients within the first 12 months after percutaneous coronary intervention (PCI). Periodic monitoring of selected, high-risk asymptomatic patients for restenosis, graft occlusion, or disease progression.

---

*Although not listed as high risk in ACC/AHA guidelines, patients with these conditions have worse long-term outcomes postrevascularization.

Class III: Localization of ischemia for determining site of intervention (i.e., an imaging test is necessary for this). Routine, periodic monitoring of asymptomatic patients after PCI or CABG without specific indications.

Exercise ECG Testing for Investigation of Heart Rhythm Disorders

Class I: Identification of appropriate settings in patients with rate-adaptive pacemakers.

Class IIa: Evaluation of patients with known or suspected exercise-induced arrhythmias. Evaluation of medical, surgical, or ablative therapy in patients with exercise-induced arrhythmias (including atrial fibrillation).

Class IIb: Investigation of isolated ventricular ectopic beats in middle-aged patients without other evidence of CAD. Investigation of prolonged first-degree atrioventricular block or type I second-degree Wenckebach, LBBB, RBBB, or isolated ectopic beats in young patients considering participation in competitive sports.

Class III: Investigation of isolated ectopic beats in young patients.

Noninvasive Stress Testing Before Noncardiac Surgery

Class IIa: For patients with elevated surgical risk and excellent (>10 METs) functional capacity, it is reasonable to forgo further exercise testing with cardiac imaging and proceed to surgery.

Class IIb: For patients with elevated surgical risk and unknown functional capacity, it may be reasonable to perform exercise testing to assess for functional capacity if it will change management. For patients with elevated risk and moderate to good (≥4 METs to 10 METs) functional capacity, it may be reasonable to forgo further exercise testing with cardiac imaging and proceed to surgery. For patients with elevated risk and poor (<4 METs) or unknown functional capacity, it may be reasonable to perform pharmacologic testing with cardiac imaging to assess for myocardial ischemia if it will change management.

Class III: Routine screening with noninvasive stress testing is not useful for patients at low risk for noncardiac surgery.

Indications for Diabetic Patients

Because of a disproportionate burden of CAD in diabetic patients, the American Diabetes Association (ADA) has developed indications for cardiac testing in diabetic patients. They include the following:

1. Patients with typical or atypical cardiac symptoms
2. Patients with an abnormal resting ECG, especially if suggestive of ischemia or infarction

The ADA has recognized additional risk factors for obstructive CAD in diabetic patients, including renal disease (40% risk of coronary event in 5 years), evidence of other atherosclerotic disease (90% of their deaths are due to CAD), cardiovascular autonomic neuropathy (e.g., tachycardia, bradycardia, orthostatic hypotension, inadequate heart rate acceleration with exertion), older age, and female sex. Some experts recommend stress testing in all diabetics about to embark on a vigorous exercise program; however, no outcome studies have compared that approach versus encouraging light exercise initially with gradual increases in exertion.

Indications in the Emergency Department

Patient has or had chest pain and fulfills the following requirements:

1. Two sets of negative cardiac markers from each of two different types of assays (troponin, myoglobin, or creatinine kinase MB) at 4-hour intervals.
2. Preexercise 12-lead ECG shows no significant changes compared with original ECG at the time of presentation to the emergency department.
3. Absence of baseline (resting) ECG abnormalities that would preclude accurate assessment of the ET.

4. From admission to the time that results are available from the second set of cardiac markers, the patient has become asymptomatic, has had lessening of chest pain symptoms, or has had persistent atypical symptoms.
5. Absence of ischemic chest pain at the time of ET.

Indications for Firefighters

The following guidelines have been recommended by the National Fire Protection Association (NFPA) since 2000:

1. At age 40 years, periodic treadmill testing should be performed. The frequency should increase with age, but at a minimum the test should be done every 2 years.
2. At age 35 years, periodic treadmill testing should be performed for individuals with one or more coronary risk factors (premature family history [<55 years], hypertension, diabetes mellitus, cigarette smoking, and hypercholesterolemia [total cholesterol >240 mg/dL or high-density lipoprotein <35 mg/dL]).

Indications Before Noncardiac Surgery

Half of serious complications related to noncardiac surgery are cardiovascular. Although older patients have the highest risk of a cardiovascular complication with surgery, they also make up the largest group of patients undergoing surgery. Consequently, as the population ages, the cardiovascular risk of surgery will increase. Guidelines are available for screening patients before noncardiac surgery, and the ACC/AHA guidelines have been studied from an outcomes perspective. Box 74.2 provides some shortcuts for determining the need for noninvasive testing. Patients considered at low risk for surgery (<1% risk; e.g., especially those undergoing low-risk surgeries such as endoscopic, superficial, cataract, breast, ambulatory surgery) or with at least a fair functional/exercise capacity do not need further testing. If the patient has undergone revascularization, a thorough evaluation of the coronary arteries (e.g., ET, CT, or invasive angiogram) within the past 1 year, and there has not been a change in symptoms suggestive of ischemia, then according to ACC/AHA guidelines, no further testing is necessary. Conversely, for those considered at elevated risk for surgery (especially those undergoing high-risk surgery such as vascular surgery) with poor functional capacity (<4 METs) or unknown functional capacity, pharmacologic stress testing is reasonable if the results will change the management. If it will not

---

BOX 74.2 Shortcuts to Determine Indicators for Noninvasive Testing Before Noncardiac Surgery

No testing necessary if "Yes" to any of these four questions:
1. Is this low-risk surgery (i.e., estimated risk <1%)?
2. Does the patient have at least fair functional/exercise capacity (≥4 metabolic equivalents) and no symptoms?
3. Has the patient undergone revascularization within past 1 yr without a change in symptoms indicating ischemia?
4. Has the patient had a thorough cardiac evaluation (e.g., normal stress test, normal CT or invasive angiogram) within past 1 yr without a change in symptoms indicating ischemia?

Conversely, if elevated risk (>1%) and poor (<4 metabolic equivalents) or unknown functional/exercise capacity, noninvasive testing is reasonable if the results will change the management.

From 2013 Multimodality appropriate use criteria for the detection and risk assessment of stable ischemic heart disease. *J Am Coll Cardiol.* 2014;63(4):380–406, and ACC/AHA: 2014 Guidelines on perioperative cardiovascular evaluation and management of patients undergoing noncardiac surgery.

change the management, surgery should proceed following guideline directed medical therapy. It should be kept in mind that the goal of perioperative cardiac assessment is to detect the patient who would benefit from revascularization anyway, not just to get him or her through surgery. (See also Chapter 71, Preoperative Evaluation.)

Indications Before and After Revascularization (Percutaneous Coronary Intervention or Coronary Artery Bypass Graft)

In recent years, at least nine studies (BARI, CABRI, RITA-1, EAST, GABI, Toulouse, MASS, Lausanne, ERACI) have been published comparing PCI with CABG in patients with symptomatic CAD. Most were smaller studies, but BARI (the Bypass Angioplasty Revascularization Investigation) included 1829 patients, CABRI (Coronary Angioplasty vs. Bypass Revascularization Investigation) 1054 patients, and RITA-1 (first Randomized Intervention Treatment of Angina trial) 1011 patients. Although these trials differ slightly in their design and in the sort of patients who were included, the findings have all been remarkably consistent. At almost any point after initial treatment, whether the patient was treated with PCI or CABG, the rates of death or nonfatal MI are essentially the same. However, at the time of these trials, patients undergoing PCI usually received percutaneous transluminal coronary angioplasty (PTCA). Consequently, the reintervention rate was much higher among patients initially treated with PCI than for those undergoing CABG. There have been several additional trials (ERACI II, ARTS, and SOS) using stents for PCI and comparing outcomes with CABG. Although the reintervention rate remains higher with PCI than CABG, it has been significantly reduced with the use of stents. Mortality and nonfatal MI rates have again remained basically the same whether the patient is treated with PCI or CABG. The BARI trial 10-year follow-up data are now published; overall, the annual mortality rate was 2.8%. Consequently, there are going to be many patients having undergone revascularization living a long time.

From the BARI trial, we also learned about ET postrevascularization. Per protocol, at years 1, 3, and 5, 1388, 1208, and 1097 patients, respectively, underwent ET (Krone, 2001). Only 9% experienced angina when taking the ET, consistent with the "protocol-not symptom-driven" indication for ET. Overall, patients taking ET during the first 3 years of the study not only had a very low risk of mortality or MI, but very rarely did ET results affect management. The authors concluded that their study supported prior ACC/AHA guidelines, which do not recommend routine testing for 3 to 5 years after successful revascularization. The authors also speculated that exercise imaging would not have been helpful because such a low-risk population would have likely produced a large percentage of false-positive results. Consequently, only a fraction of those with a significant perfusion or echocardiographic defect would have had a subsequent event.

From the BARI trial, we also learned about risk stratification postrevascularization, including the risk of not undergoing ET according to protocol. In the asymptomatic population that did not follow the protocol, *not taking the ET* was a stronger predictor of mortality than the results of the ET in those who followed the protocol. Overall, nonexercisers had a 3- to 10-fold increased risk of mortality compared with exercisers. Diabetic nonexercisers who had undergone CABG had a 30% 5-year mortality rate. Even more striking, diabetic nonexercisers who *had undergone PTCA had a 52.4% 5-year mortality rate!*

We have long known that patients with CAD and poor functional or exercise capacity (<4 METs) are at high risk for cardiovascular events, and that is one of the criteria for considering ET or other noninvasive testing when evaluating patients before surgery. Such a low exercise capacity may correlate with what the BARI investigators found to be nonexercisers. Regardless, clinicians

should be aware that patients unable to exercise are at high risk postrevascularization.

How then should we monitor patients postrevascularization? Interestingly, of the nine studies comparing PCI with CABG, most used ET at various points to monitor patients for safety. Although the ACC/AHA guidelines suggest that an exercise imaging test is the preferred method of evaluating patients postrevascularization, the experts designing these trials considered ET to be adequate. Regardless, ACC/AHA guidelines also list certain situations where ET may or may not be helpful in the revascularized patient.

A reasonable use for ET in the revascularized patient is after discharge for activity counseling or exercise training as part of a cardiac rehabilitation program (indication: class IIa). Although the evidence is less well established, ET may be considered for the detection of restenosis in the first months after PTCA in selected, high-risk (Box 74.3), asymptomatic patients (indication: class IIb). And although the evidence is likewise less well established, ET may be considered for periodic testing for restenosis, graft occlusion, or disease progression in selected, high-risk (see Box 74.3), asymptomatic individuals postrevascularization (indication: class IIb).

What about the patient who has remained asymptomatic? The AHA/ACC suggests it may be appropriate to use a stress test 2 years after PCI and 5 years after CABG. They consider it rarely appropriate to perform stress testing or any other type of testing prior to these time frames if the patient remains asymptomatic. Fig. 74.5 incorporates the ACC/AHA guidelines for these patients as well as most asymptomatic patients postrevascularization. If the patient becomes symptomatic postrevascularization during these time frames, an ET or CT angiogram may be appropriate, but the preferred would be a stress imaging test. Fig. 74.6 provides an algorithm for these patients. As multislice CT angiography becomes more readily available, combining it with an ET may be the screening and diagnostic procedure of choice for revascularized patients.

Determination of Pretest Likelihood

If the goal of the ET is to exclude CAD, determining pretest likelihood will help decide whether ET is the indicated and proper procedure. For diagnostic purposes, ET is most valuable for patients with an intermediate (20% to 70%) pretest likelihood. Simple graphs and tables are available that require only three variables to estimate pretest likelihood in symptomatic individuals (see Fig. 74.4 and Table 74.1). With a pretest likelihood in the 20% to 70% range, an abnormal or positive ET result provides strong justification for additional studies, including invasive studies. A negative ET may provide justification for merely close observation with frequent follow-up visits.

The value of using this range (20% to 70%) is further demonstrated with a graph of post-test likelihood of CAD (Fig. 74.7). From this graph, the clinician should be able to see that the most information is obtained from patients with an intermediate pretest likelihood. In other words, for Fig. 74.7 the vertical gap is largest between what would be a positive ET and a negative ET for patients in the intermediate pretest range. In this group, positive studies are most clearly delineated from negative studies; therefore, the most information is obtained. For example, a patient with a pretest likelihood of 40% with 2 mm or more of ST segment depression now has more than an 85% post-test likelihood of CAD. Such a post-test likelihood would justify an invasive procedure. However, in the same patient, less than 1 mm of ST segment depression (a negative ET) lowers the risk of CAD to less than 20%. Close follow-up of this patient may be adequate.

For patients with a low (<20%) pretest likelihood, although there may be other benefits of performing ET (e.g., customized exercise prescription), positive studies are more likely to be bothersome false-positive results that lead to unnecessary patient anxiety and further expensive diagnostic testing. On the other hand, a negative test in the high pretest likelihood group (>70%) may not be sufficient to exclude CAD. For the young or very active

BOX 74.3 Criteria for High-Risk Patients Postrevascularization

Multivessel coronary artery disease
Proximal left anterior descending coronary artery disease
Personal or family history of sudden cardiac death
Diabetes
Hazardous occupations
Suboptimal results from the revascularization
Saphenous vein graft*
Congestive heart failure*

---

* Although not listed as high risk in ACC/AHA guidelines, patients with these conditions have worse long-term outcomes postrevascularization compared with other patients.

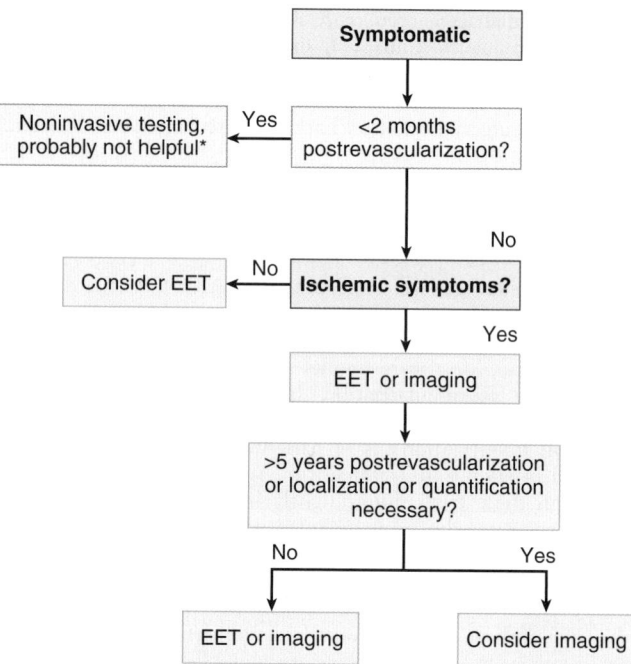

Fig. 74.6 Algorithm for exercise ECG testing (EET) in the symptomatic patient postrevascularization.*However, computed tomographic angiography may be helpful (≥16-slice post–coronary artery bypass graft; ≥32-slice post–percutaneous coronary intervention).

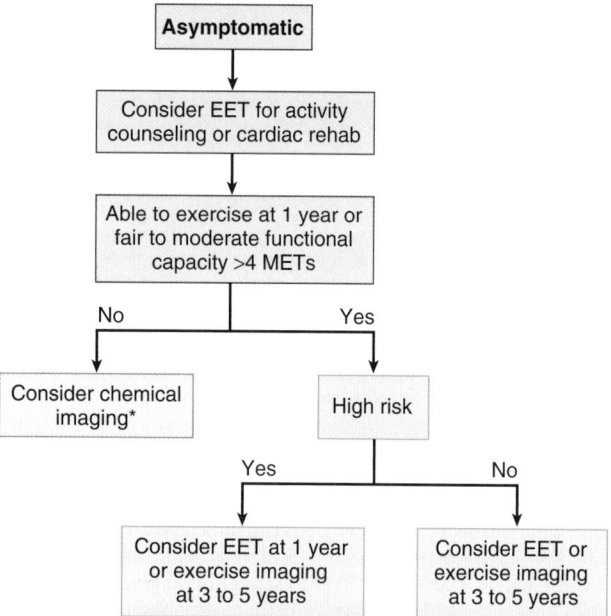

Fig. 74.5 Algorithm for exercise ECG testing (EET) in the asymptomatic patient postrevascularization. *Especially those with prior MI and/or renal insufficiency. MET, Metabolic equivalents.

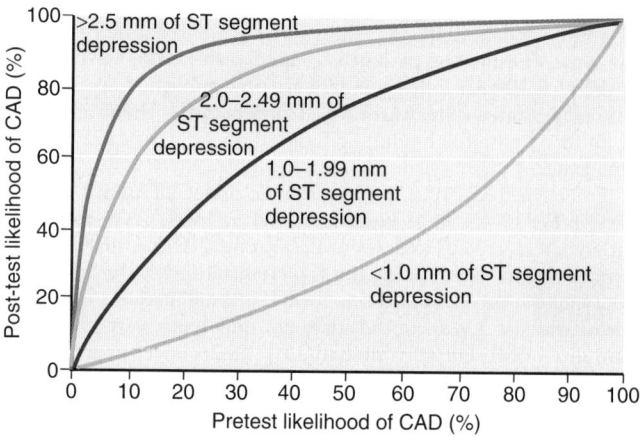

Fig. 74.7 Posttest likelihood of coronary artery disease (CAD) with positive (>1 mm ST segment depression) and negative (<1 mm ST segment depression) test results. (Modified from Epstein SE. Implications of probability analysis on the strategy used for noninvasive detection of coronary artery disease: role of single or combined use of exercise electrocardiographic testing, radionuclide cineangiography and myocardial perfusion imaging. *Am J Cardiol.* 1980;46:491–499.)

individual with a high pretest likelihood, coronary angiography is diagnostic and might be a more appropriate study. Again, to use an example, a patient with a pretest likelihood of 90% who has a positive study (>2 mm ST segment depression) has approximately a 96% post-test likelihood (using Fig. 74.7). This is only a 6% gain in probability, which is very little information. If the ET is negative, the patient still has a 75% likelihood of CAD. For diagnostic purposes, this probability certainly does not rule out CAD, so ET has apparently been of little value. (Again, even in patients for whom little diagnostic information is gained with ET, performing it may be helpful for other reasons, such as for managing CAD.)

Pretest likelihood can be estimated by a description of the chest pain and the patient's sex and age. *Typical angina* is described (Diamond and Forrester, 1979) as substernal, exertional, and relieved by rest or nitroglycerin. Chest discomfort with two of these three characteristics is *atypical angina*; with only one it is *nonanginal chest pain*. Using these three descriptions, pretest likelihood tables and their corresponding graphs (see Fig. 74.4 and Table 74.1) can be readily applied to determine pretest likelihood.

Although Fig. 74.4 and Table 74.1 also include asymptomatic patients, in general asymptomatic patients never reach an

intermediate (20%) pretest likelihood. This is why mass screening of the asymptomatic population with ET is not recommended. It should be kept in mind that the data for Fig. 74.4 and Table 74.1 were compiled from a community with an average number of risk factors (at the time, not many individuals had multiple risk factors). Therefore, for an individual patient with severe abnormalities in each of the risk categories, such as severe hypertension, heavy smoking, and severe hypercholesterolemia, or possessing multiple risk factors, pretest likelihood should be increased even if he or she is asymptomatic. Tables similar to Table 74.1 have been developed that attempt to adjust for severity of risk factors, but few experts use them because they have mostly been developed from patients seen in referral centers as opposed to the community.

In the asymptomatic group, the AHA risk calculator (available at http://hp2010.nhlbihin.net/atpiii/calculator.asp) can also be used to help quantify risk. Although the AHA risk calculator is designed to estimate absolute risk of a coronary event over the next 10 years, combining this result with clinical gestalt, clinicians can estimate which asymptomatic patients with risk factors would possibly reach the 20% pretest likelihood and benefit from ET. As newer risk factors (e.g., chronic kidney disease; elevated homocysteine, ferritin, high-sensitivity C-reactive protein, fibrinogen, apolipoprotein B, low-density lipoprotein [LDL] particle number, or lipoprotein A levels) are studied, the clinician may again have to use clinical judgment or gestalt to correctly estimate pretest likelihood for an individual with these risk factors.

CONTRAINDICATIONS

Absolute

- Very recent acute MI (within 2 days) or other acute cardiac event
- High-risk unstable angina
- Severe symptomatic LV dysfunction or uncontrolled symptomatic CHF
- Potentially life-threatening or uncontrolled cardiac arrhythmias causing symptoms or hemodynamic compromise
- Acute pericarditis, myocarditis, or endocarditis
- Symptomatic severe aortic stenosis
- Acute aortic dissection
- Acute pulmonary edema, embolus, or infarction

Relative

- Left main coronary stenosis
- Moderate stenotic valvular heart disease
- Third-degree atrioventricular block or second-degree Mobitz type II block without pacemaker
- Tachyarrhythmias or bradyarrhythmias
- Severe arterial hypertension (resting >200 mm Hg systolic or >110 mm Hg diastolic)
- Hypertrophic cardiomyopathy or other form of outflow obstruction
- Acute thrombophlebitis, deep venous thrombosis, or intracardiac thrombi
- Electrolyte abnormality
- Acute or serious general illness or infection
- Neuromuscular, musculoskeletal, or arthritic condition that precludes exercise
- Uncontrolled metabolic disease, such as diabetes, thyrotoxicosis, or myxedema
- Medication intoxication from drugs such as digoxin, sedatives, or psychotropic agents
- Patient inability or lack of desire or motivation to perform the test, including severe emotional distress
- Unavailability of advanced cardiac life support (ACLS) equipment or of an individual certified to perform ACLS

NOTE: In selected cases, a skilled cardiologist may perform testing for patients with one of these diagnoses (generally in a referral center). All are contraindications to ET in the office.

Contraindications in the Emergency Department

- New or evolving abnormalities on the resting ECG
- Abnormal cardiac markers
- Patient inability to perform exercise
- Worsening or persistent ischemic chest pain symptoms from admission to the time of ET
- Clinical risk profiling indicating coronary angiography is likely
- Any routine contraindications from the previous section

Additional Relative Contraindications

There are certain conditions that produce a study that is difficult to interpret or that will have results that add very little clinical information. Such relative contraindications include:

- Ventricular aneurysm
- Chronic infectious disease (e.g., mononucleosis, hepatitis, advanced human immunodeficiency virus infection)
- Fixed-rate pacemaker (rarely used)
- Advanced or complicated pregnancy
- Frequent or complex ventricular ectopy

EQUIPMENT

- A treadmill with adjustable speed and grade and adequate weight capacity: This is by far the most common equipment used for ET in the United States. Advantages include the ability to test most patients under the actual physiologic conditions of exercise. The most common types of exercises performed in the United States are walking and running. In addition, patient motivation wavers less during the treadmill test than with the bicycle ET. Disadvantages include the fact that the treadmill may be difficult to use for patients with lower extremity or low-back problems or for patients who are very obese. The equipment is also more expensive, causes more motion artifact, and is noisier than a bicycle ergometer.

  NOTE: If a treadmill is chosen, it should have a warm-up speed of about 0.5 to 1.5 mph, with testing speeds ranging from 2.0 mph up to 12 mph. For elite athletes, the speed may need to reach 15 mph. The slope or grades possible should range from 0% (flat) to 20%. If testing elite athletes, the grade may need to reach 25%. It should also be able to accommodate the patient's weight; capacity for some models is now 500 pounds.

- Bicycle ergometers: Bicycle ergometers use adjustable resistance and pedal frequency to exert the patient (Fig. 74.8). Advantages with the bicycle ergometer include easier-to-obtain BP measurements and the ability to terminate the test instantly. Many patients feel more secure sitting on the bicycle. Unfortunately, in the United States leg fatigue is common because most patients do not bike. In fact, as a result of leg fatigue the procedure often fails to determine VO_2 max. Bicycle ergometry also depends on motivation throughout its duration. As a result, if the patient can tolerate the treadmill, most US clinicians prefer it.
- Arm ergometer: The arm ergometer (Fig. 74.9) enables patients with severe orthopedic problems to be tested. However, muscle fatigue often occurs before the maximum heart rate is achieved.
- Continuous ECG monitor: A three- to six-lead model with a screen-freeze or capture/replay option is desirable (Fig. 74.10). Although previous models provided only 3 or 4 beats in each lead if 6 or more leads were monitored, most equipment now allows clear simultaneous monitoring of all 12 leads.
- 12-Lead ECG recorder: With modern equipment, the recorder also runs the treadmill. Recent developments for primary care offices (e.g., wider wheelbase) allow the recorder to be wheeled from room to room for routine ECGs. Interpretive packages for 12-lead ECGs are also convenient. Most equipment is now digital, allowing data to be filtered to provide a smooth baseline. However, it is important to avoid overfiltering the data and, in so doing, filtering out ST segment depression. Most models are now personal computer-based and can use either thermal paper or a laser printer. Many are compatible with electronic medical records.
- Sphygmomanometer, including various cuff sizes: A gauge manometer is adequate because the most important readings are those relative to resting pressures (not the absolute pressures).

  EDITOR'S NOTE: While automated equipment is available, most use the auscultatory method of measuring BP and do not know how to adjust to physiologic decreases in Korotkoff sounds as

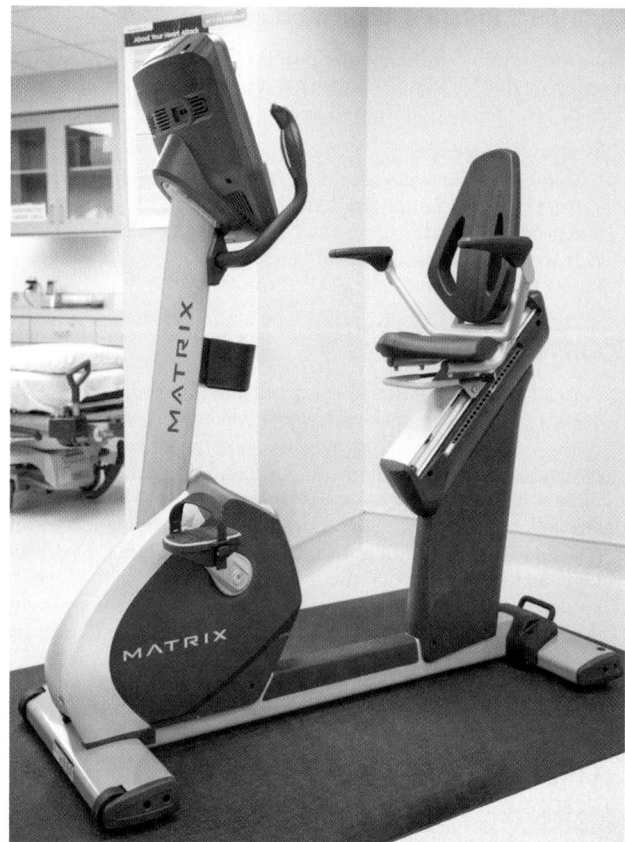

Fig. 74.8 Bicycle ergometer.

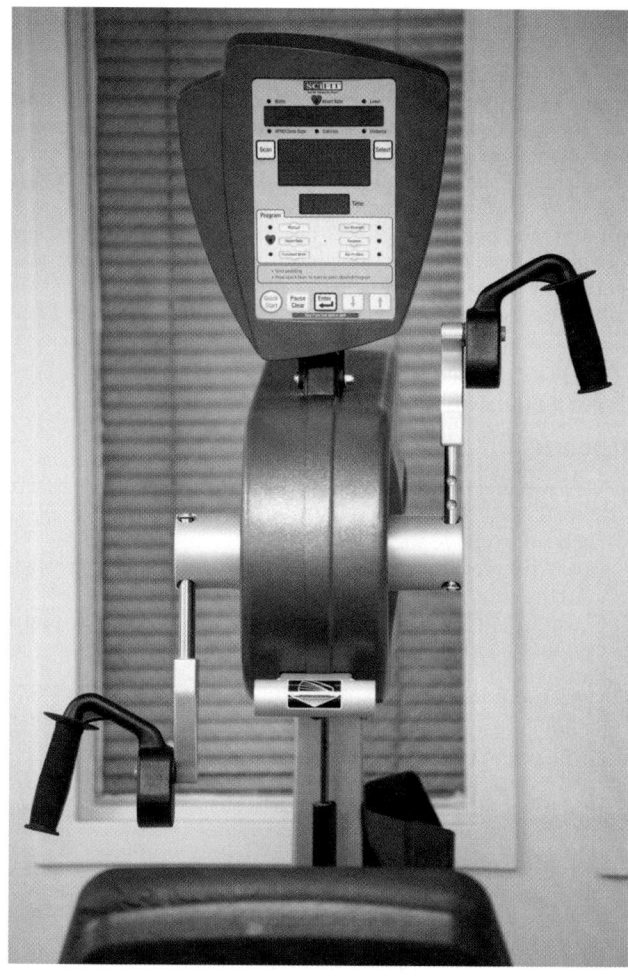

Fig. 74.9 Arm ergometer.

discussed previously. Consequently, most experts recommend measuring BPs manually.

- Stethoscope.
- Razor, rubbing alcohol, skin abrasive.
- Stress ECG electrodes: Disposable electrodes designed for ET (regular ECG electrodes are not adequate and will cause artifacts).
- Cables and belt: A disposable or washable belt is preferred because patients usually sweat.
- Emergency equipment (see Fig. 212.4 in Chapter 212, Anaphylaxis): Defibrillator; oxygen; airway, intubation, and suction equipment; and an emergency drug kit containing intravenous fluids, tubing, and medications to support ACLS protocols.

NOTE: It is also helpful to have a trained technician (Fig. 74.11) to assist during the procedure. Technician certification for ET is available through the American College of Sports Medicine. In many centers the technician prepares the patient; monitors the ECG, the patient's response to exercise, the heart rate, and the BP; and prepares the results for interpretation. For low-risk patients, the technician may actually perform the entire study without a physician being present (see ACC/AHA Clinical Competence Statement, 2000, which defines high risk patients for which a physician should be present). Otherwise, the clinician should examine the patient before, during, and after the procedure, confirm which protocol to use, and terminate the study. If present, the clinician should monitor the ECG tracing when the technician is taking BP readings. The clinician should interpret the final results.

Written Procedure Protocols

- Informed consent (see Appendix B for an explanation of the process and the sample consent form "Cardiac ET" available at www.expertconsult.com)
- Medical history, physical examination, handwritten report form (Fig. 74.12)

- Criteria for stopping ET (see the section on Test Termination Criteria, later)
- Emergency response plan (should be designed for every office and kept on file in the event of a complication from ET)
- Quality assurance plan, including calibration and testing of equipment

NOTE: All emergency equipment should be checked daily and medications should be checked weekly to monthly, depending on their use. The ET equipment should be inspected and calibrated periodically, based on manufacturer recommendations. ACLS certification cards should be kept on file along with the information and protocols listed previously.

PREPROCEDURE PATIENT PREPARATION

Deconditioned patients or those anticipated to have a poor exercise capacity (see the Veterans Administration [VA] Specific Activity Questionnaire, Fig. 74.1):

- In the debilitated, geriatric, or physically inactive population, it is safe to exercise to a heart rate of 100 beats/min, regardless of age, without prior testing. In those anticipated to have very poor exercise capacity, if they are not in urgent need of a cardiovascular intervention, it may be reasonable to help them increase their exercise capacity before undergoing an ET. This may be achieved with a walking program for several weeks or even months, four or five times a week, with a target heart rate of 100 beats/min. In this manner it may be possible to avoid some uninterpretable or incomplete tests.

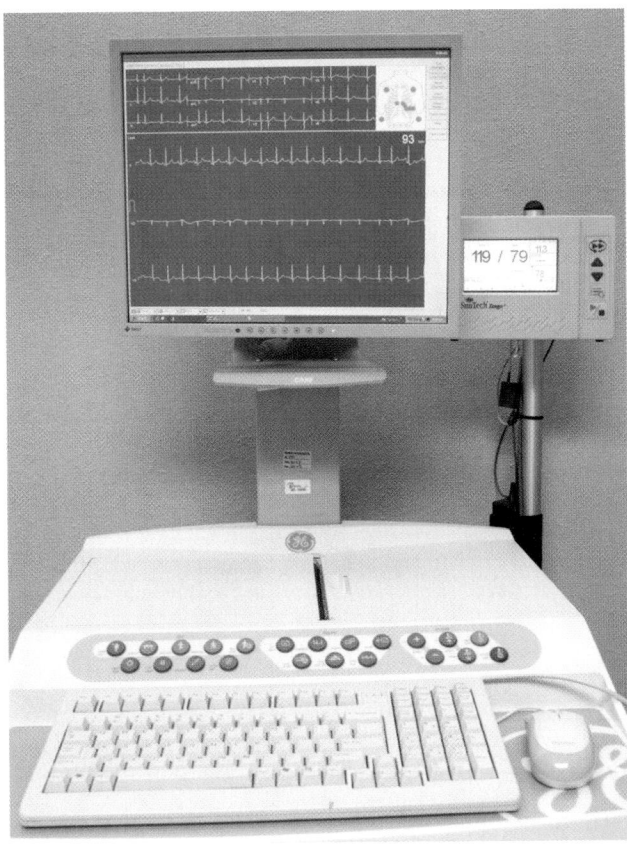

Fig. 74.10   ECG monitor.

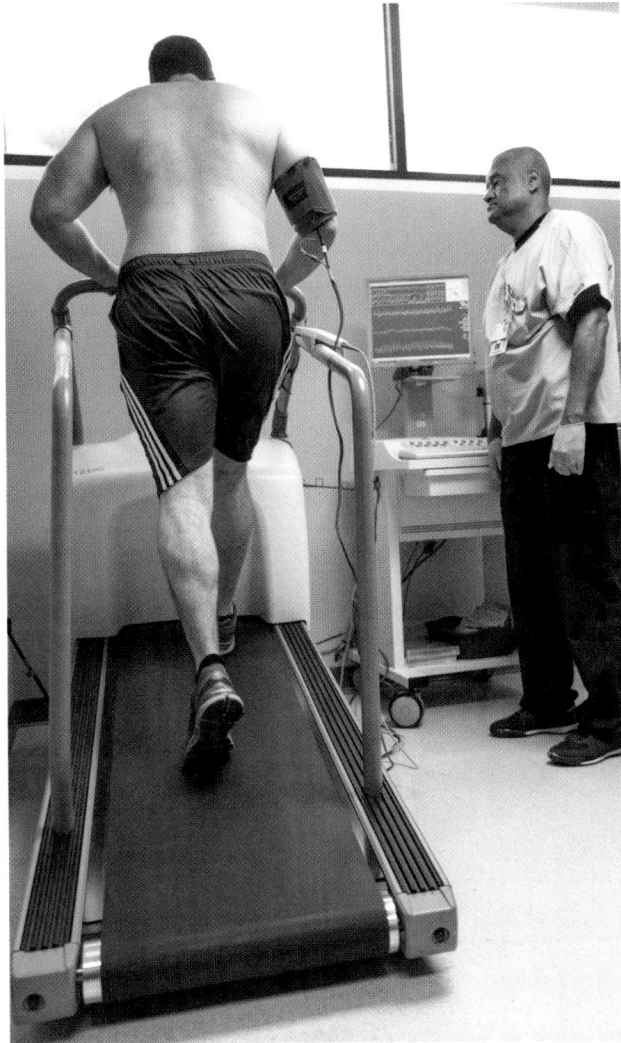

Fig. 74.11   Trained technician monitoring patient. (Courtesy JPS Health Network.)

Before arrival:

• The patient should be instructed to minimize consumption of alcohol, over-the-counter medications, and caffeine, both the day before and the day of the procedure. The patient should be encouraged to get a good night's sleep the night before the procedure. Patients should not eat for 2 hours before the test. It might be advisable for the most recent meal to be a small liquid meal. To minimize the risk of patient fatigue, many clinicians prefer performing ET in the morning (the exception being overnight workers). They then instruct the patient to avoid breakfast or to have only a liquid breakfast that day.

• The procedure should be rescheduled, if possible, if the patient has a cold or other viral illness or is not feeling well in general.

• If the indication for the test is to diagnose CAD (as opposed to managing CAD) or to screen for CAD, the clinician should instruct the patient to avoid taking β-blockers (or rate-limiting calcium channel blockers) the day of the test.

NOTE: Digoxin can cause artifacts even at therapeutic doses. If possible, digoxin should not be taken for 2 weeks before a test, the amount of time necessary for its elimination. However, a negative ET in a patient taking digitalis is a good study. Estrogen and tricyclic antidepressants can have similar effects and can be managed the same way. β-Blockers can suppress the heart rate and prevent determination of the MHR. Patients who discontinue β-blockers should watch closely for "rebound" symptoms and, if they develop, should restart their β-blockers. Because angiotensin-converting enzyme inhibitors or angiotensin receptor blockers have little or no effect on performance of an ET, frequently they may be used as a substitute antihypertensive. If necessary, they can be taken on the day of the test and usually work within an hour. Clonidine may be used in the same manner.

• If the indication for the test is to determine pharmacologic efficacy in patients with CAD, obviously β-blockers, calcium channel blockers, and nitrates should be taken the day of the study.

• The clinician should instruct the patient to bring shoes and clothing that are comfortable for walking and possibly for jogging. Bras with underwiring are contraindicated; sports bras work well.

• To minimize patient worry and stress (which often cause an elevated resting SBP), the clinician should explain that the risk of death for patients being tested using a treadmill is very small, and even less in an office setting (<1 per 10,000 patients).

After arrival:

• The clinician should again explain the reasons for the test and answer any questions.

• The procedure should be explained again to the patient (e.g., how frequently the workload will be increased, how BP measurements will be taken, how the PES works).

• The patient should be assured that close monitoring will take place and reassured that although the procedure exerts the heart, it is a relatively safe procedure (<1:10,000 mortality rate in properly selected patients).

• The patient should know what symptoms to report during the test.

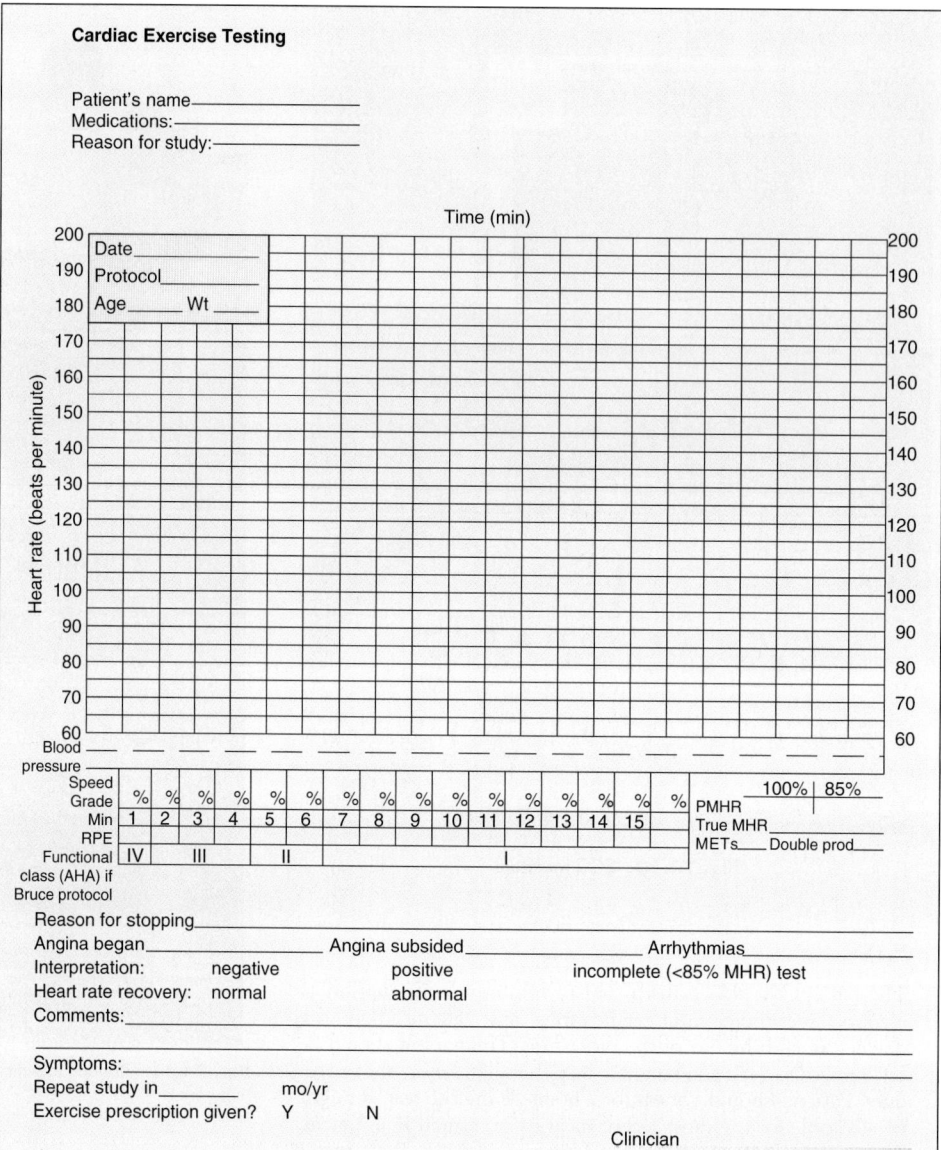

Fig. 74.12 Exercise test results form. METs, Metabolic equivalents; PMHR, predicted maximum heart rate (220 − age). (Modified from Evans CH, Karunaratne HB. Exercise stress testing for the family physician: part I. Performing the test. *Am Fam Physician* 1992;45:121–132.)

- The clinician should explain to the patient how to terminate the procedure should he or she have severe symptoms or an emergency.
- Signed, written informed consent should be obtained (see sample available at www.expertconsult.com).

DETERMINING PROTOCOL

There are many excellent protocols available; the choice usually depends on the patient's predicted exercise capacity and clinician preference. The VA Specific Activity Questionnaire (see Fig. 74.1) may be very helpful for predicting exercise capacity and deciding between a regular protocol and a modified (less aggressive) protocol. If a patient can walk up a flight of stairs carrying a bag of groceries, he or she should be able to tolerate a regular Bruce or Balke protocol. Choose a protocol that starts at a low level of exertion (2 to 3 METs) and then gradually increases.

1. A protocol with stage durations of at least 3 minutes (2 minutes for bicycle ergometer) allows more physiologic adaptation to the workload of each stage.
2. Workload increases that are no greater than 1 to 3 METs per stage also allow more physiologic adaptation.

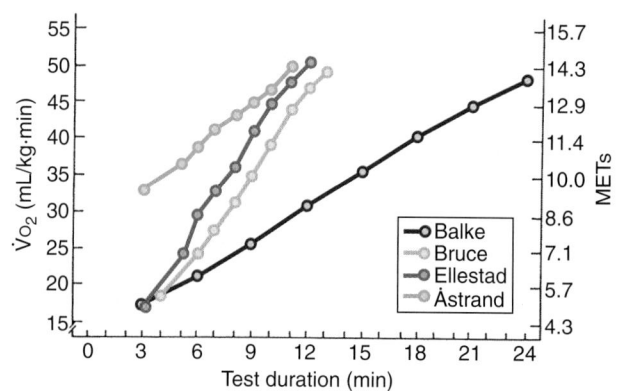

Fig. 74.13 Oxygen uptake measured according to time of exercise on four different protocols. MET, Metabolic equivalents. (From Pollock MI, Bohannon RL, Cooper KH, et al. A comparative analysis of four protocols for maximal treadmill stress testing. *Am Heart J.* 1976;92:39–46.)

TABLE 74.2   Standard Bruce Protocol

Stage*	Speed (mph)	Grade (%)	Metabolic Equivalents	Oxygen Consumption (mL/kg/min)
I	1.7	10	4	13
II	2.5	12	6.6	25
III	3.4	14	10	34
IV	4.2	16	14.2	46
V	5.0	18	17.2	58
VI	5.5	20	20.5	70

*Each stage lasts 3 min.

From Fowler GC, Evans CH, Altman MA. Office procedures: Exercise testing. *Prim Care* 1997;24:375–406.

3. Choose a protocol (Fig. 74.13) with a target of completing the ET in less than 15 minutes (even more preferable is 10 minutes or less). ETs that last more than 15 minutes may produce fatigue and overheating, which can independently affect results.

The Bruce protocol (Table 74.2) is the most frequently used protocol and has been the most extensively studied and validated. It is especially useful in active patients and takes less time than other protocols because it rapidly increases workload. Conveniently, the number of METs the patient will achieve is about the same as the number of minutes it takes to complete an ET using the Bruce protocol. A formula is available for estimating maximal exercise capacity in METs for the Bruce protocol. In men, this is METs = (2.94 × [min Bruce] + 7.65)/3.5. For women, the formula is METs = (2.95 × [min Bruce] +3.74)/3.5.

The Bruce protocol also has its disadvantages; by the fourth or fifth stage, the patient will usually need to run, which increases artifact. In addition, the patient often experiences difficulty accommodating increases in both slope and speed at the same time. Elderly patients usually have decreased proprioception in their toes and some degree of impairment in both vision and balance, making it especially difficult for them to adjust to changes in slope and speed at the same time.

In general, most "modified" protocols, such as the modified Bruce or modified Balke protocols, have a reduced progression of workload and are better tolerated by debilitated patients. Modified protocols usually maintain the same speed and vary only the elevation. Gradual but continuously increasing workload protocols (e.g., ramp) are also available. Table 74.3 indicates various protocols and Fig. 74.13 graphically compares METs per minute and VO_2 max as measured for four protocols. If the clinician chooses the ramp protocol, the VA questionnaire is helpful for estimating VO_2 max in METs; most clinicians program the equipment to reach maximal predicted METs in about 10 minutes.

With additional equipment that measures expired gases (e.g., oxygen, carbon dioxide) and total ventilation, the clinician can do four things: (1) actually measure the maximal aerobic capacity; (2) determine the anaerobic threshold (i.e., the point during exercise when marked lactic acid production begins); (3) give a more accurate exercise prescription; and (4) decide if impaired exercise capacity is due to a pulmonary condition or a cardiac cause (more common). Such equipment is becoming smaller and more affordable, which broadens the indications for ET in the office and (some experts say) increases the potential for greater reimbursement (see the Suppliers section). To avoid large capital equipment costs, there are service companies that will bring portable equipment to your office for this procedure and split the fees.

TECHNIQUE

1. Review the patient's interval medical history and examine the patient. Based on the history and reexamination, make sure no contraindication has developed since the last time the patient was seen.
2. Select the mode of ET (e.g., treadmill, bicycle ergometer, arm ergometer), based on the individual's ability to exercise.
3. Select the protocol.
4. Obtain the resting BP.
5. Prepare the patient for the ECG leads and apply them.
   - Locate sites on the chest for electrode placement, which are the same as for the office ECG (see Chapter 70, Office Electrocardiograms), except that the arm electrodes are placed in the infraclavicular fossae (mid-clavicle) and the leg electrodes are placed on the lower abdomen above the beltline (Fig. 74.14).
   - Cleanse the skin at these sites with an alcohol prep and let the sites dry thoroughly.
   - Shave any hair from the electrode sites. The cornified outer layer of skin should then be removed with gentle dermabrasion. Fine sandpaper or other abrasives are usually provided in the preparation kit for this purpose.
   - Apply electrodes to these sites.
   - Attach lead wires from the octopus to the appropriate electrodes. (An ECG octopus is the set of leads usually provided by the equipment manufacturer.)
   - Stabilize the ET octopus with a belt around the patient's waist. The octopus can be bundled and affixed to the patient with extra expansion loops to allow variation in distance from the ECG machine and to minimize motion artifact. Fortunately, most equipment is now digital and can use filters to minimize motion artifact.
   - If desired, for female patients, a gown or loose-fitting shirt can be worn over the lead wires. Jog bras work well; bras with underwire should be avoided.
6. Obtain the supine, resting ECG. Because a recent MI is a contraindication to ET, if there is even the remote chance of a recent MI or an interval MI since the last clinician visit, a routine ECG must be repeated. For maximal diagnostic sensitivity, this supine routine ECG should be obtained with the leads in the standard limb positions to allow for comparison with any prior standard ECGs. If this ECG reveals no changes, the limb leads can then be moved back to the exercise positions to obtain the baseline supine preexercise ECG.

NOTE: In an occasional patient, hyperventilation alone will produce ST segment depression. Because patients naturally hyperventilate during exercise, if there is ST segment depression during the procedure, it may be difficult to determine whether hyperventilation caused it or if there is true ischemia. However, hyperventilation artifact is rare enough that most authorities now recommend hyperventilating only those patients with a positive ET, after recovering them, to determine if hyperventilation caused the ST segment deviation. This technique of hyperventilating only those patients with a positive result saves not only time but expense, including the expense of ECG paper. This method is especially effective in the office setting, where fewer positive results typically occur.

Treadmill ECG Testing

7. Have the patient stand and obtain an ECG. This is the resting standing ECG, which becomes the baseline ECG. If the equipment is digital, it will often take 15 to 20 seconds to acquire the resting standing ECG. During this time, the equipment is acquiring an average of 15 to 20 seconds of ECG tracings to provide the "signal average" that it measures against for later comparison.

NOTE: Occasionally, ST segment depression is provoked by having the patient stand. Therefore, the isoelectric standard against which ST segment depression is measured during exercise is the resting standing baseline ECG before the ET.

TABLE 74.3 Various Exercise Protocols

AHA Functional Class	Clinical Status	O₂ Cost (mL/kg/min)	METs	Bicycle Ergometer (1 W 6.1 kpm/min; For 70 kg body weight kpm/min)	Bruce 3-min stages (Mph / percent grade)	Balke-Ware (Percent grade at 3.3 mph, 1-min stages)	USAFSAM (mph / percent grade)	"Slow" USAFSAM (mph / percent grade)	McHenry (mph / percent grade)	Stanford (Percent grade at 3 mph / at 2 mph)	ACIP (mph / Percent grade)	CHF (mph / Percent grade)	METs
Normal and I	Healthy, Dependent on Age, Activity	56.0	16	1500		26							16
		52.5	15		5.5 / 20	25	3.3 / 25		3.3 / 21		3.4 / 24.0		15
		49.0	14		5.0 / 18	24							14
		45.5	13	1350	4.2 / 16	23	3.3 / 20		3.3 / 18	22.5	3.1 / 24.0		13
		42.0	12			22		2 / 25		20	3.0 / 21.0		12
	Sedentary Healthy	38.5	11	1200	3.4 / 14	21	3.3 / 15		3.3 / 15	17.5	3.0 / 17.5	3.4 / 14.0	11
		35.0	10	1050		20	3.3 / 10	2 / 20	3.3 / 12	15		3.0 / 15.0	10
		31.5	9	900		19				12.5	3.0 / 14.0	3.0 / 12.5	9
		28.0	8	750		18		2 / 15	3.3 / 9	10	3.0 / 10.5	3.0 / 10.0	8
		24.5	7		2.5 / 12	17	3.3 / 5	2 / 10		7.5 / 17.5	3.0 / 7.0	3.0 / 7.5	7
II	Limited	21.0	6	600	1.7 / 10	16				5 / 14.0		2.0 / 10.5	6
III		17.5	5	450	1.7 / 5	15		2 / 5	3.3 / 6	2.5 / 10.5	3.0 / 3.0	2.0 / 7.0	5
		14.0	4	300	1.7 / 0	14		2 / 0	3.3 / 3	0 / 7.0	2.5 / 2.0	2.0 / 3.5	4
	Symptomatic	10.5	3			13	3.3 / 0			3.5	2.0 / 0.0	1.5 / 0.0	3
IV		7.0	2	150		12	2.0 / 0					1.0 / 0.0	2
		3.5	1			11							1
						10							
						9							
						8							
						7							
						6							
						5							
						4							
						3							
						2							
						1							

MET, metabolic equivalents.

From Froelicher VF: *Exercise and the Heart: Clinical Concepts.* 3rd ed. St Louis: Mosby; 1993.

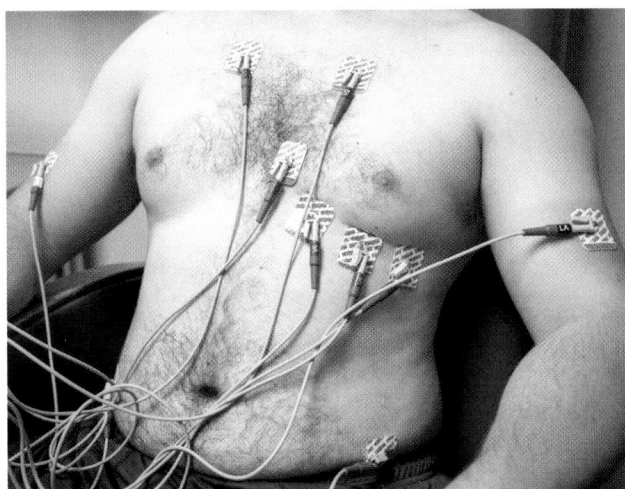

Fig. 74.14 **Patient with electrodes attached.** (Courtesy JPS Health Network.)

8. Begin the ET using the selected protocol. Try to discourage the patient from gripping the handrail during the study because this will falsely elevate the maximal exercise capacity; it may also increase ECG artifact and falsely elevate BP. Time may be saved if a staff member demonstrates the procedure and allows the patient to practice before the clinician arrives. Staff should show the patient how to rest two fingers or the wrists on the handrail while walking near the front of the treadmill and looking straight ahead. (If the patient looks down, dizziness often results.)

Bicycle Ergometer ECG Testing

7. After completing steps 1 through 6 for the treadmill ET, have the patient sit on the bicycle and obtain a sitting ECG.
8. Begin the ET using the preselected protocol. The usual protocol starts at 25 W of resistance and increases by 25 W every 2 minutes.

For Both Treadmill and Bicycle Ergometer ECG Testing

9. Monitor and record the patient's symptoms, overall condition, heart rate, and ECG at all times. *Instruct the patient to try to give adequate warning before he or she needs to stop the test.* With the exception of submaximal testing, encourage the patient to go as far and as long as possible.
10. Record a 12-lead ECG at the end of each stage, at any time an abnormality is noted on the monitor, immediately on stopping, and every minute postexercise during recovery.
    NOTE: Real data are obtained only from a hard copy of the 12-lead ECG. The monitor merely provides ongoing information, estimates of ST segment changes, and allows the clinician to monitor for arrhythmias. If there is any question regarding ST segment changes, print a hard copy for measurement and interpretation.
11. During each stage, at the start of the final minute, ask the patient if there is any chest discomfort, the point that he or she has reached on the PES, and whether he or she wants to continue into the next stage. Also record the BP and heart rate near the end of each stage or at the time of any problems.
    NOTE: For most patients, their perceived exertion (see Box 74.1) is reproducible at a given level of exercise and tracks fairly linearly with their heart rate. Ask patients to indicate on a scale of 0 to 10 how hard they feel they are working at each stage. On average, most patients feel they increase by 2 to 3 on the PES with each stage in the early part of the study. PES then usually increases more rapidly, from 7 to 9, near the end of the study. Rarely will anyone declare a 10. Individuals with good perception may not have to

measure their pulse as frequently while following their exercise prescription. They can simply be instructed to exercise to the level of perceived exertion that matched their appropriate heart rate for the aerobic range (60% to 80% MHR). On the other hand, patients who highly underestimate their effort must be taught to measure their pulse before receiving an exercise prescription.

12. After completion of the ET, if it has been done for diagnostic purposes and the study has been negative, immediately ask the patient to lie down. Although this may not be comfortable for certain patients, especially if they are overweight or having slight difficulty breathing, it minimizes false-positive results during recovery. Make sure to record the heart rate at 1 minute as HRR.
13. If the ET is positive or being performed for CAD management purposes, keep the patient exercising for 3 to 4 minutes during recovery at a very low workload to prevent venous pooling and to minimize the risk of an arrhythmia. The patient may then either sit or lie down for the remainder of recovery.
    NOTE: For positive studies—even for those profoundly positive—very rarely is it necessary to administer medications. Simply stopping the exertion and having the patient sit up to improve oxygenation should be adequate. If there is strong suspicion that a plaque has been destabilized (MI has occurred), aspirin, if not contraindicated, is the best choice for a medication. In the absence of contraindications, oxygen may also be considered. Sublingual nitroglycerin is risky in a vasodilated patient without intravenous access because it may drop the BP. Sublingual calcium channel blockers are contraindicated.
14. Monitor the BP, heart rate, any symptoms, and the ECG tracing during recovery.
15. The patient should be monitored for at least 8 minutes in recovery or until symptoms or ECG abnormalities have resolved (some clinicians monitor only for 4 minutes postexercise for negative ETs in low-risk patients, such as those being tested as part of a wellness program).

Test Termination Criteria

A good rule of thumb for stopping an ET is after the necessary information is obtained and before there is a complication. In the young or fit individual, when he or she reaches the predicted MHR (220 − age), it may be prudent to explain that all the necessary information has been obtained; however, the patient may continue to exercise for as long as he or she desires. (Allowing the patient to make this choice is also indirectly obtaining informed consent.)

NOTE: In the past, authorities denoted two possible definitions of a maximal ET: (1) achieving a target heart rate of greater than 85% of the predicted MHR for that patient's age (i.e., roughly 85% of 220 − age); or (2) exercise to the point of symptoms or maximal voluntary fatigue. *Most authorities now encourage patients to exercise to the point of symptoms or maximal voluntary exertion or fatigue.*

Predicted MHR (220 − age) is not patient specific and is frequently a poor prediction. Predicted or calculated MHR tends to overestimate true MHR in older patients and underestimate it in younger adults. The only contraindications to going to the point of symptoms are for debilitated or elderly patients or if a submaximal test is indicated. Maximal voluntary fatigue/maximal effort is usually indicated by maximal perceived exertion and the inability to continue at that workload.

Benefits to using the point of symptoms as the end point include the ability to measure true exercise capacity and to determine the patient's true MHR. It also gives the clinician knowledge about a patient's cardiac response at a level of exercise beyond what the patient is likely to reproduce on his or her own. This is certainly reassuring to the clinician when giving an exercise prescription (i.e., it should be safe for the patient to exercise at a lower level of exertion). Disadvantages include discomfort for the patient, especially if he or she is significantly deconditioned.

How does the clinician know if the patient gave a maximal effort? Following the PES is often helpful. Also, an RPP greater than 25,000 generally indicates that the patient has given a good effort. Many other physiologic parameters have been studied in an attempt to predict maximal effort (e.g., heart rate, respiratory rate, BP response), and none has been found to be predictive. However, if patients are aware that it is important to give maximal effort to exclude heart disease, they are usually motivated.

Absolute Indications to Terminate a Study

- As exertion increases during ET, if SBP drops below the resting standing value, especially after the first minute or two of the ET (most dangerous if it reflects LV dysfunction; in that situation there is a high risk of life-threatening arrhythmias).
- Worsening anginal chest pain (severe enough that the patient desires to stop); it is not prudent for patients to exercise beyond the point where they obtain their "usual" amount of chest discomfort. In other words, there is no reason for the patient to demonstrate his or her worst chest pain while performing the study.
- Central nervous system symptoms (e.g., dizziness, disorientation).
- Signs of poor perfusion (e.g., cyanosis, pallor) or severe ventricular dysfunction (e.g., dyspnea).
- Serious arrhythmias (e.g., three or more premature ventricular contractions [PVCs] in a row [e.g., a salvo, ventricular tachycardia] is an indication to terminate the test), increasingly frequent PVCs associated with ischemia (chest pain or ST segment changes), or atrial arrhythmia with cardiovascular compromise.
- Technical problems with equipment, ECG monitor, or SBP monitoring.
- Marked ECG changes (>3 mm of horizontal or downsloping ST segment depression, or 1 mm of ST segment elevation).
- When maximal voluntary exertion/maximal effort has been attained.
- Patient wants to stop the test (especially elderly patients, where there may be little warning of a complication about to happen).

Relative Indications to Terminate a Study

- Worrisome ST or QRS segment changes (e.g., excessive junctional depression, marked axis shift)
- Significant fatigue, shortness of breath, wheezing, leg cramps, or intermittent claudication
- Worrisome appearance (especially important in the elderly, where stability can deteriorate very rapidly; poor perfusion may be indicated solely by a loss of color in an elderly patient)
- Elevated BP (SBP >250 mm Hg, DBP >120 mm Hg)
- Less serious dysrhythmia, including supraventricular tachycardia
- Development of a bundle branch block pattern that cannot be distinguished from ventricular tachycardia or an ST segment elevation MI

INTERPRETATION

Incomplete Exercise ECG Tests

Failure to attain at least 85% of the age-predicted MHR is an incomplete ET.

Medications (e.g., β-blockers, rate-limiting calcium channel blockers) are a common cause of this; therefore, another reason to withhold such medications is if the ET is being performed for diagnostic purposes. If the ET is being performed to manage CAD, use of β-blockers may increase the patient's exercise capacity, which is also a goal of cardiac rehabilitation. One hopes that increased exercise capacity is a surrogate marker for improved prognosis. If the ET is being performed for diagnostic purposes and is deemed incomplete due to a medication, options at this point include an exercise imaging test, a pharmacologic (e.g., regadenoson, adenosine, dipyridamole, dobutamine, arbutamine; see Chapter 76, Stress Echocardiography, for a dobutamine echo protocol) imaging test,

cardiology consultation, or getting the patient on an exercise program and repeating the ET in 3 to 6 months. Given the choice, many patients will choose to start an exercise program.

Normal ECG Responses to Exercise

- P-wave amplitude increases.
- T-wave amplitude often increases.
- RR and PR intervals decrease in length.
- Below a heart rate of 150 beats/min, the R-wave amplitude is unchanged or increased; above 150 beats/min or near maximal exercise, the R wave in a healthy heart usually decreases in amplitude, and the overall QRS amplitude also usually decreases, especially in the lateral leads (the so-called Brody effect).
- J-point (i.e., the junction between the S wave and ST segment) is depressed in the lateral (possibly all) leads, especially at maximum exercise, and gradually returns to normal during recovery.
- The P–Q junction is also usually depressed (Fig. 74.15).
- ST segment slope is usually upsloping; however, from the J-point, the tracing rapidly returns to baseline. In other words, at 0.04 to 0.06 second after the J-point, the final position of the ST segment is at the baseline level.

ST Segment Analysis

- A positive ET is determined by ECG criteria. However, the ET results should not be labeled simply as normal, positive, or abnormal, but rather the specific responses to exercise should be identified and documented.
- Age and risk factors for CAD should be taken into account when interpreting results.
- Many conditions and circumstances can cause a false-positive or a false-negative ET (Box 74.4).
- The lateral leads (e.g., V_4, V_5, and V_6) are the most important leads to monitor for ischemia. Their electrodes are located directly over the left ventricle and are the most likely to show ischemic ST segment changes. Although it is always recommended to use at least three leads, studies have found that lead V_5 is the most sensitive lead if a single lead were to be used.
  NOTE: The actual data are the hard copy printouts of the 12-lead recordings. It is recommended that these be interpreted separately, in a quiet room, scanning the entire printout, before giving the patient the results and recording them.

1. An ET is considered positive when 1 mm of ST segment depression occurs in at least three beats in a row, in more than one lead, and in an area of the tracing where the baseline is relatively flat. If it is truly positive, ST segment depression usually occurs in almost all of the leads; in most cases it will continue more than 1 minute into recovery. In fact, the ST segment depression may worsen in recovery, especially if the patient is asked to lie down immediately after exercise is discontinued (usually recommended if ET is being performed for diagnostic purposes).
2. ST segment deviation (depression or elevation) should be measured down or up from the level of the PQ junction. A line drawn horizontally from the PQ junction denotes the isoelectric line (see Fig. 74.15).
3. ST segment deviation (depression or elevation) should be measured at the J-point (i.e., ST zero, also known as the beginning of the ST segment or end of the QRS complex).
4. Most experts now consider the study positive only if the slope for 80 ms after the J-point is horizontal or downsloping. The ACC/AHA guidelines suggest this is the best definition of a positive ET. Other experts also consider a slow upsloping ST segment pattern as positive, although this was based on much older data from the 1970s (Fig. 74.16). They will consider a slow upsloping pattern positive if the tracing fails to reach within 1.5 mm of the

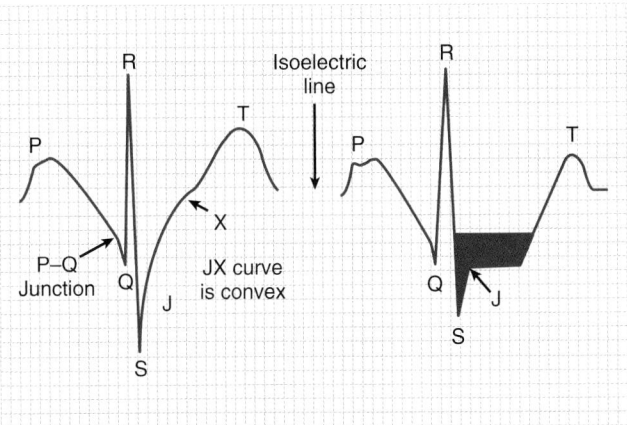

Fig. 74.15 Left, Normal exercise ECG complex. Note that the P-Q junction is deflected below the resting isoelectric line. This point is considered to be the baseline for determining ST segment deviations. Right, A horizontal ST segment depression of 2.0 mm as measured from the P-Q junction. (From Ellestad MH. *Stress Testing: Principles and Practice.* 4th ed. Philadelphia: FA Davis; 1996.)

baseline level of the PQ junction at 80 ms after the J-point. It should be understood that although a slow upsloping pattern may be positive, it is much more likely to be a false-positive result or represent insignificant CAD; however, accepting this pattern as a possible positive result slightly increases the sensitivity of the test for CAD. Therefore, increased sensitivity must thus be weighed against the increased likelihood of a false-positive result. A slow upsloping pattern is more likely to be a true-positive result if it persists beyond 1 minute into recovery and is seen not only in the inferior leads (i.e., II, III, aVF), but in other leads. If the proper technique of immediately laying the patient down during recovery is followed, slow upsloping ST segments that truly represent ischemia usually convert to flat or downsloping ST segments with depression. So a slow upsloping pattern during the test may be predictive of a true positive in recovery.

5. Although occasionally ST segment elevation (i.e., transmural ischemia) can indicate the vessel involved, ST segment depression does not localize ischemia. In other words, it cannot detect which blood vessel is involved. Subendocardial ischemia is a "global" phenomenon (i.e., for significant CAD, ST segment changes will be seen in most leads).

6. If ST segment elevation occurs over or adjacent to diagnostic Q waves, it may be caused by a ventricular aneurysm or a wall motion abnormality. If it occurs in a patient with a normal resting ECG or without a history of previous infarction, it probably indicates transmural ischemia and the test should be stopped. Transmural ischemia is extremely arrhythmogenic.

7. If downsloping or a flat-pattern ST segment depression occurs, and it is less than 1 mm or only in recovery, it may be indicative of early CAD. This is an "equivocal" result. Management options are discussed in a following section.

ET Indicators of Significant or Extensive CAD (Three-Vessel CAD with LV Dysfunction or Left Main CAD)

- Markedly positive ST segment response in multiple leads (>2.5 mm downsloping or horizontal ST segment depression)
- Early positive ST segment response (stage 1 or 2 of Bruce protocol or at ≤4 to 5 METs)
- Unable to complete stage 2 of the Bruce protocol (especially if unable to complete stage 1)
- Typical angina chest pain, especially if associated with ST segment depression

- Worrisome ventricular arrhythmias (especially if associated with ST segment depression or at a heart rate <130 beats/min)
- Fall in exercise SBP (>10 mm Hg below resting standing baseline), especially when associated with angina or significant ST segment changes
- Prolonged positive ST segment response (>6 minutes of recovery)

ST Segment Analysis in Special Situations

Baseline Abnormalities

When the ST segments are abnormal on the resting ECG, certain experts use new criteria to declare a test positive. For example, if there is already 1 mm of flat ST segment depression at rest, they only

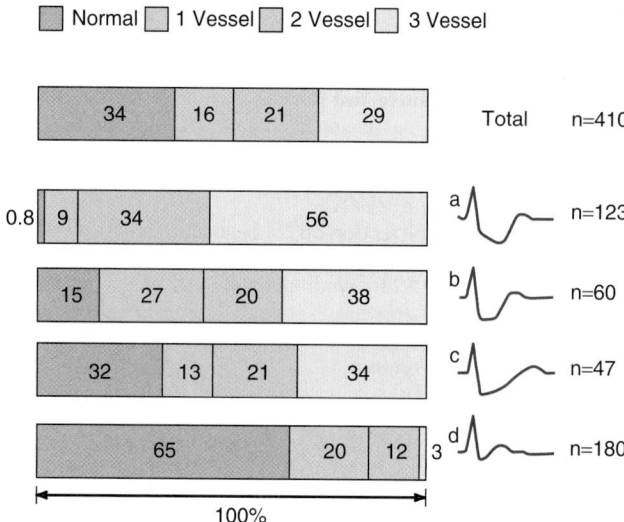

Fig. 74.16 Three patterns of ST segment depression. Although the downsloping pattern, a, usually represented three-vessel disease (56%) and the flat pattern, b, occasionally represented three-vessel disease (38%), the slow-uploading pattern, c, had three-vessel disease in 34% and at least one-vessel disease in 68% (these usually convert to flat or downsloping in recovery). The rapid-upsloping pattern, d, has been accepted as the normal physiologic pattern. (Modified from Goldschlager N, Selzer A, Cohn K. Treadmill stress tests as indicators of presence and severity of coronary artery disease. *Ann Intern Med.* 1976;85:277–286.)

declare the test positive when there is 2 mm of flat or downsloping ST segment depression during exercise or recovery. The clinician should be sure that this abnormal ECG is not due to a recent acute coronary event. Otherwise, the ST segment depression at rest is most likely due to orthostatic ST changes. These can be seen when the baseline *resting standing* ECG is obtained before the test and can be a normal variant.

ST Segment Analysis in Women

False-positive results are less common in women older than 50 years. The following data are from a study by Pratt (1989).

- True-positive results are associated with four factors:
  1. Absence of mitral valve prolapse
  2. An exercise duration of less than 5 minutes
  3. The ability to reach the target heart rate
  4. The ST segment takes 6 minutes or more to normalize (in recovery)
- False-positive results are associated with two factors:
  1. The ability to exercise to stage 3 of the Bruce protocol
  2. Rapid (<4 minutes) normalization of the ST segment shift after cessation of exercise

NOTE: In general, if slow upsloping ST segments are used to define a positive ET, they are associated with a high false-positive rate in women. If the proper technique of laying the patient down during recovery is followed, slow upsloping ST segments that truly represent ischemia usually convert to flat or downsloping ST segments with depression.

Scenarios With Decreased Sensitivity and False-Positive and False-Negative Results

- If LBBB or WPW syndrome is present, ST segment depression does not necessarily indicate ischemia.
- If RBBB is present, the ST segments can be analyzed only in V_4, V_5, or V_6, and the sensitivity of the test may be decreased.

NOTE: Recent data indicate that the presence of complete RBBB on the resting ECG is associated with a 50% greater risk of death

over the next 20 years, a rate similar to that of LBBB. The mechanism underlying the relationship is unclear.

- If ST segment depression occurs only in inferior leads II, III, or aVF and not in the lateral leads, it is usually a false-positive result caused by atrial repolarization. When reviewing, these patients frequently have a short PR interval on the resting ECG (the atrial repolarization wave, which is negative, "pulls down" the ST segment when superimposed). Also, the ST segment depression often returns to normal in less than 1 minute of recovery in the false-positive cases.
- If coronary artery bypass surgery has been performed, sensitivity of the test may be decreased.
- If anterior or lateral Q waves or both are present (after MI), the sensitivity of the test may be decreased.
- See Box 74.4 for a complete listing of causes of false-positive and false-negative test results.

Arrhythmias

- Prognosis in supraventricular and ventricular arrhythmias appears to be more related to underlying or coexisting conditions, especially ischemia or LV dysfunction. Patients who are symptomatic should be treated or referred.
- If the arrhythmia is associated with signs or symptoms of ischemia, in most cases management should be directed at treating the ischemia to minimize the arrhythmia.
- PVCs are common. They are ominous only in patients with LV dysfunction, severe ischemia, valvular heart disease, a cardiomyopathy, or a family history of sudden cardiac death.
- Three unifocal PVCs in a row is defined as a "salvo" and an indication to terminate the test. Interestingly, asymptomatic, nonsustained ventricular tachycardia in an individual with a normal ejection fraction is not associated with increased cardiovascular mortality. However, a Holter monitor, echocardiogram, or both may be indicated.
- Young (i.e., <40 years) but otherwise healthy individuals with no CAD risk factors may have frequent PVCs at rest that resolve with exercise. If the ET is negative and they have a normal echocardiogram, further evaluation is often not necessary. PVCs that go away with exercise in this population are almost always benign.

Exercise Capacity and Heart Rate Recovery

- The ability to achieve 15 METs indicates an excellent prognosis, even in those with known three-vessel CAD. The ability to achieve 10 METs indicates that medical management is reasonable, even in patients with a positive ET. An inability to achieve 5 METs indicates a poor prognosis, especially if the ET is positive.
- VO_2 max can be estimated from various exercise protocols using standard formulas, tables, or graphs. Using estimated VO_2 max, an individual's approximate level of aerobic conditioning can be determined using age- and sex-matched tables. Fig. 74.17 also estimates the exercise capacity based on the number of METs a patient can achieve.
- Failure of the heart rate to decrease 12 beats/min in the first minute of recovery is an abnormal HRR. This data has been challenged recently, because it may not be reproducible in the same patient, but it was originally thought to indicate a fourfold increased risk of mortality over the next 5 years. At a minimum, it may be worth monitoring these patients more closely over time.
- As mentioned previously, in patients where ECG changes during ET could not be used to predict prognosis (e.g., baseline ECG abnormalities, digoxin use)—in other words, the DTS could not be used—Diaz (2001) found exercise capacity and HRR to be better predictors of risk over 6.7 years than radionuclide imaging in

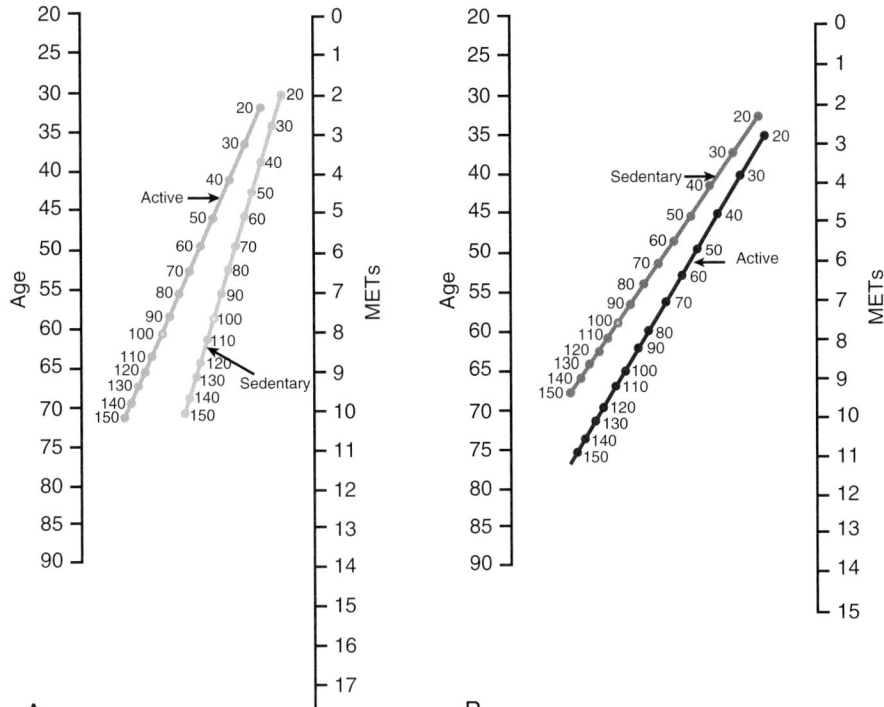

A

B

Fig. 74.17 Nomograms of percentage normal exercise capacity. (A) Percentage of normal in healthy men. (B) Percentage of normal in referred men. MET, Metabolic equivalents. (Modified from Kenney WL, ed. *ACSM's Guidelines for Exercise Testing and Prescription.* 5th ed. Baltimore: Williams & Wilkins; 1995.)

nonrevascularized patients (again, this data has been challenged as not reproducible). Gulati also found exercise capacity alone in women to be predictive of prognosis, separate from the DTS.

Other Parameters Followed

- *Heart rate:* Failure to obtain a heart rate of 120 beats/min is chronotropic incompetence with a resultant poor prognosis (approximately 15% per year will experience a coronary event) often due to cardiomyopathy; it may also indicate early sick sinus syndrome.
- *BP:* As exertion increases during ET, if the SBP drops below the resting standing baseline, it predicts either a poor prognosis or severe CAD. In one study, men with a maximal exercise SBP of less than 140 mm Hg also had a 15-fold increase in the annual rate of sudden death compared with those whose pressures exceeded 200 mm Hg. A DBP increase of more than 10 mm Hg, an SBP greater than 214 mm Hg, or failure of DBP and SBP to return to normal 3 minutes into recovery is a *hypertensive response to exercise.* In otherwise healthy individuals, a hypertensive response to exercise increases the likelihood that they will develop hypertension over the next few years. It may also increase their long-term risk of CV events and mortality (systolic BP >210 mm Hg in men, >190 mm Hg in women [Schultz, 2013]). However, ET should not be used to screen for hypertension because ambulatory BP monitoring is much more effective. In individuals with known hypertension, a hypertensive response to exercise may indicate poorly treated hypertension. Poorly treated hypertension may have a negative impact on exercise tolerance.
- *BP and heart rate in diabetic patients:* Diabetes can cause an elevated resting heart rate; BP and heart rate responses are frequently blunted in diabetic patients.
- *Symptoms:* Substernal chest pain in men being tested on a treadmill, even without ECG changes, is 90% predictive of CAD in studies from a few decades ago.
- *Lack of symptoms:* Painless ST segment depression (i.e., silent ischemia) is common in diabetic patients and those older than 70 years.

DETERMINING PROGNOSIS

Normal ECG Responses and Negative ECG Testing (Prognosis Is Excellent)

- Absence of any change in the ST segment at maximal or near MHR.
- Junctional or J-point depression with rapidly rising ST segment slope.
- Development of isolated T-wave inversion without ST segment displacement.
- Ventricular ectopic beats occur infrequently, especially those occurring at heart rates exceeding 130 beats/min and not associated with any evidence of ischemia.
- Although rare, even a poorly controlled atrial arrhythmia without cardiovascular compromise has a good prognosis.
- Although rare, development of RBBB with exercise still usually has a good prognosis.

Patients can be reassured that if they achieve a heart rate of 160 beats/min (regardless of age) and achieve 13 METs (basically equivalent to completing 12 minutes on the Bruce protocol), even with some ECG evidence of ischemia, they have a very good 4- to 5-year prognosis. They basically have less than a 1% per year risk of a cardiac event for that time span. The same is true if they achieve an RPP greater than 35,000; they are extremely unlikely to have significant CAD. Even for positive studies, periodic evaluation with a retest in 6 to 12 months may be the most aggressive management needed.

Positive and Abnormal ECG Testings

To obtain prognosis data for abnormalities of heart rate or BP, see Other Parameters Followed in the previous section. Otherwise, prognosis is poor for patients unable to achieve 5 METs or for patients demonstrating a positive ET at less than 5 METs. For those patients in whom an intervention is appropriate or if the clinician is unsure of the diagnosis, prognosis, or management, a cardiologist should be consulted.

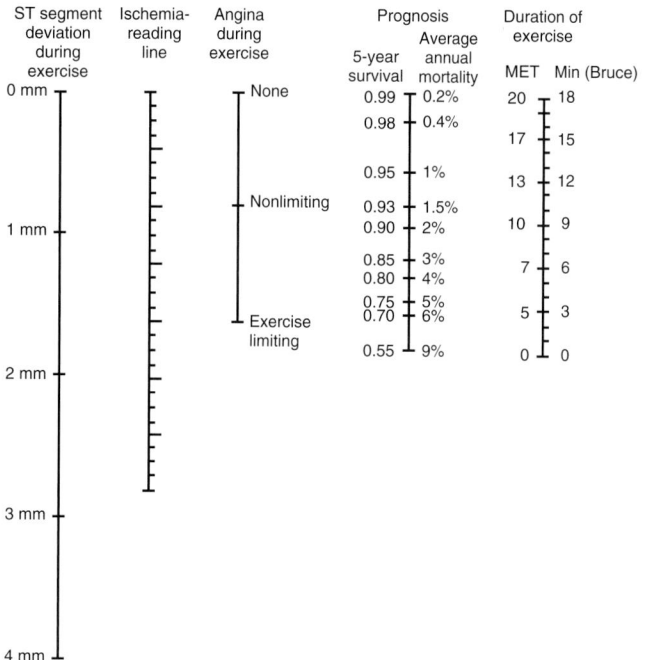

Fig. 74.18 Nomogram for Duke University Prognostic Score. (Modified from Mark DB, Shaw L, Harrell FE, et al. Prognostic value of a treadmill exercise score in outpatients with suspected coronary artery disease. *N Engl J Med.* 1991;325:849–853.)

For those patients with a positive ET and able to achieve 5 METs, a heart rate of 120 beats/min, and an RPP of more than 25,000, a nomogram is available for determining prognosis, counseling, and follow-up. As opposed to other similar nomograms available, women (although not as many) were included in the studies resulting in the nomogram in Fig. 74.18. Therefore, this nomogram can be used when counseling women.

Most large coronary artery bypass surgery centers have known or published complication rates. The AHA's website (www.americanheart.org) also has excellent data for predicting complications from coronary artery bypass surgery. Using the nomogram (see Fig. 74.18), patients can evaluate their annual risk of a cardiovascular event with medical management versus a surgical intervention. These are very powerful tools for what is usually a very important decision for patients to make.

Based on several studies, for patients with CAD and able to achieve 10 METs, which is basically the level of exertion necessary to complete approximately 9 minutes of a Bruce protocol, medical management is prudent or reasonable. It is also very unlikely that these patients have significant disease if they achieve an RPP of 25,000 or greater. With an outstanding exercise capacity, even patients with multivessel CAD do well. One study revealed that in patients with known three-vessel CAD and able to complete 15 minutes of a Bruce protocol, the 5-year survival rate was 100%.

COMPLICATIONS

- Hypotension
- Congestive heart failure exacerbation
- Severe cardiac arrhythmia
- Cardiac arrest
- Acute MI
- Acute central nervous system event, such as syncope or stroke
- Death

NOTE: The overall safety of ET has been confirmed in multiple studies. For patients being tested on a treadmill, the mortality rate in modern times is approximately 1 in 10,000; it should be less in properly selected patients, which is what must be done for office testing.

POSTPROCEDURE PATIENT EDUCATION

Patients should be informed that ET, just like any other noninvasive study for diagnosing CAD, is not 100% accurate. Individuals with a change in symptoms or symptoms of chest discomfort, palpitations, or any other symptoms that could be caused by CAD should be evaluated by their clinician regardless of the result of the ET.

In patients with CAD or a high probability of CAD, counseling should be directed at modifying risk factors. Exercise prescriptions should be given and discussed.

Giving an Aerobic Exercise Prescription

- Exercise capacity or endurance is increased by performing regular aerobic exercise at least three times per week. For primary prevention, although a fourth episode further increases exercise capacity, after the fourth episode per week, the incremental benefit is less. The greatest benefit of additional episodes of exercise per week is to assist with weight loss. For secondary prevention, there continues to be improvement in exercise capacity with additional episodes per week. Consequently, most cardiac rehabilitation programs recommend exercising most days of the week for an hour a day.
- For primary prevention, aerobic exercise can be performed 3 days in a row to maintain fitness; however, the risk of an injury increases without adequate rest between episodes. It is therefore recommended that individuals exercise, at an aerobic level, every other day. Participating in a less intense walking program on intervening days may also assist with weight loss.
- Aerobic exercise involves raising the heart rate to a specified point (60% to 80% of MHR) and maintaining that level of exercise for 30 to 45 minutes per session. Three 10-minute episodes in the same day accomplish the same effect as one 30-minute episode.
- After ET, a safe aerobic training range is at a heart rate of 60% to 80% of MHR. This range is called the *target heart rate*. A PES of 5 to 7 can also be used in most patients; however, some patients have a poor perception of level of exertion, and therefore PES cannot be used.
- Patients should avoid dehydration and weather extremes. Unlike what was done if the ET was performed for diagnostic purposes, they should warm up and cool down after each episode, especially older patients.
- A repeat ET can evaluate the improvement after implementation of an aerobic exercise program. After introduction of an exercise program, it takes approximately 12 weeks of regular exercise to achieve a new level of exercise capacity.
- To avoid boredom, it is recommended that an exercise prescription include more than one kind of aerobic exercise (e.g., swimming, biking, race walking, jogging, and aerobic dance).
- An exercise prescription should include a target heart range or level of PES, duration of exercise sessions, frequency of sessions, and types of exercises that can be used to achieve the goals of cardiovascular conditioning (aerobic). For new exercise prescriptions, the rate of progression needs to be explained.
- Competitive athletes want to use their training program to raise their anaerobic threshold (i.e., level of exercise at which they can no longer oxygenate all tissues). Anaerobic thresholds are now best measured with ventilator-expired gas analysis ET.

PATIENT EDUCATION GUIDES

See the sample patient consent form available at www.expertconsult.com.

CPT/BILLING CODES

93000   Electrocardiogram, routine ECG with at least 12 leads; with interpretation and report

93015   Cardiovascular stress test using maximal or sub-maximal treadmill or bicycle exercise, continuous ECG monitoring, and/or pharmacologic stress; with physician supervision, with interpretation and report

93016   Physician supervision only, without interpretation and report

93017   Tracing only, without interpretation and report

93018   Interpretation and report only

ICD-10-CM DIAGNOSTIC CODES

I25.2   Old MI (healed; past MI diagnosed on ECG, but currently no symptoms)

I20.8   Other and unspecified angina pectoris

I25.10   Coronary atherosclerosis, of native coronary artery w/o angina

I25.719   Coronary atherosclerosis, of autologous vein bypass graft unspecified angina

I25.709   Coronary atherosclerosis, of artery bypass graft unspecified angina

I25.799   Coronary atherosclerosis, of unspecified type of bypass graft

I25.9   Chronic coronary insufficiency

I49.49   Ventricular premature beats, contractions, or systoles

R00.2   Palpitations

R07.2   Precordial chest pain

SUPPLIERS

(See contact information available at www.expertconsult.com.)

NOTE: Most manufacturers in the following list also sell defibrillators. Purchasing these as part of a package is often cost effective.

Stress Testing Equipment
General Electric Healthcare
Burdick Quinton Mortara
Welch Allyn Schiller
Emergency/ACLS medication kits
Banyan International Corp.
Expired gas analysis or cardiopulmonary exercise testing
Medical Graphics

RECOMMENDED READING

2014 ACC/AHA. Guideline on Perioperative Cardiovascular Evaluation and Management of Patients Undergoing Noncardiac Surgery. *Circulation.* 2014;130:278–333.

ACC/AATS/AHA/ASE/ASNC/SCAI/SCCT/STS 2017 Appropriate Use Criteria for Coronary Revascularization in Patients With Stable Ischemic Heart Disease. A Report of the American College of Cardiology Appropriate Use Criteria Task Force, American Association for Thoracic Surgery, American Heart Association, American Society of Echocardiography, American Society of Nuclear Cardiology, Society for Cardiovascular Angiography and Interventions, Society of Cardiovascular Computed Tomography, and Society of Thoracic Surgeons. *J Am Coll Cardiol.* 2017;69:2212–2241.

ACC/AHA. Clinical competence statement on stress testing: A report of the American College of Cardiology/American Heart Association/American College of Physicians-American Society of Internal Medicine Task Force on Clinical Competence. *Circulation.* 2000;102:1726. Also available at http://circ.ahajournals.org/content/102/14/1726. Accessed April 21, 2018.

ACC/AHA/ASNC. Guidelines for the clinical use of cardiac radionuclide imaging—Executive summary. *Circulation.* 2003;108:1404.

ACCF/ASE/AHA/ASNC/HFSA/HRS/SCAI/SCCM/SCCT/SCMR. 2011 Appropriate Use Criteria for Echocardiography. *J Am Soc Cardiol.* 2011;24:229–267.

BARI Investigators. The final 10-year follow-up results from the BARI randomized trial. *J Am Coll Cardiol.* 2007;49:1600–1606.

Bourque JM, Charlton GT, Holland BH, Belyea CM, Watson DD, Beller GA. Prognosis in patients achieving ≥ 10 METS on exercise stress testing: was SPECT imaging useful? *J Nucl Cardiol.* 2011;18(2):230–237.

Diamond GA, Forrester JS. Analysis of probability as an aid in the clinical diagnosis of coronary-artery disease. *N Engl J Med.* 1979;300:1350–1358.

Diaz LA, Brunken RC, Blackstone EH, et al. Independent contribution of myocardial perfusion defects to exercise capacity and heart rate recovery for prediction of all-cause mortality in patients with known or suspected coronary heart disease. *J Am Coll Cardiol.* 2001;37:1558–1564.

Duvall WL, Savino JA, Levine EJ, Hermann LK, Croft LB, Henzlova MJ. Prospective evaluation of a new protocol for the provisional use of perfusion imaging with exercise stress testing. *Eur J Nucl Med Mol Imaging.* 2015;42(2):305–316.

Ellestad MH. *Stress Testing: Principles and Practice.* 5th ed. New York: Oxford University Press; 2003.

Evans CH. Exercise testing. *Prim Care Clin Off Pract.* 2001;28.

Evans CH, Karunaratne HB. Exercise stress testing for the family physician. Part I: performing the test. *Am Fam Physician.* 1992;45:121–132.

Evans CH, Karunaratne HB. Exercise stress testing for the family physician. Part II: interpretation of the results. *Am Fam Physician.* 1992;45:679–688.

Fletcher GF, Ades PA, Kligfield P, et al. American Heart Association Exercise, Cardiac Rehabilitation, and Prevention Committee of the Council on Clinical Cardiology, Council on Nutrition, Physical Activity and Metabolism, Council on Cardiovascular and Stroke Nursing, and Council on Epidemiology and Prevention. Exercise standards for testing and training: a scientific statement from the American Heart Association. *Circulation.* 2013;128(8):873–934.

Garner KK, Pomeroy W, Arnold JJ. Exercise stress testing: indications and common questions. *Am Fam Physician.* 2017;96(5):293–299.

Fowler G, Altman M. Exercise testing after bypass or percutaneous coronary intervention. In: Evans CH, White RD, eds. *Exercise Stress Testing for Primary Care and Sports Medicine Physicians.* New York: Springer-Verlag; 2009:231–254.

Fowler GC, Evans CH, Altman MA. Exercise testing. *Prim Care.* 1997;24:375–406.

Froelicher VF, Myers J. *Exercise and the Heart.* 5th ed. Philadelphia: Saunders; 2006.

Froelicher VF, Quaglietti S. *Handbook of Exercise Testing.* Boston: Little, Brown; 1996.

Gibbons RJ, Balady GJ, Bricker JT, et al. ACC/AHA 2002 guideline update for exercise testing: summary article: a report of the American College of Cardiology/American Heart Association Task Force on Practice Guidelines (Committee to Update the 1997 Exercise Testing Guidelines). *Circulation.* 2002;106:1883–1892.

Gibbons RJ, Hodge DO, Berman DS, et al. Long-term outcome of patients with intermediate-risk exercise electrocardiograms who do not have myocardial perfusion defects on radionuclide imaging. *Circulation.* 1999;100:2140–2145.

Greenslade JH, Parsonage W, Ho A, et al. Utility of routine exercise stress testing among intermediate risk chest pain patients attending an emergency department. *Heart Lung Circ.* 2015;24(9):879–884.

Gulati M, Pandey DK, Arnsdorf MF, Lauderdale DS, Thisted RA, et al. Exercise capacity and the risk of death in women: the St. James women take heart project. *Circulation.* 2003;108:1554–1559.

Klocke FJ, Baird MG, Lorell BH, et al. ACC/AHA/ASNC guidelines for the clinical use of cardiac radionuclide imaging: Executive summary. A report of the American College of Cardiology/American Heart Association Task Force on Practice Guidelines (ACC/AHA/ASNC Committee to Revise the 1995 Guidelines for the Clinical Use of Cardiac Radionuclide Imaging). *Circulation.* 2003;108:1404–1418.

Knox MA. Optimize your use of stress tests: a Q&A guide. *J Fam Pract.* 2010;59:262–268.

Krone RJ, Hardison RM, Chaitman BR, et al. Risk stratification after successful coronary revascularization: the lack of a role for routine exercise testing. *J Am Coll Cardiol.* 2001;38:136–142.

Mark DB, Shaw L, Harrell FE Jr, et al. Prognostic value of a treadmill exercise score in outpatients with suspected coronary artery disease. *N Engl J Med.* 1991;325:849–853.

Mattera JA, Arain SA, Sinusas AJ, et al. Exercise testing with myocardial perfusion imaging in patients with normal baseline electrocardiograms: cost savings with a stepwise diagnostic strategy. *J Nucl Cardiol.* 1998;5:498–506.

Myers J, Prakash M, Froelicher V, Do D, Partington S, Atwood JE. Exercise capacity and mortality among men referred for exercise testing. *N Engl J Med.* 2002;346(11):793–801.

Napoli AM. The association between pretest probability of coronary artery disease and stress test utilization and outcomes in a chest pain observation unit. *Acad Emerg Med.* 2014;21(4):401–407.

Nishime EO, Cole CR, Blackstone EH, et al. Heart rate recovery and treadmill exercise score as predictors of mortality in patients referred for exercise ECG. *JAMA.* 2000;284:1392–1398.

Pescotello LS, Arena R, Riebe D, Thompson BD, eds. *ACSMs Guidelines for Exercise Testing and Prescription.* 9th ed. Philadelphia: Wolters Klower; 2014.

Peterson PN, Magid DJ, Ross C, et al. Association of exercise capacity on treadmill with future cardiac events in patients referred for exercise testing. *Arch Intern Med.* 2008;168(2):174–179.

Pratt CM, Francis MJ, Divine GW, Young JB. Exercise testing in women with chest pain: are there additional exercise characteristics that predict true positive test results? *Chest.* 1989;95:139–144.

Schultz MG, Otahal P, Cleland VJ, Blizzard L, Marwick TH, Sharman JE. Exercise-induced hypertension, cardiovascular events, and mortality in patients undergoing exercise stress testing: a systematic review and meta-analysis. *Am J Hypertens.* 2013;26(3):357–366.

Scott AC, Bilesky J, Lamanna A, et al. Limited utility of exercise stress testing in the evaluation of suspected acute coronary syndrome in patients aged less than 40 years with intermediate risk features. *Emerg Med Australas.* 2014;26(2):170–176.

Shaw LJ, Mieres JH, Hendel RH, et al. WOMEN Trial Investigators. Comparative effectiveness of exercise electrocardiography with or without myocardial perfusion single photon emission computed tomography in women with suspected coronary artery disease: results from the What Is the Optimal Method for Ischemia Evaluation in Women (WOMEN) trial. *Circulation.* 2011;124(11):1239–1249.

Stein RA, Chaitman BR, Balady GJ, et al. Safety and utility of exercise testing in emergency room chest pain centers: an advisory from the Committee on Exercise, Rehabilitation and Prevention, Council on Clinical Cardiology, American Heart Association. *Circulation.* 2000;102:1463–1467.

Thomas GS, Wann LS, Ellestad MH. *Ellestad's Stress Testing, Principles and Practice.* 6th ed. New York: Oxford; 2018.

Wolk MJ, Bailey SR, Doherty JU, et al. American College of Cardiology Foundation Appropriate Use Criteria Task Force. ACCF/AHA/ASE/ASNC/HFSA/HRS/SCAI/SCCT/SCMR/STS 2013 multimodality appropriate use criteria for the detection and risk assessment of stable ischemic heart disease: a report of the American College of Cardiology Foundation Appropriate Use Criteria Task Force, American Heart Association, American Society of Echocardiography, American Society of Nuclear Cardiology, Heart Failure Society of America, Heart Rhythm Society, Society for Cardiovascular Angiography and Interventions, Society of Cardiovascular Computed Tomography, Society for Cardiovascular Magnetic Resonance, and Society of Thoracic Surgeons. *J Am Coll Cardiol.* 2014;63(4):380–406.

Young LH, Wackers FJ, Chyun DA, et al. DIAD Investigators. Cardiac outcomes after screening for asymptomatic coronary artery disease in patients with type 2 diabetes: the DIAD study: a randomized controlled trial. *JAMA.* 2009;301(15):1547–1555.

CHAPTER 75

ECHOCARDIOGRAPHY

Grant C. Fowler • Terry Reynolds

The prevalence of heart disease will continue to increase in the United States as the population ages. The proportion of heart disease managed by primary care clinicians will also continue to increase. In many cases both the management and prognosis of heart disease are based on the amount of remaining viable myocardium. This is especially true for patients with congestive heart failure (CHF), cardiomyopathy, arrhythmias, and ischemic heart disease. One method of quantifying the remaining viable myocardium is to assess the ejection fraction. In fact, the most common reason echocardiography is performed in the United States is to determine the ejection fraction.

Many common symptoms, signs, and diagnoses of heart disease (e.g., palpitations, cardiomegaly on electrocardiogram [ECG] or chest radiograph, atrial fibrillation, and CHF) are evaluated or managed using echocardiography (Table 75.1). In certain situations the more readily available the echocardiogram, the better the management. For example, acute chest pain is managed differently when echocardiography is immediately available. Even extracardiac causes of acute chest pain, some of which can be life threatening (e.g., pulmonary embolus, aortic dissection), can be diagnosed with echocardiography. In the setting of an acute myocardial infarction (MI), risk stratification can be performed immediately. Complications from an acute MI can also often be diagnosed early.

Other common diagnoses that can be made or evaluated in the primary care clinician's office with echocardiography include mitral valve prolapse, dilated left atrium (important for patients with atrial fibrillation), left ventricular hypertrophy, syncope, transient ischemic attack, and ischemic heart disease. Whether in the clinician's office, the hospital, or the emergency department, a rapid diagnosis of pericardial tamponade or pericardial effusion may be lifesaving. Furthermore, if pericardiocentesis is needed, the risk of complications is significantly reduced if it is performed under ultrasound guidance (see Chapter 230, Pericardiocentesis).

Improvements in image quality, portability, and affordability for real-time sonography have allowed it to become a valuable adjunct for the clinician in the office, hospital, or emergency department. Training courses are now more readily available. Consequently echocardiography has seen some of the most rapid growth among procedures performed by primary care clinicians (see Chapter 76), Stress Echocardiography. For those clinicians with a large number of adult patients, two-dimensional (2D) and M-mode echocardiography may be welcome additions to their practice. If the primary care clinician is uncomfortable performing echocardiography, contractors are available to provide sonographers. Overreading services are also available (see the "Suppliers" section). This chapter predominately describes the performance of 2D/M-mode echocardiography with a brief summary of common findings. Since color and Doppler flow imaging are helpful for almost all echocardiograms, especially for those assessing the hemodynamic severity of an abnormality, they are also discussed briefly. For a discussion of ultrasound principles and concepts and for information regarding limited echocardiography, see Chapter 214, Emergency Department, Hospitalist, and Office Ultrasound (POCUS). Electromechanical dissociation (EMD), pericardial effusion, pericardial tamponade, and the assessment of intravascular volume status, right ventricular strain/dysfunction, and acute pulmonary hypertension (e.g., pulmonary embolism) are briefly discussed in that chapter. (Assessing for possible pulmonary hypertension is also discussed in the "Interpretation" section of this chapter.)

Two-dimensional echocardiography provides the clinician with cross-sectional, real-time images of various cardiac structures. Using 2D, cardiac chambers, walls, valves, and other structures can be observed as they move through the cardiac cycle. Freeze-framing and the use of calipers allow the clinician to measure certain structures, if needed, at various points during the cardiac cycle.

M-mode echocardiography produces graphic images in which time makes up the horizontal axis and the structures in motion being scanned compose the vertical axis. In other words, wherever the cursor is placed on the image, a linear beam of ultrasound is directed through the corresponding tissue and movement of the structures is graphically imaged over time. The resultant M-mode tracing can then be used to look at excursion and contraction patterns as well as to precisely measure distances from the various horizontal structures over time. Chamber dimensions, wall thicknesses, and valve excursions can be measured precisely throughout the cardiac cycle. From chamber dimensions, an ejection fraction can be estimated.

Doppler flow imaging is used to measure the velocity of blood flowing over certain structures. Using the Bernoulli equation, pressure gradients (e.g., across a valve) can also be determined. As with M-mode, time and the cardiac cycle are graphed along the horizontal axis, whereas the vertical axis shows blood velocity in meters per second. By convention, flow *toward* the transducer is depicted above the baseline and flow *away* from the transducer is depicted below the baseline. Pulsed-wave (PW) technology and measurements use tiny three-dimensional sample volumes to detect the exact location of any abnormalities. However, PW Doppler is limited when there is high-velocity flow. Continuous wave (CW) technology uses two crystals (one continuously emitting sound waves, the other continuously listening for echoes) and can measure high velocities (e.g., stenotic valves). However, it is of limited use for localizing abnormalities. Because of these limitations, both PW and CW should be used with every valve. Color-flow Doppler is a special adaptation of PW technology. It uses thousands of sampling volumes to produce a color image of velocities. By convention, flow *away* from the transducer is *blue* and flow *toward* the transducer is *red*. The intensity of the color increases with the velocity.

INDICATIONS

- Determine ejection fraction (most common indication)
- Acute chest pain
- Acute or old MI
- Atrial fibrillation, sustained supraventricular tachycardia
- Cardioversion preparation
- Cardiomegaly on chest radiograph
- Congestive heart failure
- Dyspnea (possibly of cardiac origin) or of unknown origin for perioperative evaluation

TABLE 75.1	Common Symptoms and Differential Diagnosis for Echocardiography
Reason	**Differential Diagnosis**
Chest pain	Aortic dissection
	Coronary artery disease: acute myocardial infarction or angina
	Hypertrophic cardiomyopathy
	Pericarditis
	Pulmonary embolism
	Valvular stenosis
Heart failure	Dyspnea
	Hypotension
	Left ventricular diastolic dysfunction
	Left ventricular systolic dysfunction (global or segmental)
	Pericardial disease
	Right ventricular dysfunction
	Valvular heart disease
Palpitations	Congenital heart disease (e.g., atrial septal defect, Ebstein's anomaly)
	Left ventricular systolic dysfunction
	Mitral valve disease
	Pericarditis
	Structural cardiac disease
Murmur: systolic	Aortic stenosis, subaortic obstruction, hypertrophic obstructive cardiomyopathy
	Flow murmur (valve abnormality)
	Mitral regurgitation
	Pulmonic stenosis
	Tricuspid regurgitation
	Ventricular septal defect
Murmur: diastolic	Aortic regurgitation
	Mitral stenosis
	Pulmonic regurgitation
	Tricuspid stenosis
Cardiomegaly on chest radiograph	Dilated cardiomyopathy
	Pericardial effusion
	Specific chamber enlargement (e.g., left ventricle in chronic aortic regurgitation)
Systemic embolic event	Aortic valve disease
	Left atrial thrombus (only diagnostic if seen, otherwise transesophageal echo needed)
	Left ventricular systolic function and segmental wall motion abnormalities (aneurysms)
	Left ventricular thrombus
	Mitral valve disease
	Patent foramen ovale
	Pulmonary embolism

Modified from Otto CM. *Textbook of Clinical Echocardiography*. 2nd ed. Philadelphia: WB Saunders; 2000.

- Embolus (systemic or pulmonary)
- Frequent premature ventricular contractions or exercise-induced premature ventricular contractions
- Hypotension (possibly of cardiac origin)
- Hypertensive heart disease
- Ischemic heart disease
- Mitral valve prolapse
- Murmur or click when there is suspicion of valvular or structural heart disease
- Palpitations
- Pericardial effusion, EMD, or suspected pericardial tamponade
- Severe deceleration injury or chest trauma (e.g., suspected valvular injury, pericardial effusion)
- Suspected cardiomyopathy
- Suspected infectious endocarditis
- Suspected left ventricular hypertrophy (e.g., let ventricular hypertrophy [LVH] on ECG)
- Syncope
- Murmur

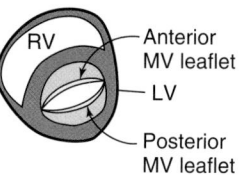

Fig. 75.1 Parasternal short-axis view at the level of the mitral valve (MV). *LV,* Left ventricle; *RV,* right ventricle. (From Reynolds T. *The Echocardiographer's Pocket Reference.* 2nd ed. Phoenix: School of Cardiac Ultrasound at Arizona Heart Institute; 2000.)

- Transient ischemic attack
- Valvular defect, stenosis, regurgitation, or insufficiency
- Ventricular arrhythmias (with suspected cardiac structural abnormality)

CONTRAINDICATIONS

- Patient too unstable or too uncooperative to be scanned
- Patient needs Doppler flow imaging or a color Doppler scan and the equipment does not have this capability

PREPROCEDURE PATIENT PREPARATION

Indications for the study and possible findings should be explained to the patient. The patient should be prepared to change positions, if possible, while being scanned. The patient should be prepared for adequate gel and pressure from the transducer to be applied to the parasternal, apical, suprasternal, and, possibly, subxiphoid areas of the chest and abdominal walls. The patient should be gowned and in the supine or left lateral decubitus position.

EQUIPMENT

- For best images, an ultrasound machine with several probes of different frequency should be available. Among these probes, a low-frequency (e.g., 2.5 MHz) probe with 2D, M-mode, and cardiac Doppler capabilities is preferred. An ultrasound machine with harmonic imaging ensures high-quality images. A method of recording and storing the data (e.g., server, DVD, VCR) is also needed for documentation. For limited scans in emergency situations, a machine without Doppler capability can be used.
- Ultrasonic jelly (and towels to clean up after scanning).
- Patient gown.

TECHNIQUE

Two-Dimensional Echocardiography

Viewing the front of the chest, if the 12 o'clock position is considered cephalad and the 6 o'clock position caudal, the axis of the heart is usually located in a line drawn between the 10 o'clock and the 4 o'clock positions. Placing the marker dot of the transducer at about the 10 o'clock position usually produces the long-axis view of the heart, especially if the probe is located parasternally. A line drawn between the patient's right shoulder and left hip also approximates the long axis of the heart. If described in the conventional terminology of ultrasound for the remainder of the body, the long-axis view is essentially the longitudinal view of the heart. Rotating the marker dot almost 90 degrees, or perpendicular to the long axis, to the 2 o'clock position, produces the short-axis view of the heart. This is essentially a transverse view of the heart (Fig. 75.1). A line drawn between the left shoulder and the right hip also approximates this axis.

Because the patient is usually lying in the left lateral decubitus position while being scanned and the transducer is placed on the anterior chest wall (or abdominal wall for the subxiphoid view), the transducer edge will be noted at the top of the image. Posterior cardiac structures will be located at the bottom (inferior aspect) of the

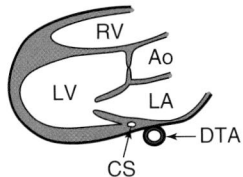

Fig. 75.2 Parasternal long-axis view. *Ao,* Aortic root; *CS,* coronary sinus; *DTA,* descending thoracic aorta; *LA,* left atrium; *LV,* left ventricle; *RV,* right ventricle. (From Reynolds T. *The Echocardiographer's Pocket Reference.* 2nd ed. Phoenix: School of Cardiac Ultrasound at Arizona Heart Institute; 2000.)

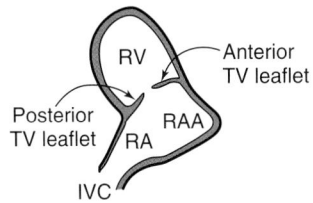

Fig. 75.3 Parasternal long-axis view of the right ventricular inflow tract. *IVC,* Inferior vena cava; *RA,* right atrium; *RAA,* right atrial appendage; *RV,* right ventricle, *TV,* tricuspid valve. (From Reynolds T. *The Echocardiographer's Pocket Reference.* 2nd ed. Phoenix: School of Cardiac Ultrasound at Arizona Heart Institute; 2000.)

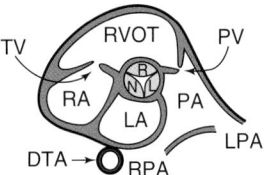

Fig. 75.4 Parasternal short-axis view at the level of the aortic valve. *DTA,* Descending thoracic aorta; *L,* left coronary cusp; *LA,* left atrium; *LPA,* left pulmonary artery; *N,* noncoronary cusp; *PA,* pulmonary artery; *PV,* pulmonary valve; *R,* right coronary cusp; *RA,* right atrium; *RPA,* right pulmonary artery; *RVOT,* right ventricular outflow tract; *TV,* tricuspid valve. (From Reynolds T. *The Echocardiographer's Pocket Reference.* 2nd ed. Phoenix: School of Cardiac Ultrasound at Arizona Heart Institute; 2000.)

image. With the usual orientation, if the directional marker is noted on the right side of the image, objects to the right of the screen will correspond to objects near the marker dot on the transducer.

1. With the patient in the left lateral decubitus position, attempt to scan by first placing the transducer in the parasternal location (third to fourth intercostal space, next to the sternum) or the apical location (inferolateral to the left nipple at the point of palpated maximal cardiac impulse [PMI]). These same two traditional auscultatory points are used for a stethoscope. If the best window is found at the apical location, skip to step 12.

2. When scanning parasternally, the probe will be rotated so that the marker dot is either in the 10 o'clock (long-axis) or 2 o'clock (short-axis) position. The short-axis view at the level of the mitral valve is often a good view for assessing the adequacy of the window, since the mitral valve is usually prominent and easily located (see Fig. 75.1).
   NOTE: Some ultrasound equipment places the marker dot 180 degrees away from this standard orientation (i.e., the 4 o'clock position is what would typically be the 10 o'clock position) even when using the echo transducer. With this equipment, the marker dot will be on the left side of the image. To determine the orientation of the probe, the directional marker on the image should be found. It corresponds to the marker dot on the probe and should be displayed on the right side of the display for standard or conventional cardiac imaging. It should be noted that this orientation is unique to echocardiography; the marker dot is usually located on the left side of the image for all other ultrasound scanning.

3. Small changes in patient position (e.g., rolling the patient further onto his or her left side) or working with the patient's breathing may improve the quality of the image. These adjustments cause the lingula of the lung to fall away from the heart, often providing a better window.

4. For unresponsive patients, those who cannot be moved, patients with chronic obstructive pulmonary disease, or other technical difficulties impairing the use of ultrasound in the parasternal position, the subxiphoid position will often provide a good window. Place the transducer directly below the xiphoid and angle it toward the patient's left shoulder, with the marker dot toward the patient's left side. If this is the only location where an adequate window can be obtained, skip to step 16.

5. If a good window can be found at the parasternal short-axis view, rotate the transducer 90 degrees to the parasternal long-axis view (Fig. 75.2). (The marker dot will be directed toward the 10 o'clock position). With this view, observe the anterior and posterior leaflets of the mitral valve as it is scanned lengthwise. With prolapse, the leaflets will close beyond 90 degrees or cross the plane of the mitral annulus. True prolapse is often associated with thickened valves. Also with this view, the right ventricle is seen at the superior portion of the image, and the interventricular septum is noted as the inferior border of the right ventricle. Beneath the interventricular septum, to the left of the image, is the left ventricular chamber bordered by its posterior wall. Note that the ventricular walls thicken during systole, reducing the size of the ventricular cavity. Very little of the apex can be visualized with this view, because it is beyond the left side of the image. The left atrium is to the right side of the image, immediately in-

ferior to the aortic root. The left atrial diameter should be about the same as the aortic root diameter. If either is markedly larger than the other or more than 4 cm in their anteroposterior diameter, they are considered dilated. The descending thoracic aorta is noted behind the left atrium. Rotate the transducer slightly clockwise if a better longitudinal view of the aorta is desired.

6. To obtain the long-axis view of the right ventricular inflow tract (RVIT) view from the parasternal long-axis view, tilt the transducer inferomedially or toward the right hip. This is a good view in which to study the tricuspid valve, right atrium, and right ventricle (Fig. 75.3). The posterior and anterior tricuspid leaflets separate the right atrium from the right ventricle. In fact, this is about the only view where the posterior leaflet of the tricuspid valve can be seen. Liver tissue is usually noted adjacent to the diaphragmatic wall of the right ventricle.

7. After angling the probe back again to the parasternal long-axis view, rotate the transducer 90 degrees so that the marker dot is at the 2 o'clock position. This will produce the parasternal short-axis view again (see Fig. 75.1). Note the appearance in real time of the opening and closing mitral valve. Some have likened this image to that of a "fish mouth" opening and closing, especially if there is any stenosis. Without stenosis, the lateral and medial commissures of the valve are easy to distinguish. At this level, the ventricular wall can be divided into six segments, and the contractility of all of the segments should be observed (see step 10). In the normal heart, the segments should be contracting uniformly and symmetrically. The tricuspid valve may be seen above and to the left of the mitral valve.

8. Next, without actually moving or rotating the transducer, merely angle it more cephalad toward the base of the heart to observe the aortic valve (Fig. 75.4). In this transverse view of the aortic valve, a characteristic "Y sign" is produced when the leaflets are closed. If the valve itself is viewed as the face of a clock, the commissures are noted in the 2, 6, and 10 o'clock positions at the edges of the Y. When the valve is open in systole, it should produce a triangular shape. If it produces an oval shape with opening, the aortic valve is bicuspid. This is one of the most common abnormal findings on adult echocardiography, occurring in 1% to 2% of the population. If it is found, the patient should also be scanned for coarctation of the aorta, because 50% to 80% of

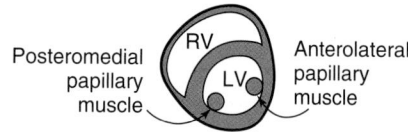

Fig. 75.5 Parasternal short-axis view of the left ventricle at the level of the papillary muscles. *LV,* Left ventricle; *RV,* right ventricle. (From Reynolds T. *The Echocardiographer's Pocket Reference.* 3rd ed. Phoenix: School of Cardiac Ultrasound at Arizona Heart Institute; 2007.)

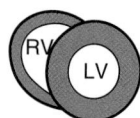

Fig. 75.6 Parasternal short-axis view at the level of the apex. *LV,* Left ventricle; *RV,* right ventricle. (From Reynolds T. *The Echocardiographer's Pocket Reference.* 2nd ed. Phoenix: School of Cardiac Ultrasound at Arizona Heart Institute; 2000.)

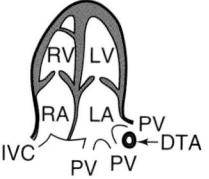

Fig. 75.7 Apical four-chamber view. *DTA,* Descending thoracic aorta; *IVC,* inferior vena cava; *LA,* left atrium; *LV,* left ventricle; *PV,* pulmonary vein; *RA,* right atrium; *RV,* right ventricle. (From Reynolds T. *The Echocardiographer's Pocket Reference.* 2nd ed. Phoenix: School of Cardiac Ultrasound at Arizona Heart Institute; 2000.)

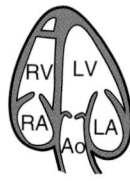

Fig. 75.8 Apical five-chamber view. *Ao,* Aortic root; *LA,* left atrium; *LV,* left ventricle; *RA,* right atrium; *RV,* right ventricle. (From Reynolds T. *The Echocardiographer's Pocket Reference.* 2nd ed. Phoenix: School of Cardiac Ultrasound at Arizona Heart Institute; 2000.)

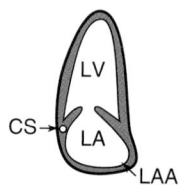

Fig. 75.9 Apical two-chamber view. *CS,* Coronary sinus; *LA,* left atrium; *LAA,* left atrial appendage; *LV,* left ventricle. (From Reynolds T. *The Echocardiographer's Pocket Reference.* 2nd ed. Phoenix: School of Cardiac Ultrasound at Arizona Heart Institute; 2000.)

those with aortic coarctation will have a bicuspid aortic valve (see the suprasternal notch view, step 21). At this level of the parasternal short-axis view, the right ventricular outflow tract can be seen curving above and around the aortic valve. The tricuspid valve is noted to the left of the aortic valve and the pulmonary valve is located superiorly and to the right. The right ventricle is located between the two. The right atrium is located in the inferior portion of the image to the left of the aortic valve. The left atrial appendage can often be seen to the far right of the aortic valve, and the left atrium is noted inferior or posterior to the aortic valve. Part of the atrial septum can be noted between the atria. The three cusps of the aortic valve are labeled the right, left, and noncoronary cusps. The right cusp is located next to the right ventricular outflow tract, the noncoronary cusp closest to the right atrium, and the left coronary cusp next to the left atrium. In a normal heart, the corresponding right and left coronary arteries originate from the same-labeled cusps.

9. Tilting the transducer yet more superiorly, beyond the aortic valve, the aortic root can be visualized in its short axis (transversely). At this level, on the right side of the image of the aortic root, the pulmonary artery can often be noted to bifurcate into the right and left pulmonary arteries.

10. Next, angle the probe back through the mitral valve, down to the level of the papillary muscles (Fig. 75.5). This level provides an excellent view for assessing left ventricular wall motion and the severity of left ventricular hypertrophy if it is present. At this level, the left ventricular wall can again be divided into six segments—the anterior, anteroseptal, anterolateral, inferolateral (posterolateral), inferoseptal (posteroseptal), and inferior (posterior) segments—which are all visualized. This same segmentation system can be used on the parasternal short-axis view at the level of the mitral valve. Each of the segments should contract in a uniform manner. With coronary artery disease, determining which wall becomes hypokinetic with ischemia may predict which coronary artery is obstructed (see the section titled "Findings and Interpretation," further on). Usually two papillary muscles are visualized at this level, one located anterolaterally and the other posteromedially. At this level, only part of the right ventricle can usually be visualized, and it will be to the left of the image.

11. Next, slide the transducer slightly toward the apex and obtain a short-axis view of the ventricles at the apex (Fig. 75.6). By convention, the left ventricular wall is divided into only four segments (anterior, lateral, septal, and inferior [posterior]) at this level. In the normal heart, all four segments will contract uniformly.

12. By moving the transducer to the apex, which can be located by palpating the maximal cardiac impulse inferolateral to the left nipple, the apical four-chamber view can be obtained

(Fig. 75.7). At this position, the majority of scanning is usually performed with the marker dot at the 3 o'clock position. Angle the transducer back up toward the base of the heart to obtain the best possible four-chamber image. To confirm the orientation while scanning, note that the septal leaflet of the tricuspid valve is closer to the apex than the anterior leaflet of the mitral valve. By convention, the tricuspid valve and the right ventricle should be on the left side of the image. The right ventricle can usually be distinguished from the left ventricle because the right ventricle has the echogenic moderator band extending from the apex to the septal wall. Again, the right ventricular wall is more trabeculated than the left ventricular wall. With this view, again observe the ventricular wall motion for uniformity of contraction. From this transducer position, observe the valves again for abnormalities.

13. Tilt the transducer slightly anteriorly, toward the anterior chest wall (tail of transducer is tilted downward slightly), from the apical four-chamber view to obtain the apical five-chamber view (Fig. 75.8). This view provides an excellent image of the left ventricular outflow tract as well as an excellent view to exclude hypertrophic obstructive cardiomyopathy.

14. Return to the apical four-chamber view and rotate the transducer 90 degrees counterclockwise and tip it slightly laterally to obtain the apical two-chamber view (Fig. 75.9). The left ventricle and atrium will be visualized, separated by the mitral valve. With this image, the full length of the inferior wall of the left ventricle can be visualized. Observe this wall, along with the anterior wall of the left ventricle, for uniform contractility.

15. Rotate the transducer counterclockwise so that the sector plane passes through the long axis of the heart to obtain the apical

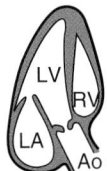

Fig. 75.10 Apical long-axis view. *Ao*, Aortic root; *LA*, left atrium; *LV*, left ventricle; *RV*, right ventricle. (From Reynolds T. *The Echocardiographer's Pocket Reference*. 2nd ed. Phoenix: School of Cardiac Ultrasound at Arizona Heart Institute; 2000.)

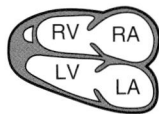

Fig. 75.11 Subxiphoid four-chamber view. *LA*, Left atrium; *LV*, left ventricle; *RA*, right atrium; *RV*, right ventricle. (From Reynolds T. *The Echocardiographer's Pocket Reference*. 2nd ed. Phoenix: School of Cardiac Ultrasound at Arizona Heart Institute; 2000.)

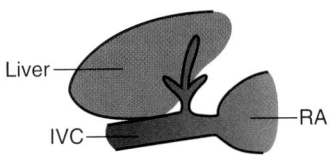

Fig. 75.12 Subxiphoid long-axis view of inferior vena cava. *IVC*, Inferior vena cava; *RA*, right atrium. (From Reynolds T. *The Echocardiographer's Pocket Reference*. 2nd ed. Phoenix: School of Cardiac Ultrasound at Arizona Heart Institute; 2000.)

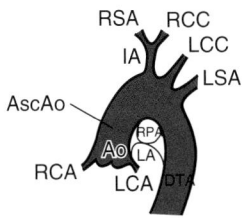

Fig. 75.13 Suprasternal notch long-axis view of aortic arch. *Ao*, Aortic root; *AscAo*, ascending aorta; *DTA*, descending thoracic aorta; *IA*, innominate artery; *LA*, left atrium; *LCA*, left coronary artery; *LCC*, left common carotid; *LSA*, left subclavian artery; *RCA*, right coronary artery; *RCC*, right common carotid; *RPA*, right pulmonary artery; *RSA*, right subclavian artery. (From Reynolds T. *The Echocardiographer's Pocket Reference*. 2nd ed. Phoenix: School of Cardiac Ultrasound at Arizona Heart Institute; 2000.)

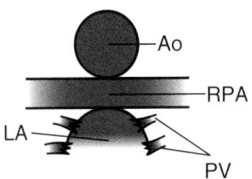

Fig. 75.14 Suprasternal notch short-axis view of aortic arch. *Ao*, Aortic root; *LA*, left atrium; *PV*, pulmonary veins; *RPA*, right pulmonary artery. (From Reynolds T. *The Echocardiographer's Pocket Reference*. 2nd ed. Phoenix: School of Cardiac Ultrasound at Arizona Heart Institute; 2000.)

long-axis view (Fig. 75.10). The aortic root can be evaluated, whereas the aortic valve is noted to be contiguous with the base of the anterior mitral leaflet. This view is very similar to the parasternal long-axis view, but the apex is visualized from this position. With this image, the anterior interventricular septum and the inferolateral ventricular wall can be inspected for uniform contractility.

16. Moving the transducer to below the xiphoid, the subxiphoid (subcostal) four-chamber view (Fig. 75.11) can be obtained with the marker dot to the patient's left side. Usually a portion of the liver is used as a window. The ventricles will be to the right side of the image and the atria to the left side. The left ventricle and atrium will be located behind (below) the right ventricle and atrium. Inspect both the mitral valve and the tricuspid valve and observe wall motion for uniformity of contraction.

17. From the subxiphoid four-chamber view, by tilting the transducer anteriorly, visualize the aortic valve lengthwise. This will again provide an image similar to that seen with the parasternal long-axis view. This technique of imaging may be very valuable if the standard parasternal long-axis image cannot be obtained because of technical difficulties.

18. From the subxiphoid four-chamber view, it is also possible to angle the transducer to visualize the entire atrial septum. This position is the most reliable for evaluating patients for atrial septal defects and patent foramen ovale.

19. From the subxiphoid view, the inferior vena cava (IVC) can be imaged (Fig. 75.12) and its diameters measured. The diameter of the IVC can be used to estimate right atrial pressure (RAP). With the marker dot toward the patient's feet and the transducer located in the midline, the long-axis view of the IVC can be obtained by angling slightly to the patient's right side. Normally the IVC is less than 2 cm in diameter and collapses more than 50% with inspiration. It will also normally collapse with pressure from the transducer. If it does not collapse, the formula in the "Findings and Interpretation" section can be used to es-

timate RAP. The IVC is thin-walled compared with the aorta, and it may appear to pulsate as a result of pulsations transmitted through solid tissue from the aorta. When it collapses with inspiration, these pulsations will be minimized.

20. In addition to what has been described, almost all of the parasternal short-axis views can be obtained scanning from the subxiphoid position. However, because of the depth of tissue necessary to scan from this position, there is usually some loss of resolution. This is especially true when compared with scanning from the parasternal position.

21. Placing the transducer in the suprasternal notch with the marker dot to the patient's left side, scan the aortic arch in its long axis (Fig. 75.13) to provide what some call the "candy cane" view. With this image, the ascending aorta, its horizontal arch, and the proximal descending thoracic aorta can often be visualized. The origins of the left subclavian and left carotid arteries off the aorta can usually be visualized, and occasionally the origin of the brachiocephalic artery can be seen. The right pulmonary artery is usually noted in the short-axis view beneath the arch. This is the best view for excluding coarctation of the aorta.

22. From the suprasternal view, by angling the transducer anteriorly and to the patient's right, the aortic root can often be visualized.

23. Further clockwise rotation can be used to obtain short-axis views from the suprasternal notch (Fig. 75.14). The right pulmonary artery can often be visualized in this manner. The right pulmonary artery is located between the aorta and the left atrium. It may be possible to visualize where the pulmonary veins drain into the left atrium.

NOTE: With the incidence of abdominal aortic aneurysm (AAA) increasing (5% to 7% of individuals over the age of 60), there is a strong correlation between individuals having an AAA and having an echocardiogram for other indications. With the patient already gowned and covered with jelly, it may be an excellent opportunity to screen for an AAA, even if no one is charged for the service.

M-Mode Echocardiography

From the parasternal position, with either the long-axis or the short-axis view, M-mode images are usually obtained at three different levels: the level of the aortic valve, the level of the mitral valve, and the

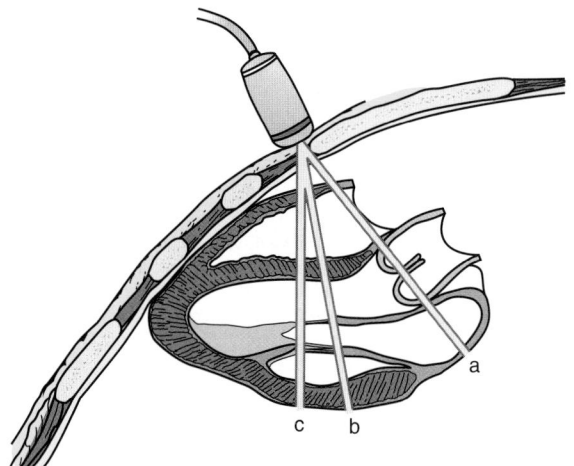

Fig. 75.15 Levels to obtain M-mode images: Level of aortic valve *(a)*; level of mitral valve *(b)*; level of papillary muscle *(c)*. (From Reynolds T. *The Echocardiographer's Pocket Reference.* 2nd ed. Phoenix: School of Cardiac Ultrasound at Arizona Heart Institute; 2000.)

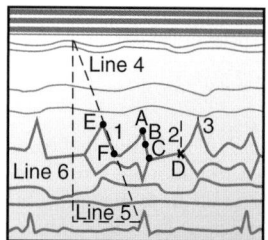

Fig. 75.16 M-mode at the level of the mitral valve. *E*, E-point, point of anterior leaflet maximal early opening); *Line 1, MV E–F*, Mitral valve, E to F slope; *Line 2, MV EXC*, vertical distance, mitral valve excursion (normal range 18 to 28 mm); *Line 3, EPSS*, E-point septal separation (normal range 2 to 7 mm); *A*, atrial systole; *B*, See text for explanation; *C*, Valve fully closed; *D*, Leaflets separate (valve opens). See text for explanation of lines 4, 5, and 6 and how to calculate E-to-F slope. (From Reynolds T. *The Echocardiographer's Pocket Reference.* 2nd ed. Phoenix: School of Cardiac Ultrasound at Arizona Heart Institute; 2000.)

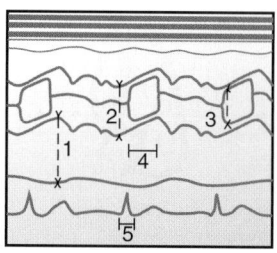

Fig. 75.17 M-mode at the level of the aortic valve. *1, LA,* Left atrium, end-systolic dimension (normal range 1.9–4 cm; *2, AoR*, aortic root, end-diastolic diameter (normal range, 2 to 3.7 cm); *3, ACS,* aortic cusps separation in systole (normal range, 1.5 to 2.6 cm); *4, LVET*, left ventricular ejection time; *5, PEP*, preejection period. (From Reynolds T. *The Echocardiographer's Pocket Reference.* 2nd ed. Phoenix: School of Cardiac Ultrasound at Arizona Heart Institute; 2000.)

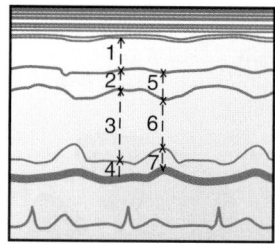

Fig. 75.18 M-mode at the level of the mitral valve chordae tendineae. *1, RVIDd,* Right ventricular internal diameter in diastole; *2, IVSd,* interventricular septal thickness in diastole; *3, LVIDd*, left ventricular internal diameter in diastole; *4, LVPWd,* left ventricular posterior wall thickness in diastole; *5, IVSs,* interventricular septal thickness in systole; *6, LVIDs*, left ventricular internal diameter in systole; *7, LVPWs,* left ventricular posterior wall thickness in systole). (From Reynolds T. *The Echocardiographer's Pocket Reference.* 2nd ed. Phoenix: School of Cardiac Ultrasound at Arizona Heart Institute; 2000.)

level of the papillary muscles in the left ventricle (Fig. 75.15). The subxiphoid transducer position can also be used for M-mode scanning when there is difficulty obtaining the standard parasternal images.

1. At the mitral valve level, the anterior mitral leaflet makes an M-shaped pattern. The posterior leaflet moves as its mirror image to make a W-shaped pattern. The point of maximal early opening excursion is labeled E (Fig. 75.16). Next, the rapid filling phase of early diastole occurs, and then the valve closes partially. While it is closing partially, the valve moves along the E-to-F slope. Note that this slope will be flatter if there is any condition impairing left ventricular filling. The E-to-F slope is followed by the remainder of diastole. During this phase, the A point indicates atrial systole. After atrial systole, the valve moves to the fully closed position labeled C. The closed leaflets then move together in ventricular systole until they separate at the D point. The B point is labeled but does not exist for normal patients. It occurs only if the A-to-C line is interrupted due to elevated left end-diastolic pressure or diastolic dysfunction (see Fig. 75.16). To determine the E-to-F slope, first draw diagonal line 4 through line 1 (i.e., basically a continuation of line 1). Draw a horizontal line (line 5) near the bottom of the tracing where line 4 intersects one of the time lines on the tracing. Draw line 5 horizontal to the left for a distance corresponding to exactly 1 second on the tracing. Next, draw a vertical line (line 6) from line 5 to where

it intersects line 4. Line 6 should be perpendicular to line 5. The length of line 6 in millimeters is the E-to-F slope of the anterior leaflet in millimeters per second (normal range 70 to 150 mm/s). The E-point septal separation (EPSS) is the vertical distance between the E-point and the septal wall. It is enlarged for dilated cardiomyopathy and suggests a reduced ejection fraction.

2. With M-mode imaging at the aortic valve level (Fig. 75.17), typically only two aortic cusps are identified. At the onset of systole, they separate abruptly; at the end of systole, they close abruptly, producing a square box on the image. Because normal aortic valves are very thin and often difficult to follow throughout the M-mode tracing, if the cusps are easily visualized, they may in fact be thickened. Following closure of the valve, the cusps normally remain opposed (closed) throughout diastole. The image at the level of the aortic valve is the most difficult to obtain with M-mode. Measurements of the left atrium, the aorta, and the valve cusp separation (opening diameter) are also taken at this level.

3. To obtain measurements of systolic time intervals, calipers can be used. The left ventricular ejection time (LVET) is the time from the opening of the aortic valve until it closes. The preejection period (PEP) is the time from the onset of the QRS to the onset of aortic valve opening (see Fig. 75.17).

4. Left ventricular measurements (e.g., systolic and diastolic dimensions) are best made slightly above the level of the papillary muscles, at the level of the chordae tendineae (Fig. 75.18). This is also an excellent view and level for obtaining right ventricular internal dimensions. Precise measurements of the thickness of all walls can also be made, in both diastole and systole.

5. For tricuspid valves, usually only one leaflet is traced with the M-mode for normal individuals. The RVIT view is an excellent view for tracing this single tricuspid leaflet. The pattern of motion for a single leaflet is similar to that of a mitral leaflet.

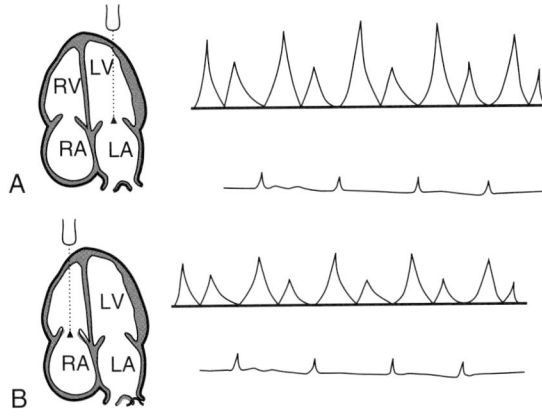

Fig. 75.19 Normal Doppler tracings. (A) Left ventricular inflow tract (mitral valve). (B) Right ventricular inflow tract (tricuspid valve). *LA*, Left atrium; *LV*, left ventricle; *RA*, right atrium; *RV*, right ventricle. (From Reynolds T. *The Echocardiographer's Pocket Reference.* 2nd ed. Phoenix: School of Cardiac Ultrasound at Arizona Heart Institute; 2000.)

6. For pulmonary valve M-mode tracings, the parasternal short-axis view at the level of the aortic valve can be used. Once again, usually only one leaflet is traced for normal individuals. Because normal tricuspid cusps are very thin, it is often difficult to follow the leaflet motion throughout the cycle.

Color and Doppler Flow Echocardiography

Multiple views can be used for this application, but inevitably the apical four-chamber view provides the best view for evaluating three of the valves. The parasternal short-axis view is often utilized to complete the evaluation of the valves. As each valve is being studied, the transducer should be placed so that it is as close as possible to being in line with the maximal flow across the valve. Transducer positioning can be guided by the resultant 2D image, by obtaining the maximal velocity on graphic image, by maximizing the sound, or by all three. Each operator develops his or her own technique for performing a complete examination and he or she should follow this technique with every evaluation (Fig. 75.19). A sample technique is provided here.

1. From the apical position, evaluate the left ventricular inflow tract with PW. Next, evaluate the left ventricular outflow tract.
2. The right ventricular or tricuspid inflow tract should then be evaluated. Next, either continuing to use the apical four-chamber view or shifting to the parasternal short-axis view at the level above the aortic valve, the right ventricular/pulmonary outflow tract should be evaluated.
3. Repeat the evaluation with CW.
4. If available, repeat the evaluation with color Doppler.

FINDINGS AND INTERPRETATION

Two-Dimensional and M-Mode Echocardiography

Overview of Study

The quality of every study should be described in the report (e.g., good, fair, poor). This determination often depends on the quality of the window, the equipment used, and the body habitus of the patient. Every report should also have at least a *qualitative* comment about the ejection fraction and segmental wall motion (e.g., normal, mildly impaired, moderately impaired, severely impaired). These parameters can also be measured *quantitatively*.

TABLE 75.2	Ventricular Volumes for Calculating Ejection Fraction

Ventricular volumes (EDV and ESV) calculated from ventricular dimensions (LVIDd and LVIDs, respectively) using the formula of Teichholz:

$$Volume = \frac{7}{2.4 + D} \times D^3$$

Dimension	Volume	Dimension	Volume	Dimension	Volume
2.0	13	4.0	70	7.0	254
2.1	14	4.1	74	7.1	265
2.2	16	4.2	79	7.2	272
2.3	18	4.3	83	7.3	280
2.4	20	4.4	88	7.4	288
2.5	22	4.5	92	7.5	300
2.6	25	4.6	97	7.6	307
2.7	27	4.7	103	7.7	315
2.8	30	4.8	107	7.8	327
2.9	31	4.9	113	7.9	336
3.0	35	5.0	118	8.0	343
3.1	38	5.1	123	8.1	356
3.2	41	5.2	129	8.2	364
3.3	44	5.3	135	8.3	372
3.4	47	5.4	142	8.4	385
3.5	51	5.5	148	8.5	393
3.6	55	5.6	155	8.6	407
3.7	59	5.7	159	8.7	415
3.8	62	5.8	166	8.8	429
3.9	66	5.9	174	8.9	439
		6.0	180		
		6.1	187		
		6.2	194		
		6.3	202		
		6.4	209		
		6.5	216		
		6.6	224		
		6.7	232		
		6.8	240		
		6.9	246		

EDV, End-diastolic volume; *ESV*, end-systolic volume; *LVIDd*, left ventricular internal diameter in diastole; *LVIDs*, left ventricular internal diameter in systole. From Teichholz LE, Cohen MV, Sonnenblick EH, Gorlin R. Study of left ventricular geometry and function by B-scan ultrasonography in patients with and without asynergy. *N Engl J Med.* 1974;291:1220.

EJECTION FRACTION

With 2D, if the equipment software is capable of tracing the ventricular cavity, the ejection fraction can be calculated by summing a series of discs. It can also be calculated using M-mode measurements applied to Table 75.2.

$$Ejection\ fraction = [(EDV - ESV)/EDV] \times 100$$

End-diastolic volume (EDV) and end-systolic volume (ESV) are both obtained from Table 75.2 using the left ventricular internal diameter in diastole and then the left ventricular internal diameter in systole (LVIDs) as the dimension in the table. Left ventricular internal diameter in systole is measured at the lowest vertical point of the septum. (See Table 75.3 for normal ranges.)

NOTE: At the Arizona Heart Institute, M-mode echocardiography is no longer used for determining the ejection fraction. Instead, at the end of every 2D study, the ejection fraction is either quantitatively measured using calipers or cavity tracings or estimated as normal (60%), moderately impaired (40%), or severely impaired (20%). As it turns out, various studies have compared qualitative estimates of ejection fraction with calculated ejection fractions, especially for those patients with suboptimal imaging. Qualitative estimates have been found to be fairly accurate.

TABLE 75.3   Normal M-Mode Measurements

	Mean	Range
Mitral Valve		
E–F slope	80 mm/sec	70–150 mm/sec
D–E excursion	20 mm	18–28 mm
EPSS	5 mm	2–7 mm
Aortic Root and Valve		
Root diameter	2.7 cm	2–3.7 cm
Root index	1.5 cm/m²	1.2–2.2 cm/m²
Valve systolic separation	1.9 cm	1.5–2.6 cm
Left Atrium		
LA diameter	2.9 cm	1.9–4 cm
LA index	1.6 cm/m²	1.2–2.2 cm/m²
LA/Ao ratio	1	0.87–1.11
Left Ventricle		
LVIDd	4.7 cm	3.7–5.6 cm
LVIDd index	2.6 cm/m²	1.9–3.2 cm/m²
LVIDs	3.1 cm	2–3.8 cm
LVIDs index	1.6 cm/m²	1.3–1.9 cm/m²
Interventricular Septum and Left Ventricular Posterior Wall		
IVS diastolic thickness	0.9 cm	0.6–1.1 cm
IVS excursion	0.7 cm	0.44–1.2 cm
LVPW diastolic thickness	0.9 cm	0.6–1.1 cm
LVPW excursion	1.2 cm	0.9–1.4 cm
Maximum velocity of LVPW excursion	61 mm/sec	40–78 mm/sec
IVS/LVPW ratio	<1.3:1	<1.5:1 hypertensive patient
Right Ventricle		
RVIDd (left lateral)	1.7 cm	0.9–2.6 cm
RVIDd index	0.9 cm/m³	0.4–2.5 cm/m²
RVIDs	1.8 cm	1.5–2.2 cm
RVIDs index	0.9 cm/m²	0.7–1.1 cm/m²
RV free wall excursion	0.9 cm	0.7–1 cm
RV free wall systolic thickening	50	30–38
RV velocity of systolic free wall excursion	41 mm/sec	36–55 mm/sec
RV wall thickness	0.5–0.8 cm	
Pulmonary Valve		
"A" dip		2–7 mm
E–F slope		6–115 mm/sec
Left Ventricular Systolic Function		
IVS % thickening*	46%	27%–70%
LVPW % thickening†	45%	25%–80%
Fractional shortening‡	33%	28%–41%
Ejection fraction§	62%	45%–90%
Mean circumferential fiber shortening¶	1.2 circ/sec	1–1.9 circ/sec
Relative wall thickness¶	37	30–45
Left Ventricular Mass		
American Society of Echocardiography 1.04 [(LVIDd + IVSd + LVPWd)³ − (LVIDd³)] 0.8 + 0.6 g		
Penn Convention 1.04 [(LVIDd + IVSd + LVPWd)³ − (LVIDd³)] − 13.6 g		

*IVS % thickening = [(IVSs − IVSd)/IVSd] × 100

†LVPW % thickening = [(LVPWs − LVPWd)/LVPWd] × 100

‡Fractional shortening = [(LVIDd − LVIDs)/LVIDd] × 100

§Ejection fraction = [(EDV − ESV)/EDV] × 100

¶Mean Vcf = (LVIDd − LVIDs)/(LVIDd × LVET)

¶¶Relative wall thickness = 2 LVPWd/LVIDd or IVS + LVPWd/LVIDd

Ao, Aortic root; *EDV*, end-diastolic volume; *EPSS*, E-point septal separation; *ESV*, end-systolic volume; *IVS*, interventricular septum; *IVSd*, interventricular septal thickness in diastole; *LA*, left atrium; *LVIDd*, left ventricular internal diameter in diastole; *LVIDs*, left ventricular internal diameter in systole; *LVPW*, left ventricular posterior wall; *RV*, right ventricle; *RVIDd*, right ventricular internal diameter in diastole; *RVIDs*, right ventricular internal diameter in systole.

From Reynolds T. *The Echocardiographer's Pocket Reference*. 2nd ed. Phoenix: School of Cardiac Ultrasound at Arizona Heart Institute; 2000.

Segmental Wall Motion

The American Society of Echocardiography has established the convention of dividing the heart into 17 segments (Fig. 75.20). These segments are distributed across three levels. Anything above the level of the head of the papillary muscle, where it joins the mitral leaflet, is defined as the basal level of the heart. The mid-level of the heart is defined by the entire length of the papillary muscle. Anything below the level of the base of the papillary muscle, where it attaches to the ventricular wall, is designated the apical level.

Each wall segment has a corresponding coronary artery that perfuses it. In general the anterior and anteroseptal walls and the entire apex are supplied by the left anterior descending coronary artery.

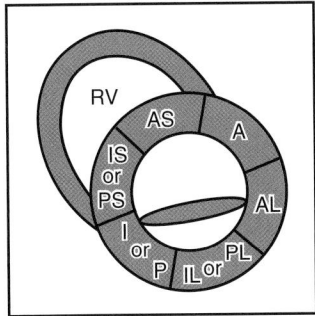

Base

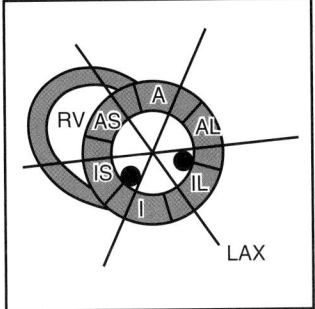

Mid

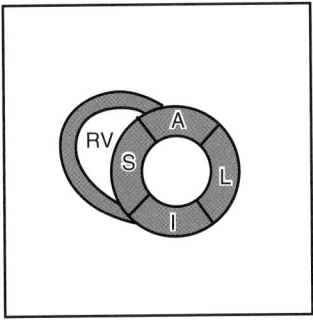

Apex

Fig. 75.20 American Society of Echocardiography 17-segment model of the heart. *A,* Anterior; *AL,* anterolateral; *AS,* anteroseptal; *I,* inferior; *IL,* inferolateral; *IS,* inferoseptal; *L,* lateral; *LAX,* long axis; *P,* posterior; *PL,* posterolateral; *PS,* posteroseptal; *RV,* right ventricle; *S,* septal. (From Reynolds T. *The Echocardiographer's Pocket Reference.* 2nd ed. Phoenix: School of Cardiac Ultrasound at Arizona Heart Institute; 2000.)

Therefore, even though the apex is divided into four segments—anterior, lateral, septal, and inferior (posterior) segments—all of these segments are usually perfused by the left anterior descending coronary artery. Both the mid-level of the heart and the basal level are divided into six segments. The inferior (posterior) wall and the inferoseptal (posteroseptal) walls at the basal and mid levels are supplied by septal perforators (posterior descending artery) from the dominant coronary artery on the inferior (posterior) surface of the heart. The lateral walls of the ventricle (anterolateral and inferolateral [posterolateral]) above the apex are supplied by the left circumflex artery.

Wall motion in each segment is scored based on the recommendations of the American Society of Echocardiography:

Normally contracting segment (or hyperkinetic segment) = 1
Hypokinesia = 2
Akinesis = 3
Dyskinesis = 4
Aneurysmal segment (i.e., deformed during diastole) = 5

The wall motion score index (WMSI) is derived from the sum of all scores divided by the number of segments visualized. A normally contracting left ventricle has a WMSI of 1 (i.e., each of the 17 segments receives a wall motion score of 1; thus, the total score is 17 and the WMSI is 17/17 = 1). Patients at increased risk for future cardiac events after an acute MI can be identified in part by a high WMSI (≥1.7).

Multiple views should be obtained with 2D echocardiography to compare the wall motion between various segments and to obtain the wall motion scores. Hypokinesis is defined as a less than 30% increase in wall thickening during systole and akinesis is defined as a less than 10% increase in thickening. Dyskinesis is present when the wall moves paradoxically outward when systolic thickening should be occurring. Comments should be made about wall motion, but more important, the walls should be scanned carefully for systolic thickening, which can be blunted by ischemia or infarction. Although wall motion scores may slightly overdiagnose the severity of an acute MI (e.g., severe ischemia can mimic an infarction), echocardiography is still much more accurate than an ECG. Of note, M-mode echocardiography has limited value in scanning for ischemia.

Acute Myocardial Infarction

In the setting of acute MI, 2D is very helpful because it provides immediate information, is noninvasive, and can be performed at the bedside. It can usually determine not only the location of the infarct but also its extent. Because 2D is noninvasive, serial scans can be performed to track progression. An abnormal wall motion score or evidence of a complication on 2D is valuable prognostic information. These patients should be triaged for aggressive therapy as opposed to patients who can be safely discharged early. In comparison, when using an ECG to determine risk (either high or low), the severity or location of the lesion cannot be predicted by ECG changes. Although an ECG may be helpful for diagnosing the acuity of an infarct, 2D is usually much more helpful overall because it can be used to actually stratify the patient's risk.

Mechanical complications of an acute MI that can be diagnosed early with 2D include pericarditis, pericardial effusion, pericardial tamponade, EMD, ventricular aneurysm, acute ischemic cardiomyopathy, mural thrombus, rupture of a papillary muscle (posteromedial much more commonly than anterolateral), and rupture of the ventricular free wall or septum.

Atrial Fibrillation

A left atrial dimension of greater than 4.5 cm indicates an increased risk of developing atrial fibrillation as well as a high probability of unsuccessful cardioversion. For more than 20 years, left atrial dilation in conjunction with mitral stenosis and atrial fibrillation has been associated with an increased risk of peripheral embolism and stroke. Such a finding should be managed aggressively with anticoagulation if not contraindicated.
NOTE: Atrial appendage thrombi are best excluded by transesophageal echo.

Cardiac Tumors

Cardiac tumors are seen as echogenic masses, and the majority (75% to 80%) of primary cardiac tumors are benign and curable. Thirty percent of benign tumors are myxomas, and they are usually attached by a stalk to the interatrial septum. They often prolapse partially or completely into the left ventricle during diastole.

Cardiac Tamponade and Pericardial Effusion

Cardiac tamponade and pericardial effusion (as well as EMD) are discussed in Chapter 214, Emergency Department, Hospitalist, and Office Ultrasound (POCUS).

Cardiomyopathy

DILATED CARDIOMYOPATHY: Cardiomyopathy is defined as a primary disease of the myocardium and, by definition, is not due to ischemia or valvular disease. Dilated cardiomyopathy is by far the most common type of cardiomyopathy. It is characterized by dilation of all four chambers and reduced systolic function in both ventricles.

Left ventricular dimensions (end-diastolic and end-systolic) and volumes are increased, whereas wall thicknesses are usually normal or slightly decreased. There will be a spherical configuration to the left ventricle with decreased left ventricular posterior wall and interventricular septal wall systolic thickening. As a result, there will be a decreased left ventricular ejection fraction. On M-mode, the LVET will be shortened, with a resultant prolonged preejection period / LVET ratio (>0.40). The distance of the anterior mitral leaflet from the septal wall (E-point septal separation) is increased. The presence of a B-bump on the mitral valve tracing indicates increased left ventricular end-diastolic pressure (>15 mm Hg). There may be pulmonary hypertension, and for an ejection fraction less than 35%, an echogenic mural thrombus (in either ventricle) must be excluded. Mitral regurgitation is present to some degree in most patients with dilated cardiomyopathy.

HYPERTROPHIC CARDIOMYOPATHY: This form is much less common than dilated cardiomyopathy and is an autosomal dominantly inherited disease with variable penetrance. The hypertrophy is usually asymmetric and the interventricular septum is often involved (asymmetric septal hypertrophy). Less commonly, the left ventricular free wall or the apex can be asymmetrically involved. Asymmetric septal hypertrophy can also be associated with obstruction of the left ventricular outflow tract, frequently as a result of the proximity of the anterior mitral leaflet to the septal wall (hypertrophic obstructive cardiomyopathy). Anterior motion of this leaflet during systole (systolic anterior motion [SAM]) can be noted on real-time or M-mode echocardiography to obstruct the outflow tract. Ventricular chambers are usually small. Most patients have mitral regurgitation as a result of systolic anterior motion. On M-mode, midsystolic closure of the aortic valve can also be noted.

RESTRICTIVE (NONDILATED/NONHYPERTROPHIC) CARDIOMYOPATHY: This type is rare and is characterized by normal ventricular wall thicknesses and cavity size at initial presentation. The systolic function is normal and the heart failure is due to a stiff, hypertrophied ventricle with resultant impaired diastolic function. Biatrial enlargement is usually noted. The etiology is usually a fibrotic or infiltrative process such as hemochromatosis, sarcoidosis, or hypereosinophilic syndrome. As the disease progresses, the patient can develop a dilated cardiomyopathy. Although amyloid heart has a definition separate from fibrotic or restrictive, it can appear very similar on echocardiography. It is common to find an associated pericardial effusion with amyloid heart.

Ischemic Heart Disease

Ischemic heart disease is assessed by looking at (1) global ventricular function (quantified with an ejection fraction) and (2) segmental wall function. Both should be assessed because both ischemia and infarction can cause significant segmental wall dysfunction without markedly affecting the ejection fraction. The most common cause of CHF in the United States is coronary artery disease; therefore it is common to see evidence of ischemic heart disease in patients with CHF.

Left Ventricular Hypertrophy

A common cause of LVH is hypertensive heart disease, initially with concentric hypertrophy, increased left ventricular mass, impaired diastolic function, and normal systolic function. As LVH progresses toward end-stage heart disease, systolic dysfunction develops and the left ventricle dilates. The left atrium will eventually dilate because of decreased left ventricular compliance and possibly mitral regurgitation. (A left atrial dimension greater than 4.5 cm indicates an increased risk of developing atrial fibrillation.) Frequently the aortic root will dilate and there will be associated aortic valve sclerosis. There may also be mitral annular calcification.

Concentric Hypertrophy

With concentric hypertrophy there is an equally distributed (uniform or globular) increase in ventricular wall thicknesses with normal ventricular dimensions (e.g., patients with valvular aortic stenosis (AS) or systemic hypertension). Left ventricular mass can be calculated to follow progression of LVH (see Table 75.3).

Eccentric Hypertrophy

Eccentric hypertrophy is commonly seen with aortic or mitral regurgitation. There is a spherical configuration to the left ventricle with normal wall thicknesses.

Mitral Valve Prolapse

In past years, MVP was overdiagnosed with echocardiography. As a result, a more formal definition was developed. Because the mitral valve, when closed, bulges normally or is "saddle shaped" in the plane of the mitral annulus, true prolapse should be diagnosed only if a portion of the anterior leaflet prolapses beyond this plane. By new criteria, it must prolapse more than 2 mm beyond the mitral annular plane on the parasternal long-axis view or more than 1 cm on the apical four-chamber view. Posterior leaflet prolapse is diagnosed if the leaflet prolapses beyond the mitral annular plane in the parasternal long-axis view, the apical four-chamber view, or by more than 2 mm on the apical two-chamber view. The mitral annular plane is defined by drawing an imaginary line from the base of the anterior leaflet to the base of the posterior leaflet.

Myxomatous degeneration is the result of an increase in the middle layer of the valve, the spongiosa. With proliferation, the spongiosa replaces part of the fibrosa layer and the valve is weakened. Eventually the valve becomes thickened, redundant, and elongated. In fact, it can develop the physical appearance of a hemorrhoid in its short-axis view. Myxomatous degeneration is usually diagnosed with 2D echocardiography; however, the thickness of the valve can be measured with either 2D or M-mode. The leaflets are considered redundant if they are 5 mm or more thick on the parasternal long-axis view during diastole or more than 1.4 times the wall thickness of the posterior wall of the aorta during diastole. On M-mode, the thickness is considered abnormal if 5 mm or greater.

Preliminary 2D and M-Mode Scanning Before Using Color and Doppler Flow

Diastolic function is best determined with color and Doppler flow imaging. As mentioned previously, color and Doppler flow imaging also assist in determining the hemodynamic severity of lesions and are therefore helpful for assessing valvular abnormalities. Color-flow Doppler also produces jets that are characteristic of certain abnormalities. Eccentric jets are very helpful for aligning CW Doppler in attempting to optimize the spectrum. Such spectrum analysis is helpful for further quantifying regurgitant lesions.

NOTE: In assessing tricuspid valve regurgitation (TR) with color- and Doppler flow imaging, note that TR is very common (90% of population). Therefore the regurgitation itself does not always have to be assessed. More importantly, the severity of the tricuspid regurgitation can be used to determine right-sided ventricular pressures. Pulmonary valve regurgitation is less common than TR, and mitral regurgitation is much less common. Aortic valve regurgitation is somewhat rare and its presence is always considered pathologic.

Despite the fact that the following disorders are best scanned with color and Doppler flow imaging, some information is usually obtained during preliminary 2D/M-mode scanning before using Doppler. This preliminary scanning is usually performed while 2D/M-mode measurements are being taken (see Table 75.4 for normal values).

TABLE 75.4	Normal Echo Measurements by Transthoracic Echocardiography
Structure	**Measurement by TTE**

Normal Values of the Right Heart Chambers

RV anteroposterior, diastole (cm)	2.5–3.8
RV anteroposterior, systole (cm)	2–3.4
RV mediolateral, diastole (cm)	2.1–4.2
RV mediolateral, systole (cm)	1.9–3.1
RV area, diastole (cm^2)	11–36
RV area, systole (cm^2)	5–20
RV ejection fraction (%)	>40
RV free-wall thickness (mm)	2–5
RV outflow tract, systole (cm)	1.8–3.4
RA anteroposterior, systole (cm)	—
RA mediolateral, systole (cm)	2.9–4.6
RA volume (mL)	15–58 in men, 14–44 in women
RA area (cm^2)	8.3–19.5

Normal Measurements of the Left Heart Valves and Great Vessels

Mitral valve area (cm^2)	4–6
Mitral annulus, diastole (cm)	2–3.4
Mitral leaflets thickness (mm)	4
Mitral regurgitation (overall %)	38–45
Pulmonary veins (mm)	8–15
Aortic valve area (cm^2)	3–5
Aortic annulus, systole (cm)	1.4–2.6
Aortic regurgitation (overall %)	0–2
Aortic root sinuses, diastole (cm)	2.1–3.5
Aortic root tubule, diastole (cm)	1.7–3.4
Aortic arch (cm)	2–3.6
Descending aorta (cm)	

Normal Measurements of the Right Heart Valves and Great Vessels

Tricuspid valve area (cm^2)	4–6
Tricuspid annulus, diastole (cm)	2–4
Tricuspid leaflet thickness (cm)	4
Tricuspid regurgitation (overall %)	15–78
Superior vena cava (cm)	—
Proximal inferior vena cava (cm)	1.2–2.3
Hepatic vein (cm)	0.5–1.1
Coronary sinus (cm)	—
Pulmonic valve area (cm^2)	3–5
Pulmonic valve annulus (cm)	1–2.2
Pulmonic regurgitation (overall %)	28–88
Right ventricular outflow tract, systole	1.8–3.4
Main pulmonary artery	1–2.9
Right or left pulmonary artery	0.7–1.7

Normal Values of the Left Heart Chambers

LV anteroposterior, diastole (cm)	3.5–5.7
LV anteroposterior, systole (cm)	2.5–4.3
LV mediolateral, diastole (cm)	3.7–5.6
LV mediolateral, systole (cm)	2.5–4.8
LV volume, diastole (mL)	59–157
LV volume, systole (mL)	16–68
LV area, diastole (cm^2)	18–47
LV area, systole (cm^2)	8–32
LV fractional shortening (%)	30–35
LV ejection fraction (%)	55
LV interventricular septal thickness, diastole (cm)	0.6–1.1
LV posterior wall thickness, diastole (cm)	0.6–1
LV mass (g)	<294 in men, <198 in women
LV outflow tract, systole (cm)	1.8–3.4
LA anteroposterior, systole (cm)	2.2–4.1
LA mediolateral, systole (cm)	2.5–4.5
LA volume (mL)	20–77 in men, 15–59 in women
LA area (cm^2)	9–23
LA appendage length (cm)	—
LA appendage diameter (cm)	—

LA, Left atrial; *LV*, left ventricular; *RA*, right atrial; *RV*, right ventricular; *TTE*, transthoracic echocardiography.
From Reynolds T. *The Echocardiographer's Pocket Reference*. 2nd ed. Phoenix: School of Cardiac Ultrasound at Arizona Heart Institute; 2000.

Aortic Stenosis

AS is usually the result of a degenerative process, rheumatic heart disease, or a bicuspid valve. With *degenerative/rheumatic AS*, the aortic cusps are usually thickened and there is associated concentric left ventricular hypertrophy, a dilated aortic root, a dilated left atrium, mitral annular calcification (50%), and a decreased mitral valve E–F slope.

As discussed earlier, the most common congenital abnormality in adult echocardiography is a bicuspid aortic valve. With AS resulting from a *bicuspid valve*, thickened leaflets are often noted as well as the characteristic oval shape of the valve opening. All of the findings of rheumatic/degenerative AS are also seen except for the mitral annular calcification.

Aortic Regurgitation

With aortic regurgitation, all of the findings of bicuspid AS can be seen except that the aortic root may not be dilated. Additional findings include premature closure of the mitral valve and premature opening of the aortic valve. Ventricular hypertrophy may be noted, either the eccentric or the globular type. There may also be an anatomic reason for the regurgitation (e.g., ascending aortic aneurysm, bicuspid aortic valve, valvular vegetation).

Mitral Stenosis

Mitral stenosis causes a decreased E–F slope and a decreased A wave on the M-mode tracing. The mitral leaflets may be thickened or they may be noted to have decreased mobility. In addition, the mitral valve opening orifice may be decreased, giving it the appearance of a "fish mouth" on 2D. The clinician should attempt to determine the degree of commissural and subvalvular involvement with the stenosis and scan for calcification of either the valve or the annulus. Possible associated findings include atrial dilation, a steep A–C slope, pulmonary hypertension, and an atrial septal defect. If the atrium is dilated, the clinician should scan for the presence of an echogenic thrombus. There may be right ventricular hypertrophy or dilation and evidence of right-sided volume overload. Clinicians should also scan for involvement of other valves. Doppler is needed to determine the orifice's opening diameter when the leaflets are densely calcified, when there is an inadequate parasternal short-axis image, there has been a surgical commissurotomy, or there is extensive subvalvular involvement (e.g., a secondary orifice located below the valve).

Mitral Regurgitation

With mitral regurgitation, there is usually echocardiographic evidence of left atrial and left ventricular volume overload patterns as well as an associated right-sided overload pattern. Pulmonary hypertension may be noted. LVH may be present, and serial scans may be needed to monitor the progression of LVH. In addition, the mitral annulus may be dilated (normal 2.3 ± 0.5 cm) on the apical four-chamber view. There may be an anatomic basis for the regurgitation: myxomatous degeneration of the valve with subsequent prolapse is the leading cause of regurgitation in the United States, but flail leaflets, annular calcification, or LV dysfunction (e.g., from ischemia) can be noted. The clinician should scan carefully to exclude flail leaflets.

Pulmonary Hypertension

With pulmonary hypertension, RAP will be elevated. The dimensions of the IVC can be used to estimate RAP (Table 75.5). There will also usually be evidence of right ventricular hypertrophy (>5 mm thickness), especially if it is chronic pulmonary hypertension. This hypertrophy may cause impingement on the left ventricle, resulting in a D-shaped left ventricle. The right atrium and pulmonary artery may also be dilated. The interatrial septum may be deviated toward the left atrium.

On M-mode, mitral valve disease may be diagnosed. Paradoxic septal motion as well as an increased septal wall thickness may be noted. There will also be abnormalities of the pulmonary valve cusp motion.

TABLE 75.5	Estimating Right Atrial Pressure	RAP (mm Hg)
IVC <2 cm diameter and collapses >50% with inspiration		5
IVC <2 cm diameter and collapses <50% with inspiration		10
IVC >2 cm diameter and collapses <50% with inspiration		15
IVC >2 cm diameter and does not collapse with inspiration		20

With pulmonary hypertension, RAP will be elevated. The dimensions of the IVC can be used to estimate RAP.
IVC, Inferior vena cava; *RAP*, right atrial pressure.

Tricuspid Regurgitation

With pathologic TR, there is usually evidence of a right ventricular volume overload pattern, including right atrial dilation. A B-bump of the anterior tricuspid leaflet is often noted on M-mode. The tricuspid valve annulus may be dilated (3.4 cm diameter in systole, ≥3.2 cm in diastole). There may be signs of pulmonary hypertension. For regurgitation, there may be an anatomic etiology (e.g., valvular vegetation, ruptured chordae tendineae).

Tricuspid Stenosis

With tricuspid stenosis, thickened valve leaflets may be noted. The right atrium is usually dilated, as well as the IVC (normal 1.2 to 2.3 cm) on M-mode. There will be decreased tricuspid valve excursion (D–E) and a decreased or absent A wave of the anterior leaflet.

Color and Doppler Flow Imaging

A complete listing of all of the possible findings and interpretation with color and Doppler flow imaging is beyond the scope of this book. However, there are some rules of thumb:

- Any velocity greater than 2 m/sec in the heart must be explained. Something as simple as a hyperdynamic heart from anemia can cause it; however, pathologic causes should be excluded.
- The Bernoulli equation can be used to determine pressure drops across values:

$$\Delta P \,(mm\,Hg) = 4 \times [velocity\,(m/sec)]^2$$

- An approximation for right ventricular systolic pressure (RVSP) is RVSP (mm Hg) = 4 Δ P [tricuspid valve (mm Hg)] + 10 mm Hg
  The actual method of calculating RSVP is:

$$RSVP\,(mm\,Hg) = 4 \times (TR\,peak\,velocity)^2 + RAP$$

  See the earlier "Pulmonary Hypertension" section for the estimation of RAP; for most patients, RAP can be approximated at 10 mm Hg.
- Normal aortic and pulmonary valves produce a bullet-shaped pattern on spectral analysis. Normal mitral and tricuspid valves produce an M-shaped pattern on spectral analysis.
- Laminar flow produces linear spectral analyses, but turbulent flow fills in the area under the curve. Regurgitant flow is always turbulent.
- With color Doppler, a green hue indicates turbulent flow. Highly turbulent flow is mosaic in appearance.

COMPLICATIONS

- Failure to provide an adequate scan
- Failure to diagnose
- Clinical deterioration while scanning in the acute setting

CPT/Billing Codes

93307 Echocardiography, transthoracic, real-time with image documentation (2D), includes M-mode recording, complete, without spectral or color Doppler echocardiography
93308 Follow-up or limited study
93320 Doppler echocardiography, pulsed wave and/or continuous wave with spectral display (list separately in addition to codes for echocardiographic imaging); complete
93321 Follow-up or limited study

ICD-10-CM Diagnostic Codes

D17.4 Myxolipoma, intrathoracic organs
I05.0 Mitral stenosis, rheumatic
I05.1 Mitral stenosis with insufficiency, rheumatic
I11.9 Hypertensive heart disease or hypertensive LVH, benign, without CHF
I11.0 Hypertensive heart disease, benign, with CHF
I21.09 Acute myocardial infarction, of anterolateral wall
I21.19 Acute myocardial infarction, of inferolateral wall
I21.29 Myocardial infarction, acute, unspecified site and episode
I25.2 Old myocardial infarction
I25.10 Coronary atherosclerosis, native coronary artery w/o angina pectoris
I25.709 Coronary atherosclerosis, of artery bypass graft(s) w/unspecified angina
I25.9 Ischemic heart disease, chronic unspecified
I25.3 Aneurysm of heart wall
I26.99 Iatrogenic pulmonary embolism and infarction
I27.0 Pulmonary hypertension, primary, chronic
I27.21 Pulmonary hypertension, secondary, chronic
I30.9 Pericardial effusion, acute
I30.0 Pericarditis, acute, idiopathic
I30.1 Pericarditis, acute, purulent* (use additional code for infectious agent)
I40.9 Myocarditis, acute
I31.2 Hemopericardium
I31.4 Cardiac tamponade* (Code first underlying cause)
I31.9 Pericardial effusion, unspecified disease of pericardium
I34.0 Mitral valve disorders, nonrheumatic (incompetence, insufficiency, regurgitation, prolapse)
I35.0-I35.9 Aortic valve disorders (incompetence, insufficiency, regurgitation, stenosis)
I42.5 Other restrictive cardiomyopathy (NOS)
I42.6 Cardiomyopathy, alcoholic
I44.7 Left bundle branch block, unspecified
I45.10 Right bundle branch block unspecified
I46.9 Cardiac arrest cause unspecified
I48.91 Atrial fibrillation unspecified
I50.9 Heart failure unspecified
I50.1 Left ventricular failure unspecified
I50.40 Combined systolic and diastolic heart failure
I50.21 Systolic heart failure, acute
I50.22 Systolic heart failure, chronic
I50.31 Diastolic heart failure, acute
I51.5 Myocardial degeneration
I51.7 Cardiomegaly
I23.0 Mural thrombus (atrial, ventricular) acquired following myocardial infarction
I66.9 Cerebral embolism
G45.8 Cerebral ischemia, transient
G45.9 Transient ischemic attack
I71.01 Aortic dissection, thoracic
R00.2 Palpitations
R07.9 Chest pain, unspecified

Suppliers

Several manufacturers have products ranging from the basic to the very sophisticated. Small handheld machines are now available. Acuson Siemens, Esaote, General Electric Healthcare, Samsung Medison, Phillips, and Toshiba all offer a range of devices from handheld to research-oriented (see the "Suppliers" section in Chapter 142, Obstetric Ultrasound, for contact information for many manufacturers). An excellent way to review the equipment is to visit the company websites. Used equipment is also available, but the cost and inconvenience of service and repairs are often a disadvantage. Overreading services are also available.

Online Resources

Mayo Clinic (CME online videos and DVDs on echocardiography): https://cveducation.mayo.edu/store/online/search.

Recommended Reading

ACC/AHA. Clinical competence statement on echocardiography. *Circulation.* 2003;107:1068–1089.

ACC/AHA/ASE. Guideline update for the clinical application of echocardiography: summary article: a report of the American College of Cardiology/American Heart Association Task Force on Practice Guidelines (ACC/AHA/ASE Committee to Update the 1997 Guidelines for the Clinical Application of Echocardiography). *Circulation.* 2003;108:1146–1162.

ACCF/ASE/AHA/ASNC/HFSA/HRS/SCAI/SCCM/SCCT/SCMR. 2011 Appropriate use criteria for echocardiography. *J Am Soc Cardiol.* 2011;24:229–267.

Armstrong WF. *Feigenbaum's Echocardiography.* 8th ed. Philadephia: Lippincott: Williams & Wilkins; 2018.

Chavey WE, Hogikyan RV, Van Harrison R, Nicklas JM. Heart failure due to reduced ejection fraction: medical management. *Am Fam Physician.* 2017;95(1):13–20.

Gazewood JD, Turner PL. Heart failure with preserved ejection fraction: diagnosis and management. *Am Fam Physician.* 2017;96(9):582–588.

King M, Kingery J, Casey B. Diagnosis and evaluation of heart failure. *Am Fam Physician.* 2012;85(12):1161–1168.

Otto CM. *Textbook of Clinical Echocardiography.* 5th ed. Philadelphia: Elsevier; 2013.

Reynolds T. *The Echocardiographer's Pocket Reference.* 4th ed. Phoenix: Arizona Heart Foundation; 2013.

CHAPTER 76

STRESS ECHOCARDIOGRAPHY

Grant C. Fowler • Al Smith

One of every four deaths in the United States is caused by heart disease, and almost half a million deaths a year are due to coronary artery disease (CAD); these are the leading causes of death in both genders. However, we are doing a better job of keeping these patients alive. Consequently primary care clinicians will continue to manage an increasing number of patients with known CAD. Stress echocardiography (stress echo) is not only a safe, cost-effective, and noninvasive method for diagnosing CAD, but it is also helpful for managing CAD, including determining the prognosis. Some clinicians also use stress echo to screen high-risk asymptomatic individuals or to stratify risk in preoperative evaluations. With medical management of CAD more successful than ever, primary care clinicians' skills in diagnosing and managing CAD have become more important. Performing stress echo is one method of maximizing these skills.

With improved ultrasound technology and image quality, adequate imaging can now be produced in 85% to 90% of patients undergoing stress echo. Improved digital imaging also makes it easier to compare preexercise and postexercise stress echo images side by side. The cost of echo equipment has decreased significantly; at the same time, more training programs have become available. Consequently echo has seen some of the most rapid growth in utilization among primary care clinicians who perform procedures.

Adding a cardiac imaging test to an exercise electrocardiography (ECG) test (EET) or a pharmacologic stress test is indicated when there is need to define the location, overall extent, or functional significance of CAD. Differing from an EET, which cannot predict which obstructed coronary artery is causing a positive test, stress echo is able to determine which artery is obstructed by noting which ventricular wall becomes ischemic (Table 76.1). Although coronary angiography may not be the best method for determining the functional significance of CAD, it can be used as the gold standard in comparing the accuracy of nuclear myocardial perfusion imaging with stress echo. In the revascularized patient, several meta-analyses compared the accuracy of these two tests for the detection of restenosis (Chin, et al, 2003, Dori, et al, 2003, Garzon, et al, 2001). Based on results showing very similar sensitivities, specificities, and accuracies for the diagnosis of CAD, the choice of imaging for CAD after revascularization will likely depend on clinician experience and other local factors, such as availability and expertise. Regarding prognosis for patients with CAD, several other meta-analyses have compared stress echo with myocardial perfusion imaging and demonstrated comparable results (Fleischmann KE, et al, 1998, Mahajan N, et al, 2010, Metz, et al, 2007). If the echo images obtained are excellent, stress echo may be more accurate than myocardial perfusion imaging.

When evaluating patients for cardiac problems, stress echo has another added benefit, that of diagnosing other possible causes—such as hypertrophic cardiomyopathy, aortic dissection, valvular heart disease, diastolic dysfunction, and pericardial effusion. This sets it apart from myocardial perfusion imaging. Stress echo is also faster to complete, is less expensive, and does not require radiation.

In addition to greater convenience to the patient, benefits for primary care clinicians performing stress echo (especially in the office setting) include having test results immediately available, improving communication and referral patterns to cardiologists, and improving their echo reading skills. Clinicians performing stress echo also naturally improve their understanding of CAD pathophysiology as well as exercise physiology. With immediately available results, patient satisfaction is usually improved and liability for the clinician from failure to diagnose should be decreased.

PHYSIOLOGY OF STRESS ECHOCARDIOGRAPHY

Normally, as the heart rate increases with exercise, the walls of the left ventricle increase contractility, increase endocardial excursion (>5 mm), become hyperdynamic, and thicken in systole. Depending on the exercise protocol utilized, the ejection fraction will also normally increase. Consequently the end-systolic volume, which is the actual size of the left ventricle at end-systole, decreases. In the patient with obstructive CAD, a threshold is eventually reached with increasing exercise, at which point the heart's demand for oxygen exceeds the supply. At this threshold, the heart becomes ischemic, first regionally or in segments and then often globally. Although it is best to obtain echo images within the first minute of discontinuing exercise, this blunting of wall motion will typically persist for 3 to 5 minutes, depending on the severity and duration of the preceding ischemia. Interpretation of a stress echo test consists of quantifying these transient regional wall motion abnormalities (Fig. 76.1) as well as the global function (i.e., ejection fraction/end-systolic volume). Transient ischemia is assessed and quantified by comparing pre- and postexercise echo images. (Depending on the protocol, images are also sometimes obtained at maximal exertion.)

From an ECG perspective, the patient with subendocardial ischemia usually demonstrates ST segment depression (i.e., a positive exercise EET; see Chapter 74, Stress ECG Testing) in several leads. Usually this depression is followed by chest discomfort (i.e., angina) as the "ischemic cascade" progresses. The term "ischemic cascade" describes the predictable sequence of events that occur after the onset of ischemia. With stress echo, earlier aspects of this ischemic cascade can be noted. Soon after the metabolic abnormalities are produced by ischemia, diastolic abnormalities appear, which can be seen with stress echo. The appearance of these abnormalities is rapidly followed by myocardial perfusion defects and, in turn, by wall motion abnormalities again seen on stress echo. In other words, ischemic changes can be seen on perfusion imaging and stress echo prior to the development of ECG changes on EET. Eventually chest pain may develop, the exception being patients who experience "silent angina" (typically patients >70 years of age, often earlier in diabetics). In patients with silent angina, dyspnea or dyspnea with exertion is a common presentation of an anginal equivalent.

Exercise capacity is an important separate predictor of outcome from a cardiovascular perspective; for those patients able to exercise, therefore, exercise echo is recommended over pharmacologic stress echo. For those able to walk on a treadmill, it is probably the preferred mode of exercise testing because the workload achieved as well as the maximal heart rate is usually higher than with a bicycle.

510

TABLE 76.1	Left Ventricular Wall Segments and Corresponding Coronary Artery Supply	
Echocardiographic Segment	**Coronary Artery**
Basal, mid, and apical anterior	LAD
Basal, mid, and apical anterior septum	LAD
Apical lateral	LAD
Basal and mid-anterolateral	LAD/LCA
Basal and mid-inferior	RCA
Basal and mid-inferior septum	RCA
Apical inferior	RCA/LAD
Basal and mid-inferolateral	LCA

LAD, Left anterior descending artery; *LCA,* left circumflex artery; *RCA,* right coronary artery.

The most common forms of exercise in the United States are walking and jogging, so patients are often more comfortable with a treadmill, and it is possibly less effort or motivation dependent. However, the maximal blood pressure achieved is usually higher on a bicycle than with a treadmill, and images can be obtained during exercise and at peak workload with use of a supine bicycle. A bicycle is also often the preferred form of exercise for patients with orthopedic problems.

INDICATIONS

NOTE: The American College of Cardiology (ACC)/American Heart Association (AHA) and others suggest that for the patient capable of exercise with no baseline ECG abnormalities affecting the ability to monitor or interpret an EET (e.g., left bundle branch block [LBBB], digitalis effect, Wolff-Parkinson-White [WPW] syndrome, left ventricular hypertrophy [LVH], >1 mm ST-segment depression), EET is the preferred method of evaluation to exclude CAD. Not every patient needs to be evaluated with imaging. Even

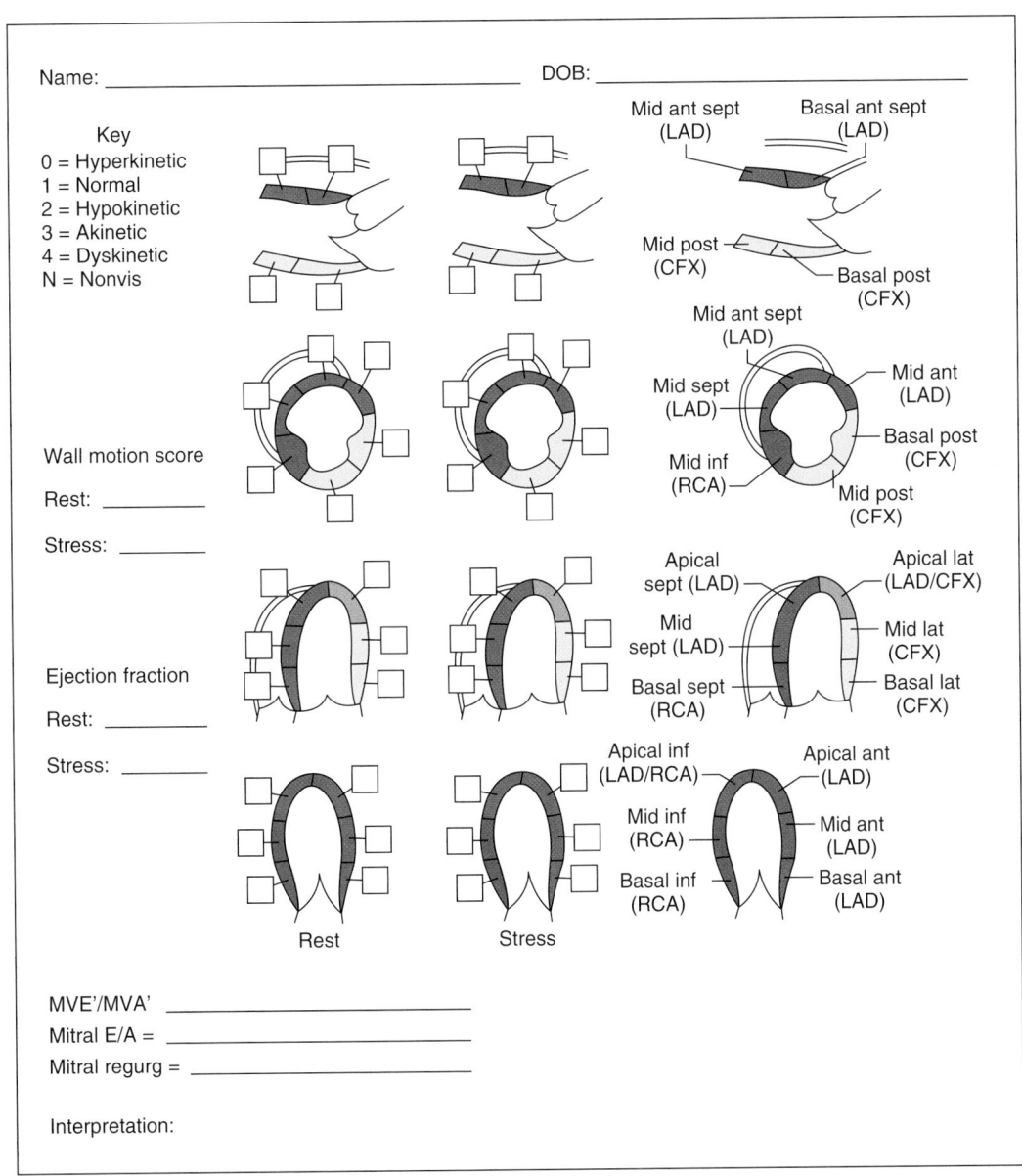

Fig. 76.1 Stress echocardiography test score form. *CFX,* Circumflex coronary artery; *DOB,* date of birth; *LAD,* left anterior descending coronary artery; *MVA´,* mitral valve annulus velocity; *MVE´,* mitral inflow velocity; *RCA,* right coronary artery.

in the patient with an intermediate pretest probability of disease, the ACC/AHA recommend a stepwise strategy for diagnosing CAD; in these patients, an EET is the preferred initial test. That said, there are plenty of indications for stress echo:

- Detection of CAD.
- Dyspnea possibly due to CAD.
- Equivocal, uninterpretable, or suspected false-positive EET.
- High probability of false-positive EET (e.g., women, mitral valve prolapse).
- Baseline ECG abnormalities that would affect the ability to monitor or interpret an EET (e.g., LBBB, digitalis effect, WPW syndrome, LVH, >1 mm ST segment depression).
- New-onset atrial fibrillation or heart failure, especially if there is an intermediate pretest probability of CAD.
- Need to define extent, location, or functional significance of CAD.
- Risk stratification/prognostic assessment in patient with known CAD (preoperative, post–myocardial infarction).
  NOTE: Dobutamine echo is probably the preferred method of evaluating a patient preoperatively for high-risk or vascular surgery. See Box 76.1 for shortcuts to determine indications for noninvasive testing prior to noncardiac surgery. (See also Chapter 71, Preoperative Evaluation.)
- Risk stratification after coronary revascularization (percutaneous coronary intervention or coronary artery bypass graft) procedures.
- Viability assessment in candidate for revascularization.
- Radionuclide perfusion imaging not available.
- High probability of false-positive radionuclide perfusion imaging (e.g., correction software package not available for perfusion imaging when likely to have attenuation artifact due to nearby adipose tissue, as in women or large-chested men).
- Asymptomatic patients with multiple risk factors for CAD or high-risk coronary calcium score from electron beam computed tomography (EBCT) or on ambulatory ECG (Holter or event) monitoring (see Chapter 73, Ambulatory Electrocardiography: Holter and Event Monitoring).
- Incomplete EET (failure to achieve 85% of predicted maximal heart rate; pharmacologic testing may be indicated).

BOX 76.1 Shortcuts to Determine Indicators for Noninvasive Testing Before Noncardiac Surgery

No testing necessary if the answer is *yes* to any of these four questions:

1. Is this low-risk surgery (i.e., estimated perioperative risk <1%)?
2. Does the patient have at least fair functional/exercise capacity (≥4 METs) and no symptoms?
3. Has the patient undergone revascularization within last 1 year without a change in symptoms indicating ischemia?
4. Has the patient had a thorough coronary evaluation (normal stress test, normal CT or invasive coronary angiogram) within last 1 year without a change in symptoms indicating ischemia?

Conversely, if elevated risk (>1%) and poor (<4 METs) or unknown functional/ exercise capacity, noninvasive testing is reasonable if the results will change the management.

CT, Computed tomography; METs, metabolic equivalents.
From ACCF/AHA/ASE/ASNC/HFSA/HRS/SCAI/SCCT/SCMR/ STS. 2013 Multimodality appropriate use criteria for the detection and risk assessment of stable ischemic heart disease. *J Am Coll Cardiol.* 2014;63(4):380–406 and ACC/AHA: 2014 Guidelines on perioperative cardiovascular evaluation and management of patients undergoing noncardiac surgery. *Circulation.* 2014;130:278–333.

- A pharmacologic agent may be indicated with stress echo (dobutamine or arbutamine preferred for stress echo over vasodilator infusion; vasodilator infusion usually preferred for myocardial perfusion imaging) in patients unable to exercise (e.g., peripheral artery disease, orthopedic problems, low exercise tolerance, contraindications to exercise [acute coronary syndrome with negative serial cardiac markers, equivocal aortic stenosis with low cardiac output]). Vasodilator (e.g., adenosine, dipyridamole, regadenoson) infusion produces only mild to moderate increases in heart rate and a mild decrease in blood pressure.
- Contrast study may be indicated with stress echo if two or more segments are not seen on noncontrast images.
- Permanent or transesophageal pacing may be indicated with stress echo (the pacing rate can be increased until the desired heart rate is achieved; however, these techniques are beyond the scope of this chapter).
- Mitral and aortic valve stenosis and regurgitation can be assessed, usually involving color Doppler (these techniques are beyond the scope of this chapter).
- Careful assessment of aortic stenosis by noting rapid change in pre– and post–aortic valve peak pressures.

Results of a comprehensive, expert survey are available regarding the appropriate use of stress echo. The most common and appropriate indications for primary care clinicians include diagnosing CAD (especially when EET is uninterpretable or equivocal or there is a high risk of a false-positive EET or myocardial perfusion imaging test) and managing CAD (especially when it is necessary to define the extent, location, or functional significance of CAD, as in the revascularized patient). These guidelines also cover special situations in which stress echo is useful (e.g., dyspnea, pulmonary hypertension, valvular stenosis, new-onset atrial fibrillation, or heart failure), especially if combined with intermediate probability of CAD. The use of stress echo often sorts out whether the symptom or problem is coming from CAD or another source. As previously discussed, clinicians should recall that by the age of 70 (often earlier for diabetics), the most common symptom for presentation of an acute myocardial infarction (MI) is dyspnea as opposed to chest pain. This is similar to the "silent angina" or anginal equivalent that patients often develop, resulting in dyspnea with exertion.

Indications for Diabetics

Because of a disproportionate burden of CAD in diabetic patients, the American Diabetes Association has suggested indications for cardiac testing in diabetic patients. Although these indications have varied over the years, two indications have persisted:

1. Typical or atypical cardiac symptoms
2. Abnormal resting ECG (especially if suggestive of ischemia or myocardial infarction)

Many diabetic patients are unable to undergo an EET due to peripheral artery disease or neuropathy. Such patients are generally at higher risk for cardiovascular events than those able to undergo an EET. Dobutamine stress echo has been shown to provide independent prognostic information in this group.

Determination of Pretest Probability

Determining pretest probability may help the clinician decide if stress echo is the indicated and proper diagnostic procedure. Stress echo is probably not indicated in patients with a low pretest probability of CAD (<10%) if they are able to exercise and have an interpretable ECG (i.e., absence of baseline ECG abnormalities such as LBBB, digitalis effect, WPW syndrome, LVH, >1 mm ST-segment depression).

Pretest probability can be estimated by a description of the chest pain and the patient's gender and age. *Typical angina* is described as substernal, exertional, and relieved by rest or nitroglycerin. Chest discomfort with two of these three characteristics is *atypical angina*. Chest discomfort with only one of these characteristics is considered *nonanginal chest pain*. Use of these three descriptions, pretest probability tables, and their corresponding graphs (see Table 74.1 and Fig. 74.4 in Chapter 74, Stress ECG Testing) can be readily applied to determine pretest probability. Determining pretest probability may also be helpful in assessing prognosis.

CONTRAINDICATIONS

- Unable to obtain adequate resting echo images
- Very recent acute MI (within 2 days) or other acute cardiac event (submaximal testing may be indicated unless patient has undergone angioplasty or stent placement)
- High-risk unstable angina
- Severe symptomatic left ventricular dysfunction or uncontrolled symptomatic heart failure
- Potentially life-threatening or uncontrolled ventricular arrhythmias causing symptoms or hemodynamic compromise
- Third-degree atrioventricular block or second-degree Mobitz type II block without pacemaker
- Acute pericarditis, myocarditis, or endocarditis
- Severe aortic stenosis, hypertrophic cardiomyopathy, or other form of outflow obstruction (can be excluded by performing echo prior to test)
- Suspected dissecting aneurysm
- Severe arterial hypertension (resting >200 mm Hg systolic or >115 mm Hg diastolic)
- Electrolyte abnormality
- Acute pulmonary edema, embolus, or infarction
- Acute thrombophlebitis, deep vein thrombosis, or intracardiac thrombi
- Acute or serious general illness or infection
- Neuromuscular, musculoskeletal, or arthritic condition that precludes exercise (pharmacologic testing may be an option)
- Uncontrolled metabolic disease such as diabetes, thyrotoxicosis, or myxedema
- Medication intoxication from drugs such as digoxin, sedatives, or psychotropic agents
- Advanced or complicated pregnancy
- Patient inability or lack of desire or motivation to perform the test, including severe emotional distress
- Nonavailability of advanced cardiac life support (ACLS) equipment or of an individual certified to perform ACLS

NOTE: Some of these contraindications are relative. In selected cases, a skilled cardiologist may perform testing for patients with these diagnoses (generally in a referral center). All are contraindications to testing in the office.

EQUIPMENT

- For best images, an ultrasound machine with several probes of varying frequency should be available. Among these probes, a low-frequency (e.g., 2.5 MHz) probe with two-dimensional (2D), M-mode, and cardiac Doppler capabilities is necessary. An ultrasound machine with harmonic imaging ensures high-quality images. A method of recording the examination (e.g., server, DVD, VCR) is also needed for documentation.
- Ultrasonic jelly and towels to clean up after scanning.
- Patient gown.
- A treadmill with adjustable speed and grade (see Fig. 74.11 in Chapter 74, Stress ECG Testing); this is the most common equipment used for stress echo. Advantages include the ability to test most patients under the actual physiologic conditions of exercise. Disadvantages include the fact that the treadmill may be difficult to use for patients with lower-extremity or lower-back problems or for patients who are very obese. The equipment is also more expensive, causes more motion artifact, and is noisier than a bicycle ergometer.
- Bicycle ergometers (see Fig. 74.8 in Chapter 74, Stress ECG Testing) use adjustable resistance and pedal frequency to exercise the patient. Advantages with the bicycle ergometer include the ability to terminate the test instantly. If a bicycle ergometer is utilized, images can be obtained at peak workload, especially if a supine bicycle is used. These images are especially useful for evaluating diastolic and valvular dysfunction, especially with use of color Doppler. Many patients feel more secure sitting on the bicycle. This method is also associated with less artifact, and blood pressure (BP) measurements are easier to obtain. Unfortunately, in the United States, leg fatigue is common because most patients do not cycle. In fact, as a result of leg fatigue, the procedure often fails to determine VO_2max. Bicycle ergometry is also dependent on motivation throughout its duration. As a result, in the United States if the patient can tolerate the treadmill, most clinicians prefer to use it.
- Arm ergometer (see Fig. 74.9 in Chapter 74, Stress ECG Testing). This enables patients with severe orthopedic or leg problems to be tested. However, muscle fatigue often occurs before the maximal heart rate is achieved.
- ECG machine (see Fig. 74.10 in Chapter 74, Stress ECG Testing). A continuous monitor is needed (at least a three-channel model with continuous tracing, and a screen-freeze option is desirable) as well as a 12-lead ECG recorder. With modern equipment, the recorder also runs the treadmill. Most equipment is now digital, allowing data to be filtered to provide a smooth baseline.
- Electrodes, cables, and belt. A disposable or washable belt is preferred because patients usually sweat.
- Sphygmomanometer, including various cuff sizes. A gauge manometer is adequate because the most important readings are those relative to resting pressures (not the absolute pressures).
- Stethoscope.
- Razor, rubbing alcohol.
- Intravenous setup and medications for pharmacologic testing, if planned, including atropine.
- Emergency equipment (see Fig. 212.4 in Chapter 212, Anaphylaxis) including a monitor/defibrillator; oxygen; airways, intubation, and suction equipment; and an emergency drug kit containing intravenous fluids and tubing (available drugs should be able to support ACLS protocols).

All emergency equipment should be checked daily, and medications should be checked weekly to monthly, depending on their use. The exercise testing equipment should be inspected and calibrated periodically based on manufacturer recommendations. ACLS certification cards should be kept on file along with any other information or written protocols.

NOTE: It is also helpful to have a trained technician assisting (see Fig. 74.11 in Chapter 74, Stress ECG Testing). Technician certification for exercise testing is available through the American College of Sports Medicine. In many centers the technician prepares the patient; monitors the ECG and the patient's response to exercise, his or her heart rate, and BP; obtains the pre- and postexercise echo images; and prepares the results for interpretation. For low-risk patients, the technician may actually perform the entire study without the presence of a clinician. Otherwise, if present, the clinician should examine the patient before, during, and after the procedure; confirm which protocol to use; and terminate the study. The clinician should also monitor the ECG tracing when the technician is taking BP readings, and the clinician should interpret the final results.

PREPROCEDURE PATIENT PREPARATION

Before Arrival

- The clinician should instruct the patient to minimize alcohol, over-the-counter medications, and caffeine consumption the day before and the day of the procedure. The patient should be encouraged to get a good night's sleep the night before the procedure and instructed to not eat for 2 hours before the test. It might be advisable for the most recent meal to be a small and predominately liquid meal. To minimize the risk of patient fatigue, many clinicians prefer performing exercise testing in the morning. They then instruct the patient to avoid breakfast or to have only a liquid breakfast that day.
- The procedure should be rescheduled, if possible, if the patient has a cold or other viral illness or is not feeling well in general.
- If the indication for the test is to screen for disease or to make the diagnosis of CAD, the clinician should instruct the patient to avoid taking β-blockers or rate-limiting calcium channel blockers the day of the test.
  NOTE: β-Blockers can suppress the heart rate, diminish segmental wall contractility, and prevent determination of the maximal heart rate (MHR). Patients who discontinue β-blockers should watch closely for "rebound" symptoms and, if they develop, should restart their β-blockers. Because angiotensin-converting enzyme (ACE) inhibitors have little or no effect on the performance of a stress test, they can be used as a substitute for other antihypertensive agents. If necessary they can be taken on the day of the test and usually work within an hour. Clonidine may be used in the same manner.
- If the indication for the test is to determine pharmacologic efficacy in patients with CAD, obviously β-blockers and calcium channel blockers should be taken the day of the study.
- Depending on the exercise protocol or mode of stress anticipated, the clinician may want to instruct the patient to bring shoes and clothing that are comfortable for walking, possibly for jogging, or for riding a bicycle.
- To minimize patient worry and anxiety (which often cause an elevated resting systolic BP), the clinician should explain that the risk of complications or death for patients being tested using a treadmill is very small. The patient should be assured of close monitoring and reassured that although the procedure stresses the heart, the mortality risk is less than 1:10,000 for exercise; there is 1:2000 event rate for dobutamine infusion (basically the risk of MI or ventricular fibrillation). Because exercise testing in an office setting is an elective procedure, patients should never be exposed to excess risk (i.e., patients should be chosen very carefully to ensure that the actual risk of death is much less than even 1:10,000). Although higher risk than with EET, dobutamine infusion has been shown to be somewhat safe even in patients with left ventricular dysfunction, aortic and cerebral aneurysms, and implantable cardioverter defibrillators.
- With dobutamine infusion, the patient may experience palpitations, nausea, headache, chills, urinary urgency, and anxiety. Symptoms related to high or low blood pressure or chest pain may also be experienced. Patients should know that it is very rare for the symptoms to be severe enough to stop the test.

After Arrival

- The clinician should again explain the reasons for the test and answer any questions.
- The procedure should be explained again to the patient (e.g., how frequently the workload will be increased or what to expect with pharmacologic infusion, how BP measurements will be taken, when the echo images will be obtained, how the perceived exertion scale [PES] works; see Box 74.1 in Chapter 74, Stress ECG Testing).
- The patient should know what symptoms to report during the test.

- The clinician should explain how the patient can terminate the procedure should he or she have severe symptoms or an emergency.
- A signed, written consent form should be obtained (see a sample consent form [Chapter 74] available at www.expertconsult.com).
- Confirm the mode of exercise (e.g., treadmill, bicycle ergometer, arm ergometer) or method of evoking stress (e.g., pharmacologic) based on the individual's ability to exercise or any contraindications to exercise.
- If using exercise, select the protocol. There are many excellent protocols in use; the choice is usually dependent on the patient's predicted exercise capacity and on clinician preference. The Veterans' Administration (VA) Specific Activity Questionnaire (see Fig. 74.1 in Chapter 74, Stress ECG Testing) may be very helpful for predicting exercise capacity and helping decide between a standard protocol and a less aggressive, modified protocol. One MET is the amount of oxygen consumed while sitting quietly at rest, or basal oxygen consumption, and it can be used as a conversion unit for exercise capacity (e.g., 2 METs is an exercise capacity that consumes twice the amount of oxygen as basal consumption). If the patient can walk up a flight of stairs, he or she has an exercise capacity of approximately 4 METs. If the patient can walk up a flight of stairs carrying a sack of groceries, he or she can probably tolerate a regular protocol. Otherwise a modified protocol will probably be necessary. Choose a protocol that starts at a low level of exertion (2 to 3 METs).
- A protocol with stage durations of at least 3 minutes (2 minutes for bicycle ergometer) allows more physiologic adaptation to the workload of each stage.
- Workload increases that are no greater than 1 to 3 METs per stage also allow more physiologic adaptation.

The Bruce protocol (see Table 74.2 in Chapter 74, Stress ECG Testing) is the most frequently used protocol with stress echo; overall, it has been the most extensively studied and validated. The number of predicted METs is usually about the same as the number of minutes an individual can complete on the Bruce protocol. The Bruce protocol is especially useful in active patients and takes less time than other protocols because it rapidly increases workload. It does have its disadvantages: By the fourth or fifth stage, the patient usually must run, which increases artifact on the EET. In addition, patients often experience difficulty in accommodating increases to both slope and speed at the same time. This difficulty is especially seen in elderly patients because they usually have decreased proprioception in their toes, impaired balance, and some degree of impairment of vision. In general, most modified protocols, such as the modified Bruce or modified Balke protocol, have a reduced progression of workload and are better tolerated by elderly or debilitated patients. Modified protocols usually maintain the same speed and vary only the elevation. Table 74.3 in Chapter 74, Stress ECG Testing, indicates various protocols, and Fig. 74.15 graphically compares METs per minute and $VO_{2\,max}$ as measured for four protocols.

- Prepare the patient for the ECG machine to be used in the test. Locate sites on the chest for electrodes, which are the same locations as for the office ECG (see Chapter 70, Office Electrocardiograms), except that the arm electrodes are placed in the infraclavicular fossae (midclavicle) and the leg electrodes are placed on the lower abdomen just above the belt line (see Fig. 74.14). The location of the lateral leads may have to be adjusted to allow application of the ultrasound transducer to sites for the parasternal and apical windows.
- Prepare the patient for the echo after exercise or dobutamine infusion. The patient should know that it is very important to obtain the recovery images within the first minute, so it will be very important to move in a safe and timely manner to the echo examination table. The patient will then have to lie fairly still in the supine position until the images have been obtained.

TECHNIQUE

Getting Started and Resting Echo

1. Review the patient's interval medical history and examine the patient. Based on the history and reexamination, make sure that no contraindication has developed since the last time the patient was seen. Again, determine that in this particular clinical scenario stress echo is the preferred technique for testing.
2. With the patient lying down, obtain and record the resting heart rate, BP, and ECG.
3. Using the left parasternal and apical windows, obtain the supine resting 2D echo images. A screening assessment should be made of ventricular function, chamber sizes, wall motion thicknesses, aortic root, and valves unless this assessment has already been performed. Severe aortic stenosis should be excluded.
4. Perform the exercise or pharmacologic stress test (see Chapter 74, Stress ECG Testing, about performing and monitoring the standard EET).

Exercise Treadmill Echocardiography

1. With the patient standing beside the treadmill, an ECG should be obtained. At this point, most equipment records data to provide the signal-averaged ECG for future monitoring.
2. Begin the exercise treadmill test using the preselected protocol.
3. Monitor the patient's symptoms, overall condition, pulse rate, and ECG at all times. *Instruct the patient to give adequate warning if the test has to be stopped.* With the exception of submaximal testing, encourage the patient to go as far and as long as possible.
4. Record a 12-lead ECG at the end of each stage, at any time when an abnormality is noted on the monitor, immediately on stopping, and every minute for 8 minutes during recovery.
5. During each stage, at the start of the final minute, ask the patient if there is any chest discomfort, what point he or she has reached on the PES, and whether he or she wants to continue into the next stage. Also record the BP and heart rate near the end of each stage or at the time of any problems.
   NOTE: For most patients, their perceived exertion (see Box 74.1 in Chapter 74, Stress ECG Testing) is reproducible at a given level of exercise and correlates fairly well with their heart rates. Ask patients to indicate on a scale of 0 to 10 how hard they feel they are working with each stage. On average, most patients feel they increase by 2 to 3 on the exertion scale with each stage in the early part of the study. PES usually increases more rapidly, from 7 to 9, near the end of the study. Rarely will anyone declare a 10. Use of the PES will not only help the clinician plan for gathering data during the stress echo but may also help with giving an exercise prescription (see Chapter 74, Stress ECG Testing, for additional information about giving a customized exercise prescription).
6. After completion of the exercise treadmill test, immediately ask the patient to lie down. Be aware that this step may be uncomfortable for certain patients, especially if they are overweight or having even slight difficulty breathing; reassure them that they will not be required to lie down for very long. Obtain the needed images within 1 minute and then record the BP and heart rate. If an assistant is available, it is best to obtain the vital signs at the same time as the images.

Exercise Bicycle Ergometer Echocardiography

1. With the patient sitting on the bicycle, an ECG should be obtained. At this point, most equipment records data to provide the signal-averaged ECG for future monitoring. There may be value in again explaining to the patient the importance of moving safely and rapidly to the echo examination table immediately after the exercise has stopped in order to obtain the images.
2. Begin the exercise test using the preselected protocol. The usual bicycle protocol starts at 25 W of resistance and increases by 25 W every 2 minutes. (A higher initial workload may be appropriate for younger patients or those with a higher estimated exercise capacity.) If images are to be obtained during exercise, many clinicians obtain them at a workload of 25 W and again at peak exercise.
3. Monitor the patient's symptoms, overall condition, pulse rate, and ECG at all times. *Instruct the patient to give adequate warning if the test has to be stopped.* With the exception of submaximal testing, encourage the patient to go as far and as long as possible.
4. Record a 12-lead ECG at the end of each stage, at any time an abnormality is noted on the monitor, immediately on stopping, and every minute for 8 minutes during recovery.
5. During each stage, at the start of the final minute, ask the patient if there is any chest discomfort, what point he or she has reached on the PES, and whether he or she wants to continue into the next stage. Also record the BP and heart rate near the end of each stage or at the time of any problems.
6. After completion of the upright bicycle exercise test, immediately ask the patient to lie down. Be aware that this step may be uncomfortable for certain patients, especially if they are overweight or having even slight difficulty breathing; reassure them that they will not be required to lie down for very long. Obtain the needed images within 1 minute and then record the BP and heart rate. If an assistant is available, it is best to obtain the vital signs at the same time as the images.

Dobutamine Stress Echocardiography

NOTE: Vasodilator infusion (e.g., adenosine, dipyridamole, regadenoson) can be used in a similar manner for perfusion imaging using contrast stress echo; however, dobutamine is usually preferred.

1. The patient can remain in the supine position for dobutamine infusion. Begin the dobutamine infusion following the standard or low-dose protocols. Dobutamine can be initiated at the standard rate of 5 µg/kg per minute and increased in 3-minute intervals to 10, 20, 30, and 40 µg/kg per minute. (For patients with moderate to severely depressed left ventricular function, multivessel disease, or at high risk for an arrhythmia, a low-dose protocol can be used with the infusion initiated at 2.5 µg/kg per minute and increased more gradually to 5, 7.5, 10, and 20 µg/kg per minute.) At the Mayo Clinic, echo images are obtained at lower doses (5 to 10 µg/kg per minute), prepeak, and at peak dose (or after administration of atropine).
2. Vigilant monitoring is indicated with the use of dobutamine, especially in patients with moderately to severely depressed left ventricular function or multivessel disease, because of the high risk for an arrhythmia. Monitor the patient's symptoms, overall condition, pulse rate, and ECG at all times. Record a 12-lead ECG at any time an abnormality is noted on the monitor.
3. The test is terminated if the target heart rate is achieved (85% of predicted MHR; predicted MHR = 220 – age) or with the appearance of new or worsening wall motion abnormalities of moderate degree, significant arrhythmias, hypotension, severe hypertension, or intolerable symptoms. If the test is being done to assess viability (low-dose protocol), it should be terminated if there is no functional improvement in segments that are akinetic at baseline. Likewise, worsening of function in hypokinetic segments should trigger termination of the test. Conversely, if there is improvement in function using the low-dose protocol and no untoward side effects, the dose can be escalated to match the high-dose protocol (up to 40 µg/kg per minute).
4. If the target heart rate is not readily achieved, atropine can be given intravenously in divided doses of 0.25 to 0.5 mg to a total of 2 mg. The minimal dose of atropine needed to obtain the target heart rate should be used to minimize the risk of the rare

complication of central nervous system toxicity. Use of atropine increases the sensitivity of the test in patients taking β-blockers or those with single-vessel CAD.

NOTE: Patients given atropine at the stage of dobutamine infusion of 30 μg/kg per minute reach the target heart rate more quickly and with fewer side effects.

5. Obtain the needed images and then record the BP and heart rate. If an assistant is available, it is best to obtain the vital signs at the same time as the images. For persistent symptoms, tachycardia, or severe tachycardia, short-acting intravenous β-blockers (e.g., metoprolol, esmolol) are effective at reversing the dobutamine effects.

After Exercise or Pharmacologic Stress Testing

1. Immediately after exercise or pharmacologic testing, the patient can be placed in the left lateral recumbent position. Obtain the apical four-chamber images, then the two-chamber images, and finally the parasternal long-axis followed by short-axis images (some laboratories obtain the parasternal images first). Observe the recovery of ischemic wall motion abnormalities (usually 3 to 5 minutes after exercise).
2. Monitor the BP, heart rate, any symptoms, and the ECG tracing during recovery. Observe the patient in recovery until symptoms, echo, or ECG changes have resolved completely (or for at least 8 minutes if symptoms, echo, or ECG changes resolve earlier).

Test Termination Criteria

A good rule of thumb for stopping the study is after the necessary information has been obtained and before there is a complication. In young or fit individuals, when they reach their predicted maximal heart rate (again, predicted MHR = 220 − age), it may be prudent to explain that all the necessary information has been obtained; however, they may continue to exercise for as long as they desire. (Allowing the patient to make this choice is also indirectly obtaining informed consent.) In older, less fit, or more debilitated patients, those with multivessel disease, and those with a positive test, obtaining at least 85% of predicted MHR is usually adequate for a stress echo. The benefit of going beyond predicted MHR is the ability to give patients a customized exercise prescription based on their true MHR.

NOTE: In the past, authorities denoted two possible definitions of a maximal stress exercise test: (1) achieving a target heart rate greater than 85% of the predicted MHR for that patient's age (i.e., roughly 85% of [220 − age]) or (2) exercise to the point of symptoms. Most authorities now encourage patients to exercise to the point of symptoms (usually generalized or voluntary fatigue or the usual amount of chest pain).

Predicted MHR is not patient-specific and is frequently inaccurate. Proceeding to the point of symptoms is contraindicated only for debilitated or elderly patients or if a submaximal test is indicated. Maximal effort is usually confirmed by the patient reaching maximal perceived exertion and the inability to continue at that workload. Also, for stress echo, a rate pressure product (RPP = systolic blood pressure × heart rate) greater than 20,000 indicates to the clinician that the patient has made a good effort.

Indications to terminate a study include the following:

- Significant elevated BP (systolic blood pressure >250 mm Hg, diastolic blood pressure >115 mm Hg) occurs.
- Significant heart rate abnormalities (inability to obtain 120 beats/min or excessive high heart rate for level of exertion) appear.
- Systolic blood pressure drops more than 20 mm Hg below resting value, especially after the first minute or two of the study (most dangerous if it reflects LV dysfunction; in that situation there is a high risk of life-threatening arrhythmias).

- Anginal chest pain worsens (severe enough that the patient desires to stop); it is not prudent for patients to exercise beyond the point at which they obtain their "usual" amount of chest discomfort. In other words, there is no reason for the patient to demonstrate his or her worst chest pain while performing the study.
- Central nervous system symptoms (e.g., dizziness, disorientation) appear.
- Signs of poor perfusion (e.g., cyanosis, pallor) or severe ventricular dysfunction (e.g., dyspnea) occur. Remember that in the elderly, stability can deteriorate very rapidly; poor perfusion may be indicated solely by a loss of color in an elderly patient.
- Serious arrhythmias develop.
- Target heart rate has been attained.
- Patient wants to stop the test (especially elderly patients, in whom there may be little warning of a complication about to happen).
- Technical problems with equipment (e.g., ECG monitor, systolic blood pressure monitor) occur.

INTERPRETATION

Chapter 74, Stress ECG Testing, discusses interpretation of the EET. ECG criteria are used to determine whether the EET is positive or negative. The test result can also be abnormal because of other responses (e.g., BP, symptoms). Rather than just labeling the result as normal, positive, or abnormal, the specific responses to exercise should be identified and documented. It should be noted that occasionally the EET is falsely positive or falsely negative; if the echo images are good, the results of the stress echo take precedence over the EET results.

Normal Echocardiographic Responses to Exercise

- Myocardial segments visualized have normal contraction at rest and become hyperdynamic with exercise or infusion of dobutamine.
- A normal stress echo is defined as normal left ventricular wall motion at rest and with stress.
- Ejection fraction normally increases with exercise.
- Left ventricular end-systolic volume normally decreases with exercise.

Abnormal Echocardiographic Responses to Exercise

- Cardiac segment changes from normal to hypokinetic, from hypokinetic to akinetic, and from akinetic to dyskinetic are considered wall motion abnormalities.
- Resting wall motion abnormalities that are unchanged with stress are classified as "fixed" and most often represent regions of prior infarction. Fixed wall motion abnormalities that develop new or worsening abnormalities are indicative of ischemia.
- Typical patterns are seen with normal, ischemic, and prior infarction responses to stress echo (Table 76.2).
- Function in each segment is graded at rest and with stress as normal or hyperdynamic, hypokinetic, akinetic, dyskinetic, or aneurysmal. (Table 76.3 provides a scoring system.)
- Images from low or intermediate stages of supine bicycle ergometry or dobutamine infusion should be compared with peak stress images to maximize the sensitivity for detecting CAD.
- Stress-induced changes in left ventricular shape, increase in cavity size, and lack of increase in global contractility indicate ischemia.
- Ischemia also delays the onset of contraction and relaxation and decreases the maximum amplitude of contraction.

TABLE 76.2 Typical Rest and Stress Wall Motion Responses

Rest	Stress	Interpretation
Normal	Hyperkinetic	Normal
Normal	Hyperkinetic/akinetic	Ischemic
Akinetic	Akinetic	Prior infarction
Hypokinetic	Akinetic/dyskinetic	Ischemic or prior infarction
Hypokinetic/akinetic	Normal	Viable

TABLE 76.3 Wall Motion Scoring

Description	Score
Hyperkinetic (hyperdynamic)	0
Normal	1
Mildly hypokinetic*	1.5
Hypokinetic	2
Severely hypokinetic*	2.5
Akinetic	3
Dyskinetic	4
Aneurysm	5

*Optional scores used by some clinicians.

Segmental Wall Motion Analysis

- One expert (Ellestad) feels the standard four-chamber view provides the most information.
- The American Society of Echocardiography (ASE) suggests that either a 16- or 17-segment model of the left ventricle (see Fig. 75.20 in Chapter 75, Echocardiography) be used for segmental wall motion analysis. The extra segment in the 17-segment model is the "apical cap," which is the portion of the left ventricle located below where the ventricular cavity is seen.
- Although there is some variability in data reported when segmental wall analysis is used to evaluate stress echo results (i.e., thresholds from calculated sum ratios of wall motion abnormalities used to define patients at high risk have been variable), the authors still use Fig. 76.1 to quantify the results. Each segment is evaluated and scored at rest and during stress (bicycle or pharmacologic) or after stress (treadmill). The sum of all the segments from the stress echo is divided by the sum of the resting segments. Patients considered at high risk have a score greater than 1.4.
- Stress-induced wall motion abnormalities involving more than two segments or two coronary beds indicate that a patient is at high risk. Small stress-induced wall motion abnormalities involving one or two segments and only one coronary bed indicate a patient at intermediate risk. A normal stress echo or no change in limited resting wall motion abnormalities during stress indicates a patient at low risk.

Ejection Fraction and End-Systolic Volume Analysis

The ejection fraction should increase on the postexercise echo images and the end-systolic volumes should decrease (with the exception of recumbent bicycle protocol). On these images, no change in the ejection fraction or end-systolic volume, a decrease in the ejection fraction, and an increase in the end-systolic volume (i.e., induced LV dilation) are all indicative of CAD and increase the patient's risk of a cardiovascular event.

Other Parameters Followed

- *Heart rate.* Failure to obtain a heart rate of 120 beats/min is chronotropic incompetence with a resultant poor prognosis

(approximately 15% per year will experience a coronary event); while it may indicate early sick sinus syndrome it may also indicate a poor prognosis due to cardiomyopathy or multivessel CAD (often small-vessel CAD).
- *Heart rate recovery.* Failure of the heart rate to decrease 12 beats/min in the first minute of recovery is an abnormal heart rate recovery. Although preliminary studies suggested that this indicated a two- to fourfold increased risk of death over the next 5 years, there were problems with reproducibility of the result. But such a finding probably indicates a higher-risk individual.
- *Blood pressure.* If the systolic BP drops below resting during exercise, it may predict either a poor prognosis or severe CAD. In one study, men with a maximal exercise systolic blood pressure below 140 mm Hg had a 15-fold increase in the annual rate of sudden death as compared with those whose BPs exceeded 200 mm Hg.

False-Positive Results

Box 76.2 lists causes of false-positive results on stress echocardiography. Advanced age, marked hypertension, a cardiomyopathy, or taking a β-blocker can blunt the normal hypercontractile response to exercise.

False-Negative Results

Box 76.2 also lists causes of false-negative results on stress echocardiography. Suboptimal stress is a primary cause of false-negative tests. An adequate level of stress is frequently defined as achievement of 85% or more of the patient's age-predicted maximal heart rate for exercise or dobutamine stress or a rate pressure product of 20,000 or more for exercise testing.

DETERMINING PROGNOSIS

Normal Stress Echocardiogram

A negative stress echo is very reassuring because prognosis is excellent. Such patients have less than a 1% annual risk of death, MI, or cardiac events, which is equivalent to that of an age- and sex-matched population (Box 76.3). These patients do not require further diagnostic evaluation unless there is a change in signs or symptoms. Patients with a negative pharmacologic stress echo have a slightly higher risk of cardiovascular events, perhaps due to their inability to exercise, other comorbidities, or typically older age at the time of testing. However, a negative pharmacologic stress echo still implies less than a 2% annual risk of MI or cardiac death (see Box 76.3).

Uninterpretable or Incomplete Exercise Test Results

This result is caused by failure to attain at least 85% of the age-predicted MHR, with absence of ischemic changes in a well-motivated patient (β-blockers are a common cause of this).

Positive and Abnormal Studies

In addition to segmental wall analysis and evaluation of the ejection fraction/end-systolic volumes, other factors are known to affect risk (Box 76.4). Although the degree to which each of these factors affects risk is variable, we know that the more factors a patient possesses, the higher the risk. Certain investigators also attempt to combine the results of the EET to estimate risk using the Duke Treadmill Nomogram (see Fig. 74.18 in Chapter 74, Stress ECG Testing). This nomogram is most accurate for those patients with a positive study who are able to achieve 5 METs, a heart rate of 120 beats/min, and an RPP of more than 25,000. Box 76.3 is utilized for further quantifying those patients considered high risk (greater than fourfold increased risk over the low-risk group previously defined).

BOX 76.2 Causes of False-Positive and False-Negative Results on Stress Echocardiography

Causes of False-Positive Results
- Hypoxemia or anemia—can cause ischemia unrelated to CAD
- Apical hypokinesis due to LVH—can cause wall motion abnormalities
- Hypertension (poorly controlled)—can cause ischemia or wall motion abnormalities
- Cardiomyopathy—idiopathic cardiomyopathy can cause ischemia; other cardiomyopathies can cause wall motion abnormalities
- Long-standing hypertension—can cause wall motion abnormalities, even without resting left ventricular dysfunction and in the absence of LVH
- Mitral valve prolapse syndrome and valvular heart disease
- Coronary spasm (Prinzmetal or variant angina)
- Mitral valve replacement or annulus calcification can lead to decreased motion of the basal inferior and basal inferoseptal segments due to tethering
- Left bundle branch block, right ventricular pacing, and previous open heart surgery can lead to decreased septal wall motion (abnormal septal motion usually present at rest)
- Inadequate recording equipment, incorrect criteria, improper interpretation, or improper transducer placement
- Technical or observer error
- Advanced age
- β-Blocker therapy

Causes of False-Negative Results
- Failure to achieve an adequate workload (heart rate >85% of age-predicted maximal heart rate for exercise or pharmacologic stress, or rate pressure product of at least 20,000 for exercise echo)
- Single vessel, especially left circumflex, CAD (supine bicycle testing has higher sensitivity)
- Concentric remodeling or LVH (especially for dobutamine stress, because affected patients have increased relative wall thickness and smaller left ventricular cavity volume)
- Significant aortic or mitral valve regurgitation (due to resulting hyperdynamic state)
- Failure to use other information (e.g., exercise electrocardiography testing results, systolic blood pressure drop, symptoms, dysrhythmia, heart rate response) in test interpretation
- Inadequate recording equipment, incorrect criteria, improper interpretation, or improper transducer placement
- Technical or observer error

CAD, Coronary artery disease; *LVH,* left ventricular hypertrophy.

BOX 76.3 Stress Echocardiography Predictors of Risk

Low Risk (<1% Annual Death or MI)
- Normal exercise echo and good exercise capacity (≥7 METs in men, 5 METs in women)
- Normal stress or no change of limited resting wall motion abnormalities during stress

Low to Intermediate Risk (<2% Annual Death or MI)
- Normal pharmacologic stress echo (defined as heart rate >85% of age-predicted maximal heart rate for dobutamine stress echo and low to intermediate pretest probability*)

Intermediate Risk (1% to 3% Annual Death or MI)
- Mild/moderate resting LV dysfunction (left ventricular ejection fraction 35%–49%) not readily explained by noncoronary causes
- Inducible small wall motion abnormality involving 1 to 2 segments and only 1 coronary bed

High Risk (>3% Annual Death or MI)
- Severe resting LV dysfunction (ejection fraction <35%) not readily explained by noncoronary causes
- Severe stress-induced LV dysfunction (peak exercise ejection fraction <45% or drop in ejection fraction by 10% with stress)
- Stress-induced LV dilation
- Inducible wall motion abnormality (involving >2 segments or 2 coronary beds)
- Multivessel ischemia or left main coronary artery disease
- Wall motion abnormality with low-dose dobutamine (<10 μg/kg per minute) or at low heart rate (<120 beats/min)

---

* See Determination of Pretest Probability in Indications section in this chapter.
METs, Metabolic equivalents; *MI,* myocardial infarction.
From Pellikka PA, Nagueh SF, Elhendy AA, et al. American Society of Echocardiography recommendations for performance, interpretation and application of stress echocardiography. *J Am Soc Echocardiogr.* 2017;20:1021–1041 and ACC/AATS/AHA/ASE/ASNC/SCAI/SCCT/STS 2017 Appropriate Use Criteria for Coronary Revascularization in Patients With Stable Ischemic Heart Disease. *J Am Coll Cardiol.* 2017;69:2212–2241.

BOX 76.4 Factors Increasing Risk in Patients With Normal Stress Echocardiography Results*

- Increasing age
- Male sex
- Diabetes
- High pretest probability†
- History of dyspnea or congestive heart failure
- History of myocardial infarction
- Limited exercise capacity
- Inability to exercise
- Exercise electrocardiography testing demonstrates ischemia
- Resting wall motion abnormalities
- Left ventricular hypertrophy
- Ischemia on stress echo
- Baseline reduced ejection fraction
- No change or increase in end-systolic volume with exercise
- No change or decrease in ejection fraction with exercise
- Increasing wall motion score with stress

---

* The degree to which each factor increases risk is variable.
† See Determination of Pretest Probability in Indications section of this chapter (>90% by calculations in that section).
From Pellikka PA, Nagueh SF, Elhendy AA, et al. American Society of Echocardiography recommendations for performance, interpretation and application of stress echocardiography. *J Am Soc Echocardiogr.* 2007;20:1021–1041.

Viability Studies

The highest sensitivity of the dobutamine test for viability is noted when there is improvement in wall motion with the low-dose protocol. Viability is defined by improvement by at least one grade in two or more wall segments (see Table 76.3). Patients with a large area of viable myocardium (>25% of the left ventricle) have a greater chance of improving ejection fraction and a better outcome (decreased remodeling, persistent improvement in heart failure, lower incident of cardiac events) when revascularized.

COMPLICATIONS

- Hypotension
- Congestive heart failure exacerbation
- Severe cardiac arrhythmia

- Cardiac arrest
- Acute MI
- Acute central nervous system (CNS) event, such as syncope or stroke
- Death

POSTPROCEDURE PATIENT EDUCATION

Patients should be counseled appropriately regarding their risk and whether consultation with a cardiologist is indicated. Patients should be informed that stress echocardiography, just like any other noninvasive study for diagnosing CAD, is not 100% accurate. However, it usually diagnoses those coronary arteries with greater than 70% obstruction. Medical management is probably best for those vessels with less than 70% obstructions, and the patient should probably be reassured that this is already ongoing (i.e., management of diabetes, hypertension, lipids). Nevertheless, individuals with a future change in symptoms or symptoms suggestive of coronary ischemia—such as chest discomfort, palpitations, or shortness of breath with exertion—should be evaluated by their clinician regardless of the result of the stress echocardiogram.

In patients with CAD or a high probability of CAD, counseling should be directed at modifying risk factors and medical management unless an intervention is indicated. Exercise prescriptions should be given and discussed. See Chapter 74, Stress ECG Testing, for how to give an aerobic exercise prescription if not contraindicated. A cardiac rehabilitation program should be considered.

CPT/BILLING CODES

93016   Cardiovascular stress testing using maximal or submaximal treadmill or bicycle exercise, continuous ECG monitoring, and pharmacologic stress; physician supervision only, without interpretation and report
93017   Tracing only, without interpretation and report
93018   Interpretation and report only
93350   Echocardiography, transthoracic, real-time with image documentation (2D), with or without M-mode recording, during rest and cardiovascular stress test using treadmill, bicycle exercise, and pharmacologically induced stress, with interpretation and report (Stress testing codes 93016 to 93018 should be reported, when appropriate, in conjunction with 93350 to capture the cardiovascular stress portion of the study. Do not report 93015 in conjunction with 93350.)
93351   Including performance of continuous electrocardiographic monitoring, with physician supervision (Do not report 93351 in conjunction with 93015 to 93018, 93350.)

ICD-10-CM DIAGNOSTIC CODES

I05.0   Mitral stenosis, rheumatic
I05.1   Mitral stenosis with insufficiency, rheumatic
I11.99 Hypertensive heart disease or hypertensive LVH, benign, without congestive heart failure (CHF)
I11.0   Hypertensive heart disease, benign, with CHF
I21.09 Acute MI, of the anterolateral wall
I21.19 Acute MI, of the inferolateral wall
I21.29 MI, acute, unspecified site and episode
I25.2   Old MI (healed or no symptoms)
I20.9   Other and unspecified angina pectoris
I25.10 Coronary atherosclerosis, native artery w/o angina pectoris

I25.719 Coronary atherosclerosis, of autologous vein bypass graft w/unspecified angina
I25.709 Coronary atherosclerosis, of artery bypass graft w/unspecified angina
I25.799 Coronary atherosclerosis, of unspecified type of bypass graft
I25.9   Chronic ischemic heart disease, unspecified
I25.3   Aneurysm of heart wall
I27.0   Pulmonary hypertension, primary, chronic
I27.21   Pulmonary hypertension, secondary, chronic
I30.9   Pericardial effusion, acute
I30.0   Pericarditis, acute, idiopathic
I40.9   Myocarditis, acute
I30.9   Pericardial effusion, unspecified disease of pericardium
I34.0   Mitral valve disorders, nonrheumatic (incompetence, insufficiency, regurgitation, prolapse)
I35.0-I35.9 Aortic valve disorders (incompetence, insufficiency, regurgitation, stenosis)
I42.5   Other restrictive cardiomyopathy, NOS
I42.6   Cardiomyopathy, alcoholic
I44.7   Left bundle branch block, complete or NOS
I45.10   Right bundle branch block
I46.9   Cardiac arrest unspecified
I48.91   Atrial fibrillation unspecified
I49.3   Ventricular premature beats, contractions, or systoles
I50.9   Heart failure unspecified
I50.1   Left ventricular failure unspecified
I50.40   Combined systolic and diastolic heart failure
I50.21   Systolic heart failure, acute
I50.22   Systolic heart failure, chronic
I50.31   Diastolic heart failure, acute
I51.5   Myocardial degeneration
I51.7   Cardiomegaly or cardiac dilation or hypertrophy
I23.0   Mural thrombus (atrial, ventricular) acquired following myocardial infarction
I71.01   Aortic dissection, thoracic
R00.2   Palpitations
R07.9   Chest pain, unspecified
R07.2   Precordial pain

SUPPLIERS

(For full contact information go to www.expertconsult.com.)

For stress testing equipment, see the Suppliers section in Chapter 74, Stress ECG Testing. Most manufacturers on that list also sell defibrillators. Purchasing these as part of a package is often cost-effective. For echo equipment, there are several manufacturers with products ranging from the very basic to the very sophisticated. Small handheld machines are now available. Acuson Siemens, Esaote, General Electric Healthcare, Medison, Phillips, and Toshiba all offer a range of devices from handheld to research-oriented (see the Suppliers section in Chapter 142, Obstetric Ultrasonound, and the Suppliers listings in Appendix D, Supplier Information , for the Internet and mailing addresses and the phone numbers for many manufacturers). An excellent way to review the equipment is to visit the company websites. Used equipment is also available, but the cost and inconvenience of service and repairs are often a disadvantage. To avoid large capital equipment costs, service companies will bring portable echocardiography equipment to the clinician's office for this procedure and split the fees. Over-reading services are also available.

Emergency/ACLS medication kits
Banyan International Corp.

RECOMMENDED READING

ACC/AHA. Guideline on Perioperative Cardiovascular Evaluation and Management of Patients Undergoing Noncardiac Surgery. *Circulation.* 2014;130:278–333.

ACC/AATS/AHA/ASE/ASNC/SCAI/SCCT/STS. 2017 Appropriate Use Criteria for Coronary Revascularization in Patients With Stable Ischemic Heart Disease. A Report of the American College of Cardiology Appropriate Use Criteria Task Force, American Association for Thoracic Surgery, American Heart Association, American Society of Echocardiography, American Society of Nuclear Cardiology, Society for Cardiovascular Angiography and Interventions, Society of Cardiovascular Computed Tomography, and Society of Thoracic Surgeons *J Am Coll Cardiol.* 2017;69:2212–2241.

ACC/AHA. Clinical competence statement on stress testing: a report of the American College of Cardiology/American Heart Association/American College of Physicians-American Society of Internal Medicine Task Force on Clinical Competence. *Circulation.* 2000;102:1726.

ACC/AHA. Clinical competence statement on echocardiography. *Circulation.* 2003;107:1068–1089.

ACC/AHA/ASE. Guideline update for the clinical application of echocardiography: summary article: a report of the American College of Cardiology/American Heart Association Task Force on Practice Guidelines [ACC/AHA/ASE Committee to Update the 1997 Guidelines for the Clinical Application of Echocardiography]. *Circulation.* 2003;108:1146–1162.

ACC/AHA/ASNC. Guidelines for the clinical use of cardiac radionuclide imaging—executive summary. *Circulation.* 2003;108:1404.

ACCF/AHA/ASE/ASNC/HFSA/HRS/SCAI/SCCT/SCMR/STS. 2013 Multimodality Appropriate Use Criteria for the Detection and Risk Assessment of Stable Ischemic Heart Disease. *J Am Coll Cardiol.* 2014;63(4):380–406.

ACCF/ASE/AHA/ASNC/HFSA/HRS/SCAI/SCCM/SCCT/SCMR. 2011 Appropriate Use Criteria for Echocardiography. *J Am Soc Cardiol.* 2011;24:229–267.

Scientific Statement AHA. Exercise standards for testing and training: a statement for healthcare professionals from the American Heart Association. *Circulation.* 2001;104:1694.

American Diabetes Association. Consensus development conference on the diagnosis of coronary heart disease in people with diabetes. *Diabetes Care.* 1998;21:1551–1559.

Armstrong WF. *Feigenbaum's Echocardiography.* 8th ed. Philadephia: Lippincott: Williams & Wilkins; 2018.

Chin AS, Goldman LE, Eisenberg MJ. Functional testing after coronary artery bypass graft surgery: a meta-analysis. *Can J Cardiol.* 2003;19:802–808.

Dori G, Denekamp Y, Fishman S, Bitterman H. Exercise stress testing, myocardial perfusion imaging and stress echocardiography for detecting restenosis after successful percutaneous transluminal coronary angioplasty: a review of performance. *J Intern Med.* 2003;253:253–262.

Ellestad MH. *Stress Testing, Principles and Practice.* 5th ed. New York: Oxford University Press; 2003.

Fleischmann KE, Hunink MGM, Kuntz KM, Douglas PS. Exercise echocardiography or exercise SPECT imaging? A meta-analysis of diagnostic test performance. *JAMA.* 1998;280(10):913–920.

Fowler G, Altman M. Exercise testing after bypass or percutaneous coronary intervention. In: Evans CH, White RD, eds. *Exercise Stress Testing for Primary Care and Sports Medicine Physicians.* New York: Springer Verlag; 2009.

Froelicher VF, Myers J. *Exercise and the Heart.* 5th ed. St Louis: Mosby; 2006.

Garcia MJ. Prior evaluation: functional testing and multidetector computed tomography. In: Topol EJ, Teirstein PS, eds. *Textbook of Interventional Cardiology.* 7th ed. Philadelphia: Elsevier; 2016.

Garzon PP, Eisenberg MJ. Functional testing for the detection of restenosis after percutaneous transluminal coronary angioplasty: a meta-analysis. *Can J Cardiol.* 2001;17:41–48.

Mattera JA, Arain SA, Sinusas AJ, et al. Exercise testing with myocardial perfusion imaging in patients with normal baseline electrocardiograms: cost savings with a stepwise diagnostic strategy. *J Nucl Cardiol.* 1998;5:498.

Mahajan N, Polavaram L, Vankayala H, Ference B, Wang Y. Diagnostic accuracy of myocardial perfusion imaging and stress echocardiography for the diagnosis of left main and triple vessel coronary artery disease: a comparative meta-analysis. *Heart.* 2010;96:956–966.

Metz LD, Beattie M, Hom R, Redberg RF, Grady D, et al. The prognostic value of normal exercise myocardial perfusion imaging and exercise echocardiography: a meta-analysis. *J Am Coll Cardiol.* 2007;49(2):227–237.

Nguyen P. Stress echo. In: Evans CH, White RD, eds. *Exercise Stress Testing for Primary Care and Sports Medicine Physicians.* New York: Springer Verlag; 2009.

Otto CM. *Textbook of Clinical Echocardiography.* 5th ed. Philadelphia: Saunders: Elsevier; 2013.

Pellikka PA, Nagueh SF, Elhendy AA, et al. American Society of Echocardiography recommendations for performance, interpretation and application of stress echocardiography. *J Am Soc Echocardiogr.* 2007;20:1021–1041.

Reynolds T. *The Echocardiographer's Pocket Reference.* 4th ed. Phoenix: Arizona Heart Foundation; 2013.

Roldan CA, Abrams J. *Evaluation of the Patient with Heart Disease. Integrating the Physical Exam and Echocardiography.* Philadelphia: Lippincott: Williams & Wilkins; 2002.

Noninvasive Venous and Arterial Studies of the Lower Extremities

Grant C. Fowler

The accuracy of noninvasive vascular studies depends not only on the skills of the operator and the interpreter, but also on the quality of the equipment and the lab. That being said, with state-of-the-art equipment and laboratory tests, many clinicians will manage anticoagulation therapy on the basis of noninvasive venous studies alone; some vascular surgeons use noninvasive studies to guide angiography and arterial surgery.

The literature has clearly demonstrated the accuracy and benefit of compression ultrasound, or duplex ultrasound if it is available, in the emergency department. Compression ultrasound is often performed by emergency medicine clinicians to exclude deep venous thrombosis (DVT). As a result, ultrasound has basically become the standard of care for excluding DVT in the emergency department (see Chapter 214, Emergency Department, Hospitalist, and Office Ultrasound [POCUS]). As more primary care clinicians become comfortable performing duplex scanning, there is little doubt that they will extend its use into arterial and other studies.

Outside of the emergency department and in vascular laboratories, duplex and/or color Doppler ultrasound have become the standard for evaluation of lower extremity veins; noninvasive arterial studies remain the standard for initial evaluation of arteries, although computed tomography (CT) or magnetic resonance angiography (MRA) have become much more available. Venography has also essentially been replaced by duplex scanning; consequently, the risk of complications from invasive techniques and contrast dye has decreased. However, it should be noted that many vascular laboratories continue to use older noninvasive techniques for veins because duplex or color Doppler ultrasound are not always available, especially after hours. Many centers can afford only one or two duplex units, and they are often kept very busy. In some settings, the cost of equipment for even one duplex or color Doppler ultrasound unit is prohibitive. In the meantime, very sensitive D-dimer assays have become available with algorithms that can be used to effectively rule out DVT. These algorithms can be implemented using older noninvasive diagnostic techniques; consequently, these older techniques remain in this chapter. Older noninvasive techniques may yet see a resurgence in popularity because not only is there evidence supporting their use, but they are very cost effective and less operator dependent. In fact, they may find permanent use as a preliminary screening test to determine if a patient should undergo compression ultrasound, duplex, or color Doppler scanning.

NONINVASIVE VENOUS STUDIES

Each year in the United States, approximately 200,000 patients die from a pulmonary embolus. DVT can be found in about 80% of patients with a pulmonary embolism. See Fig. 77.1 for the most common sites for DVT. The incidence of DVT increases with age, and it is more common in women. One-third to one-half of patients older than 40 years who experience an acute myocardial infarction

(MI), hip fracture, major surgery (especially orthopedic, pelvic, or urologic), or a stroke develop venous thrombi. Box 77.1 lists traditional risk factors for DVT in hospitalized patients. Lower limb DVT affects 1% to 2% of hospitalized patients. In addition, as a result of previous DVT, the prevalence of postphlebitic sequelae in the adult population is estimated to be 5%.

Early diagnosis of DVT is important because approximately 50% of untreated proximal DVT cases will result in a pulmonary embolism (PE). Diagnosis of DVT is also important to minimize long-term complications such as venous stasis or ulceration from chronic venous insufficiency. Accurate diagnosis is crucial to limit anticoagulation therapy to those who really need it. Venous thrombi usually arise at bifurcations and in valve cusps. An aging thrombus can adhere to the vein wall and damage or destroy nearby valves. The two most important valves for controlling venous hydrostatic pressure are those of the proximal superficial femoral and distal popliteal veins. Destruction of these valves is more likely to lead to sequelae. The goal is to diagnose DVT before a thrombus either embolizes or becomes extensive enough to permanently damage these or other valves.

Clinical diagnosis of acute DVT, without the benefit of radiographic or noninvasive techniques, has been reported to be notoriously inaccurate for years, with only about a 50% accuracy rate. However, this accuracy rate was probably underestimated because it was based on older studies performed on seriously ill, hospitalized patients. Since then, various scoring systems have been developed in an attempt to predict pretest likelihood of DVT in ambulatory patients. The best known and most studied is the Wells scoring system, which was first proposed in 1995 and updated in 2003. Although patients in this study were ambulatory, they were seen in either the emergency department or hospital, so these data may not be as applicable to patients in a primary care clinic. The Wells system was again updated in 2006 after evaluating 1082 ambulatory patients presenting to five major academic medical centers. Of these, 495 patients were thought likely to have DVT, whereas 587 were categorized as unlikely. Diagnostic evaluation followed by 3 months of observation confirmed DVT or PE in 28% of those thought likely to have DVT and in only 5.5% of those deemed unlikely to have DVT (Table 77.1). Combining the Wells system with further diagnostic studies can be used to virtually exclude DVT. For instance, a negative high-sensitivity D-dimer in those thought unlikely to have DVT effectively excluded DVT (<1%) during the 3-month follow-up.

Alternatives for Diagnosis of Deep Venous Thrombosis, Their Limitations, and Evidence Supporting Their Use

1. *Contrast venography* was once regarded as the gold standard for diagnosis of DVT; however, it was not without its own risks, including allergic reactions, congestive heart failure, acute kidney

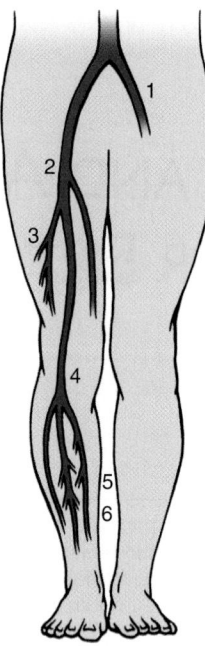

Fig. 77.1 Six most common sites of deep venous thrombosis in the lower body. *1*, Left iliac vein; *2*, common femoral vein; *3*, termination of deep femoral vein (profunda femoris); *4*, popliteal vein at adductor canal; *5*, posterior tibial vein; *6*, intramuscular veins of calf.

BOX 77.1 Traditional Risk Factors for Deep Venous Thrombosis (Especially in Hospitalized Patients)

- Acute myocardial infarction
- Acute respiratory failure
- Acute stroke with paresis
- Behçet syndrome
- Blood type (persons with type A may be at higher risk than those with type O)
- Fractures, especially spine, pelvis, long bone fractures, or multiple fractures
- Heart disease, especially congestive heart failure
- Heparin-induced thrombocytopenia
- Hypercoagulable states
- Local injury to veins
- Malignancy
- Mechanical ventilation
- Myeloproliferative disorders
- Nephrotic syndrome
- Obesity
- Oral contraceptive use
- Paroxysmal nocturnal hemoglobinuria
- Persons older than 40 years
- Persons with paralysis or otherwise immobilized
- Postoperative state from major surgery
- Pregnancy or postpartum, especially postcesarean section
- Previous deep vein thrombosis or pulmonary embolism
- Trauma
- Inflammatory bowel disease
- Venous stasis

---

injury, and postvenography syndrome. (Postvenography syndrome affects 10% to 20% of patients following a venogram. Although it usually causes only transient discomfort in the calf for 24 to 48 hours, and in most cases resolves without treatment, it could actually progress to frank DVT.) In addition, venography is not easily repeated, and is usually performed only in one limb. Venography may be impossible to perform in patients with poor venous

---

TABLE 77.1 Wells Scoring System for Predicting DVT

Clinical Variable	Score*
Active cancer (ongoing treatment or active within the last 6 mo or palliative care for cancer)	1
Paralysis, paresis, or recent plaster immobilization of the lower extremities	1
Recently bedridden for 3 or more days, or major surgery within the last 12 weeks requiring regional or general anesthesia	1
Localized tenderness along the distribution of the deep venous system	1
Entire leg swelling	1
Calf swelling at least 3 cm larger in circumference than that of the asymptomatic leg, measured 10 cm below the tibial tuberosity	1
Pitting edema confined to the affected leg	1
Distended collateral superficial veins (not varicosities)	1
Previously documented DVT	1
Alternative diagnosis at least as likely as DVT	−2

*Scoring method: if ≤1, DVT unlikely; if ≥2, DVT likely.
DVT, Deep venous thrombosis.
From Wells PS, Owen C, Doucette S, et al. Does this patient have deep vein thrombosis? *JAMA.* 2006;295:199–207.

access, especially obese patients and those with severe edema or cellulitis. It may also be difficult to perform in urgent situations without proper support staff. Furthermore, contrast venography cannot be performed in 20% to 25% of patients because of previous DVT. Although a study of postmortem contrast venograms reported a sensitivity rate of 95% and a specificity rate of 97% for diagnosis of DVT, a more recent multicenter study evaluating the degree of interobserver variation failed to verify those high sensitivities and specificities. For these reasons, as well as the fact that compression and duplex ultrasound have become more readily available, they and magnetic resonance venography (MRV) have replaced contrast venography for making the diagnosis of DVT.

2. *Compression ultrasound imaging (high-frequency, B-mode, real-time)* has limitations in obese and asymptomatic postoperative patients. Ultrasound's ability to visualize the venous system above the inguinal ligament (i.e., pelvic, iliac veins) or distal to the popliteal vein is also limited. However, for symptomatic proximal DVT, sensitivities ranging from 93% to 100% and specificities ranging from 97% to 100% have been reported since the 1980s (Appelman, 1987; Vogel, 1987; Cronan, 1987; Lensing, 1989). Compression ultrasound is less operator dependent than duplex scanning, and this may explain why it is the most common technique used in large urgent/emergent care centers and after hours in hospitals. Because it is a less expensive technique, many centers have developed algorithms; they either use compression ultrasound alone in low-risk patients, or as a screen to determine whether a duplex scan is needed. Although approximately 10% of isolated calf DVTs will be missed with compression ultrasound, calf DVT by itself is not life-threatening and may only need to be followed to exclude proximal progression. Benefits of compression ultrasound include the ability to actually visualize the veins, valves, and thrombus. Compression ultrasound may be necessary in special cases in which (other than obese or asymptomatic postoperative patients) impedance plethysmography (IPG) has unclear results or limitations. Compression ultrasound is also usually performed during duplex scanning.

3. *Duplex ultrasound scanning* combines velocity measurements using Doppler technology with ultrasound imaging. Duplex scanning may be used to confirm findings from compression ultrasound, and is accurate and reproducible; compared with venography, its sensitivity and specificity for DVT are more than 90%. Both the positive and negative predictive values for DVT are in the 90% to 95% range. Studies have shown that color enhancement of the Doppler velocities also improves accuracy in areas where compression may be difficult, such as at the inguinal ligament,

the adductor canal, or in the calf veins. It may also be used to determine patency of the pelvic and iliac veins and inferior vena cava.

4. *Electrical IPG* was previously the most extensively studied and most commonly used noninvasive technique. It remains the least expensive and least operator-dependent alternative to venography. IPG provides a functional evaluation of the venous system for outflow obstruction. Compared with contrast venography, sensitivities and specificities of 92% and 95%, respectively, were reported from studies in the 1990s. However, the range for sensitivity dropped to 66% in one study. High false-positive rates are found in the presence of certain conditions (e.g., obesity, congestive heart failure, external venous compression from gravid uterus in pregnancy) and with chronic DVT. Diagnosis with IPG is inaccurate for thrombi in calf veins, profunda femoris, or internal iliac veins. It is limited for diagnosing nonoccluding DVT, asymptomatic or moderately symptomatic DVT, and, therefore, postoperative DVT; and is limited for diagnosing clots in paired veins or determining the progression of disease. For these situations, duplex or color Doppler has mostly replaced IPG. However, it should be noted that a number of prospective studies (Hull, 1985; Huisman, 1986; Heijboer, 1993) demonstrated that serial negative IPGs are sufficiently sensitive to justify withholding anticoagulation therapy, even in symptomatic patients.

5. *Hand-held (pocket) Doppler* (with or without recorded velocities) can be used to assess venous function. Pooled data from several studies found an overall sensitivity of 84% and specificity of 88% for detection of lower extremity DVT in symptomatic outpatients. However, individual studies report sensitivities ranging from 31% to 100% and specificities ranging from 59% to 100%, thereby indicating the shortcoming of this technique and the fact that it is very operator dependent (Turnbull, 1989). Consequently, hand-held Doppler is probably most useful when combined with another study such as compression ultrasound or IPG and was, therefore, included in the protocols of many of the original noninvasive venous studies. When combined with compression ultrasound or IPG, hand-held Doppler can add important information about the calf veins.

6. *D-dimer assay* is another useful test. D-dimer, a degradation product of cross-linked fibrin, is usually elevated in patients with DVT. After determining Wells pretest likelihood, the results of a high-sensitivity D-dimer assay can be used in place of IPG, ultrasound, or duplex scanning in patients unlikely to have DVT. This test is especially useful in symptomatic patients with a suspected first episode of DVT. It can also be checked in addition to IPG, ultrasound, or duplex scanning. A D-dimer test is most effective in excluding DVT in outpatients because hospitalized patients frequently have other conditions that cause an elevated result (i.e., false positives). Increasing age also creates a higher likelihood of false-positive results. Although there are at least seven commercial assays available, the enzyme-linked immunosorbent assay (ELISA) and semiquantitative and immunoturbidimetric assays are considered high-sensitivity tests. From a meta-analysis (Wells, 2006), a negative high-sensitivity D-dimer test combined with a low-probability score (pretest likelihood) resulted in a 0.1% likelihood of DVT during 3-month follow-up *without using ultrasound*. Although semiquantitative slide agglutination assays are probably not accurate enough to use for exclusion of DVT (low sensitivity), newer quantitative agglutination methods (moderate sensitivity) have increased the accuracy to acceptable levels (<0.5% during 3-month follow-up) in patients unlikely to have DVT by the Wells scoring system. Likewise, bedside assays that use whole blood are also now available and are considered to be of moderate sensitivity and useful when combined with the Wells scoring system (Fig. 77.2).

7. *Radionuclide scintigraphy or magnetic resonance venography (MRV)* may be useful in selected patients. Scintigraphy uses radiolabeled albumin or tagged red blood cells as the contrast for venography.

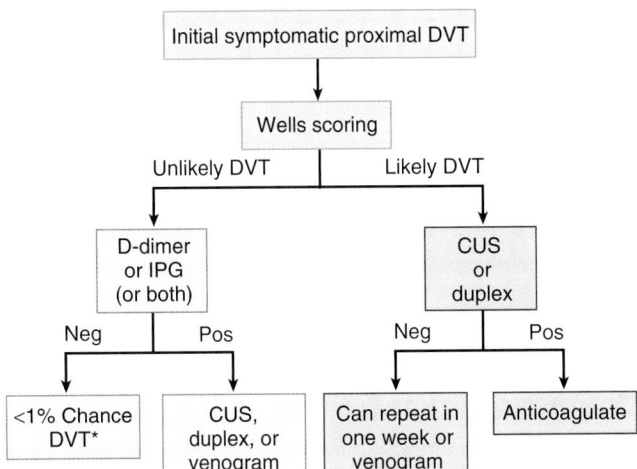

Fig. 77.2 Algorithm for incorporating Wells scoring system into testing for deep venous thrombosis (DVT). (1) If DVT is unlikely (see Table 77.1) and the moderate or high-sensitivity D-dimer test (or impedance plethysmography [IPG], or both) result is negative, no further testing is required. (2) Symptomatic patients with an abnormal compression ultrasound (CUS) or duplex study result can be treated without any further testing, or (3) if the patient has a negative CUS or duplex study result, yet DVT is likely, options include venography or serial CUS or duplex studies (i.e., repeat in 1 week). This algorithm provides a safe and cost-effective manner of excluding DVT. *Because this algorithm has not been studied prospectively and there is some subjectivity in using the Wells scoring system, some clinicians will always perform another noninvasive test before excluding DVT. *Neg*, Negative; *Pos*, positive.

However, it may be unreliable in the calf and not helpful in those with previous DVT. Radiolabeled autologous platelets or peptides can also be used to detect active thrombus formation. These techniques may be helpful in symptomatic patients with a previous history of DVT. MRV is particularly useful in the diagnosis of portal, inferior vena caval, pelvic, or calf vein DVT. However, MRV is highly operator dependent, expensive, and not always available in urgent situations. It should probably be reserved for cases in which scintigraphy is contraindicated. Both radionuclide scintigraphy and MRV are beyond the scope of this chapter.

Indications

Nongravid

- Verification of clinically suspected acute DVT. (This may require serial studies if calf thrombosis is suspected, and especially if IPG or compression ultrasound is the diagnostic study used. Neither of these techniques is highly sensitive for calf thrombosis, and serial studies are recommended to monitor for more proximal progression of a thrombus, which will occur in approximately 25% of patients. Asymptomatic calf vein thrombosis seems to progress proximally as frequently as that in symptomatic thrombosis, but some experts use risk stratification methods in this situation.)
- Diagnosis of recurrent DVT.
- Evaluation before discontinuing anticoagulation therapy for DVT. (e.g., IPG has been used to verify collateral flow or lysis of the thrombus by repeating every 4 to 6 weeks until the results return to normal. However, it should be noted that insurers often reimburse only for symptomatic patients.)
- Venous evaluation of a patient with known PE.
- Preoperative study before saphenous vein stripping.
- Preoperative study before venous sclerotherapy.
- Venous insufficiency.

Gravid

- Gravid patients with superficial venous thrombosis should be evaluated thoroughly because up to 17% will also have DVT. A gravid patient with DVT is at a very high risk for PE. (One review of maternal deaths revealed that PE was the second leading cause of death.)

- Special consideration should be given when LEFt criteria are present (left leg pain [L], calf circumference difference >2 cm [E for edema], first trimester [Ft]: if two are present, 16% risk of DVT; if three present, 58% risk of DVT).

Considerations

- Unilateral or unexplained edema of the lower extremity, especially if associated with pain in the area.
- Screening of certain high-risk patients (e.g., postoperative, especially with multiple risk factors; see Table 77.1.)

COMPRESSION ULTRASOUND

Real-time, B-mode ultrasound in the higher frequency ranges (5 to 10 MHz) allows direct visualization (imaging) of the venous system, and it allows the technician or clinician to search for a thrombus. Sound waves are best transmitted in fluid; therefore, large veins and arteries are easily visualized with the proper probe and adequate acoustic gel interface. Arteries are differentiated from veins by their thicker walls and pulsatile nature. They are also not as easily compressed when pressure is applied on the leg with the probe. In addition, arteries do not engorge with a Valsalva maneuver, vary with respiration, diminish with slight proximal occlusion, or increase flow with distal compression.

Compression ultrasound is currently the most widely used noninvasive test for diagnosis of DVT. In certain situations, such as after 5:00 PM in some emergency departments, compression ultrasound is the only diagnostic modality available. Studies of such situations have indicated that accuracy of diagnosis of DVT by compression ultrasound approaches that of venography.

Personnel and Equipment

- A clinician or technician familiar with venous anatomy (Fig. 77.3), as well as ultrasound technology
- 5- to 10-MHz probe (transducer) and scanner (2- to 3.5-MHz probe in obese patients)
- Acoustic gel

Technique

1. Place the patient in the supine position with the lower extremities lowered about 20 or 30 degrees (reverse Trendelenburg), slightly separated and externally rotated. This position increases the fluid volume in the veins and facilitates scanning. The patient should be relaxed and, comfortable to avoid venous compression by tense muscles.

2. Apply ample acoustic gel. With the probe perpendicular to the vessel and beginning at the groin, scan the common femoral vein, the saphenofemoral junction (SFJ) (the most common location for a thrombus to extend from superficial to deep veins), and then the deep and superficial femoral veins. Scan distally in the longitudinal and transverse dimensions. Longitudinal scanning is usually best for locating and following the vein, whereas transverse scanning is used to check for compressibility. Have the patient perform a Valsalva maneuver, which should expand the veins and enhance visualization as far distal as the popliteal veins. Echogenic matter (which appears white) within the vessels is the hallmark of a thrombus; if uncertain, it should be studied carefully to exclude a possible thrombus. Presence or absence of thrombus should be recorded. Partially obstructing thrombi may be confused with scarred, thickened venous walls; therefore, it is important to record and comment on wall thickness. If a thrombus is found in a femoral vein, attempt to scan the iliac vein and inferior vena cava for additional thrombi.

3. If no thrombus is visualized, turn the probe transversely and apply gentle pressure to compress the vessel walls. Compressions should be made every 3 to 5 cm, progressing distally. If the vein is not compressible, continue to apply increasing pressure until the diameter of the adjacent artery is reduced slightly. At this pressure, if the vein is not compressible, an early thrombus is preventing compression; it may not have become organized or dense enough to be visualized or to cause echoes. Compressibility of the vein walls (or lack thereof) should be recorded.

4. Proceed distally and continue scanning vessels in the longitudinal and transverse dimensions to the mid-medial, and then distal, thigh. In the distal thigh, fascial planes at the adductor hiatus (Hunter canal) may obscure the superficial femoral vein.

5. Next, scan the popliteal vein either with the patient in this same position or by having them roll into the prone position with the

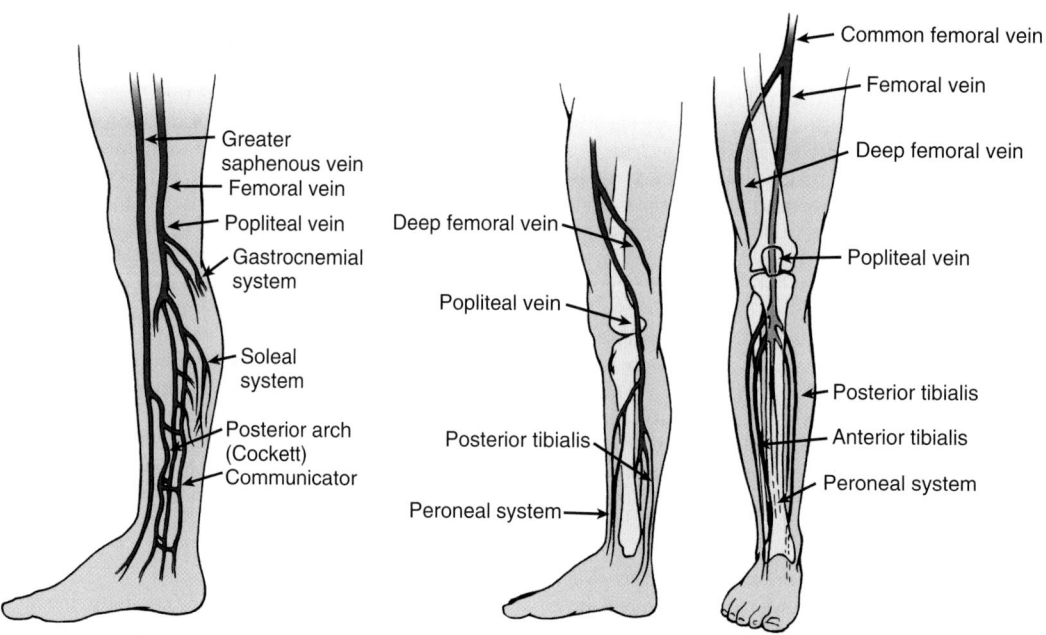

Fig. 77.3 Venous system of the lower extremity.

knees flexed 20 or 30 degrees. A pillow placed under the feet may facilitate this position and enhance patient comfort.

6. In about 30% of patients, infrapopliteal vessels can be scanned, with the anterior and posterior tibial veins visualized more easily than the peroneal veins. Sitting the patient up and allowing his or her legs to dangle over the edge of the bed may enhance imaging of the calf veins.

7. Valve thickness and motion should be recorded when observed.

8. Vein response to a Valsalva maneuver and deep inspiration should be recorded at the level of the common femoral, superficial femoral, and popliteal veins.

Interpretation

- Visualization of an intraluminal thrombus is diagnostic. A thrombus is further confirmed when a Valsalva maneuver produces minimal changes in vein diameter and the vessel wall is incompressible. Early studies indicate that these diagnostic criteria are superior to all other techniques, except venography, for diagnosing DVT. In a symptomatic patient, treatment (anticoagulation) can be initiated with the visualization of a thrombus alone.

- A *probable positive* study is one in which the veins are incompressible or do not distend with a Valsalva maneuver. Consider duplex scanning for confirmation if a thrombus is not visualized during compression ultrasound. The accuracy and outcomes of duplex scanning have been studied extensively, and it produces diagnostic results similar to venography in cases in which a thrombus is not visualized.

- Occasionally an acute thrombus can be differentiated from a chronic thrombus. Acute thrombi usually have low-level echoes, if any, and tend to have a homogeneous texture; they can be free-floating and are somewhat compressible, while the vein is often dilated. A chronic thrombus increases in echogenicity and decreases in size. With a chronic thrombus, although the vein is usually back to its normal diameter (i.e., the same diameter as the corresponding vein on the contralateral side), it still contains an echogenic clot partially obstructing the lumen. Lateral (collateral) veins will often form alongside. Chronic thrombi usually are not compressible, have heterogeneous echogenicity, and are firmly attached to the walls. These thrombi are stable, so the sonographer need not worry about dislodging them by scanning.

- Increased wall thickness, especially compared with veins of the contralateral extremity, can be due to previous or chronic DVT, or to a partially obstructing thrombus. All of these possibilities should be strongly considered in a symptomatic patient because all of these scenarios also place the patient at risk for DVT.

- At least one published study indicates safety in withholding treatment with a negative compression ultrasound scan. This result should be weighed against the pretest likelihood of DVT and the availability of duplex scanning. However, even in patients likely to have DVT by the Wells scoring system, two negative compression ultrasound studies, performed a week apart, reduces the risk of DVT to less than 1% (see Fig. 77.2).

- Although superficial thrombophlebitis is not life-threatening, patients with saphenous vein phlebitis should be scanned very thoroughly; one prospective study found 33% of patients with a thrombus in the above-knee segment of the greater saphenous vein (GSV) had a documented episode of PE. Likewise, although isolated calf vein thrombosis is not life-threatening, it will propagate proximally into the popliteal vein and thigh in approximately 25% of patients, so there is value in repeating the scan in 1 week. If the result is negative, it reduces the risk of proximal DVT to less than 2%. The risk of proximal propagation is apparently as high in asymptomatic calf vein thrombosis as in symptomatic. There are some experts that go ahead and anticoagulate patients with calf vein thrombosis, especially if they are symptomatic and they are at low risk of complications to anticoagulation. On the other hand, these same experts often withhold anticoagulation with calf vein thrombosis if the D-dimer is

normal in an outpatient with no prior history of DVT and the patient is asymptomatic.

- Because of the lack of a validated clinical model, making the diagnosis of recurrent DVT can be challenging. The diagnosis is easier if it occurs in a new location or in the contralateral extremity. However, if it recurs in the same venous segment of prior DVT, it requires comparison with a prior study. Clearly, a newly noncompressible segment confirms recurrent DVT. Certain experts consider an increase of greater than 2 mm in the compressed diameter (or >4 mm in the uncompressed diameter) of the previously thrombosed venous segment to be diagnostic for recurrent DVT. An extension of the length of the thrombus by 9 mm is also considered recurrent DVT by most sonographers. Conversely, fully compressible deep veins or no significant increase in diameter usually excludes recurrent DVT.

DUPLEX SCANNING

Duplex scanning adds another parameter—venous blood velocity—to the data obtained from compression ultrasound. With duplex scanning, Doppler technology is incorporated into the ultrasound probe. The drawbacks to duplex scanning include its cost to the patient (averaging $300 to $600 per study), the cost and nonportability of equipment, the time required for a complete examination, and the experience required for the technician or clinician to perform and interpret the study. In many centers duplex scanning is not available at all hours or in urgent situations. As with compression ultrasound, the ability to study the venous system above the inguinal ligament, and occasionally the superficial femoral and tibial veins at the adductor hiatus, is poor compared with IPG.

Duplex scanning has advantages over compression ultrasound in areas where the vein cannot be compressed because of physical restrictions, such as with smaller vessels (e.g., infrapopliteal). With duplex scanning, other measurable or demonstrable parameters of venous function can be evaluated if a suspected thrombus is not clearly visualized with compression ultrasound.

Technique

The technique of duplex scanning is the same as for compression ultrasound, except that most of the velocity data are gathered with the probe turned longitudinally along the vein. Duplex scanning allows the evaluation of venous physiologic parameters, and there are four additional criteria for a positive result: (1) the absence of phasicity (i.e., variation) during quiet respiration, (2) the absence of spontaneous blood flow, (3) the absence of augmentation of flow when the limb is compressed distal to the site of probe placement and (4) the absence of reversal of this augmentation when the distal compression is relaxed or compression is applied proximal to the probe. The effect of a Valsalva maneuver should also be observed (e.g., should reduce venous flow to the heart). Even with a thrombus that is clearly visualized, confirmation by an alteration or absence of these four factors or the loss of the Valsalva effect can be reassuring diagnostically (by demonstrating secondary effects of a thrombus) before anticoagulation therapy is initiated. In addition, duplex scanning allows valve function to be assessed; functional valves should not allow augmentation of reverse flow with proximal compression. The extent of valve function at the level of the common femoral, femoral, and popliteal veins should be routinely recorded. They should also be evaluated and recorded as far distally as possible.

Interpretation

Treatment decisions in most large centers are based on duplex scans alone. Occasionally, venography and duplex results differ. If clearly abnormal findings on a duplex scan are contradicted by normal findings on venography, the disparity may be due to the presence of a duplicate vein (up to 20% of patients), which may appear normal on venography despite the presence of a thrombus in the other vein.

Also, thrombosis of a superficial femoral or popliteal vein can be missed by a venogram. Therefore, for a patient with a normal venogram despite significant symptoms, and a clearly abnormal duplex scan, treatment can still be considered.

ELECTRICAL IMPEDANCE PLETHYSMOGRAPHY

Various plethysmography techniques are available to study a change in physical function as a result of a change in volume (e.g., strain gauge, air, IPG). Electrical IPG records the impedance (the inverse or reciprocal of conductivity) of the lower extremity as the blood volume varies. When venous return is restricted in the lower extremity by a cuff, venous volume in the lower extremity increases. Because blood is a good conductor of electricity, conductivity in the lower extremity also increases (i.e., resistance or impedance decreases). This is evaluated by administering a weak electrical current that is imperceptible to the patient, and then measuring the current's strength after it passes through the area. When the cuff is released, conductivity should rapidly decrease if the deep venous system is patent. In patients with a thrombus, the rate of change of electrical conductivity is reduced, especially if the thrombus is in the popliteal or more proximal vein. IPG has been proven to be safe, painless, reliable, and cost effective (cost to the patient is about the same as for an electrocardiogram, usually $50 to $100).

Relative Contraindications

* Patients with risk of false-positive result (e.g., patients with significant pain [involuntary muscle restriction], full bladder [especially elderly patients] or the inability to relax [involuntary muscle restriction], congestive heart failure [elevated central venous pressure], external vein occlusion [pregnancy, popliteal cyst or mass], obesity, or chronic DVT). In these patients, the risk of a false-positive result is increased and initiation of anticoagulation should be weighed against the risks of waiting for the availability of another, more accurate venous study.
* Patients who are unable to remain supine, such as those with severe orthopnea.

Personnel and Equipment

* A clinician or technician trained to perform and record IPG
* A clinician trained to interpret IPG
* IPG recorder
* Appropriate 8-inch cuff and electrodes

Technique

1. Place the patient in the supine position, with the leg to be examined elevated 25 to 30 degrees (Fig. 77.4). This can be accomplished by placing a pillow under the calf and heel. All tight garments should be removed, and the leg to be studied should be well exposed. To relax the patient, the leg is allowed to rotate externally at the hip. The knee is slightly flexed—10 to 20 degrees—to prevent compression of the popliteal vein.
2. Place an 8-inch-wide pneumatic cuff around the thigh and place electrodes circumferentially around the calf.
3. After the instrument has been electrically balanced and a stable baseline has been obtained, inflate the cuff to the manufacturer's specification, which is usually 50 mm Hg. This blocks the venous outflow but does not impair arterial inflow.
4. After the cuff has been inflated for 2 minutes and the pressure tracing has reached a stable plateau, suddenly release the pressure in the compression cuff.
5. The total rise of the IPG tracing during cuff occlusion and the fall during the first 3 seconds of deflation are now plotted on a two-way graph (Fig. 77.5 shows normal and abnormal IPG tracings, and Fig. 77.6 shows plotting).

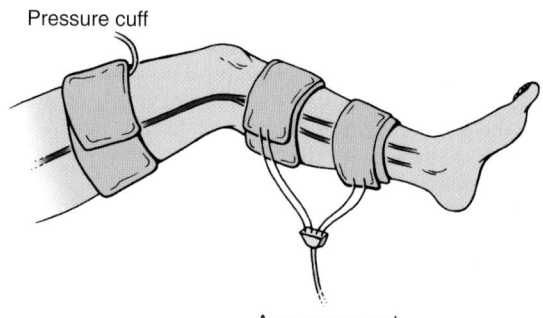

Fig. 77.4 For impedance plethysmography testing, elevate the leg 25 to 30 degrees. Apply electrodes around the calf and place a pressure cuff around the thigh.

Interpretation and Sources of Error

Overall, the major shortcoming of IPG is a false-positive rate of approximately 5%. Sensitivity increases in the symptomatic patient and is reduced during evaluation for silent proximal thrombosis, such as with postoperative screening. The error rate can be minimized by a clinician with experience who takes into consideration the following factors:

* Positive predictive accuracy is improved for those with a high pretest likelihood of DVT (see Table 77.1).
* If the first result falls below the discriminant line, it is not necessarily abnormal. With repeated testing, the values may fall above the discriminant line, where they are considered normal. In the presence of true outflow obstruction, the result remains fixed. To improve the accuracy of IPG, a five-test sequence can be used with occlusion times of 45, 45, 120, 45, and 120 seconds.
* The closer the result falls to the discriminant line on either side, the more likely that it is abnormal. Such test results (close to the line) should be confirmed with either duplex scanning or venography.
* Some experts suggest that if abnormal results are found with both lower extremities, they are likely false-positive results; therefore, the patient should be evaluated further with another technique.
* Excessive tightness of the cuff, particularly in obese patients, may cause tension on the skin during cuff occlusion and thus a false-positive result.
* Any systemic disease limiting arterial inflow or venous outflow will interfere with results.

HAND-HELD VENOUS DOPPLER

Hand-held Doppler studies (without imaging) can be used to qualitatively assess the venous system. The hand-held Doppler probe translates the velocity of venous blood into an audible signal or onto a chart recorder. Velocities are evaluated while the patient undergoes various maneuvers. This technology has not been studied as extensively as IPG or duplex scanning. Advantages to hand-held Doppler studies include inexpensive and, in most cases, more portable equipment. However, the safety of withholding anticoagulant treatment in patients with normal hand-held Doppler results has never been evaluated formally. For anyone performing noninvasive venous studies, a working knowledge of this technique is important to understand basic venous physiology.

Indications

Practical indications are slightly different than those previously discussed. For example, hand-held Dopplers may be used alone when other diagnostic methods are unavailable to confirm proximal DVT in a symptomatic patient, or they may be used to diagnose postphlebitic syndrome. This technique can also be used to screen patients

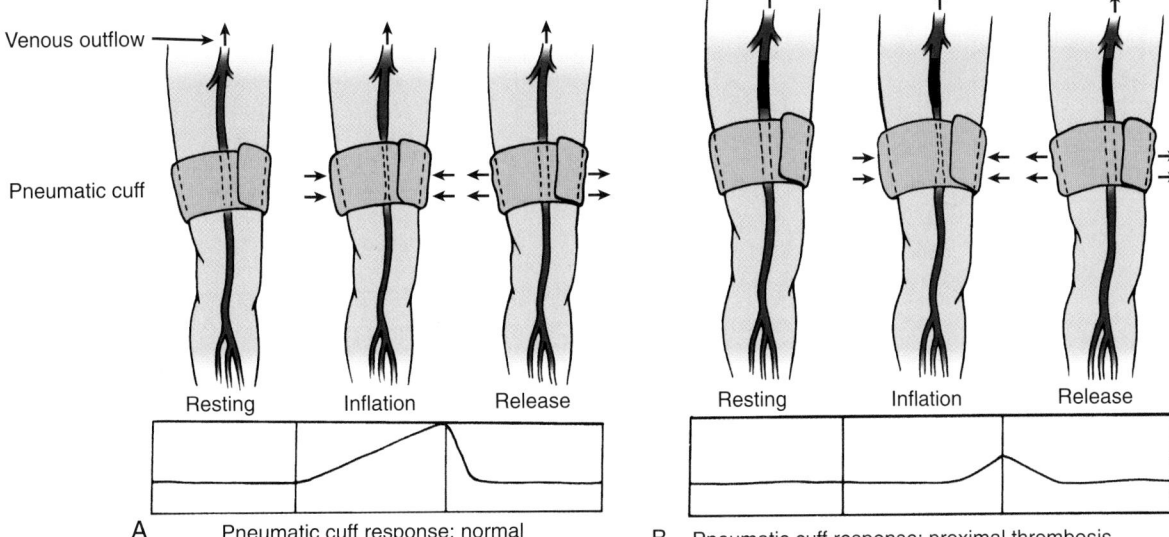

Fig. 77.5 Normal (A) and abnormal (B) impedance plethysmography tracings.

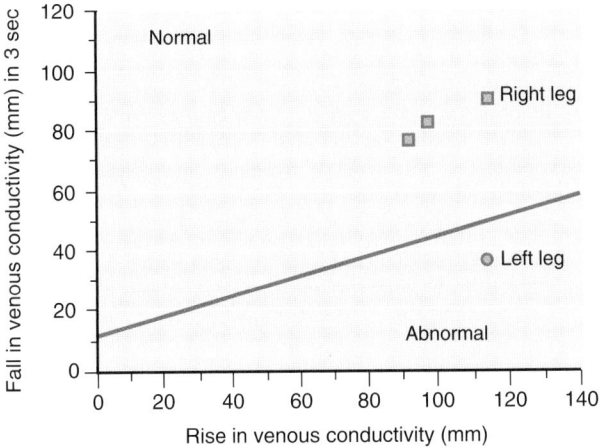

Fig. 77.6 Typical result of impedance plethysmography. This reading suggests deep venous obstruction in the left leg, with normal venous function in the right leg.

for determining whether duplex scanning or IPG is indicated, especially if those studies are not readily available. If the screening test is positive, the additional cost or effort of obtaining a duplex or IPG study may be warranted. A hand-held Doppler is more reliable than IPG for the diagnosis of DVT in patients with severe arterial insufficiency or with a leg in traction. Used alone, a hand-held Doppler provides mainly qualitative evidence of venous function.

Relative Contraindications

Obese patients and patients with massive leg swelling may be difficult to study.

Personnel and Equipment

- A clinician or technician familiar with venous anatomy and Doppler ultrasound technology. (Because the vein cannot be visualized with this technique, a better knowledge of anatomy is required than with compression ultrasound [see Fig. 77.3]. Operator experience significantly increases the accuracy of this examination.)

- 5- to 10-MHz hand-held Doppler with audio. It can often be used for listening to fetal heart tones as well.
- Acoustic gel.

Technique

1. Prepare the room and patient. The room temperature should be warmer than 70°F to prevent vasoconstriction. Place the patient in the supine position with the head slightly elevated. All tight garments should be removed and the leg well exposed (tight-fitting garments may interfere with venous return). The leg should be slightly abducted, externally rotated, and somewhat flexed at the knee; it should also be relaxed to prevent compression of the deep veins. Support the knee with a pillow for better muscle relaxation.
2. Locate the common femoral vein by first finding the artery and then moving the probe medially until the characteristic venous flow or tone is found. The best tone is usually obtained with the probe angled toward the heart (in the direction of venous flow). Use minimal probe pressure to keep from compressing the vein. Arterial flow is characterized by a high-pitched, usually abrupt, tone. Venous flow is usually lower pitched and more continuous.
3. Evaluate the patient with the Doppler from the level of the common femoral vein distally to the superficial femoral, popliteal, and posterior tibial veins (Fig. 77.7). When the level of the popliteal vein is reached, the patient may be rolled to the prone position with knees slightly flexed. Rest the patient's feet on two pillows.
4. Compare the sound or tracing from one leg with that of the other leg at each level of the examination and record the results.

Interpretation

Four characteristics describe *normal venous flow (physiology)*:

- It is *patent* if flow is heard at the anatomic level of the vein.
- It is *spontaneous* if it can be heard at all levels of the vein.
- It varies with respiration, or is *phasic*.
- It is *augmented* by distal compression of the limb or by release of proximal compression.

Patent

Rarely does the flow completely disappear with DVT because some flow is usually preserved around a thrombus or through collateral vessels. Differences between one side and the other may be more

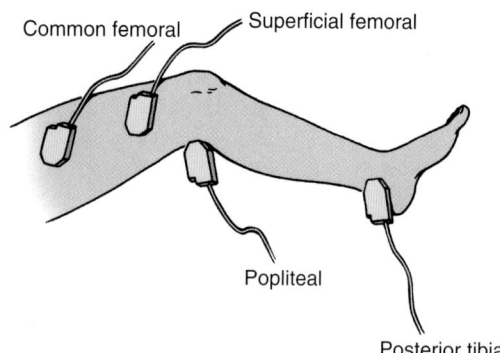

Fig. 77.7 Doppler sonographic examination. The patient is supine with the head slightly elevated. Examine the common femoral, superficial femoral, popliteal, and posterior tibial veins sequentially.

diagnostic, and DVT is frequently associated with a continuous, high-pitched signal. A pulsatile tone that varies with the cardiac cycle is not normal and indicates increased venous pressure.

Spontaneous

DVT causes loss of spontaneous flow. Other causes of loss of spontaneity include anything leading to vasoconstriction. As previously stated, low ambient room temperature or patient anxiety can cause vasoconstriction. The posterior tibial vein may not have a spontaneous signal in normal individuals. Spontaneity is usually found when venous flow is phasic.

Phasic

This characteristic variation of flow with respiration may be lost with DVT. With normal veins, a Valsalva maneuver should decrease the signal, whereas a deep breath should augment the signal.

Augmented

Firm, gentle compression of the limb for a few seconds distal to the vein should cause augmentation of the flow. Release of proximal compression should also result in augmentation. DVT causes a more abrupt and shorter augmentation—if augmentation remains present at all—compared with that of a normal leg. Presence of augmentation provides support that the vein is patent. Reverse augmentation produced by proximal compression or after releasing distal compression indicates valvular incompetence.

False-negative results may occur in patients with incomplete venous obstruction by thrombi, and false-positive results may be caused by extrinsic venous compression. When treatment decisions are made, the fact that no outcome studies are available using hand-held Doppler alone must be weighed against the availability of compression ultrasound, duplex ultrasound, IPG, or contrast studies. Abnormal Doppler results are frequently confirmed with another technique. It should be noted that portable hand-held Doppler equipment, similar to various types of plethysmography equipment (other than electrical IPG), is relatively inexpensive. Either can be used alone, but in combination they may complement each other and provide additional types of quantitative data. These supplementary studies may be helpful to the clinician when determining which patients need further evaluation.

NONINVASIVE ARTERIAL STUDIES

Peripheral artery disease (PAD) affects 29% of patients in a PCP's office who are older than 70 years (or older than 50 years with a history of diabetes or smoking). Although only a small proportion of individuals with PAD and intermittent claudication develop skin breakdown or limb loss, the associated pain and disability from PAD often restrict ambulation. The restriction of ambulation not only interferes with the quality of life, it may interfere with the ability to prevent or treat coronary artery disease (CAD) with exercise. PAD can progress to pain at rest, ulceration, and gangrene. Men are affected more frequently than women. Diabetic patients and smokers develop this disease more frequently and at an earlier age, and the prognosis is grave because PAD almost always progresses in these patients. Diabetic patients also have a greater incidence of vessel involvement between the knee and ankle. Diabetic PAD is responsible for about half of all amputations.

A history of intermittent claudication and absent or diminished peripheral pulses are unreliable signs or symptoms of PAD. The superficial femoral and popliteal arteries are most frequently involved, followed by the distal aorta and iliac arteries, in order of decreasing frequency. The absence of a posterior tibial pulse is a more useful finding on examination than the absence of a dorsalis pedis pulse because 10% to 15% of persons have congenitally absent dorsalis pedis pulses. However, neither finding is very accurate.

Multiple noninvasive techniques are available for the diagnosis of lower extremity PAD. A comprehensive history and physical examination and a combination of at least two noninvasive tests should be performed to both confirm the diagnosis and to determine the location of the lesion. If the location of a hemodynamically significant lesion is known, the risks associated with tests involving contrast dye can be minimized; this knowledge can also guide the approach for the radiologist, cardiologist, or surgeon for optimal contrast visualization. Different and sometimes more useful information can be gained from noninvasive studies than from contrast studies. A simple ankle-brachial index (ABI) technique [described later] has 90% sensitivity and 98% specificity for diagnosing greater than 50% arterial stenosis in the lower extremity. Although it can be very operator dependent for a small artery (e.g., popliteal artery), the accuracy of MR or CT angiography is similar to that of a contrast study. Contrast studies may also be avoided if noninvasive studies fail to demonstrate a hemodynamically significant lesion consistent with the patient's symptoms.

NOTE: The clinician must always consider the possibility of cardiac and cerebrovascular disease in patients with PAD. Intermittent claudication is often the first sign or symptom of generalized atherosclerosis, and these patients most frequently succumb to MI or stroke. National guidelines consider PAD a cardiovascular risk equivalent, meaning the patient with PAD has at least as high a risk of an MI over the next decade (i.e., 20%, if not higher) as a patient who has previously experienced an MI. Using routine coronary angiography in patients with claudication, CAD was identified in 90% of patients, and severe CAD in 28% of patients. The Framingham Study demonstrated a 10% risk of fatal stroke in patients with claudication. Therefore, treatment should be targeted to prevent MI and stroke as much as to prevent complications of PAD.

Regarding screening, although noninvasive studies are more accurate than physical examination, the literature does not demonstrate a benefit to early detection of PAD. Even though noninvasive diagnosis of PAD may be one of the easiest methods to diagnose generalized atherosclerosis, additional data are needed before noninvasive testing should be considered for routine screening.

Risk Factors

- Older age
- Gender (greater risk factor for men)
- Diabetes
- Cigarette smoking
- Hypertension (greater risk factor for women)
- Hyperlipidemia (not a consistent independent risk factor for claudication)
- Family history of PAD (although a risk factor for CAD, this may not be a risk factor for claudication)
- Homocystinemia, hyperfibrinogenemia, hypercoagulable states (probable risk factors)

Indications (Especially in Diabetic Patients)

- Intermittent claudication
- Nonhealing foot ulcer
- Exertional leg pain of unknown etiology
- Possible trauma to an artery

Considerations

- To screen before lower extremity surgery in a diabetic patient.
- To screen patients with neuropathy who may have ischemia without symptoms (numbness from neuropathy).
- To follow a patient after reconstructive arterial surgery or percutaneous intervention (angioplasty or stent) or for whom nonoperative therapy is selected.

It has been said that an experienced clinician can diagnose PAD in most patients by using the history and physical examination alone. However, many clinicians who evaluate patients with extremity pain are neither experienced nor current in the management of vascular disease. Noninvasive studies provide an objective, definitive diagnosis so that clinicians can either rule in PAD or search for another cause for the symptoms.

SEGMENTAL PRESSURE MEASUREMENT

The segmental pressure study is the most generally accepted and widely applied noninvasive arterial test. Segmental pressures are often evaluated as the initial test for a possible arterial abnormality.

Personnel and Equipment

- A clinician or technician familiar with arterial anatomy of the foot and Doppler ultrasound technology.
- 5- to 10-MHz hand-held Doppler probe (transducer) with audio.
- Acoustic gel.
- Blood pressure (BP) monitor.
- Four cuffs for each leg (they can be of the same diameter; if eight are available, study time is considerably reduced).

With arterial stenosis, and especially with collateral flow, arterial resistance is significantly increased. This increased resistance leads to a large or asymmetric drop in arterial BP over the particular arterial segment with obstruction. The brachial pressure can also be used as a standardized reference for the pressures of the lower extremity. At a minimum, brachial pressure should always be recorded along with its ratio to the pressure at the ankle (i.e., ABI).

When using an automatic BP machine or monitor, calibration is not a concern if the same monitor is used throughout the study (ratios and gradients are the values obtained rather than absolute BP measurements). Likewise, the same cuff widths can be used throughout the lower extremities without concern for cuff artifact. (Interpretation has taken cuff artifact into account.) In most cases, this technique produces a high-thigh systolic pressure greater than the brachial artery pressure, which is acceptable for calculating ratios.

Technique

1. With the patient in the supine position, and rested for at least 15 minutes, measure systolic pressures in both arms and record them.
2. On one lower limb apply four segmental cuffs (Fig. 77.8). The systolic values recorded refer to the cuff level rather than the artery studied.
3. Using the hand-held Doppler, evaluate the three major arteries of the foot (dorsalis pedis, posterior tibial, and peroneal) for the strongest signal. Use this artery for the remainder of the study. When determining pressures, hold the hand-held Doppler probe consistently over the artery at the angle and in the direction that produces the strongest signal.

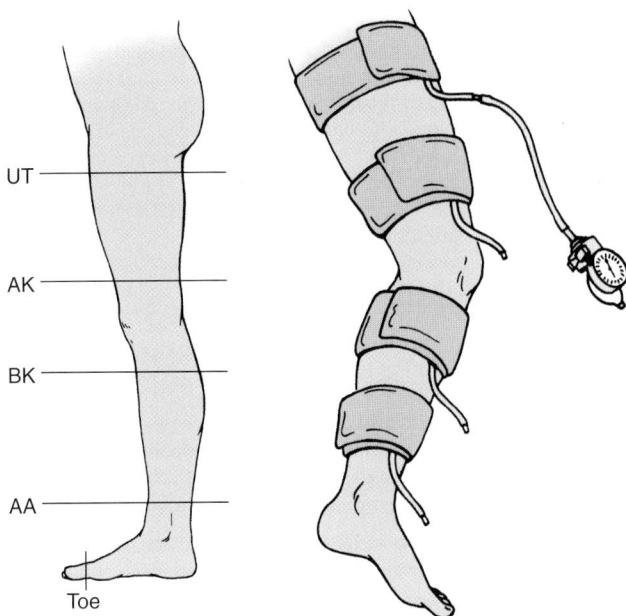

Fig. 77.8 Segmental arterial pressure measurement. Cuff positions: *AA,* above ankle; *AK,* above knee; *BK,* below knee; *UT,* upper thigh.

4. Using the same BP monitor throughout, attach it to a cuff and inflate the cuff until the Doppler signal in the foot disappears.
5. Deflate the cuff slowly until the first signal is audible in the foot and record this systolic pressure for that cuff level.
6. Sequentially inflate and deflate, then record the systolic pressures for each cuff level. Repeat at the same four levels on the other lower extremity.
7. Calculate the ABI, which is the highest ankle systolic pressure divided by the highest brachial systolic pressure.

Sources of Error

Most errors arise when the examiner moves the probe off the artery while inflating the cuff. Another limitation of this technique is that, even though it is fairly sensitive for diagnosing PAD, it is not as helpful for localizing lesions.

Vessel calcification, such as that found in patients with diabetes and chronic renal failure, may lead to an arterial segment that is compressible only at very high pressures (e.g., >300 mm Hg) and may produce unusual results. In fact, segmental pressures may appear to follow a reverse gradient. Suspect vessel calcification when the ABI is higher than 1.3, and this is considered a high ABI. It is estimated that 1.4% of the US population older than 40 years has a high ABI; it is also associated with increased risk of cardiovascular disease, almost increased as much as those with a low ABI. For these individuals, arterial Doppler waveform analysis or pulse volume waveform recordings may be necessary to assess arterial circulation.

With an ABI less than 1.0, always consider the possibility of an obstructed aorta or bilaterally obstructed iliac arteries. Because of cuff artifact, high-thigh pressures may be greater than brachial pressures, and thus mask aortic or iliac obstruction.

With an abnormal study result, consider comparing the systolic pressures in all the arteries of the foot. This would prevent the potential artifact caused by localized obstruction of just one pedal artery.

Interpretation

The single best method of quantitative screening for PAD is an ABI determined by hand-held Doppler. Normally, the ankle pressure is equal to or slightly greater than the arm pressure. An ABI less than 0.95 is abnormal. Typically, patients with rest claudication or gangrene have ABIs less than 0.5, which often indicates multisegmental disease. Patients with intermittent claudication usually have ABIs between 0.5 and 0.9, generally associated with single-segment disease.

During a follow-up evaluation, a change in the ABI of more than 0.15 is considered clinically significant. A decrease in this amount usually indicates disease progression or a problem with a reconstructive procedure. An increase suggests improvement in circulation resulting from the development of collaterals. There is no current consensus on how often studies should be repeated.

A high-thigh pressure less than the arm pressure, any pressure drop of 20 mm Hg or more from one segment to the next, or a difference of 20 mm Hg or more between extremities at the same segmental level signifies a probable obstruction in that segment. Some asymmetry of results in the lower extremities is normal. Remember that pressure drops may represent the sum of more than one lesion. Having a normal high-thigh pressure somewhat excludes obstruction proximal to the femoral artery bifurcation; conversely, a high-thigh pressure less than arm pressure suggests the patient has a lesion at, or proximal to, the bifurcation of the common femoral artery.

NOTE: Many clinicians use the ABI alone to screen for PAD, and studies have verified its value for use in this manner (Hirsch, 2001); however, it requires staff time to perform, document, and interpret the findings. This must be weighed against the fact that although Medicare and other insurers now reimburse for this procedure (CPT-93922), many insurers reimburse only for symptomatic patients. Beckman (2006) demonstrated that an automatic BP cuff (using the oscillatory technique) can be used to check ABI (and save time), with a sensitivity of 88%, specificity of 85%, and a negative predictive value of 96%. If normal, a screening ABI performed in this manner probably does not need to be repeated more than once every 5 years.

WAVEFORM ANALYSIS

Velocity waveform analysis or pulse volume waveform analysis are indicated whenever there is an abnormal ABI or segmental pressure study. These studies can confirm each other and assist in localization of the obstruction.

VELOCITY WAVEFORM ANALYSIS

Personnel and Equipment

- A clinician or technician familiar with arterial anatomy of the lower extremity and Doppler ultrasound technology.
- 5- to 10-MHz probe (transducer) with audio and chart recorder.
- Acoustic gel.

NOTE: The same equipment can often be used as that for venous Doppler studies.

Technique

1. Prepare the room and patient. The room temperature should be greater than 70°F to prevent vasoconstriction. The patient should rest in the supine position for at least 15 minutes. The leg should be well exposed, slightly abducted, externally rotated, and slightly flexed at the knee. Supporting the knee with a pillow may increase patient comfort.
2. Beginning at the common femoral artery, apply acoustic gel and auscultate with the probe for maximal tone and amplitude on the recorder. The best tone is usually obtained with the probe pointed away from the heart in the direction of arterial flow. Arterial flow is characterized by a high-pitched, usually abrupt, tone. This should be differentiated from the sound of venous flow, which is usually lower pitched and more continuous.
3. Obtain tracings from common femoral, popliteal, and posterior tibial arteries. For the popliteal arteries, the patient may be

turned to a prone position with knees slightly flexed and feet resting on two pillows if this position is more comfortable.
4. Compare the sound and tracing from one leg to the other leg at each level of the examination, and record.

Sources of Error

- Dense objects or tissue (e.g., local excess fat, hematoma, scar tissue, plaque on the anterior wall of the vessel) may significantly interfere with ultrasound transmission, making it more difficult to obtain a tracing.
- Prosthetic vessels are almost impossible to study.
- In severe disease, tracings may be unattainable in spite of being able to hear a tone, especially in distal extremities.
- With an incorrect probe angle, the multiphasic components of a tracing can be missed or lost.

Interpretation

The normal arterial velocity signal is multiphasic, characterized by one systolic and one or more diastolic components. With a directional Doppler study, the diastolic component should at first be briefly negative, followed by a positively directed systolic flow component (Fig. 77.9). The diastolic component may be decreased in a vasodilated individual and increased in a vasoconstricted individual.

The arterial velocity signal produced *just proximal* to an occlusion is usually of low amplitude and short duration (Fig. 77.10A). The arterial velocity signal produced *over* a stenotic segment is characteristically high pitched with less prominent diastolic components (Fig. 77.10B). The arterial velocity signal produced *distal* to a stenotic segment usually lacks a diastolic component and has a dampened systolic signal. It is not as high pitched as the stenotic signal (Fig. 77.10C). The arterial signal *far distal* to a stenotic segment is like the poststenotic segment, but is likely to have an even lower amplitude. *Collateral* signals are high pitched and nearly continuous.

To differentiate the contour of normal arterial signals from the contour of obstructed arterial signals, clinicians often describe them as "teepees" and "igloos." "Teepee" refers to the shape of the velocity tracing of a normal artery with its rapid upstroke and resultant high amplitude. The sluggish upstroke tracing with minimal amplitude, as seen with the typical postobstructed artery, might well be described as an "igloo."

A rule of thumb: the presence of a *multiphasic* Doppler signal in a distal vessel, such as that of the foot, strongly suggests that the proximal artery is normal.

PULSE VOLUME WAVEFORM ANALYSIS

Pulse volume recordings (PVRs) are less operator dependent, are not limited by calcification of the vessel walls, and are readily and rapidly obtained using the same cuffs already in place for segmental pressure measurements. This is a quantitative measurement that allows reasonably accurate localization of a lesion or lesions. It is probably the noninvasive test of choice (in place of an ABI) for patients with likely arterial calcinosis, and therefore high ABIs.

Personnel and Equipment

- A clinician or technician familiar with PVR technology
- Pulse volume recorder
- Four cuffs for each leg (they can be of the same diameter; if eight are available, the study time is reduced)

Technique

1. Place the patient in the supine position for at least 15 minutes. Cuffs are placed in the same locations as for segmental pressure determinations and are inflated to 65 mm Hg.
2. Record the PVR at each level.

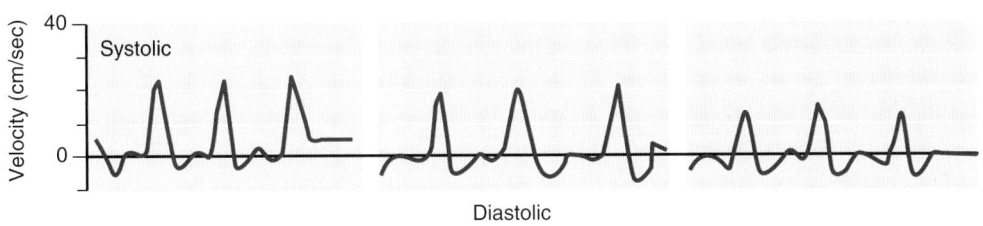

Fig. 77.9   Normal arterial Doppler velocity tracings.

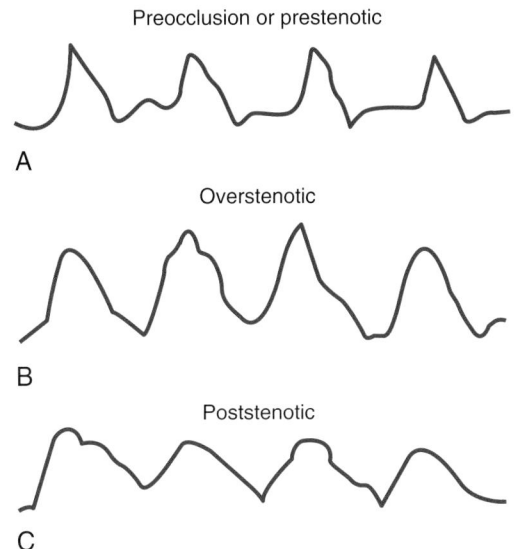

Fig. 77.10   Examples of prestenotic (A), overstenotic (B), and poststenotic (C) tracings.

Source of Error

With severe proximal disease it may be difficult to assess the degree of distal disease because the PVRs are often flat throughout the extremity.

Interpretation

Changes in waveforms with progression of PAD are shown in Fig. 77.11. First noted is the loss of the reflected diastolic wave. Next, with more progressive disease, a decrease is seen in the rate of fall of the catacrotic limb, or the downsloping portion. Finally, a further delay in the rise of the anacrotic limb, or the upsloping initial portion of the wave, is noted. With moderate to severe disease, an "igloo" is the predominant feature.

OTHER STUDIES

For the patient with a history of claudication or intermittent claudication, and yet normal vascular studies, additional testing is available.

1. Vascular treadmill stress testing is probably the most commonly used next study. Because of the cost of equipment, a referral to a vascular laboratory may be necessary. For those with a treadmill, after recording ankle systolic pressures, have the patient walk at a speed of 2 miles per hour with a 12% grade until pain begins, or 5 minutes has elapsed. Patients older than 50 years should have continuous electrocardiographic monitoring. The time it takes to induce pain is noted as the maximal walking time. Once the pain begins, or 5 minutes has elapsed, the patient is placed in a supine position and the ankle systolic pressure is again recorded. It should be recorded every minute until it returns to baseline. In healthy individuals, strenuous exercise causes a transient fall in

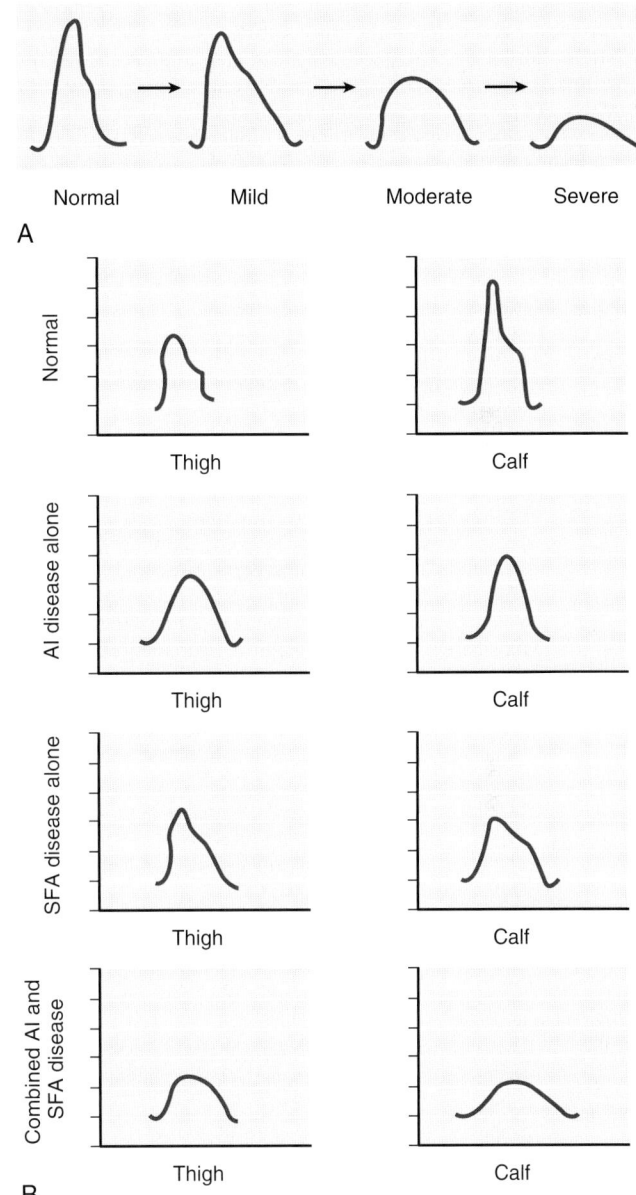

Fig. 77.11   (A) Alterations seen in pulse volume waveform as arterial occlusive disease progresses from mild to moderate to severe. (B) Various thigh and calf waveform patterns characteristic of aortoiliac and superficial femoral arterial occlusive disease. In the normal example, notice the contour of both the thigh and calf waveforms as well as the characteristic increase in amplitude of the calf pulse volume recordings. *AI,* Aortoiliac; *SFA,* superficial femoral artery.

ankle systolic pressure, which quickly returns to baseline at rest. In contrast, when a patient with PAD exercises, pain usually commences before 5 minutes and the ankle pressure falls precipitously, often to unrecordable levels. It usually does not recover for several minutes. A fall in systolic pressure of more than 20 mm Hg from baseline and a recovery time of more than 3 minutes are considered abnormal. (Note that when using the resting brachial pressure to calculate a postexercise ABI, some sources consider a postexercise ABI abnormal if it falls more than 20% from baseline and remains low for more than 3 minutes.) If a postexercise ABI returns to normal in 5 minutes, it suggests a single PAD lesion; delays of more than 10 minutes suggest multilevel PAD.

2. Toe raises, up to 50 repetitions, have been substituted in many vascular laboratories for treadmill walking with good results, and this can be performed in the office setting.

3. MRA—although sometimes a long, complex, and expensive procedure, some clinicians have replaced invasive angiography with MRA and perform invasive angiography only while they are performing a percutaneous intervention (angioplasty or stent).

4. Multislice CT angiography—although it requires considerable radiation and as much contrast dye as an invasive angiogram, CT angiography is often used to justify need for percutaneous invasive angiography.

CPT/BILLING CODES

93922	Limited noninvasive physiologic studies of upper or lower extremity arteries, 1-2e levels, bilateral (e.g., ankle/ brachial indices, Doppler waveform analysis, volume plethysmography, transcutaneous oxygen tension measurement)
93923	Complete noninvasive physiologic studies of upper or lower extremity arteries, 3 or more levels or with provocative functional maneuvers, complete bilateral study (e.g., segmental blood pressure measurements, segmental Doppler waveform analysis, segmental volume plethysmography, segmental transcutaneous oxygen tension measurement, measurements with postural provocation tests, and measurements with reactive hyperemia)
93924	Noninvasive physiologic studies of lower extremity arteries, at rest and following treadmill stress testing, complete bilateral study
93925	Duplex scan of lower extremity arteries or arterial bypass grafts, complete bilateral study
93926	Duplex scan of lower extremity arteries or bypass grafts; unilateral or limited study
93965	Noninvasive physiologic studies of extremity veins, complete bilateral study (e.g., Doppler waveform analysis with responses to compression and other maneuvers, phleborheography, impedance plethysmography)
93970	Duplex scan of extremity veins including responses to compression and other maneuvers; complete bilateral study
93971	Duplex scan of extremity veins including responses to compression and other maneuvers; unilateral or limited study

ICD-10-CM DIAGNOSTIC CODES

I26.99	Pulmonary embolism, other
I70.209	Atherosclerosis of native arteries of the extremities, unspecified
I70.219	with intermittent claudication
I70.229	with rest pain
I70.25	with ulceration
I70.399	of unspecified graft
I70.499	of autologous vein bypass graft
I80.00	Phlebitis and thrombophlebitis, superficial vessels, lower extremity
I80.10	femoral vein
I80.209	other
I80.219	iliac vein
I87.009	Postphlebitic syndrome
I87.1	Edema, leg, resulting from venous obstruction
I87.2	Venous (peripheral) insufficiency, unspecified
L97.909	Chronic ulcer of skin, lower extremity
M79.609	Pain, leg
R60.9	Edema, legs

SUPPLIERS

(See contact information available at www.expertconsult.com.)

For compression and duplex ultrasound suppliers and equipment, see Chapter 214, Emergency Department, Hospitalist, and Office Ultrasound (POCUS).

Hand-held (pocket) Dopplers
MedaSonics (Cooper Surgical)
Vascular equipment, including duplex and hand-held Dopplers
Cardinal Health (Viasys Healthcare/Nicolet Vascular/IMEX)
Parks Medical Electronics

RECOMMENDED READING

Anderson DR, Kovacs MJ, Kovacs G, et al. Combined use of clinical assessment and D-dimer to improve the management of patients presenting to the emergency department with suspected deep vein thrombosis (the EDITED Study). *J Thromb Haemost*. 2003;1:645–651.

Appelman PT, De Jong TE, Lampmann LE. Deep venous thrombosis of the leg: US findings. *Radiology*. 1987;163:743–746.

Beckman JA, Higgins CO, Gerhard-Herman M. Automated oscillometric determination of the ankle-brachial index provides accuracy necessary for office practice. *Hypertension*. 2006;47:35–38.

Bourque JM, Kramer CM. Noninvasive imaging of atherosclerosis. In: Ho VB, Reddy GP, eds. *Cardiovascular Imaging*. Philadelphia: Elsevier; 2011:1193–1214.

Brodsky CM, Martin R. Ultrasound and Doppler examination of veins and arteries. *Atlas Off Proced*. 2000;3:421.

Chan WS, Lee A, Spencer FA, et al. Predicting deep venous thrombosis in pregnancy: out in "LEFt" field? *Ann Intern Med*. 2009;151(2):85.

Creager MA, Beckman JA, Loscalzo J, eds. *Vascular Medicine: A Companion to Braunwald's Heart Disease*. 2nd ed. Philadelphia: Elsevier; 2013.

Cronan JJ, Dorfman GS, Scola FH, et al. Deep venous thrombosis: US assessment using vein compression. *Radiology*. 1987;162:191–194.

Ergun E, Turgut AT, Ergun AS, Dogra VS. Vascular ultrasonography: physics, instrumentation and clinical techniques. In: Ho VB, Reddy GP, eds. *Cardiovascular Imaging*. Philadelphia: Elsevier; 2011:1033–1046.

Heijboer H, Büller HR, Lensing AW, et al. A comparison of real-time compression ultrasonography with impedance plethysmography for the diagnosis of deep-vein thrombosis in symptomatic outpatients. *N Engl J Med*. 1993;329:1365–1369.

Heit JA, O'Fallon WM, Petterson TM, et al. Relative impact of risk factors for deep vein thrombosis and pulmonary embolism: a population-based study. *Arch Intern Med*. 2002;162:1245–1248.

Hirsch AT, Criqui MH, Treat-Jacobson D, et al. Peripheral arterial disease detection, awareness, and treatment in primary care. *JAMA*. 2001;286:1317–1324.

Huisman MV, Büller HR, ten Cate JW, Vreeken J. Serial impedance plethysmography for suspected deep venous thrombosis in outpatients: the Amsterdam general practitioner study. *N Engl J Med*. 1986;314:823–828.

Hull RD, Carter CJ, Jay RM, et al. Diagnostic efficacy of impedance plethysmography for clinically suspected deep-vein thrombosis: a randomized trial. *Ann Intern Med*. 1985;102:21–28.

Hunt D. Determining the clinical probability of deep venous thrombosis and pulmonary embolism. *South Med J*. 2007;100:1015–1021.

Lensing AW, Prandoni P, Brandjes D, et al. Detection of deep-vein thrombosis by real-time B-mode ultrasonography. *N Engl J Med.* 1989;320:342–345.

Pellerito JS, Polak JF. *Introduction to Vascular Ultrasonography.* Philadelphia: Elsevier; 2012.

Sermsathanasawadi N, Suparatchatpun P, Pumpuang T, et al. Comparison of clinical prediction scores for the diagnosis of deep vein thrombosis in unselected population of outpatients and inpatients. *Phlebology.* 2015;30(7):469–474.

Turnbull TJ, Dymowski JJ. Emergency department use of hand-held Doppler ultrasonography [review]. *Am J Emerg Med.* 1989;7:209–215.

Vogt MT, Cauley JA, Newman AB, et al. Decreased ankle/arm blood pressure index and mortality in elderly women. JAMA. 1993;270:465.

Vogel P, Laing FC, Jeffrey Jr RB, Wing VW. Deep venous thrombosis of the lower extremity: US evaluation. *Radiology.* 1987;163:747–751.

Wells PS, Anderson DR, Rodger M, et al. Evaluation of D-dimer in the diagnosis of suspected deep-vein thrombosis. *N Engl J Med.* 2003;349:1227–1235.

Wells PS, Owen C, Doucette S, et al. Does this patient have deep vein thrombosis? JAMA. 2006;295:199–207.

CHAPTER 78

SCLEROTHERAPY

Jerry Ninia

Sclerotherapy is a technique used to eliminate unwanted veins (both varicosities and spider veins). This is accomplished by injecting a noxious agent into the lumen of the vein, which causes destruction of the endothelium with an inflammatory response. When used with compression, it results in obliteration of the vessel. The goal of treatment is to eradicate abnormal veins while preserving healthy ones.

BACKGROUND

Ancient physicians, scholars, and poets, including Hippocrates and Homer, recognized varicose veins. Improvements in syringes and needles and the development of more effective and safe sclerosing solutions have allowed sclerotherapy to become a modern and effective method of treatment. Clinicians still use sclerosants developed in the 20th century (e.g., hypertonic glucose, hypertonic saline, sodium morrhuate, chromated glycerin, ethanolamine oleate, and stabilized polyiodide iodine). However, the most popular agents are sodium tetradecyl sulfate (Sotradecol, Fibrovein), polidocanol (Asclera), and hypertonic saline (Table 78.1). Sodium tetradecyl sulfate and polidocanol are detergents that work by denaturing cellular proteins and causing endothelial destruction. Hypertonic saline dehydrates endothelial cells, resulting in cell death. It can burn or sting with use; the newer agents are advertised as being less painful.

Organizations worldwide—including the American College of Phlebology and the American Venous Forum in the United States—have been formed to develop further research and education in venous disease. In 2006, The American Medical Association recognized phlebology as a separate and distinct medical specialty.

ANATOMY

The venous system is divided into three levels: *deep, perforating,* and *superficial* veins. The veins treated with sclerotherapy are the perforating and the superficial veins.

Deep veins are encased in fascia and muscle. In ascending order, they are the anterior and posterior tibial veins, the peroneal vein, the tibioperoneal trunk, the popliteal vein, the superficial femoral vein, the deep femoral vein, the common femoral vein, and the iliac vein. These veins convey blood from the lower limb back to the heart (Fig. 78.1).

The superficial venous system is confined to the veins above the fascia in the subcutaneous tissue; they include the great and small saphenous veins and their tributaries in addition to the lateral subdermal veins (of Albanese) around the knee (Figs. 78.2 and 78.3).

Approximately 150 perforating veins connect the superficial and deep systems. Many of these veins are eponymous with the anatomists who demonstrated them (Fig. 78.4). In the middle area of the thigh are the Hunterian perforators, and in the distal thigh are the Dodd perforators. These veins connect the thigh portion of the great saphenous vein to the femoral vein. Below the knee is Boyd's perforator, connecting the great saphenous vein to the popliteal vein. The infrapopliteal perforating veins along the medial aspect of the leg connect a major branch of the saphenous vein, the posterior tibial arch vein, to the posterior tibial vein.

There are also important perforating veins along the posterior aspect of the calf that connect the small saphenous system to the tibial venous system. In addition, perforators along the lateral aspect of the knee connect the lateral subdermal plexus of Albanese to the deep venous system.

Finally, there are important connections from the superficial venous system to the deep femoral vein. The posterior thigh perforator connects the superficial veins of the posterior thigh to the deep femoral vein. Similarly, the inferior gluteal vein and the veins of the medial thigh connect through the internal pudendal system to the deep pelvic veins. It is this last system that results in the vulvar varicosities seen frequently in pregnancy. Although it is not necessary to remember all of the proper names of these perforators, it is important for the clinician to have knowledge of their location so that sclerotherapy can be carried out in a logical and effective manner.

In general, unwanted veins are referred to as *telangiectases, reticular varicosities,* or *varicose veins* (Table 78.2).

PHYSIOLOGY

Primary Varicose Veins

The veins of the lower limb carry blood against the force of gravity back to the heart. This is accomplished by two principal means. When the muscles of the calf contract, they compress the soleal sinuses and the deep veins encased in fascia and muscle, achieving a pressure of up to 300 cm H_2O. Because the veins of the lower limb have valves that allow blood to flow only in a proximal direction, the column of blood is forced into the valveless veins of the abdomen.

If a person is standing still, the pressure of the veins on the dorsum of the foot will equal the distance from the foot to the right heart. This results in an average pressure of approximately 70 to 80 cm H_2O. As evidenced by the pressure relationship mentioned previously, the pressure exerted by the contraction of the calf muscles is sufficient to overcome the effects of gravity and propel blood in a proximal direction. The flow of venous blood from the calf back to the heart may be considered the systolic phase. During this phase, blood is prevented from going into the superficial venous system by the valves of the perforating veins. During the relaxation phase, when the pressure in the calf compartment is diminished, blood can flow from the superficial veins through the perforators into the deep veins. Therefore the superficial venous system may be likened to an atrium of the heart and the deep veins of the calf likened to a ventricle.

This physiologic system breaks down when the walls of the veins dilate, causing the valves to become incompetent. The manner in which veins become incompetent is somewhat controversial. The belief has been that the problem is initiated by a malfunctioning valve. Phlebitis can destroy the valve structure, so this may be the inciting event. The incompetent valve allows blood to flow in a reverse direction as gravity pulls it down toward the foot. The resulting increase in venous pressure causes the veins to dilate and sequentially creates incompetence in the more distal valves. However, it now seems likely that the initiating event is dilation of the vein itself.

Agent	Food and Drug Administration Approval	Supply	Maximum Dose Per Visit	Indications	Companies	Comments
Sodium tetradecyl sulfate (Sotradecol, STS)	Yes	2-mL ampules (1%, 3%)	10-mL 3% solution	0.1%–0.25% up to 2 mm; 0.25%–0.5% reticular; 0.5%–1% <4 mm; 1%–3% >4 mm	Mylan USA	Painless; can cause extravascular necrosis
Hypertonic saline	Yes, off label	30-mL ampules (23.4%); dilute as needed with lidocaine 1% (may be stored dilute for up to 12 wk)	10 mL; more can cause leg cramps, significant salt load	11.7% <2 mm (especially for matting); 23.4% >2 mm (many use the 18.7% solution for all vessels; see text)	Major advantages: no anaphylaxis and inexpensive; some discomfort on injection	
Polidocanol (Asclera)	Yes, spider veins and varicose veins 1 to 3 mm in diameter	2-mL ampules (0.5%, 1%)	2 mg/kg	0.25%–1% telangiectases and reticulars up to 3 mm	Merz North America	Painless; less extravascular necrosis

TABLE 78.1 Most Common Sclerosing Agents in the United States

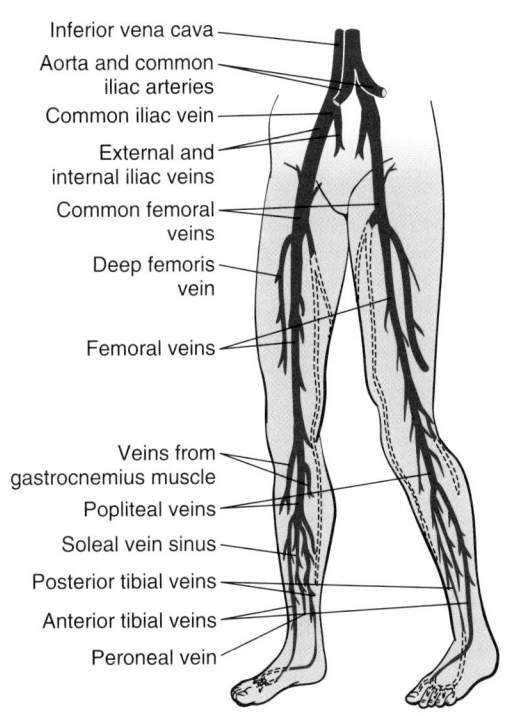

Fig. 78.1 Main venous conduits formed by the deep veins of the lower limbs; numerous branch veins join these.

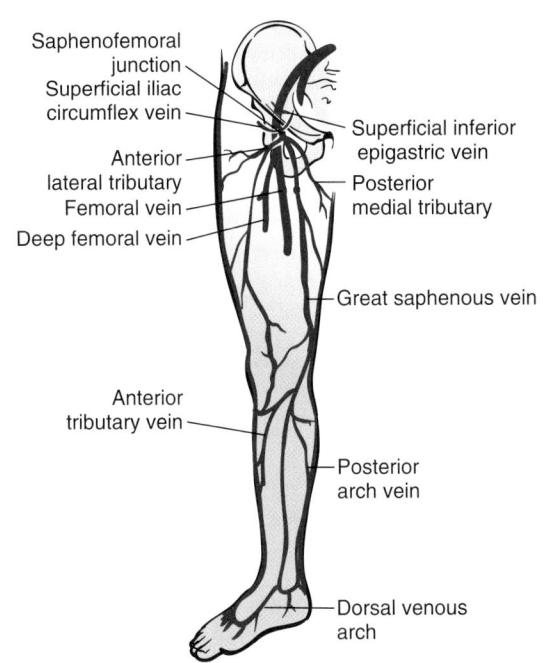

Fig. 78.2 Normal anteromedial superficial venous anatomy. The great saphenous vein ascends from the dorsal venous arch and dominates the anteromedial superficial drainage system. It receives the posterior arch vein (vein of Michelangelo). It also receives variable anterior and posterior tributary veins in the anteromedial calf just below the knee. As the saphenous vein reaches its termination, it receives important tributaries medially and laterally. These tributaries are commonly visualized in duplex ultrasound examinations, which may identify reflux in one or both of these vessels.

The most proximal valve of the superficial system is at the saphenofemoral junction. This valve normally allows blood to flow from the great saphenous vein into the common femoral vein. When it becomes incompetent, blood will flow from the common femoral vein into the great saphenous vein, causing progressive dilation of the saphenous vein. This dilation can affect more distal valves, in turn causing them to become incompetent. Thus a cycle is begun that eventually causes dilation of the entire saphenous system.

Another mechanism for the development of varicose veins is incompetence of the perforating vein valves. Normally, when the calf muscles contract and their valves close, blood is prevented from flowing through the perforating veins into the superficial system. If a valve is not working properly, blood will flow from the deep veins into the superficial venous system. The flow of blood from the deep system into the superficial system diminishes the blood flow back to the heart,

which greatly increases the venous pressure in the leg. This increase in venous pressure, termed *venous hypertension*, is the cause of many of the sequelae seen in chronic venous insufficiency, such as edema, stasis dermatitis, pigmentation from hemosiderin, and ultimately the development of lipodermatosclerosis and venous ulceration.

Secondary Varicose Veins

Secondary varicose veins can occur as a result of a superficial or deep venous thrombosis (DVT) or from an arteriovenous fistula with resulting high venous pressure. All of these conditions may cause venous dilation and lead to valve incompetence.

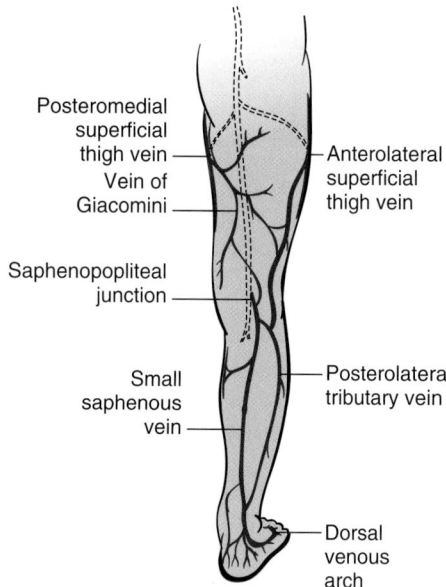

Fig. 78.3 The small saphenous vein dominates posterolateral superficial venous drainage. It originates in the dorsal venous arch; at the posterolateral ankle, it is intimately associated with the sural nerve. Note the important posterolateral tributary vein and the posterior thigh vein; it ascends and connects the small saphenous venous system with the great saphenous venous system. The anterolateral superficial thigh vein and the posterolateral tributary vein can be very important in congenital venous anomalies, such as Klippel-Trénaunay syndrome.

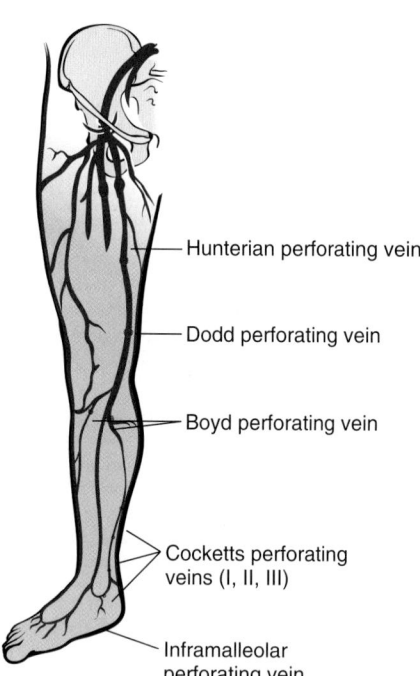

Fig. 78.4 Locations of the most important perforating veins associated with the great saphenous system. Note that the Cocketts and inframalleolar perforating veins are actually separate from the great saphenous system. The Boyd perforating vein is constantly present, but it may drain the saphenous vein or its tributaries. Perforating veins in the distal third of the thigh are referred to as *Dodd perforators*, whereas those in the middle third of the thigh are referred to as *Hunterian perforators*.

TABLE 78.2 Vessel Classification

Type	Vessel Classification	Characteristics	Color
I	Telangiectases ("spider veins")	0.1–1 mm	Red
Ia	Telangiectatic matting	<0.2 mm, very fine; can occur after injection or surgery	Red
II	Venulectasia	1–2 mm	Violaceous
III	Reticular veins	2–4 mm	Blue
IV	Nonsaphenous varicosities (second-degree incompetent perforators)	3–8 mm	Blue
V	Saphenous varicosities	7–8 mm	Blue

INDICATIONS

- Small bulging varicose veins up to 0.6 cm in diameter (Some phlebologists treat even larger veins.)
- Venulectasia
- Telangiectasia (commonly called *spider veins*)
- Pain, itching, burning, tiredness, and heaviness in the lower limb (Previously mentioned indications, regardless of size, may cause these symptoms.)
- Cosmesis in the absence of other symptoms
- Venous stasis ulcer
- Venous stasis pigmentation
- Recurrent bleeding of a vessel of any size

Injection of facial telangiectases has been done and reported and is efficacious. However, venous sinus thrombosis (in the brain) has occurred. Radiofrequency ablation or various laser/light methodologies are often equally helpful without the associated risks.

CONTRAINDICATIONS

- Saphenofemoral junction or saphenopopliteal junction reflux. (Reflux from deep into the superficial system creates high venous pressure, making it difficult to obliterate a vein.)
- Veins larger than 0.6 cm in diameter. If the vein has a large diameter, it will be difficult to obtain coaptation of the intimal surfaces for permanent obliteration; it is more likely that a thrombus will develop within the lumen of the vein and recanalize over time. (Some practitioners do inject these large vessels, but recurrence and complications are more common and phlebectomy might be a wiser treatment choice.)
- Arterial insufficiency.
- Ankle-brachial index below 0.7 or other signs of inadequate arterial flow.
- Diabetic neuropathy.
- Acute superficial or deep thrombophlebitis.
- Massive obesity.
- Coagulopathy or anticoagulated patient.
- Obstruction of the deep venous system.
- Severe systemic disease (especially collagen vascular disease, malignancy, or severe cardiac problems).
- Pregnancy.
- Lack of mobility, as seen in stroke, arthritis, or other musculoskeletal disorders.
- Unwillingness to comply with a program of compression.
- Acute febrile illness.

NOTE: The clinician should use caution in patients with asthma or numerous allergies (unless hypertonic saline is used) to avoid potential hypersensitivity. Age is not a contraindication if the patient is active and has reasonably good skin turgor.

EQUIPMENT

- Camera for pictures (optional).
- Examination table. (A power table is helpful but not mandatory.)
- Patient stand. (The examination can be performed more optimally if the patient's feet are 24 inches off the floor. Usually this requires a made-to-order stand that includes a strong railing. The stand can be used for both examination and treatment.)
- Good lighting. (A gooseneck lamp is sufficient; however, some therapists use a more intense light source, such as a headlamp.)
- Magnification loupes (3×).
- Syringes (3.0 and 1.0 mL); half-inch 30-gauge needle.
- Handheld Doppler probe.
- Sclerosing solution:
  - *Sodium tetradecyl sulfate* (preferred by the author) in dilutions of 0.2%, 0.5%, 1.0%, and (rarely) 3.0%. It is commercially available in dilutions of 1% and 3%.
  - *Hypertonic saline* in a dilution of 18.7% is also commonly used (and preferred by the author). It can be prepared by injecting 2 mL of 2% lidocaine into a 30-mL multiple-dose vial of 23.4% saline (0.5 mL of this solution is injected per site). It is sterile and can be left diluted for up to 12 weeks.
  - *Polidocanol* is another common sclerosant; it is commercially available in dilutions of 0.5% and 1%.

NOTE: The assistant should have 5 to 10 1-mL syringes drawn up for use, depending on the sclerosant and the number of veins to be injected. Each agent has benefits and risks. Hypertonic saline is effective and there are no allergic reactions; however, it causes pain and the risk of extravasation necrosis of the skin is significant (Box 78.1). Polidocanol (0.5% and 1%) is a weak sclerosant, but it works well on small veins. Allergic reactions are possible but rare (Box 78.2 and Table 78.3). Sodium tetradecyl sulfate is medium in potency and relatively painless, but it must be injected carefully to avoid skin necrosis. Allergy and anaphylaxis can occur, although this is rare (see Table 78.1).

- Cotton balls with benzalkonium chloride (Zephiran) or isopropyl alcohol.
- Tape (1 in wide). (Some patients require paper tape.)
- Compression stockings. Some clinicians stock them in the office. Patients can also be given a prescription to purchase them at a medical supply store (with proper measurements noted on the prescription), or they may be fitted at certain retail establishments. Pantyhose, full-length stockings, thigh-high stockings, or calf-high stockings are selected based on the areas being injected. Rubber gloves are helpful for donning the stockings.
- Elastic wraps (4 to 6 in wide; e.g., Ace bandages).
- Nonsterile gloves and equipment to follow universal blood and body fluid precautions.

NOTE: Additional instruments that may be helpful but are not necessary include a photoplethysmograph, light-reflection rheograph, and a duplex scanner. Duplex ultrasound has become very important in phlebology, especially in the proper evaluation and treatment of patients with advanced venous disease.

PREPROCEDURE PATIENT PREPARATION

It is best if the patient receives patient education materials before the office visit (see the patient education handouts online at www.expertconsult.com). An initial visit is scheduled for 30 minutes. The patient is evaluated, venous testing is done, the legs are measured for hose, and counseling is completed. Future visits of 15 to 30 minutes are scheduled. Although the package insert says that polidocanol injections can be repeated in 1 to 2 weeks, most

BOX 78.1 Hypertonic Saline Description

- True allergic reactions are nonexistent, but side effects are more common.
- The degree of endothelial damage is directly proportional to the concentration used.
- Dilution with heparin or anesthetics can decrease effectiveness, depending on amounts.
- It destroys *all* cells: endothelium and red blood cells (RBCs).
- Significant extravasation can produce cutaneous necrosis.
- Hemolysis of RBCs can cause cutaneous hemosiderin staining.

BOX 78.2 Polidocanol

- Originally developed as a topical anesthetic under the trade name Sch 600.
- Belongs to the urethane group of local anesthetics.
- Generally classified as a weak detergent solution.
- Should be diluted with distilled sterile water.
- Patients should be warned about an Antabuse-alcohol reaction.
- Elimination half-life is 4 hours, with 90% elimination within 12 hours; it does not cross the blood-brain barrier.
- Injection is painless, and cutaneous necrosis is difficult to produce.

TABLE 78.3 Maximum Daily Doses of Polidocanol*

Concentration	Dose (mL) Based on Patient Body Weight				
	50 kg	60 kg	70 kg	80 kg	90 kg
0.5%	20	24	28	32	36
1.0%	10	12	14	16	18

*10 mL per session is the FDA-approved maximum.

clinicians repeat injections at 2- to 4-week intervals. It is best not to reinject the same area any sooner than 3 to 4 weeks. Most patients will require three 30-minute injection visits.

A careful history and physical examination must be performed (Fig. 78.5), and problems that might affect treatment with sclerotherapy (e.g., anticoagulation, history of phlebitis, vein surgery, arterial disease, bleeding problems, diabetes, history of severe allergic reactions) should be sought.

Physical examination must include a careful evaluation of the pedal pulses. If they are not readily felt, an ankle-brachial index must be obtained. The only equipment needed for this is a blood pressure cuff, stethoscope, and handheld Doppler probe.

It is essential to look for the presence of saphenofemoral or saphenopopliteal reflux, also known as *axial vein reflux*. Its presence is a contraindication to sclerotherapy, and many insurance companies will not cover sclerotherapy if it is present. This determination can be made with a careful handheld Doppler examination. The patient must be standing. The tip of the Doppler probe is held at the saphenofemoral or saphenopopliteal junction while the calf muscle is firmly and sharply compressed. This creates a sound when the blood is propelled forward. As the muscle is released, there should be no retrograde flow; only silence. If flow is heard, it means that there is reflux at these junctions. In that situation, newer techniques are indicated, including saphenous vein ablation with a radiofrequency or laser catheter (see Chapter 80, Endovenous Vein Ablation).

Patients are often screened with *photoplethysmography* (PPG) and *light reflection rheography*. These are means of measuring the venous refilling time of the lower limb. A transducer is used to shine a certain wavelength of light into the skin about 10 cm proximal to the medial malleolus. Hemoglobin specifically absorbs this wavelength. While seated, the patient dorsiflexes the foot 8 to 10 times. This compresses and empties the normal dermal venous plexus. The light that is not absorbed by hemoglobin is reflected back to the transducer and measured. This reflection back is greater when the veins are empty (less hemoglobin to absorb the light) and decreases when the veins are full. The instrument then records how long it takes for the blood of the dermal plexus to return to baseline. A refilling time of less than 25 to 30 seconds indicates that the venous plexus is filling partially in a retrograde fashion; this confirms incompetence of the venous system. If the test result is abnormal, a tourniquet should be applied just above and then below the knee. The test is then repeated; if values normalize, it suggests that the problem is within the superficial venous system (Figs. 78.6 to 78.8) and that sclerotherapy can proceed. If the filling time does not normalize with above- and below-knee tourniquets, it suggests deep venous insufficiency and further evaluation (i.e., duplex ultrasound) may be indicated.

The results of PPG have been found to correlate well with venograms for the determination of DVT. In this instance, the outflow of blood is blocked and thus the tracing is flat.

A duplex scan performed when the patient is standing enables an estimate of the location of venous reflux and its magnitude. The clinician can also look for DVT, venous obstruction, and incompetent perforators. Duplex ultrasound has emerged as the most reliable, cost-effective, reproducible way to evaluate the venous system of the lower extremity. In recent years, units have become less expensive and training in ultrasonography is available.

Photographs of the lower limbs may be necessary. Some insurance companies require them. More importantly, photographs provide baseline information to which the patient's limbs can be compared as treatment progresses. Many phlebologists first draw the veins in on diagrams (see Fig. 78.5).

The technique of sclerotherapy must be carefully explained to the patient, including possible complications and what will happen over the course of treatment. The patient must be cautioned not to expect perfection. A well-educated patient is more cooperative and satisfied.

TECHNIQUE

Before injecting the patient, obtain a signed consent (see the sample patient consent form online at www.expertconsult.com).

Wipe the area to be injected with benzalkonium chloride or alcohol. This not only cleanses the area but improves visualization of the vessels. Use a small syringe (1 or 3 mL). Stretch the skin surrounding the vessel with the nondominant hand. It is helpful to bend the tip of the 30-gauge needle up to about 20 to 30 degrees to cannulate these tiny veins (Fig. 78.9).

Patient Questionnaire/Evaluation: Vein Injection (Sclerotherapy)

Date _____ Name _____ Birthdate _____ Age _____
Sex _____ Height _____ Weight _____
Referred by: _____

1. How many years have you noticed this problem? ___
2. Have you ever been previously treated for this problem?
   Yes _____ No _____
   By whom and when? _____
   _____

   With what method?
   Injection _____
   Electrocautery _____
   Laser _____
   Surgery _____

3. When did the problem with your veins occur?
   Age _____
   Before pregnancy _____
   After pregnancy _____
   After trauma
      or Premarin therapy _____
   Other _____

4. Is there a family history of varicose or spider veins?
   Mother _____
   Father _____
   Sister _____
   Brother _____
   Children _____
   Aunts _____
   Uncles _____

5. Do you have a history of
   Smoking _____
   Blood clots _____
   Lupus _____
   Bleeding disorders _____
   Easy bruisability _____
   Dark spots after
      skin injury or surgery _____
   Easy scarring _____

6. Are you developing new veins? _____
7. Are your present veins getting bigger? _____
8. After prolonged standing or sitting do your legs ache? _____
9. Do your legs or veins ache before menses? _____
10. Does walking or exercise relieve or aggravate the pain? (circle)
11. Describe any symptoms you have from your veins: _____
    _____
12. Are you required to be on your feet for long periods? _____
13. Do you jog, run, jump rope, or do aerobics? (circle)
    How often per week? _____
14. Are you pregnant or planning a pregnancy soon? _____
15. Did you read and understand the patient education
    materials given to you? _____
16. Do you understand the risks and benefits as well as
    possible complications to vein injection? _____
17. Are you prepared to wear hose on a regular basis
    as described? _____
18. Is your problem cosmetic or medical? _____

PMH: MI: _____
      ALL: _____
      MEDS: _____
      FH: _____

Fig. 78.5 Patient questionnaire for sclerotherapy. (Modified from Mitchel P. Goldman, MD, Dermatology Associates of San Diego County, Inc., La Jolla, CA.)

Continued

Patient Questionnaire/Evaluation: Vein Injection (Sclerotherapy)

Varicosities
    R   L
   Vulvar
   Groin
   Thigh
   Below knee

Pulses
    R   L
   Femoral
   Popliteal
   Dorsalis pedis
   Posterior tibial

Presence of
    R   L
   Edema
   Stasis pig
   Cellulitis
   Active ulcer
   Healed ulcer
   Venules
   Tenderness

PPG   R   L
PRG
Doppler

Impression: _____

Plan: Discussed
• Method
• Cost
• Complications
  hyperpigmentation
  blistering
  recurrence
  pain
  phlebitis
  matting
• Stockings
• Number of anticipated visits

Measurements
Ankle _____
Calf _____
Thigh _____
Length _____
Shoe size _____
Type:
  Panty
  Thigh high
  Knee high
  20/30 or 30/40

cc: _____
Physician signature   Date

Fig. 78.5, cont'd

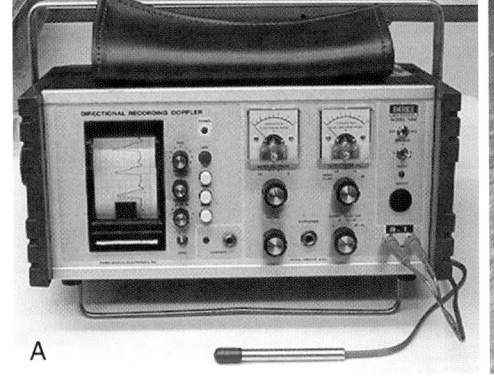
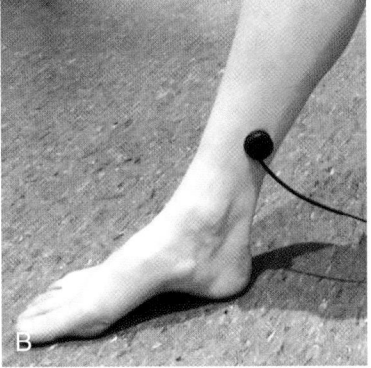

Fig. 78.6 (A) Photoplethysmography (PPG) machine. (B) PPG machine attached to a patient. (PPG has been important in the vascular laboratory, but in a clinical setting PPG has been largely replaced by duplex ultrasound.) (B, Courtesy the Whiteley Clinic, Guildford, UK.)

Direct cannulation of the vein is absolutely essential, since extraluminal injections may lead to skin necrosis. For the treatment of veins 2 mm in diameter or less, 0.2% sodium tetradecyl sulfate or polidocanol 0.1% is used. Although some therapists suggest a concentration of 0.1% sodium tetradecyl, it is not necessary to decrease the concentration (Table 78.4). Aspiration of blood from the small vessels cannot be accomplished. If a small wheal forms at the time of injection, the needle is not in the lumen and injection must be stopped. If the needle is properly inserted, the vessel should blanch. Once the blanching stops, withdraw the needle and go to the next vessel. More is not better unless new vessels continue to blanch. The injection is carried out with extremely gentle pressure, and only 0.1 to 0.3 mL is used. Too much pressure can rupture the vein and lead to unnecessary inflammation.

For the injection of veins 3 to 5 mm in diameter, 3% sodium tetradecyl sulfate is used in a quantity of 0.5 mL to a maximum of 1.0 mL. Because a stronger solution is being used, it is more likely that

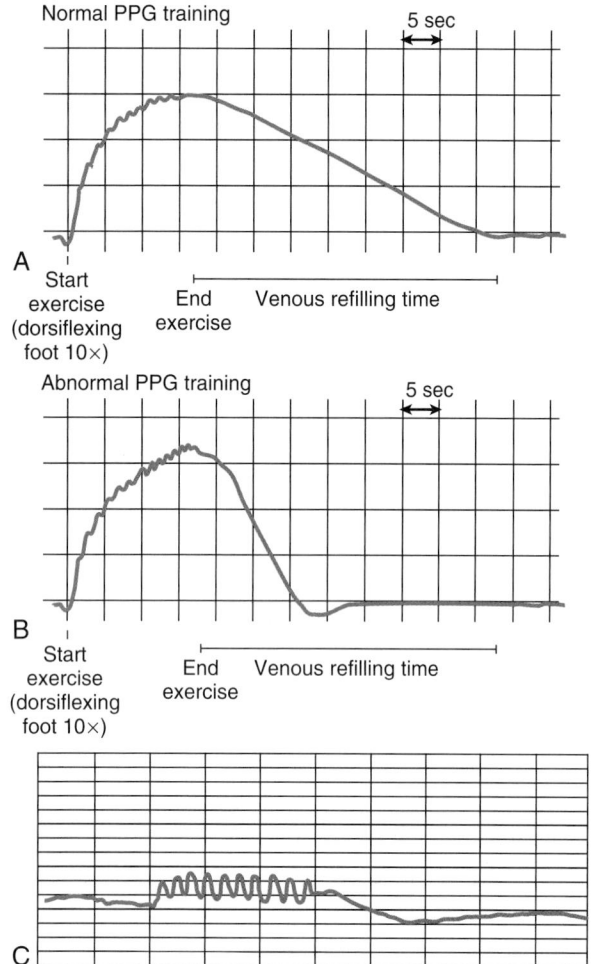

Fig. 78.7 Tracings of photoplethysmography (PPG) readings. (A) Normal. After dorsiflexing the foot 10 times, the blood has been "squeezed out" of the ankle, so less light is absorbed and more is reflected back. This gives a higher reading. As the veins refill with blood, more light is absorbed so less is reflected back. Thus, a lower amplitude is recorded. A refill time over 25 seconds is normal. (B) Abnormal. Rapid refill indicating venous insufficiency. Refill time is only 15 to 17 seconds. (Without tourniquets, this could be deep or superficial; if tourniquets are in place, this is most likely indicative of deep venous insufficiency.) (C) Abnormal. No indication of emptying, suggesting deep venous obstruction or marked insufficiency ("picket fence" pattern).

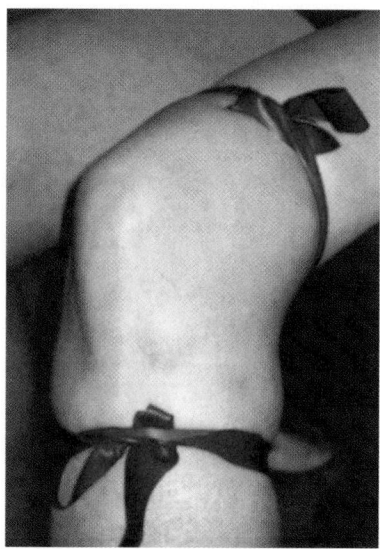

Fig. 78.8 Placement of tourniquets above and below the knee when the photoplethysmogram is abnormal. If the tracing normalizes, it indicates superficial venous incompetence. If it remains abnormal with rapid refilling, deep venous insufficiency is suggested.

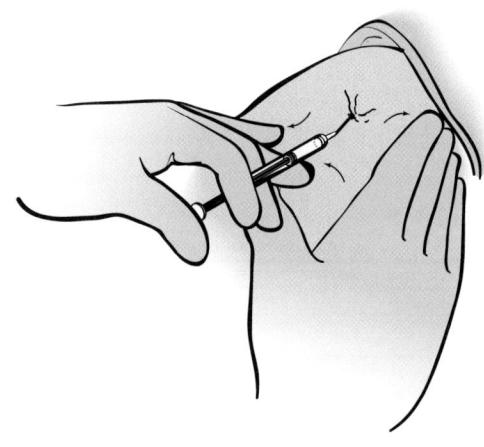

Fig. 78.9 Proper injection technique. The nondominant hand stretches the skin around the vessels. The needle bevel is up and the needle itself is bent 30 degrees upward.

subcutaneous injection may lead to tissue necrosis. Therefore aspiration of blood into the hub of the needle is recommended before the injection of sclerosant.

For veins 5 to 6 mm in diameter, 3% sodium tetradecyl sulfate is used with a volume of 0.5 mL to a maximum of 1.0 mL (see Table 78.4). Aspiration before injection is essential.

All of the previously mentioned procedures can be performed with the patient supine. Spider veins will remain visible, but sometimes it may be difficult to cannulate large veins in a supine patient because the veins are not dilated and collapse when the patient lies down. In this case the patient should be asked to stand and the vein cannulated with a no. 27 butterfly that is taped in place. The patient can then be placed in a supine position and the vein injected as previously described. Alternatively, the veins are marked with a skin-marking pen with the patient standing and the vein can be injected when the patient lies down.

A compression dressing consisting of a folded piece of gauze is placed over each site and covered with a piece of Dermicel or similar tape. Paper tape is necessary for some patients to avoid allergic responses. A cotton ball and tape are used by many phlebologists and work well. The limb is then compressed either by elastic wraps or compression stockings, as discussed in the section on compression.

NOTE: It is often quicker and easier to just wrap Coban or Co-Flex around the entire leg, followed by the compression hose. This keeps the blood off the hose and makes it easier to get the hose on the leg. These rolls are 4 in wide and 9 yd long.

A complete note should be dictated (or a form used) for at least the first injection visit (Fig. 78.10). After this, we recommend flow sheets to save time (Fig. 78.11).

PEARLS

Injection sclerotherapy using hypertonic saline solution or sodium tetradecyl sulfate is a safe, relatively painless method of ablating small varicose veins, reticular venules, and spider telangiectases with a minimum of complications. The clinician will have better results and happier patients if the following important concepts are kept in mind:

- Although spider veins may be symptomatic, most patients seek treatment because they are unhappy with the appearance of their legs. The clinician should be cautious and conservative to avoid creating a blemish worse than what the patient already has.

TABLE 78.4 Rapid Guide for Selection of Sclerosing Solution by Vessel Type*

Vessel	Solution/Concentration	Volume (per Injection Site)
Telangiectatic matting (after previous treatment)	Hypertonic saline, 11.7% **Sodium tetradecyl sulfate, 0.1%** **Polidocanol, 0.1%–0.2%** (Go slow, with low injection pressures)	**0.1–0.2 mL**
Telangiectasia (up to 1 mm)	Hypertonic saline, 11.7%† **Sodium tetradecyl sulfate, 0.1%–0.2%** **Polidocanol, 0.1%–0.2%**	**0.1–0.3 mL**
Venulectasia (1–2 mm)	Hypertonic saline, 11.7%–23.4%† **Sodium tetradecyl sulfate, 0.1%–0.25%** **Polidocanol, 0.1%–0.2%**	**0.2–0.5 mL**
Reticular veins (2–4 mm, subcutaneous blue veins)	Hypertonic saline, 18.7%–23.4%† **Sodium tetradecyl sulfate, 0.33%–0.5%** **Polidocanol, 0.1%–0.2% (up to 3 mm)**	0.5 mL (may increase to 1 mL if filling of reticular vein is observed)
Nonsaphenous varicose veins (3–8 mm)	Hypertonic saline, 18.7%–23.4% **Sodium tetradecyl sulfate, 0.5%–1.0%**	0.5 mL (may increase to 1 mL per injection site in large-capacity vein)
Saphenous varicose trunks (usually >5 mm)	Hypertonic saline, 18.7%–23.4% **Sodium tetradecyl sulfate, 1.0%**	0.5 mL (low-volume injection critical at high concentrations)

*Solutions in bold approved by the Food and Drug Administration.
†Many use standard 18.7% for all these indications.

Sclerotherapy Treatment Note

Name: _____   Birthdate: _____ .
Referring physician: _____   Date: _____
Chief Complaint: Sclerotherapy injection

S: The patient has thought over what we have discussed on the last visit and has read over multiple patient education materials supplied. He/she has elected to go ahead and have the sclerotherapy performed today. We explained again the nature of the complications: hyperpigmentation, matting, recurrence, slight ulceration, phlebitis, and blebs. He/she understands these and has elected to go ahead and have the injections done. There were no further questions and subsequently we proceeded.

O: Venous sclerotherapy

Areas: _____
Sclerosant: _____
Amount: _____ mL
Number of complexes injected: _____
Complications: None or _____

Procedure Note: The patient was once again examined in the supine position. The complexes of veins that were to be injected were noted. These areas were all wiped with Zephiran. Individual 1-mL syringes were used with 30-gauge needles. Each syringe was used no more than 3 to 4 times and no more than 0.5 mL of the solution was injected per vein site. In the majority of cases the vein was cannulated but in a few areas there was minimal extravasation of the sclerosant. After injection, a rolled 4 × 4 was immediately placed over the area and secured with paper tape. Upon completion of injection of the various veins, the Sigvaris/MediUSA/Jobst pantyhose/ thigh high/above the knee support stockings, which were measured for the patient, were used to hold the pressure dressings in place. They were of the 20/30 gradient type. The patient tolerated this well and was discharged home.

Changes to routine: _____

Impression:
1. _____
2. _____

P: The patient will wear the stockings for at least __ days and __ nights without removing them. Cool baths can then soak off the tape making it easier to remove the pressure dressings. He/she is to wear the support hose for at least 4 weeks during the day but may remove them at night. After injection, he/she is to walk at least 30 minutes. Hot baths are to be avoided for at least 2 weeks. It is best to wear some type of support hose for the rest of his/her life since venous disease is an ongoing problem and the source of the problem is not resolved by the injections. It may be necessary to come back every 1–2 years to have "touch-ups" on new or recurrent veins. There may be some pigmentation from the veins. The patient should call should there be any significant problems. Follow-up in _____ weeks for a recheck and for any possible further injections.

Other: _____
cc: _____   _____   _____
                                          Physician signature   Date

Fig. 78.10 Sample sclerotherapy treatment note. (Courtesy The National Procedures Institute, Midland, MI.)

Follow-up Sclerotherapy

Patient :_____ DOB: _____ Date: _____
Initial evaluation: _____ Referring physician: _____
PPG: _____ Sclerosant:

Working diagnosis: Support hose/Ace wrap/other:

Date	Subjective/Examination	Treatment	Impression	Plan

Fig. 78.11 Sample flow sheet for follow-up sclerotherapy appointments. (Courtesy The National Procedures Institute, Midland, MI.)

- Sclerotherapy should be viewed as a semicosmetic procedure, and the patient's expectations must be carefully considered.
- A careful preinjection discussion of risks must occur so that patients are fully aware of the protracted and tedious nature of sclerotherapy, as well as the potential complications.
- The effect of gravity and incompetent venous valves must always be remembered. Varicose veins and spider veins tend to recur. The wearing of compression stockings in the immediate postinjection period is mandatory. Compression stockings worn on a long-term basis will significantly reduce recurrence.
- Meticulous technique is essential in sclerotherapy.
  - The clinician must be sure that the needle is in the vein.
  - The solution should be injected slowly.
  - A maximum of 0.5 mL of solution should be used per injection and large bolus injections should be avoided.
  - The clinician should watch the needle tip and stop injecting if there is any extravasation.
- The larger vessels should be injected first.
- The clinician should begin injections proximally and work down the leg. If injections are started distally, the proximal vessels often go into spasm and become very difficult to inject.
- Telangiectases will be visible when the patient lies down, but varicosities may disappear. It helps to mark them with a marking pen while the patient is standing. Some clinicians recommend Doppler ultrasound guidance for injection if the varicosity is not palpable when the patient is supine.
- The clinician should not attempt to withdraw blood before injecting telangiectases; however, it is essential to withdraw blood before injecting larger vessels to be sure that the needle is in the lumen.
- If a wheal is seen, the clinician should stop injecting immediately. The magnification loupes help to identify this early in the procedure. If recognized early and the injection is stopped, the small blebs that occur generally do not lead to any tissue necrosis. Older texts recommend diluting the area with saline for extravasation, but this is not needed with these small amounts.

NOTE: With careful and precise technique, the majority of small telangiectatic (i.e., spider) veins can be eliminated. Patient satisfaction with the procedure is high.

COMPRESSION

The amount and duration of compression used with sclerotherapy remain somewhat controversial. Initially, Irish sclerotherapists who were treating large, bulging varicose veins used 6 weeks of continuous compression, a regimen that was quite difficult for the patient to follow. Later studies suggested that 3 weeks of compression for large veins was adequate. Whether compression should be used for 24 hours a day or only while the patient is standing is still an unsettled issue.

When spider veins are being injected, elastic compression bandages (4 in wide) can be used for the first 24 hours. The patient then removes the elastic bandage and the underlying dressings and wears lightweight, measured compression pantyhose (15 mm Hg gradient hose). Many therapists use 20 to 30 mm Hg gradient hose or even 30 to 40 mm Hg gradient hose. The patient is asked to wear the hose during the course of treatment whenever he or she is out of bed. If the patient has sclerotherapy appointments every 2 to 3 weeks, for example, and requires three visits, he or she will wear the stockings for 9 or 10 weeks. After the last treatment, the clinician can suggest that the patient wear the stockings while out of bed for at least 10 more days (preferably for 3 weeks). A recent review confirmed that wearing support hose continuously for 3 days and then while ambulatory for 3 more weeks markedly reduced complications and recurrence. The package insert for polidocanol recommends compression for 2 to 3 days for spider veins and for 5 to 7 days for reticular veins.

When larger veins are injected, 30- to 40-mm Hg gradient compression hose are recommended. The type of stocking depends on the areas being injected. If the thighs and both lower limbs are involved, pantyhose are best. Otherwise a full-length stocking, thigh-high stocking, or calf-high stocking can be used if it compresses the areas that were injected. The clinician can prescribe the stocking at the time of the patient's initial visit and the patient can then bring it to the first therapeutic session. Many of the stocking companies are quite good in supplying clinicians' offices with stockings and providing prompt, next-day delivery service. Ancillary personnel can learn to measure the patient for ready-made or custom stockings. The patient may then receive the stockings from the clinician's office.

It is recommended that patients wear lightweight compression pantyhose as much as possible on an indefinite basis to diminish the recurrence of varicose veins or the development of new ones; however, many patients are resistant to such a regimen. Compression stockings are also used in the management of patients with postthrombotic syndrome, healed venous ulcers, lymphedema, and other problems. Although patients can purchase cheaper over-the-counter hose, these generally provide only uniform compression and not a gradient of more to less pressure as the hose goes up the leg.

COMPLICATIONS

- *Bruising*. Patients must understand that they will look worse before they look better. It may take 4 to 8 weeks before the postsclerotherapy changes have resolved.
- *Hemosiderin staining (hyperpigmentation)*. This occurs transiently in almost every case. It is considered a complication when it lasts for more than several weeks. In about 5% to 10% of patients, it can take up to 1 year to diminish. The discoloration follows the outline of the previously injected vein and can also be seen after stripping or phlebectomy. The larger the vein, the more likely it will occur, especially if compression hose are not worn long enough. Unfortunately, in spite of trying many bleaching creams, little can be done to hasten resolution. If clots are evident, their removal lessens the duration of pigmentation. Prevention (with the use of compression hose) is the key.

- *Matting (neoangiogenesis)*. This is the development of tiny vessels at or near the site of previous injection and occurs in 3% to 10% of patients. It may result from an injection under too high a pressure (causing rupture of the vessel) or because either the volume of the sclerosing solution was too large or the solution was too strong. Matting probably develops as part of the inflammatory response due to these errors in technique. However, even with excellent technique, matting may occur. It may disappear in a few months. If it does not, the clinician should make a very careful search for a reticular vein leading into the area and try to obliterate it. Sometimes the matting itself can be injected or treated with light therapy, such as PhotoDerm or laser. If reinjection is done, the clinician should use a low concentration of sclerosants and inject slowly.
- *Skin slough with ulceration*. Usually this is related to extravasation of the solution. It may occur because of improper placement of the needle, rupture of the vein, having only part of the needle in the lumen, or injection of an arteriole. A tiny arteriole may also connect to a vein. In these cases, closure of the arteriole can cause a skin infarct. Ulcerations can even occur with a perfectly performed injection when the solution erodes through the wall of the vein into unhealthy skin. The ulceration often takes 4 to 8 weeks to resolve.
- *Arterial injection*. This is a dreaded complication. It will result in a large slough and even limb loss if a large artery it is injected. It is more likely to occur around the ankle, especially in the area of the posterior tibial artery.
- *Syncope*. This is more common if injections are done with the patient standing. At times, standing is necessary when butterfly needles are being inserted; following insertion, have the patient assume a recumbent position for the injection of large veins.
- *Allergic reaction*. This will not occur with hypertonic saline, and it occurs extremely rarely with sodium tetradecyl sulfate (approximately 0.3%). When it does occur, it is usually a mild response, although anaphylaxis has been reported. Necessary equipment to treat this problem—such as an Ambu-bag, artificial airways, epinephrine for injection, steroid for injection, and an injectable anticonvulsant—should be available (see Chapter 212, Anaphylaxis). Pretreatment of allergic patients with 50 mg of diphenhydramine (Benadryl) will obviate this problem.
- *Superficial thrombophlebitis*. Injection of sclerosant creates a chemical thrombophlebitis that is controlled and affects only the treated area. However, sometimes the solution can travel proximally or distally and create an area of thrombus within the veins. The area overlying this often becomes red and tender. In most cases, careful technique using only a small amount of solution (0.5 to 1 mL) will prevent this outcome. It is more likely to occur when larger veins are injected. When it does occur, the patient must be reassured that nothing serious has happened. Treatment consists of compression and an anti-inflammatory drug (e.g., ibuprofen).
- *Thrombus formation*. Clots can form in small veins or especially in the larger ones. They can be aspirated with a needle or incised and drained. Usually, for the larger ones, a small amount of lidocaine is injected, then a No. 11 blade is used to open the skin over the area. Pressure will expel the clot. No suture is needed. Thrombi are more common when larger veins are injected and if compression is not optimal postinjection. If a clot has been present for more than 4 weeks, it often organizes and then is difficult to remove.
- *Postinjection itching and pain*. Patients often complain of a transient itching after injection; some phlebologists apply steroid cream immediately after injection, but this is not necessary. The sites of injections may become painful. Over-the-counter pain medication, including nonsteroidal antiinflammatory drugs (NSAIDs), is adequate to control this and does not interfere with the effectiveness of treatment. Pain during the injection is minimal and well tolerated.

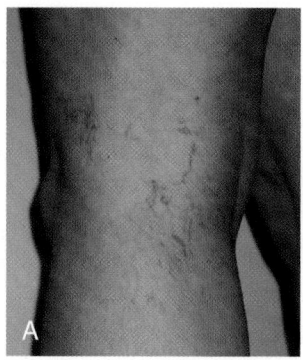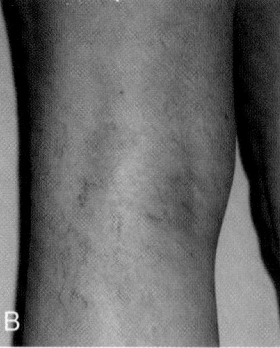

Fig. 78.12 Telangiectasia treatment with hypertonic saline. (A) Administration of treatment. (B) Appearance 2 months after procedure.

- *DVT and pulmonary emboli.* Fortunately this is a rare complication. It is most likely to occur if too much solution is used and it gets into the deep system. Patients who have had a prior venous thromboembolic event or who have an underlying thrombophilia are more likely to have this problem. Birth control pills and estrogen may slightly increase the tendency to develop this complication, but it is rare and their use does not contraindicate sclerotherapy. DVT may be reduced or eliminated by having the patient walk for 20 to 30 minutes after the injection of large veins to avoid pooling in the deep venous system.

POSTPROCEDURE PATIENT EDUCATION

Patients are asked to walk immediately after a session of sclerotherapy. Some therapists recommend 30 minutes, but even 15 to 20 minutes seems to be enough. Walking diffuses the solution that may have gone into the deep system and, more important, increases circulating fibrinolysins. (See the sample patient education form available at www.expertconsult.com.)

The same area should not be injected again for 3 weeks (Fig. 78.12). The patient can return at weekly intervals for treatment of alternate sites until treatment is complete. Patients should be able to resume normal activities, including high-impact aerobics and jogging, 24 hours after injections for spider veins; however, some therapists would further restrict patients for 1 week. No good prospective studies indicate the effect of robust activity on sclerotherapy.

CONCLUSION

Sclerotherapy, when practiced properly, is a highly effective means of treating small to medium-sized varicose veins and telangiectases. Many therapists treat even large varicosities in this manner. Laser and other forms of light therapy are not as efficient and effective in most instances. At best they are useful for treating veins 3 mm in diameter or smaller. Equipment and methods may improve the results of light therapy, but sclerotherapy remains the gold standard for treating such veins. Careful workup and management of patients, with special attention to proper technique, should provide good to excellent results in more than 90% of cases.

PATIENT EDUCATION GUIDES

See patient education and consent forms available at www.expertconsult.com.

CPT/BILLING CODES

Injections for telangiectasia, even if symptomatic, are rarely covered by insurance. Coverage for varicosities is quite variable. It is often necessary to document that conservative therapy (e.g., use of compression stockings) has failed. Frequently preapproval and photographs will be required.

Most sclerotherapists do not deal with insurance companies and ask the patient to pay at the time of service. Some will charge by the number of injections and others by the amount of solution used; still others will inject for a certain time period (15 to 30 minutes). There are no routine standards.

10140	I&D, hematoma
10160	Puncture aspiration, hematoma
36468	Single or multiple injections, sclerosing solutions; spider veins (telangiectasia), limb or trunk
36469	Face (see caution in the "Indications" section)
36470	Injection of sclerosing solution, single varicose vein
36471	Injection of multiple varicose veins, same leg
-50	Modifier for bilateral procedure
93965	Impedance plethysmography
93970	Duplex scan

ICD-10-CM DIAGNOSTIC CODES

I78.0	Spider vein/telangiectasia
I78.8	Capillary vein
I83.10	Varicosity with inflammation
I87.2	Stasis dermatitis
I83.209	Varicosity with ulceration
I83.90	Varicose vein, leg
I89.0	Lymphedema
I87.009	Postphlebitic syndrome
I87.2	Chronic venous insufficiency
L81.9	Dyschromia of skin (hyperpigmentation)
M79.609	Pain in leg
M79.89	Swelling in leg
R20.3	Burning, hyperesthesia
R60.9	Edema
S70.10XX	Hematoma, lower extremity

Acknowledgment

The editors recognize the contributions of Stanley A. Hirsch, MD, and John L. Pfenninger, MD, to this chapter in a previous edition of this text.

SUPPLIERS

(See contact information available at www.expertconsult.com.)

Headlamp and ocular loupes
Luxtec
Welch Allyn
Hypertonic saline
Delasco
Patient education materials
American Academy of Dermatology Association
Contemporary Health Communications
MJD Patient Communications: www.mjdpc.com
Polidocanol
Mertz North America
Pharmacy Specialists for compounding (Sam Pratt, RPh)
Sodium tetradecyl sulfate
Mylan Pharmaceuticals
Support hose
BSN-Jobst Institute, Inc.
MediUSA
Sigvaris

Syringes and needles
Air-Tite Products Company

Venous noninvasive diagnostic equipment (e.g., PPG, Doppler) and assistance with all sclerotherapy supplies
Wagner Medical (Sam Wagner) (NOTE: This is a superb resource.)

RECOMMENDED READING

Almeida JI, Boatright C. Injection treatment of lower extremity varicose veins. In: Stanley JC, Veith FJ, Wakefield TW, eds. *Current Therapy in Vascular and Endovascular Surgery*. 5th ed. Philadelphia: Elsevier Saunders; 2014:911–913.

Duffy DM. Sclerotherapy. In: Dover JS, ed. *Procedures in Cosmetic Dermatology Series: Treatment of Leg Veins*. 2nd ed. Philadelphia: Elsevier Saunders; 2011:65–94.

Conrad P, Malouf GM, Stacey MC. The Australian polidocanol (Aethoxysklerol) study: results at 2 years. *Dermatol Surg*. 1995;21:334–336.

Goldman MP, Beaudoing D, Marley W, et al. Compression in the treatment of leg telangiectasia: a preliminary report. *J Dermatol Surg Oncol*. 1990;16:322–325.

Goldman MP, Bergan JJ, eds. *Ambulatory Treatment of Venous Disease*. St. Louis: Mosby; 1996.

Goldman MP, Bergan JB, Guex JJ. *Sclerotherapy: treatment of varicose and telangiectatic leg veins*. 4th ed. London: Elsevier Mosby; 2006 (NOTE: This is the "bible" and a must for anyone performing sclerotherapy.).

Goldman MP, Sadick NS, Weiss RA. Cutaneous necrosis, telangiectatic matting, and hyperpigmentation following sclerotherapy: etiology, prevention, and treatment. *Dermatol Surg*. 1995;21:19–29.

Rabe E, Breu FX, Pannier F. Sclerotherapy of varicose veins. In: Robinson JK, Hanke DW, Siegel DM, Fratila A, eds. *Surgery of the Skin: Procedural Dermatology*. 3rd ed. Philadelphia: Elsevier Mosby; 2015:581–587.

Goldman MP, Weiss RA, Brody HJ, et al. Treatment of facial telangiectasia with sclerotherapy, laser surgery, and/or electrodesiccation: a review. *J Dermatol Surg Oncol*. 1993;19:899–906.

Green D. Sclerotherapy for varicose and telangiectatic veins. *Am Fam Physician*. 1992;46:827–837.

Kanter AH. The effect of sclerotherapy on restless legs syndrome. *Dermatol Surg*. 1995;21:328–332.

Pfeifer JR, Hawtof GD. Injection sclerotherapy and CO$_2$ laser sclerotherapy in the ablation of cutaneous spider veins of the lower extremity. *Phlebology*. 1989;4:231.

Sadick NS. *Manual of Sclerotherapy*. Philadelphia: Lippincott Williams & Wilkins; 2000 (NOTE: This source is superb, concise, thorough, and practical.).

Tretbar LL. Injection sclerotherapy for spider telangiectasias: a 20-year experience with sodium tetradecyl sulfate. *J Dermatol Surg Oncol*. 1989;15:223–225.

Hsu JTS. Leg vein management. In: Kaminer MS, Arndt KA, Dover JS, eds. *Atlas of Cosmetic Surgery*. 2nd ed. Philadelphia: Elsevier; 2009:455–481.

Weiss RA, Sadick NS, Goldman MP, Weiss MA. Post-sclerotherapy compression: controlled comparative study of duration of compression and its effect on clinical outcome. *Dermatol Surg*. 1999;25:105–108.

CHAPTER 79

AMBULATORY PHLEBECTOMY

Karl S. Hubach

The treatment of venous disease has undergone considerable change in the past 2 decades. Ambulatory phlebectomy (AP) remains popular as a surgical means of removing large varicose veins. This chapter introduces the basic techniques and ideas behind AP, which is an in-office surgical technique used to remove varicose veins through multiple small incisions. It is performed using only a local anesthetic and yet provides excellent cosmetic and functional results. When the compression bandage is in place, ambulation is allowed immediately after the procedure. Because the highest (most proximal) point of reflux in the venous system must be corrected for AP to remain successful, AP is frequently done in conjunction with another procedure such as junctional ligation, ultrasound-guided sclerotherapy, an ablation procedure with laser or radiofrequency, or venous stripping (see Chapter 80, Endovenous Vein Ablation, and Chapter 78, Sclerotherapy). Clinical practice guidelines by the European Society of Vascular Surgery (2015) state that phlebectomy can be considered either as an adjunctive treatment in association with endovenous ablation, or stripping of the main refluxing truncal vein, or as the sole treatment of varicose veins. AP may be preferred for large tortuous varicosities because radiofrequency catheters cannot easily be passed along a tortuous vein. Foam sclerotherapy is another option for large tortuous varicosities, especially those with thinner walls; AP may be preferred in those with thicker walls. In a recent trial (Lane et al., 2015), those receiving AP at the same time as ablation had improved clinical outcomes, early improvements in quality of life, and less need for further procedures.

Benefits of AP include the following:

- It is performed in an outpatient setting.
- It is a convenient, safe, and cost-effective treatment for varicose veins.
- The patient is able to walk out of the office following the procedure with little to no change in his or her level of activity.
- The rate of complications is extremely low.
- The procedure can be performed without hospitalization or general anesthesia and it allows for a return to normal activity; thus the expense to the patient and the health care system is markedly reduced.

For these reasons, AP can serve as an excellent addition to the total care and treatment of varicose veins and venous disease.

INDICATIONS

- To remove veins of most sizes for symptomatic or cosmetic reasons
- Primarily used for the removal of symptomatic, visible varicose veins of the lower extremities. The pudendal veins of the groin may also respond well to this treatment.

CONTRAINDICATIONS

Absolute

- Known metastatic carcinoma
- Allergy to the local anesthetic
- Hypercoagulable state
- Severe arterial occlusive diseases (see Chapter 77, Noninvasive Venous and Arterial Studies of the Lower Extremities)
- Hemodynamically important secondary varicosities
- Poor general health
- Incapacitated elderly patient
- CREST syndrome (calcinosis, Raynaud phenomenon, esophageal involvement, sclerodactyly, and telangiectasia) involving the lower extremities

Relative

- Reflux at the saphenofemoral or saphenopopliteal junction (these should be treated with ablation prior to the procedure)
- Superficial thrombophlebitis
- Bacteremia and certain other blood-borne infectious diseases
- Pregnancy
- Propensity to keloid formation
- Significant fibrosis of the vein
- Acute deep venous thrombosis
- Overlying infection or significant skin compromise
- Deep venous insufficiency

EQUIPMENT AND SUPPLIES

- Camera
- Surgical marking pen
- Vein transilluminator (e.g., Veinlite)
- 10-mL syringe with a 25-gauge, 1.5-inch needle
- 0.5% lidocaine with epinephrine
- Povidone-iodine or chlorhexidine prep
- Sterile draping
- Sterile gloves and attire for the clinician to observe universal blood and body fluid precautions
- Set of phlebectomy hooks (Muller, Oesch, or Ramelet)
- Curved iris scissors
- Minimum of six curved micro mosquito forceps
- Four towel clamps
- Needle holder (to hold the blade at proper location to produce desired depth and length of incision [see Fig. 79.5])
- No. 11 scalpel blade (alternative, 18-gauge needle)
- 3-0 absorbable suture (e.g., Vicryl)
- 4 × 4 gauze
- Steri-Strips (plain or saturated with povidone-iodine)
- Benzoin spray
- 4-in web roll (as an absorbent wrap over the 4 × 4 dressing)

- Nonstretch compression dressing (e.g., Comprilan, Coban)
- Class II thigh-high compression stockings
- Shower bag to cover dressing when needed
- Written postoperative instructions
- Consent form

ANATOMY AND PATHOLOGY OF VENOUS DISEASE

Before proper treatment options can be determined, the clinician must have a clear understanding of the patient's underlying anatomy and disease process. The clinician should also have undertaken some advanced study of the overall anatomy and diseases of the lower extremity venous system, and should have obtained some specialized training before performing AP. This section serves only as a brief overview and is far from comprehensive. (Also see Chapter 77, Noninvasive Venous and Arterial Studies of the Lower Extremities, Chapter 78, Sclerotherapy and Chapter 80, Endovenous Vein Ablation.)

There are primarily three venous systems in the leg: the superficial venous system lies above the deep fascia, the deep venous system lies under the deep fascia, and the perforator vein system connects the superficial and deep systems (Fig. 79.1). The muscular pump of the leg produces a distal-to-proximal compression to facilitate blood flow back to the cardiopulmonary system. If the valvular system is intact, normal veins allow only unidirectional flow.

The superficial venous system consists of a network of veins that feed two primary vessels, the great and the short saphenous veins. The great saphenous vein terminates at the saphenofemoral junction after it has coursed proximally from the dorsal arch vein of the foot and medially along the medial leg and thigh. The short saphenous vein also begins with the dorsal arch vein but travels behind the lateral malleolus and along the lateral leg. After reaching the popliteal fossa, the short saphenous vein empties into the popliteal vein of the deep venous system at the saphenopopliteal junction. It should be noted that the location of this junction is variable (see Chapter 78, Sclerotherapy, Figs. 78.2 and 78.3).

Perforator veins allow blood to flow from the superficial to the deep system. By doing so, more than 90% of blood flows through the deep venous system on its way back to the heart. The importance of competent venous valves for enforcing unidirectional flow in such a low-pressure system is often unappreciated. Once venous reflux occurs through incompetent valves, normal blood flow is altered, intraluminal pressure increases, and the disease process worsens. The increased flow and pressure to the superficial system leads to dilated vessels and the development of varicosities. As chronic venous insufficiency develops, approximately one-third of patients also develop problems with superficial thrombophlebitis, dermatitis, lipodermatosclerosis, or ulceration.

It is also important for the phlebologist to have a clear understanding of the sensory nerves and lymphatic vessels of the leg. Both of these systems lie close to the superficial veins. Consequently complications can develop from damage to these structures. The most frequent nerve damage occurs to the saphenous or sural nerve or their branches. The saphenous nerve is most vulnerable at the location where it lies along the distal portion of the great saphenous vein near the dorsal foot veins. The sural nerve is vulnerable along its entire course as it runs beside the short saphenous vein (Fig. 79.2). Damage to the lymphatic vessels most commonly occurs below the medial knee in the anterior tibial region near the Boyd perforators.

PREPROCEDURE PATIENT PREPARATION

An accurate patient history and physical examination will allow the clinician to formulate a better diagnosis and treatment plan—one that is best suited to the patient's needs. The examination must also exclude any potential contraindications. Additional studies—such as an electrocardiogram, complete blood count, bleeding studies, and serum electrolytes, glucose, urea nitrogen, and creatinine levels—may be required. Fig. 79.3 shows a general history form with a focus on venous-related symptoms or diseases.

The venous examination should result in an accurate map of the veins of the lower extremities. The clinician should also note if chronic venous changes are present. Dermatitis, edema, corona phlebectatica, and lipodermatosclerosis or ulcerative disease may raise a suspicion for deep venous disease or long-standing chronic venous insufficiency.

The handheld Doppler is often referred to as the "phlebologist's stethoscope." It is an invaluable instrument for examining the patient for venous reflux. The Doppler examination is performed with the patient in the standing position, bearing his or her weight on the opposite leg. The Doppler probe is placed at a 45-degree

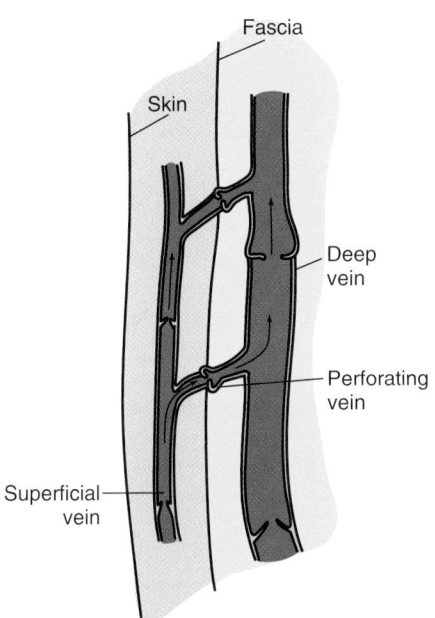

Fig. 79.1 Venous compartments of the leg consist of the superficial venous system, the deep venous system, and the perforator vein system.

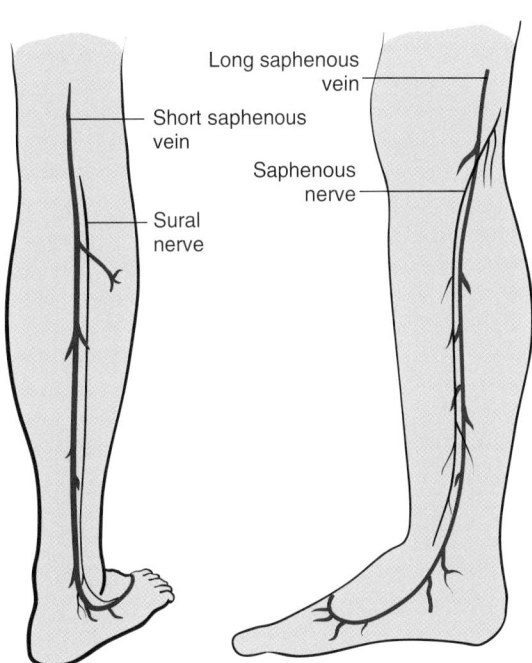

Fig. 79.2 Important sensory nerves and their location relative to vessels of the leg.

Name:_____ Date:_____ Age:_____ Ht:_____ Wt:_____
When did you first notice your enlarged or discolored veins? _____
Which leg bothers you the most?   Right_____ Left_____   Both_____
What symptoms are you having?

1. Sharp pain   Yes____ No____   8. Burning   Yes____ No____
2. Dull pain   Yes____ No____   9. Heaviness   Yes____ No____
3. Aching legs   Yes____ No____   10. Cramps   Yes____ No____
4. Swelling   Yes____ No____   11. Throbbing   Yes____ No____
5. Itching   Yes____ No____   12. Restless legs Yes____ No____
6. Leg ulcers   Yes____ No____   13. Appearance   Yes____ No____
7. Tiredness   Yes____ No____

Have you ever had any of the following:

1. Phlebitis (clots in legs)   Yes____ No____   When_____
2. Deep vein thrombosis   Yes____ No____   When_____
3. Pulmonary embolus (blood clot in lung) Yes____ No____   When_____
4. Leg or ankle ulcers   Yes____ No____   When_____
5. Painful varicose veins   Yes____ No____   When_____
6. Venogram (vein x-rays)   Yes____ No____   When_____

Have you ever been pregnant?   Yes____ No____
How many times?   _____
How many deliveries?   _____
Are you currently pregnant?   Yes____ No____

List all medicines you are currently taking (including aspirin, if applicable):

_____ _____ _____

List any hormones you are taking:

_____ _____ _____

Birth control pills: Yes____ No____

List all allergies:

_____ _____ _____
_____ _____ _____

Have you ever had any adverse reactions with scars?   Yes____ No____

Have you ever had any of the following:

AIDS or HIV positive   Yes____ No____
Diabetes   Yes____ No____
Migraine headaches   Yes____ No____
High blood pressure   Yes____ No____
Heart disease   Yes____ No____
Jaundice or hepatitis   Yes____ No____
Cancer   Yes____ No____
Recent weight change   Yes____ No____
Major injury or surgery in your legs   Yes____ No____
Leg pain at night   Yes____ No____
Leg pain caused by walking   Yes____ No____
Leg pain caused by standing   Yes____ No____
Clotting or blood problems   Yes____ No____

Fig. 79.3 Sample general patient history form with a focus on venous-related history.

Have you ever used prescription compression hose for your legs?   Yes_____ No_____ When_____

Have you ever had sclerotherapy before?   Yes_____ No_____ When_____

Have you ever smoked?   Yes_____ No_____ Packs/day_____ Number of years_____

Are you currently smoking?   Yes_____ No_____ Packs/day x years_____

List any and all family members with vein problems:

_____   _____   _____

_____   _____   _____

Whom can we thank for referring you to our office?_____

FOR DOCTOR USE ONLY

Movie seen: Yes_____ No_____

Telangiectasias: Right_____ Left_____ Severity_____

Reticulars: Right_____ Left_____ Severity_____

Varicose veins: Right_____ Left_____ Severity_____

V. V.:   Size:_____ mm

SFJ reflux: Right_____ Left_____

SPJ reflux: Right_____ Left_____

PPG: Yes_____ No_____ Right_____ Left_____ Ven_____ Art_____ Both_____

U.S.:   Yes_____ No_____ Right_____ Left_____

Appt. for sclero: Yes_____ No_____

Fig. 79.3, cont'd.

angle over the vein to be examined. Compression of the calf muscle distal to the probe induces blood flow in a proximal direction. In a diseased vein, reflux is heard as a loud rumbling sound after the sudden release of compression of the calf muscle. A normal vein has only a monophasic (unidirectional) signal. By performing this simple maneuver, the examiner can locate the highest, most proximal source of reflux. (See also Chapter 77, Noninvasive Venous and Arterial Studies of the Lower Extremities.)

Duplex ultrasound provides information useful for producing an even better venous map. The examination is typically performed with a 7.5- to 13-MHz linear probe and the patient in a standing position. Areas of venous dilation or large perforators can reveal sources of proximal venous reflux. The deep venous system can also be visualized to assess for thrombus or incompetence. Areas of reflux in the superficial system, which may be difficult to visualize or palpate, can be studied easily. Duplex

scanning also provides a hard copy (image and often a blood velocity graph) for documentation of the venous disease before and after treatment.

Many phlebologists evaluate the leg function with an additional test, photoplethysmography. This is most helpful to document normal or correctable deep venous function in those patients with evidence of stasis changes (see Chapter 78, Sclerotherapy).

Once a thorough understanding of the underlying disease process is obtained, an accurate treatment plan can be formulated. It needs to be emphasized that the highest, most proximal point of reflux must be corrected. This often requires a procedure in addition to AP. Ablation of the saphenous vein, ultrasound-guided sclerotherapy (often referred to as "chemical ablation"), or a partial stripping or ligation of the great or short saphenous vein may be needed in conjunction with AP. If the venous incompetence cannot be treated with these techniques or the clinician does not have

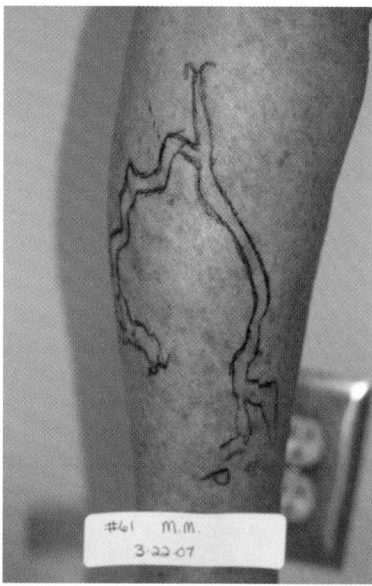

Fig. 79.4 Venous marking with surgical marking pen.

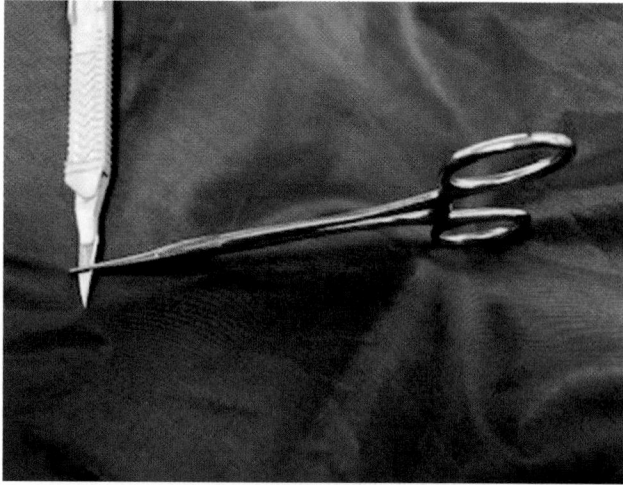

Fig. 79.5 No. 11 blade placed in needle holder in preparation for incision.

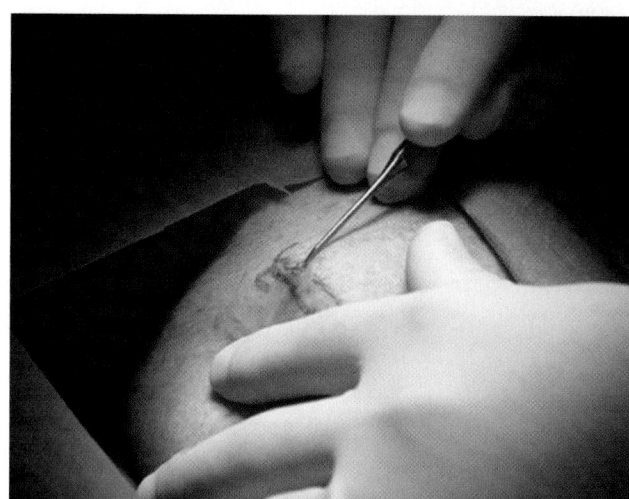

Fig. 79.6 Phlebectomy hook gently inserted through incision.

the training or skills to perform them, the clinician may choose to consult another surgeon. This consultation helps to ensure a lower recurrence rate and better relief of the symptoms from venous insufficiency. In addition, inexperienced clinicians should be very careful in the area of the popliteal fold, the dorsum of the foot, and the prepatellar and pretibial areas. These areas may be more susceptible to injury and they contain veins that can be more difficult to extract.

See the sample patient education form available at www.expert consult.com.

TECHNIQUE

1. On the night before surgery the patient should trim down the hair on his or her legs carefully and significantly, minimizing any nicking. Instead of shaving, patients (especially men) may prefer to use a product called Magic Hair Removal (a depilatory) or an electric shaver or trimmer.
2. Preoperative pictures are highly recommended.
3. Just before surgery, have the patient stand for venous marking with a surgical marking pen. Ensuring proper lighting in a warm room and having the patient stand for a period of time will maximize venous dilation and visibility. In turn, this will improve the clinician's ability to mark the veins. Some clinicians mark the most superficial and easily palpable portion of the vein with a crosshatch. A vein transilluminator (Veinlite) is helpful for ensuring accurate marking.
4. Once the visible veins have been marked, use a focused duplex examination to locate and mark the perforator veins (and any large branches along the vein) that are to be excised (Fig. 79.4).
5. Place the patient in 10 to 15 degrees of Trendelenburg to empty the veins during surgery. The foot can be propped on a pillow or cushion.
6. Prepare the area with a 5-minute povidone-iodine or chlorhexidine scrub and then apply sterile drapes to the area.
7. Inject 0.5% lidocaine with epinephrine on each side of the marked veins using a 25-gauge 1.5-inch needle.
    NOTE: Many clinicians use a tumescent technique, originally developed for use in liposuction surgery. Larger amounts of dilute local anesthetic (0.2% lidocaine with a 1:500,000 concentration of epinephrine) are instilled perivascularly with a 22-gauge spinal needle. These clinicians believe that instilling larger volumes

into the perivascular space provides additional local compression and further minimizes risk of bleeding after the procedure.
8. Starting proximally, make a small 2- to 3-mm vertical incision over or adjacent to the marked vein. A No. 11 scalpel blade or an 18-gauge needle may be used for the incision. A No. 11 blade can be held in a needle holder at the proper location to produce the desired depth and length of the incision (Fig. 79.5).
9. Gently insert a phlebectomy hook through the incision (Fig. 79.6). It may be necessary to break up adhesions and fibrous attachments to the vein before extraction by undermining the vein and surrounding skin and subcutaneous tissue with the stem of the phlebectomy hook. However, be careful not to damage any nearby structures such as nerves or lymphatics.
10. Hook the vein with a gentle rotation and retraction technique. When the vein is pulled through the incision, it will be identified by its distinguishing pearly white appearance (Fig. 79.7).
11. The vein is grasped with a set of fine curved mosquito hemostats. As the vein is exteriorized, the tension on the vein will produce a palpable cord under the skin. The next incision is made at the distal point of the palpable cord, or the next crosshatch. This distance may vary from 4 to 15 cm depending on the experience of the clinician, the size of the vein, the presence of perforators, or whether the patient has had prior sclerotherapy or phlebitis.

12. The most proximal end of the vein being excised is tied off with absorbable suture (e.g., 3-0 Vicryl). The author also chooses to tie off as many perforators as possible, and these are easily located and marked with duplex before surgery. Many phlebologists choose to simply tear the vein loose from the perforator and have an assistant apply constant pressure to the area for 5 to 10 minutes.

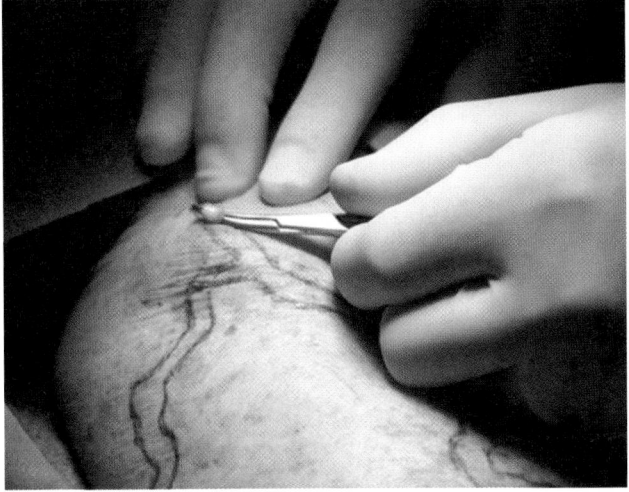

Fig. 79.7 Vein pulled through incision.

13. The vein is sequentially pulled through successive distal incisions until it is totally excised. When it is removed in pieces, these can be laid out along the course to ensure total removal of the vein (Fig. 79.8).

14. With extensive varicosities, the surgeon may choose to perform the AP in stages, separated by 7 to 14 days between each surgery. The procedure, when performed in stages, typically begins on the distal part of the limb. As the surgeon gains experience, it will take less time to remove the same length of vein. Several hours should be allowed for each surgery, and only one leg should be done at a time.

15. Clean the limb with sterile water and pat dry. Benzoin spray is used to increase adhesion of the Steri-Strips applied over the incisions.

16. Apply gauze or absorbent padding along the course of the excised vein.

17. Wrap the leg in a distal-to-proximal direction with a nonstretch compression bandage (e.g., Comprilan, Coban).

18. Place a thigh-high class II compression stocking over the dressing.

COMMON ERRORS

- Not making sure that the highest, most proximal point of reflux is corrected
- Administration of the anesthetic too deep into the tissue
- Making incisions too large, resulting in excessive scarring

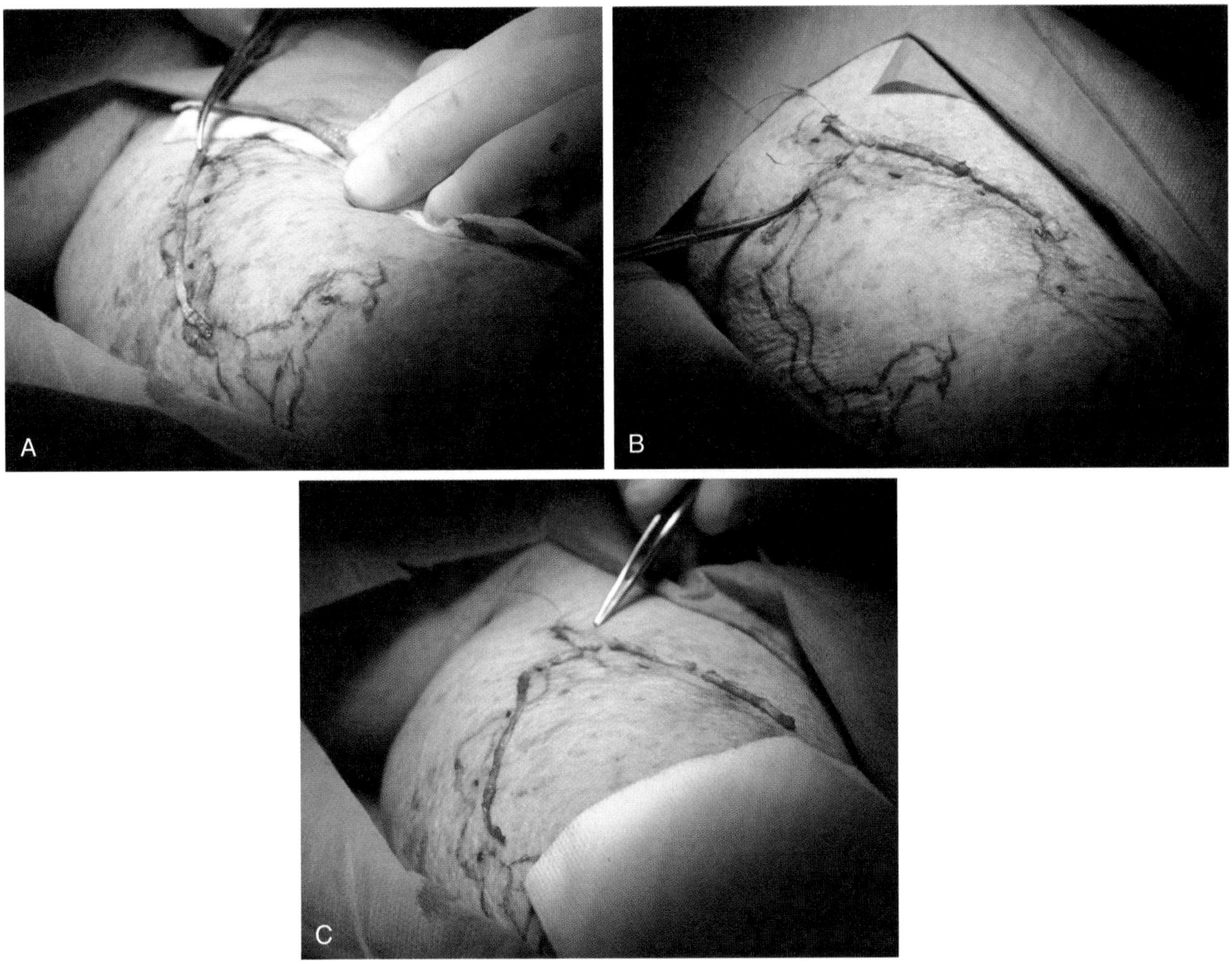

Fig. 79.8 (A to C) A vein sequentially pulled through successive distal incisions.

- Overzealous hook movement and pulling, resulting in superficial nerve or skin damage
- Poor approximation of incisions
- Not providing sufficient padding at pressure points or leaving creases under the compression dressing
- Not ensuring and stressing the importance of walking regularly after the procedure

COMPLICATIONS

Box 79.1 shows a list of complications seen in a review of the literature done by Ramelet (1997). The rate of transient, patient-perceived complications might be as high as 5% to 10%, including such things as skin blisters, hyperpigmentation, and contact dermatitis (Table 79.1). True complications that require professional attention or that have long-term sequelae arequite rare.

BOX 79.1 Complications of Ambulatory Phlebectomy

Cutaneous Complications
Skin blisters from dressing
Transient hyperpigmentation
Visible scars
Contact dermatitis
Infection
Keloid and hypertrophic scars
Tattooing with pen
Koebner phenomenon
Skin necrosis

Neurologic Complications
Postoperative pain
Paresthesia

Vascular Complications
Hematomas
Postoperative hemorrhage
Superficial phlebitis
Matting
Lymphatic pseudocyst
Lymphorrhea
Persistent edema
Deep venous thrombosis with potential pulmonary embolus

TABLE 79.1 Frequency of Complications of Ambulatory Phlebectomy

Rank	Type	No. of Events/ Phlebectomy	Percentage/ Phlebectomy
1	Blister formation	214	5.4%
2	Pigmentation (transitory)	183	4.6%
3	Telangiectasia matting	145	3.6%
4	Localized superficial phlebitis	110	2.8%
5	Temporary dysesthesia	15	0.4%
6	Lymphocele	6	0.2%
7	Extensive superficial phlebitis	5	0.1%
8	Delayed bleeding	4	0.1%
9	Hematoma	4	0.1%
10	Dimpling	3	0.07%
11	Skin necrosis	3	0.07%
12	Tattooing	3	0.07%
13	Wound infection	3	0.07%
14	Allergic reaction to wrappings	3	0.07%
15	Keloid	3	0.07%
16	Local anesthetic overload	2	0.05%
17	Deep venous thrombosis	1	0.02%
	Total	**707**	**17.79%**

Data from Olivencia JA. Complications of ambulatory phlebectomy: a review of 4000 consecutive cases. *Am J Cosmet Surg.* 2000;17:161–165.

Complications can be divided into cutaneous, vascular, and neurologic types. Most *cutaneous complications* can be avoided with the proper use and application of the postoperative dressing. The size and type of vessels operated on, the anatomic location of the surgery, and the individual patient's history of previous sclerotherapy, phlebitis, or lipodermatosclerosis will all affect the likelihood of a vascular complication. Many of the *vascular complications* are avoidable by applying adequate compression and stressing the importance of postoperative ambulation. *Neurologic complications* can occur from the local anesthetic, directly from the phlebectomy, or from the postoperative dressing. The most problematic nerve injury is damage to the sural nerve; this must be avoided by dealing carefully with the short saphenous vein. Damage to sensory nerves can often be avoided because the patient will usually complain of pain if the surgeon is too close to a nerve; this awareness allows the surgeon to avoid damaging or destroying a nerve. Excessive compression to the dorsal foot can induce a painful tarsal syndrome.

The primary care clinician does not require special training to handle the complications that occur with AP. Emphasis must be placed, however, on adequate training to perform AP and on proper understanding of the underlying pathophysiologic process.

POSTPROCEDURE MANAGEMENT AND PATIENT EDUCATION

Written and oral postoperative instructions should be provided to the patient (see the sample patient education form available at www.expertconsult.com). All patients should be encouraged to walk approximately half a mile immediately after surgery and then 1 to 3 miles per day for the next 2 weeks. They should start taking one aspirin daily for 2 weeks starting 12 to 16 hours after surgery. Strenuous workouts, heavy lifting, and standing for long periods of time should be avoided for 2 weeks. Over-the-counter ibuprofen should be sufficient to relieve any discomfort that may occur after surgery. The dressing should remain in place and be kept dry until the follow-up appointment 1 week later. At that time the dressing is removed and the incisions inspected. The compression stocking alone is worn during the day for an additional week. The Steri-Strips are removed 2 weeks after surgery, after which any further surgeries or required therapy can be scheduled.

PATIENT EDUCATION GUIDES

See the sample patient education and consent forms available at www.expertconsult.com.

CPT/BILLING CODES

37700 Ligation and division of great saphenous vein at saphenofemoral junction, or distal interruptions
37765 Stab phlebectomy of varicose veins, one extremity, 10 to 20 stab incisions
37766 Stab phlebectomy, more than 20 stab incisions
37799 Stab phlebectomy, less than 10 stab incisions. Also, use for any unlisted procedure, vascular surgery
37780 Ligation and division of the short saphenous vein at saphenopopliteal junction
37785 Ligation, division, and/or excision of varicose vein cluster(s), one leg

ICD-10-CM DIAGNOSTIC CODES

I83.891 Varicose veins of right lower extremity with other complications (inflammation)
I83.892 Varicose veins of left lower extremity with other complications (inflammation)

I83.893   Varicose veins of bilateral lower extremity with other complications (inflammation)
I83. 811   Varicose veins of the right lower extremity with pain
I83. 812   Varicose veins of the left lower extremity with pain
I83. 813   Varicose veins of the bilateral lower extremity with pain
I87.2   Venous (peripheral) insufficiency, chronic or unspecified

SUPPLIERS

(See contact information available at www.expertconsult.com.)

Sclerotherapy and phlebotomy instruments and equipment
Wagner Medical (excellent general resource)
Compression stockings
Beiersdorf-Jobst, Inc. (also manufactures Comprilan dressing)
Juzo (Julius Zorn), Inc.
Medi USA
Sigvaris
Venosan
Compression wrap
3M (Coban)
STD Pharmaceutical
Phlebectomy hooks
Aesculap
Venosan
Shower bag cover
Gill Podiatry Supply and Equipment

Acknowledgment

The editors recognize the contributions of Roger Murray, MD, to this chapter in a previous edition of this text.

OTHER RESOURCES

Phlebology Societies and Training Courses

American College of Phlebology: www.phlebology.org
The National Procedures Institute: www.npinstitute.com

RECOMMENDED READING

Brown JS. Stab-avulsion varicose veins. In: Brown JS, ed. *Minor Surgery: A Text and Atlas.* 4th ed. New York: Oxford University Press; 2000:372–377.

de Roos KP, Nieman FH, Neumann HA. Ambulatory phlebectomy versus compression sclerotherapy: results of a randomized controlled trial. *Dermatol Surg.* 2003;29:221–226.

Flynn JC. *Procedures in Phlebotomy.* 4th ed. Philadelphia: Saunders Elsevier; 2012.

Goldman MP, Weiss RA. Endovenous ablation techniques with ambulatory phlebectomy for varicose veins. In: Robinson JK, Hanke CW, Siegel DM, Sengelmann RD, eds. *Surgery of the Skin.* Philadelphia: Mosby; 2005:645–656.

Jones RH, Carek PJ. Management of varicose veins. *Am Fam Physician.* 2008;78(11):1289–1294.

Lane TR, Kelleher D, Shepherd AC, Franklin IJ, Davies AH. Ambulatory varicosity avulsion later or synchronized (AVULS): a randomized clinical trial. *Ann Surg.* 2015;261(4):654–661.

Olivencia JA. Maneuver to facilitate ambulatory phlebectomy. *Dermatol Surg.* 1996;22:654–655.

Ramelet A. Complications of ambulatory phlebectomy. *Dermatol Surg.* 1997;23:947–954.

Weiss R, Weiss M. Ambulatory phlebectomy compared to sclerotherapy for varicose and telangiectatic veins: indications and complications. *Adv Dermatol.* 1996;11:3–16.

Committee Writing, Wittens C, Davies AH, Baekgaard N, Broholm R, Cavezzi A, Chastanet S, et al. Editors' choice-management of chronic venous disease. *Eur Jrl Vasc Endovasc Surg.* 2015;49(6):678–737.

Hsu JTS. Leg vein management: In: Kaminer MS, Arndt KA, Dover JS, Rohrer TE, Zachary CB, eds. *Atlas of Cosmetic Surgery.* 2nd ed. Philadelphia: Elsevier; 2008.

CHAPTER 80

ENDOVENOUS VEIN ABLATION

Jerry Ninia

Primary venous insufficiency is characterized by the development of varicose veins of the lower extremities. The great saphenous vein (GSV) is the largest and longest vein of the superficial venous system, and reflux in the GSV is often associated with the development of large superficial varices. In addition to cosmetic issues and symptoms of leg pain and fatigue, varicose veins can give rise to ambulatory venous hypertension with its associated skin changes and ulcerations. In fact, up to 80% of leg ulcers are due to venous disease. If incompetence of the saphenofemoral junction (SFJ) or a perforator vein is detected, treatment is medically indicated. In addition, reflux in other veins such as the small saphenous vein (SSV), anterior accessory saphenous vein, and vein of Giacomini may contribute to the development of varicose veins. This chapter describes ultrasound-guided percutaneous techniques for treating patients with varicose veins who are ambulatory and whose sonographic findings include the documentation of reflux.

Knowledge of lower extremity duplex ultrasound is an absolute necessity for the performance of these procedures. The venous anatomy is described in Chapter 78, Sclerotherapy. Patients need to be evaluated before surgery with ultrasound mapping and marking, during surgery with guiding and checking, and after surgery for response to treatment. *Mapping* refers to diagramming the findings on the patient's chart. *Marking* pertains to outlining vein findings on the patient's skin. Intraoperative *guiding and checking* refers to proper performance of the procedure and proper instrumentation and application of tumescent anesthesia. Response to treatment is assessed at 1 week, 1 month, and longer intervals as needed to determine the effectiveness of the procedure.

ENDOVENOUS CHEMICAL ABLATION

Also see Chapter 78, Sclerotherapy, which discusses many of the concepts and the anatomy involved in treating venous diseases.

Commonly referred to as "ultrasound-guided sclerotherapy," *endovenous chemical ablation* (ECA) involves injecting a sclerosing solution, using ultrasound guidance, directly into the lumen of the vein being treated. Even if the vein has significant tortuosity, the sclerosant (liquid or foam) will distribute itself within the vein lumen. An example is the use of ECA in the treatment of patients with groin neovascularization—a phenomenon seen in patients who have previously undergone surgical vein stripping. As such, ECA is especially helpful in treating these patients with postsurgical recurrences and an anatomically variable SSV with its associated tortuous tributaries. Equipment needed is very similar to that used for basic injection–compression sclerotherapy, with the addition of a 7.5- to 15-MHz linear-array ultrasound transducer. Ultrasound provides real-time feedback to confirm intraluminal placement of the needle tip or catheter, intraluminal injection without extravasation, and attainment of the treatment end point (i.e., vasospasm; Fig. 80.1). Vasospasm is an indicator of the immediate efficacy of the foam injection; however, the final therapeutic effects of foam sclerotherapy should be evaluated clinically according to symptoms and follow-up duplex

ultrasound. Tumescent anesthesia is not required. Graduated class II (30 to 40 mm Hg) compression stockings need to be worn continuously for 24 to 36 hours, then during the daytime for 6 days postinjection.

The *direct needle injection* technique involves ultrasonic visualization of the vein in a longitudinal plane (Fig. 80.2). A 21- to 25-gauge, 1- to 1.5-inch needle is inserted obliquely into the lumen of the vessel with the bevel directed up. Slow aspiration is performed to verify correct needle placement. A small amount (1 to 2 mL) of sclerosant foam or liquid (1% to 3% sodium tetradecyl sulfate [STS]) is injected slowly; a "snowstorm" sonographic pattern is appreciated on injection (Fig. 80.3).

FOAM SCLEROTHERAPY

Although liquid sclerosants can be used, for larger veins the effect of sclerotherapy is enhanced by creating a sclerosant foam. Foam is created using the *Tessari technique* (Fig. 80.4). The Tessari technique involves using one syringe with liquid detergent sclerosant (e.g., STS 0.1% to 3%, polidocanol 1% to 2%, and others) and another syringe with air. The ratio of air to sclerosant is 4:1. The syringes are connected by a two- or three-way stopcock. By forcing the air and fluid back and forth numerous times, foam is created. The sclerosant is supposedly concentrated on the bubbles and thus has greater potency, leading to more efficacious treatment. The foam reconstitutes into liquid very quickly, within a matter of minutes, so it needs to be injected rather quickly. Although not mandatory, using rubber-free and silicone-free syringes (e.g., B. Braun Inkjet) prolongs the foam state. This technique is simple and economical and produces good-quality foam. Ultrasound imaging demonstrates more of a "snowstorm" pattern when foam is injected. Amounts and concentrations depend on the size and number of veins injected. Although foam can be used for telangiectases, complications may be more frequent and hence the technique is more commonly reserved for larger veins.

Whether foam or liquid is used, injections are administered with the patient supine. Injections can be administered starting 8 to 10 cm distal to the point of reflux, then proceeding from proximal to distal as previously injected segments undergo vasospasm. Alternatively, injections can be administered to the distal leg and progress proximally to the point of reflux. If 3% liquid STS is used, the maximum amount of solution during a treatment session is 10 mL. If foam is used, the volume limit is 10 mL of foam sclerosant as well, regardless of the concentration of the liquid detergent sclerosant used to create the foam (Breu and colleagues, 2008).

NEEDLE VERSUS CATHETER INFUSION

The syringe-and-needle technique is technically less difficult than the catheter infusion technique; however, it has a narrower margin of safety. This is due to the need for multiple injections and the potential for vein laceration and subsequent sclerosant extravasation.

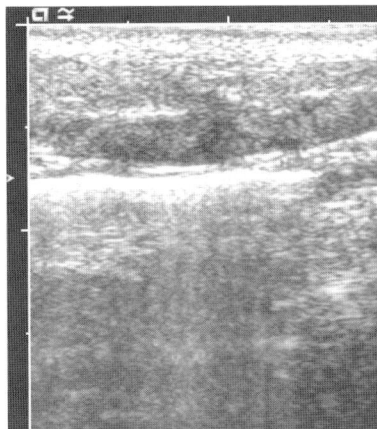

Fig. 80.1 Vasospasm end point. (Courtesy Nick Morrison, Scottsdale, AZ.)

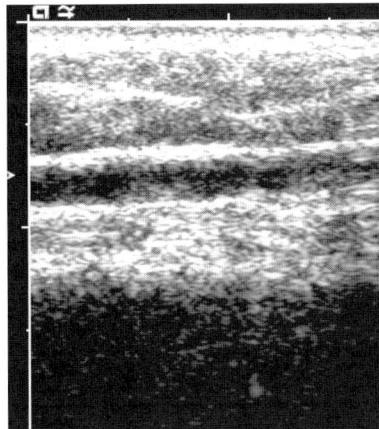

Fig. 80.2 Vein imaged longitudinally. (Courtesy Nick Morrison, Scottsdale, AZ.)

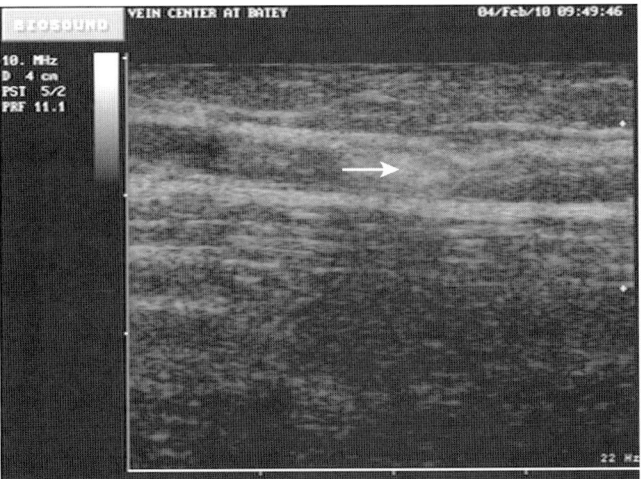

Fig. 80.3 "Snowstorm" pattern *(arrow)* after injection. (Courtesy John Mauriello, MD, Bradenton, FL.)

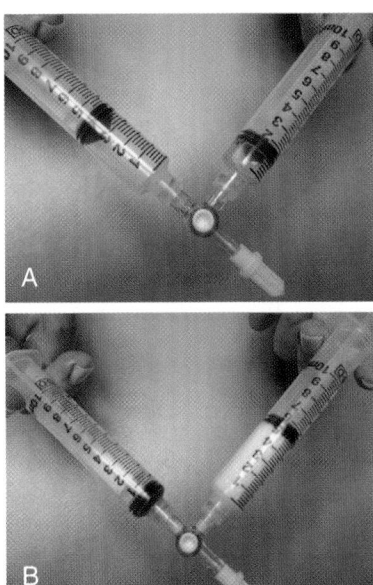

Fig. 80.4 Tessari technique. (A) A 4:1 ratio of air to liquid sclerosant. (B) Product after foam is created.

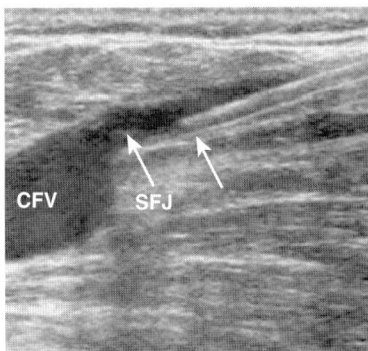

Fig. 80.5 Catheter tip *(arrow)* 1 cm below the saphenofemoral junction (SFJ). *CFV,* Common femoral vein.

The *catheter infusion technique* involves the introduction of a peripherally inserted central catheter line or a 2.5-inch, 18-gauge intravenous catheter fully inserted directly into the lumen of the vein. The catheter tip is initially located 8 to 10 cm distal to the point of reflux (Fig. 80.5). The sclerosant is injected slowly as the

catheter is withdrawn. Subsequent percutaneous catheter placements are made more distall, and injections are directed cephalad as previously injected segments undergo vasospasm. Often, incompetent perforator veins do not require direct injection because they respond to treatment of the overlying superficial vein.

When using the *syringe-and-needle technique,* injections sites move from proximal to distal, with injections also directed cephalad.

Complications of ECA include those that may occur with standard injection-compression sclerotherapy. Deep venous thrombosis (extremely rare—incidence is between 0% to 5.7%) may occur if sclerosant finds its way into the deep venous system, especially in cases of inadequate post-ECA compression and lack of ambulation. Other side effects reported after ECA include transient visual disturbances, with no long-term visual or neurologic sequelae reported to date. Intra-arterial injection—the most feared complication of sclerotherapy—has been reported more frequently in association with ECA. This can cause severe skin necrosis; limb amputations have been reported as well. Therefore, performance of ECA must not be undertaken lightly. Detailed knowledge of the vascular sonographic anatomy is essential to perform ECA properly, safely, and effectively.

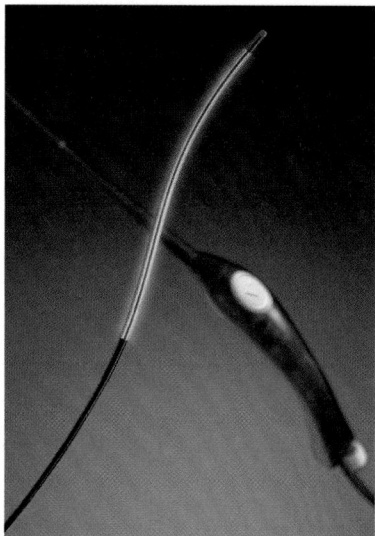

Fig. 80.6   Catheter. (Courtesy Covidien, Mansfield, MA.)

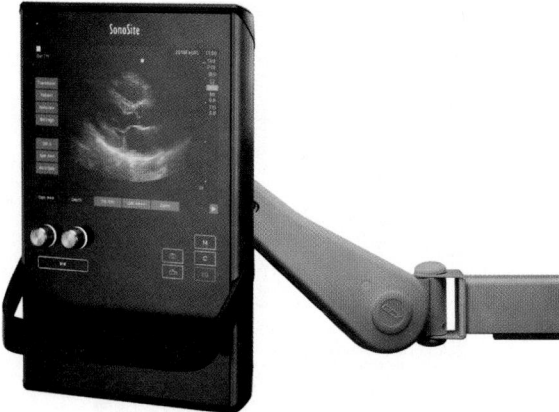

Fig. 80.7   Duplex ultrasound equipment. (Courtesy Fujifilm Sonosite, Bothell, WA.)

ENDOVENOUS RADIOFREQUENCY AND LASER ABLATION

Over the past 2 decades, in addition to ECA, newer procedures in the treatment of chronic venous insufficiency have been introduced. *Endovenous radiofrequency ablation* (RFA) and *endovenous laser ablation* (ELA) have emerged as less invasive and more effective alternatives to vein stripping. Performed in an office setting using tumescent anesthesia, these procedures can often be completed in under 1 hour. Procedure times depend on how long it takes to access the vein percutaneously, the length of the vein, and whether it is necessary to perform any ancillary procedures such as sclerotherapy or ambulatory phlebectomy. Graduated compression stockings are required post-treatment, as they are for ECA.

With RFA, radiofrequency energy is delivered to the vein lumen to heat, shrink, and occlude refluxing saphenous veins. Occlusion results from the contraction of collagen in the vein wall. VNUS ClosureFAST (VNUS Medtronic Medical Technologies) uses a specially designed catheter to treat 7-cm segments of the vein while maintaining the intraluminal temperature at 85°C to 90°C (Fig. 80.6). A 35-cm-long vein can be treated in 2 minutes. With ELA, laser energy of varying wavelengths is delivered to the vein lumen. Examples of wavelengths used for ELA include 810 nm (AngioDynamics), 980 nm (Biolitec and AngioDynamics), and 1320 nm (CoolTouch Syneron Candela). Laser treatment generates steam by heating blood inside the vein, producing fibrosis and subsequent occlusion of the vein. Deoxygenated hemoglobin is the main chromophore of the 810- and 980-nm lasers, whereas the energy of the 1320-nm laser is directed toward water in the vein wall. If treatment failure (recanalization) occurs (10%), it usually develops within the first year. If the vein is closed at 1-year follow-up, it is unlikely to recanalize.

INDICATIONS

The following are indications for RFA and ELA:

- Fully ambulatory patient without any contraindications
- Bulging varicose veins with or without symptoms (e.g., leg heaviness, throbbing, aching)
  NOTE: In some female patients, symptoms may occur only premenstrually (see Ninia, 2008).
- Bulging varicose veins with or without dermatologic signs of chronic venous insufficiency (e.g., edema, hyperpigmentation, lipodermatosclerosis, ulceration)

- Duplex ultrasound findings consistent with incompetence of the GSV or SSV
- Minimal tortuosity of the GSV or SSV to permit catheter placement

CONTRAINDICATIONS

- RFA cannot be used in patients with *pacemakers*.
- Contraindications to treatment with all methods include inability to ambulate, active superficial or deep venous thrombosis, hypoplastic deep veins, poor health, and pregnancy.

EQUIPMENT AND SUPPLIES

- Basic equipment for ELA and RFA (Total Vein Solutions; Vascular Solutions)
- Duplex ultrasound equipment, available as portable or stationary units (Fig. 80.7)
- Sterile solution (povidone–iodine or chlorhexidine) and sterile drapes
- Sterile gloves
- Equipment to follow universal blood and body fluid precautions
- Ultrasound probe cover
- 1% lidocaine without epinephrine, 5-mL syringe, and 30-gauge needle for local anesthesia before inserting the angiocatheter
- No. 11 blade
- 18-gauge angiocatheter
- Luer-Lok syringes
- Class II graduated compression stockings
- J-wire (guidewire)
- Sheath and vein dilator
- Micropuncture kits, available for veins less than 3 mm in diameter
- Protective eyewear for use during laser procedures
- Skin marking pen
- Fluid for tumescent anesthesia. Various preparations of tumescent solutions have been used, with studies showing the maximum safe dose of lidocaine to be 35 mg/kg. In general, a dilute solution of lidocaine can be prepared by taking a 250-mL bag of 0.9% normal saline, removing 15 mL, and replacing it with an equal amount (15 mL) of 1% lidocaine. A small amount (5 mL) of sodium bicarbonate can be added as a buffer to decrease the stinging sensation.

NOTE: Supplies are available commercially from various sources (e.g., Vein Solutions, Total Vascular Solutions, Cook Medical). The endolaser and radiofrequency companies preassemble kits that contain necessary supplies.

PREOPERATIVE PATIENT EDUCATION

See patient education forms available at www.expertconsult.com.

PROCEDURE

A *preoperative evaluation* is carried out, usually on a date before that of the procedure, and begins with a directed history and physical examination with an emphasis on the lower extremities of patients with varicose veins. Type and duration of symptoms along with any improvement with support stockings should be documented. Skin changes related to ambulatory venous hypertension, such as edema, hyperpigmentation, corona phlebectasia, lipodermatosclerosis, atrophie blanche, and ulceration, are best documented with photography.

1. Premedicate the patient orally with 0.5 to 1 mg of the anxiolytic lorazepam (alternatively, 2 to 5 mg diazepam) 30 minutes before the procedure.
2. Perform the ultrasound examination with the patient standing and the weight shifted onto the opposite leg (see Chapter 77, Noninvasive Venous and Arterial Studies of the Lower Extremities). For the GSV, start at the groin and work caudad along the medial thigh. The GSV is identified in its characteristic location at the SFJ and then within the fascial sheath (Fig. 80.8). Its course is marked on the skin. Vein diameter should be measured along with documentation of reflux by Doppler analysis (Fig. 80.9). Reflux is demonstrated by an audible retrograde flow of greater than 0.5 to 1 second while manually compressing and releasing the calf muscles. Significant reflux of 2 seconds or more is often associated with skin changes characteristic of venous insufficiency. Documentation of this finding is necessary to secure reimbursement as a medically necessary procedure.
3. After venous duplex mapping and marking, choose a percutaneous entry point.
4. Prepare and drape the leg in sterile fashion (e.g., povidone-iodine), and visualize the access site longitudinally with ultrasound.
5. Raise a 1% lidocaine wheal at the access site.
6. Insert an 18-gauge, 2-inch angiocatheter into the vein (Terumo). Place a 0.035-inch-diameter J-wire (guidewire) through the angiocatheter directed toward the SFJ. Remove the angiocatheter. The percutaneous entry site is slightly widened and a 5-Fr sheath with a dilator is placed over the guidewire. The sheath is positioned 1 cm below the SFJ. This serves to preserve the superficial epigastric vein. A competent superficial epigastric vein preserves venous drainage of the anterior abdominal wall and prevents the phenomenon of neovascularization—the condition associated with vein recurrences after surgical ligation and stripping. The J-wire and dilator are then removed. Venous return is confirmed by aspirating the syringe attached to the sheath.
7. At this point, introduce either an RFA or an ELA catheter into the sheath. *In the case of laser*, the aiming beam of the 600-μm laser fiber tip is transilluminated through the skin. If the aiming beam is not seen, it suggests that the laser fiber tip is incorrectly placed in the deep venous system. In this circumstance, the laser fiber and sheath need to be withdrawn until the aiming beam is visualized.
8. Administer tumescent anesthesia after the laser fiber or the RFA catheter has been inserted. It is injected manually or with the use of a mechanical pump (Klein pump, HK Surgical) perivascularly into the saphenous sheath with ultrasound guidance; the GSV is then "floated" in the anesthetic fluid (Fig. 80.10). In addition to providing anesthesia, this compresses the diameter of the GSV and causes the vein to spasm. The fluid surrounding the vein also provides for a "heat sink" to prevent injury to adjacent tissue.

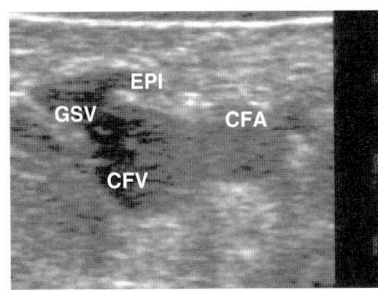

Fig. 80.8 Sonographic appearance of great saphenous vein (GSV) joining common femoral vein (CFV) at the saphenofemoral junction. *EPI,* Superficial epigastric artery; *CFA,* common femoral artery.

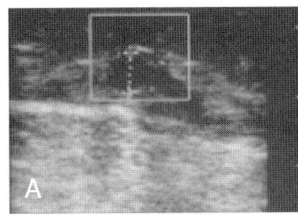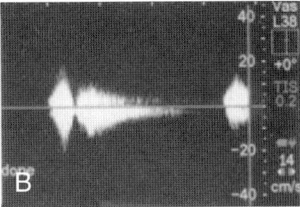

Fig. 80.9 (A) Great saphenous vein (GSV) within the fascial sheath. This vessel was measured at midthigh and noted to be approximately 0.57 cm in diameter. (B) Quantification of reflux of the GSV in (A). After manual compression of the calf muscles, reflux lasts approximately 2 seconds.

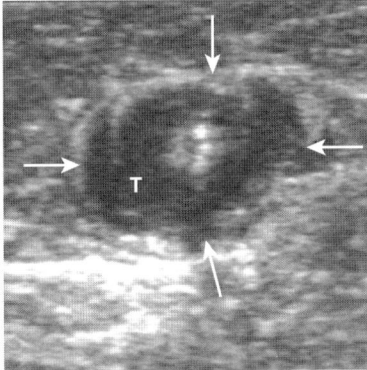

Fig. 80.10 Saphenous vein "floated" in its sheath *(arrows)* after perivascular administration of tumescent anesthetic. The "T" represents the tumescent liquid surrounding the vein. Note how, in transverse view, the vein spasms around the echogenic laser fiber after the tumescent fluid is administered. This liquid now serves as a heat sink to absorb heat energy from the laser.

9. Deliver RF or laser energy. For RF, using a "segmental heating" approach, the ClosureFAST catheter is positioned as described. The exposed 7-cm heating element portion is activated with RF energy for a 20-second heating cycle. When the cycle is complete, energy delivery is automatically terminated by the generator. The catheter is then repositioned to the next treatment zone as indicated by the markings on the catheter. Spaced at increments of 6.5 cm, the catheter shaft allows for a 0.5-cm overlap between each treated segment to ensure complete treatment along the length of the vein. In addition to speed, an advantage of RFA over ELA is that the energy delivered is controlled by the temperature sensor on the catheter. This minimizes the risk of vein perforation and associated postoperative pain and bruising.

In general, for all laser units, a minimum of 70 J/cm is needed to successfully occlude the vein. This can be accomplished by delivering 14 W of power and using a fiber withdrawal rate of

2 mm/sec. The latter is accomplished simply and accurately by using the 10-cm markings along the sheath in conjunction with the time display in seconds on the individual laser unit.

10. Immediately apply a class II (30 to 40 mm Hg) thigh-high, open-toe graduated compression stocking to the treated leg.

COMMON ERRORS

- If the vein spasms, application of a small amount of 2% nitroprusside may help correct the vasospasm. Alternatively, the patient may ambulate for 10 minutes, and venipuncture may be reattempted.
- The room temperature is too cold.
- The patient is in the wrong position (reverse Trendelenburg is correct).
- Not attending to the needs of a nervous patient. Anxiolytics (oral lorazepam 0.5 to 1 mg or oral diazepam 2 to 5 mg) work well. "Vocal anesthesia" and speaking to the patient during the procedure may also help allay anxiety.

POSTPROCEDURE PATIENT CARE AND EDUCATION

See the patient education forms available at www.expertconsult.com. Patients are encouraged to ambulate and resume their normal activities.

- The compression hose is worn overnight and then for 6 more days while the patient is up and ambulating. The stocking may be removed at bedtime and for showering.
- Ibuprofen 600 mg three times daily is prescribed for 3 days and is to be taken, then used every 6 hours as needed afterward for pain.
- Physical examination and ultrasonographic follow-up are performed 3 to 7 days post-treatment (Fig. 80.11).

The treated vein wall will be thickened and fibrotic. Adequate flow in the deep venous system should be noted (Fig. 80.12). Although a resolution of symptoms and an improved cosmetic appearance are often noted within 1 month of treatment, most patients will need additional therapy in the form of sclerotherapy or ambulatory phlebectomy of residual varices to attain maximum results. Telangiectases will need to be treated separately as well. Some operators perform these procedures at the time of the endovenous ablation procedure. Others prefer to wait 1 month postprocedure to see what, if any, additional procedures need to be performed.

COMPLICATIONS

Significant complications of RFA and ELA are rare.

- Bruising and discomfort tend to be more common with ELA.
- Local paresthesias can occur with both modalities (<5% with ELA and <15% with RFA) but typically resolve within 2 to 3 months. Application of adequate tumescent anesthesia by floating the vein at least 10 mm below the skin will reduce this risk.
- The incidence of deep venous thrombosis is reported to be less than 1% with both modalities. This is very rare, especially when immediate ambulation and compression are used.
- Failure rates for either RFA or laser are less than 2% at 5-year follow-up.

CONCLUSIONS

Results of endovenous therapies have been very encouraging. Compared with vein stripping, these office-based procedures offer the advantages of lower procedural risks and cost. Patients are awake during the procedures and remain fully ambulatory, with no downtime afterward. Over the past 2 decades there has been increased understanding and interest in the management of venous disease. It is very likely these promising minimally invasive endovenous ablative

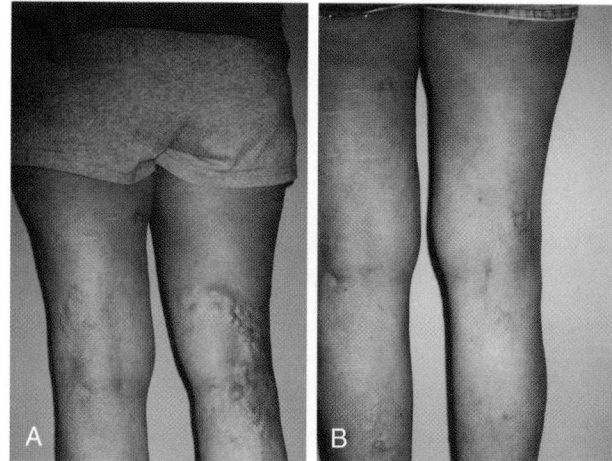

Fig. 80.11 Appearance before (A) and after (B) endovenous laser ablation.

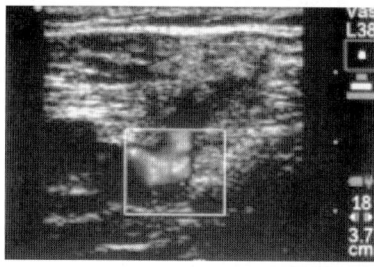

Fig. 80.12 Postprocedure blood flow in a common femoral vein (CFV). Because this is a deep vein, one would want to see blood flow in its lumen both before and after the procedure. Compromised blood flow in the CFV postprocedure raises concern over an iatrogenic deep venous thrombosis.

procedures will essentially replace vein stripping in most parts of the world.

PATIENT EDUCATION GUIDES

See sample patient education and consent forms available at www.expertconsult.com.

CPT/BILLING CODES

36475	Endovenous ablation therapy of the incompetent vein, extremity, inclusive of all imaging guidance and monitoring, percutaneous, radiofrequency; first vein treated
36476	Second and subsequent veins treated in a single extremity, each through separate access sites
36478	Endovenous laser ablation therapy of incompetent vein, extremity, inclusive of all imaging guidance and monitoring, percutaneous, laser; first vein treated
36479	Second and subsequent veins treated in a single extremity, each through separate access sites

ICD-10-CM DIAGNOSTIC CODES

I87.309	Chronic venous hypertension
I83.899	Varicose veins with complications
I83.009	Varicose veins with skin changes/ulceration
I83.90	Varicose veins lower extremity
I87.2	Venous (peripheral) insufficiency

SUPPLIERS

(See contact information available at www.expertconsult.com.)

Laser ablation
Angiodynamics
Biolitec
CoolTouch Syneron Candela
Radiofrequency ablation
VNUS Medical Medtronic
Support hose
BSN-Jobst Institute, Inc.
Carolon Health Care Products
MediUSA
Sigvaris
Ultrasonography
Esaote
Sonosite
TeraRecon
Terason
Terumo Medical Corporation

ONLINE RESOURCES

American College of Phlebology: www.phlebology.org. A good reference for frequently asked questions.

RECOMMENDED READING

Alam M, Dover JS, Nguyen TH, eds. *Procedures in Cosmetic Dermatology Series: Treatment of Leg Veins*. Philadelphia: Saunders; 2006.

Breu FX, Guggenbichler S, Wollman JC. 2nd European Consensus Meeting on Foam Sclerotherapy 2006, Tegernsee, Germany. *Vasa*. 2008;37(suppl 71):1–30.

Darte SG, Baker SJ. Ultrasound-guided foam sclerotherapy for the treatment of varicose veins. *Br J Surg*. 2006;93:969–974.

Geroulakos G. Foam sclerotherapy for the management of varicose veins: a critical reappraisal. *Phlebolymphology*. 2006;13:202–206.

Luebke T, Brunkwall J. Systematic review and meta-analysis of endovenous radiofrequency obliteration, endovenous laser therapy, and foam sclerotherapy for primary varicosis. *J Cardiovasc Surg*. 2008;49:213–233.

Merchant RF, Pichot O. Long-term outcomes of endovenous radiofrequency obliteration of saphenous reflux as a treatment for superficial venous insufficiency. *J Vasc Surg*. 2005;42:502–509.

Nesbitt C, Bedenis R, Bhattacharya V, Stansby G. Endovenous ablation (radiofrequency and laser) and foam sclerotherapy versus conventional surgery for great saphenous vein varices. *Cochrane Database Syst Rev*. 2014;(7):CD005624.

Ninia JG. Premenstrual symptoms in lower limbs and duplex scan investigations. *Phlebolymphology*. 2008;15:125.

Pavlović MD, Schuller-Petrović S, Pichot O, et al. Guidelines of the first international consensus conference on endovenous thermal ablation for varicose vein disease – ETVA Consensus Meeting 2012. *Phlebology*. 2014;30:257–273.

Rasmussen LH, Lawaetz M, Serup J, et al. Randomized clinical trial comparing endovenous laser ablation, radiofrequency ablation, foam sclerotherapy, and surgical stripping for great saphenous varicose veins with 3-year follow-up. *J Vasc Surg: Venous and Lymph Dis*. 2013;(1):349–356.

Schuller-Petrovic S, Pannier F, Pavlovic MD. Endovenous thermal ablation techniques with ambulatory phlebectomy for varicose veins. In: Robinson JK, Hanke CW, Siegel DM, Fratilla A, Bhatia AC, Rohrer TE, eds. *Surgery of the Skin: Procedural Dermatology*. 3rd ed. Philadelphia: Elsevier; 2015:588–598.

Winterborn RJ, Taiwo F, Slim F, et al. The incidence of deep vein thrombosis following ultrasound-guided foam sclerotherapy. *Br J Surg*. 2009;96(suppl 1):A10.

CHAPTER 81

PULMONARY FUNCTION TESTING

C. Mark Chassay

Pulmonary function testing (PFT) is an important tool used by clinicians to evaluate individuals for lung disease. The parameters commonly measured include lung volume, airflow (timed volume), and airway reactivity. Clinicians cannot reliably identify obstructive or restrictive patterns from history taking and physical examination alone. In one study, when clinicians were asked to predict the results of PFTs, they correctly predicted an obstructive pattern 83% of the time. However, when predicting a normal or restrictive pattern, they were correct only about half of the time. Besides identifying abnormalities, PFTs allow the severity of an abnormality to be quantified and the amount of reversibility to be determined. This ability to quantify abnormalities also allows a clinician to follow treatment in an objective manner.

A spirogram is a recording of exhaled and inhaled volume (liters) over time (seconds). Spirometric examination is the most widely used tool to assess pulmonary function in office practice. It can be used to evaluate patients suspected of having disease on the basis of clinical findings or to monitor changes in a patient over time. Although formal PFTs are more comprehensive and, if necessary, can provide an objective measure of impairment, spirometry is sufficient most of the time.

In fact, spirometry is underused. Such examinations should be readily available in most medical offices. The National Asthma Education Program (NAEP) recommends an objective measurement of lung function (either spirometry or PFTs) whenever diagnosing or managing asthma. There is evidence that patients also have inaccurate perceptions of the severity of asthma in the absence of PFTs, thereby increasing the risk of mortality. The American Thoracic Society (ATS), the European Respiratory Society, and the Global Initiative for Chronic Obstructive Lung Disease (GOLD) have published guidelines urging the use of spirometry to correctly diagnose chronic obstructive pulmonary disease (COPD). Even the National Committee for Quality Assurance, which grades quality of care, lists spirometry use in patients with newly diagnosed COPD as one indicator of clinician performance for the Health Plan Employer Data and Informed Set. Some experts suggest that spirometry should be as common as a blood pressure cuff in a primary care clinician's office, especially for patients with asthma or COPD.

NOTE: Although useful information can be obtained from spirometry and PFTs, these physiologic tools alone do not establish a diagnosis. The test results must be carefully correlated with clinical and chest radiographic findings.

DEFINITIONS AND PATHOLOGY

Common lung volumes measured by spirometry are illustrated in Fig. 81.1. The simplest test of lung function is based on a forced expiration. It is one of the most informative tests and requires minimal equipment and calculations. The *vital capacity* is the total volume of gas that can be exhaled after a full inspiration. The vital capacity measured with a forced expiration may be less than that measured with a slower exhalation, so the term *forced vital capacity* (FVC) is generally used.

Any reduction in FVC affects the ventilatory capacity. The FVC can be affected by *restrictive* conditions affecting the thoracic cage (kyphoscoliosis), diseases affecting the nerve supply to the thoracic muscles, intrinsic diseases of the muscles, abnormalities of the pleural cavity, space-occupying lesions, lung tissue pathology, or stagnation of blood flow in the lungs (as seen in congestive heart failure). In addition, chronic, severe diseases of the airways (*obstructive*) such as asthma and chronic bronchitis cause peripheral small airways to close prematurely during expiration. This limits the volume that can be exhaled rapidly.

Forced expiratory volume (FEV_1) is the volume of gas (liters) exhaled in 1 second by a forced expiration from full inspiration. The FEV_1 is affected by the airway resistance of the medium to large airways. *Forced expiratory flow* ($FEF_{25\%-75\%}$) is the flow over the middle half of the FVC, the average flow from the point at which 25% of the FVC has been exhaled to the point at which 75% has been exhaled. It is measured in liters per second and while it is probably the most variable of forced expiratory measurements, it is also the most sensitive office measurement of small airway obstruction or disease. Any increase in airway resistance reduces the ventilatory capacity.

Of note, older patients, especially those with obstructive disease, may take a long time to exhale completely for an FVC, as long as 12 to 15 seconds. Maintaining maximal expiratory effort for such a long time may cause discomfort or even lightheadedness. Consequently, certain experts suggest measuring FEV_6 (forced expiratory volume at 6 seconds) as a substitute for FVC in adults. Subsequently, FEV_6 has been shown to be equivalent to FVC for identifying obstructive and restrictive patterns in adults, and to be more reproducible and less demanding.

The flow-volume loop (Fig. 81.2) has two components: the expiratory flow-volume (top half of curve) and the inspiratory flow-volume (bottom half of curve). The top half is where 95% of the information is obtained (expiratory flow). The inspiratory flow-volume curve is not affected by anything causing dynamic compression of the airways because the pressures during inspiration always expand the bronchi. However, a large (fixed or variable) airway obstruction will cause flattening of the curve because maximal flow is limited. The expiratory flow-volume curve will also be flattened by a fixed large airway obstruction. With restrictive airway disease, the flow-volume curve will be smaller or narrower. One important place to review the inspiratory flow-volume curve is when factitious asthma is suspected. With factitious asthma, there is inappropriate vocal cord closure, also known as *vocal cord dysfunction*, and although the subsequent wheezing may mimic asthma (or exercise-induced asthma), the inspiratory curve is notched or attenuated, which does not occur in true asthma. With true asthma, only the expiratory curve is usually affected.

The expiratory flow-volume curve may take on different morphologies. Notice how the downward loop becomes more scalloped as airway obstruction increases. However, a large (fixed or variable) airway obstruction will cause flattening of the curve

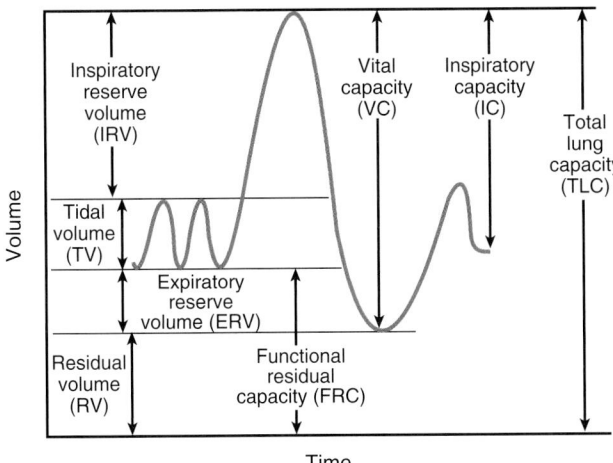

Fig. 81.1 Spirogram showing tidal breathing and the divisions of total lung capacity. The residual volume is measured by indirect techniques.

because maximal inspiratory and expiratory flow is limited. In restrictive lung disease, the flow-volume curve will be narrow (almost up-and-down), with little to no "terminal tail," such as that seen with COPD.

Two "pearls" should be borne in mind: (1) examination of the shape of the curve is just as important as the actual numerical data generated by spirometry testing; and (2) restrictive lung disease can be ruled out in 95% to 99% of cases with a normal-appearing flow-volume loop. However, if suspected on clinical grounds, formal PFTs measuring the total lung volumes are indicated. (Spirometry falsely identifies restrictive lung disease in 59% of flow-volume loops that suggest a restrictive defect.)

INDICATIONS

Diagnostic

- To evaluate symptoms, signs, or abnormal results of other diagnostic tests in individuals older than 5 years.
  - Symptoms: cough, dyspnea, wheezing, orthopnea, or chest pain
  - Signs: overinflation, expiratory slowing, cyanosis, chest deformity, wheezing, or unexplained crackles
  - Abnormal results of diagnostic tests: hypoxemia, hypercapnia, polycythemia, or abnormal chest radiographs
- To measure the effect of disease on pulmonary function.
- To screen persons at risk for pulmonary disease (e.g., persons with occupational exposure to injurious substances or who have active or passive smoke exposure). The evidence does not support the widespread use of spirometry to improve smoking cessation rates.
- To assess preoperative risk in patients with COPD or asthma. However, there are few published data comparing spirometric data with clinical data for predicting postoperative pulmonary complications in patients undergoing nonthoracic surgery. Hence, even a poor FEV_1 result is not sufficient grounds to withhold surgery in nonthoracic cases.
- To screen patients undergoing lung resection surgery.
- To assess prognosis of lung disease.
- Indirect test (as opposed to direct test with methacholine challenge; indirect test has higher sensitivity for diagnosis) for elite athletes or patients with exercise induced bronchospasm that do not respond to trial of inhaled short-acting beta₂ agonist. Can be performed in lab equipped to do exercise testing or on-site where athlete develops symptoms.

Monitoring

- To assess effectiveness of a therapeutic intervention (e.g., bronchodilator therapy, steroid treatment for asthma or interstitial lung disease). For asthma, according to NAEP guidelines, PFTs are indicated after therapy is initiated and symptoms and peak flow have stabilized, during periods of progressive or prolonged loss of control, and at least every 1 to 2 years.
- To track the course of a disease affecting lung function in patients who identify activity-limiting symptoms, especially when FEV_1 is less than 50% (e.g., obstructive airway disease, interstitial lung disease, or neuromuscular disease, such as Guillain-Barré syndrome).
- To assess current status of persons with occupational exposure to injurious substances.
- To detect adverse reactions to drugs with known pulmonary toxicity (e.g., nitrofurantoin, methotrexate, amiodarone; may be reversible if caught early and medication stopped).

Evaluation of Disability or Impairment

- To assess patients as part of a rehabilitation program (e.g., medical, industrial, vocational).
- To assess risks for an insurance evaluation (no evidence of benefit).
- To assess the condition of persons for legal reasons (e.g., Social Security or other program involving government compensation, personal injury lawsuits).

Public Health

- Epidemiologic surveys
- Derivation of normal values for PFTs

Contraindications

- Severe debilitation and excessive tiring (patients who cannot expend the required effort for testing)
- Severe or moderately severe respiratory distress
- Patients not motivated or desiring to take the test
- Children too young to conduct testing (PFTs are usually helpful if the patient is older than 5 years; however, some children cannot conduct testing adequately until after age 7 years)

Equipment

- PFT machine/spirometer
- Comfortable chair and private area of office for testing (avoids patient embarrassment)
- Nose clips (soft clips are preferred and recommended to prevent air leaks)
- Various inhalants for testing response to bronchodilators (e.g., albuterol inhaler with 90 μg/puff), if indicated

The office spirometer should conform to minimal requirements or specifications established by the ATS (Table 81.1). Not all commercially available spirometers meet these standards. Ideally, the computerized spirometer should have software that allows formulas and algorithms to be modified. Routine preventive maintenance, cleaning, and quality control measures are necessary to ensure accurate results in spirometric testing. Frequent (if not daily) calibration according to the manufacturer's instructions is highly recommended. The spirometer should also be evaluated frequently for leaks. Instructions for maintenance, as well as how to perform tests for quality control, should be provided by the manufacturer. The clinician is responsible for ensuring that the office personnel are adequately trained to carry out the recommended maintenance.

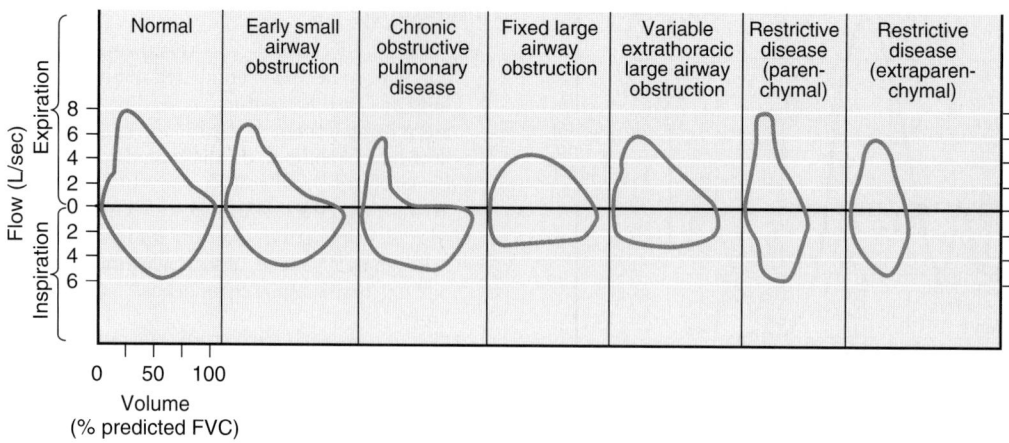

Fig. 81.2 Characteristic flow-volume curves of various types of obstructive diseases and restrictive diseases compared with normal. The top part of the curve represents maximal forced expiration, whereas the bottom represents maximal inspiration. *FVC,* Forced vital capacity.

TABLE 81.1	Minimal Recommendations (Specifications) for Diagnostic Spirometry*				
Test	**Range/Accuracy (BTPS)**	**Flow Range (L/sec)**	**Time (sec)**	**Resistance and Back Pressure**	**Test Signal**
VC	0.5–8 L ± 3% of reading or ±0.05 L, whichever is greater	0–14	30		3-L Calibration syringe
FVC	0.5–8 L ± 3% of reading or ±0.05 L, whichever is greater	0–14	15	< 1.5 cm H_2O/L per sec	24 standard waveforms 3-L Calibration syringe
FEV_1	0.5–8 L ± 3% of reading or ±0.05 L, whichever is greater	0–14	1	< 1.5 cm H_2O/L per sec	24 standard waveforms
Time zero	The time point from which all FEV_1 measurements are taken			Back extrapolation	
PEF	Accuracy: ±10% of reading or ±0.4 L/sec, whichever is greater	0–14		Same as FEV_1	26 standard waveforms
	Precision: ±5% of reading or ±0.2 L/sec, whichever is greater				
$FEF_{25\%–75\%}$	7.0 L/sec ± 5% of reading or ±0.2 L/sec, whichever is greater	±14	15	Same as FEV_1	24 standard waveforms
V	±14 L/sec ± 5% of reading or ±0.2 L/sec, whichever is greater	0–14	15	Same as FEV_1	Proof from manufacturer
MVV	250 L/min at TV of 2 L within ±10% of reading or ±15 L/min, whichever is greater	±14 ± 3	12–15	Pressure < ±10 cm H_2O at 2-L TV at 2.0 Hz	Sine wave pump

BTPS, Body temperature pressure saturated (37°C and ambient pressure); *Cal,* •••; *FEF,* forced expiratory flow; *FEV_1,* forced expiratory volume at 1 second; *FVC,* forced vital capacity; *MVV,* maximal voluntary ventilation; *PEF,* peak expiratory flow; *TV,* tidal volume; *V,* volume; *VC,* vital capacity.
*Unless specifically stated, precision requirements are the same as the accuracy requirements.
From Miller HR, Hankinson J, Brusasco V, Burgos F, Casaburi R: ATS/ERS Task Force: Standardization of lung function testing. *Eur Respir J.* 2005;26:319–338.

NOTE: Peak flow meters are advantageous for patients to use at home, but they do not provide the documentation needed in the office.

PREPROCEDURE PATIENT PREPARATION

Before performing a PFT, review the patient's respiratory history, including any medications the patient may be taking for respiratory problems. A clear explanation of the test and what is to be expected is essential to the patient's performance. The PFT has both an effort-dependent and an effort-independent portion. The best overall result is obtained when the patient gives a maximal effort. Patients with no prior experience with PFTs should make 2 to 3 practice attempts until a maximal effort is obtained. A demonstration of the test may be helpful.

The patient should plan to spend approximately 15 minutes for PFTs for adults, 15 to 30 minutes for children, and 45 minutes for prebronchodilator and postbronchodilator testing. If referred for formal PFTs, they should expect to spend at least 1 hour for measurement of lung volume, diffusion lung capacity, and so forth.

Usually the patient is seated to perform the test. The thorax should be erect and the head should be in a neutral position. Explain that this test measures lung function and that the best results are obtained when the patient takes a deep breath and then blows out as hard, as fast, and as long as possible (with the exception of older patients, for whom at least 6 seconds may be necessary to obtain a result [FEV_6]). Smokers should try to abstain from smoking for at least 1 hour before testing. To follow the diagram (see Fig. 81.1), the patient first takes several normal (tidal) breaths, after which he or she will perform a maximal inspiration to total lung capacity (TLC). The patient then exhales fast and hard, as much as he or she can (FVC or FEV_6).

TECHNIQUE

1. Prepare the equipment to test for FVC. Machine calibration and parameter setups vary between spirometers. See the individual instructions pertaining to the particular instrument for this portion of the procedure.
2. Document the patient's position (usually seated). If for some reason the patient is standing, it will increase FVC.

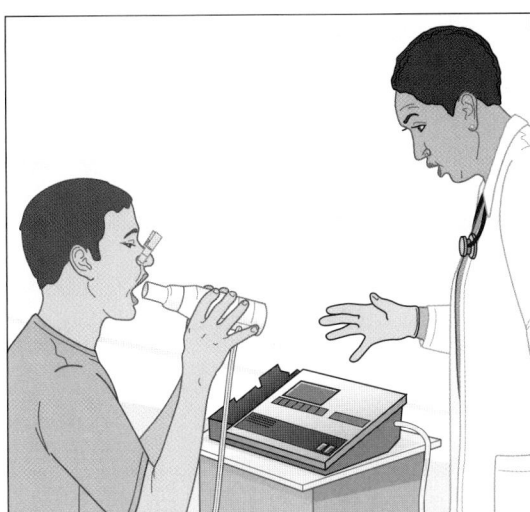

Fig. 81.3 Patient takes a deep breath, inserts the mouthpiece, and blows out as fast and as hard as possible.

3. Have the patient breathe in and out several times with the nose clips in place, to become comfortable.
4. Ask the patient to take in as deep a breath as possible, to completely fill the lungs.
5. Then have the patient quickly insert the mouthpiece. It should be between the teeth with a tight seal being held around it using the lips.
6. Next, have the patient blow out as hard, as fast, and as long as possible (try for at least 6 seconds; Fig. 81.3). Enthusiastically coach the patient to breathe out until the forced vital curve flattens out (usually 5 to 6 seconds).
7. When the lungs are completely emptied, have the patient breathe in as deeply as possible, to obtain the inspiratory parameter and complete the evaluation.
8. Repeat the test three times. A minimum of three and a maximum of eight maneuvers are performed until three acceptable curves are obtained. Two or three maneuvers that have values within a 5% difference of each other indicate reproducibility. The best effort is then saved and reported. Acceptability and reproducibility criteria are summarized in Box 81.1.
9. If prebronchodilator and postbronchodilator comparison PFTs are needed, administer a short-acting β-adrenergic agonist (e.g., albuterol 2 to 4 puffs of 90 μg/puff) or other bronchodilator through a hand-held inhaler.
10. Wait about 20 minutes for bronchodilation to occur. Then repeat the FVC (FEV_6 for older patients with obstructive disease) for the postbronchodilation measurements, as in steps 1 through 8.

INTERPRETATION

Some of the factors that influence the normal values of PFTs include the formula used to predict the normal values, test quality, height, age, weight, sex, ethnicity, posture, effort, smoking, and even circadian rhythm. The results and interpretation depend on the clinician paying careful attention to the characteristics of the equipment used, the patient's performance and clinical condition, and the reference values chosen. A patient's own baseline values will provide the best reference data for assessing a patient with chronic pulmonary disease over time.

Interpretation of PFTs can be categorized into three basic patterns: normal function, obstructive, and restrictive (Fig. 81.4). A diagnosis is then made by correlating the test results with the clinical findings from the history, physical examination, and radiographs.

BOX 81.1 Acceptability and Reproducibility Criteria Summary

Acceptability Criteria

Individual spirograms are "acceptable" if
1. They are free from artifacts, such as
   - Cough or glottis closure during the first second of exhalation
   - Early termination or cut-off
   - Variable effort
   - Leak
   - Obstructed mouthpiece
2. They have good starts
   - Extrapolated volume <5% of FVC or 0.15 L, whichever is greater; *or*
   - Time to peak expiratory flow <120 msec (optional until further information is available)
3. They have a satisfactory exhalation
   - Six seconds of exhalation or a plateau in the volume-time curve; *or*
   - Reasonable duration or a plateau in the volume-time curve; *or*
   - If the subject cannot or should not continue to exhale

Reproducibility Criteria

After three acceptable spirograms have been obtained, apply the following tests:
- Are the two largest FVCs within 0.2 L of each other?
- Are the two largest FEV_1 values within 0.2 L of each other?
- If both of these criteria are met, the test session may be concluded.
- If both of these criteria are not met, continue testing until
  - Both of the criteria are met with analysis of additional acceptable spirograms *or*
  - A total of eight tests have been performed *or*
  - The patient/subject cannot or should not continue.
  Save, at a minimum, the three best maneuvers.

FEV_1, Forced expiratory volume at 1 second; *FVC,* forced vital capacity.
From Culver BH, Graham BL, Coates AL, Wanger J, Berry CE, et al: American Thoracic Society: Recommendations for a standardized pulmonary function report. *Am J Respir Crit Care Med.* 2017; 196:1463–1472.

An obstructive process, such as asthma or COPD, is characterized by flow that is low relative to lung volume. Characteristically, timed volume (FEV_1) and flow ($FEF_{25\%-75\%}$) are decreased. A decrease in $FEF_{25\%-75\%}$ may detect obstruction in the smaller airways early in the course of the disease, before a change in FEV_1 is evident. This is especially common in smokers, and may be their best early warning before permanent lung damage. A reduction in $FEF_{25\%-75\%}$ from small airway obstruction gives the flow-volume curve a characteristic concave shape. Other causes of small airway obstructive patterns in children include cystic fibrosis, bronchiolitis, bronchiectasis, and heart disease. Causes of large airway obstructive patterns in children include a foreign body, vocal cord dysfunction, vascular rings or laryngeal webs, laryngotracheomalacia, tracheal or bronchial stenosis, enlarged lymph nodes, or tumor. In adults, causes of obstructive patterns include asthma, COPD, congestive heart failure, pulmonary embolism, mechanical obstruction of the airway (benign and malignant tumors), pulmonary infiltration with eosinophilia, vocal cord dysfunction, and cough due to medications (e.g., angiotensin-converting enzyme inhibitors).

If the patient has an obstructive defect, the clinician should determine if it is reversible based on the increase in FEV_1 or FVC after bronchodilator treatment. Distinguishing between asthma and

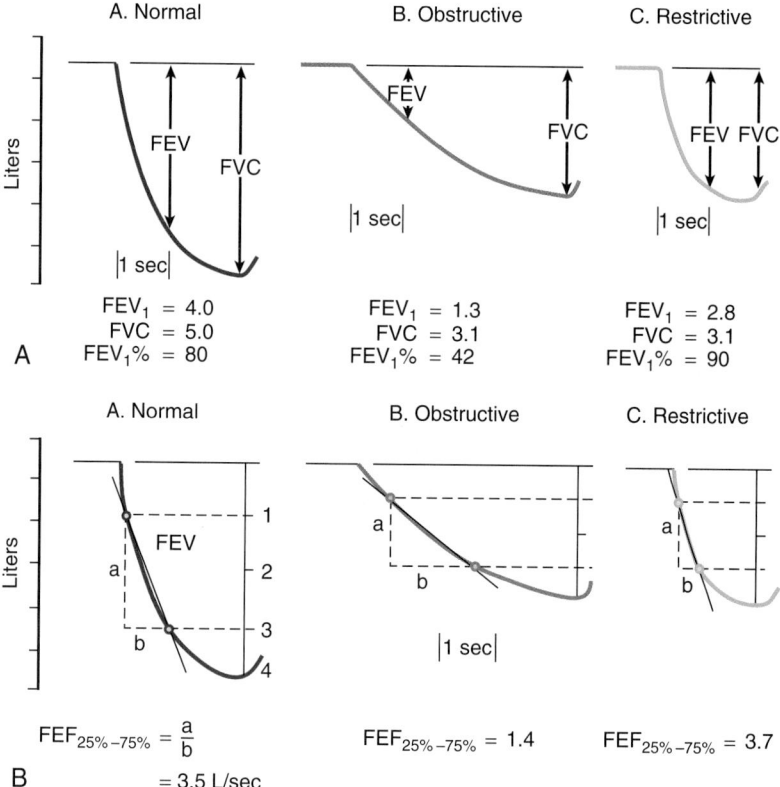

Fig. 81.4 (A) Normal, obstructive, and restrictive patterns of a forced expiration. (B) Calculation of forced expiratory flow between 25% and 75% of the FVC ($FEF_{25\%-75\%}$). FEV_1, Forced expiratory volume at 1 second; FVC, forced vital capacity. $FEV_1\% = (FEV_1/FVC) \times 100$. (From Miller HR, Hankinson J, Brusasco V, Burgos F, Casaburi R: ATS/ ERS Task Force: Standardization of lung function testing. *Eur Respir J.* 2005;26:319–338.)

COPD can be challenging; typically obstructive defects in asthma are fully reversible whereas defects in COPD are not, but there can be overlap between the two. The following points can be helpful.

For asthma:

1. The history. Diagnosis is typically picked up in childhood (although it can be missed) with cough, wheezing, dyspnea, chest tightness; occurring or worse at night; identifiable triggers (e.g., infections, stress, allergies, changes in weather, strong emotional expression [laughing or crying hard], menstrual periods); a clearly reversible component when a bronchodilator is added (e.g., increase FEV_1 >200 mL, >12% from baseline, or >10% over predicted FEV_1 in adults; >12% from baseline in patients 5 to 18 years of age).
2. FEV_1—the gold standard—<80% if moderate; also, FEV_1/FVC ratio <80%. In fact, FEV_1/FVC ratio (i.e., $FEV_1\%$) is a better measure of asthma severity than FEV_1.

For COPD:

1. The history. Almost always there will be an explanation or cause: tobacco abuse (most common, especially if at least a 20-pack-year history; note, however, that only about 20% of cigarette smokers develop clinically significant COPD), α_1-antitrypsin deficiency (accounts for 1% of COPD cases; consider if smoking history absent or very early COPD [age <55 years] in smokers), exposure to airway toxins (e.g., industrial chemicals, mineral dust, silica, dust, coal dust, and inhaled endotoxins [e.g., farm worker]).
2. COPD-related airflow obstruction is less reversible to inhaled bronchodilator challenges and less variable than asthma.
3. FEV_1/FVC ratio <70% of normal, and FEV_1 <80% of normal.

Postbronchodilator FEV_1 is also recommended for the diagnosis and assessment of severity of COPD.

Low volumes and normal flows characterize a restrictive lung process. The primary criterion for this diagnosis is a reduction in TLC; however, the presence of restriction is commonly inferred from a decreased FVC. It should be kept in mind that a decreased FVC only infers a restrictive process because FVC can also be reduced in the presence of airflow obstruction. Significant decreases in FEV_1 and the FEV_1/FVC ratio are key findings that will help differentiate an obstructive from a restrictive pattern when FVC is reduced (see Fig. 81.4A). In addition, when there is both airflow obstruction and reduced FVC, the possibility of restriction can usually be eliminated with evidence of overinflation on the physical examination or a chest radiograph. If airflow obstruction and FVC are decreased by the same amounts, the FEV_1/FVC ratio may be normal despite obstruction; however, $FEF_{25\%-75\%}$ should be helpful.

Again, spirometry falsely identifies restrictive patterns in 59% of cases in which FVC is low. Unless dictated on clinical grounds, restrictive defects should be confirmed by total lung volume measurements. Measuring TLC requires referral to a pulmonary function laboratory. Measurement of lung volume by helium dilution, nitrogen washout, or body plethysmography can definitively confirm a diagnosis of a restrictive lung condition. Although a reduced TLC defines restriction, measuring FVC has frequently been demonstrated to be more useful for following the course of the disease process. Restrictive disease is uncommon and can be divided into parenchymal and extraparenchymal etiologies. Parenchymal causes include silicosis (late), pneumoconiosis, asbestosis, berylliosis, eosinophilic pneumonia, idiopathic pulmonary fibrosis, sarcoidosis, and radiation- or drug-induced (e.g., nitrofurantoin, methotrexate, amiodarone) interstitial lung disease. Extraparenchymal disease can be due to loss of lung volume (e.g., pleural effusion, pneumothorax), chest wall deformity, extrathoracic compression (e.g., ankylosing spondylitis, ascites, kyphoscoliosis, morbid obesity), or neuromuscular problems (e.g., Guillain-Barré syndrome, myasthenia gravis, muscular dystrophy, amyotrophic lateral sclerosis, cervical spine injury, or diaphragmatic weakness or paralysis). Suspicion of restrictive disease warrants referral and probable measurement of lung volume, diffusion lung capacity testing (confirms parenchymal cause), etc. Table 81.2 summarizes the characteristic patterns of obstructive and restrictive lung diseases as measured by spirometry.

TABLE 81.2	Characteristic Patterns of Obstructive and Restrictive Lung Disease as Measured by Spirometry*	
	Obstruction	**Restriction**
FVC	Normal or ↓	↓
FEV_1	↓	Normal or ↓
FEV_1/FVC	Normal (early) or ↓	↑
$FEF_{25\%-75\%}$	↓	Normal, ↑ or ↓

FEF, Forced expiratory flow; *FEV₁*, forced expiratory volume at 1 second; *FVC*, forced vital capacity.
*Low flows with normal volumes characterize obstructive disease, whereas normal flows with low volumes characterize restrictive disease. In severe obstruction, gas trapping reduces FVC because of an increased residual volume.

Many systems are available to quantify the severity of pulmonary impairment; however, there is currently no universal standard based on differences between ethnic populations.* In practice, severity is usually described as a percentage of either predicted FEV_1 for obstructive conditions or predicted TLC for restrictive conditions. ("Normal" predicted test values are obtained by testing a large group of people who have been determined to be free of lung disease.) The test results for a given patient are then expressed as a percentage of the predicted value for age, height, sex, and race. In reality, no one set of equations will be entirely accurate for every person in a given population. For the final report, the ATS recommends that clinicians define the lower limits of normal by using calculations of the lower 95th percentiles (from the specific set of prediction equations that have been selected as standard reference values); these should be recorded, rather than just the percentages of predicted function (e.g., 80% for FEV_1/FVC%). The patient should be comparable in age, race, and sex to the reference population. In computerized equipment, it is essential for population standards to be defined in the software.

Although using percentage of predicted function to evaluate results may not be recommended, here are some guidelines the clinician can use to get a general clinical picture of pulmonary function:

Vital Capacity

FVC

80%–120% of predicted value	Normal
70%–79% of predicted value	Mild reduction
50%–69% of predicted value	Moderate reduction
<50% of predicted value	Severe reduction

Again, restrictive lung disease is characterized by reduced vital capacity and relatively normal airflow rates. If obstruction is present (see below), the reduction in vital capacity may only be reported as "probably secondary to obstruction" if the severity of the reduced vital capacity and that of the obstructive findings are approximately equal. In comparing vital capacities obtained at different times (including those obtained before and after bronchodilator administration), the expiratory time must be considered and compared. The raw curves should also be compared.

Flow Rates

FEV_1 can be plotted as the percentage of vital capacity [(FEV_1/FVC) × 100], or FEV_1%.

FEV_1%

>75%	Normal
60%–75%	Mild obstruction
50%–59%	Moderate obstruction
<50%	Severe obstruction

*There are referenced "normal" datasets on the Internet for different parts of the world. Quanjer, 2012, is used by many experts.

NOTE: For patients <25 years old, add 5% to these figures; for those >60 years old, subtract 5%.

$FEF_{25\%-75\%}$

>79% of predicted value	Normal
60%–79% of predicted value	Mild obstruction
40%–59% of predicted value	Moderate obstruction
<40% of predicted value	Severe obstruction

EDITOR'S NOTE: Most equipment uses ATS criteria for defining normal and abnormal values. A large cohort study (Mannino et al., 2007) found that using GOLD criteria for diagnosis of COPD (FEV_1/FVC <70%) in US adults age 65 years or older was more accurate than ATS for predicting COPD-related hospitalization and mortality. Another cohort study (Güder et al., 2012) looking at adults age 65 years or older found that, compared with the ATS criteria, the GOLD criteria had higher clinical agreement with an expert panel diagnosis for COPD and better identified patients with clinically relevant events (e.g., COPD exacerbation, hospitalization, mortality). Therefore many experts now recommend using the GOLD criteria to diagnose COPD in patients age 65 years or older who have respiratory symptoms and are at risk of COPD (i.e., current or previous smoker). They recommend using the ATS criteria (FEV_1/FVC ratio less than the lower limit of normal) to diagnose COPD in patients younger than 65 years (regardless of smoking status) and in nonsmokers age 65 years or older.

In most cases of obstructive lung disease, the percentage of the predicted value of the $FEF_{25\%-75\%}$ will be "worse" than the percentage of the predicted value of the FEV_1. However, the modifier used to describe the type of obstruction (i.e., mild, moderate, or severe) should be that associated with the value of the FEV_1, not the $FEF_{25\%-75\%}$. The $FEF_{25\%-75\%}$ may be separately referred to with such statements as "... particularly affecting small airways, as reflected in the $FEF_{25\%-75\%}$." Should the $FEF_{25\%-75\%}$ *alone* be abnormal, the diagnosis of obstructive lung disease should not be assumed; rather, the reduction should be interpreted as compatible with "early small airways disease." Again, for comparison over time, the raw curves should be examined to determine adequacy of effort.

Therefore, an FEV_1% less than 75% indicates some loss of elastic recoil (e.g., emphysema) or obstructive disease (e.g., asthma), whereas reduced FVC and FEV_1 (but FEV_1% >75%) indicates restrictive disease. Again, suspicion of restrictive disease warrants referral.

For the final interpretation, the flow-volume loops can be useful in conjunction with the volume-time spirogram. A flow-volume loop can help determine whether an obstruction is in the larger or the smaller airways. It can also help determine whether a restrictive pattern is due to a parenchymal or an extraparenchymal cause. Again, the most useful information obtained from flow-volume loops is usually in the expiratory portion of the flow loop (see Fig. 81.2). However, flow-volume loops may be derived only if the spirometer is accurate in displacement and time.

TABLE 81.3	Change in Spirometric Indexes Over Time		
	% Changes Required to Be Significant		
	FVC	FEV$_1$	FEF$_{25\%-75\%}$
Within a Day			
Normal subjects	≥5%	≥5%	≥13%
Patients with COPD	≥11%	≥13%	≥23%
Week to Week			
Normal subjects	≥11%	≥12%	≥21%
Patients with COPD	≥20%	≥20%	≥30%
Year to Year			
Normal subjects	≥15%	≥15%	
Patients with COPD	≥15%	≥15%	

COPD, Chronic obstructive pulmonary disease; FEF, forced expiratory flow; FEV$_1$, forced expiratory volume at 1 second; FVC, forced vital capacity.
Modified from American Thoracic Society. Lung function testing: Selection of reference value and interpretive strategies. *Am Rev Respir Dis.* 1991;144:1202–1218.

APPLICATION OF SPIROMETRY IN ASTHMA AND CHRONIC OBSTRUCTIVE PULMONARY DISEASE MANAGEMENT

The following flow rates (FEV$_1$; from NAEP Guidelines, 2007) can be used to assess asthma:

≥80%	Mild asthma (if associated with symptoms)
60% to 79%	Moderate asthma
≤60%	Severe asthma

Low FEV$_1$ is associated with increased risk of severe asthma exacerbations. However, in children, exacerbations can happen even with normal FEV$_1$. Consequently, recent emphasis has shifted to FEV$_1$% (FEV$_1$/FVC × 100, with levels of impairment listed in the Flow Rates section) because it may be a more sensitive indicator of asthma severity. Ultimately, in children and adults, treatment decisions should be based on symptoms and frequency and severity of past exacerbations, combined with PFTs as an additional guide.

Spirometry can also be very helpful in staging COPD severity. More important, it provides a basis for medical decisions based on objective data. Revised guidelines (2006) by GOLD through the National Heart Lung and Blood Institute and the World Health Organization on when to consider a clinical change to be significant are briefly summarized in Table 81.3. In this manner, the FEV$_1$ and FEV$_1$/FVC data generated in the clinician's office using a spirometer can define when to "step up" treatment. These organizations also have guidelines about which drugs to use, often in a stepwise fashion, and the clinician should stay current with them.

ERRORS AND RULES OF THUMB IN PULMONARY FUNCTION TESTING

Some technical errors and their effects in PFT include the following:

- An air leak due to a poorly fitting nose clip or mouthpiece can result in a wandering baseline, which can lead to underestimation of many spirometric measurements.
- An incomplete expiration may give a falsely low reading of FVC and a spurious increase in FEF$_{25\%-75\%}$.
- Poor initial expiratory effort may give a falsely low reading of the FEV$_1$ and FEF$_{25\%-75\%}$.

PFTs have a false-positive rate of approximately 5%. Borderline values should be interpreted cautiously. The changes in spirometric results over time for an individual can affect the interpretation of the results. Table 81.3 lists what should be considered a significant change in an individual from day to day, week to week, and year to year.

Lung function declines with age. It is estimated that vital capacity decreases 60 mL/year after peaking during young adulthood. Differentiating "real" decline in lung function from expected test variability across time can be difficult. Recommended requirements for significant spirometric changes (normal variability) have been calculated and are listed in Table 81.3.

Adolescents should not be compared with adult standards until growth and puberty are complete. This recommendation is necessary because leg length, thorax height, and total body height proportions change throughout puberty.

Other sources of error include inadequate preventive maintenance of the equipment, inadequate training of the staff, inadequate patient motivation, not correlating the results with the entire clinical picture (e.g., history, physical examination, radiographic findings), and not ordering more definitive tests when the results are unclear (e.g., obtaining a formal TLC measurement when both FVC and flow are reduced).

In the past, when managing patients with COPD, if the FEV$_1$ went below 1.0 L, the prognosis was thought to worsen dramatically (similar to a cardiac ejection fraction <20%). We now know that patients occasionally can survive for years with an FEV$_1$ less than 1.0 L if they stop smoking and have a good exercise capacity (e.g., can walk several blocks).

For final values that are confusing or do not make sense (e.g., hyperinflation on chest radiograph and abnormal PFTs, yet no history of smoking and no other risk factors for COPD), cardiopulmonary exercise testing (expired gas exercise testing) may be helpful. In addition, one of the most common causes of emphysema (or premature emphysema in nonsmokers) is α$_1$-antitrypsin deficiency. This tends to run in families and can be excluded by a simple blood test that many laboratories perform.

CPT/BILLING CODES

94010	Spirometry, including graphic record, total and timed vital capacity, expiratory flow rate measurement(s), with or without maximal voluntary ventilation
94060	Bronchodilation responsiveness: spirometry as in 94010, before and after bronchodilator administration
94375	Respiratory flow volume loop

ICD-10-CM DIAGNOSTIC CODES

J41.0	Chronic bronchitis, simple
J44.9	Chronic bronchitis, obstructive
J42	Chronic bronchitis, unspecified
J43.9	Emphysema
J45.22	Asthma, mild intermittent, without mention status asthmaticus
J45.909	Asthma, unspecified, without mention status asthmaticus
J81.0	Pulmonary edema, acute
J81.1	Pulmonary edema, chronic

Acknowledgment

The editors recognize the contributions of Michael A. Altman, MD, Edward A. Jackson, MD, and Jose Bayona, MD, to this chapter in previous editions of this text.

SUPPLIERS

(See contact information available at www.expertconsult.com.)

Henry Schein Medical
SDI Diagnostics, Inc.
Vitalograph
Welch Allyn

RECOMMENDED READING

Aaron SD, Dales RE, Cardinal P. How accurate is spirometry at predicting restrictive pulmonary impairment? *Chest*. 1999;115:869–873.

American Thoracic Society. Lung function testing: selection of reference value and interpretative strategies. *Am Rev Respir Dis*. 1991;144:1202–1218.

American Thoracic Society. Standardization of spirometry: 1994 update. *Am J Respir Crit Care Med*. 1995;152:1107–1136.

Culver BH, Graham BL, Coates AL, Wanger J, Berry CE, et al. American Thoracic Society: recommendations for a standardized pulmonary function report. *Am J Respir Crit Care Med*. 2017;196:1463–1472.

Elward KS, Pollart SM. Medical therapy for asthma: updates from the NAEPP guidelines. *Am Fam Physician*. 2010;82(10):1242–1251.

Ferguson GT, Enright PL, Buist AS, Higgins MW. Office spirometry for lung health assessment in adults: a consensus statement from the National Lung Health Education Program. *Chest*. 2000;117:1146–1161.

Güder G, Brenner S, Angermann CE, et al. GOLD or lower limit of normal definition? A comparison with expert-based diagnosis of chronic obstructive pulmonary disease in a prospective cohort-study. *Respir Res*. 2012;13(1):13.

Holzer K, Anderson SD, Douglass J. Exercise in elite summer athletes: challenges for diagnosis. *J Allergy Clin Immunol*. 2002;110(3):374–380.

Johns DP, Walters JAE, Walters EH. Diagnosis and early detection of COPD using spirometry. *J Thorac Dis*. 2014;11:1557–1569.

Johnson JD, Theurer WM. A stepwise approach to the interpretation of pulmonary function tests. *Am Fam Physician*. 2014;89(5):359–366.

Krafczyk MA, Asplund CA. Exercise induced bronchospasm: diagnosis and management. *Am Fam Physician*. 2011;84(4):427–434.

Lee TA, Bartle B, Weiss KB. Spirometry use in clinical practice following diagnosis of COPD. *Chest*. 2006;129:1509–1515.

Mannino DM, Sonia Buist A, Vollmer WM. Chronic obstructive pulmonary disease in the older adult: what defines abnormal lung function? *Thorax*. 2007;62(3):237–241.

Marseglia GL, Cirillo I, Vizzaccaro A, et al. Role of forced expiratory flow at 25–75% as an early marker of small airways impairment in subjects with allergic rhinitis. *Allergy Asthma Proc*. 2007;28:74–78.

McIvor RA, Taskin DP. Underdiagnosis of chronic obstructive pulmonary disease: a rationale for spirometry as a screening tool. *Can Respir J*. 2001;8:153–158.

Miller HR, Hankinson J, Brusasco V, Burgos F, Casaburi R. ATS/ ERS Task Force: standardization of lung function testing. *Eur Respir J*. 2005;26:319–338.

National Asthma Education Program. *National Heart, Blood, and Lung Institute: Expert Panel Report 3: Guidelines for the Diagnosis and Management of Asthma*. Bethesda, MD: Department of Health and Human Services, National Institutes of Health; 2007. http://www.nhlbi.nih.gov/guidelines/asthma/asthgdln.pdf.

Pollart SM, Elward KS. Overview of changes to asthma guidelines. *Am Fam Physician*. 2009;79(9):761–767.

Quanjer PH, Stanojevic S, Cole TJ, Baur X, Hall GL, et al. ERS Global Lung Function Initiative. Multi-ethnic reference values for spirometry for the 3–95 yr age range: the global lung function 2012 equations. *Eur Respir J*. 2012;40:1324–1343.

Qaseem A, Snow V, Fitterman F, et al. Clinical Efficacy Assessment Subcommittee of the American College of Physicians: risk assessment for and strategies to reduce perioperative pulmonary complications for patients undergoing noncardiothoracic surgery: a guideline from the American College of Physicians. *Ann Intern Med*. 2006;144:575–580.

Randolph C. Diagnostic exercise challenge testing. *Curr Allergy Asthma Rep*. 2011;11(6):482–490.

Rundell KW, Slee JB. Exercise and other indirect challenges to demonstrate asthma or exercise-induced bronchoconstriction in athletes. *J Allergy Clin Immunol*. 2008;122(2):238–246.

Smetana FW. Preoperative pulmonary evaluation. *N Engl J Med*. 1999;340:937–944.

Spahn JD, Chipps BE. Office-based objective measures in childhood asthma. *J Pediatr*. 2006;148:11–15.

Vesbo J, Hurd SS, Agustí AG, et al. Global strategy for the diagnosis, management, and prevention of chronic obstructive pulmonary disease: GOLD executive summary. *Am J Respir Crit Care Med*. 2013;187(4):347–365.

Weinberger SE, Cockrill BA, Mandel J. Pulmonary function tests: guidelines for interpretation and sample problems. In: Weinberger SE, Cockrill BA, Mandel J, eds. *Principles of Pulmonary Medicine*. 7th ed. Philadelphia: Elsevier; 2019:386–389.

SPECIAL ANATOMY
RECTAL EXAMINATION

SECTION 6

Gastrointestinal System Procedures

Section Editor: GRANT C. FOWLER

CHAPTER 82

CLINICAL ANORECTAL ANATOMY AND DIGITAL EXAMINATION

James A. Surrell

A practical knowledge of anorectal anatomy is necessary for the proper evaluation and treatment of patients with anorectal complaints, hemorrhoids, and anal fissures. A basic anorectal examination includes *visual* inspection of the perianal tissues and *digital* palpation of the anorectal area. Depending on patient complaints, anoscopy and sigmoidoscopy or colonoscopy may also be necessary. This chapter describes the practical and the clinically important features of anorectal anatomy as well as how to perform a digital examination. See Chapter 83, Anoscopy, for the anoscopic examination.

BASIC ANATOMY

Fig. 82.1 is a diagram of the anatomy of the anal canal and lower rectum.

- *Rectum:* The distal 10 to 12 cm of the colon.
- *Anus:* The outlet of the gastrointestinal tract, consisting of the distal, lower 6 to 8 cm of the bowel.
- *Anal verge:* Most distal extent of the anal canal, just at the opening.
- *Dentate or pectinate line:* The squamocolumnar junction located 2 to 3 cm proximal to the anal verge where there is an abrupt change from columnar or mucosal epithelium to squamous, sensory anoderm. There are no sensory nerve fibers above the dentate line, only visceral-type fibers that sense pressure.
- *Transitional zone.* Composed of mixed columnar and squamous epithelium, where the rectum merges with the anal canal.
- *Internal sphincter:* The innermost circular muscle, under involuntary control.
- *External sphincter:* Located outside (lateral to) the internal sphincter. Note that the external sphincter is external to the internal sphincter not only from a medial to lateral aspect, but also from a cephalic to caudal aspect at the anal verge. It is under voluntary control.
- *Puborectalis muscle (anorectal ring):* Located about 1 to 2 cm above the dentate line. The distal rectum and anal canal are surrounded by two sleeves of circular muscles. This palpable anorectal ring represents the puborectalis muscle, which encircles the very distal rectum, proceeding posteriorly from its anterior point of attachment at the pubis, and then back again to its origin.
- *Valves of Houston:* These are not really "valves" but just folds of mucosa. There are generally three located at approximately 13, 11, and 8 cm (superior, middle, and inferior, respectively) proximal to the anal verge.
- *Anal papillae:* The mucosal tips of the anal glands at the dentate line. (They can become hypertrophied and elongated and be confused with a polyp.)
- *Anal crypt:* A small pocket along the dentate line. Usually the site of cryptitis, which can lead to a fistula.
- *Anal glands:* Located at dentate line. They secrete mucus to lubricate the canal and can become infected or plugged (cryptitis).

- *Columns of Morgagni:* Folds of tissue above the anal crypts/dentate line.
- *Internal hemorrhoids:* Located at and just proximal to the dentate line.
- *External hemorrhoids:* Located distal to the dentate line at the anal verge.
- *Arteriovenous vessels:* Located above, below, or at the dentate line, or both above and below the dentate line.

PATIENT POSITION

A complete anorectal examination can be accomplished with the patient on the examining table in the left lateral decubitus position (Fig. 82.2). The patient's knees are flexed and drawn toward the chest and the buttocks are drawn toward the examiner to a point just slightly off the table (Sims' position). The patient's head and shoulders should remain well toward the middle of the examination table so that the patient is confident that he or she will not fall. This position also directs the axis of the anal canal and rectum directly toward the examiner. Alternatively, the rectum may be examined with the patient in the pelvic/ lithotomy position after a genital examination or in a flexed position while bending 90 degrees over an examination table.

EXTERNAL ANAL EXAMINATION

After appropriately advising the patient, visually inspect the external anus. Look for any signs of perianal inflammation that may suggest pruritus ani or other dermatologic conditions. Gently separate the buttocks; this will generally evert the anoderm to a sufficient degree so that a posterior or anterior anal fissure may be directly visualized. While having the patient perform a Valsalva maneuver, look for any prolapsing hemorrhoids or rectal mucosa.

If there is a sentinel skin tag present in either the posterior or anterior midline, be diligent in evaluation for a fissure, especially if the history is consistent with anal fissure (see Chapter 85, Anal Fissure, Lateral Sphincterotomy, and Anal Fistula). If present, anal skin tags, a perianal abscess, or thrombosed external hemorrhoids should be readily visible at this time. Internal and external hemorrhoids are classically located in the right anterior, right posterior, and left lateral quadrants.

Internal hemorrhoids are located at and just proximal to the dentate line. Because they are above the dentate line, any condition involving them is usually painless. *External hemorrhoids* are located distal to the dentate line at the anal verge, and pathology or treatment in this area is generally quite painful. Hemorrhoids are collections of arteries and veins that, if not enlarged, represent normal anatomy and are not considered varicosities (see Chapter 87, Office Treatment of Hemorrhoids).

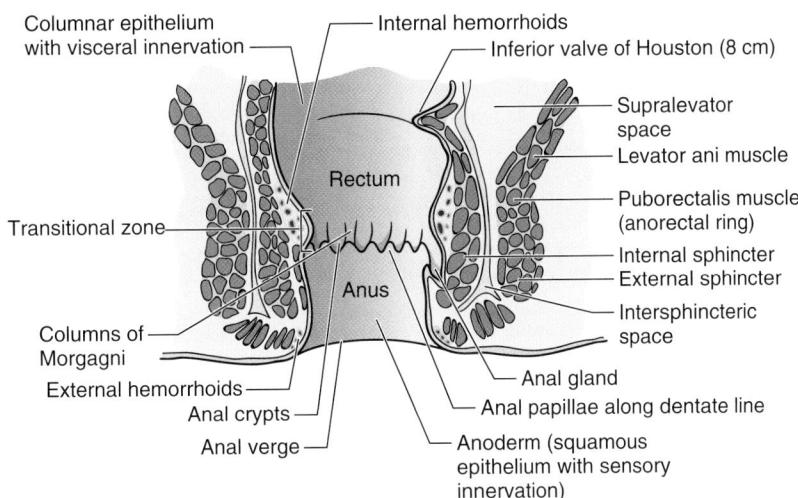

Columnar epithelium
with visceral innervation

Internal hemorrhoids

Inferior valve of Houston (8 cm)

Supralevator
space

Levator ani muscle

Rectum

Puborectalis muscle
(anorectal ring)

Internal sphincter

External sphincter

Transitional zone

Intersphincteric
space

Anus

Columns of
Morgagni

Anal gland

Anal papillae along dentate line

External hemorrhoids

Anoderm (squamous
epithelium with sensory
innervation)

Anal crypts

Anal verge

Fig. 82.1 Anal and rectal anatomy.

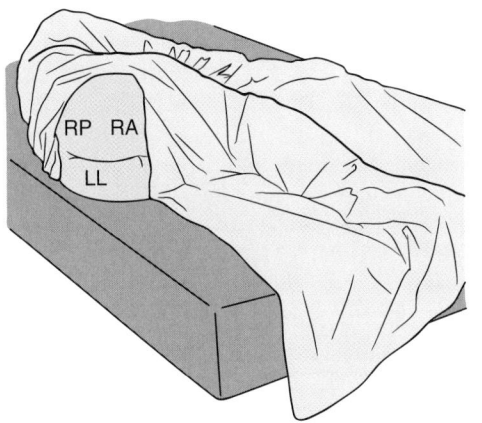

Fig. 82.2 Placing the patient in the left lateral decubitus position (Sims' position). Digital examination, flexible sigmoidoscopy, and most anorectal procedures can be performed in this position. *LL*, Left lateral hemorrhoidal quadrant; *RA*, right anterior; *RP*, right posterior.

It is recommended that clinical anorectal findings be described in terms of the anatomy (i.e., right anterior, right posterior, left anterior, left posterior, right lateral, and left lateral) to provide consistency, regardless of the position of the patient.

CONTRAINDICATIONS TO DIGITAL ANORECTAL EXAMINATION

In some extremely painful conditions, the digital anorectal examination may be postponed until the patient is anesthetized. If the presence of a sharp foreign body (e.g., broken glass) is suspected, performing a digital anorectal examination may injure the examiner, the patient or both. Although not an absolute contraindication, in patients with severe neutropenia and suspected prostatitis, an overly vigorous digital anorectal examination might provoke bacteremia.

DIGITAL ANORECTAL EXAMINATION

Inform the patient that the anus will be touched with a well-lubricated, gloved examining finger. Let them know that it will feel like they are going to have a bowel movement, but they will not. Apply gentle pressure to the anal verge to allow the examining finger to enter the anal canal. If an anal fissure is present, you may feel palpable induration, most commonly in the posterior midline and less commonly in the

anterior midline. Increased tone will also be noted. If the patient complains of severe pain, *do not persist* because you will lose the patient's confidence. You may wish to reattempt the digital examination after applying 5% lidocaine ointment to the anus and waiting 10 to 15 minutes. The most common causes of severe anal pain on examination are a deep symptomatic anal fissure or a perianal abscess. Fissures are found most commonly anteriorly and posteriorly. Rarely, you may need to consider offering the patient an examination under sedation or refer for examination under anesthesia. Otherwise, consciously palpate all around the anorectal area (360 degrees).

In men, assess the prostate gland with your gloved examining finger in the anal canal.

To assess continence and anal sphincter function, flex your index finger slightly posteriorly and ask the patient to "squeeze down" as if to try to stop a bowel movement. If the patient has normal anatomic sphincter function, you will feel the tightening of the distal extent of the external sphincter at the base of your examining finger. The puborectalis muscle of the anorectal ring will also contract, pulling the tip of the examining finger from posterior to anterior. You should then be able to sweep the examining finger around the circumference of the distal rectum at the level of the anorectal ring and note the point of fixation of the puborectalis muscle at the symphysis pubis. Advise the patient to relax as the examination continues.

In general, internal hemorrhoids and the dentate line are not palpable to the gloved examining finger. However, a large hypertrophic anal papilla present at the level of the dentate line may be palpable. If necessary, obtain a small sample of stool on the tip of the gloved examining finger for occult blood testing.

The procedure for anoscopic examination can be found in Chapter 83, Anoscopy. Anal fissures are discussed in Chapter 85, Anal Fissure, Lateral Sphincterotomy, and Anal Fistula.

ANAL CONTINENCE

The external sphincter and puborectalis muscle of the anorectal ring are the two muscles generally thought to afford *voluntary* anal continence. The external sphincter extends from the anal verge to the anorectal ring. The anorectal ring consists primarily of the puborectalis muscle, which encircles the very distal rectum. From a practical standpoint, it is generally accepted that either an intact functional external sphincter or an anorectal ring can provide near-perfect anal continence. The internal sphincter plays little role in maintaining voluntary anal continence. This is important when counseling patients about surgical treatment of anal fissures (see Chapter 85, Anal Fissure, Lateral Sphincterotomy, and Anal Fistula).

SUMMARY

A practical understanding of the anatomy of the anal canal is essential to conducting an adequate anorectal examination. Lesions commonly seen may include pruritus ani or perianal dermatitis, anal fissures, fistulas, thrombosed external hemorrhoids, prolapsing bleeding internal hemorrhoids, hypertrophic anal papillae, perianal abscess, pilonidal disease, condylomata, polyps, cancer, and others. When anal continence is an issue, the clinician must be able to evaluate the function of the external sphincter and of the puborectalis muscle of the anorectal ring on digital anorectal examination. With appropriate patient preparation and technique, the anorectal examination should not be an uncomfortable or painful experience. See Chapter 83, Anoscopy, for a description of the anoscopic examination.

RECOMMENDED READING

Coates WC. Anorectal procedures. In: Roberts JR, Custalow CB, Thomsen TW, eds. *Roberts and Hedges Clinical Procedures in Emergency Medicine.* 6th ed. Philadelphia: Elsevier; 2014:880.

Pfenninger JL, Zainea G. Common anorectal conditions: part I. Symptoms and complaints. *Am Fam Physician.* 2001;63:2391–2398.

Pfenninger JL, Zainea G. Common anorectal conditions: part II. Lesions. *Am Fam Physician.* 2001;64:77–88.

Swarz MH. The abdomen. In: Swarz MH, ed. *Textbook of Physical Diagnosis.* 7th ed. Philadelphia: Elsevier; 2014:429–467.

CHAPTER 83

ANOSCOPY

Peter L. Reynolds • Thad Wilkins

Anoscopy is a common procedure in both ambulatory and emergency medical care. It is used primarily to evaluate the patient with perianal and anal complaints. It may also be performed just before or after withdrawing the colonoscope or flexible sigmoidoscope. Chapter 82, Clinical Anorectal Anatomy and Digital Examination, includes a review of clinical anatomy. High-resolution anoscopy (HRA) is a technique to evaluate patients at high risk for complications from anal human papillomavirus (HPV) infection. This includes men who have sex with men, individuals infected with human immunodeficiency virus, transplant patients, and women who participate in anal receptive intercourse or with lower genital tract dysplasia. With HRA, the anus is stained with acetic acid and then evaluated using magnification—usually a colposcope (see Chapter 84, High-Resolution Anoscopy and Anal Pap Smear).

INDICATIONS

- Initial evaluation of rectal bleeding
- Anal or perianal pain
- Perianal itching (pruritus ani)
- Anal discharge
- Prolapse of the rectum
- External or internal hemorrhoids
- Anal fissures
- Anal fistulas
- Painful digital rectal examination
- Perianal condylomata
- Palpable masses on digital examination
- In association with sigmoidoscopy and colonoscopy (screening or diagnostic)
- Evaluation of intra-anal trauma
- Follow-up of inflammatory bowel
- Retrieval of foreign body
- Evaluation of sexual abuse
- Fecal impaction
- Anal polyps, cancer
- Screening for anal HPV in high-risk individuals

CONTRAINDICATIONS

- Unwilling patient
- Severe debilitation
- Acute myocardial infarction or similar cardiovascular condition
- Acute abdomen (relative contraindication)
- Marked anal canal stenosis or imperforate anus
- Severe pain

EQUIPMENT

- Anoscope (slotted Ives preferred, but sometimes disposable clear cylindrical is all that is available; there are now disposable, clear slotted Ives anoscopes available)
- Light source
- Gloves and equipment necessary to maintain universal blood and body fluid precautions
- Lubricant jelly (water soluble preferred)
- Large-tipped cotton swabs and 4 cm gauze pads
- Enema (optional)
- Biopsy forceps, if needed (cervical biopsy forceps or the flexible wire biopsy forceps used during sigmoidoscopy or colonoscopy work well)
- Monsel solution (ferric subsulfate solution) if biopsies performed (silver nitrate can also be used but it burns, so only apply above the pectinate line)

The anoscope consists of two parts: a hollow, gently tapering cylinder and a solid obturator that fits inside. The components are made of disposable plastic or reusable metal (Fig. 83.1). Clear plastic anoscopes may provide better visualization of the rectal and anal mucosa than opaque devices, but they do tend to compress the tissues and may obscure some findings (e.g., hemorrhoids). The size varies from 7 to 10 cm in length. They may or may not have handles. The distal diameter is approximately 2.5 cm.

Some anoscopes are readily attachable to battery-powered light sources. Others require an external light source (e.g., a gooseneck lamp or headlight).

The *Ives slotted anoscope* is usually made of metal but has an open slot on one half of the upper side of the device (see Fig. 83.1D–E). The slot provides an unobstructed view of the walls of the anal canal. This instrument is extremely useful not only for evaluation but also for use when treating various conditions. The advantage of the slotted instrument is that after the obturator is removed, the mucosa is no longer compressed; thus, small lesions and hemorrhoids may be more readily visible and treated. The diameter is also larger than most other anoscopes, and consequently instruments are more easily manipulated within the lumen. Rather than looking through the end of the tube, the operator can visualize the mucosal wall in a more direct fashion (Fig. 83.2).

PREPROCEDURE PATIENT PREPARATION

Patients dread inspection of the anal canal. They perceive this examination as unpleasant and uncomfortable, if not painful. There are always concerns of embarrassment. This mandates that the patient be prepared mentally for what is involved. However, these concerns should not dissuade the clinician from doing the examination when it is indicated. Far too often the "assumed" diagnosis by the patient or the clinician is made without completing a visual examination. This is not only unacceptable, but it can also place the patient at great risk for missed diagnoses such as cancer, inflammatory bowel disease, or other significant problems. The patient must be cooperative and relaxed. No oral bowel prep is necessary, but an enema may be helpful. Frank admission that the procedure will be unpleasant and uncomfortable, but not painful, is helpful. Explain the reasons necessitating the examination and the implications of not performing it. Reassure the patient that there are no significant complications resulting from anoscopy alone. However, if a biopsy is obtained or a lesion is removed, there may be some bleeding. If the biopsy is from below the dentate line, it will also be painful and local anesthetic will be needed.

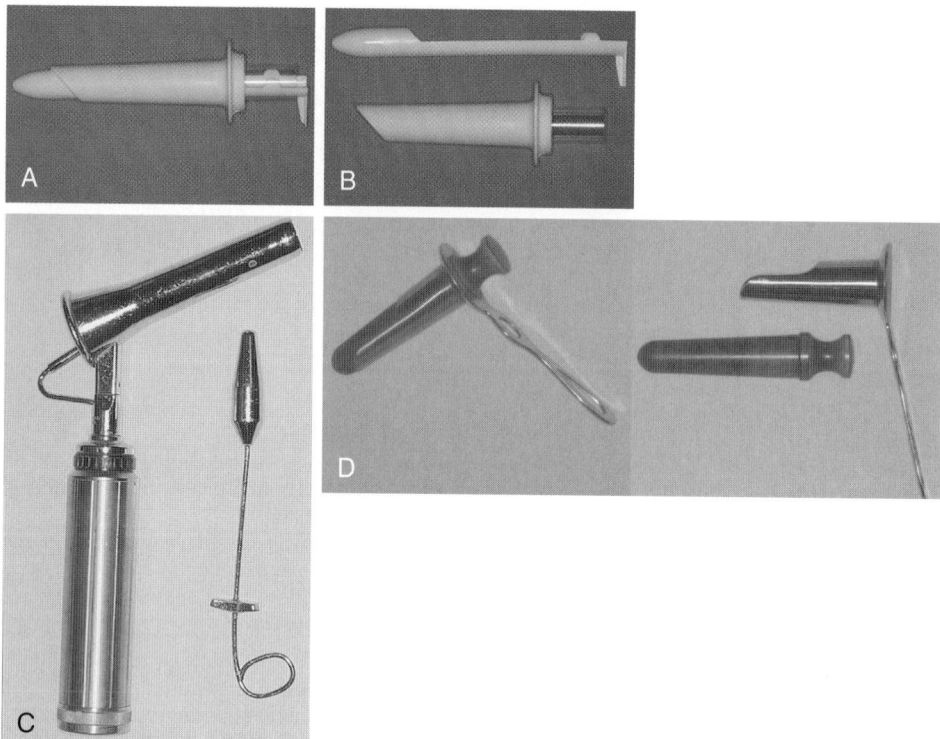

Fig. 83.1 Disposable plastic opaque anoscope requiring external light source with obturator in place (A) and obturator removed (B). Reusable type for use with battery-powered light source; inserting trocar has been removed (C). (D) Ives slotted anoscope with obturator in place *(left)* and obturator removed *(right)*. The Ives slotted anoscope provides the best visualization and the most operative space for any necessary procedures.

If the reason for the examination is to evaluate anal pain (e.g., possible fissure), patients can be extremely tender and apprehensive. In addition, the anal sphincter contracts, making the examination difficult. Application of a topical anesthetic, such as 5% lidocaine, 30 minutes before the examination can markedly reduce discomfort (see Chapter 4, Topical Anesthesia). If the pain is so severe that the examination needs to be deferred, the presumptive diagnosis is an anal fissure. But the examination, perhaps at a later date after treatment, is necessary to confirm that there is no other pathologic process.

TECHNIQUE

An assistant is helpful, and gender-appropriate chaperones are recommended. Both the clinician and assistant must wear gloves on both hands. An enema is usually not needed but may be helpful. Consider eye protection equipment necessary for universal blood and body fluid precautions.

1. Place the patient in the left lateral position and drape. This position is most comfortable for the patient and is adequate in at least 95% of situations. At times, placing the patient in stirrups or in the head-down position may be indicated.
2. Have the assistant separate the glutei laterally, allowing full visibility of the perianal area. Alternatively, have the patient pull up on their right gluteus. Check for any obvious lesions and possible fistulous tracks.
3. Inspect the tissue closely. Ask the patient to bear down, and observe for hemorrhoid or polyp prolapse.
4. Perform a careful circumferential digital examination with an index finger that has been lubricated with jelly or 2% lidocaine jelly. Note the sphincter tone. (See Chapter 82, Clinical Anorectal Anatomy and Digital Examination.)
5. In male patients, palpate the prostate for size and masses.
6. Lubricate the anoscope well with jelly with the obturator in place (see Fig. 83.1). Place a gauze pad nearby on which to place the obturator when removed.

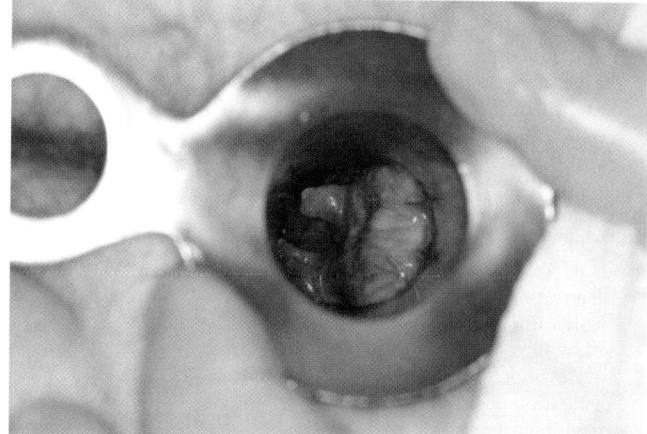

Fig. 83.2 Hypertrophic papilla found on anoscopic examination (Ives slotted anoscope). This is often palpable as a firm mass.

7. Gently insert the anoscope into the anal aperture, gradually overcoming the resistance of the sphincters. Advance the instrument in the direction of the umbilicus until the full length of the anoscope is inserted (subject to patient acceptance and tolerance). The procedure is better tolerated and accomplished by asking the patient to gently take a few deep breaths at the beginning of the procedure and to bear down just slightly. If the patient complains of pain with insertion, the quality and location should be noted and correlated with clinical symptoms. If the obturator falls out while inserting the anoscope, remove the whole instrument and start over. This will avoid pinching the mucosa by merely trying to reinsert the obturator.
8. After inserting the full length of the instrument, remove the obturator so that the mucosa of the anal canal can be visualized.

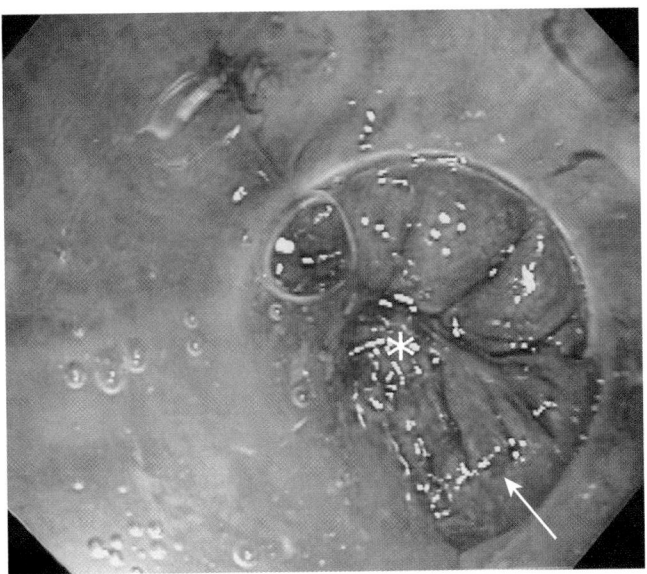

Fig. 83.3 Pectinate (dentate) line *(arrow)* and small bleeding internal hemorrhoid *(asterisk)* seen as anoscope is slowly withdrawn.

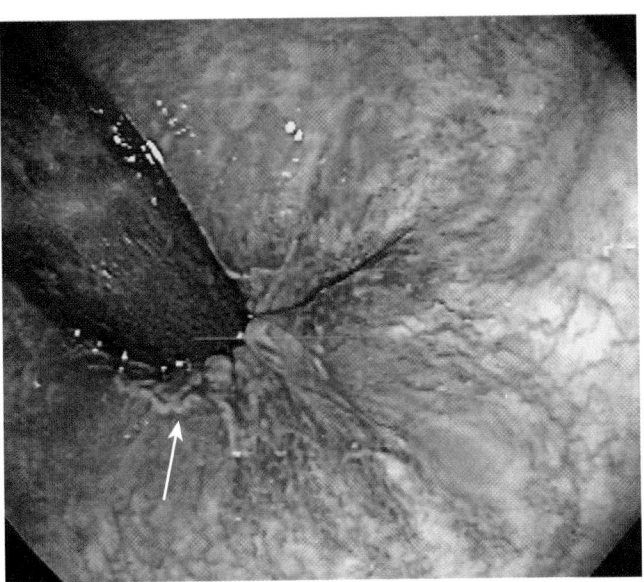

Fig. 83.4 View of same patient as in Fig. 83.3 using a retroflexed colonoscope. Pectinate line is indicated by the *arrow*. (Note that internal hemorrhoids are flattened by insufflated air.)

The obturator can be placed on a nearby gauze pad. Fecal material is often encountered and can be removed with a large swab. Note the gross appearance of the mucous membrane, the pectinate (dentate) line, and the vasculature, as well as the presence of blood, mucus, pus, ulcerations, polyps, hemorrhoidal tissue, and so forth.

9. Gradually withdraw the instrument with the obturator still removed. Observe the anal canal as the anoscope is extracted. Fig. 83.3 shows a small, bleeding internal hemorrhoid as seen through the opening of the anoscope. For reference, the same area is shown in Fig. 83.4 as visualized through a retroflexed colonoscope. With opaque devices, rotate the long-cylinder anoscopes to the right and left to ensure that the entire canal has been visualized. The Ives slotted instrument must be inserted four times so that each quadrant can be examined. Usually it is inserted with the handle at the 12, 3, 6 and 9 o'clock positions to maintain orientation for future documentation. Keeping it in place for a minute or two in each position allows any hemorrhoids that are present to engorge

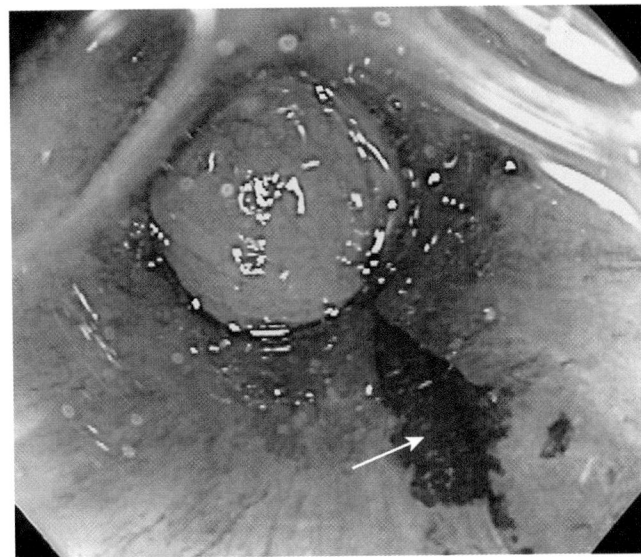

Fig. 83.5 Anal fissure seen through the wall of a clear plastic anoscope *(arrow)*.

with blood and be more readily visible. Do not rotate this instrument because it causes discomfort. The clear plastic anoscope allows the examiner to visualize the mucosa both through the anoscope as well as at the opening of the device. Fig. 83.5 shows an anal fissure as seen through the wall of the anoscope.

10. Beware of rectal spasm that can occur during the last stage of withdrawal of the anoscope. The may cause the anoscope to be expelled quickly or with some force. Use firm counterpressure to prevent such rapid expulsion.

11. If a biopsy is to be obtained, a variety of long-handled biopsy instruments can be used. The instruments used for cervical biopsy work well (obtain the smallest "bite" possible). The clinician can also use the biopsy forceps normally used for flexible sigmoidoscopy. In this case it is applied with direct visualization of the areas. Expect some bleeding, but it is usually readily controlled with Monsel solution or silver nitrate and natural pressure when the anoscope is removed. Silver nitrate burns when applied, so it may be best to avoid applying below the pectinate line. Stay superficial; only 3 or 4 mm of tissue is necessary.

11. Complete the procedure form (Fig. 83.6).

COMPLICATIONS

Anoscopy, when performed gently, has few, if any, complications. Likely or possible complications include discomfort, tearing of the perianal skin or mucosa, and abrasion or tearing of hemorrhoidal tissue. There may be bleeding, especially after biopsy, but infection almost never occurs. Note that not every anal fissure will be identified with an anoscope; they can be small and missed if the mucosa is not fully distended.

POSTPROCEDURE PATIENT EDUCATION

Thoroughly explain the findings to the patient, and use pictures and drawings in the explanation. Discuss the etiology, treatment, and course of resolution for each finding as thoroughly as possible.

CPT/BILLING CODES

46600	Anoscopy, diagnostic
46604	Anoscopy with dilation
46606	Anoscopy with biopsy, single or multiple
46608	Anoscopy with removal of foreign body
46610	Anoscopy with polypectomy, hot or bipolar forceps
46611	Anoscopy with polypectomy, snare technique

ANOSCOPY

Patient name _____ B.D. _____ Sex _____
Patient ID # _____
Procedure _____ Date _____
Chief complaint: _____
Subjective: _____
Past medical history: _____
_____
_____
Medications: _____
_____
_____
Family history: _____
_____
_____

FINDINGS
                          Normal   **Abnormal**

Perianal skin
Prostate
Sphincter tone
Anal canal
Dentate line visualized?
Mucosa
Tears/fissure
Vasculature
Tumor/polyps
Bleeding
Hemorrhoids
Imp   _____
           _____
           _____

Follow-up date _____
Clinician _____ Date _____

Fig. 83.6 Procedure form for anoscopy.

46612	Anoscopy with removal multiple polyps
46614	Anoscopy with control of bleeding
46615	Anoscopy with ablation of tumor(s), polyp(s), or other lesion(s)
46900	Destruction, lesions (e.g., condyloma), chemical
46910	Destruction, lesions, electrodessication
46916	Destruction, lesions, cryocautery
46917	Destruction, lesions, laser
46922	Destruction, lesions, excision

ICD-10-CM Diagnostic Codes

C20	Cancer, rectum
C21.0	Cancer, anus
D12.7	Benign neoplasm, colon
K64.8	Internal hemorrhoids
K64.5	Internal hemorrhoid, thrombosed
K64.9	Internal hemorrhoid, bleeding
K64.4	External hemorrhoid
K64.4	Hemorrhoidal skin tags
K50.10	Crohn disease: colon
K51.90	Ulcerative colitis
K52.0	Radiation colitis
K52.9	Colitis, nonspecific
K59.00	Constipation
K58.9	Irritable colon

K60.2	Anal fissure
K60.3	Anal fistula
K61.1	Perirectal abscess
K61.0	Perianal abscess
K61.3	Ischiorectal abscess
K61.4	Intersphincteric abscess
K62.0	Anal polyp
K62.5	Anal hemorrhage
K62.89	Anal pain
L29.0	Pruritus ani
R15.9	Stool incontinence
R19.8	Tenesmus
T18.5XX	Foreign body, anus

Add additional seventh character: A = initial, D = subsequent, S = sequela.

Online Resources

Mir F: Anoscopy: http://emedicine.medscape.com/article/79937-overview.

Recommended Reading

Abdelnaby A, Downs JM. Diseases of the anorectum. In: *Sleisenger and Fordtran's Gastrointestinal and Liver Diease*. 10th ed. Philadelphia: Elsevier; 2016:2312–2336.

Coates WC. Anorectal procedures. In: Roberts JR, Custalow CB, Thomsen TW, eds. *Roberts and Hedges Clinical Procedures in Emergency Medicine*. 6th ed. Philadelphia: Elsevier; 2014:880–883.

CHAPTER 84

HIGH-RESOLUTION ANOSCOPY AND ANAL PAP SMEAR

J. Michael Berry • Naomi Jay

High-resolution anoscopy (HRA) is the examination of the anus and perianal region using a colposcope for magnification. It is a technique pioneered at the University of California, San Francisco in the Anal Neoplasia Study to determine the natural history of human papillomavirus (HPV)–related anal neoplasia. Similar to examination of the cervix, 3% acetic acid is applied to the anus and a colposcope is used to carefully examine the anal mucosa and perianal skin. Lesions can be identified using standard colposcopic criteria and sampled for histologic confirmation.

High-risk HPV types are found in up to 93% of anal cancers. High-grade anal intraepithelial neoplasia (HGAIN), including AIN grade 2 or 3 (moderate or severe dysplasia) or carcinoma in situ, are considered potentially precancerous lesions. It is believed that identification and eradication of HGAIN may prevent anal cancer, but studies demonstrating this principle have yet to be completed (Anal Cancer HSIL (High-grade Squamous Intraapithelial Lesion) Outcomes Research Study or ANCHOR). The anus and cervix are similar biologically: both have a squamocolumnar junction, both are susceptible to the same types of HPV, and both demonstrate a similar spectrum of lesions. Because of these similarities, techniques for cervical cancer screening have been adapted for the anus.

EDITOR'S NOTE: Centers for Disease Control and Prevention currently does not recommend routine anal cancer screening with cytology in persons with human immunodeficiency virus (HIV) infection, men-who-have-sex-with-men (MSM) without HIV infection, or the general population because the data are considered insufficient. They also do not recommend anal screening for high-risk oncogenic HPV infections in MSM because of a high prevalence of anal HPV infection.

In the United States in 2018, it was estimated that there were 8300 new cases of anal cancer—2770 in men and 5530 in women. The incidence in the general population is 1.5 in 100,000. In human immunodeficiency virus–negative MSM, before the HIV epidemic, the incidence was estimated to be 35 in 100,000. Since the introduction of highly active antiretroviral therapy, studies demonstrate an incidence twice that in several cohorts of HIV-positive patients, ranging from 78.2 to 92 per 100,000. The relative risk for anal cancer is increased to 4.68 (95% confidence interval 3.87 to 5.62) in women with a history of grade 3 cervical intraepithelial neoplasia (CIN) compared with women with no history.

Anal HPV infection can be found in more than 90% of HIV-positive MSM and approximately 60% of HIV-negative MSM. HRA with biopsy of suspect lesions found HGAIN in 52% of HIV-positive MSM, and in 16% of HIV-negative MSM at baseline in a cohort of men enrolled in the University of California, San Francisco Anal Neoplasia Study between 1998 and 2000. A more recent population-based sample found rates of anal HPV infection of 57% in HIV-negative versus 88% in HIV-positive MSM. HGAIN was detected during HRA-guided biopsy in 25% and 43%, respectively.

In a study of 470 HIV-positive and 185 HIV-negative women, anal HPV was found in 80% of HIV-seropositive women compared with 50% of HIV-seronegative women. HGAIN was found in 9% of HIV-positive women and in 1% of HIV-negative women. In HIV-negative women with a history of CIN, 58% had anal HPV (slightly more than 30% had cervical HPV) and 15% had abnormal anal cytology. In women without a history of CIN who presented for sexually transmitted infection testing, 53% had anal HPV and 11% had anal squamous intraepithelial lesions. A group of 40 women with vulvar cancer were compared to 80 age-matched control women who were all examined with HRA. Coexistent HGAIN in 15 patients and 1 invasive anal cancer were found in the patients with vulvar cancer, compared with no cases of HGAIN in the control subjects.

Markov modeling demonstrated that anal cytology for anal cancer screening is cost effective every 2 to 3 years in HIV-negative MSM and every 1 to 2 years in HIV-positive MSM. In spite of these data, except for the state of New York, there are no official public health recommendations for screening programs. There are several reasons why routine screening programs have not been recommended in spite of convincing epidemiologic data. Data are just emerging demonstrating that HGAIN can progress to cancer. Currently, no controlled clinical trials (ANCHOR study) have been completed demonstrating that screening and treatment of HGAIN prevent anal cancer. Another main limiting factor for screening is the lack of providers trained and experienced in performing HRA.

Ideally, HRA should be used to identify and target lesions for treatment because these lesions are largely invisible without the application of acetic acid and magnification. Data from several papers demonstrate that HGAIN can be effectively eradicated in many patients using an office-based procedure known as *infrared coagulation* (see Chapter 87, Office Treatment of Hemorrhoids). Patients with more extensive lesions are effectively managed with a combination of targeted surgical therapy of HGAIN guided by HRA coupled with office-based infrared coagulation to manage the inevitable recurrences. There was no evidence of HGAIN in 192 of 246 (78%) patients treated with this combined approach at their last follow-up visit.

Screening HIV-positive MSM with anal cytology and referring those with any level of cytologic abnormality can be recommended based on demonstrated cost effectiveness and increased prevalence of HGAIN and anal cancer. Some providers believe that if resources are available, all HIV-positive MSM could be examined with HRA to maximize detection of HGAIN. For similar reasons, all MSM could be offered anal cytology screening. Because of the known association between high-risk HPV, high-grade CIN and vulvar intraepithelial neoplasia, and cervical and vulvar cancer, anal cytology screening may also be useful in women with these findings, followed by referral for HRA for any cytologic abnormalities.

Solid organ transplant recipients are at increased risk of anogenital cancer and may benefit from screening as well. Patients with perianal condylomata, regardless of sex or sexual orientation, may also benefit from screening.

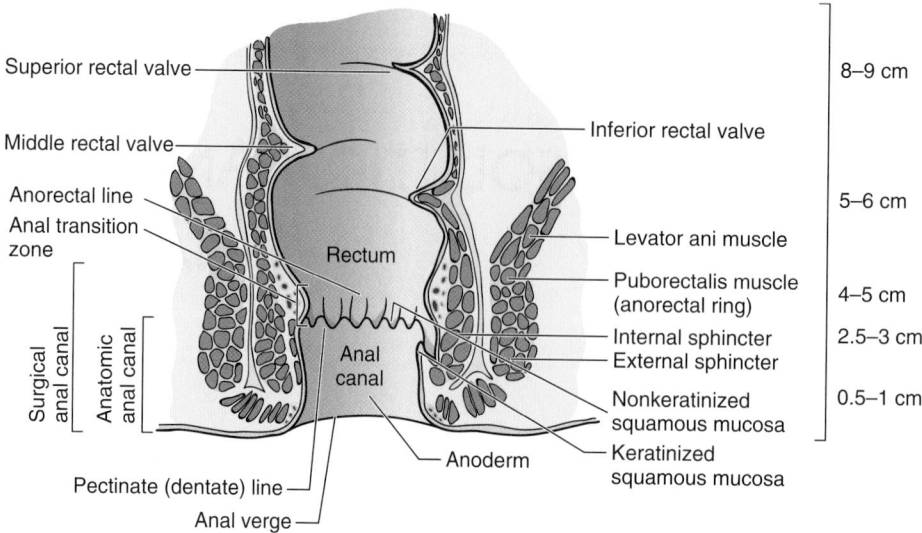

Fig. 84.1 Anal anatomy.

Anal Pap/cytology screening in patients at increased risk for anal cancer requires that providers experienced in performing HRA be available to follow up on any abnormal results. HRA is a necessary requisite for a successful program in managing anal neoplasia because in the absence of palpable or visible lesions such as condylomata or anal masses, *most HGAIN lesions are not visible or palpable.*

Formal programs for training and standards in performing HRA are in place. The first course in HRA was conducted in San Francisco in conjunction with the American Society for Colposcopy and Cervical Pathology and coupled with this group's Comprehensive Colposcopy course in August 2005. It is now offered annually.

Before learning HRA, providers should attend a formal colposcopy course and a formal didactic course in HRA, if possible. After basic colposcopy skills have been gained, attending an existing anal neoplasia clinic and spending several days observing HRA and the performance of anal biopsies in multiple patients is helpful. Further experience can be gained only by performing the procedure. Novices are advised to keep a logbook of all of their patients and to record their clinical and colposcopic impression. This can then be correlated with the cytologic and histologic results when they become available. This allows not only for patient follow-up, triage, and disposition, but for the clinician to develop and hone his or her clinical skills.

ANATOMY

Like the cervix, the anus has a *transformation zone* (AnTZ) and a *squamocolumnar junction* (SCJ), where the anal squamous mucosa is adjacent to the colonic columnar epithelium (Fig. 84.1). The SCJ is above the dentate or pectinate line. A similar process of squamous metaplasia occurs in the AnTZ, and dysplastic changes can occur during this dynamic time of transformation. When performing anal cytology, it is important to sample all areas of the AnTZ, just like in the cervix, so that cells are sampled from all areas. An adequate cytologic sample will have columnar or squamous metaplasia, which indicates that the AnTZ was sampled.

INDICATIONS

Other than for a formal screening program for those at risk (MSM, anal-receptive intercourse, women with high-grade cervical and vulvar dysplasias/cancers, and organ transplant recipients), reasons patients may be referred for HRA include the following:

- Abnormal anal Pap/cytology of any degree
- Incidentally detected condylomata or HGAIN during colonoscopy
- Before hemorrhoidectomy or surgery for other benign anorectal conditions for those at risk to rule out concurrent disease and allow treatment at the same time

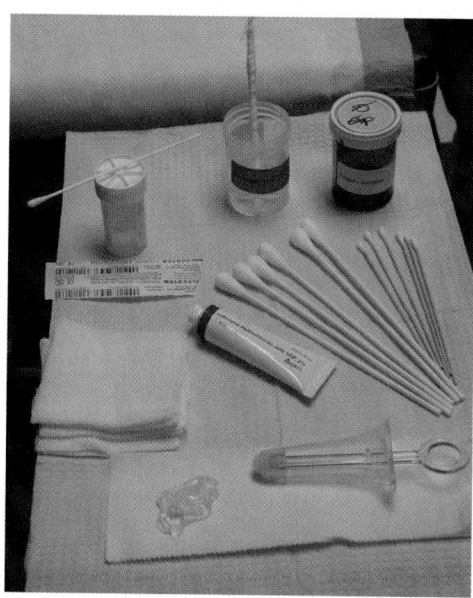

Fig. 84.2 A typical equipment tray for high-resolution anoscopy.

- Perianal lesions, including condylomata, hyperpigmented lesions typical of Bowen disease, erythematous lesions, ulcerations, or masses
- Evaluation of anal symptoms such as irritation, itching, pain with bowel movements, bleeding or discomfort with receptive intercourse
- Self-detected lump or bump
- Prior history of anal condylomata, HGAIN, or anal cancer
- CIN, vulvar dysplasia

CONTRAINDICATIONS

Severe neutropenia (<1000) is the one absolute contraindication to performing HRA. Current or past neutropenia or thrombocytopenia may indicate the need to defer biopsies or have current blood work available to determine the safety of performing biopsies.

EQUIPMENT AND SUPPLIES

Most of the equipment is the same as that used for a cervical examination (see Chapter 124, Colposcopic Examination). A procedure tray for HRA is shown in Fig. 84.2. The tray includes the following:

- Cytology liquid medium (or conventional slide with fixative solution)
- Dacron swab (Q-tip) (not on wooden or prescored stick)
- Anoscope (disposable plastic or sterilized metal)
- 3% acetic acid
- Nonsterile cotton swabs
- Nonsterile Scopettes
- Nonsterile 4 × 4 gauze pads
- Lugol solution
- Water-soluble lubricant jelly mixed with 1% to 5% lidocaine gel
- A 4 × 4 gauze wrapped around a cotton swab

Additional Equipment for Biopsies

- Formalin bottles
- Baby Tischler or mini-Townsend cervical punch biopsy or endoscopy forceps
- Monsel solution or silver nitrate

Additional Equipment for Perianal Biopsies

- 1% lidocaine with epinephrine and sodium bicarbonate (2 mL per 10 mL of lidocaine)
- 22-gauge needle (to fill syringe)
- 30-gauge needle (for injection)
- 1-mL syringe
- Small pickup Adson forceps, generally without teeth, punch biopsy
- Silver nitrate used for hemostasis

Colposcope

The following specifications are helpful for performing HRA with a colposcope:

- Double objective lens with magnification up to 25×
- Angled eyepieces (the straight-on view is ergonomically difficult for HRA unless the height of the table is adjustable)
- Side-swing arm

PREPROCEDURE PATIENT EDUCATION

Patients should be told to refrain from inserting anything per anus for 24 hours before the procedure. This includes anal sex and insertion of any toy, medication, or enemas.

When discussing the procedure with patients, explain that a normal examination with biopsies will take 10 to 20 minutes. There are no pain nerve endings in the anal canal above the dentate line, only below it. The majority of lesions are above the dentate line and so biopsies are rarely felt beyond a sensation of minor pressure. The examination itself is not painful, but often there is mild discomfort associated with the pressure of the anoscope on the sphincter. Incontinence is rare, but patients should be told that the pressure will make them feel as if they need to have a bowel movement.

Medical history should include prior anal diseases, including abnormal cytology results, diagnoses of condylomata, low-grade anal intraepithelial neoplasia (LGAIN), HGAIN, or cancer, and any treatments used. In women, prior or current genital HPV-associated disease is important. A history of rectal abscesses, fistula tracts, fissures, or hemorrhoids can help determine potential sources of pain, bleeding, and scar tissue. Evaluate for history of immunosuppression or immune-suppressing drug therapy for organ transplantation, lupus, Crohn disease, or any disease requiring ongoing steroid therapy.

Complications such as severe bleeding and infection are rare. Scant bleeding after a biopsy may occur over a 1- to 2-day period and is not cause for alarm. Vasovagal reactions occur rarely.

PROCEDURE

Anal Pap/Cytology

Anal cytology results are categorized according to the Bethesda classification system using terminology similar to that for cervical cytology. Anal cytology sensitivity for detection of anal neoplasia is comparable to that of cervical cytology, with a 25% or higher miss rate. The goal of anal cytology screening is to identify patients with HGAIN, who can then be treated. Cytology should be repeated every 2 to 3 years in low-risk patients and more frequently in high-risk patients (Fig. 84.3).

Anal cytology is used to identify those populations and individuals most likely to have HPV-associated disease. An anal cytology result of ASCUS (atypical squamous cells of undetermined significance) or higher grade is considered abnormal, and HRA is advised based on research showing that the sensitivity for cytology screening improved when ASCUS was used as the threshold for abnormal. The cytology result is considered a screening test and is not diagnostic. The diagnosis will be provided through HRA-identified and sampled lesions. Fig. 84.3 provides a screening and HRA algorithm.

Performing Anal Pap/Cytology

The anal cytology specimen should be obtained before HRA and any digital examination to obtain the highest yield of cells without interference from lubricants.

1. The left lateral position provides adequate comfort for the patient and good visualization for the clinician. However, the lithotomy position can be used, and if a proctology table is available, patients can lean forward and lie prone.
2. Gently separate the buttocks. Patients can hold their buttock to facilitate the view.
3. Insert a moistened Dacron swab approximately 4 to 5 cm into the anus. For most patients this will ensure adequate sampling of the AnTZ. (However, the depth for location of the AnTZ and SCJ varies in individuals. In some it is a significant distance in [5 to 6 cm], whereas in others it is just inside the anal verge.) The swab should be inserted just past the internal sphincter until it abuts the rectal wall. If initial resistance is encountered, change the angle of the swab and reinsert. Then insert until resistance is felt above the internal sphincter. It should be possible to insert the swab with very little discomfort. Use a nonscored, plastic Dacron swab because the scored swabs can break when pressure is applied (Fig. 84.4).
4. While slowly withdrawing the swab, apply pressure against the anal sidewalls and sample the entire circumference of the canal, going in a circular motion. This facilitates sampling cells from all aspects of the canal. A slight bending in the "stick" while removing the swab indicates that adequate pressure is being used. Count slowly to 10 as you remove it to maximize the yield of exfoliating cells.
5. Preserve the sample quickly on slides for a conventional smear, or in liquid medium. Fewer cells exfoliate from the anal canal than the cervix, and air-dried artifacts can be more problematic. If using conventional slides it is better to quickly immerse the slides in cytology fluid rather than spraying them.
6. Digital rectal examination may be the most sensitive way of detecting an actual cancer and therefore should be performed in all patients after a cytologic sample has been obtained.

Performing High-Resolution Anoscopy

After an abnormal cytology result, or for a routine baseline examination in an at-risk individual, HRA is used to inspect the AnTZ, SCJ, anal canal, anal verge, and perianal areas. The clinician identifies lesions based on clinical impression and obtains biopsies to determine the level and extent of disease for treatment.

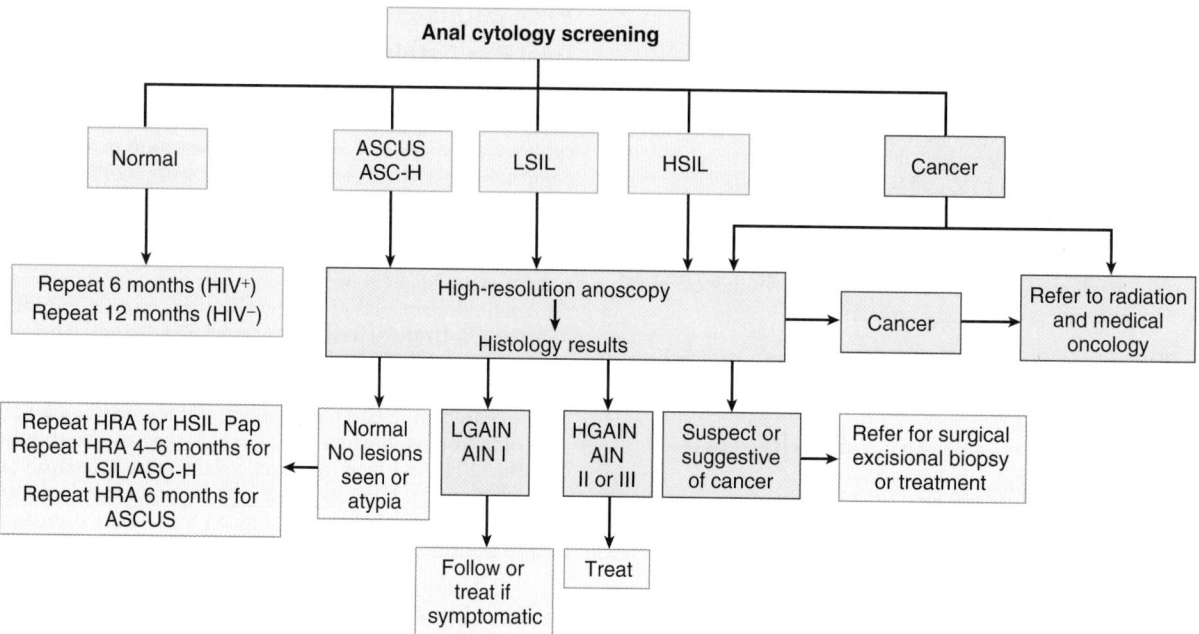

Fig. 84.3   Anal cytology screening triage algorithm. *AIN*, Anal intraepithelial neoplasia; *ASC-H*, atypical squamous cells, cannot exclude high-grade lesion; *ASCUS*, atypical squamous cells of undetermined significance; *HGAIN*, high-grade anal intraepithelial neoplasia; *HIV*, human immunodeficiency virus; *HRA*, high-resolution anoscopy; *HSIL*, high-grade squamous intraepithelial lesion; *LGAIN*, low-grade anal intraepithelial neoplasia; *LSIL*, low-grade squamous intraepithelial lesion.

Although basic colposcopy skills form a foundation for HRA, there are several unique differences in the skill sets required to accurately recognize lesions and to manage anal neoplasia. Mucosal folds and hemorrhoidal bulges make visualization of the entire SCJ difficult; unfortunately it is common for lesions to be hidden within the folds. Additional acetic acid must be applied during the examination to the entire SCJ and canal. Lesions may be more subtle in their presentation compared to colposcopy, with variations of acetowhitening and epithelial changes. Similar to colposcopy, having a low threshold for taking biopsies is necessary, particularly in the early stages of learning HRA.

1. The same position can be used for HRA as for the cytologic collection. If a cervical examination is also being performed, the lithotomy position can be used, but most women prefer to switch to the left lateral position for HRA. A prone position can be used if an overhead colposcope is available. If in the lithotomy position, patients should lie as close to the bottom edge of the table as possible to ensure adequate focusing of the colposcope. In the left lateral decubitus position, they should lie as close to the edge of the table as possible with the anus directed at the examiner. A power table facilitates the use of a colposcope.

2. After a cytologic sample has been obtained (if indicated), perform a digital rectal examination. Lubricate the anal canal with water soluble jelly mixed with 2% to 5% lidocaine gel. Palpate for warts, masses, ulcerations, fissures, and focal areas of discomfort or pain. The presence of hard, fixed, or painful lesions should increase your index of suspicion for cancer because warts and hemorrhoids do not usually present in these ways. Make note of scar tissue, which will feel less elastic and may have thickening, ridges, and firm areas. Prior abscess, fistula repair, and surgery for warts are possible causes for scarring.

3. Insert a well-lubricated anoscope and remove the obturator (see Chapter 83, Anoscopy). Wrap a 4 × 4 gauze that has been soaked in acetic acid around a cotton swab and insert it through the anoscope. Remove the anoscope, leaving the cotton swab–wrapped gauze inside (Fig. 84.5).

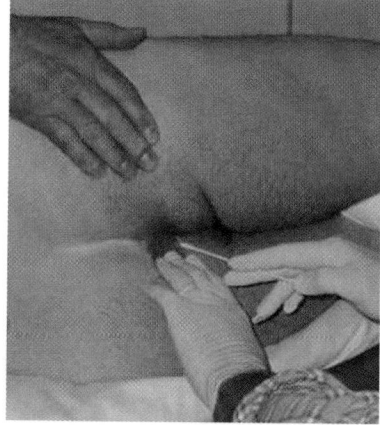

Fig. 84.4   Insertion of Dacron swab for anal cytology. Retracting the buttocks facilitates more comfortable insertion of the swab.

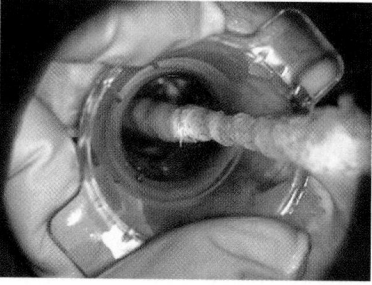

Fig. 84.5   Insertion of the acetic acid–soaked gauze through the anoscope. The anoscope is then withdrawn, leaving the gauze in place.

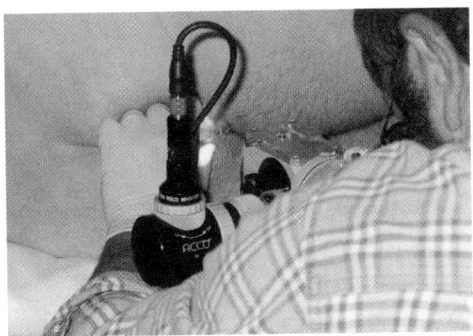

Fig. 84.6 The colposcope is focused with one hand while the other hand holds the anoscope in place.

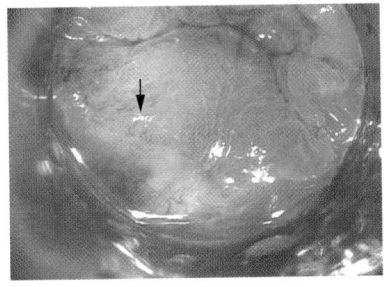

Fig. 84.7 The anal transformation zone is seen as a thin white line adjacent to the columnar epithelium. The anal mucosa is lighter than the colon, which is darker red.

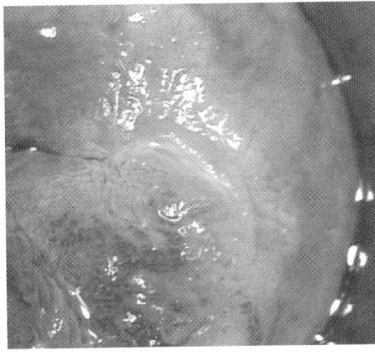

Fig. 84.8 This high-grade anal intraepithelial neoplasia is faintly acetowhite with a mosaic pattern noted in the bottom edge of the lesion.

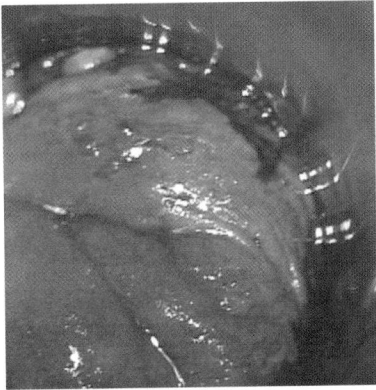

Fig. 84.9 High-grade anal intraepithelial neoplasia is more clearly delineated with application of Lugol staining.

4. Allow the acetic acid to soak for 1 to 2 minutes; 3% acetic acid is better tolerated in the anus but 5% can be used.
5. Remove the gauze and reinsert the anoscope with the obturator. Remove the obturator. Control the anoscope with one hand, while focusing the colposcope with the other hand (Fig. 84.6).
6. Observe through the anoscope as you slowly withdraw it. Focusing the colposcope requires manipulating the anoscope and colposcope simultaneously so that the anus is always in focus.
7. Withdraw the anoscope until the AnTZ comes into focus. The AnTZ is rarely viewed in its entirety in one field of view. Adjusting and re-angling the anoscope as well as using cotton swabs to manipulate the folds, hemorrhoids, or prolapsing mucosa will allow all aspects of the AnTZ to be viewed (Fig. 84.7).
8. A thorough examination requires reapplication of acetic acid to the entire SCJ multiple times. Not only does the staining of the abnormalities fade, it is essential that all areas, including those between the folds, be stained.
9. Lugol solution may be applied judiciously to help better define lesions or their margins. Normal glycogenated squamous epithelium stains dark mahogany. *Abnormal lesions lack glycogen and may stain partially or not at all.* Columnar epithelium and scar tissue also will not stain with Lugol's. We do not use Lugol solution on the fully keratinized perianal area because the staining patterns are not sensitive enough. It is important to observe directly through the colposcope while the Lugol solution is applied to differentiate areas not expected to pick up the Lugol stain from true nonstaining areas that are lesions. Most HGAIN lesions will be Lugol negative. As much as half of LGAIN lesions also are Lugol negative. Conversely, lesions that are partially or positively stained with Lugol solution are rarely HGAIN. As such, choosing a Lugol's-negative lesion to sample may help increase the yield for HGAIN (Figs. 84.8 and 84.9).
10. Once the entire AnTZ has been observed, continue the examination of the anal canal as the anoscope is slowly withdrawn. Continue to apply more acetic acid using a scopette or cotton-tipped swabs. Lesions seen at the SCJ may radiate distally into the canal and even to the verge. A complete evaluation includes assessment of the extent of all lesions so that a treatment recommendation can be made.
11. Examine the verge and perianal skin applying additional acetic acid. By consensus, the perianal area is considered to radiate 5 cm beyond the verge. Perianal lesions are more difficult to evaluate and may require applying a gauze soaked in 5% acetic acid for 3 to 5 minutes (Fig. 84.10).

Performing Anal Biopsy

1. Biopsies are directed at areas thought to represent the highest grade of abnormality (see Chapter 124, Colposcopic Examination, which reviews colposcopic findings) to determine (1) the severity of the disease present and (2) the extent of involvement to determine treatment options. If there are many different lesions, sampling multiple areas will help define the extent of HGAIN or LGAIN to clarify therapeutic options.
2. Anal biopsies are smaller than cervical biopsies. Forceps no larger than 2 to 3 mm should be used, such as the baby Tischler or mini-Townsend.
3. Insert the forceps through the anoscope while it is closed. Directly visualize the area for biopsy to determine that the correct area is being sampled. *A common mistake of novice providers* is to look around instead of through the colposcope to visualize the lesion during biopsy.
4. Sample lower lesions first so that bleeding does not obscure other lesions (which can happen if superior lesions are sampled first).
5. When the lesion is visualized, adjust the forceps so it is partially open and adjacent to the lesion. A partially opened forceps will provide an adequate specimen and only minimal bleeding. Open

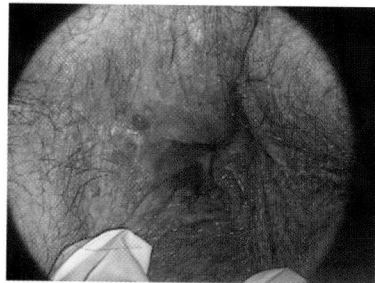

Fig. 84.10 Perianal high-grade anal intraepithelial neoplasia with acetowhite changes, shallow ulcerations, and hyperpigmentation.

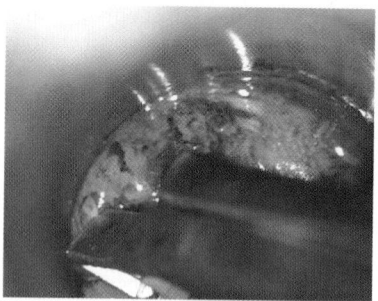

Fig. 84.11 Opening the forceps partially is wide enough for an anal specimen and will help minimize bleeding.

it in the direction that allows the forceps to grasp the tissue most easily. For some lesions the forceps must be positioned sideways or upside down (Fig. 84.11).

6. The normal pressure of the anus after removing the anoscope is often sufficient to stop bleeding, but a small amount of Monsel solution or silver nitrate can be applied to promote hemostasis. Do not use Monsel solution until all biopsies are complete because it can interfere with the pathology reading.

7. HRA-directed biopsy is a one-handed procedure because one hand will always be holding the anoscope. It takes practice to adeptly manipulate the specimens into the formalin containers with one hand while holding the anoscope in place for the remainder of the procedure. If available, an assistant can place biopsy specimens in containers.

8. Anal biopsies do not require anesthesia. Perianal biopsies, however, are similar to vulvar biopsies and require a small amount of injectable 1% lidocaine with epinephrine. Buffering the lidocaine with sodium bicarbonate (2 mL NaHCO$_3$:10 mL lidocaine) improves the comfort of the procedure.

High-Resolution Anoscopy Observations

1. Squamous epithelium usually appears lighter and pinker compared with columnar or rectal epithelium, which is darker and redder. In most people, the anoscope is longer than the anal canal and, if inserted fully, the colonic mucosa will be noted first as the obturator is removed.

2. The anal canal of most women is shorter compared with men. The AnTZ is much closer to the verge in some women and it may seem as if the anoscope is nearly outside before the AnTZ is viewed. In people with anal prolapse, the AnTZ may also be noted at the verge or at times seen externally. Those who have had surgery may also present with the SCJ closer to the verge. Acetic acid is still helpful in delineating the AnTZ and SCJ.

3. If the AnTZ does not appear readily, generously apply acetic acid while manipulating the anoscope. Eventually, a thin white line should begin to appear. Once an area of the AnTZ has been located, the remainder should be visible with manipulation of the anoscope and continued application of acetic acid.

4. Clinical/colposcopic terminology for describing anal lesions is similar to that for cervical lesions. Lesions are described by color (acetowhite), contour (raised or flat), surface vascularity (punctation, mosaic patterns, atypical vessels), margins (distinct and indistinct), and Lugol staining (negative, partial, positive). Lesion margins are not very well defined in anal mucosa. Frequently one or more parts of the lesion margins are not observed, especially adjacent to the columnar epithelium.

5. Lesions appear as demarcated acetowhite areas with characteristics similar to those seen on the cervix. Refer to the Chapter 124, Colposcopic Examination, for a more thorough discussion of lesion characteristics.

6. A typical LGAIN lesion is acetowhite and raised, has warty, looped capillary vessels and papillae, and is often partially stained with Lugol solution. A typical HGAIN lesion is acetowhite and flat, has punctation and mosaic patterns, and is Lugol negative (Table 84.1 and Figs. 84.12 and 84.13).

7. Be consistent when describing the location of the lesions. The anal "clock" is different from the cervical "clock." By convention, the 12:00 position is posterior in the anus if the patient is standing and bent over a table, but anterior if in the lithotomy position. Because referrals are frequently made to colorectal surgeons it is helpful to provide the locations anatomically (posterior, anterior, left or right lateral; Fig. 84.14).

COMMON ERRORS

- Applying lubricant or doing a digital examination before obtaining cytology
- Not sampling the entire AnTZ when obtaining cytology
- Not being persistent and examining the entire AnTZ with the colposcope
- Looking around (not through) the colposcope when obtaining biopsies
- Obtaining too large a sample for biopsy, causing excessive bleeding

INTERPRETATION OF RESULTS

Cytology is considered a screening test and is not diagnostic. Diagnosis is based on the histologic result. HGAIN is considered the cancer precursor lesion, and LGAIN is considered a benign abnormal lesion. Results that are described as "atypia suggestive of LGAIN" are considered atypical but not abnormal. "Atypia cannot rule out HGAIN" is also an atypical finding and an indicator for HRA. A higher grade on cytology than the biopsy histologic grade suggests that the lesion was not seen on HRA and the examination may have to be repeated. Repeat HRA examination is indicated if HGAIN was found on cytology but not on biopsy.

Reasons for discordant results include inadequate examinations due to obscuring hemorrhoids or warts (diffuse circumferential warts may obscure smaller areas of HGAIN) or that the highest-grade lesions were missed on HRA because of lack of adequate staining. The learning curve for HRA is steeper than for cervical colposcopy because of differences between anal and cervical anatomy. Discordant results are not unusual for novices and occur even for experienced providers.

A thorough discussion of treatment is beyond the purview of this chapter. The threshold for treatment depends on the situation (see Fig. 84.2). LGAIN can be treated when it is symptomatic, when the patient requests it to be removed, and when it is diffuse and obscures the ability to perform an adequate examination. HGAIN should be treated unless the patient is medically fragile or treatment is otherwise contraindicated. These patients should be followed carefully by cytology and digital rectal examination every 3 to 4 months. Most HGAIN can be treated as an office procedure using the infrared coagulator. Diffuse circumferential disease or patients who cannot tolerate long procedures may require referral to a colorectal surgeon for surgical removal or ablation.

TABLE 84.1	Typical Features of Anal Intraepithelial Neoplasia and Cancer on High-Resolution Anoscopy			
DRE	Surface Characteristics	Epithelial Characteristics	Vascular Characteristics	Lugol Staining
LGAIN	Granular, soft warty nodularity	Raised or flat	Papillae, micropapillae	Fine or coarse punctation, warty vessels	Negative, partial or complete
HGAIN	Nonpalpable or subtle thickening	Flat or slightly raised	Smooth	Coarse punctation, mosaic patterns, increased vascularity	Negative
Cancer	Firm mass, indurated or distinct thickening	Raised, ulcerated, occasionally flat	Peeling or denuded, heaping edges	Atypical, large, nonbranching vessels, grossly dilated, friable	Negative

DRE, Digital rectal examination; *HGAIN,* high-grade anal intraepithelial neoplasia; *LGAIN,* low-grade anal intraepithelial neoplasia.

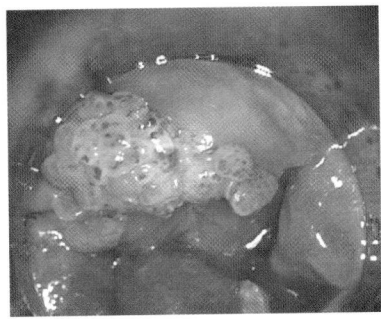

Fig. 84.12 Typical low-grade anal intraepithelial neoplasia.

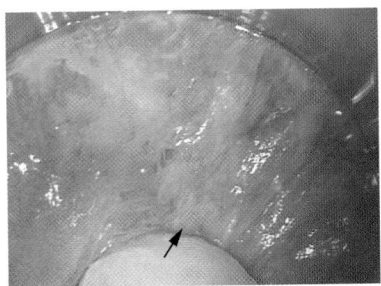

Fig. 84.13 Typical high-grade anal intraepithelial neoplasia.

Anal clock in the left lateral HRA position

Posterior = 12:00   Anterior = 6:00

R lateral   R lateral

Post.   Ant.   Post.   Ant.

L lateral   L lateral

Internal   **External**

Fig. 84.14 The "anal clock" from the perspective of the left lateral high-resolution anoscopy (HRA) position. Note that posterior = 12 o'clock, and that this is the opposite of the "cervical clock."

Ablation is the mainstay of therapy. Office ablation techniques include cryotherapy (only for external lesions), trichloroacetic acid or bichloroacetic acid for small-volume disease, and electrocautery or infrared coagulation for larger-volume disease. Small lesions can

sometimes be excised with the forceps or snipped off using sharp tissue scissors such as Metzenbaums. Laser has been used for both office and surgical ablation but requires a smoke evacuator. In surgery, most patients receive fulguration or electrocautery.

CPT/BILLING CODES

46600	Anoscopy
46601	Anoscopy, high resolution (use G6027 for Medicare patients), with collection of specimens by brushings or washing
46606	Anoscopy with biopsy
46607	Anoscopy, high resolution (use G6028 for Medicare patients), with single or multiple biopsies
46610	Anoscopy with polypectomy
46614	Anoscopy with destruction
46900	Destruction, chemical, simple
46910	Destruction, electro, simple
46916	Destruction, cryosurgical, simple
46922	Destruction, surgical excision
46924	Destruction, extensive lesions
46937	Cryosurgical destruction, benign rectal tumor

ICD-10-CM DIAGNOSTIC CODES

B20	HIV infection
A63.0	Condyloma
C21.1	Anal cancer
D12.9	Benign neoplasm of anus (low-grade squamous intraepithelial lesion or AIN 2)
D01.3	Carcinoma in situ of anal canal (AIN 3)

ONLINE RESOURCES

For providers: American Society for Colposcopy and Cervical Pathology: Sponsors courses in colposcopy and HRA: www.asccp.org.

For patients: University of California at San Francisco (UCSF) Anal Neoplasia Research and Treatment Group: Describing approach to patients at UCSF and listing providers: www.uucsfhealth.org/conditions/anal_cancer/ and analcancerinfo.ucsf.edu/hra-provider-list.

RECOMMENDED READING

Apgar BS, Brotzman GL, Spitzer M, eds. *Colposcopy: Principles and Practice. An Integrated Textbook and Atlas.* 2nd ed. Philadelphia: Saunders; 2008.

Bower M, Powles T, Newsom-Davis T, et al. HIV-associated anal cancer: has highly active antiretroviral therapy reduced the incidence or improved the outcome? *J Acquir Immune Defic Syndr.* 2004;37:1563–1565.

Chin-Hong PV, Berry JM, Cheng SC, et al. Comparison of patient- and clinician-collected anal cytology samples to screen for human papillomavirus-associated anal intraepithelial neoplasia in men who have sex with men. *Ann Intern Med.* 2008;149:300–306.

Cranston RD, Hirschowitz SL, Cortina G, Moe AA. A retrospective clinical study of the treatment of high-grade anal dysplasia by infrared coagulation in a population of HIV-positive men who have sex with men. *Int J STD AIDS.* 2008;19:118–120.

D'Souza G, Wiley DJ, Li X, et al. Incidence and epidemiology of anal cancer in the multicenter AIDS cohort study. *J Acquir Immune Defic Syndr.* 2008;48:491–499.

Edgren G, Sparen P. Risk of anogenital cancer after diagnosis of cervical intraepithelial neoplasia: a prospective population-based study. *Lancet Oncol.* 2007;8:311–316.

Goldie SJ, Kuntz KM, Weinstein MC, et al. The clinical effectiveness and cost-effectiveness of screening for anal squamous intraepithelial lesions in homosexual and bisexual HIV-positive men. *JAMA.* 1999;281:1822–1829.

Goldie SJ, Kuntz KM, Weinstein MC, et al. Cost-effectiveness of screening for anal squamous intraepithelial lesions and anal cancer in human immunodeficiency virus-negative homosexual and bisexual men. *Am J Med.* 2000;108:634–641.

Goldstone SE, Hundert JS, Huyett JW. Infrared coagulator ablation of high-grade anal squamous intraepithelial lesions in HIV-negative males who have sex with males. *Dis Colon Rectum.* 2007;50:565–575.

Goldstone SE, Kawalek AZ, Huyett JW. Infrared coagulator: a useful tool for treating anal squamous intraepithelial lesions. *Dis Colon Rectum.* 2005;48:1042–1054.

Hessol NA, Holly EA, Efird JT, et al. Anal intraepithelial neoplasia in a multisite study of HIV-infected and high-risk HIV-uninfected women. *AIDS.* 2009;23:59–70.

HPV associated cancers and precancers. In: *Sexually Transmitted Diseases Treatment Guidelines.* MMWR. 2015;64(3):93.

Jay N, Berry JM, Hogeboom CJ, et al. Colposcopic appearance of anal squamous intraepithelial lesions: relationship to histopathology. *Dis Colon Rectum.* 1997;40:919–928.

Joseph DA, Miller JW, Wu X, et al. Understanding the burden of human papillomavirus-associated anal cancers in the US. *Cancer.* 2008;113(suppl 10):2892–2900.

Leeds IL, Fang SH. Anal cancer and intraepithelial neoplasia screening: a review. *World J Gastrointest Surg.* 2016;8(1)41–51.

Moscicki AB, Darragh TM, Berry-Lawhorn JM, et al. Screening for anal cancer in women. *J Low Genit Tract Dis.* 2015;19(suppl 3):S27–S42.

Ogunbiyi OA, Scholefield JH, Robertson G, et al. Anal human papillomavirus infection and squamous neoplasia in patients with invasive vulvar cancer. *Obstet Gynecol.* 1994;83:212–216.

Palefsky JM, Holly EA, Efirdc JT, et al. Anal intraepithelial neoplasia in the highly active antiretroviral therapy era among HIV-positive men who have sex with men. *AIDS.* 2005;19:1407–1414.

Palefsky JM, Shiboski S, Moss A. Risk factors for anal human papillomavirus infection and anal cytologic abnormalities in HIV-positive and HIV-negative homosexual men. *J Acquir Immune Defic Syndr.* 1994;14:415–422.

Patel P, Hanson DL, Sullivan PS, et al. Incidence of types of cancer among HIV-infected persons compared with the general population in the United States, 1992–2003. *Ann Intern Med.* 2008;148:728–736.

Pineda CE, Berry JM, Jay N, et al. High-resolution anoscopy targeted surgical destruction of anal high-grade squamous intraepithelial lesions: a ten-year experience. *Dis Colon Rectum.* 2008;51:829–835; discussion 35–37.

Pineda CE, Berry JM, Welton ML. High resolution anoscopy and targeted treatment of high-grade squamous intraepithelial lesions. *Dis Colon Rectum.* 2006;49:126.

Scholefield JH, Castle MT, Watson NF. Malignant transformation of high-grade anal intraepithelial neoplasia. *Br J Surg.* 2005;92:1133–1136.

Stier EA, Goldstone SE, Berry JM, et al. Infrared coagulator treatment of high-grade anal dysplasia in HIV-infected individuals: an AIDS malignancy consortium pilot study. *J Acquir Immune Defic Syndr.* 2008;47:56–61.

Stier EA, Sebring MC, Mendez AE, et al. Prevalence of anal human papillomavirus infection and anal HPV-related disorders in women: a systematic review. *Am J Obstet Gynecol.* 2015;213(3):278–309.

Watson AJ, Smith BB, Whitehead MR, et al. Malignant progression of anal intra-epithelial neoplasia. *ANZ J Surg.* 2006;76:715–717.

CHAPTER 85

Anal Fissure, Lateral Sphincterotomy, and Anal Fistula

James A. Surrell

ANAL FISSURE

Anal fissure is defined as a painful linear ulcer (tear) of the distal anal canal, located just inside the anal opening and extending cephalad toward the dentate line (Fig. 85.1). The most common cause of an anal fissure is the passing a large, firm or hard, forced bowel movement. Diarrhea with trauma from multiple bowel movements can also cause a fissure, as can trauma from a digital rectal exam, endoscopy, a foreign body, or receptive anal intercourse. The history of a patient with an anal fissure is so characteristic that the diagnosis can usually be made based on history alone. Patients complain of moderate to severe pain during and after bowel movements and have a variable amount of bleeding. The painful symptoms nearly always resolve within 15 to 30 minutes of the bowel movement. Rarely, the patient with an anal fissure complains of severe and constant pain, but this is usually seen only with a severe, deep anal fissure with associated significant anal spasm. Although a small amount of bleeding with bowel movements is common ("just on the toilet paper"), frank bleeding is rare.

The severe pain, "like glass is cutting me," is thought to be secondary to the fissure's tearing open and associated internal anal sphincter spasm. Avoiding constipation and keeping the bowel movements soft or "mushy," along with relieving the anal muscle spasm, are the goals of therapy.

The *internal* anal sphincter is a totally involuntary muscle and responds to pain by contracting, which leads to more pain and a smaller opening through which the stool must pass, thus creating a vicious cycle. The *external* sphincter generally acts in an involuntary fashion but is also under voluntary control. Both sphincters form a ring of muscle around the anus (Fig. 85.2).

The history must include whether the fissure is acute or chronic. *Chronic fissure* can arbitrarily be defined as one that has been present with signs and symptoms of pain or bleeding for more than 3 months. Unless the symptoms are extremely disabling, all fissures should be given a trial of conservative or medical management, as discussed later. If conservative or medical management fails, lateral internal sphincterotomy is the procedure of choice for treatment of an anal fissure.

Once the history suggests an anal fissure, the diagnosis can usually be made by simple visual examination of the external anus and a gentle digital examination. The left lateral decubitus position is recommended for patients undergoing anorectal examination. With gentle eversion of the anoderm, one can usually see the fissure. By touching the fissure with a cotton-tipped applicator, the diagnosis can be confirmed if this reproduces the painful symptoms experienced with bowel movements. If necessary, a digital examination with good lubrication will confirm not only pain but markedly increased sphincter tone due to spasm. Finally, if the diagnosis is in

doubt, the anoscopic examination can provide more direct visualization. In classic cases, insertion of the anoscope can be so painful that it should be deferred. However, it should be performed at a later date to exclude other possible diseases.

Anal fissures occur most commonly in the posterior midline. Approximately 90% of fissures are in this location, although they can be found in conjunction with an anterior midline fissure or solely in the anterior midline position in a small percentage of patients (10%). If the clinician sees an anal fissure in any location other than the anterior or posterior midline, a thorough gastrointestinal workup will be necessary to rule out the presence of inflammatory bowel disease (IBD) or other very rare causes such as tuberculosis, syphilis, occult abscess, leukemic infiltrates, carcinomas, herpes, or acquired immunodeficiency syndrome.

If present, IBD with an atypical fissure is most commonly Crohn disease. Another physical examination feature that should raise the suspicion of perianal Crohn disease is the presence of fleshy, edematous skin tags (see Chapter 88, Removal of Perianal Skin Tags [External Hemorrhoidal Skin Tags]). If the examiner suspects IBD, upper gastrointestinal and small bowel x-ray films are necessary, as well as colonoscopy or barium enema radiography combined with flexible sigmoidoscopy. Magnetic resonance imaging enterography may also be used to evaluate for Crohn disease and other bowel lesions.

EDITOR'S NOTE: Although not every anal fissure is visible on exam (e.g., they can be obscured by hemorrhoids or small or partially healed lesions), the exam is useful for excluding other causes of similar symptoms.

Treatment

If the patient has symptoms of moderate to severe pain or bleeding during and after bowel movements, he or she probably has an anal fissure. As noted, the initial goal of therapy is to keep the bowel movements soft or "mushy" and easy to pass while providing pain relief. If the symptoms are severe, disabling, and constant, surgical intervention should be considered sooner rather than later.

However, for most fissures, a 1- to 3-month trial of conservative management is indicated. This management includes sitz baths, a high-fiber diet of at least 30 g of dietary fiber, six to eight glasses of water, and 3 to 6 g of commercially available fiber supplements per day. (If the patient is not consuming enough water with fiber, the stools can remain hard.) Polyethylene glycol is available in commercial laxatives and can be combined with fiber; the dose should be increased until the patient's stools are mushy. If the fissure pain is severe, consider prescribing 5% lidocaine ointment to be applied on arising and at bedtime, as needed throughout the day, and again after bowel movements. Commercially available nonprescription hemorrhoid ointments and creams are minimally effective

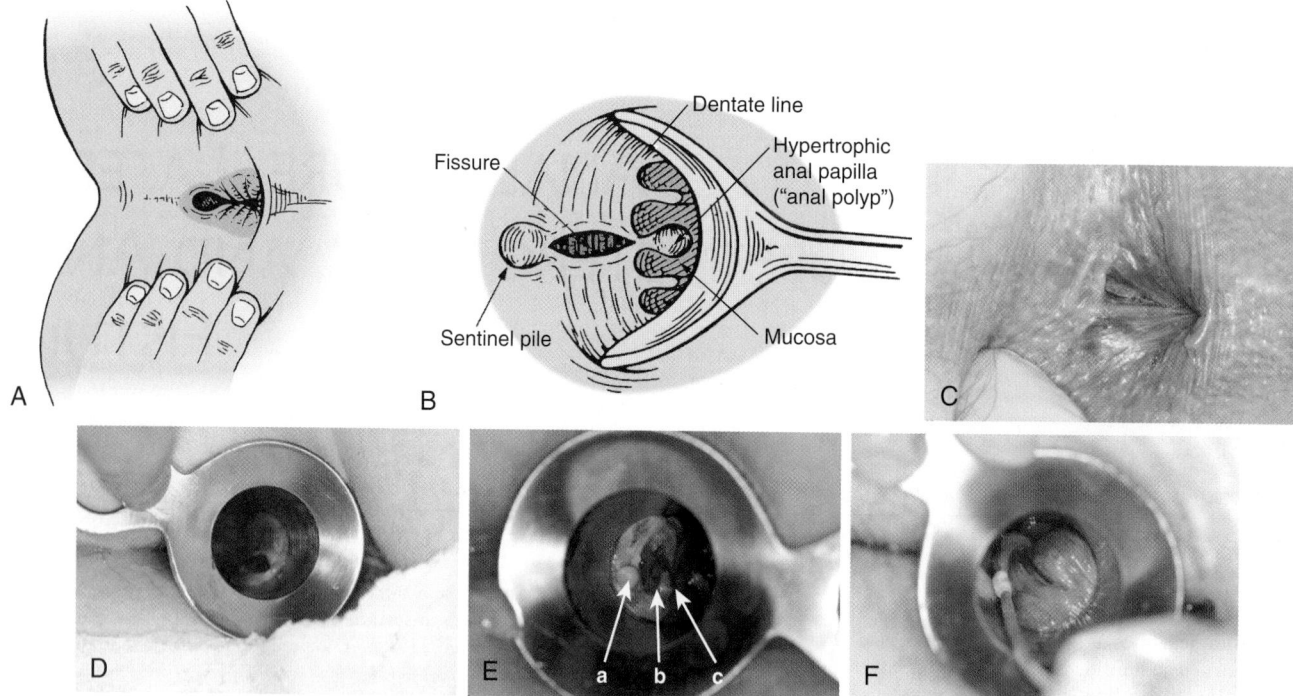

Fig. 85.1   Anal fissures. Patient is in the left lateral decubitus position. (A) External examination. Gentle eversion of the buttocks reveals a posterior midline anal fissure. (B) Anoscopic examination. Chronic posterior anal fissure with a distal sentinel pile/tag and a proximal hypertrophic anal papilla at the level of the dentate line. (C) Superficial anal fissure visualized easily with manual retraction of perianal tissues. (D) Acute anal fissure diagnosed with use of an Ives slotted anoscope. (E) Chronic anal fissure. *Arrows* point to sentinel tag (*a*), fissure (*b*), and anal polyp (*c*). (F) Large acute anal fissure obscured by hemorrhoids until fold retracted with cotton-tipped applicator. ([C–F] Courtesy The Medical Procedures Center, Midland, MI.)

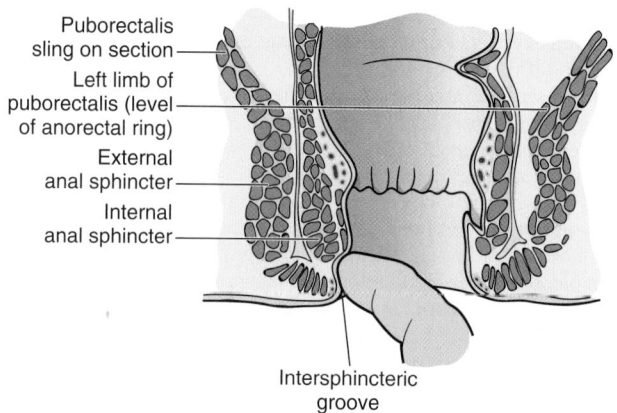

Fig. 85.2   Sagittal section of the anal canal to illustrate palpation of the intersphincteric groove by the surgeon's examining finger. (Also see Chapter 82, Clinical Anorectal Anatomy and Digital Examination.)

in the treatment of anal fissures. They may, however, be used to lubricate the anal canal for bowel movements. Steroid preparations may or may not be helpful, but they are not intended for long-term use.

Specifically advise patients not to use any ointment or cream with a rectal tube-tipped applicator or any suppositories because these products and devices tend to worsen the symptoms of an anal fissure. Advise patients to apply a small amount of any recommended ointment or cream directly to the fissure with a finger because an anal fissure is always located just inside the anal verge. The application of silver nitrate to the fissure or the use of electrocautery on the fissure site is not recommended and may even exacerbate the symptoms. Anal dilators should not be used because of the unpredictable disruption of the anal sphincters and the potential for causing incontinence.

For persistent fissures, a trial of 0.2% to 0.5% nitroglycerin ointment or jelly may be tried. A small amount of this ointment (about

the size of a pencil eraser) should be applied directly to the fissure three to four times a day; it can be gently rubbed onto the fissure instead of just applying it superficially. Patients must be cautioned that if they experience headache, they are using too much nitroglycerin ointment. Using a lesser amount, at least initially, may lessen or eliminate the headaches. The 0.2% to 0.5% nitroglycerin ointment can be compounded by a pharmacy with a physician's prescription and is also now commercially available (0.4%, Rectiv by Allergan). The prescription usually reads as follows: "Rx: 0.2% nitroglycerin ointment, DISP: 60 g, SIG: apply small amount to anal fissure, as directed, two to four times a day for 6 to 8 weeks for anal fissure pain." (Be sure to clarify 0.2%, not 2.0%.) Most studies use soft white paraffin to dilute it, or lidocaine or Anusol ointment. If headache does occur, the patient should take an aspirin 1 hour beforehand and lessen the volume applied.

Some practitioners now question the efficacy of nitroglycerin and have switched to using nifedipine gel 0.2%. The mixture is rubbed in two to three times a day. (Nifedipine gel 0.2%. Mix #10, 20-mg capsules of nifedipine in 100 mL surgical lubricant. Apply to rectal area qid [100 mL].) Some add bethanechol to make 0.1%. Diltiazem has been used in a similar manner. K-Y Jelly or 2% lidocaine jelly can be used instead of surgical lubricant.

These medications pharmacologically relax the anal sphincter to reduce spasm and pain and to assist with the healing process (a "chemical sphincterotomy"). Patients should notice an improvement in symptoms in several days to a week. Full results may not be obtained for 4 to 6 weeks. The patient should be reevaluated at that point. In those patients with resolution of symptoms but persistent fissure on exam, it is appropriate to use topical therapy for another 4 to 6 weeks.

Botulinum toxin (Botox) injected into the anal sphincter is also an option for the medical management of anal fissures. The mechanism of action appears to be inhibition of anal sphincter spasm. Initial response is favorable, but long-term follow-up in some studies shows a high recurrence rate. Botox is contraindicated in pregnant and nursing patients and those with neuromuscular disease.

Botulinum Toxin Type A Injection Technique

Botulinum toxin type A (Botox) is generally available in 100-U aliquots. (See storage and mixing instructions, Chapter 47, Botulinum Toxin.) The dosage most commonly used for anal fissures is a total of 40 U, with half injected on the right and the remainder injected into the left lateral side of the anal verge. (Remember, most "routine" anal fissures are located anteriorly and posteriorly.) Although various techniques are used, the best results are apparent when the botulinum toxin is injected away from the fissure. Usual and customary sterile technique is used, and the perianal area is prepared with povidone-iodine. A local anesthetic injection is not recommended because this will likely cause a similar amount of discomfort as the botulinum injection itself. This procedure may be done with or without an anoscope. If the patient is not in too much pain from the anal fissure, a small and well-lubricated anoscope is gently placed into the anal canal in the usual fashion. It is recommended that an open-sided anoscope (Ives slotted anoscope) be used to facilitate palpation of the intersphincteric groove on the right and left sides (see Fig. 85.2). This will obviously require withdrawal and replacement of the anoscope to identify the intersphincteric groove on the contralateral side and may cause significant pain. Each side must be injected. The specific technique is to inject a total of 20 U of botulinum toxin into the intersphincteric groove using a 30-gauge needle at a depth of approximately 1 cm. (Some choose to inject directly into the internal sphincter.) The two sites of injection are in the middle of both the right and left perianal tissues, directly within the intersphincteric groove. The intersphincteric groove is palpable and usually easily identified on digital examination by slowly withdrawing the gloved examining finger from just within the anal canal out onto the perianal area. In this manner, one should be able to identify this palpable groove without difficulty. It is important to accurately identify the intersphincteric groove for the appropriate injection site.

The effect of botulinum toxin (relaxing the internal sphincter) is not permanent and lasts only 2 to 4 months. If the patient also follows a high-fiber diet and keeps the stools mushy, however, this is usually enough time for the fissure to heal. If there is relief but the fissure persists, a second injection can be tried. If there is little relief, a second injection can be made with a smaller dosage of toxin 4 to 6 weeks after the first.

Mild, transient incontinence of gas or feces is not uncommon with this treatment.

Lateral Internal Sphincterotomy

Indications

Lateral internal sphincterotomy is indicated if conservative management has been recommended, the patient has complied for approximately 1 to 3 months, and the symptoms of pain or bleeding are still present without improvement during and after bowel movements.

Contraindications

- An atypical location of the fissure (other than anterior or posterior) until a workup for secondary causes is completed (see previous discussion)
- Preexisting anal incontinence, although the coexistence of an anal fissure and incontinence is uncommon

Equipment

The only equipment required for lateral internal sphincterotomy is an assortment of various-sized anoscopes, surgical forceps (pickups) or an Allis clamp, Metzenbaum scissors, a No. 11 blade scalpel or a surgical electrocautery unit. The Hill-Ferguson anal retractor is available in small, medium, and large sizes. Any modern electrosurgery device with a cutting and coagulation setting should suffice. Local anesthesia with epinephrine may help with hemostasis during the procedure and minimize patient discomfort during recovery.

Preprocedure Patient Preparation

Although some will perform a lateral sphincterotomy in the office, most procedures are performed in day surgery. They take approximately 15 minutes and can be performed in either the left lateral decubitus knee-chest position or in the dorsal lithotomy (pelvic) position.

Inform the patient that lateral internal sphincterotomy is a procedure to divide only the fibers of the involuntary internal sphincter so as to allow the anal canal to relax during bowel movements. The external sphincter remains intact and allows for anal control. There is an approximate 5% recurrence rate and a 3% to 5% infection rate. Patients should expect mild to moderate postprocedure pain, which usually is well controlled with oral analgesics. Generally no more than 1 or 2 days is required for recovery, and postoperative pain is minimal compared with the preoperative discomfort from the fissure. There will be minimal bleeding and spotting for up to 6 weeks after the procedure. With proper technique combined with a thorough understanding of anal sphincter anatomy, alteration of anal continence is uncommon; less than 1% of patients develop true permanent anal incontinence.

As always, before any surgical procedure patients should be made aware of nonoperative treatment options, as discussed previously. If the fissure is not resolved with either conservative or surgical treatment, the patient generally experiences intermittent, persistent symptoms. Fibrosis of the internal anal sphincter can lead to anal stenosis. A subcutaneous fistula originating through the base of a long-standing anal fissure may develop, but this is not common.

Technique

This is an outpatient procedure, usually performed in the operating room under monitored anesthesia care using intravenous sedation and local anesthesia. Complete familiarity with the anorectal anatomy is essential.

1. Place the patient on the operating table in the left lateral decubitus position with the buttocks just off the edge of the table and the knees flexed. Identify the intersphincteric groove between the internal and external sphincters so that only the fibers of the internal sphincter are divided (see Fig. 85.2); this is done to preserve anal continence for both flatus and feces.
2. Use the scalpel or electrocautery unit to make a superficial 1-cm radial incision just distal and parallel to the palpable intersphincteric groove in the left lateral quadrant of the anal area (Fig. 85.3). Local anesthesia with epinephrine can be infiltrated prior to the incision for hemostasis and to reduce patient discomfort during recovery.
3. Grasp the skin edge and clearly identify the intersphincteric groove using the dissecting scissors. The darker-red external sphincter should not be divided or damaged in any way. The lighter-colored internal sphincter is bluntly elevated with an Allis clamp or forceps. It normally extends 1 to 1.5 cm into the canal.
4. Divide the full thickness of the internal sphincter from its distal margin up to the level of the dentate line, which is visible in the anal canal. The internal sphincter is immediately subjacent to the internal hemorrhoidal vessels; these should be avoided or significant bleeding may occur. If proper hemostasis cannot be obtained by using pressure or electrocautery, figure-of-eight suture ligation of these vessels may be necessary for persistent bleeding (rare).
5. It is very important to leave the primary incision site open and allow it to close secondarily, because this technique will almost completely eliminate the chance of a postoperative infection at the operative site. If there is a prominent sentinel skin tag ("pile") *distal* to the fissure site or a prominent hypertrophic anal papilla *proximal* to the fissure site, the tag or the papilla may be excised with the dissecting scissors, scalpel, or electrocautery unit at the time of the sphincterotomy procedure, leaving a 3-mm rim of skin above the tag (see Chapter 88, Removal of Perianal Skin Tags [External Hemorrhoidal Tags]). Generally no specific operative treatment is performed at the fissure site itself. The average operative time is 15 minutes or less.

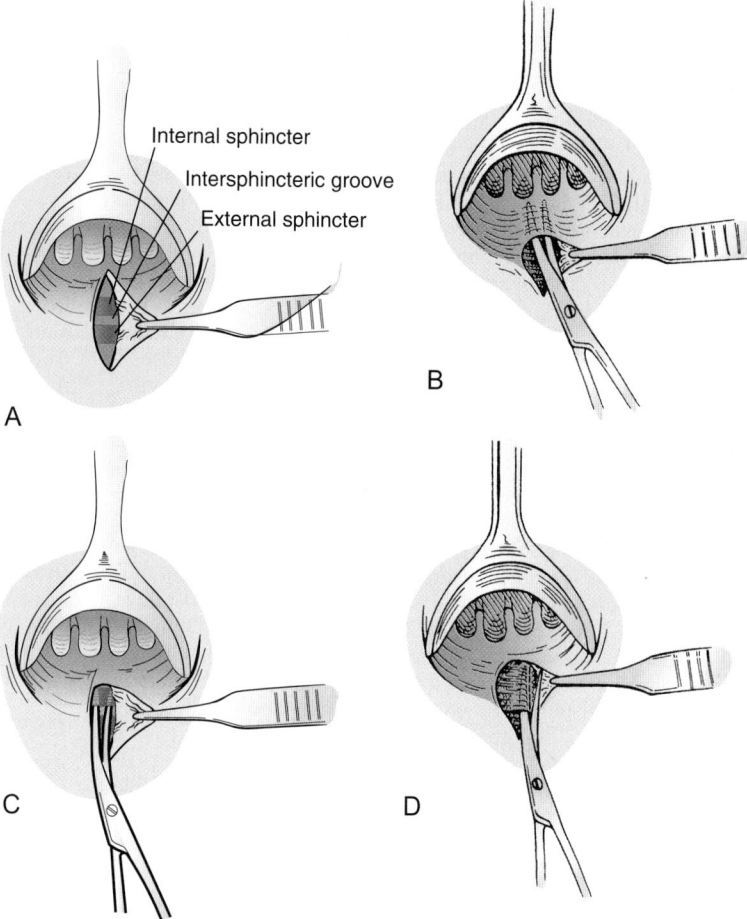

Internal sphincter
Intersphincteric groove
External sphincter

A

B

C

D

Fig. 85.3 Lateral internal anal sphincterotomy using the open technique. The patient is placed in the lateral or the prone (jackknife) position. (A) A radial incision is made across the left lateral intersphincteric groove. A narrow Hill-Ferguson retractor is in place. (B–C) The internal sphincter is separated from the anoderm by blunt dissection. (D) The internal sphincter is divided. The wound is then left open.

Postprocedure Patient Education

After lateral internal sphincterotomy, provide a prescription for nonconstipating pain medication (e.g., ibuprofen). The patient should continue to follow a high-fiber diet of at least 30 g of dietary fiber per day and to use psyllium-based powder fiber supplements once or twice a day. He or she can add enough polyethylene glycol–containing laxative to keep the stools mushy. Sitz baths after each bowel movement and before bed may be helpful. The patient should expect some discomfort, slight bleeding, and discharge from the operative site because the wound is generally left open. Bed rest is not recommended, inasmuch as the pain from the sphincterotomy is often minimal and may even be less than that due to a severe fissure.

Complications

- Approximately 5% of patients have nonhealing fissures after sphincterotomy and may need repeat sphincterotomy.
- Various studies have shown a postoperative infection rate of approximately 3% to 5%, and a very small percentage of these patients will go on to develop an associated anal fistula.
- The most morbid long-term complication is the development of anal incontinence, either of flatus or feces. Postoperative anal incontinence can result from technical operative error during the procedure, whereby muscle fibers other than those of the internal sphincter muscle are divided. Another factor that can contribute to postoperative anal incontinence is unrecognized preexisting anal incontinence.

PATIENT EDUCATION GUIDES

See the sample patient education handout available at www.expertconsult.com.

CPT/BILLING CODES

46080   Anal sphincterotomy

ICD-10-CM DIAGNOSTIC CODES

K60.2   Anal fissure

SUPPLIERS

(See contact information available at www.expertconsult.com.)

Anal retractors
Allegiance Healthcare Corp.
CareFusion

Anoscope product codes are SU180, SU181, and SU182.

Davol Surgical Electrocautery Unit
Davol, Inc.

Also see Chapter 25, Radiofrequency Surgery (Modern Electrosurgery).

ANAL FISTULA

Fistula is the Latin word for "pipe." The medical definition of fistula is an abnormal "pipe-like" communication between any two anatomic body parts that do not normally communicate. Anal fistulas are caused by (1) infection, (2) an inflammatory process, or (3) malignancy. The most common cause of a fistula is infection, usually as a secondary complication from a perianal abscess (see also Chapter 86,

Perianal Abscess Incision and Drainage). Fortunately not all patients who present with a perianal abscess develop a subsequent anal fistula. The diagnosis of anal fistula, like most medical conditions, is made based on a focused history, followed by a careful anorectal examination. Because of the pain involved, if a perianal abscess is present, the assessment for an anal fistula should be deferred unless an examination is being conducted under anesthesia. The abscess is treated first; if symptoms persist, further evaluation is needed.

Anatomy

A perianal abscess is adjacent to the anal canal and slowly enlarges to cause increased tissue damage. The abscess likely started as a superficial infection at the dentate line in one of the crypts ("cryptitis"), but rather than spontaneously draining into the anal canal without consequence, the infection spread laterally into the perianal tissues. This now becomes a potential tract, or "pipe," that may develop into a fistula. Risk of development of both perianal abscesses and anal fistulas is increased in the immune-compromised patient (e.g., on steroids) and in patients with IBD (specifically, Crohn disease), diabetes, status postperianal radiation, and other conditions. However, fewer than 20% of patients who develop a single perianal abscess will ever develop an anal fistula. If, however, a patient presents with a recurrent perianal abscess, one must strongly consider the presence of an anal fistula. In this situation, the odds of a fistula being present are at least 50% and even higher if the perianal abscess is in the same anatomic location.

An anal fistula may be simple or complex. A simple anal fistula is generally defined as a single tract, as noted in Fig. 85.4. A complex fistula has multiple tracts and may involve more than two anatomic locations. The discussion here focuses on the more common simple anal fistula.

An anal fistula always has an internal opening and an external opening. By definition, the external opening of a simple anal fistula is located on the perianal skin, usually within 3 cm of the anal opening (anal verge), and can be readily visualized on gross examination (see Fig. 85.4). The internal opening is within the anal canal and is most commonly located at the level of the dentate line, which is located within 2 cm proximal to the anal verge (Figs. 85.4 and 85.5). The external opening of the fistula may appear to be inflamed, and often there is a varying degree of discharge. In fact, this discharge may be the symptom that brings the patient in for evaluation and represents a chronically draining infection. As long as the external opening remains patent, a perianal abscess does not develop. The chance of an established anal fistula spontaneously closing without surgical intervention is essentially zero.

Three anal muscles provide anal continence: the internal anal sphincter, the external anal sphincter, and the puborectalis muscle (anorectal ring). Furthermore, the external anal sphincter has three components: subcutaneous, superficial, and deep. In general involuntary anal continence is provided by the internal sphincter and voluntary anal continence by the external sphincter and the puborectalis muscle, the latter essentially constituting the anorectal ring. It is very important to understand this anatomy thoroughly, to identify these three muscles clearly, and to establish the extent of their involvement in any fistulous tract before performing anal fistulotomy.

History and Physical Examination

A focused patient history is very important. The patient likely will have a history of a perianal abscess with a nonhealing, chronically draining site, usually at the location of the previous perianal abscess. The external opening may not always be active and may swell and drain only infrequently. Typically, however, a patient with an anal fistula presents with a small palpable firm nodule within 3 cm of the anal verge. This site will periodically swell, cause minor discomfort, and drain. The frequency of these symptoms is highly variable.

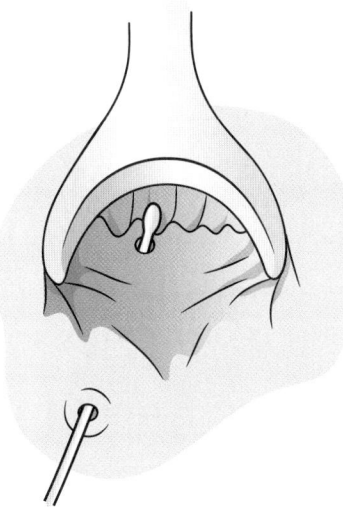

Fig. 85.4   Simple fistula tract with blunt fistula probe in place.

On physical examination, the examiner should carefully and gently palpate all around the anal verge and perianal area. Ask the patient where he or she can feel any swelling, discomfort, or site of drainage. The external opening will not necessarily appear as a true opening, or "hole"; it may appear only as a small erythematous papule (see Fig. 85.5A). Usually the external opening will feel indurated, and this firmness may extend for several centimeters from the external opening. Palpate for a subcutaneous tract leading from the external opening toward the anal canal. If present, this suggests a superficial fistula tract and will feel like a small, firm "pipe" just under the skin.

A digital anorectal examination should be completed, with careful palpation all around the level of the dentate line to feel for any induration or scar tissue; this may suggest the location of the internal opening. Carefully evaluate the anal canal and anoderm with the specific goal of locating any internal opening. Finding the location of the internal opening is ultimately necessary for treatment but is not entirely necessary to establish the diagnosis.

Very gently attempt to pass a blunt fistula probe into the external opening to assess for an established tract. This is usually a small, malleable 1- to 2-mm-diameter "silver probe" with a tiny bulbous end. The wooden end of a cotton-tipped applicator can also be used but may cause more pain. However—and this cannot be emphasized strongly enough—do not pass the fistula probe against any resistance. The creation of a false tract will worsen the situation and make treatment much more difficult. If a fistula probe is used, it is most commonly done with the anoscope in the anal canal to offer concurrent visualization of the anoderm and dentate line. The fistula probe is touched to the area of the suspected external opening, and minimal pressure is applied. If this is a true fistula, the probe will literally "drop" into the opening. If it passes easily toward the anal canal, there is really no need to probe further at this time. The suspected anal fistula diagnosis has now been confirmed (see Figs. 85.4 and 85.5).

See Chapter 82, Clinical Anorectal Anatomy and Digital Examination, and the previous discussion of anal fissure and lateral sphincterotomy.

Anal Fistulotomy or Seton

The treatment for anal fistula is anal fistulotomy. It is essential to precisely locate both the internal and external openings of a simple fistula before fistulotomy can be performed. Once these are established, the examiner must carefully assess how much anal sphincter muscle will be divided as a result of simple fistulotomy. If the

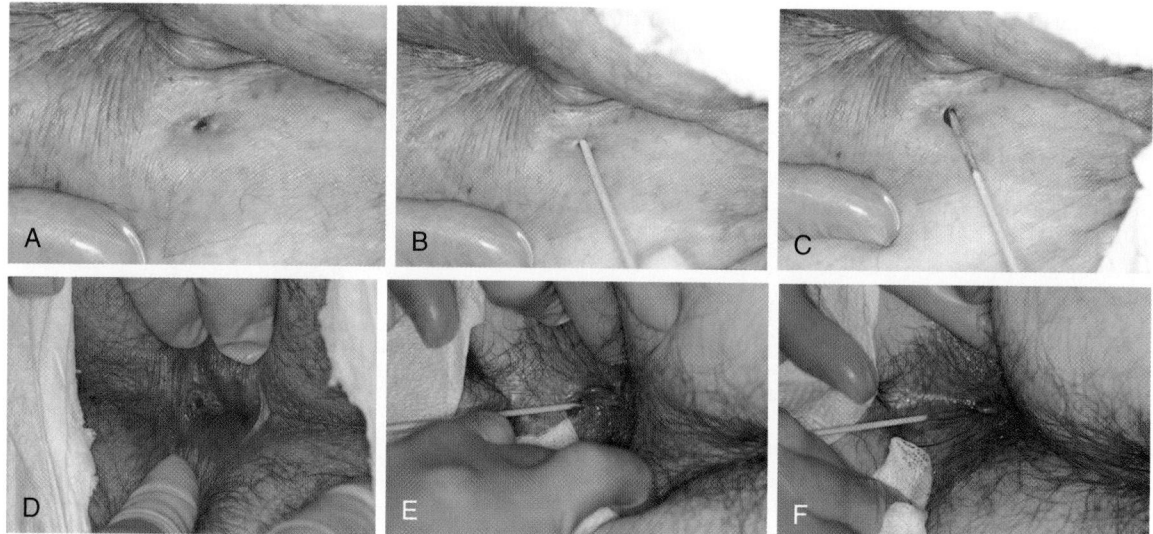

Fig. 85.5 The clinical appearance and confirmation of a suspected fistula using a blunt probe. (A) Papular, small, pustular-appearing lesion in left buttock. (B) Blunt wooden end of cotton-tipped applicator is easily and gently inserted into the fistula. The probe is inserted only a short distance to the confirm diagnosis. (C) The blood on the wooden probe shows that the fistula is at least 2 cm deep. (D) Another clinical presentation under an anal tag. (E) Probe inserted. (F) Probe removed. Blood staining shows depth probe was inserted to confirm diagnosis. (Courtesy The Medical Procedures Center, Midland, MI.)

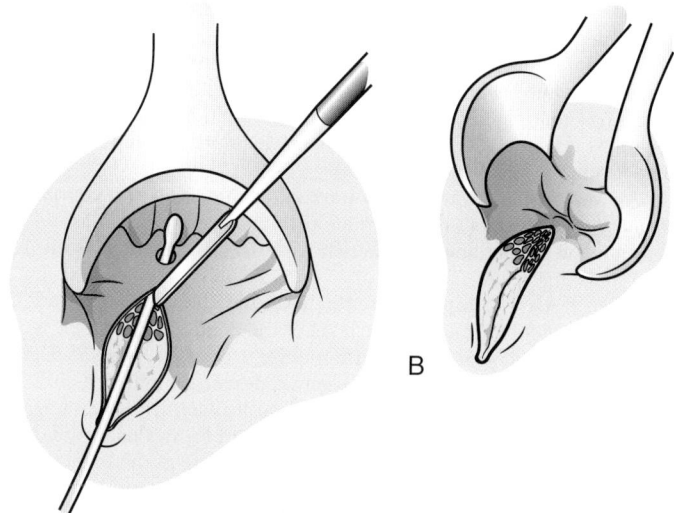

Fig. 85.6 Performing a fistulotomy. (A) Use of electrocautery to perform simple fistulotomy. (B) Completed fistulotomy with wound left open to heal by secondary intention.

internal opening is at or distal to (below) the dentate line, a simple fistulotomy may be performed with little to no likelihood of altering anal continence. During fistulotomy, one can generally divide the fibers of the subcutaneous and superficial portions of both the external and the internal sphincters, with little impact on anal continence.

Anal fistulotomy is usually performed under sedation with monitored anesthesia care. In the left lateral decubitus knee-chest position, with the patient's buttocks just off the edge of the operating room table and with the anoscope in place, local anesthetic with epinephrine is injected along the sides of the fistula tract. This is used primarily for hemostasis and early postoperative comfort. Once the anatomy of the fistula tract has been accurately identified, the blunt fistula probe is placed into the tract with an anoscope in place so that both the internal and external openings are clearly visualized (see Figs. 85.4 and 85.5). Fistulotomy may now be performed with a scalpel or electrocautery to divide the tissue overlying the fistula probe positioned within the fistula tract. Essentially an infected "pipe" is being converted into an open "ditch." Bleeding points are cauterized. This chronically infected wound is then always left open to heal by secondary intention. Dry sterile dressings are applied.

A nearly completed simple fistulotomy performed with electrocautery is shown in Fig. 85.6A. The resulting wound after simple fistulotomy is left open to heal by secondary intention (see Fig. 85.6B).

Although a seton (a suture placed into the fistula and tied into place) can also be used for simple fistulas, it is usually reserved for the treatment of complex ones. If the course of the fistulous tract is lateral to the external sphincter or the internal opening extends above the dentate line, this is not a simple anal fistula and complete fistulotomy should not be performed. This is now a complex fistula, and, because of the potential for altering anal continence, surgical treatment should be performed only by an experienced surgeon thoroughly trained in anorectal surgery.

If the internal opening to the fistula tract extends above the dentate line near the anorectal ring, then the fistulotomy becomes a staged operation and will almost certainly involve the use of a seton. The seton is usually a nonabsorbable doubled heavy silk suture (Fig. 85.7A) placed into the fistula tract and tied around it to itself to permit a slow "cutting through" of the fistula tract. The seton is placed into the fistula tract using a blunt fistula probe with an "eye" on the leading end. The probe is first inserted, then the long silk seton is threaded through this eye. The probe is then pulled through

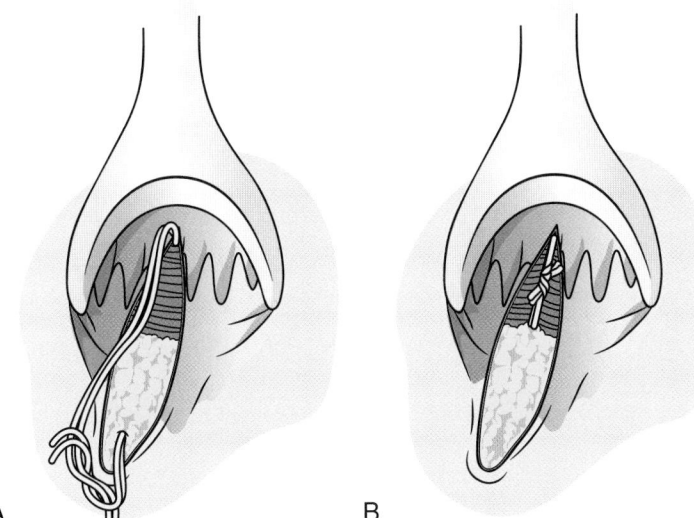

A   B

Fig. 85.7 Placement of a seton for complex fistula. (A) The doubled heavy silk suture is threaded through the fistula and tightly tied to put some tension on the skin, (B) Six weeks later, the overlying remaining tissue is separated using electrocautery and the suture is removed.

the fistula tract, leaving the doubled suture within the tract. The two ends of the seton are now snugly tied together, as noted in Fig. 85.7B, to permit continuous slow "cutting" through the overlying muscle. After the seton (doubled suture) is tied, the probe should be outside the knot; the suture outside the knot is cut to remove the probe. This also produces an inflammatory response and scarring. The few remaining fibers of muscle that overlie the fistula are then fully divided, usually with cautery, no sooner than 6 weeks later. The sphincter muscle will not retract and separate now because of the scarring, thereby preserving anal continence.

Contraindications

- Immunocompromised patient
- History of radiation to fistula location
- Uncontrolled diabetes
- Recent steroid use
- Significant medical comorbidities such as severe cardiac or respiratory disease

Common Errors and Potential Complications

- Dividing excess muscle overlying the fistula tract, leading to varying degrees of anal incontinence
- Not recognizing as-yet-undiagnosed perianal Crohn disease
- Not diagnosing and draining an associated occult perianal abscess
- Not recognizing a complex fistula with multiple tracts
- Creating a false fistula tract with overly aggressive use of the fistula probe

Postoperative Management

After fistulotomy, the patient will have an open wound extending into the anal canal. Patients are often fearful of this wound becoming infected because of its exposure to fecal material, but an open wound cannot become infected. The patient should take sitz baths, shower, or tub bathe to irrigate the wound twice a day for the first week, then once a day for 3 to 4 weeks, and apply dry dressings to absorb the expected discharge. The wound will attempt to close prematurely, and the usual wound care measures should be taken to make sure that the wound closes from "the inside out." The skin edges must be the last portion of the wound to close; this will dramatically minimize the chance of recurrence. If the skin edges close before the fistula tract is totally closed down by the healing and scarring process, another fistula, often more superficial, has been created. The patient must be

instructed that efforts must be made to keep the wound open as long as possible, with complete healing usually occurring within 4 to 6 weeks. The patient should be seen on a weekly basis to ensure proper healing.

CPT/BILLING CODES

46020	Placement of seton
46030	Removal of anal seton
46270	Surgical treatment of anal fistula (fistulectomy/fistulotomy); subcutaneous
46275	Intersphincteric (submuscular)
46280	Transphincteric, suprasphincteric, extrasphincteric, or multiple (complex), including placement of seton, when performed

ICD-9-CM DIAGNOSTIC CODES

565.1	Anal fistula

RECOMMENDED READING

American Gastroenterological Association medical position statement. Diagnosis and care of patients with anal fissure. *Gastroenterology.* 2003;124:233–234.

Baraza W, Boereboom C, Shorthouse A, Brown S. The long-term efficacy of fissurectomy and botulinum toxin injection for chronic anal fissure in females. *Dis Colon Rectum.* 2008;51:239–243.

Brisinda G, Cadeddu F, Brandara F, et al. Randomized clinical trial comparing botulinum toxin injection with 0.2 per cent nitroglycerin ointment for chronic anal fissure. *Br J Surg.* 2007;94:162–167.

Carapeti EA, Kamm MA, Evans BK, Phillips RK. Topical diltiazem and bethanechol decrease anal sphincter pressure without side effects. *Gut.* 1999;45:719–722.

Clinical practice guideline for the management of anorectal abscess, fistula-in-ano, and rectovaginal fistula. The Clinical Practice Guidelines Committee, The American Society of Colon and Rectal Surgeons. *Dis Colon Rectum.* 2016;59(12):1117–1133.

Corman ML. *Corman's Colon and Rectal Surgery.* 6th ed. Philadelphia: Wolters Klower Lippincott Williams & Wilkins; 2013.

Corning C, Weiss EG. Anal fissure. In: Cameron JL, Cameron AM, eds. *Current Surgical Therapy.* Philadelphia: Elsevier; 2011:571–577.

Fruehauf H, Fried M, Wegmueller B, et al. Efficacy and safety of botulinum toxin injection compared with topical nitroglycerin ointment for the treatment of chronic anal fissure: a prospective randomized study. *Am J Gastroenterol.* 2006;101:2107–2112.

Minguez M, Herreros B, Espi A, et al. Long-term follow-up (42 months) of chronic anal fissure after healing with botulinum toxin. *Gastroenterology*. 2002;123:112–117.

Nelson RL, Thomas K, Morgan J, Jones A. Nonsurgical therapy for anal fissure (review). *Cochrane Database Syst Rev*. 2012;(2):CD003431.

Nelson RL, Chattopadhyay A, Brooks W, Platt I, Paavana T, Earl S. Operative procedures for fissure in ano. *Cochrane Database Syst Rev*. 2011;(11):CD002199.

Richard CS, Gregoire R, Plewes EA, et al. Internal sphincterotomy is superior to topical nitroglycerin in the treatment of chronic anal fissure: results of a randomized, controlled trial by the Canadian Colorectal Surgical Trials Group. *Dis Colon Rectum*. 2000;43:1048–1057.

Schouten WR, Briel SW, Auwerda JJA, de Graaf EJR. Ischemic nature of anal fissures. *Br J Surg*. 1996;83:63–65.

Steele SR, Hull TL, Read TE, Saclarides TJ, Senagore AJ, Whitlow CB. *The ASCRS Textbook of Colon and Rectal Surgery*. 3rd ed. Cham, Switzerland: Springer; 2016.

Witte ME, Klaase JM. Botulinum toxin A injection in ISDN ointment-resistant chronic anal fissures. *Dig Surg*. 2007;24:197–201.

CHAPTER 86

PERIANAL ABSCESS INCISION AND DRAINAGE

James A. Surrell

A perianal abscess is one of the most painful anal conditions seen in the outpatient setting. Often associated with severe, disabling, and progressive pain, usually the only relief is with spontaneous rupture of the abscess or with incision and drainage (I&D). The most common etiology of perianal abscess is thought to be an infection originating at the dentate line in the anal crypts (see Chapter 82, Clinical Anorectal Anatomy and Digital Examination). This infection then usually migrates through the path of least resistance to the perianal tissues, where there is a closed-space environment ideal for proliferation of mixed bacterial flora.

The four locations where abscesses usually occur and their relative incidences are shown in Fig. 86.1. The most common site of an abscess is in the tissues immediately adjacent to the anal verge (60%). If the abscess is more than 2 to 3 cm away from the anal verge, it is most likely in the ischiorectal location (25%), just outside the anal sphincters. An intersphincteric abscess occurs in the intersphincteric plane, between the internal and external sphincters. An abscess in this location may not be externally visible or palpable. The pain of an abscess is present, but the diagnosis will be confirmed only on digital anorectal examination, where the fluctuant mass is palpable. The least common abscess in this area is in the supralevator location and is more correctly identified as a *perirectal* abscess as opposed to a *perianal* abscess. Most experts agree that if a supralevator abscess is diagnosed, an intra-abdominal or pelvic source should be sought. A supralevator abscess may be associated with appendicitis, diverticulitis, pelvic inflammatory disease, or other pelvic or abdominal disease. These patients typically have deep rectal or gluteal pain, dysuria, or other urinary symptoms.

Patients with a perianal abscess may develop an associated fever and often have a marked leukocytosis, depending on the severity of the infection. Once the diagnosis of perianal abscess is made, it is essential to proceed with adequate I&D treatment without delay. This is especially important in any patient who may be immunocompromised, on steroids, or has diabetes or any other debilitating comorbidity. The treatment of choice for a perianal abscess is clearly I&D—not antibiotic therapy. If adequate I&D of a perianal abscess is not performed, patients can rapidly develop severe infectious problems such as necrotizing fasciitis or perineal sepsis, both of, which can become life-threatening. Perineal sepsis is a medical emergency identified with the classic triad of pain, fever, and inability to void.

INDICATIONS

Nearly every perianal abscess should be incised and drained. The only reason not to perform this procedure would be if spontaneous drainage has occurred and if, in the judgment of the examining clinician, adequate drainage has resulted. These abscess cavities can have multiple loculations, and if spontaneous drainage has occurred, the abscess cavity must still be explored with a digital examination or hemostats to break down any loculations.

CONTRAINDICATIONS

Patients with underlying hematologic diseases may have perianal abscesses. Such hematologic diseases include leukemia, granulocytopenia, and lymphoma. The infecting organisms seen with this type of perianal abscess may be quite different from those seen with an otherwise uncomplicated abscess. In those patients with an associated hematologic disorder—for example, with leukemia under poor control—conservative treatment with antibiotics combined with local radiation therapy may be advised. Other clinicians recommend aggressive surgical management of perianal abscess in patients with hematologic disorders, but clearly this is never to be attempted in the outpatient setting.

EQUIPMENT

A minor surgical instrument setup includes the following:

- Local anesthesia (2% lidocaine with epinephrine)
- 25- to 30-gauge, 1.5-inch needle with 5-mL syringe
- Hemostats
- No. 11 or 15 blade scalpel
- 4 × 4 gauzes
- Penrose drain, iodoform gauze or de Pezzer catheter
- Suction may be needed if the abscess is large
- Surgical electrocautery unit is often helpful to achieve hemostasis at the I&D site of the infected and hyperemic tissue
- Ives slotted anoscope or various-sized Hill-Ferguson rectal retractors to facilitate visualization (available from most medical supply companies)

PREPROCEDURE PATIENT PREPARATION

Advise the patient that, in all likelihood, rather dramatic pain relief will follow the procedure. Further advise the patient that, unless adequate I&D is accomplished, further tissue damage may result as well as life-threatening infections. Clearly, the most effective way to afford adequate pain relief and avoid other complications is to drain the abscess. Recurrence, bleeding, and pain are all possible. Further work-up may also be necessary to rule out other disease processes, such as inflammatory bowel, once the infection is controlled.

TECHNIQUE

These patients have a clear need for prompt pain relief. Local anesthesia may be used in an attempt to anesthetize the skin at the intended I&D site, but this is often only marginally effective. The infected perianal tissues usually do not respond well to local anesthetic agents because of the highly acid environment and the indurated

593

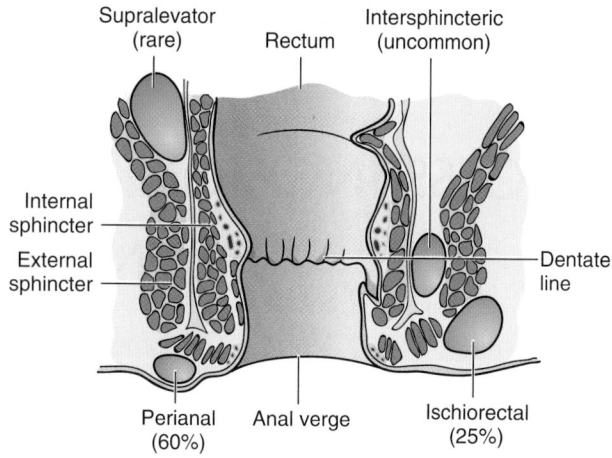

Fig. 86.1 Anatomic locations of anorectal abscesses.

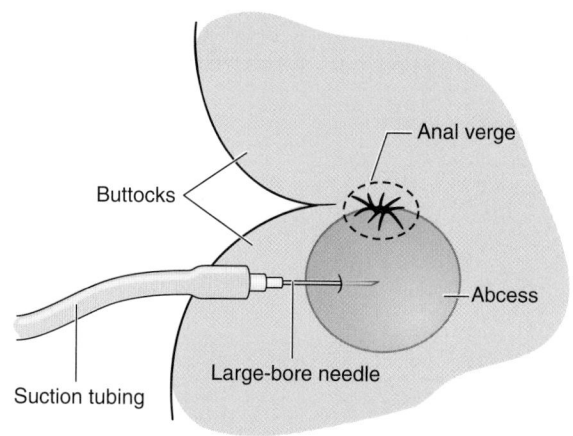

Fig. 86.2 Needle (16 gauge or larger) and suction aspiration of a perianal abscess.

skin surrounding the area. Either spinal or general anesthesia may be required, depending on the size of the abscess and the specific patient circumstances. Before the actual I&D of the abscess, it is appropriate, if not essential, to perform anoscopy to look for an internal opening of a fistula tract feeding the abscess cavity; having adequate anesthesia is important for this step. The advantage of doing the anoscopy before I&D is that with gentle pressure on the abscess cavity the clinician may see pus expressed from an internal opening at the level of the dentate line. This then clearly establishes the diagnosis of an associated anal fistula. Textbooks of colon and rectal surgery vary widely on the incidence of associated fistula with perianal abscess, but most experts would agree that it is at least in the 50% range.

1. Anesthetize the area using 2% lidocaine with epinephrine and a 27- or 30-gauge needle.
2. Make an incision over the fluctuant area near the anal canal in a plane radial to the circumference of the anal canal. The advantage of this type of incision is that it can be extended easily to perform anal fistulotomy if indicated. Extend the incision to remove an ellipse of tissue such that you can easily place a gloved examining finger into the abscess cavity (if it is that large) to break down any loculations and to place drains. Benefits of having removed an ellipse include preventing the wound from closing too early and allowing room to remove and change packing over the subsequent days. (Some clinicians perform a cruciate incision instead, for the same reasons.) At this time, express all of the purulence. Cultures may be obtained in the more complicated cases, if desired. Use of de Pezzer catheters have been described as an alternative to repeatedly packing the wound; this alternative results in equivalent rates of subsequent fistula surgery, less need for general anesthesia, and shorter postoperative hospital stay.
3. Irrigate the abscess cavity and, if deemed necessary, place a Penrose drain loosely into the abscess cavity and suture it at the skin edge level. A Penrose drain will not adhere to surrounding tissue, which makes its subsequent removal generally painless. (Alternatively, pack small wounds with 0.25- or 0.5-inch iodoform gauze.)
4. Remove the Penrose drain within 24 to 48 hours. With a small perianal abscess, in the office setting, the iodoform gauze is removed in 10 to 14 days. Earlier removal may lead to recurrence of the abscess.
5. In selected patients with a well-defined, fluctuant perianal abscess, drainage can be accomplished without anesthesia by placing a large-bore, 16-gauge needle (attached to suction or a large syringe) into the abscess (Fig. 86.2). This can be an effective temporizing measure to afford dramatic and prompt pain relief if

definitive surgical treatment is not readily available. The disadvantage of this needle suction technique is that evaluation for an associated anal fistula becomes more difficult.
6. Postoperative antibiotics are generally not required. Consider them in immunocompromised patients or if there is extensive cellulitis or sepsis.

COMPLICATIONS

Recurrence is the most common complication after I&D of a perianal abscess. The most common cause of recurrence is an unrecognized, and therefore untreated, associated fistula. The patient with a recurrent perianal abscess must be thoroughly evaluated for the presence of an anal fistula. Another possible cause of recurrent perianal abscess is inflammatory bowel disease, most commonly Crohn disease. Postprocedure bleeding and excess pain are rare complications.

POSTPROCEDURE PATIENT EDUCATION

After an adequate drainage procedure of a perianal abscess, advise the patient to take sitz baths for 10 to 15 minutes two to four times a day. Spend some time with the patient and his or her family to reinforce the fact that the infected wound must heal from the inside out. Most patients understand that they must keep the wound from closing with either sitz baths or showering along with the gauze packing. Explain that daily wound irrigations may be needed (if gauze is not used) to prevent the skin edges from closing prematurely before the abscess cavity has resolved. This will help to avoid a secondary infection and a recurrent abscess. These instructions usually serve as adequate motivation to follow the recommended postprocedure care. Patients should also know to call the clinician for high fevers, chills, or recurrence of severe pain.

CPT/BILLING CODES

45000	Transrectal drainage of pelvic abscess
45005	Incision and drainage, submucosal rectal abscess
45020	Incision and drainage of deep supralevator, pelvirectal, or retrorectal abscess
46040	Incision and drainage of ischiorectal and/or perirectal abscess
46045	Incision and drainage of intramural, intramuscular, or submucosal abscess, transanal under anesthesia
46050	Incision and drainage of superficial perianal abscess

ICD-10-CM Diagnostic Codes

K61.1   Perirectal abscess
K61.0   Perianal abscess
K61.3   Ischiorectal abscess
K61.4   Intersphincteric abscess

RECOMMENDED READING

Clinical practice guideline for the management of anorectal abscess, fistula-in-ano, and rectovaginal fistula. The Clinical Practice Guidelines Committee, The American Society of Colon and Rectal Surgeons. *Dis Colon Rectum*. 2016;59(12):1117–1133.

Corman ML. *Corman's Colon and Rectal Surgery*. 6th ed. Philadelphia: Wolters Kluwer Lippincott Williams & Wilkins; 2013.

Ferng M, Headley RC. Perianal abscess incision and drainage. In: Reichman EF, ed. *Emergency Medicine Procedures*. 2nd ed. New York: McGraw-Hill; 2013:722–728.

Gordon P, Nivatvongs S. *Principles and Practice of Surgery for the Colon, Rectum, and Anus*. 3rd ed. New York: Informa Health; 2007.

Holtzman LC, Hitti E, Harrow J. Incision and drainage. In: Roberts JR, Custalow CB, Thomsen TW, eds. *Roberts and Hedges Clinical Procedures in Emergency Medicine*. 6th ed. Philadelphia: Elsevier; 2014:745–747.

Steele SR, Hull TL, Read TE, Saclarides TJ, Senagore AJ, Whitlow CB. *The ASCRS Textbook of Colon and Rectal Surgery*. 3rd ed. Cham, Switzerland: Springer; 2016.

Steele SR, Johnson EK, Armstrong DN. Anorectal abscess and fistula. In: Cameron JL, Cameron AM, eds. *Current Surgical Therapy*. Philadelphia: Elsevier; 2011:586–590.

Pfenninger JL, Zainea G. Common anorectal conditions: part I. Symptoms and complaints. *Am Fam Physician*. 2001;63:2391–2398.

Pfenninger JL, Zainea G. Common anorectal conditions: part II. Lesions. *Am Fam Physician*. 2001;64:77–88.

CHAPTER 87

OFFICE TREATMENT OF HEMORRHOIDS

George G. Zainea • John L. Pfenninger

Hemorrhoids are present in approximately 50% to 80% (some say 100%) of the US population. Although hemorrhoids are rarely fatal, they do account for a great deal of human concern, and possibly discomfort, pain, and suffering (only about 4.4% of the population become symptomatic due to their hemorrhoids). Internal hemorrhoids are the most common cause of lower gastrointestinal bleeding. Nonetheless, it is imperative for the clinician to confirm that bleeding is indeed originating from hemorrhoidal disease and not from a more proximal lesion (e.g., adenoma, cancer). Occasionally, bleeding can be severe and is associated with anemia.

Most hemorrhoidal symptoms can be managed with medical therapies that include suppositories, topical agents, and fiber supplementation. A Cochrane review (Alonso-Coello et al, 2005) showed fiber can consistently relieve symptoms and bleeding for patients with hemorrhoids. Those who do not respond to medical therapies are appropriate candidates for in-office treatments of hemorrhoids. Only a minority of individuals require definitive treatment for severe symptomatic hemorrhoids with a surgical hemorrhoidectomy or hemorrhoidopexy. A hemorrhoidectomy requires general or regional anesthesia and is associated with significant discomfort and loss of time from work and usual activities after surgery.

Rubber-band ligation is a time-tested and proven method for treating *internal hemorrhoids*. However, other approaches have been developed, with infrared photocoagulation (IRC) being used most frequently and, rarely, sclerotherapy. Direct-current (Ultroid) and radiofrequency (Bicap) techniques have been previously described. Bicap is no longer available, and although Ultroid has recently been reintroduced to the market, the time required and the cost of the probes make it less likely to be used. Cryotherapy was also used in the past but not currently because of the availability of more cost-effective modalities. These therapies can be used selectively or in combination depending on the extent and severity of internal disease. Lasers have also been used for the treatment of internal disease. The treatment for *external hemorrhoid disease* has been unchanged for decades.

Two meta-analyses have been reported on the treatment of internal hemorrhoids. One concludes that band ligation is best, whereas the other supports IRC. In both instances, hemorrhoid symptoms resolved in 80% to 90% of properly selected cases.

The clinician must know the anorectal anatomy (see Chapter 82, Clinical Anorectal Anatomy and Digital Examination) and must be able to perform a thorough anoscopic examination (see Chapter 83, Anoscopy) to appropriately assess and treat hemorrhoids.

After completion of any of these procedures, a medical program to regulate bowel habits should be implemented to prevent recurrence, which is as important as the surgical intervention itself.

EDITOR'S NOTE: Patient education is very important for hemorrhoids; often reassurance is all that is needed. A hemorrhoid is very similar to a varicose vein; while it can be unsightly, it rarely causes a problem. As we age, muscle atrophy or sarcopenia is normal or physiologic. As the anal sphincter atrophies, having soft, pliant hemorrhoids to help maintain a seal is probably a good thing. Reassure patients that most of us, if not all of us, have hemorrhoids and that our goal should probably not be to rid ourselves of them completely.

At most, we may need to control them. Unfortunately, most patients have heard stories about dreaded complications of hemorrhoids or their surgical removal; these patients will also require reassurance. Fortunately, we now have much better methods to treat hemorrhoids in the office. The equivalent to surgical varicose vein stripping is open surgical hemorrhoidectomy; fortunately, with new varicose vein procedures available (e.g., sclerotherapy) we rarely perform vein stripping any more. This is the same with hemorrhoids. And no matter which method is used to treat varicose veins or hemorrhoids, including surgical removal, they can recur. Fortunately, we often have options for retreating them in the office instead of repeating the surgery.

CLASSIFICATIONS AND SYMPTOMS

Hemorrhoids are enlarged arteriovenous vessels within fibrous tissue and are classified according to their origin either above or below the dentate (pectinate) line. Those developing from *above the dentate line are internal hemorrhoids*; those from *below are external hemorrhoids*. It should be clear that classification depends on *origin*, not on the location of the most distal portion of the hemorrhoid (Fig. 87.1).

Hemorrhoids above the dentate line—*internal hemorrhoids*—are covered by mucosa and do not have somatic sensory innervation. Thus, internal hemorrhoids are well suited for treatment in the office setting without anesthesia because they lack pain fibers. Those below the dentate line—*external hemorrhoids*—are covered by skin (anoderm) and are extremely sensitive. Treatment of external hemorrhoids requires some form of anesthesia. *Mixed hemorrhoids* refers to those vessels that originate right at the dentate line or to the presence of both internal and external hemorrhoidal tissue in continuity.

The anal canal can be divided into eight segments. With the patient lying in the left lateral decubitus position, they are as noted in Fig. 87.2A. Internal hemorrhoids usually occur in three major positions based on the vascular architecture of the anal canal: the right anterior, right posterior, and left lateral positions (see Fig. 87.2B). However, they can occur anywhere and even be circumferential. They also seem to shift with insertion of the anoscope, so absolute position is not that critical.

Internal hemorrhoids are also characterized by their size and degree of prolapse from grades I to IV, as noted in Table 87.1 and Fig. 87.3. Symptoms of internal hemorrhoids include *painless* bleeding, prolapse, aching after defecation, and discharge. The key step in diagnosis and classification of internal hemorrhoids is anoscopic examination (see Chapter 83, Anoscopy). External hemorrhoids can form clots that are painful; patients then present with a "painful lump."

Hemorrhoidal skin tags are residual fibrotic masses of stretched skin. Their size can vary significantly. They are generally asymptomatic except for occasional pruritus. Most commonly, when larger, they can cause problems with hygiene.

Approximately 25% of internal hemorrhoid symptoms do not respond adequately to medical treatment and require further therapy. Most thrombosed external hemorrhoids require evacuation or excision to provide symptomatic relief.

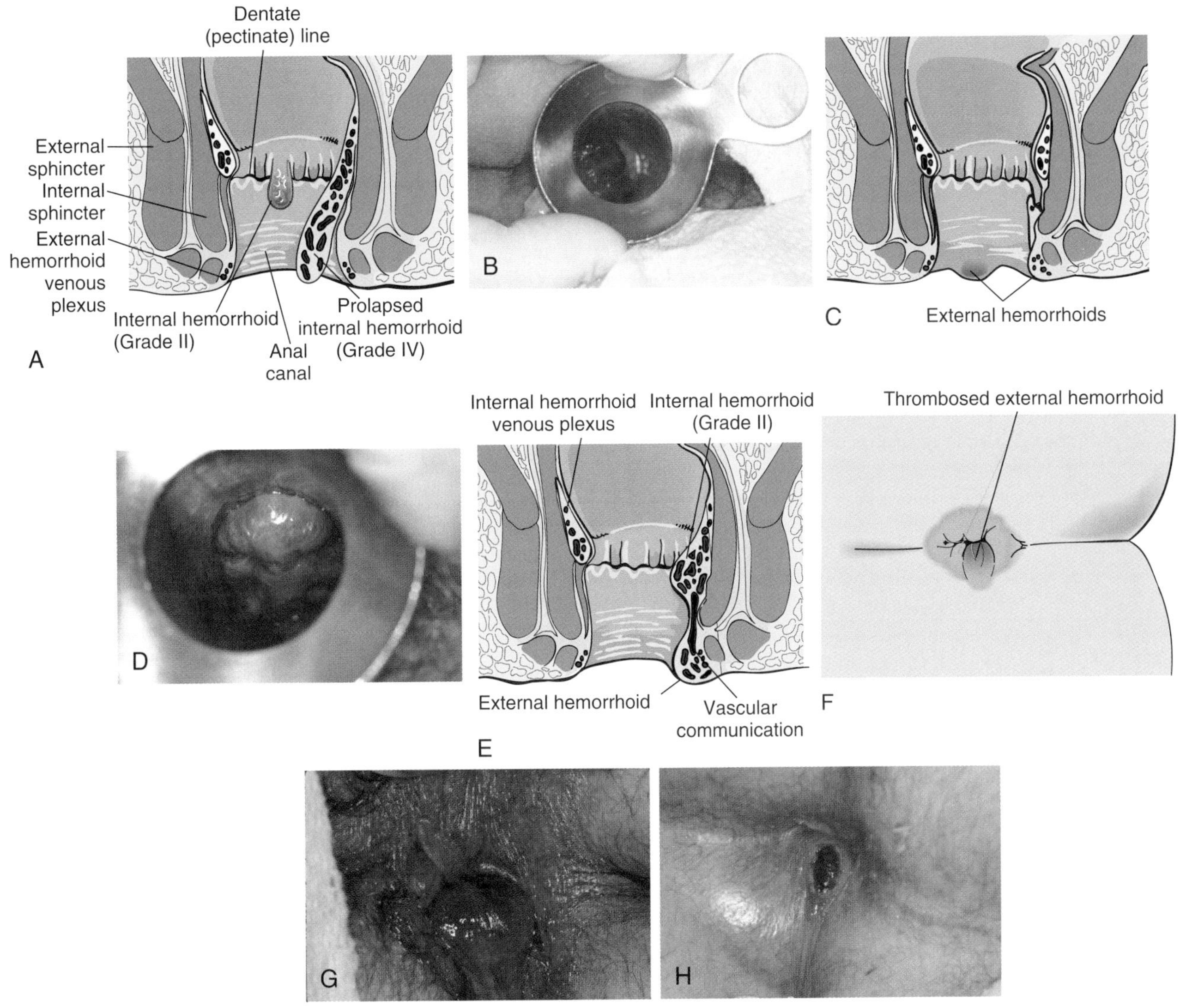

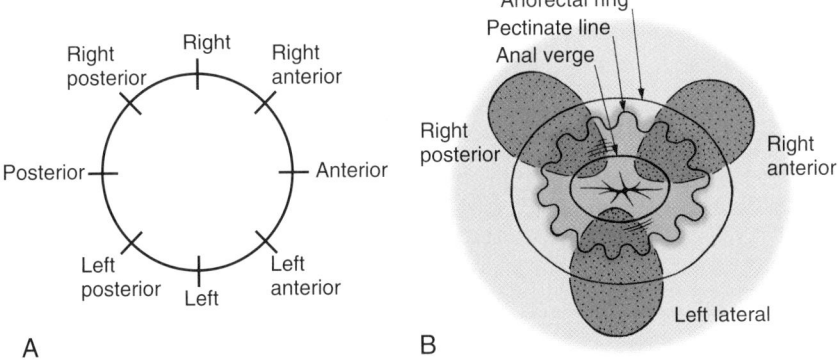

Fig. 87.1 Various types of hemorrhoids. (A) Internal hemorrhoid. Note that although an internal hemorrhoid may be visible "externally" (grade IV), it is classified by its origin, which, as shown here, is above the dentate line. (B) Internal hemorrhoid as seen through the Ives slotted anoscope. (C) External hemorrhoids. (D) External hemorrhoid as seen through the Ives anoscope. (E) Mixed hemorrhoid disease (both internal and external hemorrhoids with a vascular communication). (F) Thrombosed external hemorrhoid. (G) Large acute thrombosed hemorrhoid. (H) Normal progression of a thrombosed external hemorrhoid 4 to 5 days after occurrence. The skin over the top becomes necrotic and appears to be a thin membrane. (A, C, E, and F, Modified from Pfenninger JL, Surrell J. *Nonsurgical treatment options for internal hemorrhoids. Am Fam Physician.* 1995;52:821–837. Original art copyrighted by Steve Oh. B, D, G, and H, Courtesy John L. Pfenninger, MD, The Medical Procedures Center, Midland, MI.)

Fig. 87.2 (A) Eight segments in the rectum as seen through a slotted (Ives) anoscope, with the patient in the left lateral decubitus position. (B) Usual three primary hemorrhoidal groups.

INTERNAL HEMORRHOIDS

Indications

Bleeding or other symptomatology, such as prolapse, from internal hemorrhoids that has failed medical management (i.e., bulk agents, suppositories, topical preparations, and sitz baths) is an indication for treatment.

NOTE: The mere presence of hemorrhoids alone, without symptoms, is not necessarily an indication for treatment.

Contraindications

- Bleeding diathesis (relative). If on warfarin, the international normalized ratio should be in the therapeutic range. There is always an increased risk of bleeding if the patient is on aspirin, clopidogrel, or another oral anticoagulant (apixaban, dabigatran, and rivaroxaban) but generally this is not a contraindication to treatment.
- Pregnancy or immediately postpartum (<8 weeks).
- Inflammatory bowel disease.
- Anorectal fissures.
- Active anorectal infections.
- Acquired immunodeficiency syndrome or other immunodeficiency states.
- Portal hypertension (relative).
- Rectal wall mucosal prolapse.
- Anorectal tumors.

Recommendations for antibiotic subacute bacterial endocarditis prophylaxis have been updated (see Chapter 69, Antibiotic Prophylaxis).

TABLE 87.1	Classification of Internal Hemorrhoids
Grade	**Description**
I	Small, do not prolapse
II	Medium, prolapse and return spontaneously
III	Large, prolapse but reduce manually
IV	Largest, prolapse, not reducible

Basically, antibiotics are not indicated for hemorrhoidal procedures. For those in the very-high-risk categories, they would be optional.

Preprocedure Patient Preparation

1. Give the patient one or two enemas before the procedure. Although using an enema is not absolutely necessary, it is aesthetically helpful and improves visualization of the anatomy.
2. Ask the patient to avoid aspirin or clopidogrel and other oral anticoagulants for 1 week before treatment in low-risk situations.
3. Provide a patient education handout to ensure informed consent (see the sample patient education handouts available at www.expertconsult.com).
4. A complete history of the complaints as well as the pertinent past medical history and physical examination are essential. Record these on the sample encounter forms (go to www.expertconsult.com) that summarize the information.
5. The patient may be examined and treated in the left lateral decubitus position (which is usually more comfortable), the prone jackknife position, or even in the customary stirrups. The latter two positions can be used when exposure is difficult. No sedation is necessary for a patient having only anoscopy and internal hemorrhoid treatment. The patient may take four ibuprofen 200-mg tablets 1 to 2 hours before the office visit. Before performing anoscopy, perform an external visual and a digital anorectal examination. Ask the patient to perform a Valsalva maneuver (bearing down) to rule out full-thickness rectal prolapse. (Occasionally, examination with the patient sitting on the commode is necessary to assess for this.)

NOTE: Only internal hemorrhoids are treated by IRC, banding, or sclerotherapy. Treatment of external hemorrhoids requires excision and is associated with pain, so at least local anesthetics are needed.

Treatment

Rubber-band ligation (Barron or McGivney ligation), IRC, and sclerotherapy for internal hemorrhoids are discussed in the following sections. A summary of techniques and their indications is found in

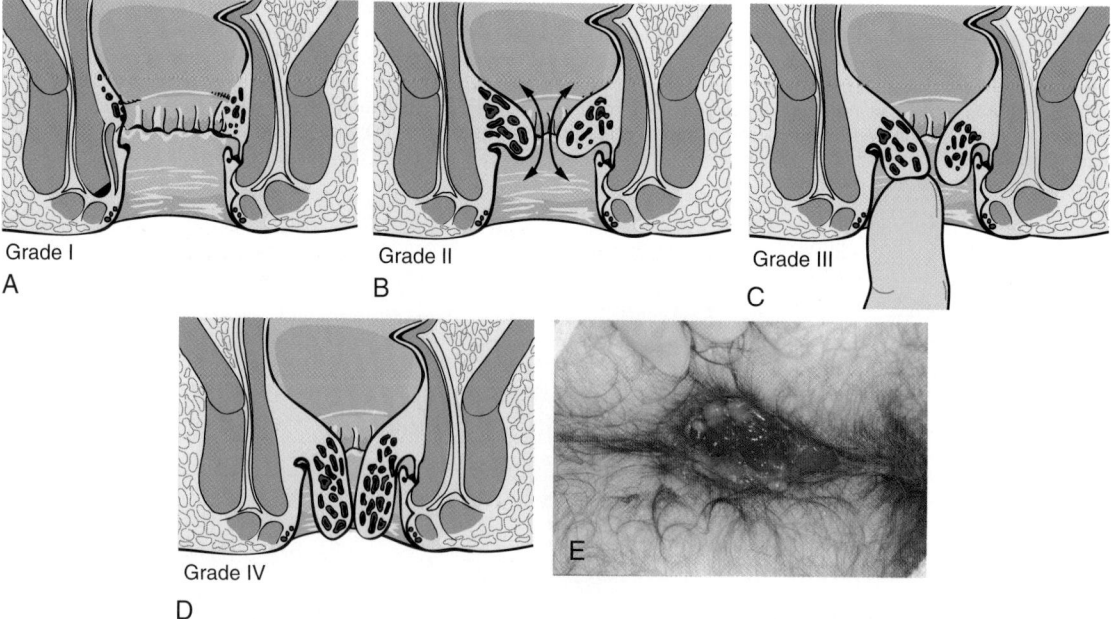

Fig. 87.3 Grading of *internal* hemorrhoids. (A) Grade I hemorrhoids are present and identifiable. (B) Grade II hemorrhoids prolapse with a bowel movement but return spontaneously. (C) Grade III hemorrhoids prolapse and can be replaced manually. (D) Grade IV hemorrhoids remain prolapsed in spite of all efforts at reduction and are often associated with varying amounts of mucosal prolapse. (E) Grade IV prolapsed internal hemorrhoid. (A–D, From Pfenninger JL, Surrell J. Nonsurgical treatment options for internal hemorrhoids. *Am Fam Physician*. 1995;52:821–837. Original art copyrighted by Steve Oh.)

	Grade				Ease of		
Method	**I**	**II**	**III**	**IV**	**Performance**	**Complications**	**Location**
Infrared coagulator	+++	+++	±	−	+++	Rare	Office
Rubber band	±	+++	+++	−	++	Some	Office
Sclerotherapy	++	+++	±	−	+	Common	Office
Stapled hemorrhoidopexy	−	−	+++	+++	+	See text	OR
Surgical excision	−	−	++	+++	+	Common	OR

TABLE 87.2 Comparison of Therapeutic Modalities for Treatment of Internal Hemorrhoids

OR, Operating room.
Scale: −, not recommended (does not work); +++, easiest (best suited).

Table 87.2. The treatment of external hemorrhoids is covered later in this chapter and the treatment of perianal skin tags is dealt with separately in Chapter 88, Removal of Perianal Skin Tags (External Hemorrhoidal Skin Tags). Because of the associated discharge and poor patient acceptance, cryotherapy is not covered in this discussion. The clinician should follow universal blood and body fluid precautions when performing any of these procedures.

Rubber-Band Ligation

Rubber-band ligation involves placing a rubber band around the base of an internal hemorrhoid. The ensnared tissue undergoes necrosis and sloughs. Rubber-band ligation is used for treatment of second- or third-degree bleeding or prolapsing internal hemorrhoids. A Cochrane review (Shanmugam, 2005) comparing rubber-band ligation to excisional hemorrhoidectomy showed banding to be as efficacious for complete resolution of hemorrhoidal symptoms as excision for grade II, but not grade III hemorrhoids. More recent studies, however, showed good long-term results for banding of grade III hemorrhoids.

EQUIPMENT:

- Slotted Ives anoscope (see Chapter 83, Anoscopy, Fig. 83.1).
- McGivney ligator with bands (or an acceptable alternative device; Fig. 87.4) is the traditional applicator. Alternatively, a disposable hemorrhoid ligator is available, the O'Regan Hemorrhoid Banding System (Fig. 87.5).
- Alligator forceps (similar to long-handled Allis clamp).
- External light source.
- Large obstetric/gynecologic cotton swabs.
- Equipment to follow universal blood and body fluid precautions.

TECHNIQUE: See Fig. 87.6.

1. Load the ligating drum with two bands. Insert the cone into the drum and slide the bands over it. A small amount of liquid soap on the cone will facilitate this. Hold the handle with the other hand to prevent the inadvertent sliding of the outer drum over the inner drum of the ligator while loading.
2. Insert the anoscope and visualize the hemorrhoid to be ligated. Treat the largest hemorrhoid group, or the obviously bleeding source, first. Have an assistant stabilize the anoscope.
3. With one hand, draw the hemorrhoidal tissue into the ligating drum with an alligator forceps. If the patient experiences pain, grasp the hemorrhoidal tissue more proximally. Pull only hemorrhoidal tissue into the ligator; avoid excessive mucosa.
4. With the other hand, grasp the handle of the ligator and push forward slightly. Squeeze the handle. The outer drum slides over the inner drum, displacing the rubber bands around the hemorrhoid.
5. Reposition or withdraw the anoscope. Patient tolerance is highest if only one hemorrhoid group is treated per visit. However, some clinicians treat more than one segment per visit. Avoid circumferential ligation because it may increase pain, and the tension on the mucosa may lead to nonhealing fissures.

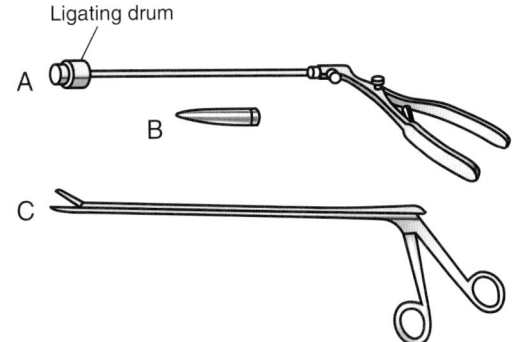

Fig. 87.4 McGivney ligator. (A) Ligator. (B) Cone to load bands. (C) Forceps to grasp hemorrhoid.

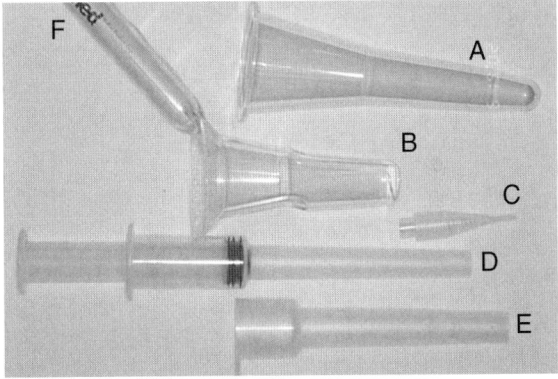

Fig. 87.5 O'Regan disposable banding unit. *A,* Trocar for insertion of anoscope; *B,* anoscope; *C,* loading cone for bands; *D,* syringe for suction to pull up hemorrhoid; *E,* sleeve that fits over syringe apparatus that pushes bands off onto hemorrhoids; *F,* penlight inserted into anoscope handle for light.

COMPLICATIONS:

- Spotting can be expected for 8 to 10 days. Profuse bleeding, although rare, occurs 1 to 2 weeks after the procedure, when the hemorrhoidal tissue sloughs. Bleeding can be significant and occasionally requires active intervention.
- Patients may experience a dull ache for 2 days after the procedure. If severe pain is experienced during the procedure, the band will need to be removed with scissors. It was applied too far distally.
- Thrombosis of external hemorrhoids occurs rarely and is treated symptomatically or with excision.
- Sepsis with pelvic cellulitis (perineal sepsis) is a serious complication, but it rarely occurs. Patients complain of fever, increasing perineal pain, swelling, inability to urinate, or dysuria. Treatment

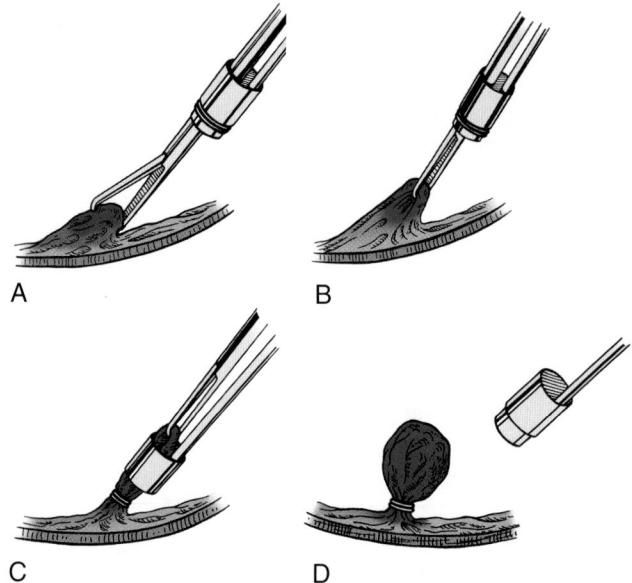

Fig. 87.6 Rubber-band ligation. The hemorrhoid is gently grasped (A) and brought into the drum of the ligator (B). Two rubber bands are released (C). Appearance of the ligated hemorrhoid after equipment is removed (D). If the patient tolerates the grasping of the hemorrhoid with forceps, ligation can be performed with minimal or no discomfort.

requires hospitalization, broad-spectrum antibiotic administration, and debridement.

- Slow healing or nonhealing of the treatment site can lead to formation of an anal fissure.

ADVANTAGES:

- The instrument itself is inexpensive, and there are no disposable tips to replace.
- Higher grades of hemorrhoids can be treated.
- The procedure is quick.
- The procedure is easy to learn.

DISADVANTAGES:

- The procedure is somewhat more uncomfortable than other techniques, and significant complications have been reported (e.g., perineal sepsis).
- Two people are needed to perform the procedure (the operator and the assistant, who holds the anoscope).

Postprocedure Patient Education

See the patient education handouts available at www.expertconsult.com.

- Inform the patient that mild aching discomfort may be experienced over the next 2 days.
- Ask the patient to report any excessive bleeding, fever, dysuria, inability to urinate (a sign of perineal sepsis), or increasing pain.
- Ask the patient to follow up in 4 to 6 weeks for reexamination and further banding, as needed.
- Patients should be on a lifetime regimen of enough fiber and fluids in their diet to keep their stools soft or mushy.

Infrared Coagulation

EQUIPMENT:

- Infrared coagulator (Redfield Corporation; Fig. 87.7).
- Slotted Ives anoscope (Redfield Corporation; see Chapter 83, Anoscopy, Fig. 83.1).
- External light source.
- Large obstetric/gynecologic cotton swabs.
- Equipment to follow universal blood and body fluid precautions.

NOTE: IRC units are not submersible for cleaning. Instead, they use a disposable sheath that is changed for each visit (see Fig. 87.7B). It is imperative not to immerse the newer units (in contrast to the older units) in sterilizing solutions.

TECHNIQUE: Infrared light is applied to the *base* of the internal hemorrhoid, forming a white coagulum that ulcerates and then forms a scar. The diameter of burn correlates with the size of the probe tip, which is usually 6 mm. The depth of penetration correlates with the time of the pulse, which is generally 1.5 to 2 seconds. Infrared coagulation is used for first- and second-degree and smaller third-degree internal hemorrhoids. It can be used for larger hemorrhoids (use a 2- to 2.5-second setting), but treatment may need to be repeated in 4 to 6 weeks. It is a painless procedure, and although more than one hemorrhoid group is sometimes treated, most clinicians begin by treating only one complex to determine patient tolerance. Treatment of more than one complex of hemorrhoids at a time may increase posttreatment discomfort and the other complications, especially bleeding. A teaching DVD/video describing this technique is available from Redfield Corporation.

1. With the patient in the left lateral decubitus position, insert the Ives slotted anoscope and identify the hemorrhoid to be treated. Insert the 6-mm IRC probe.
2. Press the probe tip onto the hemorrhoid itself, or preferably on the most proximal portion of the hemorrhoid. Only light pressure is needed.
3. Pull the trigger and keep it compressed. The unit has an incorporated time switch that limits exposure and will turn off automatically. The typical setting is 1.5 seconds. Generally, four to six separate applications are made for each hemorrhoid group. One group is treated per visit at 4- to 6-week intervals. For the first treatment, select the hemorrhoid that is bleeding or that is the largest. Larger hemorrhoids and grade III hemorrhoids may require more than one treatment session or a longer exposure (2 seconds).
   CAUTION: Do not overlap treatment sites. Overlapping increases the depth of burn. Place the probe adjacent to a previous site in a linear fashion or in a diamond shape, but do not overlap if possible (Fig. 87.8). If overlapping does occur, it rarely causes a significant problem, but purposely avoid it if possible.
4. Wipe off the tip with saline-soaked gauze between applications. This allows the tip to cool and cleans the end. If a loud "pop" is heard, there is debris or mucus between the tip and the mucosa. No damage is done, but the sudden noise can be frightening to the patient (and the clinician). It will sound much like a small firecracker.
5. Realign the anoscope and apply treatment to another hemorrhoidal group if more than one group is to be treated.
6. Remove the tip and the anoscope. No special aftercare is needed.

COMPLICATIONS:

- Patients may experience a mild, dull, aching pain lasting up to 2 days after treatment.
- Minor bleeding may be encountered for up to 2 weeks after the procedure. More bleeding can be expected at 10 to 14 days when the eschar sloughs. This can usually be managed conservatively but very rarely will require topical astringents or maybe even a suture.
- Rarely, patients experience a thrombosed external hemorrhoid in the area after treatment.
- Rarely, slow-healing ulcers can be encountered.
- Slow healing or nonhealing of the treatment site can lead to formation of an anal fissure.

ADVANTAGES:

- It is an essentially painless procedure.
- There have been no reported cases of perineal sepsis.
- The procedure is quick, simple to learn, and cost effective.

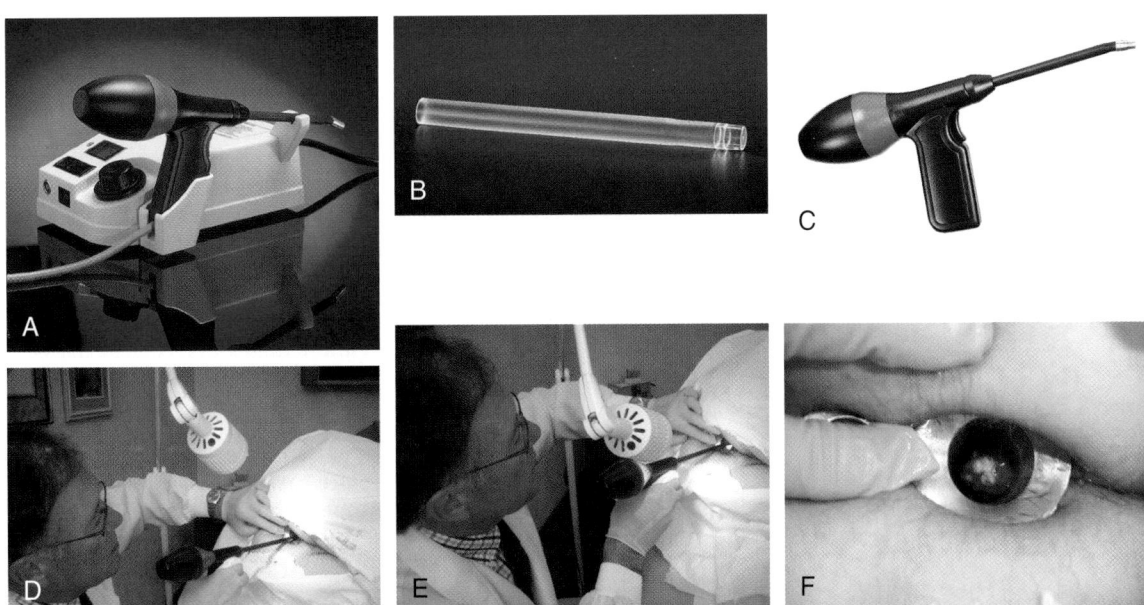

Fig. 87.7   Infrared coagulator (IRC) unit (A), sheath (B), and handpiece (C). The tip of the IRC is inserted through the Ives slotted anoscope and placed on the base of the hemorrhoid (D). When the unit is activated (E), a light is visible (noted here in the bulb of the handpiece) that automatically shuts off after the programmed time, usually 1.5 to 2 seconds. The internal hemorrhoid appears white over the treated area (F). (A–C, Courtesy Redfield Corporation, Rochelle Park, NJ. D–F, Courtesy John L. Pfenninger, MD, The Medical Procedures Center, Midland, MI.)

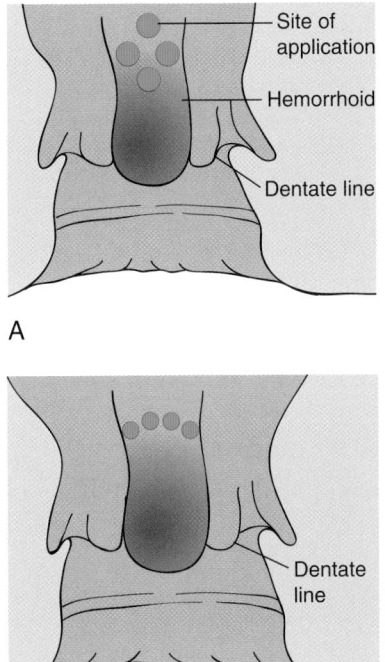

Fig. 87.8   Treatment of base (proximal portion) of the internal hemorrhoids using infrared coagulation. (A) Diamond shape. (B) Linear method. Each circle indicates a single application for 1.5 to 2 seconds. Up to six applications per visit may be needed per hemorrhoid segment.

- The procedure is well tolerated by patients.
- There are no costs for disposable probes, but disposable vinyl sheaths are used.
- It can be used in patients with pacemakers.
- The unit can also be used to remove tattoos, reduce nasal turbinates, stop bleeding from biopsy and hair donor sites, and treat verrucae and condylomata. Its use is being explored for treating anal dysplasia.

- The unit is well made and requires little maintenance.

DISADVANTAGES:

- The procedure is not very effective for advanced third-degree hemorrhoidal disease and works poorly for fourth-degree hemorrhoidal disease.
- The unit costs more than the materials for band ligation.

POSTPROCEDURE PATIENT EDUCATION: See the patient education handouts available at www.expertconsult.com.

- Ask the patient to follow up in 4 to 6 weeks to treat residual disease or another group of hemorrhoids. In the elderly or compromised patient (e.g., diabetes), it is best to wait longer.
- Ask the patient to report any severe symptoms of pain, fever, or inability to urinate.
- They should be on a lifetime regimen of enough fiber and fluids in their diet to keep their stools soft or mushy.

Sclerotherapy

Sclerotherapy is used for treatment of first- or second-degree internal bleeding hemorrhoids. Injection of 1 to 2 mL of sclerosant into the internal hemorrhoid causes sclerosis and fixation of the submucosa to the underlying muscularis. This technique is relatively quick. All three major hemorrhoidal groups can be treated at one sitting. It is a useful technique for a patient on warfarin. Unfortunately, it has not been as effective as other modalities and has been associated with impotence, the reason for which is unknown.

EQUIPMENT:

- Ives slotted anoscope
- 5-mL syringe
- 21-gauge spinal needle
- Sclerosant (sodium morrhuate, sodium tetradecyl sulfate, hypertonic saline, or phenol in almond oil)
- Equipment to follow universal blood and body fluid precautions

TECHNIQUE: See Fig. 87.9.

1. Insert the anoscope and visualize the hemorrhoid group to be injected.
2. Insert the spinal needle into or immediately above the hemorrhoid group in the submucosal space. Withdraw the plunger of

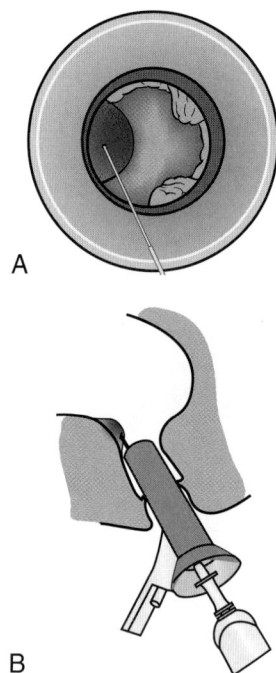

Fig. 87.9 (A) Sclerotherapy as viewed through the anoscope. If a wheal is not produced, the injection is too deep and the needle should be withdrawn. An injection that is too superficial will produce necrosis of the anal canal lining. (B) Injection technique.

the syringe and aspirate for blood to ensure that the sclerosant will not be injected directly into a vein.
3. Inject 1 to 2 mL of sclerosant. *A wheal should be noted during injection.* Take care to inject well above the level of the dentate line.
4. Document the location of the injection and the amount of sclerosant used.
5. Reposition the anoscope to visualize the next hemorrhoid group to be treated.

COMPLICATIONS:

- The procedure is painful if the sclerosant is injected below the level of the dentate line.
- Thrombosis of internal or external hemorrhoids may occur, causing pain. Thrombosis is managed with topical creams, analgesics, and sitz baths.
- Bleeding is usually the result of injection into the mucosa rather than the submucosa. Necrosis and ulceration with bleeding occur 2 to 3 weeks after injection. Healing usually occurs in 3 to 6 weeks.
- Abscess occurs very rarely.
- Anaphylaxis from the sclerosant is rare.
- Impotence has been reported, but the etiology is uncertain.

ADVANTAGES:

- The procedure is effective.
- It can be used in a patient on warfarin.
- The equipment cost is minimal.
- It can be used concomitantly with banding or other therapies.

DISADVANTAGES:

- The procedure is associated with more significant complications than other methods.
- The technique is harder to master.

POSTPROCEDURE PATIENT EDUCATION: See the sample patient education handouts available at www.expertconsult.com.

- Inform the patient that mild rectal discomfort may occur after treatment and tell the patient to report any severe symptoms.

- Instruct the patient to return to the office in 4 weeks for repeat examination and further treatments if necessary.
- Patients should be on a lifetime regimen of enough fiber and fluids in their diet to keep their stools soft or mushy.

Stapled Hemorrhoidopexy

Recently, stapled hemorrhoidopexy (SH), or procedure for prolapse and hemorrhoids (PPH), has been introduced as a novel method of correcting third- and fourth-degree hemorrhoids. During this procedure, a specialized stapling device reduces hemorrhoidal prolapse by excising a circumferential band of prolapsed mucosa and submucosa between the distal rectum and proximal anal canal (Fig. 87.10). This procedure interrupts the terminal branches of the hemorrhoidal arteries and resuspends the anal canal mucosa to a more physiologic location. The stapling device is known as the PPH 03 and is manufactured by Ethicon Endo-Surgery.

INDICATIONS: This procedure can be used with minimally symptomatic external disease. Other clinicians will perform PPH and add single- and multiquadrant excision or external hemorrhoids or tags.

CONTRAINDICATIONS:

- Anal stenosis
- Large external hemorrhoids or tags
- Gangrenous or strangulated hemorrhoids
- Perianal sepsis
- Full-thickness rectal prolapse
- Anal-receptive intercourse

ADVANTAGES:

- Less postoperative pain and more rapid return to normal activities than with a surgical hemorrhoidectomy
- No external wounds to care for
- Less incontinence and constipation reported than with conventional hemorrhoidectomy

COMPLICATIONS:

- Anal stenosis
- Secondary bleeding
- Urinary retention
- Pelvic sepsis
- Incontinence
- Prolonged, intractable pain

POSTPROCEDURE PATIENT EDUCATION:

- There are usually no external wounds to care for. This is case dependent.
- Prescribe an oral analgesic.
- Discomfort lasts for 1 to 2 weeks.
- Warm tub soaks may relieve discomfort.
- Patients should be on a lifetime regimen of enough fiber and fluids in their diet to keep their stools soft or mushy.

THROMBOSED EXTERNAL HEMORRHOIDS

External hemorrhoids occur below the dentate (pectinate) line. Patients with thrombosed external hemorrhoids have a painful, tender, swollen, bluish lump at the anal orifice. If the patient is seen within 48 hours of the onset of symptoms, the thrombosed hemorrhoid should be incised or excised. After 48 to 72 hours, symptoms have usually improved and symptomatic care is recommended if the pain is minimal, especially for smaller lesions. However, if the patient is still experiencing significant pain, the hemorrhoid can be surgically relieved at any time.

There are three basic surgical approaches: (1) excise an ellipse over the clotted hemorrhoid and evacuate the clot, (2) excise the hemorrhoid completely, or (3) make a simple incision over the clot and express the contents.

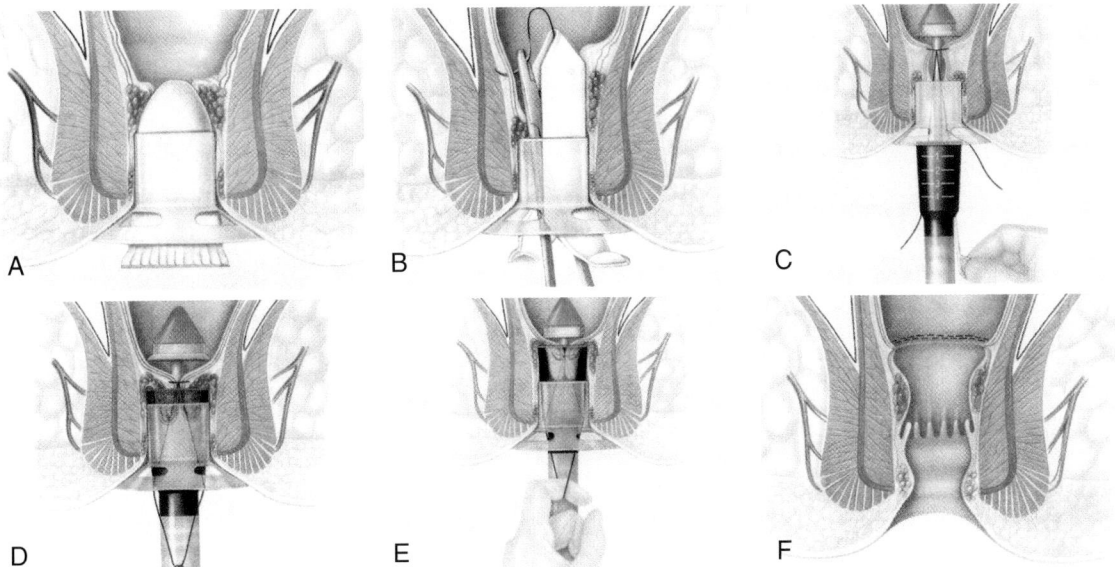

Fig. 87.10 Procedure for prolapse and hemorrhoids, or stapled hemorrhoidopexy. (A) Circular anal dilator/obturator is inserted into the anal canal to push the prolapse back and lift the hemorrhoidal tissue into place. (B) Internal hemorrhoids are held back while a purse-string suture is prepared in the rectal mucosa/submucosa approximately 4 to 6 cm from the dentate line. (C) A fully opened hemorrhoidal circular stapler is inserted beyond the purse-string suture. The purse-string is tied around the anvil to secure the excess mucosal tissue. With the suture threader, each limb of the suture is brought through the channel of the instrument. (D) After the ends of the retraction suture are knotted, the stapler is tightened and gently pushed into the anal canal. Moderate traction on the purse-string must be maintained so that the prolapse is drawn into the stapler casing. (E) The stapler is then closed completely, fired in one fluid motion, and withdrawn gently. The anal canal wall is reconnected and restored, and the hemorrhoidal artery's terminal branches, which feed internal hemorrhoids, are interrupted. (F) Successful completion of the procedure for prolapse and hemorrhoids corrects the prolapse, restores internal hemorrhoids to their normal anatomic position, and alleviates the patient's symptoms. (From Senagore AJ, Abcarian H, Chiu YSY, Ellis CN. Current treatment options for patients with grades III and IV hemorrhoids. *Contempt Surg Supplement*. 2006:S5–S11.)

Equipment

- No. 11 blade and tissue scissors
- Mosquito hemostats
- Fine tissue forceps
- Lidocaine (2%) with epinephrine; 27-gauge, 1.5-inch needle, and 3-mL syringe
- Antiseptic solution
- 4-0 or 5-0 absorbable suture (if closure is desired, but best if left open)
- Equipment to follow universal blood and body fluid precautions

Technique

See Figs. 87.11 and 87.12.
1. Cleanse the perianal area with antiseptic solution.
2. Infiltrate the skin over the thrombosed external hemorrhoid with lidocaine with epinephrine (1 to 2 mL).
3. Excise the entire hemorrhoid as an ellipse or perform an elliptical excision over the top of the hemorrhoid and remove the skin. Be sure to evacuate all clots.
4. Control any bleeding with electrocautery or silver nitrate sticks if pressure alone is not adequate.
5. The wound is best left open to heal by secondary intention, which it usually does without adverse sequelae. The skin edges may also be approximated with interrupted, fine absorbable suture (unless silver nitrate was used), but this is generally discouraged.
6. Alternatively, after anesthesia, the base of the clotted hemorrhoid can be clamped (under the clot) with a hemostat. The tissue over the hemostat is excised with a blade. With the hemostat still in place, a suture is placed proximal to the tip. If interrupted sutures are used, leave the ends of the first stitch long and use them for traction to pull down the upper portion of the incision. If a running stitch is used, the long end can be used in the same manner. Then remove the hemostat and complete the clo-

sure. This ensures that the entire excisional site has been sutured closed.
7. As an additional alternative, some clinicians simply incise over the thrombus and evacuate the clot. If this is done, it is imperative that all clots be removed. After the incision is made, express the clot, and then explore the cavity with hemostats to break down any septa. Another incision inside the cavity may be necessary. Frequently more than one clot will be evacuated. Reexpress the area to be sure all clots have been removed. This technique is quicker but warn the patient that there is a higher likelihood of reaccumulation with this approach. Consider this method when the clot has been present for several days and the acute clotting process has resolved.

Complications

- Bleeding
- Pain
- Recurrence
- Chronic fissure
- Infection

Postprocedure Patient Education

See the sample patient education handouts available at www.expertconsult.com.

- Recommend that the patient take sitz baths two to three times per day for 1 week.
- Oral analgesics, topical anesthetic cream/ointment (e.g., lidocaine 5%), and stool softeners are helpful.
- A follow-up examination should be scheduled for 4 weeks.
- Emphasize that the patient avoid prolonged sitting on the toilet to prevent recurrent thrombosis. Also, avoid excesses of any activity (e.g., weight lifting) that induces a Valsalva maneuver.
- Patients should be on a lifetime regimen of enough fiber and fluids in their diet to keep their stools soft or mushy.

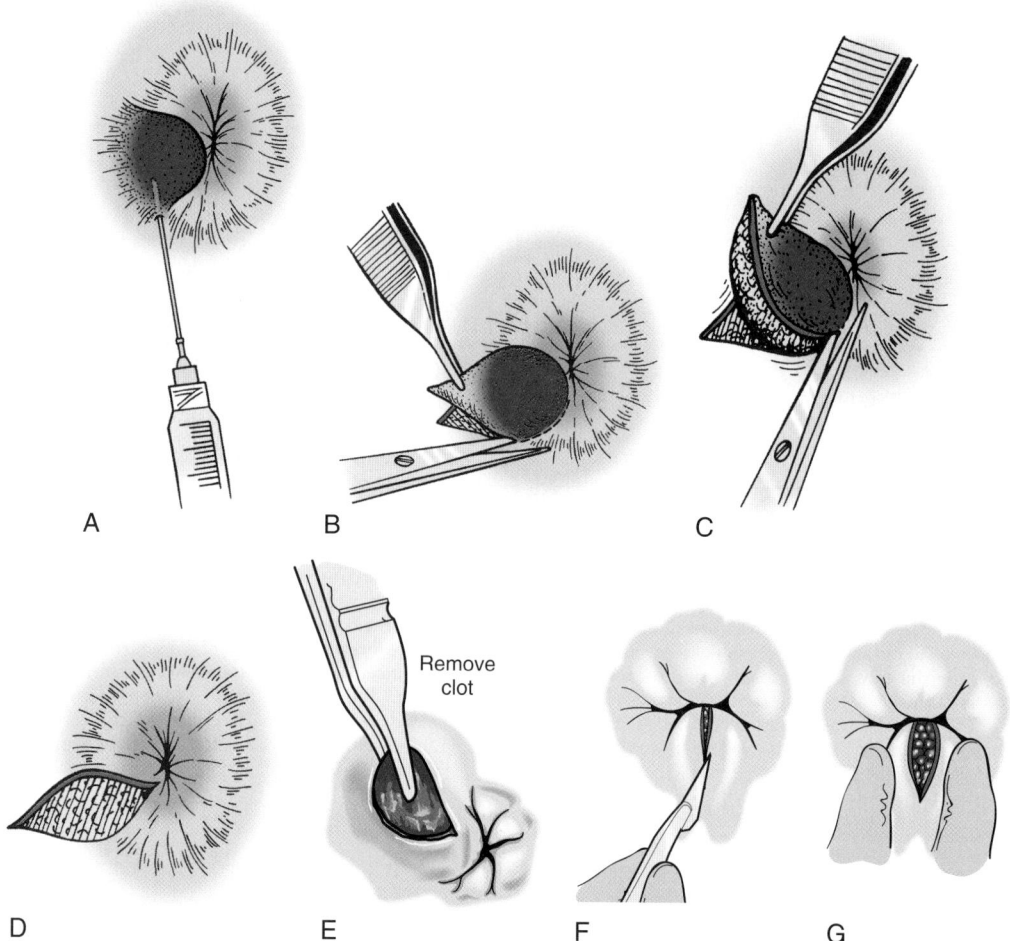

A   B   C

D   E   F   G

Remove clot

Fig. 87.11 Excision of a thrombosed hemorrhoid. (A) The area is infiltrated with 2% lidocaine with epinephrine. (B–C) The thrombosed hemorrhoid is excised along with a small wedge of skin. (D) Skin edges are sufficiently separated to permit adequate drainage, thereby preventing clot reaccumulation. They can also be closed with fine absorbable suture. (E) Instead of removing the entire hemorrhoid, a small elliptical incision is made over the hemorrhoid and the clot is expressed. No suture closure is needed. (F) A simple incision and drainage with expression of all clots can also be performed. Multiple clots are often present and should be removed. (G) After the initial clot is removed, spread the incision to expose the base of the hemorrhoid to remove other thrombi. The disadvantage of this approach is that the incision can seal over, allowing the clot to reaccumulate.

EXTERNAL HEMORRHOIDAL TAGS

See Figs. 87.13 and 87.14 (also see Chapter 88, Removal of Perianal Skin Tags [External Hemorrhoidal Skin Tags]).

External hemorrhoidal tags are usually the result of previous external hemorrhoidal disease. Occasionally, a patient has experienced a thrombosis that resolved spontaneously but the skin remains stretched out. These lesions no longer have dilated vessels and are often quite fibrotic. The major symptoms include pruritus and problems with cleanliness. Generally, when removed in the office, only one area is removed at a visit unless the attachments are quite small.

Equipment

- Alcohol wipe
- 3% to 5% lidocaine with epinephrine
- No. 15 scalpel blade
- Monsel solution to control bleeding
- Cautery (ball electrode or bipolar forceps)
- 5% lidocaine ointment
- Ives slotted anoscope
- Lubricant
- Nonsterile gloves and equipment to follow universal blood and body fluid precautions

- Formalin pathology jar

Indications

Symptomatic as noted previously.

Contraindications

The treatment is contraindicated if the patient is unwilling to tolerate pain for several days.

Technique

1. Place the patient in left lateral decubitus position. Perform digital and anoscopic examinations.
2. Identify the lesion to be removed and wipe with alcohol or other antiseptic.
3. Inject the lidocaine in a field block pattern. Be careful not to tent up the area too much under the tag, which may lead to excision of too much tissue.
4. If using a radiofrequency unit, set at cut and coag (level 3, or 30 W) and use either a Vari-Tip wire or a loop and remove the lesion. Control the bleeding with Monsel solution or cautery.

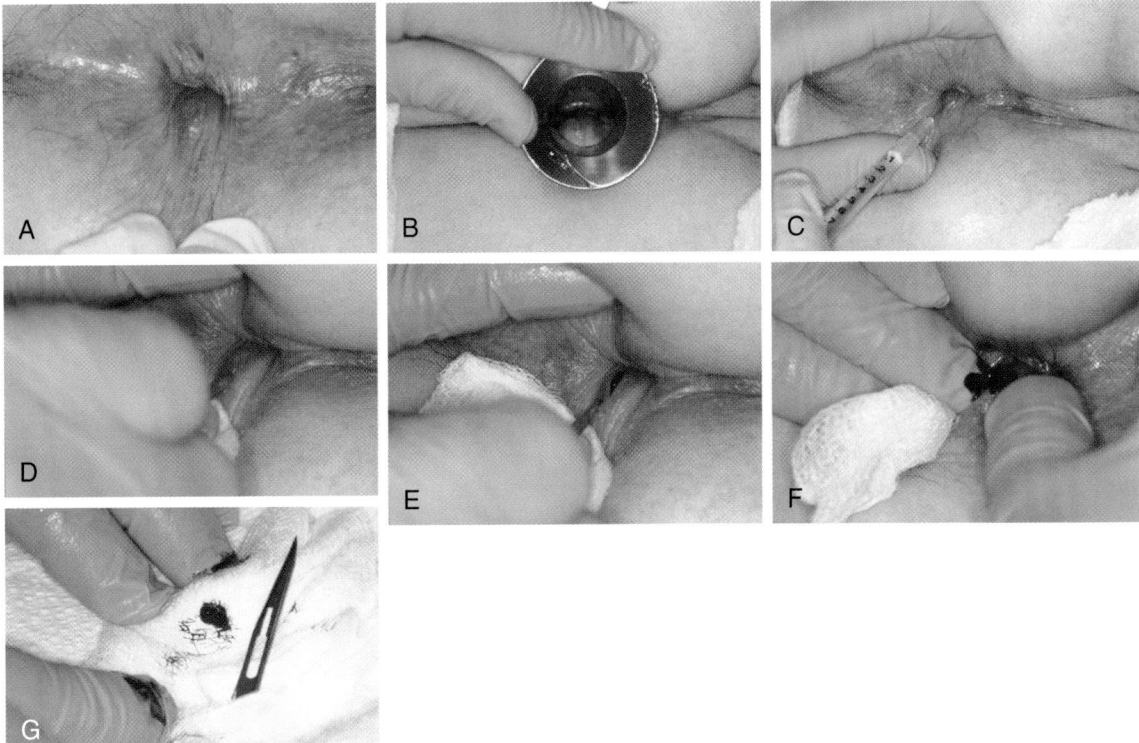

Fig. 87.12 Incision and drainage of thrombosed external hemorrhoid using small ellipse technique. (A) Thrombosed external hemorrhoid. (B) View through Ives slotted anoscope. (C) Injection of 1 mL 2% lidocaine with epinephrine. (D) Initial incision with No. 11 pointed blade. (E) Forming the ellipse. (F) Expressing the clot. (G) Clot and No. 11 blade. (Courtesy John L. Pfenninger, MD, The Medical Procedures Center, Midland, MI.)

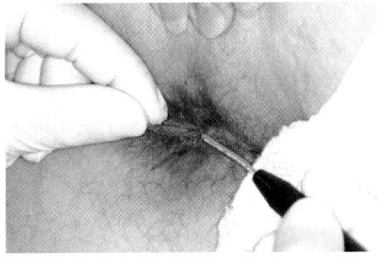

Fig. 87.13 Removal of small hemorrhoidal tag using radiofrequency loop after anesthetic injection. (Courtesy John L. Pfenninger, MD, The Medical Procedures Center, Midland, MI.)

5. Alternatives are to use a blade or scissors to remove the lesion. There may be more bleeding with this method. If the base of the tag is quite large, a hemostat can be applied and left in place for several minutes, and then the tissue excised. This ensures approximation of the skin margins. No sutures are placed because they increase the chances of infection. Control bleeding as indicated previously.
6. Apply antibiotic ointment mixed with 5% lidocaine ointment.

Complications

- Pain
- Bleeding
- Infection
- Chronic fissure

Postoperative Patient Care

Nonsteroidal antiinflammatory drugs are the mainstay for pain control. Narcotics can cause constipation. Lidocaine 5% ointment is helpful to control and reduce abrasive rubbing of clothes or other skin. Sitz baths are very helpful and the area should be cleansed three to four times a day. It may be best to stay off work for 2 to 3 days, depending on the size of the lesion. Patients should be on a lifetime regimen of enough fiber and fluids in their diet to keep their stools soft or mushy.

CPT/Billing Codes

46083	Incision and drainage of thrombosed external hemorrhoid
46220	Excision, single anal tag or papilla
46221	Hemorrhoidectomy, by simple ligature (e.g., rubber band)
46230	Excision of external hemorrhoid tags and/or multiple papillae
46250	Hemorrhoidectomy, external, 2 or more columns/groups
46255	Hemorrhoidectomy; internal and external, single column/group
46260	Hemorrhoidectomy; internal and external, 2 or more columns/groups
46320	Enucleation or excision of external thrombosed hemorrhoid
46500	Injection of sclerosing solution, hemorrhoids
46600	Anoscopy
46930	Destruction of hemorrhoids by thermal energy (e.g., IRC, cautery, radiofrequency)
46945	Hemorrhoidopexy (e.g., prolapsing internal hemorrhoids) by ligation other than rubber band, single column/group
46946	Two or more columns/groups

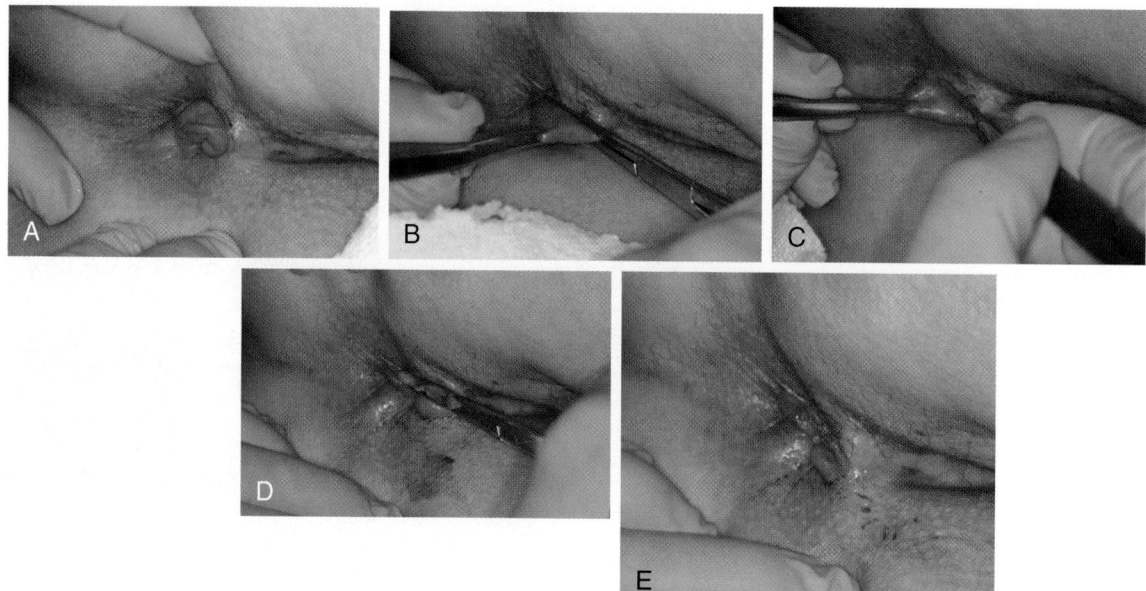

Fig. 87.14 Removal of hemorrhoidal tag with large base. (A) Tag. (B) Applying large clamp or hemostats. (C) Electrosurgical cutting/removal of tag. (D) Appearance after removal of tag with clamp in place. (E) No sutures are used to close the wound. (Courtesy John L. Pfenninger, MD, The Medical Procedures Center, Midland, MI.)

ICD-10-CM DIAGNOSTIC CODES

K64.8	Internal hemorrhoids
K64.5	Internal hemorrhoids, thrombosed
K64.9	Internal hemorrhoids, bleeding
K64.9	External hemorrhoids
K64.5	External hemorrhoids, thrombosed
K64.4	Hemorrhoid tag

SUPPLIERS

(See contact information available at www.expertconsult.com.)

Band ligator
Redfield Corporation
Infrared coagulator (IRC)
Redfield Corporation
Ives slotted anoscope
Redfield Corporation
O'Regan Hemorrhoid Banding System
CRH O'Regan System: http://physicians.crhsystem.com/order-product/
Sclerosing agents
See Table 92.1.

RECOMMENDED READING

Alonso-Coello P, Guyatt GH, Heels-Ansdell D, et al. Laxatives for the treatment of hemorrhoids. *Cochrane Database of Sys Rev.* 2005:CD004649.

Bleday R, Pena JP, Rothenberger DA, et al. Symptomatic hemorrhoids: current incidence and complications of operative therapy. *Dis Colon Rectum.* 1992;35:477–481.

Bullock N. Impotence after sclerotherapy of haemorrhoids: case report. *BMJ.* 1997;314:419–420.

Corman ML, ed. *Colon and Rectal Surgery.* 5th ed. Philadelphia: Lippincott Williams & Wilkins; 2004.

Dennison AR, Whiston RJ, Rooney S, Morris DL. The management of hemorrhoids. *Am J Gastroenterol.* 1989;84:475–481.

Devine R, Ory S. Treatment of hemorrhoids in pregnancy. *J Fam Pract.* 1992;17:65.

Gordon P, Nivatvongs S, eds. *Principles and Practice of Surgery for the Colon, Rectum, and Anus.* 3rd ed. New York: Informa Healthcare; 2007.

Johanson JF, Rimm A. Optimal nonsurgical treatment of hemorrhoids: a comparative analysis of infrared coagulation, rubber band ligation, and injection sclerotherapy. *Am J Gastroenterol.* 1992;87:1600–1606.

MacRae HM, McLeod RS. Comparison of hemorrhoidal treatment modalities: a meta-analysis. *Dis Colon Rectum.* 1995;38:687–694.

Pfenninger JL. Modern treatments for internal haemorrhoids. *BMJ.* 1997;314:1211–1212.

Pfenninger JL, Surrell J. Nonsurgical treatment options for internal hemorrhoids. *Am Fam Physician.* 1995;52:821–837.

Pfenninger JL, Zainea GG. Common anorectal conditions: part I. Symptoms and complaints. *Am Fam Physician.* 2001;63:2391–2398.

Pfenninger JL, Zainea GG. Common anorectal conditions: part II. Lesions. *Am Fam Physician.* 2001;64:77–88.

Rossi DC, Bastawrous AL. Hemorrhoids. In: Bailey HR, Billingham RP, Stamos MJ, Snyder MJ, eds. *Colorectal Surgery.* Philadelphia: Elsevier; 2013:95–116.

Russell TR, Donahue JH. Hemorrhoidal banding: a warning. *Dis Colon Rectum.* 1985;28:291–293.

Shanmugam V, Hakeem A, Campbell KL, et al. Rubber band ligation versus excisional haemorrhoidectomy for haemorrhoids. *Cochrane Database of Sys Rev.* 2005: CD005034.

Simon T. Minor office procedures. *Clin Colon Rectal Surg.* 2005;18:225–260.

Smith LE. Hemorrhoidectomy with lasers and other contemporary modalities. *Surg Clin North Am.* 1992;3:665–679.

Standards Task Force of the American Society of Colon and Rectal Surgeons. Practice parameters for the treatment of hemorrhoids. *Dis Colon Rectum.* 1993;36:1118–1120.

Templeton JL, Spence RA, Kennedy TL, et al. Comparison of infrared coagulation and rubber band ligation for first and second degree haemorrhoids: a randomised prospective clinical trial. *BMJ.* 1983;286:1387–1389.

Walker AJ, Leicester RJ, Nicholls RJ, Mann CV. A prospective study of infrared coagulation, injection and rubber band ligation in the treatment of haemorrhoids. *Int J Colorectal Dis.* 1990;5:113–116.

Zinberg SS, Stern DH, Furman DS, Wittles JM. A personal experience in comparing three non-operative techniques for treating internal hemorrhoids. *Am J Gastroenterol.* 1989;84:488–492.

CHAPTER 88

REMOVAL OF PERIANAL SKIN TAGS (EXTERNAL HEMORRHOIDAL SKIN TAGS)

James A. Surrell

Perianal skin tags represent a stretching and enlargement of the normal perianal skin (Fig. 88.1). As such, they are not true external hemorrhoids. Perianal skin tags are believed to occur as a result of large external hemorrhoids that have receded. A "sentinel" skin tag can occur at the site of an anal fissure, usually located directly posterior or occasionally anterior (for the most common sites for an anal fissure, see Chapter 85, Anal Fissure, Lateral Sphincterotomy, and Anal Fistula). A previously thrombosed external hemorrhoid may also leave redundant skin after resolving. Patients most often seek treatment for them when they begin to interfere with anal hygiene. It is important to note that perianal skin tags do not cause pain, bleeding, or a discharge. If these symptoms are present, then another source must be sought as the cause of these symptoms.

INDICATIONS

- Large perianal skin tags limiting anal hygiene
- Perianal skin tags that annoy the patient or are symptomatic (e.g., pruritus)

NOTE: The only time anal skin tags cause itching is when the patient is doing excessive perianal cleansing, thereby irritating the skin tag and the surrounding perianal tissues.

Generally, a conservative approach to the management of perianal skin tags is recommended because the vast majority of these benign lesions are asymptomatic. If the patient is bothered by pruritus, try local measures first. (See patient education form available at www.expertconsult.com.)

CONTRAINDICATIONS

- If the patient with perianal skin tags complains of pain, bleeding, or a discharge, then another source for these symptoms must be sought. Skin tag excision will not relieve these symptoms. Even when the patient complains of pruritus "from the tag," be sure he or she is following proper hygiene practices noted in the aforementioned patient education handout because the tag itself may not be the cause of symptoms.
- If the perianal skin tags have a fleshy, edematous appearance, a diagnosis of anal Crohn disease must be strongly considered. Nearly all patients with anal Crohn disease will develop fleshy, edematous skin tags and have associated signs and symptoms of pain, bleeding, discharge, and atypical anal fissures (see Chapter 85, Anal Fissure, Lateral Sphincterotomy, and Anal Fistula). Excision of perianal skin tags in Crohn disease may lead to significant morbidity because of the creation of an indolent, nonhealing wound.

EQUIPMENT

- 2% lidocaine with epinephrine, 3 to 5 mL (this can be buffered with 0.25 mL 7% to 10% sodium bicarbonate to take some of the sting out; see Chapter 5, Local Anesthesia)
- 25-gauge, 0.5-inch to 30-gauge, 0.5-inch needle
- 4 × 4 gauze pads
- Hemostat, straight not curved
- Pickups
- No. 10 or No. 15 blade scalpel or sharp tissue scissors (alternatively, a radiofrequency/electrocautery unit)
- Monsel solution (ferric subsulfate)
- Cautery unit in case of bleeding
- Absorbable suture in case of uncontrolled bleeding
- Lidocaine 5% ointment or antibiotic ointment
- Feminine Peri-Pad

Because the perianal skin tags are external to the anal canal, no anal retractor is needed. Any standard surgical forceps are adequate to grasp the skin tag. If available, the electrocautery unit should have both coagulation and cutting capability. (See Chapter 25, Radiofrequency Surgery [Modern Electrosurgery], and Chapter 127, Loop Electrosurgical Excision Procedure for Treating Cervical Intraepithelial Neoplasia, for listings of suppliers of various modern electrosurgery units.)

PREPROCEDURE PATIENT PREPARATION

Most patients should be discouraged from having their perianal skin tags excised. Because perianal skin tags per se usually cause no significant symptoms, question the patient in depth about his or her reasons for wanting the skin tags excised. Advise the patient that there will be some mild to moderate "burning" postoperative pain at the site of the excision for up to 2 weeks, possibly more. Postoperative bleeding is usually negligible but can be a problem, and infection is rare because the cauterized operative site is usually left open. The chances for infection increase if the site is sutured (Vicryl, chromic).

TECHNIQUE

1. Place the patient in the left lateral decubitus position on the procedure table.
2. Infiltrate the base of the skin tag with approximately 1 or 2 mL of local anesthetic (e.g., 2% lidocaine with epinephrine). To minimize discomfort, inject the anesthetic solution (at room temperature; it can be buffered) very slowly at the base of the skin tag with a 25- or 30-gauge, 0.5-inch hypodermic needle. When performed properly, this injection technique affords min-

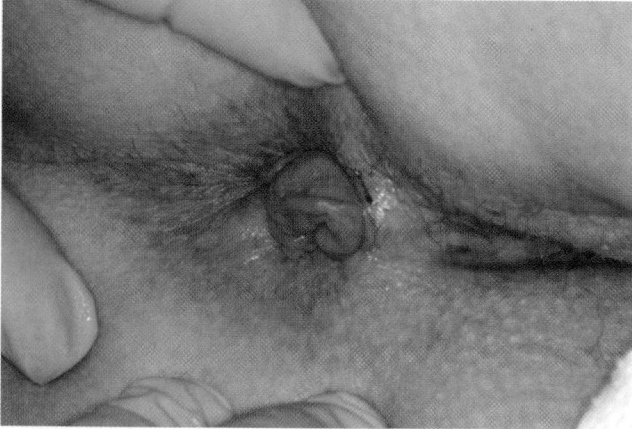

Fig. 88.1   Large perianal tag.

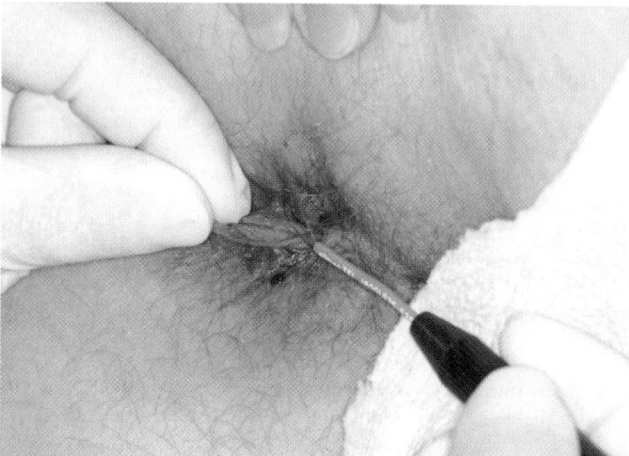

Fig. 88.2   Removing perianal tag using cutting electrosurgery.

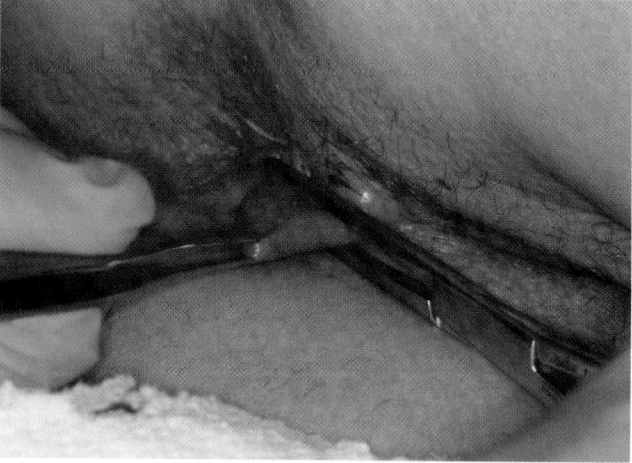

Fig. 88.3   Clamping the base of tag for hemostasis.

imal discomfort to the patient. Do not use too much volume because this will distort the area to be excised and may leave an excessively large wound. Alternatively, do a field block around the lesion to maintain undisturbed anatomy near the tag.

3. After approximately 1 minute, grasp the skin tag with a 4 × 4 gauze pad between the thumb and index finger and compress it to reduce the edema caused by infiltration of the local anes-

thetic. This also restores the skin tag to its "normal" anatomy, so the site of excision can be identified properly.

4. Grasp the skin tag with forceps (which will confirm that appropriate anesthesia has been induced) and hold it perpendicular to its base on the perianal skin. Care must be taken not to put any undue tension on the skin tag because this will also serve to "tent up" and broaden the base of the skin tag and create an excision site that is much larger than needed.

5. Excise the skin tag, using the scalpel, scissors, or electrocautery unit in the cutting or blend mode. The site of excision should be approximately 3 mm above or beyond the normal perianal tissues because there will be electrocautery tissue destruction below the site of excision. In other words, after the tag is excised, there should be an approximate 3 mm rim of normal skin tissue remaining; when the patient sits on this, it will form a nice, natural "bandage" over at least a portion of the wound. If the skin tag is held taut or excised right at the level of the perianal skin, the resulting wound defect and patient discomfort will be greater than needed (Fig. 88.2); when the patient later sits on the excised area, local pressure may force the wound to open up.

6. Cauterize any residual small bleeding sites. No more than three perianal skin tags are recommended to be excised during any one procedure.

7. Leave the site of excision open because suture closure contributes to an increase in postoperative pain and a greater likelihood of perianal abscess.

8. For larger tags, apply a straight hemostat at the base of the lesion, being careful not to grasp too much tissue. Leave it in place several minutes to control potential bleeding. Shave off the excess tissue using desired method. Remove clamp (Figs. 88.3 to 88.6).

9. Control bleeding.

10. Apply lidocaine or antibiotic ointment to soothe the area and prevent it from drying/sticking to clothing.

11. Give the patient a Peri-Pad to prevent blood from reaching clothing.

12. It is probably best to excise only one tag at a time if the procedure is being done in the office. This limits pain and the potential for bleeding, and decreases tension on the healing wound. This is especially true with larger-based lesions.

COMPLICATIONS

* A perianal abscess can develop at the site of excision of a skin tag, although this is uncommon and occurs less than 1% of the time. If an abscess does occur, appropriate incision and drainage will be necessary.
* If the skin tag excision site is very close to the anal verge, a chronic fissure may develop, although this is also very uncommon.
* Perianal cellulitis can rarely occur. Should this be diagnosed, appropriate antibiotic therapy should be instituted. Topical antibiotics can be used with the lidocaine ointment to minimize this potential.
* Bleeding or hematoma may occur within the first 24 hours after the procedure. Usually, applying ice or having the patient sit on a rolled-up washcloth provides enough pressure to tamponade a bleeder. Occasionally, a suture(s) may be required.
* Thrombosed external hemorrhoid (rare)

Excision of skin tags should not alter anal continence because of the lack of involvement of this procedure with the anal sphincter.

POSTPROCEDURE PATIENT EDUCATION

Wash the area gently three to four times a day and after defecation with mild soap and water. Sitz baths can also be used. Lidocaine

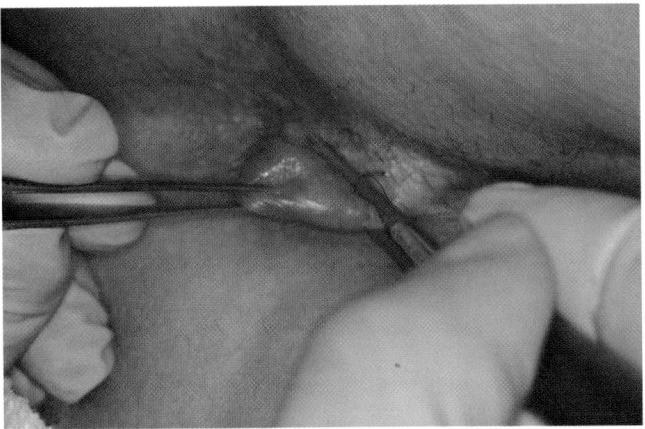

Fig. 88.4 Scalpel excision of tag.

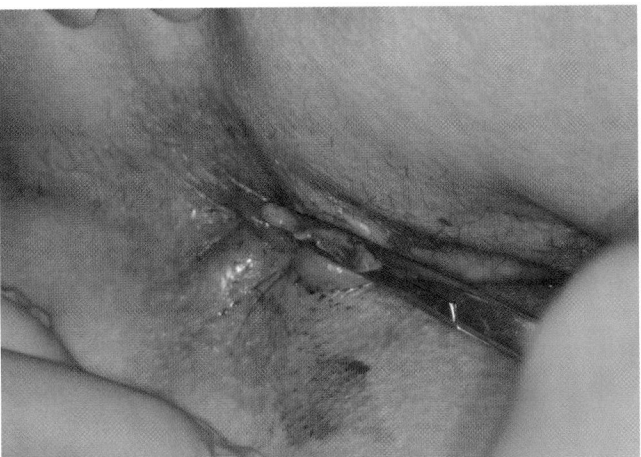

Fig. 88.5 Appearance immediately after removing tag.

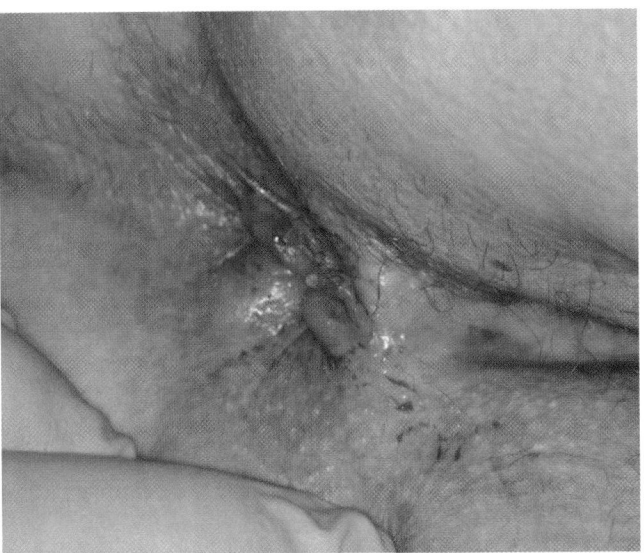

Fig. 88.6 Final result. No sutures are used for closure.

ointment 5% or an antibiotic ointment may be used to decrease discomfort. Prescribe a nonconstipating pain medication (e.g., ibuprofen). Further advise the patient to follow a high-fiber diet with commercial fiber supplements and four to six glasses of water per day. Polyethylene glycol laxative can also be used, as much as necessary, for the patient to keep their stools "mushy." Time off from work is usually minimal and would range from 0 to 3 days, depending on the extent of excision. Total healing time may take up to 6 weeks for complete new skin coverage. Perianal discomfort is usually present for 1 week or less.

PATIENT EDUCATION GUIDES

See patient education form available at www.expertconsult.com.

CPT/BILLING CODES

46220   Excision of single external papilla or tag, anus
46230   Excision of multiple external papillae or tags, anus

ICD-10-CM DIAGNOSTIC CODES

K64.4   Hemorrhoidal tag

RECOMMENDED READING

Bailey HR, Billingham RP, Stamos MJ, Snyder MJ. *Colorectal Surgery*. Philadelphia: Elsevier; 2013.
Corman ML. *Corman's Colon and Rectal Surgery*. 6th ed. Philadelphia: Wolters Klower Lippincott Williams & Wilkins; 2013.
Gordon P, Nivatvongs S. *Principles and Practice of Surgery for the Colon, Rectum, and Anus*. 3rd ed. New York: Informa Healthcare; 2007.
Pfenninger JL, Zainea GC. Common anorectal conditions: part I. Symptoms and complaints. *Am Fam Physician*. 2001;63:2391–2398.
Pfenninger JL, Zainea GC. Common anorectal conditions: part II. Lesions. *Am Fam Physician*. 2001;64:77–78.

CHAPTER 89

FLEXIBLE SIGMOIDOSCOPY

Bethany N. Norberg • Michael B. Harper

At one point, the flexible sigmoidoscope was a standard instrument in the primary care clinician's office to detect and prevent colorectal cancer (CRC). Using it made sense because approximately two-thirds of colon polyps are found in the left side of the colon, which is reachable with this instrument. Recently, its availability in the United States has declined. However, it should be noted that the Canadian Task Force on Preventive Health Care recently (2016) recommended that adults 50 to 59 years (weak recommendation) and 60 to 64 years (strong recommendation) be screened with guaiac-based fecal occult blood test (gFOBT) or fecal immunochemical test (FIT) every 2 years, or flexible sigmoidoscopy every 10 years. While the American College of Gastroenterology and the National Comprehensive Cancer Network recommend colonoscopy every 10 years as the preferred screening strategy, if colonoscopy is not available or is unacceptable to the patient, sigmoidoscopy is one of the acceptable alternatives. For the American College of Physicians and the United States Preventive Services Task Force (USPSTF), use of flexible sigmoidoscopy to screen is one of several options.

EDITOR'S NOTE: If we ever get serious in the United States about providing cost-effective health care, whether it is in underserved settings or elsewhere, use of sigmoidoscopy combined with gFOBT, FIT, or FIT-DNA (a multitargeted stool, blood, and DNA test like Cologard) is an effective screen for the entire colon. It is not only cost-effective due to avoiding anesthesia, but also due to avoiding the operating room (and can be performed in the office setting). Sigmoidoscopy also avoids the risk of anesthesia, and if biopsies are rarely performed, has a decreased risk of perforation compared with colonoscopy. In this manner, some experts use sigmoidoscopy as a "Pap smear of the colon." If something abnormal is seen on the cervix when performing a Pap smear, colposcopy is probably warranted. If a polyp is noted during sigmoidoscopy, they stop the procedure; full colonoscopy, the risk of anesthesia, and polypectomy is now warranted. Such a protocol would also avoid biopsy with sigmoidoscopy, thereby markedly decreasing the risk of perforation.

Approximately 144,000 cases of CRC occur each year in the United States, with 51,000 deaths. It is the second-highest cause of cancer deaths in this country, but the numbers are decreasing; it is one of the cancer screening successes of modern history. The sigmoidoscope is one method to decrease morbidity and mortality of CRC, either through early detection or by preventing it by removing precursor polyps. Well-designed, case-controlled studies have demonstrated the effectiveness of using sigmoidoscopy to screen for CRC, and sigmoidoscopy combined with annual gFOBT, FIT, or FIT-DNA (optionally every 3 years) can be expected to yield an 80% (or more) reduction in mortality from CRC. In addition to screening for CRC, the sigmoidoscope is a valuable tool in evaluating symptomatic patients.

All major sources of guidelines for preventive medicine recommend screening for CRC, and clinicians who fail to perform or recommend screening face medicolegal issues. Debate continues, however, regarding the best method of screening. Previously, fecal occult blood test (FOBT) and sigmoidoscopy were the most commonly used methods of screening for CRC in average-risk patients. While screening colonoscopy has become very popular, especially in high-risk patients, direct evidence of mortality reduction is lacking. An extensive review of the literature (Frazier et al, 2000) concluded that the best and most cost-effective method for CRC screening in average-risk patients was flexible sigmoidoscopy every 5 years, along with gFOBT every year. In another screening model, colonoscopy once every 10 years was more cost-effective than sigmoidoscopy every 5 years, but this model did not combine sigmoidoscopy with gFOBT (Sonnenberg et al, 2000). A more recent study demonstrated that screening flexible sigmoidoscopy performed only once on people between ages 55 and 64 years conferred a substantial (31%) reduction in mortality and long-lasting protection from CRC (Atkin et al, 2010).

Studies have concluded that patients will undergo whatever test their clinician recommends. Unfortunately, even though the number is increasing, only 67% of adults in the United States in 2016 had been screened by currently recommended methods. *It is imperative for clinicians to implement and encourage proper screening.*

INDICATIONS

- Screening: The American Cancer Society now recommends initiation of screening at 45 years for everyone. The American Society of Gastroenterology, the American College of Physicians, the National Cancer Institute, the American College of Obstetricians and Gynecologists, the American Academy of Family Physicians, and the USPSTF all recommend routine screening of not-at-risk patients 50 years of age and older for colon polyps and colon cancer. Note that no one is considered at "low risk" for screening purposes. The 2016 clinical summary of the USPSTF recommendations for screening for CRC are included in Table 89.1.
- Surveillance after previous polypectomy.
- Surveillance for effectiveness of treatment for ulcerative colitis/Crohn disease.
- Abdominal pain.
- Rectal bleeding (bright red or occult).
- Constipation or diarrhea.
- Persistent change in usual bowel habits.
- Unexplained weight loss, fever, or anemia.
- Suspected inflammatory bowel disease or antibiotic-associated colitis.
- Anorectal symptoms. (Note, however, that hemorrhoids alone are not an absolute indication for flexible sigmoidoscopy or air-contrast barium enema [ACBE] and must be put into the context of the entire patient history and examination. Medicare does not reimburse for an endoscopy procedure with the sole diagnosis of hemorrhoids.)
- Evaluation of radiographic abnormality or to confirm a radiologic finding with a biopsy.

Although flexible sigmoidoscopy may be used for the initial evaluation of some complaints, it is limited by the amount of colon it can evaluate. Certainly with selected symptoms, if the sigmoidoscopy is negative, a more extensive workup is still indicated. Thus, for many patients, obtaining a colonoscopy as the primary procedure may be more cost effective. On the other hand, availability and cost concerns may lead to sigmoidoscopy as the initial procedure of choice.

TABLE 89.1   Screening for Colorectal Cancer: Clinical Summary of U.S. Preventive Services Task Force Recommendation*

	50–75 Yr[†]	76–85 Yr[†]	>85 Yr[†]
Recommendation	Screen with high-sensitivity gFOBT, FIT, FIT-DNA, sigmoidoscopy, CT colonography or colonoscopy Grade: A	Do not screen routinely Grade: C	Do not screen Grade: D
Screening tests	High-sensitivity gFOBT, sigmoidoscopy with gFOBT, FIT or FIT-DNA, CT colonography, and colonoscopy are effective in decreasing colorectal cancer mortality. The risks and benefits of these screening methods vary. Colonoscopy and flexible sigmoidoscopy (to a lesser degree) entail possible serious complications.		
Screening test intervals	Intervals for recommended screening strategies: Annual screening with high-sensitivity gFOBT, FIT, or FIT-DNA (or FIT-DNA can be every 3 yr) Sigmoidoscopy every 5 yr CT colonography every 5 yr Sigmoidoscopy every 10 yr with FIT annually Colonoscopy every 10 yr		
Balance of harms and benefits	The benefits of screening outweigh the potential harms for 50- to 75-yr-olds.	The likelihood that detection and early intervention will yield a mortality benefit declines after age 75 yr because of the long average time between adenoma development and cancer diagnosis.	
Implementation	Focus on strategies that maximize the number of individuals who get screened. Practice shared decision making; discussions with patients should incorporate information on test quality and availability. Individuals with a personal history of cancer or adenomatous polyps are followed by a surveillance regimen, and screening guidelines are not applicable.		
Relevant USPSTF recommendations	The USPSTF found adequate evidence that aspirin use reduces the incidence of CRC in adults after 5–10 yr of use. https://www.uspreventiveservicestaskforce.org/Page/Document/RecommendationStatementFinal/aspirin-to-prevent-cardiovascular-disease-and-cancer. Accessed July 24, 2018.		

CRC, Colorectal cancer; *FIT*, fecal immunochemical test; *FIT-DNA*, FIT combined with multitargeted stool DNA (Cologuard); *gFOBT*, guaiac-based fecal occult blood testing; *USPSTF*, US Preventive Services Task Force.
*This document is a summary of the 2016 recommendation of the US Preventive Services Task Force (USPSTF) on screening for colorectal cancer. For a summary of the evidence systematically reviewed in making these recommendations, the full recommendation statement, and supporting documents, go to: https://www.uspreventiveservicestaskforce.org/Page/Document/RecommendationStatementFinal/colorectal-cancer-screening2#tab.
[†]These recommendations do not apply to individuals with specific inherited syndromes (Lynch syndrome or familial adenomatous polyposis) or those with inflammatory bowel disease.
From U.S. Preventive Services Task Force, Bibbins-Domingo K, Grossman DC. Screening for Colorectal Cancer: U.S. Preventive Services Task Force Recommendation Statement. *JAMA.* 2016;315(23):2564–2575.

Because of redundant loops of sigmoid colon and because the insertion tube that is used for barium enema can obscure a lesion, flexible sigmoidoscopy (or, at the minimum, anoscopy) is generally needed, along with ACBE if the entire bowel must be visualized. Individual circumstances dictate whether a flexible sigmoidoscopy alone or in conjunction with an ACBE is needed. ACBE is no longer recommended alone in the United States as a screening procedure for colon cancer.

CONTRAINDICATIONS

Absolute

- Acute abdomen
  - Suspected perforation abscess
  - Peritonitis or intraabdominal sepsis
  - Diverticulitis
  - Bowel infarct
  - Fulminant colitis
- Severe cardiopulmonary disease
- Inadequate bowel preparation
- Uncooperative patient
- Marked bleeding disorder

Relative

The following conditions require additional caution before performing flexible sigmoidoscopy:

- Pregnancy
- Recent abdominal surgery
- Distorted pelvic anatomy
- History of pelvic irradiation

- Recent barium enema (if still passing barium because it can occlude the scope's port)
- When colonoscopy is indicated, such as in high-risk patients (e.g., inflammatory bowel disease who should receive a colonoscopy 8 years after the diagnosis was first made and every 5 years thereafter; for follow-up of polyps and colon cancer; for patients with familial polyposis syndromes)

EQUIPMENT

The flexible sigmoidoscope is available as either a fiberoptic endoscope or video endoscope. Although the fiberoptic scope has been the most commonly used version, the video sigmoidoscope is state of the art and uses computer chip and video technology. The image from the tip of the scope is transmitted to a video monitor. This equipment facilitates video recording, sound narration, and other patient information storage.

The following basic equipment is necessary to carry out routine flexible sigmoidoscopy:

- 60- to 70-cm-long submersible scope consisting of the body with controls (Fig. 89.1) and the shaft of the scope with tip and apertures (Figs. 89.2 and 89.3)
- Light source (most have air supply and wash bottle attached; Fig. 89.4)
- Suction apparatus (Fig. 89.5)
- Biopsy forceps (Fig. 89.6)
- Water-based lubricant (e.g., K-Y Jelly)
- 4 × 4 gauze pads
- Nonsterile gloves
- Shielded glasses and other equipment necessary to follow universal blood and body fluid precautions
- Anoscope (Ives slotted anoscope preferred; see Chapter 83, Anoscopy)

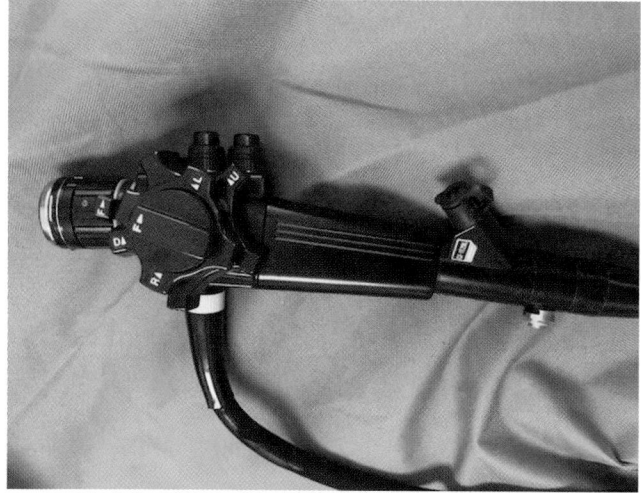

Fig. 89.1   Control head and body of the fiberoptic sigmoidoscope.

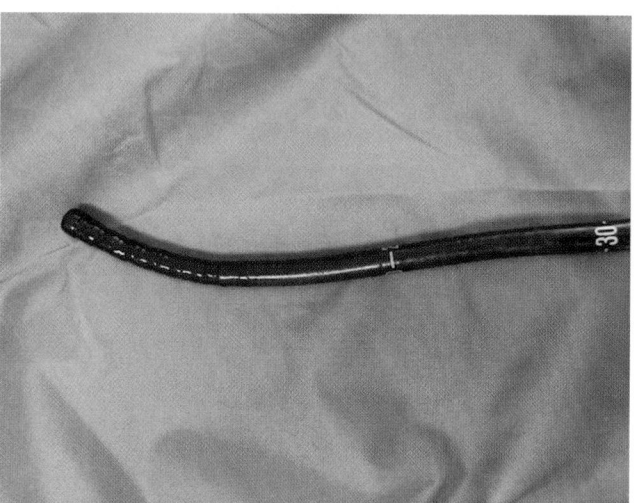

Fig. 89.2   Tip of the sigmoidoscope.

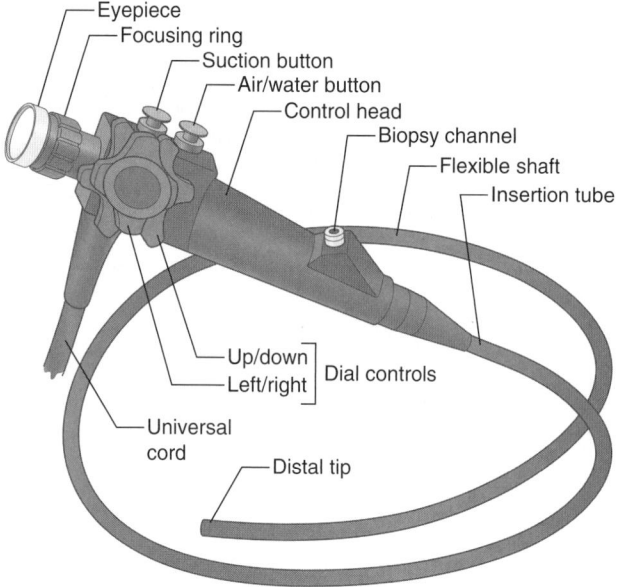

Fig. 89.3   Schematic diagram of a fiberoptic sigmoidoscope.

Eyepiece
Focusing ring
Suction button
Air/water button
Control head
Biopsy channel
Flexible shaft
Insertion tube
Up/down ⎫
Left/right ⎭ Dial controls
Universal cord
Distal tip

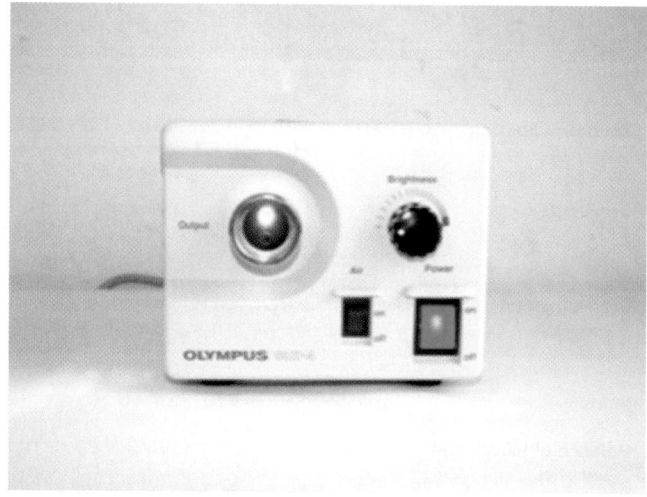

Fig. 89.4   Light source with air supply.

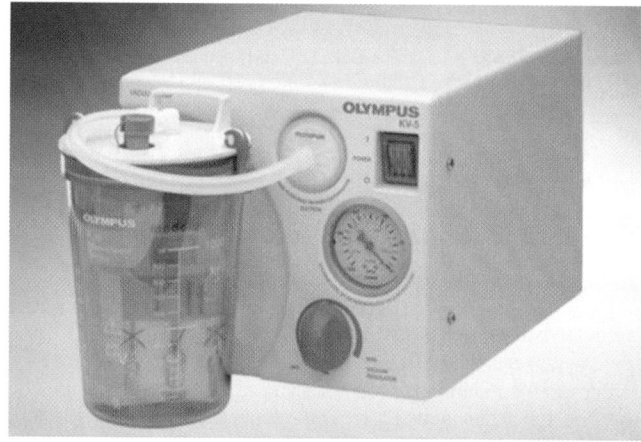

Fig. 89.5   Suction apparatus.

- Basin of soapy water (immediately on completion of the procedure, suction water through the scope, then place the scope in the basin)
- Formalin jars
- Disinfecting cleanser
- Nursing assistant (to assist with equipment and procedure)
- Video unit and monitor (for video endoscopes only)

PREPROCEDURE PATIENT PREPARATION

A good history (present and past) is essential before performing any procedure. Not only should the patient's overall medical risk status be determined, but the risk for CRC and any associated symptoms must be assessed to ensure that flexible sigmoidoscopy is indeed the proper procedure and that there are no contraindications to performing it.

Flexible sigmoidoscopy in most patients is easily performed in less than 15 minutes. However, for some patients, the very thought of a tube in the rectum provokes anxiety, apprehension, and reluctance. This makes it necessary for the clinician to reassure the patient and allay apprehension and anxiety with a thorough explanation. Use simple words with the aid of charts and figures. Explain the procedure to be performed, why and how it will be done, and the possible complications. The components of this patient education process include the following:

1. Bowel cleansing instructions (usually two enemas; see the sample patient education handout online at www.expertconsult.com)
2. Equipment used
3. Anatomy of the colon

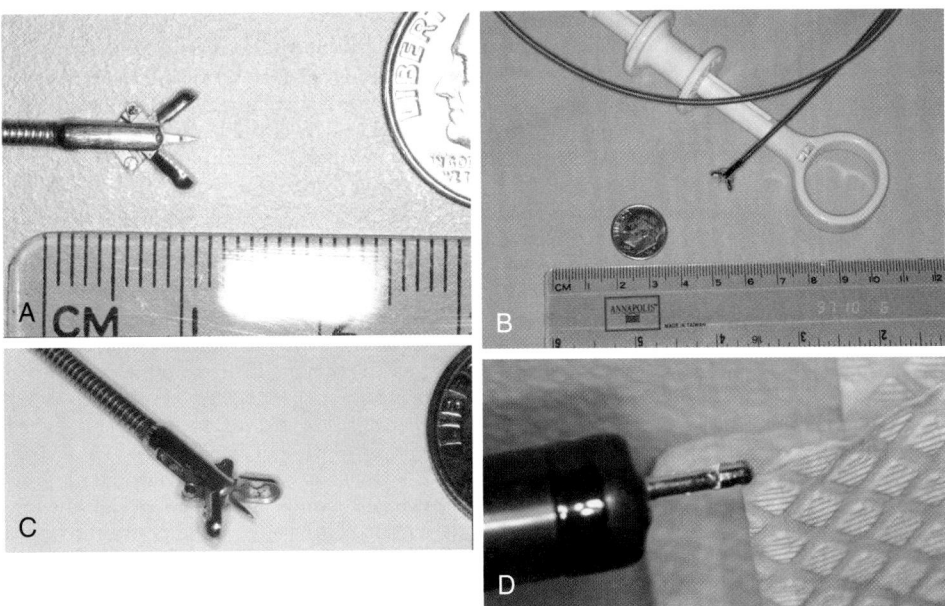

Fig. 89.6 Biopsy forceps. (A) Relative size of forceps. (B) Control handle. (C) Stabilizing needle. (D) Biopsy forceps protruding from end of scope, closed on a piece of paper. (Courtesy John L. Pfenninger, MD, The Medical Procedures Center, Midland, MI.)

4. Explanation of procedure
5. Discomfort experienced during the procedure ("crampy distention," especially at the second curve around 40 cm and with insufflation of air, similar to when the patient has excess "gas"). Giving patients permission to pass this gas while the procedure is being performed will often keep them more comfortable. Although at first they may feel embarrassed, remind them that this is just clean air that has been inserted.
6. Complications that are remotely likely (e.g., perforation, bleeding)
7. Possible diseases likely to be detected
8. Biopsy technique, if needed
9. Whether photography or video will be used
10. Management of any findings
11. The need to continue all prescribed medications

It is highly advisable to have the patient sign the informed consent form for this procedure after reading the patient information materials. (See the sample patient education handout and consent form online at www.expertconsult.com.)

Flexible sigmoidoscopy is well tolerated by the vast majority of patients. Mild analgesia or sedation, whether given orally or intramuscularly, is rarely needed. Oral diazepam or ibuprofen can be used as needed in the individual situation. Atropine 0.5 mg intramuscularly can be given for those who have a tendency to faint or experience vasovagal symptoms. If needed, this dose can usually be repeated safely in larger adults.

Patient Bowel Preparation

Simple enemas (tap water, Fleet Phospho-Soda) administered until clear fluid is passed is the only requirement. This usually entails two enemas (occasionally three) 30 to 60 minutes before the procedure. Patients are allowed to take their medications and eat normally. If the patient tends to be constipated, a laxative should be given the day before the procedure. Keeping the regimen simple is more likely to ensure compliance.

In one study (Sharma and Chockalingham, 1997), two Fleet enemas given on arrival to the endoscopy suite were compared with one bottle of magnesium citrate and two Dulcolax tablets the evening before the procedure. Both patients and endoscopists preferred the oral method. Another study (Manoucheri et al, 1999) showed no difference in results comparing four bowel preparation regimens. Some clinicians use the same preparation as for colonoscopy to ensure adequate visualization.

Antibiotic Prophylaxis

Antibiotics for subacute bacterial endocarditis prophylaxis are no longer recommended for lower endoscopy procedures with or without the performance of biopsies, even in high-risk patients (see Chapter 69, Antibiotic Prophylaxis).

TECHNIQUE

A specific terminology has developed around the procedure of flexible sigmoidoscopy. Box 89.1 summarizes this "language" that must be understood before learning the procedure.

1. Before beginning the procedure, all functions of the endoscope must be checked. The light source should be turned on and clarity of view confirmed. White balance must be performed for videoscopes. The button to insufflate air and the water button are the same (see Fig. 89.2). Just covering the air/water button (often colored blue) introduces air, whereas pushing it down all the way ejects a small amount of water to clean the lens. This button is the one closest to the patient. The second button, closer to the eyepiece (often colored red), is for suction. Remember: the button closest to the patient puts things in and is usually colored blue; the button closest to the endoscopist "sucks" things out and is usually colored red. Air function is confirmed by inserting the scope tip in water and seeing bubbles when the air port is occluded. Suction is confirmed by suctioning a small amount of water through the endoscope. Tip deflection is checked by rotating both control wheels fully in both directions while observing and feeling for free movement. After checking all functions, the fiberoptic unit may be turned off temporarily. Many video endoscopes have to be white balanced each time they are turned off, so leaving them on is preferable.
2. If sedation is to be used, record the patient's temperature, pulse, respiration, blood pressure, and results of heart/lungs auscultation and abdominal examination.
3. Position the patient in the left lateral Sims position (see Chapter 82, Clinical Anorectal Anatomy and Digital Examination, and Fig. 82.2).
4. The endoscopist and assistant should follow universal blood and body fluid precautions. They should wear nonsterile gloves on both hands. The endoscopist should double glove the right hand. (Re-

BOX 89.1   Flexible Fiberoptic Sigmoidoscopy Terminology

Tip: Distal end of the shaft of the sigmoidoscope (see Fig. 89.2).

Dials: Tip control knobs. Large inner dial moves the tip up and down. Small outer dial moves the tip left and right (see Fig. 89.3). The clinician should note the neutral position for future reference when in the bowel.

Biopsy channel: The slot through which the biopsy forceps and also the brush wire are passed through the body and shaft of the scope (see Figs. 89.1, 89.3, and 89.6D).

Suction control button (nearest the operator): When pressed all the way down, this button allows the suction to operate continuously.

Air insufflation/lens cleaner (water) button (farthest from the operator): This button has a small opening that can be occluded to allow air to pass into the colon continuously (see Fig. 89.3). Pressing the button completely down will squirt water across the lens at the tip and will clear away debris.

Suction, air, and water connection ports: The location of tubes connecting on the bottom of the handpiece that go to suction, air, and water sources.

Slide-by: A technique of passing the flexible sigmoidoscope where the advancing tip of the scope is advanced proximally into the colon without complete visualization of the lumen. As the scope advances, the practitioner sees the vascular mucosa "slide by." This maneuver is often unavoidable but should be used very sparingly, and the scope should be advanced only 5 to 10 cm. If the lumen is not fully visualized or if pressure, resistance, or pain is encountered, the clinician should pull back and look again for the lumen.

Pullback: Withdrawing the shaft of the scope to diminish or eliminate whiteout, redout, stretching, or looping.

One-on-one: As the scope is advanced into the rectum, there is an equal advance of the scope into the segment of colon (versus just stretching the colon without true advancement).

Redout: The tip of the scope lies flat against the mucosal surface, resulting in a red appearance through the lens.

Whiteout: The mucosal surface is stretched by the tip of the scope pressing against the mucosal surface. The vessels are thus blanched, giving a white appearance.

Tip deflection: The tip can be directed in four directions by rotating the dials: up ("north"), down ("south"), left ("west"), and right ("east"). The deflection should always be moderate and gentle. Alternatively, the head of the scope itself can be rotated right and left to turn the tip to the right or left after being flexed up or down.

Dithering: A to-and-fro advance-and-withdrawal process performed with an amplitude of 5–6 cm and repeated every 2–4 sec, coupled with a clockwise torque on the shaft on the pullback motion and a counterclockwise torque on the inward motion. This maneuver helps straighten the sigmoid colon, allowing it to compress like an accordion over the scope (see Fig. 89.9).

Jiggling: A to-and-fro, 5- to 6-cm inward-and-outward motion of the shaft performed every 2–4 sec. It helps in the visualization of a segment of colon and can often aid scope advancement (see Fig. 89.10).

Alpha maneuver: Used only after much practice by the experienced endoscopist to assist in shortening or pleating the segments of the colon (see Fig. 89.11 and text for explanation).

Torquing: Twisting the distal shaft of the scope by rotating the head either clockwise or counterclockwise.

Retroflexion: Maximally flexing the tip of the scope, enabling it to look back on itself. This is often used to evaluate the rectum.

---

move the extra glove after the tip has been lubricated, the rectal examination performed, and the scope initially inserted.) Place the body and shaft of the scope on the cart. Lubricate the distal 3 to 4 cm of the shaft tip with K-Y Jelly (avoid the lens). Notice where the dials are positioned when the shaft is completely straight.

5. Separate the gluteal folds laterally with the hands to expose the anal area and the anal aperture for inspection. Perform a digital rectal examination with K-Y Jelly or lidocaine ointment to ensure there is no obstruction or stool in the anal canal. In male patients, examine the prostate carefully. A painful examination should alert the endoscopist to a fissure, proctitis, or colitis. The examination is uncomfortable but should not be painful if it is done gently. The digital examination helps relax the sphincter and lubricates the anal canal. (See Chapter 82, Clinical Anorectal Anatomy and Digital Examination.)

6. Now hold the body of the scope in your left hand (Fig. 89.7). Hold the end of the scope shaft in the right hand, and with the index finger alongside and stabilizing the shaft tip, gently insert it. Hold the tip at an oblique angle pointing posteriorly, and stretch the sphincter as the tip is slipped into the anal canal. The shaft tip can be blindly inserted 10 to 20 cm. Stop when resistance is felt. Remove the second glove on the right hand.

7. With the distal 10 cm or more of the scope in the anal canal, switch on the light source, air, and suction, if these had been turned off. Check the view in the eyepiece or on the video screen.

8. Keep holding the body of the scope in your left hand so that your thumb controls the large dial and your index finger controls the suction, irrigation, and air valves. Hold the shaft and advance it with your right hand, which is also available to control the small dial. Alternatively, an assistant may advance the scope, and you may use your right hand to manipulate both dials. The assistant must be cautioned never to advance the scope against resistance and to advance the scope only when told to

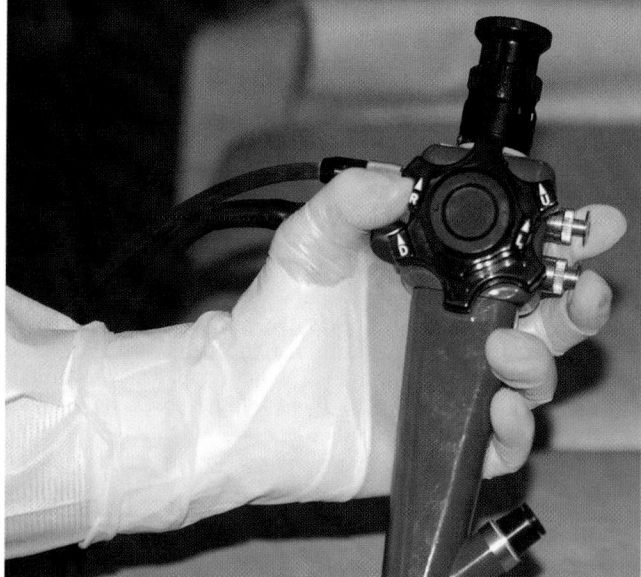

Fig. 89.7 Control head of the sigmoidoscope should be held in the left hand so that the thumb rests on the up/down control dial and the index finger can regulate the suction and air/water buttons. (*Courtesy Michael B. Harper, MD.*)

do so. This latter method is easier and faster for some clinicians, but solo operation may allow for better coordination of movements of the shaft and deflecting tip. Use the technique that accomplishes the procedure in the fastest manner with minimal patient discomfort.

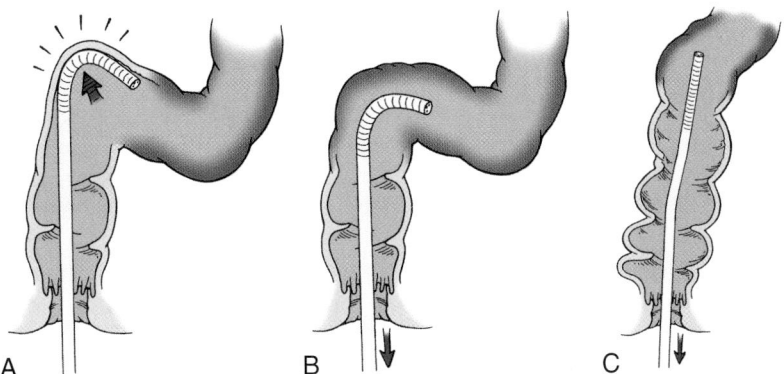

Fig. 89.8 Method of advancement at the rectosigmoid junction. Various maneuvers are needed. (A) The scope is entering into the anus, but the view from the end of the sigmoidoscope is not changing. There is no one-on-one advancement; rather, the segment of colon is merely being stretched, often causing pain. (B) Try the simple hook-and-pullback technique initially. (C) Pulling back on the scope causes an accordion effect and straightens the curve.

EDITOR'S NOTE: One study demonstrated a faster learning curve (fewer procedures necessary to demonstrate competence) for colonoscopy when trained with use of an assistant advancing the scope as opposed to performing the procedure solo.

9. Insufflation advance technique
   - Air is needed to maintain patency of the lumen and to obtain a clear view adjacent to the tip and a few centimeters beyond. Remember, the air button and water button are the same. Just covering the button introduces air, whereas pushing it down all the way diverts air into the water bottle and ejects a stream of water across the lens to clean it while also irrigating the colon. A sufficient amount of air must be used to expand the bowel, but too much air may cause cramping or, in extreme cases, even perforation. Excess air also lengthens the bowel and may cause sharper bends. Use patient comfort as a guide. With a clear view ahead, gently advance the shaft forward. The scope is usually advanced up to 15 to 18 cm without difficulty. There are three "valves" that are encountered in the rectum—the valves of Houston. These are semilunar in shape, are not really valves, and are located 6, 9, and 12 cm from the anal verge. Negotiating advancement into the rectosigmoid can be hampered by these folds, and the tip needs to be deflected away from the fold and toward the lumen to avoid redout or whiteout. The clinician can get "lost" in the vast arena of the rectal vault and have difficulty in locating the rectosigmoid orifice. This is more likely if too much air is insufflated, which causes the ampulla to expand upward.
   - There is always a question of how much air to use. The answer: enough! In general, as long as the patient is not sedated, he or she will tell if too much pressure is being generated. Some clinicians are too timid and will never see the lumen if "enough" air is not used.
   - At this stage, you do not need to attempt to visualize the entire circumference of the bowel. Rather, the primary goal is to insert the scope as far and as fast as possible. Deflect the tip only enough to clearly see the direction of the lumen. By minimizing tip deflection, the force of insertion will be directed more toward the tip and the tendency to form a loop is decreased. It is critical that the complete circumference of the bowel be closely inspected, lest a lesion be missed, but this is usually performed during withdrawal of the scope.
   - It is ideal if the scope is passed only when the lumen is seen, but practically speaking, the slide-by method is used commonly and is safe as long as the scope passes easily and the patient (unsedated) is not feeling excessive pain (see Box 89.1). To perform this maneuver, first determine the direction of the lumen. If you do not see the lumen, it is easily located by moving the controls toward neutral, then releasing the controls and slowly withdrawing the scope (this is a basic maneuver to find the lumen with any gastrointestinal endoscopy). The lumen will usually come into view after withdrawing only a few

centimeters. Once the lumen direction is determined, deflect the tip toward the lumen and gently advance the scope while watching for movement of mucosa. Continue to advance as long as the patient is comfortable and you see mucosal movement. The lumen should come back into view after advancing a few centimeters. Stop the slide-by if you have a redout or whiteout, or cause excessive patient discomfort.

10. Advancing the scope into the sigmoid and descending colon may require using different maneuvers in the presence of redundancy, adhesions, angulation, and loops. At times, especially in young persons, the scope can be advanced all the way up to the transverse colon without any difficulty. In older patients, especially those who have had abdominal or pelvic surgery, the presence of adhesions may make further advancement difficult. The rectosigmoid junction is at 15 to 18 cm. Advancement may be hampered here by the angulation of the bowel toward the left into the left iliac fossa. The length of the sigmoid itself varies from 20 to 45 cm. Certain maneuvers—individually or in combination—can then be attempted to advance the scope through the descending colon and into the distal portion of the transverse colon.
    - Advancement by hook, rotation, and pullback. When the scope will not advance, deflect the tip of the shaft 30 to 90 degrees behind a mucosal fold (Fig. 89.8) and withdraw the shaft 5 to 10 cm, pulling the segment of the colon downward, twisting the head of the scope to the right, and creating a pleating and straightening-out effect. Repeat this maneuver several times as needed to achieve the desired goal of compressing the bowel over the shaft of the scope, similar to an accordion. It should be done very gently with minimal (if any) resistance. When you cannot go forward, flex the tip down, torque to the right, and withdraw. It is a difficult concept to master, but to go forward you must pull back, as noted.
    - Dithering-torque maneuver (Fig. 89.9). The dithering-torque maneuver is a to-and-fro advance-and-withdrawal process performed with an amplitude of 5 to 6 cm every 2 to 4 seconds. It is coupled with a clockwise torque of the shaft of about 45 to 60 degrees on the pullback motion and a counterclockwise torque on the inward motion. This process "accordionizes" the colon onto the shaft of the scope, thereby shortening the colon and enabling a larger length of the colon to be traversed and examined. Gentle tip deflection of 30 degrees with the torque motion is recommended. The clockwise torque tends to loop the sigmoid, whereas the counterclockwise torque tends to straighten it. This is an effective maneuver in shortening the sigmoid, and it is of greatest use in a redundant sigmoid colon. Excessive tip deflection can become a hindrance to further advancement; therefore it should be kept to the minimum to maintain visualization of the lumen. If the tip needs greater deflection at the moment, it should be straightened soon after the lumen is located.

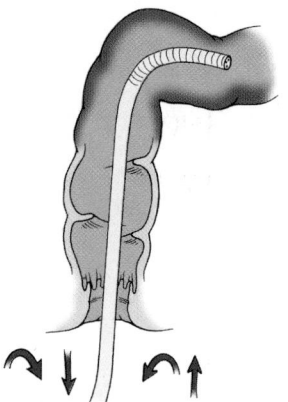

Fig. 89.9 Dithering maneuver. Rotate counterclockwise when withdrawing and clockwise when inserting.

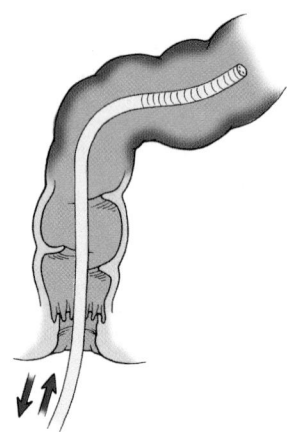

Fig. 89.10 Jiggle maneuver.

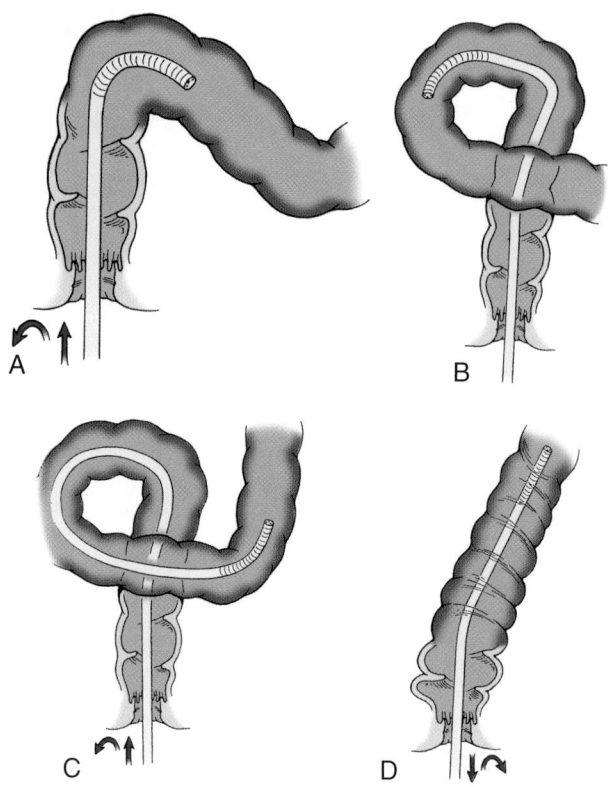

Fig. 89.11 (A)–(D) Alpha maneuver.

- Jiggling is merely an in-and-out motion while deflecting the tip slightly, trying to get the scope to advance. In performing flexible sigmoidoscopy, it is best to keep the scope moving in some manner to maximize the opportunity of seeing the lumen (Fig. 89.10).
- Alpha maneuver (for experienced endoscopists). Advance the scope into the sigmoid. At about 25 to 30 cm, deflect the tip to visualize the lumen anteriorly, and then torque the shaft counterclockwise about 145 to 180 degrees (Fig. 89.11A). This swings the proximal part of the sigmoid over the distal part, so that the sigmoid colon forms a loop over itself (see Fig. 89.11B–C). Here, minimally deflect the tip to locate the lumen and then straighten it as much as possible. Further advancement of the scope will lead it into the descending colon. If resistance is encountered, rotate the shaft clockwise and withdraw to "accordionize," or shorten, the sigmoid (see Fig. 89.11D). The shaft can then be advanced into the descending colon, to the splenic flexure (Fig. 89.12D). The alpha maneuver is rarely needed but may be necessary in the redundant bowel. It should be used only by the experienced endoscopist.

11. Opinions vary as to whether changing patient position will improve visualization or aid in advancement of the scope. Many will roll patients onto their backs. Try it if other maneuvers do not work.
12. Once past the "second curve," the scope is generally advanced with minimal manipulation into the descending colon by jiggling, hooking, and pulling back; simply maintaining mild inward pressure on the shaft usually suffices. The area of the splenic flexure can often be recognized by the bluish hue superiorly, which represents the transmitted vascularity of the spleen sitting on the colon exteriorly. The colon takes a turn anteriorly and to the patient's right at this point, and the triangular lumen and folds of the transverse colon can be identified easily (see Fig. 89.12E).
13. Inspection: Withdrawal of the scope is easy but probably the most important part of the procedure. Using a combination of tip deflection and torquing in both directions, gradually withdraw the shaft, visually inspecting the entire circumference of the intubated colon. Pay careful attention to all areas of the mucosal surface, particularly behind mucosal folds. Make note of diverticula and any masses. (See the "Biopsy" section.) If any segment is not seen completely, advance and withdraw again. Continue withdrawing until the rectum is reached. After a segment has been completely visualized, suction can be used to remove some of the air. This will make the patient more comfortable; it may also cause a small polyp hidden behind a fold to "pop" into the lumen. However, caution should be taken to avoid removing too much air, which could decrease or collapse the lumen for the remainder of the withdrawal.
14. Retroflexion: The anal canal and distal rectum must be inspected thoroughly in one of two ways: by using an anoscope, or by completely deflecting the sigmoidoscope tip to look back on itself (i.e., retroflexion; see Fig. 89.12N–Q). Either procedure is performed after completing the examination of as much proximal bowel as possible with the sigmoidoscope. The sigmoidoscope can simply be withdrawn completely and the anal canal examined with the anoscope. Or, to accomplish the retroflexion maneuver, withdraw the endoscope to the anal verge. Then, gently advance the scope about 10 to 12 cm while rotating it and simultaneously turning both control knobs counterclockwise to full deflection. You will soon be looking back onto the shaft of the scope and will see it passing through the anal canal. By torquing the shaft, you can perform a 360-degree visual inspection of the distal rectal vault and the inner aspect of the anal canal and papillae to detect masses and hemorrhoids (although these are much better appreciated with an Ives slotted anoscope).

After completing the examination, straighten the tip and withdraw it very slowly. Grasp the tip of the scope as it slips out of the anus so that it does not drop on the table, damaging its delicate tip (with videoscopes, the camera is in the tip).

15. Remove all the air: You may do this before completely removing the scope or reinsert the scope 5 to 6 cm. Apply intermittent suction and use a to-and-fro motion with rotation to prevent the mucosa from being drawn into the suction port, thus occluding it (see Step 16). After the patient indicates that the air is gone, remove the scope and immediately draw soapy water through the suction port. Also, occlude the air port to "blow out" any accumulated debris. The latter two steps will enhance cleaning and preserve proper functioning of the scope.

16. Removing colonic fluid and air. Other than polyps, do not attempt to suction any solid material through the scope. The channels are extremely small and are easily plugged. When suctioning (button closest to the endoscopist), intermittently push the button all the way down while instilling air and moving the scope back and forth a few centimeters. Constant suctioning at one position will suck mucosa into the scope, causing what appears to be a polyp ("suction polyp" or "pseudopolyp"). This artifact should disappear or flatten if the bowel lumen is expanded with air, but may temporarily leave a circular mark on the mucosa. Keeping the scope in motion and compressing the suction button intermittently will help avoid unnecessary biopsy procedures and confusing findings.

17. The scope should be cleaned and disinfected as soon as possible after the procedure is completed (see later discussion).

Biopsy

There are many opinions about when and if biopsies should be obtained during flexible sigmoidoscopy. Some points of view with countering arguments include the following:

- Primary care clinicians should not perform a biopsy on any lesion. (Counter: The biopsy technique is simple and virtually without complication when only the cold [without electrocautery] biopsy forceps are used. It samples only 2 to 3 mm of the mucosa, and unless the tissue is pulsating, ulcerated, or inside a diverticulum, perforation is almost impossible.)

- It is useless to obtain a biopsy sample because the colonoscopist will need to remove the polyp anyway. And if the patient has an adenomatous polyp, the entire colon should be screened with colonoscopy. (Counter: If the biopsy result shows only a hyperplastic polyp [see Fig. 89.12H], there is no need for colonoscopy. Documentation of an abnormality aids in categorizing the patient's risk status and reinforces the clinician's rationale for the patient to have the often-resisted colonoscopy performed. It also confirms the diagnosis for the colonoscopist and mandates that the lesion be found.)

- Do not perform a biopsy on small polyps (<5 mm). (Counter: It is precisely these lesions that are difficult to diagnose accurately with an endoscope, so they require biopsy to determine if they are adenomatous and thus require full colonoscopy. Even very small, "diminutive" polyps that appear to be benign can be advanced adenomas [villous histology or high-grade dysplasia], and cause the patient to be in the same high-risk group as patients with larger adenomatous polyps [Schoen et al, 2006].)

- Performing a biopsy may increase malpractice insurance. (Counter: Not doing it may miss a crucial diagnosis. In general, premiums are not increased for this very-low-risk diagnostic procedure. If the lesion is not sampled and the colonoscopist cannot find it on a later examination, it may prolong the procedure, and the patient's actual status remains unknown.)

- Performing a biopsy provides pathology, which in turn provides feedback to the endoscopist, and increases the learning curve for clinical diagnoses in the future.

EDITOR'S NOTE: It is our practice to perform a biopsy on essentially all nonvascular lesions. No complications have been encountered. If it does not look like the mucosa on the inside of your mouth, if it is not pulsating, if you are not inside a diverticulum, and if you do not know what it is, perform a biopsy! For flat polyps, injecting saline submucosally may raise the polyp and minimize the risk of perforation.

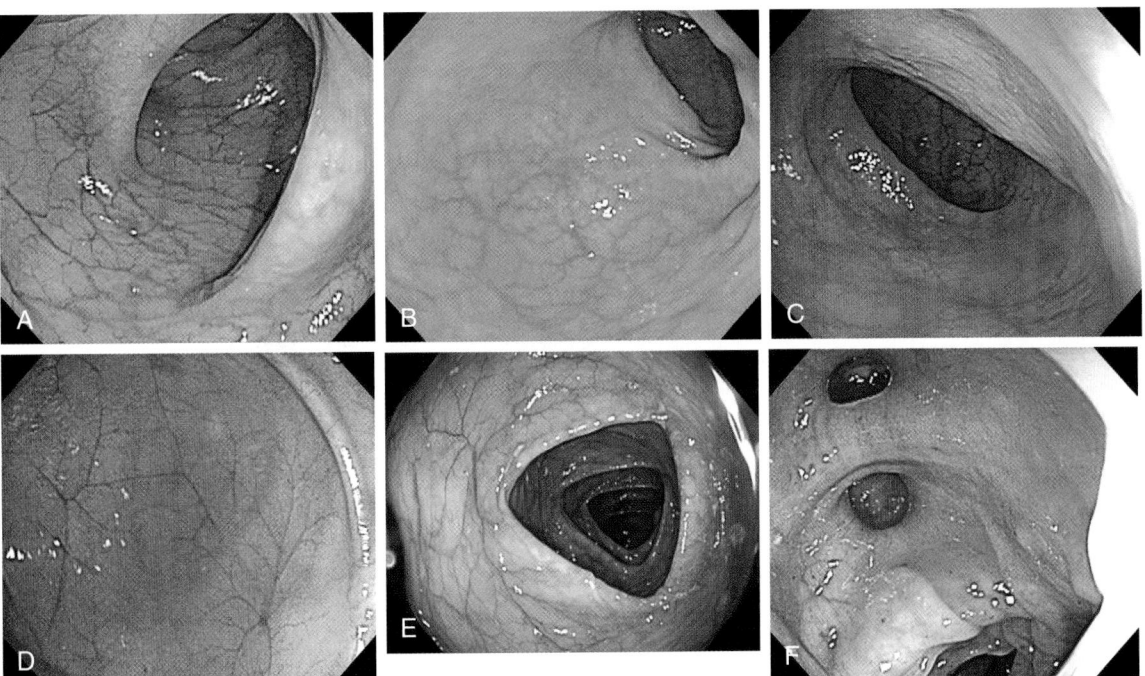

Fig. 89.12 Normal and abnormal findings during sigmoidoscopy. (A) Semilunar valves of Houston. (B) Rectosigmoid area. (C) Sigmoid colon. (D) The splenic flexure. The spleen projects a cyanotic hue through the colon wall. (E) The transverse colon with characteristic triangular appearance of the lumen and folds. (F) Diverticulosis.

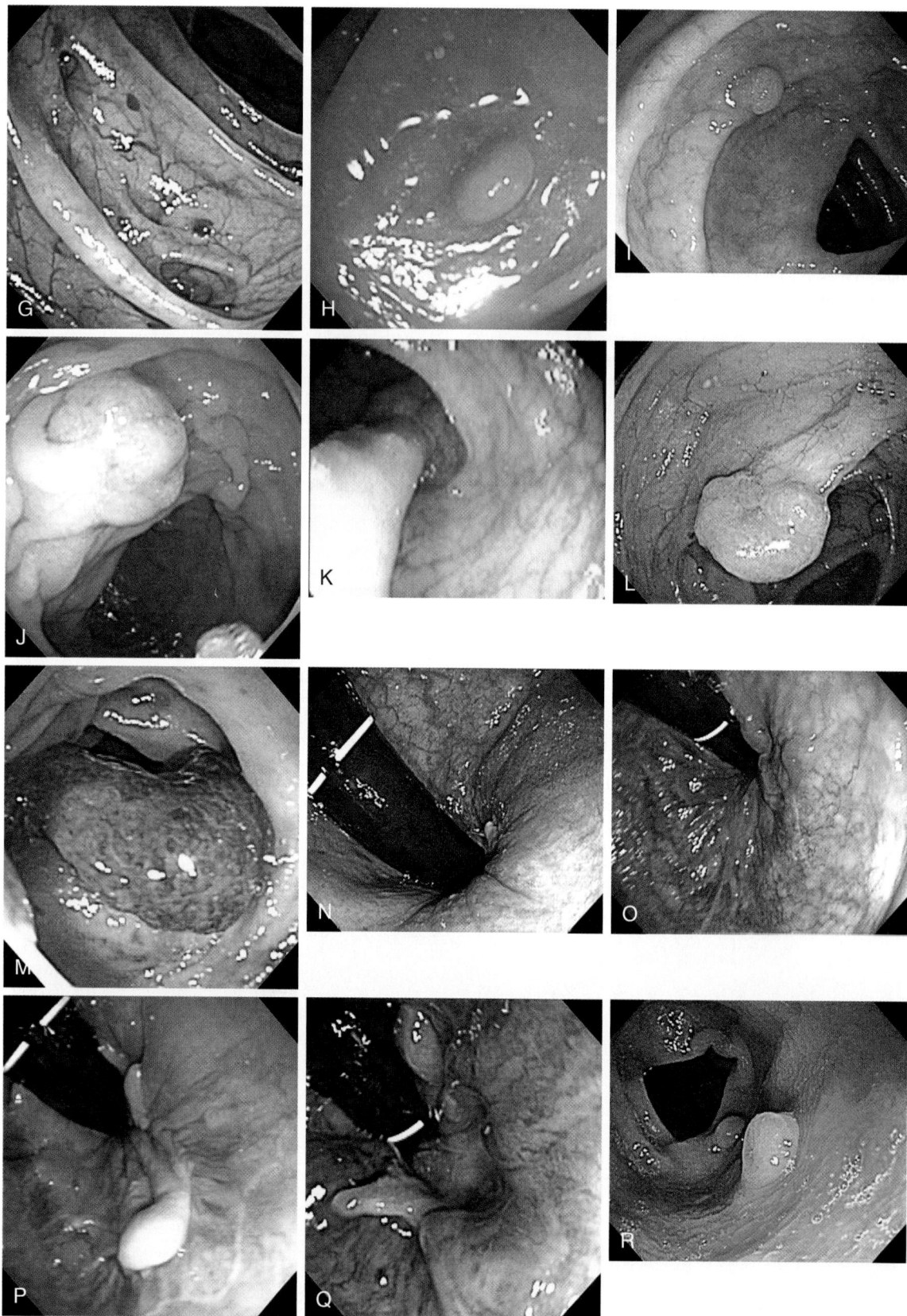

Fig. 89.12, cont'd (G) Multiple diverticula. (H) Small polyp that was hyperplastic on biopsy. (I) Small adenomatous polyp at the splenic flexure. The scope is looking across the transverse colon, which can be identified by its triangular shape. (J) Pedunculated polyp. (K) Another pedunculated polyp. (L) Large sessile polyp in the sigmoid colon. (M) Large colon mass that was a cancer on biopsy. (N) The retroflexion maneuver in a normal rectum performed just before the scope is totally removed. Note that the scope is turned upon itself in a large U shape and the view is of the scope coming through the anus. Note the normal vascular pattern of the bowel. (O) Internal hemorrhoids seen on retroflexion. (P) Hypertrophied anal papilla. (Q) Hypertrophied papilla along the dentate line. Internal hemorrhoids also present. (R) Everted diverticulum, confirm by probing with closed forceps, do not snare these. (K, Courtesy John L. Pfenninger, MD, The Medical Procedures Center, Midland, MI.)

Precautions

The following are some caveats regarding biopsy (see Chapter 90, Colonoscopy, for additional precautions):

- A vascular lesion (especially if pulsating!) may best be left for later biopsy under more controlled situations.
- Do not perform electrosurgical removal of a polyp except in a fully prepared bowel (bowel gases in the colon can explode). Use of electrosurgery on flat polyps increases the risk of later perforation. Recent studies in animal bowel suggest thermal damage carries much further than visualized when cautery is applied to a flat lesion.
- After the procedure, ensure and document that all bleeding has stopped.
- Document the location from which each polyp was removed (either the distance into the colon as seen on the scope or the segment of the colon) and, except for small polyps in close proximity to each other, place each polyp in a separate specimen container.

Biopsy Technique

Position the scope tip so that the selected biopsy site is 2 to 4 cm away and at 6 o'clock on video endoscopes or opposite the black triangle on fiberoptic scopes. Pass the closed forceps down the biopsy channel while keeping the lumen in view to avoid the risk of damaging the bowel wall. The assistant should maintain gentle pressure on the forceps controls to keep the jaws closed. Excessive closing pressure causes the forceps to become stiff and can make passage through a deflected tip difficult or damage the endoscope. Once the forceps tip has emerged from the distal tip of the scope, ask the assistant to open the jaws of the forceps. Advance the open forceps against the desired site and ask the assistant to close the jaws. Gently pull out on the forceps to "tent" the mucosa and confirm the desired site is in the jaws, and then sharply withdraw the forceps to remove the tissue by applying a quick jerk to the line. The biopsy sample is removed from the scope and placed in formalin. The site is then observed for bleeding. Occasionally, a second or even a third biopsy sample of the lesion may be indicated (see Fig. 89.5). If the forceps have a central needle, a second biopsy can often be obtained on a single passage.

FINDINGS

See Fig. 89.12.

- Polyps (iatrogenic "suction polyps," hyperplastic, and adenomatous [tubular, tubulovillous, and villous adenomas])
- Cancer
- Inflammation (inflammatory bowel [Crohn's and ulcerative colitis], antibiotic-associated colitis)
- Diverticula (90% of us by the age of 90 have these)
- Melanosis coli
- Arteriovenous malformations
- Foreign bodies
- Condylomata
- Hemorrhoids (internal)

Documentation

It is important that all findings be noted and documented. A comment should be made on each of the following: scope used, distance inserted by anatomic location and centimeters, quality of bowel preparation, patient tolerance, vascular and mucosal patterns, size of any polyps identified and location where they were found, ease of biopsy and control of any bleeding, final impression, and follow-up recommendations (Fig. 89.13).

Significance of Various Polyps

It is beyond the scope of this chapter to provide an extensive discussion of the significance of various polyps. More information is included in Chapter 90, Colonoscopy. In brief, all adenomatous (neoplastic) polyps (serrated, tubular, tubulovillous, and villous lesions) have a malignant potential. Recent articles document the reduction of CRC if all neoplastic polyps are removed. Most experts agree that hyperplastic polyps have little prognostic significance. Colonoscopy is not recommended for hyperplastic polyps, whereas it is essential with neoplastic polyps.

COMPLICATIONS

- Bowel perforation (very rare, <1:20,000)
- Bleeding (more likely if a biopsy sample was obtained, but still very uncommon)
- Abdominal distention and pain, often due to the insufflated air (be sure it is all removed)
- Infection (although very rare, inadequate cleaning of scopes can transmit disease)
- Vasovagal symptoms
- Missed disease

Complications from flexible sigmoidoscopy are very rare. Their incidence is higher in patients with previous bowel or pelvic surgery, or irradiation. These patients have more adhesions, which tether the bowel to a fixed position, predisposing it to perforation. If the scope is advanced blindly, without seeing the lumen, the risk of perforation also increases. However, at times this is necessary and safe as long as no resistance is felt and the patient is not overly uncomfortable.

Care must be taken in the presence of diverticulosis. The mouth of the diverticulum can be interpreted as the bowel lumen, and if the scope is inserted, perforation can occur.

Missed disease can occur if the endoscopist is unable to adequately insert the endoscope. This problem occurs more commonly in women and elderly patients (Walter et al, 2004). Disease in the rectum can also be missed if retroflection or anoscopic examination is not performed.

CLEANING AND DISINFECTION OF SCOPES

The various instrument representatives will detail the exact cleaning mechanism for each brand of scope. Tremain et al (1991) presents an excellent review, and reading of this article is strongly encouraged. Jackson and Ball (1997) also summarize the essential steps in disinfecting scopes. It is essential that the clinician's staff pay meticulous attention to cleaning directions for the scope. The orifices are very small, and a small amount of debris can prevent optimal functioning.

POSTPROCEDURE PATIENT EDUCATION

After completion of the procedure, explain the following to the patient:

- Findings.
- Where the biopsy samples have been taken from and the necessity for pathologic evaluation.
- Further management or referral, and future surveillance plans.
- Implications of the presence of cancer or polyps for the patient's siblings and children.
- The necessity of reporting any excessive bleeding or abdominal pain.
- Reinforce that proximal lesions are certainly possible and that if any symptoms develop (or persist if present), then further evaluation is necessary.

Flexible Sigmoidoscopy

Name: _____ Birth date: _____ Phone: (H) _____
                                          Age: _____   (W) _____

Your usual doctor: _____   Send a copy of report to him/her?   Y   N
Blood pressure: _____   Received and understood handouts?   Y   N

SYMPTOMS/HISTORY

Frequency _____   Pain: Abdomen   Rectum   w/BM
Consistency: Loose   Formed   Hard   Anemia _____
Change in stools _____   Weight loss _____
Diarrhea _____   Fever _____
Constipation _____   Polyps _____
Blood _____   Hemorrhoids _____
Black stools _____   F.H. _____

TESTS

Hemoccult: Date _____
                                             positive/negative   not done
Previous sigmoidoscopy/colonoscopy: Date _____
                                             Findings _____
Previous barium enema: Date _____
                                             Findings _____

PMH

Bleeding problems?   Yes   No
Artificial joints?   Yes   No
Artificial heart valve?   Yes   No
Heart murmur needing prophylaxis?   Yes   No

Allergies _____
Other medical problems? _____
Medications? _____
Health maintenance? _____

PROCEDURE   Scope: OSF-3
Abdominal exam: Megaly Y   N   Mass Y   N   Tenderness Y   N
Preparation: Adequate/Inadequate   Fleet given in office Y   N
Rectal: _____
Depth: _____
Reason for stopping: Limits of scope or _____
Tolerance: _____
Complications: none or _____
Findings: _____
Biopsy: _____ cm _____ cm _____ cm   Bleeding controlled   Y   N
Proctoscopy: _____

IMPRESSION: _____
RECOMMENDATIONS: _____
Daily aspirins, vitamins, diet, estrogen
Repeat exam _____
cc: _____   _____   _____
                        Physician's signature   Date

Fig. 89.13   Sample procedure form for flexible sigmoidoscopy. (Courtesy John L. Pfenninger, MD, The Medical Procedures Center, Midland, MI.)

- Primary prevention methods include the use of a nonsteroidal anti-inflammatory drug such as aspirin, not smoking, and a high-bulk, low-fat diet with at least five helpings of fruits and vegetables a day. A multivitamin a day (folic acid and vitamin D), estrogen use, and statins may also reduce the incidence of CRC. The USPSTF has found adequate evidence that aspirin use reduces the incidence of CRC in adults after 5 to 10 years of use.

CPT/BILLING CODES

45330   Sigmoidoscopy, flexible fiberoptic; diagnostic with or without collection of specimen by brushing or washing
45331   Sigmoidoscopy with biopsy, single or multiple
45332   Sigmoidoscopy with removal of foreign body
45333   Sigmoidoscopy with removal of polypoid lesion(s) by hot biopsy forceps or bipolar cautery
45334   Sigmoidoscopy with control of bleeding (e.g., electrocoagulation)
45335   Sigmoidoscopy with directed submucosal injection(s) any substance
45338   Sigmoidoscopy with removal of polypoid lesion(s) by snare technique
45339   Sigmoidoscopy with ablation of tumor, polyp, or other lesion not amenable to removal by hot biopsy, or snare technique
46600   Anoscopy; diagnostic (separate procedure)

Medicare will pay for screening flexible sigmoidoscopy after 47 months have passed since the previous flexible sigmoidoscopy or barium enema. The code GO104 should be used. If a biopsy is taken and polypectomy (etc.) performed, then the code 45331, 45338, 45339, and so on with PT modifier, not the "G" code, should be used. If the PT modifier is used, then the first diagnostic code should be for screening, the second for whatever lesion is treated. If two separate procedures (e.g., biopsy, snare polypectomy, directed submucosal injection) are performed, and it is well-documented that they are performed on separate lesions, the modifier 59 can be used.

ICD-10-CM Diagnostic Codes

A63.0	Condyloma
C18.6	Cancer, colon—descending, left
C18.7	Cancer, colon—sigmoid
C20	Cancer, rectum
C21.0	Cancer, anus
C18.9	Cancer, colon, unspecified
D12.6	Benign neoplasm, colon
D12.9	Benign neoplasm, rectum/anus
K64.8	Internal hemorrhoids
K64.9	Internal hemorrhoids, bleeding
K50.90	Crohn disease—colon
K51.90	Ulcerative colitis
K52.0	Radiation colitis
K52.9	Colitis, nonspecific noninfective
K57.90	Diverticulosis without hemorrhage unspecified
K57.91	Diverticulosis with hemorrhage unspecified
K57.92	Diverticulitis with hemorrhage
K59.00	Unspecified constipation
K58.8	Irritable colon other
K60.2	Anal fissure
K61.1	Perirectal abscess
K62.0	Anal polyp
K62.5	Anal and rectal hemorrhage
K62.89	Anal pain
K63.3	Ulcer, colon
K55.20	Angiodysplasia, colon
K92.1	Melena
K92.2	Gastrointestinal hemorrhage, hematochezia
R63.4	Weight loss
R19.2	Hyperperistalsis
R15.9	Stool incontinence
R19.8	Tenesmus
R10.9	Abdominal pain unspecified
R93.3	X-ray abnormality, gastrointestinal tract
Z85.038	Personal history colon cancer (not primary diagnosis)
Z80.0	Family history colon or other GI cancer (not primary diagnosis)
Z83.71	Family history colon polyps
Z83.79	Family history other gastrointestinal disorders (not primary diagnosis)

Acknowledgment

The editors recognize the contributions of John L. Pfenninger, MD, to this chapter in a previous edition of this text.

Suppliers

(See contact information available at www.expertconsult.com.)

Sigmoidoscopes
Fujinon, Inc.
Pentax Medical

Olympus America has limited new sigmoidoscopes available, but used equipment is very durable in most cases. (Also see the "Used or refurbished equipment" list in the Suppliers section of Chapter 90, Colonoscopy.)

Online Resources

American Association for Primary Care Endoscopy: www.aapce.org
American Gastroenterological Association (AGA): www.gastro.org
American Society of Colon and Rectal Surgeons: www.fascrs.org
CA: A Cancer Journal for Clinicians (American Cancer Association): www.ca-journal.org
The DAVE Project—Gastroenterology: http://daveproject.org/index.cfm

RECOMMENDED READING

Anderson ML, Pasha TM, Leighton JA. Endoscopic perforation of the colon: lessons from a 10-year study. Am J Gastroenterol. 2000;95:3418–3422.

Atkin WS, Edwards R, Kralj-Hans I, et al. Once-only flexible sigmoidoscopy screening in prevention of colorectal cancer: a multicentre randomised controlled trial. Lancet. 2010;375:1624–1633.

Brill JR, Baumgardner DJ. Establishing proficiency in flexible sigmoidoscopy in a family practice residency program. Fam Med. 1997;29:580–583.

Brooks DD, Winawer SJ, Rex DK, et al. Colonoscopy surveillance after polypectomy and colorectal cancer resection. Am Fam Physician. 2008;77:995–1002.

Esber EJ, Yang P. Retroflexion of the sigmoidoscope for the detection of rectal cancer. Am Fam Physician. 1995;51:1709–1711.

Frazier AL, Colditz CA, Fuchs CS, et al. Cost-effectiveness of screening for endorectal cancer in the general population. JAMA. 2000;284:1954–1961.

Gatto NM, Frucht H, Sundararajan V, et al. Risk of perforation after colonoscopy and sigmoidoscopy: a population-based study. J Natl Cancer Inst. 2003;95:230–236.

Holman JR, Marshall RC, Jordan B, Vogelman L. Technical competency in flexible sigmoidoscopy. J Am Board Fam Pract. 2001;14:424–429.

Jackson FW, Ball MD. Correction of deficiencies in flexible fiberoptic sigmoidoscope cleaning and disinfection technique in family practice and internal medicine offices. Arch Fam Med. 1997;6:578–582.

Siegel RL, Miller KD, Jemal A. Cancer statistics. 2017 CA Cancer J Clin. 2017;67(1):7–30.

Levin TR, Conell C, Shapiro JA, et al. Complications of screening flexible sigmoidoscopy. Gastroenterology. 2002;123:1786–1792.

Levin TR, Palitz A, Grossman S, et al. Predicting advanced proximal colonic neoplasia with screening sigmoidoscopy. JAMA. 1999;281:1611–1617.

Lieberman DA, Rex DK, Winawer SJ, Giardiello FM, Johnson DA, Levin TR. Guidelines for colonoscopy surveillance after screening and polypectomy: a consensus update by the US multi-society task force on colorectal cancer. Gastroenterology. 2012;143(3):844–857.

Lin OS, Schembre DB, McCormick SE, et al. Risk of proximal colorectal neoplasia among asymptomatic patients with distal hyperplastic polyps. Am J Med. 2005;118:1113–1119.

Loeve F, Brown ML, Boer R, et al. Endoscopic colorectal cancer screening: a cost-saving analysis. J Natl Cancer Inst. 2000;92:557–563.

Manoucheri M, Nakamura DY, Lukman RL. Bowel preparation for flexible sigmoidoscopy: which method yields the best results? J Fam Pract. 1999;48:272–274.

Pfenninger JL, Zainea GG. Common anorectal conditions: part I. Symptoms and complaints. Am Fam Physician. 2001;63:2391–2398.

Pfenninger JL, Zainea GG. Common anorectal conditions: part II. Lesions. Am Fam Physician. 2001;64:77–88.

Provenzale D, Garrett JW, Condon SE, Sandler RS. Risk for colon adenomas in patients with rectosigmoid hyperplastic polyps. Ann Intern Med. 1990;113:760–763.

Roetzheim RG, Pal N, Gonzalez EC, et al. The effects of physician supply on the early detection of colorectal cancer. J Fam Pract. 1999;48:850–858.

Schoen RE, Weissfeld JL, Pinsky PF, Riley T. Yield of advanced adenoma and cancer based on polyp size detected at screening flexible sigmoidoscopy. Gastroenterology. 2006;131:1683–1689.

Screening for Colorectal Cancer. U.S. Preventive Services Task Force Recommendation Statement. JAMA. 2016;315(23):2564–2575.

Sharma V, Chockalingham S. Randomized, controlled comparison of two forms of preparation for screening flexible sigmoidoscopy. Am J Gastroenterol. 1997;92:809–811.

Sonnenberg A, Delco F, Inadomi JM. Cost-effectiveness of colonoscopy in screening for colorectal cancer. *Ann Intern Med.* 2000;133:573–584.

Tremain SC, Orientale E, Rodney WM. Cleaning, disinfection, and sterilization of gastrointestinal endoscopes: approaches in the office. *J Fam Pract.* 1991;32:300–305.

UK Flexible Sigmoidoscopy Screening Trial Investigators. Single flexible sigmoidoscopy screening to prevent colorectal cancer: baseline findings of a UK multicentre randomised trial. *Lancet.* 2002;359:1291–1300.

U.S. Preventive Services Task Force. Screening for Colorectal Cancer: U.S. Preventive Services Task Force Recommendation Statement. *JAMA.* 2016;315(23):2564–2575.

Walter LC, de Garmo P, Covinsky KE. Association of older age and female sex with inadequate reach of screening flexible sigmoidoscopy. *Am J Med.* 2004;116:174–178.

CHAPTER 90

COLONOSCOPY

*Jason P. Brewington • John Bartels Pope**

Colonoscopy is a procedure that allows for visual inspection of the entire large bowel from the distal rectum to the cecum. The procedure is generally well accepted by patients and, in the proper hands, is a safe and effective means of screening for colon cancer. A well-trained endoscopist can usually perform a total colonoscopy in 20 to 30 minutes, achieving cecal intubation in greater than 95% of attempted procedures under optimal conditions (excellent bowel preparation, high-quality equipment, technical support, appropriate sedation, and low-risk patient population).

Colonoscopy has a greater sensitivity and specificity for the detection of colonic polyps and colorectal cancers (CRCs) than fecal immunochemical testing, fecal immunochemical testing-fecal DNA testing (Cologard), guaiac fecal occult blood testing, Septin9 testing, air-contrast barium enema, capsule colonoscopy, or computed tomographic (CT) colonography (virtual colonoscopy), and greater sensitivity than flexible sigmoidoscopy because more of the colon is visualized. Colonoscopy is the procedure of choice in the work-up of most cases of lower gastrointestinal bleeding. A significant advantage of colonoscopy over radiologic evaluation of the large intestine is the ability to perform additional diagnostic and therapeutic measures, such as biopsy, polypectomy, and control of bleeding. Although traditionally performed in the hospital, colonoscopy can also be performed in free-standing offices or ambulatory endoscopy centers.

It is widely accepted that the vast majority of colon cancers arise from adenomatous (neoplastic) polyps. It has been shown that the removal of adenomatous polyps by colonoscopic polypectomy can reduce the incidence of CRC by 76% to 90%. Colonoscopy thus provides an opportunity to greatly influence the incidence of CRC by allowing the removal of polyps throughout the entire colon, especially advanced adenomas. Advanced adenomas are defined as those greater than 1 cm in diameter or having high grade dysplasia or villous elements. Nonadvanced adenomas have a lower risk of being precancerous and if they do become malignant, have a much longer lag time; however, both types should be removed when encountered if possible.

ANATOMY

The colon is approximately 150 cm in length from anal verge to cecum.

Anus

- The outlet to the gastrointestinal tract

Rectum

- Dentate (pectinate) line demarcating junction between pain-sensitive squamous epithelium of anus and pain-insensitive columnar epithelium of rectum

---

* Much of the information in Chapter 89, Flexible Sigmoidoscopy, is very pertinent to colonoscopy. Material from that chapter is not repeated here. The reader is encouraged to review that chapter in conjunction with this chapter.

- Approximately 15 cm in length with capacious lumen
- Prominent folds (valves of Houston) that may create potential blind spots
- Mucosal transparency with prominent hemorrhoidal venous plexus visible

Sigmoid Colon

- Variably mobile (key to successful colonoscopy)
- Loops anteriorly, then posteriorly where it is retroperitoneal
- 35 to 45 cm in length

Descending Colon

- Fixed, straight course up left paracolic gutter
- Narrowest portion of colon
- Retroperitoneal
- Approximately 20 to 30 cm in length

Transverse Colon

- Longer than the distance it traverses and may sag into umbilical region
- Lumen generally has a triangular appearance
- Approximately 45 to 55 cm in length

Ascending Colon

- Capacious lumen with straight course
- Retroperitoneal into right paracolic gutter
- Terminates at ileocecal valve, which demarcates beginning of cecum
- Approximately 10 to 20 cm in length

Cecum

- Variable mobility and capacious lumen
- Landmarks include ileocecal valve, appendiceal orifice, and terminal portion of taeniae coli ("crow's foot")
- Transillumination is frequently seen
- Approximately 5 to 8 cm in length
  - Intraperitoneal (important for cancer staging, complications in event of perforation)
- Superior rectum, inferior sigmoid, transverse colon

NOTE: The importance of retroperitoneal versus intraperitoneal location of the colon includes the fact that a retroperitoneal malignant polyp in the rectum may need a colorectal surgeon, whereas an intraperitoneal lesion can often be handled by a laparoscopic or general surgeon. Tattooing the area where lesions are removed in the proximal rectal area may be useful for the same reason, to help determine intraperitoneal versus extraperitoneal. In the event that it happens, a retroperitoneal perforation somewhat confines the fecal material, often resulting in less risk of abscess or complications compared with intraperitoneal.

INDICATIONS

Screening

- Screening in the average-risk population (>50 years of age) and in the increased-risk groups (Table 90.1). In 2018, the American Cancer Society recommended screening average risk individuals starting at age 45; if colonoscopy is used, it should be re-

peated every 10 years. For several years, the American College of Gastroenterology has recommended beginning screening for African Americans at age 45; the American College of Physicians recommends beginning screening African Americans at age 40 years.
- Screening for neoplastic disease in patients with a family history of CRC or adenomatous (neoplastic) or advanced serrated polyps before age 60 years; screening should begin at 40 years of age or 10 years before the age of discovery in a relative.
- Screening and surveillance for neoplastic disease in hereditary cancer syndromes
  - Familial adenomatous polyposis (FAP) syndrome. Gene carri-

TABLE 90.1 Guidelines for Screening for Colorectal Adenomas and Cancer in Individuals at Increased Risk or at High Risk

Risk Category	Age to Begin	Recommendation	Comment
Increased Risk—Patients With History of Polyps at Prior Colonoscopy			
Patients with small rectal hyperplastic polyps	—	Colonoscopy or other screening options at intervals recommended for average-risk individuals	An exception is patients with hyperplastic polyposis syndrome. They are at increased risk for adenomas and colorectal cancer and need to be identified for more intensive follow-up.
Patients with 1 or 2 small tubular adenomas with low-grade dysplasia	5 to 10 years after the initial polypectomy	Colonoscopy	The precise timing within this interval should be based on other clinical factors (such as prior colonoscopy findings, family history, and the preferences of the patient and judgment of the physician).
Patients with 3 to 10 adenomas or 1 adenoma (including sessile serrated) >1 cm or any adenoma with villous features or high-grade dysplasia or any sessile serrated adeonma with dysplasia or traditional serrated adenoma	3 years after the initial polypectomy	Colonoscopy	Adenomas must have been completely removed. If the follow-up colonoscopy is normal or shows only 1 or 2 small, tubular adenomas with low-grade dysplasia, then the interval for the subsequent examination should be 5 years.
Patients with >10 adenomas on a single examination	<3 years after the initial polypectomy	Colonoscopy	Consider the possibility of an underlying familial syndrome.
Patients with sessile adenomas that are removed piecemeal	2 to 6 months to verify complete removal	Colonoscopy	Once complete removal has been established, subsequent surveillance needs to be individualized based on the endoscopist's judgment. Completeness of removal should be based on both endoscopic and pathologic assessments.
Increased Risk—Patients With Colorectal Cancer			
Patients with colon and rectal cancer should undergo high-quality perioperative clearing	Perioperative, or at 3 to 6 months after cancer resection in the event of obstructive colorectal cancer	Colonoscopy	In the case of nonobstructing tumors, this can be done by preoperative colonoscopy. In the case of obstructing colon cancers, CTC with intravenous contrast or DCBE can be used to detect neoplasms in the proximal colon.
Patients undergoing curative resection for colon or rectal cancer	1 year after the resection (or 1 year following the performance of the colonoscopy that was performed to clear the colon of synchronous disease)	Colonoscopy	This colonoscopy at 1 year in addition to the perioperative colonoscopy for synchronous tumors. If the examination performed at 1 year is normal, then the interval before the next subsequent examination should be 3 years. If that colonoscopy is normal, then the subsequent colonoscopies should be at 5 year intervals
Increased Risk—Patients With a Family History			
Either colorectal cancer or adenomatous polyps in a first-degree relative before age 60 yr or in 2 or more first-degree relatives at any age	Age 40 yr or 10 yr before the youngest case in the immediate family	Colonoscopy	Every 5 yr
Either colorectal cancer or advanced adenoma (villous or high-grade dysplasia or >1 cm) or advanced serrated adenoma (dysplasia or traditional serrated adenoma or >1 cm) in a first-degree relative ≥age 60 yr	Age 40 yr	Screening options at intervals recommended for average-risk individuals	Screening should begin at an earlier age, but individuals may choose to be screened with any recommended form of testing
High Risk			
Genetic diagnosis of FAP or suspected FAP without genetic testing evidence	Age 10–12 yr	Annual FSIG to determine if the individual is expressing the genetic abnormality and counseling to consider genetic testing	If the genetic test is positive, colectomy should be considered

TABLE 90.1	Guidelines for Screening for Colorectal Adenomas and Cancer in Individuals at Increased Risk or at High Risk—cont'd			
Risk Category	**Age to Begin**	**Recommendation**	**Comment**
Genetic or clinical diagnosis of HNPCC (Lynch) or individuals at increased risk of HNPCC Family Colon Cancer Syndrome X	Age 20–25 yr or 10 yr before the youngest case in the immediate family Begin 10 yr before age of youngest case in the immediate family	Colonoscopy every 1–2 yr and counseling to consider genetic testing Colonoscopy every 3–5 yr	Genetic testing for HNPCC should be offered to first-degree relatives of persons with a known inherited MMR gene mutation. It should also be offered when the family mutation is not already known, but 1 of the first 3 of the modified Bethesda Criteria is present
Serrated polyposis syndrome Inflammatory bowel disease, chronic ulcerative colitis, and Crohn colitis	1 yr after intial polypectomy Cancer risk begins to be significant 8 yr after the onset of pancolitis or 12–15 yr after the onset of left-sided colitis	Colonoscopy Colonoscopy with biopsies for dysplasia	Every 1–2 yr; these patients are best referred to a center with experience in the surveillance and management of inflammatory bowel disease

FAP, Family adenomatous polyposis; *FSIG,* flexible sigmoidoscopy; *HNPCC,* hereditary nonpolyposis colon cancer; *MMR,* mismatch repair.
From Kahi CJ, Boland CR, Dominitz JA, Giardiello FM, Johnson DA, et al. Colonoscopy surveillance after colorectal cancer resection: recommendations of the US Multi-Society Task Force on Colorectal Cancer. *Gastroenterology.* 2016;150:758-768 and Rex DK, Boland R, Dominitz JA, et al. Colorectal cancer screening: recommendations for physicians and patients from the U.S. Multi-society task force on colorectal cancer. *Gastrointest Endosc.* 2017;86(1):18–33.

ers or at-risk family members who have not had genetic testing or are from families in whom the gene test is uninformative should be offered a flexible sigmoidoscopy or colonoscopy every 12 months starting at around 10 to 12 years of age and continuing until 35 to 40 years of age if negative. Colonoscopy is necessary in attenuated FAP, where the usual presentation of thousands of polyps is reduced to less than 100 polyps, which may be more proximally located.

- Hereditary nonpolyposis colon cancer syndrome (HNPCC, Lynch). HNPCC is defined as CRC in three or more family members, two of whom are first-degree relatives of the third, with at least two generations involved and at least one person diagnosed with CRC before 50 years of age. Use of the term *nonpolyposis* is a misnomer. Polyps do indeed occur in HNPCC, just not to the extent seen with FAP. Individuals at risk for HNPCC should undergo colonoscopy every 1 to 2 years starting at 20 to 25 years of age or 10 years younger than the age of the earliest diagnosis of cancer in the family, whichever is earlier. For a version of Lynch, Family Colon Cancer Syndrome X, colonoscopy is recommended every 3 to 5 years.
- Serrated polyposis syndrome is defined by the World Health Organization as occurring in individuals with one of the following criteria: five serrated polyps proximal to sigmoid, or two or more serrated polyps of 1 cm or greater, or 20 serrated polyps of any size throughout the colon, or any serrated polyps proximal to sigmoid with family history of serrated polyposis syndrome. These individuals should undergo yearly colonoscopy.

Diagnostic

- Total colon evaluation after the finding of adenomatous polyps, especially high-risk polyps (i.e., those >1 cm, small polyps with advanced histopathology, or multiple small adenomatous polyps), during flexible sigmoidoscopy.
- Evaluation of abnormal or equivocal barium enema.
- Evaluation of overt or occult colonic or rectal bleeding.
- Evaluation of abnormal findings on CT colonography.
- Evaluation of iron-deficiency anemia of undetermined cause.
- Surveillance of neoplastic disease after removal of polyps or cancer.
- Evaluation and surveillance of inflammatory bowel disease (after 8 years in pancolitis and after 12 years in left-sided colitis).
- Evaluation of chronic diarrhea of undetermined cause.
- Intraoperative evaluation of polypectomy site, bleeding lesions, or anastomotic leaks.
- Endosonography for local staging (primary tumor, regional nodes, and metastasis [TNM]) of CRC.

- Evaluation of significant weight loss.
- Evaluation of abdominal pain.

NOTE: Colonoscopy is often of little benefit in determining the causes of chronic lower abdominal pain or changes in bowel habits in the absence of rectal bleeding, weight loss, or anorexia.

Therapeutic

- Biopsy of suspect lesion
- Polypectomy
- Therapy of bleeding lesions
- Removal of foreign body
- Reduction of sigmoid volvulus
- Decompression of pseudo-obstruction of colon
- Dilation of colonic strictures and placement of colonic stents
- Laser therapy of lesions

CONTRAINDICATIONS
Absolute

- Acute abdomen
- Suspected peritonitis
- Acute diverticulitis with systemic symptoms
- Acute exacerbation of inflammatory bowel disease
- Documented or suspected bowel perforation
- Patient refusal
- Risk to patient outweighs benefits of procedure

Relative

- Unstable cardiopulmonary status
- Recent myocardial infarction or pulmonary embolism
- Significant pelvic or abdominal adhesions
- Blood coagulation abnormalities
- Recent (within 1 week) bowel surgery
- Hyperplastic polyps on flexible sigmoidoscopy with no other indication
- Poorly prepared patient
- Uncooperative patient
- Metastatic adenocarcinoma of unknown primary site in the absence of colonic symptoms when it will not influence management
- Severe neutropenia
- Pregnancy (second or third trimester)
- Large abdominal aortic aneurysm
- Splenomegaly

EQUIPMENT

Basic equipment necessary to perform colonoscopy includes the following:

- Fiberoptic or video colonoscope
- Light source (i.e., halogen or xenon)
- Suction apparatus
- Biopsy forceps
- Polypectomy snares
- Endoscopic subcutaneous injection needle, normal saline
- Endoscopic clips
- Electrosurgical unit
- Equipment to follow universal blood and body fluid precautions
- Moderate (conscious) sedation setup (see Chapter 1, Procedural Sedation and Analgesia)
- Nitrogen gas system for insufflation (possibly better tolerated than air and less risk of ileus)

Additional instruments that may be useful include India ink for injection/tattooing, heater probe or multipolar cautery probe, polyp retrieval baskets and three-prong grasping forceps. Lubricating jelly, gauze pads, saline, sterile water, protective gowns, and protective eyewear are also recommended.

The colonoscope is similar in design to the sigmoidoscope, only longer. The outside diameter of the insertion tube varies from 11 to 13 mm, and the length of the shaft varies from 105 to 185 cm. The narrower scopes are typically used in pediatric settings and are generally lighter with a more flexible shaft. Their use may result in less postprocedure discomfort in small individuals. Video scopes are monitored on a screen; only those remaining fiberoptic scopes have an eyepiece with focusing controls. Scopes have control wheels to deflect the tip through a range of positions, including deflection over 180 degrees; a biopsy port; suction and air and water control knobs; and locking levers to fix control wheels in a particular position (see Chapter 89, Flexible Sigmoidoscopy).

Most colonoscopies are now performed with video endoscopes. Videoscopes are fiberoptic devices; however, they use a charge-coupled device to convert light energy into electronic signals that can be converted by a computer processor into images. Videoscopes provide photo documentation or recording capability of entire procedures, and they allow the transmission of images to remote sites. Videoscopes also provide for a more comfortable posture for the endoscopist during the procedure. Newer video colonoscopes offer optional features such as variable stiffness capability, forward water jet, high-resolution imaging, narrow-band imaging, close focusing, and 170-degree field of view. Video endoscopy setups are significantly more expensive than conventional setups.

Cleaning and disinfecting the instrument and equipment are very important to prevent iatrogenic infections. Strict adherence to appropriate cleaning protocols virtually eliminates these risks. The American Society for Gastrointestinal Endoscopy (ASGE) provides practice guidelines for infection control during gastrointestinal endoscopy. Company representatives also provide excellent guidelines and videotapes demonstrating the process.

PREPROCEDURE PATIENT PREPARATION

Informed consent is a necessary component of colonoscopy. Consent should be obtained by the clinician and should include discussion of the nature of the procedure (how it is performed), expected benefits of the procedure, risks of the procedure (including those from sedation, procedure complications [perforation and bleeding], and the possibility of missed lesions), and alternatives to the procedure. The consent process may be facilitated with the use of patient education videos (e.g., https://www.asge.org/home/for-patients/videos) or written materials available from various organizations (e.g., ASGE, Society of American Gastrointestinal Endoscopic Surgeons, National Procedures Institute). Sample patient education handouts are also available at https://www.sages.org/publications/patient-information/patient-information-for-colonoscopy-from-sages/.

A focused history should be obtained before the procedure to ensure that an appropriate indication exists for the procedure and to identify factors that may influence safe and effective performance of the procedure and subsequent management of the patient. Pertinent history should include present illness, past medical and surgical history (hysterectomy or abdominal surgeries may increase colon intubation difficulty), current medications, allergies, and tobacco and alcohol use. The patient should also be asked about any previous complications from anesthesia, as well as any history of coagulation abnormalities or chronic use of narcotics or tranquilizers, which may influence the ability to achieve proper sedation (Fig. 90.1). An adequate history for determining American Society of Anesthesiologists score may be necessary for supervision of moderate sedation.

Physical examination should include (as a minimum) assessment of vital signs, sensorium, and heart, lung, and abdominal examination. Additional examination criteria may be needed prior to the supervision of moderate sedation (e.g., Mallampati score).

Laboratory testing is not routinely performed before colonoscopy; however, in specific circumstances testing may be warranted (e.g., severe anemia with anticipation of polypectomy, known fluid and electrolyte abnormality, anticoagulation).

A clean bowel is essential for colonoscopy. Four of the most common and effective preparations for cleansing the bowel include the following:

1. Split dose: Half of a 4-L polyethylene glycol (PEG) solution is taken orally (GoLYTELY, Colyte, MoviPrep, generics) starting 4 to 6 PM the night before the procedure, with the other half of the prep taken the morning of the procedure at least 4 to 6 hours prior to the procedure.
2. Single bolus dose: PEG solution (4 L) is taken orally (GoLYTELY, Colyte, MoviPrep, generics) over a 1- to 3-hour period starting at 4 PM the evening prior to the procedure.
3. Gatorade: A less-expensive, better-tasting alternative preparation combines 238 g of over-the-counter PEG laxative (MiraLax powder) with 0.5 gallon of Gatorade or similar drink. Half is consumed over 1 to 2 hours starting at 4 to 6 PM. The other half is consumed the morning of the procedure at least 4 to 6 hours prior to the procedure.
4. Magnesium citrate solution: 10 oz is taken with four bisacodyl tablets (5 mg) the afternoon of the day before the procedure; the magnesium citrate is repeated the morning of the procedure.

Although commonly used in the past, aqueous phosphosoda (NaP) colon preparations (e.g., Fleet) are no longer approved for that purpose by the U.S. Food and Drug Administration because of the risk of renal toxicity and renal failure. The over-the-counter Fleet preparation is no longer manufactured. Tablet formulations of NaP (Visicol, Osmoprep) are available by prescription, but now carry a black-box warning. Caution should be used when administering any phosphosoda-type preparation to patients with renal insufficiency, ascites, or congestive heart failure. Acute renal failure has been reported with these preparations. The use of NaP preparations is declining, and future use should probably be avoided in light of the current restrictions and risk.

PEG bowel preparations should usually be administered starting at from 4 to 6 p.m. the day before colonoscopy (usually completed early enough to get a good night's sleep). If split dose, the other half is taken in the morning, 4 to 6 hours prior to the procedure. After beginning the preparation, the patient can have only clear liquids until midnight, then NPO. One or two tap water enemas administered 1 or 2 hours before the procedure may also be helpful if particulate matter or dark-colored bowel contents are still present. In general, enemas should be avoided because they are unpleasant for the patient and may cause punctate erosions/inflammation in the colonic mucosa, falsely suggesting colon pathology. This phenomenon also can be seen when NaP preparations are used.

Colonoscopy, Biopsy, and Polypectomy

Name: _____ DOB _____ Age _____

Telephone (H) _____ (W) _____

Your referring doctor: _____

Primary care doctor: _____ Want a copy sent to him/her?   Y   N

Blood pressure: _____ Received, read, and understood handouts?   Y   N

SYMPTOMS/HISTORY:

Reason for consult: _____

787.99 Change in stools	564.0 Constipation
285.9 Anemia, NOS	780.6 Fevers
578.9 Blood	578.1 Black stools
783.2 Weight loss	562.11 Diverticulitis/diverticulosis
455.6 Hemorrhoids, NOS	787.91 Diarrhea
780.9 Chills	211.3 Polyps
Frequency _____ daily _____ weekly	V10.05 Personal Hx colon Ca
Pain: 780.9 Abdomen Where? _____	V16.0 Family Hx Colon Ca
569.42 Rectum	Who? _____
w/BM	Age _____

Hemoccults: Date _____   Neg   Pos   Not done

Previous sigmoid: Date _____   Who? _____   OR findings: _____

Findings: _____
_____

Previous barium enema: Date _____   Findings _____
_____

Previous abdominal surgery: _____

Hysterectomy (for women)   Y   N

PMH:

Bleeding problems	Coronary artery disease
Artificial joints	Heart murmur needing prophylaxis
Artificial heart valve	COPD
Asthma	Smoker _____ PPD 3 _____ years
Other medical problems: 1. _____	2. _____
3. _____	4. _____

Medications _____

Allergies _____

OBJECTIVE:

General:

Neck:

Lungs:

Cor:

Abd:

IMPRESSION: _____
_____
_____

COUNSELING:

Indications

Sedation

Bowel prep   Mag Citrate-Dulcolax-Fleet or GoLYTELY

Alternatives   Not performing examination/flex sig and ACBE

Risks   Bleeding
               Perforation
               Infection
               Need for hospitalization
               Sedation related

Expected results

Monitoring: BP Pulse Oxygen concentration

RECOMMENDATIONS:

1. Mag Citrate-Dulcolax-Fleet bowel prep or GoLYTELY bowel prep
2. Driver when receiving sedation
3. Sedation type   IV _____   oral _____
4. _____
5. _____

_____   _____
Clinician   Date

Fig. 90.1   Sample patient counseling form for colonoscopy, biopsy, and polypectomy.

It is important for the clinician to individualize the preparation for each patient and to take time to explain the reasons for the bowel cleansing preparation. If patients are chronically dependent on laxatives or have had a previous inadequate bowel preparation, it may be advisable to add an additional day of clear liquids before beginning the preparation. Four bisacodyl tablets are taken about 2 hours before drinking the preparation the afternoon before the procedure. Optimal examination may be better accomplished if the patient has received a PEG solution (i.e., GoLYTELY, Colyte, MoviPrep, generics); however, many clinicians claim "less is best." PEG solutions may be more palatable when taken chilled or mixed with a sugar-free drink mix (red-colored mixes should be avoided). Smaller-volume PEG-type preparations (e.g., Half-Lytely) are now available that reduce the volume necessary for the patient to consume, and add a mild laxative agent to the process.

EDITOR'S NOTE: A meta-analysis in 2015 (Martel et al., 2015) found the split-dose prep to be superior to the single day before bolus dose. In my experience (G.C.F.), Half-Litely resulted in half-prepped (inadequately prepped) patients; I no longer use it.

It is important to maintain adequate hydration of the patient before, during, and after the administration of any colon preparation to minimize possible adverse events. This is especially important in older individuals and in those with known renal disease or who are on medications that may predispose to fluid and electrolyte disturbances.

Diabetic patients will be NPO for an extended time during the colon preparation and should generally refrain from taking their diabetes medications beginning the day of the preparation. It also is advisable to withhold iron therapy beginning 4 to 5 days before the preparation because iron tends to darken and thicken the stool, thereby decreasing preparation effectiveness.

Bowel cleansing is essential, not only to provide an unobstructed view but to minimize the rare, but possible, risk of combustion from methane gas should cautery be used during polypectomy or to stop bleeding. Good bowel preparation may also help improve surgical outcomes in the case of perforation and subsequent repair.

ANTIBIOTIC PROPHYLAXIS

The American Heart Association, the American College of Cardiology, and the Standards of Training and Practice Committee of the ASGE no longer recommend periprocedural antibiotic prophylaxis for the prevention of infective endocarditis for any gastrointestinal endoscopic procedure, regardless of the patient's cardiac risk status. When used, antibiotic prophylaxis regimens usually include ampicillin and gentamicin, or vancomycin in penicillin-allergic patients.

ANTICOAGULATION

The Standards of Practice Committee of the ASGE has developed practice guidelines for the use of colonoscopy in conjunction with anticoagulated patients. Management is determined by establishing risk of bleeding versus risk of thromboembolic events. Colonoscopy with polypectomy is considered a high-risk procedure for bleeding; mucosal biopsy is considered low risk. Conditions considered high risk for thromboembolic events are chronic atrial fibrillation with associated valvular heart disease, a mechanical valve in the mitral position, an older aortic mechanical valve and prior thromboembolic event. High-risk procedures (i.e., colonoscopy with polypectomy) performed in high-risk conditions should be managed by discontinuing warfarin 3 to 5 days before the procedure. Heparin should be considered while the international normalized ratio is below the therapeutic level. Or the use of low-molecular-weight heparin bridge therapy may be necessary for individuals with chronic atrial fibrillation or valvular heart prostheses in order to prevent the risk of embolic events. However, as a result of the BRIDGE study (Douketis, 2015), which showed a higher risk of bleeding and no decrease in thromboembolic events by bridging patients with atrial fibrillation (average CHADS$_2$ score of 2.3) with Lovenox, many experts performing colonoscopy with or without biopsy or polypectomy no longer use bridging therapy. Instead, they just stop the warfarin 5 days before the procedure. This higher risk of bleeding had also been seen in a meta-analysis of patients bridged with heparin (Siegal et al., 2012). ASGE guidelines do not recommend bridging therapy unless the CHA2DS2-VASc score is greater than or equal to 2, there is a mechanical aortic heart valve that is not bileaflet or a mechanical mitral valve, there is recent cerebrovascular accident, or there is a thromboembolic risk factor (prior venous thromboembolism on

anticoagulation, recent [last 6 months] transient ischemic attack or cerebrovascular accident).

EDITOR'S NOTE: As an alternative to bridging therapy, although no guidelines have been written to support it, certain experts use oral dabigatran (Pradaxa), apixaban (Eliquis) or rivaroxaban (Xarelto), and withhold them 2 days prior to major surgery or 1 day for less significant surgery. Since apixaban is taken twice a day due to its shorter half-life, it would seem quicker to reverse by withholding it.

High-risk procedures in patients with low-risk conditions require only discontinuation of warfarin 3 to 5 days before the procedure without use of heparin. Low-risk procedures, such as colonoscopy with mucosal biopsy, do not require discontinuation of anticoagulation. Some experts do not discontinue anticoagulation even if polypectomy is anticipated; instead, they utilize more hemostatic clips. The ASGE no longer considers recent aspirin or nonsteroidal antiinflammatory drug use a contraindication to colonoscopy with polypectomy in the absence of a preexisting bleeding disorder.

ANTIPLATELET MEDICATIONS

Recent coronary or carotid stent placement presents specific issues related to the risk of early stent thrombosis. Dual antiplatelet therapy (aspirin plus an adenosine diphosphate receptor inhibitor such as clopidogrel, prasugrel, or ticagrelor) is recommended in patients who have recently received coronary or carotid stents to prevent early stent occlusion until epithelialization has occurred. Decisions regarding the risk of bleeding in a particular procedure versus the risk of stent closure must be made when evaluating a patient preoperatively. It is best that the decision to continue or discontinue dual antiplatelet therapy in stented patients be made in partnership with the surgeon, anesthesiologist, cardiologist, and patient.

American Heart Association guidelines from 2014 suggest delaying elective noncardiac surgery for a month in patients with a bare metal stent, and a year for patients with a drug-eluting stent. However, it may be acceptable to do elective surgery 180 days after a drug-eluting stent if at that point the risk of delaying surgery further is greater than the risk of stent thrombosis. In an update in 2016, there is some evidence that even shorter durations for drug-eluting stents may be acceptable. For nonelective, urgent, or emergent surgery at less than 4 to 6 weeks from stent placement, they recommend continuing dual antiplatelet therapy unless the risk of bleeding is greater than the risk of stent thrombosis. If dual antiplatelet therapy is discontinued, aspirin should be continued if possible, and dual therapy restarted as soon as safely possible.

Again, according to ASGE guidelines, colonoscopy, including mucosal biopsy, is considered low-risk for bleeding in patients taking anticoagulants (including dual antiplatelet therapy) and, therefore, can be performed without the adjustment of antiplatelet medications prior to the procedure by clinicians extremely familiar with colonoscopy and biopsy technique. For those therapeutic procedures performed with colonoscopy considered high-risk procedures for bleeding (i.e., polypectomy, endoscopic ultrasound–guided fine-needle aspiration, laser ablation, coagulation, and possibly dilations) adjustment of antiplatelet therapy is suggested. The exception to this would be those patients also at high risk for thromboembolic complications in which dual therapy may be continued. It should be noted that other than polypectomy, these procedures are beyond the scope of this chapter.

SEDATION

Most colonoscopic examinations are performed while the patient is under moderate (conscious) sedation (see Chapter 1, Procedural Sedation and Analgesia), although unsedated colonoscopy is possible in some circumstances with motivated patients. Sedation may allow for a more thorough examination of the colon because of increased patient comfort and decreased anxiety. Appropriate equipment includes cardiac, blood pressure, pulse oximetry, and respiratory monitors. Nasal capnography is frequently monitored if general anesthesia is administered. During colonoscopy, it is mandatory to have an assistant available to monitor the patient. Intravenous (IV) access should be established and maintained during the entire procedure in patients receiving IV sedation.

Benzodiazepines are the drugs most commonly used for sedation and include midazolam (Versed) 2 to 5 mg or diazepam (Valium) 5 to 10 mg. Meperidine (Demerol) 25 to 100 mg or fentanyl (Sublimaze) 25 to 100 μg is often used in conjunction with benzodiazepines to achieve optimal analgesia with sedation. These medications should be administered slowly through the IV route. Dangerous side effects can be reversed with flumazenil (Romazicon) or naloxone (Narcan), although properly titrating these medications will minimize the need for reversal drugs. It should be noted that these patients need to be monitored much longer in recovery because the half-life of the reversal agent may be much shorter than the agent being reversed. This can result in delayed, dangerous, profound sedation. Propofol (Diprivan) given as repeated boluses (10 to 20 mg) IV is becoming more commonly used as a sedation agent in colonoscopy because of its rapid, profound sedative effect and subsequent clearance, with faster patient recovery time. However, most institutions require propofol be administered by an anesthetist or anesthesiologist. Endoscopists should be thoroughly familiar with the pharmacology of all these drugs. Further discussion is found in Chapter 91, Esophagogastroduodenoscopy, and Chapter 1, Procedural Sedation and Analgesia.

A "crash cart" should be immediately available in case of cardiopulmonary arrest. See Chapter 212, Anaphylaxis, and the discussion regarding Banyan kits for the office.

TECHNIQUE

Colonoscopy

The procedure for colonoscopy is as follows (also see Chapter 89, Flexible Sigmoidoscopy, because the technique is virtually identical for the first 70 cm):

1. Place the patient on the examining table in the left lateral decubitus position.
2. Check all of the equipment for proper functioning.
3. Universal blood and body fluid precautions should be followed. After appropriately sedating the patient, perform a digital anorectal examination with a well-lubricated, gloved, examining finger.
4. Lubricate the shaft of the colonoscope and gently insert its tip into the anal canal. The lumen of the bowel should be directly visualized at all times during the colonoscopy procedure.
5. Insufflate air into the rectum until the lumen becomes readily apparent. The three "valves" of Houston (i.e., prominent mucosal folds) are often seen as consistent landmarks. The plexus of blood vessels is usually very apparent in the rectal mucosa (Fig. 90.2). The scope can usually be advanced without difficulty as far as the rectosigmoid junction at 15 to 18 cm.
6. Enter the sigmoid colon by passing the scope through the rectosigmoid angle. The sigmoid colon is the most common site of

difficulty in passage of the instrument. There may be fixation of the bowel from diverticular disease or adhesions from prior surgery, including a hysterectomy. The sigmoid colon also is the most common site of perforation during colonoscopy. Successful passage through the sigmoid colon may require a series of maneuvers including torquing to the right and withdrawing the scope to reduce loops, applying abdominal pressure, repositioning the patient (even into a supine position), or deflating the lumen of excess air. An essential but difficult lesson to learn is that when passage of the scope is impeded, torque the shaft to the right and withdraw the scope to straighten out the bowel. Although intubation should optimally occur while the lumen is being visualized, occasionally a "slide-by" technique is used to negotiate abrupt angulations in the bowel. In these acute turns the lumen cannot be well visualized without extreme deflection of the scope tip. Exaggerated deflections of the scope tip may provide complete views of the lumen, but they often impair forward intubation. In the slide-by technique, the lumen view is partially sacrificed to allow the scope to be gently advanced while the mucosa is seen to slide past the scope tip. The endoscopic view of the mucosa appears reddish from the underlying vasculature. A blanching of the mucosa could indicate excessive pressure against the bowel wall, and further insertion should be discontinued as the bowel is straightened using other techniques described previously. Although most endoscopists use the slide-by technique occasionally, it should not characterize the intubation technique.

7. The descending colon can be recognized by a relatively straight passage through the circular-shaped bowel (Fig. 90.3) to the splenic flexure. Traversing the angle of the splenic flexure may resemble passage through the rectosigmoid junction because this angle may be abrupt and may require a small degree of slide-by for passage. The transverse colon can be recognized by its characteristic triangular appearance (Fig. 90.4), and it generally has a fairly straight configuration. The hepatic flexure is often recognizable

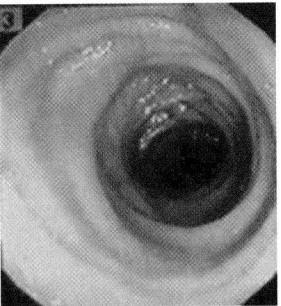

Fig. 90.3 Endoscopic view of descending colon.

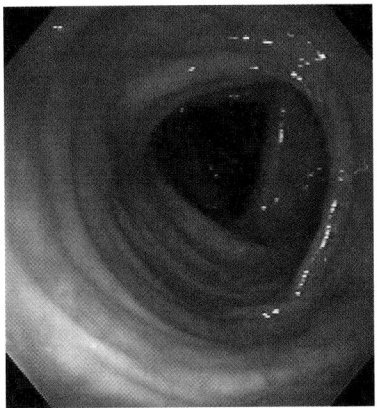

Fig. 90.4 Endoscopic view of transverse colon.

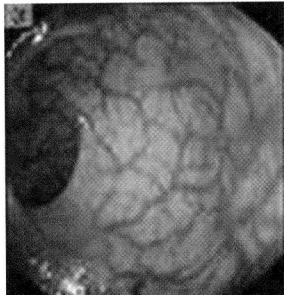

Fig. 90.2 Endoscopic view of hemorrhoidal plexus of blood vessels in normal rectum mucosa.

by the "liver shadow" (Fig. 90.5), which appears as a bluish-brown area where the liver is in direct contact with the external bowel wall. The hepatic flexure is seen as another angle to traverse with the scope. The ascending colon may also appear triangular.

8. Advance the scope into the cecum by pulling back, keeping the tip of the scope in the center of the lumen, and applying full suction to pull the cecum toward the scope tip. Positioning the scope tip in the middle of the lumen when applying suction for this maneuver often works best; otherwise, the scope just sticks to the sidewall. The cecal landmarks, which may or may not be prominent, include the ileocecal valve (Fig. 90.6) and the appendiceal orifice (Fig. 90.7). Convergence of the terminal portion of the taenia coli in the cecum forms a characteristic appearance known as the "crow's foot" or cecal strap (see Fig. 90.6). Other methods to ascertain if the cecum has been reached are to check for ballottement externally above the right inguinal canal, or for transillumination in the right lower quadrant (less consistent findings).

9. Intubate the terminal ileum by advancing the tip just beyond the ileocecal valve and then deflecting the tip toward the valve as the scope is carefully withdrawn. As the tip of the scope meets the valve opening, torque the scope gently clockwise to allow

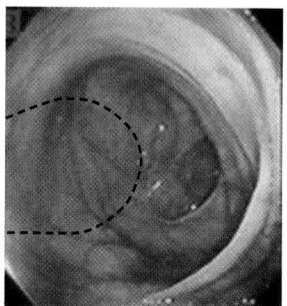

Fig. 90.5 Endoscopic view of hepatic flexure. The characteristic liver shadow is outlined by the *dashed line*.

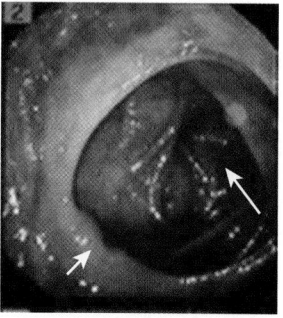

Fig. 90.6 Endoscopic view of ileocecal valve (*small arrow*) and "crow's foot" (*large arrow*) in cecum.

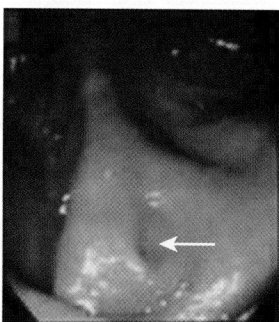

Fig. 90.7 Endoscopic view of appendiceal orifice (*arrow*).

the tip to advance briefly into the terminal ileum. Retroflexion of the scope in the ascending colon may increase the yield of polyps in that area; photo documentation of this maneuver, if performed, would be appropriate.

10. Carefully inspect the entire colon wall as the scope is withdrawn. Use a circular motion of the tip to inspect behind every mucosal fold. Lavage with water any areas of the bowel with inadequate preparation and carefully reinspect. While not currently required, photo documentation of certain landmarks, such as the appendiceal orifice, terminal ileum, and retroflexion in the rectum, may someday become part of quality metrics. Applying suction to remove the correct amount of air when withdrawing the scope will decrease patient discomfort following the procedure; it also often allows for better visualization behind folds. Such suctioning of air may cause a polyp to pop out from behind a fold. The correct amount of air to remove with suctioning results in the collapse of just the distal lumen, but not all the way to the scope, which might impair visualization with further withdrawal of the scope. The use of narrow-band imaging in the ascending colon may help identify flat polyps; it is becoming more accepted, and may become the standard of care. Obtain any necessary biopsy specimens and remove polyps during this portion of the procedure. Taking photo documentation of abnormal tissue, mucosa, polyps, or biopsy sites has become the standard of care. Endoscopists use various combinations of the techniques described in the foregoing discussion in a time-efficient manner to safely intubate the colon to the cecum in a high percentage of cases. It is important to recognize that not every colonoscopy can safely be completed to the cecum. Most colonoscopies take an average of 20 to 30 minutes, although this is variable. Time spent examining the colon during withdrawal may be a more important indicator of quality than overall procedure time. It has been suggested that withdrawal time should be at least 8 minutes because data have shown a lower polyp detection rate when withdrawal time is shorter than this. Withdrawal time should be documented.

11. Inspect the distal rectum and anorectal junction before completely withdrawing the scope. As the tip of the scope passes the dentate line, reinsert the scope approximately 5 to 10 cm while simultaneously rotating both control wheels counterclockwise to completely deflect the tip back upon itself (retroflexion or turnaround maneuver). Torque the shaft to inspect all around the anorectal junction. Obtaining an image of the scope and the rectum when the scope is retroverted not only documents good technique, it also documents the absence of polyps or cancers in an area traditionally known as a "blind spot" for endoscopy. Such practice with retroversion is also helpful in the event that such a maneuver is necessary to reach a polyp for removal from behind a fold elsewhere in the colon. Make sure the retroversion is relaxed and the scope straightened out before withdrawal at the end of the procedure to avoid rectal trauma.

Alternatively, use an anoscope (Ives' slotted anoscope is recommended) to complete the examination of the rectal area.

General principles for safe and efficient intubation of the colon to the cecum include the following:

- Minimize air insufflation.
- Keep the instrument straight most of the procedure.
- Avoid loop formation (pull back frequently).
- Avoid advancing the scope blindly (i.e., slide-by technique) when at all possible.
- Do not sedate the patient more than is necessary to maintain comfort.

Polypectomy and Biopsy

Polyps may be sessile (i.e., broad-based polyps) or pedunculated (i.e., with a stalk; Figs. 90.8 and 90.9). Almost all pedunculated polyps can be easily removed with the electrocautery snare with a low risk of perforation and bleeding. Risk may be higher in larger polyps (the larger the polyp looped, the deeper the biopsy goes), and in those located in the right colon where the mucosa is thinner. Sessile polyps may also be removed with smaller snares or hot or cold forceps (Fig. 90.10). There may be a benefit in "raising up" sessile polyps with submucosal injection of saline to minimize the risk of perforation. The patient experiences no pain with polypectomy.

There has been recent attention in the literature to the concept of "flat" or "depressed" polyps. These polyps are not exophytic and may actually lie below the regular surface of the mucosa, often making their detection difficult during colonoscopy. There is concern that these lesions may have a higher likelihood of malignant degeneration, and yet may go undetected. Careful inspection of the mucosa is imperative as well as insistence on a high-quality bowel preparation

to improve early detection of these lesions. Novel techniques are in development, which may assist in the detection of these lesions, including the use of high-magnification colonoscopes with mucosal stains (chromoscopy) and narrow-band imaging. As mentioned previously, the use of narrow band imaging in the ascending colon may help identify flat polyps; it is becoming more accepted, and may become the standard of care.

Biopsies of mucosal lesions are commonly obtained during colonoscopy as well as from normal-appearing mucosa when indicated. Generally, 4 to 6 biopsy specimens should be obtained of mucosal abnormalities and 8 to 10 biopsy specimens should be obtained from larger mass lesions. Pathologic interpretation is generally more sensitive if specimens are obtained from the junction of normal and abnormal mucosa. Avoid sampling areas of apparent necrosis or deep ulceration because these areas tend to provide poorer tissue specimens. For large sessile polyps or any other area of concern, India ink can be injected into the submucosa for later localization of the area. This "tattooing" can usually be found either when repeating endoscopy or by the surgeon during laparoscopy or laparotomy. (See Chapter 91, Esophagogastroduodenoscopy, for mucosal biopsy techniques for use on sessile polyps.)

EDITOR'S NOTE: Recent research suggests that cautery on flat lesions or in flat areas of the mucosa causes thermal damage to a much larger and deeper area than expected or visualized. Some experts therefore avoid cautery on flat lesions and instead use clips to obtain adequate hemostasis.

The procedure for polypectomy is as follows:

1. Position the scope so that the polyp can be visualized approximately 2 to 3 cm beyond the tip of the colonoscope. Positioning the polyp at the 5 o'clock position where the port for the electrocautery snare exits can be helpful for biopsy and polypectomy.
2. Under direct vision at all times, pass the electrocautery snare catheter through the colonoscope port. Position the tip of the sheath of the snare near the polyp, advance the wire loop, and open it, always under direct vision. Manipulate the snare and maneuver the tip of the colonoscope to place the snare around the polyp. Slowly secure the wire loop around the pedicle or polyp base as the snare catheter is advanced toward the stalk to avoid excessive pull on the stalk or a tangential cut. Maneuver the colonoscope to draw the polyp and snare away from the bowel wall to avoid excess burn injury and possible perforation.
3. Apply the electrocautery current (coagulation only) until a white eschar forms around the polyp stalk. Use the least amount of current necessary to achieve the eschar in 2 to 3 seconds (amount varies with the diameter of the stalk and with each electrocautery unit, but generally set at 10 to 15 W). Tighten the snare as coagulation continues until the stalk is transected.
4. Retrieve the excised polyp using suction or forceps, or simply regrasp the polyp with the snare. At times this may require removal

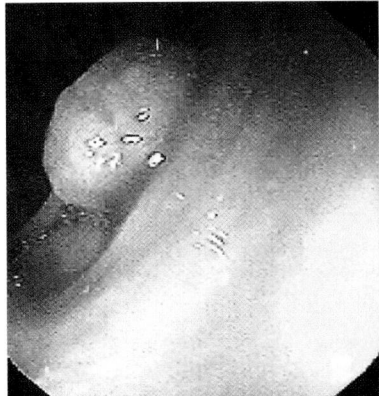

Fig. 90.8   Endoscopic view of sessile polyp.

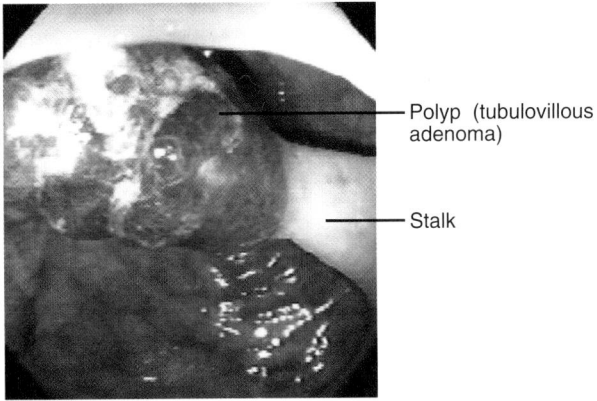

Polyp (tubulovillous adenoma)

Stalk

Fig. 90.9   Endoscopic view of pedunculated polyp.

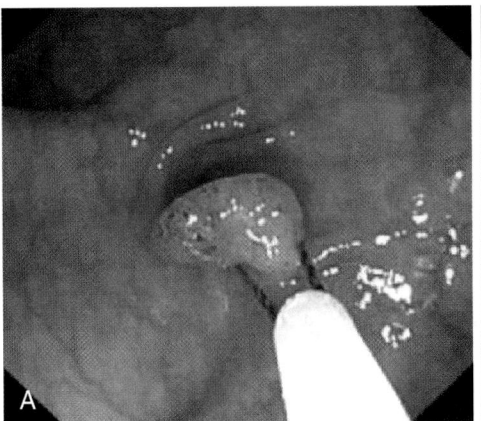
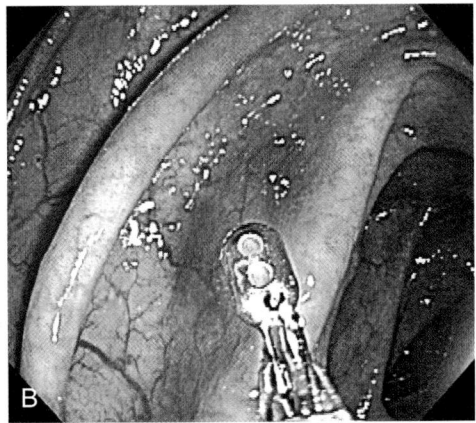

Fig. 90.10   (A) Polyp being snared. (B) Polyp being removed with cold forceps.

TABLE 90.2	Boston Bowel Prep Assessment (Applied to Each of Three Broad Segments of Colon: Right, Transverse, Left)
0	Unprepared colon segment with mucosa not seen due to solid stool that cannot be cleared
I	Portion of mucosa of the colon segment seen, but other areas of the colon segment not well seen due to staining, residual stool, and/or opaque liquid
2	Minor amount of residual staining, small fragments of stool, and/or opaque liquid, but mucosa of colon segment seen well
3	Entire mucosa of colon segment seen well with no residual staining, small fragments of stool, or opaque liquid

and reinsertion of the entire colonoscope. Unretrieved polyps may occasionally need to be retrieved later by straining stools after further bowel preparation solutions and cathartics are given, although recovery of polyps using this method is often unsuccessful. Large polyps may require multiple snare-resection excisions. Tissue desiccation without prior biopsy should be avoided because it is very important to have pathologic diagnosis of all colonic lesions.

5. Cancerous polyps do not need further resections if the tumor is well differentiated, if there is no lymphatic or vascular invasion, and if there is at least 2 mm between the tumor and the line of resection. With an obvious advanced colon cancer that is friable or ulcerated, biopsies will usually provide sufficient tissue for diagnosis. However, because only tiny samples can be obtained, the cancer may occasionally be missed and the specimens reveal only benign adenomatous tissue. If a strong clinical suspicion of cancer exists, the lesion should be reexamined and resampled. Surgical consultation may be warranted.

OPERATIVE REPORT

A well-documented procedure note is essential. The quality of the bowel preparation should be assessed and noted (e.g., Boston bowel preparation scale, Table 90.2). Procedure notes can be dictated (Fig. 90.11) or hand-written on standardized endoscopy forms (Fig. 90.12). Endoscopy report templates are available for use with electronic medical records. Procedure notes should include clear recommendations for future management and surveillance of the patient, based upon results of the procedure and any pathology, and this information should be imparted to the referring clinician and the patient.

QUALITY INDICATORS FOR COLONOSCOPY

Medicare established a Quality Payment Program in 2015 through the Medicare Access and CHIP Reauthorization Act. Starting in 2017, to implement the Merit-Based Incentive Payment System, quality measures must be reported. Since 2017, six quality measures, five advancing care measures, and four improvement activities must be reported to remain billing neutral. For exceptional performance, a bonus may be distributed. It should be kept in mind that perfect adherence to any quality measure is not expected; what is expected is the ability to follow the metrics and to report them. As an example, quality indicators that should be met in greater than 98% of colonoscopies include documented informed consent, documented quality of the prep, scope withdrawal time recorded and reported, and attempted removal of pedunculated polyps and large (<2 cm) polyps before surgical referral. It is expected than the appropriate indication for colonoscopy is documented 80% of the time, that the bowel prep is adequate in 85%, the cecum in intubated in greater than or equal to 95%, and that the average withdrawal time is greater than or equal to 6 minutes (preferred ≥8 or 9 min). In addition, reporting is expected of an adenoma detection rate of 25% (30% in men, 20%

in women), a perforation rate of less than 1 in 1000 and postpolypectomy bleeding in less than 1%. The appropriate interval should be recommended in 90% of patients for repeat colonoscopy after the procedure has been completed and the histology of the pathology report reviewed. Systems should be in place to record and report such quality measures to avoid Medicare penalties in the form of reduced payment. It will also be expected that some, if not all, of these measures will eventually be reported publicly.

COMMON ERRORS

- Failure to properly insufflate the colon with air
- Failure to identify landmarks
- Failure to monitor the patient during and after the procedure
- Failure to terminate the procedure when appropriate (lack of progression despite optimal technique, patient instability or intolerance, or risk outweighs benefit)
- Failure to adequately inspect the colonic mucosa
- Failure to straighten the sigmoid loop during insertion
- Failure to ensure an adequate preparation
- Failure to document adequately for quality measures

COMPLICATIONS

Complications occur infrequently with diagnostic colonoscopy and only slightly more frequently with therapeutic colonoscopy. Major complications include the following:

- Cardiopulmonary—over 60% related to sedation and medications used
  - Vasovagal reactions (i.e., hypotension, bradycardia)
  - Arrhythmias (including ventricular tachycardia and fibrillation)
  - Myocardial infarction
- Colon perforation
- Postpolypectomy bleeding
- Postpolypectomy syndrome
- Missed lesions
- Painful experience for patient

Other rare complications include the following:

- Preparation complications
  - Aspiration
  - Dehydration
  - Hyperphosphatemia, hyponatremia
  - Toxic megacolon
  - Renal failure
- Infections without perforation
  - Bacteremia
  - Scope transmission of infectious agent
- Sigmoid or cecal volvulus
- Splenic rupture
- Pancreatitis
- Diverticulitis
- Incarcerated snare or colonoscope

Perforation of the colon occurs at a rate of 0.1% to 0.8% (approximately) for diagnostic colonoscopy and 0.3% to 3% for therapeutic colonoscopy. Perforations can occur for a number of reasons but are most commonly caused by excessive force of insertion of the endoscope tip or with the side of the scope during slide-by, loop formation, loop reduction, or advancement despite the presence of fixating lesions. Other causes of perforation include rupture of diverticulum, rupture of stricture site, transmural injury with electrocautery current with subsequent perforation, or polypectomy- and biopsy-induced perforations. Perforations may also rarely occur from pneumatic rupture of the proximal colon.

Perforations are more common with patients who are oversedated or who are under general anesthesia. It is uncommon for

Procedure: Colonoscopy
Equipment: Olympus Colonoscope
Pre-op diagnosis: History of previous colon polyps
Post-op diagnosis: Diminutive polyp
Endoscopist:
Assistant:

HPI:
Patient is a 71-year-old African-American male who was seen by Dr. Smith on 6-26-2015 and scheduled for screening colonoscopy. The patient was asymptomatic at the time. The patient had a history of colonic polyps dating back to 1996. The patient was found on that colonoscopy to have a colonic polyp reported as an adenoma by pathology report. Patient was recommended at that time to have a repeat colonoscopy every 3 to 5 years. The patient denied any history of colon cancer. Patient had no iron-deficiency anemia. Patient received one half gallon of GoLYTELY yesterday and one half gallon early this morning, and the patient was NPO for the procedure today.

Informed consent was obtained from the patient after a full discussion of the risks, benefits and alternatives to the procedure. Patient was also advised of the risk of missed lesions with this procedure. He expressed an understanding of these issues and desired to continue with the colonoscopy. All questions were answered.

Medications: Moderate sedation was obtained with 50 mg of Demerol IV push with Versed 1 mg IV push. Moderate sedation was maintained throughout the procedure.

Procedure: After moderate sedation was obtained, the patient was placed in the left lateral position. Digital rectal examination was performed, which showed normal sphincter tone, no masses, no external hemorrhoids. Prostate gland was not enlarged. After rectal examination was performed, the regular colonoscope was introduced via the anus and advanced inside the colon into the cecum. The procedure was difficult as a result of redundancies of the colon. External compressions of the abdomen and multiple changes in the position of the patient were required throughout the procedure in order to advance into the cecum. The bowel preparation was adequate. The extent of the exam was to the cecum. The cecum was identified by the ileal-cecal valve, and the appendiceal orifice was clearly visualized. After reaching the cecum, the scope was slowly withdrawn with careful inspection of all aspects of the colon in a circular fashion. Retroflexion was performed inside the rectum before completely straightening the scope, and the scope was subsequently removed from the patient. Patient was transported to recovery area and monitored for 30 minutes until return to baseline state was observed.

Complications: None

Findings: There was a diminutive polyp approximately 3 mm in size in the ascending colon that was removed with cold-force biopsy forceps. The colonic mucosa was otherwise normal. Neither diverticula nor internal hemorrhoids were seen.

Impression: Diminutive polyp

Recommendation: Given the small size of this polyp and patient's previous history, I would recommend that the patient repeat colonoscopy in 5-10 years. Other methods of colon cancer screening would not be necessary over this 10-year period (i.e., no need for checking fecal occult blood test). Patient will return to the primary care doctor for follow-up, and I have ordered Metamucil, 1 Tbsp mixed with a glass of water once a day for constipation. This can be increased to twice a day if needed.

Fig. 90.11 Sample procedure note for colonoscopy.

the scope tip to actually penetrate the bowel, but this type of perforation is usually noticed immediately. More frequently the perforation is small and occurs away from the scope tip. It may go unrecognized until the patient later experiences abdominal pain, fever, and distention. A radiographic film of the abdomen or chest will show pneumoperitoneum. If pneumoperitoneum is not apparent on a plain radiograph, CT of the abdomen is more sensitive for making this diagnosis. In the majority of perforations, immediate surgery is indicated. Laparoscopic surgery may be adequate. With fecal soiling, a diverting colostomy or ileostomy is needed; however, in the absence of obvious contamination, primary closure may be sufficient. Perforation can occur even in experienced hands and does not, per se, imply negligence on the part of the endoscopist.

Bleeding postcolonoscopy and postpolypectomy occurs in approximately 1 in 1000 procedures. Bleeding may occur immediately or up to 4 weeks postprocedure. Most cases of bleeding resolve spontaneously, but some may require repeat colonoscopy with attempts to place a clip or coagulate the area (i.e., epinephrine injection followed by multipolar cautery, a heater probe or argon-assisted cautery) or laparotomy. Avoiding aspirin prophylaxis for 10 days postpolypectomy may decrease late bleeding risk.

Postpolypectomy syndrome is caused by a transmural thermal injury (i.e., burn) resulting in full-thickness bowel necrosis, which may lead to serosal inflammation. Postpolypectomy syndrome may be accompanied by fever, leukocytosis, and localized and rebound tenderness over the polypectomy site without evidence of intraperitoneal air. A conservative approach generally leads to a good outcome.

Missed neoplastic lesions have been shown to occur even with "expert" endoscopists. In one study, colonoscopy detected 95% of all lesions present. Of the 5% missed, half were not appreciated because of the inability to pass the scope far enough; however, in the other half, lesions were passed without being seen. Other studies report a miss rate for advanced lesions (>1 cm) of 12% to 17% for skilled colonoscopists using CT colonography as a reference standard (Pickhardt et al., 2004; Van Gelder et al., 2004).

POSTPROCEDURE MANAGEMENT

After colonoscopy, monitor the patient (i.e., clinical assessment, blood pressure, pulse, oxygen saturation) for at least 30 minutes and until a return to baseline cognitive function has occurred. Explain the results of the procedure to the patient, including the treatment plan and follow-up appointments. Patients may resume a normal diet on discharge even when polypectomy has been performed. Clearly explain precautions concerning possible delayed bleeding or unrecognized perforation when clinically indicated. Patients should be cautioned not to drive, operate heavy machinery, or sign legal documents for 24 hours after conscious sedation.

INTERPRETATION AND FOLLOW-UP OF RESULTS

Table 90.3 explains the current recommendations for follow-up of polyps. Pathology results should be communicated to the patient and the referring clinician, and appropriate follow-up or surveillance should be arranged based on the findings.

Procedure Note
Date:
Patient Name:
Identification Number:
Procedure:
Equipment:

Pre-op diagnosis:

Post-op diagnosis:

Endoscopist:

Assistant:

HPI:

Informed consent:

Medications:

Procedure:

Complications:

Findings:

Impression:

Recommendations:

Signature

Fig. 90.12 Sample procedure form for colonoscopy.

Learning Colonoscopy

For a basic overview of colonoscopy principles and technique, the reader is directed to Canard's *Gastrointestinal Endoscopy in Practice*, which contains excellent diagrams, photographs, tips, and techniques. Additional information on endoscopic technique is found in Waye's *Colonoscopy: Principles and Practice*. Chun's *Clinical Gastrointestinal Endoscopy: A Comprehensive Atlas*, and Wilcox's *Atlas of Clinical Gastrointestinal Endoscopy* contain excellent photographs of colorectal pathology as well as information on gastrointestinal diseases. For a review of colonoscopic polypectomy, see Chapter 37 of Chandrasekhara's *Clinical Gastrointestinal Endoscopy*.

Before attempting to perform colonoscopy, it would be useful to become proficient and skilled in flexible fiberoptic sigmoidoscopy; however, sigmoidoscopy is rarely performed in the United States any more. (And that is unfortunate because the instrument controls and techniques used for flexible sigmoidoscopy are identical to those used to perform colonoscopy.) Endoscopy simulators and plastic models are now available as an alternative to flexible sigmoidoscopy and as an adjunct in basic colonoscopy training, particularly when used before actual experience with colonoscopy in patients. Simulators have improved in haptic (touch) feedback technology and also offer various polypectomy simulations. Simulators are manufactured by the Immersion Corporation (www.immersion.com) and others.

Formal (CME) courses are available to teach colonoscopy concepts, skills, and techniques through the American Academy of Family Physicians (AAFP; phone: 800-274-2237), The National Procedures Institute (phone: 866-674-2631), the American Association for Primary Care Endoscopy (phone: 913-906-6000, ext. 6707) and the American Society for Gastrointestinal Endoscopy (ASGE, phone: 630-573-0600.).

One method often used for obtaining colonoscopy skills in the postresidency environment is to form a teaching relationship with a proficient endoscopist willing to act as a preceptor until proficiency is obtained. Colonoscopy can be mastered without fellowship training. Studies show that high-quality care and complication rates essentially identical to those for fellowship-trained gastroenterologists can be attained (Hopper et al., 1996; Wilkins et al., 2009), and that physician assistants and nurses may also become qualified to perform colonoscopy (Lieberman and Ghormley, 1992; Lomas, 2009). The AAFP has published, and continues to update, a position paper on family physicians performing colonoscopy. It can be found on the organization's website (www.aafp.org/about/policies/all/colonoscopy.html) and includes guidelines for establishing and maintaining proficiency and suggestions for obtaining privileges in colonoscopy. ASGE videos on endoscopy technique can be ordered through ASGE at www.asge.org/TrainingEducationIndex.aspx?id=410. Free endoscopy technique and pathology videos may be viewed at The DAVE Project—Gastroenterology (see Atlases, under Online Resources).

Obtaining Hospital Privileges

Most hospitals have credentialing standards regarding colonoscopy privileges. Hospitals vary widely in those standards but generally require a minimum number of procedures and possible proctoring of applicants until competency is established. In general, credentialing becomes more restrictive where a high number of specialists perform colonoscopy in the hospital. It is advisable to carefully document all endoscopy experience and related experience, and to provide a plan for continued medical education and quality assurance when applying for colonoscopy privileges.

TABLE 90.3 Surveillance Protocols for History of Colonic Neoplasia

Finding	Colonoscopy Interval
Small (<1 cm) hyperplastic polyps in rectum and sigmoid	10 yr
1–2 tubular adenomas (<1 cm) and only low-grade dysplasia	5–10 yr
3–10 adenomas, or villous elements, or high-grade dysplasia, or >1 cm	3 yr
>10 adenomas	<3 yr
Large sessile adenomas (especially if removed piecemeal)	2–6 mo
Sessile serrated polyp(s) (<1 cm), no dysplasia	5 yr
Sessile serrated polyp(s) with dysplasia, traditional serrated adenoma, >1 cm	3 yr
Serrated polyposis syndrome (formerly hyperplastic polyposis syndrome)	1 yr
Negative follow-up examination	No earlier than 5 yr
Previous colon cancer	High-quality clearance at or around time of resection followed by colonoscopy at 1 yr, then 3 yr and 5 yr if normal

From Lieberman DA, Rex DK, Winawer SJ, Giardiello FM, Johnson DA, Levin TR. Guidelines for Colonoscopy Surveillance After Screening and Polypectomy: A Consensus Update by the US Multi- Society Task Force on Colorectal Cancer. *Gastroenterology.* 2012;143(3):844–857; and Kahi CJ, Boland CR, Dominitz JA, et al. Colonoscopy surveillance after colorectal cancer resection: recommendations of the US multi-society task force on colorectal cancer. *Gastroenterology.* 2016;150(3):758–768.e11.

BOX 90.1 Overview of Colonoscopy Privileges

From the American Academy of Family Physicians Position Paper

- "It is the position of the American Academy of Family Physicians (AAFP) that clinical privileges should be based on the individual clinician's documented training and/or experience, demonstrated abilities and current competence, and not on the clinician's specialty."
- In 2011, more than 1846 family physicians across the United States reported performing colonoscopy in the hospital setting.
- In the 2017 AAFP Practice Profile Survey, 1420 family physicians reported performing colonoscopy in their offices.
- According to a 2004 survey, 48% of family practice residencies offered training in colonoscopy, 18% reported actually training one or more residents in the procedure.
- "Skills for performing colonoscopy are most often acquired during 3 yr of family practice residency training. Another possible route to acquire colonoscopy skills is through preceptorship with a physician who already has such training and privileges. Established experience in flexible sigmoidoscopy examination is helpful in developing colonoscopy skills."
- The American Society for Gastrointestinal Endoscopy (ASGE) recommends that clinicians perform a minimum of 140 diagnostic colonoscopies and 30 snare polypectomies as a threshold before competency can be assessed. However, this recommendation was based on expert opinion, not scientific data.
- Based upon recent studies, the AAFP has determined that the standard of fifty (50) cases as the primary operator be used as a basis for determination of basic competency.
- "…the AAFP strongly believes that all medical staff members should realize that there is overlap between specialties, and that no one department has exclusive rights to privileges."
- "A legal opinion on privileges for endoscopy submitted to the AAFP in 1993 stated the following:
  A. Hospitals and peer review participants risk liability un-

BOX 90.1 *Overview of Colonoscopy Privileges—cont'd*

der state law if they base credentialing decisions solely on whether or not a physician has obtained specialty certification.

B. The Council on Ethical and Judicial Affairs of the AMA has issued the opinion that competitive factors must be disregarded in making decisions about credentials and privileges.

C. There is no evidence that only board-certified gastroenterologists are qualified to perform endoscopic procedures.

D. Hospitals violate the Medicare Conditions for Participation if they base credentialing decisions solely on specialty board certification.

E. Hospitals and peer review participants risk loss of federal and state immunity from liability by basing credentialing decisions solely on whether or not a physician has obtained specialty certification."

From the American Medical Association Clinical Privileges

Regarding clinical privileges, AMA E-4.07 Policy says "The mutual objective of both the governing board and the medical staff is to improve the quality and efficiency of patient care in the hospital. Decisions regarding hospital privileges should be based upon the training, experience, and demonstrated competence of candidates, taking into consideration the availability of facilities and the overall medical needs of the community, the hospital, and especially patients. Privileges should not be based on numbers of patients admitted to the facility or the economic or insurance status of the patient. Personal friendships, antagonisms, jurisdictional disputes, or fear of competition should not play a role in making these decisions. Physicians who are involved in the granting, denying, or termination of hospital privileges have an ethical responsibility to be guided primarily by concern for the welfare and best interests of patients in discharging this responsibility."

From the 2010 AMA H-230.998 Policy on Hospital Privileges: "Our AMA believes that clinical departments of family

practice should be established where appropriate with duties comparable to any other specialty department of the medical staff."

From the 2015 AMA H-225.997 Policy on Physician-Hospital Relationships: "Although final authority for granting, denial, termination, or limitation of hospital staff privileges is vested in the governing board of the hospital, it is expected that the judgment of the organized medical staff will be relied upon in the evaluation of the professional competence, education, experience, and qualifications of all physicians, including the hospital-associated medical specialists."

From the American Society for Gastrointestinal Endoscopy

- "Competency is the minimum level of skill, knowledge, and/or expertise, attained through training and experience, required to perform a procedure safely and proficiently."
- "Departments often develop criteria for recommending privileges and, not surprisingly, these suggested criteria may vary significantly depending on the particular departmental discipline and whether the department represents mainly generalists or specialists."
- "Highly motivated family physicians or internists can acquire a level of training adequate to perform endoscopic examinations of high quality."

AAFP, American Academy of Family Physicians; *AMA*, American Medical Association.
Modified from AAFP Colonoscopy [Position Paper] https://www.aafp.org/about/policies/all/colonoscopy.html. Accessed 12.08.2018. American Medical Association. Clinical privileges. In AMA *Policy Finder*. Chicago: American Medical Association https://policysearch.ama-assn.org/policyfinder. Accessed August 17, 2018; and American Society of Gastrointestinal Endoscopy (ASGE): President's message, October 1999.

See the AAFP Colonoscopy Position Paper for further information (Box 90.1). For articles that may assist in obtaining colonoscopy privileges, see the AAFP Position Paper. A position paper on endoscopy privileging is available from the American Association of Primary Care Endoscopists (AAPCE; www.aapce.org). The AAPCE recommends that 50 colonoscopies be used as a target number for hospitals requiring a certain number before privileging, which is also in accord with AAFP and surgical society recommendations.

Wherever the colonoscopy is performed, it is important to keep current with most recent national quality standards such as documenting scope withdrawal time, and adenoma detection rate.

PATIENT EDUCATION GUIDES AND ADDITIONAL RESOURCES

See patient education and patient consent forms available at www.expertconsult.com. Patient videos are also available at (e.g., https://www.asge.org/home/for-patients/videos). Sample consent forms and patient education handouts are also available at https://www.sages.org/publications/patient-information/patient-information-for-colonoscopy-from-sages/.

CPT/BILLING CODES

45378*	Colonoscopy beyond splenic flexure
45379*	Colonoscopy with foreign body removal

45380*	Colonoscopy with biopsy (single or multiple)
45382*	Colonoscopy with control of bleeding (any method)
45383*	Colonoscopy with ablation of tumor
45384*	Colonoscopy with removal of lesion by hot forceps or bipolar cautery
45385*	Colonoscopy with removal of lesion by snare technique
G0105	Screening colonoscopy in patients at high risk for CRC, if 23 months since last screening colonoscopy or barium enema (Medicare)
G0121	Screening colonoscopy in patients at least 50 years of age at average risk for CRC, if 119 months since last screening colonoscopy or barium enema (Medicare)
Modifier-59	Use of this modifier will allow reimbursement for more than one procedure (e.g., biopsy [45380] and polypectomy [45385]) if performed on separate, discrete lesions
Modifier-PT	Use combined with diagnostic procedure CPT code to indicate the procedure began as a screening procedure; this allows for conversion to diagnostic procedure if biopsy, polypectomy, or other procedure is needed, usually without copayment being charged for diagnostic instead of screening procedure

---

*The Health Care Financing Administration (HCFA) allows additional payment for a tray for this procedure when performed in a physician's office. Charge appropriately using code "99070—surgical tray."

If colonoscopy is abnormal, the applicable CPT and ICD-10-CM codes (not G-codes) should be used. If a biopsy is taken, polypectomy, etc. performed, the code 45380, 45384, 45385, etc. with PT modifier, not the "G" code, should be used. If the PT modifier is used, the first diagnostic code should be for screening, the second for whatever lesion is biopsied or removed. If two separate procedures (e.g., biopsy, snare polypectomy, directed submucosal injection) are performed, and it is well documented that they are performed on separate lesions, the modifier 59 can be used. Moderate (conscious) sedation is considered part of the colonoscopy and is not billed separately unless it is performed by a different provider.

ICD-10-CM DIAGNOSTIC CODES

C18.3	Ca, colon-hepatic flexure
C18.4	Ca, colon-transverse
C18.6	Ca, colon-descending
C18.7	Ca, colon-sigmoid
C18.0	Ca, colon-cecum
C18.2	Ca, colon-ascending
C20	Ca, rectum
C20	Benign neoplasm, colon, or familial adenomatous polyposis (FAP)
D12.8	Benign neoplasm, rectum-anus
K64.8	Internal hemorrhoids
K64.9	External hemorrhoids
K50.10	Crohn disease, colon
K51.90	Ulcerative colitis
K52.89	Colitis, nonspecific
K57.30	Diverticulosis
K57.31	Diverticulosis with hemorrhage
K59.00	Unspecified constipation
K59.1	Functional diarrhea
K55.20	Angiodysplasia
K92.2	GI hemorrhage
R15.9	Stool incontinence
R10.9	Abdominal pain
R93.3	Radiographic abnormality, GI tract
Z12.11	Screening, cancer, colon (to be used with G-codes; see previous discussion)

SUPPLIERS

(See contact information available at www.expertconsult.com.)

Extensive marketing and technical information about colonoscopy equipment is readily available. When selecting a supplier, the clinician should consider local availability for education, equipment service, and technical support. It may be desirable to ask for local references from suppliers.

New equipment
Fujinon Corp.
Olympus Corp.
Pentax Corp.

Used or refurbished equipment
B-Met Endoscopic, Inc.
Cardinal Health
Corthel, Inc.
Endoscopy Support Services, Inc.
Instrument Specialists, Inc.
Integrated Medical Systems, Inc.
Karl Storz Endoscopy–America
Matlock Endoscopic
Medical Optics
Mobile Instrument Service

Nuell, Inc.
Spectrum Surgical Instruments
SterilMed Johnson and Johnson
Surgical Optics LLC
Surgical Repair Technologies
United Endoscopy
Universal Endoscopic Services
Used Medical Equipment and Devices Medline

ONLINE RESOURCES

American Association for Primary Care Endoscopy: www.aapce.org.
American College of Gastroenterology: www.acg.gi.org.
American Gastroenterological Association: www.gastro.org.
American Society for Gastrointestinal Endoscopy: www.asge.org.

ATLASES

Atlas of Gastrointestinal Endoscopy: www.endoatlas.com
The DAVE Project—Gastroenterology (good video library): http://dave1.mgh.harvard.edu/
El Salvador Atlas of Gastrointestinal Video Endoscopy: www.gastrointestinalatlas.com/index.html
Gastrolab. www.gastrolab.net/.
Jackson/Siegelbaum Gastroenterology: Images of the colon: www.gicare.com/Endoscopy-Center/Images-Colon.aspx

RECOMMENDED READING*

Ackermann RJ. Performance of gastrointestinal tract endoscopy by primary care physicians: lessons from the US Medicare database. *Arch Fam Med.* 1997;6:52–58.

American Association for Primary Care Endoscopy. *AAPCE Policy on Credentialing for Gastrointestinal Endoscopy.* Leawood, KS: 2009.

American Medical Association. Clinical privileges. In: *AMA Policy Compendium.* Chicago: American Medical Association; 1993.

American Society for Gastrointestinal Endoscopy (ASGE). Standards of Practice Committee: antibiotic prophylaxis in endoscopy. *Gastrointest Endosc.* 2008;67:791–798.

American Society for Gastrointestinal Endoscopy (ASGE). Standards of Practice Committee: guideline on the management of antithrombotic agents for patients undergoing GI endoscopy. *Gastrointest Endosc.* 2016;83(1):3–16.

American Society for Gastrointestinal Endoscopy. the Society of American Gastrointestinal Surgeons. and the American Society of Colorectal Surgeons: principles of privileging and credentialing for endoscopy and colonoscopy. *Gastrointest Endosc.* 2002;55:145–148.

American Society of Gastrointestinal Endoscopy, Eisen GM, Baron TH, Dominitz JA, et al. Methods of granting hospital privileges to perform gastrointestinal endoscopy. *Gastrointest Endosc.* 2002;55:780–783.

Atkin WS, Whynes DK. Improving the cost-effectiveness of colorectal cancer screening. *J Natl Cancer Inst.* 2000;92:513–514.

Bittner 4th JG, Marks JM, Dunkin BJ, et al. Resident training in flexible gastrointestinal endoscopy: a review of current issues and options. *J Surg Educ.* 2007;64:399–409.

Brunelli SM, Feldman HI, Latif SM, et al. A comparison of sodium phosphosoda purgative to polyethylene glycol bowel preparations prior to colonoscopy. *Fam Med.* 2009;41:39–45.

Bull-Henry K, Al-Kawas FH. Evaluation of occult gastrointestinal bleeding. *Am Fam Physician.* 2013;87(6):430–436.

Canard JM, Letard JC, Palazzo L, Penman I, Lennon AM. *Gastrointestinal Endoscopy in Practice.* Philadelphia: Elsevier; 2011.

Chandrasekhara V, Elmunzer J, Khashab MA, Muthusamy VR. *Clinical Gastrointestinal Endoscopy.* 3rd ed. Philadelphia: Elsevier; 2019.

Corley DA, Jensen CD, Marks AR, et al. Adenoma detection rate and risk of colorectal cancer and death. *N Engl J Med.* 2014;370:1298–1306.

---

*For additional pertinent references, also see Chapter 1, Procedural Sedation and Analgesia, and Chapter 89, Flexible Sigmoidoscopy.

Cotton PB, Connor P, McGee D, et al. Colonoscopy: practice variation among 69 hospital-based endoscopists. *Gastrointest Endosc.* 2003;57:352–357.

Douketis JD, Spyropoulos AC, Katz S, Becker RC, Caprini JA, et al., and the BRIDGE study group. Perioperative bridging anticoagulation in atrial fibrillation . *N Engl J Med.* 2015; 373:823–833.

Eckert LD, Short MW, Domagalski JE, Jaboori KA, Short PA. Assessing colonoscopy training outcomes using quality indicators. *J Grad Med Educ.* 2009; 1(1):89–92.

Frazier AL, Colditz GA, Fuchs CS, Kuntz KM. Cost-effectiveness of screening for colorectal cancer in the general population. *JAMA.* 2000;284:1954–1961.

Friedland S, Sedehi D, Soetikno R. Colonoscopic polypectomy in anticoagulated patients. *World J Gastroenterol.* 2009;15:1973–1976.

Giardiello FM, Allen JI, Axilbund JE, et al. Guidelines on genetic evaluation and management of Lynch syndrome: a consensus statement by the US Multi-Society Task Force on colorectal cancer. *Gastroenterology.* 2014;147:502–526.

Harper MB, Pope JB, Mayeaux EJ. Colonoscopy experience at a family practice residency: a comparison to gastroenterology and general surgery services. *Fam Med.* 1997;29:575–579.

Hopper W, Kyker K, Rodney WM. Colonoscopy by a family physician: a 9-year experience of 1048 procedures. *J Fam Pract.* 1996;43:561–566.

Imperiale TF, Glowinski EA, Lin-Cooper C, et al. Five-year risk of colorectal neoplasia after negative screening colonoscopy. *N Engl J Med.* 2008;359:1285–1287.

Kahi CJ, Boland CR, Dominitz JA, et al. Colonoscopy surveillance after colorectal cancer resection: recommendations of the US Multi-Society Task Force on Colorectal Cancer. *Gastroenterology.* 2016;150:758–768.e11.

Kim DH, Pickhardt PJ, Taylor AJ, et al. CT colonography versus colonoscopy for the detection of advanced neoplasia. *N Engl J Med.* 2007;357:1403–1412.

Knox L, Hahn RG, Lane C. A comparison of unsedated colonoscopy and flexible sigmoidoscopy in the family medicine setting: an LA net study. *J Am Board Fam Med.* 2007;20:444–450.

Kolber M. Outcomes of 1949 endoscopic procedures performed by a Canadian rural family physician. *Can Fam Physician.* 2009;55:170–175.

Leung FW. *Unsedated colonoscopy—Question: Is it worth Staying Awake for: Answer: Yes, for those Who Know What It Is.* Washington, DC: Presented at the Digestive Disease Week; 2007.

Leung FW. Promoting informed choice of unsedated colonoscopy: patient centered care for a subgroup of U.S. veterans. *Dig Dis Sci.* 2008;53:2955–2959.

Leung FW, Aharonian S, Guth PH, et al. Unsedated colonoscopy: time to revisit this option? *J Fam Pract.* 2008;57:E1–E14.

Lieberman D, et al. Standardized colonoscopy reporting and data system: report of the quality assurance task group of the National Colorectal Cancer Roundtable. *Gastrointest Endosc.* 2007;65:757–766.

Lieberman DA, Ghormley JM. Physician assistants in gastroenterology: Should they perform endoscopy? *Am J Gastroenterol.* 1992;87:940–943.

Lieberman DA, Holub JL, Moravec MD, et al. Prevalence of colon polyps detected by colonoscopy screening in asymptomatic black and white patients. *JAMA.* 2008;300:1459–1461.

Lieberman DA, Rex DK, Winawer SJ, Giardiello FM, Johnson DA, Levin TR. Guidelines for colonoscopy surveillance after screening and polypectomy: a consensus update by the US Multi-Society Task Force on Colorectal Cancer. *Gastroenterology.* 2012;143(3):844–857.

Lieberman DA, Weiss DG. One-time screening for colorectal cancer with combined fecal occult-blood testing and examination of the distal colon. *N Engl J Med.* 2001;345:555–560.

Lin OS, Kozarek RA, Schembre DB, et al. Screening colonoscopy in very elderly patients: prevalence of neoplasia and estimated impact of life expectancy. *JAMA.* 2006;295:2357–2365.

Lomas C. Endoscopy nurses "equal" doctors. *Nurs Times.* 2009;11(Feb 16):56. http://www.nursingtimes.net/whats-new-in-nursing/endoscopy-nurses-equal-doctors/1991298.article. Accessed August 15, 2018.

Martel M, Barkun AN, Menard C, Restellini S, Kherad O, Vanasse A. Split-dose preparations are superior to day-before bowel cleansing regimens: a meta-analysis. *Gastroenterology.* 149(1):79–88.

Newman RJ, Nichols DB, Cummings DM. Outpatient colonoscopy by rural family physicians. *Ann Fam Med.* 2005;3:122–125.

Pickhardt PJ, Nugent PA, Mysliwiec PA, et al. Location of adenomas missed by optical colonoscopy. *Ann Intern Med.* 2004;141:352–359.

Pierzchajlo RP, Ackermann RJ, Vogel RL. Colonoscopy performed by a family physician: a case series of 751 procedures. *J Fam Pract.* 1997;44:473–480.

Rex DK, Boland R, Dominitz JA, et al. Colorectal cancer screening: recommendations for physicians and patients from the U.S. Multi-society task force on colorectal cancer. *Gastrointest Endosc.* 2017;86(1):18–33.

Rex DK, Petrini JL, Baron TH, et al. Quality indicators for colonoscopy. *Gastrointest Endosc.* 2006;63(suppl 4):S16–S28.

Roetzheim RG, Pal N, Gonzalez EC, et al. The effects of physician supply on the early detection of colorectal cancer. *J Fam Pract.* 1999;48:850.

Schoenfeld P, Cash B, Flood A, et al. Colonoscopic screening of average risk women for colorectal neoplasia. *N Engl J Med.* 2005;352:2061–2068.

Screening for Colorectal Cancer: U.S. Preventive Services Task Force Recommendation Statement. *JAMA.* 2016;315(23):2564–2575.

Sedlack RE, Baron TH, Downing SM, Schwartz AJ. Validation of a colonoscopy simulation model for skills assessment. *Am J Gastroenterol.* 2007;102:64–74.

Siegal D, Yudin J, Kaatz S, Douketis JD, Lim W, Spyropoulos AC. Periprocedural heparin bridging in patients receiving vitamin K antagonists: systematic review and meta-analysis of bleeding and thromboembolic rates. *Circulation.* 2012;126:1630–1639.

Silverstein FE, Tytgat G. *Atlas of Gastrointestinal Endoscopy.* 3rd ed. London: Mosby; 1997.

Singh H, Turner D, Xue L, et al. Risk of developing colorectal cancer following a negative colonoscopy examination: evidence for a 10-year interval between colonoscopies. *JAMA.* 2007;295:2366–2373.

Soetikno RM, Kaltenbach T, Rouse RV, et al. Prevalence of nonpolypoid (flat and depressed) colorectal neoplasms in asymptomatic and symptomatic adults. *JAMA.* 2008;299:1027–1035.

Trindale AJ, Lichtenstein DR, Aslanian HR, Bhutani MS, Goodman A, et al. Devices and methods to improve colonoscopy completion. *Gastrointest Endosc.* 2018;87(3):625–634.

Van Gelder RE, Nio CY, Florie J, et al. Computed tomographic colonography compared with colonoscopy in patients at increased risk for colorectal cancer. *Gastroenterology.* 2004;127:41–48.

Volkers N. How can physicians define and improve procedural competency? *Ann Intern Med.* 1996;125:I39.

Wilcox CM. *Atlas of Clinical Gastrointestinal Endoscopy.* 3rd ed. Philadelphia: Elsevier; 2012.

Wilkins T, LeClair B, Smolkin M, et al. Screening colonoscopies by primary care physicians: a meta-analysis. *Ann Fam Med.* 2009;7:56–62.

Wilkins T, McMechan D, Talukder A, Herline A. Colon cancer screening and surveillance in individuals at increased risk. *Am Fam Physician.* 2018;15(2):111–116. 97.

Wilkins T, Reynolds PL. Colorectal cancer: a summary of the evidence for screening and prevention. *Am Fam Physician.* 2008;78:1385–1392. 1393–1394.

Wilkins T, Wagner P, Thomas A, et al. Attitudes toward performance of endoscopic colon cancer screening by family physicians. *Fam Med.* 2007;39:578–584.

Waye JD, Rex DK, Williams CB, eds. *Colonoscopy: Principles and Practice.* 2nd ed. Oxford: Wiley Blackwell; 2009.

Xirasagar S, Hurley TG, Sros L, Hebert JR. Quality and safety of screening colonoscopies performed by primary care physicians with standby specialist support. *Med Care.* 48:703–709.

CHAPTER 91

ESOPHAGOGASTRODUODENOSCOPY

Mark A. Koch • Edward G. Zurad

During the past 4 decades, performing flexible esophagogastroduodenoscopy (EGD), or gastroscopy, has diagnosed and clarified many conditions and diseases of the upper gastrointestinal (GI) tract for primary care clinicians, surgeons, and gastroenterologists. Refinements in equipment and technology have dramatically improved these procedures, as well as their diagnostic capabilities. Advancements have also permitted any interested clinician, in a variety of settings, to evaluate and treat patients with both simple and complex problems of the esophagus, stomach, and duodenum. Rapid diagnosis of upper GI pathology with appropriate pharmaceutical and surgical management assures a high level of cost-effective care that any primary care clinician can provide.

EGD is relatively quick procedure and can usually be completed within 5 to 20 minutes. The procedure can be performed in various clinical environments, including the office, outpatient endoscopy suite, hospital, or surgical center. It can even be performed in the intensive care unit or emergency department setting with a portable endoscopy cart. One study (Rodney et al., 1990) indicated that when primary clinicians performed EGD, it was associated with enhanced management and improved diagnostic accuracy in 89% of cases. While use of flexible sigmoidoscopy has declined, primary care clinicians increasingly perform EGD and colonoscopy, even sometimes in their offices.

With EGD, a small flexible endoscope is introduced through the mouth (or with newer thinner diameter scopes, through the nose) and advanced through the pharynx, esophagus, stomach, and usually into the second portion of the duodenum. Both the fiberoptic and video gastroscopes are similar in construction to the flexible sigmoidoscope, the device with which many primary care clinicians previously developed preliminary skills. (With decreased sigmoidoscopies being performed in the United States, primary care clinicians now often develop initial endoscopy skills performing colonoscopy.) Most modern endoscopes use a video chip (charge coupled device) for higher definition imaging, as opposed to the older endoscopes, in which fiberoptics were used for image transmission. The tip of all of these scopes can be moved in multiple directions. The endoscope has channels for air insufflation, air aspiration, biopsy, and water instillation.

EDITOR'S NOTE: While EGD and colonoscopy can be learned at the same time, it is this editor's opinion (G.C.F.) that becoming familiar and comfortable with colonoscopy before attempting EGD is a good idea. There are certain maneuvers, such as intubating the pylorus, which may take much longer if the clinician does not already have solid preliminary endoscopy skills. There is also generally much less risk of airway compromise when performing colonoscopy under monitored anesthesia care (MAC) than with EGD under MAC, making it less stressful, in some ways, to perform.

EGD is usually performed while the patient is under procedural mild or moderate (conscious) sedation, often with MAC, although it can be completed with only topical anesthesia (a common practice in Asia). General anesthesia is often available but usually reserved for a select group of patients who are difficult to sedate because of chronic narcotic drug usage or who may have allergies to the very effective agents now available for procedural sedation.

The EGD technique is also utilized to remove esophageal foreign bodies (see Chapter 94, Esophageal Foreign Body Removal). Likewise, EGD is used when performing endoscopic ultrasound (EUS) and other endoscopic interventions that are outside the realm of this chapter, including endoscopic retrograde cholangiopancreatography and transthoracic echocardiography.

INDICATIONS

Symptoms

In many instances, it is one of the following symptoms that prompt the clinician's decision to consider an EGD:

- Dyspepsia (abdominal pain)
- Dysphagia (difficulty swallowing)
- Odynophagia (painful swallowing)
- Early satiety
- Recurrent regurgitation or gastroesophageal (GE) reflux disease
- Epigastric pain
- When swallowing, sensation of food sticking or a foreign body
- Severe indigestion
- Chronic nausea and vomiting
- Substernal or paraxiphoid pain
- Severe weight loss
- Persistent anorexia
- Noncardiac chest pain

Because over-the-counter proton pump inhibitor and histamine-2 antagonist therapies are available, many patients initiate therapy on their own for their upper GI symptoms. They often present to their primary care clinician only after failing a self-directed trial of these agents. Many patients may have also tried antacids or other agents for their upper GI symptoms; if all of these have failed, patients are often concerned and wanting to know the cause of recalcitrant symptoms. EGD usually provides an answer and reassurance following direct endoscopic assessment of the esophagus, stomach, and duodenum. Furthermore, EGD permits the clinician to retrieve tissue specimens for pathologic analysis during this brief invasive procedure.

Signs

- Unexplained anemia
- Gross or occult GI bleeding or melena
- Radiographic abnormality of the upper GI tract
- Weight loss
- Abdominal mass
- Hematemesis

Preexisting Conditions

Conditions that require further evaluation or surveillance with direct EGD include the following:

- Patients at high risk for cancer (e.g., those with Barrett esophagitis, gastric or familial polyposis, pernicious anemia)
- Esophageal stricture

- Acute or chronic duodenitis
- Acute or chronic esophagitis
- Acute or chronic gastritis
- Symptomatic hiatal hernia
- Gastric ulcer monitoring
- Gastric retention
- Duodenal ulcer disease
- Pyloroduodenal stenosis
- Esophageal or gastric varices
- Angiodysplasia in other area of the GI tract

CONTRAINDICATIONS

There are relatively few contraindications to the performance of EGD. The diameter of the currently available endoscopes is similar to the diameter of the large nasogastric (NG) tubes that are inserted on a daily basis in most hospitals. The safety of both of these procedures is readily acknowledged. Most primary care clinicians have inserted NG tubes during their medical training. Recalling the simplicity of these experiences should help clinicians feel more confident about the insertion of an EGD scope.

Contraindications to EGD are described below.

Absolute

- History of a bleeding disorder (e.g., platelet dysfunction, hemophilia) that is not reversed
- History of profusely bleeding esophageal varices
- Cardiopulmonary instability from any cause
- Recent myocardial infarction
- Suspected perforated viscus
- Uncooperative patient
- Absence of informed consent

Relative

Anticoagulants

Diagnostic EGD, including mucosal biopsy, is considered low risk for bleeding in patients taking anticoagulants and, therefore, can be performed without adjustment of properly monitored or administered anticoagulants prior to the procedure. However, in this situation, EGD should only be performed by clinicians *extremely* familiar with EGD technique. Familiarity with the technique is important because difficult or traumatic intubation of the scope could result in cricopharyngeal hematoma, which could theoretically cause carotid artery occlusion. A risk of retropharyngeal hematoma also may be present in patients with severe coagulation abnormalities.

Conversely, certain therapeutic procedures performed with EGD (i.e., polypectomy, percutaneous gastrostomy, endoscopic sphincterotomy, EUS-guided fine-needle aspiration, laser ablation, coagulation, and possibly dilations) are considered *high-risk procedures for bleeding*, and adjustment of anticoagulation is suggested.

In the past, bridging therapy was recommended for patients with a high risk of thrombotic events, artificial valves, or atrial fibrillation. However, for patients with atrial fibrillation, as a result of the BRIDGE study (Douketis et al., 2015), which showed a higher risk of bleeding and no decrease in thromboembolic events by bridging patients with atrial fibrillation (average CHADS2 score of 2.3) with Lovenox, many experts performing EGD no longer use bridging therapy. Instead, they just stop the warfarin 3 to 5 days before the procedure. This higher risk of bleeding had also been seen in a meta-analysis of patients bridged with heparin (Siegal et al., 2012). American Society for Gastrointestinal Endoscopy (ASGE) guidelines do not recommend bridging therapy unless the CHADS2-VASc score is 2 or greater, there is a mechanical aortic heart valve that is not bileaflet or a mechanical mitral valve, there is recent cerebrovascular accident, or there is a thromboembolic risk factor (prior venous thromboembolism on anticoagulation or recent [last 6 months] transient ischemic attack or cerebrovascular accident).

EDITOR'S NOTE: As an alternative to bridging therapy, although no guidelines have been written to support it, certain experts convert briefly oral dabigatran (Pradaxa), apixaban (Eliquis), or rivaroxaban (Xarelto), and withhold them 2 days prior to major surgery or 1 day for less significant surgery. Since apixaban is taken twice a day due to its shorter half-life, it would seem quicker to reverse by withholding it. Many endoscopists do not stop anticoagulation at all; they just plan on using more endoscopy clips to stop bleeding if needed.

Antiplatelet Medications

Recent coronary or carotid stent placement presents specific issues related to the risk of early stent thrombosis. Dual antiplatelet therapy (aspirin plus an adenosine diphosphate receptor inhibitor such as clopidogrel, prasugrel, or ticagrelor) is recommended in patients who have recently received coronary or carotid stents to prevent early stent occlusion until epithelialization has occurred. Decisions regarding the risk of bleeding in a particular procedure versus the risk of stent closure must be made when evaluating a patient preoperatively. It is best that the decision to continue or discontinue dual antiplatelet therapy in stented patients be made in partnership with the surgeon, anesthesiologist, cardiologist, and patient.

AHA guidelines from 2014 suggest delaying elective noncardiac surgery for a month in patients with a bare metal stent, and a year for patients with a drug-eluting stent. However, it may be acceptable to do elective surgery 180 days after a drug-eluting stent if at that point the risk of delaying surgery further is greater than the risk of stent thrombosis. In an update in 2016, there is some evidence that even shorter durations for drug-eluting stents may be acceptable. For nonelective, urgent, or emergent surgery at less than 4 to 6 weeks from stent placement, they recommend continuing dual antiplatelet therapy unless the risk of bleeding is greater than the risk of stent thrombosis. If dual antiplatelet therapy is discontinued, aspirin should be continued if possible, and dual therapy restarted as soon as safely possible.

Again, according to ASGE guidelines, diagnostic EGD, including mucosal biopsy, is considered low risk for bleeding in patients taking anticoagulants (including dual antiplatelet therapy) and therefore can be performed without adjustment of antiplatelet medications prior to the procedure by clinicians extremely familiar with EGD technique. For those therapeutic procedures performed with EGD considered high-risk procedures for bleeding (i.e., polypectomy, percutaneous gastrostomy, endoscopic sphincterotomy, EUS-guided fine-needle aspiration, laser ablation, coagulation, and possibly dilations), adjustment of antiplatelet therapy is suggested. The exception to this would be those patients also at high risk for thromboembolic complications in which dual therapy may be continued. It should be noted that these procedures are beyond the scope of this chapter.

EQUIPMENT

Endoscopes are produced by several different manufacturers (e.g., Olympus, Pentax, Fujinon). The typical esophagogastroscope consists of an "umbilical cord" (containing transmitted light and imaging capabilities), control head (with hand-operated wheels for up/down and left/right, air/water control buttons, and a suction button), and the long insertion tube, which is approximately 100 cm long and 7.8 to 11 mm wide. The bending section at the tip of the scope allows up to 180 degrees of deflection for retroflexion of the tip of the endoscope. (However, modern scopes often only allow retroflexion to 180 degrees in one direction, in the other direction, retroflexion is only to 90 degrees.)

The endoscope contains a lumen for insufflation of air and water, a working channel of 2 to 3 mm diameter (larger channel diameter for therapeutic endoscopes) used for suctioning and passage of instruments, control wires for moving the tip of the endoscope, and the imaging system that is either fiberoptic (rare these days) or video (widely available). The endoscope light source and imaging source (either video monitor or direct-view through the eyepiece) are critical aspects of the scope. Images and video can be recorded and printed, depending on the equipment used.

Flexible ultrathin fiberoptic and video endoscopes can be used without sedation for office-based EGD. These endoscopes are inserted transnasally or perorally and have a working length of 925 to 1100 mm, an external diameter of 5.3 to 6 mm, and a working channel diameter of 2 mm. With interventional scopes, multiple instruments have been developed that can be introduced through the working channel of the endoscope. These instruments include biopsy forceps, snares, sclerotherapy needles, heater probes, electrocautery probes, balloon-dilation devices, nets, and baskets. Guidewires can be placed, and when the endoscope is withdrawn, wire-guided bougie dilators can be utilized. Devices can also be placed onto the end of the endoscope for banding of esophageal varices and endoscopic mucosal resection.

Some of the newer endoscopes provide high resolution and magnification. Such scopes are used for the evaluation of certain upper GI diseases. The upper endoscope is also used to guide endoscopic treatment of GE reflux disease, such as with the Bard EndoCinch endoscopic suturing device and the NDO full-thickness plicator. One of the more recent advances in video endoscopy is narrow band imaging (NBI). NBI uses optical filters and high relative intensity of blue light for imaging and assessment of mucosal morphology and topography, such as mucosal and superficial vascular patterns. NBI has been studied in patients with Barrett esophagus, early gastric tumors, and colorectal lesions with promising results. Its full clinical utility has yet to be realized. In addition to the endoscope, other important equipment should be in operational order prior to starting an EGD:

- Light source (halogen light source versus xenon)
- Camera source
- Color video printer
- Video monitor (optional, but preferred)
- Video recorder (optional, but preferred)
- Biopsy forceps/brush
- Endoscopy clips
- Endoscopy table/cart
- Intravenous (IV) stand and IV sets
- Mouth guard
- Stool with wheels for the endoscopist (if sitting during the performance of the procedure)
- Sphygmomanometer versus continuous blood pressure monitor
- Stethoscope
- Electrocardiogram (ECG) machine or continuous cardiac monitor if sedation is going to be used
- Oxygen saturation monitor (pulse oximeter) if sedation is going to be used (consider Welch Allyn system that performs all necessary monitoring functions)
- Capnography monitor (if sedation is going to be used)
- Dextrose 5% and 0.45% sodium chloride solution (1 L) or lactated Ringer solution
- Suction equipment and tubing
- Specimen jars with formalin solution
- Syringes and needles
- K-Y Jelly (water-soluble) scope lubricant
- Protective gloves (remember latex sensitivity in sensitive patients) and equipment to follow universal blood and body fluid precautions
- Rapid urease test (CLO test) materials
- Anesthetic, sedative, and narcotic medications (see Chapter 1, Procedural Sedation and Analgesia)
- Oxygen and delivery mask or nasal cannula if sedation is going to be used
- Crash cart supplies (consider the Banyan kit—"a crash cart in suitcase"—if procedure is being performed in the office)

- Toothpicks to remove tissue from biopsy forceps
- Dictation capabilities or computer for immediate completion of the procedural record
- Proper supplies for cleaning the scope, as recommended by the manufacturer

Cleaning Supplies

- Plastic containers for the endoscope tube
- Surgical scrub solution and water (follow the manufacturer's recommendations)
- Enzyme solution
- 70% isopropyl alcohol
- Glutaraldehyde soaking solution (follow the manufacturer's recommendations)
- Brushes and various channel insertion devices provided by manufacturer for internal channel cleaning

NOTE: Methods may vary by manufacturer. Follow the recommendations to ensure patient safety and endoscope longevity.

PREPROCEDURE PATIENT PREPARATION

As with any procedure, EGD needs to be explained to the patient in detail prior to the procedure. The possible risks, benefits, and complications must be reviewed. It is wise to include a patient education handout and instructions for the patient to follow before the procedure (see the patient education handout available at www.expertconsult.com). The patient should also be given a copy of these to take home to share with a spouse or other family members.

Informed consent must be obtained before performance of EGD (see the patient consent form available at www.expertconsult.com). A preprocedure video or DVD that the patient and spouse or family member can view will reduce anxiety regarding the upcoming EGD. This video, which can be obtained from various pharmaceutical or equipment companies free of charge, will also introduce the subject of procedural sedation and review contraindications to the procedure. Figs. 91.1 to 91.6 show other helpful forms for office use.

ANTIBIOTIC PROPHYLAXIS

According to American Heart Association guidelines, antibiotic prophylaxis for endoscopy with or without GI biopsy is not recommended (see Chapter 69, Antibiotic Prophylaxis). No published data demonstrate a conclusive link between procedures of the GI tract and the development of bacterial endocarditis. No studies exist that demonstrate that the administration of antimicrobial prophylaxis prevents endocarditis in association with procedures performed on the upper GI tract.

SEDATION

See Chapter 1, Procedural Sedation and Analgesia, and Chapter 2, Pediatric Sedation and Analgesia.

EGD has traditionally been performed in a hospital procedure room specializing in GI disorders (a GI suite). It has also commonly been performed in the emergency department, outpatient surgery facility, or hospital operating room specially equipped for endoscopic procedures. Facility fee costs and sedation fees exceed clinician reimbursement several-fold. Many clinicians perform the procedure in their office simply using a topical anesthetic spray (Table 91.1).

Most clinicians who perform EGD in their offices use a combination of a benzodiazepine and a narcotic to achieve appropriate mild sedation and pain control for EGD. An angiocath is usually placed when IV medications are to be used during the performance of EGD. If IV analgesia or sedation is given, in addition to the clinician performing the procedure, a nurse or clinician with knowledge of IV sedative and analgesic medication should be available to monitor

Staff Gastroscopy Instructions Guidelines

1. Be sure the patient has a copy of the patient teaching guides and that he or she understands and has read the instructions.
2. Advise the patient that the purpose of the study is to insert a tube through the mouth into the stomach and into the beginning of the small intestine in order to inspect the upper GI tract. We will be looking for inflammation, ulcers, growths, bleeding points, a hiatal hernia, and abnormal growths.
3. The following medications will probably be used: a "Caine" topical anesthetic, Demerol, and Valium or Versed. Be sure to inquire about sensitivity or allergy to any of the medications just mentioned. These medications act to depress the central nervous system. The patient's current medications, particularly tranquilizers, sedatives, sleeping pills, and muscle relaxants, must be reviewed, and their effects when taken with preprocedure medication must be considered.
4. Possible serious side effects are extremely unlikely, but they include bleeding, perforation of the GI tract, tearing of the vocal cords (voice box), aspiration of stomach contents into the lungs, tearing of the mucosa, or even death from a severe reaction (e.g., to medications).
5. All patients will have gagging, but very few (if any) will experience any discomfort with gagging if they take the full prep. Patients who take the full prep will be groggy, sleepy, or lethargic for a variable period after the procedure. They must not drive or do anything "delicate" for at least 4 hours following the procedure if they received a prep. If grogginess persists, they should wait until they are fully alert. We recommend waiting 8 hours, if possible. If patients have a medical condition that affects medication metabolism, the wait will most likely be longer.
6. The procedure can be performed in a highly motivated patient without any preparation, but the gagging is uncomfortable and tends to persist throughout the procedure. It does, however, decrease after the scope is partially inserted. A topical anesthetic spray will greatly decrease gagging in the patient who chooses to not have IV sedation.

EGD Checklist

Be sure to be aware of the following:

Recent use of:	ASA	Persantine	Motrin	Advil	NSAIDs	Warfarin, apixaban, rivaroxaban, dabigatran	Clopidogrel, prasugrel, ticagrelor
Preexisting disease:	Asthma	Heart disease	COPD	Phlebitis	Prosthetic valves or joints		

If plans to deal with any of the above medications or preexisting diseases are not recorded in the chart, please discuss with the endoscopist how to handle the situation.

Notes:_____
_____
_____

Fig. 91.1   Sample form of instruction guidelines for gastroscopy staff. (From The Medical Procedures Center, Midland, MI.)

the patient during and following the procedure. The angiocath is connected to an IV line with IV fluids. It is essential that resuscitation equipment and reversal drugs are readily available throughout the course of the procedure. A benefit of using only mild anxiolysis or sedation is that the patient can help advance the scope by swallowing during intubation. When moderate or deep sedation is used, the scope must be entirely advanced by the clinician performing the procedure.

Many endoscopists now routinely use oxygen delivered through nasal cannula at 2 L/min to prevent any likelihood of hypoxemia that can occur during EGD, resulting from the mechanical nature of the tube in the upper airway region. This allows for a continuous source of oxygen delivery. The patient can be stimulated to inhale by simply advising him or her to take a deep breath. If oxygen is not used in a continuous fashion during the performance of the procedure, oxygen must be available in the event that hypoxemia occurs. It should be noted that the use of supplemental oxygen may affect the ability to use pulse oximetry as a warning device. This is why many endoscopists use capnography for all cases. Hyperoxygenated healthy adults and adolescents will only desaturate after prolonged apnea; the time required to desaturate to 90% averages 6 minutes. While high flow oxygen has been found to decrease the incidence of hypoxia in patients undergoing propofol sedation, lesser amounts of oxygen (≤3 mL/min) only marginally decrease risk of hypoxia with propofol and not at all with lighter levels of sedation.

Midazolam (Versed) is a sedative/hypnotic commonly used for sedation. The peak effect of midazolam is seen within 3 to 5 minutes. It has a duration of action of 1 to 3 hours. Some of the major adverse effects include respiratory depression, hypotension, and rarely seen paradoxic agitation. The typical starting dose is 0.5 to 1 mg IV, which can be titrated to achieve a desirable level of sedation (usually in 1-mg increments every 2 to 3 minutes). Lower doses of midazolam should be administered to elderly patients with cardiopulmonary problems to avoid serious respiratory depression.

Diazepam (Valium) may be used instead of midazolam for sedation during EGD, but many centers prefer midazolam (over diazepam) because of its well-received amnestic effect and reduced tendency to cause local vein phlebitis. Diazepam is initiated at 1 to 2 mg IV and titrated at 2-mg doses given every 1 to 2 minutes. This agent can also cause respiratory depression and should be used carefully in elderly patients. Paradoxic excitation can be seen with this sedative.

Benzodiazepines can rarely cause paradoxic excitement. If it occurs, however, pure narcotics can usually be used to complete the procedure. In extreme cases, cancel the procedure and reschedule it when assistance with sedation is available.

Meperidine (Demerol) is a narcotic analgesic that has mild sedative properties, slow onset of action, long duration, and long recovery time. When coadministered with benzodiazepines, potential complications include respiratory depression and sedation. The peak effect of meperidine is approximately 10 minutes, with a duration of action of 2 to 3 hours. Adverse effects include respiratory depression, hypotension, nausea, and vomiting. The typical starting dose is 12.5 to 50 mg IV, with subsequent doses not to exceed 25 mg/dose.

Fentanyl (Sublimaze) is a mildly sedative narcotic analgesic that has a rapid onset of action and short recovery time. In many endoscopy centers, fentanyl is the preferred agent for outpatient EGD. The peak effect is 5 to 8 minutes, and the duration of action is 1 to 3 hours. One of the major adverse effects is respiratory depression. The typical starting dose is 20 to 50 µg IV, with subsequent doses of 25 µg/dose.

Counseling for Office EGD (Upper Endoscopy)

Name: _____ DOB_____ Age_____

Telephone (H)_____ (W)_____

Your referring doctor:_____

Primary care doctor:_____ Want a copy sent to him/her?_____

Blood pressure_____ Received, read, and understood handouts?_____

SYMPTOMS/HISTORY: Reason for consult: _____

Nausea	Previous gastric ulcer	Food getting stuck
Vomiting	Duodenal ulcer	Black, tarry stools
Heartburn	Esophagitis	Anemia
Need for antacids/H2 blockers	Bloating	Belching
Early satiety	Pain with swallowing	Atypical chest pain
Positive *H. pylori* test	Difficulty swallowing	
Family Hx of stomach Ca	Who?_____	

PAST MEDICAL HISTORY:

Ulcer treatment	Other medical problems	Current Medications
Ex-smoker–quit	(1)_____	(1)_____
Aspirin use	(2)_____	(2)_____
NSAID use	(3)_____	(3)_____
Bleeding problems	(4)_____	(4)_____
Pulmonary disease	(5)_____	(5)_____
Heart disease		
Allergies _____		

OBJECTIVE:
General
Mouth   Dentures or partials   Teeth: chips
Neck: ability to hyperextend
Lungs
Heart
Abdomen

IMPRESSION:
(1) Good candidate for EGD
(2)
(3)
(4)

COUNSELING:

Bleeding	Sore throat
Aspiration	Infection
Perforation	Medication reaction

Sedation options:
Halcion/Stadol vs. IV sedation (Demerol/Versed) or topical only. Other_____
Driver if sedated

PLAN:
(1) Halcion 0.25 mg 2 tablets PO 1 hr PRN with sip of water   or IV sedation   or topical
(2) NPO after midnight
(3) Driver if sedation
(4) Scheduled for EGD
(5)
(6)

_____Date_____
Endoscopist's signature

Fig. 91.2 Sample form for esophagogastroduodenoscopy *(EGD)* counseling. (From The Medical Procedures Center, Midland, MI.)

Guidelines for Monitoring the Patient Receiving Sedation and Anelgesia for Gastrointestinal Endoscopy: A Summation

1. Patient monitoring is one aspect of the overall quality assurance program for the endoscopy unit.
2. A well-trained gastrointestinal assistant, working closely with the endoscopist, is the most important part of the monitoring process.
3. The use of equipment to monitor patients may be a useful adjunct to patient surveillance, but it is never a substitute for conscientious clinical assessment.
4. Although changes in blood pressure, pulse, cardiac rhythm, and oxygen saturation do occur during endoscopy, no controlled studies address the question of whether noninvasive monitoring with equipment decreases complications.
5. The amount of monitoring should be proportional to the perceived risk of the patient undergoing the procedure. It may vary from one procedure to the next.
6. The minimal clinical monitoring advised for all sedated patients should include the determination of heart rate, blood pressure, and respiratory rate before sedation, during the procedure, immediately after the procedure, and when the patient is released from the endoscopy area.
7. The proper role for pulse oximetry and continuous electrocardiographic monitoring during endoscopic procedures is controversial and unsettled.
8. Given the cost of the equipment and the manpower to use it, the best decision as to whether such monitoring should be used would be based on data showing an effect on clinical outcome. Such data do not exist; however, in those situations in which the individualized need of the patient indicates that measurement of cardiac rhythm or oxygen saturation will complement the clinical assessment, the use of cardiac monitoring or pulse oximetry may be beneficial.

Fig. 91.3 Sample form of monitoring instructions for gastroscopy staff. (From Fleischer D. Monitoring the patient receiving conscious sedation for gastrointestinal endoscopy: issues and guidelines. *Gastrointest Endosc.* 1989;35[2]:262–262.)

EGD Nursing Checklist

Patient_____ Date_____ Age_____

Notify the endoscopist if an unexpected, unusual, or negative answer is obtained.
Have the patient change into a gown.
Orient the patient to the room and the equipment.
Confirm the patient read the handouts and took oral medication at home.
Consent signed.
NPO since_____
Someone is present to drive the patient home.
Current meds_____
Drug allergies_____
Recent use of anticoagulants
Preexisting and/or existing disease: None   Heart   Lung   Other
Biopsy forceps, specimen cups, and slides ready.
Gloves, lubricant, and 4x4s available.
Resuscitation equipment available and ready, including oxygen.
Scope leakage tested.
Suction and water bottles prepared and connected.
If needed: IV 500 mL D5W /D5½ NS /NS started in LUE/RUE with #_____ Intracath/butterfly
by_____ at_____ AM/PM.
Assist with obtaining and processing biopsies.
Secure the safety of the patient after the procedure.
Print record of vital signs and disconnect monitoring equipment.
Vital signs record attached.
Clean the equipment.
Disconnect IV fluids if used.
Prepare the patient for the clinician meeting or conference.
Escort patient out with instruction sheets.

	Time
Patient in room	
Sedation started	
Procedure started (scope inserted)	
Procedure ended	
Patient discharged	

Medications	Dosage	Time

Fig. 91.4 Sample form of esophagogastroduodenoscopy (EGD) nursing checklist. (From The Medical Procedures Center, Midland, MI.)

EGD Procedure

Name:_____ BD:_____ Date:_____

The patient gave informed consent for the procedure. Intravenous access was obtained in the R/L upper extremity. Topical anesthesia was used in the pharynx. The patient was placed in the left lateral position, and the neck flexed to the chest. The bite block was placed gently, and the scope lubricated and passed through the bite block over the tongue. The hypopharynx was visualized, the vocal cords visualized, and the scope passed through the cricopharyngeus. The scope was passed into the distal esophagus with the GE junction seen and diaphragmatic indentation noted by the sniff test. The scope was advanced into the stomach and the gastric lake suctioned. The scope was passed through the pylorus and maneuvered into the descending duodenum. The duodenum and duodenal bulb were visualized and the scope brought back into the stomach. A biopsy for CLO testing was obtained. The scope was retroflexed to view the cardia. The scope was pulled into the esophagus and the esophagus closely examined. The scope was withdrawn, and the patient tolerated the procedure well. Monitoring showed normal cardiac/oxygen status. The patient was informed of the procedure results. Pulse oximetry monitoring was used throughout the procedure to evaluate the patient for hypoxemia. A printed report is attached.
Changes to above procedure: None or _____
_____
_____

Anesthesia: Versed_____ mg IV   Monitoring: Oximetry
                     Demerol_____ mg IV   Cardiac monitoring
                     Topical Cetacaine spray   Blood pressure
                     Xylocaine 2% liquid

Complications: _____
Areas not well visualized:_____
Abnormalities noted:
Bleeding   Erythema   Friability   Erosion   Polyp   Tumor
Ulcer, gastric   Ulcer, duo   Barrett's   Diverticula   Gastric bile   Varices
Dilation   Hiatal hernia   Carcinoma   Stenosis   Scarring   Angiodysplasia
Biopsies performed:_____

Diagnoses:
535.00   Gastritis, acute   531.00   Gastric ulcer, acute with hemorrhage
530.81   Esophageal reflux   535.60   Duodenitis
532.00   Duodenal ulcer   553.3   Hiatal hernia, acute with hemorrhage
530.1   Esophagitis, reflux   Other

Plan: _____   Stop smoking   Low fat diet
      _____   Avoid NSAIDs   Elevate head of bed 4–6 inches
                                                  Avoid chocolate/mints   Do not eat 2 hours before bedtime
                                                  Avoid offending foods

cc:_____ Endoscopist_____

Fig. 91.5   Sample form for the esophagogastroduodenoscopy (EGD) procedure. (From The Medical Procedures Center, Midland, MI.)

When IV sedation is used, the end point to be titrated is slurred speech with the patient still able to be aroused. (Many endoscopists use the Ramsey sedation scale to monitor depth of sedation.)

Several agents are used as reversal agents for mild or moderate sedation. Clinicians employing moderate (conscious) sedation should be very familiar with these agents. If reversal agents are used, it should be noted that these patients need to be monitored much longer in recovery because the half-life of the reversal agent may be much shorter than the agent being reversed. This can result in delayed, dangerous, profound sedation. Naloxone (Narcan) reverses opioid-induced analgesia, central nervous system effects, and respiratory depression. Naloxone has a peak effect of 1 to 2 minutes and a potential duration of action of 1 to 3 hours. Adverse effects include pain, agitation, nausea, vomiting, arrhythmias, sudden death, pulmonary edema, and withdrawal syndrome in patients with chronic opioid abuse. The typical dose is 0.04 mg IV for reversal of analgesia/sedation and 0.4 mg for narcotic overdose and respiratory arrest.

Flumazenil (Romazicon) is typically used for reversal of benzodiazepine-induced sedation and respiratory depression. Flumazenil has a peak effect of 3 to 5 minutes and a duration of action of 1 to 2 hours. Potential adverse effects include resedation and seizures. The typical dose is 0.2 to 0.5 mg IV for reversal of sedation (up to 1 mg total) and 1 to 3 mg IV for benzodiazepine overdose. This agent must be used with care in patients who are chronic anxiolytic users because it could cause the onset of seizures.

The use of MAC and propofol (Diprivan) has developed widespread patient acceptance because of the short recovery time required for the patient. Such an approach is typically utilized in outpatient surgical centers, hospitals, or GI endoscopic suites. Many institutions have special guidelines regarding the use of propofol and who may administer it (usually only anesthesia, emergency medicine, or critical care clinicians) due to its possible potent adverse effects, which include apnea and hypopnea.

Sufficient anesthesia or sedation can often be accomplished without IV drug administration, using new approaches that are called non-IV moderate (conscious) sedation. With this technique, a patient can be given diazepam 10 mg orally 1 hour before the procedure, or lorazepam 1 to 2 mg sublingually 30 to 60 minutes before the procedure. Alprazolam (Halcion), 0.5 mg orally, can also be used. An optional intramuscular dose of ketorolac (Toradol) 60 mg may be given 30 to 60 minutes before the procedure.

Butorphanol tartrate (Stadol), 1 to 2 sprays (intranasally), can be added if needed to the preceding regimen, or used alone. It generally provides both sedation and analgesia sufficient to carry out EGD. In many countries, EGD is performed with topical anesthesia only. Topical anesthesia with a benzocaine and tetracaine mixture (Cetacaine) or lidocaine has the advantages of requiring less time for the overall procedure, eliminating the risks of moderate (conscious) IV sedation, and decreasing the cost of the procedure by reducing or eliminating recovery time and nursing staff and anesthesia personnel. The spray is directed toward the posterior oropharynx while advising the patient to avoid breathing during the application. Inhaling the spray can cause significant coughing and gagging.

Role of the Assistant

The well-trained and motivated assistant makes the EGD examination a pleasant task for the endoscopist. It is not necessary for the attendant to attend a special course, but it is necessary to spend time learning each step of the procedure. Representatives from the endoscope manufacturer will assist in training assistants in the cleaning and care of the scopes. It is important to have assistants trained in CPR.

Before the patient arrives for the procedure, the assistant must do the following:
1. Prepare the room.
2. Have the IV set up, medications, endoscope, and the resuscitation equipment ready (but not opened).
3. Prepare the paperwork.

When the patient arrives, the assistant must do the following:
1. Bring the patient to the procedure room.
2. Orient the patient to the room and the equipment.
3. Make sure consent forms are signed, and that the patient has read and understands the instructions.
4. Verify that the patient is properly prepared (NPO, has a qualified adult to accompany the patient home). Check patient allergies.

Review and record current patient medications.
5. Review the EGD procedure with the patient.
6. Record baseline vital signs.
7. Place EKG monitor pads and initiate oximetry and cardiac monitoring if indicated.
8. Initiate IV fluids at KVO if IV sedation used.
9. Give the patient topical anesthesia within 3 to 5 minutes of starting the procedure.

During the procedure, the assistant must do the following:
1. Record vital signs every 15 minutes during the procedure.
2. Assist the endoscopist with the scope, if needed.
3. Watch the monitoring equipment, and notify the endoscopist of changes in patient status.
4. Assist with obtaining multiple biopsies and brushings.
5. Receive and process biopsy specimens and paperwork.

After the procedure, the assistant must do the following:
1. Monitor the patient's vital signs for 15 minutes.
2. Secure the safety of the patient, raise the gurney rails, etc.
3. Complete the paperwork associated with the procedure.
4. Remove monitoring equipment from the patient.
5. Clean the equipment.
6. Discontinue the IV fluids, if used.
7. Clean the room for the next procedure.
8. Prepare the patient for the endoscopist meeting or conference.
9. Give the patient the instruction sheets.
10. Inform the person accompanying the patient of signs to observe.

Fig. 91.6 Sample form detailing the role of the assistant. (From The Medical Procedures Center, Midland, MI.)

EDITOR'S NOTE: Due to several reported cases of methemoglobinemia, many centers no longer use topical benzocaine.

The disadvantages of using only topical anesthesia are patient discomfort and problems in performing the procedure on an uncooperative patient. An alternative choice for topical anesthesia is the "popsicle stick" method. In this scenario, lidocaine ointment (2%) is squeezed on a tongue blade that is covered with the patient's favorite food flavoring, and this is placed into the back of the patient's throat. The patient sucks on the tongue blade while vital signs are completed and the patient is prepared for the procedure. A tongue blade can be pressed into the posterior oral pharynx to ascertain that appropriate topical anesthesia has been obtained before insertion of the endoscope. Lack of a gag reflex ensures the desired effect. With the cost-saving trends in medicine, and with the newer, smaller scopes, EGD without sedation will likely become more commonplace in the future. With the introduction of the previously described smaller caliber endoscopes that can be passed through the nose, EGD without sedation may be more acceptable to patients.

Currently available small-diameter scopes allow for a comfortable examination with little manipulation or trauma to the cricopharyngeal region. As stated previously, the diameter of the scope is similar to that of an NG tube inserted daily by hospital nursing staffs.

It is important to select patients wisely for office-based EGD. This is a critical step. In individuals who are in the high-risk group

(Box 91.1), the clinician should consider performing EGD in a facility where complications can be handled and more aggressive monitoring procedures can be carried out. The utilization of MAC is suggested in such cases.

MONITORING

The current move to office endoscopy was initiated because of its many benefits, including safety and cost effectiveness. There is little proven benefit for continuous ECG monitoring or continuous pulse oximetry for low-risk patients under mild sedation. More extensive monitoring becomes necessary under the following conditions:

- Procedures that last longer than 30 minutes
- Large-bore scopes
- High-risk patients (see Box 91.1)
- Situations in which more than light or mild sedation is used

In these scenarios, more extensive clinical monitoring, including continuous ECG monitoring, pulse oximetry, and capnography, is wise. All patients should have clinical monitoring of skin color, degree of sedation, loss of reflexes, blood pressure, pulse, and respiratory rate in a well-lighted room.

TABLE 91.1	Drugs Used for Esophagogastroduodenoscopy
Medication	**Dose**
Narcotics	
Meperidine (Demerol) IV	10–75 mg (0.5–1 mg/kg)
Fentanyl (Sublimaze) IV	20–50 µg
Butorphanol tartrate (Stadol nasal spray)	1–2 mg (1–2 sprays in nostril)
Propofol	Variable*
Benzodiazepines	
Diazepam (Valium) IV	1–10 mg
Midazolam (Versed) IV	2–5 mg (0.035–0.1 mg/kg)
Lorazepam (Ativan) SL (onset in 10 min)	1–2 mg
Triazolam (Halcion) PO	0.5 mg
Anticholinergic	
Glycopyrrolate (Robinul)	0.002 mg (0.01 mL/kg) IM 1 hr before procedure or 0.1 mg (0.5 mL) repeated every 2–3 min as needed
Miscellaneous	
Simethicone (Mylicon) drops	0.6 mL (30–40 mg) in 30 mL of water PO (can also be flushed through the gastroscope with 5 mL of water)
Ketorolac (Toradol)	60 mg IM; 15 mg IV
Topical Local Anesthetics	
Lidocaine 2% viscous solution gargle	
Benzocaine 20% (Hurricane) spray	
Benzocaine 14% and tetracaine 2% (Cetacaine)	
Antagonists	
Naloxone (Narcan) IV	0.2–0.8 mg
Flumazenil (Romazicon) IV	0.2–1 mg (start with 0.2 mg; repeat every 60 sec to a maximum of 1 mg or until reversal of benzodiazepine effect has been achieved)
Nalmefene hydrogen chloride (Revex)	1–2 mL IV

*Sedation may be initiated by infusing propofol at 100 to 150 mcg/kg per min (6 to 9 mg/kg/h) for a period of 3 to 5 min and titrating to the desired clinical effect while closely monitoring respiratory function. *IM*, Intramuscular; *IV*, intravenous; *PO*, orally; *SL*, sublingually.

BOX 91.1	High-Risk Groups for Esophagogastroduodenoscopy

Agitated, uncooperative patient
Barium administration within a few hours of the procedure
Cardiopulmonary instability of any type
Current active bleeding
Older than 70 years
Prosthetic cardiac valves
Recent cerebrovascular accident
Significant bleeding disorder or coagulopathy
Significant chronic obstructive pulmonary disease
Significant valvular heart disease
Uncontrolled coronary artery disease
Younger than 12 years

TECHNIQUE

It is essential to ensure that if a procedure at high risk for bleeding is being performed with EGD, unless contraindicated, clopidogrel (Plavix), prasugrel (Effient), or ticagrelor (Brilinta) have been discontinued at least 7 days before the procedure (see earlier section on

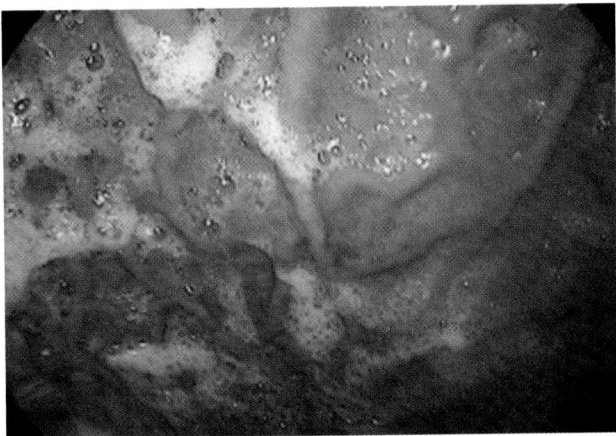

Fig. 91.7 Bubbles in the stomach.

Antiplatelet Medications). The patient must take nothing by mouth after midnight on the day of the examination (or at least 8 hours must have elapsed since eating).

The assistant should initiate the IV angiocath and connect it to the IV line. If pulse oximetry and continuous ECG monitoring are to be utilized, connect them at this time. If it is going to be used, a capnography monitor should be available. Blood pressure, pulse, and respiration monitoring can also be started at this time and recorded. Universal blood and body fluid precautions should be followed by all clinicians involved in the procedure.

1. Examine the oral cavity while the patient is in a sitting position. Any dentures or foreign objects should be removed.
2. Some clinicians ask the patient to swallow 40 mg of simethicone in 30 mL of tap water before the initiation of the procedure. This tends to minimize the reflective bubbles in the stomach (Fig. 91.7) that can present considerable impediment to visibility during the procedure. Alternatively, simethicone can be used only if needed during the procedure (0.6 mL of simethicone liquid can be injected down the gastroscope followed by 5 mL of water, or it can be mixed in the water being used to flush).
3. The topical anesthesia should be completed at this point, as noted previously.
4. After good topical anesthesia is ensured, the patient should be placed in the left lateral decubitus position, especially if sedated. Unsedated EGDs are often performed in the sitting position with the patient bent 45 degrees forward at the waist. The head should be in the "sniffing" position used to insert an NG tube.
5. Lubricate the distal 10 cm of the scope with a minimal amount of water-soluble gel (an excessive amount may induce coughing or sneezing).
6. Insert the mouth guard into the patient's mouth; the teeth should grip this guard. The guard not only protects the patient's teeth, tongue, and oral mucosa, but it also prevents the patient from damaging the scope. Introduce the scope through the mouth guard and direct it across the superior aspect of the tongue into the posterior oral pharynx. Grasping the scope at about the 15 cm mark in the operator's right hand and putting a slight downward curve on the tip usually facilitates the next step. In the edentulous patient, the mouth guard can be placed over the scope, and the scope can then be introduced through a channel created by placing the left second and third fingers of the examiner's hand over the back of the tongue. Guide the scope across the back of the tongue into the cricopharyngeal region. This is usually the first point of resistance encountered (approximately 17 cm from the incisor teeth and at the level of the vocal cords) (Fig. 91.8). Under direct vision (or blindly if the patient is sedated and unable to swallow), ask the patient to swallow repeatedly while applying gentle pressure. The scope

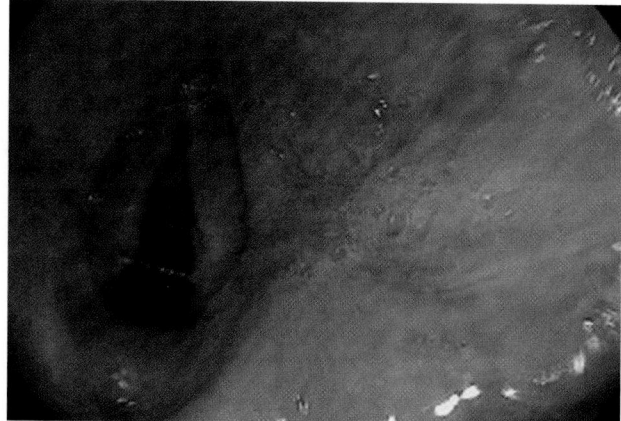

Fig. 91.8   Open vocal cord.

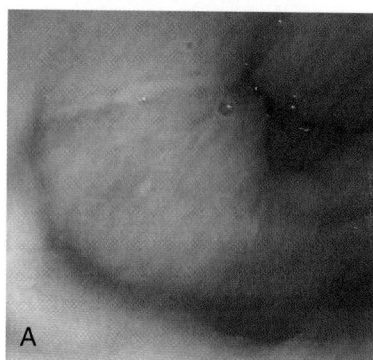

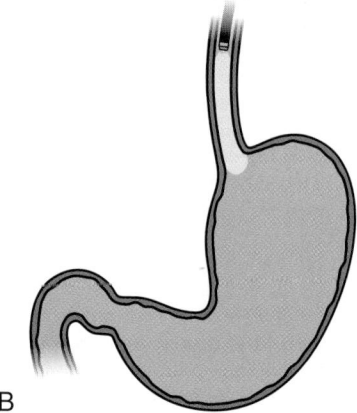

Fig. 91.9   (A) Proximal esophagus. (B) Unshaded area is seen by lighted scope.

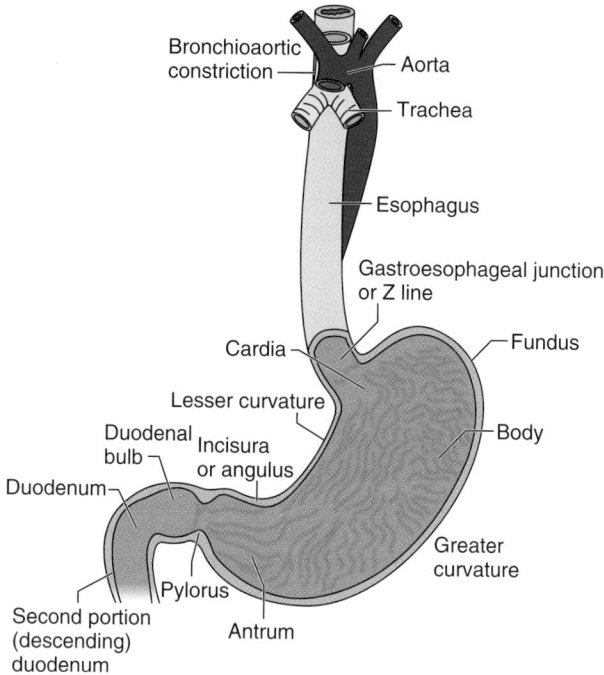

Fig. 91.10   Relevant anatomy for gastroscopy. The *cardia* is that portion of the stomach immediately surrounding the esophageal opening. The *gastroesophageal junction* is also known as the GE junction, the Z line, ora serrata, or gastric rosette. The upper end or dome of the stomach is the *fundus*. The upturn of the J of the stomach is separated from its vertical portion by the *angular notch* (also known as the angulus, angularis, or incisura). The *antrum* lies to the right of the angulus and ends at the *pylorus*, or greatly thickened muscular wall. The *duodenum* lies beyond the pylorus. The *lesser curvature* is the upper right border of the stomach, whereas the *greater curvature* is the left inferior margin.

will easily pass through the cricopharyngeus region without difficulty and can then be advanced down through the esophagus (Fig. 91.9A and B).

7. Never use force as the scope passes the cricopharyngeus region. The patient's normal swallowing mechanism will assist in advancing the endoscope. If the patient is more than mildly sedated, the operator should advance the scope in a manner similar to an NG tube. If there is difficulty passing the scope, the head may need to be repositioned into the "sniffing" position in the sedated patient.

8. Once the tip of the endoscope has entered the esophagus, insufflate a small puff of air to open the esophagus to easily visualize the mucosa throughout the cylindric esophagus. Additional air will need to be insufflated after the scope reaches the stomach and duodenum.

NOTE: Identify the lumen in front of the scope before attempting to pass the scope to prevent injury to the patient. The lumen should always be seen during EGD.

The endoscope should be advanced quickly but gently through the esophagus. The first landmark seen is the bronchoaortic constriction (Fig. 91.10).

9. As the scope is advanced, the GE junction (Z line) is typically found at approximately 40 cm from the incisor teeth. This distance should be noted. It is essential to evaluate the esophagus and GE junction during this first pass, and to obtain images, because the mucosa may become irritated by the passage of the scope. This irritation can distort the appearance of the GE junction (Fig. 91.11A and B). There is a typical mucosal color demarcation that occurs at the GE junction, with the esophageal lining being pale pink and the gastric mucosa represented by a darker pink or orange hue.

10. At this time, ask the patient to sniff through his or her nose (i.e., the sniff test) if the patient is partially conscious. As the patient sniffs, the crura of the diaphragm extrinsically compress the GE junction at the esophageal hiatus. If the Z line is visualized above the level of the extrinsic compression seen from the crura of the diaphragm, then the patient is suffering from a hiatal hernia. Repeat the sniff test when viewing the Z line from below, while the scope is in the stomach in a retroflexed position.

NOTE: Use air, water, suction, and mini-withdrawals as needed to pass the scope and to fully evaluate all surfaces of the mucosa.

11. After passing through the GE junction, the endoscope is inserted into the stomach. After the scope reaches the stomach, the gastric lake, which is a collection of fluids in the dependent portion of the stomach, will typically impair visibility (Fig. 91.12A and B). Air should be insufflated sufficiently to spread the mucosal walls apart so that this fluid can be aspirated. Some clinicians aspirate the gastric fluid and test the pH of the fluid to record the acidity of the gastric lake.

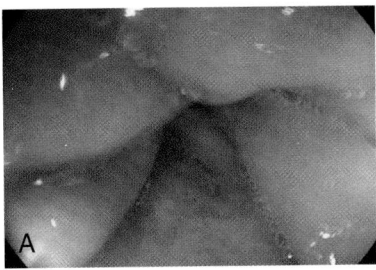

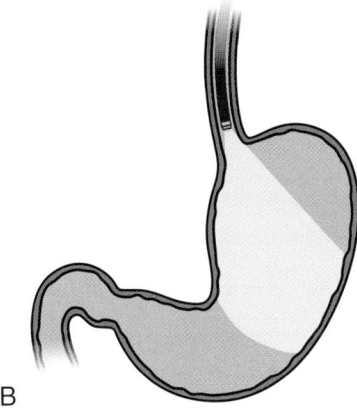

Fig. 91.11   (A) Distal esophagus Z line. (B) Unshaded area is seen by lighted scope.

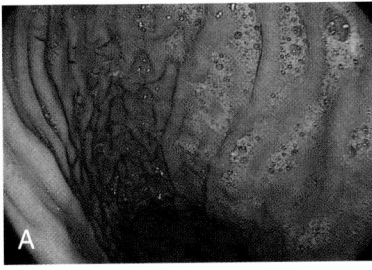

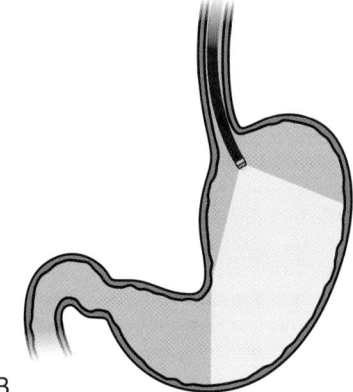

Fig. 91.12   (A) Gastric lake with reflective bubbles/fluid seen from 1 to 3 o'clock. (B) Unshaded area is seen by lighted scope.

After the fluid is removed and the lumen again is clearly visualized, the scope can rapidly be advanced following the rugae along the lesser curvature to the angular notch. The rugae are typically very linear. The scope is subsequently passed below the angularis, then into the antrum and up to the pylorus (Fig. 91.13A–E, and see Fig. 91.10).

NOTE: The scope should be adjusted so that the small black arrow is at the top of the field and so it corresponds with the

incisura. This adjustment provides proper orientation with the patient in the left lateral position. This is also a good time to obtain and image of the pylorus prior to any potential trauma that could occur with intubation.

12. Guide the endoscope through the relaxed pyloric sphincter into the duodenal bulb (Fig. 91.14A and B). Do not attempt to pass the scope through a tightly closed pylorus. The repetitive trauma of attempting to do this will simply cause greater pylorospasm and prevent good evaluation of the duodenum. When the scope is passed through the pylorus into the duodenal bulb, it is common to encounter a white-out or a red-out. This is because the scope typically tends to rapidly advance to the junction of the first and second portions of the duodenum and press against the mucosal. At this point, it is wise to withdraw the scope very slowly to reestablish the lumen and complete the duodenal examination. Biopsies are rarely needed in this area.

13. The second portion of the duodenum tracks behind the peritoneum (i.e., becomes retroperitoneal). Thus it is wise to rotate the scope clockwise and pass the scope upward so that it can enter the second portion of the duodenum (see Fig. 91.13). Retroflexion of the scope while rotating the scope clockwise will usually facilitate this maneuver. The second portion of the duodenum is recognizable because of the vertical, cylindric nature of the viscera in this region. In addition, the Kerckring folds (Fig. 91.15A) will readily appear. The ampulla of Vater (see Fig. 91.15B) can be seen along the medial aspect of the second portion of the duodenum 20% to 30% of the time. It is not essential to evaluate this area for the completion of an EGD. Never biopsy near the ampulla of Vater unless adequately trained; permanent damage can occur.

14. The scope can be advanced occasionally into the third portion of the duodenum or the horizontal portion of the duodenum.
    NOTE: At this point of the procedure, the insertion portion is complete, and it is time to withdraw the scope.

15. Withdraw the endoscope slowly with the attempt to evaluate the entire 360-degree circumferential portion of the mucosal surface. The second and sometimes the third portions of the duodenum can be evaluated readily.

16. The duodenal bulb is difficult to assess because as it is being withdrawn, the scope typically tends to rapidly retract through the pyloric junction, back into the stomach. It is therefore necessary to reinsert it through the pylorus so that the duodenal bulb mucosa can be closely examined to rule out disease.

17. Once back into the stomach, it is helpful to deflect the scope tip up and down as the control head is rotated right and left to ensure that the entire gastric mucosal surface has been evaluated. In the United States, if present, *Helicobacter pylori* seems to prefer the antrum (worldwide it is often distributed throughout the stomach). Many clinicians will therefore biopsy the antrum twice to evaluate for *H. pylori*. Next, withdraw the scope out of the antrum and, if not previously performed, retroflex the scope so that it is viewing itself and observe the GE junction. Examine the cardia and fundus (Fig. 91.16A–D). Withdraw the scope and rotate it slightly while it is retroflexed to more closely examine the GE junction. This is a good location from which to take images of a hiatal hernia. The scope can also be rotated on itself 180 degrees by grasping the scope with the right hand at the same time as the left holding the knobs is rotated to obtain another view of the GE junction.

18. Straighten the deflected scope tip before removing the scope through the GE junction. One way to do this is to align the letters on the large inner wheel (up/down control) and the small outer wheel (left/right control) before withdrawing the instrument. (Some scopes have arrows which should be pointing upward.) If the scope is withdrawn with the tip retroflexed, it could result in mucosal damage of the GE junction or an esophageal tear. Suction any remaining fluid out of the stomach, which

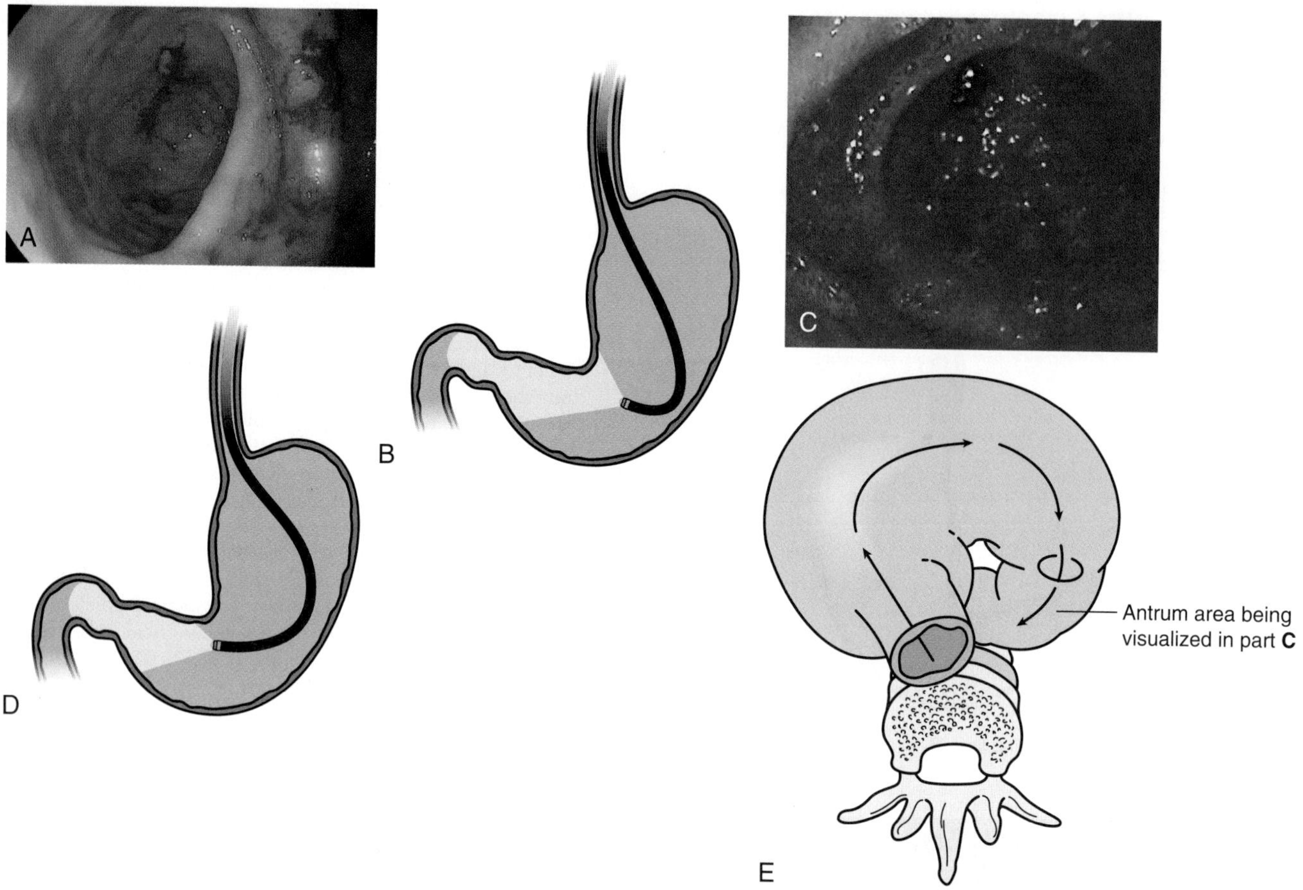

Antrum area being
visualized in part **C**

E

Fig. 91.13 (A) Angularis is along the right side of visual field. Pylorus is in the distance but cannot be seen due to angularis obstructing the view. Prepyloric ulcer is seen at 11 o'clock. (B) Unshaded area is seen by lighted scope. (C) Antrum at the 6 o'clock position. Pyloric opening and angularis at the 12 o'clock position. (D) Unshaded area is seen by lighted scope. (E) To reach the pylorus, the clinician should make a clockwise spiral around the vertebral column.

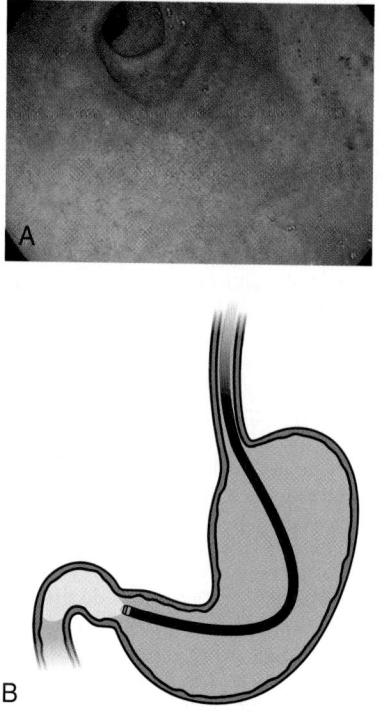

Fig. 91.14 (A) Duodenal bulb. (B) Unshaded area is seen by lighted scope.

might follow the scope back upward as it is withdrawn; the scope somewhat acts as a wick for fluid into the glottis, which can result in aspiration. Suction any remaining air out of the stomach before observing the GE junction.

19. The scope is withdrawn through the GE junction slowly. Again, close evaluation of the GE junction is completed. Complete a sniff test at this region one final time.
20. As the procedure is being carried out, images can be obtained on a continuing basis, both during the initial insertion and during withdrawal.
21. Biopsies of the GE junction are completed as the scope is withdrawn to prevent significant downstream bleeding that can impair visibility of the mucosal surface (see the Biopsy section). Observe the esophageal mucosa closely for abnormalities for the entire distance that the scope is being withdrawn.
22. It is important to record the appearance of the vocal cords before the scope is completely withdrawn. The documentation of an attempt to view the vocal cords is an important component of EGD before the removal of the scope, even if they cannot be seen because of coughing or gagging.
23. The assistant should complete the monitoring process of the patient after the scope is withdrawn. The mouth guard should also be removed, and the clinician may want to reexamine the patient before discharge from the facility. A 30-minute observation period after the procedure is typical if minimal sedation is used (Box 91.2).
24. Discuss the findings with the patient (and the person who has accompanied the patient to the office) before discharge. If the patient has received significant administration of benzodiazepines, such as midazolam (Versed), he or she may be amnestic

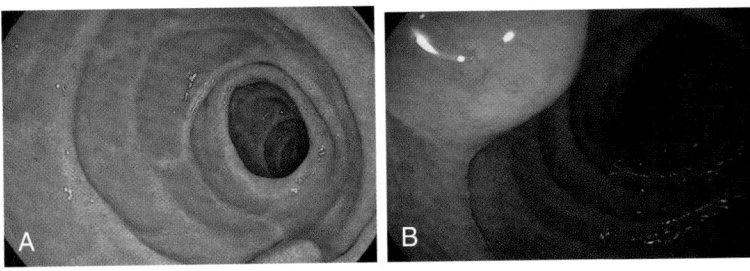

Fig. 91.15   (A) Folds of Kerckring. (B) Ampulla of Vater.

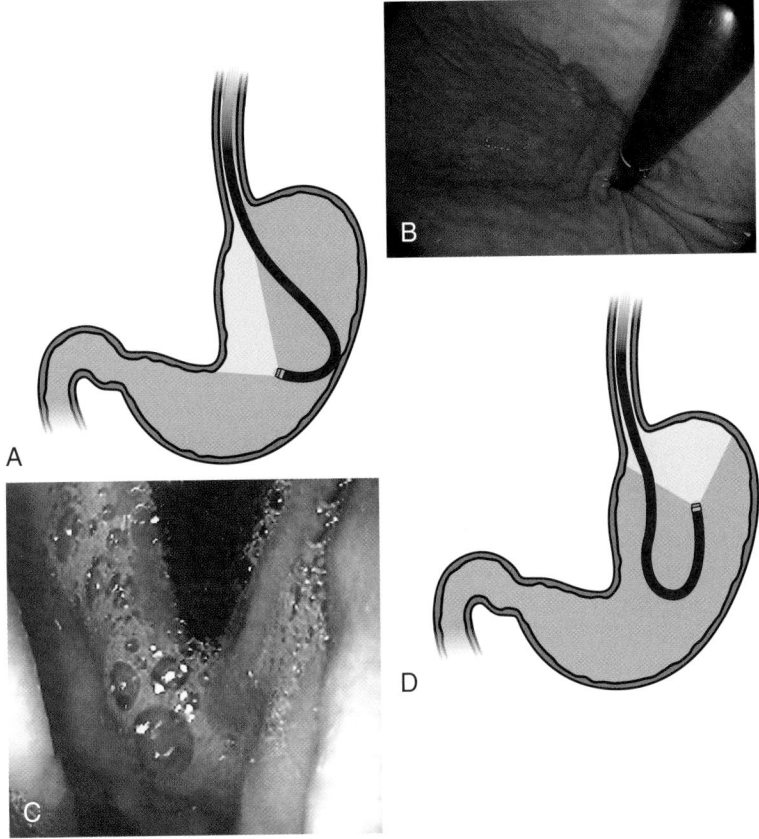

Fig. 91.16   (A) A 180-degree angulation retroflexes the tip to see the lesser curve. (B) Retroflexion view. (C) and (D) Reflexion view of the cardia.

and forget any information provided by the clinician. Providing printed images of the findings, along with graphic demonstration or written comments, are extremely helpful in reviewing the results of the procedure with the patient and his or her family. Complete and review all monitoring forms.

25. The GI assistant should document the condition in which the patient was discharged.
26. It is helpful to call the patient at home at the end of the day (before the office closes) to document that the patient is not experiencing any untoward effects after the completion of EGD.

UNSEDATED TRANSNASAL ESOPHAGOGASTRODUODENOSCOPY

With the advent of newly developed ultrathin diameter endoscopes (5.1- to 6-mm insertion tube), unsedated transnasal EGD (T-EGD) has become possible. Unsedated EGD obviously eliminates the danger of medication-related complications from sedative drugs. More than half of the morbidity and mortality attributed to EGD is due to cardiopulmonary complications from sedation effects.

Significant cost reduction is associated with the absence of fees for sedation and monitoring equipment. This alone has become a significant motivational factor to encourage office-based T-EGD.

Previously, either the patient or the clinician may have opted for an empiric therapeutic trial of medications for a myriad of upper GI complaints, rather than having an EGD. Such choices may have been based on patient anxiety or clinician concerns about the procedure. Such a delay in diagnosis is no longer necessary because T-EGD can be completed easily and rapidly in the office, eliminating the need for nursing time and anesthesia personnel. Also, preoperative, concurrent, and postoperative monitoring with a pulse oximeter are no longer issues.

Other hidden costs can also be eliminated. Such costs include the drain on the economy's workforce associated with the current need for family members or friends taking time off to assist and transport patients for EGD. Patient convenience is enhanced, because endoscopies can be performed during office hours. No lengthy recovery period or check-in or discharge time is required. Patients can return to work almost immediately following T-EGD. Clinicians can perform more endoscopies in less time after they are trained and familiar with the unsedated technique.

BOX 91.2 Intravenous Sedative Administration Recovery Nursing Documentation Parameters

- Note and record level of consciousness on arrival.
- Note and record response and anxiety level.
- Note and record patency of airway, spontaneous respiratory effort.
- Note and record status of intravenous (IV) access site (redness or edema).
- Note and record respiratory effort and degree of chest movement.
- Note and record vital signs every 5 min.
- Place the cardiac monitor.
- Place the pulse oximeter and capnography.
- Note and record body temperature.
- Administer oxygen at 2 L through a nasal cannula.
- Raise head of the bed 30–45 degrees.
- Note and record skin turgor.
- Note and record quality of speech (clarity and ease of speech).
- Note and record presence or absence of nausea, gagging, spasmodic coughing, and ability to swallow.
- Note and record presence or absence of abdominal distention or tenderness.
- Note and record quality of bowel sounds.
- Note and record expulsion of gas.
- Note and record abdominal cramping.
- On admission, perform an assessment of the patient's medical conditions.
- Note and record any untoward symptoms as they occur.
- Note and record the patient's condition after 15 min.
- Note and record discharge status.
- Record vital signs every 5 min and post monitor strips, with a simple explanation, every 15 min or when there is an unusual occurrence.
- Report any unusual responses immediately to the endoscopist.

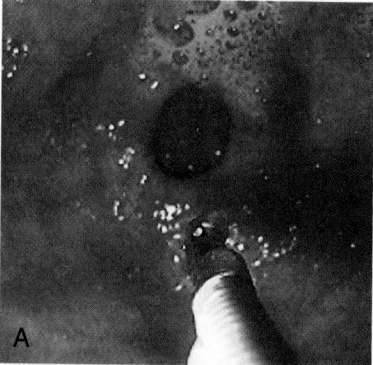

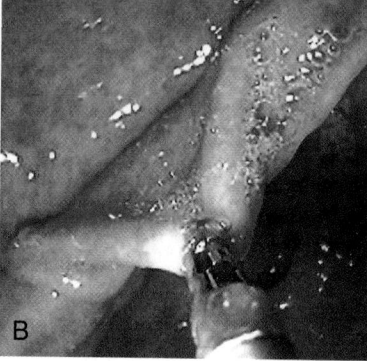

Fig. 91.17 (A) Closed biopsy forceps. (B) Tenting of the mucosa during biopsy.

A remaining hurdle is the fact that most patients experiencing EGD have come to expect that they will sleep through their procedure and awaken with little or no awareness of what was done. Patient apprehension can be a major obstacle. This concern can be overcome with good patient education (such as videos of actual procedures), which will increase acceptability and tolerance. Patients can actually watch their anatomy on the screen and actively communicate (talk during the procedure), providing feedback to the clinician. Immediate demonstration and explanation of the pathology are possible with a conscious patient who is viewing the procedure as it occurs. Biopsies can now be performed with newer generation transnasal endoscopes to allow for tissue retrieval.

BIOPSY

Biopsy samples are taken when visible changes are seen in the stomach or esophagus. Routine, blind biopsy specimens of the esophagus or duodenum are not indicated. In addition, routine biopsies of the antrum may reveal *H. pylori* that was undetectable by direct visualization. The clinician should perform a biopsy on any other GE abnormality, unless it is vascular in appearance (i.e., pulsating or bluish in color). Any intended areas of biopsy should be approached with a closed biopsy forceps to assess the vascularity and induration of the subject area. The clinician should ensure that the intended biopsy site can be successfully reached with the scope in its current position. Biopsy of duodenal ulcers is rarely necessary because the risk of cancer is extremely small in this region of the world.

During biopsy, the forceps are advanced through the end of the scope by the examiner, and the assistant is in charge of the operating controls. The closed forceps are directed at the area to be biopsied (Fig. 91.17A).

After reaching the desired site with the closed forceps, the forceps are withdrawn a few centimeters, the assistant is advised to open the forceps, and the forceps are passed directly into the biopsy area. The examiner asks the assistant to close the forceps. A gentle tug is given, and the biopsy forceps are pulled through the opening of the scope by the examiner. Tenting of the mucosa can be seen with the removal of the tissue (see Fig. 91.17B).

The assistant then retrieves the tissue by opening the biopsy forceps over a container with formalin. A toothpick is placed into the teeth of the open biopsy forceps, dislodging the tissue material into the formalin container.

For gastric ulcers, the clinician should biopsy all four quadrants at the edges. Removal of tissue from the center of the ulcer will not result in adequate tissue examination. If diffuse intestinal gastritis is present, multiple biopsies are indicated. Because the biopsies are small, there is generally minimal bleeding. In most cases bleeding from esophageal biopsies stops within 4 to 5 minutes.

It is unnecessary to continuously monitor a biopsy site during the performance of the procedure. Commonly, the examiner can complete the examination by looking at other areas of the upper GI tract and then return to reevaluate a biopsy site before the completion of the procedure. If bleeding does occur and is profuse, it must be controlled before withdrawing the scope and noted on the operative report. In most cases, the acidic milieu of the stomach coagulates bleeding sites. Occasionally the distal esophagus will bleed more persistently after the completion of a biopsy; therefore, many examiners perform brush "biopsies" in this region rather than the surgical biopsy.

Gastric antrum biopsies are also commonly done to obtain tissue samples for CLO tests or for histologic analysis for *H. pylori*. *H. pylori*–associated gastritis often cannot be diagnosed by endoscopic appearance alone. When assessing a patient with chronic dyspepsia, the clinician should remember that normal-appearing gastric mucosa may exhibit marked histologic gastritis.

When performing the CLO test, the examiner should warm the slide to room temperature before the endoscopy. The absence of bismuth preparations and a 4-week abstinence from antibiotics should be documented before the performance of the procedure.

As mentioned previously, when performing *H. pylori* biopsies, the clinician should obtain tissue samples from the normal-appearing portions of the gastric antrum. The normal-appearing area of the mucosa is chosen because *H. pylori* may be scarce in areas where the epithelium is eroded or where the mucous layer is denuded.

Many clinicians read and interpret the results of a CLO test (a simple color change) themselves. However, the tissue can be sent to a pathologist. Some clinicians collect two specimens: one for a CLO test and one for histologic analysis (the histologic analysis specimen is sent only if the CLO test is negative but there is a strong suspicion of *H. pylori*). A single biopsy has a sensitivity of approximately 95%, whereas two biopsies approach 100% sensitivity. *H. pylori* have a patchy distribution.

COMPLICATIONS

The complication rate of endoscopy performed by primary care clinicians from eight clinical sites was 0.0014 (1 in 717). All cases were collected sequentially from the beginning of each clinician's experience (Rodney et al., 1990). The complication rate in large subspecialty populations is 0.0013 (1.3 in 1000). Therefore, complications from EGD are extremely rare. Sixty percent of the adverse effects associated with EGD are due to cardiopulmonary complications that arise directly from the conscious sedation used in the procedure. True complications might include the following:

- Perforation
- Bleeding secondary to trauma or biopsy
- Infection
- Cardiopulmonary complications from conscious sedation
- Inadequate interpretation

The risk of perforation is increased when therapeutic procedures (not discussed in the text) are performed at the time of endoscopy. Risk increases as follows:

- Esophageal dilation, 0.5%
- Esophageal dilation for achalasia, 1.7%
- Endoscopic thermal therapy, 1% to 2%
- Endoscopic variceal sclerotherapy, 1% to 6%
- Endoscopic laser therapy, 5%
- Photodynamic therapy, 4.6%
- Esophageal stent placement, 5% to 25%

COMPLETION OF THE ESOPHAGOGASTRODUODE-NOSCOPY REPORT

The final EGD report can be completed on a preconstructed template (Fig. 91.18) or a computer template macro, or it can be dictated into a transcription system. The report should include the diagnosis and the symptoms or signs that led to the performance of the EGD. Inclusion of the sedative agents and doses is important to incorporate, especially if future endoscopy is contemplated. All of the findings should be detailed. A listing of the final diagnoses and treatment plan is essential to include. The clinician should also note the number of biopsies and the location from which they were obtained.

TRAINING

Most clinicians who are performing primary care endoscopy have received training either in a residency situation or in short courses, such as those through the National Procedures Institute. Both of these training situations provide excellent introduction to the technique of EGD, the use of mild to moderate sedation, practice on lifelike models, and the interpretation of common pathologic conditions seen with the endoscope.

It is essential for the clinician to obtain preceptor training from a skilled endoscopist who can assist with the proper insertion technique and the proper interpretation of anatomic findings during the performance of EGD.

There is no common agreement concerning how many EGD procedures a clinician who is already competent at other endoscopic procedures (e.g., flexible sigmoidoscopy, colonoscopy) should perform before performing EGD without supervision. In 2009, the Residency Review Committee for General Surgery changed their requirements: all surgery residents should obtain 50 colonoscopies during their training and 35 upper endoscopies. At that point, the American Academy of Family Physicians started recommending 50 colonoscopies for all family physicians wanting to obtain colonoscopy privileges. Many skilled primary care endoscopists believe that approximately 5 to 15 EGDs under supervision are adequate. This number is significantly less than a specialist who will be doing more advanced therapeutic/interventional care rather than diagnostic evaluation.

OBTAINING HOSPITAL PRIVILEGES

Hospital privileges remain a strongly contested area; the debate over who should receive these privileges is primarily motivated by subspecialty concerns. There are absolutely no study-supported data in the literature denoting a minimal number of procedures that should be supervised before obtaining hospital privileges. Although many numbers are reported by subspecialty organizations as a proposed minimum, these numbers are subject to debate and are not in any way a demonstration of individual competency. Thus it is essential to have a skilled endoscopist act as preceptor to an individual to ascertain adequate hand-eye coordination and good visual-spatial skills. For more information, the clinician should review the American Academy of Family Physicians' position paper on endoscopy, as referenced later.

PATIENT EDUCATION GUIDES

See the sample patient education and consent forms available at www.expertconsult.com.

CPT/BILLING CODES

36000	Introduction of needle or intracatheter, vein
43200*	Esophagoscopy with or without brush
43202*	Esophagoscopy with biopsy, single or multiple
43215*	Esophagoscopy foreign body removal
43234*	Simple upper endoscopy
43235*	EGD with or without brushings
43239*	EGD with biopsies
43247*	EGD with foreign body removal
90780	IV therapy 1 hour
90781	IV therapy each additional hour
90784	IV injection
94761	Oximetry
99070	Surgical tray/IV tubing/supplies

*Health Care Financing Administration (HCFA) allows additional payment for a tray for this procedure when performed in a physician's office. Charge appropriately using code "99070—surgical tray."

ICD-10-CM DIAGNOSTIC CODES

C15.3	Carcinoma (Ca), esophagus, upper third
C15.4	Ca, esophagus, middle third
C15.5	Ca, esophagus, lower third
C16.4	Ca, stomach, pylorus

Upper Endoscopy Report—EGD

Date:_____ Referring Clinician: _____

Endoscopist:_____

Indications/preprocedure diagnosis: _____

_____

Physical Exam:

Neurologic Status: ❑ Alert   Airway: ❑ patent   Dentures Y/N

Heart: ❑ RRR ❑ No murmur

Lungs: ❑ Normal breath sounds

Abdomen: ❑ Nondistended ❑ Nontender ❑ No masses

_____

Medications: Versed _____mg Demerol _____mg Fentanyl_____ mcg

Propofol_____mg

Findings: endoscope passed to _____ part of duodenum _____

Vocal Cords:

Esophagus:

Sniff Test:

Stomach:

Cardia

Fundus

Body

Antrum

Pylorus

Duodenum:

Bx for H. pylori ___x4

Pyloritek results ____

Complications:_____

Impression:

_____
_____
_____

Recommendations:

_____
_____

_____

Signature of Endoscopist (____dictated)

cc _____   _____

Endoscopist

Fig. 91.18 Upper endoscopy report.

C16.3	Ca, stomach, antrum	D13.1	Benign lesion, stomach
C16.1	Ca, stomach, fundus	D13.2	Benign lesion, duodenum
C16.2	Ca, stomach, body	J04.0	Acute laryngitis
C17.0	Ca, duodenum	J37.1	Chronic laryngotracheitis
D13.0	Benign lesion, esophagus	K22.10	Esophageal ulcer

K22.2	Esophageal stricture
K22.5	Esophageal diverticulum
K22.6	Mallory-Weiss tear
K20.9	Esophagitis, unspecified
K21.0	Esophagitis, reflux
K20.9	Acute esophagitis
K21.9	Esophageal reflux
K22.6	Esophageal hemorrhage
K22.9	Esophageal leukoplakia
K25.0	Gastric ulcer, acute with hemorrhage (hem)
K25.4	Gastric ulcer, chronic with hem
K25.9	Gastric ulcer, chronic
K26.0	Duodenal ulcer, acute with hem
K26.4	Duodenal ulcer, chronic with hem
K26.7	Duodenal ulcer, chronic
K56.699	Other intestinal obstruction
K29.00	Acute gastritis
K29.01	Acute gastritis with hem
K29.40	Atrophic gastritis
K29.80	Duodenitis
R11.10	Persistent vomiting
K30	Dyspepsia
K31.4	Gastric diverticulum
K44.9	Hiatal hernia
K92.0	Hematemesis
R49.8	Hoarseness
R06.89	Wheezing
R07.9	Chest pain
R11.2	Nausea and vomiting
R12	Heartburn (i.e., pyrosis)
R13.10	Dysphagia
R14.2	Belching
R10.9	Abdominal pain
R93.3	X-ray abnormality, GI tract
Z80.0	Family history, GI tract Ca (not primary diagnosis)
Z83.79	Family history, GI disorders (not primary diagnosis)

SUPPLIERS

Full contact information is available at www.expertconsult.com.

CME courses
ASGE VideoGIE: www.asge.org/quicklinks/gie-videogie

The National Procedures Institute (for hands-on training with simulators): www.npinstitute.com

American Association for Primary Care Endoscopy (annual meeting for excellent, up-to-date lectures): www.aapce.wildapricot.org/

Gastroscopes and transnasal esophagoscopes
Fujinon Medical

Olympus America

Pentax Medical Company

Patient education materials
ASGE (online videos)

The National Procedures Institute (DVDs)

Vital signs monitor
Welch Allyn

RECOMMENDED READING

American Academy of Family Physicians. *EGD, Training and Credentialing of Family Physicians in*; 2017 (Position Paper), originally approved 2002, updated. https://www.aafp.org/about/policies/all/egd-training.html.

American Society for Gastrointestinal Endoscopy (ASGE). Standards of Practice Committee: guideline on the management of antithrombotic agents for patients undergoing GI endoscopy. *Gastrointest Endosc.* 2016;83(1):3–16.

American Society for Gastrointestinal Endoscopy (ASGE). Methods of granting hospital privileges to perform gastrointestinal endoscopy. *Gastrointest Endosc.* 2002;55:780–783.

Bittner JG, Marks JM, Dunkin BJ, et al. Resident training in flexible gastrointestinal endoscopy: a review of current issues and options. *J Surg Educ.* 2007;64:399–409.

Bull-Henry K, Al-Kawas FH. Evaluation of occult gastrointestinal bleeding. *Am Fam Physician.* 2013;87(6):430–436.

Council of Academic Family Medicine (CAFM). *Consensus statement for procedural training in family medicine residency.* https://afmrd.socious.com/d/do/966. Accessed July 29, 2018.

Deitch K. Systemic analgesia and sedation for procedures. In: Roberts JR, Custalow CB, Thomsen TW, eds. *Roberts and Hedges Clinical Procedures in Emergency Medicine and Acute Care.* 6th ed. Philadelphia: Elsevier; 2019:594–619.

Douketis JD, Spyropoulos AC, Katz S, Becker RC, Caprini JA, the BRIDGE study group, et al. Perioperative bridging anticoagulation in atrial fibrillation. *N Engl J Med.* 2015;373:823–833.

Eisen GM, Dominitz JA, Faigel DO, et al. An annotated algorithmic approach to acute lower gastrointestinal bleeding. *Gastrointest Endosc.* 2001;53:859–863.

Fashner J, Gitu AC. Diagnosis and treatment of peptic ulcer disease and H. pylori infection. *Am Fam Physician.* 2015;91(4):236–242.

Hernandez-Diaz S, Rodriguez LA. Incidence of serious upper gastrointestinal bleeding/perforation in the general population: review of epidemiologic studies. *J Clin Epidemiol.* 2002;55:157–163.

Huang JQ, Sridhar S, Hunt RH. Role of Helicobacter pylori infection and non-steroidal anti-inflammatory drugs in peptic ulcer disease: a meta-analysis. *Lancet.* 2002;359:14–22.

Kelly BF, Sicilia JM, Forman S, Ellert W, Nothnagle M. Advanced procedural training in family medicine: a group consensus statement. *Fam Med.* 2009;41(6):398–404.

Layke JC, Lopez PP. Gastric cancer: diagnosis and treatment options. *Am Fam Physician.* 2004;69:1133–1140, 1145–1146.

Lewis JD, Brown A, Localio AR, Schwartz JS. Initial evaluation of rectal bleeding in young persons: a cost-effectiveness analysis. *Ann Intern Med.* 2002;136:99–110.

Practice Guidelines for Moderate Procedural Sedation and Analgesia, 2018. A Report by the American Society of Anesthesiologists Task Force on Moderate Procedural Sedation and Analgesia, the American Association of Oral and Maxillofacial Surgeons, American College of Radiology, American Dental Association, American Society of Dentist Anesthesiologists, and Society of Interventional Radiology. *Anesthesiology.* 2018;128:437–479.

Reed W, Kilkenny J, Dias D, Wexner S, SAGES EGD Outcomes Study Group. a prospective analysis of 3525 esophagogastroduodenoscopies performed by surgeons. *Surg Endosc.* 2004;18:11–21.

Rodney WM, Hocutt Jr JE, Coleman WH, et al. Esophagogastroduodenoscopy by family physicians: a national multisite study of 717 procedures. *J Am Board Fam Pract.* 1990;3:73–79.

Siegal D, Yudin J, Kaatz S, Douketis JD, Lim W, Spyropoulos AC. Periprocedural heparin bridging in patients receiving vitamin K antagonists: systematic review and meta-analysis of bleeding and thromboembolic rates. *Circulation.* 2012;126:1630–1639.

Sharma VK, Coppola AG, Raufman JP. A survey of credentialing practices of gastrointestinal endoscopy centers in the United States. *J Clin Gastroenterol.* 2005;39:501–507.

Society of American Gastrointestinal Endoscopic Surgeons. *Granting of Privileges for Gastrointestinal Endoscopy.* SAGES Publication No. 0011; 2001.

The Joint Commission. *Joint Commission Comprehensive Accreditation and Certification Manual for 2017.* Oak Brook, IL: Joint Commission Resources; 2017.

Wilkins T, Khan N, Nabh A, Schade RR. Diagnosis and management of upper gastrointestinal bleeding. *Am Fam Physician.* 2012;85(5):469–476.

PERCUTANEOUS ENDOSCOPIC GASTROSTOMY PLACEMENT AND REPLACEMENT

Stephen L. Twyman • Paul W. Davis

Percutaneous endoscopic gastrostomy (PEG) is the placement of a percutaneous gastrostomy tube with the aid of an endoscope. The PEG technique has largely replaced surgical gastrostomy as the procedure of choice for patients who require long-term enteral nutrition. It was first described in 1980 by Gauderer and colleagues for use in children but has since gained wide acceptance for use in patients of all ages. Along with other necessary supplies, commercial PEG tube kits usually contain the PEG tube, an internal bolster (to seal the gastric mucosa), and an external bolster (to stabilize and prevent migration of the tube). Choices for the internal bolster include a balloon, a soft dome, crossbars, a T-bar, a flange, a disk, a three-leaf retainer, and others; most are soft to avoid irritating the gastric mucosa.

The actual PEG placement procedure requires two trained individuals, one of whom must be skilled in esophagogastroduodenoscopy (EGD). See Chapter 91, Esophagogastroduodenoscopy, for a full discussion of EGD; this chapter will be limited to the application of EGD for PEG placement. The procedure can be performed in the operating room, the endoscopy suite, or at the bedside. Normally, the procedure is performed under moderate sedation (see Chapter 1, Procedural Sedation and Analgesia, and Chapter 2, Pediatric Sedation and Analgesia), with a local anesthetic such as lidocaine also used at the cutaneous site (see Chapter 5, Local Anesthesia). However, if intravenous sedative agents are unlikely to be effective because of a history of prescribed or illicit controlled substance use, or if the patient is at risk of respiratory compromise secondary to oropharyngeal anatomy, risk of aspiration, or a history of obstructive sleep apnea, a third skilled provider will be needed to provide sedation and monitor the airway. Indeed, endotracheal intubation may be advisable because these patients often have underlying conditions that impair handling of secretions. In these circumstances, the assistance of an anesthesiologist, nurse anesthetist, or trained primary care colleague is advantageous.

After PEG placement, there is no reason for routine removal; however, occasionally they require replacement owing to accidental dislodgement or because they have become obstructed, worn out, kinked, or fractured. Although most of these problems can be avoided with diligent care, this chapter also briefly discusses PEG replacement.

INDICATIONS

Placement

The decision for PEG placement has to be made on a case-by-case basis, especially when rapidly progressive and incurable diseases are present. Certainly, this includes the various forms of severe dementia.

Most commonly, PEG tube placement is performed for patients who are unable or unwilling to ingest food orally. The usual conditions include major head and neck trauma, esophageal cancer, oropharyngeal cancers, cerebrovascular accidents, esophageal dysmotility, as well as other irreversible neurologic conditions such as amyotrophic lateral sclerosis. When used for provision of nutrients, the choice of PEG placement necessarily requires a functioning gastrointestinal tract and optimally involves a prior discussion with the patient or family concerning prognosis and underlying comorbid conditions. Other uses for the PEG procedure include treatment of gastric volvulus, decompression of patients with an intestinal obstruction or peritoneal carcinomatosis, administration of unpalatable medications to pediatric and mentally impaired patients, and enhanced enteral feeding of patients with hypercatabolic states, such as burn patients.

In brief, PEG tubes have two primary indications: enteral access for feeding or medication administration and decompression of the gut.

Replacement

- Accidental PEG dislodgement or removal
- PEG blockage or obstruction
- PEG damage (e.g., worn out, kinked, fractured)

CONTRAINDICATIONS

Placement

Absolute

In general, any contraindication to endoscopy will apply to PEG insertion as well. In addition, the absence of one of three prerequisites for safe PEG placement is a good reason to abort the procedure. These prerequisites include ability to distend the stomach endoscopically with air, endoscopically visible finger invagination of the anterior gastric wall, and transillumination of the anterior abdominal incision site. Additional absolute contraindications include the following:

- Pharyngeal obstruction (cannot perform EGD, surgery or interventional radiology may be options)
- Esophageal obstruction (cannot perform EGD, surgery or interventional radiology may be options)
- Active coagulopathy
- Peritonitis
- Sepsis
- Recent myocardial infarction
- Hemodynamic instability

Relative

Either esophageal or oropharyngeal cancer is considered a relative contraindication because there is a theoretical potential for seeding of the gastrocutaneous tract with cancer cells. Although this hazard is rare, it is primarily seen with untreated oropharyngeal cancers, with an incidence of less than 1% in one reported series (Cruz and colleagues, 2005). Some have advocated use of the Russel or "poke" technique (see later), radiographically placed, or surgically placed gastrostomy tubes as more appropriate in this setting. With these techniques, the PEG tube is not drawn down the esophagus for placement.

The presence of gastroesophageal reflux with its attendant risk of aspiration has long been considered a contraindication to PEG. Historically, a surgically placed or, more recently, a radiologically placed jejunostomy tube has been preferred. However, jejunostomy does not prevent gastroesophageal reflux and it is now known that PEG placement may actually decrease reflux because the PEG effectively creates an anterior pseudogastropexy.

Other relative contraindications include the following:

- Portal hypertension
- Moderate or massive ascites
- Gastric varices
- Prior abdominal surgery
- Peritoneal dialysis
- Hepatomegaly or splenomegaly
- Large hiatal hernia
- Large ventral hernia
- Open abdominal wound
- Prior subtotal gastrectomy
- Morbid obesity
- Anorexia nervosa
- Infiltrative or malignant disorders of the stomach
- Limited life expectancy
- Short-term (<30 days) need for enteral feeding

Replacement

Absolute

- Immature PEG tract (e.g., <4 weeks after PEG placement)
- Existing PEG tube not removable with gentle, constant traction (endoscopic guidance necessary)
- Nonreplaceable catheter (e.g., needle jejunostomy with 5- to 7-Fr catheter)

Relative

- Jejunostomy (the tract can be stented with a replacement catheter, but more information should be obtained before resuming feedings)
- Witzel gastrostomy (these use a more circuitous tunnel and a smaller tube and may be difficult to maneuver)

EQUIPMENT AND MATERIALS

Placement

The equipment list in Chapter 91, Esophagogastroduodenoscopy, applies equally to the endoscopy needs of PEG placement. This includes topical benzocaine (e.g., Cetacaine, Hurricaine) spray, if desired. In addition, the following equipment and supplies are recommended (usually included in commercial PEG kits):

- Gloves and equipment necessary for clinician to follow universal blood and body fluid precautions
- Lidocaine 1% to 2% for local anesthesia of the skin and abdominal wall
- 22- and 25-gauge needles
- 50- or 10-mL syringe
- Antiseptic preparation solution such as povidone–iodine or chlorhexidine
- Scalpel with No. 11 blade
- 4 × 4 gauze sponges
- Fenestrated drape
- Introducer trocar
- Guidewire (standard or looped end, depending on technique used)
- Disposable snare for gastroscope
- Abdominal binder (for confused or impaired patients)
- PEG tube with external bolster
- Surgical jelly for PEG tube lubrication
- Large, 50- to 70-mL (e.g., Toomey) syringe to aspirate gastric contents
- Adapter to attach Foley catheter to feeding assembly or to cap it off
- Jejunal tube (if warranted)
- Low-profile device (Fig. 92.1)

Replacement

- Gloves and equipment necessary for clinician to follow universal blood and body fluid precautions
- Antiseptic preparation solution such as povidone–iodine or chlorhexidine

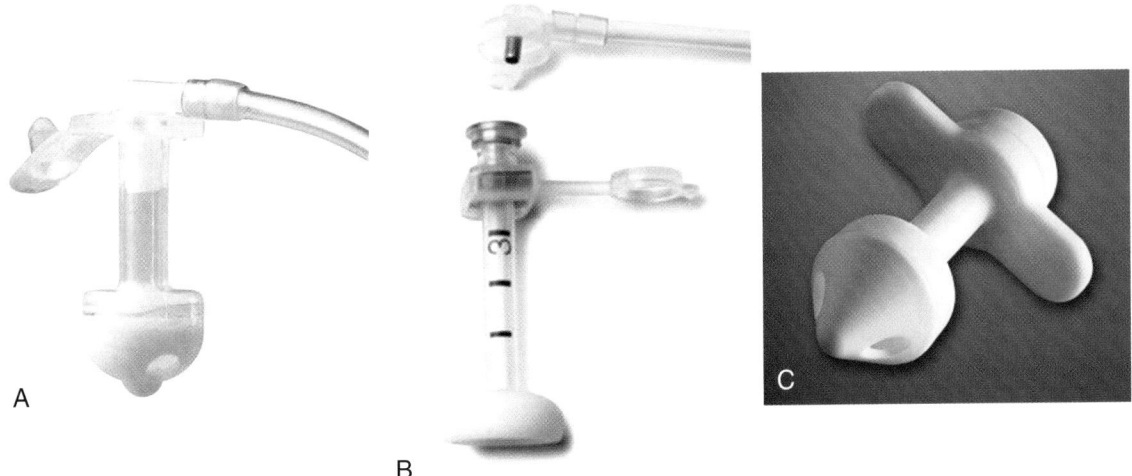

Fig. 92.1 Low-profile devices (LPD). (A) Bard Button. (B) Bard Gauderer "Genie." (C) Cook LPD.

- 4 × 4 gauze sponges and adhesive tape
- Surgical jelly for PEG tube lubrication
- Foley catheter or commercial PEG replacement kit with PEG tube of similar diameter to the original PEG
- External bolster (Options include a retainer for a nasogastric tube, a short length [3 cm] of latex or silicone tubing [cut from a Foley catheter or feeding tube] and a plastic cable tie to form a T-bar, or a 0 or 2-0 silk suture. Commercial bolster kits are available; however, they are expensive, are not always available, and often do not properly fit the replacement PEG tube.)
- Large, 50- to 70-mL (e.g., Toomey) syringe to aspirate gastric contents
- Adapter to attach Foley catheter to feeding assembly or to cap it off
- Low-profile device (see Fig. 92.1)

PREPROCEDURE PATIENT PREPARATION

The patient or legal guardian or family member who will be caring for the patient and assisting with tube feedings should be given a general description of EGD and the PEG placement or replacement procedure. Any available alternatives should be discussed. The possible risks and complications of these procedures need to be explained along with the symptoms and signs that might suggest late complications and problems. It is very important that caregivers be included in this conversation because patients requiring PEG frequently suffer from cognitive or neurologic impairments. Informed consent forms should be signed before EGD and PEG placement. It is prudent to provide a patient education handout and instructions to follow before the procedure(s). Diagrams and photographs are particularly useful for helping patients and families understand the anatomy and altered feeding pathway proposed with PEG placement.

Before PEG replacement, there may be an opportunity to explore with the patient or family whether PEG feeding is still the desired method of nutritional support. There may also need to be a discussion about PEG care to avoid the need for future replacement. The patient should experience minimal discomfort with PEG replacement; if there is more than minimal discomfort, the PEG should not be manipulated. Small children or anxious patients may benefit from mild sedation.

For PEG placement, it is essential to know if the patient is taking any anticoagulants or platelet-inhibiting medications and to withhold these for an appropriate interval before the procedure to minimize any risk of bleeding. The patient must have all solids and liquids withheld for at least 8 hours before the procedure to minimize risk of esophageal reflux and aspiration. Solids may need to be withheld for longer if diabetic gastroparesis or a similar neuropathic condition is present. The presence of a large phytobezoar in the gastric lumen may impair visualization of the gastric indentation by the assistant's finger as well as the sounding needle.

Antibiotic Prophylaxis

Although antibiotic prophylaxis is neither necessary nor recommended for endoscopic procedures according to the most recent American Heart Association guidelines (see Chapter 69, Antibiotic Prophylaxis), preprocedure antibiotic administration is recommended before PEG insertion because of the risk of infection of the gastrocutaneous tract from oropharyngeal and cutaneous flora. It is important to recognize that PEG placement is a "clean" procedure, not a sterile procedure, and every effort should be made to make it as clean as possible. Usually, a cephalosporin or fluoroquinolone is satisfactory unless special considerations are present, such as methicillin-resistant *Staphylococcus aureus* (MRSA) or *Enterococcus* colonization of the skin or oropharyngeal cavity. Refer to recommendations later in the discussion of abscess and wound infection in the section on "Postprocedure and Late Complications."

Consensus panels most often recommend cefazolin (1 or 2 g for most patients, 3 g for patients >120 kg), another cephalosporins, or

a fluoroquinolone because they meet the aforementioned criteria. If methicillin resistant *S. aureus* (MRSA) is a possibility, vancomycin should be considered. There may be benefit of preprocedure screening for MRSA if endemic. Different considerations should be made if resistant *Enterococcus* is possible. To maximize its effectiveness, intravenous perioperative prophylaxis should be administered within 30 to 60 minutes before the surgical incision. Antimicrobial prophylaxis should be of short duration to decrease toxicity and antimicrobial resistance and to reduce cost. However, repeat dosing should be considered for procedures lasting longer than 2 half-lives of the drug or in which there is excessive blood loss.

TECHNIQUE
Placement
Patient Positioning

1. The head of the patient's bed or gurney should be elevated 30 degrees to decrease the risk of aspiration of oral or gastric secretions.
2. The patient may be placed in either the left lateral decubitus or the supine position. Although the supine approach offers an added challenge for the endoscopist to identify the larynx and esophagus, this is more than compensated for by not having to rotate the patient after scope insertion.

Anesthetic Administration

3. At this point, moderate (conscious) sedation can be achieved with appropriate intravenous medications. Depending on the endoscopist's preference, the posterior oropharynx and hypopharynx can be anesthetized with a topical anesthetic such as benzocaine spray.

Endoscope Insertion and Evaluation

4. Before introducing the gastroscope, it is essential to examine the oral cavity and oropharynx for food, debris, and retained secretions, which are quite common in patients undergoing this procedure. It is important to manually remove or suction this material to prevent aspiration during the procedure.
5. The gastroscope is then introduced and passed into the hypopharynx. Esophageal intubation can be difficult because of underlying pathology or the patient's inability to follow commands to swallow. One technique that can be helpful is to pass a snare catheter through the working channel of the scope and then into the proximal esophagus posterior to the arytenoid cartilages on either side of the visualized vocal cords. The gastroscope is then advanced over the closed snare catheter into the esophagus. The catheter is then retracted into the working channel before proceeding with the procedure.
6. It is prudent to perform a complete diagnostic examination of the esophagus, stomach, and duodenum before PEG placement. One study from the 1990s found that 36% of patients scheduled for PEG tube placement had endoscopic findings, such as peptic ulcer disease or gastric outlet obstruction, that ultimately led to major changes in management or abandonment of the procedure. If a lesion is discovered that will require biopsy or some other therapy, this should be done after PEG placement.
7. Once the gastroscope is in the stomach, all residual fluid and food should be suctioned so that the stomach is completely empty. Occasionally, the standard-caliber endoscope cannot be passed beyond an esophageal stricture or tumor; use of a pediatric, slim, or ultrathin endoscope may be necessary. Rarely will esophageal dilation be required to advance the scope beyond an obstruction.

Identification of Percutaneous Endoscopic Gastrostomy Abdominal Insertion Site

8. Once the gastroscope is in the stomach, the second endoscopist (or trained assistant) can expose the anterior abdominal wall and carefully examine it for signs of transillumination. If necessary, the high light intensity feature on the light source can be used to help identify the insertion site. The assistant may also

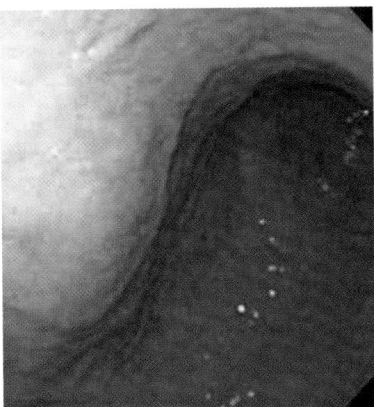

Fig. 92.2 Endoscopic visualization of finger indentation.

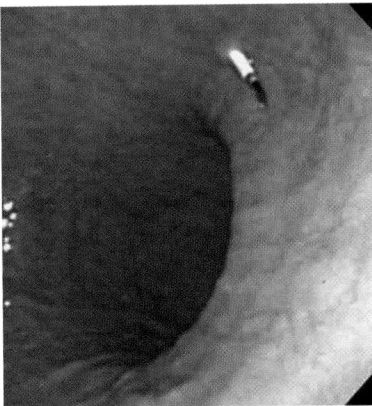

Fig. 92.3 Introducer trocar visualized entering the gastric lumen.

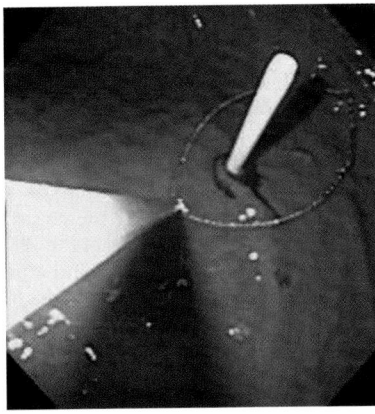

Fig. 92.4 The snare is advanced through the working port of the gastroscope and is seen looping around the introducer catheter.

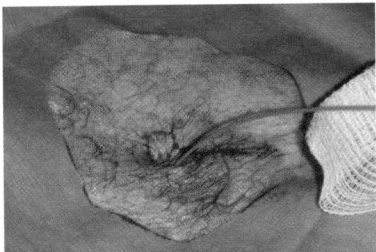

Fig. 92.5 The guidewire is advanced through the introducer catheter and the catheter is subsequently removed.

use a finger to palpate and indent the anterior abdominal wall; the endoscopist should then be able to visualize the corresponding indentation in the anterior wall of the stomach (Fig. 92.2).
NOTE: If a suitable site is not identifiable by either transillumination or finger palpation (preferably both), the procedure should be abandoned.

9. By convention, a PEG entry site is sought in the left upper quadrant of the abdomen, although a site to the right of midline is satisfactory as well. A site located a few centimeters below the costal margin will be more comfortable for the patient in the long run and will help prevent inadvertent laceration of the liver or spleen. Many endoscopists prefer a more distal site, in the anterior antrum. If the initial or subsequent plan is to convert the PEG to a jejunal enteral tube (PEG-J), an antral entry site will facilitate its advancement through the pylorus and beyond the ligament of Treitz, a measure found to minimize the risk of retrograde migration of the jejunostomy tube.

10. The assistant then prepares the anterior abdomen with an antiseptic solution, changes into sterile gloves, and covers the chosen site with a fenestrated sterile drape. Commercial PEG kits usually include a local anesthetic such as lidocaine along with a syringe, a 22-gauge needle, and a 25-gauge needle. The anesthetic can be drawn up into the syringe using the 22-gauge needle and the smaller needle can be used to raise a skin wheal at the proposed entry site. The longer 22-gauge needle can then be reattached to the syringe.

11. As the assistant then passes the sounding needle through the abdominal wall into the stomach, the endoscopist watches for entry of the needle through the gastric wall. Some endoscopists recommend keeping slight negative pressure on the syringe plunger while the needle is advanced; if air enters the syringe before visualization of the needle in the gastric lumen, it can be presumed that the needle has entered another hollow viscus such as the colon or a loop of small intestine. The needle is then withdrawn and another insertion site sought.

Percutaneous Endoscopic Gastrostomy Tube Placement

12. Once a suitable PEG insertion site has been identified, the assistant injects an additional 3 to 5 mL of anesthetic intradermally, and a No. 11 scalpel blade is used to make a horizontal or vertical skin incision.

13. While the assistant obtains the needle catheter from the PEG kit, the endoscopist can advance the snare catheter through the working channel of the gastroscope and into the gastric lumen.

14. The assistant then inserts the catheter rapidly through the skin incision and into the gastric lumen (Fig. 92.3), making certain that the catheter is directed at the same angle with respect to the skin as was just used with the sounding needle. This rapid "poke" should not be too slow or cautious; an assertive poke is necessary to ensure that the tip of the catheter successfully penetrates the tough gastric serosa instead of merely rebounding from the gastric wall.

15. As soon as the tip of the needle catheter enters the gastric lumen, the endoscopist snares it to hold it in place (Fig. 92.4). The assistant then withdraws the inner needle, leaving the outer plastic "introducer catheter" in place.

"PULL" TECHNIQUE: This is the most commonly used method of PEG placement, accounting for approximately 90% of PEGs.

16. A looped guidewire is threaded through the catheter (Fig. 92.5) and this is grasped with the snare.

17. The endoscope, along with snared guidewire, is withdrawn through the esophagus and out of the mouth under direct visualization.

18. The looped guidewire is then released and looped to the wire guide for the gastrostomy tube included in the kit.

19. The "skin" assistant pulls on the guidewire where it enters the abdominal wall to advance the gastrostomy tube through the mouth, esophagus, and into the stomach.

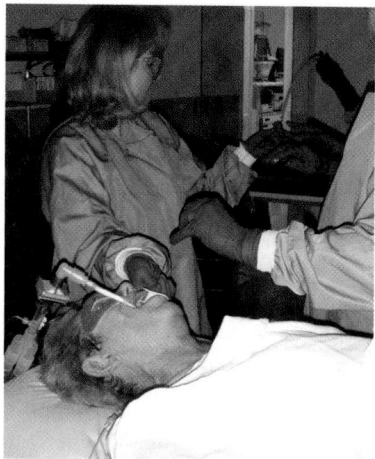

Fig. 92.6 Threading the "push" percutaneous endoscopic gastrostomy tube over the guidewire.

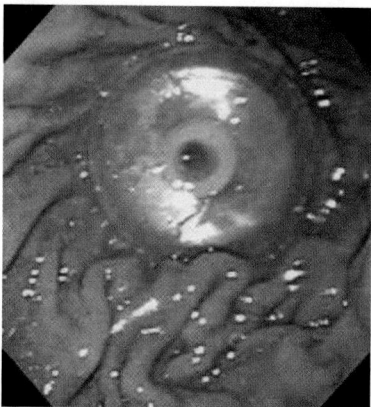

Fig. 92.7 Endoscopic image of proper placement of internal bolster.

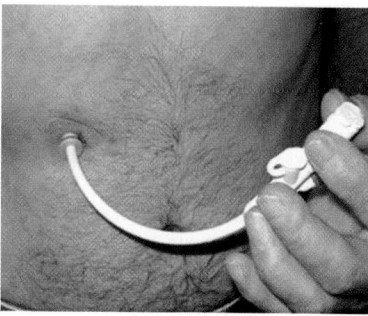

Fig. 92.8 Final result with percutaneous endoscopic gastrostomy tube in place after tract has healed completely.

20. As the guidewire exits the abdominal incision, the tapered gastrostomy tip will follow. It should be advanced until the terminal bumper is snug against the anterior gastric wall.
21. Finally, the assistant disconnects the looped guidewire from the gastrostomy tube assembly.

"PUSH" TECHNIQUE: Alternatively, the "push" (or Sacks-Vine) technique can be used.

16. A standard (nonlooped) guidewire is threaded through the catheter (see Fig. 92.5) and grasped with the snare.
17. The endoscope and snared guidewire assembly is withdrawn as a unit through the esophagus and out of the patient's mouth. Enough of the guidewire has to be threaded out of the mouth

to enable the gastrostomy tube to be completely threaded over the guidewire (Fig. 92.6) so that it extends beyond the internal bolster on the proximal end.

18. Both ends of the guidewire are then grasped in such a fashion as to create slight tension. The endoscopist maintains a firm grasp on this proximal end of the guidewire while the "skin" assistant maintains control of the abdominal end.
19. The endoscopist then advances the gastrostomy tube over the taut guidewire, through the patient's mouth, esophagus, and stomach, eventually pushing the internal bolster into the patient's mouth until the dilating tip protrudes through the abdominal wall.
20. The assistant then pulls the gastrostomy tube through the abdominal wall until the internal bolster is snug against the anterior gastric wall.
21. Finally, the guidewire is removed from the abdominal end.

Postprocedure Endoscopy

22. The endoscope is reinserted after the gastrostomy has been pulled or pushed into place. This allows careful examination of the esophagus, stomach, and visible surrounding structures for any mucosal or other trauma caused during the procedure as well as confirmation of proper placement of the internal bolster adjacent to the anterior gastric wall (Fig. 92.7). A photograph is taken and any necessary biopsies are performed at this time.

Post–Percutaneous Endoscopic Gastrostomy Placement

23. Once appropriate positioning of the internal bolster is confirmed, the endoscope is removed and an external bolster is slipped into place with the aid of some lubricant applied to the protruding gastrostomy tube.
   NOTE: Extra care must be taken when placing the external bolster to make sure it is not too tight. This will prevent such complications as PEG site infection, tissue necrosis, PEG entry site leakage, and "buried bumper syndrome" (see section on "Postprocedure and Late Complications"). Optimal external bumper placement allows the clinician's gloved index finger to slip easily between the abdominal entry site and the bumper.
24. If necessary, trim excess PEG tubing with scissors, leaving enough tubing to be looped around and taped to the skin of the abdomen, about 13 to 15 cm. This is also an ideal length to allow a jejunal tube to be inserted through the PEG and advanced beyond the ligament of Treitz, if necessary.
25. After a few minutes have passed, allowing the stomach to decompress from air introduced during the procedure, a feeding adapter is placed into the external end of the PEG tube.
26. The PEG site is then cleaned with soap and water and a split 4 × 4 gauze sponge placed around the PEG tube but *over* the external bolster. This dressing is not placed under the bolster because this will only cause more pressure on the healing wound. Dressings are changed daily and the wound is kept clean until complete healing has occurred. Dressings are changed as needed thereafter (Fig. 92.8).
27. Orders should be written to initiate tube feedings, medication administration, and tube irrigation 4 hours after placement.

Special Considerations

Patients with unresected esophageal or oropharyngeal malignancies deserve special consideration; using either the "pull" or "push" technique raises the potential for seeding the abdominal wall with tumor cells. This is particularly true of oropharyngeal tumors. In many cases, long-term survival is not expected so the PEG can be placed in the usual fashion. If the PEG is to be placed for nutritional support before the planned tumor resection and there is a chance for long-term survival or cure, some endoscopists recommend the Russel or "introducer" method using a dilator with a peel-away sheath. This technique uses the Seldinger technique and fluoroscopy for placing an inflatable gastrostomy tube with an internal balloon bolster.

The endoscope is used for direct visualization as well as to provide mucosal counterpressure during PEG insertion. The balloon tip is then inflated and an external bolster placed to secure the device. Advantages include the low risk of direct contamination of the tract with oral flora or malignant cells as well as a single passage of the gastroscope during the procedure and the avoidance of mucosal injury by the PEG tube during transesophageal passage (Vargo and Ponsky, 2000).

Obese patients present a special challenge. Transillumination of the abdominal wall may not be successful and the thickness of the subcutaneous layer may preclude successful sounding of the gastric lumen with the 1.5-inch, 22-gauge needle. In this case, the PEG entry site can be identified by finger palpation alone, the skin and subcutaneous tissue anesthetized with lidocaine, and a transverse incision made with the scalpel down through the subcutaneous layer to the fascia. Transillumination should be possible at the base of the incision. Use of the high light intensity feature may be necessary and the stomach is then sounded with the 22-gauge needle, with additional local anesthetic provided for the patient's comfort.

Prior abdominal surgery is not an absolute contraindication to PEG placement but a PEG entry site should be found that is away from the surgical scar. Careful sounding can be performed using the technique described previously to identify an interposed air-filled viscus. If air enters the syringe before the sounding needle is seen in the gastric lumen by the endoscopist, the procedure should be aborted. Otherwise, a safe tract is confirmed by endoscopic visualization of the intragastric needle tip and concurrent aspiration of air from the syringe.

Technique

Replacement

Perhaps more commonly than placing a PEG tube, primary care clinicians may be called on to replace one. This may be due to the PEG becoming dislodged (which is more common in confused or uncooperative patients) or nonfunctional (due to blockage or obstruction, fracture, or leaking). Techniques for attempting to clear blockage are discussed in a following section. Partial dislodgement presents a unique diagnostic challenge and can present as pain, buried bumper syndrome, or PEG tube blockage. Diagnostic approaches are also described for those complications in the section on "Postprocedure and Late Complications." The management approach depends on the timing of dislodgement because the gastrocutaneous tract takes about 4 weeks to heal and mature. Therefore as much information as possible should be gathered about the existing or prior PEG tube, especially regarding the procedure used to place the PEG, how long ago it was placed, and the type of PEG and internal bolster.

Dislodged Percutaneous Endoscopic Gastrostomy, Closed Mature Tract (≥4 Weeks After Placement)

Depending on the age, maturation, and diameter of the PEG, tracts begin to close as soon as the tube is removed; therefore every effort should be made to replace a dislodged PEG tube as soon as possible. A lost tract may require a repeat procedure. Dilation of a closing PEG tract has been described using filiform catheters and followers adapted from urology (see Chapter 96, Bladder Catheterization [and Urethral Dilation]); however, consultation with a gastroenterologist or surgeon may be beneficial.

Dislodged Percutaneous Endoscopic Gastrostomy, Open Mature Tract (≥4 Weeks after Placement)

1. If the original PEG tube is in good condition, after the balloon is deflated it can simply be reinserted. Alternatively, a Foley catheter of similar diameter can be used. Either tube will act as a stent until a permanent replacement can be found.
2. Lubrication should be applied liberally to the tube being used for replacement, and it should then be gently inserted through the existing tract. This can be done without endoscopy.

NOTE: Do not advance the tube against significant resistance; advancement against anything more than mild resistance can result in complications. Replacement should be painless and not require dissection or force. If these conditions occur, the procedure should be aborted.

3. Make sure that the balloon is well within the gastric lumen, and then slowly and carefully reinflate it with saline. Gentle external traction on the PEG tube should then be used to draw the balloon snugly against the anterior gastric wall. Plans for a permanent replacement PEG tube can then be made.

NOTE: Inflation of the balloon within the gastrocutaneous tract can result in pain, hemorrhage, disruption of the tract, and even peritonitis.

4. Unless changes are deemed necessary, a permanent replacement PEG tube, often found in a commercial kit, should be similar in diameter and function to the original. Placement of a low-profile PEG tube (see Fig. 92.1) may prevent recurrence of dislodgement. Alternatively, a standard PEG tube can be used and an abdominal binder and mittens placed to prevent the patient from pulling the tube out again.

5. After any replacement, aspirate gastric contents with a large syringe or use gravity drainage of gastric contents to confirm placement. After the balloon is reinflated, pull the catheter snug to lodge the internal bolster against the anterior gastric wall, immediately behind the anterior abdominal wall. If there was any difficulty with replacement of the PEG tube, or if the return of gastric contents is equivocal, a water-soluble contrast study should be obtained before resuming feedings. This will also ensure proper positioning of the internal bolster. A small amount of water-soluble, radiopaque contrast material is injected through the PEG tube, and a flat plate radiograph of the abdomen obtained. It should show intraluminal distribution of the contrast material.

NOTE: If the patient is known to have a jejunostomy tube, after stenting the tract with a replacement catheter, more information should be obtained before resuming feeding.

6. Perhaps more important than for the original PEG tube, unless a low-profile version is used (see Fig. 92.1), special attention should be paid to securing the external bolster for a replacement PEG. After bolstering, the catheter should be at approximately 90 degrees to the skin and anterior abdominal wall. It should be fixated to prevent internal migration of the catheter. Initially, 4 × 4 gauze sponges can be stacked several inches to create a pyramid-shaped dressing and taped to the skin and PEG catheter. Another temporary option is to use the same equipment provided to secure a nasogastric tube. However, temporary bolsters should usually be converted to a more permanent bolster. One option is to wrap a short (3-cm) segment of latex tubing (cut from another Foley catheter or nasogastric tube) around the base of the PEG tube and secure it with a plastic cable tie. This short segment should be wrapped perpendicularly around the PEG tube at the skin level, and the resultant friction between the tubes should prevent PEG slippage or migration. Alternatively, a T-bar can be made from such a short segment by folding it in half and cutting small nicks from the two folded corners. After unfolding the segment, the tip of a hemostat can be inserted through the resulting two diamond-shaped holes, and across the short segment. The hemostat can then be used to grasp the distal end of the PEG tube and draw it through two diamond-shaped holes in the T-bar. Make sure the diamond-shaped holes are large enough to avoid compressing the PEG tube lumen. The T-bar can then be drawn to the appropriate location on the PEG tube, approximately 0.5 to 1 cm from the skin surface, to act as a bolster. As a final alternative, placing a suture in a manner similar to that used to secure a chest tube may also be effective. Take a large bite of skin adjacent to the PEG exit site; tie a loose square knot at skin level, and then wrap the loose ends of the remaining suture several times in opposite directions around the PEG tube, finally securing the suture to the PEG tube in a snug fashion with another knot. The resultant tube fixation should be firm but allow some slack to prevent pressure necrosis if the patient changes position.

7. After placement is confirmed and the PEG tube is bolstered, the end of the tube should be clamped, capped, or fitted with the appropriate feeding adapter.

Dislodged Percutaneous Endoscopic Gastrostomy, Immature Tract (<4 Weeks After Placement)

Management of early dislodgement (<4 weeks) is different. The stomach may have separated from the anterior abdominal wall, resulting in free perforation with spillage of gastric contents, peritonitis, fever, or sepsis. In this event, broad-spectrum antibiotics should be administered, a nasogastric tube placed, and surgical consultation obtained. If the stomach has not separated from the anterior abdominal wall, a PEG tube can be replaced endoscopically, either through the same site or through a new one. Alternatively, the tract may be allowed to close spontaneously and a replacement PEG placed in 7 to 10 days if the patient remains stable.

Nonfunctioning Percutaneous Endoscopic Gastrostomy Needing Replacement

Again, as much information as possible should be gathered about the existing PEG tube, especially regarding the procedure used to place the PEG, how long ago it was placed, and the type of PEG and internal bolster.

1. If the PEG has a balloon for an internal bolster, deflation of the balloon should allow removal and replacement. If the balloon will not deflate, which is not unusual in long-standing PEG tubes, the inflation port may be clogged or damaged. Careful insertion of a guidewire into the balloon port may unclog it. If this attempt is unsuccessful, slightly further insertion of the guidewire may rupture the balloon. Alternatively, the balloon can be drawn close to the anterior abdominal wall by putting tension on the PEG tube. A needle inserted through the PEG tube can then be used to rupture the balloon. If these fail, endoscopic rupture of the balloon may be necessary. Another option is to cut the PEG tube close to the ports, which may allow the balloon to deflate on its own. After cutting, a firm external grip must be maintained with a clamp or hemostat on the portion of PEG tube remaining within the patient to prevent migration down the gastrointestinal tract; such migration may require endoscopic or surgical retrieval. If the PEG tube gets away and migrates, the majority of tubes will pass the gastrointestinal tract without incident and they can often be followed with plain radiographs every 48 hours, but there are reported cases of bowel obstruction and perforation. Endoscopic or surgical retrieval may be necessary for hardware that does not pass within 2 to 3 weeks or if the patient experiences obstructive symptoms. The risk of obstruction increases in children younger than 6 years or weighing less than 40 kg.
2. If the type of internal bolster cannot be determined or if it is thought to be soft or pliable, the application of constant, gentle external traction often results in PEG removal. Most PEGs can be removed in this manner.

   NOTE: Never apply more than gentle traction when attempting to remove a PEG tube; either the internal bolster has become embedded in the gastric wall or it was not intended to be removed externally and will likely need to be removed endoscopically.

COMPLICATIONS

Although deaths are not often directly attributable to the procedure, perioperative and postprocedure survival after PEG placement is exceedingly poor. In one study of 714 patients, 5.6% of patients died within 7 days of the procedure, whereas 22%, 31%, and 48% were dead at 30 days, 60 days, and 1 year from the procedure, respectively. The primary hospitalization mortality rate was 11%, with 50% of these patients dying within 1 week of PEG placement. Preprocedure predictors of mortality include older age, hemodialysis, mechanical ventilation, cancer, and coronary artery disease. Median survival for patients older than 70 years was less than 6 months, with length of survival decreasing rapidly with older age (Smith and colleagues, 2008).

It is important to emphasize to patients and caregivers that studies suggest PEG placement does not significantly alter survival. On retrospective review, many patients could have been fed or hydrated through a nasogastric tube until recovery or death. Thus when obtaining informed consent, it is essential that the clinician emphasize both the direct technical risks of the PEG as well as the anticipated natural course of the patient's underlying medical condition(s). This being said, complications can be as high as 10% with PEG placement, with significant events ranging from 2% to 10%. These can be discussed in three categories: (1) complications of upper endoscopy, (2) direct complications of PEG placement, and (3) postprocedure complications.

Complications Associated with Endoscopy

The most common complications associated with endoscopy include aspiration, hypoxemia, hypotension, acute myocardial infarction, hemorrhage, and esophageal perforation. The cardiopulmonary complications are actually primarily related to moderate (conscious) sedation. Refer to the respective chapters for a full discussion, including prevention, identification, and treatment. Reported mortality rates for upper endoscopy are exceedingly low, on the order of 0.005% to 0.01%, but these studies primarily include healthy patients, not the severely debilitated and poorly nourished patients requiring PEG feeding tubes. Because the possible complications are serious, a careful and complete discussion with the patient or legal guardian before the procedure is essential.

Direct Complications of Percutaneous Endoscopic Gastrostomy Placement and Replacement (to a Lesser Degree)

- *Pneumoperitoneum:* This finding is very common (35% to 50% incidence) and usually follows a benign course. It results from air escaping from the stomach during the course of a prolonged EGD during PEG placement, possibly compounded by multiple abdominal needle punctures and excessive air insufflation. Conservative management is usually acceptable. If the patient develops signs of increasing intra-abdominal air, sepsis, peritonitis, a systemic inflammatory response, or air in the portal or mesenteric veins, surgical consultation will be necessary (Vargo and Ponsky, 2000).
- *Abdominal wall bleeding:* This is usually identified soon after PEG placement and is caused by nicking or puncturing an abdominal wall blood vessel. Risk can be minimized by avoiding a tract near the midline through the rectus abdominis muscle. Hemostasis can often be obtained by tightening the external bolster against the abdominal wall to provide compression. Care must be taken to loosen the bolster again within 48 hours to prevent skin and mucosal maceration and ulceration. If bleeding is significant, standard resuscitative measures should be used. A standard crash cart should always be immediately available whenever an endoscopic procedure is performed.
- *Intraperitoneal and retroperitoneal bleeding:* Symptoms and signs that this has occurred include hypotension, decreasing hemoglobin or hematocrit, abdominal pain, a rigid abdomen, and an absence of blood seen endoscopically. It can occur from laceration of the liver, spleen, or a deep blood vessel. Diagnosis is confirmed by point of care ultrasound (POCUS) or computed tomography (CT) imaging and treatment is by immediate surgery. Surgical consultation with possible evacuation of the hemoperitoneum, repair of any solid organ injury, control of bleeding, and revision of the gastrostomy is indicated.
- *Colon injury:* Prior abdominal surgery or anatomic variation may result in the transverse colon being displaced over the anterior gastric wall. Careful attention to the special instructions provided

previously for PEG placement will minimize this complication. The usual presentation is peritonitis and the appropriate intervention is usually intravenous antibiotics and surgery. Occasionally, nonoperative management can be considered if the patient is hemodynamically stable and there are no signs of sepsis.

- *Hepatic injury:* This complication has been described only rarely and can be prevented by careful attention to the precautionary steps during placement. Close observation is often all that is necessary unless there is associated hemorrhage.
- *Splenic injury:* Splenic perforation or rupture has never been reported with PEG placement but has occurred rarely with other upper endoscopic procedures. It should be suspected if the patient develops hypotension or abdominal pain and resuscitation should immediately be initiated intravenously with crystalloid solution until blood is available. If the patient is hemodynamically stable, confirmation can be made by POCUS or CT. Immediate surgical consultation with laparotomy and splenectomy is necessary if the patient becomes unstable.
- *Small bowel injury:* Small bowel perforation is often occult and difficult to diagnose early. Fortunately, this complication is rare because the small intestine is protected by the greater omentum, which prevents it from migrating into the upper abdomen. However, if the patient has postoperative adhesions or the omentum has been previously resected, this injury can occur. It becomes clinically significant if there is intra-abdominal leakage and consequent peritonitis or if an enterocutaneous fistula develops. Fistulas often come to light only after the PEG is manipulated or replaced.
- *Gastro-colo-cutaneous fistula:* This is a rare complication of PEG placement and occurs when the PEG is inserted directly through the lumen of the large bowel into the stomach, usually near the splenic flexure. The patient may have transient ileus or fever but often remains asymptomatic for months, the diagnosis being made only after gastrostomy tube replacement. In most cases, there is no evidence of stool leakage or fistula formation. If the replacement tube is inserted into the colon rather than the stomach, diarrhea becomes evident when feedings are restarted. This complication is prevented by careful attention to the details outlined in the Technique section. Good transillumination and finger palpation are paramount to avoidance. The diagnosis is made radiographically by introducing contrast through the PEG tube. Most can be managed nonsurgically by removing the PEG and allowing the fistula to close spontaneously. A surgeon can be consulted if an abscess forms or peritonitis develops.

Postprocedure and Late Complications Related to Percutaneous Endoscopic Gastrostomy Placement and Replacement

- *Pain at the PEG site:* This complication is also the primary presenting symptom of many of the complications listed in this section. Careful attention to proper technique during PEG placement and proper cleanliness and care after placement are essential to preventing pain and discomfort. An attentive and prudent diagnostic approach to uncover the cause of pain will usually be rewarded.
- *PEG tube blockage or obstruction:* This problem is extremely common, occurring in up to 45% of patients. Prevention is the key, with liberal PEG tube flushing using 30 to 60 mL of water every 4 hours with a large syringe. This should also be performed after feeding and medication administration, as well as after checking residual volumes. Saline solutions should be avoided because the salt tends to crystallize in the channel and gradually form a blockage. Liquid formulations of medication are preferred and bulking agents such as psyllium seed and resins such as cholestyramine should be avoided. A variety of treatments are effective for unclogging PEG tubes. Plain warm water has been shown to be the best irrigant, with carbonated beverages also proving effective. Pancreatic enzymes mixed with bicarbonate have been effective for dissolving more resistant proteinaceous blockages,

with the solution being allowed to sit in the tube for several hours before flushing copiously with warm water. If these methods prove ineffective, commercially available plastic brushes can be used to manually clear the tube. Bionix Medical Technologies supplies tube decloggers in two lengths and several diameters for clearing clogs in gastrostomy and jejunostomy tubes. Wires and metal brushes should be avoided because of risk of perforation. Endoscopic snares, biopsy forceps, or Fogarty catheters have been used successfully; however, consultation with a gastroenterologist or surgeon may be helpful. Before any of these maneuvers, make sure the tube is not kinked at the bolster; merely unkinking it may correct the blockage.

NOTE: Do not force irrigation fluid into the PEG tube because it may rupture and injure the patient.

- *Abscess and wound infection:* Peristomal wound infection is common in patients not receiving perioperative antibiotics. The incidence is 18% and can be reduced to about 3% with appropriate antibiotic prophylaxis. MRSA has emerged as a significant pathogen, and at least one study has shown that nasopharyngeal decontamination before planned PEG insertion can result in a significant reduction in the incidence of wound infections (Horiuchi and colleagues, 2006). If the patient has been hospitalized or institutionalized for a prolonged period or if there is any suspicion of colonization, a nasopharyngeal culture and sensitivity should be performed. A 10-day course of an appropriate antibiotic (trimethoprim/sulfamethoxazole, clindamycin, or vancomycin) is recommended before PEG placement. A confirmatory test to ensure MRSA eradication should be performed before the procedure.
- *Peristomal leakage:* This is a very common and significant problem that is often seen in patients with diabetes, immunodeficiency, and malnutrition. Other factors that have been implicated include wound infection, peristomal abscess, hypersecretory syndromes, traction on the PEG tube, and buried bumper syndrome. Treatment is aimed at correcting these underlying conditions as well as using barrier creams such as zinc oxide. If hypersecretion is thought to be a contributing factor, agents such as hyoscyamine or glycopyrrolate can be administered. Replacing the PEG tube with a tube of larger diameter should be avoided because this frequently only exacerbates the problem. If all else fails, the PEG tube can be removed for a few days, any infection treated, and the tract allowed to heal, scar, and partially close before a new tube is placed. Alternatively, the PEG tube can be removed completely and a new PEG site chosen.
- *Diarrhea:* Diarrhea is common among patients receiving enteral feeding, occurring in 10% to 20% of patients. The possible causes are manifold, including infection, protein malnutrition, medications, and administration of hyperosmolar enteral solutions. Patients can also have other dietary contributors, including lactose intolerance, fat malabsorption, or celiac disease. Common pharmaceutical culprits include magnesium-containing antacids, proton pump inhibitors (PPIs), antibiotics, prokinetic agents such as metoclopramide, and hyperosmolar drug solutions. Management involves identifying the etiology and treating the patient accordingly. Protein malnutrition may require nutritional supplementation and delivery of isotonic feedings in the interim. Discontinuing unnecessary medications, using intravenous alternatives, and changing to a different brand or class of medication are all useful strategies. Antidiarrheals such as loperamide are useful for some patients with medication-associated diarrhea. It is important to rule out pseudomembranous colitis and the rare cases of enterocutaneous or gastro-colo-cutaneous fistula if diarrhea persists in spite of standard diagnostic and therapeutic measures.
- *Gastrointestinal bleeding and ulceration:* Gastrointestinal bleeding is a relatively infrequent late complication and occurs in about 2% of patients. It is caused by esophagitis, peptic ulcer disease, gastric pressure ulcers, and, rarely, erosion of the PEG tube into a gastric wall blood vessel. Once endoscopic diagnosis is

determined, bleeding caused by a punctured gastroepiploic vessel in the stomach wall can be treated by tightening the external bolster against the abdominal wall, thus internally compressing the bleeding vessel. Care should be taken to loosen the bumper again within 48 hours to prevent pressure necrosis. Esophagitis and peptic ulcers can both be prevented and treated with PPIs; histamine type 2 receptor antagonists have not been noted to be very effective, especially in the former case. Gastric pressure ulcers are caused by the PEG tube and can occur either anteriorly, from direct pressure of the internal bolster, or posteriorly, caused by tall internal bolsters or protruding tips from Foley-type PEG tubes. Treatment is removal of the offending tube and replacement, which can often be done nearby (Fig. 92.9). Use of a low-profile device or a balloon-tipped device with a short (<3 mm) protruding tip for the replacement may minimize risk of recurrence. Use of a PPI alone will often be insufficient to heal these ulcers.

- *Ileus and gastroparesis:* Occasionally, postprocedure gastroparesis develops and can take longer than the usual 3 to 4 hours to resolve. Metoclopramide, erythromycin, or domperidone can be administered with good results in most cases. However, if persistent vomiting or abdominal distention occurs, the PEG should be unclamped to allow decompression and feedings should be discontinued for 24 to 48 hours. If abdominal distention and pain persist, an ileus should be suspected and perforation and peritonitis need to be ruled out. Often the cause is merely excessive pneumoperitoneum from the PEG procedure. Treatment often consists of nasogastric tube decompression, discontinuance of contributing medications, and clinical support. Intravenous broad-spectrum antibiotics and surgical consultation may be required if perforation is suspected. Prolonged ileus can occur in up to 1% of cases (Lin and colleagues, 2001).

- *Aspiration:* The risk of aspiration during the PEG procedure has already been discussed. The risk of aspiration, however, is much greater as a late complication and increases with supine positioning, use of sedative agents, advanced age, and neurologic impairment. Unfortunately, these are precisely the risk factors that predispose patients to need PEG placement. Again, prevention is superior to treating the sequelae of aspiration. The primary clinician is advised to avoid excessive use of sedative agents and the patient/caretaker is instructed to keep the head of the bed elevated for several hours after feedings.

- *Gastric outlet obstruction:* The presenting complaint is usually intermittent vomiting or upper abdominal cramping and the cause is generally distal migration of the PEG tube. It is much more common with Foley-type gastrostomy tubes with the balloon lodging in the pyloric channel or duodenum, creating an intermittent obstruction. In children, a displaced internal bolster can get wedged in the gastric outlet. Prevention is the best approach by ensuring proper placement of the external bolster which prevents internal bolster migration. Diagnosis can be made by an upper gastrointestinal series or endoscopically. With the Foley-type tube, the balloon can be deflated and the tube repositioned and reinflated with proper external bolster positioning.

- *Buried bumper syndrome:* This is a rare (1% to 2%) but potentially serious complication that occurs late after PEG insertion, after an average of 4 months, but reported from 2 months to 7 years after PEG placement (Schrag and colleagues, 2007). The internal bumper retracts into the anterior gastric wall (Fig. 92.10) and becomes lodged at some point along the gastrocutaneous tract, resulting in either a partial or complete PEG obstruction. The gastric mucosa can completely reepithelialize the internal stoma, resulting in an inability to infuse feedings or medication. This is the usual presenting complaint, along with abdominal pain at the PEG site. Diagnosis can be made radiologically, endoscopically, by ultrasound, or by endoscopic ultrasound. The buried bumper should be removed regardless of whether the patient is symptomatic. Removal can be achieved surgically, endoscopically, or through a combination of approaches. Endoscopically, use of a

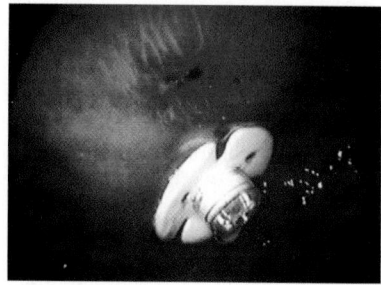

Fig. 92.9 Healing pressure ulcer at previous percutaneous endoscopic gastrostomy site with tube placed at new site.

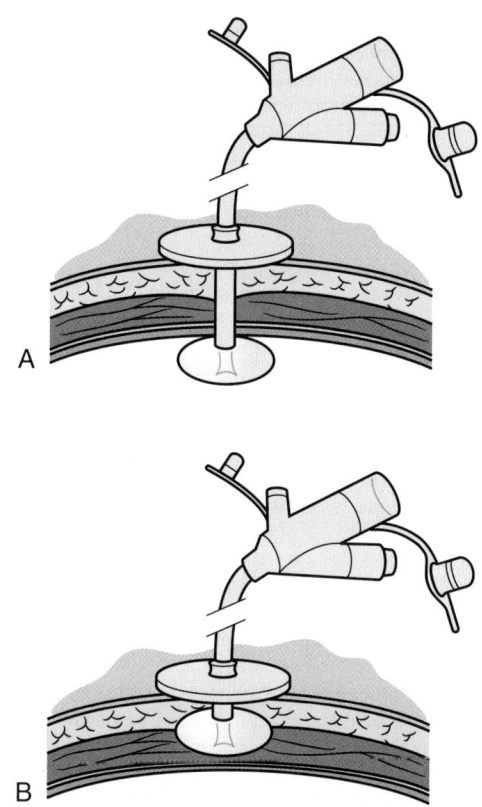

Fig. 92.10 Buried bumper syndrome. (A) Proper percutaneous endoscopic gastrostomy tube placement. (B) Buried bumper with regrowth of gastric mucosa over gastrocutaneous tract.

needle knife through the biopsy port has been found to be effective. A mucosal incision is made over the buried bumper to allow its mobilization and removal. A fresh PEG tube can then be inserted under endoscopic guidance. Occasionally, a more extensive surgical procedure is required.

- *Necrotizing fasciitis:* As noted earlier, pressure from the PEG tube and external bumper on the peristomal site can lead to this lethal complication. Patients who are diabetic, malnourished, or otherwise immunocompromised are predisposed and at increased risk, as are those with wound infections. Prevention is by proper placement and adequate spacing of the external bolster. There is good evidence that multiple aerobic and anaerobic organisms are synergistically responsible for necrotizing fasciitis. Treatment involves wide surgical debridement, broad-spectrum antibiotics, and planned operative reevaluation. Patients require transfer to the intensive care unit with extensive multisystem support.

- *PEG site herniation:* This complication has been reported only once in the literature and was a late sequela of deep ulceration. The diagnosis should be suspected whenever there is a peristomal bulge noted with Valsalva maneuver. It is confirmed by CT and repair, if indicated, is surgical.

- *Volvulus around PEG tube:* This rare complication is seen primarily in the pediatric population and can involve the small intestine, transverse colon, or stomach. It is more common if the PEG is introduced through the posterior wall of the stomach, which can lead to rotation of the gut and consequent volvulus. Prevention is by careful attention to placing the PEG through the anterior wall of the stomach with proper external bolster placement in order to achieve close apposition of the anterior gastric wall to the parietal peritoneum. Treatment requires surgical consultation with exploratory laparotomy, reduction of the volvulus, and repositioning of the gastrostomy. Gastropexy to the anterior abdominal wall may decrease the incidence of recurrence.

- *Tumor implantation in PEG tract:* As already mentioned, this late complication is extremely rare, occurring primarily in patients with oropharyngeal tumors and in less than 1% of this group. Direct seeding during the PEG placement is the accepted primary mechanism, although hematogenous or lymphatic spread is also thought to occur. This complication offers an exceedingly poor prognosis, with a 0% 1-year survival. Placement of the PEG after primary tumor resection or by using the Russell technique (non-endoscopic, using a peel-away catheter) is a reasonable approach to lowering the risk of seeding (Cruz and colleagues, 2005).

- *PEG tubes and pregnancy:* PEG tubes can be used successfully during pregnancy, although persistent emesis has been reported. Conversion of the PEG to a PEG-J may be attempted and has been reported to be successful in this condition (Wejda and colleagues, 2003).

- *Failure to provide adequate nutrition:* This can occur in a patient that is hypercatabolic, whether due to underlying malignancy or other hypercatabolic states. This can also occur in terminal dementia, despite provision of what should be adequate nutrition through a functioning PEG tube. It is due to unknown mechanism; however, as the brain fails, it makes sense that there would be denervation of catabolic or metabolic pathways.

POSTPROCEDURE CARE

The external visible portion of the PEG tube can be cleaned with soap and water using a clean 4 × 4 sponge. Antibacterial ointment is not required and could result in inflammation caused by an allergy to one of the ingredients. A split 4 × 4 tracheostomy sponge is then placed over the external bolster—not between the bolster and the skin, which will cause excessive compression of the skin of the abdominal wall and possibly result in ostomy breakdown or buried bumper syndrome. The PEG tube is then looped back over the bolster and taped to the skin. If the patient is confused or unreliable, an abdominal binder, and perhaps mittens, can be placed to prevent manipulation and inadvertent removal of the tube. After 6 to 8 weeks, when the gastrocutaneous tract has healed and matured, the PEG can be removed and replaced with a low-profile device (see Fig. 92.1). This device is level with the skin with no permanent tubing extending from the abdominal wall, thus minimizing the opportunity for the patient to dislodge it.

Dressings over the PEG site are changed daily until there is no longer any drainage. The tube and ostomy site can be cleansed daily or as needed with soap and warm water, taking care to debride excessive granulation tissue and dried secretions. Tube feeding, medication administration, and water flushes can be initiated 4 hours after placement. An example of postprocedure orders is available at www.expertconsult.com.

PATIENT EDUCATION GUIDES

The following materials are available at www.expertconsult.com:

- Sample post-PEG procedure instructions
- Sample patient consent form

Also see the patient education handouts for Chapter 1, Sedation and Analgesia, and Chapter 91, Esophagogastroduodenoscopy.

CPT/BILLING CODES

36000	Introduction of needle or intracatheter, vein
43234	Simple upper gastrointestinal endoscopy examination
43235	EGD, diagnostic, with or without brushings
43239	EGD, diagnostic, with biopsies
43246	EGD with directed placement of PEG tube
43760	Change of gastrostomy tube
94761	Noninvasive pulse oximetry for oxygen saturation; multiple determinations
96365	IV therapy, initial, up to 1 hour
96367	IV therapy each additional hour
96374	IV push, single or initial substance/drug
96376	IV push, each sequential new substance/drug

ICD-10-CM DIAGNOSTIC CODES

C15.5	Ca, esophagus, lower third
C15.4	Ca, esophagus, middle third
C15.3	Ca, esophagus, upper third
E43	Severe malnutrition unspecified
E44.1	Malnutrition, protein-calorie, moderate
E44.0	Malnutrition, protein-calorie, mild
E46	Malnutrition, protein-calorie, unspecified
K22.2	Esophageal stricture
K22.10	Esophageal ulcer without bleeding
K22.11	Esophageal ulcer with bleeding
K20.9	Esophagitis unspecified
K21.0	Esophagitis, reflux
K21.9	Esophageal reflux

SUPPLIERS

(See contact information available at www.expertconsult.com.)

FASTRAC "Pull" Gastric Access Port Kit
Bard Access Systems, Inc.
Gastroscopes
Fujinon Corp.
Olympus Corp.
Pentax Corp.
Patient education materials
American Society for Gastrointestinal Endoscopy
Bard Access Systems, Inc.
Wilson-Cook Medical Inc.

RECOMMENDED READING

Blum CA, Selander C, Ruddy JM, Leon S. The incidence and clinical significance of pneumoperitoneum after percutaneous endoscopic gastrostomy: a review of 722 cases. Am Surg. 2009;75(1):39–43.

Cosby KS. Gastrostomy tube replacement. In: Reichman E, Simon R, eds. Emergency medicine procedures. New York: McGraw-Hill; 2004:456–466.

Cruz I, Mamel JJ, Brady PG, Cass-Garcia M. Incidence of abdominal wall metastasis complicating PEG tube placement in untreated head and neck cancer. Gastrointest Endosc. 2005;62:708–711.

DeLegge MH. The experts corner: percutaneous endoscopic gastrostomy. Am J Gastroenterol. 2007;102:2620–2623.

Dormann AJ, Huchzermeyer H. Endoscopic techniques for enteral nutrition: standards and innovations. Dig Dis. 2002;20:145–153.

Gauderer MWL, Ponsky JL, Izant Jr RJ. Gastrostomy without laparotomy: a percutaneous endoscopic technique. J Pediatr Surg. 1980;15:872–875.

Horiuchi A, Nakayama Y, Kajiyama M, et al. Nasopharyngeal decolonization of methicillin-resistant *Staphylococcus aureus* can reduce PEG peristomal wound infection. *Am J Gastroenterol.* 2006;101:274–277.

Lin HS, Ibrahim HZ, Kheng JW, et al. Percutaneous endoscopic gastrostomy: strategies for prevention and management of complications. *Laryngoscope.* 2001;111:1847–1852.

McClave SA, Chang WK. Complications of enteral access. *Gastrointest Enosc.* 2003;58:739–751.

McClave SA. Techniques in enteral access. 3rd ed. *Clin Gastrointest Gastrosc.* 2018;42:467–487.e2.

Samuels LE. Nasogastric and feeding tube placement. In: Roberts JR, Custalow CB, Thomsen TW, eds. *Roberts and Hedges Clinical Procedures in Emergency Medicine.* 6th ed. Philadelphia: Elsevier; 2019: 828–851.

Schrag SP, Sharma R, Jaik NP, et al. Complications related to percutaneous endoscopic gastrostomy (PEG) tubes: a comprehensive clinical review. *J Gastrointest Liver Dis.* 2007;16:407–418.

Smith BM, Perring P, Engoren M, Sferra JJ. Hospital and long-term outcome after percutaneous endoscopic gastrostomy. *Surg Endosc.* 2008;22:74–80.

Vargo JJ, Ponsky JL. Percutaneous endoscopic gastrostomy: Clinical applications. *Medscape General Medicine.* 2000;2(4). www.medscape.com/viewarticle/407957.

Vargo JJ. Preparation for and complications of GI endoscopy. In: Feldman M, Friedman LS, Brandt LJ, eds. *Sleisenger and Fordtran's Gastrointestinal and Liver Disease.* 10th ed. Philadelphia: Elsevier; 2016:677–685.

Wejda BU, Soennichsen B, Huchzermeyer H, et al. Successful jejunal nutrition therapy in a pregnant patient with apallic syndrome. *Clin Nutr.* 2003;22:209–211.

CHAPTER 93

VIDEO CAPSULE ENDOSCOPY*

Matti Waterman • Edward G. Zurad • Ian M. Gralnek

Video capsule endoscopy (VCE) of the small bowel is one of the major advances in small bowel imaging over the last 2 decades. As it turns out, resolution with VCE is better than with most conventional endoscopes. Compared with other existing imaging modalities, VCE has been demonstrated to have the highest yield in the diagnosis of gastrointestinal (GI) hemorrhage of obscure origin, iron-deficiency anemia, small bowel tumors, suspected or early Crohn disease (CD), and several other medical conditions involving the small intestine. This relatively easy-to-use, minimally invasive procedure, requiring limited or no patient preparation and no sedation, has acquired enormous worldwide popularity since its clearance by the US Food and Drug Administration (FDA) in 2001. The original wireless capsule endoscope was the M2A small bowel capsule (now called Pillcam SB; Given Imaging Medtronic). The current version is the Pillcam SB3, which has improved resolution and a variable frame rate. In September 2007, the FDA cleared the Olympus Corporation's EndoCapsule; subsequently MiroCam from South Korea was approved. Capsocam is now also available; the OMOM capsule from the People's Republic of China has not yet received FDA approval. Pillcam ESO is now available to visualize the esophagus, and Pillcam COLON is available for patients who have failed colonoscopy. By 2008, it was estimated that over 600,000 capsules had been ingested worldwide and over 600 scientific articles regarding VCE had been published. Its popularity and simplicity make VCE a viable option in the office workup by primary care clinicians of patients with suspected small bowel disease. This chapter discusses indications for the procedure (Box 93.1), the procedure itself, the image reviewing process, the interpretation of common findings, patient instructions, and procedure-related complications and how to minimize them. Capsule endoscopy for the esophagus and the colon is still not as widely accepted and practiced; therefore these procedures are not discussed.

Obscure Gastrointestinal Bleeding

The source of GI bleeding remains unidentified in approximately 5% of patients and is thus referred to as "obscure." Obscure GI bleeding may be overt, as evidenced by clinical signs (melena or hematochezia), or occult and manifested as positive fecal occult blood testing or iron- deficiency anemia. By definition, obscure GI bleeding occurs when esophagogastroduodenoscopy (EGD) and colonoscopy are negative. In such cases further workup is required. The role of VCE in this diagnosis has been validated in two meta-analyses and is outlined in Fig. 93.1. In patients presenting with iron-deficiency anemia, VCE has a less validated role (Fig. 93.2). As has been shown in the aforementioned meta-analyses, VCE is the most sensitive diagnostic modality and is considered the first line in the diagnostic workup for obscure GI bleeding. Fig. 93.3 shows an example of bleeding in the small bowel as captured by the Pillcam.

Crohn Disease

Crohn disease (CD) is an idiopathic inflammatory disease involving the small bowel in approximately 75% of cases. Because no diagnostic gold standard exists, the diagnosis of CD in the small bowel is based on clinical, endoscopic, radiologic, and histologic findings. However, available diagnostic modalities are neither sensitive nor specific. As a result, appropriate drug therapy may be delayed. Furthermore, available endoscopic procedures (e.g., push enteroscopy) fail to visualize the entire small bowel distal to the ligament of Treitz; thus significant small bowel involvement may be missed. VCE has a role both in diagnosing suspected CD (Fig. 93.4) and in determining the extent of small bowel involvement in CD. VCE also has been shown to be more sensitive than other imaging modalities in detecting small bowel mucosal breaks and thus is very helpful in diagnosing early CD (Fig. 93.5) and in assessing mucosal healing after drug treatment and disease recurrence after surgery.

Small Bowel Tumors

The advent of VCE has resulted in a major shift in the diagnosis of small bowel tumors (Fig. 93.6). In the past, such tumors were usually diagnosed only during the workup of persistent abdominal pain or when obstructive symptoms appeared. Today approximately 80% of small bowel tumors that are detected by VCE are from referrals to for obscure GI bleeding evaluation. The estimated prevalence of small bowel tumors in VCE for obscure bleeding is 6.3% to 12.3%. There is preliminary evidence that VCE favorably changes the clinical outcome in such cases. Note that when small bowel obstructive symptoms are present, the initial workup should be push enteroscopy or double-balloon enteroscopy rather than VCE.

Inherited Polyposis Syndromes

The lifetime risk of duodenal and small bowel tumors in familial adenomatous polyposis may be as high as 5% to 12%. Other polyposis syndromes, including Peutz-Jeghers syndrome and juvenile polyposis, also portend increased risk for small bowel and duodenal cancers, with a relative risk of 13% for small bowel tumors in Peutz-Jeghers syndrome. This risk has led to a recommended screening schedule including EGD or small bowel barium series every 1 to 3 years. VCE has been shown be a sensitive surveillance tool for detecting small bowel polyps in this high-risk population, with a reported sensitivity of over 90%.

Celiac Disease

Celiac disease has a prevalence of approximately 1% in the general population and is diagnosed by clinical suspicion, serologic and histologic findings obtained by small bowel biopsy (biopsy results ranging from partial to total villous atrophy), and patient response

*Drs. Waterman, Zurad, and Gralnek have been consultants of Given Imaging, Yoqneam, Israel, the maker of Pillcam SB.

Abdominal pain
Celiac disease
Crohn disease
    Assessment of small bowel mucosal healing and evaluation
      of treatment
    Identification of postoperative disease recurrence
    Indeterminate colitis
    Suspected Crohn disease
Evaluation of abnormal small bowel imaging
Evaluation of drug-induced small bowel injury
Obscure gastrointestinal bleeding (most common indication)
    Iron-deficiency anemia
Occult (positive fecal occult blood test)
Overt (hematemesis, coffee-ground vomiting, melena, hema-
    tochezia)
Suspected small bowel tumor
Surveillance of inherited polyposis syndromes

to a gluten-free diet. VCE, which provides a high-resolution magnified view of the small bowel mucosa, can detect mucosal changes such as scalloping, mosaic pattern, loss of normal villous architecture, loss of small bowel folds, and nodularity (Fig. 93.7). These findings by capsule endoscopy have been correlated with the typical histologic findings of celiac disease. Moreover, VCE has been shown to have good sensitivity and excellent specificity in the diagnosis of celiac disease even in the detection of more subtle histologic changes. It appears that VCE has a role in the diagnosis of celiac disease when there is a strong clinical suspicion (typical symptoms or positive serology) and EGD with small bowel biopsy is either negative or inconclusive, or the patient does not tolerate or is unwilling to undergo EGD. Furthermore, when patients with diagnosed celiac disease on a strict gluten-free diet develop worrisome symptoms—such as weight loss, anemia, fever, bleeding, abdominal pain, or recurrence of malabsorption—or when results of abdominal imaging are abnormal (except for stricture), VCE is indicated to evaluate for small bowel malignancy or enteropathy-associated lymphoma. However, the diagnosis of the typical injury pattern seen with VCE in celiac disease requires considerable expertise, and such patients should probably be referred to specialized centers.

Monitoring Small Bowel Drug Effects or Side Effects

Several studies have shown that VCE is a sensitive tool to demonstrate small bowel injury caused by nonsteroidal antiinflammatory drugs (NSAIDs). In fact, VCE can readily detect erythema, erosions, ulcerations, and web-like strictures caused by NSAIDs even in asymptomatic subjects. There have also been recent reports of VCE being used to monitor response to immunosuppressive therapy to manage intestinal graft-versus-host disease.

CONTRAINDICATIONS

- Patients with known or suspected GI obstruction, strictures, or fistulas based on the clinical picture or preprocedure testing
- Intestinal pseudo-obstruction
- Gastroparesis (relative contraindication, endoscopy can be used to place VCE in the duodenum [see Equipment section for AdvanCE endoscopic delivery device])
- Extensive and active Crohn disease of the small bowel with or without strictures (relative contraindication)
- Patients with cardiac pacemakers, cardiac defibrillators, or other implanted electromedical devices (relative contraindication; the 2017 Canadian Association of Gastroenterology guidelines no longer consider it contraindication)

- Patients with swallowing disorders (relative contraindication, endoscopy can be used to place VCE in the duodenum)
- Young children (<10 years, relative contraindication; some indications now approved for children as young as 2 years)
- Women who are pregnant (relative contraindication)
- Extensive intestinal diverticulosis (relative contraindication)
- Previous abdominal or pelvic surgery (relative contraindication)
- Dementia (relative contraindication in advanced stages, that is, patients who cannot cooperate with swallowing of the capsule or who may inadvertently damage the equipment)

EQUIPMENT AND OVERVIEW OF THE VIDEO CAPSULE ENDOSCOPY SYSTEM

The capsule (Pillcam SB2) is a disposable device (11 × 26 mm) composed of a light source, lens, metal oxide semiconductor imager, battery, and transmitter (Fig. 93.8). The capsule has a slippery coating that allows easy ingestion and transit with normal intestinal peristalsis. The capsule coating also prevents adhesion of luminal contents and obstruction of the visual field. The battery life is approximately 7 to 8 hours, during which two images per second are acquired and transmitted to a recording device worn by the patient (Fig. 93.9). The images are acquired through the optical dome, creating a visual field of 140 to 176 degrees and a magnification of 8:1. In total, 50,000 to 60,000 images are acquired and transmitted by a sensor array (8 sensors)—located on the patient's chest and abdominal wall—to the recording device worn on the patient's belt (see Fig. 93.9). After 7 to 8 hours, the recorder and sensors are removed from the patient and the images are downloaded into a reporting and processing of images and data (RAPID) computer workstation (Fig. 93.10). A continuous video movie is thus created. Additional features that are currently used include an approximate localization system for each image, a blood detector, an image magnifier, and simultaneous viewing of two to four images.

In summary, the required equipment to perform small bowel VCE includes the following:

- Capsule endoscope
- Computer workstation including a data recorder, battery-charging cradle for the data recorder (Fig. 93.11), a sensor array set with disposable adhesive sleeves for sensor placement on the patient's abdominal wall, and color printer
- A diagram that describes how to locate the sensors on the patient's abdominal wall according to anatomic landmarks
- Drinking water and (disposable) cups for capsule ingestion
- Dark/dimmed light viewing room with a comfortable chair
- AdvanCE endoscopic VCE delivery device (US Endoscopy; optional)

PREPROCEDURE PATIENT PREPARATION

Although VCE is a minimally invasive procedure, there are potential procedure-associated risks that must be explained to the patient in detail before performing the procedure. Emphasis should be put on the *risk of capsule retention* (see later), *incomplete procedure*, and *missed diagnosis*. Time should be spent discussing the capsule ingestion procedure (mainly to reduce patient anxiety at swallowing a large capsule). For further information, the patient may be referred to several Internet sites (e.g., www.givenimaging.com). The patient should also be provided with a detailed information sheet explaining the VCE procedure (available at www.expertconsult.com). Immediately before the procedure, explain the alternatives and risks and have the patient sign an informed consent document (available at www.expertconsult.com).

Any history of dysphagia or neuromuscular disease that may interfere with swallowing the capsule should be carefully sought before capsule ingestion. History of bowel obstruction or symptoms suggesting partial obstruction—such as postprandial cramps,

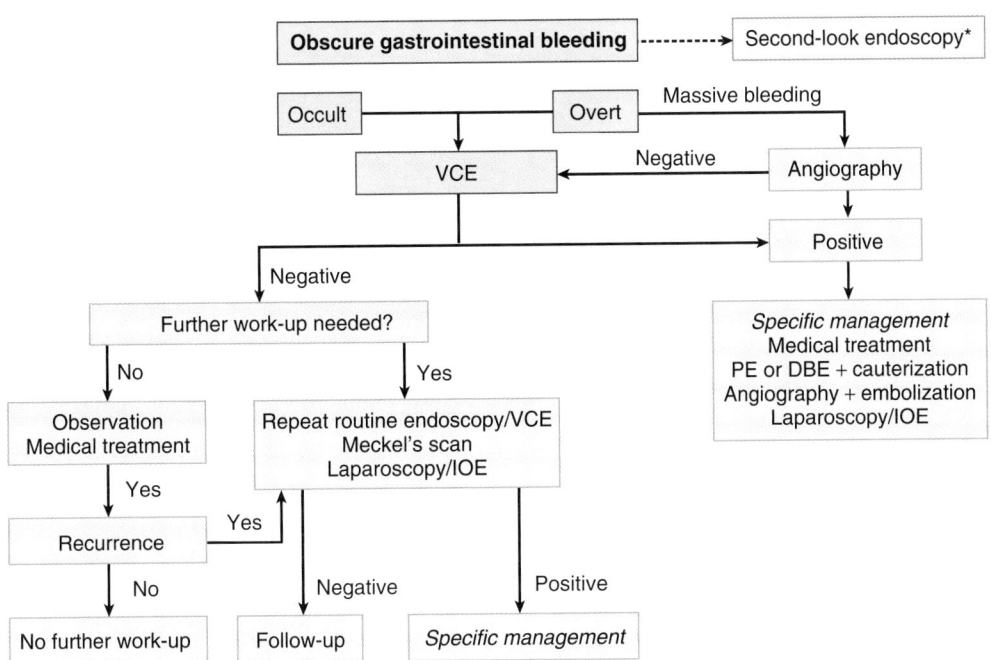

Fig. 93.1 Diagnostic algorithm of obscure gastrointestinal hemorrhage. *DBE*, Double-balloon enteroscopy; *IOE*, intraoperative enteroscopy; *PE*, push enteroscopy; *VCE*, video capsule endoscopy. *Some experts suggest a second-look endoscopy before capsule endoscopy to ensure that no pathology was missed.

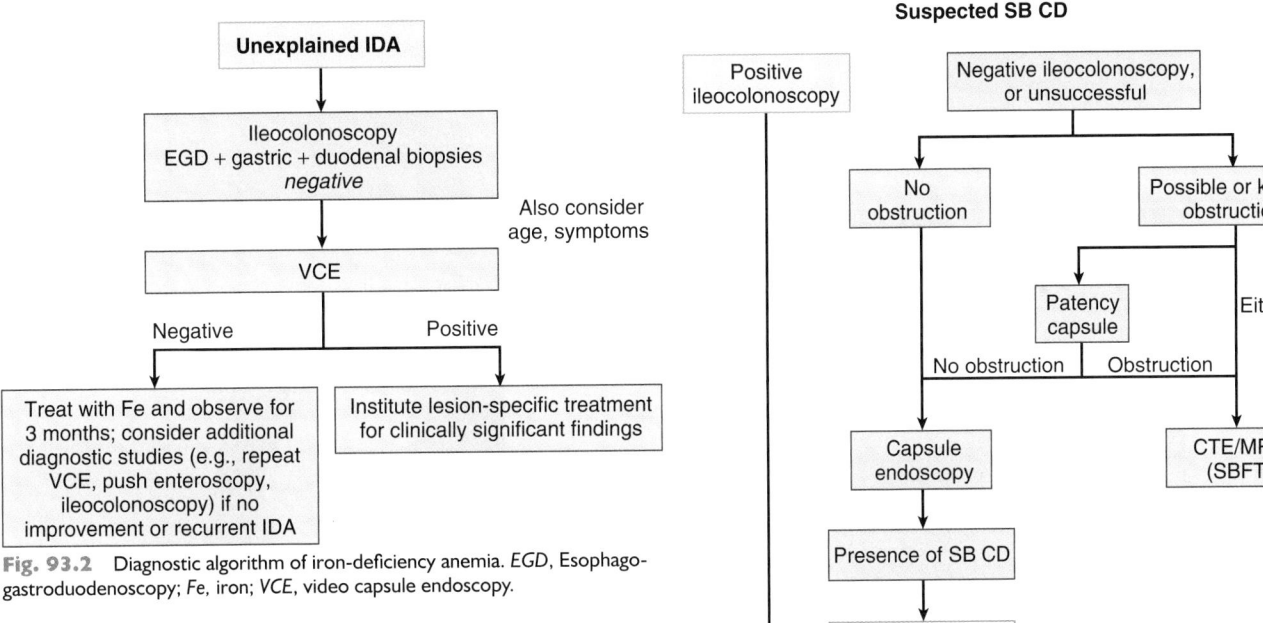

Fig. 93.2 Diagnostic algorithm of iron-deficiency anemia. *EGD*, Esophagogastroduodenoscopy; *Fe*, iron; *VCE*, video capsule endoscopy.

Fig. 93.4 Role of capsule endoscopy in the diagnosis of Crohn disease. *CTE*, Computed tomographic enterography; *MRE*, magnetic resonance enterography; *SB CD*, small bowel Crohn disease; *SBFT*, small bowel follow-through.

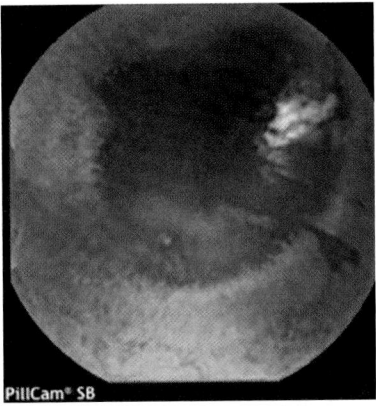

Fig. 93.3 Active small bowel bleeding.

bloating, nausea, or vomiting—should be reviewed with the patient. If any positive history exists, a small bowel barium series should be obtained looking for possible strictures or fistulas. Similarly, any history of prior small bowel or other intraabdominal surgery and any abnormal findings on small bowel imaging suggesting obstruction, stricture, or fistula should be carefully sought and addressed before capsule ingestion.

Before capsule ingestion the patient should adhere to the following regimen:

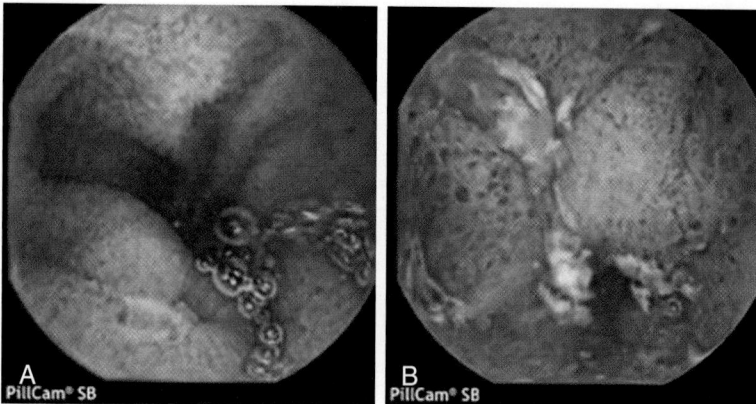

Fig. 93.5 Small bowel Crohn disease. (A) Aphthous ulcer. (B) Inflammatory stricture.

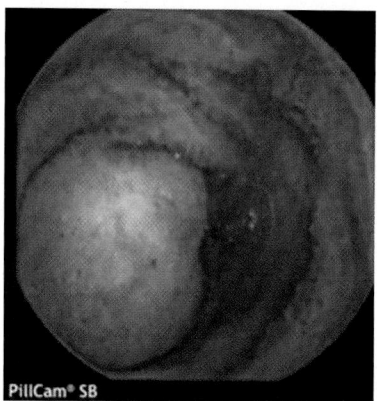

Fig. 93.6 Small bowel tumor.

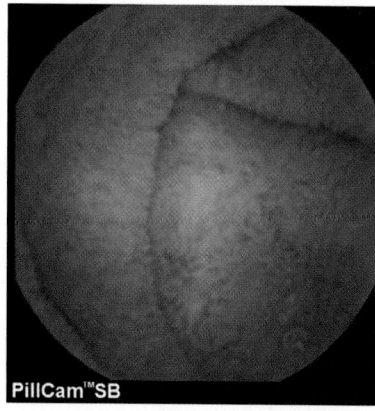

Fig. 93.7 Celiac disease: mucosal scalloping.

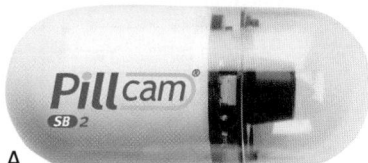

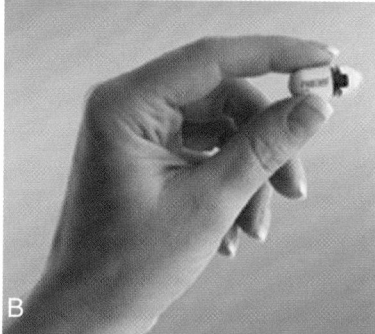

Fig. 93.8 (A) PillCam SB2. (B) Capsule size. (A, Courtesy Given Imaging Medtronic, Yoqneam, Israel.)

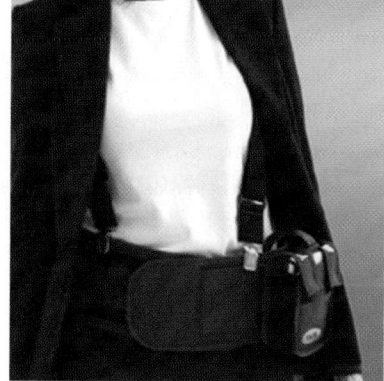

Fig. 93.9 Recorder and belt.

- Refrain from aspirin or NSAID therapy for a minimum of 14 days before capsule examination. (Even the sporadic use of NSAIDs has been shown to cause erosions and bleeding. Indeed, erosions, aphthous ulcers, and strictures mimicking CD have been reported at VCE in patients who have used NSAIDs. NSAID therapy may not be reported (or even considered) by the patient because many of these medications are sold over the counter or not believed to be significant by patients. Thus the clinician should specifically ask about regular or sporadic NSAID use in the weeks before VCE and recommend that it be discontinued if not mandatory.)
- Refrain from ingesting oral iron therapy, including iron-containing multivitamins, in the 7 days before the VCE procedure.

- Refrain from eating seeds, nuts, or grains the day before VCE. It is also advisable to refrain from dairy products and any other dark-colored or high-fiber foods. Ample intake of clear fluids the day before the procedure is also recommended.
- Fast for 10 hours.
- Consult the clinician regarding regular medication (e.g., insulin and other diabetes-related medications, antihypertensives) use before VCE examination.

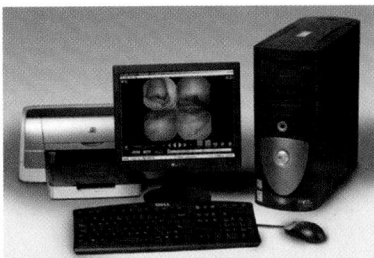

Fig. 93.10   Reporting and processing of images and data computer workstation.

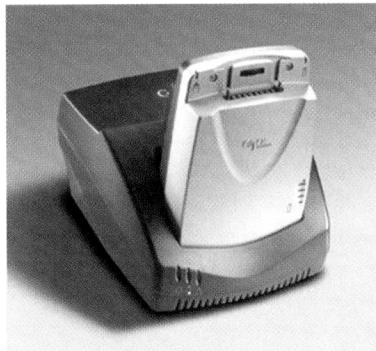

Fig. 93.11   Data recorder and charging cradle.

Use of Prokinetics, Laxative, and Osmotic Bowel Preparations

It has been reported that in as many as 20% of VCE examinations, incomplete small bowel imaging (defined as the capsule not reaching the ileocecal valve/cecum) may occur because of decreased gastric emptying or prolonged small bowel transit time. Furthermore, turbid or dark intraluminal contents of the small bowel may interfere with the quality of the examination, particularly in the distal ileum. Prokinetics are medications given with the aim of accelerating gastric emptying or small bowel transit time, thereby improving the proportion of cases in which the cecum is reached. Bowel preparations are medications given with the primary aim of cleansing the small bowel.

In 2006, the International Conference on Capsule Endoscopy (ICCE 2006) concluded that small bowel preparation (e.g., polyethylene glycol, Phospho-Soda, clear liquids) before VCE may not significantly improve small bowel cleanliness and that there is no definitive evidence that such preparations increase the diagnostic yield of small bowel VCE. A meta-analysis in 2018 reached the same conclusion. Therefore, at present, *there is no convincing evidence for recommending the routine use of bowel preparations in clinical practice.* However, if the use of a bowel preparation is desired by the practitioner, there are several regimens that may be used (Table 93.1). The 2017 Canadian Association of Gastroenterology guidelines recommend a bowel preparation but fail to distinguish between using simethicone or polyethylene glycol.

Prokinetic agents (e.g., metoclopramide and erythromycin) may shorten gastric emptying and small bowel transit times, but study results have been inconsistent, so no recommendation for their use can be made. Simethicone, an oral antifoaming agent/defrothicant, 400 mg may be given at 6 PM the night before the procedure in its liquid suspension form to improve visualization of the bowel mucosa. Although older age, diabetes mellitus, and inpatient status may be predictive factors for prolonged gastric emptying or small bowel transit time, no firm evidence supports the use of prokinetics or bowel preparation even in these patient subgroups. Delayed gastric emptying may be less of a problem in newer models, as the battery life of VCEs is being extended from 7 or 8 hours to 12 hours or more.

TABLE 93.1	Bowel Preparation Regimens
Medication	**Dosing**
Sodium phosphate*	90 mL the night before the procedure
PEG	2 L ingested 16 h before the procedure
PEG	4:3 L ingested the evening before + 1 L ingested 3 h immediately before the procedure
Simethicone	400 mg ingested 6 PM the night before the procedure

*Sodium phosphate preparations should not be used in patients with renal or cardiac insufficiency/failure and are to be avoided in older patients because of the increased risk of hyperphosphatemia.
PEG, Polyethylene glycol.

TECHNIQUE

It is mandatory to verify that the patient has completed the following steps:

- Fasted for the 10 hours immediately preceding the capsule study
- Maintained a clear liquid diet since lunch the day before the procedure
- Stopped oral iron therapy 7 days before the procedure and refrained from aspirin/NSAID use for 14 days before the procedure
- Signed the informed consent form

The clinician should verify, preferably by a checklist or a structured preprocedure visit form, that the indication for VCE is clear and that no contraindications to the procedure exist.

Preparing the Equipment

Because the procedure takes approximately 7 to 8 hours to complete, it is convenient to schedule the patient for VCE examination first thing in the morning. Therefore disconnecting the sensor array and downloading the data recorder will take place in the middle to late afternoon. The following items should be readily available at the time of patient presentation:

- A fully charged data recorder (as indicated by the battery indicator light), after the patient check-in procedure has been launched using the RAPID workstation
- PillCam SB in its original sealed package
- One disposable cup of water, a sensor array with adhesive sleeves, a sensor location diagram for correct sensor placement on the abdomen, and a belt for the data recorder

Getting Started

The patient should lie supine and the sensor array should be placed on the abdomen at the locations indicated by the sensor location diagram. Care should be taken to make sure that the sensors are firmly attached in the correct location. The patient should then stand, wearing his or her clothes, and make sure that no discomfort is caused by the sensors. The belt, with the data recorder in place, is worn over the patient's clothing (see Fig. 93.9). The capsule should then be removed from its packaging. Once the capsule is detached from its cell (and magnet), it is important to verify that the eight light-emitting diodes (LEDs) start to work (lights on the capsule will begin to flash immediately on detachment) and that the capsule transmission indicator on the data recorder starts flashing blue. This indicates that the data recorder is acquiring the signal from the capsule. The patient then takes the capsule (see Fig. 93.8), taking great care not to drop it, and places it in his or her mouth (the orientation of the capsule in the mouth is not important). The patient is then instructed to swallow the capsule while drinking a full glass of water. In cases when swallowing is unsuccessful, a repeat attempt should be made. If further attempts are unsuccessful, the capsule should be put back into its cell and magnet so that battery life is preserved.

Endoscopic placement of the capsule into the stomach or duodenum is possible using a video endoscope and a dedicated capsule-holding suction cup, snare, or endoscopic net (AdvanCE). However, this procedure should be performed only by an experienced endoscopist and as soon as possible, because the battery may not completely stop and the capsule's battery life span may be shortened.

After capsule ingestion the patient should be instructed as follows:

- Remain in the clinic area for approximately 15 to 30 minutes to make sure that no technical problems occur.
- Pay attention that the flashing blue light-emitting diode on the data recorder is on.
- Treat the data recorder with the utmost care.
- Refrain from being near areas of magnetic fields such as magnetic resonance imaging machines, security gates, and the like. Certain industrial magnetic fields may interfere with transmission of the images.
- Refrain from liquid intake for 2 hours and food intake for 4 hours after capsule ingestion.
- Contact the medical staff in case of severe abdominal pain, nausea, or vomiting.
- Note capsule excretion. In case of any doubt, any symptoms of bowel obstruction, or before magnetic resonance imaging, an abdominal radiograph should be performed to verify capsule excretion. For patients who do not visualize/observe capsule excretion and in whom the colon is not visualized on the video imaging, an abdominal radiograph should be performed on day 14 to identify those with capsule retention.

Video Reviewing

General Information

- The average reviewing time for small bowel VCE is usually 30 to 60 minutes.
- Video reviewing should take place in a semidarkened room and, because video reviewing requires considerable concentration, no visual distractions should be allowed. However, listening to music is possible.
- Before attempting to review VCE videos, it is imperative to be familiar with the software and to have experience in the interpretation of VCE findings. We strongly encourage attending capsule endoscopy courses such as those provided by the American Society for Gastrointestinal Endoscopy (www.asge.org). Furthermore, we strongly recommend reviewing the initial 10 to 20 capsule videos with proctoring from a colleague experienced in VCE.

Video Reviewing Procedure

- We recommend using the simultaneous two-picture viewing mode (Fig. 93.12), setting the video speed to 18 to 22 in the manual mode (M-mode preferable) or lower speed using the automated mode (A-mode).
- It is of utmost importance to determine and mark the following anatomic landmarks:
  - First image of the gastric folds
  - First duodenal image (identified by the first image where villi on the mucosa are seen [Fig. 93.13]; usually passage of the capsule through the pylorus is seen immediately before this point of transit)
  - First cecal image (the first image where villi are absent, fecal matter is dominant, and typically where there is a lack of the characteristic peristalsis of the small bowel)
- Capsule findings should be reported by creating a thumbnail from the image. Preferably each pathologic finding should be defined and noted in the thumbnail's comment. In cases where the nature of the finding is unclear, refer to the image atlas in

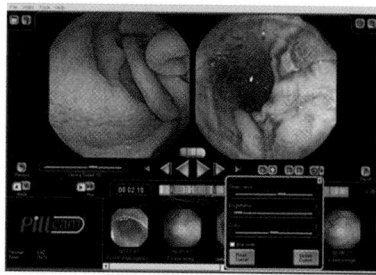

Fig. 93.12 Reporting and processing of images and data viewing screen.

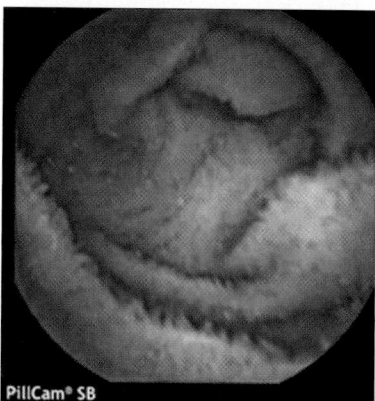

Fig. 93.13 Small bowel: normal villi.

the product software or an endoscopic atlas or VCE atlas (e.g., Keuchel et al., 2006).

- Capsule transit time through the stomach and small bowel is another aspect of video interpretation. Transit delays may suggest stricture or obstruction and should be noted. If the capsule fails to reach the ileocecal valve or did not traverse the ileocecal valve into the cecum during the time of recorded video, this should be noted in the report. Careful follow-up of these patients is warranted to verify capsule excretion in the following days and that no symptoms or signs of small bowel obstruction appear. A capsule present for more than 14 days after the capsule examination is considered to be retained.
- Use of the suspected blood identification system. The RAPID software provides an accessory tool for detecting blood in the small bowel. This software tool has limited sensitivity and specificity. The blood detector does not replace careful reviewing of the entire video for bleeding and bleeding sources.
- Localization of findings. Each clinically significant finding detected during video reviewing should be considered for further management (e.g., referral for surgery, enteroscopy, or ileocolonoscopy). This is usually done by referring to the anatomic landmarks. Although the software system provides an estimated location for each image by using the localization system, exact localization of findings in the small bowel is difficult. It is useful to use terms such as *duodenum, proximal jejunum, distal jejunum/proximal ileum, distal ileum,* and *terminal ileum* in describing the location of a finding. This description is completed using noted anatomic landmarks, transit times, and the timing of each thumbnail; but because of the variable speed of the capsule's peristaltic movement through the intestine, this method is not very accurate.
- Creating the report
  - Verify that the patient demographic details and reasons for capsule endoscopy referral are reported and inserted into the appropriate report fields during patient check-in. If not, you may do this while creating the VCE report.

- A brief summary of the VCE findings (e.g., gastric and small bowel) should be typed in the box specified for procedure information and findings.
- The final diagnosis and recommendations for further workup or treatment should be stated and typed in the appropriate field.

COMPLICATIONS

Clinical Complications

Clinical complications include complications of capsule ingestion, capsule retention, incomplete examination, and missed lesions. Capsule retention for 14 days after capsule ingestion is by far the most serious of these and, as previously mentioned, this occurs in 1% to 2% of cases. A large case series of 2300 VCEs performed for various indications noted an incomplete examination rate as high as 20% (Hoog et al, 2012). A systematic review of a larger number of cases found an incomplete rate of 12% (Liao et al., 2010). Consequently, there will also be risk of missed lesions. That said, cases have been reported in which, despite a negative VCE, malignant small-bowel pathology was identified by double-balloon enteroscopy, which should be considered when there is a high index of suspicion. The increasing battery lives of VCE capsules will eventually decrease the incompletion rate. The safety of VCE has not been examined systematically in pregnant women, therefore we do not recommend its use in this setting by primary care. Although it has been found safe in children as young as 2 years, smaller intestinal size may increase risk of retention, so we do not recommend the use of VCE by primary care clinicians in children younger than 10 years.

Capsule Retention

The most recent definition of capsule retention is failure to reach the colon during its recording time; this occurs in about 16% of procedures (this number will decrease as battery life is extended). However, of greater concern is more prolonged capsule retention. At the 2005 ICCE, capsule retention was defined as an endoscopic capsule remaining in the digestive tract for more than 14 days. Capsule retention has been further defined as failure of the capsule to be excreted unless surgical, endoscopic, or medical interventions are performed. The prediction of this serious complication is difficult in that no single modality, including small bowel follow-through, may accurately predict it. However, experts believe that obtaining a careful history is perhaps the best single method of identifying high-risk patients. Important clues to possible small bowel stricture/stenosis include the following:

- Chronic NSAID use
- Suspected or known CD
- History of intestinal surgery
- Suspected small bowel tumor
- History of abdominal radiation therapy
- Suspected mesenteric ischemia

Symptoms such as pain, nausea or vomiting, and abdominal distention may also indicate increased potential for capsule retention. The overall incidence of capsule retention is 1% to 2%, with two-thirds of capsule retentions occurring in CD-related strictures. The relative incidence rates of capsule retention are shown in Table 93.2.

PREVENTION OF CAPSULE RETENTION:

- Careful history taking and risk stratification according to the aforementioned groups.
- Small bowel follow-through: This is currently the best way to establish the presence of small bowel strictures. Possible disadvantages include false-negative results and radiation exposure.
- Patency capsule (Agile Patency System; Given Imaging Medtronic): Made of lactulose, this capsule is specifically designed to dissolve spontaneously after 40 hours in the bowel. The capsule has a radiopaque tag, a timer, and a radiofrequency identification tag.

TABLE 93.2 Capsule Retention Rates According to Video Capsule Endoscopy Indication

Indication	Retention Rate (%)
Healthy volunteers	0
All comers	0.75
Suspected Crohn disease	1.4
Obscure gastrointestinal bleeding	Up to 5
Known Crohn disease	Up to 8
Suspected bowel obstruction	21

Modified from Eliakim AR. Video capsule endoscopy of the small bowel (PillCam SB). *Curr Opin Gastroenterol.* 2006;22:124–127.

It is readily detected by plain abdominal radiographs and by the detection device of the Agile System, thus enabling localization of the stricture causing the obstruction. The patency capsule disintegrates completely after 80 to 100 hours. Current experience with the patency capsule is that it is no more sensitive than small bowel follow-through or computed tomographic enteroclysis in detecting small bowel strictures. Moreover, 2 of 22 (11%) patients who swallowed the patency capsule developed small bowel obstruction that required surgery. Thus, given the comparable sensitivity and the risk for capsule-associated bowel obstruction, we do not recommend the use of the patency capsule in the workup of a suspected small bowel stricture.

MANAGEMENT OF CAPSULE RETENTION:

- Immediate referral to plain abdominal radiographs and possible surgery in cases of clinical symptoms and signs of small bowel obstruction.
- Extraction of the retained capsule by means of push enteroscopy, double-balloon enteroscopy, or surgery. Because most patients with capsule retention are asymptomatic, the extraction is not urgent. Thus referral for further evaluation by a gastroenterologist or a surgeon is warranted promptly but not urgently.
- A prokinetic agent such as metoclopramide or erythromycin may also be prescribed to accelerate the small bowel transit time and induce capsule passage.

Swallowing Disorders

Inability to swallow the capsule or (rarely) aspiration of the device has been reported in up to 1.5% of VCE procedures. Difficulty in swallowing may be overcome by introduction of the capsule by means of an oroesophageal overtube, by EGD with a snare with a basket or foreign object retrieval device, or by the AdvanCE device. If this equipment is not available or the primary care clinician is not skilled at using it, patients who are unsuccessful in swallowing the capsule may need to be referred to a center dedicated to VCE. Aspiration of the capsule can usually be overcome simply by coughing. In cases of suspected aspiration, referral for a chest radiograph or bronchoscopy is indicated.

Technical Complications

In a large series, Rondonotti and colleagues (2005) reported an overall 9% technical failure rate in 733 patients. These technical failures included gaps in image recording; shortened battery operation; malfunction of the battery package; and failure of capsule activation, image downloading, and the localization system. In 33% of cases with technical problems, the diagnosis was hampered. Overall, a total of 3% of all hampered diagnoses were attributed to technical problems. Interference with communication between the capsule and recorder is also a technical problem. This interference may be caused by nearby electromagnetic devices such as cardiac pacemakers, electronic article surveillance systems, and cellular telephones. Because radiofrequency electrosurgery and cellular telephones have been reported to interfere with cardiac pacemaker functioning, the presence of an implantable cardiac device is considered a relative contraindication to VCE. However, a small series of patients with pacemakers who underwent VCE have been reported to have no arrhythmias or pacemaker malfunction on Holter electrocardiographic monitoring during VCE. Similarly, the pacemakers did not interfere with VCE in these patients. Leighton and colleagues (2005) have reported similar results in a small series of five patients with an implantable cardiac defibrillator.

CURRENT AND FUTURE DEVELOPMENTS IN VIDEO CAPSULE ENDOSCOPY

Since the FDA's approval of the first M2A capsule in 2001, many new developments have been put to clinical use. Newer capsules, such as PillCam ESO with double-sided cameras and acquisition of 14 frames per second for the detection of esophageal diseases, including Barrett esophagus and esophageal varices, are available. However, even PillCam ESO is being replaced by PillCam Upper with a 90-minute battery life. PillCam COLON with double-sided cameras and PillCam SB2 with better illumination technology and a wider visual field of 156 degrees for improved accuracy in the diagnosis of small bowel diseases have long been approved by the FDA for clinical use. PillCam SB3 is replacing PillCam SB2 because it has even better resolution and a variable frame rate. Endocapsule is being replaced by Endocapsule 10, which has higher resolution and three-dimensional location software. Improvements in the diagnostic software allow for simplified viewing modes and shorter video review time, making this procedure even easier to use and more widely accepted. Extended battery life is also becoming more common. It is therefore imperative for any clinician involved in VCE to be familiar with current and future developments in this rapidly evolving technology.

CPT/BILLING CODES

91110   Gastrointestinal tract imaging, intraluminal (e.g., capsule endoscopy), esophagus through ileum, with physician interpretation and report

ICD-10-CM DIAGNOSTIC CODES

C17.0-C17.9   Malignant neoplasm of duodenum Malignant neoplasm of small intestine, unspecified
C78.4   Secondary malignant neoplasm of small intestine
D01.40-   Carcinoma in situ of unspecified part of intestine
D01.49   Carcinoma in situ of other parts of intestine
D12.0-D12.6   Benign neoplasm of cecum Benign neoplasm of colon, unspecified
D13.2-D13.39   Benign neoplasm of duodenum Benign neoplasm of other parts of small intestine
D37.1-37.5   Neoplasm of uncertain behavior of stomach Neoplasm of uncertain behavior of rectum
D50.0   Iron deficiency anemia secondary to blood loss (chronic)
D50.9   Iron deficiency anemia, unspecified
D62   Acute posthemorrhagic anemia
E34.0   Carcinoid syndrome
K50.00-   Crohn disease of small intestine without complications Crohn disease of small intestine with rectal bleeding
K50.011
K50.013-   Crohn disease of small intestine with fistula
K50.019   Crohn disease of small intestine with unspecified complications
K50.80-   Crohn disease of both small and large intestine without complications Crohn's disease of both small and large intestine with rectal bleeding
K50.811

K50.813-   Crohn disease of both small and large intestine
K50.911   with fistula Crohn disease, unspecified, with rectal bleeding
K50.913-   Crohn disease, unspecified, with fistula Crohn
K50.919   disease, unspecified, with unspecified complications
K52.0-K52.1   Gastroenteritis and colitis due to radiation Toxic gastroenteritis and colitis
K52.81-K55.9   Eosinophilic gastritis or gastroenteritis Vascular disorder of intestine, unspecified
K57.11   Diverticulosis of small intestine without perforation or abscess with bleeding
K57.13   Diverticulitis of small intestine without perforation or abscess with bleeding
K57.51   Diverticulosis of both small and large intestine without perforation or abscess with bleeding
K57.53   Diverticulitis of both small and large intestine without perforation or abscess with bleeding
K63.5-K63.81   Polyp of colon Dieulafoy lesion of intestine
K90.0-K90.1   Celiac disease Tropical sprue
K90.89-K90.9   Other intestinal malabsorption Intestinal malabsorption, unspecified
K92.1-K92.2   Melena Gastrointestinal hemorrhage, unspecified
R19.5   Other fecal abnormalities
Z85.068   Personal history of other malignant neoplasm of small intestine

RECOMMENDED READING

Bailey AA, Debinski H, Appleyard M, et al. Diagnosis and outcome of small bowel tumors found by capsule endoscopy: a three-center Australian experience. *Am J Gastroenterol.* 2006;101:2237–2243.

Cave D, Legnani P, de Franchis R, et al. ICCE consensus for capsule retention. *Endoscopy.* 2005;37:1065–1067.

Cellier C, Green PH, Collin P, et al. ICCE consensus for celiac disease. *Endoscopy.* 2005;37:1055–1059.

Clinical practice guidelines for the use of video capsule endoscopy. *Gastroenterology.* 2017;152(3):497–514.

Delvaux M, Soussan EB, Laurent V, et al. Clinical evaluation of the use of the M2A patency capsule system before a capsule endoscopy procedure, in patients with known or suspected intestinal stenosis. *Endoscopy.* 2005;37:801–807.

Eisen GM, Eliakim R, Zaman A, et al. The accuracy of PillCam ESO capsule endoscopy versus conventional upper endoscopy for the diagnosis of esophageal varices: a prospective three-center pilot study. *Endoscopy.* 2006;38:31–35.

Eliakim R, Fireman Z, Gralnek IM, et al. Evaluation of the PillCam Colon capsule in the detection of colonic pathology: results of the first multicenter, prospective, comparative study. *Endoscopy.* 2006;38:963–970.

Eliakim R, Sharma VK, Yassin K, et al. A prospective study of the diagnostic accuracy of PillCam ESO esophageal capsule endoscopy versus conventional upper endoscopy in patients with chronic gastroesophageal reflux disease. *J Clin Gastroenterol.* 2005;39:572–578.

Fischer D, Schreiber R, Levi D, Eliakim R. Capsule endoscopy: the localization system. *Gastrointest Endosc Clin N Am.* 2004;14:25–31.

Gay G, Selby W. *Tumors, ICCE Consensus;* 2006.

Gkolfakis P, Tziatzios G, Dimitriadis GD, Triantafyllou K. Meta-analysis of randomized controlled trials challenging the usefulness of purgative preparation before small-bowel video capsule endoscopy. *Endoscopy.* 2018; epub ahead of print.

Goldstein JL, Eisen GM, Lewis B, et al. The use of capsule endoscopy to prospectively assess the incidence of small bowel lesions with celecoxib, naproxen plus omeprazole and placebo. *Clin Gastroenterol Hepatol.* 2005;3:133–141.

Graham DY, Opekun AR, Willingham FF, Qureshi WA. Visible small intestinal mucosal injury in chronic NSAID users. *Clin Gastroenterol Hepatol.* 2005;3:55–59.

Gralnek IM. Obscure-overt gastrointestinal bleeding. *Gastroenterology.* 2005;128:1424–1430.

Ho KK, Joyce AM. Complications of capsule endoscopy. *Gastrointest Endosc Clin N Am.* 2007;17:169–178.

Hoog CM, Bark LA, Arkani J, Gorsetman J, Brostrom A, Sjoqvist U. Capsule retentions and incomplete endoscopy examinations: an analysis of 2300 examinations. Gastroenterol Res Pract. 2012;51718.

Holden JP, Dureja P, Pfau PR, et al. Endoscopic placement of the small-bowel video capsule by using a capsule endoscope delivery device. Gastrointest Endosc. 2007;65:842–847.

Hopper AD, Sidhu R, Hurlstone DP, et al. Capsule endoscopy: an alternative to duodenal biopsy for the recognition of villous atrophy in coeliac disease? Dig Liver Dis. 2007;39:140–145.

Itzkowitz SH, Rochester J. Colonic polyps and polyposis syndromes. In: Feldman M, Friedman LS, Brandt LJ, eds. Sleisenger and Fordtran's Gastrointestinal and Liver Disease: Pathophysiology, Diagnosis, Management. 8th ed. Philadelphia: Saunders; 2006:2741–2743.

Keuchel M, Hagenmueller F, Fleicher DE, eds. Atlas of Video Capsule Endoscopy. Heidelberg: Springer-Verlag; 2006.

Krunic AL, Wang LC, Soltani K, et al. Digital anesthesia with epinephrine: An old myth revisited. J Am Acad Dermatol. 2004;51:755–759.

Leighton J, Sharma V, Srivathsan K, et al. Safety of capsule endoscopy in patients with pacemakers. Gastrointest Endosc. 2004;59:567–569.

Leighton J, Srivathsan K, Carey E, et al. Safety of wireless capsule endoscopy in patients with implantable cardiac defibrillators. Am J Gastroenterol. 2005;100:1728–1731.

Lewis B. How to prevent endoscopic capsule retention. Endoscopy. 2005;37:852–853.

Liao Z, Gao R, Xu C, et al. Indications and detection, completion, and retention rates of small-bowel capsule endoscopy: a systematic review. Gastrointest Endosc. 2010;71:280–286.

Maiden L, Thjodleifsson B, Theodors A, et al. A quantitative analysis of NSAID-induced small bowel pathology by capsule enteroscopy. Gastroenterology. 2005;128:1172–1178.

Marmo R, Rotondano G, Rondonotti E, et al. Capsule enteroscopy vs. other diagnostic procedures in diagnosing obscure gastrointestinal bleeding: a cost-effectiveness study. Eur J Gastroenterol Hepatol. 2007;19:535–542.

Mergener K, Ponchon T, Gralnek I, et al. Literature review and recommendations for clinical application of small-bowel capsule endoscopy, based on a panel discussion by international experts. Consensus statements for small-bowel capsule endoscopy, 2006/2007. Endoscopy. 2007;39:895–909.

Mishkin DS, Chuttani R, Croffie J, et al. ASGE technology status evaluation report: wireless capsule endoscopy. Gastrointest Endosc. 2006;63:539–545.

Neumann S, Schoppmeyer K, Lange T, et al. Wireless capsule endoscopy for diagnosis of acute intestinal graft-versus-host disease. Gastrointest Endosc. 2007;65:403–409.

Payeras G, Piqueras J, Moreno J, et al. Effects of capsule endoscopy on cardiac pacemakers. Endoscopy. 2005;37:1181–1185.

Rockey DC. Gastrointestinal bleeding. In: Feldman M, Friedman LS, Brandt LJ, eds. Sleisenger and Fordtran's Gastrointestinal and Liver Disease: Pathophysiology, Diagnosis, Management. 8th ed. Philadelphia: Saunders; 2006:289–290.

Rondonotti E, Herrrerias J, Pennazio M, et al. Complications, limitations, and failures of capsule endoscopy: a review of 733 cases. Gastrointest Endosc. 2005;62:712–716.

Rondonotti E, Spada C, Cave D, et al. Video capsule enteroscopy in the diagnosis of celiac disease: a multicenter study. Am J Gastroenterol. 2007;102:1624–1631.

Sachdev MS, Leighton JA, Fleischer DE, et al. A prospective study of the utility of abdominal radiographs after capsule endoscopy for the diagnosis of capsule retention. Gastrointest Endosc. 2007;66:894–900.

Schoofs N, Deviere J, Van Gossum A. PillCam colon capsule endoscopy compared with colonoscopy for colorectal tumor diagnosis: a prospective pilot study. Endoscopy. 2006;78:971–977.

Schulmann K, Hollerbach S, Kraus K, et al. Feasibility and diagnostic utility of video capsule endoscopy for the detection of small bowel polyps in patients with hereditary polyposis syndromes. Am J Gastroenterol. 2005;100:27–37.

Schwartz GD, Barkin JS. Small bowel tumors detected by wireless capsule endoscopy. Dig Dis Sci. 2007;52:1026–1030.

Selby W. Complete small-bowel transit in patients undergoing capsule endoscopy: determining factors and improvement with metoclopramide. Gastrointest Endosc. 2005;61:80–85.

Sharma P, Wani S, Rastogi A, et al. The diagnostic accuracy of esophageal capsule endoscopy in patients with gastroesophageal reflux disease and Barrett's esophagus: a blinded, prospective study. Am J Gastroenterol. 2008;103:525–532.

Signorelli C, Villa F, Rondonotti E, et al. Sensitivity and specificity of the suspected blood identification system in video capsule enteroscopy. Endoscopy. 2005;37:1170–1173.

Travis AC, Saltzman JR. Wireless capsule endoscopy & deep small bowel enteroscopy. In: Greenberger NJ, Blumberg RS, Burakoff R, eds. Current Diagnosis and Treatment: Gastroenterology, Hepatology & Endoscopy. 3rd ed. New York: McGraw Hill; 2016. Chapter 34.

Triester SL, Leighton JA, Leontiadis GI, et al. Meta-analysis of the yield of capsule endoscopy compared to other diagnostic modalities in patients with obscure gastrointestinal bleeding. Am J Gastroenterol. 2005;100:2407–2418.

Triester SL, Leighton JA, Leontiadis GI, et al. A meta-analysis of the yield of capsule endoscopy compared to other diagnostic modalities in patients with non-stricturing small bowel Crohn's disease. Am J Gastroenterol. 2006;101:954–964.

Yakoub-Agha I, Maunoury V, Wacrenier A, et al. Impact of small bowel exploration using video-capsule endoscopy in the management of acute graft versus host disease. Transplantation. 2004;15:1697–1701.

CHAPTER 94

ESOPHAGEAL FOREIGN BODY REMOVAL

Grant C. Fowler

Esophageal foreign bodies are encountered most often in children, psychiatric patients, prisoners, edentulous adults, and in patients with underlying esophageal pathology. In the emergency department, children account for 75% to 85% of esophageal foreign bodies, with the peak incidence occurring between 18 and 48 months of age. Most objects (80% to 90%) pass spontaneously, but 10% to 20% require removal using endoscopy or another technique. Approximately 1% require surgical removal.

If an object makes it into the stomach and is less than 6 cm in length and 2 cm in diameter, it will likely pass through the remainder of the gastrointestinal tract. If it makes it into the stomach and is larger than this, a gastroenterologist or surgeon should be consulted.

Occasionally, a foreign body in the pharynx or upper esophagus can cause respiratory distress or arrest. In this situation, the Heimlich maneuver may be appropriate (see Chapter 215, Heimlich Maneuver). For all other patients, the method for removal depends upon the type, shape, and size of the object, as well as where it gets impacted in the esophagus.

A plain radiograph can often help verify and localize an esophageal foreign body if it is radiopaque. It may also help to determine the configuration. Computed tomography (CT) may be needed to help localize nonradiopaque foreign bodies. Contrast-enhanced esophagrams have somewhat been replaced by CT and endoscopy, which are better and more cost effective at confirming and localizing an esophageal foreign body. Use of contrast in esophagrams also raises the risk of aspiration; it may also result in a coated esophageal mucosa and foreign object which may compromise subsequent removal.

This chapter will discuss five major categories of esophageal foreign bodies: smooth, blunt, or round objects; sharp or angulated objects; button batteries; magnets; and food bolus. Each is managed slightly differently. Regardless of the configuration, if a foreign body is impacted, it must be removed.

There are a variety of maneuvers possible to remove smooth, blunt or round objects such as using Magill forceps, pharmaceutical maneuvers, a Foley catheter, a bougienage (bougie), or an orogastric magnet (if available, useful for small metallic objects). Endoscopy is also always an option. Sharp or angulated objects cause the majority of complications; the appropriate removal technique for them is generally under direct visualization with endoscopy.

Button batteries and magnets warrant special attention. Fortunately, most button batteries (96%) are small (<15 mm in diameter) and almost never lodge in the esophagus. The larger button batteries (>20 mm in diameter) are usually responsible for severe esophageal injuries. Liquefaction necrosis of the esophageal mucosa and perforation can occur very rapidly due to an impacted battery. On x-ray, button batteries are radiopaque, round densities similar in appearance to a coin but may demonstrate a "double-contour" configuration. A button battery lodged in the esophagus is an emergency, and immediate removal is indicated.

If the foreign object is a single small magnet, it should be treated like any other blunt, nonsharp small foreign body. If multiple magnets are noted on a radiograph, this is an emergency; they need to be retrieved if in the esophagus or stomach. If they have passed the pylorus, a surgeon should be consulted. Multiple magnets tend to attract each other and trap bowel between them. This can result in pressure necrosis and perforation.

Meat or food boluses generally impact in the distal esophagus. Early removal is recommended; if there is a delay, the bolus may soften and make extraction more difficult. The risk of complications also increases significantly if a food bolus remains impacted for more than 12 hours.

TECHNIQUES

In children, the most common esophageal foreign body is an ingested coin; the most common location for it to become lodged is at the level of the cricopharyngeus muscle. Although it requires sedation, success rates as high as 95% to 100% have been reported with simple removal using Magill forceps. This is best performed with a laryngoscope or video-assisted guidance (e.g., Glidescope; see Chapter 222, Tracheal Intubation).

The lower esophageal sphincter is the narrowest portion of the entire gastrointestinal tract; therefore, if an object can get beyond the sphincter, it will likely pass through the remainder of the gastrointestinal tract. Pharmacologic relaxation of the sphincter may enhance such passage. Although diazepam, meperidine, and atropine have all been tried, they universally failed in such efforts. Conversely, glucagon, nitroglycerine, nifedipine, possibly sumatriptan, and gas-forming agents have been found to be effective. Gas-forming agents alone, or in combination with pharmacologic relaxation of the sphincter, may help an esophageal foreign body or food bolus to pass into the stomach. All of these agents can be used in combination with an esophageal bougienage (bougie), and some of the agents can be used with the endoscopic push technique (see Technique: Endoscopy).

Another way to remove foreign bodies is with a small Foley catheter. The catheter is passed beyond the foreign body, and the balloon inflated. Then the catheter is gently withdrawn, hopefully retracting the foreign body with it (Fig. 94.1). This technique is classically used for a small child brought to the clinic or hospital shortly after swallowing a coin. However, it may be used for any smooth, blunt foreign body in patients of any age. Success rates as high as 85% to 100% have been reported with complication rates of 0% to 2%. It has also been used successfully for retrieval of button batteries and food boluses. Fluoroscopic guidance may be helpful, if available. For smooth, metallic foreign bodies, an orogastric tube magnet is sometimes available to use in a similar manner. It has a magnet sealed in the distal end of an orogastric tube and is best guided by fluoroscopy.

The esophageal bougie technique is a similar technique, but instead of withdrawing the foreign body, a nasogastric or orogastric tube or esophageal bougie is used to dislodge and push the object into the stomach. This is effective for smooth, blunt esophageal foreign bodies. Because it is generally performed blindly, it is especially useful for esophageal impacted coins. Success rates as high as with the endoscopic technique have been reported, at 10% or less of the cost. The necessary criteria for bougienage are a single, smooth foreign body

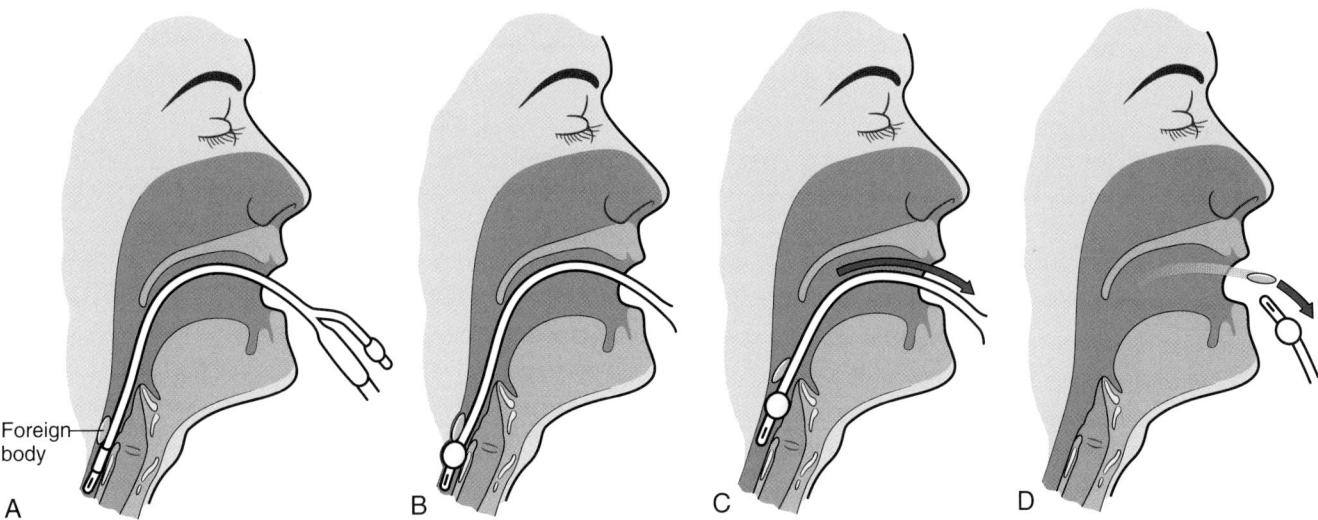

Fig. 94.1   Foley catheter removal of esophageal foreign body. (A) Insert the catheter tip past the foreign body. (B) Inflate the balloon. (C) Gently retract the catheter. (D) When it reaches the mouth, either grasp the foreign body or have the patient spit it out.

lodged less than 24 hours in a patient with no respiratory distress or history of esophageal disease or prior esophageal surgery. The foreign body must also be able to pass beyond the stomach and through the gastrointestinal tract with no problems. One advantage of this technique over some of the others is that because the foreign body will not be withdrawn, there is no risk of aspiration.

When all else fails, or when the object is sharp, angulated, or a battery, it can be retrieved endoscopically. For sharp, pointed objects, an experienced endoscopist is needed. Less expertise is needed to use the push technique. In the situation where multiple intubations will be necessary, overtubes are available that will protect the mucosa and airway. They are generally made of semirigid plastic, are slightly larger in diameter than the endoscope, and have a tapered, soft tip. Shorter tubes (20 to 25 cm) can be used when multiple intubations of the esophagus are needed and longer tubes (at least 50 cm) when multiple intubations of the stomach are necessary.

Guidelines recommend emergent endoscopic removal (preferably within 2 hours, at latest within 6 hours) for complete esophageal obstruction, sharp objects, or batteries. Urgent endoscopic removal, within 24 hours, is recommended for other esophageal foreign bodies without complete obstruction.

INDICATIONS

Magill Forceps

- Smooth or blunt foreign body (e.g., coin) lodged at cricopharyngeus muscle level

Esophageal Pharmacologic Maneuvers

- Smooth or blunt foreign body
- Food bolus
- Additional relaxation needed with bougie or endoscopic push techniques

EDITOR'S NOTE: Some guidelines suggest that pharmacologic maneuvers should not delay endoscopic removal, especially not in urgent situations.

Foley Catheter, Orogastric Magnet, and Bougienage

- Smooth or blunt foreign body (must be metallic for magnet to work)

Esophagoscopy

- Angulated, abrasive or sharp foreign body
- Impacted esophageal foreign body, including food bolus
- Button battery impacted in esophagus or multiple magnets

CONTRAINDICATIONS

- Angulated, abrasive or sharp foreign body contraindicated except with direct visualization using endoscopy
- Esophageal perforation (CT recommended when suspected or to verify)
- Total obstruction for Foley removal (cannot get Foley past object)
- Multiple objects for Foley removal (relative)
- Food bolus impaction for bougie because these typically have underlying esophageal pathology
- Endoscopic removal is not recommended for concealed packets of drugs (body packing)

EQUIPMENT AND SUPPLIES

- Nonsterile gloves and equipment to follow universal blood and body fluid precautions

Magill Forceps Technique

- Laryngoscope or video-assisted laryngoscope (e.g., Glidescope; see Chapter 222, Tracheal Intubation)
- Magill forceps
- Procedural sedation

Pharmacologic Technique

- Glucagon, nifedipine, nitroglycerine, sumatriptan, gas-forming agents
- Intravenous (IV) access for glucagon

EDITOR'S NOTE: Papain should not be used to dissolve a food bolus. It can dissolve the esophageal lining, resulting in severe damage or perforation, especially if the lining is ischemic from an impacted bolus.

Foley Catheter Technique

- 10- to 16-Fr Foley catheter in children

Orogastric Magnet Technique

- Orogastric tube with sealed magnet in tip

Bougienage Technique (Bougie)

- Nasogastric, orogastric tube or esophageal bougienage (bougie, often used for intubation of difficult airways)

Esophagoscopy Technique

- Esophagogastroduodenoscope, with instruments (e.g., snare, forceps, grasper, basket, latex hood for sharp objects) including overtube if needed
- Procedural sedation

PREPROCEDURE PATIENT EDUCATION AND FORMS

The chosen procedure should be explained to the patient or his or her representative. Risks and benefits should be explained, alternatives if available. Appropriate consent should be obtained, including for procedural sedation if anticipated.

TECHNIQUE: McGILL FORCEPS

1. The patient should be supine with the head slightly extended in the "sniffing" position. Ensure adequate sedation and appropriate monitoring are in place (see Chapter 1, Procedural Sedation and Analgesia).
2. Insert the laryngoscope or video-assisted laryngoscope (e.g., Glidescope, see Chapter 222, Tracheal Intubation). Visualize the upper part of esophagus where the foreign body is normally impacted. Suction should be available for use as necessary.
3. Grasp the foreign body with the Magill forceps; slowly and steadily remove it.
4. Following removal, scan the esophagus with the scope for any other foreign bodies, injuries, erosions, or bleeding.
5. Recover the patient from sedation.

TECHNIQUE: PHARMACOLOGIC REMOVAL

Glucagon:

1. The patient should be in the seated position.
2. After obtaining IV access, a small test dose of glucagon can be given to check for hypersensitivity. If not allergic, the therapeutic dose (0.25 to 2 mg) is then administered IV.
3. Glucagon has a rapid onset and short duration of action. If no results are seen in 10 to 20 minutes, a second administration of 0.25 to 2 mg can be tried. A small volume of oral fluid can be given to enhance the activity of glucagon.
4. Some clinicians always combine glucagon with gas-forming agents (see section, Gas Forming Agents) or even carbonated beverages (100 mL), especially if glucagon alone is not successful. Glucagon can also be combined with nitroglycerine, nifedipine, or sumatriptan.

Nitroglycerine or nifedipine (although not studied extensively, **sumatriptan** is known to reduce fasting fundic tone, prolong fundic relaxation, and delay gastric emptying):

1. The patient should be in the seated position and adequately hydrated to avoid hypotension. IV fluids maybe helpful for this, and if used, IV access should be maintained.
2. If not contraindicated, sublingual nitroglycerine (one or two 0.4-mg tablets), or 1 to 2 inches nitroglycerine paste, or nifedipine (5 to 10 mg) can be given. (Do not use both of these agents simultaneously due to risk of hypotension.)
3. The patient should be monitored for hypotension.

Gas-forming agents:

1. The patient should be in the seated position.
2. A solution of 15 mL of tartaric acid (18.7 g/100 mL) followed by 15 mL of sodium bicarbonate solution (10 mg/ 100 mL). Alternatively, 1.5 to 3 g of tartaric acid and 2 to 3 g of sodium bicarbonate can be dissolved in 15 mL of water and ingested. Carbonated beverages (100 mL) alone have been successful in disimpacting foreign bodies and are more readily available in the clinic or emergency department.

TECHNIQUE: FOLEY CATHETER

1. The patient should be placed in the Trendelenburg, lateral decubitus, or prone position. Light sedation or topical oropharyngeal anesthesia may be used (although this increases the risk for aspiration).
2. Insert the uninflated catheter until the tip is past the foreign body (see Fig. 94.1A). This can be confirmed under fluoroscopy or as measured on a plain radiograph. Inflate the balloon (see Fig 94.1B) with 3 to 5 mL of saline (or contrast material if under fluoroscopy). Stop inflating the balloon if the patient complains of increased pain.
3. Gently withdraw the catheter using steady, constant traction (see Fig. 94.1C). Once the foreign body and the tip of the catheter reach the mouth, instruct the patient to spit it out (see Fig 94.1D) or the clinician can grasp it with the forceps.
4. If the catheter slips past the foreign body, reinsert it and reinflate it with 5 to 8 mL of fluid and make one additional attempt at withdrawal with gentle, steady traction.
5. If this is not being performed under fluoroscopy and no foreign body is retrieved, obtain another radiograph. In 10% to 20% of cases, the catheter will have pushed the foreign body into the stomach.

TECHNIQUE: BOUGIENAGE (BOUGIE)

1. Measure the length of necessary bougie dilator by placing the tip at the corner of the mouth, running the dilator over the earlobe and to a point 3 to 4 cm below the costal margin. Mark this distance with tape.
2. Spray the oropharynx generously with topical anesthetic. Insert the bougie in one smooth motion until the tape is at the corner of the mouth.
3. Remove the bougie and confirm by x-ray that the object is now in the stomach.
4. The bougie technique may be repeated if the first attempt is not successful. The bougie should never be advanced against significant resistance.

TECHNIQUE: ENDOSCOPY

1. After the patient is adequately sedated, an endoscope is passed to visualize the object or bolus directly. For a meat bolus, the entire object may be able to be removed slowly with a polypectomy snare. While retracting the bolus, as the endoscope reaches the level of the cricopharyngeus muscle, extend the patients head and quickly remove the scope.
2. For a soft food bolus, a piecemeal approach may be necessary. Several passages of the endoscope can be made through an overscope.
3. For a blunt object such as a coin, a snare, forceps, or basket can be used. Grasp the object very firmly before withdrawal. Take care to not let the object become dislodged as it moves through areas of anatomic narrowing. An object that dislodges from the scope along the way can result in aspiration unless an overscope is being used. Long objects should be grasped with a snare on the proximal end so the object will align with the esophagus as it is being withdrawn. Likewise, sharp objects should be grasped with the sharpest point trailing during withdrawal to avoid perforating anything along the way.

4. Another endoscopic technique is the push technique. A small-caliber scope is used so that it can be passed beyond the food bolus to inspect the area distal to the obstruction. After passing beyond the bolus, withdraw the scope tip to above the bolus. From the right side of the bolus, use the scope to gently push the food bolus into the stomach. Pushing from the right side is especially useful in patients with a hiatal hernia, because the gastroesophageal junction usually takes a left turn as it enters the stomach.

COMPLICATIONS

- Aspiration of an object being withdrawn, with risk of airway occlusion.
- If procedural sedation or analgesia is not used, nausea, vomiting, coughing, and laryngospasm
- Mucosal abrasions, lacerations, esophageal stricture, and necrosis.
- Esophageal perforation (from the foreign body or the procedure to remove it), which can be life threatening.
- Overinflation of a Foley balloon can rupture the esophagus.
- A foreign body present for more than 24 hours can cause pressure necrosis which increases risk of perforation.
- Mediastinitis, lung abscess, pericarditis, cardiac tamponade, pneumothorax, pneumomediastinum, aortoesophageal, or tracheoesophageal fistula. These are all usually due to delay in diagnosis of esophageal perforation.
- Anesthetic or sedation complications (see appropriate chapters).

POSTPROCEDURE MANAGEMENT AND PATIENT EDUCATION

The patient should be restricted to liquids for 12 to 18 hours. If that is well tolerated, the patient can be advanced to a soft diet. Patients with a prior food bolus should know to take small bites and chew them completely before swallowing. They should return to the clinic, urgent care center, or emergency department for any chest pain, abdominal pain, dysphagia, odynophagia, fever, hematemesis, melena, or for any concerns or questions.

CPT/BILLING CODES

43247   Esophagogastroduodenoscopy with removal of foreign body

There is no other specific CPT code for esophageal foreign body removal.

99356   Prolonged physician service in the inpatient or observation setting, requiring direct (face-to-face) patient contact beyond the usual service first hour
99357   Each additional 30 minutes (list separately in addition to code for prolonged service)
99358   Prolonged evaluation and management service before and/or after direct (face-to-face) patient care (e.g., review of extensive records and tests, communication with other professionals and/or patient/family); not face-to-face care; first hour
99359   Each additional 30 minutes

ICD-10-CM DIAGNOSTIC CODES

T18.100A   Unspecified foreign body in esophagus causing compression of trachea
T18.108A   Unspecified foreign body in esophagus causing other injury
T18.190A   Other foreign body in esophagus causing compression of trachea
T18.198A   Other foreign body in esophagus causing other injury
T18.2XXA   Foreign body in stomach
T18.3XXA   Foreign body in small intestine
T18.9XXA   Foreign body of alimentary tract, part unspecified

RECOMMENDED READING

ASGE guideline. Management of ingested foreign bodies and food impactions. *Gastrointest Endosc.* 2011;73(6):1085–1091.

Attar BM. Esophageal foreign body removal. In: Reichman EF, ed. *Emergency Medicine Procedures.* 2nd ed. New York: McGraw-Hill; 2013:401–407.

Birk M, Bauerfeind P, Deprez PH, et al. Removal of foreign bodies in the upper gastrointestinal tract in adults. European Society of Gastrointestinal Endoscopy (ESGE) Clinical Guideline. *Endoscopy.* 2016;48:1–8.

Munter DW. Esophageal foreign bodies. In: Roberts JR, Custalow CB, Thomsen TW, eds. *Roberts and Hedges Clinical Procedures in Emergency Medicine and Acute Care.* 7th ed. Philadelphia: Elsevier; 2019:807–827.

CHAPTER 95

INGUINAL HERNIA REDUCTION

George G. Zainea

The *indirect inguinal hernia*—occurring lateral to the inferior epigastric vessels—is the most common type of groin hernia. The hernial sac passes through the internal inguinal ring and is associated with patency of the processus vaginalis. This type of hernia is typically seen in children and young adults (Figs. 95.1 and 95.2).

The *direct inguinal hernia*—more commonly seen in adults (see Figs. 95.1 and 95.2)—occurs medial to the inferior epigastric vessels and protrudes through the posterior inguinal floor. The risk of incarceration is less than that of an indirect inguinal hernia.

Femoral hernias, usually found in adult women, are seen far less commonly. The protrusion occurs beneath the inguinal ligament just medial to the femoral vessels in the upper thigh. The risk of incarceration and strangulation is high with this type of hernia (see Figs. 95.1 and 95.2).

DIAGNOSIS

Diagnosis involves palpation with the patient both supine and standing. An incarcerated groin hernia manifests as a nonreducible, painful groin bulge. Associated intestinal obstruction may also be present.

In a true hernia, a Valsalva maneuver (grunting or coughing) allows the examiner to appreciate a palpable impulse, and auscultation may reveal bowel sounds. Transillumination can be performed to assist with the diagnosis.

DIFFERENTIAL DIAGNOSIS

The history and physical examination usually allow the clinician to exclude other disorders that may mimic an incarcerated groin hernia, such as an inflamed lymph node, which is usually evident by history and on palpation; a dilated varicose vein, which may appear as a bulge in the inguinal region; a large lipoma; or a hydrocele of the spermatic cord, which typically is not tender, does transilluminate, and is rarely associated with an acute presentation. Malignancy is a consideration in older children. Other disorders to consider include testicular torsion, which manifests as extreme scrotal pain and swelling. With torsion, pain may be intensified with scrotal elevation, and swelling is usually confined to beneath the pubic tubercle. Finally, an undescended testicle may appear as an isolated groin bulge. This should be suspected if the gonad is not present in the scrotal sac.

INDICATIONS

Nonstrangulated hernia—although strangulation can occur in an incarcerated hernia without the usual signs and symptoms, reduction in the case of most incarcerated hernias is safe if no signs or symptoms of strangulation are present. One prospective study (Askew et al., 1992) showed that clinicians are usually correct in deciding when to reduce an incarcerated hernia and when to defer reduction of a strangulated hernia. Harmful outcomes are also unlikely with attempted reduction in unrecognized strangulated hernias (Kauffman and O'Brien, 1970).

CONTRAINDICATIONS

Strangulated hernia—if a strangulated hernia is reduced, necrotic bowel may be introduced into the abdomen, resulting in the patient's clinical deterioration.

TECHNIQUE

By definition, a hernia that is nonreducible is *incarcerated*. Incarceration usually involves either the bowel or the omentum. The practitioner may see intestinal obstruction with bowel incarceration; however, the most feared complication of incarceration is strangulation. With strangulation, the blood supply to the intestine is compromised, which may result in ischemic necrosis and gangrene.

The decision to reduce an incarcerated hernia requires clinical judgment. If strangulation is suspected, the situation is best dealt with immediately in the operating room. Patients with strangulation typically appear ill and may be febrile. The bulge is extremely tender, and overlying skin erythema may be present.

If strangulation is not suspected, the clinician may attempt closed reduction as follows:

1. Place the patient in the supine Trendelenburg position. This allows gravity to assist with reduction. A cool compress or ice pack applied to the area may help to reduce the swelling and facilitate reduction of the hernia.
2. Administer a narcotic for analgesia and an intravenous benzodiazepine for muscle relaxation. After sedation, allow for passive reduction of the hernia over a 30- to 40-minute period. In children, passive, spontaneous reduction has been reported in up to 80% of inguinal hernias over a 2-hour period without manipulation.
3. If the attempt at passive reduction is unsuccessful, proceed with an attempt at active reduction. Place one warm hand over the neck of the hernial sac to guide its contents into the peritoneal cavity. Use the other hand to provide gentle and steady distal-to-proximal compression over the hernia (Fig. 95.3). This part of the procedure can take 5 to 15 minutes. Reduce the hernia in the opposite order from which the contents protruded, meaning that the proximal contents of the hernial sac should be guided back through the defect first. Too much distal pressure too soon can cause ballooning around the fascial opening and prevent reduction.

EDITOR'S NOTE: Children can be placed in the unilateral frog-leg position with the ipsilateral leg externally rotated and both the hip and knee flexed. This position may facilitate opening the internal and external inguinal rings.

Using these techniques, the clinician should be able to reduce one-third to one-half of incarcerated groin hernias. Patients with irreducible groin hernias or incarcerated femoral hernias (which are seldom reducible) should be referred to a surgeon immediately.

Infants and children who successfully undergo closed reduction of incarcerated inguinal hernias should be admitted to the hospital

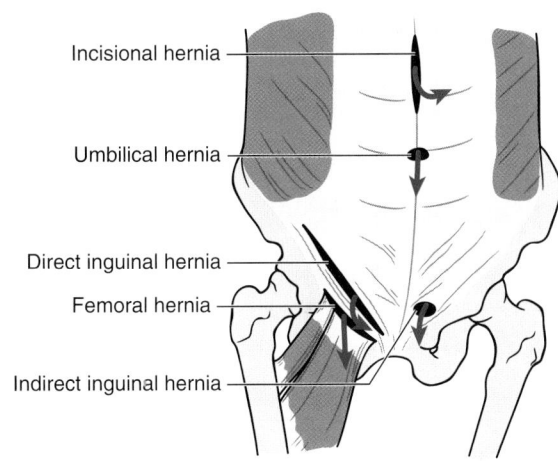

Fig. 95.1 Hernia locations in the abdominal wall.

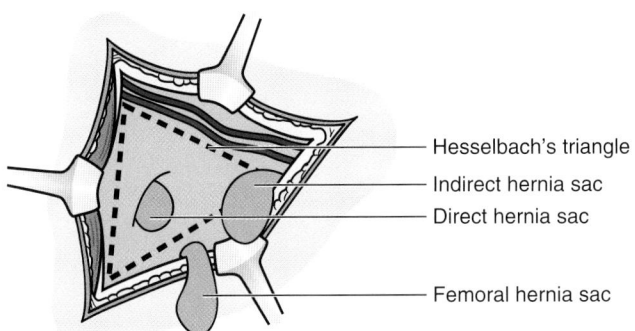

Fig. 95.2 Operative view of inguinal and femoral hernias.

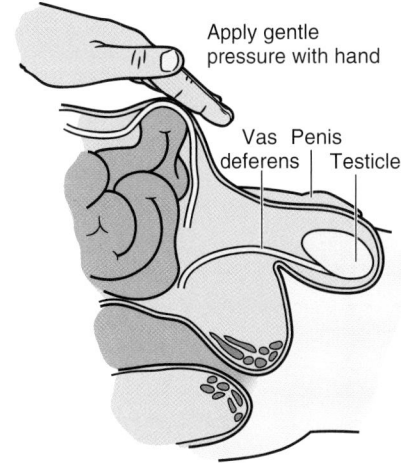

Fig. 95.3 Application of gentle pressure to reduce an inguinal hernia.

for surgical repair within 24 to 48 hours because of the risk for recurrent incarceration. An adult patient with suspected compromised bowel in the reduced hernia should be admitted to the hospital for observation. Adults who undergo successful closed reduction and return home should soon thereafter undergo elective hernia repair. A truss should be used only temporarily to prevent recurrent protrusion before surgery can be performed.

CPT/Billing Codes

There is no specific CPT code for inguinal hernia reduction. If documentation is adequate, it may be possible to bill for procedural or moderate sedation. Otherwise, billing is for prolonged physician services.

99356 Prolonged physician service in the inpatient or observation setting, requiring direct (face-to-face) patient contact beyond the usual service first hour
99357 Each additional 30 minutes (list separately in addition to code for prolonged service)
99358 Prolonged evaluation and management service before and/or after direct (face-to-face) patient care (e.g., review of extensive records and tests, communication with other professionals and/or patient/family); not face-to-face care; first hour
99359 Each additional 30 minutes

ICD-10-CM Diagnostic Codes

K40.2   Bilateral inguinal hernia, without obstruction or gangrene
K40.20 Not specified as recurrent
K40.21 Recurrent
K40.9   Unilateral inguinal hernia, without obstruction or gangrene
K40.90 Not specified as recurrent
K40.91 Recurrent

RECOMMENDED READING

Askew G, Williams GT, Brown SC. Delay in presentation and misdiagnosis of strangulated hernia: a prospective study. *J R Coll Surg Edinb.* 1992;37(1):37–38.

Fitch MT, Manthey DE. Abdominal hernia reduction. In: Roberts JR, Custalow CB, Thomsen TW, eds. *Roberts and Hedges Clinical Procedures in Emergency Medicine.* 6th ed. Philadelphia: Elsevier; 2014:873–897.

Fitzgibbons RJ, Giobbie-Hurder A, Gibbs JO, et al. Watchful waiting vs repair of inguinal hernia in minimally symptomatic men: a randomized clinical trial. *JAMA.* 2006;295:285–292.

Kauffman HM, O'Brien DP. Selective reduction of incarcerated inguinal hernia. *Am J Surg.* 1970;119:660–673.

O'Dwyer PJ, Norrie J, Alani A, et al. Observation or operation for patients with an asymptomatic inguinal hernia: a randomized clinical trial. *Ann Surg.* 2006;244.

Urinary System Procedures

Section Editor: GRANT C. FOWLER

CHAPTER 96

BLADDER CATHETERIZATION (AND URETHRAL DILATION)

Robert E. James • Grant C. Fowler

Bladder catheterization may be performed for diagnostic or therapeutic indications (or both). This procedure is the most common retrograde manipulation performed in the urinary tract. Familiarity with the anatomy of the urethra and the available catheters will increase the ease and success of this procedure. Like all procedures in urology, this should be performed in a gentle fashion; instruments need not be forced. This is considered by patients to be among the five most painful emergency procedures, so adequate lubrication and, whenever possible, anesthetic jelly should be used.

In the adult male patient, there are two points where obstruction is commonly encountered when passing a catheter. The first is at the point of acute upward angulation located between the bulbous and the membranous urethra. The second is at the bladder neck, where a bladder neck stenosis or an enlarged median lobe of the prostate gland may be present (Fig. 96.1). In younger male patients, urethral folds or valves may resist the insertion of a catheter. Other possible sources for resistance to passage are also found along the entire course of the urethra, such as meatal stenosis, a urethral disruption or stricture, a false urethral passage, an enlarged prostate, a malignant process, an inflammatory process, or a bladder neck contracture or obstruction.

In the female patient, the urethra is much shorter, averaging only 2 inches in an adult. The angle between the urethra and the bladder neck increases with age. Consequently, in the older patient, the urethra is normally directed toward the sacrum, whereas in the younger patient it is angled toward the umbilicus. Keeping these urethral angles in mind will improve the clinician's technique, thereby increasing patient comfort and facilitating passage of the catheter. Catheter size is measured in French units. As the number increases, the size increases (i.e., a 16 Fr catheter is larger than a 12 Fr catheter). One "French unit" is approximately 0.33 mm.

INDICATIONS

Indications and contraindications for infants and children are basically the same as for adults. Since urinary tract infections are the most common healthcare-associated infections and account for more than 30% of infections reported in acute care hospitals, it is important to make sure a catheter is truly indicated and not just inserted for the convenience of a busy emergency department, hospital ward, or long-term care facility. It is also important that catheters be well-maintained and removed as soon as no longer needed. (See Box 96.1 for methods to minimize catheter associated urinary tract infection).

Short-Term Catheterization

- Acute urinary retention
- Collection of uncontaminated urine specimen for analysis, culture, and sensitivity, only if the patient is not able to spontaneously void
- Diagnostic studies of the lower urinary tract (e.g., cystogram, voiding cystourethrogram, urodynamics)
- Monitoring of urinary output
- Measurement of postvoid residual urine volume
- Irrigation of the bladder or instillation of medication
- Surgery on the urinary tract or adjacent structures
- Bladder drainage during and after surgical procedures requiring anesthetics
- Intermittent (in and out) catheterization for neurogenic bladder

Long-Term Catheterization

- Chronic urinary retention
- Neurogenic bladder in patient with the inability to intermittently self-catheterize
- Incontinence complicated by skin breakdown
- Patient requires prolonged immobilization (e.g., potentially unstable thoracic or lumbar spine, multiple traumatic injuries such as pelvic fractures).
- As a comfort measure for the terminally ill or severely disabled patient with incontinence

NOTE: A 2005 Cochrane review found that patients requiring catheterization for up to 14 days had less discomfort, bacteriuria, and need for recatheterization when suprapubic catheters were used compared with urethral catheters. Similarly, in a meta-analysis of patients having abdominal surgery, suprapubic catheters were found to cause less bacteriuria and discomfort and were preferred by patients (see Chapter 99, Suprapubic Catheter Insertion and/or Change). However, a more recent (2015) Cochrane review found the evidence to be inconclusive regarding which type of catheter had the lowest risk for urinary tract infections.

CONTRAINDICATIONS

- Known or suspected urethral disruption resulting from pelvic trauma (be suspicious if there is blood at the urethral meatus, a perineal hematoma, or a high-riding prostate)
- Recent reconstructive surgery of the urethra or bladder neck (relative contraindication, but should consult urology)
- Known urinary tract obstruction, such as a urethral stricture (relative contraindication, may be able to dilate)
- A combative or uncooperative patient (relative contraindication; see Chapter 1, Procedural Sedation and Analgesia)
- An acute infection of the prostate and/or urethra (relative contraindication)

EQUIPMENT

- Urethral catheters
  - *Robinson catheter:* A straight, rounded-tip catheter used for short-term catheterization; one version is the red rubber catheter. Low-friction, hydrophilic-coated catheters have been

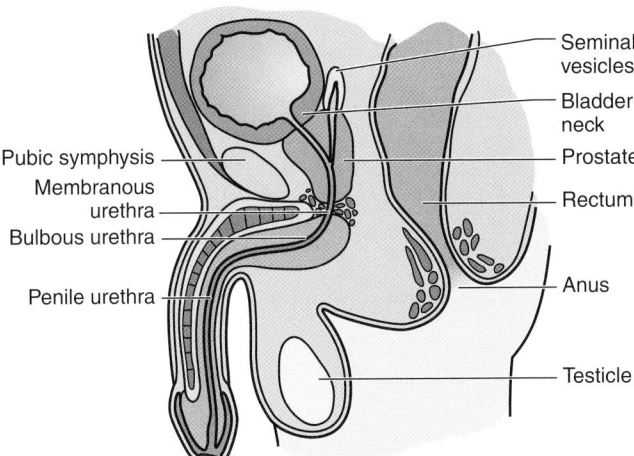

Fig. 96.1   Male urethral anatomy.

(Labels, clockwise:) Seminal vesicles; Bladder neck; Prostate; Rectum; Anus; Testicle; Penile urethra; Bulbous urethra; Membranous urethra; Pubic symphysis

found to increase patient satisfaction and decrease urinary tract infection and hematuria in patients who practice clean, intermittent self-catheterization.

• *Foley catheter:* A straight, self-retaining catheter that may have two or three lumina. While urine flows through the main, large lumen, and the secondary, smaller lumen is connected to a port used to inflate the retaining balloon (Fig. 96.2A), a Foley with a third lumen may be selected if irrigation will be necessary, such as for ongoing hematuria. A 16- to 18-Fr Foley catheter may be used for adults or adolescents (smaller sizes are used for infants and children) who require either a temporary or a chronic indwelling catheter. Foley catheters have short- or long-nose tips. Silicone or silicone-coated versions tend to be preferred over rubber catheters for long-term use because they produce less tissue reaction, have less encrustation, and have a larger lumen. By design, the retaining balloons can be overinflated, if necessary, to twice their stated capacity.

• *Coudé catheter:* This catheter is similar to a Foley catheter with some slight variations: the last 2 inches at the tip are curved upward (*coudé* is the French word for "elbow"; Fig. 96.2B) and there is a small ball on the tip. This catheter is used in adult men for whom a Robinson or Foley catheter cannot be inserted because of an enlarged median lobe of the prostate or an elevated bladder neck. Some clinicians advocate using a coudé catheter in all men older than 50 years of age. Coudé catheters are available with or without a self-retaining balloon. A 16- to 18-Fr catheter is normally used.

• *Filiforms and followers:* Filiforms are very thin, very pliable solid catheters that range in size from 1 to 6 Fr and are used to dilate a male urethral stricture. They may be straight or pig-tailed, or have a coudé tip, but they all have a female screw tip on the opposite end for attachment of followers. Followers are larger in diameter (12 to 30 Fr), have a male screw tip to attach to the filiforms, and are usually hollow with an open end. (Avoid the solid or closed-end followers; it may be impossible to tell when the forward tip has reached the bladder, so significant damage can occur. With the hollow, open-ended followers, you can tell when you are in the bladder because urine starts to flow.) Both filiforms and followers have a smooth-coated surface and are made of plastic or have a woven fiber core.

NOTE: Silastic catheters are available for latex-sensitive patients. In addition, although a Cochrane review found that silver alloy–impregnated catheters compared with standard catheters were associated with decreased rates of urinary tract infections; this is considered controversial and they are expensive.

• Lubricant—either a water-soluble lubricant (K-Y Jelly) or a lubricant with a local anesthetic (2% lidocaine jelly)—may be used. When available, the latter is preferred; 10 mL is sufficient for adult and adolescent female patients and 10 to 20 mL for adult and adolescent male patients, with smaller amounts for infants and children.
• Sterile towels and gloves
• Sterile cotton-tipped applicators
• Antiseptic solution
• Closed urinary drainage system (bedside overnight drainage bag, leg bag, or abdominal drainage system [belly bag])

PREPROCEDURE PATIENT PREPARATION

The specific indications for catheterization, as well as the risks, benefits, alternatives, and technique, should be reviewed with the patient, parent, or caregiver. Long-term catheter care should be discussed if the catheter is to remain in place. (See the sample patient education form available at www.expertconsult.com.) Informed consent is not always necessary for catheterization; however, at least verbal consent should be obtained and documented in the chart. Self-catheterization should be taught to the patient (or parent or caregiver) with the neurogenic bladder. Adequate lubrication and sufficient frequency are more important than sterile conditions if the patient is going to intermittently self-catheterize. If dilation is necessary, the patient should also understand the risks, benefits, alternatives, and technique. Informed consent should be obtained. It may be comforting to reassure the patient that everything possible will be done to maintain his or her modesty.

TECHNIQUE

Bladder Catheterization

1. The *female patient* is placed in the dorsal lithotomy (preferred) or the supine position with the legs abducted (i.e., frog-legged position). The *male patient* is placed in the supine position; the legs may be either abducted slightly or straight. The clinician should observe universal blood and body fluid precautions.
2. Identify the urethral meatus. For men, the penis should be grasped by the clinician's nondominant hand and positioned pointing toward the umbilicus. Although the meatus should be easily identified in the circumcised man, gentle retraction of the foreskin (prepuce) may be necessary to identify the meatus in the uncircumcised man. Lateral and outward traction on the labia by the clinician's nondominant hand may help identify the meatus in women. Recall the female anatomy; after lateral retraction of the labia minora exposes the vaginal vault, the clitoris is found at the anterior junction of the labia minora. The three orifices tracking posteriorly from the clitoris are the urethral meatus, the vagina and the rectum. Applying downward pressure with the posterior bill of a vaginal speculum may also be helpful in women. In female infants or girls, hymenal folds may obscure the meatus, but again, lateral traction by the nondominant hand will usually help identify the meatus. If not, downward pressure with a cotton-tipped applicator placed over the introitus will usually improve visualization. Women who will be self-catheterizing can be taught to identify the meatus with a mirror. For repeat catheterizations in women, a finger inserted into the vagina can help guide the catheter.

NOTE: Most of the difficulty regarding insertion of a catheter in women results from poor knowledge of or confusion related to the external genitalia. The clitoris is often mistaken for the urethral meatus which can result in unnecessary catheter-related trauma, patient discomfort, frustration, and bleeding.

3. Cleanse the urethral meatus and surrounding area with antiseptic solution, and isolate the genitalia with sterile drapes or towels. Maintain sterile technique throughout the remainder of the procedure.

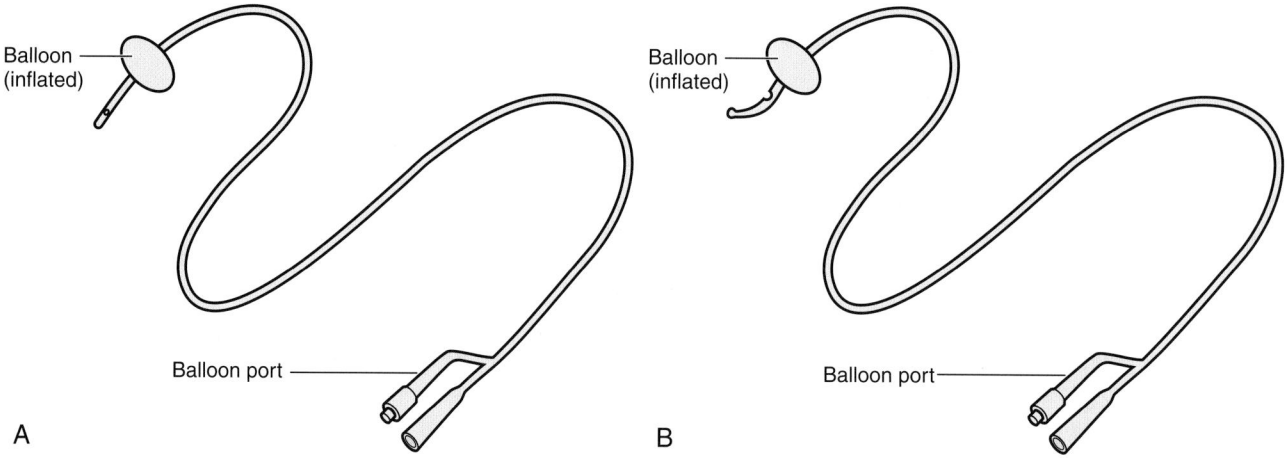

Balloon (inflated)

Balloon port

A

Balloon (inflated)

Balloon port

B

Fig. 96.2 (A) Foley catheter with balloon inflated. (B) Coudé catheter with balloon inflated.

NOTE: As previously mentioned, bladder catheterization is considered by patients to be among the top five most painful emergency procedures. If possible, anesthetic jelly should be used.

4. Insert the lubricant into the urethra with a syringe. If anesthetic jelly is used, leave it in place for approximately 5 to 10 minutes (longer is better to maximize effect). Some manufacturers place the lubricant in a syringe with a smooth conical end that can be inserted into the urethra. Otherwise, draw it into a 10-mL syringe. Place the end of the syringe (without a needle) gently inside the urethral meatus and inject the jelly into the urethra. Less lubricant is needed for infants, children, and women because the urethra is shorter. An alternative to injecting anesthetic jelly into the female urethra is to place it on a sterile cotton-tipped applicator and insert it gently into the urethra. This method allows the clinician to also determine the angle of the urethra to follow for later insertion of the catheter. After injecting the jelly, the male patient should be asked to compress the mid-urethra between his index finger and thumb to prevent the jelly from leaving the urethra.

5. Insertion technique for male and female patients:
   - For adult or adolescent female patients, select a 16- or 18-Fr Foley or Robinson catheter (use appropriately sized pediatric feeding tubes in female newborns and infants; smaller Foley or Robinson catheters can be used in larger girls). Following the anticipated course of the urethra, pass the catheter into the bladder. Catheter placement is confirmed when urine is obtained, and this is usually after advancing about 3 inches in adults (less for infants and children). For a Foley catheter advance the catheter at least another inch beyond where urine is obtained to allow room for inflation of the balloon. When certain that the tip and balloon are inside the bladder, inflate the balloon, with 5 mL of normal saline or water. The catheter is then gently pulled outward until the balloon rests against the bladder neck.
   - For adult or adolescent male patients younger than 50 years of age, a 16- or 18-Fr Foley or Robinson catheter may be used (use appropriately sized pediatric feeding tubes in male newborns and infants, smaller Foley or Robinson catheters in larger boys). With the nondominant hand, hold the penis taut while directing it toward the umbilicus to straighten the urethra. With the dominant hand, pass the catheter into the bladder the full length, up to the junction of the Foley catheter and the inflation port for the balloon (Fig. 96.3), or until it reaches the hub of a Robinson catheter.

CAUTION: In male patients, if the penis is not held taut, the catheter may get misdirected at the base of the penis and cause urethral damage. Also, if the Foley is not passed all the way to the port, the balloon may be inflated within the urethra, causing significant damage. The balloon is normally inflated with 5 mL of normal saline or water. In male or female patients, the balloon does not inflate easily, or if the patient experiences discomfort

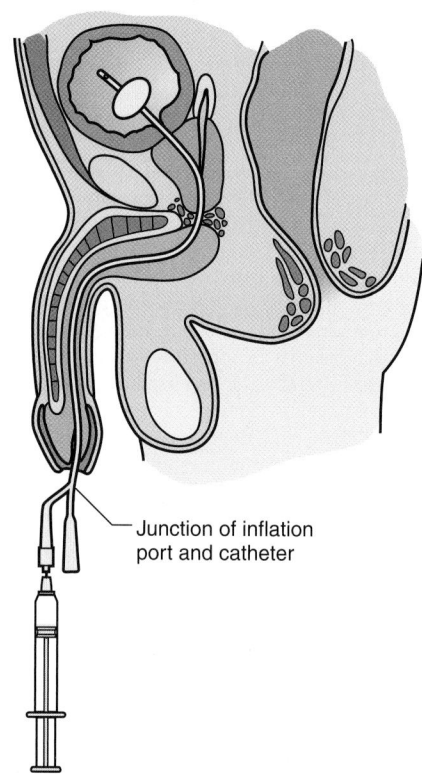

Junction of inflation port and catheter

Fig. 96.3 In the male patient, the Foley catheter is passed into the bladder until the junction of the catheter and the inflation port for the balloon is met.

in the perineum or penis as the balloon is being inflated, you should suspect that the balloon is located within the urethra. In such a case, the balloon should then be deflated and the catheter reinserted.

Once the balloon has been inflated, the catheter is then gently pulled outward until the balloon rests against the bladder neck.
   - For male patients older than 50 years, consider a coudé catheter. The curve at the tip of the catheter should be directed at the 12 o'clock (anterior) position. This will permit the catheter to glide over an enlarged median lobe of the prostate gland or an elevated bladder neck. If the catheter does not pass easily, it should be removed and the procedure repeated. Occasionally, the tip of the catheter will rotate as it is being inserted. If this occurs, the catheter will not pass through the prostatic urethra into the bladder. If you cannot pass a 16-Fr Foley or coudé catheter into the male urethra, there is usually

a urethral stricture, bladder neck stenosis, or very large median lobe of the prostate gland. *Or*, if the prostatic urethra has been previously resected, the tip of the catheter may hang up at the widened outlet of the prostatic urethra. In any of these cases, you may consider using a 12-Fr Foley or coudé catheter. The catheter tip may also be caught in a posterior urethral fold, right before it can enter the prostatic urethra. Upward pressure with three fingers from the nondominant hand on the perineum, between the scrotum and the rectum, may direct the catheter tip upward enough to enter the urogenital diaphragm on its way into the prostatic urethra. Alternatively, if the patient has an enlarged prostate, directing the catheter tip into the prostatic urethra with the dominant hand while a gloved finger from the other hand is in the rectum may also be helpful. If the smaller catheter does not pass after these maneuvers, either dilation with filiform and followers is necessary or a urology consultation should be sought. Once a Foley catheter is fully inserted, inflate the balloon and gently pull back on the catheter until the balloon is securely in place.

6. With the catheter in place, it needs to be secured to the leg with tape or other means to prevent trauma to the urethra. If urine does not flow freely, the tip of the catheter may be obstructed by lubricating jelly. Suprapubic pressure on a full bladder will usually flush the lubricant from the lumen. If the bladder is not full, gentle flushing from below with a 60-mL syringe full of sterile saline may open the lumen. It may take more than one syringe full in a dehydrated patient, but there should be return of fluid with gentle aspiration after injecting sterile saline. If not, remove the catheter from the urethra and repeat the procedure.

Difficult Catheterizations

WOMEN: Postmenopausal women with a narrow introitus, obese women, or women with a recessed or high-riding urethra may be very difficult to catheterize because the urethral meatus is difficult to visualize. In these cases, the following technique is usually successful. After preparing the patient as previously described, identify the urethral meatus with the tip of one of your index fingers. Then, slide a 16-Fr catheter along the index finger and into the urethra. If this cannot be accomplished, the patient may have a stenotic meatus. Applying the same technique, use a 12-Fr Foley or coudé catheter. If this attempt is unsuccessful, a urology consult is advised.

MEN: In uncircumcised male patients, to avoid the complication of a paraphimosis, always reduce the foreskin after catheter placement. In men with a severe phimosis, the foreskin cannot be retracted enough to see the urethral meatus. If the os of the foreskin is large enough to pass a catheter, you may be successful using the following technique. Fix the glans penis in its normal position with the meatus at the 6 o'clock position. Using a coudé catheter, rotate the catheter tip to the 6 o'clock (posterior) position. The tip of the catheter will be directed through the os of the foreskin in this position. Once the catheter has entered the the outermost portion of urethra, it may be rotated until the tip is pointed up, at the 12 o'clock position. To avoid damaging the urethra, make sure only the distal tip is in the urethra; it should rotate very easily. The catheter may then be advanced from there all the way into the bladder. If the os of the foreskin will not permit the passage of a catheter, a dorsal slit of the foreskin may be performed (see Chapter 104, Dorsal Slit for Phimosis) and the catheter inserted. Otherwise, a suprapubic catheter may need to be inserted. To minimize the risk of stricture formation in male patients with a long-term indwelling catheter, the catheter should be secured to the anterior abdominal wall (i.e., abdominal drainage system or belly bag).

The optimal amount of time to leave a catheter in place for men with benign prostatic hyperplasia (BPH) is unknown. For men catheterized to relieve acute urinary retention due to BPH, up to 70% will have recurrent urinary retention within a week if the bladder is simply drained. However, the use of α-adrenergic blockers (e.g., alfuzosin, tamsulosin) for 3 days starting at the time of catheter insertion has been shown to increase the likelihood of a successful voiding

trial without a catheter at 2 to 3 days after catheter removal. American Urological Association guidelines recommend at least one attempted trial of voiding after catheter removal before considering surgical intervention. Prevention of acute urinary retention in BPH may be achieved by long-term treatment (4 to 6 years) with dutasteride, finasteride, or a combination of finasteride and doxazosin. The American Urological Association guidelines recommend using only the 5-α-reductase inhibitors finasteride and dutasteride in men with demonstrable prostate enlargement by digital rectal examination.

Filiforms and Followers

After unsuccessful Foley and coudé catheterization attempts in male patients, these methods are available.

1. Reinstill anesthetic jelly into the urethra of the patient who has already been prepared and draped for prior catheterization attempts.
2. With the nondominant hand, hold the penis taut while directing it toward the umbilicus to straighten the urethra. With the dominant hand, grasp a filiform, dip it into anesthetic jelly, and gently insert it into the urethra. Advance the filiform into the urethra until resistance is met. The filiform should be rotated slightly while it is being advanced. Grasp a second filiform, dip it into anesthetic jelly, and advance it likewise into the urethra, while rotating it, until resistance is again met. Attempt to advance the first filiform further. If the first filiform will not advance, insert a third filiform after dipping it in anesthetic jelly, and advance it with slight rotation until it meets resistance. Attempt to advance the first and second filiforms, again. At this point, the filiform tips are either in a false lumen or the resistance is due to a fold or stricture. Inserting additional filiforms will either dilate the stricture or pass the fold or false lumen. Continue to insert filiforms, while each time attempting to advance the previously inserted filiforms, until one advances. Advance this filiform until only approximately 1 inch remains outside the penis. Remove all other filiforms except this one.
3. Lubricate a follower catheter and attach it to the inserted filiform. Use only a hollow, open-ended follower catheter so that you can tell when the bladder has been reached or entered. When the bladder has been reached by the follower, urine should flow through it spontaneously. Gently advance the follower into the bladder until only 1 or 2 inches remains outside the penis. (The tip of the filiform will curl up inside the bladder for the follower to advance.) If resistance is met, withdraw the tip connected to the filiform until it is an inch or more outside the penis. Select, lubricate, and attach a follower that is 1 or 2 Fr smaller than the previous one, and attempt to insert this gently into the bladder. Continue this process until a follower is able to be inserted into the bladder (i.e., up to the point where only 1 or 2 inches remains outside the penis). The urethra may then need to be dilated using the process described in the next step.
4. If the follower catheter is 16 or 18 Fr in diameter, remove it and insert a Foley catheter. If it is less than 16 Fr, the urethra must be dilated. Withdraw the tip connected to the filiform until it is 1 or 2 inches outside the penis. Select, lubricate, and attach a follower that is 1 or 2 Fr larger than the previous one, and attempt to gently insert this into the bladder. Continue this process until a 16- or 18-Fr follower can be inserted and then converted to a Foley.

Catheter Management

With indwelling catheters, many patients experience discomfort at the junction of the urethral meatus with the catheter. This may be mitigated by applying petroleum jelly or vitamin E ointment to the meatus daily. (Otherwise, daily meatal care should be avoided because it has been associated with increased risk of infection.) Changing indwelling catheters or drainage bags at routine, fixed intervals is no longer recommended. Rather, it is suggested to change catheters and drainage bags based on clinical indications such as infection, obstruction, or when the closed system is compromised. Robinson and non–self-retaining coudé catheters need to be secured to the penis. Clinicians should note that tape should never be applied circumferentially around the penis because it may cause ischemia. Instead, three thin strips of tape applied along the penis and attached to the catheter will usually prevent inadvertent removal. Maintenance of a closed drainage system is important for the prevention of infections. Keep the collecting bag below the level of the bladder at all times. Keep the catheter and collecting tube free from kinking. Empty the collecting bag regularly using a separate clean collecting container per patient. Prevent splashing and contact between the spigot and the nonsterile collecting container. Consider using a portable ultrasound device to assess urine volume in patients undergoing intermittent catheterization to assess urine volume and to reduce unnecessary catheter insertions.

Antibiotic Therapy

If a urinary tract infection is suspected, a urine culture and sensitivity should be obtained and the patient treated with appropriate antibiotics for at least 3 days.

COMPLICATIONS

- Urinary tract infection (see Box 96.1 for prevention guidelines)
- Transient hematuria
- Creation of a false passage urethral tear or perforation resulting from the use of a small catheter or excessive force, or the presence of a urethral stricture
- Conversion of a partial urethral tear into a complete tear in a trauma patient with urethral injury
- Urethral stricture
- Obstruction of flow
- Epididymitis, pyelonephritis, and urosepsis are often seen with prolonged catheterization. Increased mortality was found in nursing home patients with an indwelling catheter at 1 year, but that statistic is probably confounded by other factors such as protein-calorie malnutrition.

PATIENT EDUCATION GUIDES

See the sample patient education form available at www.expertcosult.com.

CPT/BILLING CODES

51700	Bladder irrigation, simple, lavage and/or instillation
51701	Insertion of nonindwelling bladder catheter (e.g., straight catheterization for residual urine)
51702	Insertion of temporary indwelling bladder catheter; simple (e.g., Foley)
51703	Insertion of temporary indwelling bladder catheter; complicated (e.g., altered anatomy, fractured catheter/balloon)
53620	Dilation of urethral stricture by passage of filiform and follower, male; initial

ICD-10-CM DIAGNOSTIC CODES

G83.4	Neurogenic bladder, with cauda equina syndrome
N32.0	Bladder neck obstruction, acquired
N31.9	Neurogenic bladder, NOS
N35.014	Male urethral stricture, caused by trauma
N35.9	Urethral stricture, unspecified
N13.9	Urinary obstruction, unspecified
N40.0	Prostatism, hypertrophy (benign) of prostate
N40.1	Hyperplasia of prostate, unspecified, with urinary obstruction
N42.89	Prostatic stricture
N47.1	Phimosis
N39.3	Stress urinary incontinence, female or male
Q64.31	Bladder neck obstruction, congenital
R33.9	Urinary retention or stasis, unspecified
R32	Urinary incontinence, unspecified

SUPPLIERS

(See contact information available at www.expertconsult.com.)

General
  Bard Medical
  Cook Medical
Catheters and closed drainage systems
  Rusch, Inc. (Teleflex Medical)

ONLINE RESOURCES

Weiner D. Bladder Catheterization: Male and Bladder Catheterization: Female. www.proceduresconsult.com/medical-procedures/procedure-results.aspx?search=bladder.
Figler BD: Bladder catheterization. www.merckmanuals.com/professional/genitourinary-disorders/genitourinary-tests-and-procedures/bladder-catheterization#v23033632.

RECOMMENDED READING

Cravens DD, Zweig S. Urinary catheter management. *Am Fam Physician.* 2000;61:369–376.

BOX 96.1 Centers for Disease Control and Prevention Guidelines for the Prevention of Catheter-Associated Urinary Tract Infection

Category I: Strongly Recommended
Catheterize only when necessary.
Educate personnel in the correct techniques of catheter insertion and care.
Emphasize handwashing.
Insert the catheter using an aseptic technique and sterile equipment.
Secure the catheter properly.
Maintain closed sterile drainage.
Obtain urine specimens aseptically.
Maintain unobstructed urine flow.

Category II: Moderately Recommended
Periodically reeducate personnel in catheter care.
Use smallest suitable catheter bore.
Avoid irrigation unless needed to prevent or relieve obstruction.
Refrain from daily meatal care.
Do not change catheter at arbitrary intervals.

From Gould DV, Umscheid CA, Agarwal RK, Kuntz G, Pegues DA, and the Healthcare Infection Control Practices Advisory Committee: CDC Guideline for prevention of catheter associated urinary tract infections; 2009. Updated November 2017. Also see Cravens DD, Zweig S. Urinary catheter management. *Am Fam Physician.* 2000;61:369–376.

Davis JE, Silverman MA. Urologic procedures. In: Roberts JR, Custalow CB, Thomsen TW, eds. *Roberts and Hedges Clinical Procedures in Emergency Medicine.* 6th ed. Philadelphia: Elsevier; 2014:1113–1154.

Gould DV, Umscheid CA, Agarwal RK, Kuntz G. *Pegues DA and the Healthcare Infection Control Practices Advisory Committee: CDC Guideline for Prevention of Catheter Associated Urinary Tract Infections;* 2009. Last updated 2017.

Kidd EA, Stewart F, Kassis NC, Hom E, Omar M. Urethral (indwelling or intermittent) or suprapubic routes for short-term catheterisation in hospitalised adults. *Cochrane Database Syst Rev.* 2015;(12):CD004203.

Jahn P, Beutner K, Langer G. Types of indwelling urinary catheters for long-term bladder drainage in adults. *Cochrane Database of Syst Rev.* 2012;10:CD004997.

Lam TBL, Omar M, Fisher E, Gillies K, MacLennan S. Types of urethral catheters for management of short-term voiding problems in hospitalised adults. *Cochrane Database of Syst Rev.* 2014;9:CD004013.

McPhail MJ, Abu-Hilal M, Johnson CD. A meta-analysis comparing suprapubic and transurethral catheterization for bladder drainage after abdominal surgery. *Br J Surg.* 2006;93:1038–1044.

Moore KN, Kelm M, Sinclair O, Cadrain G. Bacteriuria in intermittent catheterization users: the effect of sterile versus clean reused catheters. *Rehabil Nurs.* 1993;18:306–309.

Niel-Weise BS, van den Broek PJ. Urinary catheter policies for short-term bladder drainage in adults. *Cochrane Database Syst Rev.* 2005; 3:CD004203.

Selius BA, Subedi R. Urinary retention in adults: diagnosis and initial management. *Am Fam Physician.* 2008;77:643–650.

Robinson RD, Reichman EF. Urethral Catheterization. In: Reichman EF, ed. *Emergency Medicine Procedures.* 2nd ed. New York: McGraw-Hill; 2013:953–962.

CHAPTER 97

DIAGNOSTIC CYSTOURETHROSCOPY

Grant C. Fowler

The construction of the cystoscope has progressed from the original tube and candle, first described in the early 1800s, to the flexible fiberoptic cystoscope currently available. The standard rigid cystourethroscope is composed of three components: the telescope, sheath, and bridge. (Rigid urethroscopes are also available, designed exclusively for evaluation of the urethra, and are a modification of the cystoscope.) Once the sheath is in place, the telescope can be removed and changed as needed for different lenses to view different aspects of the bladder. Various instruments useful for procedures (e.g., biopsy, cautery, injection), both rigid and flexible, can also be inserted. The rigid nature of the scope also allows more to be done with one hand; this frees the other hand to manipulate ancillary instruments.

Unlike the rigid cystoscope, the flexible cystoscope combines the optical systems and irrigation/working channel into a single unit. The flexible cystoscope also has a smaller diameter and a tip that can be deflected as much as 290 degrees in a single plane; it can be used without a working sheath and is generally more comfortable for the patient. The active tip deflection allows for a more complete inspection of the bladder; it may also be easier to negotiate around the median lobe of the prostate or an elevated bladder neck. The patient can be in the recumbent position as opposed to the dorsal lithotomy position. This makes it ideal for use in the office or outpatient setting. However, although they are continuing to improve, the image from a flexible cystoscope is not generally as clear as that obtained with a rigid cystoscope. Because the diameter of the flexible cystoscope is also smaller, operative and diagnostic procedures are limited by the decreased capacities of the irrigating and working channels. Because there is no sheath, the flexible cystoscope has to be removed completely to change the lens and reinserted to assess residual urine and to reevacuate the irrigant. Therefore the flexible cystoscope is used more commonly in the office setting for routine diagnostic viewing of the bladder and urethra (hematuria or tumor surveillance, double-J stent retrieval) as opposed to operative procedures. That said, either type of cystoscope, rigid or flexible, can be useful in the diagnosis of various conditions ranging from urinary incontinence to pain syndromes.

EDITOR'S NOTE: It might be helpful to review Chapter 96, Bladder Catheterization (and Urethral Dilation), along with this chapter.

INDICATIONS

- Urethral stricture or diverticulum on radiograph (for diagnostic or therapeutic purposes; e.g., using the rigid cystourethroscope or urethroscope, a cold knife incision of a limited stricture can be performed or a catheter placed into a diverticulum for localization during open surgical repair)
- Suspected urethral calculi (rare), foreign body, or condylomata (for diagnosis or removal)
- Urinary incontinence
  - Intrinsic sphincter deficiency (cystourethroscopy confirms the diagnosis and allows treatment with periurethral bulking agents)
  - Obstructive or irritative voiding symptoms (e.g., urgency, frequency, urge incontinence) unresponsive to conservative measures
- Suspected or known bladder diverticulum or fistula, or ectopic ureter (e.g., seen on radiograph)
- Gross or microscopic hematuria
- Known or suspected urogynecologic malignancy
  - Staging or surveillance for bladder, cervical, or endometrial cancer
- Recurrent urinary tract infections
- Pelvic pain symptoms
  - Dyspareunia
  - Suspected interstitial cystitis, urethritis, or trigonitis (see also Chapter 98, Office Testing and Treatment Options for Interstitial Cystitis [Painful Bladder Syndrome])
  - Endometriosis of the bladder
- Traumatic injury to the lower genital tract
- Intraoperative assessment of the bladder or urethra
  - Exclusion of inadvertent intraluminal suture placement or bladder trauma after incontinence or prolapse correction procedures
  - Assessment of coaptation of the urethra after suburethral sling procedures
  - Evaluation of ureteral patency with intravenous indigo carmine dye

CONTRAINDICATIONS

- Acute cystitis, prostatitis, or pyelonephritis should be treated before cystourethroscopy is performed, because sepsis has been reported after cystoscopy in an infected patient.
- Anticoagulated patient or patient with coagulopathy (either the anticoagulation/coagulopathy should be reversed or urology consulted).

EQUIPMENT

- Rigid cystoscope and sheath (Fig. 97.1).
  - Sterile rigid telescopes with 0-, 30-, 70-, and 120-degree lenses.
  - The 0-degree lens (forward looking) is useful for intraurethral work, the 30-degree lens (forward oblique) is useful for evaluation of the urethra and bladder, the 70-degree lens (lateral) is useful for inspecting the interior of the bladder, and the 120-degree lens (retrograde) is useful for retrograde viewing of the bladder neck.
  - Sterile sheath of 17- to 26-Fr diameter with inflow and outflow ports.
  - Sterile scope-to-sheath bridge. This bridge may have one or two operative ports that admit the passage of biopsy instruments or urethral catheters.
  - A light cable and light source compatible with the telescope.
  - Urethral dilators, including a range from 14 to 32 Fr.
- Flexible cystoscope and light source.

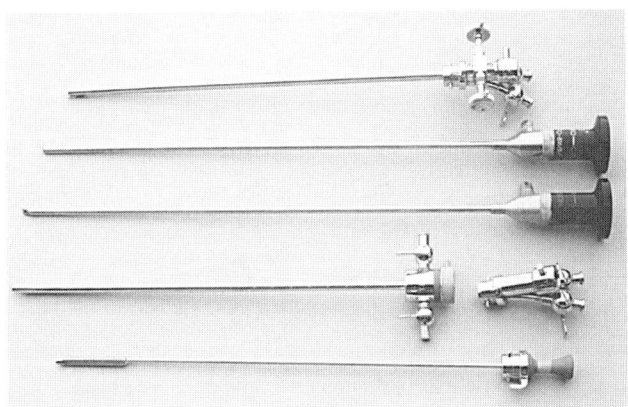

Fig. 97.1 *Top to bottom:* Cystoscope components, including operative sheath, telescopes (two), sheath and bridge, and obturator.

EDITOR'S NOTE: Digital scopes using a camera are now available. Studies comparing digital with fiberoptic scopes found the high-definition digital scopes to have significantly better resolution and depth of field. Illumination was found to be significantly better with the fiberoptic scopes. Durability was comparable; the only damage that occurred during the studies was not during use of the scopes, but rather when the scopes were being placed in a storage case.
- Irrigation tubing.
- Distension medium in 500-mL to 3-L bags. Saline or Ringer lactate may be used if electrocautery is not anticipated. If electrocautery is anticipated, then a nonconductive medium such as sterile water, mannitol, sorbitol, or glycine should be used, with water having the advantages of increased visibility and, because it is hypotonic, lysing tumor cells.
- Cotton balls moistened with an antiseptic solution (e.g., povidone-iodine).
- Sterile gloves.
- Sterile cotton-tipped applicators.
- 1% or 2% lidocaine (Xylocaine) gel.
- Blue towel for tray top.
- Basin to capture irrigation runoff.
- Necessary equipment to observe universal blood and body fluid precautions.

Although optional and expensive, video equipment, such as a camera, high-resolution monitor, video recorder, and printer, has its advantages. Video equipment provides a magnified, binocular view, allows the clinician the ability to maintain a more comfortable position when performing the procedure, is helpful for teaching or when an assistant is available, and provides the clinician greater eye protection from body fluids. Two studies that allowed men to observe during the procedure found that they tolerated the procedure better than those not allowed to observe; there was no difference when the same study was performed in women undergoing cystoscopy.

PREPROCEDURE PATIENT PREPARATION

Indications for, alternatives to, and risks of cystourethroscopy should be explained to the patient and informed consent obtained before the procedure. The patient should be informed of the possibility of discomfort during and after the procedure, as well as the potential for postprocedure urinary tract infection.

If a urinary tract infection is suspected, a urine culture and sensitivity should be obtained and the patient placed on a broad-spectrum antibiotic for at least 3 days. The American Urologic Association does not recommend antibiotic prophylaxis for routine diagnostic procedures in the absence of risk factors (Box 97.1). If the patient is not allergic to fluoroquinolones or sulfas,

BOX 97.1	Risk Factors Requiring Antimicrobial Prophylaxis

Advanced age
Anatomic anomalies of the urinary tract
Chronic corticosteroid use
Colonized endogenous or exogenous material
Distant coexistent infection
Immunodeficiency
Poor nutritional status
Prolonged coexistent infection
Smoking

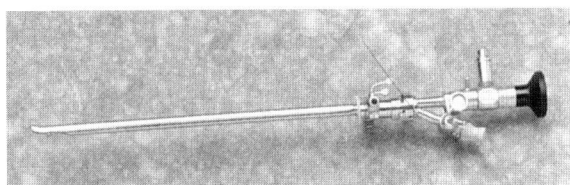

Fig. 97.2 Assembled cystoscope with telescope, bridge, and sheath.

a fluoroquinolone or trimethoprim-sulfamethoxazole for less than 24 hours is recommended for therapeutic procedures (see also Chapter 69, Antibiotic Prophylaxis). Second-line alternatives include an aminoglycoside with or without ampicillin, a first- or second-generation cephalosporin, or amoxicillin/clavulanate.

TECHNIQUE

Before routinely performing cystoscopy, clinicians should familiarize themselves with the equipment and feel comfortable recognizing abnormalities or pathology on visualization of the urethra or bladder. Universal blood and body fluid precautions should be followed throughout the procedure.

Preparation

1. After the patient has emptied the bladder, *cleanse the urethral meatus* with an antiseptic solution.
2. Generously *lubricate the cotton-tipped applicator* with 1% or 2% lidocaine gel, and insert it into the urethral meatus to the level of the bladder neck. Observe the angle of the urethra as an aid to inserting the cystoscope.

NOTE: Use sterile technique and wear sterile gloves from this point onward throughout the procedure.

Rigid Cystourethroscopy

3. Prepare the cystourethroscope as follows:
   - *Assemble the cystourethroscope* by attaching the 0-degree telescope to the bridge and sheath (Fig. 97.2).
   - *Attach the light cable* to the cystourethroscope and the light source. Turn on the light source before insertion to ensure proper illumination.
   - *Attach the infusion tubing* to the infusion port on the sheath, and attach this in turn to the appropriate instillation medium hung on a nearby intravenous pole. The tubing is then flushed.
4. *Lubricate the distal portion of the cystoscope* sheath with 1% or 2% lidocaine gel. Remove the applicator. After ensuring that all ports are in the closed position, *start the flow of the infusion medium* by opening the stopcock of the inflow port. The operator should have sole control of the fluid infusion through this port.

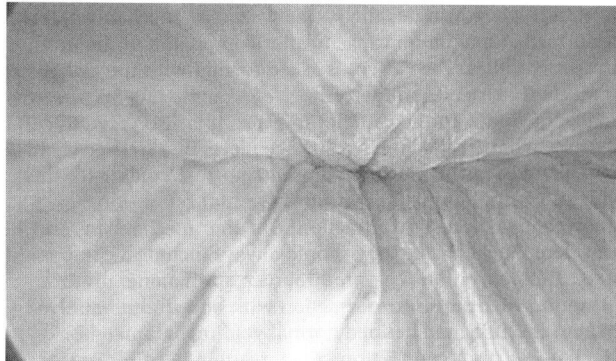

Fig. 97.3   View of normal urethral mucosa.

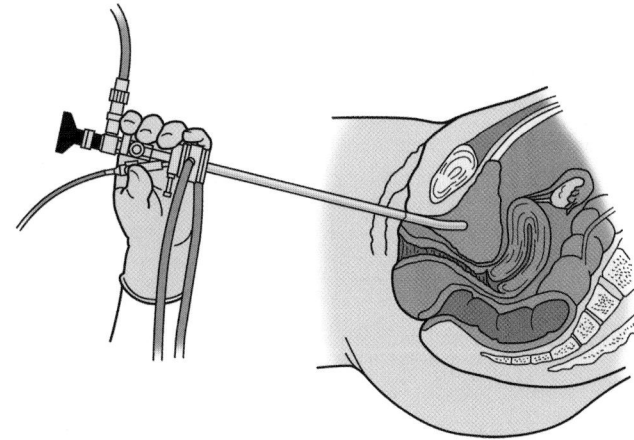

Fig. 97.4   Technique of cystoscopy using angled telescopic lens.

Urethroscopy

5. *Insert the lighted and assembled cystoscope* into the urethral meatus, following the line of the urethra. Initial insertion may be achieved using fluid as the obturator. Fluid is infused during inspection to a maximum of 350 to 500 mL or until the patient is uncomfortable. If resistance is encountered, the scope should not be forced; rather, the angle of insertion of the cystoscope should be reassessed. Continued difficulty in inserting the cystourethroscope may be an indication for urethral dilation before proceeding. Dilation can be performed serially using urethral dilators beginning with 14 Fr and dilating up to 32 Fr. Alternatively, a smaller-sized sheath can be used.

6. *Advance the cystoscope* under direct visualization into the bladder lumen. Then withdraw it slowly until the internal urethral meatus is visualized. While slowly withdrawing the cystourethroscope, examine the entire length of the urethral mucosa for pathology (Fig. 97.3). Gentle palpation of the anterior vaginal wall during withdrawal may help to identify a urethral diverticulum, which tend to occur on the posterior aspect of the urethra.

Cystoscopy

7. *Remove the cystoscope* and discontinue the infusion flow. *Replace the 0-degree telescope with an angled-lens (30- or 70-degree) telescope and reinsert* the reassembled cystoscope as described previously. For adequate cystoscopy, the bladder should be filled to approximately 250 mL or greater. If the patient notes discomfort from overdistention of the bladder, open the outflow port on the sheath and drain an appropriate amount of fluid from the bladder.

8. *Perform a systematic examination of the bladder lumen*, apply suprapubic pressure to facilitate visualization, and identify a small air bubble, which is usually present at the bladder dome. With this as a landmark, examine the anterior and lateral sidewalls in a stepwise fashion. To visualize the entire bladder dome, rotate the angled lens about the long axis of the telescope while keeping the camera in a fixed orientation (Fig. 97.4). Lateral torque, with the urethral meatus as the fulcrum, can cause pain and should be avoided. Intraluminal pathology, including the presence of tumor, endometriosis, trabeculations, stones, chronic cystitis, or hemorrhage, should be noted (Fig. 97.5). The bladder should be examined at various levels of filling; glomerulations and ecchymoses are frequently seen only with full distention. Intraluminal sutures inadvertently placed at the time of a previous urethropexy are generally identified on the lateral sidewalls at the 2 and 10 o'clock positions.

9. *Visualize the trigone*, located posteriorly just proximal to the internal urethral meatus at the 6 o'clock position. Any abnormalities should be noted. Rotating the scope 20 to 30 degrees to each side will allow visualization of the ureteral orifices. If one orifice is visualized, identification of the interureteric ridge will lead to the contralateral orifice. (In patients with large cystoceles, reduction

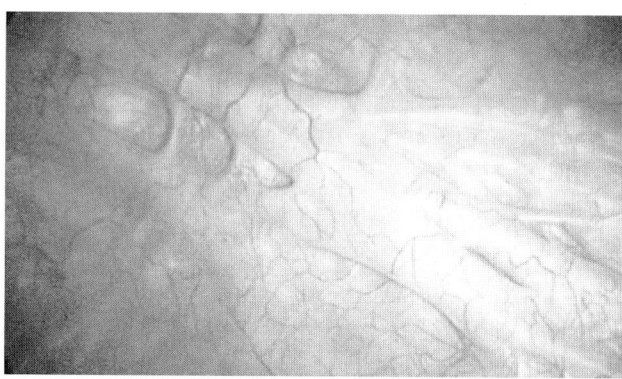

Fig. 97.5   Cystoscopic evaluation of bladder lumen demonstrating coarse trabeculations (ridges).

of the prolapse may be necessary to see the orifices.) If possible, identify ureteral peristalsis with efflux of urine.

10. Concurrent vaginal examination in women may be helpful for evaluating a cystocele. A concurrent rectal examination in men may be useful for assessing prostate size and length of the prostatic urethra.

11. For patients with pelvic pain or interstitial cystitis, bladder distention with at least 600 to 1000 mL may be therapeutic but usually requires general anesthesia because of poor tolerance in the office as a result of severe pain.

12. After completing the procedure, *turn off the infusion of distention medium and drain the patient's bladder* with the ancillary port on the cystoscope sheath. Samples of this drainage can be sent for cytologic analysis if desired (e.g., patient with prior history of malignancy). Remove the cystoscope and turn off the light source to prevent accidental injury from the hot light.

13. Disassemble the cystoscopic telescopes, bridge, and sheaths, and clean them by immersion in glutaraldehyde solution (Cidex) for 20 minutes before reuse.

Flexible Cystoscopy

14. Lubricate the distal portion of the cystoscope with 1% or 2% lidocaine gel.

15. Advance the cystoscope under direct visualization into the bladder lumen. (The flexible cystoscope is passed in a manner similar to a Foley catheter, except the lumen is visualized as it is passed.) Flex and torque the instrument to obtain a view of the same structures as visualized with rigid cystourethroscopy. The same maneuvers may be used as with rigid instruments to enhance visualization of various structures and pathology.

16. Withdraw the cystoscope slowly until the internal urethral meatus is visualized. While slowly withdrawing the cystoscope, examine the entire length of the urethral mucosa for pathology. The prostatic urethra will not be seen as clearly as with rigid instruments, but a general impression of prostatic size can be obtained.

17. Clean the flexible cystoscope and flush all channels and ports with soap and water. This should be followed by immersion in glutaraldehyde solution (Cidex) for 20 minutes before reuse.

BIOPSY

Bladder or *urethral mucosa biops*y is useful for evaluation and histologic confirmation of suspect lesions, including possible interstitial cystitis or malignancy. Although it can be performed in the office, bladder biopsy usually requires a larger sheath to accommodate the biopsy forceps, is associated with patient discomfort, and occasionally requires electrocautery to control bleeding. Given these considerations, it is recommended that cystoscopic biopsies be performed in the ambulatory surgical suite. Flexible biopsy forceps are available for the rigid scopes and may be helpful for reaching areas of the bladder that are difficult to reach with rigid forceps such as the dome and anterior wall; however, rigid biopsy forceps can remove tissue samples up to 5 mm in diameter, whereas the size of fragments obtained with flexible biopsy forceps is usually less than 2 mm.

COMPLICATIONS

- Bacteriuria
- Sepsis
- Urethral or bladder neck trauma
- Bleeding
- Pain

Complications after cystourethroscopy are rare. The reported rate of bacteriuria after this procedure is 2% to 7%. Rare cases of systemic sepsis associated with performance of cystoscopy in the presence of untreated infection have been reported. Rarely, trauma to the urethra and bladder neck can result from instrumentation.

INTERPRETATION OF RESULTS

A complete review of abnormal findings at the time of cystoscopy is beyond the scope of this chapter. However, the clinician who routinely performs cystoscopy should be familiar with the normal appearance of the bladder and urethra. Abnormal anatomic findings should correlate with the patient's symptoms. In patients with overactive bladder symptoms (urgency, frequency, nocturia, enuresis, or urge incontinence), the urethra should be inspected for a stricture or diverticulum and the bladder inspected for trabeculations, infectious changes, and foreign bodies.

For the evaluation of incontinence, cystoscopy is useful in the evaluation of intrinsic sphincter deficiency (the internal urethral meatus is open at rest) and vesicovaginal and urethrovaginal fistulas. In patients with genitourinary pain syndromes, the urethra may appear atrophic and the bladder may reveal petechial hemorrhages, ecchymoses, glomerulations, or Hunner ulcers consistent with interstitial cystitis (see also Chapter 98, Office Testing and Treatment Options for Interstitial Cystitis [Painful Bladder Syndrome]). Bladder distention, which is often therapeutic, can be accomplished at the time of cystoscopy with instillation of 600 to 1000 mL of solution.

Cystoscopy is useful for evaluation of lower urinary tract injury. Cystoscopy may reveal a bladder laceration or penetration of the bladder by sutures placed during surgery. To assess ureteral integrity and patency, patients can be given 5-mL intravenous indigo carmine at the time of cystoscopy. Both ureteral orifices should be noted to eject dye 5 to 10 minutes after intravenous injection. In some cases, dye spillage may be delayed up to 15 minutes.

POSTPROCEDURE PATIENT EDUCATION

Each patient should be provided with instructions concerning expected postprocedure symptoms. A preprinted informational handout may be useful for this purpose. Specific information should include the following:

1. Patients should take antibiotic prophylaxis, if prescribed. They should be instructed to follow up immediately if dysuria, pyuria, or fever greater than 100.4°F develops within 72 hours of the procedure.

2. A small amount of transient hematuria within the first few hours after cystoscopy is normal. If it persists or is excessive, the patient should be instructed to follow up immediately.

3. The patient may have some discomfort after the procedure. A short course of the bladder analgesic, phenazopyridine, may be used to alleviate this. If the discomfort persists, the patient should be instructed to follow up for evaluation.

CPT/BILLING CODES

52000	Cystourethroscopy (separate procedure)
52005	Cystourethroscopy, with ureteral catheterization
52204	Cystourethroscopy, with biopsy
52260	Cystourethroscopy, with dilation of bladder for interstitial cystitis; general or conduction (spinal) anesthesia
52281	Cystourethroscopy, with calibration and/or dilation of urethral stricture or stenosis
52285	Cystourethroscopy for treatment of the female urethral syndrome with any or all of the following: urethral meatotomy, urethral dilation, internal urethrotomy, lysis of urethrovaginal septal fibrosis, lateral incisions of the bladder neck, and fulguration of polyp(s) of urethra, bladder neck, and/or trigone

ICD-10-CM DIAGNOSTIC CODES

N20.1	Calculus: ureteral
N21.1	Calculus: urethral
N30.10	Interstitial cystitis chronic without hematuria
N30.20	Other cystitis chronic without hematuria
N32.2	Vesical fistula: bladder, not elsewhere classified
N34.1	Urethritis, unspecified
N34.3	Urethral syndrome, not otherwise specified
N35.12	Urethral stricture due to infection NOC female
N35.119	Urethral stricture due to infection NOC male
N36.0	Fistula: urethral
N36.1	Diverticulum: urethral
R31.9	Hematuria unspecified
N39.3	Incontinence: stress (female) (male)
N32.0	Bladder neck obstruction
R30.0	Dysuria
R33.9	Urinary retention, unspecified
R39.14	Incomplete bladder emptying
R32	Incontinence: unspecified
N39.41	Incontinence: urge
N39.46	Incontinence: mixed
N39.45	Incontinence: continuous leakage
R35.0	Urinary frequency
S37.20XA	Injury: bladder, initial encounter
S37.30XA	Injury; bladder, initial encounter

Acknowledgment

The editors recognize the contributions of Andrew C. Steele, MD, and Neeraj Kohli, MD, to this chapter in a previous edition of this text.

SUPPLIERS

(See contact information available at www.expertconsult.com.)

Gyrus ACMI Corporation (Olympus)
Karl Storz Endoscopy-America, Inc.
Stryker

ONLINE RESOURCES

Gyrus ACMI Olympus (leading supplier of endoscopic equipment): http://medical.olympusamerica.com. This site also has a number of instructional videos available on performing cystoscopy.

Karl Storz (major supplier of endoscopy equipment): www.karlstorz.com

National Institute of Diabetes and Digestive and Kidney Diseases: www.niddk.nih.gov. (Information on a wide range of topics on urologic conditions from the National Kidney and Urologic Diseases Information Clearinghouse and National Institutes of Health.)

RECOMMENDED READING

American College of Obstetricians and Gynecologists. Practice bulletin no. 155. Urinary incontinence in women. *Obstet Gynecol*. 2015;126(5): 66–81.

American College of Obstetricians and Gynecologist. Practice bulletin no. 104. Antibiotic prophylaxis for gynecologic procedures. *Obstet Gynecol*. 2009;113:1180–1189.

Duty BD, Conlin MJ. Principles of urologic endoscopy. In: Wein AJ, Kavoussi LR, Partin AW, Peters CA, eds. *Campbell-Walsh Urology*. 11th ed. Philadelphia: Elsevier; 2016:136–152.

French LM, Bhambore J. Interstitial cystitis/ painful bladder syndrome. *Am Fam Physician*. 2011;83(10):1175–1181.

Grossfeld GD, Litwin MS, Wolf Jr JS, et al. Evaluation of asymptomatic microscopic hematuria in adults: The American Urological Association best practice policy—part II. Patient evaluation, cytology, voided markers, imaging, cystoscopy, nephrology evaluation, and follow-up. *Urology*. 2001;57:604–610.

Sharp VJ, Barnes KT, Erickson BA. Assessment of microscopic hematuria in adults. *Am Fam Physician*. 2013;88(11):747–754.

Office Testing and Treatment Options for Interstitial Cystitis (Painful Bladder Syndrome)

Stephen A. Grochmal

Interstitial cystitis (IC), also known as *painful bladder syndrome* (PBS, which is actually a slightly broader category of disorders), is characterized by bladder pain of varying intensity, lasting over a prolonged period. IC is more prevalent in women but also can affect men, and the overall prevalence appears greater than was previously estimated. It may affect more than 1 million persons in the United States. Identification, diagnosis, and treatment of IC are controversial, similar to other medical conditions of unknown etiology that are difficult to treat.

Anatomy

The urinary and reproductive systems are related embryologically, and both systems develop from the intermediate mesoderm of the embryo. The endoderm that ultimately gives rise to the epithelium of the bladder trigone and urethra is the same as that which develops into the lower third of the vagina and vestibule. Therefore conditions that affect the bladder throughout life may also produce a variety of vaginal or vulvar symptoms, and vice versa.

The superior surface of the bladder is covered with peritoneum that separates it from the coils of the ileum and the sigmoid colon. As the bladder fills (maximum capacity is about 500 mL), this superior surface bulges upward into the abdominal cavity and the covering peritoneum separates from the lower part of the anterior abdominal wall. As a result, the bladder comes into direct contact with the anterior abdominal wall.

A glycosaminoglycan layer normally coats the urothelial bladder surface and renders it impermeable to any solutes. Defects in this layer may permit urinary irritants to penetrate the urothelium and activate the underlying nerve and muscle tissues. This process can lead to additional tissue damage, hypersensitivity, and pain. This ongoing bladder damage also may be propagated by mast cells in the bladder.

The pelvic floor and bladder are both innervated from sacral nerve roots S2, S3, and S4. These nerve roots include motor/efferent and sensory/afferent pathways of both the visceral and somatic systems.

Because of the proximity of the bladder to other surrounding structures, including the bowel, pelvic floor musculature, and reproductive organs, it is not surprising that if one of the pelvic organs becomes diseased the other pelvic organ systems may exhibit similar symptoms. This should be kept in mind when evaluating pelvic pain of bladder origin.

Clinical Presentation

IC is defined by chronic pelvic or suprapubic pain, pressure, or discomfort related to bladder filling, and at least one other urinary symptom, usually urinary frequency, urgency, or nocturia. This should be in the absence of proven infection or other obvious pathologic process. Furthermore, the term *interstitial cystitis* is reserved for patients with PBS symptoms who also have characteristic (but not pathognomonic) cystoscopic findings or histologic evidence during bladder hydrodistention.

Patients may also describe chronic pelvic pain, not due to their bladder pain, but associated with other ongoing symptoms or disorders such as dysmenorrhea, endometriosis, adenomyosis, vulvodynia, irritable bowel syndrome, and fibromyalgia.

Although the etiology of IC is clearly multifactorial, evidence has suggested a strong correlation between IC and (1) dysfunctional, abnormal bladder epithelial permeability, and (2) increased mast cell activity. The abnormal bladder epithelial permeability appears to be due to changes found in the bladder mucous layer. This layer contains defective glycosaminoglycans that increase the permeability of the urothelium to irritants, especially potassium. It is still unclear whether mast cells play a causative or a secondary role in the disease.

IC is expressed as a continuum from mild to severe disease, and can persist for decades. The mild to moderate stages are often associated with symptom flares and remissions. Flares may occur in association with sexual intimacy or before menses, complicating the process of distinguishing IC from other gynecologic disorders. Subsequently, women often consult multiple clinicians (an average of five over a period of 4 or more years) before the correct and precise diagnosis is made; unfortunately, the causes of IC or any associated chronic pelvic pain cannot always be determined with a simple gynecologic examination.

Additional factors known to cause IC exacerbations include allergies, emotional or physical stress, exercise, remaining seated for prolonged periods (e.g., air travel), and ingestion of foods and drinks with a high potassium content (e.g., oranges, strawberries, coffee). Most patients in the early stages of IC complain of urgency and frequency; however, dysuria and dyspareunia can also be seen. The symptoms may vary from day to day but are usually gradual in onset and worsen over a period of months. Pain of increasing severity often becomes the predominant complaint.

IC or PBS symptoms can be associated with chronic pain and fatigue, a disturbance of the patient's home and work life, and a decreased overall quality of life. From a review of multiple surveys, up to 70% of patients claim sleep disturbance, more than 50% are unable to work full time, and almost 80% complain of dyspareunia leading to decreased sexual intimacy. More than 90% of patients surveyed claim that the symptoms of IC or PBS affect their daily activities.

PELVIC PAIN and URGENCY/FREQUENCY PATIENT SYMPTOM SCALE							
Please circle the answer that best describes how you feel for each question.							
	0	1	2	3	4	SYMPTOM SCORE	BOTHER SCORE
1 How many times do you go to the bathroom during the day?	3–6	7–10	11–14	15–19	20+		
2 a. How many times do you go to the bathroom at night?	0	1	2	3	4+		
b. If you get up at night to go to the bathroom does it bother you?	Never	Mildly	Moderate	Severe			
3 Are you currently sexually active? YES ____ NO ____							
4 a. IF YOU ARE SEXUALLY ACTIVE, do you now have or have you ever had pain or symptoms during or after sexual intercourse?	Never	Occasionally	Usually	Always			
b. If you have pain, does it make you avoid sexual intercourse?	Never	Occasionally	Usually	Always			
5 Do you have pain associated with your bladder or in your pelvis (vagina, lower abdomen, urethra, perineum, testes, or scrotum)?	Never	Occasionally	Usually	Always			
6 Do you have urgency after going to the bathroom?	Never	Occasionally	Usually	Always			
7 a. If you have pain, is it usually		Mild	Moderate	Severe			
b. Does your pain bother you?	Never	Occasionally	Usually	Always			
8 a. If you have urgency, is it usually		Mild	Moderate	Severe			
b. Does your urgency bother you?	Never	Occasionally	Usually	Always			
SYMPTOM SCORE = (1, 2a, 4a, 5, 6, 7a, 8a)							
BOTHER SCORE = (2b, 4b, 7b, 8b)							
TOTAL SCORE = (Symptom Score + Bother Score)							

Fig. 98.1   A score of 15 or greater is highly suggestive of interstitial cystitis. In some patients, especially adolescents, even a score in the range of 6 to 10 may warrant further investigation and treatment.

PATIENT INVESTIGATION AND DIAGNOSIS

The work-up for IC should include a careful pelvic examination; during this examination, care should be taken to evaluate for tenderness of the anterior vaginal wall/bladder base. A urinalysis and urine culture should be obtained to rule out hematuria and infection. Conditions for which IC may be mistaken include recurrent urinary tract infection, overactive bladder, vulvar and vaginal conditions, and abdominopelvic adhesions. It is important to be aware of signs, symptoms, and risk factors for bladder cancer. Microscopic hematuria is the main sign, and, if present, cancer should be ruled out with a thorough urologic work-up, including cystoscopy (see Chapter 97, Diagnostic Cystourethroscopy). In the absence of hematuria, the value of cytology is questionable but might still be important in patients with risk factors for bladder cancer. Risk factors include age greater than 40 years, long-standing symptoms, and smoking.

Although additional procedures such as cystoscopy/cystourethroscopy (with or without bladder hydrodistention) can be performed at the clinician's discretion, these procedures are not required for the diagnosis and treatment of IC or PBS. Bladder biopsy is not required except to rule out other disorders. Additional diagnostic tools, such as biomarkers (e.g., antiproliferative factor), may play a future role in the diagnosis of IC or PBS, but further studies are needed. Urodynamic testing does not currently have a role in the identification or diagnosis of IC or PBS.

TOOLS FOR DIAGNOSING INTERSTITIAL CYSTITIS

The majority of patients with IC or PBS, even early disease, can be identified with the Pelvic Pain and Urgency and/or Frequency (PUF) questionnaire or the optional potassium sensitivity test (PST). The O'Leary-Sant symptom and problem index score is another frequently used and validated scoring system.

Pelvic Pain and Urgency and/or Frequency Questionnaire

When the clinical presentation and physical examination suggest IC, the PUF questionnaire (Fig. 98.1) is a rapid (<5 minutes), self-administered tool available to screen for IC. The PUF has been validated against the intravesical PST in both urologic patients suspected of having IC and gynecologic patients with pelvic pain. This questionnaire has proven to be of tremendous value for identifying patients with IC. Unlike other IC questionnaires, the PUF gives balanced attention to pelvic pain, urgency/frequency, and dyspareunia. (The cut-off score for a definitive IC/PBS diagnosis based on the PUF is 15 or higher; however, some patients have IC with a PUF score of 12 or higher. It is also the author's experience that in some patients with IC, particularly adolescent women not yet sexually active, the PUF score may be much lower than 12 because these patients fall out of the questionnaire's parameters.)

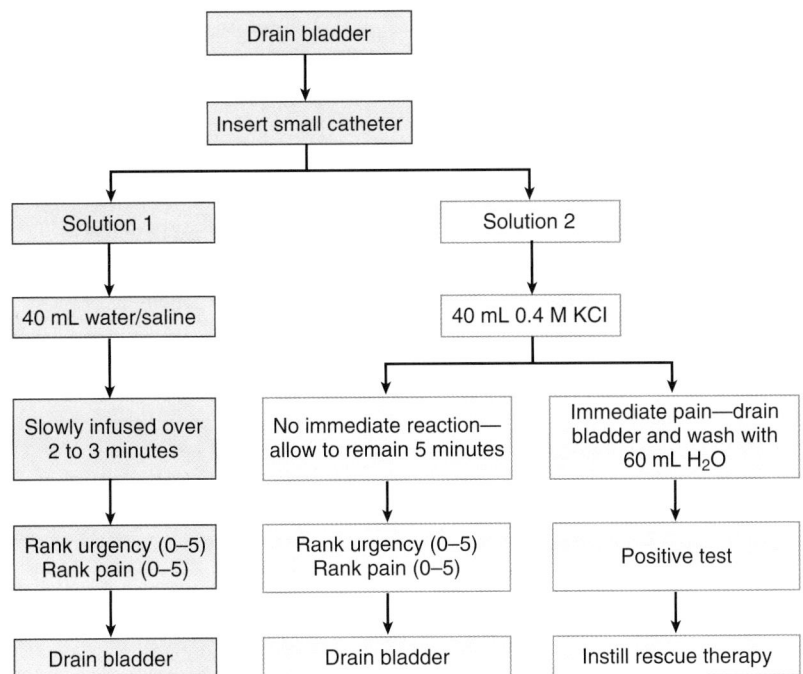

Fig. 98.2 Flow diagram of the potassium sensitivity test. The rescue solution or cocktail should be prepared in advance in the event of an uncomfortable or positive reaction to the test. The rescue solution is composed of 10,000 U heparin, 10 mL of 1% lidocaine, and 3 mL of 8.4% sodium bicarbonate in 100 mL of sterile water.

Potassium Sensitivity Test

The PST is an optional test that involves instilling potassium chloride solution into the bladder (Fig. 98.2). If the patient experiences urgency or pain, the presence of abnormal epithelial permeability is strongly suggested. During the PST, 40 mL of sterile water or saline is instilled slowly into the bladder and notation made of any associated pain. The bladder is then drained and filled equally slowly with a 40-mL solution of 0.4 M potassium chloride (40 mEq KCl/100 mL water); a finding of increased pain during this second filling is considered indicative of bladder hypersensitivity and suggestive of IC or PBS. While healthy controls can distinguish potassium chloride from sodium chloride, they do not experience severe pain. The PST can be an uncomfortable procedure; therefore an intravesical "rescue" solution should be available to alleviate symptoms provoked by the test. A less painful version has been developed, which utilizes a 0.2 M potassium chloride solution and cystometric capacity to determine infusion volume; however, further research is needed to further define its use in diagnostic or treatment algorithms.

Some studies claim that the PST should not be used routinely because its results are nonspecific for IC or PBS. Although most patients with IC have a positive PST result, a small percentage will have a negative result, and the reason for this is unknown. The hope for the PST was to identify a group of patients that would respond to a particular treatment; so far this has not happened. At least one study has found no use of PST for monitoring therapy. More important, to minimize the use of the PST, one study found an 84% correlation with positive PST findings among individuals with PUF scores of 15 or higher. This has resulted in the PUF questionnaire gaining acceptance as a sensitive and easy-to-use surrogate for the PST.

Investigators have also reported that intravesical instillation of 2% lignocaine solution is useful for excluding patients with pelvic pain originating from organs other than the bladder (Taneja, 2010). Further studies are needed to substantiate this claim.

Indications

Potassium Sensitivity Test

- Validation of patient symptom scale (PUF questionnaire)/confirmation of bladder epithelial dysfunction

- Patient seeking second opinion concerning treatment of IC previously investigated by an unremarkable cystoscopy or hydrodistention
- Confirmation for "new to treat" clinicians of their clinical impression
- Validation for suffering patients that their disease is real

Intravesical Instillation Therapy

- Provide rapid relief as needed in patients suffering with bladder pain, symptoms, or flares
- "Jump start" therapy to complement initiation of oral treatment in newly diagnosed patients
- Adjunctive second-line therapy to multimodal oral treatment regimens
- In patients unable to tolerate oral treatment or when oral therapy is ineffective
- "At home" elective intravesical instillation treatments by patients

Contraindications

- Absolute: Known allergy or sensitivity to any of the components used in the test or instillation treatment solutions (e.g., lidocaine, heparin)
- Relative: Acute urinary tract infection

Equipment and Supplies

Potassium Sensitivity Test

- Examination table with or without pelvic tilt/stirrups
- Impermeable drapes
- Surgical prep solution (e.g., povidone–iodine, chlorhexidine)
- Gloves and equipment necessary to follow universal blood and body fluid precautions
- LoFric catheter (Astra Tech Wellspect; 8 to 10 Fr, 8 inches for female patients, 12 Fr for male patients)
- Solution No. 1: 40 mL of sterile water or saline
- Solution No. 2: 40 mL of 0.4 M KCl (40 mEq of KCl/100 mL sterile water)
- One bottle of 100 mL sterile water for diluent

- Two 60-mL syringes
- 20-mL syringe
- 18-gauge needle
- Permeability Study Record Sheet (available at www.expertconsult.com)

Rescue Solution*

- 20-mL syringe
- Heparin sulfate, 10,000 U
- 10 mL lidocaine 1%
- 3 mL 8.4% NaOH (sodium bicarbonate)
- 100 mL sterile water for dilution

NOTE: 100 to 200 mg of oral pentosan polysulfate sodium (PPS) emptied from its capsule, dissolved in 10 mL of buffered normal saline per 100-mg capsule, may be substituted for heparin.†

Intravesical Instillation ("Jump Start" Therapy)

- LoFric catheter (8 to 10 Fr, 8 inches for female patients, 12 Fr for male patients)
- 20- or 30-mL syringe(s)
- 100 to 200 mg of oral PPS emptied from its capsule, dissolved in 10 mL of buffered normal saline per 100-mg capsule†
- 10 mL lidocaine 1% or 16 mL lidocaine 2%
- 3 mL 8.4% NaOH (sodium bicarbonate)
- Dimethyl sulfoxide (DMSO, is US Food and Drug Administration [FDA] approved for intravesical therapy)
- 100 mL sterile water for dilution

Technique

Potassium Sensitivity Test

1. The patient is awake and without anesthesia for this procedure.
2. Have the patient void completely.
3. Position patient in the dorsal position, preferably in stirrups.
4. Place an impermeable, waterproof drape under the patient's buttocks.
5. Cleanse/prepare the vulvar/urethral area as if you were inserting a Foley catheter. This is a clean, not sterile procedure. Universal blood and body fluid precautions should be followed.
6. Insert the straight catheter, drain any residual urine, and attach the syringe filled with solution No. 1 (see Fig. 98.2).
7. Instill solution No. 1, slowly over 2 to 3 min, wait, and record observations on the Permeability Study Record Sheet (available at www.expertconsult.com).
8. Drain the bladder.
9. Attach the second syringe, instill solution No. 2 slowly, over 2 to 3 minutes, into the subject's bladder, and wait 5 minutes.
10. Record the patient's degree of provoked urgency and pain. Patients are rated on a scale of 0 to 5 (with 0 = no provocation and 5 = severe provocation). A score of 2 or more in the pain or urgency scale is considered a positive test. If the patient's bladder is abnormally permeable, the PST will provoke urinary urgency or pain well above the patient's baseline levels.
11. If necessary (e.g., if the patient has an immediate reaction to solution No. 1 on instillation or after the test is concluded and patient voids), instill rescue solution immediately and have patient lie semi-upright for approximately 10 to 20 minutes or until bladder discomfort dissipates.
12. Make a notation in the patient's records regarding the outcome of the test, any reaction, and the administration of rescue solution, if used, and maintain a copy of the Permeability Study Record Sheet.

---

*Prepare this solution in advance of performing the PST. Use sterile water to bring volume up to at least 20 mL
†Intravesical administration of PPS is an off-label use of the drug.

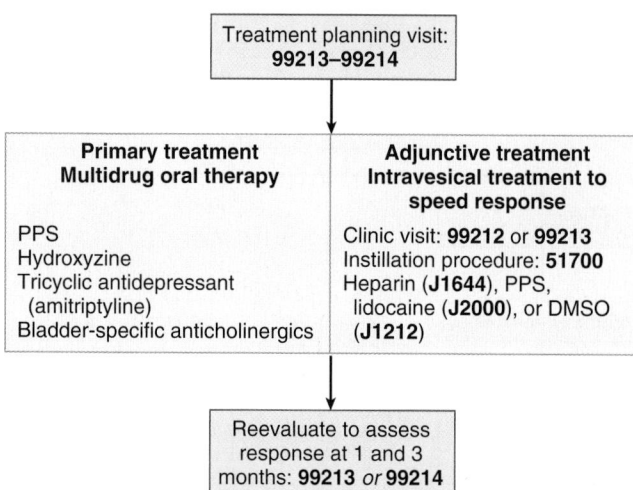

Fig. 98.3 Synopsis of treatment options with appropriate codes. *DMSO,* Dimethyl sulfoxide; *PPS,* pentosan polysulfate sodium.

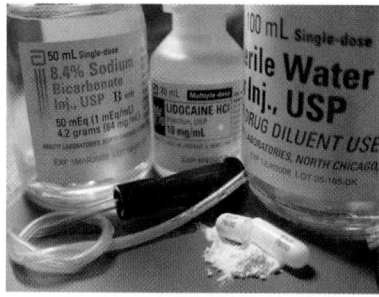

Fig. 98.4 Example of components used for intravesical instillation, including 8-Fr catheter and open capsule of pentosan polysulfate sodium.

TREATMENT OPTIONS FOR INTERSTITIAL CYSTITIS OR PAINFUL BLADDER SYNDROME

Because of the multiple possible etiologies for IC or PBS, therapy should generally use a multimodal approach. The foundation of oral therapy for IC is PPS (Elmiron), 100 mg three times a day. Additional medications are added as needed. Currently, PPS is the only oral medication approved by the FDA for the treatment of IC; it has been evaluated in five placebo-controlled trials. PPS is a compound that mimics the glycosaminoglycan layer on the surface of the bladder and is believed to help correct the dysfunctional bladder epithelium. Hydroxyzine (25 mg/day in the evening, 50 to 100 mg/day during allergy season) is prescribed to control histamine discharge associated with allergic flares, which can, in turn, provoke exacerbations of IC or PBS. Amitriptyline (25 mg/day at bedtime) can be added to block both peripheral and central neural activity. Use of amitriptyline in this manner is supported by a small randomized controlled trial of 4 months' duration. Occasionally, an anticholinergic (oxybutynin) is also used to control severe urinary urgency complaints. Extended-release nifedipine, 30 to 60 mg per day, in a very small study of 10 patients demonstrated a 50% decrease in symptoms scores in five patients at 4 months. In another small study of 10 patients taking 10 mg of montelukast (a mast cell stabilizer) daily, dramatic improvement in symptoms was noted in eight patients at 3 months. A small randomized controlled trial found oral cimetidine improved symptoms of suprapubic pain and nocturia. Cyclosporine has also been utilized with some benefit. In many patients with IC or PBS, PPS must be administered for at least 3 to 6 months before its full effectiveness can be realized (Fig. 98.3).

If a more rapid treatment response is needed, intravesical "jump start" therapy can be initiated at the time of diagnosis. This consists of various therapeutic "cocktails" made from heparin, PPS,

8.4% sodium bicarbonate, lidocaine, or DMSO (Fig. 98.4). These cocktails are instilled directly into the bladder through a catheter to facilitate immediate relief, as opposed to the several weeks to months it may take for PPS alone to take effect. If use of a bladder infusion provides symptom relief, it is also helpful diagnostically in that it confirms the patient's symptoms originate in the bladder. It should be noted that DMSO is the only FDA-approved medication for intravesical instillation. The current use of all other combinations of medications for intravesical therapy is considered off-label.

Evaluation of ongoing treatment can be accomplished with a repeat PUF questionnaire, looking for a change (decrease) in score as treatment progresses. Another form that may be useful is the patient overall rating of improvement of symptoms. This form helps in assessing patient progress with long-term treatment regimens, and should be maintained as part of the patient record (available at www.expertconsult.com).

Surgical intervention is rarely indicated or beneficial unless characteristic Hunner lesions are noted on cystoscopy. Resection of Hunner lesions has been associated with symptomatic improvement. In addition to pharmacologic therapy, various supportive or behavioral measures may be helpful. Effective self-care options for patients with IC or PBS include stress reduction and comfort activities such as pet therapy, meditation, and even prayer. Improvement in IC symptoms has been reported using self-hypnosis and posthypnotic suggestion in patients refractory to conventional medical treatments.

Technique for Intravesical Instillation Therapy

1. Prepare the therapeutic cocktail solution in a single syringe.
2. Follow steps 1 through 5 as described in the PST Technique section.
3. Place catheter into bladder (10 Fr, 8 inches for female patients, 12 Fr for male patients).
4. Drain the bladder.
5. Attach the syringe and instill the therapeutic solution.
6. Have the patient retain the instilled solution for 10 to 20 minutes.
7. Remove the catheter.
8. Direct the patient to void the solution.
9. Make a notation in the patient's record of the solution used, the amount, and the patient's tolerance for the procedure.

Assuming that the bladder is the source of pain in the patient with IC, direct treatment of the bladder surface with a therapeutic solution may result in immediate and profound relief and in improvement of symptoms. This symptom improvement resulting from the instillation therapy may aid in differentiating bladder-based pain from other forms of pelvic discomfort. Some clinicians use a purely anesthetic cocktail, such as lignocaine or bupivacaine with 2% lidocaine jelly, for this purpose.

COMMON ERRORS

- Mix-up between solutions nos. 1 and 2 during the PST (label each syringe after preparation and before use).
- Incorrect quantities of components for cocktail solutions (record components as you prepare the solution).
- Failure to record the patient reactions during the PST (keep the record sheet handy during the PST).
- Failure to have the rescue solution available at the start of the PST (it should be prepared along with testing solutions).
- Failure to observe the patient at least 15 minutes post-PST voiding for any delayed response of pain or discomfort requiring you to administer the rescue solution.

COMPLICATIONS

- Rarely, an expected adverse effect may include a worsening of symptoms when the effects of the rescue solution or therapeutic solution have ceased. Reassure the patient that this exacerbation will dissipate within a few hours.

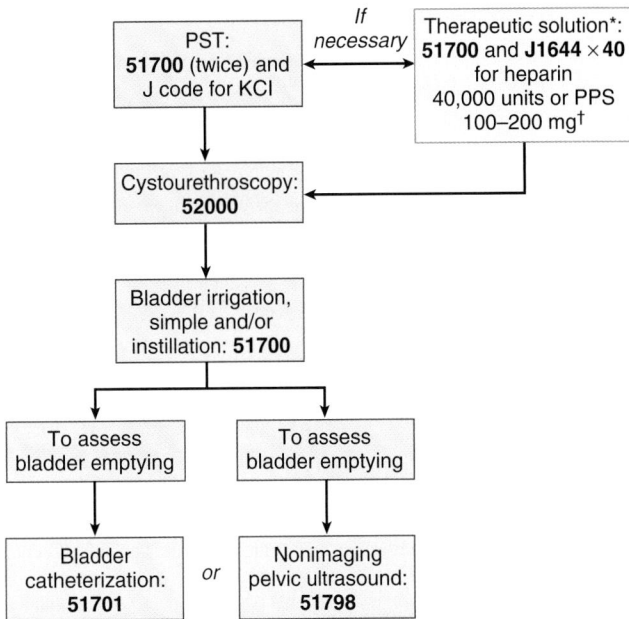

Fig. 98.5 Listed CPT and J codes for the potassium sensitivity test (*PST*), catheterization, and cystourethroscopy procedures performed in-office. *KCl*, potassium chloride; *PPS*, pentosan polysulfate sodium. *Solution also includes 10 mL of 1% lidocaine or 16 mL of 2% lidocaine and 3 mL of 8.4% sodium bicarbonate (not billable). †PPS 100 to 200 mg (not billable) may be substituted for heparin. Intravesical instillation of PPS is an off-label use of this product.

- Rarely, urinary retention. Treat as needed with catheterization to relieve discomfort.

CPT/BILLING CODES

For all newly diagnosed patients with IC there are specific codes for these procedures listed on the flow chart in Fig. 98.5.

Laboratory Testing

81000	Urinalysis
87086, 87088, 87181, 87184, P9612	Urine culture
51700	(twice) and J code for KCl Potassium sensitivity test

Therapeutic Solution

51700	Bladder irrigation, simple and/or instillation
J1644 (×40)	Heparin

NOTE: 8.4% NaOH is not billable.

J2000	Lidocaine (for rescue cocktail)

Ancillary Procedures

51701	Bladder catheterization
52000	Cystourethroscopy
A4123	Syringes
A4351	Catheter supplies, home use
J1212	DMSO

ICD-10-CM DIAGNOSTIC CODES

| N30.10 | Chronic interstitial cystitis |
| N32.9 | Bladder pain |

SUPPLIERS

(See contact information available at www.expertconsult.com.)

LoFric catheter (8 to 10 Fr for female patients, 12 Fr for male patients)
  Astra Tech Wellspect, Urology Division
Pentosan polysulfate sodium 100-mg capsules
  Ortho-McNeil-Janssen Pharmaceuticals
Lidocaine (1% or 2%), 8.4% sodium bicarbonate, heparin 10,000-U vials, sterile water diluent, DMSO, 60-mL syringes
  Moore Medical

ONLINE RESOURCES

Grochmal SA: How to Perform the PST (video for physicians): Endorepro gyne@aol.com
Interstitial Cystitis Association (ICA): www.ichelp.org
Interstitial Cystitis Network (ICN): www.ic-network.com
Ortho-McNeil-Janssen Pharmaceuticals (Elmiron): https://www.orthoelmiron.com

RECOMMENDED READING

Abrams L, Cardozo M, Fall M, et al. The standardisation of terminology of lower urinary tract function: report from the Standardisation Subcommittee of the International Continence Society. *Am J Obstet Gynecol.* 2002;187:116–126.

Chung MK, Chung RR, Gordon D, Jennings C. The evil twins of chronic pelvic pain syndrome: endometriosis and interstitial cystitis. *JSLS.* 2002;6:311–314.

Dell JR, Grochmal SA, Chandakas S, et al. Intravesical "jump start" therapy using a therapeutic cocktail for the treatment of interstitial cystitis. *JSLS.* 2006;10:S1–S77.

Fleischmann JD, Huntley HN, Shingleton WB, Wentworth DB. Clinical and immunological response to nifedipine for the treatment of interstitial cystitis. *J Urol.* 1991;146:1235–1239.

Forrest JB, Mishell Jr DR. Breaking the cycle of pain in interstitial cystitis/painful bladder syndrome: toward standardization of early diagnosis and treatment. Consensus panel recommendations. *J Reprod Med.* 2009;54:3–14.

French LM, Bhambore J. Interstitial cystitis/ painful bladder syndrome. *Am Fam Physician.* 2011;83(10):1175–1181.

Grochmal SA, Shulman L, Dell JR, et al. Continued chronic pelvic pain in adolescent women with failed treatment for endometriosis: identification and treatment outcome in patients with bladder origin of CPP (interstitial cystitis). *J Minim Invasive Gynecol.* 2006;13(suppl 5):S151.

Hanno PM. Bladder pain syndrome (interstitial cystitis) and related disorders. In: Wein AJ, Kavoussi LR, Partin AW, Peters CA, eds. *Campbell-Walsh Urology.* 11th ed. Philadelphia: Elsevier; 2016.

Henry R, Patterson L, Avery N, et al. Absorption of alkalized intravesical lidocaine in normal and inflamed bladders: a simple method for improving bladder anesthesia. *J Urol.* 2001;165:1900–1903.

Langenberg PW, Wallach EE, Clauw DJ, et al. Pelvic pain and surgeries in women before interstitial cystitis/ painful bladder syndrome. *Am J Obstet Gynecol.* 2010;202:286.e1–e286.e6.

Lynch Jr DF. Empowering the patients: hypnosis in the management of cancer, surgical disease and chronic pain. *Am J Clin Hypnosis.* 1999;2:122–130.

Marszalek M, Wehrberger C, Temml C, et al. Chronic pelvic pain and lower urinary tract symptoms in both sexes: analysis of 2749 participants of an urban screening project. *Eur Urol.* 2009;55:499–508.

Mulholland SG, Hanno P, Parsons CL, et al. Pentosan polysulfate sodium for therapy of interstitial cystitis: a double-blind placebo-controlled clinical study. *Urology.* 1990;35:552–558.

Nickel JC, Barkin J, Forrest J, et al. The Elmiron study group: randomized double-blind, dose-ranging study of pentosan polysulfate sodium for interstitial cystitis. *Urology.* 2005;65:654–658.

Papandreau C, Skapinakis P, Giannakis D, et al. Antidepressant drugs for chronic urological pelvic pain: an evidence-based review. *J Urol.* 2009;174:1–9.

Parsons CL. Argument for the use of the potassium sensitivity test in the diagnosis of interstitial cystitis. *Int Urogynecol J Pelvic Floor Dysfunct.* 2005;16:430–431.

Parsons CL. The role of the urinary epithelium in the pathogenesis of interstitial cystitis/prostatitis/urethritis. *Urology.* 2007;69(suppl 4):S9–S16.

Parsons CL, Bullen M, Kahn BS, et al. Gynecologic presentation of interstitial cystitis as detected by intravesical potassium sensitivity. *Obstet Gynecol.* 2001;98:127–132.

Parsons CL, Dell JR, Stanford JL. Increased prevalence of interstitial cystitis: previously unrecognized urologic and gynecologic cases identified using a new symptom questionnaire and intravesical potassium sensitivity. *Urology.* 2002;60:573–578.

Parsons CL, Housley T, Schmidt JD, et al. Treatment of interstitial cystitis with intravesical heparin. *Br J Urol.* 1994;73:504–507.

Parsons CL, Mulholland SG. Successful therapy of interstitial cystitis with pentosan-polysulfate. *J Urol.* 1987;138:513–516.

Sairanen J, Tammela TL, Leppilahti M, et al. Cyclosporine A and pentosan polysulfate sodium for the treatment of interstitial cystitis: a randomized comparative study. *J Urol.* 2005;174(6):2235–2238.

Sant G, Theoharides TC. The role of the mast cell in interstitial cystitis. *Urol Clin North Am.* 1994;21:41–53.

Sidman J, Lechtman MD, Lyster EG. A unique hypnotherapeutic approach to interstitial cystitis: a case report. *J Reprod Med.* 2009;54:523–524.

Taneja R. Intravesical lignocaine in the diagnosis of bladder pain syndrome. *Int Urogynecol J.* 2010;21:321–324.

Thilagarajah R, Witherow RO, Walker MM. Oral cimetidine gives effective symptom relief in painful bladder disease: a prospective, randomized, double-blind placebo-controlled trial. *BJU Int.* 2001;87(3):207–212.

Traut JL, Macdonald ES, Spangler ML, Saxena S. Montelukast for symptom control of interstitial cystitis. *Ann Pharmacother.* 2011;45:e49.

van Ophoven A, Hertle L. Long-term results of amitriptyline treatment for interstitial cystitis. *J Urol.* 2005;174:1837–1840.

Webster DC, Brennan T. Self-care effectiveness and outcomes in women with interstitial cystitis: implications for mental health clinicians. *Issues Ment Health Nurs.* 1998;19:495–519.

CHAPTER 99

SUPRAPUBIC CATHETER INSERTION AND/OR CHANGE

Robert E. James • James R. Palleschi

Suprapubic catheters are normally used to provide short-term urinary drainage. If the patient's age or comorbid conditions preclude corrective surgery, the temporary catheter may be left in place or, with the aid of an exchange wire and appropriate dilators, may be replaced with a permanent suprapubic catheter.

INDICATIONS

- An impassable urethral stricture, bladder neck contracture, or obstruction (see Chapter 96, Bladder Catheterization (And Urethral Dilation))
- Inability to pass a urethral catheter over an elevated bladder neck or an enlarged median lobe of the prostate gland
- Urethral trauma
- Recent urethral or bladder neck reconstructive surgery
- Inability to tolerate a urethral catheter and unwilling or unable to perform intermittent self-catheterization
- Bladder drainage required in the presence of a significant urethral or prostate infection
- Severe phimosis precluding the insertion of a urethral catheter (see Chapter 104, Dorsal Slit for Phimosis)
- Some surgeons place suprapubic catheters to keep pressures and flow normal while performing transurethral surgery.
- Any other contraindication to urethral catheterization.

CONTRAINDICATIONS

- Uncooperative patient
- Anticoagulated patient or patient with coagulopathy (either the anticoagulation/coagulopathy should be reversed or urology consulted)
- Cellulitis over the insertion site
- Presence of a vascular graft near the insertion site
- Surgical scar in suprapubic area, or bladder or pelvic anatomic abnormality from previous surgery, cancer, irradiation, or trauma (small bowel may be interposed in the retropubic space; however, ultrasound guidance may be helpful for avoiding the small bowel; see Chapter 214, Emergency Department, Hospitalist, and Office Ultrasound [POCUS])

EQUIPMENT

- Local anesthetic: 10-mL lidocaine 1% to 2%
- 10-mL syringe
- 1.5- to 2.5-inch, 22- to 27-gauge needle for anesthesia
- 4-inch, 22-gauge spinal needle
- Antiseptic skin preparation (e.g., povidone-iodine or chlorhexidine)
- Sterile towels or drapes
- Sterile saline, to possibly fill the bladder, irrigate the catheter, or inflate a Foley bulb

- Mask, sterile gloves and equipment needed to observe universal blood and body fluid precautions
- Mounted scalpel blade (No. 11 or No. 15)
- Suture scissors, needle holder, and 2-0 nylon suture
- Closed urinary drainage system
- Suprapubic catheter set

NOTE: There are many manufacturers of suprapubic catheters and insertion kits, including the Bonnano catheter (Becton-Dickinson Corp.) and the Stamey percutaneous suprapubic catheter set (Cook Medical/Urological). Peel-away catheters are also available, such as the Simplastic suprapubic catheter/SupraFoley suprapubic catheter introducer (Teleflex Medical) and two from Cook, which are advanced over a guidewire (e.g., the Rutner). A Foley is then advanced through the peel-away sheath that was introduced using the Seldinger technique.

The principal components of each set, except for those with the peel-away catheters, are a metal obturator and the suprapubic catheter. The metal obturator is placed down through the suprapubic catheter and is subsequently removed when the catheter is appropriately positioned within the bladder. The end of the catheter may consist of a coudé tip (with balloon), Malecot tip, or Foley. Unlike the red rubber catheter (also known as the Robinson), which is not self-retaining, all of these catheters are equally effective in retaining themselves within the bladder (Fig. 99.1).

PREPROCEDURE PATIENT PREPARATION

Explain the indications for, the alternatives to, and the risks of the procedure to the patient. Informed consent should be obtained. The patient should know what to expect during the procedure, including the need for an injection of local anesthetic before the procedure. Also explain to the patient that mild to moderate suprapubic discomfort may be experienced for a few hours to days after this procedure.

TECHNIQUE

1. Place the patient in the supine position. If the bladder is not palpable, either the procedure should be delayed until the bladder can be easily identified or else the insertion should be completed with ultrasound guidance. If the patient has a bladder or pelvic anatomic abnormality from previous surgery, cancer, or trauma, the procedure should be performed only with the aid of ultrasound guidance. (see Chapter 214, Emergency Department, Hospitalist, and Office Ultrasound [POCUS]).
2. Maintain sterile technique and observe universal blood and body fluid precautions. Prepare the suprapubic skin with an antiseptic solution and drape with sterile towels. Inject the local anesthetic into the skin overlying the abdominal wall, into the subcutane-

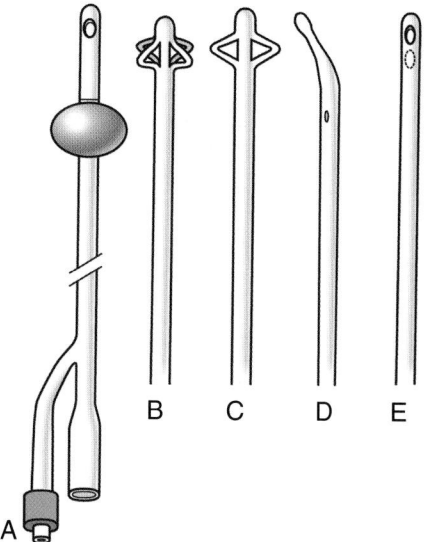

Fig. 99.1 Commonly used catheters. (A) Foley-type balloon catheter. (B) Malecot self-containing, four-wing urethral catheter. (C) Malecot self-retaining, two-wing catheter. (D) Coudé hollow, olive-tip catheter. (E) Robinson urethral catheter.

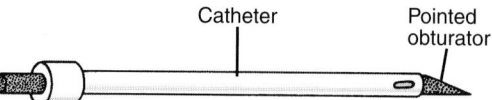

Fig. 99.2 Suprapubic catheter with obturator in place.

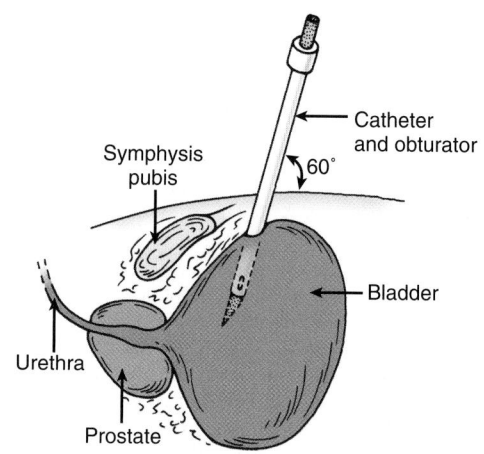

Fig. 99.3 Insertion and advancement of the catheter and obturator.

ous layer, into the fascia, and down to the dome of the bladder. After penetrating the subcutaneous layer, aspirate before injection to avoid intravascular injection.

3. With the scalpel, make a 1-cm horizontal skin incision (some clinicians also incise the anterior rectus fascia) 5 cm above the symphysis pubis in the midline (in both adult and pediatric patients). At this point, some clinicians prefer to pass a 22-gauge spinal needle down and into the bladder. The needle should be angled caudal, down into the pelvis, at about a 60-degree angle to the skin of the upper abdomen, or about 30 degrees off of the vertical. This will verify the bladder location before the suprapubic catheter is inserted. If the bladder is distended, this procedure is not necessary. If the bladder is not distended sufficiently to guide the obturator, the long needle can also be used to fill the bladder with sterile saline solution. Alternatively, ultrasound can be used to determine if the bladder is full and for guidance.

4. Once the incision has been made, and the bladder has been located, place the metal obturator into the lumen of the suprapubic catheter, with the sharp oblique end of the obturator extending beyond the tip of the catheter (Fig. 99.2). Advance the obturator and catheter together through the incision at a 60-degree caudal angle toward the bladder neck (approximately the mid-perineal area; Fig. 99.3). With momentary pressure, advance the catheter through the rectus sheath and muscle and into the dome of the bladder. This requires inserting it a total of approximately 5 cm below the skin in adults.

5. Advance the catheter and obturator an additional 5 cm in adults to ensure appropriate positioning. Remove the obturator; urine will be seen passing from the suprapubic catheter. After the obturator is removed, the wings of the Malecot type of catheter (Stamey suprapubic catheter) will expand, or the pigtail tip of the Bonnano catheter will coil inside the bladder to prevent it from falling out. If the catheter has a balloon tip, once it has been appropriately positioned within the bladder, inflate the balloon with sterile saline.Alternatively, the SupraFoley suprapubic catheter introducer consists of a plastic sheath, through which a sharp, plastic obturator is inserted. Advance the obturator through the incision and the rectus sheath, into the bladder. Then remove the obturator and advance a Foley catheter down through the plastic sheath into the bladder. The balloon is filled with 5 to 10 mL of water or saline. A tab is located on the top edge of the plastic sheath; pull down and remove it. This removes

a strip of the sheath, allowing, in turn, the removal of the whole sheath and leavingthe catheter in place in the bladder. Using the systems from Cook, a guidewire is advanced through the locating spinal needle. The needle is removed, and a small incision is made next to the guidewire. A dilator and then an introducer sheath are advanced over the guidewire and then the guidewire is removed. Finally, a Foley catheter is introduced through the sheath, the balloon inflated, and the introducer peeled away.

6. Pull back the catheter until the wings, coil, or balloon is resting against the dome of the bladder.

7. Secure the catheter in place externally with a nylon suture.

8. Using sterile saline, irrigate the catheter to ensure appropriate drainage and position.

9. Connect a drainage bag to the catheter, using an overnight or bedside drainage bag, leg bag, or abdominal drainage system (belly bag).

COMPLICATIONS

- Perivesicular bleeding
- Gross hematuria
- Failure to drain
- Infection
- Intraperitoneal or extraperitoneal extravasation
- Ureteral catheterization
- Intestinal perforation (more likely when the bladder is not distended; when the normal anatomy is distorted by previous surgery, cancer, irradiation, or trauma; or when the obturator and catheter are not introduced at the correct angle; normally, a small perforation will seal spontaneously without consequence)
- Through and through bladder penetration with associated rectal, vaginal, or uterine injury
- Occasionally, despite the best intentions, the suprapubic catheter comes out or cannot be maintained successfully; pIgtail or looped catheters are more likely to dislodge than balloon-tipped catheters
  EDITOR'S NOTE: Surrounding organ damage is the most serious complication; it occurs in less than 1% to 2.7% of procedures.

SUPRAPUBIC CATHETER REPLACEMENT

Usually, a suprapubic catheter is replaced every 4 to 6 weeks, or whenever it is not draining properly. If the catheter has been in place for several weeks and a mature tract is established, the existing catheter may be removed and replaced with a similar catheter. First, place an obturator in the new catheter. Next, fill the bladder with sterile saline or water, and remove the catheter. The sterile water or saline will begin to pass through the suprapubic catheter site, and, consequently, the catheter needs to be replaced promptly. Advance the new catheter with obturator down the tract until the sterile water or saline begins to exit through or around the catheter. Usually a local anesthetic is not required.

If the catheter needs to be replaced before the tract is mature, the bladder should be filled with sterile saline or water before removing the catheter. If the catheter is obstructed, it should be removed and another catheter inserted once a distended bladder can be palpated. At that time, a new catheter may be inserted in the same tract, using the technique described previously. Ultrasound guidance should be used if the bladder cannot be positively identified or palpated.

With a Malecot or winged-tip catheter, frequently the wings are soft enough that they will retract as the catheter is removed. If there is difficulty removing the catheter, insert the obturator in the catheter to straighten the wings before removing the catheter. The tension in the pigtail is maintained by a silk suture that runs through the catheter and exits near its end. There it is tied around a small post. When the suture is cut or released, the pigtail will uncurl and the catheter can be removed.

If an open suprapubic cystotomy has been performed, a mature tract between the skin and the bladder is usually formed within 4 to 6 weeks. If the catheter must be replaced, select a similar-sized catheter. Normally, a catheter guide or obturator is not required. The new catheter should be introduced into the bladder immediately after removing the original one. After inflating the balloon with 5 to 10 mL of sterile saline, irrigate the bladder to ensure that the catheter is draining properly.

After catheter replacement, connect an overnight or bedside drainage bag, leg bag, or abdominal drainage system (belly bag).

USE OF ANTIBIOTICS

For suprapubic catheter placement, if a urinary tract infection is suspected, or the patient is at high risk of infection or a poor outcome from endocarditis (see Chapter 69, Antibiotic Prophylaxis), a urine culture and sensitivity should be obtained and the patient placed on a broad-spectrum antibiotic for at least 3 days. If the patient is not allergic to fluoroquinolones, ciprofloxacin or levofloxacin is an appropriate choice or trimethoprim/sulfamethoxazole.

Prophylactic antibiotic therapy is not required when changing a suprapubic catheter. If a clinically significant urinary tract infection is suspected, a specimen of urine should be obtained for a culture and sensitivity, and an oral antibiotic ordered until the culture results are available. Appropriate choices, depending on the patient's allergy history, include nitrofurantoin or a fluoroquinolone or trimethoprim/sulfamethoxazole.

POSTPROCEDURE PATIENT EDUCATION

Explain again to the patient that mild to moderate suprapubic discomfort may be experienced for a few hours to days after this procedure. As long as the catheter is in place, intermittent hematuria and irritating voiding symptoms may be present. The patient should know to take good care of the catheter system, to keep it clean and dry, and not to let the bag drag on the floor. Review additional catheter care, including the use of an overnight or bedside drainage bag, leg bag, or abdominal drainage system (belly bag). Once a day, the patient should wash his or her hands with soap and water and then use a clean, soapy washcloth to clean the catheter and the skin around it. Hydrogen peroxide should be useful for removing any crustiness that does not come off with soap and water. After washing with soap or peroxide, the catheter should be rinsed with clean water then patted dry. The patient should take care not to pull too much on the catheter. If the patient wants it, a slit gauze can be placed over the catheter. Tell the patient to contact the clinician if increasing pain, excessive bleeding, a temperature greater than 101°F, or a nonfunctioning catheter is noticed.

After the catheter is removed, patients should be aware that they will have lost some of the ability to sense a full bladder; therefore, they should urinate every 2 hours for 1 to 2 weeks, even after going to bed. They should drink plenty of fluids, but not force them, and they should refrain from fluids for 2 hours before going to bed. Patients should expect the site to drain small amounts of urine for a few days, so they should keep it covered with gauze. They should clean the site with soap and water at least once a day.

CPT/BILLING CODES

51040	Cystostomy, cystostomy with drainage
51102	Aspiration of bladder; by needle with insertion of suprapubic catheter
51705	Changing a cystostomy tube (suprapubic catheter), simple

ICD-10-CM DIAGNOSTIC CODES

N32.0	Bladder neck contracture/obstruction
N31.9	Neurogenic bladder, NOS
N34.2	Urethritis, unspecified
N35.9	Urethral stricture, unspecified
N13.9	Urinary obstruction, unspecified
N40.1	Hyperplasia of prostate, unspecified, with urinary obstruction

Use additional code for associated symptoms when specified.

N41.0	Acute prostatitis
N42.89	Prostatic stricture
N47.1	Phimosis
S37.30XX	Urethral injury, with no open wound
S37.20XX	Bladder injury, with no open wound
S37.30XX	Urethral injury, laceration
S37.20XX	Bladder injury, laceration

Use additional seventh character: A = initial, D = subsequent, S = sequela.

SUPPLIERS

(See contact information available at www.expertconsult.com.)

BD Bonnano suprapubic trays and kits
Becton-Dickinson Corp.
Stamey percutaneous suprapubic catheter kit and many other suprapubic catheter sets including peel-away
Cook Medical/Urological
Simplastic, SupraFoley suprapubic catheters and introducers
Teleflex Medical

ONLINE RESOURCES

Cincinnati Children's Hospital: Kidney, Bladder and Genitals Home Care (patient education): www.cincinnatichildrens.org/health/info/urinary/home/suprapubic.htm.
Medline Plus: Urinary catheters (patient education): https://medlineplus.gov/ency/article/003981.htm.

RECOMMENDED READING

Davis JE, Silverman M. Urologic procedures. In: Roberts JR, Custalow CB, Thomsen TW, eds. *Roberts and Hedges Clinical Procedures in Emergency Medicine*. 6th ed. Philadelphia: Elsevier; 2014:1144–1146.

McPhail MJ, Abu-Hilal M, Johnson CD. A meta-analysis comparing suprapubic and transurethral catheterization for bladder drainage after abdominal surgery. *Br J Surg.* 2006;93:1038–1044.

Niel-Weise BS, van den Broek PJ, da Silva EMK, Silva LA. Urinary catheter policies for long-term bladder drainage. *Cochrane Database Syst Rev.* 2012;8:CD004201.

Robinson RD, Hsu S, Reichman EF. Suprapubic bladder aspiration. In: Reichman EF, ed. *Emergency Medicine Procedures.* 2nd ed. New York: McGraw-Hill; 2013:968–976.

Tapper AD. Suprapubic aspiration. *Emedicine.* 2017. http://emedicine.medscape.com/article/82964-overview.

Wein AJ, Kavoussi LR, Partin AW, Peters CA, eds. *Campbell's Urology.* 11th ed. Philadelphia: Elsevier; 2016.

Wolf JS, Bennet CJ, Dmochowski RR, Hollenbeck BK, Pearle MS, et al. Best practice policy statement on urologic surgery antimicrobial prophylaxis. *J Urol.* 2008;180(5):2262–2263.

CHAPTER 100

SUPRAPUBIC TAP OR ASPIRATION

Robert E. James • James R. Palleschi

Suprapubic aspiration is a valuable diagnostic procedure and may occasionally be a valuable therapeutic tool. In most cases suprapubic aspiration can be performed safely at the bedside or in the clinician's office. (For insertion of suprapubic catheters, see Chapter 99, Suprapubic Catheter Insertion and/or Change. See also Chapter 168, Pediatric Suprapubic Bladder Aspiration for the same procedure in children.)

To review the anatomy, clinicians should be aware that the dome of the bladder has peritoneal attachments and that needle penetration into this area can cause injury to bowel or an intraperitoneal bladder perforation. The colon lies posterior and inferior to the bladder, so the clinician should avoid advancing the needle through both walls of the bladder. Alongside the bladder, in the pelvis, lie significant vascular structures, including the common iliac and hypogastric vessels. Aspiration in this area may lead to inadvertent and significant hemorrhage.

A properly directed needle will penetrate only the skin and subcutaneous tissue of the lower anterior abdominal wall, the rectus sheath, the peritoneum, and the anterior bladder wall.

INDICATIONS

- Collection of a urine specimen for analysis, culture, and sensitivity using sterile technique
- Temporary relief of acute urinary retention in a patient not able to be catheterized (e.g., urethral stricture, urethral trauma)

CONTRAINDICATIONS

- Anticoagulated patient or patient with coagulopathy (either the anticoagulation/coagulopathy should be reversed or urology consulted)
- An uncooperative patient (see Chapter 1, Procedural Sedation and Analgesia)
- Infection or cellulitis of the suprapubic area
- Full bladder not palpable*
- Patient not able to lie supine or have his or her bladder palpated*
- Surgical scar in suprapubic area or bladder or pelvic anatomic abnormality from previous surgery, cancer, or trauma (small bowel may be interposed in the retropubic space)*
- Abnormalities of genitourinary anatomy, enlargement of pelvic organs (e.g., ovarian cysts, uterine fibroids, bladder tumor), distention or enlargement of abdominal viscera (including intestinal obstruction)*

EQUIPMENT

- Protective equipment to provide universal blood and body fluid precautions
- Antiseptic skin preparation (povidone-iodine or chlorhexidine)

- Sterile gloves
- Local anesthetic: 10 mL lidocaine 1%
- Needles:
  - *For anesthetic:* 0.5-inch 25- to 30-gauge needle
  - *Localization needle:* 4-inch 22-gauge spinal needle
  - *Aspiration needle:* In most cases, the localization needle will be sufficiently large to obtain an adequate urine specimen. If not, an 18- or 20-gauge spinal or intravenous needle may be used.
- 10-mL syringe
- Microscope slide for direct examination, methylene blue, and Gram stain
- Sterile urine culture collection container

PREPROCEDURE PATIENT PREPARATION

Review the purpose of the procedure, risks, alternatives, and the technique with the patient and family. The patient may experience some pain in the suprapubic area with injection of the local anesthetic and during the procedure. He or she may also experience some hematuria for 24 to 48 hours after this procedure. Obtain informed consent.

TECHNIQUE

1. Place the patient in the supine position on the examination table. Examine the suprapubic area by palpation and percussion to identify the distended bladder. If the distended bladder cannot be identified positively, the procedure should be delayed until the bladder can be identified, or the procedure may be performed with ultrasound guidance.
2. Don protective gear. Cleanse the suprapubic area with an antiseptic solution, put on sterile gloves, and drape the area in a sterile fashion. Maintain the sterile technique and observe universal blood and body fluid precautions.
3. In the midline, anesthetize the skin approximately 2 in above the symphysis pubis. Next, inject sequentially down to the fascia and bladder, aspirating each time before injection. In the adult, usually 10 mL is required to anesthetize the skin, abdominal wall, and abdominal bladder. In a child, the same can be accomplished with 3 to 5 mL of anesthetic.
4. Direct the 22-gauge needle caudad into the pelvis toward the bladder neck. If the spinal needle is being used, the obturator should be in place (Fig. 100.1). Direct the needle through the anesthetized skin at a 60-degree angle to the skin of the upper abdomen. If the bladder is distended, the needle will enter the abdominal bladder after it has been advanced approximately 2 in in the adult.
5. Remove the obturator and connect a sterile syringe (Fig. 100.2) to aspirate urine from the bladder. If urine is not obtained, slowly advance the needle, applying continuous suction on the syringe. If the specimen cannot be obtained after advancing the needle an additional 2 in, terminate the procedure and start again, as described previously, but direct the needle at a 50-degree angle

*Ultrasound guidance may allow suprapubic aspiration to be performed in these situations and may be helpful for avoiding complications (see Chapter 214, Emergency Department, Hospitalist, and Office Ultrasound [POCUS]).

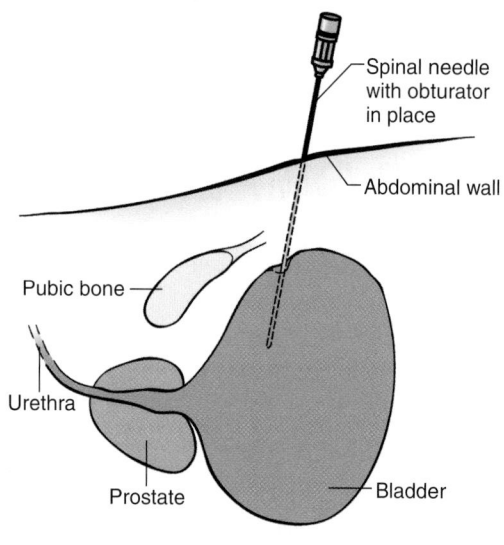

Fig. 100.1   Insertion of the spinal needle with the obturator in place. This is made at an angle of 60 degrees to the skin of the upper abdomen, angling into the pelvis.

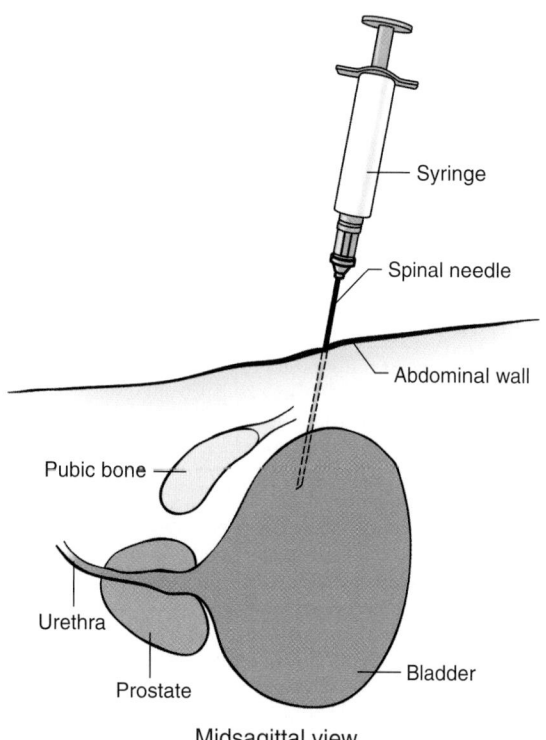

Fig. 100.2   Connection of the syringe to aspirate urine from the bladder.

to the skin. If you are unsuccessful a second time, the procedure should be delayed until the bladder is further distended, or the procedure should be performed with ultrasound guidance. If continued difficulties are encountered, a urology consultation should be obtained.

COMPLICATIONS

- Transient hematuria
- Perivesicular hematoma
- Intestinal perforation (if this occurs with a 22-gauge needle, it should seal spontaneously and not be a problem)

POSTPROCEDURE PATIENT EDUCATION

The patient may have some discomfort or soreness in the area for a day or so, which should be relieved by acetaminophen or a nonsteroidal antiinflammatory drug. The patient should notify the clinician in case of persistent (lasting longer than 2 days) or increasing blood in the urine, increasing abdominal pain, difficulty urinating, or a temperature above 101°F.

CPT/BILLING CODES

51100   Suprapubic bladder aspiration by needle

ICD-10-CM DIAGNOSTIC CODES

N39.0   Urinary tract infection, site not specified
Use additional code B95-B97 to identify infectious agent
R50.9   Fever
R33.9   Urinary retention or stasis, unspecified
A41.9   Sepsis unspecified organism
R65.20   Severe sepsis (acute organ dysfunction) without septic shock

RECOMMENDED READING

Davis JE, Silverman M. Urologic procedures. In: Roberts JR, Custalow CB, Thomsen TW, eds. *Roberts and Hedges Clinical Procedures in Emergency Medicine*. 6th ed. Philadelphia: Elsevier; 2014:1142–1143.
Nguyen HT. Bacterial infections of the genitourinary tract. In: Tanagho EA, MacAninch JW, eds. *Smith's General Urology*. 17th ed. New York: McGraw-Hill; 2008:203–227.
Robinson RD, Hsu S, Reichman EF. Suprapubic bladder aspiration. In: Reichman EF, ed. *Emergency Medicine Procedures*. 2nd ed. New York: McGraw-Hill; 2013:963–968.
Tapper AD. Suprapubic aspiration. *Emedicine*. 2017. http://emedicine.medscape.com/article/82964-overview.

CHAPTER 101

BEDSIDE URODYNAMIC STUDIES

Tricia C. Elliott • Reena R. Mathews

The diagnosis and management of urinary incontinence and voiding dysfunction (e.g., frequency, dysuria, and retention) are often challenging. Urinary incontinence has many etiologies, but it is most often the result of urethral incompetence (*genuine stress incontinence*), detrusor instability (*urge incontinence*), a combination of both (*mixed incontinence*), or poor bladder emptying (*overflow incontinence*). Urodynamic testing, specifically the cystometrogram, is used to demonstrate and differentiate among these conditions. Establishing the correct diagnosis is critical for developing an effective management plan. Although the patient history and physical examination may provide preliminary data regarding the underlying cause of incontinence or other urinary tract dysfunction, urodynamic testing provides an objective assessment while increasing the sensitivity and specificity of the diagnostic work-up.

Urodynamics is the study of the hydrodynamics and muscle activity of the lower urinary tract, with cystometry and uroflowmetry being the mainstays. Cystometry assesses the filling–storage phase by measuring the pressure–volume relationship of the bladder as it distends and contracts. It helps diagnose abnormalities of detrusor activity, sensation, capacity, and compliance. In contrast, uroflowmetry evaluates the voiding phase by measuring the urine volume voided over time. The combination of cystometry and uroflowmetry allows detection of both anatomic (obstructive) and physiologic (functional) voiding abnormalities.

Studies have shown that bedside (simple) urodynamic testing has a sensitivity of up to 75% for the correct diagnosis in the evaluation of urinary incontinence. It is easy to perform and cost effective in the office setting, and is frequently performed by the office personnel. A correlation of these test results with the patient history and physical examination usually determines the cause of urinary incontinence or other voiding dysfunction. Most conservative management protocols can be initiated on the basis of these results alone, without the need for formal multichannel urodynamic studies.

However, in certain patients, greater sensitivity or specificity or more precise measurements may be needed. Examples include patients with diabetes; individuals with neurologic disorders; and patients needing surgery for incontinence, especially if they are at high surgical risk (i.e., to clearly warrant the risk). Male patients also frequently require multichannel urodynamic testing. Additional examples include following pelvic radiation or surgery or for patients with incontinence and a confusing diagnosis or with a mixed etiology. Incontinence after failed surgery for incontinence or failing routine treatment or where the treatment progress needs to be monitored quantitatively may require more precise measurements. For all of these situations, formal uroflowmetry or formal cystometry is indicated, each being a part of formal multichannel urodynamic testing.

EDITOR'S NOTE: While urodynamic testing has been found to be safe and feasible, even in frail nursing-home patients (Resnick, 1989), there is no evidence that cystometric or urodynamic testing changes the clinical outcomes. A Cochrane review (Clement et al, 2013) found that while urodynamic testing did change clinical decision making, there was some evidence that this testing did not result in better outcomes following treatment. In other words, an empiric trial of therapy is reasonable in many, if not most, patients prior to or in lieu of urodynamic testing.

INDICATIONS

From an evidence-based perspective, these indications are most valuable when history, physical examination, or simple tests are not sufficient to make an accurate diagnosis or to institute therapy.

- Urinary incontinence
- Overactive bladder symptoms (urgency, frequency, nocturia, enuresis)
- Urinary retention or incomplete bladder emptying (ultrasound can also be used to determine postvoid residuals; see Chapter 214, Emergency Department, Hospitalist, and Office Ultrasound [POCUS])
- Pelvic pain
- Painful voiding syndromes
- Isolated stress urinary incontinence is unusual in older women; therefore before undergoing a potentially obstructive surgical procedure, it may be worthwhile to assess overall voiding function
- Evaluate impact of disease that has potential to cause serious long-term urologic damage despite minimal symptoms (e.g., spinal cord damage, multiple sclerosis, radiation cystitis)

CONTRAINDICATIONS

- Active cystitis
- Recurrent cystitis or gross hematuria (after cystoscopy and imaging have ruled out malignancy and stones, bedside urodynamics may be helpful)
- Intolerance of urethral catheterization
- Uncooperative patient
- Formal, multichannel urodynamic testing indicated

Patients with active cystitis, recurrent cystitis, or gross hematuria should be evaluated and treated before urodynamic testing. Caution should be taken in patients with uterine or pelvic prolapse, and certainly in those with a cystocele. Patients unable to tolerate urethral catheterization in the office or who are uncooperative are not candidates for bedside urodynamic testing.

EQUIPMENT

See Fig. 101.1.

- Nonsterile gloves
- Stopwatch
- Graduated voiding container (emesis bag with volume markings)
- Antiseptic (povidone iodine or chlorhexidine) swabs or solution
- Water-based lubricating gel (nonanesthetic)
- 14-Fr red rubber urinary catheter
- Sterile urine specimen container

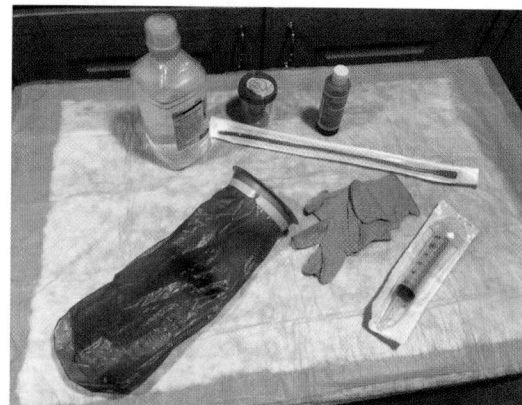

Fig. 101.1　Equipment used for urodynamic testing.

- Urinalysis Chemstrips
- 50-mL catheter-tip syringe with bulb or plunger removed
- 500 mL of room-temperature sterile saline or sterile water
- Sterile cotton-tipped swab with anesthetic gel

PREPROCEDURE PATIENT PREPARATION

All patients should be counseled regarding the indications, techniques, alternatives, and complications associated with urethral catheterization and bedside urodynamics. Clear communication and instructions should improve patient comfort during testing and thereby improve the results obtained. Patients should be instructed to come to the office with a full bladder to maximize information obtained from initial uroflowmetry. Each step of the procedure should be explained to the patient before proceeding.

TECHNIQUE

Clinicians should follow universal blood and body fluid precautions when performing this procedure.

Simple Uroflowmetry

1. The patient's bladder should be very full. If not, provide fluids and time for the patient to fill the bladder. Because urine flow parameters depend on the volume voided, the patient needs to be able to void at least 200 mL for this test to be reliable.
2. In a relaxed, private setting, tell the patient to void into a graduated container in hand or placed over the commode. The total time to void is recorded with the stopwatch, the total volume voided measured, and both are documented.

Simple Cystometry

3. After the patient has voided, clean the external urethral meatus with antiseptic swabs and insert the lubricated tip of the urinary catheter into the bladder lumen. Drain the residual urine into the sterile specimen container and record the postvoid residual volume. After completion of the cystometry and cough stress test, perform a urinalysis on this specimen to rule out urinary tract infection. In patients with a positive urinalysis, send the specimen for urine culture.
4. With the urinary catheter in place, attach the 50-mL syringe (with bulb or plunger removed) to the proximal end of the urinary catheter and hold it approximately 15 cm above the pubic symphysis. Fill the bladder by slowly pouring the sterile saline or sterile water through the open-top syringe in increments of 50 mL (Fig. 101.2). Take care to keep the tip of the catheter within the bladder lumen (i.e., avoid withdrawing it into the urethra).

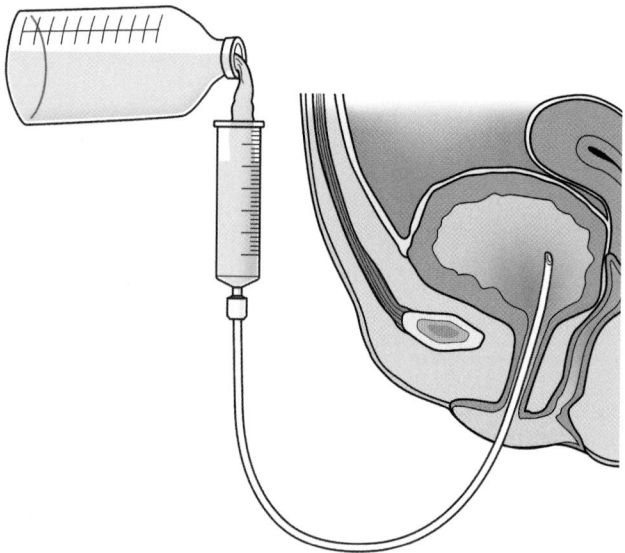

Fig. 101.2　Cystometry.

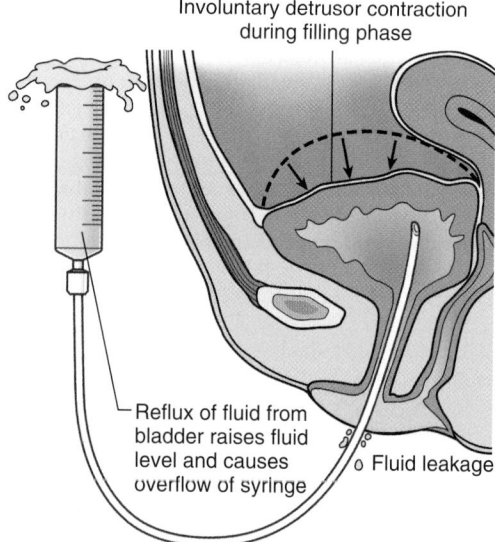

Fig. 101.3　Involuntary detrusor contraction.

5. During filling, ask the patient to report when he or she feels the first sensation of fullness and then the first urge to void, as well as when he or she has reached maximum bladder capacity. Record the total volume infused for each of these sensations.
6. Observe the water level in the syringe during filling; it should fall steadily. A sudden rise in the water level with or without associated urgency or incontinence may indicate an uninhibited detrusor contraction or detrusor instability (Fig. 101.3). Other causes of a "water hiccup" may be artifact (e.g., Valsalva maneuver, cough by the patient) or the catheter tip slipping into the proximal urethra.

Cough and Valsalva Stress Tests

7. After the bladder is filled to maximum capacity, remove the catheter and examine the patient in the supine dorsolithotomy position. The patient is asked to cough or perform a Valsalva maneuver, and the external urethral meatus is observed for

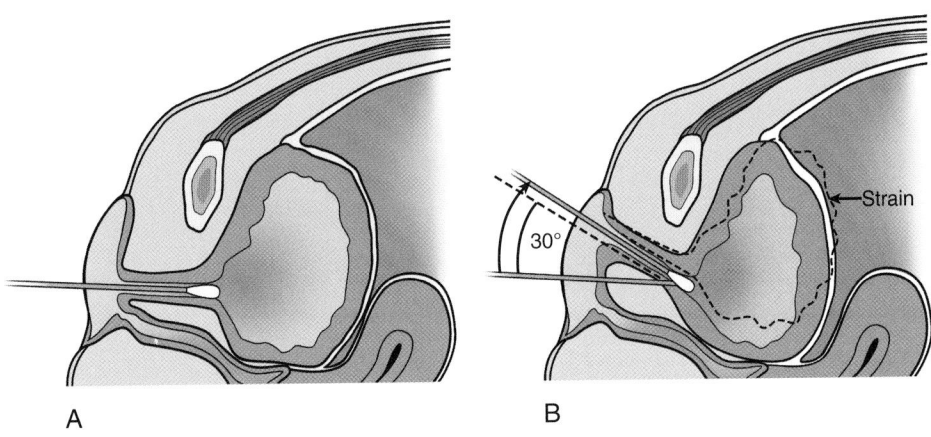

Fig. 101.4 Cotton swab test for ureterovesical junction mobility. (A) Cotton swab at rest. (B) Cotton swab with strain (Valsalva).

signs of urine leakage. Abrupt urine leakage with a cough suggests *stress urinary incontinence*, whereas prolonged leakage after cessation of the cough indicates cough-induced *detrusor instability*. In women, if urinary leakage is observed in the vagina from the anterior vaginal wall, a *vesicovaginal fistula* should be considered.

8. Repeat the test with the patient standing.

Cotton Swab Test (Q-Tip Test) for Women

9. After the supine and standing cough stress test, place the patient in the supine dorsolithotomy position and reexamine her. Insert a cotton-tipped swab with anesthetic gel into the urethra until resistance is overcome; this indicates its position at the bladder neck. Record the swab resting angle relative to the horizontal plane. Ask the patient to cough or perform a Valsalva maneuver again, and measure the maximum angle of deflection. The difference between this value and the resting angle is the *angle of change*. An angle of change of greater than 30 degrees indicates *urethral hypermobility* (Fig. 101.4).

Measurement of Postvoid Residual

10. Next, instruct the patient to void into the graduated container. Measure and record the amount voided (total void).
11. Determine a second postvoid residual by subtracting the measured total void from the maximum bladder capacity noted on filling cystometry.

COMPLICATIONS

- Urinary tract infection (rare)
- Transient gross hematuria
- Urethral discomfort, transient
- Pelvic pain, transient

Bedside urodynamics are associated with few complications. In rare cases, patients may develop a urinary tract infection after the procedure. These patients should be treated accordingly. Routine prophylactic antibiotics after the procedure are not usually indicated.

Transient gross hematuria may be noted after the procedure, especially after a difficult catheterization in a postmenopausal woman with urethral atrophy. This usually resolves spontaneously within 48 hours. Some patients may complain of urethral discomfort or pelvic pain after testing. These symptoms are usually self-limited, but these patients may benefit from a short course of phenazopyridine (Pyridium). Cystoscopy-urethroscopy should be considered in patients with hematuria or lower urinary tract pain that persists beyond 48 to 72 hours (see Chapter 97, Diagnostic Cystourethroscopy).

INTERPRETATIONS OF RESULTS

Uroflowmetry with measurement of a postvoid residual assesses bladder emptying and evaluates for overflow incontinence. Most experts consider uroflowmetry to be normal if the patient voids at least 200 mL in the course of 15 to 20 seconds. More specific normal flow rates have been determined by age and sex (Abrams and Torrens, 1979). For men younger than 40 years, between 40 and 60 years, and older than 60 years, normal rates are 22 mL/sec, 18 mL/sec, and 13 mL/sec, respectively. In women younger than 50 years, the flow rate be should be greater than 25 mL/sec; for women older than 50 years, it should be greater than 18 mL/sec. The normal flow pattern (volume over time) is bell-shaped and continuous. Prolonged voiding times may indicate an obstructed voiding pattern resulting from increased outlet resistance (e.g., urethral obstruction, external sphincter dyssynergia) or poor propulsive force (detrusor dysfunction). An interrupted pattern suggests straining to void or lack of coordination between detrusor muscle contraction and sphincter relaxation.

Cystometry evaluates bladder function, including sensation, compliance, and detrusor activity during filling. Most patients experience a first sensation of filling at 100 to 150 mL, first urge to void at 200 to 350 mL, and maximum bladder capacity at 400 to 550 mL. Urge incontinence should be considered in patients with reduced bladder capacity, with or without a spontaneous detrusor contraction and coexisting overactive bladder symptoms. Patients with increased bladder capacity should be evaluated for a neurogenic bladder. Urge incontinence from detrusor instability is documented when an involuntary contraction results in an overflow of the filling syringe (see Fig. 101.3). A cystometrogram is the best method for differentiating between bladder outlet obstruction and poor detrusor muscle contractility.

Normal values for a postvoid residual are not universally established, but various experts have defined it as less than 200 mL and less than 20% of the total void. Patients with urinary frequency or incontinence and a normal postvoid residual have a bladder storage problem, and this can result from disorders of bladder compliance, involuntary bladder contractions, bladder hypersensitivity, or bladder outlet abnormalities. Bladder outlet abnormalities can be due to lack of support, fibrosis, or neurologic insult.

A positive cough stress test indicates *genuine stress incontinence* (GSI). In patients with GSI and a positive Q-Tip test, urethral hypermobility is suspected. In patients with GSI and a fixed urethra on Q-Tip test, intrinsic sphincter deficiency is the presumed diagnosis. These patients require complex multichannel urodynamics for further evaluation.

POSTPROCEDURE PATIENT EDUCATION

The results of the testing and various management options should be discussed in detail with the patient. Patients should be instructed to call the clinician's office for pain or hematuria lasting longer than 48 hours and for symptoms of a urinary tract infection. Patients with persistent incontinence despite conservative therapy are candidates for complex urodynamics.

CPT/BILLING CODES

51725	Simple cystometrogram (e.g., spinal manometer)
51736	Simple (nonelectronic) uroflowmetry (e.g., stopwatch flow rate, mechanical uroflowmeter)
81000	Urinalysis, by dip stick or tablet reagent

ICD-10-CM DIAGNOSTIC CODES

N30.00	Cystitis, acute without hematuria
N82.0	Vesicovaginal fistula
N39.3	Incontinence, stress, female
N94.89	Unspecified symptom associated with female genital organs (i.e., pelvic pain)
R30.0	Dysuria
R39.14	Incomplete bladder emptying
R32	Urinary incontinence, unspecified
N39.41	Incontinence, urge
N39.3	Incontinence, stress, male
N39.46	Incontinence, mixed (male or female)
N39.44	Nocturnal enuresis
R35.0	Urinary frequency

Acknowledgment

The editors recognize the contributions of Jeffrey R. Dell, MD, Neeraj Kohli, MD, and Judy Wynn Neff, RN, BSN, to this chapter in a previous edition of this text.

ONLINE RESOURCES

Agency for Health Care Research and Quality: Urinary Incontinence in Adults: Clinical Practice Guideline Update (patient information on incontinence from the AHCRQ): www.ahrq.gov/clinic/uiovervw.htm.

National Institute of Diabetes and Digestive and Kidney Diseases (information on a wide range of topics on urologic conditions from the National Kidney and Urologic Diseases Information Clearinghouse and National Institutes of Health): www.niddk.nih.gov.

RECOMMENDED READING

Abrams PH, Torrens MJ. Urine flow studies. *Urol Clin North Am.* 1979;6:71–79.

Berni KC, Cummings JM. Urodynamic evaluation of the older adult: bench to bedside. *Clin Geriatr Med.* 2004;20:477–487.

Clement K, Lapitan M, Omar M, Glazener CMA. Urodynamic studies for management of urinary incontinence in children and adults. *Cochrane Database Syst Rev.* 2013. Art. No.:CD003195.

Fantl A, Newman DK, Colling J, et al. *Urinary Incontinence in Adults: Acute and Chronic Management. Clinical Practice Guideline No. 2, 1996 Update.* AHCPR Publication no. 96-0682. Rockville, Md: Agency for Health Care Policy and Research, U.S; 1996. Department of Health and Human Services.

Holroyd-Leduc JM, Tannenbaum C, Thorpe KE, Straus SE. What type of urinary incontinence does this woman have? *JAMA.* 2008;299:1446–1456.

Kohli N, Karram MM. Urodynamic evaluation for female urinary incontinence. *Clin Obstet Gynecol.* 1998;41:672–690.

Nager CW, Brubaker L, Litman HJ, et al. A randomized trial of urodynamic testing before stress-incontinence surgery. *N Engl J Med.* 2012;366:1987–1997.

Nitti VW, Brucker BM. Urodynamic and video urodynamic evaluation of the lower urinary tract. In: Wein AJ, Kavoussi LR, Partin AW, Peters CA, eds. *Campbell-Walsh Urology.* 11th ed. Philadelphia: Elsevier; 2016:1718–1742.

Resnick NM, Yalla SV, Laurino E. The pathophysiology of urinary incontinence among institutionalized elderly persons. *N Engl J Med.* 1989;320:1–7.

Wagg A. Urinary incontinence. In: Fillit HM, Rockwood K, Young J, eds. *Brocklehurst's Textbook of Geriatric Medicine and Gerontology.* 8th ed. Philadelphia: Elsevier; 2018:895–903.

SECTION 8

Male Reproductive System

Section Editor: GRANT C. FOWLER

CHAPTER 102

ADULT CIRCUMCISION

*John R. Holman**

Adult circumcision is a procedure about which little is written, even in the urologic literature. It is often performed for reasons that are not purely medical, yet it also has clearly defined medical indications. Some patients have their own nonmedical reasons.

General anesthesia may be necessary, but usually local anesthesia is sufficient in the outpatient setting, including the properly equipped office. Informed consent should be obtained after a thorough discussion with the patient (and partner, if appropriate), during which the indications, procedure, postprocedure care, and potential complications are explained. (See the sample patient education and consent forms available at www.expertconsult.com.) Consent is required for all patients, and it must always be documented to serve as a record of the authenticity of the patient's presenting symptoms. Thorough documentation is important because individual clinicians may vary in their judgment of surgical necessity. The clinician must make sure that the patient's reasons for requesting circumcision are medically sound and that the patient's expectations of the results are realistic. There is evidence that circumcision does not change sexual experience or satisfaction.

EDITOR'S NOTE: despite many of us having been trained to perform *newborn* circumcision, *adult* circumcision is not a common procedure performed by primary care clinicians in the United States. However, there are many more primary care clinicians performing adult circumcision overseas while doing missionary work (the original impetus for including the procedure in this book). Lately, more primary care clinicians in the United States have been performing adult circumcision in the office for patients lacking insurance or having high deductibles. It should also be noted that the Gomko clamp is available in adult sizes for those of us originally trained with this clamp.

ANATOMY

Identify normal male anatomy before proceeding. Patients with an occult hypospadias or epispadias should be referred to a urologist.

INDICATIONS

- Phimosis (tightness of the foreskin so that it cannot be drawn back from over the glans); possibly related to complaints of pain with erections and intercourse
- Paraphimosis (retraction of a narrow, inflamed foreskin that cannot be replaced or reduced)
- Penile hygiene; recurrent balanitis (inflammation of the glans penis)
- Posthitis (inflammation of the prepuce) not relieved by medical treatment
- Preputial neoplasms (e.g., erythroplasia of Queyrat, which is severe squamous dysplasia)
- Excessive foreskin redundancy
- Frenular tears

- Patient or partner preference after informed discussion
- Dissatisfaction with "beagle ear" or "dog ear" appearance of foreskin (Fig. 104.3)

Patients may also have social, religious, or personal reasons for requesting a circumcision. Exploration of these reasons ensures a thorough understanding of the risks and benefits as well as alternatives to the procedure. Circumcision can reduce the rate of human immunodeficiency virus infection by 50% to 60% and decreases penile human papillomavirus infection. However, it does not appear to prevent other sexually transmitted infections.

EDITOR'S NOTE: Performing a dorsal slit procedure (see Chapter 104, Dorsal Slit for Phimosis) is an option for circumcision for phimosis and other indications, either urgently or electively, especially for the patient who is not concerned about the cosmetic result.

CONTRAINDICATIONS

Relative

- Psychiatric disorder or history (relative contraindication; these patients must be screened carefully)
- Bleeding dyscrasias (evaluate appropriately)
- History of penile surgery, significant trauma, or unusual-appearing or ambiguous genitalia (consider a referral to a specialist)

Absolute

- Active inflammation in the genital area
- Infection in the genital area

EQUIPMENT AND SUPPLIES

EDITOR'S NOTE: the Gomko clamp is available in adult sizes. See Chapter 167, Newborn Circumcision and Office Meatotomy, for equipment and supplies needed for this technique.

- 10-mL syringe with a 1- to 1.5-inch 27-gauge needle and a 0.5-inch 30-gauge needle
- Prep bowl with a dozen 4 × 4 gauze sponges
- Povidone-iodine solution, chlorhexidine, or other antiseptic for scrub
- Pack of sterile 4 × 4 gauze bandages
- One fenestrated drape
- 6-in segment of 0.5-inch Penrose drain
- Six straight mosquito forceps
- One large straight forceps
- One curved Mayo scissors
- One medium-size straight Metzenbaum scissors
- One suture scissors
- 5-inch needle holder
- One Brown-Adson thumb forceps
- 4-0 or 5-0 absorbable suture (e.g., catgut, chromic, Vicryl, Dexon) or cyanoacrylate glue
- Petrolatum gauze

---

*The opinions contained herein are those of the author and should not be construed as official or as reflecting the views of the Departments of the Navy or Defense.

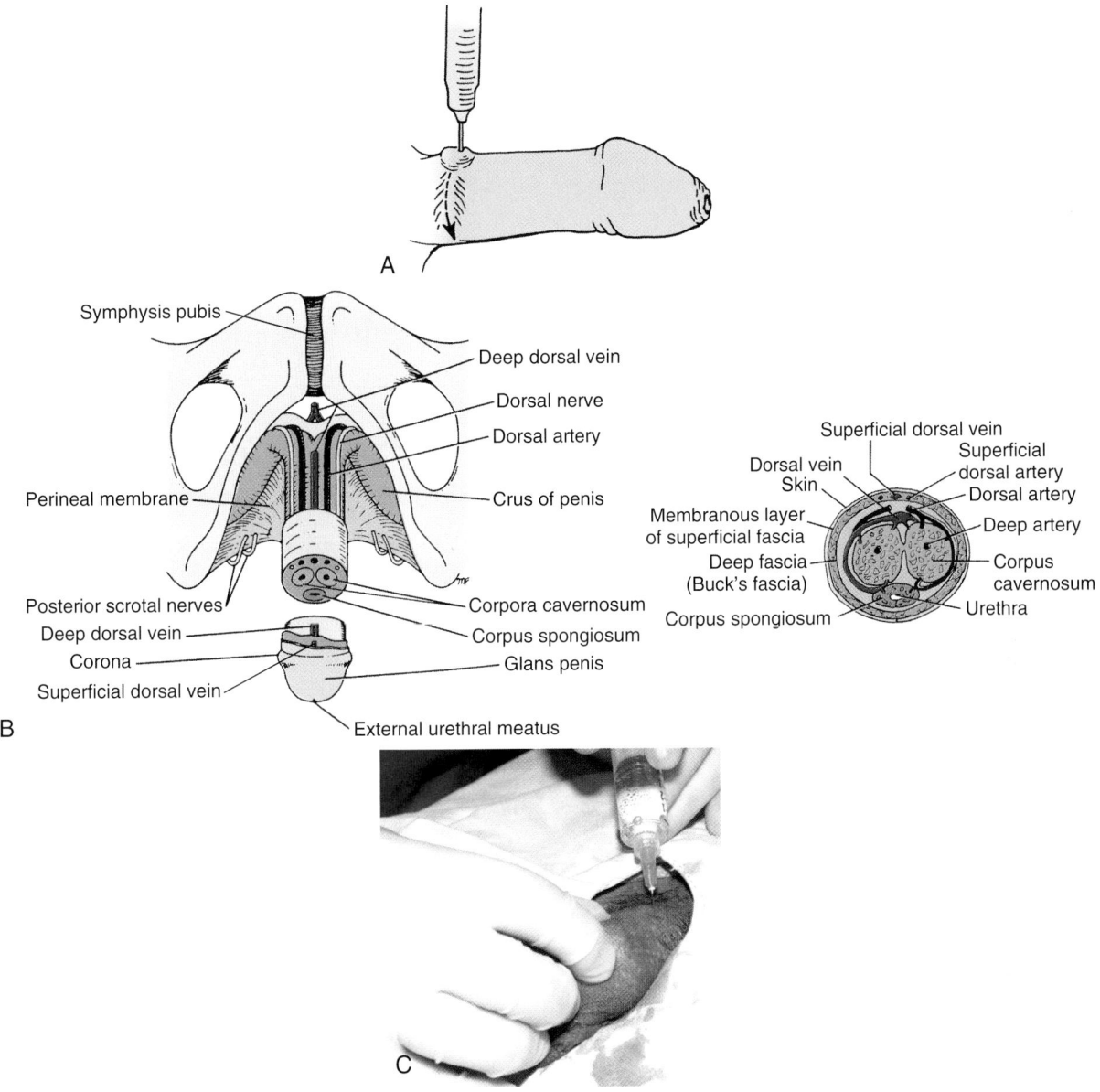

Fig. 102.1 Ring block of the penis. (A) Site of initial injection over dorsal vein. (B) Cross-sectional view of the penis. (C) Operative view.

- 1-in Kling or Kerlix bandage
- One malleable 4- to 6-inch silver probe (optional)
- Needle-tip electrocautery unit
- Sterile marking pen

PREPROCEDURE PATIENT EDUCATION AND FORMS

The patient should be properly counseled and evaluated before the surgery. A patient education handout is provided and a consent form is signed. (See the sample patient education and consent forms available at www.expertconsult.com.) If the patient is anxious, a preprocedural dose of an oral, sublingual, intramuscular, or intravenous anxiolytic (e.g., diazepam 10 mg) may be administered. If such a dose is used, someone must drive the patient home after the procedure. (See the sample patient education handout available at www.expertconsult.com.)

PROCEDURE

The patient should be supine and comfortable. Shaving and clipping of hair should be avoided to minimize the risk of infectious complications.

Surgically prepare the entire genitalia, scrotum, and pubic area with an appropriate antiseptic solution. Use a fenestrated drape.

Anesthesia

Ring Block

1. Using a 10-mL syringe filled with 1% lidocaine without epinephrine and a 1-in 27-gauge needle, inject 0.5 to 1 mL subcutaneously over the superficial dorsal vein so that a wheal is raised at the junction of the penis and pubis (Fig. 102.1).
2. Without withdrawing the needle completely, redirect it downward and laterally on both sides of the dorsal vein and inject additional lidocaine.
3. Extend the needle subcutaneously downward to the deep fascia of the penis—an area of firm resistance—and continue injecting circumferentially, staying close to the deep fascia of the penis. The penile skin is loose; therefore complete circumferential deployment of the anesthetic agent can be accomplished and the ventral surface can be reached from both sides. This is called a *ring block*. Inject approximately 4 mL in this manner on each side. Do not penetrate the fascia.

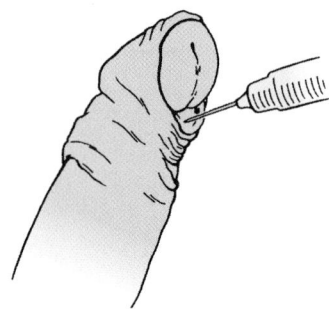

Fig. 102.2 Additional anesthetic injected into the frenulum.

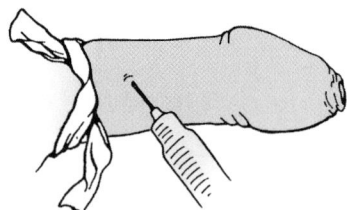

Fig. 102.3 Injection of anesthetic into the corpora cavernosa with tourniquet applied.

4. Wait a few minutes and then inject 1 mL of the local anesthetic subcutaneously into the frenulum using a 0.5-inch 30-gauge needle (Fig. 102.2).
5. Wait several more minutes and then test the depth of local anesthesia by cautiously grasping the edge of the foreskin with a mosquito hemostat. Should more anesthesia be required, use a Penrose drain as a tourniquet around the midportion of the penis. Tie the tourniquet tightly or hold the Penrose drain with a clamp to obstruct venous return. Inject an additional 2 mL of lidocaine into both corpora cavernosa just distal to the tourniquet (Fig. 102.3).
6. After approximately 5 minutes, retest for anesthesia; if anesthesia is adequate, remove the tourniquet.

Dorsal Penile Nerve Block

As an alternative to or in addition to the ring block, the surgeon may perform a dorsal penile nerve block. The dorsal penile nerve is blocked by injecting local anesthetic solution deep to the Buck's fascia, where the nerves emerge from under the pubic bone (see Fig. 102.1B).

1. The patient is placed in the supine position.
2. After preparation of the skin, two injection sites are identified over the inferior edge of the pubic bone at approximately the 10 and 2 o'clock positions relative to the base of the penis.
3. A 27-gauge (1.5-inch) needle is inserted directed ventrally until the pubic bone is contacted.
4. The needle is "walked" caudad off the pubis and through the Buck's fascia.
5. After aspiration, 5 mL of local anesthetic is injected at each site. A mixture of equal volumes of 0.5% bupivacaine (Marcaine) and 1% or 2% lidocaine without epinephrine provides a rapid onset of anesthesia of suitable duration for circumcision.

Dorsal Slit Technique

EDITOR'S NOTE: the Gomko clamp is available in adult sizes. See Chapter 167, Newborn Circumcision and Office Meatotomy for this technique.

The dorsal slit technique is preferred if the patient has phimosis or paraphimosis. An assistant is of considerable help in carrying out this procedure.

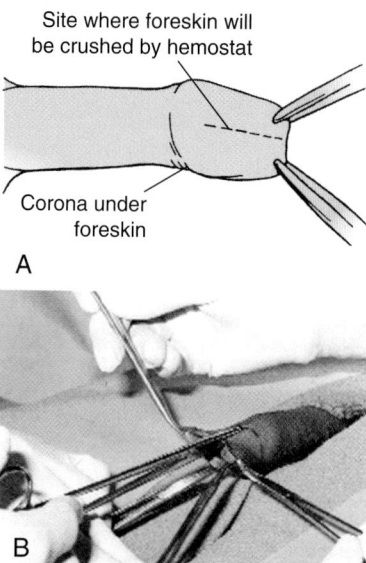

Fig. 102.4 Straight hemostats (four) applied at the dorsal and ventral aspects of the tip of the foreskin at the 11, 1, 5, and 7 o'clock positions. (A) Schematic. (B) Operative view with the large straight hemostat in crush position at 12 o'clock.

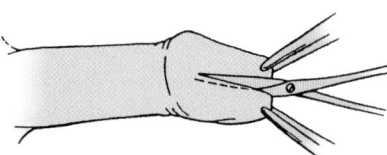

Fig. 102.5 Cutting through crushed tissue.

1. Using small straight hemostats, grasp the distal foreskin at the 11, 1, 5, and 7 o'clock positions and gently pull the foreskin over the glans.
2. Use a malleable silver probe or the hemostats on the undersurface of the dorsal foreskin, tenting it up slightly, to determine a point 1 cm distal to the corona.
3. Place a large straight hemostat at the 12 o'clock position, close it firmly, and compress and crush the foreskin to the point that you previously determined with the silver probe (Fig. 102.4). Repeat this procedure of clamping at the 6-o'clock position, going up to the base of the frenulum.
4. After the dorsal and ventral areas have been clamped, mark a line where the circumferential excision of the foreskin is to occur. Use a marking pen to connect the dorsal point with the inferior point on each side.
5. After 5 or more minutes (time it by the clock), remove the forceps and use a straight Metzenbaum scissors to incise through the center of the crushed areas (Fig. 102.5). Crushing the tissue reduces bleeding from this incision.
6. Using a curved Mayo scissors, carefully excise these two lateral tissue flaps, maintaining a 1-cm margin from the corona except at the frenulum, where the foreskin is tapered to only 2 to 3 mm remaining (Fig. 102.6). Fulgurate all bleeders or tie with a 5-0 plain catgut.
7. If the large dorsal vein is cut, ligate with absorbable sutures.
8. After complete hemostasis, sew the outer layer of skin just proximal to the glans to the underlying mucosal layer (1-cm skin remnant of prepuce) with multiple 4-0 or 5-0 absorbable sutures (Fig. 102.7). If performing the procedure alone, leave some sutures long dorsally. These can be used (and cut off later) for retraction to stabilize the penis when suturing ventrally. Use hemostats to fix the long suture to the drape.

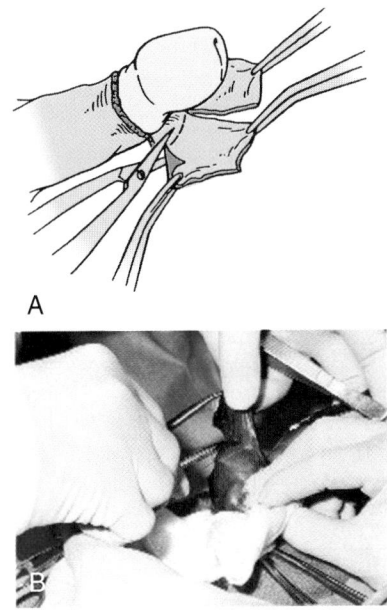

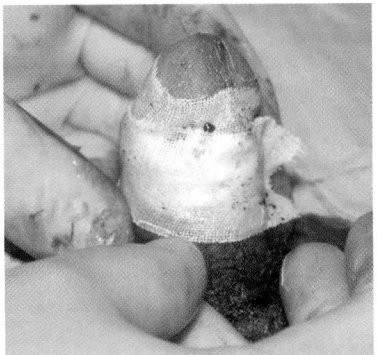

Fig. 102.8   Suture covered with gauze dressing.

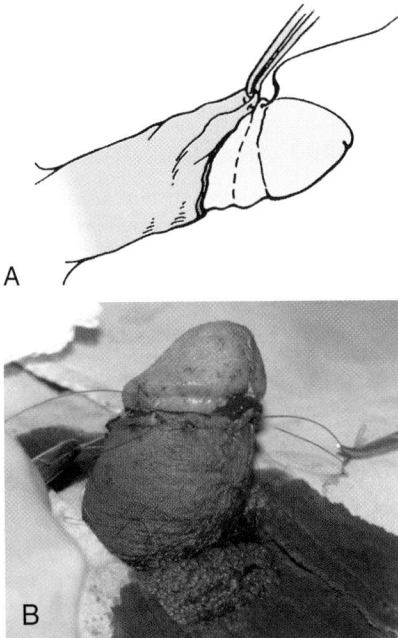

Fig. 102.6   Excision of foreskin. (A) Schematic. (B) Operative view.

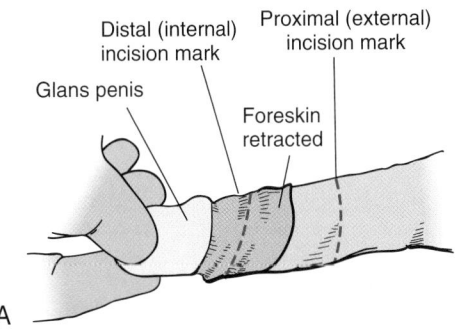

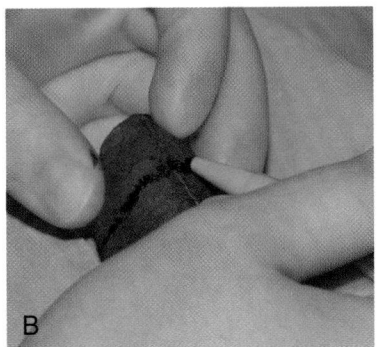

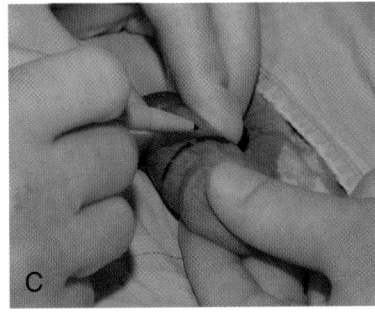

Fig. 102.7   Suturing of the skin to the shaft mucosa just proximal to the corona. (A) Schematic. (B) Operative view.

Fig. 102.9   External and internal preputial skin incision sites are marked. (A) Schematic. (B) Operative view, internal incision mark. (C) Operative view, external incision mark. (A, Modified from Holman JR, Stuessi KA. Adult circumcision. *Am Fam Physician.* 1999;59:1514–1518.)

EDITOR'S NOTE: some surgeons are now using cyanoacrylate glue in children, adolescents, and adults (Millard, Tiwari) instead of absorbable sutures to make this mucocutaneous approximation. Adequate amounts should be applied, just at the ends to attach to the mucosal layer under the glans. Avoid splashing it on the glans, as it could cause a slight burn and later denudement.

9. Place two layers of petrolatum gauze dressing, which is nonadherent, over the suture line around the entire circumference and overlay with a light layer of Kerlix or Kling (Fig. 102.8).

Sleeve Technique

The sleeve technique uses two circumferential incisions. One is made on the internal aspect of the foreskin distally, near the coronal sulcus. The other is made on the external part of the foreskin proximally and defines the amount of prepuce to be removed. A "sleeve" of tissue between the two incisions will be excised.

1. The external preputial incision is outlined with a marking pen at the level of the corona (Fig. 102.9A–B).
2. After retracting the foreskin, the internal preputial incision is marked with the pen approximately 1 cm proximal to the coronal sulcus. It is important to apply gentle downward

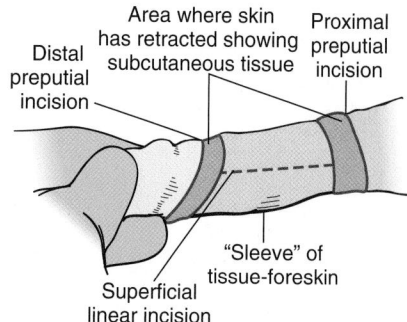

Fig. 102.10 After incisions are made, a "sleeve" of preputial skin remains. The shaded *(pink)* areas show where the skin has retracted, revealing subcutaneous tissue. (Modified from Holman JR, Stuessi KA. Adult circumcision. *Am Fam Physician*. 1999;59:1514–1518.)

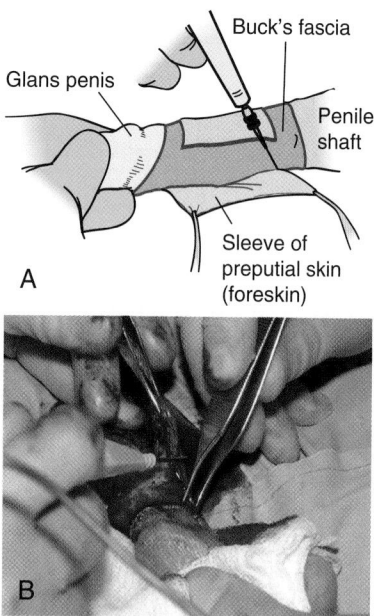

Fig. 102.11   Sleeve excised with electrocautery, tissue scissors or scalpel. (A) Schematic. (B) Operative view. (A, Modified from Holman JR, Stuessi KA. Adult circumcision. *Am Fam Physician*. 1999;59:1514–1518)

pressure on the prepubic fat pad at the base of the penis while making the initial outlines to remove the correct amount of skin (see Fig. 102.9A and C).
3. The external proximal circumferential preputial incision is made with the scalpel and carried to the Buck's fascia.
4. After retracting the foreskin, a second circumferential incision is made in the inner prepuce at the previous mark. The internal incision is carried straight across the frenulum ventrally.
5. A sleeve of tissue now exists between the two incisions (Fig. 102.10). This sleeve is the foreskin. Hemostats are placed dorsally for traction.
6. After making a superficial linear incision on the sleeve with the electrocautery tool, tissue scissors or a scalpel, subcutaneous attachments are separated between Buck's fascia and the prepuce. The sleeve is excised with electrocautery (Fig. 102.11), tissue scissors, or scalpel.
7. The frenulum is reapproximated initially with the "U" stitch.
8. Four quadrant sutures are placed on the dorsum and both sides, and the remaining interrupted sutures are placed at 4- to 7-mm intervals (see Fig. 102.7).

EDITOR'S NOTE: some surgeons are now using cyanoacrylate glue in children, adolescents, and adults instead of absorbable sutures

to make this mucocutaneous approximation. Adequate amounts should be applied, just at the ends, to attach to the mucosal layer under the glans. Avoid splashing it on the glans, as it could cause a slight burn and later denudement.

9. A sterile dressing of petroleum gauze can be applied (see Fig. 102.8).

SAMPLE OPERATIVE REPORT

See the sample operative report available at www.expertconsult.com.

COMMON ERROR

Removal of too much or too little foreskin is a common error. Correct planning of the incision is crucial to avoid this mistake.

COMPLICATIONS

- Bleeding: direct pressure, cautery, or suture ligature can be used.
- Hematoma: avoid with management of bleeding before skin closure. Apply pressure.
- Infection: sterile technique during surgery is important.
- Pain with erection: prevented by leaving an adequate "cup" (1-cm margin) of coronal skin (see step 6 under section "Dorsal Slit Technique").
- Stricture and scarring (rare).
- Dehiscence resulting from nocturnal erections (see next section).

POSTPROCEDURE MANAGEMENT

- Prescribe 5 days' worth of adequate analgesics appropriate for the patient's pain tolerance. A combination product containing codeine (such as Tylenol 3), a nonsteroidal antiinflammatory drug, or a similar product will suffice. Topical 5% lidocaine ointment can also be helpful.
- Instruct the patient to soak in a tub of warm water 24 to 36 hours later, to remove all the dressing at that time, and to replace the dressing daily after soaking off.
- One ampule of amyl nitrate (crush and inhale one to six times as needed; may be repeated once after 5 minutes) can be used as abortive therapy for erections during the 1-week recovery period.

EDITOR'S NOTE: Following trauma to the penis, erections are usually less common for a while. Likewise, with local discomfort from the sutures, erections will somewhat abort themselves until the sutures are removed. Patients should obviously be instructed to avoid erotic materials, direct penile stimulation, and erectile dysfunction meds. Although amyl nitrate ("poppers") is legal in the United States and may abort erections in some individuals, it might offend other patients to ask them to obtain it in the places where it is available over the counter ("smoke shops" or adult "toy" stores). If the patient has any history of substance abuse, recommending amyl nitrate might not be a good idea either, because its use can cause a brief euphoria.

POSTPROCEDURE PATIENT EDUCATION

- Instruct the patient on how to replace the petroleum gauze and Kling or Kerlix gauze, which should be done every day until the patient returns to the office for the follow-up visit in 1 week.
- Tell the patient to call if there is any undue pain, active bleeding, or sign of infection (e.g., streaks of redness, fever, purulent drainage).
- Instruct the patient to avoid sexual arousal and sexual intercourse for about 4 weeks.

PATIENT EDUCATION GUIDES

See the sample patient education, operative report, and consent forms available at www.expertconsult.com.

CPT/BILLING CODES

54161   Circumcision, surgical excision other than clamp device, or dorsal slit, other than newborn

ICD-10-CM DIAGNOSTIC CODES

N47.1   Phimosis and paraphimosis
N48.1   Balanitis(use additional code to identify infectious agent)
N48.9   Penile pain
F52.9   Psychosexual dysfunction

RECOMMENDED READING

Holman JR, Stuessi KA. Adult circumcision. *Am Fam Physician.* 1999;59(6):1514–1518.
MacLean R. Odds of penile HPV are reduced for circumcised men and condom users. *Int Fam Plan Perspect.* 2005;31:42.

Mehta SD, Moses S, Agot K, et al. Adult male circumcision does not reduce the risk of incident Neisseria gonorrhoeae, Chlamydia trachomatis, or Trichomonas vaginalis infection: results from a randomized, controlled trial in Kenya. *J Infect Dis.* 2009;200:370–378.
Millard P, Fumo A, Sabino E. Minimally invasive childhood and adult circumcision. *Tropical Doctor.* 2012;42(1).
Phillips R. Adult male circumcision cuts HPV viral load. *Nat Rev Urol.* 2014;11:603.
Pienkos EJ. Circumcision at the 121st Evacuation Hospital: report of a questionnaire with cross-cultural observations. *Mil Med.* 1989;154:169–171.
Pories WJ, Thomas FT. *Office Surgery for Family Physicians.* Stoneham, Mass: Butterworth; 1985.
Senkul T, Iseri C, Sen B, et al. Circumcision in adults: effect on sexual function. *Urology.* 2004;63:155–158.
Tiwari P, Tiwari A, Kumar S, et al. Sutureless circumcision, an Indian experience. *Indian J Urol.* 2011;27(4).
Wakefield SE, Elewa AA. Adult circumcision under local anaesthetic. *Br J Urol.* 1995;75:96.
White RG, Glynn JR, Orroth KK, et al. Male circumcision for HIV prevention in sub-Saharan Africa: who, what and when? *AIDS.* 2008;22:1841–1850.

CHAPTER 103

ANDROSCOPY

John L. Pfenninger

Androscopy is an office procedure mainly used to identify condylomata. It examines the male genitalia under magnification after acetic acid has been applied. It can be used to evaluate any dermatologic disorder/lesion in the genital areas, and to ensure complete removal of lesions. Another term for this procedure is *penoscopy*.

The scientific evidence has confirmed that the human papillomavirus (HPV) is the cause of almost all cervical dysplasia and cervical cancer. HPV is the necessary, if not the single, sufficient cause for cervical cancer; it is also associated with vulvar, vaginal, anal, penile, and oropharyngeal cancers. HPV is very contagious and it is most readily spread through sexual contact. It is the most common sexually transmitted infection. Intromission is not necessary because skin-to-skin contact is enough. It may also be transmitted in yet-unknown ways in a minority of cases. Fomites do not transmit the disease. Condoms provide only partial protection from HPV but do help prevent spread.

The clinical significance of condylomata and HPV in men is less serious than it is in women, but men act as carriers and may transmit the disease to sexual partners. Although penile cancer is rare, HPV can cause it. Anal-receptive homosexual men have 50 times the rate of anal carcinoma compared to the incidence in the average population. An increased rate of anal carcinoma in anal-receptive women also can be anticipated, but there is no literature to document this.

There are over 150 types of HPV. Of these, 8 to 10 characteristically infect the genital areas. Condylomata acuminata, the visible lesions that are commonly seen, are caused by noncarcinogenic strains, such as types 6 and 11. The subclinical types, identified only by examination under magnification after acetic acid staining, are more likely to cause neoplastic changes; frequently these are types 16 and 18. (See Chapter 124, Colposcopic Examination, Chapter 121, Human Papillomavirus DNA Typing, and Chapter 138, Treatment of Noncervical Condylomata Acuminata.)

There is no evidence that treatment of male partners of women who have dysplasia lessens the likelihood of persistence or recurrence in the woman. It is uncertain why condom use is beneficial because the infection is a regional disease. In men, it is present on the penis, scrotum, perineum, and perianal areas. What is visible is only a focal manifestation of a diffuse involvement. In women, it is present on the cervix, vagina, vulva, and the perineal and perianal areas. However, Winer and colleagues (2006), in a well-designed study, showed significant protection in women with consistent condom use by their male partners.

Some clinicians question the value of carrying out an androscopic examination. However, identification and treatment of condylomata is not the only reason to perform androscopy. Patient education is perhaps the most valuable aspect of this procedure. Men can spread the disease even when visible lesions are not apparent. Only through education can they be made aware of the risk of spreading it. That said, infection with HPV is common, and in most individuals, the body can clear the infection by itself.

EDITOR'S NOTE: In their most recent guidelines (2015), the Centers for Disease Control (CDC) do not recommend the routine use of applied mild (3% to 5%) acetic acid to detect mucosal changes due to HPV. This is because the results do not often influence the clinical management. However, there are providers trained in the technique that still utilize acetic acid with androscopy.

Men who have HPV can affect their partners in several ways. Not only do they spread the virus by skin-to-skin contact, but also HPV has been shown to be present in the semen and in the spermatozoa. Men who smoke have nicotine and its byproducts in their ejaculate as well as on their hands (important during manual stimulation), which may be a cofactor in HPV persistence. Those who are subject to passive smoking have lower folate levels—a known risk factor for cervical cancer.

The common factors for penile carcinoma include lack of hygiene, smoking, and HPV infection. Clinically differentiating mild, moderate, and severe dysplasia of the penis (penile intraepithelial neoplasia) is nearly impossible without obtaining biopsy samples. Anorectal cancer frequently contains the HPV, and some now recommend obtaining a Papanicolaou (Pap) smear of the pectinate (dentate) line on a regular basis to detect anal dysplasias in high-risk individuals. High-resolution anoscopy, which uses magnification (usually a colposcope) and acetic acid staining, can identify precursor lesions for treatment (see Chapter 84, High-Resolution Anoscopy).

INDICATIONS

- Visible condylomata on the penis, scrotum, or anus. Staining and examination with magnification will identify smaller lesions that are easier to treat and often not visible to the naked eye. This is likely to decrease recurrences. Androscopy also confirms that the entire lesion has been removed when surgical or ablative therapies are used. Early and complete treatment may reduce the recurrence of the disease. Fig. 103.1 shows an example of large condylomata. Examination under magnification will aid in completing removal once the bulk of the lesion has been removed and in identifying any smaller lesions that are not immediately obvious. Completing the removal under magnification helps in limiting the depth of excision because penile skin is so thin.
- Partner with recurrent or persistent condylomata acuminata or cervical dysplasia. There is some evidence that if the male partner presents with a high viral load, the immune system response of his partner may be overwhelmed by the virus. High viral load may exist if the man has extensive visible acuminate lesions or a diffuse acetowhite staining of the penis (Fig. 103.2).
- Psychological reassurance.
- Chronic perineal or perianal irritation.
- Recurrent condylomata. This could be from incomplete previous removal or failure to identify smaller lesions.
- Medicolegal examinations in child abuse cases.
- History of other sexually transmitted infections. Although rarely performed for this reason, androscopy with a negative result helps reassure patients that currently there are no HPV lesions.

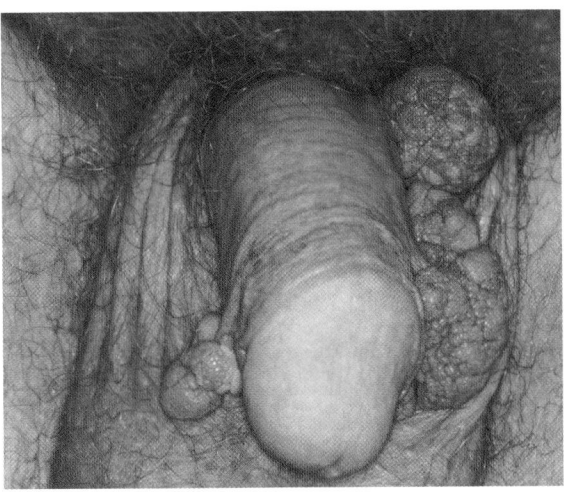

Fig. 103.1 Large condylomata. (Courtesy John L. Pfenninger, MD, The Medical Procedures Center, Midland, MI.)

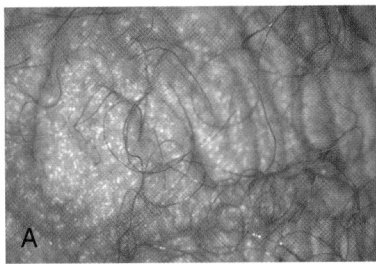

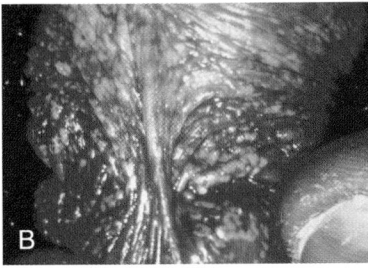

Fig. 103.2 (A) White epithelium seen on the scrotum after application of 5% acetic acid. (B) Condylomata seen on the penis after application of 5% acetic acid. Lesions were not visible before staining. (Courtesy John L. Pfenninger, MD, The Medical Procedures Center, Midland, MI.)

- Necessity for patient education. Performing a procedure is better received by the patient than just "coming in to talk." A biopsy-proven diagnosis speaks a thousand words of reinforcement.
- Penile lesions of uncertain significance.

EDITOR'S NOTE: As mentioned previously, the CDC does not recommend the routine use of applied mild (3% to 5%) acetic acid to detect mucosal changes due to HPV. This is because the results do not often influence the clinical management. However, there are providers trained in the technique that still utilize acetic acid with androscopy.

EQUIPMENT

- Spray bottle with 5% acetic acid (white vinegar).
- Colposcope (or a high-quality hand-held magnifying lens).
- High-quality fine tissue scissors (e.g., 5-inch curved Metzenbaum scissors) or sharp dermal curettes to obtain a biopsy/remove lesions.
- Pickups.
- Formalin jars.

- Aluminum chloride (Drysol) for hemostasis. Monsel solution may cause an extended period of hyperpigmentation but is also acceptable.
- 1- to 5-mL lidocaine 1% or 2% without epinephrine.
- 30-gauge needle.
- 1- to 5-mL syringe (depending on size and number of lesions).
- Radiofrequency unit with smoke evacuator, 85% trichloroacetic acid (TCA), or an infrared coagulator if condylomata are to be treated. (See Chapter 138, Treatment of Noncervical Condylomata Acuminata.)

PREPROCEDURE PATIENT PREPARATION

It is always best if the patient is well informed about the nature of the disease before the procedure. Provide the patient with educational material. Prior to the visit, encourage the patient to read about HPV online at www.cdc.gov/std/hpv/stdfact-hpv-and-men.htm) which includes a discussion about the implications of HPV infection in men. Reading this information before the procedure will help the patient focus on questions that he or his partner may have, and it will allow the practitioner to avoid repetitive explanations of the same counseling information. Written handouts are also available from many organizations. No preoperative medication is needed for the procedure, and the patient can be reassured that there will usually be minimal discomfort, even if biopsies are obtained. However, more discomfort may be experienced should treatment be undertaken.

TECHNIQUE

Although the examination may take only 10 minutes, patients frequently have numerous questions and concerns. Unless the patient is well known to the practitioner, at least 20 minutes should be allotted for this examination—longer if treatment is undertaken.

1. After the patient is placed in the examination room, the nurse instructs him to spray the entire genital and anal area with 5% acetic acid (white vinegar) and allow it to soak for 5 minutes.
2. Obtain a detailed sexual history (Fig. 103.3, Androscopy Encounter Form).
3. Place the patient on an examination table with stirrups, and position as a woman is positioned for a Pap smear. Conduct a visual inspection first and note any lesions.
4. Spray the entire genital and perineal area again. Allow the solution to run freely over the perineum and anus.
5. Inspect the entire anogenital area under magnification, including the meatus of the penis. Generally, a colposcope is used on low power (3× to 5×). Move the penis and scrotum forward and back to bring them into focus (unlike colposcopy, where the cervix is stationary and the scope is adjusted into focus). There is no study comparing good hand-held magnification to colposcopy.
6. Grossly apparent warts that were previously seen will generally turn white with the acetic acid. Previously unseen, small, "flat," or subclinical lesions will also now be identifiable on the penis, scrotum, perineum, or rectum. They will show up as white areas, referred to as *acetowhite changes* (see Fig. 103.2).
7. Sample any atypical lesions with an unusual vascular pattern (mosaicism or punctation; see Chapter 124, Colposcopic Examination) or pigmentation. The pigmentation in lesions that predicts dysplasia will look different from that of a freckle or nevus; it will be a nondiscrete, brownish discoloration (Fig. 103.4). If no atypical lesions are seen, sample one or two of the acuminate lesions or the acetowhite areas to document the presence of HPV; also check that there is no dysplasia (Fig. 103.5). It is very convincing to have the pathology report confirm your clinical diagnosis, which reinforces the findings to the patient. Also, it is not always possible to clinically tell what the lesions are.
8. A penile biopsy specimen is easily obtained by using sharp tissue scissors. (A punch biopsy is not needed—you are not sampling

Androscopy Patient Encounter Form

Patient to fill out:

Name_____ Date_____

Birth date_____ Age:_____ Referring clinician_____

Phone_____ Reason for exam_____

History   History of sexual abuse   Y   N
   Smoker   Y   N   History of genital warts   Y   N
      Packs per day_____ Since_____   Treated previously
   Age at first intercourse _____   How?_____
   No. of sexual partners (Total in lifetime)_____   Visible warts now   Y   N
   Family history of cancer   Y   N   Partners with warts   Y   N
                                              Previous partners w/abnormal Pap Y   N

Other history of venereal disease (circle):   Gonorrhea   Syphilis   AIDS   Herpes   Hepatitis
Do you desire testing for any of the above diseases: Y   N   Advised:_____
Other_____

Clinician Section

Illnesses: _____
_____

Medications: _____
Allergies: _____
Health maintenance: _____
Family history: _____

Procedure:

   Gross inspection:
   5% acetic acid and
      examination with colposcope: penis
                                          urethra
                                          scrotum
                                          groin
                                          perineum
                                          rectum

Biopsy:_____
Impression:_____
Treatment._____

Plan: Discourage smoking
         Counseling regarding safer sex, cause for cancer, reporting penis lesions, partner evaluation, vaccines
         Instruction sheets on androscopy/HPV?   Y   N   Videos viewed?   Y   N
         Consider other VD testing?   Y   N
         Follow-up in _____ weeks

Clinician signature: _____   Date _____

cc: _____

Fig. 103.3   Patient encounter form. (Courtesy John L. Pfenninger, MD, The Medical Procedures Center, Midland, MI.)

the cavernosa) If only one or two small lesions are to be sampled, simply tent up the skin by pinching it at its base (Fig. 103.6). Looking through the colposcope, obtain a 3- to 4-mm sample with the sharp tissue scissors or remove the entire lesion. No anesthetic is required if only one to two small lesions will be sampled, and this method is often less painful than the injection with anesthesia. Only a very superficial sampling is needed. If the lesions are larger, or more than two samples are to be obtained, it is best to anesthetize with 1% to 2% lidocaine without epinephrine. Using a 30-gauge needle minimizes any discomfort. Alternatively, a 3- to 4-mm, disposable, sharp

dermal curette can be used for the biopsy or removal. This is a particularly effective method for small lesions, but the curette *must be sharp*. Use disposable units because the reusables are never sharp enough.

9. If the condylomata are numerous (see Fig. 103.5), diffuse, or large, they may need to be treated with radiofrequency fine loop surgical removal, ball electrocautery, 85% TCA (Fig. 103.7), cryosurgery, 5-fluorouracil (Efudex; Valeant Pharmaceuticals), imiquimod (Aldara and Zyclara; Medicis Valeant Pharmaceuticals), podofilox (Condylox; Valeant Pharmaceuticals), the infrared coagulator, laser, or excision-

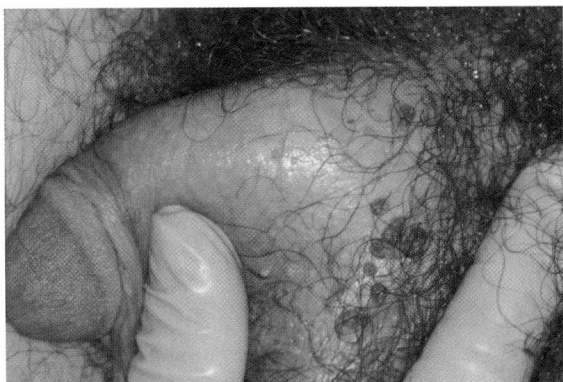

Fig. 103.4 Pigmented condylomata. These lesions are more likely to be dysplastic. (Courtesy John L. Pfenninger, MD, The Medical Procedures Center, Midland, MI.)

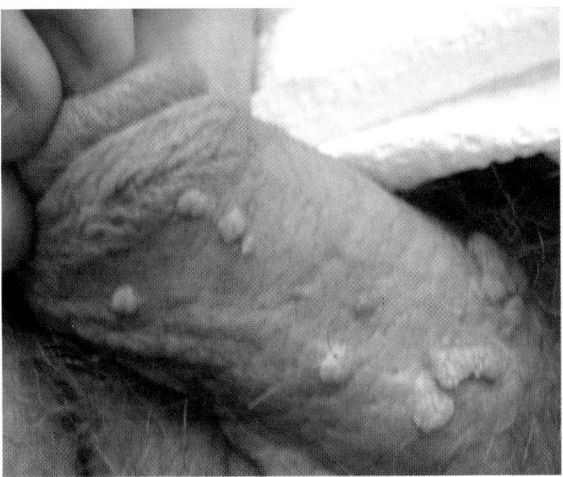

Fig. 103.5 Extensive condylomata. (Courtesy John L. Pfenninger, MD, The Medical Procedures Center, Midland, MI.)

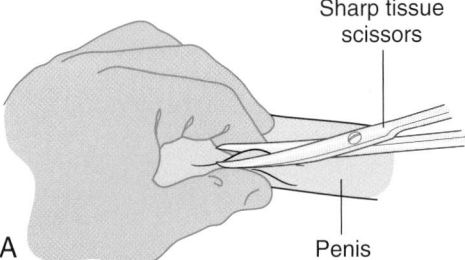

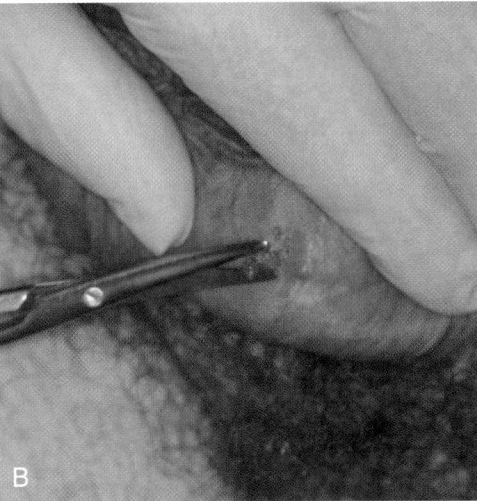

Fig. 103.6 (A) Tenting up the penile skin to obtain a biopsy. (B) Penile biopsy using curved Metzenbaum scissors.

al (shave) therapy; there are many options. A dorsal penile nerve block may facilitate removal. (See Chapter 138, Treatment of Noncervical Condylomata Acuminata.) Excision with suture closure is generally not only unnecessary, it is contraindicated.

10. Aluminum chloride (Drysol; Person & Covey), ferric subsulfate (Monsel solution), or light electrocautery/desiccation may be needed as an astringent to limit postoperative bleeding.
11. If only flat, asymptomatic acetowhite changes appear on the penis, anus, or scrotum, biopsies may be necessary to confirm HPV.
12. Unless the patient has had an extensive area of warts treated, he can return to full activity with no modification of his daily routine.
13. Sample any lesion of uncertain significance. The differential of penile and anal lesions and the approach to evaluation are noted in Box 103.1 and Fig. 103.8.
14. Cystoscopy and anoscopy are not routinely recommended for men with condylomata. If lesions are present around the anus, and if the man is not anal receptive (which occurs very frequently), treat all perianal lesions first. Anoscopy is indicated but only after resolving the external lesions. Frequently, more lesions will be found proximally around the dentate line; these can be removed as biopsies, treated with 85% TCA, frozen, or ablated with ball electrocautery (see Chapter 84, High-Resolution Anoscopy).

PRECAUTION

Not everything that turns acetowhite (white epithelium) is HPV. Chronic irritation, tinea, and other similar conditions can also appear white after the application of acetic acid.

COMMON ERRORS

- Not allowing enough time during the visit to counsel the patient and partner adequately.
- Not performing a complete examination, including retracting the foreskin (Fig. 103.9).
- Sampling or treating a normal variant of the corona, pearly penile papules (Fig. 103.10).
- Failing to perform a biopsy and continuing to treat lesions when they do not respond (Fig. 103.11).
- Using expensive prescription topicals when a simple surgical procedure or application of TCA will quickly and more cost-effectively treat the lesion.
- Not using magnification when removing lesions, which increases the likelihood of incomplete removal or missing smaller lesions, thereby increasing the likelihood of recurrence/persistence. Without magnification, it is also more common to perform any removal too deeply, leading to scarring.
- Treating all acetowhite lesions. Even when biopsies confirm the presence of HPV, if the lesions are totally asymptomatic and not visible to the naked eye, treatment is probably unnecessary. Remember that treatment does not eliminate the virus, but only the external manifestations of the disease. It is likely that the virus persists at a subclinical level. There is no evidence that treatment of the male partner in such cases reduces recurrences in female partners.

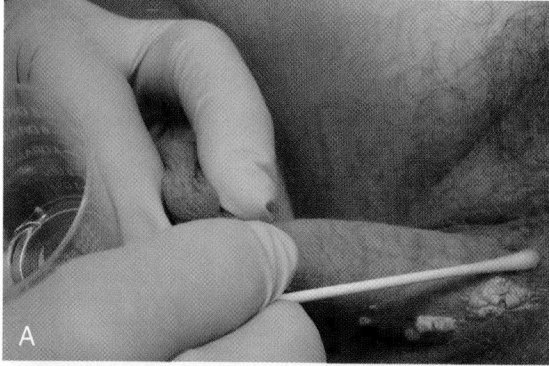
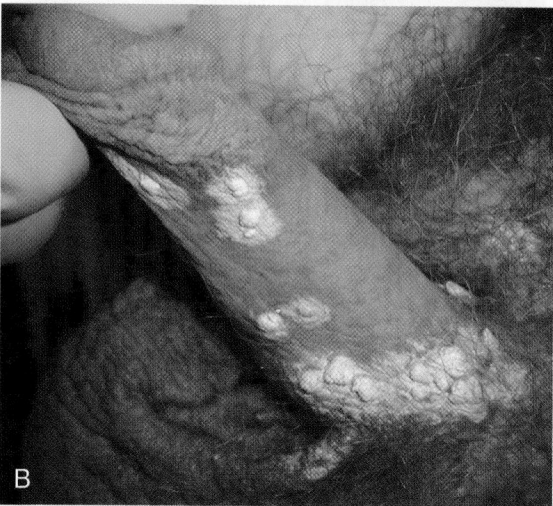

Fig. 103.7 (A) Application of 85% trichloroacetic acid (TCA) with a cotton-tipped applicator. (B) Appearance of condylomata immediately after application of 85% TCA. (Courtesy John L. Pfenninger, MD, The Medical Procedures Center, Midland, MI.)

BOX 103.1   Differential Diagnosis of Anogenital Lesions in Men

Infectious Lesions
Chancre
Condylomata acuminate
Condylomata lata
Herpes simplex virus
Molluscum contagiosum
Syphilis
Tinea pubis

Noninfectious Benign Lesions and Conditions (Including Normal Variants)
Anal polyp
Contact dermatitis
Cyst
Nevus
Normal-variant, papular lesions of the corona (pearly penile papules)
Normal-variant, papular lesions of the frenulum
Seborrheic keratosis
Sentinel "polyp" or "tag" on a chronic fissure
Skin tags

Preneoplastic and Neoplastic Lesions
Bowen disease (severe dysplasia)
Bowenoid papulosis
Cancer (squamous cell carcinoma of the penis and anus, prolapsing adenocarcinoma of the rectum)
Erythroplasia of Queyrat (squamous cell cancer in situ)
Penile intraepithelial neoplasia (PIN I, PIN II, PIN III)

From Pfenninger JL. Androscopy: examination of the male partner. In: Apgar B, Brotzman G, Spitzer M, eds. *Colposcopy: Principles and Practice. An Integrated Textbook and Atlas.* 2nd ed. Philadelphia: Saunders; 2008:483–496.

POSTPROCEDURE PATIENT CARE

Topical 5% lidocaine ointment not only soothes the area but prevents treated sites from adhering to the undergarments. A nonsteroidal antiinflammatory drug is recommended to reduce pain and swelling if more than just a biopsy was done.

No definite recommendations can be made regarding treatment of dysplastic lesions on the penis because studies with long-term follow-up have not been conducted. Between 1% and 5% of the sampled lesions will be reported as mild or moderate bowenoid dysplastic change. Rarely, a severe dysplasia will be found. (Unlike dysplastic cervical lesions in women, it is difficult to predict the degree of dysplastic change observed during the clinical examination, even with magnification, in the man.) In such situations, the patient should return for reexamination in 6 weeks to confirm that the entire dysplastic lesion(s) was removed. The patient should report any unusual growths or ulcerations at once, and he should discuss his HPV history with his clinician during future examinations. Sexual partners should be examined and should obtain regular Pap smears. Smoking is strongly discouraged. Supplemental vitamins with folic acid may reduce recurrences. See Chapter 138, Treatment of Noncervical Condylomata Acuminata, for posttreatment patient instructions.

COMPLICATIONS

Complications are minimal. There may be some depigmentation, scarring, pain, or bleeding, regardless of the technique used. The penile skin is very thin and the biopsy/removal should be kept very superficial. Condylomata acuminata can be confused with other lesions, such as condylomata lata, molluscum contagiosum (commonly seen), keratoses, bowenoid dysplasia, nevi, hemorrhoidal tags, and other nondescript papular lesions. Care must be taken that men do not experience undue psychological difficulty because of HPV infection, but at the same time know that each new sexual partner is at risk of contracting the wart virus if they have not been previously exposed.

CONCLUSION

Androscopy is a simple procedure to perform, which enhances the evaluation and treatment of genital lesions in the male patient. The colposcope is expensive, but if it is available in the office for colposcopic examinations, it can also aid male patients. Studies have not been completed using simple magnification devices, but they may also be an aid. An HPV vaccine (Gardasil) is now approved for men and women age 9 to 45 years.

PATIENT EDUCATION GUIDES

See patient education and consent forms available at www.expertconsult.com.

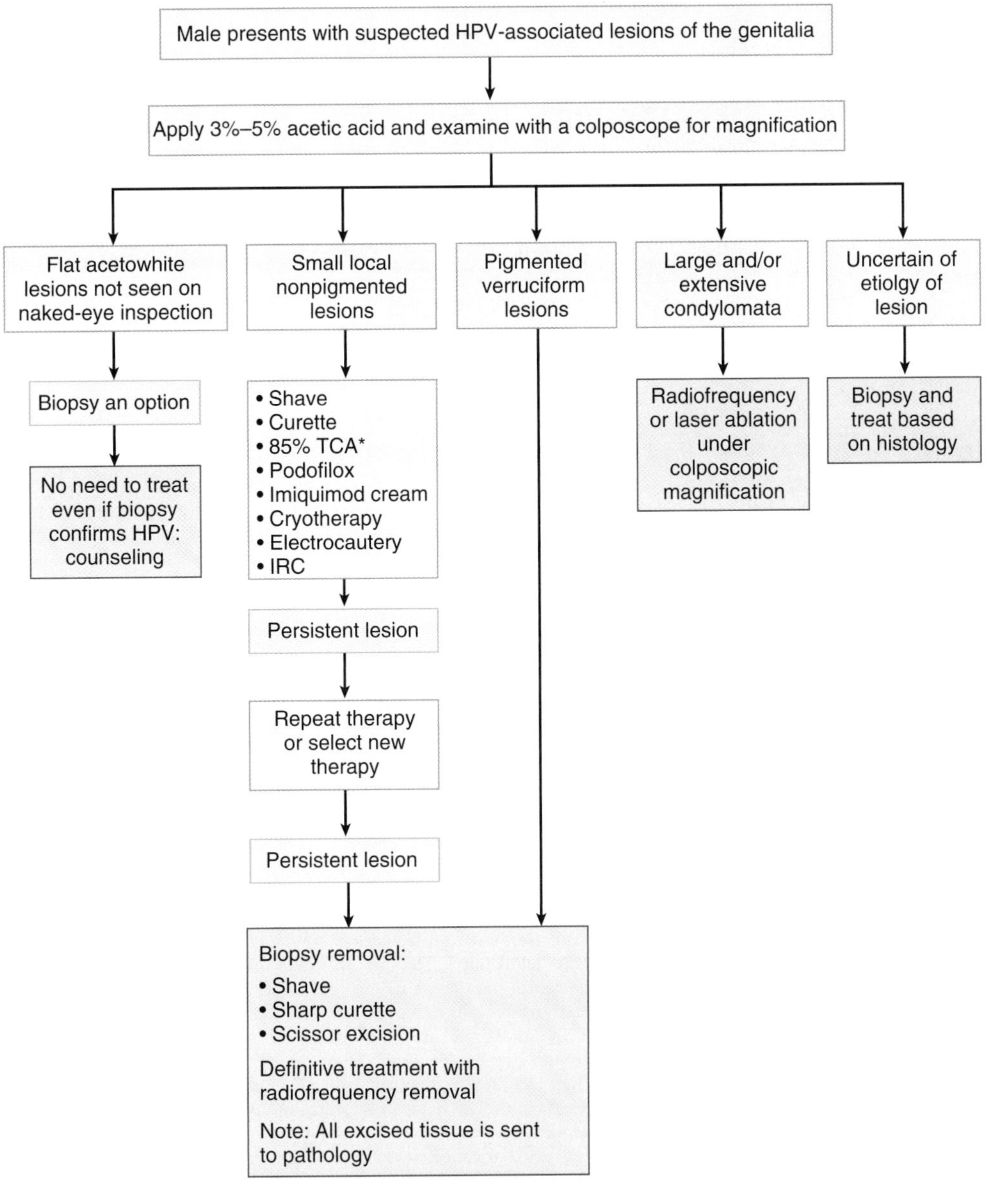

Male presents with suspected HPV-associated lesions of the genitalia

↓

Apply 3%–5% acetic acid and examine with a colposcope for magnification

| Flat acetowhite lesions not seen on naked-eye inspection | Small local nonpigmented lesions | Pigmented verruciform lesions | Large and/or extensive condylomata | Uncertain of etiolgy of lesion |

Flat acetowhite lesions not seen on naked-eye inspection
↓
Biopsy an option
↓
No need to treat even if biopsy confirms HPV: counseling

Small local nonpigmented lesions
↓
• Shave
• Curette
• 85% TCA*
• Podofilox
• Imiquimod cream
• Cryotherapy
• Electrocautery
• IRC
↓
Persistent lesion
↓
Repeat therapy or select new therapy
↓
Persistent lesion
↓
Biopsy removal:
• Shave
• Sharp curette
• Scissor excision

Definitive treatment with radiofrequency removal

Note: All excised tissue is sent to pathology

Large and/or extensive condylomata
↓
Radiofrequency or laser ablation under colposcopic magnification

Uncertain of etiolgy of lesion
↓
Biopsy and treat based on histology

Fig. 103.8 Summary of evaluation and treatment options for lesions of the male genitalia. *85% trichloroacetic acid (TCA) is often a first choice for therapy. It is effective 70% of the time, is quick acting, and can treat extensive lesions during the office visit if they are not too large. It is inexpensive compared with other treatments; however, it does burn for 5 minutes after application. HPV, Human papillomavirus; IRC, infrared coagulation. (Modified from Pfenninger JL. Androscopy: examination of the male patient. In: Apgar BS, Brotzman GL, Spitzer M, eds. *Colposcopy: Principles and Practice. An Integrated Text and Atlas.* 2nd ed. Philadelphia: Saunders; 2008:483–496.)

CPT/BILLING CODES

There currently is no CPT code for androscopy. Use 55899, unlisted procedure, male genital system (documentation suggested). Insurance companies still rarely pay. Consider charging for a more extended visit with a higher category E&M code (if a new patient or a consult) and for treatment of warts or penile biopsy rather than for "androscopy."

54100	Biopsy, penis, cutaneous
54050	Simple destruction of penile lesions: chemical
54055	Simple destruction of penile lesions: electrosurgical
54056	Simple destruction of penile lesions: cryocautery
54057	Simple destruction of penile lesions: laser
54060	Simple destruction of penile lesions: excision
54065	Destruction of penile lesions, extensive, any method
54105	Biopsy of penis, deep (generally not applicable with HPV)

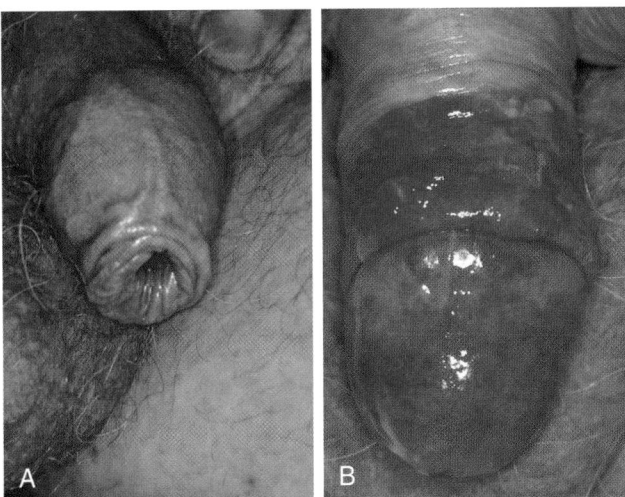

Fig. 103.9 (A) Appearance of uncircumcised penis on presentation. (B) Erythroplasia of Queyrat (bowenoid carcinoma in situ) after retraction of foreskin. A biopsy can easily be obtained with the technique noted previously using sharp tissue scissors after local anesthesia. (Courtesy John L. Pfenninger, MD, The Medical Procedures Center, Midland, MI.)

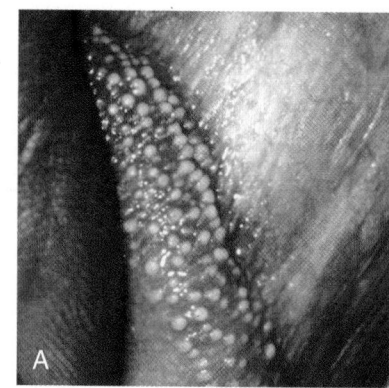
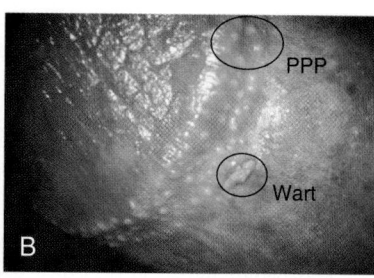

Fig. 103.10 Pearly penile papules (PPP) of the penile corona. (Courtesy John L. Pfenninger, MD, The Medical Procedures Center, Midland, MI.)

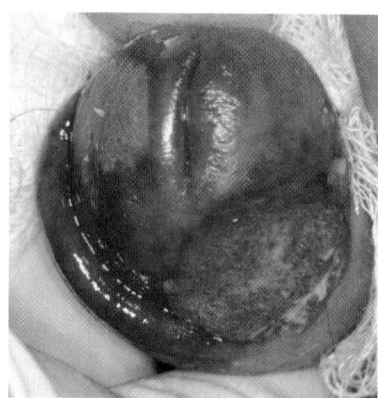

Fig. 103.11 Penile squamous cell carcinoma appearing as a "simple condyloma" clinically. Patient was referred for definitive treatment after being treated four times with 85% TCA and cryotherapy. (Courtesy John L. Pfenninger, MD, The Medical Procedures Center, Midland, MI.)

ICD-10-CM DIAGNOSTIC CODES

| A63.0 | Anogenital (venereal) warts; Condyloma |
| N48.9 | Penile pain |

Skin Lesions

C21.0	Anus, primary malignancy
C60.9	Penis, primary malignancy
C63.2	Scrotum, primary malignancy
C79.82	Penis, scrotum, metastatic
C78.5	Anus, metastatic
D12.9	Anus, benign
D01.3	Anus, cancer-in-situ
D07.4	Penis, cancer-in-situ
D07.61	Scrotum, cancer-in-situ
D29.0	Penis, benign
D29.4	Scrotum, benign
D40.8	Penis, uncertain
D37.8	Anus, uncertain
D49.0	Anus, unspecified
D49.59	Penis, scrotum, unspecified

RECOMMENDED READING

Barrasso R, DeBrux J, Croissant O. High prevalence of papillomavirus-associated penile intraepithelial neoplasia in sexual partners of women with cervical intraepithelial neoplasia. *N Engl J Med.* 1987;317:916–923.

Brinton LA, Li JY, Rong SD, et al. Risk factors of penile cancer: results from a case-control study in China. *Int J Cancer.* 1991;47:504–509.

Burmer GC, True LD, Krieger JN. Squamous cell carcinoma of the scrotum associated with human papillomavirus. *J Urol.* 1993;149:374–377.

Centers for Disease Control and Prevention. Sexually transmitted diseases treatment guidelines 2015. *MMWR.* 2015;64:1–137.

Christopher A. Hearing addresses condoms for HPV prevention. *J Natl Cancer Inst.* 2004;96:985.

Darragh TM, Berry TM, Jay M, Palefsky J. Anal disease. In: Apgar B, Brotzman G, Spitzer M, eds. *Colposcopy: Principles and Practice. An Integrated Textbook and Atlas.* 2nd ed. Philadelphia: Saunders; 2008:45M82.

Demeter LM, Stoler MH, Bonnez W, et al. Penile intraepithelial neoplasia: clinical presentation and an analysis of the physical state of human papilloma DNA. *J Infect Dis.* 1993;168:38–46.

Epperson WJ. Androscopy for anogenital HPV. *J Fam Pract.* 1991;33:143–146.

Frisch M, Fenger C, van den Brule AJ, et al. Variants of squamous cell carcinoma: cancer of the anal canal and perianal skin and their relation to human papillomavirus. *Cancer Res.* 1999;59:753–757.

Goldie SJ, Kuntz KM, Weinstein MC. The clinical effectiveness and cost-effectiveness of screening for anal squamous intraepithelial lesions in homosexual and bisexual HIV-positive men. *JAMA.* 1999;281:1822–1829.

Holmes KK, Levine R, Weaver M. Effectiveness of condoms in preventing sexually transmitted infections. *Bull World Health Org.* 2004;82:454–461.

Krebs HB, Helmkamp F. Does the treatment of genital condylomata in men decrease the treatment failure rate of cervical dysplasia in the female sexual partner? *Obstet Gynecol.* 1990;76:660–663.

Krogh G. Clinical relevance and evaluation of genito-anal papillomavirus infections in the male. *Semin Dermatol.* 1992;11:229–240.

Malek RS, Goellner JR, Smith T, et al. Human papillomavirus infection and intraepithelial, in-situ, and invasive carcinoma of the penis. *Urology.* 1993;42:159–170.

Palefsky JM. Anal cancer and its precursors: an HIV-related disease. *Hosp Physician.* 1993;29:35.

Palefsky JM, Holly EA, Gonzales J, et al. Detection of human papillomavirus DNA in anal intraepithelial neoplasia and anal cancer. *Cancer Res.* 1991;51:1014–1019.

Patton D, Rodney WM. Androscopy of unproven benefit. *J Fam Pract.* 1991;332:135–136.

Pfenninger JL. Androscopy: technique for examining men for condyloma. *J Fam Pract.* 1989;29:286–288.

Pfenninger JL. Letter to the editor. *J Fam Pract.* 1991;33:566.

Pfenninger JL. Androscopy: Examination of the male partner. In: Apgar B, Brotzman G, Spitzer M, eds. *Colposcopy: Principles and Practice. An Integrated Textbook and Atlas.* 2nd ed. Philadelphia: Saunders; 2008:483–496.

Pineda CP, Berry JM, Welton ML. High resolution anoscopy and targeted treatment of high-grade squamous intraepithelial lesions. *Dis Colon Rectum.* 2006;49:126.

Poblet E, Alfaro L, Fernander-Segoviano P, et al. Human papillomavirus-associated penile squamous cell carcinoma in HIV-positive patients. *Am J Surg Pathol.* 1999;23:1119–1123.

Rosemberg SK. Sexually transmitted papillomaviral infections: IV. The white scrotum. *Urology.* 1989;33:462–464.

Teichman JMH, Mannas M, Elston DM. Noninfectious penile lesions. *Am Fam Physician.* 2018;97(2):102–110.

Tokudome S. Semen of smokers and cervical cancer risk [letter]. *J Natl Cancer Inst.* 1997;89:96.

von Krogh G. Clinical relevance and evaluation of genitoanal papilloma virus infection in the male. *Semin Dermatol.* 1992;11:229–240.

Weiner JS, Liu ET, Walther PJ. Oncogenic human papillomavirus type 16 in association with squamous cell cancer of the male urethra. *Cancer Res.* 1992;52:5018–5023.

Whidden P. Cigarette smoking and cervical cancer [letter]. *Int J Epidemiol.* 1994;23:1099.

Wikström A, Hedblad MA, Johansson B, et al. The acetic acid test in evaluation of subclinical genital infection: a competence study on penoscopy, histopathology, virology and scanning electron microscopy findings. *Genitourin Med.* 1992;68:90–99.

Winer RL, Hughes JP, Feng Q, et al. Condom use and the risk of genital human papillomavirus infection in young women. *N Engl J Med.* 2006;354:2645–2654.

Winer RL, Lee SK, Hughes TP, et al. Genital human papilloma virus infection: rates and risk factors in a cohort of female university students. *Am J Epidemiol.* 2003;157:218–226.

Xi LF, Critchlow CW, Wheeler CM, et al. Risk of anal carcinoma-in-situ in relation to human papillomavirus type 16 variants. *Cancer Res.* 1998;58:3839–3844.

Zabbo A, Stein BS. Penile intraepithelial neoplasia in patients examined for exposure to human papillomavirus. *Urology.* 1993;41:24–26.

CHAPTER 104

Dorsal Slit for Phimosis

Morteza Khodaee • Gary Yen

Although the exact definition of phimosis is still controversial, this condition has been recognized since ancient times. American literature describes phimosis as "scar formation of the foreskin secondary to any injury or inflammatory condition, with the inability to retract the foreskin over the glans penis" (Wein and colleagues, 2007). Phimosis can be physiologic, congenital, or acquired as a result of inflammation or infection. About 90% of boys have a fully retractable foreskin by the age of 3 years. Only 1% of boys have physiologic phimosis that persists until age 17 years. Poor hygiene, balanitis, balanoposthitis (infection of glands and foreskin), diabetes, malignancy, and zipper injuries are conditions that may increase the risk of phimosis. *Acute phimosis* may occur with infection or as a complication of various treatments (e.g., 85% trichloroacetic acid, electrocoagulation) for conditions such as verrucae, which can cause inflammation.

Phimosis may lead to urinary retention or infection as well as *paraphimosis* (nonreducible retracted foreskin), which may require urgent or emergent intervention (Fig. 104.1). A debate exists over the medical versus surgical management of paraphimosis. In countries where circumcision is not widely practiced, nonsurgical and conservative surgical methods are most often used. Recent worldwide studies demonstrate the efficacy of topical steroids (0.05% betamethasone cream once or twice a day for 4 to 6 weeks).

Surgical options for phimosis include dorsal slit, ventral slit, preputioplasty, and circumcision. Various preputioplasty techniques (including sutureless prepuceplasty, triple incision plasty, La Vega slit) have been developed to accomplish better cosmetic results. These techniques usually involve a longitudinal incision in an attempt to release the tight prepuce ring; the incision is then often reapproximated. Dorsal slit is a simple procedure involving a single cut along the dorsal foreskin that is left open and allows rapid access to the urethral meatus and glans penis.

INDICATIONS

- To gain emergency access to the urethral meatus for bladder catheterization in the presence of phimosis if noninvasive and less invasive techniques have failed
- To prevent recurrent balanitis with abscess formation (as an alternative to circumcision)
- As an adjunctive treatment before circumcision or after phimotic ring incision for paraphimosis

CONTRAINDICATIONS

- Active infection of the genitalia
- Anatomic abnormalities of the external genitalia (refer to a urologist)

EQUIPMENT

- 10-mL syringe with 1-inch 27-gauge needle
- 1% to 2% lidocaine without epinephrine

- Three small straight hemostats
- Straight iris or small Metzenbaum scissors
- Suture scissors
- Absorbable suture (4-0) on small reversed cutting needle
- Needle driver
- Fenestrated drape
- Povidone-iodine solution or other antiseptic scrub
- Preparation bowl with 4 × 4 gauze sponges
- Adson forceps

PREPROCEDURE PATIENT PREPARATION

Provide appropriate information to the patient about the procedure while obtaining informed consent (see the sample patient education and consent forms available at www.expertconsult.com).

Risks include pain, bleeding, infection, hyperesthesia with intercourse (temporary or permanent), damage to the glans, poor cosmetic result, and hematoma formation. Benefits include resolution of phimosis, prevention of paraphimosis, increased ease of hygiene, decreased risk of urinary retention, and eventually decreased pain with intercourse.

Place the patient in a comfortable supine position on an examination table in a well-lit room. Using sterile technique, surgically prepare the genital area with an antiseptic solution. Place the penis through a fenestrated drape and onto the surgical field.

TECHNIQUE

Anesthesia

1. *Dorsal penile nerve block, ring block* (see Chapter 166, Subcutaneous Ring and Dorsal Penile Block for Newborn Circumcision and Chapter 102, Adult Circumcision), or modified ring block is used to obtain anesthesia after preparing and draping the penis. A dorsal penile nerve block anesthetizes the right and left dorsal nerves where they branch from the pudendal nerve from under the pubic bone. The lateral and ventral portions of the penile shaft are innervated by branches arcading from the dorsal midline, radiating toward the ventral surface. The axons innervating the glans are in a constant dorsal midline location along most of the penile shaft.
2. A 27-gauge 1-inch needle is inserted at the base of the penis just under the pubic bone and into the Buck's fascia at the 2 o'clock and 10 o'clock positions (Fig. 104.2A–B).
3. After aspirating, inject 3 to 5 mL of lidocaine into the base of the penis at the 2 o'clock and 10 o'clock positions deep to the Buck's fascia at the inferior edge of the pubic bone.
4. Wait 5 minutes and test for the adequacy of anesthesia by grasping the dorsal foreskin with a hemostat.
5. A *modified ring block* can be used if anesthesia is incomplete. This is performed by interconnecting the two positions across the dorsal midline at the base of the penis in a subcutaneous fashion (Fig. 104.2C).

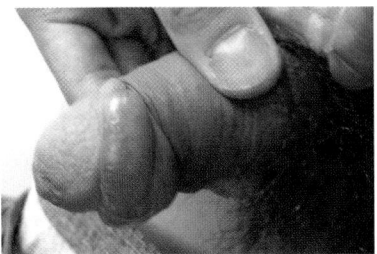

Fig. 104.1   Paraphimosis.

Procedure

1. After achieving local anesthesia, the operator grasps the distal dorsal foreskin in the 2 o'clock and 10 o'clock positions with two of the small straight hemostats (see Fig. 104.2D). Use the instruments to apply countertraction when performing the procedure.
2. Identify the corona of the glans with the foreskin in a relaxed position or with just gentle straightening. The corona determines the proximal extent of the dorsal slit.
3. Gently retract the foreskin and attempt to identify the urethral meatus.
4. A closed small straight hemostat is horizontally introduced into the opening of the foreskin between the inner layer of the foreskin and the glans penis. Advance it proximally to the coronal sulcus. Avoid entering the urethral meatus.
5. Tent up the foreskin and spread open the hemostat. Make sure you can palpate or visualize the tips of the hemostat beneath the

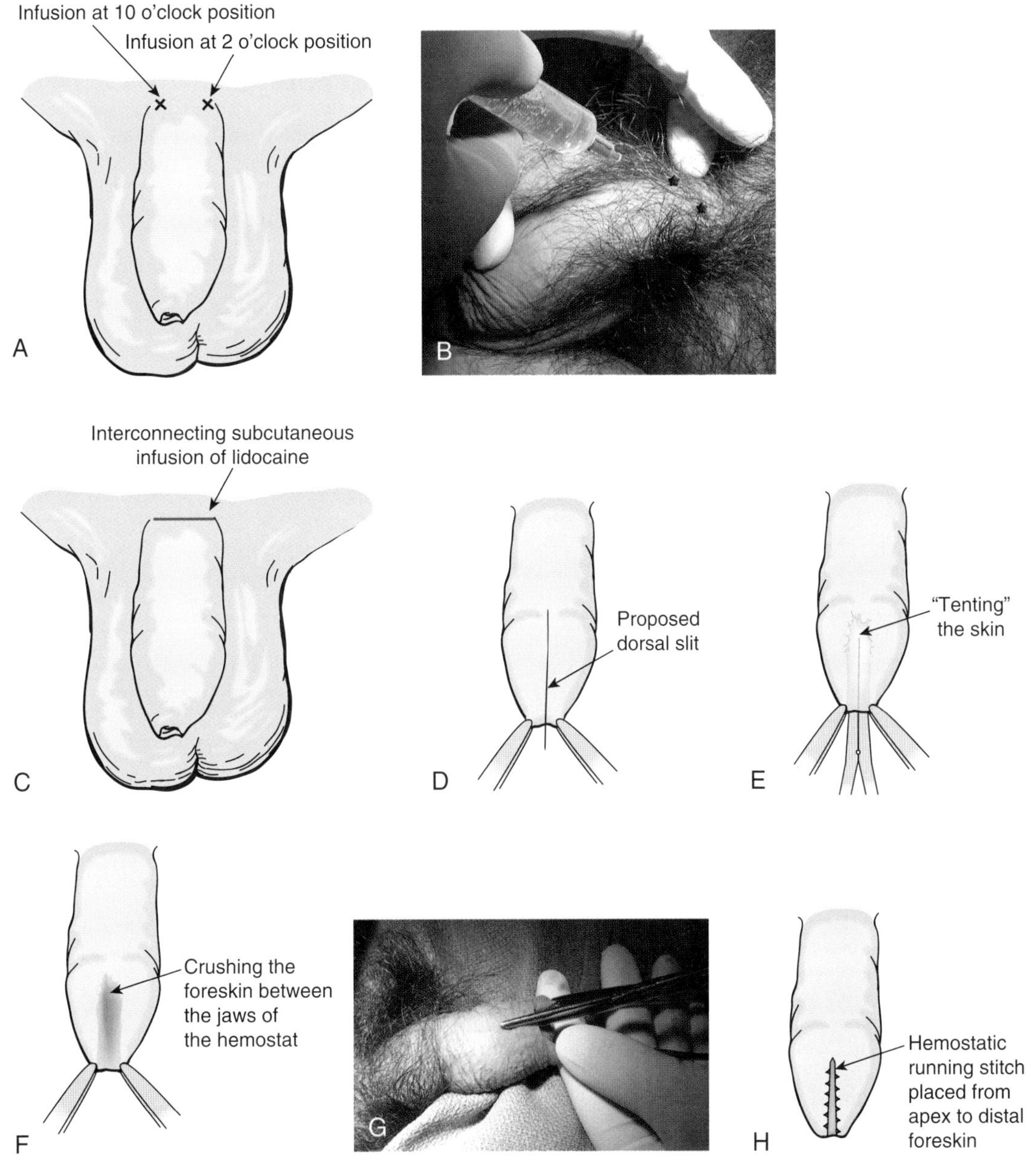

Infusion at 10 o'clock position
Infusion at 2 o'clock position

A

B

Interconnecting subcutaneous infusion of lidocaine

C

Proposed dorsal slit

D

"Tenting" the skin

E

Crushing the foreskin between the jaws of the hemostat

F

G

Hemostatic running stitch placed from apex to distal foreskin

H

Fig. 104.2   Dorsal penile nerve block. (A–B) Inject at the 10 o'clock and 2 o'clock positions. (C) Partial ring block. (D) Grasp foreskin at the 10 o'clock and 2 o'clock positions. Attempt to identify urethral meatus. (E) Lyse adhesions, again making certain to avoid the urethral meatus. Separate the "tented up" foreskin from the glans by spreading while withdrawing the hemostat. The tips of the hemostat should be somewhat visible or palpable beneath the foreskin that it is tenting up. (F–G) Place tented up clamp longitudinally in the 12 o'clock position. (H) If needed, place sutures to control bleeding.

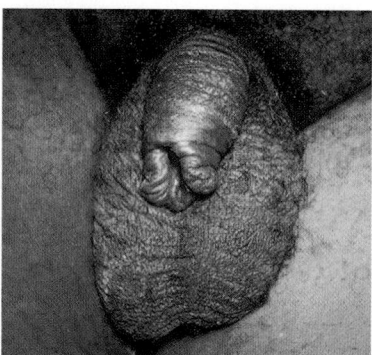

Fig. 104.3 "Beagle-ear" appearance resulting from the dorsal slit procedure. If desired, a formal complete circumcision can be performed after the inflammation has resolved. (From Roberts JR, Hedges JR, eds. *Clinical Procedures in Emergency Medicine*. 6th ed. Philadelphia: Elsevier; 2014.)

foreskin; if not, the hemostat should be withdrawn, as it may be in the urethra. If the tips are palpable or visible, withdraw the instrument slightly and twist to the right and left to break up adhesions around the circumference of the glans (see Fig. 104.2E). When lysis of the adhesions is complete, the hemostat is withdrawn.

EDITOR'S NOTE: At this point, if the preputial opening has been significantly stretched with the hemostat, the surgeon can consider one last attempt to insert a urinary catheter and thus avoid the dorsal slit procedure.

6. Reinsert the hemostat in the open position with one jaw of the hemostat in the plane between the glans and the inner layer of the foreskin while the other is placed on the outer skin. This should be at the 12 o'clock position with the instrument in a longitudinal position. Advance the instrument to the level of the coronal sulcus, tent it up again to palpate or visualize the tip and thus make sure that it is not in the urethra, and clamp it tightly. This crushes the interposed anesthetized foreskin (see Figs. 104.2F and G).
7. Remove the hemostat and cut the foreskin longitudinally with iris or Metzenbaum scissors along the entire distance of the serrated, crushed foreskin, being careful to leave 1 or 2 mm of crushed tissue at the apex. If uncrushed skin is incised, it can lead to significant bleeding.
8. If crush hemostasis is inadequate or if the incision extends too far and there is bleeding after cutting the dorsal slit, absorbable sutures should be used to obtain adequate hemostasis. This is performed by placing two running 4-0 Vicryl or Dexon sutures beginning at the apex of the dorsal slit and running distally to reapproximate the two layers of each side of the incision of the foreskin (see Fig. 104.2H).
9. Application of sterile petroleum jelly or antibiotic ointment on the wound edges will prevent the dressing from adhering to the wound.

COMPLICATIONS

- *Bleeding.* Late bleeding can be controlled with direct pressure, Monsel solution, Gelfoam, or the placement of hemostatic ligatures.
- *Injury to the urethral meatus or glans.* When the procedure is being performed, avoid blind introduction of hemostat and scissors so as to prevent injury to the urethral meatus or glans. All instrumentation should be performed on the dorsal aspect of the penis to avoid the ventral meatus.
- *Infection.* Antibiotics can be used to control infection, which is commonly due to skin pathogens such as *Streptococcus* or *Staphylococcus*.
- *Pain.* Hyperesthesia with intercourse may occur.
- *Anesthesia complications.* There may be hematoma formation at the site of injection.

- *Poor cosmetic result.* Elective circumcision (see Chapter 102, Adult Circumcision) may be recommended if the patient is not satisfied with the "beagle ear or dog ear" appearance of the foreskin (Fig. 104.3).

POSTPROCEDURE PATIENT EDUCATION

- After successful dorsal slit surgery for phimosis, the prepuce is easily retracted to access the urethral meatus and cleanse the glans penis.
- After completion of catheterization or cleansing, the foreskin should be reduced to avoid iatrogenic paraphimosis.
- Between 3 and 5 days of analgesics should be prescribed for postprocedure pain.
- The patient should wear loose briefs and gently cleanse the wound for 5 to 7 days with soap and water three to four times a day.
- The patient should avoid intercourse or masturbation for 4 to 6 weeks to prevent disruption of the wound.
- The patient should be instructed to return for a postprocedure wound check in 1 to 2 weeks and to return immediately if excessive bleeding occurs.
- Instruct the patient on signs of infection, which should not be confused with fibrinous exudate (a straw-colored exudate) that is part of normal healing.

PATIENT EDUCATION GUIDES

See the sample patient education form available at www.expertconsult.com.

CPT/BILLING CODES

54001   Slitting of prepuce, dorsal or lateral (separate procedure), except newborn

ICD-10-CM DIAGNOSTIC CODES

N47.1   Phimosis
N47.2   Paraphimosis

Acknowledgment

The editors recognize the contributions of Scott A. Cota, MD, to this chapter in a previous edition of this text.

RECOMMENDED READING

Christianakis E. Sutureless prepuceplasty with wound healing by second intention: an alternative surgical approach in children's phimosis treatment. *BMC Urol.* 2008;8:6.
Cuckow PM, Rix G, Mouriquand PD. Preputial plasty. A good alternative to circumcision. *J Pediatr Surg.* 1994;29:561–563.
Esposito C, Centonze A, Alicchio F, et al. Topical steroid application versus circumcision in pediatric patients with phimosis: a prospective randomized placebo controlled clinical trial. *World J Urol.* 2008;26:187–190.
Holman JR, Stuessi KA. Adult circumcision. *Am Fam Physician.* 1999;59:1514–1518.
Munro NP, Khan H, Shaikh NA, et al. Y-V preputioplasty for adult phimosis: a review of 89 cases. *Urology.* 2008;72:918–920.
Davis JE, Silverman MA. Urologic procedures. In: Roberts JR, Custalow CB, Thomsen TW, eds. *Roberts and Hedges Clinical Procedures in Emergency Medicine.* 6th ed. Philadelphia: Elsevier; 2014:1126–1129.
Reichman EF, Peres N. Phimosis reduction. In: Reichman EF, ed. *Emergency Medicine Procedures.* 2nd ed. New York: McGraw-Hill; 2013:995–998.
Roldan CJ. Dorsal slit of the foreskin. In: Reichman EF, ed. *Emergency Medicine Procedures.* 2nd ed. New York: McGraw-Hill; 2013: 998–1001.

Terlecki RP, Kim ED: Phimosis, adult circumcision and buried penis. eMedicine last updated November 18, 2015. www.emedicine.com/med/topic2873.htm.

Steadman B, Ellsworth P. To circ or not to circ: indications, risks, and alternatives to circumcision in the pediatric population with phimosis. *Urol Nurs*. 2006;26:181–194.

Szmuk P, Ezri T, Ben Hur H, et al. Regional anaesthesia for circumcision in adults: a comparative study. *Can J Anaesth*. 1994;41:1181–1184.

Wein AJ, Kavoussi LR, Partin AW, et al., eds. *Campbell-Walsh Urology*. 11th ed. Philadelphia: Elsevier Saunders; 2016.

Yang CC, Bradley WE. Neuroanatomy of the penile portion of the human dorsal nerve of the penis. *Br J Urol*. 1998;82:109–113.

CHAPTER 105

PROSTATE MASSAGE

Robert E. James • James R. Palleschi

Prostate massage has been used therapeutically and diagnostically in the management of recurrent or chronic prostatitis, prostatosis (congested, sterile), and prostatodynia for over a century. However, with the introduction of the scientific method in the 1960s, its role was relegated to that of a diagnostic tool. At present its primary benefit is to aid in the diagnosis of chronic prostatitis. However, owing to the failure of standard medical therapy in many patients with refractory symptoms of chronic prostatitis and prostatosis, prostate massage is regaining popularity as a treatment. Although a systematic review of the literature (Mishra and colleagues, 2008) found that evidence for repetitive prostate massage (two to three times a week for 4 to 6 weeks) as an adjunct to the treatment of chronic prostatitis is at most "soft," the authors concluded that it could be considered as part of multimodal therapy in select patients. (As it turns out, frequent ejaculation may achieve the same function as prostate massage [Yavascaoglu et al, 1999]). Hennenfent and colleagues (2006) also demonstrated, in a very small study, that repetitive prostate massage in addition to medical therapy may delay the need for transurethral resection of the prostate.

INDICATIONS

- Diagnosis of chronic or subacute prostatitis.
- Chronic urinary tract infection.
- Management of chronic prostatitis, prostatosis, and prostatodynia.
- Possibly useful in combination with medical management for benign prostatic hyperplasia.
- Although still considered experimental and expensive, the urinary PCA3 test is offered by some facilities as screen for prostate cancer.

CONTRAINDICATIONS

- Acute prostatitis, especially in immunocompromised patients
- Prostatic abscess
- Significant difficulty voiding

EQUIPMENT

- Examination glove and water-soluble lubricant
- Microscope
- Sterile culture container

PREPROCEDURE PATIENT PREPARATION

Tell the patient that he may have an urge to urinate and may feel rectal pressure for 15 to 60 minutes after prostatic massage. Tell the patient to contact the clinician or the nearest emergency department if he experiences chills, myalgia, rigors, or a temperature above 10°F.

TECHNIQUE

1. Place the patient in a comfortable position for the prostate examination. A variety of positions may be used: the knee-chest position, left lateral decubitus position, or bent over the examination table. (With this position, the patient should place his elbows on the examination table and spread his heels apart. The patient is thus immobilized, which facilitates the prostate examination and the subsequent massage.) In addition, the patient may assist you in collecting the expressed prostatic fluid by holding the microscope slide below the urethral meatus of the glans penis.

2. Apply a generous amount of lubricant to the anus and to your gloved index finger. The examination will be more comfortable for the patient if he performs a mild Valsalva maneuver as the finger passes through and into the anal opening. In patients with a high-riding prostate, a Valsalva maneuver may bring the gland down to the examining finger.

3. For the prostate massage, press the pad of your index finger into the substance of the prostate. Start on the superior and lateral aspect of the prostate and move your index finger toward the midline or median sulcus. Gradually work from the base or superior aspect of the prostate gland down to the inferior portion or apex (Fig. 105.1), carrying this motion out several times bilaterally. Last, massage the median furrow, or mid-aspect, of the prostate gland from the base to the apex. This is the technique followed whether or not secretions will be collected. If secretions are to be collected, by following this pattern, the prostatic secretions are massaged toward the prostatic urethra. They then pass through the distal urethra and can be collected for microscopic examination and culture and sensitivity if desired. Normally you will have to repeat the prostatic massage for a period of 30 to 90 seconds before any secretions are obtained. The quantity collected may vary from a few drops to 2 to 3 mL. Some patients will not discharge any secretions (despite correct performance of the prostate massage as described) or may have discomfort sufficient to abort the procedure. Clinically, more than 15 white blood cells per high-power field suggest an infectious process.

COMPLICATIONS

- Rarely, bacteremia or urosepsis may occur after a prostate massage. These problems can be avoided by not performing prostate massage on a patient suspected of having acute prostatitis or a prostatic abscess.
- Occasionally a patient with significant prostatism resulting from prostatic hypertrophy may develop prostatic edema after a massage, leading to temporary difficulty urinating or to urinary retention.

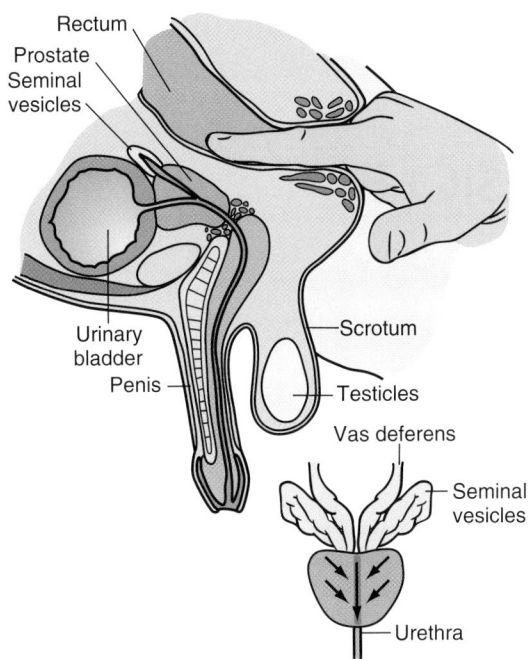

Fig. 105.1 Technique of prostatic massage. The glandular substance is compressed from its lateral edges to the urethra, which lies in the center. The *arrows* in the inset drawing show the direction of pressure. The seminal vesicles are then stripped from above downward.

• Hematuria and hematospermia occur infrequently after a prostate massage.

NOTE: Any manipulation or trauma to the prostate gland may elevate a patient's serum prostate-specific antigen (PSA) for several weeks. Therefore, after performing a digital rectal examination, I wait 1 week before performing a PSA; after a prostate massage, I wait 2 weeks. An acute prostatitis or prostate infarct may cause an elevated PSA for up to 6 weeks.

CPT/BILLING CODES

| 87205 | Prostatic smear |

There is no CPT code for prostate massage.

ICD-10-CM DIAGNOSTIC CODES

N41.1	Prostatitis, hypertrophic
N41.9	Prostatitis
N41.0	Prostatitis, acute
N41.1	Prostatitis, subacute or chronic
N41.3	Prostatocystitis
N42.83	Abscess of prostate (avoid prostate massage)
N42.1	Congestion or hemorrhage of prostate
N42.81	Unspecified disorder of prostate, prostatodynia

RECOMMENDED READING

Nickel JC. Inflammatory and pain conditions of the male genitourinary tract: prostatitis and related pain conditions, orchitis, and epididymitis. In: Wein AJ, Kavoussi LR, Partin AW, eds. *Campbell-Walsh Urology.* 11th ed. Philadelphia: Elsevier; 2016.

Hennenfent BR, Lazarte AR, Feliciano AE. Repetitive prostate massage and drug therapy as an alternative to transurethral resection of the prostate. *MedGenMed.* 2006;8(4):19.

Meng MV, Tanagho EA. Physical examination of genitourinary tract. In: McAninch JW, Lu TF, eds. *Smith and Tanagho's General Urology.* 18th ed. New York: McGraw-Hill; 2013:44–46.

Mishra VC, Browne J, Emberton M. Role of repeated prostate massage in chronic prostatitis: a systematic review of the literature. *Urol.* 2008; 72(4):731–735.

Shoskes DZ, Zeitlin SI. Use of prostatic massage in combination with antibiotics in the treatment of chronic prostatitis. *Prostate Cancer Prostatic Dis.* 1999;2(3):159–162.

Wei JT, Feng Z, Partin AW. Can urinary PCA3 supplement PSA in the early detection of prostate cancer? *J Clin Oncol.* 2014;32:4066–4072.

Yavascaoglu I, Oktay B, Simsek U, et al. Role of ejaculation in the treatment of chronic non-bacterial prostatitis. *Int J Urol.* 1999;6:130–134.

CHAPTER 106

PROSTATE AND SEMINAL VESICLE ULTRASONOGRAPHY AND BIOPSY

Philip J. Aliotta • Grant C. Fowler

Transrectal ultrasound of the prostate (TRUSP) and seminal vesicles (SVs) is an essential tool in the assessment of these organs. Useful for defining anatomy, evaluating blood flow, and diagnosing and treating benign and malignant diseases of these glands, it is now the standard in most urologists' practices.

Although TRUSP-SV has proved helpful in the investigation of the infertile couple, more importantly, the introduction of TRUSP-SV has improved the accuracy of prostate tissue sampling. Even though a digital rectal examination (DRE)-guided fine-needle or core (e.g., Tru-Cut, Biopty) biopsy may confirm cancer, it is not as useful for excluding cancer; DRE is more helpful for guiding the biopsy of a palpable nodule. TRUSP-SV improves the ability of the clinician to exclude cancer in more regions of the gland and has somewhat become the standard for evaluation of possible prostate cancer.

One important recent development for TRUSP-SV, especially for underserved areas, is that technicians or sonographers are making services available on-site for primary care clinicians. They can also be very useful when using TRUSP-SV for guiding biopsy. Over-reading services for TRUSP-SV by a radiologist are available over the Internet (see the Suppliers section). This may revolutionize the management of suspected prostate cancer.

Although large studies in the United States and Europe have failed to clarify whether men benefit from screening for prostate cancer, most organizations recommend at least a discussion of this topic with their clinician, especially in men younger than 75 years and with at least a 10-year life expectancy. A prostate biopsy may be indicated if the examination or laboratory result is suspicious for cancer (Fig. 106.1). Although certain ethnic groups (e.g., African Americans) were thought to be at increased risk of prostate cancer in the past, more contemporary analyses suggest that this discrepancy is decreasing. Much of any remaining variation may be more strongly related to education, insurance status, and access to health care.

GENERAL ANATOMY

An understanding of anatomy is necessary before scanning or biopsy. The prostate can be described by its general, vascular, zonal, tissue, or ultrasonographic anatomy. Fig. 106.2 shows the general anatomy of the prostate and SVs.

Prostate

The prostate is a chestnut-shaped gland surrounded by a pseudocapsule of dense fibrous tissue and smooth muscle that connects with the muscular layers of the prostatic urethra. The pseudocapsule cannot be separated from the gland itself. It has anterior, posterior, and lateral surfaces. The prostate base is contiguous with the bladder superiorly. The apex of the prostate is contiguous with the striated urethral sphincter. Lateral to the prostate is the pubococcygeal portion of the levator ani and endopelvic fascia. The Denonvilliers fascia, which separates the prostate from the rectum, is posterior to the prostate.

Vas Deferens and Seminal Vesicles

Arising from the tail of the epididymis, the vas deferens consists of a tortuous proximal portion and a dilated terminal portion called the *ampulla*. The ampulla is capable of storing sperm and lies posterior to the bladder. Bordering the base of the bladder, posteriorly, are the SVs. They also lie adjacent to the ampullae of the vasa deferentia and the distal ureters.

VASCULAR ANATOMY

The prostatic artery is a branch of the internal iliac artery. It divides into capsular and urethral arteries. The capsular arteries supply two thirds of the gland; the urethral arteries supply the remaining third. Branches of the inferior vesical artery supply the SVs, and occasionally the base of the prostate gland. The neurovascular bundles located posterolaterally (at the confluence of the SV and prostate bilaterally) provide the main neurovascular supply and drainage system of the prostate.

ZONAL ANATOMY

Traditionally, the prostate was divided into five major lobes (anterior, middle, posterior, and two lateral lobes) and two minor lobes (trigonal and subcervical lobes). McNeal derived a three-dimensional model of the prostate, as illustrated in Fig. 106.3.

TISSUE ANATOMY

The normal prostate consists of a combination of glandular tissue and fibromuscular structures.

Glandular Tissue

Glandular tissue accounts for about 66% of the prostate. There are four identified glandular zones, each with a distinct ductal system draining into a specific part of the urethra. The first three zones share similar histologic and embryologic origin. The fourth zone is the central zone (CZ) and differs histologically from the rest of the gland. It is derived from the Wolffian duct.

1. Peripheral zone (PZ; as much as 75% of the glandular tissue). The largest area of glandular tissue is in the PZ, which comprises the lateral and most of the posterior aspect of the prostate (except at the base). The PZ ducts drain into the distal urethral segment. The majority (>65%) of prostate cancers occur in the PZ.

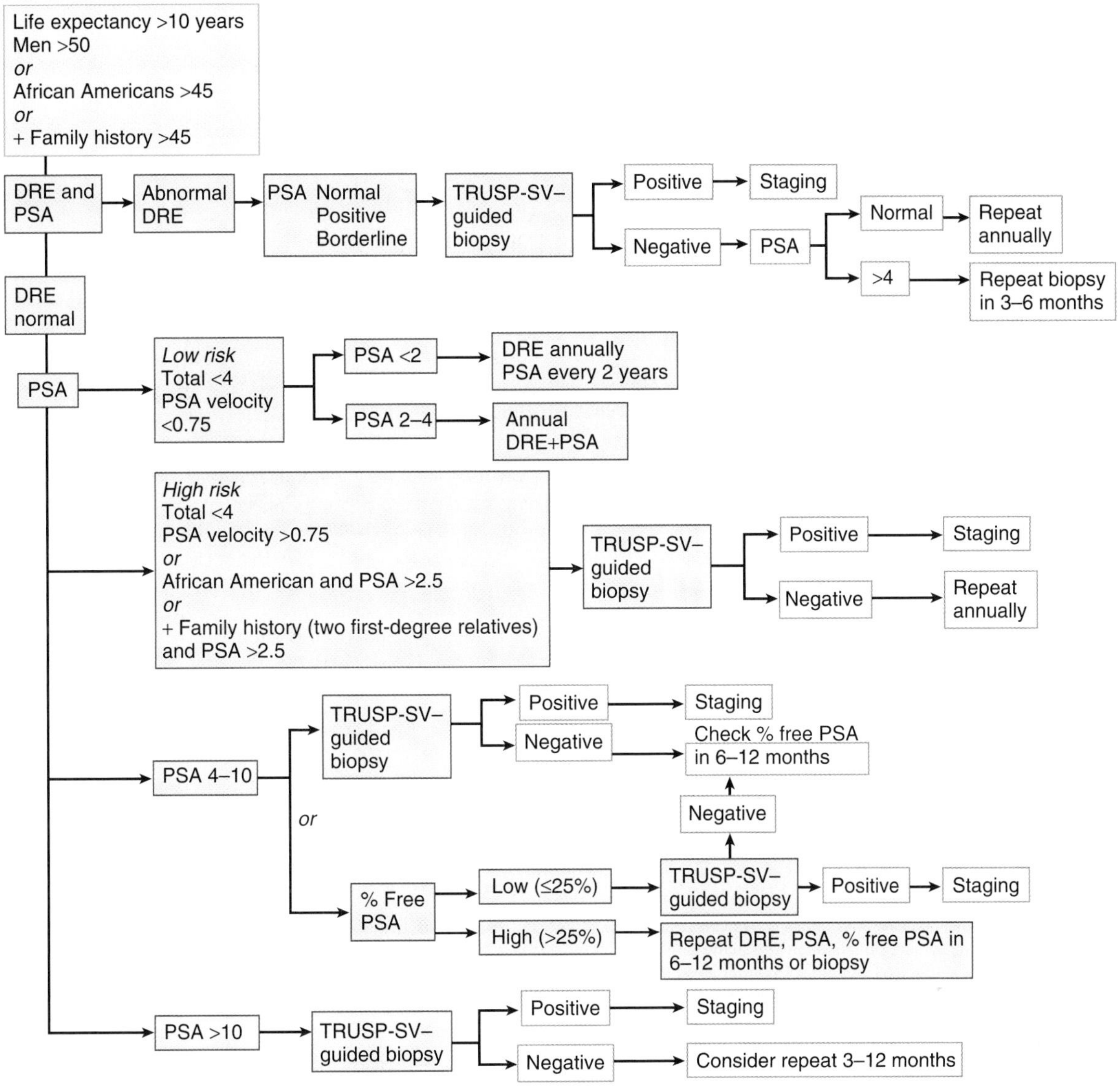

```
Life expectancy >10 years
Men >50
or
African Americans >45
or
+ Family history >45
```

DRE and PSA → Abnormal DRE → PSA Normal Positive Borderline → TRUSP-SV–guided biopsy → Positive → Staging
TRUSP-SV–guided biopsy → Negative → PSA → Normal → Repeat annually
PSA → >4 → Repeat biopsy in 3–6 months

DRE normal

PSA → Low risk Total <4 PSA velocity <0.75 → PSA <2 → DRE annually PSA every 2 years
Low risk → PSA 2–4 → Annual DRE+PSA

High risk Total <4 PSA velocity >0.75 or African American and PSA >2.5 or + Family history (two first-degree relatives) and PSA >2.5 → TRUSP-SV–guided biopsy → Positive → Staging
→ Negative → Repeat annually

PSA 4–10 → TRUSP-SV–guided biopsy → Positive → Staging
→ Negative → Check % free PSA in 6–12 months

or

% Free PSA → Low (≤25%) → TRUSP-SV–guided biopsy → Positive → Staging
→ Negative
% Free PSA → High (>25%) → Repeat DRE, PSA, % free PSA in 6–12 months or biopsy

PSA >10 → TRUSP-SV–guided biopsy → Positive → Staging
→ Negative → Consider repeat 3–12 months

Fig. 106.1 Sample algorithm for men who desire early cancer detection after discussion of pros and cons with their clinician. Contemporary analyses of African-American men suggest that ethnic discrepancies are disappearing. Much of any ethnic variation still noted may be more strongly related to education, insurance status, and access to health care rather than ethnicity. *DRE*, Digital rectal examination; *PSA*, prostate-specific antigen; *TRUSP-SV*, transrectal ultrasonography of the prostate and seminal vesicles. (Modified from Braunwald E, Fauci AS, Kasper DL, et al, eds. *Harrison's Principles of Internal Medicine.* 15th ed. New York: McGraw-Hill; 2001.)

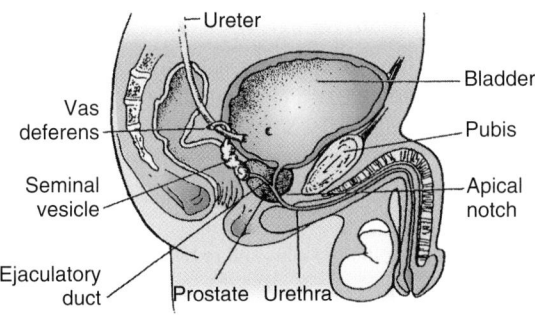

Fig. 106.2 General anatomy of prostate and seminal vesicles. (From Brooks JD. Anatomy of the lower urinary tract and male genitalia. In: Walsh PC, Retik AB, Vaughan ED Jr, Wein AJ, eds. Campbell's Urology. 7th ed. Philadelphia: WB Saunders; 1998:112–117.)

2. Transition zone (TZ; 5% to 10% of the glandular tissue). The TZ comprises two small lobules on either side of the proximal urethral segment just lateral to the periprostatic sphincter. The TZ is the origin of most symptomatic benign prostatic hyperplasia (BPH) and approximately 20% of carcinomas.
3. Periurethral glands (PUGs; 1% or more of the glandular tissue). These glands are embedded in the smooth muscle wall of the urethra, entirely within the preprostatic sphincter (PPS). Involved in the BPH process, these glands can give rise to an enlarged middle lobe.
4. CZ (as much as 25% of the glandular tissue). The CZ is cone-shaped and surrounds the ejaculatory ducts. The major distinction between the CZ and the PZ is that the CZ is relatively resistant to the development of cancer. Only 10% of cancers occur in the CZ. Interestingly, BPH does not seem to occur in the CZ.

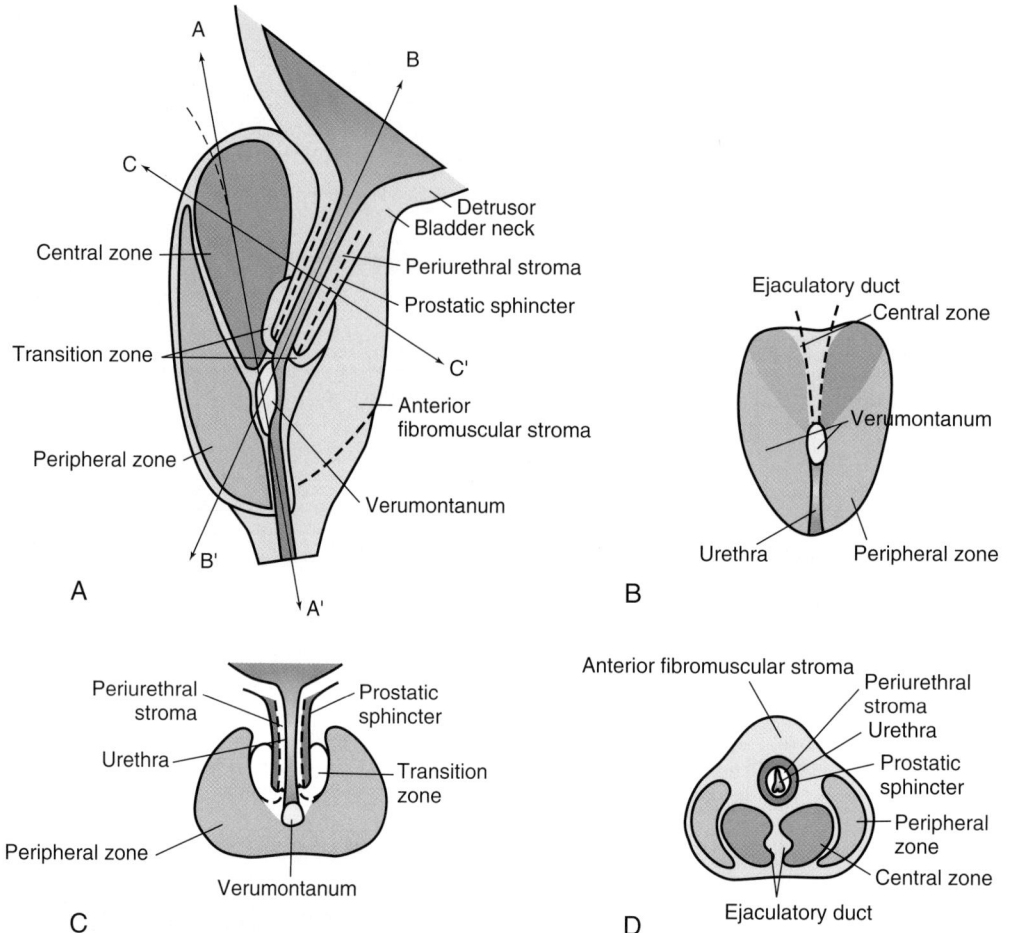

Fig. 106.3   Anatomy of the prostate. (A) Midsagittal plane. (B) Coronal section (through the plane A-A′ in A). (C) Oblique coronal section (through the plane B-B′ in A). (D) Transverse section (through the plane C-C′ in A). (A, Modified from McNeal JE. Normal and pathologic anatomy of prostate. *Urology.* 1981;17[suppl 3]:11–16. B–D, Modified from Muldoon LD, Resnick MI. Normal anatomy of the prostate. In: Resnick MI, ed. *Prostatic Ultrasonography.* Philadelphia: BC Decker; 1990.)

Fibromuscular Structures

Fibromuscular structures make up 33% of the prostate. There are four fibromuscular structures:

1. Anterior fibromuscular stroma
   - A continuation of the detrusor muscle
   - Covers the anterior and anterolateral aspects of the glandular tissue from base to apex
2. Preprostatic sphincter (PPS)
   - Smooth muscle fibers of the lower ureters and superficial trigone
   - Intimately related to the TZ
   - Prevents pooling of urine in the proximal segment of the urethra
   - Prevents retrograde ejaculation
3. Postprostatic sphincter
   - The proximal extension of the striated external urethral sphincter muscle covering the anterior and lateral aspects of the distal urethra
   - Contributes to continence
4. Longitudinal smooth muscle
   - Part of the urethra

The key to understanding prostate tissue anatomy is to understand the anatomy of the prostatic urethra, which is approximately 3 cm long. It should be used as a primary reference point. After traveling through the proximal prostate, the urethra takes a 35-degree turn, angling anteriorly. The point of angulation divides the urethra into its proximal and distal urethral segments. The proximal urethral segment is related to two tiny glandular regions, the TZ and PUG, and to the PPS. The verumontanum lies entirely in the distal segment. In addition, the distal urethral segment is related to the function of ejaculation. The ejaculatory ducts and the excretory ducts (PZ and CZ) empty into the distal urethral segment.

ULTRASOUND ANATOMY

(For definitions of *hyperechoic, isoechoic,* and *hypoechoic,* see the Interpretation section.)

With ultrasound, the anatomy is divided into two general areas that are immediately obvious to the examiner:

1. The outer area, or *outer gland,* is close to the rectum and generally described as isoechoic.
2. The inner area, or *inner gland,* is more hypoechoic in appearance.

Composition of the Inner and Outer Glands

Inner Gland

- Anterior fibromuscular stroma
- Preprostatic sphincter

- PUGs
- Longitudinal smooth muscle
- Postprostatic sphincter

Outer Gland

- Transition zone
- Central zone
- Peripheral zone

BASIC ULTRASOUND PHYSICS

Ultrasound imaging is based on the pulse echo principle, whereby a short burst of ultrasound is emitted from a transducer and directed into the tissue. Echoes are produced as a result of the interaction of sound with tissue, and some of these echoes travel back to the transducer. By timing the period elapsed between the emission of the pulse and the reception of the echo, the distance between the transducer and the echo-producing structure can be calculated and an image produced (see Chapter 214, Emergency Department, Hospitalist, and Office Ultrasound [POCUS]).

Sound consists of longitudinal vibrations that propagate through a medium such as water or soft tissue. It consists of the repetitive (or periodic) production of such compressions, which travel in regular succession. The number of compressions produced each second is the *frequency* (measured in hertz [Hz]), and the distance between successive compressions, which depends on the speed at which the sound travels in the medium, is the *wavelength* (measured in millimeters). Tissues that are very elastic, dense, or compressible tend to transmit sound waves through them (fluid). Inelastic, less dense, or noncompressible tissues (bone or stones) tend to reflect the sound waves.

Gain adjustment refers to the amount of amplification applied to a returning echo signal. *Contrast and brightness* adjustments can also be made to provide a homogeneous midrange echo pattern of the normal PZ.

Sound Frequency

The characteristics of sound transmission are as follows:

- The lower the frequency, the longer the wavelength.
- The higher the frequency, the shorter the wavelength.
- The lower the frequency of sound, the greater the ability to penetrate tissue, but the poorer the quality (resolution) of the ultrasonographic picture obtained.
- The higher the sound frequency, the poorer the tissue penetration by sound, but the better the quality (resolution) of the picture.

The ideal frequency for imaging the prostate is about 7 MHz. Although a 10-MHz probe provides better resolution of smaller objects, it has a more limited field or depth of view—it shows only the part of the prostate closest to the rectum. A 3-MHz probe, with its lower frequency, delivers higher penetration, but the image quality and resolution usually suffer (Fig. 106.4).

INDICATIONS

TRUSP-SV

- Suspicion of prostatic abscess
- Azoospermia
- Brachytherapy
- Prostatitis
  - Acute
  - Chronic
  - Prostatitis with an elevated prostate-specific antigen (PSA)
- Chronic pelvic pain syndrome
- Prostate volume study
- Detection of posttreatment prostate cancer recurrence
- Prostatic intraepithelial neoplasia on prior biopsy

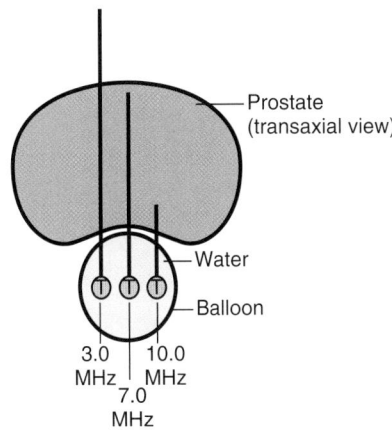

Fig. 106.4 Ideal frequency for imaging the prostate is about 7 MHz. (From Cooner WH. Physical principles of prostate ultrasonography. *Monogr Urol.* 1990;11:18.)

- Prostate cancer staging
- Adenosis on prior biopsy

NOTE: In the patient with cancer, when attempting to determine the extent of local disease, TRUSP-SV is generally restricted to determining whether the tumor has invaded the SVs.

TRUSP-SV and Prostate Biopsy

- Evaluation of a palpable prostatic nodule or induration
- Abnormal PSA (Fig. 106.1 shows an algorithm combining PSA, free PSA, PSA velocity, and TRUSP-SV.)
  - Elevated PSA
  - Low free PSA (<25%) in individual with PSA in the range of 4 to 10 ng/mL
  - Elevated PSA velocity (doubling in <6 months or >0.75 ng/mL rise in PSA per year; optimally these have been done by same laboratory)
  - Elevated PSA density (>0.1 to 0.15 ng/mL)
- Detection of posttreatment prostate cancer recurrence
- Prostatic intraepithelial neoplasia on prior biopsy

CONTRAINDICATIONS

TRUSP-SV and Prostate Biopsy

- Bleeding disorders
- Anticoagulant therapy
- Significant rectal disease
  - Obstructing lesions
  - Fissures
  - Thrombosed hemorrhoids
  - Proctitis
- Untreated bacterial urinary tract infection
  - Cystitis
  - Prostatitis
- Operator not familiar with the procedure, the anatomy, or the interpretation of TRUSP-SV
- Patient life expectancy less than 10 years, or age 75 years or greater (relative contraindications)

NOTE: If a hypoechoic area is seen on transrectal ultrasound (TRUSP-SV), it probably should be sampled for biopsy, regardless of PSA. Therefore, some experts warn against performing TRUSP unless a biopsy is indicated; it should probably not be used for screening. The primary role of ultrasound is to ensure accurate sampling of any lesions and of the entire gland during biopsy.

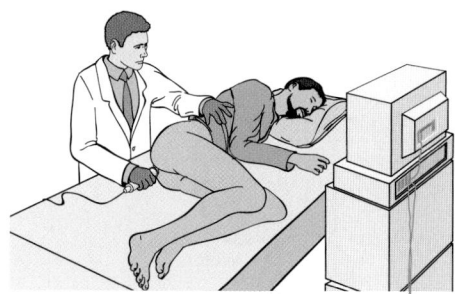

Fig. 106.5 Positioning of patient.

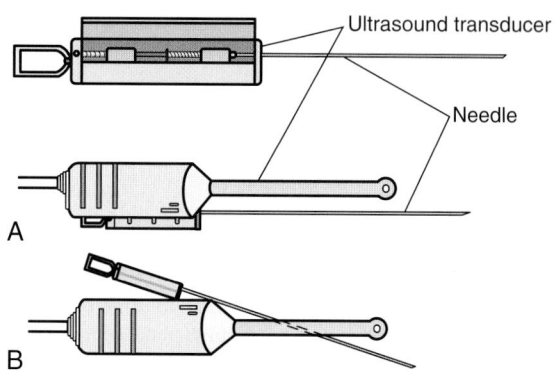

Fig. 106.6 Biopsy instrument can be introduced through an internal (A) or an external (B) needle guide or puncture guide. (Modified from Brackman J, Denis LJ. Prostate ultrasound and needle biopsy. In: Graham SD Jr, ed. *Glenn's Urologic Surgery*. 5th ed. Philadelphia: Lippincott-Raven: 1998.)

PREPROCEDURE PATIENT PREPARATION

1. Serum PSA on record
2. Documented DRE
3. Informed consent signed and copy on chart
4. Fleet enema 1 to 2 hours before the procedure
5. Fluoroquinolone therapy
   - The authors prefer a 3-day regimen using a quinolone the day before, the day of, and if a biopsy is performed, the day after for all patients, with or without risk factors.
   - For patients undergoing repeat TRUSP-SV and biopsy (for persistent abnormalities in PSA despite negative biopsies and normal DRE), use a 5-day protocol of quinolone therapy, extending the quinolone for 3 days after the biopsy. Also, add metronidazole 500 mg twice a day by mouth for 3 days after the biopsy.
   - The American Urological Association guidelines (2014) added first-, second-, and third-generation cephalosporins, trimethoprim-sulfamethoxazole, an aminoglycoside, or aztreonam as alternatives to fluoroquinolones. An intramuscular route is acceptable for all of these agents; only the fluoroquinolones are recommended orally. When an aminoglycoside or aztreonam is used, neither metronidazole nor clindamycin are necessary. For patients at risk of endocarditis or an infected prosthetic joint, pacemaker, implantable defibrillator, prophylaxis should consist of intravenous ampicillin and gentamicin preoperatively followed by 3 days of a fluoroquinolone (see also Chapter 69, Antibiotic Prophylaxis). A Cochrane (2011) meta-analysis of nine trials found that prophylactic antibiotics prior to prostate biopsy significantly reduced the risk for bacteriuria, bacteremia, fever, urinary tract infection, and the need for hospitalization. However, they concluded there is no definitive data to confirm that antibiotics for long-course treatments (3 days) are superior to short-course treatments (1 day), or that multiple-dose treatment is superior to single-dose.
6. Patient vital signs before procedure
7. Patient positioning options
   - Knee-chest
   - Lithotomy
   - Left lateral decubitus with knees flexed 90 degrees (Fig. 106.5)

Indications, alternatives, risks, potential benefits, and expected results should be discussed with the patient and signed informed consent obtained. The patient should expect some discomfort with either TRUSP-SV or biopsy. He should also expect some discomfort with injection of the local anesthetic and the prostate biopsy. Let the patient know he will be warned before a biopsy. It will also be important for him to remain very still during certain portions of the procedure.

EQUIPMENT

An available assistant is useful to help with the equipment, especially if a biopsy is to be performed.

TRUSP-SV

- Transducer sheath or condom (should be sterile if biopsy is to be performed)
- Nonsterile gloves (also sterile gloves if biopsy is to be performed)
- Ultrasonic gel
- Eye protection, gown (sterile gown if biopsy is to be performed), and equipment necessary to maintain universal blood and body fluid precautions

Types of Prostate Ultrasound

- Transabdominal
- Transperineal
- Endourethral
- Transrectal (with and without color flow Doppler enhancement)

Transperineal ultrasound may be preferred in diabetic males who are at high risk for sepsis because it can be done aseptically. It may be required in an individual without a rectum. An increased rate of urinary retention is noted in the transperineal approach. The transperineal approach to biopsy is more painful.

Types of Transducer Design

Original ultrasound technology:
- Radial array (with cephalocaudad or right-to-left oscillation)
- Linear array (piezoelectric crystals are placed in a line, and each crystal fires and receives echoes in sequential order)

More recent developments in ultrasound technology:
- Biplanar probe transducers
- Single probe to image the gland in both the transverse and sagittal planes
- A single probe that can have one of the following:
  - Two perpendicularly positioned transducers
  - A single transducer that can rotate
  - An end-fire transducer that can provide either a transverse or sagittal view by merely rotating the probe 90 degrees

Prostate Biopsy

- Biopsy instrument, usually spring-loaded, and needle guide (Fig. 106.6)
- Sterile tray and sterile drapes for patient
- Bottles containing specimen preservative (formaldehyde)
- Lidocaine 1%, 22-gauge, 15- to 20-cm spinal needle, and 10-mL syringe (optional)

TECHNIQUE

TRUSP-SV

General Principles

The performance of prostate ultrasound requires the examiner to know which aspects of the procedure are operator-dependent so that the best possible study can be obtained. No mandatory technical standards exist for performance of prostatic ultrasound. The examination sequence remains a matter of personal preference. Practitioners should develop a technique that is thorough and reproducible, and with which they are comfortable.

Prostate ultrasound and examination should be carried out in at least two planes:

1. Transaxial–transverse (across the long axis; Fig. 106.7). Images from this orientation offer several advantages in the assessment of the prostate:
   * Increased information about the lateral margins
   * Assessment of capsular integrity
   * Accurate volume assessment
2. Longitudinal-sagittal (parallel to the body axis or long axis). Images from this orientation provide more information about the apex and base of the prostate and facilitate biopsy.

Procedure

1. Observing universal blood and body fluid precautions, perform a DRE before insertion of the probe. This procedure serves many purposes:
   * Dilates the anal sphincter, reducing discomfort from probe insertion.
   * Assesses the gland for size, shape, and areas of irregularity or suspicion. This enables the sonographer to associate palpable lesions with what is being viewed during the study.
   * Rules out a rectal obstructive process of either benign or malignant etiology.
2. Position the patient. Various positions will work, but the left lateral decubitus position is often more comfortable for the patient and may reduce bowel gas interference (see Fig. 106.5).
3. Prepare the probe. A small amount of ultrasonic gel is placed either in the tip of the probe sheath or on the tip of the probe. The cover or sheath is then inserted over the probe. Any air bubbles over the tip of the probe should be smoothed away.
4. Have the patient perform a slight Valsalva maneuver during probe insertion to relax the sphincter and further facilitate probe insertion.
5. After insertion, while scanning in the transaxial mode, advance the probe to the level of the SVs. Making parallel images (cuts), scan from superior to inferior (Fig. 106.7). Examination of the SVs should focus on the following:
   * Symmetry
   * Size
   * Echo pattern
   * Any masses
   * Cystic changes
   Because the SVs do not always lie symmetrically in the body, it is occasionally difficult to comment on their symmetry on a cut-by-cut basis. Often they must be studied and their images interpreted as they appear in their entirety. If prostate cancer is present, it is important to determine whether there has been local invasion to the SVs (see the Interpretation section).
6. From the SVs, the probe is withdrawn to the level of the base of the prostate, and all areas from the base to the apex should be scanned. Evaluate the prostate for symmetry, its lateral margins, and the integrity of the capsule. Assess the inner and outer gland for irregularities. The periprostatic "environment" is also assessed at this time. Normal PZ echogenicity represents the *baseline* or is

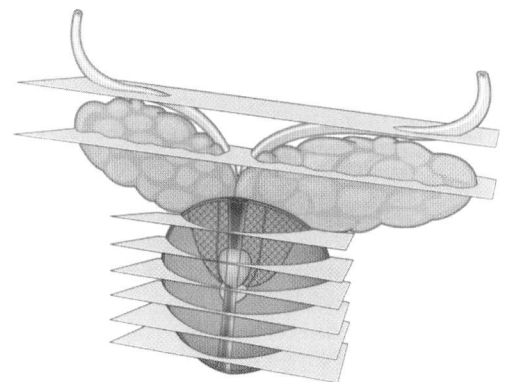

Fig. 106.7 Ultrasonographic transaxial examination of the seminal vesicles and prostate using parallel images from superior to inferior. (From Rifkin MD. *Ultrasound of the Prostate: Imaging in the Diagnosis and Therapy of Prostatic Disease.* 2nd ed. Philadelphia: Lippincott-Raven; 1997.)

isoechoic. Any lesion that is less echogenic is labeled *hypoechoic;* anything giving rise to more echoes is *hyperechoic.*

7. The probe should then be rotated (or a perpendicular plane in the probe activated) to scan the prostate longitudinally. The clinician should be thorough and evaluate the entire prostate and surrounding tissue in each longitudinal plane. Particular emphasis should be placed on scanning and evaluating the apex and base of the prostate.
8. Volume determination should be performed. Various software applications or technical features of individual ultrasound machines enable the examiner to estimate prostate volume. An option is a formula for calculating estimated prostate volume: prostate volume (mL) = (π/6) × (anterior-posterior diameter [cm]) × (transverse diameter [cm]) × (sagittal diameter [cm]). Regardless of technique used, the error in measuring prostate volume may approach 25%.

Prostate Biopsy

1. With eye protection in place, the clinician is gowned in a sterile manner and the patient draped likewise. Universal blood and body fluid precautions should continue to be followed. A small amount of ultrasonic gel should be placed either on the tip of the probe sheath or on the tip of the probe. The needle guide and transducer are then covered with the sterile sheath. The sterile sheath often has an extension that can be unrolled over the transducer cord. Any air bubbles located over the probe tip should be smoothed away.
2. After having the patient perform a slight Valsalva maneuver, the probe is inserted in the same manner as for TRUSP-SV.
3. *Prostate anesthetic block:* It is our opinion that providing a local anesthetic block with 1% lidocaine before prostate biopsy is beneficial. It not only may reduce anxiety and discomfort, but it may enhance patient compliance (especially if a repeat biopsy is ever necessary). After the probe is in the rectum, a 22-gauge, 15- to 20-cm spinal needle is introduced through the needle guide on the probe. The needle is then advanced into the Denonvilliers fascia and the area adjacent to the apex in the longitudinal plane. Lidocaine is injected between the gland and the rectum. The authors usually inject 4 mL of local anesthetic in the apical region and then switch to the horizontal plane to inject the remaining 3 mL into the right and left neurovascular bundles. After waiting 5 to 10 minutes for the anesthetic to take effect, one can proceed with the biopsy. At this point, some clinicians also use moderate (conscious) sedation (see Chapter 1, Procedural Sedation and Analgesia).
4. The biopsy instrument, usually a spring-loaded biopsy gun, is then inserted until the tip of the instrument can be seen at the

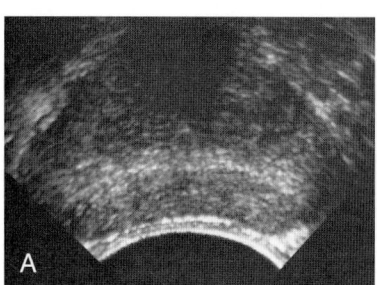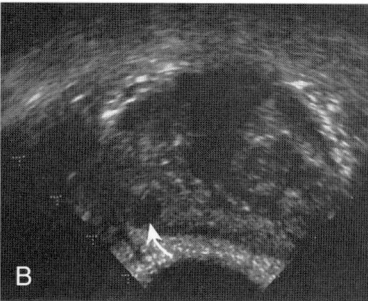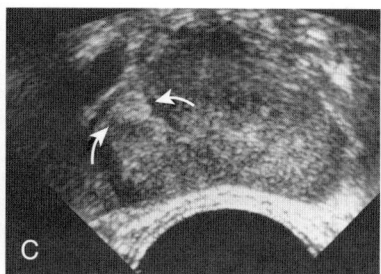

Fig. 106.8   Echogenic patterns of the prostate. (A) Isoechoic patterns. The images are typically produced by the glandular areas of the prostate and appear as low-level gray. The images are in a midrange and a medium percentage of sound waves are reflected back to the transducer. (B) Hypoechoic patterns *(arrow)* are seen typically in the fibrous and muscular structures of the prostate, and with cancers of the prostate. With hypoechoic patterns, fewer echoes are reflected back and more actually pass through the tissues, making them appear darker. (C) Hyperechoic patterns *(arrows)* result when more sound waves are reflected back to the transducer, producing images that are light gray to white. The periprostatic fat is hyperechoic, as are some cancers. (From Rifkin MD. *Ultrasound of the Prostate: Imaging in the Diagnosis and Therapy of Prostatic Disease.* 2nd ed. Philadelphia: Lippincott-Raven; 1997.)

edge of the prostate. For an *outer gland lesion*, the tip of the instrument is placed just in front of the lesion, at the edge of the mass and before the prostatic capsule is penetrated. For an *inner gland lesion*, the tip of the instrument must first penetrate the capsule and outer gland before it is placed just in front of the lesion, at the edge of the mass.

5. If the patient is awake, to avoid any surprises, he should be warned just before the instrument is fired. The instrument is then fired. Any additional suspect areas on TRUSP-SV should likewise be sampled.

6. Additional random passes are then made, obtaining biopsies in the superior, central, and inferior portions of the prostate. Emphasis should be placed on obtaining tissue from the PZ. The specific number of biopsies varies by clinician, but the current literature recommends 12 to 18 passes (6 to 9 on each side). Various systems are used to label the biopsies, with "1" or "A" commonly used to label the right superior gland, "2" or "B" for right middle, "3" or "C" for right inferior (apex), "4" or "D" for left superior, "5" or "E" for left middle, and "6" or "F" for left inferior. When in doubt about which system to use, the clinician can merely be descriptive with the labeling (e.g., "right superior").

INTERPRETATION AND EVALUATION OF THE PROSTATE

Interpretation

From the prostate, three types of echogenic patterns are described: isoechoic (Fig. 106.8A), hypoechoic (see Fig. 106.8B), and hyperechoic (see Fig. 106.8C). Unfortunately, no single finding on ultrasound provides universal distinction between malignant and benign conditions. That said, most cancers are hypoechoic. Cancers less than 5 to 7 mm, those that are well differentiated, and those located in the TZ are difficult to distinguish from a normal prostate.

Evaluation

- General appearance
- Inner gland status
- Outer gland status
- Anterior prostate status
- Any focal intraprostatic abnormalities
- Status of the internal architecture
  - Normal
  - Disrupted
- Integrity of capsule
- Urethral position

- Focal lesion(s)
  - Number
  - Location
  - Echogenic pattern: hypoechoic, isoechoic, hyperechoic, mixed, anechoic
  - Margin of the focus: well defined, poorly defined
  - Calculi
  - Cysts
- Ejaculatory duct status
  - Normal
  - Dilated
  - Infiltrated
- Neurovascular bundles present?
- Lymph nodes visible?
- Seminal vesicles
  - Overall, symmetric, or asymmetric
  - Size
  - Shape
  - Echo pattern
  - Cystic changes
  - Solid mass effect
- Rectal wall integrity

Normal Ultrasound Appearance of the Prostate Gland

- The PZ is isoechoic and the transitional zone hypoechoic.
- The appearances change with enlargement—the PZ becomes thinner.
- The gland shape depends on the type of TRUSP-SV probe used.
- The CZ is not identifiable as a separate area.
- The prostatic capsule, although seen, is not a true capsule.
- Flow on color Doppler is symmetric.

Abnormal Ultrasound Appearance of the Prostate Gland

Most prostate cancers appear as a hypoechoic lesion in the PZ.

Hints for Staging

- Findings consistent with extracapsular extension of prostate cancer include bulging of the prostate contour and an angulated appearance of the lateral margin.
- Findings consistent with SV invasion include a posterior bulge of the prostate contour at the base of the SV and asymmetry of echogenicity in the SVs associated with hypoechoic areas at the base of the prostate.

COMPLICATIONS

TRUSP-SV and Prostate Biopsy

- Rectal bleeding from the following:
  - Hemorrhoidal vessels
  - Rectal wall laceration
  - Arteriovenous malformation
- Hematuria
- Hematospermia
- Urinary retention
- Urosepsis
- Bacteremia
- Vasovagal response with or without seizure

Prostate Biopsy (Rare)

- Perirectal or pelvic hematoma or hemorrhage
- Needle tract seeding of cancer

POSTPROCEDURE PATIENT EDUCATION

Postprocedure vital signs should be performed and fluids offered or provided (e.g., sports drink, fruit juice). The TRUSP-SV findings and any instructions should be reviewed with the patient. A follow-up appointment should be made. If biopsies were performed, the results will be discussed with the patient at the follow-up appointment. Patients should be aware that even with a negative biopsy, they may have microscopic cancer in a small area of the prostate. If the biopsy was for an abnormal PSA and it remains abnormal, a repeat biopsy may be necessary at a later date. After TRUSP-SV or biopsy, the patient should call the facility for difficulty urinating, rectal bleeding, high fever, or further questions.

PATIENT EDUCATION GUIDES

See the sample patient education and consent forms available at www.expertconsult.com.

CPT/BILLING CODES

55700	Prostate biopsy; needle or punch, single or multiple, any approach
76872	Ultrasound, transrectal
76942	Ultrasonic guidance for needle placement (e.g., biopsy, aspiration, injection, localization device), imaging supervision and interpretation

ICD-10-CM DIAGNOSTIC CODES

C61	Malignant neoplasm of prostate
C63.7	Malignant neoplasm of seminal vesicles
N40.0	Hypertrophy (benign) of prostate without urinary obstruction
N40.1*	Hypertrophy (benign) of prostate with urinary obstruction
N40.2	Nodular prostate without urinary obstruction
N40.3*	Nodular prostate with urinary obstruction
N40.0	Benign localized hyperplasia of prostate without urinary obstruction
N40.1	Benign localized hyperplasia of prostate with urinary obstruction
N41.0*	Prostatitis, acute
N41.1*	Prostatitis, chronic
N42.0	Calculus of prostate
N42.30	Dysplasia of prostate unspecified
R36.1	Hematospermia

*Use additional code.

Acknowledgment

The editors recognize the contributions of Robert S. Tan, MD, to this chapter in a previous edition of this text.

SUPPLIERS

(See contact information available at www.expertconsult.com.)

Transrectal ultrasound units with needle guides
Available from most ultrasound equipment manufacturers (see Chapter 142, Obstetric Ultrasound, and Chapter 171, Musculoskeletal Ultrasound, for lists of manufacturers).
Bard biopsy cut instruments and needle
Bard Peripheral Technologies
Overreading services
Nighthawk Radiology Services (www.nighthawkradiology.com)

NOTE: These services require T1 internet access; DSL is not compliant with the Health Insurance Portability and Accountability Act [HIPAA]).

Probes and scans
See Figs. 106.9 to 106.14.

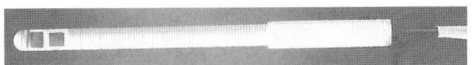

Fig. 106.9 Biplane probe. (From Rifkin MD. *Ultrasound of the Prostate: Imaging in the Diagnosis and Therapy of Prostatic Disease.* 2nd ed. Philadelphia: Lippincott-Raven; 1997.)

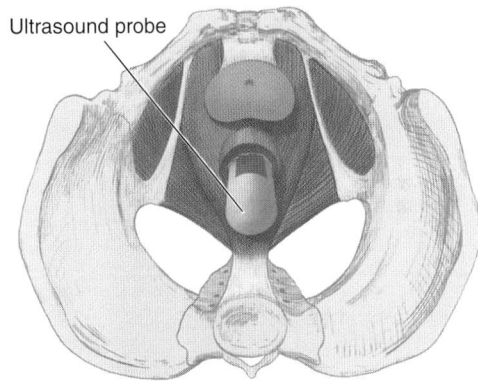

Ultrasound probe

Fig. 106.10 Endorectal scan. Note probe is located very near and posterior to prostate. (From Rifkin MD. *Ultrasound of the Prostate: Imaging in the Diagnosis and Therapy of Prostatic Disease.* 2nd ed. Philadelphia: Lippincott-Raven; 1997.)

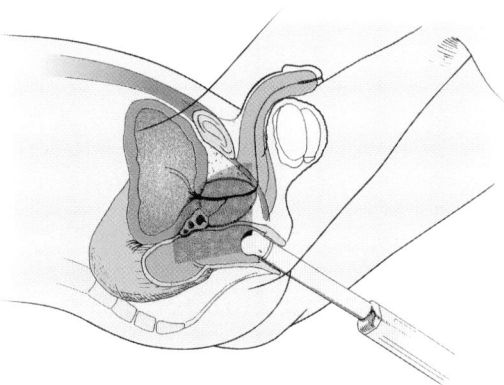

Fig. 106.11 End-fire endorectal probe scanning longitudinally. (Modified from Rifkin MD. *Ultrasound of the Prostate: Imaging in the Diagnosis and Therapy of Prostatic Disease.* 2nd ed. Philadelphia: Lippincott-Raven; 1997.)

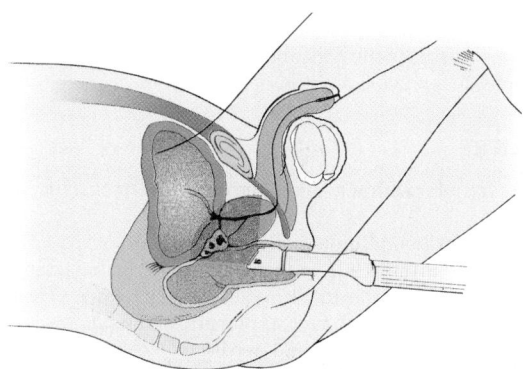

Fig. 106.12 **Oblique end-fire probe scanning longitudinally.** (From Rifkin MD. *Ultrasound of the Prostate: Imaging in the Diagnosis and Therapy of Prostatic Disease.* 2nd ed. Philadelphia: Lippincott-Raven; 1997.)

Fig. 106.13 **Side-fire probe.** (From Rifkin MD. *Ultrasound of the Prostate: Imaging in the Diagnosis and Therapy of Prostatic Disease.* 2nd ed. Philadelphia: Lippincott-Raven; 1997.)

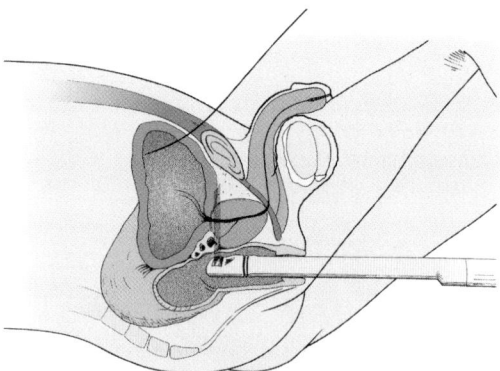

Fig. 106.14 **Side-fire probe scanning transaxially.** (From Rifkin MD. *Ultrasound of the Prostate: Imaging in the Diagnosis and Therapy of Prostatic Disease.* 2nd ed. Philadelphia: Lippincott-Raven; 1997.)

RECOMMENDED READING

Bieker T, Ledwidge ME. Prostate: prostate carcinoma, benign prostatic hypertrophy. In: Sanders RC, Hall-Terracciano B, eds. *Clinical Sonography: A Practical Guide.* 5th ed. Philadelphia: Wolters Klower; 2016:747–756.

Brawer MK. Techniques of examination in prostatic ultrasonography. In: Resnick MI, ed. *Prostatic Ultrasonography.* Philadelphia: BC Decker; 1990.

Brooks JD. Anatomy of the lower urinary tract and male genitalia. In: Walsh PC, Retik AB, Vaughan Jr ED, Wein AJ, eds. *Campbell's Urology.* 7th ed. Philadelphia: WB Saunders; 1998:112–117.

Cooner WH. Physical principles of prostate ultrasonography. *Monogr Urol.* 1990;11:18.

Gomella LG, Halpern EJ, Trabulsi EJ. Prostate biopsy: techniques and imaging. In: Wein AJ, Kavoussi LR, Partin AW, Peters CA, eds. *Campbell-Walsh Urology.* 11th ed. Philadelphia: Elsevier; 2016.

Kaye KW. Ultrasound of the normal prostate. *Contemp Urol.* 1991;3:64–75.

McNeal JE. The prostate gland: morphology and pathology. *Monogr Urol.* 1988;9:36.

Muldoon LD, Resnick MI. Normal anatomy of the prostate. In: Resnick MI, ed. *Prostatic Ultrasonography.* Philadelphia: BC Decker; 1990.

Patel U, Rickards D. *Transrectal Ultrasound & Biopsy of the Prostate.* London: Martin Duntz; 2002.

Presti Jr KC, Kane CJ, Shinohara K, Carroll PR. Neoplasms of the prostate gland. In: Tanagho EA, McAninch JW, eds. *Smith's General Urology.* 17th ed. New York: McGraw-Hill; 2008:367–385.

Rifkin MD. *Ultrasound of the Prostate: Imaging in the Diagnosis and Therapy of Prostatic Disease.* 2nd ed. Philadelphia: Lippincott-Raven; 1997 (This book is a must-read for the individual who is serious about prostate ultrasonography.).

Zani EL, Clark OAugusto Camara, Rodrigues Netto Jr N. Antibiotic prophylaxis for transrectal prostate biopsy. *Cochrane Database of Systematic Reviews.* 2011;(2):CD006576.

CHAPTER 107

SELF-INJECTION THERAPY FOR THE TREATMENT OF ERECTILE DYSFUNCTION

Robert E. James • James R. Palleschi

Significant advances have been made over recent decades in the diagnosis and treatment of erectile dysfunction. Although the introduction of oral drugs has decreased the need for and use of injection therapy, it is still indicated in some patients. The self-injection of vasoactive agents into the corpora cavernosa enables many patients to resume satisfactory sexual activities without surgery.

Oral medications (avanfil, sildenafil, tadalafil, and vardenafil) are most effective in patients with mild to moderate impotence. This category would include men who are able to obtain a good erection but cannot maintain it and those who have an erection that is at least a 5 out of 10 in rigidity, where "10" is defined as the best erection they can remember.

The *transurethral form of alprostadil* (MUSE, Meda Pharmaceuticals) has about a 50% response rate (it is effective in about 50% of males) and is most effective in men who have difficulty maintaining an erection and in those who have a partial erection, or 5 out of 10 in rigidity.

Despite advances in the treatment of erectile dysfunction, *vacuum erection devices* remain an option or adjunct. These devices are attractive to patients who have failed oral therapy and decline or fail intraurethral or intracavernosal alprostadil. Patients using intracavernosal therapy who want to have intercourse more than three times a week usually meet their goal by using vacuum erection devices (see Chapter 108, Vacuum Devices for Erectile Dysfunction).

In the treatment of moderate to severe erectile dysfunction, intracavernosal therapy with vasoactive agents still has a very important role. Efficacy for this treatment option is reported as high as 87% to 93%.

It has been two decades since the US Food and Drug Administration (FDA) approved *injectable alprostadil (prostaglandin E$_1$ [PGE$_1$])* for the treatment of organic erectile dysfunction. The American Urological Association's guidelines for the treatment of erectile dysfunction recommend alprostadil as the drug of choice, and it is the only intracavernosal vasoactive agent approved by the FDA. (Use of an FDA-approved injection may make it more likely to be covered or reimbursed by insurance.)

There is also *papaverine hydrochloride*, a nonspecific smooth muscle relaxant. In addition to alprostadil, which is a vasodilator and a smooth muscle relaxant, papaverine hydrochloride may be used with *phentolamine mesylate*, a smooth muscle relaxant that enhances the effect of papaverine. These agents have been used extensively for impotence for many years, although this remains an unlabeled indication.

These vasoactive agents induce an erection by increasing arterial blood flow, relaxing the sinusoidal spaces within the cavernosal tissue, and increasing venous resistance. An excellent erection that lasts for 30 to 90 minutes usually occurs in patients with mild to moderate arterial insufficiency, mild to moderate venous incompetence, psychogenic impotence, neurogenic impotence, and medication-induced impotence.

INDICATIONS

- Impotence resulting from arterial insufficiency
- Impotence resulting from mild to moderate venous incompetence
- Psychogenic impotence (Patients with performance anxiety may be treated with counseling, oral agents, short-term intracavernosal agents, or a combination of these methods.)
- Neurogenic impotence
- Medication-induced impotence, when drug therapy cannot be altered or terminated
- Diagnostic erection
- Intolerance to or ineffective oral drugs

CONTRAINDICATIONS

- Blood dyscrasia, coagulation disorder, or anticoagulation drug therapy
- Unstable cardiovascular disease or hypotension
- Impaired manual dexterity or vision
- Presence of a prosthetic penile device
- Intolerance to the test dose of the vasoactive agent
- Patients taking monoamine oxidase inhibitors
- Patients with a propensity toward secondary forms of priapism, such as individuals with sickle cell disease or trait, leukemia, or multiple myeloma
- Prior history of priapism *(relative, depends on suspected cause)*

NOTE: If a clinician elects to prescribe intracavernosal pharmacotherapy to treat erectile dysfunction in men with Peyronie disease, a special informed consent is advised.

EQUIPMENT

- 1- to 3-mL syringes with ½-inch, 27- and 30-gauge needles
- Alcohol swabs
- Vasoactive agents
  - *Papaverine HCl* 30 mg/mL is available in 10-mL multidose vials.
  - *Papaverine and phentolamine* solution: Inject 5 mg (or 10 mg) of phentolamine (Regitine; Novartis) into a 10-mL vial of papaverine 30 mg/mL. The (approximate) concentrations will be papaverine 30 mg/mL and phentolamine 0.5 or 1.0 mg/mL.
  - *PGE$_1$ (alprostadil)*: Two proprietary forms of injectable alprostadil for the treatment of erectile dysfunction are available

in the United States: Caverject (Pfizer) and Edex (Actient). The clinical dose range varies from 2 to 40 µg per injection. Each manufacturer has provided alprostadil in a ready-to-use, easily assembled syringe that does not require refrigeration. The syringes are meant for single use only. Generic alprostadil is also now available.

- PGE_1 *(alprostadil)* is also available in 1-mL ampules from Pfizer as Prostin VR Pediatric 500 µg/mL. For the desired concentration, inject 0.2 mL of this preparation into each of five 10-mL vials of bacteriostatic normal saline for injection. Each vial will contain PGE_1 10 µg/mL.
- *Bimix* (alprostadil 20 µg/mL plus phentolamine 0.5 mg/mL) and *trimix* (alprostadil 10 µg/mL plus papaverine 30 mg/mL plus phentolamine 1 mg/mL) are available.

When Bennett and coworkers first developed *a trimix combination therapy* for the treatment of erectile dysfunction (1991). Their three-drug mixture contained 2.5 mL of papaverine (30 mg/mL), 0.5 mL of phentolamine (5 mg/mL), and 0.05 mL of alprostadil (500 µg/mL). They found patients require less than 0.25 mL per injection. A *quadmix combination* has also been described containing papaverine, phentolamine, alprostadil, and atropine. Use of alprostadil alone seems to have fewer systemic side effects and to cause less fibrosis than seen with the other medications as well as a lower incidence of priapism. If the alprostadil alone is ineffective or becomes ineffective over time, it is usually worthwhile to try a mix. Proposed additional benefits of using a mix include not only less cost but also less pain; pain is the most common side effect when alprostadil is used alone. Use of a mix allows for a reduction in dose of alprostadil. When the mixes are compounded, cost per dose is about one-third the cost of brand-name alprostadil. Compounded generic alprostadil alone should cost even less.

Open vials or compounded solutions should be refrigerated to maintain sterility and effectiveness. A 30-day expiration date is recommended; however, sufficient effectiveness has been reported for up to 3 months.

Alpha-adrenergic agents will cause vasoconstriction and thus will usually result in prompt detumescence should priapism occur. Some of the available agents include *ephedrine sulfate, epinephrine,* and *phenylephrine hydrochloride* (Neo-Synephrine). (See the section titled "Treatment of the Persistent Erection [Priapism]" for dilutions and use.)

PREPROCEDURE PATIENT PREPARATION

Discuss the self-injection program, alternatives, and potential complications with the patient and, when possible, his partner. The patient's partner may have to be taught how to perform injections if the patient is unable. Patients using this program may experience *bruising* at the injection site and local or systemic infection (<0.05% incidence). *Chronic fibrosis* at the injection site may occur with repeated injections, which may result in *pain or penile curvature*. Papaverine may elevate the results of *liver function tests*. Consequently patients should obtain pretreatment liver function tests and should be retested every 3 months while using papaverine. If the liver function test values begin to rise, the medication should be discontinued. If the initial liver function test results are elevated, use PGE_1 instead of papaverine. Approximately 20% of patients using PGE_1 may experience an *ache or pain in the penis* that may last for several hours and that may recur with each injection. This seems to be more common in the postprostatectomy patient, especially during the first 2 years following surgery. *Priapism,* an erection lasting longer than 4 hours, may occur in up to 10% of patients receiving any of the vasoactive agents, but it reportedly occurs less frequently with PGE_1. Systemic side effects, such as dizziness and orthostatic hypotension, occur in 2% of patients receiving these vasoactive agents and are believed to be secondary to penile venous incompetence.

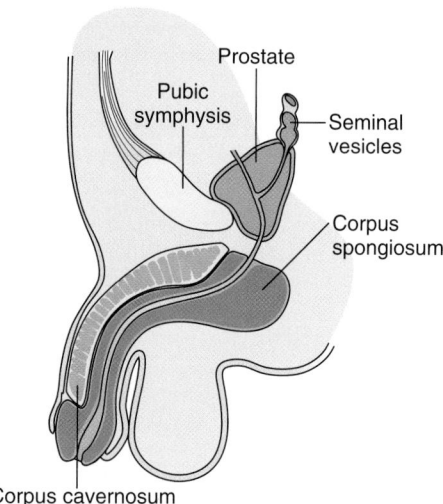

Fig. 107.1   Side view of penis and scrotum.

Instruct the patient to contact the clinician if he experiences a significant erection that persists for more than 3 hours. This condition will have to be treated promptly to prevent intracorporeal fibrosis and failure to respond to future therapy.

TECHNIQUE

1. Complete the patient's history and physical examination to provide a preliminary diagnosis.
2. Select the agent and the dose. If psychogenic or neurogenic impotence is suspected, use a smaller dose of the vasoactive agent. In patients with psychogenic impotence, one-fourth of the maximal dose should be used; in patients with neurogenic impotence, no more than one-sixth of the maximal dose should be used initially. The maximal dose of *papaverine* is 60 mg and that of PGE_1 is 20 µg. To reduce the risk of priapism and prevent other untoward reactions, even when vascular disease is suspected as the cause of impotence, the initial dose should not exceed 30 mg of papaverine or 10 µg of PGE_1. If a satisfactory erection does not occur, the dose may be appropriately increased at the time of the next office appointment. Although the usual dose of *alprostadil* is between 10 and 20 µg, urologists have used up to 40 µg in some cases. In patients with psychogenic or neurogenic impotence, you should begin with 2 to 5 µg and gradually increase the dose as needed. Otherwise the usual starting dose is 10 µg in men above 65 years of age. If the patient has had a prostatectomy in the preceding 2 years and/or is under 65 years of age, a starting dose of 5 µg may decrease the risk of associated pain. Some experts even start as low as 2.5 µg in patients below 55 years of age who have had a prostatectomy in the preceding year.
3. Once the desired dose of the vasoactive agent has been selected, extend the patient's penis and prepare the lateral surface with an alcohol swab. Locate the neurovascular bundle at the 12 o'clock position and the urethra at the 6 o'clock position (Figs. 107.1 and 107.2). Select as the injection site an area between these two structures (1 to 5 o'clock on the patient's left, 7 to 11 o'clock on the patient's right) in which there are no superficial veins. The injection site may be anywhere between the base of the penis and just proximal to the glans penis. It is strongly recommended that only Caverject or Edex be used. With the patient supine, gently direct the penis to the left or the right to expose its lateral surface. Introduce a 27- or 30-gauge needle perpendicular to the skin and tunica albuginea and into the corpus cavernosum. Normally the needle is advanced 0.5 inch. Inject the vasoactive agent rapidly as a bolus into the corpus cavernosum. The medication

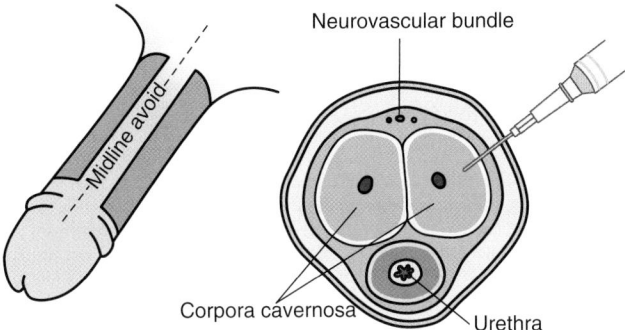

Fig. 107.2   Intracavernous injection site. The clinician grasps the glans and pulls firmly outward to tense penis without rotating it.

will enter the opposite corpus cavernosum through cross-circulation. If resistance is met as the medication is injected, withdraw the needle slowly as you continue to inject. The resistance normally occurs because the needle is against the opposite wall of the corpus cavernosum. To prevent injection of the medication into the subcutaneous space, *advance the needle the entire 0.5 inch and then withdraw it slowly.*

4. Once the injection has been completed, have the patient apply pressure to the injection site for 2 minutes.
5. Evaluate the condition of the patient periodically during the first 15 minutes after the injection. The patient's comfort, presence of side effects, and the quality of the erection should be evaluated at 15-minute intervals for 30 to 60 minutes. To evaluate the quality of the erection the patient will experience with sexual stimulation, you may ask the patient to apply manual stimulation. The patient may be discharged from the office within 30 to 60 minutes after the injection provided that he is comfortable and not experiencing any side effects. Instruct the patient to contact you if priapism occurs. Once the appropriate dose has been determined and the patient is skilled and comfortable with self-injection therapy, he may perform it independently but *no more than three times per week or more than once in 24 hours.* Priapism rarely occurs after the appropriate dose has been determined unless the patient independently increases the dose.

Treatment of the Persistent Erection (Priapism)

Patients should be instructed to come to the clinic (during working hours) or the emergency department for erections lasting more than 3 hours. Some clinics prescribe terbutaline 5 mg, one or two tabs orally, and wait approximate 45 minutes to see if the erection resolves. If this is unsuccessful and the patient does not have significant hypertension or unstable cardiac or cerebrovascular disease, an intracavernosal alpha-adrenergic agonist, which is safe and very effective in the treatment of priapism, may be used (see later section). Priapism is defined as an erection that lasts more than 4 hours. If the intracavernous α-adrenergic injection is unsuccessful, you should attempt to treat the priapism by aspirating blood from the corpus cavernosum followed by reinjecting/irrigating with saline. Inject the skin over the aspiration site (shaft of the penis) with 0.5 to 1 mL of local anesthetic (1% to 2% lidocaine) prior to aspiration and irrigation. If that is ineffective, the patient may benefit from a penile block with 1% to 2% lidocaine and intravenous morphine sulfate. Then aspirate/irrigate using aseptic technique with a 30-mL syringe and a 16- to 18-gauge needle. Insert the needle 0.5 inch into the midlateral corporal body aspirate 20 to 30 mL of corporal blood and irrigate with 10 to 30 mL of saline. Repeat the cycle; a visible change from venous blood (dark red) to arterial (bright red) indicates success. If the priapism does not resolve after aspirating/irrigating with 250 to 500 mL of saline, proceed

with injection of ephedrine, epinephrine, or phenylephrine, as discussed in the following section.

The following agents may be considered for the treatment of priapism:

- *Ephedrine sulfate:* A vial contains 50 mg (25 mg/mL). Initially inject 10 to 25 mg into the corpus cavernosum. If detumescence does not begin within 15 to 30 minutes, the dose may be repeated. A maximum of 50 mg may be given. Ephedrine is the drug of choice because of its efficacy, simplicity, and safety. If ineffective, consider aspiration/irrigation technique and a urology consult is advised.
- *Epinephrine:* Inject 1 mL of diluted epinephrine (10 to 20 μg/mL) slowly into the corpus cavernosum every 5 to 10 minutes. This may be repeated twice, and if satisfactory detumescence does not occur, consider aspiration/ irrigation technique and a urology consultation should be obtained. (To prepare the proper dilution, use epinephrine 1:10,000 solution. For 10 μg/mL, dilute 0.1 mL of epinephrine with 0.9 mL of normal saline. For 20 μg/mL, dilute 0.2 mL of epinephrine with 0.8 mL of normal saline. Some experts use as high as 100 μg/mL concentration.)
- *Phenylephrine hydrochloride (Neo-Synephrine) 1%:* Inject 1 mL slowly into the corpus cavernosum every 5 to 10 minutes. If satisfactory detumescence does not occur after the third dose, consider aspiration/ irrigation technique and obtain a urology consultation. (To prepare the proper dilution, use phenylephrine hydrochloride 0.1 mL diluted with 0.9 mL of normal saline for 100 μg/mL. Use phenylephrine hydrochloride 0.2 mL diluted with 0.8 mL of normal saline for 200 μg/mL. Some experts use as high as 500 μg/mL concentration.)
- *Lidocaine 2% with epinephrine (1: 100,000):* Inject 1 mL into each side or 2 mL into one side.)

These medications should be given individually and never in combination. Monitor the blood pressure and pulse closely in all patients if given the higher concentrations. Cardiac arrhythmias and significant hypertension may occur. However, there is literature supporting patients self-administering such injections (minimally invasive technique) for home treatment of recurrent priapism. If these measures are ineffective, at home or in the office, consider the aspiration/ irrigation technique and obtain a urology consultation. Surgical intervention may be required at this time.

COMPLICATIONS

- Priapism (an erection that lasts over 4 hours)
- Infection
- Subcutaneous ecchymosis or hematoma
- Fibrosis to the corpus cavernosum with repeated injections
- Curvature of the penis occurring after repeated injections
- Painful erections
- Dizziness or postural hypotension
- Myocardial infarction, stroke, or both in patients with unstable cardiac or cerebrovascular disease
- Elevated liver function test results (papaverine)

POSTPROCEDURE PATIENT EDUCATION

As many as 50% of men using self-injection therapy will discontinue this treatment within 1 year. There may be many reasons for this cessation, including lack of a suitable partner; fear of needles; inadequate response to therapy; fear of complications; lack of sexual spontaneity; and the desire for alternative therapy, including a permanent solution, such as a penile prosthesis. Consequently the patient should be seen periodically and should be asked about his sexual activity and satisfaction with self-injection therapy.

PATIENT EDUCATION GUIDES

See the sample patient education form available at www.expertcon
sult.com.

CPT/BILLING CODES

54235	Injection of corpus cavernosum
54250	Nocturnal tumescence and/or rigidity test

J-Codes

J0170	Epinephrine, adrenalin up to 1 mL
J0270	Alprostadil injection 1.25 μg
J0275	Alprostadil urethral suppository
J2370	Phenylephrine HCl up to 1 mL
J2440	Papaverine HCl up to 60 mg

ICD-10-CM DIAGNOSTIC CODES

F52.21	Impotence (sexual, psychogenic)
N52.9	Impotence, organic origin NEC

ONLINE RESOURCES

Caverject Impulse: www.caverject.com
Viagra: www.viagra.com
Sexual Medicine Society of North America: www.smsna.org

RECOMMENDED READING

Bennett AH, Carpenter AJ, Barada JH. An improved vasoactive drug combination for a pharmacological erection program. *J Urol.* 1991;146:1564–1565.

Burnett AL. Evaluation and management of erectile dysfunction. In: Wein AJ,
Kavoussi LR, Partin AW, Peters CA, eds. *Campbell-Walsh Urology.* 11th ed.
Philadelphia: Elsevier Saunders; 2016:643–668.

Davis JE, Silverman MA. Urologic procedures. In: Roberts JR, Custalow CB,
Thomsen TW, eds. *Roberts and Hedges Clinical Procedures in Emergency Medicine and Acute Care.* 7th ed. Philadelphia: Elsevier; 2019:1141–1185.

Floth A, Schramek P. Intracavernous injection of prostaglandin E$_1$ in combination with papaverine: enhanced effectiveness in comparison with papaverine plus phentolamine and prostaglandin E$_1$ alone. *J Urol.* 1991;145:56–59.

Fritsche HMA, Usta MF, Hellstrom WJG. Intracavernous, transurethral, and
topical therapies for erectile dysfunction in the era of oral pharmacotherapy.
In: Broderick GA, ed. *Oral Pharmacotherapy for Male Sexual Dysfunction:
A Guide to Clinical Management (Current Clinical Urology).* Totowa, NJ:
Humana Press; 2005:253–277.

Kulmala RV, Tamella TL. Effects of priapism lasting 24 hours or longer
caused by intracavernosal injection of vasoactive drugs. *Int J Impot Res.*
1995;7:131–136.

Lee M, Cannon B, Sharifi R. Chart for preparation of dilutions of alpha-
adrenergic agonists for intracavernous use in treatment of priapism. *J Urol.*
1995;153:1182–1183.

Lue TF. Priapism after transurethral alprostadil. *J Urol.* 1999;161:725–726.

Lui SM-C, Lin JS-N. Treatment of impotence: comparison between the
efficacy and safety of intracavernous injection of papaverine plus
phentolamine (Regitine) and prostaglandin E$_1$. *Int J Impot Res.* 1990;
2(suppl):147–151.

Montague DK, Jarow JP, Broderick GA, Dmochowski RR, Heaton JPW,
Lue TF, et al. *The Management of Erectile Dysfunction (2005) (Reviewed
and Validity Confirmed, 2011.* American Urologic Association; 2011.

Roberts JR, Price C, Mazzeo T. Intracavernous epinephrine: a minimally invasive treatment for priapism in the emergency department. *J Emerg Med.*
2009;36:285–289.

Sundaram CP, Thomas E, Pryor LB, et al. Long-term follow-up of patients
receiving injection therapy for erectile dysfunction. *Urology.* 1997;
49:932–935.

Virag R, Shoukry K, Floresco J, et al. Intracavernous self-injection of vasoactive drugs in the treatment of impotence: 8-year experience with 615 cases.
J Urol. 1991;145:287–292.

CHAPTER 108

VACUUM DEVICES FOR ERECTILE DYSFUNCTION

John R. Holman

Erectile dysfunction is a common medical problem occurring in nearly 30 million American men. Vacuum devices to promote erection are safe and have overall clinical success rates of approximately 90%, but they are considered second-line therapy given the efficacy, favorable side-effect profile, and ease of use of phosphodiesterase inhibitors. That said, vacuum devices can be useful in nearly all men with erectile dysfunction except those with severe cavernous fibrosis. Therapy depends on the ability to transfer blood into the corpus cavernosa, which is limited if fibrosis is present.

A number of devices are available for use. The majority have three common components: a *vacuum chamber* or *cylinder*, a *vacuum pump* that creates a negative pressure within the chamber, and an *elastic constriction band*.

The devices create a nonphysiologic erection by trapping blood in both the intracorporeal and extracorporeal compartments of the penile shaft by means of the negative-pressure vacuum. The constrictor band is then placed below the chamber, over the proximal shaft, constricting blood flow into and out of the penis and maintaining an erection for sexual intercourse. Erection is maintained distal to the constricting band. Most manufacturers recommend that the vacuum-induced erection be maintained for less than 30 minutes because penile distention, edema, and cyanosis may ensue with prolonged use. The American Urologic Association, in its erectile dysfunction clinical practice guideline, updated in 2009 recommends that only vacuum constriction devices containing a vacuum limiter–relief valve should be used, whether purchased over the counter or procured with a prescription.

INDICATIONS

- Penile rehabilitation following prostate surgery (the only therapy shown to preserve penile length after radical prostatectomy)
- Erectile dysfunction resulting from
  - Vascular disorders
  - Prostate or colon cancer
  - Neurologic disorders
  - Psychogenic disorders
  - Hormonal disorders
  - Medications, when the medication cannot be altered or terminated

CONTRAINDICATIONS

- Sickle cell anemia or blood dyscrasias, coagulation disorders, or anticoagulation drug therapy
- Impaired manual dexterity; unable to operate the device (relative contraindication)

EQUIPMENT

- Vacuum erection device, including chamber, vacuum pump, and constriction bands (Fig. 108.1A). Battery-operated suction devices may be preferable in patients with impaired manual dexterity or after debilitating neurologic events such as stroke or quadriplegia. Constriction bands come in a variety of sizes to fit the penile shaft.
- Lubricant as needed.

PREPROCEDURE PATIENT PREPARATION

Discuss use of the suction device, alternatives, relative benefits, and potential complications with the patient and, when possible, his partner. The patient should be aware that a vacuum-induced erection, unlike a physiologic erection, causes rigidity distal to the constrictor band and may allow the penis to pivot at its base, requiring positioning for vaginal penetration. Although it is generally well tolerated, patients using this device may experience *painful ejaculation, penile pain, ecchymoses, hematomas, petechiae,* and *decreased penile temperature or numbness* distal to the constriction band. Most men have normal ejaculations with vacuum devices. Delayed or painful ejaculations have been reported in 10% to 15%, along with a feeling of trapped semen during ejaculation. The use of constriction rings with a "cut out" on the ventral aspect of the ring can help to prevent this (see Fig. 108.1B). Otherwise the semen drains out the penile meatus once the constriction band has been removed. Hematomas have been reported in 9.8% and local skin injury in 2.2% of long-term users. These complications can be reduced or eliminated by increased experience with the device and by emphasizing the need to remove the constriction band after 30 minutes. Most manufacturers provide instructional materials, videos, and customer service availability by phone to assist with use of their equipment.

TECHNIQUE

1. Complete the patient's history and physical examination to establish a diagnosis of erectile dysfunction.
2. Select a desired device for use.
3. Apply the open end of the vacuum chamber over the penis. A seal should be made with the skin at the base of the penis, usually with the help of lubricant jelly.
4. Activate the vacuum pump to create negative pressure within the chamber, thereby drawing blood into the penis and producing an erection-like state. Most devices have release valves in the chamber that prevent the formation of excessive pressure (see Fig. 108.1C).
5. Once adequate tumescence has been achieved, slide the constrictor band at the base of the chamber onto the penile shaft. This effectively traps blood in the penis to maintain the erection. The chamber and pump may now be removed. Constrictor bands are available in a variety of sizes.

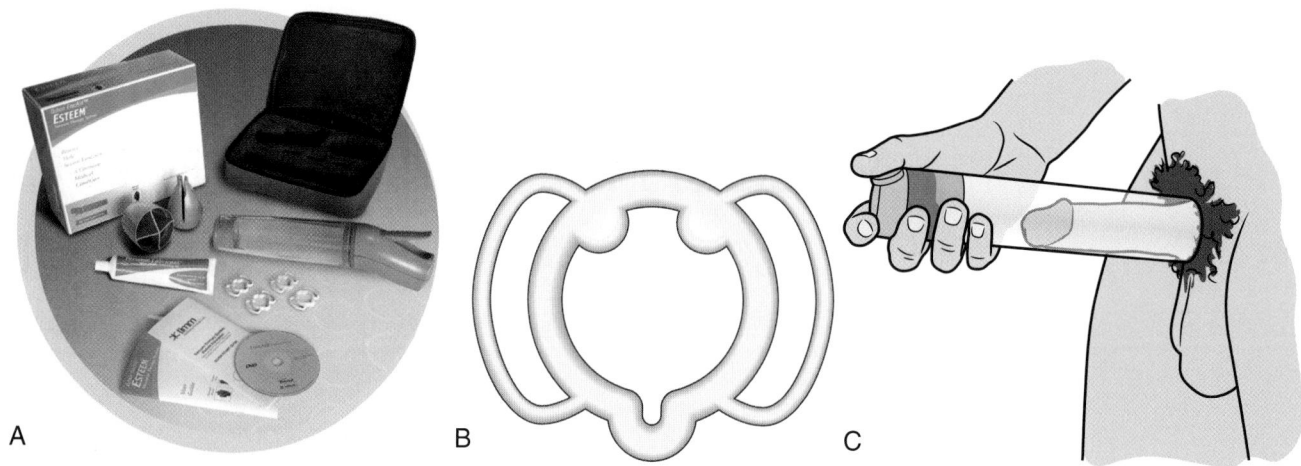

Fig. 108.1   (A) Typical vacuum device for the treatment of erectile dysfunction. (B) Constricting rings on device, cross-sectional view. (C) How to activate the pump. (A, Courtesy TIMM Medical Technologies, Eden Prairie, MN. B, Modified from TIMM Medical Technologies.)

6. After intercourse, remove the band from the penile shaft. The vacuum-induced erection will then subside.
7. Inspect the penis for evidence of injury.
8. After use, submerge all parts of the suction devices except the vacuum pump in soapy water for cleaning.

COMPLICATIONS

- Decrease in penile temperature or numbness distal to the constriction band.
- Local skin injury.
- Painful or no ejaculation.
- Penile pain.
- Subcutaneous ecchymoses, petechiae, or hematoma.
- With prolonged use (>30 minutes), progressive penile distention, edema, and cyanosis may occur.

PATIENT EDUCATION GUIDES

See the sample patient education and consent forms available at www.expertconsult.com.

CPT/BILLING CODES

55899   Unlisted procedure, male genital system (documentation suggested)

ICD-10-CM DIAGNOSTIC CODES

F52.21   Psychosexual dysfunction
N52.9   Impotence of organic origin

Acknowledgment

The editors recognize the contributions of Chad J. Smith, DO, to this chapter in a previous edition of this text.

SUPPLIERS

(See contact information available at www.expertconsult.com.)

Encore
Encore Medical
ErecAid
TIMM Medical Technologies
Post-T-Vac
Post-T-Vac Medical
SOMAerectSTF
Augusta Medical Systems

RECOMMENDED READING

Burnett AL. Evaluation and management of erectile dysfunction. In: Wein AJ, Kavoussi LR, Partin AW, Peters CA (eds). *Campbell-Walsh Urology.* 11th ed. Philadelphia, Elsevier, 2016;643–668.

Heidelbaugh JL. Management of erectile dysfunction. *Am Fam Physician.* 2010;81(3):305–312.

Montague DK, Jarow JP, Broderick GA, et al. *for the American Urological Association Erectile Dysfunction Update Panel: The Management of Erectile Dysfunction: An update*; 2007. www.auanet.org/content/guidelines-and-quality-care/clinical-guidelines/main-reports/edmgmt/content.pdf.

Raina R, Agarwal A, Alamaneni SS, et al. Sildenafil citrate and vacuum constriction device combination enhances sexual satisfaction in erectile dysfunction after radical prostatectomy. *Urology.* 2005;65:360–364.

Wylie KR, Jones RH, Walter S. The potential benefit of vacuum devices augmenting psychosexual therapy for erectile dysfunction: a randomised controlled trial. *J Sex Marital Ther.* 2003;29:227–236.

Yuan J, Hoang AN, Romero CA, Lin H, Dai Y, Wang R. Vacuum therapy in erectile dyfunction-science and clinical evidence. *Int J Impot Res.* 2010;22:211–219.

CHAPTER 109

IMPLANTABLE HORMONE PELLETS FOR TESTOSTERONE DEFICIENCY IN ADULT MEN

John Harlan Haynes III • *Terrance S. Hines*

Testosterone is responsible for the normal growth and development of the male sex organs and maintenance of secondary sex characteristics. As the primary androgenic hormone, its production and secretion are the end products of hormonal and biochemical interactions. Gonadotropin-releasing hormone is secreted by the hypothalamus and controls the pituitary secretion of luteinizing hormone (LH) and follicle-stimulating hormone (FSH). LH regulates production of testosterone by the testes, and FSH stimulates spermatogenesis. Testosterone can be converted in the body either to dihydrotestosterone by 5-α reductase or to estradiol by aromatase. Dihydrotestosterone preferentially binds to androgen receptors and becomes the more active form involved in hair growth and sebum production. Estradiol may be important in maintaining libido and bone mass but may also contribute to truncal obesity and feminine characteristics.

Testosterone deficiency is common, occurring in 1 in 200 men. The prevalence increases with age as testosterone levels decrease and sex hormone–binding globulin levels increase (causing a further decrease in free or bioavailable testosterone). Some experts suggest that more than 50% of men older than 55 years of age have low testosterone, increasingly referred to as *andropause*. Treatment should be considered in all men with testosterone deficiency as long as contraindications do not exist. Adherence to testosterone therapy is notoriously low; only 17% of prescriptions are filled more than once, and discontinuation rates are reported to be high (Schoenfeld et al, 2013).

Abnormally low testosterone levels are associated not only with sexual dysfunction but also with other comorbid conditions such as lipid disorders, cardiovascular disease, insulin insensitivity, osteoporosis, and cognitive and mood changes. Testosterone deficiency may be a cause of sarcopenia, a condition of aging senescence characterized by muscular weakness and atrophy.

In general, there are two basic types of testosterone deficiency:

1. *Primary*, or hypergonadotropic, hypogonadism is the result of primary testicular failure. In this situation, testosterone levels will be low and levels of pituitary gonadotropins (LH or FSH) will likely be high normal or elevated.
2. *Secondary*, or hypogonadotropic, hypogonadism is the result of inadequate secretion of pituitary gonadotropins. In addition to a low testosterone level, LH or FSH levels will be low or low normal.

Satisfactory replacement of testosterone is possible regardless of the type of deficiency.

Hypogonadism is defined as a free testosterone level that is below the lower limit of normal for young adult control subjects. Age-related decreases in free testosterone were once accepted as "normal." Currently they are not considered normal. No agreement exists on the exact normal level of testosterone as men age or on the serum testosterone level at which a man loses his sexual function.

The definition of *relative hypogonadism* is also uncertain. Many men have perfectly normal sexual function even if their testosterone levels decline into the age-adjusted lower normal range. Patients with low-normal to subnormal testosterone levels may warrant a clinical trial of testosterone. The threshold of response to and dosage of testosterone varies with age. If LH is increased and the testosterone level is low, the patient will have decompensated primary testicular failure. Testosterone replacement therapy can be essential to maintaining physiologically normal levels. Testosterone replacement improves sexual function and mood, increases lean muscle mass and strength, and decreases fat mass in hypogonadal men.

A positive effect of testosterone on endothelial function in men is supported by studies on the effects of intravascular administration of physiologic doses of testosterone on coronary blood flow in men with coronary artery disease. Studies have shown an increase in coronary vasodilation and blood flow in the testosterone test subjects.

EDITOR'S NOTE: Several recent publications have raised concern that testosterone replacement therapy in men may increase cardiovascular risk. Consequently, the US Food and Drug Administration (FDA) released a statement in 2015 that only men with low testosterone due to certain medical conditions and confirmed laboratory tests should receive testosterone therapy. They recommend that men receiving therapy be made aware of possible increased cardiovascular risks and be taught for which symptoms they should seek immediate medical attention, such as those for heart attack or stroke. Meanwhile, the American Association of Clinical Endocrinologists/American College of Endocrinology released a position statement (2015) indicating that there is no compelling evidence that testosterone therapy either increases or decreases cardiovascular risk. They also called for large-scale prospective randomized controlled trials focusing on cardiovascular benefits and risks.

HEALTH IMPLICATIONS OF TESTOSTERONE DEFICIENCY

Testosterone deficiency can result in the following:

- Anemia
- Decreases in or loss of libido and erectile function
- Absence or regression of secondary sexual characteristics
- Oligospermia or azoospermia
- Decrease in energy, increased fatigue
- Depressed mood
- Increase in fat mass
- Progressive decrease in lean body mass and muscle strength
- Decrease in bone density and increased risk of osteopenia/osteoporosis

Men with testicular failure may suffer from sexual dysfunction as well as osteoporosis, muscle weakness, depression, and lassitude, which is the clinical spectrum of hypogonadism. The sexual dysfunction, especially decreased libido and decreased erectile capacity, often reverses with testosterone replacement therapy. Ideally, testosterone therapy should provide physiologic-range testosterone levels (400 to 800 ng/dL). The variability of response in some patients may be related to comorbid medical illnesses, vascular dysfunction causing erectile dysfunction at the penile level, or psychologic factors (Box 109.1).

MEN AT INCREASED RISK FOR TESTOSTERONE DEFICIENCY

- Decreased secondary sexual characteristics
- Erectile dysfunction or reduced libido
- An unexplained decrease in energy or increased muscle weakness
- Unexplained osteopenia or osteoporosis
- Testicular atrophy
- Human immunodeficiency virus infection/acquired immunodeficiency syndrome with weight loss
- Long-term systemic glucocorticoids
- Chronic alcoholism or substance abuse
- Chronic systemic diseases (e.g., chronic renal failure, chronic inflammatory diseases)
- Recent-onset gynecomastia
- Morbid obesity
- Family history of endocrine failure
- Hypothyroidism

DIAGNOSIS OF TESTOSTERONE DEFICIENCY

In symptomatic men, these suggested guidelines may be followed:

- Measure total testosterone (total T) by blood measurement taken between 7 and 10 AM
- A total T above 400 ng/mL is considered normal.
- If total T is between 300 and 400 ng/mL, use the free or bioavailable testosterone level and clinical judgment to guide therapy.
- If total T is less than 300 ng/dL
  - Rule out treatable endocrine causes and transient hypogonadism due to reversible illness, drugs, or nutritional deficiency.
  - Repeat the test and measure free or bioavailable testosterone, LH, and FSH levels.
- If repeat total T or free T is confirmed as low, consider initiating testosterone replacement therapy.

BOX 109.1 Testosterone Deficiency Screening Questions

The "low-testosterone syndrome," often seen in healthy older men, is thought to play a role in a number of clinical problems seen in the growing elderly male population. A checklist has been developed to help raise awareness of the presence of testosterone deficiency in the older man. Clinicians may find the following questions helpful in screening their older patients:
1. Do you have a decrease in libido (sex drive)?
2. Do you have a lack of energy?
3. Do you have a decrease in strength or endurance?
4. Have you lost height?
5. Have you noticed a decreased "enjoyment of life"?
6. Are you sad or grumpy?
7. Are your erections less strong?
8. Have you noted a recent deterioration in your ability to play sports?
9. Are you falling asleep after dinner?
10. Has there been a recent deterioration in your work performance?

- LH, FSH, or both, are measured to distinguish between primary (testicular) and secondary (pituitary hypothalamic) hypogonadism.
- If FSH and LH are low or normal, this is secondary hypogonadism, and in the presence of very low total T (<150 ng/dL), a prolactin level and other pituitary hormones should be obtained. If the prolactin level is elevated or other signs of a tumor mass exist, obtain magnetic resonance imaging of the sellar and pituitary region to rule out a pituitary tumor. Referral to an endocrinologist is indicated for further evaluation.
- With a low total T and a high FSH and LH, primary hypogonadism is likely but Klinefelter syndrome must also be considered. Klinefelter syndrome is a somewhat common identifiable cause of primary testicular failure and may be diagnosed by obtaining a karyotype.
- A dual-energy x-ray absorptiometry scan may considered to evaluate bone mineral density in men with severe androgen deficiency and fracture risk.

CONTRAINDICATIONS

- Known or suspected prostate cancer or breast cancer
- Palpable prostate nodule or induration
- Prostate-specific antigen (PSA) greater than 4 ng/mL (or >3 ng/mL in men at high risk, such as those with a first-degree relative having prostate cancer or African Americans) without further urologic evaluation
- Severe benign prostatic hypertrophy (BPH)-related bladder outlet obstruction or other urinary tract symptoms (International Prostate Symptom Score >19)
- Erythrocytosis (hematocrit >50%)
- Treatment desired to improve athletic performance, body building, or short stature
- Untreated sleep apnea
- Untreated, severe or poorly controlled congestive heart failure
- Desire for fertility

Patients in Whom Treatment Requires Careful Monitoring

- Prostate problems and uncorrected obstructive symptoms caused by BPH
- Edema, fluid retention
- Gynecomastia
- Polycythemia or exacerbated erythropoiesis
- Hypogonadal adolescent boys because treatment may increase physical aggression
- Anyone whose epiphyses have not yet closed because premature closure and permanent short stature can result from treatment

NOTE: It is important to closely monitor those patients with a family history (i.e., presence in a first-degree relative) of prostate cancer, although the relationship between the cancer and testosterone replacement therapy is controversial. A double-blind randomized placebo-controlled trial of 237 men aged 60 to 80 years conducted in the Netherlands from 2004 to 2005 and published in the *Journal of the American Medical Association* (Emmelot-Vonk and colleagues, 2008) showed an increase in lean body mass, a decrease in fat mass, increased insulin sensitivity, and no short-term negative effects on the prostate or on cognition. In a review of the literature in the *New England Journal of Medicine* (Rhoden and Morgentaler, 2004), prospective studies demonstrated a low frequency of prostate cancer in association with testosterone replacement therapy. The conclusion was that there is no compelling evidence at present to suggest that men with higher testosterone levels are at greater risk of prostate cancer or that the treatment of men who have hypogonadism with exogenous androgens increases this risk. It should be recognized that prostate cancer becomes more prevalent at exactly the time of a man's life when testosterone levels decline.

TREATMENT

Testosterone should be administered only to men who are testosterone-deficient as evidenced by distinctly subnormal serum testosterone levels (<400 ng/dL or subnormal based on the specific assay used). The Endocrine Society's 2010 Clinical Practice Guidelines recommend testosterone therapy for symptomatic men with androgen deficiency who have low testosterone levels in order to induce and maintain secondary sex characteristics and to improve their sexual function, sense of well-being, muscle mass and strength, and bone mineral density.

The principal goals of testosterone therapy are to alleviate symptoms and to reduce health risks by restoring the serum testosterone concentration to the normal range.

The currently acceptable modes of testosterone delivery are transdermal, intramuscular (IM), implantable, and buccal.

NOTE: *Oral androgens* (methyltestosterone, fluoxymesterone) are not as effective as other treatments; they are also associated with a significant risk of hepatotoxicity (e.g., cholestatic jaundice, peliosis hepatis, and hepatoma) and are therefore not recommended.

Transdermal testosterone (Testoderm, Androderm): Unlike the original patches applied to scrotal skin, Androderm is worn on the arm or torso and delivers approximately 5 mg in 24 hours. Transdermal therapeutic systems are replaced every 24 hours. Transdermal preparations provide a relatively stable concentration of testosterone compared with other routes. Serum levels of testosterone peak 2 to 8 hours after application of a patch. Anecdotally, as much as one-third of men do not tolerate this route because of severe skin rash. This rash may be prevented by pretreatment with a topical corticosteroid.

Testosterone gel (AndroGel, Testim, Fortesta, Axiron) 5-mg packs or tubes: Applied daily to skin, "T gel" is a translucent hydroalcoholic gel that may cause less skin irritation and lower discontinuation rates compared with the transdermal patch. These positive results occur within 30 days. Because of the amount of skin to which the gel is applied, the serum concentrations are more even and higher over 24 hours than with the patch. Testim is dosed at 50 to 100 mg and has a musky aroma. All T-gel formulations have a warning about secondary exposure because virilization has been reported in children who were secondarily exposed to testosterone gel. The black box warning states that children should avoid contact with unwashed or unclothed application sites in men using testosterone gel and that health care providers should advise patients to strictly adhere to recommended instructions for use. Generic versions produced by compounding pharmacies may help offset the cost of these preparations.

Injectable testosterone esters: The principal esters available in North America are testosterone enanthate and testosterone cypionate. Injections of testosterone enanthate or testosterone cypionate may be given at intervals ranging from 7 to 14 days. Dosing typically is 100 mg IM per week to 300 mg IM per 3 weeks. A weekly injection of 100 mg causes less variation outside of the normal range. Although it is biologically effective, disadvantages of this route include the need for frequent deep IM administration and pronounced fluctuations in energy, mood, and libido (particularly as the dosing interval is increased). Testosterone undecanoate (Nebido) is available in several countries and is dosed at 100 mg every 3 months.

Implantable hormone pellets (Testopel): The implantable pellets are perhaps the most convenient, dependable, and best-tolerated method of testosterone delivery. Subcutaneous pellets are viewed as a more cost-effective and convenient therapy with potentially much greater compliance and tolerance than other methods. Placed subcutaneously in the buttocks through a special trocar device, 8 to 10 pellets (600 to 750 mg) usually provide sustained adequate physiologic blood levels (e.g., 400 to 800 ng/dL) for 4 to 6 months (Box 109.2). **NOTE:** Due to their long-acting effect, it may be best to use pellets in men for whom the beneficial effects and tolerance of testosterone replacement have already been proven.

Buccal tablet: Striant (30 mg, twice a day, Endo Pharmaceuticals) is placed in a depression in the gum above the upper incisors.

Finally, although not an androgen, human chorionic gonadotropin (hCG) stimulates the production of testosterone and sperm by the testes.

MONITORING PATIENTS ON TESTOSTERONE REPLACEMENT

- Clinical symptoms and signs of testosterone deficiency
- Frequency and duration of erections
- Acne and oiliness of skin, breast size and tenderness
- Possible skin irritation with transdermal therapy
- Serum testosterone levels
- Lipid profiles, liver function, and hematocrit
- Sleep apnea

Transdermal testosterone delivery systems: Serum testosterone should be drawn 8 to 12 hours after application or per patch label instructions. Because concentrations fluctuate in an unpredictable way when the gel preparation is used, at least two measurements should be obtained. Skin irritation at the site of the patch is common.

Injectable or implantable testosterone: Monitor nadir testosterone levels at 3 months (implants) or before the next injection/implantation. Levels that exceed 800 ng/dL or are less than 200 ng/dL require adjustment of the dose or frequency.

Digital rectal examination (DRE) and PSA: DRE should be performed and a PSA level checked in all men before initiating treatment, again at 3 months, and then annually in men older than 40 years of age. An abnormal DRE, a confirmed increase in PSA of more than 1.4 ng/mL in any 1-year period, a total PSA of more than 4.0 ng/mL, or a PSA velocity of greater than 0.4 ng/mL per year (beginning 6 months after therapy initiation) requires evaluation by a urologist. Exacerbations of obstructive uropathy related to BPH are a concern, and, if warranted, urine flow rate and postvoid residuals should be measured.

Hematocrit: Testosterone replacement therapy has been associated with increased hematocrit and hemoglobin. The hematocrit should be checked at baseline, then at 3 months and yearly. A hematocrit of more than 52% warrants evaluation for hypoxia and sleep apnea or a reduction in the dose of testosterone therapy. Testosterone is known to stimulate erythropoiesis.

Sleep apnea: Screening for sleep apnea includes interrogation of symptoms (e.g., excessive daytime sleepiness, snoring, or witnessed apnea) and polysomnography when indicated.

BOX 109.2 Insurance Criteria for Reimbursement for Testosterone Pellets

Aetna, US Healthcare, BlueCross/Blue Shield, and Medicare cover FDA-approved implantable testosterone pellets (Testopel pellets) subject to the following patient selection criteria only:

- As *second-line testosterone replacement therapy* in men with congenital or acquired endogenous androgen absence or deficiency associated with primary or secondary hypogonadism when neither transdermal nor intramuscular testosterone replacement therapy is effective or appropriate.
- Primary hypogonadism includes conditions such as testicular failure as a result of cryptorchidism, bilateral torsion, orchitis, vanishing testis syndrome, inborn errors in testosterone biosynthesis, or bilateral orchiectomy.
- Secondary hypogonadism (hypogonadotropic hypogonadism) includes conditions such as gonadotropin-releasing hormone deficiency and pituitary-hypothalamic injury as a result of surgery, tumors, trauma, or radiation, and is the most common form of hypogonadism seen in older adults.

Liver function, cholesterol, and high-density lipoprotein (HDL) cholesterol: Levels should be checked periodically. Testosterone lowers total cholesterol, low-density lipoprotein, and HDL.

Breast examination: Regular breast examinations are recommended.

Bone mineral density: Measurement of bone mineral density of the lumbar spine or the femoral necks at 1-year intervals may be considered in hypogonadal men with osteopenia, especially those younger than 80 years of age.

EQUIPMENT

- Trocar implanter kit (includes the trocar and stylet plunger)
- Disposable 5-cm trocar pellet implanter (3.2-mm bore diameter)
- Forceps
- Stainless steel tray
- Sterile gloves
- 1% lidocaine with epinephrine 2 to 3 mL
- 3-mL syringe; 27-gauge 1.5-in needle
- No. 11 scalpel blade
- 75-mg testosterone pellets (Testopel; Endo Pharmaceuticals), 3 × 8 mm (most common total dose for 4 to 6 months is 10 pellets, manufacturer's recommended dose is 2 to 6 pellets, every 3 to 6 months), in individual sterile glass tubes
- Lidoderm 5% patch or topical anesthetic placed 15 minutes before the procedure at site of insertion (optional)
- 2.0 chromic suture or Steri-Strips and tincture of benzoin

NOTE: The disposable trocar should be sterile and individually packaged. If an older stainless steel trocar is used, it should be sterilized by steam in an autoclave at 121°C for a minimum of 15 minutes. The standard procedures for sterilizing surgical instruments should be followed.

PREPROCEDURE PATIENT PREPARATION

All potential risks, benefits, and alternatives to testosterone replacement therapy should be discussed, specifically the potential complications regarding trocar insertion subcutaneously (including infection and bleeding). The patient should understand that once the pellets have been inserted, they are not typically removed unless the risks outweigh the benefits. The pellets slowly dissolve and the effects last for 3 to 6 months.

TECHNIQUE

The office procedure usually takes approximately 15 minutes. The testosterone pellets should be implanted into the subdermal fat of the buttocks using a special trocar implanter under sterile conditions and a local anesthetic. The 75-mg pellets are fat soluble and therefore are implanted subcutaneously. In most men, an area on either lateral buttock between the gluteus maximus and the tensor fasciae latae muscle is preferred. In this location, implantation is made below the skin and above the muscle and fascia, just inferior to the iliac spine, directed inferiorly along the line of the femur. The skin is marked 3 cm below the halfway mark between the iliac crest and the sacroiliac joint and the line is extended about 10 cm inferiorly parallel to the femur. Basically, the final location is in the upper outer quadrant of the hip. Anecdotally, pellets implanted more superiorly near the belt line or in the buttock on the side under the wallet pocket have been subject to inadvertent extrusion (Fig. 109.1A).

Preparation

1. Place patient comfortably in the lateral jackknife or fetal position.
2. Cleanse the skin over the insertion site with Hibiclens, alcohol, and povidone-iodine (see Fig. 109.1B).

3. Sterile technique is used, and universal blood and body fluid precautions should be followed.
4. Create a skin wheal using lidocaine 1% with epinephrine (1:100,000; see Fig. 109.1C).
5. Inject 2 to 3 mL of 1% lidocaine with epinephrine along the intended tract of the trocar insertion to a depth of 2 cm.

Implantation

1. Place pellets as indicated in the sterile container (the most common dose is ten 75-mg pellets).
2. After adequate local anesthesia is ensured, make a small (4-mm) puncture incision with a No. 11 scalpel blade (see Fig. 109.1D).
3. Insert the trocar with sharp stylet (solid rod in metal sheath with pointed end); direct it subcutaneously pointed at a 45-degree angle to the skin surface and advance it inferiorly to a depth of 2 cm into the subcutaneous fat.
4. The trocar and sharp stylet are then angled horizontal toward the skin surface and advanced beneath the skin through the subcutaneous tissue above the muscle and parallel to the trajectory of the femur. The trochar implanter should be inserted completely, (about 5 cm) until reaching the pellet slot (Fig. 109.2A).
5. The pointed, sharp stylet is then removed, and, using sterile tissue forceps, pellet implants are carefully placed in the slot of the hollow tube of the implanter. Usually three to five pellets per tract are placed (see Fig. 109.2B). (A sterile tray or cup may be held beneath the implanter as a "safety net" to catch pellets that may be inadvertently misplaced.)
6. The blunt stylet is then inserted into the trocar to be used as a plunger. The implanter is stabilized with one hand as the pellets are pushed through the bore and advanced within the hollow trocar sheath. The stylet is advanced inside the trocar as the trocar is slowly withdrawn, and the pellets are pushed out and deposited into the fatty tissue (see Fig. 109.2C).
7. This insertion process may be repeated through the same incision in a fan-like fashion until the total dose (usually 6 to 10 pellets) is deeply inserted. As the trocar is reinserted, swap back to the sharp stylet. Change back to the blunt stylet for pellet insertion. Extrusions may be minimized by placing pellets in tracts arranged in a fan-like pattern (e.g., three, four, and three at 45, 90, and 135 degrees, respectively).
8. After all the pellets have been inserted, the stylet is advanced within the trocar and the trocar is withdrawn using a clockwise–counterclockwise twisting motion.
9. Give the patient a dry pressure dressing to apply pressure for a few minutes.
10. Clean and then close the puncture site using Steri-Strips or a chromic suture and cover with an adhesive bandage (see Fig. 109.2D). Cold compression using body weight on an ice pack is advised for 10 minutes.

The pellets are slowly absorbed and are not removed. The procedure may be repeated on the opposite buttock in 3 to 6 months, depending on the adequacy of serum testosterone. Have the patient return in 3 months to check for efficacy and tolerability.

COMPLICATIONS AND RISKS

The chief adverse reactions with testosterone pellets include the following:

- Pellet extrusion
- Minor bleeding (typically insignificant and controlled by applying pressure to the surgical wound)
- Infection (infrequent and may also result in pellet extrusion)

The use of povidone-iodine skin disinfectant before the procedure appears to lower pellet extrusion rates. The likelihood of pellet

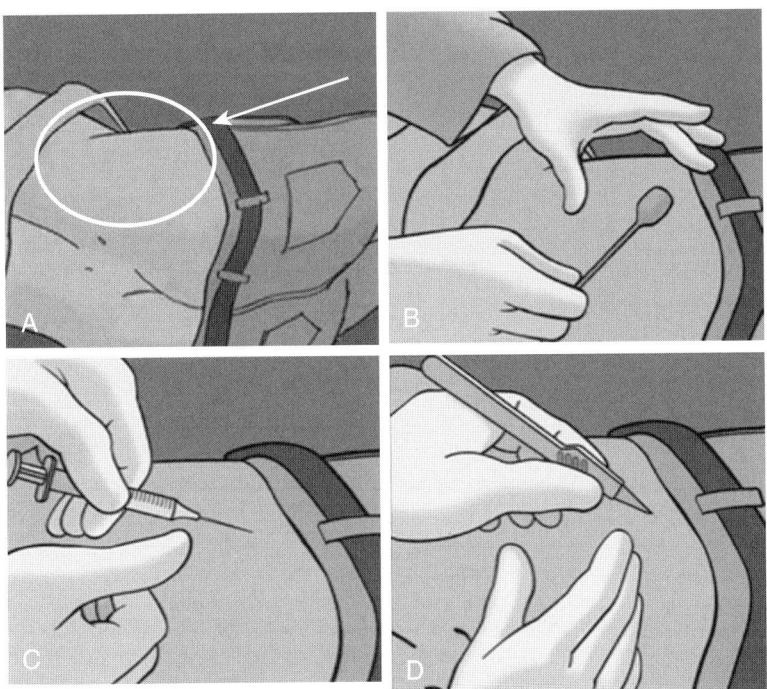

Fig. 109.1 Preparation for implantation of testosterone pellets. (A–B) Cleanse skin with Hibiclens, alcohol, and povidone-iodine. (C) Create skin wheal using lidocaine 1% with epinephrine. (D) Make small incision with No. 11 blade. (Modified courtesy Endo Pharmaceuticals, Inc., Malvern, PA.)

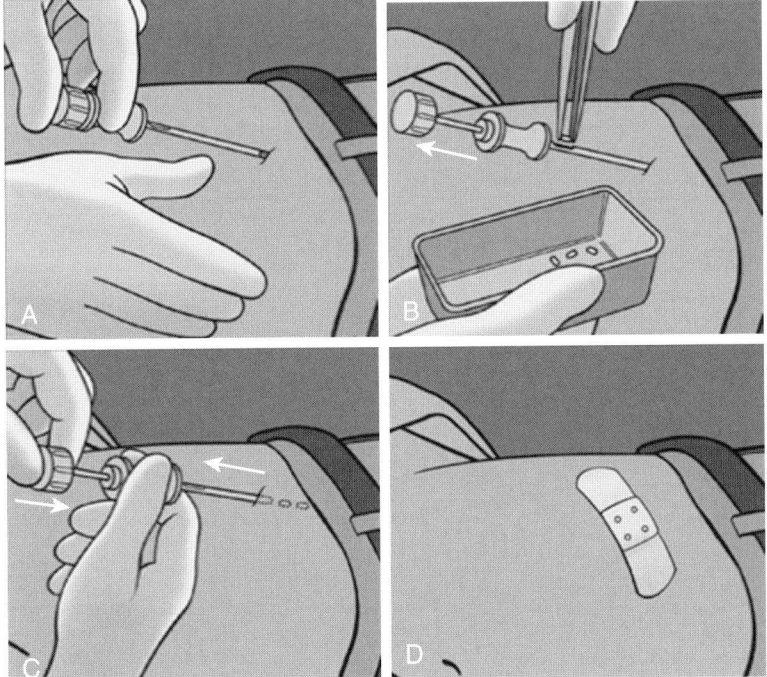

Fig. 109.2 Implantation of testosterone pellets. (A) Insert the trocar implanter with the stylet in place and direct it subcutaneously to the depth of the bolt (about 5 cm). (B) Remove the sharp stylet and place all the pellets in the lumen of the implanter with sterilized tissue forceps. (C) Insert the blunt stylet and, while stabilizing and slowly pulling back the implanter, push the pellets through the bore and into the fatty tissues. (D) Close the puncture site. (Modified courtesy Endo Pharmaceuticals, Inc, Malvern, PA.)

extrusion may decline with increasing operator experience. Preoperative and postoperative oral antibiotics (e.g., cephalexin 1000 mg) may reduce the incidence of infection. Some patients develop fibrosis (scarring, nodules) around implantation sites, but this typically does not prevent further implantations.

Other, rare, complications include the following:

- Pain at insertion site
- Increased fluid retention
- Gynecomastia
- Worsening sleep apnea
- Increased hematocrit

- Worsening prostate symptoms
- Testicular atrophy
- Mood swings
- Oligospermia or azoospermia

POSTPROCEDURE PATIENT EDUCATION

Most patients return to work the day of or the day after implantation but are advised to avoid bending or vigorous physical activity. For the first 24 hours, the patient should keep a dry pressure bandage on the insertion site and limit strenuous activity. He should watch for any complications, as noted previously.

REGULATIONS

Testopel pellets are classified as a Schedule III controlled substance under the Anabolic Steroids Act of 1990. Clinicians should restrict usage to avoid long-term on-site storage. As with other Schedule III substances, it is necessary to strictly follow state pharmacy and federal Drug Enforcement Agency regulations and always to document and copy. A prescription may be written and the patient may obtain the pellets and bring them to the clinic for insertion, or the pellets and trocar may be ordered directly from Endo Pharmaceuticals. Endo has an updated website for additional reference (www.Testopel.com).

CPT/BILLING CODES

S0189   Testosterone pellet (75 mg)
11980   Subcutaneous implantation of testosterone pellets

ICD-10-CM DIAGNOSTIC CODES

E23.0   Pituitary hypogonadism
E29.1   Male hypogonadism, testicular, primary or secondary
E29.8   Other testicular dysfunction
E23.0   Hypogonadotropic hypogonadism

SUPPLIERS

(See contact information available at www.expertconsult.com.)
Endo Pharmaceuticals

RECOMMENDED READING

Bhasin S, Cunningham GR, Hayes FJ, et al. Testosterone therapy in adult men with androgen deficiency syndromes: an Endocrine Society clinical practice guideline. *J Clin Endocrinol Metab.* 2010;6:2536–2354.
Cavender RK. Subcutaneous pellet implantation procedure for treatment of testosterone deficiency syndrome. *J Sex Med.* 2009;6:21–24.
Cavender RK, Fairall M. Subcutaneous testosterone pellet implant (Testopel) therapy for men with testosterone deficiency syndrome: a single-site retrospective safety analysis. *J Sex Med.* 2009;6:3177–3192.

Emmelot-Vonk MH, Verhaar HJ, Nakhai Pour HR. Effect of testosterone supplementation on functional mobility, cognition, and other parameters in older men: a randomized controlled trial. *JAMA.* 2008;299:39–52.
Goodman N, Guay A, Dandona P, Dhindsa S, Faiman C, Cunningham G. American Association of Clinical Endocrinologists and American College of Endocrinology position statement on the association of testosterone and cardiovascular risk. *Endocr Practice.* 2015;21:1066–1073.
Handelsman DJ, Mackey MA, Howe C, et al. An analysis of testosterone implants for androgen replacement therapy. *Clin Endocrinol (Oxf).* 1997;47:311–316.
Jockenhovel F, Vogel E, Kreutzer M, et al. Pharmacokinetics and pharmacodynamics of subcutaneous testosterone implants in hypogonadal men. *Clin Endocrinol (Oxf).* 1996;45:61–71.
Mäkinen J, Järvisalo M, Pöllänen P, et al. Increased carotid atherosclerosis in andropausal middle aged men. *J Am Coll Cardiol.* 2005;45:1603–1608.
McCullough A. A review of testosterone pellets in the treatment of hypogonadism. *Curr Sex Health Rep.* 2014;6(4):265–269.
Petak SM, Nankin HR, Spark RF, et al. *AACE Clinical Practice Guidelines for the Evaluation and Treatment of Hypogonadism in Adult Male Patients: 2002 Update (Developed by the American Association of Clinical Endocrinologists and the American College of Endocrinology).* 2002. http://www.aace.com/pub/pdf/guidelines/hypogonadism.pdf.
Rhoden EL, Morgentaler A. Risks of testosterone-replacement therapy and recommendations for monitoring. *N Engl J Med.* 2004;350:482–492.
Rosano GM, De Ziegler D, Pagnotta P, et al. Plasma testosterone levels in males with coronary disease. *Eur Heart J.* 1998;19(suppl):141. [abstract].
Schoenfeld MJ, Shortridge E, Cui Z, Muram D. Medication adherence and treatment patterns for hypogonadal patients treated with topical testosterone therapy: a retrospective medical claims analysis. *J Sex Med.* 2013;10:1401–1409.
Surampudi P, Swerdloff RS, Wang C. An update on male hypogonadism therapy. *Expert Opin Pharmacother.* 2014;15:1247–1264.
Tenover JL. Male hormone replacement therapy including "andropause." *Endocrinol Metab Clin North Am.* 1998;27:969–987.
Wang C, Swerdloff RS, Iranmanesh A, et al. Transdermal testosterone gel improves sexual function, mood, muscle strength, and body composition parameters in hypogonadal men. *J Clin Endocrinol Metab.* 2000;85:2839–2853.
Webb CM, McNeill JG, Hayward CS, et al. Effects of testosterone on coronary vasomotor regulation in men with coronary heart disease. *Circulation.* 1999;100:1690–1696.

CHAPTER 110

SPERM BANKING

Dan B. French • Edmund S. Sabanegh

Men with certain medical conditions or those undergoing various surgeries or medical therapy (e.g., chemotherapy, radiation therapy) face the real possibility of temporary or permanent infertility. An option to preserve fertility is to freeze (cryopreserve) sperm before the medical condition progresses or they undergo surgery or treatment. Cryopreservation of sperm, or sperm banking, involves the freezing of sperm in liquid nitrogen followed by long-term storage for future use. Unfortunately patients who may benefit from cryopreservation of sperm are not always aware of their options or, considering the stress of their immediate situation, may not even be contemplating their future fertility. Therefore a well-informed health care provider who is able to appropriately discuss cryopreservation with the patient is an invaluable resource.

Cryopreserved sperm were first used to achieve a successful pregnancy in 1953. Because of the moral controversy surrounding assisted reproductive techniques at that time, it took another 10 years for the use of cryopreserved sperm for artificial insemination to become generally accepted. A technique using liquid nitrogen for freezing of sperm was developed in 1963. Over the years other technical developments, such as the addition of cryoprotectants and the advancement of assisted reproductive techniques, have been introduced. With the advent of in vitro fertilization and intracytoplasmic sperm injection, even men with very few and poor-quality sperm can achieve fertility, with pregnancy rates approaching 50% per cycle.

INDICATIONS

One of the most important patient populations that may need this service is reproductive-age men who will undergo gonadotoxic chemotherapy for malignancy. Testicular cancer, leukemia, and lymphoma are the most common malignancies that may have reproductive consequences, either from the treatment or the disease itself. Cytotoxic chemotherapeutic regimens often result in acute azoospermia, as defined by the absence of sperm in the ejaculate. Depending on the regimen used, only some 50% of these men will recover spermatogenesis, and there is no precise way to predict who will do so. Even before receiving cytotoxic therapy, these patients often have suboptimal semen quality as a result of their systemic disease; therefore every effort should be made to cryopreserve any sperm they might have before initiating chemotherapy.

Radiation therapy, often used for certain testicular tumors and Hodgkin disease, is also gonadotoxic, and appropriate individuals should be offered sperm cryopreservation before treatment. Even if the radiation is administered to distant sites and the testes are shielded, fertility can be impaired owing to scatter radiation.

Nonmalignant conditions may also require gonadotoxic treatment or otherwise result in infertility. Conditions such as autoimmune disorders, inflammatory bowel disease, and organ transplants may require immunosuppressive or cytotoxic therapies that impair fertility (e.g., methotrexate and sulfasalazine may impair sperm production or quality). Men with other testicular or prostate diseases

or those about to undergo surgery that may affect the ability to ejaculate (e.g., prostatectomy, retroperitoneal lymph node biopsy, colon surgery) may wish to preserve sperm. Certain other medical conditions may also eventually affect the ability to ejaculate (e.g., multiple sclerosis, diabetes). These patients should be offered sperm banking if it is known that their treatment, surgery, or disease may lead to infertility.

Because up to 5% of men receiving a vasectomy will eventually request restoration of their fertility, it is reasonable to offer sperm banking to all those planning on this procedure. Men who are undergoing vasectomy reversal may choose to have sperm extracted at the time of reconstructive surgery in the event that the vasa reconstruction should fail. Men who are about to enter a line of work where they may be exposed to reproductive toxins or those with hazardous occupations (e.g., law enforcement, the military) may want to consider sperm banking.

Men with a history of spinal cord injury may require electroejaculation or surgical extraction for sperm retrieval. They may also choose to have sperm banked as a matter of convenience instead of undergoing repeated procedures.

CONTRAINDICATIONS

The main contraindication to sperm cryopreservation is the *presence of a disease communicable through the sperm*. For this reason, donors are screened for human immunodeficiency virus, hepatitis B and C, chlamydial infection, gonorrhea, syphilis, cytomegalovirus, and human T-lymphotropic virus. Specimens are incubated for 6 months to confirm the absence of these conditions before use.

Although not a contraindication, it should be noted that sperm with damaged DNA do not thaw as well as healthy sperm. With the development of in vitro fertilization/intracytoplasmic sperm injection, even semen samples with elevated levels of sperm DNA damage or severe oligospermia can be used effectively. Among the thousands of conceptions that have occurred from frozen sperm, the incidence of birth defects has been no different than that among children conceived through intercourse.

PROCEDURE

The patient will complete various forms, including a consent form, agreement of fee schedules, and, most important, a legal document clearly outlining the fate of the sperm should the patient die or otherwise become incapacitated. Blood samples are drawn for screening for various sexually transmitted infections. Before freezing, a semen analysis is performed to assess the concentration, total number, and quality of sperm. The sample is then mixed with cryoprotectants such as egg yolk or glycerol.

Sperm can be collected for banking from various sources depending on the clinical circumstances. These include ejaculated semen specimens, sperm recovered from the bladder in patients with retrograde ejaculation, and surgically retrieved specimens from either the epididymis or testicular tissue. If the specimen is an ejaculate, it should be produced by masturbation at the collection site or at least brought to the collection site immediately after collection. The donor should not have had any ejaculations within the preceding 48 to 72 hours if at all possible. Depending on semen quality, several collections separated by 48 to 72 hours of abstinence may be required. Once collected, the sample is allowed to liquefy at room temperature.

The specimen is labeled with the pertinent data, including but not limited to patient name, identification number, and date of collection. This information is verified by the donor. Sometimes photographs of the donor are used as an additional security feature. The sample is divided into a certain number of straws or vials for freezing based on the concentration of sperm. One of these aliquots is thawed the next day to assess for viability following thaw. This test is used as a predictor of future viability for the entire batch. Once preserved, samples can be stored for many years (at least up to 12 years) without fear of deterioration.

The cost of sperm cryopreservation varies between institutions. Cost for an initial analysis and freezing ranges from $150 to $600. The price is even higher when specimens must be shipped, usually using a commercial cryobank. Most cryobanks assess annual storage fees ranging from $50 to $365.

CONCLUSION

The incidence of cancer in reproductive-age men has been increasing worldwide over the past 25 years. Although cancer cure and the management of acute toxicities remain the paramount issues for both the medical professional and the patient, future fertility is a major concern for many patients. With advances in both cryopreservation technology and assisted reproductive techniques, cryopreservation of sperm has become a valuable tool in the treatment of male infertility. Men of reproductive age embarking on gonadotoxic treatments for cancer as well as other selected groups of patients need to be aware that cryopreservation of sperm is an option, and it is incumbent on the provider to educate them about this. The procedure is relatively simple and affordable and, unfortunately, remains underutilized.

CPT/BILLING CODES

89259	Sperm cryopreservation
89343	Storage per year, sperm
89353	Thawing of cryopreserved sperm/each aliquot

ICD-10-CM DIAGNOSTIC CODES

Z98.52	Status vasectomy
Z51.89	Other aftercare; status post chemotherapy
C62.90-C62.92	Testicular tumor
C81.9	Hodgkin's Lymphoma unspecified
C85.90-C85.99	Lymphoma non-Hodgkin's unspecified
C95.90-C95.92	Leukemia unspecified
N46.02	Azoospermia due to extratesticular causes
N46.01	Organic azoospermia
N46.12	Oligospermia due to extratesticular causes
N46.11	Organic oligospermia

ONLINE RESOURCES

American Society for Reproductive Medicine: www.asrm.org
CryoChoice: www.cryochoice.com (for information on sperm cryopreservation using the mail system)
RESOLVE: The National Infertility Association: www.resolve.org
Society for the Study of Male Reproduction: www.ssmr.org
Sperm Bank Directory: www.spermbankdirectory.com (for a listing of local sperm banks)

RECOMMENDED READING

Agarwal A, Sidhu RK, Shekarriz M, Thomas Jr AJ. Optimum abstinence time for cryopreservation of semen in cancer patients. *J Urol.* 1995;154:86–88.

Anger JT, Gilber BR, Goldstein M. Cryopreservation of sperm: indications, methods and results. *J Urol.* 2003;170:1079–1084.

Goldstein M, Schlegel PN. *Surgical and Medical Management of Male Infertility.* New York: Cambridge University Press; 2013.

Kliesch S, Kamischke A, Nieschlag E. Cryopreservation of human semen. In: Nieschlag E, Behre HM, eds. *Andrology: Male Reproductive Health and Dysfunction.* 2nd ed. Berlin: Springer; 2000:349–356.

Nalesnik JG, Sabanegh Jr ES, Eng TY, Buchholz TA. Fertility in men after treatment for stage 1 and 2a seminoma. *Am J Clin Oncol.* 2004;27:584–588.

Peterson PM, Giwercman A, Skakkebaek NE, Rorth M. Gonadal function in men with testicular cancer. *Semin Oncol.* 1998;25:224–234.

Wald M, Prins GS. Sperm banking: indications and techniques. In: Lipshultz L, Howards SS, Niderberger C, eds. *Infertility in the Male.* 4th ed. New York: Cambridge University Press; 2009:593.

CHAPTER 111

Vasectomy

Charles L. Wilson

Vasectomy is a safe, relatively inexpensive, permanent form of contraception. One percent of men aged 25 to 49 years have a vasectomy annually in the United States, totaling between 500,000 and 600,000 procedures per year. In comparison, one recent survey found that female tubal ligation was performed two to three times more often. This is a phenomenon that has occurred over the last 50 years; it was only in the early 1970s that permanent female sterilization surpassed male sterilization in the number of procedures performed in the United States. Worldwide, vasectomy is performed as often or more often than tubal ligation in only eight nations: Austria, Bhutan, Canada, Denmark, Korea, the Netherlands, New Zealand, and the United Kingdom. This is unfortunate, because unlike tubal ligation, vasectomy is usually performed in an office setting, is less expensive, and is associated with fewer and less severe complications. No mortality from vasectomy has been reported in the contemporary United States, whereas approximately 10 women die annually from complications of tubal ligation. Although both procedures have low failure rates, a failure of tubal ligation is discovered only when pregnancy occurs, whereas failure of vasectomy can be detected by routine postvasectomy semen testing. Thus vasectomy offers high efficacy, lower morbidity and lower cost, and the ability to verify success yet it continues to be underused.

The decision process that leads up to the choice of vasectomy often starts with a general discussion of birth control options and family planning, which may involve the primary care clinician or the partner's gynecologic care provider. It is essential that these providers be knowledgeable and prepared to provide accurate information about vasectomy to the man and his partner.

Patient education handouts for this procedure are available at www.expertconsult.com or www.engenderhealth.org. Explicit patient instructions are imperative, especially for this procedure. The patient education handouts are highly recommended for this purpose.

Vasectomy can be performed in many ways. In the mid-1980s, EngenderHealth (formerly AVSC International) helped popularize the no-scalpel vasectomy (NSV), a method devised in China by Dr. Li Shunqiang. China was at that time struggling against a 2:1 bias favoring tubal ligation over vasectomy. Dr. Li designed a vas fixation clamp and sharp dissecting forceps (SDF), which allowed him to perform vasectomy in a "refined" and less-invasive manner. NSV became widely accepted by Chinese men. Whether NSV is, in practice, less invasive than the traditional methods depends entirely on the training, skills, and experience of the surgeon. Certainly, it has been demonstrated in some hands to be a quick, virtually bloodless, and often painless procedure. It therefore lends itself a significant psychological advantage with the apprehensive patient.

Similarly, the "no-needle, no-scalpel vasectomy," or more simply, no-needle vasectomy (NNV) technique, devised by the author in 1999, replaces the previous skin wheal and vasal block anesthetic with a jet injection. This helps relieve patients' fear of needle administration of anesthetic in this sensitive area (Wilson, 2001).

In any case, the no-needle and no-scalpel approaches simply define methods of anesthesia and of entry and access to the vas deferens. How the vas deferens is then occluded is variable and a matter of preference.

The term *laser vasectomy* has been used to refer to the minimally invasive techniques, but in reality there is no practical use or value for a laser in the vasectomy procedure.

The long-sought goal of a completely reversible vas occlusion method has spawned experimental models of occlusion without dividing the vas deferens. Such methods include simply clamping the vas with metal vascular clips, the plastic VasClip (no longer available) or the spring ligation Pro-Vas clip (no longer available), injecting glues or scarifying agents into the lumen, implanting silicone plugs, or simply cauterizing a length of the lumen transcutaneously. None of these methods has proven sufficiently successful or reversible.

ANATOMY

The *scrotal epidermis* is very thin and the *dermis* is supported by the thick and elastic dartos muscle. These layers are well endowed with blood vessels, which makes them susceptible to bleeding and ecchymosis; however, they are also particularly resistant to infection and are capable of rapid healing after surgical incision. The *scrotum* can vary widely among patients in its size, shape, and texture (from that of a full, round, tense, cyst-like structure that resists palpation, to a thin, smooth, droopy sac with nearly visible contents, or a flat, rugose thickening along the dependent fold of an abdominal panniculus). Individual anatomy plays the largest role in determining whether a vasectomy will be easy or difficult to perform. A *septum* separates the left and right sides of the scrotum, and loose connective tissue cushions the scrotal contents. In single-incision vasectomy, the septum does not present a practical barrier, and bleeding risk is less than that with two separate incisions.

The *epididymis* is a soft, comma-shaped attachment on the testis that originates at the superior pole and wraps around the back posterior aspect down to the inferior pole, clinging to the smooth, firm surface of the testis, but separated by a sulcus. (See patient education worksheet available at www.expertconsult.com.)

The *vas deferens* originates as a convoluted, tenuous duct from the tail of the epididymis at the inferior pole of the testis. As it courses cephalad along the posteromedial aspect of the spermatic cord, it becomes straight and sturdy, with thick walls of smooth muscle tissue, which give it a dense, almost gritty texture to palpation. In a cross-section of the scrotum above the level of the testicles, the vas is a prominent tubular structure surrounded by tiny vasal nerves and supplied by its own small deferential artery (Fig. 111.1). It is deep within the scrotum, separated from the skin surface by nine tissue layers, the deepest of which is the *internal spermatic fascia*, which also contains the testicular artery, lymphatics, and nerves, and the pampiniform plexus. At that level, the vas is usually distinctly palpable and firm, about 3 mm in thickness, like a hard-cooked spaghetti noodle or a ball-point pen refill. But anatomic variation accounts for vasa that may be as thin as 1.5 mm or as thick as 4.5 mm. Occasionally, the convoluted portion extends all the way to the inguinal

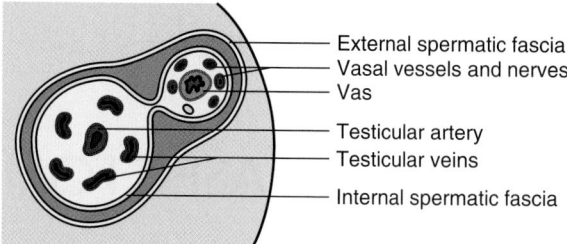

External spermatic fascia
Vasal vessels and nerves
Vas
Testicular artery
Testicular veins
Internal spermatic fascia

Fig. 111.1   Schematic coronal view of spermatic cord and internal structures. Note location of vas deferens with its associated vessels and nerves, as well as the testicular artery and veins, all located within the internal spermatic fascia.

canal. Some patients have congenital absence of the vas on one side, although they are rarely aware of it.

Sensation in the anterior scrotum is mediated by the ilioinguinal nerves and the perineal nerves arising from the pudendal nerves. Complete anesthesia for vasectomy depends on blocking not only these somatic sensory paths, but also the autonomic afferents that supply the vas deferens with its visceral sensation. Fortunately, there are few sensory nerves (there is little sensation) in the fascia between the scrotal skin and the vas deferens. Most sensation is in the immediate perivasal fascia, so that is where the focus should be when injecting or administering the local anesthetic after numbing the scrotal skin.

INDICATIONS

* Vasectomy is appropriate for a man when he (and usually his partner) have decided they do not wish to have children, or to have any more children.
* For some couples there is a medical contraindication to pregnancy in the female partner or a commitment to adopt children in lieu of having their own.
* Occasionally a man seeks vasectomy as extra assurance even though his partner has had a tubal ligation or a history of infertility.
* A man diagnosed with a genetic contraindication to fathering a child may desire vasectomy.

CONTRAINDICATIONS

Absolute

* Bacterial skin infection
* Uncontrolled coagulation disorders
* Inability to palpate and elevate both vasa
* Hypersensitivity to palpation, precluding isolation of the vas
* Lack of adequate informed consent
* Depression, psychosexual impairment, or impaired decision making

Relative

* Anticoagulant or antiplatelet therapy. Aspirin, clopidogrel, prasugrel, and ticagrelor should ideally be stopped for 5 days before the surgery and for 2 to 3 days afterward. Other oral anticoagulants should also be discontinued before surgery. Warfarin (Coumadin) should ideally be stopped for 5 days before surgery and held for 2 to 3 days afterward. Dabigatran (Pradaxa) should be stopped for 1 to 2 days (longer if creatinine clearance <50 mL/min), rivaroxaban (Xarelto) for 24 hours and apixaban (Eliquis) for 24 to 48 hours prior to surgery. These can be restarted as soon as adequate hemostasis is confirmed; it should be noted that their time to onset of therapeutic effect is short. Each case should be evaluated individually and if the medications cannot be stopped, meticulous hemostasis must be ensured at the time of surgery.

* Impending infertility, such as menopause or hysterectomy in partner.
* Unresolved conflict or stress; for example, recent childbirth, marital discord, divorce, or financial setback.
* Inappropriate expectations of vasectomy (e.g., improving a troubled marriage, curing sexual problems).
* Excessive, unreassured concerns regarding sexual functioning after the vasectomy.

Preprocedure Patient Preparation

Patient education materials and handouts are widely used and are of great value in preparing the patient for vasectomy. The vasectomy questionnaire, patient education handouts, and patient consent forms help achieve fully informed consent. (See all of these forms available at www.expertconsult.com.)

Schedule a preoperative consultation and evaluation at least several days before the scheduled procedure. This allows time for the patient and his partner to think about the decision and the information provided before the procedure. This appointment will generally take 15 minutes if prior patient education material has been reviewed by the patient or if he has reviewed a counseling video. Without these materials, it may take 30 minutes to properly inform the patient and answer all questions.

Many now recognize the educational value of patient education DVDs or online streaming videos. The patient can review the material several times privately at home. A vasectomy counseling DVD is available from Creative Health Communications through The National Procedures Institute (see the section "Suppliers"). With portable DVD players, the patient can easily view the material in the office before seeing the clinician.

The patient should sign the formal consent form. The consent form may be titled "Request for Vasectomy" to emphasize the patient's role in decision making. The clinician still retains responsibility to help the patient make a decision that will be in his best long-term interest. It is wise to include the wife or partner, if any, in the consent process; however, a man has the right to choose vasectomy even in the absence of spousal consent. Similarly, a patient who is young, unmarried, or without children should not be denied vasectomy on these grounds alone.

The preprocedure counseling visit can be documented using the encounter form, which reviews the patient's pertinent history, physical examination, and counseling points, and documents the follow-up semen specimen checks. The form can be found online at www.expertconsult.com.

At the conclusion of the session, perform a careful genital examination, noting any anomalies of the area and especially the size, texture, and position of the vasa deferentia as they course through the upper scrotum. Be alert to the possible absence of a vas or presence of a third or fourth vas, although such cases are extremely rare. Make a mental note of the ease or difficulty of mobilizing each vas to the anterior midline, and make a final decision whether to proceed with this vasectomy or stop and refer. Check for testicular masses, varicoceles, inguinal hernias, and possible granulomas. Note any tenderness to palpation. Groin rashes should be resolved before surgery.

Also helpful is the Patient Education Worksheet, available at www.expertconsult.com. This is a checklist of the counseling material to be reviewed with the patient. The original sheet is for the patient and a copy is made for the chart. Not only is it a good summary of all points covered, but it serves as a reminder for the patient of what to do just before and after the surgery.

The clinician should note the questions, "How well do you tolerate pain?" and "Do you have a tendency to faint?" on the encounter form. If the patient tolerates pain poorly or has a tendency to faint, atropine 0.5 mg may be given intramuscularly on arrival to the office before surgery to reduce vasovagal effects of nausea, bradycardia, and syncope. This optimizes the vasectomy experience for both the patient and clinician. *Oral sedation* with either diazepam 10 mg or alprazolam 1 mg 1 hour before surgery may be used in addition to the atropine or alone to help relax the nervous patient. However, sedation requires that he avoid driving and other activities requiring alertness for the rest of the day. One may plan to prescribe a narcotic analgesic for patients who indicate above-average sensitivity to pain based on their prior experiences. However, acetaminophen 650 mg taken up to an hour prior to surgery is usually adequate and safe. Some now use tramadol (Ultram) 100 mg. The patient should be reassured that after the anesthesia is administered, they will feel nothing sharp. They may experience some pressure or dull discomfort when the clamp is placed around the vas, similar to if they were ever "racked," and it may radiate into the abdomen on the appropriate side. But they should not feel anything sharp after the anesthesia is administered. While every man's anatomy is different, when asked after the procedure, some patients say they felt nothing sharp or dull, basically nothing more than their body parts being maneuvered.

To minimize the risk of bleeding complications, patients on antiplatelet therapy should have their platelet function restored by the time of surgery. This requires abstaining from aspirin-containing products, clopidogrel, prasugrel, and ticagrelor for 5 days. Nonsteroidal antiinflammatory drugs (NSAIDs) in very rare instances are associated with bleeding. If a patient does have a questionable history, NSAIDs should be withheld for 48 hours before and after surgery. If the patient is taking any other oral anticoagulant, the guidelines noted above under Relative Contraindications should be followed. If there is no history of bleeding disorder or prior complications of surgery, normal platelet function can usually be assumed.

Federal agencies require that a specific consent form be executed for the clinician to be compensated. These are usually available from local health departments or the state Medicaid agency. Forms must be completed fully and accurately to avoid denial of payment. Note that consents are valid only for surgery performed more than 30 days and less than 180 days after the counseling session at which the form is signed.

EQUIPMENT AND SUPPLIES

The preparation for vasectomy includes gathering the necessary equipment and supplies and arranging the sterile items on a surgical tray (Fig. 111.2). Each setup depends on the surgical setting and the surgeon's preferred technique and choice of available supplies. A checklist for the staff to use in preparing for the procedure is a good way to avoid omissions and oversights.

- Vas-fixing forceps (VFF; one or two pairs) are locking clamps used to secure the vas during puncture and dissection (Fig. 111.3A). Historically, sharp or blunted towel clips have been popular. The Wilson vasectomy forceps (Advanced Meditech International [AMI]; Marina Medical; Zinnanti Surgical) provide a secure yet atraumatic grasp of the vas for incisional vasectomy, and work equally as well as VFF in the no-scalpel technique. The Li vasectomy forceps (AMI, Integra Miltex) were introduced in China as VFF for NSV. They feature a cantilever design to limit closing force on the tip.
- SDF (AMI, Integra Miltex, Marina Medical) are the key to atraumatic dissection of the vas and are used to puncture the skin instead of a scalpel incision and to hook and deliver the vas. They are essentially sharp-pointed hemostats (see Fig. 111.3B and C).
- Small dermatologic skin hook (optional).
- If a scalpel will be used for incision or sharp dissection, include a disposable scalpel or scalpel handle with a No. 15 blade.
- Cautery unit, either an electrocautery unit and handpiece, with a fine-needle electrode (unit should be set at the lowest level that quickly cauterizes small "bleeders"), or a battery unit. Battery-powered thermal cautery units with disposable sterile sheaths and disposable specialized vasectomy tips are available from AMI (Fig. 111.4). Based on Schmidt's (1992) findings, a battery-powered cautery unit may be the instrument

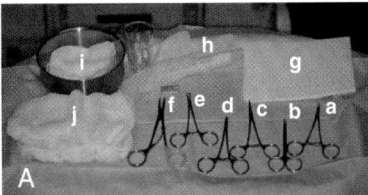
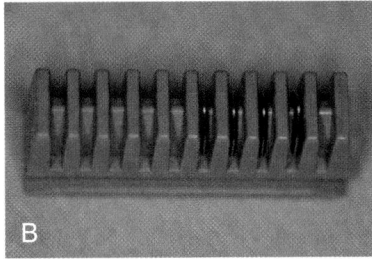

Fig. 111.2 (A) The surgical tray: (a) sharp dissecting forceps; (b) scissors; (c) straight mosquito hemostats; (d) curved mosquito hemostats; (e) Wilson vasectomy forceps; (f) hemoclip applicator with clips; (g) pack of 4 × 4 gauze; (h) battery cautery in sterile glove; (i) basin of wet gauze pads; (j) large number of "fluffed-up" gauze pads to place inside scrotal supporter. (B) Close-up of hemoclip pack with four clips remaining.

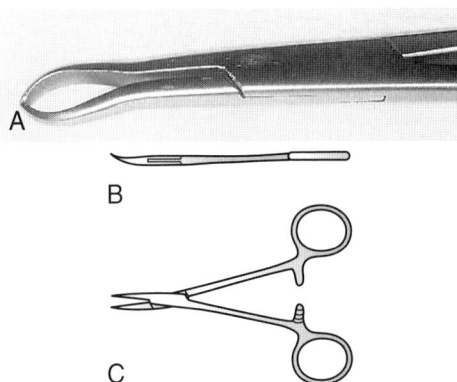

Fig. 111.3 No-scalpel instruments. (A) Wilson vasectomy forceps. (B–C) Sharp dissecting forceps. (B–C, From Li SQ, Goldstein M, Zhu J, Huber D. The no-scalpel vasectomy. J Urol. 1991;145:341–344.)

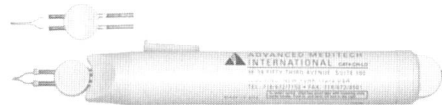

Fig. 111.4 Battery-operated cautery unit with disposable tip. (Courtesy Advanced Meditech International, Flushing, NY.)

of choice for optimal sealing of the vas ends compared with an electrosurgical unit.
- Three or four mosquito hemostats.
- Adson tissue forceps (1 × 2 teeth) with suture platform for holding the vas or fascia.
- Tissue scissors for dividing or hemitransecting the vas.
- Method to seal vas sheath: Either a needle holder with a 4-0 absorbable plain, chromic, or polyglycolic acid suture on an atraumatic needle or a medium hemoclip applicator with clips (Teleflex Pilling Weck; Ethicon). Silk ties (2-0 or larger) can also be used.
- A method to anesthetize the area: Traditionally, a 10-mL syringe (1.5-inch, 27-gauge needle) with lidocaine (2%) without epinephrine (10 mL) was used. In the NNV anesthesia technique

(see later discussion), an instrument called the MadaJet is used to administer the lidocaine. Only 0.1 mL of lidocaine is used per side with this instrument, but it requires at least 1 mL in the chamber to prime and function correctly.

- Sterile sodium bicarbonate solution to mitigate pain during anesthetic infiltration if needle injection is used (optional). Just before injection of the anesthetic, the clinician should draw up 1 mL of sodium bicarbonate with 9 mL of the lidocaine. This reduces the sting and burning associated when lidocaine is injected. Sodium bicarbonate is not needed if the MadaJet is used.
- Large pack of 4 × 4 gauze.
- Warmed povidone-iodine (Betadine) or chlorhexidine (Hibiclens) preparation (A povidone-iodine or chlorhexidine containing disposable surgical scrub brush soaked in warm tap water works well).
- Fenestrated sterile drape and nonfenestrated drape.
- Sterile gloves and mask.
- Single sterile glove (into which the cautery device is placed if the sterile cautery sheaths are not used). This is not needed if a sterile cautery handset is used.
- Pair of nonsterile gloves for preparation.
- Specimen jars with formalin.

No-Needle Vasectomy Anesthesia Technique

In the NNV technique, the traditional vasal block method is replaced by the no-needle technique. This is accomplished using a piston-like instrument (MadaJet 401UR; Mada Medical.; Fig. 111.5A), which uses the force of fluid under pressure to "push" the anesthetic into the tissues. The jet injection is a fine stream (about 0.006 inch in diameter) that instantly penetrates about 4 mm through the skin and vas deferens, producing an almost immediate and complete anesthetic effect (see Fig. 111.5B). It is also fairly quiet. It may be helpful to fire the gun once over the sink, before application, so everyone can hear that it is not very loud, and to avoid any chance that the patient might be startled; this may be reassuring.

The vas should be isolated as described later in step 3 of the No-Scalpel Vasectomy Procedure section. However, now both the index and middle fingers are placed behind the scrotum with the thumb in front. The straight segment of vas spans a small "safe" space between the index and middle fingers. The MadaJet is cocked and the tip is then placed firmly over the vas next to the thumb, directed into the "safe" space, and actuated by pushing the button. Each injection will be 0.1 mL of lidocaine. When beginning, it may help to mark the intended site of the scrotum with a marking pen and then isolate the vas to this spot for anesthesia. The marked spot will make it easier to bring the other vas to the same location. It also identifies where the opening should be made. A second application can be made over each vas to ensure a good block if desired. The total amount of anesthetic will then be 0.2 to 0.4 mL. Usually the clinician can reassure the patient that the anesthetic is working because the patient will feel the second application less than the first.

CAUTION: Be careful not to have fingers positioned behind the vas in line with the jet injection stream. Lidocaine can penetrate through the patient's tissues and into the surgeon's fingers. This is the reason for the special finger positions for NNV.

The MadaJet 401UR is supplied with the proper settings for NNV and comes with a stainless-steel spacer, which is notched to conform to the vas. The MadaJet design incorporates air space between the tip of the injector and the skin, so it does not require disposable parts like other injectors do. However, it does demand careful attention to cleaning, sterilization, and maintenance procedures between uses, according to the manufacturer's instructions.

After each patient use, the tip should be changed to a different, sterile tip. After each use, careful sterilization of the MadaJet is essential. The entire MadaJet may be routinely autoclaved, but that is not necessary between patient uses. After use, the device is fired once to clean the exit port, then the tip, the spacer, and the body

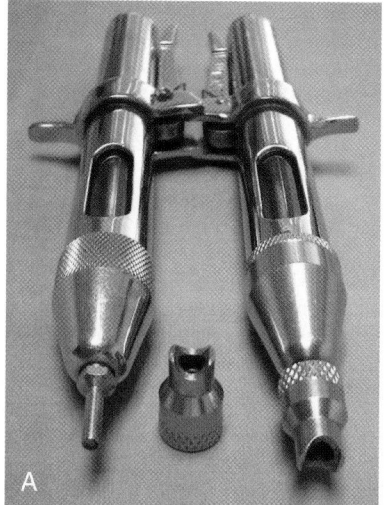

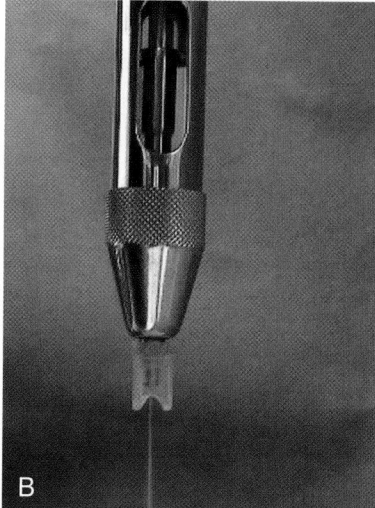

Fig. 111.5 (A) MadaJet model 401UR with metal sheath that fits over the nozzle tip to align the stream with the vas. (B) Stream of lidocaine emitted from the MadaJet orifice.

are cleaned, and the entire tip end of the device is cold sterilized by immersion in Madacide-FD solution for at least 10 minutes. The reservoir tube holds 4 mL of lidocaine, enough for about 40 actuations. At the end of each day, the MadaJet is disassembled, cleaned, and autoclaved. Periodic maintenance, at least annually, is required and is performed by the manufacturer.

There are several advantages to NNV. First, no needle penetrates the skin, reducing the risk of bleeding complications related to needle damage. Second, needlestick risk for surgical personnel is avoided, and medical waste is reduced. Third, it relieves the patient of fears they may have about needles—this benefit cannot be overestimated. (The jet injector is very efficient. In over 11,000 NNVs by the author, 97% required only one injection for each vas. That is only 0.2 mL of lidocaine per patient, or about 1/30 the usual amount required for the complete vasectomy. It is so effective that even "slow responders" to local anesthetics experience rapid numbness.)

The major limitation of NNV is the small area of numbness, about the size of a dime. With advanced skills and precision in the NSV technique, a clinician can incorporate the no-needle anesthetic technique successfully. Otherwise, more injections to include adjacent tissues will be required to keep the patient comfortable.

Clinicians will find a myriad of other applications for the MadaJet among the procedures they perform in the office. No-needle anesthesia will be embraced by many patients in addition to men undergoing vasectomy. A single snap suffices for a punch biopsy, injecting scars with steroids, skin tag excision, or skin anesthesia before needling for joint aspiration or injection, or fine-needle aspiration of the breast, to name a few examples. A special dermatologic tip is needed for these applications.

TECHNIQUE VARIATIONS

Traditional Vasectomy versus No-Scalpel Vasectomy Technique

In both techniques, the anesthetized vas is manipulated to lie under the skin of the scrotum where the opening will be made. (Wherever incisions or punctures will be made should also be anesthetized.) Traditional technique may involve two separate anterolateral incisions (one for each vas) in the scrotum, although increasingly a single midline entry is used. The NSV technique specifies a single opening located in the anterior midline of the scrotum, between the upper one-third and the lower two-thirds of the scrotum.

The essential difference is in the method of entry through the skin and in the delivery of the vas. In the traditional technique, a typical surgical incision 1 to 2 cm long is made in the skin with a scalpel, then carried through the dartos and fascial layers sequentially until the vas is exposed and bluntly dissected free of the fascia. Bleeding is controlled at each layer, as needed, usually with cautery. If the incision is kept to 1 cm or less, it can be considered a minimally invasive technique, which is recommended by recent American Urological Association (AUA, 2015) guidelines.

In the NSV technique, the method of entry is reduced to three smooth, precise movements, eliminating most of the operating time, tissue trauma, bleeding, and hemostatic maneuvers of traditional vasectomy. The key is the SDF. It is held and used in a precise manner to puncture the skin, all layers of fascia, and the anterior wall of the vas deferens in one smooth motion. It is then used to dilate the resulting 2-mm tract by stretching, not cutting, all layers at once. Finally, the tip of the SDF is precisely placed in the vas and rotated to hook the vas and deliver it cleanly from the fascial sheath, minimizing dissection. The overall entry wound is less than 1 cm in length, so this is also considered a minimally invasive technique as recommended by the AUA.

Once the vas is delivered, there is no distinction between traditional and NSV in how one proceeds with occlusion of the vas, and alternatives are discussed in the following section. After occlusion of the vasa, traditional scalpel incisions are usually closed with one or two sutures, whereas the small stretched opening of NSV or any minimally invasive technique usually contracts and rarely requires closure.

Occlusion Methods

A number of occlusion techniques have been used, with varying degrees of success, but existing evidence is insufficient to recommend one specific technique (AUA guidelines, 2015; Sokal and Labrecque, 2009).

Traditional division of the vas and suture ligation of both ends has a 1% to 3% failure rate and is discouraged at this time. However, the AUA guidelines note that certain surgeons have personal training or experience with this technique, which allows them to have successful results with failure rates less than 1%.

Intraluminal/mucosal cautery alone is superior to ligation of the vas in every way, regardless of whether cautery is also used. In other words, ligation or placing a hemoclip over the *vas itself* is discouraged.

Interposing fascia between the cut and cauterized ends results in very low failure rates of 0.1% to 0.5%. The fascia can be closed with absorbable suture or with hemoclips. The latter are quicker and avoid the bleeding seen occasionally when placing a suture.

The AUA guidelines (2015) endorse three techniques using various combinations:

1. Intraluminal/mucosal cautery with fascial interposition and without ligatures or clips applied on the vas

2. Intraluminal/mucosal cautery without fascial interposition and without ligatures or clips applied on the vas
3. Open-ended vasectomy leaving the testicular end unoccluded while using intraluminal/mucosal cautery on the abdominal end of the vas with interposing fascia.

There is also a Marie Stopes International method using extended nondivisional electrocautery of the vas. This technique yields acceptable results but is beyond the scope of this text. For an excellent discussion of various techniques, see the AUA guidelines, 2015. (See also Lipshultz and Benson [1980]; although it is a dated article, the material remains an excellent review.)

Excision of a vas segment greater than 4 cm is 100% successful, but causes excess morbidity and leaves little possibility of reversal. Labrecque and colleagues (2002) found that excising a longer (>15 mm) segment of vas did not improve recanalization rates over shorter excisions. In some settings, specimens for pathologic examination may be required by policy; however, there is little or no benefit, and substantial added cost, in having histologic confirmation. The optimal length of excised segment is thought to be 1 to 2 cm. Experienced surgeons may not remove any tissue once they are able to identify the vas in vivo with certainty, and are certain of their cautery and fascial interposition techniques. The AUA guidelines (2015) have stated that sending vas segments for histologic confirmation is not necessary. Instead of sending the segments for histologic examination, some clinicians give the 1-cm vas segments in formalin to the patient and instruct him to keep the segments in a medicine cabinet, away from children, until he has had two negative semen checks. The patient can then dispose of the segments once sterility is confirmed. Considering that 500,000 vasectomies are performed each year in the United States, that each pathology specimen costs between $150 and $200 to process, and that some clinicians put each side in separate bottles, clinicians can save the health care system $75 million to $150 million/year by not sending the vas segments to the laboratory! If the patient keeps the specimens, and if the vasectomy should fail (which is rare), the patient can then submit the tissue to the laboratory for evaluation, if desired.

Open-Ended versus Closed-Ended

The "open-ended" technique uses cautery only on the prostatic end of the cut vas, along with closing the fascia over that end. It differs from other techniques in that the testicular end of the vas remains unoccluded, or "open." The open-ended technique was first recommended and used more than 50 years ago. Errey and Edwards (1986) reported an improvement in postoperative complaints. The technique is assumed to minimize back-pressure on the testicle, which could be associated with long-term pain in the occasional patient (i.e., postvasectomy pain syndrome). The trade-off is that symptomatic sperm granulomas and vasectomy failure could be increased because of the open pathway from the testicle. Careful attention to the proper technique of cautery and fascial interposition helps prevent failure; however, most surgeons still routinely cauterize both the prostatic and testicular ends in the belief that this "closed-ended" method is the best assurance against failure. Some surgeons use the open-ended technique only for men younger than 30 years on the basis that they may be more likely to request reversal, which would then be theoretically easier; they use the closed-ended technique in those older than 30 years.

NO-SCALPEL VASECTOMY PROCEDURE

1. *Examination and positioning of patient:* Have the patient lie down undressed but draped from the waist down. As described earlier, it is recommended that a genital examination be performed at the conclusion of the counseling process. Review those findings and, if necessary, reexamine the patient to be

confident about the position and mobility of each vas. Clip any remaining excess scrotal hair.

2. *Skin anesthesia* (this step is not required with NNV): After cleaning the site with an alcohol wipe, the anesthetic may be administered before the sterile preparation and draping. Use 0.5 to 1 mL of lidocaine to raise a wheal in the median raphe. The small volume helps prevent distortion at the site of entry. Lidocaine may be mixed with sodium bicarbonate to reduce the brief burning sensation during injection. Epinephrine is generally not used in the deep injection to avoid arterial constriction. However, some clinicians prefer to use lidocaine with epinephrine in the skin wheal because the area of anesthesia is later identified by the resulting blanching.

3. *Isolating the vas with the three-finger technique*: The right-handed surgeon stands at the patient's right side. The left-handed surgeon will use reverse handedness throughout. Identify the left vas in the upper third of the scrotum by palpating from the midline laterally. The vas is dense and firm to compression and about the diameter of a cooked spaghetti noodle or a ball-point pen refill. It is the only thing this dense and firm in the scrotum. Use the three-finger fixation method to secure the vas, as follows. Reaching across the patient, place the middle finger of the left hand (if right-handed) under the scrotum and press up from behind the scrotum, elevating the vas to the anterior surface. Press down from the front of the scrotum with both the thumb and index finger, securing the vas in place (Fig. 111.6A). The space between the thumb and index finger is where you will access the vas.

Although the vas can be occluded close to the epididymis (even in the convoluted portion), it is desirable to choose a site more distal (i.e., closer to the groin), where the straight segment of vas is more easily mobilized, less likely to spontaneously recanalize, and more amenable to surgical reanastomosis. Secure the vas then in the midline between the upper one-third and the lower two-thirds of the scrotum.

4. Anesthetizing the vas: Use NNV (see earlier discussion) or the following traditional vasal block technique (Fig. 111.7): With needle and syringe, enter the skin from the anesthetized midline spot, advance the needle tip several centimeters cephalad along the vas, and inject 3 to 5 mL around the vas high on the left. If the needle tip lies very close to the vas, the anesthetic will flow around the vas, within the internal spermatic fascia, and it will effectively block the perivasal nerves without having to repeatedly insert the needle. (Do not inject into the vas; rather, inject the lidocaine along and around the vas.) The anesthetic effect will extend along the vas toward the epididymis without distorting the tissues where you will be dissecting the vas. Let the vas fall back, then grasp the right vas (see Fig. 111.6B). Here the three-finger fixation method does not require reaching across the patient, but directly placing the left middle finger behind the right side of the scrotum to elevate the right vas, and applying counter-pressure with the thumb and index finger anteriorly. Reinsert the needle through the midline, advance the tip along the right vas, and inject another 3 to 5 mL around and along the vas.

5. Surgical preparation and draping: The anesthetic will have time to take effect while the preparation is taking place. Nonsterile gloves are used with warm disinfectant solution. Warm solutions will help relax the scrotum, which allows easier palpation of the vas. A 50% solution of chlorhexidine (Hibiclens) smooths the skin during palpation of the vas, unlike the stickier povidone–iodine solutions. Prep the skin well down onto the perineum because the hands will often be in this area when manipulating the vas. Also prep the skin over, around, and along the penis to prevent it having to be retracted or taped out of the field. Cover the area with sterile surgical drapes. A fenestrated drape usually goes over the scrotum, whereas a nonfenestrated drape may be placed over the thighs.

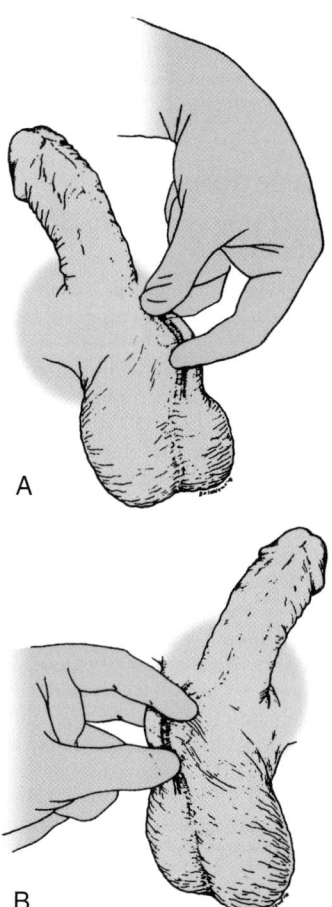

Fig. 111.6 (A) Three-finger fixation of the left vas beneath the skin in the midline. (B) Three-finger fixation of the right vas. (From Li SQ, Goldstein M, Zhu J, Huber D. The no-scalpel vasectomy. *J Urol.* 1991;145:341–344.)

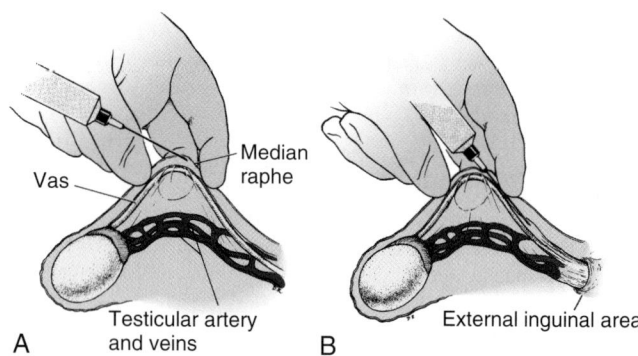

Fig. 111.7 Technique of vasal block anesthesia, using the traditional syringe and needle method. (A) To anesthetize the skin, a wheal of anesthetic is placed intradermally in the median raphe. (B) To anesthetize the vas, the 1.5-inch needle is inserted through the midline wheal and advanced along the vas toward the inguinal area. The anesthetic diffuses around the vas. This is then repeated with the other vas. (From Li SQ, Goldstein M, Zhu J, Huber D. The no-scalpel vasectomy. *J Urol.* 1991;145:341–344.)

6. Fixing the vas in the clamp: Isolate the left vas using the three-finger technique described in step 3. Next, use the VFF to pinch the skin to demonstrate for both you and the patient the effect of the anesthetic. (If necessary, reposition your grasp or inject more lidocaine.) Now spread the tips of the VFF approximately

4 mm and place them against the skin, straddling the vas, which is in the space between your thumb and index finger. Gradually increase downward pressure against your middle finger. Warn the patient that he will feel pressure for the next few seconds. When you feel the pressure of the two tips of the forceps distinctly on the pad of your middle finger, begin slowly closing the VFF. Just before locking the forceps closed, slightly relax the downward pressure, so as not to pinch the posterior scrotum, but while completely encircling the vas in the grasp of the VFF (Fig. 111.8A).

7. Repositioning your grasp: At this point, release the three-finger grasp and reposition your left hand to hold only the VFF in the manner shown (see Fig. 111.8B). Note that there are no fingers behind the scrotum at this point. The tips of the VFF are elevating the vas and the handles are lowered.

8. Penetrating the skin: While holding the vas firmly fixed in position in the VFF, use the SDF with the tips spread apart to pierce the skin where it is tensed over the vas, penetrating down into the lumen of the vas with one of the tapered tips (see Fig. 111.8C). This tract will be dilated to deliver the vas to the surface. So, carefully slip the single tip out of the tract, close the forceps, and reinsert the two tips while closed together to the depth of the tract. Alternatively, a 3 to 10 mm incision can be made through the skin with the scalpel, and it is still considered a minimally invasive technique.

9. Exposing the vas: While keeping the tips deep in the tract, spread the handles of the SDF widely to spread the tips 4 to 8 mm, dilating all layers of skin and fascia down to the vas in one step. This mode of dissection is remarkably free of bleeding compared with a layer-by-layer approach or sharp dissection using a scalpel. The vas is distinguishable as grayish-white, slightly translucent tissue with a low-sheen surface. A very shiny surface indicates the vas is still covered by a layer of fascia. In that case, pierce again and spread just the thin fascia to reveal the bare vas. It is not necessary to expose more than a few millimeters of vas to proceed with delivery (see Fig. 111.8D).

10. Delivering the vas: Now open the SDF with the curve facing down and the handles held below the level of the tips. Insert one jaw, the far tip of the SDF, into the vas just 1 to 2 mm. Using care to keep the tip buried in the vas, rotate clockwise about the long axis of the instrument. As the curve of the SDF points upward, the vas will rise through the skin (see Fig. 111.8E). With the vas poised in this position, use your left hand to unlock and remove the VFF (see Fig. 111.8F). Provided that the fascia has been adequately dissected and there are no fascial adhesions from previous infections, trauma, or surgery, a bare loop of vas will slide out of the fascia. Now regrasp the vas by pinching it at the top of the loop with the VFF. Avoid encircling the vas at this point; rather, grasp into the vas tissue itself (see Fig. 111.8G). If a loop of vas does not slide out easily, replace the VFF around (vs. through) the vas once again and try removing any adherent fascia by inserting the closed SDF under the vas fascia and spreading the tips against the vas surface. Alternatively, try passing the closed SDF or hemostat through the minimally invasive incision and under the vas to elevate about a 1-cm section.

11. Baring a loop of vas: With the vas held securely, create a "window" in the "web" of fascia under the loop. Start near the top of the loop by passing one tip of the SDF through the loop, close enough to the vas that the deferential artery and all fascial vessels are cleanly separated from the vas. The artery often may not be visible, but meticulous dissection at this step will be rewarded with a bloodless field. Dilate the opening by spreading the two tips of the SDF within the loop to "strip" the tissue off about 1 cm of vas (see Fig. 111.8H).

12. Securing the loop: A measure of safety may be added by applying hemostats to the fascia at one or both ends of the isolated vas segment (see Fig. 111.8I).

13. Accessing the vas lumen: If a segment of vas is going to be removed, hemitransect the vas but do not cut completely through, making two partial incisions 1 to 1.5 cm apart (see Fig. 111.8J). If a portion of the vas is not going to be removed, the lumen of the vas may be accessed through the initial puncture of the vas if it is visible, or through an incision (see Fig. 111.8K). Alternatively, the wall of the vas may be penetrated using a sharp electrocautery needle or a hot thermal cautery tip.

14. Cauterizing the vas: Cauterize the lumen of the prostatic end only (open-ended technique) or of both ends of the vas (closed-ended technique) by inserting the cautery tip 10 mm into the lumen, activating the cautery unit, and then withdrawing the tip (see Fig. 111.8L). Whether using electrocautery or thermal cautery, the objective is to create a graduated injury to the duct lining, minimal at the upper portion and maximal at the cut tip so that fibroblasts are stimulated to form scar tissue that will occlude the vas somewhere in between. If a section of vas is excessively desiccated to the point that the muscular wall is devitalized, the entire tip may slough.

15. Completing transection/removing segment of vas: With the hemostats still in place, complete the transection through the entire vas. If a segment of vas is to be removed, it is placed in formalin (see Fig. 111.8M).

16. Creating fascial interposition: With 4-0 chromic, create a purse-string closure and draw the fascia over the prostatic end of the vas, being careful that the open testicular end does not fall back into the sheath (see Fig. 111.8N). Alternatively, a medium hemoclip is applied (only on the fascia). This is quicker and may cause less bleeding (see Fig. 111.8O). In a similar alternative, the edges of fascia may be approximated with a hemostat and then ligated with a free tie, avoiding the use of a suture needle. Release the hemostat only from the prostatic end at this point. (There is little research evidence to conclude which side should have the fascial interposition to optimize results, or if it really makes a difference.) **NOTE:** The suture is placed only through the fascia, not on the vas itself. Ligating the vas itself is not recommended because if it is not tight enough, the suture serves no purpose, allowing sperm to pass through. If it is too tight, the end necroses, often leaving an open tip.

17. Releasing the vas: Lower the vas into the scrotum while still grasping the fascia with one hemostat. This can reveal a bleeder that was not previously evident owing to constriction by the tight skin edges. After hemostasis is ensured, drop the vas back into the scrotum. If a bleeding point is identified at any time during the procedure, use the least amount of cautery necessary to control it. For bleeding from the vasal artery, clamp and ligate with suture or a hemoclip. Often the bleeding will be from the skin opening and not the deeper tissues, so check this area closely. In general, skin edge bleeding can be ignored until the end of the procedure, and then managed with 5 minutes of gently pinching the wound closed.

18. Repeat the entire procedure on the right side: Now identify the right vas. (If a second incision is made, provide additional anesthesia on the skin.) Isolate the right vas in the VFF. Confirm that it is the right vas by tugging gently to move the right testicle. The procedure that was carried out on the left side is now carried out on the right.

19. Care for the scrotal opening: The scrotal incision may occasionally require a suture if it gapes or continues to bleed from the skin edge after cautery or 10 minutes of firm pinching between gauze. A single 4-0 absorbable suture should suffice. Tell the patient to expect the suture knot to fall off after the period of absorption.

20. Dressing: Antibiotic ointment on the wound is optional. Several 4 × 4 gauze pads provide a loose dressing, held in place with the patient's tight briefs or an athletic supporter.

21. Postoperative instructions: Give the patient appropriate instructions for care. Provide one or two containers for semen samples, and caution the patient to use alternative birth control until a semen check is clear.

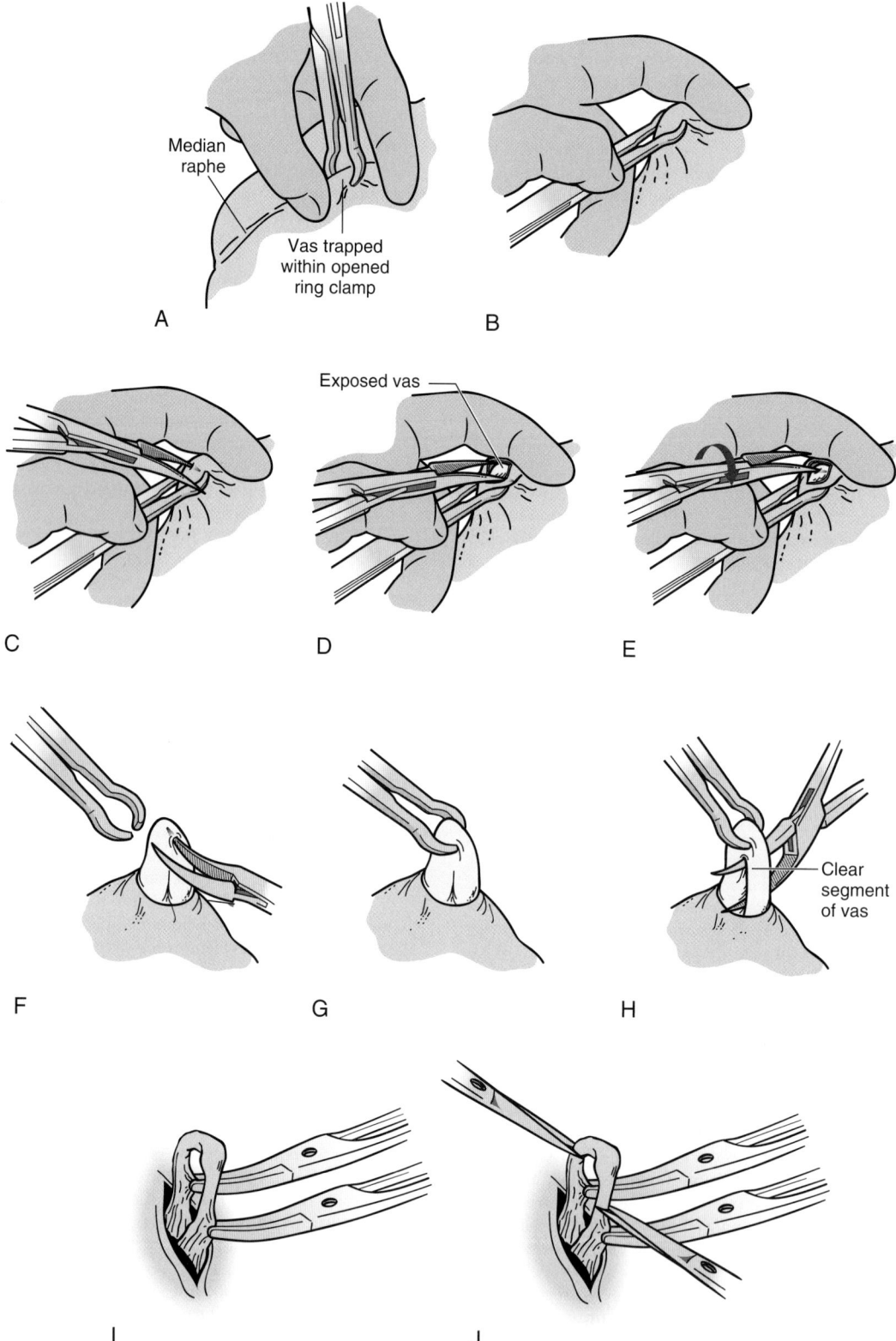

Fig. 111.8 (A–H) Sequence of the no-scalpel vasectomy procedure. (A) Percutaneous clamping with Li forceps. (B) Tenting up vas. (C) Incising with single jaw of dissecting forceps. (D) Spreading perivasal tissue down to vas. (E) Inserting single jaw into vas. (F) Holding vas. (G) Grasping through with clamp. (H) Further stripping of perivasal tissue. (I–O) Several alternatives for occlusion. See text for details. (I) Grasping perivasal tissue just below intended resection sites. (J) Hemisection of vas at intended sites of resection. (K) Open-ended technique (cauterize only the prostate end, no piece removed). (L) Cauterizing both ends (piece to be removed). (M) Removing a 1.5-cm segment of vas. (N) Using the purse-string suture to close the perivasal tissue. (O) Alternatively, a medium hemoclip occludes the fascia over the vas end.

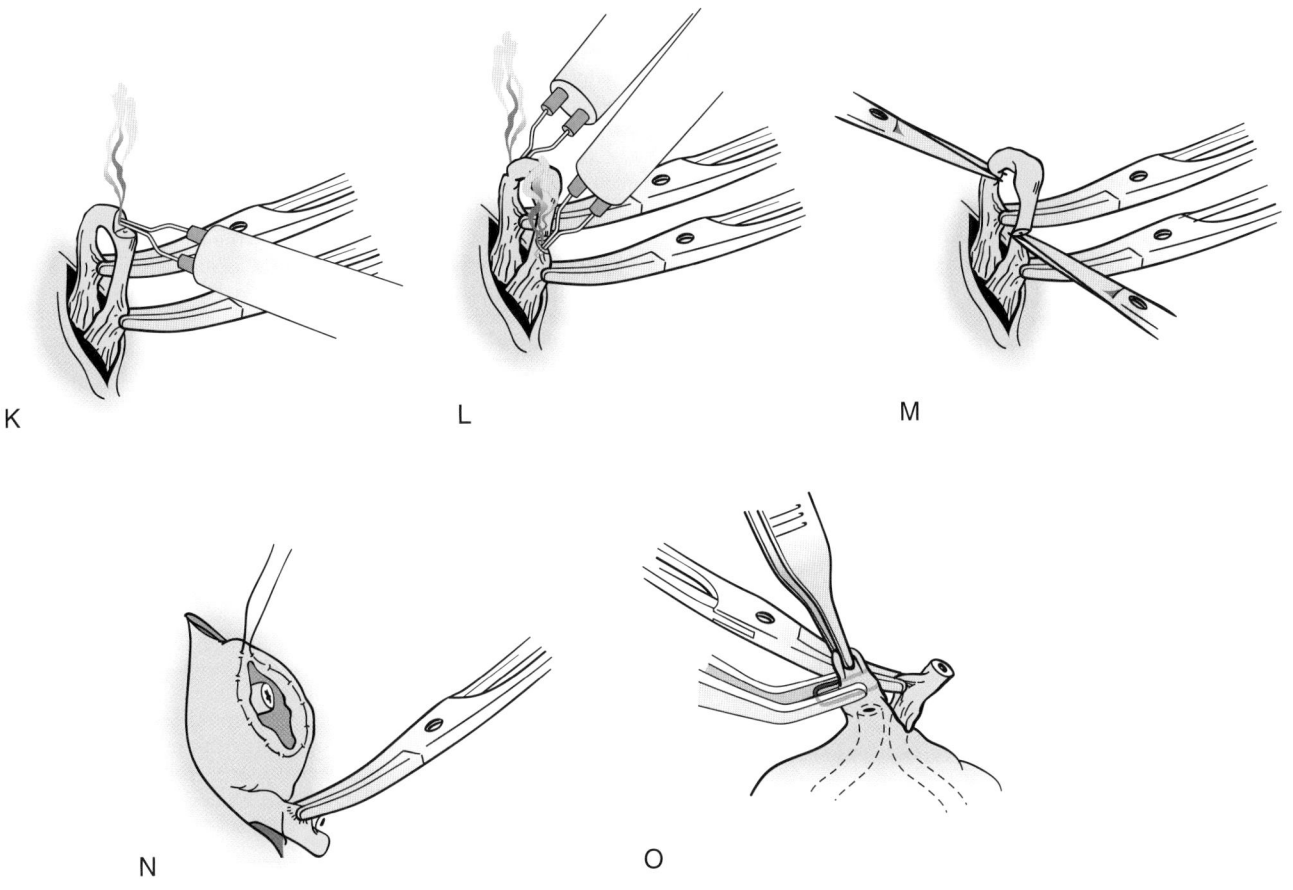

Fig. 111.8, cont'd.

22. Discharge the patient once he is ambulatory with no lightheadedness.
23. Document the procedure with the appropriate operative report (Box 111.1).

Clinical photographs of the procedure are shown in Figs. 111.9 to 111.11.

CAUTERY INSTRUMENT STERILITY

Sterile, disposable, single-use, battery-powered thermal cautery units are available and inexpensive for use in vasectomy. More environmentally friendly reusable units are provided with replaceable tip elements and sterile sheaths to envelop the handle.

For electrocautery users, sterile single-use, or reusable autoclavable handle and cord sets are available, but a clean, nonsterile cord set and handle can be safely reused, if the cord is maintained out of contact with the sterile field and the surgeon's sterile gloves. After the clinician is gloved, have an assistant lower the cautery handle into a spare sterile glove by holding the cord (Fig. 111.12). Place a sterile electrode tip into the handpiece right through the glove. The handpiece can now be safely placed on the sterile tray. Reusable battery-powered units can be used in a similar fashion.

POSTPROCEDURE PATIENT CARE

All of this information should be discussed with the patient during the preoperative counseling session. It is important to reinforce it on the day of surgery.

No routine postprocedure office visit is necessary. For the clinician who is just beginning to perform vasectomy procedures, it may be advisable to see the patients in 1 to 2 weeks to gain an appreciation for the normal postprocedure changes.

An uneventful recovery thus depends on the patient following good self-care principles and the specific written instructions he received in the office. Sample postoperative handouts can be found at www.expertconsult.com. These sample instructions describe expected conditions and those that should prompt a call to the clinician. It is always best to thoroughly review the instructions with the patient, as well as providing them in written format for later reference.

Patients usually report minimal to mild discomfort after NSV. Severe pain is rare enough that it should prompt a call to the clinician. NSAIDs such as naproxen sodium (Aleve) or ibuprofen (Motrin, Advil) will keep most patients comfortable and may be routinely taken the day of surgery, if there is no sign of active bleeding, and the first day after surgery. They can be continued if the patient is feeling an ache or fullness. Some patients will simply rest easier knowing they have a prescription analgesic medication on hand, should they need it. Narcotics (rarely needed) can supplement, but should not replace antiinflammatory medication, except when the latter is contraindicated.

Most men will do better if they use tight underwear (as opposed to boxer shorts) or a scrotal supporter (jock strap) for a few days. These are often reinforced with gauze or a washcloth to provide more support/pressure.

Activity should be limited. The day of surgery, it is best to relax with the feet up such as in a recliner. It is permissible to go to the bathroom and to the table to eat, but otherwise the feet should be up.

BOX 111.1 No-Scalpel Vasectomy Operative Report

Patient _____

DOB: _____ Date _____

The patient comes in today for a vasectomy. He understands the risks, benefits, and possible complications. He has read over the handouts and viewed the instructional tapes. All questions were answered before the start of the procedure. He does understand that alternative contraceptive choices are available and that vasectomy must be considered a permanent procedure. He has no further questions, and subsequently we proceeded.

Procedure note:

Procedure: Bilateral no-scalpel, no-needle vasectomy.

Surgeon: _____

Assistant: _____

Present in the room: wife, partner, friend, family member

Driver: _____

Anesthesia:

_____ mL of a 50/50 mixture of 2% lidocaine with epinephrine and 1% lidocaine without epinephrine

Or

_____ mL of 2% lidocaine with epinephrine using the MadaJet.

Premedication: 650 mg acetaminophen, valium 10 mg, atropine 0.5 mg

Tolerance (*circle one*): Excellent Good Poor

Estimated blood loss: _____ mL

Complications: None or _____

_____

The patient was laid supine and the anterior scrotum was prepped with alcohol. The left vas was grasped and 0.1 mL of 2% lidocaine with epinephrine was deposited around the vas in the upper scrotum using the MadaJet technique, in the midline. Similarly, a vasal block was carried out on the right. The entire scrotum, penis, and suprapubic and inguinal areas were then prepped with Betadine. Sterile draping was carried out.

Betadine was wiped clear of the scrotum. The left vas was identified, brought to the midline, and isolated with the ring forceps. The skin over the vas was then punctured using the sharp dissecting vas forceps. A small opening was made and the perivasal tissue was stripped clear. The sharp dissecting forceps were then inserted under the vas and the ring clamp removed and replaced through the vas itself for stabilization. Dissection of the perivasal fascia was completed providing 1 to 1.5 cm of vas deferens. The vas was then hemitransected on both sides of the elevated loop. The

proximal and distal ends of the vas were cauterized using the battery cautery unit. The proximal vas (testicular end) was then fully transected and allowed to retract below the fascial tissues. The fascia over the proximal vas was then occluded using a medium metal hemoclip. The clip was placed up to, but not on, the distal vas. This completed a good fascial interposition between the two ends. The distal vas end protruded above the hemoclip. The distal end was then fully transected and the tissues returned to the scrotum. The 1 cm of transected vas was placed in formalin. Good hemostasis was noted. Attention was then turned to the right side where the vas was isolated and brought through the same midline opening. The same technique was carried out. The right vas was confirmed by gently tugging the vas and noting testicular movement on the right.

After completion of the procedure, the scrotum was washed with sterile saline. Good hemostasis was noted at the skin site. Antibiotic ointment was placed over the entry wound and gauze applied. An athletic supporter was placed.

The patient was given postoperative instructions and will watch for signs of infection and report any excessive pain or bleeding. Guidelines for complete rest today with gradual increase in activity were reviewed. Acetaminophen and ibuprofen are to be used for discomfort. Ice is to be applied to the scrotum until the evening. Gauze packing should be used inside the scrotum until the morning. The athletic supporter should be used for at least 48 hours. The patient should refrain from heavy lifting, straining, running, jogging, and sexual activity for 1 week. He is aware that live sperm may be present in the ejaculate for up to 2 months. It was emphasized to use contraception until a negative sperm evaluation at 8 weeks or later shows no sperm. Containers were given to the patient and methods of collection were explained. The patient shall keep the two pieces of transected vas in the medicine cabinet, in the formalin jars, until the two negative semen checks. At that time, he can dispose of them. The patient should call if there are any other problems. Postoperative instruction sheets were also given. Once again, the patient had no further questions.

Changes to procedure: None or _____

_____

Impression: Uncomplicated no-scalpel, no-needle vasectomy

Other instructions: _____

_____

Cc: _____

Clinician: _____

Date: _____

On the first postoperative day the patient may walk around inside the house. A cool shower is acceptable. On the second postoperative day limited activities outside the house, such as going to church, to a movie, or to a restaurant, are permitted. On the third day, most activities can be resumed, except for strenuous ones, such as jogging, riding a bike, weight lifting, and having sex. These should be delayed for a week. Most men can return to work and gradually ease back into their usual activities.

Be sure to reinforce that the patient must use another form of contraceptive until he has a negative semen check at 8 weeks. Samples can be obtained by self-stimulation, collecting secretions from a condom, or withdrawing after intercourse and collecting the ejaculate. It is best to examine the specimen within 2 hours of collection.

A routine telephone call to the patient on the first or second day after the vasectomy can provide valuable reassurance, promote compliance with activity restrictions, and address any questions or concerns that might have arisen on the part of the patient or his partner.

COMPLICATIONS

Minor

Minor complications, causing discomfort and inconvenience, but no serious threat to health, occur in 5% to 10% of vasectomy patients.

- Swelling and discomfort are prevented by routinely using an ice pack, mild analgesic (acetaminophen or ibuprofen), tight underwear, or a tight athletic supporter packed with gauze or a wash cloth, and bed rest. The ice is usually placed over the supporter but may need to be applied directly to the skin if bleeding is suspected.
- Bleeding from the skin incision is normally nil or less than a 3-cm spot on the gauze overnight. Persistent bleeding is controlled with pressure by pinching the skin incision between gauze for 10 minutes.
- Ecchymosis, a purple discoloration, makes the scrotum look bad but is harmless. Careful cautery of any bleeding, especially on the

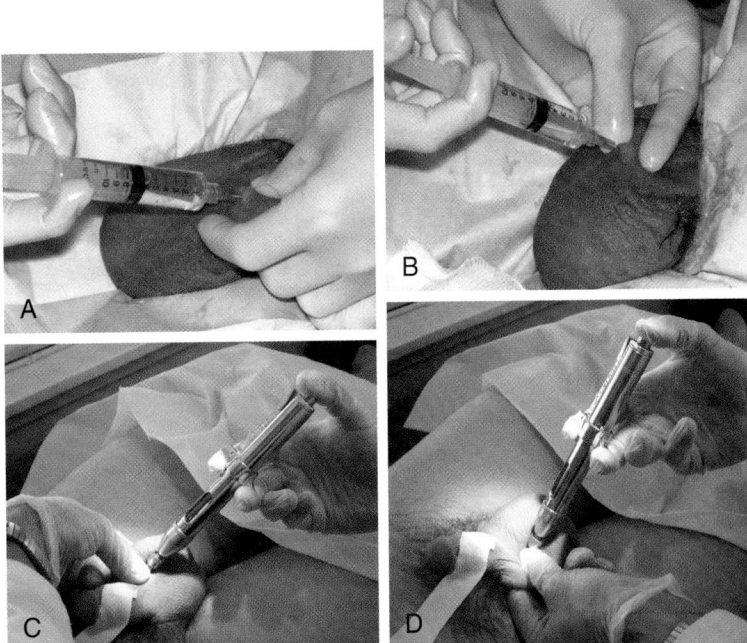

Fig. 111.9 Vasectomy anesthesia: vasal block of left vas (A) and right vas (B). No-needle anesthetic using MadaJet to left vas (C) and right vas (D).

skin margins of the incision, usually prevents it. Ecchymosis may become extensive, involving the entire scrotum, and can extend to the penis and even to the groin and thighs. It may present in the first day or several days later. It will be alarming to the patient, but in the absence of a hematoma (see later discussion), ecchymosis is harmless and usually painless, and results from minor amounts of blood extravasated into the skin or subcutaneous layers. The color may evolve through red, yellow, and green as the blood is resorbed. Prevention is by meticulous hemostasis. Icing the area intermittently during the first day may be effective.

- Superficial wound infection is rare because of the excellent blood supply to the scrotum. A minimal infection responds to local treatment and oral antibiotics. The key to prevention may lie in dissuading the curious patient from touching the wound.
- Skin reaction to the surgical antiseptic solution may present with rash and itching.
- Neuroma is a tender nerve ending buried in scar tissue, where a small sensory nerve was severed or damaged. It is rarely reported after vasectomy and is more often a curiosity than a hindrance to normal activities. A single injection of procaine combined with an equal dose of reassurance can provide a definitive cure.
- Suture rejection can present weeks after vasectomy. Absorbable plain gut suture may prove the least reactive for fascial closure.
- Hemospermia occurs very rarely in the first few months after vasectomy. It clears up spontaneously and has no clinical significance.
- Sperm granuloma is a reaction to sperm leakage into the tissue at the site of the vas division or a rupture in the epididymis. Although such leakage is common, only about 1.5% of patients report finding a tender nodule there. Treatment is an NSAID and reassurance. Rarely, the nodule will require excision or injection with steroids. Abstaining from sexual stimulation in the first week is thought by some to reduce the incidence of sperm leaking from an unhealed vas, but data are lacking on the question. Patients with open-ended vasectomy do not present more frequently with this complaint, suggesting that leakage and scarring are not factors.
- Congestive epididymitis usually presents with a new, unilateral, or occasionally bilateral, tenderness and achy pain localized to the epididymis and radiating to the ipsilateral groin, aggravated by movement. It can occur weeks or years after the procedure. The epididymis feels enlarged and boggy to palpation and may be somewhat tender. It is self-limited, but may linger for 1 to 3 weeks if untreated. It responds within 48 hours to a full regimen of NSAIDs, such as naproxen sodium 1100 mg/day or ibuprofen 800 mg three times a day, and sexual abstinence for 10 to 14 days.
- Postvasectomy pain syndrome is a term applied to various types of chronic pelvic and scrotal pain in men who have previously had a vasectomy. The incidence is low and, in most cases, the symptoms eventually abate spontaneously. Its causation and relationship to vasectomy and to chronic pain that occurs in men without vasectomy are unknown. Management may be enhanced by a supportive, multidisciplinary approach, including urologic evaluation, psychological support, and pain clinic management of medications and therapies (an extremely rare occurrence). Surgery has provided little if any benefit to patients with postvasectomy pain syndrome.
- Persistent sperm in the ejaculate. Depending on the study and technique used, vasectomy failure rates vary from 1/100 to 1/1200. The latter efficacy is usually obtained by using resection of 1 cm of vas, cautery of the ends, and fascial interposition. Most often failure is due to the process of spontaneous recanalization, by which a channel forms between the cut ends of a vas and conducts fresh sperm from the testicle. If recanalization occurs, it generally takes place in the first few weeks after surgery and is detectable by routine semen testing (see later discussion). In half of these cases the channel will close permanently and sperm will disappear from the semen as the scar around the vas matures. However, if motile sperm persist over time, a repeat vasectomy is performed on each vas.
- If a true surgical failure is suspected based on semen analysis, it may be advisable to have the patient produce a specimen in the office before proceeding with repeat vasectomy. However, genetically proven paternity has occurred with men whose semen tests were clear of visualized sperm both before and after impregnation. Couples dealing with unexplained postvasectomy pregnancy should be made aware of such rare possibilities.
- One of the most common causes of persistent sperm in the ejaculate is not having had at least 20 ejaculations before the check. Even then, sperm that may have refluxed into the prostate and seminal vesicles can persist for 8 to 10 weeks or more.

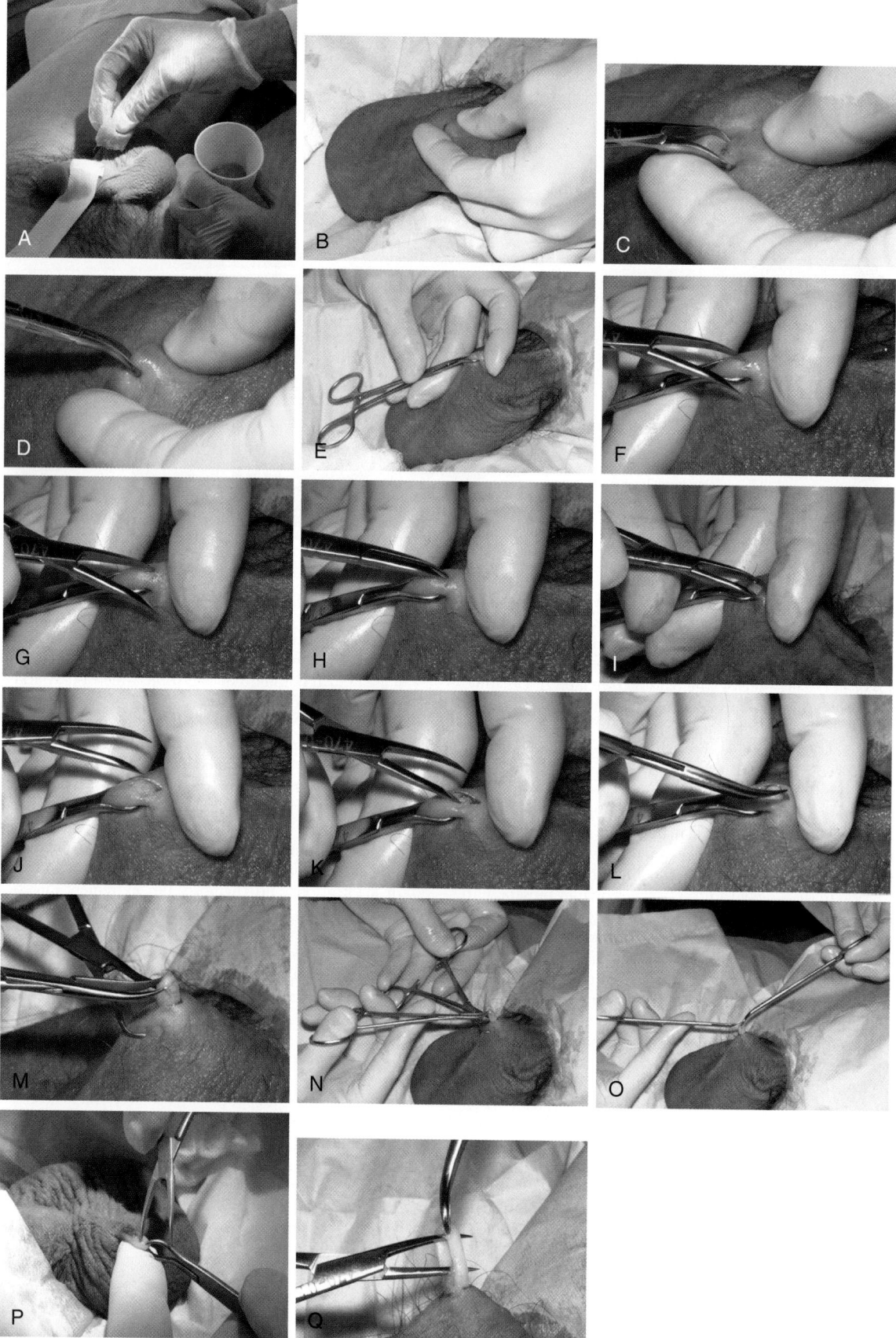

Fig. 111.10 The no-scalpel vasectomy procedure. (A) Warmed chlorhexidine (Hibiclens) preparation. (B) Three-finger grasp of left vas. (C) Straddling left vas with vas-fixing forceps (VFF). (D) Vas is securely fixed in place with the VFF. (E) Regrasping the VFF, the handles are lowered and skin is tensed over the prominent segment of the vas. (F) Sharp dissecting forceps (SDF) poised over vas. (G) SDF tip in the lumen of vas. (H) Both tips now in lumen. (I) Spreading all layers, skin to vas, in one motion. (J–K) The SDF tip is placed into the lumen. (L–M) The hand is rotated palm up, so the SDF tip hooks and delivers the vas. (N) The VFF is unlocked and released. (O) The vas loop is then regrasped. (P) The fascia is sharply dissected from loop. (Q) Fascia is stripped from a bare loop of vas, allowing occlusion to proceed with no bleeding from the plethora of fascial vessels.

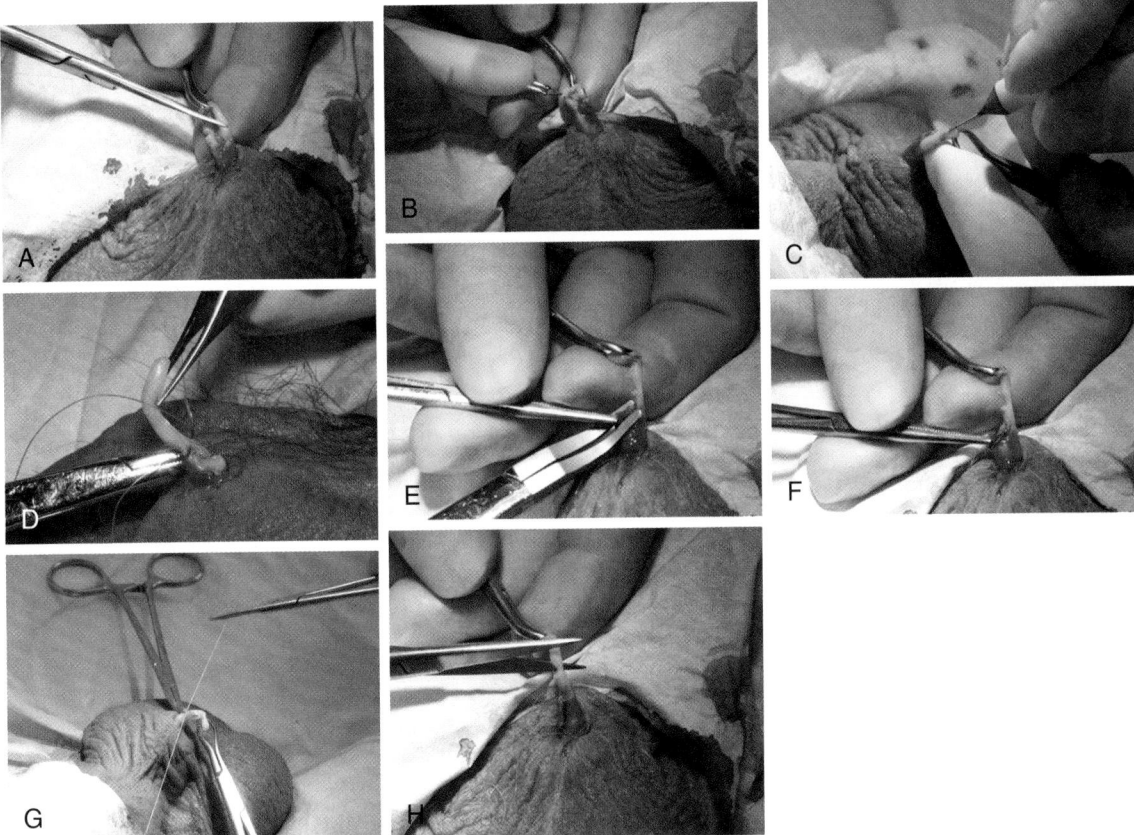

Fig. 111.11 Various occlusion steps. (A) Hemitransecting the vas in two areas approximately 1.5 cm apart. (B) Cauterizing the two ends of the hemitransected vas. (In the open-ended technique, only the prostatic end would be occluded.) Here, a battery cautery unit within a sterile glove is being used. (C) Intraluminal electrocautery. The sharp tip has penetrated the vas wall and 1 cm of the needle electrode lies within the lumen before the current is applied and the electrode is gradually withdrawn. (D) Fascial interposition may be accomplished using a purse-string suture to close the edges of the fascial opening. (E) Here the fascia is approximated with a hemostat, covering over the vas end. A hemoclip is then applied to secure fascial closure. (F) Note the hemoclip does not include the vas. (G) Alternatively, the fascial closure is secured with a free tie. (H) Excising the segment of vas by completing the other hemitransection. (A, B, E, F, and H, Courtesy Jan Drlik, MD, The Medical Procedures Center, Midland, MI.)

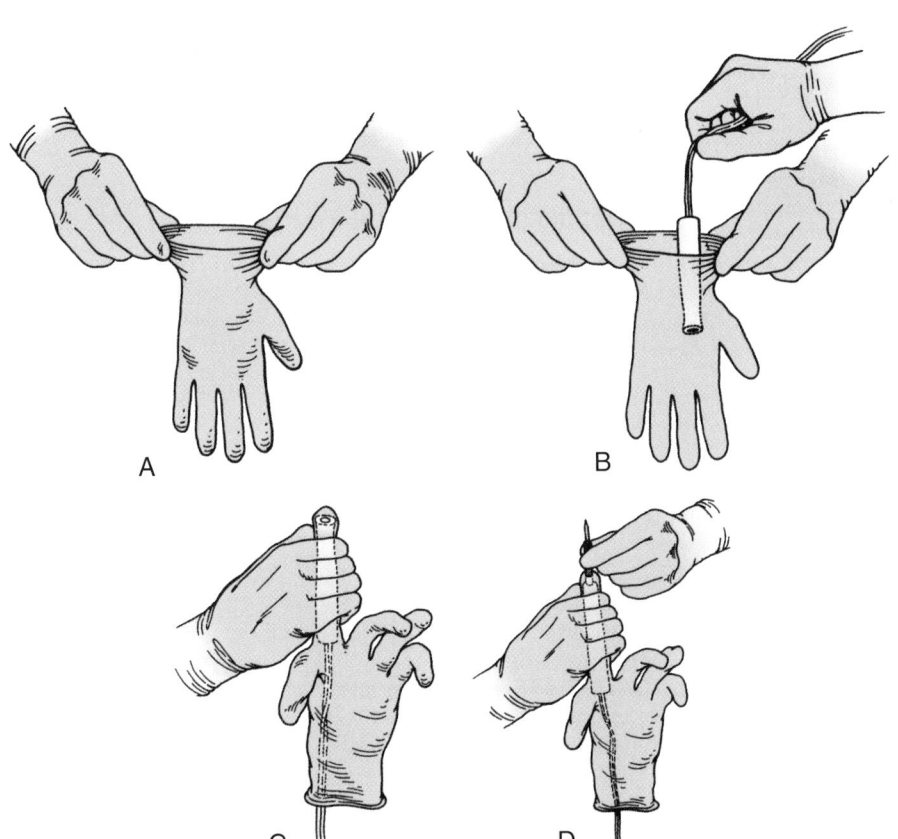

Fig. 111.12 Maintaining a sterile cautery instrument. (A) Gloved clinician holds the sterile glove. (B) Assistant holds the cautery handpiece without the tip by the cord and carefully drops it into a finger of glove. (C) Gloved clinician grasps the cautery handle inside the glove finger. (D) Sterile tip is punctured through rubber glove. The unit can now be handled in a sterile fashion; the clinician is careful not to contaminate the surgical field with the cord. (If it is a battery unit without wire, the unit can be activated so that the tip will burn through the glove to be exposed for use.)

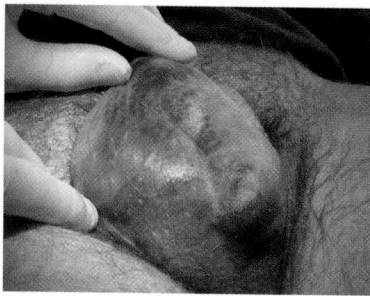

Fig. 111.13 Left hemiscrotal hematoma postvasectomy.

- Misidentification of one or both of the vasa deferentia (very rare) could be detected by submitting excised specimens for histologic examination by a pathologist. This is advisable when any doubt exists at the time of surgery. However, when gross tissue identification is certain, histologic examination is not cost effective and does not provide assurance against failure. The AUA guidelines (2015) state that routine histologic examination is not required.
- Despite hearsay evidence of vasectomies failing because of a third vas deferens, documented cases of supernumerary vasa are extremely rare.
- Prematurely abandoning other contraceptive methods before achieving a clear test can result in pregnancy with a successful vasectomy as well as with a failed vasectomy. If two clear semen checks are obtained (no sperm seen), the incidence of late (secondary) failure is very rare, and pregnancy risk is even lower.

Major

Major complications, which cause temporary disability and require medical or surgical intervention, occur in less than 1% of patients and include scrotal hematoma and infection.

- Hematoma is a mass of blood accumulated in the scrotum from a leaking blood vessel. It is a major concern because the loose connective tissue of the scrotum may allow a hematoma to expand from a few centimeters to the size of a grapefruit (Fig. 111.13). Thus, early (nonsurgical) intervention is critical. It is generally not possible to apply direct pressure on the site of internal bleeding, but the supporter can be packed tight with gauze or a washcloth. Strict bed rest, elevating the scrotum on a folded towel, and applying ice packs intermittently (30 minutes on and 15 to 20 minutes off to prevent injury) will usually stop progression. Attempts at surgical evacuation is usually unwise because clots are not easily extracted and surgical trauma to neurovascular structures may contribute to excess morbidity. Close monitoring for signs of infection is combined with progressive mobilization with scrotal support. Complete resolution may take from several weeks to many months. Prevention is by meticulous surgical hemostasis during the surgery and by limiting patient activity after surgery. With the current NNV methods, patients feel so good after surgery that they tend to overdo it. Proper postoperative rest and care cannot be stressed enough.
- Scrotal infection after vasectomy is a rare but potentially serious complication. AUA guidelines (2015) do not recommend prophylactic antibiotics for vasectomy unless the patient is high risk for infection. That said, fever, chills, redness, warmth, swelling, and induration are signs of infection. Prompt evaluation and early consultation are important. Very localized signs around the incision with an otherwise negative scrotal examination and no systemic symptoms might safely be treated on an outpatient basis with oral antibiotics and warm packs, if careful observation for progressive symptoms and follow-up within 48 hours is ensured. Signs of cellulitis or the presence of systemic symptoms would usually warrant parenteral antibiotics. If fluctuance is detected,

surgical drainage of an abscess should not be delayed. Preexisting skin infections, diabetes mellitus, smoking, prolonged hospitalization, poor nutritional status, and immunodeficiency contribute to risk of infection. Careful attention to sterile techniques is essential to prevention. Also important is reducing tissue trauma in surgery by handling tissues gently, minimizing cautery and suture ligation, and using atraumatic forceps. Early recognition and careful evaluation of symptoms are keys to correct diagnosis. A low threshold for hospitalization and for parenteral antibiotic use to arrest an infection may prove critical to the management of resistant infections.

Regardless of one's surgical skills, some complications cannot be avoided. The most important thing is to be prepared to handle them properly to minimize the adverse effect on your patient.

Be sure patients know to call you if symptoms arise, and ensure that you, or someone equally knowledgeable, are available to take their calls.

Stay in touch, providing open communication that is compassionate, informative, and honest. Even when a consultant is making treatment decisions, be sure to stay involved and obtain information on your patient. Contribute to his care through active listening and ensuring his needs are met. He should know that you care about his recovery. Even a patient who has a good outcome may become resentful and litigious if he feels neglected or uncared for. On the other hand, a patient who has suffered a major complication may advocate for his clinician if he feels genuinely well cared for throughout the experience. Remember, too, the common wisdom that one patient's unhappiness can have widespread repercussions with other men considering vasectomy in the community.

In large, long-term studies of vasectomy, no increase in mortality or incidence of chronic disease, including, among other entities, hypertension, diabetes, autoimmune diseases, cardiovascular diseases, and prostate cancer, has been found. There is no decreased libido or sexual experience. Basically, what is present before the procedure will persist after the procedure. The AUA guidelines (2015) state that clinicians do not need to routinely discuss prostate cancer, coronary artery disease, stroke, hypertension, dementia, or testicular cancer in pre- or postvasectomy counseling because vasectomy is not a risk factor for these conditions.

Studies show that patients are 98% to 99% satisfied with the vasectomy decision. However, some regret having the procedure, either because of the complications discussed previously or the later desire for children.

POSTOPERATIVE SEMEN TESTING

A postoperative semen check is a waived Clinical Laboratory Improvement Amendments test. The AUA guidelines suggest only one postoperative semen check at 8 to 16 weeks and if azoospermia is noted or only rare (<100,000 sperm/mL) nonmotile sperm, and no motile sperm, the procedure has been a success. At this point, the AUA suggests the couple can stop using other methods of contraception. Many experts require two postprocedure semen tests. Because sperm can persist in the ejaculate for many weeks, the first specimen is tested after 8 weeks and the second after 3 months. If recanalization occurs, it most often happens during the first 3 months.

Allow the freshly collected (within 2 hours) semen specimen to stand at room temperature for 30 minutes (or 10 minutes at body temperature) until the viscous mucus component is autolyzed by enzymes in the semen. The clinician places a drop of unspun fresh ejaculate onto a slide (no staining is necessary). The sample is covered with a coverslip and examined under high power (40× magnification) for the presence of live or dead sperm (higher power with oil immersion is not necessary). Fig. 111.14 shows the appearance of many sperm in one high-power field in a failed vasectomy (no sperm should be seen).

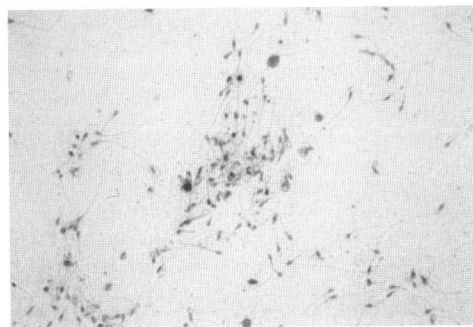

Fig. 111.14 Postoperative semen check: the appearance of sperm in the ejaculate of a failed vasectomy. (Courtesy Nicholas Hruby, MD, Saginaw, MI.)

Some define a positive specimen as having any visualized sperm under high power (unspun specimen). Sequential semen testing in a study of 364 patients showed that a single sample with severe oligospermia (<100,000 sperm/mL) at 12 weeks predicted success of vasectomy with 99.7% accuracy. That would correspond to seeing approximately one sperm per high-power field using the aforementioned technique. However, observing live or motile sperm after 8 weeks suggests that a second specimen should be examined.

The AUA guidelines (2015) define a vasectomy failure when motile sperm are noted at 6 months. If greater than 100,000 nonmotile sperm/mL are noted at 6 months, then trends of repeat sperm counts can be used by the surgeon to decide whether the vasectomy has failed. Factors in deciding whether to repeat the vasectomy when nonmotile spermatozoa are present can include the patient's preference and their tolerance for the risk of pregnancy. Again, if less than 100,000 nonmotile sperm/mL are noted, and no motile sperm, the AUA suggests the couple can stop using other methods of contraception.

NOTE: The author's approach is to require that a single specimen pass an examination of 100 high-power fields with no more than 2 sperm seen (approximately 10,000/mL) and no motile sperm. Specimens are accepted up to 24 hours after collection to improve patient compliance. The editor prefers two samples at 8 and 12 weeks. A few dead sperm are acceptable at 8 weeks but usually are not seen. If any sperm persist at 12 weeks, another sample is requested. Any live sperm after 12 weeks should be regarded as a possible failure. Unprotected intercourse is allowed after the two consecutive negative checks.

An early pregnancy does not mean a failed surgical technique. Pregnancy can occur either because contraception was not used until the sperm were cleared, or because of spontaneous recanalization in spite of the proper technique.

Semen tests are included as part of the vasectomy procedure code (55250) if performed in the clinician's office. (They are separately billable if performed by an independent laboratory.)

REVERSAL

With fully informed consent, patient and partner satisfaction with vasectomy is extremely high. (Rosenfeld and colleagues [1993] showed it is the only contraceptive method with which 100% of women are satisfied. For tubal ligation, the method with next-highest acceptance rate, only 78% of women are satisfied.) Occasionally, however, patients request vasectomy reversal, usually because a new partner wishes to have children. Reversal can be accomplished using either a macroscopic or microscopic approach and results in pregnancy approximately 50% to 80% of the time. The sooner it is reversed, and the longer the testicular remnant of the vas, the better the chances of reversal. Observation of live sperm from the testicular vas end at the time of surgery is another good prognosticator. Although patency is often achieved, the presence of sperm antibodies that persist after reversal can inactivate sperm efficacy to impregnate the egg. Intracytoplasmic sperm injection

can be used, but is much more costly. The use of previously frozen sperm is the least expensive option, if available (see Chapter 110, Sperm Banking).

PATIENT EDUCATION GUIDES

See the following forms available at www.expertconsult.com:

- Patient Consent
- Patient Education
  - Preoperative
  - Postoperative
  - Postsedative
  - Worksheet
- Vasectomy Questionnaire

CPT/BILLING CODES

55250	Vasectomy, unilateral or bilateral (separate procedure), including postoperative semen examination(s)
89321	Semen analysis, presence and/or mobility of sperm (if vasectomy performed elsewhere)
99203	Counseling visit(s), new patient
99214	Counseling visit(s), established patient

Other routine office visit codes can also be used for the counseling sessions.

ICD-10-CM DIAGNOSTIC CODES

Z30.09	Contraceptive management/family planning advice
Z30.09	Sterilization advice
Z30.8	Other specified contraceptive management, postvasectomy sperm count
Z30.49	Contraceptive surveillance, unspecified
Z48.816	Sterilization status (vasectomy)

Acknowledgment

The editors recognize the contributions of George C. Denniston, MD, to this chapter in a previous edition of this text.

SUPPLIERS

(See contact information available at www.expertconsult.com.)

Battery-operated cautery
Advanced Meditech International (AMI)
Ellman
NOTE: Most medical suppliers also carry battery-operated cautery equipment.
Hemoclips and clip applicators
Advanced Meditech International (AMI)
Ethicon, Inc.
Teleflex Pilling Weck
No-needle instruments
Mada Medical, Inc.
No-scalpel instrument suppliers
Advanced Meditech International (AMI)
Integra Miltex, Inc.
Marina Medical (Wilson clamp and dissecting forceps)
Zinnanti Surgical Instruments
Other patient information
Advanced Meditech International (AMI)
EngenderHealth
Teaching models
Advanced Meditech International (AMI)
The National Procedures Institute (NPI)

Technique videos for clinicians
Advanced Meditech International (AMI)
American Academy of Family Physicians
Creative Health Communications
EngenderHealth
Health Sciences Center for Educational Resources, University of Washington
The National Procedures Institute (NPI)

Videos for patient education
Creative Health Communications
EngenderHealth
The National Procedures Institute (NPI)

Written patient education handouts
Advanced Meditech International (AMI)
American Urological Association
EngenderHealth
Krames Communications
Procter & Gamble Pharmaceuticals

ONLINE RESOURCES

www.vasectomy.com: This website provides balanced, well-written information for patients on vasectomy, no-needle vasectomy, and vasectomy reversal. One can locate doctors nearby who provide services.

www.VasectomyMedical.com: An excellent resource on vasectomy and vasectomy reversal that includes clinician directories for providers. This popular site walks the prospective patient through the decision-making process, explaining in simple, understandable language all that should be considered.

RECOMMENDED READING

Alderman PM. Complications in a series of 1224 vasectomies. *J Fam Pract.* 1991;33:579–584.

Alderman PM. Standard incision in non-scalpel vasectomy. *J Fam Pract.* 1999;48:719–721.

Barone MA, Irsula B, Chen-Mok M, Sokal DC. The Investigator Study Group: Effectiveness of vasectomy using cautery. *BMC Urol.* 2004;4:10.

Benger JR. Persistent spermatozoa after vasectomy: a survey of British urologists. *Br J Urol.* 1995;76:376–379.

Denniston GC. The effect of vasectomy on childless men. *J Reprod Med.* 1978;21:151–152.

Denniston GC. Vasectomy by electrocautery: outcomes in a series of 2,500 patients. *J Fam Pract.* 1985;21:35–40.

Denniston GC, Kuehl L. Open-ended vasectomy: approaching the ideal technique. *J Am Board Fam Pract.* 1994;7:285–287.

Edwards IS. Early testing after vasectomy, based on the absence of motile sperm. *Fertil Steril.* 1993;59:431–436.

Errey BB, Edwards IS. Open-ended vasectomy: an assessment. *Fertil Steril.* 1986;45:843–846.

Giovannucci E, Tosteson TD, Speizer FE, et al. A long-term study of mortality in men who have undergone vasectomy. *N Engl J Med.* 1992;326:1392–1398.

Greenberg MJ. Vasectomy technique. *Am Fam Physician.* 1989;39:131–138.

Hartanto VH, Chenven ES, DiPiazza DJ, et al. Fournier gangrene following vasectomy. *Infect Urol.* 2001;14:80–82.

Haws JM, Feigin J. Vasectomy counseling. *Am Fam Physician.* 1995;52:1395–1399.

Hendry WF. Vasectomy and vasectomy reversal. *Br J Urol.* 1994;73:337–344.

Kendrick JS, Gonzales B, Huber DH, et al. Complications of vasectomy in the United States. *J Fam Pract.* 1987;25:245–248.

Labrecque M, Hoang D, Turcot L. Association between the length of the vas deferens excised during vasectomy and the risk of postvasectomy recanalization. *Fertil Steril.* 2003;79:1003–1007.

Labrecque M, Nazerali H, Mondor M, et al. Effectiveness and complications associated with 2 vasectomy occlusion techniques. *J Urol.* 2002;168:2495–2498.

Labrecque M, St-Hilare K, Turcot L. Delayed vasectomy success in men with a first postvasectomy semen analysis showing motile sperm. *Fertil Steril.* 2005;83:1435–1441.

Leslie TA, Illing RO, Cranston DW, Guillebaud J. The incidence of chronic scrotal pain after vasectomy: a prospective audit. *BJU Int.* 2007;100:1330–1333.

Li PS, Li SQ, Schlegel PN, Goldstein M. External spermatic sheath injection for vasal nerve block. *Urology.* 1992;39:173–176.

Li SQ, Goldstein M, Zhu J, Huber D. The no-scalpel vasectomy. *J Urol.* 1991;145:341–344.

Lipshultz LI, Benson GS. Vasectomy—1980. *Urol Clin North Am.* 1980;7:89–105.

McKay W, Morris R, Mushlin P. Sodium bicarbonate attenuates pain on skin infiltration with lidocaine, with or without epinephrine. *Anesth Analg.* 1987;66:572–574.

O'Brien TS, Cranston D, Ashwin P, et al. Temporary reappearance of sperm 12 months after vasectomy clearance. *Br J Urol.* 1995;76:371–372.

Pfenninger JL. Complications of vasectomy. *Am Fam Physician.* 1984a;30:111–115.

Pfenninger JL. Preparation for vasectomy. *Am Fam Physician.* 1984b;30:177–184.

Raspa RF. Complications of vasectomy. *Am Fam Physician.* 1993;48:1264–1268.

Reynolds RD. Vas deferens occlusion during no-scalpel vasectomy. *J Fam Pract.* 1994;39:577–582.

Reynolds RD. Evaluating vasal occlusion methods for vasectomy. *Am Fam Physician.* 2008;78:697.

Rosenfeld JA, Zahorik PM, Saint W, Murphy G. Women's satisfaction with birth control. *J Fam Pract.* 1993;36:169–173.

Schmidt SS. The vas after vasectomy: comparison of cauterization methods. *J Urol.* 1992;40:468–470.

Sharlip ID, Belker AM, Honig S, Labrecque M, Marmar JL, et al. Vasectomy: AUA guidelines. *J Urol.* 2012;188(suppl 6):2482–2491 (amended 2015).

Sokal D, Irsula B, Hays M, et al. Vasectomy by ligation and excision, with or without fascial interposition: a randomized controlled trial. *BMC Med.* 2004;2:6.

Sokal D, Labrecque M. Effectiveness of vasectomy techniques. *Urol Clin North Am.* 2009;36:317–329.

Stockton MD, Davis LE, Bolton KM. No-scalpel vasectomy: a technique for family physicians. *Am Fam Physician.* 1992;46:1153–1167.

Wilson CL. No-needle anesthesia for no-scalpel vasectomy [letter]. *Am Fam Physician.* 2001;63:1295.

Wilson CL. *No-scalpel vasectomy: A self-study program for the family physician.* Videotape/DVD. Leawood, Kan: American Academy of Family Physicians; 2002.

Wilson CL. Re: no-needle jet anesthetic technique for no-scalpel vasectomy [letter]. *J Urol.* 2005;174:1504–1505.

Vasectomy. Procedures for your practice. *Patient Care.* 1991;24:116.

CHAPTER 112

MANUAL TESTICULAR DETORSION

Grant C. Fowler

Testicular torsion is a surgical emergency affecting 1 in 4000 males younger than 25 years annually. It usually has a bimodal distribution in the neonatal period and early teens, often near puberty. However, it can affect an adult or geriatric patient. Treatment is expedient detorsion or surgery. That said, of boys going to surgery for this, it unfortunately results in an orchiectomy in 42%.

Testicular torsion occurs when the vascular supply of the testicle is compromised as a result of the testicle twisting around its axis. This is usually associated with a "bell-clapper" deformity, the result of congenital incomplete fusion of the tunica along the epididymis. As a consequence, the testicle is incompletely attached to the scrotum and remains in a more horizontal suspension in the sac, predisposing to torsion. In the event of torsion, persistent horizontal suspension is often noted on physical examination, along with the absence of a cremasteric reflex. Absence of a cremasteric reflex should prompt the clinician to compare with the contralateral side for confirmation. Conversely, the presence of a cremasteric reflex on the affected side suggests, but does not confirm, the absence of torsion.

If expedient detorsion is not successful, expedient surgery improves outcomes. A meta-analysis of 1140 patients in 22 series demonstrated a greater than 90% salvage rate with surgery within 6 hours of pain onset (Visser and Heyns, 2003). The clinician should keep in mind that the testis may torse, detorse, and retorse; consequently, caution is advised regarding the assignment of an exact time as the time of onset. An incorrect time assignment may result in the incorrect diagnosis of a nonviable testis thereby missing the opportunity for timely and valuable urologic consultation.

Many urologists prefer confirmation of diagnosis with imaging prior to exploratory surgery; however, this is only useful if imaging can be provided expediently while preparing for surgery. As color flow Doppler ultrasound quality and availability has improved, including at the bedside (see Chapter 214, Emergency Department, Hospitalist, and Office Ultrasound [POCUS]), it has become the imaging procedure of choice. However, false negative ultrasound results have been reported. That said, when radionuclide scintigraphy and color flow Doppler ultrasound have been compared, (Nussbaum et al, 2002) similar sensitivity, as well as false-negative rates, for the diagnosis of testicular torsion have been seen. If only plain ultrasound is available, there are other sonographic signs of a torsioned testicle (again, see Chapter 214, Emergency Department, Hospitalist, and Office Ultrasound [POCUS]).

INDICATIONS

- If surgery is not an immediate option
- While awaiting surgery

CONTRAINDICATIONS

- There are no absolute contraindications other than if this procedure will delay surgery.
- If an alternative cause of acute scrotal pain is likely.

- If the testis has become fixed to the scrotal wall.
- If the degree of pain and swelling prevent the examiner from applying firm pressure on the testicle (consider analgesic administration)
- If the testicle has been torsed more than 24 hours, fertility in the contralateral testicle may be better preserved by orchiectomy without detorsion in the affected testicle.

EQUIPMENT AND SUPPLIES

- Nonsterile gloves
- If local anesthetic is to be utilized, a 5- to 10-mL syringe, 25- to 27-gauge needle, 5 to 10 mL of 1% plain lidocaine, antiseptic solution (e.g., povidone iodine, chlorhexidine), and proper equipment to follow universal blood and body fluid precautions
- If available, bedside color flow Doppler ultrasound (also ultrasound gel, warm towels) for assessing pre- and postprocedure intratesticular blood flow

PREPROCEDURE PATIENT EDUCATION AND FORMS

The procedure should be explained to the patient or their representative. Review the patient's medical record. Potential complications include continued pain, increased pain, increased ischemia, or the inability to detorse the testicle. Systemic analgesia or light sedation may be offered, if appropriate (see Chapter 1, Procedural Sedation and Analgesia and Chapter 2, Pediatric Sedation). However, it should be explained that giving medication to reduce the pain may interfere with the ability to determine if the detorsion has been successful. That said, many experts recommend the use of local anesthesia injected into the spermatic cord. Analgesia or anesthesia may help the patient better tolerate the procedure as well as relax the cremasteric response, facilitating the clinician's efforts at detorsion. Risks and benefits of the analgesia, anesthesia, or detorsion procedure and alternatives are discussed with the patient or their representative while obtaining informed consent. The patient should be kept NPO in case detorsion is unsuccessful; emergent operative intervention may be necessary.

TECHNIQUE

1. The patient should be in the supine or semirecumbent position. If the patient is placed in the lithotomy position, it prevents them from retreating due to pain. Universal blood and body fluid precautions should be followed if injections are to be performed.
2. If spermatic cord local anesthetic is to be used, after application of antiseptic solution, grasp the spermatic cord between thumb and index finger of the nondominant hand. Inject 5 to 10 mL directly into the cord from the proximal aspect. This is usually performed at the level of the external inguinal ring. If the cord is not palpable due to swelling or if the testicle is very high-lying, it can usually be palpated as it passes over the pubic tubercle. It can be injected at that level.

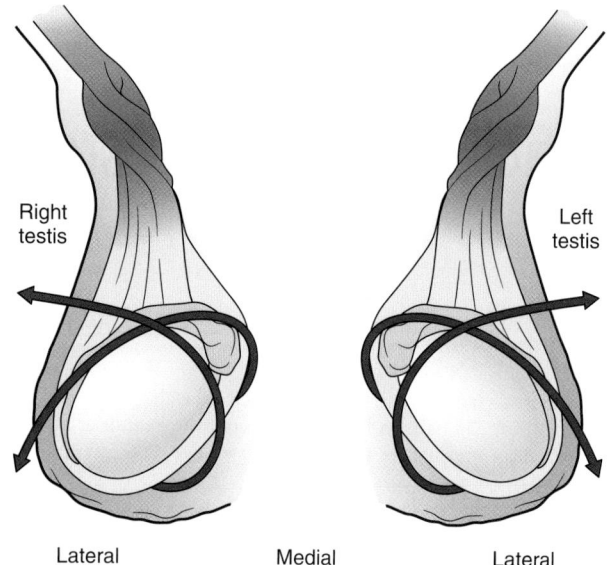

Fig. 112.1 Manual detorsion of a testicle. The *arrows* represent direction that will successfully detorse two-thirds of testicles. Reverse direction is needed in the remaining one-third.

3. To attempt detorsion, if the clinician is right-hand dominant, they should be on the right side of the patient. If left-hand dominant, they should be on the patient's left side.
4. The initial attempt at rotation should be in an outward, medial to lateral direction (correct direction for two-thirds of patients, Fig. 112.1). It is usually described as "detorse as you would open a book." Attempt 180 degrees of rotation.
   EDITOR'S NOTE: A normal testicle should not be adversely affected by a 180-degree rotation; hence, the initial attempt should start with only a 180-degree rotation.
5. If significant resistance is felt, pain increases, or mechanical difficulty is encountered, attempt rotation in the opposite direction (correct direction in one-third of patients).
6. If the initial attempt is successful, more than one rotation may be required; the testicle is often torsed more than 360 degrees (studies suggest a range from 180 to 1080 degrees, median of 360 to 540 degrees). The desired end point is relief of pain and return of intratesticular blood flow on ultrasound. While manual detorsion may re-establish blood flow, it should be kept in mind that even 180 degrees of remaining torsion can still infarct a testicle. Hence, the scrotum should be surgically explored even if the blood flow has been re-established.
   EDITOR'S NOTE: Altered vascular flow patterns and relative hyperemia in a newly revascularized testicle may occasionally obscure color flow Doppler ultrasound results (Kapoor, 2008).
7. Proceed with urologic surgery; the testicle should be pexed permanently with nonabsorbable suture. The other testicle will also likely need to be pexed, and nonabsorbable suture should be utilized.

COMPLICATIONS

- The procedure is painful and if attempts at detorsion are in the wrong direction, it will initially increase the patient's discomfort.
- Anesthetic complications, see appropriate chapters.

POSTPROCEDURE MANAGEMENT AND PATIENT EDUCATION

Whether the manual detorsion effort is successful or not, all patients with testicular torsion should be admitted to the hospital and urology

consulted. If the detorsion is successful, the timing of the operative intervention is changed from emergent to urgent. A bell-clapper deformity is almost always bilateral; consequently, the patient must undergo bilateral orchipexy with permanent suture.

With successful detorsion, systemic analgesics can be provided as needed. The time that it takes for the edema and induration to resolve depends on how long the torsion has been present as well as its severity. Several authors have commented that the edema and induration typically resolve in 3 to 4 hours.

CPT/BILLING CODES

There is no specific CPT code for testicular detorsion.

55899	Unlisted procedure, male genital system

This unspecified code can be attempted or it is possible to code this as an increased acuity of care using office, emergency department, or hospital evaluation and management (E/M) codes. Time is not a descriptive component for the emergency department levels of E/M services.

99354	Prolonged service in the office or other outpatient setting, requiring direct (face-to-face) patient contact beyond the usual service; first hour
99355	Each additional 30 min (list separately in addition to code for prolonged service, 99354)
99356	Prolonged physician service in the inpatient or observation setting, requiring direct (face-to-face) patient contact beyond the usual service first hour
99357	Each additional 30 minutes (list separately in addition to code for prolonged service, 99356)
99358	Prolonged evaluation and management service before and/or after direct (face-to-face) patient care (e.g., review of extensive records and tests, communication with other professionals and/or patient/family); not face-to-face care; first hour
99359	Each additional 30 min (list separately in addition to code for prolonged service, 99358)

ICD-10-CM DIAGNOSTIC CODES

N44.00	Torsion of testis, unspecified

RECOMMENDED READING

Davis JE, Silverman MA. Urologic procedures. In: Roberts JR, Custalow CB, Thomsen TW, eds. *Roberts and Hedges Clinical Procedures in Emergency Medicine and Acute Care*. 7th ed. Philadelphia: Elsevier; 2019:1141–1185.

Go S. Manual testicular detorsion. In: Reichman EF, ed. *Emergency Medicine Procedures*. 2nd ed. New York: McGraw-Hill; 2013:1001–1004.

Kapoor S. Testicular torsion: a race against time. *Int J Clin Pract*. 2008;62(5):821–827.

Nussbaum AR, Bulas D, Shalaby-Rana E, et al. Color Doppler sonography and scintigraphy of the testis: a prospective, comparative analysis in children with acute scrotal pain. *Pediatr Emerg Care*. 2002;18:67–71.

Palmer LS, Palmer JS. Management of abnormalities of the external genitalia in boys. In: Wein AJ, Kavoussi LR, Partin AW, Peters CA, eds. *Campbell-Walsh Urology*. 11th ed. Philadelphia: Elsevier; 2016:3368–3398.

Sharp VJ, Kieran K, Arlen AM. Testicular torsion: diagnosis, evaluation, and management. *Am Fam Physician*. 2013;88(12):835–840.

Visser AJ, Heyns CF. Testicular function after torsion of the spermatic cord. *BJU Int*. 2003;92:200–203.

SECTION 9

Gynecology and Female Reproductive System

Section Editor: DEEPA IYENGAR

CHAPTER 113

PREGNANCY TERMINATION: FIRST-TRIMESTER SUCTION ASPIRATION

Lawrence Leeman • Emily Godfrey

First-trimester surgical termination of pregnancy (suction aspiration) is one of the safest surgical procedures performed in the United States, with 1.2 million procedures performed each year. By the time a woman reaches 45 years of age, approximately one in three will have had an abortion. About half of these are performed at 8 weeks or less in gestational age, and 88% are completed in the first trimester of pregnancy. Although abortion has been legal in all 50 states since the 1973 *Roe v. Wade* Supreme Court decision, many states have imposed laws, such as parental consent for minors, mandatory waiting periods, and compulsory state-directed counseling, that may limit availability of the procedure or discourage a woman from having an abortion. *Therefore, clinicians performing abortion must be aware of any state and local restrictions that govern it.*

Virtually all first-trimester surgical abortions are accomplished with vacuum aspiration. This chapter contains specific information about uterine aspiration using manual vacuum aspiration (MVA) and electric suction abortion in the first trimester. The most commonly used MVA device is a 60-mL syringe with locking valves and a plunger that provides identical suction pressure (26 inches of mercury) as an electric pump until the cylinder reaches approximately 80% capacity. The aspirator can be quickly emptied and reused if more capacity is needed. It is small, portable, and quiet, and thus very practical for a variety of settings, including offices, emergency departments, and hospital-based locations. Although there is still some suction sound, there is no mechanical noise. When MVA and electric suction have been compared in studies, some patients prefer MVA because the sound of electrical suction can be disquieting. Clinicians may prefer MVA for aspiration at early gestational ages because it causes less disruption of the gestational sac, the presence of which confirms a successful aspiration procedure. Electrical suction may be preferred for later first-trimester gestational ages because of the larger amounts of products of conception (POC) and the need for repeat passes if MVA is used.

The suction technique described in this chapter for first-trimester abortion also can be used for surgical completion of spontaneous abortion, including missed and incomplete abortion. Many institutions use operating room settings for the completion of spontaneous abortion. However, in most circumstances, spontaneous abortion treatment can be integrated into outpatient settings. Expectant management to await spontaneous passage of the POC and medical management with misoprostol are also safe options. The highest patient satisfaction is achieved when patients can make their own choice of a management plan. The relative and absolute contraindications to first-trimester abortion would also apply to treatment of spontaneous abortion.

ANATOMY

Anatomic variations can increase the likelihood of complications occurring during uterine aspiration. A vaginal septum may interfere with visualizing and accessing the cervix. Cervical stenosis may

occur and can be caused by prior surgical procedures including loop electrical excision, cryotherapy, and cold knife cone biopsy. Dilation may be more difficult in nulliparous teenagers because of a tight cervical os, particularly at early gestational ages. Mullerian anomalies including uterus didelphys, bicornuate uterus (Fig. 113.1), and an intrauterine septum may interfere with successful uterine aspiration. Intraoperative ultrasonography can facilitate the procedure. Adnexal masses or uterine fibroids may result in inaccurate gestational age dating; fibroids can interfere with cervical dilation.

INDICATIONS

- Elective abortion up to 12 weeks estimated gestational age
- Treatment of early pregnancy failure or spontaneous abortion for uterine sizes up to 12 weeks
- Postabortal hematometra
- Backup for medical abortion (mifepristone/misoprostol or methotrexate/misoprostol; see Chapter 114, Pregnancy Termination: Medication Abortion)

CONTRAINDICATIONS

Medical contraindications are rare. It is important for clinicians to be aware that some clinical scenarios require stabilization before abortion or that the procedure be performed in a hospital setting.

Absolute

Absolute contraindications to first-trimester abortion in an outpatient setting include the following:

- Hemodynamic instability
- Active pelvic infection

Relative

Relative contraindications include the following:

- Uncontrolled hypertension
- Uncontrolled diabetes
- Molar pregnancy (based on gestational age)
- Coagulopathy or patient taking anticoagulants

EQUIPMENT AND SUPPLIES

- Medium Graves speculum (size and type vary based on patient habitus).
- Single-tooth or atraumatic tenaculum.
- Syringe with 22- to 27-gauge, 3-inch spinal needle, or 22- to 27-gauge needle on 3-inch needle extender.

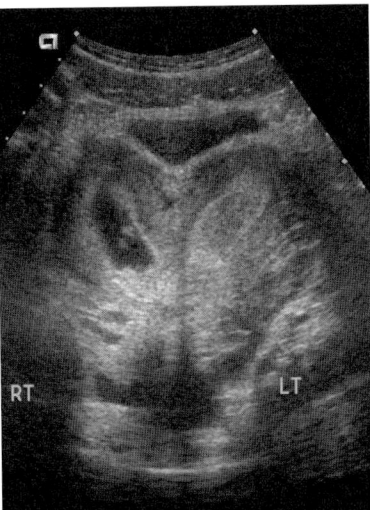

Fig. 113.1 Ultrasound scan of bicornuate uterus with gestational sac in the right horn.

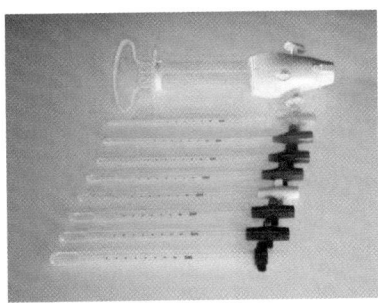

Fig. 113.2 Ipas Plus syringe with flexible plastic cannulas for manual vacuum aspiration. (Courtesy Association of Reproductive Health Professionals, www.arhp.org.)

- Anesthetic agent for cervical block (e.g., 0.5% or 1% lidocaine with epinephrine or vasopressin).
- Rigid cervical dilators for mechanical dilation: Pratt, Hegar, or Denniston (see Chapter 136, Cervical Stenosis and Cervical Dilation).
- Osmotic dilators: Sterilized seaweed stem (*Laminaria japonicum*) available in a variety of sizes (2 to 10 mm); when used, they should be inserted into the cervical os 6 to 18 hours before the procedure (see Chapter 126, Cervical Stenosis and Cervical Dilation).
- Cervical softening agents: misoprostol (prostaglandin E_1 analog), available in 100-µg and 200-µg doses.
- Povidone-iodine, chlorhexidine or other antiseptic solution or sterile water.
- Ring forceps.
- 4 × 4 gauze pads.
- Manual vacuum syringe (Ipas MVA Plus; Fig. 113.2).
- Disposable suction cannulas, which come in a variety of sizes or flexibility, including flexible, semiflexible, or rigid (curved and straight; see Fig. 113.2). It is essential that the clinician identify which cannula produces adequate seal and suction with the type of MVA device that is being used.
- Suction machine with tubing as an alternative to MVA syringe (Fig. 113.3).
- Metal bowl for POC (if using MVA).
- Medium-sharp uterine curette
- Formalin jar (POC may be sent to pathology; however, many physicians performing aspiration abortion examine their own POC)

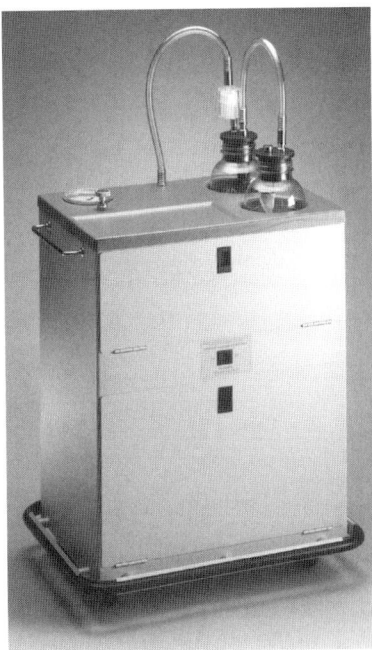

Fig. 113.3 Berkeley Synevac vacuum curettage machine.

- Intravenous (IV) solutions, tubing, and oxytocics (for treatment of excessive bleeding)
- Equipment necessary to follow universal blood and body fluid precautions

PRECAUTIONS

With the availability of portable office ultrasound, pregnancies can be detected at very early gestational ages. In the past, women were frequently asked to defer pregnancy termination until they were at least 7 weeks' gestation, when a change of uterine size can be detected on physical examination and cervical softening occurs naturally. Now that these pregnancies can be verified earlier with ultrasound and cervical softening agents are available, women can routinely be offered uterine aspiration or medical abortion as soon as a gestational sac is identified on transvaginal ultrasonography. Women who present for a first-trimester abortion with a positive urine pregnancy test in whom ultrasound cannot confirm an intrauterine pregnancy can pose a management dilemma. In these cases, an algorithm has been suggested by Creinin and Edwards (Fig. 113.4). Outpatient uterine aspiration under local analgesia with a cervical block works well for most women. Some women, including those with a history of anxiety disorder, substance abuse, or poor tolerance to gynecologic examinations may be best cared for in clinical sites where conscious sedation or general anesthesia is provided. These patients should be identified during options counseling and offered referral to a clinic that can offer a greater range of anesthetic options.

PREPROCEDURE PATIENT EDUCATION

It would be impossible provide a full discussion of counseling here, but several techniques and general principles can be outlined.

1. *Explore the patient's feelings.* This may be done by asking non-judgmental and open-ended questions as well as through active listening. The clinician should empathize and help the patient reflect on her own feelings. Ambivalence should be acknowledged and discussed.
2. *Explore options.* The patient's options regarding her pregnancy include terminating or continuing the pregnancy. If she chooses to continue the pregnancy, she has the additional option of

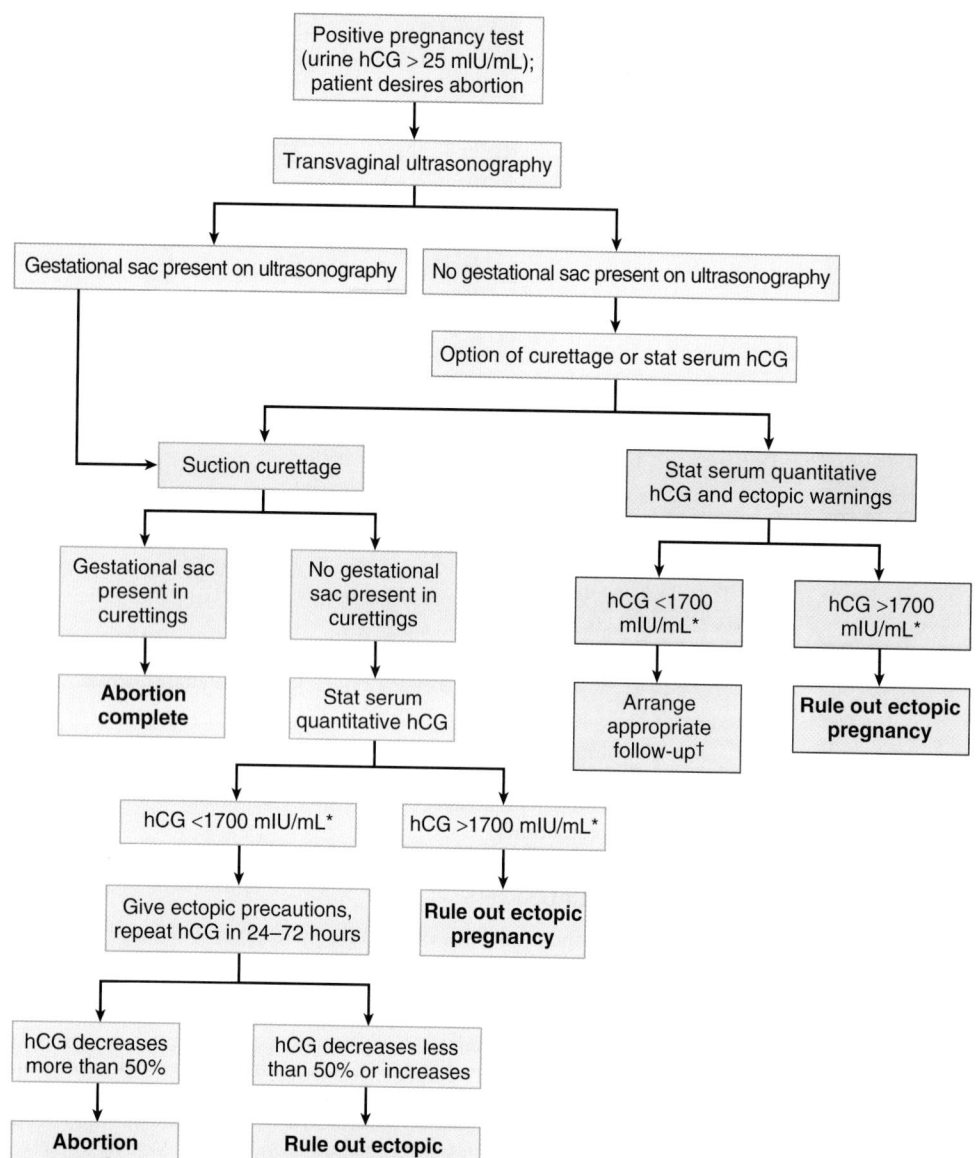

Fig. 113.4 Algorithm for early surgical abortion. hCG, Human chorionic gonadotropin. *Discriminatory zone. †The timing of follow-up serum quantitative hCG test or ultrasonography (or both) may vary according to the patient's risk factors for ectopic pregnancy. (Modified from Creinin MD, Edwards J. Early abortion: surgical and medical options. *Curr Probl Obstet Gynecol Fertil.* 1997;20:1–32.)

parenting or making an adoption plan. The risks, advantages, and disadvantages of each option should be explored in the context of the woman's particular life situation. If she chooses pregnancy termination, appropriate options based on gestational age should be discussed. The option of medication abortion should be discussed.

3. *Make decisions.* Strategies for decision making and the need for any additional counseling may be explored. The patient should be encouraged to seek advice from others she trusts: partner, parents, siblings, friends, teachers, or spiritual counselors. It is imperative that a timetable for decision making be established based on the gestational age.

4. *Screen for special problems.* Extreme anxiety, ambivalence, drug or alcohol use, medical problems, or psychological problems may require special and individualized measures.

5. *Obtain informed consent.* The risks of the procedure must be reviewed and any questions answered. The patient's ability to give informed consent must be reviewed with regard to her age, mental status, and any possibility of coercion. A support person may be present during any procedure.

6. *Consider postprocedure issues.* These include the need for any additional counseling, contraception, follow-up visits, and reporting any complications. Emerging evidence indicates that increasing use of contraceptive implants and intrauterine devices (IUDs) could reduce repeat pregnancy among adolescent mothers and repeat abortions among women seeking induced abortion. IUDs can be inserted immediately after a first-trimester surgical abortion.

7. *Prescribe antibiotics.* The patient should obtain periprocedure antibiotics (doxycycline 100 mg twice daily for 3 days or metronidazole 500 mg orally, twice daily for 2 days). The patient should be offered testing for chlamydia and gonorrhea, but this should not delay the procedure. Empiric treatment of chlamydia may be considered for patients with history, signs, or symptoms of current infection.

PROCEDURE

Before starting the procedure, the following steps must be completed:

1. *Pregnancy must be confirmed.* A home pregnancy test may not have been performed correctly, and therefore it is best to confirm a pregnancy with an in-office urine pregnancy test or ultrasonography demonstrating an intrauterine pregnancy.

2. *Gestational age must be determined.* This can be accomplished by correlating weeks from the last normal menstrual period with a pelvic examination to size the uterus. Abnormal bleeding in pregnancy, contraception use, menstrual irregularities, and poor recall of dates, denial, and even the possibility of falsification may hinder a clinician in calculating an accurate gestational age from historical data. A pelvic examination to size the uterus requires practice and may be complicated when a patient is obese or uncooperative, has uterine fibroids or adnexal masses, or has a retroverted uterus. As a rough guideline, up to the sixth week of pregnancy, the uterus is the size of a plum in nulliparous women and the size of a pear in parous women. By 8 to 9 weeks the uterus is the size of a small orange but is softer and often asymmetrically enlarged. By 10 weeks the uterus is the size of a medium orange. By 12 weeks the uterus is as large as a grapefruit and becomes palpable suprapubically in thin or normal-weight women. A retroverted uterus will pop forward out of the pelvis between 12 and 13 weeks. By 15 or 16 weeks the uterus is the size of a cantaloupe. Ultrasonographic examination is highly accurate in dating a pregnancy, regardless of historical data or results of the physical examination. Ultrasonography also sheds light on several important complications of pregnancy such as first-trimester fetal demise, ectopic pregnancy, and gestational trophoblastic disease, or molar pregnancy. Many clinicians routinely perform a dating ultrasonographic examination before planning abortion by uterine aspiration. Ultrasonography can also be useful during or after the procedure to confirm completion of the procedure. Intraoperative ultrasonographic guidance is recommended for women with uterine anomalies or fibroids. It can also be used if the clinician has difficulty with dilation or uterine aspiration.

3. Perform a *hematocrit or hemoglobin* test if there is a history or clinical suspicion of anemia.

4. *Optional testing,* depending on patient risk factors, the nature of the practice, and financial considerations, includes wet prep, Papanicolaou smear, gonorrhea and chlamydia screening, and blood tests for syphilis and human immunodeficiency virus.

5. *Determine Rh factor status (mandatory).* Rh-negative women who have been pregnant less than 13 weeks should receive a 50-μg dose of D immunoglobulin (MICRhoGAM 50 μg) within 48 hours of the procedure. It is ideally given during the procedure or immediately after. Some give the MICRhoGAM injection intracervically at the anterior lip where the cervical block was placed.

6. *Premedication* is recommended 30 to 60 minutes before the procedure with a nonsteroidal antiinflammatory medication such as ibuprofen 600 to 800 mg orally. Diazepam (5 or 10 mg) or an oral narcotic may be given an hour before the procedure in selected cases.

7. Establishment of an IV line generally is unnecessary in an outpatient setting. Oxytocin, methylergonovine (Methergine), and other injectable drugs must be readily available should an unexpected hemorrhage occur. They can be administered intramuscularly when an IV line is not in place.

8. *Conscious sedation may be offered.* It is important that clinicians be aware of the rules and regulations regarding conscious sedation at their institutions before instituting this level of care. A simple and effective regimen is midazolam (Versed) given IV at the rate of 1 mg/min up to 5 mg, accompanied by fentanyl 50 to 100 μg IV. The patient should be monitored for respiratory depression with a pulse oximeter and frequent vital signs, and a crash cart should be available (see Chapter 1, Procedural Sedation and Analgesia).

9. Atropine 0.4 mg may be given IV or subcutaneously in patients with a history of a vagal reaction to prior cervical manipulations (e.g., bradycardia, fainting/loss of consciousness, diaphoresis, nausea).

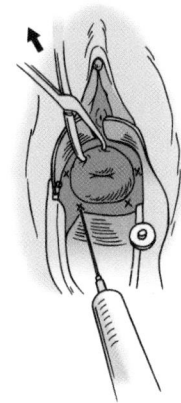

Fig. 113.5 Paracervical block technique. "x" marks the locations where submucosal injections can be made. Ten milliliters of local anesthetic (1% lidocaine or 2% chloroprocaine) are injected with a 22-gauge needle into four sites at the 3, 5, 7, and 9 o'clock positions. (Some clinicians prefer to inject in the 4 and 8 o'clock positions only.) Ideally, the injection should be given submucosally, near the junction of the cervix and vagina. The injection should be superficial enough to raise a bleb or wheal under the mucosa. Because the area is vascular, care must be taken not to inject the anesthetic directly into a vessel. The tenaculum may be used to elevate the cervix and hold it to either side for better exposure of the injection sites.

10. *Prophylactic antibiotics* are a standard of care. A common regimen is doxycycline 100 mg twice daily for 3 days. Metronidazole (500 mg orally, twice daily for 2 days) is an option if the patient is allergic to doxycycline. Special consideration must be given to women with active infections and other very high-risk conditions (see Chapter 69, Antibiotic Prophylaxis).

Initial Steps

1. Position the patient in the dorsal lithotomy position using stirrups. The patient should have her buttocks at or slightly beyond the edge of the table.

2. If not already done, assess the shape, size, and position of the uterus by performing a bimanual examination. The clinician should follow universal blood and body fluid precautions.

3. Remove osmotic dilators, if placed previously.

4. After inserting the speculum, cleanse the cervix with sterile water or other antiseptic solution such as povidone–iodine.

PARACERVICAL BLOCK

1. Paracervical block (see Chapter 153, Paracervical Block, for additional information) is a simple, safe, and effective means of providing local anesthesia for abortion in the office setting (Fig. 113.5). The technique can vary, including the site of injection, the type of anesthetic, and the quantity of solution injected. Most clinicians limit the total amount of 1% lidocaine injected to 20 mL (or 0.5% lidocaine to 40 mL) to avoid lidocaine toxicity.

Cervical Preparation

The cervix may be dilated mechanically with plastic or metal dilators, or with the assistance of preprocedural prostaglandins such as misoprostol. Prostaglandins cause softening and dilation of the cervix as well as some uterine cramping. Misoprostol is the prostaglandin of choice because it is inexpensive, stable at room temperature, and effective in a variety of dosing routes, and has been shown to be effective in first-trimester abortion. Several studies show that misoprostol, given vaginally, is more effective than given orally; buccal and sublingual dosing have also been documented as effective, but they both have more unwanted side effects than the vaginal route.

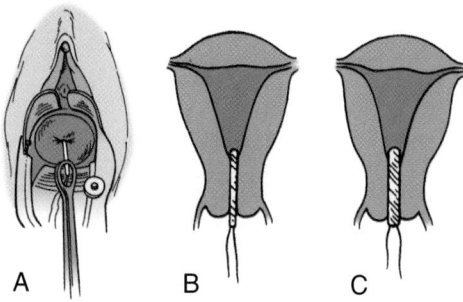

Fig. 113.6 (A) Insertion of the laminaria. (B) Immediately after insertion. (C) Twelve to 24 hours after insertion.

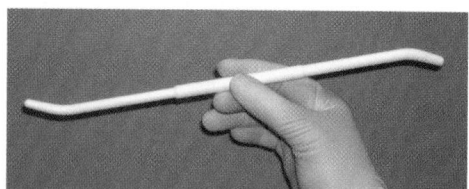

Fig. 113.7 Denniston dilator held using the "no-touch" technique.

Studies examining various doses found that 400 μg (vaginal or sublingual) is most effective and that higher doses were not necessary. Although not well studied, 400 μg by the buccal route is a commonly used alternative. Optimal dosing occurs when misoprostol is given 2 to 4 hours before the procedure; however, administration as late as 1 hour before the procedure can be helpful with cervical softening. Patients commonly experience some cramping and bleeding before the actual surgical procedure with this drug.

Laminaria is an option for dilation but it is less popular because it requires two visits to the office (Fig. 113.6). Some clinicians routinely use misoprostol for all women undergoing uterine aspiration in the outpatient setting regardless of gestational age. Other providers prefer laminaria for primiparous women over 10 to 12 weeks and for multiparous women with an estimated gestational age of 12 weeks or greater. The Society of Family Planning guidelines for first-trimester abortion state that cervical ripening be considered for all adolescents and is recommended for any women at 12 to 14 weeks or if an initial attempt at dilation has been unsuccessful.

"No-Touch" Technique

Bacteria invariably contaminate the vagina and perineum during outpatient uterine aspiration procedures despite attempts at cleansing with povidone-iodine or other preparations. The operator's fingers are likely to become contaminated from the vagina and perineum during the introduction of the speculum despite the use of sterile gloves. The "no-touch" technique is based on the operator not touching the parts of the instruments that will enter the cervix. The dilators are grasped only in their midportion (Fig. 113.7), the cannula tip is not touched, and care is taken to prevent used instruments from contaminating unused instruments.

Mechanical Dilation with Surgical Dilators

1. Apply a single-tooth tenaculum to the anterior or posterior cervical lip.
2. Gradually open the cervix by introducing progressively larger dilators (Fig. 113.8). Hold the dilator with a delicate pencil grip, in the middle of the dilator, using the no-touch technique.
3. Pull gently on the cervix using the tenaculum to straighten out the endocervical canal while moving instruments into the uterus.
4. Apply enough pressure to move the dilator forward through the os and feel for a slight "pop" or giving sensation as the dilator passes through the internal os (see Fig. 113.8). Sometimes this

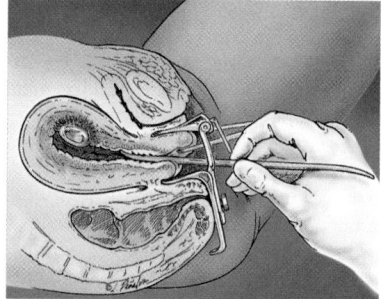

Fig. 113.8 Dilation is needed when the cervical canal will not permit passage of a cannula of the appropriate size. (Courtesy Association of Reproductive Health Professionals, **www.arhp.org**.)

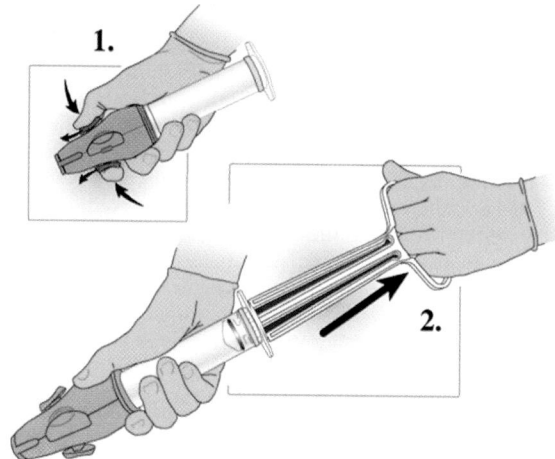

Fig. 113.9 (1) Begin with the valve buttons open and the plunger pushed all the way into the barrel. Close the valve by pushing the buttons down and forward until they lock into place. (2) Pull the plunger back until its arms snap outward over the end of the syringe barrel. Make sure the plunger arms are positioned over the wide edges of the barrel. (Modified courtesy Ipas, www.ipas.org.)

sensation is not present if the patient has already undergone cervical ripening with misoprostol or laminaria.
5. Each dilator should be left in place for a few seconds before going to the next larger one.
6. Dilation is complete when the size of dilator matches the intended size of curette. Many clinicians prefer a cannula size with the millimeter diameter equal to or one size smaller than the gestational age of the patient. For example, if the patient is 9 weeks gestational age, an 8- or 9-mm cannula is used. Most patients experience some cramping during dilation.

Manual Vacuum Aspiration

A key component of MVA is the preparation and use of the syringe (Fig. 113.9).

1. Place the cannula into the cervical os of the uterus (Fig. 113.10). Take care to maintain the no-touch technique by touching only the end of the cannula that attaches to the aspirator, being careful not to touch the tip of the cannula with the hands, the perineum, or the vagina.
2. With the Ipas-type MVA, suction is created by first pushing the buttons on the unit down and forward (see Fig. 113.9).
3. Draw back the plunger using a moderate amount of force to create the vacuum, until the wings of the plunger spring outward over the end of the syringe barrel (see Fig. 113.9). This preserves the vacuum until the valve is opened.

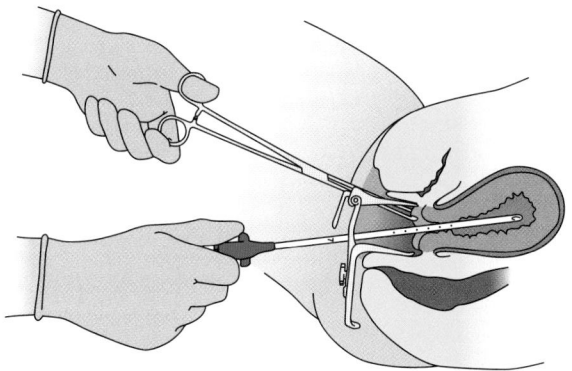

Fig. 113.10 The cannula is inserted through the cervix with traction on the tenaculum to straighten the endocervical canal. (Modified courtesy Ipas, **www.ipas.org**.)

4. Attach the aspirator to the cannula that has been placed into the uterus (Fig. 113.11).
5. Releasing the buttons in a backward direction activates the vacuum (Fig. 113.12).
6. Uterine aspiration is performed by holding the cylinder of the MVA device and using a combination of quick rotation and gentle back-and-forth movements (Fig. 113.13).
7. Watch the tissue that appears in the cannula and MVA cylinder to confirm correct cannula placement. Frequently, clear fluid is noted initially, followed by light tan, "fluffy" material, which is the remnants of the placenta and decidua mixed with blood. The appearance of abnormal tissue (such as omental fat or bowel) in the cannula is a sign of perforation. Absence of tissue is also important to note.
8. Withdraw the cannula and break suction to clear tubing. Empty the contents of the MVA cylinder into a metal bowl or emesis basin. The MVA device is emptied by pushing the plunger down through the cylinder.
9. The cannula can be reinserted into the cervical os, should an additional pass be desired. The MVA device can be recharged and attached to the cannula for additional passes into the uterus for aspiration.
10. Aspiration should be repeated until there is no tissue noted in the cannula or syringe.
11. As the uterus is evacuated, it tends to clamp down, creating a gritty sensation with the cannula. Patients will experience more discomfort at this point.
12. If the abortion is not complete based on clinical or ultrasonographic diagnosis, then a medium-sharp uterine curette can be used to curette and feel all quadrants of the uterine cavity. A clean uterus will have a firm, slightly gritty or rough feel. Additional tissue adherent to the uterine walls feels spongy or slippery. Alternatively, a small ring forceps or stone polyp forceps may be used to grasp within the uterine cavity for any additional tissue. Particular caution should be used to avoid perforation when placing metal instruments into the uterus.
13. If sharp curettage is used, a final pass with the cannula and MVA device should be done to remove any debris or blood.
14. Follow-up transvaginal ultrasonography may be performed immediately after the procedure to demonstrate that the gestational sac and POC have been removed from the uterus.
15. The procedure is now complete. Remove the tenaculum and clean the vagina with gauze and check for signs of bleeding or cervical tears.
16. Once the vaginal check is complete, the speculum should be removed and the perineum should be wiped down to clear any blood or other fluids that may have collected from the procedure.
17. Observe the patient for 10 to 15 minutes for bleeding or any unusual reaction. If sedation or general anesthesia was

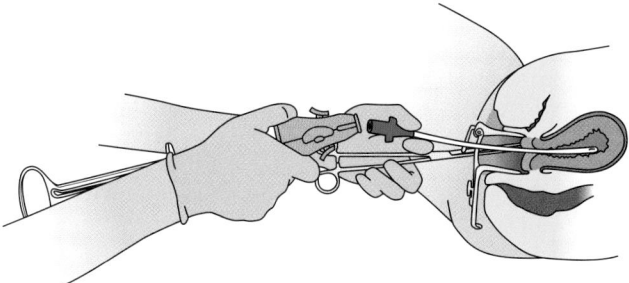

Fig. 113.11 Aspirator is attached to the cannula. Alternatively, the cannula may be attached to the aspirator at the time of initial insertion of the cannula. (Modified courtesy Ipas, **www.ipas.org**.)

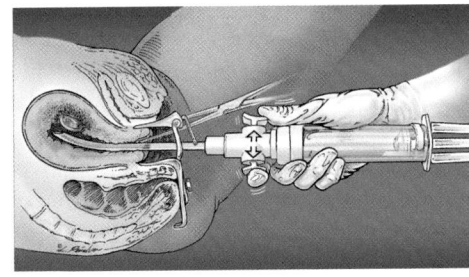

Fig. 113.12 Releasing the pinch valve transfers the vacuum through the cannula to the uterus. (Courtesy Association of Reproductive Health Professionals, **www.arhp.org**.)

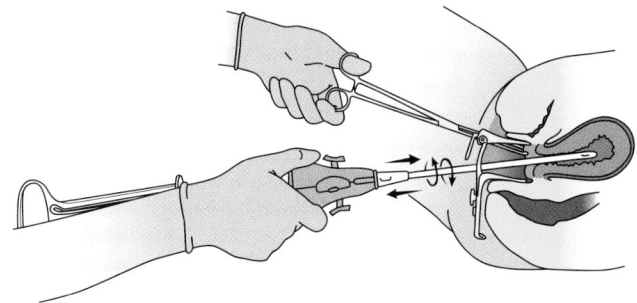

Fig. 113.13 Rotating the syringe moves the cannula gently back and forth. Do not withdraw cannula aperture(s) beyond cervical os. Do not grasp syringe by the plunger arms. Blood, tissue, and bubbles will flow through the cannula into the syringe. (Modified courtesy Ipas, **www.ipas.org**.)

used, follow the appropriate guidelines for postprocedure monitoring.
18. The patient is then free to leave, with appropriate follow-up information (see the sample patient education handout, "Instructions after Termination of Pregnancy," online at www.expertconsult.com).
19. Examine all tissue using the float test to identify POC immediately after the procedure. This step is particularly important in very early abortions, procedures in which scant tissue is obtained, and in patients who are at risk for ectopic pregnancy. The tissue obtained should be washed free of blood with saline or tap water in a strainer. Fragments of tissue can then be suspended in any clear fluid—saline, tap water, and formalin all work—and carefully inspected. Placental tissue has a characteristic "fronding" or finely arborized appearance because of the villi. Backlighting and low-power magnification, with a colposcope or a magnifying glass, for example, is helpful. With a little practice, the gestational sac and placental tissue can be distinguished easily from decidua and clot (Fig. 113.14).
20. In some states, the uterine contents must be sent for confirmation of tissue by a pathologist. It is important that clinicians be aware of the laws in their states.

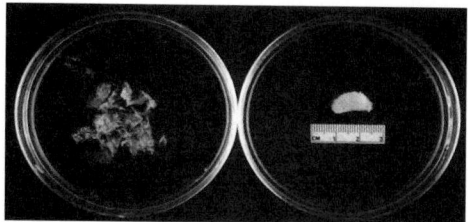

Fig. 113.14 Five-week gestational sac aspirated by electric *(left)* or manual *(right)* vacuum aspiration. Note that the sac appears intact after manual vacuum aspiration. (Courtesy Association of Reproductive Health Professionals, www.arhp.org.)

Suction Abortion (Electrical Pump)

An electrical vacuum pump is the predominant mode of aspiration in many US clinics. Electric power allows for constant flow of suction, which many providers find convenient—particularly for later first-trimester gestations. Rigid disposable plastic cannulas are usually used with machine suction. The disadvantages of machine suction are the cost of the machine itself, which may not be affordable in offices that perform uterine aspiration only periodically, as well as the noise, which may not be acceptable in some clinical settings. Performing uterine aspiration with machine suction is similar to using MVA, except that the machine creates suction with an electrical pump.

1. Attach the suction machine to the cannula by means of the tubing. Do not activate the suction yet. The suction is controlled with the slide control on the handle. It is not necessary to turn the machine on and off. Insert the cannula into the uterus.
2. Close the valve on the handle to create intrauterine suction. A suction pressure of 55 to 75 mm Hg or greater is required to accomplish the procedure. If suction is inadequate, there is probably a leak in the system, which should be identified and corrected.
3. Rotate the handle on the tubing as you would with the MVA, and watch the tissue that appears in the curette and tubing.
4. After several rotations in each direction, remove the curette while the suction is still on. Reinsert it into the uterus with the suction off. Turn the suction back on, rotate, and remove it again, repeating this until no further tissue is seen in the curette. Even with disposable rigid cannulas, the uterus should feel smaller at the end of the procedure and the operator should feel some sense of "grittiness," although not as great as felt when using MVA.
5. Inspect the uterine contents as described in step number 19 under MVA.

SAMPLE PROCEDURE NOTE

The patient presents to clinic today requesting an elective abortion. She is a G**P** with an LMP of (date) and estimated gestational age (weeks). She is Rh+. The patient was counseled on all of her options and she is sure of her decision. The patient was informed of the risks and benefits of the MVA procedure and all questions were answered. The patient was informed about the possibility of perforation, infection, bleeding, pain, and missing some tissue. Diazepam (Valium) 10 mg PO and ibuprofen 800 mg PO were given preoperatively. Patient was taken to the procedure room and placed in the dorsal lithotomy position. Bimanual exam revealed an anteverted uterus measuring about 8 weeks' gestation. Speculum placed without difficulty. Cervix cleansed with povidone-iodine. Approximately 2 mL of 1% lidocaine with epinephrine was injected at the anterior lip. A sharp-tooth tenaculum was placed on the anterior lip. Another 8 mL of lidocaine was injected at the cervicovaginal junction at 4 o'clock and 8 mL placed at 8 o'clock. Cervix was dilated with Dennison dilators to 8 mm. An 8-mm cannula was inserted without difficulty and uterine contents were aspirated without incident. The uterine

cavity was explored with forceps and no residual tissue was found. Tenaculum removed. Minimal bleeding at tenaculum site. Patient tolerated procedure well. No complications. Estimated blood loss = 30 mL.

Gross inspection of the POC revealed villi and gestational sac consistent with 8-week gestation. POC were then placed in sterile urine cup with formalin and sent to pathology.

Patient recovered in procedure room for 20 minutes after procedure. Vital signs were reassessed and were stable, and patient reported minimal cramping. Patient was released to home at (time) and given printed instruction sheets as well as emergency numbers of the clinic. She was also given an oral contraceptive pill prescription to start this evening. (Alternatively, the Copper T 380A IUD was inserted without difficulty.) Patient agreed with plan and verbalized understanding of instructions. Patient is to follow up for a postoperative visit in 1 to 2 weeks or if experiencing any problems whatsoever.

COMMON ERRORS

1. *Poor speculum placement* is a common error that can make the procedure more cumbersome than necessary. A speculum placed too anterior to the cervix elongates and narrows the working space needed to perform the procedure. In addition, it can lead to expulsion of the speculum, which can be problematic, particularly if instruments are already on or in the cervix.
2. *Inadequate traction on the tenaculum* placed on the cervix. Tenaculum traction is essential so the endocervical canal can straighten and decrease the angle between the cervix and the uterine cavity during dilation. This is important to decrease the risk of creating a false passageway or a uterine perforation. Some clinicians fear traction will cause the patient to feel pain or cause the tenaculum to rip away from the cervix. It is important that the tenaculum is placed with a large enough "bite" so that there is adequate tissue to hold it. A vertical placement of the tenaculum through the cervical os often provides a firm purchase on the cervix when it is short.

COMPLICATIONS

Less than 0.5% of women experience a complication during a first-trimester surgical abortion, and the risk of death is about one-tenth that during childbirth. However, complications can and do occur, including those resulting in major disability or even death. Careful attention to technique and constant vigilance for complications are mandatory. Complications may occur before the uterine aspiration procedure (misdiagnosis, problems with laminaria, or problems with a paracervical block), during the process of dilation and aspiration (hemorrhage, uterine perforation, inability to evacuate the uterus), or after the patient has returned home (infection, retained POC, hematometra).

Preprocedure Complications

- *Misdiagnosis* may occur when a woman presenting for a first-trimester abortion procedure has an ectopic pregnancy, a miscarriage, or advanced gestational age. *Ectopic pregnancy* may be suspected when preprocedure ultrasonography does not show a gestational sac with a yolk sac or fetal pole and the float test of the tissue obtained from such a procedure shows only decidua and not the actual POC. In these cases, additional studies, such as ultrasonography and serial quantitative β-human chorionic gonadotropin (hCG) determinations, are indicated.
- *Miscarriage* or early pregnancy failure occurs in about 15% of clinically diagnosed pregnancies. Symptoms include bleeding, cramping, and passage of tissue. Modern means of diagnosing miscarriage in the first trimester include transvaginal ultrasonography and serial quantitative hCG determinations. Patients who are already bleeding may request an abortion and may want to

have uterine aspiration even if a nonviable pregnancy is diagnosed or suspected. Alternatively, a woman may elect to initiate expectant management for miscarriage and defer uterine aspiration.

- *Advanced gestational age* can become a complication if the practitioner initiates a procedure that is beyond his or her training or clinical setting because of inaccurate gestational age dating based on the misinterpretation of ultrasonographic or bimanual examination findings. Adnexal masses or uterine fibroids may render bimanual examination less accurate. Fortunately, this will usually result in an overestimation of gestational age rather than underestimation.
- If laminaria have been placed they may fall out, migrate up into the uterus, or fragment. If the laminaria falls out before dilation is effected, mechanical dilation or replacement of the laminaria will be required. Occasionally, the internal os will be stenotic and the laminaria may assume an hourglass configuration, which makes it difficult to remove because the part of the laminaria that is in the intrauterine space is larger than the narrowed, stenotic os. If migration or fragmentation (a piece breaks off and remains intrauterine) is suspected, a careful search of the uterine cavity must be carried out to remove it. Occasionally, a patient will change her mind after the laminaria has been placed. The laminaria can be removed at any time, and in most cases the pregnancy will continue unaffected. However, the patient must be warned of the risk of miscarriage.
- Some patients may experience a *vasovagal reaction* during laminaria placement or at other times during or after the procedure. Vasovagal reactions involve bradycardia, diaphoresis, nausea, and (rarely) convulsions. Atropine may be administered for treatment and prevention (0.4 mg IV or subcutaneously); the patient's legs should be elevated and her head lowered. If the patient admits to having a low pain threshold or tendency to faint easily, atropine may be given prophylactically 15 to 30 minutes before laminaria placement or the aspiration procedure. Alternatively, atropine may be added to the paracervical block.

Procedural Complications

The minor complications reported in a large review of 170,000 procedural abortions performed at Planned Parenthood clinics included mild infection (incidence, 0.46%); the need for reaspiration (incidence, 0.18%); and a cervical tear (incidence, 0.01%). The overall incidence of these complications was reported as 0.846%.

Complications requiring hospitalization were very rare but included incomplete abortion (incidence, 0.028%); sepsis (incidence, 0.021%); uterine perforation (incidence, 0.009%); and vaginal bleeding (incidence, 0.007%). The overall incidence of these complications was 0.071%. In this review the procedures were performed using an electric vacuum machine and included patients with pregnancies up to 14 weeks gestational age. A recent meta-analysis examined the complication rates of EVA versus MVA for first-trimester procedural abortion and concluded that MVA may be marginally safer.

- The *paracervical block injection can cause some bleeding* at the sites of injection. Intravascular injection is common despite efforts to prevent it. Patients may experience dysphoria, tinnitus, an unusual taste in the mouth, and visual disturbances. These sensations are transient. Severe reactions, such as convulsions or allergic reactions, are rare.
- The clinician may be *unable to successfully dilate the cervix* and enter the uterine cavity. A decision can be made to defer the procedure until after the placement of laminaria or the use of misoprostol for cervical ripening.
- *Uterine fibroids* may prevent or limit access to the uterine cavity. Performing the procedure under ultrasonographic guidance may be the only recourse. *Duplication anomalies of the female genital tract* result from the failure of the uterus to fuse completely during embryonic development; these anomalies range from arcuate uterus to total duplication of the cervix and uterus in uterus didelphys. The critical point in abortion in a woman with a duplicated system is determining the location of the pregnancy and gaining access to it. Rarely, a pregnancy in a hemiuterine horn is inaccessible to surgical evacuation. Mifepristone medical abortion might be the preferred method in women at less than 63 days estimated gestational age with complex uterine anomalies or fibroids preventing easy access to the uterine cavity.
- *Uterine perforation* is an uncommon but feared complication that occurs in less than 1 per 1000 procedures. It is generally asymptomatic if caused during the dilation phase. If it occurs with suctioning, then *the perforation may be* identified by increased pain, hemorrhage, or signs of an acute abdomen. Fat or bowel tissue observed in the suction apparatus is diagnostic, as is passing a blunt instrument up through the perforation. Visualization of the cul de sac by transvaginal or abdominal ultrasonography may point to the possibility of internal bleeding. A culdocentesis is another option to help confirm bleeding (see Chapter 126, Cervical Stenosis and Cervical Dilation). Treatment must be individualized and depends on whether the abortion is complete and whether there is the likelihood of intra-abdominal injury. Minimum treatment includes close observation for 2 to 4 hours or overnight in an inpatient setting. Outpatient observation is reasonable if the perforation did not result in fat or bowel tissue aspiration and there is no abdominal pain or rebound tenderness, or evidence of intra-abdominal bleeding. If the risk of hemorrhage or visceral injury is great, laparoscopy or laparotomy may be necessary. If perforation occurs before the uterus is emptied, the procedure may be completed under laparoscopic guidance.
- *Hemorrhage* occurring during the procedure suggests *laceration* or *perforation* or, more commonly, *uterine atony* with incomplete evacuation of the uterus. Coagulopathy is an uncommon cause of hemorrhage. Lacerations of the cervix can sometimes occur on the ectocervix because of a tenaculum tearing off during the process of cervical dilation. These are usually quite superficial, and bleeding will usually stop with tamponade. Suturing is rarely needed. Puncture sites on the cervix can also bleed briskly and respond to tamponade with the clamping of the ring forceps for a few minutes. Monsel solution or silver nitrate may be applied to achieve hemostasis if bleeding does not resolve with pressure or packing.
- *Atony* occurs infrequently but the risk increases when the pregnancy is greater than 10 weeks gestation. Methylergonovine (Methergine) 0.2 mg intramuscularly or orally may be helpful, and some clinicians use methylergonovine routinely when terminating pregnancies of 8 to 10 weeks and beyond. Misoprostol may be given in an 800-µg dose by rectal or buccal route for atony. Carboprost tromethamine injection (Hemabate; Pharmacia-Upjohn Pharmaceuticals [Pfizer]) given intramuscularly or directly into the cervix is indicated if atony is severe. Retained POC because of incomplete evacuation may be present along with atony. The procedure must be repeated if retained POC are suspected. If bleeding is severe, repeating the procedure may require deeper anesthesia to ensure complete evacuation of all tissue.

Postprocedure Complications

- *Excessive bleeding* in the days or weeks after the abortion suggests incomplete abortion, which may be accompanied by infection. Alternatively, a hematometra may have developed in which blood clots gradually fill the uterine cavity and are unable to easily pass through the cervix. Repeating the procedure is the best course for retained POC or hematometra.
- *Postabortal infection*, or endometritis, is relatively common but not usually severe. Symptoms of endometritis include uterine tenderness, lower abdominal pain, fever, and elevated white

blood cell count. Oral antibiotics may be prescribed; however, repeat suction curettage may be required. Rarely, a patient will have severe sepsis or septic shock and require aggressive treatment, including hospital admission, broad-spectrum IV antibiotics (e.g., gentamicin and clindamycin), fluids, and even hysterectomy.

• Late sequelae, such as *infertility, premature labor, and incompetent cervix*, have been studied extensively and are not thought to be associated with first-trimester aspiration procedures using modern methods. Asherman syndrome is the formation of intrauterine or cervical adhesions after curettage. Because uterine aspiration has replaced curettage as the primary technique of first-trimester abortion Asherman syndrome is a very uncommon complication and usually involves cervical rather than intrauterine adhesions. The cervical adhesions can be treated by using small dilators to reopen the endocervical canal.

POSTPROCEDURE MANAGEMENT

Doxycycline 100 mg orally twice a day for 3 days is recommended as routine surgical prophylaxis, with the first dose given before or soon after the procedure. Methylergonovine 0.2 mg administered orally every 6 hours for six doses is occasionally given to assist in contracting the uterus and preventing bleeding in women having aspiration abortion after 10 to 12 weeks gestational age or experiencing postprocedure bleeding because of uterine atony. If the provider is concerned that the patient may have more bleeding than usual, misoprostol can be given, although the U.S. Food and Drug Administration has not approved its use in this manner. Effective contraception should be offered to the patient and prescribed or provided the same day the abortion is performed. IUDs may be placed immediately after the conclusion of a first-trimester uterine aspiration abortion. Hormonal contraceptives may be started the same day of an abortion procedure.

POSTPROCEDURE PATIENT EDUCATION

No sexual activity is advisable for 1 week. Also see the sample patient education form available at www.expertconsult.com.

INTERPRETATION OF RESULTS

The POC must be examined after the procedure either by the float test or by sending them to a laboratory for pathology. In states that do not require pathologic examination, many operators will defer sending POC for pathologic analysis. If scant tissue is noted or a molar pregnancy is suspected based on ultrasonographic findings or gross review of the POC, evaluation by a pathologist should be considered. If the pathology is read as consistent with a molar or partial molar pregnancy, then appropriate follow-up with a clinician skilled in the management of gestational trophoblastic disease is essential. In addition, a pathology report that notes trophoblastic tissue inconsistent with preprocedural gestational age assessment requires follow-up. The patient should be contacted and reassessed with a repeat bimanual examination, ultrasonography, or serial quantitative hCG determinations, as indicated.

PATIENT EDUCATION GUIDES

See the sample patient education and consent forms available at www.expertconsult.com.

CPT/BILLING CODES

59200   Insertion of cervical dilator (e.g., laminaria, prostaglandin)
59812   Treatment of incomplete abortion, any semester, completed surgically

59820   Treatment of missed abortion, completed surgically, first trimester
59821   Treatment of missed abortion, completed surgically, second trimester
59830   Treatment of septic abortion, completed surgically
59840   Induced abortion, by dilation and curettage
59841   Induced abortion, by dilation and curettage and evacuation
59855   Induced abortion, by one or more vaginal suppositories (e.g., prostaglandin) with or without cervical dilation (e.g., laminaria), including hospital admission and visits, delivery of fetus

ICD-10-CM DIAGNOSTIC CODES

N88.2   Cervical stenosis
O02.1   Abortion, missed
O03.4   Abortion, spontaneous, incomplete
O03.9   Abortion, spontaneous, complete
Z33.2   Abortion, elective
O03.9   Abortion, inevitable
O03.4   Abortion, incomplete
O03.9   Abortion, complete
O20.0   Abortion, threatened, unspecified
O26.20   Abortion, habitual or recurrent

Acknowledgment

The editors recognize the contributions of Steven H. Eisinger, MD, to this chapter in a previous edition of this text.

SUPPLIERS

(See contact information available at www.expertconsult.com.)

All special equipment, including suction machines,* hosing, curettes, dilators, laminaria, and ancillary instruments
   Berkeley Medevices, Inc.
Manual vacuum aspiration syringes
   HPSRx Enterprises, Inc.
   Ipas
Most instruments are available from general medical suppliers or the following sources:
   Cheshire Medical Specialties, Inc.
   Gynex
   MedGyn
   Wallach Surgical Devices, Inc.
Portable ultrasonography
   SonoSite Inc.

ONLINE RESOURCES

Additional Resources for Clinicians

Advancing New Standards in Reproductive Health (ANSIRH), Early Abortion Project: group that has developed training resources for primary care clinicians learning to provide abortion care. Online and downloadable versions of the Early Abortion Training Workbook are available at www.ansirh.org/training/workbook.php.

Association of Reproductive Health Professionals (ARHP) (www.arhp.org): offers up-to-date slide presentations and Internet presentations on the use of MVA for the treatment of miscarriage or induced abortion.

---

*A Gomco suction unit, which many offices have for other purposes, also can be used. The pressure is set between 50 and 60 mm Hg.

Center for Reproductive Health Education In Family Medicine (RHEDI) (www.rhedi.org): dedicated to the goal of integrating high-quality comprehensive abortion and family planning training into U.S. family medicine residency programs.

Ipas (www.ipas.org): provides additional information regarding MVA and electrical aspiration.

National Abortion Federation (NAF) (www.prochoice.org): provides many resources for physicians providing abortion services. Information on surgical abortion services and the NAF Clinical Practice Guidelines is available at www.prochoice.org/education/resources/surgical.html.

Reproductive Health Access Project (www.reproductiveaccess.org). Website includes guidelines, office forms, consents, and other resources for primary care clinicians offering abortion services.

Society of Family Planning (www.societyfp.org): provides evidence-based insight to improve clinical care in the areas of contraception and abortion. Evidence-based clinical guidelines are available.

Counseling Resource for Patients

Exhale (www.4exhale.org): talk line for women to discuss their experience with abortion (available in other languages, including Spanish, Vietnamese, Chinese).

RECOMMENDED READING

Allen R, O'Brien BM. Use of misoprostol in obstetrics and gynecology. *Rev Obstet Gynecol.* 2009;2:159–168.

Allen RH, Goldberg AB. Board of society of family planning: cervical dilation before first trimester surgical abortion (<14 weeks' gestation). *SFP Guideline 2007. Contraception.* 2007;76:139–156.

American College of Obstetricians and Gynecologists. *Antibiotic Prophylaxis for Gynecologic Procedures. ACOG Practice Bulletin No. 104.* Washington DC: ACOG; May 2009.

American College of Obstetricians and Gynecologists. Misoprostol for post-abortion care. ACOG Committee Opinion No. 427. *Obstet Gynecol.* 2009;113:465–468.

Blumenthal PD, Remsburg RE. A time and cost analysis of the management of incomplete abortion with manual vacuum aspiration. *Int J Gynaecol Obstet.* 1994;45:261–267.

Fiala C, Gemzell-Danielssson K, Tang OS, von Hertzen H. Cervical priming with misoprostol prior to transcervical procedures. *Int J Gynaecol Obstet.* 2007;99(suppl 2):S168–S171.

Goldberg AB, Dean G, Kang MS, et al. Manual versus electric vacuum aspiration for early first-trimester abortion: a controlled study of complication rates. *Obstet Gynecol.* 2004;103:101–107.

Keder LM. Best practices in surgical abortion. *Am J Obstet Gynecol.* 2003;189:418–422.

Lichtenberg ES, Shott S. A randomized clinical trial of prophylaxis for vacuum abortion: 3 versus 7 days of doxycycline. *Obstet Gynecol.* 2003;101:726–731.

Lyus RJ, Gianutsos P, Gold M. First trimester procedural abortion in family medicine. *J Am Board Fam Med.* 2009;22:169–174.

Macisaac L, Grossman D, Balistreri E, Darney P. A randomized controlled trial of laminaria, oral misoprostol, and vaginal misoprostol before abortion. *Obstet Gynecol.* 1999;93:766–770.

National Abortion Federation. *Clinical Policy Guidelines.* Washington, DC: National Abortion Federation; 2018. https://prochoice.org/resources/clinical-policy-guidelines/.

Panchal HB, Godfrey EM, Patel A. Buccal misoprostol for cervical ripening prior to first trimester abortion. *Contraception.* 2010;81:161–164.

Paul M, Lichtenberg S, Borgatta L, et al., eds. *Management of Unintended and Abnormal Pregnancy: Comprehensive Abortion Care.* San Francisco: Wiley-Blackwell; 2009.

Goodman S. *Flaxman G, for the TEACH Trainers Collaborative Working Group: Early Abortion Training Workbook.* 5th ed. San Francisco: UCSF Center for Reproductive Health Research & Policy; 2016.

Policar MJ, Pollack AE. *Clinical Training Curriculum in Abortion Practice.* Washington, DC: National Abortion Federation; 1995.

Sawaya GF, Grady D, Kerlikowske K, et al. Antibiotics at time of induced abortion: the case for universal prophylaxis based on a meta-analysis. *Obstet Gynecol.* 1996;87:884–890.

Stubblefield PG, Carr-Ellis S, Borgatta L. Methods for induced abortion. *Obstet Gynecol.* 2004;104:174–185.

Swingle HM, Colaizy TT, Zimmerman MB, Morriss Jr FH. Abortion and the risk of subsequent preterm birth: a systematic review with meta-analysis. *J Reprod Med.* 2009;54:95–108.

CHAPTER 114

PREGNANCY TERMINATION: MEDICATION ABORTION

Ruth Lesnewski • Linda Prine

Medication abortion is the elective termination of a pregnancy using pharmaceuticals. Since 2000, when mifepristone became available in the United States, mifepristone/misoprostol has been the most commonly used medication abortion regimen. Alternate regimens use methotrexate/misoprostol or misoprostol only and are not used as frequently. The US Food and Drug Administration (FDA) recently approved the use of mifepristone for elective termination of pregnancy through 70 days of gestation (previously approved through day 49), which means that approximately twice as many women now qualify. Medication abortion has proven to be remarkably safe and effective; it also provides women with an alternative to surgical abortion.

SELECTING MEDICATION OR SURGICAL ABORTION

Women with unintended pregnancy often present to their primary care provider for pregnancy diagnosis and counseling, treatment, or referral. Clinicians who do not offer abortion in the office can counsel women about the factors influencing selection of medication or aspiration abortion methods. Table 114.1 provides an overview of both methods. Although aspiration abortion is quicker and slightly more effective, medication abortion offers women more privacy, less instrumentation, and a feeling of control over the experience (see Chapter 113, Pregnancy Termination:

First-Trimester Suction Aspiration). Because medication regimens involve cramping and bleeding at home, women who choose medication abortion should have a safe, supportive environment available to them. Women who select medication abortion must agree to return for a follow-up visit and to have an aspiration procedure if the medications fail.

INDICATION

- Elective termination of pregnancy (through 70 days of gestation)

CONTRAINDICATIONS

- Ectopic pregnancy (mifepristone/misoprostol protocols)
- Uncertain gestational age (must establish gestational age before procedure)
- Inherited porphyrias
- History of allergy or anaphylaxis to mifepristone or misoprostol or other prostaglandins
- Chronic adrenal failure
- Severe asthma
- Long-term systemic glucocorticoid therapy
- Intrauterine contraceptive device in place (must be removed before procedure)
- Hemorrhagic disorders, coagulopathy, or the use of anticoagulation therapy

EQUIPMENT AND SUPPLIES

Risk evaluation and mitigation strategy (REMS): The FDA recommends use of REMS to ensure the safe use of Mifeprex (mifepristone). Under the REMS:

- Mifeprex must be ordered, prescribed, and dispensed in clinics, medical offices, and hospitals by or under the supervision of a health care provider who prescribes and meets certain qualifications.
- Health care providers who wish to prescribe Mifeprex must complete a prescriber agreement form prior to ordering and dispensing Mifeprex.
- The health care provider must obtain a signed patient agreement form before dispensing Mifeprex.

Health care providers who prescribe Mifeprex are required under FDA regulations to provide the patient with a copy of the Mifeprex Medication Guide (FDA-approved information for patients; available at www.earlyoptionpill.com). Routine ultrasonography is not required. However, clinicians need access to ultrasonography (either in office or by referral) for women with an uncertain last menstrual period, size/dates discrepancy, or increased risk of ectopic pregnancy.

TABLE 114.1	Comparison of Medication and Aspiration Abortion	
Medication Abortion	**Aspiration Abortion**
Suitable for early pregnancy only	Suitable for early and later pregnancy
Medications only	Surgical procedure
Higher level of patient involvement	Lower level of patient involvement
Abortion may take place in the clinician's office (FDA protocol) or at home (updated protocol)	Occurs in office, clinic, or hospital
Takes two to three visits over several days; sometimes longer	Takes one to two visits; the actual procedure is brief
High success rate (>96%) but some chance of failure	Very high success rate (>98%)
Requires careful patient follow-up	Requires follow-up
Oral pain medication over several hours	Local or intravenous sedation or general anesthesia
Treats missed abortion	Treats missed abortion
Does not treat ectopic pregnancy (mifepristone/misoprostol)	Does not treat ectopic pregnancy
Resembles miscarriage	Surgical procedure
May be more private	Requires office or clinic visits during surgical hours; may be less private

FDA, US Food and Drug Administration.

Preprocedure Patient Education

Patients who undergo mifepristone/misoprostol abortion must read the Medication Guide (see the guide available at www.earlyoptionpill.com/userfiles/file/Med%20Guide%204-22-09%20Final.pdf) produced by Danco Laboratories, mifepristone's sole US manufacturer (see Online Resources). Patients must then sign Danco's Patient Agreement (Fig. 114.1). Clinicians must also provide patients with an office-specific consent form (Fig. 114.2; see also at www.expertconsult.com), which describes the risks, benefits, and possible complications as well as the correct dosing and administration of both mifepristone and misoprostol. After obtaining informed consent, the clinician should have the patient sign the consent form. Clinicians should also carefully review the misoprostol aftercare instructions (Figs. 114.3 and 114.4) with their patients to make sure that they understand the guidelines for administering misoprostol at home and that the practitioner's contact information is clear.

PATIENT AGREEMENT
Mifeprex (mifepristone) Tablets

1. I have read the attached MEDICATION GUIDE for using Mifeprex* and misoprostol to end my pregnancy.
2. I discussed the information with my health care provider.
3. My provider answered all my questions and told me about the risks and benefits of using Mifeprex and misoprostol to end my pregnancy.
4. I believe I am no more than 49 days (7 weeks) pregnant.
5. I understand that I will take Mifeprex in my provider's office (Day 1).
6. I understand that I will take misoprostol in my provider's office two days after I take Mifeprex (Day 3).
7. My provider gave me advice on what to do if I develop heavy bleeding or need emergency care due to the treatment.
8. Bleeding and cramping do not mean that my pregnancy has ended. Therefore, I must return to my provider's office in about 2 weeks (about Day 14) after I take Mifeprex to be sure that my pregnancy has ended and that I am well.
9. I know that, in some cases, the treatment will not work. This happens in about 5 to 8 women out of 100 who use this treatment.
10. I understand that if my pregnancy continues after any part of the treatment, there is a chance that there may be birth defects. If my pregnancy continues after treatment with Mifeprex and misoprostol, I will talk with my provider about my choices, which may include a surgical procedure to end my pregnancy.
11. I understand that if the medicines I take do not end my pregnancy and I decide to have a surgical procedure to end my pregnancy, or if I need a surgical procedure to stop bleeding, my provider will do the procedure or refer me to another provider who will. I have that provider's name, address and phone number.
12. I have my provider's name, address and phone number and know that I can call if I have any questions or concerns.
13. I have decided to take Mifeprex and misoprostol to end my pregnancy and will follow my provider's advice about when to take each drug and what to do in an emergency.
14. I will do the following:
    - Contact my provider right away if in the days after treatment I have a fever of 100.4°F or higher that lasts for more than 4 hours or severe abdominal pain.
    - Contact my provider right away if I have heavy bleeding (soaking through two thick full-size sanitary pads per hour for two consecutive hours).
    - Contact my provider right away if I have abdominal pain or discomfort, or I am "feeling sick," including weakness, nausea, vomiting or diarrhea, more than 24 hours after taking misoprostol.
    - Take the MEDICATION GUIDE with me when I visit an emergency room or a provider who did not give me Mifeprex, so that they will understand that I am having a medical abortion with Mifeprex.
    - Return to my provider's office in 2 days (Day 3) to check if my pregnancy has ended. My provider will give me misoprostol if I am still pregnant.
    - Return to my provider's office about 14 days after beginning treatment to be sure that my pregnancy has ended and that I am well.

Patient Signature: _____
Patient Name (print): _____
Date: _____

The patient signed the PATIENT AGREEMENT in my presence after I counseled her and answered all her questions. I have given her the MEDICATION GUIDE for mifepristone.

Provider's Signature: _____
Name of Provider (print): _____
Date: _____

After the patient and the provider sign this PATIENT AGREEMENT, give 1 copy to the patient before she leaves the office and put 1 copy in her medical record. Give a copy of the MEDICATION GUIDE to the patient.
Rev 2: 7/19/05

*Mifeprex is a registered trademark of Danco Laboratories, LLC.

Fig. 114.1   Patient agreement form. (Courtesy Danco Laboratories, New York, NY.)

Consent for Mifepristone/Misoprostol Abortion

Write your initials before each statement to show that you understand and agree with it.

___ I understand that this consent form differs from the Mifeprex patient agreement.

___ I understand that my three choices for this pregnancy are parenthood, adoption and abortion.

___ "Medication abortion" means an abortion using drugs. A suction abortion uses instruments to empty the uterus or womb. I know that I should not begin a medication abortion unless I am sure that I want to end my pregnancy. I am willing to have a suction abortion if the medication abortion fails.

___ I understand that medication abortion must be done within the first 9 weeks of pregnancy. A physical exam, a blood test and/or an ultrasound exam will be done to confirm the size of my pregnancy.

___ I will take 2 medications. The first is mifepristone, which blocks a hormone needed to continue a pregnancy. I will take a 200 mg dose because research shows this dose is effective. The second drug is misoprostol. It causes the cramps which expel the pregnancy.

___ Before I take these medications, I may have blood tests to check for anemia and to check my Rh type. If I am Rh negative, I will get a shot of MICRhoGAM.

___ I will swallow the mifepristone tablet before I leave the health center. I know that this can cause some nausea and diarrhea, and later cramps.

___ I know that I will take 4 misoprostol tablets home with me.

___ BUCCAL MISOPROSTOL: I will put 2 misoprostol tablets in each cheek no sooner than 24 hours after I swallow the mifepristone, but before 48 hours have passed.

or

___ VAGINAL MISOPROSTOL: I will put 4 misoprostol tablets in my vagina no sooner than 6 hours after I swallow the mifepristone, but before 72 hours have passed.

___ I will receive prescriptions for pain medications.

___ I understand that 1 to 6 hours after I insert the misoprostol, I will have cramping and bleeding. The cramping can be very strong for a few hours, but usually not for more than 24 hours. The bleeding can be quite heavy with clots for a few hours. I may see some pregnancy tissue (usually white or gray in color).
If the heavy bleeding lasts for more than 12 hours, or if I soak more than two maxi pads each hour for two hours in a row, I should call my provider. I know that I should also call if I do NOT bleed within 24 hours of inserting the misoprostol.

___ If I start to feel very ill, I will call the health center. Very rarely, women have had "toxic shock" type illness after a medication abortion.

___ I know that I should return for my one-week check-up to be sure that the abortion is complete. At this visit, an ultrasound or a blood test may be done. If the abortion is not complete, I may need a vacuum aspiration (a suction procedure to empty the uterus) to end the pregnancy.

___ The abortion must be complete because misoprostol can cause serious birth defects if a pregnancy continues.

___ I have read this form and have had time to think about it. I have had all of my questions answered.

___ If a complication occurs, I request and allow the physician to do whatever is necessary to protect my health and welfare.

___ I hereby consent that _____ give me the medications mifepristone and misoprostol for an early medication abortion.

Signature of patient: _____

Date:_____

Witness: _____

Date: _____

Fig. 114.2 Patient consent form.

PROCEDURE

Mifepristone and Misoprostol

Mifepristone is a progestin blocker that causes decidual necrosis. Misoprostol is a prostaglandin analog that causes uterine contraction and expulsion of pregnancy. Mifepristone/misoprostol abortion involves several steps and at least two office visits. The clinician determines—by history, ultrasound, or bimanual sizing with a quantitative human chorionic gonadotropin (hCG) level—that the age of the pregnancy is less than 70 days. After pregnancy dating confirmation, counseling regarding options, selection of method, and completion of the necessary paperwork, the patient can take mifepristone in the office. Danco sought and in March 2016 received a label change on mifepristone dosage from the FDA. The current regimen is to take 200μ of mifepristone in the office followed by buccal administration of four tablets each consisting of 200 μg of misoprostol (total of 800 μg) 24 to 48 hours later at home (Table 114.2). Soon after taking misoprostol, the patient will experience cramping and bleeding. At first the cramps can be quite intense, often requiring a combination of a nonsteroidal anti-inflammatory drug and a mild narcotic to relieve the pain. The bleeding that follows may be heavy, with large clots. The patient should call

---

Medication Abortion (Vaginal Misoprostol) Patient Aftercare Sheet

Today, _____, you took mifepristone to end your pregnancy. You took 200 milligrams of mifepristone at ____am/pm. You may have some vaginal bleeding after taking this pill.

Any time from 6 to 72 hours from now, _____am/pm, you must take another medicine, misoprostol (also called Cytotec). **Choose a time when you have had a good meal and plenty of rest.** Swallow one ibuprofen pill one hour before you take the misoprostol—this will help decrease your cramps. You must take the misoprostol even if you have started to bleed.

Each misoprostol pill is 200 micrograms. **Place 4 misoprostol pills in your vagina.** Lie down for 30 minutes. It's OK if the pills fall out after 30 minutes.

What to expect
Misoprostol causes cramping and bleeding, often with clots. The cramps and bleeding may be much more than you get with a period. The cramps usually start 2 to 4 hours after you insert the pills, and may last for 3 to 5 hours. This heavy bleeding means that the treatment is working. The bleeding often lasts 1 to 2 weeks, and it may stop and start a few times.

You may have a lot of pain or cramps—if so, take pain medicine. You can take ibuprofen (Motrin or Advil) up to 800 milligrams every 8 hours and/or hydrocodone up to 2 pills every 4–6 hours. You can also use a heating pad to relieve the pain. Some women get nausea, diarrhea or chills. This should get better in a few hours.

You should call me if
• Your bleeding soaks through more than 2 maxi pads per hour for 2 hours.
• You do **not** bleed within 24 hours after inserting the misoprostol.
• You start to feel very ill after the heavy cramping and bleeding are over.

To reach me
Call my 24-hour number: _____. If you have any questions or think something is going wrong, call this number and I will call you back. It may take me 10 to 15 minutes to return your call. No question is too small. **Please feel free to call me.**

Follow-up
You have an appointment to come back to my office on _____at _____ am/pm. At this visit I will make sure that the abortion is complete.

Birth control
If you want to use birth control pills, patch, or ring, I have given you a prescription. You should start these on _____, even if you are still bleeding.

Fig. 114.3 Aftercare information for vaginal misoprostol.

her clinician if she bleeds enough to soak through more than two pads per hour for 2 consecutive hours. Cramps and bleeding decrease in intensity after the first few hours but can persist in a milder form for 3 weeks or more. Bleeding sometimes lasts long enough to blend into the woman's next menstrual period.

Rh-negative women should receive Rh immune globulin. A 50-μg dose (MICRhoGAM) should be given before using misoprostol or within 72 hours of bleeding. Patients should be informed that this medication is a human blood derivative. Patients who refuse the injection should sign a statement documenting their decision.

Four to 14 days after the initial visit, the patient returns for follow-up. At this visit, the clinician confirms the procedure's success by history and by either repeating the ultrasound examination or repeating the hCG test (depending on which was done at the initial visit). The clinician also revisits the woman's choice of an ongoing contraceptive method. If the hCG test is repeated, it will drop by 75% from the previous week, indicating the success of the medication abortion. New changes in the legislation, which may differ in each state (check with your state jurisdiction authorities), have eliminated the need for unnecessary follow-up visits and exams in order to simplify the process of ensuring abortion completion. The use of low-cost and self-administered home pregnancy tests and symptom checks—via telemedicine communication with the provider—has been approved in some states to confirm the completion of medical abortion in lieu of a follow-up office visit. Legislative challenges to evidence-based medical abortion practice still persist, making access to these services difficult.

Methotrexate and Misoprostol and Misoprostol-Only Regimens

Of the three most commonly used medication abortion regimens, mifepristone/misoprostol has the highest efficacy and best side-effect profile. Methotrexate/misoprostol, used in the United States before mifepristone's release, works over weeks rather than days, requires multiple office visits, and can be used only in pregnancies of less than 8 weeks' gestation. Methotrexate has the advantage of treating early ectopic pregnancy, whereas mifepristone and misoprostol regimens do *not* terminate ectopic pregnancies. Misoprostol-only regimens require several doses, each with significant side effects. This regimen has widespread lay use in countries where abortion remains legally restricted or is too expensive.

SAMPLE PROCEDURE NOTES

See Initial Visit Note and Follow-up Visit Note (Figs. 114.5 and 114.6) for examples of documentation for the mifepristone/misoprostol regimen.

COMPLICATIONS

Mifepristone causes far fewer side effects than misoprostol. Misoprostol's side effects include nausea, vomiting, fever, chills, and uterine cramping. Vaginal or buccal administration causes fewer side effects than oral administration. Misoprostol is believed to be a teratogen

Medication Abortion (Buccal Misoprostol) Patient Aftercare Sheet

Today, _____, you took mifepristone to end your pregnancy. You took 200 milligrams of mifepristone at ____am/pm. You may have some vaginal bleeding after taking this pill.

Any time from 12 to 48 hours from now, _____am/pm, you must take another medicine, misoprostol (also called Cytotec). **Choose a time when you have had a good meal and plenty of rest.** Swallow one ibuprofen pill one hour before you take the misoprostol—this will help decrease your cramps. You must take the misoprostol even if you have started to bleed.

Each misoprostol pill is 200 micrograms. **Place 2 misoprostol pills in each cheek.** Leave them in your cheeks for 30 minutes. After 30 minutes, swallow the pills with water.

What to expect
Misoprostol causes cramping and bleeding, often with clots. The cramps and bleeding may be much more than you get with a period. The cramps usually start 2 to 4 hours after you insert the pills, and may last for 3 to 5 hours. This heavy bleeding means that the treatment is working. The bleeding often lasts 1 to 2 weeks, and it may stop and start a few times.

You may have a lot of pain or cramps—if so, take pain medicine. You can take ibuprofen (Motrin or Advil) up to 800 milligrams every 8 hours and/or hydrocodone up to 2 pills every 4–6 hours. You can also use a heating pad to relieve the pain. Some women get nausea, diarrhea or chills. This should get better in a few hours.

You **should** call me if
• Your bleeding soaks through more than 2 maxi pads per hour for 2 hours.
• You do **not** bleed within 24 hours after taking the misoprostol.
• You start to feel very ill after the heavy cramping and bleeding are over.

To reach me
Call my 24-hour number: _____. If you have any questions or think something is going wrong, call this number and I will call you back. It may take me 10 to 15 minutes to return your call. No question is too small. **Please feel free to call me.**

Follow-up
You have an appointment to come back to my office on _____at _____ am/pm. At this visit I will make sure that the abortion is complete.

Birth control
If you want to use birth control pills, patch, or ring, I have given you a prescription. You should start these on _____, even if you are still bleeding.

Fig. 114.4 Aftercare information for buccal misoprostol.

TABLE 114.2 Medication Abortion Protocol Comparison

Protocol	FDA Regimen	Updated Regimen Vaginal Misoprostol	Buccal Misoprostol
Maximal gestational age	49 days from LMP	63 days from LMP	63 days from LMP
Mifepristone dose	600 mg orally in office	200 mg orally in office	200 mg orally in office
Misoprostol dose	400 µg orally (2 tablets)	800 µg vaginally (4 tablets)	800 µg buccally (4 tablets)
Misoprostol timing	48 hr after mifepristone	6–72 hr after mifepristone	24–36 hr after mifepristone
Misoprostol location	Clinician's office	Home	Home
Follow-up visit	14 days after mifepristone	4–14 days after mifepristone	4–14 days after mifepristone
Minimal number of office visits	Three	Two	Two
Cost	Higher	Lower	Lower

FDA, US Food and Drug Administration; *LMP,* last menstrual period.

when administered in early pregnancy if abortion should fail to occur.

Although all are uncommon, the major complications of mifepristone/misoprostol abortion are continuation of the pregnancy, retained products of conception, heavy bleeding, and infection. Continuation of pregnancy may occur slightly more often with later gestational age. Overall, the rate of continuing pregnancy is under 1%. Incomplete abortion—that is, failure to expel all pregnancy tissue with medications alone—occurs in 0.6% to 3% of women. The rate depends in part on clinicians' and patients' threshold for resorting to an aspiration procedure. Cramping and bleeding are expected

with medication abortion, but bleeding heavy enough to require emergency care (or heavy enough to require transfusion) occurs in fewer than 0.1% of patients. The treatment for continuing pregnancy, retained products of conception, and heavy bleeding is the same: a uterine aspiration procedure.

Endometritis after medication abortion is extremely rare. The rate varies from 0.09% to 0.5%, and treatment requires broad-spectrum antibiotics. Over the past few years, five North American women have died because of toxic shock after mifepristone/misoprostol abortion. Four of these deaths were associated with the pathogen *Clostridium sordellii.* The death rate associated

---

Medication Abortion Initial Visit Note

Subjective:

_____ is here with an unintended pregnancy. We fully discussed all of her options. The patient has indicated that this is not a good time for her to become a parent and would like to end the pregnancy. The options, including medication abortion, suction abortion with local anesthesia, and referral for suction abortion under general anesthesia, were discussed. She has chosen a medication abortion with mifepristone and misoprostol.

Past Medical History:

Past Surgical History:

G___P___

Her obstetric and gynecologic history is _____. Her prior methods of contraception: _____.

She ❏ IS   ❏ IS NOT in a safe situation at home and ❏ DOES   ❏ DOES NOT   describe a situation that might be high risk for abuse.

The patient ❏ DOES   ❏ DOES NOT   meet the following criteria: There is no IUD in place, she is not allergic to prostaglandins/mifepristone, there is no chronic adrenal failure, no long-term systemic corticosteroid use, no concurrent anticoagulant therapy, and no hemorrhagic disorders.

Rh status: ___

Physical examination
Vital signs:

General appearance: _____

Uterus: ___ weeks size

ULTRASOUND (limited study for the purpose of determining gestational age):
Performed: ❏ YES   ❏ NO   ❏ Not applicable
Gestational sac: ❏ YES   ❏ NO   ❏ Not applicable
Yolk sac: ❏ YES   ❏ NO   ❏ Not applicable
Crown–rump: ❏ YES   ❏ NO   ❏ Not applicable, ___mm
Gestational age: _____ days by ultrasound

Assessment
_____ is a good candidate for medical abortion with a pregnancy at less than 63 days gestational age. She has no medical contraindications. She understands the protocol and possible side effects, the need for a follow-up visit, and the need for a suction procedure if the medical abortion fails. She knows how to contact me in case of an emergency.

Plan
Mifeprex medication guide given: ❏ YES   ❏ NO
Mifeprex provider / patient agreement signed: ❏ YES   ❏ NO
Updated consent form signed: ❏ YES   ❏ NO
Pain medication prescribed as per orders.
Mifeprex lot number recorded: by nursing, see nursing note.
Dispensed 4 tablets of misoprostol (200 mcg each) for home use.
Patient information sheet given; this sheet details the self-insertion of the misoprostol and the expected bleeding patterns.
RhoGAM given: ❏ YES   ❏ NO   ❏ Not applicable
The certificate of induced termination was sent to the health department   ❏ YES   ❏ NO   ❏ Not applicable
The sonogram (if done) is to be scanned into the record along with the Mifeprex and alternative consent form.
She has chosen _____ as her ongoing contraceptive method and has been instructed on when to begin this method. (OCP users to start one or two days after the insertion of the misoprostol)

Quantitative hCG level ordered: ❏ YES   ❏ NO
Follow-up visit scheduled in approximately 1–2 weeks

Fig. 114.5 Procedure note for initial visit. *IUD*, Intrauterine device.

with medication abortion remains exceedingly low—under 1 in 100,000—and very little is known about the risk factors for C. *sordelli* infection. However, after these deaths, many clinicians began to advise buccal rather than vaginal administration of misoprostol.

POSTPROCEDURE MANAGEMENT AND EDUCATION

The mifepristone aftercare instruction sheets explain misoprostol administration, use of pain medications, and initiation of contraception (see Figs. 114.3 and 114.4).

Medication Abortion Follow-up Visit Note

_____ presents for follow-up after medical abortion.
Within 24 hours after taking misoprostol, she had cramping and bleeding.
Bleeding now reported as: _____
She has no symptoms of pregnancy.

Objective
Vital signs:
General appearance:
Ultrasound (if done) shows absence of gestational sac and thickening of the endometrial lining:
❑ YES   ❑ NO   ❑ Not applicable

Assessment
Abortion completion assessed by:
History: ❑ YES   ❑ NO
Sonogram: ❑ YES   ❑ NO   ❑ Not applicable

Plan
Contraception plan reviewed: ❑ YES   ❑ NO
Repeat hCG level ordered: ❑ YES   ❑ NO   ❑ Not applicable
Discussed duration of bleeding and potential complications.
No restrictions on activity.

Fig. 114.6 Procedure note for subsequent visit. *hCG,* Human chorionic gonadotropin.

PATIENT EDUCATION GUIDES

See the medication guide for Mifeprex at www.earlyoptionpill.com/userfiles/file/Med%20Guide%204-22-09%20Final.pdf.

See the consent form available at www.expertconsult.com. See Figs. 114.1 through 114.4 for patient information.

CPT/BILLING CODES

Visit 1

The first visit includes verification of pregnancy and pregnancy date, counseling, and administration of mifepristone.

CPT 99204 or 99214	Level 4 new or established patient E/M visit
J8499	Prescription drug, oral, nonchemo, not otherwise specified *Or*
J3490	Unclassified drug

If J codes are not accepted by insurance carrier, use 99070 (a cost-of-materials CPT code) or S0190 for mifepristone. *Each insurance carrier may reimburse for mifepristone using a different code.* The name of the drug (mifepristone), the dosage (200 mg), and the 11-digit national drug code from the drug package must accompany this claim. In addition, submit a copy of the drug invoice to show the cost of the drug.

76815	Limited ultrasound, pregnant uterus *or*
76817	Transvaginal ultrasound, pregnant uterus

In addition, submit codes for appropriate laboratory tests or MICRhoGAM (90385) if done in office.

Visit 2

The second visit is to verify that the pregnancy has ended.

CPT 99213 or 99214	Level 3 or 4 E/M visit for established patient
76817 or 76815	Ultrasound

ICD-10-CM DIAGNOSTIC CODES

Z33.2	Legally induced abortion without mention of complication, complete

ONLINE RESOURCES

Association of Reproductive Health Professionals (www.arhp.org): resource for clinical education in reproductive health topics.
Center for Reproductive Health Education in Family Medicine (www.rhedi.org): resource for family medicine residency programs expanding their reproductive health education and services.
Gynuity Health Projects (www.gynuity.org): research and technical assistance organization.
Mifepristone information (Danco Laboratories): www.earlyoptionpill.com.
Mifepristone medication guide: www.earlyoptionpill.com/userfiles/file/Med%20Guide%204-22-09%20Final.pdf.
National Abortion Federation (www.prochoice.org): medication abortion information.
Reproductive Health Access Project (www.reproductiveaccess.org): resource for community family physicians offering medication abortion.

RECOMMENDED READING

American College of Obstetricians and Gynecologists. Medical Management of Abortion. *ACOG Practice Bulletin No. 143.* 2014. Reaffirmed 2016 http://www.acog.org/Womens-Health/Abortion/.
American College of Obstetricians and Gynecologists. ACOG Committee Opinion no. 450: increasing use of contraceptive implants and intrauterine devices to reduce unintended pregnancy. *Obstet Gynecol.* 2009;114:1434–1438.
Blanchard K, Shochet T, Coyaji K, et al. Misoprostol alone for early abortion: an evaluation of seven potential regimens. *Contraception.* 2005;72:91–97.
Borgatta L, Burnhill MS, Tyson J, et al. Early medical abortion with methotrexate and misoprostol. *Obstet Gynecol.* 2001;97:11–16.
Creinin MD. Medical abortion regimens: historical context and overview. *Am J Obstet Gynecol.* 2000;183(suppl 2):S3–S9.
Jones RK, Boonstra HD. *The Public Health Implications of the FDA Update to the Medication Abortion Label.* https://www.guttmacher.org/article/2016-/06/public-health-implications-fda-update-medication-abortion-label/.
Kulier R, Kapp N, Gülmezoglu AM, et al. Medical methods for first trimester abortion. *Cochrane Database Syst Rev.* 2011;(4):CD002855.
Swingle HM, Colaizy TT, Zimmerman MB, Morriss Jr FH. Abortion and the risk of subsequent preterm birth: a systematic review with meta-analysis. *J Reprod Med.* 2009;54:95–108.

CHAPTER 115

EMERGENCY CONTRACEPTION

Steven H. Eisinger • Eric A. Smith

Emergency contraception (EC) is treatment intended for women who have had unprotected intercourse and wish to avoid pregnancy. Ingestion of high doses of sex steroids administered within 120 hours of exposure is known to prevent pregnancy. The mechanism remains unclear but appears to involve either the inhibition or delay of ovulation. Some regard this as a form of abortion, but others believe that abortion occurs only after implantation. Evidence suggests that EC cannot prevent the implantation of a fertilized ovum and hence is not an abortifacient. Current commercially available medical EC taken by an already pregnant patient does not interrupt the pregnancy and there is no proven harm to the developing fetus. Three types of oral EC are currently available in the United States: a progestin-only pill, an antiprogestin pill (ulipristal acetate), and combined estrogen/progestin pills.

Lack of knowledge of EC, lack of knowledge that EC is not an abortifacient, and lack of access appear to be the major barriers to the provision of EC. Both clinicians and patients are often unaware of the possibility of EC. Critical delays in treatment may occur when clinicians require an office visit before prescribing or the patient has to search for a pharmacy that carries the prescription. Even though there may still be efficacy with a delay up to 120 hours, efficacy tends to decrease over time, as discussed later. For these reasons, the American College of Obstetricians and Gynecologists has advocated the practice of discussing EC with all patients who are sexually active and at risk for a contraceptive failure. In the primary care setting, this should include both female and male patients of reproductive age. Telephone prescribing appears to be safe.

The cost of EC varies from $21 to $50 retail. Availability has been sporadic in the past. Indeed, the excellent safety profile of the progestin-only method led the US Food and Drug Administration (FDA) to approve Plan B (Duramed Teva Pharmaceuticals) for nonprescription sale to adults in August 2006; in 2009 a generic version was made available. In June 2011, the FDA approved Plan B One-Step and similar formulations for nonprescription sale to any woman of childbearing age; however, the Secretary of Health and Human Services disagreed with the FDA and required a prescription for women under the age of 17.

INDICATIONS

Women who have had unprotected intercourse within 5 days, whose method of contraception failed (e.g., a broken condom) or who have been victims of sexual assault are candidates for EC if they are at risk for pregnancy. Women at the midmenstrual cycle who may be near ovulation are at greatest risk, but risk exists at any time in the cycle and EC need not be "timed" to coincide with the menstrual cycle. See Fig. 115.1 for an approach to the use of EC.

CONTRAINDICATIONS

The progestin-only method (Plan B One Step, Next Choice, or their equivalent) has no known medical contraindications. The World Health Organization has stated that the only contraindication to EC is an ongoing pregnancy. No teratogenic effects have been identified, however. Medical contraindications to oral contraceptives, such as severe hypertension and history of thromboembolism, should be considered but have not been shown to be significant with the short dosage schedule.

PRECAUTIONS

An accurate time line of exposure is critical to the use of EC. A pregnancy test can be considered before administration. Testing for and treatment of sexually transmitted infections should be offered and encouraged. An adequate plan for contraception after EC use should be recommended.

PREPROCEDURE PATIENT EDUCATION

Because the product is available over the counter, preprocedure counseling may not be possible. If the patient contacts her clinician before taking EC, she should be informed of the risks and benefits of the medication as outlined in this chapter and the patient education handout. Educating patients about the availability of EC at health maintenance visits may be appropriate.

PROCEDURE

Medical

Plan B One Step, Take Action, My Way, Next Choice, and other generic forms are available over the counter without age restriction for women and men. Plan B One Step consists of one double-dose tablet containing 1.5 mg of levonorgestrel. Plan B and Next Choice (both being phased out) consist of two tablets, each containing 0.75 mg of levonorgestrel. Following the FDA-approved regimens, the first or single pill is taken as soon as possible within 72 hours after exposure and, if it is part of the prescription, the second pill is taken 12 hours later. An alternate and equally effective regimen to the two-pill prescription is to take both tablets (1.5 mg levonorgestrel) as a single dose. Research conducted since FDA approval has demonstrated effectiveness up to 120 hours (5 days) after exposure, with declining success as delay increases.

A dual-hormone brand of EC known as Preven is no longer available by prescription, but hormones found in certain common oral contraceptives, including a number of generic preparations, can be used to replicate it. It may be advantageous to know about the dual-hormone ("Yuzpe") method because it may be more readily available and less expensive than commercially available EC, especially if the patient already has access to oral contraceptive pills. Two widely used forms of progestin can be used: levonorgestrel (such as Plan B, Plan B One Step, and Next Choice) and norgestrel. Twice as much norgestrel is required for the same therapeutic effect (0.75 mg levonorgestrel or 1.50 mg norgestrel per dose). Determining the correct number and color of active pills available to the patient may require help from the local pharmacy (Table 115.1). The antiprogestin ulipristal (ella; Watson Pharmaceuticals) is available by prescription as a micronized EC tablet effective up to 120 hours after intercourse.

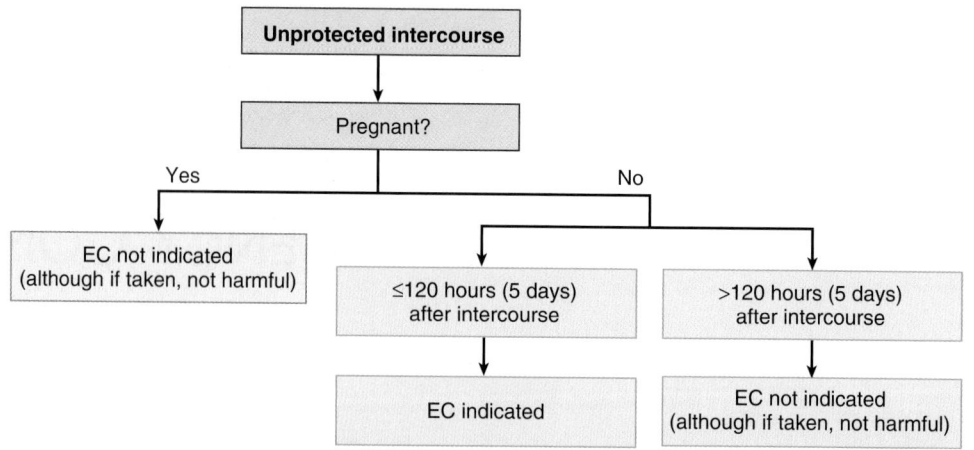

Fig. 115.1 Emergency contraception (EC) decision pathway.

| TABLE 115.1 | Oral Contraceptives That Can Be Used for Emergency Contraception in the United States |

Brand	Company	First Dose*	Second Dose* (12 hr Later)	Ulipristal Acetate Per Dose (mg)	Ethinyl Estradiol Per Dose (μg)	Levonorgestrel Per Dose (mg)†
Ulipristal Acetate (Dedicated EC Pills)						
ella	Afaxys	1 white pill	None	30	–	–
Progestin-Only (Dedicated EC Pills)						
Aftera†	Teva	1 white pill	None	–	–	1.5
AfterPill‡	Syzygy	1 white pill	None	–	–	1.5
EContra Ez§	Afaxys	1 white pill	None	–	–	1.5
Levonorgestrel Tablets	Perrigo	2 white pills	None*	–	–	1.5
My Way	Gavis	1 white pill	None	–	–	1.5
Next Choice One Dose	Actavis	1 peach pill	None	–	–	1.5
Plan B One-Step	Teva	1 white pill	None	–	–	1.5
Take Action	Teva	1 white pill	None	–	–	1.5
Combined Progestin and Estrogen Pills (Regular Oral Contraceptive Pills)						
Altavera	Sandoz	4 peach pills	4 peach pills	–	120	0.60
Amethia	Actavis	4 white pills	4 white pills	–	120	0.60
Amethia Lo	Actavis	5 white pills	5 white pills	–	100	0.50
Amethyst	Actavis	6 white pills	6 white pills	–	120	0.54
Aubra	Afaxys	5 white pills	5 white pills	–	100	0.50
Aviane	Teva	5 orange pills	5 orange pills	–	100	0.50
Camrese	Teva	4 light blue-green pills	4 light blue-green pills	–	120	0.60
CamreseLo	Teva	5 orange pills	5 orange pills	–	100	0.50
Chateal	Afaxys	4 white pills	4 white pills	–	120	0.60
Cryselle¶	Teva	4 white pills	4 white pills	–	120	0.60
Enpresse	Teva	4 orange pills	4 orange pills	–	120	0.50
Introvale	Sandoz	4 peach pills	4 peach pills	–	120	0.60
Jolessa	Teva	4 pink pills	4 pink pills	–	120	0.60
Lessina	Teva	5 pink pills	5 pink pills	–	100	0.50
Levora	Actavis	4 white pills	4 white pills	–	120	0.60
Lo/Ovral¶	Akrimax	4 white pills	4 white pills	–	120	0.60
LoSeasonique	Teva	5 orange pills	5 orange pills	–	100	0.50
Low-Ogestrel¶	Actavis	4 white pills	4 white pills	–	120	0.60
Lutera	Actavis	5 white pills	5 white pills	–	100	0.50
Lybrel	Wyeth	6 yellow pills	6 yellow pills	–	120	0.54
Nordette	Teva	4 light-orange pills	4 light-orange pills	–	120	0.60
Ogestrel¶	Actavis	2 white pills	2 white pills	–	100	0.50
Portia	Teva	4 pink pills	4 pink pills	–	120	0.60
Quasense	Actavis	4 white pills	4 white pills	–	120	0.60
Seasonale	Teva	4 pink pills	4 pink pills	–	120	0.60
Seasonique	Teva	4 light-blue-green pills	4 light-blue-green pills	–	120	0.60
Sronyx	Actavis	5 white pills	5 while pills	–	100	0.50
Trivora	Actavis	4 pink pills	4 pink pills	–	120	0.50

ella and the levonorgestrel EC products listed in the top section are dedicated products specifically marketed for emergency contraception. The regular oral contraceptives listed have been declared safe and effective for use as emergency contraceptives by the US States Food and Drug Administration. Outside the United States, about 100 emergency contraceptive products are specifically packaged, labeled, and marketed. Levonorgestrel-only ECPs are available either over the counter or from a pharmacist without having to see a clinician in 60 countries. In the United States, progestin-only ECs, such as Plan B One-Step, are available on the shelf with no restrictions. ella is available by prescription only.

EC, Emergency contraception.

*The label for levonorgestrel tablets says to take one pill within 72 hours after unprotected intercourse and another pill 12 hours later. However, research has found that both pills can be taken at the same time. All of the brands listed here may be effective when used within 120 hours after unprotected sex, but they should be taken as soon as possible.

†Aftera is sold exclusively at CVS stores.

‡Afterpill is sold at www.afterpill.com.

§EContra EZ is sold at family planning clinics and at www.kwikmed.com.

¶The progestin in Cryselle, Lo/Ovral, Low-Ogestrel, and Ogestrel is norgestrel, which contains two isomers, only one of which (levonorgestrel) is bioactive; the amount of norgestrel in each tablet is twice the amount of levonorgestrel.

From the Office of Population Research at Princeton University. Answers to frequently asked questions about effectiveness. http://ec.princeton.edu/questions/dose.html.

The prescription regimen is similar for all the options: the first dose is taken immediately, and, when indicated, the second dose is taken 12 hours later. Only Plan B has been proven to be equally effective if both tablets are taken as a single dose and thus received FDA approval for Plan B One Step. Evidence shows that early administration enhances efficacy. The greatest efficacy occurs when the regimen starts within 24 hours of exposure, but the treatment may be initiated up to 120 hours after exposure.

In a head-to-head randomized, blinded study, the progestin-only method had an efficacy up to 89%, whereas the dual-hormone method had an efficacy of 43% to 55%. Thus progestin-only EC, when available, is the better option.

Female patients may be given a prescription to be held in reserve in case of an exposure.

Intrauterine Contraceptive Device

Another approach to EC is the placement of a copper intrauterine device (IUD), ParaGard (Teva Pharmaceuticals). The IUD is effective up to 1 week after exposure and is significantly more effective than oral methods, with a reduced risk of pregnancy by 99% if inserted within 5 days of unprotected intercourse. IUD insertion has its own risks and disadvantages, but placement for EC has the advantage of immediate and continuous contraception. See Chapter 135, Intrauterine Device Insertion, for a full discussion of IUD insertion.

COMPLICATIONS

With the dual-hormone method, nausea and vomiting are common problems. Therefore a prophylactic antiemetic is recommended before the hormones are administered. Breast tenderness may also occur. Side effects are less frequent with the progestin-only methods. Menses may be early, on time, or delayed after treatment. If the menstrual delay is 21 days or more from the date of treatment, a pregnancy test should be performed. If the medication is vomited within the first hour of ingestion, repeat administration with an antiemetic is indicated. If vomited more than 1 hour postingestion, repeat administration is still advised.

POSTPROCEDURE MANAGEMENT

Discuss a post-EC plan for contraception and make sure that the patient understands that EC is not an effective method of continuous contraception. If the patient has no menses within 21 days,

test for pregnancy. Screen for sexually transmitted infections when indicated.

PATIENT EDUCATION GUIDES

See the patient education form available at www.expertconsult.com.

CPT/BILLING CODES

There is no specific CPT code for EC. The appropriate office visit or telephone consultation should be documented and billed.

ICD-10-CM DIAGNOSTIC CODES

Z30.012	Emergency contraception
Z30.430	IUD insertion
Z30.40	Contraceptive surveillance unspecified
Z72.51-Z72.53	High-risk sexual behavior

ONLINE RESOURCES

Association of Reproductive Health Professionals: Emergency Contraception: www.arhp.org/ec.
The Emergency Contraception Website: http://ec.princeton.edu and www.not-2-late.com.

RECOMMENDED READING

Emergency contraception. Practice Bulletin No. 112. American College of Obstetricians and Gynecologists. *Obstet Gynecol.* 2010;115:1100–1109.

Office of Population Research at Princeton University. Answers to frequently asked questions about effectiveness. http://ec.princeton.edu/questions/dose.html.

Trussel J, Raymond EG, Cleland K. *Emergency Contraception, a Last Chance to Prevent Unintended Pregnancy*; 2017. Updated http://ec.princeton.edu/questions/ec-review.pdf.

Cheng L, Gülmezoglu AM, Piaggio GGP, et al. Interventions for emergency contraception. *Cochrane Database Syst Rev.* 2008;2:CD001324.

Grimes D, Raymond E, Jones B. Emergency contraception over-the-counter: the medical and legal imperatives. *Obstet Gynecol.* 2001;98:151–155.

Ngai SW, Fan S, Li S, et al. A randomized trial to compare 24 h versus 12 h double dose regimen of levonorgestrel for emergency contraception. *Hum Reprod.* 2005;20:307–311.

CHAPTER 116

BARRIER CONTRACEPTIVES: CERVICAL CAPS, CONDOMS, AND DIAPHRAGMS

Beth A. Choby

Cervical barriers are relatively safe and inexpensive options for contraception. They are immediately effective and reversible, and have few side effects. Barrier methods are options for women who have contraindications to hormonal contraceptives, do not desire or cannot tolerate intrauterine devices, do not want to use natural family planning, or are not ready for sterilization. Additional benefits include ease of transportability, safety during lactation, and the convenience of flexible timing of insertion. Of the methods available, only the FemCap and diaphragm require prescriptions. Current barrier methods are 80% effective in preventing pregnancy when used correctly and consistently. Table 116.1 lists various barrier options, contraceptive failure rates, and costs.

Although more options for barrier contraception are available today than ever before, the percentage of women choosing barrier methods is small. Currently, only about 0.3% of women use a diaphragm for contraception; in the 1980s, 8.1% of women selected this method. A possible protective effect against sexually transmitted infection (STI) has focused renewed attention on barrier contraception. Protection is thought to occur through mechanical blocking of exposure to semen and bodily fluids. Most barrier devices are used in combination with nonoxynol-9, the only spermicide available in the United States, but patients need to know that the spermicide itself does not enhance protection against STIs; in fact, it may increase risk slightly. The Centers for Disease Control and Prevention recommends that women at high risk for human immunodeficiency virus (HIV) infection avoid nonoxynol-9-containing spermicides because they offer no protection against STIs and may slightly increase the risk of HIV infection. While the mechanism is not known, nonoxynol-9 is a mild detergent that disrupts the cellular membrane of spermatozoa; in so doing, it can also slightly disrupt the vaginal epithelium thereby possibly decreasing a natural barrier to HIV.

CERVICAL CAPS

The only cervical cap currently available in the United States is the FemCap (Fig. 116.1). The FemCap is silicone based and shaped like a sailor's hat with the upturned brim that lies against the vaginal walls around the cervix. Initial efficacy studies of the FemCap were based on the first-generation product, which is no longer available. A Cochrane Database Review comparing the first-generation FemCap with the diaphragm found that the FemCap was less effective in preventing pregnancy. During the first year with typical use 14% of nulliparous women using the FemCap became pregnant; and parous women had a 29% failure rate. The first-generation FemCap, with which most of these data were obtained, is now considered obsolete and has been replaced with a second-generation design. Although research on the effectiveness of the second-generation FemCap is limited, the typical failure rate is estimated to be 7.6%. Failure rates with perfect use are less (2% to 4%). Dislodgement of the

first-generation device occurred in one-third of users; the second-generation FemCap dislodgement rate is estimated at 2%. Future studies should better clarify long-term efficacy. The cap has a high level of patient acceptability, and FemCap users may have decreased risk of urinary tract infections compared with women using a diaphragm. Although small trials do not link cytologic abnormalities with FemCap use, baseline Papanicolaou screening (Pap smear) and annual surveillance are reasonable in women choosing this method.

Anatomy

The FemCap has a dome that fits over the cervix. An asymmetric brim flares outward to fit against the vaginal fornices (see Fig. 116.1).

Indications

Prevention of pregnancy
Possible protection against STIs

Contraindications

- Allergy to silicone/spermicide
- Less than 10 weeks postpartum
- History of toxic shock syndrome
- History of recent cervical surgery or abortion
- Cancer of the vulva, vagina, cervix, or uterus
- Anatomic abnormalities of the vagina, uterus, or cervix
- Uterine prolapse
- Patient unable to be properly fitted
- Patient unable to understand the instructions for use or proper insertion/removal of the device
- Current genital tract infection
- Poor vaginal muscle tone
- Vaginal or cervical tissue breakdown

Equipment and Supplies

The FemCap is a clear silicone device that covers both the cervix and vaginal fornices. A strap over the dome augments removal. Spermicide is applied in the groove between the brim and the dome. The cap is available in three sizes. Determining the correct size depends in general on the user's childbearing history:

- 22 mm (small): use in nulliparous women
- 26 mm (medium): use in women with a previous abortion or cesarean delivery
- 30 mm (large): use in women with history of vaginal delivery

The FemCap kit contains the device, clinician instructions for fitting, and a patient education DVD/video detailing product use. Cost of the kit averages $65.

TABLE 116.1	Comparison of Female Barrier Contraceptives						
Method	Over-the-Counter	Multiuse/Reusable	1-Year Failure Rate With Typical Use (%)	Timing of Insertion (Maximum Hours Prior to Intercourse)	Time to Be Left in after Intercourse (Hours)	Maximum Duration of Use (Hours)	Cost (US$)
Diaphragm	No	Yes	16	6	6	24	50*
FemCap	No	Yes	7.6†	40	6	48	65: includes video/DVD, device and instructions*
FC2 female condom	Yes	No	21	8	Remove after intercourse	One-time use	2.50
Sponge	Yes	No	13–17	24	6	30	7.50–9 for pack of 3
Male condom	Yes	No	18	Prior to intercourse	Remove after ejaculation		0.50

*Does not include costs for spermicide.
†Based on limited-duration trials of second-generation FemCap.

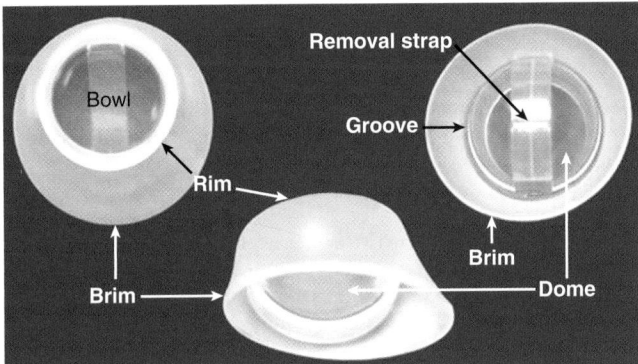

Fig. 116.1 FemCap cervical cap. (Courtesy FemCap, Inc., Del Mar, CA.)

Precautions

- Perform a pelvic examination before a cervical cap fitting. A Pap smear is recommended at baseline and then annually. Cervical cultures should be obtained in women at risk for STIs.
- Cervical cap fitting is contraindicated during pregnancy or the postpartum period (10 weeks).

Patient Education: Cervical Cap Use for Contraception

- Before use, one-third of the inner side of the dome should be filled with spermicidal jelly.
- The jelly should not be applied to the inner surface of the rim.
- The cap may be inserted at any time from immediately before intercourse up to 40 hours before intercourse. It is most easily inserted in a squatting or semireclining position.
- The cap should be left in place for at least 6 hours following intercourse.
- The cap may be left in place for up to 48 hours.
- If intercourse occurs more than once while the cap is in place, no additional spermicide is needed. However, the wearer should check for correct positioning of the cap before each episode.
- An additional contraceptive method should be used the first three times the cap is worn during intercourse (to ensure protection should the cap become dislodged). If dislodgement occurs, cap use should be discontinued and the cap should be refitted.
- The cap should not be used during menses.
- Refitting is necessary after abortion or childbirth.
- The cap should not be used in the presence of vaginal infection, discharge, pain, or odor. If these occur, medical evaluation is necessary.

- If lubrication is needed for intercourse, only water-based lubricants should be used. (Spermicide works well for this purpose.)
- The cap should be washed carefully after use with soap and water. If an odor develops, it can be soaked in vinegar or a cup of water with a teaspoon of lemon juice. Alternatively, the cap can be cleaned with a 25% bleach solution for 20 minutes, after which it should be rinsed thoroughly.
- If the initial Pap smear is negative, then a Pap smear should be obtained every year thereafter.
- The cap should be replaced yearly (sooner if thin spots or tears occur). The patient should make an appointment with her physician to check if it still fits adequately.
- If the device is left in too long, infections can occur, so the patient must follow the previously listed guidelines.

Procedure

1. Review the instructions from the FemCap kit.
2. Put on gloves, follow universal blood and body fluid precautions, and select the appropriate size of FemCap (described in the equipment section).
3. Lubricate the edges of the device, compress it, and insert vaginally. The FemCap should be inserted with the long brim first and pushed into the vagina until the dome fits snugly over the cervix (Fig. 116.2).
4. The cap should cover the entire cervix and adhere to it by self-generated suction.
5. The rim of the cap should fit evenly around the circumference of the vaginal fornices.
6. No gaps should be felt between the rim of the cap and the cervix.
7. Tug gently on the removal strap to guarantee that the cap will not dislodge.
8. If the cap does not fit satisfactorily, try one of the other two sizes.
9. Remove the cap by gripping the strap and rotating the FemCap. Push on the dome to break the suction and pull the cap out using the strap.
10. Have the patient repeat the insertion and removal process to demonstrate understanding.

Complications

- Pregnancy is possible if the cap dislodges during intercourse. This was one of the major reasons women discontinued the first-generation cervical cap, although dislodgement is much less common with the second-generation FemCap. Counseling patients about emergency contraception and providing a prescription for emergency use may be a desired option for certain women (see Chapter 115, Emergency Contraception).

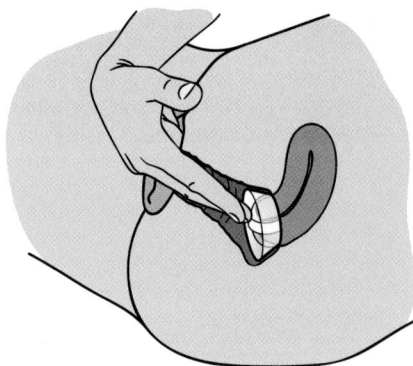

Fig. 116.2 Proper placement and positioning of the FemCap. (Courtesy FemCap, Inc., Del Mar, CA.)

- Vaginal odor or discharge occurs in 5% to 27% of users.
- Vaginal or cervical lacerations and abrasions are possible if the cap is left in place too long.
- Vaginal discomfort occurs in less than 3% of users.
- Toxic shock syndrome is uncommon.

Postprocedure Management

The patient should sit and ambulate to ensure that the cap does not dislodge. No discomfort should be noted when the cap is correctly applied.

Postprocedure Patient Education

- The FemCap should be used with a one-quarter teaspoon of spermicide. Spermicide should be applied in the dome and spread over the brim.
- The FemCap must be placed before intercourse.
- The cap must be left in place for 6 hours after intercourse.
- It may be safely worn for up to 48 continuous hours.
- After removal, the FemCap should be washed with mild soap and water and allowed to air dry.
- FemCaps generally last approximately 1 year.

DIAPHRAGM

Diaphragms were first produced in the United States in 1925, and current diaphragm design is not significantly different. Of the four models currently available, two are made of latex and two of silicone. Contraceptive efficacy studies of newer barrier methods are usually judged against the diaphragm. Although diaphragms are traditionally used with spermicidal jelly, a recent Cochrane Review was unable to distinguish a difference in effectiveness when diaphragm use with spermicide was compared with diaphragm use alone.

Barrier contraceptive efficacy is highly dependent on proper and consistent use. Of 100 women using the diaphragm, 16 become pregnant annually with typical use. Perfect use of the diaphragm has a 6 per 100 failure rate.

INDICATIONS

- Pregnancy prevention
- Contraception for women with contraindications to other methods and who do not desire to be sterilized
- Desire for additional STI protection in combination with other contraceptive methods that do not confer protection

CONTRAINDICATIONS

- Latex or spermicidal jelly allergy/hypersensitivity (relative; may not be required)

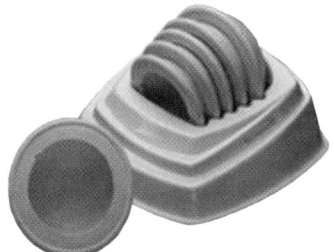

Fig. 116.3 Diaphragm fitting kit. (Courtesy CooperSurgical, Inc., Trumbull, CT.)

- Postpartum (<6 weeks)
- Vaginal stenosis or significant pelvic abnormalities
- Recurrent urinary tract infections
- Aversion to manipulation of the genitals
- Uterine prolapse
- Significant cystocele or rectocele

Equipment

- Diaphragms (sizes 65 to 90) are of four types:
  1. *Arching spring*: Molded one-piece spring and firm-rimmed dome that form an arc when the rim is compressed in the center. It requires no introducer and is recommended for women with decreased pelvic support, cystocele or rectocele, or retroverted uterus. Most women find it the easiest to insert and it is the most popular type in the United States.
  2. *Coil spring*: Molded one-piece with spring, dome, and a softer, more flexible rim. It may be used with an introducer and is recommended for women with good vaginal support and no cystocele, rectocele, or pelvic floor relaxation; the cervix should be midplane or anterior.
  3. *Flat spring*: Molded one-piece with spring, dome, and a softer, more flexible rim than either the arching or the coil spring. It has flat-plane flexibility, may be used with an introducer, and is recommended for smaller women with a narrow or shallow pelvic shelf. It is excellent for nulliparous women or athletic women with strong pelvic musculature.
  4. *Wide seal rim*: A silicone version, which is best for latex allergic women. It comes in arching or coil spring versions.
- Fitting ring kit. Kits can be obtained from most diaphragm manufacturers at minimal to no cost. The rings are graduated sizes that differ by increments of 5 mm. Fitting with domed rings provides a more realistic sensation for the patient as to how a diaphragm will feel (Fig. 116.3).
- Diaphragm introducer (optional).
- Spermicidal jelly.

Precautions

- Poor vaginal tone, a shallow vaginal shelf, or a cystocele or rectocele may prevent effective use of the diaphragm.
- Refitting is often necessary after pregnancy, pelvic surgery, or weight gain of more than 15 pounds.
- Women with a latex allergy are candidates for the wide seal rim diaphragm or any other silicone version (latex free).

Preprocedure Patient Education and Forms

Diaphragm fitting by a health care provider is required. The fitting process should be discussed with the patient. Efficacy rates and the proper and consistent use of the diaphragm should be stressed. Please refer to the patient education form available at www.expertconsult.com.

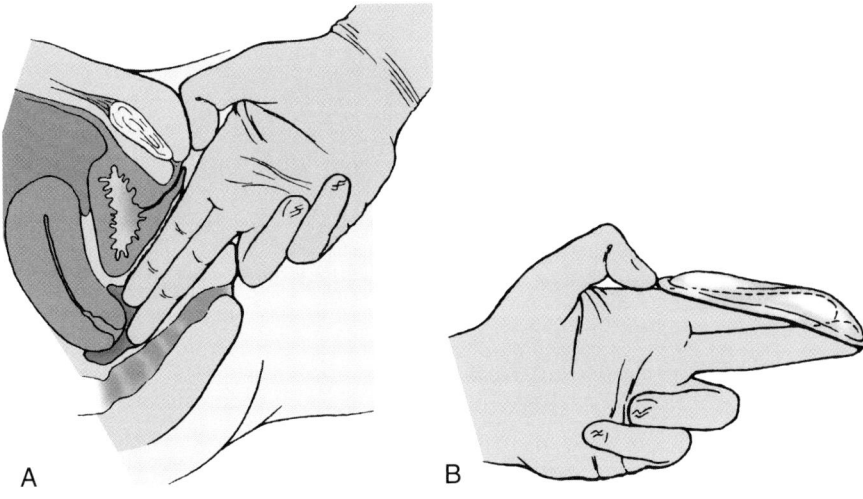

A   B

Fig. 116.4 Clinical examination to determine proper diaphragm size. (A) Insert the gloved index and middle fingers into the vagina, aiming for the posterior fornix with the middle finger. Mark the spot on the glove where the index finger touches the inferior pubic symphysis. (B) Place the fitting ring or diaphragm over the end of the middle finger, and place the opposite side of the ring over the line marked on the gloved index finger.

Procedure

1. Place the patient in dorsal lithotomy (pelvic) position.
2. Don examination gloves and apply surgical lubricant to the index and middle fingers. Observe universal blood and body fluid precautions.
3. To estimate the size of the diaphragm, insert the gloved index and middle fingers into the vagina. Aim for the posterior fornix with the middle finger (Fig. 116.4A).
4. Note the spot where the index finger touches the inferior pubic symphysis.
5. Mark this spot on the glove using either a marker or instrument, or your thumb.
6. Remove the fingers from the vagina.
7. Place the fitting ring or diaphragm over the end of the middle finger.
8. Place the opposite side of the ring over the line marked on the gloved index finger (75 mm is a common size; see Fig. 116.4B).
9. Apply surgical lubricant to the outer surface of the fitting ring (only) that most closely approximates the determined diameter.
10. Fold this fitting ring in half by pressing the sides together with the thumb and fingers (Fig. 116.5A).
11. Insert the folded diaphragm vaginally while the other hand holds open the vulva. Direct the diaphragm toward the posterior fornix (see Fig. 116.5B).
12. Check for correct positioning by feeling for the cervix through the dome of the fitting diaphragm or in the center of the fitting ring (see Fig. 116.5C).
13. Gently manipulate the anterior rim until it rests directly behind the pubic symphysis.
14. Have the patient perform a Valsalva maneuver and squat to confirm the fit.
15. Remove the diaphragm by hooking the index finger up and around the anterior rim and pulling the diaphragm down and out through the introitus (Fig. 116.6).
16. The patient should demonstrate proper technique for both insertion and removal of the diaphragm. Check that the patient can feel the cervix through the diaphragm dome and confirm placement of the anterior rim behind the pubic symphysis.
17. Describe the proper application of spermicide to the diaphragm. One tablespoon of spermicidal jelly is applied to the concave side of the dome (for use) in addition to around the rim.

Common Errors

- Improper fitting. A diaphragm that is too small does not lodge behind the pubic symphysis and falls out. An inappropriately large diaphragm protrudes out in front of the pubic symphysis.

- Failure to leave the diaphragm in place for a minimum of 6 hours after intercourse. Patients should be counseled not to douche or remove the diaphragm immediately after coitus.

Complications

- Continuous diaphragm use for longer than 24 hours increases the risk of toxic shock syndrome (incidence of 2.4 per 100,000 women).
- Ulceration can result from excessive pressure of the diaphragm against the vaginal sidewalls with a poorly fitting device.
- Urinary tract infections and bacterial vaginosis are the most frequent side effects of diaphragm use.

Postprocedure Patient Education

- Patients should be shown and should practice diaphragm insertion and removal techniques, including how to apply spermicidal jelly to the rim and the dome. One tablespoon should be applied to the concave surface of the dome and the rim of the diaphragm so that the uterus is sealed off mechanically and chemically.
- Make sure that the diaphragm rim is firmly in place behind the pubic bone and below and behind the cervix. The patient should feel for the cervix through the dome of her diaphragm to ensure correct placement.
- Warn the patient not to douche or remove the diaphragm for 6 hours after intercourse. Leave the diaphragm in place and apply more spermicide if additional coitus occurs during this time.
- The patient should walk around the examination room with the diaphragm in place to ensure a comfortable fit.
- The diaphragm prescription should include the manufacturer's name, the type, and the size. A refill can be prescribed in case a new diaphragm is needed and the provider is unavailable.

Please refer to the sample patient education form available at www.expertconsult.com.

SPONGES

The sponge is a nonprescription, single-use barrier contraceptive made of polyurethane foam impregnated with spermicide (nonoxynol-9). The concave side fits against the cervix, whereas the loop on the opposite side augments sponge removal. Although the Protectaid sponge is available in Canada, the Today Sponge is the only contraceptive sponge currently available in the United States (Fig. 116.7).

Sponges are sold in packs of three ($7.50 to $9). The effectiveness rate is 89% to 91% for perfect use and 84% to 87% with typical

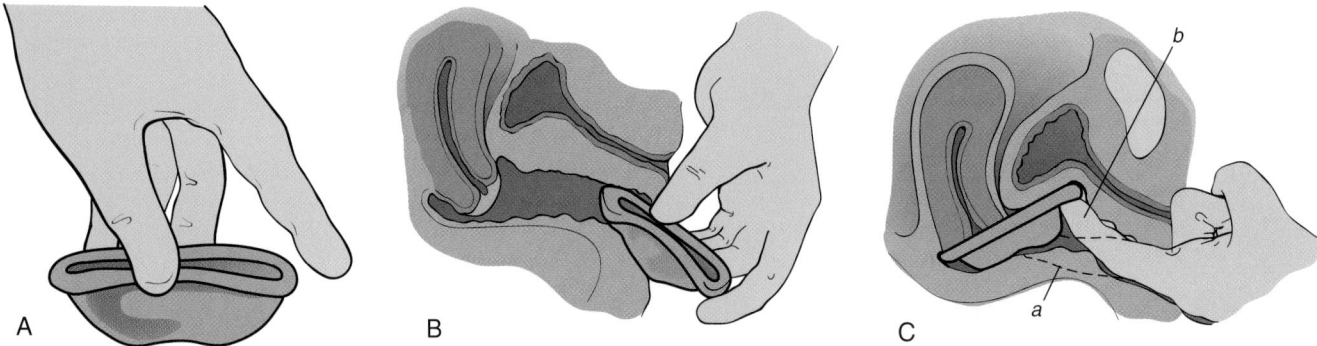

Fig. 116.5 (A) Diaphragm is folded for insertion. (B) Insertion of the folded diaphragm. (C) Proper diaphragm position: The cervix is palpable behind the diaphragm (*a*); the rim fits snugly behind the symphysis pubis (*b*).

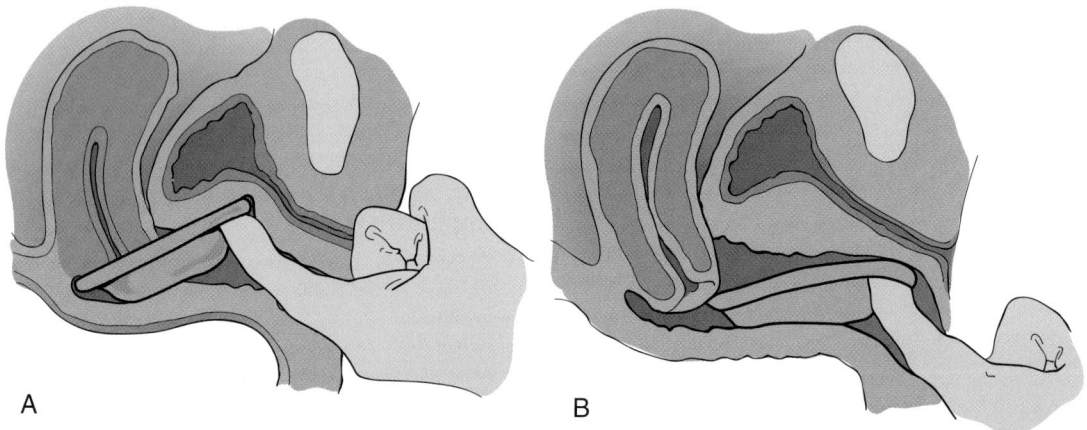

Fig. 116.6 Removal of the diaphragm. (A) Finger is hooked under the rim. (B) Diaphragm is pulled through the introitus.

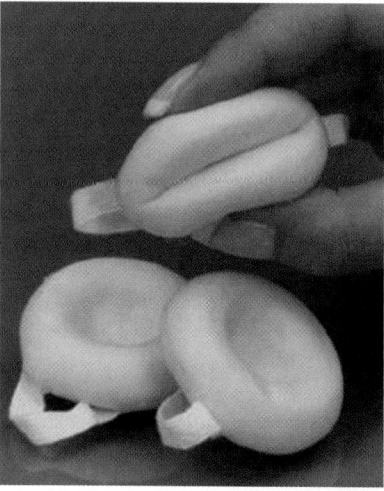

Fig. 116.7 Today Sponge. (Courtesy Allendale Pharmaceuticals Mayer Laboratories, Sonoma, CA.)

use. Parous women may have higher rates of failure than women who have not been pregnant. The sponge does *not* reduce the risk of STIs or HIV/acquired immunodeficiency syndrome; in fact, it may slightly increase the risk of HIV in women at high risk of HIV, due to the mild vaginal irritation caused by spermicide.

Anatomy

The sponge is inserted transvaginally and placed with the concave side covering the cervix.

Indications

- Prevention of pregnancy
- Contraception for women who are breast-feeding, especially after 6 months postpartum or if they are not amenorrheic
- Birth control for women with contraindications to other methods or who need backup for the pill

Contraindications

- Allergies to polyurethane, nonoxynol-9, or medications containing sulfa
- History of toxic shock syndrome
- History of recent delivery, miscarriage, or abortion (<8 weeks)
- Vaginal obstruction/anatomic abnormalities
- Current menstruation
- Active genital tract infection
- Patient difficulty in understanding instructions for use
- Patient difficulty correctly inserting or removing the sponge
- Patient discomfort touching genitals

Precautions

The sponge offers no protection against STIs or HIV/acquired immunodeficiency syndrome, and in fact may increase risk slightly in women at high risk of HIV due to possible mild vaginal irritation caused by spermicide.

Procedure

1. The patient should read the package insert before use.
2. Wash hands with soap and water.

3. Wet the sponge with a minimum of two tablespoons of clean water.
4. Squeeze the sponge to help activate the spermicide.
5. Fold the sponge in half with the loop toward the outside.
6. Slide the folded sponge into the vagina and push it inside until the cervix is covered. The sponge will unfold.
7. Check sponge placement by sliding a finger around the edge to guarantee that it covers the cervix. The loop should be palpable.
8. Insert up to 24 hours before intercourse; the sponge must be left in place for 6 hours after intercourse.
9. Remove the sponge after 30 hours of continuous use.
10. *To remove*, insert a finger intravaginally and pull the sponge out using the loop.

Common Errors

- Failure to hydrate the sponge before use. The spermicide is most effective if the sponge is dampened with at least two tablespoons of water and then squeezed.
- Failure to place the correct side of the sponge directly against the cervix. After placement, check that the sponge edges are well applied against the fornices and that the loop is on the side that faces the vagina.

Postprocedure Patient Education

The sponge should be left in for a minimum of 6 hours after intercourse. It should not be left in place for longer than 30 continuous hours. Sponges are for one-time use only. Used sponges should be disposed of in a trash receptacle and not in a toilet.

MALE AND FEMALE CONDOMS

The male condom is a barrier contraceptive device that covers the penis and isolates sperm. It is unrolled onto the erect penis while leaving a space at the end to contain the ejaculate. Although most modern male condoms are made of latex, 2% to 4% of individuals are latex allergic (higher risk in those frequently exposed to latex, such as health care workers). Animal-product and polyurethane- or isoprene-based prophylactics are available for the latex allergic; all are relatively inexpensive and available without a prescription. While latex condoms are quite elastic, they do not conduct heat well, so they can feel almost cold. Polyurethane conducts heat better than latex and is also thinner; however, it is slightly more expensive than isoprene. Isoprene is the material used in latex-free surgical gloves; it conducts heat well, is soft and stretchy, feels more like a natural material, but it is slightly thicker than polyurethane.

The clinician should discuss appropriate use with patients because male condoms are frequently used incorrectly, and patients are often reticent about asking questions. When used correctly and consistently, the first-year failure rate is 2%; however, with typical use the failure rate is 18%. Male condoms serve as a barrier and can decrease the transmission of STIs. However, it should be noted that animal-product condoms may be porous enough to transmit human papilloma and herpes simplex viruses and HIV.

The FC Female Condom is an over-the-counter, FDA-approved condom for women (Fig. 116.8). It is one size and does not require fitting. Made of soft, flexible polyurethane, it is a lubricated sheath with flexible rings on each end. The sealed ring is inserted into the vagina like a diaphragm, whereas the open ring rests against the vulva. Female condoms made of nitrile (FC2 condoms) are one-third the cost of the polyurethane condom, but are not available in the United States. Of 100 women who use female condoms, 21 become pregnant within 1 year with typical use; perfect use has a 5 in 100 failure rate.

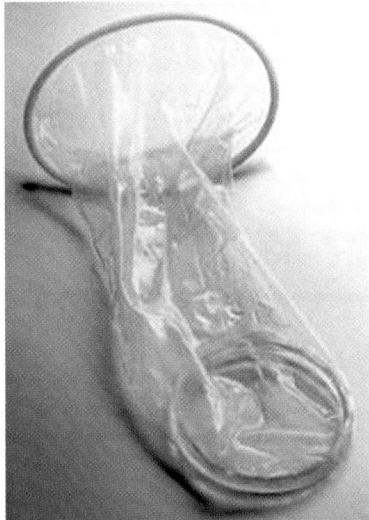

Fig. 116.8 **FC female condom.** (Courtesy The Female Health Company, Chicago, IL.)

Indications

- Pregnancy prevention
- Prevention of STIs
- Adjunct to other contraception for STI prevention

Contraindications

- Allergy or hypersensitivity to latex (latex condoms)
- Allergy or hypersensitivity to spermicide (condoms containing spermicide)
- Allergy to polyurethane (female condom and some male condoms)

Precautions

The availability of emergency contraception should be discussed.

Preprocedure Patient Education and Forms

The male condom is applied immediately before use. The female condom can be inserted up to 8 hours before intercourse but usually is inserted immediately before use. The FC2 condom is available over the counter and is for one-time use only. The cost is around $2.50 per condom.

Please see the patient education form available at www.expertconsult.com.

Procedure (Female Condom)

1. Detailed instructions for use are available in the product packaging.
2. Squeeze the sides of the inner ring (closed end of condom) and insert it into the vaginal vault.
3. Push the inner ring until it encircles the cervix.
4. Let the outer ring overlap an inch over the perineum.
5. For condom removal, squeeze and twist the outer ring to keep semen from leaking out. Pull the condom from the vagina and dispose of it in the trash.

Common Errors

- Condom efficacy is decreased with the use of certain lubricants or oil-based compounds (Box 116.1).

BOX 116.1   Common Oil-Based Preparations That Adversely Affect Condom Efficacy

Baby oil
Butoconazole (Femstat)
Butter
Cocoa butter
Cold cream
Conjugated estrogens (Premarin) cream
Estradiol (Estrace) cream
Hand lotion
Lubricants
Medications
Miconazole (Monistat)
Mineral oil
Petroleum jelly
Shortening
Suntan oil
Tioconazole (Vagistat-1)
Vegetable oil

- Use of old/outdated condoms may result in contraceptive failure. Keep condoms properly stored and use by the expiration date printed on the wrapper.

Complications

- Vaginal irritation with female condom use.
- Condom rupture can result in pregnancy. Emergency contraception may be considered if the risk of pregnancy is high (see Chapter 115, Emergency Contraception).
- Hypersensitivity or allergy to latex or polyurethane. Male and female condoms made from plastic or nitrile are an option.

CPT/Billing Codes

57170   Diaphragm or cervical cap fitting with instructions

ICD-10-CM Diagnostic Codes

Z30.09   Encounter for contraceptive advice and management
Z30.018   Encounter for initial prescription of other contraceptives (diaphragm)
Z30.40   Surveillance of a previously prescribed unspecified contraceptive
Z30.9   Unspecified contraceptive management

Suppliers

(See contact information available at www.expertconsult.com.)

Cervical cap
FemCap
Diaphragm
Milex Wide-Seal silicone diaphragm, Milex Products, Inc.
Ortho All-Flex Arcing Spring and Ortho Coil Spring diaphragms, Ortho-McNeil Janssen Scientific Affairs, LLC
Female condoms
FC Female Condom, Female Health Company
Sponges
Today Sponge contraceptive, Mayer Laboratories

Online Resources

American Academy of Family Physicians patient education material including topics on birth control in general, how to use your diaphragm, etc.: familydoctor.org
Association of Reproductive Health Professionals: https://www.arhp.org/
Cervical Barrier Advancement Society (CBAS): www.cervicalbarriers.org/information/methods.cfm
Female Health Company: www.femalehealth.com/theproduct.html
FemCap News: https://www.femcap.com/resources/
Planned Parenthood: Birth control: https://www.plannedparenthood.org/learn/birth-control

Recommended Reading

Allen R. Diaphragm fitting. *Am Fam Physician.* 2004;69:97–100. 103, 105–106.
Cook L, Nanda K, Grimes D. Diaphragm versus diaphragm with spermicides for contraception. *Cochrane Database Syst Rev.* 2003;1:CD002031.
Gallo M, Grimes D, Schulz K. Cervical cap versus diaphragm for contraception. *Cochrane Database Syst Rev.* 2002;4:CD003551.
Kuyoh M, Toroitich-Ruto C, Grimes D, et al. Sponge versus diaphragm for contraception. *Cochrane Database Syst Rev.* 2002;3:CD003172.
Minnis A, Padian N. Effectiveness of female controlled barrier methods in preventing sexually transmitted infections and HIV: current evidence and future research directions. *Sex Transm Infect.* 2005;81:193–200.
Nelson AL. Family planning: reversible contraception, sterilization, and abortion. In: Hacker NF, Gambone JC, Hobel JC, eds. *Hacker and Moore's Essentials of Obstetrics and Gynecology.* 6th ed. Philadelphia: Elsevier; 2016:327–335.

CHAPTER 117

FERTILITY AWARENESS–BASED METHODS OF CONTRACEPTION (NATURAL FAMILY PLANNING)

William Ellert

Fertility awareness–based (FAB) methods of contraception are frequently referred to as *natural family planning*. FAB methods are an approach to contraception that identifies the days of the menstrual cycle when couples should avoid unprotected intercourse as determined by the normal physiology of the menstrual cycle and the life expectancy of sperm and ovum. Studies in multiple countries have shown that couples choose this method of contraception for a variety reasons, the most common of which are health issues and concerns about side effects of other methods. Other reasons include financial concerns, religious beliefs, and the view that "natural" is better.

Currently, in referring to FAB methods of contraception, seven major methods are discussed. Two are considered historical methods, and five other methods are currently considered more practical for clinical use.

Historical methods are:

- Calendar rhythm
- Basal body temperature

Other current FAB methods are:

- Standard days method
- Ovulation method
- Two-day method
- Symptothermal method
- Lactational amenorrhea

PHYSIOLOGY

The standard days method is based on hormonal studies indicating that a woman is generally fertile 5 days before ovulation and 24 hours after ovulation. This conclusion is based on the viability of the sperm after sexual intercourse being no more than 5 days and the viability of the egg after ovulation being less than 24 hours. These data indicate that the probability of pregnancy from unprotected intercourse is as follows:

- 4% 5 days before ovulation
- 25% to 28% for the 2 days before ovulation
- 8% to 10% for the 24 hours after ovulation
- 0% for the remainder of the cycle

Three current methods of FAB contraception rely on interpretation of the physiologic signs of fertility. Before ovulation, estradiol levels increase and cause the production of characteristic cervical secretions. The environment created by estradiol production is conducive to the transportation of sperm to the ovum. After ovulation, progesterone produced by the corpus luteum causes a distinct change in the secretions. There is a typical, obvious pattern to the secretions. No noticeable vaginal secretions are present for approximately 3 to 4 days after menstruation. After this, there is a distinctly sticky, elastic secretion that lasts for approximately 3 to 4 days. The secretions then turn clear and wet for about another 3 to 4 days. Following this there is again an absence of secretions for approximately 11 to 14 days before the next menstrual cycle. This pattern is seen in the typical menstrual cycle lasting 26 to 32 days (Fig. 117.1).

The fourth modern method of FAB relies on the fact that breastfeeding women who remain amenorrheic are infertile for 6 months.

INDICATIONS

FAB methods of preventing pregnancy are indicated for those couples who wish to avoid hormonal and surgical methods of contraception, who wish to minimize the use of barrier methods of contraception, and who are able to avoid unprotected intercourse on fertile days. These methods require the active participation of both partners and a willingness to assess the signs of fertility daily. The ability to use modern methods of FAB contraception relies ultimately on the acceptance of the techniques by clinicians as legitimate and effective methods of family planning. The availability of trained instructors and other resources that readily convey the needed information is also crucial. These methods of fertility awareness are also very helpful for couples who desire pregnancy.

CONTRAINDICATIONS

Unless pregnancy is absolutely contraindicated, there are no absolute contraindications to these methods of contraception. Relative contraindications are related to an unreliable hormone status and include the following:

- Breastfeeding
- Recent menarche
- Recent childbirth
- Recent discontinuation of some hormonal contraceptives
- Perimenopause
- Menstrual cycles that are frequently shorter than 26 days or longer than 32 days (for the Standard Days method)
- Persistent reproductive tract infections that affect the signs of fertility
- An inability to interpret the signs of fertility correctly

Most of these relative contraindications can be overcome through more extensive counseling and follow-up.

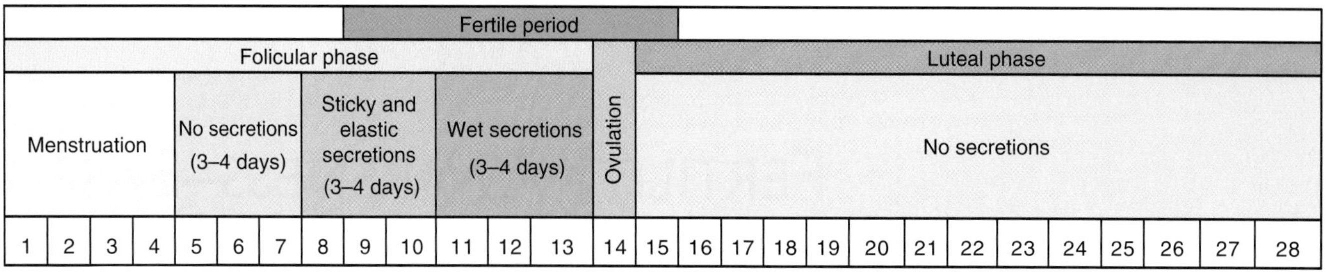

							Fertile period																					
Folicular phase														Ovulation	Luteal phase												
Menstruation				No secretions (3–4 days)			Sticky and elastic secretions (3–4 days)			Wet secretions (3–4 days)					No secretions												
1	2	3	4	5	6	7	8	9	10	11	12	13	14	15	16	17	18	19	20	21	22	23	24	25	26	27	28

Fig. 117.1 Physical signs associated with days of the typical 28-day menstrual cycle.

METHODS

Historical Methods

The *calendar rhythm method* and the *basal body temperature method* are rarely recommended today by practitioners familiar with more current FAB methods of contraception. The calendar rhythm method consists of recording the length of six cycles. Eighteen days are subtracted from the number of days in the shortest cycle and 11 days are subtracted from the number of days in the longest cycle. This determines the period in which sexual intercourse should be avoided. For example, if the shortest cycle is 23 days and the longest cycle is 31 days, then the fertile period is from day 5 until day 20.

The basal body temperature method is based on the fact that in a normal cycle a woman's basal body temperature is approximately 0.5°F (0.3°C) higher in the luteal phase than in the follicular phase. This method requires avoiding unprotected sexual intercourse from the beginning of the cycle until 3 days of elevated temperatures have occurred. Thus the daily monitoring of temperature is required before any activity or consumption of food.

Other Current Methods

Standard Days Method

- Screening: The standard days method is appropriate for women whose cycles are usually between 26 and 32 days long. Women who have more than one cycle outside of the 26- to 32-day range in a 12-month period should be encouraged to use another method.
- Instructions: Avoid unprotected intercourse from day 8 of the cycle through day 19. Day 1 is defined as the first day of menstrual bleeding.

Ovulation Method

The Billings ovulation method is the oldest method of observing cervical secretions for fertility awareness. A variant of the Billings ovulation method, the Creighton Model, requires that the woman score the secretions according to a multiple-characteristic scale.

- Screening: This method is appropriate for women regardless of their cycle length. Women who are breastfeeding, have recently used hormonal contraception, or are perimenopausal require more detailed counseling and instructions.
- Instructions: This method requires women to observe, record, and interpret their cervical secretions at the vulva several times each day, generally before each urination. Women are taught to chart the days of their menses, the days with secretions (including the characteristics of secretions), and the days when pregnancy is likely. Unprotected intercourse is to be avoided at the following times:
  - During menses (because menstrual bleeding can obscure the presence of secretions).
  - On preovulatory days after days with intercourse (because of the possible confusion with semen).
  - On all days with fertile secretions (see description in "Physiology" section).

Two Day Method

- Screening: The screening criteria for this method are identical to those for the ovulation method.
- Instructions: This method is very similar to the ovulation method, but it is much simpler. The two-day method also requires women to determine the presence or absence of cervical secretions. Two questions are then asked: "Were there any secretions today?" and "Were there any secretions yesterday?" If the patient notes 2 consecutive days without secretions, she is deemed to be in a nonfertile period. If the answer to either of those questions is yes, the woman is potentially fertile on that day.

Symptothermal Method

- Screening: The screening criteria for this method are identical to those for the ovulation method.
- Instructions: The symptothermal method provides several different "rules" for avoiding pregnancy. Each rule recognizes the appearance of cervical mucus at the vulva or vagina as the first sign of fertility. In determining the end of the fertile window, couples may choose to emphasize the observation of mucus over that of temperature (and vice versa). The most conservative rule recognizes both observations equally. For example, postovulatory infertility commences after the third day (or more) of a thermal shift (>0.4°F), which is cross-checked by 4 or more days of "drying up" of the cervical mucus. This allows the couple to personalize their method and focus on a marker they prefer while still using an alternative to "back up" their primary marker.

Lactational Amenorrhea

- Lactational amenorrhea is 92% to 100% effective at preventing pregnancy in women who exclusively breastfeed their infants. This method is effective for 6 months postpartum provided that menstruation does not resume.

NEW ADVANCES

There are several devices that can help women to identify their fertile days. These include minimicroscopes that allow women to observe the ferning of saliva or of cervical mucus (e.g., PG53, Ovatel, Maybe Baby) and handheld computers that measure cycle length and correlate the day of the cycle with basal body temperature (e.g., Babycomp, Ladycomp, Bioself 2000, Cyclotest 2 Plus). Studies that have assessed the contraceptive efficacy of computing devices are inconclusive. Studies of women using the Clearblue Easy Fertility Monitor indicate that the device provides accurate information about the fertile window, particularly when it is used with a calendar-based formula to double check the beginning and end of the fertile phase. This approach is referred to as the Marquette model.

Computer and phone applications (apps): Many fertility apps are essentially digital platforms that support a woman's use of an existing FAB method, such as the symptothermal method, the ovulation method, or the Standard Days method. Such apps replace the traditional paper-and-pencil charts associated with these methods. If an app accurately represents the FAB method on which it is based, it can be assumed that its effectiveness for pregnancy avoidance would be the same as that for the underlying method. Duane and colleagues (2016) evaluated multiple apps, finding that most were not founded on an evidence-based FAB method. Some fertility apps use algorithms, the majority of which are proprietary and have not been methodologically evaluated in the peer-reviewed literature. However, there was at least one app in every category of FAB method (except the symptohormonal method) that had a perfect accuracy score.

EFFICACY

The effectiveness of FAB methods of contraception when taught and used correctly ranges from 97% to 100% in all published studies. It must be emphasized, however, that these methods rely on the ability of the couple to abstain from genital contact during periods of fertility; the actual "use effectiveness" rate typically approaches about 80%.

CONCLUSION

FAB methods of avoiding pregnancy (or facilitating pregnancy) are very useful tools for women to become more aware of and knowledgeable about the physiologic changes that occur during their menstrual cycle. Frequently this awareness can serve to facilitate communication between partners regarding mutual reproductive responsibility. The personal decision of a couple to use this method of contraception should be supported by primary care providers in a responsible and informed manner.

ICD-10 ICM DIAGNOSTIC CODES

N89.8	Vaginal discharge
N92.6	Irregular menses
Z30.02	Counseling and instruction in natural family planning to avoid pregnancy
Z30.09	Family planning advice
Z30.40	Contraception, maintenance/examination
Z30.40	Unspecified contraceptive management

ONLINE RESOURCES

Ovulation Method—USA (BOMA), Billings Ovulation Method—USA (BOMA): www.boma-usa.org
Couple to Couple League: http://ccli.org/
Fertility Awareness Center: www.fertaware.com
Institute of Reproductive Health (Georgetown University): www.irh.org/
Marquette University (the Marquette Model): http://nfp.marquette.edu
Pope Paul VI Institute: www.popepaulvi.com

RECOMMENDED READING

Duane M, Contreras A, Jensen ET, White A. The performance of fertility awareness-based method apps marketed to avoid pregnancy. *J Am Board Fam Med.* 2016;29:508.

Alliende ME, Cabezon C, Figueroa H, Kottmann C. Cervicovaginal fluid changes to detect ovulation accurately. *Am J Obstet Gynecol.* 2005;193:71–75.

Arevalo M, Jennings V, Nikula M, Sinai I. Efficacy of the new TwoDay method of family planning. *Reprod Endocrinol.* 2004;82:885–891.

Febring R, Kitchen S, Shivanandan M. *An Introduction to Natural Family Planning [booklet].* Washington, DC: Diocesan Development Program for Natural Family Planning, National Conference of Catholic Bishops. 1999.

Guida M, Tommaselli GA, Pellicano M, et al. An overview on the effectiveness of natural family planning. *Gynecol Endocrinol.* 1977;11:203–219.

Howard M, Stanford J. Pregnancy probabilities during use of the Creighton Model Fertility Care System. *Arch Fam Med.* 1999;8:391–402.

Jennings V. Fertility awareness-based methods of pregnancy prevention. In: Rose BD, ed. *UpToDate. Waltham, Mass, UpToDate.* 2007. www.uptodate.com.

Pallone SR, Bergus GR. Fertility awareness-based methods: another option for family planning. *J Am Board Fam Med.* 2009;22:147–157.

Sinai I, Jennings V, Arevalo M. The importance of screening and monitoring: the standard days method and cycle regularity. *Contraception.* 2004;69:201–206.

Smoley BA, Robinson CM. Natural family planning. *Am Fam Physician.* 2012;86(10):924–928.

BARTHOLIN CYST AND ABSCESS: WORD CATHETER INSERTION MARSUPIALIZATION

Michael L. Tuggy

The Bartholin glands are located at the vaginal opening between the hymenal ring and labia minora (at approximately the 5 and 7 o'clock positions). Simple incision and drainage (I&D) of a Bartholin duct cyst or gland abscess, which occurs in 2% of women, may produce immediate results and significant pain relief, but recurrence after such a procedure is common. Bartholin cysts and abscesses are best treated using a Word catheter to induce the formation of an epithelialized tract from the vulvar vestibule to the cyst. This allows continued functioning of the Bartholin gland, proper drainage, and minimal risk of recurrence (2% to 15%). The Word catheter has a short latex stem with an inflatable bulb at the distal end (Fig. 118.1); it can be used for both conditions. The stem of this rubber catheter is 1 inch long and the diameter is that of a No. 10 Fr Foley catheter; the small inflatable balloon tip holds up to 3 or 4 mL of saline.

For patients with noninflamed and recurrent Bartholin cysts, marsupialization is a permanent cure. The procedure can be performed in the office but often is done as a same-day surgical procedure. It is very well tolerated by patients, with a rapid healing time and minimal postprocedure discomfort. Complications are rare and the technique is easily learned, especially by clinicians familiar with perineal repairs.

INDICATIONS

* Treatment of symptomatic Bartholin duct cyst (painful, growing)
* Treatment of Bartholin gland abscess

CONTRAINDICATIONS

Any condition that would preclude normal I&D of a vulvar cyst or abscess would preclude the use of the Word catheter. Small, asymptomatic glands do not have to be drained. A Word catheter should not be used in a patient with latex allergy. Marsupialization should not be performed in the patient with cellulitis.

EQUIPMENT

* Word catheter (Rusch and Milex; most medical suppliers will have these on hand)
* 3-mL syringe (for catheter inflation)
* 22- to 25-gauge 1-inch needle (for catheter inflation)
* 2% lidocaine for anesthesia, usually with epinephrine
* 27- to 30-gauge 1.5-inch needle (for anesthesia)
* 3-mL syringe (for anesthesia)
* No. 11 blade scalpel
* Pickups (Adson) with teeth
* Two small hemostats
* 4 × 4 gauze pads
* Normal saline for irrigation
* Antiseptic solution (povidone-iodine if not allergic)
* 4-0 Vicryl suture (if marsupialization is done)
* Needle holder (if marsupialization is done)
* Silver nitrate or electrocautery may be needed (if marsupialization is done)

PREPROCEDURE PATIENT EDUCATION

The clinician should explain the procedure to the patient and obtain informed consent. A nonnarcotic oral analgesic may be administered before the procedure if desired.

PROCEDURE

Word Catheter Placement

1. Place the patient in the dorsal lithotomy position.
2. Prepare the labia and vagina with the antiseptic solution. It is preferable to enter the cyst (Fig. 118.2A) or abscess from the vaginal side of the introitus, just inside the labia majora and outside the hymenal ring, unless this would require a much deeper incision (see Fig. 118.2B). Inject lidocaine over the intended site of entry. If the incision is to be made external to the introitus where the abscess is "pointing," plan to insert the catheter approximately in the area of the original duct orifice, immediately external and adjacent the hymenal ring (see Fig. 118.2C).
3. Grasp the cyst to stabilize it with the nondominant hand. With dominant hand, lance or incise the cyst or abscess with a No. 11 scalpel blade (see Fig. 118.2C). It is essential that the stab wound penetrate both the mucosa and the cyst or abscess wall, which will be evidenced by the free flow of pus or mucus. *Culture* the contents if indicated. Although the majority of simple cysts are sterile, abscesses are typically polymicrobial, and many others contain *Neisseria gonorrhoeae*. Culture usually will not change initial management. The stab wound must be just large enough for the catheter to be inserted, usually 3 to 4 mm.

It may be difficult to insert the catheter into the cyst cavity after the incision has been made, the contents have been extruded, and the cyst/abscess has collapsed. Attempts to insert the catheter blindly may create a false tract and the catheter may not be in the cyst/abscess itself, where it should be. To avoid creating a false tract and to ensure proper placement of the catheter, incise carefully through the skin until the cyst/abscess fluid drains. Before removing the blade but after the incision has been made, insert a closed hemostat down the side of the blade, open the hemostat, and break up any adhesions. Remove the hemostat and now insert open pickups

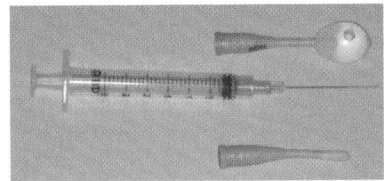

Fig. 118.1 Word catheter (*bottom*). Three-mL syringe filled with water and 25-gauge needle (*middle*). Word catheter inflated with water (*top*).

(Adsons with teeth) down the side of the blade, one arm into the lumen and the other outside. Use the pickups to gently grasp the sidewall of the cyst and surrounding tissue (see Fig. 118.2D). This stabilizes the tissue and identifies the cavity. Remove the blade and insert the Word catheter (see Fig. 118.2E).

4. Once the catheter has been inserted, inflate the catheter's bulb by injecting 2.5 to 4 mL of saline through the sealed-stopper end (see Fig. 118.2F). Use just enough saline to ensure that the catheter will not fall out with normal activity (usually 2.5 to 4 mL). Do *not* use air to inflate the catheter. Remove the pickups (see Fig. 118.2G).

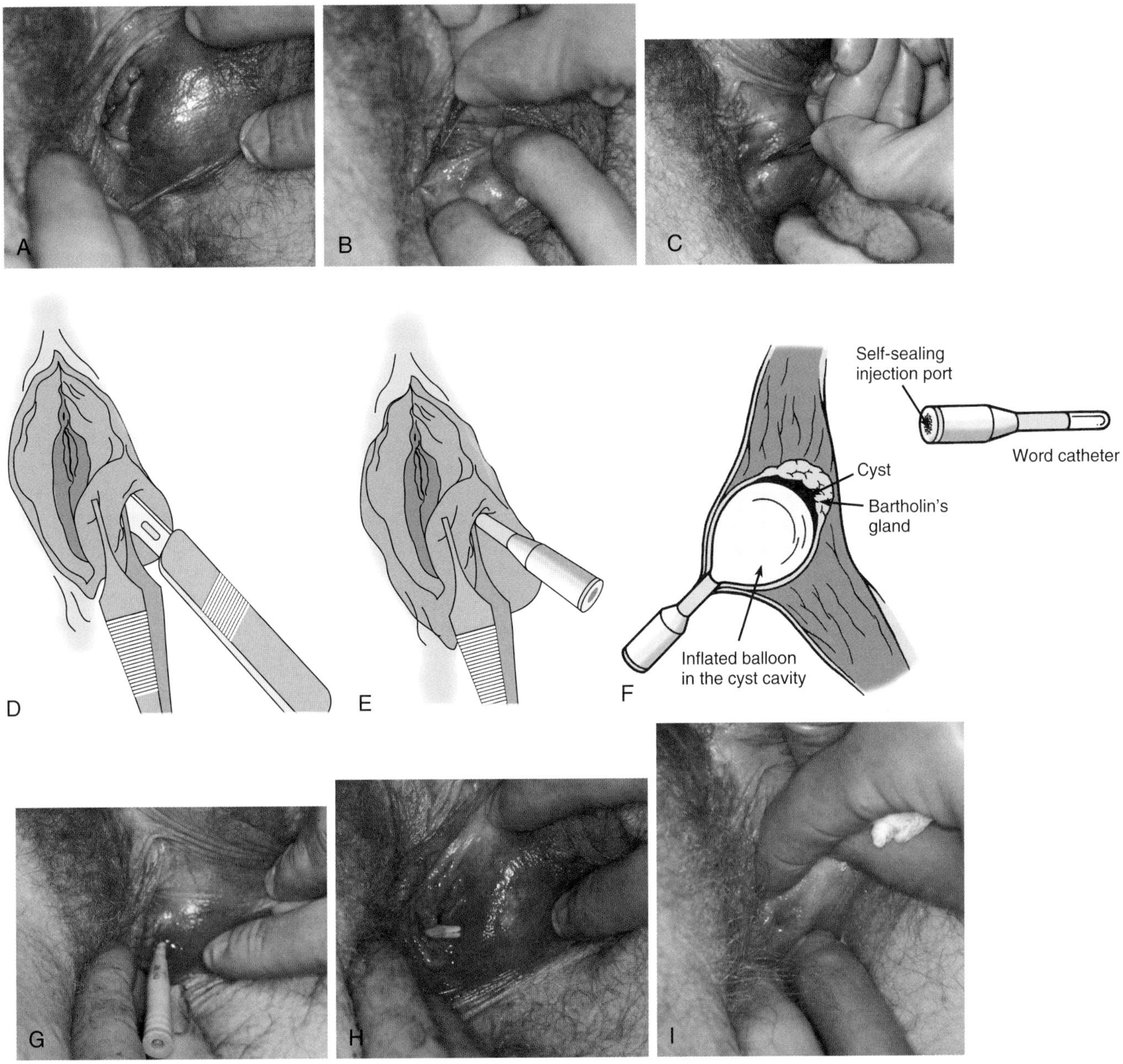

Fig. 118.2 Insertion of Word catheter. (A) Bartholin cyst on patient's left vaginal sidewall after local anesthetic was injected superficially. (Note vaginal orifice viewed slightly to left of cyst.) (B) No. 11 blade points to ideal location inside the hymenal ring for the incision. However, the cyst is more prominent externally, so incision will be made there. (C) Incising the cyst. Make the opening just large enough for the uninflated Word catheter tip to enter. (D) Slide Adson forceps with teeth along the blade (which is in the cyst/abscess) and gently grasp the tissue. This will define the tract into the cyst. If this is not done, especially in smaller cysts, a false cavity may be created when the catheter is inserted. (E) The blade is removed but the forceps are kept in place. Insert the catheter along the forceps. (F) Remove the forceps. Inflate the balloon with saline. Gently tug the catheter after inflation to make sure that it does not fall out of the opening. (G) The balloon is inflated within the cavity of the cyst so that it will not fall out through the stab wound. (H) Tuck the exposed portion of the catheter into the vagina. (I) Appearance of the area immediately after removal of the catheter.

5. If the incision was made inside the hymen, tuck the catheter stem into the vagina, where it will rest perpendicular to the perineum (see Fig. 118.2H). If the incision was made just outside the hymen, it can still be tucked into the vaginal canal. With the catheter in the vagina, the patient has freedom of movement and activity without the added awareness of protrusion of the catheter stem, which can occur if an external incision site is used. Most patients tolerate the catheter without discomfort if excessive amounts of saline are not introduced into the catheter bulb.

6. The catheter can be removed in 4 to 6 weeks after withdrawing the saline, leaving a small ostium for the gland (see Fig. 118.2I). The gland may eventually scar shut, which has no adverse consequences.

Bartholin Cyst Marsupialization

1. Place the patient in the dorsal lithotomy position. Block the incision site with local anesthetic with 2% lidocaine with epinephrine or use a pudendal block with 2% lidocaine without epinephrine. Some patients may prefer spinal or general anesthesia, but this requires that the procedure be done in a same-day surgery center.

2. Clean the perineum with povidone-iodine solution (if the patient is not allergic).

3. Inspect the external genitalia to determine the extent of the duct cyst. Retract the labium laterally to identify the incision site, internal to the hymenal ring. Make the incision longitudinal with respect to the vagina (Fig. 118.3). Incisions can also be done vertically, following the circumferential folds of the vaginal mucosa, but these will lack the natural tension of the mucosa and could lead to premature closure and incomplete marsupialization. Generally a fusiform incision 1 or 2 cm in width at the center is needed to allow for removal of a substantial portion of the Bartholin cyst wall. Avoid excising any portion of the external skin (vs. mucosa). Excise the mucosal fusiform segment first, and if the cyst wall is still intact, excise a fusiform section of the exposed cyst wall in the same manner.

4. During excision of the mucosal fusiform segment, the cyst wall will usually be entered, the contents will spill, and the cyst wall will collapse. Therefore the mucosa over the cyst should be excised first, so it can be clearly defined. Next, the exposed cyst wall should be grasped with two small hemostats before the cyst wall fusiform segment is removed. Explore the remaining cyst with small hemostats and remove any attached loculations. Patients above 40 years of age are at higher risk for cancer in the Bartholin gland, so look for any signs of neoplastic appearing epithelium on the cyst wall being removed and the remaining cyst wall (Fig. 118.4). The removed tissue should be sent for pathology.

5. Thoroughly irrigate the cyst cavity with normal saline.

6. When the Bartholin cyst wall is being sutured, approximate the cut edge of the cyst wall to the adjacent edge of the vaginal mucosa. This allows for more rapid transformation of the Bartholin cyst wall into a normal mucosal lining that will blend into the vaginal mucosa. Interrupted sutures will be placed around the excisional margins using 4-0 Vicryl.

7. Place an anchoring stitch with long tags proximally to grasp and stabilize the tissue. Pass the interrupted stitches from the inside through just the Bartholin cyst wall. Bring the needle to the surface between the cyst wall and the submucosal layer. Now insert the needle under the vaginal epithelium and pull it to the surface of the vaginal wall. This effectively imbricates the two layers (cyst wall and vaginal mucosa) over the submucosal tissue, which allows them to heal together (Fig. 118.5). The intent is to suture the cyst cavity open.

8. After the entire site has been sutured open, irrigate the wound and inspect it for bleeding. There should be a gap of at least 1 cm across the open marsupialization. Normally no dressing is needed. A pad is placed to allow for the collection of blood or drainage from the wound. Pressure, silver nitrate, or electrocautery can be used to deal with any bleeding. For persistent bleeding, the entire incision can be closed with suture for 20 to 30 minutes, if necessary, for hemostasis. After 20 to 30 minutes, the suture can be removed and any persistent bleeding treated with pressure, silver nitrate, or electrocautery.

9. Instruct the patient to perform sitz baths daily for 3 or 4 days and to return for follow-up in about a week (see the postoperative patient handout available at www.expertconsult.com). At that time, the cavity will be probed for patency. Use of prophylactic antibiotics is unnecessary in most cases; the need for this should be assessed individually. Excessive induration in the local tissue or risk factors for infection, such as pregnancy or diabetes, may prompt the need for antibiotic therapy. The sutures will be absorbed without further intervention.

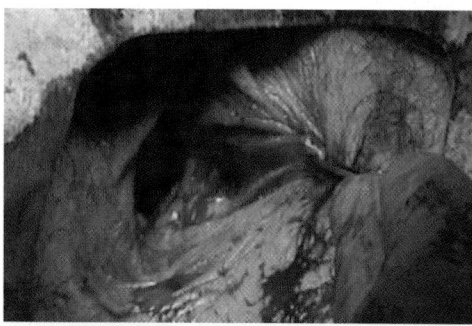

Fig. 118.4 Bartholin cyst opened with roof removed.

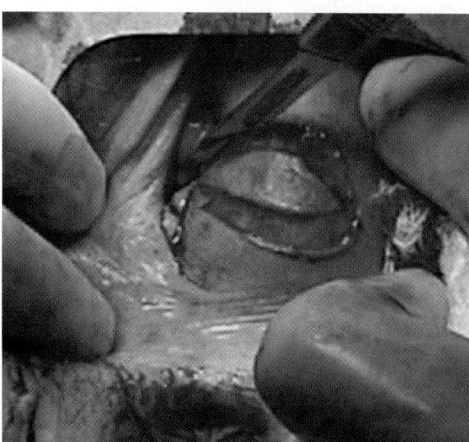

Fig. 118.3 Fusiform longitudinal incision for marsupialization on patient's left vaginal sidewall (retracted).

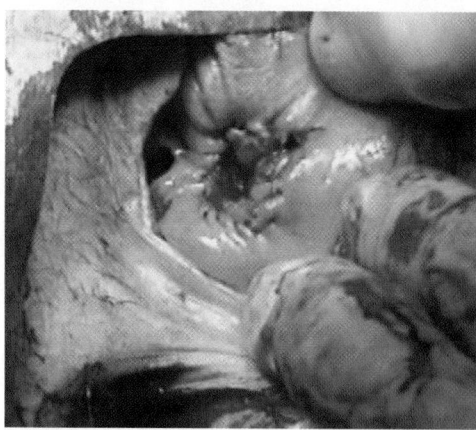

Fig. 118.5 Marsupialized Bartholin cyst with sutures in place. (Note vaginal orifice viewed slightly to the left of the marsupialized cyst.)

COMMON ERRORS

- Creating a false tract for the catheter placement (see earlier).
- Catheter falls out before it is time for it to be removed. This may lead to recurrence of the cyst/abscess. The error occurs after the balloon is inserted into the cyst/abscess and after the fluid is injected into the balloon (but the syringe is still in the port), when the clinician releases the pressure on the syringe plunger to check the tightness of the balloon in the cavity by tugging on it. Although it may seem secure then, the increased pressure in the balloon will push some saline back up into the syringe (unless pressure is maintained on the plunger). The balloon then, in effect, deflates to a smaller size and the catheter may inadvertently fall out prematurely. To prevent this from occurring, maintain pressure on the syringe plunger while checking the bulb placement and snugness in the cavity. The catheter could also fall out because of too large a stab wound.
- Continuous pain after insertion of the Word catheter may occur. The bulb may be too large for the cyst cavity, which may be corrected by withdrawing some of the fluid, thus reducing the size of the bulb. Also, if the bulb is not in the true cavity but in the space between the fascia and the cyst wall, the patient will complain of significant pain. In this case, catheter removal and reinsertion will have to be repeated under local anesthesia.
- With an abscessed Bartholin gland, there may be cellulitis around the vulvar opening of the duct. Insertion of the catheter may not correct the cellulitis and antibiotics may have to be administered for 48 to 72 hours after insertion of the catheter. If *N. gonorrhoeae* is cultured, appropriate actions must be taken.
- If the needle used to introduce the saline into the catheter punctures the stem, the catheter will gradually deflate and fall out before epithelialization is complete.
- If the stab wound is too large, the catheter will fall out. It may be necessary to suture the stab wound around the catheter to keep it in place. If the catheter falls out in less than 4 weeks, the likelihood of recurrence is high. If there is only partial formation of a new tract, placement of another Word catheter may be indicated, but that may not be possible because of constriction of the opening.
- Marsupialization can fail due to inadequate fusiform excision, circumferential instead of longitudinal fusiform excision, or improper placement of sutures.

COMPLICATIONS

- Excessive bleeding (rare)
- Discomfort (usually lasting only a few days)
- Recurrence
- Scarring (usually minimal)
- Infection
- Premature expulsion of the catheter

POSTPROCEDURE PATIENT EDUCATION

Word Catheter

- Tell the patient to expect a discharge because the catheter will allow for drainage of the cyst or abscess.
- The Word catheter is left in place for 4 to 6 weeks until epithelialization of the new tract is complete.
- Advise the patient that sexual activity may be resumed after 2 weeks but that it may increase the risk of expulsion of the catheter. If this happens, another catheter may have to

be inserted. It is best to defer sexual activity until the catheter has been removed.
- Encourage daily showers or tub baths.
- Schedule a return visit in 4 to 6 weeks. At that time the catheter is removed by inserting a needle into the catheter's sealed stopper end and drawing out the saline. The catheter is then withdrawn from the incision.

Marsupialization

- Daily sitz baths are encouraged for 3 to 5 days.
- Sexual activity is to be avoided until after the first postoperative check at 1 week, although waiting for an additional week would be prudent to allow for more complete healing.

CPT/BILLING CODES

56405	I&D of vulvar or perineal abscess
56420	I&D of Bartholin's gland cyst/abscess
56440	Marsupialization of Bartholin's gland cyst
56740	Excision of Bartholin's gland or cyst

ICD-10-CM DIAGNOSTIC CODES

N75.0	Bartholin's cyst
N75.1	Bartholin's abscess
N76.4	Other vulvar abscess

Acknowledgment

The editors recognize the contributions of Barbara S. Apgar, MD, to this chapter in previous editions of this text.

SUPPLIERS

(See contact information available at www.expertconsult.com.)

Word Bartholin gland catheter
Milex Products, Inc.
Rusch, Inc.

RECOMMENDED READING

Goldberg JE. Simplified treatment for disease of Bartholin's gland. *Obstet Gynecol.* 1970;35:109–110.

Folashade O, Simmons BJ, Hacker Y. *Am Fam Physician.* 2003;68(1):135–140.

Holtzman LC, Hitti E, Harrow J. Incision and drainage. In: Roberts Jr, Custalow CB, Thomsen TW, eds. *Roberts and Hedges Clinical Procedures in Emergency Medicine.* 6th ed. Philadelphia: Elsevier; 2014:739–744.

Kilpatrick CC. Bartholin gland abscess or cyst incision and drainage. In: Reichman EF, ed. *Emergency Medicine Procedures.* 2nd ed. New York: McGraw-Hill; 2013:930–935.

Omole F, Simmons BJ, Hacker Y. Management of Bartholin's duct cyst and gland abscess. *Am Fam Physician.* 2003;68:135–140.

Tuggy M, Garcia J. Bartholin's Gland: Marsupialization. http://www.proceduresconsult.com/medical-procedures/bartholins-gland-%E2%80%93-marsupialization-FM-023-procedure.aspx.

Wechter MD, Wu JM, Marzano D, Haefner H. Management of Bartholin duct cyst and abscesses: a systematic review. *Obstet Gynecol Surv.* 2009;64:395–404.

Word B. New instrument for office treatment of cyst and abscess of Bartholin's gland. *JAMA.* 1964;190:777–778.

CHAPTER 119

BREAST BIOPSY

Helen A. Pass

An open excisional breast biopsy is a technically straightforward outpatient procedure readily performed with the patient under local anesthesia. With appropriate training and experience, primary care clinicians can become qualified to perform most simple breast biopsies. The challenge is to correctly identify which lesions are amenable to biopsy and which require referral to a breast (general) surgeon. The goals in the management of a patient with a breast mass should be to obtain the diagnosis in the most expedient manner, to achieve good cosmesis, and to preserve all therapeutic options if the mass is unexpectedly found to be malignant at biopsy.

The only definitive method for ensuring that a mass is benign is to remove tissue for pathologic examination. The missed or delayed diagnosis of a breast mass that ultimately proved to be cancerous is currently the most litigious aspect of medical practice. Failure to be impressed with physical examination findings was cited as the most common reason for the delay in the diagnosis of breast cancer. Malignant lesions are usually hard, immobile, fixed to surrounding tissue, and have poorly defined margins. Benign masses are usually smooth, well-circumscribed (round), soft to firm, do not cause skin changes, and are freely mobile; however, many cancers (e.g., colloid, medullary, and expansive intraductal) may mimic this presentation. Similarly, even though the incidence of breast cancer rises dramatically after age 65 years, 63% to 80% of lawsuits resulted from the missed diagnosis of cancer in women younger than 50 years. In addition, whereas the presence of a significant positive family history increases the suspicion that a palpable abnormality may prove to be malignant, two thirds of all women with the diagnosis of breast cancer have no identifiable risk factor. Nevertheless, it is important to remind our patients and ourselves that not all breast masses are cancerous.

That said, if a patient describes a mass but no mass is palpable on examination, it is reasonable to either repeat the examination in 1 to 2 months or to refer the patient to a subspecialist.

The role of mammography in women with a breast mass is twofold. First, it can offer clues as to the degree of suspicion that the mass may be malignant. Worrisome mammographic features include the findings of a spiculated lesion, a mass associated with pleomorphic microcalcifications, or dermal edema and retraction. Second, it allows assessment of the remainder of the breast parenchyma in both the involved and contralateral breasts. Before proceeding with excisional biopsy, a baseline mammogram must be obtained to rule out the presence of an occult synchronous lesion that may alter the surgical approach. Moreover, if the mass is highly suspect, referral to a surgeon may be indicated to facilitate management of a presumed breast cancer. *It is crucial to realize that failure of mammography or ultrasonography to visualize a discrete, palpable abnormality should not be construed as evidence of the benignity of the lesion.* Up to 10% of breast cancers are radiographically occult. Thus a lesion should be removed if it meets the criteria for biopsy based on the clinical breast examination, regardless of the breast imaging characteristics. Likewise, if a woman identifies an area of change in her breasts, the complaint should be taken seriously.

In addition to highly suspect lesions, referral to a breast (general) surgeon should be considered for an additional small subset of patients. Masses in prepubertal or pubescent girls (prepubertal gynecomastia) could represent the forming breast buds and must not be sampled for biopsy unless highly suspect because lifelong cosmetic deformity may result. Masses greater than 4 cm are best approached by core biopsy, provided that if the lesion proves to be malignant, consideration should be given to neoadjuvant chemotherapy. In addition, if the lesion is benign, special surgical techniques will be necessary to minimize the cosmetic deformity associated with subsequent removal. Finally, biopsy of lesions requiring preoperative mammographic localization with wire placement should be performed by clinicians who have received specific training in this technique.

Consideration should be given to performing fine-needle aspiration (FNA) before core or excisional biopsy (see Chapter 68, Fine-Needle Aspiration Cytology and Biopsy). FNA is both diagnostic and therapeutic for simple cysts, thereby avoiding unnecessary anxiety and surgery. If the mass is solid, a specimen for cytologic examination can be obtained, and breast cancer can be diagnosed before excisional biopsy. The false-negative rate of FNA is 0.4% to 35%, and the false-positive rate is less than 1%. Thus concordance among the clinical breast examination, the breast imaging, and the FNA (the triple test) must be established, especially if the decision is made not to proceed to biopsy.

As it turns out, with improvement in skills and access of percutaneous needle biopsy (i.e., core-needle biopsy, FNA), less than 35% of breast biopsies now utilize the open excisional technique in the United States. Although open excisional biopsy was once considered the gold standard, a 2014 systematic literature review found similar sensitivity and specificity for ultrasound- and stereotactic-guided biopsies compared with open biopsies. Prior to this, an expert panel at the 2009 International Breast Cancer Consensus Conference III recommended percutaneous needle biopsy replace open surgical biopsy as the new gold standard and best practice for the initial diagnostic workup for breast lesions. Further recommendations from the panel include limiting the rate of open surgical biopsy as the initial diagnostic biopsy for breast lesions to less than 5% to 10% of a surgeon's practice. That said, there are large parts of the United States and the remainder of the world where percutaneous breast biopsy is not available.

ANATOMY

Anatomically, the breast extends superiorly to the level of the clavicle, inferiorly to the sixth or seventh rib, medially to the lateral border of the sternum, and laterally to the border of the latissimus dorsi muscle. The glandular structure sits atop the pectoralis major muscle, and deep breast biopsies may extend to the level of the fascia. The blood supply originates from the internal mammary, axillary, and intercostal arteries. The venous outflow parallels this arterial supply. The only innervation to the breast is cutaneous, extending from the plexus of nerves in the neck for the superior half of the breast and the intercostal nerves for the lower half of the breast. There is no direct innervation to the glandular structure. The lymphatic vessels in the breast drain to the axilla and the internal mammary lymph nodes.

In the center of the breast is the nipple and areolar complex. Surrounding the edge of the areolar complex are Montgomery tubercles, which provide lubrication important for breastfeeding.

The breast mound itself is composed of fat and glandular milk-producing tissue. About 15 to 20 ducts converge to exit the nipple. Cooper ligaments run from the deep fascia to the dermis, traversing the breast gland and serving as suspensory ligaments of the breast. The lack of named structures within the breast glandular tissue simplifies breast biopsy because hemostasis usually is readily achieved with electrocautery. Except with circumareolar incision placement, numbness is rare in the peri-incisional area.

INDICATIONS

- The presence of a palpable, dominant abnormality in a male or female patient
- A cystic lesion if
  - The FNA contained bloody fluid
  - A palpable abnormality remains after FNA
  - The cyst recurred after two FNAs
- After an FNA that was equivocal, nondiagnostic, or not concordant with the clinical breast examination or breast imaging
- Unresolved patient anxiety and a desire for removal of the mass
- Clinician uncertainty about the true nature of the lesion

CONTRAINDICATIONS

- Mass that is highly suspect for breast cancer (refer to breast or general surgeon).
- Mass greater than 4 cm (consider diagnosis by core biopsy or referral to surgeon).
- Mass in a prepubertal or pubescent female (consider referral).
- Lesion requiring preoperative mammographic localization (i.e., it is nonpalpable; consider referral).
- Uncorrected bleeding disorder or other unstable medical condition is an absolute contraindication.

EQUIPMENT AND SUPPLIES

- Surgical marking pen
- Povidone–iodine or other antiseptic skin preparation solution
- Fenestrated drape
- Local anesthetic (the addition of 1 mL of 8.5% sodium bicarbonate solution to each 10 mL of 1% lidocaine without epinephrine creates a buffered solution with a more neutral pH, allowing less discomfort during infiltration and a more rapid onset of action)
- Sterile 4 × 4 gauze
- Scalpel with No. 15 blades
- Two curved hemostats
- Needle driver
- Adson pickups
- DeBakey pickups (optional)
- Metzenbaum tissue scissors
- Allis clamp
- Small self-retaining retractor (e.g., mastoid retractor or small Weitlaner retractor) (optional)
- Army-Navy or Senn retractor
- Electrocautery unit
- 3-0 or 4-0 Vicryl suture
- 4-0 or 5-0 Monocryl or polydioxanone suture
- Steri-Strips or Dermabond
- Jobst postoperative brassiere (optional)

PRECAUTIONS

Immediately before any planned procedure, the woman must be examined. The surgeon must verify with the patient that the palpable abnormality still persists, concur on its location, and mark it with indelible ink. As with any surgical procedure, standard presurgical clearances and permits should be obtained.

PREPROCEDURE PATIENT PREPARATION

All women older than 30 years should have a preprocedure mammogram. Provide calm reassurance to the patient, because the discovery of a breast mass and the knowledge that biopsy is necessary is a highly stressful event for the patient. Provide detailed explanations of the procedure supplemented by written educational material.

PROCEDURE

The abnormality should be identified and marked before the procedure with the patient's assistance. Determining the optimal placement of the incision for an excisional breast biopsy is a balance between achieving the most desirable cosmetic result and preserving further surgical options should the lesion prove to be cancerous. Use of preoperative FNA or core biopsy can minimize the number of breast masses unexpectedly found to be malignant. In general, incisions placed along Langer lines—the natural lines of skin tension and creasing—produce the best cosmetic result (Fig. 119.1A). However, a radial incision may be preferable in the most medial part of the breast (much easier to reexcise if a mastectomy is subsequently required) or in the lower half of the breast if the mass is larger, or subsequent removal of skin will be required (e.g., with reexcision lumpectomy; see Fig. 119.1B). A better cosmetic result is achieved in the lower half of the breast by narrowing the breast when removing breast volume through a radial incision than by shortening the distance between the areolar complex and inframammary fold with a curvilinear incision. In a young woman in whom the mass is likely benign, consideration may be given to placing the incision in a circumareolar location.

Benign lesions may be either enucleated or removed with a small rim of normal tissue. Care should be taken to ensure that the mass is not morcellated. The specimen should be oriented for pathologic examination in case it is found to be malignant and reexcision is necessary.

After removing the breast mass, most surgeons no longer reapproximate the remaining deep breast parenchyma ("dead space"). This eliminates the breast distortion with poorer cosmesis and greater mammographic distortion that occurs when the "dead space" is reapproximated. Meticulous hemostasis must be achieved to avoid hematoma formation. Drains should not be used. Closure of the superficial fascia provides good restoration of the breast contours. The skin is then closed in a subcuticular fashion.

1. Obtain written informed consent.
2. Using sterile technique, cleanse and drape the breast.
3. Using a surgical marking pen, outline the incision and the borders of the mass (Fig. 119.2).
4. Give local anesthesia (1% lidocaine without epinephrine mixed 10:1 with 8.5% sodium bicarbonate). Infiltrate the incision with the local anesthetic to create a dermal wheal. Use the anesthetized wheal for all subsequent needle inserts, and infiltrate circumferentially around the lesion to be removed. Excess local anesthetic directly overlying the mass may obscure palpation of the nodule, hindering identification. (Alternatively, do a field block by injecting circumferentially around the lesion but not over the lesion itself. This allows easier palpation of the mass in the center of the field without the distortion created by the volume of anesthetic [Fig. 119.3].)

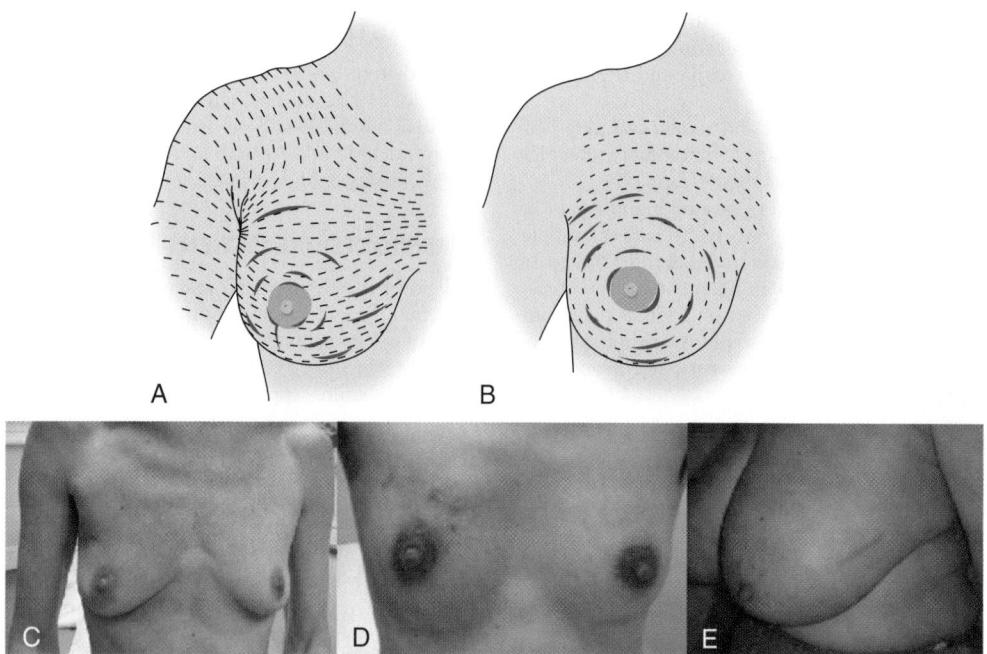

Fig. 119.1 Proper planning of incisions limits postoperative scarring. (A) Langer lines: naural lines of skin tension and creasing. (B) Radial incision is preferable in certain cases. (C–E) Outcome examples.

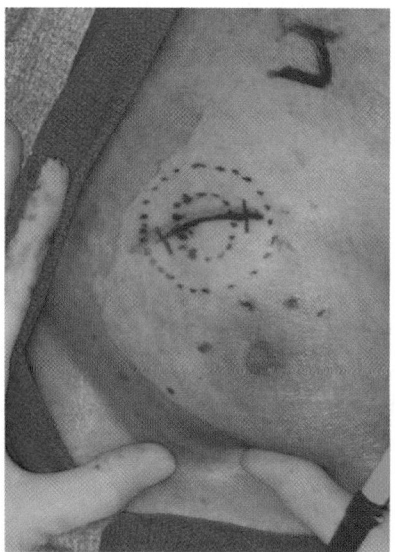

Fig. 119.2 Palpable lesion marked for biopsy.

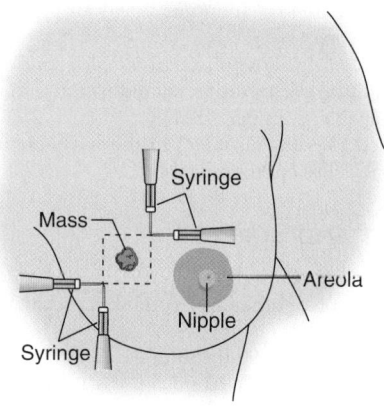

Fig. 119.3 Field block local anesthesia technique to preserve the ability to palpate the lesion in the center of the field. Infiltration of excessive amounts of local anesthetic directly over the mass makes palpation of the abnormality difficult.

5. Incise the skin with a No. 15 blade, making sure to hold the blade at right angles to the skin edges to avoid beveling the incision. Carry the incision vertically to the subcutaneous layer.
6. Use tissue scissors or cautery to dissect down to the level of the mass (Fig. 119.4).
7. Cauterize bleeders with the electrocautery.
8. Circumferentially excise the specimen using the tissue scissors, a No. 15 blade, or the electrocautery unit (Fig. 119.5). Exercise care to avoid harming the skin edges. An Allis clamp may be used on the mass to provide countertraction, facilitating removal of the mass. Provide more local anesthesia in the deeper layers as needed.
9. Orient the specimen for pathologic evaluation using marking sutures (this can facilitate localization of inadequate margins, should the lesion be found to be an incompletely excised malignancy).
10. Submit all specimens for pathologic evaluation. Use of frozen-section analysis is optional because hormone receptor analysis is now routinely performed on paraffin-embedded tissue in case of malignancy.
11. Obtain meticulous hemostasis with electrocautery.
12. Reapproximate the subdermal tissue with buried interrupted Vicryl sutures. To prevent deformity, do not reapproximate the deep tissues, and do not incorporate excessively large amounts of tissue because this may lead to dimpling (Fig. 119.6).
13. Close the skin with a running subcuticular suture of 4-0 or 5-0 Monocryl or polydioxanone (Fig. 119.7).

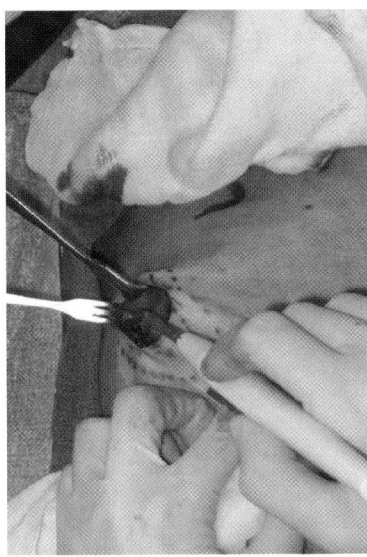

Fig. 119.4   Dissection with electrocautery.

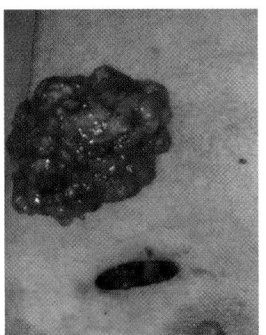

Fig. 119.5   Lesion excised.

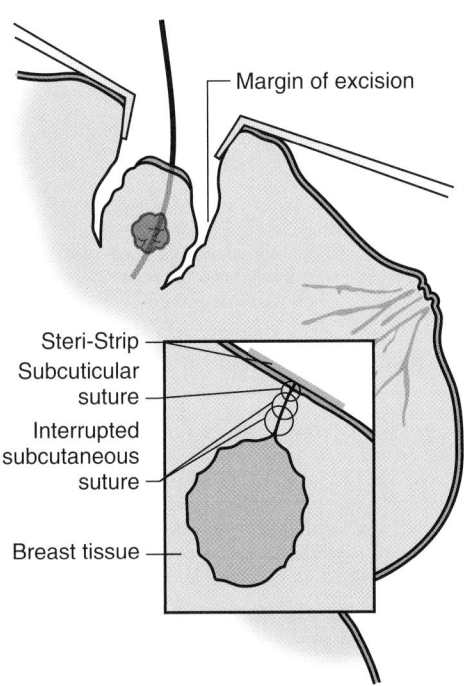

Margin of excision

Steri-Strip

Subcuticular suture

Interrupted subcutaneous suture

Breast tissue

Fig. 119.6   Schema for closure technique.

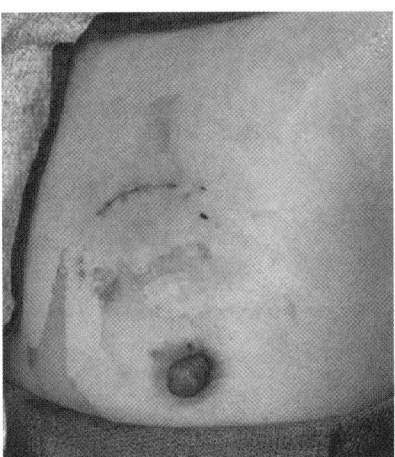

Fig. 119.7   Cosmetic closure: appearance on completion of the surgery.

SAMPLE OPERATIVE REPORT

See the sample operative report available at www.expertconsult.com.

COMMON ERRORS

- Failure to sample a palpable, dominant mass because the lesion is radiographically occult. *Resolution:* Because up to 10% of cancers can be radiographically occult, biopsy must be performed if clinical examination confirms the presence of a dominant mass.
- Failure to obtain a mammogram before biopsy. *Resolution:* All women older than 30 years should have a recent mammogram before biopsy to rule out the presence of occult synchronous lesions that may modify the surgical approach.
- Poor orientation of the surgical incisions. *Resolution:* Proper planning can ensure a better cosmetic outcome and allow for subsequent surgery if malignancy is identified (see Fig. 119.1).

COMPLICATIONS

- Hematoma (may mimic recurrence of the mass). *Resolution:* (1) Confirm patient does not have an unsuspected bleeding diathesis. (2) If the hematoma is symptomatic, reoperate with evacuation of the hematoma. Search for and cauterize or ligate of any site of bleeding. Use a compressive dressing. (3) If asymptomatic, reassurance, use of a supportive brassiere, and passage of time will allow spontaneous resolution.
- Infection (cellulitis or abscess formation). *Resolution:* Seroma aspiration can differentiate between cellulitis and cellulitis with abscess formation (send fluid for Gram stain, culture, and sensitivity even if the fluid is clear). Cellulitis without abscess formation usually responds to oral antibiotic therapy. Resolution is usual with the use of a first-generation cephalosporin. If no response is obtained in 7 to 10 days, culture and sensitivity data may be helpful. For cellulitis with abscess formation, drainage of the abscess is necessary. Complete aspiration under ultrasonographic guidance and initiation of oral antibiotic therapy may be tried initially. If abscess recurs, drain placement with or without surgical evacuation and irrigation may be necessary. Again, culture and sensitivity data can help with antibiotic selection.
- Scarring or skin distortion. *Resolution:* Be sure the patient understands that a fine scar should be expected. If the patient tends to form hypertrophic or keloid scars, a small amount of triamcinolone (10 mg/mL) can be used with the local anesthesia in the incision tract. Avoid scarring with appropriate preoperative planning. After surgery, silicone sheeting, Mederma cream application, or cross-scar massage may improve appearance of scarring.

- Pain (usually minimal). *Resolution:* The use of oral analgesics, use of supportive brassiere, and topical application of ice or heat should provide adequate relief.
- Fluid collection (seroma). *Resolution:* May require aspiration but only if symptomatic. The presence of an asymptomatic seroma is not an indication for drainage.
- Failure to identify the correct mass or incomplete removal of the lesion. *Resolution:* Can be avoided by proper preoperative localization, marking, and patient confirmation. Before closure, palpate the biopsy bed to confirm the absence of residual palpable abnormality. If it is recognized after surgery, prompt reoperation is indicated.
- Need for subsequent surgery. *Resolution:* If the mass is malignant or incompletely excised, promptly refer to a breast (general) surgeon.

POSTPROCEDURE MANAGEMENT

Wash off any remaining skin preparation solution, and then apply Steri-Strips and a sterile bandage or use a cyanoacrylate surgical glue (e.g., Dermabond [Ethicon]). If adequate hemostasis has been ensured, there is no need for bulky, pressure dressings. A surgical brassiere may be used to enhance postoperative comfort.

The patient must be provided with prescriptions for adequate analgesia by mouth, emergency phone numbers, and written postoperative instructions.

The patient may remove the dressing in 24 to 48 hours and resume showering. If Dermabond or Opsite (Smith & Nephew) is used over gauze-covered Steri-Strips, the patient may shower immediately. Submersion of the incision (e.g., swimming) and vigorous exercise should be avoided for 1 week. The sutures will dissolve and should not require removal.

POSTPROCEDURE PATIENT EDUCATION

Give the patient written instructions regarding removal of the dressing, resumption of showering, and follow-up appointment. The patient should report excessive pain, drainage from the wound, redness, fever, or abnormal swelling. A follow-up appointment will ensure the lesion has been removed, although induration may be palpable for several weeks. See the patient education form available at www.expertconsult.com.

SPECIAL CONSIDERATIONS

- The appearance of the incision is all the patient sees; your surgical skill will be judged by the scar left on the breast. Plan the incision carefully and use plastic surgical technique for skin closure.
- It is imperative to communicate the pathology results in a timely manner and to refer to specialists if necessary.
- Avoid biopsy of large or complicated lesions; refer instead.
- Management of breast complaints is very litigious. Adequately document the workup. Obtain informed consent. Diligently follow up on all biopsy results, and recognize when referral is appropriate.

CONCLUSION

Accurate interpretation of the clinical breast examination can be difficult. Any persistent palpable abnormality or asymmetric finding must be evaluated with physical examination, breast radiologic imaging (mammography or ultrasonography), and tissue diagnosis. All findings must be concordant; if they are not, workup must proceed even if the mammogram is negative. With sufficient training and experience, most primary care practitioners can perform excisional breast biopsies in the office setting expeditiously and with a good cosmetic outcome. Complex or highly suspect masses may prompt referral to a breast specialist.

PATIENT EDUCATION GUIDES

See patient education and patient consent forms available at www.expertconsult.com.

CPT/BILLING CODES

10021	Fine-needle aspirate (FNA)
10022	Fine-needle aspiration with imaging guidance
19000	Needle aspiration, cyst—one
19001	Needle aspiration, each additional cyst
19100	Biopsy of breast, core needle
19101	Biopsy of breast, open incisional
19081	Biopsy of breast with placement of localization device, when performed, and imaging of the biopsy specimen, when performed, percutaneous; first lesion, including stereotactic guidance
19082	Each additional lesion
19120	Excision of cysts or breast lesions
19125	Excision of breast lesion identified by preoperative placement of radiological marker
19126	Each additional lesion separately identified by a preoperative radiologic marker

ICD-10-CM DIAGNOSTIC CODES

C50.919	Malignant neoplasm of breast (female), unspecified
D24.9	Benign neoplasm of the breast
N63.0	Lump or mass in the breast unspecified
R92.8	Abnormal mammogram, unspecified
R92.0	Mammographic microcalcification
R92.8	Other abnormal findings on radiological examination of the breast

SUPPLIERS

(See contact information available at www.expertconsult.com.)

Jobst postoperative brassiere
   Fredericks-Jobst Institute, Inc.

ONLINE RESOURCES

National Comprehensive Cancer Network: www.nccn.org (breast cancer screening and diagnosis guidelines, updated annually)
Susan G. Komen for the Cure: www.komen.org (medically reviewed material on screening, diagnosis, and treatment of breast diseases authored by the largest breast cancer patient advocacy group)

RECOMMENDED READING

Cady B, Steele GD, Morrow M, et al. Evaluation of common breast problems: guidance for primary care providers. *CA Cancer J Clin.* 1998;48: 49–63.
Dahabreh IJ, Wieland LS, Adam GP, et al. *AHRQ Comparative Effectiveness Reviews. Core Needle and Open Surgical Biopsy for Diagnosis of Breast Lesions: An Update to the 2009 Report.* Rockville, MD: Agency for Healthcare Research and Quality; 2014.
Donegan WL. Evaluation of a palpable breast mass. *N Engl J Med.* 1992;327:937–942.
Gamble WG. Breast surgery. In: Benjamin RB, ed. *Atlas of Outpatient and Office Surgery.* 2nd ed. Philadelphia: Lea & Febiger; 1994.
Klein S. Evaluation of palpable breast masses. *Am Fam Physician.* 2005;71(9):1731–1738.

Layfield LJ, Glasgow BJ, Cramer H. Fine-needle aspiration in the management of breast masses. *Pathol Annu.* 1989;24:23–62.

Obeng-Gyasi S, Grimm LJ, Hwang S, Klimberg VS, Bland KI. Indications and techniques for biopsy. In: Bland K, Copeland EM, Klimberg VS, Gradishar WJ, eds. *Breast: Comprehensive Management of Benign and Malignant Diseases.* 5th ed. Philadelphia: Elsevier; 2018: 377–385.

Physician Insurers Association of America. *Breast Cancer Study.* Lawrenceville, NJ: Physician Insurers Association of America; 1990.

Salzman B, Fleegle S, Tully AS. Common breast problems. *Am Fam Physician.* 2012;86(4):343–349.

Silverstein MJ, Recht A, Lagios MD, et al. Special report: consensus conference III. Image-detected breast cancer: state-of-the-art diagnosis and treatment. *J Am Coll Surg.* 2009;209:504–520.

CHAPTER 120

PAP SMEAR AND RELATED TECHNIQUES FOR CERVICAL CANCER SCREENING

Gary R. Newkirk

The incidence of cervical cancer in the United States has decreased by more than 50% in the past 30 years. In 1975, the rate was 14.8 per 100,000 women; by 2014 it had decreased to 6.8 per 100,000 women. Similar to incidence, mortality from the disease has decreased from 5.55 per 100,000 women in 1975 to 2.3 per 100,000 women in 2014. From 2005 to 2014, the death rate decreased by 0.8% per year. In the United States in 2017, it is estimated that 12,820 cases of invasive cervical cancer will be diagnosed and that 4210 women will die of the disease. These improvements in incidence and mortality have been attributed largely to widespread screening with the Papanicolaou (Pap) test. The only variance noted so far from the improvement curve was from 2008 to 2012; during this time, incidence rates quit going down and instead stabilized in women younger than 50 years. It continued to decrease by 3.0% per year among women aged 50 years or older. The most common cervical cancers are squamous cell carcinoma and adenocarcinoma.

Cervical cancer is much more common worldwide, particularly in countries without screening programs, with an estimated 527,624 new cases of the disease and 265,672 resultant deaths each year. When cervical cancer screening programs have been introduced into communities, marked reductions in cervical cancer incidence have followed. Despite the controversies surrounding cervical Pap smear testing, it remains an effective tool for cancer prevention and detection. That said, this potentially preventable disease has not been eradicated. The current cervical cancer detection system relies on a complex system of clinical and laboratory procedures that have potential for error at numerous points. Koss' (1989) landmark discussion summarizes major sources of error, including (1) problems with the initial clinical examination, (2) inappropriate smear collection technique, (3) laboratory errors in sample preparation and interpretation, (4) errors in report interpretation, (5) failure of the clinician to understand or appropriately respond to Pap smear–generated data, and (6) failure of the patient to follow the clinician's recommendations.

Compelling data link cervical intraepithelial neoplasia (CIN) with human papillomavirus (HPV) infection; sexually transmitted high-risk HPV likely causes more than 99% of cervical cancers. Epidemiologic data further document the somewhat ubiquitous nature of new genital HPV infections in sexually active individuals younger than 30 years. Box 120.1 summarizes risk factors for cervical dysplasia. Most women who are exposed to HPV have transient infections and do not develop cervical cancer. It generally takes the immune system 6 to 24 months to clear an HPV infection (Rodríguez et al., 2008). Patients with the persistence of HPV as detected by either abnormal cytologic features (Pap) with or without positive high-risk HPV testing or by direct high-risk HPV testing alone (see Chapter 121, Human Papillomavirus DNA Typing) are the subgroup of women who remain at greatest risk for developing cervical cancer.

Despite the success of Pap smear screening methodology, numerous studies indicate that there remains a 20% to 50% false-negative rate for a single Pap smear in identifying patients with cervical dysplasia (20% for high grade intraepithelial lesion, greater than 20% for glandular lesions or invasive cancer). Consequently, the sampling devices, method of preparation, and transport systems for Pap samples have also evolved. Liquid-based Pap systems such as ThinPrep and SurePath, approved by the Food and Drug Administration (FDA) as alternatives to conventional slide smear techniques, have been developed to decrease the risk of false negative Pap smears (although, as discussed later, evidence may not support such an improvement). Liquid-based systems also allow simultaneous submission of material for high-risk HPV testing (as well as other sexually transmitted infections). This is usually at the request of the clinician or as a "reflex" test dependent on the cytologic interpretation (see Chapter 121, Human Papillomavirus DNA Typing and the ASCCP Guidelines in Appendix K, Management Guidelines for Abnormal Cervical Cancer Screening Tests and Histologic Findings). *Reflex testing* means the high-risk HPV testing is automatically performed if ASC-US (atypical squamous cells of undetermined significance) is found on Pap smear. However, reflex testing can also be ordered for cytology for those positive for high-risk HPV. When HPV is ordered as an adjunct to the Pap smear, it is called *cotesting*.

Two high-risk HPV tests are now FDA approved as the primary screening test in place of the Pap. As a result of these advancements and a better understanding of HPV screening, cervical cancer screening guidelines have been reconsidered. Interim Guidelines (2015) for Primary High-Risk HPV Screening were developed by representatives from the Society of Gynecologic Oncology (SGO), the American Society of Cytopathology, and the College of American Pathologists (ASCCP), in addition to the American College of Obstetricians and Gynecologists and all groups authoring the 2012 Screening Guidelines. The Interim Guidelines state that because of equivalent or superior effectiveness, primary high-risk HPV screening can be used as an alternative to cytology. They did not recommend primary HPV screening in women younger than 25 years, and rescreening should not be repeated more frequently than every 3 years. In addition, although more research is necessary, the Interim Guidelines suggest that the best management of high-risk HPV-positive women is to triage positive tests with genotyping for 16 of 18 to colposcopy and to use reflex cytology for women positive for the 12 other high-risk genotypes.

Multiple studies provide mounting evidence for the utility of HPV testing as primary screening and may continue to lead to further changes in guidelines, particularly as the actual impact of new screening guidelines on cancer prevention is investigated. For example, a 2017 Cochrane review found that when screening for CIN2 or CIN3, testing primarily and only for high-risk HPV is less likely to miss those with CIN2 or CIN3 than a Pap smear alone. However, HPV tests are more likely to lead to additional procedures or referrals. That said, a negative HPV test is more reassuring than a negative cytologic test because the cytologic test is more likely to be falsely negative, which could result in a delay in treatment. Despite these data, and largely because of the frequently transient nature of HPV, the American College of Obstetricians

and Gynecologists, the American Academy of Family Physicians, the American Cancer Society (ACS), and the US Preventive Services Task Force do not recommend use of the high-risk HPV tests until age 30, unless used as reflex testing for abnormal cytology on Pap.

Clinicians are advised to keep current regarding the seemingly ever-changing cervical cancer screening recommendations because these guidelines will continue to evolve as new evidence-based and outcome data become available. At the present time, clinicians can continue to make significant contributions to cancer prevention in women by refining their method of Pap smear sampling, enhancing their understanding of Pap smear interpretation, clarifying their recommendations for patient management, and making sure that their efforts are implemented by an effective follow-up and intervention system. Clearly, efforts to prevent cervical cancer are inconsequential if mechanisms for follow-up and quality assurance are not developed. Unfortunately, nearly 90 years after the advent of Papanicolaou's revolution with cervical cancer prevention, almost 50% of the women who develop cervical cancer in the United States have never had a single Pap test, and another 10% have not had a Pap smear for 5 years prior to their diagnosis! This is unacceptable in this modern age of medical care.

This chapter focuses on a contemporary approach to Pap smear screening; it is assumed that basic pelvic examination skills have been mastered. Box 120.2 offers a brief summary of the terminology used throughout this discussion.

BOX 120.2   Terminology and Definitions

Atypical glandular cells (AGC): In the past these were called AGC-US (atypical glandular cells of undetermined significance), but because the incidence of significant pathology is so high with this finding (10% cancers and 25% high-grade lesions), the "US" was dropped by Bethesda 2001. All AGC reports need further investigation.

Atypical squamous cells (ASC): Bethesda 2001 divided these into ASC-US (atypical squamous cells of undetermined significance) and ASC-H (atypical squamous cells, cannot exclude HSIL).

Carcinoma in situ (CIS): Dysplasia involves the entire squamous epithelium but does *not* penetrate the basement membrane. Included in CIN 3 and HGSIL designations.

Cervical intraepithelial neoplasia (CIN): See "Dysplasia." *CIN 1* refers to mild dysplasia, *CIN 2* to moderate dysplasia, and *CIN 3* to severe dysplasia, including carcinoma in situ (CIS).

Columnar epithelium: Single-layer, mucin-secreting epithelium on the surface of the endocervix. It can often be seen on the ectocervix and is proximal to the SCJ.

Cotesting: Adjunct HPV testing with cytology.

Dysplasia: Premalignant change in the cervical epithelium displaying proliferation of parabasal cells with disordered polarity, loss of cellular junctions, coarse nuclear chromatin clumping, abnormal nuclear cytoplasmic ratio, and high mitotic index. Reported as *mild, moderate,* and *severe* dysplasia. Usually refers to histologic features.

Ectocervix (also called exocervix): The flat portion of the cervix that is readily visible. The cervical os is located centrally.

Endocervical cells: Glandular, columnar-shaped cells obtained from the endocervical (columnar) epithelium in the endocervical canal.

Endocervix: The area within the endocervical canal.

Exocervix: See Ectocervix.

Frankly invasive squamous cell carcinoma of the cervix: Invasion greater than 3 mm (or 5 mm, depending on classification used) below the basement membrane.

Koilocytotic or koilocytic: Equivalent terms include condylomatous atypia and human papillomavirus (HPV) effect; these

terms describe cells that have perinuclear halos or vacuoles that vary in shape and configuration, and that show a distinct zone of clearing between the nucleus and cytoplasmic membrane. The abnormal nuclei are characterized by wrinkling, variation in size and shape, binucleate forms, and hyperchromasia. Usually indicative of HPV infection.

Microinvasive cervical cancer: Invasion 3 mm or less below the basement membrane. Some terminologies allow 5 mm of invasion and include other descriptive factors.

Reflex HPV testing: Automatically obtaining HPV test for patients that have an ASC-US report. If HPV testing is used as primary, reflex testing for cytology can be performed to determine the need for colposcopy.

Squamocolumnar junction (SCJ): The line where the squamous epithelium of the ectocervix joins the mucus-secreting columnar epithelium of the endocervix.

Squamous cells: Epithelial cells on the surface of the ectocervix. These cells appear smooth and pink on the cervix.

Squamous intraepithelial lesion (SIL): Reported as either low-grade (LGSIL, LSIL) or high-grade (HGSIL, HSIL), corresponding to increasing severity of dysplasia (Bethesda terminology). Originally referred to cytologic diagnosis, but now often used to describe histologic findings as well.

Squamous metaplasia: A type of tissue present where the columnar epithelium is being replaced (transformed) by squamous epithelium. This normal tissue occurs within the cervical transformation zone, and the transformation of columnar to squamous epithelium is a totally normal process.

Transformation zone (TZ): Area of transformation or replacement of the cervical columnar epithelium by squamous epithelium through a process called metaplastic change. The *active* TZ goes from the outermost gland to the SCJ. The TZ is the principal site of origin for precancerous and invasive squamous cell carcinomas of the cervix.

See Figs. 120.1 and 120.2, and Chapter 124, Colposcopic Examination.

ANATOMY

Fig. 120.1 depicts the anatomy involved. Successful Pap smear technique requires sampling from the active transformation zone in women with an intact cervix or from the vaginal cuff for those who have undergone hysterectomy. Fig. 120.2 provides a graphic representation of the changes involved with preinvasive and invasive disease of the cervix as well as a depiction of histologic and cytologic correlates. (Refer to Chapter 124, Colposcopic Examination, for further discussion of anatomy.)

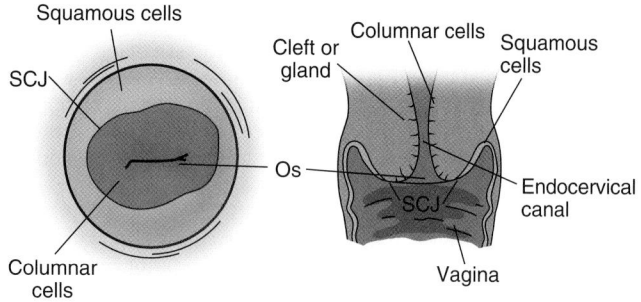

Age 12 (puberty)

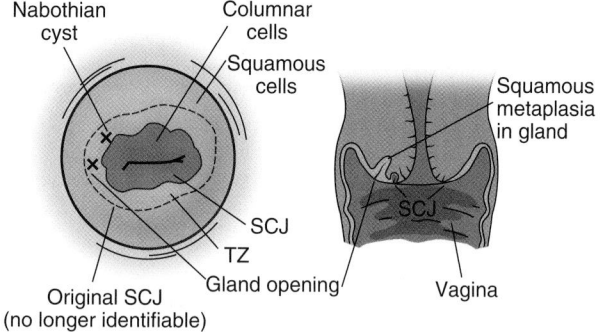

Age 21 (reproductive)

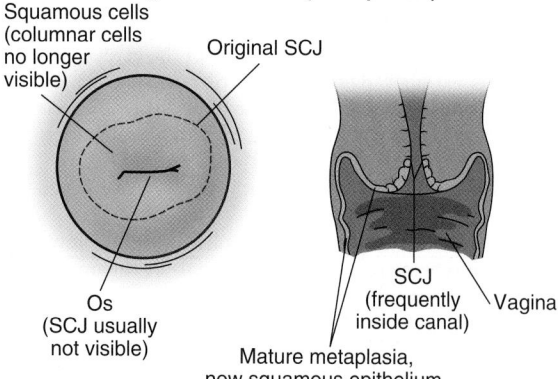

Age 50 and older (menopausal)

Fig. 120.1 Appearance of cervix in various age groups. The area most at risk in all age groups is the transformation zone (TZ), including the squamocolumnar junction (SCJ). Note how location varies with age. The SCJ and TZ are readily visible in younger women and may be quite large. The SCJ migrates inward with aging, and by menopause, it is usually within the canal and is not visible. The entire TZ must be sampled to maximize efficacy of the Papanicolaou smear. Also see Fig. 124.2 (Chapter 124, Colposcopic Examination) for cervical photographs showing these findings and developmental changes.

INDICATIONS

- Cervical cancer screening should not begin at age less than 21 years, regardless of age of sexual initiation or other risk factors.
- Women who have been vaccinated for HPV should follow these same recommendations (long-term effectiveness of vaccine unknown).
- Women aged 21 to 29 years should be tested with cervical cytology alone, and screening should be performed every 3 years. Cotesting should not be performed in women less than 30 years.
- For women aged 30 to 65 years, cotesting with cytology and HPV testing every 5 years is preferred; screening with cytology alone every 3 years is acceptable.
- Screening by any modality should be discontinued after age 65 years in women with evidence of adequate negative prior screening test results and no history of CIN 2 or higher. Adequate negative prior screening test results are defined as three consecutive negative cytology results or two consecutive negative cotest results within the previous 10 years, with the most recent test performed within the past 5 years.
- Women with a history of CIN 2, CIN 3, or adenocarcinoma in situ (AIS) should continue screening for a total of 20 years after spontaneous regression or appropriate management of CIN 2, CIN 3, or AIS, even if it extends screening past age 65 years.
- Women who have had a hysterectomy with removal of the cervix (total hysterectomy) and have never had CIN 2 or higher, routine cytology screening and HPV testing should be discontinued and not restarted for any reason.
- ACS, American Society for Colposcopy and Cervical Pathology (ASCCP), American Society for Clinical Pathology guidelines, all in 2012.
- Women who are at high risk of cervical cancer because of a suppressed immune system (e.g., from HIV infection, organ transplant, or long-term steroid use) or because they were exposed to diethylstilbestrol in utero may need to be screened more often. They should follow the recommendations of their health care team (ACS guidelines).
- Older ACS guidelines: Women with any of the following risk factors may require more frequent cervical cancer screening than recommended in the routine screening guidelines, which were intended for average-risk women:
  - Women who are infected with HIV
  - Women who are immunocompromised (such as those who have received solid organ transplants)
  - Women who were exposed to diethylstilbestrol in utero
- In women 25 years and older, the FDA-approved primary HPV screening test can be considered as an alternative to current cytology-based cervical cancer screening methods. Cytology alone and cotesting remain the options specifically recommended in current major society guidelines. If screening with primary HPV testing is used, it should be performed as per the SGO, ASCCP 2015 interim guidance (SGO and ASCCP, 2015).
- See also Box 120.3 for ACS and reasonable statements from older guidelines. Clinicians are advised to consider these guidelines in relation to the patient population they serve and their practice and patient resources.
- Follow-up after treatment for cervical dysplasia, malignancy: See the ASCCP Guidelines in Appendix K, Management Guidelines for Abnormal Cervical Cancer Screening Tests and Histologic Findings. All women with a history of cervical dysplasia remain at significant risk for disease recurrence and should undergo Pap smear testing, as recommended by guidelines such as those of the ASCCP. There are numerous schemes for follow-up after treatment for cervical carcinoma; the recommendations of the treatment team should be followed.
- Victims of rape, incest, abuse: Pap smear is part of the initial workup. Intact spermatozoa may be seen several days later on a Pap smear. Evaluations in these circumstances require

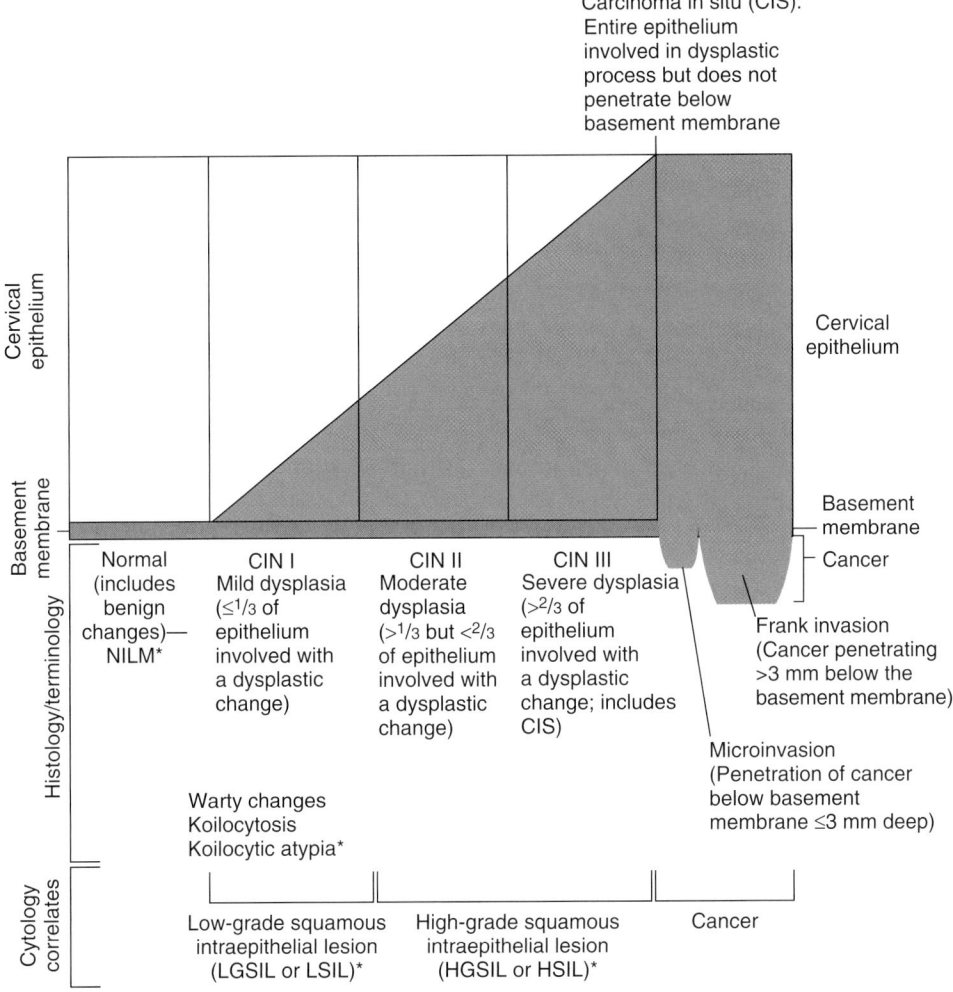

Carcinoma in situ (CIS):
Entire epithelium
involved in dysplastic
process but does not
penetrate below
basement membrane

Cervical
epithelium

Basement
membrane
Cancer

Frank invasion
(Cancer penetrating
>3 mm below the
basement membrane)

Microinvasion
(Penetration of cancer
below basement
membrane ≤3 mm deep)

Cervical epithelium

Basement membrane

Histology/terminology

Normal
(includes
benign
changes)—
NILM*

CIN I
Mild dysplasia
(≤¹/₃ of
epithelium
involved with
a dysplastic
change)

CIN II
Moderate
dysplasia
(>¹/₃ but <²/₃
of epithelium
involved with
a dysplastic
change)

CIN III
Severe dysplasia
(>²/₃ of
epithelium
involved with
a dysplastic
change; includes
CIS)

Warty changes
Koilocytosis
Koilocytic atypia*

Cytology correlates

Low-grade squamous
intraepithelial lesion
(LGSIL or LSIL)*

High-grade squamous
intraepithelial lesion
(HGSIL or HSIL)*

Cancer

Fig. 120.2 Histologic and cytologic correlations of various terms used to describe preinvasive and invasive squamous cell disease of the cervix. Also see Box 120.2 for further description of the terms. The degree of epithelial involvement correlates with the severity of cytologic findings as well as the total degree of involvement of the dysplastic tissue in relation to the thickness of the cervical squamous epithelium. On histologic examination, involvement below the basement membrane supports a diagnosis of invasive cancer. *CIN*, Cervical intraepithelial neoplasia, *NILM*, negative for intraepithelial lesion or malignancy. *Atypical squamous cells (ASC), atypical squamous cells of undetermined significance (ASC-US), and atypical squamous cells that cannot exclude HSIL (ASC-H) are not depicted here because they include a variety of histologic diagnoses. Note, too, that glandular cell abnormalities include atypical glandular cells (AGC), endocervical adenocarcinoma in situ (AIS), and adenocarcinoma, and are also not depicted in this graph.

expertise and strict adherence to medical/legal chain of evidence. (See Chapters 140, Treatment of the Adult Victim of Sexual Assault, and 170, Management of the Young Female as Possible Victim of Sexual Abuse.)

EDITOR'S NOTE: The Pap smear is a screening test only; it is not diagnostic. Thus, if an abnormality is seen or palpated at the time of the pelvic examination, it should be examined with a colposcope and a directed biopsy performed. *The clinician cannot rely on the Pap smear alone to be diagnostic for an observed lesion.*

CONTRAINDICATIONS

Absolute

There are no absolute contraindications to obtaining a Pap smear.

Relative

Relative contraindications include clinical circumstances in which sample collection is difficult to obtain or difficult to interpret (e.g., active vaginitis or cervicitis, pelvic inflammatory disease, or menses). The clinician must weigh the benefits versus the risk of obtaining the screening Pap smear under these circumstances. For instance, if a woman presents with abnormal vaginal bleeding, a Pap smear is advised, despite the presence of blood. (The liquid-based Pap systems are less vulnerable to blood interfering with accuracy.) This contrasts with a patient who comes in for a routine Pap smear screening and has begun to menstruate. In the latter instance, because the presence of red blood cells can affect the result, the Pap smear can be

deferred to a more favorable time. See the sample patient education handout available at www.expertconsult.com, which includes advice on what women can do to optimize Pap smear results.

EQUIPMENT

- Examination table appropriate for placing the patient in the lithotomy position
- A warm, well-lit examination room
- Various-sized speculums: Graves (metal); Pederson (metal); plastic, disposable (Welch Allyn, Inc.)
- Water-soluble lubricant (e.g., K-Y Jelly)
- Nonsterile examination gloves
- Large swabs for gently blotting excess discharge
- Cotton swabs
- Method for warming the speculum (warm water or speculum drawer warmer [light bulb])
- Sampling devices (see Fig. 120.5)
  - Wooden spatulas (Cervical Scraper No. 7, Hardwood Puritan Products) or plastic spatula (Cervical Scraper [8.5 inch], Milex CooperSurgical Products) for ectocervical sample
  - Cytobrush Plus for endocervical sample (Medscand CooperSurgical)
  - As an alternative to taking two samples, a "broom" device can be used for both the ectocervical and endocervical samples (Cervex-Brush, CooperSurgical; Papette, Wallach Surgical Devices)
- Microscope slides, fixative (consult with reference laboratory performing cytologic evaluation for its preference), or medium for liquid-based testing

---

BOX 120.3 American Cancer Society Guidelines for the Early Detection of Cervical Neoplasia and Cancer, Updated 2016 (and Some Older Worthwhile Recommendations)

- Women aged 21–29 years should have a Pap test every 3 years. HPV should not be used as a screening test in this age group (but it may be used in follow-up of abnormal Pap).
- Beginning at age 30 years, the preferred way to screen is with a Pap test combined with an HPV test every 5 years. This is called cotesting and should continue until age 65 years. Another reasonable option for women aged 30–65 years is to get tested every 3 years with just the Pap test.
- Women who are age 65 and older with an intact cervix and who have had three or more documented consecutive technically satisfactory, normal/negative cervical cytologic tests, and no abnormal/positive cytologic tests (such as CIN2 or CIN3) within the last 20 years may cease cervical cancer screening. Women with a history of CIN2 or CIN3 should continue to have testing for at least 20 years after the abnormality was found.
- Women who are at high risk of cervical cancer because of a suppressed immune system (e.g., from HIV infection, organ transplant, or long-term steroid use) or because they were exposed to DES in utero may need to be screened more often. They should follow the recommendations of their health care team.
- When comorbid or life-threatening illnesses are present, Pap smears are not needed.*
- Screening should be continued for women older than 70 years*:
  If they have not been previously screened
  When previous Pap smear screening information is unavailable
  If there was in utero exposure to DES
  For immunocompromised women (including those with HIV-seropositive status)
  For women older than 70 years who have tested positive for HPV DNA
- After a total hysterectomy with removal of the entire cervix for benign lesions, Pap smears and HPV screens are not indicated. (The presence of CIN 2/3 is not considered a benign lesion, so continued screening would be indicated.)
- Women who have had a subtotal hysterectomy (the cervix remains) should continue cervical cancer screening.
- Women with DES exposure or history of cervical carcinoma should continue screening after hysterectomy as long as they are in reasonably good health and do not have a life-limiting chronic condition.*
  - Women of any age should NOT be screened every year by any screening method.
  - Women who have been vaccinated against HPV should still follow these guidelines.
- Adolescents who may not need a Pap test should still obtain appropriate preventive health care, including contraception and education, other screening, and treatment of sexually transmitted diseases.*

Additional Recommendations*

- Patients need to be educated (especially teens) that a pelvic examination does not equate with a cytologic (Pap) test. They still need regular health care visits.
- No recommendation was made regarding pelvic and rectal examinations. They are not effective in detecting cervical cancer early enough, but there are other reasons to consider them. These should be discussed on an individual basis with the primary care clinician.
- Health insurance coverage for new cervical screening technology is not uniform. Patients should be advised of this by their primary care provider.
- There is considerable clinical evidence with the use of the Cytobrush in pregnant women with no apparent complications.
- Cervical broom instruments and other single sampling instruments are comparable to the spatula and brush.
- An endocervical swab is less sensitive than an endocervical brush and its use is discouraged. It may be considered for pregnant women.

---

* Included in the 2009 guidelines and still makes sense.
CIN, Cervical intraepithelial neoplasia; DES, diethylstilbestrol; FDA, Food and Drug Administration; HIV, human immunodeficiency virus; HPV, human papillomavirus; Pap, Papanicolaou.
Modified from the 2016 American Cancer Society Guidelines for the Prevention and Early Detection of Cervical Cancer and Smith RA, Cokkinides V, Brawley OW. Cancer screening in the United States, 2009: a review of current American Cancer Society guidelines and issues in cancer screening. CA Cancer J Clin. 2009;59(1):27–41.

- Appropriate patient identification, history forms to accompany Pap smear and other tests
- Culture or transport media and swabs as necessary for detection of gonorrhea, chlamydia, herpes, and fungal infection, and KOH/wet mount
- Cervical tenaculum or cervical hook (rarely needed)
- Ring forceps
- Materials and solutions for liquid-based Pap smears (e.g., ThinPrep, SurePrep)
- Equipment to follow universal blood and body fluid precautions

Sampling Devices

Concern over the frequency and occurrence of false-negative Pap smears has led to the development of newer Pap smear sampling, preparation, and processing techniques. Despite the higher costs for the newer sampling devices (nominally $0.40 to $0.80 each), the increased quality of smears, the improved detection rates, and ultimately the fewer patients who must return for "inadequate" repeat smears more than justify this added expense. The routine use of the Cytobrush, Cervex-Brush, Papette, or similar devices is recommended (see later discussion of liquid-based technologies). A Pap smear consists of sampling the endocervical canal and the entire transformation zone (Figs. 120.3 and 120.4). At times, the broom device will not be wide enough to sample the entire area at risk (the transformation zone). Additional sampling of the missed area is then required. Clinicians should not be locked into using a single method of transformation zone sampling. A good strategy for obtaining ideal Pap smears is to have several types of sampling devices such as the brush and broom available. One-size-fits-all strategies are less effective than using the sampling device that matches the patient's particular cervical anatomy.

The Pap smear test samples "exfoliated" cells. As such, the transformation zone need not be denuded of its mucosa to obtain an adequate sample. There are enough cells from one Cytobrush and a wooden spatula sample, for instance, to provide material for cytologic interpretation for five slides. Sharp, fine-edged plastic devices are advocated by some clinicians; however, wood works fine for sampling of the ectocervix. Both should be accompanied by brush sampling of the endocervical canal. A bloody Pap smear sample decreases detection rates. Fig. 120.5 illustrates several of the common sampling devices that achieve satisfactory sampling.

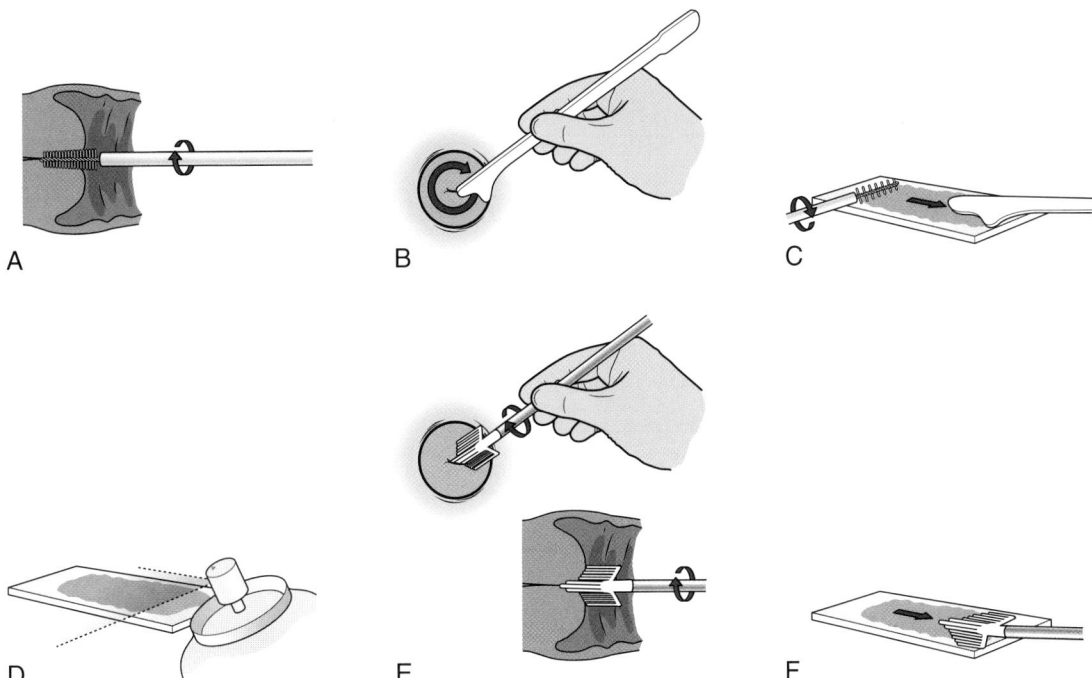

Fig. 120.3 Obtaining the Papanicolaou smear. (A) Endocervical sample with Cytobrush; rotate 90 to 180 degrees. (B) Ectocervical sample obtained with a wooden or plastic spatula. (C) A single-slide technique is preferred. First, the spatula sample is spread, which is then followed by "unrolling" of the brush sample directly over the first sample. (D) Immediate fixation of the slide with cytologic fixative. (E) Alternatively, a single sampling device may be used (Papette, Cervex-Brush, or "broom") to obtain both ectocervical and endocervical samples at the same time. Rotate 360 degrees 5 times. (F) Spreading the sample from broom device onto the slide.

Liquid-Based Pap Smears

In the United States there are two FDA-approved liquid-based Pap smear systems available. Both rely on a method of sampling the cervix that is similar or identical to conventional slide prepared smears, but they differ in the transport media and the technical methods of cytologic preparation. With liquid-based Pap smears, the same principles apply regarding collection of cells. The sample, however, instead of being spread on a glass slide, is "swished" in a vial of liquid that is subsequently processed to eliminate blood and other debris.

Prior study suggested that liquid-based Pap testing is more sensitive and specific than conventional slide methods; however, a recent systematic review and meta-analysis indicated that liquid-based Pap smear testing is neither more sensitive nor more specific for high-grade CIN when compared with the conventional Pap test. A clearer advantage of the liquid-based technique is that the residual cytologic material left over after the cytologic examination is completed in the laboratory can be used for HPV DNA testing. (Refer to Chapter 121, Human Papillomavirus DNA Typing, and Appendix K, Management Guidelines for Abnormal Cervical Cancer Screening Tests and Histologic Findings, to guide when HPV testing may be useful.) In particular, the data support that reflex HPV testing will enhance management of women with ASC-US cytologic findings, separating those who need colposcopy (HPV DNA high-risk positive) from those who can be returned to standard screening (HPV DNA negative). If the HPV testing is performed automatically (reflex) based upon ASC-US cytologic findings, the patient need not return for a separate HPV screening visit. Data support the cost-effectiveness of this strategy. Furthermore, the combined use of liquid-based cytologic examination and same-time HPV testing has immediate advantage for management of women over age 30 and women in certain posttreatment categories (see Chapter 121, Human Papillomavirus DNA Sampling, and the ASCCP Guidelines in Appendix K, Management Guidelines for Abnormal Cervical Cancer Screening Tests and Histologic Findings).

In addition to the reflex HPV testing potential, liquid-based Pap techniques are also directly adaptable to computer-based automated screening devices. Development of automated screening devices has been driven more by the need to reduce labor costs than the need for accuracy. It is not clear that they will improve traditional human review of light microscopy samples. Currently these computer systems are used for either repeat evaluation of previously read Pap smears or for selecting certain cells for technicians to view. Computers can interpret only liquid-based preparations at the present time.

PREPROCEDURE PATIENT PREPARATION

The patient should understand the reason for performing the Pap smear. The Pap smear is best performed during midcycle. The patient should avoid douching, vaginal medications, and intercourse for 24 hours prior to the procedure. In most instances, the examination should be rescheduled if the patient is actively menstruating. The patient should void before undressing for the examination. Make sure the room is warm enough and the speculum is warmed as well. Question the patient regarding her concerns. Not infrequently, women are hesitant to discuss symptoms related to the genitals, such as vaginal dryness, itchiness, or discharge, unless the clinician asks. The patient should know that the clinician will explain each step of the pelvic examination prior to proceeding. Inform the patient of the mechanisms that you use to follow up on test results (Pap smear, cultures, etc.). (See the sample patient education handout available at www.expertconsult.com.) They should be informed if they will be checked for anything in addition to the Pap smear (e.g., guidelines suggest screening for chlamydia in all women younger than 25 years; they may not know this). Such an explanation may be very helpful if someone else may see the bill from the lab or insurance company.

TECHNIQUE

1. Obtain history (especially sexual aspects of age at first intercourse, number of sexual partners, and history of sexual abuse or rape), perform review of systems, and answer questions. Clarify the patient's risk factors for cervical dysplasia. Review past Pap results if available.

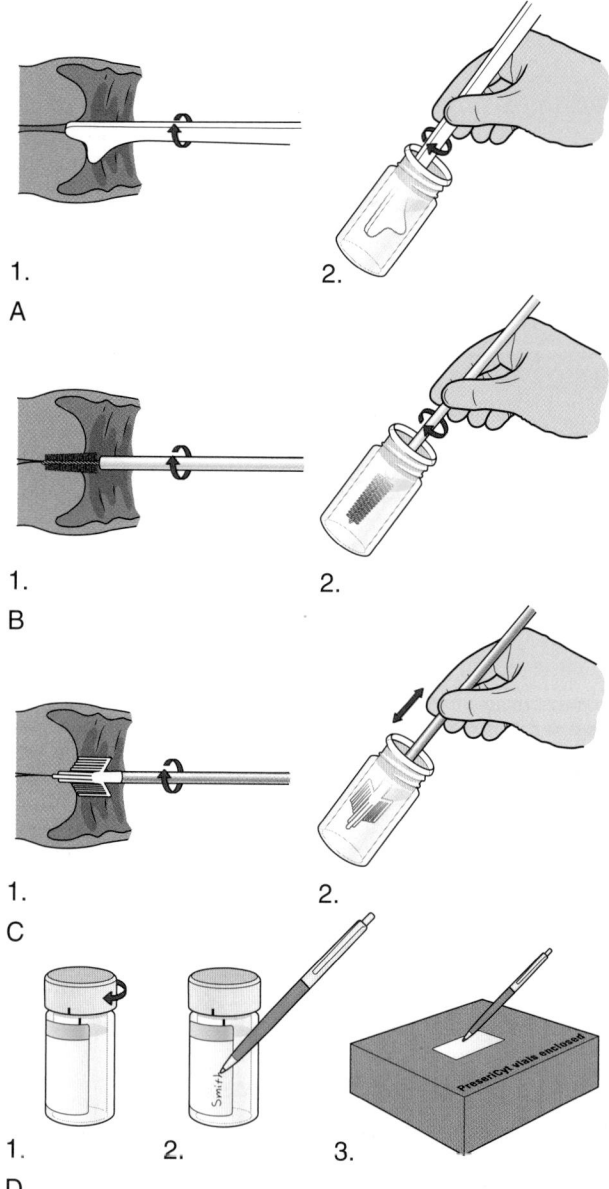

1.
A

1.   2.
B

1.   2.
C

1.   2.   3.
D

Fig. 120.4 Liquid-based (ThinPrep, SurePath) methods using plastic spatula (A), endocervical brush (B), or broom-like device (C). (D) Shows the final three steps for each method. (A) *1,* Obtain an adequate sampling from the ectocervix using a plastic spatula. *2,* Rinse the spatula as quickly as possible into the PreservCyt Solution vial by swirling the spatula vigorously in the vial 10 times. Discard the spatula. (B) *1,* Obtain an adequate sampling from the endocervix using an endocervical brush device. Insert the brush into the cervix until only the bottommost fibers are exposed. Slowly rotate one-quarter or one-half turn in one direction. *Do not overrotate. 2,* Rinse the brush as quickly as possible into the PreservCyt Solution by rotating the device in the solution 10 times while pushing against the PreservCyt vial wall. Swirl the brush vigorously to further release material. Discard the brush. (C) *1,* Obtain an adequate sampling from the cervix using a broom-like device. Insert the central bristles of the broom into the endocervical canal deep enough to allow the shorter bristles to fully contact the ectocervix. Push gently, and rotate the broom in a clockwise direction 5 times. *2,* Rinse the broom as quickly as possible into the PreservCyt Solution vial by pushing the broom into the bottom of the vial 10 times, forcing the bristles apart. As a final step, swirl the broom vigorously to further release material. Discard the collection device. Be sure entire transformation zone has been sampled. (D) *1,* Tighten the cap so that the torque line on the cap passes the torque line on the vial. *2,* Record the patient's name and ID number on the vial, and record the patient information and medical history on the cytology requisition form. *3,* Place the vial and requisition in a specimen bag for transport to the laboratory. (Courtesy CYTYC Hologic Corp., Boxborough, MA.)

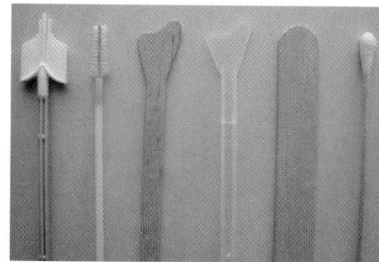

Fig. 120.5 Papanicolaou sampling devices. *Left to right:* Cervex-Brush, Cytobrush, wooden spatula, plastic spatula, tongue blade, and cotton swab. Use of the swab and tongue blade is discouraged.

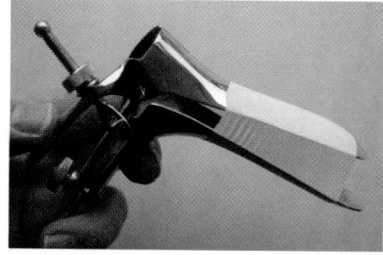

Fig. 120.6 Vaginal speculum stent. To aid in the visualization of the cervix, a single finger of a latex examination glove can be cut off and placed over the blades of a standard vaginal speculum. This is helpful if there is redundant vaginal mucosa, as seen with pregnancy, obesity, or multiparity.

2. Proceed with the general medical examination, leaving the pelvic examination for last.

3. Label the frosted end of the glass slide or the liquid Pap vial with the patient's name and other identifying data prior to applying the sample.

4. Place the patient in the lithotomy position, and begin the examination. Wear nonsterile gloves and follow universal blood and body fluid precautions. Inspect the vulva, and assess hair pattern, anatomy, estrogen effect, discharge, and any abnormal areas. Ask the patient if she has any concerns.

5. Place a small amount of water-soluble lubricant or even just warm water on the warmed speculum and insert it. Carefully advance the speculum, applying gentle pressure posteriorly. In patients whose vaginal walls prolapse and obstruct view, consider using a vaginal "stent." This can be fashioned by cutting off both ends of a single finger of a latex rubber glove and placing it over the blades of the speculum (Fig. 120.6). Vaginal sidewall retractors are also available. For those who are very obese or have excessively deep vaginas, a special, long "snowman" speculum is available from CooperSurgical, Inc. and other manufacturers.

6. Adjust the speculum to obtain adequate visualization of the cervix, and tighten the screw or lock the speculum open.

7. Determine whether the vagina or cervix appears inflamed or infected. Avoid rubbing or otherwise traumatizing the cervix.

8. Identify cervical landmarks, including the transformation zone with its squamocolumnar junction. Note the nature of the cervical mucus. Markedly excessive mucus or discharge may be gently blotted, not rubbed, from view. However, mucus may actually contain the exfoliated cells needed for the microscopic examination. So, unless truly necessary, do not remove this mucus; include it in the sample. Note any gross cervical lesions, such as erosions (ulcerations), leukoplakia (white areas), nabothian cysts, or condylomas. Examine the vaginal fornices for obvious abnormalities.

9. Obtain the Pap smear by using an endocervical sampling device (Cytobrush, Papette, or Cervex-Brush). Q-Tips are not to be used. If the Cytobrush is used, first insert the Cytobrush into the canal and rotate it 90 to 180 degrees. Do not rotate it more than this,

because that may cause bleeding, which can wash away or obscure abnormal cells. Follow this by a gentle sampling of the entire transformation zone using a spatula device, rotating it 360 degrees. If broom devices (Papette, Cervex-Brush) are used, insert and rotate them 360 degrees 5 times. The broom will obtain both endocervical and ectocervical samples at the same time but must be rotated multiple times to collect an adequate number of cells.Sampling the vaginal pool has little advantage during Pap smear screening, unless the patient has had a hysterectomy. In this instance, be sure to sample the vaginal cuff itself. If vaginal abnormalities are seen, another Pap smear of these areas (using a spatula) may be submitted on a separate slide. Areas that appear abnormal on visualization will ultimately require colposcopy and biopsy.

10. Glass slide method:
    - If a one-slide smear technique is suggested by your reference laboratory (check with your pathologist), withhold smearing the endocervical Cytobrush sample on the slide until the ectocervical spatula sample is smeared on the slide first. Once this is done, then quickly roll out the Cytobrush sample (which is less subject to drying artifact) right over the spatula smear material and spray immediately with cytofixative.
    - If a two-slide smear technique is used, each sample (ectocervical and endocervical) is evenly applied to different slides immediately after sampling, and then the slide is sprayed or dipped in preservative within 5 seconds. (The broom devices will provide only a single slide because they sample both the ectocervical and endocervical areas at the same time.)
11. If a thin-layer liquid-based technology Pap smear method is utilized, follow the instructions of the manufacturer, which usually require rinsing the Pap sample (collected on the brush, broom, or spatula) directly into a vial of transport liquid rather than smearing the sample on glass slides. (See later discussion under "ThinPrep Pap Smears.")
12. Perform the appropriate cervical cultures after cytologic sampling, if indicated. (The Centers for Disease Control recommends that all sexually active females under age 25 be routinely screened for chlamydia. If treated, they should be rechecked after treatment is completed.)
13. Examine the vagina by slowly withdrawing the speculum, which is held slightly open, allowing the vagina to collapse over the blades. Note abnormalities.
14. Lubricate the gloved hand as necessary and proceed with the bimanual examination. Pay particular attention to palpated abnormalities of the introitus, vagina, fornices, and cervix. Palpate the areas of the Skene and Bartholin glands. Ask your patient to bear down, and observe for uterine or pelvic floor prolapse and for leaking of urine. Having her cough facilitates assessment of pelvic support.
15. Complete the remainder of the bimanual examination, noting the size, contour, tenderness, and mobility of the uterus and adnexal structures.
16. Perform a rectal examination on women with rectal complaints, or who are over age 40. Be sure to put on a new glove before the rectal examination, which may prevent the spread of HPV or other infectious agents to the anus. For women who have had abnormal high-grade Pap or biopsy results, a rectal examination may be indicated at any age because high-risk HPV viruses also cause anal cancers.
17. Allow the patient to dress.
18. Make sure the Pap smear requisition form includes all pertinent data regarding your patient. Include clinical findings, patient risk factors, or your concerns as part of this "referral" (Bethesda recommendation).

ThinPrep Pap Smears

1. Use a nonwooden spatula or supplied sampling device.
2. The Cytobrush should not be rotated more than 180 degrees, and only in one direction.

3. The collecting devices are then swished along the inner surface of the fluid container at least 20 times around.

SurePath Pap Smears

1. A cervical broom is provided with the transport fluid and vial.
2. Insert the central or longest bristles into the cervical canal.
3. Apply gentle pressure to allow the outer bristles to contact the cervix.
4. Rotate the broom five full turns in one direction, making sure it samples the entire transformation zone.
5. Pop the broom head off into the transport vial.

Pap Smears During Pregnancy

During pregnancy, the cervix progressively enlarges, the squamocolumnar junction displaces outward, the mucus becomes thicker and more abundant, and the cervix becomes much more vascular. Extra care must be used to gently blot off excess mucus and when applying the Pap sampling device to collect the sample, especially after 20 weeks' gestation. Despite these changes, the Pap smear in a pregnant woman maintains a similar sensitive and specific profile when compared with the nonpregnant state. Pregnancy itself does not accelerate or worsen cervical dysplasia. In most women, the first trimester cervix appears very similar to the nonpregnant cervix. The active transformation zone everts, or externalizes, progressively with advancing gestation, so there is little need to probe or sample the cervical canal, especially with wire tip brush devices. (In the author's opinion, broom or spatula devices are preferred in pregnancy, and the brush is avoided to reduce the risk of bleeding.)

1. Ideally, obtain the Pap smear as early in pregnancy as possible to avoid exaggerated spotting. Patients are also more uncomfortable in the lithotomy position with an advanced gestation.
2. Although there is controversy with using brush devices in pregnancy, the broom or spatula devices make excellent sampling devices and are preferred.
3. Be gentle when rotating the brush because bleeding is more common in pregnancy.

SAMPLE PROCEDURE NOTE

This 32-year-old G3P3 white female is here for a screening Pap smear. She had a tubal ligation 4 years ago. Last Pap smear was 2 years ago. Prior Pap testing has been reviewed and is normal. With a chaperone present and the patient in the lithotomy position, the external genitalia were inspected and found to be free of abnormality. A speculum was lightly lubricated and gently inserted. The cervix was manipulated into view and found to be free of inflammation, infection, and abnormal discharge. The squamocolumnar junction was seen in its entirety and was about 10 mm in diameter. A Cytobrush sample and spatula sample were obtained, sampling the entire visible transformation zone, and quickly smeared and fixed on a single identified glass slide or in the liquid medium. Cultures were not deemed necessary by history and examination. Bimanual examination revealed a smooth, midline, freely mobile, nontender uterus that was not enlarged. Ovaries and adnexal structures were of normal size and position and were not painful. No pelvic masses were identified. The vagina and cervix were normal on palpation.

COMMON ERRORS

1. Lack of understanding of the basic anatomy of the cervix, including the squamocolumnar junction and the transformation zone, can lead to incorrect sampling.
2. Inadequate exposure of the cervix with the speculum can lead to incomplete sampling of the transformation zone.
3. Failure to review the patient's history for prior abnormal Pap smears or cervical treatment. The patient may require colposcopy

(see the ASCCP Guidelines in Appendix K, Management Guidelines for Abnormal Cervical Cancer Screening Tests and Histologic Findings).

4. Failure to inform or follow up with patients with Pap results, especially if abnormal.
5. Not obtaining recent contact information from the patient, confounding attempts to notify the patient of Pap smear results.
6. An aggressive approach to Pap smear sampling can lead to unnecessary bleeding, patient concern, and potentially less than satisfactory sample.
7. Obtaining cervical cultures or DNA probes for sexually transmittable infections prior to the Pap smear may cause bleeding or remove valuable cytologic material from the Pap smear sample.
8. Relying on the Pap smear result even when the cervix appears abnormal. An abnormal-appearing cervix warrants colposcopy regardless of the Pap smear result.
9. Interpretative confusion on the part of the clinician regarding the recommended follow-up of cytologic examination indicating atypical glandular cells versus atypical squamous cells (AGC vs. ASC-US, Bethesda 2001).
10. Inappropriately ordering DNA testing in women younger than 30 years of age for routine screening.

COMPLICATIONS

The Pap smear is only a screening test. False-negative rates are high (20% to 50%, with an average of 25%), and significant disease can be missed or underestimated. More frequent Pap smear screening or colposcopy may be indicated, depending on patient history and risks of having or developing genital malignancy. Minor spotting and occasional uterine cramps can commonly follow Pap smear sampling. Many of the shortfalls of Pap smear screening can be addressed by adhering to the following "golden rules":

- Identify cervical landmarks and gross abnormalities, and sample both the endocervical canal and the entire transformation zone. Choose a transformation zone sampler that fits your patient.
- All Pap smears reported as abnormal require some form of intervention. A report of dysplasia warrants colposcopy. Many clinicians also recommend colposcopy for reports of ASC, especially in patients with numerous risk factors. At the least, repeat Pap smear is indicated, or DNA typing is needed to determine which ASC Pap sample has high-risk HPV. AGCs definitely need further evaluation. (See Chapter 124, Colposcopic Examination, and Appendix K, Management Guidelines for Abnormal Cervical Cancer Screening Tests and Histologic Findings.)
- Clarify your patient's risk factors for having HPV infection and cervical dysplasia as part of the routine examination. Anyone with substantial risks requires at least annual Pap smears.
- An observed abnormality on the cervix that cannot be readily explained by normal variants (e.g., nabothian cysts) warrants colposcopic examination. A normal Pap smear report in the face of an observed abnormal cervix should *not* dissuade the clinician from performing colposcopy and biopsy.
- Know your cytopathologist. Interpretive problems should be discussed directly with the pathologist, who can address your questions, including the option to review the cytologic findings at issue.
- The optimal way to reduce morbidity and mortality rates from cervical cancer may not be new technology, but rather convincing women who have not been screened for large intervals, or at all, to have a Pap smear.

POSTPROCEDURE MANAGEMENT

Most of the postprocedure management issues with the pelvic examination including Pap smear sampling can be addressed by environmental issues and having an informed patient. Inform the patient to expect minor spotting or cramping. This is especially important for Pap smears during pregnancy, when these symptoms can be very concerning. Make sure that you have accurate follow-up contact information and patient preferences for contact methods. Take time to explain when you feel the next Pap smear is due. With the new Pap smear screening recommendations, which may include HPV testing, patients and clinicians alike are often confused regarding what is recommended. Clearly document your recommendation.

INTERPRETATION OF RESULTS

Adequacy

The Pap smear report should indicate whether the smear was adequate. Unless the patient has had a hysterectomy, the report should include cytologic evidence that the transformation zone was sampled. Ordinarily, the reporting of endocervical cells along with squamous cells implies adequate sampling. Many cytologists attribute the same significance to "squamous metaplasia" as the reporting of "endocervical cells present." Either is considered objective evidence that the transformation zone was sampled, which implies an adequate sample. Many reports will in some way use or check the word "adequate" on a form. The Bethesda system further delineates adequacy.

Interpretation System

The Bethesda system, named after the national consensus conference for Pap smear interpretation, provided a uniform nomenclature for Pap smear cytologic interpretation and attempts to address much of the confusion regarding Pap smear terminology. In September 2001, the Bethesda consensus conference convened for the third time and provided revisions of the reporting system, with general recommendations as follows:

- The Pap smear report should use terminology that is understood by the clinician.
- The clinician should be able to discuss the Pap smear report with the cytopathologist if questions arise.
- All abnormal Pap smears require some form of intervention in addition to the routine yearly screening interval.
- See the discussion in the following section regarding findings in postmenopausal women.

Follow-up Recommendations

A consensus group hosted by the American Society of Colposcopy and Cervical Pathology met in Bethesda, MD, in 2012, to revise the 2006 American Society for Colposcopy and Cervical Pathology Consensus Guidelines. The group's goal was to provide revised evidence-based consensus guidelines for managing women with abnormal cervical cancer screening tests, CIN, and AIS following adoption of cervical cancer screening guidelines incorporating longer screening intervals and cotesting. These recommendations use the terminology of the 2001 Bethesda interpretation system and are applicable to clinical circumstances. (See also Chapter 124, Colposcopic Examination.) The ASCCP guidelines are summarized with algorithms that can be found in Appendix K, Management Guidelines for Abnormal Cervical Cancer Screening Tests and Histologic Findings. These algorithms can guide clinicians through evidence-based recommendations for the majority of abnormal Pap smear scenarios. Participants at the consensus conference affirmed that the 2006 ASCCP guidelines for the management of abnormal cervical cancer screening tests and CIN or AIS remain valid, with the exception of the specific areas reviewed.

1. Essential Changes from Prior Management Guidelines (www. ASCCP.org/ascp-guidelines) and Cytology reported as negative but lacking endocervical cells can be managed without early repeat.

2. CIN 1 on endocervical curettage should be managed as CIN 1, not as a positive ECC.
3. Cytology reported as unsatisfactory requires repeat even if HPV negative.
4. Genotyping triages HPV-positive women with HPV type 16 or type 18 to earlier colposcopy only after negative cytology; colposcopy is indicated for all women with HPV and ASC-US, regardless of genotyping result.
5. For ASC-US cytology, immediate colposcopy is not an option. The serial cytology option for ASC-US incorporates cytology at 12 months, not 6 months and 12 months, and then if negative, cytology every 3 years. HPV-negative and ASC-US results should be followed with cotesting at 3 years rather than 5 years. HPV-negative and ASC-US results are insufficient to allow exit from screening at age 65 years.
6. The pathway to long-term follow-up of treated and untreated CIN 2+ is more clearly defined by incorporating cotesting.
7. More strategies incorporate cotesting to reduce follow-up visits. Pap-only strategies are now limited to women younger than 30 years, but cotesting is expanded even to women younger than 30 years in some circumstances. Women aged 21 to 24 years are managed conservatively. Prior management guidelines were from the "2006 Consensus Guidelines for the Management of Women With Abnormal Cervical Screening Tests" and remain the same, as follows:
   a. Less aggressive management of adolescents with abnormal Pap smears.
   b. A recommendation to avoid HPV screening in adolescents and those younger than 30 years of age.
   c. Options to use HPV testing for follow-up of ASC-US cytologic findings with reflex testing preferred if liquid-based Pap techniques are already used for cytologic evaluation.
   d. Specific suggestion for management of pregnant women with abnormal cytologic features.
   e. Preferred recommendations for follow-up of both adolescent and nonadolescent women with low-grade squamous intraepithelial lesion.
   f. Suggested workup of women with initial and subsequent AGCs.
   g. Use of HPV testing for screening and management of results in women age 30 years and older.
   h. Reconfirmation that all women with high-grade squamous intraepithelial lesion will require colposcopy. However, follow-up for high-grade dysplasias may differ for adolescent and nonadolescent women.
   i. A statement that although these guidelines are based on available evidence, they remain only guidelines, and clinicians are advised to utilize them as they may apply to a specific patient and are encouraged to consider alternative management or follow-up strategies based on the social, economic, risk stratification, and other factors that may influence management decisions.

A report describing *glandular* or *adenomatous atypia* (also called *atypical glandular cells* [AGC], and previously termed *atypical glandular cells of uncertain significance*, which is to be differentiated from squamous atypia) warrants immediate colposcopy with endocervical curettage to rule out a high-grade lesion and cervical adenocarcinoma. Furthermore, *endometrial carcinoma* may be suggested by abnormal cytologic findings detected by a Pap smear. In such instances, formal endometrial sampling is mandated in patients older than 40 years of age if no cervical abnormality is found. In postmenopausal women who are not on estrogen replacement, a report of estrogen effect or endometrial cells on the Pap smear is not normal. Evaluate the ovaries and uterus. If the findings of adenomatous atypia or of estrogen effect/endometrial cells (in a postmenopausal woman not on estrogen) are definite, conization, pelvic ultrasound, and even laparoscopy may be indicated.

PATIENT EDUCATION GUIDES

See the sample patient education handout available at www.expertconsult.com.

CPT/BILLING CODES

Q0091	Screening Papanicolaou smear; obtaining, preparing, and conveyance of cervical or vaginal smear to laboratory*
57500	Biopsy of cervix[†]
57505	Endocervical curettage[†]
88150	Pap smear interpretation[‡]
99201–99215	For a Pap smear, use office visit codes

*One Pap test is covered by Medicare every 2 years for low-risk patients and every 1 year for high-risk patients. Q0091 can be reported with a separate E&M code for Medicare patients.

[†]The majority of cervical biopsies and the endocervical curettage (ECC) will be performed as part of the formal colposcopic examination. Refer to Chapter 124, Colposcopic Examination, for appropriate billing information.

[‡]This code is used by the cytopathologist for billing. Very few clinicians (i.e., nonpathologists) interpret their patients' cytologic findings.

ICD-10 DIAGNOSTIC CODES

C53.9	Malignant neoplasm of the cervix, unspecified
D26.0	Neoplasm of the cervix, benign
D06.9	Cervical carcinoma in situ, severe dysplasia of cervix
N86	Cervical ulcer
N88.0	Cervical leukoplakia
N84.1	Cervical polyp
N88.8	Cervical atrophy
N87.9	Cervical dysplasia, unspecified
N87.0	Mild dysplasia of cervix
N87.1	Moderate dysplasia of cervix
N93.9	Abnormal vaginal bleeding
N93.9	Uterine bleeding
R87.619	Abnormal Pap smear (some insurances will not reimburse for this code)
Z91.89	Other specified personal history presenting hazards to health; other (for high-risk patients)
Z12.4	Special screening for malignant neoplasms; cervix
Z12.72	Special screening for malignant neoplasms; vagina

SUPPLIERS

Full contact information is available at www.expertconsult.com.

Becton Dickinson Diagnostics (SurePath)
Milex CooperSurgical, Inc.
Hologic Cytyc Corp. (ThinPrep)
Hardwood Puritan Products Co. (Cervix Brush, spatulas)
Wallach Surgical Devices, Inc. (Brush device, spatulas)

ONLINE RESOURCES

Agency for Healthcare Research and Quality Clinical Guidelines and Recommendations: US Preventive Services Task Force recommendations: www.ahcpr.gov/clinic/uspstf/uspscerv.htm
American Cancer Society recommendations: https://www.cancer.org/healthcare-professionals/american-cancer-society-prevention-early-detection-guidelines/cervical-cancer-screening-guidelines.html
American Society for Colposcopy and Cervical Pathology: Consensus guidelines for abnormal cytology: www.ASCCP.org/asccp-guidelines
National Cancer Institute Cervical Cancer Screening (PDQ): https://www.cancer.gov/types/cervical/hp/cervical-screening-pdq#section/_1
Tuggy M, Garcia J: Procedures Consult: Colposcopy. http://www.procedures-consult.com/medical-procedures/colposcopy-FM-028-procedure.aspx.

RECOMMENDED READING

ACOG Practice Bulletin Number 157. Screening for cervical cancer. *Obstet Gynecol.* 2016;128(4):111–130.

Apgar BS, Brotzman GL, Spitzer M. *Colposcopy. Principles and Practice.* 2nd ed. Philadelphia: Saunders; 2008.

Arbyn M, Bergeron C, Klinkhamer P, et al. Liquid compared with conventional cervical cytology. *Obstet Gynecol.* 2008;111:167–177.

Castle PE, Glass AG, Rush BB, Scott GR, Wentzensen N. Clinical human papillomavirus detection forecasts cervical cancer risk in women over 18 years of followup. *J Clin Oncol.* 2012;30(25):3044–3050.

Huh WK, Ault KA, Chelmow D, Davey DD, Goulart RA, et al. Use of primary high-risk human papillomavirus testing for cervical cancer screening: interim clinical guidance. *Gynecol Oncol.* 2015;136(2):181.

Koliopoulos G, Nyaga VN, Santesso N, Bryant A, Martin-Hirsch PPL, Mustafa RA, et al. Cytology versus HPV testing for cervical cancer screening in the general population. *Cochrane Database of Systematic Reviews Issue.* 2017;8:CD008587.

Koss LG. The Papanicolaou test for cervical cancer detection: a triumph and a tragedy. JAMA. 1989;261:737–743.

Rerucha CM, Caro RJ, Wheeler VL. Cervical cancer screening. *Am Fam Physician.* 2018;97(7):441–448.

Rodríguez AC, Schiffman M, Herrero R, et al. Rapid clearance of human papillomavirus and implications for clinical focus on persistent infections. *J Natl Cancer Inst.* 2008;100(7):513–517.

Schlichte MJ, Jacqueline Guidry J. Current cervical carcinoma screening guidelines. *J Clin Med.* 2015;4(5):918–932.

Solomon D, Davey D, Kurman R, et al. The 2001 Bethesda system: terminology for reporting results of cervical cytology. JAMA. 2002;287:2114–2119.

CHAPTER 121

HUMAN PAPILLOMAVIRUS DNA TYPING

Gary R. Newkirk

Papanicolaou cervical screening (the Pap test) has dramatically reduced the incidence of cervical cancer in developed countries. For over 20 years a relationship between human papillomavirus (HPV) infection and cervical cancer has been recognized. HPV is a sexually transmitted DNA virus that causes over 99% of cervical cancer. Of the 120 HPV types, at least 40 are known to infect the anogenital tract, causing genital warts or dysplasia (Table 121.1). HPV types have unique biologic potential and often prefer specific sites of infection (e.g., hands, feet, genitals). Among the types that infect a given target tissue, such as the cervix, specific types are more likely to predispose to cancer. HPV types that infect the genitalia can be categorized as high, low, and intermediate risk based on their predilection for causing severe dysplasia.

Other cancers have also been linked to the high-risk HPV viruses, including anorectal, vulvar, vaginal, oropharyngeal, bladder, and nonmelanoma skin cancers, among others. Sophisticated new tests for the detection of HPV hold great promise for improving both the sensitivity and specificity of cervical cancer screening. These new tests have also supported the development of triage mechanisms to help identify women who are at greatest risk for the development of high-grade cervical intraepithelial neoplasia (CIN) or recurrence of disease after treatment for CIN.

Current HPV tests that have been cleared by the US Food and Drug Administration (FDA) detect viral nucleic acid (DNA) or messenger RNA. Testing for HPV relies on the detection of viral DNA. The first test approved by the FDA for the detection of HPV DNA was the Hybrid Capture 2 (HC2) system (Qiagen Digene Corporation). This commercially available test uses a liquid hybridization format to detect 13 high-risk HPV types (HR HPV) (genotypes 16, 18, 31, 33, 35, 39, 45, 51, 52, 56, 58, 59, and 68). This test does not distinguish individual HPV types but rather identifies "the group." Other HPV tests have also received FDA approval since then. The cobas 4500 (Roche) uses a standardized polymerase chain reaction-based technique to detect 14 oncogenic HPV DNA types and can also detect individual types HPV 16 and 18. The Cervista HPV 16/18 DNA test detects only oncogenic HPV types 16 and 18. The APTIMA HR HPV (Hologic Gen-Probe) test detects 14 oncogenic HPV types of HPV messenger RNA. The Aptima HPV 16/18/45 test is also FDA-cleared to triage the pooled Aptima HR HPV test further. The most recently approved is Onclarity (Becton Dickinson) which detects 14 HPV strains including 16, 18, and 45. Table 121.2 lists the different FDA-approved HPV tests with their intended use. HPV testing can be performed as both a stand-alone test or combined with Pap testing when a liquid-based Pap test is used (see Chapter 120, Pap Smear and Related Techniques for Cervical Cancer Screening). Two HPV tests are now approved as the primary test in place of cytology. "Reflex" HPV testing refers to an automatic HPV DNA analysis on a liquid-based Pap test based on the cytologic diagnosis, such as atypical squamous cells of undetermined significance (ASCUS). In this setting, because the same sample aliquot is used, the patient need not return for a separate HPV sample collection examination.

HPV is very common among sexually active women. Nearly 75% of women are infected by age 30. Because most HPV infections are transient and do not always progress to severe dysplasia or cancer, there is controversy regarding whether isolated finding of HPV by current technology offers sufficient predictive value to replace current cytologic Pap screening. That said, the FDA recently approved currently available HPV DNA tests as a sole primary method for cervical cancer screening. The cobas HPV test was approved as the primary screening method at 3-year intervals and appears to provide cancer protection very similar to that of cotesting at 3-year intervals or annual cytology and superior protection relative to cytology at 3-year intervals. The Onclarity HPV test has also been approved as the primary screening method. In response to FDA approval, Interim Guidelines (2015) for primary high-risk HPV screening were developed by representatives from the Society of Gynecologic Oncology (SGO), the American Society of Cytopathology, and the College of American Pathologists (ASCCP) in addition to the American College of Obstetricians and Gynecologists (ACOG) and all groups that authored the 2012 Screening Guidelines. The Interim Guidelines state that because of equivalent or superior effectiveness, primary high-risk HPV screening can be utilized as an alternative to cytology. Primary HPV screening should not be implemented among women younger than 25 years of age and rescreening after a negative primary high-risk HPV test should not take place more frequently than every 3 years. In addition, although more research is necessary, the Interim Guidelines suggest that the best management of high-risk HPV-positive women is to triage positive tests with genotyping for 16/18 to colposcopy and to utilize reflex cytology for women positive for the 12 other high-risk genotypes. Multiple studies provide mounting evidence for the utility of HPV testing as primary screening and may continue to lead to further changes in recommendations, particularly as the actual impact of new screening guidelines on cancer prevention is investigated. Since the issuance of these Interim Guidelines, ACOG, the American Cancer Society (ACS), and the US Preventive Services Task Force (USPSTF) have decided against recommending HPV testing as a primary screen until age 30. This is largely due to the transient nature of HPV infection in younger women.

A recent (2017) Cochrane review found that when screening for CIN 2 or CIN 3 is being done, HPV primary testing is less likely to miss; however, HPV tests are more likely to lead to additional procedures or referrals. That said, a negative HPV test is more reassuring than a negative cytologic test because the cytologic test is more likely to be falsely negative, which could result in a delay in treatment.

At present, testing for HPV is used mainly to triage patients with ASCUS (see Chapter 120, Pap Smear and Related Techniques for Cervical Cancer Screening, Box 120.2, Terminology and Definitions, and Appendix K: Management Guidelines for Abnormal Cervical Cancer Screening Tests and Histologic Findings), screening otherwise healthy women over age 30, and posttreatment or postcolposcopy follow-up. HPV testing has clearly been shown to be a useful tool in screening women with ASCUS cytologic features, especially if performed as a "reflex" test after liquid-based Pap smears. Current HPV tests detect over 90% of high-grade CIN; a negative test greatly reduces unnecessary colposcopy and treatment. Current evidence supports lengthening the screening interval for women over age 30 to 5 years when both Pap and HPV tests are normal. Combined cytologic and HPV DNA testing in women aged 30 years and older is highly sensitive and cost-effective, reducing overall costs by 30%. HPV testing also can be used for postcolposcopy and posttreatment follow-up. Patients with an ASCUS, atypical squamous cells (high-grade squamous intraepithelial lesion [ASC-H] cannot be excluded), or low-grade squamous intraepithelial lesion Pap test result who are diagnosed with CIN 1 after colposcopy can be screened either by repeat cytology at 6 and 12 months or with a single HPV test

at 12 months. Likewise, women who are treated for CIN 2/3 can be followed by a repeat Pap test with HPV testing at 6 months. If both these tests are negative, the patient can safely return to routine screening. An abnormal HPV or Pap test result necessitates follow-up colposcopy. Of note, HPV testing can be performed on tissue samples (in situ sampling) to help correlate histologic finding with the presence of HPV. Currently testing for low-risk types of HPV is not recommended. HPV testing is not approved for males.

Again, if HPV testing is used as the primary, ASCCP and SGO 2015 Interim Guidelines suggest starting at age 25. If that test is negative, it should not be repeated for 3 years. Patients whose results are positive for HPV 16 and 18 should go for colposcopy. Those whose results are positive for the 12 other high-risk HPVs should have reflex cytology performed. The ASCCP and the SGO 2015 Interim Guidelines as well as the ASCCP 2012 Consensus Guidelines for the management of both cytologic and histologic cervical abnormalities are presented as algorithms in Appendix K: Management Guidelines for Abnormal Cervical Cancer Screening Tests and Histologic Findings.

At present (2018), neither the ACS nor ACOG recommend using the HPV high-risk assays as primary cervical cancer screening tools until age 30. From age 21 through 29, HPV testing may be used as part of a follow-up of an abnormal Pap. Both groups as well as the USPSTF recommend a Pap smear alone every 3 years from age 21 through 29. At age 30, preferred testing for ACS and ACOG is cotesting (Pap and HPV high risk) every 5 years through age 65. A reasonable alternative is Pap smear cytology alone every 3 years. At this point, women who have been vaccinated against HPV are still recommended to follow these same guidelines. Women who are immunocompromised or were exposed in utero to diethylstilbestrol are at higher risk; they should not follow these guidelines

TABLE 121.1 Human Papillomavirus Types Associated with Various Lesions

Lesion	HPV Type
Common wart	2
Planar	4
Butcher	7
Flat	3
Plantar	1
Epidermodysplasia verruciformis	3, 5, 8, 9, 10, 12, 14, 15, 17, 19, 26, 27
Respiratory	11, 16, 30, and others
Genital	
Low risk	6, 11, 42, 43, 44
High risk	16, 18, 31, 33, 35, 39, 45, 51, 52, 56, 58, 59, 68

HPV, Human papillomavirus.

TABLE 121.2 US Food and Drug Administration Approved Human Papillomavirus Tests

Instrument (Manufacturer)	Summary of Test	Test Principle	Intended Use
Onclarity HPV Assay (Becton Dickinson)	Used with the Becton Dickinson Viper LT machine, identifies genetic DNA from 14 HPV strains including high-risk strains 46, 18, and 45 in cervical cells.	Uses polymerase chain reaction amplification and detection.	Used as primary screening test. Follow-up test for when a Pap smear is abnormal. Used in combination with a Pap. Collected in SurePath preservative fluid.
Hybrid Capture 2 High-Risk HPV DNA test (Digene)	Identifies genetic DNA from HPV in cervical cells.	Uses a DNA-Probe-Hybrid immunoassay technique and is used combined when a woman's Pap test results are mildly abnormal.	Detection of high-risk HPV (HR-HPV). Follow-up test when a PAP smear is mildly abnormal.
Cervista HPV HR and Genfind DNA Extraction (Hologic)	Identifies DNA from 14 high-risk genital HPV types commonly associated with cervical cancer.	Uses DNA-probe technology.	Determines a patient's risk for developing cervical cancer.
Cervista HPV 16/18 (Hologic)	Identifies HPV types 16 and 18 in cervical samples.	Uses specific DNA-probe technology and may be used in combination or as a follow-up to the Cervista HPV HR test.	Determines a patient's risk for developing cervical cancer. Used for women age 30 and over or any age with borderline cytology results to determine the need for additional follow-up procedures.
cobas HPV test (Roche Molecular Systems)	Used on the cobas 4800 system to identify DNA from 14 high-risk genital HPV types commonly associated with cervical cancers. Specific for HPV types 16 and 18 but also identifies other high-risk types.	Uses fluorescent-labeled DNA probes.	Provides information on a patient's risk for developing cervical cancer; now also used as primary screening test including those specimens collected in SurePath preservative fluid. For women age 30 or over or women age 21 and older with borderline cellular results to assess the need for additional follow-up and diagnostic procedures.
APTIMA HPV Assay (Hologic Gen-Probe)	Used with the Tigris DTS system to identify RNA from 14 high-risk genital HPV types commonly associated with cervical cancer. Detects messenger RNA from two HPV viral oncogenes, E6 and E7.	Uses RNA capture and amplification of HPV RNA.	Determines a patient's risk for developing cervical cancer. Used for women age 30 and over or any age with borderline cytology results to determine the need for additional follow-up procedures.

HPV, Human papillomavirus; HR, high-risk.
Modified from Lab CE by Media Lab, www.labce.com/spg761630_fda_approved_hpv_tests.aspx.

but rather be counseled individually. The USPSTF recommends against using HPV testing for primary screening in women under the age of 30.

ANATOMY

Cervical testing requires sampling the same area targeted by the Pap smear, namely, the active transformation zone (see Chapter 120, Pap Smear and Related Techniques for Cervical Cancer Screening, Figs. 120.3 and 120.4, and Chapter 124, Colposcopic Examination).

INDICATIONS

- Adjunct to triage of ASCUS cytologic finding
- In combination with Pap testing for women over age 30 years
- For follow-up of women who have colposcopic/histologic findings consistent with CIN 1 without treatment
- For follow-up of women who have had treatment of the cervix for CIN 2/3
- To evaluate for the presence of HPV-related abnormal histologic findings (in situ testing)

HPV testing can potentially be useful for the evaluation of persistent low-grade cytologic changes in the postmenopausal patient, potential cases of child abuse, and cases of disease in the anal canal.

There are no indications at present for testing noncervical lesions for HPV. Some men who have sex with men are now being screened with Pap smears of the anal canal, and HPV testing may become an adjunctive test in these individuals.

CONTRAINDICATIONS

There are no absolute contraindications. Because this procedure is frequently performed at the time of a Pap smear, see Chapter 120, Pap Smear and Related Techniques for Cervical Cancer Screening, for contraindications to collection of the sample.

EQUIPMENT AND SUPPLIES

There are several FDA-approved HPV testing kits available from clinical reference laboratories for the collection and transport of the sample material. When used in combination with the Pap smear, both the cervical sampling and HPV DNA testing sample can be obtained with the same sampling device. Either a brush- or broom-type sampler may be used. ThinPrep and the Sure-Path are the liquid-based Pap smear systems that are approved by the FDA for reflex HPV testing.

- The HPV cervical sampling kit with brush, transport tube, and medium is used for stand-alone HPV DNA testing when a liquid-based Pap is not performed.
- Cervical biopsies (or other genital biopsies) are taken with the usual biopsy equipment and placed in the tube with the specimen transport medium.
- Tissue biopsies from lesions located anywhere on the body can also be placed in standard formalin for transport, although the specimen transport medium is preferred.
- Pap smear specimens can be collected with either broom or brush devices and placed in the Cytyc PreservCyt (Hologic Cytyc Corporation) or SurePath (Becton Dickinson) solution.

PROCEDURE

Cervical Sample Without Pap Smear Collection

1. The cervix is placed in view as for collecting a Pap specimen (see Chapter 120, Pap Smear and Related Techniques for Cervical Cancer Screening, Fig. 120.3).

2. Blot and gently remove excess cervical mucus.
3. The special cervical conical brush supplied in the specimen collection kit is inserted into the cervical os until the outer or widest bristles make contact with the cervix or reasonable resistance is encountered for further advancement (Fig. 121.1).
4. There is no need to advance the brush farther than 10 to 15 mm.
5. Rotate the brush three full turns in a counterclockwise direction.
6. Insert the brush into the bottom of the transport tube, snap off the shaft at the scored line, and cap securely.

Cervical Sample at the Time of Liquid-Based Pap Testing

1. The cervix is sampled with the broom or brush (see Chapter 120, Pap Smear and Related Techniques for Cervical Cancer Screening, Fig. 120.4), which is then rinsed thoroughly in Hologic Cytyc PreservCyt or SurePath solution for use in transporting material for the ThinPrep Pap process.
2. The ThinPrep Pap preparation produces a slide for cytologic evaluation. The remaining supernatant must be at least 4 mL and is processed with the HPV test protocol.
3. The sampling kit is used for HPV sampling at the time of a Pap smear (i.e., either in addition to the liquid-based Pap or with conventional Pap testing); the HPV DNA sample should be taken *after* the Pap sample is taken.
4. If HPV DNA sampling is performed at the time of colposcopy, the HPV sample should be collected *before* the use of any applied solutions such as saline, acetic acid, or Monsel solutions and prior to cervical biopsies.

Biopsy Testing for Human Papillomavirus

1. Biopsies may be taken from the cervix, vagina, rectum, vulva, or any other anatomic location and placed in the Hologic Digene or SurePath Specimen Transport Medium. Because there is no other preservative, this sample must be frozen immediately.
2. Biopsy specimens can be tested for in situ hybridization in formalin-preserved and paraffin-prepared histologic blocks.
3. Clinicians should check with their reference laboratory regarding the sampling, preparation, and handling of biopsy samples. Opinion differs on the ideal manner to handle this tissue for the somewhat rare in situ hybridization protocols.

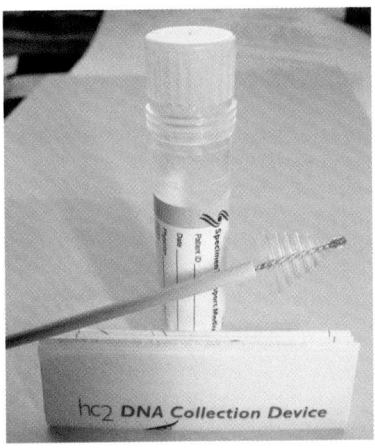

Fig. 121.1 Qiagen Digene Hybrid Capture 2 human papillomavirus (HPV) DNA kit (Qiagen Digene) tests for the 13 most common HPV types known to be associated with high-grade cervical dysplasia and cervical cancer. The kit includes a transport vial with fluid medium and a special conical sampling brush, which is rotated three times in the cervical os and then placed in the transport tube, snapped off, and sealed.

COMPLICATIONS

None have been reported. Minor spotting as per routine Pap testing is normal.

POSTPROCEDURE MANAGEMENT

The ASCCP guidelines suggest management based on the results of HPV testing. These guidelines will be appropriate for most patients but are not a substitute for clinical judgment in the management of cervical dysplasia.

NOTE: Operative report, complications, and postprocedure management are identical to those of the Pap smear protocol (see Chapter 120, Pap Smear and Related Techniques for Cervical Cancer Screening).

INTERPRETATION OF RESULTS

The HPV test is reported as positive or negative. A positive test indicates the presence of one or more of the 13 high-risk HPV viral types in the test. The overwhelmingly most common type causing a positive result is type 16. A negative test indicates either absence of these types or an amount of viral DNA deemed clinically irrelevant. Appendix K, Management Guidelines for Abnormal Cervical Cancer Screening Tests and Histologic Findings, presents the Interim 2015 Guidelines as well as the ASCCP 2012 Consensus Guidelines, which offer suggested evidence-based management interventions based on a positive HPV test.

CPT/BILLING CODES

87621   HPV amplified probe technology interpretation

There is no specific code for collection of the specimen.

SUPPLIERS

Full contact information is available at www.expertconsult.com.

Digene HC2 HPV DNA Kit; Qiagen, Inc.
Aptima and Cervista HPV HR/HPV 16/18 and Cytyc preservative; Hologic
Cobas HPV; Roche Molecular Systems
Clarity and SurePath preservative; Becton Dickinson

ONLINE RESOURCES

Hologic Digene patient education: www.thehpvtest.com/
Centers for Disease Control and Prevention: https://www.cdc.gov/std/tg2015/hpv-cancer.htm
American College of Obstetrics and Gynecology; http://www.acog.org/Womens-Health/Human-Papillomavirus-HPV

RECOMMENDED READING

ACOG Practice Bulletin Number 157. Screening for cervical cancer. *Obstet Gynecol.* 2016;128(4):111–130.
Apgar BS, Brotzman GL, Spitzer M. *Colposcopy: Principles and Practice.* 2nd ed. Philadelphia: Saunders; 2008.
ASCUS-LSIL Triage Study Group (ALTS). Results of a randomized trial on the management of cytology interpretations of atypical squamous cells of undetermined significance. *Am J Obstet Gynecol.* 2003;188:1383–1392.
Castle PE, Glass AG, Rush BB, Scott GR, Wentzensen N. Clinical human papillomavirus detection forecasts cervical cancer risk in women over 18 years of followup. *J Clin Oncol.* 2012;30(25):3044–3050.
Huh WK, Ault KA, Chelmow D, Davey DD, Goulart RA, et al. Use of primary high-risk human papillomavirus screening for cervical cancer: interim clinical guidance. *Gynecol Oncol.* 2015;125(2):330–337.
Koliopoulos G, Nyaga VN, Santesso N, et al. Cytology versus HPV testing for cervical cancer screening in the general population. *Cochrane Database Syst Rev.* 2017;8:Art. No.: CD008587. https://doi.org/10.1002/14651858.CD008587.pub2.
MJ Schlichte, Jacqueline Guidry J. Current cervical carcinoma screening guidelines. *J Clin Med.* 2015;4(5):918–932.

CHAPTER 122

WET SMEAR AND POTASSIUM HYDROXIDE PREPARATION

Gary R. Newkirk

Abnormal vaginal discharge is a common complaint. In fact, vaginitis is the most common gynecologic diagnosis in primary care. Vulvovaginal candidiasis, bacterial vaginosis (BV), and trichomoniasis (trich) account for over 90% of abnormal vulvovaginal symptoms and discharge. About 25% of cases are mixed infections where several pathogens may coexist. Office-based wet smear, potassium hydroxide (KOH) preparation, and vaginal secretion pH can be used to ensure a more accurate diagnosis and effective treatment of vaginitis. Recently the Affirm VPIII Microbial Identification Test (Becton Dickinson) has been developed for the detection and identification of *Candida* species, *Gardnerella vaginalis*, and *Trichomonas vaginalis* from vaginal fluid specimens in both symptomatic and asymptomatic patients. In many offices, this has become the standard. Affirm VPIII utilizes a standardized, rapid RNA probe technology that differentiates and confirms the etiology of infectious vaginitis. The Affirm VPIII assay simultaneously detects the presence of clinically significant levels of *Trichomonas*, *Gardnerella*, and *Candida* from vaginal specimens and is easy to read. Total hands-on time is approximately 5 minutes and test results are available in less than 1 hour. An extended specimen transport option, Affirm VPIII Ambient Temperature Transport System, is also available; it extends specimen stability to 72 hours at ambient temperature. Each of these test characteristics is important, since the assay was developed for use in a clinician's office as well as the clinical laboratory. The BD Affirm VPIII diagnosis is not affected by factors such as douches, lubricants, or menses; these factors are present in 50% of specimens and will obscure microscopic examinations. Recent study has shown that the Affirm VPIII test is a more sensitive diagnostic test for the detection and identification of symptomatic vaginitis/vaginosis than conventional clinical examination and wet mount testing. Empiric treatment for vulvovaginal symptoms including vaginal discharge should be avoided until appropriate testing is performed to make a specific diagnosis.

ANATOMY

Obtaining vaginal or vulvar samples to determine the cause of vulvovaginal symptoms and discharge requires familiarization with lower female genital anatomy and the basic skills of pelvic examination. Chapter 124, Colposcopic Examination, and Chapter 120, Pap Smear and Related Techniques for Cervical Cancer Screening, review the anatomy and basic steps of the pelvic examination.

INDICATIONS

- Abnormal vaginal discharge
- Vulvar or vaginal itching, burning, or pain
- Discomfort with intercourse

CONTRAINDICATIONS

- Active menses (relative contraindication; clinician should not postpone evaluation for significant discharge or vulvovaginitis during menses)
- Recent douching (relative contraindication; not for the VPIII Affirm testing)
- Recent application of vaginal creams or lubricants (relative contraindication; not for the VPIII Affirm testing)

EQUIPMENT AND SUPPLIES

- Vaginal speculum
- Small cotton-tipped applicators
- Small test tubes
- Normal saline
- 10% KOH solution
- Glass slides and coverslips
- pH test tape (narrow range needed: Micro Essential laboratory)
- Microscope
- Equipment to follow universal blood and body fluid precautions

PRECAUTIONS

- In some instances, women with extremely inflamed vulvovaginitis cannot tolerate speculum insertion. The clinician should be prepared to perform a limited examination by obtaining samples from the distal vagina or vulva.
- The clinician should maintain a high index of suspicion for a primary cervical infection with either *Chlamydia trachomatis* or *Neisseria gonorrhoeae* in patients who have an observed mucopurulent cervicitis or are at risk for those infections.

PREPROCEDURE PATIENT PREPARATION

- Discuss the need for pelvic (speculum) examination and testing requirements that may incur additional costs.
- Written consent is not required, although women should be informed if testing for *Neisseria gonorrhoeae* or *C. trachomatis* is performed (it will show up on their bill).
- Educate women during annual pelvic examinations regarding the avoidance of douching, creams, and lubricants prior to the evaluation of abnormal discharge.

PROCEDURE

1. With the patient in the lithotomy position, begin with a careful examination of the vulva for inflammation, ulcers, lesions, and discharge.

2. While observing universal blood and body fluid precautions, insert a warm lubricated speculum and expose the cervix.

3. Inspect the cervix, vaginal walls, and fornices. Perform cervical sampling for *N. gonorrhoeae*, *C. trachomatis*, or herpes as deemed appropriate. Consult with your laboratory on the detection methodology (culture, DNA testing) and technique for sample collection, preparation, and transport.

4. Collect secretions from both the vaginal fornices and lateral vaginal walls by gently rubbing with a cotton-tipped applicator. Place the cotton-tipped applicator with sample in a patient-identified small test tube that contains 1 mL of 0.9% (normal) saline. Leave the applicator in the test tube until the wet smear is performed in the laboratory. Remove the speculum from the vagina.

5. To properly prepare the slide for review, vigorously mix the swab in the saline solution. Remove the swab from the tube and depress it on the slide to express a small amount of fluid. Apply a coverslip over the sample. The slide ("wet prep" or "wet smear") is then immediately examined with the microscope under low power (10×) for vaginal squamous cells, white blood cells, lactobacilli, clue cells, and trichomonads. Examine under low and high power (40×). If a KOH slide is needed, prepare another slide exactly as previously described. Before placing the coverslip, put one drop of a 10% KOH solution on the sample. Apply a coverslip. Allow to air- or flame-dry and examine under low power for hyphae, mycelial tangles, or spores. The "whiff test" is performed when KOH is applied to the sample (see later discussion).

6. A pH test of vaginal secretions can improve diagnostic specificity. A vaginal secretion pH of 3.8 to 4.5 is considered normal in premenopausal women; above 4.5 suggests BV or trichomoniasis. A piece of the pH test tape may be directly applied to the moist vaginal wall or to the vaginal secretions adhering to the speculum when it is removed from the vagina. Standard nitrazine paper is not accurate; a narrower pH range test method should be used (narrow-range test paper: Micro Essential Laboratory). Cervical mucus, semen, douche solutions, and blood are alkaline and can interfere with pH testing.

7. Cultures of vaginal secretions can be obtained for *Candida* and non-*Candida* yeast, aerobic vaginitis, or trichomoniasis. DNA testing is available for candidiasis or trichomoniasis. Cultures are recommended when microscopy and pH testing fail to document a cause for recurrent vaginitis.

PROCEDURE FOR VP III AFFIRM COLLECTION AND TRANSPORT

1. Place the patient in position for a pelvic examination. Insert an unlubricated speculum (without jelly or water) into the vagina to permit visualization of the posterior vaginal fornix.

2. Using a sterile swab, obtain a sample from the posterior vaginal fornix. Twist or roll the swab against the vaginal walls two or three times, ensuring that the entire circumference of the swab has touched the vaginal wall. Swab the lateral vaginal wall while removing the swab.

3. Immediately place the swab in the sample collection tube (SCT). With the swab touching the bottom of the collection tube, grasp the prescored handle of the swab just above the top of the tube and bend it until the swab breaks.

4. When the swab is fully inserted in the collection tube, the score mark on the swab is approximately 1 cm above the top of the collection tube. Discard the broken handle into an infectious waste container.

5. Place the cap over the exposed end of the swab and firmly press the cap onto the tube. The cap will snap onto the tube when it is properly seated. Label the SCT with the patient identification information. Include the time at which the sample was collected.

6. Place the capped SCT into the plastic sample transport bag for transport and testing with the Affirm VPIII Microbial Identification Test.

COMMON ERRORS

- Not obtaining cervical cultures for *N. gonorrhoeae*, *C. trachomatis*, or herpes in settings where this may be probable. These infections often cause vaginal discharge as well.
- Not obtaining samples from the vaginal wall as well as the cervical fornices.
- Not performing a careful history of patient-directed treatment, such as douching or over-the-counter treatments that can interfere with testing, prior to examination.
- Failure to consider the contribution of chronic douching, spermicidal compounds, or condom-related latex allergy as contributors of vaginal irritation and discharge.
- Failure to treat BV in women about to undergo a gynecologic procedure or pregnant women at high risk of preterm labor

COMPLICATIONS

The most common complication is allowing confusing or conflicting results to lead to misguided or "shotgun" treatment. Women with BV undergoing a gynecologic procedure require treatment regardless of symptoms in order to prevent postprocedural complications.

POSTPROCEDURE MANAGEMENT

- Offer general education regarding the relationship of vulvovaginitis to self-treatment, douching, use of female "deodorant" or cleansing, latex, or spermicidal products.
- Offer specific instructions regarding the treatment modalities recommended such as intravaginal creams with applicator, oral medications, and side effects (e.g., metronidazole for BV).

Interpretation of Results

At least five different microscopic fields should be surveyed to observe an adequate number of representative fields. Initially low (10×) and high (40×) power should be used.

Findings: Saline Examination ("Wet Prep" or "Wet Smear")

- *Lactobacillus* species are normal vaginal flora. Lactobacilli are large, long bacillary rods. Their absence or decrease, coupled with an abundance of clue cells and a vaginal pH greater than 4.7, may be consistent with the clinical findings observed in BV (Fig. 122.1).
- Leukocytes at a concentration of more than 5 to 10 cells per high power field may indicate infection. If the number of leukocytes exceeds the number of squamous cells, an inflammatory process should be suspected.
- Parabasal cells may indicate a low estrogenic state.
- Trichomonads (*Trichomonas vaginalis*) distinctively appear as actively motile protozoans with whipping flagella (Fig. 122.2). They are about the same size as epithelial cells.
- Clue cells are epithelial cells with indistinct borders often described as "fuzzy" or "dirty" caused by abundant adherent multiple coccobacilli organisms. Clue cells are indicative of BV (see Figs. 122.1 and 122.2).

Findings: Potassium Hydroxide Examination

Hyphae or buds suggest candidiasis (Figs. 122.3 and 122.4). The absence of hyphae but presence of budding spores suggests infection with a non-*albicans* type of *Candida*, such as *C. glabrata* (Fig. 122.5). While the addition of KOH increases the sensitivity of the test, it

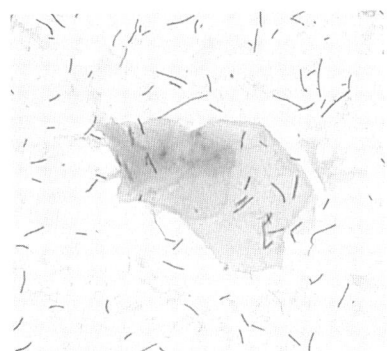

Fig. 122.1 *Lactobacillus* species. The large rods are normal flora. (From Morse SA, Moreland A, Holmes K. *Atlas of Sexually Transmitted Diseases and AIDS.* 2nd ed. London: Gower Medical; 1996.)

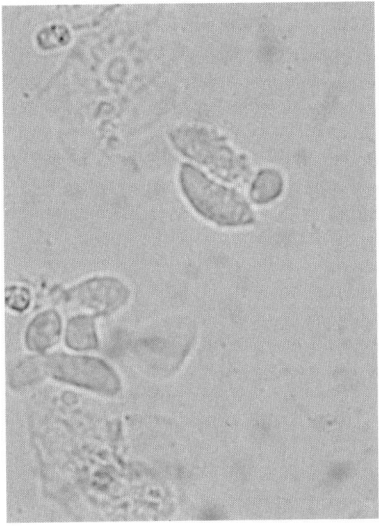

Fig. 122.2 Microscopic examination of a wet mount reveals multiple motile trichomonads. They are about same size as epithelial cells. (From Zitelli BJ, Davis HW. *Atlas of Pediatric Physical Diagnosis.* 4th ed. St Louis: Mosby; 2002.)

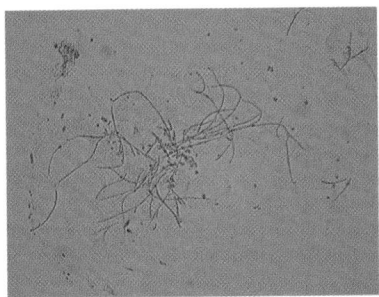

Fig. 122.3 Low-power view of potassium hydroxide (KOH) preparation showing the ghost-like appearance of disintegrating epithelial cells from the KOH and the fungal mycelia and spore forms becoming evident. (Courtesy Gary R. Newkirk, MD.)

should be kept in mind that at least one-third of patients with symptomatic candidiasis will have negative findings.

pH Test

The range of values will be determined by the color of the tape.

Normal flora	pH 4.5
Candidiasis	pH 3.8 to 4.5
BV	pH 4.7
Trichomoniasis	pH above 4.5

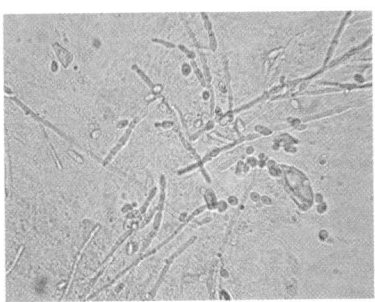

Fig. 122.4 Higher-power (40×) view of mycelia, budding yeast, and spores supporting the diagnosis of yeast vaginitis. (Courtesy Gary R. Newkirk, MD.)

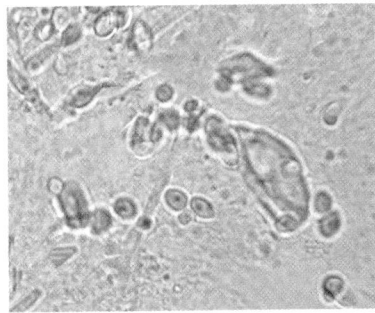

Fig. 122.5 High-power view of potassium hydroxide preparation with predominately spore forms suggesting *Candida glabrata* yeast vaginitis. (Courtesy Gary R. Newkirk, MD.)

NOTE: Combined infections such as yeast and BV can produce variable pH results.

Whiff Test

The presence of a strong amine or "fishy" odor after application of 10% KOH implicates BV. A positive whiff test was predictive of positive culture results for anaerobic flora such as *Bacteroides* species with 67% sensitivity, 94% specificity, and a positive predictive value of 95%. The whiff test is usually negative with trichomoniasis.

CPT/BILLING CODES

58999	Unlisted procedure, female genital system (wet smear and KOH preparation)
87220	Tissue examination by KOH slide from skin, hair, or nails
87480; 87510; 87660	VPIII Affirm collection and testing

ICD-10-CM DIAGNOSTIC CODES

B37.3	Monilial vulvovaginitis (candidiasis)
A59.01	Trichomonal vaginitis
N76.0	Vaginitis and vulvovaginitis, unspecified (includes BV)
N89.8	Vaginal discharge
N94.89	Unspecified symptom associated with female genital organs
N95.2	Atrophic vaginitis

Acknowledgment

The editors recognize the contributions of Barbara Apgar, MD, to this chapter in a previous edition of this text.

ONLINE RESOURCES

Centers for Disease Control: Diagnosis and treatment of vaginitis: http://www.cdc.gov/std/treatment/2006/vaginal-discharge.htm

Affirm instructions: http://www.healthcare.uiowa.edu/path_handbook/extras/BD_AffirmKit_Instructions.pdf

RECOMMENDED READING

Brown HL, Fuller DD, Jasper LT, Davis TE, Wright JD. Clinical evaluation of affirm VPIII in the detection and identification of Trichomonas vaginalis. Gardnerella vaginalis and Candida species in vaginitis/vaginosis. *Infect Dis Obstet Gynecol.* 2004;12(1):17–21.

French L, Horton J, Matousek M. Abnormal vaginal discharge: using office diagnostic testing more effectively. *J Fam Practice.* 2004;53:805–814.

Sobel JD. Vaginitis. *N Engl J Med.* 1997;337:1896–1903.

Swygard H, Cohen MS. Approach to the patient with a sexually transmitted infection. In: Goldman L, Schafer AI, eds. *Goldman Cecil Medicine.* 25th ed. Philadelphia: Elsevier; 2016:1876–1881.

Usatine RP. *The Color Atlas of Family Medicine.* New York: McGraw-Hill; 2009.

Wiesenfeld HC, Macio I. The infrequent use of office-based diagnostic tests for vaginitis. *Am J Obstet Gynecol.* 1999;181:39–41.

CHAPTER 123

CERVICAL POLYPS

Beth A. Choby

Cervical polyps affect 4% of women. Although their etiology is poorly understood, polyps are associated with obstructed cervical blood vessels, pregnancy, chronic inflammation, and an abnormal response to increased estrogen. Women with diabetes or recurrent vaginitis may be at increased risk. Most cervical polyps are benign, although 1% of lesions undergo malignant transformation. A recent study (Levy, 2016) reported that as high as 3.7% of polyps had clinically significant histologic findings (although most were likely reactive or inflammatory changes). Because of these risks, polyps are generally removed and histologically examined to rule out precancerous change.

The incidence of cervical polyps increases with age. They are rarely seen in girls who have not reached menarche but are fairly common in parous women in their 20s. Diagnosis is often made during a routine speculum examination. Multiparous women 30 to 50 years of age and perimenopausal women are most often affected. The influence of hormone therapy on the progression of cervical polyps is not well defined. Postmenopausal cervical polyps are often associated with endometrial polyps and are more prone to be symptomatic. Women taking tamoxifen who have a cervical polyp are significantly more likely to have concomitant endometrial polyps. Evaluation with hysteroscopy is indicated in this situation.

Most cervical polyps are asymptomatic and found by chance during routine gynecologic examination. When present, symptoms are usually vague and include vaginal spotting or bleeding after exercise, douching, or intercourse. Vascular congestion and edema can cause ulceration of the polyp tip and postcoital bleeding. Larger polyps are associated with intermenstrual spotting. Defecation or straining can cause bleeding. Abnormal menses or nonpurulent vaginal discharge is sometimes noted. When cervical polyps cause postmenopausal vaginal bleeding, further workup to exclude malignancy is mandatory.

Cervical polyps range in size from a few millimeters to several centimeters. Polyps on longer pedicles (stalks) sometimes protrude from the vaginal orifice. Large endocervical polyps cause cervical dilation and pain.

The differential diagnosis for cervical polyps is given in Box 123.1. Because cervical polyps often coexist with endometrial polyps, hysteroscopy has been suggested as the first-line therapy in the management of cervical polyps. Older recommendations include performing a suction dilation and curettage with all cervical polypectomies. Current literature fails to support either intervention as substantially improving outcomes compared with routine simple polyp removal. In low-risk, asymptomatic women, most clinicians still proceed with in-office cervical polypectomy.

ANATOMY

Cervical polyps are pedunculated tumors arising from endocervical or ectocervical tissue. *Endocervical* polyps originate within the endocervical canal, are most common in premenopausal women, and can prolapse through the cervix (Fig. 123.1). *Ectocervical* polyps more often affect postmenopausal women (Fig. 123.2). Polyps are bright red to pink and appear spongy. Most often they are solitary, although multiple polyps are sometimes encountered.

Endometrial polyps are sometimes confused as being of cervical origin. Endometrial polyps can protrude through the endocervical canal. Management of endometrial polyps is more complicated because the polyp's blood supply is usually more extensive and the attachment is much higher up (Fig. 123.3). Likewise, a pedunculated uterine fibroid can be mistaken for a cervical polyp.

Although some lesions can mimic cervical polyps and be benign (Fig. 123.4), malignant conditions such as adenocarcinoma can also masquerade as a polyp. Histologic study is often the only way to be certain of the true nature of the lesion.

INDICATIONS FOR REMOVAL

- Asymptomatic cervical polyps found on routine gynecologic examination
- Cervical polyps associated with pain, bleeding, or other symptoms

CONTRAINDICATIONS

- Patient unwilling/unable to consent to procedure
- Patient unwilling/unable to cooperate with vaginal examination
- Endometrial polyps or cervical polyps with a dense, thick pedicle and strong blood supply (However, these can be clamped and then ligated, just clamped, or sutured at the base if visible and then removed.)
- Polyps larger than several centimeters (may be better removed in a surgical suite)
- Pregnancy
- Blood dyscrasias
- High likelihood of multiple polyps (consider hysteroscopy)

EQUIPMENT AND SUPPLIES

- Nonsterile gloves and equipment necessary to maintain universal blood and body fluid precautions
- Vaginal speculum
- Colposcope (optional)
- Ring forceps (a Kelly clamp is an alternative, especially if the base is small)

BOX 123.1 Differential Diagnosis of Cervical Lesions
Cervical malignancy
Cervical polyp
Condyloma
Endometrial polyp
Nabothian cyst
Prolapsed fibroid/ myoma
Retained products of conception
Sarcoma
Squamous papilloma

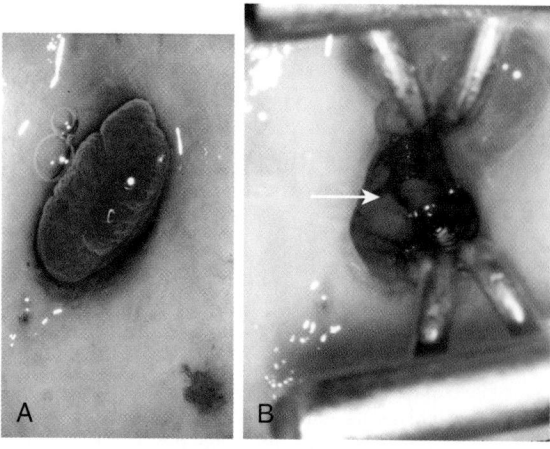

Fig. 123.1 (A) Endocervical polyp. (B) Identification of polyp base *(arrow)* using an endocervical speculum. (Courtesy Duane Townsend, MD.)

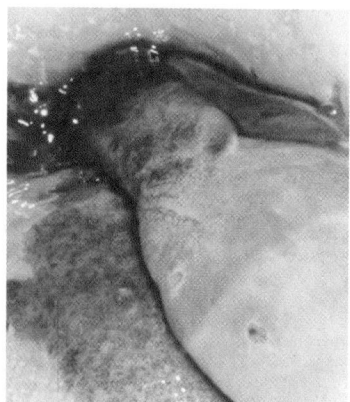

Fig. 123.3 Dysplastic endometrial polyp. Stalk originates in endometrial cavity. (Courtesy Duane Townsend, MD.)

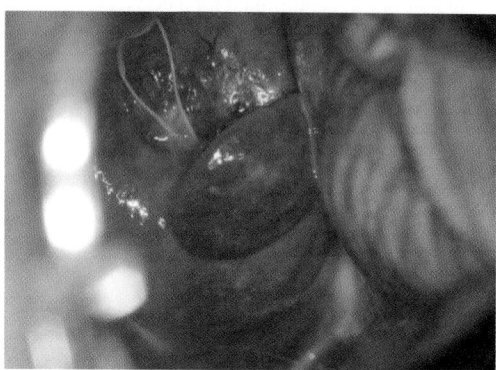

Fig. 123.2 Ectocervical polyp. The stalk is attached to the ectocervix. Note the strings of the intrauterine device. (Courtesy The Medical Procedures Center, Midland, MI.)

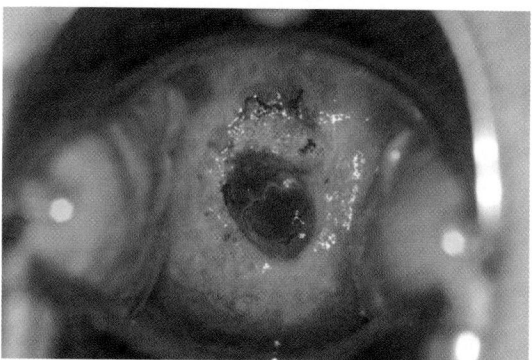

Fig. 123.4 Suspected cervical polyp, which is actually a large nabothian cyst. (Courtesy The Medical Procedures Center, Midland, MI.)

- Cervical biopsy forceps (may not be needed)
- Endocervical curette (Kevorkian)
- Pathology specimen containers
- Silver nitrate sticks
- Topical anesthetic (lidocaine jelly or benzocaine solution), though this is usually not needed
- Kogan endocervical speculum

PRECAUTIONS

- Identify the base of the polyp stalk to exclude an endometrial polyp. Endometrial polyps are often larger, with more vascular stalks. Suspect an endometrial polyp if the stalk extends into the cervix or remains visible after polypectomy. Endometrial polypectomy is most often done by hysteroscopy.
- Cervical polyps have increased vascularity during pregnancy. Asymptomatic polyps that do not change in size or appearance may be observed and removed after delivery. If bleeding necessitates removal during pregnancy, electrocautery or a loop electrosurgical excision procedure is sometimes required.
- Remove large cervical polyps in an outpatient surgical suite. Hysteroscopy is useful for confirming the size and origin of polyps found deeper inside the endocervical canal.

PREPROCEDURE PATIENT EDUCATION AND FORMS

Naproxen (500 mg) or a similar nonsteroidal anti-inflammatory drug can be given orally 1 hour before the procedure. Although menstruation is not a contraindication, the procedure should not be scheduled during menses. Discuss the risks and benefits of the procedure with the patient and obtain informed consent. See the consent form available at www.expertconsult.com.

PROCEDURE

1. While observing universal blood and body fluid precautions, don nonsterile gloves and insert a vaginal speculum. If a recent Pap examination has not been performed, it can be completed before the procedure.
2. Visualize the polyp. The use of a colposcope may improve visualization.
3. Gently manipulate the cervical os using closed ring forceps to identify the polyp base. Use of a Kogan endocervical speculum may be helpful if the stalk extends into the endocervical canal.
4. Determine whether the polyp is cervical or endometrial in origin.
5. Remove the polyp using one of the following methods:
   - Grasp the polyp with the ring forceps and twist the forceps around the stalk until it comes off. Patients may complain of mild discomfort (preferred and most commonly used technique).

   NOTE: If multiple twists have been performed, and the polyp still has not come off, it is likely a prolapsed uterine fibroid. Although it may cause more bleeding, the cervical biopsy forceps may be helpful for cutting the stalk.
   - Cut through the tissue at the base of the polyp using cervical biopsy forceps (optional technique, may cause more bleeding).

- If the polyp is small, scrape it off in its entirety using a sharp curette (optional technique, may cause more bleeding, but best suited when polyp too small to grasp with ring forceps).
6. Place the cervical polyp and stalk into a specimen container with formalin.
7. Perform an endocervical curettage using a Kevorkian curette (see Chapter 124, Colposcopic Examination). Although this step is optional, it ensures that all of the abnormal tissue has been removed. Place the tissue in a separate specimen container from that containing the cervical polyp.
8. Bleeding is usually minimal. Control bleeding, if necessary, using silver nitrate, Monsel solution, or cautery. Silver nitrate also destroys residual polyp tissue and minimizes the chance of recurrence.

SAMPLE OPERATIVE REPORT

See the sample operative report available at www.expertconsult.com.

COMMON ERRORS

- Failure to remove the polyp, stalk, and base entirely. The use of a colposcope to identify the origin of the polyp before excision may facilitate complete removal. If it is a very high polyp, hysteroscopy may be the procedure of choice. For a very large high polyp, a gynecologist can use a laser to split the posterior wall of the cervix to improve access and remove the polyp.
- When multiple polyps are present, it is best to thoroughly curette the endocervical canal.
- If the patient is postmenopausal, has irregular bleeding, or takes tamoxifen, a dilation and curettage or hysteroscopy may be a better option.
- Misidentification of a prolapsed endometrial polyp or prolapsed uterine fibroid as a cervical polyp.
- Occasionally pathology will report a "pseudopolyp." This can be managed according to Pap smear results.

COMPLICATIONS

- Postprocedure bleeding or spotting
- Postprocedure pain
- Recurrence

POSTPROCEDURE MANAGEMENT

- Monitor the patient for vasovagal reactions.
- Provide the patient with a sanitary pad.
- Advise the patient to take a nonsteroidal antiinflammatory drug for 24 hours as needed for abdominal cramping.

POSTPROCEDURE PATIENT EDUCATION

Patients should avoid tampon use, douching, or sexual intercourse for 1 week after cervical polypectomy. Active vaginal bleeding warrants timely reevaluation. Patients can be followed up at 6 to 8 weeks. Because polyps are generally benign and no further treatment usually needed, routine gynecologic surveillance is appropriate.

PATIENT EDUCATION GUIDES

See patient education and consent forms and sample operative report available at www.expertconsult.com.

CPT/BILLING CODES

There is no separate CPT code for cervical polyp removal.

57500	Biopsy of the cervix, single or multiple, or local excision of lesion, with or without fulguration
57505	Endocervical curettage (not performed as part of dilation and curettage)

ICD-10-CM DIAGNOSTIC CODES

A63.0	Condyloma acuminatum
D26.0	Benign neoplasm of the cervix (adenomatous polyp of the cervix)
D39.0	Neoplasm of uncertain behavior: uterus
N84.0	Polyp endometrium/uterus NOS
N84.1	Polyp of cervix NOS
N94.89	Unspecified symptoms associated with female genital organs
N92.6	Metrorrhagia. Bleeding unrelated to menstrual cycle; irregular intermenstrual bleeding
N95.0	Postmenopausal bleeding

ONLINE RESOURCES

Martin E. Cervical polyp. Discovery Health: Diseases and Conditions. http://health.discovery.com/encyclopedias/illnesses.html?article=1991

MedlinePlus Encyclopedia: Cervical polyps. www.nlm.nih.gov/medlineplus/ency/article/001494.htm

RECOMMENDED READING

Baggish MS. Cervical polypectomy. In: Baggish MS, Karram MM, eds. *Atlas of Pelvic Anatomy and Gynecologic Surgery*. 4th.ed. Philadelphia: Elsevier; 2016:519–522.

Tarney CM, Han J. Postcoital bleeding: a review on etiology, diagnosis and management. *Obstet Gynecol Int*. 2014;192087.

Bajo J, Moreno-Calvo F, Uguet-de-Resayre C, et al. Contribution of transvaginal sonography to the evaluation of benign cervical conditions. *J Clin Ultrasound*. 1999;27:61–64.

Hassa H, Tekin B, Senses T, et al. Are the site, diameter and number of endometrial polyps related with symptomatology? *Am J Obstet Gynecol*. 2006;194:718–721.

Levy RA, Kumarapeli AR, Spencer HJ, Quick CM. Cervical polyps: is histologic evaluation necessary? *Pathol Res Pract*. 2016;212(9):800–803.

Neri A, Kaplan B, Rabinerson D, et al. Cervical polyp in the menopause and the need for fractional dilatation and curettage. *Eur J Obstet Gynecol Reprod Biol*. 1995;62:53–55.

Speiwankiewicz B, Stelmachow J, Sawicki W, et al. Hysteroscopy in cases of cervical polyps. *Eur J Gynaecol Oncol*. 2003;24:67–69.

CHAPTER 124

COLPOSCOPIC EXAMINATION

Gary R. Newkirk

Colposcopy is the examination of the cervix, vagina, and genital organs with light and magnification to identify abnormal areas for biopsy, so that the patient can be managed or triaged to appropriate care. The topical application of saline, acetic acid, and iodine solutions helps identify biopsy sites.

Addressing the widespread human papillomavirus (HPV) and genital epithelial dysplasia epidemic requires mastery of the skills to perform colposcopy, cervical biopsy, and endocervical curettage (ECC). The most frequent indications for these procedures include the evaluation of an abnormal Papanicolaou (Pap) smear (see Chapter 120, Pap Smear and Related Techniques for Cervical Cancer Screening), visible cervical abnormalities, evidence of clinical HPV infection, and follow-up of prior cervical treatment. Most cases of cervical dysplasia can be managed entirely in the outpatient setting. Successful colposcopy requires strict compliance with established protocol and often the support of the pathologist. Occasionally, the support of a gynecologist will also be helpful. Mechanisms for excellent documentation and rigorous follow-up are mandatory. Clinicians who assimilate colposcopy skills into their practices will respond to a major public health problem and enhance their patients' access to care.

The colposcope is essentially a stereoscopic, portable operating microscope (3× to 40×) with a focal distance appropriate to examine the genitalia and cervix. The colposcopic examination serves to (1) identify normal landmarks, (2) identify abnormal areas in relation to these landmarks, (3) facilitate directed biopsy of abnormal areas for histologic diagnosis, and (4) rule out invasive cancer. Based on the findings, patients are managed or triaged for observation, for procedures (e.g., cryotherapy, loop electrosurgical excision procedure [LEEP], cervical cold conization), or for definitive staged therapy for invasive carcinoma.

Colposcopic-directed biopsy provides histologic clarification of abnormal Pap smears; this is mandatory before definitive therapy. Premalignant and malignant cervical conditions produce colposcopically identifiable epithelial changes that are often characteristic and generally occur within the transformation zone (TZ), which can be examined carefully during the colposcopic examination. Ultimately, the pathologist is the one who provides the histologic diagnoses for abnormalities identified during the colposcopic examination. Therefore, the major challenge for the colposcopist is to distinguish the normal from the abnormal and to sample the most abnormal-appearing changes for histologic confirmation. When there is any question about the colposcopic impression, biopsy should be undertaken. The ECC, or other cervical assessment methods such as endocervical brushing techniques, is performed as part of the routine colposcopic examination (contraindicated in pregnancy) to confirm the absence of occult disease in the endocervical canal. Nearly all agree that traditional ECC should be performed (1) if there is any question of invasive disease within the canal, (2) before ablative therapy such as cryotherapy or laser ablation, (3) as part of the work-up for atypical glandular cell abnormalities, (4) when either the initial or follow-up cytology indicates a high-grade squamous intraepithelial lesion and colposcopy of the cervix does not yield a clear source, and (5) when the entire TZ/squamocolumnar junction (SCJ) cannot be evaluated (previously known as "unsatisfactory," but now known as "not fully visualized" or "inadequate" colposcopy). Other common reasons for performing a traditional ECC include follow-up of the treatment of severe dysplasia, especially when a cone resection (including LEEP) was performed and histology indicates positive margins with significant dysplasia, or if the ECC immediately after a cone resection was positive.

Colposcopy itself, without the benefit of histologic confirmation, is not considered a diagnostic tool. Even though colposcopically defined visual abnormalities correlate with cervical dysplasia or frank carcinoma, the ultimate diagnosis rests on the traditional histologic interpretation of submitted samples and not with the visual pattern recognition.

Even with biopsy, it turns out that the accuracy and reproducibility of colposcopy can be limited. One study (Massad, 2003) found that colposcopic impression of a high-grade lesion only identified 56% of cervical intraepithelial neoplasia (CIN) grade 2 or higher. There is also a risk of false negative biopsy (Zuchna, 2010). Taking multiple biopsies (more than four) seems to increase the likelihood of making the correct diagnosis. Accordingly, diagnostic accuracy requires that the colposcopist perform liberal biopsy of the abnormal cervix. In the United States, there are also limitations, which are often due to the lack of standardized terminology, the lack of recommendations for colposcopic practice and procedures, and the lack of quality assurance measures. A lack of experience by the colposcopist can also affect the false-negative rate (missed high-grade lesion/invasive cancer); this ranges from 13% to 69%. In an attempt to improve the standardized terminology, the International Federation for Cervical Pathology and Colposcopy (IFCPC) adopted revised colposcopic terminology in June 2012 based on the world congress in Rio de Janeiro in July 2011. In turn, these guidelines were used as a template to modify the terminology to fit colposcopic practice in the United States by the American Society for Colposcopy and Cervical Pathology (ASCCP, Khan) in 2017 (Table 124.1). These terms should be used to describe findings during the colposcopic examination. A comparison of the two guidelines is seen in Table 124.2. Both of these guidelines were designed based upon our improved understanding of the epidemiology and science of cervical carcinoma, which has been developed over the last decade.

COLPOSCOPIC ANATOMY AND FINDINGS

The prudent colposcopist must be completely familiar with the normal findings and the visual abnormalities that correlate with dysplasia and malignancy on the cervix. Basic Pap smear terminology and cervical anatomy are reviewed in Chapter 120, Pap Smear and Related Techniques for Cervical Cancer Screening. Colposcopy terminology is summarized in Table 124.1. It is also important to consider the appearance of the cervix in different age groups because the anatomy varies developmentally in response to hormonal stimulation (Figs. 124.1 to 124.3).

TABLE 124.1   Standardized Colposcopic Terminology (ASCCP)

Category	Features/Criteria	Details
General assessment	Visualization of the cervix	Fully visualized Not fully visualized due to: ____
	Visualization of the SCJ	Fully visualized Not fully visualized
Acetowhite changes	Any degree of whitening after application of 3%–5% acetic acid	Yes/no
Normal colposcopic findings	Original squamous epithelium: mature, atrophic	
	Columnar epithelium	
	Ectopy/ectropion	
	Metaplastic squamous epithelium	
	Nabothian cysts	
	Crypt (gland) openings	
	Deciduosis in pregnancy	
	Submucosal branching vessels	
Abnormal colposcopic findings	Lesion(s) present (acetowhite or other)	Yes/no
	Location of each lesion	Clock position At the SCJ (yes/no) Lesion visualized (fully/not fully) Satellite lesion
	Size of each lesion	No. quadrants the lesion involves Percentage of surface area of TZ occupied by lesion

	Low-grade features	Acetowhite:
		  Thin/translucent
		  Rapidly fading
		Vascular patterns:
		  Fine mosaic
		  Fine punctation
		Margins/border:
		  Irregular/geographic contour
		  Condylomatous/raised/papillary
		  Flat

	High-grade features	Acetowhite:
		  Thick/dense
		  Rapidly appearing/slowly fading
		  Cuffed crypt (gland) openings
		  Variegated red and white
		Vascular patterns:
		  Coarse mosaic
		  Coarse punctation
		Margins/border:
		  Sharp border
		  Inner border sign (internal margin)
		  Ridge sign
		  Peeling edges
		Contour: flat
		Fused papillae

	Suspicious for invasive cancer	Atypical vessels Irregular surface Exophytic lesion Necrosis Ulceration Tumor or gross neoplasm A suspicious lesion may not be acetowhite
	Nonspecific	Leukoplakia Erosion Contact bleeding Friable tissue
	Lugol staining	Not used Stained Partially stained Nonstained
Miscellaneous findings	Polyp (ectocervical or endocervical)	
	Inflammation	
	Stenosis	
	Congenital TZ	
	Congenital anomaly	
	Posttreatment consequence (scarring)	
Colposcopic impression (highest grade)	Normal/benign	
	Low grade	
	High grade	
	Cancer	

ASCCP, American Society of Colposcopy and Cervical Pathology; SCJ, squamocolumnar junction; TZ, transformation zone.
Modified from Khan M, Werner CL, Darragh TM, et al. ASCCP colposcopy standards: role of colposcopy, benefits, potential harms, and terminology for colposcopic practice. J Low Genit Tract Dis. 2017;21(4):223–229.

TABLE 124.2	Comparison Between 2011 IFCPC and 2017 ASCCP Guidelines	
	ASCCP	**IFCPC**
General assessment: cervix visibility	Fully/not fully visible	Adequate/inadequate
General assessment: squamocolumnar junction visibility	Fully/not fully visible	Completely/partially/not visible
General assessment: transformation zone type	Not used	Transformation zone types 1, 2, 3
Abnormal colposcopic findings	Low-grade features	Grade 1 (minor)
	High-grade features	Grade 2 (major)
Excision type	Not used	Excision types 1, 2, 3

ASCCP, American Society of Colposcopy and Cervical Pathology; *IFCPC*, International Federation for Cervical Pathology and Colposcopy.

Normal Colposcopic Findings

See Figs. 124.1 and 124.2.

Original Squamous Epithelium

This is a featureless, smooth, pink epithelium on the outer aspects of the ectocervix going back to the cervicovaginal reflection. There are no features suggesting columnar epithelium, such as gland openings or nabothian cysts. The epithelium was "always" squamous and was not transformed from columnar to squamous after birth.

Columnar Epithelium

This is a single layer of mucus-producing, tall epithelium that extends between the endometrium and the cervical squamous epithelium. Columnar epithelium appears irregular, with stromal papillae and clefts. With acetic acid application and magnification, columnar epithelium has a grapelike or "sea anemone" appearance. It turns mildly acetowhite. Columnar epithelium is found in the endocervix, surrounding the cervical os, and is generally visible on the ectocervix in the reproductive age group.

Transformation Zone

As a woman ages, and under the influence of various hormones, the columnar epithelium that is originally found on the ectocervix is covered and transformed into squamous epithelium. The TZ is the geographic area between where the original squamous epithelium ended medially and where the outer lateral edge of the columnar epithelium currently exists. It is occupied by metaplastic epithelium in varying degrees of maturity because the columnar epithelium is being "transformed" into squamous epithelium. There is no way to discern where the original squamous epithelium was and what has been transformed. What can be identified is the active TZ, which contains gland openings, nabothian cysts, and, typically, islands of columnar epithelium surrounded by metaplastic squamous epithelium. The recognizable TZ is the area of most active metaplasia and transformation. The active TZ then extends from the SCJ (see later) laterally to the outermost visible gland. For all practical purposes, when the term "TZ" is used, it is generally referring to the active TZ because that is where disease processes occur. The progression, then, from central to lateral, is columnar epithelium, SCJ, active TZ, squamous epithelium that has been transformed, and original squamous epithelium.

Squamous Metaplasia

Columnar epithelium on the ectocervix is transformed over time into mature squamous epithelium by undergoing squamous metaplasia. Squamous metaplasia typically occupies the TZ to varying degrees. Metaplasia appears as a "ghost white" film when acetic acid is applied, and it looks like a denser line of this white where the columnar epithelium and squamous epithelium meet.

Squamocolumnar Junction

Generally, this is a clinically visible line seen on the ectocervix or within the distal canal (e.g., postcryotherapy or in the postmenopausal age group) that demarcates endocervical tissue from squamous tissue. Conceptually, the SCJ is comparable with the vermilion border around the mouth and the dentate or pectinate line in the rectum, where the mucosa meets squamous epithelium. The SCJ is the inner (medial) border of the TZ.

Abnormal Colposcopic Findings

See Fig. 124.3.

Atypical Transformation Zone

A TZ with findings suggesting cervical dysplasia or neoplasia is considered abnormal. Usually, acetic acid (3% to 5% vinegar) is applied and the cervix is viewed under magnification with the colposcope. The new nomenclature addresses location of the lesion relative to the original SCJ. "Inside" location means medial to the original SCJ (toward the cervical os) and vice versa. The border of a lesion is a sharp border that is a straight edge of an acetowhite cervical lesion. Other edge definitions are a feathered or geographical margin, usually associated with a low-grade lesion, and rolled peeling edges that may be associated with a high-grade lesion. The *inner border sign* is a sharp demarcation between a thin and dense acetowhite area within the same lesion (Fig. 124.4). The *ridge sign* is an opaque protuberance at the area of white epithelium within the TZ (Fig. 124.5).

1. *Acetowhite epithelium* (AWE): Epithelium that transiently whitens after the application of acetic acid. Areas of acetowhite correlate with higher nuclear density. The white staining fades within minutes. The more abnormal the changes, the more quickly they will turn white, the denser they will be, and the longer they will last. All AWE is not necessarily abnormal because metaplasia also has a higher nuclear ratio owing to a more rapid growth rate and turns white with acetic acid.
2. *Punctation:* A stippled appearance of capillaries viewed end-on; often found within acetowhite areas, where they appear as fine-to-coarse red dots. In general, the coarser the punctation the more severe the dysplasia.
3. *Mosaicism:* An abnormal change made up of small red blood vessels appearing in linear form, suggesting a confluence of tile or chicken-wire patterns. This is best viewed after staining with acetic acid under magnification. In general, the coarser the mosaicism the more severe the dysplasia.
4. *Leukoplakia (hyperkeratosis):* Typically, an elevated white plaque seen before the application of acetic acid. There is generally no change, or the area becomes more densely white, after application of acetic acid.
5. *Abnormal blood vessels:* Atypical, irregular, true vessels with abrupt courses and patterns; often appear as commas, corkscrews, or spaghetti-like shapes. No definite pattern is recognized, as there is with punctation or mosaicism. Abnormal blood vessels are seen in cancer and occasionally in advanced dysplasias.
6. *Iodine-negative epithelium:* Estrogenized epithelium will stain with Lugol solution to a deep brown. Abnormal tissue and nonestrogenized tissue do not stain.

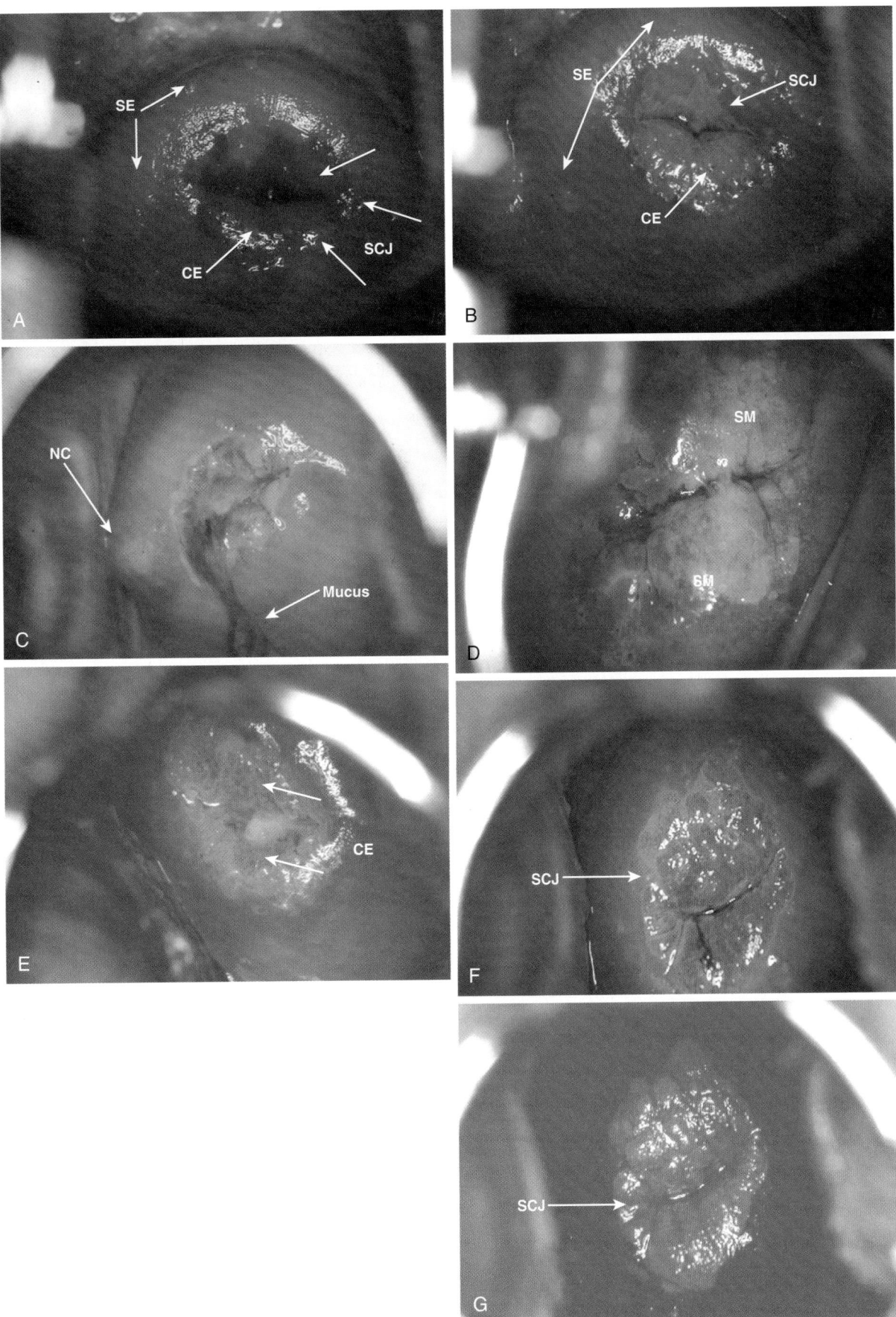

Fig. 124.1 Normal colposcopic findings. (A) Normal cervix showing squamous epithelium (SE), columnar epithelium (CE), and the squamocolumnar junction (SCJ). (B) Cervix after application of acetic acid. (C) Normal cervix with nabothian cyst (NC) and mucus. (D) Predominant squamous metaplasia (SM) after application of acetic acid. (E) Columnar epithelium (CE). (F) Cervix before application of Lugol solution. (G) Cervix after application of Lugol solution. Estrogenized squamous epithelium will stain dark.

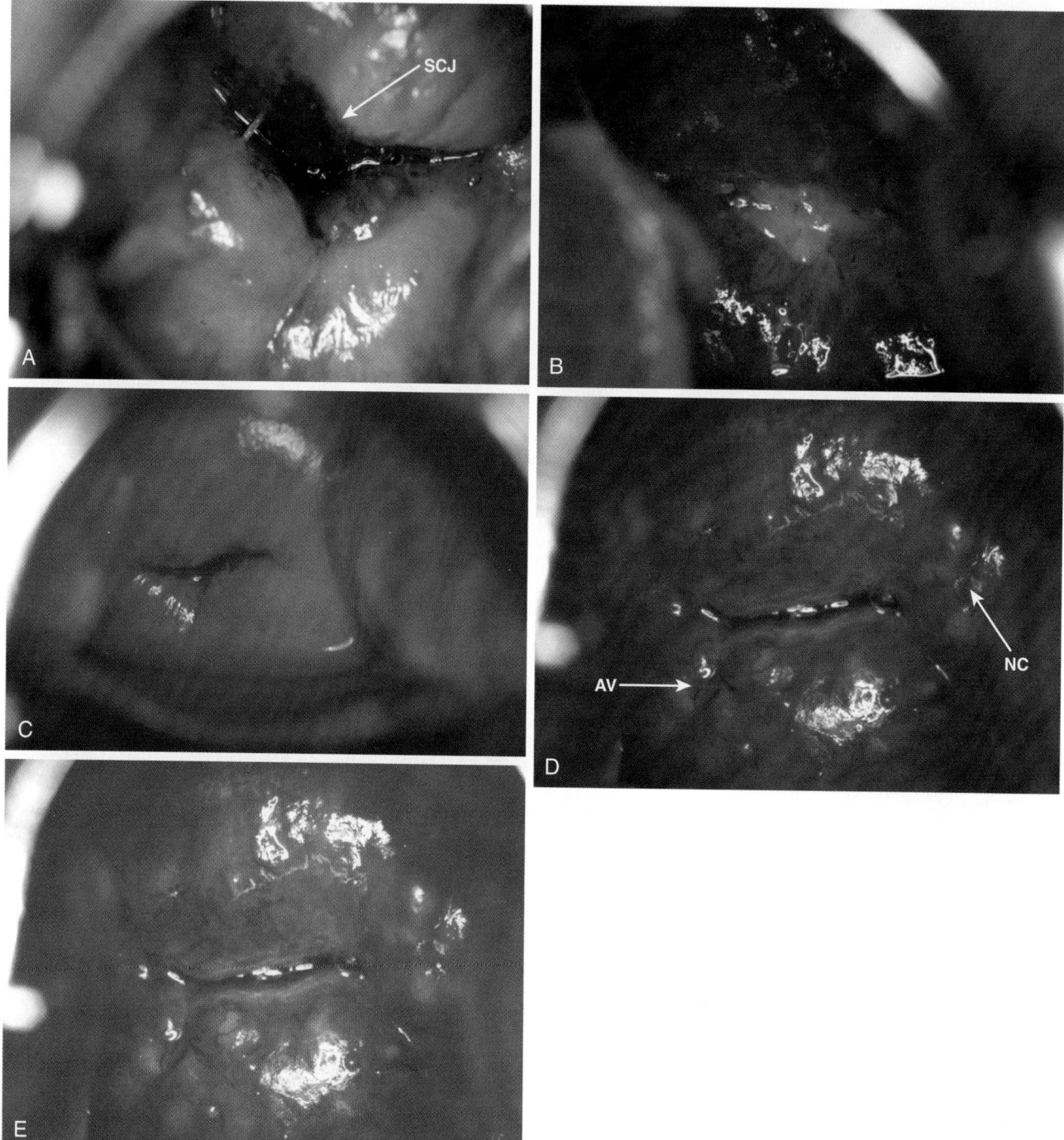

Fig. 124.2 Normal colposcopic variants. (A) Cervix with irregular contour due to birth trauma. (B) Pregnant cervix with mucus, thin, bluish epithelium, and metaplasia. (C) Squamocolumnar junction (SCJ) unable to be seen (often encountered after treatment and in older patients). (D) Prominent vessels can overlie nabothian cysts (NC), some of which may appear atypical. Biopsy is recommended if there is any doubt. (E) Blue/green filter can enhance visualization of vessels, allowing the red vessels to appear black against a greenish background. *AV,* Atypical vessel.

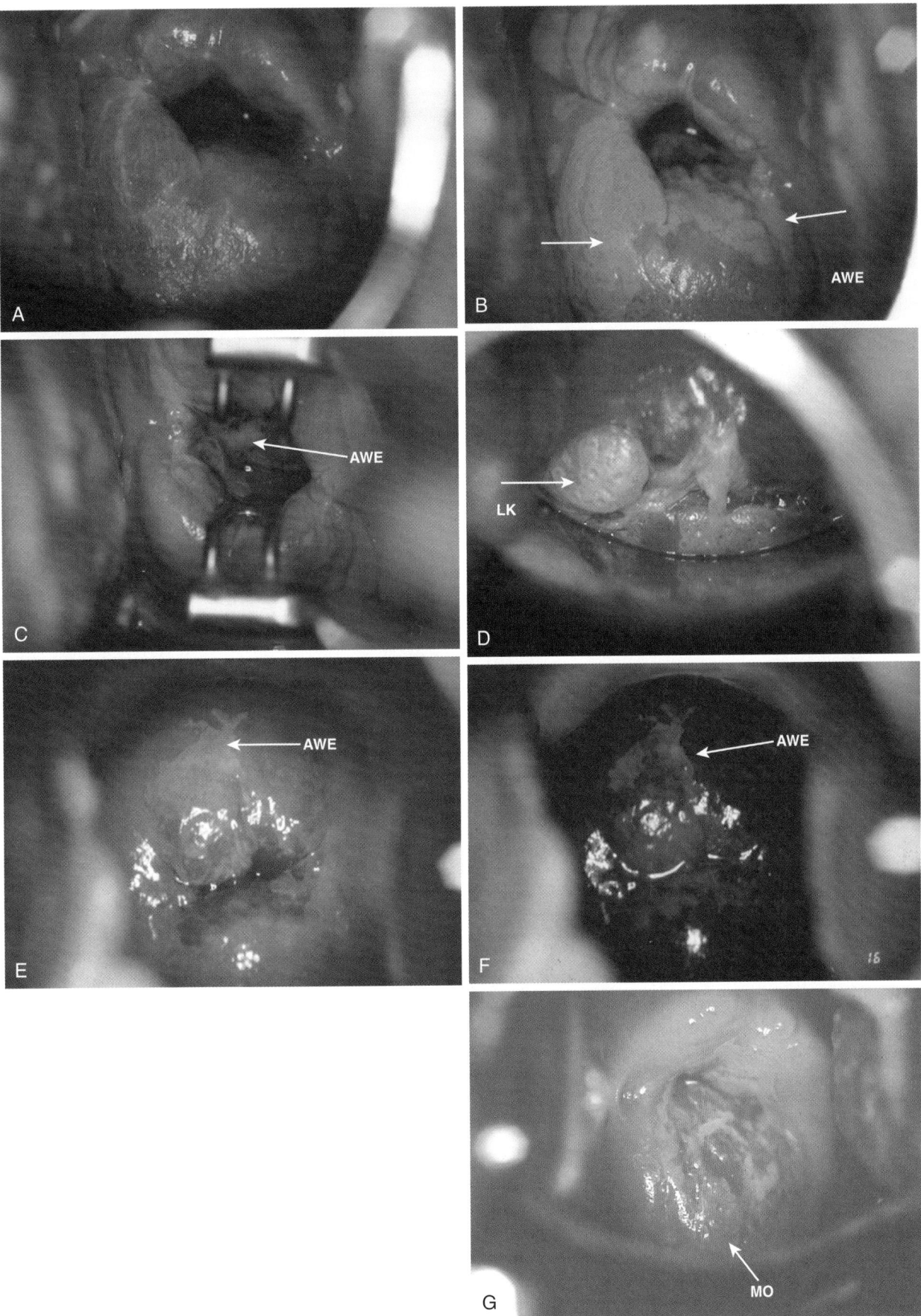

Fig. 124.3 Abnormal colposcopic findings. (A) Cervix before application of acetic acid. (B) Cervix after application of acetic acid, showing acetowhite epithelium (AWE) extending into cervical canal. (C) Use of Kogan forceps to demonstrate AWE in the endocervical canal. (D) Leukoplakia (LK), a white lesion seen before application of acetic acid. (E) AWE lesion before application of Lugol solution. (F) After application of Lugol solution, the same AWE is now iodine negative. (G) AWE with mosaic pattern (MO) and endocervical involvement. (H) AWE with endocervical involvement seen with Kogan endocervical dilators. (I) AWE showing a coarse mosaic pattern before green light application. (J) AWE showing a coarse mosaic pattern after green light application. (K) Large, protruding lesion with coarse punctation (PT). (L) Friable, peeling cervical epithelium and atypical vessels (AV) suspect for invasive carcinoma are seen in this example of invasive cervical carcinoma. (M) Grossly deformed mass replacing the cervix consistent with invasive carcinoma. (N) Colposcopic view of the vulva with both condylomata and vulvar intraepithelial neoplasia (VIN). Remember, colposcopy includes inspection of the vulva. (O) Central cervical polyp.

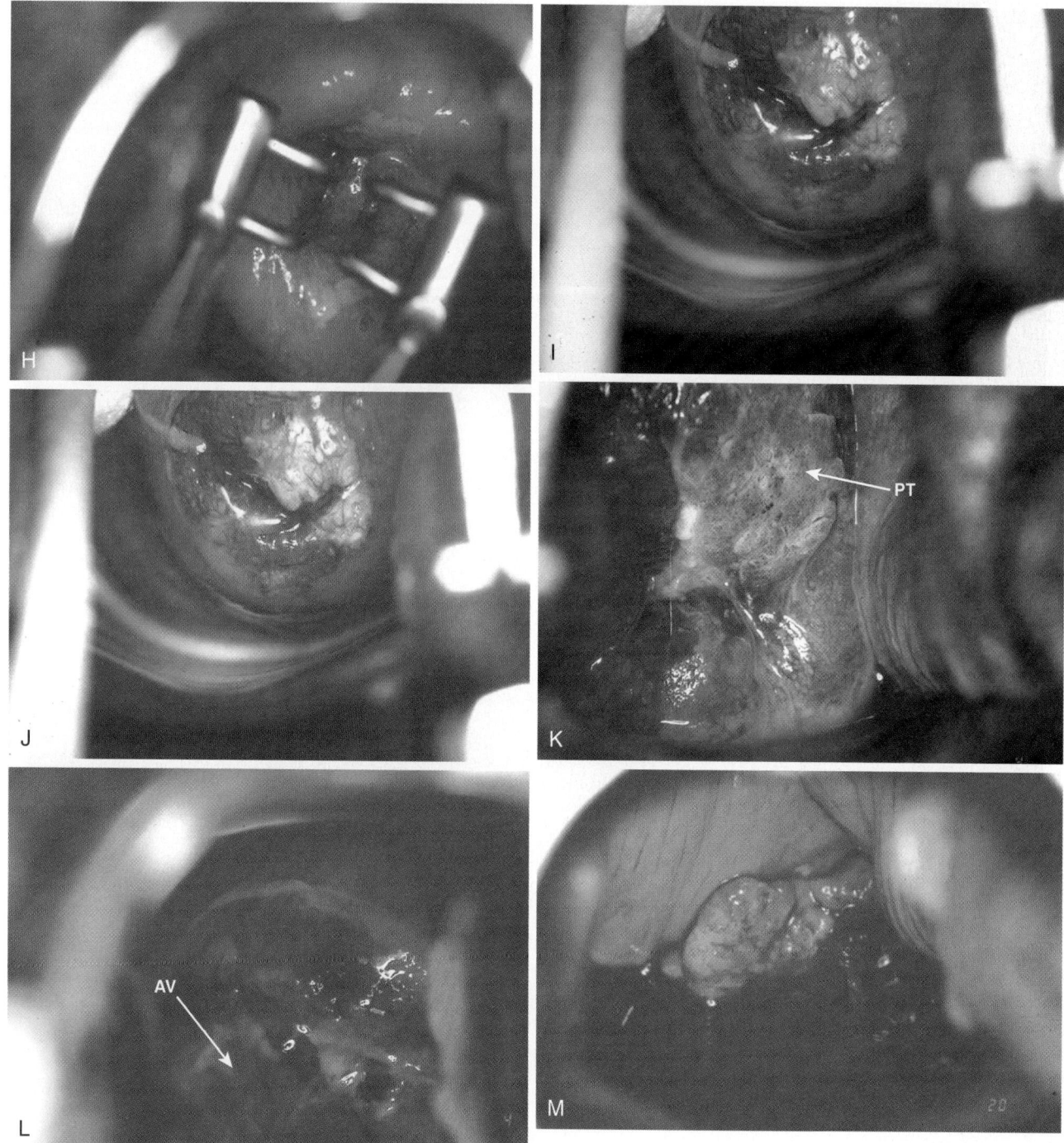

Fig. 124.3, cont'd.

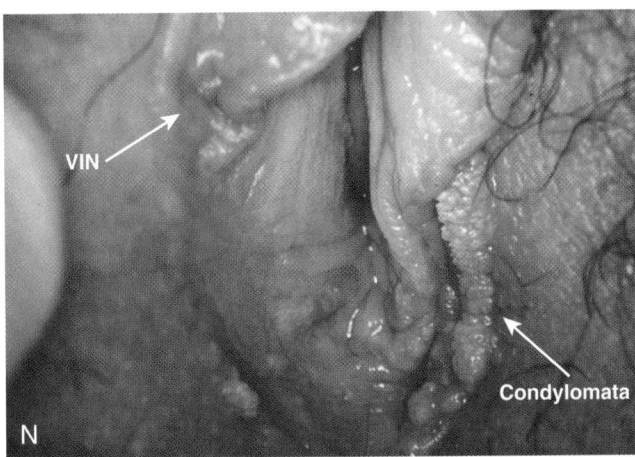

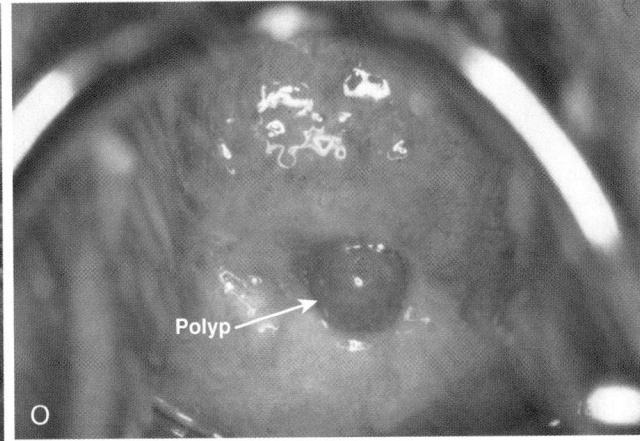

Fig. 124.3, cont'd.

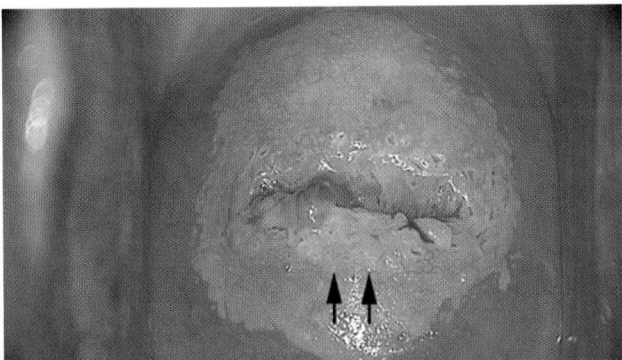

Fig. 124.4 The inner border sign is a sharp demarcation between a thin and a dense acetowhite area within the same lesion, which is suggestive of high-grade dysplasia.

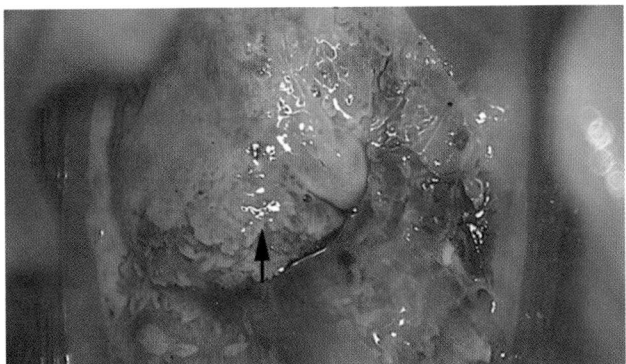

Fig. 124.5 The ridge sign is an opaque protuberance at the area of a white epithelium within the transformation zone; it is suggestive of high-grade dysplasia.

Suspect Invasive Cancer

A complex pattern consisting of roughened, irregular cervical epithelium, typically with abundant abnormal vessel patterns and dense acetowhite change, often with a dense eggshell-white or slightly yellowish hue. It may also appear as ulcerated, friable, necrotic tissue. There may be a bulk effect or tumor-like appearance.

Not Fully Visualized/Inadequate (Previously Unsatisfactory) Colposcopy

The popular terms "satisfactory colposcopy" and "unsatisfactory colposcopy" were abandoned by the new nomenclature. Unsatisfactory, not fully visualized (ASCCP, 2017) SCJ or inadequate (IFCPC,

2012) examination suggests colposcopy that needs to be repeated. IFCPC guidelines assess the colposcopic examination by three variables. The first is the "adequate or inadequate for the reason…" in which the cause of inadequacy should be explained; for example, the cervix is obscured by inflammation, bleeding, or scarring. The second variable is "SCJ visibility," which can be described as "completely visible," "partially visible," or "not visible." The reason that the visibility and site of the SCJ are so important is that they dictate both the ability to do an adequate examination, and the treatment is indicated, based on the extent and type of excision. The third parameter was retained from the 2002 IFCPC nomenclature, and involves assigning a TZ type. Proper examination also can be hampered if an active inflammatory process is present, if the patient is not estrogen primed (e.g., postmenopausal without hormone replacement therapy, on progesterone-only type contraception, lactation), or if heavy menses is present. In the ASCCP guidelines, the SCJ junction is either fully visible or not visible and the TZ is not typed, it is merely described. This description of the TZ should also include whether it is fully visible or not fully visible. There has been no evidence that typing the TZ improves prediction or management of cervical disease.

Other Colposcopic Findings

- Vaginocervicitis
- Traumatic erosion
- Atrophic epithelium
- Endocervical polyps
- Changes from diethylstilbestrol
- Abnormal pigmentation
- Nabothian cysts
- Posttraumatic clefts, deformities from birth or treatment
- Vaginal, vulvar, perineal, perianal lesions

Guidelines regarding visual colposcopic findings help ensure sampling of the most advanced sites of cervical dysplasia. The classic hallmark of cervical dysplasia includes the change that dysplastic epithelium undergoes after the application of 3% to 5% acetic acid (vinegar) or Lugol (concentrated iodine) solution.

After the application of acetic acid to estrogenized tissue, dysplastic epithelium typically turns whiter than the surrounding normal epithelium AWE. More advanced dysplasia typically appears more densely white, thicker, and smoother with raised borders. The surface of advanced dysplasia often becomes rougher or thicker as the severity of dysplasia advances and satellite lesions (multiple small abnormal areas) are less common. There may begin to be a "yellowish" hue. Changes in the vasculature pattern also correlate with cervical dysplasia. These abnormal patterns, which often occur in an acetowhite or leukoplakia patch, include *punctation, mosaicism,* and frankly *abnormal vessel variations.* The coarser the punctation or mosaicism the more severe the dysplasia (see Table 124.1). Fine mosaicism and punctuation are now categorized as *low-grade* features with the new ASCCP guidelines; course mosaicism and punctuation are *high-grade* features, which increases the likelihood of severe dysplasia. Frankly abnormal vessel patterns imply severe dysplasia or potential invasive carcinoma.

After the application of Lugol solution to estrogenized tissue, there is an immediate blackening (staining) of normal epithelium (iodine uptake is high in normal cells that are rich in cytologic glycogen). Abnormal dysplastic tissue, which has cells that contain much less intracellular glycogen, are not stained by iodine (Lugol-negative epithelium) and remain white or faint yellow. The same pattern is seen if there is little or no estrogen stimulation.

Squamous metaplasia, a normal finding, may appear slightly acetowhite and may take up Lugol solution incompletely; therefore, this tissue can cause some degree of confusion for the colposcopist. Squamous metaplasia is the physiologically normal tissue present where the columnar epithelium is being transformed into mature squamous epithelium. This occurs in the TZ—the same site where dysplasia generally occurs. Squamous metaplasia is especially prominent with certain conditions, such as active cervicitis, and where healing and reparative activities occur, such as after treatment. *Questionable areas always warrant biopsy.* If squamous metaplasia without dysplasia is reported on biopsy, but the Pap smear was abnormal, the prudent colposcopist must look elsewhere to explain the finding of dysplasia on the Pap smear (see Appendix K, Algorithms for the Evaluation of Abnormal Pap Smears and Treatment of Colposcopic Findings). A report of squamous metaplasia among other biopsies revealing dysplasia reflects the difficulty encountered by the colposcopist in evaluating this normal variant of acetowhite change. (Indeed, appendices removed for an acute abdomen are not always the source of the pain!) The only other common areas that normally turn slightly white with acetic acid are the endocervical (columnar) cells, which are typically located in the cervical canal and extend a variable distance onto the exocervix. Endocervical tissue usually can be differentiated from abnormal areas by colposcopic examination because of its grape-like appearance on high-power magnification. Biopsy is still warranted if there is any confusion.

This chapter focuses on the evaluation of the abnormal Pap smear as it typically relates to cervical disease. The complete examination also includes the colposcopic examination of the remainder of the genital system in women. The colposcope also can be used for other purposes, such as to examine male genitalia or the anus, and to evaluate sexual abuse victims (see Chapter 84, High-Resolution Anoscopy, Chapter 103, Androscopy, and Chapter 140, Treatment of the Adult Victim of Sexual Assault). Ultimately, the patient's cytologic, colposcopic, and histologic data are used in concert to direct appropriate management. A well-managed colposcopy program provides effective evaluation and treatment for all patients with identified abnormalities of the cervix and genital tract.

Many colposcopists keep their scopes immediately available to augment the routine Pap and pelvic examination, especially if abnormalities are seen and both time and patient preference are favorable. Although complete formal colposcopic examination and biopsy can be performed when visual abnormalities are identified, many clinicians prefer to reschedule patients for full colposcopic examination at a later date. This allows more time for patient education and thorough evaluation.

INDICATIONS

Refer to Appendix K, Algorithms for the Evaluation of Abnormal Pap Smears and Treatment of Colposcopic Findings, for the 2012 Updated Consensus Guidelines for the Management of ASCCP. The most common indications for colposcopy include:

- Pap smear consistent with dysplasia or cancer (see Chapter 120, Pap Smear and Related Techniques for Cervical Cancer Screening, for detailed recommendations regarding abnormal Pap smears)
- Pap smear with atypical glandular cells (always perform colposcopy)
- Worrisome history despite normal Pap smear findings (e.g., postcoital bleeding)
- An atypical Pap smear in which the patient tests positive for high-risk HPV
- Suspect visible lesion or palpable lesion of the cervix
- Abnormal vaginal bleeding, especially if postcoital, regardless of Pap smear status
- History of intrauterine diethylstilbestrol (DES) exposure
- Evaluation or follow-up of previously treated or high-risk patients

The colposcope can be used for other reasons, such as removal of a cervical polyp, to find a lost intrauterine contraceptive device string, or to evaluate a rape victim, but in these instances a full colposcopic examination protocol is generally not indicated.

CONTRAINDICATIONS

There are no absolute contraindications to colposcopy. Most contraindications relate to temporary or treatable conditions that alter the timing of the colposcopic examination rather than absolutely prevent it from occurring. The adequate colposcopic examination requires excellent visualization with a compliant and cooperative patient.

Relative

- Active inflammatory cervicitis
- Uncooperative patient
- Heavy menses (may prevent adequate examination)

NOTE: Pregnancy is not a contraindication to colposcopy, including biopsy, although a slightly different protocol is used and more bleeding can be expected from the biopsies.

EQUIPMENT AND SUPPLIES

The equipment and supplies used during routine colposcopy should be within easy reach in the colposcopy examination room (Figs. 124.6 to 124.8).

- Colposcope: variable fixed-power or zoom lens (3× to 7× low power to 15× to 40× high power).

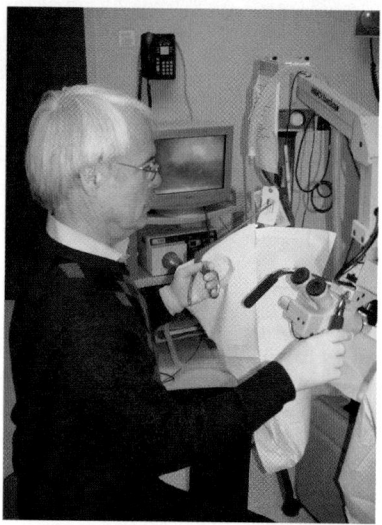

Fig. 124.6 A contemporary colposcopy suite with motorized table with leg stirrups, boom-mounted video colposcope, and available loop electrosurgical excision procedure unit.

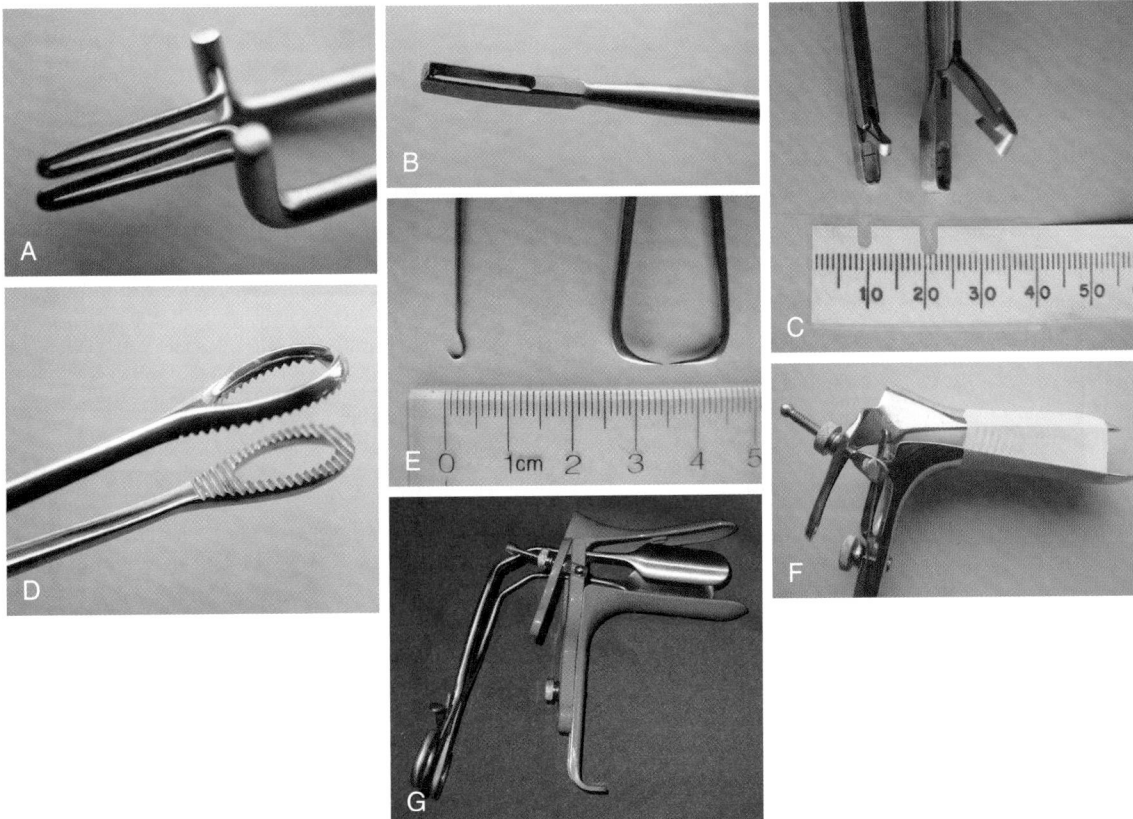

Fig. 124.7 (A) Narrow Kogan endocervical speculum. (B) Kevorkian endocervical curette without basket. (C) Tischler "wide jaw opening" biopsy forceps in both the large and small ("baby") options. (D) A 1-cm ring forceps used to apply vinegar with folded gauze or cotton balls, or assist in visualizing the vaginal fornices and manipulating the cervix. (E) A small cervical hook and tenaculum to help move the cervix (rarely needed). (F) Vaginal speculum with glove finger applied and used as vaginal wall retractor. (G) Vaginal speculum with vaginal wall retractor inserted.

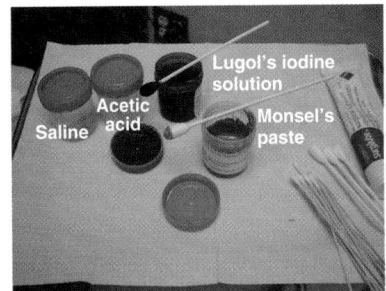

Fig. 124.8 Common items on the colposcopy tray in addition to the equipment in Fig. 124.6: cups of normal saline, acetic acid, Lugol solution, Monsel solution that has dehydrated to a paste, small and large swabs, lubricant. Formalin bottles and Pap smear supplies are not included here.

- Biopsy forceps* (e.g., Tischler, baby Tischler, mini-Townsend, Kevorkian).
- Endocervical curette* (Kevorkian, no basket or disposable).
- Endocervical speculum† (Kogan, both narrow and wide types).
- Ring forceps.*
- Tenaculum† (rarely used).
- Cervical hook† (rarely used).
- Pap smear materials.†
- Vaginal speculums (e.g., metal Graves or disposable plastic spec-

ulum) in various sizes and lengths (use largest tolerated), or a clear, lighted, plastic speculum setup (e.g., Welch Allyn) for selected cases.
- Acetic acid solution 3% to 5% (white vinegar; 4 to 6 oz, or 120 to 180 mL).‡
- Full-strength Lugol iodine solution (30 mL) (not always necessary after experience is gained but must be readily available). †§
- Monsel solution (ferric subsulfate), 1 mL.§ Monsel solution is a topical astringent and is used to control bleeding after biopsy. It should be thoroughly shaken in its original bottle and then allowed to evaporate in a separate container until it is the consistency of a thick, yellowish-brown paste; this renders it a potent astringent to control biopsy-induced bleeding. Monsel solution should be prepared several days in advance to achieve proper consistency. If the solution becomes too thick, it can be diluted with liquid solution from the original bottle.
- Cotton- or rayon-tipped swabs (8 to 10)
- Junior scopettes/OB-GYN applicators (6 to 10)
- 4 × 4-inch gauze
- Urine or sputum cups for vinegar
- Vaginal sidewall retractor
- Underpads ("chuck pads") (17 × 24 inch)
- Cotton balls (15 to 20)
- Power-assisted patient examination table that can be raised or lowered. (Minimum height should be no more than 24 inches from floor, or older and disabled patients will have a difficult time getting on to it.)

*Included in the "colpo pack." These must be sterilized before procedures. A "no-touch" technique is used on the ends of instruments touching the patient. Reusable instruments are sterilized, but colposcopy is not a "sterile" procedure per se.
† Available in colposcopy room but not used at every procedure.

‡Grocery store or mix to make 3% to 5% acetic acid.
† Available in colposcopy room but not used at every procedure.
§ Hospital pharmacy.

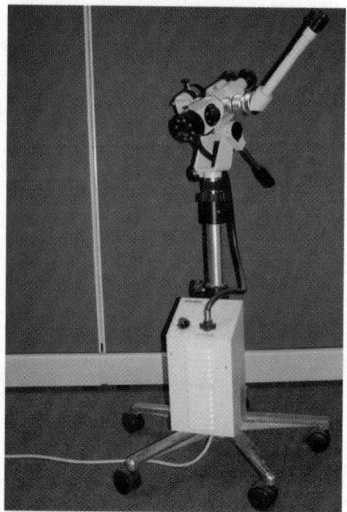

Fig. 124.9 A pedestal-mounted colposcope with teaching head attached and fiberoptic light source.

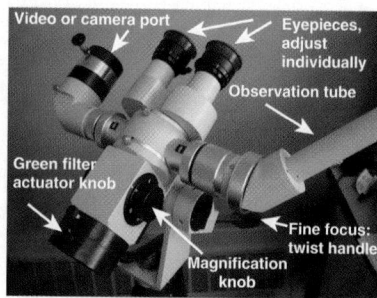

Fig. 124.10 Features of the colposcopic head: fixed magnification knob, green filter knob, twisting handle for fine focus. Magnification changes are available between 4× and 25× in five steps. The camera/video port and observation (teaching) tube are optional features.

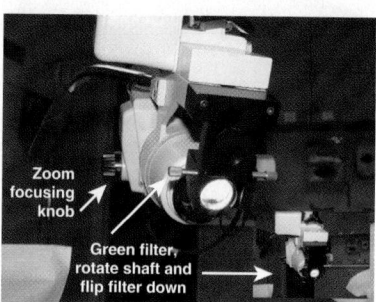

Fig. 124.11 A zoom power colposcope head with green filter and zoom focus knob. Magnification smoothly zooms from 3× to 20×.

Optional items include a preprocedural dose of an oral nonsteroidal anti-inflammatory agent, aromatic ammonium capsules ("smelling salts") for vasovagal responses, and a camera-video attachment.

Some clinicians now use a Pap smear sampling or similar brush to obtain the endocervical assessment instead of performing a formal ECC. Disposable ECC devices are also available and may be substituted for the reusable Kevorkian device.

Colposcopes come in a variety of "shapes and sizes" (Figs. 124.9 to 124.12), but all are basically the same. The stand may be a pedestal, may be on rollers, or may project out on an arm. There is a knob for changing magnification and another for fine focusing. The eyepieces also focus independently. A simple mechanism is usually available for inserting a green filter into the visual field, which makes identifying vascular abnormalities easier. The unit is turned on to the highest light intensity and then used essentially as a three-dimensional, short-range set of binoculars, but with an intense light source and variable magnification.

Some scopes have video options that project the image on a screen instead of using the binocular option (i.e., Welch Allyn; see Fig. 124.9). Most other scopes can be adapted for video use. In teaching situations, some type of video mode or teaching head adapter is mandatory. It is not necessary to take pictures or video for routine colposcopic examinations.

PREPROCEDURE PATIENT EDUCATION AND FORMS

Providing educational materials to the patient and the patient's partner before the procedure can help alleviate the fear and uncertainty surrounding not only the procedure, but all of the issues surrounding HPV infection. Brochures are available from the American College of Obstetricians and Gynecologists, ASCCP, and several other organizations (see the sample patient education handout available at www.expertconsult.com). An excellent patient education videotape is available from The National Procedures Institute (Midland, MI). By providing materials beforehand, the clinician can focus on questions rather than try to take the time to explain a very complex topic with every patient.

- Discuss the indications for colposcopy with the patient. The patient should acknowledge the importance of long-term follow-up. The patient should advise the clinician's clinic of change of address or telephone number.
- Instruct the patient to continue contraceptive practices before and after the colposcopic examination until treatment or man-

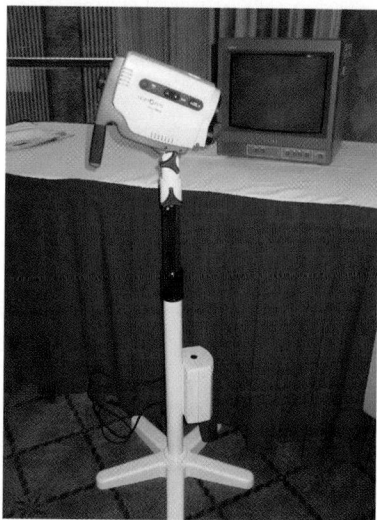

Fig. 124.12 A dedicated video colposcope with traditional binocular optical viewing replaced with a monitor for viewing. (Courtesy Welch Allyn, Skaneateles Falls, NY.)

agement decisions have been made. There is no evidence that any type of contraception or estrogen replacement therapy causes progression of cervical dysplasia.
- Explain to the patient that a pregnancy test may be performed on the day of the procedure if pregnancy is a possibility, but colposcopy with or without biopsies carries very low risk in the pregnant woman. ECC is contraindicated in pregnancy.
- Instruct the patient to consume a regular diet on the day of the procedure and not to skip a meal before the procedure. This lessens the possibility of a vasovagal episode.
- Advise against taking aspirin, or medications containing aspirin,

for 7 days before the procedure. Aspirin consumption within the past week does not ordinarily contraindicate colposcopy with biopsy, but you should be aware of the potential for more bleeding. Normally, nonsteroidal antiinflammatory drugs, such as ibuprofen, do not significantly prolong bleeding; therefore they may be taken before the procedure for pain control.

- Review the medical history with particular attention to in utero exposure to DES; drug allergies; asthma; diabetes mellitus; history of vagal sensitivity (frequent fainting); bleeding disorder; recent symptoms of cervicitis or pelvic inflammatory disease; symptoms or history suggesting pregnancy; symptomatology suggestive of an endometrial disorder that may require endometrial sampling; and history of prior cervical treatment, including conization, laser therapy, or cryotherapy. Latex or iodine allergy history would contraindicate the use of latex gloves or iodine-containing solutions (Lugol or povidone-iodine).
- Explain that the procedure will take about 20 to 30 minutes. Most clinics ask patients to arrive at least 15 minutes early to allow for appropriate education, a pregnancy test, and questions.
- If pictures will be taken, inform the patient and establish consent before the actual procedure.
- Review the risks before the procedure: pain, infection, bleeding, discharge, and missed disease. Menstrual-type cramping and limited discharge are common, but persistent pain, bleeding, or infection is rare.
- Explain that colposcopy with biopsy ordinarily renders a diagnosis and is not a therapeutic procedure per se. Definitive therapy will be determined by correlation of historical, colposcopic, cytologic, and histologic data.
- Discuss treatment options. Ordinarily, cervical cryotherapy, if indicated, is performed after the cervix has had time to heal from the biopsy and pathology reports are available. This typically can be performed as early as 2 weeks after colposcopy or after the next menstrual cycle.
- If applicable, inform the patient that she will probably receive a separate bill for the interpretation of the pathology samples obtained during the biopsy procedure.
- Subacute bacterial endocarditis prophylaxis is not necessary.

PROCEDURE

Fig. 124.13 includes forms for documenting the colposcopic examination for both initial and follow-up visits. Clinicians are also advised to either dictate or record their findings in the medical record to supplement the colposcopic examination form, if necessary.

In addition to the necessary technical skills, the successful colposcopy program requires close attention to data interpretation and careful patient follow-up. The patient who has an abnormal Pap smear and who ultimately has biopsy-confirmed cervical dysplasia remains at an increased lifetime risk for recurrence of genital malignancy.

1. Prepare the colposcopy room. Make sure the room is warm. Some patients benefit from quiet background music. Have all necessary solutions and equipment ready at hand. Make sure the appropriate culture media, potassium hydroxide (KOH), and wet preparation materials are in the room. Keep all sizes of specula in your colposcopy room; prewarming is appreciated.
2. Prepare the patient. Mail information before the procedure. Answer her questions. (See section on Preprocedure Patient Education.) Ibuprofen 800 mg may be offered 30 minutes before the procedure. Check for medication, latex, and iodine allergies.
3. Obtain informed consent. Before the office visit, allow the patient to review a written description of the procedure, its risks, and complications (see the sample patient education handout available at www.expertconsult.com). Address questions and concerns. Obtain informed consent, which should include a signed consent.
4. Obtain a pregnancy test as necessary. ECC is contraindicated in pregnancy. Unexpected early pregnancy at the time of colposcopy is common. Even if ECC is performed, it rarely, if ever, has any adverse consequence.
5. Perform a bimanual examination if one has not been done recently. If a Pap smear is to be collected/repeated, complete that before the bimanual examination. The bimanual examination can also be performed after the colposcopy, but it may be more difficult if biopsies are taken. Care should be taken not to traumatize the cervix. Is the uterus enlarged or tender? What position is the cervix? Can the cervix be moved? How long is the vagina? Are there palpated abnormalities of the introitus, vagina, fornices, or cervix? Examine the vulva for obvious condylomata.
6. Warm and insert the speculum. Colposcopy requires the widest speculum the patient can comfortably tolerate. The examination requires greater cervical and vaginal exposure than a screening Pap smear. Because of the relative duration of the colposcopic examination, the vaginal walls may migrate inward, which makes visualization more difficult. A carefully inserted, wide, large Graves speculum is far more comfortable in the long run than constant prodding and manipulating of the vagina to move the vagina out of the field of view if an inappropriately narrow speculum is used. If necessary, use a vaginal sidewall retractor. Alternatively, a surgical glove finger or condom can be stretched over the speculum blades and the end cut before insertion of the speculum to facilitate visualization. A thin layer of water-soluble vaginal lubricant can be applied on the speculum. This thin coating significantly facilitates the insertion and removal of the speculum and does not interfere with biopsy or Pap smear interpretation. Use both thumbscrew dimensions of the speculum to gain maximum exposure. Ideally, the colposcopic examination is facilitated by having the cervix facing anteriorly and virtually "suspended" between the blades of the speculum.
7. Grossly (using the naked eye) examine the cervix and vaginal fornices. Does the cervix appear inflamed or infected? An active cervicitis confuses colposcopic detail. Characterize the vaginal and cervical discharge. Are there areas of obvious vessel atypia? Scan the cervix for gross leukoplakia before applying acetic acid. Although acetic acid greatly enhances the elucidation of diseased areas, its mild vasoconstricting properties can render significant vessel detail less obvious. Use magnification to quickly scan the unstained cervix to identify landmarks, such as the TZ with its SCJ, and identify any possible abnormalities.
8. Obtain specimens for cultures, KOH and wet preparations, HPV DNA probe, and Pap smear, as necessary (see Chapter 121, Human Papillomavirus DNA Typing, Chapter 151, Pap Smear and Related Techniques for Cervical Cancer Screening, and Chapter 122, Wet Smear and KOH Preparation). Even a correctly performed Pap smear irritates the cervix, may cause bleeding, and may change fine colposcopic detail. The Pap smear may need to be repeated because the original Pap smear was performed at a different laboratory; because more than 3 months have elapsed since the last Pap smear; because the patient is pregnant (Pap smears are less reliable during pregnancy and because colposcopy is more difficult, it is important to maximize clinical assessment); and because of the need to allay any concern or confusion regarding the adequacy or interpretation of the original Pap smear results. Once the Pap smear, KOH, or wet preparation is obtained as deemed necessary, it is permissible to gently blot (not rub) excess secretions to view the cervix more clearly.
9. Apply 3% to 5% acetic acid. One method is to use 4 × 4 gauze rolled up tightly and held longitudinally in a ring forceps. This saturates the cervix with vinegar quickly and without trauma. Cotton balls or large swabs also work well. Use large swabs to repeat the application. Refer to acetic acid as "vinegar" or simply

COLPOSCOPY

PATIENT INSTRUCTIONS: Please complete questions down to "Procedure."

Date_____ Age_____ Birthdate_____

Name_____ Referring physician_____

Phone (home)_____(work)_____ Reason for colposcopy_____

HISTORY

Previous abnormal Paps?	Y	N
History of previous cryocautery (freezing)?	Y	N
History of previous cervical surgery?	Y	N
Personal history of cancer?	Y	N
Family history of cancer?	Y	N
History of venereal diseases (circle)		

   • gonorrhea   • AIDS   • herpes   • syphilis

Do you desire testing for any of these diseases?	Y	N
History of genital warts?	Y	N
Visible warts now?	Y	N
Previously treated?	Y	N

   If so, how?_____

Age of first Pap_____ How often_____

Number of pregnancies_____ Children_____

Date of last menstrual period_____

Type of contraception_____

Number of sexual partners (lifetime)_____

Age at first sexual intercourse_____

Do you smoke?	Y	N
Partner(s) with warts?	Y	N
History of sexual abuse?	Y	N

Other PMH:

Meds:_____

Allergies:_____

Other: _____

PROCEDURE (Doctor will fill out)

Observation without staining: _____

Pap repeated?	Y	N
SCJ seen?	Y	N
Endo spec needed?	Y	N
EGG done?	Y	N
Entire lesion seen?	Y	N

Vaginal vault:

Urethra:

Labia:

Perineum:

Rectum:

LK = Leukoplakia
WE = While epithelium
PN = Punctation
MO = Mosaicism
ATZ = Abnormal transformation zone
AV = Abnormal vessel
BE = Bulk effect
AG = Atypical glands
X = Biopsy sites

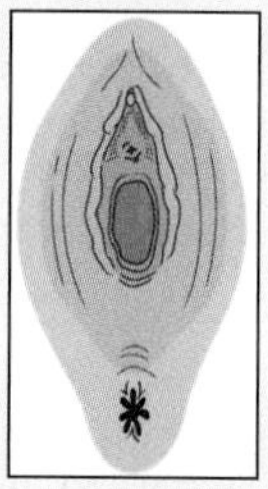

IMPRESSION: Adequate colposcopy?   Y   N

RECOMMENDATIONS:

Cryocautery	Y	N	Tip: _____
Referral to specialist	Y	N	
LEEP	Y	N	
Other:			

cc:_____

PLAN:

Discourage smoking

Partner needs information

Need at least annual Paps for rest of life no
    matter what others say

Handout on cryocautery/LEEP/Andro/HPV/
    vitamins/smoking

Physician's Signature

Fig. 124.13   **Examples of initial colposcopy procedure and follow-up documentation forms.** (Courtesy John L. Pfenninger, MD, The Medical Procedures Center, Midland, MI.)

Follow-up Colposcopy Visits

Name_____ Referred by_____

Initial colposcopy date:_____ Findings: Cervix _____

                                               ECC _____

                                               Other _____

                    Laser

                    Cryo

Treatment date: _____ TCA

                    Efudex

                    LETZ: Ecto _____ Endo _____ ECC _____

Problem: _____

Partner evaluated? Y N   Viewed tapes: Self? Y N

                                            Partner? Y N

Smoker?   Y N

Diet: _____

Vitamins?   Y N

Date	History Findings/Treatments	Pap/Bx's: Done	Pap/Bx's: Results	Plan	Copy Sent

_____

Physician

Fig. 124.13, cont'd.

as "douche solution" when discussing it with the patient. Warn her of brief stinging and coldness. Repeat application as necessary, usually every few minutes because the changes fade rapidly.

10. Perform the colposcopic examination. Start with low power (typically 5×). Scan the entire cervix with bright white light. Use a vinegar-soaked, cotton-tipped swab to help manipulate the cervix and TZ into view. It is almost never necessary to use the tenaculum to move the cervix. The cervical hook can

be used; however, it is rarely needed. The Kogan endocervical speculum aids in the examination of the distal endocervical canal. It should be used when either the entire SCJ or the entire lesion cannot be seen because it (or they) is inside the endocervical canal. Use this instrument gingerly to prevent bleeding and pain. (Proper application of the Kogan endocervical speculum, although generally not needed, requires skill and practice. Using it routinely, especially for those new to colposcopy, will assist in learning the technique for when it is needed.) Now use higher magnification to carefully document abnormal findings. The entire TZ, including the SCJ, must be seen and evaluated. Abnormalities will usually turn white (AWE).

11. Use the green filter to enhance vascular detail. The green filter helps highlight vascular detail by rendering the red vascular patterns as black against a greenish background, similar to its use with the ophthalmoscope during the funduscopic examination. All abnormal areas require biopsy.

12. Consider the use of Lugol solution. Lugol solution aids with the identification of abnormal (dysplastic) areas, but its use is not mandatory (it is unnecessary and messy). Both dysplastic and reparative (metaplastic) tissue will incompletely stain with concentrated iodine because of low levels of cellular glycogen (compared with the staining of healthy, mature squamous epithelium). The sharply outlined borders afforded by Lugol staining can be dramatic, and this can help clarify biopsy sites. Iodine staining does not interfere with histologic investigation. However, Lugol solution will obscure the underlying vascular pattern. It should be used when further clarification of potential biopsy sites is necessary or when no lesion is seen with acetic acid. Applying Lugol solution will also help delineate the SCJ for the beginning colposcopist (endocervical cells do not stain with it), and Lugol solution is used for performing cervical (LEEP, large loop excision of the TZ) because its effects last longer than those of acetic acid. Lugol solution is also helpful in the examination of the vagina because acetowhite changes there can be more subtle.

13. Mentally map the cervix. The main goal of colposcopy is to identify areas for biopsy. The colposcopist must be able to differentiate normal tissues from abnormal. Tips on the findings include the following:
   - Acetowhite areas that are unifocal; have sharp, flat, straight borders; stain white quickly; and appear thick or raised, are likely to be more abnormal histologically.
   - The presence of coarse punctation or mosaic patterns, or of frankly abnormal vessels, is associated with a more severe degree of dysplasia. Ultimately, however, the histopathologist is the one who makes the diagnosis from biopsy samples.

   Be prepared to draw a careful record of what is observed and where biopsy samples were taken. The colposcopic impression of severity of disease must be recorded to compare and correlate later findings. Coppleson (1986) proposed scoring indexes to help discern colposcopically identifiable lesions. Many clinicians find these helpful when beginning colposcopy (Reid, 1993), but their utility and ability to predict the degree of disease present have been called into question.

14. Is the colposcopic examination adequate? The entire TZ, including all the SCJ, must be visualized. The borders of all lesions must be seen in their entirety (lesions should not disappear into the canal, for example). Patients who are uncooperative or who have a severely flexed uterus with inadequate visualization are potential "real-world" causes of inadequate colposcopy. An inadequate colposcopic examination coupled with cytologic evidence of significant dysplasia may necessitate a cervical conization for evaluation. It is a very important principle that all criteria be met to have an adequate examination. In summary, then, the adequate colposcopic examination requires:
   - Visualizing the entire TZ, including the SCJ
   - Identifying the area of abnormality producing the abnormal Pap smear
   - Confirming that the limits of all abnormal areas are clearly seen
   - Obtaining a biopsy sample of all abnormal areas
   - Verifying no colposcopic evidence of malignancy

15. Perform the ECC. Some colposcopists elect to omit ECC in instances where a clear source of cervical dysplasia is identified on the ectocervix, the SCJ is clearly seen, and the canal appears colposcopically clear of dysplasia. This is especially true if a low-grade squamous intraepithelial lesion is the indication for colposcopy, the colposcopic examination supports CIN 1 or less, and visual inspection of the canal is negative. Others consider replacing ECC with careful endocervical brush sampling of the canal at the time of the colposcopic examination. Nonetheless, most colposcopists still perform ECC as a necessary component of the colposcopic examination, especially for a high-grade squamous intraepithelial lesion on a Pap smear, a marginally adequate colposcopy, a canal that is impossible or difficult to evaluate, suspicion of any degree of atypical adenomatous or glandular dysplasia, and always when ablative therapy, such as cervical cryotherapy, may be performed later (see Chapter 125, Cryotherapy of the Cervix, and Appendix K, Algorithms for the Evaluation of Abnormal Pap Smears and Treatment of Colposcopic Findings). Usually, neither local nor topical anesthesia is necessary.
   - Use a Kevorkian curette without a basket (or other appropriate curette). Insert gently until the internal cervical os is reached, about 1.5 to 2 cm within the canal. This can be manifested by a slight puckering of the cervix with further advancement. In multiparous women the internal os is not well defined; the curette should not be advanced farther than 2 cm. Scrape the entire lining of the canal (360 degrees) twice. The procedure may be done with or without colposcopic observation. Use caution that the curette does not sample any tissue on the ectocervix and thus provide a false impression that there is disease within the canal. The curetted sample appears as a coagulum of mucus, blood, and small gray or tan tissue fragments. Sometimes a Cytobrush is used to retrieve the remnants of the ECC sample, which may persistently remain stuck in the canal. Submit the ECC sample in a separate bottle on a piece of paper towel, lens paper, or Telfa. Ordinarily, it is not necessary to place a sample pad in the posterior vaginal fornix, as it is with formal dilation and curettage.
   - Do *not* perform an ECC on pregnant patients or patients with evidence of active cervicitis or pelvic inflammatory disease. All other patients must have a documented negative ECC before ablative therapy.
   - Some clinicians prefer to perform ECC after the cervical biopsy samples are obtained because (a) bleeding caused by the ECC can obscure lesions on the lower lip (but a cervical biopsy can bleed and "wash away" or dilute the curettage sample), and (b) the ECC, which takes only 30 seconds, is still the most uncomfortable part of the procedure. If performed first, however, the patient can be reassured early on that "the worst is over." Also, the chance of including dislodged tissue from a previous biopsy in the ECC specimen is minimized. This could again cause a false-positive ECC result, leading to more invasive treatment.

16. Obtain cervical biopsy samples. Sample the posterior (lower) areas first to prevent blood from dripping over future biopsy sites. Select the areas that appear most abnormal. "Blind random biopsies" are generally discouraged. The average number of biopsies taken is often in the range of two to five, but may be as few as one or as many as six or seven. It all depends on experience and the size, appearance, and number of lesions. The cervix can be manipulated with a cotton-tipped swab (preferred) or a hook (rarely) to provide an adequate angle for obtaining the biopsy sample. A 3-mm-deep sample is all that is necessary. It is *not* necessary to include normal-appearing tissue with biopsy samples (i.e., to include the margins of lesions in the sample). Beginning colposcopists can enhance their skills by placing samples from different biopsy sites in separate bottles and subsequently correlating them with colposcopic impression. After sufficient experience, colposcopists can place all biopsy samples together. The cervix will be treated based on the most severe lesion as well as the size of the lesion. *Putting different biopsies in*

separate containers only increases cost; it does not change therapy. For anyone, to enhance the learning experience, an unusual or atypical-appearing lesion may be placed in a separate container to provide better feedback. If bleeding is profuse from a particular site and more samples are needed, hold a cotton-tipped swab to the area and proceed with obtaining the next sample. (To control persistent bleeding, see the Complications section.) Do not apply Monsel solution until all samples are obtained. Monsel solution in a biopsy specimen can affect the histologic interpretation. As noted previously, some clinicians prefer to obtain the cervical biopsy samples before the ECC.

17. Apply Monsel solution to bleeding areas after all biopsies have been obtained. To be most effective, the Monsel solution should be as thick as toothpaste. This consistency can be achieved by allowing the solution to evaporate down to a pasty consistency. Once bleeding is controlled, swab out the excess solution and bloody debris in the posterior vaginal vault, which appears as a black mass of coagulum that may alarm the patient when it appears as a black discharge and irritates the vulva. Observe the cervix until all evident bleeding ceases.

18. Examine the vagina while removing the speculum. Reapply acetic acid to the vaginal sidewalls. Gently retract the speculum with a back-and-forth twisting motion to the right and left and observe through the colposcope as the vaginal wall collapses around the receding blades. Are abnormal vaginal areas apparent? If there is any question, Lugol solution may help clarify the situation because condylomata and dysplasia (vaginal intraepithelial neoplasia) do not stain. Be sure to colposcopically examine any vaginal areas that felt abnormal during the bimanual examination. Biopsies of the vagina can be obtained with the same biopsy forceps but are placed in separate containers. It is not necessary to take deep bites.

19. Examine the vulva and anus. Acetic acid application will produce an acetowhite effect in most sites with condylomata or dysplasia (vulvar intraepithelial neoplasia). It is mandatory to do a careful vulvar colposcopic examination with acetic acid in these women who are at high risk for vulvar dysplasia, especially those with unexplained vulvar itching or other symptoms, smokers older than 40 years, those with abnormal-appearing areas of vulvar tissue, and those with human immunodeficiency virus infection. The easiest way to examine the vulva is to begin superiorly. Use two hands to separate the vulva and slowly raise the power table with the foot pedal. Examine carefully from clitoris to anus. The finding of perianal condylomata warrants anoscopy, especially if they have been persistent. The Ives slotted anoscope is ideal (see Chapter 83, Anoscopy). If condylomata are grossly visible, it may be best to resolve the external lesions first before inserting the anoscope and risking spread internally. Acetic acid can be used in the anal canal but is rarely necessary. Small anal canal condylomata can usually be palpated. For the technique for sampling the vulva, see Chapter 139, Vulvar Biopsy. For high-resolution anoscopy, which is a colposcopic examination of the anal area, see Chapter 84, High-Resolution Anoscopy.

20. Allow the patient to recover. Have the patient rest supine for at least several minutes, then sit up slowly and rest again. Offer juice or cookies, especially if the patient has a history of syncope or missed the meal before her colposcopy.

21. Document your findings. Carefully draw a picture of lesions and biopsy sites. Photographs of the cervix do not replace accurately drawn diagrams of the colposcopic cervical findings. These should be included regardless of whether the colposcopic examination is considered adequate.
Chart whether the colposcopic impression supports outpatient cervical cryotherapy or if excisional treatment will be needed, and which cryotip or loop electrode should be used (size and shape). This is not a decision based solely on colposcopic appearance. It requires correlation of cytologic, colposcopic, and histologic data to define the appropriate therapeutic interven-

tion. Factors such as lesion location, grade of dysplasia, and number and size of lesions also dictate treatment options. For instance, large lesions (>25 mm in diameter, >15 mm from the os, or involving more than two cervical quadrants), even if they are only mildly dysplastic, are treated more appropriately with loop excision or laser therapy, as opposed to a small focal severe dysplasia, which may respond to ambulatory cryotherapy very well. (See Chapter 125, Cryotherapy of the Cervix, and Chapter 127, Loop Electrosurgical Excision Procedure for Treating Cervical Intraepithelial Neoplasia.) In general, the patient is a candidate for ablative therapy if the colposcopy is adequate (see earlier) and the following criteria are met:
- No lesion extends more than 5 mm into the canal
- The ECC is negative
- There is no colposcopic evidence of malignancy
- Any high-grade lesion is only focal in size (<1 cm)
- There is correlation between the Pap smear findings, the colposcopic impression, and the histology

22. *Discuss the findings and give postprocedure instructions. After the patient has recovered and is dressed, review your impressions but withhold the specific diagnosis until the histology report has returned and all the clinical data have been examined. Provide careful postprocedure instructions (see the sample patient education handout available at www.expertconsult.com). Advise abstaining from intercourse for 24 hours and using tampons for 5 days. Instruct the patient to return if she experiences unusual vaginal odor, discharge, pelvic pain, or fever. Make a specific agreement as to how the results of the biopsy are to be reported. Unless a problem arises, the patient does not need a follow-up pelvic examination. Discussing the results of the biopsy sampling and subsequent treatment options on the telephone may be an appropriate follow-up mechanism for some patients; however, most will appreciate a visit to the clinician for this important interaction.*

SAMPLE OPERATIVE NOTE

A prepared colposcopy procedure form, including patient identification materials, history, and a written diagram of findings, is an excellent way to document and archive findings (see Fig. 124.13).

COMMON ERRORS

1. Losing track of patients who have a significantly abnormal Pap smear or biopsy-proven dysplasia, and for whom treatment is necessary. This can place the patients at risk for delayed management and treatment. "No-shows" are a significant problem. Develop a follow-up tracking system.
2. Finding an abnormal-appearing cervix on visual inspection when obtaining a Pap smear but then relying on the Pap result to determine if colposcopy is needed. Visual abnormalities take precedence over the Pap report as an indication for colposcopy. If the cervix appears to be abnormal, colposcopy with biopsy is indicated.
3. Omitting the ECC in patients for whom cervical ablative treatment may be an option, especially for high-grade dysplasia (see Chapter 125, Cryotherapy of the Cervix).
4. Failing to inspect the vulva, cervical fornices, and vagina during colposcopy. Significant dysplasia can be a comorbid condition to cervical disease.
5. Performing too few biopsies, especially for large, high-grade appearing lesions where there is risk of missing invasive cancer. Studies continue to emphasize the importance of obtaining enough biopsies.
6. Canceling colposcopy in women who are having routine menses. Colposcopy can be performed in most patients regardless of bleeding.
7. Trying to perform colposcopy with an active cervicitis. Culture and reschedule soon.

8. Failing to take the time to address all the emotional issues surrounding HPV and other sexually transmitted infections, and condylomata/abnormal Pap smear concerns.
9. Putting biopsies in separate formalin containers. This usually is not necessary.

COMPLICATIONS

- Bleeding. Most biopsy or ECC bleeding is minimal and handled readily with Monsel solution. Rarely, the patient experiences a fresh, bloody discharge. Often, a simple reapplication of Monsel solution is all that is necessary. Silver nitrate sticks may also be used to cauterize small areas of bleeding (see Chapter 199, Topical Hemostatic Agents). Some clinicians will saturate the end of a vaginal tampon with Monsel solution and insert this to provide pressure and astringent action for persistent cervical oozing. The tampon can then be removed several hours later by the patient. Very rarely, a simple stitch of 4-0 absorbable suture across a particularly deep biopsy site may be required. At times, it may be necessary to cauterize the biopsy site. An effective way to control fairly brisk bleeding is to inject 1 to 2 mL of 2% lidocaine with epinephrine into the bleeding site. This will either stop or reduce the bleeding enough to effectively apply Monsel solution or to cauterize the site. Use a needle extender (see Chapter 127, Loop Electrosurgical Excision Procedure for Treating Cervical Intraepithelial Neoplasia) or a spinal needle to reach the cervix. If possible, try to avoid obtaining a cervical biopsy sample immediately before the menses; subsequent bleeding may be confused with menstrual flow. This may not be very practical in the busy daily routines.
- A foul cervical discharge, fever, or pelvic pain may indicate postprocedure infection. Infection is almost unheard of, but typically occurs on the third or fourth day after the biopsy sample has been taken. A cervical biopsy should be avoided if there is clinical evidence of significant, extensive cervicitis identified by erythematous changes and marked friability. Not only will pathology be more difficult to interpret, but bleeding can be quite brisk.
- Despite the correct technique, there is the potential risk that the most advanced cervical disease may be missed by the colposcopist at the time of the biopsy sampling, or potentially by the histologist at the time of tissue analysis. Careful, timely transport of all samples to a reputable laboratory is important. The ECC sample should remain separate from cervical biopsies. The colposcopist is well advised to be liberal in obtaining biopsies of all abnormal-appearing areas of the cervix for histologic interpretation; costs can be controlled by placing all biopsies in one container. Widespread, four-quadrant cervical disease challenges the colposcopist to identify areas most likely to contain cervical carcinoma. Lack of correlation between the Pap cytologic results and subsequent histologic findings can suggest a situation in which potentially the worst area has not been sampled. The main goal of colposcopy is to rule out invasive cervical cancer and to select patients who are candidates for outpatient treatment. When the colposcopist cannot safely accomplish this goal, cervical conization—rarely, but importantly—is the only way of accomplishing this task. "Blind biopsies" in which random samples are obtained are, again, generally discouraged.
- Some women will experience vaginal discharge that often looks like coffee grounds after a cervical biopsy sample is obtained. This will typically last 1 or 2 days and should diminish with time. It is often due to the Monsel solution used to control bleeding.
- Cervical biopsy sampling typically causes brief pain and discomfort. Ordinarily, this pain is well tolerated by most women. Careful explanation of the procedure, a warm room, and a caring, careful manner all minimize the discomfort. Studies have shown preoperative oral nonsteroidal antiinflammatory drugs decrease

discomfort associated with the procedure. Topical anesthetics generally are not left on long enough to make any difference.
- Rarely, vasovagal reactions occur with the procedure but are much more likely to occur with cervical cryotherapy.

POSTPROCEDURE PATIENT EDUCATION

See the sample patient education handout available at www.expertconsult.com.

- Agree on a time to discuss and interpret biopsy findings by phone or follow-up visit.
- Explain that mild vaginal discharge may occur after a cervical biopsy procedure, especially if Monsel solution was used to control bleeding. This discharge is often grainy and black, such as coffee grounds, which is the result of Monsel solution mixing with mucus and blood. This discharge may last approximately 24 hours.
- Advise the patient that she may have spotting for at least 48 hours. Although there may be some spotting, it is safe to resume intercourse after 24 to 48 hours.
- Instruct the patient to report passage of clots, onset of fresh, profuse bleeding, foul vaginal odor, fever, or pelvic pain. Women with these complaints after a cervical biopsy procedure require evaluation.
- Encourage the patient to continue contraception.
- Patients rarely require vaginal creams after a cervical biopsy has been obtained. Nonetheless, some women may have vaginitis caused by organisms such as yeast, bacteria, or *Trichomonas*, and therapy aimed at these pathogens may be helpful and is not contraindicated after biopsy.
- Emphasize the importance of returning for definitive therapy. Reemphasize the relationship of cervical dysplasia with sexually transmissible disease, poor diet, smoking, and nonmonogamous sexual practices. Be sure the patient understands the lifelong risks of HPV infection.

INTERPRETATION OF RESULTS

If at all possible, the same pathologist (or at least the same group of pathologists) should interpret both the cytologic and histologic results for a given patient. The clinician should be concerned if a significant discrepancy is found between the Pap smear cytology, the colposcopic appearance of the cervix, and the biopsy histology. In general, a report that a more advanced lesion was found on the biopsy compared with the Pap smear (e.g., Pap = CIN 2; biopsy = CIN 3) is common and acceptable. However, the clinician should be concerned if biopsy-generated histology results are significantly less advanced than the Pap cytology. In general, most will accept a biopsy diagnosis one degree less, but if it is two degrees the discrepancy must be explained. For instance, a cytology smear indicating carcinoma in situ, with biopsy samples of only mild dysplasia, might indicate that the worst area was missed on evaluation and that the patient may have in situ or invasive carcinoma in another site. The clinician is advised not to freeze or ablate any cervix until the discrepancy between histology and cytology has been explained adequately and sufficiently. Repeating colposcopy with biopsy to reconcile the difference is indicated. Freezing invasive cancer is never acceptable.

A negative ECC sample will show strips or fragments of orderly, benign columnar epithelium with mucus and blood. Lack of identifiable endocervical tissue constitutes an inadequate ECC sample. An inadequate ECC sample is not uncommon, and in the overwhelming majority of patients it simply means that the ECC must be repeated before definitive ablative therapy. If the ECC sample indicates dysplasia, it is a positive ECC and is an indication for an excisional procedure (see Chapter 128, Cervical Conization, and Chapter 127, Loop Electrosurgical Excision Procedure for Treating

Cervical Intraepithelial Neoplasia). Current protocol does not support freezing the canal with a long, narrow probe to treat endocervical dysplasia. Some "positive" ECCs result from contamination with dysplastic lesions at the verge of the os. Nonetheless, do not assume this! The beginning colposcopist must remain comfortable referring patients with equivocal or problematic colposcopic, cytologic, and histologic correlation. Know your limitations and seek help.

PATIENT AND CLINICIAN EDUCATIONAL RESOURCES

(See full contact information available at www.expertconsult.com under "Suppliers.")

American College of Obstetricians and Gynecologists: www.acog.org
American Social Health Association: www.healthinaging.org
American Society for Colposcopy and Cervical Pathology: www.asccp.org (national society for promotion of quality education and patient care for cervical/vaginal disease)
National Procedures Institute: www.npinstitute.com (DVDs)
Krames Communications: www.kramesstore.com

CPT/BILLING CODES

56605	Biopsy of vulva, single
56606	Biopsy of vulva, each additional
56820	Colposcopy of the vulva
56821	Colposcopy of the vulva; with biopsy(s)
57100	Biopsy of vaginal mucosa, simple
57105	Biopsy of vaginal mucosa, extensive
57420	Colposcopy of the entire vagina, with cervix if present
57421	Colposcopy of the entire vagina, with cervix if present; with biopsy(s) of vagina
57452	Colposcopy of the cervix including upper/adjacent vagina
57454	Colposcopy of the cervix including upper/adjacent vagina with biopsy(s) of the cervix and endocervical curettage
57455	Colposcopy of the cervix including upper/adjacent vagina with biopsy(s) of the cervix
57456	Colposcopy of the cervix including upper/adjacent vagina; with endocervical curettage
57460	Colposcopy of the cervix including upper/adjacent vagina with loop electrode biopsy(s) of the cervix
57461	Colposcopy of the cervix including upper/adjacent vagina; with loop electrode conization of the cervix (do not report 57456 in addition to 57461)
57500	Biopsy of cervix only, single or multiple (also use this code for removal of a cervical polyp since there is no other specific code)
57505	Endocervical curettage (not done as part of a D&C)
57510	Electrocautery of cervix
57511	Cryosurgery of cervix
57513	Laser ablation of cervix
57520	Conization of cervix, laser or cold knife
57522	Conization, LEEP technique

ICD-10-CM DIAGNOSTIC CODES

A63.0	Condyloma acuminatum
C53.9	Cervical neoplasm, malignant (excludes carcinoma in situ)
D26.0	Benign neoplasm, cervix
D06.9	Carcinoma in situ, cervix
D06.9	CIN III
D07.2	Vagina dysplasia, severe
D07.1	Vulvar dysplasia VIN III
N72	Cervicitis
N76.0	Vaginitis
N86	Cervical ectropion
N88.8	Cervical erosion/ulcer
N88.9	Cervical atypia
N88.0	Cervical leukoplakia
N88.2	Cervical stenosis
N84.1	Cervical polyp
N88.4	Cervical atrophy
N88.8	Nabothian cyst
N87.9	Cervical dysplasia (unspecified)
N87.0	CIN I
N87.1	CIN II
N89.3	Vagina, dysplasia
N89.4	Vaginal leukoplakia
N89.8	Vaginal leukorrhea
N84.2	Vaginal polyp
N89.8	Vaginal cyst
N90.0	Vulvar dysplasia, leukoplakia VIN I
N90.1	Vulvar dysplasia VIN II
N90.5	Vulvar atrophy
N84.3	Vulvar or labial polyp
R87.619	Abnormal Pap

SUPPLIERS

(See contact information available at www.expertconsult.com.)

Colposcope and instrument manufacturers
Carl Zeiss Surgical, Inc.
CooperSurgical, Inc. (acquired Leisegang)
Gyne-Tech Instrument Corp.
Gyrus ASMI Distributor (Olympus)
MedGyn
Seiler Colposcope
Wallach Surgical
Welch Allyn, Inc.

Other colposcopy equipment and supplies
CooperSurgical (Medscand [Cytobrush])
Delasco
Milex
Wallach Surgical (Papette, Pap smear samplers)
Welch Allyn, Inc.

Also see Chapter 125, Cryotherapy of the Cervix, and Chapter 127, Loop Electrosurgical Excision Procedure for Treating Cervical Intraepithelial Neoplasia.

ONLINE RESOURCES

American Society for Colposcopy and Cervical Pathology (ASCCP): Available at www.asccp.org.

RECOMMENDED READING

American Academy of Family Physicians. *Colposcopy (position paper), originally approved 1998, updated*; 2015. https://www.aafp.org/about/policies/all/colposcopy.html.
Apgar BS, Kaufman AJ, Bettcher C, Parker-Featherstone E. Gynecologic Procedures: colposcopy, treatment of cervical intraepithelial neoplasia, and endometrial assessment. *Am Family Physician.* 2013;87(12):836–843.
Apgar BS, Brotzman GL, Spitzer M, eds. *Colposcopy: Principles and Practice.* 2nd ed. Philadelphia: Saunders; 2008.

Bornstein J, Bentley J, Bösze P, et al. 2011 Colposcopic terminology of the International Federation for Cervical Pathology and Colposcopy. *Obstet Gynecol*. 2012;120:166–172.

Coppleson M, Pixley E, Reid B, The tissue basis of colposcopic appearances. *Colposcopy: A Scientific and Practical Approach to the Cervix, Vagina, and Vulva in Health and Disease*. 3rd ed. Springfield, IL: Charles C. Thomas; 1986.

Ferris DG, Cox JT, O'Connor DM, et al. Modern colposcopy: textbook and Atlas. In: *American Society for Colposcopy and Cervical Pathology*. 2nd ed. Dubuque, IA: Kendall/Hunt; 2004.

Hacker NF. Cervical dysplasia and cancer. In: Hacker NF, Gambone JC, Hobel JC, eds. *Hacker and Moore's Essentials of Obstetrics and Gynecology*. 6th ed. Philadelphia: Elsevier; 2016:429–439.

Khan M, Werner CL, Darragh TM, et al. ASCCP colposcopy standards: role of colposcopy, benefits, potential harms, and terminology for colposcopic practice. *J Low Genit Tract Dis*. 2017;21(4):223–229.

Massad LS, Collins YC. Strength of correlations between colposcopic impression and biopsy histology. *Gynecol Oncol*. 2003;89(3):424–428.

Massad LS, Einstein MH, Huh WK, et al. 2012 update consensus guidelines for the management of abnormal cervical screening tests and cancer precursors. *J Low Genit Tract Dis*. 2013;17(5 supp 1):S1–S27.

Newkirk GR, ed. *Colposcopy for the Family Physician*. 2nd ed. Kansas City, MO: American Academy of Family Physicians *[includes video instruction on colposcopy, cryotherapy, and LEEP]*; 2005.

Reid R. Biology and colposcopic features of human papillomavirus–associated cervical disease. *Obstet Gynecol Clin North Am*. 1993;20:123–151.

Tatti S, Bornstein J, Prendiville W. Colposcopy: a global perspective: introduction of the new IFCPC colposcopy terminology. *Obstet Gynecol Clin North Am*. 2013;40(2):235–250.

Tuggy M, Garcia J. Procedures Consult. Colposcopy. www.proceduresconsult.com/medical-procedures-colposcopy-FM-028-procedure.aspx.

Wentzensen N, Walker JL, Gold MA, et al. Multiple biopsies and detection of cervical cancer precursors at colposcopy. *J Clin Oncol*. 2015;33:83–9.

World Health Organization. *Comprehensive Cervical Cancer Control: A Guide to Essential Practice*. 2nd ed. Geneva: World Health Organization; 2014.

Zuchna C, Hager M, Tringler B, et al. Diagnostic accuracy of guided cervical biopsies: a prospective multicenter study comparing the histopathology of simultaneous biopsy and cone specimen. *Am J Obstet Gynecol*. 2010;203(4):321.e1–e6.

CHAPTER 125

CRYOTHERAPY OF THE CERVIX

Madeline R. Lewis • John L. Pfenninger

Cryotherapy is the treatment of choice for select small cervical intraepithelial lesions (cervical intraepithelial neoplasia [CIN] 1, 2, and 3 or mild, moderate, and severe dysplasia). This procedure is easy to learn, is well tolerated by the patient, is less expensive than other therapies —including the large loop electrical excision procedure (LEEP) and laser—and has a similar success rate. It requires a refrigerant gas under pressure, such as nitrous oxide, and an applicator probe. The cryoprobe allows rapid freezing of cervical tissue, causing a controlled destruction of the transformation zone and the epithelial lesion. Cellular destruction is greatest when a rapid freeze, slow thaw, and refreeze method is used. This efficacious procedure has few complications, can be performed quickly, is low in cost, and preserves cervical tissue.

Basically the only negative aspect is that there is no tissue specimen available to confirm removal of all abnormalities. However, considering that up to 18% of patients experience pregnancy complications after LEEP, cryotherapy should be strongly considered for women who meet the criteria for treatment.

Cryotherapy treats cervical dysplasia by destroying the lesion and the transformation zone. Cell death occurs as a result of ice crystal penetration into the intracellular space. The depth of destruction is directly proportional to the lateral spread of the freeze, which is measured by the size of the ice ball that forms around and beyond the tip of the cryoprobe. An ice ball of 5 to 7 mm will result in adequate cellular destruction and is necessary, because severe dysplasia (CIN 3) can extend to a depth of 3 to 5 mm into the glands in the transformation zone. The frequency and depth of gland involvement seem to be directly proportional to the grade of the squamous intraepithelial lesion. However, the overall success of cryotherapy is related more to the size than the grade of the lesion. Small high-grade lesions (<1 cm) may be adequately treated with cryotherapy. Low-grade lesions should be less than 3 cm in diameter (some recommend <2 cm). All lesions should involve no more than two quadrants of the cervix and extend no more than 5 mm into the endocervical canal. Large high-grade lesions (>1 cm), microinvasive lesions, and invasive lesions need more aggressive treatment such as LEEP, conization, or even hysterectomy.

Treatment failures may occur with cryotherapy as with any other treatment modality. "Cure rates" have been in the 95% range for CIN 1 and CIN 2, which is consistent with other modalities. For CIN 3, the cure rate drops to 89% overall, but this has been correlated more with lesion size and depth, not to severity of disease. High-grade lesions are often larger and extend deeper into the glands, making them more difficult to treat.

EDITOR'S NOTE: The mere presence of CIN itself may increase the risk of preterm labor, perhaps due to treatments for it. The more procedures a woman has undergone to treat CIN, the higher the risk of preterm labor. If an excisional method is chosen to treat CIN, the deeper the cone depth, the higher the risk of prematurity. Therefore when women likely to become pregnant in the future are being treated, consideration should be given to using an ablative method such as cryotherapy rather than LEEP, provided the colposcopy is satisfactory and there is no suspicion of occult invasive cancer.

A 2017 Cochrane review found ablative therapy to be associated with less risk of preterm delivery than excisional therapy.

ANATOMY

Cervical anatomy is discussed in detail in Chapter 124, Colposcopic Examination.

INDICATIONS

Also see the current recommendations of the American Society for Colposcopy and Cervical Pathology in Appendix K, Algorithms for the Evaluation of Abnormal Pap Smears and Treatment of Colposcopic Findings.

Cryotherapy may be used for the treatment of squamous dysplasia that has been confirmed with a biopsy after a complete and adequate colposcopic examination and if all criteria noted later have been met. It is essential that the Pap smear results, the appearance of the cervix on colposcopic examination, and the histologic report from the biopsy do not vary by more than one degree of severity. That is, colposcopic impression and histologic findings can be only one degree less severe than the Pap smear findings. If there is lack of correlation, this must be resolved or a LEEP or conization of the cervix is indicated because it is presumed that the most advanced lesion has not been identified. It is common for histology to be worse than the Pap smear because the Pap smear is a screening test only. However, the Pap smear is essentially never two grades worse than tissue pathology or biopsy. If the correlation principle is met, the patient would then be treated based on biopsy findings. Cryotherapy may be used to treat low-grade squamous intraepithelial lesions (LSILs) and small focal high-grade intraepithelial lesions (HSILs). Large high-grade lesions usually have deeper gland involvement, and these patients usually need to have an excisional treatment, such as LEEP or conization. *Cryotherapy is not appropriate for any invasive lesion.* The practitioner must be sure to differentiate between carcinoma in situ and microinvasive cancer. Although select patients with carcinoma in situ who meet the criteria may be treated with cryotherapy, *microinvasive lesions should never be treated this way.* Patients with microinvasive disease need a conization procedure to determine the true extent of the disease.

Criteria for cryotherapy of the cervix include the following:

- Complete colposcopic examination with good correlation between Pap smear results, visual examination, and histologic biopsy report.
- The entire squamocolumnar junction and entire lesion must be visible ("adequate colposcopy" or "satisfactory exam").
- Lesions should be less than 2 to 3 cm in diameter and involve no more than two quadrants of the cervix.
- The probe tip must be able to cover the entire lesion and the entire transformation zone.
- The lesion does not extend more than 5 mm into the endocervical canal.
- The endocervical canal sampling is negative for dysplasia.
- The cervix should be relatively flat, without large crevices.

- There should be no significant glandular involvement on biopsy.
- The patient must be reliable for follow-up.

Cryotherapy may also be useful to treat patients with chronic cervicitis that is culture-negative and unresponsive to antibiotic therapy and has negative colposcopy and biopsy findings. External genital human papillomavirus lesions may be treated with cryotherapy, although a different freezing technique is used (see Chapter 14, Cryosurgery, and Chapter 138, Treatment of Noncervical Condylomata Acuminata).

EDITOR'S NOTE: It is important for anyone performing cervical cryotherapy to keep up with the guidelines. Recent guidelines from the World Health Organization (WHO) suggest that it is reasonable to just follow biopsy-proven low-grade squamous intraepithelial lesions (LGSILs) up to CIN1 without active treatment because many will regress spontaneously. However, active treatment is always indicated for HSILs of CIN2 or greater. The American Society for Colposcopy and Cervical Pathology (ASCCP) 2012 guidelines recommend treatment of HSILs and persistent CIN1.

CONTRAINDICATIONS

Absolute

- Patients with colposcopic or histologic findings more than one degree less severe than the Pap smear findings. (This means the lesion causing the abnormal Pap smear was likely missed or overlooked on colposcopy.) These patients need to have a complete reevaluation before any treatment (see previous discussion).
- Positive endocervical curettage or other canal sampling that is positive (dysplasia or cancer).
- Large lesion that the cryoprobe will not cover completely.
- Lesion extends into the endocervical canal more than 5 mm.
- Large high-grade lesions or carcinoma in situ (>1 cm). LEEP is the treatment of choice for most of these lesions and will result in a better cure rate than cryotherapy.
- Invasive lesions (including microinvasion); these will need more aggressive treatment.
- Pregnancy.
- Cryoglobulinemia.
- Significant glandular involvement on endocervical curettage or biopsy.

Relative

- Patient is within 1 week of menses or is having heavy menstrual flow. The resulting canal edema from cryotherapy could obstruct the normal menstrual outflow.
- Acute cervicitis. In these patients it is best to treat the acute infection before cryotherapy.
- Immunosuppressed patients.
- Women exposed to diethylstilbestrol (DES) in utero because they are at greater risk for cervical stenosis.
- Markedly irregular cervix where the indentations are too deep to be reached by the cryoprobe.
- Noncompliant patient (consider doing a definitive excisional procedure).

Many would suggest that all CIN III lesions (i.e., carcinoma in situ) be treated with conization procedures. However, the data strongly support the efficacy of properly performed cryotherapy for small lesions that meet the aforementioned criteria. Cryotherapy is much more cost-effective than alternatives, with potentially fewer and less significant complications.

EQUIPMENT AND SUPPLIES

- Nitrous oxide 20-lb tank with a pressure gauge and gas cutoff valve (Figs. 125.1 and 125.2).
- Flexible tubing from tank to probe.

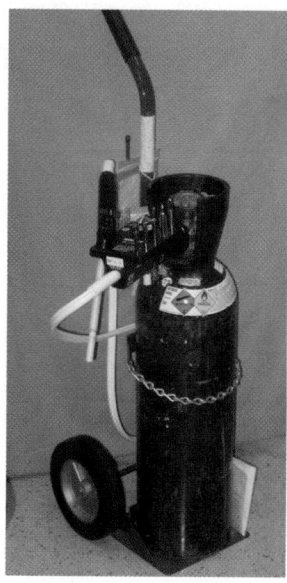

Fig. 125.1   Nitrous oxide tank with yoke adapter for the cryogun. Several cryotips are attached.

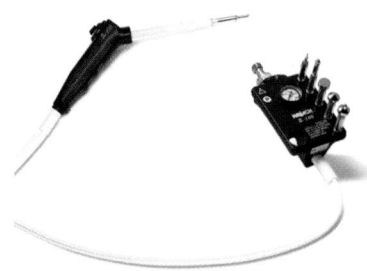

Fig. 125.2   Closeup views of yoke adapter with pressure gauge, cryogun, and cryotips. (Courtesy Wallach Surgical Devices, Milford, CT.)

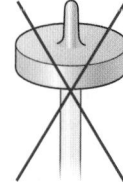

Fig. 125.3   Older cryotherapy tips with endocervical nipples longer than 5 mm should be avoided.

- Probe handle.
- Probe tips: 19 and 25 mm in diameter, slightly coned or flat; do not use any tips with nipples that are more than 5 mm in length (Fig. 125.3).
- Water-soluble lubricant, such as K-Y Jelly.
- Vaginal speculum.
- A minute timer.
- Vaginal sidewall retractors or glove to place over the speculum (to prevent injury to vaginal sidewalls in patients with redundant vaginal walls. (See the Technique section of Chapter 120, Pap Smear and Related Techniques for Cervical Cancer Screening, for instructions on how to retract sidewalls with a homemade device.)

- O-ring supply for some older cryotherapy units. These are round rubber washers that attach at the base of the probe tip. They may crack over time, which could result in leakage of the refrigerant at the joint between the probe and the rod tip. They are easily and quickly replaced by simply removing the old one and sliding on the new one.
- Injectable local anesthetic (1% lidocaine with epinephrine), needle and syringe setup, oral benzocaine spray (optional).

PREPROCEDURE PATIENT EDUCATION

- Provide the patient with a patient education handout (see the patient education handout available at www.expertconsult.com).
- Discuss the risks, benefits, and possible complications of cryotherapy.
- Before the procedure, review the indications with the patient.
- Obtain written informed consent.
- Confirm that this patient is willing to return for follow-up.
- Update the menstrual history and do a pelvic examination if one has not been done within the previous few months.
- Verify that the patient is not pregnant; perform a pregnancy test if there is any doubt.
- Confirm the biopsy report, confirm a negative endocervical curettage and note any area where disease is concentrated to make sure that the cryoprobe will readily cover the area.
- Premedicate the patient on her arrival to the office (if appropriate) with ibuprofen 800 mg or another nonsteroidal antiinflammatory drug (NSAID) to reduce cramping that may occur with the procedure (if not already taken). For maximal effectiveness, the NSAID should be taken approximately 30 to 60 minutes before the procedure.

EDITOR'S NOTE: Although a Cochrane review in 2016 found no benefit to giving an NSAID prior to cervical procedures, most clinicians recommend one. Optimal therapy for painful cervical procedures appears to be intracervical injection of local anesthetic with a vasoconstrictor (e.g., lidocaine with epinephrine), and this can be done prior to this procedure. Some minimally invasive gynecologists spray topical oral benzocaine (e.g., Americaine, Hurricane spray) before any cervical procedure, but there is no evidence to support this.

PROCEDURE

Prepare Equipment

1. Ensure that the tank has adequate pressure; for most tanks the needle on the pressure gauge will be in the "green zone."
2. Ensure that the O-ring (the small rubber washer) at the base of the probe tip is intact, if applicable (mainly on older units).
3. Select the proper size and shape of probe tip. If the 19-mm tip covers the entire lesion and the entire transformation zone, it can be used. If all areas are not covered, use the larger, 25-mm tip. If the lesion is near the os or extends slightly (<5 mm) into the os, use the conical tip. If the lesion and squamocolumnar junction are well out on the ectocervix, a flat probe tip may be more appropriate to use. Avoid tips with long extensions because these may cause cervical stenosis (see Fig. 125.3).
4. Select the proper size vaginal speculum; the entire cervix and transformation zone must be well visualized, so consider using the largest speculum the patient can tolerate.

Prepare the Patient

1. Place the patient in a comfortable dorsal lithotomy position in stirrups.
2. In select cases, consider using a submucosal cervical injection with lidocaine. (See Chapter 127, Loop Electrosurgical Excision

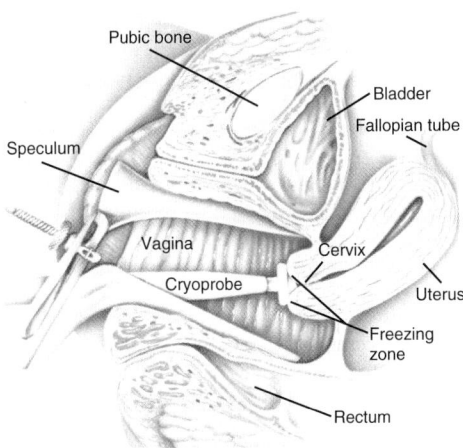

Fig. 125.4 Proper application of the cryotip to the cervix.

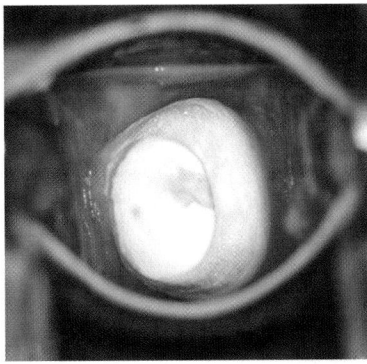

Fig. 125.5 Appearance of the cervix immediately after cryotherapy. (Courtesy John L. Pfenninger, The Medical Procedures Center, Midland, MI.)

Procedure for Treating Cervical Intraepithelial Neoplasia.) Some clinicians use topical anesthetics (e.g., oral benzocaine spray), but unless they are in place for 20 to 30 minutes, they have little effect.
3. Insert the speculum. If necessary, use a speculum cover or vaginal sidewall retractor to prevent vaginal injury in patients with redundant mucosa.

Perform Cryotherapy

1. Apply water-soluble lubricant (e.g., K-Y Jelly) to the cryoprobe tip.
2. Turn on the gas valve (pressure gauge in the "green zone").
3. Apply the probe firmly to the cervix and begin freezing by pulling the trigger or pushing the freeze button. The tip will adhere in about 3 to 5 seconds (Fig. 125.4). After the tip adheres, pull back slightly. *Avoid the tendency to push in on the probe*, which would stretch the uterosacral ligaments and cause discomfort. Pulling back slightly will cause the vagina to billow out, reducing the likelihood of the probe sticking to the sidewalls.
4. Watch the probe tip carefully to monitor the rim of ice. A 5- to 7-mm ice ball around the perimeter of the tip is required for adequate cellular destruction (Fig. 125.5). This usually takes at least 3 minutes to form. A timed freeze alone is not recommended because the size of the tip used, the amount of cervical vascularity and fibrous tissue, and the pressure in the nitrous tank all alter the length of time required to form the 5- to 7-mm ice ball. In the majority of cases, at least a 3-minute freeze is

used, after which the cervix is inspected to judge the size of the ice ball around the tip. If there is any question, continue the freeze. Overfreezing generally does not cause a significant problem.

5. When the ice ball around the probe tip reaches 5 to 7 mm, defrost by pushing the defrost button (on most machines) or releasing the freeze button. The probe tip will detach in about 15 seconds. Do not try to pull the probe off until it has thawed, because that may result in the laceration of cervical tissue. (The "active" defrost requires that the gas be left on—do not turn off the gas valve on the tank itself. A "passive" defrost takes at least 5 minutes just for the probe to release from the tissues.) If the probe does not easily release, check to make sure that no one has turned off the gas. Switch back and forth between freeze and defrost. Sometimes the valve can stick.

6. Allow for a complete thaw of the cervix, which is seen when the cervix resumes a normal pink color. This may take 8 to 10 minutes. The patient often feels "flushed" during this period. Now refreeze; the second freeze may take less time. Again, a 5- to 7-mm ice ball is required. A rapid freeze, slow defrost, and rapid refreeze technique has been shown to be the most efficacious method of treatment.

7. Thaw as described previously.

8. Remove the speculum and turn off the tank.

9. Have the patient sit up slowly to avoid any vasovagal symptoms, such as light-headedness or flushing. These may occur up to 10 minutes after completing the procedure.

10. Give the patient follow-up information. She will have a profuse, watery, or blood-tinged discharge for 2 to 4 weeks. The next Pap smear should be scheduled for 6 months after this procedure (see the sample patient education handout available at www.expertconsult.com).

A 2015 Cochrane review found no evidence for the best surveillance strategy following treatment for CIN. The next visit, whenever it occurs, will provide an opportunity to reinforce prevention methods, such as not smoking. It is important to check for cervical stenosis. The os is easier to dilate early rather than waiting for a more mature scar. (See Chapter 126, Cervical Stenosis and Cervical Dilation/)

11. Consider prescribing a vaginal cream to aids in healing the cervix and potentially decrease the discharge. Such a cream was previously available as Amino-Cerv Vaginal Crème, but it is no longer offered. It now must be compounded with the following ingredients:
    - Urea 8.34% (6.672 g)
    - Sodium propionate 0.50% (0.4 g)
    - Methionine 0.83% (0.664 g)
    - Cysteine 0.35% (0.28 g)
    - Inositol hexanicotinate 0.83% (2.988 g)

    These ingredients are buffered to pH of 5.5 in a water-miscible emollient cream base to make 80 g. Prescribe one vaginal application at bedtime for 2 weeks.

COMMON ERRORS

- The patient may experience vasovagal symptoms after the procedure; avoid this by having the patient sit up slowly and rest a while before standing. Caution her to sit down immediately if she feels light-headed.
- The anticipated postprocedure copious vaginal discharge can be mistaken for cervicitis.
- Turning off the gas at the tank before the probe has been released from the cervix.
- Timing of the application as the sole criterion for the length of freeze. The size of the ice ball is the most important factor.
- Not emphasizing adequately to the patient that there will be

a copious discharge but that this temporary inconvenience is worth it to avoid other, more severe complications associated with other methods of treatment.

COMPLICATIONS

- *Vaginal mucosal injury* is possible; avoid this by being certain that the cryoprobe does not touch the vaginal sidewalls. Use a speculum cover or vaginal wall retractors if necessary. If small areas are frozen, there are usually no significant adverse outcomes. If it appears that large areas of mucosa are being frozen, stop the procedure, take measures to protect the sidewalls, and start over.
- *Pain and cramping* may occur during cryotherapy; medicate patients with an NSAID about 30 to 40 minutes before the procedure. On rare occasions an anxiolytic may be helpful. In an especially anxious patient, consider a mucosal block. Avoid aggressive pulling on the cryoprobe during freezing, because this may cause more intense cramping.
- The *profuse watery discharge* that follows cryotherapy is the most unpleasant consequence. It usually begins within the first day or two and lasts at least 2 weeks. The compounded cream noted earlier may help and may be used for a total of 4 weeks. Do not confuse this discharge, which always occurs, with an infection.
- A *cervicitis* is possible after therapy. If the discharge is not improving after 2 weeks, consider oral metronidazole.
- A *pelvic inflammatory infection* is extremely rare. Consider it if there is extreme pelvic tenderness and fever.
- If the patient unexpectedly starts her period within 4 to 5 days of cryotherapy, she may *retain menses*, causing severe discomfort. The cervix can be probed with a cotton-tipped applicator, which will usually release the blood.
- A very rare complication is *cervical stenosis*; using the proper probe tip should prevent this. Avoid any cryotip with projections greater than 5 mm. (See Chapter 126, Cervical Stenosis and Cervical Dilation if it occurs.)
- *Asymmetric freeze of the cervix*. If the cervix is very irregular in shape, consider freezing in segments, starting with the small, slightly nippled tip and then using the flat tip to cover the remaining areas.
- *Treatment failure*. Close follow-up is essential.

It is important to reassure the patient that there have been no documented long-term follow-up complications with future pregnancies after cryotherapy treatment.

POSTPROCEDURE MANAGEMENT

See the patient education handout available at www.expertconsult.com.

1. Give the patient written follow-up information. She will have a profuse watery or blood-tinged discharge for 2 to 4 weeks.
2. Consider a compounded cream to decrease the discharge (see earlier discussion). A peri-pad will be needed for a few weeks.
3. Regular bathing is acceptable. Showers are preferable over baths.
4. Tampons should be avoided because they can irritate the friable cervix and cause bleeding.
5. Intercourse should be avoided for 2 to 3 weeks to allow adequate cervical healing and prevent infection.
6. As previously mentioned, there is no evidence supporting when to follow up. The World Health Organization recommends follow-up with a Pap smear only in a year and then going back to routine Pap screening. An exception to this rule is if the original CIN being treated was CIN3 or greater; in that situation, follow-up Paps should be yearly for 3 years. Many other experts perform a follow-up Pap 6 months after cryotherapy, which

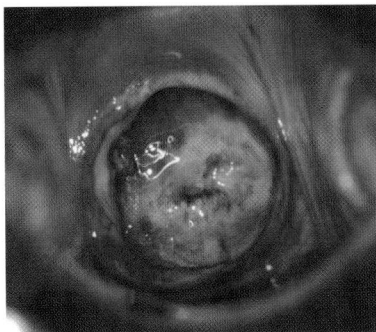

Fig. 125.6 Appearance of the cervix with large eschar 10 days after cryotherapy. (Courtesy John L. Pfenninger, The Medical Procedures Center, Midland, MI.)

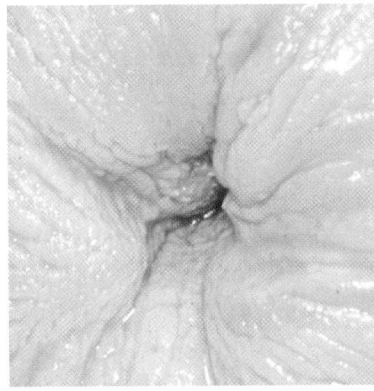

Fig. 125.8 Appearance of the cervix 8 to 10 weeks after cryotherapy. Note radial striations. (Courtesy Duane Townsend, MD, Park City, UT.)

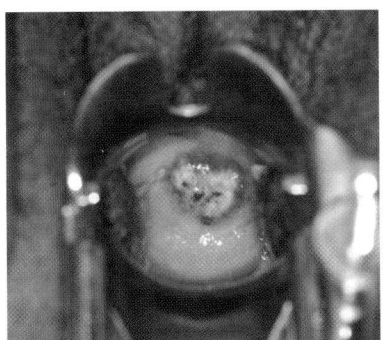

Fig. 125.7 Appearance of the cervix 6 weeks after cryotherapy. (Courtesy Duane Townsend, MD, Midway, UT.)

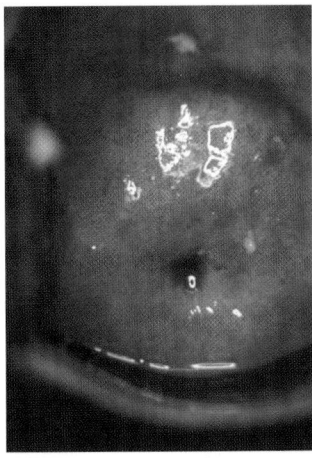

Fig. 125.9 Appearance of the cervix 8 months after cryotherapy. Note the smooth ectocervix and lack of ectocervical transformation zone. The squamocolumnar junction is located right at the os. (Courtesy Duane Townsend, MD, Park City, UT.)

allows adequate time for the cervical tissues to recover. If that Pap smear is normal, the test should be repeated in another 6 months. Colposcopy or human papillomavirus DNA testing may be performed along with either of these Pap tests and may be especially useful if the patient had an initial high-grade lesion (see the American Society for Colposcopy and Cervical Pathology Guidelines in Appendix K). If follow-up laboratory results are normal, routine Pap examinations are resumed. Most recurrences appear within the first year after cryotherapy. If any of the postcryotherapy test results are abnormal, a complete reevaluation should be performed, including colposcopy, biopsy—especially endocervical sampling—and treatment. The cervix will have an altered appearance after cryotherapy, taking up to 4 months to return to a totally normal appearance (Figs. 125.6–125.10).

NOTE: Although some authors previously recommended bringing a patient back to the office after 2 to 7 days to "debride the cervix" in order to reduce the discharge, this procedure has been found to be of little or no value.

PATIENT EDUCATION GUIDES

See the patient education and patient consent forms available at www.expertconsult.com.

CPT/BILLING CODES

57511   Cryocautery of cervix, initial or repeat

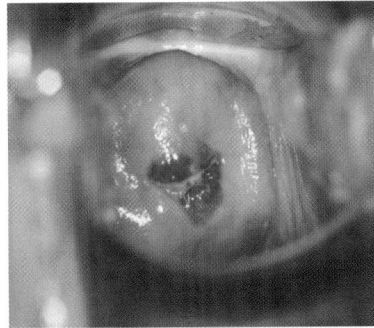

Fig. 125.10 Inadequate cryotherapy because the transformation zone has not been eliminated. Repeat treatment is not necessary unless significant abnormalities recur.

ICD-10-CM DIAGNOSTIC CODES

A63.0	Condyloma acuminatum
N87.0	Mild dysplasia of cervix (CIN 1)
N87.1	Moderate dysplasia of cervix (CIN 2)
D06.9	CIN 3/carcinoma in situ of cervix
N72	Chronic cervicitis (use additional code B95–B97 to identify infectious agent)

SUPPLIERS

(See contact information available at www.expertconsult.com.)

CooperSurgical, Inc.
Wallach Surgical Devices, Inc.

RECOMMENDED READING

Apgar BS, Kaufman AJ, Bettcher C, Parker-Featherstone E. Gynecologic procedures: colposcopy, treatment of cervical intraepithelial neoplasia, and endometrial assessment. *Am Family Physician*. 2013;87(12):836–843.

Castro W, Gage J, Gaffikin L, et al. *Effectiveness, Safety and Acceptability of Cryotherapy: A Systematic literature Review*. Seattle, WA: Program for Appropriate Technology in Health; 2003.

Denny L, Kuhn L, De Souza M, et al. Screen-and-treat approaches for cervical cancer prevention in low-resource settings: a randomized controlled trial. JAMA. 2005;294:2173–2181.

Gajjar K, Martin-Hirsch PPL, Bryant A, Owens GL. Pain relief for women with cervical intraepithelial neoplasia undergoing colposcopy treatment. *Cochrane Database Syst Rev*. 2016;(7):Art. No.:CD006120.

Hacker NF. Cervical dysplasia and cancer. In: Hacker NF, Gambone JC, Hobel JC, eds. *Hacker and Moore's Essentials of Obstetrics and Gynecology*. 6th ed. Philadelphia: Elsevier; 2016:429–439.

Kyrgiou M, Athanasiou A, Kalliala IEJ, et al. Obstetric outcomes after conservative treatment for cervical intraepithelial lesions and early invasive disease. *Cochrane Database Syst Rev*. 2017;(11):Art. No.: CD012847.

Luciani S, Gonzales M, Munoz S, et al. Effectiveness of cryotherapy treatment for cervical intraepithelial neoplasia. *Int J Gynaecol Obstet*. 2008;101:172–177.

Sherris J, Wittet S, Kleine A, et al. Evidence-based, alternative cervical cancer screening approaches in low-resource settings. *Int Perspect Sex Reprod Health*. 2009;35:147–154.

Spitzer M, Brotzman GL, Apgar BS. Practical therapeutic options for treatment of cervical intraepithelial neoplasia. In: Apgar BS, Brotzman GL, Spitzer M, eds. *Colposcopy: Principles and Practice*. 2nd ed. Philadelphia: Saunders; 2008:505–520.

World Health Organization. *Comprehensive Cervical Cancer Control: A Guide to Essential Practice*. 2nd ed. Geneva: World Health Organization; 2014.

Massad LS, Einstein MH, Huh WK, et al. 2012 update consensus guidelines for the management of abnormal cervical screening tests and cancer precursors. *J Low Genit Tract Dis*. 2013;17(5 supp 1):S1–S27.

van der Heijden E, Lopes AD, Bryant A, Bekkers R, Galaal K. Follow-up strategies after treatment (large loop excision of the transformation zone (LLETZ)) for cervical intraepithelial neoplasia (CIN): impact of human papillomavirus (HPV) test. *Cochrane Database Syst Rev*. 2015;1:Art. No.: CD010757.

CHAPTER 126

CERVICAL STENOSIS AND CERVICAL DILATION

Linda Prine

Cervical stenosis is a stricture or narrowing of the cervix; it is diagnosed by the inability to pass a 2-mm dilator into the uterus. Cervical stenosis can be either congenital or acquired. Acquired stenosis can result from postoperative scarring (from conization, whether it be cold knife, large loop electrosurgery, or laser; cautery; or cryotherapy of the cervix), cancer (endometrial or endocervical), radiation complications, infections, or atrophy from lack of estrogen (most common). In acquired cases the external os is most frequently affected (Fig. 126.1). In congenital cases, seen most often in nulliparous cervices, the stenosis is usually at the internal os.

Narrowing of the cervical canal can impede menstrual flow, causing increased intrauterine pressure during menses. Premenopausal women with cervical stenosis may have pelvic pain, dysmenorrhea, amenorrhea, infertility, or abnormal bleeding. In some cases retrograde menstrual flow may occur, causing endometriosis. Women may have a soft, slightly tender midpelvic mass as a result of hematometra. Postmenopausal women may have pyometra, which is highly suspect for endometrial carcinoma.

Ultrasound can be used to assess canal anatomy while also evaluating the patient for hematometra and pyometra. Most often cervical stenosis is discovered when the clinician is attempting to enter the uterus for a Pap smear, hysteroscopy, intrauterine device (IUD) insertion, endometrial biopsy, uterine aspiration for elective or spontaneous abortion, or placement of Essure birth control devices.

CERVICAL DILATION

Treatment of cervical stenosis consists of dilation by using (1) progressive metal or plastic dilators, (2) osmotic dilators, (3) prostaglandin analogs, or a combination of these.

Cervical dilatation is an unpleasant procedure; cervical priming prior to operative procedures not only improves the tolerance but also facilitates the operation and reduces the risk of cervical injury and uterine perforation. Agents commonly used for this purpose include osmotic dilators (e.g., laminaria sticks or tents, synthetic osmotic dilators) and various prostaglandin preparations. Osmotic dilators are more effective than prostaglandins for priming the cervix, but a combination of the two is also very effective. Laminaria sticks or tents (e.g., Dilatera) are made from the dried stems of seaweed, usually *Laminaria japonica*. Self-expanding synthetic osmotic cervical dilators (e.g., Dilapan) that resemble laminaria sticks can also be used. Once the dilators are placed into the endocervical canal, they rehydrate and expand, thereby causing dilation of the cervical canal (Figs. 126.2 and 126.3). Laminaria sticks should not be used if pyometra is present or infection is suspected. The os and canal must be patent enough to admit the osmotic dilators, which are available in several diameters. Some mechanical dilation may be necessary to allow their placement. Another option for the treatment of external os stenosis is the use of the carbon dioxide laser or a small radiofrequency loop excision. These last two methods can remove a stricture that is readily visible externally.

Clinicians now also use misoprostol for softening and dilating the cervix. Although misoprostol is most effective on the pregnant uterus and very small doses are often all that is needed, efficacy has been shown in nonpregnant uteri, especially in women of reproductive age. Studies of misoprostol's effectiveness in postmenopausal women are conflicting; fortunately pretreatment with vaginal estrogen for 2 weeks before dilation may augment the effect of misoprostol. In nonpregnant uteri or in the first trimester, two to four 200-μg tablets administered vaginally, buccally, or sublingually 1 to 2 hours before the procedure is usually effective. Patients can also take the same dose the night before. Women should be warned of the side effects of misoprostol, including diarrhea, cramping, uterine bleeding, and fever.

Injection of dilute vasopressin (0.05 U/mL) into the cervical stroma has also been found to decrease the force needed to dilate the cervix (Phillips, 1997). In this case a dilute solution (4 U of 0.05 U/mL in 80 mL of normal saline) was injected intracervically, 10 mL each at the 4 o'clock and 8 o'clock positions, immediately before the dilation. When used in conjunction with hysteroscopy, it had the added benefits of decreased procedure time, fluid intravasation, and operative blood loss.

The majority of dilations can be performed in the office. For extremely anxious patients or if pain cannot be controlled easily, the procedure may need to be performed in the operating room. Although a Cochrane review (Tangsiriwatthana, 2013) found that women had less pain with cervical dilation and uterine instrumentation following a paracervical block than with placebo injection, the investigators found that clinically this may be unimportant. There was no evidence that paracervical block reduced pain compared with regional or systemic anesthesia.

INDICATIONS

- Symptomatic stenosis (e.g., dysmenorrhea)
- Inability to obtain adequate Pap smears
- IUD insertion
- To perform an indicated endocervical curettage or dilation and curettage
- To perform an aspiration abortion
- If needed for hysterosalpingography
- Before hysteroscopy
- Before endometrial ablation
- To perform an endometrial biopsy
- To insert an Essure device for mechanical tubal occlusion

CONTRAINDICATIONS

The procedure is absolutely contraindicated in a patient who is trying to become pregnant.

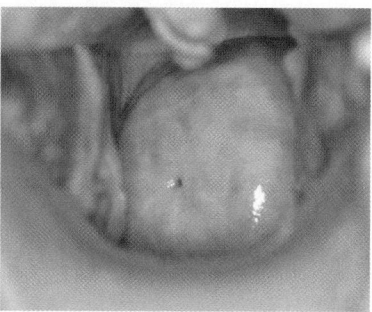

Fig. 126.1   External os stenosis after loop electrosurgical excision procedure.

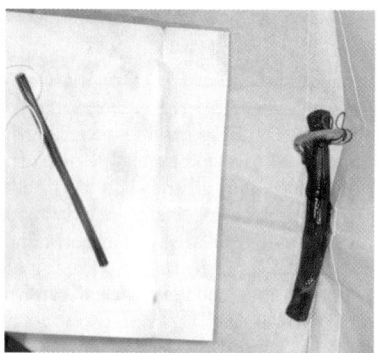

Fig. 126.2   *Left,* Laminaria before insertion. *Right,* Expanded laminaria after removal.

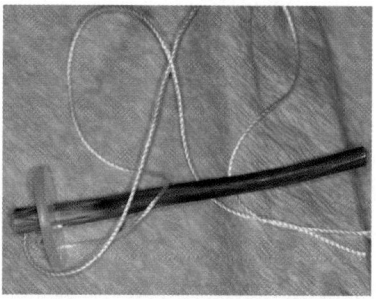

Fig. 126.3   Closeup of laminaria in Fig. 126.2A.

- Laminaria tents are not to be used in cases of pyometra or prior allergic reaction to laminaria (very rare).
- Pelvic inflammatory disease; vaginal or cervical infections (treat before dilation).

EQUIPMENT

- Table that allows the patient to be placed in the lithotomy position
- Needle extender or long spinal needle to provide local anesthesia if needed (see Chapter 127, Loop Electrosurgical Excision Procedure for Treating Cervical Intraepithelial Neoplasia)
- 5 mL 1% lidocaine
- Adequate light source
- Appropriately sized vaginal speculum
- Nonsterile gloves; use sterile gloves if a procedure entering the uterus is to be performed
- Equipment to follow universal blood and body fluid precautions
- Ring forceps
- Uterine sound—plastic or malleable metal preferred

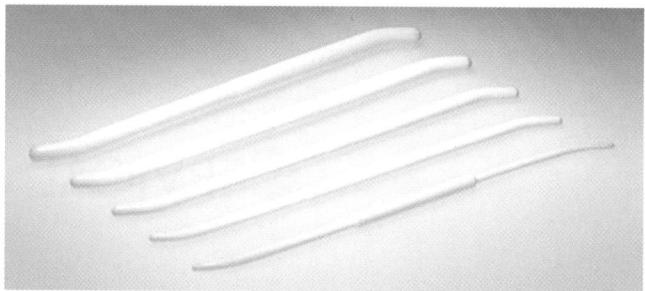

Fig. 126.4   Denniston plastic dilators, 5 to 14 mm sizes.

- Denniston plastic (1 to 8 mm; Fig. 126.4) or metal (e.g., Hegar, Hank, Pratt, 1 to 6 mm) dilators and/or osmotic stick or tent (various sizes; see Fig. 126.2)
- OS Finder, os locator, or very small silver probe (like an ophthalmic lacrimal duct probe)
- Cervical single-tooth tenaculum
- Paracervical block kit with 10 mL 1% lidocaine in a 10-mL syringe with a 6-in 20-gauge needle; may be helpful if dilation of more than 4 to 6 mm is done (see Chapter 153, Paracervical Block)
- 4 × 4 inch gauze pads; povidone-iodine or chlorhexidine solution
- Ultrasound machine with abdominal probe if needed for guidance (optional)

PREPROCEDURE PATIENT EDUCATION

- Obtain informed consent from the patient. (See the patient consent form available at www.expertconsult.com.)
- The patient can take 400 to 800 µg of misoprostol orally or insert the same dose vaginally at home the night before the procedure or an hour or two before the procedure; the clinician can also insert it at the time of the procedure when the stenosis is discovered. For postmenopausal women, pretreatment with vaginal estrogen for 2 weeks before dilation may augment the effect of misoprostol.
- Generally 800 mg of ibuprofen 1 hour before the procedure helps with pain management. Consider diazepam 10 mg by mouth for the anxious patient.
- If further sedation is needed, see Chapter 1, Procedural Sedation and Analgesia.

PROCEDURE

1. Place the patient in the lithotomy position.
2. Following universal blood and body fluid precautions, perform a pelvic examination to evaluate the size and position of the uterus.
3. Prepare the cervix and vagina with povidone-iodine (or diluted chlorhexidine if the patient is allergic to povidone-iodine).
4. Try to cannulate the cervical canal with a small silver probe, the 2-mm dilator, or the OS Finder or os locator (Fig. 126.5). If the patient becomes uncomfortable, administer 5 mL of a local anesthetic submucosally at the 12, 3, 6, and 9 o'clock positions on the cervix (see Chapter 127, Loop Electrosurgical Excision Procedure for Treating Cervical Intraepithelial Neoplasia), or use a paracervical block with 5 mL lidocaine at the 4 and 8 o'clock positions (see Chapter 153, Paracervical Block). Aspirate for blood before injecting to ensure that the needle is not in a blood vessel. The use of a local injection into the cervix may obviate the need for the more complicated and uncomfortable paracervical block.
5. If the cervix is too mobile, place a tenaculum at the 12 o'clock or 6 o'clock position and use it to apply traction on the cervix while dilating it (Fig. 126.6). The straightening action of

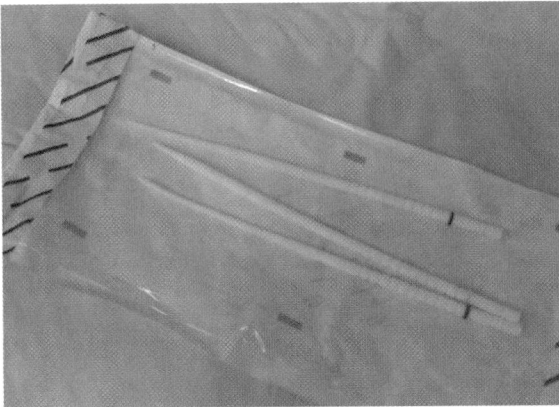

Fig. 126.5 Os finder.

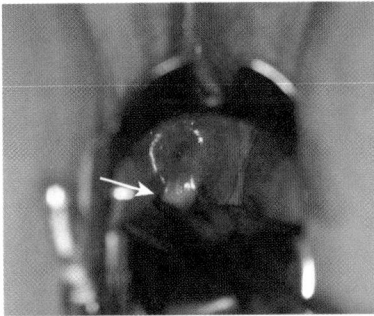

Fig. 126.6 Single-tooth tenaculum placed posteriorly *(arrow)* on the cervix.

placing traction on the cervix (Fig. 126.7) is often the solution to the problem of uteri with extremes of anatomic flexion. Use progressively larger dilators and proceed slowly.

6. Once the external os has been entered, the most difficult part of the procedure is passing through the internal os. If the sound/dilator does not pass readily, apply the tenaculum if this has not already been done. The OS Finder or os locator usually enters the lumen without creating a false passage. It often takes firm, steady pressure on the dilators to penetrate the internal os. Be patient with this; sometimes it takes 10 to 20 seconds of firm, steady pressure before the internal os finally gives way. To avoid perforation, the plastic Denniston dilators are strongly recommended. (This step causes significant anxiety in the clinician!) The clinician should be able to feel the smooth contour of the cervical canal. A rough surface as the dilator advances is a strong indicator that a false passage is being created. (If the roughness is felt, this would be a good time to confirm orientation with ultrasonography if this is not already in use.) As the tenaculum is pulled outward, the dilator is pushed forward until a "give" is felt. Insert the dilator finder just through the internal os.

7. Gradually insert larger dilators until the degree of dilation needed for the particular procedure is attained.

8. If needed, a plastic, malleable, or metal uterine sound can be inserted to determine the size of the uterine cavity. If a metal sound is used, bend it to conform to the position of the uterus as determined on the pelvis (anteverted or retroverted). The sound should pass easily before resistance is felt. For the normal-sized uterus, this should be no more than 10 cm (possibly 12 cm). If the sound goes beyond this, suspect perforation unless the clinical examination or ultrasonography suggested a large uterus. If a perforation occurs, stop further efforts. (See later discussion.)

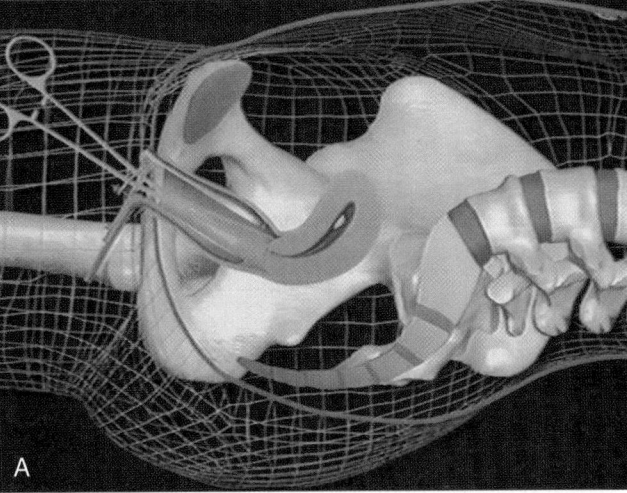

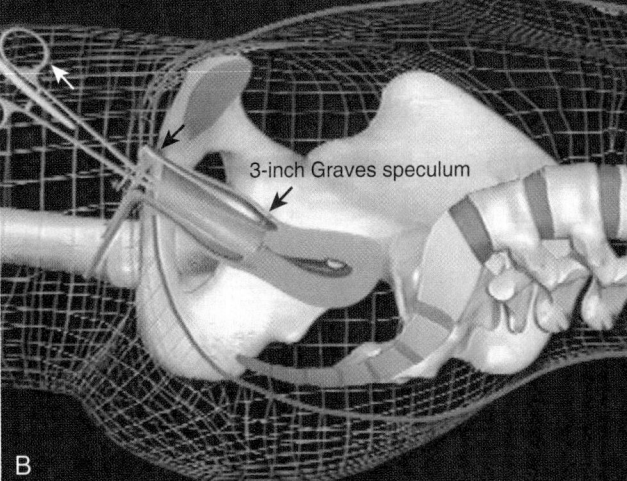

3-inch Graves speculum

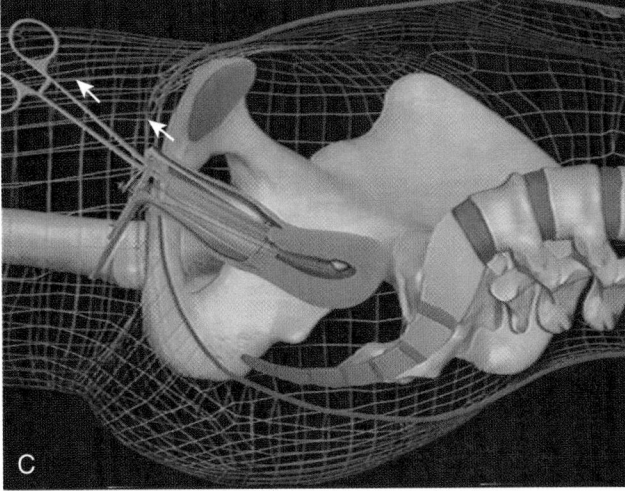

Fig. 126.7 Application of traction to the cervix is often the solution to the problem of uteri with extremes of anatomic flexion. (A) A tenaculum has been applied to the cervix of an anteroflexed uterus. (B) By applying outward traction *(arrows)* on the tenaculum, the uterus is straightened. (C) Dilators can now be inserted. Additional pressure on the speculum against the perineum is sometimes needed for the acutely ante-flexed uterus in order to create a straightened passageway.

9. Dilation to 4 to 6 mm is sufficient for most non–pregnancy-related procedures and is usually readily accomplished in the office. When inserting the dilator, rest your fourth and fifth fingers

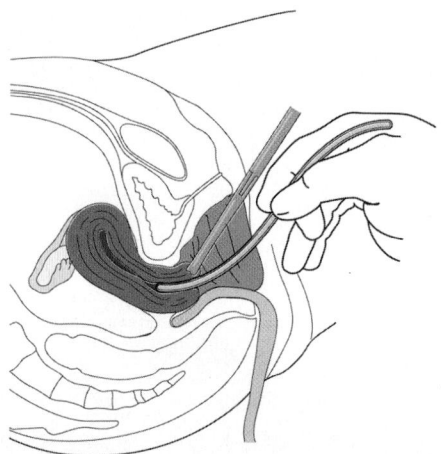

Fig. 126.8 Cervical dilation using a Hegar dilator. During the procedure, the fourth and fifth fingers rest against the perineal area in order to prevent uncontrolled movements of the dilator, which can lead to uterine perforation. A weighted speculum is in the posterior vagina. The tenaculum is applied to the anterior lip of the cervix.

on the perineum and buttocks to prevent uncontrolled movements of the dilator (Fig. 126.8).
10. Perform the procedure indicated.

LAMINARIA TENT OR SYNTHETIC OSMOTIC DILATOR PLACEMENT

1. For laminaria tents or synthetic osmotic dilators to be used, the external os must be patent. Subsequently, they are used either for internal os stenosis or for a gradual dilation of the canal for larger procedures. They come in various sizes, and more than one may be inserted for greater dilation if needed.
2. Prepare the patient and cervix as described previously.
3. Sound the endocervix if possible.
4. Grasp the cervix with the tenaculum, if necessary, and use it to apply traction on the cervix (see Fig. 126.6).
5. Hold the string end of the osmotic dilator with ring forceps and insert it into the os, ensuring that the dilator does not extend into the uterine cavity. If using laminaria, choose the largest tent that will fit into the os. Sometimes this may be quite small. If you are unable to insert the synthetic osmotic dilator, you may have to dilate the os further before its insertion (Figs. 126.9 and 126.10).
6. Osmotic dilators are quite long and usually protrude out of the cervix for several millimeters.
7. Cover the cervix and the inserted osmotic dilator with a sterile 4- × 4-inch gauze pad that has been dipped into dilute povidone-iodine solution and tuck the edges into the fornices. Then place several dry 4- × 4-inch gauze pads over the first one to hold the laminaria tent in place (Fig. 126.11).
8. Remove the speculum while holding the gauze pads in place with the ring forceps.
9. To prevent infection, the dilator should be removed within 24 hours by grasping it with a ring forceps, rotating it 360 degrees, and pulling it out. Lesser procedures may require a wait of only 8 to 12 hours. Often the osmotic dilator is inserted at the end of the day and removed the next morning. Alternatively, the patient can be the first one seen during the morning, with the osmotic dilator removed when she is seen again as the last patient of the day. It may be necessary to replace an initial small laminaria with a larger one if the dilation is not adequate on removal. If there is difficulty removing the dilator, misoprostol can be helpful, especially if it was not used before.

10. Dilation can cause significant cramping; ibuprofen 600 mg every 6 hours is advised.

COMMON ERRORS

- The most common error is failure to straighten the uterus. This occurs by not placing sufficient traction on the tenaculum or by using a speculum with long blades, trapping a flexed uterus in its flexed position. Failure to make this adjustment can result in uterine perforation, the most common complication of a difficult dilation.
- The osmotic dilator may fail to dilate the canal because it has not been inserted far enough. Sounding the canal and marking the dilator will aid in knowing when it has been inserted far enough (see Fig. 126.9C).
- The osmotic dilator can be inserted too far, making it difficult to remove because of a bulbous swelling inside the uterine cavity (see Fig. 126.9D).

COMPLICATIONS

- Pain.
- Hemorrhage.
- Infection (especially if the laminaria tent is left in over 24 hours).
- Anaphylaxis or allergic reaction to the laminaria tent or misoprostol (rare).
- Inability to dilate the os.
- Laminaria tents can break or separate on removal, making retrieval of the pieces difficult.
- Inability to remove the luminaria tent because of an excessively deep placement.

Many clinicians are fearful of a perforation, but it is generally uneventful unless it is not recognized. The perforation can be complicated if further procedures are attempted and the instruments are introduced beyond the uterine cavity. If perforation is suspected, no further instrumentation should be done. Explain to the patient what is suspected. After 30 minutes of observation, if vital signs are stable and there is no pain, she can go home. She should report any fever, pain, or excessive bleeding. A follow-up visit or phone call within 24 hours is advisable. Repeat cannulation or dilation can be attempted after 6 to 8 weeks.

POSTPROCEDURE PATIENT EDUCATION

See also Chapter 162, Dilation and Curettage.

- If a laminaria tent or synthetic osmotic dilator is placed, the patient should be instructed to return within 24 hours for removal; 8 to 12 hours is often adequate.
- The patient should not engage in sexual intercourse while the dilator is in place.
- If dilation was performed for cervical stenosis causing hematometra or pyometra or after an excisional procedure, the patient should be instructed to return in 4 to 6 weeks for repeat examination and possible repeat dilation.
- The patient should return or call for fever, abdominal or pelvic pain, purulent vaginal discharge, or bleeding.
- In postmenopausal women not on estrogen replacement or those with low estrogen states (e.g., Depo-Provera or Implanon users), estrogen cream helps maintain patency of the os. This is especially important if dilation was done for postsurgical (conization) scarring complications.

CONCLUSION

Cervical stenosis may require cervical dilation several times on a monthly basis to keep the os patent. Pregnancy and vaginal delivery

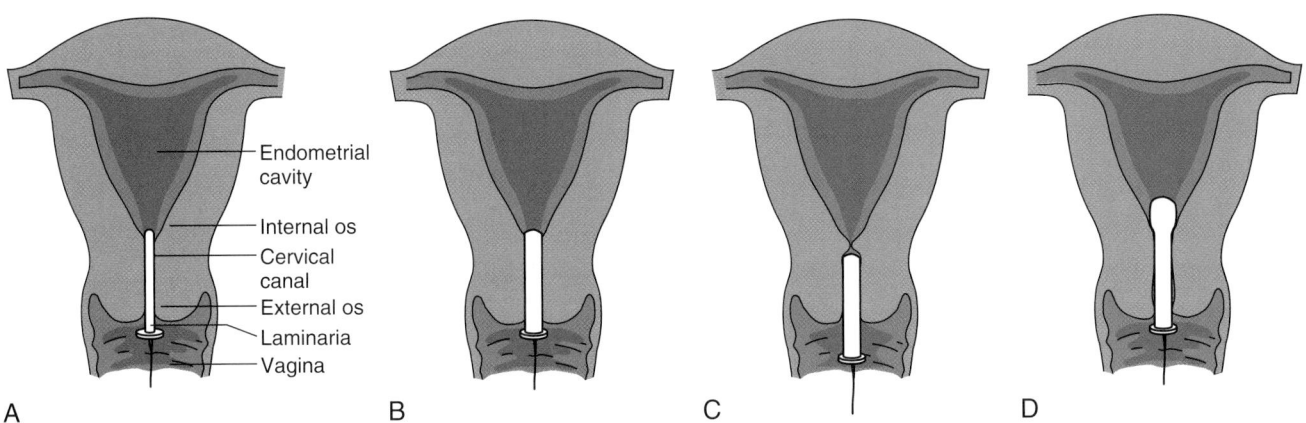

A   B   C   D

Fig. 126.9 Insertion of a laminaria tent. (A) The laminaria tent immediately after placement. Note that the upper end is just through the internal os. It is difficult to determine this optimal position, and it is not possible to obtain it with internal os stenosis. (B) The laminaria tent 24 hours later. (C) The laminaria tent not placed far enough to dilate the internal os. (D) The laminaria tent inserted too far, making it difficult to remove.

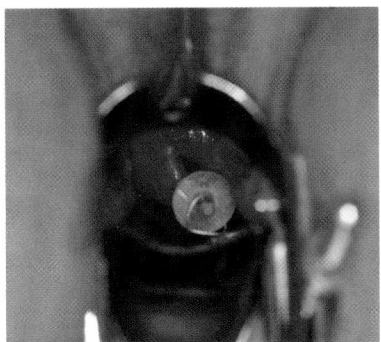

Fig. 126.10 Inserted laminaria tent. It is difficult to appreciate that the tent actually protrudes 2 mm outside the cervix.

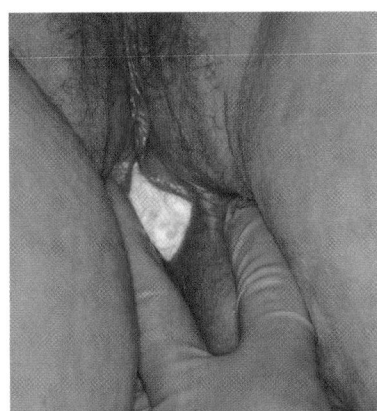

Fig. 126.11 Laminaria held in place with 4- ×4-inch gauze inserted in the vagina. Patients tolerate this surprisingly well.

may actually lead to a more lasting cure. As long as the patient is menstruating and is asymptomatic and a Pap smear can be obtained, clinician intervention is not needed.

PATIENT EDUCATION GUIDES

See patient education and consent forms available at www.expertconsult.com.

CPT/BILLING CODES

57505	Endocervical curettage
57800	Dilatation of cervical canal, instrumental
58120	Dilation and curettage, diagnostic and/or therapeutic (nonobstetric)
59200	Insertion of cervical dilator (e.g., laminaria, prostaglandin), separate procedure

ICD-10-CM DIAGNOSTIC CODES

N88.2	Cervical stenosis

Acknowledgment

The editors recognize the contributions of Kathleen T. Dor, MD, to this chapter in a previous edition of this text.

SUPPLIERS

(See contact information available at www.expertconsult.com.)

Laminaria
 Norscan Medical
Laminaria, mechanical dilators, os locator, canal finder
 MedGyn, Cooper Surgical
Synthetic osmotic dilators (Dilapan)
 MPM Medical Supply

ONLINE RESOURCES

The Indian Health Service provides a good review of the topic: http://www.ihs.gov/medicalprograms/MCH/m/documents/MisoIUD4306.doc

RECOMMENDED READING

Gkrozou F, Koliopoulos G, Vrekoussis T, et al. A systematic review and meta-analysis of randomized studies comparing misoprostol versus placebo for cervical ripening prior to hysteroscopy. *Eur J Obstet Gynecol Reprod Biol.* 2011;158(1):17–23.
Hammoud AO, Deppe G, Elkhechen SS, Johnson S. Ultrasonography-guided transvaginal endometrial biopsy: a useful technique in patients with cervical stenosis. *Obstet Gynecol.* 2006;107:518–520.
Kapp N, Lohr PA, Ngo TD, Hayes JL. Cervical preparation for first trimester surgical abortion. *Cochrane Database Syst Rev.* 2010:Art. No:CD007207.
Nada AM, Elzayat AR, Metwally AA, Taher AM, Ogila AL, et al. Cervical priming by vaginal or oral misoprostol before operative hysteroscopy: a double-blind randomized controlled trial. *J Minim Invasive Gynecol.* 2016;7:1107–1112.

Ngai SW, Chan YM, Liu KL, Ho PC. Oral misoprostol for cervical priming in non-pregnant women. *Hum Reprod.* 1997;12:2373–2375.

Philips DR, Nathanson HG, Milim SJ, Haselkorn JS. The effect of dilute vasopressin solution on the force needed for cervical dilation: a randomized controlled trial. *Obstet Gynecol.* 1997;89(4):507–511.

Tangsiriwatthana T, Sangkomkamhang US, Lumbiganon P, Laopaiboon M. Paracervical local anaesthesia for cervical dilatation and uterine intervention. *Cochrane Database Syst Rev.* 2013;9:Art. No.: CD005056.

LOOP ELECTROSURGICAL EXCISION PROCEDURE FOR TREATING CERVICAL INTRAEPITHELIAL NEOPLASIA

Thomas C. Wright

A variety of techniques can be used to treat cervical intraepithelial neoplasia (CIN), although excisional (e.g., loop electrosurgical excision procedure [LEEP], cold knife conization) and ablative (e.g., cryotherapy, laser, electrocautery) techniques have about the same outcomes for the eradication of CIN. Excisional methods are associated with an increased risk of adverse obstetric outcomes, such as preterm labor and low birth weight. That said, the appropriateness of a particular technique to treat a particular lesion depends on a number of factors, including lesion size, location, extension into the endocervical canal, and desire for future pregnancy. Many clinicians now use LEEP to treat most women with biopsy-confirmed CIN 2 or CIN 3. With LEEP, thin wire loop electrodes are used to excise the entire cervical transformation zone (TZ). This procedure is referred to by a number of different names, including LEEP, large loop excision of the transformation zone, and loop excision. Many clinicians subdivide LEEP into two procedures: (1) routine LEEP, which is used to excise lesions confined to the exocervix (or visible portion of the cervix), and (2) LEEP conization, which is used when lesions extend into the endocervical canal. LEEP has a number of advantages over other treatment modalities for CIN, including the following:

- The equipment is less expensive than laser equipment.
- The entire lesion is excised and can be assessed histologically to rule out invasive cancer.
- Patients can be diagnosed and treated in a single office visit.
- It allows cervical conization to be performed in the office at a significantly reduced cost (LEEP conization).
- Complications are few for the procedure itself, but it can affect future pregnancies.

LEEP uses an electrosurgical cutting setting that achieves some coagulation while cutting by blending both cutting and coagulation electrical currents. This combination of electrical currents is called *blended cutting*. The type of coagulation used in in LEEP is called *fulguration*. Fulguration is achieved using a 5-mm ball electrode. The ball electrode does not touch the tissue; the activated current sprays multiple sparks between the ball, electrode, and tissue.

ANATOMY

The anatomy relevant to LEEP is reviewed in detail in Chapter 124, Colposcopic Examination. As the procedure involves complete removal of the TZ, it is important to understand the anatomy of the cervix, including normal and abnormal appearances. In most circumstances, a colposcopy will be completed prior to LEEP to define the anatomy of the cervix.

INDICATIONS

The following indications are based on the 2012 American Society for Colposcopy and Cervical Pathology guidelines, which are reproduced in Appendix K. Several options are given for the treatment of most of these indications. This chapter presents the possible indications for LEEP.

Routine Loop Electrosurgical Excision Procedure

- Biopsy-confirmed CIN 2 or CIN 3 and a satisfactory colposcopy
- High-grade squamous intraepithelial lesion (HSIL) on referral cytologic examination that is immediately treated in a patient over age 20 ("screen and treat")
- Persistent HSIL on screening for 6 to 12 months (without CIN 2 or 3 documented by biopsy)
- CIN 1 on biopsy after screening result of HSIL or atypical glandular cells–not otherwise specified

When several treatment options exist within the treatment guidelines, LEEP is preferred over ablative therapies such as cryotherapy in the following conditions:

- High-grade lesion involving three or more quadrants.
- Complex-appearing CIN 2 or CIN 3 with prominent abnormal vessels.
- Lesion is not covered by cryoprobe.
- Ectocervix is irregular.
- Patients have recurrent CIN after previous therapy (e.g., cone biopsy, LEEP, cryotherapy).

Loop Electrosurgical Excision Procedure Conization

- Unsatisfactory colposcopy in women with biopsy-confirmed CIN of any grade (e.g., cannot see entire lesion, squamocolumnar junction, or TZ)
- HSIL on referral cytologic examination and unsatisfactory colposcopy
- HSIL on referral cytologic examination with satisfactory colposcopy and either no CIN or only CIN I identified ("lack of correlation principle")
- Positive endocervical sampling (e.g., neoplasia of any grade present)
- Microinvasive lesions on cervical biopsy

CONTRAINDICATIONS

Absolute

- Pregnancy
- Clinically apparent invasive carcinoma of the cervix
- Lack of expertise to control potential severe cervical bleeding

Relative

- Bleeding diathesis
- Patient exposed in utero to diethylstilbestrol
- Patient is fewer than 12 weeks postdelivery
- Equivocal cervical abnormalities
- Heavy menses
- A preexisting short cervix (clinician should consider referral)
- Patients with pacemakers (special precaution necessary)
- Severe cervicitis

EQUIPMENT AND SUPPLIES

- Electrosurgical generator or unit (ESU) (Fig. 127.1) with the following features:
  - Minimum output capability of 50 W in both cutting and coagulation modes
  - Rapid-start features
  - Patient grounding pad monitor (beneficial if the patient is under anesthesia)
  - Isolated circuitry

  EDITOR'S NOTE: Although the Ellman Surgitron does not meet some of these qualifications, it has been used extensively for LEEP.

- Loop electrodes of the appropriate size and a ball electrode for fulguration (Fig. 127.2). (These electrodes can be either of the disposable or reusable variety.)It is recommended that clinicians use only the shallow loop electrodes (i.e., either 0.8 or 1.0 cm deep) for routine LEEP. Larger electrodes can be used with large cervices or when lesions extend into the endocervical canal (e.g., LEEP conization). A variation is the Fischer electrode, which provides a true "cone" specimen.
- Electrode handle and a patient return electrode (grounding pad or antenna).
- Nonconductive speculum (either coated with a nonconductive material or made of plastic) capable of being used in conjunction with a smoke evacuator (Fig. 127.3).
- Smoke evacuator equipped with an adequate viral and odor filter.
- Colposcope capable of low magnification (4× to 7.5×).
- Nonsterile gloves and equipment to follow universal blood and body fluid precautions.
- Acetic acid (5%).
- Full-strength aqueous Lugol solution.
- Cotton balls and large ob-gyn applicators.
- Ring forceps.
- Syringe (5-mL) with 4-inch needle extender and 1.5-inch 25-gauge needle as well as 5 mL of 2% lidocaine with epinephrine or dental type of syringe equipped with a 25- to 27-gauge needle at least 1.5 inches long with two 1.8-mL ampules of 2% lidocaine with 1:100,000 epinephrine (Fig. 127.4).
- Topical benzocaine oral spray (e.g., Americaine, Hurricane) (optional).
- Coated vaginal sidewall retractor (see Fig. 127.3).
- Kevorkian endocervical curette.
- Monsel paste, which is made by allowing Monsel solution to evaporate until it forms a thick yellow paste.
- Containers of histologic fixative (usually 10% formalin).

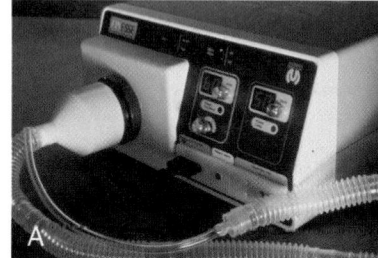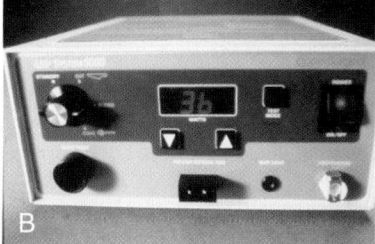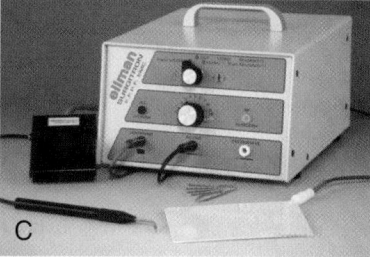

Fig. 127.1 Electrosurgical units used for loop electrosurgical excision procedure (LEEP). (A) Utah Medical electrosurgical unit. The smoke evacuator is included in the basic unit. (B) CooperSurgical LEEP unit. (C) Ellman Surgitron with handpiece, electrodes, antenna plate, and foot pedal. (A, Courtesy Utah Medical Products, Inc., Midvale, UT. B, Courtesy CooperSurgical, Trumbull, CT. C, Courtesy Ellman Cynosure, Hicksville, NY.)

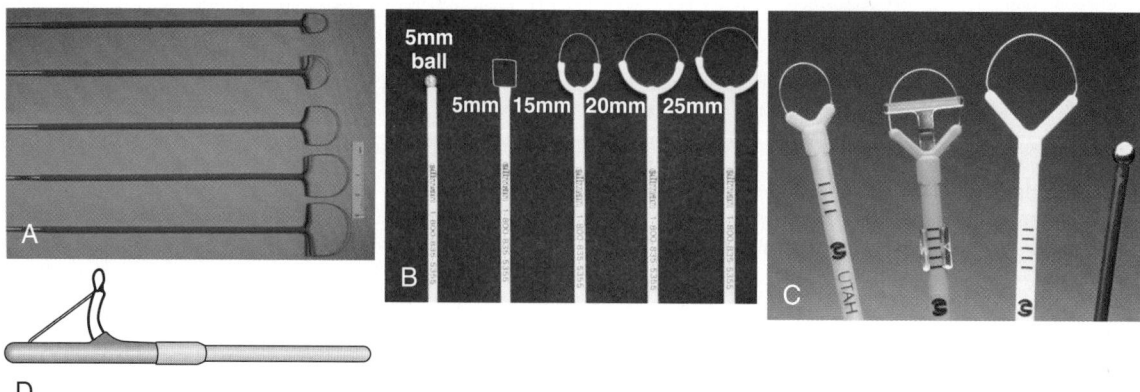

Fig. 127.2 Wire loop electrodes for loop electrosurgical excision procedure. (A) Loop electrodes come in a variety of sizes and shapes. (B) Ellman electrodes. (C) Utah Medical electrodes with an optional adjustable stop to limit depth (*middle*, green-handled loop). (D) Fischer electrode, which removes more of a conical piece. (A–C, Courtesy John L. Pfenninger, MD, Courtesy The Medical Procedures Center, Midland, MI.)

- A 12-inch needle holder and 2-0 Vicryl suture material together with a vaginal pack in the event that large-vessel bleeding occurs.
- Power examination table with adjustable height (recommended).

PRECAUTIONS

It is imperative that LEEP not be used to excise the TZ indiscriminately in women with atypical Papanicolaou (Pap) smears. The procedure should be reserved to treat advanced lesions as per the established indications, not just atypical Pap smears or CIN 1. CIN 1 has a high rate of regression and should usually be observed or treated with less invasive options. Cryotherapy is less expensive; has fewer complications, especially related to future pregnancies; and has equal outcomes in properly selected patients (while at the same time removing less tissue) (see Chapter 125, Cryotherapy of the Cervix). Cold-knife conization is preferred when conization is being performed for a glandular abnormality.

PREPROCEDURE PATIENT EDUCATION

- Provide a patient education handout (see the sample patient education handout available at www.expertconsult.com).
- Instruct the patient to take 600 to 800 mg of ibuprofen or a preferred nonsteroidal antiinflammatory drug 1 to 2 hours before the procedure.
  EDITOR'S NOTE: Although a Cochrane review in 2016 found no benefit to nonsteroidal anti-inflammatory drugs prior to the procedure, most clinicians recommend one. Optimal therapy appears to be intracervical injection of local anesthetic with a vasoconstrictor (e.g., lidocaine with epinephrine).
- Obtain informed consent.

Procedure

The procedure is best performed immediately after menses so that any vaginal bleeding is not confused with menses.

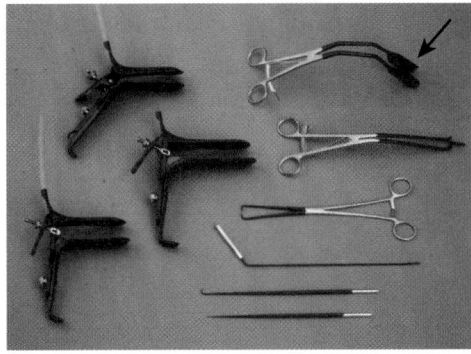

Fig. 127.3 Coated instruments to prevent electrical shocks. Vaginal sidewall retractors *(arrow)* are essential in many cases to avoid lacerating the vaginal walls. Three different vaginal speculums are on the left, each with a vented tube to attach to the smoke evacuator tubing.

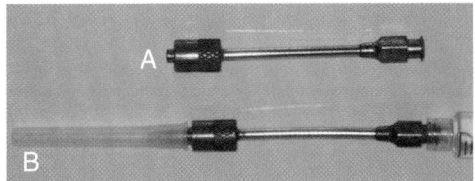

Fig. 127.4 (A) Needle extender (5-inch). (B) Needle extender placed on the end of a 5-mL syringe with a 25-gauge 1.5-inch needle attached. *(Courtesy John L. Pfenninger, MD, The Medical Procedures Center, Midland, MI.)*

1. Have the patient undress from the waist down and lie on the gynecologic examination table. It is important that the patient not move, cough, or change position once the excision is started. Thus a cooperative patient is essential.
2. Attach the patient return electrode grounding pad to the patient's thigh and connect the grounding pad to the ESU (or place the "antenna plate" under the hip). The clinician should follow universal blood and body fluid precautions.
3. Insert a nonconductive speculum with the smoke evacuator attachment into the vagina and connect it to the smoke evacuator. It is important that the speculum be large enough to allow complete, unobstructed visualization of the cervix. If the vaginal sidewalls remain in the way, use a vaginal sidewall retractor (Fig. 127.5, and see Fig. 127.3).
4. Apply the acetic acid solution, examine the cervix colposcopically, and identify all lesions and the TZ.
5. Apply full-strength Lugol solution to the cervix (this lasts longer than acetic acid). Use cotton balls or a large ob-gyn applicator.
6. Although there is little evidence to support it, some minimally invasive gynecologists spray the cervix with topical oral benzocaine before injecting or applying instruments. Next, inject approximately 0.5 to 1.5 mL of 2% lidocaine with epinephrine 1:100,000 intracervically (submucosally) at each of the 12, 3, 6, and 9 o'clock positions (to a total of 2 to 6 mL), usually just outside the TZ. Take care to inject the cervix superficially, only 3 to 5 mm deep. Additional injections may be needed at intervals between those noted previously, depending on the size of the cervix.
   EDITOR'S NOTE: a 2016 Cochrane review of the literature found this to be optimal therapy for pain prior to LEEP.
7. Although loops of many different sizes are available from various manufacturers, a round loop 2 cm wide by 0.8 cm deep (R2008) is most frequently used for CIN lesions confined to the portio. For a small, nulliparous cervix, use a 1.5- × 0.7-cm loop (R1507). For LEEP conizations when lesions extend into the endocervical canal, a 1- × 1-cm loop electrode can be used to excise the endocervical canal itself. This can be performed after the ectocervical excision has been completed to perform a "cowboy hat" type of procedure (see Fig. 127.7C). The power required will depend on the ESU used and the diameter of the loop. In general, a 2.0- × 0.8-cm loop will require between 35 and 45 W of power, whereas a 1- × 1-cm loop will require only 20 to 30 W of power. For LEEP, the use of a blended (cut and coagulate) current provides the combination of minimal tissue artifact and minimal amounts of bleeding. However, many use a pure cutting setting, which provides even less burn artifact for the pathologist while still controlling bleeding. It also allows for the use of less power so that less tissue is damaged. Three different types of cervical LEEP excisions can be performed, depending on the size and location of the CIN lesion: (1) LEEP

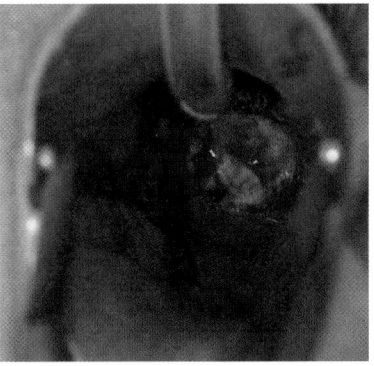

Fig. 127.5 Cervix as seen through a coated vaginal speculum with coated, nonconductive sidewall retractors in place.

for small lesions confined to the exocervix, (2) LEEP for large lesions confined to the ectocervix, and (3) LEEP conization for lesions extending into the endocervix. For small lesions confined to the ectocervix, the following is suggested:

- Select a loop electrode 1.5 to 2.0 cm wide and 0.8 cm deep.
- Place the loop several millimeters lateral to the edge of the CIN lesion and make a test pass over the lesion to ensure that the path is clear.
- Hold the loop just above the surface, activate the loop, and then gradually push it perpendicularly into the tissue to a depth of about 4 mm.
- While pushing the loop deeper into the cervical stroma to the full depth of 8 mm, draw it laterally and through the endocervical canal. Pull it to the other side several millimeters past a lesion or several millimeters beyond the TZ, whichever is more lateral, before removing it (Fig. 127.6).
  NOTE: In most instances the entire CIN lesion and the TZ can be removed in a single pass. This produces a donut-shaped specimen with the endocervical canal in the center.

For larger lesions confined to the ectocervix, the following technique is advised:

- In some instances, CIN lesions may be too extensive to be removed in a single pass. In this event, remove the central portion of the lesion using a 2-cm-wide loop electrode, as previously described.
- Then excise the remaining CIN and TZ with additional, more superficial passes using the same loop electrode. Alternatively, the remaining tissue can be ablated using electrocoagulation with a ball electrode (Fig. 127.7).

For CIN extending into the endocervical canal, LEEP conizations are performed and lesions are removed in a two-step procedure that uses a 2-cm-wide exocervical electrode in conjunction with a 1- × 1-cm loop or square endocervical electrode to produce a cowboy-hat type of excision. For this procedure, one of two methods can be used:

- The first method involves excising the endocervical portion of the lesion first using the 1- × 1-cm endocervical electrode. Once the endocervical portion of the lesion has been excised, the exocervical portion is excised using a standard 2.0- × 0.8-cm loop electrode (Fig. 127.8A).
- In the second method, the large ectocervical portion is excised first, followed by the smaller endocervical portion (see Fig. 127.8B). Care should be taken not to excise the endocervical canal too deeply. Both approaches leave a cowboy hat–shaped excision on the cervix (see Fig. 127.8C). The endocervical and exocervical excisional specimens should be submitted for pathologic assessment in separate containers.

After the specimen has been excised, some pathologists prefer that it be removed from the cervix using forceps, opened along one side, and placed in a plastic holder to allow it to fix in formalin in the proper orientation. Other pathologists prefer the specimen to be tagged at a certain location. Clinicians should check with the particular pathologist to determine preferences. Generally "tagging" the tissue to provide location provides little practical information. Although some clinicians want to know whether or not the endocervical margin of the specimen is involved with CIN, this can be difficult to evaluate because of tissue orientation on the histology slide and thermal damage. An endocervical curettage (ECC) taken immediately after LEEP can also be used to evaluate whether the CIN lesion has been removed in its entirety. In most instances, when the margin or post-LEEP ECC is positive, the patient should simply be followed up 4 to 6 months later with cytologic examination and a repeat ECC (see the section "Complications").

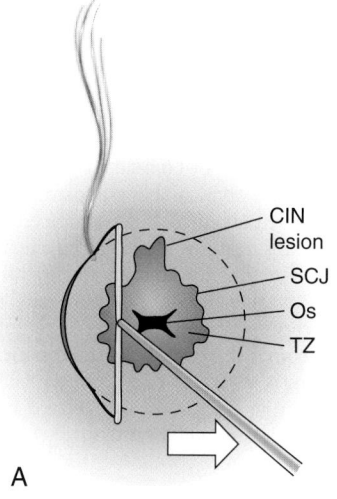

A

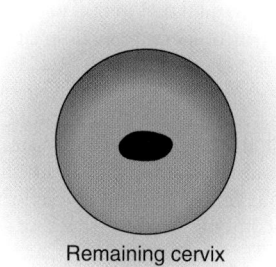

Remaining cervix

B

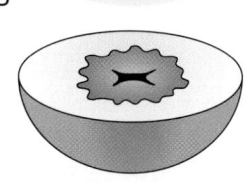

Portion removed

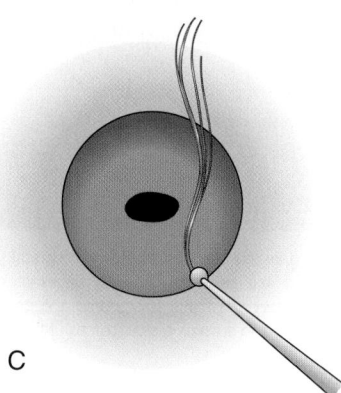

C

Fig. 127.6 Standard loop electrosurgical excision procedure for cervical intraepithelial lesions that can be removed in a single pass. After painting the cervix with Lugol solution and injecting lidocaine, the clinician uses an ectocervical loop (2 cm wide and 0.8 cm deep) to resect the entire lesion. (C) The crater base is then coagulated using a 5-mm ball electrode followed by the application of Monsel paste. *CIN,* Cervical intraepithelial neoplasia; *SCJ,* squamocolumnar junction; *TZ,* transformation zone.

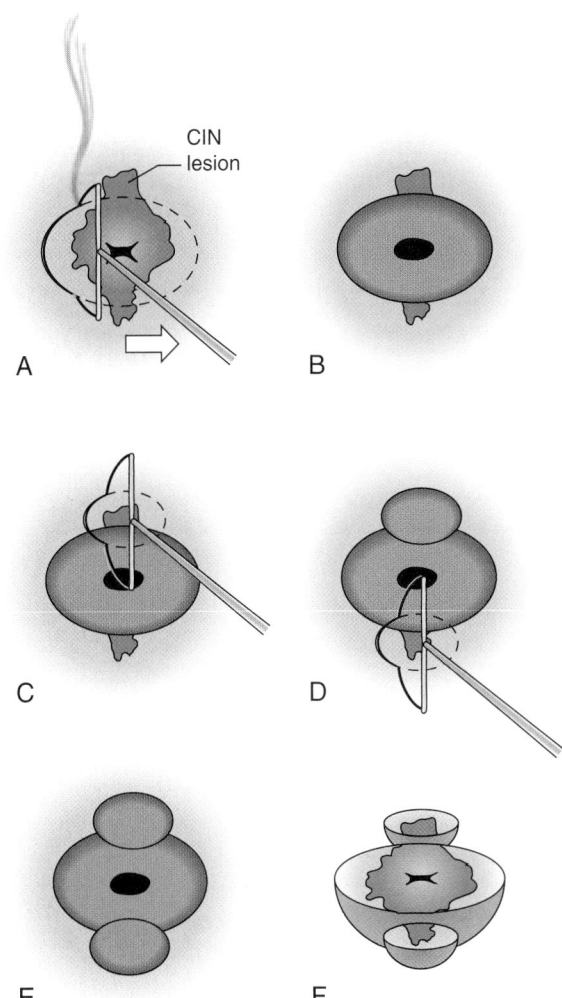

Fig. 127.7 (A–B) For lesions too large to be removed in a single pass, the clinician uses a 2- × 0.8-cm loop electrode to resect the central portion of the lesion. (C–E) Remaining tissue is then resected with additional passes using the same electrode. (F) Tissue specimens are placed in the same bottle of formalin. *CIN*, Cervical intraepithelial neoplasia.

8. Inspect the ectocervix and the endocervical canal to ensure that all nonstained (iodine negative) ectocervix and all acetowhite epithelium (AWE) in the canal has been excised. (More acetic acid may have to be applied to the canal with a cotton-tipped applicator.) If AWE remains in the canal (often identified by a thin rim of white along the margin of the os), another excision should be carried out and the process repeated until there is no AWE remaining. Care should be taken not to interpret thermal cautery effect in the endocervical canal as residual neoplasia.
9. Perform an ECC above the excisional base. This helps to confirm that there was no dysplasia above the excision.
10. Fulgurate any bleeding points at the base of the excision using a ball electrode with the "coagulation" setting on the ESU. For 5-mm ball electrodes, power settings of 40 to 55 W are usually required to obtain adequate arcing between the electrode and the tissue. (Excessive bleeding is more frequent in patients with severe cervicitis and in those less than 12 weeks postdelivery.) Frequently the entire base of the excision is lightly coagulated. Perform the coagulation up to the endocervical canal but take care not to insert the electrode into the canal. Excessive coagulation is not warranted and may be detrimental to optimal healing. See the section "Complications" for a technique of injecting vasopressin.

11. Apply Monsel paste to the entire area. Fig. 127.9A to E shows the typical cervix on completion of the procedure with Monsel applied (A) and 4 months after the procedure (B). Part C shows another cervix after the cowboy-hat procedure as seen through a coated vaginal speculum. Part D shows the average tissue specimen from LEEP. Part E is a microphotograph showing the minimal amount of thermal tissue damage from LEEP.

If the diameter of a lesion exceeds the width of the largest loop or triangle electrode, the lesion may be removed by multiple passes in separate pieces. The central part of the lesion is removed first, followed by the peripheral parts. If the lesion has extensive endocervical involvement, triangle electrodes can remove a cone-shaped specimen with a depth of 1.5 cm. If an even deeper removal of the endocervix is warranted, a smaller curvilinear loop can excise the endocervix on top of the initial "cone." In most cases excision with a triangle loop guarantees endocervical lesion removal and usually guarantees excision of the lesion and the TZ. Using a triangle loop as the preferred initial loop is recommended in most cases. Lesions with vaginal extensions require fulguration onto the vaginal portion in addition to LEEP. Do not use loop electrodes on the vagina unless with extreme caution and very superficially. Otherwise excisions on the vaginal wall may extend to nearby tissue (such as bladder and rectum) and result in perforation, fistula formation, or damage to other nearby structures.

SAMPLE OPERATIVE REPORT

Preoperative diagnosis: CIN 3
Postoperative diagnosis: CIN 3
Surgeon: Dr. _____
Anesthesia: Local, 1% lidocaine with epinephrine, 5 mL
Procedure: LEEP
Indications: The patient is a 35-year-old female with a history of several abnormal Pap smears including the most recent with HSIL. She underwent colposcopy with biopsy revealing a large CIN 3 lesion. After a discussion of the options for treatment, the patient preferred LEEP.
Procedure: Informed consent was obtained and prior colposcopic findings were reviewed. The patient was placed in the dorsal lithotomy position and an insulated vaginal speculum was introduced with good visualization of the cervix. Acetic acid was applied and the previously noted lesion at 3 o'clock was again visualized under colposcopic magnification, as was the entire squamocolumnar junction. No other abnormalities were noted. Lugol solution was applied and the cervix again visualized with the colposcope. Anesthesia was provided with injections of 1% lidocaine with epinephrine at 3, 6, 9, and 12 o'clock just peripheral to the TZ. Approximately 5 mL was used in total. After adequate anesthesia had been confirmed, a round 2.0-by 0.8-cm loop electrode was used on a pure cutting setting at 35 W to remove the entire TZ in one pass. The edges of the lesion were visualized and included in the excision. There was minimal bleeding, which was controlled with coagulation using a ball electrode. Monsel solution was applied prior to removing the speculum. The patient tolerated the procedure with minimal discomfort.
Estimated blood loss: Negligible
Specimen removed: One cervical specimen removed and sent to pathology
Complications: None

COMMON ERRORS

- The patient experiences an electric shock. Using a coated nonconductive speculum prevents electric shock, which is caused by touching the speculum with the electrode during the procedure. A "shock" sensation can make the patient jump, causing significant injury.

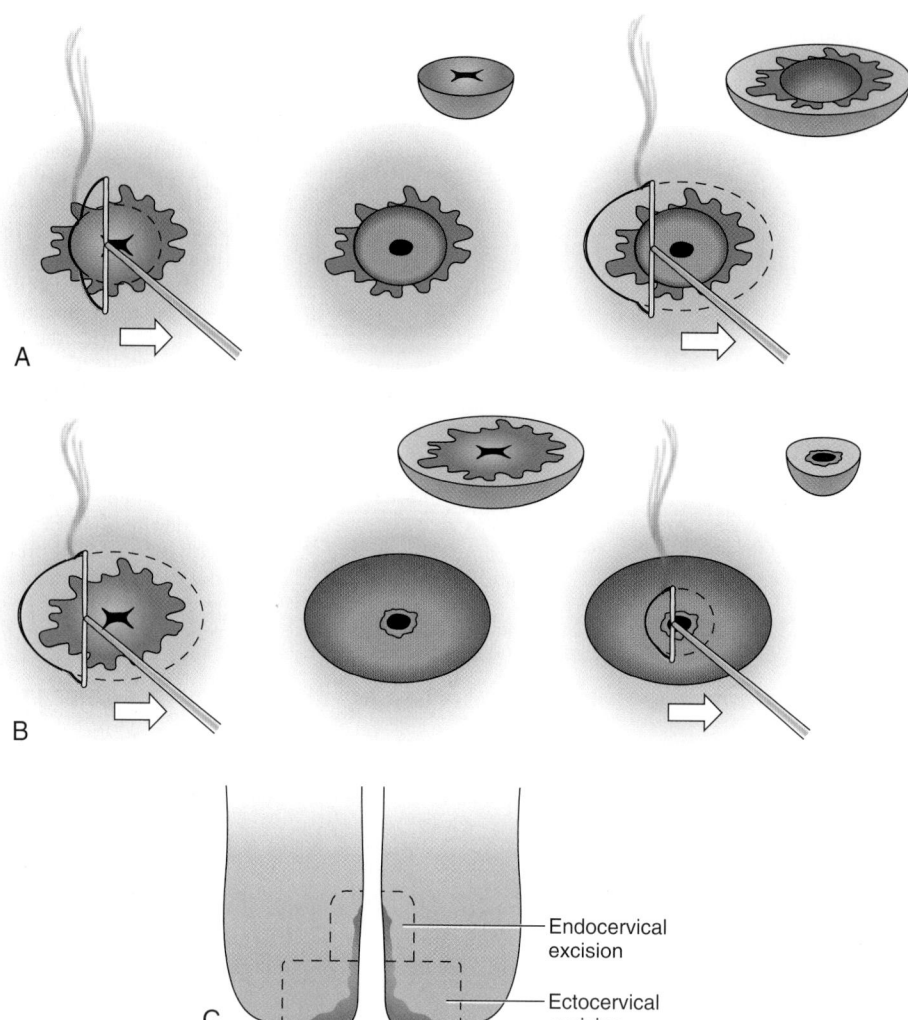

Fig. 127.8 Two methods for obtaining an endocervical sample with the loop electrosurgical excision procedure. (A) The clinician resects the endocervical portion of the lesion using a 1- × 1-cm loop. A 2.0- × 0.8-cm loop is then used to resect additional cervical intraepithelial neoplasia extending onto the portio. (B) In some cases it may be necessary to excise the ectocervical portion first. Excising to a depth greater than 1.5 cm into the canal increases the chances of significant bleeding. (C) Longitudinal section showing the "cowboy hat" procedure.

Endocervical excision

Ectocervical excision

- The loop electrode "stalls" as it is going through the tissue. Possible causes include the following:
  - If using a reusable loop, it must be free of carbon. Use a piece of fine sandpaper to shine the loops before the procedure. When using disposable loops, this will not be a problem.
  - The operator is moving the loop too quickly through the tissue. Go fast enough to prevent excessive tissue damage but slow enough to maintain a cutting function.
  - The cutting power is too low on the unit. Often, a pure cutting current will be easier to use than the "cut and coag" mode.
  - The unit has an automatic shutoff and the patient is not grounded. Check that the grounding pad is securely inserted to the main unit and attached to the patient.
    If a stall occurs for any reason, withdraw the electrode and either try passing it through the same tissue again after the problem has been corrected or approach from the other side.
- The electrode won't "cut" when touching the cervix. The electrode has not been activated before touching the patient or the tissue is too dry. In order for the electrode to cut, the tissue must be moist. Apply some acetic acid. Always activate the unit before touching the tissue with the loop.
- Pathologist reports excessive thermal damage on the tissue. Turn down the power on the unit or switch to the pure cutting mode for future procedures.

COMPLICATIONS

- Significant *intraoperative bleeding* is an uncommon but potentially serious complication. It sometimes occurs when the electrode is inserted too deeply into the tissue at the 3 and 9 o'clock positions (where the cervical branches of the uterine artery are located) or when the patient has severe cervicitis. The most effective way to control bleeding is to first apply pressure directly to the bleeding site using a large cotton-tipped applicator. Once the bleeding has slowed, the ball electrode is then placed in direct contact with the bleeding site and tissue is "desiccated" using coagulation current. If the bleeding is not controlled with pressure, the clinician should inject 1 to 2 mL of 2% lidocaine with epinephrine into the bleeding site. With the bleeding slowed or stopped, the ball electrode may then be effective. Vasopressin is now being used more for excessive bleeding during gynecologic surgery. A solution of vasopressin diluted in saline (0.1 U/mL) can be injected directly into the cervix, 10 mL each at the 4 o'clock and 8 o'clock positions. (It is probably best to limit use to ≤3 units of vasopressin.) For rare cases of persistent bleeding a figure of eight hemostatic stitch can be placed or the vagina and cervix can be packed tightly with 4- × 4-inch gauze and the patient transported to the emergency room.
- *Postoperative bleeding* occurs in less than 5% of patients. These patients experience a modest amount of bleeding 4 to 10 days after LEEP. It can usually be managed by electrofulguration or by packing the crater base with Monsel paste. Minimal spotting is to be expected up to 14 days after the procedure and after initial intercourse.
- Posttreatment *cervical stenosis* (Fig. 127.10) is an uncommon complication (<1%) and occurs more commonly in postmenopausal women and those lacking estrogen stimulation (postmenopausal women; Implanon and Depo-Provera users; lactating women).

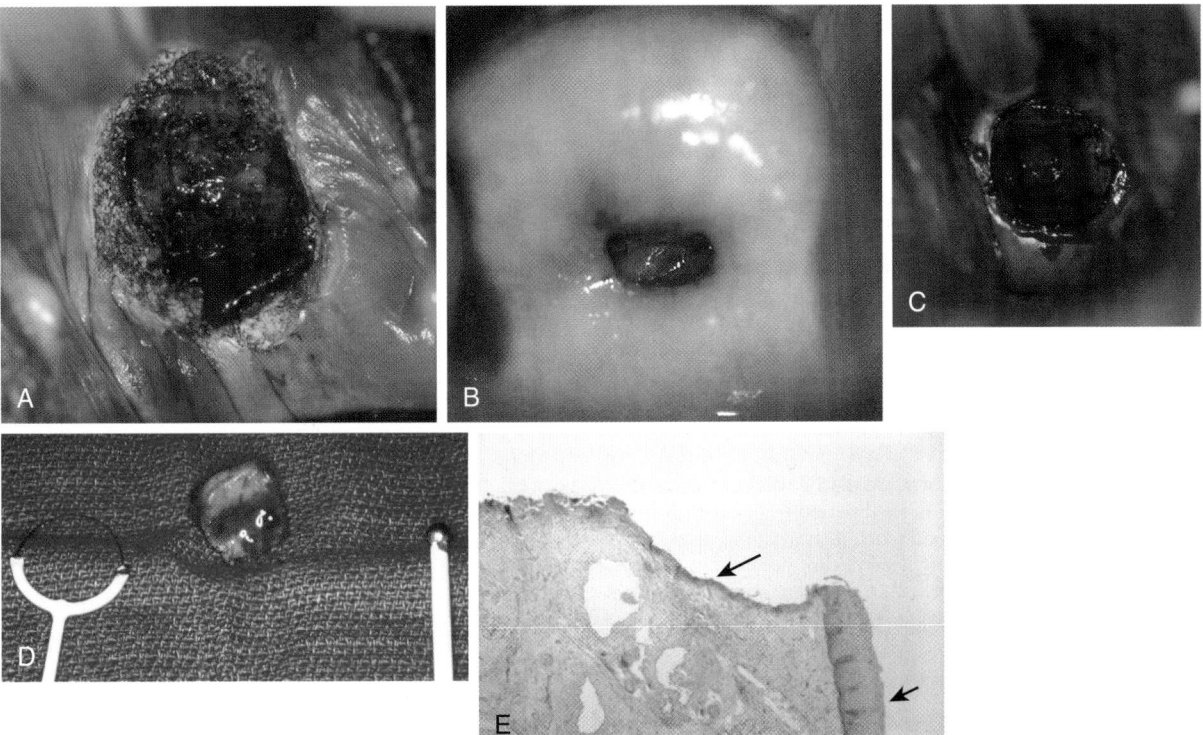

Fig. 127.9 (A) Appearance of the cervix as seen through a nonconductive speculum immediately after the loop electrosurgical excision procedure (LEEP). (B) Appearance of cervix 4 months after LEEP. Note the absence of an ectocervical transformation zone. (C) Appearance of cervix immediately after the "cowboy hat" LEEP procedure (ectocervical and endocervical excision). Coated speculum and smoke evacuator tubing are in place. (D) Tissue specimen from a single-pass LEEP procedure. (E) Microscopic view of the removed tissue. Note the minimal tissue damage on the resected edge *(arrows)*. (Courtesy John L. Pfenninger, MD, The Medical Procedures Center, Midland, MI.)

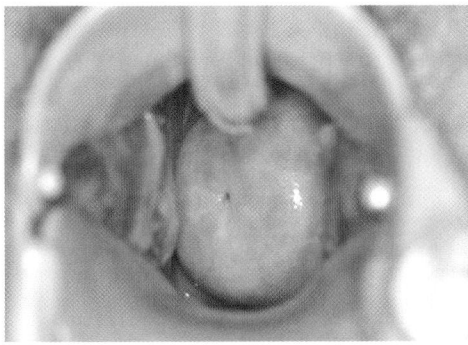

Fig. 127.10 Cervical stenosis following a loop electrosurgical excision procedure. (Courtesy John L. Pfenninger, MD, The Medical Procedures Center, Midland, MI.)

For postmenopausal patients and hypoestrogenic states, consider replacement estrogen for 2 to 3 weeks after the procedure (one applicator of estrogen cream in the vagina every night).

- *Inadvertent burns or lacerations* to the lateral vaginal wall or other sites can occur but are rare. The clinician should instruct the patient not to move. Ureters, bowel, and bladder are only millimeters away from the vaginal sidewalls.
- *Pain and discomfort* are minimal and generally can be controlled with nonsteroidal anti-inflammatory drugs.
- *Infection* is rare. Metronidazole or doxycycline can be used.
- *Recurrence or persistence* of disease occurs in 5% to 10% of cases.
- *Heat or diathermy artifact.* In unskilled hands, this may make histologic interpretation or the removed specimen impossible.
- *Cervical incompetence.* Although it is generally recognized that cold-knife conization is associated with adverse obstetric

outcomes, most of the studies published in the early 1990s showed little impact of LEEP on obstetric outcomes. Since that time, larger studies have indicated that all forms of excisional procedures used to treat CIN produce similar obstetric risks. A meta-analysis of these published trials found that LEEP has a significant association with preterm delivery (11% risk in treated women versus 7% risk in untreated women), low-birth-weight infants (8% in treated women vs. 4% in untreated women), and premature rupture of membranes (5% in treated women vs. 2% in untreated women). In fact, the presence of CIN itself may increase the risk, perhaps due to treatments for it. The more procedures a woman has undergone to treat CIN, the higher the risk of preterm labor. The deeper the cone depth, the higher the risk of prematurity. Therefore, when treating women likely to become pregnant in the future, consideration should be given to using an ablative method such cryotherapy rather than LEEP provided that the colposcopy is satisfactory and there is no suspicion of occult invasive cancer. A 2017 Cochrane review found ablative therapy to be associated with less risk of preterm delivery than excisional therapy.

POSTPROCEDURE MANAGEMENT

A 2015 Cochrane review found no evidence for the best surveillance strategy following treatment for CIN. That said, most clinicians recommend that patients be seen 4 to 6 weeks after the procedure for a review of the pathology report and a brief postoperative check. This visit helps to reassure the patients and decreases their anxiety about how well they have healed. It also provides an opportunity to reinforce prevention methods, such as not smoking. It is important to check for cervical stenosis. The os is easier to dilate early rather than waiting for a more mature scar (see Chapter 126, Cervical Stenosis and Cervical Dilation).

I recommend that the clinician reevaluate the patient using either a program of repeat cytologic examination at 6 and 12 months, a single HPV DNA test for high-risk types of HPV at 6 to 12 months, or a combination of cytologic examination and colposcopy at 6 and 12 months. If a program of repeat cytologic examination is used for follow-up, patients with a cytologic result of atypical squamous cells or higher classification should be referred for colposcopy. If HPV DNA testing at 6 to 12 months is used, patients with high-risk types of HPV identified should be referred for colposcopy.

POSTPROCEDURE PATIENT EDUCATION

See the sample patient education handout available at www.expertconsult.com.

- The clinician should instruct the patient to avoid vaginal intercourse, douching, use of tampons, and heavy exercise (especially weight lifting) for 3 weeks.
- If significant bleeding persists for more than 2 weeks (if the volume is comparable to that of a normal period or greater), if the patient begins passing large blood clots, if the vaginal discharge becomes foul-smelling, or if there is significant pelvic pain (especially if it is associated with a fever), the patient should call the physician or return to the clinic.

INTERPRETATION OF RESULTS

The specimen removed during LEEP should be sent to pathology, as previously discussed. The pathologic diagnosis should confirm the prior biopsy and examination findings. The extent of dysplasia and involvement of the margins of resection will be reported. If invasive carcinoma is present, immediate reevaluation and follow-up are essential and the patient is generally referred to a gynecologic oncologist. Ideally the lesion should be completely excised and the margins clear of any abnormal findings. If the ectocervical or endocervical excisional margins are positive on histologic examination or if the ECC is positive for neoplasia, the patient is at higher risk for recurrence. However, even in these situations, less than one-third of lesions will persist. The cautery and inflammatory response appear to resolve most of these. In these cases it is prudent to perform colposcopy with ECC and repeat cytologic examination approximately 3 to 4 months after the initial LEEP. In some instances, especially in high-risk and postmenopausal patients, consideration should be given to performing a repeat diagnostic conization procedure (e.g., either a cold-knife or LEEP conization) once the cervix has healed.

PATIENT EDUCATION GUIDES

American College of Obstetrics and Gynecology (ACOG): https://www.acog.org/Patients/FAQs/Loop-Electrosurgical-Excision-Procedure-LEEP?IsMobileSet=false
American Society of Colposcopy and Cervical Pathology (ASCCP)
Krames Communications: http://www.asccp.org/store-detail?pid=e6fa1a37-6b25-4e34-be89-1049b599b148

CPT/BILLING CODES

57460	Colposcopy with loop electrode excision or excisions of the cervix (LEEP)
57461	Colposcopy with loop electrode conization of cervix (LEEP cone)
57500	Cervical biopsy
57505	Endocervical curettage
57522	Cervical conization using loop electrode technique (LEEP cone)
99070	Supplies and materials for kits and electrodes (a surgical tray charge is generally allowed for an office LEEP)

ICD-10-CM DIAGNOSTIC CODES

C53.9	Cervical cancer
D06.9	CIN 3 (severe dysplasia, carcinoma in situ)
N87.0	CIN 1
N87.1	CIN 2
R87.613	HSIL
R87.619	Atypical glandular/endocervical cells

SUPPLIERS

(See contact information available at www.expertconsult.com.)
Bovie Medical Corporation
ConMed
CooperSurgical
Ellman Cynosure
ERBE USA, Inc.
MedGyn Products, Inc.
Premier Medical Products
Utah Medical Products, Inc.
Valleylab, Inc.
Wallach Surgical Devices, Inc.
Welch Allyn

PATIENT EDUCATION GUIDES

See the sample patient education handout available at www.expertconsult.com.

RECOMMENDED READING

American College of Obstetricians and Gynecologists. Cervical cancer in adolescents: Screening, Evaluation and management. Committee Opinion No. 463. *Obstet Gynecol.* 2010;116:469–472.

American College of Obstetricians and Gynecologists. Management of abnormal cervical cytology and histology. Practice Bulletin No. 99. *Obstet Gynecol.* 2008;112:1419.

Apgar BS, Kaufman AJ, Bettcher C, Parker-Featherstone E. Gynecologic procedures: colposcopy, treatment of cervical intraepithelial neoplasia, and endometrial assessment. *Am Family Physician.* 2013;87(12):836–843.

Brockmeyer AD, Wright JD, Gao F, et al. Persistent and recurrent cervical dysplasia after loop electrosurgical excision procedure. *Am J Obstet Gynecol.* 2005;192:1379.

Crane JM. Pregnancy outcome after loop electrosurgical excision procedure: a systematic review. *Obstet Gynecol.* 2003;102:1058.

Dunn TS, Bajaj JE, Stamm CA, et al. Management of the minimally abnormal Papanicolaou smear in pregnancy. *J Low Genit Tract Dis.* 2001;5:133.

Gajjar K, Martin-Hirsch PPL, Bryant A, Owens GL. Pain relief for women with cervical intraepithelial neoplasia undergoing colposcopy treatment. *Cochrane Database Syst Rev.* 2016;7:Art. No.: CD006120.

Hacker NF. Cervical dysplasia and cancer. In: Hacker NF, Gambone JC, Hobel JC, eds. *Hacker and Moore's Essentials of Obstetrics and Gynecology.* 6th ed. Philadelphia: Elsevier; 2016:429–439.

Kyrgiou M, Koliopoulos G, Martin-Hirsch P, et al. Obstetric outcomes after conservative treatment for intraepithelial or early invasive cervical lesions: systematic review and meta-analysis. *Lancet.* 2006;367:489.

Kyrgiou M, Tsoumpou I, Vrekoussis T, et al. The up-to-date evidence on colposcopy practice and treatment of cervical intraepithelial neoplasia: the cochrane Colposcopy and cervical cytopathology collaborative group (C5 group) approach. *Cancer Treat Rev.* 2006;32:516.

Martin-Hirsch PPL, Bryant A. Interventions for preventing blood loss during the treatment of cervical intraepithelial neoplasia. *Cochrane Database Syst Rev.* 2013;12:Art. No.: CD001421.

Massad LS, Einstein MH, Huh WK, et al. 2012 update consensus guidelines for the management of abnormal cervical screening tests and cancer precursors. *J Low Genit Tract Dis.* 2013;17(5 supp 1):S1–S27.

Mossa MA, Carter PG, Abdu S, et al. A comparative study of two methods of large loop excision of the transformation zone. *Br J Obstet Gynaecol.* 2005;112:490.

Paraskevaidis E, Arbyn M, Sotiriadis A, et al. The role of HPV DNA testing in the follow-up period after treatment for CIN: a systematic review of the literature. *Cancer Treat Rev.* 2004;30:205.

Paraskevaidis E, Kalantaridou SN, Paschopoulos M, et al. Factors affecting outcome after incomplete excision of cervical intraepithelial neoplasia. *Eur J Gynaecol Oncol.* 2003;24:541.

Pfenninger JL. Good things still come in old packages: cryosurgery vs. loop electrosurgical excision procedure. *J Am Board Family Pract.* 1999;12:416.

Spitzer M, Brotzmon GL, Apgar BS. Practical therapeutic options for treatment of cervical intraepithelial neoplasia. In: Apgar BS, Brotzman GL, Spitzer M, eds. *Colposcopy Principles and Practice.* 2nd ed. Philadelphia: Saunders; 2008:505–509.

van der Heijden E, Lopes AD, Bryant A, Bekkers R, Galaal K. Follow-up strategies after treatment (large loop excision of the transformation zone [LLETZ]) for cervical intraepithelial neoplasia (CIN): impact of human papillomavirus (HPV) test. *Cochrane Database Syst Rev.* 2015;1:Art. No.: CD010757.

World Health Organization. *Comprehensive Cervical Cancer Control: A Guide to Essential Practice.* 2nd ed. Geneva: World Health Organization; 2014.

Wright TC, Richart RM, Ferenczy AF. *Electrosurgery for HPV-Related Lesions of the Anogenital Tract.* New City, NY: Arthur Vision; 1992.

CHAPTER 128

CERVICAL CONIZATION

Lydia A. Watson

In most cases, proper evaluation of abnormal Pap smears and cervical lesions includes colposcopy, multiple-punch biopsy sampling, and endocervical curettage. However, conization of the cervix plays an important role in both the diagnosis and the management of abnormalities of the cervix. Cold-knife conization (CKC) is considered the gold standard by which all other outpatient techniques are critiqued. "Cold knife" refers to a surgical blade versus the old "hot-wire" cone, or the loop electrosurgical excision procedure (LEEP) procedure.

Conization of the cervix consists of the removal of a cone-shaped wedge of tissue from the cervix uteri. To be considered an adequate specimen, the tissue removed must include the entire transformation zone with the squamocolumnar junction and the entire lesion surrounded by uninvolved margins. CKCs have decreased considerably in frequency following the wide acceptance of LEEP, which yields equivalent results, is more cost effective, and appears to cause less intraoperative and postoperative bleeding. However, the cold-knife approach may be preferable in situations in which evaluation of the margins is particularly critical or in situations in which the use of a diathermic loop is impossible because of the proximity of the exocervical margin to the vaginal fornix. The large loop electrical excision procedure is described in Chapter 127, Loop Electrosurgical Excision Procedure for Treating Cervical Intraepithelial Neoplasia. A review of Chapter 124, Colposcopic Examination, and Chapter 125, Cryotherapy of the Cervix, is also recommended.

CKC and LEEP are considered excisional methods of treating CIN versus the ablative techniques (e.g., cryotherapy, laser, electrocautery). All of these techniques have about the same outcomes for the eradication of CIN; however, excisional methods are associated with an increased risk of adverse obstetric outcomes, such as preterm labor and low birth weight. That said, CKC is still considered the gold standard in certain situations.

INDICATIONS

A conization may be indicated for diagnosis or treatment, or both. Usually any conization method can be used interchangeably, although using a knife blade causes less tissue or heat artifact (pathologic distortion) than other methods and may allow a better histologic examination.

FOR DIAGNOSIS

- Inadequate colposcopic evaluation of the cervix
  - The lesion is not seen on colposcopic examination, but Pap smear is significantly abnormal
  - Incomplete visualization of a lesion that extends into the endocervical canal (ECC) on colposcopic examination
  - Inadequate visualization of entire transformation zone, including the squamocolumnar junction (e.g., goes into the os, where it cannot be evaluated)
- Positive endocervical curettings (i.e., dysplasia or cancer)
- Inconsistencies between cytologic findings, histologic diagnoses, and colposcopic impression (e.g., a Pap smear that is at least two stages worse than colposcopic biopsy)
- Inability of colposcopic examination to exclude invasive cancer

For Therapy

- Cytology or biopsy specimen suggests microinvasive carcinoma of the cervix (clinician must rule out frank invasion to define the proper treatment; in this case, procedure may also be therapeutic)
- High-grade dysplasia (i.e., moderate or severe dysplasia by biopsy) greater than 2 cm or in more than two quadrants
- Cervical cryotherapy is contraindicated (see Chapter 125, Cryotherapy of the Cervix)
  - Lesion too large for cryotip
  - Markedly irregular surface of cervix with crevices that cryotherapy will not reach
  - Glandular involvement on biopsy (relative)
  - Lesion extends more than 5 mm into the os
- Noncompliance (e.g., patient unlikely to be compliant with follow-up after cryotherapy and during attempts to monitor lesser cervical intraepithelial neoplasia without treatment)
- Correction of cervical stenosis (although the os is more likely to be opened using a shallow LEEP than a CKC)

CONTRAINDICATIONS

Absolute

- Known frank invasive carcinoma of the cervix or endocervix (*Carcinoma in situ* is not a cancer, but rather a severe dysplasia. With microinvasive cancer, a conization procedure must be performed to rule out frank invasion.)
- Patient with contraindications to general or regional anesthesia
- Unstable medical conditions (rarely is conization an emergency)

Relative

- Unstable bleeding disorders
- Inflammatory cervicitis (causes increased bleeding)
- Heavy menses at time of surgery (makes the procedure more difficult)
- Pregnancy

NOTE: Although pregnancy is not an absolute contraindication to conization, only a well-trained clinician capable of managing complications should perform the procedure on a pregnant patient (see section "Complications").

PREPROCEDURE PATIENT EDUCATION

- The procedure and potential complications should be explained to the patient, and written informed consent should be obtained. (See the patient education handout titled "CKC of the Cervix [Cone Biopsy]" available at www.expertconsult.com.)

- The need for general, local, or regional anesthesia should be explained.
- All options for treatment and evaluation should be explained.

EQUIPMENT

- Povidone-iodine or chlorhexidine
- Colposcope with green filter
- Acetic acid (4%) and full-strength Lugol solution
- Vasopressin 20 U in 20 mL of normal saline for infiltration of the cervix
- Long scalpel handle with No. 11 blade
- Long, fine-tooth forceps
- Kevorkian endocervical curette
- Electrocautery unit
- 0-chromic or 0-Vicryl suture (or Surgicel, Gelfoam, or Avitene) for hemostasis; long needle holders
- Large Graves speculum
- Uterine sound
- Equipment to follow universal blood and body fluid precautions

PROCEDURE

1. *Special considerations:* Most lesions are found on the ectocervix in premenopausal women, so the cone should have a broad base and the top should have a wide angle (Fig. 128.1A). In postmenopausal women, the specimen will be long and narrow, with an acute angle at the cone top. The squamocolumnar junction in these patients has generally moved inside the ECC, and lesions are more likely to be endocervical. The transformation zone in older women is usually quite small (see Fig. 128.1B).
2. Administer general, local (intrastromal), or regional anesthesia to the patient, and obtain adequate exposure of the cervix. The bladder should be drained.
3. Apply full-strength Lugol solution to the cervix to aid in determining the width of the cone base. All areas that do not stain will be removed. Alternatively, perform colposcopy using acetic acid (4%) and the green filter to demarcate the lesion and the transformation zone.
4. Obtain hemostasis by circumferentially infiltrating the cervical stroma with a solution of 5 U of vasopressin diluted in 20 mL of normal saline (Fig. 128.2).

   NOTE: Hemostatic retention sutures are no longer routinely used.

5. Gently sound the uterine canal to determine position and size of the uterus.
6. Incise the cervix in a circular fashion, making the incision outside of the Lugol-negative or acetowhite area. Begin at the 6 o'clock position. This will prevent the blood that runs down from obscuring the incision line (Fig. 128.3A). Angle the blade centrally to the width and depth desired.
7. Use a fine-tooth forceps to elevate the cone away from the underlying bed. Avoid damaging the cervical epithelium (see Fig. 128.3B).
8. Mark the 12 o'clock position of the specimen for the pathologist with a single suture placed into the cervical stroma. Consider measuring the specimen because it may shrink before it is measured by the pathologist.
9. Curette the remainder of the ECC with a small curette to rule out disease above the upper margins of the cone.
10. Perform a dilation and curettage, if indicated, at this time.
11. Obtain hemostasis with superficial electrocoagulation by using a ball electrode or individual suture ligatures to control bleeding. The cone site may also be packed with an absorbable gelatin sponge (e.g., Gelfoam) or similar hemostatic material. Most apply Monsel solution to the base of the excision after coagulation.

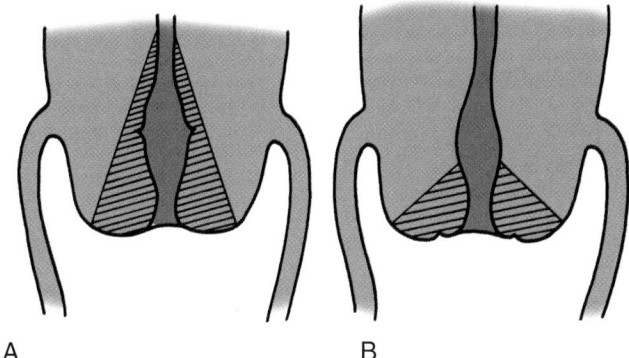

Fig. 128.1 Variation in size and shape of cervical tissue removed during conization. (A) For large ectocervical lesion. (B) For canal lesions.

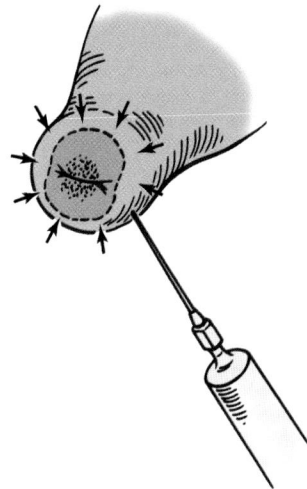

Fig. 128.2 Intracervical injection.

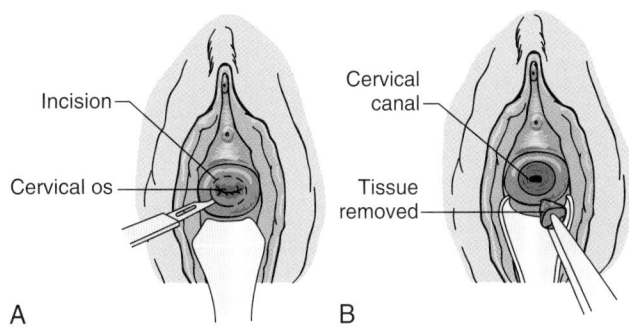

Fig. 128.3 Conization technique. (A) Incision. (B) Removal of tissue.

12. Place the cone specimen in fixative to send for pathologic interpretation. Some evidence indicates that conization performed during the first, rather than the second, half of the menstrual cycle is less likely to be associated with significant blood loss.

COMPLICATIONS

Complications for the nonpregnant patient include the following (overall complication rate 10%):

- Pain and cramping (generally minimal).
- Immediate or delayed hemorrhage. (Eschar sloughs in 7 to 10 days. Delayed hemorrhage can occur at this time; some spotting

is to be expected for 10 to 14 days.) If bleeding is excessive at the time of surgery, inject 1 mL of 2% lidocaine with epinephrine into each bleeding spot. This will usually slow bleeding enough to allow electrocoagulation. Alternatively, and rarely, a figure-of-8 stitch may need to be placed over the bleeding vessel.

- Cervical stenosis (<3 mm) that prevents menses or obtaining a good endocervical Pap smear.
- Uterine perforation.
- Pelvic cellulitis (very rare) or cervicitis.
- Damage to the bladder or rectum. (This is usually seen in cases of significant vaginal atrophy with shallow vaginal fornices.)
- Cervical incompetence (see Chapter 127, Loop Electrosurgical Excision Procedure for Treating Cervical Intraepithelial Neoplasia for a further discussion on possible effects on future pregnancy.)
- Infertility caused by loss of mucus-producing endocervical glands.
- Anesthetic complications.
- Positive margins or positive ECC. (If ectocervical margins show only dysplasia, the patient should be followed closely but a repeat cone is not indicated. Usually the lesion will resolve during the inflammatory healing process. A repeat cone may be indicated in older patients who are at a high risk and do not desire pregnancy, those who have had pelvic irradiation, or in whom both the margins and ECC are positive. If the ECC above the excisional site is positive with a high-grade lesion, repeat conization should be considered.)
- Missing the lesion (rare).
- In addition to the complications mentioned for the nonpregnant patient, complications for the pregnant patient include the following:
- Fetal loss rate of 10% (secondary to rupture of the membranes, premature labor, and excessive hemorrhaging).
- Postoperative hemorrhage rate of 30%.

POSTPROCEDURE MANAGEMENT

- A follow-up appointment should be scheduled for 4 to 6 weeks.
- The patient should be instructed to avoid intercourse, douching, and tampon use until follow-up examination confirms healing.
- The patient should be asked to notify the clinician of elevated temperature, excessive vaginal bleeding, or purulent discharge.
- The first follow-up Pap smear should be scheduled in 3 to 4 months if all margins are clear.

NOTE: A 2015 Cochrane review found no evidence for the best surveillance strategy following treatment for CIN. The World Health Organization only recommends follow-up with Pap smear in a year, and then going back to routine Pap screening. An exception to this rule is if that the original CIN being treated was CIN3 or greater; in that situation, followup Pap smears should be yearly for 3 years.

PATIENT EDUCATION GUIDES

- See the sample patient education handout, "CKC of the Cervix (Cone Biopsy)," available at www.expertconsult.com.
- See the sample patient consent form, "Cervical Conization," available at www.expertconsult.com.

CPT/BILLING CODES

57520	Conization, with or without fulguration, with or without dilation and curettage (D&C), with or without repair, cold knife or laser
57522	Conization, loop electrode
57505	Endocervical curettage (not done as part of D&C)
99070	Surgical tray

ICD-10-CM DIAGNOSTIC CODES

A63.0	Condyloma
B97.7	Human papillomavirus as the cause of diseases classified elsewhere
C53.9	Cervical neoplasm, malignant (excludes carcinoma in situ)
D26.0	Benign neoplasm, cervix
D06.9	Carcinoma in situ, cervix (includes CIN III, severe dysplasia of cervix)
N86	Cervical erosion or ulcer
N87.0	Dysplasia of cervix mild [CIN I],
N87.1	Dysplasia of cervic moderate [CIN II])
N88.0	Cervical leukoplakia
N88.2	Cervical stenosis
N84.1	Cervical polyp

RECOMMENDED READING

Apgar BS, Kaufman AJ, Bettcher C, Parker-Featherstone E. Gynecologic Procedures: Colposcopy, Treatment of Cervical Intraepithelial Neoplasia, and Endometrial Assessment. *Am Family Physician.* 2013;87(12):836–843.

Hacker NF. Cervical dysplasia and cancer. In: Hacker NF, Gambone JC, Hobel JC, eds. *Hacker and Moore's Essentials of Obstetrics and Gynecology.* 6th ed. Philadelphia: Elsevier; 2016:429–439.

Narducci F, Occelli B, Boman F, et al. Positive margins after conization and risk of persistent lesion. *Gynecol Oncol.* 2000;76:311–314.

Pfenninger JL. Good things still come in old packages: Cryosurgery vs LEEP. Loop electrosurgical excision procedure. *J Am Board Fam Pract.* 1999;12:416–418.

Reich OP, Lahousen M, et al. Cervical Intraepithelial neoplasia III: long-term outcome after cold-knife conization with clear margins. *Obstet Gynecol.* 2001;97(3):428–430.

Ryan KJ, Berkowitz R, Barbieri RL, eds. *Kistner's Gynecology: Principles and Practice.* Chicago: Mosby–Year Book; 1990.

Turner RJ, Cohen RA, Voet RL, et al. Analysis of tissue margins of cone biopsy specimens obtained with "cold knife," CO2 and Nd:YAG lasers and a radiofrequency surgical unit. *J Reprod Med.* 1992;37:607–610.

White CD, Cooper WL, Williams RR. Cervical intraepithelial neoplasia extending to the margins of resection in conization of the cervix. *J Reprod Med.* 1991;36:635–638.

World Health Organization. *Comprehensive Cervical Cancer Control: A Guide to Essential Practice.* 2nd ed. Geneva: World Health Organization; 2014.

CHAPTER 129

ENDOMETRIAL BIOPSY

Beth A. Choby

Endometrial biopsy (EMB) is a safe and cost-effective diagnostic method of evaluating the endometrium. EMB is an office-based procedure most commonly used in perimenopausal and postmenopausal women to investigate abnormal uterine bleeding (AUB) and to rule out endometrial cancer. Endometrial cancer is the most common invasive gynecologic malignancy, and endometrial hyperplasia is sometimes a precursor. EMB may be considered in any woman with risk factors for endometrial hyperplasia or cancer (Box 129.1). Grand multiparity and use of combined oral contraceptives for 1 or more years are protective against endometrial cancer.

Although EMB is sensitive enough to diagnose hyperplasia or cancer, it is less useful for detecting abnormalities such as endometrial polyps or the changes of endometrial atrophy. It can also be difficult to obtain an adequate sample; one study (Elsandabesee, 2005) showed that only 34% of patients had an adequate sample using the Pipelle. (This is compared with earlier studies showing a 79% to 99% adequacy rate.) However, the false-negative rate for EMB is 5% to 15% when an adequate sample is obtained. In fact, when an adequate sample is obtained, the Pipelle method has a high diagnostic accuracy, with a positive predictive value of 81.7% and a negative predictive value of 99.1% (Saso, 2011). One predictor of obtaining an adequate sample is endometrial thickness on transvaginal ultrasound; the likelihood rises to 60% when evaluating women with an endometrial thickness of at least 5 mm. Although EMB recently became the preferred initial procedure for evaluating AUB and had mostly replaced dilation and curettage, it is often combined with transvaginal ultrasound to measure endometrial thickness. It can also be combined with sonohysteroscopy. Transvaginal ultrasound and sonohysteroscopy may also be combined in lieu of EMB (see Chapter 130, Hysteroscopy). Because EMB is cost effective, efficient, and readily available in the outpatient setting, it continues to be an important diagnostic tool.

ANATOMY

The EMB involves transcervical sampling of the endometrial lining. An endocervical curettage of the cervical canal is performed as part of the EMB.

INDICATIONS

- Evaluation of postmenopausal AUB, regardless of volume (including spotting and staining). Transvaginal ultrasound may be an alternative in appropriately selected women
- Evaluation of abnormal endometrial thickness on transvaginal ultrasound in postmenopausal women
- Work-up of infertility, especially short luteal phase or anovulation
- Assessment of the effects of hormone therapy
- Investigation of atypical glandular cells of endometrial origin, atypical glandular cells of any origin if older than 35 years and risk factors for endometrial cancer, or endometrial cells on Papanicolaou (Pap) smear in women older than 40 years who also have AUB or risk factors for endometrial cancer

- Failure to respond to medical treatment of AUB
- Surveillance in women previously diagnosed with endometrial hyperplasia
- AUB in women with risk factors for endometrial cancer (see Box 129.1)
- Women with an intact uterus receiving unopposed estrogen therapy
- Evaluation for endometrial carcinoma or precancerous changes
- Identification of causes of dysfunctional uterine bleeding
- Evaluation of uterine enlargement in conjunction with ultrasound
- Screening in hereditary nonpolyposis colon cancer (HNPCC) syndrome (HNPCC, Lynch syndrome, familial colorectal cancer syndrome X). The lifetime risk of endometrial cancer in women with HNPCC ranges between 40% and 60%. Annual or biennial EMB or transvaginal ultrasound is recommended in women with HNPCC beginning at 30 to 35 years of age. Recommendations are based on expert opinion because the effectiveness of gynecologic surveillance is not definitive. Diagnosis of HNPCC requires histologically confirmed colorectal cancer in three relatives, at least one of whom must be a first-degree relative. Two successive generations must be affected and one case has to be diagnosed before 50 years of age. Screening is appropriate in known carriers of this autosomal dominant gene or in cases where there is strong suspicion of HNPCC type syndromes.

CONTRAINDICATIONS

Absolute

- Pregnancy
- Bleeding diathesis/coagulopathy

Relative

- Use of anticoagulant therapy
- Active vaginal, cervical, uterine, or pelvic infection
- Cervical stenosis (see Chapter 136, Cervical Stenosis and Cervical Dilation)
- Morbid obesity
- Significant pelvic relaxation with uterine prolapse

EQUIPMENT

A variety of instruments are available for EMB. The more popular methods are described for comparison. Equipment common to all methods is listed here; additional items required with specific aspirators are listed in the aspirator descriptions.

- Large Graves vaginal speculum
- Povidone-iodine solution in nonallergic patients, chlorhexidine in those allergic to iodine
- Cotton balls

> **BOX 129.1   Risk Factors for Endometrial Hyperplasia and Cancer**
>
> Age >50 years
> Atypical endometrial hyperplasia
> Chronic anovulation
> Polycystic ovary syndrome
> Diabetes
> Hypertension
> Thyroid disease
> Infertility
> Early menarche, menopause after age 55 years
> Nulliparity
> Obesity*
> Tamoxifen
> Unopposed estrogen therapy
> Family history of endometrial cancer
> Lynch syndrome, hereditary nonpolyposis colorectal cancer, familial colorectal cancer syndrome X, Cowden syndrome
>
> ---
>
> *21–50 lb overweight (relative risk three times that of <50 lb overweight)

- Ring forceps
- Uterine sound
- Single-tooth tenaculum
- Endocervical curette without basket (e.g., Kevorkian curette, or disposable plastic one)
- Buffered formalin specimen containers with patient identification labels (two)*
- Endometrial sampler (special equipment requirements by method)
  - Disposable flexible plastic endometrial aspirator (e.g., Pipelle, Pipet Curet, Pipette, Endocell)
  - Scissors *or* reusable stainless steel curette (Novak or Randall) *or*
  - 20-mL syringe *or*
  - Disposable endometrial aspirators with syringe suction and more rigid curettes (Karman type Cannula-Curette, Uterine Explora, Explora II) *or*
  - Tis-U-Trap endometrial curette or a Vabra aspirator (disposable) *or*
  - External suction pump *or*
  - Brush sampler (Tao Brush)

Cervical dilators should be kept available (see Chapter 136, Cervical Stenosis and Cervical Dilation).

PRECAUTIONS

- The previous Pap smear should be reviewed before the procedure. If no recent smear report is available and it is indicated, obtain one before proceeding with the EMB.
- A bimanual examination identifies extreme uterine anteversion or retroflexion. There is an increased risk of uterine perforation when sounding the uterus or collecting the EMB if significant angulation is present between the cervical neck and uterus.
- The use of small cervical dilators is often necessary in women found to have cervical stenosis, so they should be available. Methods for managing cervical stenosis are described in Chapter 136, Cervical Stenosis and Cervical Dilation.

PREPROCEDURE PATIENT EDUCATION AND FORMS

- Obtain a thorough history, and review pertinent clinical records (see encounter form available at www.expertconsult.com). Explain

---

*The Tao Brush uses CytoRich Red solution instead of buffered formalin for specimen preservation.

to the patient the indications for the procedure, the process itself, side effects, and potential complications so that she may provide informed consent. See the sample patient education handout and the sample patient consent for EMB available at www.expertconsult.com.

- Nonsteroidal antiinflammatory drugs (NSAIDs) effectively decrease uterine cramping during EMB. Patients can be instructed to take 600 to 800 mg of ibuprofen orally 30 to 60 minutes before the procedure unless they are allergic to aspirin or NSAIDs. Other NSAIDs have similar efficacy.
- In extremely anxious patients, premedication with an oral anxiolytic such as 10 mg of oral diazepam (Valium) 1 hour before the EMB is an option. Patients receiving these medications should be counseled to bring a family member to drive them home.
- In the patient who faints easily, having 0.5 mg atropine available to give IM may be useful to avoid the vasovagal effects of nausea, bradycardia, and syncope. Some clinicians give 0.5 mg IM upon arrival in a patient with this history or at the first signs of vasovagal. It may be worthwhile to have another 0.5 mg available, just in case an additional dose is needed.
- The American Heart Association does not recommend antibiotic prophylaxis against bacterial endocarditis before EMB because the procedure is unlikely to cause bacteremia. No current studies specifically stratify this risk.
- Postmenopausal women can be scheduled for EMB at any time, although significant bleeding episodes are best avoided to optimize sample size.
- EMB in reproductive-age women is best performed on day 22 or 23 after the first day of the last menstrual period. The presence of secretory glands confirms that ovulation has occurred. Avoid EMB during menses because stromal breakdown can be misinterpreted as cell fragmentation and hemorrhage due to malignancy.

PROCEDURE

The initial steps for EMB are similar for the various methods. These are listed first (steps 1 through 8) and followed by descriptions of individual endometrial aspirators and specific instructions for their use. *Confirm that the patient is not pregnant, if appropriate, before beginning the procedure.*

1. The patient is placed in stirrups in dorsal lithotomy position (after the Pap smear is obtained, if indicated), and a bimanual examination is performed to determine the size and position of the uterus. The provider wears nonsterile gloves for this portion of the procedure.
2. Insert a large Graves speculum vaginally. Visualize the cervix, and remove any mucus or debris.
3. Change into sterile gloves.
4. Prepare the cervix and vagina with povidone-iodine–soaked cotton balls using the ring forceps.
5. Perform an endocervical curettage in cases where neoplasm is suspected (see Chapter 137, Colposcopic Examination). Insert a Kevorkian curette without basket or a disposable curette into the endocervical canal. Manipulate the curette 360 degrees circumferentially around the entire canal, scraping in and out for two full rotations. Warn the patient about cramping. Collect all of the available material. Use ring forceps to collect any blood or secretions draining from the os. Place all the material on lens paper, and then place it in formalin. (Disposable plastic endocervical curettage equipment is also available, usually made by same manufacturers who make plastic endometrial curettage equipment.)
6. If insertion of the curette is difficult, use a single-tooth tenaculum to grasp the cervix at 12 o'clock while having the patient cough (or whichever position gives best exposure without blocking access to the curette, except not the 3 or 9 o'clock positions). Traction on the tenaculum straightens the cervical neck and allows for easier endocervical curettage. Avoid grasping the 3 and

9 o'clock positions because of the presence of arteries at these points. Topical benzocaine gel (20%) or benzocaine spray (Hurricaine) may be applied to the tenaculum site to decrease pain. If used, the anesthetic needs to be in place several minutes before it has an effect. A submucosal injection of lidocaine works well (see explanation in Chapter 149, Loop Electrosurgical Excision Procedure for Treating Cervical Intraepithelial Neoplasia).

7. Once a gritty sensation is noted, remove the curette. Collect all tissue obtained, and place it in formalin.

8. Proceed with EMB using one of the following techniques. With all EMB techniques, insert the sterile sampling device through the cervical os without touching the vulva or vaginal walls. Do not touch or contaminate the part of the sampler that is placed into the uterus. Sterile gloves and speculum are not necessary if a "no-touch" technique is used.

Plastic Endometrial Aspirators (e.g., Endocell, Pipelle, Pipet Endometrial Aspirator)

Disposable flexible endometrial sampling devices are the most popular method for EMB (Fig. 129.1A–B). The device is made of a clear, flexible polypropylene tube with an inner plunger. This functions as a piston and creates negative pressure when retracted quickly. A 2.4-mm distal side port allows for tissue sampling. The stiffer-tipped aspirators are more useful when cervical stenosis is present. More flexible types may be "stiffened" by placing them in a freezer for 10 to 15 minutes.

The Pipelle samples 5% to 15% of the endometrial surface. Several types are calibrated and can be used to sound the uterus (6.5 to 10 cm is normal). If the endometrial thickness is adequate, 79% to 99% of specimens obtained using the Pipelle are adequate for histopathologic diagnosis.

The procedure for flexible endometrial aspirators follows, continued from previous steps 1 through 8.

9. Sound the uterus using either a calibrated flexible aspirator with the piston fully inserted or a metal sound (when using an uncalibrated product). Document the depth of the endometrial cavity (usually 6.5 to 10 cm). If the sound cannot be inserted, use a tenaculum to grasp the cervix at 12 o'clock while having the patient cough (or whichever position gives best exposure without blocking access to the curette, except not the 3 or 9 o'clock positions, as discussed earlier). Outward traction straightens the cervical neck and allows the sound to pass through the cervical os. If the sound still will not pass, cervical dilation may be necessary (see Chapter 136, Cervical Stenosis and Cervical Dilation).

10. Introduce the aspirator, with internal piston fully inserted, into the endocervix. Pass it through the cervix and into the uterine cavity. Stop once the fundus is reached or resistance is encountered (Fig. 129.2A).

11. Stabilize the sheath with one hand while the piston is drawn back with the other hand. Negative pressure builds up in the lumen of the tube (see Fig. 129.2B).

12. Rotate the sheath 360 degrees between the thumb and index finger. At the same time, withdraw the aspirator going from the fundus to the internal os. Most of the endometrial cavity can be sampled with a minimum of four complete in-and-out, fundus to internal os, circumferential passes. As the aspirator completes a helical arc against the uterine walls, negative pressure within the sheath draws the sheared-off endometrial tissue through the distal port and into the lumen. The aspirator must be kept within the cervix or suction is lost (see Fig. 129.2C).

13. Withdraw the entire device from the uterus, with the piston pulled back the full distance. Avoid contaminating the tip. *Do not* push the piston back into the sheath before removal because the tissue sample will be lost.

14. Expel the sample into formalin by advancing the piston into the sheath (see Fig. 129.2D to F). If insufficient tissue is obtained

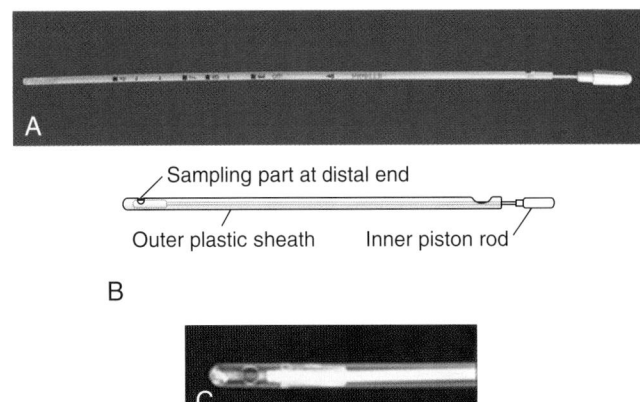

Fig. 129.1 (A) Pipelle endometrial sampler. (B) Pipelle sheath and piston. (C) Opening at the end of the Pipelle. (Courtesy CooperSurgical, Inc., Trumbull, CN, with permission.)

or if the aspirator fills with blood or other material before four complete passes have been made, a second insertion may be attempted using the same catheter as long as it has not touched the formalin or vaginal sidewalls. The manufacturers often recommend that the tip of the catheter be cut off using scissors before the sample is expelled into formalin, although this is unnecessary. Additional sampling would then require an additional unused aspirator.

15. Remove the speculum from the vagina.

Reusable Stainless Steel Curette (Novak or Randall) and Disposable Endometrial Aspirators with Syringe Suction (Cannula Curette, Uterine Explora, Explora II)

The Novak curette is made of stainless steel and has been available for more than 50 years (Fig. 129.3A). The cannula is rigid and is attached to a 10- to 20-mL disposable plastic syringe. When the syringe plunger is pulled, the negative pressure generated draws endometrial tissue into the cannula. Both the Novak and Randall curettes are reusable after sterilization. A disadvantage of this method is that patients complain of greater pain than with flexible plastic aspirators.

Several disposable methods allow easier use of suction by connecting a locking syringe to the end of the plastic aspirator. The Cannula-Curette, Uterine Explora, and Explora II combine the benefits of a rigid cannula with disposability. Both Explora models are nylon with a sharp Randall-type cutting edge (see Fig. 129.3B). The Explora has one distal port, whereas the Explora II has two distal ports on opposing sides of the aspirator. Tissue is obtained with suction using a scraping and peeling action. In women with large endocervical canals, the Cannula Curette may be a better option (Fig. 129.4). It comes in sizes ranging from 3 to 7 mm, whereas the Explora and Explora II are available only in 3- and 4-mm sizes. When AUB is present, the larger-diameter Cannula Curette is less likely to clog than the smaller curettes. Sensitivity and specificity of these types of endometrial samplers are similar to those for the flexible plastic endometrial aspirators. These type aspirators may be more likely to get tissue in the premenopausal woman or one who is having menstrual bleeding at the time of the procedure.

After completing previous steps 1 through 8, the procedure for the reusable stainless steel curette (Novak or Randall) and disposable endometrial aspirators with syringe suction (Cannula Curette, Uterine Explora, Explora II) is as follows:

9. Apply a tenaculum to the anterior or posterior tip of the cervix, depending on the direction of flexion of the uterus. Grasp

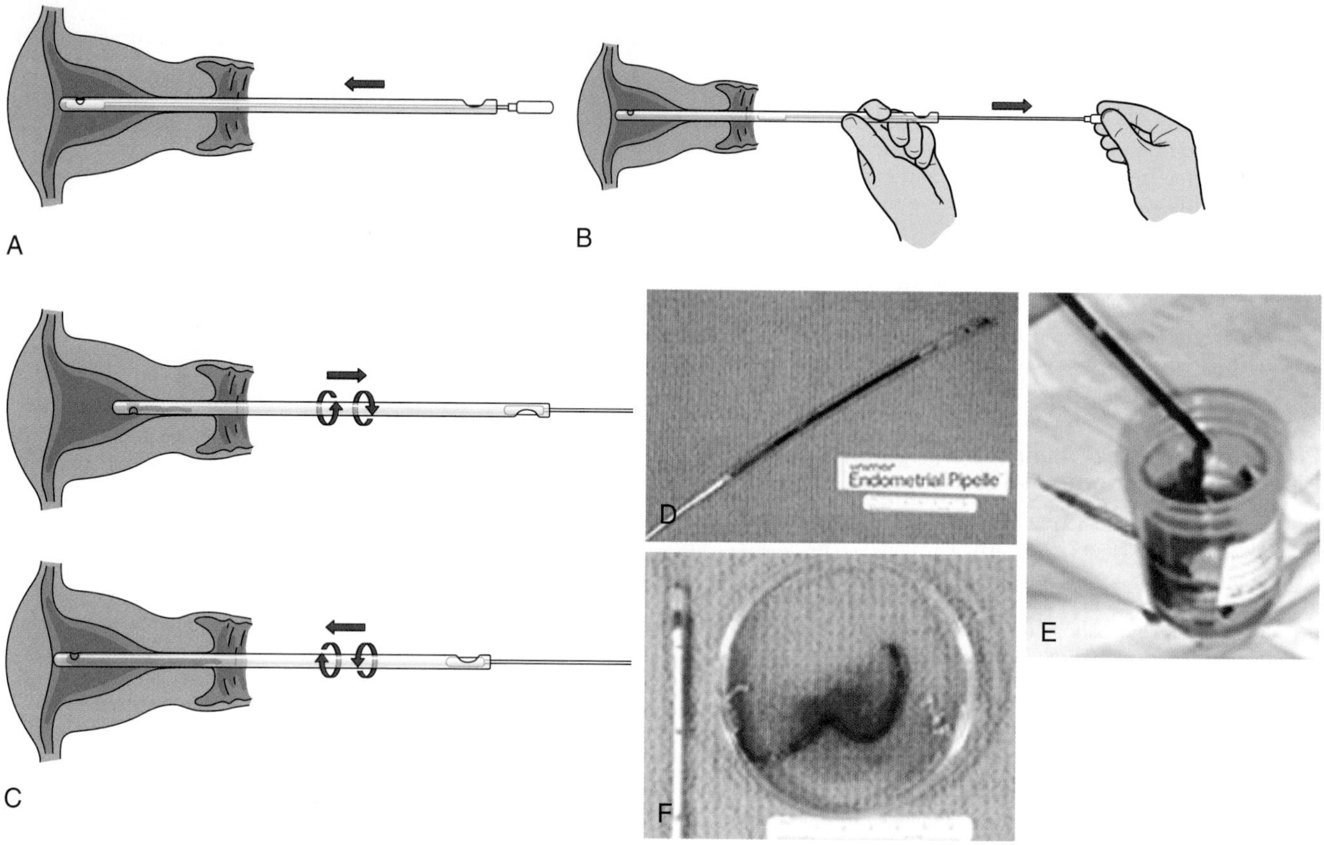

A

B

C

D

E

F

Fig. 129.2   (A) With the piston fully advanced in the sheath, insert the aspirator transcervically into the endometrial cavity. (B) Hold the outer sheath with one hand while simultaneously pulling back the piston to create negative pressure. (C) Roll the sheath between the fingers while simultaneously moving the sheath in and out from the fundus to the internal os. Complete a minimum of four passes. (D) Appearance of tissue in the sampler. (E) Expressing the tissue into the formalin bottle. (F) Sample as it appears in the formalin container.

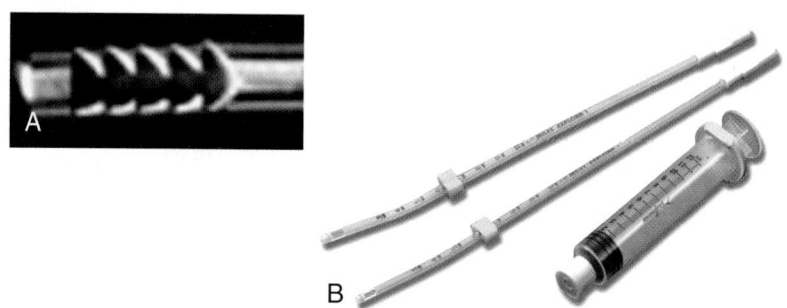

Fig. 129.3   (A) Close-up of the end of the Novak stainless steel curette. (B) Uterine Explora and Explora II endometrial aspirators. (Courtesy CooperSurgical, Inc., Trumbull, CN.)

the cervix with the tenaculum teeth in the horizontal position. Grasping the cervix at the 3 or 9 o'clock position with the tenaculum in the vertical plane decreases the diameter of the external os. Local anesthesia (2 mL of 2% lidocaine solution or spray) where the tenaculum teeth are applied decreases patient discomfort (optional).

10. Insert a uterine sound into the cervix while applying gentle traction to the tenaculum. Halt when the fundus is reached, and note the insertion measurement in centimeters. Remove the sound from the patient. If stenosis is present, cervical dilation may be necessary (see Chapter 126, Cervical Stenosis and Cervical Dilation).

11. Gently insert the curette into the endometrial cavity while applying traction with the tenaculum. Stop insertion once the curette is at the depth that was sounded.

12. Before attaching the curette, draw up 1 to 2 cm of air into the syringe. This will be used to evacuate the curette when the procedure is completed.

13. Attach a 20-mL syringe to the curette hub. Pull the syringe back to the 10- to 15-mL mark to create suction. The Explora models recommend pulling the syringe back to 1 or 2 mL to avoid discomfort.

14. Apply pressure against the uterine sidewalls, and perform four to six single-strip curettages. Sample from the fundus to the lower uterine segment, and obtain at least one sample from each quadrant. More sampling can be done if the patient is tolerating the procedure well.

15. Release the pressure on the syringe, withdraw the curette from the uterus, and express the sample into the formalin bottle by pushing the plunger of the syringe toward the curette. Label the formalin bottle.

16. Remove the speculum from the vagina.

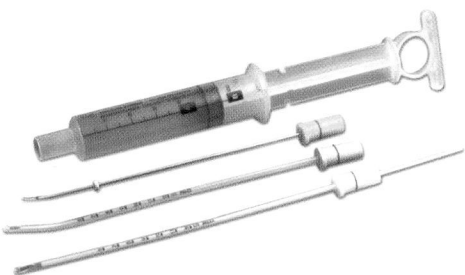

Fig. 129.4 Cannula curette endometrial aspirator. (Courtesy CooperSurgical, Inc., Trumbull, CN.)

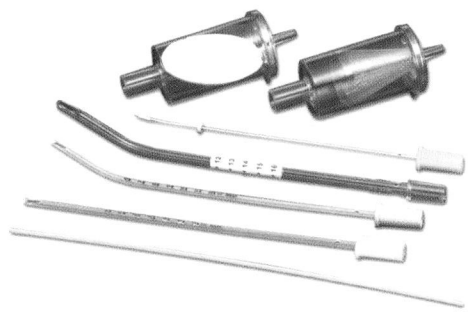

Fig. 129.5 Tis-U-Trap plastic disposable aspirator, including flat and cone-shaped collection chamber, sound, and endometrial curettes. (Courtesy CooperSurgical, Inc., Trumbull, CN.)

Tis-U-Trap, Vabra Aspirator, and Karman Cannula

The sterile and disposable Tis-U-Trap is a clear plastic tissue collection chamber (Fig. 129.5). It comes with a funnel, two sealing caps, a resealable bag, and either a flat or cone-shaped tissue trap. The Tis-U-Trap is used with one of several types of endometrial curettes. The trap is attached to an external suction source such as a pump or wall suction. Endometrial tissue is aspirated directly into the collection chamber, eliminating the need to transfer the tissue sample into another container. The design of the collection chamber permits easy visualization of the tissue collected and simplifies routine tissue handling for pathology.

The Vabra aspirator uses a 4-mm disposable curette or 2- to 3-mm stainless steel curette with an external vacuum pump. The vacuum pump is noisy, and this method is less commonly used than those listed previously. Tissue collected is gathered from a trap and placed in formalin.

The Karman cannula is made of flexible plastic and comes in diameters of 4 to 6 mm. It can be attached to a reusable syringe or external vacuum pump.

These devices are usually less comfortable for the patient due to the larger diameter and often require use of a tenaculum, dilation, and a paracervical block. However, they yield large amounts of tissue, similar to that of a dilation and curettage (D&C). They are particularly useful in women with moderate menstrual bleeding; they often allow the clinician to circumvent the clots and obtain tissue.

After completing previous steps 1 through 8, follow these steps for using the Tis-U-Trap, Vabra aspirator or Karman cannula-curette:

9. Apply a tenaculum to the anterior or posterior lip of the cervix.
10. Using a metal sound, carefully measure the depth of the endometrial cavity. Measurements usually range between 6.5 and 10 cm. If stenosis is present, cervical dilation may be necessary (see Chapter 126, Cervical Stenosis and Cervical Dilation).
11. Attach the device to the external suction pump (or large syringe for Karman cannula-curette).
12. Insert the curette through the cervical os, and gently advance until the fundus is reached. The depth should coincide with the uterine sound measurement.
13. Activate the pump to 55 cm H$_2$O.
14. Initiate suction by covering the suction hole with a finger (Fig. 129.6A).
15. Carefully curette the entire endometrium using a circumferential in-and-out movement. Keep the curette within the uterine cavity. The tissue passes through the curette and into the trap, where it collects on the grid.
16. When sufficient tissue accumulates in the trap, halt suction and then remove the curette from the uterus.
17. Turn the suction pump off, and disconnect the curette from the trap.
18. Add formalin to the trap, and ensure that all tissue is exposed. Cap and label the trap for submission to pathology (see Fig. 129.6B).
19. Remove the speculum from the vagina.

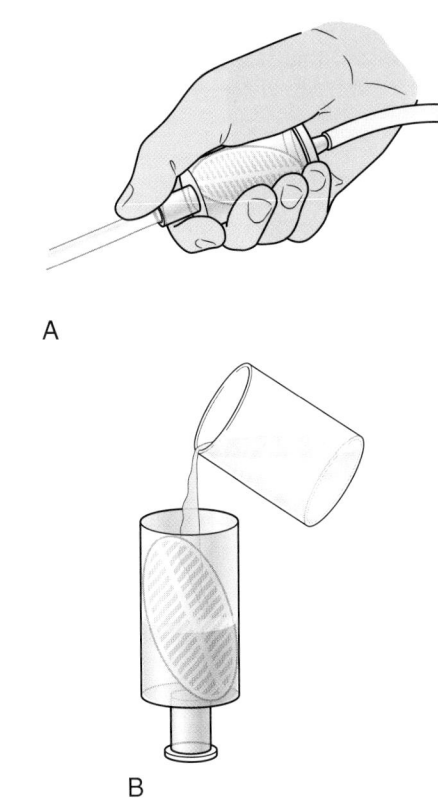

Fig. 129.6 (A) Initiate suction by covering the hole on the curette. (B) Remove the curette from the trap and cap the outlet. Pour formalin into the trap to cover all tissue and then seal.

Tao Brush

The Tao brush sampler consists of a tube with a distal brush (Fig. 129.7A). The brush is covered by a 26-cm, 9.0-Fr vinyl sheath. By keeping the brush covered during insertion, the sheath allows for sampling of endometrial cells only, without contamination from the vagina or cervix, because the brush is uncovered only once when it is in the uterine cavity. The brush obtains an adequate sampling from the entire endometrium. It is supplied in a sterile package and intended for one-time use only. The Tao brush may be used alone or before or after use of a plastic aspirator. In one study (Del Priore) of 101 women, the combination of the brush with a plastic aspirator had a sensitivity and specificity of 100% for diagnosis of endometrial hyperplasia or cancer. The manufacturer also suggests it can be used at the time of a routine Pap smear.

After following previous steps 1 through 8, the Tao brush procedure is as follows:

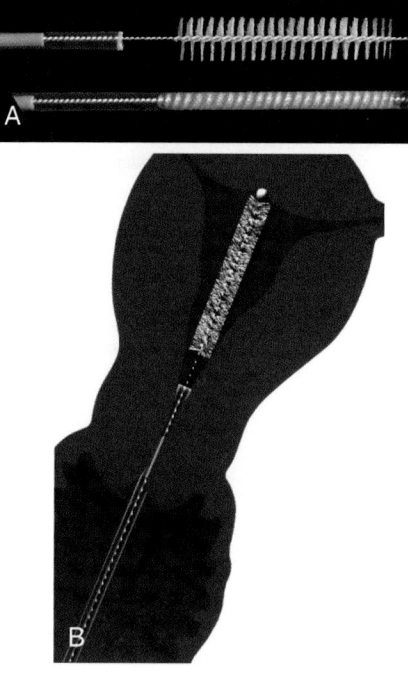

Fig. 129.7 Tao brush. (A) Endometrial sampler with sheath. (B) Brush inserted in the endometrial cavity with sheath retracted to allow for sampling. (Courtesy Cook Women's Health, Spencer, IN.)

9. Sound the uterus (up to 10 cm is normal). If stenosis is present, cervical dilation may be necessary (see Chapter 126, Cervical Stenosis and Cervical Dilation).
10. Insert the Tao brush with the outer sheath covering the brush. Gently advance it until the fundus is reached, based on the initial sounding depth.
11. Slide back the outer sheath to expose the plastic bristles and rotate 360 degrees once clockwise and then once counterclockwise against the uterine walls (see Fig. 129.7B).
12. Slide the sheath back in to cover the brush, and then remove the Tao brush and speculum.
13. Place the brush into the supplied CytoRich Brush Cytology Preservative. Rotate the brush in the preservative. Pull the sheath back and forth 10 times to dislodge the endometrial tissue. CytoRich Brush Cytology Preservative allows the pathologist to prepare a "thin-layer" sample (liquid-based cytology).

SAMPLE OPERATIVE REPORT

See the sample encounter form available at www.expertconsult.com.

COMMON ERRORS

- Inability to develop suction with a Pipelle or Novak/Randall-type endometrial aspirator. If the endocervical canal is large, change to a larger-diameter cannula and reattempt aspiration.
- Loss of suction during the biopsy. If the distal port of the Pipelle or syringe suction aspirator is pulled too far outside the endocervix, suction is lost as air is pulled in. To avoid this error, concentrate on keeping the aspirator within the uterine cavity and endocervix until the sample is obtained.
- Use of a small-diameter cannula in the setting of significant uterine bleeding. Large clots clog the cannula and make obtaining an adequate sample (rather than just blood) challenging. Switch to a larger-diameter cannula or Karman cannula-curette, Tis-U-Trap or Vabra aspirator, and reattempt aspiration.

COMPLICATIONS

- Uterine perforation occurs in 0.1% to 1.3% of EMBs. Perforation most often occurs with the use of rigid devices, while sounding the uterus, or when the cervix is stenotic. If the uterine sound passes more than 12 cm in a uterus that does seem that large on palpation, perforation is suspected. Stop the procedure, and withdraw all instruments. Observe the patient closely for bleeding. No other intervention is indicated unless symptoms develop. Patients may be discharged home with close follow-up if bleeding is minimal and vital signs are stable after 30 minutes of observation. Precautions regarding infection and bleeding should be discussed before release. Repeat biopsy can be attempted in 6 to 8 weeks.
- Excessive uterine bleeding is possible, especially in patients with undiagnosed coagulation disorders or perforation.
- Missed pathology is possible because only a small area of the endometrium is sampled. Although the sensitivity of EMB is estimated to be high as 96%, it may miss up to 18% of focal lesions. Fibroids and polyps will also not be identified.
- A vasovagal response occurs in an estimated 10% of patients after EMB. As previously discussed, use of IM atropine may help to minimize the risk of this complication.
- Although most women experience cramping during the endocervical curettage, pain after the procedure is usually minimal. Pain lasting longer than 24 hours should be reported to the provider.
- Bacteremia, septicemia, and endocarditis have been reported after EMB, although they are exceedingly rare. The patient should report any fever or foul discharge.

POSTPROCEDURE MANAGEMENT

- Patients should remain semirecumbent for 10 minutes after the EMB has been taken. Assess for vasovagal reaction.
- Painful uterine cramps (if present) usually subside rapidly or are relieved with NSAIDs.
- Patients with minimal cramping and bleeding may be discharged home.
- Although a follow-up visit is usually not necessary, it may be needed to discuss pathology findings. If AUB persists, further evaluation with a repeat EMB, D&C, hysteroscopy, or pelvic ultrasound is indicated.

POSTPROCEDURE PATIENT EDUCATION

Bleeding and cramping usually resolve within 24 to 48 hours. Fever, cramping lasting longer than 48 hours, or bleeding heavier than a normal period should be reported. NSAIDs can be used for pain or cramping. Sexual relations may be resumed after bleeding has stopped.

INTERPRETATION OF RESULTS

1. When submitting an EMB, conveying adequate clinical history to the pathologist is essential. The patient's age, clinical indication for biopsy, menopausal status, and date/length of last menstrual period in premenopausal women are important. Exogenous hormones, hormonal contraceptives, and drugs such as tamoxifen can alter the morphology of the endometrium and cause false-positive or false-negative results (Fig. 129.8).
2. Biopsy interpretation is based on the status of the functionalis layer located in the upper two thirds of the endometrium. The basalis layer usually shows minimal change. Atrophic, denuded, or scarred endometrium may not yield sufficient tissue for diagnosis. Inadequate samples are possible in biopsies immediately after menses, with hypoestrogenism, with prolonged bleeding, or with intrauterine adhesions/synechiae. Menopausal status has a greater effect on specimen adequacy than the type of instrument used (Box 129.2).

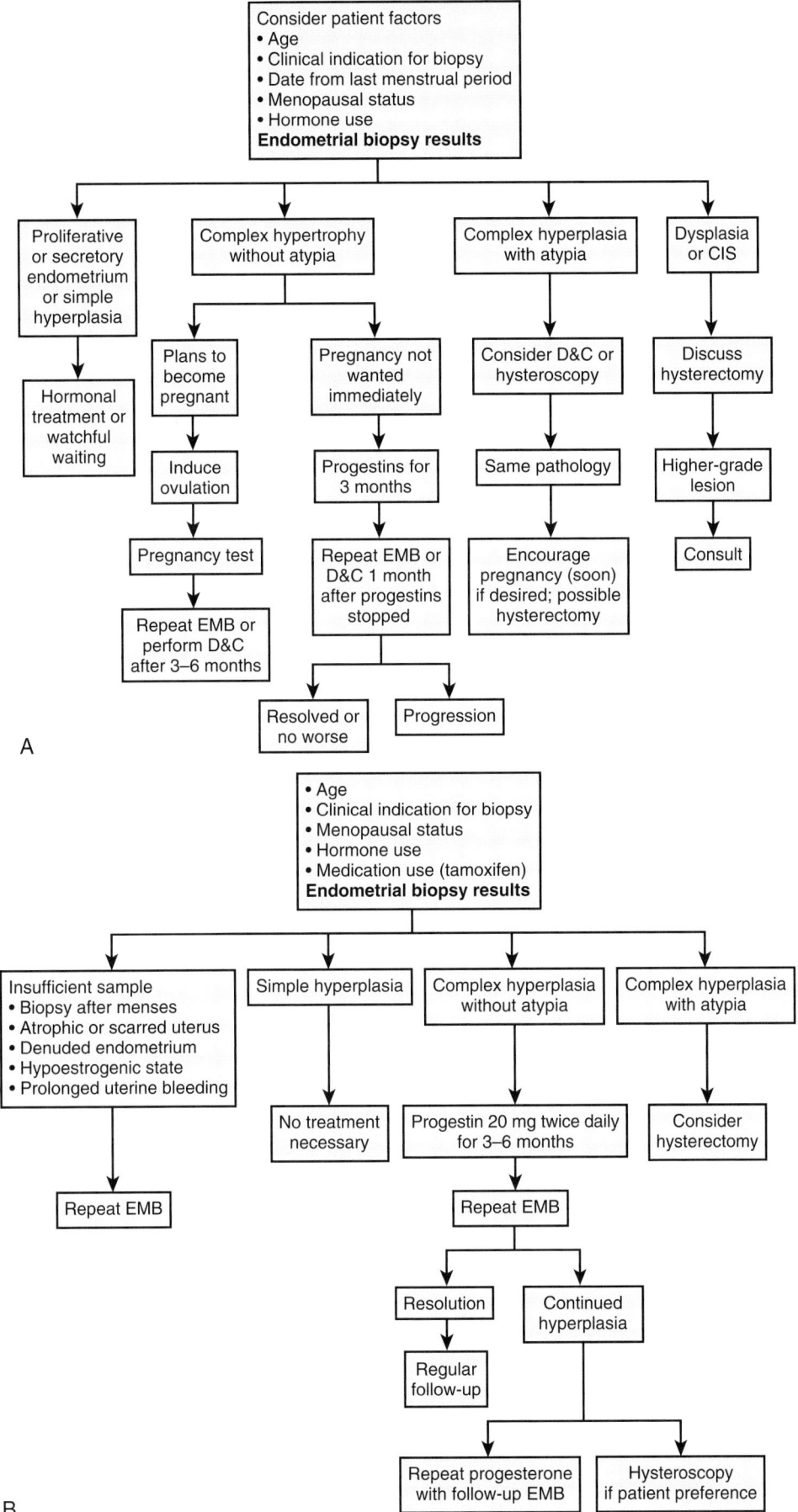

Fig. 129.8 Management options after endometrial biopsy in premenopausal (A) and postmenopausal (B) women. *CIS*, Carcinoma in situ; *D&C*, dilation and curettage; *EMB*, endometrial biopsy.

> **BOX 129.2 Findings on Endometrial Biopsy Sampling**
>
> **Insufficient Tissue**
> Follow-up depends on clinical situation; may need to repeat or use other diagnostic techniques
>
> **Normal**
> Proliferative endometrium
> Secretory endometrium
> Atrophic endometrium
>
> **Pregnancy Related**
> Retained products of conception
> Decidua (consider an ectopic or missed abortion)
>
> **Infectious Etiology**
> Endometritis, treat as indicated
>
> **Abnormal**
> Rarely, endometrial polyp
> Simple (cystic) hyperplasia
> * Risk for progression to cancer extremely small; little need for follow-up unless symptoms present.
> Complex (adenomatous) hyperplasia
> * Low but some risk for progression to cancer
> * Treat with progestational agents and follow up with tissue sampling in 6 months
> Atypical hyperplasia (simple and complex)
> * Significant risk for progression to cancer
> * Consider hysterectomy because of significant risk of progression to invasion and need for long-term follow-up to detect progression. If childbearing is not complete, treat with progestational agents and follow with frequent biopsies. Referral and consultation should be strongly considered.
> Adenocarcinoma
> * Referral indicated for appropriate work-up and treatment
> If the endocervical curettage is positive for dysplasia, a conization is indicated. If symptoms persist in spite of treatment, regardless of biopsy results, further evaluation is indicated.

3. The classification of endometrial hyperplasia is made according to guidelines from either the International Society of Gynecological Pathologists or the World Health Organization (Box 129.3). Endometrial hyperplasia covers a spectrum of alterations in the stroma and glands of the endometrium. Changes range from hyperplasia to atypical hyperplasia to carcinoma. Both hyperplasia and atypical hyperplasia are further categorized as either simple or complex:

   * Simple hyperplasia describes an increased glandular-to-stromal ratio without evidence of glandular crowding or cellular atypia. Cystic hyperplasia is an older term that is no longer used. There is no clinical significance to this finding, and no treatment is needed.
   * In complex hyperplasia, infolding and budding of the glands is noted. Glands are crowded in comparison with simple hyperplasia, but no atypia is noted. The older term adenomatous hyperplasia is no longer in use.
   * In atypical hyperplasia, cytologic atypia is divided into simple or complex categories depending on the glandular architecture. Large nuclei of varying shape and size, increased nuclear-to-cytoplasm ratio, and prominent nucleoli are commonly described.

4. Endometrial hyperplasia without cytologic atypia is usually managed with progestins; 10 to 20 mg medroxyprogesterone acetate given daily is prescribed for 3 to 6 months. EMB is repeated after therapy, and complete reversal of lesions is often noted. If hyperplasia without atypia is again confirmed, a repeat course of progestin with follow-up EMB or hysteroscopy can be performed. Some patients may opt for a hysterectomy at this point.

> **BOX 129.3 International Society of Gynecological Pathologists Classification for Endometrial Hyperplasia**
>
> **Endometrial Hyperplasia**
> Simple
> Complex
>
> **Endometrial Hyperplasia With Atypia**
> Simple
> Complex

5. Hyperplasia with cytologic atypia is best managed with a hysterectomy because of the risk of progression to adenocarcinoma. Approximately 10% of women with postmenopausal bleeding have endometrial cancer.

6. Histology determines management. Severity of endometrial hyperplasia and the probability of cancer cannot be determined by the amount of bleeding, at what point during the menstrual cycle the bleeding occurs, the gross appearance of the sample, or the tissue volume obtained by biopsy. Histopathology must be determined. Transvaginal endometrial thickness measurement is never a substitute for histologic tissue assessment in symptomatic women.

PATIENT EDUCATION GUIDES

See the patient education and consent forms available at www.expertconsult.com.

CPT/BILLING CODES

57505	Endocervical curettage not done as part of dilation and curettage
57800	Dilatation of cervical canal, instrumental
58100	Endometrial sampling (biopsy) with or without endocervical sampling, without cervical dilation, any method
59200	Insertion of cervical dilator (e.g., laminaria)

ICD-10-CM DIAGNOSTIC CODES

C54.9	Ca uterus
D26.9	Benign neoplasm of uterus
D07.0	Ca in situ, endometrium
D39.8	Neoplasm of uncertain behavior, uterus
N84.0	Polyp of endometrium
N85.2	Hypertrophy of uterus; bulky or enlarged uterus
N85.00	Endometrial hyperplasia unspecified
N85.01	Endometrial hyperplasia without atypia
N85.02	Endometrial hyperplasia with atypia
R87.619	Atypical glandular cells
N94.89	Pain associated with female genital organs (requires a fourth digit and must be as specific as possible)
N94.9	Unspecified symptoms associated with female genital organs
N92.3	Ovulation bleeding (regular intermenstrual bleeding)
N93.9	Metrorrhagia (bleeding unrelated to menstrual cycle; irregular intermenstrual bleeding)
N93.8	Dysfunctional uterine bleeding
N93.9	Unspecified uterine bleeding
N92.4	Premenopausal menorrhagia
N95.0	Postmenopausal bleeding
Z79.890	Postmenopausal HRT

Z85.40   Personal history of cancer of female genital organ, unspecified

Z85.41   Personal history of cancer of cervix, uteri

SUPPLIERS

(See contact information available at www.expertconsult.com.)

Plastic endometrial aspirator (often also make plastic endocervical aspirator)

Endocell endometrial sampler, Wallach Surgical

Endocervical curette with Vac-Loc syringe, Pipelle de Cornier, Pipet Curet; Cooper Surgical

EndoSampler and Pipette, MedGyn Products

Rigid Plastic Cannulas

Karman-type Cannula-Curette with 60-mL Handyvak Locking Syringe, Explora Models I and II; Milex CooperSurgical, Inc.

Tis-U-Trap Sampler Device, endometrial suction curette (flat trap and cone trap)

Milex CooperSurgical, Inc.

Vabra aspirator

Berkeley Medevices

Tao Brush

Cook Medical Women's Health

Acknowledgment

The editors recognize the contributions of Barbara S. Apgar, MD, and John L. Pfenninger, MD, to this chapter in previous editions of this text.

ONLINE RESOURCES

National Cancer Institute

For practitioners: Endometrial Cancer Treatment (PDQ)–Health Professional Version: https://www.cancer.gov/types/uterine/hp/endometrial-treatment-pdq

For patients: Uterine cancer: www.cancer.gov/types/uterine

RECOMMENDED READING

American College of Obstetricians and Gynecologists. 2009 American College of Obstetricians and Gynecologists. Antibiotic prophylaxis for gynecologic procedures. Practice Bulletin no. 104. *Obstet Gynecol.* 2009;113:1180–1189.

American College of Obstetricians and Gynecologists. The role of transvaginal ultrasonography in the evaluation of postmenopausal bleeding. Committee Opinion no. 426. *Obstet Gynecol.* 2009;113:462–464.

Apgar BS, Kaufman AJ, Bettcher C, Parker-Featherstone E. Gynecologic procedures: colposcopy, treatment of cervical intraepithelial neoplasia, and endometrial assessment. *Am Family Physician.* 2013;87(12):836–843.

Braun MM, Overbreek-Wager AE, Grumbo JR. Diagnosis and management of endometrial cancer. *Am Fam Physician.* 2016;93(6):468–474.

Del Priore G, Williams R, Harbatkin CB, Wan LS, Mittal K, Yang GC. Endometrial brush biopsy for the diagnosis of endometrial cancer. *J Reprod Med.* 2001;46(5):439.

Elsandabesee D, Greenwood P. The performance of Pipelle endometrial sampling in a dedicated postmenopausal bleeding clinic. *J Obstet Gynaecol.* 2005;25(1):32–34.

Hill DA. Abnormal uterine bleeding: avoid the rush to hysterectomy. *J Fam Pract.* 2009;58:136–142.

McCluggage W. My approach to the interpretation of endometrial biopsies and curettings. *J Clin Pathol.* 2006;59:801–812.

Renkonen-Sinisalo L, Butzow R, Leminen A, et al. Surveillance for endometrial cancer in hereditary nonpolyposis colorectal cancer syndrome. *Int J Cancer.* 2006;120:821–824.

Saso S, Chatterjee J, Georgiou E, et al. Endometrial cancer. *BMJ.* 2011;343:d3954.

Sierecki AR, Gudipudi DK, Montemarano N, Del Priore G. Comparison of endometrial aspiration biopsy techniques: specimen adequacy. *J Reprod Med.* 2008;53:760–764.

Smith R, Cokkinides V, Eyre HJ. American Cancer Society Guidelines for early detection of cancer, 2006. *CA Cancer J Clin.* 2006;56:11–25.

Sweet MG, Schmidt AT, Weiss MP, Mdsen PK. Evaluation and management of abnormal uterine bleeding in premenopausal women. *Am Fam Physician.* 2012;85(1):35-43.

Tanriverdi H, Barut A, Gün B, Kaya E. Is Pipelle biopsy really adequate for diagnosing endometrial disease? *Med Sci Monit.* 2004;10:CR271–CR274.

HYSTEROSCOPY

Stephen A. Grochmal • Lydia A. Watson • Dale A. Patterson

Hysteroscopy is one of the oldest endoscopic procedures described in the medical literature and was first performed in 1807 by Bozzini. Unfortunately, few gynecologists and even fewer primary care physicians perform office hysteroscopy today. The hysteroscope is an extremely valuable tool for viewing the endocervical canal and uterine cavity, and hysteroscopy is now recognized as the method of choice for diagnosing, sampling, and treating intrauterine disorders. Hysteroscopy provides an immediate direct visualization of the topography and contents of the uterine cavity, resulting in a more accurate diagnosis than that obtained from a dilation and curettage (D&C) or blind endometrial biopsy. More importantly, a hysteroscopic inspection increases the accuracy of diagnosis when there is an abnormally shaped endometrial cavity or other pathologic condition present. Visually directed biopsies (via hysteroscopy) are preferable to D&C, especially for focal rather than global disease. Direct visualization provided by the hysteroscope confirms that the suspicious pathology has been sampled appropriately. Hysteroscopy can be performed in the office or in an operating room and typically is most easily accomplished when performed during the proliferative phase of the menstrual cycle, when the endometrium is the thinnest.

ANATOMY

The uterus is a muscular organ that is partially covered by peritoneum. The cavity of the uterus is lined by the endometrium. The uterus resembles a flattened pear in shape and consists of two major but unequal parts: an upper triangular shaped portion referred to as the *body* or *corpus* and a lower fusiform or cylindrical portion, the *cervix*. The demarcation line between these two portions is known as the *isthmus*. The anterior surface of the uterus is practically flat, whereas the posterior surface is distinctly convex. The fallopian tubes emerge from the *cornua* of the uterus at the junction of the superior and lateral margins. The visible openings of the fallopian tubes are referred to as *ostia*. The upper or "top" portion of the uterus between the points of insertion of the fallopian tubes is called the *uterine fundus*. The cervical canal openings are called the *external os* and the *internal os*. The external os opens into the vaginal vault. The internal os is an important anatomic landmark during hysteroscopy because it marks the boundary between the uterine cavity and the endocervical canal, the location at which the main blood supply, the *uterine arteries and veins*, enters the uterus. Manipulation of the scope during hysteroscopy should cease when this landmark is reached. Overly vigorous operative procedures or activity in this area may result in excessive bleeding; they can even cause an unsuspected perforation during cervical dilation.

The wall of the body of the uterus is composed of three layers: (1) the outermost layer, the *serosa*, (2) the middle and thickest layer, the *myometrium*, and (3) the innermost portion, which lines the entire uterine cavity, the *endometrium*. The endometrium is a thin, pale pink, velvet-like membrane normally measuring in thickness from 0.5 to 5 mm, depending on cyclic changes that occur throughout the reproductive life of a woman. The endometrium is perforated by a large number of tiny openings, referred to as *uterine gland ostia*, which are easily visualized during a hysteroscopy.

Hysteroscopic findings should be described schematically, mentioning both negative and positive findings at the different levels of anatomy of the uterine cavity: cornua and tubal ostia, fundus, isthmus, internal cervical os, and the endocervical canal. A description of the appearance of the endometrium and endocervical mucosa also should be included.

INDICATIONS

- Unexplained abnormal uterine bleeding (AUB; premenopausal or postmenopausal)
  - Endometrial polyps
  - Submucous leiomyoma
  - Hyperplasia/malignancies
  - Endometritis
  - Adenomyosis
- Evaluation of selected infertility cases
  - Abnormal hysterosalpinogram
  - Foreign body (e.g., lost intrauterine device)
  - Uterine adhesions (Asherman syndrome)
  - Occluded tubal ostia (proximal tube can be cannulated; however, this is often performed in conjunction with laparoscopy for distal tube evaluation)
  - Suspected müllerian anomalies
  - Repeated pregnancy loss
  - Recurrent miscarriage
  - Abnormal uterine cavity (i.e., septum or another uterine anomaly)
  - Retained products of conception
- Preprocedural evaluation of uterine cavity (i.e., endometrial ablation [any method])
- Visually directed insertion of tubal occlusion contraceptive device
- Essure microinsert hysteroscopic sterilization procedure (see Chapter 132, Insertion of Essure [Contraceptive Implant] [Hysteroscopically Assisted Female Sterilization])
- Localization of lost intrauterine device

CONTRAINDICATIONS

Absolute
- Cardiac or pulmonary instability
- Acute pelvic infection

Relative
- Pregnancy
- Coagulopathies: idiopathic thrombocytopenic purpura, von Willebrand disease
- Previous uterine perforation or recent surgery or synechiae
- Known cervical or uterine carcinoma

- Morbidly obese patients
- Acute uterine bleeding
- Medical comorbidity that could be exacerbated by intravascular volume expansion (e.g., saline infusion)

EQUIPMENT

In order to perform hysteroscopy safely the mindset of the clinician should be the same, whether the procedure is performed in the office or in an operating room. The choice of equipment is important, especially if the clinician plans to perform operative procedures after gaining proficiency with simple diagnostic hysteroscopies.

The *basic* hysteroscope is a simple rigid (solid rod lens) device (Fig. 130.1). The diameter of the scope preferably is no greater than 5 to 5.5 mm when the introducing sheath is over the scope (used to protect the scope from breaking and provides a channel for continuous flow for fluid distention or an instrument). Size is important because the smaller the diameter of the scope, the less cervical dilation is required, and the more comfortable the procedure is for the patient. The angle of view for the scope is commonly 0 degrees, which provides a panoramic view once inside the uterine cavity; this is ideal for an all-around hysteroscope. Some surgeons prefer a 30-degree downward-looking view; other surgeons consider this more limiting.

Currently, the most commonly used device is the *flexible hysteroscope* (Fig. 130.2). The flexible distal tip can improve maneuverability once inside the uterine cavity because of the ability to deflect from 90 degrees to over 120 degrees. These flexible scopes are small in diameter (3.5 to 5 mm), do not require an outer sheath, and possess an operating channel. The latest generations have moved from fiberoptic bundle technology to digital chip-on-the-tip camera sensors (Fig. 130.3).

All newer flexible hysteroscopes are designed to accommodate instrumentation for office procedures such as the Essure sterilization. These flexible scopes are more costly than a rigid system. The high initial cost may be offset by the increased reimbursement achieved with the variety of procedures that can be performed with the flexible scope. The clinician may also choose to perform the procedure in a surgery center instead of investing in an office scope.

A *light source* ranging from 100 to 300 watts is needed. A halogen light is acceptable, but a xenon light source is preferred because it emulates natural daylight and provides superior illumination of the uterine cavity.

In addition, a *simple grasping forceps, biopsy forceps,* and *scissors* will round out the special instrumentation necessary to perform simple operative procedures such as endometrial biopsy, polyp removal, and removal of retained intrauterine devices.

An optional piece of equipment is a *video endoscope* (Fig. 130.4). A camera eliminates the need to look through the eyepiece of the hysteroscope and improves the working position, comfort, and visualization. It also allows the patient to observe the hysteroscopic evaluation as it is performed. Some vendors now offer systems with all these components in one stand-alone unit (Fig. 130.5).

Additional video equipment provides the ability to record and document the procedure so that photographic documentation of findings can be included in the patient's operative report. It also allows the clinician to send detailed information back to a referring colleague. These pictures should be maintained as an integral part of the patient's chart.

Choose a distention medium. Uterine distention is crucial to the success of any hysteroscopic procedure. Most office hysteroscopic procedures are performed with saline. CO_2 distention is mainly used for diagnostic hysteroscopy. Hyskon is a mixture of Dextran and dextrose, designed for use with hysteroscopy, but it is difficult to use and is messy. CO_2 is more difficult for the novice because of the tendency for troublesome gas bubbles to form, and it cannot be used if any bleeding occurs. For this reason, it is not useful if biopsies are performed. Sorbitol and glycerin are for use with electrical

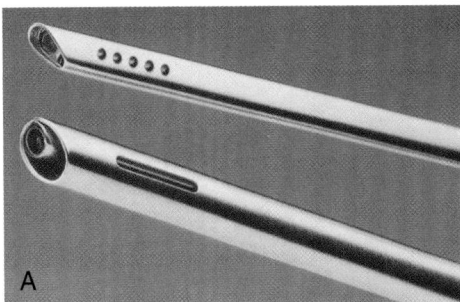
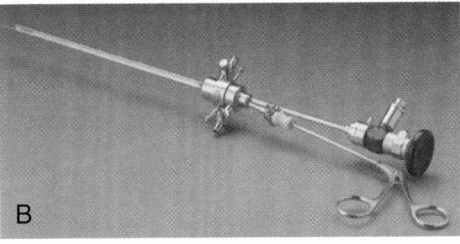

Fig. 130.1 (A) Diagnostic hysteroscopes with continuous-flow outer sheaths. The fenestrations on the distal tip of the sheath improve circulation of the liquid distention media. When using CO_2 distention, a single-flow sheath may be preferable. (B) Example of a diagnostic rigid hysteroscope and continuous-flow operating sheath with an operating channel used to pass a biopsy forceps or other instrumentation.

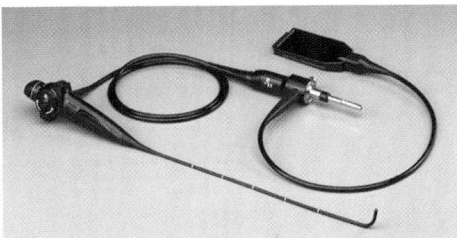

Fig. 130.2 Flexible small-diameter hysteroscopes are easy to manipulate and are comfortable for patients but may lack a large-diameter operating channel for the passage of biopsy instruments, tubal sterilization inserts, or other procedure instrumentation. (Courtesy Olympus Surgical America.)

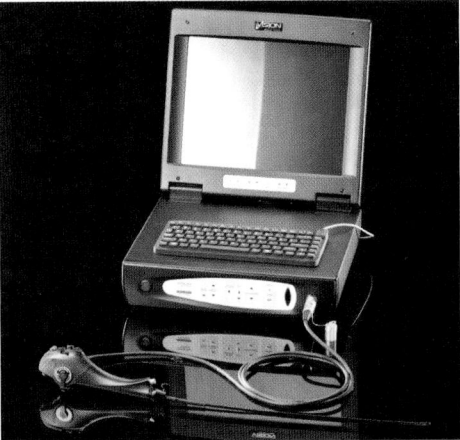

Fig. 130.3 Technologic advances in electronics and hysteroscope designs have produced all-in-one systems that contain a camera controller, light source, documentation digital photo/video recorder, and, in this example, a flexible hysteroscope. These systems are small and portable, allowing them to fit easily on a countertop. (Courtesy Medtronics VisionSciences.)

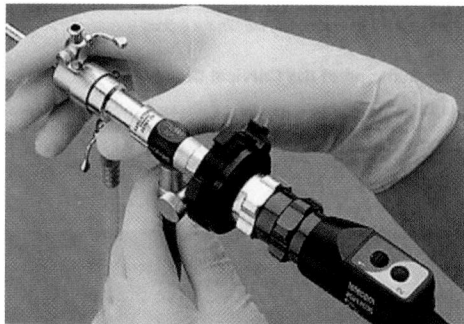

Fig. 130.4 Video cameras can directly attach to the eyepiece of the hysteroscope, dramatically improving visualization of the uterine cavity.

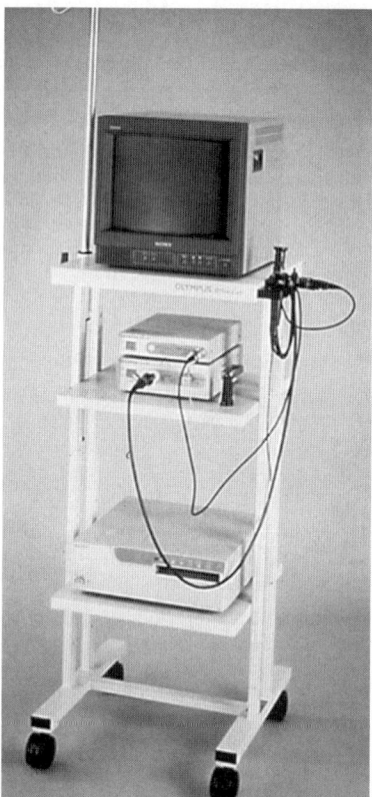

Fig. 130.5 New electronic equipment designs for office hysteroscopy have resulted in systems that allow the hysteroscope (in this case a flexible design) to connect directly to one unit, which contains the camera controller, light source, documentation recorder, and LCD monitor.

(bipolar) operative procedures. Consequently, saline is the consensus gold standard for office hysteroscopy. It is safe, physiologic, and inexpensive. A gravity flow system can be used for the majority of diagnostic procedures, providing more than adequate uterine distention (Fig. 130.6). A method for monitoring the amount of fluid used to distend the uterus is needed. It is uncommon to have fluid and electrolyte complications if less than 1 L of fluid is used during the procedure. Commercial systems are available to control the flow and accurately record the fluid deficit during hysteroscopy. Intraoperative fluid management is an important aspect of hysteroscopy. Both the American Congress of Obstetricians and Gynecologists, and the American Association of Gynecologic Laparoscopists recommend the use of an automated fluid management system. These systems provide real-time information about the fluid deficit and can actively manage intrauterine pressures. A staff person should be designated to call out the deficit when it reaches 500 mL; they should also call out every additional 100 mL. For short diagnostic procedures, the

amount of fluid used to distend the uterus is usually 500 mL or less. For slightly larger volumes, monitoring the amount of fluid used and collecting the residual in a pouched drape for subsequent measurement is an option. Carbon dioxide is also commonly used with few complications (Fig. 130.7). Instructions on the use of both normal saline and carbon dioxide are noted later.

A standard tray for hysteroscopy includes instruments for anesthesia and cervical dilation (Fig. 130.8A–B):

- Antiseptic solution (e.g., povidone-iodine, chlorhexidine)
- Large cotton-tipped swabs
- Vaginal speculum (unhinged one side, open-sided Graves, or disposable illuminated types) (see Fig. 130.8C)
- Cervical tenaculum
- Ring forceps
- Uterine sound
- Cervical dilators (see Chapter 126, Cervical Stenosis and Cervical Dilation)
- Topical 2% benzocaine solution or spray (e.g., Hurricaine, Americaine)
- Lidocaine without epinephrine 1% to 2% (optional but helpful); anesthesia can be accomplished with topical and local anesthetic
- 10-mL syringe with 4-inch needle extender and 25- to 27-gauge needle, or a dental syringe, if anesthetic is to be given into or near the cervix (see Chapter 127, Loop Electrosurgical Excision Procedure for Treating Cervical Intraepithelial Neoplasia, and Chapter 153, Paracervical Block)
- Endocervical curette
- Equipment to maintain universal blood and body fluid precautions

PRECAUTIONS

Poor visualization increases the risk of complications. Larger uteri may take a bit longer to achieve adequate distention. Plan ahead for adequate time with each patient to ensure adequate distention and visualization.

- Be aware that not all insufflators, light sources, and scopes are interchangeable. Mixing and matching may be dangerous. Check compatibility issues with your suppliers.
- A pregnancy test is advised in all reproductive-age patients prior to the procedure.
- Cervical cultures should be obtained for patients at high risk for pelvic infections before hysteroscopy is performed.
- Avoid hysteroscopy during menses or heavy bleeding if possible—it is more difficult to see uterine contents and landmarks.
- As with any in-office invasive procedure, proper emergency resuscitation equipment and action plan should be readily available (see discussion of the Banyan kit in Chapter 212, Anaphylaxis).

PREPROCEDURE PREPARATION

- The patient should be provided with a patient education handout or pamphlet prior to the procedure.
- A consent form for diagnostic hysteroscopy with or without endometrial biopsies should be obtained.
- Document the last menstrual period, contraceptive method, and pregnancy test (if indicated) results on every patient.
- Preprocedure antibiotics are not required.
- Nonsteroidal antiinflammatory drugs (NSAIDs) (e.g., ibuprofen 800 mg) administered 30 minutes before the procedure can significantly diminish discomfort.

PROCEDURE

There are multiple variations of how to perform a hysteroscopy. The steps listed here are one such method.

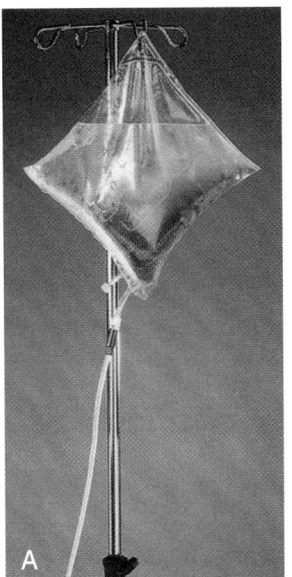
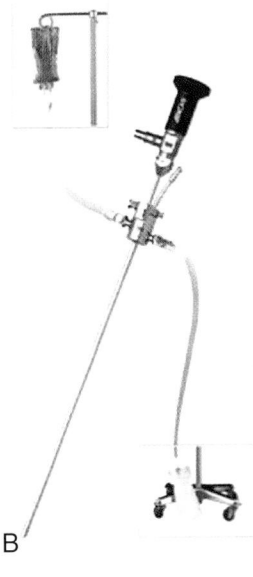
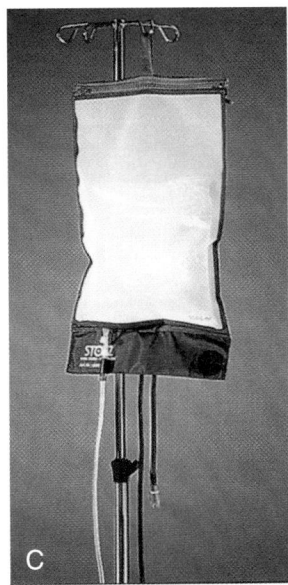

Fig. 130.6 Systems used to achieve distention of the uterine cavity during diagnostic hysteroscopy. (A) A 1000-mL bag of saline with large-bore tubing used for gravity flow distention. (B) A closed system designed to capture the outflow distention fluid. (C) A simple pressure cuff used to increase flow of distention medium; it offers no control of intrauterine pressure. (B, Courtesy Gynex.)

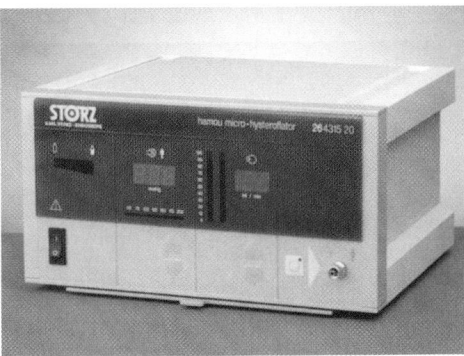

Fig. 130.7 Use of CO_2 as a distention medium for diagnostic hysteroscopy mandates an appropriate device for instillation of the CO_2 gas. Intrauterine pressure must be precisely maintained to avoid passage of distention media into the fallopian tubes and subsequently into the abdominal cavity. (Courtesy Karl Storz.)

1. Throughout the procedure, attempt to maintain a sterile environment, especially with equipment and instrumentation that are inserted into the uterus. The vaginal component of the procedure is considered a "clean" field, but it is a good habit to maintain sterile technique throughout the entire procedure. Follow universal blood and body fluid precautions.
2. With the patient in dorsal lithotomy position and preferably on an electric-powered examination table, perform a bimanual pelvic examination to ascertain the size, shape, and position of the uterus. Failure to do this may result in a uterine perforation during cervical dilation or initial insertion of the hysteroscope.
3. Insert a disposable illuminated vaginal speculum or a reusable open-sided Graves speculum.
4. Prep the cervix and vagina with antiseptic solution.
5. Insert a large cotton applicator under the cervix and spray a small amount of topical 2% benzocaine oral anesthetic (Hurricaine, Americaine) solution on the cervix. The cotton applicator will absorb the anesthetic. Allow the applicator to remain in contact with the cervix as you talk to the patient and prepare your instruments. Remove the applicator.
6. Infiltration of the paracervical tissue with a local anesthetic is common for hysteroscopy. A paracervical block can decrease the pain of tenaculum placement, cervical dilation, and hysteroscope insertion through the cervix. However, paracervical

anesthesia has less effect on the pain of uterine distension. One must balance the expected pain of the hysteroscopic procedure with the pain and potential side-effects of the paracervical block, which can include bradycardia and hypotension. For these reasons, many providers choose to forgo this step, especially for brief diagnostic procedures. If chosen, local anesthesia of the cervix is obtained using a dental-style cartridge syringe with ampules of 2% lidocaine (or another anesthetic) and a 25- to 27-gauge dental needle. Place a minimum of 1 mL (maximum amount per quadrant is 2 mL) of anesthetic at the 3, 6, 9, and 12 o'clock positions of the cervix into the subserosal layer. (For more detailed instructions, see chapters noted earlier.)

7. Grasp the anterior (or posterior, depending on uterine position) lip of the cervix with a tenaculum.
8. Perform an endocervical curettage if indicated.
9. Sound the uterus to determine depth and direction of the central uterine axis.
10. Dilate the cervical canal. Using a set of Silastic or metal graduated dilators, insert the os finder or a 3 mm dilator into the cervix, and, feeling for resistance, pass this through to the internal os, if possible. Continue progressive dilation up to a size 1 mm over the diameter of the hysteroscope. Dilation should be done slowly with a constant gentle pressure, especially in the nulligravid patient. Multiparous patients are generally easier to dilate. You may leave this dilator in the cervix to maintain patency as you reach for the hysteroscope. For stenotic patients, see Chapter 126, Cervical Stenosis and Cervical Dilation.
11. Remove the dilator.
12. The saline is suspended 60 cm above the uterus and will enter the cavity with a pressure of 45 mm Hg (see Fig. 130.6). The maximum uterine pressure via any distention method should not exceed 70 mm Hg, which is below the capillary pressure of 100 mm Hg. Varying the height of the saline bag will alter this infusion pressure. If a pressure sleeve is placed around the bag of saline, additional pressure required to increase flow rate of the distention medium can be achieved by inflating the sleeve as needed. This is a useful technique in patients with a larger uterus or when a faster flow of distention medium is required to clear the field of view (see Fig. 130.6C). If carbon dioxide is used, begin insufflation once the scope engages the external os. Use the instillation port on the scope at an initial rate of 30 mL/min. As the hysteroscope traverses the endocervical canal, the carbon dioxide will create a visual space ahead of the scope. Advance the scope only if the view is clear. The internal os is seen

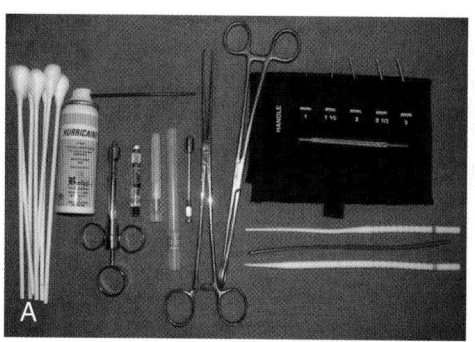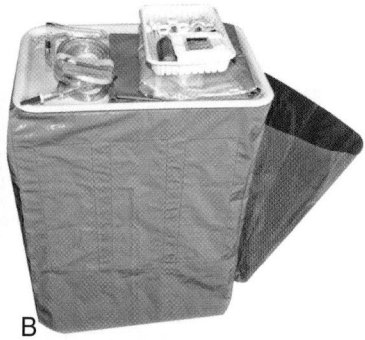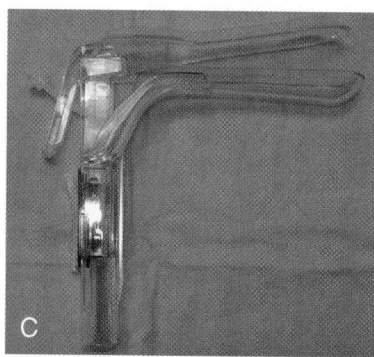

Fig. 130.8 (A) Typical instrument setup for office diagnostic hysteroscopy. (B) Disposable office packs make procedure setup and clean-up simple. These packs contain all the necessary items required to perform an office hysteroscopy. (C) Example of a disposable, self-illuminating LED, open-sided speculum. (B–C, Courtesy OBP Medical, Inc.)

as a narrow constriction at the upper portion of the endocervical canal. Increase the carbon dioxide insufflation rate to 40 to 60 mL/min when the isthmus of the uterus is entered. The carbon dioxide insufflation must be critically controlled during the procedure. If the gas is instilled too quickly, obstructive bubbles of carbon dioxide will form. The maximum flow rate should not exceed 100 mL/min and a maximum pressure of 100 mm Hg. The risk of gas embolism is proportional to the flow rate of the infused gas. Embolization of small amounts of CO_2 is not dangerous, and over 50% of CO_2 hysteroscopies have some amount of carbon dioxide embolization.

If saline is used, the hysteroscope is inserted under direct visualization, advancing the scope slightly into the endocervical canal. Start the distention fluid (e.g., normal saline) flowing and continue to gently advance the scope until you feel a slight resistance. You are now at the uterine fundus. Pause to confirm that the distention fluid is flowing into the cavity. Using a continuous flow hysteroscope and a bag of saline hanging from an intravenous (IV) pole approximately 60 cm above the patient, the distention fluid flow rate will range between 125 and 200 mL/min with an average intrauterine pressure of approximately 45 mm Hg; this rate creates no problems. This flow rate may vary based on parameters such as the diameter of the tubing used, exact height of the IV pole, if suction aspiration is used on the outflow side of the hysteroscope, and if a pressure cuff is employed around the saline bag.

13. Withdraw the scope ever so slightly from the fundus and wait. As the distention fluid clears, the fundus will come into view. If you have successfully reached this point, the hysteroscopy is 75% complete and all that remains is the visual inspection of the cavity. Remember, failure to achieve adequate distention and repeated attempts to do so increase the risk of procedure failure and complications. If the uterus cannot be easily distended, consider stopping the procedure. It is important to recognize when to stop!

14. Inspect the uterine cavity. Withdraw the scope slightly and look at the fundus. Move the hysteroscope to the patient's right, then left. You can move the scope in or out, up or down, and rotate it to achieve the best views (Figs. 130.9 and 130.10). The central point of müllerian duct fusion projects down from the fundus. The cornua are located on both sides of this fused tissue. Evaluate the tubal ostia. Continue to withdraw the hysteroscope down into the lower segment of the uterine cavity. Visualize the anterior, posterior, and lateral walls of the cavity, maneuvering the scope ever so slightly when needed. Document any findings with photo or video recording as the procedure is performed. Continue to withdraw the scope until a "ring" appears over the scope. This is the level of the internal os of the cervix and the start of the endocervical canal. It is an important landmark to document and confirm the completion of the uterine cavity inspection (Figs. 130.11 and 130.12).

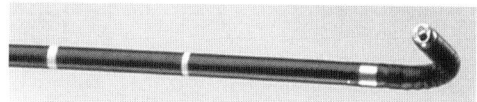

Fig. 130.9 Mobile tip at the end of the hysteroscope. (Courtesy Olympus Corp., Melville, NY.)

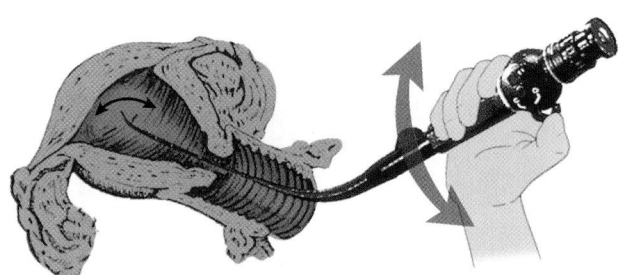

Fig. 130.10 Hysteroscopic examination of the uterine cavity.

15. Biopsy any suspicious areas. If hysteroscopy is being performed to evaluate endometrial polyps or other intrauterine pathology, tissue samples can be obtained with hysteroscopic forceps followed by a D&C after hysteroscopy. The hysteroscopy can be repeated after the D&C to confirm complete tissue removal. Remove stalked endometrial polyps with grasping forceps. Generally, any bleeding will stop on its own and no cautery or chemicals are needed. All biopsies are taken after a complete inspection of the uterine cavity and prior to terminating hysteroscopy. Bleeding from the biopsies, even minimal, may decrease visualization regardless of the distention medium selected. With CO_2, this will decrease the view and may not allow re-entry into the cavity and require terminating any further observation. With saline, the clouding will dissipate as fluid continues to flow through the uterine cavity. The field generally clears, allowing the procedure to continue if necessary, but this may not always be the case.

16. When the diagnostic survey is complete, the hysteroscope is slowly withdrawn. Careful inspection during removal provides one final chance to inspect the endocervical canal. A complete diagnostic hysteroscopy should take approximately 10 to 15 minutes. Continue to withdraw the scope through the endocervical canal, observing and documenting when necessary. You have now completed what is referred to as a retrograde diagnostic hysteroscopy. Shut off the distention flow and remove the scope from the vagina. Remove the tenaculum and observe for any bleeding. Remove all other instrumentation and the procedure is complete.

17. Clean the scope.

18. Dictate an operative report.

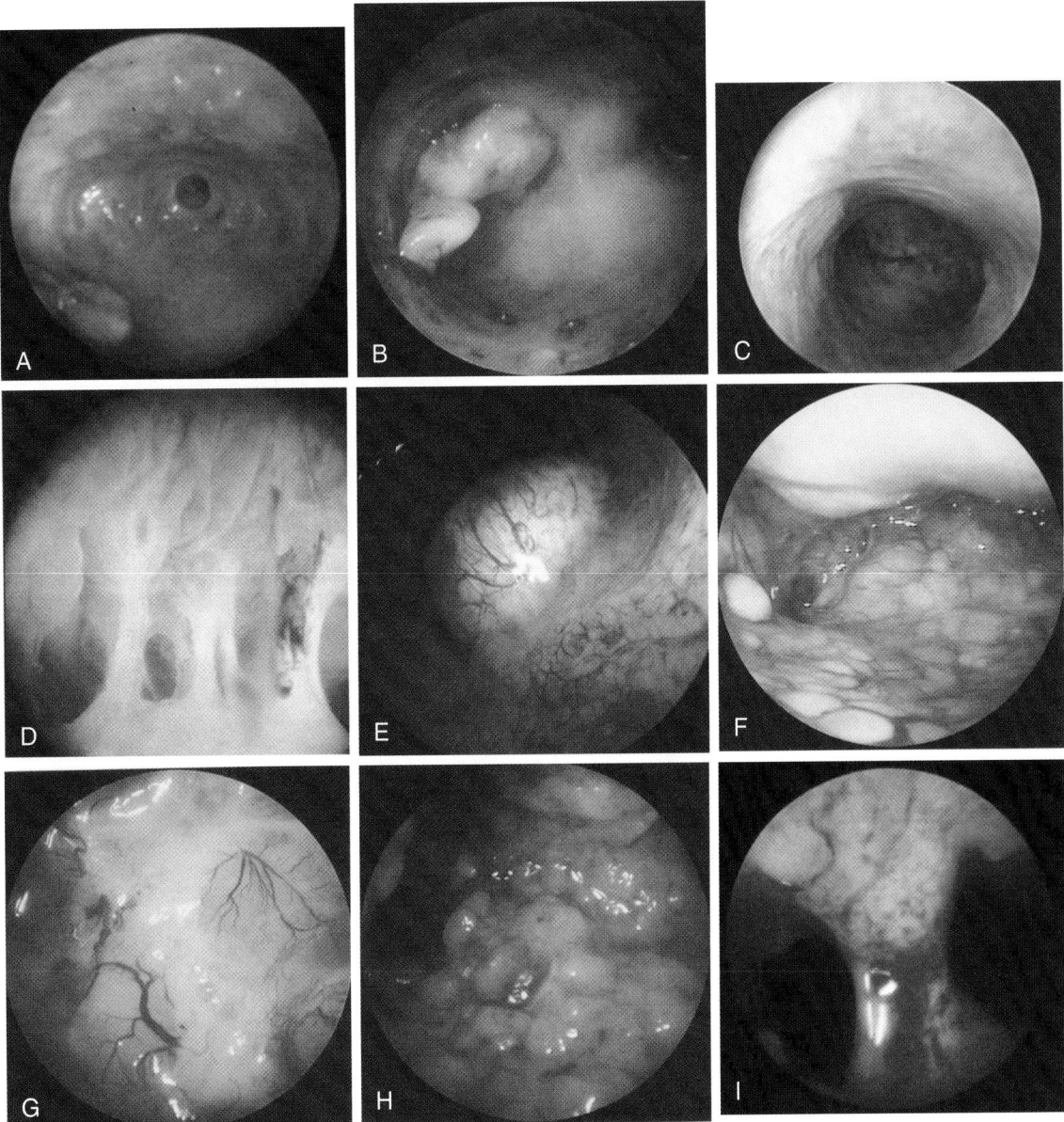

Fig. 130.11 Typical uterine anatomy and pathology seen during diagnostic hysteroscopy. (A) Tubal ostium (normal). (B) Benign polyp in right cornua of uterine cavity. (C) Atrophic endometrium. (D) Uterine adhesions (synechiae). (E) Submucosal fibroid. (F) Benign endometrial hyperplasia (cystic). (G) Endometrial hyperplasia (high risk). (H) Endometrial cancer. (I) Uterine septum (side-by-side double-barrel shotgun appearance).

SAMPLE OPERATIVE REPORT

Preoperative diagnosis: Abnormal uterine bleeding
Procedure performed: Diagnostic hysteroscopy with endometrial biopsies; endocervical curettage
Postoperative diagnosis: Endometrial polyps, hypertrophic endometrium
Surgeon: Dr. _____
Assistant: _____ (Dr.'s name, assistant's name, or none)
Estimated blood loss: Nil
Complications: None
Findings: _____
Total distention fluid instilled: Approx. 350 mL of normal saline
Total fluid recovered: Approx. 300 mL

With the patient on the procedure table in dorsal lithotomy position and in Allen stirrups, the patient was prepped and draped for

hysteroscopy. Bimanual examination revealed a normal size, anteverted uterus and no significantly palpable adnexal masses.

An illuminated speculum was inserted into the vagina and the cervix was cleansed with povidone iodine solution. Topical benzocaine (e.g., Hurricaine, Americaine) was applied to the cervix and the run-off collected by a sponge stick. After waiting a few minutes for the topical anesthetic to take effect, an intrastromal cervical block was performed. Approximately 1.8 mL of 2% lidocaine without epinephrine per quadrant was injected at 12, 3, 6, and 9 o'clock positions on the cervix with a 27-gauge needle and Tubex syringe. The anterior lip of the cervix was grasped with a single-tooth tenaculum and an endocervical curettage was performed, followed by uterine sounding. Progressive dilation of the cervix with graduated dilators was carried out up to 6 mm. The uterus sounded to 10 cm. Thereafter, a 30-degree hysteroscope with diagnostic/operating sheath was inserted into the uterus under direct visualization and gently brought to bear against the fundus of the uterus. Using a

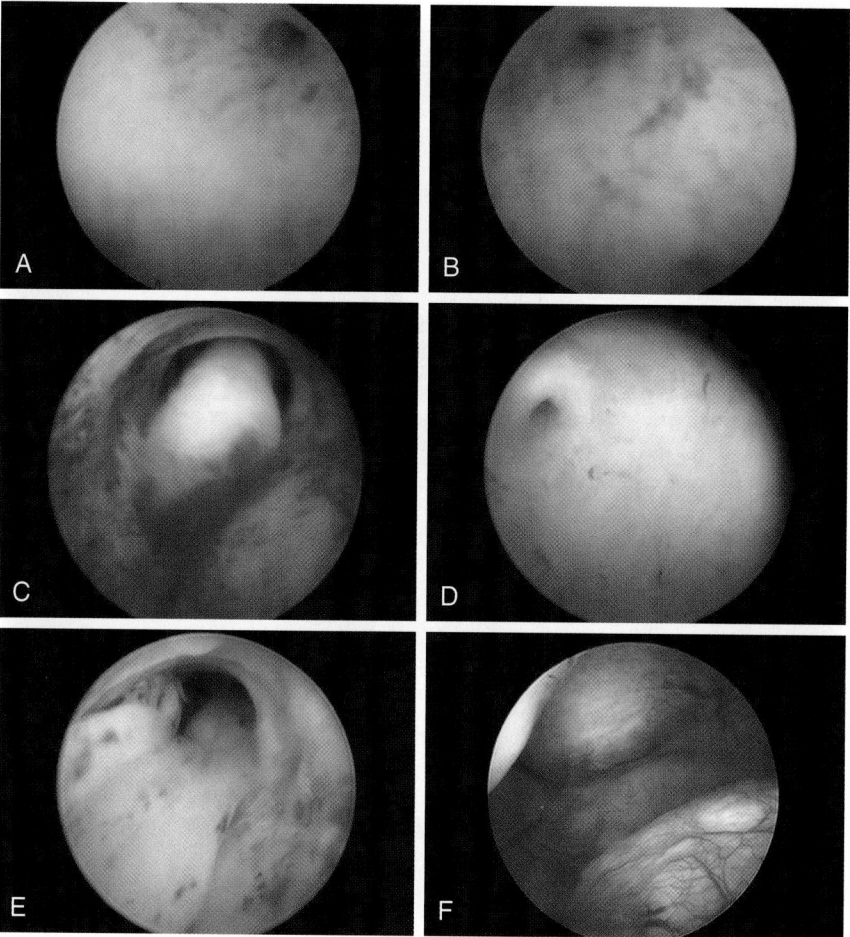

Fig. 130.12 (A–B) Fallopian tube. (C) Endometrial polyp arising from fundus (seen on entrance into uterus). (D) Fallopian tube. (E) Attachment site of endometrial polyp at fallopian tube. (F) Uterine fibroids.

gravity flow saline distention, the uterine cavity was distended until a clear image was achieved. [Optional to mention: video footage or digital photos were taken.] The hysteroscope was withdrawn gradually from the fundus until both tubal ostia could be visualized; both appeared normal. As the hysteroscope was withdrawn further into the uterine cavity, the entire fundus and upper portion of the cavity were visualized. Inspection of the cavity did not reveal the presence of any adhesions, submucous fibroids, or abnormal configuration. Of note were areas with visible large vessels coursing superficially beneath the thickened, hypertrophic endometrium. Multiple biopsies were taken with the biopsy forceps via the operating channel and individually marked according to their location. As the hysteroscope was withdrawn further, the level of the internal os was clearly identified. Three small endometrial polyps, the largest measuring approximately 0.5 cm, were seen. [Mention that a photograph or video was taken.] The hysteroscope continued to be withdrawn in a retrograde fashion under direct visualization through the endocervical canal, which was unremarkable. The hysteroscope was then removed from the vagina and the saline distention discontinued. Any residual fluid was evacuated from the vagina and the cervical tenaculum removed. No bleeding was noted from the cervix. Any remaining instruments were then removed from the vagina to complete the procedure. The patient tolerated the procedure well; after a 15-minute recovery they left the office feeling well and in good condition.

COMMON ERRORS

- Attempting procedure with inadequate distention of the uterus.
- Performing the procedure under poor visualization. If the distention fluid is murky or bloody, stop until the field clears. Then

proceed slowly. If the field is still cloudy, check your distention connection tubing and bag of fluid. If this problem continues, stop the procedure and reschedule the patient. Do not perforate!
- If you suspect a perforation, just stop. Remove all instruments. Place the patient in a semi-upright position and observe her for changes in vital signs, pallor, complaint of pain, or vaginal bleeding. Be prepared to consider a diagnostic laparoscopy. Most perforations are uneventful and the puncture closes readily, but always err on the side of caution. Repeat hysteroscopy can be performed in 6 weeks.
- Performing a biopsy prior to completing inspection of the entire uterine cavity may cause bleeding, thus clouding the visual field and resulting in the inability to complete the uterine cavity evaluation.

COMPLICATIONS

- Cervical laceration secondary to forceful dilatation.
- Uterine perforation.
- Infection.
- Fluid overload (usually not a concern with diagnostic hysteroscopies; most only require 250 to 350 mL of distention medium).
- Complications related to carbon dioxide insufflation (if used) are rare with the use of a constant-flow insufflator. Acidosis and hypercarbia are rare events. Patients can experience shoulder pain due to irritation of the diaphragm from the CO_2 (rare, 2% to 5% of cases). If the patient complains of shoulder pain, keep her lying flat and ask her to breathe deeply. The pain may last up to 20 minutes before dissipating.
- Inability to perform the procedure secondary to cervical stenosis
- Vasovagal reactions occur in less than 1% of patients, but clinicians should be prepared to manage these reactions and symptomatic bradycardia.

POSTPROCEDURE MANAGEMENT

- Keep the patient in a semiupright position for about 15 minutes.
- Observe for any watery discharge or excessive bleeding.
- Suggest NSAIDs as needed for any postprocedure discomfort.
- Patient resumes normal activity within 4 to 6 hours.

POSTPROCEDURE PATIENT EDUCATION

- Patients may notice mild cramping after the procedure. Reassure them that it is transitory and to use NSAIDs for relief.
- Some watery or blood-tinged discharge is normal for up to 2 to 3 hours. Instruct the patient to use a sanitary pad and to report any prolonged episodes of vaginal discharge, bright red bleeding, fever, or excessive abdominal pain.
- Instruct patients to avoid inserting anything in the vagina for 24 hours. They may resume intercourse after 24 hours.
- Patients generally will return to their daily lifestyle activities within 8 hours after the procedure with no restrictions on physical activity.
- Patients should call if there is any foul odor or discharge, which could signal an infection.

INTERPRETATION OF FINDINGS

- *AUB* is probably the most common symptom investigated by hysteroscopy. Endometrial biopsy or D&C can be carried out at the end of the hysteroscopic examination. The main causes of AUB are submucous myomas, endometrial polyps, endometrial atrophy, and postpregnancy metrorrhagia.
- *Submucous myomas* can vary in appearance. At times they have a regular, smooth surface covered by a homogeneous endometrium similar to that of the remainder of the uterine cavity. If there is extensive intracavitary progression, then the ensuing compressed endometrium may give rise to ulceration and necrosis near the apex of new growth. At times, the surface of the myoma appears lobulated, pearly white in color, and grooved with one or more large blood vessels (see Fig. 130.11E).
- *Endometrial polyps* are exophytic, usually sessile mucous lesions varying in shape, number, size, and appearance. Their surface is typically similar to that of the surrounding endometrium; they are usually soft in consistency upon contact with biopsy forceps or a hysteroscope. Pedunculated polyps have a variable length to their pedicle consisting of vascularized connective tissue. These lesions have cubic, short, cylindrical epithelium interspersed with hypertrophic blood vessels. Polyps can be associated with glandular endometrial hyperplasia (EH) and can remain latent for long periods (see Fig. 130.11B).
- *Endometrial atrophy* is a postmenopausal physiologic change that may cause bleeding. The hysteroscopic image is quite characteristic; since the endometrial mucosa is quite thin, it often appears transparent, revealing the underlying vascular structures. The presence of hemorrhagic petechiae is very typical. With severe endometrial atrophy, the epithelium is smooth and pale, nearly white (see Fig. 130.11C).
- *Postpregnancy metrorrhagia.* In patients with postpartum or postabortal bleeding, hysteroscopy may be used to confirm evacuation or removal of all abortive debris from the uterine cavity. The overall appearance is that of an atrophic endometrium infused with hemorrhagic areas and petechiae along with dangling pedicles and fragments of benign, shredded endometrium.
- *Intrauterine adhesions.* Hysteroscopically, synechiae may be centrally or marginally located and may be classified as endometrial, myometrial, or connective fiber synechiae. Endometrial synechiae often grow from abortive tissue and create filmy adhesions, which are easy to remove. Myometrial synechiae appear buttress-like, are usually marginally located throughout the cavity, and are

distinct organized structures. Connective fiber adhesions often change the normal morphology and structure of the uterine cavity (see Fig. 130.11D).
- *Uterine cavity septum* appears as either arcuate (involves the fundus) or as an incomplete or complete septum. The latter two are generally discovered upon entry into the uterine cavity just past the internal os. The appearance is likened to looking at a double barrel shotgun head-on or a pig's snout. The septum generally has the same appearance as the surrounding endometrium. The arcuate type is usually visualized as a bulge in the top of the fundus protruding downward into the uterine cavity. The surface area may appear more atrophic than the rest of the uterine cavity endometrium (see Fig. 130.11I).
- *Endometrial carcinoma and precursors.* AUB is the first symptom in over 90% of cases, so early detection is relatively straightforward if proper procedures are performed. In fact, 75% of endometrial cancers are diagnosed as stage I.

Hysteroscopic findings include the following:

- EH is a precursor of endometrial cancer. The hysteroscopic appearance generally resembles normal glandular epithelium, and the thickness of the mucosa can be determined by pressing with the hysteroscope (see Fig. 130.11F).
- Low-risk EH often shows a specific pattern of widened glandular ostia with cystic-glandular formations about 1 mm in diameter. The same formation can be found in an endometrium of reduced thickness where their presence indicates cystic atrophy. Aside from the cystic form, EH is characterized by a variety of other hysteroscopic changes such as increased endometrial thickness, nonhomogeneous endometrial regeneration, increased vascularization, presence of ciliated epithelium, cystic dilation, polypoid formations, irregularly arranged glandular orifices, and necrotic areas. If one or more of these elements are found, hyperplasia must be suspected and endometrial biopsies should be performed.
- High-risk EH presents with a varied hysteroscopic image; a polypoid appearance and vascularization are usually clearly evident. This vascularization takes on an arborescent appearance, sometimes described as like a corkscrew in that it surrounds groups of glandular ostia. The appearance of the mucosa could also be described as cerebroid due to the abnormal growth and vascularization, similar to the irregular surface of brain tissue (see Fig. 130.11G).
- Endometrial neoplasia. Hysteroscopy is an extremely reliable technique for the diagnosis of endometrial neoplasia. The hysteroscopic images of cancer are usually so clear and obvious that it would be hard to confuse them with other lesions. In its initial stage, adenocarcinoma presents a germinative scenario, with irregular, polylobular, delicate excrescences, which may be bleeding or necrotic; vascularization is irregular or anarchic. In some instances, the involved area may be clearly demarcated from the normal endometrium. In other cases, it may be possible to see focal lesions. These can be located on the tubal cornua or sporadic implants can be found throughout the uterine cavity (see Fig. 130.11H).

CPT BILLING CODES

57505	Endocervical curettage, not with D&C
57800	Dilation; cervical canal, instrumental
58555	Hysteroscopy, diagnostic
58558	Hysteroscopy with biopsy of endometrium or polypectomy with or without D&C.
58559	With lysis of intrauterine adhesions
58560	With division or resection of intrauterine septum
58561	With removal of leiomyomas

58562	With removal of impacted foreign body
58563	With endometrial ablation, any method
58565	Hysteroscopic sterilization (Essure, Adiana)

ICD-10-CM DIAGNOSTIC CODES

C54.8	Malignancy, corpus uteri except isthmus
C54.0	Malignancy, isthmus of uterus
D25.0	Submucous leiomyomas, uterus
D25.1	Intramural leiomyoma
D28.2	Uterine neoplasm, benign
D07.0	Carcinoma in situ, unspecified part of uterus
N84.0	Polyps, uterine
N85.00	Hyperplasia of endometrium, unspecified
N85.6	Adhesions, intrauterine (synechiae)
N88.2	Stricture and stenosis of cervix
N84.1	Mucous polyp of cervix
N94.6	Dysmenorrhea
N91.2	Absence of menstruation
N92.0	Excessive or frequent menstruation
N92.6	Irregular menstrual cycle
N92.1	Metrorrhagia
N92.4	Premenopausal menorrhagia
N95.0	Postmenopausal bleeding

SUPPLIERS

(See contact information available at www.expertconsult.com.)

Conventional rigid and flexible hysteroscopes, graspers, biopsy forceps and scissors, endoscopic cameras, light sources and video monitors, and recording systems:
CooperSurgical
Karl Storz Endoscopy-America, Inc.
Olympus America, Inc.
Pentax Precision Instruments Corporation
Richard Wolf Medical Instruments Company
Stryker

Disposable endoscopes and hysteroscopes:
Micro-Imaging Solutions, Inc.

Disposable side-opening speculum with built-in LED light source, office "all-in-one" pack/procedure kits for office hysteroscopy (includes custom Mayo drape with built-in instrument pockets and trash container, disposable side-opening speculum with built-in LED light, 1.2-mm endoscopic double sealing seal, inflow and outflow tubing with Luer-Lok adapters, under buttocks drape with graded drain bag, and a drawstring for easy postprocedure disposal):
OBP Medical, Inc.

EndoSheath sterile, disposable single-use sheaths (diagnostic and therapeutic designs):
Medtronic Vision-Sciences, Inc.

IV saline bags, TURP tubing, Gyn applicators, topical anesthetics, gauze, disinfectant solutions, Welch Allyn Kleenspec disposable vaginal speculum, power examination tables, Mayo stands, and vital signs monitors:
Moore Medical

Special open-sided speculum, large speculum, cervical dilators and os finders, dental syringe and supplies, needle extenders and topical anesthetics, drapes, tenaculum, long forceps, sponge sticks and specialized fluid collection devices:
Gynex

ONLINE RESOURCES

Patient Education Information and Brochures

American College of Obstetricians and Gynecologists Hysteroscopy Patient Education/Brochure: http://acog.org/publications/patient_education/bp084.cfm. To order pamphlets: 800-762-2264.
American Association of Gynecologic Laparoscopists Hysteroscopy Patient Information: http://www.aagl.org.
Krames Online, Hysteroscopy: www.geisinger.kramesonline.com/HealthSheets/3,S,82976.

Hysteroscopy "How to" and Procedure Videos

American Association of Gynecologic Laparoscopists: www.aagl.org.
Conceptus: www.essuremd.com.
Karl Storz: www.karlstorz.de/cps/rde/xchg/SID-388011F6-05A9997C/karl-storz-en/hs.xsl/7239.htm.
Office Hysteroscopy Procedure Videos: SA Grochmal (endoreprogyne@aol.com).
Richard Wolf USA: www.richardwolfusa.com/specialties/gynecology/officehysteroscopy.html.

RECOMMENDED READING

ACOG releases guidelines on management of abnormal uterine bleeding associated with ovulatory dysfunction. *Am Fam Physician.* 2014;89(12):987–988.

ACOG technology assessment no. 7: hysteroscopy. *Obstet Gynecol.* 2011;117(6):1486–1491.

AAGL practice report: practice guidelines for management of intrauterine synechiae. *J Minim Invasive Gynecol.* 2010;17:1–7.

American College of Obstetricians and Gynecologists. Antibiotic prophylaxis for gynecologic procedures. ACOG Practice Bull. No. 104; 2009. Washington, DC.

Bradley LD. Assessment of abnormal uterine bleeding: three office-based tools. *J Fam Pract.* 2004;15:1–11.

Bradley LD. Instrumentation in office hysteroscopy: flexible hysteroscopy. In: Bradley LD, Falcone T, eds. *Hysteroscopy.* Philadelphia: Mosby; 2009:7–18.

Bradner P, Neis KJ, Ehmer C. The etiology, frequency, and prevention of gas embolism during hysteroscopy. *J Am Gynecol Endosc.* 1999;6:421–428.

Brooks PG. In the management of abnormal uterine bleeding, is office hysteroscopy preferable to sonography? The case for hysteroscopy. *J Minim Invasive Gynecol.* 2007;14:12–15.

Buchanan EM, Weinstein LC, Hillson C. Endometrial cancer. *Am Fam Physician.* 2009;80:1075–1080.

Carlson SM, Goldberg J, Lentz GM. Endoscopy: hysteroscopy and laparoscopy: indications, contraindications, and complications. In: Lobo RA, Gershenson DM, Lentz GM, Valea FA, eds. *Comprehensive Gynecology.* 7th ed. Philadelphia. Elsevier; 2017:190–204.

Garry R. Uterine distention methods and fluid management in operative hysteroscopy. In: Grochmal SA, ed. *Minimal Access Gynecology.* Oxford: Radcliffe Medical Press; 1995:301–315.

Grochmal SA. Office hysteroscopy: the time has come. *Female Pat.* 2007;32:15.

Hill D, Maher P, Wood C, et al. Complications of operative hysteroscopy. *Gynaecol Endosc.* 1992;1:185–189.

Hill DA. Abnormal uterine bleeding: avoid the rush to hysterectomy. *J Fam Pract.* 2009;58:136–142.

Hulf JA. Blood carbon dioxide changes during hysteroscopy. *Fertil Steril.* 1979;32:193–196.

Itzkowic DJ, Laverty CR. Office hysteroscopy and curettage—a safe diagnostic procedure. *Aust NZ J Obstet Gynecol.* 1990;30:150–153.

Fergusson RJ, Lethaby A, Shepperd S, Farquhar C. Endometrial resection and ablation versus hysterectomy for heavy menstrual bleeding. *Cochrane Database Syst Rev.* 2013:CD000329. Pub2.

Levie MD, Chudnoff SG. Prospective analysis of office-based hysteroscopic sterilization. *J Mini Invasive Gynecol.* 2006;13:98–101.

Loffer FD. Complications of hysteroscopy—their cause, prevention and correction. *J Am Assoc Gynecol Laparosc.* 1995;3:11–26.

Loffer FD, Bradley LD, Brill AI, et al. Hysteroscopic training guides. *J Am Assoc Gynecol Laparosc.* 2000;7:165.

Nagele F, O'Connor H, Baskett TF, et al. Hysteroscopy in women with abnormal uterine bleeding on hormone replacement therapy: a comparison with postmenopausal bleeding. *Fertil Steril.* 1996;65:1145–1150.

Nichols M, Carter JF, Fylstra DL, Childers M. for the Essure System U.S. Post-Approval Study Group. A comparative study of hysteroscopic sterilization performed in-office versus a hospital operating room. *J Minim Invasive Gynecol*. 2006;13:447–450.

Presthus JB. Office-based hysteroscopy: getting started now. *Contemp Obstet Gynecol*. 2006;15:1–6.

Raimondo G, Raimondo D, D'Aniello G, et al. A randomized controlled study comparing carbon dioxide versus normal saline as distension media in diagnostic office hysteroscopy: is the distension with carbon dioxide a problem? *Fertil Steril*. 2010;94(6):2319–2322.

Sagiv R, Sadan O, Boaz M, et al. A new approach to office hysteroscopy compared with traditional hysteroscopy: a randomized controlled trial. *Obstet Gynecol*. 2006;108:387–392.

Shah J. Endoscopy through the ages. *BJU Int*. 2002;89:645–652.

Uenol J, Ikeda F, Carvalho FM, et al. Routine hysteroscopy with endometrial biopsy in an infertility clinic. *J Minim Invasive Gynecol*. 2009;16:118–120.

Vilos GA, Edris F, Abu-Rafea B, et al. Miscellaneous uterine malignant neoplasms detected during hysteroscopic surgery. *J Minim Invasive Gynecol*. 2009;16:318–325.

Wang JH, Zhao J, Lin J. Opportunities and risk factors for premalignant and malignant transformation of endometrial polyps: management strategies. *J Minim Invasive Gynecol*. 2010;17:53–58.

Weekes A, Voss E. Complications of office hysteroscopy. In: Grochmal SA, ed. *Minimal Access Gynaecology*. Oxford, UK: Radcliffe Medical Press; 1995:370–381.

CHAPTER 131

PERMANENT FEMALE STERILIZATION (TUBAL LIGATION)

Gary R. Newkirk

In the United States, voluntary sterilization remains one of the most widely used contraceptive methods. According to the National Survey of Family Growth (2002), 10.3 million women (27%) rely on female sterilization for birth control, whereas 3.5 million women (9.2%) rely on vasectomy in their partners for contraception. Primary care clinicians skilled with basic surgical technique are in an ideal position to discuss and perform permanent sterilization procedures for both men and women. Approximately 600,000 tubal ligations are performed each year in the United States, half of which are performed within 48 hours postpartum. While some data say a similar number of vasectomies are carried out, there are conflicting data (Eisenberg and Lipshultz, 2010) that say two to three times the number of women undergo sterilization in the United States as men. This has been a phenomenon since the 1970s when permanent female sterilization surpassed male sterilization in number of procedures performed. Worldwide, in only eight nations is vasectomy performed as often or more often than tubal ligation: Austria, Bhutan, Canada, Denmark, Korea, the Netherlands, New Zealand, and the United Kingdom.

Why is this important? No man has died from the vasectomy procedure itself in the contemporary United States, whereas between 10 and 14 women die each year (in the United States) from tubal ligation. The failure rate for vasectomy is somewhere between 1 in 500 and 1 in 1200 in the United States, whereas tubal ligation failures occur in 1 in 200 procedures within the first year and may increase in frequency over time. Although vasectomy allows detection of failures, no simple technique allows the surgeon to find tubal ligation failures. The cost of a tubal ligation is five to six times that of an office vasectomy. When a patient asks about permanent contraception, it behooves the primary care clinician to point out the benefits of vasectomy over a tubal ligation. Even the American College of Obstetricians and Gynecologists agrees that, all things considered, a vasectomy is the procedure of choice. Nevertheless, when vasectomy is inappropriate for any reason, tubal ligation remains an excellent choice for permanent surgical contraception.

Despite numerous variations, female sterilization consists of two basic steps: (1) exposing the fallopian tubes, and (2) partially resecting or occluding the tubes to prevent conception. This chapter discusses the minilaparotomy approach to permanent female sterilization, both as an interval and as a postpartum procedure.

Box 131.1 outlines basic terminology related to permanent female sterilization methodology. Minilaparotomy and laparoscopy are abdominal surgical approaches that are considered safe, quick, and readily available.

Table 131.1 shows advantages and disadvantages of the minilaparotomy and the laparoscopic techniques. Despite the recognized advantages of laparoscopy for certain situations, minilaparotomy—because of its reliance on readily available surgical equipment, fewer technical demands, and applicability to both interval and postpartum periods—is the method of choice for many primary care clinicians. Box 131.2 summarizes the more common methods for ligating the tubes.

This chapter outlines the minilaparotomy approach and the modified Pomeroy or "Parkland" method for ligation (Figs. 131.1 and 131.2). The ideal method is still under debate; however, the modified Pomeroy and Parkland methods (with their variations) remain popular in the United States. Prudent clinicians should identify patients who may benefit by referral, either for alternative methods that the referring clinician cannot offer because of a lack of skill, training, equipment, or facility or because of the patient's clinical condition.

ANATOMY

Fig. 131.3 demonstrates the anatomy relevant to a tubal ligation.

INDICATIONS

- Desire for permanent sterilization
- Medical conditions that place the patient at significant risk for irreversible morbidity or death if she should become pregnant
- Known severe inheritable genetic disease (that makes childbearing undesirable)

CONTRAINDICATIONS

Absolute

- Active peritoneal infections
- Severe chronic heart, lung, or metabolic disease (abdominal insufflation [laparoscopy] and the head-down [Trendelenburg] position can cause acute cardiopulmonary decompensation)
- Any unstable medical condition (including unstable postpartum condition)
- Lack of informed consent
- Inability to tolerate necessary anesthesia
- Patient unsure of desire for permanent sterilization

Relative

- Prior significant pelvic or abdominal infection: minilaparotomy or laparoscopy may be more difficult. (Laparotomy may be necessary.)
- Severe obesity, especially with a history of pelvic or abdominal infection.
- Chronic heart disease, irregular pulse, uncontrolled hypertension, pelvic masses, uncontrolled diabetes, bleeding disorders, severe nutritional deficiencies, severe anemia, and umbilical or hiatal hernia. (The risks of future pregnancies must be weighed against the risks of permanent sterilization procedures.)

BOX 131.1 Female Sterilization Terminology

Colpotomy: A vaginal approach to tubal ligation through the posterior vaginal fornix.

Interval tubal ligation: Tubal ligation performed at times other than during the immediate postpartum period—generally 6 weeks or more after delivery.

Laparoscopy: Involves inserting an illuminated telescope-like instrument into the abdomen that allows visualization of the fallopian tubes to accomplish electrocoagulation or application of clips or rings. For open laparoscopy, a small incision is made within or just below the umbilicus to allow passage of a special cannula, around which the skin makes an airtight seal. The cannula allows for insufflation of the abdomen, passage of the laparoscope and instruments, and occlusion of the tubes. Open laparoscopy is considered safer than traditional closed laparoscopy, especially in women with prior pelvic or abdominal surgery or infection. With the closed laparoscopic procedure, the laparoscope is inserted blindly through the abdominal wall.

Laparotomy: A relatively large abdominal incision performed to optimize surgical exposure for a variety of intra-abdominal surgeries.

Minilaparotomy: Sometimes referred to as a *minilap*; involves a small abdominal incision, usually less than 5 cm (2 inches).

Postpartum tubal ligation: Tubal ligation performed within 72 hr of delivery.

Technical failure: Inability to complete the planned sterilization during the operation, which results in a change of method or failure to perform the sterilization.

TABLE 131.1 Advantages and Disadvantages of Minilaparotomy and Laparoscopy

	Advantages	Disadvantages
Minilaparotomy	Easy to learn Basic surgical training and skill Inexpensive instruments Complications are usually minor Can be performed as a postpartum or interval	Takes longer than laparoscopy Difficult to perform on patients who are obese or who have pelvic scarring or adhesions Scar slightly larger More pain from the abdominal incision Higher infection rate than laparoscopy procedure
Laparoscopy	Very low complication rate Quick procedure (10–15 min) Very small incision Useful for other diagnostic and therapeutic purposes Less painful	Complications may be serious Requires abdominal insufflation, with its added risk More difficult to learn; requires specialized training for clinician and staff Equipment is more expensive and requires more maintenance and repair Not recommended as a postpartum procedure

EQUIPMENT

- A laparotomy pack contains most of the instruments necessary for basic abdominal surgery and is available in most hospital outpatient and inpatient surgical suites.
- Suction catheter: Generally, suction is not used during a routine minilaparotomy tubal ligation. Suction is available on demand at most surgical suites; it is mandatory if complications such as bleeding develop.

BOX 131.2 Common Tubal Ligation Methods

Minilaparotomy ("Open" Procedure)

Electrocoagulation: A bipolar probe is passed through a small segment of tube to cauterize and obstruct the lumen.

Fimbriectomy: This method is accomplished by the complete removal of the fimbriated end of the tube. The procedure appears to have a higher pregnancy failure rate, and reversal is unlikely.

Irving technique: An extremely effective, though more difficult, method that cannot be reversed easily. The tube is cut and the uterine end buried beneath the peritoneum within the wall of the uterus. The remaining end is buried within the mesosalpinx.

Laparoscopy clips: Under laparoscopic guidance, clips are applied to occlude the tubal lumen. Hulka (spring-loaded) and Filshie clips (titanium and silicone rubber) are commonly used. Clips destroy less than 1 cm of tissue, and reversals are considered much easier.

Parkland technique: A small length of tube is separated from the mesosalpinx and ligated at each end, about 2 cm apart; the free segment between the ligatures is removed (see Fig. 131.2).

Modified Pomeroy technique: The most common procedure performed for both interval and postpartum tubal ligations. Absorbable catgut sutures are used to tie the base of a loop of midportion (ampullary) tube. The ligated loop of tube is then removed. As the suture absorbs, the ends pull apart and are obstructed by the healing and scarring process. From 3- to 6-cm of the tube is destroyed (see Fig. 131.1).

Tubal ring: A small Silastic ring is stretched and placed over a loop of fallopian tube and then released. The tube is blocked by compression. Usually a 2- to 3-cm segment of the tube is involved. Reversal is more successful than with the electrocauterization, Irving, or Uchida techniques.

Uchida technique: A technically demanding, yet extremely effective, method that is becoming more popular in the United States. The tube is severed and the uterine end is buried within the mesosalpinx.

Vaginal Approaches

Ligation, clips, and electrocoagulation rings: Two varieties have been used.
1. *Colpotomy*, which involves a surgical incision in the posterior vaginal fornix through which the tube is delivered and occluded by ligation, clips, or rings.
2. *Culdoscopy*, in which a culdoscope is passed through a smaller colpotomy incision to allow identification of the tubes and application of the electroprobe, clips, or rings. Both of these less popular methods share higher complication and failure rates. They are not postpartum methods.

Transcervical Approaches

Essure: In the fall of 2002, the Food and Drug Administration approved a new method, called Essure, whereby a device with a small stainless steel inner coil and superelastic outer coil (4 cm × 0.8 mm, after release 4 cm × 1.5–2 mm) is inserted hysteroscopically into the fallopian tubes for permanent sterilization. (See Chapter 132, Insertion of Essure [Hysteroscopically Assisted Female Sterilization].)

Others: Still considered experimental procedures, these methods of blocking the tubes from a transcervical-intrauterine approach continue to evoke interest. One method is to use Silastic "plugs" placed under hysteroscopic guidance. Various techniques are under development to provide a reversible sterilization by "pulling the plugs" when a pregnancy is desired.

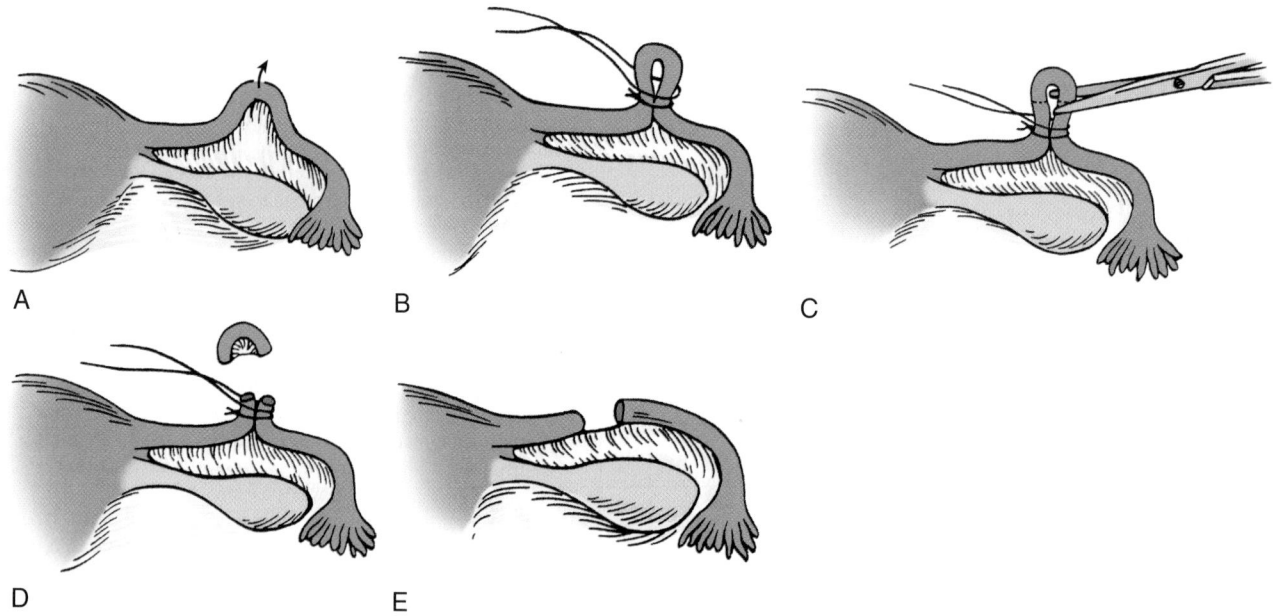

Fig. 131.1 Modified Pomeroy technique. (A) Lift loop. (B) Double ligation 0 or 2-0 plain gut suture, no crushing. (C) Each limb of tubal loop is cut separately. (D) Loop is cut off. (E) Later results.

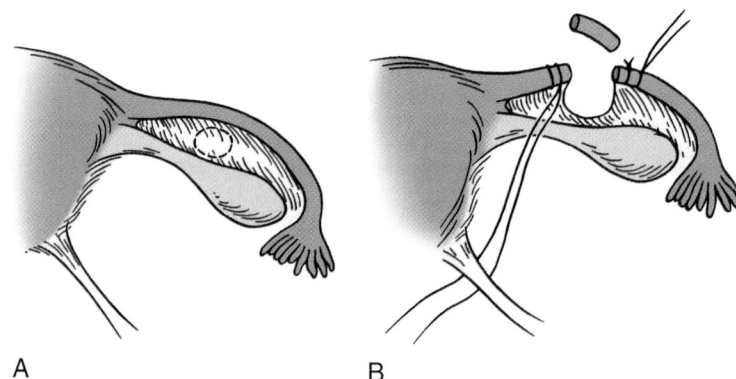

Fig. 131.2 Parkland method of tubal ligation. (A) A relatively avascular area of the mesosalpinx is identified within the isthmic portion of the tube. (B) A segment of tube is isolated and removed after double ligation with chromic suture.

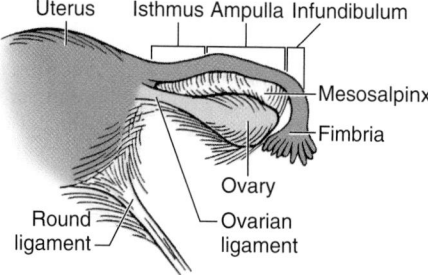

Fig. 131.3 Basic anatomy of the parauterine structures.

- Coagulation device: Most operative suites have a Bovie or similar coagulation device available. Some surgeons prefer to have this available for all cases; others use this electively, or when complications develop. Because a Bovie requires grounding, it should be set up in advance. A ground plate can be attached before the patient is draped and scrubbed.
- Sutures
  - Anatomic site suture
  - Tubal ligation 0 plain or chromic
  - Peritoneum 2-0 chromic

- Fascia 0 Dexon
- Scarpa's fascia 2-0 chromic
- Skin Metal clips, 4-0 Dexon
- 8-inch Babcock forceps to separate and retract fallopian tube (Fig. 131.4A)
- Ring sponge (a ring forceps holding a tightly folded gauze pad)
- Small Richardson or Army-Navy retractors for holding the incision open (see Fig. 131.4B)
- Adson tissue forceps with teeth for skin manipulation (see Fig. 131.4C)
- Metzenbaum scissors for general tissue blunt dissection and incision (see Fig. 131.4D)
- Kelly clamps for blunt dissection, and for grasping and tagging suture, bleeders, or tissue planes (fascia, peritoneum)
- Uterine manipulators for use with the cervical tenaculum or the newer uterine manipulators (see Fig. 131.4E)
- 5-mL, 0.5% bupivacaine (Marcaine) (optional)

PRECAUTIONS

Tubal ligation is elective surgery and should be performed when optimal preparation of both the patient and surgical environment are at hand. Patients must be competent to offer informed consent or the appropriate arrangements (legal guardianship for health care

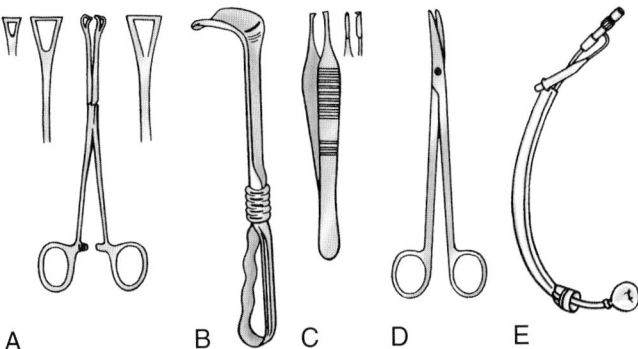

Fig. 131.4 Instruments for tubal ligation. (A) Babcock forceps; (B) small Richardson retractor; (C) Adson tissue forceps; (D) Metzenbaum scissors; (E) uterine manipulator (Also see Chapter 134, Hysterosalpingography and Sonohysterography).

decisions) made to assure legal basis to proceed with permanent sterilization. As with all elective surgeries, the patient's medical condition should be optimized for the stress of regional or general anesthesia to allow for this intra-abdominal surgery. It is not uncommon to postpone a postpartum tubal ligation (PTL), which was planned well in advance, because of intrapartum complications such as unexpected blood loss or unstable condition of the newborn. In these instances, delaying a PTL as well as reevaluation for other contraceptive options may be prudent and appropriate.

PREPROCEDURE PATIENT PREPARATION

Preprocedure Visits

Preprocedure evaluation and counseling for women who want permanent sterilization warrant focused attention. A special visit should be scheduled to discuss contraceptive options, risks, technique, and follow-up demands of sterilization surgery. (See the sample patient education form available at www.expertconsult.com.) In addition, many insurance companies require preauthorization, which should be obtained at this visit. The counseling session should not be hurried or added to the end of a visit for an acute illness. Written materials should be given to the patient at this time. Federal payment programs require that counseling precede surgery by at least 30 days and not more than 180 days. Special forms need to be signed, and the patient must be at least 21 years of age. If the patient is involved in a monogamous relationship, it is wise to have the partner present during the consultation to address any concerns. Partner written consent is not mandatory, but if there is disagreement with this decision, it should be discussed and the reasons explored. It is also important to address the issues and benefits of vasectomy (refer to the opening paragraph of this chapter).

A preprocedure examination, which requires a reasonable amount of time, should occur within 10 days (some hospitals require <5 days) of anticipated surgery. Review the patient's complete medical history, paying particular attention to prior pelvic or abdominal surgery and infection. Are there drug allergies or drug intolerances? Are there medications (such as aspirin) that should be stopped? Is the patient on chronic anticoagulants? Is there a history of heart disease, diabetes, bleeding disorder, endometriosis, or dysfunctional uterine bleeding? Is other concomitant surgery necessary (e.g., dilation and curettage [D&C], breast biopsy, or procedure for urinary incontinence)? Is the Pap smear normal? Discuss the method of anesthesia that is to be used. Carefully review anticipated postprocedure morbidities (e.g., pain, the necessity of limited lifting). Remain mindful of the risk factors for regret (see later discussion under General Information). Review current contraceptive methods. Is pregnancy a possibility at the time of surgery? If the patient smokes, can she quit before surgery?

Preprocedure examination should be thorough. Focus on the heart, lung, breast, and abdominal examinations. During the pelvic examination, assess for the presence of vulvar, vaginal, or cervical disease. Obtain specimens for culture (e.g., gonorrhea, chlamydia) as necessary. Assess the degree of uterine prolapse and urinary incontinence; have the patient bear down and cough. Perform a bimanual examination to assess uterine size, shape, and tenderness. Palpate the ovaries for enlargement. Pay particular attention to uterine mobility. Can the uterus be brought out of the pelvis easily, or is it frozen in a particular direction? Estimate the degree of abdominal wall obesity. Show the patient the location and size of the anticipated abdominal incision and eventual scarring.

Perform laboratory tests as necessary. Typically, hospitals require hemoglobin levels and a urinalysis as the minimum prerequisites for general anesthesia. Perform a pregnancy test if there is any question of pregnancy. If there is clinical evidence of cervicitis or pelvic inflammation, obtain specimens for culture, and treat the condition accordingly. In this case, schedule the surgery only when treatment and clinical response have been adequate.

Many same-day and outpatient surgery services offer preanesthesia counseling. The patient can meet with the anesthesia clinician to discuss anesthesia, risks, time to arrive at the hospital, how long to fast before surgery, and other issues. This counseling should be used whenever it is available; for many hospitals, it is a requirement.

Call the hospital surgery personnel with any special requests for the anticipated surgery. Will a D&C be performed? (If so, it should be done after minilaparotomy.) Is a uterine manipulator necessary, and what type will be used?

General Information

- Minilaparotomy is the safest sterilization method in the postpartum period, with a complication rate approaching that of interval sterilization, which is usually less than 3%. Laparoscopy is not as safe during the immediate postpartum period as at other times.
- Average rates for tubal sterilization failures are 1 in 250 at 1 year.
- Postpartum and postabortion sterilization appears to be somewhat less effective than interval sterilization.
- Of the women who have tubal sterilization, 1% to 2% seek reversal; however, sterility is not easily reversed. Only 30% to 70% of these women are candidates for reversal surgery (this broad range for reversal success is related to the original method of the tubal ligations), and pregnancy occurs in about 50% of those who do undergo reversal procedures. Insurance will frequently not cover reversal. Reversal is most successful if less than 3 cm of the tubes was originally damaged or removed. The most "reversible" techniques include those that do not involve electrocautery and those in which the smallest segment is removed from within the isthmic portion of the tube. Women with the following risk factors for regret should not necessarily be denied surgery; however, the prudent clinician should counsel these patients before performing sterilization.
  - Marital disharmony at the time of sterilization. (Remarriage is the reason 90% of women request reversal.)
  - Age less than 30 years at the time of sterilization. (Some clinicians debate whether this is a significant risk factor.)
  - Religious, socioeconomic, and educational backgrounds show much less correlation with regret. Low parity or number of live children is also less well correlated.
  - Regret may be slightly more prevalent after postpartum sterilization procedures; however, as a risk factor, this is less well defined.
  - Regret is more likely when sterilization is chosen because of financial difficulties, health, or emotional problems.

PROCEDURE

Fig. 131.5 illustrates the procedure for tubal ligation. According to the latest American College of Obstetricians and Gynecologists and

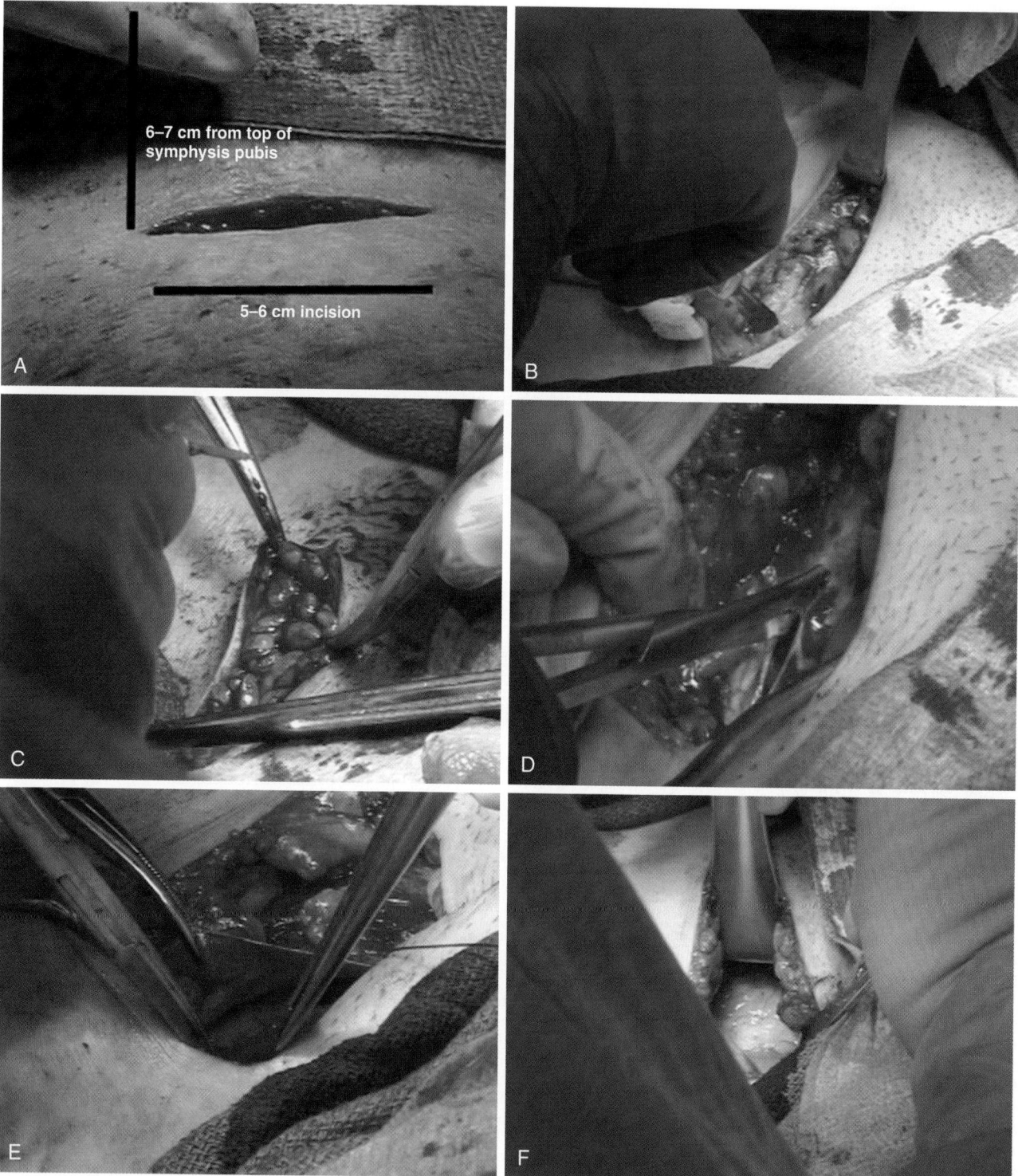

Fig. 131.5 Procedure for tubal ligation. (A) A transverse abdominal incision is made about 6 cm above the top of the symphysis pubis and about 5 cm wide. (B) A small retractor is used to part the incised tissue and improve exposure as the incision is carried through the abdominal wall. (C) Small bleeders encountered can be grasped with a hemostat and coagulated by touching the electrosurgical coagulator to the hemostat. (D) As the fascia is encountered, it is carefully divided transversely and the incision is carried down to the peritoneum. (E) The peritoneum is identified by its thin, translucent quality and is divided entering the abdominal cavity. (F) A small Richardson retractor with counter-retraction by the surgeon's fingers improves visual access to the abdominal contents. (G) The Babcock clamps are used in pairs to carefully retrieve the fallopian tube and follow it to the fimbriated end and ovary confirming its identification. (H) Here a single Babcock clamp retracts the tube and demonstrates the widened fimbriated end. (I) A loop of suture on a reel is used to tie off a loop of fallopian tube in the simple Pomeroy procedure. With the modified Pomeroy technique, a hemostat is passed through the center of the tied-off loop of fallopian tube and is used to guide suture material to individually tie off each side of the fallopian loop. (J–L) Scissors are used to cut through the fallopian tube just above where the prior ties were seated. The incision is made at the crush mark left by the hemostats that were used to cross-clamp the tube. (M–O) The severed end is retracted and the opposite side of the loop is cut, freeing a 2- to 3-cm section of fallopian tube. (P) It is critical to completely close the fascial layers identified by their white, thick, and tough nature.

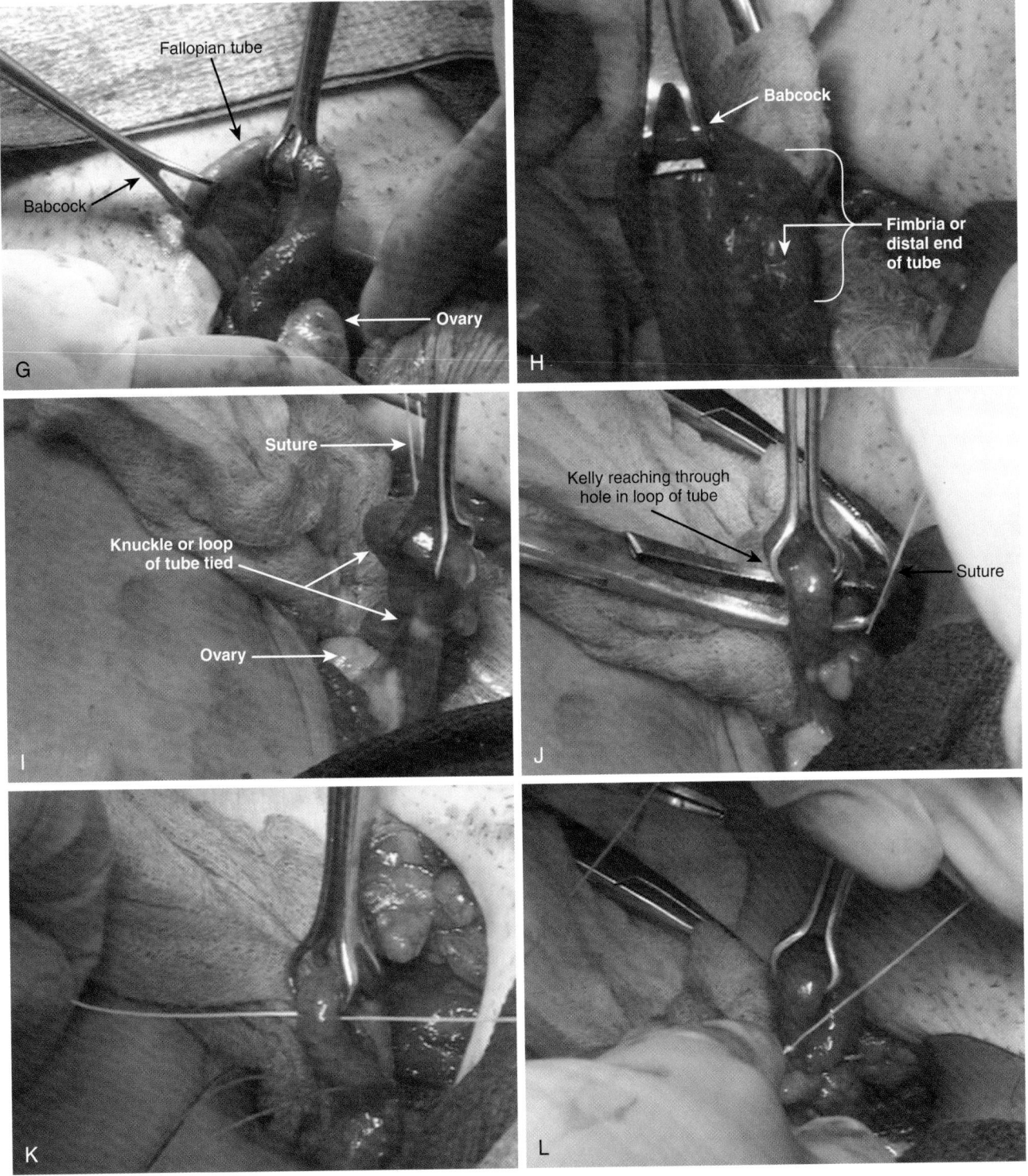

Fig. 131.5, cont'd

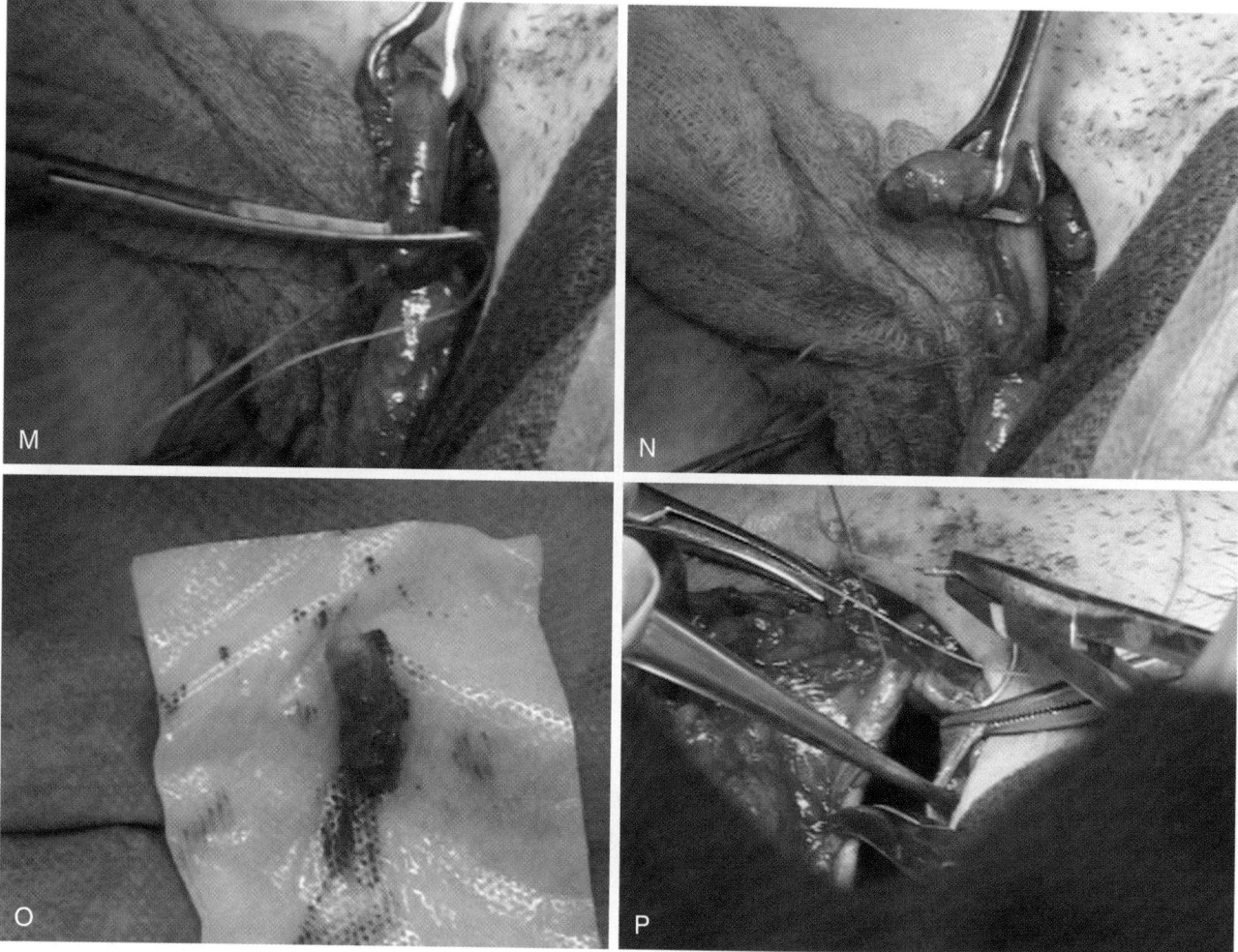

Fig. 131.5, cont'd

American Heart Association guidelines, prophylactic antibiotics are not indicated for laparoscopy or laparotomy sterilization procedures.

Check in with the preoperative holding area. Is the patient's chart complete and informed consent form available and signed? Are the laboratory values within normal range? Does your patient have any questions? Is the family in the waiting room?

Tell the operating room scrub or float nurse what equipment and sutures you will need. Clarify the position that the patient will be placed in for the surgery (e.g., lithotomy, frog-legged, or standard supine position). Request a specific cleansing agent for patients who are allergic to iodine.

1. Cleanse the vulva and vagina. A vaginal prep is necessary if the bladder is to be catheterized or a uterine manipulator is to be applied.
2. Drain the bladder. Perform a quick, gentle, straight catheterization to decompress a distended bladder from the operative field. Catheterization of the bladder is not universally performed. This is particularly true for patients under local anesthesia who can void sufficiently just before anesthesia. However, when the surgeon is new to this technique or when delay is anticipated in completing the abdominal entry (obesity, prior pelvic surgery, or infection), bladder injury is more likely. Draining the bladder helps reduce this risk. "Fluid blousing" at the time of general anesthesia induction is common, and the bladder can fill quickly.
3. Apply the uterine manipulator (for interval minilaparotomy) as deemed necessary. Traditional devices include acorn or Hulka devices. Adaptations, such as CooperSurgical's uterine manipulator (see Fig. 131.4E), are easy to apply and are rarely

traumatic. Many clinicians use manipulators routinely; others reserve them for anticipated problems with adequate exposure (abdominal obesity, prior pelvic surgery or infection, or retroversion or flexion of the uterus). Less-experienced surgeons will find them helpful. The patient must be in either the lithotomy or the frog-leg position, and general anesthesia is required.
4. Sterile gloves may be used without formal gowning for insertion of the uterine manipulator or for straight catheterization of the urinary bladder. In fact, it is advisable for the surgeon not to perform these procedures with the same formal gowning and gloving worn for the minilaparotomy, because contamination is likely when the patient is in the lithotomy position.
5. Prepare and scrub the abdomen. Minilaparotomy should not be performed through pubic hair. Depending on patient pubic hair distribution, shaving a small strip of pubic hair over the operative site may be necessary.
6. After thorough surgical scrub and gowning, perform the procedure.
7. Apply surgical drapes as for abdominal surgery.
8. Locate the site for the incision. Palpate three fingerbreadths above the symphysis pubis. With one hand on the abdomen above the symphysis, move the uterine manipulator. Often the uterus can be felt with the abdominal hand, which offers reassurance that the incision will provide ready access to the uterus and adnexa. Using the skin scalpel with a No. 10 blade, make a transverse incision. There is no need to arc this incision. Often the linea nigra, the faint line demarcating the midline, can be visualized. The incision should be no more than 5 cm long, and often a smaller incision will suffice (see Fig. 131.5A).

9. Switch to the deep knife (new No. 10 blade) and progress through Scarpa's fascia (within the fat) until the rectus sheath is encountered (see Fig 131.5B). Often, once Scarpa's fascia is divided, the sub-Scarpa's fat can be brushed away with a sponge, using a wiping motion. Bleeders can be cauterized using the electrocoagulator. Do not tunnel the incision, especially in the obese abdomen; this can be prevented by ensuring that the subcutaneous fat has been divided all the way to both edges of the skin incision. The subcutaneous fat presents an excellent opportunity to test the power on the Bovie before entering the abdomen. The Bovie device should never be used for the first time on intra-abdominal tissue, in case the power is set dangerously high (see Fig. 131.5C).

10. Once the rectus fascia is identified by its dense, white fibrous appearance, make a small transverse incision on each side of the linea alba. Using a Metzenbaum scissors, carefully extend the fascial incision to the lateral margin of the skin incision and across the midline (see Fig. 131.5D). Place two Kelly clamps on the incised lower fascial edge and gently retract and elevate the fascia. Gently place the index finger (preferably) or the blunt end of the scalpel along the midline under the incised fascial edge, and gently roll it toward the lateral margins, freeing the sheath from the underlying rectus muscle. In the midline, the pyramidalis remains adherent; use the Metzenbaum scissors to carefully cut along the inferior linea alba, freeing the muscle and making more room. Apply Kelly clamps to the upper segment of the anterior rectus sheath, and free the underlying muscles in a similar fashion. You do not need to roll the index finger under the rectus sheath any further than the skin incision. Perforating vessels arise more laterally and can be ruptured. Carefully use cautery to control bleeding.

11. Using blunt dissection with the index finger or the blunt end of the knife, separate the rectus muscles from the transversalis fascia and peritoneum in the midline. A gentle rolling action of the index finger (or the blunt end of the scalpel) under each lateral band of rectus muscles ensures adequate room.

12. Using two Kelly clamps or pickups, opposing each other, lift the transversalis and peritoneum, thereby tenting these layers away from underlying abdominal structures. Using either the scalpel or Metzenbaum scissors, make a small buttonhole incision between the two clamps. This incision should be well above the symphysis pubis, favoring the cephalad (toward the umbilicus) portion of the wound to avoid the bladder. At this point, use a Kelly clamp to enter the small incision, and with a combination of blunt dissection and retraction of tissues, enter the abdomen. The key maneuver is to maintain this elevation of the incision edges to expose abdominal viscera. The obese abdomen may contain a significant amount of fat below the peritoneum, which requires special care when dissecting. It may be difficult to distinguish this tissue from omentum or mesenteric fat that may be adherent in the lower pelvis, especially in women with a history of abdominal surgery or infection. The peritoneal incision may be extended either transversely (preferred) or vertically. The edges of the incised peritoneum are grasped and elevated and the incision inspected to ensure the abdominal cavity has been entered (see Fig. 131.5E).

13. Place the small Richardson retractors, and with gently opposed and elevating retraction, lift the abdominal wall and inspect the abdominal cavity (see Fig. 131.5F). If the small intestine obscures the view, place the patient in the reverse Trendelenburg position (head down) to allow the bowel to gravitate cephalad out of view. Use a gauze pad rolled tightly on a ring clamp to brush the bowel and adnexal structures aside if they are obstructing the view. Using Babcock forceps, identify the adnexal structures. Once the fallopian tube is identified, use Babcock forceps to gently retract the tube until the ovary and fimbriated end are clearly identified (see Fig. 131.5G). Apply further slight traction on the Babcock to deliver the tube through the

incision. Note the glistening white ovary, which assures the surgeon that the fallopian is being grasped (see Fig. 131.5H). Gentle traction is always advised because the tube can be adherent to vascular structures, which may bleed if torn. Use the uterine manipulator to help with visualization and exposure.

14. For the traditional Pomeroy tubal ligation technique, the Babcock forceps delivers a knuckle of tube, which is tied off with the 2-0 chromic suture. A second suture around this isolation knuckle of tube is often applied to achieve a tight, hemostatic construction before the knuckle of tube is excised (see Fig. 131.5I).

15. For the modified Pomeroy tubal ligation procedure, carefully elevate the fallopian tube and identify a relatively avascular area of the mesosalpinx. Using a Kelly clamp to gently penetrate or the Bovie on "coag" (not "cutting") to avoid making too large of a hole, make a small hole through the mesosalpinx (see Fig. 131.5J). Then clamp the tube with a Kelly, placing one jaw through this hole and the other across the tube. Place another Kelly clamp 2 cm distal to the first one, isolating a segment of tube. Using a 2-0 chromic suture on a needle, place a stick-tie on the uterine side of the tube so that the suture encircles the tube next to the portion of the tube that connects to the uterus Kelly clamp (see Fig. 131.5K). Tag this tie (Kelly is placed on the suture to maintain control). Most surgeons place a second tie on the same side and cut (see Fig. 131.5L). Place a similar tie on the fimbriated side of the tube. Remove the Kelly clamps. Incise through each of the two crush marks made by the Kelly clamps that lie on the side of the encircling suture toward the excised piece of tube; remove the segment of the tube (see Fig. 131.5M and N). Place the cut segment of tube on a piece of Telfa, note right or left side, and submit for pathologic evaluation when the surgery is completed (see Fig 131.5O). Lightly cauterize the exposed mesosalpinx if bleeding is observed. Cut the tags and repeat this procedure on the other tube. Current evidence supports the use of preemptive analgesia using infiltration of the incised skin and uterine tubes at cut ends with 0.5% bupivacaine. Postoperative pain, nausea, vomiting, and cramping were significantly lessened by this practice.

16. Perform a sponge count and, if it is correct, close the abdomen.

17. Identify and hold the edges of the peritoneum with Kelly clamps or pickups (see Fig. 131.5E). Use a running 3-0 chromic suture to reapproximate the cut edges. Identify and tag the fascial sheath edges with Kelly clamps. Close this sheath with a running 0 Dexon suture (see Fig. 131.5P). Palpate the closure to make sure there are no buttonhole defects in the fascial repair that could later manifest as incisional hernias. If there is more than 1 cm of subcutaneous fat, close Scarpa's fascia with interrupted 2-0 chromic sutures. The skin may be closed with staples or by running a subcuticular stitch of 3-0 chromic suture on a Keith needle.

18. Cleanse the surgical site with normal saline and apply a gauze dressing.

19. Take the patient to the recovery room. She may be discharged when she is awake, is tolerating oral liquids, and is ambulatory. Send the tubal segments for routine pathologic examination; place them in separate bottles marked "right" and "left." Write a brief operative note in the chart. State any complications, blood loss, and other findings. Dictate a complete operative report immediately after surgery. The patient is generally seen in the office within 7 to 14 days or at any time a complication develops. Review the tubal histologic report.

POSTPARTUM TUBAL LIGATION

PTL has many similarities to interval tubal ligation, but there are also major differences. Despite the convenience, cost savings, and ultimate desires of the patient, PTL remains an elective surgery. Numerous contraindications include maternal fever, pregnancy-related hypertension, uncontrolled diabetes mellitus, and excessive blood loss. Concerns regarding the viability and health of the newborn must be considered as well. Women who must postpone their postpartum sterilization should be reassured that interval tubal ligation as early as 6 weeks after delivery is also an excellent method of sterilization surgery. PTL can readily be performed during cesarean section; however, never assume that PTL remains the patient's desire if the cesarean section was performed because of concern over the condition of the fetus. (See the sample patient education form available at www.expertconsult.com.)

Technique

Review the technique described earlier for interval tubal ligation.

1. PTL can often be performed with the same block (epidural, caudal) that was used during labor. If this is not desirable or possible, there are many advantages to allowing the patient to rest and recover from labor and to schedule the PTL procedure for the next morning. A repeat hemoglobin determination will be much more meaningful after equilibration of fluid, especially if there is concern over blood loss during delivery. This delay also allows more time to observe the condition of the newborn.
2. The bladder should be drained either by having the patient void immediately before surgery or by straight catheterization (preferred method). Prepare the abdomen in the immediate umbilical area. Surgical scrub and draping are required.
3. Make a curved infraumbilical incision in the abdomen with the skin knife (No. 10 blade) (Fig. 131.6). Gentle inferior retraction on the abdominal skin at the time of this incision ensures that the scar will be close to or within the umbilical crater.
4. Carry the incision deeper with the deep knife (No. 10 blade). Once the skin and subcutaneous fat have been divided, enter the abdomen by favoring the inferior portion of the wound. (Dissecting through the substance of the umbilicus can be frustrating because tissue planes are not well defined.) Blunt dissection with Kelly clamps, which can probe and spread, is the preferred method for exploring and defining the portal of entry into the abdominal cavity. Some surgeons prefer to grasp each lateral side of the incision with towel clamps and elevate the entire incision away from underlying structures, such as the bowel and the uterus, when entering the peritoneum. Once the abdominal cavity is identified, the incision through the fascia and peritoneum can be extended, but it rarely needs to be longer than 4 to 5 cm.
5. Push the uterus gently to one side to rotate the adnexal structures into view. Use Babcock clamps to identify the fallopian tube, which in the postpartum period is typically swollen and engorged compared with the nonpregnant state. Follow each tube until the fimbriated ends and ovaries are identified. Extremely gentle traction is warranted because vessels within the mesosalpinx can be huge and easily damaged by traction. Tears in these vessels can cause profound bleeding.

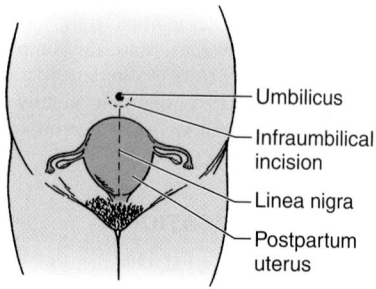

Fig. 131.6 Postpartum tubal ligation by minilaparotomy requires a small transverse infraumbilical incision.

6. Once the tube has been identified clearly, perform a tubal ligation as described previously for the interval sterilization technique. If the mesosalpinx is extremely fragile, many clinicians prefer the more traditional modified Pomeroy technique. The loop, tie, and cut features of the Pomeroy render a quick hemostatic procedure that can minimize the traction injuries or raw cut edges of the mesosalpinx produced by other procedures. Remember that if the tube cannot be delivered through the incision for a tubal ligation procedure, clips may be applied to the correctly identified fallopian tube.
7. Close the abdomen in a layered fashion as previously described. With periumbilical incisions, it is sometimes difficult to clearly redefine the peritoneal edges for closure. However, closure of the fascia is crucial and time should be spent clearly identifying the edges of this layer for definitive suturing.
8. The patient is generally seen within 2 weeks of PTL. At this time, the histology report should be reviewed.

SAMPLE OPERATIVE REPORT

Identifying data: Patient is a 36-year-old white G2P2 who requests sterilization
Procedure performed: Minilaparotomy tubal ligation
Preoperative diagnosis: Elective permanent sterilization
Postoperative diagnosis: Bilateral tubal ligation
Estimated blood loss: Less than 5 mL
Complications: None
Operation performed: Modified Parkland excision of tubal segments
Surgeon: Dr. _____
Assistant: Dr. _____
Anesthesia: General with intubation

Procedure: The patient's preoperative examination and consent were obtained with prior office visit. The preoperative hematocrit and urinalysis are normal and the pregnancy test negative. The patient was identified by me prior to surgery. The patient was placed in the lithotomy position and a bimanual examination demonstrated a normal-sized, mobile uterus without abnormality. A Foley catheter was placed. The vulva and vagina were cleansed with Betadine, the cervix identified, and a Hulka intrauterine manipulator applied. The patient was then prepped and draped in the usual fashion. An incision site was identified three fingerbreadths above the pubic symphysis. A 4-cm transverse incision was performed and advanced, layer by layer, into the abdomen. Richardson retractors were used for exposure. The uterine manipulator was used to help identify the right tube. The tube was confirmed by inspecting its length distally to the right ovary. Babcock forceps were used to gently deliver a loop of tube through the abdominal incision. A relatively avascular window in the mesosalpinx was identified, the tube was cross-clamped on each side of this window. Stick-ties with 2-0 chromic suture were placed on each side of the clamps encircling the tube. Double ties were placed on the uterine side. A 2-cm section of the tube was removed and sent for pathologic evaluation. Minor bleeding was controlled with minimal coagulation. A similar procedure was performed for the left tube. The instrument and sponge count was correct and the incision was closed layer by layer with 2-0 chromic on the peritoneum, 0 Dexon suture on the fascia, 2-0 chromic on Scarpa's fascia, and a 3-0 chromic running subcuticular suture on the skin. The urine was noted to remain clear during and after the procedure. The Foley catheter and uterine manipulator were removed. The patient was extubated and taken to the recovery room in stable condition.

COMMON ERRORS

1. Incomplete preoperative assessment overlooking medications (e.g., aspirin), prior pelvic surgeries (e.g., appendectomy), medical morbidities (e.g., poorly controlled diabetes).

2. Failure to have a contraception plan to prevent pregnancy prior to the tubal ligation.
3. Performing procedure when the patient's ability to make the decision for permanent sterilization is questioned (e.g., mentally challenged, unstable emotional or psychiatric status, consider legal and/or psychiatric consultation).
4. Attempting interval tubal ligation by minilaparotomy in women with significant abdominal obesity.
5. Failing to discuss alternatives to permanent sterilization.
6. Failing to review the postprocedure pathology report. Are there two segments of tube resected?

COMPLICATIONS

Minilaparotomy and laparoscopy have similar complication rates.

Major

- Major factors related to the development of complications include clinician inexperience, patient obesity, prior pelvic or abdominal surgery, and other medical problems such as diabetes mellitus, heart disease, asthma, bronchitis, and emphysema.
- Major complications occur in less than 2% of all procedures and may require prolonged hospitalization (0.3% requiring three or more nights in the hospital) or laparotomy (0.02% to 1.2% in large studies) to resolve complications.
- Delayed complications requiring readmission to the hospital occur after less than 1% of procedures.
- Female sterilization causes very few deaths (10 to 15 deaths per 500,000 procedures per year in the United States), and most are related to anesthetic complications (overdose or drug reaction), infection, and hemorrhage. Mortality rates from sterilization are far lower than with childbirth.
- Rare complications of tubal litigations include pregnancy (intrauterine and ectopic) and luteal phase pregnancy.
- Failure occurs due to surgical errors such as failure to remove the tube (e.g., removed part of round ligament instead) or only partial transection of the tube. A spontaneous fistula may also form or spontaneous reanastomosis occur between the severed stumps. Defective current from electrocautery may contribute to failure. An insufficiently occlusive clip using the laparoscopic technique can also cause failure.

Minor

- There is a twofold increased risk of functional ovarian cysts following tubal sterilization (Holt et al., 2003).
- Minilaparotomy appears to have a higher rate of minor complications (12% vs. 7%) and a longer average operating time when compared with laparoscopy. Minilaparotomy convalescence appears to be slightly longer and more painful. Higher complication rates have been reported when laparoscopy is performed by inexperienced clinicians.
- Minor minilaparotomy complications include wound infections, slight blood loss, uterine perforation by uterine manipulation instruments, and bladder injury. Most minor injury complications are immediately recognized and managed intraoperatively.
- Laparoscopy complications include those of minilaparotomy, as well as unique problems related to insertion of the instrument and gas insufflation of the abdomen. These complications include gas embolism, subcutaneous emphysema, and cardiac arrest. Vessel or organ laceration may occur. Open laparoscopy may make some of these complications less likely.
- Pain occurs after both minilaparotomy and laparoscopy. Chest and shoulder pain is common after laparoscopy and is caused by trapped gas under the diaphragm after insufflation of the abdomen. Most postprocedure and recovery pain can be managed with oral drug therapy, and narcotics are rarely necessary after the third postprocedural day.

- There is no compelling evidence that female sterilization causes menstrual cycles to change significantly, but abnormalities may persist if they existed before surgery. Among women who do experience menstrual changes, about half observe improvements and half experience irregular cycles or increased bleeding.
- Sterilized women do not appear to have different rates of pelvic inflammatory disease, cervicitis, hysterectomy, or D&C. Ovarian cancer may be diminished.
- Sterilized women are no more likely to experience severe psychiatric problems than unsterilized women.

POSTPROCEDURE MANAGEMENT

The surgeon is advised to check in on the recovery of the patient prior to leaving the hospital. Speak with family members in the waiting room, if available. Postoperative instructions can often be reviewed at this time. In most circumstances, patients can resume normal activities within 5 days following tubal ligation. Until then, heavy lifting and vigorous activities, such as jogging or weight training, should be postponed for about 5 days or until comfortable. Baths or hot tubs should be avoided for 10 days. Showers are recommended. A postoperative visit in the office in 7 to 10 days is advised. At this time, recovery experience, tubal pathology report, and other questions can be explored.

POSTPROCEDURE PATIENT EDUCATION

Give the patient postprocedure instructions and inform the family of any follow-up instructions. (See the sample patient education form available at www.expertconsult.com.)

INTERPRETATION OF PATHOLOGY RESULTS

The surgeon must review the pathology report, which is generally available within 7 to 14 days following the procedure. Two segments of fallopian tube with evidence of complete resection of their diameter should be obtained. Failure to document two segments requires that the patient be informed and appropriate steps be initiated to prevent pregnancy and allow time for evaluation. In most instances, waiting 8 weeks to allow for internal healing and performance of a hysterosalpingogram will help assess whether or not both tubes are indeed blocked or, in fact, whether the wrong structures, such as the round or ovarian ligaments, were removed. Avoid performing the hysterosalpingogram prior to 8 weeks to allow for adequate healing. Each patient requires individual management in this circumstance. Some may opt for repeat procedures while others will reconsider other options of contraception.

PATIENT EDUCATION GUIDES

See the sample patient education form available at www.expertconsult.com.

CPT/BILLING CODES

58600	Interval tubal ligation
58605	Postpartum tubal ligation
58670	Laparoscopic tubal ligation
58671	Laparoscopic tubal clipping or banding

ICD-10-CM DIAGNOSTIC CODES

Z30.09	General counseling and family planning advice
Z30.2	Sterilization; admission for interruption of fallopian tubes or vas deferens

SUPPLIERS

(See contact information available at www.expertconsult.com.)

HUMI Intrauterine Manipulators
CooperSurgical, Inc.

RECOMMENDED READING

American College of Obstetricians and Gynecologists guidelines at a glance. Benefits and risks of sterilization. *Contemporary Ob/Gyn*. 2013;58(10):2013.

American College of Obstetricians and Gynecologists. Antibiotic prophylaxis for gynecologic procedures. ACOG Practice Bulletin No. 104. *Obstet Gynecol*. 2009;113:1180–1189.

American College of Obstetricians and Gynecologists. Benefits and risks of sterilization. *Practice Bulletin No*. 2013;133.

Cunningham, F Gary. In: Cunningham F, Leveno KJ, Bloom SL, et al.*Williams Obstetrics*. 24th ed. New York: McGraw-Hill; 2013, Chapter 39.

Eisenberg ML, Lipshultz LI. Estimating the number of vasectomies performed annually in the United States: Data from the national survey of family growth. *The Journal of Urology*. 2010;184:2068.

Hillis SD, Marchbanks PA, Tylor LR, Peterson HB. Poststerilization regret: Findings from the United States Collaborative Review of Sterilization. *Obstet Gynecol*. 1999;93:889–895. 1999.

Holt VL, Cushing-Haugen KL, Daling JR. Oral contraceptives, tubal sterilization, and functional ovarian cyst risk. *Obstet Gynecol*. 2003;102:252.

Kuilier R, Boulvain M, Walker D, et al. Minilaparotomy and endoscopic techniques for tubal sterilization. *Cochrane Database Syst Rev*. 2004: CD001328.

Nelson A. Family planning: reversible contraception, sterilization and abortion. In: Hacker NF, Gambone JC, Hobel JC, eds. *Hacker and Moore's Essentials of Obstetrics and Gynecology*. 6th ed. Philadelphia: Elsevier; 2016:327–335.

Peterson HB, Xia Z, Hughes JM, et al. The risk of ectopic pregnancy after tubal sterilization: U.S. Collaborative Review of Sterilization Working Group. *N Engl J Med*. 1997;336:762–767.

Peterson HB, Xia Z, Hughes JM, et al. The risk of pregnancy after tubal sterilization: findings from the U.S. Collaborative Review of Sterilization. *Am J Obstet Gynecol*. 1996;174:1161–1168.

Peterson HB. Sterilization. *Obstet Gynecol*. 2008;111:189–203.

Rulin MC, Davidson AR, Philliber SG, et al. Long-term effect of tubal sterization on menstrual indices and pelvic pain. *Obstet Gynecol*. 1993;82:118–121.

CHAPTER 132

INSERTION OF ESSURE (HYSTEROSCOPICALLY ASSISTED FEMALE STERILIZATION)

Stephen A. Grochmal • Lydia A. Watson • Dale A. Patterson

EDITOR'S NOTE: As of July 2018, Essure has been voluntarily withdrawn from the market by Bayer Corporation. However, it is still available in other countries.

Female tubal sterilization remains the most widely used method of permanent contraception worldwide. Approximately 700,000 female sterilizations are performed annually, and approximately half of these are completed within 48 hours postpartum. The remaining 345,000 sterilizations are "interval" procedures, meaning they do not occur immediately following pregnancy. Until recently, the majority of interval sterilizations in the United States were performed laparoscopically, under general anesthesia or intravenous (IV) conscious sedation, in either the hospital or an out-patient surgery setting. Although the laparoscopic approach is considered safe and effective, it is not without complications, including infection, anesthesia complications, vascular damage, failure, and injury to internal organs; and occasionally, as a result of a failed laparoscopic attempt, an unintended laparotomy may occur. Annually, an average of 14 women die in the United States from complications of tubal ligation surgery, and there is a reported 1 in 200 failure rate. Sterilization rates have remained the same for men and women over the past 45 years; however, the types of surgical procedures used have changed, influenced by improvements in medical device technologies and anesthesia.

Historically, the concept of hysteroscopic or transcervical occlusion of the fallopian tubes (using electrocoagulation) was first described by Schroeder in 1927. Unfortunately, there was sporadic interest in this hysteroscopic "incisionless" or "scarless" tubal ligation procedure, and further progress to find an acceptable method was plagued by numerous attempts and failures. An innovative technique was approved by the US Food and Drug Administration (FDA) in November 2002 as the first hysteroscopic tubal occlusion device for permanent female sterilization in the United States. Now in its third generation, the Essure (ESS305, Bayer Conceptus, Inc.) is a less-invasive, incisionless alternative to tubal ligation that provides significant advantages, such as decreased morbidity, rapid patient recovery, ability to detect failures, decreased expense, and a high level of patient satisfaction when compared with tubal ligation.

Transcervical sterilization lends itself nicely to the office setting because it can be performed with little to no anesthesia or sedation in a standard gynecologic examination room. Patients describe only minimal postoperative discomfort and have a high tolerance for the procedure. A recent survey reported that more than 97% of patients who underwent the procedure would recommend it to a friend. Now, more than 15 years after its introduction, transcervical hysteroscopic sterilization (Essure) has proven to be an enduring technology, making it increasingly popular as the option of choice for permanent interval female sterilization.

An investigation of the trends in female sterilization between January 1, 2002, and December 31, 2007, at the Detroit Medical Center, Michigan, revealed a significant decrease in the percentage of interval laparoscopic sterilizations and postpartum tubal ligations performed after vaginal delivery. Of the interval sterilizations performed, the percentage of hysteroscopic sterilizations (Essure) increased significantly from 0% to 51.3% of all procedures performed. Although not indicative of a universal shift in trends across the United States, this study suggests that a minimally invasive, incisionless procedure is an appealing alternative choice for many patients.

The Essure sterilization procedure entails one office visit, followed by a postprocedure low-pressure hysterosalpingogram (HSG) 3 months later. (See sample Essure Confirmation Test checklist available at www.expertconsult.com.) The placement of the Essure microinserts can be accomplished in approximately 9 minutes with a 97% to 99% successful bilateral placement rate and little to no patient discomfort and downtime.

If the clinician is proficient with basic diagnostic office hysteroscopy, then performing the Essure procedure (after attending a certified device user course) would be a logical "next step" office procedure. Currently, many gynecologists and a few primary care physicians perform hysteroscopic sterilizations. Increased awareness and available training for hysteroscopic sterilization for "seasoned" practitioners or recent residency graduates will continue to increase the popularity and availability of this permanent contraception option to patients.

A second method of transcervical sterilization became available in July, 2009. However, there was a patent infringement suit, and manufacturing of Adiana Permanent Contraception System (Hologic, Inc.) was discontinued in 2012.

ANATOMY

The anatomy relevant to Essure placement is identical to that described in Chapter 130, Hysteroscopy.

INDICATION

- Any woman who desires permanent elective sterilization

CONTRAINDICATIONS

Absolute

- Pregnancy or suspected pregnancy
- Less than 6 weeks after delivery or abortion
- Inability to observe both tubal ostia during hysteroscopy

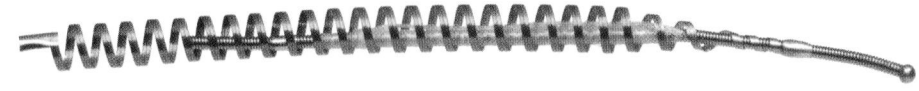

Fig. 132.1   Essure microinsert. (Courtesy Bayer Conceptus, Inc., Mountain View, CA.)

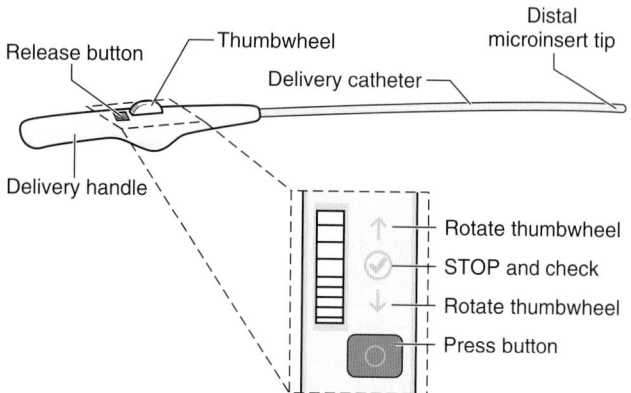

Fig. 132.2   Delivery system. (Modified courtesy Bayer Conceptus, Inc., Mountain View, CA.)

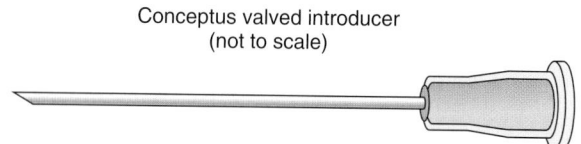

Fig. 132.3   Valved DryFlow introducer for the Essure ESS305. (Redrawn from images courtesy Bayer Conceptus, Inc., Mountain View, CA.)

* Patients who have previously undergone a tubal ligation
* Radiologic contrast allergy (according to FDA protocol; although ultrasound has been used to confirm placement it would be considered off-label)

Relative

* Active or recent pelvic infection
* Uterine anomalies
* Immunosuppressive therapy

EQUIPMENT AND SUPPLIES

* Materials for a paracervical block (see Chapter 153, Paracervical Block)
* Powered examination table
* The standard hysteroscopic equipment already available in the physician's office (see Chapter 130, Hysteroscopy) or surgery center

The third-generation Essure system (ESS305) consists of two Essure microinserts (Fig. 132.1) (one insert per disposable delivery catheter) and two disposable introducers (Fig. 132.2). A standard hysteroscope with a 5-Fr operating channel, preferably with continuous flow and an angle of view between 12 and 30 degrees is required equipment necessary for this procedure. The only uterine distention medium recommended for hysteroscopic sterilization is normal saline using a gravity flow system (see Chapter 130, Hysteroscopy).

Each Essure insert (see Fig. 132.1) consists of a Nitinol (nickel-titanium alloy) outer coil, a 316L stainless steel inner coil wrapped in polyethylene terephthalate (PET) fibers, platinum marker bands (2), and a silver-tin solder. The wound-down insert is approximately 4 cm in length and 0.8 mm in diameter. The insert is designed with a 15-degree angle at the tip to facilitate entry into the fallopian tube. When released, the outer coil expands up to 2.0 mm in diameter, conforming itself to the varied diameters and shapes of the fallopian tube. The microinserts do not contain or release hormones. Once inserted, the PET fibers stimulate a local, benign tissue growth that surrounds and infiltrates the device over the course of several weeks, leading to occlusion of the tubal lumen.

The disposable delivery device handle contains a delivery wire, release catheter, and delivery catheter housing the microinsert. An ergonomic, single-use handle provides effortless control of the

microinsert deployment via a button-thumbwheel combination built in to the handle (see Fig. 132.2). The valved, DryFlow introducer permits passage of the Essure introducer catheter into the operating channel without any valve manipulation on the hysteroscope, thus preventing backflow of fluid (Fig. 132.3). The ESS305 has a new gold band where the notch used to be on the previous version, making it easier to visualize and correctly place the device into the tubal ostia. The release catheter has a contrasting green color to improve visibility. In addition, the device has an automatic release mechanism on the handle that eliminates the need, as was required with the previous generation, for counterclockwise rotations to disconnect the introducer catheter from the actual implanted insert.

PRECAUTIONS

* Patient must use an alternative form of contraception until an HSG is done to confirm both placement and tubal occlusion.
* Essure does not prevent sexually transmitted diseases.
* Essure is considered permanent and irreversible.
* Caution should be used when performing surgeries with electrosurgical or radiofrequency devices in the pelvis because Essure microinserts may conduct energy and potentially injure the patient.
* If both tubal ostia cannot be visualized, the procedure cannot be performed.
* If patient has a known prior history of intrauterine disease, previous surgical procedure, or uterine anomaly, consideration should be given to performing a "presterilization" diagnostic hysteroscopy to rule out any abnormal uterine conditions prior to the day of the planned hysteroscopic sterilization.
* The presence of an intracavitary lesion may obstruct the view of the tubal ostia and the Essure procedure may be technically difficult to perform. Removal of the lesion (e.g., submucous fibroid, endometrial polyp) may be necessary before the Essure microinserts can be placed.

PREPROCEDURE PATIENT EDUCATION

Presurgical counseling is important. The patient should understand that she is contemplating a permanent procedure. This is particularly important in young patients, who may later regret their decision to be sterilized. A history of nickel allergy is no longer a contraindication to the procedure. Patients should be queried about an allergy to contrast dye because the HSG is still required postprocedurally by the FDA protocol. If an allergy exists to dye, ultrasound is a useful alternative and is equally effective at confirming tubal occlusion; however, the patient must be told that this postprocedure evaluation of her fallopian tubes will be a deviation from the recommended FDA protocol.

It is important to schedule the patient during the early proliferative phase of her cycle. If needed, medical preparation of the endometrium with low-dose oral contraceptives or norethindrone (5 mg) or medroxyprogesterone (10 mg) can begin around day 4 or 5 of the cycle and continue until the procedure date. This

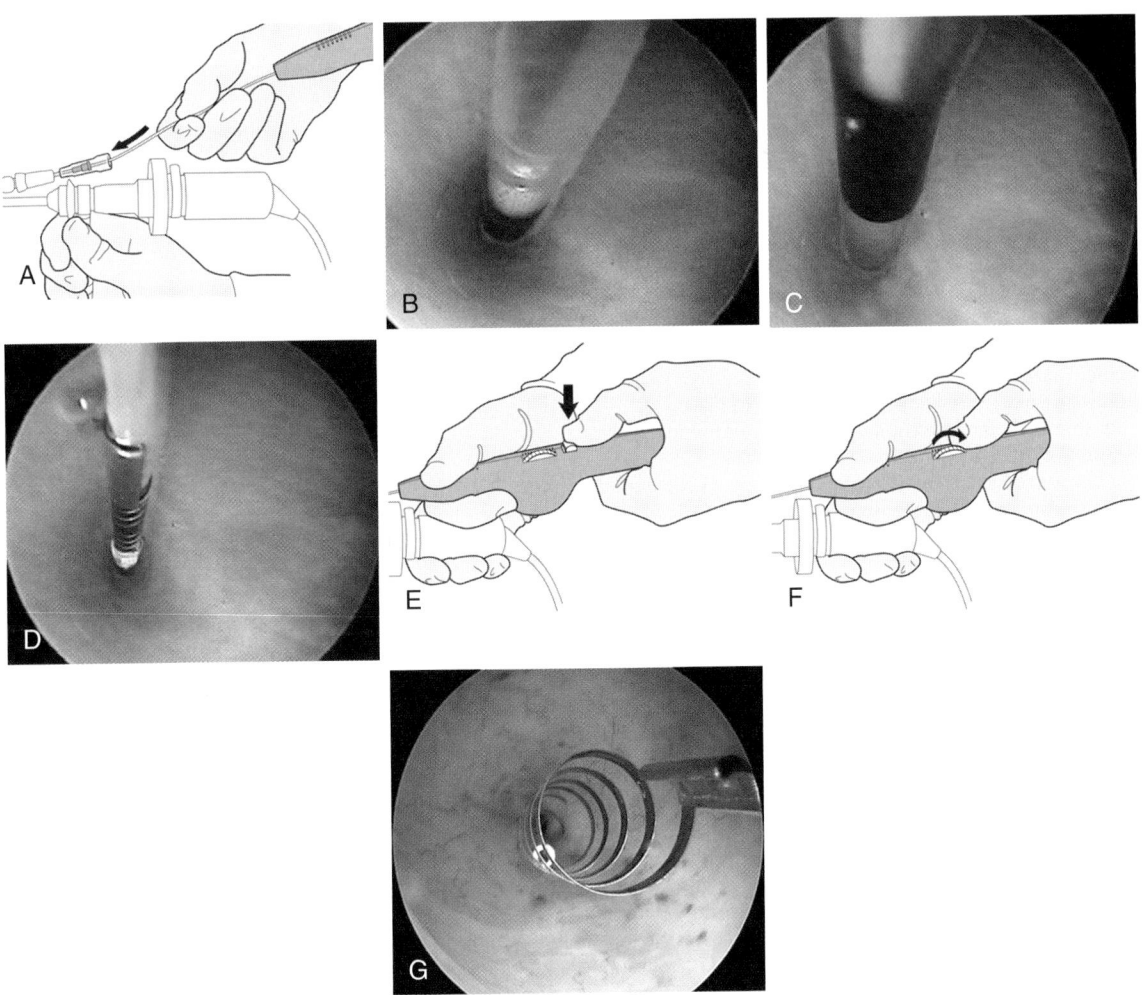

Fig. 132.4 (A–G) Essure placement steps for procedure. See text for details. Note especially how the inserter device is stabilized with the hand on the hysteroscope.

helps to prevent menstruation and produces a temporary atrophy of the uterine endometrium, which should improve visualization and manipulation within the uterine cavity during the hysteroscopic procedure. Hysteroscopic sterilization may be successfully performed in patients with a Mirena intrauterine device in place within the uterine cavity. The IUD's presence may be advantageous by allowing more flexibility in the timing of the Essure procedure, providing continuous contraceptive effect until confirmation of tubal occlusion at 12 weeks.

The risks of hysteroscopy (see Chapter 130, Hysteroscopy) and an unlikely but small risk of tubal perforation should be discussed with the patient. The sterilization procedure is 99.74% effective in preventing pregnancy after 5 years of follow-up. It should again be emphasized that a backup birth control method must be used until bilateral tubal occlusion and correct placement are confirmed by HSG. (See sample consent form available at www.expertconsult.com.)

The recently updated Discussion Checklist, along with the Patient Information Booklet, is designed to support appropriate patient counseling and to facilitate a patient's understanding of birth control options and benefits and risks associated with Essure, as well as what to expect during and after the Essure procedure. The patient should know that she will need to obtain a low-pressure modified HSG 3 months after the procedure.

PROCEDURE

Fig. 132.4 illustrates the insertion procedure. The Essure procedure is made up of two components: the Essure insert placement

procedure and the Essure Confirmation Test. Both are equally important. Because the procedure is short, there is no need for conscious sedation or general anesthesia. A paracervical block (see Chapter 153, Paracervical Block) and nonsteroidal premedication (recommended to prevent tubal spasm) are all that is needed to keep the patient comfortable during the procedure. Some minimally invasive gynecologists spray the cervix with oral benzocaine spray (e.g., Americaine, Hurricane) before applying a tenaculum. The average office visit time start to finish is approximately 30 minutes, with only approximately 9 to 10 minutes of actual hysteroscopy time to place the microinserts.

1-8. Follow universal blood and body fluid precautions. The procedure begins with insertion of the hysteroscope. (Steps 1 to 8 are identical to the procedure described in Chapter 130, Hysteroscopy. See also Chapter 126, Cervical Stenosis and Cervical Dilation if priming or dilation of the cervix is needed.) Once both tubal ostia have been identified, the insertion procedure begins as outlined in Fig. 132.4.

9. Identify both tubal ostia, and ensure that they are normal in appearance.

10. Insert the introducer through the working channel of the hysteroscope (see Fig. 132.4A).

11. Advance the catheter through the introducer to the tubal ostium on one side. There is a black marker on the introducer to signify the correct location of the catheter at the ostium (see Fig. 132.4B).

12. Stabilize the device handle on the hysteroscope.

13. Roll the thumbwheel on the inserter handle back so that the black positioning marker on the catheter moves toward you until reaching a hard stop. The handle is marked with a "1" and an arrow at this location (see Fig. 132.4C).
14. Check the placement of the microinsert by locating the gold band, which should be just outside the ostium with the green release catheter in view (see Fig. 132.4D).
15. Deploy the insert by pressing the button on the handle. The microinsert will not yet expand, allowing for any final positioning adjustments for the insert at this time (see Fig. 132.4E).
16. Expand and detach the microinsert by rolling the thumbwheel back to a second hard stop (see Fig. 132.4F).
17. Document visualization of the coils at the ostium to show proper placement (see Fig. 132.4G).
18. Withdraw the catheter, leaving the introducer in place.
19. Insert another catheter into the hysteroscope, and repeat steps 11 to 18 on the other tubal ostium.
20. Remove the introducer. Then remove the hysteroscope from the uterine cavity under direct visualization.

When inserted, the device is placed in the proximal fallopian tube in the contracted state (Fig. 132.5A) and then deployed to an expanded state once correctly positioned in the interstitial portion of the tubal lumen. After release, the outer coil expands to 1.5 to 2.0 mm in diameter, anchoring and embedding the microinsert in each fallopian tube (see Fig. 132.5B). The trailing coils of the microinsert are easily visualized at each tubal ostium, ensuring "on-site" confirmation of proper placement within the fallopian tubes. Once the inserts are in place, the PET fibers elicit tissue in-growth. The PET fiber mesh and the microinsert act as scaffolding into which the tissue grows, further embedding the microinsert within the proximal uterotubal junction, thus resulting in sterilization (see Fig. 132.5C).

The Essure Confirmation Test is an integral part of the Essure permanent birth control procedure. The test must show either bilateral satisfactory insert location (when using a transvaginal ultrasound [TVU]) or both bilateral satisfactory insert location and occlusion (when using a modified HSG) in the fallopian tubes before the patient can rely on Essure for contraception (see Fig. 132.5D).

An Essure Confirmation Test should be performed 3 months after insert placement to evaluate insert retention and location. The Essure Confirmation Test may be performed with TVU or modified HSG, although the FDA protocol only uses modified HSG.

The Essure Confirmation Tests (TVU or modified HSG) should be performed only by an experienced health care provider, including gynecologist, ultrasonographer, and/or radiologist who knows how to perform the appropriate Essure Confirmation Test. Training and educational materials on the Essure Confirmation Test are available through Bayer Conceptus.

SAMPLE OPERATIVE REPORT

Identifying data: Patient is a 36-year-old white G2P2 who requests sterilization by Essure microinserts
Preoperative diagnosis: Elective permanent sterilization
Postoperative diagnosis: Bilateral Essure insertion
Estimated blood loss: None
Complications: None
Operation performed: Hysteroscopically guided bilateral tubal sterilization with Essure microinserts
Surgeon: Dr. _____
Anesthesia: Paracervical block
Procedure: The patient's preoperative examination and consent were obtained with a prior office visit. A negative urine pregnancy test was confirmed prior to starting the procedure. The patient was placed in the dorsolithotomy position, and a bimanual examination demonstrated a normal-sized, mobile uterus without abnormality. An open-sided self-illuminating speculum was inserted into the vagina and the cervix identified and prepped with

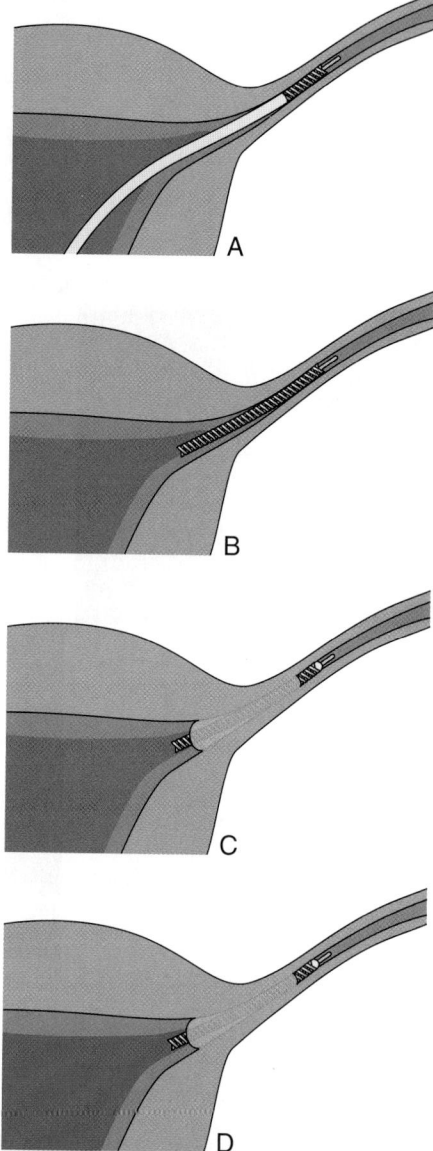

Fig. 132.5 Essure procedure for permanent birth control. (A) Using a hysteroscope, the Essure microinsert is inserted into the fallopian tube using a small catheter. (B) Once deployed, the Essure microinserts expand to fit the fallopian tube, which anchors them in place. (C) Approximately 12 weeks after procedure, tissue grows into the Essure microinserts, forming a permanent natural barrier, which occludes the fallopian tube. (D) At 3 months, low-pressure hysterosalpingography is performed. The radiologic study documents that injected dye remains in the uterine cavity and does not pass through the fallopian tubes, confirming tubal occlusion. (Courtesy Bayer Conceptus, Inc., Mountain View, CA.)

antiseptic solution. A paracervical block was performed with approximately 5 mL of 1% lidocaine. The anterior lip of the cervix was grasped with a single-tooth tenaculum. The cervix was progressively dilated to approximately 6 mm. The hysteroscope was inserted under direct visualization into the uterine cavity. The uterine cavity was distended with normal saline via a gravity flow system. The uterine fundus was well visualized. Both tubal ostia were identified and appeared normal. The tip of the hysteroscope was brought within close proximity of the patient's left tubal ostium. The Essure microinsert was advanced through the operating channel of the hysteroscope and maneuvered easily into the left fallopian tube. Under direct visualization, the microinsert was deployed without difficulty. After release, the trailing coils of the microinsert were easily visualized at the tubal ostium. The preceding technique was repeated, resulting in a successful, confirmed placement of a microinsert into the patient's right fallopian tube. The hysteroscope was withdrawn under direct visualization. All instrumentation was removed from the vagina. The patient tolerated the procedure well.

COMMON ERRORS

- Performing sterilization on a patient who is uncertain about future childbearing. Be certain to discuss the permanent nature of the procedure.
- Failure to obtain HSG 12 weeks after the procedure. Be certain to arrange follow-up for this portion of the procedure to ensure efficacy and proper placement. Alternatively, ultrasonography (two or three dimensional) can be used to determine successful bilateral placement because the microinserts are highly echogenic on pelvic ultrasound.
- Failure of clinician to properly reinforce patient compliance regarding the importance of back-up contraception until the HSG confirms both correct placement and tubal occlusion. Should the HSG be inconclusive, the patient must continue back-up contraception until a final determination is reached.
- Microinsert removal should not be attempted hysteroscopically once the microinsert has been placed and detached from the delivery wire. Attempted removal of a microinsert having fewer than 18 coils trailing into the uterine cavity may result in tubal perforation or other patient injury. Consult product Instructions for Use guide for complete details and exceptions.
- The radiologist must know to perform a modified, low-pressure HSG. There are reported cases when the HSG is ordered, the radiologist was unaware of the presence of an Essure. In an attempt to open what was seen as an obstructed fallopian tube, the HSG infusion pressure was increased significantly and the Essure was expelled.

COMPLICATIONS

In November 2016 the FDA introduced a Boxed Warning listing adverse events that have been reported either in clinical studies or through postmarket surveillance. The boxed warning reads "Some patients implanted with the Essure System for Permanent Birth Control have experienced and/or reported adverse events, including perforation of the uterus and/or fallopian tubes, identification of inserts in the abdominal or pelvic cavity, persistent pain, and suspected allergic or hypersensitivity reactions. If the device needs to be removed to address such an adverse event, a surgical procedure will be required. This information should be shared with patients considering sterilization with the Essure System for Permanent Birth Control during discussion of the benefits and risks of the device."

Failure Rates

Evaluation of all available clinical data from 2001 to 2009 reveals 503 reported pregnancies with 372,112 Essure systems sold commercially. Most pregnancies are avoidable and occur as a result of physician/patient noncompliance with recommended follow-up or misinterpreted confirmation test.

Although no major complications are associated with transcervical sterilization, short-term complications reported in the Instructions for Use or clinical studies include the following:

- Inability to place two microinserts in the first procedure, approximately 3.1% (Levie, 2009).
- An initial tubal patency rate of 3.5% at 3 months and 0% at 6 months.
- Expulsion rate of 2.9%.
- Unsatisfactory device location, 0.6%.

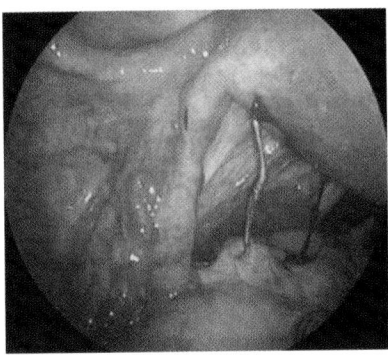

Fig. 132.6   Perforation by Essure microinsert of left side of the proximal tube. The microinsert remains attached to the tube by its distal portion while the proximal end rests on the fatty tissue of the sigmoid colon. (Courtesy V. Thoma, MD.)

- Risks related to the insertion procedure itself include cramping (29.6%) and pain (12.9%) on the day of the procedure, dizziness (8.8%), bleeding or spotting (6.8%), and vasovagal response/fainting (1.3%). The majority of patients actually consider the procedure painless or scarcely painful. Cramping pain during the procedure was reported comparable to or less than menses.
- Tubal perforation rate of 1.1%. Tubal perforation (Fig. 132.6) may often go undiagnosed during the procedure or even at the HSG 3 months after the sterilization. The microinsert may perforate into the peritoneal cavity and be entrapped by the omentum, causing chronic pain, or can lead to complications such as hemorrhage, infection, or bowel injuries and compromise the contraceptive efficiency of Essure. Therefore, in the case of a suspected perforation into the abdominal cavity, the prudent option is to investigate sooner rather than later. The possible need for a laparoscopic evaluation (carried out elsewhere if procedure is office-based) should always be discussed prior to the procedure as part of the informed consent. Alternatively, the use of fluoroscopy and two- or three-dimensional ultrasound have been suggested as useful tools in locating microinserts dislodged into the abdominal cavity.

The Essure Instructions for Use and Patient Information Booklet have been updated with additional information on safety (contraindications, warnings, and precautions), clinical data, and instructions. Important modifications have been made to the patient counseling and device removal sections of the Instructions for Use to provide physicians with additional guidance in these areas.

The inclusion of a Patient-Doctor Discussion Checklist within the Patient Information Booklet should help to minimize complications.

POSTPROCEDURE MANAGEMENT

- Patients return to work in 1 day, and most resume their daily activities the same day as the procedure.
- Patients should be counseled to use an alternative form of contraception until HSG confirmation of placement and occlusion of tubal lumen.
- Patients should be educated to inform their health care providers of the presence of Essure microinserts prior to undergoing any future medical or surgical procedure.

Concomitant Hysteroscopic Sterilization and Global Endometrial Ablation

Initially, FDA approval was granted for a Thermachoice endometrial ablation (see Chapter 133, Endometrial Ablation) to be performed concomitantly on those women who had a transcervical microinsert hysteroscopic sterilization. After evaluation of postapproval study data, the FDA later recommended a modification to the microinsert procedure label stating that the Thermachoice treatment should not be performed until after the completion of the 3-month HSG. As it turns out, Thermachoice is no longer being manufactured.

Until recently, little was known about concomitant use of global endometrial ablation (GEA) methods for endometrial ablation (e.g., balloon, cryoablation, hydrothermablation microwave, or radiofrequency energy) and hysteroscopic sterilization with microinserts. Studies assessing Thermachoice and Essure in a perihysterectomy setting demonstrated no interference with achieving a uniform ablation effect and no conduction of heat via the Essure microinsert to the serosal surface of either fallopian tube or cornua. Another retrospective study of concomitant use of Thermachoice, NovaSure, and hydrothermablation demonstrated an 85% patient satisfaction rate and no adverse events, leading to the conclusion that performance of combined GEA and hysteroscopic sterilization is effective in the treatment of menometrorrhagia.

Although current data support that it is feasible and effective to perform GEA and hysteroscopic sterilization at the same session, long-term data are still needed. Either the Essure insertion or ablation can be performed first, depending on the topography of the uterine cavity, surgeon's expertise, and the type of energy used for the ablation.

- Remember that, if a concomitant procedure is planned, you must inform the patient that this is an off-label, non-FDA approved use of these combined technologies.
- It would be prudent that, taking into consideration all of the preceding information, until a level of proficiency is reached with office hysteroscopic sterilization, any endeavor to perform a concomitant procedure should be carried out with particular caution.

CPT/Billing Codes

Physician reimbursement for this procedure is substantially greater if the procedure is performed in the office rather than the hospital.

57800   Dilatation of cervical canal, instrumental
58340   Catheterization and introduction of saline or contrast material for saline infusion sonohysterography or hysterosalpingography
58565   Hysteroscopy, with bilateral fallopian tube cannulation to induce occlusion by placement of permanent implants
59200   Insertion of cervical dilator (e.g., laminaria, prostaglandin), separate procedure

ICD-10-CM Codes

Z30.09   Encounter for family planning advice
Z30.2   Encounter for sterilization
Z30.40   Contraceptive surveillance, unspecified

Suppliers

(See contact information available at www.expertconsult.com.)

Essure ESS305 microinsert device, patient education, clinician information, procedure videos, and training/credentialing information: http://essuremd.com.
For hysteroscopy equipment, disposable illuminated vaginal speculums, distention media, miscellaneous supplies, see Chapter 130, Hysteroscopy.

Acknowledgment

The authors thank Jeanne Ballard, MD, for her assistance with this chapter.

Recommended Reading

American College of Obstetrics and Gynecology. Use of hysterosalpingography after tubal sterilization. Committee Opinion No. 458. Obstet Gynecol. 2010;115:1343–1345.
Arjona JE, Mino M, Cordon J, et al. Satisfaction and tolerance with office hysteroscopic tubal sterilization. Fertil Steril. 2008;90:1182–1186.
Guiahi M, Goldman KN, McElhinney MM, Olson CG. Improving hysterosalpingogram confirmatory test follow-up after essure hysteroscopic sterilization. Contraception. 2010;81:520–524.
Levie M, Chudnoff S. Office hysteroscopic sterilization compared with laparoscopic sterilization: a critical cost analysis. J Minimal Invasive Gynecol. 2005;12:318–322.
Levie M, Weiss G, Kaiser B, et al. Analysis of pain and satisfaction with office-based hysteroscopic sterilization. Fertil Steril. 2010;94(4):1189–1194.
Nichols M, Carter JF, Fylstra DL, et al. A comparative study of hysteroscopic sterilization performed in-office versus a hospital operating room. J Minimal Invasive Gynecol. 2006;13:447–450.
Ory EM, Hines RS, Cleland WH, Rehberg JF. Pregnancy after microinsert sterilization with tubal occlusion confirmed by hysterosalpingogram. Obstet Gynecol. 2008;111:508–510.
Shavell VI, Abdallah ME, Shade GH, et al. Trends in sterilization since the introduction of essure hysteroscopic sterilization. J Minimal Invasive Gynecol. 2009;16:22–27.
Syed R, Levy J, Childers ME. Pain associated with hysteroscopic sterilization. JSLS. 2007;11:63–65.
Tatalovich JM, Anderson TL. Hysteroscopic sterilization in patients with a Mirena intrauterine device: transition from interval to permanent contraception. J Minimal Invasive Gynecol. 2010;17:228–231.
Valle RF. Tubal perforation by Essure microinsert: clearly not a tubal perforation but a cornual-uterine perforation. J Minimal Invasive Gynecol. 2006;13:487–488.
Veersema S, Vleugels MP, Timmermans A, Brölmann HA. Follow-up of successful bilateral placement of essure microinserts with ultrasound. Fertil Steril. 2005;84:1733–1736.

CHAPTER 133

ENDOMETRIAL ABLATION

Thomas A. Kintanar

For over a century clinicians have attempted a variety of methods to control abnormal uterine bleeding as an alternative to hysterectomy. It is estimated that nearly 50% of women will have significant, heavy menstrual bleeding during their lifetime, particularly during the fifth and sixth decades of life. In the late 1880s there was a report of a physician placing a uterine sound into the endometrial cavity of patients and attaching the sound to a series of batteries. It was noted that women who did not have uterine fibroids had significant improvement in their heavy bleeding. However, because of the lack of suitable equipment and delivery systems, interest in endometrial ablation remained essentially nonexistent. During this time, the technique of dilation and curettage (D&C) was introduced and subsequently became the gold standard for the treatment of abnormal bleeding, even though it continues to be ineffective. More recently, different methods of hormone manipulation have been used with success. The levonorgestrel-containing intrauterine devices (IUDs) provide not only a comparable reduction in menstrual blood loss, but they also provide contraception. Consequently, we are seeing fewer ablation procedures.

Modern methods of achieving endometrial coagulation by heat had their beginning when Goldrath successfully used the neodymium-doped yttrium-aluminum garnet (Nd:YAG) laser in the early 1980s. His technique was quickly followed by other methods in which a urologic resectoscope was used to remove the endometrial lining. Resection was soon followed by rollerball endometrial ablation, in which the lining is not removed, but is destroyed by cauterization. For a decade, the Nd:YAG laser, uterine resection, and rollerball ablation were the primary methods used to control abnormal bleeding when hysterectomy was not desired and hormones were ineffective.

Endometrial ablation is safe, effective, efficient, and readily learned. It allows patients to address problematic vaginal bleeding from the endometrium while allowing them to keep their uterus. Methodologies that use hysteroscopy for visualization of the uterus are considered invasive. Newer techniques were developed which obtained US Food and Drug Administration (FDA) approval and did not require the use of hysteroscopy; they were termed *minimally invasive* or *second-generation nonhysteroscopic methods for endometrial ablation*. This chapter covers these approaches to endometrial ablation with a historical discussion of the classic techniques of rollerball, hysteroscopic methods of resection, and laser. At the end of the discussion, a table highlighting the FDA comparative data on the three remaining second-generation approaches is provided (Table 133.1). These data reflect the FDA Manufacturer and User Facility Device Experience database review. Unfortunately, these newer techniques are more expensive than older techniques; with insurance deductibles being very high these days, and the possible need to repeat endometrial ablation, hysterectomy is again being chosen increasingly to treat abnormal uterine bleeding in those who cannot or do not want to use an IUD.

ADVANTAGES

- Minimal anesthesia (cryoablation)
- Short operating time
- Performed in outpatient facility (rollerball and thermal balloon ablation) or office (radiofrequency, cryoablation)
- Few complications
- Rapid postoperative recovery and return to normal activity
- Highly effective in controlling bleeding (95% success rate)
- Highly effective in controlling or eliminating associated symptoms (e.g., premenstrual syndrome, dysmenorrhea, moodiness)
- Easily mastered (radiofrequency, cryoablation)

INDICATIONS

The ideal candidate for endometrial ablation meets all of the following criteria. However, there are differences in indications and contraindications depending on which technique is used.

- Menorrhagia or heavy menstrual bleeding (defined as blood loss >80 mL/cycle; bleeding for longer than 8 days; blood loss or symptoms that interfere with normal activities; or blood loss sufficient to cause anemia)
- Pharmaceutical treatment (including levonorgestrel-containing IUD) contraindicated, failed, refused, or created adverse effects
- Desire to avoid hysterectomy, especially in those with significant medical problems and surgical risks

PREREQUISITE CONDITIONS

- Absence of any precancerous or cancerous lesions of the endometrium or cervix; normal Papanicolaou (Pap) smear and negative endometrial biopsy or hysteroscopy.
- Uterine size less than 12 weeks of gestation and uterine cavity less than 12 cm in length (with the cryoablation technique, large uterine size does not preclude performing the procedure).
- Other potential causes of excessive menstrual bleeding that could be treated medically or by other alternative forms of surgery have been excluded.
- No underlying uterine lesions requiring surgery.
- Childbearing has been completed.
- No active pelvic infection.

CONTRAINDICATIONS

Absolute

- Current or planned pregnancy
- Presence of cervical or endometrial cancer or precancer
- Myomas in uterus larger than 4 cm
- Previous uterine surgeries such as myomectomy, classic cesarean section (excluding low transverse cesarean section), or any uterine surgery that would render the myometrium thin (e.g., deep myomectomy)
- Clotting or bleeding disorders, ongoing anticoagulant therapy
- Adnexal masses

TABLE 133.1	Comparative Data From 2001 US Food and Drug Administration Trial of Five Remaining Second-Generation Endometrial Ablation Devices		
Device Characteristic	**Cryotherapy**	**Radiofrequency**	**Hydrothermal**
Operating principle	Probe with transfer media creates ice ball at −100°C to −120°C	Bipolar, radiofrequency ablation at 180 W	Hydrothermal circulation of saline at 90°C
Average treatment time	10–18 min	90 sec	10 min
Average procedure time	30 min	4.2 min	30 min
Direct visualization	Ultrasonography	None required; visualization before and after procedure	Hysteroscopy
Pretreatment	Leuprolide acetate	None required	In the FDA trial, patients received a 7.5-mg dose of leuprolide acetate administered 3 wk before ablation; other trials used 3.75-mg dosages. Treatment occurred on days 19–27 after injection.
Safety features	Ultrasonographic visualization provides guidance for ice ball progression	Tests for perforations; terminates procedure at proper tissue impedance	Automatic shut-off at fluid loss of 10 mL or increase of 20 mL
Patients enrolled in the FDA trial: selected inclusion criteria	Uterine sound measurement of <10 cm Uterine volumetric measurement <300 mL	Uterine sound measurement of 6–10 cm Polyps <2 cm Submucous fibroids that did not distort the uterine cavity	Endometrial cavity measuring <10.5 cm
Patients enrolled in the FDA trial: selected exclusion criteria	Intramural myomas >2 cm diameter Intrauterine polyps Pedunculated fibroids Septate uterus	Abnormal/obstructed uterine cavity as confirmed by hysteroscopy, saline-infused sonogram, or hysterosalpingogram Specifically, septate or bicornuate uterus, pedunculated submucosal leiomyomata, or polyps (>2 cm) likely to cause menorrhagia Previous uterine surgery interrupting integrity of uterine wall	Intramural fibroids >4 cm on sonography contributing to menorrhagia Uterine anatomic anomaly Previous endometrial ablation procedure Classical cesarean section

FDA, US Food & Drug Administration.
Data from Sanfilippo JS, ed. *Options in Endometrial Ablation. Supplement to OBG Management.* www.obgmanagement.com/mededlibr/PDFs/1205Suppl_EA.pdf; 2005.

Relative

- Uterine size greater than 12 cm (this may vary depending on the procedural approach of the surgeon).
- Total cervical stenosis.
- Previous endometrial ablation.
- Unusual anatomic variation that may preclude adequate ablation, such as congenital uterine abnormalities. If there is a septate or bicornuate uterus, both cavities must be ablated separately; in the case of hydrothermablation (HTA), this may constitute a relative contraindication. Clinical consideration and procedural approach must be considered before proceeding with the ablation procedure of choice.

EQUIPMENT AND SUPPLIES

Because there are different systems that use supplies specific to the particular procedure, the following equipment/supply list provides the supplies to perform the majority of the procedures. A list of equipment/supplies germane to each procedure is listed with each particular section.

- For hysteroscopy-based ablation, a rigid (0-, 12-, or 30-degree viewing angle) hysteroscopic resectoscope (Fig. 133.1)
- Uterine sound
- Cervical dilators (e.g., Denniston, Hegar, Hank, Pratt) and possibly osmotic dilators (e.g., luminaria or synthetic) (see Chapter 126, Cervical Stenosis and Cervical Dilation)
- Tenaculum
- Vaginal bivalve speculum
- Antiseptic solution
- Lidocaine 1% with 10-mL syringe and 4-inch needle extender, 25-gauge needles (optional)
- Light source
- Uterine distention system (CO_2 or fluid) for hysteroscopy-based systems (see Chapter 130, Hysteroscopy)
- Energy source and ablative attachments (laser or cautery, ther-

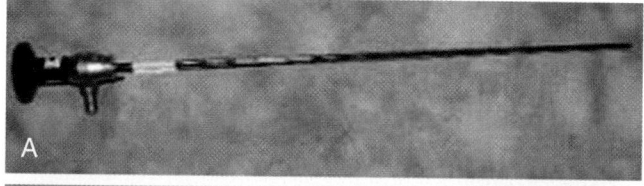
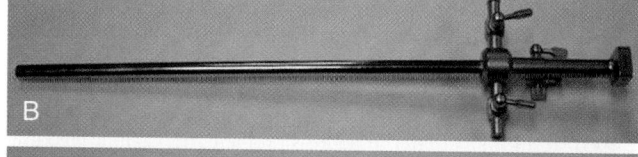
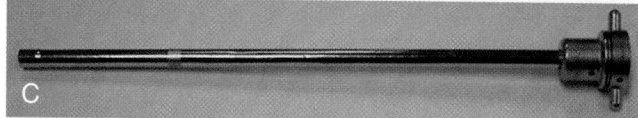

Fig. 133.1 Full resectoscope kit. (A) Hysteroscope. (B) Operating sheath. (C) Continuous-flow sheath.

mal balloon, and cryosurgical ablation techniques do not require these components)
- Video camera and display monitor for hysteroscopy-based systems
- Equipment necessary to follow universal blood and body fluid precautions

PRECAUTIONS

Endometrial ablation does not exclude the possible future development of endometrial cancer or pregnancy. Although the risks of these are low, patients should be made aware of this before undergoing the procedure. If a patient is on estrogen therapy after endometrial ablation, progestin supplementation is still necessary to prevent the development of atypical endometrium.

If the patient is still of childbearing age and pregnancy is a distinct although distant possibility, contraceptive measures should be taken to ensure pregnancy is prevented.

PREPROCEDURE PATIENT EDUCATION AND FORMS

Endometrial ablation is such a life-altering procedure that it is the surgeon's obligation to provide the patient with all of the information needed to understand all of the possible outcomes (see the example patient education form available at www.expertconsult.com). Some key elements of discussion are to emphasize that ablation may induce sterility but does not guarantee that pregnancy will not occur. Another element is that sexual desire should not be affected by the procedure. Because the endometrium is the only focus of treatment, and not the ovaries, hormonal cycles will continue if the patient is premenopausal.

PREPROCEDURE PATIENT PREPARATION

- In most instances, the patient will have already had endometrial sampling performed in the investigation of her abnormal bleeding. If this has not been done, endometrial sampling should be performed in advance of the procedure to verify the absence of malignant or premalignant lesions.
- Screening for cervical cancer (Pap smear) should also be up to date.
- Pregnancy should be excluded at the time of the procedure.
- Preoperative ultrasonography is helpful to ascertain the endometrial thickness and assess the uterine anatomy. The ideal thickness of the endometrium for ablation is less than 3 to 4 mm. There are several ways to reach this goal:
  - Physiologically, the late menstrual or early proliferative phase of the cycle will provide the ideal setting for proceeding without the use of pharmacologic agents.
  - Another simple approach would be to perform the ablation immediately after curettage.
  - To produce an atrophic, thin endometrium before the surgery, pharmacologic agents may be used. This will allow for more efficient ablation and lessen bleeding to decrease postoperative anemia. Agents available are either antiestrogenics, such as danazol (600 to 800 mg daily for 3 to 12 weeks), or gonadotropin-releasing hormone agonists, such as leuprolide acetate (two 3.75-mg intramuscular injections administered 3 to 4 weeks before surgery), or goserelin (3.6 mg injected subcutaneously 3 to 4 weeks before surgery). Pharmacologic preparation is not required with use of the NovaSure.
- Laminaria tent placement and/ or misoprostol the day before the procedure will enhance cervical dilation (see Chapter 126, Cervical Stenosis and Cervical Dilation). However, care must be taken to limit cervical dilation owing to concerns regarding the seal that the cervix can provide during the procedure, as in the case of the HTA procedure or the NovaSure.
- Antibiotic prophylaxis is unnecessary in most cases.

Preoperative preparation in this manner can decrease surgical time, lessen fluid absorption, and improve safety and surgical outcome for the patient.

Appropriate anesthesia for these procedures varies with the procedure, patient, clinician, and clinical setting. Paracervical block, sedation, regional anesthesia, general anesthesia, or a combination of these should be considered.

PROCEDURE

The following descriptions summarize the procedures in the most succinct manner. However, the focus is on the more contemporary techniques, with as much detail as possible. Inclusion of the rollerball and laser ablation is of more historical rather than practical value given the advent of the more contemporary ablative techniques. Some of the new-generation techniques for endometrial ablation do not require the use of the hysteroscope and are termed *minimally invasive nonhysteroscopic methods for endometrial ablation*. Discussion of long-term success rates regarding issues such as amenorrhea, patient satisfaction, and the eventual need for hysterectomy is well covered in the references provided. Universal blood and body fluid precautions should be followed during these procedures.

Anesthesia

The anesthesia provided for the rollerball and laser procedures is usually general anesthesia, but with the new procedural approaches, paracervical block along with oral analgesics may be all that is required to effect adequate clinical comfort. The paracervical block is used in several of the new techniques (see Chapter 153, Paracervical Block).

Technique of Hysteroscopic Endometrial Ablation With Rollerball

A rigid (0-, 12-, or 30-degree viewing angle) hysteroscopic resectoscope (see Fig. 133.1) is necessary for this procedure.

The objective of this procedure is to ablate the basal layer of the endometrium as well as the first few millimeters of the myometrium in order to ensure endometrial destruction. The first pass of the rollerball ablates to a depth of approximately 3 mm, exposing the base of the endometrial glands. The second pass ablates 2 to 3 mm of myometrium.

For the surgeon to adequately visualize the entire uterine cavity, it must be distended with liquid. Operative hysteroscopy usually uses a low-viscosity medium that continuously flows into and out of the uterus, clearing out surgical debris and blood and improving the surgeon's field of view. An inflow pressure of 80 to 110 mm Hg ensures optimal distention and continuous irrigation. An automated irrigation delivery system may be used, or a bag of distending medium is hung 1 m above the patient and produces distention through gravity. Distention media used during endometrial ablation include hypotonic agents such as glycine (1.5%), sorbitol (3%), or mannitol; isotonic agents such as normal saline; or the high-viscosity agent, dextran 70 (a viscous solution of 32% dextrose). Infused and collected fluid volumes are measured every 5 minutes, and consideration should be given to terminating the procedure if the fluid accumulation exceeds 1 to 1.5 L.

Procedure

Under sterile conditions, perform a standard bimanual pelvic examination to ascertain uterine position.

1. Insert bivalve speculum to expose the cervix. Another alternative would be to place a weighted speculum in the posterior vaginal cavity and use an anterior retractor to expose the cervix, thus maximizing exposure of the cervix.
2. Grasp anterior lip of cervix with a fine-tooth tenaculum.
3. Gently sound the uterus with a uterine sound. The tenaculum can be used to provide uterine stability.
4. Use Hegar or other dilators to gradually dilate the cervix (usually 8 to 12 mm to provide enough width to advance the resectoscope component of the hysteroscope). Also, be careful to not overdilate the cervix because this may induce leakage of distention media, thus limiting the view. If this does occur, a fine-tooth tenaculum may be used to approximate the loose cervical edges.
5. Assemble the resectoscope, making sure the advance and retraction capability is in order. (There is a paradoxical mechanism in all resectoscopes. Pulling the trigger advances the rollerball and gently relaxing pressure retracts the rollerball. The pushing and pulling of the trigger create the extension/retraction of the

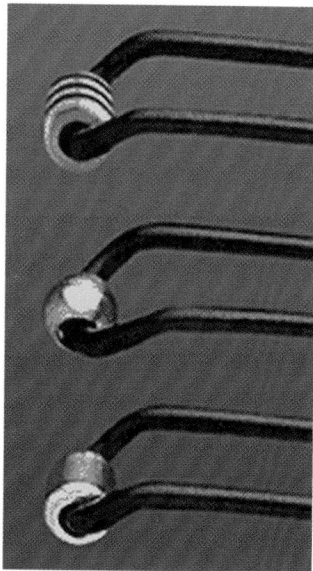

Fig. 133.2 Examples of rollerball ablation probes.

rollerball, which effects the row-like destruction of the endometrium. The rollerball is a spherical or barrel-shaped electrode that rolls over the endometrium at a speed of 10 to 15 mm/sec [Fig. 133.2].)

6. Insert the resectoscope by gentle advancement under direct visualization, following the lumen, with the irrigating fluid flowing (very similar to advancing a rigid sigmoidoscope).

7. Identify landmarks (bilateral tubal ostia and fundal area; see Chapter 130, Hysteroscopy).

8. Gently advance the rollerball by pulling the trigger until it approximates the proximal segment of the internal os. About 1.5 cm below (distal to) the internal os, set the end-point line of demarcation for ablation. Cauterize the entire circumference of this area by placing the rollerball directly on the segment by gently maneuvering the resectoscope. This creates a ring-like area of destruction that marks the eventual end point for the rollerball retraction.

9. Activate the cautery source by the foot pedal, set to a coagulating power of 50 to 80 W. There are differing viewpoints on the average power. Some operators use up to 200 W. There are also recommendations to start at 60 W to destroy the endometrial tissue for the first layer of endometrial destruction, followed by an increase to 80 to 100 W for subsequent passes. Visualize the entire distended uterine fundus and then start ablating the fundus by contacting the rollerball with the fundal tissue in a right-to-left manner. When performing ablation on the fundus, the rollerball is extended to near its maximum. The rollerball "paints" the fundus in a right-to-left manner in rows until the fundal area is entirely ablated. The ostia are handled in a similar fashion. However, because the ostial area is spherical, the rollerball must be rotated within the resectoscope to contact the tissue, consistent with the anatomy being ablated. After the line of demarcation has been established at the internal os, the corpus is ablated with the rollerball fully extended, starting at the fundus at around the 6 o'clock position. Advance the rollerball to the fundus to ablate the entire fundal and periosteal area. Gently advance the rollerball to full or nearly full extension to the fundus, then retract in a linear fashion while activating the energy source to destroy the endometrium. A count of 3 seconds should be used to effect a subjective but fairly accurate time for contact of the rollerball with the tissue during the ablation process. Continue this in a row-by-row fashion, destroying 360 degrees around the entire endometrial cavity two to three times, ending once again at the 6 o'clock position.

10. On completion of the procedure, check the fluid balance to confirm minimal risk of postoperative fluid overload.

11. Remove all instruments and transport the patient to recovery.

Common Errors

- Equipment malfunction or poor assemblage of the equipment
- Poor endometrial preparation resulting in less than optimal long-term outcomes
- Fluid leakage resulting in inaccurate fluid balance estimation

Complications

The media used to distend the uterine cavity during hysteroscopy can cause fluid overload, allergic reactions, and other toxic reactions. Fluid overload is associated with prolonged operating times and the use of high distending pressures.

- Absorption of excess amounts of hypotonic distending solution results in increased central venous pressure and hyponatremia that, if untreated, lead to pulmonary edema, hypotension, cerebral edema, and potentially fatal cardiovascular collapse. To avoid these complications, intraoperative fluid use must be strictly monitored during the procedure and the patient observed for signs and symptoms of fluid overload. Most clinicians will stop a hysteroscopic procedure at a 1- to 1.5-L fluid deficit when using glycine, sorbitol, or mannitol to avoid hyponatremic hypovolemia. A lower threshold may be required for older patients or those with preexisting cardiovascular problems. Dextran 70 has been associated with fluid overload, pulmonary edema, intravascular coagulopathy, renal insufficiency or failure, rhabdomyolysis, and anaphylactoid reactions. Glycine can result in hyperammonemic encephalopathy and transient blurred vision and blindness.
- Mechanical complications include air embolism, cervical laceration, perforation of the uterus, and severe hemorrhage.
- Thermal damage to the bowel, although rare, may occur with rollerball or laser ablation.
- Endometrial cancer may persist if occult presence is not diagnosed before the ablation, making diagnosis afterward very difficult.
- Pregnancy, although rare, is possible. With a very thin posttreatment endometrium, there is a higher risk of ectopic pregnancy as well as poorly sustained placenta and embryonic implantation.
- Infection.

Postprocedure Management

Consideration should be given to the use of postoperative antiemetics and pain medication. Options for pain control include nonsteroidal antiinflammatory drugs (NSAIDs), opiates, and acetaminophen. The patient should be instructed to have a return appointment at the surgeon's office within 1 to 2 weeks and be apprised of possible postoperative complications such as prolonged bleeding, vaginal discharge, infection, and abdominal discomfort.

Endometrial Laser Ablation

A resective hysteroscope with Nd:YAG laser attachment is necessary for this procedure.

Endometrial laser ablation is performed as an inpatient or outpatient procedure under general or regional anesthesia. A distention medium, usually normal saline, is delivered into the uterus by peristaltic pump, sphygmomanometer, or gravity, and uterine pressure is maintained between 80 and 100 mm Hg. The amount of medium is measured so that the development of fluid overload can be monitored. The Nd:YAG 600-μm fiber can produce 17,000 W/cm² at 60-W power when maximally focused. Characteristic front-scatter, coagulation, and bubbling occur during the process. A 1200-mm microfiber at same power will produce 4200 W/cm².

Procedure

1. Repeat steps 1 to 7 from the hysteroscopic rollerball ablation section, earlier.
2. The rigid hysteroscope is placed, and the endometrium is visualized. The laser attachment is placed through the operating channel of the hysteroscope and activated at a power level of approximately 60 to 80 W delivered by a 600-μm bare quartz fiber.
3. There are two techniques used for endometrial laser ablation, the touch or drag technique and the nontouch or blanching technique. During the touch technique, the laser tip is lightly applied to the endometrial surface and gently swept across the uterine cavity. For the nontouch technique, the laser tip is brought within 1 to 5 mm of the endometrial surface but does not touch it. Compared with the touch technique, this technique reduces the potential for fluid absorption because the blood and lymphatic vessels are coagulated as opposed to being cut open. Some clinicians use a combination of the two techniques. Ablation begins at the cornual and fundal areas with the delivery of short, 5- to 10-second bursts of laser energy. The anterior wall is ablated to the level of the cervical os, followed by ablation of the lateral and posterior walls.
4. The Nd:YAG laser coagulates and denatures the endometrium to a depth of approximately 4 to 6 mm. As coagulation proceeds, tissue damage is minimized because the laser energy absorbed decreases and the amount reflected increases. Fluid balance is calculated every 5 minutes and intravenous (IV) furosemide is given if the fluid absorption exceeds 1500 mL. Endometrial laser ablation takes approximately 30 to 180 minutes. If the procedure is successful, a postablation histologic study months later will reveal a single layer of simple cuboidal epithelium devoid of endometrial glands.
5. Remove all of the instruments and transport patient to recovery.

Common Errors

Potential errors are the same as for the rollerball technique.

Complications

Complications are the same as for the rollerball technique.

Postprocedure Management

Postprocedure management is the same as for the rollerball technique.

Radiofrequency (NovaSure) Ablation of the Endometrium

Equipment and Supplies

- NovaSure endometrial ablation device and radiofrequency controller
- Miller speculum (open sided)
- Hegar or other chosen dilators in sizes up to 9 mm
- Dressing forceps
- Two single-tooth tenacula
- Uterine sound
- Paracervical block supplies (see Chapter 153, Paracervical Block)
- Optional: benzocaine spray (e.g., Americaine, Hurricane)
- Optional instrumentation: 5.5-mm diagnostic hysteroscope, weighted speculum, Simms retractor, small Deaver retractor, 16-Fr straight catheter

Appropriate resuscitative equipment is necessary and varies depending on the setting and type of anesthesia administered.

Use of the NovaSure radiofrequency device (Hologic) involves inserting a slender wand through the cervix (Figs. 133.3 to 133.5). A triangular, meshlike device (the electrode array) is then passed through the wand and expands to fit the uterus. Radiofrequency electrical energy is passed through it for about 90 seconds and the

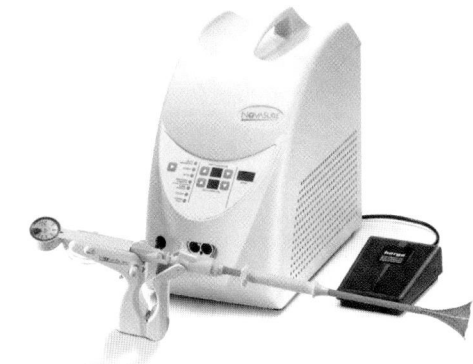

Fig. 133.3 NovaSure Controller. (Courtesy Hologic, Inc., and affiliates, Marlborough, MA.)

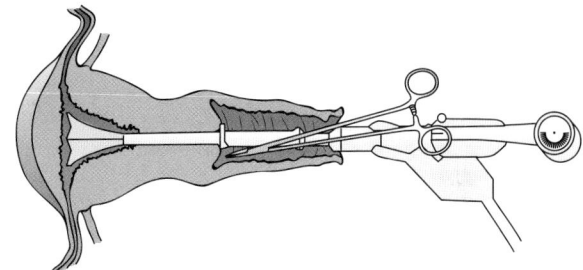

Fig. 133.4 Fully expanded NovaSure device in vaginal cavity with fully expanded bipolar electrode in the uterine cavity. (Modified courtesy Hologic, Marlborough, MA.)

mesh and wand are then withdrawn. As with many other second-generation ablation techniques, it is quick and effective and does not require pretreatment to expand the uterus.

Procedure

1. Repeat steps 1 to 3 from the hysteroscopic rollerball ablation section.
2. Anesthetic administration is similar to that for the other second-generation techniques. It can be performed in the operating room under general anesthesia or with IV sedation with paracervical block. It can also be performed in the office with NSAIDs and a paracervical block. If performed in the office, many minimally invasive gynecologists will spray oral benzocaine (e.g., Americaine, Hurricane) on the cervix before applying a tenaculum.
3. Insert the untapered Hegar or other chosen dilator until resistance is met at the internal os to measure endocervical canal length. Subtract this length from the original uterine sound length to obtain uterine cavity length. *This is a crucial measurement.*
4. Diagnostic hysteroscopy is optional.
5. Squeeze the handles of the sterile NovaSure device into the locked position to open the mesh electrode array before inserting it into uterus to ensure that it deploys. Verify that the cornual width gauge found on the instrument is greater than 4 cm. On deployment of the device, the electrode array indicator light should no longer illuminate.
6. Unlock the device and retract the array into the protective sheath by pulling back the handle using the "bow and arrow" technique.
7. Adjust the cavity length (the total uterine cavity length on uterine sounding minus the cervical cavity length) using the length-adjusting feature on the handle of the device.
8. Dilate the cervix to 8 mm with tapered Hegar dilators.

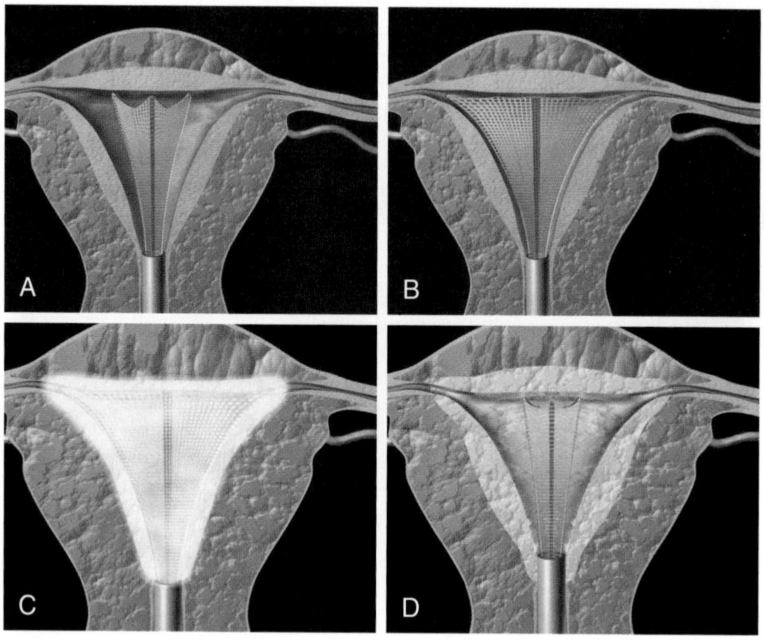

Fig. 133.5 NovaSure procedure. (A) Step 1: The NovaSure bipolar electrode expands from the slender sheath to conform to the contours of the uterine cavity. (B) Step 2: The system insufflates the uterine cavity with CO_2 to perform the cavity integrity assessment. (C) Step 3: NovaSure delivers bipolar radiofrequency energy for a complete and contoured ablation in approximately 90 seconds. (D) Step 4: The electrode array is retracted into the sheath for easy removal, leaving the uterine lining desiccated down to the superficial myometrium. (Courtesy Hologic, Marlborough, MA.)

9. Slide the cervical collar onto the sheath in its entirety. Insert the device into the cervix while holding the handle until the distal sheath reaches the fundus.
10. Tap the fundus with the array while slowly squeezing the handles, which deploys the electrode array inside the uterine cavity.
11. Seat the device by maneuvering it laterally, medially, anteriorly, and posteriorly, rotating it clockwise and counterclockwise. Pull the device backward until a decrease in value is noted on the cornual width gauge. Advance toward the fundus at this point. Repeat until maximum width is gained as demonstrated on the cornual width gauge. Input the width and length measurements into the controller (the length is the total uterine cavity length on uterine sounding minus the cervical cavity length).
12. Use one hand to stabilize the cervix with the tenaculum while holding the device. Slide the cervical collar forward to create a seal.
13. Assess the cavity integrity by stabilizing the cervical collar, then stepping on the footswitch once to activate this function on the controller. Carbon dioxide is insufflated into the uterine cavity. When the uterine cavity is insufflated to 50 mm Hg for approximately 4 seconds, the control unit (CU) must recognize no evidence of perforation. The procedure cannot proceed if perforation is evident; there is no way to override the device.
14. Once the cavity integrity is established, the controller will signal that the ablation process is enabled. The operator then steps on the footswitch once to activate the ablation cycle. The cycle using radiofrequency power lasts at least 90 seconds and not over 2 minutes. The controller signals when the cycle is complete.
15. Remove the cervical sheath and retract the array carefully.
16. Remove all instruments and transport the patient to recovery.

Common Errors

- Deployment problems with the device due to improper patient selection
- Errors in connecting and setting up the equipment properly
- Improper interpretation of measurement data, thus prolonging procedural time

Complications

Perforation, thermal burns to adjacent tissue, prolonged bleeding, infection, prolonged pain (beyond the usual expected postoperative discomfort), pregnancy, and prolonged discharge are some of the most common complications encountered.

Postprocedure Management

The usual analgesics of the surgeon's choice should be used. These include NSAIDs, opiates, and acetaminophen. There will be a vaginal discharge for 3 to 6 weeks. Uterine cramping will likely occur. The patient should return for a reevaluation appointment in 2 weeks and for possible complications, such as prolonged bleeding, pain, fever, or septic symptoms such as fever and tachycardia.

Cryoablation of the Endometrium

The Her Option Cryoablation System (Cooper Surgical) is another minimally invasive nonhysteroscopic method for endometrial ablation.

Cryoablation of the endometrium destroys tissue by the application of extreme cold through the use of the gas-cooled cryoprobe. Its operation is based on the Joule-Thomson principle, in which pressurized gas is expanded through a small orifice to produce cooling. Temperatures of −100°C to −120°C are achieved at the tip, producing an ice ball. As this ice ball grows, tissue that comes into contact with the portion of the ice ball that is −20°C or colder is destroyed. Activation of the cooling process initiates an efflux of gas through the cryoprobe; it expands at low pressure at the tip of the cryoprobe, causing an abrupt drop in temperature and freezing of the endometrium. The gas then is transported back to the compressor for recirculation.

FDA-directed studies have demonstrated the safety and effectiveness of the cryoablation system in controlling abnormal uterine bleeding. Cryoablation was found to be as effective as rollerball ablation, but is much easier to learn and causes less significant side effects. It is safer than rollerball ablation because it does not require distention of the uterus or the use of large amounts of fluid necessary with operative hysteroscopy. Moreover, cryoablation requires minimal anesthesia and can be performed in a clinician's office, although the surgical suite is still an option if dictated by clinical circumstances.

The work-up and preparation of a patient for a cryoablation procedure is similar to that for rollerball ablation, except that all patients *must have an ultrasonographic examination* performed to determine whether they have endometrial polyps or myomas. If submucous fibroids or polyps are found in the uterine cavity, the tissue should be sampled to rule out a premalignant or malignant process. This is accomplished by hysteroscopy and D&C. If the submucous myomas are greater than 3 cm in diameter or extend over halfway into the uterine cavity, the patient is not a good candidate for cryoablation. This is because the depth of tissue destruction is characteristically 9 to 15 mm. In this case, the resectoscope should be considered to remove the myomas before ablation. Pretreatment with a gonadotropin-releasing hormone agonist is not necessary.

Equipment and Supplies

The Her Option self-contained control console comes with an attached, slim 5-mm disposable cryoprobe with a two-button CU. The console also provides an audio-guided, step-by-step tutorial. A 3-L bag of 0.9% saline, a catheter that inserts into the machine, and a portable ultrasonography unit are also required.

Procedure

1. Repeat steps 1 to 3 from the hysteroscopic rollerball ablation section.
2. Provide the appropriate anesthetic. (This procedure may involve less pain because of the cryoanesthesia conferred by the instrument and procedure.)
3. Once the anesthetic is administered, a Foley catheter is inserted to instill 300 to 400 mL of saline into the bladder to facilitate ultrasonographic visualization of the uterus during the procedure.
4. Place the disposable CU over the cryoprobe. It is provided sterile, for single use only. A fuse in the disposable CU prevents function of the system if reuse is attempted. The "heat" button is used at the end of each freeze cycle to thaw the probe away from the tissue for the next freeze cycle.
5. Dilate the cervix to 5.5 mm to accept the cryoprobe.
6. Gently insert the cryoprobe into the uterine cavity (Fig. 133.6). The probe is provided with measurement markers enabling the surgeon to measure the uterine cavity. Confirm successful cannulation with ultrasonography.
7. Aim the CU toward one of the cornua and inject 5 mL of saline into the uterus through the accessory port on the cryoprobe. This will help to effect optimal tissue adherence to the cryoprobe during the freezing process.
8. Active freezing is initiated by pressing the "freeze" button on the CU (Fig. 133.7). Freezing continues until the user presses the freeze button again to pause freezing (freeze time will stop counting and resume when the user presses the freeze button again) or presses the heat button to begin heating, or until the safety time limit of 10 minutes is reached. The user presses the heat button to terminate the freeze. The heater cycles automatically to maintain a temperature of 37°C on the probe surface until the user pushes the freeze button again to complete a second freeze cycle.
9. The cornua are subjected to cryoablation first, with the process taking 4 to 6 minutes for each (Fig. 133.8). After the first cornu is finished, ultrasonography may be used to ascertain the depth of cryoablation. Ideally, the cryoablation process stops before the edge of the ice ball reaches the serosa. Ultrasonography also helps to assess the progress of the procedure and will help determine the number of passes required to effect successful ablation. Uterine size also determines the number of passes required. When the tip of the cryoprobe cools to a temperature of less than −90°C, an ice ball ellipse 3.5 to 5 cm in size forms around the probe. The edge of the ice ball is approximately 0°C and is nonlethal to the endometrial tissue. The lethal temperature for the tissue is −20°C and is found approximately 1.5 cm from the edge of the ice ball. Again, ultrasonography can be used to assess the characteristic changes in the tissue that denote adequate destruction. After satisfactory destruction of the tissue of the second cornu is completed, the heat button is pressed to pull the CU away from the destroyed endometrium. The CU is then

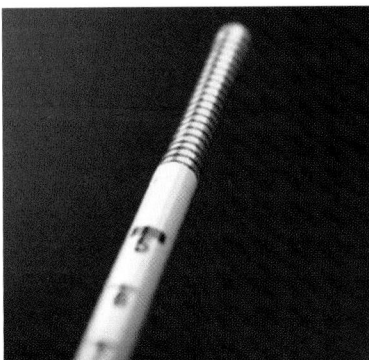

Fig. 133.6 Her Option cryoprobe tip. (Courtesy CooperSurgical, Trumbull, CT.)

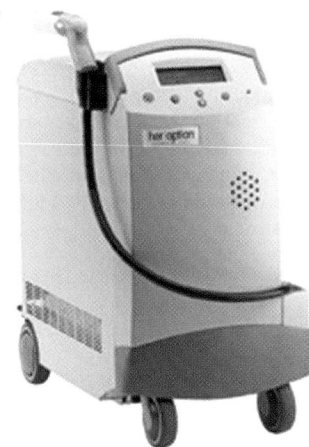

Fig. 133.7 Her Option P30 module. (Courtesy CooperSurgical, Trumbull, CT.)

reactivated at the midline in the uterus in the same manner as for the cornua. The ice ball is monitored by ultrasonography to assess destruction. Again, the procedure takes from 4 to 6 minutes, depending on the depth of destruction. Because there is no distention medium and saline is injected to effect maximal contact, both anterior and posterior components of the uterine cavity may be destroyed simultaneously. Examples of the varied options for passes made with the CU include (1) one freeze for 6 minutes in both cornua and one freeze for 6 minutes in the midline; (2) two freezes in both cornua for 6 minutes; (3) two freezes in both cornua for 6 minutes and two freezes in the midline for 4 minutes; and (4) one freeze in the midline for 4 minutes and two freezes in both cornua for 6 minutes. The number of variations depends on the anatomy and desired clinical outcome as defined by the surgeon and the ultrasonographic findings.
10. Once adequate tissue destruction is achieved, remove all instruments and transport the patient to recovery or allow recovery in the procedure suite.

Common Errors

- Inadequate assembly of equipment, thus delaying procedural start
- Operator error causing failure of equipment to perform as expected
- Insufficient freeze time to provide adequate cryoablation
- Inadequate destruction of fibroid tumors

Complications

Potential complications include adjacent tissue damage, perforation, prolonged bleeding, prolonged pain, and infection.

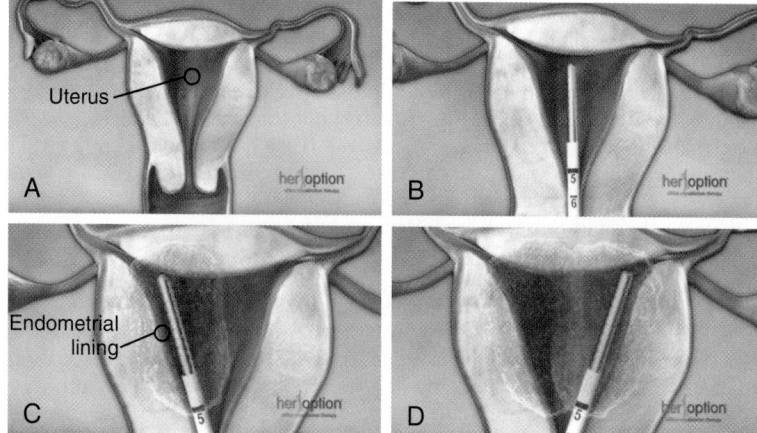

Fig. 133.8 Stages of cryoablation. (A) Uterus before cryoablation. (B) Insertion of cryoprobe. (C) Cryoablation of right cornua. (D) Cryoablation of left cornua. (Courtesy CooperSurgical, Trumbull, CT.)

Postprocedure Management

Cryoablation usually does not cause a great deal of pain because of the nature of the destruction. However, if postoperative pain does present, the usual pain medications of the surgeon's choice should be used. An NSAID, opiate, or acetaminophen is appropriate. A follow-up appointment should be scheduled for 1 to 2 weeks. The patient should be instructed to call in the event of prolonged postoperative bleeding, pain, fever, or infection.

Hydrothermablation

Equipment and Supplies

- *HTA control unit.* The CU (Genesys HTA Boston Scientific) has a microprocessor that relays a series of instructions noted on the monitor for system setup as well as providing leakage alerts. The microprocessor also monitors fluid loss and alerts the operator if a loss of 10 mL is detected at any time during the setup or ablation procedure. The CU uses room-temperature saline to purge air from the delivery system.
- A *3-L bag of sterile 0.9% saline* is suspended from an IV pole connected to the CU (ideally 115 cm above the uterus to ensure good outflow pressure).
- A *sterile procedure kit* and an *unsterile fluid management reservoir.* The one-use sterile procedure kit consists of a cassette assembly, heater canister, a disposable HTA sheath that connects to the hysteroscope, and fluid tubing. Some institutions use the heater canister 10 times, repackaging and resterilizing the unit and marking the number of sterilizations before each use and subsequent disposal.
- A *rigid hysteroscope* of the surgeon's choice is also needed (the 12-degree scope is the most versatile). If one uses the 30-degree scope, care must be taken to avoid aiming the end of the scope toward the wall of the uterine cavity so as not to traumatize the area.
- A *silicone tip* that creates the closed-loop circulation system when attached to the HTA sheath is also needed.

Procedure

1. Repeat steps 1 to 3 from the hysteroscopic rollerball ablation section.
2. With HTA, *it is essential that the cervix **not** be dilated greater than 8 mm.* It is also important *not* to use cervical dilating agents such as laminaria tents. If the cervix is dilated greater than 8 mm, the seal of the cervix around the sheath may be compromised, resulting in leakage. This may lead to thermal burns, which is a potential complication of this procedure.
3. Proceed with paracervical block (see Chapter 153, Paracervical Block).

4. Remove the HTA sterile sheath from its pouch and connect it using appropriate adapters (if needed) to the hysteroscope of choice. Be sure to use a hysteroscope with a diameter of less than 3 mm. This will ensure proper flow of the heated fluid from the HTA sheath.
5. Place the silicone tip attachment over the end of the sheath. This is crucial in maintaining the closed loop for circulating the heated fluid in and out of the uterus during the procedure.
6. Have an assistant connect the inflow and outflow tubes to the pump mechanism on the machine. Tips are color coded to ensure correct placement.
7. Press the start button. This commences the procedure, and the unit circulates saline through all of the tubing, eliminating any residual air. This takes approximately 1 minute; the main unit displays a counter until this portion of the process is complete.
8. During the countdown phase, all tubing connections and the sheath should be checked for leaks, and the light source and hysteroscope unit can be assembled in their entirety.
9. The circulation of the proper amount of saline at the proper pressure is ensured by placing the bag of saline 115 cm (45 inches) above the patient's pelvic region. This provides approximately 50 to 55 mg Hg intrauterine pressure, ample circulating pressure but below the tubal ostia opening pressure of 70 mm Hg. The circulating function begins with the pressure created by the height of the saline bag. The sheath functions as the circulating conduit for the saline. The HTA CU functions as an aspiration pump, returning saline from the uterus to the reservoir and heater canister on the CU for heating and reheating.
10. Gently insert the hysteroscope–sheath unit under direct visualization and with saline flowing into the intrauterine cavity. This procedure requires an assistant to observe the ablation process and operate the ablation control unit. The intrauterine cavity is inspected at this point.
11. Once the cavity has been evaluated, the hysteroscope–sheath unit is withdrawn to the level of the internal os to ensure the ablation treatment area remains in the uterine cavity and does not extend into the cervix. A tight uterine seal is essential to avoid the potential complication of vaginal burns from leakage of fluid onto the vaginal mucosa. This can be effected by adding one or two tenacula to the cervix to tighten the seal.
12. Commence the ablation process by starting the fluid warming cycle. Once the fluid reaches 90°C (194°F; Fig. 133.9A), the ablation cycle begins as the microprocessor on the main unit is triggered. Ablation is performed under the surgeon's direct visualization until the approximately 10-minute cycle is completed. Tissue necrosis is usually appreciated to a depth of 2 to 4 mm after 10 minutes.
13. After the ablation cycle has ended, the CU triggers a 1-minute cooling cycle to evacuate the superheated saline from the delivery system tubing. This must be completed before removing

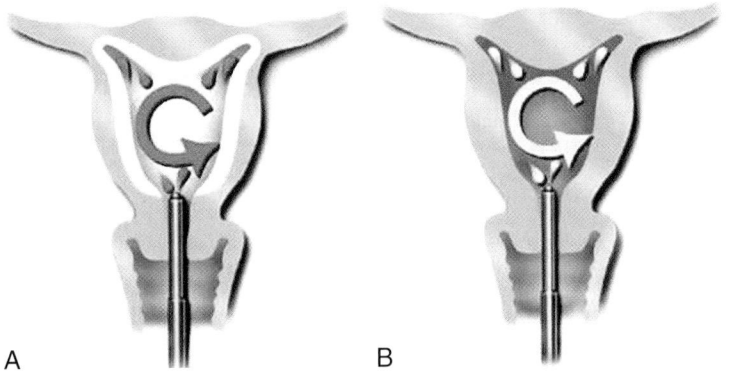

A   B

Fig. 133.9 Hydrothermablation. (A) Heating component of the ablative procedure. (B) Cooling component of the ablative procedure, showing circulation of saline.

the hysteroscope–sheath unit from the cervix (see Fig. 133.9B). Room-temperature saline flows into the uterus, which circulates the heated saline into the collection bag. When the cooling cycle is complete, the CU displays a message indicating safe conditions exist for removal of the sheath from the uterus and cervix. Again, this prevents an efflux of superheated saline into the vaginal cavity with subsequent burns to the area.

14. Before disassembling the unit, the team must wait for the entire system to cool down. This includes the canister, tubing, cassette, heater, and reservoir. This is indicated by a message in the CU when the temperature in the heater canister falls below 45°C.

Common Errors

- Improper assembly or construction of the system
- Inefficient dilation of the cervix
- Improper placement of IV tubing into the unit, thus decreasing saline pressure for HTA
- Hysteroscopy malfunction
- Improper cervical seal
- Removing the unit prematurely from the cervix before the cooling process is complete

Microwaves occupy the part of the electromagnetic spectrum between radio and infrared waves and exert their effect both directly and, in adjacent deeper layers, by thermal propagation. There currently are two FDA-approved versions of the microwave endometrial ablation device, one reusable and one disposable, each of which comprises an 8-mm OD probe attached by a reusable cable to a dedicated control module. The probe also contains an integrated thermal coupling device that transmits information about adjacent tissue temperature back to the control module for display on a screen. The surgeon controls activation and manipulation of the device. The microwave probe is inserted to the uterine fundus and, when the measured temperature of the tissue around the probe reaches 30°C, the machine is activated. The operator moves the probe across the entire endometrial surface from the fundus down as the device gradually is withdrawn. Treatment time depends, in part, on cavity size but is usually 2 to 4 minutes.

Complications

Potential complications include thermal burns from leakage of fluid into the peritoneal or vaginal cavity, perforation, postoperative infection, vaginal discharge (greater than expected), and abdominal cramping longer than expected.

Postprocedure Management

Postprocedure management is the same as for thermal balloon ablation of the endometrium.

CONCLUSION

Table 133.1 summarizes and compares the different second-generation techniques of endometrial ablation still available.

The procedure of endometrial ablation enables clinicians to serve patients who have abnormal endometrial bleeding. It has evolved from a surgical suite procedure with the hysteroscope into a potentially office-based service that provides convenience, safety, and the avoidance of hysterectomy. The particular approach depends on the clinician performing the procedure and his or her training, level of expertise, and comfort level with the service performed. Although the results from the newer procedures are similar to those with the traditional ablative techniques, complications are fewer and recovery is quicker with the newer methods.

PATIENT AND CLINICIAN EDUCATION GUIDES

Each company listed in this chapter has its own brochure for clinicians and patients. In addition, there may be descriptive instructional videos available. The company websites should be reviewed for examples.

CPT/BILLING CODES

57800	Dilation of the cervical canal, instrumental (separate procedure)
58353	Endometrial ablation, thermal, without hysteroscopic guidance
58356	Endometrial cryoablation with ultrasonic guidance, including endometrial curettage, when performed
58555	Hysteroscopy, diagnostic (separate procedure)
58558	Hysteroscopy, surgical with sampling, with or without D&C
58561	Hysteroscopy with removal of leiomyomata
58563	Hysteroscopy, surgical; with endometrial ablation (e.g., endometrial resection or electrosurgical ablation or thermoablation)
59200	Insertion of cervical dilator (e.g., laminaria, prostaglandin) (separate procedure)

ICD-10-CM DIAGNOSTIC CODES

N92.0	Excessive or frequent menstruation, menometrorrhagia, menorrhagia
N93.8	Dysfunctional uterine bleeding

Acknowledgment

The editors wish to recognize the contributions of Duane E. Townsend, MD, to this chapter in a previous edition of this text.

SUPPLIERS

(See contact information available at www.expertconsult.com.)

Bipolar cautery equipment
Hologic (NovaSure)
Cryoablation
Cooper Surgical
Hydrothermablation
Boston Scientific
Rollerball endometrial ablation: The equipment required for rollerball endometrial ablation includes a standard urologic resectoscope, a video system, and an electrocautery system.
CooperSurgical
Karl Storz Endoscopy-America, Inc.
Olympus America, Inc.
Richard Wolfe Medical Instruments Corp.

RECOMMENDED READING

American College of Obstetricians and Gynecologists (ACOG). Endometrial ablation: ACOG Practice Bulletin No. 81 (reaffirmed 2012). *Obstet Gynecol.* 2007;109:1233–1248.

Bongers MY, Bourdrez P, Willem B, et al. A prospective, double-blind, randomized, and controlled trial of two second-generation ablation devices, NovaSure GEA and ThermaChoice. *J Am Assoc Gynecol Laparosc.* 2001;8(suppl 3):S5–S6.

Carlson SM, Goldberg J, Lentz GM. Endoscopy: hysteroscopy and laparoscopy: indications, contraindications, and complications. In: Lobo RA, Gershenson DM, Lentz GM, Valea FA, eds. *Comprehensive Gynecology.* 7th ed. Philadelphia: Elsevier; 2017:190–204.

Fergusson RJ, Lethaby A, Shepperd S, Farquhar C. Endometrial resection and ablation versus hysterectomy for heavy menstrual bleeding. *Cochrane Database Syst Rev.* 2013:CD000329. Pub2.

Gurtcheff SE, Sharp HT. Complications associated with global endometrial ablation: the utility of the MAUDE Database. *Obstet Gynecol.* 2003;102:1278–1282.

Health Technology Advisory Committee—Minnesota. *Surgical Alternatives To Hysterectomy For Vaginal Bleeding.* Bethesda, MD: National Library of Medicine (US), National Center for Biotechnology Information; 2000.

Moulder J, Yunker A. Endometrial ablation considerations and complications. *Curr Opin Obstet Gynecol.* 2016;28(4):261–266.

HYSTEROSALPINGOGRAPHY AND SONOHYSTEROGRAPHY

Steven Fettinger • Linda Fanelli

Hysterosalpingography (HSG) is a radiologic examination of the female genital tract. It allows for the evaluation of the cervical canal, endometrial cavity, tubal lumen, and the periadnexal area. A basic infertility workup generally includes HSG, although some clinicians feel that it has been superseded by laparoscopy with hysteroscopy. That said, HSG remains an integral part of many other diagnostic workups. HSG is a relatively easy procedure, requires no anesthesia, and has a low complication rate. Its use as a therapeutic procedure for enhancing fertility is promoted by some clinicians. The addition of selective cannulation of the cornual ostia has not only eliminated many false positives (or blockage), but also opened new therapeutic options. Selective cannulation, however, requires special training and the use of HSG in this manner is generally limited to an infertility specialist or an interventional radiologist. Fortunately, the radiation exposure is usually minimal, in the 50 to 500 mrem range.

Saline infusion sonohysterography (SIS) is a technique for visualizing the reproductive tract using ultrasound combined with the injection of sterile normal saline as an ultrasonic contrast medium. Both the ease of this procedure and the availability of ultrasound in the office have likely contributed to its rapid increase in utilization. The discomfort involved is usually less than that of HSG, but the complications and contraindications are similar. A vaginal ultrasound probe and catheter-injected normal saline (or ultrasonic contrast medium—not yet approved by the US Food and Drug Administration [FDA] for gynecology) are used to image the anatomy. The procedure itself is simple, but the expertise and experience needed for interpretation require specialized training. The decreased accuracy in visualizing the fallopian tubes limits its use for this purpose. However, these limitations are outweighed by the ability to identify endometrial pathologic changes and to define uterine anomalies.

Many clinicians start their workup of a patient with abnormal uterine bleeding with a transvaginal ultrasonic measurement of the thickness of the endometrial stripe to rule out endometrial cancer (ACOG Committee Opinion 734, 2018). Ultrasonic evaluation of the endometrial stripe's thickness in the workup of abnormal uterine bleeding has been greatly enhanced by using SIS in combination. An endometrial thickness of 4 or 5 mm or less is thought to represent abnormal uterine bleeding. However, ethnic variations exist and cancer has been found in Japanese women with stripes only 3 to 4 mm thick. SIS is performed in patients with a double-layer endometrium thicker than 4 or 5 mm. A single-layer endometrium of 3 mm or less with no focal abnormalities on SIS is also treated as abnormal uterine bleeding (Fig. 134.1). Symmetrical thickening of the single-layer endometrium greater than 3 mm with no focal lesions is evaluated by an office endometrial biopsy. An available SIS sonobiopsy catheter allows for an immediate endometrial biopsy, if indicated, through the same catheter. A recent study (Rotenberg, 2015) found a sensitivity of 87% and specificity of 100% for detecting endometrial hyperplasia or cancer using this combination. An endometrium with focal lesions or asymmetry requires hysteroscopy

and directed biopsy (Fig. 134.2). Hormone replacement and the use of tamoxifen also affect the uterine lining, requiring the use of different discrimination thicknesses.

INDICATIONS

- Infertility (uterine)
  - Endometrial adhesions (Asherman syndrome)
  - Submucosal polyps
  - Pedunculated endometrial leiomyomas
  - Uterine anomalies
  - Diethylstilbestrol: T-shaped uterus
- Infertility (tubal)
  - Assessment of tubal patency
  - Salpingitis isthmica nodosa
  - Periadnexal adhesive disease
  - Tubal cannulation procedures
  - Follow-up after a medically or a surgically treated ectopic pregnancy
- Habitual abortions
  - Asherman syndrome
  - Uterine anomaly
  - Diethylstilbestrol changes
  - Leiomyomas
- Cervical incompetency (controversial indication, transvaginal ultrasound usually preferred)
- Preoperative and postoperative evaluation
  - Tubal reanastomosis/reimplantation, tuboplasty
  - Uterine septal resection, metroplasty
  - Myomectomy

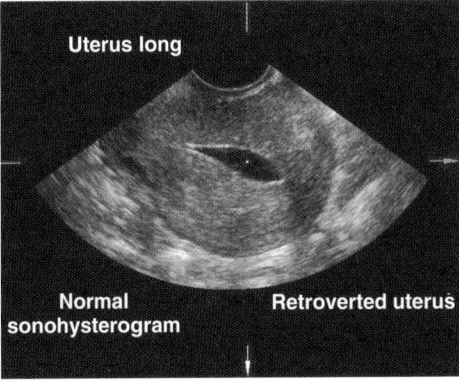

Fig. 134.1 Normal saline infusion sonohysterogram with normal thin endometrial stripe. Longitudinal view (uterus long) with fundus to the right and posterior position inferior.

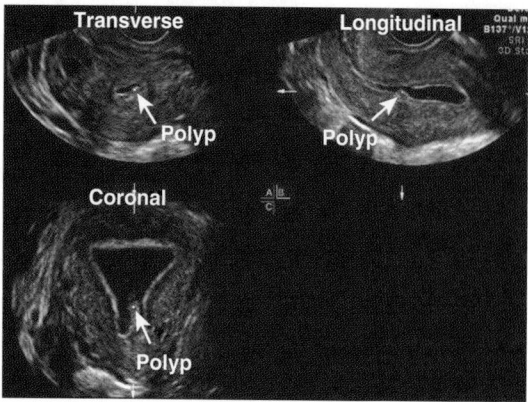

Fig. 134.2 Abnormal saline infusion sonohysterogram with thin normal endometrial stripe and a focal lesion (endometrial polyp) in three planes of view.

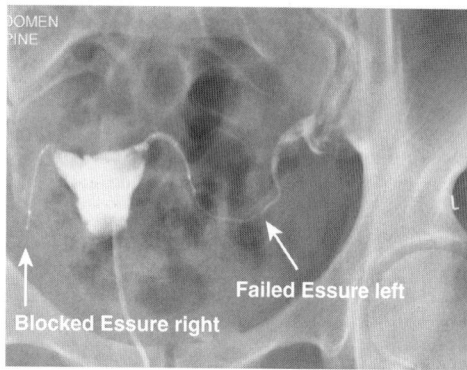

Fig. 134.3 Hysterosalpingography after an Essure cornual occlusion procedure.

- Localization of lost intrauterine contraceptive device; ultrasound alone is the procedure of choice
  - Abnormal uterine bleeding (SIS)
- Confirmation of tubal occlusion after Essure contraceptive coil insertion (Fig. 134.3)

EDITOR'S NOTE: As of 2018, manufacture of the Essure device has been discontinued by Bayer Conceptus. Previously, the Essure confirmation test (modified, low-pressure HSG) was only performed by an experienced health care provider; this may have been a gynecologist, ultrasonographer, and/or radiologist who knows how to perform the appropriate Essure confirmation test. Training and educational materials on the Essure confirmation test were available through Bayer Conceptus.

CONTRAINDICATIONS

Absolute

- Active salpingitis
- Pregnancy

Relative

- Recent dilation and curettage
- Allergy to contrast medium
- Untreated sexually transmitted disease

EQUIPMENT AND SUPPLIES

- Cannulas

Many types of HSG cannulation devices are available. The choice of catheters used may depend on the procedure and the clinician's

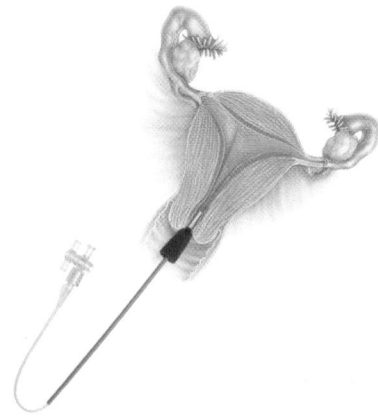

Fig. 134.4 Saline infusion sonohysterography using EZ-HSG. (Courtesy CooperSurgical, Trumbull, CT.)

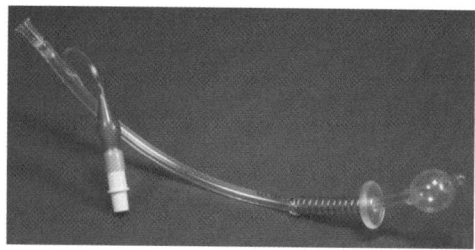

Fig. 134.5 HUI catheter. (Courtesy CooperSurgical, Trumbull, CT.)

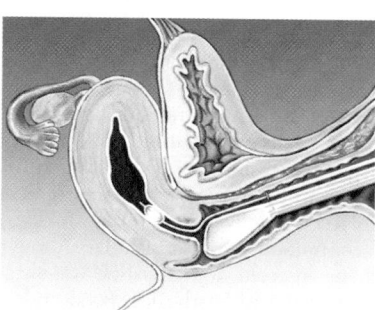

Fig. 134.6 Saline infusion sonohysterography using H/S Elliptosphere catheter. (Courtesy CooperSurgical, Trumbull, CT.)

preference. Three general types are in common use, with multiple modifications (the flexible balloon cannulas are also used for SIS):

1. *Olive-tipped cannulas.* A small cannula traverses the cervical canal and an olive- or cone-shaped seat is held against the cervical os to seal it (Fig. 134.4).
2. *Suction cannulas.* A small cannula is held in place and sealed by a suction cup on the ectocervix.
3. *Balloon cannulas.* One or two balloons are used to fix and seal the cervix. A primary intrauterine balloon is pulled down against the internal cervical os by a second balloon, a spring-loaded platform, or manual traction. The balloon catheters (including pediatric Foley catheters) obscure the lower uterine anatomy; however, the balloon can be deflated near the end of the procedure and additional contrast dye can be injected to evaluate this area (Figs. 134.5 and 134.6).

Special selective cannulation catheterization systems are available (see the "Suppliers" section). These catheters are used to selectively cannulate and evaluate a fallopian tube in special circumstances (e.g., unilateral or bilateral nonvisualization, salpingitis isthmica nodosa, or prior ectopic pregnancy). They may also be used therapeutically in some patients to open a blockage in the proximal tubes.

BOX 134.1	Common Cannulas

EZ-HSG (CooperSurgical) (see Fig. 134.4)
Goldstein sonohysterography catheter (CookMedical)
Goldstein sonobiopsy catheter (Cook Medical) (Fig. 134.7)
H/S Elliptosphere catheter set (Ackrad/CooperSurgical)
HUI catheter (CooperSurgical) (see Fig. 134.5)
HUI Mini-Flex catheter (CooperSurgical)
Hysterocath (CookMedical)
Jaco or Kuhn catheter (nondisposable)
ZUMI 2.0/4.0/4.5 catheter (CooperSurgical/Zinnanti)
  (Fig. 134.8)
Pediatric Foley catheter

TABLE 134.1	Selection of Contrast Medium	
Medium	**Advantages**	**Disadvantages**
Water soluble	Rapidly absorbed Less need for delayed films Improved visualization of details Extravasation tolerated	No enhancement of fertility
Oil based	Possible fertility enhancement	Delayed films may be needed Granuloma formation possible Embolism if extravasation occurs

SIS catheters with and without cervical sealing balloons and sponges are used for these procedures. In addition, an infusion/endometrial biopsy (sonobiopsy) catheter makes it possible to biopsy at the same time (Box 134.1).

- Contrast medium
  - HSG contrast
    Water-soluble: Salpix (Ortho McNeil Pharmaceutical), Sinografin (Bracco Diagnostics)
    Conray 60 (Mallinckrodt Pharmaceutical, Liebel-Flarsheim)
    Oil-based (Lipiodal or Ethiodol)
    Nonionic water-soluble: Hypaque-60 (Winthrop-Breon Pharmaceutical)
  - SIS contrast
    Normal saline
    Echovist (Schering-Berlin Pharmaceutical)
    Albunex (Mallinckrodt Pharmaceutical)

Both oil- and water-based iodinated contrast media are used for HSG. Most studies ultimately fail to show a difference in the diagnostic accuracy of uterine or tubal pathology with either of these media. However, water-soluble dyes have been found to provide better detail of the uterine cavity and mucosal folds of the ampullary portion of the tube and are more quickly eliminated. Oil-based dyes may be associated with less postprocedural bleeding but pose the risk of sequestration in an occluded tube and granuloma formation. That said, oil-based dyes may have increased therapeutic effect in women with unexplained infertility. Keeping all of this in mind, it may be best to have already proven the tube patent with water-based dye.

Most centers currently use water-soluble dye. Table 134.1 highlights some of the continued controversy regarding the use of water-soluble versus oil-based media. The question of ionic or nonionic water-soluble dye generally depends on the preference of the clinician. The majority of centers are using the less expensive ionic dyes except in patients with a history of an iodine allergy. Preprocedural administration of antihistamines and steroids may reduce this risk in allergic patients. Alternatively, a gadolinium radiologic contrast agent can be used in iodine-allergic patients without renal failure.

- Prep tray, including 4- by 4-inch gauze pads, ring forceps, antiseptic solution (povidone-iodine or chlorhexidine), medicine cups, lubricating jelly, and a plastic speculum (prep trays with catheters included are available)
- Vaginal speculum
  - One-armed Graves speculum (removable after placement of cannula)
  - Plastic nonradiopaque (disposable)
- Tenaculum (if needed to fixate cervix for cannula placement)
- Syringe, 10 or 20 mL
- Equipment to follow universal blood and body fluid precautions

PRECAUTIONS

- HSG should be performed in the preovulatory phase of the menstrual cycle to avoid exposing an embryo to radiation and to decrease the risk of infection (infection rates are higher if the procedure is performed during the secretory phase). SIS is performed as soon as possible after menstruation ends to minimize endometrial growth/thickness. HSG/SIS during the preovulatory phase will also avoid the possibility of dislodging a preimplantation conception and thereby theoretically prevent an ectopic pregnancy.
- Patients with a history of salpingitis require negative cultures for sexually transmitted disease and a nontender preprocedure pelvic examination. Some practitioners require a normal sedimentation rate as well.
- Patients with a history of pelvic inflammatory disease or prior tuboplasty should be treated with prophylactic antibiotics. One option shown to be effective is doxycycline 200 mg the morning of the procedure and 100 mg twice a day for 5 days following the procedure. Antibiotic prophylaxis is controversial for patients without a history of pelvic inflammatory disease or prior tuboplasty. Despite the lack of evidence in low-risk patients, many clinicians still use prophylaxis with all patients undergoing HSG. The use of prophylactic antibiotics for SIS is even less well studied, but they are used by some sonographers.

The clinician should follow universal blood and body fluid precautions.

PREPROCEDURE PATIENT EDUCATION AND PREPARATION

- Discuss the procedure, the typical findings, and alternatives to, risks of, and possible complications of the procedure with the patient (obtain informed consent).
- HSG is best performed as the patient completes her menstrual cycle, day 8 to 9 of the menstrual cycle, so the appointment should be planned accordingly.
- No special preparation is needed except that the patient will be asked to remove a tampon, if present, and to go to the toilet and empty her bladder prior to the test.
- Explain to the patient that mild discomfort will be experienced during the procedure and that spotting for up to a few days after the procedure is expected.
- Educate the patient about the warning signs of complications (e.g., increasing pain, heavy bleeding, fever).
- Preoperative medications may include a nonsteroidal anti-inflammatory agent, such as ibuprofen 600 mg, given 1 to 2 hours preoperatively, to decrease pain and cramping. The effectiveness of this premedication, however, is limited at best. Oral diazepam 5 to 10 mg 1 to 2 hours preoperatively may be given for extreme apprehension.
- A paracervical block (see Chapter 153, Paracervical Block) may increase patient comfort during the procedure. Some minimally invasive gynecologists spray the cervix with oral benzocaine spray (e.g., Americaine, Hurricane) before applying a tenaculum; however, this needs some time to take effect.

PROCEDURE

Hysterosalpingography

1. Check all equipment to ensure that the setup is complete and in proper working condition.
2. Draw up the contrast material and preload the cannula (bubbles may obscure intrauterine disease or be confused with intrauterine polyps).
3. Position the patient on a high-resolution image-intensifier fluoroscopy table in the dorsal lithotomy position. An adequate light should be available.
4. Perform a bimanual pelvic examination to assess the degree of flexion or retroflexion of the uterus and to exclude pelvic tenderness (the latter is a contraindication to HSG if there is suspected inflammation).
5. Insert the vaginal speculum.
6. Cleanse the cervix and upper vagina with antiseptic.
7. A blunt dilator may be used to dilate the cervical canal. If indicated by the cannula choice, grasp the anterior lip of the cervix with the tenaculum (slowly, to minimize pain).
8. Insert the cannula and seat it as indicated by the specific cannula:
   - Inflate the upper balloon, then the lower balloon for a double-balloon system. Alternatively, inflate the upper balloon and set the spring platform—HUI/Zinnanti (CooperSurgical) (see Figs. 134.5 and 134.8).
   - If a single balloon, inflate it and pull down—pediatric Foley and H/S Elliptosphere (CooperSurgical) (see Fig. 134.6).
   - Insert the cannula and set spring to tenaculum (Jaco).
   - Insert the cannula and seat the suction cup onto the cervix, then apply suction to the cup.
9. Remove the speculum (a nonradiopaque plastic speculum may be left in place).
10. Place the patient in the recumbent position for fluoroscopy. The following radiographic images are typically obtained:
    - Scout before contrast injection.
    - Early filling anteroposterior view of the uterus.
    - Anterolateral oblique view of one tube demonstrating spill.
    - Anterolateral oblique view of the other tube demonstrating spill.
    - En face anteroposterior view of the uterus. To achieve this view, the clinician gently pulls down on the catheter to lie the uterine cavity out in the imaging plane.
11. Inject the contrast slowly. Between 1 to 3 mL may be sufficient to show intrauterine detail; greater volumes may obscure small polyps or adhesions. The injection should be viewed concurrently and a single spot film taken. Upward or downward movement of the tenaculum will often change the degree of flexion to obtain a better view. Warming the dye preprocedurally may decrease associated cramps.
12. Continue to inject dye until the tubes start to fill. A spot film at this point may show tubal detail that will be obscured after dye spills.
    EDITOR'S NOTE: In the Essure patient, although slight injection pressure is needed to prove tubal occlusion, it should remain a low-pressure HSG. There is a case reported where the indication for the procedure was not known and, in an attempt to open the tubes, pressure was increased until the Essure device was extruded into the abdomen.
13. In the non-Essure patient, continue to inject dye until intra-abdominal spill of dye is seen bilaterally. A spot film at this point will sometimes show peritubal detail. A delayed film may be needed to confirm the location of dye in peritubal adhesions. If the tube has been proven patent with water-based dye, some clinicians will now use an oil-based dye to enhance fertility.
14. Rolling the patient from side to side during the procedure sometimes helps the clinician visualize lesions but it also increases the radiation exposure.
15. If visualization of one tube cannot be accomplished initially, try relaxing tubal spasm by relieving the pressure on the syringe and waiting 1 to 2 minutes.
16. Upon completion of the procedure, remove the instruments.
17. Observe the patient for 30 minutes for allergic reactions and heavy bleeding.
18. Selective cannulation of the ostium is briefly done as follows:
    - Preassemble coaxial catheter portions to be used or add portions as indicated for the given patient.
    - Place the cervical access catheter as previously discussed (catheter type must match the system used).
    - Introduce the uterine ostial access catheter through the cervical access catheter under radiologic guidance until the tip reaches the tubal ostium (this may be aided by the injection of a small amount of a contrast agent).
    - Pass the uterine cornual access catheter (UCAC) through the uterine ostial access catheter until the ostium is reached.
    - Advance the guidewire into the tube for a short distance, advance the UCAC over the wire, and then repeat the process until the UCAC is well within the tubal lumen.
    - While holding the UCAC in place, remove the wire.
    - Confirm placement by injecting contrast material into the UCAC.

Technical difficulties can arise during any part of the HSG examination. Some common difficulties and potential solutions include the following:

- Leaking of contrast medium: Use of a balloon catheter reduces the risk of contrast leak. If the study is being done with a cannula, using a larger cannula tip or placing additional traction on the tenaculum can resolve the leak.
- Cervical stenosis: Women with cervical stenosis can require a pediatric bladder catheter or cervical dilation (see also Chapter 126, Cervical Stenosis and Cervical Dilation).
- Air bubbles: Air bubbles can mimic filling defects in the uterus or tubes. Prior to the examination, we expel as many bubbles as possible through the catheter. During fluoroscopy, rotation of the patient can cause air bubble movement, which helps to distinguish mobile bubbles from fixed structural abnormalities. Last, aspirating and refilling the uterine cavity can remove air bubbles.
- Inadequate visualization of the uterine cavity: If the uterine cavity is inadequately visualized, we apply more outward traction on the cervix (with a tenaculum) to bring the fundus into a more axial position
- Blocked fallopian tube: Nonfilling of one or both fallopian tubes can be caused by obstruction or cornual spasm. A temporary blockage from a mucous plug or other debris can be dislodged by infusing contrast under constant pressure. If unilateral blockage is visualized, we inject 1 to 2 mL of additional contrast material. With this amount, inject until either the previously nonvisualized tube fills and spills or spillage from the patent side obscures visualization.
- Intravasation: Early intravasation into uterine and ovarian veins or lymphatics manifests as multiple thin ascending beaded channels on radiography. These channels can be identified by their anatomy, but they can sometimes be mistaken for tubal filling. To minimize the risk of intravasation, we avoid inadvertent insertion of the cannula into the myometrium and excessive pressure during the injection of contrast material.
- External artifacts: Abdominal structures (e.g., air or stool in the colon) superimposed over the uterus can mimic uterine pathology. Moving the patient onto her side and taking another radiograph can help distinguish intrauterine from extrauterine structures.

Sonohysterography

1. Using the infusion port of the catheter, fill the catheter with sterile normal saline, purging all air. Even a few tiny air bubbles can create difficulties when the images are being evaluated.
2. A brief transvaginal ultrasound should be done prior to the SIS to establish the angle of the uterus and to measure the endometrial stripe. If other than a thin endometrial stripe is noted, a pregnancy test should be ordered prior to insertion of the catheter. Tenderness noted at this point should prompt the question of inflammation and may be a contraindication to continuation with the SIS.
3. Place the patient in the lithotomy position and insert a speculum (the one-armed Graves speculum is preferred because it will be removed after placement of the catheter and before the vaginal ultrasound probe is reintroduced).
4. Prep the vagina and cervix with antiseptic.
5. Insert the SIS catheter of choice and inflate the balloon. If the patient has not had a vaginal delivery, the balloon can frequently be inflated in the endocervix instead of in the endometrial cavity, enhancing the evaluation of the lower uterine segment and decreasing the discomfort.
6. Remove the speculum and insert the transvaginal ultrasound transducer into position, taking care not to displace the cannula (see Fig. 134.6).
7. While imaging the uterus, slowly inject 5 to 10 mL of contrast agent. In some cases up to 20 mL of normal saline is necessary.
8. The uterine distention allows evaluation of the cavity for polyps or other disease.
9. Continued injection (especially if Albunex is used) fills the tubes for study; if spillage into the abdomen occurs, patency of at least one fallopian tube will be verified.
10. If an endometrial biopsy is indicated and a sonobiopsy catheter is used, the biopsy is performed without removing the catheter. The saline is removed and suction is applied to the catheter while it is moved in and out and rotated at the same time to obtain an endometrial sample (see Fig. 134.7).

COMPLICATIONS

- Infection rates may be as high as 3% in patients with a prior history of pelvic infection. Antibiotic prophylaxis is indicated in select patients (as mentioned previously) to decrease this risk.
- Tenaculum site bleeding is rare but may require suturing.
- Extravasation of dye into the intravascular space warrants discontinuation of the procedure, especially if an oil-based dye is used (there is a risk of oil pulmonary embolus).
- Granuloma formation after use of an oil-based dye is a rare late complication.
- Perforation of the uterus (or tube with selective cannulization) should prompt discontinuation.
- Rupture of a hydrosalpinx can occur.

INTERPRETATION OF RESULTS

Interpretation of results is not reviewed in this chapter, but a few points may be helpful.

- The normal HSG should show (1) a smooth triangular endometrial cavity; (2) a narrow smooth isthmic tube; (3) a progressively enlarging, increasingly convoluted ampullary tube with internal mucosal folds; and (4) spillage into the peritoneal cavity with dispersion between bowel loops.
- The correlation of HSG and laparoscopy may be as poor as 25% false positives and false negatives (the use of selective cannulation may decrease this). *Therefore absolute statements regarding tubal patency and chances for conception should be avoided.*

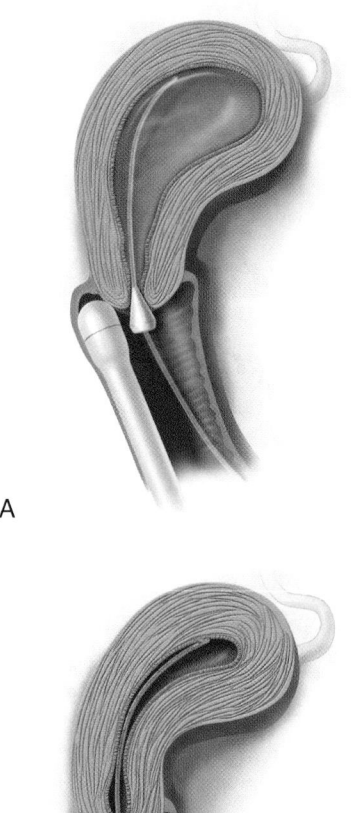

A

B

Fig. 134.7 Goldstein sonobiopsy catheters. (A) Saline infusion sonohysterography catheter. (B) Endometrial biopsy catheter. (*Copyright 2013 Lisa Clark, courtesy Cook Medical.*)

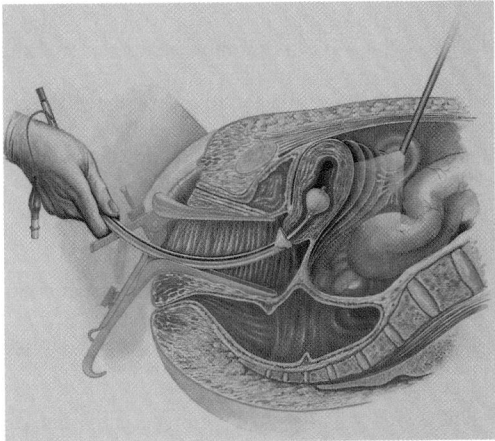

Fig. 134.8 ZUMI catheter inserted for hysterosalpingography at the time of laparoscopy. (Courtesy Zinnanti CooperSurgical, Trumbull, CT.)

- Uterine anomalies are classified according to Buttram and Gibbons; they may also require SIS or laparoscopy to fully define the abnormality. SIS has the advantage over HSG in classifying uterine anomalies because it can evaluate the myometrium as well as the endometrial cavity without the risk of anesthesia

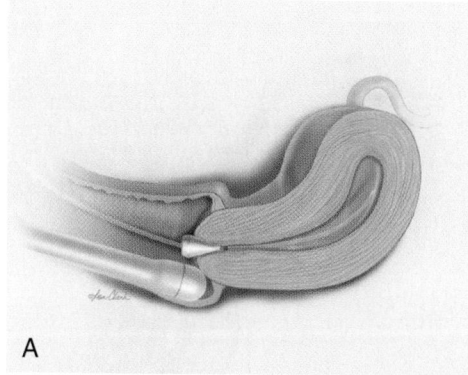 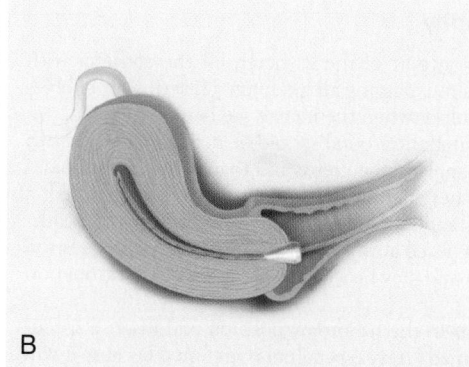

Fig. 134.9 Septate uterus diagnosed by saline infusion sonohysterography. (A) Subseptate uterus. (B) Large septum. Notice that the fundus is intact, not bicornuate, and the septum does not reach the cervix. (Copyright 2013 Lisa Clark, courtesy Cook Medical.)

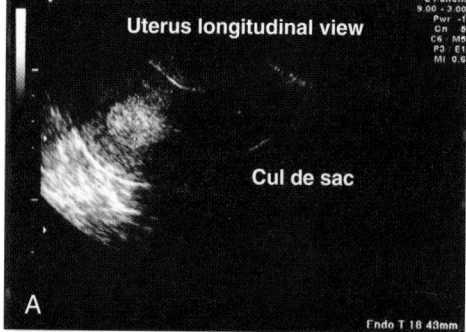

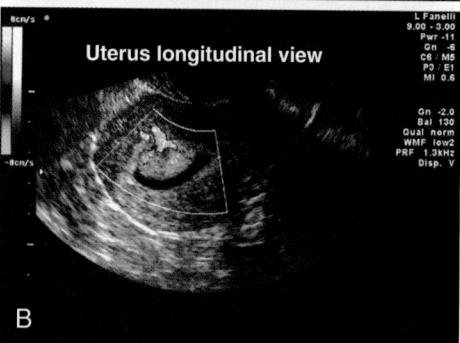

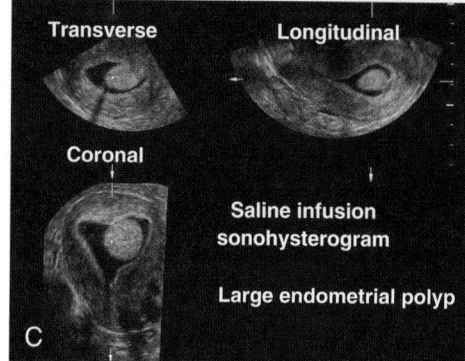

Fig. 134.10 Example of a large endometrial polyp. (A) Transvaginal ultrasound shows a thickened endometrium. (B) Saline infusion sonohysterogaphy (SIS) with Doppler shows a large polyp with its blood supply. (C) Three-dimensional reconstruction of this SIS polyp in three orthogonal planes.

or surgery. Ultrasound of the late menstrual endometrium with three-dimensional sonography allows better delineation of these uteri (Fig. 134.10).

- The association of renal with uterine developmental anomalies may be as high as 20%; therefore renal evaluation may be indicated.

The benefits of HSG over SIS are as follows:

- HSG establishes patency of both fallopian tubes.
- HSG can give the appearance of pelvic adhesions if loculations of dye occur in the adnexa.
- HSG can be "therapeutic" and increase pregnancy rates for unknown reasons if oil-based contrast agent is used (see Table 134.1).

The benefits of SIS over HSG are as follows:

- SIS enables visualization of the entire uterus, including the myometrium as well as the endometrial cavity. It is becoming the gold standard for the evaluation of uterine anomalies and can, for example, more accurately differentiate between a bicornuate and a septate uterus (see Fig. 134.9). Adding 3D ultrasound enables further evaluation, as one can reconstruct and rotate the 3D uterus for additional views (see Fig. 134.10).
- For patients with abnormal uterine bleeding, SIS will reveal global or focal thickening. If there is focal thickening—from a polyp, for example—it can determine anatomic location and size (Fig. 134.10; and see Fig. 134.2).
- SIS is helpful for evaluating fibroids, particularly if they are submucosal or intracavitary. The degree to which a fibroid extends into the endometrial cavity can be established and help to determine if hysteroscopic removal is feasible.

CPT/BILLING CODES

58340	Catheterization and introduction of saline or contrast medium for the HSG or SIS
58345	Transcervical introduction of fallopian tube catheter for diagnosis or re-establishing patency (selective catheterization)
74740	HSG, with radiologic supervision and interpretation
74742	Transcervical introduction of fallopian tube catheter for diagnosis or treatment, radiologic supervision, and interpretation
76830	Transvaginal ultrasound, nonobstetric (with radiologic interpretation)
76831	SIS (with radiologic interpretation)
99070	Supplies and materials

ICD-10-CM DIAGNOSTIC CODES

Z31.41	Fertility testing, fallopian insufflation
Z31.42	Aftercare following sterilization reversal

Z31.49	Other investigation and testing for procreative management
Z98.51	Tubal ligation status
D25.9	Uterine leiomyoma, unspecified
N84.0	Endometrial polyp
N88.3	Incompetence of cervix
N92.0	Menorrhagia or menometrorrhagia
N92.1	Metrorrhagia
N93.0	Postcoital bleeding
N93.9	Other abnormal uterine bleeding
N95.0	Postmenopausal bleeding
N96	Habitual aborter without current pregnancy
Q52.9	Congenital anomaly of genital organs

SUPPLIERS

Full contact information is available at www.expertconsult.com.

Cook Medical, Inc.
CooperSurgical (Ackrad)

RECOMMENDED READING

American College of Radiology (ACR). *ACR Practice Parameter for the Performance of Hysterosalpingography. Amended*; 2014. Resolution 39) https://www.acr.org/-/media/ACR/Files/Practice-Parameters/HSG.pdf?la=en.

American Institute for Ultrasound in Medicine (AIUM) practice parameter for the performance of sonohysterography. http://www.aium.org/resources/guidelines/sonohysterography.pdf.

Alborzi S, Dehbashi S, Khodaee R. Sonohysterosalpingographic screening for infertile patients. *Int J Gynaecol Obstet (Ireland)*. 2003;82:57–62.

American College of Obstetricians and Gynecologists. Antibiotic prophylaxis for gynecologic procedures. ACOG Committee Opinion. No. 734. *Obstet Gynecol*. 2018;131:e124–e129.

American College of Obstetricians and Gynecologists. Antibiotic prophylaxis for gynecologic procedures. ACOG Practice Bull. No. 104. *Obstet Gynecol*. 2009;113:1180–1189.

American College of Obstetricians and Gynecologists. Technology assessment in obstetrics and gynecology, No. 3. Saline Infusion Sonohysterography. *Obstet Gynecol*. 2003;102:659–662.

Buchanan EM, Weinstein LC, Hillson C. Endometrial cancer. *Am Fam Physician*. 2009;80:1075–1080.

Buttram Jr VC, Gibbons WE. Mullerian anomalies: a proposed classification. *Fertil Steril*. 1979;32:40–46.

deKroon CD, Jansen FW. Saline infusion sonography in women with abnormal uterine bleeding; an update of recent findings. *Curr Opin Obstet Gynecol*. 2006;18:653–657.

Gambone JC. Gynecologic procedures, imaging studies and surgery. In: Hacker NF, Gambone JC, Hobel JC, eds. *Hacker and Moore's Essentials of Obstetrics and Gynecology*. 6th ed. Philadelphia: Elsevier; 2016:356–368.

Gambone JC, Rodi IA. Infertility and assisted reproductive technologies. In: Hacker NF, Gambone JC, Hobel JC, eds. *Hacker and Moore's Essentials of Obstetrics and Gynecology*. 6th ed. Philadelphia: Elsevier; 2016:395–405.

Hill DA. Abnormal uterine bleeding: avoid the rush to hysterectomy. *J Fam Pract*. 2009;58:136–142.

Jansen FW, deKroon DC, van Dongen H, et al. Diagnostic hysteroscopy and saline infusion sonography; prediction of intrauterine polyps and myomas. *J Minimal Invasive Gynecol*. 2006;13:320–324.

Lee C, Salim R, Ofili-Yebovi D, et al. Reproducibility of the measurement of submucous fibroid protrusion into the uterine cavity using three-dimensional saline contrast sonohysterography. *Ultrasound Obstet Gynecol*. 2006;28:837–841.

Lindsay JT, Vitirikas RK. Evaluation and treatment of infertility. *Am Fam Physician*. 2015;91(5):308–314.

Noorhasan D, Heard MJ. Gadolinium radiologic contrast is a useful alternative for hysterosalpingography in patients with iodine allergy. *Fertil Steril*. 2005;84:1744.

Rotenberg O, Renz M, Reimers L, Doulaveris G, Gebb J, et al. Simultaneous endometrial aspiration and sonohysterography for the evaluation of endometrial pathology in women aged 50 years and older. *Obstet Gynecol*. 2015;125(2):414–423.

Salim R, Woelfer B, Backos M, et al. Reproducibility of three-dimensional ultrasound diagnosis of congenital uterine anomalies. *Ultrasound Obstet Gynecol*. 2003;21:578–582.

Simpson WL, Beitia LG, Mester J. Hysterosalpingography: a reemerging study. *Radiographics*. 2006;26:419–431.

Soares SR, Barbosa dos Reis MM, Camargos AF. Diagnostic accuracy of sonohysterography, transvaginal sonography, and hysterosalpingography in patients with uterine cavity diseases. *Fertil Steril*. 2000;73:406–411.

Steiner AZ, Meyer WR, Clark RL, Hartmann KE. Oil-soluble contrast during hysterosalpingography in women with proven tubal patency. *Obstet Gynecol*. 2003;101:109–113.

Swart P, Mol BW, van der Veen F, et al. The accuracy of hysterosalpingography in the diagnosis of tubal pathology: a meta-analysis. *Fertil Steril*. 1995;64:486–491.

Tsuda H, Kawabata M, Kawabata K, et al. Differences between Occidental and Oriental postmenopausal women in cutoff level of endometrial thickness for endometrial cancer screening by vaginal scan. *Am J Obstet*. 1995;172:1494–1495.

Watson A, Vanderkerckhove P, Lilford R, et al. A meta-analysis of the therapeutic role of oil soluble contrast media at hysterosalpingography: a surprising result? *Fertil Steril*. 1994;61:470–477.

Wittmer MH, Famuyide AO, Creedon DJ, Hartman RP. Hysterosalpingography for assessing efficacy of essure microinsert permanent birth control device. *Am J Roentgenol*. 2006;187:955–958.

CHAPTER 135

INTRAUTERINE DEVICE INSERTION AND REMOVAL

Ashley Christiani

The intrauterine contraceptive device (IUD) has been in use for more than 6 decades and is the most commonly used method of reversible birth control, with current use estimated at over 160 million women worldwide. In the United States, two major types of IUDs are available: the *ParaGard T380A*, a copper IUD containing no hormones that may be left in place for 10 years; and the *Levonorgestrel Intrauterine System* (LNG IUS), a progesterone-secreting device that is effective for 3 to 5 years. There are currently four LNG IUS hormonal IUDs available on the US market. Mirena, manufactured by Bayer Healthcare Pharmaceuticals, is the hormonal IUD that has been on the market longest and is most commonly used. It provides contraception for 5 years. In addition to preventing pregnancy, the US Food and Drug Administration (FDA) has approved use of Mirena to treat heavy menstrual bleeding. Mirena, as well as the copper IUD, are not FDA-approved for women who have not had children (who are nulliparous), but research has found that they can be provided safely and effectively to these women. Skyla, also manufactured by Bayer, is slightly smaller than the Mirena, making it a better candidate for nulliparous women. It provides contraception for 3 years. Liletta was approved in 2015. Actavis in conjunction with Medicines360, a nonprofit women's pharmaceutical company, developed Liletta specifically to be low cost and to make it available to public health clinics enrolled in the national 340B Drug Pricing Program. This program offers reduced-cost pharmaceuticals to providers that serve low-income populations. Liletta is the same size as Mirena and releases the same levonorgestrel dose, but it provides contraception for only 3 years. Kyleena, the newest IUD, was approved by the FDA in September 2016 and became available in October 2016. It is also manufactured by Bayer, provides contraception for 5 years, and contains lower levels of hormone than Mirena. **EDITOR'S NOTE:** Of all the hormonal methods available for contraception, including minidose pills, hormonal IUDs provide contraception with the lowest doses of hormone available, even lower than those in Nexplanon (see Chapter 136, Insertion and Removal of Nexplanon).

The primary mode of action of IUDs is by inhibiting sperm function (thus preventing the fertilization of ova) through the release of endometrial prostaglandins and leukocytes, enzymes, and copper ions. As a secondary effect, the endometrium is typically rendered inhospitable to embryonic implantation. The LNG IUS has additional effects related to hormonal suppression of the endometrium, the thickening of cervical mucus, and the inhibition of ovulation.

Although IUDs fell out of favor in the United States many years ago, after a reported increase in the incidence of pelvic inflammatory disease (PID) and the highly publicized Dalkon Shield lawsuits, contemporary IUDs have reemerged as an excellent option for reversible, long-term birth control owing to their well-demonstrated safety and potential therapeutic effects (Tables 135.1 and 135.2). Numerous studies demonstrate that the risk of PID and upper genital tract infection is low in properly selected patients. Features that make the IUD an attractive form of birth control for many women are an efficacy rate that rivals sterilization, a favorable safety profile, ease of use once inserted, and relative lack of systemic effects. Disadvantages include altered bleeding patterns (especially in the first few months after IUD placement), the need for a procedure to place and remove the device, cramping and pain at the time of insertion (as well as the possibility of increased dysmenorrhea with copper IUDs), risk of expulsion of the device (2% to 10% in the first year), and the risk of uterine perforation at the time of the procedure (the risk is 1 per 1000 in experienced hands).

INTRAUTERINE DEVICE INSERTION

Indications

- The ideal candidate for an IUD is a parous woman in a stable, mutually monogamous relationship, with no sexually transmitted infection (STI) risk factors, who is looking for long-term but reversible birth control. The patient should be willing to check for the presence of IUD threads on a monthly basis.
- The IUD is especially appropriate for women who have difficulty remembering to take oral contraceptives or are intolerant to them, who wish to maintain fertility, and who want to minimize or avoid systemic hormones.
- Women older than 35 years who are smokers and others with increased risk of thromboembolic events, cardiac disease, hypertension, or other contraindications to hormonal therapy are also good candidates for copper IUDs.
- Although not listed as an indication by the company, the LNG IUS may be a preferred contraceptive method in women with endometriosis, dysmenorrhea, hypermenorrhea, or significant anemia, given that menstrual bleeding and cramping generally decrease significantly within 3 to 6 months after insertion. Overall blood loss drops approximately 90%, and 20% of women experience absence of bleeding because of the localized progestin effect. Other possible off-label uses of the LNG IUS are to treat endometrial hyperplasia and for postmenopausal women on hormone replacement who are intolerant to oral progestins. The progesterone component provides suppression of the endometrial lining, thus decreasing the risk of endometrial hyperplasia and uterine cancer.
- The IUD is also acceptable for women who were once considered poor candidates for the device, including adolescents, nulliparous women, women in nonmonogamous relationships, and those with a history of PID or ectopic pregnancy. Use of the IUD in these populations is reasonable in the context of appropriate screening and counseling regarding side effects and STI prevention (Table 135.3).
- Emergency contraception may be provided with the copper IUD only.

TABLE 135.1 Rate of Continuation of Contraceptive Method at 1 Year

Method	Continuing Method After 1 Year (%)
Mirena IUD	81
ParaGard Copper IUD	79
Oral contraceptive pill	68
Depo-Provera	56
Condom	53
Diaphragm	57
Spermicide	42

IUD, Intrauterine device.
Data modified from Trussell J, Kowal D. The essentials of contraception: efficacy, safety and personal considerations. In: Hatcher RA, Trussell J, Stewart F, et al, eds. Contraceptive Technology. New York: Ardent Media; 1998:211–247.

TABLE 135.2 Annual Failure Rates for Birth Control Methods

Method	Typical Use Failure (%)	Ideal Use Failure (%)
Sterilization		
Male sterilization	0.15	0.1
Female sterilization	0.5	0.5
Hormonal Methods		
Implanon	<0.1	<0.1
Hormone shot (Depo-Provera)	3	0.3
Combined pill (estrogen/progestin) and minipill	8	0.3
Intrauterine Devices		
Copper T	0.4	0.3
LNG 20 Mirena	0.2	0.1
LNG 17.5 Kyleena	0.3	0.3
LNG 14 Skyla	0.4	0.3
LNF 18.6 Liletta	0.2	0.15
Barrier Methods		
Male latex condom*	15	2
Diaphragm†	16	6
Vaginal sponge (no previous births)‡	16	9
Vaginal sponge (previous births)‡	32	26
Cervical cap (no previous births)†	16	9
Cervical cap (previous births)†	32	26
Female condom	21	5
Spermicide (gel, foam, suppository, film)	29	18
Natural Methods		
Withdrawal	27	4
Natural family planning (e.g., calendar, temperature, cervical mucus)	25	1–9
No method	85	85

*Used without spermicide.
†Used with spermicide.
‡Contains spermicide.
Data modified from Trussell J, Kowal D. The essentials of contraception: efficacy, safety and personal considerations. In: Hatcher RA, Trussell J, Stewart F, et al, eds. Contraceptive Technology. New York: Ardent Media; 1998:211–247.

Contraindications

The World Health Organization (WHO) Medical Eligibility Criteria provide guidance in risk assessment for the IUD and LNG IUS. The full-eligibility screening tool is available at www.who.int/reproductive-health/publications/mec/iuds.html. Category 4 indicates unacceptable health risk, category 3 indicates that the risks generally outweigh the benefits, category 2 indicates that

the benefits generally outweigh the risks, and category 1 indicates no restrictions.

World Health Organization Category 4 (Unacceptable Health Risk)

ALL INTRAUTERINE CONTRACEPTIVE DEVICES:

- Congenital or acquired uterine cavity malformations that would distort the uterine cavity, making it incompatible with IUD insertion. Includes large fibroids, bicornate uterus, abnormally large or small uterine cavity (axial length <6 cm or >9 cm).
- Pregnancy or suspicion of pregnancy (except in the setting of emergency contraception).
- Immediate postseptic abortion.
- Puerperal sepsis.
- Current PID, purulent cervicitis, or infection with *Chlamydia trachomatis* or *Neisseria gonorrhoeae*.
- Known pelvic tuberculosis (insertion of IUD may substantially worsen the disease).
- Unexplained vaginal bleeding.
- Known or suspected uterine or cervical cancer (awaiting treatment).
- Malignant gestational trophoblastic disease.

LEVONORGESTREL INTRAUTERINE SYSTEM ONLY:

- Breast cancer (category 1 for copper IUD).

World Health Organization Category 3 (Risks Generally Outweigh Benefits)

ALL INTRAUTERINE CONTRACEPTIVE DEVICES:

- Severe or advanced human immunodeficiency virus (HIV) disease (WHO stage 1 or 2).
- Postpartum greater than 48 hours but less than 4 weeks
- Multiple current sexual partners, a partner who is not monogamous or is otherwise at increased risk for sexually transmitted infections (STIs), including HIV.
- Benign gestational trophoblastic disease (decreasing or undetectable β-human chorionic gonadotropin levels).
- Ovarian cancer (contraindication to IUD insertion, but existing IUD may remain in place until time of treatment if contraception needed).
- For patients taking certain antiretroviral therapies.

LEVONORGESTREL INTRAUTERINE SYSTEM ONLY:

- Liver adenoma, hepatoma, or severe (decompensated) cirrhosis (category 1 for copper IUD)
- Current deep venous thrombosis (DVT) or pulmonary embolism (category 1 for copper IUD)
- Positive for antiphospholipid (category 1 for copper IUD)
- History of breast cancer, disease-free for 5 years (category 1 for copper IUD)
- Migraines with aura, at any age (category 1 for copper IUD)
- Current or history of ischemic heart disease (category 1 for copper IUD)

COPPER INTRAUTERINE CONTRACEPTIVE DEVICES ONLY:

- Severe thrombocytopenia (category 2 for LNG IUS)

World Health Organization Category 2 (Benefits Generally Outweigh Risks)

- Past menarche but younger than 20 years.
- Nulliparity (or, more specifically, nulligravidity). Although the manufacturers list nulliparity as a contraindication to some IUDs, many authorities state that any nulliparous woman who feels confident that she can avoid STIs should be considered a possible candidate for an IUD. These women should be warned of the risk of PID and of the slightly elevated risk of IUD expulsion. These women may benefit from cervical priming with misoprostol 400 μg or osmotic laminaria before insertion. (Although

TABLE 135.3	Special Populations and Considerations
Population	**Considerations**
Adolescents	Despite increased risk of pregnancy, expulsion, and removal for bleeding or pain, the IUD is still more effective than other forms of reversible contraception in this age group, and age should not be the primary determinant of candidacy for the device. Rates of infection are similar to those in adults.
Nulliparous women	Nulliparous women have similar rates of infection and efficacy with IUD use compared with multiparous women; however, higher rates of expulsion and discomfort can limit tolerance of the device.
Fertility	Most women, including nulliparous patients, can expect a rapid return to fertility after discontinuing copper- or hormone-releasing IUDs. Contrary to common belief, use of a copper IUD does not appear to increase the risk of tubal infertility in nulligravid women in the absence of chlamydial infection.
Prior ectopic pregnancy	The IUD is protective against ectopic pregnancy and is appropriate for women with a history of an ectopic pregnancy.
Insertion after abortion	IUD insertion is safe immediately after spontaneous or induced abortion and is not associated with an increased risk of perforation or infection. Expulsion rates are higher when an IUD is inserted immediately after a second-trimester abortion.
Insertion postpartum	Postpartum insertion appears to have a higher rate of expulsion but no increase in perforation or infection. Expulsion is less likely when insertion is performed within 10 minutes of delivery of the placenta compared with 1–2 days postpartum. If immediate postpartum insertion is not done, then waiting 4–6 weeks is advisable. Only the Paragard Cu380A has approval for immediate postpartum insertion. The LNG IUS can be inserted at the 6-week postpartum visit. Breastfeeding women can safely use either device.
Use for emergency contraception	The ParaGard IUD can be inserted within 120 hr of unprotected intercourse for emergency contraception with an efficacy of 98.1% in parous women and 92.4% in nulliparous women.
Valvular heart disease	There is no contraindication to use of the IUD in women with uncomplicated valvular heart disease (including mitral valve prolapse and aortic stenosis). Even in women with complicated valvular heart disease, the benefits an IUD generally outweigh the risks. Advantages include avoidance of pregnancy risks and those associated with estrogen-containing contraceptives. Prophylactic antibiotics are recommended at the time of insertion to prevent infective endocarditis in those with high-risk valvular heart disease.
Coexistent gynecologic conditions	There is no contraindication to use of the IUD in women with irregular menses, vaginitis, cervical dysplasia or cervical ectropion, a history of benign ovarian cysts, past PID with a subsequent pregnancy, or prior cesarean delivery. In some situations, such as menorrhagia, use of the LNG IUS is therapeutic. The cause of any abnormal bleeding should be defined prior to insertion. It is best to evaluate significant abnormal Pap smears prior to insertion since performing a LEEP procedure can be difficult if not impossible to do with the strings in place.
Coexistent chronic medical conditions	There is no contraindication to use of the copper IUD in women with diabetes mellitus, cardiovascular disease, migraine headaches, breast cancer or benign breast disease, smoking, obesity, epilepsy, or liver, gallbladder, or thyroid disease. There is no increased risk of pelvic infection in women with diabetes mellitus. Neither the copper IUD nor LNG IUS adversely affects glycemic control in diabetic patients.
Immunocompromise	IUD use does not enhance the risk of HIV acquisition over that in users of other contraceptives. Limited data suggest no increased risk of PID in HIV-positive IUD users. In conjunction with appropriate condom use, the IUD may be safely used in women with or at risk for HIV infection. However, for women at risk of HIV and other sexually transmitted infections, hormonal contraception may be preferable due to its protection against ascending infections.
Cancer	Use of the copper IUD has been associated with lower risks of endometrial and cervical cancer. The LNG IUS likely reduces the risk of endometrial cancer but may increase the risk of breast cancer.
Menopausal women	An IUD inserted for contraception should be removed 1 yr after the last menstrual period in menopausal women.

HIV, Human immunodeficiency virus; *LEEP,* loop electrosurgical excision procedure; *PID,* pelvic inflammatory disease.

the use of misoprostol has been found to facilitate placement, there was no significant effect on patient discomfort and there were no procedural complications [Saav, 2007].)

- Recent second-trimester abortion (increased risk of expulsion).
- Rheumatologic disease in patient on immunosuppressant therapy.
- Minor anatomic anomalies such as cervical stenosis or laceration or small fibroids that do not distort the uterine cavity or significantly interfere with IUD insertion.
- High risk of HIV or asymptomatic or mild HIV (WHO stage 1 or 2).
- History of PID without current risk factors for STIs but without subsequent pregnancy (note that if patient has had subsequent pregnancy, risk is reduced to category 1).
- Vaginitis (including *Trichomonas* infection and bacterial vaginosis).
- Complicated valvular heart disease (pulmonary hypertension, risk of atrial fibrillation, history of subacute bacterial endocarditis). Prophylactic antibiotics may be advised for insertion (see Chapter 69, Antibiotic Prophylaxis for Prevention Endocarditis).

COPPER INTRAUTERINE CONTRACEPTIVE DEVICES ONLY:

- Endometriosis or severe dysmenorrhea, which may worsen symptoms (category 1 for LNG IUS).
- Thalassemia (category 1 for LNG IUS).
- Sickle cell disease (category 1 for LNG IUS).

- Iron-deficiency anemia (category 1 for LNG IUS).
- Heavy or prolonged uterine bleeding (includes regular and irregular patterns, category 1 of LNG IUS).

LEVONORGESTREL INTRAUTERINE SYSTEM ONLY:

- Postpartum less than 48 hours and breastfeeding.
- Diabetes, type 1 or 2 (category 1 for copper IUD).
- Gallbladder disease or a history of cholestasis (not pregnancy-related), or focal nodular hyperplasia of liver (category 1 for copper IUD).
- Multiple cardiac risk factors (e.g., older age, smoking, diabetes, hypertension, hyperlipidemia; category 1 for copper IUD).
- Hypertension where blood pressure cannot be evaluated or systolic pressure is greater than 160 mm Hg or diastolic pressure is greater than 100 mm Hg (category 1 for copper IUD).
- Known dyslipidemias (without other cardiovascular known risk factors, category 1 for copper IUD).
- History of stroke (category 1 for copper IUD).
- History of deep venous thrombosis/pulmonary embolism (DVT/PE) or DVT/PE on established anticoagulant therapy, known thrombogenic mutations (factor V Leiden, prothrombin mutation, protein S, protein C, and antithrombin deficiencies) or major surgery with prolonged immobilization (due to DVT risk; all category 1 for copper IUD).
- Migraines, without aura (category 1 for copper IUD).
- Cervical intraepithelial neoplasia (category 1 for copper IUD).

Other Contraindications

- Allergy to copper (for copper IUD); hypersensitivity to any component of the IUD, including levonorgestrel, silicone, or polyethylene; any past history of IUD intolerance.
- Wilson disease (for copper IUD).
- Desire for short-term contraceptive use (may be more cost-effective to use any other method).

EQUIPMENT

- The desired prepackaged IUD (ParaGard, LNG IUS; Fig. 135.1)
- Speculum
- Sterile basin with cotton balls moistened with a water-based antiseptic, such as povidone-iodine or chlorhexidine gluconate
- Ring forceps
- Cervical tenaculum
- Uterine sound
- Nonsterile gloves (for bimanual examination before insertion procedure)
- Sterile gloves (for IUD insertion phase)
- Sterile towel to cover tray
- Long suture scissors (to cut IUD threads after insertion)

Optional Equipment

- Nonsteroidal antiinflammatory drug (NSAID) to be taken before procedure (e.g., 800 mg ibuprofen).

EDITOR'S NOTE: Although multiple studies have failed to show any improvement in patient symptoms or comfort with the administration of preprocedure NSAIDs, many clinicians still utilize them.

- Although not generally necessary, local anesthetic may be helpful in some patients. Lidocaine 2% without epinephrine may be used to perform a paracervical or submucosal block (additional equipment includes 10-mL syringe, needle extender with a 22-gauge long needle, Monsel solution, and cotton-tipped swabs; see Chapter 153, Paracervical Block, for submucosal injection technique). Paracervical blocks seem most helpful if insertion was previously abandoned due to patient discomfort or if there is significant concern regarding patient tolerance of the procedure.
- Cervical dilators (see Chapter 126, Cervical Stenosis and Cervical Dilation).

PREPROCEDURE PATIENT PREPARATION

A separate office visit for patient counseling, consent, and preparation is advised before the IUD insertion visit. Such counseling has proven to decrease the interval removal rate of IUDs. The patient's preprocedure expectation of pain is also thought to correlate with perceived pain during IUD insertion, so reassurance at this visit is important. A separate visit gives the patient the opportunity to review the material, consider her contraceptive options, ask questions, examine sample IUDs, and plan for the procedure. This visit also gives the clinician an opportunity to review the potential risks and benefits of IUD insertion, address common myths and misconceptions regarding the device (Table 135.4), and perform the screening evaluation. After a counseling visit, it is usually easier to plan and schedule an insertion date at another time. That said, current guidelines suggest that the patient may be counseled, evaluated, and have the IUD inserted, if appropriate, on the first visit. But most patients and clinicians prefer to discuss, review, and counsel in a separate visit.

Patient Counseling and Consent

Federal guidelines require that patients be given an IUD patient information brochure as part of the consent process before IUD insertion. Brochures are provided through the manufacturers of

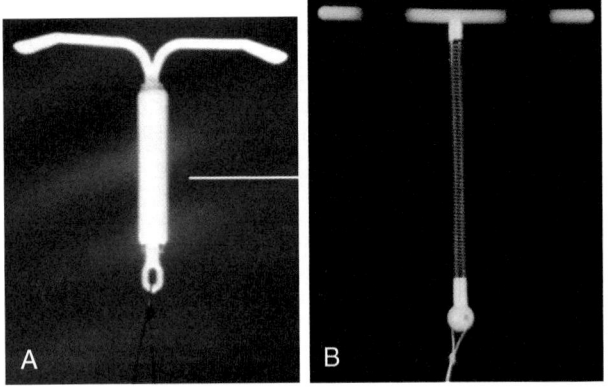

Fig. 135.1 Two types of intrauterine devices. (A) Mirena LNG IUS. (B) ParaGard T380A. Not shown are Kyleena, Liletta, or Skyla, which look very similar to Mirena. (A, Courtesy Bayer Healthcare, Whippany, NJ. B, Courtesy Teva Women's Health, Frazer, PA.)

TABLE 135.4	Myths and Misconceptions About Intrauterine Contraceptive Devices
Myth	**Fact**
IUDs are abortifacients.	IUDs prevent fertilization and thus are true contraceptives.
IUDs increase the risk of ectopic pregnancy.	IUDs significantly reduce a woman's risk of an ectopic pregnancy because the IUD prevents all types of pregnancies. Should a pregnancy occur with an IUD in place, the ratio of ectopic to intrauterine pregnancies may be increased.
IUDs expose the provider to medicolegal risk.	In past decades, product liability suits against manufacturers alleged inherently unsafe products or failure to warn of risks. Today, IUDs have been judged safe by the US Food and Drug Administration. Package inserts and patient brochures provide extensive information about risks and benefits. Hence litigation related to IUDs has virtually disappeared.
IUDs increase the risk of PID.	The IUD itself appears to have no effect on the risk of upper genital tract infection. Rather, the insertion process carries a small, transient risk in some women. The risk of PID in appropriately selected IUD candidates is so small that prophylactic antibiotics are not warranted.

From Stewart F, Gary K. Intrauterine devices (IUDs). In: Hatcher RA, Trussell J, Stewart F, et al, eds. *Contraceptive Technology*. New York: Ardent Media; 1998:511–543.

ParaGard and LNG IUSs (see the "Suppliers" section). These brochures are excellent resources and can serve as consent documents when the patient reviews the checklists and signs the forms. The clinician should confirm that the patient understands her risks, benefits, and alternatives to IUD placement and the common side effects experienced with this form of contraception. The clinician should advise the patient of the possible cramping and discomfort associated with IUD insertion as well as removal and the potential for transient nausea, dizziness, or faintness during and immediately after the procedure. Patients who experience increased pain with insertion are more commonly nulliparous, under 30 years of age, have had a longer interval since their last menses or pregnancy, and are nonlactating.

It is common to have mild spotting and cramping for a few days after the procedure and up to 8 weeks thereafter; however, if these symptoms are severe or the discomfort is not alleviated with over-the-counter analgesics, the patient will require medical evaluation.

Patients must be willing to check for the presence of IUD threads after the first menstrual period and each month thereafter. If the threads cannot be found or seem to be migrating upward, the patient must notify her clinician. Depending on menstrual cycle timing, some patients may expect reliable birth control immediately after IUD insertion; however, some authorities recommend 1 to 2 weeks of pelvic rest after the procedure to minimize risk of infection and other complications. The importance of a mutually monogamous relationship should be emphasized, with the explanation that any new partners will increase the risk of PID while the IUD is in place. Although the IUD has not been shown to increase the risk of cervical dysplasia, women using this form of contraception may be less likely to present for routine gynecologic examinations and should be specifically instructed to continue regularly scheduled pelvic examinations and Pap smears. After IUD insertion, the patient should be given an identification card or form giving the name and design of her IUD, the date of insertion, recommended date for removal, and the date of her follow-up appointment.

Screening Evaluation

Before IUD insertion, a Pap smear (within 6 months) and pelvic examination along with any appropriate STI screening should be performed and the results documented as negative. The pelvic examination should include an assessment of uterine size and position, examination for signs of cervicitis or vaginitis, and evaluation of the general morphology of the cervix and os, including signs of cervical stenosis.

Timing of Procedure

Because of higher risk of expulsion during menses (5% risk of expulsion with insertion during the first 5 days of the menstrual cycle compared with 2% risk with luteal-phase insertions) and slightly higher risk of postinsertion pain or bleeding with luteal-phase insertions, the optimal timing is the late follicular phase (day 5 to 10 of cycle). However, the IUD may be inserted at any time provided that the patient is consistently using a reliable method of contraception, has been abstinent since the last menses, or is within 5 days of a single act of unprotected intercourse and desires emergency contraception with a copper IUD.

Pretreatment

Although, as mentioned previously, there are little data supporting increased procedural comfort, patients may take ibuprofen (600 to 800 mg) or another NSAID 45 to 60 minutes before IUD insertion. Local anesthetic is usually not necessary but may be helpful in apprehensive patients, particularly those at risk for significant discomfort (nulliparas, those requiring cervical dilation, those with history of pain with prior cervical procedures) or vasovagal reaction. If desired, use lidocaine 1% to 2% without epinephrine to perform a paracervical or submucosal block (see Chapter 153, Paracervical Block, for the submucosal injection technique). Some clinicians advocate the use of topical benzocaine spray (e.g., Hurricane); however, studies with patients undergoing endometrial biopsy failed to demonstrate a pain-control benefit compared with placebo. Per current guidelines from the American College of Obstetricians and Gynecologists and American Heart Association, routine antibiotic prophylaxis for PID prevention is not recommended; however, it may be recommended in patients with severe valvular disease (see WHO guidelines and Chapter 69, Antibiotic Prophylaxis for Prevention of Endocarditis).

TECHNIQUE

The IUD insertion technique described here provides general guidelines for the procedure. For further details, the clinician should refer to the insert provided by each manufacturer in the respective packaging.

Initial Steps: All Intrauterine Contraceptive Devices

1. Make sure that the patient understands the method of and alternatives to IUD placement and that the consent form has been signed. Confirm that the patient is still a candidate for the IUD (i.e., is in a stable monogamous relationship and has not developed any contraindications as listed previously). Confirm a negative Pap smear result.
2. Confirm a negative pregnancy test if there is any question of pregnancy.
3. Reassess the need for an NSAID, antibiotic prophylaxis (not routinely recommended), heating pad (low to medium heat) for the patient's abdomen, or other special accommodations.
4. Perform a bimanual pelvic examination to reconfirm the size, position, consistency, and mobility of the uterus and to screen for the presence of any signs or symptoms of acute pelvic infection. A speculum examination may be repeated at this time if desired.
5. Change to sterile gloves and observe sterile technique from this point on in the procedure.
6. Prepare a sterile field containing the supplies discussed previously. Request an assistant if desired.
7. With the patient in the lithotomy position, insert a warm sterile speculum into the vagina. The cervix should be well visualized and the os centered in the midline.
8. Using the ring forceps, cleanse the cervix with the antiseptic-soaked cotton balls.
9. Perform a paracervical (see Chapter 153, Paracervical Block) or submucosal block if desired.
10. Clamp a single-tooth tenaculum to the anterior lip of the cervix. It may be helpful to ask the patient to cough as you apply the device or to inject 1 to 2 mL of lidocaine into the tenaculum site before placement. Apply gentle downward traction on the tenaculum to correct for any angulation and to stabilize the cervix.
11. Gently and slowly sound the uterus. Careful technique will decrease the patient's discomfort and the risk of perforation, laceration, and other complications. The uterine depth should be between 6.5 and 8.5 cm. Do not place an IUD if the depth is outside the normal range (there is an increased risk of complications in this setting). If the sound cannot be inserted because of stenosis, dilate the cervix (see Chapter 126, Cervical Stenosis and Cervical Dilation).
12. Prepare the IUD/LNG IUS for insertion. The four units are different. The *inserter tube* refers to the hollow cylinder into which the IUD fits. It may be possible to load the ParaGard IUD into the inserter while it is still in the original packaging. This is referred to as the "no touch" technique and is described in the packaging information of IUDs that provide this loading option (Fig. 135.2). Alternatively, sterile gloves are used to load the unit by folding the arms down and inserting them in the inserter tube. The inserter "rod" for the ParaGard refers to the solid trocar that fits inside the inserter tube. Fig. 135.3 is a graphic depiction of the Mirena IUS loading system, which is similar to that used by Kyleena and Skyla. Loading this system is quite different and is shown as part of the procedure in Fig. 135.5. Liletta is loaded slightly differently and is described in an individual section further on.
13. Insert the chosen IUD, using the appropriate technique for the ParaGard or LNG IUS.

ParaGard Insertion

After following the previous initial steps, insert the ParaGard IUD as follows (Fig. 135.4):

1. Make certain that the horizontal arms of the IUD are parallel to the horizontal orientation of the blue flange to ensure proper

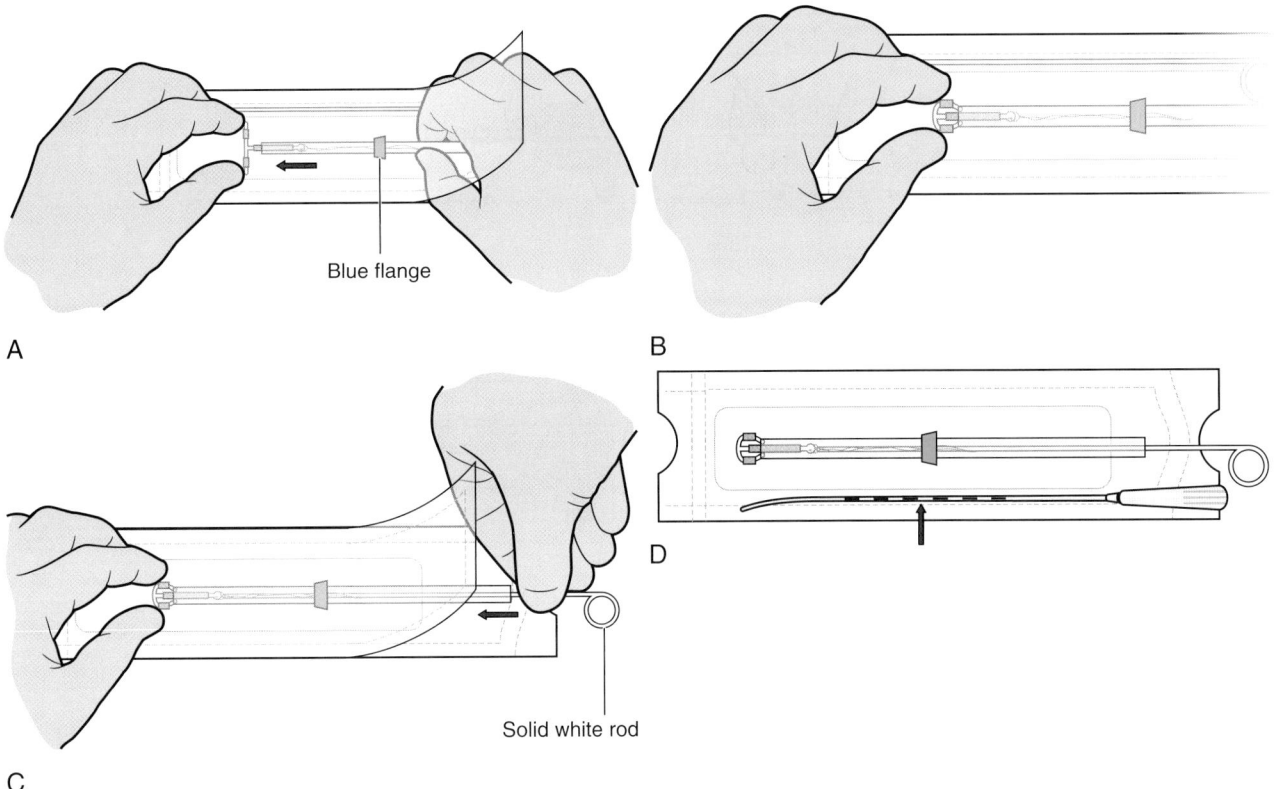

Blue flange

A

B

Solid white rod

C

D

Fig. 135.2 Loading the ParaGard intrauterine device (IUD) using the "no touch" technique just before insertion. (A) After the bimanual examination and preparation of the antiseptic solution and after the uterus has been sounded, the IUD is inserted into the hollow inserter tube. (B) The arms of the tube are bent down and inserted just far enough to retain them in the tube. (C) The solid white inserter rod is placed into the hollow insertion tube from the other end so that it just touches the bottom of the vertical arm of the IUD. (D) The blue flange is set so that the distance from the tip of the IUD to the flange is the same distance as the depth of the uterus (as determined by the uterine sound; *red arrow*). (Modified from Pfenninger JL. Techniques for inserting an IUD. *Fam Pract Recertification.* 1992;14:131–138.)

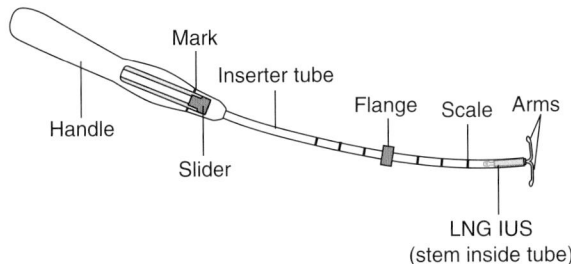

Handle
Mark
Inserter tube
Flange
Scale
Arms
Slider
LNG IUS
(stem inside tube)

Fig. 135.3 Mirena Levonorgestrel Intrauterine System (LNG IUS) and inserter. (Modified courtesy Bayer Healthcare, Whippany, NJ.)

placement in the uterus. Slide the blue flange so it is the same distance from the tip of the inserter tube as the depth the uterus sounded, maintaining the horizontal orientation.

2. Grasping the IUD inserter unit with the single-tooth tenaculum, insert it into the cervical canal up to the flange (see Fig. 135.4A). You may wish to have an assistant hold the tenaculum. With the solid white rod in your dominant hand, use the other hand to withdraw the clear plastic inserter tube toward you approximately 2 cm as the white rod is held in place (see Fig. 135.4B). This maneuver will allow the IUD to open or "fall" into place. Pushing in on the solid rod can cause a perforation. A small "pop" can often be felt as the IUD unfolds.

3. Now, while holding the white rod stable, gently and slowly push the hollow tube inserter toward the fundus until resistance is felt, to allow "high placement" of the IUD (see Fig. 135.4C[1]).

Fundal placement of the IUD decreases the risk of expulsion, accidental pregnancy, and other complications. Withdraw the solid rod only (see Fig. 135.4C[2]). Do not withdraw the tube without first removing the rod. The strings are inside the tube and compressed against the tube by the rod. Pulling both out at the same time can immediately pull out the IUD.

4. Withdraw the insertion tube (see Fig. 135.4D).

5. Complete the procedure as noted in the section Completion of Procedure.

Levonorgestrel Intrauterine System Insertion

After following the initial steps outlined previously, insert the LNG IUS (Kyleena, Mirena, Skyla) as follows (Fig. 135.5):

1. After opening the sterile package, load the IUD into the inserter by pushing the slider forward into the furthest position from you (see Fig. 135.5A). When the IUD is being loaded into the inserter, the arms will fold upward (the ParaGard arms fold down). The knobs at the ends of the arms should occlude the open end of the inserter. Do not move the slider downward at this time, as this may prematurely release the threads of the IUD. Once the slider has been moved below the mark, the IUD cannot be reloaded.

2. Set the upper end of the flange at the uterine depth measured previously (see Fig. 135.5B).

3. Hold the slider firmly with your forefinger or thumb in the furthermost position and advance the inserter into the cervical canal until the flange is about 1.5 to 2 cm from the cervix. This is a significant difference from the method of inserting the ParaGard. Keeping the

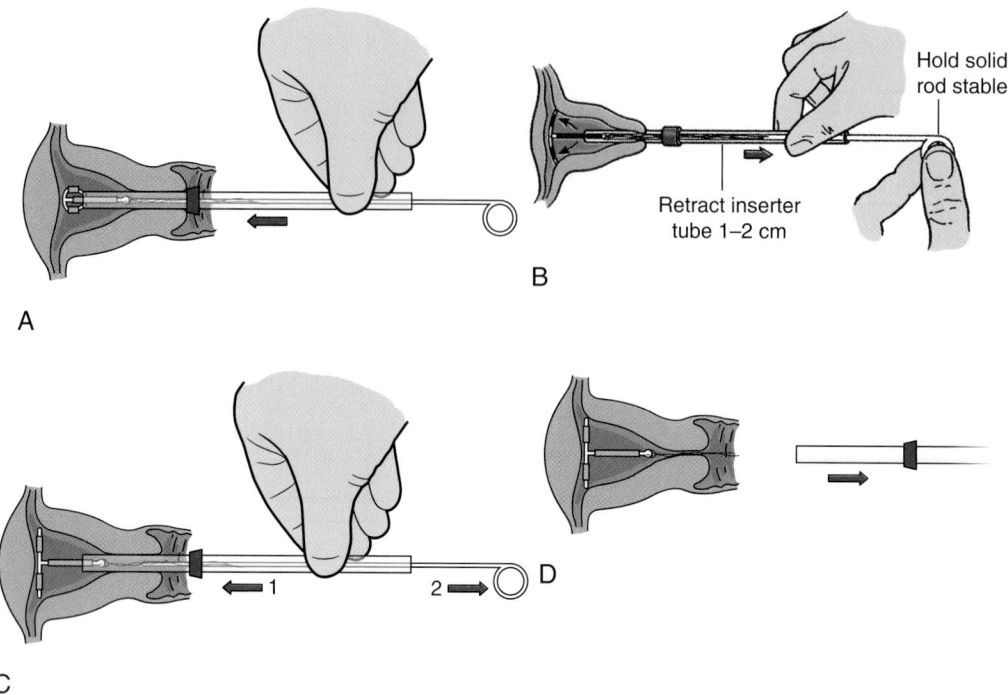

Fig. 135.4 Inserting the ParaGard intrauterine device (IUD). (A) The single-tooth tenaculum is applied to stabilize the cervix and the IUD–inserter unit is placed into the cervical canal up to the flange. (B) While an assistant holds the tenaculum, the clinician holds the solid white rod stable in the dominant hand and withdraws the insertion tube approximately 2 cm. (C) *1,* The inserting tube (with the rod held stable and still in place) is gently advanced to ensure high placement of the IUD. *2,* The solid inserting rod is withdrawn while holding the tube steady. (D) The insertion tube is withdrawn and the threads are cut, ensuring adequate length. (Modified from Pfenninger JL. Techniques for inserting an IUD. *Fam Pract Recertification.* 1992;14:131–138.)

flange 1.5 to 2 cm away from the cervical os allows sufficient space for the arms to open within the uterus (see Fig. 135.5C).

4. While holding the inserter steady, release the arms of the LNG IUS by pulling the slider back until it reaches the mark (i.e., raised horizontal line; see Fig. 135.5D). Wait 10 seconds for the horizontal arms to open completely.

5. Stabilize the slider in the current position and push the inserter gently inward until the flange now touches the cervix. The LNG IUS should now be in the fundal position (see Fig. 135.5E).

7. Holding the inserter rod steady, release the LNG IUS by pulling the slider all the way back (see Fig. 135.5F). Carefully remove the inserter from the uterus.

8. Complete the procedure as noted in the next section.

Liletta Insertion

1. Pull back the blue threads to dislodge them from the flange. Be careful not to pull the IUS down at the same time. Hold the exposed end of the insertion tube containing the IUS and threads with one hand while keeping the end of the insertion tube with the IUS inside the packaging. Remove the rod from the pouch with the other hand. Do not touch the end of the rod that will go into the insertion tube. Place the rod into the insertion tube (alongside the IUS threads) to about the 5 cm marking.

2. While holding the insertion tube and the rod firmly between your fingers and your thumb, pull downward on both blue threads with the other hand to draw the IUS into the insertion tube. The arms of the IUS should be kept in a horizontal plane, parallel to the flat side of the flange. Do not pull the IUS all of the way through the insertion tube; pull the threads only until the IUS is loaded at the top of the insertion tube. Note: If you accidentally remove the IUS completely from the insertion tube, do not use it or attempt to reload it.

3. Maintain a firm pinch of the insertion tube and rod and, with the other hand, adjust the position of the flange (through the sterile packaging if not using sterile gloves) by moving the tube to correspond to the sound measurement. The top end of the flange should be at the measurement corresponding to the sounded depth of the uterus. Position the IUS in the tube so that the knobs of the lateral arms are opposed to each other and protrude slightly above the tip of the insertion tube to form a hemispheric dome. When the IUS tips are in the correct position, pinch and hold the bottom end of the tube firmly to maintain rod position. The proximal end of the insertion tube will be approximately at the top of the first indent on the rod. Maintain a firm pinch with hand at the bottom of the insertion tube and remove the loaded IUS insertion tube from the pouch.

4. Maintain a firm pinch with the hand at the bottom of the insertion tube. With the other hand apply gentle traction on the tenaculum to straighten the alignment of the cervical canal with the uterine cavity. Slide the loaded insertion tube through the cervical canal until the upper edge of the flange is approximately 1.5 to 2 cm from the cervix.

5. Hold the insertion tube with the fingers of one hand and the rod with the fingers of the other hand and hold the rod still. Relax the firmness of the pinch on the tube, and pull the insertion tube back to the edge of the second (bottom) indent of the rod. Wait 10 to 15 seconds for the arms of the IUS to open fully. You can release the hold or traction on the tenaculum while waiting.

6. Next, apply gentle traction with the tenaculum again before advancing the IUS. With one hand still holding the bottom end of the tube, gently advance both the insertion tube and rod simultaneously up to the uterine fundus. You will feel slight resistance when the IUS is at the fundus. The flange should be touching the cervix when the IUS reaches the uterine fundus.

7. Hold the rod still with one hand while pulling the insertion tube back with the other hand to the ring on the rod. While holding the inserter tube with one hand, withdraw the rod from the insertion tube all of the way out to prevent the rod from catching on the knot at the lower end of the IUS. Next, completely remove

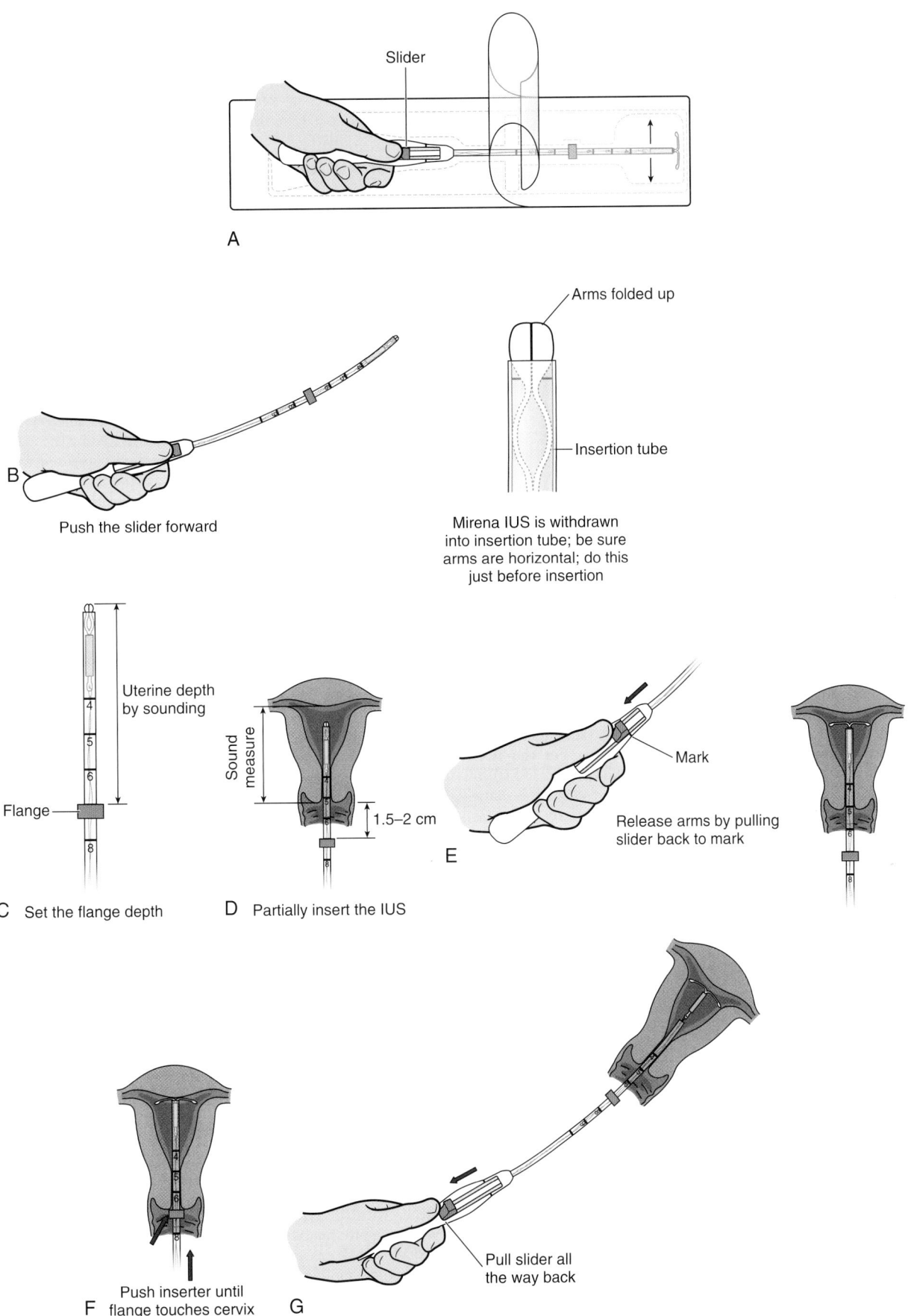

Slider

Arms folded up

Insertion tube

B Push the slider forward

Mirena IUS is withdrawn
into insertion tube; be sure
arms are horizontal; do this
just before insertion

Uterine depth
by sounding

Flange

Sound measure

1.5–2 cm

Mark

Release arms by pulling
slider back to mark

E

C Set the flange depth

D Partially insert the IUS

Push inserter until
F flange touches cervix

Pull slider all
the way back

G

Fig. 135.5 Loading and inserting the Mirena Levonorgestrel Intrauterine System (LNG IUS) using the sterile glove technique. (A–B) The package is opened. The LNG IUS is prepared for insertion. The slider is advance to the forward position, which withdraws the Mirena into the insertion tube. (C) The upper end of the flange is set at the uterine depth found with sounding. (D) The LNG IUS is inserted with the flange 1.5 to 2 cm from the ectocervix. (E), The arms are released by pulling the slider back to the mark. (F) For fundal positioning, the clinician holds the slider in position at the mark and pushes the inserter gently inward until the flange touches the cervix. The LNG IUS should now be in the fundal position. (G) Finally, the LNG IUS is released by pulling the slider all the way back, which releases the strings. The insertion tube is then removed. The strings are cut to leave 2 to 3 cm visible outside the cervix. (Courtesy the Association of Reproductive Health Professionals, Ithaca, NY, Copyright 2000. B, *right*, Modified courtesy Association of Reproductive Health Professionals, Ithaca, NY.)

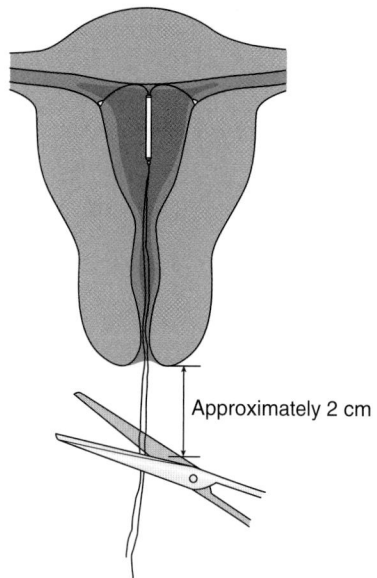

Approximately 2 cm

Fig. 135.6   The threads are cut, leaving about 2 to 3 cm visible outside the cervix. (Modified courtesy Bayer Healthcare, Whippany, NJ.)

the insertion tube. Removing the rod first and then the tube prevents the IUS from being pulled out of the uterus.

Completion of Procedure

1. After insertion, the IUD should remain within the uterine cavity. If any portion of the device is visible or protruding from the endocervical canal, the device should be removed by pulling the string; then a sterile device from a new package should be used.
2. After the inserter is removed from the uterus, cut the IUD threads to a length of 2 to 3 cm beyond the os (Fig. 135.6). It is better to leave the threads too long than too short because they can be shortened on subsequent visits if necessary, and short threads may be irritating or painful for a male partner.
3. Remove the tenaculum and observe the site for bleeding. If bleeding is seen, apply pressure or Monsel solution to achieve hemostasis.
4. Remove the speculum.
5. Provide postprocedure counseling to the patient and arrange a follow-up appointment for an IUD and symptom check after the first postinsertion menses.
6. Complete the encounter form (Fig. 135.7) or dictate a complete note.

COMMON ERRORS

- Cutting the strings too short.
- Device slips back out during the insertion process.
- Contaminating the IUD.
- Not doing a pelvic examination and determining the uterine position.
- Not using a tenaculum to straighten the cervical angle.
- The last common error that can cause a significant problem is pushing in on the inserter rod (for the ParaGard) instead of pulling back on the inserter tube (see Fig. 135.4B) to release the IUD. Pushing in on the rod could cause a perforation.

Short Strings

It is better to cut the strings too long than to risk cutting them too short. Short strings may make it difficult for the patient to check the strings and can cause discomfort to her partner (see later). If the strings are accidentally cut too short (<2 cm), the clinician should

consider inserting a new device. If the patient is able to reach the strings and prefers to keep the IUD in place, she can be monitored with instructions to return for any difficulty or complications.

Contamination of the Intrauterine Contraceptive Device

Contamination of the device most commonly occurs when the IUD or the distal tip of the insertion tube is touched with a nonsterile hand during the preparation or insertion process. If this occurs, a new package must be opened and the procedure repeated with a sterile device. The contaminated IUDs may be returned to the manufacturer for refund.

COMPLICATIONS

Placement of an IUD is a relatively safe procedure with significantly less morbidity and mortality than pregnancy and delivery. The IUD itself is generally well tolerated, as demonstrated by the 1-year continuation rate for this birth control method compared with other methods. Nonetheless it is important to counsel patients on the risk of complications and common side effects of the IUD, which are discussed in the following sections.

Vasovagal Reaction

Some women experience vasovagal reactions with instrumentation of the cervix or immediately after insertion. Such reactions may include lightheadedness, hypotension, bradycardia, nausea, or even syncope. If such symptoms occur, the patient should be kept in the supine position and given supportive care until the reaction resolves. Rarely do such symptoms persist. In severe cases a paracervical block may be done (or repeated) or atropine (0.4 to 0.6 mg) can be given intramuscularly. Occasionally the IUD may have to be removed.

Perforation

Perforation of the uterus or cervix is extremely rare (<0.1%). It generally occurs at the time of uterine sounding or occasionally with insertion. Perforation should be suspected if the sound enters the uterine cavity more than 12 cm and uterine palpation has indicated a normal size. The perforation itself is usually painless and often occurs in the setting of forceful pressure through a tight cervical os. Should perforation be suspected, the clinician should pull out the IUD (if already inserted) and observe the patient for 30 minutes. If stable, the patient can be discharged and told to report any signs of infection, abdominal pain, rapid pulse, or shortness of breath. Usually there is an uncomplicated resolution, and insertion can be attempted again in 6 to 8 weeks (no prophylactic antibiotics are indicated). Unstable patients may require immediate surgical consultation.

Uterine Bleeding and Cramping

IUD may cause abdominal or low back pain and cramping as well as irregular uterine bleeding, particularly in the first 3 months of use. Some women will have heavier bleeding and increased dysmenorrhea with the IUD, particularly when using the ParaGard. Conversely, approximately 20% of women using the Mirena and Kileena LNG IUS will cease having periods after 3 to 6 months. Menstruation returns rapidly once the device is removed.

Spontaneous Expulsion

Although uncommon, most IUD expulsions occur within the first 6 months after insertion. The patient may experience cramping, pain, vaginal discharge, abnormal vaginal spotting, dyspareunia, or lengthening of the IUD strings. However, expulsion may be

---

IUD ENCOUNTER FORM

Patient to fill out:

Name _____   Date _____

Birth date _____   Age _____

Number of pregnancies _____   Miscarriages or abortions _____

Current contraceptive method _____

Have you had:

A pregnancy in your tubes?	Y N	Are you allergic to copper?	Y N
Infection in your tubes?	Y N	How long is your usual period?	_____ days
Any venereal disease?	Y N	Have you ever had a low blood count?	Y N
An IUD before?	Y N	Number of lifetime sexual partners? _____	
Leukemia, AIDS, heart murmur?	Y N	Current number of sexual partners? _____	
Rheumatic fever, diabetes?	Y N	Last Pap smear: Date _____ Result _____	
Are you on steroids?	Y N	Did you read and understand the company handout? Y N	

For the doctor:

Company handout explained?   Y N   PMH: PMI: _____

Impression _____   All: _____

Plan _____   Meds: _____

                                              Surgeries: _____

Procedure/(Insertion):   Date _____

LMP _____

Pap: Y N   Type of IUD: ParaGard T380A

Bimanual: uterus: adnexa: Mirena IUS

Prep with tenaculum   Y N

Sound   cm

Insertion:

Patient tolerance:

Complications:

Reinforce: bleeding, pregnancy, infection, pain, expulsion

Remove on: _____

Given new company handout?   Y N

Given card?   Y N

Follow-up: _____

_____
                                              Physician Signature

cc: _____

Fig. 135.7 Sample intrauterine device encounter form. (Courtesy The Medical Procedures Center, Midland, MI.)

asymptomatic. For this reason the patient should be instructed to check for IUD strings each month after menstruation. Occasionally the IUD will become lodged in the cervical os, which may cause cramping and discomfort. In this case, the IUD should be removed and a new one placed if desired. If an IUD is spontaneously passed, is removed because of a complication, or becomes contaminated during the insertion process, it may be returned to the company for a free replacement.

Embedded or Lost Intrauterine Device String

Missing strings may indicate unsuspected perforation, spontaneous expulsion (see previous section), or migration of the IUD into the endometrial cavity. If the strings are not visible in the os, the clinician should first rule out pregnancy. Ultrasonography may quickly confirm intrauterine location. If the IUD is in place, nothing needs to be done. If the patient desires removal of an IUD whose strings are not visible in the os, special procedures may assist in recovering the IUD (see "IUD Removal" later). Occasionally the IUD may become embedded in the uterine lining, which complicates removal and may necessitate cervical dilation and instrumentation to remove the device.

Partner Discomfort Due to Intrauterine Contraceptive Device Strings

The IUD strings should be cut to a length of 2 to 3 cm from the external os. It is preferable to leave the strings slightly too long rather than to risk trimming them too short, which may cause irritation to the partner during intercourse. If the partner complains of penile discomfort (a barblike sensation), the strings can be trimmed further, or the device may need to be replaced. Strings that are too long may be trimmed. Strings that lengthen over time may be a sign of impending expulsion.

Contraception Failure

Although rare (<1%), pregnancy is possible even with the IUD in place. In this event, the patient must immediately be assessed for ectopic pregnancy. Although patients with IUDs do not have a higher ectopic pregnancy rate (the risk is actually lower), if pregnancy does occur, nearly 50% will be extrauterine. The IUD should be promptly removed if the woman is in the early stages of pregnancy regardless of whether she desires to continue the pregnancy. Although there is a risk of inducing abortion with removal of an IUD, if it is left in place there is a significant risk of premature labor, sepsis, and spontaneous abortion. Whether the IUD is removed or left in place, there is no increased risk of fetal anomalies.

Pelvic Inflammatory Disease

The risk of PID is elevated only the first 20 days after IUD insertion or in the setting of exposure to a new sexual partner. If the clinician suspects PID, it should be promptly treated according to Centers for Disease Control and Prevention guidelines, with initiation of antibiotics before IUD removal.* A new IUD may be placed 3 months after resolution of the infection. However, because of the risk of recurrent STIs and PID, other contraceptive options should be strongly considered.

Actinomyces

Actinomyces is an anaerobic gram-positive bacterium. It is more frequently found in IUD users (on routine Pap smear) and is generally asymptomatic. Most authorities recommend removal of the device and antibiotic treatment only in the presence of clinical symptoms. Rarely do the bacteria cause a systemic problem in healthy individuals, but if present or past infection is known, it is best not to insert the IUD because *Actinomyces* preferentially grows on foreign bodies.

Ovarian Cysts

Ovarian cysts may develop in patients using a LNG IUS because of hormonal stimulation. The likelihood of symptomatic cysts is low and general discontinuation as a result of symptomatic cysts was less than 1%. Enlarged follicles are seen in about 8% to 20% of LNG IUS users. Most of the cysts are asymptomatic and self-limiting, but on occasion they may cause pelvic pain or dyspareunia.

Hormonal Side Effects and Intrauterine Contraceptive Device Use During Lactation

Hormone-containing IUDs, such as the LNG IUS, may cause side effects such as mood changes, acne, headache, breast tenderness,

dysmenorrhea, nervousness, vaginitis, hypertension, and nausea. Weight gain is usually not a problem. Other forms of contraception may be preferable for lactating women.

Pap Smears and Cervical Dysplasia

Although no known association has been shown between cervical dysplasia and use of the IUD, it is essential that the Pap smear be normal before insertion. Should the patient present with abnormality on her Pap smear, the IUD may complicate the process of cervical and endocervical sampling and procedures such as the loop electrosurgical excision procedure (LEEP) or conization. Because patients using IUDs do not require annual renewal of their contraception, they are at greater risk of neglecting their regular Pap smears. When these patients are being treated, the clinician should emphasize that they must return for their routine Pap smear and pelvic examinations.

POSTPROCEDURE PATIENT EDUCATION

- Give the patient a copy of the IUD handout provided by the manufacturer, including the name and design, the date of insertion, and recommended date for removal. Discuss the following:
  - The patient should check for the presence of IUD strings after each menstruation.
  - The patient should be clear on the signs and symptoms of IUD expulsion, infection, and other possible complications. Instruct her to return for fever, worsening pelvic or abdominal pain, foul-smelling or abnormal vaginal discharge, excessive bleeding (other than spotting for a few months), pain with intercourse, prolonged amenorrhea, any type of genital lesions, or signs of STI or pregnancy.
  - Reiterate that the IUD will not protect her from infection from HIV, herpes simplex virus, human papillomavirus, *Chlamydia*, gonorrhea, or any other STI and that she must take precautions to avoid these infections.
- A routine follow-up examination to check for strings and review symptoms is scheduled for 1 to 3 months. The IUD is removed when the patient desires pregnancy or as indicated by the manufacturer. The ParaGard IUD should be replaced after 10 years, the Mirena and Kyleena LNG IUSs should be replaced after 5 years, and the Skyla and Liletta LNG IUSs after 3 years.

INTRAUTERINE DEVICE REMOVAL

Generally IUD removal is a simple and uncomplicated procedure that takes only a few minutes. The rare case in which the IUD string is not visible ("lost" IUD) presents a more challenging situation.

Indications

- Desire for pregnancy
- Postmenopause (no need for contraception)
- Pregnancy confirmed (early)
- Pelvic infection
- Before LEEP/conization (but with careful precautions, a LEEP can be performed without cutting the string)
- Patient intolerance: pain, bleeding, other
- Manufacturer recommendations
  - ParaGard T380: 10 years
  - Kileena: 5 years
  - Mirena: 5 years
  - Skyla: 3 years
  - Liletta: 3 years
- Inability to identify the strings

---

*WHO guidelines state that in resource-poor settings, it is an option to treat mild to moderate PID without removing the device.

Contraindications

- Advanced pregnancy (second or third trimester; generally contraindicated because of risk of spontaneous abortion)
- Suspected extrauterine location

PREPROCEDURE PATIENT PREPARATION

Patient Counseling and Consent

Although typically IUD insertion is a straightforward and simple procedure, patients should receive counseling on the risks, benefits, and alternatives to IUD removal and provided with a general overview of what to expect during the process. Depending on the reason for IUD removal, appropriate discussion of contraceptive options, preconception counseling, or management of menopause should be discussed. The clinician should advise of possible cramping and discomfort associated with IUD removal as well as the potential for transient nausea, dizziness, or faintness during and immediately after the procedure. Mild spotting and cramping may occur.

Pretreatment

Although no studies have found benefit, patients may consider taking ibuprofen (600 to 800 mg) or other NSAID 45 to 60 minutes before IUD removal to minimize cramping and discomfort during the procedure. Local anesthetic is usually not necessary, but may be helpful in the case of a complicated removal, particularly in patients at risk for significant discomfort (nulliparas, those requiring cervical dilation, those with history of pain with prior cervical procedures) or vasovagal reaction. In this case, lidocaine 1% to 2% without epinephrine may be used to perform a paracervical or submucosal block (see Chapter 153, Paracervical Block, for the submucosal injection technique).

TECHNIQUE

Removal With Visible Intrauterine Contraceptive Device Strings

The usual IUD removal is straightforward, and there is no need for sterile technique. Insert the speculum and visualize the IUD strings. Using ring forceps, grasp the strings and pull toward the introitus in a firm and deliberate motion until the IUD is delivered. The patient will likely experience momentary discomfort. Remove the speculum and send the patient home. Some minor spotting may be expected for a few days. There is no need to culture the IUD unless infection is suspected.

Removal When Intrauterine Contraceptive Device Strings Are Not Visible

If the speculum is inserted and IUD strings cannot be visualized after a diligent search, one of several approaches may be used. First, try using a Cytobrush or similar instrument and insert the brush portion the full depth into the cervical canal (approximately 2 cm). After insertion, rotate and extract the brush in a continuous motion. Repeat several times if needed. In one study, 24 of 27 lost strings were retrieved with this maneuver when other methods had failed.

If this fails, try a second method. Insert a long-handled alligator forceps or other hemostat-like instrument such as a uterine packing forceps into the os with the instrument opened as much as the os will allow. Close the jaws in a blind attempt to catch any strings that may be present. If the strings are indeed grasped, resistance will be felt when the instrument is removed. Carry out this maneuver four or five times in an attempt to grasp the strings. If unsuccessful or if the os is too small, other methods will be needed to find the strings.

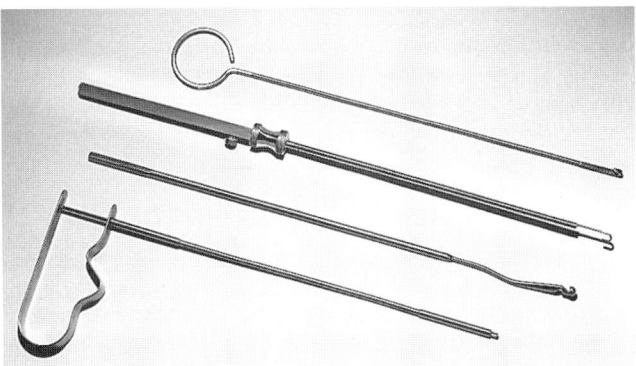

Fig. 135.8 **Intrauterine device (IUD) removal instruments.** *Top to bottom,* simple IUD hook, universal IUD hook, double IUD extractor, and flexible IUD hook. Not shown is the Cheshire IUD grasping forceps.

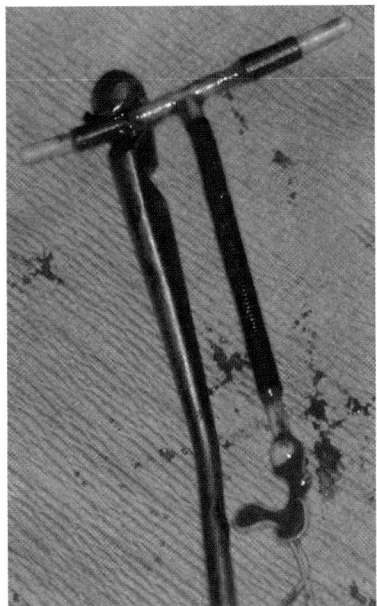

Fig. 135.9 Double intrauterine device (IUD) extractor after retrieving a "lost" IUD (ParaGard T380).

A third approach uses an endocervical speculum along with a colposcope to identify the strings. Frequently the end of the string is just within the os. Once visualized, it is much more easily grasped with forceps and removed.

Should these techniques fail, proceed with a more invasive fourth option (see Chapter 126, Cervical Stenosis and Cervical Dilation, for the instrumentation to be used). Perform a bimanual examination to identify the position of the uterus. Prepare the area with an antiseptic solution. Grasp the anterior lip with a single-toothed cervical tenaculum and apply slight traction to straighten the uterus. A uterine sound may be used to dilate the internal os if needed. An IUD remover is then used to enter the intrauterine cavity (Fig. 135.8). Using the larger-sized instruments will prevent or minimize the potential for perforation of the uterus. The double IUD extractor and flexible IUD hook are commonly used. The double IUD extractor resembles a crochet hook that hooks the IUD (Fig. 135.9). Use a twist-and-pull motion to catch the IUD. Frequent repeated passes are often needed. The flexible IUD hook is actually a forceps. Insert the stem into the uterus and compress the handle to open the jaws. When the handle is released, the jaws grasp the IUD as they close. Another forceps grasper (not shown here), which is the favorite of some clinicians, is the Cheshire IUD forceps. It is used to grasp the IUD. Whichever forceps is used, once the IUD has been grasped, slowly withdraw the unit. With any instrument, if the string or the IUD is grasped, resistance will be felt.

Embedded Intrauterine Contraceptive Devices

If the IUD has been in place for a significant length of time, it may have become embedded in the endometrium and significant force will be required to remove it. Firm pressure rarely if ever breaks the strings. If the force seems to be extreme, there is excessive pain, or there is any question of whether the IUD is still in place, it may be best to defer removal. Although a flat-plate radiograph of the abdomen will identify whether the IUD is present (IUDs are radiopaque), the x-ray film will not indicate whether the IUD is intrauterine. A pelvic ultrasound, on the other hand, will confirm whether it is present and whether it is intrauterine. If the IUD has moved to an extrauterine position, surgery will be required.

If an IUD is confirmed by ultrasonography, the patient must return for a visit when further, more aggressive attempts can be made to remove it. If all else fails, the patient may require a dilation and curettage procedure, with the IUD removed under anesthesia or with the aid of a hysteroscope.

No prophylactic antibiotics are needed.

COMPLICATIONS

Other than slight discomfort and the possibility of vasovagal reactions, there are no significant complications from routine IUD removal. If other instrumentation is required because of lost strings, rare complications include perforation, infection, and bleeding. If the IUD is being removed in the context of pregnancy, there is significant risk of miscarriage, with rates as high as 50% to 60% in some studies.

POSTPROCEDURE PATIENT EDUCATION

Provide contraception, preconception counseling, or hormone replacement and menopause counseling as appropriate. If the patient desires to continue IUD use, there is no need to delay insertion. An IUD may be removed and a new IUD (same or different type) inserted at the same visit.

CONCLUSION

The safety issues and misconceptions that plagued IUDs in the past have largely been resolved, offering patients an excellent option for long-term reversible contraception. IUDs have high efficacy; require little maintenance; provide long-term yet reversible contraception; and are cheaper than birth control pills over a 3- to 5-year period. The LNG IUS offers the benefit of decreased vaginal bleeding and may be used in hormone replacement to protect against uterine malignancy and hyperplasia. Conversely, the copper IUD offers the potential advantage of being hormone-free.

CPT/BILLING CODES

58300	Insertion of IUD, not including device
58301	Removal of IUD
J7300	Charge for cost of copper IUD (ParaGard T380A)
J7302	Charge cost Levonorgestrel-Releasing Intrauterine System (Mirena)

ICD-10-CM DIAGNOSTIC CODES

T83.39XA	Complications (lost IUD)
T83.83XA	Causing menorrhagia
Z30.430	Insertion of IUD
Z30.433	Reinsertion of IUD
Z30.433	Removal of IUD
Z30.431	Maintenance/surveillance/checking IUD

SUPPLIERS

(See contact information available at www.expertconsult.com.)

NOTE: Most companies provide videotapes and training models for their devices.

Mirena, Skyla, Kyleena
Bayer Healthcare Pharmaceuticals, Inc.
Liletta
Allergan, Medicines360
ParaGard T380A
Teva Women's Health
Removal Instruments
Cheshire Medical (hooks and grasping forceps)
CooperSurgical (those instruments shown in Fig. 135.8)

The various IUD removal instruments should be available from most medical supply firms.

RECOMMENDED READING

http://hcp.skyla-us.com/insertion-and-removal/skyla-insertion-instructions.php.
https://www.lilettahcp.com/Content/pdfs/liletta-stepbystep-insertion-guide.pdf.
American College of Obstetricians and Gynecologists. Long-acting reversible contraception: implants and intrauterine devices. *Replaces Practice Bulletin Number.* 2011;59(121):2005. Reaffirmed 2015.
American College of Obstetricians and Gynecologists. Antibiotic prophylaxis for gynecologic procedures. Practice Bulletin no. 104. *Obstet Gynecol.* 2009;113:1180–1189.
Ben-Rafael Z, Bider D. A new procedure for removal of a "lost" intrauterine device. *Obstet Gynecol.* 2011;87:785–786.
Bounds W, Hutt S, Kubba A, et al. Randomised comparative study in 217 women of three disposable plastic IUCD thread retrievers. *Br J Obstet Gynaecol.* 1992;99:915–919.
Einarsson JI, Henao G, Young AE. Topical analgesia for endometrial biopsy: a randomized controlled trial. *Obstet Gynecol.* 2005;106:128–130.
Fortney JA, Feldblum PJ, Raymond EG. Intrauterine devices: the best long-term contraceptive method? *J Reprod Med.* 1999;44:269–274.
Hatcher RA, Trussell J, Stewart F, et al. *Contraceptive Technology.* 18th rev ed. New York: Ardent Media; 2004.
Hill DA. Abnormal uterine bleeding: avoid the rush to hysterectomy. *J Fam Pract.* 2009;58:136–142.
Hov GG, Skjeldestad FE, Hilstad T. Use of IUD and subsequent fertility: follow-up after participation in a randomized clinical trial. *Contraception.* 2007;75:88–92.
Hubacher D, Lara-Ricalde R, Taylor DJ, et al. Use of copper intrauterine devices and the risk of tubal infertility among nulliparous women. *N Engl J Med.* 2001;345:561–567.
Johnson BA. Insertion and removal of intrauterine devices. *Am Fam Physician.* 2005;71:95–102.
Paladine HL, Blenning CE, Judkins DZ, Mittal S. Clinical inquiries: what are contraindications to IUDs? *J Fam Pract.* 2006;55:726–729.
Saav I, Aaronson A, Marions L, Stephansson O, Gemzell-Danielsson K. Cervical priming with sublingual misoprostol prior to insertion of intrauterine device in nulliparous women: a randomized controlled trial. *Hum Reprod.* 2007;22(10):2647–2652.
Stanford JB, Mikolajczyk RT. Mechanisms of action of intrauterine devices: update and estimation of postfertilization effects. *Am J Obstet Gynecol.* 2002;187:1699–1708.
Usatine RP. *The Color Atlas of Family Medicine.* New York: McGraw-Hill; 2009.

Walsh T, Grimes D, Frezieres R, et al. Randomised controlled trial of pro-phylactic antibiotics before insertion of intrauterine devices. IUD Study Group. *Lancet.* 1998;351:1005–1008.

World Health Organization. *Medical Eligibility Criteria for Contraceptive Use.* 5th ed. Intrauterine devices (IUDs); 2015. Accessed March 6, 2017. Or publications in general. http://apps.who.int/iris/bitstream/10665/181468/1/9789241549158_eng.pdf?ua=1. www.who.int/reproductive-health/publications/mec/iuds.html.

Zieman M, Kanal E, Copper T. 380A IUD and magnetic resonance imaging. *Contraception.* 2007;75:93–95.

CHAPTER 136

INSERTION AND REMOVAL OF NEXPLANON

Stephen A. Grochmal • Dale A. Patterson

Nexplanon is an implantable contraceptive device that functions like other progestin-based contraceptives by preventing ovulation, developing a thick cervical mucus barrier, and causing eventual atrophy of the uterine endometrium. It is the most effective method of reversible contraception. Compared with the original Implanon apparatus, Nexplanon has a simpler insertion device and also has a coating of barium sulfate, designed to help locate the device with radiographs. It can also be located with high-frequency ultrasound, computed tomography (CT), or magnetic resonance imaging (MRI). Nexplanon is designed as a single implant measuring 4 cm long with a diameter of 2 mm and an outer structural membrane composed of ethylene vinyl acetate copolymer (Fig. 136.1). This copolymer outer membrane is designed to curtail reaction with the surrounding tissue, hopefully minimizing tissue fibrosis and facilitating extraction when its content is exhausted. The implant core contains 68 mg of etonogestrel in ethylene vinyl acetate. The progestin is released initially at the rate of 60 μg/day in weeks 5 to 6 of use and then decreases to 35 to 45 μg/day at the end of the first year. The released amount of etonogestrel continues to decrease to 30 to 40 μg/day and 25 to 30 μg/day at 2 and 3 years of use, respectively. Nexplanon is effective for 3 years and has a shelf life of 5 years. The implant is placed in the subcutaneous tissue of the upper arm with a 12-gauge disposable, preloaded inserter. The insertion is a minor surgical procedure performed in the office. Nexplanon was approved in 2011 by the US Food and Drug Administration and replaced the Implanon device, which was phased out by the manufacturer. Instruction and training are required before the manufacturer will allow a clinician to order the device.

Long-acting reversible contraceptives (LARCs) include intrauterine devices (IUDs) and contraceptive implants such as Nexplanon. In 2012 the American College of Obstetricians and Gynecologists (ACOG) reversed the order of their recommendations for contraception, recommending consideration of LARCs as first line in most women, including at-risk adolescents. Although more expensive than short-acting contraceptives such as diaphragms and oral contraceptives, LARCs are more effective and have the highest continuation and satisfaction rates. This increase in effectiveness is, in part, because they require little ongoing effort by the user and can remain in place for several years. LARCs are safe and appropriate for most women needing contraception, including adolescents. It is the ACOG's opinion that adolescents at high risk for unintended pregnancy may benefit from increased access to LARCs.

INDICATIONS

To prevent pregnancy for up to 3 years (Ali [2016] found Nexplanon effective up to 4 years and possibly longer).

CONTRAINDICATIONS

Pregnancy or suspected pregnancy
Current or past history of thrombosis of thromboembolic disorders
Present or past history of breast cancer or progestin-sensitive cancers
Active hepatic disorders or liver tumors, benign or malignant
Unexplained abnormal vaginal bleeding
Hypersensitivity to the components of the product

EQUIPMENT

- Examination table
- Sterile surgical drapes and gloves, antiseptic solution (e.g., povidone-iodine, chlorhexidine), sterile skin marker (optional)
- Local anesthetic (1% lidocaine without epinephrine), syringes (3 mL), and needles (25 to 27.5 g)
- Sterile gauze, adhesive bandage (self-adhesive wrap such as Coban), pressure bandage
- Nexplanon product kit (No. 11 blade, straight and curved mosquito clamps, and forceps, preferably without teeth, are needed for removal)

PRECAUTIONS

Although progestin-containing contraceptives have not been shown to cause birth defects, it is imperative to ensure that a patient is not pregnant prior to inserting Nexplanon. If a patient is found to be pregnant or becomes pregnant after insertion, the device should be removed.

Caution is also advised in patients with bleeding disorders and patients taking anticoagulants. Nexplanon may be an appropriate contraceptive for these patients, but precautions should be taken to minimize bleeding.

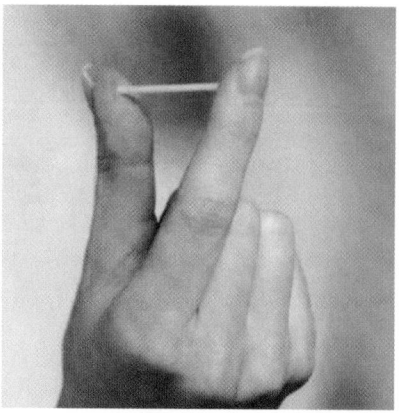

Fig. 136.1 **Nexplanon device.** (Courtesy Merck Schering-Plough Corp., Kenilworth, NJ.)

PREPROCEDURE PATIENT EDUCATION

Nexplanon is more than 99% effective, and when the device is inserted correctly, the risk of pregnancy is less than 1 per 100 women who use it. As mentioned previously, Nexplanon is the most effective method of reversible contraception. Approximately 82% of women continue to use Nexplanon for 2 or more years. Nexplanon may be less effective in women who are overweight or are taking certain types of medications. (However, Xu et al. [2012] found no decrease in effectiveness in overweight or obese women.) Contraception with progestins is very useful in patients with known hepatic disease, hypertension, psychosis, mental retardation, or a history of thromboembolism. It should be noted that the manufacturer lists thromboembolism, hepatic disorders, and breast cancer as contraindications to the use of Nexplanon; however, clinical practice has shown that progestin-based contraceptives are not only safe in these patients but also preferred over estrogen-containing products.

The implant must be removed after all the progestin is released, generally by the end of the third year. Women should be informed that Nexplanon does not protect against human immunodeficiency virus or other sexually transmitted diseases. A detailed patient consent form is available from the manufacturer's website and at www.expertconsult.com.

ADVANTAGES

- Menstrual: Menstrual and ovulatory discomfort and cramping are decreased. There is less bleeding as compared with other implant devices, with more consistent amenorrhea reported (20% at 1 year). In Nexplanon users, uterine pain was reduced or eliminated in 88% of women previously experiencing dysmenorrhea.
- Sexual and psychological: Sexual intercourse may be more pleasurable because fear of pregnancy is reduced, allowing for more spontaneity.
- Risk of cancer: None known.
- Additional factors: There was a high continuation rate reported in the clinical trials, and asymptomatic follicular cysts were less common than with users of Mirena or Norplant. The single implant permits quick removal.

DISADVANTAGES

- Menstrual: Amenorrhea and oligomenorrhea are commonly reported. A more common patient complaint is persistent irregular and less predictable menstrual bleeding (see Complications section for possible treatments).
- Sexual and psychological: The irregular bleeding may become disconcerting and possibly discourage sexual intercourse.
- Headache and acne are commonly reported side effects.
- Interactions with other medications may make Nexplanon less effective. These medications include barbiturates, griseofulvin, rifampin, phenylbutazone, carbamazepine, felbamate, oxcarbazepine, topiramate, and modafinil. Herbal remedies such as St. John's wort may also reduce effectiveness. In these situations, a secondary nonhormonal method of birth control should be considered.

PATIENT SELECTION

The Nexplanon implant is particularly useful for women with contraindications to or severe side effects from estrogen. As previously mentioned, Nexplanon candidates would include those patients with a personal history of thrombosis, coronary artery disease, cerebrovascular disease, hypertension, or hepatic disorders. Included in this list are those patients who suffer from other related estrogen side effects, including migraine headaches, previous history of drug-induced chloasma, and hypertriglyceridemia, and those women who are recently postpartum, breastfeeding, over the age of 35 years, or smoke. The published prescribing precautions are the same as for

other progestin-only pills. Patients concerned about their fertility after discontinuation of Nexplanon should be counseled that they will experience a rapid return to baseline fertility, with more than 94% of patients demonstrating ovulation within 3 to 6 weeks after removal of the implant. It is important to inform patients that irregular bleeding may be expected and might persist while the implant rod is in place. If the pattern of bleeding becomes intolerable, additional treatments can be used to make the bleeding pattern more acceptable.

PROCEDURE

Ideally, the insertion should be scheduled between day 1 and 5 of a regular menstrual period, even if still menstruating. If switching from a combination oral contraceptive, insertion should occur on the day the last active tablet is taken. When switching from a progesterone-only injection, insertion should occur on the day the next injection is due. If inserted postpartum and she is not breastfeeding, insertion should occur on day 21 to 28 postpartum. When breastfeeding, do not insert until 4th week postpartum; a barrier method of contraception should be used for first 7 days. Following a first trimester miscarriage or abortion, insertion should occur within 5 days. Following a second trimester miscarriage or abortion, insertion should occur within 21 to 28 days. If these rules are not followed, pregnancy may need to be excluded and the use of a backup method of birth control (i.e., condoms) should be recommended for 7 days after insertion.

The insertion procedure for Nexplanon is somewhat opposite that of an injection. The manufacturer has specific training seminars and onsite support available for health care providers wishing to offer this device to their patients (www.nexplanon.com). A provider must complete the manufacturer's course before being able to order Nexplanon and perform the procedure. This procedure is performed in the office setting. The Nexplanon rod and inserter should remain sterile throughout the procedure. If at any time sterility is compromised, a new device should be used.

Insertion Technique

Various YouTube videos are available from the patient's perspective, as well as demonstrating insertion for clinicians.

1. Have the patient lie on her back on the examination table with her nondominant arm flexed at the elbow and externally rotated. Her hand should be beside or next to her head (Fig. 136.2A).
2. Mark a site for insertion on the medial aspect of the nondominant arm, 8 to 10 cm above the medial epicondyle of the elbow. Avoid the sulcus (groove) between the biceps and triceps and the large blood vessels and nerves that lie there in the neurovascular bundle, deeper in the subcutaneous tissue. A second mark should be made on the same arm a few centimeters proximal (farther up the arm) to the first mark (see Fig. 136.2B).
3. Prep the insertion site with the antiseptic of choice. Apply sterile drapes as needed.
4. Anesthetize the area locally with 1 to 3 mL of 1% to 2% lidocaine with or without epinephrine (see Chapter 5, Local Anesthesia). A bleb of lidocaine should be placed where the device needle will enter the skin and the remainder placed along the tract where the rod will be inserted. Caution: Nexplanon should be inserted subdermally, just beneath the skin.
5. The clinician should now be seated beside the insertion site so as to better visualize the depth of insertion (depth might not be visible if the clinician is standing over the insertion site). Remove the inserter device from the packaging.
6. Remove the transparent shield from the device by sliding it horizontally away from the needle (see Fig. 136.2C); identify the white rod inside the needle tip.
7. It is now theoretically possible for the rod to fall out of the needle. Keep the applicator in the somewhat upright position

until insertion to minimize this risk. The needle tip and area around it should also be kept sterile. From this point, until the end of the procedure, do not touch the purple slider until you have fully inserted the needle subdermally, because it will retract the needle and prematurely release the implant from the applicator.

8. While applying countertraction to the skin (see Fig. 136.2D), puncture the skin and insert the tip of the needle bevel under the skin. The angle of insertion should be less than 30 degrees (see Fig. 136.2E).

9. After the skin is punctured, lower the applicator to a position horizontal to the skin and lift the skin up with the tip of the needle keeping the needle subdermal (see Fig. 136.2F).

10. Tent the skin and insert the needle fully into the subdermal tissue, remaining as shallow as possible. Aim for the second mark made earlier on the arm. Some resistance may be felt; the insert-

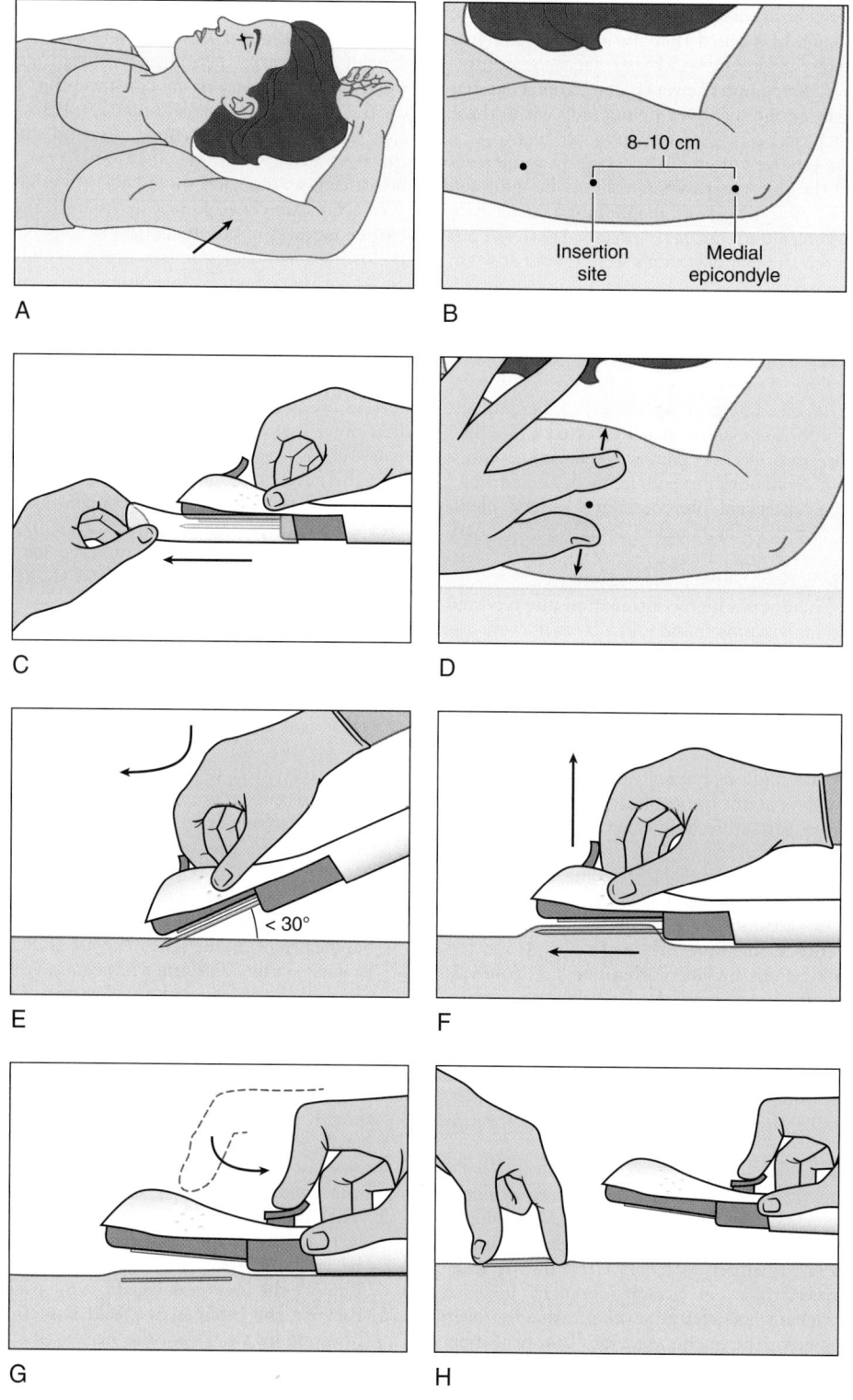

Fig. 136.2 (A–H) Insertion procedure (see text for details). (From Merck Schering-Plough Corp., Kenilworth, NJ.)

er can be rotated back and forth slightly to ease insertion. You should be able to see movement of the needle tip just beneath the skin. **The needle should not be inserted with excess force.**

11. When the needle is fully inserted, unlock the purple slider by pushing it slightly downward. Move the slider fully back; this will drop the implant in place (see Fig. 136.2G).

    Caution: Do not move the slider back until the needle is fully inserted in the skin. Moving the slider back prematurely will leave a portion of the implant hanging outside the skin; this will render that implant ineffective and require repeating the procedure with another implant.

12. Confirm placement of the implant by palpating the skin (see Fig. 136.2H). If a rod cannot be palpated, it can be seen on plain radiograph, high-frequency ultrasound, CT, or MRI. An alternative form of contraception must be used until correct placement is verified.

13. The wound can be dressed with an adhesive bandage and pressure dressing. Have the patient palpate the rod for confirmation of placement.

14. A card is provided to give to the patient with details of the device implanted and when a new one needs to be inserted.

Removal Technique

Various YouTube videos are available for Nexplanon removal.

1. Removal is performed with the patient in a position similar to that for insertion. The rod should be palpated (Fig. 136.3A) or located with ultrasound prior to removal. The removal site should also be prepared with antiseptic solution.

2. Locally anesthetize the area for removal, injecting beneath the rod tip so that the tip can still be palpable (see Fig. 136.3B). Anesthetize the area under and along the rod if another implant is going to be placed (see Chapter 5, Local Anesthesia). Most clinicians seat themselves in a comfortable position; this is helpful in the event the procedure becomes tedious.

3. Make a 2- to 3-mm incision longitudinally, along the tip of the rod, at the end of the rod closest to the elbow, using a No. 11 blade (see Fig. 136.3C).

4. Push the rod toward the incision until it is visible. It may be necessary to further dissect the tissue to visualize the device (see Fig. 136.3D). The scalpel can be used to incise or scrape fibrous tissue away from the tip (see Fig. 136.3E); caution should be taken to not incise any portion of the rod. Although the rod may appear white through fibrous tissue, when enough tissue is scraped away the rod usually becomes very white. At this point, it is usually more readily removed.

5. Grasp the device with a hemostat or forceps (see Fig. 136.3F) and remove (see Fig. 136.3G).

6. If the device is not seen, fibrous tissue beneath the rod may be grasped with one fine hemostat while tissue is further dissected with a second fine hemostat to facilitate removal. The capsule or sheath of fascia over the rod tip may need to be incised or scraped with the No. 11 blade (see Fig. 136.3E). Grasping the fibrous tissue beneath the rod may help to stabilize it so that the scalpel can be used to scrape away this fibrous sheath. Grasping the rod with a fine hemostat through the skin may also help to stabilize the tip so that the fibrous sheath can be scraped away.

7. Ensure that the entire device has been removed by measuring it (length is 4 cm).

8. A new device may be inserted into the same incision, if desired.

9. Dress the wound with an adhesive bandage and pressure dressing.

NOTE: If an implant is not palpable, it can often be located using radiography, high-frequency ultrasound, CT, or MRI. If these methods fail, call 1-877-467-5266 for information on the procedure for measuring etonogestrel blood levels.

SAMPLE OPERATIVE REPORT

Preoperative diagnosis: Elective contraception with implantable device
Postoperative diagnosis: Same
Procedure performed: Insertion of Nexplanon contraceptive device
Surgeon: Dr. _____
Blood loss: None
Complications: None

Procedure: The patient was placed in the supine position with her left arm up above her head exposing the medial (inside) portion of the upper left arm. The proper region medial to the antecubital space (avoiding the biceps/triceps sulcus) was prepped and draped. Local infiltration of the skin with 2 to 4 mL of 1% lidocaine with epinephrine was accomplished along a 3- to 4-cm line approximately two fingerbreadths from the antecubital space, using a 27-gauge needle, and satisfactory anesthetic effect was achieved. The 12-gauge preloaded insertion device was directed at a less than 30-degree angle, beveled side up, through the incision and into the subcutaneous tissue, tenting up the skin to keep the needle just under the skin. The inserter device was stabilized and the Nexplanon implant deposited into the subcutaneous space by withdrawing the needle. The implant was palpated to confirm accurate placement within the designated tissue space. The skin site was covered with an adhesive bandage, and a small sterile pressure dressing was applied. The patient then confirmed placement of the implant by palpating it. The patient tolerated the insertion procedure well and will return to the office for follow-up in 3 days.

COMMON ERRORS

* Shallow insertion, causing the implant to be clearly visible directly under the skin surface.
* More commonly, the implant is inserted too deeply, which will make it difficult to palpate and complicate the removal process.
* Inadvertent or premature release of the slider, which results in the inability to advance the implant.
* Inability to confirm proper placement of the Nexplanon device by digital palpation after the procedure may be due to placing the rod too deep in the fatty tissue (as noted earlier). Confirmation of correct placement should be attained by radiography, ultrasound, CT, or MRI. The patient must use a barrier method of contraception until proper placement is confirmed. Document this activity at the end of the operative report and in the patient's chart.

WARNINGS

Although extremely rare, Nexplanon should be removed in event of thrombosis, if the blood pressure rises significantly or is uncontrolled, or if jaundice occurs.

COMPLICATIONS

* Uterine bleeding patterns are somewhat unpredictable: 34% have infrequent bleeding, and 22% become fully amenorrheic. However, 7% experience frequent bleeding and 18% have prolonged bleeding. Ultimately, 11% discontinue Nexplanon because of bleeding. Women with lower body weight had fewer bleeding and spotting days than women with a higher body weight (ACOG, 2011). Women with a favorable bleeding pattern in the first 3 months are likely to continue Nexplanon for 2 years. Those with an unfavorable bleeding pattern had a 50% chance of improving (ACOG, 2011). To manage menstrual bleeding complications, a trial of up to 3 months of oral contraceptives (30 to 35 µg of ethinyl estradiol plus progestin) can be used. Mefenamic acid 500 mg 2 to 4 times daily for 5 days may alter or stop the bleeding (other nonsteroidal antiinflammatory drugs may also work). Another

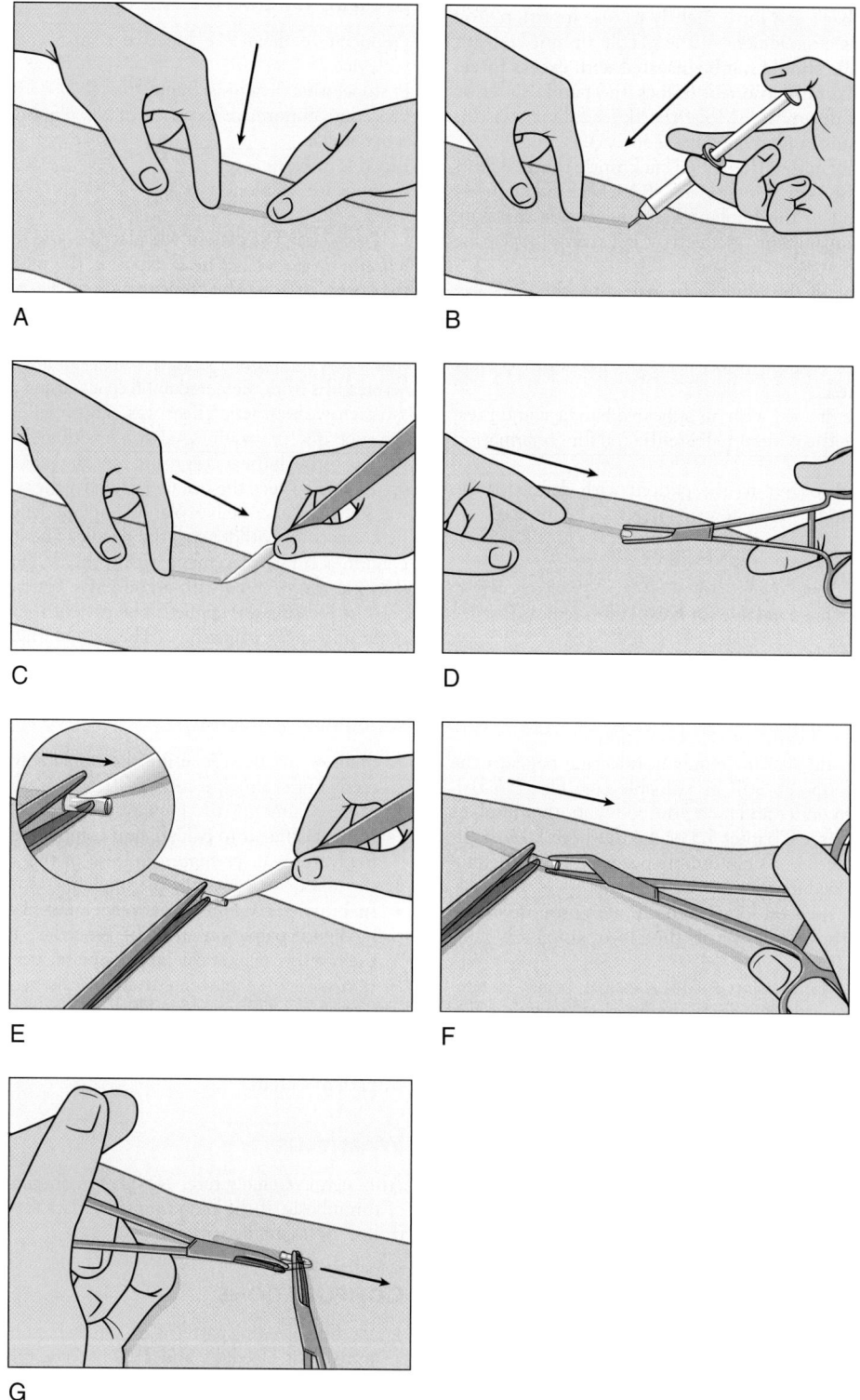

Fig. 136.3 (A–G) Removal procedure (see text for details). (From Merck Schering-Plough Corp., Kenilworth, NJ.)

option is tranexamic acid (Lysteda) 1300 mg 3 times daily for 5 days.
- Weight gain reported by 12%, but only 2% to 7% discontinue because of this. One study comparing Nexplanon with copper IUD found no difference in weight gain at 1 year (ACOG, 2017)
- Acne worsens in 10% to 14% of users, but only 2% discontinue because of this (ACOG, 2017)
- Vascular injury

- Postprocedure pain (insertion area of arm)
  - Determine if there is evidence of local nerve damage (extremely rare and unlikely).
  - Ecchymosis: confirm bandage is not applied too tightly. Apply ice packs for 24 hours.
  - Recommend nonsteroidal antiinflammatory drugs or acetaminophen as needed.
- Infection in the insertion area

- *No abscess present.* Suspect a localized cellulitis. Do not remove the rod. Clean the infected area with antiseptic solution and begin an oral antibiotic for 7 days. Evaluate in 24 hours and again after course of antibiotics is concluded.
- *Abscess is present.* Begin course of antibiotics for 7 to 10 days. Prepare infected area, incise and drain any purulent material, and remove the rod. Drain and dress the wound, and continue antibiotic therapy and wound care until resolved.
- Pap smear noncompliance. Studies have documented poor Pap smear compliance in IUD users. This will probably be the same with implants.

POSTPROCEDURE MANAGEMENT

- After insertion, apply a pressure dressing on the insertion site for 24 hours; thereafter, apply just a small bandage for approximately 3 to 5 days.
- After removal, Steri-Strips should be left in place until they fall off. The wound should be treated as a simple laceration.

POSTPROCEDURE PATIENT EDUCATION

The process of wound healing should be discussed with the patient, and she should be reminded that the device does not protect against sexually transmitted diseases. The Nexplanon website has patient education materials available (www.nexplanon.com).

CPT/BILLING CODES

11981   Insertion, nonbiodegradable drug delivery implant (11975, 11976, 11977, 11980 used for other implant types)

11982   Removal, nonbiodegradable drug delivery implant

11983   Removal with reinsertion, nonbiodegradable drug delivery implant

ICD-10-CM DIAGNOSTIC CODES

Z30.8   Insertion of implantable subdermal contraceptive

Z30.46   Surveillance of subdermal implantable contraceptive

Z97.5   Other postprocedural states, presence of contraceptive device, subdermal contraceptive implant

J-Code

J7307   Etonogestrel (contraceptive) implant system, including implant and supplies (It is necessary to include this code on CMS form 1500 to be reimbursed for the cost of the device.)

ONLINE RESOURCES

Insertion/removal form: www.expertconsult.com
Nexplanon patient support: www.nexplanon.com
Nexplanon website for health care professionals: www.merckconnect.com/nexplanon/overview.html

RECOMMENDED READING

Ali M, Akin A, Bahamondes L, Brache V, Habib N, Landoulsi S, et al. Extended use up to 5 years of the etonogestrel-releasing subdermal contraceptive implant: comparison to levonorgestrel-releasing subdermal implant. WHO study group on subdermal contraceptive implants for women. *Hum Reprod.* 2016;31:2491–2498.

American College of Obstetricians and Gynecologists: Committee on adolescent health care long-acting reversible contraception work group; committee opinion number 539, October, 2012. Reaffirmed Number 735, May 2018.

American College of Obstetricians and Gynecologists: Increasing use of contraceptive implants and intrauterine devices to reduce unintended pregnancy. Opinion no. 450. *Obstet Gynecol.* 2009;114:1434–1438.

American College of Obstetricians and Gynecologists: Long acting contraceptives: implants and intrauterine devices. Practice bulletin number 121. July 2011.

American College of Obstetricians and Gynecologists: Long acting contraceptives: implants and intrauterine devices. Practice bulletin number 186, November 2017.

American College of Obstetricians and Gynecologists: Long-Acting Reversible Contraception Work Group: clinical challenges of long-acting reversible contraceptive methods. Committee opinion number 672, September 2016.

Xu H, Wade JA, Peipert JF, Zhao Q, Madden T, Secura G. Contraceptive failure rates of etonogestrel subdermal implants in overweight and obese women. *Obstet Gynecol.* 2012;120(1):21–26.

CHAPTER 137

PESSARIES

Sandra M. Sulik

Historically pessaries have been used to correct pelvic floor deformities and dysfunctions and symptoms associated with genital prolapse, uterine retrodisplacement, and cervical incompetence in women. In addition to hanging women by their heels, physicians as early as Hippocrates reported the use of half a pomegranate soaked in vinegar and placed in the vagina for women with prolapse! In 1860, Hugh Lenox Hodge, Professor of Gynecology at the University of Pennsylvania, designed a pessary using Goodyear's newly patented vulcanized rubber. Pelvic organ prolapse is seen in up to 50% of parous women. A pessary is a device placed into the vagina to support the prolapsing vaginal walls or to provide urinary continence. Pessaries have the distinct advantage of being minimally invasive while also providing immediate relief of symptoms. Over time, technologic advances in composition and design have provided a wide variety of sizes and shapes; fitting pessaries is now somewhat of an art (Fig. 137.1).

INDICATIONS

- Stress urinary incontinence (including athletic stress urinary incontinence)
- Uterine prolapse
- Vaginal vault prolapse
- Uterine retrodisplacement
- Pelvic relaxation
- Cystocele
- Enterocele
- Rectocele
- Poor surgical candidates with significant signs and symptoms
- Prophylactic, placed postoperatively
- Preoperative diagnostic aid while awaiting surgery
- Cervical incompetence (proposed indication)

Preoperative use of pessaries as a diagnostic tool for any of the preceding indications can help to estimate the amount of normal function that may be restored after surgery. A pessary can also help to determine if the patient will develop incontinence after the prolapse is surgically corrected. Although surgery generally produces a more permanent cure, a pessary may be the treatment of choice for women who are poor surgical candidates, who want to postpone surgery indefinitely, or who prefer a nonsurgical treatment option. Pessaries may also be used postoperatively in women at risk for recurrent prolapse. Use of the pessary has been proposed as an alternative to cerclage to prevent preterm delivery. Only limited data support this indication, and it has not achieved widespread use.

CONTRAINDICATIONS

- Noncompliant patient
- Impaired mental capacity leading to inability to follow up
- Persistent vaginal ulceration/erosions (relative)
- Active vaginitis (relative)
- Any pelvic infections or lacerations (relative)
- Severe atrophic changes (relative)
- Lack of manual dexterity

Active vaginitis including atrophic changes and vaginal ulcerations should be maximally treated before pessary use. Although ulcerations are generally considered a contraindication, when they are a direct result of an exteriorized prolapse, a pessary may prevent further injury and promote healing.

EQUIPMENT AND SUPPLIES

Approximately 71% to 90% of women can be successfully fitted with a pessary. Unsuccessful fitting is more likely with a shorter vagina (<6 cm) or a wide introitus (>4 fingerbreadths), higher parity, and previous hysterectomy. Most women using pessaries are satisfied and experience improvement in their symptoms.

There are two major types of pessaries: *support* and *space-filling*. Most pessaries are made of silicone, some from rubber (avoid in latex-allergic patients), and a few from plastic. Silicone has the advantage of being nonallergenic and does not absorb odors or secretions; it is pliable and soft and therefore well tolerated.

The support pessaries are the ring, the Gehrung, and the Mar-Land; the space-occupying pessaries are the Gellhorn, the cube, and the donut. A properly fitted pessary should be comfortable for the patient; it should remain in place while walking, standing, and during provocative maneuvers (e.g., coughing, Valsalva); and it should not interfere with bladder and bowel function. The pessary should fill the vagina but should easily admit the examiner's finger between the pessary and the vaginal wall.

PESSARY SELECTION

Pessaries are available in a wide range of sizes and shapes, each with a specific indication and function. Selection depends on anatomy, symptomatology, and the overall goal of treatment. Identifying the best choice is often a trial-and-error process; clinicians and patients should not be discouraged if the first selection is unsuccessful. The most commonly prescribed pessaries are the ring, the Gellhorn and the donut. For the novice just starting to fit pessaries, obtain a fitting kit and samples of the most commonly used pessaries; this will lessen the initial difficulty of pessary fitting.

Pessaries are made with several modifications on the same theme. For example, the ring pessary has a version "with support," which has a silicone web across the central opening. This supports the bladder, effectively reducing a mild to moderate cystocele. The "ring with knob" has a bulbous portion that placed retropubically (at the pubic notch) to restore the urethral-vesical (U-V) angle and increase urethral closing pressure. The "knob" is added for stress urinary incontinence from a hypermobile U-V angle. Some devices have both modifications.

PESSARY TYPES BY INDICATION

- *Stress incontinence:* ring with knob, Hodge, Hodge with knob, Smith, Risser, incontinence ring, incontinence dish, Mar-Land, Gehrung with knob (Fig. 137.2)

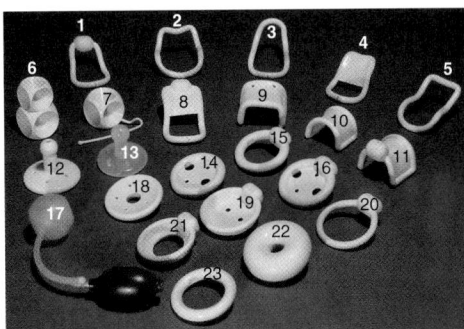

Fig. 137.1 Various types of pessaries. 1, Hodge with knob; 2, Risser; 3, Smith; 4, Hodge with support; 5, Hodge; 6, tandem cube; 7, cube; 8, Hodge with support and knob; 9, Regula; 10, Gehrung; 11, Gehrung with knob; 12, Gellhorn flexible; 13, Gellhorn rigid (acrylic silicone); 14, ring with support; 15, ring with knob; 16, ring with knob and support; 17, Inflatoball; 18, Shaatz; 19, incontinence dish with support; 20, incontinence ring; 21, incontinence dish; 22, donut; 23, ring. (Courtesy CooperSurgical, Inc., Trumbull, CT.)

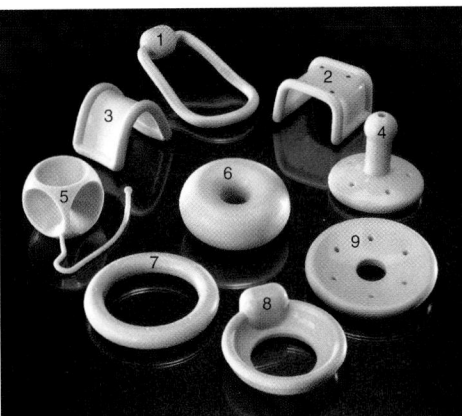

Fig. 137.2 Stress urinary incontinence pessaries (made with silicone). 1, Hodge with knob; 2, Regula; 3, Gehrung; 4, Gelhorn flexible; 5, tandem cube; 6, donut; 7, ring; 8, incontinence dish; 9, Shaatz. (Courtesy CooperSurgical, Inc., Trumbull, CT.)

- *Preoperative evaluation for Burch procedure for stress incontinence:* Hodge, Risser, and Hodge with support
- *Uterine retrodisplacement:* Smith, Risser, and Hodge
- *Uterine prolapse, first or second degree:* ring, ring with support, Shaatz, Regula, Oval, Smith, Risser, and Hodge
- *Uterine or vaginal vault prolapse, third or fourth degree:* donut, Inflatoball, cube, tandem cube, Gellhorn (not well suited for severe vaginal prolapse)
- *Stress incontinence with cystocele, first or second degree:* ring with support (with or without knob) incontinence dish with support, Gehrung with knob, and Hodge (with/without support, with/without knob), Mar-Land with support (Fig. 137.3)
- *Stress incontinence with uterine prolapse, first or second degree:* ring, incontinence ring, ring with support and knob, incontinence dish (with/without support), Mar-Land, Mar-Land with support, Hodge (with/without support, with/without knob and support)
- *Cystocele:* Gehrung, Gehrung with knob, ring with support, Gellhorn, donut, Inflatoball, cube, and tandem cube
- *Enterocele:* Gellhorn, Gehrung, donut, Inflatoball, cube, and tandem cube
- *Rectocele:* Gellhorn, Gehrung, donut, Inflatoball, cube, and tandem cube
- *Incompetent cervix:* Hodge

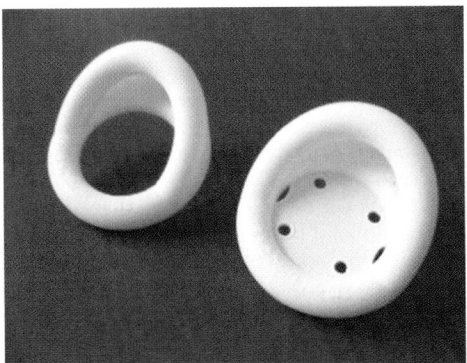

Fig. 137.3 Mar-Land pessaries with (left) and without (right) support. (Courtesy Coloplast Corporation [formerly Mentor Corporation], Minneapolis, MN.)

PROCEDURE

Fitting Pessaries

Pessaries are fitted by trial and error. Proper fitting often requires multiple sizes and or styles. Fitting can be done from fitting kits (obtained from the manufacturer) or by stocking multiple sizes so as to fit from stock. Fitting kits are available from the two largest manufacturers of pessaries in the United States: Milex Cooper Surgical and Coloplast Corporation. Milex Cooper Surgical has kits for the ring, Gellhorn, cube, and Gehrung pessaries. The Coloplast Corporation has a kit for fitting the ring pessary with a conversion chart for converting the size of the ring pessary to other types the company manufactures. Conversions of pessary sizes are difficult, however. The totally different shape of each pessary and whether the pessary fits in front of the cervix (e.g., the Gellhorn, donut, or cube), behind the cervix (e.g., the lever pessaries), or over the cervix (e.g., the Gehrung) precludes simple conversions. The manufacturer should be contacted for product information and to obtain pessary fitting kits.

When a pessary for *incontinence* is being fitted, it is best for the patient to have a full bladder. If fitting for *prolapse,* the patient should empty her bladder before the fitting process. A ring pessary is usually fitted initially, as it is easy to use and tends to be more comfortable. The pessary is folded and the leading edge is lubricated. It is inserted by directing it toward the sacrum, and it is unfolded above the pelvic floor, with the anterior edge just behind the symphysis. There should be a finger's breadth of space between the pessary (edge) and the symphysis anteriorly and between the side of the pessary and the lateral vaginal wall. The ring pessary should be turned one-quarter turn in either direction following placement to ensure the foldable edge is not placed in front of the introitus, thus potentially limiting spontaneous expulsion. Once the pessary has been fitted, the patient should ambulate in the clinic and perform activities such as squatting and the Valsalva maneuver to make sure that it will not fall out. It is necessary to make sure that patients are able to void and that they are given appropriate education before leaving the clinic with the new pessary. Ideally, the patient should insert and remove the pessary on a daily basis. The pessary can be removed at bedtime, washed with soap and water, and then replaced in the morning. If daily changing is too cumbersome, a schedule of twice weekly can be used. In this setting, an early follow-up should be arranged to assess the vaginal walls and make sure that no erosions are developing. If the patient is unable to remove her pessary regularly, most pessaries can be left in place and removed on a monthly basis, cleaned, and reinserted by the clinician. On the other hand, the cube and Inflatoball pessaries must be removed daily. An applicator containing an acidifying gel such as Trimo-San inserted into the vagina two or three times a week should be recommended to help decrease the amount and odor of vaginal discharge.

An incontinence ring is fitted by assessing the distance between the posterior cul-de-sac and the mid-urethra. Because the incontinence ring is more flexible, it will adapt to the configuration of the vagina. The health care provider must make sure that the knob is centered underneath the mid-urethra and that the proximal ring is placed in the posterior cul-de-sac and not in front of the cervix in the anterior fornix. A ring pessary with incontinence knob is placed like a regular ring, but once it is opened, the knob will be facing the sidewall: it must therefore be rotated one-quarter turn to place the knob under the mid-urethra. If the vaginal introitus is more than the width of three or four fingers, a space-occupying pessary is most likely to be successful. A Shaatz pessary is fitted similarly, with the convex portion placed anteriorly. A Gellhorn pessary is fitted by folding the disc, as described earlier, when possible with the stem folded down for ease of insertion. The stem will be directed caudally (pointing out), and it should be possible to pass a finger between the disc and the vaginal sidewall. Because of its shape, a cube pessary need not be as large as the width of the vagina (as measured with the examining fingers spread apart), but approximately half that width. Insertion simply involves compressing the edge that is introduced into the vaginal opening and pushing it up and back. Donut pessaries also require compression for insertion.

Prior to fitting the pessary, the vagina should be inspected for estrogen status, erythema, erosions, and ulcerations. A Papanicolaou (Pap) smear should be obtained if indicated. Determining pessary size for all round pessaries is similar to fitting a contraceptive diaphragm (see Chapter 116, Barrier Contraceptives: Cervical Caps, Condoms, and Diaphragms). A rough estimate of the length of the vagina is determined by measuring the distance from the posterior fornix or vaginal apex to the symphysis pubis. The second and third fingers are placed in the vagina with the third finger in the posterior fornix. The depth of insertion is marked on the second finger. The distance between the tip of the third finger and the mark on the second finger approximates vaginal depth (see Figure 116.5 in Chapter 116, Barrier Contraceptives: Cervical Caps, Condoms, and Diaphragms). This is also a good opportunity to evaluate the strength of the pelvic floor and teach the patient how to do Kegel exercises. Several pessary sizes can be tried to find the proper fit.

Once the appropriate pessary has been found, the patient should be reexamined after performing provocative maneuvers. Provocative maneuvers include coughing, standing, sitting, walking, squatting, and the Valsalva maneuver. Then the patient should try to void. If the patient is unable to void comfortably or if discomfort is noted during these maneuvers, the next smaller size of pessary should be tried. If the pessary has shifted position or falls out after these maneuvers, a larger size or different pessary should be tried.

USE OF SPECIFIC PESSARIES

Uses for specific pessaries are listed in Table 137.1.

COMPLICATIONS

- Vaginitis
- Vaginal erosion or ulceration
- Discomfort
- Obstructed defecation and/or urination
- Impaction of the pessary

It is normal for the patient to experience an increase in vaginal discharge. However, odor, itching, change in color of discharge, or bleeding should be reported to the health care provider. The use of vaginal estrogen with pessaries generally prevents vaginal erosion and ulceration. Many health care providers overlook the importance of estrogen in maintaining the acid pH balance necessary to prevent vaginitis. The vagina should be resupplied with estrogen by using vaginal estrogen cream 1 g every other night for 1 month and then two to three times a week. Alternating a pH-adjusted vaginal gel (e.g., Trimo-San gel, half applicator, two or three times a week) with the estrogen cream is beneficial as well if the pessary is left in place and

not removed nightly. In addition to atrophic changes, ulcerations may be associated with a device that is too large or not removed on a regular basis. Discomfort is usually associated with anterior displacement during a Valsalva maneuver or a device that is too large. If anterior displacement is noted, the patient should push the pessary further into the vagina. If that does not alleviate the discomfort, a smaller size should be tried. Obstruction of defecation should be promptly reported to the provider. Removal of the pessary should resolve the problem, and delay in removal may lead to obstipation. Obstruction of urination should be uncommon if voiding was performed in the office with the device in place. A smaller pessary should resolve the problem. Impaction of the device is rare and typically associated with "forgotten" pessaries. A reminder system should help to alleviate this problem and ensure appropriate follow-up.

POSTPROCEDURE MANAGEMENT

Pessary Care

Patients should remove the pessary and wash it with warm, soapy water. Soap with deodorants, perfumes, or detergents should not be used. Autoclaving (15 lb pressure for 15 minutes) is the recommended method of sterilization for pessaries from the fitting sets between fittings.

Follow-up Care

Ideally, the pessary should be removed nightly and cleaned and replaced the next morning. Realistically, women are reluctant to comply with such frequency. In many cases pessaries have been left in the vagina for months at a time without complication. (The cube and tandem cube and Inflatoball must be removed nightly because there are no holes for drainage.) The final decision is left to the health care provider and the patient and should be based on several factors: the patient's mental and physical capacity to insert and remove the device and willingness to do so on a regular basis; the health of the vaginal mucosa; the potential for complications; how well the device fits; and the patient's ability to comply with follow-up visits.

In general reevaluate the patient 1 week after the initial fitting and then at 1 month and 3 months. At a minimum the patient should be seen every 6 months thereafter. Patients unable to care for the device themselves should be seen at least every 2 to 3 months. At each visit the patient should be questioned about bowel and bladder function, symptoms associated with vaginitis, vaginal bleeding, and problems with insertion and removal. The device should be removed and the vaginal mucosa inspected for erythema, ulceration, laceration, and estrogen status. The device may be cleaned and reinserted if there are no complications. The pessary is a foreign body in the vagina. Inspection of the vaginal vault at regular intervals seems prudent and warranted.

TIPS

The following are anecdotal helpful hints and not manufacturers' recommendations.

- *Diaphragms:* A diaphragm can be very effective for mild degrees of prolapse or incontinence.
- *Stay relaxed for device removal:* The patient should keep the pelvic floor muscles relaxed and even perform a gentle Valsalva maneuver to assist with removal.
- *Estrogen:* Regular use of vaginal estrogen cream should be strongly encouraged. The Estring estradiol vaginal ring may also be used with several of the pessaries.
- *Double pessaries:* A small donut coupled with a Gellhorn pessary may be useful for patients with excessive redundant tissue. The donut is placed closest to the cervix with the Gellhorn facing out into the vagina. The stem of the Gellhorn does not fit through the hole in the donut (Fig. 137.4).
- *Pelvic floor muscle exercises/Kegel exercises:* Ongoing performance

Continued

TABLE 137.1	Use of Pessaries						
Condition	Pessary	Common Sizes	Features	Company	Insertion	Removal	Other Pessaries to Try
First- and second-degree prolapse	Ring	0–13, 2–7 most common	One of the easiest to use, requires a well-defined pubic notch for pessary to rest.	Milex Cooper Surgical, EvaCare	The device is hinged and will fold in only one direction; once inserted rotate 90 degrees to decrease chance of expulsion with Valsalva.	Insert the index finger into the notch and rotate the hinge anteriorly; pull down and out.	Gellhorn, donut, Gehrung, Shaatz, oval, Inflatoball, Regula
	Ring with support	0–13, 3–5 most common	Supports mild cystocele as well.	Milex Cooper Surgical, EvaCare	Same as ring	Same as for ring	Same as for ring
	Shaatz	1.5–3.5 inches, most common 2.5–3 inches	Utilizes levators for support, especially effective in patients for whom ring pessary does not stay in place.	Milex Cooper Surgical, EvaCare	Compress the sides and turn the device parallel to the introitus; advance until it rests against cervix; insert with concave surface facing up.	Hook the index finger in the center hole; bring device down to introitus; pull down and out.	Gellhorn, Gehrung, ring with support, oval, donut
	Regula	Most common 2–8	The pressure exerted by the prolapsed uterus/cervix on the flexible anatomically adjusting arch or bridge of the regula automatically spreads the heels outward, thereby helping to prevent the expulsion of the pessary. The patient should be forewarned that it may be necessary for her to be refitted several times.	Milex Cooper Surgical	Flexibility of the bridge, which alters the support dimensions of the pessary, must be balanced with the size of the patient's vaginal vault and the degree of uterine prolapse.	Reach in, grasp pessary and pull down toward introitus.	Gellhorn, donut, Gehrung, Shaatz, oval, Inflatoball
	Oval	Most common sizes, 1–9	Designed specifically to fit a narrow vaginal vault. Works extremely well in women with a prior history of vaginal surgery that resulted in scarring and in some cases palpable sutures from anterior repair or bladder suspension procedures.	EvaCare	Fold pessary at flexible joint; insert and rotate to fit.	Reach in, grasp pessary and pull down toward introitus.	
Third-degree prolapse	Donut	2–3.5 inches most common, also 2.5–3.5 inches	Most commonly used pessary. A space-occupying device that is useful in patients with excessive redundant tissue; works well in a vaginal vault with little or no support; most commonly used in older, postmenopausal women; works well for vaginal prolapse as well.	Milex Cooper Surgical, EvaCare	Turn the device parallel to the introitus; exert pressure posteriorly, and advance until it is fully intravaginal; then rotate until the pessary is transverse and up against the cervix.	Hook the index finger in the center hole, bring device down to introitus; pull down and out.	Gellhorn, Inflatoball, Gehrung
	Gellhorn	1.5–3.5 inches, most common 2.5–3 inches	Requires a relatively capacious vaginal vault so that the base is broad enough to rest above the levators. The stem functions to stabilize the device in the vagina and facilitates removal. A shorter stem is available by special order. Can be ordered as rigid silicone or acrylic for severe prolapse. Not well suited for severe vaginal prolapse because the walls can prolapse around the pessary.	Milex, Eva-Care	Fold the knob of the device; position the disk portion parallel to the introitus, angling downward to avoid pressure on the urethra; push posteriorly until the entire disk is within the vagina; then turn and push the knob upward toward the cervix.	Insert finger up to the disk and release the suction; pull disk towards introitus and remove. Can use a barber pole action. Can inject a small amount of water or saline into the hole in the knob to help release the suction.	Donut, Inflatoball, or Gehrung

TABLE 137.1 Use of Pessaries—cont'd

Condition	Pessary	Common Sizes	Features	Company	Insertion	Removal	Other Pessaries to Try
	Cube	0–7, most common 2–5	May be used in women with either a small or a large introitus because of its malleability. Has no area for drainage, must be removed nightly. Support is achieved by creating negative pressure on the vaginal walls. Atrophic changes increase the risk of ulceration and erosion.	Milex Cooper Surgical, EvaCare	Compress the cube and insert it high into the vagina.	The string is used to help locate the pessary; it should not be used to pull on to remove the pessary. The suction should be released by squeezing the walls of the cube and then pulling the device in a downward fashion. The pessary must be removed and cleaned daily. Regular use of estrogen cream in postmenopausal women is recommended.	Tandem cube, Gellhorn, Inflatoball, donut
	Tandem cube	The larger cube is 2 sizes bigger than the small one. 2/0–7/5, most common 4/2–7/5.	Try if single cube does not work. Can be used in young women who experience stress incontinence with vigorous exercise when other pessaries are ineffective.	Milex Cooper Surgical	Insert with larger cube toward cervix.	Same as for cube	Gellhorn, Inflatoball
	Inflatoball	Small (2 inches), medium (2.25 inches), large (2.5 inches), extra large (2.75 inches); medium and large are the most common sizes.	Can be used for mild cystocele or rectocele associated with a procidentia/prolapse. The unique design permits individualized fitting and adjustments by varying the amount of air pressure within the pessary. The fully deflated pessary is easy to insert or remove, even with a narrow introitus. Inflatoball is sometimes the only pessary the patient can tolerate. Manual dexterity is needed for use of this pessary. This is a latex rubber pessary. Must be removed daily.	Milex Cooper Surgical	Compress all the air out of the ball, insert into vagina, and position high. Inflate to the desired pressure, remove the pump, push the small ball up to keep the pessary inflated, then tuck the tube into the vagina.	Deflate by pushing the small ball down to release the air; reach into the vagina, grab the pessary, pull towards the introitus, and remove.	Gellhorn, Gehrung, donut
Incontinence pessaries	Incontinence ring (ring with knob)	0–10, 2–7 most common sizes	The device stabilizes the bladder base and increases urethral functional length and closure pressure.	Milex Cooper Surgical	Compress the ring and insert with the knob in the anterior direction; knob fits just below pubic notch.	Grasp and pull in a downward fashion.	Incontinence dish, ring with support and knob, Gehrung with/without knob, Hodge, Smith, Risser, Mar-Land Hodge with/without support, Mar-Land with support
	Incontinence dish with/without support	55–85 mm, most common 60–75 mm (Milex Cooper), 0–7 (EvaCare brand)	Continence is restored by stabilizing the bladder base, increasing urethral closure pressure, and lengthening the functional urethra. It also offers support to an accompanying mild prolapse.	Milex Cooper Surgical, EvaCare	Compress the device and turn it parallel to the introitus. Rotate the device once it is intravaginal so that the heel is posterior to the cervix and the knob is retropubic.	Hook the index finger and pull down and out or Insert index finger between the device and the symphysis; grasp between the finger and thumb, and pull down and out.	

Pessary	Sizes	Description	Manufacturer	Insertion	Removal	Related
Mar-Land with/without support	2–8, most common 2–5	An adaptation of the ring pessary; has a round Silastic base with a half-moon support that fits retropubically.	EvaCare	Compress the device and turn it parallel to the introitus. Rotate the device once it is intravaginal so that the heel is in the vault or posterior fornix and the arch is positioned retropubically. May also be inserted by folding the pessary in half so that the back ring collapses the supportive sling. The folded pessary should be in a crescent shape and inserted by directing the crescent shape downward; advance it until the device is fully intravaginal and the supportive sling is retropubic.	Hook the device with the index finger and rotate parallel while pulling down and out.	Hodge with/without support, incontinence ring, incontinence dish.
Gehrung with/without knob	0–9, most common sizes 2–5	"Saddle pessary"; manually shapeable, which allows for fit in most women. Support derived from the elevator sling. Gehrung with knob useful for cystocele coupled with stress incontinence.	Milex Cooper Surgical	Compress the sides of the device and turn it parallel to the introitus. Insert the left heel and advance until the device is fully intravaginal; rotate the anterior arch forward so that the cystocele rests on the bridge. The heels of the pessary rest on the vaginal floor.	Push the anterior arch posteriorly toward the rectum; grasp the lateral heel and fold to remove.	Hodge with/without support, incontinence ring, incontinence dish with/without support
Hodge with/without knob; Hodge with/without support	0–9, most common size 2–5	Originally designed for uterine retrodisplacement, Hodge with knob restores continence by stabilizing the bladder base and increasing urethral closure pressure and functional urethral length. Designed for patients with a shallow pubic notch. Can be used for patients with stress incontinence associated with urethral hypermobility, first- and second-degree prolapse, and uterine retrodisplacement. The Hodge can be used as a test of effectiveness of the Burch procedure for stress incontinence. Has also been used for treatment of incompetent cervix with or without cerclage.	Milex Cooper Surgical	Compress the sides and insert the rounded end into the vagina; direct the heel into the vault or posterior fornix and position the anterior portion retropubically. The device should fit snugly, should not rotate, and should remain retropubic.	Hook the device with the index finger to fold it, and pull the device down and out.	Incontinence ring, incontinence dish, or Mar-Land
Uterine retrodisplacement — Smith (designed for a patient with a well-defined pubic notch) Risser (designed for a patient with a shallow pubic notch; has a larger weight-bearing zone to support the vaginal aspect of the pubis).	Smith: 0–8, 2–5 most common; Risser: 0–9, 2–5 most common	Can be used for a number of other conditions, including dysmenorrhea when no other cause except uterine retroversion is noted, infertility if retroversion is considered the cause, and backache if attributed to uterine retroversion.	Milex Cooper Surgical	Insertion same as for Hodge.	Same as for Hodge	Hodge with/without support/knob, Mar-Land, incontinence ring, or incontinence dish

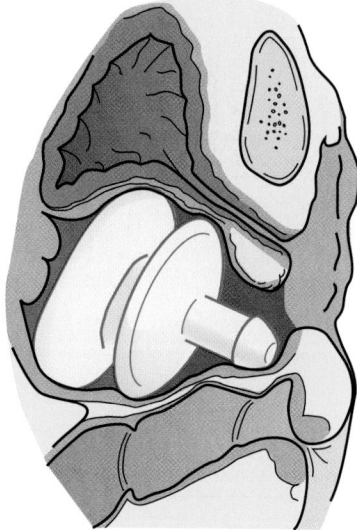

Fig. 137.4 Double pessaries in place. The donut pessary is inserted first and then the Gellhorn pessary (stem out). (Modified from Myers DL, LaSala CA, Murphy JA. Instruments and methods: Double pessary used in grade 4 uterine and vaginal prolapse. Obstet Gynecol. 1998; 91[6]:1019–1020.)

of Kegel exercises is important to maintain and improve pelvic floor tone and should be encouraged with all follow-up visits. If a patient is unable to perform Kegel exercises on her own, useful patient devices include Kegel Kones (a set of six weighted devices, which get progressively smaller and heavier). The Kegel Exersizer is an intravaginal device that measures intravaginal pressure. The cone-shaped device has an approximately 2-foot flexible hose to transmit the pressure to a gauge that gives the patient positive feedback with a proper perineal (Kegel) contraction. Some physical therapy departments have assisted patients with proper technique for Kegel exercises by using this type of device.

- *A woman with very little or no vaginal muscle tone or marked vaginal wall prolapse* may have difficulty even in retaining a donut or Gellhorn pessary. In such cases the cube pessary is indicated.
- *Sexual activity:* Some pessaries can be left in place during intercourse. Most often, women remove the pessary prior to engaging in sexual activity. A ring pessary is an effective device for women who leak urine with orgasm.
- *Pessaries and radiographs:* Some pessaries contain wire coils; these pessaries must be removed before proceeding with radiographs or magnetic resonance imaging. The face page of each pessary instructional brochure indicates whether the pessary contains metal. An instructional brochure is enclosed with each pessary.

CONCLUSION

Although surgical repair remains the treatment of choice for many urogynecologic dysfunctions, pessaries are a viable option for a variety of situations. Pessaries are useful for the rising elderly population but also for younger, active women who wish to maintain their activities without the discomfort of prolapse or leaking of urine.

PATIENT EDUCATION GUIDES

See the sample patient educaiton form available at www.expertconsult.com.

CPT/BILLING CODES

The pessary cost is considered a supply. It should be billed to the local Medicare Part B carrier or the patient's insurance company.

57160   Pessary fitting and insertion

An E/M code may also be billed with a -25 modifier depending on documented examination and decision-making complexity. Only the E/M code is to be used when the patient comes in for removal, cleaning, and reinsertion.

A4561   Rubber pessaries or intravaginal devices
A4562   Nonrubber pessaries or intravaginal devices

In some areas, the alternative for Part B providers is to write a prescription for the device, have the patient fill the prescription at a local pharmacy or medical supply store, and return with the pessary for insertion. Place of service is the home of the patient.

ICD-10-CM DIAGNOSTIC CODES

N81.89	Vaginal wall prolapse, unspecified (without uterine prolapse)
N81.11	Cystocele midline or lateral (without prolapse)
N81.6	Rectocele (without uterine prolapse)
N81.4	Uterine prolapse (without vaginal wall prolapse)
N81.3	Uterovaginal prolapse complete
N81.2	Uterovaginal prolapse, incomplete
N99.3	Posthysterectomy vault prolapse
N81.5	Enterocele, vaginal
N81.9	Unspecified genital prolapse
N81.82	Incompetence or weakening of pubocervical tissue
N81.83	Incompetence or weakening of rectovaginal tissue
N81.84	Pelvic muscle wasting
N85.4	Retroflexed uterus, symptomatic
N39.3	Incontinence, stress
O34.30	Cervical incompetence in pregnancy

Acknowledgment

The editors recognize the contributions of Edward J. Mayeaux Jr, MD, to this chapter in a previous edition of this text.

SUPPLIERS

(Full contact information is available at www.expertconsult.com.)
Estring
   Pharmacia and Upjohn Company
Pessaries, Kegel Kones, Kegel Exercizer
   Coloplast (formerly Mentor Corporation) Corporation (EvaCare Pessaries)
   Milex Cooper Surgical Products, Inc.

ONLINE RESOURCES

Society of Obstetricians and Gynecologists of Canada: Technical Update on Pessary Use. https://sogc.org/wp-content/uploads/2013/07/gui294CPG1307E.pdf.
www.webmd.com/urinary-incontinence-oab/what-are-vaginal-pessaries 1.

RECOMMENDED READING

American College of Obstetricians and Gynecologists. Pelvic Organ Prolapse. ACOG Practice Bulletin No. 185. *Obstet Gynecol.* 2017;130:234–250.
Bugge C, Adams EJ, Gopinath D, Reid F. Mechanical devices for pelvic organ prolapse in women. *Cochrane Database Syst Rev.* 2013;2:CD004010.

Gleason JL, Richter HE, Varner RE. Pelvic organ prolapse. In: Berek JS, ed. *Berek and Novak's Gynecology*. 15th ed. Philadelphia: Lippincott Williams & Wilkins; 2012:920–922.

Jones JK, Harmanli O. Pessary use in pelvic organ prolapse and urinary incontinence. *Rev Obstet Gynecol*. 2010;3(1):3–9.

Lipp A, Shaw C, Glavind K. Mechanical devices for urinary incontinence in women. *Cochrane Database Syst Rev*. 2014;3:CD001756.

Myers DL, LaSala CA, Murphy JA. Instruments and methods: double pessary use in grade 4 uterine and vaginal prolapse. *Am Coll Obstet Gynecol*. 1998;91:6.

Newcomer J. Pessaries for the treatment of incompetent cervix and premature delivery. *Obstet Gynecol Surv*. 2000;55:443.

Rosenman AE. Pelvic floor disorders: Pelvic organ prolapse, urinary incontinence, and pelvic floor pain syndrome. In: Hacker NF, Gambone JC, Hobel JC, eds. *Hacker and Moore's Essentials of Obstetrics and Gynecology*. 6th ed. Philadelphia: Elsevier; 2016:291–303.

Viera AJ, Larkins-Pettigrew M. Practical use of the pessary. *Am Fam Physician*. 2000;61:2719.

CHAPTER 138

TREATMENT OF NONCERVICAL CONDYLOMATA ACUMINATA

Harris Mones

The increased incidence of human papillomavirus (HPV) infection combined with increased public awareness of the association of HPV with cervical carcinoma has led to a greater number of patients seeking counseling and treatment for condylomata (genital warts). More than 1 million new infections occur every year in the United States, and 74% are in those 15 to 24 years of age. Although there is some evidence that treatment reduces infectivity, there is no evidence supporting the concept that treatment of condylomata (the warty lesions themselves) reduces the incidence of cervical or genital neoplasia. In the majority of cases, genital HPV infection is subclinical and resolves on its own (Fig. 138.1). HPV types 6 and 11 rarely give rise to cervical cancers and are thus considered low-risk subtypes. Infection by these genotypes is responsible for 90% of the cases of genital wart formation. In contrast, HPV types 16 and 18 are strongly associated with cervical dysplasia and are therefore considered to be high risk, oncogenic subtypes. The treatment of subclinical asymptomatic genital HPV infection, regardless of its mechanism of detection (e.g., colposcopy, biopsy, acetic acid application, laboratory testing), is not recommended. The purpose and goal of treatment are to eliminate visible warts or symptomatic infection, to identify and resolve any associated dysplasia, and to educate the patient and any partners about the disease.

HPV is a multicentric infection. Coexisting external and internal lesions, or multiple lesions involving the entire lower genital system of both men and women, may be present. They can present as totally flat or 1- to 2-mm papular lesions, or as large, 1- to 2-cm cauliflower-like growths (see Chapter 103, Androscopy, Figs. 103.1 and 103.5). Some may be detected only with magnification (e.g., a colposcope), whereas others will be detected by a white discoloration after application of acetic acid (white epithelium). Some are flesh colored, whereas others are pigmented (see Chapter 103, Androscopy, Fig. 103.4; for a differential diagnosis, see Box 103.1). Warts may be found in and around the anus and inside the mouth. Because of the risk of neoplastic transformation, a biopsy should be obtained if the clinician is uncertain about the diagnosis, lesions fail to respond or worsen during therapy, the patient is immunocompromised, or if the lesion has an atypical, suspect appearance, including pigmentation, bleeding, or ulceration.

A biopsy of suspect lesions should be performed before treatment is initiated. If biopsy is performed after treatment, it is important to communicate to the pathologist the type and amount of preceding treatment.

To date, no definitive therapy has emerged as the ideal standard of care in the treatment of genital warts, and therapy selection generally occurs in a patient-specific manner. The clinician must decide which treatment modality is best, based on clinical skill, extent of disease, cost, patient preferences, and overall chance of success. The 2015 Centers for Disease Control and Prevention Treatment Guidelines point out that there is no definite evidence suggesting any of the available treatments are better than the others or are ideal for all patients. Spontaneous resolution is a possibility, and therefore observation alone without specific treatment may be a reasonable alternative for some patients. Because there is no specific "cure" for HPV infection itself, the goal of treating it is the elimination of obvious visible or troublesome lesions (the disease caused by the virus). Treatment of HPV infection is analogous to the treatment of herpes virus infection. The virus will not be eliminated, but symptoms can be controlled.

Some infections may not be grossly visible, yet still cause anogenital pruritus, burning, vaginal discharge, or bleeding. Conversely, the treatment of asymptomatic intraurethral, intravaginal, or cervical condylomata (without dysplasia) exposes the patient to treatment risk without obvious benefit.

The patient may harbor HPV DNA for life; therefore patient education is important to prevent unreasonable expectations. Treating male sexual partners with HPV infection has not appeared to change the posttreatment failure rate in women with cervical dysplasia. These findings should not deter the clinician from appropriately counseling, examining, and treating HPV-infected men (see Chapter 103, Androscopy). All methods of treating HPV have significant failure and recurrence rates. Common modalities for treatment are noted in Table 138.1; additional information is presented in Chapter 14, Cryosurgery; Chapter 25, Radiofrequency Surgery (Modern Electrosurgery); Chapter 103, Androscopy; Chapter 124, Colposcopic Examination; and Chapter 121, Human Papillomavirus DNA Typing.

The latest in the "treatment" of HPV infection is prevention. Three HPV vaccines have been licensed by the US Food and Drug Administration (FDA) since 2006. HPV vaccine is recommended for routine vaccination of adolescents (including girls and boys) at age 11 or 12 years, and can be started at age 9 years. Bivalent HPV vaccine protects against two types of HPV, quadrivalent HPV vaccine protects against four types of HPV, and 9-valent HPV vaccine protects against nine types of HPV. Bivalent, quadrivalent, and 9-valent HPV vaccine all protect against HPV 16 and 18, the HPV types that cause about 66% of cervical cancers and the majority of other HPV-attributable cancers in the United States. Quadrivalent and 9-valent HPV vaccine also protect against HPV 6 and 11, the HPV types that cause anogenital warts. In addition, 9-valent HPV vaccine targets five additional cancer-causing types, which account for another 15% of cervical cancers. The additional five types in 9-valent HPV vaccine account for a higher proportion of HPV-associated cancers in women compared with men, and cause cervical precancers in women. Therefore the additional protection from 9-valent HPV vaccine will mostly benefit women. As of 2017, only 9-valent HPV vaccine are available in the United States.

INDICATIONS FOR TREATMENT OF HUMAN PAPILLOMAVIRUS INFECTION

- Visible, acuminate condylomata
- Symptomatic condylomata

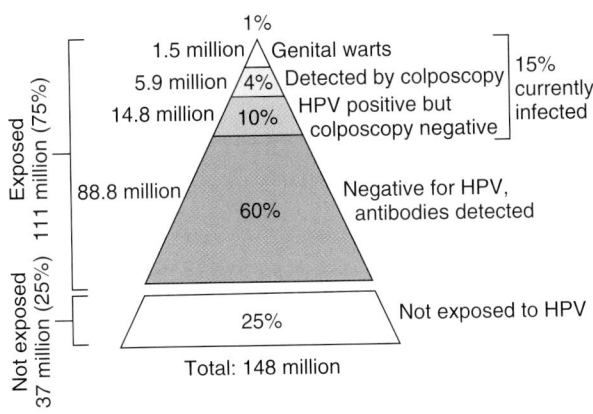

Fig. 138.1 Hierarchy of clinically apparent and subclinical human papillomavirus infections: 15 to 49 years of age, United States, 2004. HPV, Human papillomavirus. (From U.S. Census estimates of population as of July 1, 2004.)

CONTRAINDICATIONS TO TREATMENT OF HUMAN PAPILLOMAVIRUS INFECTION

- Any known adverse reactions to the selected treatment modality
- Any lesion that is possibly cancerous. (These lesions should be sampled for biopsy before treatment.)

PREPROCEDURE PATIENT EDUCATION

Explain the procedure along with the risks and benefits to the patient. If an investigational drug is to be used, such as 5-fluorouracil ([5-FU] Efudex; Valeant Pharmaceuticals), review the non-FDA-approved status and why it is still being used. Counseling and education are key components in the comprehensive management of HPV-infected individuals. It is imperative that appropriate time be taken by clinicians and staff to counsel patients and answer questions. Educational materials include pamphlets, printouts, videotapes, hotlines, and Internet sites (e.g., www.cdc.gov/std/hpv). Advise patients and sexual partners that although HPV infection itself has been associated with carcinoma, it is very common among sexually active adults and usually remains a benign disease that resolves on its own. Most sexually active adults will be exposed to the virus at some point in their lives. Penile penetration of the vagina is the most common mode of transmissions, but HPV can also be spread through nonpenetrative contact. Most sex partners are infected by the time the patient's diagnosis has been made, even though they may not have any clinical evidence of infection. HPV DNA testing is currently not indicated for partners of patients with genital warts. In female patients, if not already immunized, HPV recombinant vaccine should be administered to protect against types 6, 11, 16, and 18. Prior infection with HPV is not a reason to withhold the vaccine because it may prevent infection from HPV types other than the one(s) causing the current situation. In the past, condoms were not thought to be of much benefit in providing protection, but a 2006 study by Winer and colleagues suggests a 70% decrease in risk of new infection with consistent use.

Women who develop signs of HPV infection, or who are sexually active with a partner who has HPV, must be advised to obtain regular Pap smears because they are at higher risk for the development of dysplasia.

CRYOSURGERY

See Chapter 14, Cryosurgery, and Chapter 125, Cryotherapy of the Cervix.

Equipment

Cryosurgery may be carried out with a variety of methods, the differences being the approximate temperatures achieved (liquid nitrogen −320°F, nitrous oxide probe −95°F, canister gases −95°F):

- Cryogun with nitrous oxide tank and small dermal tips
- Liquid nitrogen and cotton-tipped applicators
- Liquid nitrogen pressurized sprayer (Wallach Ultrafreezer, Brymill Cry-Ac)
- Canister gases (Verruca-Freeze, Ellman Medi-Frig)

Techniques

General Techniques for All Methods

1. No anesthetic is required for cryotherapy, although if there are large or multiple lesions, patients may prefer it (see Chapter 4, Topical Anesthesia).
2. Place the patient in the lithotomy position and examine the vulva, perineum, and rectum (or scrotum and penis). If the lesions cover a large area, it may be prudent to treat subsections at separate visits to prevent excessive posttreatment discomfort. Treatment should be directed at the acuminate warts rather than at subclinical condylomata that cannot be seen with the naked eye. Staining with dilute acetic acid may make smaller acuminate lesions more prominent.

Nitrous Oxide

1. Select the proper size of cryotip based on the size of the lesion. The tip should cover small lesions; larger lesions may be frozen in sections or clusters.
2. Moisten the lesion with water-soluble gel before positioning the probe to improve tip-to-tissue adhesion. With the cryotip at ambient temperature, place the tip on an individual lesion. Activate the cryogun to initiate the flow of gas within the probe, which begins the freezing process. Apply gentle traction on the lesion to lift the skin away from underlying tissue as soon as ice appears on the tissue (this is especially important on the penile shaft). This traction isolates the lesion from the surrounding tissue, minimizes discomfort, and ensures cold transfer. Clumped lesions may be frozen in clusters but will require longer freezing times. Clusters also require the freeze–thaw–refreeze technique to produce the necessary cryonecrosis. (The tissue is frozen until it appears solid white, then thawed until it turns pink again, and then frozen a second time.) Stop freezing as soon as the ice extends just 2 to 3 mm beyond each lesion's border. This generally takes only 15 to 30 seconds. Some practitioners prefer a second application after the initial thaw in all cases.
3. Explain to the patient that a tingling or burning sensation is normal, especially with thawing.

Liquid Nitrogen (Cotton-Tipped Applicator and Spray)

1. Standard or large cotton-tipped applicators may be used to apply liquid nitrogen. Standard applicators (Q-Tips) work better if wisps of cotton are pulled from a cotton ball and twirled to add bulk to the end of the applicator. Pour liquid nitrogen into a Styrofoam cup. Dip the cotton-tipped applicator into the liquid nitrogen and apply immediately to the lesion. Reapply until the lesion turns white. Avoid freezing more than 2 to 3 mm beyond the border of the lesion. Thaw time should take at least 1 minute.
2. With the thermos-type containers (e.g., Wallach Ultrafreezer, Brymill Cry-Ac), spray a jet of liquid nitrogen on the lesions. Select an orifice large enough to have the site of the spray cover the lesion, but do not overspray. (This is a quick and economical use of liquid nitrogen.) Apply the liquid nitrogen until the lesion turns white. Avoid freezing more than 2 to 3 mm beyond the lesion. It generally takes only 5 to 10 seconds, depending on

TABLE 138.1   Therapies Currently Available for the Treatment of Genital Warts*

Treatment Modality	Average No. of Treatments	Success Rate (%)[†]	Recurrence <6 Months (%)	Average Length of Study Follow-up (mo)	Total Cost to Patient[‡]
Ablative Therapy					
CO$_2$ laser	1.3	89	8	13.9	$$
Cryotherapy	1.9	83	28	2.7	$$
Electrocautery	1.4	93	24	3	$$
Infrared coagulator	1.5	80	20	6	$$
Chemical-Ablative Therapy					
Topical 5-fluorouracil (Efudex)	Patient applied	71	13	10.9	$$
85% Trichloroacetic acid	4	81	36	2	$$$
Podophyllin	4.2	65	39	6	$$$
Podophyllotoxin (Condylox)	10.5 (patient applied)	61	34	3.2	$$
Chemical–Immune Enhancer Therapy					
Imiquimod (Aldara)	30 (patient applied)	56	—§	7	$$$
Interferon (local injection)	11	52	25	7.8	$$$$
Other					
Sinecatechins	300 (patient applied)	55	6	4.0	$$$$
Excisional Therapy					
Blade/scissors	1.1	93	24	8.3	$$
Radiofrequency (loop)	1	90	—§	8	$$

*Based on estimates as compiled from available English-language literature. Very small studies, study results that fell 2 standard deviations beyond the means, and very poorly designed studies were excluded.
[†]Defined as clearance of all condylomata at end of therapy or healing from therapy.
[‡]Relative cost based in office visits and cost of treatment for each method. $, low cost; $$, low-moderate cost; $$$, high-moderate cost; $$$$, high cost.
§No data or not recorded.

the size of the lesion. Thaw time should take at least 1 minute. A spray guard is available to protect surrounding skin. Alternatively, the clinician can place an ear speculum around the lesion to limit overspray.

EDITOR'S NOTE: With temperatures below −320°F achieved, the application of liquid nitrogen is basically surgery. Caution should be observed during application to avoid excessive tissue damage, scarring, hypopigmentation, etc.

Gases (Verruca-Freeze and Medi-Frig)

Verruca-Freeze and Medi-Frig work similarly to liquid nitrogen. Compressed gas in a can is sprayed into an ear speculum that should just cover the lesion. The compressed gas liquefies with spraying, and rapid evaporation results in freezing of the lesion. The use of this agent obviates the need for storing large amounts of liquid nitrogen. The speculum must be positioned so that it is perpendicular to the lesion; in this way it acts like a funnel. This position requirement may be impractical on the genitalia. Once the material is sprayed into the speculum, it is held in place until the bubbling stops. Care must be taken that the liquid does not leak out from under the speculum and freeze normal tissue. One application may suffice on small lesions. If the lesions are large, a second application may be necessary after thawing. There are also cotton-tipped applicator–like attachments that allow this device to be used in a manner similar to liquid nitrogen.

Postprocedure Patient Education

- Usually no postprocedure medication is needed. Topical anesthetic ointments may be used to minimize discomfort (e.g., lidocaine 5% ointment). Sitz baths may aid resolution when large areas are treated. Silver sulfadiazine (Silvadene) ointment or other over-the-counter antibiotic ointments (Polysporin, Bacitracin) not only may be soothing but also may reduce the possibility of superficial infection. They also help keep the denuded tissue from sticking to underclothing. No dressing is required, but some patients may request a sanitary napkin.
- Lesions that are cryonecrosed progress from erythema to edema and then turn black. They may also blister. The blister may be left intact or removed. The lesions disappear within a few days, and healing should be complete in 7 to 8 days.
- The patient should be advised to report any signs of infection or excessive discomfort.
- Treated areas should be washed with mild soap and water several times each day. Postcryotherapy management is similar to that for a second-degree burn.

Complications

- If the area treated at one visit is too large, extensive necrosis and pain may occur. It is prudent to treat large areas over multiple visits. Infection may occur at the treatment site if the area is not kept clean by normal hygienic measures.
- Recurrence or persistence of lesions is common.
- Cryotherapy is probably the safest therapy for treating HPV lesions during pregnancy.
- Nitrous oxide cryoguns are associated with a higher risk of perforation and fistula formation inside the vagina compared with the cotton-tipped applicator method.

Suppliers

See Chapter 14, Cryosurgery.

CHEMICAL CAUTERY

Equipment

- Bichloracetic acid, 85% trichloroacetic acid (TCA), or 0.5% podofilox (Condylox)
- Cotton-tipped applicators or toothpicks

Technique

1. For bichloracetic acid, TCA, or podophyllin, identify the lesions to be treated. For small lesions, use the wooden end of the cotton-tipped applicator or a toothpick to apply the solution directly on the lesion. Avoid getting the solution on normal skin. However, the wart virus is often present 3 mm beyond the obvious lesion. Do not apply petrolatum or other ointments around the lesions, as may have been the custom in the past. Besides being time consuming, it often covers the lesion itself and protects exactly what is meant to be treated. For larger lesions, use the cotton-tipped end of the applicator to apply the solution, again being careful to avoid getting the solution on normal skin. Continue in the same manner until all the lesions are treated. With high-strength acid application, the warty tissue rapidly turns white (see Chapter 103, Androscopy, Fig. 103.7A–B). Although, in the vast majority of patients, this treatment method is extremely well tolerated, patients treated with acids do experience intense, burning-like pain that subsides in about 5 minutes. In 1 to 2 days the skin will slough. Patients may need retreatment every 1 to 3 weeks until the lesions resolve. The acids can be used in pregnancy and on mucous membranes.

2. Patients may apply topical 0.5% podofilox solution or gel themselves at home. Typically, the solution is recommended for penile lesions, whereas cream or gel vehicle preparations are thought to be more comfortable for application to anal or vaginal lesions. Podofilox is a pure standardized compound of the active ingredient in podophyllin. Podofilox is indicated for topical treatment of external genital warts, but it is not indicated for the treatment of mucous membrane (urethra, rectum, vagina) condylomata. Podofilox is applied to the warts with a cotton-tipped applicator supplied with the medication. Treatment should be limited to an area less than 10 cm^2, and no more than 0.5 mL of the solution should be used each day. The solution is applied in the morning and evening for 3 consecutive days; then a 4-day waiting period is observed, during which the solution is not applied. This 1-week treatment cycle may be repeated up to four times, until there is no visible wart tissue. Remember the 2-3-4-4 rule: twice a day for 3 days, off for 4 days, used for up to 4 weeks. Later, the entire treatment can be repeated if needed. Podofilox should not be used in pregnant women, young children, and nursing mothers.

Complications

- Treatment with too much solution can lead to excessive tissue damage and prolonged healing.
- Persistence and recurrence of the warts are not uncommon.
- Systemic reactions with extensive exposure to podophyllin may include nausea, vomiting, fever, confusion, coma, renal failure, ileus, and leukopenia. Local reactions include erosions, ulcerations, scarring, balanitis, and phimosis.
- Seizures and death have occurred with the application of podophyllin to occluded mucous membranes.

Postprocedure Patient Education

- For lesions that are cauterized chemically, the healing process is usually less than 1 week but may take longer.
- Patient education sheets are supplied by the manufacturer of podofilox.

INTERFERON THERAPY

Indication

Interferon therapy is indicated for recalcitrant condylomata unresponsive to other modalities.

Contraindication

Pregnancy is the only contraindication.

Equipment

- Recombinant interferon alfa-2b
- 27- to 30-gauge needle and a 1-mL syringe

Technique

1. The manufacturer recommends that only five warts be treated at one time, making this treatment time consuming and expensive. It is rarely used.
2. The standard dose is 1 million U of interferon (0.1 mL) intralesionally three times a week for 3 weeks (total of nine injections).
3. Use a 27- to 30-gauge needle to inject the interferon directly into the center of the wart's base (intralesional).
4. Maximum response should occur within 4 to 6 weeks. If there is no clinical response after 16 weeks, a second 3-week course should be completed.

Complications

- Flu-like symptoms such as myalgias, fatigue, headache, chills, and fever may occur.
- May cause menstrual problems in adolescents.
- Treatment beyond 3 weeks may cause reversible leukopenia and liver enzyme elevations.

Postprocedure Patient Education

The patient may take an analgesic if flu-like symptoms develop.

ELECTROSURGERY OR LASER THERAPY

Treatment of warts with electrosurgery can be ablative or excisional (see later). Lesions that are small or few in number can be cauterized easily with a ball or needle electrode. Place the electrosurgical unit on coagulation (or hemostasis) with just enough power to "cook" the wart. Wipe away the debris. If viable tissue remains, touch the wart again with the electrode. Condylomata are epidermal, and there is little need to go deep. With just enough current there will be little scarring. An alternative approach is laser ablation, but this treatment is expensive. Its use is more commonly reserved for when there are extensive condylomata on the vulva or when the vagina or cervix also needs treatment (Fig. 138.2).

INFRARED COAGULATION

Infrared coagulation can also be used to ablate warts on the external genitals as well as mucous membranes. Its advantages are that it is quick and the depth of destruction is readily controlled by the automatic timer (see Chapter 87, Office Treatment of Hemorrhoids). Destruction occurs when infrared light travels down the light guide and concentrates on the lesion. There is no electrical current involved.

Technique

1. Anesthetize lesions.
2. Set timer on 1 to 1.25 seconds for the average lesion. If the lesion is quite thick, the unit can be set up to 3 seconds. The depth of penetration will be roughly 1 mm/sec.
3. Apply the Teflon-coated tip inside the disposable sheath to the lesion using slight pressure.
4. Pull the trigger and hold it in place until it automatically turns off. The light will not harm the eyes, although it is bright and uncomfortable if directly viewed.

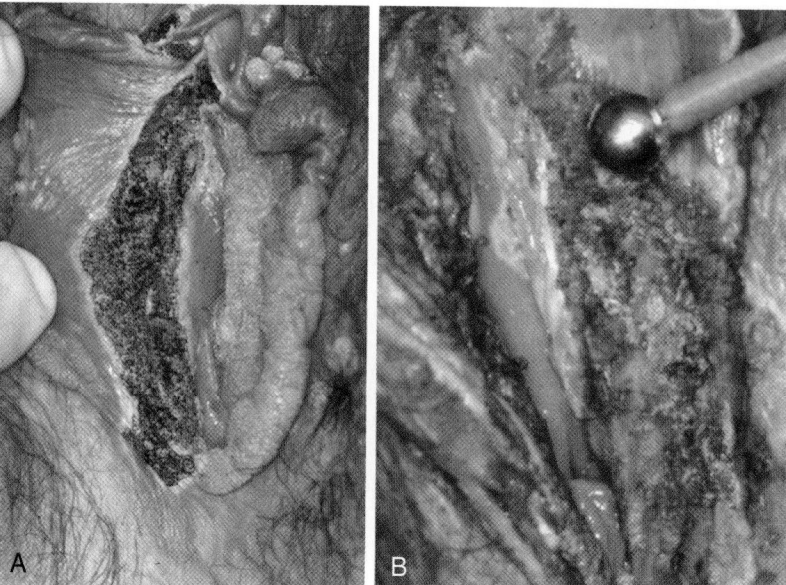

Fig. 138.2 Treatment of condyloma with laser (A) and ball electrocautery (B). (From Ferenczy A, Behelak Y, Haber G, Wright TC Jr, Richart RM. Treating vaginal and external anogenital condylomas with electrosurgery vs CO_2 laser ablation. *J Gynecol Surg* 11[1]:41–50, 1995.)

5. Wiping the tip and allowing the tip to cool for a few seconds between applications is recommended.
6. If the lesion is large, reapplication is carried out with slight overlapping.
7. Wipe away the ablated tissue with moistened gauze and determine if depth is adequate.
8. Treat the next lesion.
9. Postoperative treatment is the same as noted for other ablative treatments with electrocautery and acids.
10. Reexamine and retreat if necessary in 3 to 4 weeks. Expect slight denuding of the epithelium and mild ulceration as seen with topical acid treatments. There usually is little residual scarring.

SURGICAL REMOVAL

Condylomata can be excised surgically with sharp iris scissors (see Chapter 103, Androscopy, Fig. 103.6) or a knife blade after appropriate anesthesia. However, the penile and vulvar skin is thin; it is easy to resect too deeply, which may result in scarring. Sharp disposable curettes offer a good alternative. Warty lesions also tend to be vascular and bleed easily. Although this can be controlled with Monsel solution, it is often easier to use radiofrequency (loop) excisional surgery, especially for bigger lesions (see later discussion, as well as Chapter 25, Radiofrequency Surgery [Modern Electrosurgery]). For small pedunculated growths, scissor excision may be ideal. Flatter papular lesions can usually be easily curetted with a sharp, disposable 2- to 4-mm dermal curette.

LOOP RADIOFREQUENCY ELECTROSURGICAL EXCISION

This technique is especially useful for large condylomata, in which any type of excisional process can create excessive bleeding. Use of the radiofrequency (a type of electrosurgery) unit can readily control this excess. Using a pure cutting setting minimizes any scarring, and there is still at least a 10% coagulation current. Thus, removal is carried out quickly with minimal residual tissue destruction. Complete details of this technique are found in Chapter 25, Radiofrequency Surgery [Modern Electrosurgery].

Equipment

- Square or round/oval loop electrodes (Usually the larger oval loops work best. Use dermatology electrodes with shorter shafts rather than the longer ones used to carry out the loop electrosurgical excision procedure. The shorter shafts allow better control of depth, and the operator's hand can be stabilized against surrounding tissue.)
- Electrosurgical generator
- Colposcope or 3× to 5× magnification lens (helps to keep the loop superficial, avoiding deep excisions as well as ensuring that all the lesion has been removed)
- Grounding pad or antenna
- Smoke evacuator
- 2% lidocaine with or without epinephrine (epinephrine is generally not used on the penis)
- Syringe with 30-gauge needle
- Ball electrodes (5 mm) to cauterize any bleeders
- Antibiotic ointment (over-the-counter preparations Bacitracin and Polysporin work well)
- Virus-filtering (submicron) mask and nonsterile gloves
- 4 × 4 sterile gauze pads
- Acetic acid
- Monsel solution
- Formalin bottles
- 5% lidocaine ointment to apply after excisions completed

Suppliers

See the list of companies for radiofrequency units in Chapter 25, Radiofrequency Surgery [Modern Electrosurgery], and Chapter 127, Loop Electrosurgical Excision Procedure for Treating Cervical Intraepithelial Neoplasia.

Preprocedure Patient Preparation

Explain the procedure to the patient and obtain informed consent. The major risks are pain, bleeding, infection, recurrence, and scarring.

Technique

See Figs. 138.3 and 138.4.

1. Apply 5% acetic acid (or white vinegar) to the warts. Keep the tissue moist by repeated acetic acid application.
2. Turn on the electrosurgical generator power supply. Check the manufacturer's guidelines for proper power settings (usually around 15 to 20 W or, if using the Ellman unit, level 2).

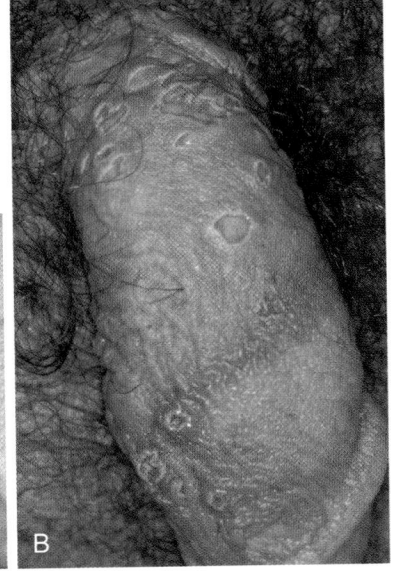

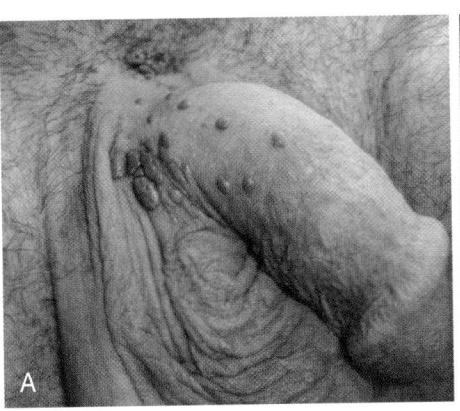

Fig. 138.3 Treatment of condyloma using radiofrequency loop excision. During (A) and immediately after (B) removal. Note lack of bleeding. (Courtesy John L. Pfenninger, MD, The Medical Procedures Center, Midland, MI.)

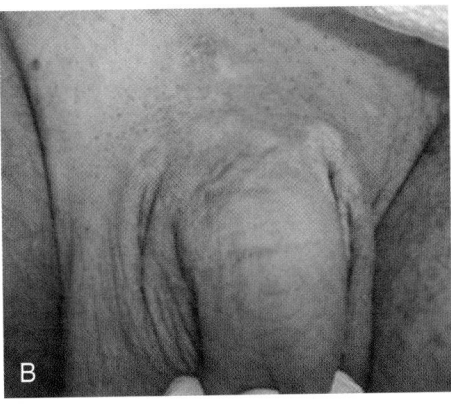

Fig. 138.4 Treatment of condyloma using radiofrequency loop excision. Appearance before (A) and 1 month after (B) removal. (Courtesy John L. Pfenninger, MD, The Medical Procedures Center, Midland, MI.)

3. Select the cutting (preferred) or blend mode on the electrosurgical generator.
4. Place the grounding pad or antenna on the patient's thigh or buttocks.
5. With a 27- to 30-gauge needle, inject 2% lidocaine under the base of the wart(s) to make a wheal that extends beyond the margin of the wart.
6. Activate the smoke evacuator and place the hose close to the excisional site.
7. Using a method of magnification allows more precise removal and assurance that small lesions are not missed. The loop should not excise deeper than 1 mm to the dermal–epidermal junction (looks like chamois cloth). Often it is best just to debulk the wart on the first pass. Then make fine, superficial feathering strokes to remove the remaining tissue. Significant bleeding may be a sign that the excision is too deep or, paradoxically, that there is residual wart tissue. To control the depth of excision and stabilize the loop, place the fifth finger of the hand holding the electrode in the pencil wand on the patient. Should the patient jump or move, the operating hand will move too, avoiding a deep cut. Hold the pencil wand close to where the electrode inserts into the wand. Use caution because the loops cut very quickly. Be especially cautious over the penis.
8. After the loop electrode has been used to excise the wart, the ball electrode may be used to coagulate any bleeders or residual tissue, although this is rarely necessary.

9. Remove the coagulated remnants with gauze sponges soaked with acetic acid (5%).
10. On completion, inspect the excised area with the colposcope to ensure that the entire wart has been removed and that no coagulated remnants are left at the base of the excised lesion. Also, be sure no small lesions have been missed.
11. Apply an antibiotic ointment and/or lidocaine ointment to the excision area and use gauze pads to cover the excision sites.
12. Although not mandatory, consider sending all tissue that was removed for histologic evaluation. Many lesions that appear totally benign and clinically are condylomata can be dysplastic or, albeit rarely, verrucous carcinoma.

NOTE: Many patients prefer this modality over chemical cautery methods because healing is often more rapid and less painful.

Complications

- Hypopigmentation may rarely occur at the excision site.
- If Monsel solution is used to control bleeding, there may be some residual ferrous pigmentation for several months. This gradually fades.
- Keloids may form on skin that has a tendency toward keloid formation.
- Postprocedure bleeding and wound infection are extremely rare.
- According to Ferenczy (1990), the treatment failure rate at 8 months (average two treatments) is 19%.

- If the procedure is performed correctly, scarring is minimal and comparable to that with laser ablation.

Postprocedure Patient Education

- Provide the patient with the sample patient education handout available at www.expertconsult.com. Instruct the patient that some postprocedure discomfort may last for up to 2 weeks. However, initial discomfort should resolve in 24 to 48 hours and is well controlled with nonsteroidal antiinflammatory drugs. When large areas have been treated, sitz baths may be taken two to three times a day during the initial recovery period. At a minimum, the area should be washed three to four times per day, followed by application of an antibiotic ointment. This is continued for 5 to 7 days until re-epithelialization has taken place. Ice packs may also be used initially. For those patients who have perianal removals, stool softeners (docusate sodium) are important throughout the entire recovery period.
- If acute discomfort persists beyond 48 hours, instruct the patient to contact the physician. Rarely, a mixture of equal parts of 20% benzocaine (Hurricaine) ointment and topical antibiotics may be used. Lidocaine ointment 5% provides excellent relief and keeps the tissues moist.
- Instruct the patient to return to the office in 4 to 6 weeks and to call if fever, chills, or purulent discharge develops.

IMIQUIMOD CREAM (ALDARA)

Use of imiquimod (Aldara) cream is a unique approach to HPV treatment. It acts as an immune stimulator by inducing multiple subtypes of interferon-α. This causes induction of several cytokines, including tumor necrosis factor and interleukins. These, in turn, activate natural killer cells, T cells, polymorphonuclear neutrophil leukocytes, and macrophages, thus increasing antitumor activity. The drug has almost no systemic side effects. The use of this drug is not indicated in children younger than 12 years of age. It can be used primarily or after other treatments to reduce recurrences. In randomized, placebo-controlled trials, 37% to 54% of treated patients showed clearance after 16 weeks. Although it is an off-label indication, imiquimod has been used with excellent results to treat extensive intravaginal condylomata.

Indications

It can be used on all external HPV-infected sites.

Contraindications

- It is a pregnancy class C drug.
- It is not approved for use on occluded mucous membranes or on the uterine cervix. However, an off-label use for extensive intravaginal lesions is to use one packet of the cream at bedtime, once a week, for 4 to 6 weeks. It is very efficacious but may cause irritation.
- It is not recommended for use with condoms or diaphragms because of possible latex damage.

Technique

The cream comes in small packets (box of 12 or 24) and is applied to the lesions three times a week for up to 16 weeks. The cream may be applied to the affected area, not strictly to the lesion itself. For best results it must be rubbed in well, not just lightly applied to the involved areas.

Complications

- Side effects can include pain, pigmentary changes at the application site, erythema, erosion, itching, skin flaking, and edema. Therapy may be temporarily halted if symptoms become prob-

lematic. Systemic symptoms have been reported but are extremely rare.

5-FLUOROURACIL

Treatment with 5-FU should be considered only for extensive, intractable condylomata resistant to other modalities or for the treatment of vaginal intraepithelial neoplasia. The FDA has not approved labeling of 5-FU for treatment of these diseases, and the patient should be advised that this is technically an investigational use. Because of the reported teratogenic potential, 5-FU should be used with extreme caution—if at all—in nonsterile women of reproductive age. If used, a signed consent form is advised indicating the patient will not become pregnant. Although commonly used historically, 5-FU use has fallen into disfavor for HPV treatment because of complications of vaginal scarring and the development of other, more acceptable methods. It is still one of the easiest and most effective treatments for male urethral/meatal lesions.

Indications

- Extensive vulvar, perianal, penile, or vaginal condylomata
- Vaginal intraepithelial neoplasia
- Vulvar intraepithelial neoplasia
- Urethral meatus lesions
- Bowenoid carcinoma in situ of the penis (erythroplasia of Queyrat)

CAUTION: Patients with blond or red hair, or with very light complexions, may be more sensitive to 5-FU. Also use cautiously in patients with known skin sensitivities such as atopic dermatitis. Mucosal areas are much more sensitive than keratinized skin.

Contraindications

- Pregnancy
- Lack of birth control method (relative contraindication)
- Lack of informed consent with regard to the absence of FDA approval

Equipment

- 5% 5-FU (Efudex, Fluoroplex) cream
- Vaginal applicator marked with dosage lines

Preprocedure Patient Preparation

- Obtain informed consent before initiating treatment.
- Advise the patient of alternative methods of treatment. Frequently when 5-FU is being considered, laser ablation or loop electrosurgical excision procedure therapy is also an option.
- The patient should know that the inflammatory response is delayed by 3 to 4 days. The patient may believe the medication is not working and so apply it more frequently, leading to complications.
- Use of 5-FU should be limited to clinicians experienced with managing side effects, which are similar to those experienced when treating the face for actinic changes (e.g., chemical burns). See the sample patient education form available at www.expertconsult.com.

Technique

For the Vagina

1. Instruct the patient to use 1.5 g of 5-FU per week for 10 weeks. A standard Ortho vaginal applicator will hold 10 mL of cream (5 g of 5-FU). Patients should then use only one third of an applicator of cream for each treatment. The 5-FU should be inserted intra-

vaginally or applied directly to any external lesions at bedtime (e.g., for perianal lesions).

2. Instruct the patient to apply zinc oxide to the vulva (where treatment is not necessary) to protect it in the event that intravaginal, perineal, or perianal 5-FU should leak out or come into contact with the vulva. This is not necessary if external condylomata exist in this area.
3. The patient may insert a small tampon into the vagina to keep the 5-FU within the introitus.
4. If there is no inflammatory response after 3 weeks, the patient may increase the frequency of application to every 5 days.

For the Urethral Meatus

Use a cotton-tipped applicator and apply a small amount of 5-FU cream into the meatus for a distance of 5 to 6 mm. Apply after voiding at bedtime and again after voiding and showering in the morning. Repeat for 7 days. Lesions will generally resolve. If not, repeat for another 7 days. Allow any inflammation to resolve before reapplication.

For the Penis (Carcinoma In Situ, Erythroplasia of Queyrat)

This lesion usually occurs under the foreskin. Because of occlusion, the effects are magnified. Although quite efficacious, the treatment can be quite painful, especially if the medication is overused. Also, these lesions generally occur in older men, so compliance can be difficult. Cream will often drip out on the scrotum, so it must be protected. A small amount of cream is applied once a week to the affected area for 6 weeks. If there is little reaction after the first week, the schedule can be increased to every 5 days for two periods. If there is still minimal response, the cream can be tried every 3 to 4 days, but must be monitored closely. Treatment for 6 weeks usually resolves the dysplasia, but longer treatment may be needed. Recheck 6 weeks after completing treatment to be sure the abnormality has resolved. Small residual spots may be treated with excision or electrocautery, or even more 5-FU.

Complications

- Pain.
- Bleeding.
- Persistence of disease.
- Persistent vaginal ulcers may develop in patients who are extremely sensitive to 5-FU or in patients who overuse the medication. For some patients, the vaginal ulcers may fail to heal with time, and the patient may have persistent vaginal discharge and bleeding (rare). Patients who fail to heal may require surgical excision of the ulcer and primary closure of the defect.
- Vaginal stenosis (rare).
- If 5-FU is to be used after cryotherapy of the cervix, wait at least 4 weeks before initiating 5-FU therapy to avoid cervical stenosis.
- Inflammation of the scrotum, if not properly protected, when treating Bowen disease (squamous cell carcinoma in situ).
- Foreskin adhesions.

Postprocedure Patient Education

Instruct the patient to contact the physician if severe inflammation or any hypersensitivity reaction occurs. Intravaginal estrogens or steroid creams may be used to decrease the inflammatory reaction. See the sample patient education handout available at www.expertconsult.com.

SINECATECHINS

Sinecatechins, a green tea extract, is approved by the FDA for the treatment of genital and perianal warts. It is a 15% ointment, produced by PharmaDerm Fougera Sandoz, and marketed as Veregen. It is approved for use in immunocompetent patients 18 years of age

or older. The recommended initial dose of the Veregen is a 0.5-cm strand applied in a thin layer over all external and perianal warts, three times a day.

In clinical trials patients applied 10% or 15% ointment three times daily for a maximum of 16 weeks or until complete resolution of the warts occurred. Complete clearance of warts was seen in 56.3% and 57.2% of patients, respectively. Partial clearance rates of at least 50% were reported for 74% and 78.4% of patients.

GUIDELINES FOR TREATING PERIANAL AND INTRA-ANAL LESIONS

Treatment of perianal and intra-anal lesions is similar to treatment for vaginal condylomata. Additional guidelines are:

- Podofilox and imiquimod should not be used on mucous membranes (i.e., inside the anus). TCA, excisional therapy, electrocautery, and infrared coagulation may be used intra-anally.
- Anoscopy should be performed on all patients with perianal lesions to rule out more proximal lesions. This is often done after resolution of the external lesions to avoid possible trauma and potential spread of the virus proximally.
- The risk of rectal carcinoma is increased 50 times in receptive homosexual men, and HPV appears to be involved in the process. Some suggest Pap smears of the dentate line of the anus to detect early dysplastic lesions just as with the cervix, followed by staining and biopsy (see Chapter 84, High-Resolution Anoscopy).

GUIDELINES FOR TREATING CONDYLOMATA IN PREGNANCY

Condylomata may grow rapidly and multiply quickly during the second-trimester immune suppression. After delivery, they may, and often do, resolve spontaneously. Women who have warts in the perineum with subsequent tears or episiotomies have a higher risk of wound dehiscence. Most clinicians recommend treatment of perineal condylomata during the third trimester. Safe modalities include cryotherapy, 85% TCA, electrocautery, laser therapy, infrared coagulation, and radiofrequency (loop) or sharp tissue scissor excision. Although cryotherapy may be used, there is often more swelling and discomfort.

It appears that HPV is in the amniotic fluid of infected mothers, so there is no indication for cesarean section unless the lesions are so large that they inhibit normal delivery.

OTHER METHODS FOR TREATING CONDYLOMATA ACUMINATA

Although Candida antigen injection is used for verrucae, there have been no published reports of its use in treating condylomata. Theoretically, there is no contraindication to its use, and it has been tried with some degree of success (editor's experience).

GENERAL CONSIDERATIONS FOR ALL METHODS

See Box 138.1 for a summary of treatment options for various locations. See Fig. 138.5 for an algorithm on treatment protocol selection.

- HPV is associated with cervical cancer, and women must be followed closely with Pap smears, HPV DNA typing, or colposcopy.
- The patient and partner must not smoke. Even passive smokers have been found to have lower folate levels—a known risk for HPV. Reducing smoking leads to a reduction in cervical dysplasia, whereas continuing to smoke encourages progression.
- The patient should consume a diet with at least five helpings of fruits and vegetables daily.

External Genital and Perianal
Cryotherapy
Electrocautery
Electrofrequency/radiofrequency excision
Imiquimod (Aldara)
Laser
Podofilox (Condylox)
Sinecatechins (Veregen)
85% TCA

Cervical
Must rule out dysplasia before treatment (perform colposcopy),
   then the following:
   Cryotherapy
   Electrocautery
   Excision with radiofrequency or multiple biopsies
   85% TCA

Vaginal
Cryotherapy
Electrocautery
5-FU (extensive disease)—not FDA approved
Imiquimod (Aldara)—not FDA approved
Laser
85% TCA

Urethral Meatus
Cryotherapy
Electrocautery

Excision
5-FU
85% TCA

Penis or Bowen Disease
Electrocautery
5-FU
Frank excision of lesion

Intra-anal
Cryotherapy
Electrocautery
Surgical
85% TCA

Oral
Cryotherapy
Electrocautery
Excision

Pregnancy
Cryotherapy
Electrocautery/excision
85% TCA

_____

5-FU, 5-fluorouracil; *FDA*, US Food and Drug Administration; *TCA*,
trichloroacetic acid.
* See text for details.

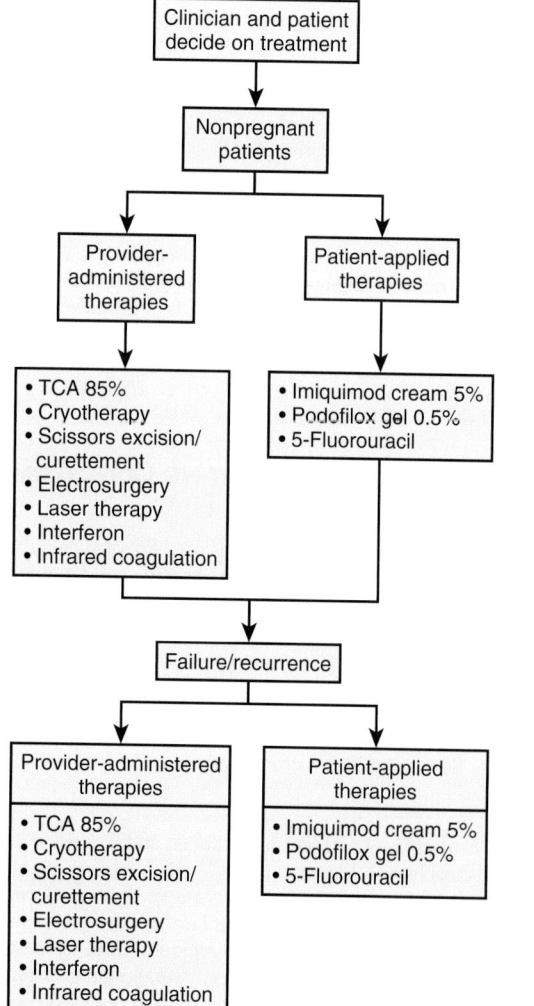

Fig. 138.5 Algorithm for treatment protocol selection for condyloma.
TCA, Trichloroacetic acid. (From Ferenczy A. External anogenital warts: old and
new therapies. *J SOGC* 1999;21[14]:1305–1313.)

- Patients must be informed that they can spread the disease at any time and that monogamy is most prudent.
- Condoms are not needed with current partners if there has been unprotected intercourse because they already have the virus; theoretically, once infected, the patient will always harbor the virus. Condoms may protect against transmission with new partners and against other sexually transmitted infections.

CPT/BILLING CODES

11900	Injection, intralesional; up to and including seven lesions (interferon)
11901	Injection intralesional; more than seven lesions

For destruction codes, if it takes less than 15 minutes, use "simple" codes. If treatment takes longer than 15 minutes, requires the use of the colposcope and an extensive examination, or is particularly complicated because of the size or extent of the condylomata, use the "extensive" codes.

46900	Destruction of lesion(s); anus (e.g., condyloma), simple; chemical
46910	Destruction of lesion(s); anus electrodesiccation, simple
46916	Destruction of lesion(s); anus cryosurgery, simple
46917	Destruction of lesion(s); anus laser surgery, simple
46922	Destruction of lesion(s); anus surgical excision, simple
46924	Destruction of lesion(s); anus, extensive; any method
54050	Destruction of lesion(s); penis (e.g., condyloma), simple; chemical
54055	Destruction of lesion(s); penis electrodesiccation, simple
54056	Destruction of lesion(s); penis cryosurgery, simple
54057	Destruction of lesion(s); penis laser surgery, simple
54060	Destruction of lesion(s); penis surgical excision, simple
54065	Destruction of lesion(s); penis, extensive, any method
54100	Biopsy, cutaneous, penis
56501	Destruction of lesion(s); vulva, simple; any method
56515	Destruction of lesion(s); vulva, extensive; any method
56605	Biopsy, vulva introitus
57061	Destruction of lesion(s); vagina, simple; any method

| 57065 | Destruction of lesion(s); vagina, extensive; any method |
| 57100 | Biopsy, vagina |

ICD-10-CM DIAGNOSTIC CODES

| B07.9 | Viral warts, unspecified |
| A63.0 | Condyloma acuminatum |

Acknowledgment

The editors recognize the contributions of Edward J. Mayeaux Jr, MD, to this chapter in a previous edition of this text.

ADDITIONAL RESOURCES

Physician Education

Centers for Disease Control and Prevention, Centers for Disease Control and Prevention: HPV Vaccine Information for Clinicians: https://www.cdc.gov/hpv/hcp/need-to-know.pdf

National Procedures Institute (www.npinstitute.com): Pfenninger JL: Removal of condyloma with radiofrequency (33 minutes)

Patient Education

Centers for Disease Control and Prevention, Centers for Disease Control and Prevention: Human Papillomavirus: https://www.cdc.gov/hpv/

National Procedures Institute (www.npinstitute.com): Pfenninger JL: Genital warts and cancer: The man's side (21 minutes)

National Procedures Institute (www.npinstitute.com): Pfenninger JL: Genital warts and cancer: The woman's side (35 minutes)

RECOMMENDED READING

Baker DA, Douglas Jr JM, Buntin DM, et al. Topical podofilox for the treatment of condylomata acuminata in women. *Obstet Gynecol.* 1990;76:656–659.

Bekassy Z, Westrom L. Infrared coagulation in the treatment of condyloma acuminata in the female genital tract. *Sex Transm Dis.* 1987;14:209–212.

Bergman A, Bhatia NN, Broen EM. Cryotherapy for the treatment of genital condylomata during pregnancy. *J Reprod Med.* 1984;29:432–435.

Centers for Disease Control and Prevention. *Sexually transmitted disease treatment guidelines;* 2015. www.cdc.gov/std/treatment/2006/genital-warts.htm#warts1.

CenterWatch. Drug information: Veregen (kunecatechins). www.centerwatch.com/patient/drugs/dru938.html.

Doorbar J. The papillomavirus life cycle. *J Clin Virol.* 2005;32(suppl 1):S7–S15.

Edwards L, Ferenczy A, Eron L, et al. Self-administered topical 5% imiquimod cream for external anogenital warts. *Arch Dermatol.* 1998;134:25–30.

Ferenczy A. Diagnosis and treatment of anogenital warts in the male patient. *Prim Care.* 1990;10:11.

Ferenczy A. External genital condyloma. In: Apgar BS, Brotzman GL, Spitzer M, eds. *Colposcopy: Principles and Practice.* 2nd ed. Philadelphia: Saunders; 2008:381–400.

Fletcher JL. Perinatal transmission of human papillomavirus. *Am Fam Physician.* 1991;43:143–148.

Friedman-Kien AE, Eron LJ, Conant M, et al. Natural interferon alfa for treatment of condylomata acuminata. JAMA. 1988;259:533–538.

Frisch M, Fenger C, van den Brule AJ, et al. Variants of squamous cell carcinoma of the anal canal and perianal skin and their relation to human papillomaviruses. *Cancer Res.* 1999;59:753–757.

Karnes JB, Usatine RP. Management of external genital warts. *Am Fam Physician.* 2014;90(5):312–318.

Krebs HB, Helmkamp BF. Treatment failure of genital condylomata in women: role of the male sexual partner. *Obstet Gynecol.* 1991;165:337–339.

Mayeaux Jr EJ, Dunton C. Modern management of external genital warts. *J Low Genit Tract Dis.* 2008;12:185–192.

Pfenninger JL. Androscopy: examination of the male partner. In: Apgar BS, Brotzman GL, Spitzer M, eds. *Colposcopy: Principles and Practice.* 2nd ed. Philadelphia: Saunders; 2008:483–496.

Richart R. Ways of using LEEP for external lesions. *Contemp Obstet Gynecol.* 1992;5:138–152.

Slattery ML, Robison LM, Schuman KL, et al. Cigarette smoking and exposure to passive smoke are risk factors for cervical cancer. JAMA. 1989;261:1593–1598.

Swinehart JM, Sperling M, Phillips S, et al. Intralesional fluorouracil/epinephrine injectable gel for treatment of condylomata acuminata: a phase 3 clinical study. *Arch Dermatol.* 1997;133:67–73.

Szarewski A, Jarvis MJ, Sasieni P, et al. Effect of smoking cessation on cervical lesion size. *Lancet.* 1996;347:941–943.

Tatti S, Swinehart JM, Thielert C, et al. Sinecatechins, a defined green tea extract, in the treatment of external anogenital warts: a randomized controlled trial. *Obstet Gynecol.* 2008;111:1371–1379.

Tyring SK, Friedman-Kien AE, Kent HL, et al. Alpha interferon in the management of genital warts. *Female Pat.* 1993;18:33–39.

Villa LL, Costa RL, Petta CA, et al. High sustained efficiency of a prophylactic quadrivalent human papilloma virus types 6/11/16/18 L1 virus-like particle vaccine through 5 years of follow up. *Br J Cancer.* 2006;95:1459–1466.

Yanofsky VR, Patel RV, Goldenberg G. Genital warts: a comprehensive review. *J Clin Aesthet Dermatol.* 2012;5(6):25–36.

CHAPTER 139

VULVAR BIOPSY

Gregory L. Brotzman

Evaluation of the vulva is an important component of a routine gynecologic examination. Although most lesions found are benign, such as skin tags, condylomata, and simple nevi, biopsy is occasionally needed to obtain a clearer understanding of the lesion present. This is especially true in older women and in those who smoke because they have a significantly increased risk of developing vulvar intraepithelial neoplasia (VIN) or cancer.

Most vulvar cancers are squamous cell carcinomas, and there are two different types. The more common type is seen in older women and usually related to long-standing lichen sclerosis. The less common type is related to smoking and human papilloma virus infection. Approximately half of women with VIN are asymptomatic; for those that are symptomatic, itching is the most common symptom. Alternatively, some patients present with palpable or visible abnormalities. Lesions are multicentric in about two-thirds of cases. Biopsy is important for differentiating lesions and diagnosing VIN or cancer.

Depth of biopsy is an important consideration. Disease of the non–hair-bearing areas of the vulva (labia minora, fourchette, interior aspect of the labia majora) is usually only 1 to 2 mm in depth. In contrast, hair-bearing areas (outer aspect of labia majora) may have disease that follows the hair shaft and may be several millimeters in depth. Deep biopsies are not necessary for non–hair-bearing vulvar skin areas, but biopsies should go down full depth to adipose tissue where hair is present. An elevated lesion can be shaved off (see Chapter 26, Skin Biopsy) if it is certain not to be a melanoma (e.g., seborrheic keratosis, condyloma, or benign nevus).

Examination of the vulva is aided by the use of a colposcope (low-power setting, 5×) or a magnifying glass after soaking the skin with 3% to 5% acetic acid (vinegar) using a spray bottle or large cotton applicators. Use of vinegar helps delineate dysplastic tissue and warty changes by turning them white (acetowhite epithelium).

Vulvar biopsy is a straightforward, easy-to-perform office skill that allows the practitioner to differentiate benign from neoplastic lesions, often being curative when the entire lesion is encompassed by the biopsy.

In addition to this chapter, see Chapters 13 and 18 through 22 on excision of lesions and follow-up repair; Chapter 26, Skin Biopsy; and Chapter 138, Treatment of Noncervical Condylomata Acuminata.

ANATOMY

Fig. 139.1 shows basic vulvar anatomy as well as the orientation of lines of skin tension. Skin tension lines are important in considering excisional or punch biopsies of the vulva. With the index finger and thumb of the nondominant hand, the skin should be stretched in the opposite direction of (perpendicular to) the tension lines, so that the excision margins form an ellipse after release. This allows an easier closure if sutures are used.

INDICATIONS

- Pigmented lesions
- Vulvar ulceration of uncertain etiology or a nonhealing ulcer

- Acetowhite epithelium (skin that turns white after the application of 5% acetic acid)
- Leukoplakia (white skin before the application of acetic acid)
- Presumed condylomata that do not readily respond to conventional therapy (if not resolved or significantly improving after two treatment attempts of any kind)
- Any skin abnormality that needs definitive diagnosis

CONTRAINDICATIONS

Absolute

- None

Relative

- Bleeding diathesis
- Allergy to local anesthetic/preservatives
- Recent (<3 weeks) chemical destruction attempts. These may result in false-positive histologic findings owing to reparative changes. It is best to wait until healing has occurred after any treatment before attempting a biopsy of such lesions.
- Infected site (if nonhealing, this may be reason for biopsy)

EQUIPMENT

- 3-mm Keyes punch biopsy (4 and 5 mm also acceptable but may require suturing, whereas 3 mm does not; Fig. 139.2A), a cervical punch biopsy forceps (see Fig. 139.2B), sharp tissue scissors

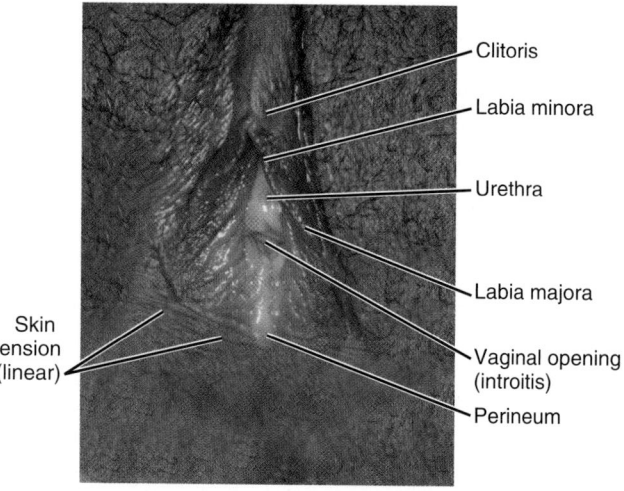

Clitoris

Labia minora

Urethra

Labia majora

Vaginal opening (introitis)

Perineum

Skin tension (linear)

Fig. 139.1 Vulvar anatomy. The vertical and horizontal lines demonstrate the lines of skin tension. When a biopsy is being performed, stretch the skin in the direction opposite to the skin tension lines so that after the biopsy is done, the skin will form an ellipse when relaxed, making it easier to close if sutures are needed.

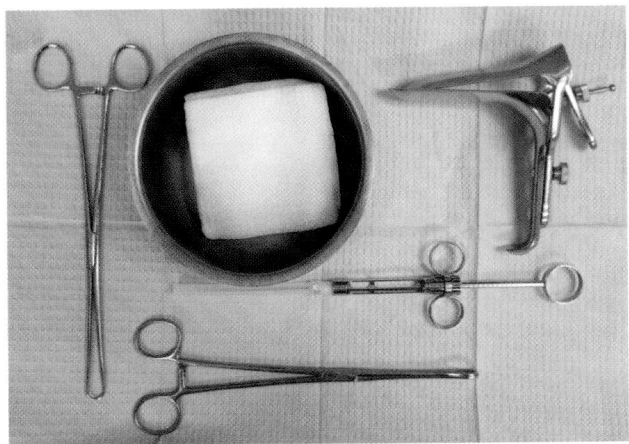

Fig. 139.2 (A) Keyes punch biopsy. (B) Cervical punch biopsy forceps. (C) Iris scissors. (D) Tissue forceps.

(see Fig. 139.2C) or a No. 15 blade for elevated or non–hair-bearing areas ("shave biopsy")
- No. 15 scalpel blade for excision
- 1% lidocaine (Xylocaine) with or without epinephrine (can mix 1:10 with sodium bicarbonate solution to decrease discomfort)
- 30-gauge, 0.5-inch needles
- 1- to 5-mL syringe
- Nonsterile gloves (sterile gloves needed if placing sutures) and equipment to follow universal blood and body fluid precautions
- Formalin containers
- Iris scissors (see Fig. 139.2C)
- Pickups (see Fig. 139.2D)
- Gauze sponges
- Povidone-iodine, chlorhexidine, or alcohol swabs
- Monsel solution (thickened ferric subsulfate solution), silver nitrate sticks, or aluminum chloride solution (Drysol)
- Small cotton-tipped applicators
- Antibiotic or petrolatum ointment
- 3-mm disposable (sharp) dermal curette

PREPROCEDURE PATIENT EDUCATION

If there are no contraindications, have the patient take 600 mg of ibuprofen 1 hour before the procedure to help with postprocedure discomfort.

PROCEDURE

There are four ways to perform a biopsy of the vulva:

1. Punch biopsy (with a Keyes punch or cervical biopsy forceps)
2. Excisional biopsy (using a No. 15 scalpel blade)
3. Shave excision (using tissue scissors or a blade)
4. Curettement using a 3-mm disposable (sharp) dermal curette

Deciding which type of biopsy technique to use depends on the size and location of the lesion (see earlier discussion). A large or deep lesion would likely require punch biopsies to sample it, or it may be possible to excise it in its entirety with an excisional biopsy technique. Frequently, small lesions can be excised completely with a punch or shave biopsy. Most punch biopsies do not require suturing, whereas excisional biopsies do. The curette technique can be used to sample a large lesion or to remove small, especially papular, lesions.

General Technique

1. Draw up 1 to 5 mL lidocaine with or without epinephrine, mixed with a 10:1 ratio of lidocaine to bicarbonate solution, 1 mEq/mL

(avoid use of epinephrine around the clitoral area). One may also use a small amount of a topical anesthetic such as 5% lidocaine cream (LMX5) applied with a cotton-tipped applicator to the area to be sampled. This is left on for 5 minutes before local anesthetic infiltration.
2. Identify the lesion.
3. Prepare the skin with a povidone-iodine or chlorhexidine swab or alcohol.
4. Following universal blood and body fluid precautions, inject around and under lesion with local anesthetic to raise the lesion (Fig. 139.3A).
5. Test skin with needle to be sure anesthesia is adequate (should be immediately effective).
6. Stretch the skin in direction opposite of skin tension lines in the vulvar area (i.e., stretch horizontally for a labial biopsy and stretch vertically for a perineal biopsy).
7. If using a blade, curette, or scissors to remove lesion, stay more superficial in non–hair-bearing areas.
8. If there is a choice of location, avoid biopsy from clitoris, labia minora, or urethra, if possible, because these are particularly sensitive areas. The closer the biopsy is taken to the rectum, the higher the risk of infection.

Technique for a Keyes Punch

The Keyes punch is a pen-sized instrument with a sharp, circular cutting edge that is used to cut tissue in a twisting motion.

1. To obtain deeper samples (e.g., hair-bearing areas), place punch over lesion perpendicular to the surface and slowly twist with minimal pressure on the punch instrument (let the cutting occur with the instrument; Fig. 139.3B).
2. Continue until you feel a give and the punch is loose from the surrounding tissues.
3. Gently grasp the edge of the lesion or the subcutaneous portion of the biopsy with the tissue forceps and lift up (avoid grasping the central portion of the lesion because this may cause crush artifact to the specimen).
4. Snip the base of the specimen with iris scissors and remove the biopsy sample (if multiple biopsies of the same lesion are obtained, each sample should be placed in its own container; Fig. 139.3C). Multiple biopsies may be necessary for a large lesion.
5. Apply a small amount of Monsel solution or aluminum chloride solution to the biopsy crater, using a small cotton-tipped applicator.
6. More resistant bleeding may be treated with a small piece of Gelfoam, silver nitrate, electrocautery, or an absorbable suture.
7. Wipe away any excess hemostatic agent or blood with saline-moistened gauze.

NOTE: After either a punch biopsy or an excisional biopsy, apply a small amount of antibacterial or petrolatum ointment to the biopsy site.

Technique for Using Cervical Punch Biopsy Forceps

1. Place the forceps jaws perpendicular to the surface of the lesion and grasp the skin. This will cause tenting of the skin (Fig. 139.3D).
2. Close the biopsy forceps to obtain the biopsy. The goal is to obtain approximately a 3-mm-wide and 3-mm-deep biopsy.
3. Apply a small amount of Monsel solution, silver nitrate, or aluminum chloride solution to the biopsy crater, using a small cotton-tipped applicator.
4. Wipe away any excess hemostatic agent or blood with saline-moistened gauze.

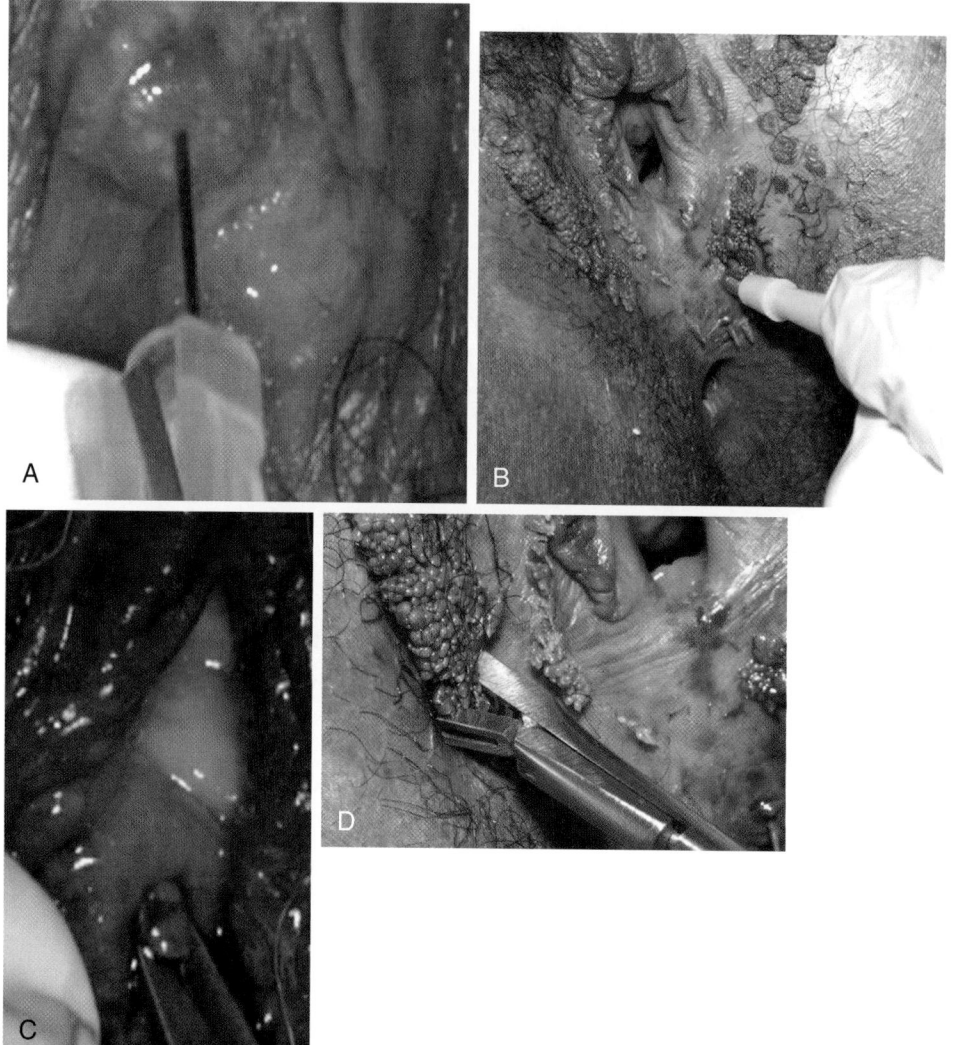

Fig. 139.3   Punch biopsy. (A) The lesion is anesthetized. (B) Biopsy is performed with a Keyes punch. (C) If a Keyes punch is used, once the skin is free from surrounding tissues, snip base with iris scissors. (D) Alternatively, biopsy is performed with a cervical biopsy forceps. (B and D, Courtesy Hope Haefner, MD.)

Technique for an Excisional Biopsy

Fig. 139.4 illustrates an excisional biopsy. See Chapter 26, Skin Biopsy, for further details on performing an excisional biopsy with repair.

COMMON ERRORS

- Not sampling the most advanced part of the lesion. If uncertain, take multiple biopsies for large lesions. An area that is more darkly pigmented and raised, or an area of leukoplakia, is usually more advanced.
- Taking too deep of a sample. Use careful technique to take only the depth of specimen necessary.

COMPLICATIONS

The following complications are extremely rare:

- Inadequate sample resulting in need to repeat procedure
- Infection
- Bleeding, hematoma, ecchymosis
- Hypopigmentation
- Pain
- Scar
- Recurrence
- Hyperpigmentation from Monsel solution (usually temporary)
- Misdiagnosis or failure to diagnose

POSTPROCEDURE PATIENT EDUCATION

Instruct the patient to perform the following after the procedure:

- Wash the area twice a day with soap and water. Showers are permitted 24 hours after a wound is sutured.
- Apply antibiotic or petrolatum ointment after each cleansing.
- Use acetaminophen or ibuprofen for discomfort (first determine any contraindications to the use of these medications in the patient).
- Take sitz baths as needed for discomfort if extensive removals are performed.
- Use ice packs as needed.
- For more recalcitrant pain, use over-the-counter benzocaine gel (toothache-type pain reliever) as needed.
- Call if there is persistent pain, redness, or swelling.
- Avoid intercourse until discomfort is gone (usually 3 to 5 days).
- Arrange a follow-up appointment or phone call to discuss biopsy results.

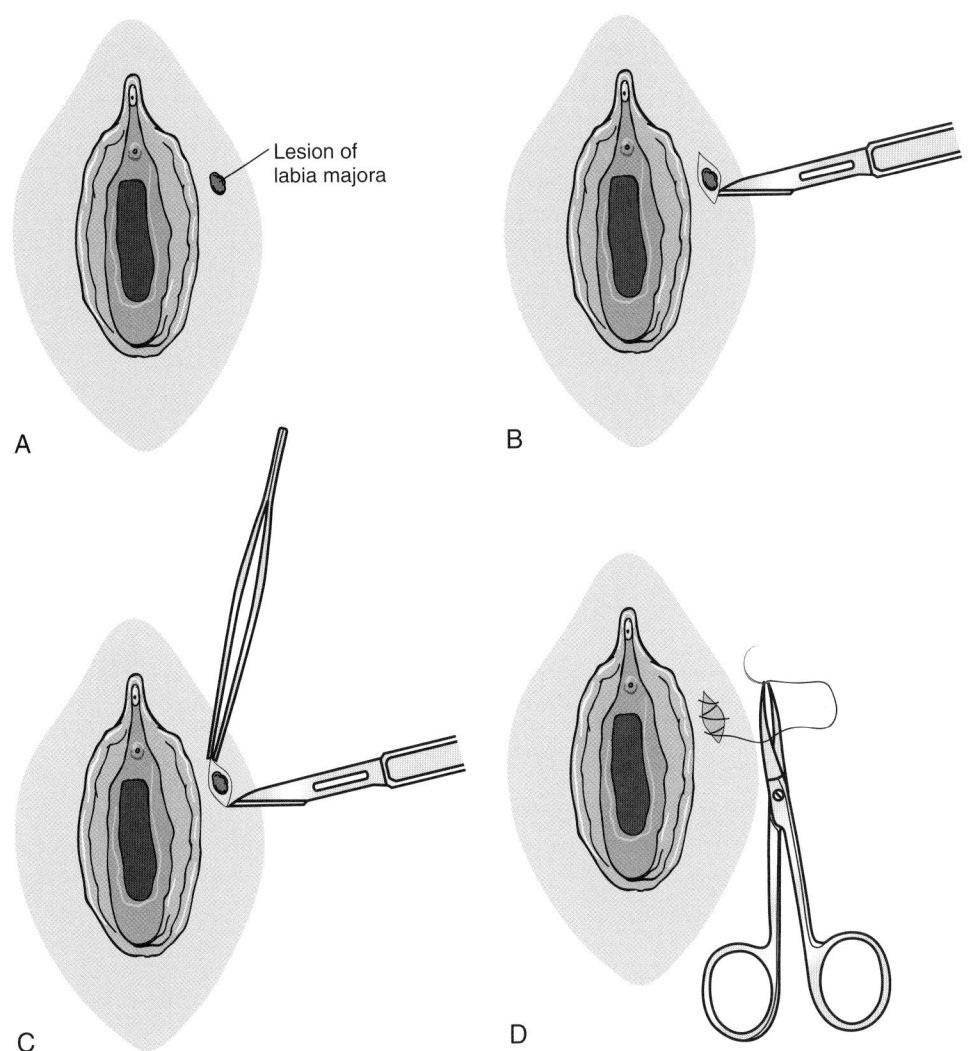

A

B

C

D

Fig. 139.4 Excisional biopsy. (A) Lesion of labia majora. (B) After anesthesia, an elliptical incision is made along skin tension lines. (C) Scalpel is used to free base from apex toward center of excised area. (D) Skin is closed with subcuticular running absorbable suture.

PATIENT EDUCATION GUIDES

See patient education and patient consent forms available at www.expertconsult.com.

CPT/BILLING CODES

56501	Destruction benign lesion vulva, single
56515	Destruction benign lesion vulva, extensive
56605	Biopsy of vulva or perineum (one lesion)
56606	Biopsy of each additional vulvar or perineal lesion

For complete excisional removals, also see excision codes.

ICD-10-CM DIAGNOSTIC CODES

A63.0	Condyloma acuminatum
D28.0	Benign vulvar neoplasm
D07.1	VIN III
N76.2	Vulvitis
N90.0	Vulvar intraepithelial neoplasia I (VIN I)
N90.1	VIN II
N90.9	Unspecified noninflammatory disorder of vulva and perineum
L91.8	Skin tag

RECOMMENDED READING

Apgar BS, Brotzman GL, Spitzer M, eds. *Colposcopy: Principles and Practice.* 2nd ed. Philadelphia: Saunders; 2008.

Apgar BS, Cox JT. Differentiating normal and abnormal finding of the vulva. *Am Family Physician.* 1996;53:1171–1180.

Bornstein J, Bogliatto F, Haefner HK, Stockdale CK, Preti M, Bohl TG, et al. The 2015 International Society for the Study of Vulvovaginal Disease (ISSVD) terminology of vulvar squamous intraepithelial lesions. ISSVD terminology committee. *Obstet Gynecol.* 2016;127:264–268.

Committee Opinion No, 675. Management of vulvar intraepithelial neoplasia. American College of Obstetricians and Gynecologists. *Obstet Gynecol.* 2016;128:178–182.

Hacker NF. Vulvar and vaginal cancer. In: Hacker NF, Gambone JC, Hobel JC, eds. *Hacker and Moore's Essentials of Obstetrics and Gynecology.* 6th ed. Philadelphia: Elsevier; 2016:449–456.

Rock J, Jones III H, eds. *Te Linde's Operative Gynecology.* 10th ed. Philadelphia: Lippincott Williams & Wilkins; 2009.

Tuggy M, Garcia J. *Procedures Consult.* Vulvar biopsy. http://www.proceduresconsult.com/medical-procedures/vulvar-biopsy-FM-021-procedure.aspx.

Wheeless Jr C, Roenneburg M. *Atlas of Pelvic Surgery.* www.atlasofpelvicsurgery.com/home.html.

CHAPTER 140

Treatment of the Adult Victim of Sexual Assault

Olasunkanmi W. Adeyinka

Current statistics indicate that a sexual assault occurs every 4 seconds in the United States. One in every four women will be sexually assaulted in her lifetime. The lifetime prevalence of sexual assault in the United States is approximately 18% to 19% in women and 2% to 3% in men. Sexual assault is the fastest-growing, most frequently committed, and most underreported violent crime in the United States. Sexual assault is a crime of violence and aggression, and encompasses a continuum of sexual activity that ranges from sexual coercion to contact abuse (unwanted kissing, touching, or fondling) to rape. In 2013, the definition of rape was changed to "penetration, no matter how slight, of the vagina or anus with any body part or object, or oral penetration by a sex organ of another person, without the consent of the victim" and has been broadened to include male victims, though this still excludes statutory rape.

Sexual assault is underreported for many reasons, including societal misconceptions about the victims of sexual assault, feelings invoked by such an assault, and the burden of reporting an assault. Misconceptions persist, despite enhanced public education, that individuals who are assaulted may have encouraged the act by their behavior, dress, lack of resistance, or previous promiscuity. Complex law enforcement and health care systems are often perceived as being impersonal and nonsupportive. An estimated 75% of victims know their perpetrators, possibly enhancing feelings of embarrassment, guilt, and fear of retribution. These feelings and misconceptions combined with inadequate support systems often prevent a victim from reporting a sexual assault.

The purpose of the medical evaluation after sexual assault is to assess the patient for physical injuries, to document injuries, and to collect the necessary evidence. The remainder of the encounter should be used to treat any injuries, to prevent pregnancy and disease, and to find the proper support services for the victim. The examination and treatment should be completed as soon as possible after the assault, especially the collection of evidence. Although an evaluation within 48 hours is preferred, victims are encouraged to see a clinician even if more than 72 hours have elapsed (this still allows a clinician to treat and prevent many problems).

Collaboration between hospitals, community services, and local law enforcement agencies for the establishment of protocols is very helpful, and such protocols will ease victims' pain and suffering. Primary care clinicians can be instrumental in ensuring that this collaboration takes place. Such collaboration is effective at not only streamlining the evaluation process but for easing the burden of reporting. Sexual assault response teams (SARTs) have become available in many communities since the 1990s. If a SART is not available, many institutions have specially trained providers available to perform a sexual assault assessment and some with a 24-hour availability of specially trained and experienced volunteers, such as a nurse on every shift. These volunteers can provide the victim continuous support during the cumbersome process of answering questions and the examination. They can also act as witnesses for the chain of evidence. A supportive volunteer system can offer such simple things as a change of clothing (victims often need to leave their clothing as evidence), which are hugely appreciated by victims.

INDICATION

Sexual assault
NOTE: Sexual assault is any form of nonconsenting sexual activity. It encompasses all unwanted sexual acts, from fondling to forcible penetration.

CONTRAINDICATION

A lack of patient consent.

EQUIPMENT AND SUPPLIES

- Camera and film (medical institutions may supply professional photographic teams; others must rely on law enforcement for photo documentation)
- Wood's light or other high wavelength light
- Sexual assault kit: Most emergency departments have a standard kit that contains a protocol for care and all the necessary specimen containers. These should be in compliance with and fulfill state laws for sexual assault (Table 140.1). In general, kits should contain the following:
  - Information for the victim
  - Consent form for the examination
  - Instructions, checklist, and chain of custody form
  - History and physical examination forms
  - Diagrams for use in documentation of injuries (Fig 140.1)
  - Specimen containers, equipment, and labels
- Toluidine dye (not always available)
- Colposcope (optional)

PREPROCEDURE PATIENT EDUCATION

If a patient calls before presenting to the emergency department, first make sure that the patient is safe. If not, encourage the patient to call the police. Next, encourage the patient not to take a bath or remove the clothing worn during the assault. If possible, they should postpone urinating, defecating, brushing their teeth, or drinking anything until samples are collected. Also, ask them to bring a change of clothing. Patients should sign for informed consent before starting the evaluation (see the patient consent form available at www.expertconsult.com).

Explain the process of the evaluation to patients. Let them know that you will explain every step of the examination before performing it. Even if they may not want to report the assault, a very thorough

TABLE 140.1	Sexual Assault Kit Equipment*	
Contents	**Purpose**
Two urine containers	Urine for microscopic urinalysis, pregnancy test, and drug screen
Fingernail clippers, file, and envelope	Fingernail clippings and scrapings
Forceps, scissors, two envelopes	Pubic hair trimming in one envelope, head hair trimming in other envelope
Plastic comb, large paper towel, two envelopes	Pubic hair combing in one envelope, head hair combing in other envelope
Vaginal speculum, aspiration pipette, red-topped test tube and stopper	Aspiration of vaginal contents
Four cotton-tipped swabs and a test tube or envelope, one slide	Vaginal (or penile) swabbing, and smear (same for rectal swabbing and smear if indicated)
Saline, 10 mL; two aspiration pipettes and bulbs; two test tubes, two slides	Vaginal washing (and rectal if indicated using second pipette and test tube)
Cervical scraper, brush, slides, Pap smear fixative	Pap smear
Four cotton-tipped swabs and a test tube or envelope, one slide	Oral swabs and smear
Two cotton-tipped swabs and a test tube or envelope	Saliva collection for secretor status
Three red-topped test tubes and stoppers, tourniquet, nonalcohol swab to prepare skin, syringe and needle	Blood samples
Labeled paper bags	Collection of clothing and dried body fluids
Necessary and helpful forms	Information, consent, and documentation
Patient education handout	
Consent form	
History and physical examination form	
Diagrams for documentation of injuries	
Chain of custody form	
Any necessary instructions	
Checklist	

*Contents should be refrigerated after collection.

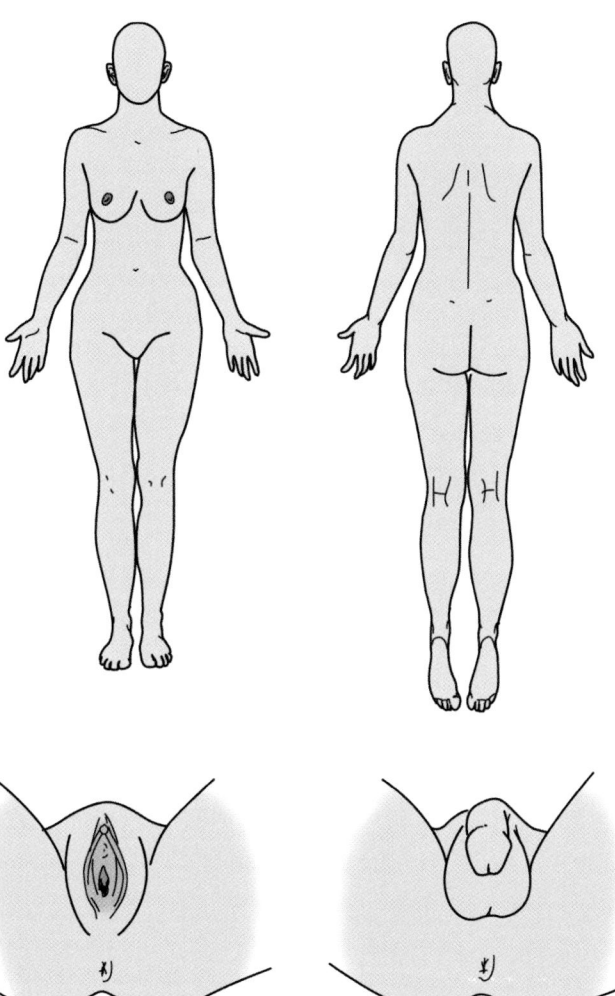

Fig. 140.1   Traumagram. Mark and label locations where there is evidence of trauma.

examination is necessary in case of a later change of mind. Continue to reassure patients that they are safe and that someone else will always be in the room to comfort them during the evaluation.

PROCEDURE

1. Open the sexual assault kit. Once the kit is opened, the chain of evidence must be maintained and evidence must not be left unattended. Signatures of those in attendance must be documented on the form for any and all evidence collected. (See Chapter 170, Management of the Young Female as a Possible Victim of Sexual Abuse, Fig 170.8, for a sample chain of evidence form.) The kit should be labeled as a biohazard. After the patient has signed the consent form, proceed with taking the history.

History

2. The history should be taken in a quiet room, with a witness present, after the patient has been assured that she or he is safe. Be cautious about the terms used in stating patient complaints. Avoid use of the word "rape" because this is a legal term. Instead, state the patient complaint as being a "sexual assault." Also, try to avoid the phrases "why didn't you …" or "you shouldn't have …" or "Did you do anything to lead them on?" In fact, try to avoid the words "why" and "alleged" altogether; "why" implies blame and "alleged" implies disbelief.

   Questions should be directed to the victim in a nonjudgmental way, and the patient should be allowed to talk about the assault at a comfortable pace, using her or his own words. It is important to observe nonverbal communication that may indicate a need for further questioning. Supportive terms worth using include "I'm glad you're alive," "You did what you needed to survive," "I'm sorry this happened to you," and "It was not your fault." Allow the victim to express her or his feelings. To build rapport, it may be worth obtaining the medical and sexual history before obtaining the assault history.

NOTE: If you have a long-term relationship with the patient, the patient may prefer to be examined in your office. However, in many jurisdictions, legally admissible evidence of a sexual assault cannot be collected without using the kit and other resources that are often available only in the emergency department. It is important for practitioners to know the assault and rape laws in their state so that they can comply with any legal requirements.

Medical and Sexual History (Gynecologic History for Women)

- Medical disease, if present, should be documented.
- Last voluntary sexual encounter up to 1 week before the assault and the race of that individual should be documented. If the encounter is less than 48 hours ago, blood and fluid samples may be requested from that individual at a later date.
- The victim's alcohol and drug intake should be documented.
- For women, the date of the victim's last menstrual period, her contraceptive use, pregnancy history, use of tampons, and any previous pelvic surgery or recent sexually transmitted infection (STI) should be documented.

Assault History

An accurate but brief description of the assault is crucial for proper collection and analysis of the physical evidence. This includes documenting the following:

- Age and identifying information for victim, and assailant(s), if available.
- Date, time, and location of the alleged assault.
- Details of sexual contact, such as actual or attempted oral, rectal, or vaginal penetration of the victim. Attempt to determine

whether there was an ejaculation, digital penetration, or penetration with foreign objects. It should be documented whether a tampon was present, or if a lubricant, contraceptive foam, a spermicide, or a condom was used. If any of these are unknown, that should be documented.

- Type of physical restraints used, if any, and whether there were any threats, weapons, drugs, or alcohol involved. Was there a loss of consciousness? Was the assailant injured during the assault?
- Activities of the victim after the assault, such as changing clothes, wiping, washing, bathing, douching, dental hygiene, urination, vomiting, smoking, eating, drinking, or defecation.

Physical Examination

Suggested terminology for describing examination findings includes the TEARS categorization: tears (defined as any break in tissue including fissures and lacerations), ecchymoses, abrasions, redness, and swelling.

3. Having a trained, experienced volunteer in the room in addition to the nurse may help distract the victim from her or his emotional and physical pain during the examination. The physical examination and collection of evidence are performed congruently. Carefully examine the entire body and photograph or make drawings of the injured areas (see Fig 140.1). The clinician should search for bruises, abrasions, or lacerations about the head, neck, back, buttocks, and extremities. A victim who was choked may have petechiae on the face and conjunctiva. Physical trauma may be greater in sexually assaulted men, perhaps because only those who have been more seriously injured are likely to report the crime.

4. Examine the oral cavity. Broken teeth, a torn frenulum of the tongue or lip, or pharyngeal trauma may indicate that the mouth was forced open. Using two swabs simultaneously, swab the oral cavity and along the teeth for evidence of semen. Do not moisten the swabs before sample collection.

   Repeat with two additional swabs. Prepare one smear on the slide by gently smearing the swabs over the surface. Allow the swabs and smear to air dry. Place swabs in envelope or test tube provided. Local law enforcement may want an additional swab for victim DNA evidence.

5. The victim's clothing should be collected and placed in a paper bag that is sealed and signed. Allow any wet clothing to air dry before packaging. If additional bags are needed, use only new paper (grocery-type) bags.

   It may be helpful to photograph the patient before she or he disrobes. Semen may appear as flaking, crusty stains on clothing and will fluoresce under a high wavelength light. Have the patient disrobe while standing on paper from the examination table. Each item of clothing should be placed in a separate paper bag. Do not use plastic bags for clothing collection because they promote bacterial growth on blood or semen. Use gloves when touching the victim's clothes to avoid contaminating the evidence with your DNA or blood type from sweat.

6. For women, a pelvic examination should be performed with the victim in the lithotomy to complete the physical examination. Using both hands, the examiner can use a technique of separation and traction to evaluate the tissues most likely injured. Lesions around the vulva or rectum may be present because of trauma from a hand, penis, or other foreign body. Superficial or extensive lacerations of the hymen and vagina, injury of the urethra, and, occasionally, rupture of the vaginal wall may be present. Swab and preserve any semen for later DNA analysis. Although historically recommended and still used in many locations, a Wood's lamp does not cause semen to fluoresce more than other commonly found substances. Al-

ternative light sources with a higher wavelength may be more effective than the traditional Wood's lamp. The procedure is as follows:

- Lubricate the speculum with water. Standard lubricants may adversely affect the results of the acid phosphatase test and alter sperm motility. Examine the vaginal wall and cervix for abrasions, ecchymoses, and lacerations. A colposcope may be helpful to document any microtrauma to the cervix or vagina. It can also be used to take photographs. The cervix should be swabbed with four swabs and a smear prepared in a manner similar to the oral swabs. The swabs should be allowed to air dry before sealing. The crime lab may recover sperm from cervical specimens up to 12 days after coitus.
- A Pap smear should be performed. Intact spermatozoa may be seen several days later on a Pap smear.
- Any fluid from the posterior fornix should be aspirated and examined under the microscope. A sample of the aspirated fluid should be saved for DNA testing, as well as for testing for acid phosphatase and blood group antigens.
- If no secretions are visible, a small amount of saline (about 5 mL) may be used to lavage the cervix and posterior fornix. Aspirate this fluid and save while using some to prepare slides. Examine the slides under the microscope for spermatozoa. Lavage with normal saline may enhance motility of spermatozoa for up to 2 hours. Motile sperm from the vagina imply intercourse within the past 6 hours (rarely within the past 12 hours) and their presence should be documented. Immotile sperm imply intercourse within the past 12 to 18 hours (in rare cases, up to 24 hours). In addition to examining for spermatozoa with a wet smear, the slide should be examined for *Trichomonas*, bacterial vaginosis, and the presence of any *Candida* species.

7. The victim's pubic hair should be combed to detect foreign bodies, as well as for perpetrator pubic hair samples. Place clean paper below the victim's buttocks with the victim in the lithotomy position and comb the pubic hair onto the paper. Fold these hairs and the comb into the paper provided and place them in the large envelope to be given to law enforcement. If present, 15 to 20 perpetrator hairs should be collected as part of the evidence. In a separate container, 15 to 20 of the victim's trimmed pubic hairs should be saved. This process should be repeated for head hair, using separate specimen containers.

8. Bimanual and rectal examinations should be performed. Anal assault is more common in men. Look for erythema, edema, bleeding, mucosal tears, fissures, a hematoma, or sphincter laxity or spasm. The digital rectal examination is usually sufficient if nothing suspect is palpated and bleeding is absent or insignificant.

9. Anoscopy or proctoscopy are difficult for the patient, but may be required if you suspect a tear. If anal intercourse is known to have occurred, four anal swabs should be used and a smear prepared in a manner similar to the oral swabs. Anal swabs can be moistened with sterile normal saline before using, if necessary. They should be allowed to air dry before sealing. (Penile swabs and smears can be performed in the same manner by swabbing the outside of the penile shaft.)

Next, wash the rectal vault with 5 to 10 mL of normal saline introduced through the anus with the hub of a syringe. Allow the saline to stand for 5 to 10 minutes, then aspirate and preserve as evidence. These samples can be examined for motile sperm, immotile sperm, and acid phosphatase. Fecal contamination precludes their use for blood group antigen analysis.

10. Toluidine dye (1% aqueous solution) is a nuclear stain that highlights areas of injury. The nucleated cells beneath denuded epithelium (from trauma) take up the dye and can enhance the examiner's ability to visualize and photographically document more subtle genital or anal injuries. It should be applied before speculum or anoscopy exam to avoid documenting inadvertent injury from these instruments. Apply the dye to the perineum or anal folds using a swab; excess dye is then removed with a cotton ball moistened with water-soluble lubricating jelly. Allow to dry for approximately a minute; any areas that retain the dye indicate a disruption of the epidermis, most likely due to injury. The dye will fade in 1 to 2 days. Do not use the dye in the vaginal vault or on mucous membranes.

NOTE: Pelvic, rectal, and proctoscopic examinations should be done gently and with careful explanation because the victim not only may experience severe discomfort because of the local trauma but may experience flashbacks.

Medical management of adult male victims of sexual violence with regard to the physical examination and medical interventions:

- Male victims of sexual violence should be triaged in the same manner as female victims.
- The same procedures for obtaining consent, taking a history, conducting the physical examination (although the genital examination will be different), and ordering diagnostic laboratory tests should be followed, that is: perform a top-to-toe examination looking for any signs of injury; conduct a thorough examination of the genitoanal area; treat any injuries (men also need to be treated for STIs, hepatitis B, and tetanus).
- Men need to be informed about, and offered, an HIV test and the option of postexposure prophylaxis, if available. Men also need to receive follow-up care for wound healing, any prescribed treatments (including those for STIs), completion of medications, and counseling.

Laboratory Tests

11. Obtain fingernail clippings and scrapings. These may harbor bits of the assailant's blood, skin, or hair. Photographs of bite marks may also be used to match dental records.

12. Saliva samples should be taken. The victim should not be allowed to smoke or eat for 30 minutes before taking a sample. If there is trauma to the mouth, this procedure should be delayed until the wound is healed. The swabs should be allowed to air dry before sealing. They should not be removed from the victim's mouth by anyone other than the victim or the examiner.

13. Guided by the history of the assault, the victim's symptoms, and any local protocol, determine which laboratory tests are appropriate. Recommended laboratory tests in all cases of sexual assault include the following:
    - The patient's blood type should be determined from blood or saliva swabs. Some crime labs will also request blood samples for DNA reference, toxicology analysis, or both.
    - For women, a urine or serum β-human chorionic gonadotropin pregnancy test at the initial examination is needed to rule out existing pregnancy.
    - The Centers for Disease Control and Prevention suggests obtaining a cervical, rectal, and oral specimen for culture, polymerase chain reaction, or both for chlamydia and gonorrhea. However, the majority of SART programs in the United States do not routinely perform these tests. STI testing during sexual assault examination can detect only infection before the assault and provides no meaningful information for the crime laboratory. Prophylaxis for sexually transmitted diseases will also going to be provided, making these tests superfluous.

Treatment

14. Treatment of major or life-threatening injuries should occur before initiating the evaluation. After the patient is stable, treatment of other physical injuries should depend on the type sustained.

15. STI prevention
    - Antibiotic prophylaxis: The current recommendation for the treatment of trichomoniasis, bacterial vaginosis, gonorrhea, and chlamydial infection is 250 mg of ceftriaxone intramuscularly or cefixime 400 mg orally and 2 g of metronidazole orally and either 100 mg of oral doxycycline twice daily for 7 days or 1 g of oral azithromycin once. Doxycycline should not be prescribed for pregnant patients.
    - Ceftriaxone treats incubating syphilis; the World Health Organization considers a 2 g dose of azithromycin effective treatment against incubating syphilis. Although the overall risk of acquiring an STI from a single sexual encounter is only 5% to 20% (gonorrhea 6% to 18%, chlamydial infection 4% to 17%, syphilis 0.5% to 3%, HIV <1%), the aforementioned treatment should be prescribed for all victims of sexual assault.
    - Hepatitis B prophylaxis: If the patient has not been immunized, hepatitis B virus vaccine should be given at the initial visit, then repeated at 1 and 6 months. Hepatitis B immunoglobulin 0.06 mL intramuscularly should be offered if the assailant is thought to be in a high-risk group for hepatitis B and the victim has experienced vaginal or anal bleeding from the assault. The same dose can be repeated in 1 month if the victim's serology is negative.
    - HIV prophylaxis is not universally recommended. However, it should be understood that if the assailant cannot be apprehended and tested (most cases), the victim's infection status may not be known for 6 months. Treatment should be tailored to the patient's needs after counseling for medication costs and potential toxicity. If the suspect is known or suspected to be HIV positive, treat with medications recommended by local infections disease experts or consider Combivir (2 times a day) or Truvada (once a day) for 28 days. If the suspect is not known to be HIV positive, there is no consensus on recommendations for treatment; clinicians must consider each patient individually. In a non–assault-related scenario, the risk of transmission of HIV from one episode of unprotected consensual receptive vaginal intercourse with an infected individual is approximately 1 in 1000. The risk with unprotected receptive anal intercourse is 8 to 32 per 1000. This may be higher in sexual assault victims because of the injuries sustained because of the violent nature of the act.
    - The human papillomavirus (HPV) vaccine is approved for females and males age 9 to 26 years, and the series can be initiated at this visit.
    - Tetanus prophylaxis is indicated for anyone not immunized in the past 5 years.
16. For women, if the pregnancy test is negative, pregnancy prevention should be offered. Pregnancy occurs in up to 4.7% of sexual assault victims. See Chapter 115, Emergency Contraception, for available methods and dosing. These treatments are most effective for prevention of pregnancy if used within 72 hours of intercourse.

NOTE: Because up to half of all victims do not report for their follow-up visits, it is very important to perform adequate prophylaxis on patients during the initial visit.

Follow-up

17. The patient should have a follow-up visit with a clinician within 72 hours to again document bruising. Follow-up counseling referrals should be made at the first visit. An additional follow-up visit should be made at 1 to 2 weeks to monitor patient progress (and to evaluate for pregnancy in women) as a result of the assault. If the patient did not receive prophylaxis for infection, STI testing should be performed or repeated at this 1- to 2-week follow-up visit. If the patient received prophylaxis, repeat testing is indicated only if the patient is symptomatic. For women who are pregnant, counseling can be initiated and appropriate options for care can be discussed. HIV, hepatitis B, hepatitis C, and syphilis testing can be repeated or performed at 4 to 6 months.

POSTPROCEDURE PATIENT EDUCATION

Sexual assault is associated with major emotional and psychologic sequelae. Most women go through the three stages of rape trauma syndrome: (1) trauma (e.g., fear of being alone, fear of men, sexual problems, depression); (2) denial (not wanting to talk about it); and (3) resolution (dealing with fears and feelings, regaining a sense of control over life). During the first two stages, patients may experience flashbacks, numbness or constriction of feeling, or hypervigilance. Mood swings, irritability, and anger are common and may indicate signs of healing. Insomnia, tension headaches, anorexia, fatigue, nausea, abdominal pain, and genitourinary symptoms are not uncommon. The last stage may take years to reach. The patient should be aware that should the case go to court, it may be necessary to gather additional evidence at a later time. Adequate follow-up and a counseling referral are an essential component of management. Men go through similar stages and need similar counseling.

Patients should receive a written outline of what was performed with the initial evaluation and what treatments were provided. They should also be given a written list of specific instructions and follow-up appointments. It should be written because most assault victims will not remember the evaluation and treatment they received, much less the instructions they were given after the treatment. Many communities have sexual assault centers that will provide advocates and support personnel for the victims during medical visits and for follow-up appointments. If this is not available or feasible, after obtaining the victim's permission, a trained counselor should be consulted. The most important contributing factor to the patient's recovery is contact with a trained advocate or counselor within the first 72 hours of a sexual assault.

The Rape, Assault and Incest National Network (RAINN; phone: 1-800-656-HOPE; website: www.rainn.org) can assist with finding local agencies and counselors trained to assist sexual assault victims.

PATIENT EDUCATION GUIDES

See the patient education and consent forms available at www.expertconsult.com.

CPT/BILLING CODES

Use E/M codes for established or new patients for the noncolposcopic portion of the examination.

57452	Colposcopy

In some states, the law enforcement agency is required to pay for the evidence collection examination in the case of a reported sexual assault. The patient should sign a consent form to allow the law enforcement agency to be billed.

ICD-10-CM DIAGNOSTIC CODES

S31.40XX	Unspecified open wound, vagina and vulva
S31.41XX	Laceration w/o foreign body of vagina and vulva
S31.42XX	Laceration w/ foreign body of vagina and vulva
T74.21XX	Adult sexual abuse confirmed
T76.21XX	Adult sexual abuse suspected
T76.11Xx	Adult physical abuse suspected
Z01.419	Encounter for gynecologic examination, (general) (routine) without abnormal findings

SUPPLIERS

(See contact information available at www.expertconsult.com.)

Sexual assault evidence collection kit
  MediTech International
  Sirchie Fingerprint Laboratories, Inc. (standardized kit available that fulfills laws for many western states)
  Lynn Peavey Company

ONLINE RESOURCES

American College of Emergency Physicians. *Evaluation and management of the sexually assaulted or sexually abused patient.* 2nd ed. Atlanta: U.S. Department of Health and Human Services; 2013. http://bookstore.acep.org/evaluation-and-management-of-the-sexually-assaulted-or-sexually-abused-patient-314500.

Centers for Disease Control and Prevention: Sexual assault and STDs. https://www.cdc.gov/std/tg2015/sexual-assault.htm.

World Health Organization Guidelines Violence and Injury Prevention, Adult Victims Sexual Violence. http://www.who.int/violence_injury_prevention/resources/publications/en/guidelines_chap4.pdf

RECOMMENED READING

Abrahams N, Devries K, Watts C, et al. Worldwide prevalence of non-partner sexual violence: a systematic review. *Lancet.* 2014;383:1648.

American College of Emergency Physicians. *Management of the Patient with the Complaint of Sexual Assault*; 2014. https://www.acep.org/content.aspx?id=29562.

Anderson A. "Don't scream, Miss Annie. Don't scream." *Am Fam Physician.* 1999;59:213–214.

Centers for Disease Control and Prevention. Sexually transmitted diseases treatment guidelines 2015. *MMWR.* 2015;64:1–137.

Dunn S. Lavage fluid in sexual assault examination. *CMAJ.* 1988;138:400.

Holmes MM, Resnick HS, Frampton D. Follow-up of sexual assault victims. *Am J Obstet Gynecol.* 1998;179:336–342.

Lenahan LC, Ernst A, Johnson B. Colposcopy in evaluation of the adult sexual assault victim. *Am J Emerg Med.* 1998;16:183–184.

Luce H, Schrager S, Gilchrist V. Sexual assault of women. *Am Fam Physician.* 2010;81:489–495.

Nelson DG, Santucci KA. An alternate light source to detect semen. *Acad Emerg Med.* 2002;9:1045–1048.

Sachs CJ, Wheeler M. Examination of the sexual assault victim. In: Roberts JR, Custalow CB, Thomsen TW, eds. *Roberts and Hedges Clinical Procedures in Emergency Medicine and Acute Care.* 7th ed. Philadelphia: Elsevier; 2019:1225–1241.

Usatine RP. *The Color Atlas of Family Medicine.* New York: McGraw-Hill; 2009.

White C. Genital injuries in adults. *Best Pract Res Clin Obstet Gynaecol.* 2013;27:113.

Young WW, Bracken AC, Goddard MA, Matheson S. Sexual assault: review of a national model protocol for forensic and medical evaluation. *Obstet Gynecol.* 1992;80:878–883.

SECTION 10

Obstetrics

Section Editor: BETH A. CHOBY

CHAPTER 141

POSTCOITAL TEST (SIMS-HUHNER TEST)

Julie M. Sicilia

The postcoital test (PCT) evaluates the survival and motility of sperm in the cervical mucus. The PCT detects whether sperm are present in the ejaculate and cervical mucus; it is not a diagnostic test for cervical factor infertility. The PCT should be used in conjunction with semen analysis, not as a substitute for it. Validity of the PCT has been questioned because of the lack of reproducibility and universal standards for obtaining and interpreting samples. The role of the PCT as part of the infertility workup is greatly debated. A 1998 randomized controlled trial concluded that routine PCT for infertile couples increased the amount of testing but did not increase the pregnancy rate for the couples. More recent studies suggest that the PCT may be helpful for identifying patients that can be offered expectant management rather than proceeding directly to intrauterine insemination (IUI) or assisted reproductive technologies.

INDICATIONS

- Investigation of the sperm and cervical mucus interaction
- Monitoring the cervical mucus during the first ovulatory cycle of treatment with clomiphene citrate for couples planning timed intercourse infertility treatment
- To assist in deciding if a couple is a candidate for expectant management versus aggressive therapy ([IUI] or in vitro fertilization [IVF]) with suspected cervical factor infertility

CONTRAINDICATIONS

- Any condition that precludes unprotected sexual intercourse followed by examination and sampling of the cervix
- Active vaginal infection

EQUIPMENT

- Nonsterile examination gloves
- Vaginal speculum (no lubricant) and swabs
- Tuberculin syringe with cap
- Ring forceps
- Microscope, slides, and coverslips
- Plastic endometrial aspirator (optional)

PREPROCEDURE PATIENT EDUCATION

- One month prior to PCT, the patient should measure daily basal body temperature (BBT) or undergo urinary luteinizing hormone ovulation testing. Review the BBT or luteinizing hormone graphs to determine optimal timing for intercourse. Have the patient watch for clear cervical mucus (more estrogenic). (See Chapter 117, Fertility Awareness–Based Methods of Contraception [Natural Family Planning].) The PCT should be performed as near as possible to ovulation. With an ideal 28-day cycle, the test is usually performed on day 12 to 14.

- The couple should abstain from intercourse or masturbation for 48 hours prior to testing. Before performing the PCT, determine that the BBT is in accord with the proper timing of the menstrual cycle for the performance of the test. Nothing (lubricants, medications, douches, etc.) should be placed in the vagina 24 hours prior to and up to the time of the PCT.
- Instruct the patient to come to the office 6 to 10 hours after intercourse.

PROCEDURE

1. Have the patient lie in dorsal lithotomy position. Insert a vaginal speculum (without lubricant) and visualize the cervix. Gently wipe the cervix with a vaginal swab.
2. Insert a tuberculin syringe (without the needle) into the endocervical canal and retract the plunger to draw the mucus into the syringe (collect at least 0.2 mL of mucus). An endometrial aspirator may make this collection easier. Place the syringe cap over the hub of the syringe once the sample is obtained so that the mucus is stored in an airtight container until it is ready for processing.
3. Record the amount and clarity of the mucus.
4. Record the degree of mucus stretchability (i.e., spinnbarkeit). A ring forceps may be used to grasp the mucus at the cervical os to measure its stretch as the forceps is removed from the vagina. The mucus can also be placed between the index finger and thumb of the examiner's hand with the stretch determined as the fingers are drawn apart. A normal mucus stretch greater than 5 to 10 cm indicates a high estrogenic state. A spinnbarkeit of less than 3 cm lessens the likelihood that sperm could penetrate through the mucus, indicating an unfavorable situation for fertilization.
5. Place a drop of the mucus from the syringe on a glass slide and immediately place a coverslip over the sample. Examine the cervical mucus under low power for the presence of sperm and other components, such as trichomonads, leukocytes, squamous cells, or *Candida*. Make a note of the number of sperm. Examine the specimen under high power. The number of sperm in at least five different fields should be averaged. Record an average number or range of numbers of sperm present. Note whether the sperm are mobile, whether they have normal or abnormal morphology, and, if possible, whether they exhibit forward progression (rotatory or shaky motion of the sperm suggest presence of antisperm antibodies). For a normal (positive) study, in specimens examined 6 to 10 hours postintercourse, there should be an average of at least 5 to 10 actively motile sperm per high-power field. Actively moving sperm are facilitated by the presence of optimal cervical mucus. A decrease in the quality of the cervical mucus and an increase in viscosity and cellularity caused by rising postovulatory progesterone levels impair sperm survival. The presence of ferning, increased elasticity, and decreased viscosity of the cervical mucus is an indirect indication of estrogen production and ovulation.

COMMON ERRORS

The primary cause of an inconclusive or abnormal (negative) PCT is failure to accurately time the test. PCTs are also usually abnormal in anovulatory cycles. If the initial PCT yields poor results, a second test should be performed 1 to 3 hours after intercourse in the next menstrual cycle month.

COMPLICATIONS

Falsely abnormal results can be due to poor timing of the menstrual cycle, poor mucus quality because of infection, coital positions not favoring vaginal sperm retention, low semen volume, or low numbers of sperm. Although a normal PCT is encouraging, an inadequate test does not necessarily preclude fertilization.

POSTPROCEDURE PATIENT EDUCATION

If the test is inconclusive or abnormal, the PCT may be repeated. IUI or IVF, although expensive, are readily available in the United States. IUI and IVF bypass cervical mucus/sperm interaction abnormalities and should be offered to couples as a treatment option when indicated, especially in couples wanting multiple pregnancies or older couples (>35 years old).

INTERPRETATION OF RESULTS

A normal result is 5 or more motile sperm per high-power field. The mucus should also be thin, clear, and have a stretch of more than 5 cm.

CPT/BILLING CODES

89300	Semen analysis; presence or motility (or both) of sperm, including Huhner test

ICD-10-CM DIAGNOSTIC CODES

N46.01	Infertility, male (due to azoospermia)
N46.11	Oligospermia
N46.9	Infertility, male, unspecified
N97.8	Infertility, female (due to cervical origin)
N97.9	Infertility, female (of unspecified origin)

RECOMMENDED READING

American Society for Reproductive Medicine. Optimal evaluation of the infertile female. A practice committee report. *Fertil Steril.* 2012;98: 302–307.

Check JH. A practical approach to diagnosing and treating infertility by the generalist in obstetrics and gynecology. *Clin Exp Obstet Gynecol.* 2015;42(4):405–410.

Glazener CM, Ford WC, Hull MG. The prognostic power of the postcoital test for natural conception depends on duration of infertility. *Hum Reprod.* 2000;15:1953–1957.

Hessel M, Brandes M, De Bruin JP, et al. Long-term ongoing pregnancy rate and mode of conception after a positive and negative post-coital test. *Acta Obstet Gynecol Scand.* 2014;93:913–920.

Oei SG, Helmerhorst FM, Bloemenkamp KW, et al. Effectiveness of the postcoital test: randomized controlled trial. *BMJ.* 1998;317:502–505.

Scholten I, Moolenaar LM, Gianotten J, et al. Long term outcome in subfertile couples with isolated cervical factor. *Eur J Obstet Gynecol Reprod Biology.* 2013;170:429–433.

Van der Steeg JW, Steures P, Eijkemans M, et al. Should the post-coital test (PCT) be part of the routine fertility work-up? *Hum Reprod.* 2004;19(6): 1373–1379.

CHAPTER 142

OBSTETRIC ULTRASOUND

Thomas A. Kintanar

Ultrasound is defined as the range of sound waves with frequencies greater than 20,000 cycles per second (Hz); it is undetectable to the human ear. Most ultrasound scanners use frequencies from 1 to 10 MHz; 3 to 5 MHz are the most common for obstetric transabdominal examinations, although 2 to 2.25 MHz may be required in patients who are obese. Higher frequencies are used for transvaginal scanning. According to natality data, use of ultrasound has gradually increased in the United States; in 1989, 48% of mothers who had live births underwent ultrasound scanning during pregnancy, and by 2002 it was 67%. These numbers will likely increase with the 2016 American College of Obstetricians and Gynecolgists (ACOG) guidelines recommending ultrasound for all pregnancies. Suggested benefits include more accurate determination of gestational age, viability, fetal number, and placental location.

Will there be any harms to this increase? Chiossi et al. (2015) found that multiple ultrasounds in low-risk private patients may increase the risk for cesarean delivery. After controlling for confounders, private patients having more than four antenatal ultrasound examinations were more likely to undergo cesarean delivery than public patients with four or fewer ultrasound assessments (five to eight prenatal scans: relative risk ratio, 3.3; 95% confidence interval [CI] 1.4 to 8; nine or more prenatal scans: relative risk ratio, 4.1; 95% CI 1.2 to 14). Conclusions were that multiple prenatal ultrasound examinations in low-risk obstetric populations appear to be an independent and potentially modifiable risk factor for cesarean deliveries.

In years past, use of ultrasound as a routine screening procedure during pregnancy was discussed at the National Institutes of Health (NIH) landmark Consensus Development Conference in 1984. The conclusion was that routine screening was not justified and ultrasound should be used only for specific indications. Until recently, those indications remained fairly constant and are similar to those listed below in the Indications section. Evidence from the 1993 RADIUS study (Ewigman, 1993, N = 15,151) reinforced the consensus findings although controversy remains regarding generalizability of the findings, as 93% of women in the study were white and 71% had at least some college education. Obviously, the current position of ACOG has changed dramatically; earlier guidelines suggested the clinician and patient could opt for screening, however, routine ultrasound in pregnancy was not recommended.

The US consensus was never a worldwide consensus; the Royal College of Obstetricians and Gynecologists and the European Committee for Ultrasound Radiation Safety long ago endorsed routine prenatal ultrasound examinations. Ultrasound has been routinely used in several European countries, including Sweden and Germany. The Canadian Task Force on Preventive Health Care in 1992 found fair evidence for routine ultrasound screening in the second trimester, even in women without clinical indications. Many US insurers have reimbursed for routine obstetric ultrasound screening for many years. The advent of three- (3D) and four-dimensional (4D) ultrasound (3D imaging is three-dimensional in appearance; 4D is 3D imaging in real time) conferred some proprietary advantages for screening in terms of the quality of fetal features appreciated (e.g.,

improved diagnosis of facial anomalies, skeletal malformations, and neural tube defects with 3D and 4D ultrasound).

EDITOR'S NOTE: Investigators long ago found routine first-trimester scanning in a high-risk population to be more accurate than last menstrual period for confirming gestational age; this is especially useful when later managing intrauterine growth restriction (IUGR) or postdate pregnancies (in two studies, postdate deliveries and inductions were reduced by more than 50%). A Cochrane review (Whitworth, 2015) further confirmed improved gestational dating may result in fewer inductions for post maturity; it also confirmed ACOG's findings of improved detection of multiple pregnancies. Such accurate dating may also alter the method of pregnancy termination; conversely, its use may improve maternal bonding.

Transabdominal, transvaginal, and transperineal approaches are available for obstetric ultrasound. Transabdominal and transvaginal scanning are much more commonly used than transperineal. Transvaginal scanning during the first trimester permits visualization of fetal structures 1 week earlier than transabdominal scanning. Second- and third-trimester transvaginal and transperineal imaging may also be useful for evaluating the cervix and endocervical areas for preterm labor, cervical insufficiency, and placenta previa.

Ultrasound can detect on average 40% (range, 15% to >80%) of major fetal malformations, with higher detection rates of anomalies seen at tertiary care centers (ACOG, 2016). A recent systematic review and meta-analysis (Karim, 2017) found detection rates of first-trimester fetal anomalies ranged from 32% in low-risk groups to more than 60% in high-risk groups. That said, sensitivity of obstetric ultrasound is highly technician and clinician dependent. Clinicians performing these procedures must have adequate training, equipment, and willingness to seek appropriate consultation for complicated cases. Although a complete survey of fetal anatomy can often be performed by the end of the first trimester, the American Institute of Ultrasound in Medicine (AIUM) suggests that such a survey is best if performed after 18 weeks (e.g., 18 to 20 weeks).

Obstetric ultrasound studies are based on three classifications: billing purposes, radiologically, and training requirements. Billing nomenclature usually classifies studies as a *standard* (survey), a *limited* ("quick look," e.g., in emergencies, to evaluate a single organ, to guide a procedure, when time does not allow for a standard scan, to answer a clinical question [e.g., "Is there fetal heart activity," or "Is there a placenta previa?"]), a *follow-up* (reassessment following a standard scan), or a *detailed* anatomic evaluation. Radiologic nomenclature uses *standard* (also termed *basic*), *limited*, or *specialized* (*targeted*) scan. The terms *level I* and *level II* scans are no longer used. A limited scan is a goal-directed search for a problem or finding; it should not be based upon limited skills of person scanning. Limited scans are appropriate when a prior standard scan has been done; it may also be appropriate if the patient has not yet received prenatal care. If a prior standard scan has not been done, a limited scan will usually be followed by a standard or specialized scan. A specialized (targeted, detailed) evaluation identifies, characterizes, or excludes fetal anomalies, often based on an abnormal history, maternal serum screening results, or abnormal standard scan, and is usually performed by individuals with special expertise.

The American Academy of Family Physicians, the Advanced Life Support in Obstetrics (ALSO) advisory board, and others classify ultrasound applications as either *basic* or *extended*. With basic applications (e.g., most of the intrapartum indications), practicing clinicians with a base of knowledge in maternal–fetal anatomy and physiology can usually master basic scanning in a 1-day workshop. For extended applications, significant additional study and supervised practice such as that obtained in residency or other training programs are necessary. More advanced applications, such as measurement of Doppler velocimetry, require specialized training and are beyond the scope of this chapter. It should be noted that a Cochrane review (Alfirevic, 2015) found no benefit to mother or baby of use of routine umbilical artery Doppler ultrasound, or a combination of umbilical and uterine artery Doppler ultrasound, in low-risk or unselected populations.

DOCUMENTATION

Adequate documentation for every ultrasound study is essential. A permanent written report, complete with the ultrasound images incorporating measurement parameters and anatomic findings, is necessary. Fig. 142.1 provides an example of an ultrasound report form. Suggested documentation (adapted from the AIUM guidelines) for first-, second-, and third-trimester imaging and intrapartum imaging is discussed in the following sections. Only standard obstetric ultrasound studies are discussed; these should include the elements described in the following sections.

First-Trimester Standard Imaging Documentation

1. Document the location of the gestational sac. The gestational sac should be examined for the presence of a yolk sac and embryo/fetus. If visible, the embryo should be identified and the crown–rump length (CRL) measured and recorded. If an embryo is not visible, the mean gestational sac diameter should be recorded and can be used for estimating gestational age (Box 142.1).

OBSTETRIC ULTRASOUND						PATIENT IDENTIFICATION				
						Name				
						Age		DOB		
						PMD				
						LMP		EDC		
Age	Gravidity	Term	Preterm	Abortion	Living	Parameter	Measurement	Gestational age	Indices	
Reason for examination						GEST SAC			CI	
Requested by						CRL			HC/AC	
Estimated gestational age at examination						BPD			FL/AC	
Number of fetuses			Presentation			OFD			FL/BPD	
Placental location			Placental grade			HC			AC/BPD	
AFI=			☐ Septum cavum pellucidum			AC			Distal femoral epiph?	
			☐ Cisterna magna ☐ Lateral ventricle ☐ Extremities			FL			Proximal humeral epiph?	
Biophysical profile score= Movement _____ Breathing _____ Tone _____ Fluid _____ NST _____			☐ 4 Chamber heart ☐ Stomach ☐ Fetal kidneys ☐ Fetal bladder ☐ Normal abd. wall			OTHER			Proximal tibial epiph?	
			☐ Normal spine ☐ 3-Vessel cord			Estimated fetal age			Other	
TOTAL _____			☐ Normal diaphragm			Estimated fetal weight	EFW	Percentile		

Birth weight (grams) chart: 5000, 4500, 4000, 3500, 3000, 2500, 2000, 1500, 1000, 500 vs Weeks gestation completed: 0 22 24 26 28 30 32 34 36 38 40 42 44 46 48 50. Percentile curves: 90%, 10%, 97%, 50%, 3%.

Impressions/recommendations:

Uterus _____

Adnexa _____

_____

_____

_____

_____

_____

_____

_____

Prepared by:

(Signature and title)

Date of examination:

Fig. 142.1 Sample obstetric ultrasound report form.

BOX 142.1 Indicated Dating Parameters Based on Gestational Age

1. <13⁶ᐟ⁷ weeks: use CRL
2. From 14⁰ᐟ⁷ to term: u.320021se average of BPD, HC, FL, and AC

AC, Abdominal circumference; *BPD,* biparietal diameter; *CI,* cephalic index; *CRL,* crown-rump length; *FL,* femur length; *GS,* gestational sac; *HC,* head circumference.

2. Report the presence or absence of fetal life (e.g., cardiac or somatic activity). Cardiac activity is usually observed once an embryo is greater than or equal to 5 mm in length on transvaginal imaging. Cardiac activity should be recorded by a two-dimensional video clip or by M-mode imaging. A later scan may be needed to document cardiac activity if this cannot be visualized.
3. Document fetal number.
4. Assess embryonic/fetal anatomy to ascertain that it is appropriate for the first trimester.
5. Evaluate the uterus (including the cervix), adnexal structures, and the cul de sac for any abnormalities.
6. Fetal nuchal translucency (NT) should be measured between 11 and 13⁶ᐟ⁷ weeks (CRL between 45 and 84 mm). Fetal translucency is present in all fetuses; a transabdominal approach with the fetus in a supine position is the best way of obtaining a NT measurement. The proper level of magnification is such that the fetal head occupies 75% of the image. A translucency width greater than 2.5 mm may indicate Down syndrome, trisomy 18, or other chromosomal or congenital abnormalities. If suspicious, absence of the nasal bone occurs on 2.5% of normal fetuses, but increases the background risk for Down syndrome about 30 times. Absence occurs in about 75% of fetuses with a chromosomal abnormality.
7. Gut extending through the anterior abdominal wall is a normal variant until about 11 weeks. From 11 to 13⁶ᐟ⁷ weeks, findings suspicious for spina bifida (e.g., absent fourth ventricle or cisterna magna, fetal head size <10th percentile) may be noted. Signs of anencephaly, cystic hygroma, gastroschisis, omphalocele, and cardiac or skeletal anomalies can also sometimes be seen after 11 weeks.

EDITOR'S NOTE: Use of a standardized anatomic imaging protocol improves the sensitivity of first-trimester ultrasound screening for all anomalies (Karim, 2017).

Second- and Third-Trimester Standard Imaging Documentation

1. Document fetal position, life (fetal and cardiac activity), and number. Cardiac activity should be recorded.
2. Report a quantitative and qualitative estimate of the amount of amniotic fluid (increased, decreased, normal; amniotic fluid index [AFI], single deepest vertical pocket, two-diameter pocket).
3. Record the placental location and determine its relationship to the internal cervical os. The umbilical cord should be imaged and the number of vessels evaluated, when possible.
4. Assess gestational age using a combination of biparietal diameter (BPD), or head circumference (HC) and femur length. Abdominal circumference can also be used to assess gestational age (see Box 142.1).
5. If a previous ultrasound has been done, assess fetal growth using the abdominal circumference. Estimate the appropriateness of the interval growth. Fetal weight should be estimated with late second- and all third-trimester scans. It can be estimated using BPD, HC, abdominal circumference, and femoral diaphysis length. Significant discrepancies between gestational age and fetal weight may suggest fetal growth abnormality, intrauterine growth restriction, or macrosomia.

6. Visualize the uterus, cervix, and adnexal structures as clinically appropriate when technically feasible.
7. The study should include, but not necessarily be limited to, the following fetal anatomy: head and neck, lateral cerebral ventricles, midline falx, cavum septum pellucidum, choroid plexus, cisterna magna, cerebellum, four-chamber view of heart (also right and left ventricular outflow tract views), spine (cervical, thoracic, lumbar, and sacral), stomach (presence, size, and site), diaphragm, kidneys, urinary bladder, umbilical cord insertion site, umbilical vessel count, extremities (presence and number), anterior abdominal wall to evaluate for gastroschisis, and fetal sex (medically indicated only in multiple gestation pregnancy to consider whether mono- or dichorioinic). The latest guidelines require a view of the upper lip on a transverse view of the face so a cleft lip or palate can be detected.

Intrapartum Standard Imaging Documentation

1. Document fetal life, number, and presentation.
2. Estimate the amount of amniotic fluid.
3. Record the placental location and its relationship to the internal cervical os.

INDICATIONS

- Confirmation of pregnancy
- Vaginal bleeding of undetermined etiology during pregnancy
- Determination of fetal presentation/presenting part
- Suspected multiple gestation
- Estimation of gestational age
- Evaluation of fetal growth, including multiple gestation
- Significant uterine size/dates discrepancy
- Pelvic mass/pain
- Suspected hydatidiform mole
- Suspected ectopic pregnancy
- Suspected fetal death (see Chapter 214, Emergency Department, Hospitalist, and Office Ultrasound [Clinical Ultrasound])
- Suspected uterine abnormality
- Intrauterine contraceptive device localization (see Chapter 214, Emergency Department, Hospitalist, and Office Ultrasound [Clinical Ultrasound])
- Ovarian follicle development surveillance for infertility
- Biophysical profile (BPP) or modified BPP (nonstress test combined with AFI)
- Suspected polyhydramnios or oligohydramnios
- Follow-up evaluation of placental location after identified placenta previa
- Suspected placental abruption
- Premature rupture of membranes or preterm labor (e.g., estimation of fetal weight and/or presentation and/or cervical dilation)
- Evaluation for cervical cerclage placement
- Evaluation of fetal condition in late registrants for prenatal care
- Observation of intrapartum events
  - Management of second twin
  - Manual removal of placenta
- Adjunct to special procedure
  - Amniocentesis
  - External cephalic version
  - In vitro fertilization/embryo transfer
  - Chorionic villous sampling
- Measure NT as part of a screening program for fetal aneuploidy
- Follow-up observation of identified anomaly*
- History of previous infant with congenital anomaly*
- Anomaly screening following abnormal maternal serum markers for aneuploidy or neural tube defects*
- Evaluation of fetal well-being by Doppler flow velocities in suspected IUGR*

*Usually a targeted examination performed by individuals experienced in this area.

CONTRAINDICATION

Maternal refusal.

EQUIPMENT

- Real-time ultrasound machine with either a 3-MHz or higher transducer for transabdominal or transperineal scans (2 to 2.25 MHz may be needed for patients who are obese) or a 5-MHz or higher transducer for transvaginal scans
- Ultrasound gel
- Towels to remove gel when study completed
- Sheaths, probe covers, or a glove for transvaginal or transperineal scanning
- Equipment necessary to follow universal blood and body fluid precautions
- Appropriate forms or software for documentation

PREPROCEDURE PATIENT PREPARATION

If the pregnancy is over 20 weeks' gestation, the bladder should be empty for transabdominal scanning. The patient's bladder should be empty or only slightly full for transvaginal or transperineal scanning. Patient position is usually either recumbent or semirecumbent for transabdominal or transperineal imaging and dorsal lithotomy for transvaginal scanning. Many patients prefer the option of self-inserting the vaginal probe during transvaginal imaging.

Issues to be discussed with patients who undergo obstetric ultrasound include the following:

- Safety: Ultrasound is considered safe for fetuses but should be used only when clinical information is required. Although current observational research suggests ultrasound energy has no deleterious effect, it likely is not completely innocuous. Future biological effects may be identified, therefore the AIUM "as-low-as-reasonably-achievable" (ALARA) guideline is important. Routine use of high-energy spectral (color-flow) Doppler for first-trimester cardiac rate auscultation should be avoided (ACOG, 2016).
- Purpose of the examination and detection of anomalies: Expectations and indications for each scan should be discussed with patients. Some may assume a complete anatomy scan is done, regardless of what is imaged. Review basic information regarding dating of the pregnancy, especially when an estimated date of confinement (EDC or "due date") might be changed. Estimated fetal weight is by definition estimated, and patients should be counseled about how the information changes basic clinical decision making. Mention that no scan can detect all anomalies; no to a scan can "make sure the baby is ok." Gender determination is not a medical indication for imaging, although sharing this information after imaging for a medical indication is reasonable if the parent requests. A preultrasound patient information handout is available at www.expertconsult.com.

TECHNIQUE

1. For transabdominal scanning, a recumbent or semirecumbent position with left tilt/left lateral hip displacement is most comfortable and less likely to cause maternal vena caval obstruction in later gestation. This position can also be used for transperineal scanning if the legs are flexed and wide apart. Apply ultrasound gel directly to the maternal abdomen. For transvaginal (and often transperineal scanning), the dorsal lithotomy position is usually used. Apply gel directly to the vaginal probe transducer tip and then cover it with a sheath or glove for transvaginal or transperineal scanning. Water-soluble lubricant is then applied on top of the sheath. Some patients may wish to insert the probe themselves, although this is less likely later in pregnancy. The clinician should observe universal blood and body fluid precautions.

2. By convention, transabdominal scanning is performed with the clinician on the patient's right. Transducer position and image orientation are described relative to the mother rather than the fetus. When the transducer marker dot/hash is located toward the mother's head, a longitudinal (sagittal) view is seen. The maternal head is "located" on the left side of the image (cranial) while her feet are on the right (caudal). When the marker dot is placed on the mother's right side, a transverse image is produced; the mother's right side is located on the left side of the screen and vice versa. (See Chapter 214, Emergency Department, Hospitalist, and Office Ultrasound [Clinical Ultrasound], for a more complete discussion of orientation.) By convention, transvaginal and transperineal scanning follow the same image orientation.

3. For transvaginal imaging, avoid inserting the transducer too far, which can cause patient discomfort and the clinician to miss the cervix and lower uterine segment (LUS). The transducer handle is gently angled to the left or right of midline to evaluate the adnexa. First-trimester transvaginal scanning often requires a lot of manipulation and can be uncomfortable; a chaperone should be present when performing a transvaginal scan.

4. For transperineal scanning, use the same transducer as for abdominal scanning. Additional gel is applied to the outside of the sheath or glove covering the transducer and the transducer is then placed against the introitus, labia, and perineum. During transperineal scanning, the vagina appears as a bright line usually meeting the cervix at a 90-degree angle. The distance from the perineum to the cervix usually places the cervix at an ideal distance for (and within) the focal zone of the transducer. Bowel gas in the rectum can sometimes obscure the external os. The image is sometimes improved if the patient is placed in left lateral decubitus position.

5. Develop a routine when performing standard imaging. A low threshold for varying from the routine may be reasonable if you see an excellent ultrasound image that requires later documentation (e.g., three-vessel cord), freeze it and record an image at that time. If an abnormality is noted, document it, but follow your usual exam flow to avoid missing things.

6. First, perform a "scout sweep" to briefly sweep the entire uterus to assess fetal viability, gross pathology, and fetal position/lie. For first-trimester scans, it is important to scan the uterus carefully to exclude multiple gestations.

7. In second- and third-trimester imaging, evaluate the LUS before the bladder fills and distorts the cervical length or its relationship to the placenta. A full bladder can sometimes press on the LUS, creating an impression of placenta previa. If this is seen, revisualize the LUS after the patient voids.

8. Find the long axis of the fetal spine. Once oriented to the direction it lies, it allows better special orientation about where to image specific fetal parts. Transverse views of various organs become easier to obtain.

9. Evaluate transverse images from fetal head to pelvis. Transverse views of the brain, spine, chest, heart, diaphragm, abdominal wall, stomach, kidneys, and bladder should be obtained. The cord insertion site should be imaged, along with the cord insertion to the placenta, if possible. Record appropriate images for documentation.

10. Longitudinal views of the spine, diaphragm, stomach, kidneys, and bladder should also be visualized. Document these images.

11. Visualize all four extremities. Record an image of a femur for measurements if a good view is obtained, although many clinicians wait and do all measurements in sequence.

12. A final sweep should be made looking over the entire fetus. In later trimesters, an overall feel for tone and movement is an important observation.

13. Evaluate the placenta and amniotic fluid volume (AFV). If the placenta has not already been localized, it is often located posteriorly. If images of the fetus are difficult to obtain, decreased amniotic fluid or oligohydramnios can be a cause. In a patient with a history of cesarean delivery, pay particular attention to placental lie. Invasive placentation (accrete, percreate, and increta) is

TABLE 142.1 Developmental Landmarks According to Abdominal Ultrasound*

Landmark	Fetal Age (From LMP)
Visualization of gestational sac	5–6 wk
Embryonic pole	6–7 wk
Fetal heart motion	7–8 wk
Fetal movement	8–9 wk
Biparietal diameter measurable	12–13 wk

*Many of these may be visualized up to a week earlier with transvaginal scanning.
LMP, Last menstrual period.

associated with an abnormality of the decidual basalis between the uterine wall and placenta. A large multicenter cohort study of women with current placenta previa and prior cesarean delivery found the risk of accreta placentation is 3%, 11%, 40%, 61%, and 67% for first, second, third, fourth, and fifth or more cesarean deliveries, respectively (Silver, 2006). When imaging a patient with prior cesarean(s), a mid-trimester ultrasound showing anterior placenta previa or low-lying placenta should prompt further search for other signs of abnormal placentation (e.g., villous myometrial invasion).

14. While scanning, measurements listed in the next section can be obtained. Techniques and formulas for obtaining specific measurements are also discussed.

Measurements

NOTE: Modern ultrasound machines calculate these values for the sonographer based on the formulas given in the text. Many also use nomograms for making estimates. Estimates on age or weight are most accurate when multiple parameters are used and the nomograms are derived from fetuses of similar ethnic or racial background living at similar altitude.

The BPD, abdominal circumference, and femur length are measured as the basis of most obstetric ultrasound evaluations for estimating gestation age from the mid-second trimester to delivery. Overall, the use of femoral length for estimating gestational age is slightly more accurate than use of BPD. CRL and gestational sac measurements are important first-trimester dating parameters. Specific early developmental landmarks provide worthwhile information for estimating gestational age (Table 142.1).

1. CRL
   - Formula: Gestational age (weeks) = (CRL [mm] +65) /10
   - The CRL is the longest length of the fetus excluding the fetal limb buds and the yolk sac. The genital tubercle and longitudinal fetal spine should be visualized in the sagittal plane. The longest straight-line distance between cranium and caudal rump is measured. Three measurements should be taken and averaged.
   - CRL is the most accurate measurement for dating less than $13^{6/7}$ weeks' gestation. Earlier scanning provides a better estimate, with imaging done prior to $8^{6/7}$ weeks' gestation being accurate to 5 days and imaging between $9^{0/7}$ weeks and $13^{6/7}$ weeks being accurate to within 7 days. Transvaginal scanning generally permits about 1 week earlier visualization of the embryo compared with transabdominal scanning (Fig. 142.2), and is generally used prior to 11 weeks; transabdominal scanning is often used between 11 and $13^{6/7}$ weeks.
2. Gestational sac (GS) diameter
   - Formula: Gestational age (weeks) = (AvgGS [mm] + 25.43)/7.02
   - The gestational sac measurement is not the best value to use for estimating gestational age, and it should be used only if other dating parameters are not available. CRL should be obtained later and compared to dates based on the GS measurement. CRL is a more precise estimate for establishing the EDC.
   - The gestational sac consists of a hypoechogenic area, which corresponds to the chorionic vesicle, and an echogenic rim (ring), which corresponds to the trophoblast. This *double echogenic ring* is often noted in a healthy pregnancy. The inner ring is the decidua capsularis plus the chorion laeve. The outer ring is the decidua vera. At the implantation site, the hyperechoic rim is thicker, and it comprises the decidua basalis and chorion frondosum (Fig. 142.3).

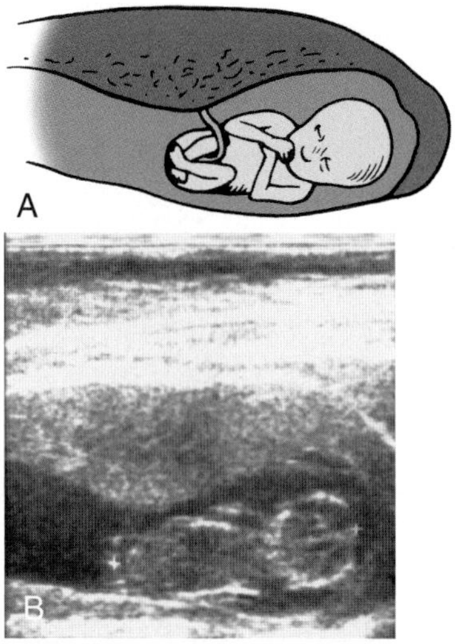

Fig. 142.2 Measurement of the crown-rump length. (A) Fetus at 12 to 13 weeks' gestation. (B) Ultrasound showing the longest length of a 12-week-old fetus. Measurement should be made from the top of the crown (head) to the bottom of the rump.

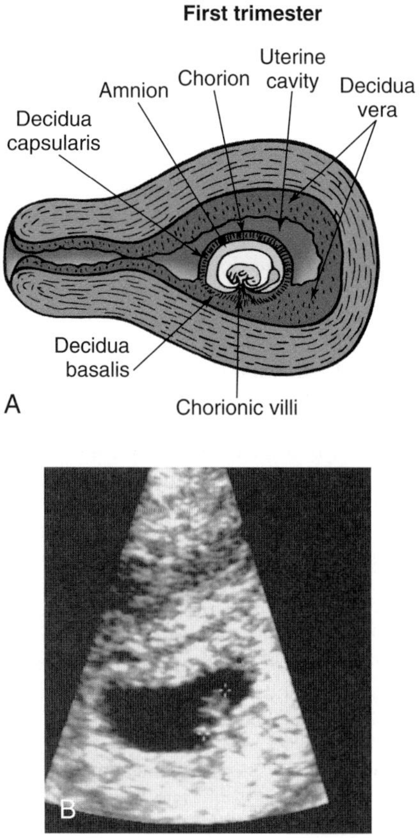

Fig. 142.3 (A) Early gestation. The decidua capsularis and the decidua vera form the double echogenic ring. (B) Ultrasound containing a fetal pole with 7-mm crown-rump length, which corresponds to 6 weeks' gestation. Pregnancies earlier than 5 weeks by transvaginal scanning and earlier than 6 weeks by transabdominal scanning generally do not show a fetal pole. Usually, only a hypoechogenic area corresponding to the chorionic vesicle is seen at this age.

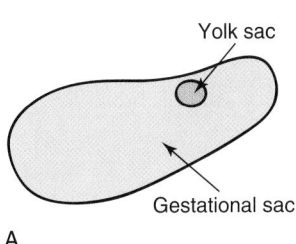

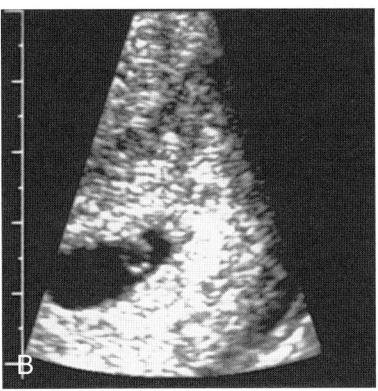

Fig. 142.4 Gestational sac with yolk sac on transvaginal ultrasound. (A) Yolk sac is generally first seen at about 5 weeks' gestation by transvaginal scanning and at 6 to 7 weeks' gestation by transabdominal scanning. Its presence confirms an intrauterine gestation but does not rule out a rare concomitant ectopic pregnancy. (B) Ultrasound of gestational sac with yolk sac demonstrated.

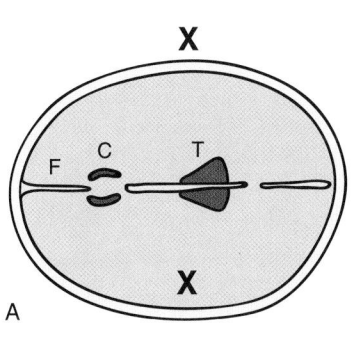

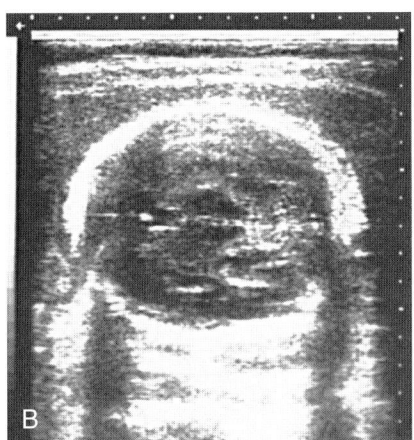

Fig. 142.5 (A) Biparietal diameter (BPD) is measured from outer to inner aspects of the skull. (B) Ultrasound of the fetal cranium at the proper level for a BPD, the level of the cavum septi pellucidi and thalamus. Note artifact behind posterior skull table. *C,* Cavum septi pellucidi; *F,* falx cerebri; *T,* thalami.

- Presence of a normal gestational sac with a yolk sac, fetal pole, or embryo (Fig. 142.4) usually confirms an intrauterine pregnancy and indirectly excludes ectopic gestation. In some cases, differentiating between a normal intrauterine gestational and a *pseudogestational sac* from ectopic pregnancy can be difficult (see the First-Trimester Standard Scan Documentation section, and Chapter 214, Emergency Department, Hospitalist, and Office Ultrasound [Clinical Ultrasound]).

  NOTE: This method of exclusion of ectopic pregnancy may be less helpful for patients taking ovulation induction medications for fertility (see the First-Trimester Standard Scan Documentation section); they have a higher risk of combination pregnancy (ectopic *and* intrauterine pregnancy), possibly as high as 1 in 100.
- The gestational sac is measured inside the hyperechoic rim, including only the anechoic (dark or fluid-filled) space. If the sac is round, only one dimension is needed; if ovoid, three measurements are taken and an average diameter calculated (Avg GS).
3. Biparietal diameter
   - The BPD is ideally measured with the fetus in occiput transverse position. Distance is measured between the outer table of the proximal fetal skull and the inner table of the contralateral side of the skull.

     NOTE: The BPD is one of the only outer-to-inner diameter measurements used in ultrasonography. Inner diameter is used due to artifact from the posterior calvarium that distorts accurate outer-to-outer diameter measurements (Fig. 142.5).
   - The most commonly accepted reference plane for BPD is a cross-section parallel to the canthomeatal line and slightly above it. This cross-sectional plane cuts through the falx cerebri, the thalamus, the cavum septi pellucidi, and the medial cerebral artery. Head shape should be oval in this plane. If the cerebellar hemispheres are visible, the probe is too steeply angled.
4. Head circumference (HC)
   - Formula: HC = 1.57 (BPD + occipital–frontal diameter [OFD]).

     NOTE: Some clinicians use HC = 1.57 (BPD + 0.3 cm + OFD) due to the manner in which BPD is measured.
   - The OFD is measured in the same plane as the BPD. The OFD diameter measurement should be made from the skull's outer-to-outer aspect.
5. Cephalic index (CI)
   - Formula: CI = BPD/OFD
   - Prenatal molding of the fetal skull is common in later pregnancy and may result in an inaccurate BPD measurement. The CI (the ratio of the BPD to the OFD) screens for cranial shape abnormalities because it is constant throughout pregnancy. The normal value is 78.3% ± 8% (±2 standard deviations [SD]). Values below this normal range indicate a dolichocephalic head (an ellipse with a BPD that is shorter than expected, or "too flat"). Values above this normal range indicate a brachycephalic head (an ellipse with a BPD that is wider than expected, or "too round").
   - If the CI is significantly above or below the normal range, the BPD may not be a reliable estimation of gestational age. Instead, the HC should be used for estimating gestational age.
6. Abdominal circumference (AC)
   - Formula: AC = 1.57 (D1+D2)

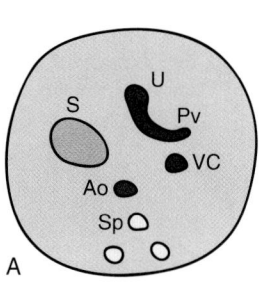

Fig. 142.6 Abdominal circumference. (A) This third-trimester cross-section of the fetal abdomen shows the junction of the umbilical vein and left portal vein. The stomach is seen on the left side of the fetus. (B) Cross-sectional ultrasound of fetal abdomen. *Ao,* Aorta; *Pv,* portal vein; *S,* stomach; *Sp,* spine; *U,* umbilical vein; *VC,* vena cava.

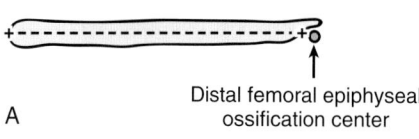

Distal femoral epiphyseal ossification center

A

Fig. 142.7 (A) Third-trimester femur is measured along the central shaft of the diaphysis. (B) Ultrasound demonstrating the echogenic distal femoral epiphyseal ossification center on the right, which indicates a gestational age of 33 weeks or more.

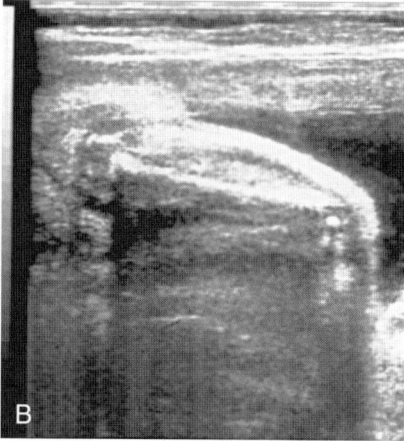

- Two diameters (D₁ and D₂), the anteroposterior abdominal diameter and the transverse abdominal diameter, are taken at the level of the stomach, the liver, and the junction of umbilical vein and left portal vein. This junction appears as an echolucent structure shaped like a hockey stick. These diameters should be at right angles to one another, and the plane in which they are taken should be at a right angle to the fetal spine. If kidneys or ribs are visualized, the plane level is too high. AC is taken in outer-to-outer diameter fashion.
- Clinical conditions that modify hepatic size can spuriously affect the abdominal circumference. Because it relies on soft tissue measurement, AC is less accurate for estimating gestational age in the early second trimester compared with BPD. That said, it is most useful for estimating gestational age in the late second and third trimesters (Fig. 142.6).

7. Femur (FL) and humerus lengths. The central diaphysis of the shaft of the femur should be measured (excluding the epiphysis). The beam should be as perpendicular to the shaft as possible (Fig. 142.7). While this is not necessarily the largest or longest measurement that can be obtained, including the femoral neck overestimates the actual FL. The lateral aspect of the femur is straight while the medial aspect is curved; therefore measuring the lateral aspect is more precise. The humeral length is now often routinely measured because shortening of the humerus is a slightly more sensitive indication of increased Down syndrome risk than femoral length shortening.

Fetal Body Ratios

1. *Cephalic index* (See previous discussion.)

2. *Head circumference/abdominal circumference.* This ratio has a positive predictive value of 62% for detecting asymmetric IUGR; negative predictive value is 98%. HC/AC is normally around 1.2 at 20 weeks' gestation. It decreases linearly to around 1 at 36 to 38 weeks' gestation. It then remains around 1 or below until delivery. Screening for an HC/AC greater than 1 after 36 weeks detects 85% of fetuses with IUGR. This method fails to detect symmetric IUGR, however.

3. *Femur length/abdominal circumference.* The FL/AC ratio does not detect symmetric IUGR, but is sensitive for asymmetric cases. This ratio has the further advantage of having normal-range values (ratios) that remain consistent after 20 weeks. The normal value for this ratio expressed as a percentage is 22% ± 2% (±2 SD). A value greater than 24% indicates IUGR. A value less than 20.5% suggests macrosomia. However, while negative predictive value is 92% to 93%, positive predictive value only approaches 18% to 20%.

4. *Femur length/biparietal diameter.* After 22 weeks' gestational age, the FL/BPD ratio is almost constant, with a normal range of 79% ± 8% (±2 SD) from 22 to 40 weeks. The predictive values of this ratio are similar to those for FL/AC. The FL/BPD has three important uses: (1) evaluation of the ultrasound examination for measurement error, (2) detection of diseases of the fetal head and limbs, and (3) classification of IUGR.

Ultrasound Dating

1. Because of biologic variability, traditional clinical methods accurately predict gestational age with 90% certainty only to within 2 weeks. These include estimated last menstrual period, date when

TABLE 142.2	Outline of Ultrasound Dating of Pregnancy	
Weeks of Gestation Based on LMP	Recommended Dating Measurement	Accuracy (±)
3–5	None	
≤8$^{6/7}$ wk	CRL	5 days
9$^{0/7}$ to 13$^{6/7}$ wk	CRL	7 days
14$^{0/7}$ wk to 15$^{6/7}$ wk	BPD, HC, AC, FL	7 days
16$^{0/7}$ wk to 21$^{6/7}$ wk	BPD, HC, AC, FL	10 days
22$^{0/7}$ wk to 27$^{6/7}$ wk	BPD, HC, AC, FL	14 days
28$^{0/7}$ wk and beyond	BPD, HC, AC, FL	>21 days

AC, Abdominal circumference; *BPD,* biparietal diameter; *CRL,* crown–rump length; *FL,* femur length; *GS,* gestational sac; *LMP,* last menstrual period.
    Modified from American College of Obstetricians and Gynecologists. Method for estimating due date. ACOG Practice Bulletin no. 611. *Obstet Gynecol.* 2014;142(4):863–866.

uterus reaches umbilicus, first heard fetal heart tones, fundal height, and quickening. Twenty-five percent to 45% of women are unable to provide an accurate menstrual history. Thus, the EDC based on last menstrual period differs by more than 2 weeks from the actual date of birth in nearly 25% of pregnancies. Addition of ultrasound dating in early pregnancy is more accurate for helping establish the EDC.

2. Measured size of certain fetal body parts correlates with gestational age. In general, growth is quite uniform in the first 20 weeks of gestation. Progressive variability makes estimation after this less accurate (Table 142.2).

3. Ultrasound estimates of gestational age have inherent uncertainty. This uncertainty or variability is usually expressed as plus or minus two standard deviations (±2 SD), which should include 95% of fetuses in a normal population. Reporting a single age estimate without considering this range gives a false impression about accuracy. ACOG recently numerically described these uncertainties throughout pregnancy (see Table 142.2).

4. Pregnancy dating involves averaging various measurements (e.g., BPD, AC, and FL). Single measurements may be technically incorrect, especially by the third trimester. It is unlikely that several measurements are incorrect in the same direction, however. When averages are used, measurement errors tend to self-cancel to provide an overall accurate estimate. Each measurement should be individually considered. If a lone measurement is significantly different from the others (e.g., fetal position precludes a good measurement but prior ultrasound measurement was normal), it can be excluded from that average.

5. When using the multiple-parameter dating approach, or an averaged estimate of age, avoiding any measurements affected by a pathologic fetal process is an important consideration (e.g., hydrocephaly, microcephaly, macrosomia, IUGR, fetal dwarfism). After 22 weeks' gestational age, potential errors are minimized by considering fetal body ratios (see the Fetal Body Ratios section). If the CI indicates a normally shaped head, the FL/BPD ratio can be calculated. If the FL/BPD ratio is less than 70%, the FL should be eliminated; if the ratio is greater than 86%, the fetal head measurements should be discarded. If the FL/BPD ratio is normal, the FL/AC ratio can be calculated. If the FL/AC ratio is less than 20%, the AC is suspect because of possible macrosomia; if the ratio is greater than 24%, the AC is of concern for possible IUGR.

6. Fetal epiphyseal ossification centers are helpful in pregnancies beyond 30 weeks. This is especially useful because dating by other ultrasound parameters has limited reliability at later gestational ages (see Table 142.2). A visible distal femoral epiphysis (see Fig. 142.7) indicates a menstrual age of at least 33 weeks, a visible proximal tibial epiphysis indicates a menstrual age of at least 35 weeks, and a visible proximal humeral epiphysis indicates a gestational age of at least 38 weeks.

Organ Survey

1. Fetal organs should be categorized as anatomically normal, abnormal, or not visualized. Cardiac anomalies are most common, followed by central nervous system defects, especially neural tube. Deviations from normal anatomy require a specialized scan.

2. The brain should be surveyed in three transverse (axial) views. The transthalamic view is used to measure BPD and HC and is at the level of the thalamus and cavum septi pellucidi. Moving slightly superiorly, with the transventricular view, the lateral ventricles and their atria are visualized, and this is where the echogenic choroid plexus is noted. (The atria are the confluence of the lateral and occipital horns.) The diameter of an atrium is normally between 5 and 10 mm from 15 weeks to term; ventriculomegaly is quantified by amount of dilation (mild: >10 mm but <15 mm; moderate to severe: >15 mm). Angling posteriorly through the posterior fossa produces the transcerebellar view. The cisterna magna and cerebellum are usually measured. The cerebellar diameter in millimeters is roughly equivalent to the gestational age in weeks up to 20 weeks (accurate enough to help establish gestational age in late registrants; tables are available for after 20 weeks). Note: the view at which cerebellar diameters are obtained is also usually an excellent view for measuring NT.

3. The entirety of the spine should be surveyed in both longitudinal and transverse views. Neural tube defects result from incomplete closure by 6 weeks. In 90% of cases of spina bifida, not only is there an opening in the vertebrae through which the meninges protrude (meningocele), but the sac also contains neural elements (meningomyelocele). One or more additional defects are classically associated with spina bifida (e.g., small BPD, ventriculomegaly, frontal bone scalloping, elongation and downward displacement of the cerebellum, and effacement or obliteration of the cisterna magnum).

4. The lungs are best visualized from 20 to 25 weeks and should be homogeneous. Cystic or solid lesions require further evaluation. Ninety percent of diaphragmatic hernias are located on the left side and posteriorly; almost half are associated with other major anomalies or aneuploidy. The heart may be pushed to the middle or right side of the thorax, the stomach bubble may be missing from the abdomen, and the AC may be decreased.

5. The basic survey of the heart should include a four-chamber view, rate, and rhythm. It can usually be viewed by turning the transducer 90 degrees from the longitudinal view of the spine at the level of the heart. The four-chamber view is obtained with this transverse view immediately above the diaphragm. The two atria should be about the same size, as should the two ventricles. The apex of the heart should form a 45-degree angle with the left anterior chest wall; abnormalities of axis should be followed with a specialized scan. Thirty percent to 40% of cardiac defects are associated with chromosomal abnormalities. An attempt should be made to evaluate the left and right ventricular outflow tracts by turning the transducer slightly oblique to the four-chamber view.

6. The stomach is visible in 98% of fetuses after 14 weeks. Nonvisualization could be the result of various abnormalities (e.g., esophageal atresia, abdominal wall defects, diaphragmatic hernia), so ultrasound should be repeated in a week, possibly with a specialized scan. The liver, spleen, gallbladder, and intestine are visible in many second- and third-trimester scans. After visualizing the stomach, the abdominal wall should be scanned because defects are quite common. Gastroschisis is typically located to the right of the umbilical cord insertion, and bowel herniates into the amniotic cavity. In over half of cases, an omphalocele is associated with other major anomalies or aneuploidy.

7. The kidneys and urinary tract should be scanned. Kidney are visualized as early as 14 weeks and nearly always by 18 weeks. Renal agenesis or cysts in the kidneys (infantile polycystic kidney disease, multicystic dysplastic kidney disease) should

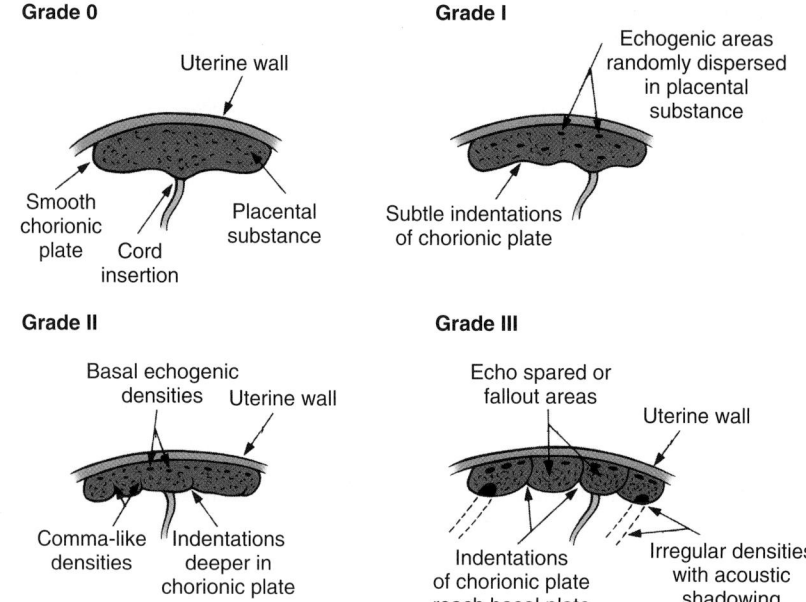

Fig. 142.8 Grades of placental maturity. (Modified from Grannum P, Berkowitz R, Hobbins J. The ultrasonic changes in the maturing placenta and their relation to fetal pulmonic maturity. *Am J Obstet Gynecol.* 1979;133:915–922.)

be noted. After 16 to 20 weeks, most of the amniotic fluid is produced by the kidneys, so oligohydramnios should prompt a careful look at these areas. A normal AFI indicates that at least one side of the urinary tract is patent and functioning. A normal renal pelvis diameter is less than 4 mm before 20 weeks; if it is enlarged, ultrasound should be repeated at 34 weeks, and if it is greater than 7 mm at that point, neonatology should be consulted. Pyelectasis is dilation at the level of the renal pelvis, and two-thirds of infants with pyelectasis greater than 7 mm will have a renal abnormality. Duplicate collecting ducts occur in 4% of the population, and the classic finding is pyelectasis of the upper pole. Reflux of the lower pole is common, so antimicrobial therapy from birth onward may reduce the incidence of urinary tract infections. Posterior urethral valves in a male fetus will result in dilation of the bladder and proximal urethra; associated oligohydramnios portends a poor prognosis because of pulmonary hypoplasia.

Placental Imaging

1. Maturational changes of the placenta occur in its three basic anatomic areas (the amniochorionic plate, the placental body, and the basal layer) and form the basis for the following grading system of placental maturity (Fig. 142.8):
   EDITOR'S NOTE: Placental grading based upon the amount of placental calcification is no longer used clinically because it does not correlate with lung maturity; however, calcification within the placenta prior to 36 weeks usually indicates that the fetal lungs are mature. The more complete placental grading system remains in this chapter to demonstrate somewhat normal maturation stages.

Grade 0: Placenta has a chorionic plate that is very smooth. The placental substance is homogeneous and without calcifications.
Grade I: There is some undulation and some indentations in the chorionic plate. There are also scattered echogenic areas, which represent calcifications in the placental substance.
Grade II: The chorionic plate has more indentations, but they do not reach the basal plate. The grade II placenta is characterized by a straight line of echoes with calcifications present along the axis of the basal plate. These echoes are high-amplitude, bright, white, and linear or comma-shaped.

Grade III: The chorionic plate indentations reach the basal plate. There is complete compartmentalization of the placenta with extensive echogenic areas representing calcifications. They may cast shadows.
   NOTE: In a third-trimester transabdominal scan, if the placenta has not been located by the time measurements have been obtained, it is usually located posteriorly, having been obscured by fetal body parts.

2. Grade 0 is most common in the first trimester; grade I appears after 14 weeks' gestation and is most common until around 34 weeks. Grade II may appear after 26 weeks' gestation and is most common around 36 weeks. Grade III most commonly appears after 35 weeks' gestation. Even with a grade III placenta, there is a 4% chance of fetal pulmonary immaturity.
3. A grade II placenta prior to 26 weeks or a grade III placenta before 35 weeks is abnormal.
4. IUGR, oligohydramnios, and hypertension are associated with accelerated placental maturation. IUGR is usually associated with a small placenta. Diabetes mellitus and Rh sensitization are associated with delayed maturation. Preeclampsia and gestational hypertension do not affect placental maturation.
5. With second- and third-trimester bleeding, ultrasound is used to delineate the placental implantation site, to exclude placenta previa, and to attempt to determine whether there has been an abruption. Scanning transvaginally or transperineally may improve visualization of these abnormalities in the second and third trimester and during labor, although abruption remains a clinical, rather than ultrasound, diagnosis.

NOTE: Most placental abruptions are small and easy to miss on ultrasound (high false-negative risk). Placental venous lakes can also appear very similar to findings of an abruption.

Amniotic Fluid Volume

1. Estimation and documentation of AFV is the standard of care during routine ultrasound examinations. Although there is no precise method of determining AFV, there are several indirect methods of estimation.
   • Maximum vertical pocket or two-diameter: The maximal vertical pocket technique involves measuring the single deepest vertical pocket of amniotic fluid, in which segments of the

TABLE 142.3 Fetal Biophysical Profile Scoring

Variable	Score 2	Score 0
FBM	The presence of at least 30 sec of sustained FBM in 30 min of observation	<30 sec of FBM in 30 min
Fetal movement	Three or more gross body movements in 30 min of observation; simultaneous limb and trunk movements are counted as a single movement	≤2 gross body movements in 30 min of observation
Fetal tone	At least one episode of motion of a limb from a position of flexion to extension and a rapid return to flexion	Fetus in a position of semi- or full-limb extension with no return to flexion with movement; absence of fetal movement is counted as absent tone
Fetal reactivity*	The presence of two or more fetal heart rate accelerations of ≥15 beats/min and lasting ≥15 sec and associated with fetal movement	No acceleration or <2 accelerations of the fetal heart rate during observation (see Chapter 146, Antepartum Fetal Monitoring)
Qualitative amniotic fluid volume†	A pocket of amniotic fluid that measures ≥2 cm in two perpendicular planes	Largest pocket of amniotic fluid measures <2 cm in two perpendicular planes
Maximal score	10	—
Minimal score	—	0

*Most centers perform a nonstress test.
†Most centers usually determine an amniotic fluid index.
FBM, Fetal breathing movement.
Modified from Manning FA, Platt LD, Sipos L. Antepartum fetal evaluation: Development of a fetal biophysical profile. Am J Obstet Gynecol. 1980;136:787–795.

umbilical cord should not be seen. *Oligohydramnios* is defined as the absence of a pocket of fluid at least 2 cm in depth, and *polyhydramnios* is diagnosed when any pocket exceeds 8 cm. This technique is most helpful for quantitating fluid with a multiple-gestation pregnancy or in the assessment of polyhydramnios. The two-diameter method is used as part of a modified BPP. Excluding umbilical cord, there should be at least one pocket of amniotic fluid measuring 2 cm in both the horizontal and vertical planes (i.e., 2 × 2 cm), which results in a score of 2. Failure to identify a fluid pocket of at least this size results in a score of 0.

- Amniotic fluid index: This is the quantitative approach used by most centers. The uterus is divided into four quadrants. The ultrasound transducer is then held in a vertical and sagittal/longitudinal (marker dot on the probe turned toward the mother's head/cephalad) or transverse (marker dot on the probe turned toward the mother's right side) alignment (oblique views can be misleading). With the patient supine, the transducer is held perpendicular to the plane of the floor and aligned longitudinally or transversely with the mother's spine. Starting in one quadrant, the pocket of fluid with the largest vertical dimension is identified, measured, and recorded. Care must be taken not to include segments of the umbilical cord in the measurement. Coiled cord can fill the space and appear to be fluid (color Doppler can be used to identify the cord). This procedure is repeated in each quadrant and the values summed. If the sum (AFI) is less than 8 cm, perform the four-quadrant evaluation three times and average the values. From 16 weeks onward, the majority of normal pregnancies have an AFI between 8 and 24 cm.

2. Polyhydramnios
   - In women who do not have diabetes, polyhydramnios is defined as an AFI of 24 cm or more.
   - The most likely etiology is idiopathic (34.6%), followed by diabetes mellitus (24.6%), congenital anomalies (20.1%), erythroblastosis fetalis (11.5%), and multiple gestation (9.2%).
   - Once identified, a patient with an AFI of 24 cm or more should have a detailed or targeted ultrasound examination to rule out fetal anomalies.
   - Abnormal fetal lie, operative delivery, and placental abruption all occur more frequently during labor in patients with polyhydramnios.

3. Oligohydramnios

- Significant oligohydramnios is defined as an AFI of less than 5 cm.
- Excluding patients with premature rupture of membranes, approximately 83% of patients with oligohydramnios will have fetal IUGR; however, only 16% of patients with fetal IUGR will have oligohydramnios.
- Fetal weight should be estimated whenever oligohydramnios is present.
- Premature rupture of membranes can cause severe oligohydramnios or anhydramnios.
- Fetal causes of oligohydramnios are usually related to urinary tract anomalies.
- Fetal heart rate abnormalities, depressed Apgar scores, and passage of meconium all occur more frequently during labor in patients with oligohydramnios.
- In most cases, oligohydramnios in a term infant is an indication for delivery.

Fetal Assessment (Biophysical Profile)

1. A combination of biophysical variables (the BPP) was first introduced by Manning in 1980. BPP combines both acute and chronic markers of fetal and placental status (Table 142.3). Documenting the acute markers (fetal heart rate reactivity [FR; normal is reactive on nonstress test], fetal movement [FM; normal is three or more significant body or limb movements in 30 minutes], fetal breathing movement [FBM; normal is 30 seconds or more of breathing movements in 30 minutes], and fetal tone [FT; normal is extension/flexion of an extremity or spine and then return to normal position]) is very similar to performing an in-utero neurologic examination of the fetus. It can demonstrate acute oxygenation of various parts of the neurologic system. Normal acute markers result in a score of 2 each; abnormal, a score of 0. Documenting the chronic marker AFI is similar to obtaining a hemoglobin A_{1C} measurement of fetal oxygenation; it demonstrates how well the fetus has been oxygenated over the past few days, weeks, or maybe even a month. Normal AFI, maximal vertical pocket, or a two-diameter pocket results in a score of 2. Failure to identify a two-diameter fluid pocket (one at least 2 × 2 cm in diameter) results in a score of 0. Conversely, even if there is oligohydramnios using an AFI (i.e., AFI <5 cm), if there is a 2 × 2-cm diameter pocket, the score for BPP is 2. Adding the acute and chronic markers, the highest possible score for a normal fetus is 10.

2. A normal BPP is indirect evidence that each of the portions of the central nervous system that control particular activities is functioning and, therefore, oxygenated. When all of the various portions of the central nervous system are active, it indicates that overall the fetus is well oxygenated at that time. The absence of a given BPP activity, however, is difficult to interpret because it may reflect either pathologic depression or normal periodicity.

3. In chronic sustained fetal hypoxia, a protective redistribution of fetal cardiac output may occur, with blood being directed away from nonvital fetal organs (kidneys or lung) toward vital fetal organs (heart, brain, and adrenals). This redistribution leads to decreased renal perfusion and urine production, oligohydramnios, and a low AFI. A low AFI may be the earliest marker of placental insufficiency.

4. A fetal BPP score of 8 or more is reassuring of fetal well-being. It has a high negative predictive value and is associated with stillbirth risk of 0.8%. BPP of less than 8 is nonreassuring, and repeated testing or delivery is indicated (see Table 142.3). The presence of oligohydramnios constitutes an abnormal biophysical assessment regardless of the overall score. Concerns about the BPP as a screening test include that it is time consuming, intensive, and has a false-positive rate as high as 60%. The modified BPP (nonstress testing combined with AFI) has similar predictive value as the full BPP.

Fetal Size

1. Many formulas and tables are available for prediction of fetal weight. These formulas are based on a variety of combinations of BPD, HC, AC, and FL. Predictive accuracy ranges from ±14.8% to ±20.2% (±2 SD). Formulas are often compared against a commonly used table (Shepard, 1987).

2. Size-date discrepancy on clinical examination requires investigation, often done with ultrasound imaging. In early pregnancy, suspect multiple gestation, a hydatidiform mole, incorrect menstrual history, and genetic or developmental defects. Later in pregnancy, fetal malposition, IUGR, fetal dysmaturity, genetic or developmental defects, multiple gestation, fetal macrosomia, and abnormal AFV are causes to consider.

Intrauterine Growth Restriction

1. Clinical signs of IUGR include a lag in fundal height (>4 cm difference from expected fundal height) or maternal weight gain (<100 to 200 g [3.5 to 7 oz] per week in third trimester), or both. Diagnosis of IUGR by clinical factors is possible in only around one-third of pregnancies.

2. IUGR diagnosed by ultrasound is much more accurate, especially if first-trimester dating was done. A combination of clinical and ultrasound data improves the sensitivity and specificity of IUGR diagnoses.

3. The following are important ultrasound parameters for evaluating potential IUGR:
   - Oligohydramnios. In low-risk pregnancies, the sensitivity of oligohydramnios in the diagnosis of IUGR is approximately 16%. In high-risk populations, the predictive value and sensitivity of oligohydramnios are enhanced (sensitivity can exceed 85%). If oligohydramnios is present and there is no evidence of premature rupture of membranes or congenital anomalies, IUGR is the likely cause. The combination of oligohydramnios and IUGR portends a less favorable outcome, and early delivery should be considered.
   - BPD. While not a helpful sole parameter, BPD is useful for ratios. With symmetric IUGR, both head and body measurements fall off the growth curve similarly and result in an erroneous estimate of gestational age. Even with asymmetric IUGR, the BPD remains normal until late in the course.
   - Head circumference. The HC is a more shape-independent measurement of fetal head size than the BPD. In cases of cra-

nial shape abnormalities, its inclusion in the growth profile will significantly decrease the high number of false-positive results seen when BPD is used alone. However, because IUGR may not selectively affect brain and head growth, or is "relatively head-sparing," HC alone is also not a very useful measurement. The HC is most useful when it is used with another measurement as a ratio.
   - Femur length. The FL can also be misleading with IUGR. In asymmetric IUGR, FL usually parallels the gestational age as calculated from the last normal menstrual period. Therefore, for asymmetric IUGR, FL may not be helpful. In symmetric IUGR, all measurements will be small and result in an erroneously early gestational age estimate, so again FL is not helpful. Similar to HC, FL is most predictive of IUGR when it is used in a ratio.
   - Abdominal circumference. The AC is useful for assessing fetal nutritional status. The AC involves measurement of the liver, which is smaller in chronic hypoxia. With inadequate oxygen or nutrition, the liver cannot produce substrate (glycogen); thus the AC is the best single predictor of IUGR with a specificity of 89.8% and negative predictive value of 90.7% (Nardozza, 2017).
   - Calculation of fetal body ratios (see the Fetal Body Ratios section).
   - Placental grade. When fetal growth pattern and estimated weight suggest a small fetus, the finding of a prematurely grade III (before 35 weeks) placenta is further evidence of IUGR.
   - Use of fetal epiphyseal ossification centers (see the Ultrasound Dating section).

4. Suspect IUGR by ultrasound if the following occur:
   - AC falls in the lower 15th percentile. (Sensitivity of ultrasound is >95% if AC <2.5th percentile.)
   - Weight falls in the lower 15th percentile.
   - HC/AC ≥0.95 (HC/AC >1.0 after 36 weeks detects 85% of IUGR).
   - FL/AC ≥23.5%.

5. In the absence of an accurate gestational age, the assessment of risk for IUGR relies predominantly on fetal disproportionality and asymmetry. This may lead to the diagnosis of asymmetric IUGR. However, to diagnose symmetric IUGR, unless dates are very accurate, serial ultrasound studies must be performed to assess fetal growth. Some experts recommend serial scans at 2- or 3-week intervals to identify IUGR in the absence of reliable dating. Therefore, for those at risk, liberalizing the use of early ultrasound for establishing gestational age may be the best way to diagnose symmetric IUGR.

6. Newer techniques to identify IUGR are being evaluated, including Doppler velocimetry of the umbilical artery, vein or other placental vessels, M-mode echocardiography of the fetal heart or middle cerebral artery waveforms. Abnormal placental vessel Doppler velocimetry may alert the clinician to the need for an additional study such as a BPP, continuous fetal monitoring, or delivery.

Macrosomia

1. Fetal macrosomia is defined in absolute terms as a fetal weight of greater than 4000 to 4500 g, regardless of gestational age. However, macrosomia is also considered when a fetal weight is in the upper 90th percentile for any gestational age at any point during the pregnancy.

2. Symmetric macrosomia occurs when the excessive fetal weight is the result of proportionate growth of all fetal parameters. For example, the weight, length, and head size may all be above the 90th percentile for age. Symmetric macrosomia is usually the result of a postdates pregnancy or genetics (i.e., large parents). The HC/AC and the FL/AC ratios are usually within the normal range for age. This type of macrosomia is also termed large-for-gestational-age.

3. Asymmetric macrosomia generally occurs in patients with class A to C gestational diabetes mellitus. Although the values of HC and FL are higher than average, they usually fall below the 90th percentile for age. The excessive weight results from profound increases in soft tissue mass that are reflected by an AC and an estimated fetal weight above the 90th percentile.

4. Skin thickening is common in infants of diabetic mothers and when macrosomia is present. This is due to subcutaneous fat deposition, and the fetal cheeks are especially prominent. However, it may affect scalp or trunk skin. This observation should be recorded when the skin is thickened to a width of greater than 5 mm.

NOTE: Ultrasound diagnosis of macrosomia does not predict prognosis for vaginal delivery, largely because the positive predictive rate for macrosomia in postdates pregnancies is only about 50%. In fact, for suspected macrosomia, the accuracy of estimated fetal weight by ultrasound is no better than that obtained with clinical palpation (e.g., Leopold's maneuvers). As a result, ACOG guidelines state that suspected macrosomia is not a contraindication to attempted vaginal birth. It is also not an indication for induction, because induction does not improve prognosis for mother or infant. However, with an estimated fetal weight of greater than 4500 g, a prolonged second stage of labor or arrest of descent in the second stage is an indication for cesarean delivery. Cesarean delivery should usually be performed for midpelvis arrest with suspected macrosomia. One benefit of ultrasound is the ability to exclude macrosomia in the management of expected macrosomia which may help to avoid maternal morbidity.

Preterm Labor

1. Preterm labor is defined as onset of labor before a gestational age of 37 weeks. Preterm labor affects 12% of pregnancies and accounts for 70% of neonatal deaths (ACOG, 2016).

2. Ultrasound parameters that are important when evaluating the patient in preterm labor include the following:
   - Fetal number: Multiple gestations have an increased risk of preterm labor.
   - Estimated fetal weight. Preterm labor is associated with IUGR.
   - Amniotic fluid index. Preterm labor is associated with both oligohydramnios and polyhydramnios.
   - BPP: Low BPP score may contraindicate tocolysis.
   - Other possible contraindications to tocolysis include fetal malformations and evidence of concealed placental abruption.
   - Ultrasound cervical evaluation
   - Cervical shortening (present if the distance from internal os to external os [or the leading edge of the portio vaginalis] is <3 cm). Transperineal and transvaginal scanning appear to be equally accurate for making this measurement. Transvaginal scanning does not seem to increase the risk of infection in women with preterm premature rupture of membranes. A cervical length of less than 2 cm or funneling (dilation and shortening of the upper half of the cervix) has been associated with a short time interval between rupture of membranes and delivery and an indication for treatment with progesterone therapy.
   - Dilation of the endocervical canal (present if the maximal diameter of the endocervical canal exceeds 1 cm).
   - Bulging of the fetal membranes into the endocervical canal (conical or funnel-shaped rather than flat or slightly rounded shape of the internal os).
   - Thinning of the LUS (anterior wall thickness <0.6 cm).

3. Although studies have shown variable results with the use of cervical cerclage for cervical insufficiency, at least one large prospective study found that fewer women delivered before 32 weeks if a cerclage was placed in those with a cervical length of 25 mm or less at 23 weeks (see also Chapter 143, Cervical Cerclage).

Postdates Pregnancy

1. Expected date of confinement is defined as 40 weeks (280 days) from the first day of the last normal menstrual period, or 266 days after ovulation, provided cycles are regular and occur at 28-day intervals. Normal term ranges from 38 to 42 weeks.

2. A postdates pregnancy is one with a duration that has exceeded 42 weeks (294 days) from the last normal menstrual period, assuming a 28-day cycle.

3. One study showed that the incidence of postdates pregnancy was overestimated by 7.5% when gestational age was determined using just the menstrual history, but it fell to 2.6% with early ultrasound examination, and to 1.1% when both menstrual history and early ultrasound measurements were used.

4. Complications detectable by ultrasound include the following:
   - Physiologic oligohydramnios (these are detectable by AFV determination)
   - Macrosomia (this is detectable by calculation of estimated fetal weight)
   - Dysmaturity resulting from chronic uteroplacental insufficiency (this is detectable by evidence of asymmetric IUGR)
   - Congenital anomalies (these are detectable by anatomic survey)
   - Inaccurate dating (e.g., a preterm delivery could be prevented by having early estimates of gestational age)

5. The contraction stress test (CST) is still regarded as the most reliable method of antenatal surveillance for a postdates pregnancy. However, it has basically been replaced by the modified BPP (nonstress test [NST] combined with an AFI) or the BPP (which includes an NST). Studies comparing the use of twice-weekly modified BPP or BPP with a CST do not show a significant difference between the tests (see Chapter 146, Antepartum Fetal Monitoring). All are characterized by strong negative predictive value, but unfortunately high false-positive rates that lead to unnecessary interventions.

First-Trimester Scanning

See Chapter 214, Emergency Department, Hospitalist, and Office Ultrasound [Clinical Ultrasound], for a detailed description.

1. Caution should be used in making a presumptive diagnosis of a gestational sac in the absence of a yolk sac or a definite embryo. Overlooking a second or third gestational sac in first-trimester scans is also a possibility. The first trimester is the best time to determine the number of chorions for multiple gestations (monochorionic twins are at higher risk for complications such as cord entanglement).

2. First-trimester scanning is the best opportunity to evaluate the uterus (including the cervix), adnexa, and cul de sac for abnormalities.

3. The most common causes of bleeding in the first trimester include the following:
   - Idiopathic or unknown
   - Embryonic resorption/blighted ovum
   - Threatened, missed, incomplete, or complete abortion
   - Ectopic pregnancy
   - Abortion of one fetus of a multiple gestation
   - Hydatidiform mole

4. Transvaginal scanning is preferred at this gestational age. Color flow and Doppler should generally be avoided. When evaluating for ectopic pregnancy using transabdominal imaging, an extrauterine gestational sac is seen in less than 10% of cases (rates are higher with transvaginal scanning). Ultrasound is more helpful for ruling out ectopic pregnancy when an intrauterine gestation is

TABLE 142.4	Possible Outcomes Based on Ultrasound Findings and Quantitative Human Chorionic Gonadotropin Correlations		
hCG Level (mIU/mL)*	Presence/Absence of GS on TAUS	Significance
>1800	+GS	Intrauterine pregnancy; if fetal pole or yolk sac is identified, no further ultrasound is required. Ectopic pregnancy is basically ruled out. (<1:7000 risk unless patient taking fertility ovulation induction medications; see text.)
<1800	+GS	Failed intrauterine pregnancy or absorbed pregnancy; ectopic pregnancy with pseudogestational sac; or very rarely, an early pregnancy that may continue.
>1800	−GS	Suspect ectopic pregnancy.
<1800	−GS	Indeterminate. May be result of an early intrauterine pregnancy, or ectopic or failed pregnancy. Follow hCG titer every 2–4 days; for normal pregnancies, hCG should double. However, normal hCG trends occur in 15% of ectopic pregnancies. Thus, as soon as the level crosses the threshold for the practitioner's facility, repeat the ultrasound examination.

*Actual values will vary from institution to institution based on particular assay used, quality of machine, and the skill of the sonographer.
GS, Gestational sac; hCG, human chorionic gonadotropin; TAUS, transabdominal ultrasound.

visualized. When an intrauterine gestation is clearly demonstrated, the likelihood of simultaneous extrauterine and intrauterine gestations (i.e., heterotopic pregnancy) is only 1 in every 7000 to 8000 cases or 1 in 30,000 low-risk pregnancies. If a patient has had infertility treatment, the risk of heterotopic pregnancy increases. An ectopic pregnancy becomes almost certain with transvaginal scanning if (a) no intrauterine pregnancy is visualized, (b) no vaginal bleeding is present, and (c) the quantitative human chorionic gonadotropin (hCG) is greater than 2000 IU.

5. The ultrasound appearance of a gestational sac can be mimicked by the exfoliation of hyperplastic endometrium associated with an ectopic pregnancy. This finding, known as a *pseudogestational sac*, can appear very similar to a gestational sac. A pseudogestational sac occurs in 10% to 20% of ectopic pregnancies. Unequivocal diagnosis of an intrauterine pregnancy should not be made until the gestational sac contains two concentric rims, a fetal pole, and a yolk sac, or fetal heart activity can be identified within the sac.

6. In a normal pregnancy, the mean serum hCG doubling time is 1.98 days. If serial hCG titers plateau or fall, an abnormal (ectopic) or nonviable pregnancy is likely.

7. Optimally, each institution should correlate its ultrasound equipment and sonographer's skill with quantitative hCG levels obtained from its own reference laboratory. When this is accomplished, externally published quantitative hCG reference levels and expected ultrasound findings should be used only as rough guidelines. Current published quantitative hCG levels and ultrasound correlations are outlined in Table 142.4.

8. If a gestational sac is absent at an hCG value above the institution's threshold, ectopic pregnancy, recent spontaneous abortion, and early hydatidiform degeneration should be considered. Suspicion of an ectopic pregnancy should be even higher if there is significant fluid in the cul de sac.

9. Ultrasound examination is helpful for evaluating for residual products of conception following spontaneous abortion, for diagnosing the vanishing twin syndrome (abortion of one fetus of a multiple gestation), and for evaluating fetal viability in threatened abortion. It is the procedure of choice for evaluation of gestational trophoblastic disease.

10. With ultrasound examination alone, a normal gestational sac can often be distinguished from an abnormal sac doomed to miscarriage, even before the embryo is visible. A gestational sac of abnormal size or appearance correlates highly with an abnormal outcome.
   Major criteria for a normal-appearing gestational sac:
   • A sac of 25 mm or more in diameter should contain an embryo (17 mm in diameter for transvaginal scanning).
   • The sac should be round.
   Minor criteria for a normal-appearing gestational sac:
   • The gestational sac is located in the fundus of the uterus.

• A thick, echogenic decidual ring surrounds the gestational sac.
• There is evidence of the double-ring sign.

11. When a gestational sac with a mean diameter greater than 25 mm (17 mm for transvaginal scanning) lacks an embryo or is grossly distorted, abnormal pregnancy is almost certain. A single ultrasound correctly classifies 76% of abnormal pregnancies and 93% of normal pregnancies.

12. Once embryonic cardiac motion is seen on ultrasound, the likelihood of spontaneous abortion is very low (<16% for pregnancies at <8 weeks; <2% to 4% after 12 weeks).

13. NT is the maximum thickness of the subcutaneous translucent area between the skin and soft tissue that overlies the fetal spine in the sagittal plane at the neck. It can be accurately measured between 11 and 14 weeks; with several large studies ($N > 8500$ and $N > 33,000$) detecting 85% of cases of Down syndrome by ultrasound combined with serum markers, ACOG has recognized it as an acceptable option to screen for trisomy 18 and 21. Specialized training is required to perform NT evaluations.

Intrapartum Scanning

1. Limited scans can usually be performed by individuals with minimal ultrasound training to document fetal life, number, and presentation; to estimate the amount of amniotic fluid; and to record the placental location and determine its relationship to the cervical os. Several factors unique to late pregnancy may make such scanning more difficult (e.g., physical crowding due to advanced gestational age, advanced station during labor, loss of acoustic window due to fluid loss after rupture of membranes). Fetal life is usually confirmed by observing fetal cardiac motion. It can also be documented on a still image using M-mode imaging. Diagnosis of fetal demise is discussed in detail in Chapter 214, Emergency Department, Hospitalist, and Office Ultrasound (Clinical Ultrasound).
   Fetal lie is defined by the orientation of the fetal spine to the maternal spine (longitudinal, transverse, oblique). After several sweeps of the uterus with ultrasound, the fetal lie and presentation are usually apparent. If the fetal lie is transverse, it is helpful to know if the fetal spine is up or down in relation to the LUS. Choice of uterine incision for cesarean changes and risk of cord prolapse increases when the fetal spine is transverse. Methods of estimating AFV are discussed elsewhere. The placenta is generally seen while performing other parts of an intrapartum scan. If not, it is probably posterior. Uterine contractions can alter the apparent location, thickness, and appearance of the placenta. A more thorough evaluation of the placenta usually requires more comprehensive training.

2. Extended applications require additional training. They include examination for placenta previa (see section on Placental

Imaging), evaluation of preterm cervical change (see section on Preterm Labor), evaluation for procedural guidance (see appropriate chapters), and evaluation for intrapartum twin management. Such applications may also include organ survey and biometry for fetal age and weight (see sections on Ultrasound Dating, Organ Survey, Fetal Size, and Postdates Pregnancy). When evaluating for placenta previa, make sure the maternal bladder is not overdistended. This can compress the LUS and cause a false perception of placenta previa. Such scanning is probably best performed with the bladder partially full and then with an empty bladder. It should also be performed between contractions when possible.

3. When managing intrapartum twins, the initial presentation and lie of the fetuses should be determined. After delivery of the first twin, the cardiac rate and rhythm of the second twin should be observed.

Complications

Although there are theoretical risks of ultrasound damaging human fetuses, no proven harm has been documented to any human fetus or mother. Other possible complications from obstetric ultrasound are failure to diagnose an anomaly or condition, inaccurate estimate of gestational age or weight, inappropriate reassurance, or inaccurate determination of fetal sex. Because fetal anomalies can remain undetected even by the best sonographer with the best equipment, the patient should never be unequivocally assured that the fetus is "fine." However, the patient can be reassured with answers from the imaging to specific questions.

Postprocedure Patient Education

If follow-up scans or other management will be needed, the patient should receive instructions.

PATIENT EDUCATION GUIDES

See the patient education and patient consent form available at www.expertconsult.com.

CPT/BILLING CODES

76801	Ultrasound, pregnant uterus, real time with image documentation, fetal and maternal evaluation, first trimester (<14 weeks 0 days), transabdominal approach; single or first gestation
76802	Each additional gestation (List separately in addition to code for primary procedure. List 76802 in conjunction with 76801.)
76805	Ultrasound, pregnant uterus, real time with image documentation, fetal and maternal evaluation, after first trimester, transabdominal approach, single or first gestation
76810	Each additional gestation (List separately in addition to code for primary procedure. List 76810 in conjunction with 76805.)
76813	Ultrasound, pregnant uterus, real time with image documentation, first trimester fetal nuchal translucency measurement, transabdominal or transvaginal approach; single for first gestation
76814	Each additional gestation (List 76814 in conjunction with 76813.)
76815	Limited (e.g., fetal heart beat, placental location, fetal position, and/or qualitative amniotic fluid volume)
76816	Follow-up or repeat of 76815 (Report 76816 with modifier 59 for each additional fetus examined in a multiple pregnancy.)
76817	Ultrasound, pregnant uterus, transvaginal
76818	Fetal biophysical profile; with nonstress testing
76819	Fetal biophysical profile; without nonstress testing

ICD-10-CM DIAGNOSTIC CODES

N93.9	Vaginal bleeding, nonpregnant
O01.9	Hydatidiform mole
O02.89	Blighted ovum
O02.1	Missed abortion
633.9	Ectopic pregnancy, unspecified
O03.4	Abortion or miscarriage, incomplete, without complications
O03.9	Abortion or miscarriage, complete, without complications
O20.0	Threatened abortion, antepartum
O20.9	Unspecified hemorrhage in early pregnancy, antepartum
O44.00	Placenta previa complete without hemorrhage unspecified trimester
O44.10	Placenta previa complete with hemorrhage unspecified trimester
O45.90	Placental abruption unspecified trimester
O10.919	Benign essential hypertension complicating pregnancy unspecified trimester
O14.00	Mild or unspecified preeclampsia, unspecified trimester
O14.10	Severe preeclampsia, unspecified trimester
O11.9	Preeclampsia or eclampsia superimposed on preexisting hypertension, unspecified trimester
O60.14X0	Preterm labor, delivered
O60.00	Preterm labor, unspecified trimester
O48.0	Post-term pregnancy (40 to 42 weeks), antepartum
O48.1	Prolonged pregnancy (>42 weeks), antepartum
O26.849	Uterine size–date discrepancy, unspecified trimester
O24.019	Diabetes mellitus, preexisting, unspecified trimester
O24.419	Abnormal glucose tolerance (gestational diabetes)
O30.009	Multiple gestation, twins, unspecified trimester
O30.90	Multiple gestation, unspecified, unspecified trimester
O36.4XX	Maternal care for intrauterine death
O36.5990	Intrauterine growth retardation, unspecified trimester
O36.60X0	Fetal macrosomia, unspecified trimester
O40.9XX0	Polyhydramnios, unspecified trimester
O41.00X0	Oligohydramnios, unspecified trimester
P00.5	Maternal injury, fetus or newborn affected by maternal conditions

Acknowledgment

The editors recognize the contributions of Richard E. A. Brunader, MD, to this chapter in previous editions of this text.

SUPPLIERS

(See contact information available at www.expertconsult.com.)

Note that ultrasound machine technology continues to evolve. There are now probes that are compatible with USB ports or iPhones. However, the variance in pricing for the most basic equipment can be substantial.

Acuson
Esaote (Biosound), Inc.
General Electric Medical Systems
Hitachi Aloka Medical Corp.
Samsung Medison America, Inc.
Philips
Toshiba America Medical Systems

RECOMMENDED READING

Alfirevic Z, Stampalija T, Medley N. Fetal and umbilical Doppler ultrasound in normal pregnancy. *Cochrane Database Syst Rev.* 2015;(4):CD001450.

American College of Obstetricians and Gynecologists. *Fetal Macrosomia. ACOG Practice Bulletin no. 173.* Washington, DC: ACOG; 2016.

American College of Obstetricians and Gynecologists. Method for estimating due date. ACOG practice bulletin no. 611. *Obstet Gynecol.* 2014;142(4):863–866.

American College of Obstetricians and Gynecologists. Nonmedical use of obstetric ultrasonography. committee opinion no. 297. *Obstet Gynecol.* 2004;104(2):423–424.

American College of Obstetricians and Gynecologists. Ultrasonography in pregnancy. ACOG practice bulletin no. 175. *Obstet Gynecol.* 2016;128(6):e241–e256.

American Institute of Ultrasound Medicine. *AIUM Practice Parameter for Obstetric Ultrasound Examinations.* Laurel, MD: AIUM; 2013. http://www.aium.org/resources/guidelines/obstetric.pdf.

Benson CB, Douiblet PM. The history of imaging in obstetrics. *Radiology.* 2014;273(suppl 2):S92–S110.

Bhide A, Leslie K, Chandraharan E, et al. Morbid adherence of the placenta: lack of specificity should remind us that ultrasound is a screening tool. *Ultrasound Obstet Gynecol.* 2017.

Callen PW, ed. *Ultrasonography in Obstetrics and Gynecology.* 6th ed. Philadelphia: Elsevier; 2017.

Chiossi G, Palomba S, Balduzzi S, Costantine MM, Falbo AI, la Sala GB. "The more the better" paradox of antenatal ultrasound examinations in low-risk pregnancy. *Am J Perinatol.* 2016;33(07):646–657.

Delle Donne RD, Araugo Junior E, Rolo LC, et al. Reproducibility of placental maturity grade classification using a dynamic ultrasonography. *J Matern Fetal Neonatal Med.* 2016;24:1–3.

Deutchman M, Sakornbut E. Diagnostic ultrasound in labor and delivery. In: *Syllabus for Advanced Life Support in Obstetrics.* Kansas City, MO: American Academy of Family Physicians; 2010.

Everett TR, Peebles DM. Antenatal tests of fetal wellbeing. *Semin Fetal Neonatal Med.* 2015;20(3):138–143.

Ewigman BG, Crane JP, Frigoletto FD, et al. Effect of prenatal ultrasound screening on perinatal outcome: RADIUS Study Group. *N Engl J Med.* 1993;329:821–827.

Karim JN, Roberts NW, Salomon LJ, Papageorghiou AT. Systematic review of first-trimester ultrasound screening for detection of fetal structural anomalies and factors that affect screening performance. *Ultrasound Obstet Gynecol.* 2017;50(4):429.

Markham KB, Iams JD. Measuring the cervical length. *Clin Obstet Gynecol.* 2016;59(2):252–263.

Nardozza LM, Caetano AC, Zamarian AC. Fetal growth restriction: current knowledge. *Arch Gynecol Obstet.* 2017.

Peleg D, Warsof S, Wolk MF. Counseling for fetal macrosomia: an estimated fetal weight of 4,000 g is excessively low. *Am J Perinatol.* 2015;32(1):71–74.

Reddy UM, Abuhamad AZ, Levine D, et al. Fetal imaging: executive summary of a joint Eunice Kennedy Shriver National Institute of Child Health and Human Development Society for Maternal-Fetal Medicine, American Institute of Ultrasound in Medicine, American College of Obstetricians and Gynecologists, American College of Radiology, Society for Pediatric Radiology, and Society of Radiologists in Ultrasound Fetal Imaging Workshop. *Obstet Gynecol.* 2014;123:1070.

Sanders RC, Hall-Terracciano B, eds. *Clinical Sonography: A Practical Guide.* 5th ed. Philadelphia: Wolters Kluwer; 2016.

Shepard MJ, Richards VA, Berkowitz RL, et al. An evaluation of two equations for predicting fetal weight by ultrasound. *Am J Obstet Gynecol.* 1987;156:80.

Silver R, Landon MB, Rouse DJ, et al. National Institute of Child Health and Human Development Maternal Fetal Medicine Units Network. Maternal morbidity associated with multiple repeat cesarean deliveries. *Obstet Gynecol.* 2006;107:1226–1232.

Tuggy M, Garcia J. *Procedures Consult.* First-trimester obstetric ultrasound. http://www.proceduresconsult.com/medical-procedures/first-trimester-obstetric-ultrasound-FM-039-procedure.aspx.

Tuggy M, Garcia J. *Procedures Consult.* Third-trimester obstetric ultrasound. http://www.proceduresconsult.com/medical-procedures/third-trimester-obstetric-ultrasound-FM-040-procedure.aspx.

Whitworth M, Bricker L, Mullan C. Ultrasound for fetal assessment in early pregnancy. *Cochrane Database Syst Rev.* 2015;7:CD007058.

Zolotor AJ, Carlough MC. Update on prenatal care. *Am Fam Physician.* 2014;89(3):199–208.

CHAPTER 143

CERVICAL CERCLAGE

Madeline R. Lewis • Mark Lewis

Cervical insufficiency involves painless cervical dilation. It can lead to early second trimester pregnancy loss or premature delivery with neonatal complications in the third trimester. Making the diagnosis of cervical insufficiency is often difficult due to lack of objective findings or distinct diagnostic criteria. It can be based on history alone: painless cervical dilation and fetal expulsion in the second trimester (before 24 weeks) without labor, contractions, or other obvious pathology (e.g., infection, preterm rupture of membranes or bleeding [American College of Obstetricians and Gynecologists, 2014]).

Cerclage is a procedure that attempts to manage cervical insufficiency by delaying time to delivery. *History-indicated* (prophylactic) cerclage may be considered in patients with a history of unexplained second-trimester delivery in the absence of labor or abruption. Another consideration is in a patient with a history of cervical insufficiency necessitating cerclage placement in a prior pregnancy. Parturients who present with advanced cervical dilation in the absence of labor or abruption have also usually been offered *physical examination-indicated* (i.e., emergency or rescue) cerclage. With *ultrasound-indicated* cerclage, the diagnosis of short cervical length (e.g., <25 mm) is in and of itself not a specific marker for cervical insufficiency. However, studies indicate that women with a current singleton pregnancy, a history of preterm delivery (prior to 34 weeks gestation), and short cervical length before 24 weeks gestation may benefit from cerclage placement (ultrasound-indicated cerclage). Cerclage prior to 24 weeks gestation in this group is estimated to reduce preterm delivery rate (before 35 weeks gestation) by 30% (Dahlke et al., 2016).

There are various cerclage techniques, including transabdominal techniques (permanent, so cesarean delivery is required), the Shirodkar technique (which may or may not be permanent), the McDonald technique, and several variations on each. Transabdominal cerclage can now be done laparoscopically, before or during pregnancy, and is probably indicated when vaginal cerclage has failed. The most common and simplest is the vaginal McDonald procedure, which will be discussed in this chapter. The McDonald cerclage involves inserting a pursestring stitch at the cervicovaginal junction using monofilament suture. This procedure is best done as an elective procedure; it may also be performed in an urgent or emergent setting.

American College of Obstetricians and Gynecologists guidelines recommend performing an elective cerclage at 13 to 14 weeks gestation after verifying fetal viability by ultrasound. The cerclage is then removed after 36 to 37 weeks of pregnancy or at the onset of premature labor.

ANATOMY

The relevant anatomy is shown in Fig. 143.1. The area of focus is the proximal cervix, near the area where the smooth ectocervix meets the rugated mucosa overlying the bladder. Cervical orientation is important—this chapter uses the clock method for describing locations on the cervix. With the patient in the dorsal lithotomy position, the anterior cervix is defined as the 12 o'clock position.

INDICATIONS

Cervical insufficiency may be due to a variety of factors. Indications for cerclage in women with singleton pregnancies include the following:

- History of one or more second-trimester pregnancy losses related to painless cervical dilation (absence of labor or abruption).
- History of prior cerclage placement due to second-trimester painless cervical dilation.
- Painless cervical dilation in second trimester noted on physical exam.
- Surgical trauma from cone biopsy, loop electrosurgical excision procedure, obstetric laceration, or damage from surgical dilators (e.g., Hegar or Hicks) during pregnancy termination.
- Maternal congenital cervical anomalies.
- Short cervical length (<25 mm) prior to 24 weeks gestation in women with current singleton pregnancy and history of preterm delivery prior to 34 weeks gestation.
- Deficiencies in cervical collagen and elastin.
- Maternal in-utero diethylstilbestrol exposure. (Diethylstilbestrol was abandoned in 1970s, so it is no longer a congenital risk; this is listed more for historic purposes.)
- Amniotic membrane funneling into the cervical canal on ultrasound.
- Placenta previa if associated with cervical dilation. However, in the absence of cervical dilation, use of cerclage with placenta previa does not prolong pregnancy. Cerclage is not contraindicated in patients with placenta previa who otherwise are candidates for the procedure.

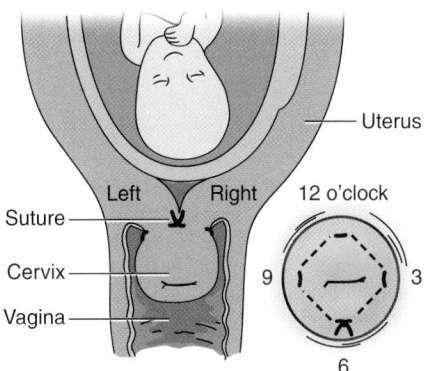

Fig. 143.1 Cervical cerclage and relevant anatomy. Note that the initial suture can be placed at 6 o'clock to allow the knot to reside in the posterior vagina.

CONTRAINDICATIONS

Absolute

- Fetal demise or conditions incompatible with survival
- Undiagnosed vaginal bleeding
- Ruptured membranes
- Active preterm labor
- Acute cervical or intraamniotic infection
- Twin pregnancy (Cerclage has been shown to increase risk of preterm birth if ultrasound-measured cervical length is <25 cm.)

Relative

- Known or suspected fetal anomalies
- Prolapse of fetal membranes through the external cervical os (increased risk of iatrogenic rupture of membranes)

EQUIPMENT AND SUPPLIES

Cerclage is considered an outpatient surgical procedure and is performed in the operating room. Sterile preparation and proper drapes and equipment are necessary. Equipment to maintain universal blood and body fluid precautions should be available. Specific instruments include the following:

- Bladder catheter (red rubber) with lubricant
- Weighted vaginal speculum (Graves)
- Retractor (Deaver or right-angle)
- Ring forceps
- Nonabsorbable suture material on a curved needle (No. 5 Mersilene band, Ethibond; [do not confuse with a 5-0 suture, which is much smaller])
- Pickups
- Metzenbaum scissors
- Needle driver

PRECAUTIONS

Be aware that urgent or emergent cerclage has an increased incidence of complications. A cerclage is best performed in a controlled setting with appropriate indications. Be certain to confirm a viable pregnancy before starting the procedure.

PREPROCEDURE PATIENT EDUCATION

- Review the risks of the procedure with the patient. Overall, there is a low risk of complications with cerclage placement; the incidence varies depending on the timing and indication for the cerclage (e.g., indicated by history, by physical exam, by ultrasound, or emergently).
  - Rupture of membranes. (Based on randomized controlled trials, the estimated intraoperative rupture of membrane rate is 0.3% for ultrasound-indicated cerclage and 0.9% for emergency-indicated cerclage [Dahlke et al., 2016].)
  - Chorioamnionitis (may occur in up to 30% of cases).
  - Increased frequency of contractions.
  - Uterine rupture (rare).
  - Need for caesarean delivery (3% risk due to inability of cervix to dilate secondary to scarring or dystocia).
  - Maternal septicemia.
  - Preterm labor and delivery.
  - Fetal loss.
  - Cerclage displacement; may need to replace cerclage if still early in pregnancy (<24 weeks).
  - Cervical laceration at time of delivery.

- Preoperative testing may be indicated to rule out cervical infection (gonorrhea/chlamydial infection).
- Ultrasound is done before the procedure to confirm a normal intrauterine pregnancy.
- The procedure is performed in an operating room and requires anesthesia (general or regional); the patient will need to have someone with her to drive her home after the procedure.
- The procedure is usually performed as an outpatient, same-day procedure. In the setting of emergency-indicated cerclage, patients are often observed in the hospital for 24 hours, although this is based on expert opinion. (There are no large studies.)
- The patient is placed on a fetal monitor before and after the procedure to document fetal viability.
- After the procedure, acetaminophen (Tylenol) usually provides adequate pain control, if necessary.
- Significant vaginal discharge may be present for weeks following the procedure.
- The patient will need to be seen more frequently throughout the remainder of the pregnancy.
- Pelvic rest is often recommended; instruct the patient to limit physical activity for at least 1 week and to abstain from vaginal intercourse for at least 1 week and up to the entire pregnancy.

PROCEDURE

1. Obtain informed consent (see sample patient consent form available at www.expertconsult.com). The clinician should follow universal blood and body fluid precautions.
2. Document intrauterine viability.
3. The patient is brought to the operating room where either general or regional anesthetic is administered. Local anesthesia or a paracervical block should be avoided because of concern for altered uterine blood flow.
4. Place the patient in the dorsal lithotomy position with feet in candy cane stirrups; prepare and drape in a sterile fashion.
5. Drain the bladder with a red rubber catheter (a Foley catheter is not necessary).
6. Place a weighted Graves speculum in the posterior vagina.
7. Insert a Deaver or right-angle retractor in the vagina to provide adequate exposure; have an assistant hold it carefully to avoid bladder trauma.
8. Using a ring forceps, grasp the anterior lip of the cervix at 12 o'clock, and displace it superiorly.
9. Place a stitch at the 6 o'clock position in the midportion of the cervix equidistant from the ectocervix and the vaginal reflection (near the cervicovaginal junction). Place the suture through the midportion of the cervical stroma, being careful not to enter the cervical canal. Sutures that are too shallow may tear out when drawn tight. Be aware of the cervical vascularity (at 3 and 9 o'clock). Direct the needle toward the 3 o'clock position within the cervical tissue.
10. Proceeding in a counterclockwise manner (clockwise if left-handed), pass the suture to the 3 o'clock position. Remove it from the cervix and then immediately loop it back into the cervix. Pass the stitch to the 12 o'clock position, again, within the tissue itself. Withdraw it and then reinsert in same area. Again, pass the stitch to the 9 o'clock position, withdraw, and reinsert. Finally, pass the stitch to the starting position (6 o'clock) and withdraw the suture (see Fig. 143.1).
11. Cinch down the suture, similar to a pursestring. Without drawing too tightly (to avoid tissue strangulation), tie it, leaving ends long enough to grasp with ring forceps for removal. By starting at the 6 o'clock position instead of the 12 o'clock position, the patient may have decreased bladder irritation from the suture because the knot rests in the posterior vagina. However, evidence does not support the superiority of this, and starting the stitch at 12 o'clock to place the knot anteriorly may make later removal of the cerclage easier.

12. Some surgeons prefer to place a second cerclage lower than the first, although no improvement in outcome has been documented. Complications such as membrane rupture or bladder perforation may be more frequent.

13. The patient then recovers while being placed on a fetal monitor to ensure fetal well-being.

14. Discharge after a period of adequate observation. Antibiotics are not recommended, and tocolytic agents have no proven benefit.

15. Complete a postoperative note indicating the type of cerclage placed (McDonald), the suture type, the anesthesia, the location of the suture placement, and the number of knots placed. A diagram is helpful. Place a copy of the operative report in the patient's medical record.

REMOVAL

The cerclage is left in place until the 36th to 37th week of pregnancy, at which time it can usually be easily removed in the office. The patient is placed in dorsal lithotomy position (stirrups), and following universal blood and body fluid precautions, the cervix is visualized using a sterile speculum. The knot is grasped with pickups (e.g., a Russian), the knot is elevated, and Metzenbaum scissors are used to cut the cerclage stitch, which is then easily removed. If difficulty arises when attempting to remove the cerclage, proceeding to the operating room may be prudent. If preterm labor is encountered later in the pregnancy and tocolysis is unsuccessful, the cerclage should be removed at that time to avoid cervical damage.

SAMPLE OPERATIVE REPORT

Procedure:	McDonald cervical cerclage
Preop diagnosis:	Cervical insufficiency at _____ wk gestation
Postop diagnosis:	Same
Surgeon:	
Anesthesia:	
Estimated blood loss:	_____ mL
Specimen:	None
Drains:	None
Complications:	None
Disposition:	To Labor and Delivery for observation

History and Indications

Patient is a _____-year-old G_____ P_____ at _____ weeks' gestation with a viable fetus. She had _____ prior second-trimester pregnancy losses, with a history suggestive of cervical insufficiency. The plan was to place a cervical cerclage at 14 weeks. Risks and benefits of the procedure were discussed with the patient, who provided informed consent. Consents are signed and included in the chart.

Procedure Note

Fetal heart tones were documented and the patient was evaluated by both the surgeon and the anesthesiologist. The patient was then taken to the operating room, where she received a spinal anesthetic by Dr. _____. She was then placed in the dorsal lithotomy position. After verifying the adequacy of the spinal anesthetic, the patient was prepped and draped in the usual manner, and her bladder was drained using a red rubber catheter.

A weighted Graves speculum was placed in the posterior vagina, and the anterior lip of the cervix was grasped with a ring forceps. No membranes protruded through the external cervical os.

A No. 5 Mersilene tape suture was placed at the 6 o'clock position at the level of the internal os with the suture exiting at the 3 o'clock position, reinserted in this same area, exiting at the 12 o'clock position. The suture was reinserted at the 12 o'clock position and removed at the 9 o'clock position, reinserted in this same area, exiting at the 6 o'clock position. The suture was tied with three knots at the 6 o'clock position. No significant bleeding was noted.

The weighted speculum and ring forceps were removed. The patient tolerated the procedure well and was transported to Labor and Delivery in stable condition.

Signature, date, and time: _____

COMMON ERROR

Placing a suture shallowly so that it pulls out when tightened is a potential error.

COMPLICATIONS

Discussed in the Preprocedure Patient Education section.

POSTPROCEDURE PATIENT CARE

- Monitor the patient until adequately recovered from anesthesia and patient is able to ambulate and void.
- Document fetal viability prior to discharge.
- Acetaminophen should provide any necessary pain relief.
- Patient discharge instructions should include the following:
  - Vaginal discharge after the procedure is normal and may continue for weeks.
  - Call the office if any leakage of fluid from the vagina, fever, severe cramping, or pain develop.
  - Pelvic rest and limited physical activity for at least 1 week for history-indicated (prophylactic) cerclage; if procedure was emergent, pelvic rest and limited activity throughout remainder of pregnancy.
- See patient frequently (weekly or biweekly) for follow-up.

POSTPROCEDURE PATIENT EDUCATION

- The patient should avoid vaginal intercourse and limit physical activity for at least the first week after the procedure. Consider no intercourse and no heavy physical activity until after delivery.
- Vaginal discharge may be normal for weeks after this procedure. The patient should contact her clinician if she experiences severe cramping, fever, or any vaginal bleeding.
- Acetaminophen is helpful for any pain or discomfort after this procedure.
- Monitor the patient closely with checks every 1 to 2 weeks.
- Advise that a second stitch may be needed if the first stitch does not remain tightly secured.
- The cerclage will be removed at around 36th to 37th week gestation in the office.

Be aware that there is little evidence to support these recommendations, and they may be modified to fit the individual situation. An emergently placed cerclage has a higher risk for complications.

CPT/BILLING CODES

59320	Cerclage
59871	Removal of cerclage suture under anesthesia (other than local)*

No CPT code exists for removal of a cerclage without anesthesia.
*If the same physician both places and removes the cerclage, removal is bundled as part of the original placement charge.

ICD-10-CM DIAGNOSTIC CODES

O34.30	Cervical insufficiency in pregnancy trimester unspecified
O34.3	Maternal care for cervical incompetence (nonbillable)
O34.30	Maternal care for cervical incompetence, unspecified trimester (nonbillable)
O34.31	Maternal care for cervical incompetence, first trimester (nonbillable)
O34.32	Maternal care for cervical incompetence, second trimester (nonbillable)
O34.33	Maternal care for cervical incompetence, third trimester
P01.0	Cervical insufficiency in pregnancy affecting fetus or newborn

Acknowledgment

The editors recognize the contributions of Charles E. Werner Jr, MD, to this chapter in previous editions of this text.

RECOMMENDED READING

American College of Obstetricians and Gynecologists: ACOG practice bulletin no. 142: cervical insufficiency. *Obstet Gynecol.* 2014;123(2):372–379.

Cunningham FG, Leveno KL, Bloom S, et al., eds. *Williams Obstetrics.* 24th ed. New York: McGraw-Hill; 2015:829–861.

Dahlke JD, Sperling JF, Chauhan SP, et al. Cervical cerclage during periviability. *Obstet Gynecol.* 2016;127(5):934–940.

Ehsanipoor RM, Seligman NS, Saccone G, et al. Physical examination-indicated cerclage. *Obstet Gynecol.* 2015;126(1):125–135.

Ludmir J, Owen J, Berghella V. Cervical insufficiency. In: Gabbe SG, Niebyl JR, Simpson JL, et al., eds. *Gabbe's Obstetrics: Normal and Problem Pregnancies.* 7th ed. Philadelphia: Elsevier; 2017:595–614.

McDonald IA. Suture of the cervix for inevitable miscarriage. *J Obstet Gynaecol Br Emp.* 1957;64:346–350.

Naqvi M, Barth WH. Emergency cerclage: outcomes, patient selection, and operative considerations. *Clin Obstet Gynecol.* 2016;59(2):286–294.

Sneider K, Christiansen OB, Sundtoft IB. Recurrence rates after abdominal and vaginal cerclages in women with cervical insufficiency: a validated cohort study. *Arch Gynecol Obstet.* 2017.

Wood SL, Owen J. Cerclage: Shirodkar, McDonald, and modifications. *Clin Obstet Gynecol.* 2016;59(2):302–310.

CHAPTER 144

Amniocentesis

Dale A. Patterson • John J. Andazola

Although genetic studies were first performed on amniotic fluid in the 1950s, before the 1970s the primary indication for amniocentesis was for evaluation of the Rh-immunized patient. Indications rapidly expanded to include evaluation of fetal lung maturity (FLM), fetal genetic diagnosis, rupture or infection of the amniotic membranes or fluid, and other factors related to fetal health. In high-risk centers, amniocentesis became a routine procedure in approximately 15% of pregnancies. However, the overall frequency of amniocentesis decreased every year from 1989 through 2003 (down to 1.7% of pregnancies). In one study examining incidence of invasive testing over the years between 2002 and 2014, there were significant declines in both chorionic villus sampling (CVS) and amniocentesis, although the decrease in amniocentesis was more marked (6.3% of cases in first third of the study vs. 1.2% in last third of the study [Khalifeh et al., 2016]). That said, amniocentesis remains the most common invasive procedure performed to diagnose fetal aneuploidy and other genetic conditions.

Benefits of CVS over amniocentesis are that results from CVS are available earlier in pregnancy (at 10 to 13 weeks), allowing safer pregnancy termination if desired. A full genetic karyotype is generally available in 7 to 10 days, with some laboratories providing preliminary results in 48 hours. CVS can be performed transcervically or transabdominally.

AMNIOCENTESIS INDICATIONS

Prenatal Diagnosis (First and Second Trimester)

Chromosomal Studies

Advances in technology have increased options for genetic screening in pregnancy. Development of noninvasive prenatal testing (NIPT) permits genetic sequencing of cell-free DNA from the maternal plasma to assess for specific aneuploidies (e.g., trisomies 13, 18, 21). This has provided a less invasive means for screening for aneuploides in high-risk women, although NIPT does not currently pick up single gene deletions and other types of genetic anomalies that diagnostic testing (e.g., amniocentesis, CVS) can detect. A joint American College of Obstetricians and Gynecologists (ACOG)/Society for Maternal-Fetal Medicine Committee Opinion states that "cell-free fetal DNA testing should not be offered to low-risk women or women with multiple gestations because it has not been sufficiently evaluated in these groups." NIPT also does not screen for neural tube defects or anterior abdominal wall defects, so maternal alpha-fetoprotein must be measured. In women who have an ultrasound indicating fetal structural anomalies, diagnostic testing (i.e., CVS or amniocentesis) is indicated. As a screening test, NIPT also has both false-positive and false-negative results. Abnormal results require follow-up with a diagnostic study such as CVS or amniocentesis. However, over the first 2 years of NIPT availability, one study found a 28% decrease in referrals for genetic counseling and prenatal diagnosis, and a significant increase in women who decline diagnostic testing following a positive screen (Williams et al., 2015). Because each

method of testing has individual strengths and weaknesses, no universal consensus exists about which to initially pursue.

Amniotic fluid contains both fetal and amniotic cells. The fetal cells include desquamated squamous cells and cells from the gastrointestinal tract, respiratory tract, and urinary system. Although it requires 7 to 10 days for karyotype results, culture of these cells allows accurate analysis for fetal chromosomal, sex-linked, and metabolic disorders. For chromosomal analysis, amniocentesis is usually performed at 15 to 18 weeks, when there are sufficient numbers of desquamated fetal cells to allow successful culture.

Although early amniocentesis (i.e., 10 to 14 weeks gestation) can be performed, CVS can also be performed at this time for similar indications. With amniocentesis, because there is very little fluid at the stage, less fluid should be withdrawn, which makes it less likely to produce cell growth. This increases the likelihood of need for a second procedure. Sac puncture is also more difficult due to lack of sac fusion to the uterine wall. Both amniocentesis and CVS at this stage carry higher risks of amniotic fluid leakage, fetal loss, and talipes equinovarus (club foot). However, the risk for talipes equinovarus with early amniocentesis is fourfold that of CVS (Philip et al., 2004). The risks and benefits of these procedures are otherwise similar but vary slightly by location and indication. Due to the increased risk of complications, ACOG recommends against the use of early amniocentesis between 10 and 14 weeks of gestation.

Indications for amniocentesis include the following:

- Advanced maternal age (35 years of age or older)
- Parent who is a carrier of a genetic disease that can be diagnosed by amniocentesis
- Mother who is a carrier of an X-linked disorder or known translocation
- History of a child with a chromosomal disorder, neural tube defect, inherited biochemical disorder, or multiple anomalies
- Mother with a history of three or more spontaneous abortions
- Follow-up after fetal abnormalities suggested by ultrasound
- Follow-up of abnormal NIPT or serum analyte testing (e.g., Quad screen)

Evaluating Fetal Health (Late Second or Third Trimester)

Bilirubin levels, measured spectrophotometrically as $\Delta OD450$, are no longer the standard of care for following the Rh or other blood group isoimmunized pregnancy. This has been replaced by Doppler ultrasound measurement of the peak velocity of systolic blood flow in the middle cerebral artery; this flow is abnormally increased in the setting of fetal anemia. The sensitivity and specificity of Doppler ultrasound have been shown to be superior to those of measurement of the amniotic fluid $\Delta OD450$. Doppler ultrasound is noninvasive and thus does not carry the risk associated with amniocentesis. It is recommended that patients with Rh alloimmunization be referred to a center where Doppler ultrasound of the middle cerebral artery is performed.

Evaluating Fetal Maturity (Third Trimester)

A common historic indication for performing amniocentesis was to assess fetal lung maturity (FLM). Lecithin (L), sphingomyelin (S), and phosphatidylglycerol (PG) are phospholipids in the newborn lung that act as surfactants and lower the alveolar surface tension. Amniocentesis to determine the L/S ratio, the presence of PG, or both, minimized the risk of delivering an infant with respiratory distress syndrome (RDS). Other methods of determining FLM include the foam stability index (FSI), fluorescence polarization, and lamellar body counts (Table 144.1).

Current guidelines for prenatal care state that in the absence of medical indications, routine delivery should not occur prior to 39 weeks gestation (ACOG, 2013). ACOG further recommends that in well-dated pregnancies, amniocentesis for determination of FLM should not be used to guide timing for delivery. Late-preterm or early-term gestations with a clear medical indication for delivery are delivered regardless of lung maturity. Conversely, if an immature FLM profile could safely delay delivery, a valid indication for early delivery is missing. The debate as to whether amniocentesis for FLM is obsolete in pregnancies with ultrasound dating prior to 20 weeks is ongoing. One indication that remains, though, is for women with late or no prenatal care where a 39-week elective induction is desired.

However, many providers will simply wait until these patients go into labor rather than pursue invasive testing. ACOG similarly recommends that these patients be induced at 41 weeks' gestation unless a medical indication for delivery occurs prior to this.

Therapeutic Interventions

- Relief of symptomatic polyhydramnios, although this is temporary because the fluid rapidly reaccumulates
- Intrauterine transfusion for Rh-hemolytic disease

CONTRAINDICATIONS

Absolute

- Abdominal wall skin infection/lesions where amniocentesis is to be performed
- Patient refusal
- Test results will not alter clinical course

Relative

- Maternal coagulopathy
- Placental abruption
- Problems not diagnosable by amniotic fluid evaluation (e.g., teratogen exposure, radiation exposure, drug use early in pregnancy, history of genetic disorders not diagnosable by amniocentesis)

EQUIPMENT AND SUPPLIES

- Real-time diagnostic ultrasound unit
- Commercial amniocentesis tray or sterile tray containing at least three plain sterile specimen tubes (5 to 10 mL each) with caps; standard-length 20- or 22-gauge spinal needle (no larger than 20 gauge should be used; standard needles are usually 9 cm long, which may need to be increased based upon body habitus); 20-mL syringe; 5-mL syringe; 1.5-inch, 22- or 23-gauge needle; sterile 4 × 4 gauze pads; sterile adhesive bandages; and sterile towels for drapes
- Skin antiseptic (e.g., povidone–iodine, chlorhexidine gluconate)
- Fetal heart rate monitor
- Sterile gloves and equipment to follow universal blood and body fluid precautions

TABLE 144.1	Commonly Used Direct Tests of Fetal Lung Maturity								
					Typical Predictive Value (%)				
					Mature	Immature			
Test*	Technique	Time and Ease of Testing†	Threshold		Negative Predictive Value	Positive‡ Predictive Value	Blood Contamination Affects Results	Meconium Contamination Affects Results	Vaginal Pool Sample
Fluorescence polarization	Fluorescence polarization with TDx FLM II	1+	≥55 mg/g of albumin§		96–100	47–61	Yes	Yes	Yes
Lecithin/ sphingomyelin ratio	Thin-layer chromatography	4+	2–3.5		95–100	33–50	Yes	Yes	No
Phosphatidyl-glycerol	Thin-layer chromatography	4+	Present (usually >3% of total phospholipids)		95–100	23–53	No	No	Yes
	Antisera with AminoStat-FLM	1+	0.5 = low positive 2 = high positive		95–100	23–53	No	No	Yes
Lamellar body counts	Counts using commercial hematology counter	2+	30,000–40,000 (still investigational)		97–98	29–35	Yes	No	Not available
Optical density at 650 nm	Spectrophotometric reading	1+	Optical density of ≥0.15		98	13	Not available	Not available	Not available
Foam stability index	Ethanol added to amniotic fluid, solution shaken, presence of stable bubbles at meniscus noted	2+	≥47–48		95	51	Yes	Yes	No

*Commercial versions are available for all tests except optical density and lamellar body counts.
†Range in complexity: 1+ indicates procedure is simple, procedure is available all the time, procedure time is short, and personnel effort is not intensive; 4+ indicates procedure is complex or difficult, time consuming, and, therefore, frequently not available at all times.
‡Positive predictive value is the probability of neonatal respiratory distress syndrome when the fetal lung maturity test result is immature.
§The manufacturer has reformulated the product and revised the testing procedure. Currently, the threshold for maturity is 55; with the original assay, it was 70.
FLM, Fetal lung maturity.

- Local anesthetic solution (e.g., 1% or 2% lidocaine, without epinephrine) (optional)
- Dilute carmine dye for twin pregnancy (optional)
- Anti-D-immune globulin (e.g., RhoGAM) for Rh-D-negative mothers

NOTE: Disposable amniocentesis trays are available through most surgical suppliers.

PREPROCEDURE PATIENT EDUCATION AND FORMS

The clinician should discuss the procedure with the patient (and significant other when available) beforehand. Discuss the risks and benefits of amniocentesis. Describe alternative modes of evaluation or treatment (if any) and obtain signed informed consent. Note the increased risk of fetal loss with amniocentesis in markedly obese mothers (body mass index ≥40 kg/m^2) or with multiple gestation as discussed in the "Complications" section. (See the sample patient education and consent forms available at www.expertconsult.com.)

TECHNIQUE

1. Have the patient lie on the examining table or bed with the head elevated 20 to 30 degrees. Alternatively, perform the procedure with the patient in slight (15 degrees) left lateral decubitus position. Monitor the fetal heart rate for 20 minutes to establish a baseline.
2. Locate a pocket of fluid with real-time ultrasound (Fig. 144.1). Try to find a pocket that the needle will be able to reach while avoiding the umbilical cord and without going near the fetal face. Ideally, the path should not transverse the placenta. The best locations (associated with low risk of cord puncture) are usually in the area of the fetal extremities. Use the ultrasound electronic calipers to measure the depth from the skin that the needle must penetrate to enter the pocket. Note the desired longitudinal angle for the needle. If not perpendicular to the abdomen, note the lateral angle of the probe used to locate the pocket. The needle should be directed at the same lateral angle. Mark the location of the puncture site on the skin using pressure from a needle hub.
   EDITOR'S NOTE: The placenta is attached to the anterior uterine wall in approximately half of pregnancies. Consequently, the amniocentesis needle transverses the placenta in approximately 60% of these cases. Fortunately, this has not been associated with increased risk of pregnancy loss.
3. Prepare the abdomen with antiseptic solution.
4. The use of local anesthetic is optional. Most women have no or mild discomfort during the procedure, and administration of anesthetic is mildly painful. (A Cochrane review found no intervention has been shown to reduce discomfort (local anesthestic, subfreezing the needle, or leg rubbing). [Mujezinovic, 2011].) If anesthetic is desired, wearing sterile gloves and following universal blood and body fluid precautions (here and during amniocentesis), raise a skin wheal with the anesthetic at the puncture site. The needle should then be advanced to anesthetize along the course of the future amniocentesis needle track to anesthetize the parietal peritoneum and serosal surface of the uterus (requires 4 to 5 mL of anesthetic solution). Remove the needle.
5. With the stylet in place and concurrent real-time ultrasound guidance (transducer in sterile plastic bag, glove, or cover), insert the 20- or 22-gauge spinal needle along the selected track (at the correct angle) to the previously measured pocket depth. A slight "pop" may be felt as the needle passes through the fascia. When it penetrates the amniotic membrane, sudden free movement is noted. Attempts should be made to penetrate or puncture the chorioamnion rather than tent it away from the uterine wall.
6. Remove the stylet. In most cases, the amniotic fluid will flow through the needle. If not, rotate the needle (this may move the tip away from membranes, fetal parts, etc.). If there is no flow of fluid, attach the empty 5-mL anesthetic syringe to the needle hub and apply gentle suction. If there is still no fluid, replace the stylet and advance the needle another 0.5 to 1 cm or until resistance is felt. Again, remove the stylet. If there is no fluid, reattach the small syringe and withdraw the needle slowly with gentle suction, rotating it as it is withdrawn.
7. Once the fluid pocket is tapped, withdraw 2 or 3 mL of fluid in the small syringe and then discard it. This minimizes the amount of maternal blood or cells in the remaining fluid sample (blood can affect laboratory results). Next, withdraw 15 to 25 mL of fluid (or the volume needed for the tests planned). A rule of thumb is to collect a volume in milliliters equivalent to the gestational age of the pregnancy in weeks. Avoid prolonged contact of amniotic fluid with the rubber grommet at the end of the syringe plunger (i.e., keep syringe in tip down position until transferred). Remove the needle, clean the excess antiseptic from the abdominal wall, and cover the puncture wound with an adhesive bandage. If the patient is unsensitized Rh-negative, administer 300 mg of Rh-immune globulin. Monitor fetal heart tones for 20 minutes after the procedure using external fetal monitoring.

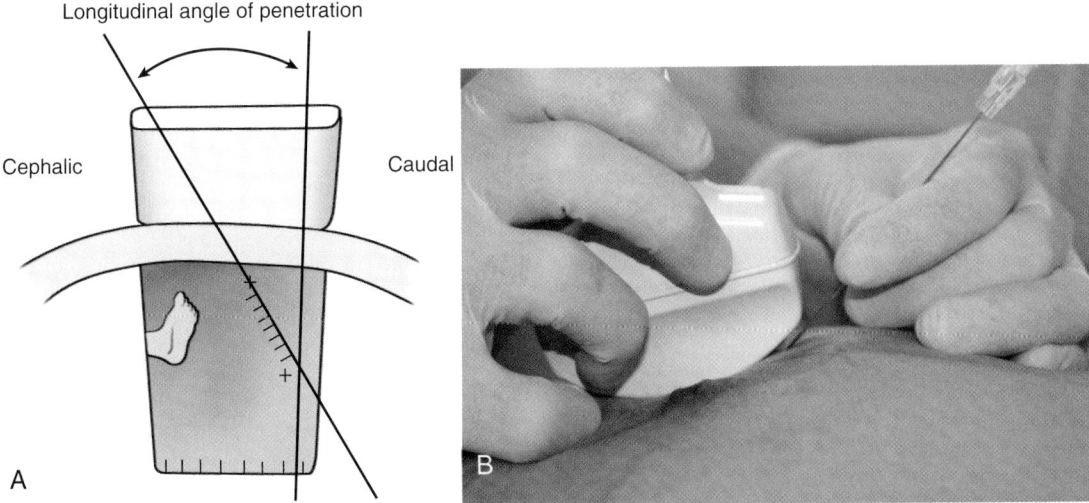

Fig. 144.1 Proper needle insertion. (A) Graphical depiction. Note measurements with calipers; the needle direction is also determined. (B) Photograph. Needle is inserted to previously measured depth at the proper angle.

8. If no amniotic fluid is obtained (dry tap), repeat the ultrasound examination and again localize a fluid pocket, its angle, and its distance from the skin; prepare the skin with antiseptic and repeat the tap (again under continuous ultrasound guidance). Many experts recommended that no more than two attempts be made because repeated attempts increase the risk of significant fetal injury or induction of labor. The procedure can be attempted again after 1 week. It is also important not to use a needle larger than 20 gauge because the incidence of complications rises with needle gauge.

9. The color and clarity of the fluid should be recorded. Normal amniotic fluid is clear and colorless or pale yellow. Dark brown or greenish fluid in a second trimester amniocentesis may indicate prior intraamniotic bleeding. Blood-tinged fluid may indicate transplacental passage of the needle, and it generally clears.

10. For twins, 2 mL of dilute indigo carmine dye was historically injected into the first sac before the needle was removed. This confirmed needle placement in the second sac when clear liquid was obtained. The dye dilution was prepared by mixing 1 mL of indigo carmine with 10 mL of sterile saline. Because of widespread shortages in indigo carmine dye, this is much less commonly done. Methylene blue dye is contraindicated due to its association with fetal anomalies. Due to a rare report of fetal jejunal atresia with use of carmine dye, the best solution for twins is to rely on ultrasound confirmation of needle placement and avoid dye altogether.

SAMPLE OPERATIVE REPORT

The patient was placed in low semi-Fowler's position, and the fetal heart tones were monitored for 20 minutes. Real-time ultrasound was used to locate a collection of amniotic fluid in the area of the fetal extremities at a depth of 5 cm. No loops of cord were noted. The overlying skin was marked, prepped with povidone–iodine solution, and draped with sterile towels. After local anesthesia with 1% lidocaine (if used), a 20-gauge spinal needle was inserted into the fluid pocket under continuous ultrasound guidance. A total of 15 mL of clear ("yellow," "green," "brown," "meconium stained," "slightly blood tinged," "grossly bloody") amniotic fluid was removed without (with) difficulty. A sterile dressing was applied to the puncture site, and the fetal heart tones were monitored for another 20 minutes; these remained reassuring. The patient felt well and was discharged with warnings and instructions for follow-up.

COMPLICATIONS

A wide variety of complications have been reported, including fetal injury or loss. Serious complications are rare, though, and the procedure is considered relatively safe in experienced hands. Complications from amniocentesis include the following:

- Pain, bruising, or infection at the puncture site.
- Maternal abdominal visceral injury.
- Uterine contractions, occasionally progressing to labor but usually self-limited.
- Occasional spontaneous abortion (fetal loss). The estimated rate of fetal loss for amniocentesis prior to 24 weeks' gestation in one series of 6752 cases done between 2004 and 2010 was 1.9% (Theodora, 2016). ACOG suggests the risk of fetal loss in midtrimester amniocentesis is 1 in 300 to 500. This loss risk may be doubled in women with marked obesity (body mass index ≥40 kg/m^2) (Harper et al., 2012). In twin pregnancies, the loss risk may be 1.8% (Cahill et al., 2009).
- Premature rupture of membranes.
- Placental separation or abruption.
- Fetal injury, such as skin scars, dimpling, eye injury, genital injury (risk increases with oligohydramnios).

- Orthopedic deformities of the newborn (more common with amniocentesis performed prior to 15 weeks gestational age, possibly due to fetal compression from less amniotic fluid).
- Cord or placental blood vessel injury with resultant fetal hemorrhage.
- Rh-factor isoimmunization.
- Uterine or amniotic fluid infection (<0.1%).
- Fluid leak with resultant oligohydramnios (rare, 1% to 2%; fetal survival with leakage is 90%).
- Transmission of maternal infectious disease (e.g., hepatitis B).

POSTPROCEDURE MANAGEMENT

After a normal successful amniocentesis, monitor the fetal heart rate and the mother's response for 20 to 30 minutes, after which the patient may leave. Prolonged monitoring for 1 to 2 hours may be indicated if there are frequent uterine contractions or if the sample was grossly bloody. Placental bleeding often can be seen on ultrasonography and monitored visually.

POSTPROCEDURE PATIENT EDUCATION

Printed instructions help patients remember follow-up precautions. Provide the patient an instruction sheet to use after amniocentesis.

INTERPRETATION OF RESULTS

In the rare case where amniocentesis may be necessary to establish FLM in a patient with unknown dates for 39-week elective induction, the following review is provided.

1. PG by itself can be used as an indicator of FLM. Blood, meconium, or vaginal secretions (as contaminants) in the amniotic fluid do not affect PG. PG appears after 35 weeks gestation. While not an absolute guarantee, PG presence provides reassurance that RDS is not likely to develop. Absence of PG is not necessarily a strong predictor of RDS after delivery. Although commercially available kits can be used to document PG presence rapidly and with considerable accuracy, several hours are needed for results. Lecithin to sphingomyelin (L/S) studies are usually more convenient due to this.

2. Around 33 weeks' gestation, the concentration of L relative to S begins to rise, and both can be measured directly. Risk of RDS is small when the L/S ratio is greater than 2; increased risk of RDS is possible when the ratio is less than 2. With some pregnancy complications (e.g., maternal diabetes; at present, it is unknown whether diabetes itself or the lack of maternal glycemic control causes this), RDS may occur despite a mature L/S ratio. The presence of blood can cause either increased or decreased ratios; meconium can produce falsely mature results.

3. The "shake test" is a rapid screening test for L/S ratio in which varying dilutions of amniotic fluid are shaken with ethanol. Ethanol is a nonfoaming, competitive surfactant that eliminates the contributions of protein, bile salts, and salts of free fatty acids to the formation of a stable foam. At an ethanol concentration of 47.5%, stable bubbles that foam after shaking are due entirely to lecithin in the amniotic fluid. Positive tests, a complete ring of bubbles at the meniscus with a 1:2 dilution of amniotic fluid, are rarely associated with RDS. The shake test, as a quick screen, is moderately successful for predicting RDS. There are problems with this test in the presence of even slight contamination; there are also frequent false negative results.

   To perform the shake test, mix 1 mL of amniotic fluid with 1 mL of 95% ethanol. This vial should be compared with a second vial of 1 mL of amniotic fluid mixed with 0.5 mL of 95% ethanol plus 0.5 mL of normal saline. After 30 seconds of vigorous shaking, a ring of bubbles in the second vial indicates an L/S ratio of 2 or greater. Bubbles in the 1:1 mix, but not in the second vial, indicate equivocal maturity.

4. The FSI is a commercially available variation of the shake test. The kit has test wells built into it containing predispensed amounts of ethanol. Amniotic fluid (0.5 mL) is added to each well and shaken. A "control" demonstrates an example of the stable foam end point. The FSI is read as the highest reading corresponding to a well in which a ring of stable foam persists. This test appears to be a reliable predictor of FLM if the FSI is 47 or higher; however, this test is unreliable if the amniotic fluid is contaminated with blood.

5. Although results are not available as rapidly as with the shake test, the fluorescence polarization test, or FLM assay, usually provides results faster than a PG assay. The FLM assesses overall surfactant activity, using polarized light to quantify the competitive binding of a probe to albumin and surfactant in amniotic fluid. An FLM result greater than 55 mg of surfactant per gram of albumin indicates maturity, from 35 to 55 indicates borderline maturity, and less than 35 indicates immaturity. A recently modified TdX-FLM II version is currently used by many hospitals with result ranges staying the same.

6. Amniotic fluid lamellar counts are also quite reliable. They are quick, inexpensive, and readily available anywhere that platelet counts are done. Clinicians experienced with lamellar counts often use them as a quick screen to decide who needs the full L/S or PG evaluation. Values of 50,000/μL or greater are consistent with FLM.

PATIENT EDUCATION GUIDES

See patient education and consent forms available at www.expertconsult.com.

CPT/BILLING CODES

The clinician should include a picture of the amniotic fluid pocket from the ultrasound examination (when possible; Fig. 144.2) and a procedure note in the documentation.

59000	Amniocentesis, diagnostic
59001	Amniocentesis, therapeutic amniotic fluid reduction (includes ultrasound guidance)
76946	Ultrasonic guidance for amniocentesis, imaging supervision and interpretation

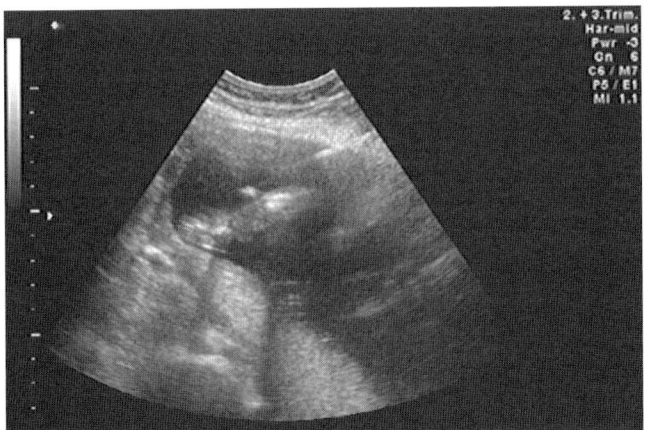

Fig. 144.2 Example of an ultrasound image for documenting the site chosen for amniocentesis. Note the large pocket of fluid and the absence of the cord. Also note needle visualization.

ICD-10-CM DIAGNOSTIC CODES

O14.10	Severe preeclampsia unspecified trimester
O60.00	Threatened premature labor (after 22 weeks)
O48.1	Prolonged pregnancy
O26.20	Habitual aborter unspecified trimester
O34.219	Previous cesarean delivery, not otherwise specified
O35.1XXX	Chromosomal abnormality in fetus
O35.2XXX	Hereditary disease in family, possibly affecting fetus
O35.8XXX	Other known or suspected fetal abnormality, not elsewhere classified
O36.099X	Rh isoimmunization
O77.9	Fetal distress
O40.9XXX	Polyhydramnios unspecified trimester
O42.00	Premature rupture of membranes
O41.1290	Chorioamnionitis
O09.529	Advanced maternal age, primiparous or multiparous

Acknowledgment

The editors recognize the contributions of Clark B. Smith, MD, to this chapter in previous editions of this text.

RECOMMENDED READING

American College of Obstetricians and Gynecologists. ACOG committee opinion no. 560: medically indicated late-preterm and early-term deliveries. *Obstet Gynecol.* 2013;121(4):908–910.

American College of Obstetricians and Gynecologists. ACOG committee opinion no. 545: noninvasive prenatal testing for fetal aneuploidy. *Obstet Gynecol.* 2012;120:1532–1534.

Cahill AG, Macones GA, Stamilio DM, Dicke JM, Crane JP, et al. Pregnancy loss rate after mid-trimester amniocentesis in twin pregnancies. *Am J Obstet Gynecol.* 2009;200(3):257.

Canadian Early and Mid-Trimester Amniocentesis Trial (CEMAT) Group. Randomised trial to assess safety and fetal outcome of early and midtrimester amniocentesis. *Lancet.* 1998;351(9098):242.

Chen T, Tenhunen H, Torkki P. Women's choice for invasive or non-invasive testing: influence of gestational age and service delivery. *Prenat Diagn.* 2016;36(13):1217–1224.

Gordon MC, Ventura-Braswell A, Higby K, et al. Does local anesthesia decrease pain perception in women undergoing amniocentesis? *Am J Obstet Gynecol.* 2007;196:55e1.

Harper LM, Cahill AG, Smith K, et al. Effect of maternal obesity on the risk of fetal loss after amniocentesis and chorionic villus sampling. *Obstet Gynecol.* 2012;119(4):745.

Khalifeh A, Weiner S, Berghella V. Trends in invasive prenatal diagnosis: effect of sequential screening and noninvasive prenatal testing. *Fetal Diagn Ther.* 2016;39(4):292–296.

Khazardoost S, Yahyazaheh H, Bornal S. Amniotic fluid lamellar body count and its sensitivity and specificity in evaluating fetal lung maturity. *J Obstet Gynecol.* 2005;25(3):257–259.

Mujezinovic F, Alfirevic Z. Analgesia for amniocentesis or chorionic villus sampling. *Cochrane Database Syst Rev.* 2011;11:CD008580.

Norton ME, Rine BD. Changing indications for invasive testing in an era of improved screening. *Semin Perinatol.* 2016;40(1):5666.

Prenatal Diagnosis. In: Cunningham F, Leveno KJ, Bloom SL, et al. *Williams Obstetrics.* 24th ed. New York: McGraw-Hill; 2013.

Philip J, Silver RK, Wilson RD, Thom EA, Zachary JM, et al. Late first-trimester invasive prenatal diagnosis: results of an international randomized trial. *Obstet and Gynecol.* 2004;103(6):1164–1173.

Theodora M, Antsaklis A, Antsaklis P, et al. Fetal loss following second trimester amniocentesis. Who is at greater risk? How to counsel pregnant women? *J Matern Fetal Neonatal Med.* 2016;29(4):590–595.

Varner S, Sherman C, Lewis D. Amniocentesis for fetal lung maturity; will it become obsolete? *Rev Obstet Gynecol.* 2013;6(3-4):126–134.

Wax JR, Chard R. Noninvasive prenatal testing: impact on genetic counseling, invasive prenatal diagnosis, and trisomy 21 detection. *Clin Ultrasound.* 2015;43(1):16.

Williams J, Rad S, Beauchamp S. Utilization of noninvasive prenatal testing: impact on referrals for diagnostic testing. *Am J Obstet Gynecol.* 2015;213(1):102.e16.

CHAPTER 145

EXTERNAL CEPHALIC VERSION

Andrew S. Coco

In 3% to 4% of pregnancies at term, the fetus is still in the breech position. The Term Breech Trial in 2000 showed a reduction in fetal morbidity and mortality with planned cesarean versus planned vaginal breech delivery. Since then, the numbers of clinicians performing vaginal breech delivery has markedly declined. Cesarean delivery (CD) has become the preferred breech delivery method in the United States, currently accounting for approximately 20% of primary CDs (Caughey, 2014). Planned cesarean also has inherent risk; increasing cesarean rates are associated with higher maternal morbidity, partly from increased risk of abnormal placentation in future gestations, uterine rupture, and maternal hemorrhage.

Practiced since the time of Aristotle, external cephalic version (ECV) is a procedure that uses external forces to rotate the fetus from a breech to a vertex presentation. Trials of ECV conducted over the past 25 years demonstrate an extremely strong safety record. Factors predictive of success and failure have been described (Box 145.1), although a validated prediction model for ECV has yet to be developed. One recent prediction model estimated ECV success at between 20% and 70% (Velzel and colleagues, 2015). A recent

---

BOX 145.1 Factors Predictive of Successful and Failed External Cephalic Version

Factors Predictive of Successful Version

Increasing parity (most consistent factor in studies)
Normal amount of amniotic fluid (may be linear correlation between success rate of ECV and AFI; i.e., higher success rate with increasing AFI)
Fetal presentation (success rate with transverse lie approaches 90%)
Unengaged fetal part
Ability to palpate fetal head
Earlier attempts at ECV (increase success rate, but also increase risk of spontaneous reversion to breech)

Factors Predictive of Failed Version

Engaged fetal presenting part*
Difficulty palpating the fetal head*
Uterus tense to palpation*
Maternal obesity
Cervical dilation
Anterior placenta
Anterior or posterior positioning of fetal spine
Descent of breech into pelvis
Decreased AFI

AFI, Amniotic fluid index; *ECV*, external cephalic version.
* The success rate is >90% if none of the factors marked by an asterisk is present and <20% if two of these factors are present. There have been no successful ECVs when all three factors are present.

Cochrane review showed a statistically significant and clinically meaningful reduction in noncephalic presentation at birth (average risk ratio [aRR], 0.42; 95% confidence interval [CI], 0.29 to 0.61), vaginal birth not achieved (aRR, 0.46; 95% CI, 0.33 to 0.62), and CD (aRR, 0.57; 95% CI, 0.40 to 0.82) when ECV was attempted versus no ECV. No significant differences were seen between groups in low Apgar scores (<7 at 1 minute or 5 minutes), low umbilical vein pH, or neonatal intensive care admission (Hofmeyr et al., 2015).

With widespread availability of ultrasound, electronic fetal monitoring, and effective tocolytic agents, there is increased interest in ECV as a method to mitigate CD rates. In addition to reducing cost and being safe and effective, the manual skills to perform ECV are easily acquired. Despite these favorable features, ECV is still underused. Successful ECV is around one-third less likely among women who delivery at hospitals with annual CD frequency greater than 35%, compared with hospitals with low CD rates (<20%) (Weiniger et al., 2016). Women who underwent successful ECV had decreased risk for developing endometritis and sepsis. Hospital charges and admission duration are also lower than with planned CD.

ECV can be performed in basically any setting that has an ultrasound machine and an experienced clinician (i.e., clinician comfortable with ultrasound and ECV). Clinicians must also be equipped and prepared for cesarean delivery if the need for emergent delivery arises. ECV is best performed in a setting with close proximity to an operating room.

INDICATIONS

- Adequately dated (e.g., dated prior to 20 weeks) low-risk singleton pregnancy at 36 weeks' gestation or greater. At 36 weeks' gestation, the likelihood of spontaneous version is low, whereas complications of immediate, iatrogenic, and preterm delivery are less significant than at earlier gestational ages (i.e., 33 to 34 weeks).
- The type of breech (e.g., frank, complete, footling) is not a factor in determining suitability. Women with a fetus in transverse lie are candidates.
- Previous CD is not associated with decreased ECV success in the current pregnancy, although the absolute risk of uterine rupture is unknown.

NOTE: When attempting ECV, the diagnosis of breech is preferably made before the patient is in active labor. The deeper the breech is engaged in the pelvis, the more difficult the procedure. Leopold maneuvers are useful for screening for fetal position both near and at term. The American College of Obstetrics and Gynecology (ACOG) recommends that because risk of adverse events with ECV are small and the CD rate is significantly lower among women with successful ECV, all women with breech presentation near term should be offered ECV if no contraindications exist.

CONTRAINDICATIONS

Absolute

- Indications for CD aside from fetal presentation (e.g., placenta previa or fetal/obstetric conditions)
- Major uterine or fetal anomaly
- Nonreassuring fetal heart tones
- Multiple gestation
- Abruptio placentae
- Ruptured membranes or severe oligohydramnios
- Hyperextended fetal head

Relative

- Suspected intrauterine growth restriction
- Decreased amniotic fluid volume
- Maternal cardiac disease
- Maternal hypertension or preeclampsia with severe features
- Previous CD (in small studies, ECV was not associated with uterine rupture in patients with previous cesarean or vaginal birth after cesarean)
- Maternal obesity

EQUIPMENT AND SUPPLIES

- Intravenous catheter with heparin lock
- Phlebotomy equipment for a complete blood count and blood type and screen
- Syringe containing 0.25 mg of terbutaline (Brethine)
- Fetal heart rate monitor
- Examination table able to position patient in Trendelenburg position (maternal head lower than feet)
- Ultrasound machine
- Ultrasound gel
- Towels
- Sterile gloves and lubricant (if vaginal examination is required)
- Rh_0 (D) immune globulin for Rh-negative patients (should be given within 72 hours of ECV)

PREPROCEDURE PATIENT EDUCATION

Counseling about risks, benefits, and alternatives to ECV is best done at a clinic visit a week or more prior to the scheduled procedure (see the sample patient education form available at www.expertconsult.com). This allows time for both the patient and her partner to make an informed decision. Consent forms can be signed at this time or the day of the visit. The procedure is ideally scheduled after 36 weeks gestation to allow the breech to spontaneously turn while also reducing risk of a more preterm neonate should ECV induce labor. ACOG recommends assessing fetal position at $36^{0/7}$ weeks gestation and then scheduling ECV at $37^{0/7}$ weeks if breech lie is detected and the patient consents. Before 36 weeks, although there is a high success rate for ECV, fetuses are more likely to spontaneously revert to breech. Prior to ECV, the patient should be instructed to take nothing by mouth for at least 4 hours after a light meal or 8 hours following a heavier meal.

The clinician should also reassure the patient that ECV generally causes only minimal discomfort. A recent meta-analysis of 9 RCTs, including 934 singleton breech gestations, found that administration of neuraxial analgesia (including spinal, epidural, and combined spinal/epidural techniques) in addition to a tocolytic had significantly increased rates of successful ECV compared with a tocolytic alone (58.4% vs. 43.1%; relative risk, 1.44; 95% CI, 1.27 to 1.64) (Magro-Malosso and colleagues, 2016). The optimal neuraxial technique and dose required for ECV has yet to be elucidated, however. A 2016 ACOG committee opinion found current data are insufficient to make a recommendation favoring spinal or epidural during ECV attempts.

TECHNIQUE

1. Using ultrasound, confirm a singleton in breech or transverse presentation, determine the amniotic fluid index, note the placental location, and rule out uterine malformations or congenital anomalies. The patient should empty her bladder after the ultrasound exam.
2. Perform a nonstress test to confirm a reassuring fetal heart rate tracing.
3. Draw blood for a complete blood count; type and screen. Establish intravenous access.
4. Administer a tocolytic agent, such as terbutaline (Brethine) 0.25 mg intravenously (slow push over 2 to 3 minutes) or subcutaneously about 15 minutes before the procedure. Evidence supports the use of parenteral tocolysis to improve ECV success.
5. Place the patient in slight Trendelenburg position to facilitate disengagement and mobility of the breech. Liberally coat the abdomen with ultrasound gel to decrease friction and lessen the chance of overly vigorous manipulation.
6. ECV may be performed by one or two operators. Determine the degree of pelvic engagement of the breech and gently disengage it, if possible. Sometimes this requires a second clinician to attempt vaginal disengagement. Successful disengagement is a key factor for successful ECV. After the fetal buttocks are elevated out of the pelvis and displaced laterally, the clinician(s) grasps each fetal pole in a hand. The fetal head should be gently stabilized to prevent it from ducking under the maternal ribs, where it may become unreachable.
   NOTE: The breech (i.e., buttocks) is what is actually manipulated during the maneuver. The fetal head is merely guided gently toward the pelvis while the breech is actively moved cephalad.
7. Attempt either a classic forward roll or a back flip. Most clinicians tend to attempt the forward roll first (Fig. 145.1). Some base their preference on whether the fetus is mostly on one side of the uterus (e.g., fetal head and spine are on the same side of the maternal midline) or not. A forward roll is opted for when the fetal head and spine are on different sides of the maternal midline, whereas a back flip (Fig. 145.2) is chosen when they are on the same side. Emphasis should be on gentle persuasion of the fetus, as opposed to forceful movements.
8. In most cases of successful ECV, repositioning is accomplished with slow and deliberate movements. If the first attempt is unsuccessful, a second attempt is made in the opposite direction. If the fetus goes into a transverse lie but does not progress to cephalic position, stop and monitor the fetal heart rate with ultrasound before attempting to complete the ECV. An attempted version should be discontinued for significant maternal discomfort or a persistently abnormal fetal heart rate. Three to four attempts may be considered if there are favorable indicators for success, although many will reschedule another ECV at a later time after two failed attempts.
9. It is important to monitor the fetal heart rate with ultrasound immediately after each ECV attempt to assess for fetal bradycardia or other abnormalities. If persistent bradycardia is noted after a successful version, some experts will return the fetus to its breech presentation in hopes of reducing umbilical cord compression. Immediate cesarean may also be indicated if continued nonreassuring heart tones are seen, although this is rare.
10. Regardless of success or failure, perform a formal nonstress test after the procedure to exclude fetal heart rate abnormalities.
11. Administer postprocedural Rh_0 (D) immune globulin to all Rh-negative patients because of a 4.1% risk of fetomaternal blood exchange.
12. If an attempt is unsuccessful and no fetal compromise is suspected, repeating ECV several days to 1 week later is safe and cost-effective.

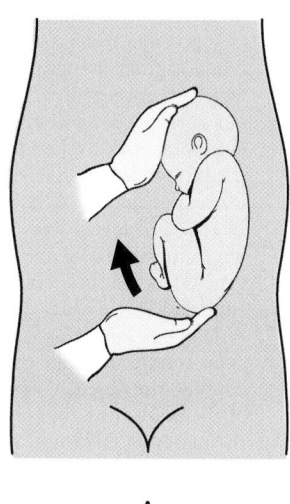
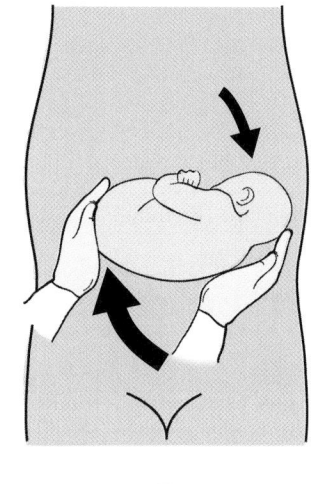
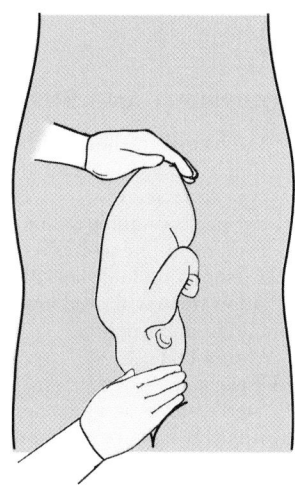

Fig. 145.1 External cephalic version using the classic forward roll. (A) The breech is mobilized. A second person is sometimes needed to vaginally disengage the fetus. (B–C) At the same time, the breech is gently pushed upward while the head is stabilized and directed into the pelvis.

Fig. 145.2 External cephalic version using the back flip. (A) As with the forward roll, the breech is mobilized, possibly using a second person to vaginally disengage the fetus. (B–C) At the same time, the breech is gently pushed upward while the head is gently directed into the pelvis.

NOTE: ECV is easier to perform with multiparous patients and when there is plenty of amniotic fluid. ECV may be worth considering, even in early labor, in willing multiparous women while en route to cesarean. It should never be performed under anesthesia unless the clinician is very experienced or is preparing for cesarean section.

SAMPLE OPERATIVE REPORT

See sample operative report available at www.expertconsult.com.

COMMON ERRORS

Attempting to turn the fetus prior to mobilizing the breech from the pelvis.

COMPLICATIONS

In general, ECV is very safe. When a protocol includes fetal heart rate monitoring, ultrasound, and ready access to operative delivery, the complication rate is around 1%. Reported adverse effects include abruption, umbilical cord prolapse, rupture of membranes, fetomaternal hemorrhage, and stillbirth, although all are rare.

- The risk of spontaneous reversion to a breech presentation after successful ECV is around 7%.

- Occasionally the procedure needs to be discontinued because of significant or excessive maternal discomfort.
- There is a small risk of premature rupture of membranes or active labor within several days after the procedure. If the ECV was unsuccessful, either of these events could lead to a cesarean for breech presentation, depending on patient and provider interest in an attempt at vaginal breech delivery.
- Transient, benign changes in fetal heart rate tracings are common. There is a small risk of more worrisome changes, such as severe variable decelerations, late decelerations, or persistent bradycardia. These changes could signify placental abruption or umbilical cord entanglement and necessitate urgent cesarean delivery.
- Nonfatal fetomaternal hemorrhage occurs in about 4% of cases. A case of fetal brachial plexus injury has been reported.
- One maternal death has been reported due to amniotic fluid embolism. There is also risk of uterine rupture.
- After successful ECV, several reports suggest that the risk of CD does not revert to institutional risk for vertex presentations. Dystocia, malpresentation, and nonreassuring heart rate patterns may be slightly more common after ECV.

POSTPROCEDURE MANAGEMENT

Follow-up visits and plans for a repeat attempt at ECV (in the event of an unsuccessful attempt) or planned cesarean are important to discuss with the patient.

POSTPROCEDURE PATIENT EDUCATION

- The clinician should review the postprocedure information on the sample patient education handout (available at www.expertconsult.com) with the patient.
- Women who have undergone successful ECV should be instructed to watch for fetal reversion to breech position. If the fetus has reverted (significant pain or perception of greater than normal fetal movement), the patient should call or return to the clinic. One study has shown that training women to make regular self-assessments of the presenting part after successful ECV improves the vaginal delivery rate. In this study, prompt, repeat ECV was performed when reversion was detected before labor.
- Patients should call for any signs of contractions, fluid leakage from the vagina, or decreased fetal movement. They should be instructed about the symptoms of both.

PATIENT EDUCATION GUIDES

See patient education and patient consent forms available at www.expertconsult.com.

CPT/BILLING CODES

59412   External cephalic version (ECV), with or without tocolysis

ICD-10-CM DIAGNOSTIC CODES

O32.1XX0   Breech presentation antepartum
O32.2XX0   Transverse or oblique fetal presentation, antepartum

ONLINE RESOURCES

The Cochrane Collaboration: www.cochrane.org (for updates on most obstetric issues).
Familydoctor.org: Breech babies: What can I do if my baby is breech? https://familydoctor.org/breech-babies-what-can-i-do-if-my-baby-is-breech/.

RECOMMENDED READING

American College of Obstetricians and Gynecologists. *External cephalic version*. Washington, DC: ACOG Practice Bulletin No. 161; 2016.

Caughey AB, Cahill AG, Guise JM, Rouse DJ. Safe prevention of the primary cesearean delivery. *Am J Obstet Gynecol.* 2014;210(3):179–193.

Hannah ME, Hannah WJ, Hewson SA, et al. Planned caesarean section versus planned vaginal birth for breech presentation at term: a randomised multicentre trial. Term breech trial collaborative group. *Lancet.* 2000;356:1375–1383.

Hofmeyr GJ. External cephalic version facilitation for breech presentation at term. *Cochrane Database Syst Rev.* 2015;4:CD000083.

Hutton EK, Hofmeyr GJ. External cephalic version for breech presentation before term. *Cochrane Database Syst Rev.* 2015;7:CD000084.

Lim S, Lucero J. Obstetric and anesthetic approaches to external cephalic version. *Anesthesiology Clin.* 2017;35:81–94.

Magro-Malosso ER, Saccone G, Di Tommaso M, et al. Neuraxial analgesia to increase the success rate of external cephalic version: a systematic review and meta-analysis of randomized controlled trials. *Am J Obstet Gynecol.* 2016.

Rosman AN, Vlemmix F, Ensing S, et al. Mode of childbirth and neonatal outcome after external cephalic version: a prospective cohort study. *Midwifery.* 2016;39:44–48.

Skupski DW, Ghidini A. External cephalic version: some tricks of the trade. *Birth.* 2016;43(3):189–192.

Velzel J, de Hundt M, Mulder FM, et al. Prediction models for successful external cephalic version: a systematic review. *Eur J Obstet Gyn Reprod Bio.* 2015;195:160–167.

Weiniger CF, Lyell D, Tsen LC, et al. Maternal outcome of term breech presentation delivery: impact of successful external cephalic version in a nationwide sample of delivery admissions in the United States. *BMC Pregnancy Childbirth.* 2016;16:150.

CHAPTER 146

ANTEPARTUM FETAL MONITORING

Stephen D. Ratcliffe

Commonly used options for fetal surveillance include fetal movement counting (FMC), the nonstress test (NST), the biophysical profile (BPP), the modified BPP (mBPP), and the contraction stress test (CST). Arterial Doppler velocimetry of the uterine artery, the middle cerebral artery, or the ductus venosus is increasingly used to evaluate fetal wellbeing in cases of intrauterine growth restriction. Most centers use varying combinations of these tests. The "best test" for antepartum monitoring has yet to be agreed upon, largely due to a lack of randomized clinical trials (RCTs); FMC, NST, mBPP, and CST are described in this chapter. Doppler velocitometry will be briefly discussed, while the BPP is covered in Chapter 142, Obstetric Ultrasound.

Whether NST, mBPP, BPP, or CST is used, a negative test is very reassuring, with negative predictive values (no fetal death within a week of the test) of 99.8% or higher. Unfortunately, overall positive predictive values are quite low, ranging from 10% to 40%, which can be problematic for the clinician. Additional challenges include deciding when to start and the frequency of testing. Most experts start testing high-risk pregnancies at 32 to 34 weeks. Pregnancies with severe complications may need testing as early as 26 to 28 weeks.

DOPPLER VELOCIMETRY

Doppler velocimetry technology can assess arterial velocity and flow. This antenatal test has been the subject of more RCTs than any other antenatal test. Fetal Doppler studies were initially used to evaluate the placenta by measuring umbilical artery outflow; normal fetuses have high-velocity diastolic flow. This flow decreases and can even reverse with increasing placental resistance. Randomized studies on the utility of umbilical artery Doppler velocimetry generally have defined abnormal flow as either absent or reversed end-diastolic flow. According to the American College of Obstetricians and Gynecologists (ACOG), to maximize interpretability, multiple waveforms should be assessed, and wall-filter settings should be set low enough (typically less than 150 Hz) to avoid masking diastolic flow. Commonly measured flow indexes, based on the characteristics of peak systolic velocity and frequency shift (S), end-diastolic frequency shift (D), and mean peak frequency shift over the cardiac cycle (A), include the following: systolic to diastolic ratio (S/D), resistance index (S-D/S) and pulsatility index (S-D/A). Guidelines from the Society of Maternal-Fetal Medicine suggest when delivery should be considered based on abnormal Doppler velocimetry results.

For high-risk pregnancies, a Cochrane review of over 10,000 high-risk gestations (Alfirevic, 2017) found that Doppler use was associated with a reduction in fetal death (relative risk, 0.71; 95% confidence interval, 0.52 to 0.98) as well as fewer labor inductions and cesareans. However, in low-risk or unselected populations, another Cochrane review (Alfirevic, 2015) found no conclusive evidence of a benefit to mother or baby with routine use of umbilical artery Doppler ultrasound, or a combination of umbilical and uterine artery Doppler ultrasound.

Antenatal testing for fetal well-being with intrauterine growth restriction (IUGR) should begin at the time of diagnosis, but not prior to fetal viability. Best testing practices have yet to be described in terms of scheduling. The American College of Radiologists gives this procedure an appropriateness rating of 6 (may be appropriate) in high-risk pregnancies and 2 (not usually indicated) in low-risk gestations. With improved technology, multivessel evaluation is possible, including the middle cerebral artery and others. The current position of the ACOG (2013) is that umbilical artery Doppler velocimetry used in conjunction with standard fetal surveillance, such as NST, or BPP, or both, is associated with improved outcomes in fetuses diagnosed with IUGR.

FETAL MOVEMENT COUNTING

Both human and animal studies indicate that a hypoxic fetus reduces oxygen requirements by reducing its activity. FMC has developed as a means of monitoring the fetus during the third trimester of pregnancy. In women who perceived decreased fetal movement, one-quarter have poor perinatal outcomes, and more than half of stillbirths are preceded by reports of decreased movement (Dutton, 2012). While FMC is commonly recommended to patients by providers, no RCT evidence supports its use.

Studies of women presenting with decreased fetal movement have produced variable results, ranging from no increase in adverse outcomes to a 3.8% perinatal mortality rate in a cohort of 599 low-risk pregnancies. The largest RCT (N = 68,000) of routine FMC use in low-risk pregnancy failed to demonstrate improved perinatal outcomes (Grant, 1989). Although the study authors did not find improved outcomes with FMC, they did conclude that maternal perceptions of decreased fetal movement were as good as formally counted and recorded fetal movement. In 2011, Saastad found increased identification of growth-restricted pregnancies when FMC was used. Warrander (2012) found increased risk of placental pathology when decreased fetal movement was noted. A more recent review of 23 publications on maternal awareness of decreased fetal movement (Winje, 2016) found insufficient evidence to recommend the introduction of FMC or any other fetal movement intervention to either a select or the total population. Indirect evidence did suggest FMC may improve perinatal outcomes, so until more rigorous evidence is available, clinicians should inform women about fetal movement awareness and reporting perceived decreased fetal movement. Another recent Cochrane review found insufficient evidence to influence our practice in terms of FMC (Mangesi, 2015). It does support being on the alert for overall decreased fetal movement.

Indications

The clinician needs to decide whether to use FMC. RCTs have not been performed to study the use of FMC in high-risk patients.

However, it is a common practice to recommend FMC as a secondary method of fetal surveillance in these pregnancies. Robust research comparing routine FMC with selective FMC is needed.

Contraindications

- Impaired mental status or significant linguistic or cultural barrier: any barrier preventing adequate communication or the proper use of FMC could cause screening errors or failures.
- Mother unable to sense fetal movements: there are cases where the clinician can actually see the fetus moving (e.g., during a routine visit, while measuring the fundal height, or otherwise observing the anterior abdomen), yet the patient cannot sense the movement. It may not be possible to use FMC with these patients.

Technique

1. The patient should be instructed in the count-to-10 method of FMC (see patient education handout online at www.expertconsult.com). The Cardiff count-to-10 method has been studied and compared with the Sadovsky method (three 30- to 60-minute counts at preset times each day) and the Rayburn method (FMC for 60 minutes, once a day). There is a higher patient compliance rate with the count-to-10 method. Instruct the patient to count 10 fetal movements (e.g., swishes, rolls, kicks). The test is complete and considered to be "reassuring" when 10 movements are counted in less than 2 hours. Tests are usually performed in the evening and are often completed within 20 minutes.
2. The patient is instructed to report to labor and delivery or to notify her clinician if 10 movements are not recorded within a 2-hour period. Such a result is a nonreassuring screening test.

Complications

Unfortunately, FMC produces frequent false-positive results. A nonreassuring FMC may be further complicated by false-positive follow-up antenatal testing results. These abnormal findings often result in the decision to induce labor, thereby exposing the mother and fetus to unnecessary risks.

Interpretation of Results

A reassuring test is described in the earlier section on Technique. Patients arriving at labor and delivery with a complaint of decreased fetal movement usually undergo NST. A normal or reactive NST is sufficient to assess fetal wellbeing. If the NST is not reassuring, then additional antenatal fetal testing is necessary, such as a BPP.

NONSTRESS TEST

The NST was introduced in the United States in the early 1970s. Despite the lack of RCT evidence to support its use, the NST is the workhorse of antenatal fetal surveillance. It is usually the first-line test to evaluate high-risk pregnancies and fetal wellbeing. The NST uses fetal monitoring to document fetal heart rate accelerations that occur in conjunction with fetal movements. Extensive clinical observations have shown a strong correlation between absent or less frequent fetal heart rate accelerations and progressive fetal hypoxia. Conversely, the presence of fetal heart rate accelerations associated with fetal movement (reactive NST) is a reassuring indicator of good fetal health. Although not a complex procedure, the clinician must be adept at the proper interpretation of the NST. Important considerations include the indication for testing, gestational age, and any known congenital anomalies or maternal medical conditions. The clinician should also know whether the patient has taken any medications (e.g., opioids, barbiturates) that might affect the reactivity of the fetal tracing.

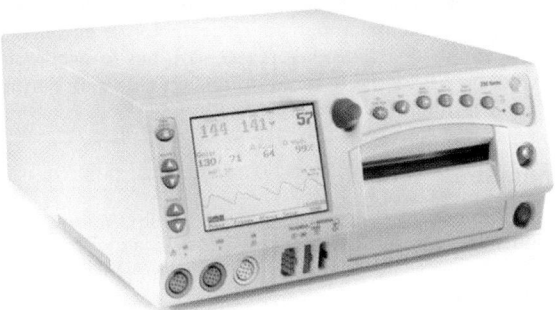

Fig. 146.1   Intrapartum fetal and uterine monitor. (Courtesy GE Medical Systems.)

Indications

Antepartum fetal surveillance results have not been definitively demonstrated to improve perinatal outcome, so all indications for antepartum testing are somewhat relative. The NST is often selected to monitor pregnancies considered high-risk as early as 32 weeks' gestation. Some of these high-risk conditions include:

- Suspected or confirmed intrauterine growth restriction (IUGR; may also use umbilical artery Doppler velocitometry)
- Preexisting or gestational diabetes
- Hypertensive disorders of pregnancy
- Prolonged or postterm pregnancy
- Decreased fetal movement
- Maternal trauma
- Other maternal or fetal condition posing risk to the fetus (e.g., cardiac, thyroid or renal disease, multiple gestation, substance abuse, cholestasis of pregnancy, history of fetal demise)

Some clinicians use the NST as early as 26 weeks' gestation. Different criteria are used to define a reactive or reassuring fetal heart rate tracing before 32 weeks (see the Interpretation of Results section). As experience has evolved with the NST, the interval between testing has shortened. Originally set rather arbitrarily at 7 days, more frequent testing is advocated for women with prolonged or postterm pregnancy, type 1 diabetes mellitus, IUGR, or gestational hypertension. In these circumstances, many experts perform twice-weekly NSTs, with more frequent testing for maternal or fetal deterioration. Some even perform NSTs daily, or more frequently, especially for preeclampsia with severe features remote from term. Cumulative research on NST accuracy suggest a 0.3% false-negative rate within 1 week of reactive NST and a 50% false-positive rate (DeVoe, 2008)

Contraindications

There are no specific contraindications to performing an NST, although the test should be aborted if the mother goes into labor or there is marked fetal intolerance of labor.

Equipment

- Fetal heart rate and uterine pressure monitor (Fig. 146.1)
- Blood pressure cuff
- Fetal stimulation device (vibroacoustic stimulator [VAS], such as an artificial larynx)
- Ultrasonic gel for monitor
- Bed or comfortable reclining chair

Preprocedure Patient Education

Before the NST is performed, the patient should be given a handout outlining the procedure and the steps to follow (see sample patient education handout online at www.expertconsult.com). Many testing centers use standardized protocols in an attempt to minimize confounding environmental variables. These protocols encourage the patient to eat about 2 hours before the NST, not to smoke or take sedative drugs before the test, and to remain sedentary during the hour before testing.

Technique

1. Place the patient in a semirecumbent (semi-Fowler's) position, tilted slightly to her left or with slight left lateral hip displacement. She can also be seated in a reclining chair at a 30- to 45-degree angle.
2. Apply external uterine and fetal monitors (tocodynamometer and Doppler) to record any uterine contractions and the fetal heart rate. Record the patient's blood pressure before the test to make sure she does not have supine hypotension, which could cause a falsely abnormal test result. Check the blood pressure every 10 to 15 minutes during the test.
3. Ask the patient to report or record any fetal movements using a button that marks when the fetus is active.
4. Monitor the patient for a 20-minute baseline period. Two additional 20-minute monitoring periods should be considered if the tracing is nonreactive.
5. If there is insufficient fetal movement in the first or second 20-minute observation period, there is strong evidence (based on multiple RCTs) supporting the use of a fetal stimulation device, such as a VAS, to induce fetal movement. According to ACOG, this can be used for 3 seconds and repeated up to three times. The use of a VAS reduces the frequency of nonreassuring NST by 40% and shortens the average time for the NST by 7 minutes (ACOG, 2014).

Complications

False-positive results can occur. Such results may lead to premature interventions that could result in iatrogenic perinatal complications, such as an unnecessary cesarean intervention with its associated complications. Variables may be noted in 50% of NSTs. If nonrecurring and brief (<30 seconds), variables are not associated with fetal compromise or the need for immediate intervention. Repetitive variables (e.g., three in 20 minutes) are associated with increased risk for cesarean due to nonreassuring intrapartum fetal heart rate.

Interpretation of Results

A fetal tracing is considered reactive if there are two or more accelerations of more than 15 beats/min above baseline that last for at least 15 seconds but not for more than 2 minutes (Fig. 146.2A). These usually occur within 20 minutes of starting the test. (It may be necessary to monitor for 40 minutes or longer due to variations of the sleep-wake cycle.) ACOG considers accelerations occurring without fetal movement to also be reactive.

Because the premature fetus has less pronounced heart rate accelerations than the more mature fetus, a 10 beats/min acceleration lasting for 10 seconds is considered a reassuring or reactive NST for fetuses before 32 weeks' gestation.

In a low-risk pregnancy, nonreactivity (see Fig. 146.2B) usually indicates that the infant is sleeping. The clinician should extend the observation period for as long as 90 minutes total to decrease the likelihood of a false-positive test result. Alternatively, the clinician may safely use VAS to induce fetal movements. In addition, make sure that the patient undergoing an NST is in a semirecumbent position to avoid supine hypotension and a false-positive (nonreactive) NST.

The clinician must consider the risk status of the patient and the indication for ordering an NST when interpreting a nonreactive NST and before proceeding with further interventions. The positive predictive value of an abnormal NST ranges from 15% for evaluating a postterm pregnancy to 69% for evaluating IUGR. Hence, false-positive tests are common.

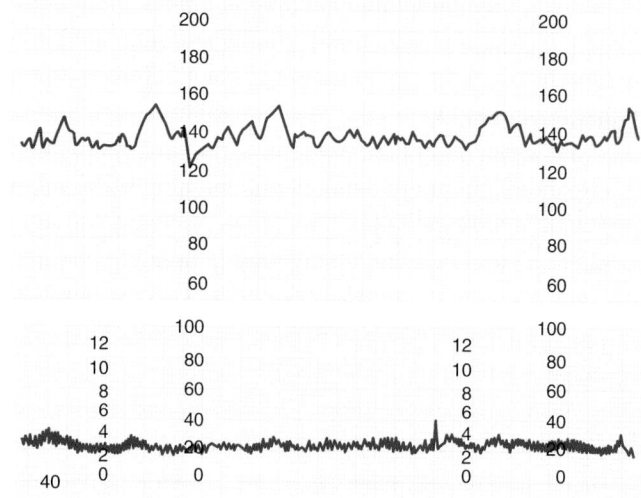

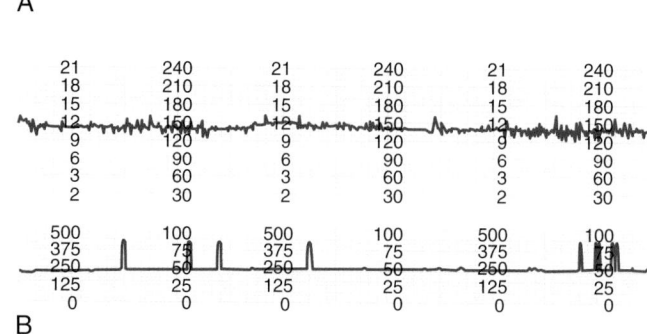

Fig. 146.2 (A) Reactive (normal) nonstress test (NST), with two or more accelerations of 15 beats/min lasting for at least 15 sec but not longer than 2 min. Note the fetal heart rate in the upper tracing accelerates with fetal movement, which is noted by the vertical marks on the lower tracing. The vertical marks are made when the mother presses the button as she perceives fetal movement. (B) Nonreactive (abnormal) NST. Although the mother perceives fetal movement, as noted by the vertical marks on the lower tracing, there are no fetal heart rate accelerations. (A, From Biophysical profile scoring. In: Rumack CM, Wilson SR, Charboneau JW, Johnson J-A, eds. *Diagnostic Ultrasound*. 3rd ed. Philadelphia: Mosby; 2005. B, From Antepartum fetal evaluation. In: Gabbe SG, Niebyl JR, Simpson JL, et al, eds. *Obstetrics: Normal and Problem Pregnancies*. 5th ed. New York: Churchill Livingstone; 2007, Fig. 11.7.)

Reactive NSTs that have no other abnormalities on the tracing (e.g., variable decelerations) have a very low false-negative rate (2 in 1000). Combining an NST with an amniotic fluid index (AFI; see Chapter 142, Obstetric Ultrasound, for a more complete discussion of evaluating amniotic fluid volume [AFV]) produces an mBPP, and results in an even more sensitive test, with a false-negative rate of 0.8 per 1000.

In addition to obtaining a modified BBP, options available for the clinician to evaluate a fetus with a persistently nonreactive NST include CST, BPP or proceeding with induction if the infant is mature (e.g., more than $37^{0/7}$ weeks gestational age) and the mother has a favorable cervix. A sample flowchart for the management of an NST is shown in Fig. 146.3. In settings that do not routinely perform mBPPs, the occurrence of repetitive variable decelerations in an otherwise reactive NST should prompt a measurement of the AFI. This subgroup of fetuses is at increased risk of cord compromise during labor.

Postprocedure Patient Education

It is essential that patients receive a detailed explanation of the results of the NST and the specific signs and symptoms (e.g., decreased fetal movement, vaginal bleeding, leakage of fluid) for which they should

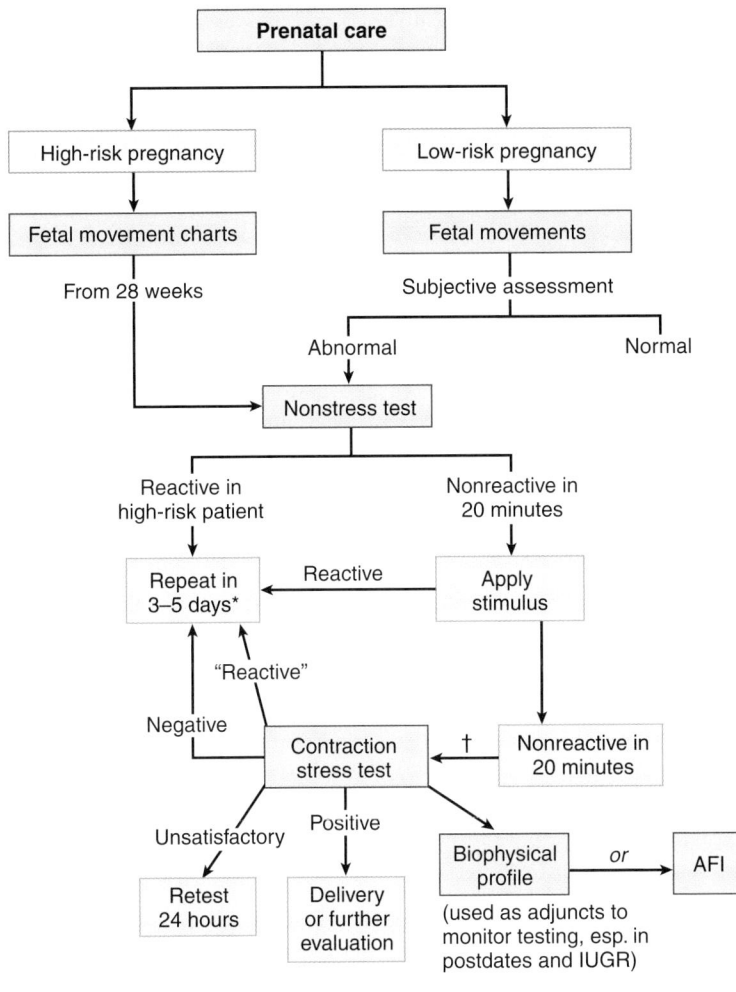

Fig. 146.3 Sample flowchart for management of the nonstress test *(NST)* and modified biophysical profile. *AFI,* Amniotic fluid index; *IUGR,* intrauterine growth retardation. *"Twice weekly" NSTs recommended. †"Prolonged" NST may be repeated in 2 to 3 hr. (Courtesy Kent Petrie, MD, Vail, CO.)

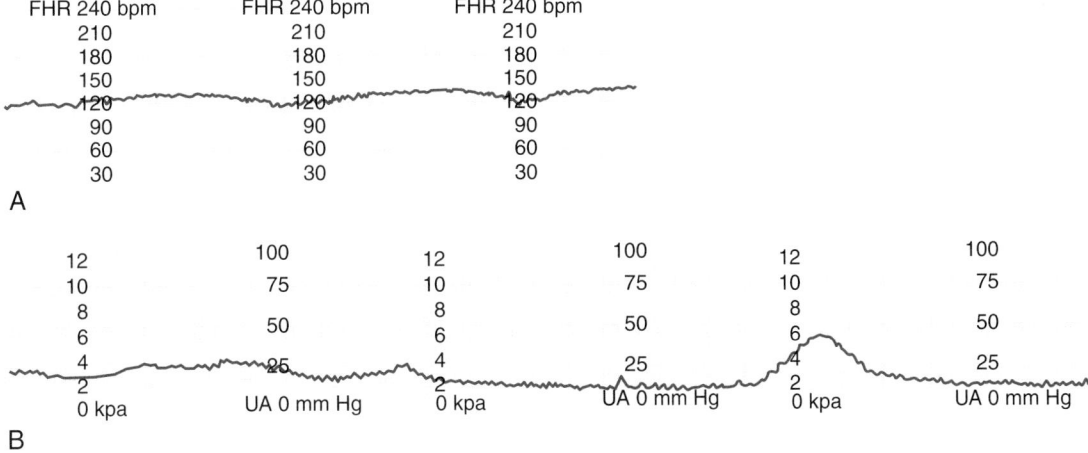

Fig. 146.4 Nonreactive positive contraction stress test. (A) Fetal heart rate (FHR). (B) Uterine activity (UA; i.e., contractions).

watch. Patients should receive explicit instructions regarding follow-up appointments and when to go to labor and delivery.

MODIFIED BIOPHYSICAL PROFILE

Although a normal weekly BPP result can somewhat ensure fetal wellbeing, this is a labor-intensive process and requires a high level of expertise—a sonographer or clinician trained to perform and interpret ultrasound scans. Therefore, the mBPP (NST combined with an AFI) was developed in the late 1980s. An AFI less than 5 cm, or oligohydramnios, is suspected to be due to decreased urine production, which is, in turn, due to decreased fetal renal blood flow; this suggests uteroplacental insufficiency. One of the early studies reported that it took only about 10 minutes to perform an mBPP when a VAS was used for the NST; if nursing staff are trained to perform an AFI, they can perform the entire mBPP. In centers using mBPPs for surveillance, most perform it twice weekly. A study of results from more than 54,000 mBPPs in 15,400 high-risk pregnancies described a false-negative rate of 0.8 per 1000 (Miller, 1996). Iatrogenic prematurity resulting from interventions based on false-positive mBPP affected 1.5% of pregnancies tested before 37 weeks. Subsequently, ACOG endorsed the mBPP as an acceptable means of antepartum monitoring.

Indications

- High-risk pregnancy, especially a prolonged or a postterm pregnancy
- A follow-up evaluation of a suspect or abnormal NST

Equipment

- Real-time ultrasound machine with a 3-MHz or higher transducer. Among state-of-the-art machines, the differences between different manufacturers are primarily subjective. (See the Suppliers section of Chapter 142, Obstetric Ultrasound.)
- Bed
- Ultrasonic gel
- Towels to remove gel when study completed
- Appropriate forms for documentation

Preprocedure Patient Education

Before the mBPP is performed, the patient should be given a handout outlining the procedure and the steps to follow (see sample patient education handout available at www.expertconsult.com). Unlike in nongravid pelvic ultrasound, the patient does not need a full bladder. The patient should be made aware that although the sonogram will visualize the fetus, it will only be evaluating the amount of amniotic fluid. See Chapter 142, Obstetric Ultrasound, for more Preprocedure Patient Education.

Technique

1. After the NST has been completed, place the patient in the recumbent or a semirecumbent (semi-Fowler's) position, tilted slightly to her left or with slight left lateral hip displacement.
2. Visualize the maternal abdomen as divided into four quadrants. Hold the ultrasound transducer in a vertical and sagittal alignment (marker dot on the probe turned toward the mother's head [cephalad]). With the patient supine, the transducer is held perpendicular to the plane of the floor and aligned longitudinally with the mother's spine. Starting in one quadrant, identify, measure, and record the pocket of fluid with the largest vertical dimension. Care must be taken not to include segments of the umbilical cord in the measurement. Coiled cord can fill the space and appear to be fluid.
3. Results of the mBPP are considered normal if the NST is reactive and the AFV is greater than 2 cm in the deepest vertical pocket seen. If either the NST is nonreactive or the AFV in the deepest vertical pocket is less than 2 cm (i.e., oligohydramnios is probably present), the mBPP is abnormal. Conversely, measuring in all four quadrants and summing the results should provide a sum of 5 or greater in normal gestations, although most studies simply use the one 2 cm pocket technique rather than obtaining an official four-quadrant AFV.

Interpretation of Results

Abnormal mBPP or NST results are generally followed up with either CST or a full BPP. The BPP is discussed in Chapter 142, Obstetric Ultrasound. A BPP score of 6 of 10 in a fetus at or past 37⁰/⁷ weeks gestation necessitates further evaluation and consideration of delivery. At gestational ages less than 37⁰/⁷ weeks, a repeat BPP is generally done in 24 hours. BPP scores of 4 usually suggest that delivery is warranted regardless of gestational age, although management must be individualized, especially in cases at risk of complications from prematurity.

CONTRACTION STRESS TEST

The CST is one of the earliest available and studied antepartum fetal surveillance tests; however, it is used infrequently today. Designed to identify fetuses at risk from uteroplacental insufficiency, it is usually performed in a hospital setting. A CST is now usually a secondary antenatal test when NST, mBPP, or BPP fail to provide the reassurance needed to continue expectant management. The basis of the test is to determine whether uterine contractions cause late decelerations in the fetal heart tracing. A secondary use of the CST is to determine if regular uterine contractions provoke recurrent variable decelerations suggestive of umbilical cord compression.

In the setting of uteroplacental insufficiency, fetal oxygen reserves are diminished. As a result, a brief hypoxic episode from a uterine contraction can cause a vagally mediated fetal bradycardia, which, in turn, produces a late deceleration. Hypoxia can also directly affect the fetal myocardium and trigger a late deceleration.

Research in the mid-1960s demonstrated that late decelerations were associated with adverse perinatal outcomes such as an increased stillbirth rate and low Apgar scores (Ray, 1972). The CST was originally described as the oxytocin challenge test and involved an infusion of synthetic oxytocin. Clinicians may choose to use spontaneous contractions or those induced by nipple stimulation in place of oxytocin administration. This simplification of the procedure has also resulted in the procedure being called the CST.

CST is the most sensitive test for antenatal fetal surveillance, with a stillbirth rate of 0.03% within 1 week of a negative CST (negative predictive value, 99.9%). Disadvantages to the CST include the time required for testing (an average of 90 minutes in one study) and the need for intravenous access when oxytocin is used.

Indications

- Suspected fetal compromise in a high-risk pregnancy
- Follow-up evaluation of a suspect or abnormal NST, mBPP, or BPP

Contraindications

Relative

Relative contraindications generally include conditions that are also contraindications to labor or vaginal delivery (preterm labor, preterm premature rupture of membranes, placenta previa, or history of uterine surgery).

Equipment

- Fetal heart rate and uterine pressure monitors (see Fig. 146.1)
- Ultrasound gel for monitors
- Blood pressure cuff
- Intravenous setup
- Terbutaline
- Bed or comfortable reclining chair

Preprocedure Patient Education

Give the patient a teaching guide explaining the CST and answer any questions she may have. Risks, benefits, and alternatives should be explained and informed consent obtained.

Technique

1. Place the patient in a semirecumbent (semi-Fowler's) position, tilted slightly to her left, or with slight left lateral hip displacement. She can also be sitting in a reclining chair at a 30- to 45-degree angle. Attach fetal and uterine monitors.
2. Take a baseline blood pressure to ensure that supine hypotension, which could cause a false-positive CST result, is not present. Repeat every 10 to 15 minutes during the test.
3. Record a baseline fetal heart rate tracing for 20 to 30 minutes to assess for reactivity. Monitor the uterus to determine whether there are spontaneous uterine contractions. Subcutaneous terbutaline, which relaxes uterine muscle in the event of serious uterine hyperstimulation and hypertonic contractions, should be readily available. If there are adequate spontaneous contractions (three or more per 10 minutes, lasting 40 seconds or longer), monitor the fetal heart rate during these contractions, and the study is completed.
4. If there are not enough adequate spontaneous contractions, after obtaining the baseline NST, ask the patient to stimulate one nipple by massaging it through her clothing for about 2 minutes (or less if a contraction starts). She can restart the stimulation in 5 minutes if three contractions do not occur in 10 minutes. If no contraction is induced after 2 minutes, have her stop the stimulation for 2 minutes before repeating the process on the other side. If intermittent stimulation does not achieve the desired uterine contractions, bilateral stimulation should be performed for about 10 minutes.
5. Once an adequate contraction pattern is achieved, nipple stimulation should be stopped. Uterine hyperstimulation (tachysystole) patterns (more than five contractions per 10 minutes or contractions lasting 90 seconds or more) occur in 3% to 4% of CSTs using nipple stimulation. Provide continuous fetal and uterine monitoring.
   NOTE: The nipple-stimulation CST is frequently used because it bypasses the need for intravenous (IV) intervention. It also reduces testing time by about one-half when successful (compared to IV oxytocin).
6. If nipple stimulation does not produce an adequate contraction pattern, administer IV oxytocin. An initial rate of 0.5 to 1.0 mU/min is appropriate. This rate may be increased every 15 minutes by increments of 0.5 to 1.0 mU/ min until regular uterine contractions are achieved. (Another published protocol doubles the infusion rate every 20 minutes.) An adequate CST is achieved once there are three contractions lasting 40 seconds or longer within a 10-minute period. If oxytocin is used, the majority of patients achieve this contraction pattern by the time infusion levels reach 4 to 8 mU/min. Uterine hyperstimulation occurs in around 1% of patients during oxytocin CST and generally responds to stopping the oxytocin infusion. If the contractions do not rapidly decrease after stopping the oxytocin, administer 0.25 to 0.5 mg of subcutaneous terbutaline.

Complications

- Uterine tachysystole often provides a false-positive CST that may lead to improper management if not correctly identified.
- Nonreassuring fetal status requiring an urgent intervention is a rare complication of uterine tachysystole. Tachysystole almost always resolves once the oxytocin infusion or breast stimulation is stopped. If this is not sufficient, subcutaneous terbutaline may be used as previously described.

Interpretation of Results

Categories for CST interpretation are listed below:

- *Negative* test results are reassuring and indicate that no late or significant variable decelerations were seen.
- *Positive*: late decelerations are seen following 50% or more of the contractions, even if the contraction frequency is less than three in 10 minutes. The reactivity of the fetal tracing is an important factor to weigh when faced with a positive CST. A *reactive*, positive CST is associated with a high incidence of false-positive results, whereas a *nonreactive*, positive CST has a much higher predictive value for identifying a compromised fetus (Fig. 165.4).
- *Equivocal-suspicious*: intermittent late decelerations or significant variable decelerations are noted.
- *Equivocal-hyperstimulatory*: fetal heart rate decelerations are seen in the presence of contractions that occur more often than every 2 minutes or last longer than 90 seconds.
- *Unsatisfactory*: either uninterpretable tracing or fewer than three contractions in 10 minutes.

A negative CST that is *nonreactive* is uncommon. This test result deserves further scrutiny to determine if the result is due to medication (e.g., opioids, phenobarbital), a fetal central nervous system defect, prematurity or actual fetal hypoxia.

A positive or suspect CST result requires careful consideration. Maternal factors that affect placental function, such as dehydration or hypotension, should be addressed. If improvement in the fetal heart rate tracing is not seen in the setting of a term pregnancy or fetal pulmonary maturity, labor is often induced.

Postprocedure Education

A CST must be interpreted in the context of the patient's overall clinical condition. Because CSTs are usually reserved for high-risk patients, clear postprocedure instructions are essential. Even patients with negative CSTs require explicit instructions for follow-up antenatal testing, prenatal visits, and any suspicious signs and symptoms. Rare fetal deaths reported after negative CST are often attributed to congenital malformations, placental abruption, or poor glycemic control in women with diabetes.

PATIENT EDUCATION GUIDES

See patient education and consent forms available at www.expertconsult.com.

CPT/BILLING CODES

59020	Fetal contraction stress test
59025	Fetal nonstress test
76818	Fetal biophysical profile; with nonstress testing
76818	(with modifier -52) Modified biophysical profile

If the patient has a diagnosis in addition to normal pregnancy, counseling for FMC is coded with an E/M code. If there is no additional diagnosis (normal pregnancy), preventive medicine codes should be used.

ICD-10-CM DIAGNOSTIC CODES

Z34.00	Encounter for supervision of normal first pregnancy unspecified trimester
Z34.90	Encounter for supervision of other normal pregnancy unspecified trimester
O10.113	Preexisting hypertension complicating pregnancy, unspecified trimester
O14.00	Mild to moderate preeclampsia, unspecified trimester
O14.10	Severe preeclampsia, unspecified trimester
O15.00	Eclampsia, unspecified trimester
O11.9	Preeclampsia or eclampsia with preexisting hypertension, unspecified trimester
O48.0	Postterm pregnancy, pregnancy over 40 completed weeks to 42 completed weeks

O48.1	Prolonged pregnancy, beyond 42 completed weeks
O26.839	Pregnancy related renal disease, unspecified trimester
O26.20	Pregnancy care habitual aborter, unspecified trimester
O24.919	Diabetes mellitus, preexisting, unspecified trimester
O99.810	Abnormal glucose complicating pregnancy
O36.4	Fetal demise, antepartum
O36.5990	Intrauterine growth restriction, unspecified trimester
P00.5	Maternal injury, fetus or newborn affected by maternal conditions

SUPPLIERS

(See contact information available at www.expertconsult.com.)

Philips Medical Systems
Corometrics, General Electric Healthcare
Ultrasound equipment: see the Suppliers section of Chapter 142, Obstetric Ultrasound.

RECOMMENDED READING

Alfirevic Z, Stampalija T, Medley N. Fetal and umbilical Doppler ultrasound in normal pregnancy. *Cochrane Database of Syst Review.* 2015;(4):CD001450.

Alfirevic Z, Stampalija T, Dowswell T. Fetal and umbilical Doppler ultrasound in high-risk pregnancies. *Cochrane Database Syst Review.* 2017:CD007529. pub4.

American College of Obstetricians and Gynecologists. Antepartum fetal surveillance. *ACOG Practice Bulletin No.* 2014;145.

American College of Obstetricians and Gynecologists. ACOG Practice Bulletin no. 134: fetal growth restriction. *Obstet Gynecol.* 2013;121(5):1122–1133.

Devoe LD. Antenatal fetal assessment: contraction stress test, nonstress test, vibroacoustic stimulation, amniotic fluid volume, biophysical profile and modified biophysical profile- an overview. *Semin Perinatol.* 2008;32:247–252.

Dutton PJ, Warrander LK, Roberts SA, et al. Predictors of poor perinatal outcome following maternal perceptions of reduced fetal movements. *PLoS ONE.* 2012;7(7):e39784.

Fetal Assessment. In: Cunningham F, Leveno KJ, et al., eds. *Williams Obstetrics.* 24th ed. New York: McGraw-Hill; 2013.

Kopel E, Hill WC. The effect of abused substances on antenatal and intrapartum fetal testing and well-being. *Clin Obstet Gynecol.* 2013;56(1):154–165.

Mangesi L, Hofmeyr GJ. Fetal movement counting for assessment of fetal well-being. *Cochrane Database Syst Rev.* 2015;15(10):CD004909.

Miller DA, Rabello Y, Paul R. The modified biophysical profile: antepartum testing in the 1990s. *Am J Obstet Gynecol.* 1996;174:812–817.

Oyelese Y, Vintzileos AM. The uses and limitations of the fetal biophysical profile. *Clin Perinatol.* 2011;38:47–64.

Saastad E, Winje BA, Stray Penderson B, et al. Fetal movement counting improved identification of fetal growth restriction and perinatal outcomes—a multi-centre, randomized, controlled trial. *PLoS One.* 2011;6(12):e28482.

Simpson L, Khati NJ, Deshmukh SP, et al. ACR appropriateness criteria assessment of fetal well-being. *J Am Coll Radiol.* 2016;13(12 Pt A):1483–1493. .

Tan KH, Smyth RM, Wei X. Fetal vibroacoustic stimulation for facilitation of tests of fetal wellbeing. *Cochrane Database Syst Rev.* 2013;7(12):CD002963.

Walton JR, Peaceman AM. Identification, assessment and management of fetal compromise. *Clin Perinatol.* 2012;39:753–768.

Warrander LK, Batra G, Bernatavicius G, et al. Maternal perception of reduced fetal movements is associated with altered placental structure and function. *PloS One.* 2012;7(4):e34851.

Winje BA, Wojcieszek AM, Gonzalez-Angulo LY, et al. Interventions to enhance maternal awareness of decreased fetal movement: a systematic review. *BJOG.* 2016;123:886–898.

Zolotor AJ, Carlough MC. Update on prenatal care. *Am Fam Physician.* 2014;89(3):199–208.

CHAPTER 147

INDUCTION OF LABOR

Scott T. Henderson

Although labor usually begins spontaneously, labor induction is a common obstetric procedure. Significant changes have occurred over the past few years regarding how induction is approached both in the United States and worldwide. Based on expert consensus from the American College of Obstetricians and Gynecologists and the National Institutes for Child Health and Human Development, nonmedical inductions prior to 39 weeks of gestation are not recommended. Substantial evidence demonstrates increased morbidity and mortality in neonates delivered in the late preterm period ($37^{0/7}$ week to $38^{6/7}$ weeks) compared with those born after 39 weeks' gestation. Risks include higher rates of respiratory failure, ventilator use, and increased risks for respiratory distress syndrome, transient tachypnea of the newborn, pneumonia, and surfactant and oscillator use (American College of Obstetricians and Gynecologists, 2013a, 2013b). Pregnancies in which a medical indication for delivery exists should be delivered prior to 39 weeks. Guidelines for suggested induction ranges for specific maternal and fetal conditions are available (Table 147.1). Amniocentesis to assess fetal lung maturity is also no longer indicated—if risk to mother or fetus is significant enough to warrant early delivery, amniocentesis is not needed to further guide management. If delivery can be safely delayed based on lung immaturity, the seriousness of the induction becomes less urgent, thus precluding early delivery.

Various institutional approaches to limit nonmedical inductions before 39 weeks have been rolled out based on these guidelines. These include hard stops (e.g., protocols that prohibit scheduling unless adequate dating can be proved); soft stops, where health care providers agree not to induce early; and educational programs

to discuss risks with clinicians. Of these approaches, the hard stop policy seems to reduce the rate of nonindicated inductions the most. US induction statistics show an impact from these changes. Between 2006 and 2012, induction rates at 38 weeks of gestation declined for all maternal age groups less than 40; overall labor induction rates showed 5% to 48% declines in 36 states and the District of Columbia (Centers for Disease Control, 2014). After nearly 20 years of consecutive increases, labor induction in singletons peaked at 23.8% in 2010, but later declined to 23.3% in 2012 (Centers for Disease Control, 2014).

Induction involves two phases: cervical ripening, followed by initiation of contractions through artificial stimulation of the uterus. Cervical status plays a vital role in success or failure. The Bishop Score is a well-established and validated tool for quantifying cervical maturity for labor (Table 147.2). A Bishop score of less than 6 correlates with increased risk of a prolonged labor or failed induction. For research purposes, a Bishop score between 4 and 6 is often used to define an unfavorable cervix. Likelihood of a successful vaginal delivery using oxytocin approaches that of spontaneous labor with a Bishop score above 8. The maximum score is 13.

When the Bishop score is not favorable, ripening methods are usually considered. Historical methods for nonpharmacologic induction include nipple stimulation, acupuncture, membrane stripping (sweeping), and intracervical placement of a Foley catheter or laminaria. With the development of artificial prostaglandins (dinoprostone [prostaglandin E_2; PGE_2] and misoprostol [PGE_1]), use of pharmacologic now surpasses nonpharmacologic methods. Once cervical ripening is undertaken or when a cervix is already favorable,

TABLE 147.1 Recommendations for the Timing of Delivery When Conditions Complicate Pregnancy at or After 34 Weeks of Gestation

Category Type	Condition	Suggested Time for Delivery
Obstetric issues	PPROM	After $34^{0/7}$
Maternal issues: diabetes	Diabetes: pregestational and well controlled	Induction prior to 39 weeks not indicated
	Diabetes: pregestational with vascular complications	$37^{0/7}$ to $39^{6/7}$
	Gestational: well-controlled on diet or medication	Induction prior to 39 weeks not indicated
Maternal issues: hypertension	Chronic, controlled without medications	$38^{0/7}$ to $39^{6/7}$
	Controlled with medication	$37^{0/7}$ to $39^{6/7}$
	Poorly controlled	$36^{0/7}$ to $37^{6/7}$
	Gestational hypertension	$37^{0/7}$ to $38^{6/7}$
	Preeclampsia, severe	At onset or after $34^{0/7}$ (if develops after 34 weeks)
	Preeclampsia, mild	At diagnosis after $37^{0/7}$ weeks
Placenta/uterine	Placenta previa	$36^{0/7}$ to $37^{6/7}$
	Suspected placental accrete, percreta or increate	$34^{0/7}$ to $35^{6/7}$
	Prior classical cesarean	$36^{0/7}$ to $37^{6/7}$
Fetal	Twins	
	Dichorionic/diamniotic	$38^{0/7}$ to $39^{6/7}$
	Monochorionic/diamniotic	$34^{0/7}$ to $37^{6/7}$
	Fetal growth restriction, singleton, otherwise uncomplicated	$38^{0/7}$ to $39^{6/7}$
	Oligohydramnios	$36^{0/7}$ to $37^{6/7}$

Modified from information in: American College of Obstetricians and Gynecologists. ACOG Committee opinion no. 560: medically indicated late-preterm and early-term deliveries. *Obstet Gynecol.* 2013;121(4):908–910.

TABLE 147.2	Bishop Scoring System				
Assessment Score	Dilation (cm)	Effacement (%)	Station	Consistency	Position of Cervix
0	Closed	0–30	−3 (engaged)	Firm	Posterior
1	1–2	40–50	−2	Moderate	Mid
2	3–4	60–70	−1/0	Soft	Anterior
3	≥5	≥80	+1/+2		

Add the score for each of the clinical assessments. If the total score is > 8, the success of induction approaches that of spontaneous labor.

amniotomy with oxytocin is a reasonable way to induce labor (see Chapter 148, Amniotomy).

Providers and nursing staff should develop team protocols for management of labor induction, including possible complications. Team protocols and written policies maximize maternal and infant safety and reduce provider and hospital liability. Protocols should outline the procedures used, the indications, and any contraindications. Special attention should be given to the protocols for induction in women with a previous cesarean delivery.

INDICATIONS

Induction prior to 39 weeks of gestation should be done only for specific medical indications, rather than patient preference, clinician convenience, or other factors. Induction is indicated if health benefits of delivery to the mother or fetus outweigh potential risks of continuing the pregnancy. Gestational hypertension, chronic hypertension, and prolonged or postterm pregnancies have historically accounted for more than 80% of reported inductions. After 39 weeks, nonmedical (elective) indications are permissible, although expectant management is also reasonable in the setting of reassuring maternal and fetal health. Reasonable medical indications for induction prior to 39 weeks include:

- Chronic hypertension, gestational hypertension, preeclampsia, or eclampsia
- Postterm pregnancy
- Abruptio placentae (unless emergent cesarean indicated)
- Abnormal antepartum testing with need for delivery
- Chorioamnionitis
- Suspected fetal compromise (e.g., severe fetal growth restriction, isoimmunization)
- Fetal demise
- Premature rupture of membranes
- Nonreassuring fetal status
- Oligohydramnios
- Maternal medical complications (e.g., poorly controlled diabetes mellitus, renal disease, chronic pulmonary disease, chronic hypertension)

Elective (without medical or obstetric indications) induction of labor after 39 weeks is an option for reasonable indications such as logistic factors (e.g., distance from the hospital), a history of rapid labor and delivery, or psychosocial issues.

CONTRAINDICATIONS

Absolute

Absolute contradictions are similar to those for spontaneous labor or delivery:

- Placenta previa
- Vasa previa
- Transverse fetal lie
- Previous myomectomy entering the endometrial cavity
- Prolapsed umbilical cord
- Previous classic cesarean incision or other longitudinal uterine scar

- Distorted pelvic anatomy
- Active genital herpes infection
- Invasive cervical carcinoma
- Nonreassuring fetal status
- Severe hydrocephalus
- Known hypersensitivity to prostaglandins (dinoprostone [PGE$_2$] or misoprostol [PGE$_1$]); other induction methods are recommended
- Previous asthma, glaucoma, or myocardial infarction (contraindication to dinoprostone)

Relative

- Multiple gestation
- Polyhydramnios
- Appreciable macrosomia
- Maternal cardiac disease
- Grand multiparity
- Previous cesarean delivery with low transverse uterine incision
- Breech presentation
- Malpresentations
- Presenting part above pelvic inlet
- Unexplained vaginal bleeding during pregnancy
- Prematurity
- Ruptured membranes

EQUIPMENT AND SUPPLIES

- External device for monitoring fetal heart rate (FHR) and uterine activity
- Sterile gloves and equipment to follow universal blood and body fluid precautions
- Sterile speculum (if membranes ruptured or using dinoprostone gel)
- Intravenous (IV) access (e.g., heparin lock, lactated Ringer's, normal saline)
- Pharmacologic induction supplies: dinoprostone (PGE$_2$) gel 0.5 mg in 2.5 mL (Prepidil) or 10 mg vaginal insert (Cervidil); misoprostol (PGE$_1$) 100-μg tablet divided into quarters; or oxytocin 10 U/mL (Pitocin)

NOTE: Dinoprostone should be stored between −20°C and −10°C. Because misoprostol is available only in a 100-μg dosage, the pharmacist should cut the tablet into quarters to ensure the correct dose.

EDITOR'S NOTE: A meta-analysis of randomized, controlled trials comparing dinoprostone with misoprostol for cervical ripening and induction of labor found the time to delivery was shorter and the rate of cesarean delivery was lower in the misoprostol group.

- Oxytocin, 60 units diluted in 1 L of lactated Ringer or normal saline (60 mU/mL), which allows the pump setting (mL/hr) to match the administered dose (milliunits/min).
- Infusion pump, if oxytocin is to be used.
- Mechanical induction device (16- to 26-Fr Foley catheter or laminaria [from the brown, cold-water seaweed *Laminaria digitata* or *japonica*], available in small, medium, and large sizes) and povidone–iodine or chlorhexidine solution, sterile 4 × 4 gauze sponges, sponge or uterine packing forceps. A blunt-tipped stylet (urologic sound) or Haney clamp may be useful with Foley insertion.

- Terbutaline 0.25 mg (At least two doses should be readily available prior to dinoprostone or misoprostol use.)

PRECAUTIONS

Before proceeding with induction, review and confirm accurate pregnancy dating:

1. Ultrasound measurement performed prior to 22 weeks of gestation supports a gestational age of 39 weeks or greater. The earlier the ultrasound is done, the more accurate the dating (see Chapter 156, Vaginal Delivery).
2. Thirty-six weeks have elapsed since a documented positive β-human chorionic gonadotropin.
3. Fetal heart tones present (documented) for 30 weeks by fetal Doppler

Before proceeding with induction in a patient who has had a previous cesarean delivery, patients should be counseled regarding the increased risk for uterine rupture, especially those who required surgery due to a prior failed trial of labor. Since some women attempting vaginal birth after a cesarean delivery may require induction, documentation of counseling and informed consent is essential. At some institutions, this is mandatory prior to scheduling a VBAC. The optimal method for labor induction in women with prior cesarean is controversial. A Cochrane meta-analysis of trials comparing oxytocin, misoprostol, and prostaglandins found insufficient information from randomized controlled trials regarding the optimal method of labor induction in women with a prior cesarean birth (Jozwiac, 2013). Although misoprostol has historically been avoided due to safety concerns about uterine rupture, a recent small retrospective cohort ($N = 208$) did not show an increased risk of uterine rupture with misoprostol when it was used as the primary induction agent in women with a prior cesarean (Stenson, 2016). More studies are needed to determine the optimal induction method for this group.

Dinoprostone should be used with caution in patients with ruptured membranes or those with a history of previous uterine hypertonia, glaucoma, myocardial infarction, or childhood asthma (even if no asthma attacks have occurred in adulthood).

PREPROCEDURE PATIENT EDUCATION AND FORMS

All patients should be counseled regarding the indications for induction, the expected results, the alternatives, and the possible adverse effects, including possible cesarean delivery, uterine hyperstimulation, and fetal distress. The US Food and Drug Administration (FDA) has approved only oxytocin and dinoprostone for labor induction. Review the possible complications with the patient (and family, if present). The clinician should be familiar with the package insert information. While the use of prostaglandins for postpartum hemorrhage can be associated with vomiting, diarrhea, or fever, no difference between the treatment and control group with prostaglandins given for cervical ripening was seen in a recent literature review. Laminaria are made from brown seaweed and act by drawing water from the cervix and swelling, which softens and then dilates the cervix. Laminaria is rarely used for labor induction due to concerns over slightly increased infection risk. Anaphylaxis has also been reported.

FDA warnings regarding misoprostol were changed in May 2002 to state that it is contraindicated for use as an antiulcer medication during pregnancy. It is not FDA approved for any obstetric indication, and warnings regarding risks with labor induction remain in the product labeling. Clinicians frequently use medications off-label, however, and there is more than a decade of research on the use of misoprostol for cervical ripening. It has become the induction method of choice in many hospitals due to its low cost, stability at room temperature, and ease of use.

TECHNIQUE

Before initiating any method of labor induction, perform a cervical assessment and calculate the Bishop score. The patient should have a nonstress test and be assessed for any regular uterine contractions (see Chapter 146, Antepartum Fetal Monitoring). If the nonstress test is nonreactive or a normal uterine contraction pattern is noted, further evaluation rather than induction is indicated. Universal blood and body fluid precautions should be followed during all cervical ripening or labor induction procedures.

Mechanical

Foley Catheter

1. Cleanse the cervix with a povidone-iodine or chlorhexidine soaked gauze sponge or swab. Introduce the Foley into the endocervix under direct visualization using a vaginal speculum. The Foley is then guided through the endocervix and into the potential space between the amniotic membrane and the lower uterine segment. Some clinicians use a stylet or curved Haney clamp to help permit passage of the Foley tip into the cervix. Care must be taken not to rupture the membranes or inadvertently traumatize the fetus.
2. Inflate the balloon reservoir with 30 to 50 mL of normal saline.
3. The balloon is then retracted so that it rests on the internal os.

The following additional steps may be taken:

4. Pressure, either constant or intermittent, may be applied by adding weights to the catheter end. Constant pressure can be achieved by attaching 1 L of IV fluid to the catheter end and suspending it from the end of the bed. Intermittent pressure can be obtained by a gentle pull on the catheter end 2 to 4 times/hr.
5. Remove the catheter at rupture of membranes. It also may spontaneously expel once the cervix dilates sufficiently (usually >4 cm).

Cook Cervical Ripening Balloon

The Cook Cervical Ripening Balloon is a silicone double-balloon catheter with an adjustable-length malleable stylet indicated for mechanical dilation prior to labor induction at term.

1. Loosen the fitting on the proximal hub of the stylet. Adjust the wire so the distal stylet tip is even with the distal tip of the balloon.
2. Twist the fitting so the wire does not move during placement, and seat the adjustable handle into the blue port labeled "S."
3. Use the stylet within the balloon to move the catheter across the cervix if necessary. Once the uterine balloon is at the level of the internal os, remove the stylet before advancing the catheter further.
4. Advance the balloon through the cervix until both uninflated balloons are through the cervical canal.
5. Inflate the uterine balloon with 40 mL of saline through the red port. Once inflated, pull the catheter back until the uterine balloon is up against the internal cervical os.
6. Inflate the vaginal balloon with 20 mL of saline using the green port.
7. Once both balloons are correctly situated, add saline to a maximum of 80 mL/balloon.
8. The balloon should be in place no longer than 12 hours prior to active labor being induced.

Laminaria

1. After cleansing the cervix with a povidone-iodine or chlorhexidine soaked swab, the anterior aspect is grasped with a tenaculum.

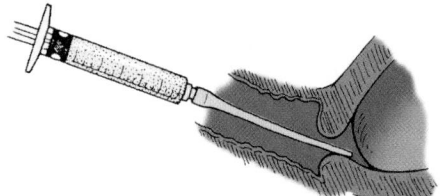

Fig. 147.1   Application of dinoprostone (PGE₂) gel.

2. Using a sponge or uterine packing forceps, a laminaria of appropriate size is inserted so that the tip rests against the internal os. The laminaria will gradually increase in diameter by three- to fourfold.

3. After 4 to 6 hours, remove the laminaria and reevaluate the cervix. If the cervix remains unfavorable, the procedure may be repeated with a second laminaria of larger diameter.

Pharmacologic

Dinoprostone Gel

1. Obtain IV access (optional).
2. Connect the appropriate shielded catheter (20 mm in length if no cervical effacement is present or 10 mm if greater than 50% effacement) to the filled syringe.
3. For proper gel administration, the patient should be in a dorsal lithotomy position. To help ensure proper placement of the gel, a speculum can be used to visualize the cervix.
4. Under sterile conditions, insert the catheter into the vagina. Use a gentle expulsion technique to express the contents of one syringe (0.5 mg) into the cervical canal just below the level of the internal os (Fig. 147.1). If the tube becomes disconnected, spread the remaining contents of the syringe onto the cervix digitally. Use the contents of one syringe for one patient only. After injection, do not attempt to administer the small amount of gel remaining in the catheter. Discard the syringe, catheter, and any unused package contents after use.
5. The patient should remain supine for at least 15 to 30 minutes to minimize leakage from the cervical canal. Monitor uterine activity and fetal heart tones for 2 hours postadministration using external FHR monitoring. Monitoring may be discontinued if there is no uterine activity or FHR abnormality during this period.
6. Reevaluate the cervix after 6 hours. If there is minimal change, the procedure may be repeated using a second dose. If needed, a third dose may be administered after 6 more hours. The maximum recommended cumulative dose for a 24-hour period is 1.5 mg of dinoprostone.
7. The package insert recommends an interval of 6 to 12 hours between the use of dinoprostone gel and oxytocin. However, some clinicians will initiate oxytocin in 4 hours if there is no uterine tachysystole.

Dinoprostone Insert

1. Obtain IV access (optional).
2. Cervidil is supplied in an individually wrapped aluminum/polyethylene package with a tear mark on one side of the package. The package should be opened only by tearing the aluminum package along the tear mark. The package should never be opened with scissors or other sharp objects, which may compromise or cut the knitted polyester pouch that serves as the retrieval system for the polymeric slab.
3. On bimanual examination, place the 10 mg dinoprostone insert transversely in the posterior vaginal fornix (Fig. 147.2). A minimal amount of water-soluble lubricant can be used to assist with insertion. The vaginal insert must not be used without its retrieval system.

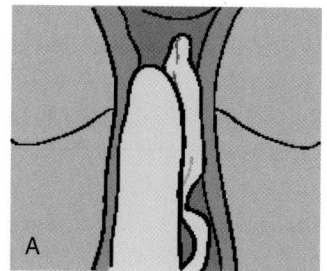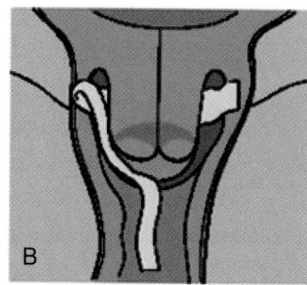

Fig. 147.2   Application of dinoprostone (PGE₂) insert. (A) Insertion, (B) Final placement. (Modified courtesy Forest Pharmaceuticals, Inc., St. Louis, MO.)

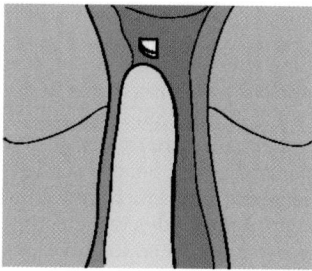

Fig. 147.3   Insertion of 25 μg Cytotec (one-fourth of a 100 μg tablet).

4. The patient should remain supine for at least 2 hours after insertion but may ambulate after this. Continue external fetal monitoring for 2 hours postadministration. Monitoring may be discontinued after 2 hours if there is no uterine activity or FHR abnormality.
5. Remove the insert at onset of labor or 12 hours after insertion. Reevaluate the cervix at that time. When removing the insert, confirm that the medication has been removed by visualizing the knitted polyester retrieval system and confirming that it contains the slab. In the rare event that the slab is not in the polyester retrieval system, perform a vaginal examination to remove the slab and prevent continued delivery of the active ingredient.
6. Remove the insert if uterine tachysystole develops and at least 30 minutes before oxytocin administration or prior to amniotomy.

Misoprostol

1. Obtain IV access (optional).
2. On bimanual examination, insert 25 μg of misoprostol (one quarter of 100-μg tablet) into the vaginal fornix (Fig. 147.3). Certain protocols recommend continuous uterine and fetal monitoring after insertion. At a minimum, maintain external fetal monitoring for 2 hours after placement.
3. Reevaluate the cervix after 4 hours. If there is minimal change, place a second dose.
4. Misoprostol should be held if two or more contractions occur in 10 minutes, a Bishop score of 8 or higher is achieved, active labor begins, or the FHR pattern is nonreassuring. Oxytocin should not be administered sooner than 2 hours after the last dose of misoprostol.
5. Misoprostol use for cervical ripening should not exceed 24 hours.

Studies have examined higher doses and shorter dosing intervals of misoprostol. Both are associated with a greater incidence of side effects such as tachysystole and FHR abnormalities. Use of buccal and oral misoprostol for cervical ripening is also becoming more common. Both oral and buccal misoprostol (25 μg given every 4 hours) seem to be safe and effective for cervical ripening. Additional studies are needed to determine the optimal dosing recommendations.

TABLE 147.3   Oxytocin Protocols

Regimen	Starting Dose (mU/min)	Incremental Increase (mU/min)	Frequency of Increasing Dosage (min)
Low dose	0.5–1	1	30–40
Alternative low dose	1–2	2	15
High dose	6	6 (max 40 mU/min)	15
Alternative high dose	4	4 (max 32 mU/min)	15

Oxytocin

Oxytocin is the preferred pharmacologic agent for labor induction when the cervix is favorable. It is administered as a dilute IV solution, with the flow rate precisely regulated by an infusion pump. Protocols vary on the number of units of oxytocin per liter of fluid (typically lactated Ringer or normal saline). Providers should be familiar with which concentrations are typically used at their institution.

As with other pharmacologic means of induction, fetal monitoring is indicated before beginning the infusion. FHR and uterine activity monitoring is indicated during oxytocin administration. If doses over 20 units are needed, consider placement of an internal fetal monitor and an intrauterine pressure catheter (see Chapter 150, Intrauterine Pressure Catheter Insertion).

Multiple protocols have been established regarding the initial dose of oxytocin and the amount and frequency of dosage increases (Table 147.3). Starting doses typically range from lower doses of 0.5 to 2 mU/min to 6 mU/min. Dosage increases range from 1 to 2 mU/min to as much as 6 mU/min, with adjustments for uterine tachysystole. Time intervals between dosage increases in protocols usually range from 15 to 40 minutes. An adequate labor pattern with contractions 2 to 3 minutes apart, 45- to 60-seconds in duration, 50- to 75-mm Hg intensity, and a normal resting tone between contractions is the goal. Regardless of protocol, approximately 90% of patients respond to 16 mU/min or less. It is unusual for a patient to require more than 20 to 40 mU/min to obtain an adequate labor pattern. In fact, higher doses may predict failure. This must be weighed against the fact that if the FHR is reassuring and labor has arrested (i.e., contractions not adequate [<200 Montevideo units]), there are no apparent risks to oxytocin doses greater than 48 mU/min. It should be kept in mind that oxytocin is a homolog to vasopressin and has significant antidiuretic properties. When infused at doses greater than 20 mU/min, renal retention of free water may result. Infusion of oxytocin in appreciable amounts can result in water intoxication and hyponatremia, leading to coma, convulsions, and even death.

COMMON ERRORS

The provider must be prepared to handle both maternal and fetal complications before an induction is initiated. Once applied (except for the dinoprostone insert, which can be removed by using its retrieval system), prostaglandins cannot be removed or quickly discontinued like oxytocin. For practical purposes, all of these ripening techniques can be performed in the evening and overnight, with planned oxytocin administration or amniotomy the following morning. The provider must also ensure that resources are available for immediate delivery (vaginal or cesarean) and newborn resuscitation, if necessary.

COMPLICATIONS

- Uterine tachysystole (defined as more than 5 contractions in a 10-minute period averaged over a 30-minute window) and possible premature separation of placenta

- Failed induction with increased risk of cesarean delivery
- Abnormalities or changes in FHR pattern
- Premature infant if dates calculated incorrectly
- Fetal acidosis
- Fetal intolerance of labor
- Neonate with low Apgar scores
- Precipitous delivery
- Prolapsed umbilical cord
- Maternal or neonatal infection
- Uterine rupture

POSTPROCEDURE MANAGEMENT

The goal of an induction is an otherwise uneventful vaginal delivery. The provider must be prepared to manage urgent situations that can occur during induction and delivery. Should tachysystole occur, assess the FHR pattern immediately. If the FHR pattern is not reassuring, initiate immediate intrauterine resuscitation. This includes an IV fluid bolus of 1000 mL, lateral positioning of the mother, and oxygen administration at 10 L/min through a nonrebreather face mask to increase fetal oxygenation. If tachysystole occurs and a dinoprostone insert is being used, it should be removed; an oxytocin drip should be turned off. Some protocols suggest restarting oxytocin (tachysystole resolved and FHR reassuring) at half the prior dose. If other pharmacologic methods are being used, they cannot be removed. Terbutaline 0.25 mg subcutaneous injection can be administered and repeated as necessary. If the FHR pattern does not respond in a satisfactory manner, proceed to an immediate operative delivery. If the FHR pattern is reassuring despite the uterine hyperactivity, the oxytocin rate should be titrated down until the contraction pattern is acceptable.

CPT/BILLING CODES

No specific CPT codes exist for labor induction. According to the CPT manual, labor that is preterm, postterm, induced, augmented, or otherwise complicated is not routine and requires additional time and resources. The clinician should code these situations with hospital Evaluation and Management codes.

99356 Prolonged physician service in the inpatient setting, requiring direct (face-to-face) patient contact beyond the usual service (e.g., maternal fetal monitoring for high-risk delivery or other physiological monitoring); first hour (list separately in addition to code for inpatient Evaluation and Management service).

99357 Each additional 30 minutes (list separately in addition to code for prolonged physician service).

And, if prolonged, but not face-to-face, care:

99358 Prolonged Evaluation and Management service before and/or after direct (face-to-face) patient care (e.g., review of extensive records and tests, communication with other professionals and/or the patient/family); first hour (list separately in addition to code[s] for other physician service[s] and/or inpatient or outpatient Evaluation and Management service).

ICD-10-CM DIAGNOSTIC CODES

O45.90	Premature separation of placenta
O10.019	Preexisting essential hypertension complicating pregnancy
O10.02	Preexisting essential hypertension complicating childbirth
O10.03	Preexisting essential hypertension complicating puerperium
O10.419	Preexisting secondary hypertension complicating pregnancy, unspecified trimester
O10.42	Preexisting secondary hypertension complicating childbirth
O10.43	Preexisting secondary hypertension complicating puerperium

O14.00	Mild or unspecified preeclampsia unspecified trimester
O14.10	Severe preeclampsia unspecified trimester
O15.9	Eclampsia unspecified
O11.9	Preeclampsia preexisting hypertension
O48.0	Postterm pregnancy, 40 to 42 weeks' gestation
O48.1	Prolonged pregnancy, beyond 42 weeks' gestation
O26.839	Pregnancy related renal disease unspecified trimester
O24.319	Unspecified preexisting diabetes mellitus unspecified trimester
O24.419	Gestational diabetes mellitus in pregnancy unspecified control
O36.019X	Maternal care Rh isoimmunization
O36.199X	Isoimmunization from other and unspecified blood-group incompatibility
O68	Fetal distress
O36.4XX	Intrauterine fetal death
O36.599X	Intrauterine growth retardation
O42.00	Premature rupture of membranes (membranes ruptured <24 hours before onset of labor)
O42.10	Delayed delivery after spontaneous or unspecified rupture of membranes (ruptured >24 hours before onset or prolonged rupture of membranes)
O41.109X	Infection of amniotic cavity
O61.1	Failed mechanical induction
O61.0	Failed medical or unspecified induction
O76	Abnormality in fetal heart rate or rhythm

ONLINE RESOURCES

Cook Medical: Cervical ripening balloon with stylet instructions: https://www.cookmedical.com/data/resources/RH-D25085-EN-F_M3_1459966992494.pdf

Esakoff TF, Kilpatrick S. The transcervical Foley balloon: A simple device for a common clinical scenario. Contemporary OB/GYN. http://www.contemporaryobgyn.net/medicine-feature/articles/transcervical-foley-balloon.

RECOMMENDED READING

American College of Obstetricians and Gynecologists. ACOG Committee opinion no. 107: induction of labor. *Obstet Gynecol.* 2009;114(2):386–397.

American College of Obstetricians and Gynecologists. ACOG Committee opinion no. 688: management of suboptimally dated pregnancies. *Obstet Gynecol.* 2017;129:e29–e32.

American College of Obstetricians and Gynecologists. ACOG Committee opinion no. 561: nonmedically indicated early-term deliveries. *Obstet Gynecol.* 2013a;121(4):911–915.

American College of Obstetricians and Gynecologists. ACOG Committee opinion no. 560: medically indicated late-preterm and early-term deliveries. *Obstet Gynecol.* 2013b;121(4):908–910.

Centers for Disease Control. National Center for Health Statistics. *Recent Declines in Induction of Labor by Gestational Age*; June 2014. NCHS Data Brief No. 155.

Dorr ML, Pierson RC, Daggy J, et al. Buccal verses vaginal misoprostol for term induction of labor: a retrospective cohort study. *Am J Perinatol.* 2018. Epub ahead of print.

Gibson KS, Waters TP. Measures of success: prediction of successful labor induction. *Semin Perinatol.* 2015;39(6):475–482.

Induction and augmentation of labor. In: Cunningham F, Leveno KJ, Bloom SL, et al., eds. *Williams Obstetrics.* 24th ed. New York: McGraw-Hill; 2013.

Jozwiak M, Dodd JM. Methods of term labor induction for women with a previous caesarean section. *Cochrane Database Syst Rev.* 2013;3:CD009792.

Jozwiak M, Bloemenkamp KW, Kelly AJ, et al. Mechanical methods for induction of labor. *Cochrane Database Syst Rev.* 2012;3:CD001233.

Marroquin GA, Tudorica N, Salafia CM. Induction of labor at 41 weeks of pregnancy among primiparas with an unfavorable Bishop score. *Arch Gynecol Obstet.* 2013;288(5):989–993.

Mozurkewich EL, Chilimigras JL, Berman DR, et al. Methods of induction of labour: a systematic review. *BMC Pregnancy Childbirth.* 2011;11:84.

Spong CY, Mercer BM, D'Alton M, et al. Timing of indicated late-preterm and early-term birth. *Obstet Gynecol.* 2011;118:323–333.

Stenson D, Wallstrom T, Sjostrand M, et al. Induction of labor in women with a uterine scar. *J Matern Fetal Neonatal Med.* 2016;20:3286–3291.

CHAPTER 148

AMNIOTOMY

Rebecca H. Gladu

Amniotomy, or artificial rupture of the membranes, is a common labor intervention. It is often used either alone or in combination with oxytocin for active labor induction management or in situations of dysfunctional labor progress. Other reasons include placement of a fetal scalp electrode or intrauterine pressure catheter monitor, or assessment for the presence of meconium in nonreassuring fetal tracings. Amniotomy is traditionally considered to shorten labor, although evidence is conflicting. One randomized controlled trial showed that early amniotomy (performed at <4 cm dilation) in nulliparous women decreased time to delivery by 2 hours, with women more likely to deliver within 24 hours compared with no amniotomy (Macones and colleagues, 2013). No statistically significant increase in cesarean rates, cord prolapse, or risk of chorioamniotis was seen. A Cochrane review found that early intervention with oxytocin and amniotomy shortened labor duration by 1.28 hours with no impact on cesarean rate or other neonatal factors. Another Cochrane review of 5500 women who underwent amniotomy to shorten spontaneous labor, conversely, showed no difference in labor duration, maternal satisfaction, or Apgar scores. Routine amniotomy is controversial. Current data suggest that in women with normally progressing labor and no evidence of fetal compromise, routine amniotomy is not needed unless required for invasive monitoring (e.g., scalp electrode or intrauterine pressure catheter placement). Expert opinion from the American College of Obstetricians and Gynecologists currently recommends amniotomy for labor dystocia, especially before cesarean delivery is considered.

Whether amniotomy increases cord prolapse risk is also incompletely understood. Performing amniotomy during the second stage of labor when the head is well engaged, avoiding amniotomy during a contraction, and tearing a small hole in the membranes have been suggested to decrease the risk of prolapse from a large amount of amniotic fluid exiting the cervix under pressure (Cohain, 2013).

EDITOR'S NOTE: Amniotomy should not be performed routinely. Some experts perform it only if there is a strong indication; in most cases, nature will run its course without an intervention. Depending on the station of the fetal head, attempts to rotate or change the position (e.g., from occiput posterior to occiput anterior) are best performed prior to amniotomy.

INDICATIONS

- Need for fetal or internal uterine pressure monitoring when membranes are intact
- Active management of labor protocol
- Concerns for meconium (postdate gestation; nonreassuring external fetal monitoring)
- Induction of labor
- Dysfunctional labor

NOTE: Although a fetal scalp electrode can be applied through the amniotic membranes, performing an amniotomy first simplifies this procedure (see Chapter 149, Fetal Scalp Electrode Application).

CONTRAINDICATIONS

Absolute

- Malpresentation
- Cord palpable below or near fetal head
- Unstable lie
- Suspected velamentous insertion of umbilical cord
- Maternal HIV positive status
- Maternal active perineal herpes infection or viral hepatitis
- Placenta previa (complete)

Relative

- Unknown fetal presentation
- Nonengaged fetal head (biparietal diameter not at ischial spines-may increase risk of cord prolapse)
- Cervix dilated less than 3 cm
- Patient not in active labor
- Patient refusal or intolerance of procedure
- Polyhydramnios (increased risk of cord prolapse if fetal head not well applied to cervix)

EQUIPMENT AND SUPPLIES

- Amniotomy hook (Fig. 148.1) or amniotomy finger cot (Fig. 148.2)
- Sterile gloves and lubricant
- Absorbent pads and towels to be placed under the patient
- Fetal monitor
- Tocolytics should be available, especially if the patient is being augmented
- Equipment for universal blood and body fluid precautions (e.g., mask, eye protection, or gown if needed)

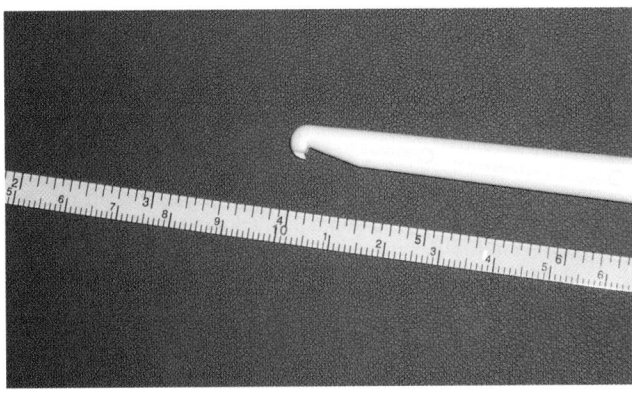

Fig. 148.1   Amniotomy hook.

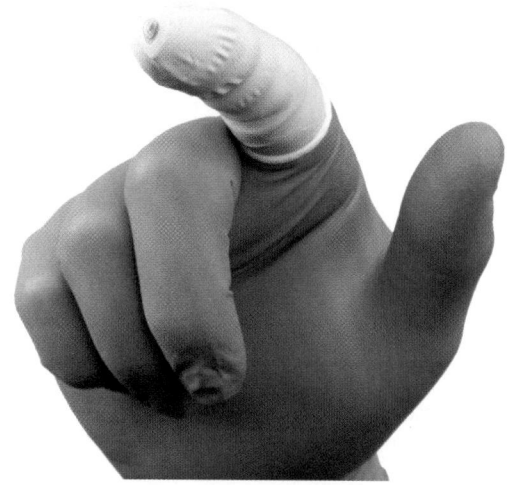

Fig. 148.2 Amniotomy glove (AROM-COT). (Courtesy Utah Medical Products.)

PRECAUTIONS

Risks to the patient and fetus include the following:

- Infection such as chorioamnionitis (especially with prolonged labor)
- Need for antibiotics (especially if labor is prolonged)
- Bleeding from maternal cervical or vaginal trauma
- Cord prolapse
- Uterine tetany
- Fetal scalp scratch or laceration

PREPROCEDURE PATIENT EDUCATION AND FORMS

The procedure should be explained to the patient, including risks, benefits, and alternatives (see patient consent form available at www.expertconsult.com). Discuss the possibility of cord prolapse and the precautions taken to avoid this and other possible complications. If the procedure is being done to stimulate labor progression, explain that amniotomy alone may not significantly reduce labor duration. Contractions may become stronger or more frequent following amniotomy, necessitating pain control in some women. Explain a possible increased risk of infection (and need for antibiotics) and bleeding. Rupture of membranes commits the patient to delivery, usually within 24 hours. After 24 hours, chorioamnionitis risk increases significantly, possibly necessitating cesarean delivery. There is a rare chance that the fetal head could be scratched or cut.

TECHNIQUE

Amniotomy Hook

1. The patient should attempt to relax in the recumbent position with feet together and hips externally rotated (i.e., frog-legged) or in stirrups. Observe universal blood and body fluid precautions when performing this procedure. Record the fetal heart rate before, during, and after amniotomy. Perform a cervical examination to confirm that the membranes are intact, the cervix is at least 3 cm dilated, and the head is well applied. The presence of an umbilical cord should be excluded.
2. Introduce the second and third digits (index and middle fingers) of the nondominant hand, palmar side up, into the vagina. Insert the fingertips past the cervical lip, into the uterus, and against the membranes. Make sure that the fingers are placed against the membranes rather than over a thin cervical lip.

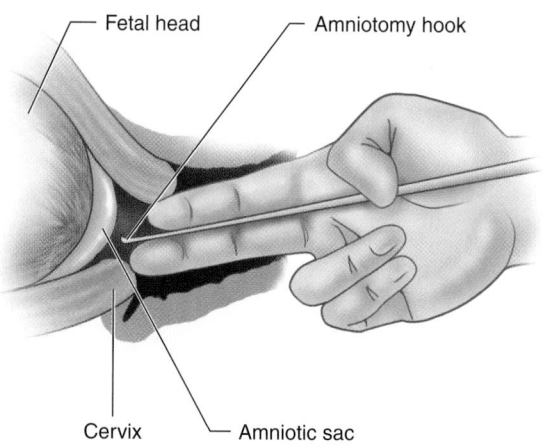

Fig. 148.3 Proper insertion of amniotomy hook.

3. Grasp the amniotomy hook with your dominant hand. Introduce the tip into the vagina and into a position between the two fingers on the nondominant hand already applied against the membranes (Fig. 148.3). The hook should be pointed downward (away from the membranes). Ask an assistant to apply fundal and suprapubic pressure to reduce the risk of cord prolapse. This maneuver may also increase the amount of fluid bulging between the membranes and the head. This bulge mimics a bag, hence the description of the mother's "bag of water." Avoid compressing the membranes too tightly against the infant's head with the nondominant hand; this may make it more difficult to hook the bag.
4. Invert the hook upward (i.e., rotate it 180 degrees), apply pressure to the bag with the hook, and rupture the bag with a single motion of the sharp hook. If successful, amniotic fluid should run from the vagina. If no fluid is seen, repeat this step two or three times until fluid is noted to flow from the vagina. If these attempts are unsuccessful, and the bag is still palpable, relax the fingertips away from the membranes and move them slightly. This will allow you to hook the bag from a different direction. Make sure the fingers of your nondominant hand are against the membranes (and not the cervix) and again attempt to rupture the bag with a single motion of the hook. The bag may be quite slippery, so redirecting several times may be required before the amniotomy is successful. Apply varying amounts of pressure against the membranes with the nondominant hand with each attempt. If unsuccessful at this point, request a new hook because the hook may be defective. If there is little fluid palpable (no bag) at the beginning of the procedure, instead of rupturing the membranes or "breaking the bag of water" with the hook, the clinician should attempt to grasp and tear the membranes with the hook. If successful, even though fluid was not apparent as a bag before amniotomy, it may still run out of the vagina. Without a full bag, the sensation of performing amniotomy is quite different; the clinician may have the sensation of merely scratching the fetal scalp with the hook. As long as the clinician is sure that the presentation is vertex and only gentle attempts are made at hooking the bag, the risk of actually scratching or lacerating the infant's scalp is small.
5. After successful amniotomy, remove the hook. Note the amount of fluid that drains. If very little fluid is seen, no prior ultrasonography was performed, and the membranes were previously thought to be intact, the diagnosis of oligohydramnios should be considered. If so, be prepared for additional resuscitative needs at delivery, especially in a growth-restricted fetus.
6. Maintain the fingers of the nondominant hand against the fetal head as fluid is allowed to leak out, noting the color of the fluid (clear or meconium stained). Be sure to confirm that the umbilical cord has not prolapsed.

7. Remove the fingers and observe the fetal monitor for any non-reassuring signs, such as fetal bradycardia or tachycardia. Prepare to respond (e.g., administer oxygen to the mother, roll her on her side, administer intravenous fluid) if an abnormal fetal heart rate persists.

Amniotomy Glove

Steps 1 and possibly 2 are the same as with the amniotomy hook, except the patient does not need to be in the recumbent or lithotomy position unless that is the most comfortable position for her. The finger cot is placed over a sterile gloved index finger with the hook pointing toward the palm of the hand, and then against the amnion to rupture it. This simplifies the procedure and prevents the clinician from having to use an instrument blindly. Whether the cot is placed on the dominant hand or the nondominant hand is based on clinician preference. No matter which hand is used for the cot, the other hand's index and middle finger can be inserted behind the cervix and against the membranes, as with the amniotomy hook. It can then be used to stabilize the head postamniotomy. Alternatively, because only one to two fingers need to be inserted into the vagina to perform the amniotomy, the other hand can be used to apply fundal or suprapubic pressure, which can then be released after successful amniotomy. Universal blood and body fluid precautions should be observed when performing this procedure.

3. Use the finger cot to apply pressure to the membranes with the sharp device. This step may be repeated until fluid is noted to flow from the vagina.
4. See steps 4 through 7 from the "Amniotomy Hook" section.

SAMPLE OPERATIVE REPORT

See the sample operative report available at www.expertconsult.com.

COMMON ERRORS

- Failure to fully rupture the amnion. Should this occur, reposition the examiner's digits and repeat the procedure. Occasionally, only one layer of the membranes is ruptured (partial amniotic tear), requiring repetition of the procedure ("a double bag").
- Mistaking an effaced thin cervical lip for the amnion. This may cause some patient discomfort if she does not have some type of anesthesia/pain control.

COMPLICATIONS

- Fetal distress
- Failure to induce or augment labor
- Increase in pain sensation with labor
- Prolapsed cord
- Infection due to prolonged rupture of membranes
- Possibly increased risk of cesarean delivery

POSTPROCEDURE MANAGEMENT

Observe the patient and fetus for signs of distress, such as fetal heart rate decelerations on the fetal monitor. Ensure that the cord did not prolapse and that the amniotomy hook did not lacerate the cervix or infant.

POSTPROCEDURE PATIENT EDUCATION

The patient should be instructed to expect vaginal fluid leakage. Should she develop any pain or bleeding after the procedure, the clinician should be notified immediately. While written postprocedure education materials are not generally provided, discussing the procedure as part of routine antepartum care in the third trimester is prudent.

CPT/BILLING CODES

Amniotomy is considered part of labor management and is not billed separately (falls under global delivery charge).

ICD-10-CM DIAGNOSTIC CODES

| O41.93XX | Disorder of amniotic fluid and membranes unspecified (Meconium-stained fluid) |
| O40.9XXX | Polyhydramnios unspecified trimester |

Use additional seventh character to identify fetus: 0 = 1, 1–5 = multiple.

O77.9	Fetal distress, not otherwise specified
O62.1	Secondary uterine inertia
O63.0	Prolonged labor, first stage
O63.1	Prolonged labor, second stage

SUPPLIERS

(See contact information available at www.expertconsult.com.)

Amniotomy hook
  AmniHook Briggs Healthcare
  CooperSurgical
Amniotomy glove (AROM-COT)
  Utah Medical Products
  Amnicot Admedus Allied Medical

RECOMMENDED READING

American College of Obstetricians and Gynecologists. Committee opinion No. 687. Approaches to limit intervention during labor and birth. *Obstet Gynceol.* 2017;129(2):e20–e28.

Archie CL. Chapter 7 normal and abnormal labor and delivery. In: DeCherney AH, Nathan L, Laufer N, Roman AS, eds. *Current Diagnosis and Treatment in Obstetrics and Gynecology.* 11th ed. New York: McGraw-Hill; 2013:203–211.

Cohain JS. The less studied effects of amniotomy. *J Mat Fet Neonat Med.* 2013;26(17):1687–1690.

Jackson S, Gregory K. Management of the first stage of labor: potential strategies to lower the cesarean delivery rate. *Clin Obstet Gynecol.* 2015;58(2):217–226.

Macones GA, Cahill A, Stamilio DM, et al. The efficacy of early amniotomy in nulliparous labor induction: a randomized controlled trial. *Am J Obstet Gynecol.* 2012;207(403):e1–e5.

Smythe RMD, Markham C, Dowswell T. Amniotomy for shortening spontaneous labor. *Cochrane Database Syst Rev.* 2013;(6):Art. No. CD006167.

Wei S, wo B, Qi H, et al. Early amniotomy and early oxytocin for prevention of, or therapy for, delay in first stage of spontaneous labour (sic) compared with routine care. *Cochrane Database Syst Rev.* 2013;(8):Art. No. CD006794.

Tuggy M, Garcia J. *Procedures Consult.* Amniotomy. http://www.procedures-consult.com/medical-procedures-amniotomy-FM-012-procedure.aspx.

CHAPTER 149

FETAL SCALP ELECTRODE APPLICATION

Beth A. Choby

Fetal heart rate monitoring is the most common obstetric procedure in the United States, with approximately 85% of fetuses being assessed with internal or external monitoring during labor. Electronic fetal monitoring (EFM) became possible in the 1950s with Edward Hon's design of an electrode that directly attached to the fetus. EFM entered widespread clinical use in the late 1960s, despite the fact that evidence supporting its benefit was nominal (i.e., limited to case reports and retrospective studies).

Intermittent auscultation and continuous EFM are both available for assessing fetal heart rate trends. To perform intermittent auscultation, a hand-held Doppler ultrasonography transducer is used at specific intervals during labor. It requires a one-to-one nurse-to-patient ratio and an explicit auscultation schedule, making intermittent auscultation both resource intensive and expensive to perform. Although the majority of professional maternity care societies believe that some type of fetal monitoring is needed during labor, no randomized, controlled trials have compared either intermittent auscultation or continuous EFM with no monitoring. Because continuous EFM is simpler and less expensive and provides more data, it has become the default method of monitoring on most labor units, especially in the United States.

Continuous EFM is available through either external or internal monitoring. With external monitoring, a cardiotachometer measuring fetal heart rate is attached across the maternal abdomen using a belt. Internal EFM technology makes use of a bipolar spiral electrode that attaches directly to the fetal scalp. An electrical circuit is created between the wire electrode that twists into the fetal scalp and the metal wing on the electrode. Vaginal fluids create a saline electrical bridge and close the circuit. The resulting voltage difference (fetal cardiac signal) is amplified and transferred to a cardiotachometer that calculates heart rate. The bipolar wires also connect to a reference electrode on the maternal thigh to minimize electrical interference.

Both internal and external EFM are hindered by poor intraobserver consistency and a high false-positive rate. Continuous EFM is usually performed with the patient in dorsal lithotomy position and likely contributes to dysfunctional labor. Widespread use of EFM is associated with higher rates of cesarean delivery, operative vaginal delivery, and litigation. Continuous EFM has limited ability to identify a truly hypoxic-ischemic fetus and fails to decrease rates of cerebral palsy. In a recent meta-analysis of 13 randomized, controlled trials, the only clinically significant benefit for routine continuous EFM was the prevention of neonatal seizures.

With older EFM technology, internal scalp electrodes provided more accurate information on fetal heart rate trends than external monitoring. Newer-generation equipment allows for better evaluation of FHR variability using the external monitor. Scalp electrodes are less frequently used as a result of these technological improvements. Because certain situations still necessitate the use of an internal monitor, understanding both the application and the use of the fetal scalp electrode (FSE) is important for maternity care providers.

NOTE: In 2008, a National Institute of Child Health and Human Development workshop standardized FHR monitoring guidelines, including a three-tiered classification system for EFM interpretation. Discussion of the subtleties of the abnormal fetal heart rate tracing is beyond the scope of this chapter, although several recent references are listed for your convenience. The comprehensive clinical picture, including stage of labor, concurrent medical problems, current medications, and availability of a physician to perform an operative delivery, should be considered when making management decisions.

INDICATIONS

Most healthy, low-risk pregnancies are safely monitored with intermittent auscultation or continuous external monitoring. Higher-risk pregnancies affected by maternal or fetal medical complications often require continuous monitoring. Although continuous external monitoring is usually adequate, the following situations warrant consideration of internal monitoring with a FSE:

- Ineffective external monitoring or inadequate fetal tracing as a result of
  - Maternal body habitus
  - Excessive maternal movement
  - Excessive fetal movement
- Inadequate staffing for provision of intermittent auscultation
- Nonreassuring fetal heart rate patterns
  - Persistent fetal bradycardia (fetal heart rate [FHR] < 110 beats/min)
  - Persistent fetal tachycardia (FHR > 160 beats/min)
  - Decreased FHR variability on external monitoring
  - Lack of FHR accelerations
  - Moderate to severe variable decelerations
  - Repetitive late decelerations

CONTRAINDICATIONS

Absolute

- Nonreassuring fetal status mandating emergent delivery
- Nonvertex presentation
- Patient refusal/uncooperative patient
- Active maternal hepatitis C, human immunodeficiency virus, or transmissible blood infection
- Placenta previa
- Vasa previa
- Head not fully engaged in maternal pelvis (membranes may rupture when applying FSE; possibility of prolapsed cord)
- Inadequate cervical dilation to allow safe placement of FSE

Relative

- Untreated group B *Streptococcus* (GBS) infection
- Imminent delivery (relative)

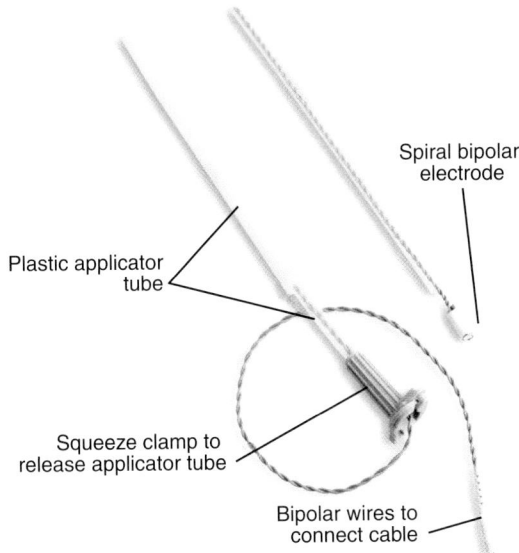

Fig. 149.1 Fetal scalp electrode with applicator tube. (Courtesy GE Healthcare, Waukesha, Wisconsin.)

Labels: Spiral bipolar electrode; Plastic applicator tube; Squeeze clamp to release applicator tube; Bipolar wires to connect cable

EQUIPMENT AND SUPPLIES

- Scalp electrode (FSE; Fig. 149.1)
- Fetal monitor
- Sterile gloves
- Connecting wires between FSE and electronic monitor
- Surgical lubricant or povidone-iodine solution

Scalp electrodes and fetal monitoring equipment are available on all labor units. Familiarity with locally available equipment is suggested.

PRECAUTIONS

- Vertex presentation
- Cervical dilation greater than 2 cm
- Ruptured membranes
- Head well engaged in maternal pelvis to decrease the risk of cord prolapse during FSE application

The fetal presentation, station, and position are determined from a sterile vaginal examination. If the placental location is unknown, bedside ultrasonography is helpful to rule out placenta previa and confirm vertex presentation. Rupturing the membranes (see Chapter 148, Amniotomy) makes applying an FSE easier, although it can be applied through the amniotic sac to create a slow leak of amniotic fluid. Rupturing membranes when the head is not fully engaged (i.e., "floating" in uterus) can result in cord prolapse. When meconium-stained fluid is encountered, fetal well-being should be closely assessed using continuous monitoring or a biophysical profile.

PREPROCEDURE PATIENT EDUCATION AND FORMS

Indications for FSE placement are discussed with the patient. Patient discomfort is generally minimal, and the procedure usually takes only a few minutes. Pain to the fetus is thought to be minimal. Showing the patient an FSE may help allay her concerns.

The patient lies in dorsal lithotomy position, and the FSE is placed after a cervical examination to confirm fetal presentation. Fundal pressure from an assistant is helpful to reduce the risk of cord prolapse. Most hospitals do not require patients to sign specific operative consents for this procedure; obtaining verbal informed consent from the patient is prudent.

TECHNIQUE

The following steps are performed when applying an FSE:

1. Read the package insert accompanying the FSE.
2. Put sterile gloves on both hands.
3. Confirm vertex presentation and assess for adequate cervical dilation (>2 cm).
4. Perform an amniotomy if membranes are intact and there are no contraindications (see Chapter 148, Amniotomy).
5. Ask an assistant to apply the adhesive pad (reference electrode) to the maternal thigh and connect the leads to the fetal electrocardiographic (ECG) monitor.
6. Holding the scalp electrode, free the tail wire to permit clockwise rotation of the electrode in the applicator tube.
7. Place the tip of applicator tube between the pads of the index and middle fingers of the hand used for vaginal examination.
8. Insert the fingers and applicator into the vagina and slide them toward the fetal vertex.
   NOTE: Be careful to avoid the fetal fontanelles. The electrode should not be placed on or near the anterior or posterior fontanelle.
9. Place the electrode against the fetal skull. Turn the outer portion of the FSE clockwise, approximately two times, until a "pop" is felt. Applying the electrode during a contraction or with fundal pressure from an assistant makes placement easier and decreases the risk of cord prolapse.
10. Ensure that the scalp electrode tip is well anchored by applying gentle, external/outward traction on the electrode applicator (which is still attached to the wires of the FSE). If the FSE holds in place with this maneuver, it is likely well anchored. If the FSE pulls loose with this maneuver, a second attempt should be made to implant the FSE nearby. Before attempting to reimplant, the FSE should be turned counterclockwise twice in the applicator (i.e., to untwist the wires). Then, while applying the FSE with slightly more pressure against the fetal skull than last time, a reassuring "pop" should be felt with two more clockwise turns of the tip. If the clinician is unable to anchor the electrode after a second attempt, the next attempt should be made using a new FSE.
11. Palpate the area around the scalp electrode to check that it is not applied to the maternal cervix or vaginal walls. Also ensure that it is not connected on or around the anterior or posterior fontanelle.
12. Unwind the wires from the clamp located on the exterior end of the scalp electrode.
13. Gently squeeze the clamp and allow the applicator to slide over the wires and out of the vagina. If the FSE pulls loose with this maneuver, it was not well anchored and should be removed. The next attempt should be made using a new FSE.
14. Have the assistant connect the red and green FSE wires to the cable that attaches to the fetal monitor.
15. Switch the fetal monitor setup from Doppler to ECG.
16. Review the ECG tracing for nonreassuring signs, including persistent tachycardia/bradycardia, decreased variability, or decelerations (discussed in Chapter 146, Antepartum Fetal Monitoring). If severe decelerations are noted, check for umbilical cord prolapse immediately. If cord prolapse is noted, the vertex should be pushed up into the uterus while an emergent cesarean delivery is arranged.
17. Consider whether placing an intrauterine pressure catheter is necessary (see Chapter 150, Intrauterine Pressure Catheter Insertion).

SAMPLE OPERATIVE REPORT

A formal note detailing the indications for FSE placement and specifics of the procedure should be documented in the chart.

Procedure: FSE placement for internal EFM
Indication: Inability to perform external monitoring due to (circle one):
    Maternal body habitus
    Maternal activity
    Fetal movement
    Poor external tracing
    Other: _____
Procedure: Risks, benefits, and alternative options were discussed with the patient/family. The patient provided informed consent and agreed to proceed. A sterile vaginal exam was performed demonstrating vertex presentation, cervical dilation of _____ cm, and a well-engaged fetal head. The membranes were/were not artificially ruptured. The FSE was applied to the fetal scalp, avoiding the fetal fontanelles. The patient and fetus tolerated the procedure well and a reassuring tracing was noted after FSE placement.

COMMON ERRORS

- Incorrect placement of the FSE onto maternal tissue
- Placement of the FSE close to the maternal cervix
- Entanglement of the FSE in fetal hair without fetal scalp attachment
- FSE attachment on or close to the fetal fontanelles
- Puncture injury to operator's finger from an extended bipolar wire

Scalp electrodes inadvertently attached to the maternal cervix or vagina do not provide an ECG tracing when connected to the monitor. FSEs placed close to the maternal cervix create pronounced vertical spikes on the tracing secondary to interference from "bumping" against the cervix. No ECG tracing is apparent if the electrode is tangled in the fetal hair. Scalp electrodes attached on or near a fontanelle or on locations other than the fetal scalp should be removed immediately. Keeping the electrode sheathed in the applicator until the fetal skull is palpated helps avoid an unintentional puncture injury to the person applying the FSE.

COMPLICATIONS

- Fetal scalp abscess (<0.1%), scalp trauma (1.2% vs. 0.9% without FSE).
- Meningitis, cerebrospinal fluid leak, or infection if an FSE is applied on a fontanelle.
- Cephalohematoma (1% vs. 0.9% without FSE), subgaleal hematoma, or subcutaneous scalp emphysema, especially if vacuum extraction is performed. The FSE should be removed before vacuum application. Depending on clinician experience, forceps may be preferred over vacuum-assisted delivery after FSE placement. A secondary analysis of data from the Consortium of Safe Labor study ($N = 171,698$), showed increased risk for scalp injury, subdural and cerebral hemorrhage, subgaleal hematoma, and cephalohematoma in deliveries with FSE use if vacuum assisted operative delivery was later performed.
- Fetal trauma if FSE is incorrectly placed or applied in nonvertex positions: ocular injury in face presentation; scrotal, labial, or buttock lacerations with breech presentation.
- Umbilical cord prolapse.
- Increased risk of neonatal GBS sepsis if intrapartum antibiotic treatment is not given to mothers with GBS infection.
- Puncture injury to the clinician applying the FSE.

POSTPROCEDURE MANAGEMENT AND PATIENT EDUCATION

Patients should be warned not to make sudden position changes or attempt to get out of bed without the hospital staff disconnecting the wire leads for the FSE. Internal monitoring generally limits patient mobility, although women may elect to sit in a rocking chair or on a birthing ball if close attention is paid to the wire leads.

REMOVING THE FETAL SCALP ELECTRODE

Indications

- Impending delivery (fetal head crowning)
- Application of vacuum-assisted device
- Cesarean delivery
- Inadvertent electrode placement on maternal tissue or nonscalp fetal parts
- Signal interference because of proximity of electrode to cervix

Technique

1. Remove the electrode when the fetal skull is visible between contractions with the head on the perineum or at the time that incorrect placement is noted.
2. Cut the wire leads with scissors approximately 2 inches from the perineum or from the FSE attachment to the fetal head.
3. Manually untwist the wires until they can be easily unwound.
4. The electrode tip spins counterclockwise and unscrews from the fetal scalp. This usually happens as the wires are being untwisted.
5. Electrodes occasionally become tangled in the fetal hair. In this situation, scissors are helpful for FSE removal.
6. During precipitous deliveries, cut the wire leads close to the perineum to prevent the electrode from catching and pulling on the fetal scalp. The electrode is easily removed after delivery.

CPT/BILLING CODES

A specific code does not exist for FSE placement.

59050	Fetal monitoring during labor by consulting physician (not attending physician) with written report; supervision and interpretation
59051	Fetal monitoring during labor by consulting physician (not attending physician) with written report; interpretation only

ICD-10-CM DIAGNOSTIC CODES

O68	Fetal distress, acid-base imbalance labor and delivery complicated
O36.519X	Maternal care for known/suspected placental insufficiency unspecified trimester
O41.90XX	Disorder amniotic fluid and membranes unspecified trimester (meconium-stained fluid antepartum)
O77.9	Fetal distress, not otherwise specified
O36.93XX	Maternal care unspecified fetal problem (umbilical cord prolapsed)
P02.29	Newborn affected by abnormality of placenta
P12.0	Cephalohematoma, because of birth injury
O77.8	Fetal distress, liveborn, during labor and delivery
O77.0	Labor and delivery complicated by meconium-stained amniotic fluid

SUPPLIERS

(See contact information available at www.expertconsult.com.)

Qwik Connect Plus fetal scalp electrodes and Abcorp belts
    Utah Medical Products, Inc.
    GE Medical

ONLINE RESOURCES

NICHD Definitions and Classifications: Applications to Electronic Fetal Monitoring Interpretation: https://www.nccwebsite.org/resources/docs/final_ncc_monograph_web-4-29-10.pdf

RECOMMENDED READING

Alfirevic Z, Devane D, Gyte G, et al. Continuous cardiotocography (CTG) as a form of electronic fetal monitoring for fetal assessment during labor. *Cochrane Database Syst Rev.* 2017:CD006066. pub 3.

Bloom SL, Belfort M, Saade G. What we have learned about intrapartum fetal monitoring trials in the MFMU network. *Semin Perinatol.* 2016;40:307–317.

Harper LM, Shanks AL, Tuuli M, et al. The risks and benefits of internal monitors in laboring patients. *Am J Obstet Gynecol.* 2013;209(38):e1–e6.

Katawuta T, Reddy UM, Landy HJ, et al. Neonatal complications associated with use of fetal scalp electrode: a retrospective study. *BJOG.* 2016;123:1797–1803.

Miller DM. Intrapartum fetal heart rate definitions and interpretation: evolving consensus. *Clin J Obstet Gynecol.* 2011;54(1):16–21.

Tuggy M, Garcia J. Procedures consult. Scalp lead placement. http://www.proceduresconsult.com/medical-procedures/scalp-lead-placement-FM-013-procedure.aspx.

CHAPTER 150

INTRAUTERINE PRESSURE CATHETER INSERTION

Beth A. Choby

The intrauterine pressure catheter (IUPC) permits direct intra-uterine monitoring of contraction strength and frequency when external tocodynamometry is ineffective. Approximately 20% of laboring patients in the United States are monitored using an IUPC, although a large randomized controlled trial of an inter-nal IUPC versus external tocodynamometry for labor monitoring showed no differences between operative delivery rates and fetal outcomes.

Although the routine use of an IUPC is not recommended, IUPC placement is appropriate for specific intrapartum indications. Maternal indications include excessive maternal movement or an elevated body mass index. IUPC use is also common with pro-tracted/dysfunctional labor or a trial of labor after a cesarean deliv-ery (TOLAC). When significant variable decelerations are present, IUPC placement allows for amnioinfusion.

Intrauterine pressure monitoring was first developed in the 1860s, using intrauterine balloons placed transabdominally to determine contraction strength. The current transcervical route for IUPC placement was developed in the late 1960s, when one clinical moni-toring unit became available that concurrently monitored fetal heart rate and contractions. Early IUPC technology determined intrauter-ine pressure using a column of water, although this was later replaced by an electronic microtip pressure sensor.

Today's IUPC technology uses either electronic pressure trans-ducer–tip catheters or air-coupled flexible balloon catheters. Both types graphically represent intrauterine pressure through mea-surements of the frequency, duration, and amplitude of contrac-tions. In women with arrest of labor, internal monitoring allows for an assessment of contraction strength with Montevideo units (MvUs). Montevideo units are calculated as the product of con-traction intensity multiplied by frequency (i.e., number of con-tractions in a 10-minute period multiplied by the mean amplitude of contractions during this time). During active labor, individual contraction amplitude ranges from 30 to 80 mm Hg; calculated Montevideo units between 180 and 220 are considered adequate. Historically a pattern of 200 MvUs for at least 2 hours during active labor has been used as a criterion for making the diagnosis of failure to progress. Some experts have proposed cutoffs for fail-ure to progress during the active phase of first-stage labor as 4 hours or more with uterine contractions greater than 200 MvUs; arrest is diagnosed after 6 or more hours if more than 200 MvUs cannot be sustained.

Whether women with a previously scarred uterus attempting TOLAC benefit from IUPC monitoring is uncertain. An elevated uterine resting tone or abnormalities in the contraction pattern may suggest uterine rupture, although the best predictor seems to be an abnormal fetal heart tracing (variable or late decelerations). Fetal indications for an IUPC include amniotic fluid sampling. Routine IUPC placement/prophylactic amnioinfusion to dilute meconium-stained amniotic fluid is not recommended (discussed in Chapter 151, Transcervical Amnioinfusion).

INDICATIONS

Eighty-five percent of patients in labor in the United States are man-aged using continuous fetal monitoring. Surveillance with external monitoring for fetal heart rate and contractions is most frequently used. When external monitoring is not possible, internal monitor-ing with a fetal scalp electrode and IUPC is sometimes necessary. Indications for an IUPC include the following:

- Inadequate contraction pattern
- Failure to progress/descend
- Arrest of labor
- TOLAC
- Ineffective external monitoring secondary to maternal motion or body habitus
  - Need for amnioinfusion
  - Amniotic fluid sampling
  - Oligohydramnios with variable decelerations

CONTRAINDICATIONS

Absolute

- Intact fetal membranes (absolute unless rupture acceptable; see Chapter 148, Amniotomy)
- Complete placenta previa

Relative

- Inadequately dilated cervix
- Partial placenta previa
- Vasa previa
- Uterine bleeding of undetermined etiology
- Nonreassuring fetal status
- Fetal anomalies (e.g., gastroschisis)

EQUIPMENT AND SUPPLIES

- Sterile gloves and equipment to follow universal blood and body fluid precautions
- Amniotomy hook if membranes are not ruptured
- Intrauterine pressure catheter (sterile; Fig. 150.1)
- Cable to join IUPC with fetal monitor (nonsterile)
- Fetal monitor
- Intravenous tubing, pole, and fluid if amnioinfusion is planned (see Chapter 151, Transcervical Amnioinfusion)

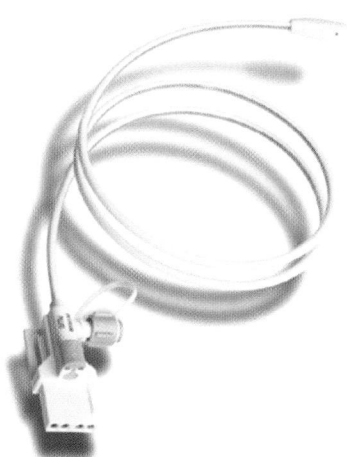

Fig. 150.1 Intrauterine pressure catheter. (Courtesy Utah Medical Products, Midvale, UT.)

PRECAUTIONS

• Assess fetal presentation to avoid traumatizing the fetus.
• Ascertain placental location to avoid traumatizing the placenta.

PREPROCEDURE PATIENT EDUCATION AND FORMS

Review the patient's medical record and progress in labor. If the placental location is unknown, bedside ultrasound can confirm whether a partial or complete placenta previa is present. Indications for IUPC placement and risks and benefits of the procedure are discussed with the patient to obtain informed consent.

The patient is placed in dorsal lithotomy position. A cervical examination is necessary to determine cervical dilation and fetal presentation. If the membranes are unruptured, artificial rupture, when indicated, may be performed during the cervical examination. IUPC placement is not usually painful, although some women experience mild discomfort during the procedure.

TECHNIQUE

1. Read the package insert to ensure familiarity with the equipment.
2. Ensure that all necessary supplies are present. Prepare a sterile field on the delivery bed or table.
3. Turn on the fetal monitor. Connect the interface cable (nonsterile) to the fetal monitor. Switch the fetal monitor from the external tocometer setting to the IUPC setting.
4. Open the IUPC package. Don sterile gloves. Remove the IUPC and plastic introducer (guide) from the package and observe the double hatch marks at 45 cm. Hand the end of the IUPC that connects to the interface cable to an assistant.
5. Establish a "0" baseline for the monitor as described by the manufacturer.
6. While observing universal blood and body fluid precautions, perform a sterile vaginal examination; assess cervical dilation and confirm that the membranes are ruptured. Place your index and third fingers posteriorly between the fetal vertex and cervix. Position the fingers away from the area above which the placenta is located.
7. Use the opposite hand to slide the IUPC/plastic introducer into the vagina over the palmar aspect of the intravaginal hand. Pass the catheter through the vagina and into the cervical os. Stop advancement of the IUPC/introducer when the tip of the IUPC rests between the fingers of the examining hand.
8. Hold the plastic introducer with the intracervical fingers and push the external (outside) part of the IUPC with the opposite hand to advance it through the introducer. The IUPC should pass the fetal vertex with minimal resistance and advance into the amniotic sac.
9. Stop advancing the IUPC when the double hatch marks (45 cm) reach the maternal introitus or when resistance is felt. IUPC advancement should proceed smoothly and without resistance. If resistance is encountered, change the direction of the catheter until insertion proceeds easily. Do not force the catheter because this increases the risk for placental, uterine, or fetal damage. IUPC insertion in an area remote from the placenta decreases the risk for iatrogenic abruption. The double hatch marks correlate with normal placement of the IUPC. Checking for a flash of amniotic fluid in the IUPC channel during insertion is recommended to guard against extramembranous placement.
10. Once the IUPC has been properly positioned, hold the external IUPC with the external hand. Remove the intravaginal hand and use it to "peel" the introducer away from the IUPC as the introducer is pulled out of the vagina. Take care not to dislodge the IUPC as the introducer is being removed.
11. Connect the distal end of the IUPC to the interface cable. Secure the IUPC to the patient's thigh using the belt or adhesive pad provided. Leave some slack between the introitus and the belt to prevent inadvertent IUPC expulsion with patient repositioning or movement. Proper IUPC placement is again confirmed by checking that the double hatch marks are at the introitus.
12. Confirm that connections between the IUPC and the reusable monitor cable and from the monitor cable to the monitor are all secure.
13. Have the patient cough or perform a Valsalva maneuver to check for proper IUPC functioning. Palpable contractions should correlate with increased intrauterine pressure on the monitor.
14. Write a brief procedural note in the chart. Chapter 151, Transcervical Amnioinfusion, provides more information for use of the IUPC when amnioinfusion is indicated.

REMOVAL OF THE INTRAUTERINE PRESSURE CATHETER

Removal of the IUPC is straightforward and usually performed before delivery. Apply traction to the IUPC between contractions. The IUPC should come out easily. If resistance is encountered, stop and redirect the catheter until it can be removed with minimal resistance.

SAMPLE OPERATIVE REPORT

See a sample operative report available at www.expertconsult.com.

COMMON ERRORS

• Extramembranous placement. This problem occurs when the IUPC is positioned between the uterine wall and the amniotic/chorionic membranes. Complications include placental perforation, uterine perforation, and abruptio placentae. Estimates of the frequency of incorrect IUPC placement range from 14% to 38% (Lind, 1999). Although uterine perforation following IUPC placement is often asymptomatic and likely underreported, several case reports of perforation necessitating emergent cesarean section are reported in the literature. If no uterine waveforms are seen after IUPC placement in the setting of a soft, nontender, contracting uterus, perforation should be considered. If vaginal bleeding or uterine hypertonicity/tachysystole is seen after IUPC placement, placental abruption should be suspected. The likelihood of intraamniotic placement increases if the clinician watches for a flash of amniotic fluid each time an IUPC is being inserted.

- Inability to thread the IUPC into the amniotic cavity. Redirect the IUPC tip and gently reintroduce. As the fetal head descends, placement becomes more challenging.
- The baseline tone on the uterine monitor is above zero. Rezero the IUPC using the slide switch on the base of the IUPC.
- No contraction pattern is evident after the IUPC is zeroed. Suspect extramembranous placement. Withdraw the IUPC and check for blood in the IUPC tip.

COMPLICATIONS

- Extramembranous (extraovular) placement of the IUPC
- Inaccurate pressure tracings
- Placental perforation
- Uterine perforation
- Fetal vessel laceration
- Fetal trauma
- Amnionitis or increased risk of maternal fever due to ascending infection from vaginal microbes with IUPC placement
- Disseminated intravascular coagulation and anaphylaxis (rare)
- Maternal cardiac failure secondary to amniotic fluid embolus (rare)

POSTPROCEDURE MANAGEMENT AND PATIENT EDUCATION

The fetal heart rate and the contraction pattern are monitored closely to ensure fetal and maternal well-being. Vaginal bleeding should be reported. Counsel the patient that mobility is limited with an IUPC. The patient can be disconnected from the monitor but should ask for assistance when she needs to get out of bed. Some providers prefer placing Foley catheters in women who have internal monitors.

CPT/BILLING CODES

Although there is no CPT code for IUPC insertion, labor that is postterm, augmented/induced, or complicated can be billed in addition to a routine delivery charge. Code this increased acuity of care using hospital evaluation and management codes. Obstetric care and delivery charges should be submitted in addition to these codes.

99356	Prolonged physician service in the inpatient setting, requiring direct (face-to-face) patient contact beyond the usual service first hour*
99357	Each additional 30 min*
99358	Prolonged evaluation and management service before and/or after direct (face-to-face) patient care (e.g., review of extensive records and tests, communication with other professionals and/or patient/family); not face-to-face care; first hour*
99359	Each additional 30 min*

*This is an add-on code and is designed to be used in addition to the E/M code.

ICD-10-CM DIAGNOSTIC CODES

O41.00X0	Oligohydramnios
O41.1090	Infection of amniotic cavity
O62.0	Abnormality of forces of labor
O63.9	Prolonged labor
O71.1	Rupture of uterus during labor
O28.9	Nonspecific abnormal findings in fluid surrounding fetus

SUPPLIERS

(See contact information available at www.expertconsult.com.)

Intran Plus IUP-400 (An electronic pressure transducer-tip catheter)
Utah Medical Products, Inc.
Koala IUPC (Air-coupled flexible balloon catheter)
Clinical Innovations, Inc.

ONLINE RESOURCES

Clinical Innovations. Koala: Essentials in IUP monitoring: https://player.vimeo.com/video/179257642.
Intran Plus intrauterine pressure catheters (Utah Medical Products): http://www.utahmed.com/intran.htm.

RECOMMENDED READING

Bakker JJ, Janssen PF, van Halem K, et al. Internal versus external tocodynamometry during induced or augmented labor. *Cochrane Database Syst Rev.* 2013;8:CD006947.
Bakker JJ, Verhoeven CJ, Janssen PF, et al. Outcomes after internal versus external tocodynamometry for monitoring labor. *N Engl J Med.* 2010;362(4):306–313.
Harbison L, Bell L. Anaphylactoid syndrome after intrauterine pressure catheter placement. *Obstet Gynecol.* 2010;115(2):407–408.
Hofmeyr G, Xu H, Eke AC. Amnioinfusion for meconium-stained liquor in labour. *Cochrane Database Syst Rev.* 2014;1:Art. No.: CD000014.
Lind B. Complications caused by extramembranous placement of intrauterine pressure catheters. *Am J Obstet Gynecol.* 1999;180:1034–1035.
Macones G, Cahill A, Pare E, et al. Obstetric outcomes in women with two prior cesarean deliveries: is vaginal birth after cesarean delivery a viable option? *Am J Obstet Gynecol.* 2005;192:1223–1229.
Rood KM. Complications associated with insertion of interuterine pressure catheters: an unusual case of uterine hypertonicity and uterine perforation resulting in fetal distress after insertion of an interauterine pressure cathether. *Case Rep Obstet Gynecol.* 2012:517461.
Wilmink FA, Wilms FF, Heydanus R, et al. Fetal complications after placement of an intrauterine pressure catheter: a report of two cases and review of the literature. *J Matern Fetal Neonatal Med.* 2008;21:880–883.

CHAPTER 151

TRANSCERVICAL AMNIOINFUSION

David G. Weismiller

Amnioinfusion is an inexpensive, minimally invasive, proven thera-peutic measure used since 1983 to restore or replace amniotic fluid during labor. During labor, amnioinfusion is indicated for the man-agement of variable or prolonged decelerations. This is performed by infusing normal saline or lactated Ringer's solution transcervically through a catheter. More recently, amniotomy has been increasingly used to prophylactically supplement amniotic fluid in pregnancies affected by preterm premature rupture of membranes, iatrogenic rup-ture of membranes after amniocentesis, or for severe oligohydram-nios in the late second and third trimesters. This chapter focuses on amnioinfusion during labor. In general amnioinfusion appears to pose little risk while offering considerable benefit in properly selected patients.

Severe, persistent, or prolonged variable decelerations increase the risk for both fetal distress and need for emergent operative deliv-ery or cesarean delivery. Artificially increasing the volume of the amniotic fluid theoretically protects the umbilical cord from com-pression, thus reducing the number and severity of variable decel-erations. Numerous randomized controlled trials provide supportive evidence for amnioinfusion for variable decelerations. Several ran-domized controlled trials have shown that the use of amnioinfusion for infants at risk of cord compression (e.g., repetitive variable decel-erations, especially in the presence of oligohydramnios or amniot-omy) decreases not only the occurrence of variable decelerations but also the rates of cesarean deliveries. A recent Cochrane review of amnioinfusion in pregnancies with chorioamnionitis found insuf-ficient evidence to fully evaluate its effectiveness or safety. One small trial demonstrated that intrauterine temperature decreases by 1°C when room-temperature saline is used (Tomlinson et al., 2012) Amnioinfusion is also associated with a reduction in postpartum endometritis in women at risk.

Previous randomized controlled trials had suggested that the pro-phylactic use of amnioinfusion for oligohydramnios in term preg-nancies might reduce the incidence of fetal distress and the need for a cesarean delivery. More recent studies show no advantage to prophylactic amnioinfusion as opposed to using amnioinfusion only when deceleration of the fetal heart rate occurs.

Amnioinfusion had historically been advocated for meconium-stained amniotic fluid in labor. Meconium passage occurs in three distinct situations: (1) as a physiologic or maturational event, (2) as a response to acute hypoxic events, and (3) as a response to chronic intrauterine hypoxia. Risk of meconium aspiration is greater in infants of mothers with thick meconium, particularly if this is asso-ciated with an episode of fetal hypoxia. In contrast, thin meconium is not associated with increased perinatal mortality or the incidence of meconium aspiration syndrome.

Although one Cochrane review suggests that amnioinfusion for meconium has benefit in perinatal outcomes only in settings where resources for perinatal surveillance are limited, current literature recommends against routine prophylactic amnioinfusion for the dilution of meconium-stained amniotic fluid. For women in labor who have thick meconium staining, amnioinfusion does not reduce the risk of moderate or severe meconium aspiration syndrome, peri-natal death, or other major maternal or neonatal disorders. Data are not available to determine whether amnioinfusion for decelerations of the fetal heart rate in the presence of meconium-stained amniotic fluid decreases meconium aspiration syndrome or other meconium-related morbidities.

Different protocols for amnioinfusion are available. All appear to be safe, easy to perform, and associated with few complications.

INDICATION

Repeated severe or prolonged variable fetal heart rate decelerations (e.g., lasting longer than the contraction) that are unresponsive to conventional therapy (e.g., left-sided labor, intravenous hydration, oxygen therapy) regardless of amniotic fluid meconium status are an indication for amnioinfusion.

EDITOR'S NOTE: Since variable decelerations are very common in labor, amnioinfusion might be a consideration in many pregnan-cies. In reality, experienced clinicians use amnioinfusion in certain selected situations. An example is the multiparous patient who is close to delivery with deep variables on fetal heart rate monitoring despite overall adequate reactivity. We have all nervously watched such a labor, fearing that these deep variables may exhaust the fetus. It is reassuring to have amnioinfusion available as a possible preven-tive measure. A similar situation may be seen with oligohydramnios or even borderline oligohydramnios. Often these infants endure a stormy labor with deep variables early in labor. Amnioinfusion may be an option in these situations. It will also be interesting to see how intra-abdominal and transcervical amnioinfusion will change practice in the case of severe oligohydramnios or preterm premature rupture of membranes in the late second and early third trimester.

CONTRAINDICATIONS

- Amnionitis
- Polyhydramnios
- Uterine hyperstimulation (tachysystole)
- Multiple gestation
- Known fetal anomaly
- Known uterine anomaly
- Severe fetal intolerance of labor
- Nonvertex presentation
- Fetal scalp pH less than 7.20
- Placental abruption or placenta previa (known or suspected)
- Patient refusal or uncooperative/unable to tolerate

EQUIPMENT

- Intrauterine pressure catheter (see Chapter 150, Intrauterine Pressure Catheter Insertion)
- Normal saline or lactated Ringer's solution at room temperature
- Fetal monitor

- Intravenous tubing
- Intravenous pump
- Fetal scalp electrode (recommended)
- Sterile gloves (for insertion of intrauterine pressure catheter [IUPC]) and equipment for universal blood and body fluid precautions
- Vaginal lubricant (for insertion)
- Fluid warmer (if the fluid is to be infused at a rate >15 mL/min)

PREPROCEDURE PATIENT PREPARATION

Before performing the procedure, discuss the risks and benefits with the patient and family. For severe repetitive or prolonged variable decelerations, amnioinfusion decreases the number of variable decelerations and cesarean deliveries and possibly the risk of postpartum endometritis. Describe alternative modes of intervention (if applicable) and obtain informed consent. Answer any questions that the patient or family may have.

TECHNIQUE

1. Perform a sterile vaginal examination to confirm cephalic presentation and that the membranes are ruptured (see Chapter 148, Amniotomy), determine cervical dilation, and exclude cord prolapse. Observe universal blood and body fluid precautions.
2. Place a fetal scalp electrode (recommended, not required; see Chapter 149, Fetal Scalp Electrode Application) or ensure adequate fetal monitoring.
3. Insert an intrauterine pressure catheter (see Chapter 150, Intrauterine Pressure Catheter Insertion) and document resting uterine tone. The resting tone should be below 15 mm Hg. Some studies have also used a pediatric feeding tube for fluid instillation.
4. Link room-temperature normal saline (or lactated Ringer's solution) to the intravenous tubing. Prime the tubing as would be done for intravenous use.
5. Attach the tubing to the infusion port of the IUPC (Fig. 151.1).
6. For patients with repetitive severe or prolonged variable decelerations,
   - Start the infusion with an initial bolus of 250 to 500 mL of fluid over 20 to 30 minutes.
   - Next, adjust the infusion rate according to the severity of decelerations. The usual infusion rate is 10 to 20 mL/min until either a total infusion of 600 to 800 mL is reached or variable decelerations improve or resolve if this occurs first. Another method begins with a 500-mL bolus of room-temperature fluid followed by a continuous infusion of 3 mL/min.
   - If variables resolve, continue the infusion for an additional 250 mL beyond the volume at which the decelerations improved.
   - Terminate the infusion if 800 to 1000 mL of saline fails to resolve decelerations. If decelerations do not resolve completely yet there is an increase in frequency and severity when amnioinfusion is discontinued, resumption of the infusion is reasonable.
7. If fluid is administered at a rate above 15 mL/min, warm the fluid to body temperature.
8. Monitor fetal heart rate and resting uterine tone continuously during the intervention; monitor intrauterine pressure using the same IUPC, a second one, or a double-lumen catheter.
9. After the initial bolus, it is very important to verify that fluid is flowing from the vagina so as to prevent volume overload.
10. Discontinue the infusion if uterine tone becomes persistently elevated or if the flow of fluid from the vagina stops. Allow the uterine pressure to equilibrate over 5 minutes and reassess resting uterine tone. Discontinue the infusion if the new resting tone remains greater than 15 mm Hg above the baseline resting tone or 30 mm Hg maximum.

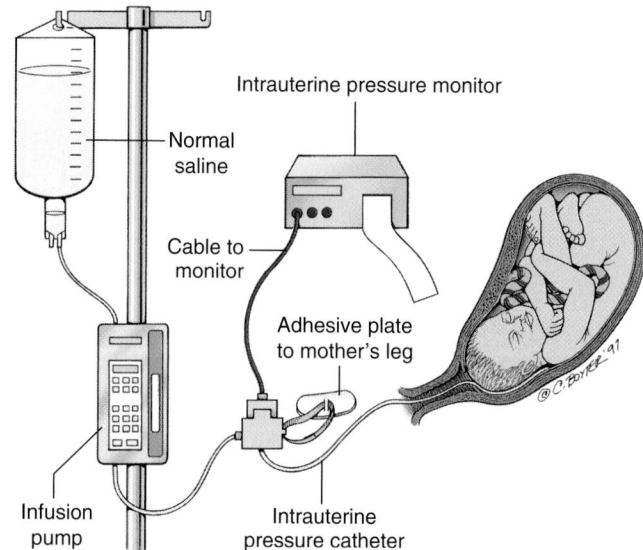

Fig. 151.1 **Procedure for amnioinfusion.** (From Weismiller DG. Transcervical amnioinfusion. *Am Fam Physician.* 1998;57:504–510.)

COMPLICATIONS

There are occasional amnioinfusion failures. Possible causes include an inadequate infusion rate or volume, rapid progression to the second stage of labor, and cord complications. However, the cause of the majority of failures is unknown.

In a teaching hospital survey intended to determine how, when, and with what results amnioinfusion is being performed in the United States, it was found that neither the method used nor the number of infusions performed appeared to significantly increase the risk for complications. The fact that the mean number of amnioinfusions performed per year is similar between centers that did and centers that did not report complications suggests that complications are generally infrequent or, perhaps, that the risk of complication decreases as clinician experience increases. (It might also indicate a reporting problem!)

- Isolated cases of umbilical cord prolapse have been reported, but they are well within the usual occurrence rate of prolapse in pregnancies with vertex presentation even when amnioinfusion is not used.
- Uterine tone may increase and hypertonus has been reported; monitoring intrauterine pressure, the total volume infused, and the continuous flow of fluid from the vagina is important. In one study, this was the most common complication.
- Abnormal fetal heart rate tracings were the second most common complication in one study.
- Prolonged fetal bradycardia has been reported after rapid administration (50 mL/min) of unwarmed fluid.
- Prophylactic amnioinfusion (although not recommended) was associated with increased intrapartum fever.
- Other reported rare complications
  - Uterine scar disruption (one reported case).
  - Iatrogenic polyhydramnios and elevated intrauterine pressure resulting in fetal bradycardia (one reported case).
  - Amniotic fluid embolism (AFE): one recent retrospective review showed a threefold higher risk of AFE with amnioinfusion (adjusted odds ratio 3.4 [1.6 to 7.6] $P < .001$), although these were still rare and based on case studies (Fong, 2014). Interestingly, fetal scalp electrode placement and IUPC placement were not associated with increased AFE risk.

- Rare complications associated with placement of an IUPC included
  - Uterine perforation
  - Umbilical cord trauma
  - Placental abruption
  - Fetal trauma
- Amnionitis is a possible complication. Prolonged use of an IUPC is also associated with an increased risk of amnionitis and perinatal infection.

NOTE: Most trials reviewed have been too small to address the possibility of rare but serious adverse maternal effects of amnioinfusion.

PATIENT EDUCATION GUIDES

See patient education and patient consent forms available at www.expertconsult.com.

CPT/BILLING CODES

59899   Unlisted procedure, maternity care and delivery

ICD-10-CM DIAGNOSTIC CODES

O68   Fetal distress, antepartum
O76   Abnormality in fetal heart rate or rhythm, antepartum
O69.2 XXX   Cord compression

RECOMMENDED READING

American College of Obstetricians and Gynecologists. *Amnioinfusion does not Prevent Meconium Aspiration Syndrome. Committee Opinion No. 346.* Washington, DC: American College of Obstetricians and Gynecologists; 2006.

Bullens LM, Heimel PJ, van der Hout-van der Jagt M, et al. Interventions for intrauterine resuscitation in suspected fetal distress during term labor: a systematic review. *Obstet Gynecol Survey.* 2015;70(8):524–539.

Dad N, Abushama M, Konje J, et al. What is the role of amnioinfusion in modern day obstetrics? *J Matern Fetal Neonat Med.* 2016;29(17):2823–2827.

Fong A, Chau C, Pan D, et al. Amniotic fluid embolism: antepartum, intrapartum and demographic factors. *J Mat Fetal Neo Med.* 2014;28(7):793–798.

Hofmeyr GJ, Eke AC, Lawrie TA. Amnioinfusion for third trimester preterm premature rupture of membranes. *Cochrane Database Syst Rev.* 2013;30(3):CD00942.

Hofmeyr GJ, Xu H, Eke AC. Amnioinfusion for meconium-stained liquor in labour. *Cochrane Database Syst Rev.* 2014;23(1):CD000014.

Hofmeyr GJ, Kiiza JA. Amnioinfusion for chorioamnionitis. *Cochrane Database Syst Rev.* 2016;24(8):CD011622.

CHAPTER 152

INTRATHECAL (SPINAL) ANALGESIA IN LABOR

Edward Anthony Yaghmour • Beth A. Choby

Intrathecal (spinal) analgesia involves injection of an opioid or a combination of an opioid and local anesthetic into the subarachnoid space. This space contains the cerebrospinal fluid (CSF). This technique provides better relief than intravenous opioids; intravenous opioids also cross the placenta and can affect fetal well-being. Pain relief with intrathecal injection is also more rapid than with epidural analgesia. Overall, intrathecal opioids permit profound analgesia without clinically significant motor or autonomic blockade. For vaginal deliveries, optimal intrathecal injection provides analgesia below the T10 dermatome.

Intrathecal fentanyl or sufentanil can be administered alone in early labor to provide significant or complete analgesia without a sympathectomy or motor blockade. This may be particularly useful in patients for whom a sudden decrease in preload (secondary to neuraxial local anesthetic–induced sympathectomy) might not be well tolerated (e.g., patient with a stenotic heart lesion).

Spinals, epidurals, and combined spinal-epidurals should be performed by individuals with adequate training and the ability to identify and manage complications that may arise. These individuals are often anesthesiologists, but certified registered nurse anesthetists or certified anesthesiologist assistants, family physicians, and other physicians with training and competence also perform these procedures, especially in rural or more remote areas of the world. Intrathecal analgesia is an option if epidural analgesia is unavailable (Box 152.1). Intrathecal analgesia may also be used in combination with epidural analgesia (combined spinal-epidural [CSE]).

Intrathecal analgesia is ideally suited for patients in the first stage of labor. Pain during the first stage of labor results from uterine contractions. This visceral pain is mediated by spinal nerves T10–L1, which innervate the myometrium. Pain during the second stage of labor is due to both uterine contractions and fetal descent and additional somatic pain from perineal stretching. Since pain during the second stage is mediated through the pudendal nerve (S2–S4), intrathecal analgesia is less effective; it does, however, continue to provide analgesia for the uterine contractions. The overall benefit for intrathecal analgesia is improved tolerance of contractions, possibly resulting in a more rested patient during the second stage of labor.

Because a single intrathecal analgesic injection has a limited duration of effect, an epidural or CSE remains the gold standard for labor analgesia.

ANATOMY

Intrathecal analgesia is produced when medications are injected directly into the subarachnoid space (CSF), just after penetrating the dura. Anatomy is identical to that for adult lumbar puncture and is described in detail in Chapter 221, Lumbar Puncture, as well as that for saddle block anesthesia, described in Chapter 155, Saddle Block Anesthesia.

INDICATIONS

- Active first stage of labor with anticipated vaginal delivery, used alone or in combination with epidural analgesia
- Epidural analgesia not available

CONTRAINDICATIONS

Absolute

- Medication allergy
- Patient refusal or uncooperative patient (unable to remain still)
- Maternal coagulopathy
- Use of anticoagulant therapy (e.g., heparin, warfarin, clopidogrel, direct thrombin inhibitor, factor Xa inhibitor); see SOAP Consensus Statement on the Anesthetic Management of Pregnant and Postpartum Women Receiving Thromboprophylaxis or Higher Dose Anticoagulants
- Refractory maternal hypotension
- Active infection at the planned injection site
- Increased intracranial pressure (except for idiopathic intracranial hypertension)
- Supratentorial mass lesion
- Untreated maternal bacteremia

Relative

- Spinal abnormalities that make the procedure technically difficult, such as marked scoliosis, prior spinal fusion in the area
- Treated active systemic infection, such as that resulting in maternal bacteremia
- Cutaneous lesion/skin abnormalities of the lower back, such as cellulitis or dermatitis

---

BOX 152.1 Advantages and Disadvantages of Intrathecal Opioids in Labor

Advantages
Superior analgesia compared with intravenous administration
No effect on expulsive forces in labor
Rapid onset of analgesia
Technique similar to lumbar puncture
Low incidence of serious side effects
Cost advantages compared with epidural anesthesia

Disadvantages
Analgesia generally inadequate for second stage of labor
No anesthesia for instrumented delivery or episiotomy
Does not provide surgical anesthesia
Risk of respiratory depression
High incidence of mild side effects
Tachyphylaxis with repeat injection; opioid ineffective for repeat dosing

---

TABLE 152.1	Duration and Onset of Action for Intrathecal Opioids		
Medication	**Dosage**	**Onset of Action (min)**	**Duration of Action (hr)**
Fentanyl	10–25 µg (usual dose 15 µg)	5	1.4–3.5
Sufentanil*	2.5 µg	5–10	1–3

*Although fetal outcomes were the same, bradycardia has been associated with higher doses of sufentanil; therefore, at Parkland Hospital, fentanyl or this dose of sufentanil is preferred.

See also Chapter 214, Emergency Department, Hospitalist, and Office Ultrasound [Clinical Ultrasound], and Chapter 221, Lumbar Puncture, for ultrasound-guided technique to use in individuals with difficult to palpate spinous processes such as those who are morbidly obese.

EQUIPMENT AND SUPPLIES

- Spinal anesthesia kit, which includes sterile preparation materials, local anesthetic, a 25-gauge or smaller atraumatic spinal anesthesia needle, and a 20-gauge introducer

NOTE: Pencil point spinal needles (Sprotte or Whitacre needles, with rounded or pencil-point, ends) decrease the risk of postdural puncture headache.

- Filter-tip needle for drawing up medications
- Opioid analgesic for injection (Table 152.1)
- Bupivacaine 0.25% to 0.5% anesthetic suitable for spinal injection, 1.25 mg to 2.5 mg
- IV ephedrine and IV phenylephrine
- Opioid antagonist (e.g., naltrexone 25 mg oral tablet or naloxone ampules 0.4 mg)
- Sterile gloves, mask, and surgical cap/bonnet
- Fenestrated drape for the skin at the level of L4
- Equipment to follow universal blood and body fluid precautions
- Equipment for continuous fetal monitoring (internal or external)
- Nurse/personnel to monitor vital signs and assess for side effects
- Pulse oximeter, blood pressure, and cardiac monitors

PRECAUTIONS

Spinals, epidurals, and CSEs should be performed by individuals with adequate training and the ability to identify and manage complications that may arise. In the absence of a medical contraindication, maternal request is a sufficient medical indication for pain relief during labor. Opioid-only intrathecal injection is not as effective for second stage labor pain. Therefore, a combination of opioid (visceral pain) and local anesthetic (somatic pain) should be used during the second stage of labor. Side effects including pruritus and nausea (associated with intrathecal opioids) may occur. Aseptic technique is critical to avoid introducing infection into the central nervous system.

PREPROCEDURE PATIENT PREPARATION

Prior to labor, provide counseling about options for analgesia and anesthesia. Informed consent should be obtained (see the sample patient consent form available at www.expertconsult.com). Address desired analgesia or anesthesia in the written birth plan. Staff providing prenatal education should be knowledgeable about analgesic options. An educational handout can be provided prior to the onset of labor (see the patient education form available at www.expertconsult.com). Analgesia/anesthesia during labor is optional, based on patient preference, and has certain risks.

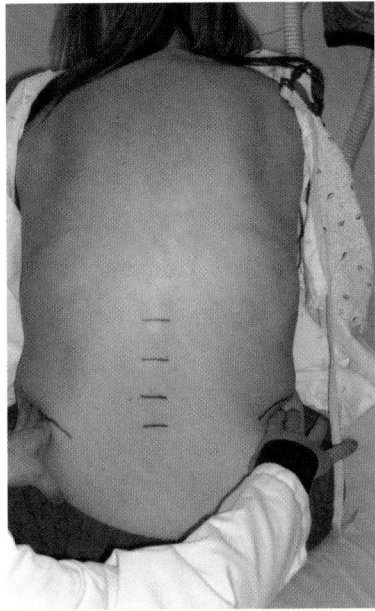

Fig. 152.1 To locate the L3–L4 or L4–L5 interspace, the iliac crests are palpated. The line between the crests intersects the L4 spinous process. The L3–L4 interspace is found slightly above (cephalic to) the L4 spinous process; the L4–L5 interspace is found below this.

Physiologic effects of severe pain during labor from increased circulating catecholamine levels cause tachycardia, increased cardiac output/myocardial workload and oxygen demand, and decreased gastric emptying. Excessive fatigue due to discomfort during labor may also affect the birth experience and the likelihood of successful spontaneuous vaginal delivery.

During labor, the clinician should again review the risks and benefits with the patient and obtain informed consent. An interval history and physical should be performed and recorded. Historically, because labor pain was feared to impair a patient's ability to adequately provide informed consent, prelabor counseling about pain control was considered best. A recent nonrandomized trial found no difference in recall between parturients who received information on neuraxial analgesia (epidural, intrathecal, or CSE), whether they were in pain or pain-free at the time of counseling; women in pain were actually found to have greater satisfaction with the informed consent process.

TECHNIQUE

1. Ensure continuous fetal monitoring is in place and verify that there are no contraindications to intrathecal analgesia.
2. Obtain informed consent and perform time out to confirm correct patient and procedure.
3. Establish intravenous access. A co-load of crystalloid (e.g., 500 mL) is recommended to help prevent the side effect of maternal hypotension (give this bolus very slowly for women with hypertensive disorders of pregnancy).
4. Have the patient assume either a seated forward leaning or left or right lateral decubitus position. Identify the spinous processes and vertebral interspaces. An imaginary line between the upper borders of the iliac crests approximates the level of L4 and the L4–L5 interspace. Locate the L4–L5 interspace (Fig. 152-1).
5. Using sterile technique, prep the skin at the selected interspace in addition to one space above and one below. Drape the patient using the fenestrated drape.
6. Draw up 3 mL of 1% lidocaine into the syringe with the 20- to 22-gauge needle. Use a 25-gauge skin needle to raise a wheal

TABLE 152.2   Side Effects and Their Management for Intrathecal Analgesia in Labor

Side Effects	Incidence (%)	Treatment
Pruritus (usually mild)*	≥50	Nalbuphine 2.5–5 mg IV or naloxone (Narcan) 0.2–0.4 mg IV
Nausea and vomiting	30–50	Ondansetron 4–8 mg IV or 4–8 mg disintegrating tablet; Decadron 4–8 mg IV
Urinary retention	4–20	In-and-out catheterization as necessary
Postdural puncture headaches	1–6	Epidural blood patch if not resolved with conservative management (rest, fluids, analgesics, caffeine)
Maternal hypotension	Up to 15	Generally transient. If systolic blood pressure <90 mm Hg or any nonreassuring fetal heart rate tracing, use IV fluid bolus, uterine displacement, and ephedrine (5–10 mg IV push) or phenylephrine 100–200 μg IV. Repeat every 5 min as necessary.
Respiratory depression	0.2–0.4	Naloxone (Narcan) 0.2–0.4 mg IV. Consider oxygen with decreased SaO_2

IM, Intramuscular; *IV*, intravenous.
*Not related to histamine release.

over the L4–L5 interspace. Inject a small amount deeper into the posterior spinous region along the tract that the spinal needle will follow.

7. Prepare the local anesthetic and adjunct for subarachnoid injection. From the kit, draw up bupivacaine 0.25% or 0.5% (1.25 to 2.5 mg) using the filter tip needle. Use of a filter tip needle prevents drawing up tiny glass particles into the syringe. Ensure that the bupivacaine is suitable for spinal anesthesia. Compared to using an opioid alone, bupivacaine shortens time of analgesia onset and increases the duration of effect. It also reduces the incidence of pruritus. This combination of medications permits rapid and prolonged analgesia after intrathecal injection.

8. Draw up the selected rapid-onset opioid adjunct (fentanyl or sufentanil) into syringe using the filter tip needle. Options include preservative-free fentanyl 15-25 μg (0.3 to 0.5 mL) or sufentanil 2.5 μg.

9. Insert the introducer needle where the skin infiltration was done. Use of an introducer, especially in patients with an elevated body mass index, improves the ability to direct the spinal needle. Spinal needles used for this procedure are thinner and less rigid than those for lumbar puncture. Narrower gauge, atraumatic needles have an advantage of reducing postdural puncture headache incidence to around 1%.

10. Insert a narrow-gauge (25 to 27 gauge), pencil-point spinal needle with stylette through the introducer through the posterior layers of the subarachnoid space. (The distinct pop or snap when passing through the ligamentum flavum tends to be less pronounced with atraumatic needles.) Whereas minimal or no fluid return is noted when passing through the epidural space, once the intrathecal space has been entered, CSF return is seen (similar to a lumbar puncture). Remove the stylette from the spinal needle and confirm that CSF flows from the hub of the needle.

11. Attach the syringe with the bupivacaine-opioid combination to the spinal needle. Aspirate a small amount (e.g., 0.25 to 0.5 mL) of CSF into the syringe (a swirl will be noted), which mixes with the medications in the syringe and confirms free CSF flow. Slowly inject the syringe contents back through the needle over 5 to 10 seconds. To guard against intravascular administration, aspirate to confirm CSF flow at the beginning and middle of medication administration. Take care to perform aspiration and injection between contractions.

12. Remove the spinal needle, introducer, and syringe as a unit from the patient's back. Position the patient on either her left or right side to prevent aortocaval compression. Monitor pulse and blood pressure every 5 minutes for 15 minutes.

13. If maternal hypotension develops (3% of cases), it usually occurs soon after medication administration (Gizzo, et al, 2014). The primary mechanism involves decreased cardiac output caused by decreased preload from venous pooling. Risk factors include obesity, hypovolemia, and age over 40 years. Hypotension should be treated with another IV fluid bolus and ephedrine 5 to 10 mg IV and/or phenylephrine 100 to 200 μg IV. Repeat dosing every 5 minutes may be necessary.

14. If pain relief diminishes before delivery, options include:
    - A supplemental intravenous opioid injection may be given. However, it is important to titrate the dose to avoid the side effect of respiratory depression.
    - Epidural analgesia can be administered.
    - CSE, in which an epidural catheter is placed at the time of the intrathecal injection for later use if operative delivery is necessary or if added pain relief is desired.

SAMPLE OPERATIVE REPORT

See a sample operative report available at www.expertconsult.com.

COMMON ERRORS

- Incorrect dosing of medications: Be certain that medications are properly labeled and dosages are verified.
- Failure to monitor patient. Risk of respiratory depression is higher in patients with intrathecal analgesia who have also received intravenous opioids for pain.
- Insufficient pain relief: Intrathecal injection works well in many instances, but is not effective in all patients. Alternative forms of analgesia may be required. If multiple routes of analgesic administration are used, monitor closely for deleterious reactions, especially respiratory depression.

COMPLICATIONS

Although serious complications with intrathecal analgesia are uncommon, the incidence of less severe side effects is relatively high (Table 152.2). Pruritus, although common, is usually not severe. About one-third of patients request treatment for pruritus. Nalbuphine (Nubain) is an opioid agonist–antagonist that can be used for pruritus. Nausea and vomiting are treated symptomatically. For postdural puncture headache, oral or IV caffeine, autologous blood patch, or intravenous fluids may be helpful. See Chapter 221, Lumbar Puncture, for these treatments.

There are no adverse fetal outcomes expected from this procedure. Transient fetal heart rate decelerations occur 10% of the time. Fetal heart rate monitoring is recommended according to institutional protocols. Intrathecal analgesia is not thought to impact duration of labor.

POSTPROCEDURE MANAGEMENT

Vital signs (respiratory rate, heart rate, and blood pressure) are monitored every 30 minutes for the duration of labor. Continued postpartum monitoring is required until the anesthestetic effect ceases. Nursing staff should assess sedation level and arousability (Table 152.3).

If moderate or somnolent sedation is noted by nursing staff, the clinician should be notified and the patient's oxygen saturation

TABLE 152.3	Sedation Scale to Monitor for Respiratory Depression from Intrathecal Opioids
Sedation Level	**Assessment**
None	Awake and alert
Minimal	Drowsy or sleeping but easily aroused
Moderate	Drowsy or sleeping but not easily arousable
Somnolent	Drowsy or sleeping and cannot be fully aroused

(SaO_2) checked. Use naloxone for treatment of respiratory depression at doses of 0.2 to 0.4 mg IV. This can be repeated every 3 minutes until respiratory depression or sedation is reversed. Administer oxygen if the oxygen saturation is diminished. Naloxone can also be given as a continuous IV infusion at 0.4 mg/hr if needed. Although the exact mechanism is unknown, respiratory depression may be caused by ascending spread of the analgesic agent. In theory, if the opioid spreads too far cephalad, it can suppress the respiratory centers in the fourth ventricle of the brain. The time of highest risk for the mother is after delivery, when respiratory drive may be decreased. Unfortunately, this is also a time when mothers are monitored less frequently. Some protocols call for postpartum continuous pulse oximetry or frequent reassessments of vital signs and mental status.

PATIENT EDUCATION GUIDES

See examples of patient education and consent forms available at www.expertconsult.com.

CPT/BILLING CODES

62273   Injection, lumbar epidural, of blood or clot patch
62322   Injection(s), of diagnostic or therapeutic substance(s) (including anesthetic, antispasmodic, opioid, steroid, other solution), not including neurolytic substances, including needle or catheter placement, includes contrast for localization when performed, epidural or subarachnoid; lumbar or sacral (caudal)

ICD-10-CM DIAGNOSTIC CODES

Z33.1   Pregnant state, not otherwise specified
O80   Normal delivery

The seventh digit (X) is added to identify the fetus in multiple gestations (use "0" for one fetus).

0	Not applicable or unspecified (single)
1-5	Fetuses 1–5
9	Other fetus
O60.10XX	Premature labor with delivery (<37 weeks)
O75.9	Other specified condition of labor (pain)
O64.1XX	Breech presentation
O66.2	Unusually large fetus causing disproportion

Codes Related to Deliveries With Forceps or Vacuum

O63.0	Prolonged first stage of labor
O63.1	Prolonged second stage of labor
O76	Abnormality in fetal heart rate or rhythm or fetal distress

Acknowledgment

The editors recognize the contributions of Thomas Howard, MD, and Renae Rasmussen, MD, to this chapter in previous editions of this text.

SUPPLIERS

(See contact information available at www.expertconsult.com.)

Disposable trays, needles
 B. Braun Medical, Inc.
 Baxter Healthcare Corporation
 Becton, Dickinson and Co.
 Rusch Inc. (Teleflex)
 Smiths Medical USA
Epidural and intrathecal block needles
 Kendall Company (Covidien)

RECOMMENDED READING

American College of Obstetricians and Gynecologists. Obstetric analgesia and anesthesia. Practice bulletin 177. *Obstet Gynecol.* 2017;129(4):e73–e89.

American College of Obstetricians and Gynecologists Committee on Obstetric Practice. Optimal goals for anesthesia care in obstetrics. ACOG committee opinion no. 433. *Obstet Gynecol.* 2009;113:1197–1199.

American Society of Anesthesiologists Practice Guidelines for Obstetric Anesthesia. An updated report by the American Society of Anesthesiologists Task Force on Obstetric Anesthesia and the Society for Obstetric Anesthesia and Perinatology. *Anesthesia.* 2016;124:270–300.

Burkle CM, Olsen DA, Sviggum HP, et al. Parturient recall of neuraxial analgesia risks: impact of labor pain vs no labor pain. *J Clin Anesthesia.* 2017;36:158–163.

Chapter 25. In: Cunningham G, Leveno KJ, Bloom SL, eds. *Williams' Obstetrics.* 24th ed. Obstetric Anesthesia and Analgesia; 2010.

El-Wahab N, Robinson N. Analgesia and anaesthesia in labour. *Obstet Gynecol Reprod Med.* 2011;21(5):137–141.

Gizzo S, Noventa M, Fagherazzi S, et al. Update on best available options in obstetrics anaestesia: perinatal outcomes, side effects and maternal satisfaction. Fifteen years systematic literature review. *Arch Gynecol Obstet.* 2014;290:21–34.

Hoefnagel A, Yu A, Kaminski A. Anesthetic complications in pregnancy. *Crit Care Clin.* 2016;38:1–28.

Minty RB, Kelly L, Minty A, et al. Single-dose intrathecal analgesia to control labour pain. *Can Fam Physician.* 2007;53:437–442.

Nag DS, Samaddar DP, Chatterjee A, et al. Vasopressors in obstetric anesthesia: a current perspective. *World J Clin Cases.* 2015;3(1):58–64.

Novikova N, Cluver C. Local anaesthetic nerve block for pain management in labour. *Cochrane Database Syst Rev.* 2012;(4):Art. No.: CD009200.

Schrock SD, Harraway-Smith C. Labor analgesia. *Am Fam Physician.* 2012;85(5):447–454.

Simmons SW, Taghizadeh N, Dennis AT, et al. Combined spinal-epidural versus epidural analgesia in labour. *Cochrane Database Syst Rev.* 2012;(10): Art. No.: CD003401.

Wong CA. Epidural and spinal analgesia/ anesthesia for labor and vaginal delivery. In: Chestnut DH, ed. *Chestnut's Obstetric Anesthesia: Principles and Practice.* 5th ed. Philadelphia: Elsevier; 2014:457–517.

CHAPTER 153

PARACERVICAL BLOCK

Scott T. Henderson

A paracervical block anesthetizes the paracervical (Frankenhäuser) ganglion. By injecting local anesthetic into the vaginal fornix submucosally (i.e., cervicovaginal junction), anesthesia during the first stage of labor can be attained. Although a paracervical block may provide adequate pain relief during the first stage, the pudendal nerves are not blocked. Additional anesthesia may be required for delivery, such as a pudendal block, because a paracervical block does not block sensory fibers from the lower vagina, vulva, or perineum. Preferred anesthetics used with paracervical block are also fairly short acting, so the procedure may need to be repeated during labor. This procedure is rarely used in the United States anymore (5% of deliveries in 1981, 2% to 3% of deliveries in 2001) because of the availability of other techniques for regional (neuraxial) analgesia and concerns about postparacervical block fetal bradycardia. However, there are situations where regional anesthesia is contraindicated, not available, or the patient may not want it, and paracervical block might be very helpful. Paracervical block is more popular in Scandinavia and was used with 17% of deliveries in Finland in 2005. One study has shown it may be more helpful in nulliparous than parous women, possibly because it does not provide adequate analgesia for the rapid descent of the presenting part in parous women. A 2012 Cochrane review found paracervical block to be more effective than intramuscular meperidine and that there was no difference in efficacy between the local anesthetics. Paracervical blocks are also often used for anesthesia for other procedures involving the cervix (e.g., hysteroscopy, cryosurgery, ablation, conization, loop electrosurgical excision procedure, pregnancy termination, dilation, and curettage). A 2013 Cochrane review found that women had significantly less pain during cervical dilation and uterine intervention with paracervical block compared with placebo injections, but concluded that clinically this may be unimportant.

ANATOMY

During the first stage of labor, pain is due to increased intrauterine pressure and cervical dilation. Pain arises from the visceral sensory nerve fibers of the uterus, cervix, and upper vagina. These pass through the paracervical ganglion to the hypogastric and then the preaortic plexuses, later entering the spinal cord at T10–T12 and L1. These same fibers are activated during cervical procedures in nongravid patients.

INDICATIONS

- First stage of labor
- Cervical ablation or conization procedures
- Dilation and curettage
- Possibly with endometrial biopsy, intrauterine device insertion, or hysteroscopy

CONTRAINDICATIONS

Absolute

- Uteroplacental insufficiency
- Preexisting fetal intolerance of labor

- Nonreassuring fetal heart tracing
- Imminent delivery
- Allergy to anesthetic agent
- Presence of local infection

Relative

- Known coagulopathy or anticoagulant therapy (e.g., heparin or its analogs, factor Xa inhibitor, thrombin inhibitor, warfarin, clopidogrel)

EQUIPMENT AND SUPPLIES

Prepackaged paracervical/pudendal block trays are available.

- 10-mL syringe (ideally with finger rings; otherwise a plain syringe may be used)
- Iowa trumpet with a 6-inch, 20-gauge needle (a must during labor); or a 3-inch needle extender on the end of a syringe with a 1.5-inch, 22-gauge needle
- Anesthesia
  - Gravid: lidocaine (Xylocaine or generic) 1% (10 mg/mL) without epinephrine, or chloroprocaine (Nesacaine or generic) 1% (10 mg/mL). (Note with lidocaine that toxicity may occur with doses greater than 1 mg/kg [70 mg or 7 mL in a 70-kg patient].) With lidocaine or chloroprocaine, toxicity may result from rapid absorption or if inadvertent intravascular administration occurs. The maximum lidocaine dosage should not exceed 4.5 mg/kg or a maximum of 30 mL of a 1% solution (300 mg); maximum dose should not be repeated in less than 2 hours. With chloroprocaine, the maximum recommended dose is 120 mg; it should not be repeated in less than 1 hour.
  - Nongravid: 1% lidocaine or 2% chloroprocaine can be used, with maximum recommended dose of 300 mg lidocaine or 120 mg chloroprocaine.
  - Gravid or nongravid: bupivacaine (Marcaine or generic) is contraindicated because of an increased risk of cardiotoxicity in healthy adults and risk of fetal bradycardia.
- Sterile gloves
- Antibacterial solution and sterile gauze pads
- Sterile ring forceps
- Sterile speculum
- Sterile tenaculum for nongravid cervix
- Fetal heart monitor (for gravid patient)

PREPROCEDURE PATIENT EDUCATION

Obtain informed consent and outline the possible complications, risks, benefits, and alternatives to anesthesia. (See the sample patient education and patient consent forms available at www.expertconsult.com.)

TECHNIQUE

1. Place the patient in the lithotomy position. (The modified lithotomy position [uterus displaced leftward] should be used for late trimester pregnancy. This can be accomplished by placing a folded pillow beneath the patient's right buttock.) Observe universal blood and body fluid precautions during this procedure. Some clinicians establish intravenous access prior to paracervical block.

2. In the gravid patient, assess the cervix and proceed if dilation is 5 to 8 cm. If the cervix is dilated greater than 7 or 8 cm, proceed with caution to avoid injecting the fetal scalp.

3. Prior to the procedure, swab the injection sites in the vaginal fornix with antibacterial solution–soaked sterile gauze pads, held in ring forceps. For a conization procedure, the entire perineal area may be prepped with an antibacterial solution, as for gynecologic surgery. The injection sites in the fornix are then swabbed with antibacterial solution–soaked sterile gauze pads held in a ring forceps.

4. Using your sterile-gloved, lubricated index and middle fingers as a guide, lay the trumpet against them and insert it into the vagina (Fig. 153.1). Use your right hand to guide the trumpet on the right side of the pelvis (patient's left side), and your left hand to guide on the left side of pelvis (patient's right side). In a nongravid cervix, paracervical block is usually performed under direct visualization, using the sterile speculum and a tenaculum placed on the anterior lip of the cervix (Fig. 153.2).

5. Place the 20-gauge needle within the trumpet (or 1.5-inch needle on an extender) through the mucosa at the cervicovaginal junction at the 4 o'clock position. Take care not to inject yourself. Avoid inserting the needle deeper than 0.4 cm into the tissue (see Fig. 153.1). Note that in the nongravid cervix and in early labor, the nerves are located at the 4 and 8 o'clock positions, respectively (see Fig. 153.2). As labor progresses, the position of the paracervical nerves migrates anteriorly with progressive cervical dilation (closer to the 3 and 9 o'clock positions, where the cervical vessels are also found).

6. To avoid intravascular injection, gently pull back on the plunger to make sure you do not aspirate blood. Inject 5 to 10 mL of the chosen local anesthetic for the gravid patient. (Alternatively, 2 to 3 mL may be placed in two or three locations around the probable location of the nerve.) After aspirating for blood in the nongravid patient, some clinicians inject at four locations (2, 4, 8, and 10 o'clock positions).

7. For the gravid patient, monitor the fetal heart rate for approximately 3 to 5 minutes after the first injection. If the tracing is reassuring (e.g., no bradycardia), inject on the contralateral side at the 8 o'clock position. Then, monitor the fetal heart rate for 20 to 30 minutes, along with maternal blood pressure and pulse. In the nongravid patient, if there no untoward reaction noted with the first injection, some proceed with the opposite side injection without waiting.

COMMON ERROR

Failure to inject at proper locations, and therefore not gaining maximum effect, is the most common error.

COMPLICATIONS

- Intrafetal injection
- Postparacervical block fetal bradycardia. The historic paracervical block method of deep injection and high-dose anesthetic were associated with serious adverse effects in fetuses and high rates of postparacervical block bradycardia. Reported in 10% to 20% of blocks, bradycardia usually occurred within 10 minutes and could last up to 30 minutes. More recent studies of the more superficial injection method and use of milder anesthetic solutions suggest a lower risk. Four Scandinavian trials (>200 patients each) using superficial injection technique found a postparacervical block bradycardia frequency of 2.2% (Volmanen, 2011). Most studies report only a small to moderate decrease in fetal heart rate of short duration (<10 minutes). Some investigators suggest that the fetal bradycardia associated with this procedure is not a sign of fetal asphyxia because it is almost always transient and the infants are usually vigorous at birth. Whether anesthetic injection causes uterine artery spasm or changes in umbilical blood flow is controversial. Paracervical block is not thought to harm maternal or fetal oxygen saturation, neonatal arterial pH, or neonatal behavior. However, there have been occasional reports of profound bradycardia, low fetal scalp pH, depressed Apgar scores, and other adverse outcomes, including fetal demise.
- Subgluteal, paracervical, parametrial, or retropsoas hematoma or infection
- Neuropathy resulting from hematoma formation or direct sacral plexus trauma
- Cardiotoxicity or neurotoxicity resulting from intravascular injection

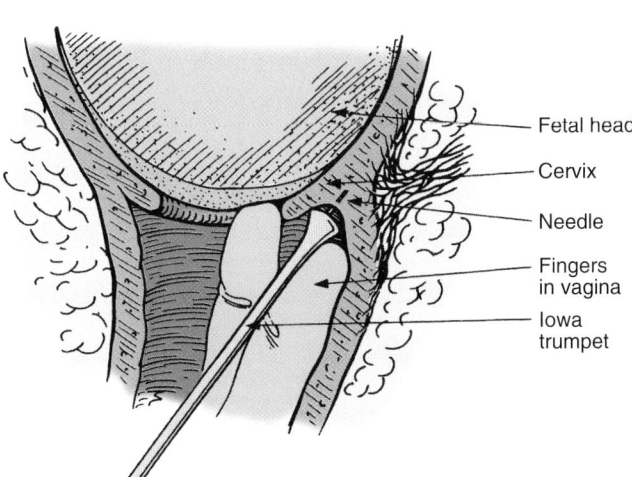

Fig. 153.1 Administering a paracervical block during labor using an Iowa trumpet.

Fetal head
Cervix
Needle
Fingers in vagina
Iowa trumpet

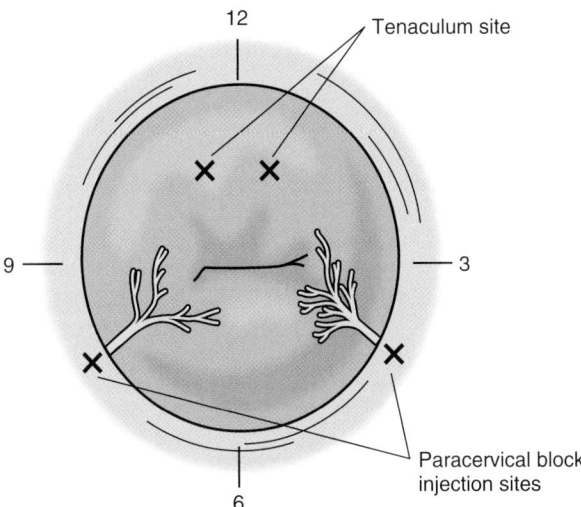

Fig. 153.2 Paracervical block location in nongravid or early-labor patient and where to place the tenaculum in the nongravid cervix.

12
Tenaculum site
9
3
6
Paracervical block injection sites

- Allergic reactions (rare)
- Vasovagal syncope
- Laceration of vaginal mucosa

POSTPROCEDURE MANAGEMENT

Continue to monitor the fetal heart rate after placing the block. It may be necessary to repeat the entire procedure, depending on the duration of activity of the anesthetic agent. A good response is generally maintained for 45 to 75 minutes. However, the effect may last only 30 minutes, or it can last as long as 90 minutes.

The patient should be advised to report any signs or symptoms suggesting postprocedural complications. The patient should report any fever, areas of numbness, vaginal bleeding, or abdominal, vaginal, or pelvic pain in the weeks following the procedure. Although the potential for complications such as paravaginal hematoma or infection exists, no cases have been reported in the literature (Volmanen, 2011).

PATIENT EDUCATION GUIDES

See patient education and patient consent forms available at www.expertconsult.com.

CPT/BILLING CODES

64435   Injection, anesthetic agent; paracervical (uterine) nerve

ICD-10-CM DIAGNOSTIC CODES

See the Diagnostic Codes sections in Chapters 113, Pregnancy Termination: First-Trimester Suction Aspiration; 162, Dilation and Curettage; 129, Endometrial Biopsy; 135, Intrauterine Device Insertion; 127, Loop Electrosurgical Excision Procedure for Treating Cervical Intraepithelial Neoplasia; and 156, Vaginal Delivery.

EDITOR'S NOTE: Colposcopy does not generally require a paracervical block, although the rest of the cervical procedures listed here do.

ONLINE RESOURCES

Military Obstetrics and Gynecology: Paracervical Block: http://www.brooksidepress.org/Products/Military_OBGYN/Textbook/LaborandDelivery/Anesthesia/paracervical_block.htm#.

RECOMMENDED READING

Althaus J, Wax J. Analgesia and anesthesia in labor. *Obstet Gynecol Clin North Am.* 2005;32:231–244.

Chestnut DH. Alternative regional analgesic techniques for labor and vaginal delivery. In: Chestnut DH, ed. *Chestnut's Obstetric Anesthesia: Principles and Practice.* 5th ed. Philadelphia: Saunders Elsevier; 2014:518–529.

Jagerhorn M. Paracervical block in obstetrics. An improved injection method. A clinical and radiological study. *Acta Obstet Gynecol Scand.* 1975;54:9–27.

Junttila EK, Karialainen PK, Ohtonnen PP, et al. A comparision of paracervical block with single-shot spinal for labour analgesia in multiparous women: a randomised controlled trial. *Int J Obstet Anesth.* 2009;18(1):15–21.

Novikova N, Cluver C. Local anaesthetic nerve block for pain management in labour. *Cochrane Database Syst Rev.* 2012;18(4):CD009200.

Renner R, Edelman AB, Nichols MD, et al. Refining paracervical block techniques for pain control in first trimester surgical abortion: a randomized controlled noninferiority trial. *Contraception.* 2016;94(5):461–466.

Tangsiriwatthana T, Sangkomkamhang US, Lumbiganon P, Laopaiboon M. Paracervical local anesthesia for cervical dilation and uterine interventions. *Cochrane Database Syst Rev.* 2013;9:CD005056.

Volmanen P, Palomaki O, Ahonen J. Alternatives to neuraxial analgesia for labor. *Curr Opin Anesthesiol.* 2011;24:235–241.

CHAPTER 154

PUDENDAL ANESTHESIA

John J. Andazola • Dolores M. Gomez

Pudendal nerve anesthesia is a common nerve block technique used in obstetrics and minor gynecologic surgery. Its advantages include its safety, ease of administration, and rapidity of onset. Pudendal nerve block can be used to provide analgesia during the second stage of labor and to facilitate pelvic floor relaxation when using outlet forceps or vacuum extraction. It also provides anesthesia for the perineum in order to create or repair an episiotomy. Pudendal nerve anesthesia can be used for minor surgery of the lower vagina and perineum. While largely supplanted by epidural anesthesia, pudendal blocks are an alternative when neuraxial blockade is not feasible, not effective, contraindicated, or declined by the patient. Although both transperineal and transvaginal approaches for pudendal blockade are options, the transvaginal approach is more practical and most often used. Therefore only the transvaginal approach is discussed here.

ANATOMY

The pudendal nerve supplies both sensory and motor innervation to the perineum. It is composed of parts of the second, third, and fourth sacral nerves, and has three branches. In a woman, these branches supply the following structures:

1. The dorsal nerve of the clitoris, which innervates the clitoris and its erectile tissues
2. The perineal nerve, which innervates the muscles of the perineum and the skin of the labia minora, labia majora, and vestibule
3. The inferior hemorrhoidal nerve, which innervates the external sphincter of the anus and perianal skin (responsible for the anal "wink" reflex)

Pudendal anesthesia attempts to block the nerve as it enters the lesser sciatic foramen, usually inferior and medial to the insertion of the sacrospinous ligament on the ischial spine. The pudendal vessels lie lateral to the nerve at this location, so care must be taken to avoid intravascular injection. Although total block of the pudendal nerve should abolish pain and sensation over this entire area, other nerves may also supply sensory innervation to the perineum. Thus "skip" areas of analgesia may be noted, and nerve blockade can be ineffective on one or both sides as frequently as 50% of the time.

While being cautious to avoid anesthetic toxicity, some clinicians perform pudendal block early, when the patient first complains of pelvic and perineal pain. This may allow a repeat block if one or both sides fail, as long as the safe maximum dose of anesthetic is not exceeded.

A 2012 Cochrane review found both paracervical and pudendal block to be more effective than intramuscular meperidine, and that there was no difference in efficacy between the various local anesthetics.

INDICATIONS

- Obstetric anesthesia for spontaneous vaginal delivery, episiotomy and episiotomy repair, repair of low vaginal lacerations, and outlet forceps or vacuum-assisted delivery

- When epidural anesthesia is incomplete, inadequate, contraindicated, or declined
- For minor surgery of the lower vagina and perineum

NOTE: Because the upper vagina, cervix, and uterus receive separate innervation from the lower thoracic nerves (i.e., ilioinguinal and genitofemoral), pudendal anesthesia alone is insufficient for midforceps application or for high vaginal, cervical, or uterine manipulation or repair. Paracervical block may be more helpful for cervical or uterine interventions (see Chapter 153, Paracervical Block).

CONTRAINDICATIONS

Absolute

- Patient refusal
- Allergy to local anesthetic agents
- Current infection in the ischiorectal space or neighboring structures, including the vagina and perineum

Relative

Coagulopathy or anticoagulant therapy (e.g., heparin or its analogs, warfarin, factor Xa inhibitor, thrombin inhibitor) or antiplatelet therapy (e.g., clopidogrel) is a relative contraindication for this procedure.

EQUIPMENT AND SUPPLIES

- Local anesthetic: 30 to 40 mL of 1% lidocaine (Xylocaine or generic) without epinephrine or 2% chloroprocaine (Nesacaine or generic; this may have lower toxicity than lidocaine but has shorter duration of effect)
- Iowa trumpet (Fig. 154.1A) or similar guide to facilitate placement of the needle
- 10-mL syringe with finger rings (see Fig. 154.1B)
- 16- to 18-gauge needle used to draw up anesthetic agent
- Needle, usually 6-inch, 22-gauge (see Fig. 154.1B) (Before the procedure, the operator should check that the needle is longer than the guiding device and equipped with a "stop" to prevent penetration of tissue deeper than 10 to 15 mm.)
- Povidone iodine or low alcohol (4%) chlorhexidine solution
- Sterile gloves

PRECAUTIONS

Care must be taken to avoid intravascular injection because the pudendal vessels lie lateral to the pudendal nerve. Toxicity may occur after inadvertent intravascular administration of greater than 1 mg/kg of 1% lidocaine without epinephrine (10 mg/mL; e.g., 70 mg or 7 mL in a 70-kg patient). Maximum dosage should not exceed 4.5 mg/kg or a maximum of 30 mL of 1% solution (300 mg), and the maximum dose should not be repeated in less than 2 hours (see Chapter 5, Local Anesthesia, for maximum dosages). A successful

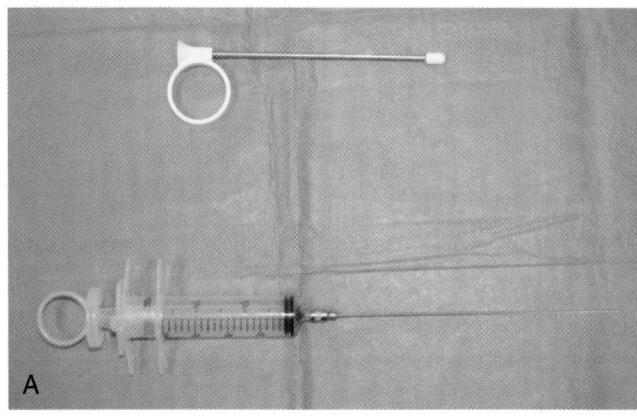
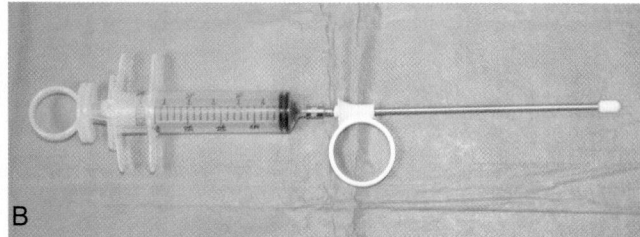

Fig. 154.1 (A) Iowa trumpet and syringe with finger rings separated. (B) Iowa trumpet and syringe with finger rings together.

pudendal block may impair some reflexive maternal pushing, which may prolong the second stage of labor in women who are ineffective at pushing.

PREPROCEDURE PATIENT PREPARATION

Potential risks and benefits should be discussed with the patient (see sections on Contraindications and Complications). This discussion should include alternatives and ideally occur by the third trimester and prior to labor. Written plans can be documented in the birth plan.

TECHNIQUE

Because a fairly large volume of anesthetic agent is given, appropriate monitoring of the patient (and, in obstetric cases, the fetus) should be considered. Adverse reactions are described in the Complications section as well as Chapter 6, Local and Topical Anesthetic Complications.

1. Timing is important for pudendal anesthesia. The anesthetic requires approximately 5 to 10 minutes to infiltrate the nerve and take effect. With obstetric indications, the anesthetic must be administered neither so early that it blocks effective reflex pushing, nor so late that it wears off before delivery. In nulliparous women, it is usually administered after the cervix has completely dilated and the head has descended to a +2 to +3 station. A pudendal block may be administered earlier in multiparous patients if rapid delivery is expected, but should be avoided until cervical dilation is greater than 5 cm because it may slow or arrest labor. The resultant anesthetic effect may last for 20 to 60 minutes.
2. Place the patient in the dorsal lithotomy position; prep the area around the bilateral ischial spines with povidone iodine or 4% chlorhexidine solution. The length of time the patient lies flat should be minimized. The fetus must be carefully monitored during and after the procedure. Universal blood and body fluid precautions should be observed.
3. Draw up 10 mL of 1% lidocaine into the syringe using a larger bore needle, attach the pudendal needle, and clear any air from the syringe and pudendal needle. Insert the needle into the Iowa trumpet or needle guide.
4. Grasp the Iowa trumpet or needle guide with your sterile-gloved, nondominant hand. The wrist should be pronated, with the thumb through the ring and the shaft between the index and middle fingers. Adequately lubricate the index and middle fingers of your other hand and use them to protect the vaginal mucosa (and, in obstetric cases, the fetal head). Insert the fingers into the vagina and direct the tip of the guide to the patient's ipsilateral ischial spine (i.e., the left hand of the right-handed operator is used to direct the guide to the patient's left ischial spine). Maintain the guide at an angle nearly parallel to the patient's back (Fig. 154.2).

5. Carefully define the anatomy to increase the likelihood of a successful injection. Attempt to delineate the ischial spine. Slightly below the spine, on its inferoposterior surface, the sacrospinous ligament is attached. Next, attempt to palpate the pudendal artery laterally. Locating these landmarks helps prevent injection of the anesthetic directly into the vessels. It also helps define the location of the nerve, which is medial to the vessels. The optimal injection site is 10 mm medial and 10 to 15 mm posterior to the ischial spine. If the anatomy is particularly difficult to define, injection just below the ischial spine should be sufficient (but only after aspirating to be certain the needle is not in a vessel).
6. With your nondominant hand grasping the syringe, use your dominant hand to direct the needle through the guide, and insert it to the appropriate depth at the desired injection site(s). The needle guide permits only 10 to 15 mm of needle to protrude past its end and varies by manufacturer

   NOTE: Aspirate for blood with the syringe before injecting anesthetic each time the needle placement is changed. If blood is aspirated, intravascular injection is likely; withdraw the needle and redirect medially, away from the vessels.

7. Inject the desired sites. Usually two to three sites are injected on each side in a fanlike fashion, with a total of 10 mL of local anesthetic injected per side. For the sacrospinous ligament (below/inferior/posterior and medial to the spine), some clinicians raise a mucosal wheal at this site with 1 mL of anesthetic and then insert the needle through the wheal until it contacts the ligament. After infiltrating the ligament with 2 to 4 mL of anesthetic, the needle is advanced through the ligament. The clinician will know that the ligament has been traversed when resistance to the plunger decreases. Another 2 to 4 mL of anesthetic can then be easily injected into the loose areolar tissue behind the ligament; another 2 to 4 mL can be injected above/superior/anterior to the ischial spine; and another 2 to 4 mL can be injected medial to the tip of the spine, for a total of 10 mL per side.

   NOTE: At each site (except when raising the mucosal wheal below the ischial spine), the needle should be inserted at least 10 mm but not more than 15 mm beyond the needle guide. Each time the needle is redirected, the tip should be drawn back into the guide, the guide redirected, and then the needle advanced to the desired depth.

8. Withdraw the needle, refill the syringe, and inject into the opposite side if bilateral anesthesia is desired. Most clinicians prefer to use the same hand for the guide; however, some claim switching hands for the opposite side is more effective. If switching hands, make sure the needle tip is withdrawn to protect yourself from a puncture wound.

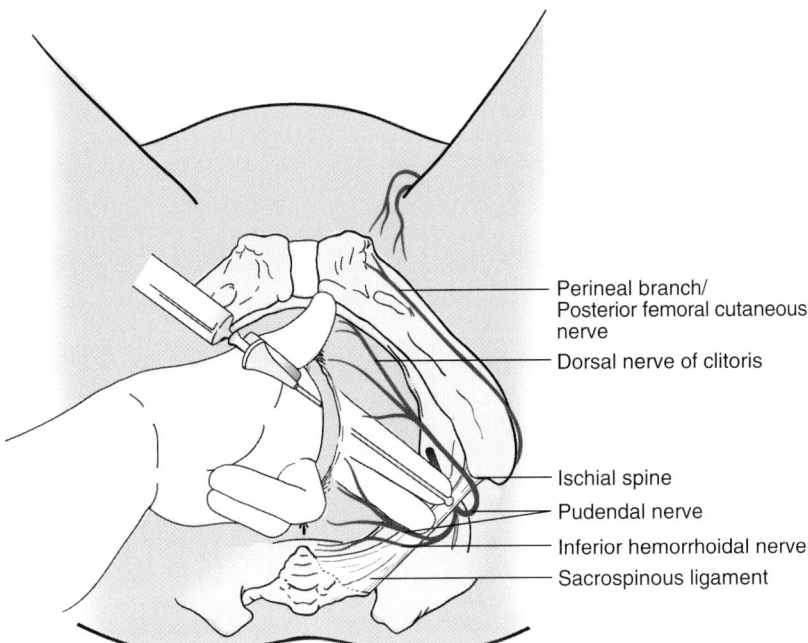

Perineal branch/
Posterior femoral cutaneous
nerve

Dorsal nerve of clitoris

Ischial spine
Pudendal nerve
Inferior hemorrhoidal nerve
Sacrospinous ligament

Fig. 154.2 Practitioner's left hand is directing guide and needle toward the patient's left pudendal nerve.

9. After 5 minutes, check the anesthesia on each side. Using an Allis forceps, gently scratch over the perineum and watch for the anal "wink" reflex. If there is no reflex to mild stimulus, confirm that the anesthesia is complete with a pinch on each side.
10. A smaller repeat dose on a side not demonstrating adequate anesthesia may be used, but care must be taken to avoid doses at which, even with slow absorption from the tissues, toxic serum levels could be reached. Local anesthesia may be used on the perineum to augment the effect, if necessary (when the pudendal block is not completely effective or if it has not had time to take full effect). For example, in the pregnant patient, if the head is descending rapidly, local anesthetic can also be infiltrated into the area where an episiotomy will be made. After the head has been delivered, the pudendal block should have had time to take effect and will usually provide anesthesia for the episiotomy repair.
11. As discussed earlier, a pudendal block does not provide pain relief from contractions and usually does not provide anesthesia for the upper vagina or cervix. This is important to remember after delivery when attempting to visualize the entire cervix and upper vagina. If manual exploration of the uterus is necessary, the addition of an intravenous opioid analgesic may be necessary.

COMPLICATIONS

*   Systemic anesthetic toxicity is rare and usually results from intravascular administration or an inappropriately high dose. Toxicity may initially cause palpitations, tinnitus, dysarthria, or drowsiness. It may progress to confusion, loss of consciousness, convulsions, hypotension, and bradycardia. Although complications are usually transient, support of the patient's oxygenation and blood pressure is essential (especially to minimize fetal complications in obstetric cases). See Chapter 6, Local and Topical Anesthetic Complications, for management of complications.
*   The most frequent complication with pudendal anesthesia is failure to provide adequate anesthesia. Local or regional (e.g., saddle block or epidural) anesthesia should be offered if available.
*   Laceration of vaginal mucosa

*   Hematomas and infections have been reported but are rare. Vaginal, ischiorectal, and retroperitoneal hematomas can occur. Infection may spread into the hip joint, the gluteal musculature, or the retropsoas space. Infections may be life-threatening and must be suspected when there is severe pain in the pelvis, back, or hip, limitation of motion, and increasing fever.
*   Despite the fact that the anesthetic reaches the neonatal bloodstream after regional anesthesia, studies have failed to demonstrate neonatal neurobehavioral effects or other adverse effects.

POSTPROCEDURE MANAGEMENT AND PATIENT EDUCATION

There is little need for specific postanesthesia instruction. Remind the patient of the rare but possible complications so that she will report to her clinician if any symptoms develop, especially pelvic, back, or hip pain, limited range of motion, or fever.

CPT/BILLING CODES

64430	Injection, anesthetic agent, pudendal nerve

ICD-10-CM DIAGNOSTIC CODES

O80	Normal delivery

Deliveries With Forceps or Vacuum

O76	Abnormality in fetal heart rate or rhythm
O63.0	Prolonged second stage of labor

Episiotomy and Episiotomy Repair, Repair of Low Vaginal Lacerations

O70.0	First-degree perineal laceration
O70.1	Second-degree perineal laceration
O72.20	Third-degree perineal laceration
O70.3	Fourth-degree perineal laceration
O70.9	Unspecified perineal laceration

Acknowledgment

The editors recognize the contributions of Donald N. Marquardt, MD, PhD, to this chapter in previous editions of this text.

RECOMMENDED READING

American College of Obstetricians and Gynecologists. Optimal goals for anesthesia care in obstetrics. Committee opinion no. 433. *Obstet Gynecol.* 2009;113:1197–1199.

Anderson D. Pudendal nerve block for vaginal birth. *J Midwifery Women Health.* 2014;59:651–659.

Chestnut DH. Alternative regional analgesic techniques for labor and vaginal delivery. In: Chestnut DH, ed. *Chestnut's Obstetric Anesthesia: Principles and Practice.* 5th ed. Philadelphia: Saunders Elsevier; 2014:518–529.

Ford JM, Owen DJ, Coughlin LB, et al. A critique of current practice of transvaginal pudendal nerve blocks: a prospective audit of understanding and clinical practice. *J Obstet Gynaecol.* 2013;33(5):463–465.

Matejcik V. Surgical location and anatomical variation of pudendal nerve. *ANZ J Surg.* 2012;82:935–938.

Novikova N, Cluver C. Local anaesthetic nerve block for pain management in labour. *Cochrane Database Syst Rev.* 2012;18(4):CD009200.

Volmanen P, Palomaki O, Ahonen J. Alternatives to neuraxial analgesia for labor. *Curr Opin Anesthesiol.* 2011;24:235–241.

CHAPTER 155

LOW SPINAL (SADDLE BLOCK) ANESTHESIA

Edward Anthony Yaghmour • Beth A. Choby

Low spinal (saddle block) anesthesia provides pain relief in the area of the perineum, buttocks, and inner thigh by using an intrathecal (spinal) injection of local anesthetic. Although a saddle block may be confused with a caudal block (injection of local anesthetic into the sacral canal through the sacral hiatus) because the resulting anesthesia is similar, the technique is much different. An ideal "saddle block" anesthetizes the area that would touch a saddle if the patient were riding a horse.

With the the increased availability of epidurals and combined spinal-epidurals (CSEs), saddle blocks are rarely used. In the past, saddle blocks were used for both surgical procedures and obstetric deliveries.

Saddle block anesthesia has been used for many years for both surgical procedures and obstetric deliveries. Past problems with profound motor block can be avoided by using lower doses of bupivacaine (e.g., 1 to 2 mL 0.25% bupivacaine with or without an opioid). Therefore, variations of saddle block anesthesia can be used midlabor or near delivery. Saddle block may be helpful for an outlet/low forceps delivery. Saddle block anesthesia is also commonly used in gynecologic, genital, anorectal, and urologic surgeries.

Clinicians administering saddle block anesthesia must have a good understanding of the anatomy, needle placement techniques, pharmacology, and physiology involved, particularly with regard to the obstetric patient. Knowledge of the American Society of Anesthesiologists (ASA) Practice Guidelines for Obstetric Anesthesia (2016) and the ASA Difficult Airway Algorithm is highly recommended for medical professionals anesthetizing obstetric patients. Saddle blocks should only be performed in hospitals, surgical centers, or facilities where drugs, equipment, and adequately trained personnel are available to manage possible complications. Available equipment should be comparable to that of the main operating room.

INDICATIONS

- For use in obstetrics when time or other circumstances do not allow the use of continuous catheter epidural or spinal anesthetic techniques (e.g., routine delivery, assisted delivery [forceps, vacuum], episiotomy or perineal repair, or other obstetric procedures)
- Genital surgery (e.g., dilation and curettage, hysteroscopy, vaginal surgery, adult circumcision, orchiectomy, or complicated vasectomy)
- Anorectal surgery (e.g., hemorrhoidectomy, fistulectomy, or rectal-anal biopsy)
- As part of a combined spinal epidural technique, when the spinal needle is placed through an epidural needle that is in the epidural space

CONTRAINDICATIONS

Absolute

- Patient refusal or uncooperative patient (unable to remain still)
- Medication allergy
- Active infection at the planned injection site
- Moderate to severe hypovolemia
- Maternal coagulopathy
- Use of anticoagulant therapy (e.g., heparin, warfarin, clopidogrel, direct thrombin inhibitor, factor Xa inhibitor); see SOAP Consensus Statement on the Anesthetic Management of Pregnant and Postpartum Women Receiving Thromboprophylaxis or Higher Dose Anticoagulants

Relative

- Cutaneous lesion/skin abnormalities of the lower back, such as cellulitis or dermatitis
- Treated active systemic infection, such as that resulting in maternal bacteremia
- Spinal abnormalities that make the procedure technically difficult, such as marked scoliosis, prior spinal fusion in the area
- Preexisting neurologic diseases (amyotrophic lateral sclerosis, other degenerative nerve diseases, poliomyelitis)

NOTE: See also Chapters 214, Emergency Department, Hospitalist, and Office Ultrasound [Clinical Ultrasound], and 221, Lumbar Puncture, for ultrasound-guided technique to use in individuals with difficult to palpate spinous processes such as those who are morbidly obese.

EQUIPMENT AND SUPPLIES

- Disposable sterile gloves
- Equipment for the clinician to observe universal blood and body fluid precautions
- Disposable spinal tray containing the following:
    - Appropriate prep solutions, swabs, and sterile 4 × 4 gauze pads
    - Disposable drapes
    - Syringes
        - 3-mL plastic Luer-Lok for local infiltration of lidocaine 1%
        - 5-mL procedural syringe for administration of intrathecal agent
    - Needles
        - 3.5-inch, 25-gauge spinal needle (pencil point [e.g., Sprotte or Whitacre] instead of cutting bevel)
        - 20-gauge introducer needle
        - 19-gauge filter tip needle for drawing solutions into the syringes
        - 25- or 27-gauge skin wheal needle

- Medications (Note that a 1% solution equals 10 mg/mL)
  - Lidocaine 1% (available in 5-mL vial) for local skin/track infiltration
  - Hyperbaric local anesthetic
  - Lidocaine 5% (preservative free) in 7.5% dextrose for intrathecal administration (2-mL vial), or
  - Bupivacaine 0.5% in 8.25% dextrose (2-mL vial)
  - Epinephrine 1:1000 (1-mL vial); addition of 0.1 to 0.2 mg (0.2 to 0.3 mL of 1:1000) epinephrine to bupivacaine will produce vasoconstriction and prolong the duration of anesthesia from 90 to 120 minutes to 100 to 150 minutes; addition to lidocaine does not significantly extend anesthetic duration, however
  - Ephedrine 5% (1-mL) in case hypotension develops (the usual dose to treat hypotension is 10 mg [0.2 mL] intravenously [IV] 5 to 10 mg in addition to phenylephrine 100 to 200 μg)
  - Fentanyl 50 μg/mL for injection
- IV fluids (Ringer lactate, normal saline)
- Continuous fetal monitoring equipment if used for labor and delivery
- Patient monitoring equipment, including automated blood pressure cuff, continuous electrocardiograph, and pulse oximeter
- Emergency and resuscitative equipment, including suction, positive-pressure breathing device (Ambu-Bag), airway equipment, oxygen, and defibrillator
- Emergency and other drugs not included in the spinal kit
  - Atropine
  - Diphenhydramine (Benadryl)
  - Ephedrine (not included in all commercial spinal kits)
  - Lidocaine for IV injection
  - Epinephrine
  - Succinylcholine
  - Propofol, and midazolam

ANESTHETIC AGENTS AND DOSES

For saddle block, the two commonly used local anesthetics are lidocaine and bupivacaine. Lidocaine produces a more rapid onset of action than bupivacaine, but has a shorter duration of action. Lidocaine generally produces adequate surgical analgesia for 45 to 90 minutes, whereas bupivacaine lasts 1.5 to 3 hours. Because intrathecal use of lidocaine has been linked with transient radicular irritation, bupivacaine is an excellent alternative; however, its increased duration of action requires a longer recovery period.

Hyperbaric solutions (solutions more dense than CSF) are used for saddle block anesthesia so that in the sitting position the anesthetic solution travels caudad, affecting only the lower levels of the spinal cord. It is important to remember that during pregnancy, inferior vena caval compression causes engorgement and distention of the vertebral venous system. As a result, the subarachnoid space has decreased CSF capacity; anesthetic dose requirements are generally reduced in the pregnant patient.

Near delivery, the usual dose of lidocaine for a saddle block is 25 to 50 mg of 5% lidocaine in 7.5% dextrose (0.5 to 1.0 mL). For spinal bupivacaine, 8 to 10 mg (1.5 to 2 mL of the 0.5% bupivacaine in 8% dextrose) should be used. In surgical procedures for the nonpregnant patient, higher doses are often given.

Confining the anesthetic to a saddle block distribution depends on the dosage and the time that the patient remains in the sitting position after administration of the anesthetic. Too little time in the sitting position (lying down too soon) may produce a higher level of anesthesia than desired, placing the patient at higher risk of hypotension and a higher level of block.

NOTE: From an anesthetic perspective, the level of anesthesia refers to an anatomic level or segment of effect (e.g., up to the level of the umbilicus [T10], the lower border of the ribs [T8], or the level of the xiphoid [T6]), whereas depth refers to the amount of remaining sensation. With saddle block, both motor and sensation are blocked; however, the level of the sensory block is usually two segments above the motor block.

PRECAUTIONS

A focused history (general maternal health, anesthetic history, allergies, relevant obstetric history, current medications, and NPO status) should be obtained. Perform a physical examination with special attention to the airway, vital signs, heart, lungs, and spinal anatomy. Look for contraindications to performing the block.

Expert witnesses in medical liability cases often note a lack of preblock examinations by the anesthesiologist. Laboratory studies are obtained on an individualized basis. The history, physical examination, and lab results should determine whether there are any contraindications to performing the block. Counsel the patient about the risks, benefits, and alternatives to analgesia and anesthesia.

PREPROCEDURE PATIENT EDUCATION AND FORMS

Prior to labor, counsel the patient about analgesia and anesthesia options and obtain informed consent (see the sample patient consent form available at www.expertconsult.com). Staff providing prenatal education should be knowledgeable about analgesic options. An educational handout can be provided prior to the onset of labor (see patient education form available at www.expertconsult.com). Analgesia/anesthesia during labor is optional, is based on patient preference, and has certain risks. Physiologic effects of severe pain during labor from increased circulating catecholamine levels include tachycardia, increased cardiac output/myocardial workload/oxygen demand, and decreased gastric emptying. Excessive fatigue due to labor discomfort may affect the birth experience and the likelihood of successful vaginal delivery.

TECHNIQUE

1. Confirm that informed consent and preblock history and physical exam documentation are signed and in order.
2. Perform time-out procedure to confirm the correct patient and procedure.
3. Establish IV access with an 18-gauge or larger catheter and give a bolus of 500 to 1000 mL of IV fluids. The patient should be well hydrated before the procedure to minimize the risk of developing hypotension.
   NOTE: Administer IV fluids slowly in women with hypertensive disorders of pregnancy.
4. For patients in labor, fetal monitoring should be used. For all patients, secure the continuous blood pressure, electrocardiograph, and pulse oximetry monitors, and record the initial values. Cycle the blood pressure monitor to take measurements at least every 2.5 minutes to monitor for hypotension. Vital signs should be recorded on the anesthesia chart at least every 5 minutes.
5. Put on mask and surgical cap or bonnet and don sterile gloves. Follow universal blood and body fluid precautions.
6. Have an assistant open the disposable spinal kit and mix the appropriate solutions. Mix the appropriate solutions using the filtered needle to draw up any solutions to be administered intrathecally.
7. Place the patient in the sitting position with the back and neck flexed and the spine straight and not rotated. An assistant should stand in front of the patient during the procedure to help the patient maintain the proper position.
8. Locate the L2–L3, L3–L4, or L4–L5 interspace. Prep around the planned injection site using sterile technique and then drape the area with the fenestrated drape.

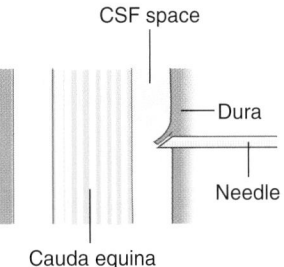

Fig. 155.2 Bevel of spinal needle occluded by a dural flap after puncture. The flap prevents free flow of cerebrospinal fluid (CSF) through the spinal needle.

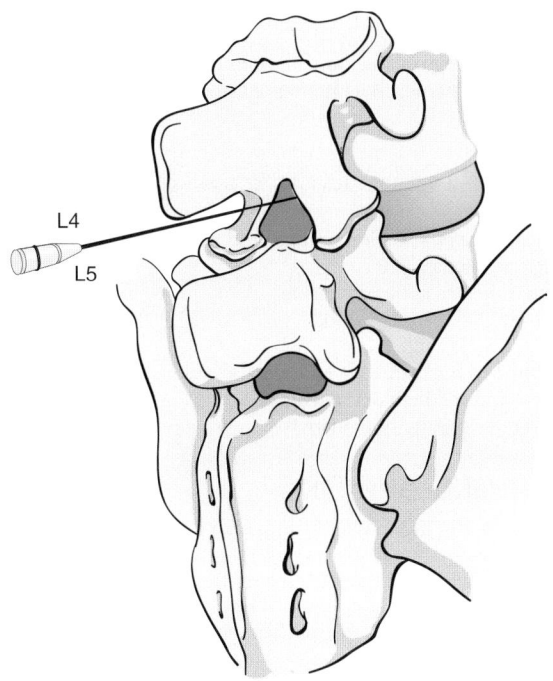

Fig. 155.1 Spinal needle introduced through the L4–L5 interspace. Note that the needle is introduced just below the inferior border of the L4 spinous process. The tip is directed at 90 degrees to the spine or slightly cranial.

9. Administer the local anesthesia (lidocaine 1%) to the interspace area by first making a skin wheal, then injecting into the deeper tissues in the same direction that the spinal needle will be advanced.
10. Insert the introducer needle into the supraspinous ligament at the proper angle to later direct the spinal needle into the subdural space.
    NOTE: The proper angle depends on which interspace is used. At the L4–L5 interspace, the proper direction for the needle tip is basically perpendicular (90 degrees) to slightly cranial, whereas it decreases to about 70 degrees (and aimed cranial) at the L2–L3 interspace. The proper location is usually just below the inferior edge of the spinous process or slightly below that level (Fig. 155.1). For saddle block anesthesia, insertion angle and location are identical to those used for epidural anesthesia; however, the depth of insertion is unique to each procedure.
11. Insert the 3.5-inch, 25-gauge spinal needle into the introducer. Next, advance the spinal needle into the intrathecal space. A "pop" is usually felt when the needle passes through the ligamentum flavum and into the space. Confirmation is obtained when CSF flows from the hub of the spinal needle (Fig. 155.2).
12. With the anesthetic solution syringe connected to the hub of the spinal needle, aspirate a small amount of CSF to confirm the placement of the needle. Slowly inject the lidocaine or bupivacaine through the spinal needle over a period of 5 to 10 seconds. Try to avoid aspiration or injection during a uterine contraction, as the patient may move.
13. Remove the spinal needle, syringe, and introducer as a unit. Have the patient remain in the sitting position for 2 to 5 minutes to allow the anesthetic to "set" as it drifts downward into the spinal canal. Allowing the patient to become recumbent or lie in the lithotomy position too soon can result in a higher level of anesthesia than desired. However, if the patient becomes hypotensive, he or she should be returned to the recumbent position immediately and treatment initiated. Otherwise, at the end of the seated period, place the patient in the lithotomy position. For pregnant women, left uterine displacement helps

minimize or avoid vena caval compression syndrome (decreased venous return to the heart combined with venous congestion around the spinal cord). In a late-trimester pregnancy, this syndrome can lead to prolonged hypotension.
13. Check sensation to sharp objects (e.g., a needle) and record the level of anesthesia on the anesthesia record. Once adequate anesthesia has been established, the patient may be prepared for delivery.

NOTE: Factors affecting the level of anesthesia include (1) the level of the lumbar puncture site, (2) the volume of solution used, (3) the rate of injection, (4) the specific gravity of the solution used, and (5) patient positioning.

COMPLICATIONS

Intraoperative and postoperative complications of saddle block anesthesia are essentially the same as for high levels of spinal anesthesia.

Intraoperative Complications

- Hypotension may occur at any time, particularly during and shortly after administration of the anesthetic. It must be quickly corrected by (1) placing the patient in a recumbent position, (2) infusing a rapid bolus of IV fluids (e.g., 500 mL), (3) rapidly administering intravenous ephedrine 10 mg (IV), and (4) relieving vena cava compression via leftward displacement of the gravid uterus. If bradycardia and hypotension occur (from blocking of cardiac accelerator nerves), rapidly administer epinephrine. If hypotension and maternal tachycardia are present, a 0.1- to 0.5-mg IV bolus of phenylephrine is acceptable.
- High spinal block with respiratory insufficiency or total spinal block with complete respiratory arrest must be treated immediately with respiratory support until resolution. Concurrent hypotension commonly occurs.
- Nausea and vomiting may also develop with a drop in blood pressure and usually are relieved with correction of the hypotension using ephedrine (10 mg IV). If accompanied by bradycardia, the nausea and vomiting may improve after treatment with atropine (0.4 to 0.6 mg IV).
- Allergic reactions: use diphenhydramine 25 to 50 mg IV.
- Systemic reactions, including cardiac arrhythmia/arrest, are rare. To treat this, routine Advanced Cardiac Life Support (ACLS) protocols should be followed.

Postoperative Complications

- Headache may occur, with an incidence around 1%. Most postspinal puncture headaches can be treated conservatively (oral analgesics, fluids, rest), but some require more aggressive treatment, including an epidural blood patch (see Chapter 221, Lumbar Puncture, for instructions on performing an epidural blood patch).

- Urinary retention, sometimes requiring catheterization
- Neurologic sequelae (rare), including arachnoiditis, meningitis, palsies, and paralysis. To minimize infection risk, injected anesthetics should only be from sterile, single use, preservative-free vials.

PATIENT EDUCATION GUIDES

See the sample patient education form available at www.expertconsult.com.

CPT/BILLING CODES

62273	Injection, lumbar epidural, of blood or clot patch
62322	Injection(s), of diagnostic or therapeutic substance(s) (including anesthetic, antispasmodic, opioid, steroid, other solution), not including neurolytic substances, including needle or catheter placement, includes contrast for localization when performed, epidural or subarachnoid; lumbar or sacral (caudal)

ICD-10-CM DIAGNOSTIC CODES

For other than pregnancy codes, see the appropriate procedure chapter for ICD-9-CM codes.

O80	Normal delivery
Z33.1	Pregnant state, NOS
Z34.00-Z34.93	Supervision of normal pregnancy
O60.10-O60.14	Preterm labor with preterm delivery
O60.20-O60.23	Term delivery with preterm labor
O64.0XX-O64.9XX	Obstructed labor due to malposition malpresentation of fetus

Use additional seventh character: A = initial, D = subsequent, S = sequela.

O64.0	O65.9 Obstructed labor due to maternal pelvic abnormality

Deliveries With Forceps or Vacuum

O76	Abnormality in fetal heart rate or rhythm or fetal distress
O63.1	Prolonged second stage of labor

Episiotomy and Episiotomy Repair, Repair of Low Vaginal Lacerations

O70.0	First-degree perineal laceration
O70.1	Second-degree perineal laceration
O70.20-O70.23	Third-degree perineal laceration
O70.3	Fourth-degree perineal laceration
O70.9	Unspecified perineal laceration

Acknowledgment

The editors recognize the contributions of Thomas H. Corbett, MD, MPH, to this chapter in a previous edition of this text.

SUPPLIERS

(See contact information available at www.expertconsult.com.)

Disposable trays, infusion pumps, and needles
B. Braun Medical Inc.
Baxter Healthcare Corporation
Becton, Dickinson and Co.
Rusch Inc. (Teleflex)
Smiths Medical USA
Epidural and saddle block needles
Kendall Company (Covidien)

RECOMMENDED READING

Al-Kazwini H, Sandven I, Dahl V, Rosseland LA. Prolonging the duration of single-shot intrathecal labour analgesia with morphine: a systematic review. *Scandinavian J Pain*. 2016;13:36–42.

American College of Obstetricians and Gynecologists. Optimal goals for anesthesia care in obstetrics. Committee opinion no. 433. *Obstet Gynecol*. 2009;113:1197–1199.

American College of Obstetricians and Gynecologists Committee on Obstetric Practice. Analgesia and cesarean delivery rates. Committee opinion no. 339. *Obstet Gynecol*. 2006;107:1487–1488.

American Society of Anesthesiologists. Practice guidelines for obstetric anesthesia (last amended on October 2015). An updated report by the American Society of Anesthesiologists task force on obstetric anesthesia. *Anesthesiology*. 2016;124(2):270–300.

American Society of Anesthesiologists Task Force on management of the difficult airway: practice guidelines for the management of the difficult airway: an updated report by the American Society of Anesthesiologists task force on management of the difficult airway. *Anesthesiology*. 2013;98:251–270.

Gerancher JC. Cauda equina syndrome following a single spinal administration of 5% hyperbaric lidocaine through a 25-gauge Whitacre needle. *Anesthesiology*. 1997;87:687–689.

Hoefnagel A, Yu A, Kaminski A. Anesthetic complications in pregnancy. *Crit Care Clin*. 2016;32:1–28.

Shon Y, Huh J, Kang S, et al. Comparison of saddle lumbar epidural and caudal block on anal sphincter tone: a prospective, randomized study. *J Int Med Research*. 2016;44(5):1061–1071.

Vittanen H, Porthan L, Vittanen M, Heula LA, et al. Postpartum neurologic symptoms following single-shot spinal block for labour analgesia. *Acta Anaesthesiol Scand*. 2005;49:1015–1022.

Wong CA. Epidural and spinal analgesia/anesthesia for labor and vaginal delivery. In: Chestnut DH, ed. *Chestnut's Obstetric Anesthesia: Principles and Practice*. 5th ed. Philadelphia: Saunders Elsevier; 2014:457–517.

CHAPTER 156

VAGINAL DELIVERY

Dale A. Patterson • Coral D. Matus • Jacob Curtis

Vaginal delivery is a natural process that has gradually become a medical procedure. Although early medical efforts were successful at decreasing maternal and fetal mortality, more recent and advanced interventions have not been as successful. Routine interventions such as electronic fetal monitoring, amniotomy, and fetal pulse oximetry have not been demonstrated to improve outcomes. Some medical interventions, such as routine episiotomy, have actually been shown to be harmful. Evidence-based practice changes are an ever-evolving aspect of modern medicine. Staying up to date is essential if attending deliveries.

Even though birth is a natural process, labor is very complex and varies widely among women. Underlying hormonal changes are incompletely understood. Exploring all of the possible variables and complications that could occur during a vaginal delivery is beyond the scope of this chapter. The focus, rather, is on uncomplicated vaginal delivery of a term vertex singleton gestation. Evidence-based recommendations regarding delivery techniques are incorporated when available. Procedures common to vaginal delivery are also described in Section 10, Obstetrics, Chapters 141 to 162.

ANATOMY AND PHYSIOLOGY

Labor is defined as the onset of regular contractions that cause progressive cervical dilation and effacement with eventual descent of the fetal presenting part. Labor involves three progressive stages. The first stage is further subdivided into two phases: latent and active. Latent labor is characterized by mild, irregular uterine contractions that cause cervical softening, effacement, and gradual dilation. *First stage active labor* is the time from labor onset to complete cervical dilation. *Second stage* involves complete cervical dilation to delivery of the neonate, while *third stage* involves placental delivery after the neonate is born.

With cervical dilation, the fetus starts its descent through the birth canal. Each contraction moves the fetal head further as it incrementally negotiates the angles of the maternal pelvis, following a standard pattern known as the cardinal movements of labor:

1. Engagement
   - Defined by descent of the biparietal diameter of the fetus to a level below the maternal pelvic inlet. The borders of the pelvic inlet are formed by the sacral promontory posteriorly and the inner pubic arch anteriorly; this diameter is also referred to as the "obstetric conjugate." In most cases, the anteroposterior (AP) diameter of the pelvic inlet is the smallest dimension. Thus, the smallest diameter of the fetal head (biparietal diameter) must align with the AP diameter of the pelvic inlet.
   - Clinically defined as when the lowest portion of the occiput (not caput) is palpable at or below the maternal ischial spines (0 station).
   - In most cases, it indicates the maternal pelvic inlet is sufficient to allow descent of the head.
   - Often occurs before the onset of labor, especially in nulliparas.
   - Verification may be difficult if the fetal head is molded or in the occipitoposterior (OP) presentation.

2. Descent (Fig. 156.1)
   - Slowly progressive process
   - Measured by station (level of presenting part) and quantified by number of centimeters the presenting part is either above (e.g., −2, −1) or below (e.g., +1, +2) the ischial spines
3. Flexion
   - The force of contractions against the cervix and maternal tissue eventually maneuvers the head into a flexed position so that the smallest diameter of the fetal head is presenting first, further aiding in descent of the presenting part (Fig. 156.2A). It remains in this position until the head reaches to the level of the perineum.
   - Normally, the posterior fontanelle is in the center of the dilating cervix, allowing for optimal "molding" of the fetal cranial bones.
   - Fetuses in an OP position often assume a more "deflexed" position due to their orientation in the maternal pelvis. This causes a less favorable alignment between the fetal head and the maternal pelvis.
4. Internal rotation
   - As the fetal head continues to descend, the fetal biparietal diameter rotates to align with the lateral diameter (intertuberous diameter between the ischial tuberosities [spines]) of the maternal pelvic outlet. Typically, this diameter constitutes the smallest dimension of the pelvic outlet. The borders of the pelvic outlet are formed by the ischial spines laterally and the angle of the pubic symphysis anteriorly.
   - The final position of the vertex is usually left occipitoanterior (see Fig. 156.2B), occipitoanterior (OA) (see Fig. 156.2C), or right occipitoanterior; in around 5% to 10% of cases, the vertex presents in an OP position, however.

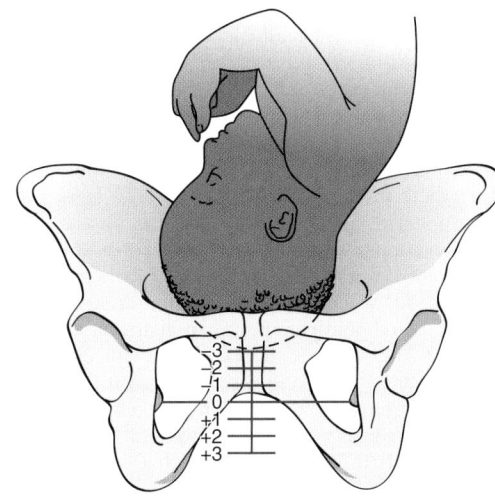

Fig. 156.1 Descent of fetal head into the pelvis. Zero station is diagnosed when the fetal vertex has reached the level of the ischial spines.

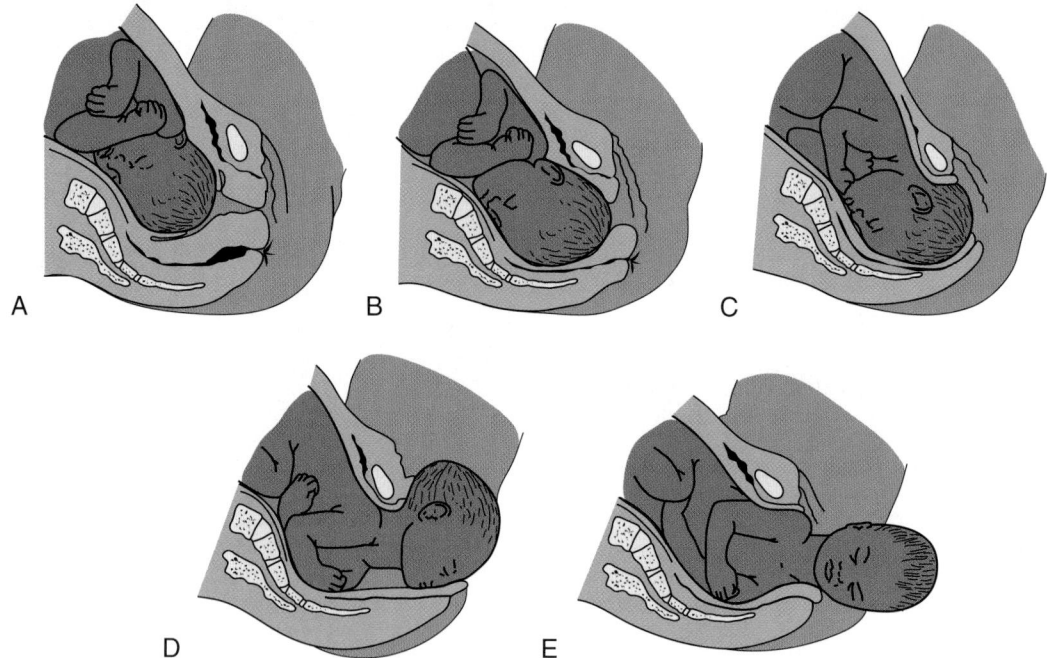

Fig. 156.2 (A) Engagement of flexed head. (B) Left occipitoanterior position. (C) Internal, anterior rotation of head to occipitoanterior position. (D) Extension of head. (E) External rotation of head. (Modified from Pernoll M. *Benson and Pernoll's Handbook of Obstetrics and Gynecology*. 9th ed. New York: McGraw-Hill; 2001.)

5. Extension
   - The outward force of uterine contractions meets the pelvic sling muscles making the pubic symphysis function as a fulcrum. This combination of forces pushes the head under and around the pubic symphysis (see Fig. 156.2D).
   - The head extends as it is crowning due to these forces.
   - Extension occurs fairly rapidly and is clinically observed as the perineum distends.
6. External rotation and restitution
   - After delivery of the head, the head rotates back to transverse and the shoulders rotate into an AP position (see Fig. 156.2E).

Although dilation and descent may occur predictably, more often the pattern of labor is irregular and erratic. The original labor curves describing duration of normal active phase labor were plotted by Friedman in the 1950s. Traditionally thought to begin at 4 cm dilation, Friedman's expected rates of cervical dilation were 1.2 cm/hr in nulliparas and 1.5 cm/hr in multiparas. Descent at 1 cm/hr or greater in nulliparas and at least 2 cm/hr in multiparas was the expectation. Protraction disorders were defined as a rate of either dilation or descent slower than these minimums. Risk of dysfunctional labor was considered to increase if no cervical change was noted in 2 hours with adequate uterine contractions (e.g., Montevideo units >200 to 220 in a 10-minute period).

Whether these numbers actually characterize labor patterns in the modern obstetric population is debatable. Retrospective data from the observational Consortium on Safe Labor study examined 228,668 singleton vaginal deliveries at 19 US hospitals between 2002 and 2008, of which 80% had epidural anesthesia. Interestingly, nulliparous and multiparous women dilated at about the same rate from 4 to 6 cm, after which multiparous women dilated more rapidly. In nulliparous women at the 95th percentile for labor progression, dilating from 4 to 5 cm required more than 6 hours, with another 3 hours required to move from 5 to 6 cm. Second-stage labor was nearly 3.6 hours in women who later had a successful vaginal delivery (Zhang et al., 2010). The National Institutes of Health and Child Development workshop on Preventing the First Cesarean recommended that rupture of membranes only be considered after a minimum of 6 cm cervical dilation. Some experts suggest that a duration of 13 to 15 hours of active labor or cervical change rate of less than 0.5 cm/hr be used to diagnose protracted labor in both nulliparas and multiparas (Millen et al., 2014). In the setting of reassuring maternal and fetal status, protracted labor should not be the sole reason for cesarean.

In an attempt to reduce prolonged labor in nulliparas, the active management of labor (AML) protocol was created and studied at the National Maternity Hospital in Dublin, Ireland in the 1970s. AML included education, labor support, and medical interventions geared toward shortening active-phase labor in nulliparas. A 2013 Cochrane review of seven randomized controlled trials found no statistically significant decrease in cesarean rates between AML and routine care, although the AML group had shorter duration of labor.

INDICATIONS

- Vertex presentation, active labor, perineal distention, and deliverable baby
- Fetal distress in a vaginally deliverable baby

CONTRAINDICATIONS

Absolute

- Cord prolapse
- Complete placenta previa or vasa previa
- Abnormal fetal lie (e.g., footling breech, transverse lie, persistent brow presentation)
- Prior classical cesarean section or transfundal uterine surgery
- Herpes simplex infection with active genital lesions or prodromal symptoms
- Untreated human immunodeficiency virus infection

Relative

- Pelvic deformities
- Fetal congenital deformities (hydrocephalus)
- Invasive cervical carcinoma

- Treated human immunodeficiency virus infection
- Macrosomia
- Malpresentation (including breech)
- Previous low transverse cesarean deliveries
- Multiple gestation

EQUIPMENT AND SUPPLIES

Although equipment setups vary by hospital, the following list is found in a standard birthing room. Equipment should be available to follow universal blood and body fluid precautions. Deliveries in an operating room additionally require a full gown, mask, shoe covers, and a surgical cap.

- Oxygen with flowmeter and tubing/cannula (one for mother and a second for infant)
- Delivery bed (should be able to break down into a modified lithotomy position and have adjustable height)
- Fetal monitoring equipment (optional, see Chapter 149, Fetal Scalp Electrode Application)
- Setup for infant (infant warmer, oxygen with bag and mask, suction, infant laryngoscope, intubation equipment, umbilical catheter, medications, and resuscitation equipment [see Chapter 163, Neonatal Resuscitation])
- Sterile equipment tray or table containing the following (Fig. 156.3):
  - 10-mL tube for cord blood
  - Two pairs of scissors (blunt Mayo-Noble straight scissors for cutting the cord; sharp scissors for cutting suture and dressings)
  - Bulb syringe
  - Plastic cord clamp (may use curved Kocher clamp for the other; some clinicians use three plastic cord clamps if cord segment needs to be sent)
  - Two curved Kocher clamps (some clinicians like to have four of these clamps, especially if cord blood gases are needed)
  - Needle holder
  - Two sets of ring forceps
  - Sterile drapes and towels (including under buttocks drape with fluid pouch)
  - Placenta basin
  - Gown and sterile gloves (latex-free recommended)
- Optional equipment (also see Chapter 158, Episiotomy and Repair of the Perineum)
  - Additional needle holder
  - Two Allis clamps (for third- or fourth-degree repair)
  - Pickups (toothed [Adson] and smooth)
  - Gelpi retractor (for added visualization during a third- or fourth-degree repair)
  - Weighted speculum (offers greater visualization of the vaginal wall and cervix)
  - 10-mL syringe
  - 22-gauge, 1.5-inch needle (for local anesthesia)
  - 1% lidocaine, without epinephrine
  - Two 3-0 absorbable synthetic sutures with tapered needles
  - Gauze pads (4 × 4 inches)
  - Sterile speculum
  - Red rubber catheter—povidone–iodine, chlorhexidine, or solution for preparation
- Emergency kit (for precipitous deliveries)
  - Sterile gloves (large size, latex-free recommended)
  - Two sterile towels
  - One pair of blunt-end scissors
  - One plastic cord clamp
  - Two curved Kocher clamps
  - Gauze pads (4 × 4 inches)
  - Bulb syringe
  - Placenta basin

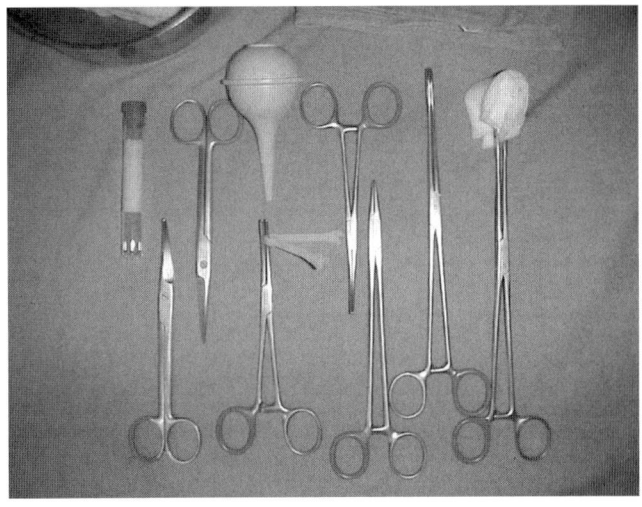

Fig. 156.3 Instruments for vaginal delivery. *Left to right:* Cord blood tube, two scissors (blunt and sharp edge), bulb syringe, plastic cord clamp, two curved Kocher clamps (one is holding plastic cord clamp), needle holder, two-ring forceps (one grasping folded 4 × 4 gauze is called a *sponge stick*).

PRECAUTIONS

Prior Cesarean: Women with a single prior low transverse uterine incision should be counseled regarding a trial of labor after cesarean. While there is no reliable prediction model for an individual's risk of uterine rupture, consideration of specific factors that are associated with uterine rupture require discussion. In one study of 15,519 women attempting trial of labor after a previous cesarean, 0.64% had uterine rupture (Smith et al., 2015). Having a prior successful vaginal delivery when attempting trial of labor after cesarean also may confirm benefit compared with women without prior vaginal delivery (rupture rate of 0.5%; odds ratio, 0.62 [95% CI:0.43–0.90] [Landon and Grobman, 2016]). Patients with a history of classical or T-incisions should avoid trial of labor due to increased uterine rupture risk.

Group B streptococcus (GBS) colonization occurs in 10% to 30% of women. The incidence of early-onset neonatal infection with GBS, the most common serious infection of the newborn period, is reduced by intrapartum chemoprophylaxis. The Centers for Disease Control and Prevention (CDC) recommends universal GBS screening at 35 to 37 weeks' gestation with rectal and vaginal swabs. Treatment with penicillin (5 million units) at least 4 hours prior to delivery and repeat doses every 4 hours (2.5 million units) is first-line therapy. The CDC has an online app for managing GBS in pregnancy (see https://www.cdc.gov/groupbstrep/guidelines/prevention-app.html). GBS bacteriuria during pregnancy and a previous neonate infection with GBS also require automatic treatment in labor, and thus do not need to be screened.

Other maternal conditions that warrant preprocedure evaluation and counseling include cardiovascular conditions, coagulopathies, diabetes, and other chronic medical conditions.

PREPROCEDURE PATIENT EDUCATION

Education is a major focus of prenatal care. Patients ideally have several months to prepare and numerous provider encounters prior to delivery. Numerous resources are available, including electronic prenatal records that incorporate education into the flowsheets. Behaviors that increase chances for a healthy pregnancy include exercise, eating a healthy diet, and avoiding tobacco, alcohol, and drugs. See the resources listed under "Continuing Education" later in this chapter.

The birth process can be intimidating for many women, especially first-time mothers. Education about the normal birth process can greatly relieve these fears and improve a woman's experience in labor. A birth plan may be helpful for the patient and the provider (Fig. 156.4). An open conversation about pain control, labor uncertainties, and the possibility of interventions, including operative vaginal delivery (vacuum or forceps), episiotomy, and cesarean delivery is important.

As the rate of operative deliveries in the United States continues to increase, more patients may express a desire for a primary elective cesarean delivery or opt for repeat cesarean delivery. Despite advances in anesthesia and surgical care, a vaginal delivery is a safer procedure than a cesarean delivery. Primary cesarean delivery on maternal request is not recommended for women who desire several children as the risk of placenta previa and accreta as well as the need for gravid hysterectomy increase with each cesarean.

TECHNIQUE

First Stage

Management of the first (latent) stage of labor is passive. Once active phase begins, labor should be monitored for progression and intervention considered if adequate progress toward delivery is not achieved. Adequacy of contractions can be assessed by inserting an intrauterine pressure catheter if adequate process is not seen (see Chapter 150, Intrauterine Pressure Catheter Insertion).

Anticipatory Guidance and Patient Preferences for Birthing Plan (Checklist Completed by Clinician)

Patient name: _____

Date: _____ Clinician: _____

Answers to the following will help determine the patient's individual preferences and amount of preparation during prenatal care, labor, and postpartum care:

Is prenatal birth education (Lamaze) planned? ☐ Yes ☐ No

   Who will attend Lamaze? _____

If no rupture of membranes has occurred (ROM), is an enema desired? ☐ Yes ☐ No

Diet preferences: ☐ Clear liquids ☐ Ice chips ☐ Nothing

IV access preferences: ☐ Hep-Lock ☐ None ☐ IV with lactated Ringer's at 100 mL/hr

Fetal assessment (low-risk patient):

   ☐ Continuous electronic fetal monitoring for 20 minutes (baseline strip); then, if baseline is reassuring, periodic auscultation every 30 minutes in first stage, then every 15 minutes in second stage (auscultation done during contraction and for 30 seconds following).

   ☐ Continuous electronic fetal monitoring.

   ☐ Scalp clip okay.

Preferences for maximizing comfort during labor (anesthesia?): _____ Position _____

Partner to be present during labor? ☐ Yes ☐ No

Female support person (doula) to be present? ☐ Yes ☐ No

Patient attitude toward episiotomy? _____ (desired) _____ (only if necessary)

Infant feeding preferences? ☐ Breast-feeding ☐ Bottle feeding

For male infant, is circumcision desired? ☐ Yes ☐ No

Preferred clinician for baby: _____

Rooming-in with baby? ☐ Yes ☐ No

Postpartum contraception preference: _____

Baby's name? _____

Hospital preregistration? ☐ Yes ☐ No

Mother has visited labor and delivery? ☐ Yes ☐ No

Encouraged intrapartum ambulation, frequent position changes? ☐ Yes ☐ No

Practiced positions for emergencies (e.g., knee chest, rolling onto hands/knees)? ☐ Yes ☐ No

If the clinician provides anticipatory guidance, it may not only improve the outcomes, but it may also give mother a greater sense of security. The results of this questionnaire should be dictated or copied, signed by the patient, and a copy given to the patient. She should bring it to labor and delivery when admitted.

Fig. 156.4 Sample birthing plan.

Second Stage

Typically, as the cervix nears complete dilation, contraction intensity increases and the patient feels the urge to push. Even if the patient has regional anesthesia, she will usually feel pressure as the fetus begins to descend more rapidly. When the cervix is completely dilated, the second stage of labor begins. Pushing prior to complete cervical dilation may cause soft tissue injury and exhaust the patient. Physiologic management of the second stage has been proposed as a method for decreasing maternal exhaustion and shortening the overall duration of pushing. In the setting of reassuring maternal and fetal status, women are encouraged to push only once the fetal head reaches the introitus and a strong desire to push occurs (i.e., laboring down). Pushing with an open rather than closed glottis and pushing based on the patient's preferences rather than proscribed instructions from providers are encouraged. Recommendations to allow a primigravida with an epidural to remain in second stage labor for as long as 4 hours and multigravidas with epidural for 3 hours also have been made as long as reassuring maternal and fetal status is seen.

Persistent OP position is one of the most common reasons for prolonged second-stage labor. On average, OP position prolongs labor by 1 hour in multiparas and 2 hours in nulliparas. "Back labor" (pain focused in the patient's back) is common. A persistent anterior cervical lip or an easily palpable anterior fontanelle may also be noted. To confirm OP position by examination, the fetal skull sutures should be followed until the posterior fontanelle can be palpated. (Recall that the anterior fontanelle is shaped like a cross or plus (+) and is usually larger than the posterior fontanelle; the posterior fontanelle is Y-shaped.) If an ear is palpable, the direction that the ear is facing can determine which direction the fetus is facing.

To rotate the fetus from the OP position, various positions and activities can be tried, such as squatting or ambulating, all fours, on her side, or with her back arched. If position changes fail to cause rotation, manual rotation can be attempted. Place the mother in the lithotomy, lateral Sims, or all fours position. With a hand in the posterior pelvis behind the occiput, attempt to rotate and flex the head, during a contraction, while the mother is pushing. If the fetus is straight OP, the clinician's dominant hand should be used. If the fetus is partially rotated, use whichever hand can most easily rotate the head the shortest distance to OA. (If a vacuum-assisted delivery is to be performed, the vacuum device can sometimes help rotate the infant from OP to OA; see Chapter 157, Forceps- and Vacuum-Assisted Deliveries.)

Preparation for delivery should begin at the onset of the second stage for the multipara and as the vertex reaches the pelvic floor in the nullipara.

Preparation

1. Put on sterile gloves and a gown. Remember to observe universal blood and body fluid precautions.
2. Prepare the delivery table.
3. Have someone turn on the warmer for the newborn isolette and notify the nursery staff. Make sure that all necessary equipment is available for a neonatal resuscitation, especially if a nonreassuring tracing or meconium is present (see Chapter 163, Neonatal Resuscitation).
4. Verify that all needed equipment is on the sterile tray or table and within reach. If the patient does not have a Foley catheter, empty the maternal bladder with a red rubber catheter.
5. Make an attempt to rotate a persistent OP vertex to an OA position if necessary.
6. Chlorhexidine vaginal irrigation in labor is inexpensive and safe, although it is associated with similar infection rates (chorioamnionitis, endometritis, and neonatal sepsis) as no vaginal prep. No evidence supports any benefit from perineal shaving or enemas prior to delivery.

Positioning

Allow the patient to find a comfortable position for pushing or laboring down (Fig. 156.5). The rationale for each position is noted here, as well as possible inconveniences or complications for each position:

1. Modified dorsal
   - Semisitting position with knees flexed and legs widely separated; the mother can grip below her knees for leverage when pushing
   - Good position for multiparous women
2. Squatting, kneeling (see Fig. 156.5A)
   - More physiologic for pushing
   - Less discomfort with pushing
   - Fewer perineal tears
   - Increased incidence of hemorrhage (>500 mL) compared with other positions
3. Lithotomy (see Fig. 156.5B)
   - Better provider access to perineum, so useful if operative vaginal delivery is needed

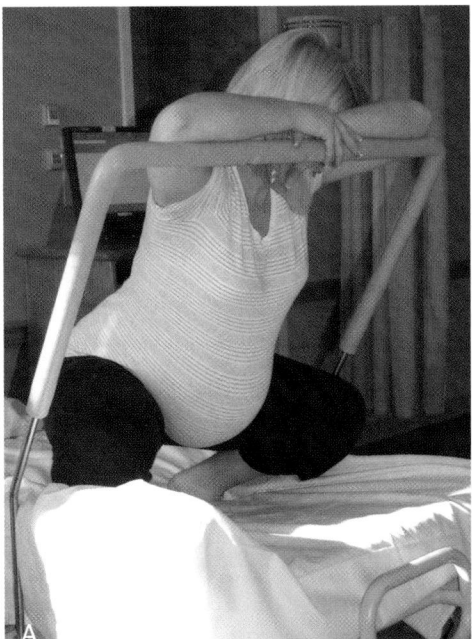
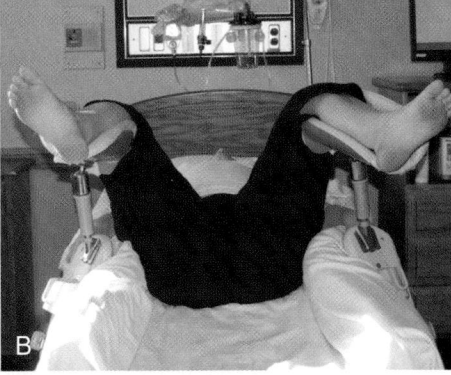
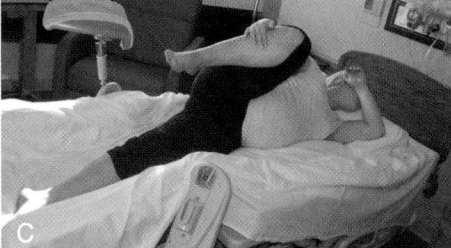

Fig. 156.5 Maternal birthing positions. (A) Squatting; (B) lithotomy; (C) left lateral.

- Difficult position for pushing (fetal head must push up and over the maternal sacrum without benefit of gravity)
- Increased risk for maternal aspiration

4. Left lateral (see Fig. 156.5C)
- Left side with knees flexed and separated
- Offers better clinician access for control of fetal head
- Need an assistant to hold upper leg

Anesthesia (Optional)

- Regional anesthesia (see Chapter 3, Nitrous oxide or Chapter 10, Epidural Anesthesia and Analgesia; Chapter 152, Intrathecal Analgesia in Labor; and Chapter 155, Saddle Block Anesthesia)
- Paracervical block, for first stage of labor to decrease the discomfort with contractions (see Chapter 153, Paracervical Block)
- Pudendal block, for perineal pain in the second stage (see Chapter 154, Pudendal Anesthesia)
- Local lidocaine infiltration if episiotomy is required (routine episiotomy is contraindicated; see Chapter 158, Episiotomy and Repair of the Perineum)

Delivery

There are many variations in technique for vaginal delivery. There is not one "right" way to deliver a vertex infant. Two commonly debated techniques are the "hands on" and "hands poised" techniques. Essentially, the "hands on" technique is a process by which the provider puts pressure on the baby's head and supports the mother's perineum throughout the delivery process. The "hands poised" technique requires the provider to allow spontaneous delivery of the head prior to any intervention. No significant differences in outcomes have been shown between the two methods and either is acceptable practice. This section will describe the hands on technique. The hands poised method is similar after delivery of the infant's head.

1. Observe the perineum for distention by the fetal head. When the head is visible (crowning), it is appropriate to apply pressure to the infant's head to control the force of delivery and to support the perineum with gentle pressure. Either hand may be used.
2. Routine episiotomy causes more posterior perineal trauma, need for suturing, healing complications, and later dyspareunia compared to restrictive episiotomy. Insufficient evidence exists as to whether there are any indications for episiotomy (e.g., operative vaginal delivery, nonreassuring fetal tracing, preterm or breech delivery, possible macrosomia, imminent tears [Berghella et al., 2008]; see also Chapter 158, Episiotomy and Repair of the Perineum).
3. As the head advances, make sure to control its progress. Maintain flexion of the head with pressure applied through a blue towel placed on the perineum. The head should be delivered slowly, in a controlled manner, as it edges forward with each contraction. Between contractions the head will gradually extend. Recall that as the head extends, it increases in diameter. Do not allow the head to extend too rapidly or the chin may tear the perineum. In other words, palpate the chin (through the towel over the perineum), and prevent it from "popping" (suddenly extending) and tearing the perineum.
4. For an OP delivery, the head is usually delivered more readily by applying flexion, not extension. Perineal tension can be very high, resulting in a third- or fourth-degree laceration. Gently controlling the amount of flexion with a hand, through the towel on the perineum, may minimize the risk of lacerations.
5. Once the head is delivered, instruct the mother to stop pushing. Wipe the mucus out of the infant's nose and mouth. There is no evidence that oronasal suctioning by a bulb or catheter is beneficial in healthy term neonates. If suctioning is performed, clear the mouth first, and then the nose, with a bulb syringe to decrease aspiration risk as newborns are obligate nose breathers.

6. After the head is delivered, check for a nuchal cord (occurs in 27% of deliveries). Although most studies fail to show adverse outcomes with nuchal cords, no guidelines exist for management (Kong et al., 2015). Reduction is best accomplished by gently sliding the cord over the neonate's head when possible. Another newer technique is to attempt a fetal "side somersault" although further study is warranted. If the nuchal cord cannot be reduced, it can be doubly clamped and cut on the perineum. Deliver the neonate without delay because blood supply and oxygenation are interrupted until fully delivered.
7. The head should rotate to transverse so the shoulders assume an AP position. Delivery of the shoulders involves slow and deliberate motions without excessive traction. Gently guide the head toward the floor (Fig. 156.6A), and once the anterior shoulder has cleared the symphysis, guide the fetal head upward (see Fig. 156.6B). Lifting the head in this way permits posterior shoulder delivery. As the posterior shoulder is delivered, it should also be prevented from "popping" through the perineum and possibly causing a third- or fourth-degree laceration. If shoulder dystocia is a concern, deliver the head and shoulders in one controlled continuous motion to prevent the anterior shoulder from becoming impacted against the symphysis.

EDITOR'S NOTE: Although management of shoulder dystocia is beyond the scope of this chapter (see "Continuing Education" section), several maneuvers used for shoulder dystocia may be useful even in the absence of dystocia. Having practiced these maneuvers during routine deliveries also may be beneficial when a shoulder dystocia finally arises. To perform the Rubin II maneuver, enter the vagina with your hand and apply two fingers against the back of the fetus's anterior shoulder. Apply pressure to rotate it toward the front of the infant and in effect "shrug" the baby's shoulders (adduct them). This will decrease their AP (bisacromial) diameter. At the same time, the clinician's other hand can be applied to the infant's posterior shoulder from the front of the infant. Applying pressure here will abduct this shoulder, and rotate it toward the

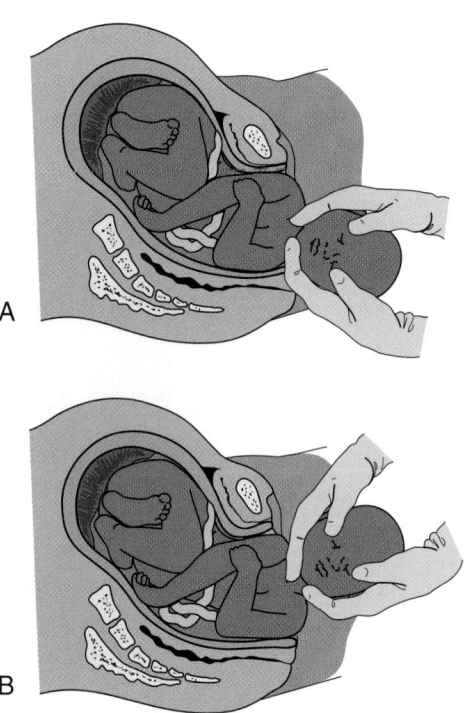

Fig. 156.6 (A) Gentle downward traction to bring about descent of anterior shoulder. (B) After anterior shoulder delivers, applying gentle upward traction delivers the posterior shoulder. (Modified from Ratcliffe S, Baxley EG, Byrd J, Sakornbut E. *Family Practice Obstetrics.* 2nd ed. Philadelphia: Hanley & Belfus; 2001.)

back of the infant. With both maneuvers applied at the same time, the infant's shoulders turning together approximates the turning of a threaded screw (Woods' screw). Attempting to deliver the posterior arm by reaching in and flexing the posterior arm at the elbow and then rotating it across the fetal torso is a third option.

8. Next, support the neonate's head and neck and place a finger in the infant's axilla to maintain lateral flexion of the trunk as the arms deliver. The trunk is easily delivered with gentle, continuous traction. Support the trunk with the hand or arm not supporting the fetal head and neck. Once the entire body is delivered, dry and stimulate the neonate. Delayed cord clamping after 30 to 60 seconds is associated with benefits in term infants, including higher birth weight, improved iron stores at 3 months, and improved transition phase, although there is also increased risk for jaundice. Keeping the neonate at a level lower than the placenta is not necessary prior to cord clamping. Some clinicians place the newborn on the mother's chest or abdomen while clamping the cord. The infant should be dried rapidly with towels while initial Apgar scores are being obtained.

If cord blood gas collection is warranted, apply two additional plastic or Kocher clamps to the cord 10 to 20 cm distal to the original Kocher clamp placed when the cord was cut. Transect between the most distal clamps and send the cord section clamped on either end to the laboratory. On-site blood gas collection is another option. Obtain one sample from the umbilical vein, as well as from one of the umbilical arteries, by drawing blood into a 1- or 2-mL heparin-flushed syringe. Samples should be immediately labeled and transported on ice to the laboratory. A delay in clamping or collection can cause inaccurate results.

Third Stage

Active management of the third stage of labor decreases maternal blood loss, postpartum hemorrhage (PPH), length of the third stage, and the need for maternal blood transfusion. Despite an increase in maternal nausea and vomiting, active management of the third stage of labor is highly encouraged.

1. Once the anterior shoulder is delivered, consider administering an oxytocic agent. Usually this is given intravenously (20 to 40 units in 1 L of isotonic solution over 8 hours). Evidence suggests that oxytocin immediately after delivery of the anterior shoulder is beneficial to the patient in terms of blood loss.
2. Release the clamp on the cord still attached to the placenta to collect 7 to 10 mL of cord blood. Verify the cord has two arteries and a vein. With a birth prevalence around 1%, single umbilical artery is the most frequent congenital anomaly (Rittler et al., 2010). Presence of a two-vessel cord is associated with increased risk of congenital malformations, especially renal, although the presence of single umbilical artery is neither diagnostically sensitive nor specific. After the cord blood is collected, the clamp may either be reapplied or the cord left to drain. Draining the cord slightly reduces the length of third stage of labor (around 3 minutes shorter) and decreases blood loss (around 75 mL), although no differences are seen in retained placenta or PPH risk (Soltani et al., 2011).
3. While waiting for the placenta to deliver, place one hand (on a sterile drape) over the fundus (Brandt maneuver) while assessing uterine tone. Apply firm traction on the cord with the other hand. Avoid overaggressive pulling which can avulse the cord. Monitor the uterus for atony or any signs of uterine inversion (see "Complications" section).
4. Placental separation occurs when the uterus becomes more globular, the cord lengthens, and a gush of vaginal blood is seen. The placenta usually separates within 5 minutes after delivery, but may take as long as 30 minutes. Once separation occurs, ask the mother to bear down gently. This normally creates enough

pressure to expel the placenta. If not, "milk" the placenta out of the birth canal by placing one hand on the fundus and using it to exert slight to moderate amount of pressure. This should propel the placenta into the vagina (Fig. 156.7). Most clinicians deliver the placenta with gentle twisting traction to help remove membranes. After the placenta has cleared the introitus, gently remove any remaining or attached membranes with ring forceps. Always examine the placenta to make sure it is intact using the basin or delivery table. Retained clots or membranes are a risk factor for PPH. If a portion of the placenta is missing, manually enter the vagina and uterus to retrieve these fragments (see manual delivery of the placenta below).

If the placenta fails to deliver within 30 minutes, consider a contracted cervical ring. This diagnosis is possible if signs of placental separation have already occurred but the placenta does not follow. The Brandt maneuver will often deliver the placenta: apply firm pressure suprapubically to hold the uterus in place, apply firm traction on the umbilical cord, and attempt to deliver the placenta.

Manual Delivery of the Placenta

Manual placenta removal is indicated if the placenta does not deliver within 30 minutes or if significant bleeding occurs and the uterus fails to clamp down. It affects 3% of vaginal deliveries. Injection of oxytocin (2 mL/20 IU in 20 mL of normal saline) into the placental side of the clamped cord (umbilical vein) may be helpful if the uterus remains boggy. It will occasionally result in uterine contraction and delivery of the placenta.

For manual removal, don sterile gloves and place the dominant hand in the vagina. Slide fingertips through the cervix to locate the intrauterine placental edge. Locate the cleavage plane between the placenta and the uterine wall. Gently follow this plane and manually separate the placenta from the uterine wall. After complete separation, cup the placenta with the dominant hand, and slowly withdraw both hand and placenta. If the cleavage plane cannot be

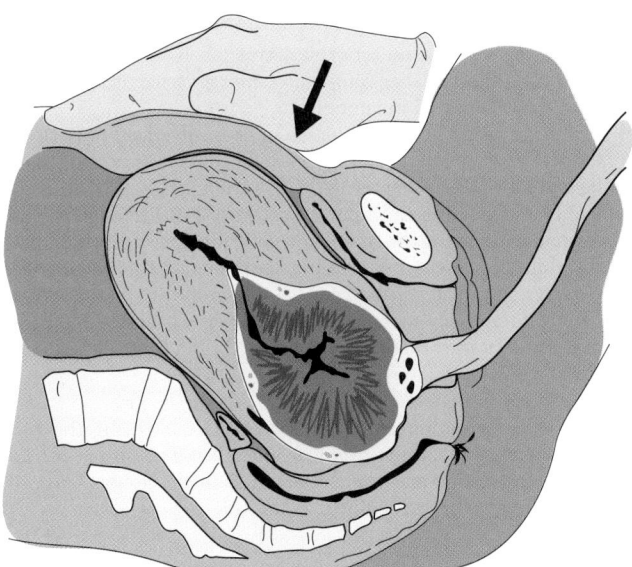

Fig. 156.7 Expression of placenta. Note that the hand is *not* trying to push the fundus of the uterus through the birth canal. As the placenta leaves the uterus and enters the vagina, the uterus is elevated (fundus pushed upward and posteriorly) by the hand on the abdomen *(arrow)* while the cord is held in position. The mother can aid in the delivery of the placenta by bearing down. As the placenta reaches the perineum, the cord is lifted, which in turn lifts the placenta out of the vagina. Adherent membranes are eased away from thin attachments to prevent their being torn off and retained in the birth canal.

separated or parts of the plane cannot be separated completely, prepare for surgical removal.

Covering the sterile glove on the inserted hand with a 4 × 4 gauze may give additional traction when sweeping the uterus. Such sweeps may also be useful in vaginal birth after cesarean patients, for those bleeding excessively, or for premature deliveries. Confirm (if not previously done) that the cord has three vessels. If not given after anterior shoulder delivery, IV oxytocin should be administered and bimanual uterine massage performed to help reduce atony. If atony and bleeding persist, intramuscular (IM) methylergonovine (0.2 mg IM [normotensive patients only]) or 15-methyl prostaglandin (250 μg IM) can be given. A 600 to 800 μg dose of misoprostol placed in the posterior vaginal fornix is another pharmacologic option for atony. After the uterus is firm, begin any necessary repair.

SAMPLE OPERATIVE REPORT

A 28-year-old G2P1 at 39 weeks' gestation by 18-week ultrasound was admitted for contractions and rupture of membranes. Epidural anesthesia was provided. Fetal heart monitoring was category 1 throughout labor. Patient progressed from 6 cm at admission to complete and pushing at 08:00. Patient delivered a viable female infant over intact perineum via normal spontaneous vaginal delivery at 08:35. Amniotic fluid was clear. Nuchal cord × 1 manually reduced. Anterior shoulder delivered without incident. IV oxytocin 40 units in 1 L of normal saline started after delivery of the anterior shoulder. Infant mouth and nose were wiped clean. Infant was vigorous, with Apgar scores of 8 and 9 at 1 and 5 minutes. Cord was clamped and cut after 1 minute and infant was placed on maternal abdomen. Placenta delivered intact with three-vessel cord. No cervical, vaginal, or perineal lacerations were noted. Estimated blood loss 300 mL. Mother and newborn were stable and remained in the delivery room.

If vacuum or forceps are applied, the delivery note should also include indication, consent, position, station, number of applications, and time of application (see Chapter 157, Forceps- and Vacuum-Assisted Deliveries).

COMMON ERRORS

- Admitting patient when not in active labor. Women in active labor have shorter labor courses and undergo fewer interventions than those admitted in latent labor.
- Failure to diagnose fetal malpresentation. If uncertainty about fetal lie exists, Leopold maneuvers and bedside ultrasound should be performed (see Chapter 142, Obstetric Ultrasound).
- Failure to recognize and address a category 2 or 3 tracing. A team approach involving the nurses and delivering providers enhances the ability to detect abnormalities in the fetal heart tracing (see Chapter 146: Antepartum Fetal Monitoring).
- Failure to actively manage the third stage of labor. Good evidence shows that this protocol decreases PPH, but it has been slow to be adopted in some settings.
- Liberal episiotomy use: episiotomy use should be rare.
- Poor documentation of labor progress. Documenting the provider's presence and involvement in the labor process is crucial. All interventions must be documented in the medical record, including fetal heart rate interpretation.

COMPLICATIONS
Maternal Complications

- Perineal pain and postpartum dyspareunia are commonly seen after vaginal delivery, especially those involving perineal or vaginal trauma. Restrictive episiotomy use has been shown to reduce the risk of more severe tears and postpartum perineal pain. When perineal repair is required, a continuous, knotless suturing technique with absorbable synthetic suture decreases postpartum analgesia needs as well as dyspareunia at 12 months.

- PPH is a leading cause of maternal death both in the United States and globally. The ACOG reVITALize program recently reclassified PPH as blood loss greater than 1000 mL, regardless of whether at vaginal or cesarean delivery. In young, healthy women, hemodynamic instability may not manifest until more than 1.5 to 2 L of blood are lost. Causes of PPHs are classified into four categories:
  1. Tone: Uterine atony is responsible for 70% to 80% of PPH. Bimanual uterine massage and prophylactic oxytocin often improve tone, with use of agents such as misoprostol, methylergonovine, and carboprost given if PPH is suspected.
  2. Trauma: Perineal, cervical, and vaginal lacerations, as well as uterine rupture or inversion, should be ruled out as causes of bleeding. These account for 20% of PPH cases.
  3. Tissue: Retained tissue and invasive placenta account for 10% of PPH. In some cases, manual placenta removal becomes necessary. In the case of undiagnosed invasive placenta (placenta accreta, increta, or percreta) at delivery, surgical consultation and intervention are required.
  4. Thrombin: Coagulation disorders are rare causes of PPH (<1%). Most are previously identified, allowing for planning and management prior to vaginal delivery. Early recognition, immediate fluid resuscitation, and identification and treatment of the underlying cause constitute usual management.
    - Endometritis after an uncomplicated vaginal delivery is more common with uterine manipulation, instrumentation, or prolonged labor and rupture of membranes. Retained products of conception (placenta or membranes) also increases infection risk.
    - Uterine inversion is an infrequent complication of vaginal delivery. Risk factors include a fundal placenta, uterine atony, and congenital weakness of the uterus. Management begins with calling for assistance, including general anesthesia, and immediately attempting to replace the uterus. If possible, it should be replaced without removing the placenta. If the uterus is not easily replaceable, tocolysis use has an 85% to 90% success rate. Oxytocin should be discontinued and the uterus relaxed with IV beta-mimetic medications or magnesium sulfate (preferred). The remaining 15% to 20% of patients require general anesthesia. After replacement, oxytocin should be restarted and any sign of PPH managed aggressively.
    - A rare complication of vaginal delivery is amniotic fluid embolism, occurring in 1 of 40,000 deliveries, with a mortality rate of 20% to 60% (Shamshirsaz and Clark, 2016). Amniotic fluid embolism presents with rapid, unexpected respiratory distress and cardiovascular collapse, leading to disseminated intravascular coagulopathy, coma, and death. Rapid clinical diagnosis and aggressive intensive care unit management can reduce mortality risk, although progression can be very rapid and difficult to reverse.

Fetal Complications

Major risks to a fetus during labor are trauma and hypoxia. Numerous problems can occur, but most newborns survive delivery without complication. Following is a partial list of possible neonatal complications:

- Respiratory distress
- Hemodynamic instability
- Neonatal sepsis
- Intracranial hemorrhage
- Brachial plexus damage
- Fractures (humerus and clavicle most commonly)
- Hypoxic ischemic encephalopathy and associated problems, although hypoxic ischemic encephalopathy may occur remote from labor from in utero insults

Management of these complications is beyond the scope of this chapter. Chapter 163, Neonatal Resuscitation, gives an overview of the acute treatment of emergent neonatal complications.

POSTPROCEDURE MANAGEMENT

Unless delivered in a labor-delivery-recovery-postpartum room, the patient is transferred to a postpartum room approximately 2 hours after an uneventful vaginal delivery. Discharge home usually occurs 24 to 48 hours later.

Assessment of uterine tone by checking the fundus transabdominally and assessing for vaginal bleeding by checking pads is usual care while in recovery stage. The uterine fundus should be firm and below the umbilicus. Vital signs should be hemodynamically stable prior to transfer. If concern for PPH or other complication exists, transfer to the postpartum floor should be delayed.

Routine postpartum care includes evaluation of vaginal bleeding or infection. The patient should be instructed regarding the normal amount of vaginal bleeding after delivery (lochia rubra), return to normal function, and the fact that nursing will cause uterine contractions. She should also be monitored for signs and symptoms of postpartum blues and depression, mastitis, venous thromboembolism, constipation, and sleep disturbance. Acetaminophen, ibuprofen, naproxen, and acetaminophen with codeine are all acceptable for pain control. For constipation, Milk of Magnesia, docusate sodium, Dulcolax suppository, or psyllium may be helpful. Routine blood count measurements are generally not indicated following an uncomplicated vaginal delivery. Prior to discharge, birth control options should be discussed and instructions given to not start estrogen-containing methods for at least a month due to increased thrombosis risk.

POSTPROCEDURE PATIENT EDUCATION

Patients should be given specific instructions about their medications and other postpartum care issues at hospital discharge. Breast care instructions should be provided whether patients are breast-feeding or not. Sitz baths, Peri-Pads, and other perineal care can be discussed. Inform patients about when to call the clinician. Pelvic rest should be maintained for at least 1 month. Make a follow-up appointment 4 to 6 weeks after the delivery. Counsel women about baby blues, postpartum depression, and postpartum psychosis. Women with gestational diabetes require glucose testing at their follow-up visit.

INTERPRETATION OF RESULTS

Although fetal acidosis at birth is uncommon in most term, low-risk deliveries, an understanding of fetal acid-base status is important. The most objective way to assess for fetal acidosis at birth is by analysis of umbilical cord blood at delivery. This information can be useful in differentiating those newborns who are "depressed" (have low Apgar scores) from those who are truly acidotic at delivery. The pH, PCO_2, PO_2, CO_2, hemoglobin, and oxygen content of the blood can be measured, and the bicarbonate concentration, oxygen saturation, and base excess/deficit calculated from these measurements. Table 156.1 shows normal values for these measurements.

The most useful lab value for assessing fetal condition is pH. Fetal pH is typically 0.1 unit lower than maternal pH. The mean arterial fetal pH is 7.28, with the 5th and 95th percentiles at 7.14 and 7.40, respectively. The risk of neonatal morbidity is inversely related to pH, with the highest risk for those with pH less than 6.9. In several studies, umbilical artery pH less than 7 was predictive of neonatal morbidity (e.g., seizures). However, it should be noted that the majority of newborns with pH less than 7 were admitted to the regular newborn nursery and had an uncomplicated neonatal course. Umbilical artery PO_2 does not predict adverse neonatal outcome.

The calculated base deficit or excess is also useful, because metabolic acidosis leads to excess production of acid, or a negative base excess (base deficit). A base deficit greater than 12 mmol/L is suggestive of neonatal complications. Fetal blood gas analysis does not distinguish between potential causes of fetal acidosis; fetal, placental, and maternal factors can all play a role.

CPT/BILLING CODES

59400	Global vaginal delivery (routine obstetric care, including antepartum care, vaginal delivery [with or without episiotomy, and/or forceps] and postpartum care)
59409	Vaginal delivery only (with or without episiotomy, and/or forceps)
59410	Vaginal delivery only (with or without episiotomy, and/or forceps) and postpartum care (no antepartum care)
59430	Postpartum care only
59610	Global VBAC delivery (routine obstetric care including antepartum care, vaginal delivery [with or without episiotomy and/or forceps] and postpartum care after previous cesarean delivery)
59612	Vaginal delivery only, after previous cesarean delivery
59614	Vaginal delivery only, after previous cesarean delivery including postpartum care
59899	Unlisted procedure maternity care and delivery (induction, etc.)

NOTE: A patient who is admitted for labor that is post-term, induced, augmented, or otherwise complicated (blood pressure problems, arrest of labor, fetal distress, etc.) is not considered a routine delivery. These types of deliveries should be coded using routine inpatient or outpatient evaluation and management codes (e.g., 99221 to 99223).

99291	Critical care, evaluation of the critically ill or critically injured patient, first 30 to 74 minutes (e.g., preeclampsia, placenta previa or abruptio, postpartum hemorrhage, pulmonary or amniotic fluid embolism)
99292	Each additional 30 minutes
99356	Prolonged physician service in the inpatient setting, requiring direct (face-to-face) patient contact beyond the usual routine service, but not in critical care unit (e.g., maternity fetal monitoring for high-risk delivery or other physiologic monitoring); first hour
99357	Each additional 30 minutes
99358	Prolonged evaluation and management service before and/or after direct face-to-face patient care (e.g., review of extensive records and tests, communication with other professionals and/or patient/family); first hour
99359	Each additional 30 minutes

NOTE: A good reference for coding is provided by the American Academy of Family Physicians at http://www.aafp.org/online/en/home/practicemgt/codingresources/codingob.html.

ICD-10-CM DIAGNOSTIC CODES

O48.0	Post-term pregnancy (40–42 weeks)
O48.1	Prolonged pregnancy (>42 weeks)
O99.210	Obesity complicating pregnancy, childbirth, or the puerperium unspecified trimester
O80	Normal delivery

TABLE 156.1	Normal Ranges for Cord Blood Gas Analysis
pH	7.27–7.28
PCO_2 (mm Hg)	49.2–50.3
HCO_3^- (mEq/L)	22–23.1
Base excess (mEq/L)	−2.7 to −3.6

O34.219	Maternal care unspecified type scar from previous cesarean section
O77.9	Fetal distress
O41.00X0	Oligohydramnios unspecified trimester
O42.00	Premature rupture of membranes unspecified weeks of gestation
O75.2	Pyrexia in labor NOC
O09.40	Supervision of pregnancy with grand multiparity unspecified trimester
O76	Abnormality in fetal heart rate or rhythm complicating labor delivery
O63.0	Prolonged first stage of labor
O63.1	Prolonged second stage of labor
O69.0X0	Prolapse of cord
069.2X0	Cord around neck, with compression
O70.1	Perineal laceration, second degree
O70.20	Perineal laceration, third degree
O70.3	Perineal laceration, fourth degree
O72.1	Postpartum hemorrhage
O73.1	Retained placenta/membranes
O28.9	Meconium staining

ONLINE RESOURCES

AAFP coding resources: https://www.aafp.org/fpm/toolBox/viewToolBox.htm

Centers for Disease Control Group B Strep online app: https://www.cdc.gov/groupbstrep/guidelines/prevention-app.html Accessed May 28, 2018.

Cochrane Collaboration: Pregnancy and Childbirth. https://pregnancy.cochrane.org/our-reviews

Patient Education from the U.S. government: www.womenshealth.gov/pregnancy

Tuggy M, Garcia J: Procedures Consult. Vaginal delivery. http://www.proceduresconsult.com/medical-procedures/vaginal-delivery-FM-011-procedure.aspx

CONTINUING EDUCATION

Advanced Life Support in Obstetrics (ALSO)

This course provides practice for both the cognitive and the manual skills for simple or complicated deliveries. Lifelike pelvic and infant mannequins allow the learner to practice in a calm environment, even using forceps or vacuum-assisted delivery equipment. Courses are taught throughout the United States as well as internationally. See https://www.aafp.org/also.

Family-Centered Maternity Care Conference

This course is designed to provide state-of-the-art, evidence-based education in the knowledge, training, and skills of caring for patients and their families during pregnancy and the birth process. It is organized by the American Academy of Family Physicians (AAFP). See https://www.aafp.org/.

RECOMMENDED READING

American College of Obstetricians and Gynecologist. Cesarean delivery on maternal request. Committee Opinion No. 559. Obstet Gynecol. 2013;121:904–907.

American College of Obstetricians and Gynecologists. Umbilical cord blood gas and acid-base analysis. Committee Opinion No. 348. Obstet Gynecol. 2006;108:1319–1322.

American College of Obstetricians and Gynecologists. Vaginal birth after previous cesarean. Practice Bulletin No. 115. Obstet Gynecol. 2010;116(2):450–463.

American Academy of Pediatrics, American College of Obstetricians and Gynecologists. Neonatal Encephalopathy and Cerebral Palsy: Defining the Pathogenesis and Pathophysiology. Elk Grove Village, IL, AAP; Washington, DC: ACOG; 2003.

Andres RL, Saade G, Gilstrap LC, Wilkins I. Association between umbilical blood gas parameters and neonatal morbidity and death in neonates with pathologic fetal acidemia. Am J Obstet Gynecol. 1999;181(4):867–871.

Berghella V, Baxter J, Chauhan SP. Evidence-based labor and delivery management. Am J Obstet Gynecol. 2008:445–454.

Brown HC, Paranjothy S, Dowswell T, et al. Package of care for antepartum management in labour for reducing caesarean section rates in low-risk women. Cochrane Database Syst Rev. 2013;9:CD004907.

Carroli G, Mignini L. Episiotomy for vaginal birth. Cochrane Database Syst Rev. 2009;1:CD000081.

Committee on Obstetric Practice. American College of Obstetricians and Gynecologists. Committee opinion No. 543: timing of umbilical cord clamping after birth. Obstet Gynecol. 2012;120(6):1522–1526.

Daoub A, Drake TM. Congenital abnormalities of the urogenital tract; the clus is in the cord? MJ Case Rep. 2014.

Hamm RF, Wang EY, Bastek JA, et al. Assessing revitalize: should the definition of postpartum hemorrhage differ by mode of delivery? Amer J Perinatol. 2017;34(05):503–507.

Kelleher J, Bhat R, Salas AA, et al. Oronasopharyngeal suction verus wiping of the mouth and nose at birth: a randomized equivalency trial. Lancet. 2013;382:326.

Kong CW, Lin WC, Kee WW. Neonatal outcome and mode of delivery in the presence of nuchal cord loops: implications on patient counseling and the mode of delivery. Arch Gynecol Obstet. 2015;292(2):283–289.

Landon MB, Grobman WA. What we have learned about trial of labor after cesarean delivery from the maternal-fetal medicine units cesarean registry. Sem Perinatology. 2016;40(5):281–286.

Landon M, Spong CY, Thorn E, et al. Risk of uterine rupture with a trial of labor in women with multiple and single prior cesarean delivery. Obstet Gynecol. 2006;108(1):12–20.

Millen KR, Kuo K, Zhao L, et al. Evidence-based guidelines in labor management. Obstet Gynecol Survey. 2014;69(4):209–217.

Osborne K, Hanson L. Labor down or bear down: a strategy to translate second-stage labor evidence to perinatal practice. J Perinat Neonat Nurs. 2014;28(2):117–126.

Rittler M, Mazzitelli N, Fuksman R, et al. Single umbilical artery and associated malformations in over 5500 autopsies: relevance for perinatal management. Pediatr Dev Pathol. 2010;13:465–470.

Shamshirsaz AA, Clark SL. Amniotic fluid embolism. Obstet Gynecol Clin North Am. 2016;43(4):779–790.

Soltani H, Poulose TA. Hutchon DR Placental cord drainage after vaginal delivery as part of the management of the third stage of labor. Cochrane Database Syst Rev. 2011;9:CD004665.

Smith D, Stringer E, Vladutiu CJ. Risk of uterine rupture among women attempting vaginal birth after cesarean with an unknown uterine scar. Am J Obstet Gyencol. 2015;213(1): 80e–80e5.

Spong C, Berghella V, Wenstrom KD, et al. Preventing the first cesarean delivery: summary of a joint Eunice Kennedy Shriver National Institute of Child Health and Human Development, Society ofMaternal-Fetal Medicine and American College of Obstetricians and Gynecologists Workshop. Obstet Gynecol. 2012;120:1181–1193.

Verani JR, McGee L, Schrag SJ. Prevention of perinatal group B streptococcal disease, revised guidelines from CDC. 2010 MMWR. 2010;59:1–32. RR-10.

Zhang J, Landy HJ, Branch DW, et al. Contemporary patterns of spontaneous labor with normal neonatal outcomes. Obstet Gynecol. 2010;116:1281–1287.

CHAPTER 157

FORCEPS- AND VACUUM-ASSISTED DELIVERIES

Carol Osborn • Jennifer Bell • Dale A. Patterson

Knowledge and experience with operative vaginal delivery (instrument-assisted forceps or vacuum extraction) are important for all obstetrics providers managing the second stage of labor, particularly for emergencies such as severe maternal or fetal compromise. In unexpected situations, competent use of operative vaginal delivery may be lifesaving and help reduce morbidity. Assisted deliveries are also a safe alternative to cesarean delivery, as long as criteria and indications are followed. Rates of operative vaginal delivery are decreasing (especially forceps deliveries), in part because incidence of cesarean delivery is increasing. Between 2005 and 2013, of 22,598,971 deliveries in the United States, 1083 (4.8%) were vacuum-assisted and 237,792 (1.1%) used forceps; overall vacuum use decreased from 5.8% to 4.1%, while forceps use decreased from 1.4% to 0.9% in this time period (Merriam, 2017).

The safe use of these procedures depends on correctly understanding and judging the station and position of the vertex. A Cochrane review comparing forceps with vacuum found slightly more deliveries with vacuum, and fewer cesarean deliveries, less maternal trauma, and less general and regional anesthesia use with vacuum. However, vacuum extraction was associated with an increase in neonatal cephalohematoma and retinal hemorrhages. Serious neonatal injury was uncommon with either form of assisted delivery or instrument. The failure rate of forceps is 7%, whereas the failure rate for vacuum extraction is 12%.

CLASSIFICATION

As operative vaginal delivery became further defined, over the past few decades, because of difficulties in estimating engagement and in defining fetal stations, the American College of Obstetrics and Gynecology further defined and classified instrumented deliveries in order to improve the safety of operative vaginal delivery.

Outlet Forceps or Vacuum

- Fetal skull has reached the pelvic floor.
- Fetal scalp is visible at the introitus between contractions without separating the labia.
- Sagittal suture is in an anteroposterior diameter (i.e., occipitoanterior [OA], right occipitoanterior, left occipitoanterior, occipitoposterior [OP], right occipitoposterior, or left occipitoposterior) that is less than 45 degrees from the midline.

Low Forceps or Vacuum

- Leading edge of the vertex is at +2 or greater station.
- Fetal head at this station fills the hollow of the sacrum.
- Head is not on the pelvic floor.
- Rotations can be less than 45 degrees or greater than 45 degrees from the midline.

Midforceps or Vacuum

- Head is engaged, although vertex is higher than +2 station.
- Advisable only in emergency situations and only for providers with demonstrated training and competence with this method.

With the classification change, the term *high forceps* was eliminated. High forceps described forceps application before engagement of the vertex. This procedure has no place in modern obstetrics because of unacceptably high morbidity rates. Mid-instrumentation is reserved for providers who are experienced with this application. If a provider is uncomfortable with the evaluation or application of forceps, a cesarean delivery is likely a safer route of delivery.

Before any operative vaginal delivery, the position and station of the vertex presentation must be determined. First, verify fetal engagement. By definition, engagement indicates that the biparietal diameter has passed the plane of the pelvic inlet. Clinically, the fetal skull is at or below the ischial spines (i.e., 0 station). Checking the amount of space between the fetal head and the symphysis gives an additional measurement of station (Fig. 157.1).

Ability to ensure complete engagement and assess descent are complicated by (1) molding, which leads to overestimation of descent or station, and (2) asynclitism or OP presentation, which also leads to overestimation of station. To avoid this miscalculation, confirm that the fetal head fills the sacral hollow. When the vertex fills the sacral hollow, there should not be room to admit the examiner's fingers on vaginal exam.

Position can be difficult to determine, especially with marked caput. The following method helps determine position:

- Anterior fontanelle is shaped like a cross or plus (+) and is usually larger than the posterior fontanelle.
- Posterior fontanelle is Y-shaped.
- When in doubt, the fetal ears help determine position by the direction in which they bend.

If the fetal position and station meet criteria for an operative vaginal delivery, the provider must consider whether to use forceps or a vacuum to assist the delivery. Risks and benefit of forceps versus vacuum extraction are described in Box 157.1.

INDICATIONS

Conditions Required for Instrumentation

- Vertex presentation (Vertex presentation is required for vacuum and outlet or low forceps applications. Breech deliveries using Piper forceps for the aftercoming head are not discussed in this chapter.)
- Complete cervical dilatation
- Ruptured membranes
- No known severe cephalopelvic disproportion

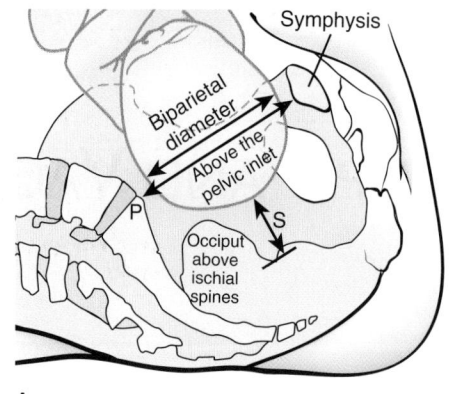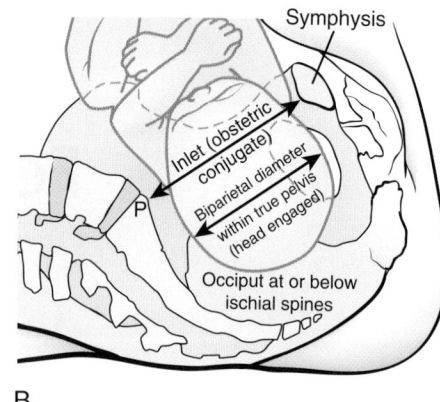

Fig. 157.1 (A) When the lowermost portion of the fetal head is above the ischial spines, the biparietal diameter of the head is not likely to have passed through the pelvic inlet and therefore is not engaged. (B) When the lowermost portion of the fetal head is at or below the ischial spines, it is usually engaged. Exceptions occur when there is considerable molding, caput formation, or both. *P*, Sacral promontory; *S*, ischial spine. (Modified from Cunningham FG, MacDonald P, Gant N, et al., eds. *William's Obstetrics*. 19th ed. East Norwalk, CT: Appleton & Lange; 1993.)

BOX 157.1   Forceps versus Vacuum Extraction

Forceps
Pros
Higher rate of successful vaginal delivery
Usually a more rapid delivery (e.g., for fetal distress)
Useful in breech (for the aftercoming head) and face presentations
Useful for rotations by experienced providers
Cons
Requires significant experience
Increased risk of neonatal craniofacial injuries
Increased risk of intracranial hemorrhage
Requires more maternal anesthesia
Associated with more cervical, vaginal, and perineal lacerations

Vacuum
Pros
Easy to apply
Teaches the provider to follow the pelvic curve
Allows autorotation from occipitoposterior and occipitotransverse positions
Less force applied to the head
Requires less anesthesia
Results in fewer cervical, vaginal, and perineal lacerations
Easier to learn
Can use if not completely sure of head position
Cons
Difficult to maintain vacuum if head is molded or infant has full head of hair
Pull only with contractions, which increases time needed for successful delivery
Associated with intracranial hemorrhage at a greater rate than spontaneous deliveries
Only useful in vertex presentations
Increased incidence of cephalohematomas and retinal hemorrhage
Slightly higher failure rate (12%) versus forceps (7%)

- Willingness to abandon procedure and proceed to cesarean delivery if unsuccessful
- Adequate anesthesia (ideally epidural, although saddle block or pudendal block are also options)

Maternal Indications for Instrument Delivery

- Maternal exhaustion. This is associated with prolonged second-stage pushing. Maternal exhaustion is especially common with nulliparous labor. The lack of a trained labor companion during the second stage is associated with a longer labor and increased use of instrumentation.
- Lack of maternal cooperation.
- Lack of informed consent for cesarean.
- Prolonged second stage or failure to progress. The average second stage is 50 minutes for primiparous patients and 20 minutes for multiparous patients. Regional anesthesia prolongs the second stage by inhibiting the maternal urge to push (Table 157.1).
- Medical conditions for which the strain of the second stage of labor would be deleterious. Examples include cardiac valvular disease, respiratory disease (e.g., active asthma), cerebrovascular disease, or deteriorating maternal medical conditions such as preeclampsia or chronic hypertension.

Maternal and Fetal Indications for Instrument Delivery

- Relative cephalopelvic disproportion
- Malposition (OP and other factors resulting in difficulty, or occiput transverse)

TABLE 157.1	Limits of the Duration of the Second Stage of Labor Before Intervention	
Parity	Without Regional Anesthetic	With Regional Anesthetic
Nullipara	3 hr	4 hr
Multipara	1 hr	2 hr

- Malpresentation (face or breech); use forceps only as vacuum is contraindicated. For breech deliveries, Piper forceps are often needed for the aftercoming head once the body has been delivered.
- Hemorrhage
- Intrapartum infection

Fetal Indications for Instrument Delivery

- Nonreassuring fetal heart tracing
- Rapid deterioration of the tracing or any condition that makes it unsafe for the fetus
- Premature placental separation

CONTRAINDICATIONS

Absolute
- Fetal head not engaged
- Position of the head not determined (forceps)

Relative

- History of a failed forceps or vacuum delivery with a macrosomic fetus
- Suspected fetal coagulation defect (e.g., hemophilia) or fetal demineralizing disease (e.g., osteogenesis imperfecta)
- Incomplete cervical dilatation (only exceptions are the urgent delivery of a second twin and a severely abnormal tracing without immediately available cesarean delivery)
- Delivery requiring excessive traction
- Prematurity (vacuum not recommended before 34 weeks' gestation because of increased risk of intracranial hemorrhage)
- Malpresentation (e.g., breech, face, brow, transverse lie)
- Prior scalp sampling (vacuum)
- Position of fetal head not precisely determined in vertex presentation (vacuum)

EQUIPMENT

Include all equipment listed for normal vaginal delivery (see Chapter 156, Vaginal Delivery). Modern vacuum extractors are available from numerous suppliers. Both rigid and soft cups are available; each has advantages over the other. Rigid cups more often result in a successful assisted delivery, but they are also more likely to be associated with complications. The operator should be familiar with the models available at the institution and should be trained in their proper use. Any associated tubing or pumps must also be available. The Mityvac is one example of a vacuum apparatus (Fig. 157.2). Tucker-McLean (Fig. 157.3) and Simpson (Fig. 157.4) forceps are commonly used in vertex presentation of term infants. Local availability and user training should determine the type of forceps employed. Both forceps and vacuum equipment should be readily available on all labor floors.

PRECAUTIONS

The US Food and Drug Administration (FDA) published a public advisory in 1998 concerning complications resulting from vacuum deliveries. The FDA found a fivefold increase in death and serious injury after vacuum deliveries. Although part of this increase may be due to the increased use of this procedure, failing to follow established protocols was a likely underlying factor. The most concerning complication is subgaleal hematoma, which can be life-threatening. The duration of vacuum application is an important factor in the development of complications. It is not recommended to apply a vacuum for more than 20 minutes.

PREPROCEDURE PATIENT EDUCATION

Discussing the possibility of the need for vacuum or forceps delivery before a patient is in labor is best, although this is not always possible. Nonetheless, the risks and benefits of the procedure should be explained to the patient in as much detail as possible prior to operative vaginal delivery. Informed consent should be obtained from the patient.

TECHNIQUE

Forceps Delivery

The forceps have interlocking parts, with a right and a left side that correspond to the side of the maternal pelvis on which they lie when applied. Each side has a handle, shank, and blade. Simpson forceps are most commonly used for low and outlet deliveries.

Initially developed by Dr. J. Bachman, the acronym *ABCDEF-GHIJ* has become part of the Advance Life Support in Obstetrics curriculum; it is useful when training for forceps- and vacuum-assisted deliveries. Except for *F*, *G*, and *H*, the acronym is essentially the same for both procedures:

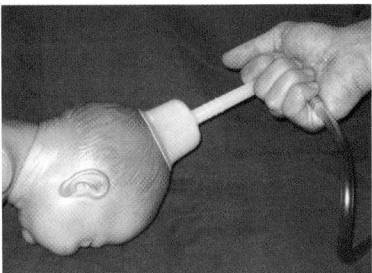

Fig. 157.2   Mityvac extractor.

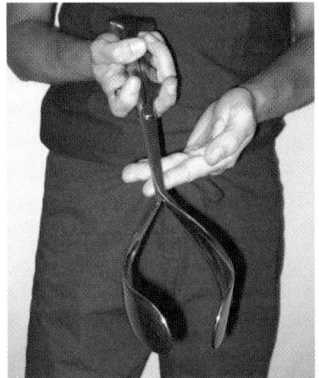

Fig. 157.3   Tucker-McLean forceps.

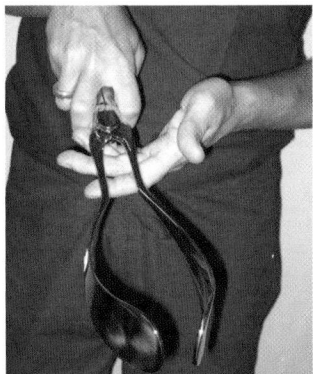

Fig. 157.4   Simpson forceps.

A. Is *anesthesia* adequate? Consider a local or pudendal block or both. *Ask* for help. (e.g., make sure enough nursing personnel and support staff are present).
B. Is the *bladder* empty? Straight catheterize if needed.
C. Is the *cervix* completely dilated?
D. *Determine* the position of the fetal head. Consider shoulder *dystocia* (i.e., why is there a delay?).
   - Anterior fontanelle is larger and forms a cross.
   - Posterior fontanelle is smaller and forms a Y.
   - Find the ear, feeling which way it bends.
   - Fetal descent should be to a +2 station, with the vertex filling the sacrum.
E. Is the *equipment* ready (e.g., cord clamp, instruments, delivery table)?
F. Are the *forceps* ready for application?
   1. Articulate the forceps to ensure a proper fit and that the right and left halves match.
   2. Disarticulate the handles and take the left handle in your left hand (holding it like a pencil with concave cephalic curve toward the vulva and the shank directed upward, perpendicular to the floor).

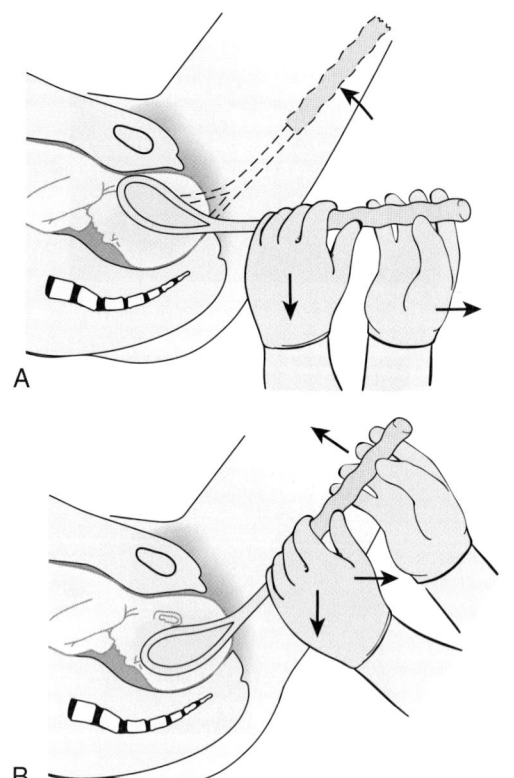

A

B

Fig. 157.5 Occiput anterior delivery by outlet forceps (Simpson). The direction of gentle traction for delivery of the head is indicated. Initially, the forceps are horizontal (A) and they are gradually rotated forward (B). Forces are as noted.

3. Begin to ease the forceps along the left side of the fetal head (OA); use your right hand to protect the maternal sidewalls and guide the blade into position. (The right thumb is placed on the heel of the blade as it is gently inserted.)
4. Right forceps handle is then held in your right hand.
5. Insertion is along the right side of the fetal head, with the left hand protecting the maternal right pelvis and guiding the blade into place.
6. If correctly applied, the handles should fit together and lock easily.
7. Check the application position for safety (posterior fontanelle, fenestration, sagittal suture).
   - Posterior fontanelle should be midway between the shanks and 1 cm above the plane of the shanks.
   - Fenestrations of the forceps should admit no more than one fingertip.
   - Sagittal suture should be midline and midway between the shanks. (For OP deliveries, the blades should be equidistant from the midline of the face and brow.)
G. Use *gentle* traction (i.e., Pajot maneuver) (Fig. 157.5).
   1. The pelvic curve from the inlet through the outlet is described as a J-shaped curve.
   2. Initially, one hand pulls the forceps handles in the same direction that the handles extend (an approximately horizontal vector, outward and away from the mother).
   3. The other hand is placed on the shaft close to the perineum and pushes in a downward vector.
   4. The summation of these two vectors creates an outward-and-downward force.
   5. As the occiput of the head moves from under the symphysis, the traction should shift toward a more upward vector. (For OP deliveries, the horizontal traction continues until the base of the infant's nose passes under the symphysis.)

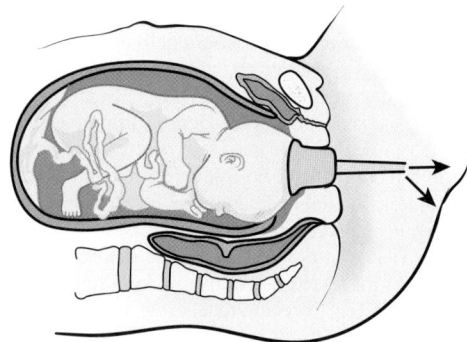

Fig. 157.6 Correct position of the vacuum cup and the correct direction of traction before the vertex clears the symphysis pubis.

H. The *handle* is elevated to follow the J-shaped pelvic curve (see Fig. 157.5B).
I. Evaluate for the need for an episiotomy *incision*. The amount of distention of the perineum will dictate the need. (For OP deliveries, there will be greater distention of the vulva, and a large episiotomy may be needed.) Routine episiotomy is not indicated, and a midline approach increases the risk of third- or fourth-degree extension (see Chapter 158, Episiotomy).
J. Remove the forceps when the *jaw* of the infant is reachable.

Vacuum Delivery

A. Is *anesthesia* adequate? *Ask* for help.
B. Is the *bladder* empty?
C. Is the *cervix* completely dilated?
D. *Determine* the position of the fetal head. Consider shoulder *dystocia* (i.e., why is there a delay?).
   - Anterior fontanelle is larger and forms a cross.
   - Posterior fontanelle is smaller and forms a Y.
   - Find the ear, feeling which way it bends.
   - Descent should be to a +2 station, with the vertex filling the sacrum.
E. *Equipment* and *extractor* ready (vacuum and tubing, infant suction bulb, cord clamp, instrument table, etc.)? When the pump is inflated against a sterilely gloved hand, does it hold pressure?
F. Insert and apply the cup over the posterior *fontanelle*.
   - Wipe vertex clean of blood and fluid.
   - Spread the labia.
   - Compress and insert the cup.
   - Place the cup over the posterior fontanelle (or over the sagittal suture up to 3 cm in front of the posterior fontanelle, toward the fetal face).
   - Sweep the finger around the cup to check for trapped maternal tissue.
   - Calibrate the vacuum dials, noting that yellow (10 mm Hg) is the resting suction and that red (50 mm Hg) is the suction pressure required for traction during contractions.
G. Use *gentle* traction (Fig. 157.6).
   1. Apply traction at right angles to the plane of the applied surface of the cup.
   2. Do not rock or torque the cup or handle. Only use gentle, steady traction.
   3. As the fetal head moves around the symphysis and extends, the vacuum handle will rise from a horizontal to a nearly vertical position. (The angles and traction are more difficult for OP deliveries, with the handle often pointing toward the floor.) Incorrect vectors cause the cup to "pop off" the fetal vertex.
   4. If the cup detaches, consider the following problems: inadequate vacuum suction, trapped maternal tissue, a fetal scalp electrode in the way, incorrect application of the extractor

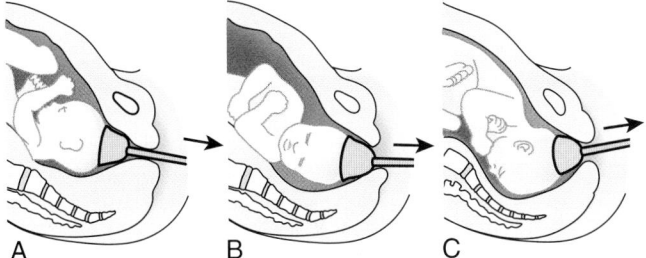

Fig. 157.7 Occipitoposterior application (A), rotation (B), and delivery (C) using vacuum extractor. (Modified from Lowdermilk DL, Perry SE, Bobak IM. *Maternity and Women's Health Care.* 7th ed. St. Louis: Mosby; 2000.)

(not over the flexion point), or bending or rotation of the shaft. Neonatal complications are not significantly different, comparing fetal scalp electrode with vacuum-assisted vaginal delivery and vacuum-assisted vaginal delivery alone.

H. *Halt* traction when the contraction is over.
  1. While vacuum pressure is traditionally reduced to 10 mm Hg between contractions, release of pressure between contractions does not seem to be associated with improved fetal outcomes (e.g. decreased cephalohematoma or fetal scalp injury) [American College of Obstetrics and Gynecology, 2015].
  2. Repeat the gentle traction cycle with the next contraction.
  3. *Halt* the procedure if the cup disengages more than three times, if no progress is noted after three consecutive pulls, or if a delivery does not occur after 20 minutes of intermittent traction. Some studies indicate increased incidence of cephalohematoma when vacuum application time until delivery exceeds 5 minutes.
  4. Use caution when attempting a forceps delivery after a failed vacuum extraction (only if the vertex is right on the perineum). A cesarean delivery is likely a better choice (intracranial hemorrhage is more common after a failed vacuum extraction followed by a forceps delivery).
I. Make an *incision* for episiotomy, if necessary. A midline episiotomy has increased risk of third- and fourth-degree perineal lacerations.
J. Remove the vacuum cup when *jaw* of the infant can be reached or is delivered.

A suction application can also be used to rotate the head from an OP to an OA position before delivery (Fig. 157.7).

SAMPLE OPERATIVE REPORT

The operative report from an operative vaginal delivery should be included in the delivery note. The actual note varies depending on the individual labor and local custom. The following is an outline of suggested topics to include in this note:

- Preoperative diagnosis (note indication for the assistance, such as maternal exhaustion)
- Postoperative diagnosis (note preoperative diagnosis and result of the procedure [e.g., vaginal delivery, term infant, weight, Apgar score, cord pH])
- Operation (note outlet forceps or vacuum extraction)
- Instrument (e.g., Simpson forceps)
- First stage (note length, interventions, any complication)
- Second stage (same information as in first stage, including type of fetal monitoring)
- Third stage (type of placenta delivery, description of placenta)
- Repairs
- Bladder
- Estimated blood loss
- Anesthesia

COMMON ERRORS

- Starting the procedure too soon: Be sure that head is engaged and position is clear prior to attempting operative vaginal delivery.
- Incorrectly positioning the instrument: Ensure proper placement of vacuum or forceps prior to pulling.
- Including vaginal tissue in the vacuum application: Circle finger around cup to make sure no maternal tissue is trapped between the cup and the head.
- Continuing with assisted vaginal delivery when success is unlikely: Be prepared to stop and proceed to a cesarean delivery if unable to deliver with 3 pulls, if vacuum pops off three times, or if delivery does not occur within 20 minutes.

COMPLICATIONS

- Cervical, vaginal, or perineal lacerations
- Postpartum hemorrhage from the lacerations
- Fetal birth trauma (e.g., fractured clavicle, cephalohematoma, lacerations, abrasions, facial nerve palsy, intracranial and retinal hemorrhage)
- Subgaleal hematoma
- Shoulder dystocia
- Neonatal scalp emphysema
- Cephalohematoma
- Hyperbilirubinemia
- Fetal cervical trauma
- Maternal discomfort at delivery
- Maternal urinary retention

EDITOR'S NOTE: A review (Ekeus et al., 2017) of complicated vacuum deliveries, where complicated was defined as greater than 15 minutes, more than 6 pulls, and more than 1 cup detachment, resulted in 4% of infants with severe complications (low Apgar score, neonatal convulsion, encephalopathy, or intracranial hemorrhage). Brachial plexus injury occurred in 1.3%. The authors concluded these complications supported the recommended guidelines for use of vacuum extraction.

POSTPROCEDURE PATIENT EDUCATION

Instrument-assisted deliveries can increase the level of maternal anxiety regarding her infant. The provider should discuss the rationale for the instrument delivery and maternal perceptions regarding the delivery on the first postpartum day. Communicating with the newborn care provider about forceps or vacuum use during the delivery is also important so the infant can be assessed for any complications. After the procedure, the mother should be advised to monitor the following and report any changes she has to the practitioner:

- Bleeding
- Fever
- Dysuria and urinary retention
- Pelvic pain (could indicate hematoma)

CPT/BILLING CODES

59400	Global vaginal delivery (antepartum, vaginal delivery with or without episiotomy and/or forceps or vacuum) and postpartum care
59409	Vaginal delivery only (with or without episiotomy and/or forceps or vacuum)
59410	Vaginal delivery only (with or without episiotomy and/or forceps or vacuum) including postpartum care
59610	VBAC (global)
59899	Unlisted procedure, maternity care and delivery (induction)

ICD-10-CM DIAGNOSTIC CODE

O66.5   Forceps or vacuum delivery, without mention of indication

RECOMMENDED READING

American College of Obstetricians and Gynecologists. ACOG practice bulletin No. 154: operative vaginal delivery. *Obstet Gynecol.* 2015;126(5):e56–e65.

Damos J. *ALSO Curriculum.* Leawood, KS: American Academy of Family Physicians; 2010.

Ekeus C, Wrangsell K, Penttinen S, Aberg K. Neonatal complications among 596 infants delivered by vacuum extraction (in relation to characteristics of the extraction). *J Matern Fetal Neonatal Med.* 2017. https://doi.org/10.1080/14767058.2017.1344631.

Hobel CJ. Obstetric procedures. In: Hacker NF, Gambone JC, Hobel JC, eds. *Hacker and Moore's Essentials of Obstetrics and Gynecology.* 6th ed. Philadelphia: Elsevier; 2016:224–233.

Hook CD, Damos RJ. Vacuum-assisted vaginal delivery. *Am Fam Physician.* 2008;78:953–960.

Kawakita T, Reddy UM, Landy HJ, et al. Neonatal complications associated with use of fetal scalp electrode: a retrospective study. *BJOG.* 2016;123(11):1797–1803.

Liabsuetrakul T, Choobun T, Peeyananjarassri K, et al. Antibiotic prophylaxis for operative vaginal delivery. *Cochrane Database Syst Rev.* 2014: CD00445.

Merriam AA, Ananth CV, Wright JD, Siddiq Z, D'Alton ME, Friedman AM. Trends in operative vaginal delivery, 2005-2013: a population-based study. *BJOG.* 2017;124(9):1365–1372. https://doi.org/10.1111/1471–0528.14553.

O'Mahony F, Hoymeyr GJ, Menon V. Choice of instruments for assisted vaginal delivery. *Cochrane Database Syst Rev.* 2010;2:CD005455. pub.

Palatnik A, Grobman WA, Hellenday MG, et al. Predictors of shoulder dystocia at the time of operative vaginal delivery. *Am J Obstet Gynecol.* 2016;215(5):e1–e624.e5.

Tuggy M, Garcia J. *Procedures Consult.* Forceps delivery. http://www.proceduresconsult.com/medical-procedures/forceps-delivery-FM-017-procedure.aspx.

Tuggy M, Garcia J. *Procedures Consult.* Forceps delivery. http://www.proceduresconsult.com/medical-procedures/forceps-delivery-FM-016-procedure.aspx.

Zhang J, Landy HJ, Branch DW, et al. Contemporary patterns of spontaneous labor with normal neonatal outcomes. *Obstet Gynecol.* 2010;116:1281–1287.

CHAPTER 158

EPISIOTOMY AND REPAIR OF THE PERINEUM

Montiel T. Rosenthal

Episiotomy is an intentional incision in the perineum used to facilitate the second stage of labor. It is performed much less often in the United States than in previous years, when routine episiotomy was common. However, clinicians in Europe use it even less often, affirming that vaginal delivery is a natural process that does not necessarily benefit from intervention. Although use of an episiotomy may slightly decrease the risk for labial and anterior vaginal lacerations, avoidance of episiotomy leads to less maternal blood loss, less overall perineal trauma, less risk of disruption of the anal sphincter (third-degree extension) or rectal mucosa (fourth-degree extension), and less delay in the patient's resumption of sexual activity. Avoidance may also decrease risk of spontaneous lacerations with future deliveries. Eight studies that compared a restrictive policy of episiotomy with a policy of its routine use were reviewed for the Cochrane Database and found less posterior vaginal or perineal trauma with a restrictive policy and less overall need for suturing. Episiotomy therefore falls into the Cochrane category of "Forms of Care Likely to Be Ineffective or Harmful," and it should not be routinely performed. However, for certain situations or indications, episiotomy may be unavoidable or extremely useful.

An episiotomy is performed to enlarge the vaginal outlet to facilitate delivery. Clinicians should be familiar with the anatomy of the vagina, introitus, and perineum (Fig. 158.1) before performing an episiotomy. In a midline or median episiotomy, the incision is made in a direct line posteriorly from the vagina, through the attachments of the bulbospongiosus muscle and the tendinous perineal body, and toward the anus. Mediolateral episiotomy directs the incision 45 degrees laterally from the midline at the base of the introitus (Fig. 158.2) or at the 5- or 7-o'clock positions. Although more commonly performed in Europe, mediolateral episiotomy is rarely performed in the United States and is associated with more bleeding, a more difficult surgical repair, complicated healing, and a higher risk of postoperative pain, including dyspareunia. The only benefit to mediolateral episiotomy is a decreased risk of extension to a third- or fourth-degree tear. Severe perineal lacerations that extend into or through the anal sphincter complex are termed *obstetric anal sphincter injuries*. This chapter focuses on the midline or median episiotomy, although a modified "hockey stick" version of the midline and the mediolateral episiotomy is also discussed. In addition to the general risk factors for midline episiotomy, risk factors for third- or fourth-degree extensions include nulliparity, arrest of second-stage labor, persistent occiput posterior position, very short perineum, use of mid- or low-outlet forceps, and use of local anesthetics.

INDICATIONS

Any situation that prolongs the second stage of labor and thereby significantly endangers the life of the mother, the integrity of her perineum, or fetal well-being could warrant episiotomy. The fact that episiotomy is a surgical procedure with attendant risks and

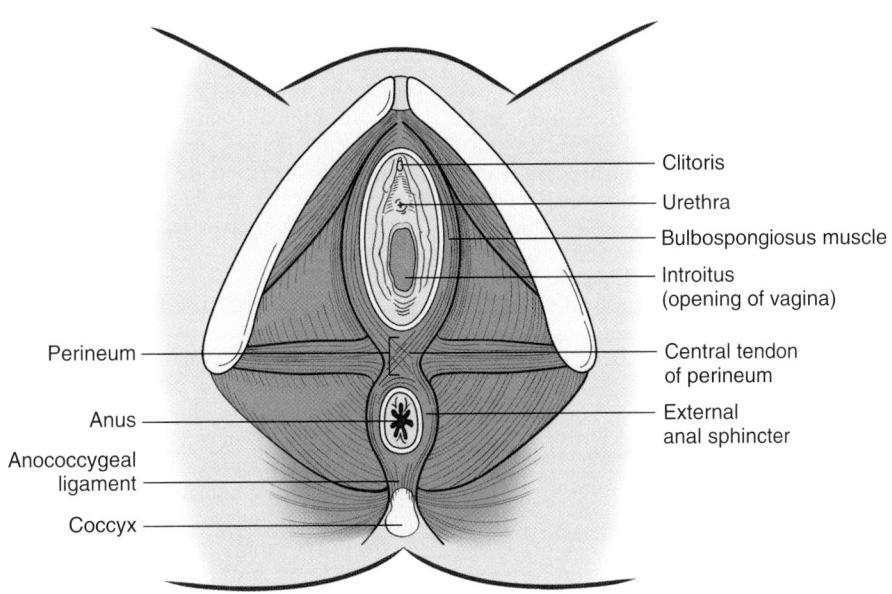

Fig. 158.1   Anatomy of the vagina, introitus, and perineum.

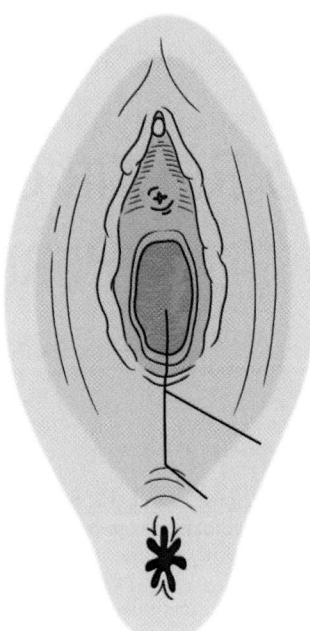

Fig. 158.2 "Hockey stick" extension of midline episiotomy versus mediolateral episiotomy.

potentially fatal complications has to be weighed against the need to shorten the second stage of labor by a few minutes. Current obstetric literature suggests that episiotomy may be indicated when vaginal delivery is anticipated and one of the following maternal or fetal indications exists.

Maternal Indications

- Significant cardiac disease (e.g., mitral stenosis)
- Risk of significant perineal trauma (e.g., large infant, use of forceps or vacuum, imminent perineal rupture)

Fetal Indications

- Significant fetal distress in second stage
- Prematurity
- Breech or face presentation
- Shoulder dystocia
- Occiput posterior position (possible benefit)

Precipitous deliveries are associated with more perineal and pelvic injuries; therefore, a timely episiotomy is critical in this situation. For all other deliveries, less invasive maneuvers (e.g., perineal massage, warm perineal compresses, sitting for delivery, breathing, hands off until crowning, and slowing delivery of fetal head—delivering the head between contractions and avoiding maternal pushing while the head is being delivered) may be helpful in alleviating second-stage complications or in reducing trauma. Again, recent evidence has suggested that episiotomy use should be restricted to instances where it is clearly indicated.

CONTRAINDICATIONS

Absolute

The only absolute contraindication is patient refusal.

Relative

- Prior fourth-degree laceration or fourth-degree repair breakdown
- Severe scarring or malformation of perineum

- Extensive or large condylomata that may lead to frank hemorrhage if incised
- Prior or concurrent fistula
- Maternal disorders that impair healing such as autoimmune disorders, diabetes, or human immunodeficiency virus infection

EQUIPMENT

- Sterile gown, gloves, drapes, and any other equipment necessary for the clinician to follow universal blood and body fluid precautions.
- Povidone–iodine solution (or chlorhexidine if patient allergic to iodine).
- Blunt-tipped straight surgical scissors (e.g., Mayo scissors; a scalpel may also be used but the editors do not recommend this because it can cause significant injury to the mother, fetus, or clinician).
- Needle holder.
- Nontraumatic forceps.
- Vaginal retractor(s).
- Ring forceps.
- 4 × 4 sterile gauze sponges.
- 2-0 or 3-0 polyglycolic braided absorbable sutures (e.g., Vicryl, Dexon, Polysorb; preferred over chromic, which is associated with an increased risk of episiotomy breakdown and more discomfort during the first 3 days of healing; however, polyglycolic sutures may more frequently cause local irritation and work themselves to the skin surface or fail to heal and have to be removed weeks later) on a large, curved cutting or tapered-point needle. Rapidly absorbable versions of polyglycolic sutures are now also available and may decrease the need for suture removal within the first 3 months after episiotomy repair.
- Allis clamps (especially for third- and fourth-degree extension repairs).
- 4-0 or 5-0 polyglycolic suture on smaller curved needle (for fourth-degree extension repairs).

NOTE: If effective regional (e.g., epidural, pudendal) anesthesia is not in place, a 10-mL syringe with a 1.5-inch, 27-gauge needle should be available to locally infiltrate the anesthetic of preference (usually 10 mL 1% lidocaine without epinephrine; use ≤30 mL lidocaine).

PREPROCEDURE PATIENT EDUCATION

Discuss potential risks and possible benefits of an episiotomy with the patient (and partner) during prenatal care, before an emergent moment of need when neither the clinician nor the patient is in an optimal situation for exchange of information. Ideally, the patient's desires are part of a birth plan, and this should be discussed and written well before the pregnancy is at term. (See also Chapter 10, Epidural Anesthesia and Analgesia, Chapter 154, Pudendal Anesthesia, and Chapter 156, Vaginal Delivery, for examples.)

TECHNIQUE

In the second stage of labor, as the fetal cranium begins to distend the maternal perineum, if time permits, effort should be directed toward assisting with the natural thinning of the perineum and dilation of the introitus (Fig. 158.3). These efforts should include applying warm compresses and placing tension on the perineum and gently stretching it from inside the introitus with the index and middle fingers. Labeling posterior as the 6 o'clock direction, rotate these fingers, under gentle tension (directed outwardly), from about the 4 o'clock to the 8 o'clock positions. Gentle exterior massage with the thumb or other hand at the same time, in this same location, may also help with thinning of the perineum.

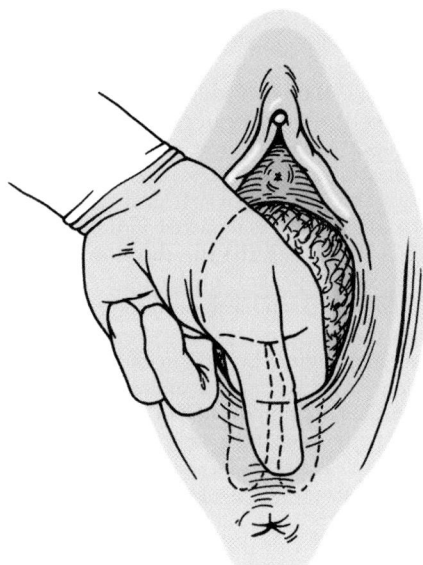

Fig. 158.3 Palpating and attempting to stretch and thin the perineum before episiotomy.

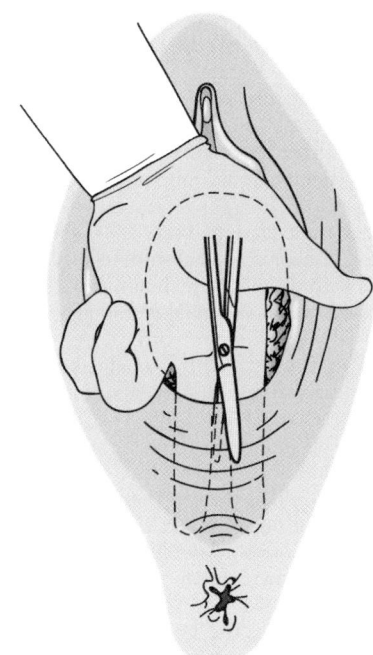

Fig. 158.4 Performing the midline episiotomy.

The decision for episiotomy is usually made after the fetal cranium (not just the caput) distends the introitus. Waiting until a minimum of 3 to 4 cm of the fetal scalp diameter is visible and delivery is imminent will prevent excessive blood loss. If the indication for episiotomy is for a forceps or vacuum delivery, most clinicians perform the episiotomy after application of the blades or vacuum device. Until this time, massaging the perineum, as described previously, may not only minimize bleeding but may provide some anesthesia by placing pressure on the local nerve endings. As the head further distends the introitus, an episiotomy may be needed if it appears that the head will not be deliverable without an episiotomy or that there will be so much tension on the perineum that it will tear (i.e., imminent rupture). An episiotomy may also be necessary for one of the other indications. If the patient is in stirrups, make sure the legs are not separated too widely or one leg placed higher than the other; this may produce excess tension on the perineum, resulting in an extension of the episiotomy into a third- or fourth-degree laceration. When performing this procedure, the clinician should follow universal blood and body fluid precautions.

EDITOR'S NOTE: A one-time intravenous dose of a second-generation cephalosporin (e.g., cefoxitin or cefotetan) prior to obstetric anal sphincter injuries repair is associated with significantly lower rates of postpartum wound complications at 2 weeks compared with no antibiotics (8% vs. 24%; $P = .04$; Duggal et al., 2008); however, the American College of Obstetricians and Gynecologists concluded that this practice has not been extensively studied.

1. With the palm of the clinician's nondominant hand facing outward, the index and middle fingers are inserted between the fetal scalp (or presenting part) and the maternal perineum, directed toward the maternal anus (toward the 6 o'clock position). The thumb should be placed on the exterior perineum. The thumb and fingers serve two functions: to protect the fetus and to palpate the anal sphincter as a reminder of its location for the clinician. The thumb defines the bottom of the episiotomy (see Fig. 158.3).
2. Check for adequate anesthesia by gently scratching the perineum with tissue forceps. If there is no anal wink reflex (i.e., sphincter contraction) with this scratching, it suggests adequate anesthesia. Further confirm anesthesia by gently pinching the perineum with the tissue forceps or an Allis clamp. Even epidural anesthesia or a pudendal block is not always effective, so be prepared

to locally anesthetize the midline of both the perineum (for a median episiotomy) and the floor of the vagina. The middle and index fingers should be in place between the fetus and the perineum/floor of the vagina to avoid fetal injection with anesthetic.
3. Insert the blunt blade of the scissors inside the introitus to cut parallel to and between the fingers. Make the incision downward after bringing the other blade of the scissors flat against the skin on the outside of the perineum (Fig. 158.4). Again, take care to protect the fetal presenting part. After the incision has passed the fetus, avoid cutting the external sphincter of the anus by keeping pressure posteriorly just above the fullness of the anus. The incision length is generally from 2 to 3 cm, depending on length of the perineum and amount of thinning. Under direct visualization, extend the incision up the vaginal mucosa an additional 2 to 4 cm, through the hymenal ring, to release tension and prevent tearing. The introitus should readily open after making the episiotomy, and delivery should proceed expeditiously to minimize blood loss.

In the patient with a very short perineum (especially if nulliparous or with prolonged second stage of labor, or the fetus is in the occiput posterior position), consider performing a variant of the median episiotomy, the hockey stick episiotomy (see Fig. 158.2). To form the hockey stick, as the midline incision is being made and before it reaches the anus, extend it laterally 1 to 2 cm. That way, if the incision extends further by tearing, it should naturally follow the L shape and avoid the anal sphincter. Another option is a mediolateral episiotomy (see Fig. 158.2). The incision is directed at a 45-degree angle to the midline of the posterior fourchette or at the 5- or 7-o'clock position, from the hymenal ring toward the ischial tuberosity. The mediolateral episiotomy is usually made on the same side of the patient as the handedness of the clinician (e.g., right side of patient at about the 7 o'clock position for a right-handed clinician). The length of the incision is not as critical as for a midline incision, but it is commonly extended to 3 to 4 cm. Keep in mind, the longer the incision, the more extensive the repair.

Repair

1. Repair the episiotomy after the third stage of labor. This allows full attention to the process of placental separation and

delivery and avoids disturbing the episiotomy repair with the delivery of the placenta. (If the episiotomy repair has already been completed, the sutures could become disrupted with delivery of the placenta, especially if a manual extraction is necessary. If the episiotomy is in the process of being repaired, delivery of the placenta often obscures the field with blood.) Again, the clinician should follow universal blood and body fluid precautions.

2. Check again for adequate anesthesia by gently scratching the perineum, and if there is no anal wink reflex, by gently pinching the perineum with tissue forceps. If not already done, a pudendal block (see Chapter 154, Pudendal Anesthesia) can again be considered, especially if a third- or fourth-degree extension needs to be repaired. Check patients with an epidural in the same manner; additional dosing may be necessary or supplemental injected local anesthesia.

3. A digital rectal examination should be performed after every delivery. After donning a clean glove and lubricating a finger with antiseptic solution, palpate the distal 6 cm of the rectal mucosa. The gloved finger should not be visible in the vaginal wound. Such a tear or "buttonhole," usually located superior to the sphincter, could later produce a rectovaginal fistula if left unrepaired. Determine whether the sphincter has sufficient bulk remaining (i.e., produces the sensation of a small doughnut being palpated). In the absence of this sensation, evaluate closely for a third-degree extension. Carefully examine the remainder of the lower urogenital tract for lacerations not contiguous with the episiotomy, repairing those that need it.

Repair of Third- and Fourth-Degree Extensions (Tears)

1. If the rectal mucosa is no longer intact (fourth-degree extension), it must be repaired to prevent fistula formation. Reapproximate the submucosa and muscularis with 4-0 or 5-0 polyglycolic on a tapered needle (Fig. 158.5A). Use running stitches placed 3 to 5 mm apart. (These are basically subcuticular stitches, but unlike subcuticular stitches placed in skin, these are placed from the other side—the back side—of the mucosa.) Interrupted sutures can be used, but create more foreign body footprint due to multiple knots. Reapproximating the submucosa and muscularis in this manner should invert the mucosa back into the lumen (see Fig. 158.5B). Doing so will eliminate the risk of sequestering rectal mucosa in overlying tissue. Sutures should begin just above the apex of the laceration and proceed distally.

NOTE: If the apex of the laceration is not visible, an interrupted suture can be placed as close as possible to the apex and used to apply gentle traction toward the clinician, bringing the apex of the wound into view. This suture can later be removed. (A similar technique can be applied to any vaginal or even a cervical laceration when there is difficulty visualizing the apex.)

The musculature of the anal canal, including the anal sphincters, basically consists of two tubes, one inside the other. The inner cylinder, closest to the rectal mucosa, contains the internal anal sphincter. This sphincter consists of smooth muscle under involuntary control and provides the resting tone noted when performing a digital rectal examination. In turn, this cylinder is surrounded by the thicker cylinder containing the external anal sphincter, which consists of skeletal muscle under voluntary control and can be used to squeeze the clinician's finger when a digital rectal examination is being performed.

2. After reapproximation of the mucosa, a second layer of running or interrupted 3-0 polyglycolic sutures should be placed to provide a reinforcing layer of fascia over the stitches in the submucosa. This layer should also close the torn ends of the internal anal sphincter, a roughly 2.5-cm-long (the most distal 2.5 cm of the anal canal) fibrous layer lying between the rectal mucosa and the external anal sphincter. It is identified as a white, glistening, fibrous structure that may have retracted laterally and need to

be retrieved with an Allis clamp for repair. These sutures should give the wound additional strength, again decreasing the chance for fistula formation.

3. The external anal sphincter (third-degree extension) is then repaired by using three or four interrupted stitches. Suturing the sphincter muscle alone will not provide sufficient strength to hold until healing is complete, so the fibrous sphincter sheath (fascia) must also be reapproximated. It is identified as a tenacious white sheath, often retracted further laterally than the muscle edges. Search for the sheath on the posterior, inferior (caudal), superior (cephalic), and anterior aspects of the muscle. Again, lateral probing and fixation with an Allis clamp may be necessary.

4. Several techniques are described in the literature for external anal sphincter repair. Four simple sutures (see Fig. 158.5C–I) can be placed in the posterior, superior (cephalic), inferior (caudal), and anterior portions of the muscle and the adjacent aspects of the torn sphincter sheath for an end-to-end repair. (Some experts place the posterior and caudal sutures first and then tie them last.)

Alternatively, the ends of the sphincter may be pulled to overlap and sutured with three sutures. Although the overlapping-type repair was initially thought to provide superior results, especially in the first year (less fecal urgency and anal incontinence), randomized trials comparing it with traditional end-to-end repair have failed to demonstrate superior anatomic or functional results at 36 months. Another method of end-to-end repair is to merely place two large transfixion sutures in the posterior and anterior aspects of the external sphincter. Usually it is easier to place the posterior transfixion suture first, followed by the anterior suture. These large transfixion sutures should also traverse the superior (cephalic) and inferior (caudal) sheaths in both locations (see Fig. 158.5J).

5. On completion, a repeat rectal examination should be performed to confirm adequate sphincter reapproximation and adequate bulk/support. The examination glove should be discarded after rectal examination.

Repair of the Episiotomy (Second Degree Laceration Repair)

1. After any injury to the rectal mucosa and anal sphincters has been repaired, carefully examine the wound. Use 2-0 or 3-0 polyglycolic suture to place a stitch above the apex on the vaginal incision. Tie there, and then run it down to the introitus and reapproximate the hymenal ring (Fig. 158.6). It is critical that these stitches provide hemostasis, close all dead space, and not enter the rectum. Although some clinicians use a subcuticular running stitch for this reapproximation, it seems that simple running sutures would be more effective at providing hemostasis and closing the dead space. Interrupted sutures can also be used with equal outcomes, but use of running sutures is faster and requires less suture material. One way to avoid entering the rectum is to take wide bites laterally on each side and then to bring the needle out at the base of the incision, ensuring that it does not go as deep as the rectum (merely piercing the rectum with a needle increases the risk of rectovaginal fistula). Either locked or unlocked running sutures may be used, although the literature suggests that unlocked sutures are associated with less pain and need for analgesia for up to 10 days postpartum and a trend for reduced dyspareunia in the 3 initial months following delivery (Kettle C, 2012). If locked sutures are used, take care to avoid too much tension, which might cause tissue ischemia and necrosis.

2. At this point, two techniques are available, either continuing with the current suture to close the perineum for the one-suture technique (Fig. 158.7), or using an additional suture for the two-suture technique (Fig. 158.8). If the one-suture technique is chosen, after approximating the hymenal ring, the needle is buried beneath the hymenal ring to exit at the apex/top of the perineal wound. From there, running stitches are placed in the deep perineal tissue, approximating the perineum (or at least taking the

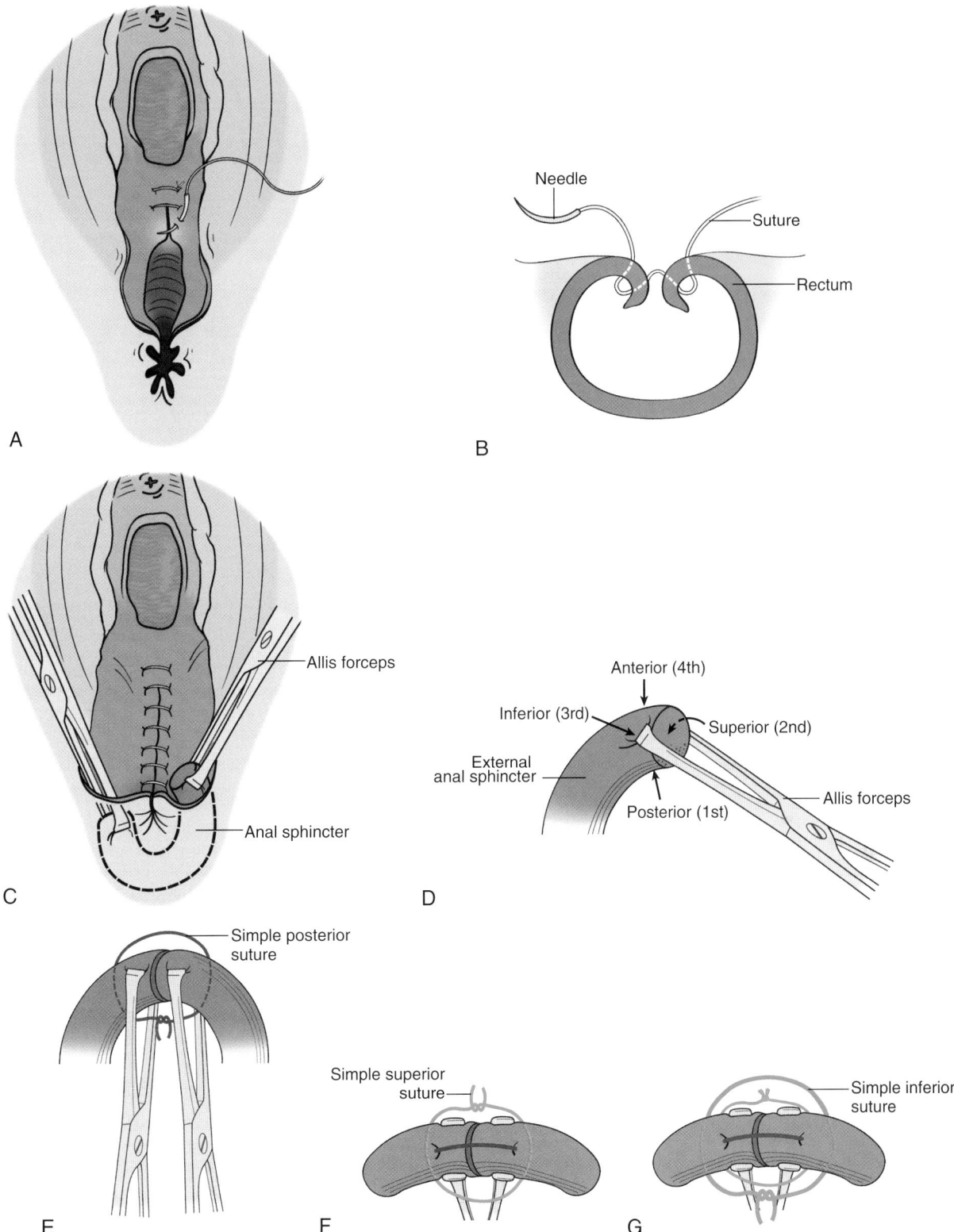

Fig. 158.5 Repair of fourth-degree extension of a midline episiotomy. (A) The rectal mucosa is repaired using interrupted submucosal stitches. (B) Cross-sectional view of rectal laceration closure, inverting mucosa. (C) The sphincter is retrieved with Allis forceps. (D) Right edge of external anal sphincter from perineal view with order of placement of sutures. The location correlates with where the knot will reside. (E) Placement of simple posterior suture (final knot in posterior position), perineal view. (F) Placement of simple superior (cephalic) suture, anterior view. (G) Placement of simple inferior (caudal) suture, anterior view. (H) Placement of simple anterior suture with removal of Allis clamps (perineal view). (I) Complete closure of external anal sphincter (perineal view). (J) Alternative technique of reapproximating external anal sphincter using two large transfixion sutures.

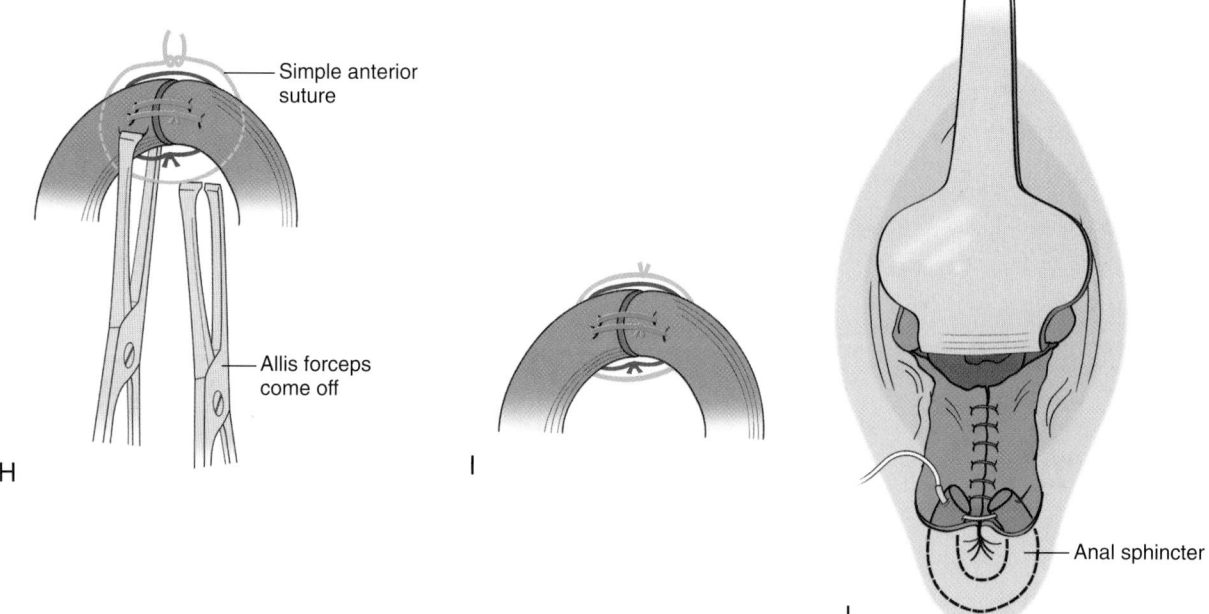

Simple anterior suture

Allis forceps come off

H

I

Anal sphincter

J

Fig. 158.5 cont'd

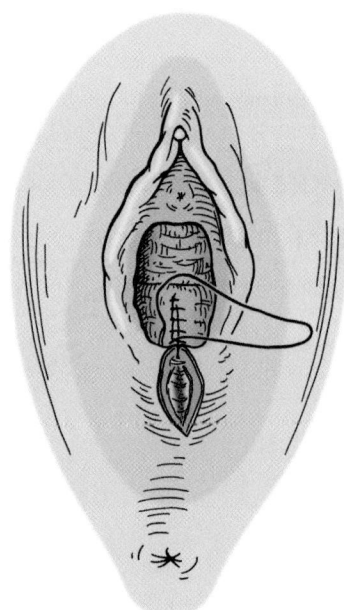

Fig. 158.6   Closure of the vaginal mucosa. The first stitch is placed *above* the apex of the wound and tied. This stitch is then usually continued as a simple or locked running stitch down to the introitus. The hymenal ring has been reapproximated and the needle is then taken to the depth of the perineum.

tension off the eventual subcuticular stitch) while proceeding to the most posterior aspect/bottom of the wound. After the deep perineal tissue has been reapproximated and the posterior aspect of the wound reached, the suture is redirected to become a running subcuticular stitch and used to close the skin of the perineum. The suture is run back up the perineum, and then the needle is again buried beneath the hymenal ring to exit through the already sutured incision in the vaginal mucosa. One final stitch is placed beneath the incision in the vaginal mucosa, to hide or invert it, a knot tied, and any remaining suture cut.

NOTE: Deep placement of the perineal subcuticular stitches (but leaving the perineal wound gaping only 2 to 3 mm) significantly decreases itching during healing with no loss of cosmesis or function. Also, avoid interrupted transcutaneous sutures when closing the perineum because they are associated with more pain in the immediate postpartum period compared with continuous subcuticular sutures.

3. If the two-suture technique is used, after the hymenal ring is approximated with the first suture, the needle is buried beneath the hymenal ring to exit into the perineal wound. The needle is then laid aside or tagged with a hemostat to keep it out of the wound and ready for later use. With the second suture, a crown stitch is placed to carefully reapproximate the perineum where the bilateral bulbospongiosus (formerly known as bulbocavernosus) muscles merge (see Fig. 158.6B). Then, either interrupted or running sutures can be placed to close the perineum from the apex/top to the posterior/bottom of the wound. If a running suture is used, after the deep perineal tissue has been reapproximated, the suture can then be redirected as a subcuticular stitch and run back up to close the skin of the perineum. At that point, when the first suture is reached, both needles are removed and the sutures tied together into an inverted knot. Alternatively, if interrupted sutures are used to repair the deep perineal tissue (see Fig. 158.8), the suture tagged after reapproximating the hymenal ring can then be used for a running subcuticular stitch to close the skin of the perineum.
4. To repair a hockey stick extension, merely follow the incision with the subcuticular suture. Fig. 158.9 diagrams the repair of a mediolateral episiotomy.
5. Once repair is complete, perform a final rectovaginal examination. Verify again that the rectal mucosa is intact and is not obstructed by suture, and that no gauze sponges or instruments remain in either the rectum or the vagina. Immediate correction, by removal of the existing repair and repeating the procedure with care, is imperative to minimize the risk of infection and fistula formation.

EDITOR'S NOTE: When managing spontaneous first- and second-degree lacerations sustained during childbirth, insufficient evidence exists to recommend surgical or nonsurgical repair (observation).

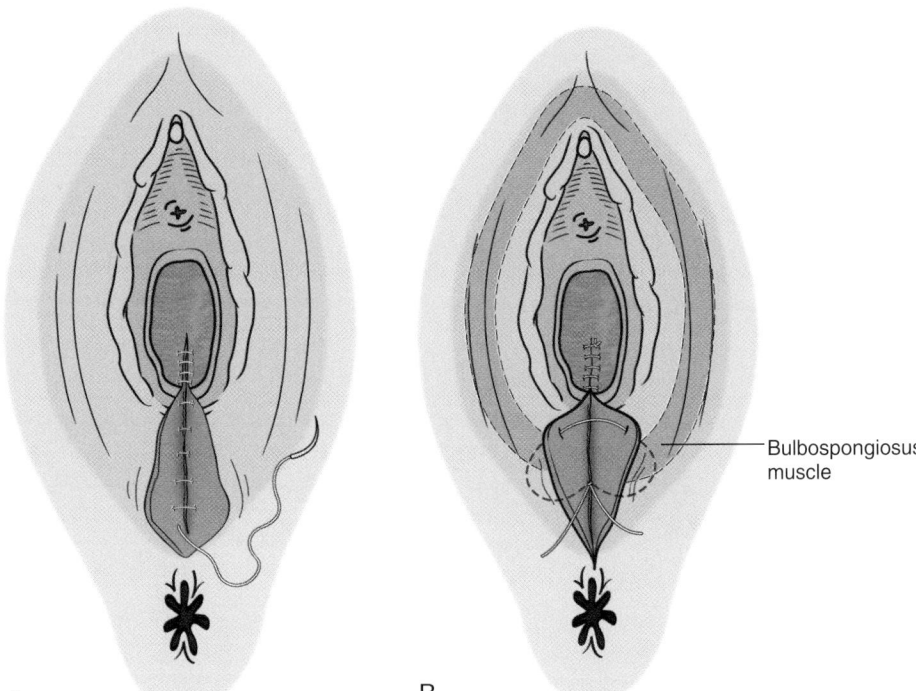

Fig. 158.7 (A) Repair of the vaginal mucosa has been completed with running stitches. The hymenal ring and perineal body have been reapproximated and a deep running layer of perineal sutures has been placed, using the same suture. Finishing the perineal closure entails running the subcuticular stitches back to the introitus. (B) Alternative closure of deep perineum after running vaginal suture. The crown stitch approximates the perineal body, where the fibers of the bulbospongiosus muscles join from either side. (*Dotted line* indicates placement of suture out of view of the person doing the repair.)

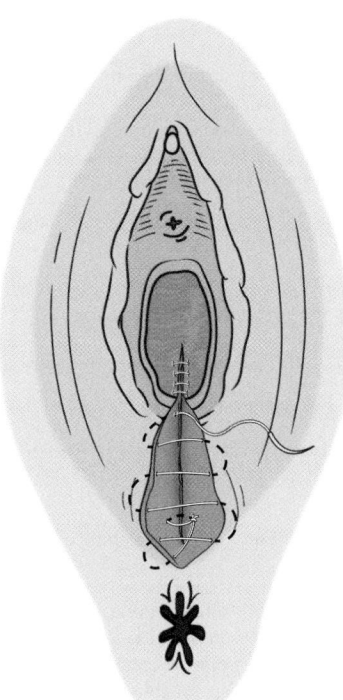

Fig. 158.8 Two-suture technique of closing the deep perineal space. The second suture is used for deep interrupted stitches. The perineal skin is closed with a subcuticular stitch using either the second suture or the remaining first suture from the vaginal repair. (*Dotted line* indicates placement of subcuticular suture.)

One randomized controlled trial comparing adhesive skin glue for closure of first-degree perineal tears without excessive bleeding found similar cosmetic and functional results at 6 weeks compared with routine suturing. The American College of Obstetrician and Gynecologists recommends that either standard suture or adhesive may be chosen to repair hemostatic first-degree lacerations or perineal skin in a second-degree laceration.

Fig. 158.10 summarizes the episiotomy and repair technique.

COMPLICATIONS

- Blood volume loss is reported to be approximately 300 mL from an uncomplicated median episiotomy, but easily may be more if there is an unexpected delay in delivery or repair. Observe the patient carefully and treat proactively, especially if other conditions threaten to compromise the patient's blood volume (e.g., intravascular hypovolemia resulting from other blood loss or preeclampsia).
- Hematoma formation with acute swelling and pain is unusual but not rare. In addition to large vulvar hematomas, paravaginal and ischiorectal hematomas can occur. If present, a hematoma may need to be opened immediately. The bleeding must then be arrested and the space either closed or drained to prevent recurrence.
- Infection is probably the most serious threat to episiotomy recovery. A range of wound infections is possible, from a minor superficial exudative wound infection to a life-threatening septic hematoma or necrotizing fasciitis. Maternal fever and unusual pain or swelling in the perineum must be evaluated thoroughly to rule out serious infection.
- Incontinence of stool or urine and flatus are possible complications of episiotomy, especially when associated with extensions.
- Rectovaginal and urogenital fistulas (vesicovaginal, vesicocervicovaginal, urethrovaginal, and ureterovaginal) may occur from either direct trauma (hence the importance of careful examination of the entire lower genital tract) or from infection or necrosis associated with suturing. Incontinence of either feces or urine starting 10 or more days after delivery should alert the clinician to the possibility of these complications.
- Pelvic relaxation and poor perineal tone, once thought to be minimized by performing an episiotomy, may actually be exacerbated by the procedure. Although not life-threatening, they may lead to a lifetime of misery and disability.

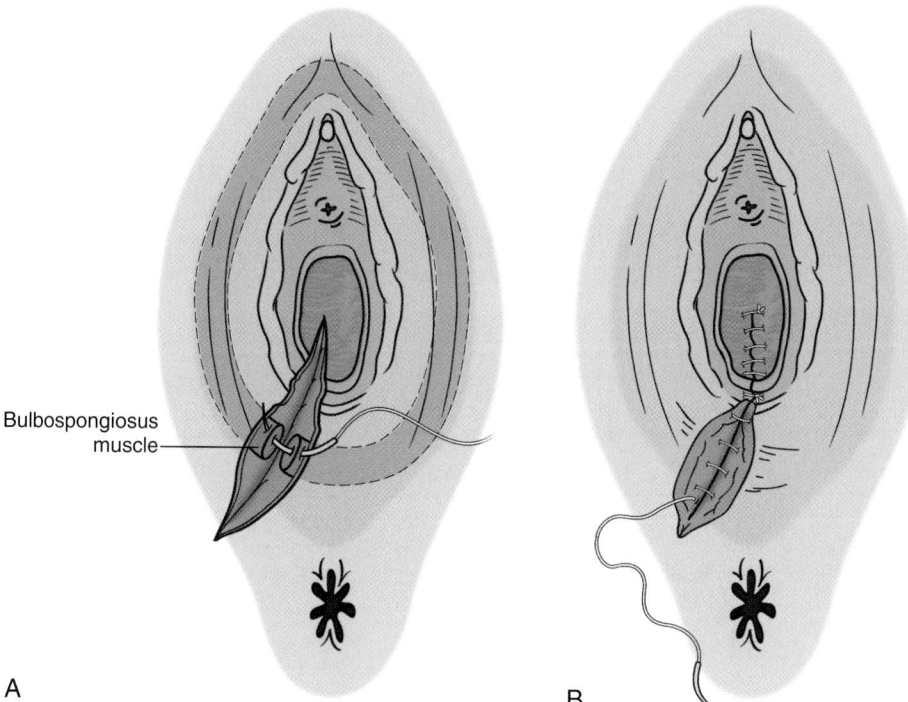

Bulbospongiosus
muscle

Fig. 158.9 Repair of a mediolateral episiotomy. (A) Similar to placing a crown stitch, the bulbospongiosus muscle is first approximated. (B) The remainder of the episiotomy is repaired in a manner similar to a midline episiotomy, using either a one- or two-suture technique.

A   B

- Local pain or wound breakdown and dyspareunia are usually self-limited complications. Bartholin duct cysts, inclusion cysts, and endometriosis at the wound site are rarely encountered but may require surgical repair.
- In addition to maternal complications, episiotomies place a nearby patient in jeopardy: the fetus. Fetal complications may range from injecting the scalp with anesthetic, to producing lidocaine toxicity, to minimal abrasions, to rare but significant lacerations on the presenting part (e.g., eyelid lacerations and even castration of a male breech infant).

POSTPROCEDURE MANAGEMENT AND PATIENT EDUCATION

After delivery, patients with sutures are less comfortable than patients without sutures, and women with episiotomies may experience more pain than women with minor lacerations. Many women will desire analgesia, and nonsteroidal antiinflammatory drugs (e.g., ibuprofen) are increasingly used instead of acetaminophen with codeine. Codeine can be constipating, which is especially problematic among women after a third- or fourth-degree repair. Stool softeners may decrease pain with defecation as well as the risk of episiotomy disruption, especially after third- or fourth-degree extensions. The application of ice packs to the perineum the first 24 hours after delivery is effective for reducing swelling and postpartum pain, whereas warm sitz baths can provide comfort beyond the immediate postpartum period. Alternatively, adding ice cubes to a lukewarm sitz bath and soaking for 20 to 30 minutes may be preferred by some patients for pain relief. Potential complications must be discussed so that she is aware of the signs and symptoms for which she must immediately contact the clinician, especially bleeding, fever, or severe or persistent pain. Patients should also know that if a suture works its way to the surface, they can return to the office for removal. Intercourse is probably best avoided for those with second degree lacerations or greater until the first postpartum visit at 4 to 6 weeks.

CPT/BILLING CODES

59300	Episiotomy or vaginal repair by other than the attending physician
59400	Routine obstetric care, including antepartum care, vaginal delivery (with or without episiotomy, and/or forceps), and postpartum care
59409	Vaginal delivery only (with or without episiotomy and/or forceps)

ICD-10-CM DIAGNOSTIC CODES

O80	Encounter for full-term uncomplicated delivery

Deliveries With Forceps or Vacuum

O76	Abnormality in fetal heart rate or rhythm
O63.1	Prolonged second stage of labor

Episiotomy and Episiotomy Repair, Repair of Low Vaginal Lacerations

O70.0	First-degree perineal laceration
O70.1	Second-degree perineal laceration
070.20	Third-degree perineal laceration
O70.3	Fourth-degree perineal laceration
O70.9	Unspecified perineal laceration

Acknowledgment

The editors recognize the contributions of Donald N. Marquardt, MD, PhD, to this chapter in previous editions of this text.

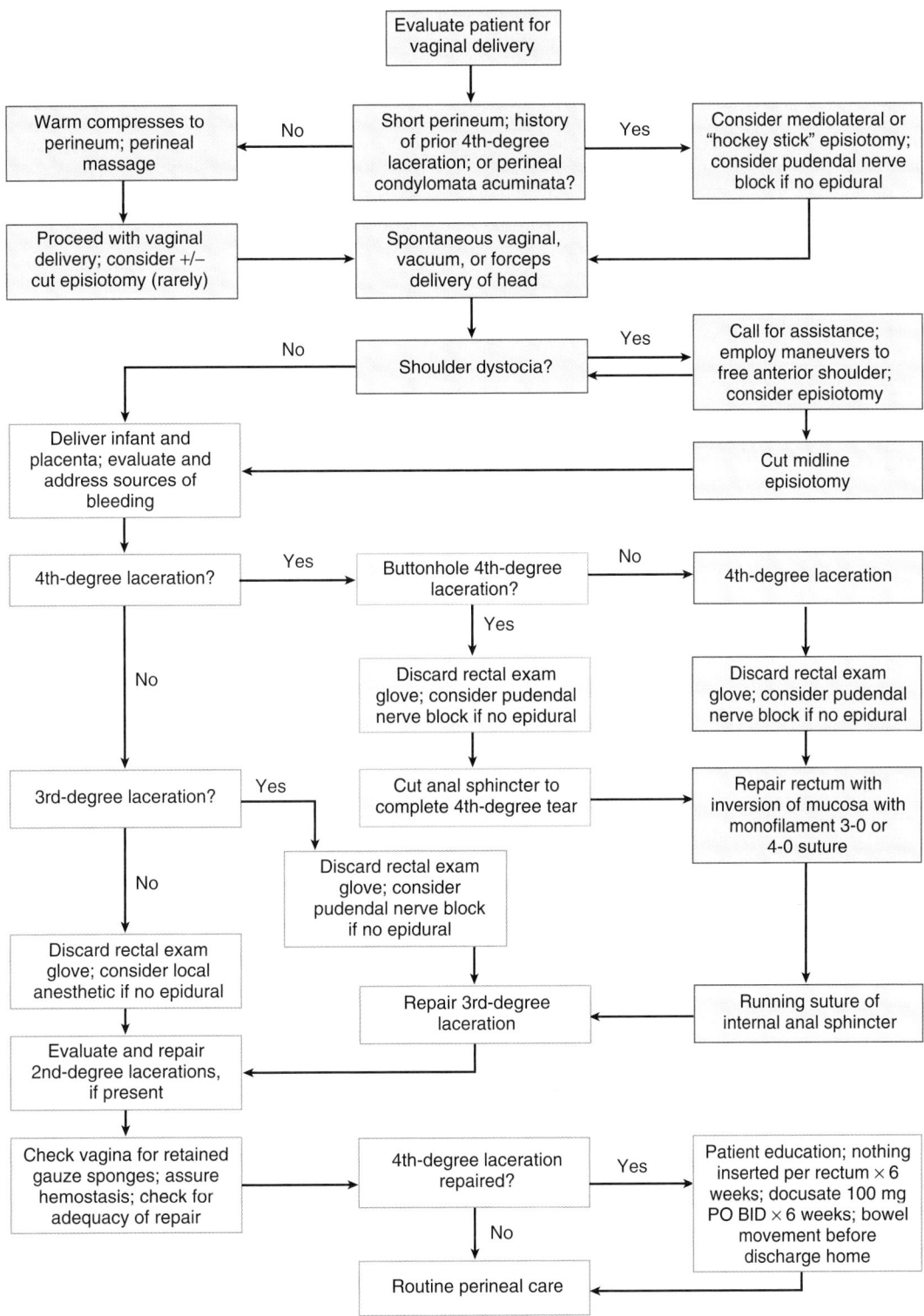

Fig. 158.10 Episiotomy and repair.

ONLINE RESOURCES

Tuggy M, Garcia J. Procedures Consult. First and second degree repair of the perineum. http://www.proceduresconsult.com/medical-procedures/first-and-second-degree-repair-of-the-perineum-FM-015-procedure.aspx.
Tuggy M, Garcia J. Procedures Consult. Third and fourth degree repair of the perineum. http://www.proceduresconsult.com/medical-procedures/third-and-fourth-degree-repair-of-the-perineum-FM-018-procedure.aspx.

RECOMMENDED READING

Asheim V, Nilsen AB, Reinar L, Lukasse M. Perineal techniques during the second stage of labour for reducing perineal trauma. *Cochrane Database Syst Rev.* 2017:CD006672. pub3.
American College of Obstreticians and Gynecologists. Prevention and management of obstetric lacerations at vaginal delivery. Practice Bulletin No. 165. *Obstet Gynecol.* 2016;128(1):e1–e15.

American College of Obstetricians and Gynecologists. Prophylactic antibiotics in labor and delivery. Practice Bulletin No. 120. *Obstet Gynecol.* 2011;117:1472–1483.

Bulchandani S, Watts E, Sucharitha A, et al. Manual perineal support at the time of childbirth: a systematic review and meta-analysis. *BJOG.* 2015;122:1157–1165.

Duggal N, Mercado C, Daniels K, et al. Antibiotic prophylaxis for prevention of postpartum perineal wound complications: a randomized controlled trial. *Obstet Gynecol.* 2008;111:1268–1273.

Feigenberg T, Maor-Sagie E, Zivi E, et al. Using adhesive glue to repair first degree perineal tears: a prospective randomized controlled trial. *Biomed Res Int.* 2014:526590.

Fernando RJ, Sultan AH, Kettle C, Thakar R. Methods of repair for obstetric anal sphincter injury. *Cochrane Database Syst Rev.* 2013;12:CD002866. pub3.

Kettle C, Dowswell T, Ismail KM. Continuous and interrupted suturing techniques for repair of episiotomy or second-degree tears. *Cochrane Database Syst Rev.* 2012;11:CD000947.

Menzies R, Leung M, Chandrasekaran N, et al. Episiotomy technique and management of anal sphincter tears: a survey of clinical practice and education. *J Obstet Gyneacol Can.* 2016;38(12):1091–1099.

Selo-Ojeme DO, Okonkwo CA, Atuanaya C. Single-knot versus multiple-knot technique of perineal repair: a randomized controlled trial. *Arch Gynecol Obstet.* 2016;294:945–952.

Vaginal delivery. In: Cunningham F, Leveno KJ, Bloom SL, et al. *Williams Obstetrics.* 24th ed. New York: McGraw-Hill; 2013.

CHAPTER 159

SYMPHYSIOTOMY

Beth Choby • Gini Ikwuezunma

Symphysiotomy is a procedure where the cartilaginous fibers of the pubic symphysis are partially divided to permit joint separation. This separation enlarges the anterior-posterior pelvic diameter of the maternal pelvis by 1 to 2 cm. It does not require an operating room and can be performed with local anesthesia. Symphysiotomy is most commonly performed for obstructed labor due to mild to moderate cephalopelvic disproportion (CPD). Combined with vacuum extraction, symphysiotomy is a life-saving procedure in areas where caesarean delivery is not feasible or immediately available (World Health Organization, 2007). The procedure involves no uterine scar, so the risk of uterine rupture in future pregnancies is not increased compared with cesarean.

Symphysiotomy as a procedure was first suggested in 1776, a time at which maternal mortality from cesarean delivery was nearly 100% (Sigualt, 1776). The first procedure was performed on a 3 foot 8 inches woman severely disfigured by rickets. The patient, who had had four prior stillbirths, survived the procedure and actually delivered a live infant. Her pelvic deformity from the rickets, likely combined with the symphysiotomy, resulted in long-term issues with both stress urinary incontinence and gait. Critics decried the procedure as dangerous. In Ireland between 1944 and 1992, approximately 1500 women underwent symphysiotomy, some without adequate consent or even knowledge of the procedure. A series of 37 women were interviewed some 40 years later; long-term complications included stress urinary incontinence and low back pain. These studies have led to controversy regarding whether symphysiotomy still has a place in modern obstetrics.

A recent meta-analysis compared symphysiotomy with cesarean in seven studies (N = 1266) of women from low- and middle-income countries. No differences were found in perinatal or neonatal mortality or hemorrhage, although an increase in later stress urinary incontinence (RR, 4.36; 95% CI, 1.07 to 16.39) and fistula formation (RR 10.04; 95% CI 3.23 to 31.21) was noted with symphysiotomy. Symphysiotomy was suggested as an alternative to cesarean in areas of the world where resources are limited (Wilson, 2016). A Cochrane review states that while symphysiotomy may be a life-saving procedure in specific circumstances, professional and global medical societies should provide evidence-based guidelines for the use (or nonuse) of the procedure based on best available evidence. Cesarean is preferable to symphysiotomy in developed nations. The question becomes whether women lacking access to immediate cesarean delivery and their fetuses are better off with symphysiotomy, a procedure that entails less surgical risk, less blood loss, and the ability to avoid a uterine scar in future gestations versus uterine rupture or fetal death from obstructed labor.

MATERNAL/FETAL INDICATIONS

The World Health Organization recommends that symphysiotomy be combined with vacuum extraction and employed as a life-saving procedure in areas where cesarean delivery is not immediately available or feasible.

- Established, obstructed labor with mild to moderate CPD with a live fetus when vacuum extraction has failed or when there is severe infection
- Entrapment of the aftercoming head during a breech delivery

FETAL INDICATIONS

- Fetus is alive.
- Fetal head is at −2 station and should not override the pubic symphysis.
- Cervix is fully dilated.

PROCEDURAL INDICATIONS

- Provider is experienced and proficient with procedure.
- Cesarean is not immediately available.

CONTRAINDICATIONS

Absolute

- Severe CPD where there is significant molding of the fetal head
- More than three-fifths of the fetal head is palpable suprapubically
- Maternal major lower limb/pelvic deformities
- Malpresentations: face, brow, or transverse lie
- History of repair of vesicovaginal fistula (elective cesarean should be performed in these cases)

Relative

- Maternal age: older patients have higher risk of severe stress incontinence compared with teenagers.
- Preexisting ambulation or gait issues (maternal).
- Previous symphysiotomy: surgical technique is more challenging due to having to divide fibrous scar tissue and possibility that urethra is adherent to the back of the symphysis pubis.
- Maternal obesity: increased risk of landmark distortions and inability to gauge fetal size; later mobility issues may be worsened.

EQUIPMENT

Standard vaginal delivery table (See Chapter 156, Vaginal Delivery) or delivery bed with ability for lithotomy positioning
Equipment needed for vacuum extraction (See Chapter 157, Forceps and Vacuum-Assisted Delivery)
Sterile gloves and equipment to follow universal blood and body fluid precautions
Skin prep (povidone iodine or chlorhexidine scrub)
10-mL syringe
18- to 22-gauge, 0.5-inch or longer needle to draw up anesthetic

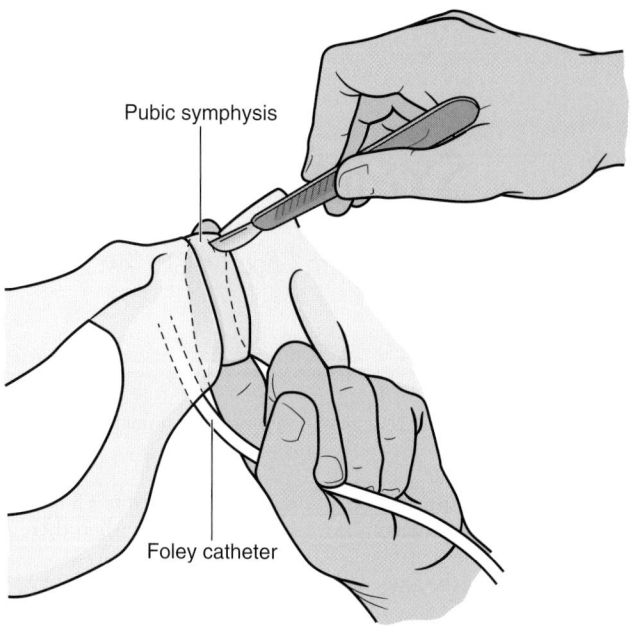

Pubic symphysis

Foley catheter

Fig. 159.1 An index finger should be placed in the vagina behind the pubic symphysis. While holding the Foley catheter to one side to protect the urethra, the scalpel is used to divide the pubic symphysis. Avoid going too deep, which could lacerate both the vagina and your finger.

22- to 27-gauge, 1-inch or longer needle to administer anesthetic
Lidocaine 1% or 2% with epinephrine
Foley catheter
Scalpel (size 20 or 21 blade)

PREPROCEDURE PATIENT EDUCATION

Symphysiotomy is often a procedure of last resort in resource limited settings where immediate cesarean is not available. It is not an elective procedure and should not be used for anticipation of CPD. Even in emergency situations, obtaining informed consent is essential. Risks and benefits should be discussed with the patient, including damage to the urethra, future risk of vesicovaginal fistula, and problems with gait.

TECHNIQUE

1. Don sterile gloves and personal protective equipment.
2. Ask two assistants to hold and stabilize patient's legs to prevent abduction past a maximum of 45 degrees from the midline. Abduction of the thighs more than 45 degrees may result in urethral damage.
3. Recheck fetal heart tones to assure that they are present.
4. Prep the mons and vulva with povidone iodine or chlorhexidine solution.
5. Place a Foley catheter using standard placement technique (see Chapter 96, Bladder Catheterization).
6. Anesthetize the vulva and skin over the mons pubis with 10 mL of 0.5% lidocaine with epinephrine. Drawing up another 10mL of lidocaine into the syringe, carry the needle down in the midline into the symphyseal joint itself. Wait at least 2 minutes and assess for adequacy of anesthesia using forceps.
7. Place your gloved, nondominant index finger into the vagina above and behind the pubic symphysis. Displace the urethra sideways to protect it in a lateral position. It may be necessary to displace the fetal head upward (Fig. 159.1).
8. With your other hand, palpate the anterior symphysis, feeling for the midline depression in the cartilage. Pierce the skin over the mons with the scalpel tip, using a stabbing motion. Carry the incision down toward the center of the joint.

9. Once the cartilage is cut, the blade pressure will be felt against the nondominant finger. Do not transect the thick band of tissue (posterior ligament) and be sure not to cut yourself with the scalpel.
10. Divide the cartilage in the lower half of the joint by gently withdrawing the blade a few millimeters and then using downward sweeping motions.
11. Withdraw the scalpel, reinsert it, and use the blade to make upward sweeping motions to divide the upper half of the cartilage.
12. Allow the pubic symphysis to separate, but do not let the maternal legs separate further than 45 degrees from the midline.
13. Strongly consider an episiotomy to enlarge the delivery passage and prevent further anterior vulvar trauma (See Chapter 158, Episiotomy and Repair of the Perineum).
14. Remove the catheter prior to delivery of the fetal head.
15. Apply the vacuum extractor to assist with delivery of the fetal head. Some providers will leave the vacuum attached while performing the symphysiotomy.
16. One or two stitches may be used to close the initial scalpel incision site.
17. Reinsert the Foley catheter.
18. Bring the maternal knees together strapping them together at the knees. Apply pressure to the symphysis pubis until bleeding is controlled.
19. Have the patient lie in left or right lateral decubitus position for 24 hours to prevent postoperative hematoma.

COMPLICATIONS

In one review of 5000 symphysiotomies performed in 28 different nations on 4 continents between 1900 and 1999, only 2 maternal deaths were directly related to the procedure (Bjorklund, 2002). Both involved maternal sepsis in the preantibiotic era, although overall morbidity from symphysiotomy was not greater than that seen with cesarean delivery. Stress incontinence, gait problems, and low back pain are main concerns, although incidence was often minimal in many of the studies. Urethral damage and osteitis from cutting into bone rather than the symphyseal cartilage are rarely encountered when appropriate surgical procedure is followed. Risk of injury to the surgeon's finger has not been reported.

POSTPROCEDURE MANAGEMENT AND PATIENT EDUCATION

Patients should wear elastic strapping across the front of the pelvis to reduce pain and stabilize the symphysis. The catheter should be left in place for a minimum of 5 days. If any hematuria is noted, consider leaving the catheter in for 10 days. Vulvovaginal fistula development following an obstructed labor sometime becomes apparent only after 72 hours, once necrotic tissue begins to break down at this time. If a fever or any signs of infection develop, intravenous ampicillin (2 g every 8 hours), gentamicin (5 mg/kg every 24 hours), and metronidazole (500 mg every 8 hours) should be given until the patient is afebrile for 48 hours. Analgesia for pain should be given based on provider preferences. Bedrest is indicated for 3 to 7 days after discharge. Patients should be encouraged to walk with assistance initially using a walker. Someone to provide assistance with walking is needed the first 2 to 3 days. Long-term concerns after symphysiotomy include stress incontinence, backache, and gait problems, although the incidence of these complications is significantly lower than previously reported in the Irish literature.

CPT/BILLING CODES

As symphysiotomy is a procedure generally done in resource-limited countries, a CPT code for delivery-related use is not available.

ICD-10-CM Diagnostic Codes

O66.9   Obstructed labor unspecified

Online Resources

World Health Organization. *Managing Complications in Pregnancy and Childbirth: A Guide for Midwives and Doctors.* Geneva: WHO; 2007:P53–P57. http://apps.who.int/iris/bitstream/10665/43972/1/9241545879_eng.pdf.

Recommended Reading

Armon P. Symphysiotomy. *Tropical Doctor.* 2015;45(2):60–67.
Bjorklund K. Minimally invasive surgery for obstructed labour. a review of symphysiotomy during the 20th century (including 5000 cases). *BJOG.* 2002;109:236–248.
Choudhury AP, Bhadra B, Roy A. Practical symphysiotomy: an overview. *J Indian Med Assoc.* 2010;108(8):498–504.

Hofmeyr GJ, Shweni PM. Symphysiotomy for feto-pelvic disproportion. *Cochrane Database Syst Rev.* 2012;10:CD005299.
Shaarani SR, van Eeden W, O'Byrne JM. The Irish experience of symphysiotomy: 40 years onwards. *J Obstet Gynaecol.* 2016;36(1):48–52.
Sigualt JR. *Discours sur les Avantages de la Section de la Symphyse.* Paris: Quillau; 1776.
Wilson A, Truchanowicz EG, Elmoghazy D, et al. Symphysiotomy for obstructed labor: a systematic review and meta-analysis. *BJOG.* 2016;123:1453–1461.

CHAPTER 160

CESAREAN DELIVERY

R. Levi Sundermeyer • Lee I. Blecher • Benjamin Mailloux

Cesarean delivery is the operative delivery of an infant and is usually performed to decrease the risk of perinatal morbidity and mortality. The term *cesarean* is considered to have been derived from the Latin verb *caedere*, meaning "to cut." The first reported case series of cesarean deliveries was published in 1591 by Rouseto and Casparo. In the United States, the rate of cesarean deliveries has been increasing every year since 1996, but in 2015, this rate decreased slightly to 32% (varying from 23% to 40%). For many years before 1960, the cesarean rate was closer to 5%.

Among family physicians in the United States, 19% actively perform vaginal deliveries and about 7% perform cesarean deliveries. These family physicians are found in a wide variety of practice settings ranging from urban teaching institutions to isolated rural practices. Several family medicine obstetrics fellowships exist to offer additional training for family physicians who choose to perform cesareans.

This chapter discusses one standard technique for performing an uncomplicated low transverse cesarean delivery. As with many surgical procedures, there is no standard technique, although there are several evidence-based recommendations based on available data. The Pfannenstiel skin/Kerr uterine approach is described in this chapter, along with a brief description of incisions of the Joel-Cohen type (Misgav Ladach approach).

INDICATIONS

Maternal Indications

- Repeat cesarean when mother declines or does not respond to a trial of labor
- Repeat cesarean when a trial of labor is not indicated (e.g., prior classical uterine incision)
- Antepartum hemorrhage/placental abruption
- Obstructive pelvic, vaginal, or vulvar tumors or condylomata
- Severe hypertension or preeclampsia with severe features remote from delivery
- Contracted pelvis (cephalopelvic disproportion)
- Medical contraindication due to maternal disease (e.g., retinal detachment or cardiac disease)
- Uterine rupture
- Active maternal herpes simplex genital infection
- Maternal exhaustion
- Failed induction of labor
- Placenta previa
- Elective on maternal request with adequate maternal counseling

Fetal Indications

- Malpresentation (e.g., brow or face presentation, transverse or breech lie)
- Nonreassuring fetal heart rate (e.g., recurrent late decelerations, bradycardia, lack of heart rate variability)
- Arrest of the active stage, including deep transverse arrest
- Fetal anomalies
- Cord prolapse
- Very low birth weight infant (<1500 g)
- Multiple gestation when the presenting fetus is nonvertex
- Failed trial of forceps or vacuum
- Macrosomia (controversial; estimated fetal weight >5000 g or >4500 g in a mother with diabetes)
- Maternal human immunodeficiency virus infection in patient with elevated viral loads or not taking highly active antiretroviral therapy

CONTRAINDICATIONS

Because cesarean delivery is a lifesaving procedure in many instances, there are no absolute contraindications other than patient refusal after the consequences have been explained clearly to the mother.

EQUIPMENT

- Intravenous antibiotic such as cefazolin 1 or 2 g or, for a penicillin-allergic patient, clindamycin 600 mg, ideally given 15 to 60 minutes prior to skin incision
- Medications: oxytocin, methylergotamine, carboprost, misoprostol, terbutaline
- Standard operating room cesarean package to include the following:

Quantity Needed	Instrument
6	Allis clamps
4	Pennington clamps (8-in)
2	Tissue forceps (toothed; 6- and 8-in)
2	Dressing forceps (smooth; 6- and 8-in)
2	Russian forceps (6- and 8-in)
4	Sponge (ring) forceps
2	Adson forceps with teeth
2	Blade handles
2	No. 10 blade scalpel
6	Curved hemostats (5.5-inch)
6	Curved Kelly clamps
2	Needle holders
4	Kocher or Ochsner clamps (7.5-inch)
1	DeLee, Fritsch, or Rochard universal retractor
3	Richardson retractors (small, medium, and large)
1	Bandage scissors (7.25-inch)
1	Metzenbaum scissors (7-in)
1	Curved Mayo scissors (6.5-inch)
1	Straight Mayo scissors (6.5-inch)
1	Suction device with Poole and Yankauer suction tips

4	Packages of suture (uterine: 2 each of No. 1 or 0 Vicryl, chromic or Monocryl; fascia: 1 of 0 Vicryl or PDS; Skin suture: 3-0 or 4-0 Vicryl or Monocryl; optional 2-0 or 3-0 Vicryl for peritoneum or subcutaneous layers)
20	Lap sponges
1	Bovie cautery device with grounding pad
2	Babcock clamps (if tubal ligation planned) (optional)
2	Army-Navy retractors (optional)
1	Surgical stapler (optional)

PRECAUTIONS

Several conditions increase surgical risk with cesarean procedures:

- Grand multiparity
- Preterm delivery
- Placenta previa (specifically with a history of any uterine scar)
- Placenta accreta
- Maternal morbid obesity
- Transverse fetal lie (specifically fetal back/shoulder presentation)
- Maternal coagulopathy
- Large uterine fibroids
- Multiple gestation
- Repeat cesarean on patient with extensive adhesions
- Maternal diseases (diabetes, hypertension, infection)

PREPROCEDURE PATIENT EDUCATION

Informed consent should be obtained, the patient's questions answered, and a consent form signed. A standard hospital consent form can be used, emphasizing the following risks to the patient and infant undergoing cesarean:

- Complications due to anesthesia
- Injury to the bladder or ureters
- Injury to the bowel
- Need for hysterectomy
- Hemorrhage requiring transfusion
- Infection
- Injury to the fetus (rare)
- Rupture of the uterus during future labor

A consent for the use of blood products in the event of hemorrhage should also be obtained. Box 160.1 shows typical preoperative orders for a cesarean section.

TECHNIQUE

There are three choices of uterine incision when performing a cesarean section: low transverse (Kerr), low vertical (Krönig), and classical. These are outlined in Table 160.1. The most popular technique, the low transverse (Kerr), is described here. Regardless of technique used, preoperative antibiotics (cefazolin 1 to 2 g IV or clindamycin 900 mg IV if patient is penicillin- allergic) should be given 15 to 60 minutes prior to skin incision. Some data suggest that additional preoperative prophylaxis with azithromycin 500 mg for cesarean delivery during labor or after membrane rupture further reduces infectious morbidity. Surgical preparation of the skin with a combination of chlorhexidine and alcohol provides the lowest risk of wound infection.

1. Create a left tilt by either tilting the operating table or placing a wedge under the patient when regional anesthesia is used. (This displaces the uterus to the left, which permits better venous return and improves fetal oxygenation.)
2. After anesthesia has been induced by a regional (epidural), spinal, or general anesthetic, test for anesthesia of the abdominal skin with the Allis clamp.

BOX 160.1 Typical Preoperative Orders for Cesarean Section

CBC without diff
Type and hold 2 units PRBCs (or type and screen)
Foley to gravity
Anesthesia preop for epidural, spinal, or general anesthesia
NPO
Lactated Ringer solution at 125 mL/hr IV
Cefazolin 1–2 g IV on call to operating room (should be given 15–60 min prior to skin incision); clindamycin 600–900 mg IV if patient is penicillin allergic
Prep abdomen per physician's preference

CBC, Complete blood cell count; *IV*, Intravenous; *NPO*, nothing by mouth; *PRBCS*, packed red blood cells.

TABLE 160.1 Types of Uterine Incisions

Incision	Advantages	Disadvantages
Low transverse	Lower uterine segment is thin and less vascular. Incision heals well, less risk of subsequent dehiscence. Most popular; >90% of all cesarean births	Risk of lateral extension into the uterine vessels
Low vertical	Useful if lower uterine segment is thick or has fibroids. Back down transverse fetal lie. Fetal anomalies such as hydrocephalus	Need for greater separation of the bladder from lower uterine segment. Need for repeat cesarean section if upper segment entered
Classical incision	Suitable for emergent cases, easiest and fastest access to the infant. Better exposure. Ability to develop a larger opening for delivery	Increased blood loss. Difficult repair (three layers). Increased risk of rupture in subsequent pregnancies. Adhesion formation between incision and abdominal organs. Eight times greater risk of dehiscence than with transverse incision

3. When anesthesia is deemed adequate, perform a Pfannenstiel skin incision by incising the abdominal skin to a width of approximately 13 to 15 cm, two fingerbreadths above the symphysis pubis, using a No. 10 blade (Fig. 160.1). Maintain hemostasis from dermal bleeding with Bovie cautery.
4. Carry the incision down through the subcutaneous fat to the fascia with the No. 10 blade. In the midline, make a 2-cm horizontal incision in the fascia with the scalpel. Lift the fascia and extend the cut edges laterally and superiorly in a curvilinear fashion with the curved Mayo scissors (Fig. 160.2).
5. Grasp the superior edge of the fascia with two Kocher clamps to elevate the fascia off of the underlying muscle, and bluntly dissect the fascia and the heavier fibers of the linea alba away from the muscle with your fingers, staying in the midline (Figs. 160.3 and 160.4). This may be more difficult in a repeat case because of adhesive scar formation. In such cases, use the Mayo scissors to cut the adhesions. Then use the Mayo scissors again to cut through the midline fibers of the linea alba. Be careful not to cut the muscle tissue or to cut a "buttonhole" through

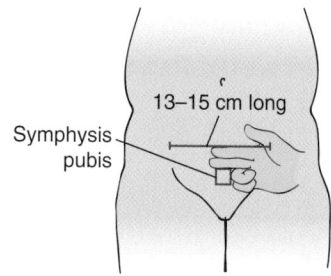

Fig. 160.1 Pfannenstiel skin incision. The horizontal incision is carried out two fingerbreadths above the symphysis pubis.

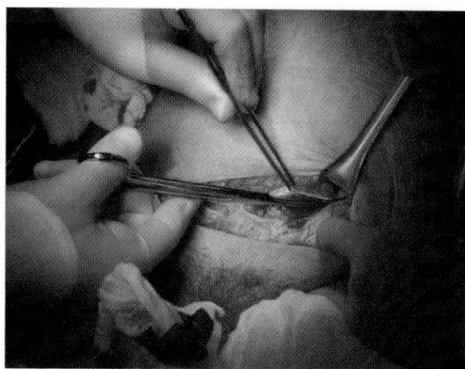

Fig. 160.2 Extending the fascia incision using curved Mayo scissors.

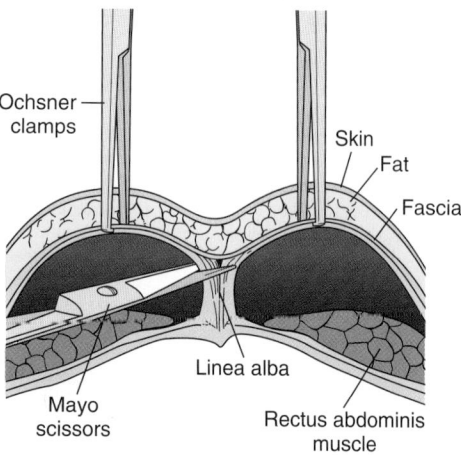

Fig. 160.3 Dissecting the linea alba.

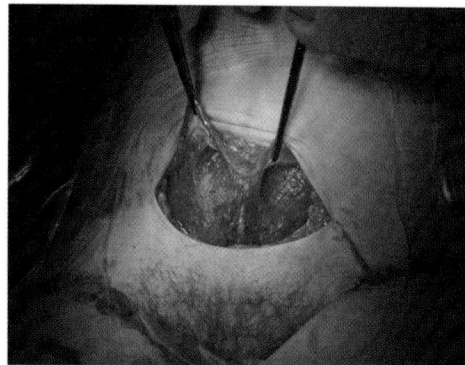

Fig. 160.4 Elevating the fascia off the underlying muscle by gripping the superior edge using two Kocher clamps.

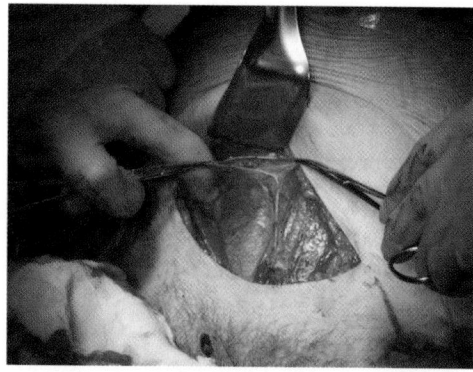

Fig. 160.5 After tenting the exposed peritoneum with two hemostats, a small incision is made before bluntly extending it.

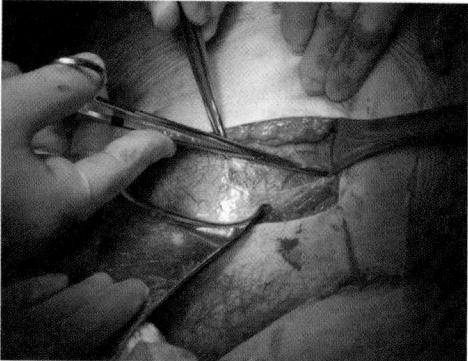

Fig. 160.6 Developing the bladder flap.

the fascia. This dissection can be repeated on the inferior edge of the fascia, bluntly and sharply dissecting the fascia away from the muscular tissue.

6. Bluntly separate the rectus muscle in the midline in a vertical fashion to expose the peritoneum. The peritoneal cavity can be entered bluntly or sharply. If it is sharply opened, grasp the peritoneum superiorly with two hemostats, tent it away from the underlying viscera, and incise with Metzenbaum scissors or the No. 10 blade (Fig. 160.5). Keep this incision above the urachus (if visualized) to make sure that you are above the bladder. Bluntly extend this incision vertically slightly, being careful not to extend to the bladder inferiorly.

7. Place the DeLee bladder blade to retract and identify the bladder.

8. *Optional step that can be safely omitted:* Develop the bladder flap (Fig. 160.6) by picking up the peritoneum over the lower uterine segment with tissue forceps and incising it laterally to make a flap approximately 12 cm long (Figs. 160.7 and 160.8). Dissect the peritoneum off the uterus bluntly with your fingers. Push fingers downward against the lower uterine segment while gently moving medial to lateral. Reapply the DeLee bladder blade to include the inferior bladder flap just created.

9. Determine the position of the lateral uterine vessels as well as the orientation of the uterus. Next, incise the lower uterine segment over the fetal head; this is known as *scoring the uterus* (Fig. 160.9). Announce "uterine incision" so that the anesthesiologist and nursery attendant can prepare for imminent delivery. It is best to use a No. 10 blade and a 2- to 3-cm incision, proceeding millimeter by millimeter in depth to avoid injuring the presenting fetal part below (Fig. 160.10).

10. Extend the uterine incision bluntly with your fingers in a cephalocaudad direction. Bandage scissors may then be used to extend the incision (protecting the fetal parts with two fingers inside

the opening) in a superior and lateral direction through the lower uterine segment for a total incision of approximately 10 to 11 cm (Fig. 160.11). However, this carries the added risk of extending the incision into the uterine arteries, so proceed with caution.

11. Rupture the membranes with the Allis clamp.

12. Deliver the fetal head by inserting a cupped hand over the head and occiput, keeping the wrist straight. Gently lift upward without flexing the wrist, bringing the head out of the incision along with your hand (Fig. 160.12). The surgical assistant will have to exert gentle fundal pressure after the occiput has cleared the incision.

NOTE: If the head is flexed tightly or stuck from excessive pushing before the procedure, as is common in arrest-of-descent cases

or true cephalopelvic disproportion, have an assistant push the head inward and upward from the vagina (Fig. 160.13). Occasionally it may be necessary to inject 0.25 mg of terbutaline subcutaneously or intravenously to relax the uterus and move the infant upward far enough to allow for delivery. Note that use of terbutaline can increase blood loss from uterine atony.

13. Deliver the anterior shoulder, the posterior shoulder, and then the rest of the infant as in a vaginal delivery. Delayed cord clamping until after 30 to 60 seconds following delivery is recommended to increase both hemoglobin levels at birth and iron stores in the first months of life. This may favorably affect developmental outcomes in both term and preterm infants. Clamp and cut the cord and hand the infant to the nurse in attendance. Obtain cord blood if necessary. The preferred method for removal of the placenta is by continuous cord traction allowing it to separate spontaneously. Manual removal increases infectious morbidity but may be indicated in the setting of excessive bleeding (Fig. 160.14). Remove the last adherent membranes with the aid of ring forceps.

14. You may choose to externalize the uterus for improved visualization and access, but this is optional. To control blood loss, two Pennington clamps can be placed at the edges of the incision where bleeding is most vigorous. Wrap the uterine fundus in a clean moist lap sponge as you massage the uterus; gently clean the inner endometrium with moist lap sponges so that it is free of any clots, membranes, and debris. Routine manual or instrumental dilation of the cervix prior to uterine closure is not necessary; the practice neither improves postoperative hemoglobin levels nor reduces maternal fever or infection.

16. The hysterotomy incision should be closed using a two-layer (double layer) closure, which theoretically reduces the risk of uterine rupture in the next pregnancy. Single-layer closure may be an option when bilateral tubal ligation is also performed during the procedure. Unless arterial bleeding is evident, nonlocking stiches are reasonable. No strong evidence supports choice of suture technique (e.g., continuous [locked vs. unlocked] versus interrupted closure). The cesarean section surgical techniques (CORONIS) randomized controlled

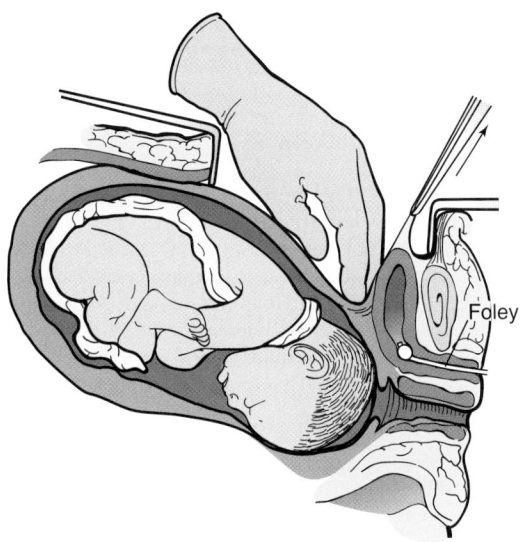

Fig. 160.7   Dissection of the bladder away from the uterus.

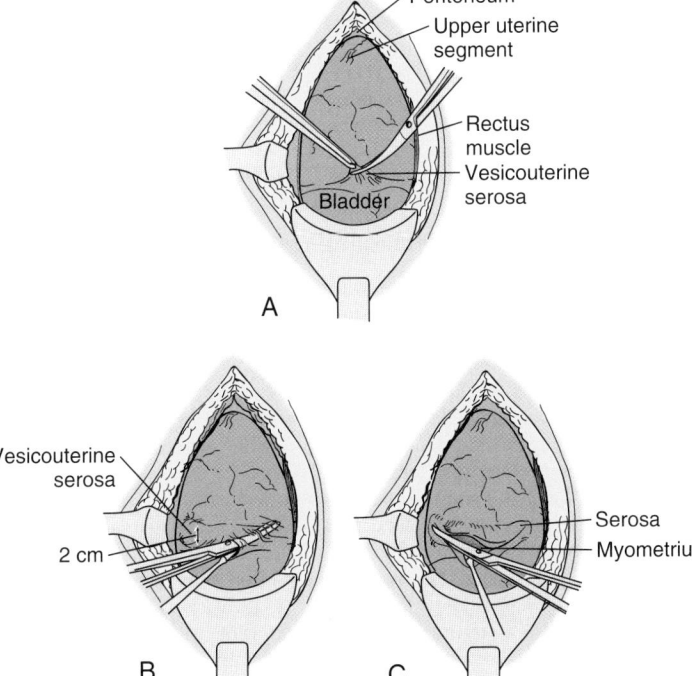

Fig. 160.8   Development of the bladder flap. (A) Tenting of the peritoneum. (B) Undermining of the peritoneum. (C) Incising the peritoneum.

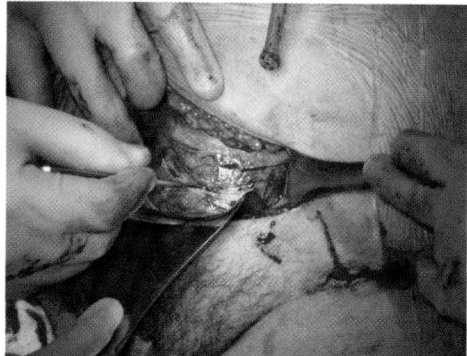

Fig. 160.9   Scoring the uterus.

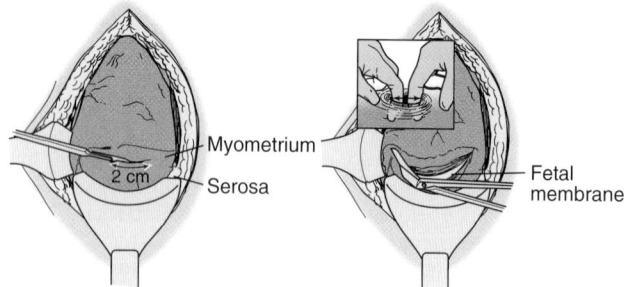

Fig. 160.10   Low transverse incision. The uterine incision is developed in a curvilinear fashion.

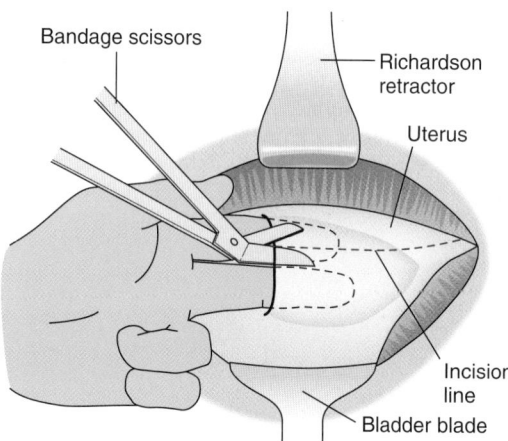

Fig. 160.11   Protecting the fetal head from the bandage scissors when the uterus is being incised. Two fingers are placed under the incision to protect the infant from the bandage scissors.

trial found that the type of suture material (chromic vs. delayed synthetic absorbables like polyglactin 910 and poliglecaprone 25) did not show statistically significant effects on maternal outcome, so choice of suture based on surgeon's preference is reasonable—No. 0 chromic, 0 Monocryl (synthetic monofilament), and 0 Vicryl (braided) sutures are commonly used in the United States (Figs. 160.15 and 160.16). One RCT of 78 term patients who underwent cesarean delivery showed a wedge-type healing defect in cases where the endometrial layer was not included in the full-thickness myometrial uterine closure; the clinical significance/long-term impact of this is unknown, however. Should an extension of the incision occur (typically inferiorly toward the cervix), the extension should be repaired first and then the hysterotomy

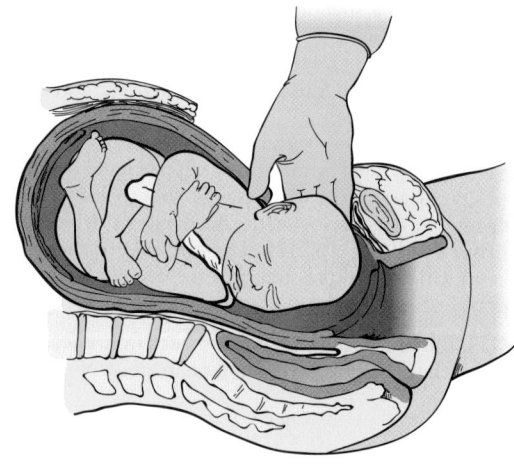

Fig. 160.12   Lifting the fetal head out of the uterus. Keep the wrist straight to avoid using the uterus as a fulcrum.

incision. Occasionally one small area of the hysterotomy incision may bleed; this can be repaired with a figure-of-eight stitch for hemostasis.
17. Inspect the uterus, tubes, and ovaries. If a bilateral tubal ligation is desired, perform it at this time.
18. Clear the pouch of Douglas of any clots and debris using moist lap sponges. Intra-abdominal irrigation does not decrease maternal morbidity beyond that seen from preoperative antibiotics and may increase maternal nausea. If the uterus was exteriorized, return it to the abdominal cavity.
19. Palpate the right and left colic gutters for abnormal structures. *Optional:* Close the bladder flap/parietal peritoneum with No. 2-0 chromic. However, most experts do not recommend closing the peritoneum because it reapproximates on its own without suturing and closure extends surgical time.
20. Close the two-layered fascia in a running stitch with No. 0 Vicryl or 0 PDS. Make sure that the sutures are placed equally across the incision and no more than 1 cm apart (Fig. 160.17).
21. Inspect the subcutaneous fat and stop any bleeding with a Bovie cautery (Fig. 160.18). Close the subcutaneous dead space if the tissue depth is 2 cm or greater. This may inhibit accumulation of blood or serum, which can cause seromas or wound breakdown. If suturing is required for closure, use interrupted sutures with absorbable suture material, such as No. 3-0 plain or chromic gut. Routine use of wound drains is not beneficial.
22. Close the skin. The skin can be closed with running subcuticular sutures (like No. 3-0 or 4-0 Vicryl or Monocryl) or with a skin stapler.

Misgav Ladach Technique (Modified Joel-Cohen Technique)

1. Cut a straight transverse incision through the skin 3 cm caudal to the anterosuperior iliac spines.
2. In the middle of the incision (2 to 3 cm), use the scalpel to incise down to the fascia.
3. Digitally take down the subcutaneous fat overlying the fascia.
4. Open the fascia using a small midline transverse incision. Extend it laterally using bandage scissors.
5. Bluntly separate the superior rectus sheath from the rectus muscle by pulling the sheath cranially and caudally using your two index fingers.
6. Bluntly open the peritoneum using one or two fingers and stretch it caudally and cranially to create a transverse window.
7. Create a transverse superficial incision in the visceral peritoneum 1 cm above the bladder reflection. Use your fingers or a swab to reflect the bladder inferiorly.

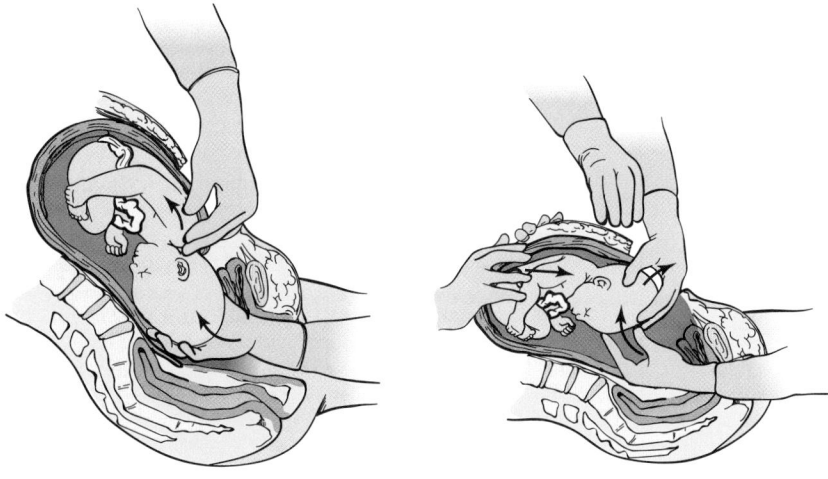

Fig. 160.13 Technique for extracting an impacted fetal head. An assistant exerts gentle upward force on the head from the vagina as the operator exerts steady upward pressure on the head and shoulders.

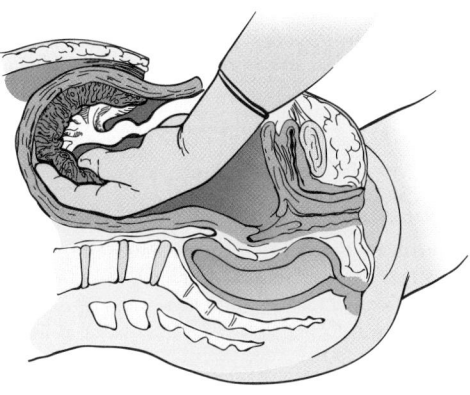

Fig. 160.14 Manual extraction of the placenta.

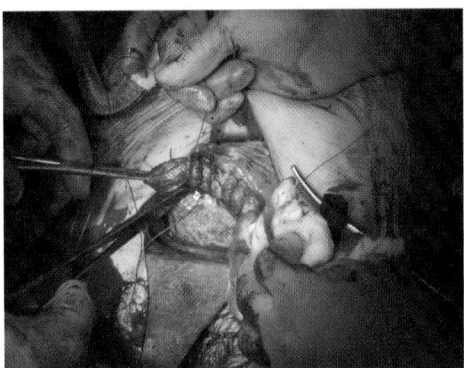

Fig. 160.16 Closing the uterus using a running locked stitch.

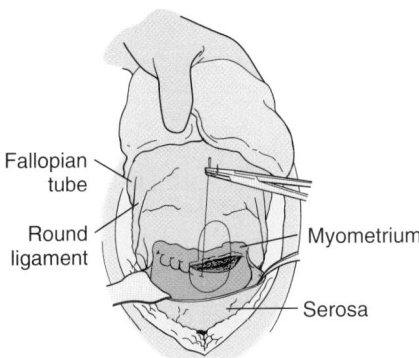

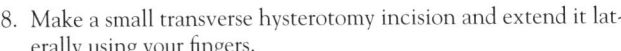

Fig. 160.15 Uterine closure with a running locked stitch of No. 0 chromic catgut suture.

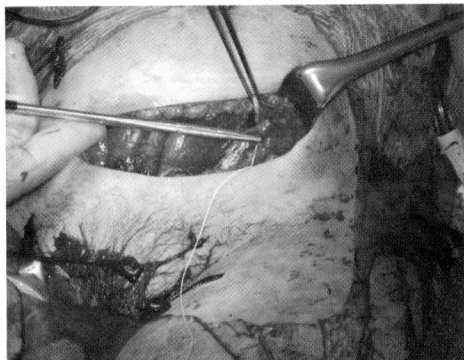

Fig. 160.17 Closing the fascia.

8. Make a small transverse hysterotomy incision and extend it laterally using your fingers.
9. Deliver the fetus and placenta as described earlier in steps 13 and 14.
10. Close the hysterotomy incision with one layer of continuous locking suture. A second layer can be placed if needed.
11. Reapproximate the fascia with the continuous running suture technique.
12. Close the skin using two or three mattress stitches.

SAMPLE OPERATIVE REPORT

The sample operative report, available at www.expertconsult.com, shows an example of an ordinary, uncomplicated case. Any complications should be added and noted in the dictation.

COMPLICATIONS

- Anesthesia-related
- Injury to the bladder, ureters, or bowel
- Uterine hemorrhage
- Neonatal injury

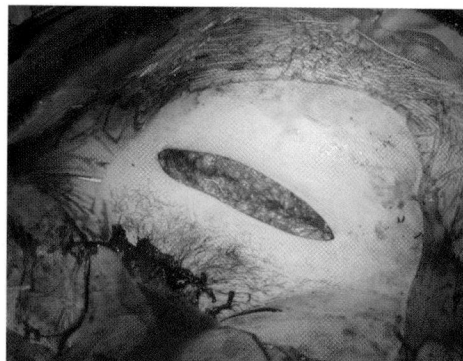

Fig. 160.18 Subcutaneous fat after closure.

POSTOPERATIVE ORDERS

Box 160.2 shows typical postoperative orders for cesarean delivery.

POSTPROCEDURE PATIENT EDUCATION

First 24 Hours

The patient should be told what to expect, such as pain control issues (e.g., patient-controlled analgesia [PCA] pump vs. intravenous opioid analgesia). Uterine cramping is expected and may occur after fundal massage by the nurses. The Foley catheter remains in place. Rooming-in with the infant as early as possible to start breastfeeding and bonding is encouraged. Most patients stay in the hospital for 48 to 72 hours after a cesarean delivery.

First Postoperative Day

Early ambulation is important to prevent atelectasis and pneumonia. The diet is advanced early to clear liquids and then full liquids as tolerated. If the patient is ambulating well and can walk to the bathroom, the Foley catheter is discontinued. Heparin lock the intravenous line and transition to oral opioid analgesia from a PCA pump, intravenous, or intramuscular opioids. The patient should note some flatus, and urination should increase from postpartum diuresis.

Second Postoperative Day

The criteria for discharge may include flatus, ability to tolerate a regular diet, lack of fever, and full ambulation on oral pain medication only. Many patients can be discharged 36 hours after a cesarean. If the skin is closed, staples can be removed and replaced with Steri-Strips. If not, this can be done at postoperative day 5 on an outpatient basis. Morbidly obese patients may benefit from leaving staples in longer.

Discharge Instructions

* No driving while on opioids.
* Intercourse can be resumed when there is mutual interest.
* Care of the surgical incision is relatively simple. Water can wash over the wound as long as there is no direct impact of water onto the wound. Keeping the wound clean and dry is important for adequate healing. This includes avoiding coverage by skin folds, which can lead to excessive moisture and infection.
* Notify the physician's office for the following problems: pus seeping out of the wound, fever, painful urination, difficulty breathing, shortness of breath, or increasing pain.
* Follow up in the office for a wound check in 1 week.

BOX 160.2 Typical Postoperative Orders for Cesarean Section

1. Admit to the service of _____.
2. Admit to recovery room, then to floor as per PACU protocol.
3. Monitor vital signs q15min until stable, then q30min until anesthesia wears off, then q4h on the floor for 24 hr, then per routine.
4. IV lactated Ringer solution with 20 U of oxytocin at 125 mL/hr × 1 L (started in OR).
5. After first liter, follow with IV lactated Ringer at 125 mL/hr.
6. Activity: out of bed as tolerated with assistance first time and PRN thereafter; deep venous thrombosis prophylaxis (SCDs or TED hose) until ambulatory (or longer if indicated)
7. Diet: clear liquids, advance as tolerated.
8. Labs: CBC in the morning on first postpartum day.
9. Foley to gravity drainage. Discontinue if urine is clear and patient is ambulating.
10. Strict intake and output every shift. Discontinue after patient voids at least 250 mL × 2, is tolerating oral intake, and IV fluids are discontinued.
11. K-Pad as needed to abdominal incision after 24 hr.
12. Call clinician for the following:
    * Temperature >100.4°F
    * Pulse >110 beats/min
    * Increasing uterine tenderness
    * Foul-smelling lochia
    * Excessive vaginal bleeding
13. Pain medication (coordinate with anesthesia)
    * PCA pump if available × 24 hr
    * If not tolerating orals—morphine 2 mg IV q6h PRN.
    * If tolerating orals—Percocet 1–2 tabs PO q4–6h PRN for pain
14. Other medications to consider:
    * Promethazine 6.25–12.5 mg IV q4h PRN for nausea.
    * Ondansetron 4 mg IV × 1 PRN for nausea.
    * Diphenhydramine 25 mg PO/IV q6h PRN for itching or as a sleep aid.
    * Simethicone 80 mg 1–2 tablets PO after meals and QHS PRN for gas.
    * Bisacodyl 10 mg PR × 1 PRN for severe gas/constipation.
    * Methylergonovine 0.2 mg PO/IM q6h PRN for excessive vaginal bleeding.
15. Breast care and lactation consult PRN.
16. Sitz bath 3–4 times daily PRN for hemorrhoids and/or perineal discomfort.
17. Patient self-administered medications to bedside:
    * Sennosides 8.6 mg and docusate 50 mg 2 capsules PO at bedtime PRN for constipation.
    * Perineal spray to perineum PRN for pain.
    * Witch hazel pads: apply 1 pad to perineum/hemorrhoids PRN for discomfort.
    * Anusol-HC ointment to hemorrhoids three times daily PRN for discomfort.
18. Provide Rh–D immune globulin if indicated (Rh D-negative mother and Rh D-positive baby).

CBC, Complete blood cell count; *IV*, Intravenous, *OR*, operating room; *PACU*, postanesthesia care unit; *PCA*, patient-controlled analgesia; *PO*, orally; *PRN*, as needed; *SCD*, sequential compression device. *TED hose*, antiembolism stockings.

---

* Limit activity to walking for the first week, back to full activity by 6 weeks.
* Arrange for interconception planning/postpartum contraception.

CPT/BILLING CODES

59510	Routine obstetric care including antepartum care, cesarean delivery, and postpartum care
59514	Cesarean delivery only
59515	Cesarean delivery only, including postpartum care
59618	Routine obstetric care including antepartum care, cesarean delivery, and postpartum care, following attempted vaginal delivery after previous cesarean delivery
59620	Cesarean delivery only, following attempted vaginal delivery after previous cesarean delivery
59622	Cesarean delivery only, following attempted vaginal delivery after previous cesarean delivery, including postpartum care

ICD-10-CM DIAGNOSTIC CODES

O44.01	Complete placenta previa without hemorrhage unspecified trimester
O45.90	Premature separation of placenta (e.g., abruptio placentae), unspecified trimester
O45.009	Premature separate of placenta with coagulation defects, unspecified trimester
O14.14	Severe preeclampsia complicating childbirth
O48.0	Prolonged pregnancy, beyond 42 completed weeks of gestation, delivered, with or without mention of antepartum complication
O98.519	Other viral diseases complicating pregnancy, unspecified trimester
O32.1XXX	Maternal care for breech presentation
O32.2XXX	Maternal care for transverse or oblique presentation
O32.3XXX	Maternal care for face or brow presentation
O33.5XXX	Maternal care for unusually large fetus
O34.219	Maternal care unspecified type scar from previous cesarean delivery complication
O77.9	Fetal distress unspecified
O61.9	Failed induction of labor unspecified
O64.8XXX	Obstructed labor, caused by malposition and malpresentation unspecified
O65.9	Obstructed labor due to maternal pelvic abnormality
O64.0XXX	Obstructed labor due to incomplete rotation of fetal head
O66.9	Obstructed labor (dystocia NOS)
O66.40	Failed trial of labor, unspecified
O66.5	Attempted application of forceps or vacuum extractor, unspecified
O62.0	Abnormality of forces of labor, primary uterine inertia, failure of cervical dilation, primary hypotonic uterine dysfunction
O62.1	Abnormality of forces of labor, secondary uterine inertia, arrested active phase of labor or secondary hypotonic uterine dysfunction
O63.0	Prolonged labor, first stage
O63.1	Prolonged labor, second stage
O69.89	Prolapse of cord, delivered, with or without mention of antepartum complication
O71.1	Rupture of uterus during labor

Acknowledgment

The editors recognize the contributions of Rebecca H. Hart, MD, to this chapter in a previous edition of this text.

RECOMMENDED READING

American College of Obstetricians and Gynecologists. Delayed umbilical cord clamping after birth. *Committee Opinion No. 684. Obstet Gynecol.* 2017;129(1):e5–e10.

Berghella V, Baxter JK, Chauhan SP. Evidence-based surgery for cesarean delivery. *Am J Obstetr Gynecol.* 2005;193:1607–1617.

Dahlke JD, Mendez-Figueroa H, Rouse DJ, et al. Evidence-based surgery for cesarean delivery: an updated systematic review. *Am J Obstet Gynecol.* 2013;209:294–306.

Dahlke JE, Mendez-Figueroa H, Shim HG, et al. Preferences in cesarean delivery surgical technique: a survey of maternal-fetal medicine fellows. *J Matern Fetal Neonatal Med.* 2015;28(1):77–81.

Dodd JM, Anderson ER, Gates S, et al. Surgical techniques for uterine incision and uterine closure at the time of cesarean section. *Cochrane Database Syst Rev.* 2014:CD004732.

Holmgren G, Sjoholm L, Stark M. the Misgav Ladach method for cesarean section; method description. *ACTA Obstet Gynecol Scand.* 1999;78:615–618.

Liabsuetrakul T, Peeyananjarassri K. Mechanical dilation of the cervix at non-labour cesarean section reducing postoperative morbidity. *Cochrane Database Syst Rev.* 2011:CD008019.

Macones GA, Cleary KL, Parry S, et al. The timing of antibiotics at cesarean: a randomized controlled trial. *Am J Perinatol.* 2012;29:273–276.

Martin JA, Hamilton BE, Osterman MJK. *Births in the United States, 2015. NCHS data brief, no 258.* Hyattsville, MD: National Center for Health Statistics; 2016.

Parantainen A, Verbeek JH, Lavoie MC, Pahwa M. Blunt versus sharp suture needles for preventing percutaneous exposure incidents in surgical staff. *Cochrane Database Syst Rev.* 2011;11:CD009170.

Yazicilgu F, Gokdogan A, Kelekci S, et al. Incomplete healing of the uterine incision after cesarean section: is it preventable? *Eur J Obstet Gynecol Repord Biol.* 2006;124:32.

CHAPTER 161

CULDOCENTESIS (COLPOCENTESIS)

Steven H. Eisinger

Culdocentesis is a procedure used to detect and sample free fluid in the peritoneal cavity of female patients. The classic application of this test is for the diagnosis of hemoperitoneum due to ruptured ectopic pregnancy, but it can also be used to detect acute pelvic inflammatory disease and to sample ascites. Modern imaging modalities, such as ultrasonography, have largely supplanted culdocentesis. Occasionally in an emergency or where imaging resources are unavailable, culdocentesis can still be extremely useful—even life-saving. Approximately 85% to 90% of patients with ruptured ectopic pregnancy have a positive culdocentesis. Even 65% to 70% of patients who have a stable presentation and unruptured ectopic pregnancy have a positive culdocentesis. If available, ultrasonography can also be used to guide culdocentesis or to confirm the presence of fluid (see Chapter 214, Emergency Department, Hospitalist and Office Ultrasound).

When compared for accuracy, the sensitivity and specificity of echogenic fluid for establishing a hemoperitoneum were 100% and 100%, respectively, compared with 66% and 80%, respectively, for culdocentesis. The negative predictive value of a nondiagnostic culdocentesis was 25% compared with 100% for echogenic fluid in the ectopic pregnancy subgroup of patients (Chen et al., 1998).

ANATOMY

The cul de sac (rectouterine pouch or pouch of Douglas) is the lowest point in the female abdominal cavity (when upright). The tissue septum between the posterior fornix of the vagina and the posterior cul de sac consists of vaginal mucosa, peritoneum, and little else. It is about 1 cm in thickness and contains no major blood vessels or organs. A needle introduced from the vagina into the cul de sac can easily access free fluid in the peritoneal cavity (Fig. 161.1).

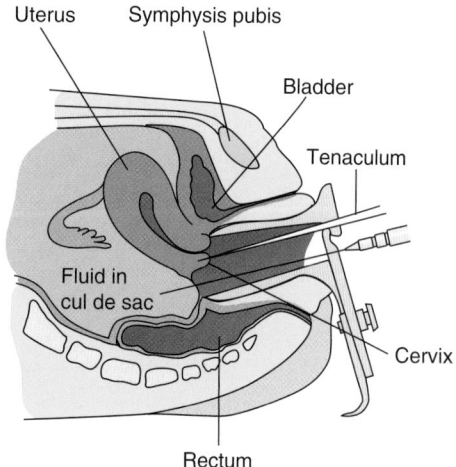

Fig. 161.1 Midline sagittal view of pelvis during culdocentesis showing anatomic relationships and position of instruments. (Modified from Eisinger SH. Procedures in family practice: culdocentesis. *J Fam Pract.* 1981;13:95–101.)

INDICATIONS

Ectopic Pregnancy

Ruptured ectopic pregnancy is the classic indication. Signs and symptoms of ruptured ectopic pregnancy include amenorrhea, abdominal pain with rebound tenderness, vaginal bleeding, shoulder pain, and a positive pregnancy test. Hemodynamic instability and acute anemia may be present. On speculum examination, the posterior fornix of the vagina may bulge into the vagina from the weight of the blood behind it. This test can be performed very rapidly to offer definitive proof of hemoperitoneum requiring immediate surgery.

Acute Salpingitis

Acute salpingitis can also be diagnosed by culdocentesis. This is the only means, short of laparotomy or laparoscopy, to obtain pus from within the abdominal cavity for diagnosis and culture.

Blunt Abdominal Trauma

Culdocentesis can be used in place of diagnostic peritoneal lavage following blunt abdominal trauma, particularly in patients with prior abdominal surgery.

Other

Ascitic fluid may be sampled for analysis such as for cytology for ovarian cancer, or even for therapeutic withdrawal (paracentesis).

CONTRAINDICATIONS

Absolute

A mass in the cul de sac whose rupture could be harmful (e.g., a neoplasm, abscess, endometrioma, or unruptured ectopic pregnancy) is an absolute contraindication. A bleeding diathesis is also a contraindication.

Relative

Severe, fixed retroversion of the uterus is a relative contraindication. Culdocentesis may be unsuccessful, as the cul de sac is obliterated and the needle will merely strike the corpus of the uterus.

EQUIPMENT AND SUPPLIES

The equipment for culdocentesis is simple and should be available in any emergency department or medical office that performs gynecologic procedures (Fig. 161.2). The following are required:

- Speculum
- Single-tooth tenaculum
- 10- or 20-mL syringe (a three-finger control syringe permits aspiration with one hand)

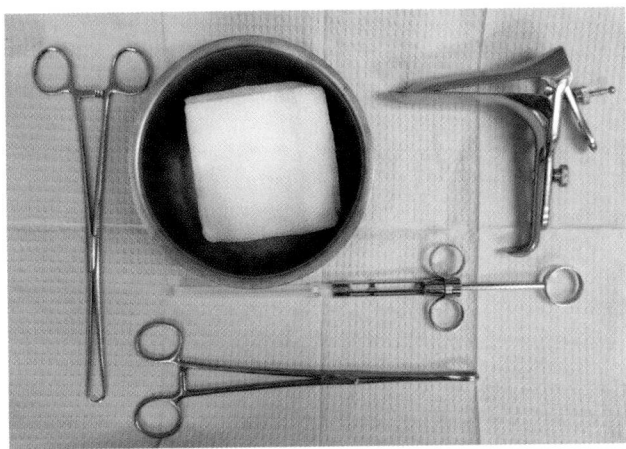

Fig. 161.2 Equipment required to perform culdocentesis.

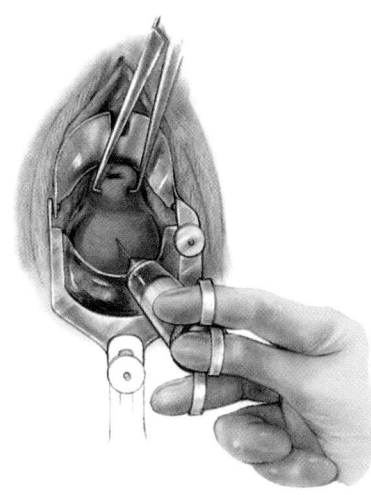

Fig. 161.3 Operator's view of culdocentesis. (From Eisinger SH. Procedures in family practice: culdocentesis. *J Fam Pract.* 1981;13:95–101.)

- 20-gauge spinal needle or a 3-inch needle extender with a 20-gauge needle attached
- Sterile swabs or sponges
- Ring forceps
- Antiseptic solution (povidone iodine, chlorhexidine)
- Local anesthetic such as 1 or 2% lidocaine for injection or 2% lidocaine gel (optional)
- Equipment necessary to observe universal blood and body fluid precautions

The instruments should be sterile and gloves should be used to perform the procedure. Drapes are unnecessary.

Precautions

Universal blood precautions should be observed.

PREPROCEDURE PATIENT EDUCATION

Verbal discussion of indications, risks, and benefits is recommended. A procedure consent form should be completed. The listed risks should include pain, bleeding, bowel perforation, rupture of a cyst, infection, and failure to detect blood (or fluid). This procedure is very similar to that performed by fertility specialists when harvesting eggs for in vitro fertilization. However, they usually use transvaginal ultrasound to direct the path of the needle.

PROCEDURE

1. *Perform a standard pelvic examination* before the procedure. During the speculum examination, vaginal cultures may be obtained or other tests performed. Bulging of the cul de sac into the posterior fornix of the vagina is a finding suggestive of the presence of intraperitoneal fluid. It is important to check for fixed masses in the cul de sac, or fixed uterine retroversion, both of which contraindicate culdocentesis.
2. *Position the patient.* After first obtaining orthostatic vital signs, ask the patient to stand or sit up for a minute before the procedure to permit blood to collect in the cul de sac. The procedure may be performed on any regular examination table with stirrups. The patient's head and shoulders should be slightly raised.
3. *Place the speculum.* A medium Graves speculum is suitable for most patients. Open it widely with the blades deeply positioned in the anterior vaginal fornix above and posterior fornix below the cervix. This placement exposes the posterior fornix below the cervix and stretches it taut, making the needle puncture easier.
4. *Cleanse the vagina and cervix* with a suitable antiseptic solution.
5. *Grasp the cervix with a tenaculum* (Fig. 161.3). The tenaculum may be placed vertically or horizontally on the anterior or posterior lip, per clinician preference. One milliliter of local anesthetic can be injected into the planned tenaculum site (optional).
6. *Choose the puncture site.* Manipulate the cervix by gently pulling either in and out or up and down using the tenaculum. This maneuver will identify the line of reflection where the mucosa sweeps off the cervix and crosses or covers the cul de sac. The needle puncture site should be about 1 cm below this reflection, in the midline.
7. *Administer anesthesia.* This step is optional. Culdocentesis is usually perceived as quite painful. Some clinicians recommend injecting a small amount of local anesthetic into the mucosa at the puncture site (e.g., 1 to 2 mL of 1% lidocaine). Lidocaine gel can also be applied. Alternatively, an intravenous sedation medication such as midazolam or hydromorphone may be given. The patient should be reassured that although the pain may be sharp, it will last only for a few seconds.
8. *Make the puncture.* Elevate the cervix in the vagina with the tenaculum to expose and stretch the mucosa of the posterior fornix. A small amount of air (1 to 2 mL) may be placed into the syringe before the puncture. The needle should be held in an approximately horizontal plane. Use a bold, smooth movement for the initial puncture, inserting the needle 3 to 4 cm through the mucosa, in the midline.
9. *Inject the air in the syringe.* Usually the air passes freely, and sometimes it can be heard bubbling through fluid. If the air does not pass freely, the needle tip is in a solid organ such as the uterus, and should be repositioned. Some practitioners may choose not to inject air to avoid the risk of inadvertent air embolism (exceedingly rare).

EDITOR'S NOTE: Transvaginal ultrasound can be used to determine the angle and depth necessary to direct the needle to obtain fluid. It can also be used to estimate the amount of fluid that is present. If transvaginal ultrasound is used, the injection of air may not be necessary. If transvaginal ultrasound is not available, transabdominal ultrasound may also be used to confirm the presence of fluid as well as to estimate the volume (see Chapter 214, Emergency Department, Hospitalist and Office Ultrasound).

10. *Aspirate by pulling back on the syringe plunger.* If blood or fluid fills the syringe, stop when it is full. If no fluid is obtained, then a

second or even third attempt may be made at a slightly different angle or location.

11. *Terminate the procedure when fluid is obtained*, or when three attempts fail to yield fluid.

12. *Examine the fluid from the cul de sac.* Observe free-flowing blood for several minutes for clotting because this may indicate a traumatic tap. Blood-tinged or frankly bloody fluid should be spun for a hematocrit. Clear or turbid fluid should be examined microscopically, and sent for aerobic and anaerobic cultures. Fluid can also be sent for cytology if indicated.

13. *A brief handwritten note* or dictated paragraph in an operative note will suffice for documentation.

SAMPLE OPERATIVE REPORT

Indication: Suspected ruptured ectopic pregnancy.
Procedure: Informed consent was obtained. Speculum placed allowing good visualization of the cervix and vagina. Area cleansed with povidone iodine swabs. Two mL of 1% lidocaine injected at aspiration site. Culdocentesis performed with 20-gauge spinal needle with insertion in the posterior fornix. First stick obtained 10 mL of free-flowing, nonclotting, bloody fluid with hematocrit of 20%. Patient tolerated procedure well with no signs of hemodynamic instability.

COMMON ERRORS

The most common error is incorrect angle or depth of needle puncture. This results in a failure to obtain fluid. This is corrected by repositioning the needle.

COMPLICATIONS

Complications of culdocentesis are rare. Bowel may be punctured on occasion. This usually resolves without sequelae. Puncturing a neoplasm or abscess is an unlikely possibility. Intra-abdominal bleeding is unlikely as long as the needle is kept in the midline, away from the great vessels of the pelvis. The most serious complication is a spurious or unclear result that prevents necessary treatment or leads to unnecessary intervention.

POSTPROCEDURE MANAGEMENT

Vaginal bleeding is usually minimal and stops quickly. Patients should be provided with appropriate postprocedure instructions related to the diagnosis made as a result of the procedure (e.g., pelvic infection, ectopic pregnancy).

INTERPRETATION OF RESULTS

Blood obtained from the cul de sac should be assessed for clotting and sent for hematocrit. Pooled blood taken from within the peritoneal cavity is usually defibrinated and will not clot. However, in exceptional cases, bleeding from a ruptured ectopic pregnancy is so brisk that the blood has not had time to become defibrinated and will therefore clot in the syringe. Peritoneal fluid may appear bloody even with a very low hematocrit. As a rough rule, a hematocrit less

than 15% suggests slight bleeding or a bloody tap, whereas a hematocrit more than 15% indicates hemoperitoneum and confirms a surgical emergency. A hemoperitoneum is signified by the aspiration of more than 2 mL of nonclotting blood. The finding of nonclotting blood with a hematocrit greater than 15% has been 70% to 97% predictive of a significant bleeding source such as an ectopic pregnancy. However 10% to 20% of ectopic pregnancies will have a negative or nondiagnostic culdocentesis. False positives occur in 2% of cases. A ruptured corpus luteum cyst is the most common cause of a false positive.

Pus or turbid fluid should be sent for Gram stain and culture. White blood cells and bacteria may be noted. Appendicitis and pelvic inflammatory disease can cause a turbid exudate.

Clear fluid may result from a ruptured cyst, ascites, or normal peritoneal fluid.

Somewhat less than half the time, no fluid can be obtained despite multiple taps. This phenomenon should be referred to as a dry tap, rather than a negative tap. No diagnostic assumptions should be made on the basis of a dry tap.

CPT/BILLING CODES

57020	Colpocentesis (culdocentesis)

ICD-10-CM DIAGNOSTIC CODES

N70.01	Salpingitis (acute)
N94.89	Other specified condition associated with female genital organs (pelvic pain)
O00.00	Abdominal pregnancy without uterine pregnancy; ruptured

RECOMMENDED READING

Chen PC, Sickler GK, Dubinsky TJ, Maklad N, Jocobi RL, et al. Sonographic detection of echogenic fluid and correlation with culdocentesis in the evaluation of ectopic pregnancy. *Am J Roentgenol.* 1998;170(5):1299–1302.

DeCherney AH, Nathan L, Laufer N, et al. *Current Diagnosis and Treatment: Gynecology.* 11th ed. McGraw-Hill; 2013.

Eisinger SH. Procedures in family practice: culdocentesis. *J Fam Pract.* 1981;13:95–101.

Hager WD, Eschenbach DA, Spence MR, Sweet RL. Criteria for diagnosis and grading of salpingitis. *Obstet Gynecol.* 1983;61:113–114.

Levine DL. Culdocentesis. In: Reichman EF, ed. *Emergency Medicine Procedures.* 2nd ed. New York: McGraw-Hill; 2013:945–948.

Mishell Jr DR. Ectopic pregnancy: Etiology, pathology, diagnosis, management, fertility prognosis. In: Stenchever MA, Droegemueller W, Herbst AL, Mishell Jr DR, eds. *Comprehensive Gynecology.* 4th ed. St. Louis: Mosby; 2001:457.

Papadakis MA, McPhee SJ, Rabow MW. *Chapter 19: Obstetrics and Obstetrics Disorders. Current Medical Diagnosis and Treatment.* 56th ed. McGraw-Hill; 2017.

Vermesh M, Graczykowski JW, Sauer MV. Reevaluation of the role of culdocentesis in the management of ectopic pregnancy. *Am J Obstet Gynecol.* 1990;162:411–413.

CHAPTER 162

DILATION AND CURETTAGE

Verneeta L. Williams • Sheila Thomas

Dilation and curettage (D&C) is a valuable diagnostic and therapeutic tool in the management of abnormal uterine bleeding (AUB) and pregnancy-related disorders. Endometrial biopsy techniques have replaced D&C in most diagnostic situations, and hysteroscopy (see Chapter 130, Hysteroscopy) is now often performed in place of the "blind" D&C when initial diagnostic and therapeutic interventions fail. (See Chapter 129, Endometrial Biopsy and Chapter 130, Hysteroscopy.) When the operator is experienced and the proper ancillary personnel are available, the office D&C proves to be a very cost-effective and safe procedure for the patient. Otherwise the procedure can be performed in the operating room. In many instances of abnormal bleeding, diagnosis is facilitated if the sampling is done just before an anticipated period (e.g., for anovulatory bleeding). Unless the procedure is pregnancy related, the clinician should ensure that the patient is not pregnant and should know the status of the Papanicolaou (Pap) smear before the surgery.

On reaching menopause, all women should be informed about the risks and symptoms of endometrial cancer and be strongly encouraged to report any unexpected bleeding or spotting to their clinician.

INDICATIONS

Diagnostic

- Evaluation of abnormal premenopausal bleeding not corrected by medical management
- Evaluation of abnormal premenopausal bleeding occurring in women older than 40 years in the setting of inadequate endometrial biopsy
- Evaluation of postmenopausal bleeding when endometrial aspiration is nondiagnostic
- Rule out cancer and adenomatous hyperplasia with atypia when complex hyperplasia (adenomatous hyperplasia) is found on endometrial biopsy
- Endometrial lining (stripe) measures more than 5 mm on ultrasound (some women may not need sampling if <5 mm).
- Evaluation of significant uterine bleeding too excessive for an endometrial biopsy
- When a reliable pelvic examination is required but cannot be obtained without anesthesia
- Debilitated or apprehensive patient when endometrial biopsy cannot be performed
- Cervical stenosis that precludes an in-office procedure
- AUB
- Atypical glandular cells confirmed on Pap smear but no cause is found after less invasive workup

Therapeutic

- Endometrial polyp removal
- Removal of retained products of conception associated with postpartum infection or hemorrhage
- Removal of retained products of conception following incomplete abortion

- Excessive hemorrhaging
- For use in combination with hysteroscopy

NOTE: Performing a D&C to resolve hormonally related AUB has been found to be ineffective.

Other

Elective termination of pregnancy (see Chapter 113, Pregnancy Termination: First-Trimester Suction Aspiration) is another indication for D&C.

CONTRAINDICATIONS

Absolute

- Unstable comorbid medical conditions (e.g., renal failure, active cardiac compromise)
- Desired viable intrauterine pregnancy

Relative

- Active pelvic infection (should be performed only in emergencies)
- Systemic coagulopathy (i.e., diffuse intravascular coagulation or severe thrombocytopenia)
- Uncertainty concerning the viability of an intrauterine pregnancy
- Patient's preference to defer procedure in anticipation of spontaneous resolution of a miscarriage
- History of Asherman syndrome (i.e., endometrial synechiae) after prior uterine procedure

NOTE: An in-office D&C should be performed only with a cooperative patient who has no significant health risks. Adequate resuscitation equipment must be readily available.

EQUIPMENT

See Fig. 162.1.

- Sterile gowns (optional)
- Sterile gloves
- Sterile drapes
- Equipment necessary to follow universal blood and body fluid precautions
- Sterile sponge gauze
- Formalin bottles
- Lens paper or Telfa pads for endocervical curettage and uterine curettage tissue (disposable endocervical curettage suction devices are available)
- Antiseptic cleansing solution
- Sterile bowl

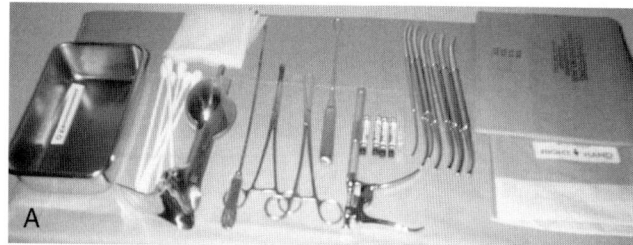

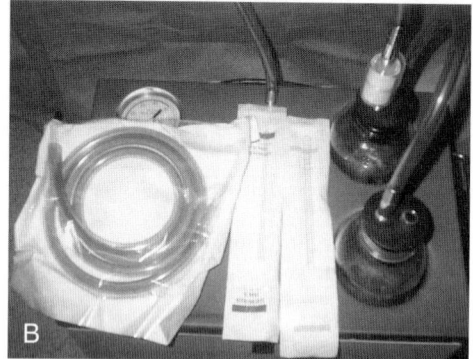

Fig. 162.1 (A) Equipment used for dilation and curettage. *Left to right:* sterile basin, 4- × 4-inch sterile sponge gauze, large obstetrics/gynecology applicators, weighted speculum, uterine sound, ring forceps, single-tooth tenaculum, curette, dental anesthesia gun, 1.8 mL of 2% lidocaine with epinephrine, uterine dilators, leggings, and sterile covering. (B) Suction device and tubing.

- Suction hosing and apparatus with pump (for some situations, especially if significant bleeding or pregnancy related)
- Ring forceps
- Single-toothed tenaculum or multitoothed (Bierer)
- Uterine sound
- Graves or weighted (Auvard) speculum
- Polyp (Stone) forceps
- Cervical dilators (Pratt or Hegar)
- Kevorkian endocervical curette for endocervical curettage
- Curved and straight suction catheters (sizes 8–12 mm) when applicable
- Sharp uterine curette
- Intravenous needle, catheter, and tubing
- Intravenous fluids (optional)
- A 20-gauge spinal needle and syringe, dental anesthesia gun, or needle extender when using local anesthesia for submucosal block
- Lidocaine 5 mL (2%) with epinephrine for submucosal block or 10 mL of lidocaine without epinephrine for paracervical block or equivalent

NOTE: Review Chapter 127, Loop Electrosurgical Excision Procedure for Treating Cervical Intraepithelial Neoplasia, for information regarding local anesthetic use (not necessary if general anesthesia is given).

- Ultrasound (optional)
- Pulse oximeter if intravenous sedation is given

PREPROCEDURE PATIENT EDUCATION

Each patient should be comfortable with the decision to undergo a D&C. The procedure, alternatives, and anticipated risks should be carefully explained so the patient can give informed consent (see the sample patient consent form available at www.expertconsult.com). If D&C is performed in an office setting with sedation, appropriate knowledge and equipment to handle possible complications or resuscitation is essential. A nurse experienced with the procedure should be available throughout to aid with patient preparation, administer intravenous medications, supply equipment, and monitor the patient during the postoperative and recovery periods. Preoperative vital signs must be stable for the clinician to perform an office D&C. If bleeding has been prolonged or heavy, obtain a hemoglobin or hematocrit. Intravenous access is also important should hemodynamic instability arise.

ANESTHESIA AND ANALGESIA

In the outpatient setting, anesthetic and analgesic options are somewhat limited. For D&C procedures performed in the hospital, the choice of sedation is broader. No matter which drug regimen is selected, personnel and equipment for resuscitation must be available should anaphylaxis, bleeding, or oversedation occur.

When anesthetic and analgesic choices for D&C are being considered, the following issues are important:

- A paracervical block prior to tenaculum placement and cervical dilation is indicated unless general anesthesia is used (see Chapter 153, Paracervical Block).
- Alternatively, a local submucosal cervical block is generally sufficient and easier to perform (see Chapter 127, Loop Electrosurgical Excision Procedure for Treating Cervical Intraepithelial Neoplasia).
- A nonsteroidal antiinflammatory drug (NSAID) taken 1 hour before the procedure reduces cramping and decreases uterine bleeding.
- Diazepam (Valium) 10 mg orally 1 hour before the procedure combined with a maximum-dose NSAID and local lidocaine are generally sufficient to accomplish a D&C.
- Intravenous medication can be used for sedation if needed (see Chapter 1, Procedural Sedation and Analgesia).

TECHNIQUE

1. Consider obtaining a hematocrit and hemoglobin, Rh, blood type, and screen if the patient's problem is pregnancy related. Platelet count, prothrombin time, partial thromboplastin time, and fibrin split products may be indicated in some situations. If pregnancy status is uncertain, obtain a pregnancy test.
2. Start an intravenous line and administer fluids. Sedate the patient if needed.
3. Prophylactic antibiotics, including subacute bacterial endocarditis prophylaxis, are not indicated for routine D&C.
4. Place the patient in the dorsal lithotomy position.
5. Determine the position of the uterine fundus by performing a bimanual examination or using ultrasound guidance if skilled in its use.
6. Expose the cervix using a Graves or Auvard speculum and cleanse the vagina, cervix, and posterior fornix with an antiseptic solution (e.g., povidone-iodine, chlorhexidine, or cyproheptadine).
7. Put on a sterile gown and gloves. The clinician should follow universal blood and body fluid precautions.
8. Place sterile drapes around the perineum.
9. Empty the bladder (if full) with an in-and-out catheter. Alternatively, ask the patient to void just prior to the procedure.
10. Perform a paracervical block (see Chapter 153, Paracervical Block) or submucosal block (Fig. 162.2). This step is omitted if the patient has general anesthesia.
11. Grasp the cervix at the 12 o'clock position and elevate it using a tenaculum (Fig. 162.3).
12. Perform an endocervical curettage unless the problem is pregnancy related or if one has been performed during a recent evaluation (see Chapter 124, Colposcopic Examination).

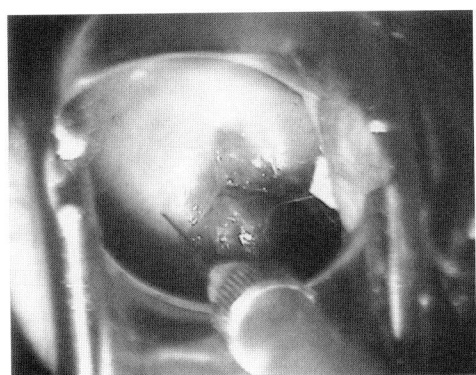

Fig. 162.2 Dental anesthesia gun used for submucosal block.

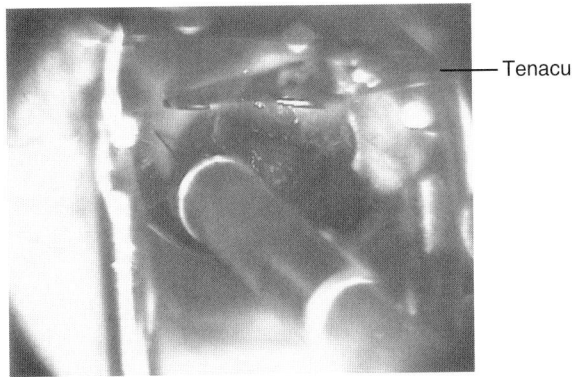

—— Tenaculum

Fig. 162.3 Dental anesthesia gun used for a paracervical block at fornix. The single-tooth tenaculum has been placed on the anterior lip of the cervix.

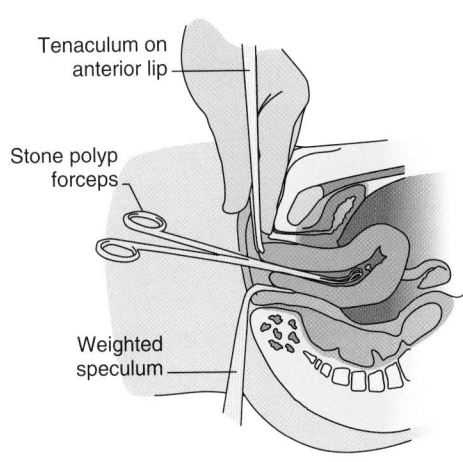

Tenaculum on anterior lip —

Stone polyp forceps —

Weighted speculum —

Fig. 162.4 Stone polyp forceps used to remove polyp from uterine cavity.

NOTE: Uterine malformations or irregularities, whether congenital (septa) or acquired (myomata), are sometimes diagnosed during this procedure.

This is called a *fractional curettage* because the endocervical canal is being evaluated separately from the uterine cavity. (A disposable suction device is available and can be used for this. It does not require the use of a Telfa pad for this portion of the procedure.)

13. Use short, firm, in-and-out strokes from the internal os to the external os, curetting in a full 360-degree circle twice.
14. Place the collected tissue on a Telfa pad or common lens paper. Send this specimen in a separate formalin container to the pathology laboratory.
15. Insert a uterine sound into the os to determine the axis of the cervix and uterine cavity as well as the depth of the uterus. Greater than 10 cm is abnormal in a premenopausal woman. Most postmenopausal uteri sound less than 8 cm. (For information regarding steps to take when either external or internal os stenosis is encountered, see Chapter 126, Cervical Stenosis and Cervical Dilation.)
16. Dilate the os to 8 to 12 mm using sequentially larger cervical dilators.
17. If using a suction method, insert the largest suction curette that can easily pass through the os and attach the other end to the suction hosing. Suction curettes range from 2 to 16 mm in diameter. Curettes less than 6 mm in diameter are flexible; large-caliber curettes are rigid. Both straight and curved versions are available.
18. Ask an assistant to attach the suction hosing to a tissue trap.
19. Slide the suction curette into the center of the endometrial cavity, turn on the suction machine, and slide the suction valve on the handle of the curette so that it is closed. A pressure of 50 to 60 cm Hg is needed to obtain adequate suction. Use a rotary, slightly in-and-out motion until an increased resistance to rotation is achieved.

20. Suction curette the entire endometrial lining, moving 360 degrees around its long axis using a to-and-fro motion. Do not pull the curette past the internal os lest suction be lost. Continue to suction until the entire cavity is sampled and there is no further return of tissue. Release the suction by sliding open the valve on the curette and remove the instrument.
21. Place a Telfa pad or large sheet of lens paper into the posterior vaginal vault.
22. Insert a sharp uterine curette and lightly scrape all sides of the uterine cavity. Collect the materials on the Telfa pad or lens paper and send for pathology in separate specimen container.
23. Using the Stone forceps, explore the uterine cavity for polyps by systematically opening and closing the forceps while moving across the dome and anterior and posterior walls of the uterus (Fig. 162.4). Remove any tissue grasped with the forceps with gentle pressure or twisting.
24. Reinsert the curette and suction out any remaining tissue (optional).

Optional Methods

- The entire procedure can be performed under ultrasound guidance (Fig. 162.5).
- Laminaria can be placed in the os the night before the procedure for dilation of the cervix. If cervical dilation over 10 mm is needed, as for second-trimester pregnancy loss or operative hysteroscopy, osmotic dilators are useful. If products of conception must be removed, dilate the cervix to a diameter (in millimeters) equal to the gestational age of the pregnancy (Chapter 126, Cervical Stenosis and Cervical Dilation).
- A sharp curette alone can be used instead of a suction curette to remove abnormal endometrial tissue.
- A curved suction curette is used if the uterus is anteflexed or retroflexed. A straight suction curette is used for a midposition uterus.

COMPLICATIONS

- *Hemorrhage*: This is very rare (<1%) unless the problem is pregnancy related. Most women have some postprocedural spotting for a few weeks afterward.
- *Infection*: This is extremely rare; broad-spectrum antibiotic with anaerobic coverage is the treatment of choice if infection develops.

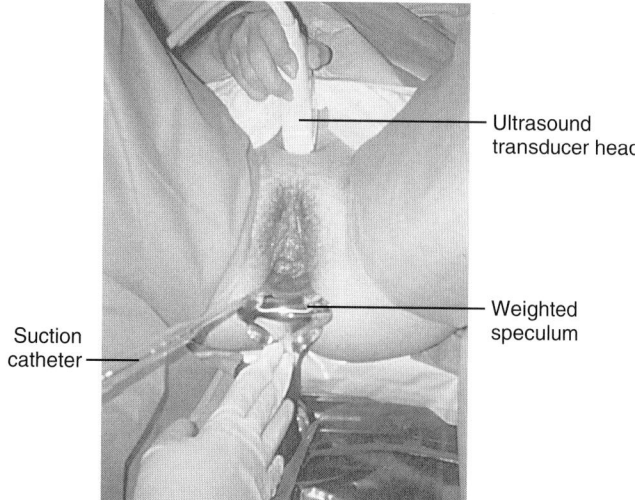

Fig. 162.5 Weighted speculum and suction equipment used in dilation and curettage. Ultrasound is used to guide the clinician during the procedure.

- *Cervical laceration.*
- *Perforated uterus:* This is more likely to occur in the presence of uterine infection, with a stenotic cervical os (especially in elderly postmenopausal women); in cases in which a sharp (as opposed to vacuum) curette is used, if there is unrecognized marked anterior or posterior flexion, and in patients who are less than 8 weeks postpartum.
  - With lateral perforation, injury to the uterine artery is possible.
  - Anteroposterior perforation is usually not serious if a small curette is used.
  - Perforation with a blunt object (usually the uterine sound) is generally uncomplicated.
  - Perforation with a sharp object is more significant.
  - In most cases, treatment for perforation is simple observation. Perforation should be suspected if the uterine sound or curette passes beyond 9 to 10 cm in women who are postmenopausal or beyond 12 cm in menstruating women (unless the uterus is actually this large on palpation). If perforation occurs, the procedure should be terminated. Before discharging the patient, the clinician should look for unstable vital signs and significant pelvic pain or bleeding. Some clinicians provide antibiotic coverage, although this is not generally done. The patient should report any fever, pelvic pain, or discharge. The risk of perforation is reduced if the D&C is carried out under ultrasonographic guidance.
- Asherman intrauterine adhesions may cause secondary amenorrhea, infertility, recurrent abortion, or other menstrual irregularities. Postoperative adhesions are more common when the D&C is performed on the puerperal uterus.
- Disease may be missed. Even in vigorous D&Cs, studies show that only 50% to 60% of the endometrial cavity is actually curetted. The patient and clinician must understand that if symptoms persist, additional diagnostic testing may be needed.

POSTPROCEDURE MANAGEMENT

Immediately After the Procedure

- After completing the D&C, observe the vital signs for any significant changes (i.e., hypotension, tachycardia, decreased oxygen saturation).
- Give 10 to 20 U oxytocin (Pitocin) IV in 1 L of lactated Ringer solution once the procedure begins. This should be con-

tinued throughout the recovery period (usually 1 to 2 hours). If continued vaginal bleeding is evident after the procedure, methylergonovine maleate (Methergine) 0.2 mg IM can be given. This is especially helpful in pregnancy-related procedures.
- If bleeding does not stop, inspect for lacerations and use ultrasonography to visualize the endometrial cavity to rule out an incomplete evacuation.
- If a significant decrease in blood volume is seen, provide normal saline or lactated Ringer solution intravenously.
- Provide RhoGAM if the patient is Rh-negative and the procedure is pregnancy-related.

Before Discharge

- The patient should be alert and ambulatory and should have stable vital signs prior to discharge.
- Consider NSAIDs for pain.
- If the patient is at risk for vaginal infection, consider oral doxycycline 100 mg twice daily for 7 to 10 days.
- Oral ergonovine 0.2 mg every 4 hours for 1 to 2 days can be given to decrease bleeding in pregnant patients.

After discharge, consider a postoperative check in 1 to 2 weeks to discuss pathologic findings and assess the patient's well-being.

POSTPROCEDURE PATIENT EDUCATION

- Instruct the patient to insert nothing in the vagina for 2 weeks. This includes sexual activity.
- The patient should call the office if bleeding is greater than one sanitary napkin per hour or if fever, purulent discharge, or significant abdominal pain develops.

INTERPRETATION OF RESULTS
Normal Findings

- Proliferative endometrium
- Secretory endometrium
- Atrophic endometrium
- Products of conception

Abnormal Findings

- Endometrial polyp
- Chronic endometritis
- Intrauterine synechiae
- Submucous leiomyoma
- Intramural leiomyoma
- Uterine enlargement
- Vaginal bleeding
- Premenopausal menorrhagia
- Postmenopausal bleeding
- Endometrial hyperplasia (adenomatous, cystic, glandular)
- Simple endometrial hyperplasia without atypia
- Complex endometrial hyperplasia without atypia
- Complex endometrial hyperplasia with atypia
- Adenocarcinoma in situ
- Endometrial carcinoma (i.e., adenocarcinoma)
- Hydatidiform mole (i.e., trophoblastic disease)
- Malignant hydatidiform mole
- Variations of cervical dysplasia (from endocervical curettage)
  - Cervical intraepithelial neoplasia (CIN) I
  - CIN II
  - CIN III

PATIENT EDUCATION GUIDES

See sample patient education and consent forms available at www.e xpertconsult.com.

CPT/BILLING CODES

59820	Treatment of missed abortion; completed surgically, first trimester
59821	Treatment of missed abortion; completed surgically, second trimester
58120	D&C (diagnostic or therapeutic but nonobstetric)
59160	D&C (postpartum)
64435	Paracervical block*
36000	Starting an IV
36415	Venipuncture
57505	Endocervical curettage*
76856	Ultrasound, complete pelvic (nonobstetric)
76857	Ultrasound, pelvic, limited or for follow-up
76830	Transvaginal ultrasound

*Considered as part of D&C bundled payment and not separately reimbursed.

ICD-10-CM DIAGNOSTIC CODES

D07.0	Adenocarcinoma in situ
N71.1	Chronic endometritis
N85.01	Complex endometrial hyperplasia w/o atypia
N85.02	Complex endometrial hyperplasia with atypia
C54.1	Endometrial carcinoma (i.e., adenocarcinoma)
N85.00	Endometrial hyperplasia (adenomatous, cystic, glandular)
N84.0	Endometrial polyp
O01.9	Hydatidiform mole (i.e., trophoblastic disease)
D39.2X	Hydatidiform mole, malignant
D25.1	Intramural leiomyoma
N8536	Intrauterine synechiae
Z85.40	Personal history of cancer of the uterus
N95.0	Postmenopausal bleeding
N92.4	Premenopausal menorrhagia
N85.01	Simple endometrial hyperplasia w/o atypia
D25.0	Submucous leiomyoma
N85.2	Uterine enlargement
N89.8	Vaginal bleeding
N87.0	Mild cervical dysplasia CIN I
N87.1	Moderate cervical dysplasia CIN II
D06.9	Carcinoma in situ cervix CIN III

RECOMMENDED READING

American College of Obstetricians and Gynecologists. Antibiotic prophylaxis for gynecologic procedures. *ACOG Practice Bulletin No. 104.* Washington DC: ACOG; May 2009.

Buchanan EM, Weinstein LC, Hilson C. Endometrial cancer. *Am Fam Physician.* 2009;80:1075–1080.

Dovnik A, Crnobrnja B, Zegura B, et al. Incidence of positive peritoneal cytology in patients with endometrial carcinoma after hysteroscopy vs. dilatation and curettage. *Radiol Oncol.* 2016;51(1):88–93.

Gambone JC. Gynecologic procedures: imaging studies and surgery. In: Hacker NF, Gambone JC, Hobel JC, eds. *Hacker and Moore's Essentials of Obstetrics and Gynecology.* 6th ed. Philadelphia: Elsevier; 2016:356–368.

Kim DH, Seong SJ, Kim MK, et al. Dilatation and curettage is more accurate than endometrial aspiration biopsy in early-stage endometrial cancer patients treated with high dose oral progestin and levonorgestrel intrauterine system. *J Gynecol Oncol.* 2017;28(1):e1.

Prine LW, MacNaughton H. Office management of early pregnancy loss. *Am Fam Physician.* 2011;84(1):75–82.

Smith RA, Andrews KS, Brooks D, et al. Cancer screening in the United States, 2017: a review of current American Cancer Society guidelines and current issues in cancer screening. *CA Cancer J Clin.* 2017;67(2):100–121.

Pediatrics

Section Editor: BAL REDDY

CHAPTER 163

NEONATAL RESUSCITATION

Robert T. Coles

The first few moments of a newborn's life can be the most critical. Failure to provide effective emergency care, particularly resuscitation, during this transition can have lifelong consequences.

Proper resuscitation requires essential equipment and knowledge of major risk factors and necessary protocols before delivery. Prior knowledge of the gestational age of the newborn is helpful in anticipating the need for resuscitation. Low birth weight and premature delivery predispose infants to the need for resuscitative efforts. Maternal infection, hypertension or diabetes, multiple pregnancy of less than 35 weeks, oligohydramnios, polyhydramnios, intrauterine growth retardation, major fetal anomaly or hydrops, prolapsed cord, placenta previa or abruption placentae, breech presentation, meconium-stained amniotic fluid, nonreassuring fetal heart rate, emergency cesarean section, general anesthesia, shoulder dystocia, vacuum or forceps delivery, and maternal opiate use are additional risk factors.

Approximately 10% of newborns require some degree of assistance to begin breathing at birth (i.e., some sort of stimulation to breathe); fortunately less than 1% require extensive resuscitation. In at least one study, the risk factors listed earlier identified approximately 80% of newborns who required resuscitation.

After birth, the use of three essential assessment questions—Term gestation? Good tone? Breathing or crying?—can generally identify those newborns that do not require resuscitation and can stay with the mother for routine care. However, if the answer to any of the three questions is no, the infant should be moved to a radiant warmer for further evaluation and management. It is here that the concept of "the golden minute" has replaced the 1-minute Apgar score to indicate the need for resuscitation.

Using the heart rate and respiratory effort as guidelines, basic resuscitative efforts (warm, position, clear secretions as indicated, dry, stimulate), reevaluation, and positive pressure ventilation (PPV) should be initiated within the first 60 seconds after birth if indicated. At some point, the Apgar scores should still be recorded.

INDICATIONS

Neonate with the following:

- Inadequate or ineffective respirations
- Inadequate heart rate (i.e., <100 beats/min)
- Central cyanosis (not a reliable method of determining oxygen saturation in the immediate neonatal period)
- Other evidence of cardiorespiratory distress, such as poor tone

EQUIPMENT

- Suction equipment, including a bulb syringe, mechanical suction device, suction catheters (6, 8, and 10 Fr) or pediatric feeding tube (8 Fr).
- Oxygen source with flowmeter, infant resuscitation bag (750 mL) with appropriately sized face masks, laryngoscope with No. 0 and 1 straight blades, and sterile newborn endotracheal tubes (2.5, 3, 3.5, and 4 mm), CO_2 monitor

EDITOR'S NOTE: Self-inflating bags reexpand after compression and may be the most useful for those with limited resources. They can be used without a gas source. If a positive end-expiratory pressure (PEEP) valve is attached, some PEEP can be delivered; however, a self-inflating bag cannot deliver continuous positive airway pressure (CPAP). A flow-inflating bag needs a continuous gas supply to inflate the bag. PEEP can be delivered by experienced operators with a PEEP valve; however, many operators find the flow-inflating bag more difficult to use than the self-inflating bag. Although CPAP can be delivered, it is very difficult to deliver reliably. A T-piece device requires a continuous gas supply. PEEP is generated by limiting flow through the ported expiratory valve. CPAP is effectively delivered while the port is open; therefore T-piece equipment may be optimal for preterm infants at birth. A T-piece device is easy to use and generally preferred by both experienced and inexperienced operators.

- Drugs, including epinephrine 1:10,000 (0.1 mg/mL) and volume expanders (normal saline or type O Rh-negative blood; Ringer lactate solution is no longer recommended)
- Orogastric tube (8 Fr) for infants undergoing prolonged PPV
- Meconium aspirator
- Pulse oximeter, sensor, and sensor cover
- Electronic cardiac monitor with leads
- Miscellaneous items, including a radiant warmer, clock with second hand, measuring tape, pediatric stethoscope, needles (25, 23, 21, and 18 gauge), syringes (1, 3, 10, and 20 mL), adhesive tape (0.5-inch width), antiseptic solution, an umbilical catheter (3.5 or 5 Fr), intraosseous needle (18 gauge), and food-grade heat-resistant plastic wrap

TECHNIQUE

As with all medical procedures, universal precautions against exposure to blood and other body fluids should be followed during this procedure. Initial measures—including proper positioning, drying, and stimulation—should be provided to all newborns. Suctioning should be reserved (including suctioning with a bulb syringe) for babies immediately after birth who exhibit obvious obstruction due to secretions or require PPV. Fig. 163.2 is a flow diagram of the protocol for neonatal resuscitation; it is explained in the following sections.

Positioning, Suction, and Stimulation

1. Newly born nonasphyxiated infants should have their temperature maintained between 36.5°C and 37.5°C. Prevent heat loss by placing the infant under a radiant heat source, then quickly drying him or her and removing the wet linen. If the infant is stable, warmed blankets or the mother's body heat will also reduce heat loss. (Recovery from acidosis is delayed by hypothermia. Cold stress also increases oxygen consumption and impedes effective resuscitation.) If the infant needs to be monitored, he or she can be placed on a warm blanket but should be left unwrapped. Being

unwrapped also enhances radiant warming. Other strategies may also be used, including increasing the room temperature, using a thermal mattress, and using warmed humidified resuscitation gases. Infants of low birth weight (<1500 g) need extra equipment and effort to keep them warm because the traditional radiant warmer and blankets are insufficient. The body, but not the head, of the infant may be covered with food-grade heat-resistant plastic wrap in addition to the provision of radiant heat. Use of this technique requires constant monitoring to make sure that

overheating does not occur. Hyperthermia (temperature greater than 38°C) can be associated with perinatal respiratory depression.

2. The infant should be placed in the supine position. Open the airway by positioning the infant with the neck in a neutral or slightly extended position (in the sniffing position). A rolled blanket or towel should be placed under the back and shoulders to elevate the torso 2 to 2.5 cm; this will help maintain head position. Avoid extreme hyperextension or flexion of the infant's neck, which may diminish airflow.

3. A soft cloth or towel can be used to gently wipe the face, mouth, and nose of a vigorous newborn. Vigorous newborns should not be routinely suctioned after delivery, even those delivered through meconium-stained fluid. As mentioned previously, suctioning immediately after birth (including bulb suctioning) should be reserved for those babies who exhibit obvious obstruction due to secretions or who require PPV. If suctioning is needed, clear the airway by suctioning the mouth and then the nose with a bulb syringe or suction catheter connected to a mechanical device. If mechanical suction is used, the pressure should not exceed 100 mm Hg. Deep or aggressive suctioning of the oropharynx may produce tissue trauma, laryngeal spasm, a vagal response, brady-

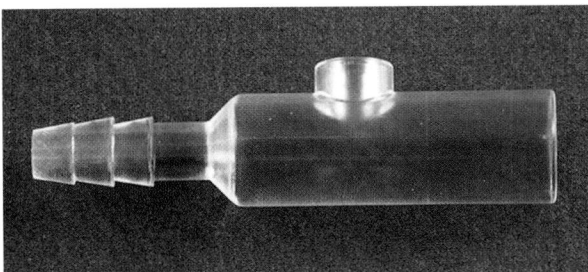

Fig. 163.1 Meconium aspirator.

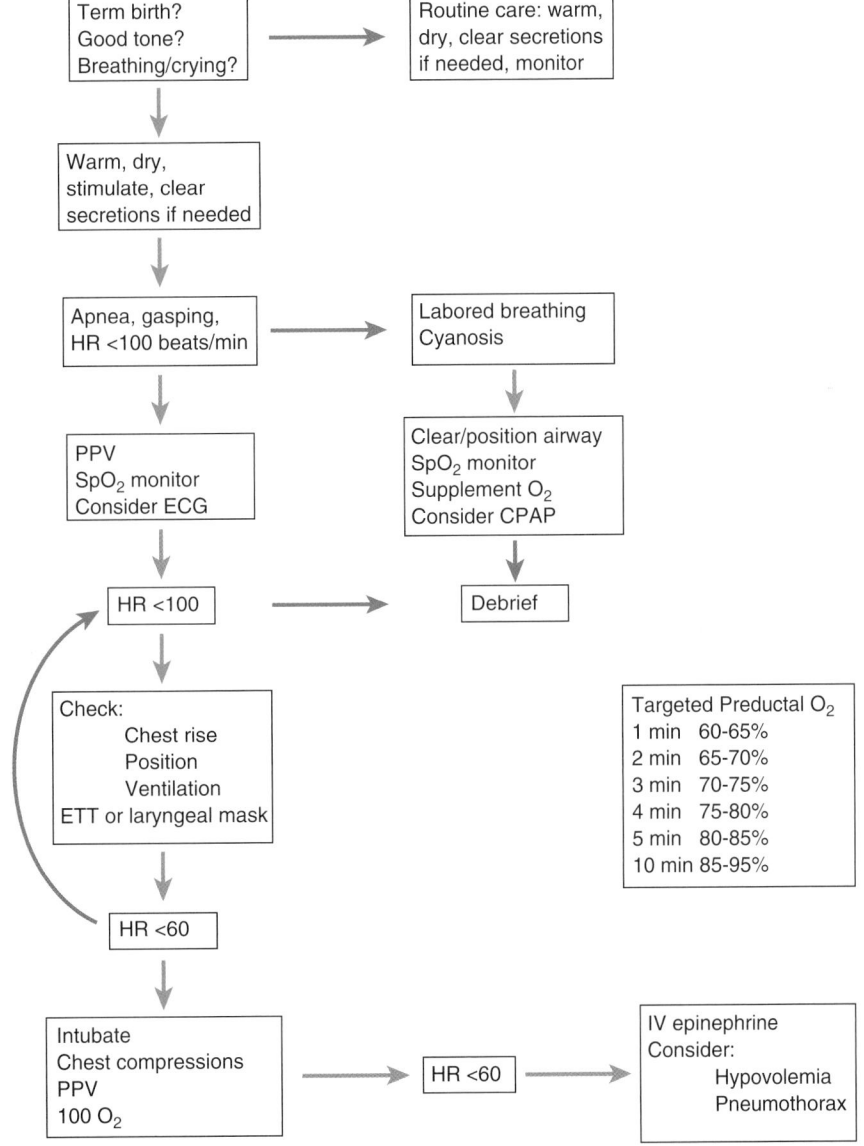

Fig. 163.2 Resuscitation flowchart. Consider endotracheal intubation if meconium is present and the infant is not vigorous. *CPAP*, Continuous positive airway pressure; *ECG*, electrocardiogram; *ETT*, endotracheal tube; *HR*, heart rate; *PPV*, positive pressure ventilation; *SpO₂*, oxygen saturation.

cardia, and apnea. Infants with meconium-stained amniotic fluid should no longer be suctioned with mechanical devices after the head is delivered and prior to the body being delivered. Endotracheal suctioning is no longer recommended for nonvigorous babies born through meconium-stained amniotic fluid. It should be carried out only if the newborn has absent or depressed respirations, a heart rate below 100 beats/min, or poor muscle tone.

4. Respiratory activity can be promoted by providing tactile stimulation (e.g., gently flicking the soles of the feet or rubbing the back, trunk or extremities).

Initial Assessment

1. Assess the infant's respiratory status and heart rate.
2. Infants with adequate respiratory and cardiac function (good ventilation and heart rate >100 beats/min) can be merely observed.
3. Infants with depressed respiratory function (shallow, slow, or absent respirations) or an abnormal heart rate should undergo further resuscitation.

EDITOR'S NOTE: experts are now aware that measuring heart rate by palpation of the umbilical cord or by listening with the stethoscope may systematically underestimate the heart rate by 15 to 20 beats/min when compared with an electrocardiogram. Electrocardiography provides data more quickly than pulse oximetry, which also may underestimate heart rate; however, both are considered more accurate than physical examination, and pulse oximetry is still needed to evaluate the newborn's oxygenation. Both are now usually available within the first 90 seconds of life; when either or both are used it is not necessary to halt resuscitative efforts in order to assess heart rate.

General Guidelines of Resuscitation

As with all resuscitations, the order of importance is airway, breathing, and circulation. The two cardinal indicators in neonatal resuscitation are respirations and heart rate. In general the initial assessment should take no more than 30 seconds; should the need for further resuscitation arise, reassessment of interventions should occur every 30 seconds. Apgar scores should still be determined and recorded at appropriate intervals. Special circumstances may arise and may be treated with procedures used in general pediatric resuscitation (e.g., chest tube for pneumothorax).

Ventilation

1. Ventilatory insufficiency produces the majority of respiratory and circulatory abnormalities during the newborn period. Rapid institution of ventilatory support in newborns with abnormalities of respiratory function or heart rate maximizes the chances of a successful outcome.
2. Positive pressure support is indicated for infants with inadequate respiratory effort despite drying, wrapping, and gentle stimulation. CPAP may be adequate to aid lung inflation and regularize breathing. This is typically first applied noninvasively with a face mask or nasal prongs and a pressure-generating device. PPV with room air is indicated for infants of 35 weeks' gestational age or more with no respiratory effort, heart rate less than 100 beats/min, or who remain hypoxic despite CPAP support.
   EDITOR'S NOTE: A substantial body of evidence now indicates that the use of 100% oxygen increases mortality rates compared with the use of room air. However, uncertainty remains regarding the long-term effect on neurodevelopment. Resuscitation in term infants should be initiated with room air (21% oxygen at sea level). Resuscitation in preterm infants should be initiated with low oxygen (21% to 30%). In both term and preterm infants, pulse oximetry should be used to guide the titration of oxygen concentration to achieve normoxia (see Table 163.1 for normal newborn oxygen

TABLE 163.1	Normal SpO$_2$, After Birth
Time Point After Birth	**SpO$_2$ Range**
1 min	60%–65%
2 min	65%–70%
3 min	70%–75%
4 min	75%–80%
5 min	80%–85%
10 min	85%–95%

TABLE 163.2	Endotracheal Tube Selection	
Infant Weight (g)	**Gestation Age (wk)**	**Endotracheal Tube Size (mm)**
<1000	<28	2.5
1000–2000	28–34	3
2000–3000	34–38	3-3.5
>3000	>38	3.5–4

saturation ranges). However, whenever chest compressions are initiated, the oxygen concentration should be increased to 100%.

3. PPV is usually accomplished with a bag and mask, using either a self-inflating bag, an anesthesia flow-inflating bag, or a T-piece device. A good seal should be maintained by using an appropriately sized face mask with a cushioned rim. A pressure gauge or pop-off valve should be used to ensure adequate ventilatory pressures.
4. Ventilate the infant at a rate of 40 to 60 beats/min with a tidal volume of 6 to 8 mL/kg. Adequate ventilation is verified clinically by observing bilateral symmetric chest expansion, the presence of bilateral breath sounds, and observing the cardiac monitor and pulse oximeter. Inadequate ventilation may indicate an inadequate face mask seal, a blocked airway, or inadequate ventilation pressure. After initial ventilations, pressures of less than 20 to 30 cm H$_2$O (20 to 25 cm H$_2$O for preterm infants) should be adequate.
5. Perform an endotracheal intubation when prolonged PPV is required, bag-and-mask ventilation is ineffective, the infant remains apneic despite adequate mask ventilation, heart rate remains less than 100 beats/min following 30 seconds of effective PPV, chest compressions are used, endotracheal delivery of medication is necessary, or diaphragmatic hernia is suspected. Select an endotracheal tube of appropriate size (Table 163.2) and insert it under direct visualization using the laryngoscope. The tip should rest above the tracheal bifurcation. Appropriate endotracheal tube location is verified clinically by the presence of bilaterally symmetric breath sounds and confirmation of expired CO$_2$. Most clinicians also confirm endotracheal tube placement with a chest radiograph.
6. Oral airways are rarely required during neonatal resuscitation but are indicated for bilateral choanal atresia, Pierre Robin syndrome, and when necessary for adequate ventilation.
7. Use of a laryngeal mask airway (LMA) (Fig. 163.3) can be an acceptable alternative when bag-and-mask ventilation and endotracheal intubation have failed. (The LMA is a substitute in certain cases for traditional endotracheal intubation.) The LMA should be used only by properly trained personnel and is not considered a routine substitute for endotracheal intubation.
8. Gastric catheter placement (8 Fr) is indicated in prolonged resuscitation efforts to prevent stomach distention—a frequent problem in newborns who are being ventilated by mask.

Chest Compressions

1. Administer chest compressions if the infant's heart rate is less than 60 beats/min after adequate PPV for 30 seconds. Chest compressions can be accomplished with the thumbs placed on the sternum and the hands encircling the chest (preferred meth-

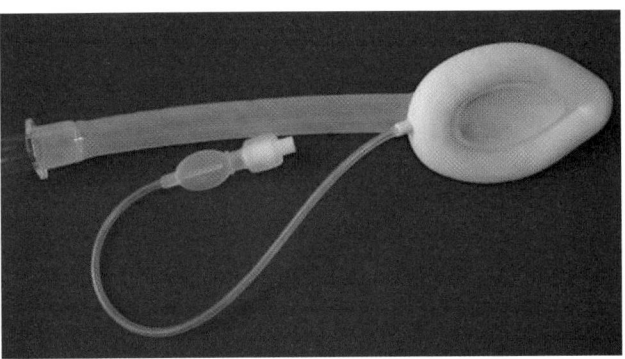

Fig. 163.3 Laryngeal mask airway. (Courtesy Legend Medical Devices, Inc.)

od) or with the tips of the middle and index fingers (Fig. 163.4). Chest compressions should be applied to the lower third of the sternum, just below the nipple line, but not over the xiphoid (to avoid damage to the liver). The sternum should be depressed one-third of the anteroposterior dimension of the chest rather than an exact depth of compression. The compression depth must be adequate to produce a palpable pulse.

2. Chest compressions should be administered at a ratio of 3:1 with PPV, at a rate of 90 compressions and 30 ventilations every minute. Reassess the pulse every 30 seconds by observing the cardiac monitor or pulse oximeter. If continuous monitor not available, the umbilical cord stump can also be used to palpate the pulse.

3. Continue chest compressions until the spontaneous heart rate is 60 beats/min or higher (see Fig. 163.2).

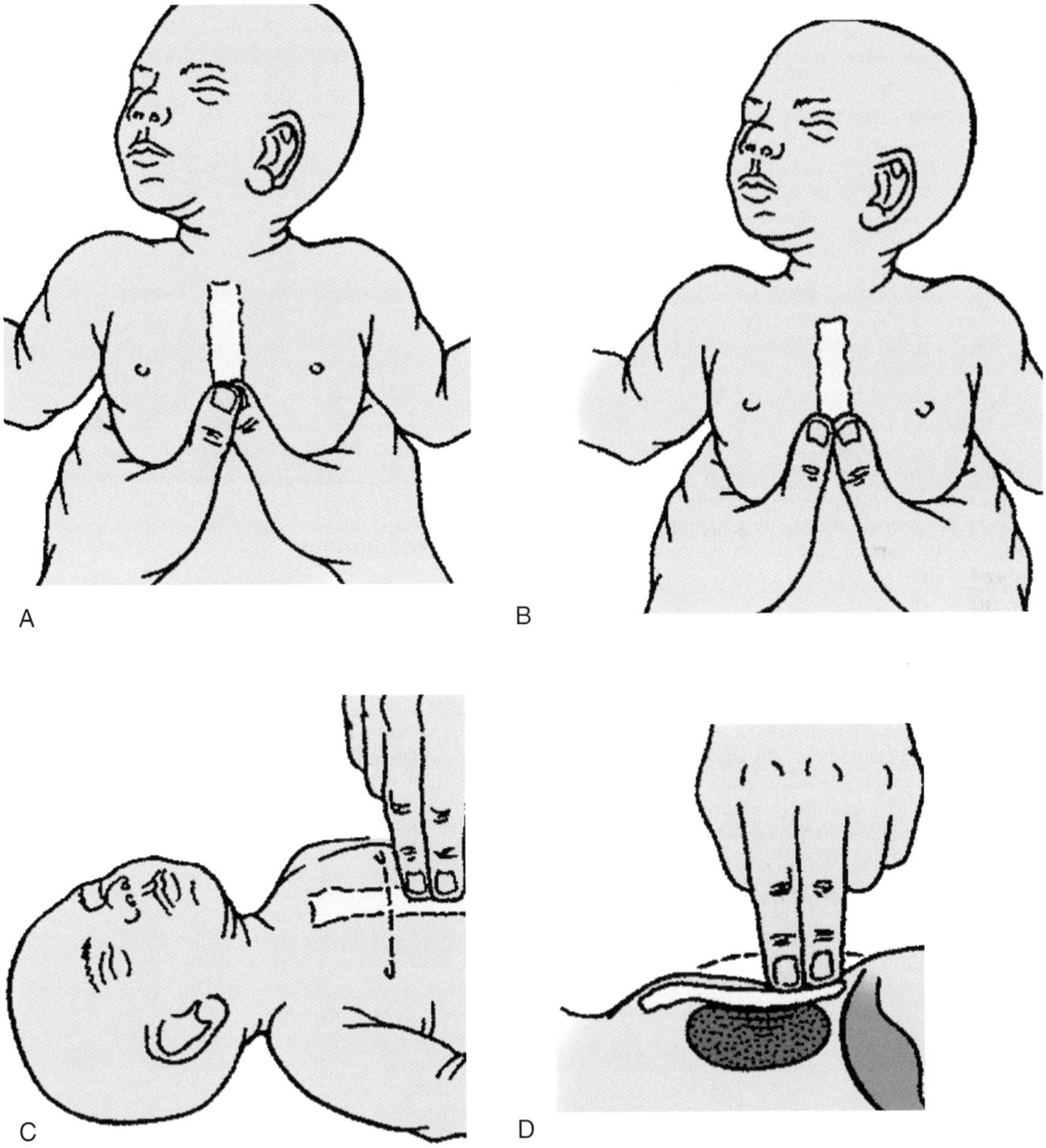

A

B

C

D

Fig. 163.4 Chest compression over lower third of sternum just below the nipple line but not over the xyphoid. Two-thumb technique with (A) thumb over thumb and (B) thumbs side by side. (C) Two-finger technique (can also use ring and middle fingers). (D) Chest compression depth is one-third to one-half of the anteroposterior diameter of the chest such that a palpable pulse is generated.

TABLE 163.3	Medications Used for Neonatal Resuscitation			
Medication	**Indication**	**Dose**	**Route of Administration**	
Epinephrine	Asystole or HR <60 beats/min despite adequate PPV and chest compressions for 30 sec	0.1–0.3 mL/kg of a 1:10,000 solution or 0.01–0.03 mg/kg	IV (preferred) or ET; can repeat every 3–5 min	
Volume expander (crystalloid or blood)	Evidence of acute blood loss with signs of hypovolemia or failure to respond to resuscitation or signs of shock	10 mL/kg	IV over 5–10 min	

ET, Endotracheal; *HR*, heart rate; *IM*, intramuscular; *IV*, intravenous; *PPV*, positive pressure ventilation.

Medications

Drugs are rarely indicated in resuscitation of the newly born infant; when needed, however, epinephrine and/or volume should be used. There is insufficient evidence to evaluate the safety and efficacy of administering naloxone to a newborn with respiratory depression after maternal opiate exposure; thus naloxone is not recommended as part of initial resuscitative efforts in the delivery room. Table 163.3 summarizes the medications used in neonatal resuscitation. Administer epinephrine and/or volume for asystole or if the heart rate remains less than 60 beats/min after adequate PPV and chest compressions for a minimum of 30 seconds. Epinephrine should be administered intravenously as soon as venous access is established, since there is a lack of supportive data for endotracheal administration. Medications may be administered through the umbilical vein with a 3.5- or 5-Fr umbilical catheter placed just below the skin. (See Chapter 165, Umbilical Vessel Catheterization.) Alternative access can be obtained through a peripheral vein or, in the event that no other access is available, by intraosseous access (see Chapter 226, Intraosseous Venous Access). Intraosseous access can be very difficult to obtain in premature infants.

Termination of Resuscitation

Discontinuation of resuscitative efforts may be appropriate if resuscitation of an infant with cardiorespiratory arrest does not produce spontaneous circulation within 10 minutes. Resuscitation of newly born infants after 10 minutes of asystole is also very unlikely to result in survival or survival without severe disability. Those involved in neonatal resuscitation should pursue local discussions to formulate guidelines consistent with local resources and outcome data.

POSTPROCEDURE PATIENT MANAGEMENT

- Maintain careful monitoring in an appropriately staffed intensive care unit (or arrange transfer to such a facility).
- Continue evaluation with serial arterial blood gases, frequent determination of fluid and electrolyte status, chest radiographs, and other modalities as indicated by clinical findings.
- Completely document the resuscitation effort in the medical record.
- Discuss situation with parents.

COMPLICATIONS

Suction

- Vagal response (bradycardia or apnea)
- Hypoxia
- Tissue trauma

Ventilation

- Pneumothorax
- Hypoxia resulting from inadequate ventilation
- Complications from intubation (see Chapter 222, Tracheal [Endotracheal and Nasotracheal] Intubation)

CPT/BILLING CODES

99460, 99463	History and examination of the normal newborn infant, initiation of diagnostic and treatment programs, and preparation of hospital records
99464	Attendance at delivery (when requested by delivering physician or other qualified health care professional) and initial stabilization of newborn
99465	Newborn resuscitation: provision of positive pressure ventilation and/or chest compressions in the presence of acute inadequate ventilation and/or cardiac output

ICD-10-CM DIAGNOSTIC CODES

I46.9	Cardiorespiratory arrest
P84	Asphyxia, hypoxemia newborn
P24.01	Meconium aspiration, with respiratory symptoms
P28.5	Respiratory failure, newborn
P28.81	Respiratory arrest, newborn
P28.89	Other respiratory problems after birth
P29.12	Bradycardia, newborn
P29.81	Cardiac arrest, newborn

Acknowledgment

The editors recognize the contributions of Marvin A. Dewar, MD, JD, and Eric M. Hugues to this chapter in previous editions of this text.

RECOMMENDED READING

Owen LS, Weiner GM, Davis PG. Delivery room stabilization, and respiratory support. In: Goldsmith JP, Karotkin EH, Keszler M, Suresh GK, eds. *Assisted Ventilation of the Neonate.* 6th ed. Philadelphia: Elsevier; 2017:275–290.

Perlman JM, Wyllie J, Kattwinkel J, et al. Neonatal resuscitation: 2015 international consensus on cardiopulmonary resuscitation and emergency cardiovascular care science with treatment recommendations. *Circulation.* 2015;132(16 suppl 1):S204–241.

Samreen V, Dobiesz VA. Emergency childbirth. In: Roberts JR, Custalow CB, Thomsen TW, eds. *Roberts and Hedges Clinical Procedures in Emergency Medicine and Acute Care.* 7th ed. Philadelphia: Elsevier; 2019:1186–1210.

Wyckoff MH, Aziz K, Escobedo MB, et al. Part 13: Neonatal resuscitation: 2015 american heart association guidelines update for cardiopulmonary resuscitation and emergency cardiovascular. *Circulation.* 2015;132:S543–S560.

CHAPTER 164

PEDIATRIC ARTERIAL PUNCTURE AND VENOUS MINI-CUTDOWN

John J. Andazola • Karyn B. Kolman

ARTERIAL PUNCTURE

Arterial blood may be needed for blood gas analysis or for routine laboratory analysis. In the infant or child, the radial artery is the most appropriate and most commonly selected site for arterial puncture. The posterior tibial and dorsalis pedis arteries are optional sites, but each has its own risk of complications. Because of the risk of thrombosis, use of the femoral artery for arterial puncture in the infant or child should be reserved for emergencies. Likewise, because of the risk of median nerve damage and the fact that the brachial artery has minimal collateral circulation, the brachial artery should be reserved for use as a last resort in emergencies. The temporal artery should probably not be used because of the high risk of neurologic complications.

The radial artery is located just medial to the styloid process of the radius. It is palpable between the radius and the tendon of the flexor carpi radialis (see Chapter 225, Arterial Puncture and Percutaneous Arterial Line Placement).

Indications

- To obtain arterial blood from the pediatric patient in respiratory distress or for other studies that require arterial blood
- To guide the management of the pediatric patient receiving ventilatory support or undergoing intensive respiratory therapy (e.g., to confirm hypoxia or hypercapnia when pulse oximetry [SaO_2] or end-tidal CO_2 [$ETCO_2$] monitoring, respectively, indicates it)
- To obtain blood for routine laboratory analysis when venous blood cannot be obtained

NOTE: The last indication is controversial. The benefit must outweigh the higher risk of obtaining an arterial sample.

Contraindications

Infection, burns, local skin damage, trauma, or severely disturbed anatomy at the site of the intended puncture are all contraindications. They are considered relative contraindications in a life-threatening situation.

Equipment and Supplies

- Commercially available heparinized arterial blood gas (ABG) syringe or 1-mL (tuberculin syringe) to 3-mL syringe (to be flushed with heparin)
- Rubber stopper or syringe plug to seal blood sample
- 23- to 27-gauge butterfly scalp vein needle or standard 23- to 27-gauge needle (the smaller the needle, the lower the risk of complications). Butterfly needles are easier to control if an assistant is present and generally allow removal of more blood.

- Antiseptic skin preparation, such as povidone-iodine or chlorhexidine, and 70% isopropyl alcohol
- Container of crushed ice for sample transport
- Sterile 4- by 4-inch gauze pads
- Sterile gloves
- Goggles or eye protection and other equipment necessary for universal blood and body fluid precautions
- Bright light source (e.g., bright penlight, otoscope) for transillumination (optional)
- 1 or 2 mL heparin, 1000 U/mL (optional, for use in nonheparinized syringe)
- In the alert patient (optional), 1% or 2% lidocaine without epinephrine and a 1- or 3-mL syringe with 25- or 27-gauge, ⅝-inch (1.6-cm) needle
- Arm or leg board (optional; it is preferable to have an assistant stabilize the arm)

Precautions

The modified Allen test is performed to ensure patency of the ulnar artery before an arterial puncture or the placement of an indwelling arterial catheter. Verification of adequate collateral circulation may reduce the risk of ischemic complications if thrombosis of the radial artery occurs. (See Chapter 225, Arterial Puncture and Percutaneous Arterial Line Placement, for a description of the modified Allen test as well as other techniques available to test for collateral circulation.)

Technique

1. Always perform a modified Allen test (or equivalent) to confirm adequate collateral circulation.
2. Attach a butterfly needle (preferred for infants and neonates) or a standard 23- to 27-gauge needle to a heparinized ABG syringe. Alternatively, draw a small amount of heparin into the syringe and eject the heparin. The heparin remaining in the syringe will prevent the sample from clotting and also decrease the dead space in the syringe. Heparin has a very low pH, so avoid using excessive heparin, which could result in falsely abnormal ABG results. If the sample will be used for another laboratory test, do not use heparin.
3. Immobilize the upper extremity by taping it to an arm board or by having an assistant stabilize it manually.
4. Grasp the wrist with your nondominant hand and identify the radial artery by dorsiflexing and slightly externally rotating the wrist and palpating over the distal volar (palmar) radius. Use of a bright light source for transillumination may help to locate the artery, especially in a newborn. Cleanse the site of intended puncture with an antiseptic solution, which can be wiped off

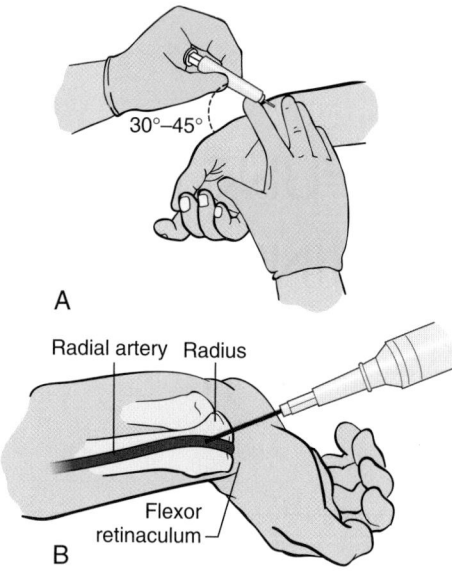

A

Radial artery Radius

Flexor
retinaculum

B

Fig. 164.1 Pediatric arterial puncture. (A) Anatomic location of the radial artery with immobilization of the wrist in hyperextension. (B) The artery is entered with the bevel up and the needle at 30 to 45 degrees from horizontal.

with an alcohol swab. If the patient is alert, the area can also be infiltrated with 1% to 2% lidocaine without epinephrine. Be aware that use of subcutaneous lidocaine may make it more difficult to palpate the artery.

5. Universal blood and body fluid precautions should be followed. Insert the needle with the bevel up, at the point of maximum pulsation, at a 30- to 45-degree angle (Fig. 164.1) to the distal skin. Usually little aspiration is needed to fill the syringe when the artery is pierced. If the syringe does not flash blood immediately, continuous gentle suction can be applied with the plunger of the syringe as the needle is removed or on the next attempt. Be aware that arterial blood may not flash into the syringe as vigorously in a child as in an adult patient. If the butterfly needle is being used, have an assistant maintain gentle suction while the needle is advanced.

6. If resistance is encountered, most likely the needle has made contact with underlying bone (radius). At this point, withdraw the needle very slowly while maintaining gentle suction on the plunger until there is blood return. If there is no blood return and the tip of the needle has been withdrawn to a point just beneath the skin, readvance the needle toward the point of maximal pulsation before withdrawing it from the skin. Although the risk of complications increases with the number of attempts, several attempts can be made in this manner, causing minimal trauma to the infant before choosing another site.

7. When arterial blood is encountered, withdraw 0.3 to 0.5 mL into the syringe before removing the needle. Leave the butterfly needle in place (with its extension tubing) if more blood is needed for other analyses. This will facilitate changing the syringe. For blood gas analysis, remove any bubbles from the syringe and then seal it. Place it on ice and immediately transport it to the laboratory.

NOTE: The total blood volume in a neonate is usually about 80 mL/kg, and the volume of blood withdrawn should not exceed 3% to 5% of this total blood volume. As an example, 8 mL is 5% of the total blood volume in a 2-kg infant, so do not exceed this amount.

8. After removing the needle, always maintain manual compression at the arterial puncture site for a minimum of 5 minutes to prevent the formation of a hematoma. Apply firm but not occlusive pressure.

TABLE 164.1		Normal Values for Arterial Blood Gases by Age		
Age	pH	PaO$_2$ (mm Hg)	PaCO$_2$ (mm Hg)	HCO$_3$ (mEq/L)
Birth	7.26–7.29	60	55	19
Birth–1 yr	7.37	70	33	20
1–2 yr	7.40	90	34	20
7–19 yr	7.39	96	37	22
>19 yr	7.35–7.45	90–110	35–45	22–26

Sample Operative Report

See the sample operative report available at www.expertconsult.com.

Complications

- Bleeding and hematoma formation (To minimize this risk, use the smallest needle possible.)
- Arterial spasm, thrombosis, and embolism (Risk increases with repeated punctures in the same location; however, arterial spasm will usually resolve spontaneously, and the artery will usually recanalize over time after thrombosis.)
- Nerve injury
- Infection
- Spurious laboratory results (see Chapter 225, Arterial Puncture and Percutaneous Arterial Line Placement, for a discussion)

NOTE: Because the radial artery is not close to a nerve or vein, its puncture usually results in fewer complications than puncture of the posterior tibial or dorsalis pedis artery. Repeated puncture at the same site increases the chance of complications but may be unavoidable.

Interpretation of Results

See Table 164.1.

VENOUS MINI-CUTDOWN

Obtaining percutaneous venous access in infants or in hypovolemic children can be a challenge. In an emergent situation, when percutaneous venous access in not easily obtainable, intraosseous line placement is the preferred alternative (see Chapter 226, Intraosseous Venous Access). If intraosseous line placement is not possible, venous cutdown can be used to gain vascular access. Venous cutdown can often be performed rapidly, usually in a matter of minutes. Chapter 227, Venous Cutdown, offers technical advice on the overall mechanics of venous cutdown. This chapter offers an abbreviated and clinically easier method for pediatric patients in emergencies: the mini-cutdown. Although standard venous cutdown takes 5 to 15 minutes (even in the hands of a skilled clinician) mini-cutdown is less complicated and can usually be performed in less than 5 minutes.

The saphenous vein is a consistent anatomic structure located a fingerbreadth (1 cm) anterior to and a fingerbreadth (1 cm) superior to the medial malleolus at the ankle in infants and 2 cm anterior and superior in older children (Fig. 164.2). Because of its superficial and consistent location, the saphenous vein is the most common site for cutdown in the pediatric patient. The saphenous nerve travels with the saphenous vein and is often transected when isolating the saphenous vein at the ankle, but fortunately it is of minimal clinical significance. In this location, there is very little subcutaneous tissue and, other than the saphenous vein and nerve, there are few other structures between the dermis and the tibial periosteum.

Indications

In an emergency, the inability to obtain needed percutaneous intravenous or intraosseous vascular access in a matter of minutes or the inability to maintain a peripheral intravenous line

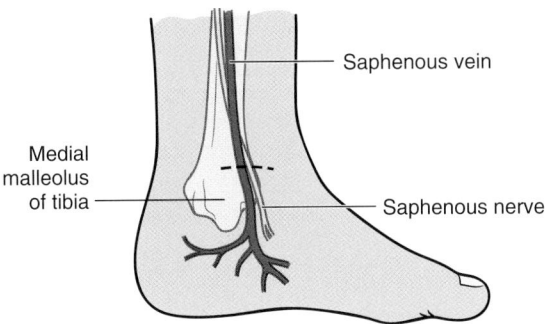

Fig. 164.2 Path of the saphenous vein as it courses anterior to the medial malleolus of the tibia. An incision (about 1– 2 cm in length) through the skin is made perpendicular to the long axis of the tibia.

Contraindications

- Vascular injury or long bone fracture proximal to the site of the intended cutdown (Proximal venous flow or vascular access may be obstructed, so this is a relative contraindication because the mini-cutdown may not work.)
- Infection, burn, trauma, or severely disturbed anatomy at the site of the intended cutdown (relative contraindication in life-threatening situation)
- Anticoagulation from bleeding disorders or anticoagulant therapy (relative contraindication in life-threatening situation)

Equipment and Supplies

- Mounted No. 15 blade scalpel
- Mosquito hemostat
- Antiseptic skin preparation, such as povidone-iodine or chlorhexidine, and 70% isopropyl alcohol
- 4-0 silk suture, 4-0 nylon skin suture
- Sterile 4- × 4-inch gauze pads
- Sterile gloves
- Goggles or eye protection and other equipment necessary to follow universal blood and body fluid precautions
- 16- to 20-gauge standard over-the-needle intravenous catheter
- Tourniquet
- Skin retractors (optional)
- Leg board (optional)
- In the alert patient (optional), 1% or 2% lidocaine without epinephrine and a 1- or 3-mL syringe with 25- or 27-gauge, ⅝-inch (1.6-cm) needle

Technique

1. Immobilize the lower extremity by securing it to a board or by having an assistant hold the patient manually. The lower extremity should be extended and slightly externally rotated. Apply the tourniquet proximal to the intended incision site.
2. Cleanse this area with an antiseptic solution. If time allows, wipe the antiseptic solution off with an alcohol pad. Follow universal blood and body fluid precautions. If time allows and the patient is alert, anesthetize the area with lidocaine.
3. Locate the medial malleolus, and at the appropriate location anterior (one to two fingerbreadths [1 to 2 cm], depending on age) and superior (1 to 2 cm, depending on age) to it, make a 1- to 2-cm transverse (perpendicular to the vein and the tibia) incision through the dermis, exposing the underlying subcutaneous tissue. (In other words, the incision should be made in the anteroposterior direction.)
   NOTE: The incision should be very superficial, limited to the skin and exposing only the subcutaneous tissue. Incising into the subcutaneous tissue may result in transection of the vein with subsequent bleeding into the surgical field, obscuring the vein.

4. Exposure of the vein is accomplished with traction on either side of the incision with your nondominant hand (or skin retractors) and blunt dissection with a mosquito hemostat. Most clinicians insert the hemostat with the tips down against the posterior tibia, down to the periosteum, and aim it in the direction of the incision (transverse to the vein) from posterior to anterior. The tips are then advanced across the tibia, with downward pressure so that they slide across the periosteum until they reach the anterior border of the tibia (the tips will slide beneath the saphenous vein). The tips are then rotated 180 degrees (until they are facing upward), and all of the tissue between the skin and the tibial periosteum should be on top of the hemostat. When the hemostat is opened wide, the saphenous vein should be visualized in this tissue (usually a scant amount of subcutaneous tissue). In older children, the saphenous nerve can frequently also be visualized and avoided.
   Alternatively, the clinician can attempt to visualize the vein by bluntly spreading the subcutaneous tissue with the hemostat tips, spreading parallel to the course of the vein (perpendicular to the incision; Fig. 164.3A). However, some experts consider this technique to take longer because it may be difficult to find the vein against the white background of the periosteum.
   With either technique, if there is difficulty visualizing the vein, the foot can be squeezed to backfill the vein. This should improve localization of the vein.
5. When the saphenous vein is identified, pass a 4-0 silk suture beneath the vessel and clamp both ends of the suture with a hemostat (Fig. 164.3B).
6. Using upward traction on the vein with the suture to stabilize it, cannulate the vessel with an intravenous catheter under direct visualization (Fig. 164.3C). Advance the catheter in the usual fashion, then attach intravenous tubing, remove the tourniquet and begin infusing fluid. As with percutaneous line placement, a steady flow of fluid indicates successful cannulation.
7. Suture the catheter in place. (With the mini-cutdown technique, the vein is not ligated after cannulation.)
8. The incision site is then sutured with nylon suture and a sterile occlusive dressing is applied. Because the mini-cutdown technique does not destroy the vein, standard cutdown can still be performed if needed.

Sample Operative Report

See the sample operative report available at www.expertconsult.com.

Complications

- Wound infection
- Local hematoma
- Phlebitis
- Sensory nerve damage
- Damage to adjacent structures from incision and dissection

NOTE: Because this is only a temporary procedure, the risk of these complications is minimal.

Postprocedure Management

A sterile occlusive dressing should be placed immediately and routine wound care provided. Once other means of vascular access have been obtained, the venous mini-cutdown catheter should be removed and the incision repaired with appropriate suture material.

CPT/BILLING CODES

36420	Venipuncture, cutdown; younger than age 1 year
36425	Venipuncture, cutdown; age 1 year or older
36600	Arterial puncture, withdrawal of blood for diagnosis

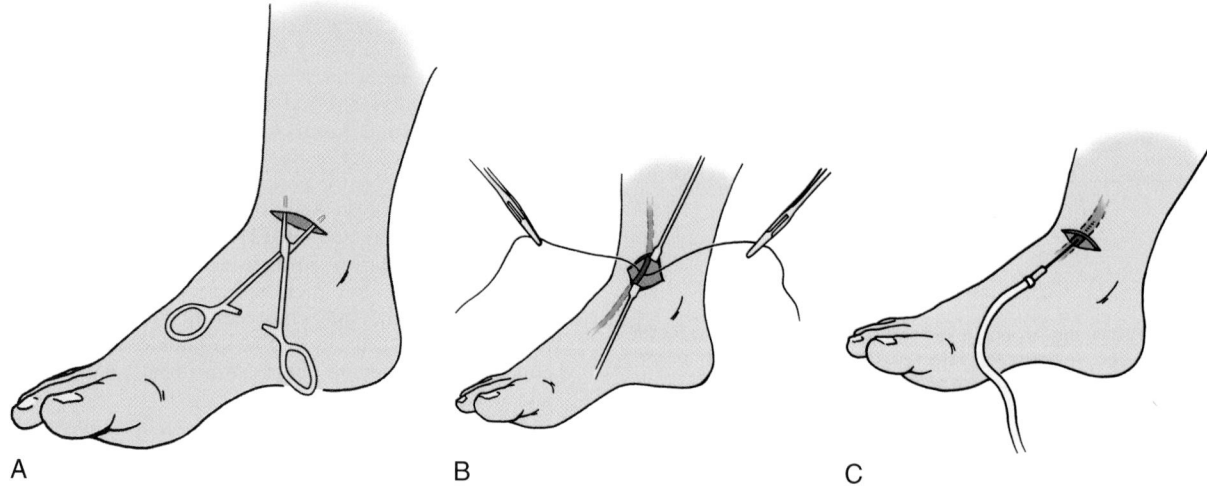

Fig. 164.3 Venous mini-cutdown. (A) Blunt dissection after a transverse incision has been made. (B) Localization of the vein. (C) Cannulation of the vein.

ICD-10-CM Diagnostic Codes

Pediatric Arterial Puncture

E11.10	Diabetic ketoacidosis
E87.2	Acidosis
E87.3	Alkalosis
E87.4	Acid-base mixed disorder
I46.9	Cardiac or cardiorespiratory arrest unspecified
I50.1	Pulmonary edema (left heart failure)
J45.20	Asthma, extrinsic, unspecified
J45.22	Asthma, extrinsic, with status asthmaticus
J45.909	Dyspnea, asthma; or asthma, unspecified
J95.821	Pulmonary insufficiency following shock, trauma, or surgery
J96.00	Respiratory failure, acute, not otherwise specified
R06.03	Respiratory distress or failure, acute
J96.10	Respiratory failure, chronic
J96.20	Respiratory failure, acute and chronic
P22.0	Respiratory distress syndrome of newborn
P24.01	Meconium aspiration syndrome
R40.20	Coma
R57.9	Shock, unspecified, without mention of trauma
R57.0	Shock, cardiogenic
R65.21	Shock, septic
R57.1	Shock, other (hypovolemic, septic)
R06.02	Shortness of breath
R06.82	Tachypnea
R06.00	Respiratory distress or insufficiency, not otherwise specified
R09.01	Asphyxia
R09.02	Hypoxemia
R09.2	Respiratory arrest
T58.94XA	Carbon monoxide, toxic effect unspecified source

Venous Minicutdown

R58	Hemorrhage, unspecified
I99.8	Venofibrosis
P54.9	Hemorrhage, in newborn, not otherwise specified
T79.4XXA	Hemorrhagic shock due to trauma

RECOMMENDED READING

Hughes H, Kahl LK, eds. *The Harriet Lane Handbook: A Manual for Pediatric House Officers*. 21st ed. Philadelphia: Elsevier; 2018.

Klofas E. A quicker saphenous vein cutdown and a better way to teach it. *J Trauma*. 1997;43:985–987.

Nobay F. Peripheral venous cutdown. In: Reichman EF, ed. *Reichman's Emergency Medicine Procedures*. 3rd ed. New York: McGraw-Hill; 2018.

Santillanes G, Claudius I. Pediatric vascular access and blood sampling techniques. In: Roberts JR, Custalow CB, Thomsen TW, eds. *Roberts and Hedges Clinical Procedures in Emergency Medicine*. 6th ed. Philadelphia: Elsevier; 2014.

Sweeney MN. Vascular access in trauma: options, risks, benefits, and complications. *Anesthesiol Clin North Am*. 1999;17:97–106.

CHAPTER 165

UMBILICAL VESSEL CATHETERIZATION

Carman H. Whiting

Being able to quickly assess and rapidly intervene in a severely ill infant is essential. Because the umbilical vessels are easily visualized, they are an excellent route for catheterization to provide central vascular access. Whereas umbilical artery catheterization allows for accurate monitoring of central arterial pressure directly through the aorta, umbilical vein catheterization allows for central venous pressure (CVP) monitoring through the inferior vena cava. Umbilical vein catheterization also provides access for rapid infusion of life-sustaining therapies (Fig. 165.1).

Primary care clinicians may need to perform umbilical vessel catheterization in the delivery room for a newborn resuscitation or in the emergency department for a newborn or infant in distress. They may also need to perform it in the nursery or neonatal intensive care unit (NICU) for an infant requiring continuous monitoring or frequent infusions of medications or fluids. In fact, both vessels are frequently catheterized in the NICU for premature infants requiring prolonged vascular access or monitoring.

Compared with the vein, the umbilical artery is a more durable vessel with higher-velocity blood flow; therefore, it is easier to visualize and there is a slightly lower risk of complications when it is catheterized. Inserting an umbilical artery catheter (UAC) or an umbilical vein catheter (UVC) is easier if performed in the first 30 to 60 minutes of the infant's life. However, a UAC may be inserted up to the seventh day of life and a UVC at up to 2 weeks of age. Despite the fact that the vessels are easily accessible, placing a UAC can be a time-consuming procedure and requires skill and experience. Contraindications or difficulty obtaining a UAC insertion may necessitate the need for a UVC for infusions because a UVC insertion is easier to perform. A UVC is also an option if peripheral intravenous access is difficult to obtain, which is likely the case in very premature infants. After the first day of life, there are few data supporting any benefit of a UAC over a UVC for infusion, although an attempt should always be made to obtain peripheral venous access before either of these is inserted, except in infants of very low birth weight (BW).

INDICATIONS

Umbilical Artery Catheterization

- Newborn resuscitation requiring monitoring for cardiorespiratory distress (e.g., arterial pressure monitoring, frequent arterial sampling)
- Newborn or infant in a NICU requiring
  - Mechanical ventilation for respiratory distress (i.e., frequent arterial sampling)
  - Oxygen hood and greater than 40% oxygen (FIO_2 >0.4) requirement with an abnormal chest radiograph (i.e., frequent arterial sampling)
  - Exchange transfusion that can be performed through a UAC (e.g., newborn weighing <1800 g)

Umbilical Vein Catheterization

- Newborn resuscitation requiring
  - Administration of drugs, blood, blood expanders, or fluids
  - Monitoring for possible cardiorespiratory distress (e.g., CVP monitoring)
- Newborn or infant in the NICU requiring
  - Greater than 12.5% dextrose to maintain blood glucose while taking nothing by mouth
  - Pressor drips, total parenteral nutrition solution, or hypertonic medications (e.g., newborn weighing <1000 g or who is critically ill)
  - Exchange transfusion or partial exchange transfusions that can be performed through a UVC (e.g., newborn weighing <1800 g)

NOTE: By convention, a newborn is defined as an infant younger than 1 month.

CONTRAINDICATIONS

- There are no contraindications during the first hours of life if the newborn has normal anatomy and no local skin infections.
- Vascular insufficiency of a lower extremity is a contraindication to UAC.
- Local infection (e.g., omphalitis, impetigo) and abdominal distention (possibly caused by intestinal hypoperfusion or necrotizing enterocolitis) are contraindications that can develop after the first few hours of life.

EQUIPMENT

- Sterile measuring tape
- 3.5- to 5.0-Fr umbilical catheter for UAC; up to 8-Fr umbilical catheter for UVC
- Surgical cap and mask; sterile gown and gloves
- Eye protection for clinician and any other equipment necessary for universal blood and body fluid precautions
- Povidone-iodine, chlorhexidine, or other antiseptic scrub solution
- Three-way stopcock (sterile); locking connectors
- Heparin for flush (1 to 2 U heparin/mL of 0.25 normal saline [NS])
- Sterile instrument tray with small hemostats, forceps (iris curved), scissors, needle holder, straight forceps, mounted No. 11 scalpel blade, and drapes
- Antibiotic ointment
- 4-0 or 5-0 silk suture with a small needle or a catheter stabilizer
- Sterile umbilical tape
- Infant radiant warmer, means of restraint, cardiac and oxygen saturation monitors, supplemental oxygen

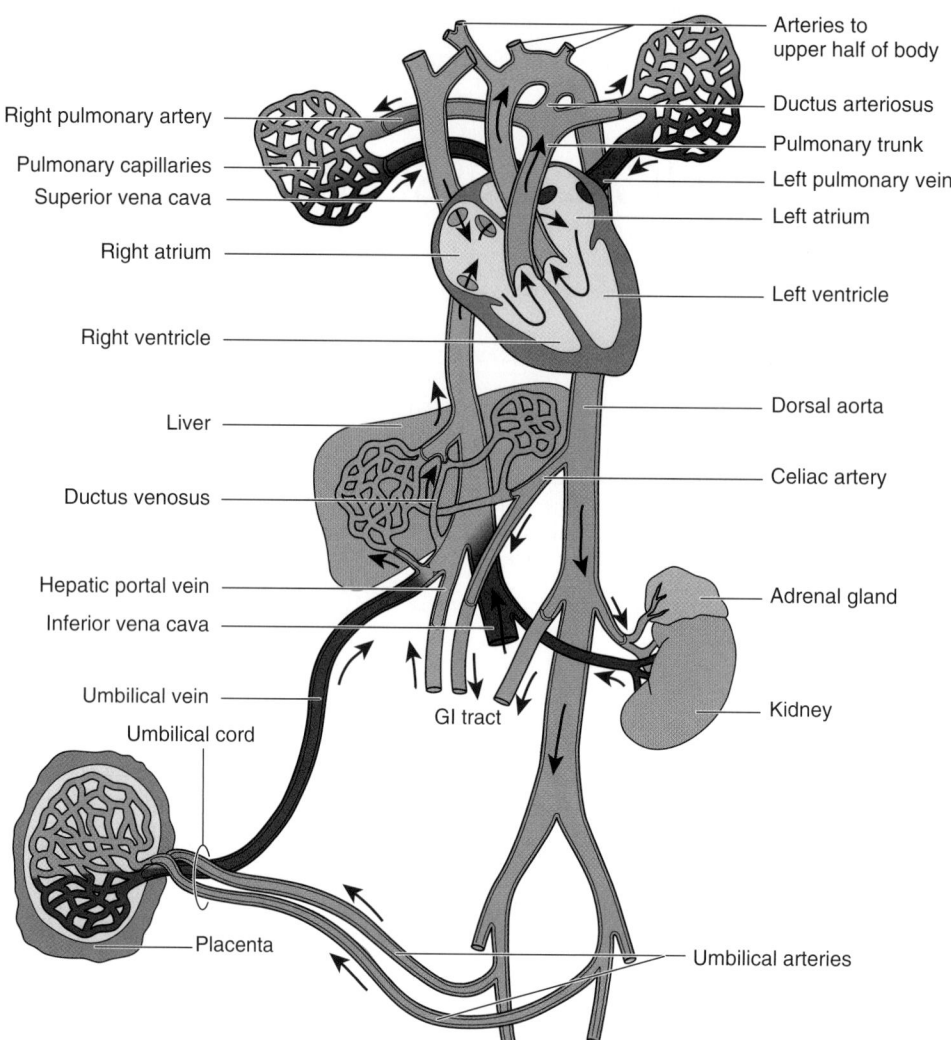

Fig. 165.1 Fetal circulation at term.

- 5% or 10% dextrose in water or NS infusion setup (use heparin 1 U/mL, unless medications are to be administered that are incompatible with heparin) with fluid chamber, 0.22-μg filter, and infusion pump
- Adhesive tape

A rule of thumb for selecting UAC size is to use a 5-Fr catheter for infants weighing more than 2000 g and a 3.5- to 4-Fr catheter for infants weighing less. Because the lumen of the vein is larger, a 5- to 8-Fr catheter can be used for UVC in term infants (>1800 g), especially infants requiring exchange transfusion. The catheter may be composed of any U.S. Food and Drug Administration–approved material; double-lumen catheters are also available.

PREPROCEDURE PATIENT PREPARATION

The newborn needing umbilical catheterization typically demonstrates signs and symptoms of cardiorespiratory distress shortly, if not immediately, after birth. If performed as an emergency procedure, implied consent and the indications should be documented in the chart. Explain the need for the procedure to the parent(s) when there is time. For less urgent insertions, obtain informed consent from the parent(s) after discussing the alternatives, risks, and potential benefits of the procedure.

TECHNIQUE

When the infant arrives at the nursery, if umbilical catheterization is probable, the umbilical stump should be left at least 4 cm long. The two thick-walled arteries and the single vein should be easily identifiable. Place the infant under an infant warmer and restrain; keeping the infant warm during the procedure is critical. The cardiac rate should be monitored, and adequate oxygenation should be provided throughout the procedure.

1. Set up the tubing, fluids, fluid chamber, 0.22-μg filter, and infusion pump. Flush and fill the tubing with heparin flush to remove air from the system.
2. Prepare the entire abdomen from xiphoid to pubis with sterile povidone–iodine, chlorhexidine, or other antiseptic scrub solution. Scrub the umbilical stump and apply sterile drapes. Observe universal blood and body fluid precautions when performing the procedure. The infant's head should be left exposed for observation.
3. Calculate the insertion length of the catheter for proper placement.
   - UAC. There are two commonly used, standard insertion depths for UAC. One results in "high" placement of the catheter tip, which is above the diaphragm at the level of the thoracic aorta (spinal level T6–T9). This site places the

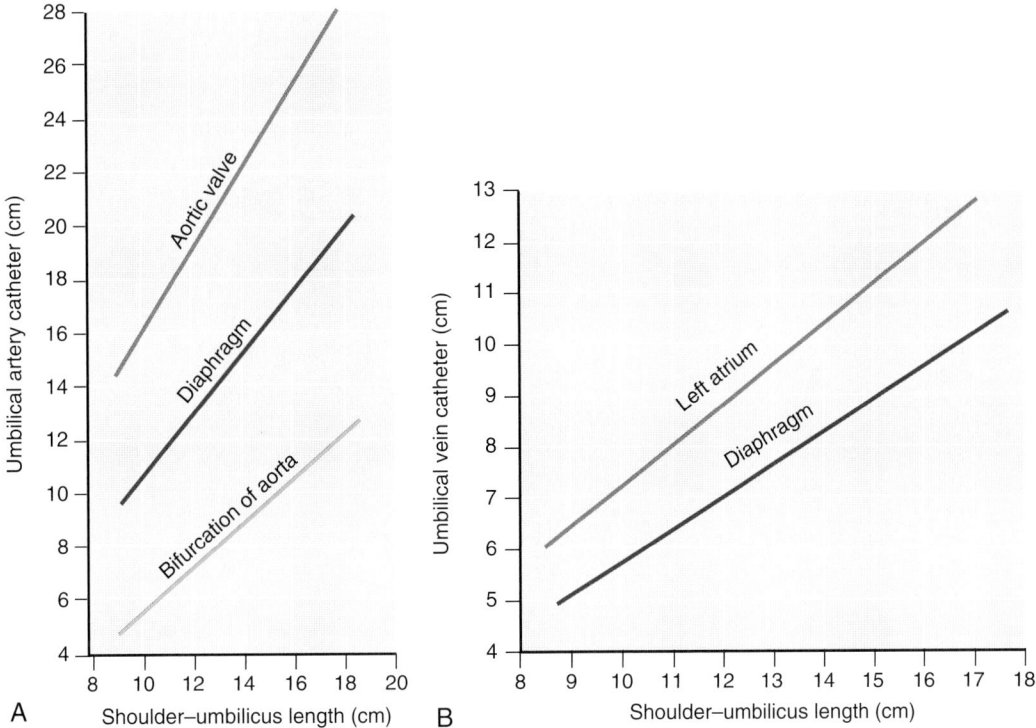

Fig. 165.2   Approximate distances for catheter insertion, with radiographic confirmation of proper placement after insertion. (A) Umbilical artery catheter (avoid inserting to level of aortic valve). (B) Umbilical vein catheter. (From Johns Hopkins Hospital; Siberry G, Iannone R, eds. *The Harriet Lane Handbook: A Manual for Pediatric House Officers*, 15th ed. St. Louis, Mosby; 2000.)

tip between the ductus arteriosus and the origin of the celiac axis. The second site results in "low" placement of the catheter tip (spinal level L3–L5), which is below the diaphragm. This site places the tip between the inferior mesenteric artery and the bifurcation of the aorta.

- For high placement: (a) Measure the axial or longitudinal distance from the level of the umbilicus to the level of the shoulder or clavicle (shoulder–umbilicus length). Then use the nomogram shown in Fig. 165.2A; or (b) calculate the length based on BW: length (cm) = (4 × BW [kg]) + 7.
- When a nomogram or the BW is not available or the situation is urgent, if the shoulder–umbilicus length is greater than 13 cm, simply add 1 cm to the shoulder–umbilicus length. This results in a reasonable estimate for the catheter insertion depth. When the shoulder–umbilicus length is less than 13 cm, insert the catheter 2 cm further than the shoulder–umbilicus length.
- For low placement: (a) Use the nomogram (see Fig. 165.2A) with the shoulder–umbilicus length, or (b) calculate the length based on BW: length (cm) = BW (kg) + 7.
- If a nomogram or the BW is unavailable or the situation is urgent, insert the catheter until blood is first encountered and then advance it 1 additional centimeter.

  NOTE: A Cochrane review meta-analysis found that high-placement UACs (compared with low-placement) have fewer acute vascular complications and no increase in permanent vascular sequelae. They saw no need to ever use low-placement.
- UVC. For CVP readings, place the catheter tip 0.5 to 1 cm above the diaphragm. The insertion depth can be estimated with a nomogram (see Fig. 165.2B) or with one of two formulas: (a) length (cm) = shoulder–umbilicus length (cm) × 0.6, or (b) length (cm) = (UAC insertion length [cm] × 0.5) + 1. If a nomogram or the BW is not available or the situation is urgent, a second option is to insert the UVC gently

for 4 to 5 cm until blood return is noted. Never insert the UVC more than 5 cm without radiographically checking the placement because the tip may be in the portal vein. If the catheter is being placed for a single-exchange transfusion, it may be inserted to just beneath the skin (3 to 5 cm), as long as good blood flow is noted and there is no leakage around the catheter.

4. Loosely tie the sterile umbilical tape around the proximal stump. It should be tight enough to control bleeding but loose enough to allow later passage of the catheter. A silk suture can be used as a pursestring ligation in the same manner.
5. Holding the cord with straight forceps, transect it with the scalpel approximately 1 cm above the umbilical tape (Fig. 165.3A). Correctly identify the arteries and the vein. Because the vein is the single vessel and has the largest lumen, it is usually the easiest to identify. It can then be distinguished from the thicker-walled arteries that are usually lateral to the vein.
6. The cord stump should be grasped with one or two hemostats (on opposite sides of the umbilicus) and the cut edge everted. Gently dilate the desired vessel with small curved forceps (see Fig. 165.3B). To do so, insert one prong, then both prongs of the iris forceps, then open the forceps prongs slightly to dilate the lumen to a depth of about 1 cm. Next, grasp the catheter approximately 1 cm from the tip with your thumb and forefinger or with the forceps. Gently insert the catheter through the vessel lumen to the length previously measured (see Fig. 165.3C).
7. Insertion
- UAC. Placing traction on the cord stump in a cranial direction usually facilitates directing the catheter caudally. With insertion, use gentle, constant pressure to overcome any resistance. Resistance is usually encountered at a depth of about 1 to 2 cm as the vessel turns caudad. Slight resistance may again occur when the catheter enters the internal iliac artery at approximately 5 to 6 cm. At this depth, the catheter must turn cephalad. Twisting the catheter slightly may

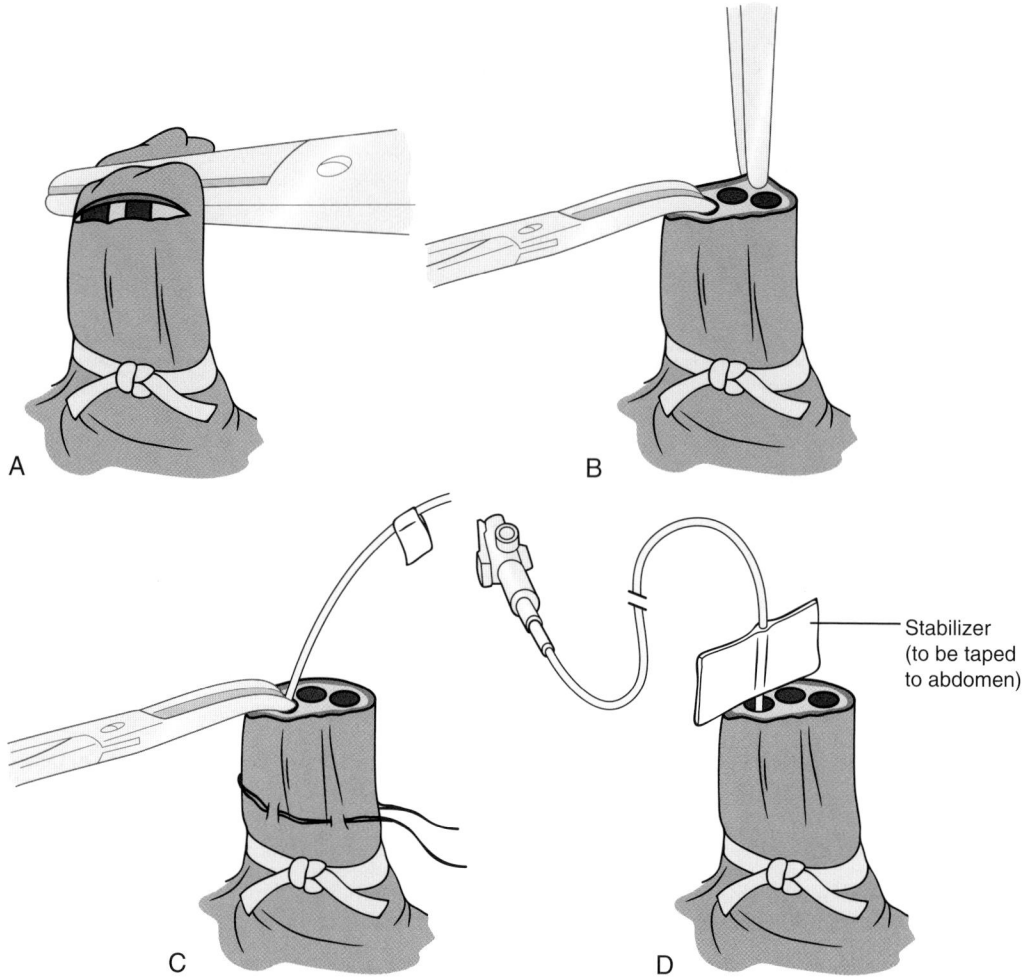

A

B

C

D

Stabilizer
(to be taped
to abdomen)

Fig. 165.3 Umbilical artery catheter placement. (A) The cord is transected approximately 1 cm above the umbilical tape. (B) The desired artery is dilated with small curved forceps. (C) The catheter is inserted through the vessel lumen to the length previously measured and secured with a silk pursestring suture. (D) Alternatively, the catheter can be secured by a stabilizer taped to the abdomen.

also help overcome resistance. Occasionally, resistance from vasospasm may be overcome by applying constant gentle pressure for 30 to 60 seconds, causing the spasm to subside. Another technique for relieving vasospasm is to fill the tip of the catheter with 2% lidocaine and then to flush some of it at the level where the resistance is noted. After waiting 1 to 2 minutes, attempt to advance the catheter again. Do not advance against significant resistance, especially at a depth of 4 to 5 cm. Resistance at this depth generally indicates that a false tract has been created. Rather than continuing to advance the catheter, withdraw it and attempt to cannulate the other artery.

- UVC. Insert in the same manner as a UAC. At the higher insertion depths (previously determined, usually 10 to 12 cm to reach above the diaphragm and into the inferior vena cava), CVP can be measured, hypertonic and hyperalimentation solutions can be administered, and high concentrations of glucose and medications can be infused. If an obstruction is encountered at a depth of 5 to 10 cm, the catheter has probably entered a branch of the portal vein of the liver and should be withdrawn. It can then be reinserted; sometimes a slight twisting motion will redirect the catheter into the inferior vena cava.

8. Secure the catheter with the umbilical tape. Also use a silk suture in a pursestring fashion (see Fig. 165.3C), or with a stabilizer (see Fig. 165.3D). Once the sterile field is taken

away, the catheter may not be advanced. For that reason, it is often more convenient to insert the catheter slightly further than necessary. (For a UAC, never exceed the distance to the aortic valve [see Fig. 165.2].) Then it can be withdrawn slightly after radiographic confirmation of the location of the tip.

NOTE: Occasionally a persistent urachus in the umbilical stump is mistaken for the umbilical vein. Catheterization of the urachus results in the return of urine instead of blood and is easily identified and corrected.

9. Apply sterile gauze over the antibiotic ointment and tape the catheter to the abdomen.

10. Obtain radiographic confirmation of proper placement. Again, the ideal location of the UAC tip is either high placement at T6–T9 (above the diaphragm and the celiac axis but below the ductus arteriosus) or low placement at L3–L5 (above the aortic bifurcation but below the inferior mesenteric artery). If radiographic confirmation is not possible, a UVC should be used instead of a UAC and should be inserted only 3 to 5 cm or until prompt return of blood is noted. For UVC, radiographs should confirm placement above the diaphragm prior to infusion of any hypertonic fluids, hyperalimentation, high concentrations of glucose, and so on.

11. Check the catheter frequently for patency and the infant for signs of infection. If signs of infection are noted, take cultures from the catheter.

12. As soon as the catheter is no longer needed, it should be removed. In addition, remove the catheter in the face of complications. When the catheter is no longer needed for arterial sampling or for CVP monitoring, in some NICUs it is simply pulled out enough to leave the tip in the midline. This maintains peripheral access if it is extremely critical or has been difficult to obtain. At that level, it then can be used for infusions.

13. If vasospasm occurs while the UAC is in place, causing ischemia of one buttock or leg, apply warm compresses to the contralateral limb in an attempt to trigger reflex vasodilation in the affected limb. If no improvement in limb color or pulse is observed in 15 minutes, the catheter should be withdrawn. An attempt can also be made to relieve vasospasm by repositioning the catheter. Withdraw it a short distance or rotate it, while observing limb color. If successful, obtain radiographic confirmation of proper placement. Other options include withdrawing the line completely and catheterizing the other artery or using a smaller catheter in the same artery.

14. For catheter removal, the stopcock should be turned off. Umbilical tape should be tied loosely around the stump. The catheter should then be gradually withdrawn over 3 to 5 minutes. If there is bleeding, tighten the umbilical tape or grasp the vessel with forceps and apply pressure until it stops.

COMPLICATIONS

- Air embolization (use a three-way stopcock and flush all tubing before connecting). Make sure the vein is rapidly secured with a suture tie upon removal of the catheter, especially if the infant is crying. Negative intrathoracic pressure induced by crying may pull an air embolism through a patent vein.
- Necrotizing enterocolitis
- Bladder rupture
- Pelvic exsanguination
- Exsanguination from disconnected tubing (use locking connectors on tubing, secure the line)
- Bacteremia or sepsis (to minimize risk, remove the catheter once the infant is stabilized or within 5 days)
- Vascular perforation or malformation
- Congestive heart failure
- Fluid around the umbilicus, if the catheter is placed too low or withdrawn too far
- Silent thrombus (difficult to diagnose without contrast studies)
- UAC complications (risk of complications is as high as 10%)
  - Ischemia or thromboembolic phenomena to bowel, liver, or other intraabdominal organ, or lower extremity
  - Systemic hypertension as a result of blockage of renal arteries, renovascular stenosis, or thrombosis
  - Embolization of catheter tip or clots causing loss of digits, organ infarcts, or skin ulceration
  - Hypoglycemia
  - Aortic aneurysm
  - Aortic thrombosis
  - Peritoneal perforation
- UVC complications (risk of complications is as high as 20%)
  - Air embolism
  - Catheter tip embolism and resultant ischemia including myocardial infarction
  - Portal hypertension
  - Pericardial perforation (if placed in the right atrium for central monitoring)
  - Arrhythmias
  - Hepatic hematoma, abscess, or necrosis
  - Malplacement
  - Pulmonary embolism

POSTPROCEDURE PATIENT EDUCATION

If the procedure is successful, this should be explained to the family. If there were any complications, this should also be explained, as well as what will be done about them. Any questions regarding the umbilical catheter should be answered. The family should be informed of the need for and value of having the catheter in place, and reassured that it will be monitored continuously for any signs of complications. They should be aware that it will be withdrawn to a safer level or removed as soon as it is no longer needed. It will also be removed at the first signs of a complication. Families also usually appreciate any other reassurances and guidance provided when they have a critically ill loved one in an intensive care setting, especially an infant.

CPT/BILLING CODES

| 36510 | Catheterization, umbilical vein, for diagnosis or therapy; newborn |
| 36660 | Catheterization, umbilical artery, for diagnosis or therapy; newborn |

ICD-10-CM DIAGNOSTIC CODES

R58	Hemorrhage, unspecified
P22.0	Respiratory distress syndrome of newborn
P24.01	Meconium aspiration syndrome
P28.89	Other respiratory problems after birth (e.g., perinatal apnea, newborn bradycardia)
P36.9	Neonatal sepsis
P51.8	Hemorrhage, in newborn, umbilical
P54.9	Hemorrhage, in newborn, NOS
P55.0	Newborn hemolytic disease caused by Rh isoimmunization
P71.8	Hypocalcemia and hypomagnesemia of newborn
P70.4	Neonatal hypoglycemia
P92.9	Feeding problems in newborn
R57.1	Hypovolemic shock
T79.4XXA	Hemorrhagic shock as a result of trauma

RECOMMENDED READING

Advanced Life Support Group. *Advanced Paediatric Life Support: The Practical Approach.* 5th ed. London: BMJ Publishing Group; 2011.

Barrington KJ. Umbilical artery catheters in the newborn: effects of position of the catheter tip. *Cochrane Database Syst Rev.* 1999;1:CD000505.

Carlson B. *Human Embryology and Developmental Biology.* 5th ed. Philadelphia: Elsevier; 2014.

Fanaroff A, Martin R, Walsh M, eds. *Neonatal-Perinatal Medicine: Diseases of the Fetus and Infant.* 8th ed. St. Louis: Elsevier; 2006.

Gomella TL, Cunningham MD. *Neonatology: Management, Procedures, On-Call Problems, Diseases, and Drugs.* 7th ed. New York: McGraw-Hill; 2013.

Johns Hopkins Hospital. In: Robertson J, Shilkofski N, eds. *The Harriet Lane Handbook: A Manual for Pediatric House Officers.* 21st ed. Philadelphia: Elsevier; 2018.

Kang I, Reichman EF. Umbilical vessel catheterization. In: Reichman EF, Simon RR, eds. *Emergency Medicine Procedures.* New York: McGraw-Hill; 2004:390–397.

Santillanes G, Claudius I. Pediatric vascular access and blood sampling techniques. In: Roberts JR, Custalow CB, Thomsen TW, eds. *Roberts and Hedges Clinical Procedures in Emergency Medicine.* 6th ed. Philadelphia: Elsevier; 2014.

Spitzer AR. *Intensive Care of the Fetus and Neonate.* 2nd ed. St. Louis: Mosby; 2005.

CHAPTER 166

DORSAL PENILE AND SUBCUTANEOUS RING BLOCK FOR NEWBORN CIRCUMCISION

Grant C. Fowler

The American Academy of Pediatrics has recommended routine use of analgesia for circumcision since 1999. A 2006 survey of residency program directors found that 97% of pediatric, family medicine, and obstetrics and gynecology programs that teach circumcision teach the administration of an anesthetic, either locally or topically. Therefore, the controversy about whether or not infants should receive analgesia or anesthesia for circumcision ended long ago; it is now considered the standard. With proper planning, the number of steps and the time required are minimal. In addition, studies have documented the safety of anesthesia as well as the improved outcomes in neonates.

Common analgesic and anesthetic techniques for circumcision include subcutaneous ring block, dorsal penile nerve block (DPNB), topical anesthesia (see Chapter 4, Topical Anesthesia), and precircumcision oral analgesics. Several studies have reported that the subcutaneous ring block is the most effective, and it has therefore basically replaced DPNB as the anesthetic technique of choice. (This is different in adults, where the most effective anesthesia for office circumcision is probably a combination of all three.) This chapter discusses subcutaneous ring block, DPNB, and an alternative technique of DPNB using a single injection. All three techniques appear to be more effective than topical or oral anesthesia, and no major complications have been reported with any of these methods. Studies have found that anesthetized infants show less crying, tachycardia, and irritability, and exhibit fewer behavior changes during the 24 hours after circumcision. They also have less variability in oxygen saturation and blood pressure during the procedure and lower serum cortisol levels after the procedure. One small study in children found that lidocaine–prilocaine (eutectic mixture of local anesthetics, or EMLA) cream applied an hour before the ring block reduced the pain of needle puncture. However, because most clinicians cannot prepare a newborn an hour before circumcision, they would have to rely on the nursing staff to apply the cream. Conversely, in adults and children who are about to undergo office circumcision under local anesthesia, waiting an hour for the lidocaine-prilocaine cream to take effect may be very worthwhile.

Nonpharmacologic proven strategies to minimize pain include addition of oral sucrose water and stimulating other sensations (e.g., gently looking at, talking to, stroking or massaging the face or back, or rocking the infant). Swaddling, positioning, and facilitated tucking, which is holding the infant's arms in a flexed position close to the chest, with or without parental assistance, decreases stress. Obviously, breastfeeding and skin-to-skin care (nude infant held against mother's skin), although proven beneficial, would be more difficult to manage at the same time as an ongoing circumcision. That said, these may be useful for other painful procedures such as an injection.

INDICATION

- Parental desire (Parents should be encouraged to consent to this procedure in any healthy newborn undergoing circumcision.)

CONTRAINDICATIONS

- Known hypersensitivity to anesthetic
- A known bleeding disorder (relative contraindication)

EQUIPMENT

- 1% lidocaine without epinephrine.
- 1-mL syringe with 27-gauge needle (some tuberculin syringes come with this combination). If the needle is removable, using a 30-gauge needle to administer the anesthetic may minimize bleeding and discomfort.
- Alcohol wipe.
- Infant restrainer (Papoose board or Circumstraint) if assistant not available to hold infant.
- Oral sucrose.
- Lidocaine–prilocaine (EMLA) cream (optional).

NOTE: There is risk of methemoglobinemia with use of EMLA cream in certain situations. However, this risk is minimized with circumcision because it is used only once on intact skin and not with other drugs known to cause methemoglobinemia (e.g., nitric oxide).

PREPROCEDURE PATIENT PREPARATION

Discuss the risks, benefits, and alternatives with the parents, and obtain informed consent. Most clinicians combine this consent with the circumcision consent.

TECHNIQUE

Before the procedure, note the anatomy as shown in Fig. 166.1. Consider giving the infant a few swallows of glucose or sucrose water or a sugar-coated pacifier to minimize distress (a Cochrane review found benefit when oral sucrose was provided before a painful procedure). In a warm room, have an assistant hold the infant or place the infant's legs in restraints. Fold back the diaper to expose the penis.

NOTE: As the clinician becomes more comfortable performing ring block or DPNB, time may be saved by performing the procedure before the infant is surgically prepared. This allows time for the anesthetic to take effect while other preparations are being made.

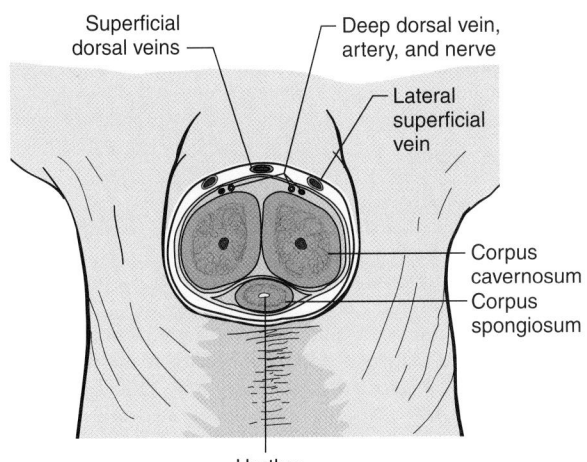

Fig. 166.1   Anatomy of the penile root (cross-section).

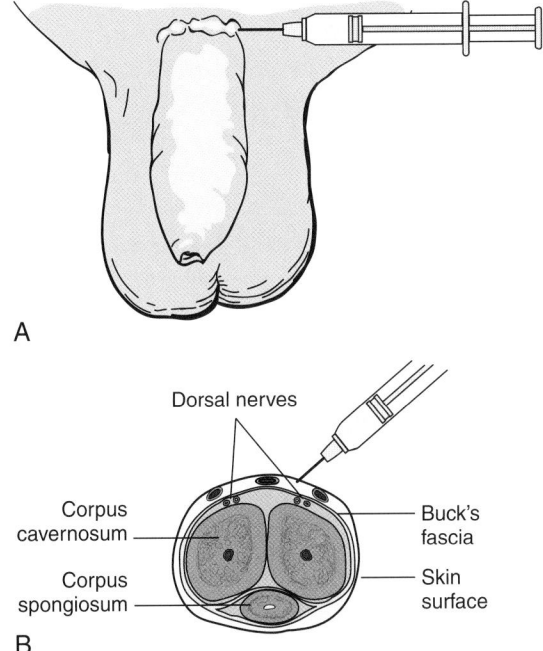

Fig. 166.2   Subcutaneous ring block. (A) Needle is inserted at base of penis and a subcutaneous bleb of lidocaine is placed. A 360-degree ring of anesthesia is completed around the penis. (B) Cross-section of penis at base showing paired dorsal nerves deep to the Buck's fascia.

Subcutaneous Ring Block

1. Prepare the skin both at the base of the penis as well as around the penis with an alcohol pad. Using aseptic technique and stabilizing the penis by gentle, slightly downward or ventral traction, insert the needle into the lateral side of the penis at the base (Fig. 166.2). Staying superficial to the Buck's fascia, place a subcutaneous bleb of lidocaine. Then advance the needle circumferentially around the base of the penis while injecting. A couple of punctures may be necessary to accomplish this.
2. After completing a 180-degree half-circle, the same procedure is followed on the opposite side of the penis. A maximum of 1 mL of lidocaine should be used to complete the 360-degree circumferential ring. Intravascular injection can be avoided by frequently aspirating with the syringe to check for any blood return prior to each 0.25 mL injected.

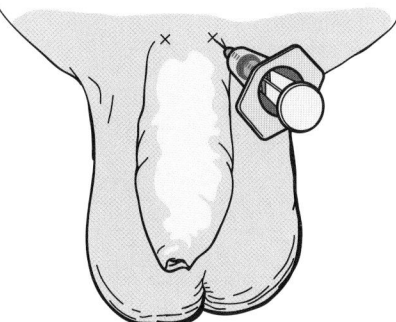

Fig. 166.3   Injection sites and direction of needle for administering dorsal penile nerve block.

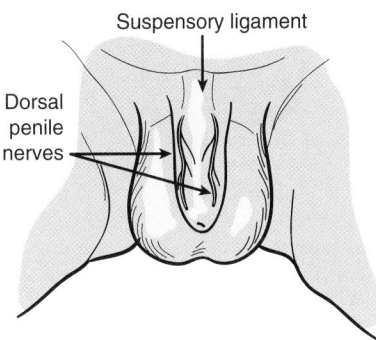

Fig. 166.4   Location of dorsal penile nerves. Note branching begins after emergence from the suspensory ligament of the penis.

Dorsal Penile Nerve Block (Two Techniques)

Standard Technique

1. Using an index finger, palpate the lateral side of the penis to determine the depth of the root of the penis, which is usually about 0.75 to 1 cm beneath the skin surface. Often it is about the size, shape, and consistency of a large blueberry and is located just under the symphysis pubis.
2. Prepare the skin at the base of the penis with an alcohol pad. Using aseptic technique and stabilizing the penis by gentle, slightly downward, or ventral traction, insert the needle at the 1 o'clock position (the dorsal or cranial direction being the 12 o'clock position, and the ventral direction being the 6 o'clock position) and direct it posteromedially (Fig. 166.3). Insert to a depth of 0.3 to 0.5 cm, which corresponds to 0.5 to 0.7 cm distal to the penile root, and this is slightly proximal to where the dorsal nerves branch (Fig. 166.4). The tip of the needle should be freely movable, indicating that it is in loose connective tissue, and this should prevent injection into the corpus cavernosum. Taking care not to inject into a blood vessel (check by aspirating), inject 0.4 mL of lidocaine. Repeat the injection at the 11 o'clock position with another 0.4 mL of lidocaine. (Avoid exceeding a total of 0.8 mL of lidocaine.)
3. In the infant whose penile root is not palpable because it is embedded in pubic fat, the anesthetic can be injected at the same locations, depths, and directions, but about 0.3 to 0.5 cm inferolateral to the penile–suprapubic skin junction (Fig. 166.5).

Alternative Technique Using Single Injection Site

1. Instead of making two skin punctures (at the 11 and 1 o'clock positions), an alternative is to insert the needle at the 12 o'clock position and angle the needle toward the 11 and 1 o'clock positions. In other words, if the 12 o'clock position is where the dorsal skin of the penis reflects onto the abdomen (penile–suprapubic skin junction), insert the needle here and angle it toward the 1 o'clock position to a depth of about 0.5 cm. The tip of the needle should be freely movable, indicating that it is

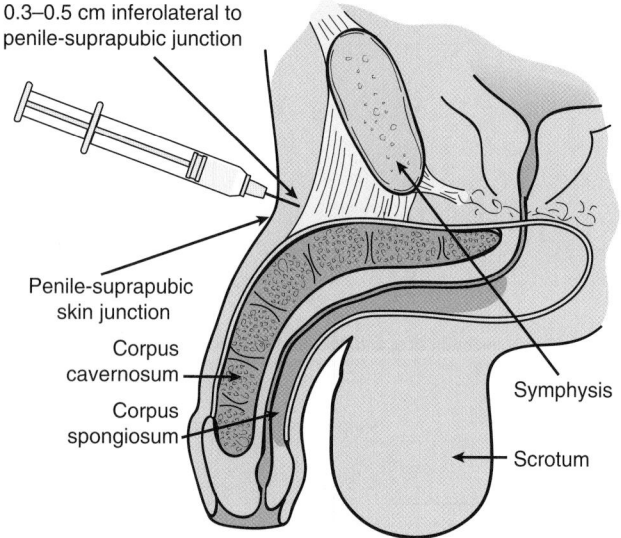

0.3–0.5 cm inferolateral to
penile-suprapubic junction

Penile-suprapubic
skin junction

Corpus
cavernosum

Corpus
spongiosum

Symphysis

Scrotum

Fig. 166.5 Sagittal view through the perineum showing anesthetic injection in a posteromedial direction at a depth of 0.3 to 0.5 mm.

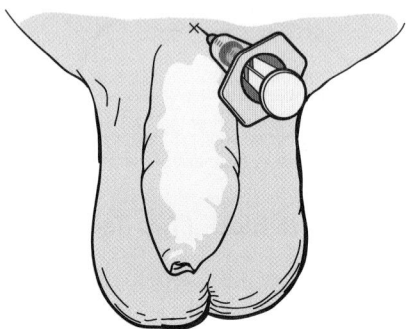

Fig. 166.6 Dorsal penile nerve block using a single injection site at the 12 o'clock position.

in loose connective tissue, and this should prevent injection into the corpus cavernosum. After aspirating to ensure the needle is not in a blood vessel, inject 0.4 mL of lidocaine.

2. Withdraw the needle until the tip is just below the skin surface, and then advance it again toward the 11 o'clock position (Fig. 166.6). The second injection can then be made, taking care not to exceed a total of 0.8 mL of lidocaine.

NOTE: A combination of ring block and DPNB has been demonstrated to be effective in adults undergoing office circumcision. Obviously, larger doses of lidocaine are used in adults.

Notes Regarding Optimal Effects

- One study in adults has found that using slower injection rates (i.e., longer injection times, such as 100 to 150 seconds) caused less pain than shorter injection times (40 to 80 seconds). Using a 30-gauge needle will not only slow the injection rate; it will increase overall patient comfort and cause less bleeding.
- Another study comparing plain and buffered lidocaine in newborns failed to demonstrate a difference in oxygen saturations, crying, heart rate, or any other measure of distress.
- Although some anesthesia will take effect in as little as 2 to 3 minutes, ideally 3 to 5 minutes should be allowed for the full effect of the anesthesia before performing circumcision. Conveniently, this is about the amount of time it takes to prepare and drape the infant and appropriately arrange the instruments.
- Avoid injecting air, which can cause pain.

COMMON ERRORS

- Insufficient time allowed for anesthetic to take effect
- Lidocaine injected in the wrong location

COMPLICATIONS

- Inadequate anesthesia
- Localized edema, bleeding, or hematoma at the injection site
- Local skin infection or necrosis
- Allergic reaction to lidocaine
- Systemic reaction to intravascular lidocaine
- Erythema and mild skin pallor observed with use of EMLA
- Penile necrosis (This is theoretical, because it has not been reported. Only lidocaine without epinephrine should be used because epinephrine can cause vasospasm of the penile arteries.)
- Methemoglobinemia with use of EMLA (very rare). Prompt recognition and treatment with methylene blue and other methods is critical.

CPT/BILLING CODES

64450-47   Nerve block, diagnostic or therapeutic, other peripheral nerve,

(Modifier 47 is used when anesthesia is provided by the surgeon. A few insurers will pay for this as a separate procedure from the circumcision.)

ICD-10-CM DIAGNOSTIC CODE

Z41.2   Routine or ritual circumcision, in absence of significant medical indication

SUPPLIERS

(See contact information available at www.expertconsult.com.)

Circumstraint
    Olympic Medical Corp. (Natus Newborn Care, Alimed)

RECOMMENDED READING

American Academy of Pediatrics. Committee statements: report of the task force on circumcision. *Pediatrics.* 1999;103:686–693.

American Academy of Pediatrics, Task Force on Circumcision. Circumcision Policy Statement. *Pediatrics.* 2012;130(3):585.

American Academy of Pediatrics, Committee on Fetus and Newborn and Section on Anesthesiology and Pain Medicine: Prevention and management of procedural pain in the neonate: an update. *Pediatrics.* 137(2): e20154271.

Brady-Fryer B, Wiebe N, Lander JA. Pain relief for neonatal circumcision. 2004;(3):CD004217.

Lander J, Brady-Fryer B, Metcalfe JB, et al. Comparison of ring block, dorsal penile nerve block, and topical anesthesia for neonatal circumcision: a randomized controlled trial. *JAMA.* 1997;278:2157–2162.

Serour F, Mandelberg A, Mori J. Slow injection of local anesthetic will decrease pain during dorsal penile nerve block. *Acta Anaesthesiol Scand.* 1998;42:926–928.

Stevens B, Yamada J, Ohlsson A, Haliburton S, Shorkey A. Sucrose for analgesia in newborn infants undergoing painful procedures. *Cochrane Database Syst Rev.* 2016;7:CD001069.

The Newborn. In: Cunningham F, Leveno KJ, Bloom SL, et al. *Williams Obstetrics.* 24th ed. New York: McGraw-Hill; 2013.

Yawman D, Howard CR, Auinger P, Garfunkel LC, Allan M, Weitzman M. Pain relief for neonatal circumcision: a follow-up of residency training practices. *Ambul Pediatr.* 2006;6(4):210–214.

CHAPTER 167

NEWBORN CIRCUMCISION AND OFFICE MEATOTOMY

Grant C. Fowler

Newborn circumcision is the most common surgical procedure performed in the United States, yet there has been much controversy over the need for the procedure. Studies have shown a lower incidence of urinary tract infection (UTI), phimosis, paraphimosis, balanoposthitis, and some sexually transmitted infections (STIs), including human immunodeficiency virus (HIV), in circumcised men. Circumcision helps prevents penile cancer and may decrease the risk of cervical cancer in the sexual partner. However, some of these problems (i.e., penile cancer, UTIs, foreskin problems, and HIV infection) are rare even in uncircumcised men.

In developed countries, where it is much less common for males to be circumcised, there is a low incidence of foreskin problems later in life. Behavioral factors also appear to be far more important than circumcision status in regard to the acquisition of STIs and HIV infection. Therefore the decision to circumcise is rarely based on scientific evidence. Rather, this decision is generally made based on cultural, familial, ethnic, or even regional preference.

There is controversy in the literature regarding the cost-effectiveness of newborn circumcision. Authors of a retrospective cost-benefit analysis of almost 15,000 newborn boys born in 1996 and insured by Kaiser Permanente Northern California (a large health maintenance organization) concluded that neonatal circumcision can be achieved at basically no cost. When total costs of newborn circumcision were weighed against total medical costs of not having it, the costs were basically equal. This was largely because postneonatal circumcision costs were about 10 times more than neonatal circumcision costs ($1921 per child vs. $165 per newborn), and circumcision was eventually medically indicated in 9.6% of uncircumcised boys. However, other cost-benefit analysis studies have reached opposite conclusions.

Clinicians performing circumcision are encouraged to remain current with guidelines and the scientific evidence. The American Academy of Pediatrics (AAP) circumcision position from March 1999, endorsed by the American College of Obstetricians and Gynecologists in 2001 and reaffirmed in 2005, found insufficient data to recommend routine newborn circumcision. Consequently there was an overall decrease in the rate of newborn circumcisions performed nationally. Since then, studies in Africa have found that performing adult male circumcision could lower the risk of HIV by half as well as lower the risk of human papillomavirus and herpes infections. These and other studies led the AAP Task Force to conclude that the health benefits of newborn male circumcision outweigh the risks, and thus access to the procedure is justified for all families who choose it. Benefits cited include the prevention of UTI, penile cancer, and transmission of some STIs, including HIV. The Task Force stopped short of recommending circumcision for *all* newborn males. In 2011, The American College of Obstetricians and Gynecologists endorsed these views.

Since these studies on the benefits of circumcision and new guidelines have become available, there has been controversy in the literature as to whether the percentage of male newborns undergoing circumcision is increasing. If that is the case, it may start becoming more of a norm. When the Centers for Disease Control last looked at the data, the trends and likelihood of having circumcision were found to be very regional. In 2010 in the northeastern United States, the circumcision rate had been somewhat flat for 32 years, basically unaffected by AAP guidelines. In the Midwest and South, the circumcision rates had fluctuated, increasing until the 1997 AAP guidelines and then decreasing; now they seem to be increasing again. In the West, rates decreased the most. However, in summary across the United States, the rate remained at about 58% through 2010; some experts are anticipating an increase with the change in the AAP guidelines.

Of note, a 2006 study found that 97% of pediatric, family medicine, and obstetrics and gynecology residency programs that teach circumcision also teach the administration of an anesthetic, either locally or topically. The AAP has recommended use of analgesia since 1997, and this has become the standard. Common methods of analgesia administration include subcutaneous ring block, dorsal penile nerve block (see Chapter 166, Dorsal Penile and Subcutaneous Ring Block for Newborn Circumcision), topical anesthesia such as lidocaine-prilocaine cream (also known as eutectic mixture of local anesthetic [EMLA]; see Chapter 4, Topical Anesthesia), and precircumcision oral analgesics. Although studies have shown lidocaine-prilocaine cream to be helpful, injected blocks appear to be more effective, and the ring block is more effective than a dorsal penile nerve block. Studies have shown that infants anesthetized with a block cry less, are less likely to have tachycardia, are less irritable, and have fewer behavior changes during the 24 hours after the procedure. They also have less variability in oxygen saturation and blood pressure during the procedure and lower serum cortisol levels after it.

Nonpharmacologic proven strategies to minimize pain include the addition of oral sucrose water and other stimulating sensations (e.g., gently looking at the infant, talking to him, stroking or massaging his face or back, or rocking him). Swaddling, positioning, and facilitated tucking—which means holding the infant's arms in a flexed position close to the chest with or without parental assistance—decrease stress. Obviously breastfeeding and skin-to-skin care (nude infant held against the mother's skin), although proven beneficial, would be more difficult to manage at the same time as an ongoing circumcision. That said, these may be useful for other painful procedures such as injections.

Three techniques of newborn circumcision are common in the United States: Mogen, Gomco, and Plastibell. Most clinicians continue to use the technique they were taught in their training. Both Gomco and Plastibell require a dorsal slit and considerable manipulation to prepare the foreskin for excision and result in the removal of a cylindrical sleeve of tissue. Both techniques carry the risk of removing too much tissue from the ventral side. In addition, Plastibell leaves behind a foreign body that may contribute to infection. One study comparing Gomco with Plastibell indicated that there was not only a higher rate of infection with Plastibell but also a slightly higher rate of bleeding.

Most clinicians who learn to use the Mogen clamp tend to prefer this technique because it is quicker and simpler, and it follows the angle of the corona so as to avoid removing excess tissue ventrally. At least two studies (Kurtis and colleagues, 1999; Kaufman and colleagues, 2002) comparing the use of the Mogen with the Gomco technique found that the Mogen procedure took about half the time and seemed to cause less discomfort (however, discomfort may be a moot point when anesthesia is used). Contrary to popular belief, the Mogen clamp is not a guillotine. It is simply a crushing device with a narrow slot that, when used appropriately, does not allow entry of the glans into the slot.

One apparent complication of circumcision is meatal stenosis (i.e., it is very rare in uncircumcised boys). Whether circumcision or a chronic inflammatory process—due to superabsorbent disposable diapers, ammonia dermatitis, or inadequate parental postprocedure care—is to blame is yet to be determined. In a prior edition of this text, a technique for newborn meatotomy was included; however, there are few data suggesting that such a procedure might decrease the later incidence of meatal stenosis. (And it must be very rare or it would be more common in uncircumcised men.) This scarcity of data exists partly because it is difficult to define meatal stenosis in a newborn. It is usually diagnosed later in life, at the time of toilet training or even later, because of its complications (e.g., painful urination that may require straining or standing, difficulty aiming the stream, blood spotting in the underwear). To make the diagnosis may require observed voiding (i.e., pinpoint meatus and a dorsally deflected, forceful urine stream of very fine caliber with a long voiding distance) because the appearance of the glans may be somewhat normal and therefore misleading. However, newborn meatotomy is included again in this edition because the risk of such a procedure is minimal compared with its potential benefits (e.g., repair in an older male patient can be somewhat psychologically traumatic). Also, in certain situations, newborn meatal stenosis is obvious; because the infant is already anesthetized for circumcision, it would seem prudent to repair it at that time.

After toilet training, a popular method of defining meatal stenosis is by the size of the feeding tube or pediatric urethral catheter that can be easily inserted. Because meatal stenosis is a possible complication of newborn circumcision, it seems appropriate to also include a technique for its later repair (i.e., office meatotomy) in this chapter. Although it might seem somewhat psychologically traumatic to repair meatal stenosis under mere topical anesthesia, boys having difficulty with urination may be strongly motivated to cooperate, especially if assured of the adequacy of topical anesthesia. Pediatric sedation may also be useful (see Chapter 2, Pediatric Sedation).

ANATOMY

The neonatal foreskin is composed of three layers: skin, loose subcutaneous tissue, and mucosa. At birth, the foreskin mucosa is adherent to the glans penis, with just a small distal opening to allow for urination. The ventral side of the mucosal surface has the highest density of nerve endings. A band of tissue called the *frenulum* attaches the foreskin along the ventral side of the penis and ends distally near the urethral meatus. The frenulum contains a small artery.

CIRCUMCISION

Indication
- Parental desire is the only necessary indication for circumcision.

Contraindications

Absolute
- Hypospadias, epispadias, or megaurethra (the foreskin is used for later repair)
- Unusual-appearing genitalia
- Inability to determine the sexual phenotype of the child (ambiguous genitalia)

Relative
- Age younger than 12 hours (physiologic adaptation requires 12 to 24 hours)
- Age greater than 6 to 8 weeks
- Severe illness
- Prematurity (until the child is ready for discharge from the hospital)

Precautions

If there is a family history of bleeding problems, appropriate laboratory studies should be performed before the procedure. If the mother is thrombocytopenic, the infant's platelet count should be checked.

By the age of 6 to 8 weeks, maternal clotting factors have been metabolized, possibly predisposing the infant to increased blood loss. The foreskin may also develop significant edema after the plane is defined and adhesions between the glans and the foreskin are broken up, making it difficult to use the Gomco clamp or Plastibell.

Preprocedure Patient and Parent Preparation

Discuss the risks and benefits of the procedure with the parents. Informed consent is obtained and a patient teaching guide is given to the parents. (See patient education and patient consent forms available at www.expertconsult.com.) The AAP also has online information (https://healthychildren.org/English/ages-stages/prenatal/decisions-to-make/Pages/Circumcision.aspx).

The parents are usually asked to leave the room during the procedure. If they want to stay, they should be given the option to look away while the procedure is being performed, because it can be disconcerting to some.

Because of the risks of regurgitation and aspiration, infants being circumcised should be at least 1 hour postprandial. Confirm that the infant has had at least one void since birth.

Equipment

Equipment Common to All Techniques
- Assistant for holding infant, infant restraint or papoose board (e.g., Circumstraint) with leg straps
- Anesthetic supplies: gloves, alcohol wipes, 1% plain lidocaine, 1-mL syringe, 30-gauge needle
- Sterile gloves and equipment necessary to follow universal blood and body fluid precautions
- Antiseptic solution (e.g., alcohol wipes, povidone-iodine, chlorhexidine) or swabsticks
- Sterile drape with 1-inch fenestration
- Sterile 2 × 2 or 4 × 4 gauze pads
- Three straight mosquito hemostats
- White petrolatum ointment (e.g., Vaseline)
- Disposable diaper
- Adequate light source
- Glucose water or sugar-coated pacifier (optional)
- Skin marking pen (optional)
- Flexible blunt probe *(optional)*
- Acetaminophen drops or solution (10 to 15 mg/kg) (optional)

Equipment for the Mogen Technique
- Mogen clamp, neonatal size (2.5-mm slot)

NOTE: The larger adult size is dangerous to use on a newborn because the glans can become trapped in the larger slot. The clinician should confirm that the neonatal size does not open more than 2.5 mm.

- No. 10 blade scalpel

Equipment for the Gomco Technique

- Straight scissors with one blunt tip
- Gomco circumcision clamps (1.1-, 1.3-, and 1.45-cm sizes)
  NOTE: The most commonly used size is 1.3 cm. The 1.1-cm size is used for a very small infant, whereas the 1.45-cm clamp usually fits a large infant. Larger sizes are available for children and adults.
- No. 10 blade scalpel
- Sterile safety pin (optional)

Equipment for the Plastibell Technique

- Straight scissors with one blunt tip
- Plastibell device (1.1-, 1.2-, 1.3-, and 1.4-cm sizes)
  NOTE: As with the Gomco technique, 1.3 cm is the most commonly used Plastibell size.
- Iris scissors

Equipment for Bleeding Complications in All Three Techniques

- Topical epinephrine
- Topical hemostatic agent of choice (e.g., Gelfoam, Surgicel, silver nitrate; see Chapter 199, Topical Hemostatic Agents)
- 5-0 absorbable suture (chromic or catgut) on a taper-point needle
- Needle holder and suture scissors

Mogen Technique

1. Consider using a skin marker to mark the coronal edge. Inspect the penis for abnormalities and for the location of the meatus on the glans. If epispadias or hypospadias is found, terminate the procedure, because the foreskin may be used for later repair by a urologist.
2. The clinician should follow universal blood and body fluid precautions. If penile anatomy is normal, anesthetize the penis with a subcutaneous ring block (see Chapter 166, Dorsal Penile and Subcutaneous Ring Block for Newborn Circumcision). Consider doing the block with the infant still in his crib to allow time for the block to take effect while the rest of the surgical preparations are made. Position the infant appropriately in a warm room. An infant may experience discomfort when his legs are extended on an infant restraint board. Therefore an assistant can hold the infant on a pillow with the knees flexed and legs abducted for adequate exposure. Most often, though, an infant restraining board is used. Leave the infant's arms free to minimize distress. Offer him a swallow or two of glucose water or a sugar-coated pacifier to calm him.
3. Using antiseptic solution or swabsticks, prepare the entire penis and a 1-inch area surrounding the penis. Wear sterile gloves when placing the fenestrated drape.
4. Grasp the very edge of the foreskin with hemostats at the 2 and 10 o'clock positions, taking care not to grasp the glans. (When describing the penis, use the dorsal midline as the 12 o'clock position. To identify the true dorsal midline, identify the ventral raphe at the frenulum, which is the 6 o'clock position, and consider the foreskin 180 degrees opposite it to be the 12 o'clock position [Fig. 167.1]. This orientation technique is important in case the penile shaft gets rotated.)
5. Place gentle traction on the foreskin by holding the two hemostats side by side in your nondominant hand. Gently insert the third hemostat with your dominant hand, closed and from be-

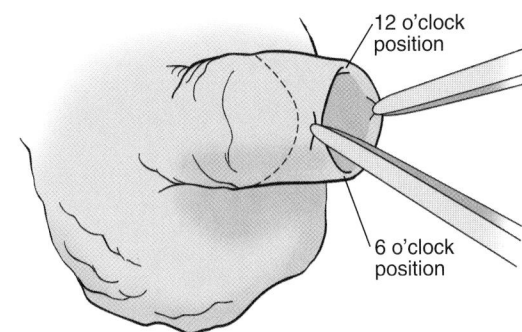

Fig. 167.1 Using 6 o'clock as the ventral position of the frenulum, 12 o'clock is the dorsal midline position.

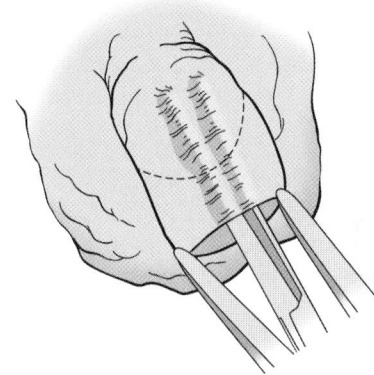

Fig. 167.2 Insert the third hemostat between the foreskin and the glans, tenting the foreskin as it is advanced. Here the surgeon is just beginning to open the hemostat to free the foreskin from the glans.

low the grasping hemostats, at the 12 o'clock position between the foreskin and the glans. Advance to the depth of the coronal sulcus (Fig. 167.2). To ensure that the meatus is not entered, keep the foreskin tented up as this hemostat is advanced. Open this hemostat and sweep it clockwise and counterclockwise to free the foreskin off the glans. This may take a number of open-close cycles starting at different places around the corona. Do not free the area from the 5 to 7 o'clock positions (the frenulum) because it contains an artery. Do not dissect beyond the depth of the coronal sulcus. As an alternative to opening and closing a hemostat, a blunt probe may be used to free the foreskin off of the glans.

6. Tent the foreskin away from the glans by gently lifting the grasping hemostats. Ensure that no part of the glans is in the way. Advance the lower blade of the third hemostat between the glans and foreskin at the 12 o'clock position to a position no less than 5 mm distal to the coronal sulcus (Fig. 167.3). Do not apply traction to the grasping hemostats as this dorsal hemostat is applied or you will remove too much foreskin. Close and lock the hemostat in place.
7. Remove the two foreskin edge-grasping hemostats.
8. Using the thumb and index finger of your nondominant hand, pinch the free foreskin underneath the dorsal hemostat while curling your other fingers of the same hand around the handles of the hemostat. This pushes the glans back out of the way of the Mogen clamp. Release any traction on the hemostat and foreskin because traction on the frenulum can dorsally rotate the glans and bring the meatus into the path of the Mogen clamp. Maintain the pinch while the Mogen clamp is placed. The tips of the pinching fingers should be slightly proximal to the tip of the grasping hemostat.

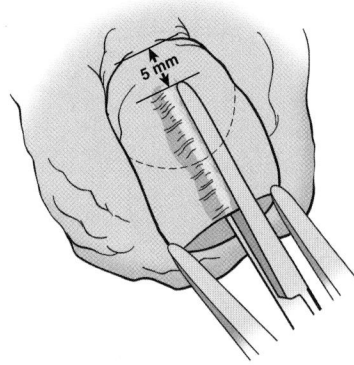

Fig. 167.3   Place a dorsal hemostat with its tip 5 mm from the corona.

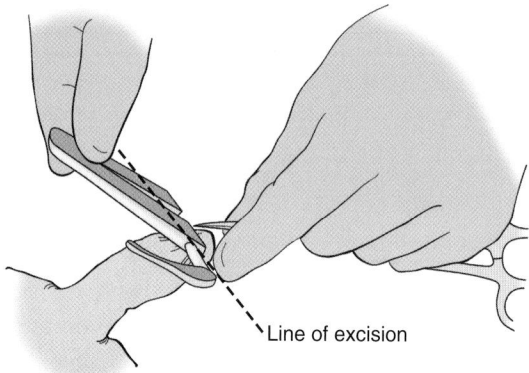

Fig. 167.4   Pinch the foreskin to push the glans back while advancing the Mogen clamp vertically along the angle of the corona.

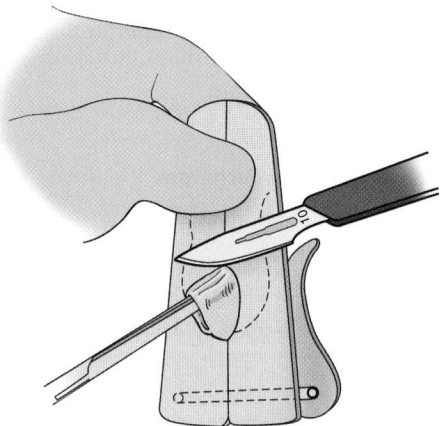

Fig. 167.5   Excise the foreskin.

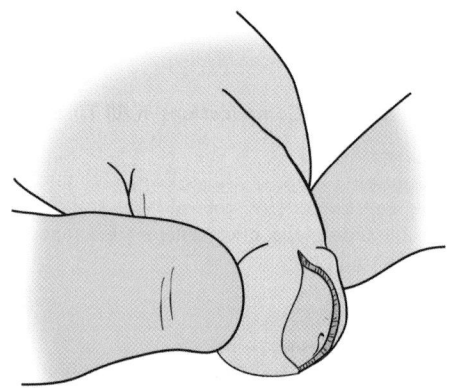

Fig. 167.6   Liberate the glans with thumb pressure.

9. Inspect the Mogen clamp to be sure that its joint is not loose and that it opens only 2.5 mm, then open it fully. Hold it so that the open end of the slot is down and the flat surface faces you. With your dominant hand, advance the Mogen slot across the foreskin, starting immediately behind the tip of the dorsal hemostat (Fig. 167.4). Angle the Mogen's advancement to remove more foreskin dorsally than ventrally, following along the angle of the corona (dorsum of the glans). Slide the clamp across the foreskin as far as it will easily go. At this point, the use of previous skin markings can ensure that an adequate but not excessive amount of foreskin is removed.

10. Before locking the Mogen clamp, drop the foreskin pinch and attempt to move the glans beneath the slot. You should be able to move the glans freely for a few millimeters up and down and side to side. If the glans is not free, do not lock the Mogen clamp.

11. Lock the Mogen clamp by moving the bar across the slot and closing the cam lever fully.

12. Use the scalpel to cut the foreskin off flush with the flat surface of the Mogen clamp (Fig. 167.5). Discard the foreskin in a biohazard waste container.

13. Unlock and remove the Mogen clamp. There is no medical rationale for leaving the clamp on for any specific length of time.

14. Gently separate the crushed edges of the foreskin to liberate the glans. Grasp the penile shaft skin at the 3 and 9 o'clock positions to pull the crush line apart (Fig. 167.6). Be sure to separate the edges fully to avoid the possibility of causing a paraphimosis. It is not unusual to have a few remaining attachments between the glans and the mucosal surface of the remaining foreskin next to the corona. The easiest way to divide these is to use the tip of a closed and locked hemostat to follow the coronal sulcus, but

a blunt probe can also be used. Do not be too vigorous or try to free the frenular area, because this will cause bleeding.

15. Check for hemostasis. To control any bleeding, apply pressure or topical epinephrine to the specific source. In rare cases of persistent bleeding, topical hemostatic agents can be applied with pressure to hasten clotting. Rarely will bleeding require suturing. In the event that it does, use an absorbable suture at the site of the bleeding, which is usually an arteriole. Persistent bleeding after circumcision is a common presenting sign for a factor-deficient bleeding disorder, such as hemophilia. If bleeding persists after following these described measures, obtain clotting studies and consider a hematology consultation.

16. Cover the glans with white petrolatum ointment and reapply the diaper.

17. Administer an oral dose of acetaminophen (10 to 15 mg/kg) (optional).

18. Document the procedure and time in the chart. To ensure continued hemostasis, do not discharge the infant for about an hour after the procedure. The infant should also have urinated before discharge.

Gomco Technique

1. Choose an appropriate-size Gomco clamp, which is 1.3 cm for most newborns. (The bell diameter should be slightly larger than the diameter of the glans; although the bell should cover the glans completely, it should just barely cover it.) Carefully inspect the clamp. If the clamp was packaged disassembled, reassemble it in the sterile field. Because there is more than one manufacturer for Gomco clamps, make sure the reassembled clamp parts fit together properly. (Disassembled parts may be

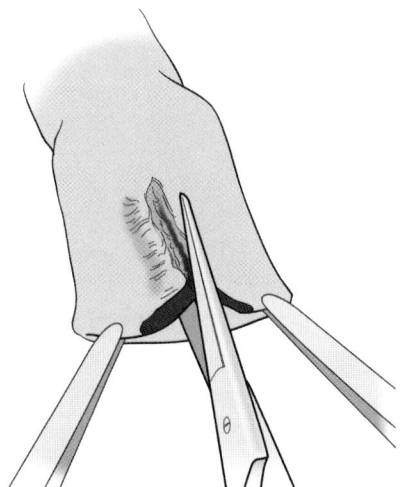

Fig. 167.7   Incise the dorsal slit.

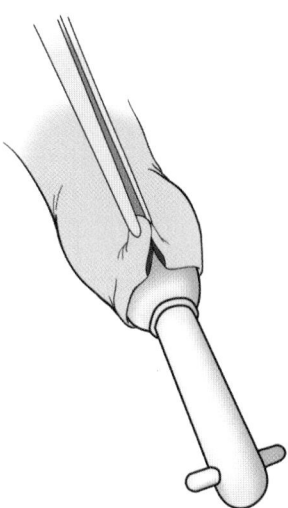

Fig. 167.8   Reapproximate the dorsal slit around the Gomco bell.

from different manufacturers.) Make sure the bell is the correct size for the clamp and that there are no defects. Lightly tighten the clamp with the bell in place. Make sure that no light can be seen around the bell where it meets the clamp at the baseplate. This ensures a complete circumferential crush for optimal hemostasis. Next, verify that the top surface of the baseplate is flat (it can become warped over time). Last, there should be at least 2 mm between the back of the lever arm and the baseplate beneath the nut before tightening. This also ensures adequate clamping.

NOTE: In 2000, the US Food and Drug Administration issued a warning because there had been some complications with newborn circumcisions in hospitals when clamps were either reassembled incorrectly or parts had been damaged from overuse. Since disassembled parts may be from different manufacturers, the clinician must verify that they all fit together correctly. Following the steps noted earlier should minimize the risk of complications from defective or mismatched clamps.

2. As in steps 1 through 5 of the Mogen technique, inspect the penis for abnormalities, consider marking the coronal edge if not already done, administer a penile subcutaneous ring block, position the infant (restrain if necessary), apply antiseptic and drapes, and free the foreskin from the glans.

3. As in step 6 of the Mogen technique, place a crushing dorsal hemostat at the 12 o'clock position but apply it only to the distal third or half of the length of the foreskin (the total length of the foreskin extends from the foreskin edge to the coronal sulcus). This hemostat is not applied more proximally than 1 cm from the coronal sulcus. Make sure that the crushing hemostat contains both the mucosal and skin layers of the foreskin.

4. The hemostat can be removed immediately after crushing. Removal reveals a crushed straight line down the dorsal aspect of the foreskin; this crushed tissue has been devitalized and therefore will not bleed when cut. Insert the blunt blade of the scissors between the foreskin and the glans, underneath the crush line, and tent the foreskin with the two edge hemostats and this blade of the scissors. The crushed dorsal line should be thin enough to let you somewhat visualize the blunt blade through it when it is tented up. With the scissors placed in this manner, cut a dorsal slit down the center of the crush line (Fig. 167.7). Be careful to cut only in the crush line; do not extend laterally or past the apex of the crush line. Venturing beyond or outside the crush line will often result in unnecessary bleeding.

5. Separate the cut edges of the foreskin; this should then allow you to retract the foreskin back from around the glans. If, at this point, you cannot fully retract the foreskin and it is due to an

inadequate incision (and not to adhesions), recrush a bit further dorsally on the foreskin and extend the dorsal slit. Lyse any remaining adhesions between the foreskin and glans with the closed tips of a locked hemostat or the blunt probe. You should be able to fully reveal the sulcus behind the corona. Be very careful when dissecting between the 5 and 7 o'clock positions to avoid the frenulum and its artery.

NOTE: If you notice hypospadias or epispadias after the dorsal slit has been made, terminate the procedure. After termination, if there is bleeding from the dorsal slit, whipstitch the edges or close the dorsal slit using fine chromic suture. Repair of penile congenital anomalies by a urologist may require foreskin tissue; do not remove any of it if possible.

6. Place the bell of an appropriate-size Gomco clamp over the exposed glans. (If the bell and Gomco are not in the same package, another package may have to be opened by an assistant and handed to you in a sterile manner.)

7. Use the two still attached edge hemostats to reapproximate the foreskin around the outside of the bell while applying gentle downward pressure on the bell's stem. Make sure that both mucosal and skin layers of the foreskin are reapproximated. The bell should occupy the space between the glans and the foreskin and sit against the coronal edge.

8. Once the Gomco bell has been appropriately placed, grasp both sides of the dorsal slit near the middle of the incision with the tips of a third hemostat. This reapproximates the foreskin around the stem (Fig. 167.8) of the bell. The approach with the hemostat is from above at a low angle, with handles up near the infant's umbilicus. This will ease the next step. (Some clinicians use a safety pin to hold the dorsal slit edges together in this step, but this increases the risk of a puncture injury to the clinician.)

9. Remove the two hemostats at the foreskin edge.

10. Place the end of the stem through the hole in the Gomco baseplate as far as it will go without dislodging the foreskin.

11. Reaching through the baseplate hole with a hemostat, grasp across the foreskin's dorsal slit just above the tips of the lower hemostat (Fig. 167.9). Remove the lower hemostat. Pull the stem and surrounding foreskin fully up through the baseplate hole. (If using a safety pin, pull the entire pin along with the bell through the baseplate hole. The safety pin will need to be turned parallel to the stem of the bell to pull it through the hole. The safety pin can then remain in place throughout the remainder of the procedure to avoid exposing its sharp tip.)

12. Assemble the Gomco clamp by grasping the wings of the bell's stem in the rocker arm's end, placing the rocker arm in its fulcrum slot and loosely placing the nut on its screw.

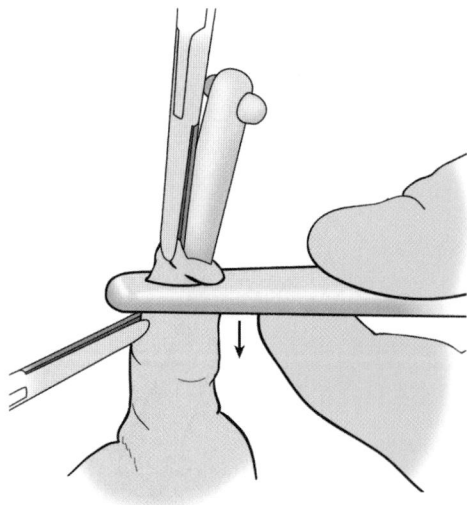

Fig. 167.9 Bring the bell's stem and foreskin through the ring by exchanging hemostats.

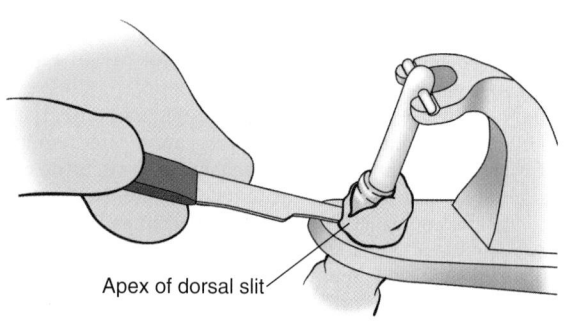

Apex of dorsal slit

Fig. 167.10 Excise the foreskin. The apex of the dorsal slit should be visible above the baseplate.

13. Make sure that the foreskin has been drawn through the hole in the Gomco clamp evenly from all sides. The apex of the dorsal slit must be above the baseplate. Using a hemostat or forceps, pull on the mucosal edge of the dorsal slit to be sure that the mucosal apex of the dorsal slit is also above the baseplate. Prior marking of the coronal edge position on the foreskin with a skin marker can be helpful at this point. When you are sure that the foreskin is evenly pulled through the Gomco clamp and the apex of the dorsal slit is visible above the baseplate, firmly tighten the clamp.
14. On the top side of the baseplate, the same side as the fulcrum, bell stem, and rocker arm, the scalpel can be used to immediately excise the foreskin. It should be excised circumferentially and completely on the top side at the junction of the baseplate and the bell (Fig. 167.10). Make sure that all skin and mucosal layers are removed. Any remaining tissue above the clamp will become necrotic and a possible source of infection. The excised ring of foreskin should be removed from the bell (it may be slid over the stem or cut away from the stem with scissors) and discarded in a biohazard waste container. Alternatively, the excised foreskin may be left on the stem until the device has been disassembled.
15. Loosen and disassemble the Gomco clamp. There is no medical rationale for leaving the clamp on for any specific length of time.

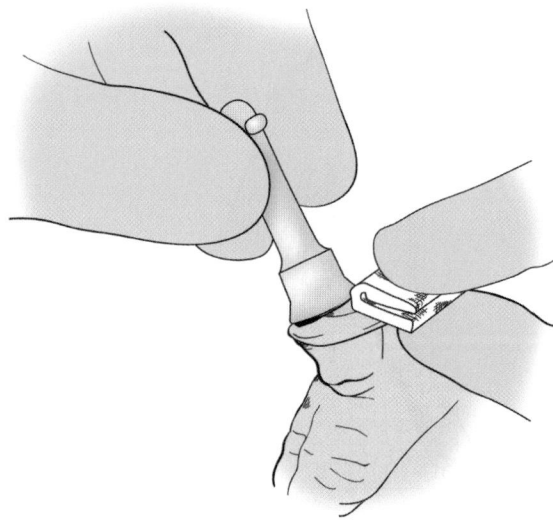

Fig. 167.11 Tease the adherent tissue off the bell edge with gauze.

16. To remove the adherent foreskin edge from the bell, gently tease it away using a piece of gauze (Fig. 167.11).
17. Follow steps 15 through 18 of the Mogen technique to check hemostasis, dress the wound, and document the procedure.

NOTE: A rare complication of using a Gomco clamp that is too large or from pulling too much foreskin through the baseplate hole is degloving of the penile shaft's skin. In this situation, after the clamp and bell have been removed, the shaft's skin will retract too far and expose the underlying tissue proximal to the coronal sulcus. Attempts to control bleeding in the usual manner often fail. If bleeding is not controlled, a primary closure with four absorbable (5-0 chromic) sutures should be made. Sutures are placed circumferentially to reposition the retracted shaft skin to a point just proximal to the corona. Care must be taken in the ventral area to avoid the urethra. Some clinicians catheterize the infant with a 5-Fr feeding tube before performing the repair. Otherwise no special aftercare is needed. If bleeding is controlled, degloving does not have to be repaired.

Plastibell Technique

1. Choose an appropriate-size Plastibell, which is 1.3 cm for most normal newborns. (The Plastibell should fit like an appropriate-size Gomco bell.) Drop the device into the sterile field.
2. As in steps 1 through 5 of the Mogen technique, inspect the penis for abnormalities, consider marking the foreskin at the coronal edge, administer a penile subcutaneous ring block, position the infant (restrain if necessary), apply antiseptic, drape, and free the foreskin from the glans.
3. As in steps 3 through 5 of the Gomco technique, place a dorsal crushing clamp and remove it, cut a dorsal slit, and retract and fully free the foreskin. Leave the two foreskin edge hemostats in place.
4. Place the Plastibell string loosely around the base of the penis and put two twists in the string to start a surgeon's knot.
5. Place the Plastibell over the glans (Fig. 167.12) with its "wishbone" vertical (along the 12 to 6 o'clock axis). The edge of the Plastibell should just touch the coronal edge. Exchange the Plastibell for one of an appropriate size if this is not the case. It is particularly dangerous to use too large a Plastibell because the glans can push through its center and cause a paraphimosis, with resultant necrosis of the glans. If the size is correct, pull the foreskin over the device by manipulating the two grasping hemostats.

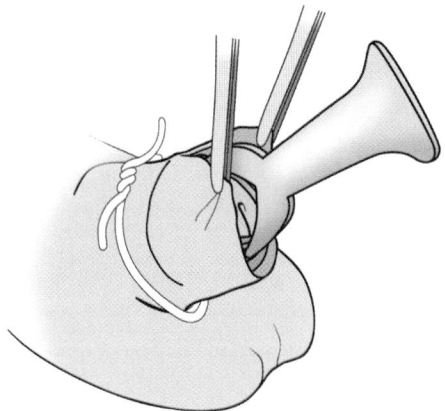

Fig. 167.12 Place the Plastibell on the glans and check for proper size.

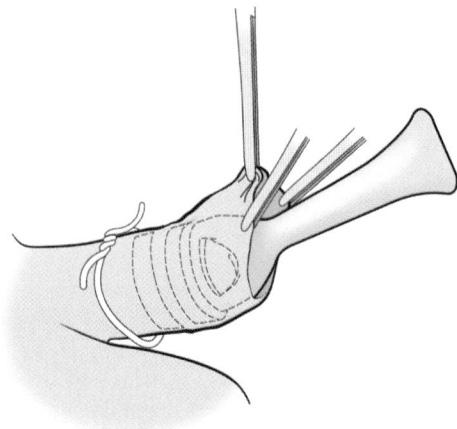

Fig. 167.13 Reapproximate the foreskin around the Plastibell and hold it in place with a hemostat.

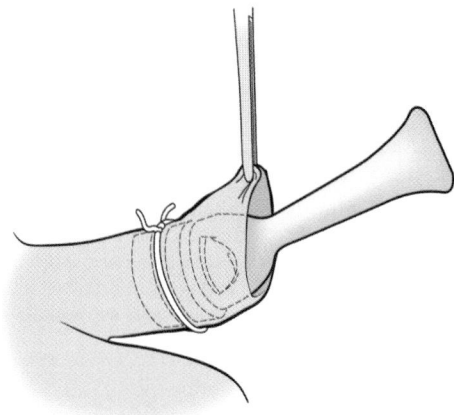

Fig. 167.14 String in the groove of the Plastibell with knot trimmed.

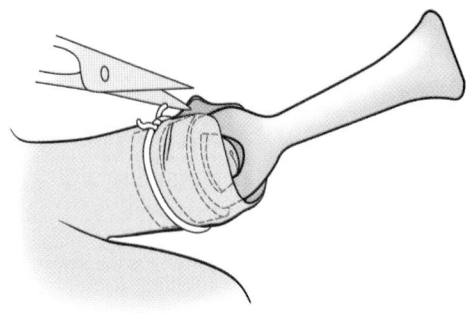

Fig. 167.15 Trim the excess foreskin with iris scissors.

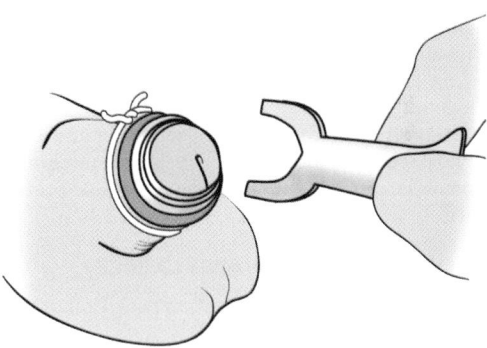

Fig. 167.16 Snap the Plastibell at the junction of the ring and the wishbone.

6. Once the Plastibell has been appropriately placed, use a third hemostat to grasp both sides of the dorsal slit with the hemostat tips at about the middle of the incision. This will reapproximate the foreskin around the device and hold it in place (Fig. 167.13).
7. Ensure that the string groove of the Plastibell is below the apex of the dorsal slit and at the appropriate place on the foreskin. Adjust the grasping hemostat if necessary. When you are certain of Plastibell placement, remove the two foreskin edge hemostats.
8. Place the string over the groove in the Plastibell and tighten the string just until it remains in place.
9. Check the placement of the string and bell again, making sure that the apex of the foreskin incision is distal to the string. Be sure that you are not removing too much foreskin and that the Plastibell can move freely on the glans.
10. Tighten the string as much as possible and hold at this tension for a few seconds. Complete the surgeon's knot in the string and trim the excess string to 0.25-inch in length (Fig. 167.14).
11. Remove the hemostat that has been approximating the dorsal slit.
12. Using iris scissors, cut the foreskin away to within 3 mm of the string. Be careful not to cut the string (Fig. 167.15). Discard the foreskin in a biohazard waste container.
13. Holding the body of the Plastibell between the index finger and thumb of one hand, bend the wishbone with the other hand until it snaps at its junction with the bell (Fig. 167.16).
14. Verify again that the Plastibell can move up and down on the glans and that the meatus is not occluded.

15. As in steps 15 through 18 of the Mogen technique, check for bleeding, cover with white petrolatum, reapply the diaper, and record the procedure in the chart.

Postprocedure Management and Parent Education

All Techniques

Parents should report any bleeding or signs of infection. It is normal to have a red, angry-looking glans, often with a yellowish crust; this may last for a week. Acetaminophen (10 to 15 mg/kg q6-8h) is given for any apparent pain or irritability. Rarely is any analgesic needed beyond 24 hours. The patient education handout includes postprocedure instructions for parents. (See the sample handout titled "Newborn Circumcision" available at www.expert consult.com.)

After a Mogen or Gomco procedure, parents are told to retract the penile shaft skin back from the corona and apply white petrolatum to the area at each diaper change. After the Plastibell falls off, this same procedure is followed. This should continue for a week to prevent adhesions from forming. To prevent the glans from sticking to the diaper, parents should apply a smear of white petrolatum to the front of the diaper for the first week. They can wash the penis with soap and water the day after surgery.

Parents are instructed to watch for meatal stenosis. Meatal stenosis appears as a pinhole urethra causing a narrow or angulated urinary stream. This can be associated with enuresis or incontinence. Meatotomy is a simple office procedure and will usually correct the problem.

Plastibell Technique

In addition to following all of the same basic instructions for patients who undergo circumcision using the Mogen or Gomco clamp, parents need to know what to expect with a Plastibell. They should know that the foreskin remaining beyond the string will turn black and necrotic and fall off along with the Plastibell within 1 week. Each Plastibell device comes with a postoperative education card that is given to the parents.

Complications

- Bleeding.
- Infection (most common with Plastibell because of the retained tissue and the presence of a foreign body).
- Trauma to the glans or urethra.
- Poor cosmetic result due to remaining adherence of mucosa to glans, removal of too much or too little foreskin, or uneven removal of foreskin. Most cosmetic problems resolve as the infant grows and the wound heals. Secondary intervention is very rarely necessary.
- Paraphimosis from inadequate opening of the Mogen crush line after the procedure has been completed or from the use of Plastibell that is too large. A Plastibell may be removed with orthopedic bone-cutting forceps.
- Degloving of penile shaft skin (Gomco only; see the Gomco technique section).
- Meatal stenosis: is a rare but possible late complication.
- Methemoglobinemia with use of EMLA (very rare). Prompt recognition and treatment with methylene blue and other methods is critical.

MEATOTOMY (NEWBORN AND OFFICE)

Indications

- Newborn (following circumcision): width of meatus less than 2 mm or less than 25% to 30% of diameter of glans
- Male infant younger than 1 year: symptoms of meatal stenosis and unable to easily insert 5-Fr feeding tube
- Male child older than 1 year and younger than 6 years: symptoms of meatal stenosis and unable to easily insert 8-Fr feeding tube

Contraindications

- The contraindications are the same as for circumcision except that the child can be older than a newborn

Preprocedure Patient Preparation

If there is a possibility that newborn meatotomy may be performed, the procedure, its alternatives, and its risks and benefits should be explained. Meatotomy is often added to the informed consent for circumcision. If office meatotomy is to be performed in an older male child, similar explanations should be made and informed consent obtained.

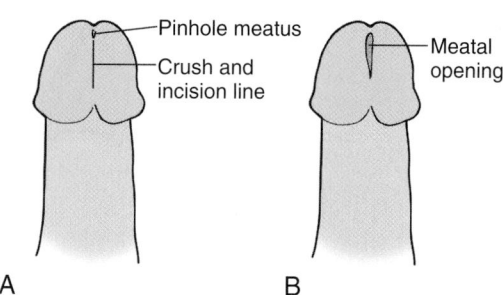

Fig. 167.17 (A) Meatal stenosis and location of crush line. (B) Meatus after meatotomy.

Equipment

- Antiseptic solution (e.g., povidone-iodine, chlorhexidine)
- Antibiotic ointment
- Fenestrated drape
- Straight mosquito hemostat
- Straight iris scissors
- Lidocaine-prilocaine cream or gauze soaked with 2% lidocaine (office meatotomy)
- 30-gauge needle with 1-mL syringe and 1% lidocaine without epinephrine (office meatotomy, alternative for anesthesia)

Technique

1. Anesthesia is usually already adequate for a newborn having just undergone circumcision. For office meatotomy, lidocaine-prilocaine cream should be smeared liberally over the entire glans, especially the ventral portion and the meatal opening. It should be secured in place with occlusive dressing and left for at least an hour of contact time before the procedure. Alternatively, a small amount of lidocaine can be injected directly into the meatal skin. For very anxious children (for 2 of 58 children in one study, ages 30 months to 10 years, a preoperative anxiolytic was used), it may be useful to use pediatric sedation (see Chapter 2, Pediatric Sedation).
2. Apply antiseptic solution to the penis and place a fenestrated drape.
3. Place one tip of the straight mosquito hemostat, lubricated with antiseptic solution, inside the meatus at the 6 o'clock position. The tip should be several millimeters inside the meatus, the distance being judged by the severity of stenosis and patient age. In the newborn, the other tip should be no farther than the frenulum.
4. Close the hemostat to obtain a crush line of hemostasis on the inferior side of the meatus. Frequently the majority of the crush line will be located on the thin, sometimes translucent inflammatory membrane that has caused the meatal obstruction.
5. Using the fine iris scissors, cut through the center of the crush line (Fig. 167.17). Be careful to cut only in the crush line; if you extend laterally or past the crush line, bleeding may occur.
6. A closed hemostat can then be inserted into the urethra to gently and blindly palpate for distal urethral webs. If webs are noted, urologic referral is indicated.
7. A small amount of antibiotic ointment is then placed on the incision.

Postprocedure Management and Parent Education

The meatotomy site should be shown to parents, and they can then be given instructions for care. Parents are instructed to insert a small dilator into the meatus daily for 2 weeks to prevent recurrence of the stenosis. Either a small eyedropper or the tip of a tube of ophthalmic antibiotic ointment may be used as the dilator. White petrolatum ointment can be used as a lubricant.

SAMPLE OPERATIVE REPORT

After most neonatal circumcisions (or meatotomies) in the United States, only a cursory operative note is made in the chart—for example, "1% lido ring block, Mogen circ without complication, infant tolerated well, parents given instructions for care." This chart is signed by the clinician, and the date and time are noted.

PATIENT EDUCATION GUIDES

See patient education form available at www.expertconsult.com.

CPT/BILLING CODES

53025	Meatotomy, infant
54150	Circumcision, using clamp or other device with regional dorsal penile or ring block
54150-52	Circumcision, using clamp or other device without regional dorsal penile or ring block, regardless of age (reduced services)
54160	Circumcision, surgical excision other than clamp, device, or dorsal slit; neonate (28 days of age or less)
54161	Circumcision, surgical excision other than clamp, device, or dorsal slit (older than 28 days of age)
64450-47	Nerve block, diagnostic or therapeutic, other peripheral nerve, (Modifier 47 is used when anesthesia provided by surgeon. A few insurers will pay for this as a separate procedure from the circumcision.)

ICD-10-CM DIAGNOSTIC CODES

Z41.2	Circumcision, routine or ritual (in the absence of significant medical indication)
N36.8	Urethral obstruction, unspecified

Acknowledgment

The editors recognize the contributions of S. Shevaun Duiker, MD, and Ron Reynolds, MD, to this chapter in previous editions of this text.

SUPPLIERS

(See contact information available at www.expertconsult.com.)

Brochures
American Academy of Pediatrics
Circumstraint
Natus Medical Incorporated
Gomco circumcision clamps (1.1-, 1.3-, and 1.45-cm sizes)
Allied Healthcare Products, Inc. (Gomco Division), Zinnanti Surgical
Mogen clamp
Mogen Instrument Co.
Plastibell device (1.1-, 1.2-, 1.3-, 1.4-, 1.5-, and 1.7-cm sizes)
Briggs Mabis Plastibell

RECOMMENDED READING

Cartwright PC, Snow BW, McNees DC. Urethral meatotomy in the office using topical EMLA cream for anesthesia. *J Urol.* 1996;156:857–858; discussion 858–859.

Castellsagué X, Bosch FX, Muñoz N, et al. Male circumcision, penile human papillomavirus infection, and cervical cancer in female partners. *N Engl J Med.* 2002;346:1105–1112.

Centers for Disease Control and Prevention. Trends in in-hospital newborn male circumcision—United States, 1999-2010. *MMWR.* 2011;60(34):1167.

Haouari N, Wood C, Griffiths G, Levene M. The analgesic effect of sucrose in full term infants: a randomized controlled trial. *BMJ.* 1995;310:1498–1500.

Kaufman GE, Cimo S, Miller LW, Blass EM. An evaluation of the effects of sucrose on neonatal pain with 2 commonly used circumcision methods. *Am J Obstet Gynecol.* 2002;186:564–568.

Kunz HV. Circumcision and meatotomy. *Prim Care.* 1986;13:513–525.

Kurtis PS, DeSilva HN, Bernstein BA, et al. A comparison of the Mogen and Gomco clamps in combination with dorsal penile nerve block in minimizing the pain of neonatal circumcision. *Pediatrics.* 1999;103:E23.

Peleg D, Steiner A. The Gomco circumcision: common problems and solutions. *Am Fam Physician.* 1998;58:891–898.

Reynolds RD. Use of the Mogen clamp for neonatal circumcision. *Am Fam Physician.* 1996;54:177–182.

Schoen EJ. The increasing incidence of newborn circumcision: data from the nationwide inpatient sample. *J Urol.* 2006;175:394–395.

Schoen EJ, Colby CJ, To TT. Cost analysis of neonatal circumcision in a large health maintenance organization. *J Urol.* 175:1111–1115,

Spach DH, Stapleton AE, Stamm WE. Lack of circumcision increases the risk of urinary tract infection in young men. *JAMA.* 1992;267:679–681.

The Newborn Circumcision. In: Cunningham F, Leveno KJ, Bloom SL, et al. *Williams Obstetrics.* 24th ed. New York: McGraw-Hill; 2013.

CHAPTER 168

PEDIATRIC SUPRAPUBIC BLADDER ASPIRATION

Carlos A. Moreno

Suprapubic bladder aspiration is a method of obtaining a sterile urine specimen from a young infant when other methods are unsatisfactory. This procedure is most successful in an infant younger than 2 years because at that age the bladder is an abdominal organ. After 2 years, as the child grows, the bladder moves into the pelvis, increasing both the difficulty of the procedure and the risk of complications. In children older than 2 years, ultrasound is recommended to determine the proper needle insertion site and direction. (See Chapter 214, Emergency Department, Hospitalist and Office Ultrasonography [Clinical Ultrasonography], for a method of confirming a full bladder and determining where to direct the needle.) For older children, see the note at end of Procedures section.

INDICATIONS

- To obtain sterile urine for culture in an infant or child younger than 2 years (e.g., suspected urinary tract infection [UTI] or sepsis). For older children, see the note at end of Procedures section later.
- To decompress the urinary bladder when there is urethral obstruction (after decompression, a referral should be made to pediatric urology)

CONTRAINDICATIONS

Absolute
There are no absolute contraindications.

NOTE: Some experts consider "blind" aspiration to be an absolute contraindication. They suggest that the bladder location should be confirmed by palpation, percussion, or transillumination or visualized with ultrasound.

Relative
- Bleeding abnormality or coagulopathy
- Infection or loss of integrity of skin or fascia at the site of needle insertion (e.g., burn, cellulitis)
- Genitourinary tract anomalies
- Bowel distention (e.g., ileus, obstruction)
- Scars from previous lower abdominal surgery that might cause adhesions

NOTE: With ultrasound-directed aspiration, the last three contraindications may be overcome (see Chapter 214, Emergency Department, Hospitalist and Office Ultrasonography [Clinical Ultrasonography]).

EQUIPMENT AND SUPPLIES

- Povidone-iodine or chlorhexidine solution
- 70% isopropyl alcohol
- Sterile 4 × 4 gauze pads
- Sterile gloves
- 3-mL sterile syringe with 1- or 1.25-inch 22- or 23-gauge needle
- Sterile urine specimen container
- Adhesive bandage
- 1% lidocaine in a tuberculin syringe with 0.5-inch 27-gauge needle (optional)
- High-frequency ultrasound (5- to 10-MHz) probe and acoustic gel (optional)

PREPROCEDURE PATIENT PREPARATION

The parent(s) should be informed of the indication(s) for suprapubic aspiration as well as alternatives and possible complications. In nonemergent situations, informed consent should be obtained. The parent(s) should be given the option to leave the room or to look away as the procedure is being performed because it can be disconcerting to some.

PROCEDURE

1. Before bladder aspiration, the infant's diaper should be dry and urination should not have occurred within the previous hour. Often the full bladder can be palpated, percussed, or transilluminated to ensure a full bladder. An alternative is to perform a quick ultrasound evaluation to confirm a full bladder.
2. Hold the infant in the supine frog-leg position. Observe universal blood and body fluid precautions.
3. Urination can be prevented by gently pinching the penis in a male or applying manual pressure in the area of the anterior rectum or urethral meatus in a female infant.
4. Cleanse the lower abdomen with povidone-iodine or chlorhexidine solution and then remove the solution with 70% isopropyl alcohol.

   NOTE: At this point, some clinicians inject a small amount (<1 mL) of a local anesthetic, such as 1% lidocaine, to raise a subcutaneous wheal in the area of the intended puncture site. However, this is considered optional by many clinicians because the discomfort caused by the lidocaine is similar to that caused by the puncture for bladder aspiration.

5. With the needle attached to a 3-mL sterile syringe, direct the needle into the midline of the abdomen at a point 1 to 2 cm above the symphysis pubis (there is usually a transverse suprapubic crease at this location). Hold the needle perpendicular to the abdominal wall or direct it slightly cephalad (Fig. 168.1).
6. Aspirate gently with the syringe while advancing the needle. To avoid puncturing the posterior bladder wall or retroperitoneal structures, do not advance the needle after urine begins to enter

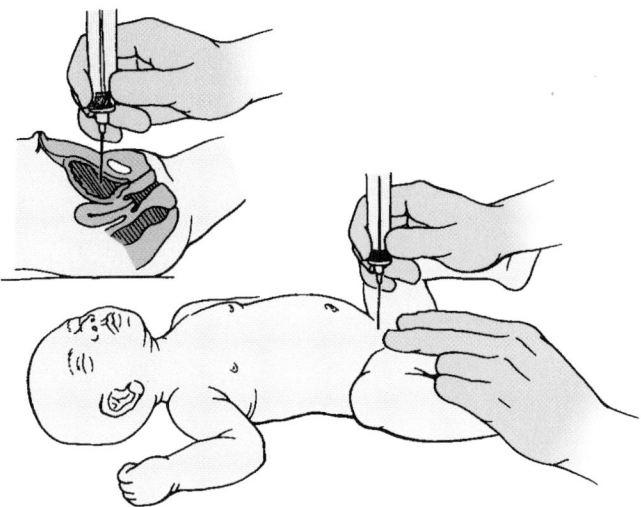

Fig. 168.1   Proper technique for suprapubic bladder aspiration.

the syringe. If the bladder is full, urine is usually obtained before the needle is inserted to its full depth.

7. If no urine is obtained, withdraw the needle without removing it from the skin and attempt bladder puncture again, angling 20 degrees more cephalad. If three attempts are unsuccessful, the bladder is considered empty. The procedure can be repeated in an hour if the patient is stable. Some urine should have accumulated over this time.

NOTE: An alternative is to catheterize the infant, especially if he or she is too unstable to wait an hour. If ultrasound is available, it can be helpful to confirm the presence of urine before subjecting the infant to catheterization and risk of iatrogenic UTI.

8. After withdrawing the needle, immediately apply pressure to the puncture site until it can be covered with a sterile gauze dressing. Next, apply mild pressure to the dressing for a minute. After a minute, if there is adequate hemostasis and no urine draining from the puncture site, pressure can be discontinued and the bandage applied.

9. Transfer the aspirated urine to a sterile container and transport to the laboratory for analysis, culture, and sensitivity.

NOTE: For older children, the positioning of the patient should be the same. The use of ultrasound is recommended to determine the proper needle location site and the angle of direction. The bladder of the older child may be in the abdomen or may have migrated to the pelvis.

COMPLICATIONS

- Microscopic hematuria (typically transient, resolving without specific treatment)
- Iatrogenic UTI (risk is minimized by the use of sterile technique)

- Perforation of the bowel (rare and may be managed by close observation and, if necessary, antibiotic administration. Simple penetration of the bowel with a needle is considered an innocuous event and requires no specific treatment)
- Retroperitoneal hematoma or damage to retroperitoneal structures (very rare)
- Infection of the abdominal wall
- Bacteremia (very rare)

POSTPROCEDURE PATIENT EDUCATION

The parent(s) should be given instructions to keep the site clean and to seek medical care for fever, nausea, vomiting, or infection at the puncture site.

CPT/BILLING CODES

51100-51102	Aspiration of bladder by needle
76942	Ultrasonic guidance for needle placement, imaging supervision, and interpretation

ICD-10-CM DIAGNOSTIC CODES

N30.00	Acute cystitis without hematuria
N30.01	Acute cystitis with hematuria
P36.8	Other bacterial sepsis of the newborn

Use additional code from B96 to identify organism

P39.3	Neonatal urinary tract infection
P36.9	Bacterial sepsis of newborn unspecified
R33.9	Urinary retention, unspecified
R39.14	Feeling of incomplete bladder emptying

Acknowledgment

The editors recognize the contributions of Marvin A. Dewar, MD, JD, to this chapter in a previous edition of this text.

RECOMMENDED READING

Davis JE, Silverman MA. Urologic procedures. In: Roberts JR, Custalow CB, Thomsen TW, eds. *Roberts and Hedges Clinical Procedures in Emergency Medicine.* 6th ed. Philadelphia: Elsevier; 2014:1142–1143.

Hoekelman RA, ed. *Primary Pediatric Care.* 4th ed. St. Louis: Mosby; 2001.

James DM. Suprapubic bladder aspiration and placement of a suprapubic catheter. In: James DM, ed. *Field Guide to Urgent and Ambulatory Care Procedures.* Philadelphia: Lippincott Williams & Wilkins; 2001:189–193.

Robertson J, Shilkofski N, eds. *The Harriet Lane Handbook.* 20th ed. St. Louis: Elsevier; 2015.

Stokes S, Kulkarni A. Suprapubic bladder aspiration. In: Reichman EF, Simon RR, eds. *Emergency Medicine Procedures.* 2nd ed. New York: McGraw-Hill; 2013:963–968.

CHAPTER 169

TONGUE-TIE SNIPPING (FRENOTOMY) FOR ANKYLOGLOSSIA

Gary R. Newkirk • Mary Jane Newkirk

"Tongue-tie," or ankyloglossia, results from underdevelopment of the lingual frenum (frenulum) and occurs in nearly 5% of infants. Infants differ substantially in the degree to which the frenum attaches to the tongue. Most cases of tongue-tie are thought to resolve spontaneously by adulthood with little likelihood of feeding or speech development problems. If symptomatic, the infant usually has issues with breastfeeding or similar problems (e.g., acting irritably or fussy, even after feeding; poor weight gain or weight loss; problems latching onto the nipple; maternal nipple pain). However, the condition is often not noticed until later in life and has been associated with speech defects (e.g., a lisp), dental problems (especially with the lower teeth), and the accumulation of food in the floor of the mouth. If such problems are noticed in an infant or child, the parents are usually the ones to bring ankyloglossia to the clinician's attention (Fig. 169.1). The condition is often overlooked during the newborn examination because infants typically retract and roll the tongue downward when their mouth is open, effectively hiding the frenum from view. Furthermore, newborns rarely stick their tongues out for more than brief periods, so no one notices that the tongue cannot be protruded due to ankyloglossia.

Although the cause of tongue-tie is unknown, genetics probably plays a role; the condition tends to run in families. Since ankyloglossia is a fairly common and often unnoticed condition that lacks a precise definition, until recently there have been few formal outcome studies comparing frenotomy with conservative management. On one side of the debate, problems with sucking, breastfeeding, chewing, swallowing, dentofacial growth and development, gingival hygiene, and speech have clearly been attributed to being tongue-tied. Alternatively, some researchers feel that the parents, not the child, have the problem. These issues should be weighed against the fact that partial frenotomy, also referred to as *tongue-tie snipping*, remains a quick, easy, and safe procedure with benefits even if

performed for cosmetic reasons or parental "disease." Clinicians are more likely to perform partial frenotomy if they believe that ankyloglossia contributes to poor infant sucking and other breastfeeding problems, such as insufficient infant weight gain or sore nipples/recurrent mastitis in the mother. Although there are few data to support prophylactic frenulotomy, there is now evidence that it may be beneficial with problematic breastfeeding, especially if it is likely attributable to ankyloglossia (Brookes and Bowley, 2014). A Cochrane review did not find a consistent positive effect of frenulotomy on breastfeeding; however, it did find a benefit for maternal nipple pain (O'Shea et al., 2017). The authors also called for more studies. In the meantime, simple frenotomy for infants and small children with partial ankyloglossia can be performed safely in the outpatient setting.

The best method and timing for frenotomy remain debatable. When ankyloglossia *severely* interferes with lingual function (e.g., "frozen tongue"), few would argue the need for reduction, but in this case formal Z-plasty is necessary. The patient should be referred to an experienced surgeon because this procedure requires general anesthesia and sometimes a complicated reconstruction.

Anatomically, the frenum of the tongue is a triangular fold of mucous membrane extending back from the lower midline gingival tissue along the floor of the mouth and then arching to the midline of the undersurface of the tongue. The extent to which the tongue portion of the frenum extends along the undersurface to the tip of the tongue is variable. Tongue-tie occurs when two situations coexist: the frenum continues distally (abnormally) toward the tip of the tongue and the height/length of the frenum is short. This combination prevents normal elevation or protrusion of the tongue.

INDICATIONS

Clinical evidence of short lingual frenum in an infant with resultant perceived speech problems or inhibited tongue protrusion, feeding, or swallowing.

RELATIVE AND ABSOLUTE CONTRAINDICATIONS

- Lack of clinical evidence or suspicion that ankyloglossia is a problem
- Unstable medical conditions, such as a bleeding disorder (In many cases this can be reversed.)
- Evidence of dental or oral infection (The procedure should be postponed until the infection is adequately treated or resolves.)
- Severe ankyloglossia, which requires frenectomy under general anesthesia (Usually this procedure involves Z-plasty or a similar plastic surgery procedure.)
- Orofacial abnormalities (It is recommended that infants or children with ankyloglossia combined with other orofacial abnormalities be referred.)

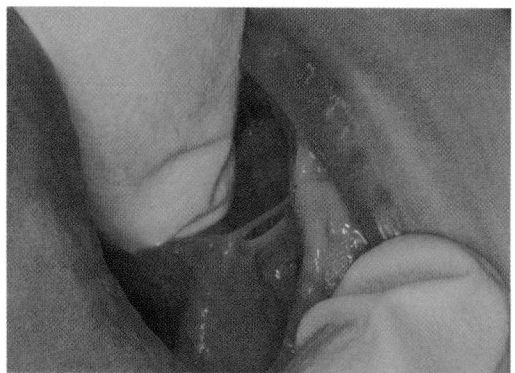

Fig. 169.1 Ankyloglossia in a 2-week-old infant experiencing feeding difficulties.

Equipment

- Straight or curved mosquito hemostat
- Surgical scissors (some clinicians prefer iris or other straight scissors, others use curved Metzenbaum scissors)
- Tongue retractor (e.g., small spoon, wooden tongue blade)
- Ice, ice chips, popsicle, or frozen teething ring (optional)
- Topical anesthetic (e.g., viscous lidocaine, benzocaine [Cetacaine spray or Hurricaine syrup]) (optional)
- Infant restraint (e.g., swaddling sheets, circumcision, or immobilization board) (optional)
- Lidocaine with epinephrine to control bleeding afterward (optional)

PREPROCEDURE PATIENT EDUCATION

Describe the risks to the parents, including discomfort; possible medication reaction (if used); recurrence of ankyloglossia during or after healing; injury to tongue or sublingual mucosa or tissue; infection; or bleeding. A parent may help by holding a small child in his or her lap and, while doing so, holding the child's head still and the child's mouth open. However, for newborns and infants—for the same reasons as in a circumcision—parents may want to leave the room. After examining the child, if more than one technique is possible, the clinician should explain the various techniques to the parents and attempt to obtain their input on the desired technique. Parents should be aware that whereas performance of partial frenotomy may improve tongue function, it does not prevent all tongue, feeding, or speech problems.

TECHNIQUE

1. With assistance as necessary, position or hold small infants or children in such a way that they will remain still. Wrapping an infant with sheets or a blanket is a very effective method of immobilization. A parent can still hold an infant that is swaddled in this manner in his or her lap. A circumcision board is effective if an assistant also stabilizes the head.
   NOTE: Crying often improves exposure of the frenum.
2. Identify the frenum, the abnormal portion of the frenum (causing ankyloglossia), and the necessary degree of surgical lysis. A limited snipping of the lucent, membranous portion of the distal frenum is usually all that is required.
3. Many clinicians snip a lucent membranous or very thin fibrinous distal frenum without topical agents or the use of a hemostat, especially in infants younger than 4 months. Although this technique may increase local bleeding, for a thin membrane there should be no more bleeding than when a child falls and bites his or her lip or tongue. This technique may also cause less overall trauma than with the use of a hemostat. If the child is old enough not to aspirate, have him or her suck on ice, ice chips, or a popsicle before and after the procedure for a certain degree of anesthesia and to minimize bleeding. Younger children may appreciate a frozen teething ring.
4. For a thicker or coarser frenum, topical anesthesia may be beneficial. For example, a cotton-tipped swab can be moistened in benzocaine syrup or sprayed with benzocaine (Fig. 169.2) and focally applied to the lower mouth and bottom of the tongue (Fig. 169.3). Viscous lidocaine or benzocaine spray can be applied directly to the area in the same manner. Mild sedation may also be beneficial (see Chapter 2, Pediatric Sedation).
5. If necessary, retract and gently elevate the tongue. A small spoon or wooden tongue blade may be helpful. A wedge cut out of the end of the tongue blade may be beneficial for retracting the tongue.

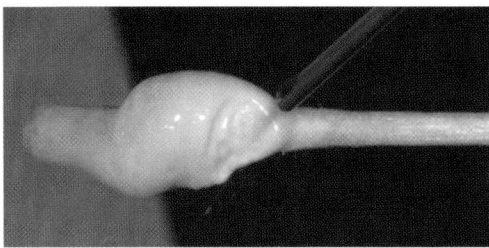

Fig. 169.2 Spraying topical anesthetic on a cotton-tipped applicator.

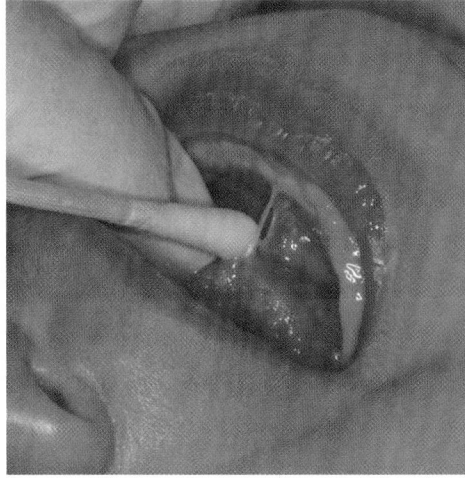

Fig. 169.3 Applying topical anesthetic to the frenum and surrounding area.

6. As an option, with the tip of the mosquito clamp, grab and crush the frenum to the depth and at the position where the scissor snip will be made (Fig. 169.4A). After the discomfort from crushing the tissue has resolved, a certain degree of anesthesia is experienced in the crushed area.
7. Snip the crushed portion of the frenum (see Fig. 169.4B). *Warning:* If tissue is snipped outside or beyond the crushed area of the frenum, it will result in more bleeding and pain.
   NOTE: Although crushed tissue is somewhat anesthetized, the patient experiences some discomfort at the time of the crush. A child's immediate memory of pain as the result of an instrument being placed in the mouth may make it difficult to open the mouth again to snip the crushed frenum. This is why some clinicians perform the procedure by simply snipping (Fig. 169.5) without using a hemostat (especially when the frenum is very thin). However, for a thicker and coarser frenum, crushing the tissue with a hemostat will be necessary. For older children, there may be value in telling them that the painful part of the procedure is over once the hemostat has been applied and removed.
8. Use a dry cotton-tipped swab or one moistened with 1% lidocaine with epinephrine to control any bleeding or oozing. Ice, a popsicle, or an iced teething ring may also help to control oozing. Fig. 169.6 shows the appearance of the completed procedure.

SAMPLE OPERATIVE REPORT

See a sample operative report available at www.expertconsult.com.

POSTPROCEDURE PATIENT EDUCATION

- No special care of the surgical site is necessary.
- Ask the patient (or parent) to report significant bleeding or signs of infection.

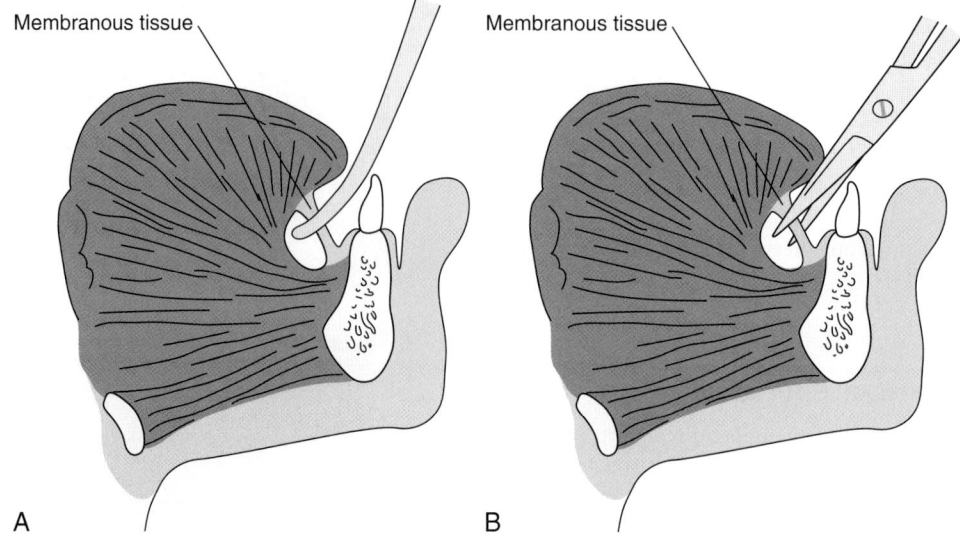

Membranous tissue   Membranous tissue

A   B

Fig. 169.4   Tongue-tie snipping technique. (A) Crush the abnormal portion of the frenum where the snip is to be made. (B) Cut through the crushed area.

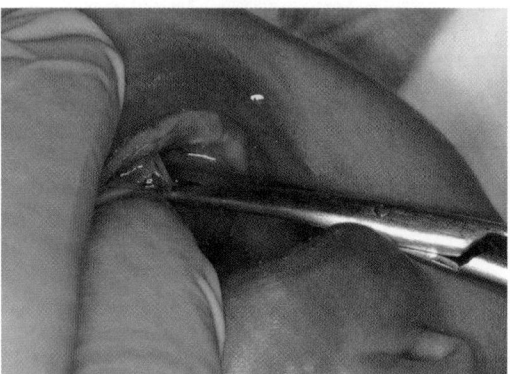

Fig. 169.5   Incising the abnormal portion of frenum (causing ankyloglossia) using curved Metzenbaum scissors.

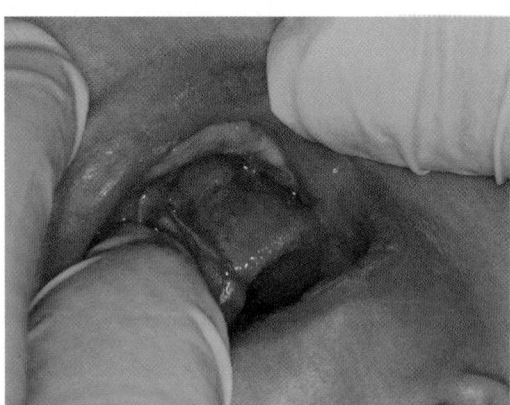

Fig. 169.6   Appearance of the normal remaining frenum after partial frenotomy has been completed.

- Instruct the parent to allow infant or child to resume normal feeding habits immediately.
- Ice chips, an ice cube, or a popsicle for children old enough to not aspirate, or a frozen teething ring for infants, may help stop any later bleeding or oozing.

- Ask the patient (or parent) to report any feeding difficulties or significant swelling.
- Inform the patient (or parent) to return for follow-up in 2 weeks, or sooner if complications arise.

CPT/BILLING CODES

41010   Incision of lingual frenum (frenotomy)

Q38.1   Ankyloglossia

SUPPLIERS

(See contact information available at www.expertconsult.com.)

Hurricaine Syrup
Beutlich LP Pharmaceuticals

ONLINE RESOURCES

MedlinePlus: Tongue tie: www.medlineplus.gov/ency/article/001640.htm
Tongue Tie: From Confusion to Clarity: www.tonguetie.net

RECOMMENDED READING

Brookes A, Bowley DM. Tongue tie: the evidence for frenotomy. *Early Hum Dev.* 2014;90(11):765–768.

Hogan M, Westcott C, Griffiths M. Randomized, controlled trial of division of tongue-tie in infants with feeding problems. *J Paediatr Child Health.* 2005;41:246–250.

Messner AH, Lalakea ML, Aby J, et al. Ankyloglossia: incidence and associated feeding difficulties. *Arch Otolaryngol Head Neck Surg.* 2000;126:36–39.

Murtagh J. Release of tongue tie (frenulotomy). *Murtagh J: Practice Tips.* 7th ed. Sydney: McGraw-Hill; 2017:205.

O'Shea JE, Foster JP, O'Donnell CPF, et al. Frenotomy for tongue-tie in newborn infants. *Cochrane Database of Systematic Reviews.* 2017:Art. No. CD011065. https://doi.org/10.1002/14651858.CD01165.pub2.

Ricke LA, Baker NJ, Madlon-Kay DJ, et al. Newborn tongue-tie: prevalence and effect on breast feeding. *J Am Board of Fam Pract.* 2005;18:1–7.

CHAPTER 170

MANAGEMENT OF YOUNG FEMALE AS POSSIBLE VICTIM OF SEXUAL ABUSE

David B. Bosscher

Sexual abuse is so common that primary care clinicians should consider it as a possibility, even during routine office visits. The prevalence is estimated to be 22% for girls and 9% for boys. Unfortunately, more than half of sexually abused children do not disclose their abuse until they are adults. A history of childhood sexual abuse can have lifelong deleterious effects on a child's physical and mental health. Although child advocacy centers are increasingly available in many regions and communities, the generalist clinician is often the critical first line of evaluation. In some regions, they may be the only available expert. If a specialized abuse-related service (e.g., a child advocacy center or hospital-based child protection program) is not available, the clinician must educate themselves about childhood genital and anal examinations, and how to interview children to obtain enough information to make important decisions regarding reporting to children protective service agencies and referral to counseling agencies. The American Academy of Pediatrics (AAP) offers a variety of educational materials on child abuse for clinicians including continuing education courses, textbooks, and a comprehensive video. The 2013 guidelines provided by the AAP is available online and is an excellent reference. This chapter is provided only to enhance such guidelines and as a start for those obtaining competence in this area or as a reminder for those that do not perform such examinations very often.

In young females, common initial complaints include itching, redness, burning, irritation, discharge, or bleeding at the vagina. The abuse may be disclosed initially or discovered later. Occasionally, the abuse will be discovered when a parent wants a child examined after their use of sexually explicit language, demonstration of a sexual act on their doll, or other overtly sexual behavior. Because children may be exposed to sexually explicit media, the examiner must carefully sift through such allegations and concerns. Often the complaints are nonspecific and parents hope that a medical test can prove or disprove abuse. Unfortunately, in the majority of cases, children are seen long after the incident may have occurred. If, however, the alleged incident took place within 72 hours of complaint, immediate examination using a carefully structured protocol (e.g., a rape kit; see Chapter 140, Treatment of the Adult Victim of Sexual Assault) is mandatory.

When a parent brings up the possibility of sexual abuse, the child should be immediately excluded from the discussion. Children, particularly young children, might be influenced by hearing their parents' concerns. During this exclusion, it may be helpful to determine which terms the family uses to describe bathroom activities and private parts for later use if an examination is necessary. At some point, the parent(s) will also need to be excluded from the interview, if at all possible. Parents can subtly or not-so-subtly influence the child's statements. Separation of the child from the parent is particularly important if they are a potential perpetrator or are supportive of the suspected perpetrator. The child should be reassured that the parent will be present during the examination if that is the child's preference.

As this data is being gathered, five issues should be at the forefront of the clinician's thinking. The foremost issue is the child's safety. Is the child safe to go back home? Is the perpetrator still there, and will the child be harmed or punished for disclosing the abuse? If there is no imminent danger, does child protective services need to be contacted? In most localities in the United States and Canada, it is mandated that suspected child abuse or neglect be reported. Next on the list of considerations is the child's mental health. This can be a very stressful time for the child and the family. Is emergency referral warranted for mental health for either the child or the parent? If sexual abuse is suspected, the need for a thorough physical examination to rule out injury has likely been confirmed. At this point, the decision should be made whether there is need for collection of forensic evidence.

A careful physical examination for children with allegations of sexual abuse is imperative, either in the clinician's office or through a regional child advocacy center. Nonetheless, only about 4% of physical examinations result in positive findings. A negative finding does not negate the claim of abuse, but does make interviews with social workers and other trained interviewers critically important to sort out allegations.

Although this chapter focuses on females, it is not meant to deny the possibility of abuse in males. If abuse is suspected in a young male, many of the same principles apply. It is important to know local laws regarding collection of evidence because they vary by location. The examiner should be certain to follow local standards for collection of forensic specimens. Typically a child will prefer to have the same-sex parent in the room, if possible.

INDICATIONS

- Suspicion of sexual abuse after initial questioning or preliminary physical examination
- Referral from teacher, parent, or other responsible person alleging sexual abuse

CONTRAINDICATIONS

- Lack of the instruments or supplies needed to carry out the examination
- Lack of forms to preserve the chain of evidence
- Lack of a witness for the examination to preserve the chain of evidence
- Lack of consent to examine or treat a minor if a parent or guardian is not present

EQUIPMENT

- Either a hand-held lens with an adequate examination light or a colposcope to examine details. One major benefit of a colposcope is that it allows the clinician to use both hands for the examination. If a hand-held lens is used, an assistant will be needed.

- Camera (helpful but not mandatory). In specialty centers, photos or videos are often taken. If taken in primary care office, they should be treated as a confidential part of the medical record and care taken to label them for proper identification.
- A rape kit should be available in case it is necessary to document rape. If alleged sexual contact was within the past 72 hours, consider using the rape kit to collect evidence in an organized manner (see Chapter 140, Treatment of the Adult Victim of Sexual Assault).
- Chain of evidence form (see Fig. 170.8).

EQUIPMENT ON A MAYO STAND

- Room-temperature culture media for gonorrhea or culture transport media from your reference laboratory
- Chlamydia and herpes culture media or culture transport media from your reference laboratory
- Materials for wet prep and potassium hydroxide (KOH) prep
- Cotton swabs, calcium alginate swabs (Calgiswab) or equivalent

NOTE: A recent multicenter study found commercially available nucleic acid amplification tests (NAATs) to be not only highly sensitive but also highly specific for diagnosing *Chlamydia trachomatis* and *Neisseria gonorrhoeae*. Urine tests using NAATs were performed, as well as vaginal swabs to detect infections in both prepubertal and postpubertal girls. All positive tests were confirmed, resulting in a high positive predictive value. This led investigators to conclude that these tests provide a better alternative than culture as a forensic standard. Consequently, the AAP recommends the use of NAATs when evaluating children and adolescents for suspected genital infections with these organisms. At this time, the use of NAATs for diagnosing other genital infections, such as those involving *Candida* species, *Gardnerella vaginalis,* and *Trichomoniasis vaginalis,* is not recommended for forensic purposes because they have not been studied extensively in children. In its 2015 guidelines, the CDC says there is inadequate data to suggest use of NAATs is adequate for testing in boys or in extragenital sites for girls and boys. At this point, the CDC still recommends cultures for these sites. Regardless, all positive specimens in suspected abuse should be retained by the laboratory for additional testing. Consultation may be needed with an expert to decide whether confirmatory testing is necessary.

PREPROCEDURE PATIENT PREPARATION

Explain the entire procedure to the caregiver and the child at a language level that both will understand. The child needs to know that she will be asked a lot of questions and that some may seem "silly." Explain that after the questions, the child will be examined.

It is often helpful to allow a young girl to maintain her sense of control over the process. After establishing rapport with the child, assure her that she will be allowed to be as active a participant as possible. If possible, she should know that she will be asked for permission before proceeding with any part of the examination.

Issues of privacy and confidentiality are important when examining older children. Although most young girls will prefer to have a parent (usually the mother) in the room at all times, in some cases it will be helpful to later spend time alone with the child. When alone with an examiner, a child may disclose abuse or other concerns. Letting her and the parent(s) know ahead of time (before the examination) that the clinician will be spending time alone with her may increase her comfort. Allowing that time alone may give her a greater sense of control and a feeling of responsibility for her own health. Consideration should be given to having a second person in the room with the patient and examiner at all times to serve as an assistant, chaperone, and witness. If the examiner is male, having a female assistant in the room may make the patient more comfortable.

Parents should be reassured that the child's hymen will not be altered in any way by the examination. Anatomic diagrams may be helpful for demonstration.

TECHNIQUE

Taking the History

1. Assuming that a social worker or trained interviewer is responsible for taking a detailed history, the primary care clinician should take sufficient history to perform all pertinent portions of the examination. If no trained interviewer is available, a complete history should be taken in an unhurried and comfortable setting. Consider setting aside separate visits for the history and the physical examination.
2. Take some time to establish rapport. Ask about the current family structure, recent life changes, and which activities she enjoys, as well as about school and friends. Take notes while obtaining the history. It is often complicated. Obtain the names of persons potentially involved.
3. Document the descriptions of any potential sexual abuse in the child's own words. When the meaning of a word is unclear, ask clarifying questions. Document the meaning of the word in her terms. For example, if the child mentions *sex*, ask her what that means (e.g., because of depictions on television, children often think that sex means just being naked and in bed with another person).
4. Do not be any more leading in questioning than is absolutely necessary. Begin with very general questions and go to more specific ones if the child does not offer sufficient information. For example, ask "Has anyone touched you in a way that made you feel funny or bad?" before asking "Has anyone touched your bottom?" Leading questions cannot only misdirect the child and, subsequently, the examiner; they can also be neutralized by a defense attorney.
5. Do not allow the caregiver(s) to adopt a coaching role. Such a role may negate the clinician's testimony as well as the child's.
6. Young children have an incomplete concept of numbers and time. They often cannot tell how many times something occurred, but can often specify in general terms: "a lot," "once in a while," or "one time." Likewise, regarding time, small children do not understand the difference between "3 months ago" and "8 months ago."

Preparing for the Vaginal Examination

1. Again, take time to establish a comfortable setting. A child-friendly, compassionate medical assistant or nurse can be very helpful in using a toy, book, or stuffed animal to distract the child during the examination.
2. Explain the examination to the caregiver and the child at a language level they will comprehend. This is an important step toward reinforcing the child's sense of control over the examination. Begin by describing familiar portions of the examination ("I'm going to listen to your heart and then feel your tummy"). Then simply state that you are going to examine her genitalia ("Then I'm going to look at your bottom").
3. Explain to the child that the most important part of the examination is when the examiner merely "looks" around and that it is important for her to communicate with the examiner during the examination. Reassure the child that the examination should not hurt.
4. Perform the physical examination except for the vaginal-rectal portion. The examination should proceed from the least to the most intrusive while gaining the confidence of the child with each step.
5. Before performing the vaginal examination, it is helpful to recall normal anatomy (Fig. 170.1).

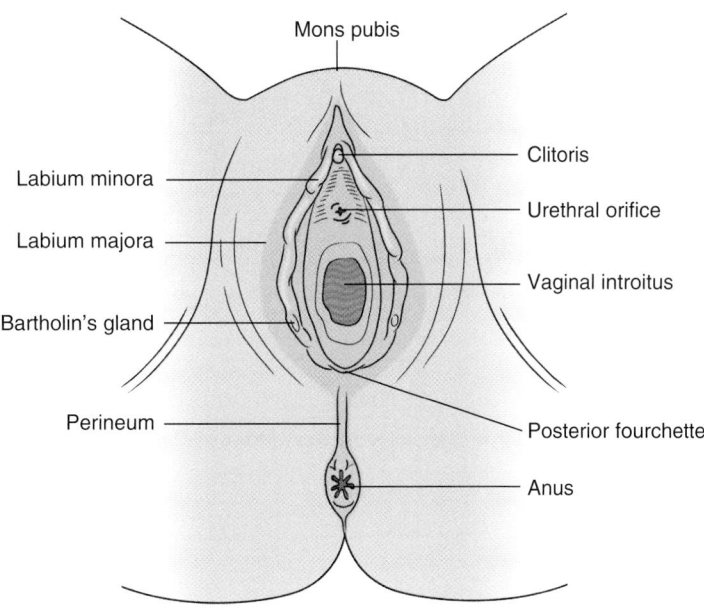

Fig. 170.1   Anatomy of genitalia in prepubertal girl.

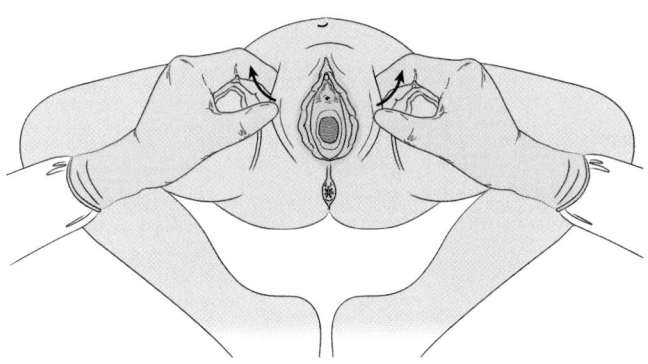

Fig. 170.2   Frog-leg position for examining labia. Note gentle traction on posterior labia to enhance visualization.

Performing the Vaginal Examination

1. Talk constantly ("verbal anesthesia"). A calm, quiet, confident voice can be reassuring. A relaxed and unhurried approach may decrease the child's anxiety. Having the parent sit close by or hold the child's hand may also provide comfort. If the child is provided a hand mirror, it may distract her, promote education, and allow her to participate more actively in the process.
2. Tell the child that it is acceptable to undress because she is in a clinician's office. For the male exam, the majority of the exam will focus on the scrotum, penis, and rectal area, looking for signs of trauma.
3. Frog-leg examination
   • Begin with the frog-leg examination. The child is supine with knees apart and feet touching in the midline with buttocks at the end of the table (Fig. 170.2). Alternatively, the mother may assist with the frog-leg position (Fig. 170.3). Older children may be placed in adjustable stirrups (Fig. 170.4).
   • Inspect the vulva and areas lateral to it. Use the colposcope or a hand lens with adequate lighting to best visualize the introitus.
   • Gently open the labia by applying gentle lateral and posterior traction just lateral to the vulva at the level of the posterior introitus. Do not force the labia open; they will usually open

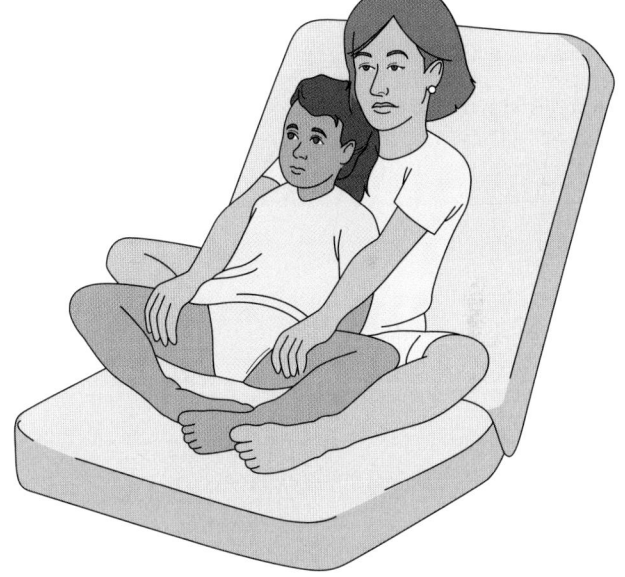

Fig. 170.3   Frog-leg position with mother's assistance.

with persistent gentle traction, or the child may assist by holding her labia apart.
   • Examine carefully the entire circumference of the introitus and hymen. Normal hymenal variants are illustrated in Fig. 170.5. Look carefully for asymmetry, for notching in the posterior hymen, and for posterior hymenal attenuation (thinning; Fig. 170.6). These findings are usually caused by sexual abuse, and rarely by accidental trauma. The significance of the diameter of the hymenal orifice is controversial; do not worry about measurements. If the hymen cannot be fully visualized, ask the child to cough or take a deep breath. Pull the labia gently forward and down or laterally. A colposcope is helpful at this stage. A hand lens can also be used if an assistant can help with the examination. Box 170.1 can be useful for differentiating normal accidental trauma from suspected sexual abuse.

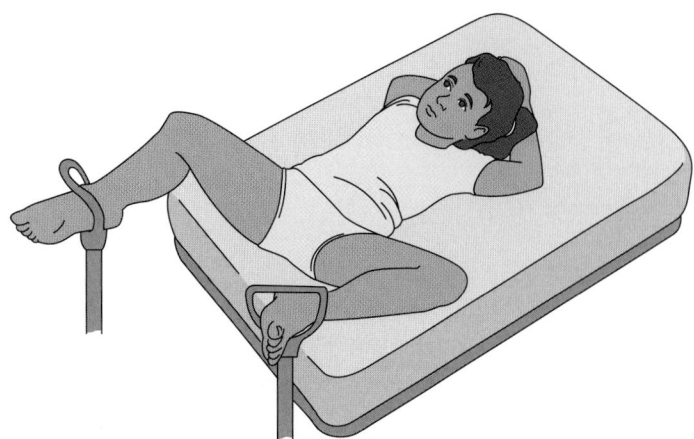

Fig. 170.4 Lithotomy position with use of stirrups.

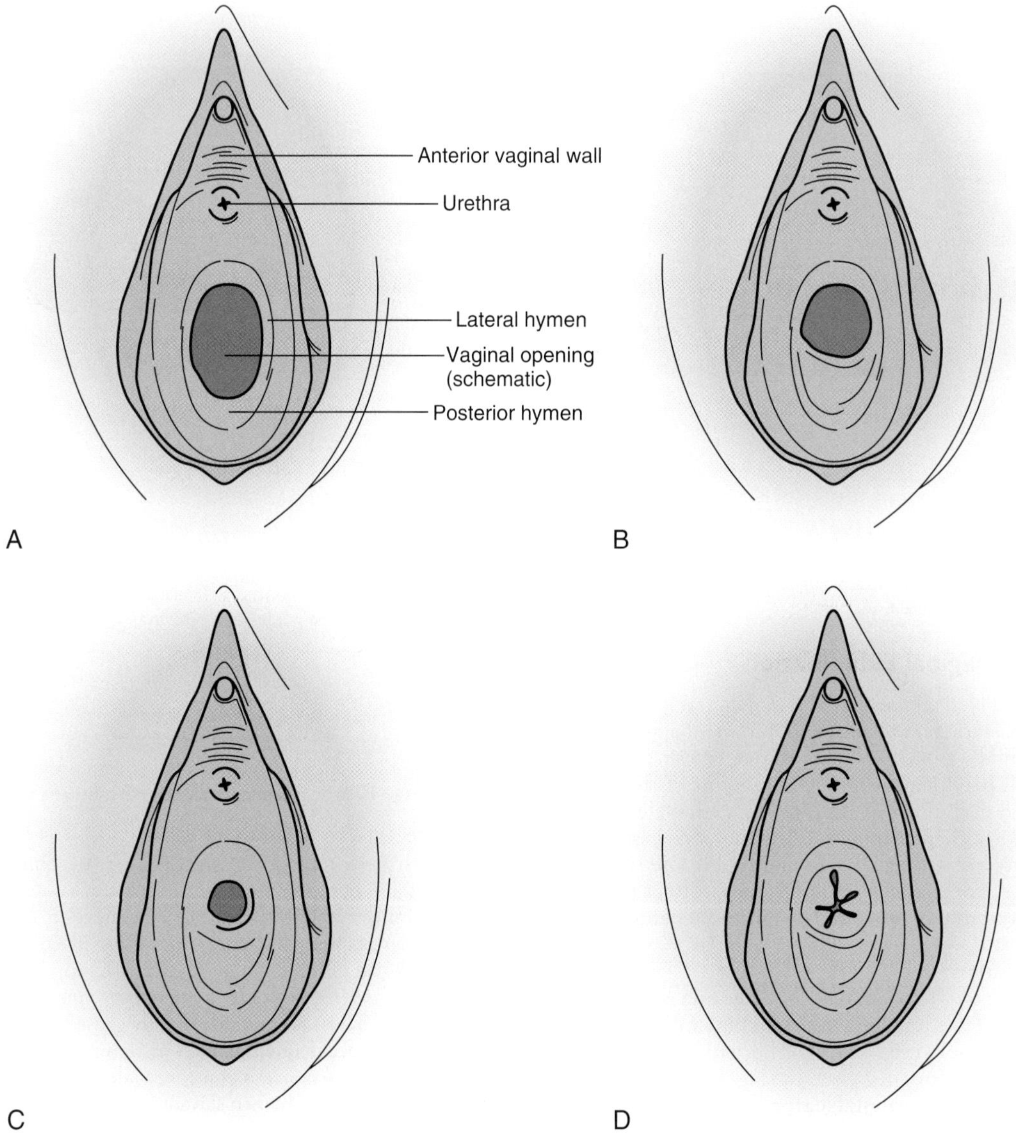

Anterior vaginal wall

Urethra

Lateral hymen

Vaginal opening (schematic)

Posterior hymen

A

B

C

D

Fig. 170.5 Variants of normal hymen. (A) Normal hymen. (B) Posterior rim or crescentic hymen. (C) Circumferential or annular hymen. (D) Fimbriated or redundant hymen.

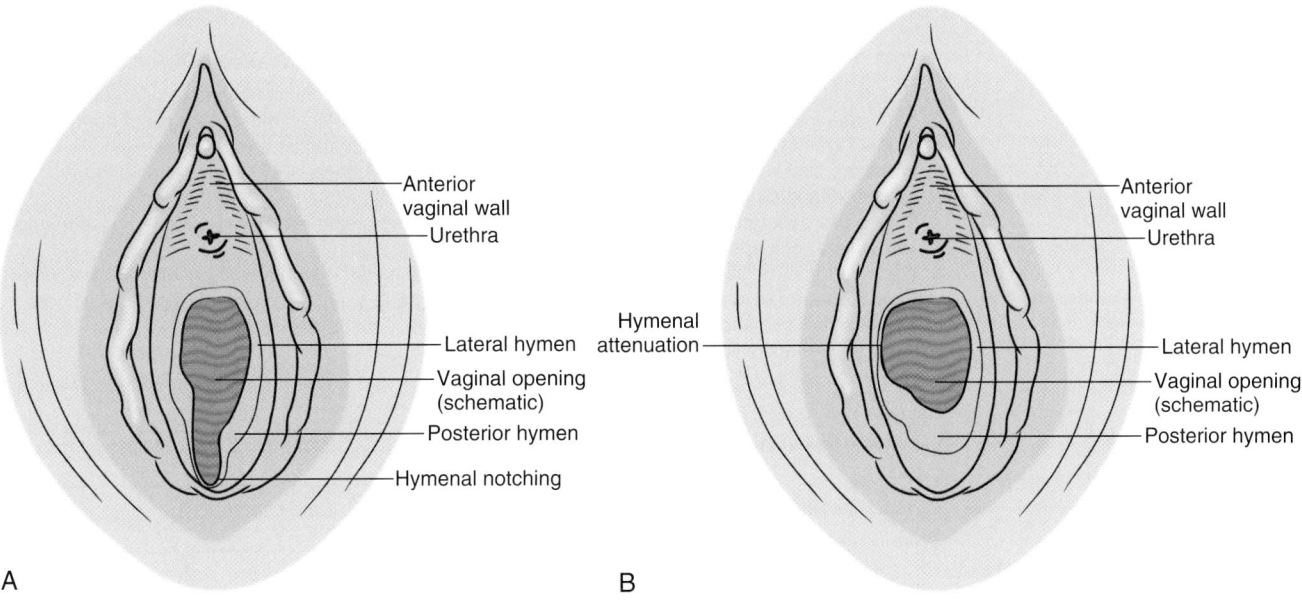

Fig. 170.6   (A) Hymenal notching. (B) Hymenal attenuation.

BOX 170.1   Acute Findings on Examination of Accidental versus Diagnostic of Sexual Contact in Children

Acute Trauma to External Genital/Anal Tissues, Which Could Be Accidental or Inflicted

- Acute laceration(s) or bruising of labia, penis, scrotum, perianal tissues, or perineum
- Acute laceration of the posterior fourchette or vestibule, not involving the hymen
- Residual (healing) injuries to external genital/anal tissues (These rare findings are difficult to diagnose unless an acute injury was previously documented at the same location.)
- Perianal scar
- Scar of posterior fourchette or fossa

Injuries Indicative of Acute or Healed Trauma to the Genital/Anal Tissues

- Bruising, petechiae, or abrasions on the hymen
- Acute laceration of the hymen, of any depth; partial or complete
- Vaginal laceration
- Perianal laceration with exposure of tissues below the dermis
- Healed hymenal transection/complete hymen cleft (a defect in the hymen between 4 o'clock and 8 o'clock that extends to the base of the hymen, with no hymenal tissue discernible at that location)
- A defect in the posterior (inferior) half of the hymen, wider than a transection, with an absence of hymenal tissue extending to the base of the hymen

From Adams JA, Kellogg ND, Farst KJ, et al: Updated guidelines for the medical assessment and care of children who may have been sexually abused. *J Pediatr Adolesc Gynecol.* 2:81–87, 2015.

- Acute trauma from sexual abuse is evidenced by the presence of hematomas, abrasions, lacerations, hymenal transections, or vulvar erythema. These conditions usually resolve within 10 to 14 days.
- Cultures can be taken at this time (assuming the child is comfortable) or after the knee–chest examination.

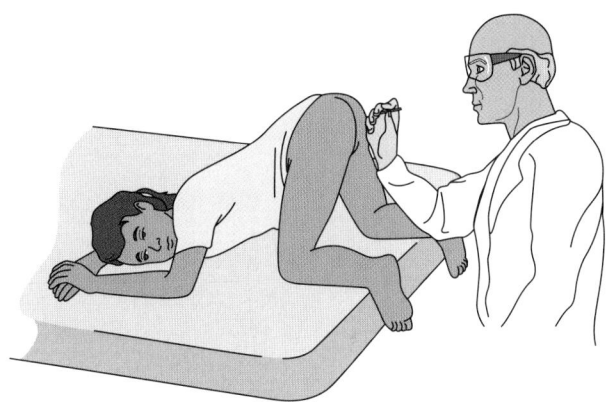

Fig. 170.7   Knee-chest position.

4. Knee-chest examination (for children older than 2 years)
   - Most young children readily adopt this position with a little encouragement. Buttocks should be higher than the back, with knees approximately 25 cm (12 inches) apart. The child can rest her head to one side on her folded arms or pillow (Fig. 170.7).
   - Gentle traction laterally will often open up the labia. Ask the patient to take 10 slow, deep breaths, because this will also relax the perineal structures.
   - Use the colposcope (or hand lens with an assistant) to look at the posterior hymen. The knee–chest position is the preferred position for detecting small but significant abnormalities of the hymen. Again, look for asymmetries, notching, or attenuation. Take photographs or carefully document if abnormalities are seen.
   - The lower vagina may be visualized in this position, and the upper vagina and cervix in 80% to 90% of prepubertal girls. Also, examine the rectum in this position.
5. Resume the frog-leg position if cultures are needed. Perform the following only if vaginal discharge or pain is noted, if there is genital itching or odor or urinary symptoms, or if there are genital ulcers or lesions. Consider cultures if the prevalence of sexually transmitted infections (STIs) in the community is high, if a sibling or another child or adult in the household has an STI, or a known assailant has an STI or is at high risk.

Chain of Evidence Form

* PLEASE COMPLETE CAREFULLY—THIS FORM IS REQUIRED FOR LEGAL PURPOSES

1. Use this LOG to document specimen transfer so that "chain of evidence" can be preserved.
2. Each time the specimen changes hands, the new carrier-technologist must place his or her initials on the form in the appropriate location and must mark the date and time.
3. When the final laboratory report is prepared, staple securely to the LOG before sending the report to the ordering clinician.
4. Please use separate forms if specimens of different types are submitted (e.g., blood specimen and GC culture) or if specimens are sent to different labs.
5. If you perform the laboratory test in your office, have each staff member who handles the specimen initial the form. Anyone in attendance during the history and examination should sign as a witness at the bottom of the form.
6. If you have questions, call the ordering clinician.

Patient's name: _____ Date: _____

Laboratory test(s) ordered (circle): RPR Urine culture Culture for GC/Chlamydia HIV
Other: _____

Patient's medical record number: _____ Date of birth: _____
Ordering clinician: _____

Each person handling the specimen should *place initials in the first column, then mark the time and date.*

1. Specimen collected by _____   1. Date _____ Time _____
2. Delivered to lab by _____   2. Date _____ Time _____
3. Received in lab by _____   3. Date _____ Time _____
4. Processed by _____   4. Date _____ Time _____
5. Processed by _____   5. Date _____ Time _____
6. Final report prepared by _____ 6. Date _____ Time _____

Witnesses to examination:

1. _____ 1. Date _____ Time _____
2. _____ 2. Date _____ Time _____
3. _____ 3. Date _____ Time _____
4. _____ 4. Date _____ Time _____
5. _____ 5. Date _____ Time _____
6. _____ 6. Date _____ Time _____

Fig. 170.8 Chain of evidence form.

- Culture for *Chlamydia*. Collect the specimen as deeply in the posterior vagina as you can. Use a cotton or calcium alginate swab. If possible, it should be moistened with nonbacteriostatic saline to minimize the discomfort. Before inserting, allow the child to feel a similar swab on her skin. Avoid touching the hymen when obtaining the culture. It may also be helpful to ask the child to cough in order to distract her and open the hymen. A male urethral swab may also be used to gently scrape the vaginal wall.
- Alternatively, a vaginal wash and aspiration can be obtained. Using a small feeding tube attached to a small syringe, insert the tube into the vagina and inject and aspirate 0.5 to 1 mL of sterile saline. A soft plastic or glass eyedropper with 4 to 5 cm of intravenous plastic tubing attached can also be used in the same manner. Insert the catheter into the vagina and inject and then aspirate the saline.
- For gonorrhea (gonococci), use a cotton or calcium alginate swab to obtain samples from the following: throat, deep in the posterior vagina, and rectum. Place them on a single plate partitioned into thirds. (This is done to reduce the number of cultures needed.) If any area of the plate is actually positive, you will need to reculture each area separately to confirm the location. A false-positive chlamydial or gonococcal culture is very rare, so it should be investigated.
- Obtain a herpes culture if it is suspected.

- Cultures for other organisms can be obtained by placing the calcium alginate swab into a transport Culturette II (contains medium) or by sending the aspirated fluid to your local hospital laboratory for direct plating.
- Obtain a wet prep or KOH prep if indicated.
- Note and document the presence of any condylomata.

NOTE: Cultures are the standard for forensic evidence for boys and for boys and girls in extragenital sites. NAATs may, however, be helpful in other instances. See the note in the equipment section.

6. In addition to the aforementioned studies, consider a urine culture, syphilis serology, and hepatitis B and human immunodeficiency virus testing on all patients because of the paucity of clinical findings with these diseases. Parents may also be reassured by doing these studies.
   NOTE: Foreign bodies are often found as the cause of a discharge. Removal may be possible with a cotton-tipped applicator or by lavaging the vagina with saline or warm water. Viscous lidocaine may be useful for anesthesia at the introitus.
7. Send all cultures and other laboratory studies to the laboratory, using chain of evidence form and precautions (Fig. 170.8).
8. After the examination, congratulate the child for his or her cooperation. Discuss the results and the diagnosis and management

TABLE 170.1   Implications of Commonly Encountered STIs in Prepubertal Children

STD Confirmed	Sexual Abuse	Suggested Action
Gonorrhea	Certain	Report
Syphilis	Certain	Report
Chlamydial infection	Probable	Report
Condylomata	Probable	Report
Trichomoniasis	Probable	Report
Herpes simplex type 1 (on genitals)	Possible	Report
Herpes simplex type 2	Probable	Report
Bacterial vaginosis	Uncertain	Medical follow-up
Candida infection	Unlikely	Medical follow-up

STD, Sexually transmitted disease; *STI*, sexually transmitted infection.
Modified from American Academy of Pediatrics Committee on Child Abuse and Neglect: Guidelines for the evaluation of sexual abuse of children. *Pediatrics* 87:254–260, 1991.

TABLE 170.2   Guidelines for Making the Decision to Report Sexual Abuse of Children

History	Physical Examination	Laboratory Abnormality	Level of Concern About Sexual Abuse	Action
None	Normal	None	None	None
Behavioral changes	Normal	None	Low	Possibly report, follow closely
None	Nonspecific	None	Low	Possibly report, follow closely
Nonspecific history by child or history by parent only	Nonspecific	None	Possible	Possibly report, follow closely
None	Specific findings	None	Probable	Report
Child's clear statement	Specific findings	None	Probable	Report
None	Normal, nonspecific, or specific findings	Positive culture for gonococci, *Chlamydia*, or *Trichomonas*, +RPR, presence of sperm Positive NAAT in girls	Definite	Report
Behavioral changes	Nonspecific changes	Other sexually transmitted infections	Probable	Report

RPR, Rapid plasma reagin test.
Modified from American Academy of Pediatrics Committee on Child Abuse and Neglect: Guidelines for the evaluation of sexual abuse of children. *Pediatrics* 87:254–260, 1991.

plan with the child and her parent(s) after she is dressed. Because the results of the examination are often inconclusive, help the parent(s) understand that a careful and complete investigation includes protective services or law enforcement officials, or both.
9. Implications of positive laboratory findings are set out in Table 170.1. Table 170.2 contains guidelines for making reporting decisions.

Uncooperative Patients

The uncooperative patient calls for patience and artistry on the part of the examiner. Often (but not always), proceeding through the examination slowly will result in a satisfactory examination. Leaving the room and returning when she is ready often allows a child to regain control.

Nasally administered midazolam (Versed), a short-acting benzodiazepine (dosage 0.2 to 0.4 mg/kg of the injectable solution) can enhance cooperativeness. When administered by this route (use a tuberculin syringe without a needle), the drug will be effective within 15 minutes. Side effects are rare. Versed syrup is available as another option, but therapeutic onset is longer. The child must be observed by a knowledgeable parent or by your staff for about 1 to 2 hours after the drug is given. This anxiolytic technique requires no intensive monitoring (see Chapter 2, Pediatric Sedation).

Antibiotics are rarely indicated. Usually, the alleged abuse occurred long ago.

PATIENT EDUCATION GUIDES

See the patient education form available at www.expertconsult. com. To find a regional child advocacy center, consult the National Children's Alliance website at www.nca-online.org.

CPT/BILLING CODES

Use E/M codes for the noncolposcopic portion of the examination.

57452   Colposcopy

ICD-10-CM DIAGNOSTIC CODES

Z04.41   Rape, alleged, observation or examination, victim or culprit
S31.40XA   Open wound vagina and vulva, initial encounter
S31.41XA   Laceration wound vagina and vulva, initial encounter
S31.42XA   Open wound, vagina and vulva with foreign body initial encounter
T74.22XA   Child sexual abuse, confirmed
T76.22XA   Child sexual abuse, suspected

RECOMMENDED READING

Adams JA, Kellogg ND, Farst KJ, et al. Updated guidelines for the medical assessment and care of children who may have been sexually abused. *J Pediatr Adolesc Gynecol.* 2015;2:81–87.
American College of Emergency Physicians. *Evaluation and Management of the Sexually Assaulted or Sexually Abused Patient.* 2nd ed. Atlanta: U.S. Department of Health and Human Services; 2013. http://bookstore.acep. org/evaluation-and-management-of-the-sexually-assaulted-or-sexually-abused-patient-314500.

Black CM, Driebe EM, Howard LA, et al. Multicenter study of nucleic acid amplification tests for detection of *Chlamydia trachomatis* and *Neisseria gonorrhoeae* in children being evaluated for sexual abuse. *Pediatr Infect Dis J.* 2009;28(7):608–613.

Berkoff MC, Zolotor AJ, Makoroff KL, et al. Has this prepubertal girl been sexually assaulted? *JAMA.* 2008;300:2779–2792.

Centers for Disease Control and Prevention. Sexually transmitted diseases treatment guidelines 2015. *MMWR.* 2015;64:1–137.

Jenny C, Crawford-Jakubiak JE, for the American Academy of Pediatrics committee on child abuse and neglect. The evaluation of children in the primary care setting when sexual abuse is suspected. *Pediatrics.* 2013;132(2):558–568.

McDonald KC. Child abuse: approach and management. *Am Fam Physician.* 2007;75:221–228.

O'Connell BJ. Evaluation of the sexually abused child, including the role of colposcopy. *J Low Genit Tract Dis.* 2001;5:87–93.

Sachs CJ, Wheeler M. Examination of the sexual assault victim. In: Roberts JR, Custalow CB, Thomsen TW, eds. *Roberts and Hedges Clinical Procedures in Emergency Medicine and Acute Care.* 7th ed. Philadelphia: Elsevier; 2019:1225–1241.

SECTION 12

Orthopedics and Sports Medicine

Section Editor: FRANCIS G. O'CONNOR

CHAPTER 171

MUSCULOSKELETAL ULTRASOUND

John Hill • Mark Lavallee • Grant C. Fowler

Ultrasound (US) has been used to assess the musculoskeletal system since the 1980s. The diagnostic and interventional aspects of this imaging modality were once the sole province of radiologists, and it was used primarily in Europe (especially the United Kingdom) and Canada for these applications. This technology was not largely embraced by radiologists in the United States because it was overshadowed by the growth of computed tomography and magnetic resonance imaging. However, additional innovations in instrumentation, advances in clinical applications, and availability of clinician training programs have led us out of the infancy of musculoskeletal ultrasound (MSK US). These technologic improvements, combined with increasing recognition of the benefits over traditional computed tomography and magnetic resonance imaging (e.g., less cost, higher patient satisfaction, ease of use, immediate results, dynamic capabilities including guiding interventions), have led to a resurgence of interest. Primary care clinicians, particularly those skilled in sports medicine, are applying their knowledge of anatomy and pathophysiology to use this diagnostic tool as an extension of the history and physical examination. Training in MSK US is now required (beginning 2016) in all accredited primary care sports medicine fellowships. The diagnostic applications for MSK US in the upper and lower extremities and for special populations, including pediatric patients, are immense. There are also a significant number of procedural applications. To cover every joint and procedural application of MSK US would be beyond the scope of this book; therefore this chapter addresses some of the more common clinical uses.

TECHNOLOGY AND TERMINOLOGY

Various terms are used to describe US equipment and images. *B-mode US* refers to brightness mode, and it allows real-time imaging. B-mode US is the precursor to grayscale US and is somewhat limited beyond differentiating fluid from solid; consequently, it has largely been replaced by *grayscale US*. Grayscale US differentiates between intensities of echoes and displays them in black, white, and various shades of gray, which improves not only the resolution of the images but also the ability to distinguish between different types of tissue. However, even grayscale US cannot differentiate between fibrous synovial tissue and active synovitis; such a differentiation requires characterization of blood flow. *Color Doppler US* uses the principle that sound waves *increase* in frequency when they reflect from objects moving *toward* the transducer and *decrease* when they reflect from objects moving *away*. This is combined with real-time imaging to indicate the presence and direction of blood flow. Red signals indicate flow toward the transducer, and blue signals indicate blood flow away from the probe (some use Blue Away, Red Toward as mnemonic). *Power Doppler US* has increased sensitivity for imaging small vessels and slow blood flow, which better demonstrates hyperemia and can help to differentiate between inflammatory (hyperemic) and scar tissue. Power Doppler US may help to visualize neovascularization or angiogenesis in inflamed or otherwise affected tissues (e.g., chronic tendinosis). Both color and power Doppler US allow one to clearly differentiate cystic lesions from vessels. (See also

Chapter 214, Emergency Department, Hospitalist, and Office Ultrasound [Clinical Ultrasound], for discussions of principles of US, beginner scanning, quality assurance, credentialing, and liability.)

MSK US should be performed with a high-resolution linear-array transducer with frequencies between 7.5 and 20 MHz. The lower frequencies allow visualization of the deeper structures (e.g., hip joint), whereas the higher frequencies are better for superficial structures (e.g., finger joints). In addition to grayscale US, machines with tissue harmonic imaging or compound imaging are useful for musculoskeletal applications. Advances in US equipment mirror changes in computer technology, and the actual machine used does not have to be the latest version. Although the newer machines have more features and are more portable, they are more expensive. To reduce startup costs, instead of purchasing a new machine, it may be possible to purchase a high-frequency linear-array transducer for a machine already owned or to purchase a used machine when someone else upgrades his or her equipment. Standoff probe attachments are available to enhance resolution in certain older equipment; they are also useful with most equipment when scanning very superficial structures.

ORIENTATION AND ANATOMY

US scans are defined by two views oriented perpendicular to one another, the *transverse/axial/short-axis view* and the *longitudinal/long-axis view* (Fig. 171.1). Long-axis images are further defined as *sagittal* or *coronal*. Understanding anatomy as viewed by US is a learned skill that takes both patience and practice to acquire. One must keep two principles in mind. First, three-dimensional structures are seen on a screen in only two dimensions. Second, a 90-degree turn of the probe will change the orientation of a two-dimensional view from axial (short axis) to longitudinal (long axis) or vice versa.

SCANNING

The position of the probe in the practitioner's hand is variable; many hold it like a large pencil or a computer mouse (Fig. 171.2). Artifact is minimized by keeping the probe as perpendicular as possible to the tissue being scanned. By convention, solid or echogenic tissue or structures are whiter on the image, whereas fluid or fluid-filled tissue or structures are darker, hypoechoic, or echolucent. Table 171.1 shows some common superficial anatomic structures seen with MSK US and the common views used to scan these structures.

INDICATIONS

See Table 171.2.

PRECAUTIONS AND CONTRAINDICATIONS

Diagnostic MSK US is a safe imaging modality with no exposure to radiation, no risks of a large magnet disrupting vascular clips, and no issues related to claustrophobia. The fact that US has been used for years

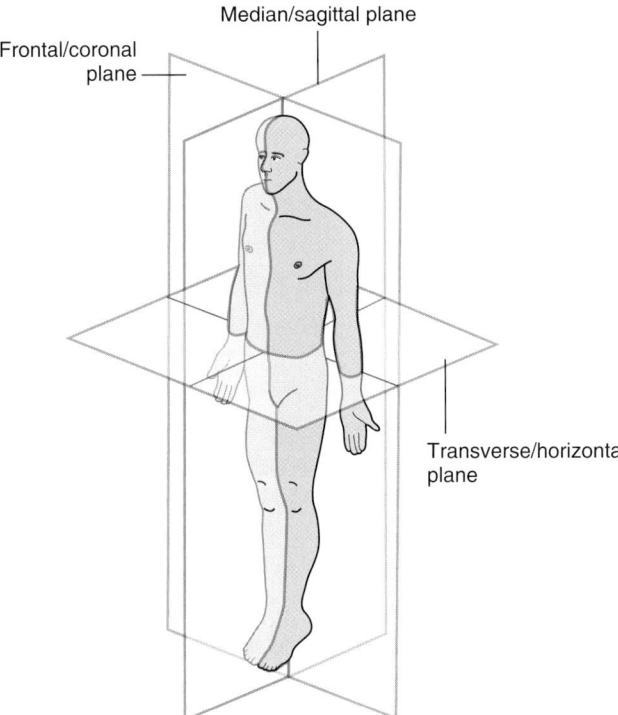

Fig. 171.1 Short-axis (transverse/axial) and long-axis (longitudinal/sagittal/coronal) views in ultrasound scanning.

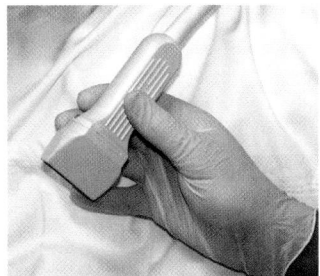

Fig. 171.2 Hand and probe position.

in maternal-fetal medicine with no documented ill effects speaks to its safety. Therefore the major precaution is related to the imaging abilities; this procedure is highly operator and interpreter dependent. The sensitivity and specificity are related to the ability to visualize the individual structures and, once these are seen, to distinguish normal from abnormal anatomy. It is quite easy to visualize and diagnose an inflamed biceps tendon; however, it can be quite difficult to differentiate between chronic hamstring inflammation and a high hamstring injury. Clinicians must know their limitations, and caution must be used to avoid scanning, diagnosing, or performing procedures beyond their skills.

Although procedures performed using US guidance are safer than blindly performing injections and aspirations, whenever a needle enters the skin there are inherent risks of pain, bleeding, infection, and damage to underlying or surrounding tissues. No absolute contraindications to MSK US exist, but similar to all procedures, using good judgment and proper techniques will protect you and your patient.

EQUIPMENT

- US machine with a high-frequency (7.5 to 20 MHz), high-resolution, linear-array transducer able to capture images (see the section on "Suppliers"). Standoff disks are available to artificially increase the transducer frequency.
- Printer paper for images.
- Ultrasonic gel.
- Towels to drape the area and for cleanup afterward.
- Equipment necessary to perform procedure such as sterilizing solution (e.g., alcohol, povidone-iodine, chlorhexidine), sterile needles, local anesthetic, or any necessary instruments.

NOTE: Linear-array transducers do have one significant limitation: they accentuate anisotropy. Anisotropy is artifact. In particular, this hypoechogenic artifact of the tendon insertions can look like a tendon tear (Fig. 171.3). It is more likely to occur when the probe is not perpendicular to structure being scanned (due to the lack of divergent beam geometry). Anisotropy can be proven to be artifact with careful scanning: rocking the probe, attempting to get perpendicular to what is being scanned, and it goes away (a tear should not disappear).

PREPROCEDURE PATIENT EDUCATION AND PREPARATION

Diagnostic US, and any possible US-guided procedure, should be briefly explained to the patient (or representative) before obtaining consent verbally and often in writing. The approximate length of time to accomplish the procedure, the few risks involved (e.g., irritation from ultrasonic gel, having to remain still during the examination, missed diagnosis), the amount of discomfort to expect from an US-directed procedure, the benefits of having this procedure, and any alternatives should be explained. For an US-guided procedure, any additional risks should be explained (e.g., risks of infection, injury to a nearby structure such as a vessel or nerve, scar formation, tendon rupture, hematoma), as well as any alternatives. Any other aspects should be addressed, depending on the practitioner's personal style (e.g., some clinicians curtail use of nonsteroidal anti-inflammatory drugs or aspirin before certain procedures [e.g., dry needling a tendon]; other clinicians use topical ethyl chloride "cold" spray before needling instead of injecting an anesthetic). The cost should also be explained, especially for Medicare patients; a Medicare waiver should be signed. There may be benefit to discussing postprocedure expectations at this point, especially those regarding activity, physical therapy, and restrictions. The patient should know that the room lights will be dimmed to improve visualization of the screen. (See the sample forms available at www.expertconsult.com for checklists for diagnostic and US-guided procedures.)

TECHNIQUE

Overall

1. There are several prerequisites essential to performing adequate MSK US; these should be ensured before scanning. Enough time should have been allocated to provide the imaging and perform the procedure (10 to 60 minutes). There must be adequate support staff, and they can help to prepare the patient (e.g., obtain informed consent, appropriately uncover the body part to be imaged), turn on the machine, and record the patient's demographic information. Often an assistant is needed to operate the machine during a procedure because the clinician's hands may be occupied with the probe and needle. Both the patient and clinician should be positioned in a manner that will be comfortable for the duration of the procedure. Any additional questions should be answered before starting the procedure.

TABLE 171.1   Common Superficial Anatomic Structures Seen with Musculoskeletal Ultrasound

Structure	Probe/Setting	Best Views	Example
Skin/integument (dermis and epidermis at *large arrow*)	Linear/high resolution/2D and Doppler	Transverse and longitudinal	
Patellar tendon (*large arrow*)	Linear/midresolution/2D	Transverse and longitudinal	
Achilles tendon (*large arrow*)	Linear/midresolution/2D	Transverse and longitudinal	
Vasculature, femoral artery in right groin (*large arrow*)	Linear/high resolution/Doppler	Transverse and longitudinal	
Supraspinatus tendon, longitudinal view (*large arrow*)	Linear/low resolution/2D	Transverse and longitudinal	

TABLE 171.1   Common Superficial Anatomic Structures Seen with Musculoskeletal Ultrasound—cont'd

Structure	Probe/Setting	Best Views	Example
Biceps tendon, axial view (large arrow)	Linear/midresolution/2D	Transverse and longitudinal	
Biceps tendinopathy, hypoechoic fluid surrounding thickened tendon (large arrow)	Linear/midresolution/2D	Longitudinal and axial	
Bursa, right subacromial (large arrow)	Linear/high resolution/2D	Transverse and longitudinal	
Muscle, pectoralis major (relaxed)	Linear/mid–low resolution/2D	Longitudinal defect in pectoralis major	
Muscle, pectoralis major (contracted)	Linear/mid–low resolution/2D	Longitudinal	
Joint capsule/synovial fluid acromioclavicular joint	Linear/high resolution/2D	Transverse and longitudinal	

Continued

TABLE 171.1	Common Superficial Anatomic Structures Seen with Musculoskeletal Ultrasound—cont'd		
Structure	**Probe/Setting**	**Best Views**	**Example**
Nerves, carpal tunnel	Linear/high resolution/2D	Transverse/axial or longitudinal	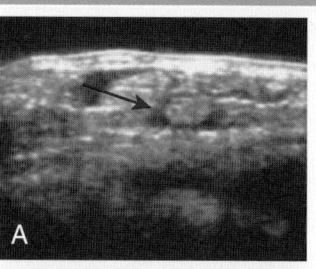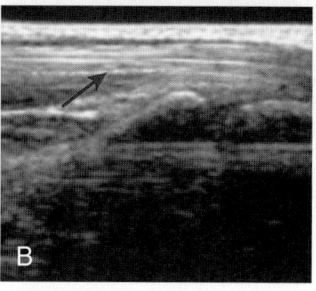

2D, Two-dimensional.

TABLE 171.2	Summary of Musculoskeletal Ultrasound Uses

Indications, Examples, and Interventional Uses of Musculoskeletal Ultrasound

General Indications	Specific Applications	Ultrasound-Guided Interventional Technique
Traumatic ligament tears	UCL sprain (skier's thumb)	Stress testing
Chronic tendon injury	Partial- vs. full-thickness rotator cuff tear	Motion testing
Calcific tendinopathy	Calcific supraspinatous	Steroid injection or needle debridement
Chronic tendinopathy	Proximal hamstring overuse	Dry needling, ABI, or PRPI
Bursitis	Trochanteric bursitis	Steroid injection
Effusion/infection	Hip effusion/septic joint	Aspiration/arthrocentesis/viscous supplementation
Cysts and masses	Popliteal cyst	Aspiration (avoiding popliteal aneurysm)
Wound/abscess management	Abscess vs. cellulitis	Abscess aspiration
Elbow pain	Lateral epicondylitis	Dry needling, ABI, or PRPI
Muscle tear versus hematoma	Quadriceps muscle tear	Hematoma aspiration
Neuropathy	Carpal tunnel syndrome	Steroid injection (avoiding nerve)
Foot/heel pain	Plantar fasciitis	Needle tenotomy/Injection

Specific Indications by Joint, Abnormality, or Procedure

Joint	Indication
Shoulder	Shoulder pain or dysfunction
Elbow, wrist and hand, hip, knee, ankle, and foot	Soft tissue injury, tendon or ligament pathology, arthritis, loose intra-articular body, soft tissue mass, nerve entrapment, joint effusion, foreign body, bone injury
Prosthetic hip	Joint effusion and extra-articular fluid collection (often for ultrasound-guided aspiration)
Foot	Morton neuroma, plantar fasciitis
Peripheral nerves	Compression neuropathies, neuritis, nerve mass, nerve trauma, nerve subluxation
Soft tissue mass	Differentiating cystic from solid mass; determining size, vascularity, margins, and relationship to adjacent structures
Soft tissue foreign body	Detection and localization of foreign body, especially nonradiopaque foreign body from wood, plastic, or certain types of glass
Interventional ultrasound/ultrasound-guided procedures	Aspiration of cysts, fluid collection or abscess; arthrocentesis or insertion of drain; injection of medication, ABI, PRPI, or contrast; ultrasound-guided biopsy or foreign body removal; lavage or aspiration of tendon calcification

ABI, Autologous blood injection; *PRPI,* platelet-rich plasma injection; *UCL, ulnocollateral* ligament.

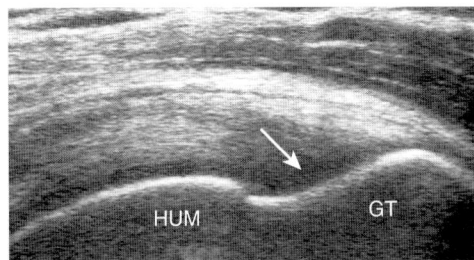

Fig. 171.3 Anisotropy *(arrow)* artifact of supraspinatus insertion on greater tuberosity *(GT)*. It appears (falsely) like a tear; scanning carefully and moving the probe to more perpendicular position should make it disappear. *HUM*, Humerus.

2. Apply ultrasonic gel to the patient's skin. If planning an US-guided percutaneous procedure, certain additional steps should be taken to minimize the risk of infection. The provider must ensure that the skin around the needle point entry is sterile throughout the procedure. There is tremendous controversy over preparation of the transducer prior to the procedure, with recommendations varying from the use of an antiseptic cleaner prior to and after each procedure, to including a sterile condom cover. Critically, the provider must know the manufacturer's recommendations to ensure not only sterility, but no harm to the probe.
   - Consider applying a sterile cover (e.g., probe condom, Tegaderm) over the probe/transducer (a sterile glove can be used). Some clinicians apply a small ribbon of gel to the probe before applying the sterile cover.
   - Cleanse the area of skin with antiseptic solution.
   - Apply to the area any of the following:
     - Sterile ultrasonic gel
     - Betadine-impregnated gel (if you are not using a disposable probe cover, this will stain the transducer)
     - Apply sterile probe to site (a sterile cover should preferably be over the probe).
3. Capture basic images (Table 171.3 shows some common sonographic pathologic findings):
   - Identify large and obvious structures first.
   - Get into the habit of viewing most structures in both transverse and longitudinal planes.
   - When needed, capture images of the area in question in both static and dynamic positions (i.e., relaxed and contracted or flexed and extended).
   - Consider using color or power Doppler to look for blood flow in low- to high-flow states to assess for inflammation or neovascularization or to differentiate between a cyst and a vessel.
   - When performing percutaneous needling (aspiration/injection or dry needling), try to obtain and document images. Because the clinician's hands will be occupied with the probe and syringe (Fig. 171.4), an assistant may be needed to run the machine.
4. Postprocedure: Once the procedure is completed, wipe the ultrasonic gel off of the patient and the probe.
   - It is important to remove the gel before it dries.
   - If a percutaneous procedure has been performed, remove and discard the sterile cover. Clean the probe head with manufacturer's approved cleaning solution.
   - If blood, body fluids, or povidone-iodine somehow gets onto the probe surface, wash it with soap and water and then follow the manufacturer's recommendation to disinfect the probe. (**NOTE:** Povidone-iodine, if allowed to stay on the probe even for a short length of time, will discolor the probe and may shorten its working life.)
   - Complete and save any documentation on the US unit and in the patient's chart.

Specific

Shoulder

1. To examine the biceps tendon, the patient's hand should be in the supine position and resting on the thigh or a pillow on the examination table with the arm slightly rotated externally. To localize the tendon, it can be scanned transversely, from where it emerges under the acromion, and followed distally to where it inserts. It runs between the lesser tuberosity (on medial side) and the greater tuberosity (on lateral side). The tendon should then be scanned longitudinally. While scanning, determine whether the tendon is properly located in the bicipital groove or if it can be subluxated or dislocated. In addition, attempt to determine whether it is torn or disrupted.
2. To scan the subscapularis tendon, the patient's elbow should be by his or her side and the arm externally rotated. The tendon should be scanned transversely and then longitudinally. The majority of subscapularis tears occur within 1 cm of its insertion onto the lesser tuberosity. It may be helpful to observe the tendon longitudinally as the patient moves the arm from externally to internally rotated. It will be the tendon moving if the probe is oriented transversely near the origin of the biceps tendon.
3. To scan the supraspinatus tendon, ask the patient to place the hand in his or her back pocket on the same side. In this position, the elbow will be flexed, the arm extended posteriorly, and the palm of the hand placed against the posterior pelvis (iliac wing). The tendon should be scanned longitudinally and then transversely. The majority of supraspinatous tears occur within 1 cm of its insertion onto the greater tuberosity. The infraspinatus tendon can be scanned with the arm in the same location. The probe can be placed anteriorly and posteriorly to get longitudinal scans of both tendons and will usually need to be angled 45 degrees to the sagittal plane, or in between the sagittal and coronal planes, to obtain good views. Transverse images are then obtained by rotating the probe 90 degrees. Sweep the transducer over the tendons laterally from the acromion to their insertion on the greater tuberosity of the humerus.
4. The arm is then returned to rest supinated on the thigh. In this position, the most posterior aspect of the infraspinatus tendon can be scanned, as well as the posterior teres minor tendon. Internal and external rotation of the arm will help identify the infraspinatus tendon. The probe will usually need to be directed inferiorly to evaluate the entire teres minor tendon.
5. Scan also the posterior aspect of the glenohumeral joint below the scapular spine, perhaps while internally and externally rotating the arm. Small joint effusions may be noted with the transducer in this position. The depth setting on the probe may need to be changed to scan deeper to obtain this image.
6. When scanning the rotator cuff tendons, comparison with the contralateral side may be useful. In addition, be on the alert for tendon calcification, bursal thickening, or loose bodies. Compression of the cuff may help to identify nonretracting tears.

Elbow

1. For scanning, the elbow is divided into anterior, posterior, medial, and lateral quadrants. The patient should be sitting or lying with the hand supine and the arm extended.
2. To scan the anterior elbow, the bicipital tendon can first be followed down to its insertion on the radial bicipital tuberosity. Next, assess the articular cartilage and cortical bone while scanning the anterior humeroradial and humeroulnar joints and the coronoid and radial fossae, both longitudinally and transversely. Also look for joint effusions, synovial thickening, or loose bodies. Note the brachialis muscle, the adjacent radial and brachial nerves and vessels, and the median nerve. While the patient is supinating and pronating the forearm, scan the annular recess of the neck of the radius.

TABLE 171.3   Common Sonographic Pathologic Findings

Diagnosis	Views Needed	Characteristics	Example
Full-thickness supraspinatus tear	Coronal, adduction, and abduction	Retraction of supraspinatus muscle, disrupted tendon	
Calcific tendinopathy of supraspinatus	Longitudinal and axial	Intense echogenic mass within tendon; shadowing below mass similar to bone shadows	
Chronic, partial-thickness supraspinatus tear	Coronal, adduction, and abduction	Hypoechoic defect within supraspinatus tendon, but no complete disruption	
Lateral epicondylitis (tennis elbow)	Longitudinal and axial	Hypoechoic (edema) and thickening within normal tendon	
Thumb, UCL partial-thickness tear (skier's thumb)	Longitudinal and stress	Hypoechoic thickened tendon with joint laxity on stress	
Soft tissue abscess	Longitudinal and axial	Hypoechoic cystic structure with bright internal echoes	
Long head of biceps tendon rupture (large arrow)	Longitudinal and axial	Tendon disrupted and hypoechoic fluid replacement within tendon sheath	

TABLE 171.3 Common Sonographic Pathologic Findings—cont'd

Diagnosis	Views Needed	Characteristics	Example
Achilles tendinosis (large arrow)	Longitudinal and axial	Thickened, mixed echogenicity of focal site within tendon	
Hematoma in muscle (large arrows)	Longitudinal and axial	Hypoechoic fluid-filled pocket within muscle	
Fracture of distal radius (large arrow)	Longitudinal	Defect in appearance of cortex ± angulation	
Ganglion cyst (large arrow)	Longitudinal and axial	Complex, multiloculated cystic structure	
Vasculature	Transverse and longitudinal	Radial artery next to ganglion cyst	
Finger/hand	Longitudinal	Hematoma on dorsum of hand	

Continued

TABLE 171.3 Common Sonographic Pathologic Findings—cont'd

Diagnosis	Views Needed	Characteristics	Example
Joint space, acromioclavicular joint	Transverse and longitudinal	Cyst Acromioclavicular joint	
Ligaments, lateral collateral	Longitudinal	Lateral collateral ligament disruption	

UCL, Ulnocollateral ligament.

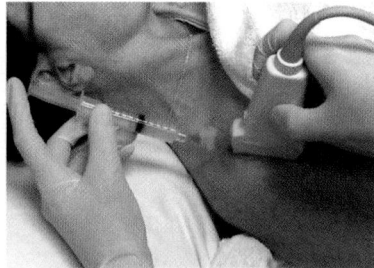

Fig. 171.4 Example of positioning for an ultrasound-guided injection.

3. To scan the lateral elbow, have the patient put both palms together if sitting; if lying, have him or her place the forearm across the abdomen. Scan the lateral epicondyle and the attachments of the common extensor tendon, extensor carpi radialis longus, and brachioradialis. The radial collateral ligament is then scanned by having the patient pronate the hand while the transducer is on the posterolateral aspect of the elbow.
4. The medial elbow is scanned with the hand in the supine position. The medial epicondyle, common flexor tendon, and ulnar collateral ligaments should be scanned in longitudinal and transverse planes. While scanning, the integrity of the ulnar collateral ligament can be tested by applying valgus stress with the elbow slightly flexed. Scan the ulnar nerve in the cubital tunnel between the olecranon process and the medial epicondyle. Test for ulnar nerve subluxation by scanning while the patient flexes and extends the elbow.
5. Scan the posterior elbow by placing the palm down on the examination table (if the patient is sitting) or by placing the forearm across the abdomen with the elbow flexed 90 degrees (if the patient is lying). Scan the posterior joint space, the triceps tendon, the olecranon process, and the olecranon bursa in both longitudinal and transverse planes.

Wrist

1. The wrist is scanned from volar, ulnar, and dorsal locations.

2. To scan the volar wrist, the hand is placed on the examination table (if the patient is sitting) or pillow (if the patient is lying) with the palm up. Slight dorsiflexion may facilitate scanning. Scan from the wrist crease distally to the thenar muscles in both longitudinal and transverse planes. Within the carpal tunnel, the flexor retinaculum, the flexor digitorum profundus, the superficialis tendons, and the adjacent flexor pollicis longus tendons should be identified. The median nerve lies superficial to these tendons but deep to the retinaculum. Flexion and extension of the fingers will demonstrate normal motion of these tendons and, to a lesser degree, the median nerve. Superficial to the retinaculum is the palmaris longus tendon. On the ulnar side of the wrist, branches of the ulnar nerve and artery lie within the Guyon canal. The flexor carpi ulnaris tendon borders the ulnar aspect of the Guyon canal. On the radial side of the wrist, the flexor carpi radialis longus tendon lies in its own canal. Whichever tendon is clinically indicated should be scanned for integrity, both longitudinally and transversely, to its site of insertion. Occult ganglion cysts can occasionally be noted originating from the radiocarpal joint capsule.
3. On the ulnar side, the triangular fibrocartilage can be scanned in its long axis by placing the transducer in a transverse position and scanning distal to the ulnar styloid. Rotating it 90 degrees allows for scanning the cartilage in short axis. The meniscus homolog lies distal to the triangular fibrocartilage and deep to the extensor carpi ulnaris longus tendon. This tendon should also be scanned for subluxation by pronating and supinating the wrist.
4. Dorsal scanning may be facilitated by placing the wrist in slight volar flexion. Structures on the dorsal wrist are very superficial, and the extensor retinaculum divides the dorsal wrist into six compartments. These compartments contain nine tendons that should be scanned longitudinally and transversely, at rest and in motion, to their point of insertion, as clinically indicated. With the transducer turned transversely, the scapholunate ligament can be scanned distal to the Lister tubercle. This is a common site for ganglion cysts and ligamen-

tous tears. Otherwise, the remaining intercarpal ligaments are not routinely assessed. With an inflammatory arthritis, the metacarpophalangeal joints and, if symptomatic, the proximal interphalangeal joints can be scanned, both longitudinally and transversely. The clinician should look for effusions, synovial hypertrophy, or bony erosion. Color and power Doppler may be useful for detecting synovial hyperemia. Because the structures on the dorsal wrist are very superficial, a standoff pad may be helpful.

Hip

1. The hip can be scanned from anterior, posterior, medial, or lateral locations. In adults, a lower-frequency probe may be necessary for adequate tissue penetration; however, use the highest-frequency probe that will allow visualization of the deeper structures.
2. To scan from the anterior location, the patient should be supine with the hip rotated slightly externally. Scan longitudinally along the femoral head and neck. Evaluate the joint for any signs of an effusion, and then evaluate the labrum, the iliopsoas tendon and bursa, and the sartorius and rectus femoris muscles. These structures should also be scanned in short-axis views. The femoral vessels can be scanned. An anterior "snapping hip" is sometimes caused by the iliopsoas muscle tendon where it passes over the superior pubic bone.
3. To scan from the lateral location, rotate the patient to the lateral decubitus position with the symptomatic side up. Scan the greater trochanter, the greater trochanteric bursa, the tensor fascia lata, and the glutei medii, maximi, and minimi, all longitudinally and then transversely. Another type of snapping hip can be diagnosed when scanning from this position if the iliotibial tract snaps when passing over the greater trochanter while the hip is being moved from extension to flexion, or vice versa.
4. To scan from the medial location, the hip is placed in the frog-leg position (externally rotated with 45 degrees of knee flexion). The abductor muscles can be scanned longitudinally, as well as the distal iliopsoas tendon, and then in their short-axis plane. The pubic bone and symphysis, as well as the distal insertion of the rectus abdominis on the pubic bone, should be scanned from this position.
5. To scan from the posterior position, the patient should be turned to the prone position with the leg extended slightly. The glutei, hamstrings, and sciatic nerve can be scanned longitudinally and then transversely. The glutei can be scanned from origin to insertion on the greater trochanter (minimus and medius) or linea aspera (maximus). The sciatic nerve can be followed from its exit under the greater sciatic foramen, deep to the gluteus maximus muscle, and then distally to where it lies superficial to the quadratus femoris muscle. Along its course, it lies midway between the ischial tuberosity and the greater trochanter. It should be scanned both longitudinally and transversely.
6. The prosthetic hip is typically scanned for the presence of an effusion or extra-articular fluid collection. It is usually scanned from the anterior or lateral location, as described previously, and effusions are usually located at the prosthesis-bone junction. Any effusions should be measured and documented. The greater trochanteric and iliopsoas bursae should also be scanned for the presence of fluid.

Knee

1. The knee is also divided into anterior, medial, lateral, and posterior quadrants when scanning.
2. To scan the anterior knee, the patient is usually supine with the knee flexed 30 degrees. Longitudinal and transverse scans are obtained of the quadriceps and patellar tendons, the patellar retinacula, and the suprapatellar recess. The prepatellar, superficial, and infrapatellar bursae should also be evaluated. The patella can be scanned for occult injury if clinically indicated. With the knee in maximal flexion and the transducer in the transverse plane,

the suprapatellar recess can be scanned and the distal femoral cartilage assessed. This cartilage can also be assessed using longitudinal scans over the medial and lateral condyles, if indicated. While maintaining the knee in maximal flexion, the distal anterior cruciate ligament can be followed longitudinally with the probe to its insertion into the anteromedial tibial plateau.
3. To scan the medial knee, the patient remains supine with the knee slightly flexed and the hip slightly externally rotated. Alternatively, the patient can be in the lateral decubitus position with the affected knee located inferiorly. Scan the medial joint space in both longitudinal and transverse planes. The medial collateral ligament, the pes anserine tendons and bursa, and the medial patellar retinaculum should be evaluated. The anterior body and horn of the medial meniscus can be scanned from this position, possibly facilitated by the application of some valgus stress.
4. To scan the lateral knee, the patient may remain supine with the ipsilateral leg internally rotated or in the lateral decubitus position with the affected knee located superiorly. Placing a pillow between the knees may increase patient comfort. Scanning longitudinally and transversely, and moving from posterior to anterior, the popliteus tendon, fibular collateral ligament, iliotibial band, and bursa should be evaluated. The lateral patellar retinaculum can also be assessed from this location. The lateral meniscus can be evaluated by scanning in the joint line.
5. The posterior knee is scanned with the patient lying prone and the leg slightly extended. Scanning both longitudinally and transversely, the popliteal fossa and the semimembranosus and medial and lateral gastrocnemius muscles, tendons, and bursae can be assessed. The posterior horns of both menisci can be assessed by scanning transversely from this location, and the posterior cruciate ligament can be followed longitudinally. The superior aspect of the anterior cruciate ligament can be assessed somewhat when scanning transversely in the intercondylar region. To confirm a popliteal cyst, it should be demonstrated to originate from the posterior joint capsule between the medial head of the gastrocnemius tendon and the semimembranosus tendon when scanning transversely.

Ankle

1. The ankle is divided into the anterior, medial, lateral, and posterior quadrants.
2. To scan the anterior quadrant, the patient lies supine with the knee flexed and the foot flat on the examination table. From medial to lateral, the tibialis anterior, extensor hallucis longus, extensor digitorum longus, and peroneus tertius (occasionally congenitally absent) tendons are scanned in longitudinal and transverse planes. They should be followed from their musculotendinous origins to their distal insertions. The anterior joint recess is scanned for effusions, loose bodies, and synovial thickening. It may need to be compared with the contralateral side joint recess. The anterior joint capsule is attached to the anterior tibial margin, superiorly, and the neck of the talus, inferiorly. The cartilage of the talus appears as a thin, hypoechoic line. Assess the anterior tibiofibular ligament by moving the transducer over the distal tibia and fibula, superior and medial to the lateral malleolus, and scanning in an oblique transverse plane.
3. The medial ankle can be scanned with the patient in the same position. Scanning from anterior to posterior with the transducer in the transverse position, the posterior tibial, flexor digitorum longus, and flexor hallucis longus tendons can be located proximal to the medial malleolus. They can then be scanned transversely and longitudinally from their muscle of origin above the malleolus to their distal insertions. The probe angle may need to be varied to follow the tendon around the medial malleolus. The tibial nerve can then be identified at the level of the malleolus where it travels between the tendons of the flexor digitorum, anteriorly, and flexor hallucis longus, posterior to it. The nerve can be followed proximally and distally. The flexor hallucis longus

can also be scanned in the posterior position, where it lies medial to the Achilles tendon. The deltoid ligament is then scanned longitudinally from the medial malleolus to its attachments on the navicular, talus, and calcaneus bones.

4. The ankle is scanned from the lateral location with the patient in the same position. Slight inversion of the foot may facilitate scanning. Scanning transversely, proximal to the lateral malleolus, the peroneus brevis and longus tendons are usually easy to identify. They can then be scanned transversely and longitudinally from their proximal muscle of origin to their distal insertion. The peroneus longus tendon can be followed to the cuboid groove, where it turns to course medially along the plantar aspect of the foot to insert at the base of the first metatarsal and medial cuneiform. The peroneus brevis tendon is followed to its insertion on the base of the fifth metatarsal. These tendons should be assessed for subluxation by scanning while dorsiflexing and everting the foot. The lateral ligament complex is then assessed by placing the transducer on the tip of the lateral malleolus. From this position, the transducer will need to be turned out of the strict sagittal plane to scan and follow the anterior and posterior talofibular and calcaneofibular ligaments longitudinally.

5. The posterior ankle is scanned with the patient supine and the foot extended over the end of the examination table. Scan the Achilles tendon longitudinally and transversely from its origin, the medial and lateral heads of the gastrocnemius and soleus muscles, to its insertion on the posterior surface of the calcaneus. Plantar flexion and dorsiflexion of the foot while scanning may assist in the diagnosis of a tear. Along the medial aspect of the Achilles, the plantaris tendon may be noted to insert on the posteromedial calcaneus. Although absence of this tendon may be a normal variant, it often remains intact despite a full-thickness Achilles tendon tear. The retrocalcaneal bursa deep to the Achilles tendon can also be scanned. The plantar fascia should be scanned transversely and longitudinally from its origin on the medial calcaneal tubercle to where it divides distally and merges with soft tissue.

Foot

1. Similar to the hand, in patients with inflammatory arthritis, the metatarsophalangeal joints can be scanned, as well as the proximal interphalangeal joints if symptomatic, looking for effusions, synovial hypertrophy or hyperemia, or bony erosions. These joints, as well as any other symptomatic joints in the foot, should be scanned longitudinally and transversely. They can be scanned from dorsal or plantar locations.

2. The interdigital spaces of the foot can be scanned from either dorsal or plantar locations. Starting at the level of the first interdigital space, with the transducer in the longitudinal orientation, the interdigital spaces are scanned while moving the transducer laterally. The same areas should also be scanned transversely. The intermetatarsal bursa lies on the dorsal aspect of the interdigital nerve, so care must be taken to differentiate it from a Morton neuroma. Pressure can be applied to reproduce the symptoms with a Morton neuroma.

Peripheral Nerves

1. Common peripheral nerve problems include entrapment and subluxation. The most common locations for entrapment are within fibro-osseous tunnels such as the cubital or Guyon tunnel for the ulnar nerve, the carpal tunnel for the median nerve, the tarsal tunnel for the tibial nerve, or the tunnel formed by the fibular neck and the common peroneal nerve. The most common subluxating nerve is the ulnar nerve in the cubital tunnel.

2. Nerves course adjacent to tendons and vessels, and Doppler US can be used to distinguish them from vessels. Tendons can be distinguished by the fact that they move much more readily than nerves with flexion or extension of the nearest joint. Surrounded longitudinally by hyperechoic fascicles, nerves are usually hypo-

echoic and may be interspersed with hyperechoic endoneurium or further surrounded by hyperechoic epineurium. It may be easier to follow the course of a nerve and to differentiate it from nearby tendons by scanning transversely, at first, and then scanning longitudinally.

3. For an entrapment neuropathy, after locating the nerve in the tunnel, nearby tissues (e.g., tendons, soft tissue, bones) should be scanned in an attempt to identify the source of entrapment. US features suggesting potential entrapment include hypoechoic swelling of the involved nerve at the entrapment site and compression distally. Many times, direct transducer pressure (sonopalpation) on the affected nerve reproduces the patient's symptoms.

4. A statically dislocated nerve is usually readily identified with US; however, an intermittently subluxating nerve may need to be imaged during flexion or extension of a nearby joint.

Soft Tissue Masses

A soft tissue mass should be scanned longitudinally and transversely and diameters measured in three planes. Cysts should be differentiated from solid masses, and nearby structures should be determined, particularly neurovascular bundles, bones, tendons, and joints. Compressibility of the mass should be determined. Vascularity can be evaluated using Doppler.

Foreign Bodies

When scanning a foreign body, the approximate size, location, and nearby structures should be determined. Most foreign bodies larger than a certain diameter (depending on the frequency and quality of the probe) will cast an acoustic shadow or a comet tail artifact. A standoff pad may be needed for the probe to scan very superficial foreign bodies in subcutaneous tissues. (See also Chapter 214, Emergency Department, Hospitalist, and Office Ultrasound [Clinical Ultrasound].)

Interventional Ultrasound

1. US provides direct visualization of the needle pathway, and if the probe is equipped with a needle guide, it may provide direct visualization of the needle and show the position of the needle as it enters the target area.

2. Nearby structures should be evaluated, in an attempt to avoid them, and the shortest pathway to the interventional site is usually determined. For US-guided biopsy, focal areas of vascularity may indicate viable tissue.

3. US-guided procedures can be performed either statically or in real time. For statically guided interventions, the insertion site, angle, and depth are initially identified with US and then the probe is laid aside while the procedure is performed. For real-time guidance, the procedure is performed with simultaneous US imaging. Either a one-person or two-person technique can be used for US-guided procedures. (See also Chapter 214, Emergency Department, Hospitalist, and Office Ultrasound [Clinical Ultrasound].)

SAMPLE OPERATIVE REPORT

Diagnostic: Patient (or patient's proxy) was informed about the protocol and the risks of having a diagnostic US. Written informed consent was obtained. Longitudinal and axial views were captured, reviewed, measured, and archived. Doppler US views were also obtained and the following vascular structures were identified. The following anatomic structures were seen via US, and noted caliper measurements were archived. Images of the area in question were viewed both in a relaxed (or static) phase and also in a contracted (or dynamic) phase, captured, and archived. No complications were noted from this scan, and the patient tolerated the procedure well. Results were explained to the patient before discharge from the office. (Finally, the impression should state a defined diagnosis, and the plan should include any pertinent instructions.)

TABLE 171.4	Additional Documentation Needed for Percutaneous Needling Procedure		
Aspiration	**Cortisone**	**PRP/Autologous Blood**	**Dry Needling**
Anesthetic and amount	Anesthetic and amount	Anesthetic and amount	Anesthetic and amount
Gauge needle	Gauge needle	Gauge needle	Gauge needle
Amount of fluid removed	Amount/type of steroid	Location of blood/plasma	Amount of needling
Description of fluid		Amount injected	
Fluid sent for analysis?		Amount of needling	

PRP, Platelet-rich plasma.

Percutaneous needling: Patient (or patient's proxy) was informed verbally about the protocol and the risks of having this procedure performed, as well as having a diagnostic US. Written informed consent was obtained. Topical ethyl fluoride or local lidocaine was used for anesthesia. Normal sterile preparation of both patient and equipment was done using antiseptic solutions and sterile barrier devices. Prepercutaneous and postpercutaneous images were reviewed, measured, and archived. Images of the needle in the appropriate location were viewed and documented (Table 171.4).

There were no complications, adverse reactions, or premature termination of this procedure. (Finally, the impression should state a defined diagnosis and the result of the procedure, and the plan should include any pertinent instructions.)

NOTE: Images should be saved when billing for an US-guided procedure.

COMMON ERRORS

MSK US is often considered the most operator-dependent imaging technique available. In other words, the most common errors in using this tool are using it incorrectly and incorrectly interpreting the images. In Europe, standardized training courses are available, taught by experienced sonographers, and a set preceptorship period is established after the introductory course. At the conclusion of training, individuals are assessed on their ability to make US diagnoses; thus interoperator variability is minimized. Standardized teaching methods are lacking in the United States; however, it will now be part of all primary care sports medicine fellowships. The American Institute of Ultrasound in Medicine has a set of practice guidelines for the performance of MSK US. These guidelines have been developed to provide practitioners with the minimum requirements for performing diagnostic procedures. Although it is not possible to detect every abnormality, by using a standardized approach one can maximize the ability to detect most problems. These guidelines specifically address examinations of the shoulder, elbow, wrist, hand, hip, knee, ankle, foot, peripheral nerves, and soft tissue masses, as well as the performance of interventional MSK US.

To avoid obvious errors, general scanning principles should be followed that require axial/transverse and longitudinal views of each structure. In an axial scan, one might see a structure that looks like a fluid-filled cyst; however, in the longitudinal image it will be obvious that the structure is in fact a vessel. A full understanding of the underlying anatomy and common abnormalities that might be relevant will increase the operator's scanning sensitivity and accuracy. Attempt to hold the probe perpendicular to structures being scanned to minimize anisotropy artifact.

COMPLICATIONS

US is generally a safe procedure; the main complication is misdiagnosis. If, when evaluating a shoulder injury, an acute full-thickness supraspinatus tendon tear is missed, surgery could be delayed, which could ultimately lead to a less-than-ideal outcome. If performing a US-guided injection, one must follow the usual standards for all interventional procedures: appropriate consent, sterile technique, and, to avoid damage to nerves and vessels, proper positioning of the needle.

POSTPROCEDURE MANAGEMENT AND PATIENT EDUCATION

The patient should be repositioned into a comfortable position and the results of the US examination explained. At this point, some clinicians review the images with their patients. Future patient care management should also be discussed based on the results.

If a US-guided procedure was performed, the postprocedure plan should be reviewed with the patient. The patient should know to watch for signs of infection, increasing pain or swelling, or fever and know how to reaccess medical personnel if necessary. After aspiration, the patient should know to watch for reaccumulation of aspirated fluid. A pressure dressing for 1 to 3 days may prevent this. Depending on the clinician, restrictive dressings, bracing, immobilizers, sterile bandages, and limits on bathing or activity may be recommended. These are best communicated in writing and shared with the patient and his or her responsible friend or family member. Certain procedures may benefit from a 24 to 48 hours' postprocedure check in the office to assess for pain control, development of a hematoma, or signs of infection. As with many procedures in musculoskeletal medicine, certain home exercises and formal physical therapy protocols may be initiated depending on the clinician's personal protocol. Discuss with patients how to control their pain and give them appropriate medications. Many clinicians now avoid nonsteroidal antiinflammatory drugs or aspirin in the postprocedure phase because of their antiplatelet effects and inhibition of the normal physiologic inflammatory cycle.

Specific instructions may be warranted with certain procedures:

Injection: Look for local reaction to the injected substance (e.g., cortisone, lidocaine, autologous blood, platelet-rich plasma) or development of a hematoma. A pressure dressing for 1 to 3 days may prevent this. Restrictions and expectations should be discussed.

Dry needling and tenotomy: Look for excessive swelling or new-onset hematoma. A pressure dressing for 1 to 3 days may prevent this. Sometimes elevation of the limb, compression dressing, and ice may be needed post procedure. Limited, short-term extremity immobilization is often recommended when extensive needling is done, to protect against tendon/ligament rupture. The role of physical therapy is crucial when dealing with long-standing injuries that have had needling. Restrictions and expectations should be discussed.

INTERPRETATION AND RESULTS

See Table 171.3.

CPT/BILLING CODES

20550	Injection, single tendon sheath, or ligament
20551	Injection, single tendon origin/insertion
20552	Injection(s), single or multiple trigger point(s), one or two muscles
20553	Injection(s), single or multiple trigger point(s), three or more muscles
27096	Injection into sacroiliac joint

76880   Diagnostic ultrasound examination of extremity, nonvascular, including image documentation

76942   Ultrasound-guided biopsy, aspiration, injection, localization device

93922   Color or spectral waveform Doppler of upper or lower extremity arteries, single level

Modifiers

25   To be used with separate Evaluation and Management (E&M) code
50   Bilateral procedures
51   Multiple procedures

Coding Example

If a patient is referred from another clinician for consultation on shoulder pain, you can bill for an office consultation (99243, although Medicare abandoned this code in 2010, some Medicaid and managed care plans still reimburse) or an E&M code (99202 or 99213) for the initial evaluation. If it is determined that you need, on another date, to perform a diagnostic MSK US (76880), you can bill for this. If you then determine the patient has a long head of the biceps tendinopathy and would benefit from an US-guided injection of the tendon sheath, then you can add 76942 and 20550 to your procedures and use the modifier 51 for more than one procedure performed on the same date.

76881   Ultrasound, extremity, nonvascular, real-time with image documentation; complete
76882   Ultrasound, extremity, nonvascular, real-time with image documentation; limited
76942   Ultrasonic guidance for needle placement (e.g., biopsy, aspiration, injection, localization device), imaging supervision and interpretation

Procedures that may be ultrasound guided (report 76942 in addition):

20526   Injection, therapeutic (e.g., local anesthetic, corticosteroid), carpal tunnel
20527   Injection, enzyme (e.g., collagenase) palmar fascial cord (Dupuytren cord) post enzyme injection
20550   Injection(s) single tendon sheath, or ligament, aponeurosis (e.g., plantar "fascia")
20551   Injection(s) single tendon sheath, or ligament, aponeurosis (e.g., plantar "fascia") single tendon origin/insertion
20552   Injection(s), single to multiple trigger point(s) one or two muscle(s)
20553   Injection(s), single to multiple trigger point(s) three or more muscle(s)
20612   Aspiration and/or injection of ganglion(s) cyst any location

Procedures that include ultrasound guidance (do not report 76942 in addition):

10022   Fine-needle aspiration; with imaging guidance
20604   Arthrocentesis, aspiration and/or injection; small joint or bursa (e.g., fingers, toes) with ultrasound guidance, with permanent recording and reporting
20606   Arthrocentesis, aspiration and/or injection; intermediate joint or bursa (e.g., temporomandibular, acromioclavicular, wrist, elbow or ankle, olecranon bursa) with ultrasound guidance, with permanent recording and reporting
20611   Arthrocentesis, aspiration and/or injection; major joint or bursa (e.g., shoulder, hip, knee joint, subacromial bursa) with ultrasound guidance, with permanent recording and reporting

ICD-10-CM DIAGNOSTIC CODES

G56.01   Carpal tunnel syndrome right upper limb
G56.02   Carpal tunnel syndrome left upper limb
G56.21   Cubital tunnel syndrome right upper limb
G56.22   Cubital tunnel syndrome left upper limb
G57.51   Tarsal tunnel syndrome right lower limb
G57.52   Tarsal tunnel syndrome left lower limb
G57.61   Morton neuroma right lower limb
G57.62   Morton neuroma left lower limb
G58.8   Mononeuritis of unspecified site (e.g., compression neuropathy)
L03.90   Other cellulitis and abscess, unspecified site
M24.10   Articular cartilage disorder, site unspecified
M24.00   Loose body in joint, site unspecified
M25.40   Effusion of joint, site unspecified
M25.50   Pain in joint, site unspecified
R29.898   Other symptoms referable to joint, site unspecified (e.g., snapping hip)
M77.9   Enthesopathy unspecified
M71.811   Other specified bursopathies right shoulder
M71.812   Other specified bursopathies left shoulder
M70.21   Olecranon bursitis right elbow
M70.22   Olecranon bursitis left elbow
M70.41   Prepatellar bursitis right knee
M70.42   Prepatellar bursitis left knee
M76.891   Enthesopathy of right lower extremity
M76.892   Enthesopathy of left lower extremity
M67.40   Ganglion of joint or tendon sheath unspecified
M71.21   Baker cyst right knee
M71.22   Baker cyst left knee
M66.9   Nontraumatic rupture of unspecified tendon
M75.121   Complete rupture of rotator cuff right shoulder non-traumatic
M75.122   Complete rupture of rotator cuff left shoulder non-traumatic
M66.821   Spontaneous rupture of tendon right biceps
M66.822   Spontaneous rupture of tendon left biceps
M66.241   Spontaneous rupture of extensor tendons of right hand and wrist
M66.242   Spontaneous rupture of extensor tendons of left hand and wrist
M66.341   Spontaneous rupture of flexor tendons of right hand and wrist
M66.342   Spontaneous rupture of flexor tendons of left hand and wrist
M66.251   Spontaneous rupture of right quadriceps tendon
M66.252   Spontaneous rupture of left quadriceps tendon
M66.261   Spontaneous rupture extensor tendon right lower leg
M66.262   Spontaneous rupture extensor tendon left lower leg
M66.361   Spontaneous rupture right Achilles tendon
M66.362   Spontaneous rupture left Achilles tendon
M67.01   Short Achilles tendon right ankle
M67.02   Short Achilles tendon left ankle
M71.40   Calcium deposits bursa unspecified
M65.20   Calcific tendinitis, unspecified site
M24.20   Disorder ligament unspecified site
M35.7   Hypermobility syndrome
M62.10   Rupture of muscle, nontraumatic, unspecified site
M79.5   Residual foreign body in soft tissue
M79.89   Swelling of limb

SUPPLIERS

(See contact information available at www.expertconsult.com.)

General Electric Medical Systems (including handheld Vscan)
Mindray Medical International
MySono/SamsungMedison/Sonoace America

Siemens/Acuson
SonoSite
Sonoscape USA
Toshiba America

ONLINE RESOURCES

American Institute of Ultrasound in Medicine: www.aium.org
European Society of Musculoskeletal Radiology Technical Guidelines. Ankle: https://essr.org/content-essr/uploads/2016/10/ankle.pdf. Elbow: https://essr.org/content-essr/uploads/2016/10/elbow.pdf. Hip: https://essr.org/content-essr/uploads/2016/10/hip.pdf. Shoulder: https://essr.org/content-essr/uploads/2016/10/shoulder.pdf. Wrist: https://essr.org/content-essr/uploads/2016/10/wrist.pdf
Sonosite Institute (online training modules): www.sonositeinstitute.com/

RECOMMENDED READING

American Institute of Ultrasound Medicine (AIUM). *AIUM Practice Parameter for the Performance of a Musculoskeletal Ultrasound Examination.* American Institute of Ultrasound in Medicine; 2012. www.amssm.org/Content/pdf%20files/AIUM_Practice_Parameter_Preform_MSKUS.pdf. Accessed February 6, 2017.
Bianchi S, Martinoli C. *Ultrasound of the Musculoskeletal System.* New York: Springer; 2007.

Bryun GAW. Musculoskeletal ultrasonography: nomenclature, technical considerations, validation, and standardization. In: Shmerling RH, ed. *UpToDate.* 2015. Waltham, MA. www.uptodate.com.
Bryun GAW. Musculoskeletal ultrasonography: guided injection and aspiration of joints and related structures. In: Shmerling RH, ed. *UpToDate.* 2015. Waltham, MA. www.uptodate.com.
Finnoff JT, Hall MM, Adams E, et al. American Medical Society for Sports Medicine: American Medical Society for Sports Medicine position statement: interventional musculoskeletal ultrasound in sports medicine. *Clin J Sport Med.* 2015;25(1):6–22.
Jacobson JA. *Fundamentals of Musculoskeletal Ultrasound.* 2nd ed. Philadelphia: Elsevier; 2013.
McNally EG. *Practical Musculoskeletal Ultrasound.* 2nd ed. Philadelphia: Churchill Livingstone; 2014.

CHAPTER 172

EXTENSOR TENDON REPAIR

David T. Bortel

The superficial location of extensor tendons makes them very vulnerable to trauma; consequently, acute extensor tendon injuries are common. Fortunately, with the proper equipment, most such injuries can be addressed as an outpatient procedure in an acute care setting. The specialized elastic fatty tissue that allows tendons to glide over the hand, forearm, or dorsum of the foot is called *paratenon*. This vascularized, filmy connective tissue envelops the extensor tendon and does not readily separate when lacerated. Fortunately, this makes these injuries more amenable to repair with less need for significant dissection compared with flexor tendons. However, the practitioner should not ignore the complexity of the extensor mechanism. In the hand, most experts consider finger extension to be more of an intricate act than that of finger flexion. To extend a finger requires the use of two separate and neurologically independent (yet interdependent) systems: the extrinsic extensor system, originating from the forearm and innervated by the radial nerve, and the intrinsic extensor system, originating in the hand and innervated by the median and ulnar nerves (Fig. 172.1).

For years, extensor injuries have been classified by zones of injury (Kleinert zones; Fig. 172.2), with each zone having unique injury patterns and different modes of treatment. Greater than 50% of extensor tendon injuries are accompanied by another injury (e.g., fracture, dislocation/ligamentous injury, capsular damage, or flexor tendon injury).

PRINCIPLES

Penetrating trauma to the dorsum of the hand first needs to be examined carefully for any loss of the neurovascular status or motor/tendon function. The wound should then be anesthetized and explored to visualize the potentially involved tendon; the wound should be extended, if necessary, to understand the characteristics of the specific injury (Fig. 172.3). When a tendon is completely transected, the cut ends can retract a considerable distance. Because a partial tendon laceration might appear to have full function on examination, the wound must be evaluated judiciously. Unrepaired partial tendon lacerations can result in delayed rupture one to several days after the initial injury. Observe the entire tendon complex through the full range of motion at the injury location; its function should be compared with that of the unaffected same finger on the opposite hand. Most practitioners believe a repair is warranted if 50% or more cross-sectional damage has occurred. After closure, a tendon repair must have healthy padded skin over it to retain viability, or tissue grafting will be necessary. Wounds older than 6 to 8 hours need aggressive cleansing; the clinician should also consider leaving the wound open for a later staged irrigation or debridement and subsequent closure. During this interval, exposed bone, joint, and tendon tissue should be loosely covered with native tissue or a damp sterile gauze followed by a bulky dressing and an anterior-posterior splint, extending from fingertip to forearm. With such protection in place, tendon repair may be delayed up to 7 days.

A repaired tendon develops a fibroblastic bulbous connection during the first 2 weeks. Tendon collagen usually does not begin to form until the third week. At the end of the fourth week, swelling and vascularity will decrease. Once the junction becomes strong, the tendon can tolerate active gliding; therefore physical therapy and rehabilitation can be initiated. Knowledge of appropriate splinting and necessary therapy is essential when caring for these injuries. Repaired tendons should usually be immobilized to promote healing and to prevent tendon rupture. After hand extensor tendon repair, the splint typically can be placed on the dorsal surface from the forearm to the fingertips to protect and prevent active extension. The digits and wrist may be slightly flexed within the tolerances of the splint. These joints must be protected against flexion when changing dressings or splints. After a 3-week period of immobilization, depending on the particular circumstances, passive motion can generally be initiated under the guidance of a skilled hand therapist. Reasonable strength may return to this repaired tendon as early as 6 weeks after the injury, again depending on the patient's reliability and health status (e.g., neurologic status, tobacco use, metabolic and rheumatologic issues). Protected, nonloaded motion with a dynamic splint under the supervision of a hand therapist is increasingly chosen for postoperative care.

The vast majority of flexor tendon injuries should be treated by a clinician trained to repair them in an appropriate surgical suite. In particular, flexor tendon injuries located in "no-man's land" (between the proximal palmar crease and the proximal interphalangeal [PIP] joint) are a significant challenge. Results of tendon repair are consistently better when fixed primarily (within 7 days) rather than secondarily (after 7 days or delayed). Familiarity with the sources referenced is encouraged if managing tendon injuries (Cannon, 2017; Colzani and colleagues, 2016; Harper and colleagues, 2013; Strauch, 2017).

CONTRAINDICATIONS

- Less than 50% of the extensor tendon is lacerated, and the finger functions as well as the same finger on the unaffected opposite hand.
- Clinician is unfamiliar with the anatomy of the hand or lacks the skills necessary for these repairs (in this situation, the wound should be loosely closed, the hand splinted, and the patient referred).
- There is an open joint space, a bony fracture, or inadequate soft tissue or skin to cover the defect or the subsequent repair (generally in this situation, the wound should be loosely closed, the hand splinted, and the patient referred).
- By zone (see Fig. 172.2)
  - Zone I open laceration: extensor tendon remnants are too short to repair.
  - Zone II (except in the thumb), III: extensor tendon remnants are usually too thin to repair.
  - Zones IV, V, and VI: consider referral if tendon laceration has actual or potential joint or lateral band involvement.

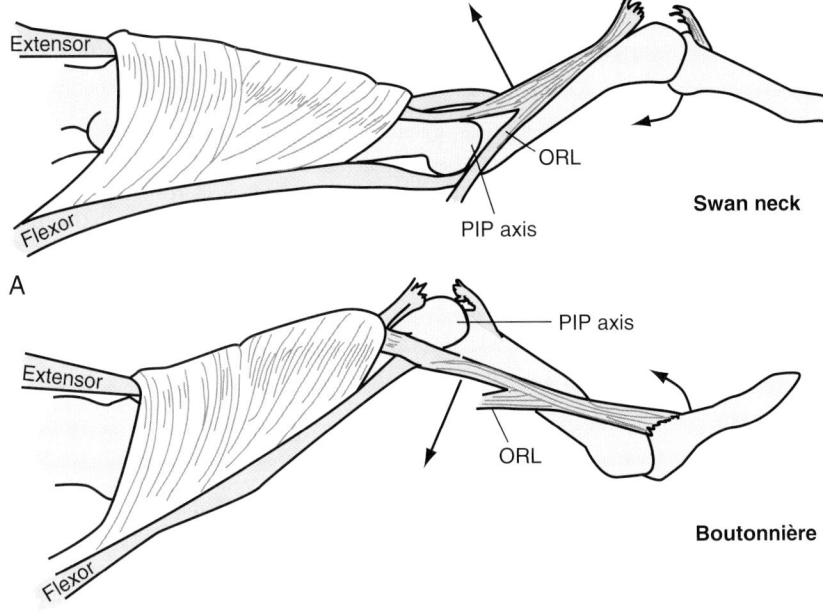

Fig. 172.1 Note the intimate working relationship of the intrinsic and extrinsic extensor mechanisms. (Note that the flexor is not shown.) (A) Mallet finger (zone I injury) that has resulted in a swan neck deformity because the oblique retinacular ligament (ORL), also known as the conjoined lateral bands, has subluxated dorsal to the axis of rotation at the level of the proximal interphalangeal (PIP) joint. (B) A zone III injury allows the ORL to subluxate volar to the axis of rotation at the PIP joint, resulting in a boutonnière deformity.

- Zone VII: consider referral if there is actual or potential extensor retinaculum involvement.
- Zone VIII: consider referral if there is actual or potential need for tendon transfer.

In these situations requiring referral, the wound should be loosely closed, the hand splinted, and the patient referred.

EQUIPMENT

- Surgical prep solution (e.g., povidone-iodine, chlorhexidine; from hand to elbow with particularly thorough cleansing of the contaminated tissues)
- Ruler marked in centimeters
- Irrigation device for contaminated wounds: 30-mL syringe with 18-gauge angiocatheter or commercially manufactured splash shield device (see Chapter 19, Laceration and Incision Repair, Fig. 19.1) and sterile saline
- Appropriate anesthetic (see Chapter 5, Local Anesthesia, and Chapter 7, Peripheral Nerve Blocks and Field Blocks)
- 3- to 20-mL syringe
- 27-gauge, 1.25-inch needle (small-gauge needles are preferred to administer anesthesia)
- Additional 27-gauge, 1.5-inch needles (useful to pierce and stabilize tendon end; optional)
- Sterile drapes; fenestrated drape applied over the lesion; appropriate larger barrier as indicated
- 4 × 4 gauze sponges; sterile cotton-tipped applicators are also useful
- Sterile pack containing 4.5-inch needle holder; curved dissecting scissors; one or more mosquito hemostats; suture scissors; Adson forceps with and without teeth; skin hooks; small self-retaining retractor (e.g., Alm, Holzheimer, Weitlaner)
- Additional small (micro) instruments (may be helpful depending on the size of structures)
- No. 15 blade for excisions or wound lengthening with blade handle (or single disposable scalpel)
- Pack of folded sterile towels for patient arm positioning and clinician wrist support
- Appropriate suture: usually a 4-0 braided, nonabsorbable suture such as Tycron, Mersilene, or Ethibond for the tendon; a fine monofilament (e.g., 5-0 to 7-0 nylon) suture for closing the epi-

tenon (see following text for specifics); also a monofilament (e.g., 4-0 to 5-0 nylon) suture for closing the skin (see Chapter 21, Laceration and Incision Repair: Suture Selection)
- Allis forceps for removal of deeper masses (optional)
- Skin-marking pen
- Electrocautery unit
- Specimen jar (if necessary)
- Sterile gloves
- Mask
- Protective glasses with shield
- Sterile gown
- Arm board
- Mayo or instrument holding stand draped in a sterile manner
- 0.25-inch Penrose drain (to tag and protect critical structures)
- Appropriate finger or arm tourniquet (with routine use precautions; the maximum time for tourniquet application is generally 2 hours)
- Comfortable chair
- Operative microscope or magnifying loupes, particularly if considering neurovascular repair (optional)

Suture Material Considerations

Suture preferences can be quite variable among clinicians who perform tendon repairs. Currently, experienced clinicians usually choose nonabsorbable suture. (Absorbable materials such as Vicryl can precipitate an inflammatory response, which might lead to excessive tendon adhesion formation. Furthermore, an absorbable suture tends to break down while the tendon is very weakened and prone to failure.) If the tendon is of sufficient size with a transected pattern, most clinicians will place one or two "core sutures" using a braided, nonabsorbable material such as Tycron, Mersilene, or Ethibond (usually 4-0 is a good size for the repair, depending on the tendon size). If a running or interrupted epitenon repair is performed, ideally a fine monofilament material is implemented. This commonly will range from a 5-0 to a 7-0, with nylon being a frequently used material. Other suture material can be considered, depending on the clinician's preference and experience. Appropriate suture for the wound closure will also be needed (see Chapter 21, Laceration and Incision Repair: Suture Selection).

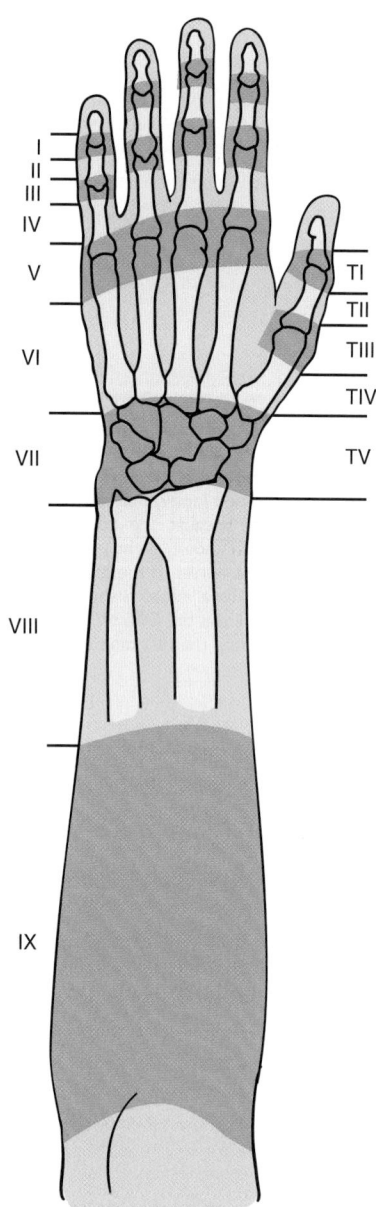

Fig. 172.2 Zones of extensor injury (Kleinert zones). The extensor mechanism can be injured from the fingertip to the proximal forearm. Corresponding zones in the thumb are referred to as "T" plus the zone number.

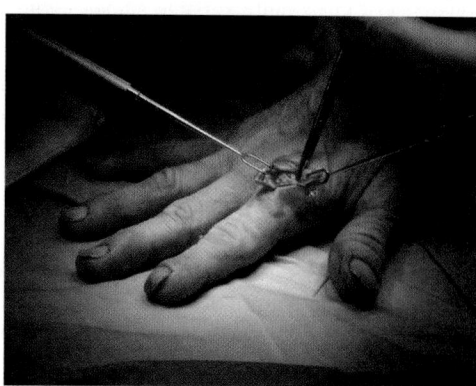

Fig. 172.3 Exploration of an extensor tendon injury over the metacarpophalangeal joint with wound extension for appropriate visualization. (Courtesy John Lubahn, MD.)

PREPROCEDURE PATIENT PREPARATION

The risks, benefits, alternatives, and actual procedure should be explained to the patient. Informed consent should be obtained. If irrigation is necessary, this should be explained to the patient, as well as the fact that he or she may feel some discomfort when the local anesthetic is being injected. Patients should understand the importance of remaining still during the procedure. They should be placed in a comfortable position, generally supine, in which they can remain still throughout the procedure.

TECHNIQUE

Radiographic evaluation of the injured area is useful to rule out any residual foreign material in the soft tissues. Sometimes, depending on the mechanism, an unsuspected fracture might also be present. This information might influence the treatment plan. Ultrasound is an additional and evolving imaging strategy that is increasingly being used to assist in the assessment of tendon integrity; see Chapter 171, Musculoskeletal Ultrasound. After verifying appropriate anesthesia (usually a digital or wrist block; see Chapter 7, Peripheral Nerve Blocks and Field Blocks) and completion of a thorough preparation and draping, the wound should be explored carefully to further delineate the injury. The clinician should follow universal blood and body fluid precautions. An additional irrigation and debridement might be necessary, depending on the nature of the injured tissues and if further foreign material is discovered. Any nonviable tissue must be removed. One should have little reluctance to extend the wound proximally and distally to understand the extent of the trauma, to satisfactorily visualize the damaged tissues, and to gain access to proximal and distal segments of the involved tendon(s). Electrocautery and a tourniquet are most useful to ensure appropriate hemostasis (although the maximal time for tourniquet application is generally 2 hours, most clinicians should not be performing a procedure that takes this long in the outpatient setting). Because these repairs can be quite tedious, most clinicians will perform them seated in a comfortable chair with the patient's arm positioned out to the side on an arm board. The primary surgeon will usually have his back facing the patient's head, allowing greater access to the extensor portion of the forearm and hand. With a large sterile field including the elbow through the hand and a sterile-gowned clinician, contamination is less likely when positioning the patient and providing stable wrist supports.

Ragged tendon ends should be trimmed to allow a clean and direct reapproximation. It is imperative that the clinician be familiar with the associated anatomy for consideration of possible neurovascular injury. If a neurovascular injury is discovered, further referral to an experienced upper extremity surgeon is warranted. If critical structures are near the repair area, the clinician should take special precaution to protect these structures. Incomplete tendon lacerations can be repaired directly or debrided if considered an insignificant portion of the tendon. Occasionally, a tendon is lacerated in an oblique fashion, which is usually amenable to a direct repair with a fine nonabsorbable material. Most clinicians recommend a direct end-to-end (rather than side-to-side) repair of transverse extensor tendon lacerations. If a tendon has adequate substance, a "core" suture, particularly with a braided, nonabsorbable material is implemented. Typically one or two core sutures are placed. The stitch ideally has a buried knot (Fig. 172.4). A Kessler or Bunnell stitch or their modifications is commonly used, and these sutures redirect the force of the tendon perpendicular to the longitudinal axis to allow it to heal. Although no study has determined the optimal stitch for repair in each zone of injury, the modified Kessler and modified Bunnell stitches have been shown to produce the greatest strength for a core-type tendon repair. Although the literature supports the use of these modified core-type stitches, certain experts find them less useful in zones II and III because the tendons are so thin. These core-type stitches are most useful when repairing rounder, thicker tendons.

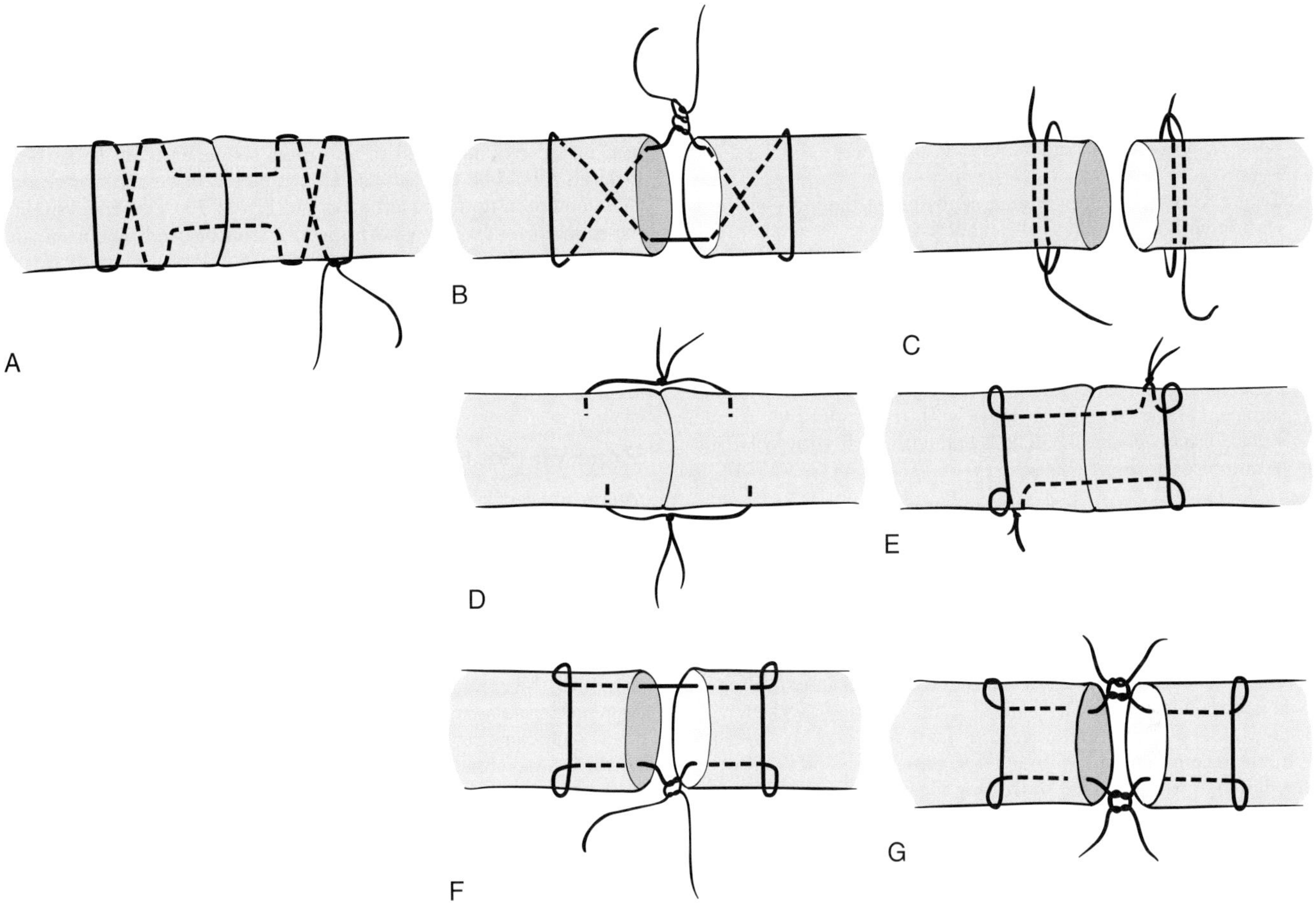

Fig. 172.4 Commonly used techniques for end-to-end tendon suture. (A) Conventional Bunnell stitch. (B) Crisscross stitch (modified Bunnell) with buried knot. (C) Mason-Allen (Chicago) stitch. (D) Mason-Allen (Chicago) stitch after knots tied. (E) Kessler grasping stitch. (F) Modified Kessler stitch with single buried knot. (G) Tajima modification of Kessler stitch with double buried knots. *Note:* In A, B, E, F, and G, *dotted lines* mean stitch passes into and through tendon, the *vertical solid lines* indicate the stitch is passed around behind the tendon. If the tendon is large enough, it can be passed directly and transversely through the tendon (i.e., in that case, vertical *solid lines* would be *dotted lines*). See text for details. (Modified from Strickland JW. Flexor tendon injuries: I. Foundations of treatment. *J Am Acad Orthop Surg.* 1995;3[1]:44–54.)

NOTE: If the tendon is not very thick, a loop of suture can be passed around the tendon (the solid vertical lines in Fig. 172.4A, B, E, F, and G). Granted that this loop outside the tendon may later interfere with the tendons ability to glide in its sheath, it may also be what is needed to best reapproximate the lacerated ends. If the tendon is thick enough, the core suture can be passed directly and transversely through the tendon (in that case, the solid vertical lines in Fig. 172.4A, B, E, F, and G would be drawn as dotted vertical lines), which is how many experts have been suturing tendons for years.

Many clinicians use an epitenon running suture with or without a core stitch. The epitenon repair usually is with a fine, monofilament, nonabsorbable material that is appropriate for the size of the structures being repaired (Fig. 172.5). Simple interrupted sutures commonly fail by pulling through the tendon ends and fraying the tendon because of the fiber alignment. When the sutured tendon ends are brought together, a secured knot is present with minimal trauma to the tendon ends. During the repair, the tendon ends should be handled in an atraumatic technique with minimal tissue crushing. (Ideally, the tendon ends should be handled only by the clinician's fingers. Nontoothed forceps can also be quite helpful. A 27-gauge needle can be used to pierce the tendon perpendicularly and stabilize it, as can a single suture placed temporarily through the tendon. Traumatizing the tissue can result in disruption to the vascular and nutritional supplies and subsequent adhesions.) The approximated tendon ends should not buckle or be compressed excessively. A flat end repair promotes proper healing and return

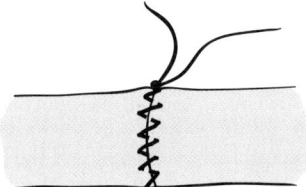

Fig. 172.5 Simple running suture used for peripheral epitenon tendon repair. A locked running suture can also be used for greater strength.

of the proper gliding action to the tendon. Particular considerations regarding the anatomic zones are detailed in the following sections.

BY THE ZONES

Zone I: Distal Interphalangeal Joint

An extensor tendon disruption in this zone is by definition a "mallet finger" (flexion deformity at the distal interphalangeal [DIP] joint; see Fig. 172.1) unless the laceration is incomplete. These sometimes will progress to a "swan neck" deformity as the conjoined lateral bands subluxate dorsally, resulting in PIP joint hyperextension with the associated mallet deformity (see Fig. 172.1). Zone I injuries are commonly missed, especially when not associated with an open/laceration injury. These injuries usually occur when an athlete or manual laborer "jams" the fingertip. These frequently have a poor outcome, often needing a tendon graft or DIP fusion because the incomplete extensor mechanism at the unstable DIP joint interferes with dexterity and leads to subsequent arthritic changes at this joint.

Zone I injuries are classified into four subtypes:

- Type I: Closed or blunt trauma with loss of tendon continuity with or without a small avulsion fracture
- Type II: Laceration proximal to the DIP joint with loss of tendon continuity
- Type III: Deep abrasion with loss of skin, subcutaneous cover, and tendon substance
- Type IV: (1) Transepiphyseal plate fracture in children, (2) hyperflexion injury with fracture of 20% to 50% of the articular surface, (3) hyperextension injury with fracture of the articular surface usually greater than 50% and with fairly early volar subluxation of the distal phalanx

A radiograph should be obtained with the lateral projection of the DIP joint being scrutinized. Fractures (typically interarticular) should be stabilized appropriately. Commonly, the fracture will need to be pinned.

Treatment

If not open, all zone I injuries should be splinted in extension or even hyperextension across the DIP joint (a digital block may be needed). Open lacerations can be repaired with care to avoid the vulnerable germinal nail matrix. These patients should be directed to a clinician who is skilled in treating these injuries. A temporary, retrograde, buried pin in full extension is often better tolerated than external splinting.

Zone II: Middle Phalanx and Thumb Proximal Phalanx

Zone II injuries typically can be treated similarly to zone I injuries, with the exception being the thumb. The extensor tendon in the thumb in this zone may be large enough to repair. Many of these injuries are associated with a crush. The splint must be extended to include the PIP joint.

Zone III: Proximal Interphalangeal Joint

An injury at this location frequently will lead to a boutonnière deformity (see Fig. 172.1). A zone III deformity and the previously noted mallet finger are the most commonly missed closed injuries of the hand. The central slip is injured and the lateral bands can migrate in a volar direction past the axis of rotation at the PIP, resulting in a PIP flexion contracture with or without hyperextension at the DIP joint. Many patients have an associated collateral ligament or volar plate injury. If not recognized and treated early, no good salvage operation can restore normal function to these injuries.

Treatment

The PIP should be splinted in extension, possibly incorporating the DIP joint in extension. The patient should be referred to a clinician trained in these complex problems to have definitive care initiated within 7 days.

Zone IV: Proximal Phalanx

These injuries are normally easy to identify. The lateral band extension is rarely completely transected. A repair using a nonabsorbable suture is typically performed, followed by protected motion while the PIP joint is splinted in extension. Consider a bite wound (see next section, Zone V).

Zone V: Metacarpophalangeal Joint

Zone V injuries are frequently from a human tooth. Obtain a radiograph to rule out a fracture or foreign body. If there is any chance of a bite wound, it should be cleansed aggressively and left open with consideration of appropriate antibiotic coverage. Frequently, the metacarpophalangeal joint capsule is penetrated. Thus these wounds should be opened, carefully explored in flexion and extension, and then normally left open (see Fig. 172.3). The hand should be splinted for later wound inspection and delayed tendon repair. An experienced practitioner can repair the wound primarily if it is considered noncontaminated and not associated with a bite wound.

NOTE: At this level of injury, disruption of the sagittal bands of the extensor hood may occur (e.g., dislocation of the extensor tendon) acutely or spontaneously. These injuries should be splinted and directed to a clinician skilled in managing hand and tendon injuries.

Zone VI: Metacarpal Level

A primary repair can be pursued routinely. Buried core sutures are the typical technique used. The practitioner must oversee a careful splinting and therapy program. Again, consider a bite wound.

Zone VII: Wrist Extensor Retinacular Area

Zone VII injuries may be repaired similarly to zone VI injuries, realizing that the extensor retinaculum is involved and may need repair or resection. Posttraumatic adhesions are not uncommon; hence many clinicians refer all zone VII injuries for retinaculum repair. These injuries should be managed with added diligence during hand therapy.

Zone VIII: Distal Forearm

Zone VIII injuries may be treated similarly to zone VI and VII injuries. At this level, adjacent structures can easily be injured, retracted, and difficult to appreciate. Sensory cutaneous nerves (radial branches and the antebrachial cutaneous nerve) should be protected carefully if in the field and repaired if observed to be lacerated.

Zone IX: Proximal Forearm

Zone IX injuries are frequently associated with neurovascular trauma. These injuries should be explored in an operating room by a clinician skilled in treating these problems.

If the practitioner has experience with extensor tendon injuries and is comfortable with splinting and therapy programs, repairs of zones IV through VI and maybe VIII can be addressed in an emergency department or an appropriately equipped office, if the inherent problems of each zone are understood. The remaining zones might be repaired in these settings relative to the clinician's experience and available equipment. The potential complications associated with these injuries and their repairs must be followed carefully. Complications can be quite significant, including primary failure of the repair, secondary later rupture of the tendon, stiffness, contractures with limited range of motion from resultant adhesions, residual pain, residual overlying tissue problems, infection, and problems related to other adjacent structures. The practitioner will never be faulted for leaving a wound open and splinted after an *aggressive* irrigation and debridement, especially over the metacarpophalangeal joint, and then referring. Ideally, tendon, bone, and joint tissues are kept moist in the wound with a damp sterile dressing to protect against desiccation of these vulnerable structures.

Extensor tendon lacerations to the feet occur less frequently than in the upper extremities because of activity patterns and the protection that shoes and pants can provide. However, when these injuries do occur, they commonly are associated with additional significant trauma to other tissues, including fractures. The clinician must be diligent to rule out other possible injuries by considering associated anatomic structures and obtaining appropriate radiographs. Isolated lower extremity extensor tendon injuries otherwise might be managed in a similar fashion to upper extremity injuries, taking into account the correlating anatomic zones (e.g., a tendon injury at the ankle under the retinacular tissues would correlate to a zone VII injury in the upper extremity). Foot flexor tendons should be addressed by a clinician skilled in these areas. (It is not uncommon for an isolated flexor tendon laceration to be relatively well tolerated without repair.)

Clinicians normally will give an appropriately dosed first- or second-generation cephalosporin for a clean open injury, which should provide satisfactory coverage for most gram-positive skin organisms. Consideration for gram-negative and anaerobic coverage should be entertained for contaminated wounds, especially if occurring at a farm. *Pseudomonas* coverage usually is wise for foot lacerations. Continued antibiotics are typically unnecessary unless there is gross contamination or a subsequent infection develops. It is safest to reevaluate these wounds and repairs 2 to 3 days later for possible early infection. Adjustment of antibiotic management might be necessary, especially when considering the patient's particular circumstances.

PATIENT EDUCATION GUIDES

See patient education and patient consent forms available at www.expertconsult.com.

CPT/BILLING CODES

25270	Repair, tendon or muscle, extensor, forearm and/or wrist; primary, single, each tendon or muscle
25272	Repair, tendon or muscle, extensor, forearm and/or wrist; secondary, single, each tendon or muscle
26410	Repair, extensor tendon, hand, primary or secondary; without free graft, each tendon
26418	Repair, extensor tendon, finger, primary or secondary; without free graft, each tendon
26432	Closed treatment of distal extensor tendon insertion, with or without percutaneous pinning (e.g., mallet finger)
28208	Repair, tendon, extensor, foot; primary or secondary, each tendon

ICD-10-CM DIAGNOSTIC CODES

M66.241	Spontaneous rupture of tendon, extensor tendons of right hand and wrist
M66.242	Spontaneous rupture of tendon, extensor tendons of left hand and wrist
M66.871	Spontaneous rupture of tendon other tendons of right foot and ankle
M66.872	Spontaneous rupture of tendon other tendons of left foot and ankle
M20.011	Mallet finger right
M20.012	Mallet finger left
S66.829X	Laceration specified muscles, fascia and tendons at wrist and hand
S96.929X	Laceration specified muscles, fascia and tendon at ankle foot

Add additional seventh character: A = initial D = subsequent S = sequela.

Acknowledgment

The editors recognize the contributions of Thomas J. Zuber, MD, and John L. Pfenninger, MD, to this chapter in a previous edition of this text.

RECOMMENDED READING

Cannon DL. Flexor and extensor tendon injuries. In: Azar FM, Beaty JH, Canale ST, eds. *Campbell's Operative Orthopaedics*. 13th ed. Philadelphia: Elsevier; 2017:3348–3402.

Carl HD, Forst R, Schaller P. Results of primary extensor tendon repair in relation to the zone of injury and the pre-operative outcome estimation. *Arch Orthop Trauma Surg*. 2007;127:115–119.

Colzani G, Tos P, Battiston B, Merolla G, Porcellini G, Artiaco S. Traumatic extensor tendon injuries to the hand: clinical anatomy, biomechanics, and surgical procedure review. *J Hand Microsurg*. 2016;8(1):2–12.

Dabezies EJ, Schutte JP. Fixation of metacarpal and phalangeal fractures with miniature plates and screws. *J Hand Surg Am*. 1986;11:283–288.

Harper J, Harper S, Kalimuthu R. Extensor tendon repair. In: Reichman EF, ed. *Emergency Medicine Procedures*. 2nd ed. New York: McGraw-Hill; 2013:490:495.

Kleinert HE, Verdan C. Report of the Committee on Tendon Injuries (International Federation of Societies for Surgery of the Hand). *J Hand Surg Am*. 1983;8:794–798.

Mohammadrezaei N, Seyedhosseini J, Vahidi E. Validity of ultrasound in diagnosis of tendon injuries in penetrating extremity trauma. *Am J Emerg Med*. 2017;(17): pii: S0735-6757(17)30077-3.

Newport ML, Blair WF, Steyers Jr CM. Long-term results of extensor tendon repair. *J Hand Surg Am*. 1990;15:961–966.

Strauch RJ. Extensor tendons injuries. In: Wolfe SW, Hotchkiss RN, Pederson WC, Kozin SH, Cohen MS, eds. *Green's Operative Hand Surgery*. 7th ed. Philadelphia: Elsevier; 2017:152–182.

CHAPTER 173

NURSEMAID'S ELBOW: RADIAL HEAD SUBLUXATION

Russell D. White • Christopher F. Adams

Nursemaid's elbow (radial head subluxation) or "pulled elbow" is a common injury to children younger than 7 years old. Although this injury can occur in children in the age ranges from less than 6 months to the preteens, the majority occur between 1 and 3 years of age. The mechanism of injury is usually sudden axial traction of the outstretched, pronated forearm. It often occurs when a parent picks the child up and suspends the child's entire weight while holding only his or her hands. Alternatively, the child may have asked to be "swung around" while holding his or her hands. At times, the injury occurs unobserved by an adult. Regardless of mechanism, the child initially complains of pain and then refuses to use the arm; this is when concerned parents usually seek medical attention.

The elbow consists of the articulation of the humerus, ulna, and radial head. While the radius and ulna can flex and extend against the humerus, the radial head also rotates against the ulna and capitellum (humerus) to permit forearm pronation and supination. Held in place against the proximal ulna and capitellum by the annular ligament and joint capsule, the radial head is usually quite stable. However, in infants and young children, sudden traction on the distal forearm is sometimes more than the annular ligament can sustain; consequently, the radial head slides distally and partially dislocates or subluxes. If the annular ligament or synovial tissue becomes interposed between the radial head and capitellum, there is persistent discomfort and the radial head is prevented from spontaneous reduction.

DIAGNOSIS

Often the history suggests the diagnosis. Typical scenarios for radial head subluxation include a caregiver pulling a child out of harm's way, a reluctant child being pulled along by the hand, a child suddenly falling or dropping to the floor while being held, or a child being swung playfully by the arms. It is also not uncommon for the subluxation to occur unwitnessed; in that case, the child may provide the history of having fallen or rolled over in bed. At presentation, the child expresses acute pain, refuses to move the affected extremity, and holds the elbow in a pronated and slightly flexed position (the nursemaid's position). Examination reveals no deformity and little if any swelling around the elbow. (Having the parent question the child and examine for areas of tenderness, with the clinician's guidance, may be less threatening than being examined by an unknown clinician.) The child resists range of motion at the elbow, including further flexion or extension as well as supination and further pronation.

Some tenderness is noted over the radial head but not the supracondylar regions. Neurovascular compromise is rare with this injury. Not infrequently, as previously mentioned, the child has no known traction injury but holds the arm against the chest, refuses to use it, and has no significant deformity, swelling, or neurovascular compromise. In fact, a small retrospective study found that a third of the 45 cases of nursemaid's elbow in the emergency department did not have a history of axial traction.

RADIOGRAPHIC STUDIES

The clinician should take standard elbow radiographs, including three views (anteroposterior, lateral, and oblique). Comparison radiographs of the contralateral elbow are essential in the young child because incomplete ossification increases the difficulty in evaluating the immature elbow as well as its alignment. Radiographs of nursemaid's elbow are usually normal or reveal longitudinal misalignment of the radial head with the capitellum. The subluxation is occasionally reduced by the technician when taking the radiographs; the child is often distracted while being positioned for three radiographs, and this may allow the elbow to be supinated and flexed. The child then returns to the clinical area using the affected extremity.

The clinician should evaluate the radiographs for the presence of a "fat pad sign" (joint effusion, and a contraindication to this procedure), location and alignment of epiphyseal growth centers, and the longitudinal alignment of the radial head with the capitellum. The fat pad sign is positive if a radiolucent stripe is visible at the posterior distal aspect of the humerus on the lateral view of the elbow and not visible on the comparison view of the other elbow. The fat pad sign is produced when periarticular fat is displaced posteriorly by an increase in intraarticular joint fluid, making it visible in the lateral view. This is a nonspecific finding. A positive fat pad sign associated with a history of trauma suggests a bloody joint effusion and intraarticular injury. In this case, immediate orthopedic referral is recommended. A nursemaid's elbow usually lacks the fat pad sign; in fact, the diagnosis is usually made by ruling out a fat pad sign.

Misalignment of the ossification centers suggests a growth plate injury. Orthopedic referral is recommended for a growth plate injury or other obvious fracture. Elbow fractures have a high complication rate.

We would never recommend manipulation of the patient, even with classic symptoms, before a radiographic study has been performed, although some clinicians do.

INDICATIONS

- A child holding his or her arm in a pronated, partially flexed position, refusing to use it, often with a history of axial traction compatible with radial head subluxation (but not always), and negative radiographs

CONTRAINDICATIONS

- Edema or ecchymoses over the site
- Fracture (visible fracture or a fat pad sign on radiograph, or suspicion of a fracture if no radiographs obtained)

- Mechanism of injury inconsistent with radial head subluxation (unless radiographs negative)
- Presence of distal neurologic or vascular compromise (orthopedic consultation recommended)

PREPROCEDURE PATIENT EDUCATION

The procedure, as well as any risks and alternatives, should be explained to the patient and caregivers. Informed consent should be obtained. The patient can be sitting or supine on an examination table or sitting in a parent's lap. No preprocedure medications are generally required.

TECHNIQUE

Supination and flexion of the forearm has been the classic method described in modern literature, including the first edition of this text, to reduce radial head subluxation. More recently, a method of hyperpronation with flexion has been evaluated as a safe and effective alternative technique and has been shown in small studies to be a less painful method of reduction. A recent meta-analysis and systematic review (Bexkens et al., 2017) found that hyperpronation was more effective in terms of success rate and appeared to be less painful compared to the supination-flexion maneuver. The techniques differ in the direction the forearm is rotated. Some clinicians have always preferred the hyperpronation technique, saying that because the child often presents in pronation, the additional pronation (hyperpronation) required may need less force than forced supination.

Supination and Flexion Method

Fig. 173.1 illustrates the supination and flexion method.

1. The elbow is held in one of the operator's hands (usually the nondominant hand) with either the thumb or second and third fingers exerting constant gentle pressure over the radial head in a medial direction.
2. While applying slight distal traction with the operator's other hand, the patient's wrist is supinated.
3. The patient's forearm is then rapidly raised toward the upper arm, flexing the elbow past 90 degrees. This should all be done in one smooth motion, and a click may be felt by the finger held over the radial head as it is reduced.

4. The forearm is moved so that the elbow is in 90 degrees of flexion and released.
5. The success of the manipulation is often tested by offering the child his or her favorite toy or a piece of candy on the side of the affected arm. If the child reaches with the affected arm, the manipulation was successful.
6. The child should be using the forearm normally within 30 minutes or else a repeat manipulation can be attempted. Using the alternative method of hyperpronating the forearm and rapid flexion has been successful even when repeat supination and flexion has failed.

Pronation and Flexion Method (Hyperpronation)

Fig. 173.2 illustrates the pronation and flexion method.

1. The elbow is held with one of the operator's hands with the thumb or second and third fingers again exerting constant gentle medial pressure on the radial head.
2. While the operator applies slight distal traction, the patient's wrist is hyperpronated with the operator's other hand.
3. Rapid flexion at the elbow is performed; this should all be done in one smooth motion. Sometimes a click, snap, or satisfying clunk of the radial head may be felt, indicating reduction.
4. The elbow is extended to 90 degrees and released.
5. The success of manipulation is tested as noted previously.

EDITOR'S Note: there are two variations on the hyperpronation technique. The first technique merely hyperpronates the forearm without any additional flexion at the elbow. This may be all that is needed; if unsuccessful, obviously additional maneuvering can be performed.

DIFFERENTIAL DIAGNOSIS

If there is concern regarding the possibility of a growth plate injury, generally the best approach is to obtain an orthopedic consultation. Rarely, an arthrogram is needed to determine the extent of injury. Sedation or general anesthesia is often required to complete that study. The radiographic contrast material can help to outline articular surfaces and give the examiner a better understanding of the nonossified anatomy.

Alternative diagnoses include osteomyelitis or clavicular, distal humeral, stress, or radial head fracture. Joint aspiration can be performed if there is concern regarding the possibility of more significant trauma or infection in the elbow (see Chapter 180, Joint and Soft Tissue Aspiration and Injection [Arthrocentesis]). Bloody fluid

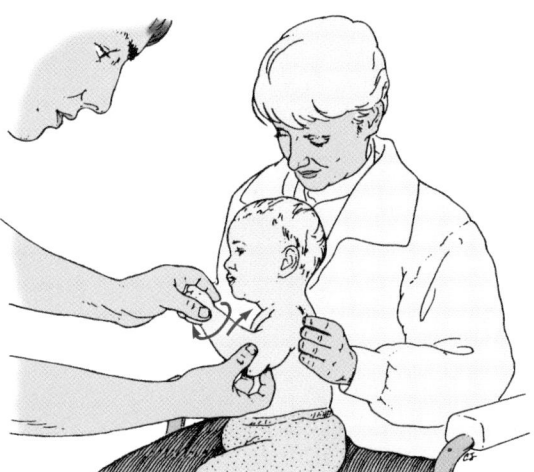

Fig. 173.1 The reduction maneuver for a subluxed radial head (nursemaid's elbow) involves gentle supination of the forearm and flexion of the elbow. The examiner's thumb can be placed over the child's elbow to help palpate the radial head during the reduction process.

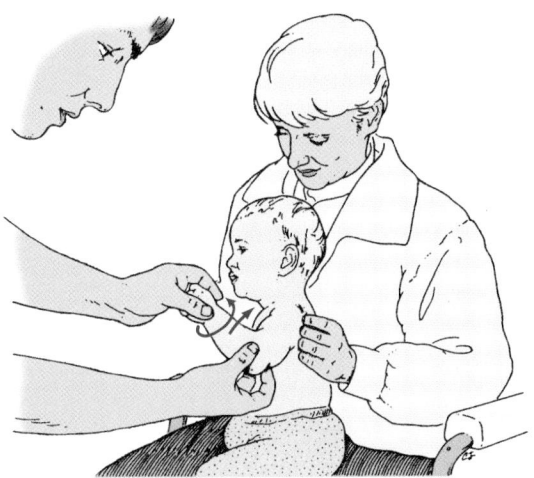

Fig. 173.2 Pronation and flexion method.

confirms the presence of a traumatic intracapsular injury, such as a fracture. Purulent material confirms the diagnosis of septic arthritis. Routine elbow aspiration is not recommended for a nursemaid's elbow; it is merely an adjunctive procedure that can be used in difficult diagnostic situations. Sedation or general anesthesia may be required. If any of the preceding diagnoses are being considered, an orthopedic surgeon should be consulted.

POSTPROCEDURE PATIENT EDUCATION

After successful reduction of a subluxed radial head, the provider should tell the child (and caregivers) to rest the limb for several days. The child should then be reevaluated with clinical and possible radiographic examination if symptoms do not totally resolve in 24 to 48 hours. If reduction is delayed more than 8 hours from the time of injury, it may take the full 24 to 48 hours to recover. A small percentage of patients will resublux the radial head within a few days of reduction, although the number and risk factors are not well defined. In a small randomized prospective study, immobilization in a flexed, supinated position with a posterior splint reduced the recurrence rate from 13% to zero ($P < .05$) at follow-up 2 days after manipulation (Taha, 2000). Children who remain reluctant to use their elbow in a normal fashion should be splinted from shoulder to hand. Follow-up evaluation in 2 or 3 days is recommended to determine normal joint function. If not normal at that point, orthopedic referral should be considered. Patients with splints should not remove the splint until the short-term follow-up examination.

In general, children will let their symptoms be their guide in regard to activity level; once they are comfortable, they will resume their activities. It may take several days for them to do so. The long-term prognosis of nursemaid's elbow is generally favorable; the caregivers generally need assurance that the child has suffered nothing serious. Occasionally the child will have several episodes of subluxation, but the incidence drops off significantly after age 7. Caregivers should be educated regarding the mechanism of injury and how to avoid future subluxations. Long-term functional or growth problems are rare after appropriate treatment of this injury. Congenital radial head dislocation is a separate entity and is not related to the common pediatric problem of nursemaid's elbow.

CPT/BILLING CODES

>24640	Closed treatment of radial head subluxation in child, nursemaid's elbow, with manipulation
29105	Splint, arm, long (shoulder to hand)

ICD-10-CM DIAGNOSTIC CODES

S53.031X	Nursemaid's elbow right elbow
S53.032X	Nursemaid's elbow left elbow

Add seventh character: A = Initial D = Subsequent S = Sequela

Acknowledgment

The editors recognize the contributions of Fred M. Hankin, MD, and James L. Telfer, MD, to this chapter in previous editions of this text.

RECOMMENDED READING

Bexkens R, Washburn FJ, Eygendaal D, van den Bekerom MP, Oh LS. Effectiveness of reduction maneuvers in the treatment of nursemaid's elbow: a systematic review and meta-analysis. *Am J Emerg Med.* 2017;35(1):159–163.

Green DA, Linares MYR, Garcia-Peña BM, et al. Randomized comparison of pain perception during radial head subluxation reduction using supination-flexion or forced pronation. *Pediatr Emerg Care.* 2006;22:235.

Kling MP, Reichman EF. Radial head subluxation ("nursemaid's elbow") reduction. In: Reichman EF, ed. *Emergency Medicine Procedures.* 2nd ed. New York: McGraw-Hill; 2013:553–557.

Macias CG, Bothner J, Wiebe R. A comparison of supination/flexion to hyperpronation in the reduction of radial head subluxations. *Pediatrics.* 1998;102:e10.

McDonald J, Whitelaw C, Goldsmith LJ. Radial head subluxation: comparing two methods of reduction. *Acad Emerg Med.* 1999;6:715.

Sacchetti A, Ramoska EE, Glascow C. Nonclassic history in children with radial head subluxations. *J Emerg Med.* 1990;8:151.

Taha AM. The treatment of pulled elbow: a prospective randomized study. *Arch Orthop Trauma Surg.* 2000;120:336.

CHAPTER 174

SHOULDER DISLOCATIONS

Jeffrey V. Smith

Dislocations of the shoulder are quite common. Approximately 50% of shoulder injuries in the emergency department are dislocations. Anterior dislocations are far more common than posterior dislocations. The four types of anterior dislocations account for 96% of all shoulder dislocations.

Of the four types of anterior dislocations, subcoracoid dislocations occur three times more frequently than all the others (subglenoid, subclavicular, and thoracic) combined. This chapter deals only with the care of subcoracoid anterior dislocations. All others should be treated with the assistance of an orthopedic surgeon.

The shoulder is the most flexible joint in the human body; consequently it is the most unstable and most commonly dislocated joint. It is designed to enable a wide range of motion of the upper extremity in all directions. To accomplish this feat, the actual bony articulation occupies only a very small part of the overall functional area of the joint. The glenohumeral joint surface and capsule are small sliding structures without significant fixed ligamentous limitations. The tendons around the joint, making up the rotator cuff (Fig. 174.1), are the structures primarily responsible for the integrity of the joint and its complex function.

EDITOR'S NOTE: Contrary to what many of us were taught in anatomy class, the shoulder joint is not a ball-and-socket joint; it is more like a ball-and–quarter-socket joint or even a joint with only a shallow bowl. If it had a complete socket, its range of motion would be very limited, perhaps no more than an arc of 45 degrees. To obtain the full 360 degrees arc of motion, the articular surface of the glenoid fossa must be fairly flat. Consequently the humerus is held in place predominantly by muscles, tendons, and ligaments.

When the normal joint capsule and rotator cuff restraints are exceeded, the shoulder moves out of joint. Most frequently the clinician encounters a dislocation in which the humeral head has been pulled out of the joint and is then held anteriorly and medially by a spasm of the muscles of the anterior chest wall. This is the subcoracoid anterior shoulder dislocation, usually occurring when an abducted, extended, and externally rotated upper extremity takes a major jolt. (Picture the arm in overhead position for spiking a volleyball or in the overhead crawl swim; this is the vulnerable position for forces to dislocate a shoulder if such forces are placed on the hand in a posterior direction.) The resulting lever forces the proximal humerus anteriorly out of the glenoid fossa. After the humeral head comes to rest under the coracoid process, the patient usually presents to the clinician in extreme pain with a nonfunctional arm. Dislocations may also occur during a seizure. With recurrent dislocations, the mechanism can be surprisingly minor. If the first dislocation happens before 20 years of age, there is an 80% to 92% rate of recurrence. If the first dislocation occurs after 40 years of age, the recurrence rate is 10% to 15%.

The patient will have a loss of the normal shoulder contour, with a step-off where the deltoid muscle used to be prominent. Instead, the acromion becomes very prominent. The contour of the humeral head may be noted in the region of the anterior chest wall. Clinically a hollow can be appreciated beneath the acromion process due to the missing humeral head. The arm will frequently be held in a slightly abducted, externally rotated posture. Inability to place the palm of the hand of the affected side on the uninjured shoulder is consistent with an anterior dislocation; after reduction, this maneuver should be possible. A neurologic deficit, most frequently involving the axillary nerve (provides innervation for shoulder abduction and sensation over the deltoid), may be noted on careful examination. Additional neurovascular compromise may be evident, but this is uncommon with subcoracoid anterior dislocations.

Radiographs should be obtained; it is important to determine the presence (24% of anterior dislocations) or absence of a fracture before attempting to reduce the shoulder. Obtain standard radiographs of the shoulder. A single anteroposterior view of the shoulder will usually demonstrate the abnormal location of the humeral head. Another view at approximately 90 degrees will not only confirm the direction of humeral head movement but also help to exclude a fracture or posterior dislocation. A lateral transcapular or Y-type view will provide this information; an axillary view (Fig. 174.2) is preferred by some clinicians, but it is often difficult to get the patient to move his or her arm into the necessary position. Alternatively, in some obese individuals, a computed tomography (CT) scan may be necessary to determine the direction of the shoulder dislocation and the presence of concomitant fractures. Point-of-care ultrasound is emerging as an effective tool in managing anterior shoulder dislocations in the emergency room.

EDITOR'S NOTE: The Hill-Sachs deformity produces a groove on the posterolateral aspect of the humeral head. It is often seen with repeated dislocations and rarely has any clinical significance other than that it may result in a loose body within the joint.

INDICATIONS

A subcoracoid anterior shoulder dislocation

CONTRAINDICATIONS

The following findings or conditions should generate an immediate orthopedic consult:

- A shoulder dislocation other than a subcoracoid anterior dislocation
- Any fracture dislocation of the shoulder
- Dislocations that are more than a few days old (higher risk of vascular injury, especially in older patients)
- Other fractures of the shoulder, neck, ribs, or upper extremity
- Prior orthopedic surgery for chronic or recurrent shoulder dislocations
- Shoulder dislocations in children (if ossification centers are not fused, there is usually an associated Salter-Harris fracture)

EDITOR'S NOTE: A neurologic deficit does not preclude closed reduction; however, multiple forced attempts at reduction should be avoided. A patient with neurovascular compromise (other than a mild axillary nerve sensory defect) due to shoulder dislocation should undergo immediate reduction. Although it is beyond the

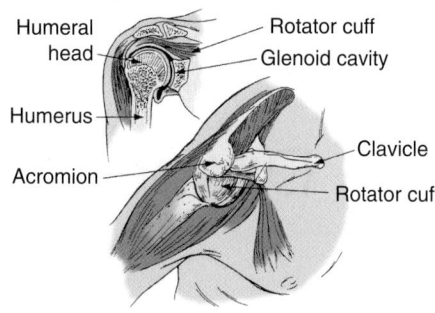

Fig. 174.1 Anatomy of the shoulder joint and how the tendons of the muscles (supraspinatus, infraspinatus, subscapularis, and teres minor) form the rotator cuff. Also see Chapter 171, Musculoskeletal Ultrasonography, and Chapter 180, Joint and Soft Tissue Aspiration and Injection (Arthrocentesis).

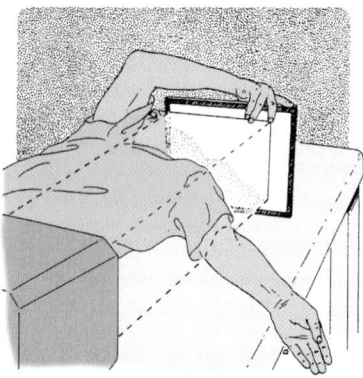

Fig. 174.2 Radiographs should include a view at 90 degrees from the anteroposterior view, such as this axillary view. This projection helps to document the direction (anterior vs. posterior) of the shoulder dislocation.

scope of this book, even inferior or posterior shoulder dislocations should undergo immediate reduction if the distal pulse is compromised. Although immediate orthopedic assistance is optimal, it may not always be available.

EQUIPMENT AND SUPPLIES

- Stretcher
- Washcloth or small towel
- Soft restraints such as sheets or blankets
- Cloth tape, gauze or elastic bandage, padded wrist restraint or commercially available device for hanging weights from wrist
- Weights (5 to 15 lb) or bucket (0.5 to 1 gallon in size and adequate tap water or intravenous fluid
- Intra-articular anesthetic (10 to 20 mL of a 50:50 mixture comprising 1% or 2% lidocaine with sterile saline), antiseptic solution (e.g., chlorhexidine, povidone-iodine), 10- to 20-mL syringe, 25-gauge 2.5-inch needle
- Procedural sedation forms, consent, equipment (see Chapter 1, Procedural Sedation and Analgesia) and medications (e.g., analgesia, muscle relaxant, narcotics, benzodiazepines, reversal agents)
- Shoulder immobilizer or sling and swath

PREPROCEDURE PATIENT PREPARATION

Patients should be informed about the indications for shoulder reduction as well as any alternatives and possible complications. They should know what to expect and try to relax as much as possible. If a local anesthetic injection will be used, the patient can be

reassured that this should decrease the discomfort. Informed consent should be obtained appropriate for the procedure(s) to be performed.

PRECAUTIONS

To be successful, this procedure usually takes some time and relaxation—on the part of both the patient and the clinician. The procedure is easy, but trying to rush it may result in an unsuccessful episode. One exception is the dislocation witnessed by the sports medicine clinician; if the dislocation is not associated with high-energy forces, some clinicians will reduce the shoulder immediately, field side, without radiographs and before the muscular spasm can occur.

TECHNIQUE

There are a number of available techniques, all designed to apply gentle and persistent tension on the spasmodic chest wall muscles to elongate them and to reestablish the mobility of the humeral head. Once this has been done, the humeral head will usually track or be gently manipulated back into the glenoid fossa. The patient is probably best served by the simplest technique, the one that minimizes both operator and patient stress. Typically this is the Stimson technique, wherein weight loading and time can be used to gently stretch the muscles and reduce the joint. Certainly this is the least traumatic technique for the shoulder and should help minimize the chances of a fracture developing in relation to the reduction process.

Other techniques may also be successful. Although many have been described in the literature, all of the listed techniques have been tested and are effective in a situation where the clinician is willing to take enough time with the reduction. Experience suggests that the clinician should not attempt more than two reduction procedures. If the second attempt is unsuccessful, the resultant muscle spasm will likely prevent closed reduction in a safe manner. An orthopedic surgeon should be called if the second attempt is unsuccessful.

Intra-articular Anesthetic

Some experts recommend the injection of intra-articular anesthetic with every shoulder reduction (see also Chapter 180, Joint and Soft Tissue Aspiration and Injection [Arthrocentesis]). It can be performed under ultrasound guidance and can be used in place of procedural sedation or if procedural sedation is contraindicated. A recent meta-analysis (Jiang, 2014) and Cochrane review (Wakai, 2011) showed that the use of intra-articular lidocaine had success rates similar to those of procedural sedation; it also led to lower costs and emergency department lengths of stay.

1. Identify the hollow area where the humeral head used to be located, 2 cm (two fingerbreadths) directly inferior to the lateral border of the now prominent acromion process. Apply antiseptic solution to the skin over this area and allow it to dry.
2. Using sterile technique, insert the 25-gauge 2.5-inch needle into this area, perpendicular to the skin, to a depth of 2 cm. Inject 10 to 20 mL of a 50:50 mixture of local anesthetic and sterile saline solution.

Stimson Technique

1. With this technique procedural sedation is often unnecessary; some experts use the injected local intra-articular anesthetic. Also, there are reports of a 96% success rate, and there is no need for an assistant. Conversely, the prone position may be impossible to use because of other injuries; procedural sedation is also not recommended because the prone position may interfere with respiration. Procedural sedation is even relatively contraindicated because of the prolonged nature of this technique.

2. The patient is placed in the prone position on a stretcher with the affected arm hanging over the side. A rolled-up washcloth or small towel can be placed beneath the coracoid process and pectoralis major muscle as needed for comfort. The clinician may want to wrap soft restraints (sheets or blankets) around the bed and the patient at the hips to prevent him or her from falling off the stretcher. A weight (usually from 5 to 15 lb) is affixed to the wrist to provide sustained longitudinal traction. Wrapping tape, a gauze or elastic bandage, or a padded wrist restraint around the wrist should provide secure fixation of the weight to the limb. Commercial devices are also available for securing and hanging a weight from the wrist. A bucket of water can be used if weights are not available; the disadvantage for the patient is having to hold the bucket for a considerable length of time. Intravenous fluid can be used to gradually increase the traction as the bucket fills up (Fig. 174.3).

3. With time (usually 15 to 30 minutes) and relaxation, the shoulder will usually reduce itself. Occasionally (perhaps after 30 minutes), the clinician will have to facilitate the reduction by grasping the forearm and gently twisting it, externally first and then internally, while the arm is still under traction. The patient, the clinician, or both may feel a "clunk" as the joint is reduced, and there may be brief fasciculations of the deltoid muscle. However, the reduction may be more subtle; if the patient can touch his or her nose or the opposite shoulder with the index finger of the hand on the affected side, it usually indicates a successful reduction.

4. After the shoulder has been reduced, the limb is held in internal rotation against the abdomen and adduction (humerus against the lateral trunk) with a shoulder immobilizer or sling and swath device. A careful postreduction neurovascular assessment is then required.

5. While keeping the shoulder immobilized, obtain appropriate postreduction radiographs to determine whether adequate reduction of the joint surfaces has been achieved. A congruous-appearing joint without significant distraction (interposed tissue) between the glenoid and the humerus should be noted. Occasionally comparison shoulder radiographs or a postreduction CT scan may be required. Some recent studies question the value of postreduction imaging, but in most communities it is still the standard of care.

Scapular Manipulation Technique

The patient may or may not require analgesia or injected anesthesia for this technique because somewhat less manipulation is required (and less chance of injury) than with most other techniques. Using this technique, the glenoid fossa is repositioned rather than just the humeral head. Scapular manipulation may be performed with the patient prone, sitting, or supine. When the patient is prone or supine, traction is applied to the arm by an assistant (or by attached weights if the patient is prone). The shoulder is gently and gradually flexed by an assistant to a 90-degree position, and from 5 to 15 lb of traction is required. The clinician then uses one hand to rotate the inferior aspect of the scapula upward and medially and the other hand to rotate the superior aspect laterally (Fig. 174.4). When the patient is sitting, an assistant provides forward traction on the affected arm with countertraction against the head of the humerus to obtain the same 90 degrees of flexion. From behind the patient, the clinician manipulates the scapula as described previously. If reduction does not occur within 1 to 3 minutes, a small degree of dorsal displacement of the inferior scapular tip may be helpful. At this point, slight external rotation of the humerus by an assistant while traction is maintained on the humerus and the scapula is being manipulated may also be helpful. Complications from using this technique have never been reported; however, it is a cumbersome process. Reduction may also be very subtle when accomplished by this technique, without a perceived "clunk." This technique may be used when other injuries limit repositioning the patient.

Hennepin Technique

The Hennepin technique is named after the Hennepin County Emergency Medical Center (Minnesota), where the technique was first described. It is preferred by some authors for anterior shoulder dislocations. There is less manipulation than with most other techniques, a lower probability of neurovascular or musculoskeletal

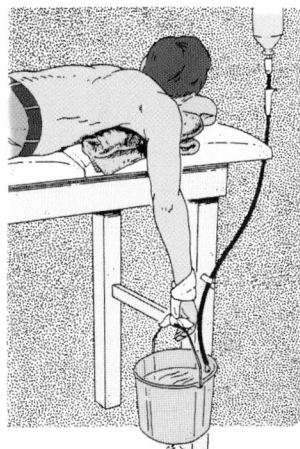

Fig. 174.3 Gentle sustained distal traction can provide an effective means for closed reduction of an anterior dislocation. As the intravenous fluid slowly empties into the bucket, the traction force gradually increases.

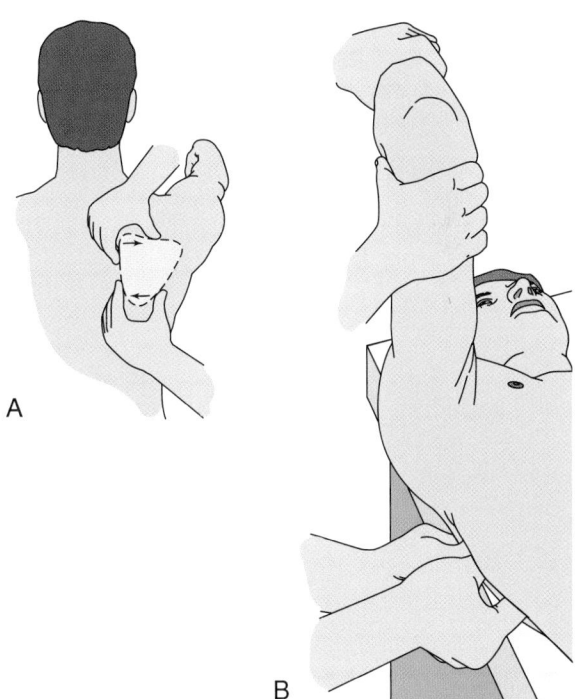

Fig. 174.4 Scapular manipulation technique. (A) An assistant flexes the patient's arm (or if the patient is prone, it can be flexed by gravity and weights, as with the Stimson technique). It must be slowly brought to a 90-degree position. The clinician then rotates the inferior scapular tip upward and medially and the superior aspect laterally (clockwise on the right shoulder when viewed from back, counterclockwise on the left shoulder). (B) The same technique with the patient in supine position. With the patient's shoulder and elbow both flexed 90 degrees and the shoulder adducted, gentle upward pressure is maintained by an assistant while the scapula is manipulated as described.

damage, and little or no need for analgesia (although an injection of intra-articular anesthesia may be beneficial). The patient is seated upright, reclining at 45 degrees, or supine. With the clinician stabilizing the elbow joint of the affected arm with one hand, the clinician's other hand is used to grasp the patient's wrist. Slowly (it can take up to 10 minutes to accomplish this) the patient's forearm is then externally rotated until there is 90 degrees of external rotation (Fig. 174.5). The procedure should be stopped if the patient experiences pain or discomfort, but the arm must not be released or allowed to return to its original position. Usually, after allowing the musculature or spasm to relax, the procedure can be continued without analgesia. If pain or discomfort persists, the patient may require analgesia. The reduction usually occurs by the time the forearm has reached 90 degrees of external rotation; if it has not, the arm is slowly elevated. Occasionally it will have to be elevated to the level where the patient can touch his or her contralateral ear (over the head) with the hand of the affected side. If reduction still does not occur, the humeral head is gently manipulated toward the glenoid until it reduces.

Modified Kocher Maneuver

The modified Kocher maneuver is similar to the Hennepin technique. The patient is placed supine with the arm of the affected shoulder over the edge of the gurney and analgesia or injected anesthesia is provided if necessary. The patient's forearm, with the elbow

held at 90 degrees, is then rotated externally (abducting superiorly) over at least a 5-minute period (see Fig. 174.5), with simultaneous gentle downward pressure applied on the dislocation. After the arm reaches 120 degrees of rotation, it is brought back to internal rotation, at which time the reduction usually occurs.

Milch Technique

With the patient sitting or supine, the arm is moved to 10 to 20 degrees of forward flexion with slight abduction. One of the clinician's hands, using slight traction, is then used to gently guide the patient's arm (grasping at the elbow) in this slightly abducted position until it is directly overhead (Fig. 174.6). The patient may be able to move the arm without assistance to this position; however, there is usually too much pain and spasm. While this is occurring, the clinician's other hand is placed on the humeral head to prevent it from moving downward. When the arm is located directly overhead, the rotator cuff muscles are all in alignment, and all cross stresses are eliminated. Using just his or her thumb, the clinician should be able to direct the humeral head superiorly over the rim of the glenoid and into the fossa. Otherwise, abduction of the arm and outward traction at the shoulder are increased and the arm is brought through a full lateral downward arc. Reduction is usually signified by an audible or palpable "clunk."

Fulcrum Technique

With the patient supine or sitting, a firmly rolled towel, sheet, or blanket 6 to 8 inches long is placed as a fulcrum within the axilla of the affected shoulder. The distal humerus is used as a lever and

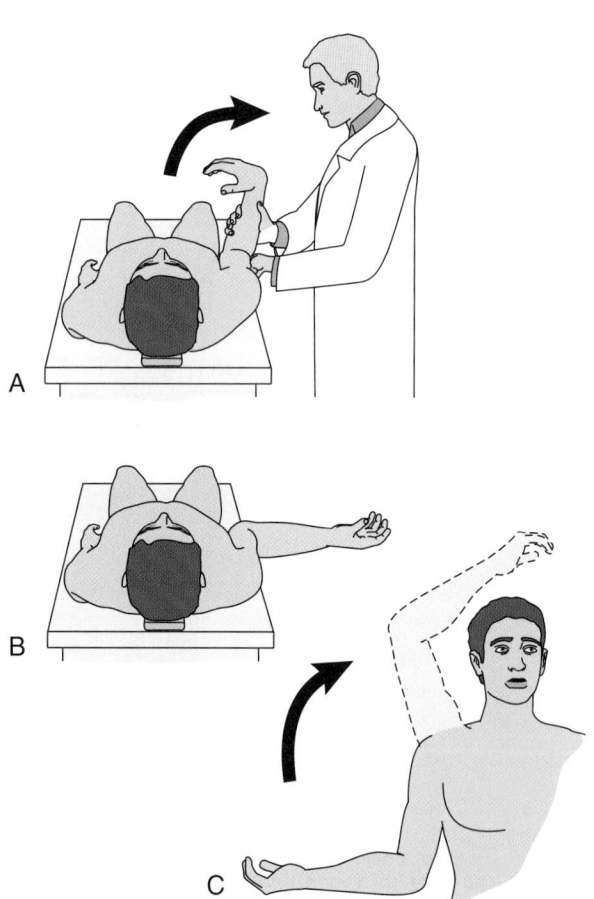

Fig. 174.5 Hennepin and modified Kocher techniques. Both techniques start with the elbow flexed to 90 degrees (A) and then fully externally rotated (B). For the modified Kocher, the forearm is then returned to complete internal rotation while gentle pressure is applied to the shoulder joint. The Hennepin technique (C) is continued from (B), if necessary, with elevation of the arm and manipulation of the joint posteriorly until the arm is overhead and the dislocation is reduced.

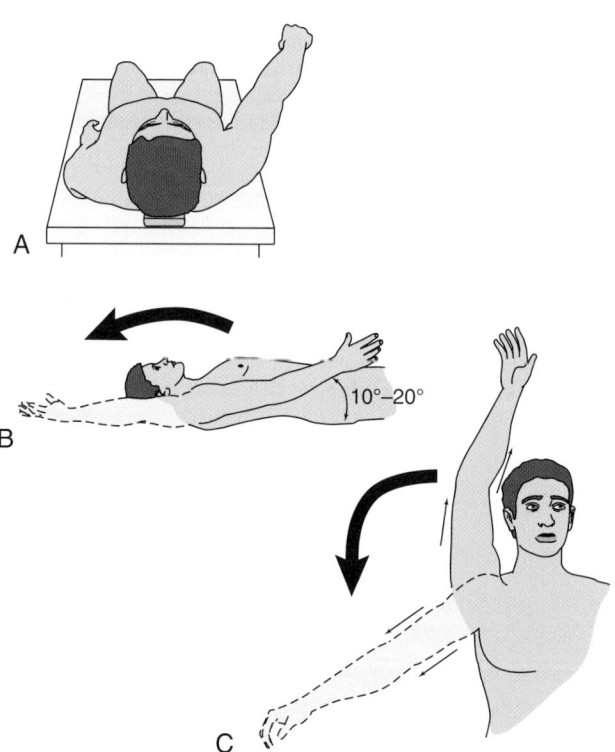

Fig. 174.6 Milch technique. (A) The arm is started at 10 to 20 degrees of flexion and slight abduction. (B) Elevation continues slowly, with slight distal traction, until the arm is directly overhead. The patient may be able to raise the arm on his or her own. The head of the humerus should be held immobile at this stage of maneuver. (C) If no reduction occurs with gentle, direct manipulation of the head of the humerus, the arm is then slowly brought through a full, lateral downward arc, maintaining constant outward traction until reduction occurs. Note that this is the only step of the procedure in which outward traction is maintained.

is adducted gently, with simultaneous posterolateral manipulation of the humeral head. This technique increases the forces applied; therefore the risk of complications is increased.

Boss-Holzach-Matter Technique

The patient sits against the maximally raised head of a gurney and wraps his or her forearms around the ipsilateral knee, which is flexed at 90 degrees. The head of the gurney is then lowered. The patient is asked to hyperextend his or her neck while leaning back and shrugging the shoulders anteriorly. This technique reportedly does not require analgesia.

Hippocratic Technique

Because the Hippocratic technique is no longer recommended, it is included only for historical interest. The clinician places his or her foot against the chest wall to provide countertraction and then manipulates the arm. This technique can cause serious neurovascular trauma.

COMPLICATIONS

If the shoulder dislocation proves irreducible, an orthopedic surgeon should be consulted and the use of general anesthesia considered. Fracture (due to the dislocation or reduction [iatrogenic]) and neurovascular damage are ever-present risks. Up to 50% of anterior dislocations have the previously mentioned Hill-Sachs deformity, an impaction fracture defect in the posterolateral portion of the humeral head. A Bankart lesion may also be noted, which is an avulsed fragment of the glenoid labrum with contiguous bone. Both lesions tend to get worse the longer the humeral head remains dislocated. Many clinicians obtain postreduction radiographs to document reduction of the joint, any injury associated with the reduction, and any bony abnormalities such as the aforementioned lesions.

Even nerve injuries following reduction in the operating room generally have a good prognosis; but the patient should be informed of the findings, the need to follow up, and that the symptoms may take many months to resolve.

Another risk after a shoulder dislocation is redislocation. In patients followed for 10 years, age at initial dislocation was the only predictor of recurrence; duration of subsequent immobilization had no effect. Rotator cuff tears and hemarthroses are more common with inferior dislocation and in patients above 60 years of age. To avoid serious complications of procedural sedation, adequate respiratory support measures and monitoring should be available. Patients must be observed after such sedation to make sure that they are awake, alert, and oriented before discharge.

POSTPROCEDURE EDUCATION AND CARE

Patients may need oral analgesic medications, possibly even narcotics, for a few days. Those below 20 years of age should be immobilized for 3 weeks; patients aged 20 to 40 years should be immobilized for 1 to 2 weeks; and patients above 60 years should have less than 1 week of immobilization. Appropriate clinical, neurologic, and radiographic follow-up examinations should be made throughout this time to confirm maintenance of the reduction. After the designated period of immobilization, a gentle strengthening program should be assigned with particular emphasis on the shoulder's internal rotators. Unrestricted external rotation, abduction, and lifting activities are usually not permitted for a period of 3 months. Even combing the hair involves external rotation and abduction and should be avoided indefinitely on the side of the dislocation. With recurrent dislocations, an arthrogram, CT arthrogram, magnetic resonance imaging, or arthroscopy might be warranted to help identify an anatomic variant that might make the patient more prone to redislocation. Patients with peripheral neuropathies, syringomyelia, and psychiatric histories may be more liable to dislocate their shoulders; therefore these underlying conditions should be considered in patients with repeated dislocations.

CPT/BILLING CODES

| 23650 | Closed treatment of shoulder dislocation, with manipulation, without anesthesia |
| 23655 | Closed treatment of shoulder dislocation, with manipulation, requiring anesthesia |

ICD-9-10-CM DIAGNOSTIC CODES

M24.119	Articular cartilage disorder, unspecified shoulder
M24.019	Loose body in joint, unspecified shoulder
M24.419	Recurrent dislocation of joint, unspecified shoulder
S43.006A	Dislocation unspecified of unspecified shoulder

Acknowledgment

The editors recognize the contributions of Fred M. Hankin, MD, and J. Mark Wiedemann, MD, MS, to this chapter in previous editions of this text.

RECOMMENDED READING

Akyol C, Gungor F, Akyol AJ, et al. Point-of-care ultrasonography for the management of shoulder dislocation in ED. *Am J Emerg Med.* 2016;34(5):866–870.

Doyle WL, Ragar T. Use of the scapular manipulation method to reduce an anterior shoulder dislocation in the supine position. *Ann Emerg Med.* 1996;27:92–94.

Eiff MP, Hatch RL. *Fracture Management for Primary Care.* 3rd ed. Philadelphia: Saunders Elsevier; 2012.

Jiang N, Hu YJ, Zhang KR, et al. Intra-articular lidocaine versus intravenous analgesia and sedation for manual closed reduction of acute anterior shoulder dislocation: an updated meta-analysis. *J Clin Anesth.* 2014;26:350.

Naples RM, Ufberg JW. Management of common dislocations. In: Roberts JR, Custalow CB, Thomsen TW, eds. *Roberts and Hedges Clinical Procedures in Emergency Medicine and Acute Care.* 7th ed. Philadelphia: Elsevier; 2019:980–1026.

Ng VK, Hames H, Millard WM. Use of intra-articular lidocaine as analgesia in anterior shoulder dislocation: a review and meta-analysis of the literature. *Can J Rural Med.* 2009;14:145–149.

Reichman EF. Shoulder joint dislocation reduction. In: Reichman EF, ed. *Emergency Medicine Procedures.* 2nd ed. New York: McGraw-Hill; 2013:531–549.

Stimson LA. An easy method of reducing dislocations of the shoulder and hip. *Med Rec.* 1900;57:356–357.

Tuggy M, Garcia J. *Atlas of Essential Procedures.* Philadelphia: Elsevier; 2010.

Wakai A, O'Sullivan R, McCabe A. Intra-articular lignocaine versus intravenous analgesia with or without sedation for manual reduction of acute anterior shoulder dislocation in adults. *Cochrane Database Syst Rev.* 2011;2:CD004919.

CHAPTER 175

ANKLE AND FOOT SPLINTING, CASTING, AND TAPING

Gregory A. Marolf

Primary care clinicians encounter a wide variety of acute and chronic foot and lower leg injuries that may benefit from immobilization. The value of immobilization as an initial means of therapy has been known for centuries. Treatment of foot and ankle injuries involves an accurate clinical evaluation and, when indicated, radiographic assessment of potential fractures, avulsions, or instability. Casting and cast splinting are commonly used in acute situations and fractures (see Chapter 178, Fracture Care), whereas splinting and taping are probably best used to control chronic instabilities and as adjuncts in rehabilitation. PRICES (protect, rest, ice, compression, elevation, splint) is the mnemonic often used when acute immobilization is indicated. It should also be noted that rapid remobilization is an important part of the rehabilitation for most soft tissue injuries to the ankle.

INDICATIONS

Soft Tissue Injuries

- Ankle sprains: Treatment options include use of a sugar-tong splint, taping, and braces (stirrup or lace-up type) for support as the patient returns to weight bearing.
- Plantar fasciitis: Immobilization can be achieved with a nocturnal posterior leg splint, which provides a constant stretch to the plantar fascia (see Chapter 185, Podiatric Procedures, for other treatments, including customized orthotics) or by taping.

Fractures

- Tibial or fibular: Stable distal tibial or fibular fractures, including malleolar fractures, can be immobilized with a splint or short-leg walking cast (see Chapter 178, Fracture Care).
- Fifth metatarsal: Immobilize avulsion fractures with a postoperative shoe, posterior splint, or short-leg cast (see Chapter 178, Fracture Care).
- Other: Primary care clinicians may also encounter fractures of the tarsals, or first through fourth metatarsals. When these fractures are nondisplaced and stable, immobilization alone may be appropriate; otherwise, surgical referral may be necessary (see Chapter 178, Fracture Care).

Prophylaxis Against Injuries

Ankle taping or bracing may be used as prophylaxis against injury in ankles that need additional stabilization and improved proprioception.

CONTRAINDICATIONS

- Early (premature) casting: Casting before maximal swelling has occurred can cause necrosis and compartment syndrome.

- Open wound: Never place a cast over an open wound because of the potential for infection. If the wound is not too large, a window may be cut in the cast to monitor it.
- Unstable fractures: These fractures need surgical repair; splint only until definitive treatment can be provided.

BENEFITS OF DIFFERENT TYPES OF IMMOBILIZATION

The type of immobilization used may vary with the location and severity of the injury, patient or clinician preference, and the plan of treatment. The following list of benefits for each option may help when making decisions.

Splinting or Bracing

- Stability for soft tissue injuries
- Pain relief
- Easily removable to apply ice, massage, etc.
- Provides temporary support for patients needing surgery

Casting

- Marked stability
- Significant pain relief
- Immobilization for hard-to-treat soft tissue injuries and fractures

Taping

- Supports acutely injured ankles
- Supports chronically weak or injured ankles or a chronically injured plantar fascia
- Enhances proprioception
- Prophylaxis against injury

EQUIPMENT

Casting

Fig. 175.1 illustrates the materials needed for casting.

- Stockinette: 4-inch stockinette is appropriate for most patients, but 3-inch stockinette may be needed for smaller patients
- Cast padding: 3- or 4-inch rolls (depending on patient size), soft cotton (e.g., Webril) or synthetic (e.g., polyester)
- Synthetic waterproof cast liner (e.g., Gore Procel, Scotchcast Wet or Dry, Delta-Dry, Waterpruf) (optional)
- Cast material: 3- or 4-inch rolls, depending on patient size, plaster or synthetic (e.g., fiberglass)
- Rubber heels (for walking cast, but may not be needed for fiberglass cast)

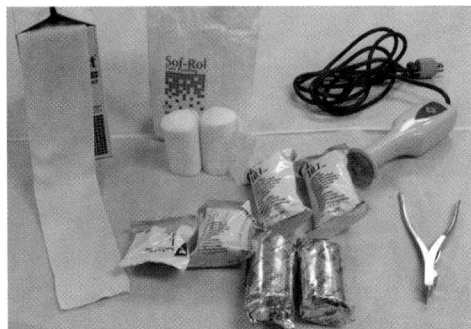

Fig. 175.1 Materials needed for casting: cast padding, casting material, cast spreader, cast cutter, and stockinette.

- Gloves, nonsterile
- Gown and shoe covers for the clinician
- Patient towels or drapes
- Water bucket with tepid water (if using plaster, should have traps in drains)
- Foot stand (optional)
- Scissors
- Cast cutter
- Cast spreader
- See Chapter 176, Cast Immobilization and Upper Extremity Splinting, if cast removal protective strips (e.g., De-Flex) indicated or desired to protect skin from cast saw during removal

Splinting

- Most of the foregoing supplies for casting or premade splint material (plaster or synthetic)
- Compression wrap elastic bandage (Ace bandage)

Taping for Ankle

- Skin preparation (benzoin)
- Lubricant (optional)

  NOTE: The lubricant may be applied to the skin at sites of potential friction or irritation.

- Underwrap
- 1.5- or 2-inch athletic tape
- Pressure pads or moleskin

Taping for Plantar Fasciitis

Equipment is similar to that used for the McConnell method of taping for patellofemoral knee pain:

- 2-inch dressing retention sheet (skin tape, white)
- 1.5-inch patellofemoral adhesive tape (high-tensile strength tape, brown; some of the original work with McConnell taping was rumored to have used duct tape!)
- Alcohol swabs
- Commercial adhesive remover

PREPROCEDURE PATIENT PREPARATION

Obtain verbal or written consent. Possible complications should be explained to the patient. For example, the patient should be aware that there will be a temporary loss of flexibility following immobilization, especially in the foot. In some cases, a partial loss of flexibility can become permanent. Place the patient in a seated or supine position. Some clinicians prefer a prone position with the knee flexed 90 degrees.

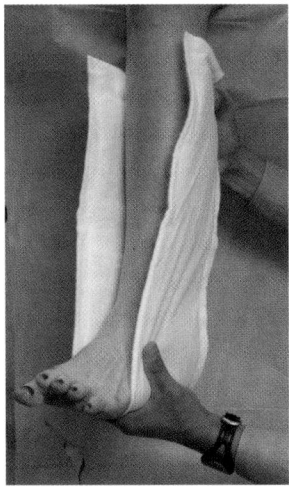

Fig. 175.2 Splint material in the shape of a U (sugar tong). The splint allows for swelling while providing medial and lateral support.

TECHNIQUE

Splinting

Most clinicians have access to premade splinting materials that are fixed or inflatable (e.g., Aircast). However, inexpensive splints can be made from a plaster cast roll and cast padding:

1. Estimate the length of the splint you plan to use.
2. Unroll cast material into layers, making 11 to 13 layers.
3. In a similar fashion, unroll cast padding into layers, making 6 to 8 layers.
4. Unroll a single layer of cast padding for the outside of the splint.
5. The plaster cast material will be placed between the inner and outer layers of cast padding. The inner layers (6 to 8 layers) are placed between the splint and the skin, while the single outer layer of cast padding is placed on the outside of the splint. The latter is used to prevent the Ace bandage from adhering to the plaster.

Generally, when making a splint from casting materials, plaster is used. With this type of splint, the padding will not be wet. The casting material is immersed in water separately. Premade splints may be plaster or fiberglass. With premade materials, the padding will be wet. Premade splint material can also be simulated by rolling a stockinette over the outside of the 11 to 13 layers of cast materials. Fold over the ends of the stockinette and tape them to keep the splint neat. Both the stockinette and the casting materials are then immersed in water together. Both will be wet when applying. Several layers of cast padding are then placed between the patient's skin and this splint to prevent skin breakdown.

Two types of ankle splints will be discussed: sugar tong and posterior. Application depends on the indication and degree of stabilization desired. The sugar-tong (stirrup) splint may be used in ankle sprains to prevent inversion or eversion.

Sugar-Tong (Stirrup) Splint

1. Measure from the fibular head (at the knee) to the calcaneus, double that measurement, and cut the splint material and padding to size.
2. Wet the splint material and remove excess water by applying gentle pressure across the width of the splint material.
3. Place the padding against the patient's skin and have the patient or an assistant hold it in place.
4. Apply the splint material against the lateral aspect of the leg, starting just distal to the fibular head (2 fingerbreadths below). Wrap the splint under the heel, and return it up the medial side of the leg to just below the knee (Fig. 175.2). (It is U-shaped, similar to a long sugar tong; the anterior and posterior aspects are open.)

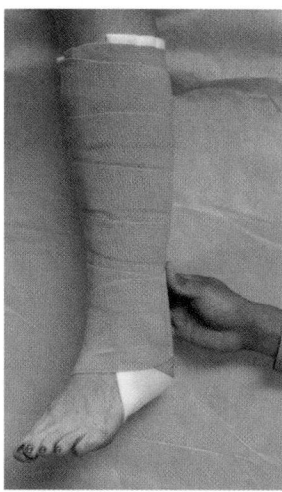

Fig. 175.3   Finished sugar-tong splint held in place with a compression wrap.

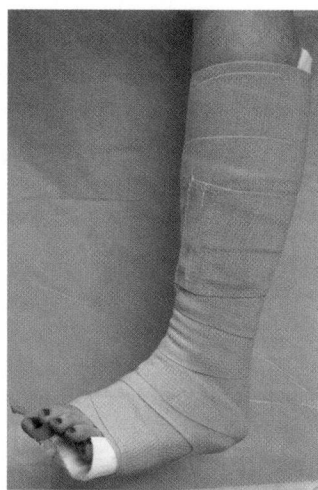

Fig. 175.5   Finished posterior splint held in place with a compression wrap.

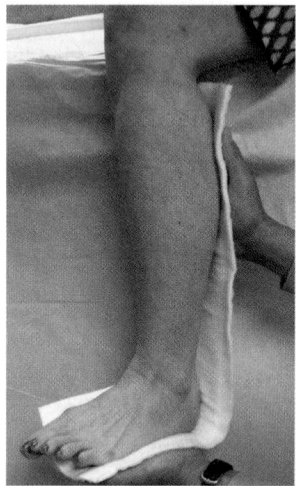

Fig. 175.4   Cast material runs along the posterior aspect of the lower leg and the plantar surface, providing immobilization for ankle dorsiflexion and plantar flexion.

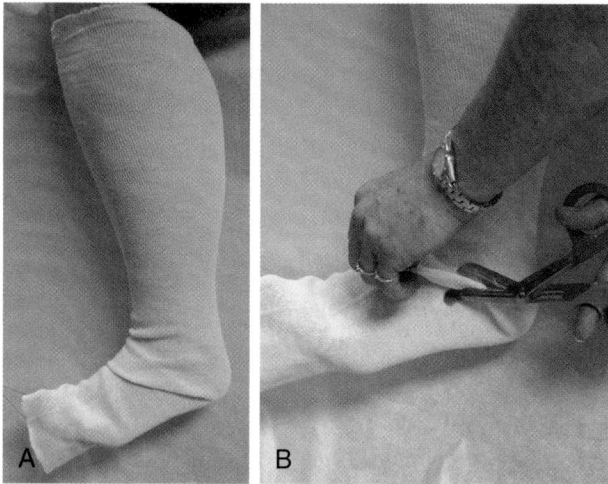

Fig. 175.6   (A) Stockinette is placed on the lower leg from the knee to the toes. (B) The transverse crease formed at the ankle should be removed.

5. Mold the splint material to support the ankle and heel.
6. Place a layer of padding over the splint.
7. Wrap the splint material to hold it in place with an elastic bandage or a roll of cast padding (Fig. 175.3).

Posterior Splint

The posterior splint may be used with stable tibial or fibular fractures and plantar fasciitis to restrict dorsiflexion or plantar flexion of the foot-and-ankle complex.

1. Measure from the metatarsal heads to just distal to the popliteal fossa (2 fingerbreadths above), and cut the splint material and padding to size.
2. Wet the splint material and remove excess water.
3. Place the padding against the patient's skin and have the patient or an assistant hold it in place.
4. Apply the splint material over the padding and against the plantar aspect of the foot and along the posterior aspect of the leg. Extend the splint from the metatarsal heads to just distal to the popliteal fossa (Fig. 175.4).
5. Mold the splint material to support the ankle and heel.
6. Place a layer of padding over the outside of the splint.

7. Wrap the splint material to hold it in place with an elastic bandage or a roll of cast padding (Fig. 175.5).

Casting

Short-Leg Cast

A short-leg cast may be used for stable tibial or fibular fractures, fifth metatarsal fractures, or severe ankle sprains (after acute swelling subsides).

1. Measure from the metatarsal heads to the knee and cut the stockinette to length. Be sure to allow extra stockinette to fold over the ends of the cast.
2. Slide stockinette on and smooth all wrinkles or folds. The crease that will be formed at the anterior ankle should be trimmed away (Fig. 175.6).
3. Place the ankle in a neutral position (90 degrees). Failure to flex it to 90 degrees may lead to difficulty in ambulating and to Achilles tendon shortening. A foot stand may be useful to support the foot.
4. Wrap the cast padding over the stockinette, starting at the foot. The padding should overlap 50% with each consecutive wrap. The padding should extend from the metatarsal heads to just

distal to the fibular head. Care should be taken to provide adequate padding around the heel, the malleoli, the metatarsal heads, the proximal fibula, and the anterior tibia (Fig. 175.7).

5. Wet the cast material. Wrap the foot and ankle with the cast material in a manner similar to that already done with the cast padding. It should be wrapped over the cast padding. Maintain moderate tension, and overlap the rolls by 50% (Fig. 175.8).
6. Mold the cast to ensure a neutral position of the ankle at 90 degrees.
7. Fold the stockinette over the ends of the cast to provide a smooth edge (Fig. 175.9).
8. Apply a final layer of cast material over the initial layer and the folded-down edge of the stockinette at the ends (Fig. 175.10). For a walking cast, 6 to 8 layers of reinforcing strips may be placed under the heel and foot prior to the final cast layer. These are shaped similar to an L and go from the metatarsal heads to the midcalf to provide additional support.
9. Allow 10 minutes for the cast to set, and instruct the patient not to bear weight for at least 24 hours. Provide crutches for ambulation.
10. A walking boot may be fitted to ease ambulation. Again, wait 24 hours for the cast to set before allowing weight bearing. A cast check by the clinician the next day can assure a proper fit.

NOTE: A walking heel is unnecessary for a fiberglass cast.

Cast Removal or Bivalving

1. When splitting the cast, both the medial and lateral sides should be cut.
2. Starting at the top of the cast, make straight cuts that run posterior to the malleoli. Use a finger to stabilize the saw against the cast and to control the depth of the cut.

NOTE: When using a cast saw, make plunging cuts along the length of the cut. Do not attempt to steadily drag the saw along the length of the cut, as this will cause the blade to heat up, and may burn the patient.

3. Next, make cuts along the medial and lateral sides of the foot that intersect with the initial cuts. Take care to avoid cutting over bony prominences (Fig. 175.11).
4. After the cuts are complete, a cast spreader is inserted into the cut and spread to widen the cut.
5. The cast padding and stockinette are then cut with blunt-tipped scissors.
6. The cast may then be opened and removed, or wrapped with a compression bandage to serve as a splint.

NOTE: When wrapped with a compression bandage, the resultant splint provides almost as much support as a cast; therefore a clinician should have a low threshold for bivalving a cast to minimize complications. The same saws can be used for both plaster and fiberglass.

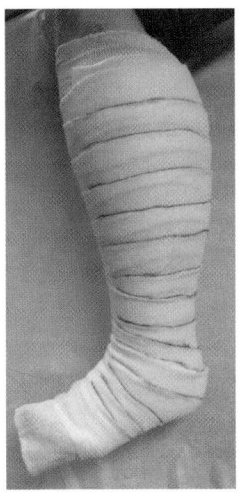

Fig. 175.7   Cast padding is applied with 50% overlap on each turn.

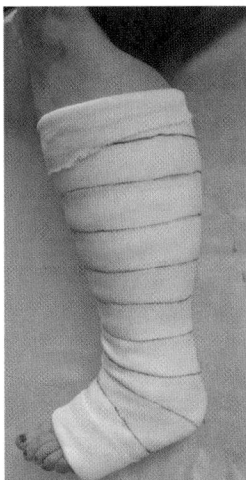

Fig. 175.9   After the first roll of cast material is placed, the stockinette is folded back over the ends.

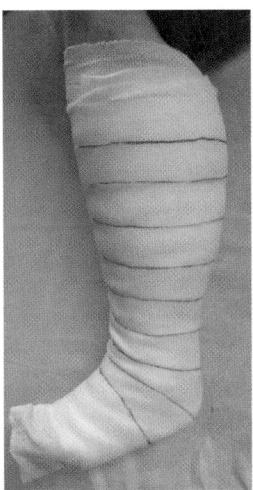

Fig. 175.8   Application of cast material with 50% overlap on each turn.

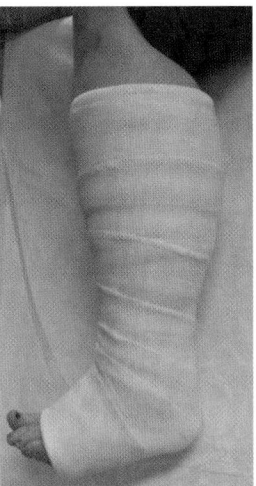

Fig. 175.10   Finished short-leg cast.

Bracing

Ankle bracing may be used prophylactically (to prevent injury), therapeutically, after an acute injury, or after injury to prevent reinjury. Commercial premade braces come in several styles. All styles may be used for any of these indications. Consider patient comfort and stability in choosing a brace. If the patient does not tolerate one style, consider a different one. Available styles include a lace-up, stirrup, or hinged brace.

Taping

Plantar Fasciitis

For this procedure, two pieces of skin tape will be applied followed by two pieces of high-tensile adhesive tape placed over them. The first three pieces of tape are simply applied smoothly and without wrinkles or any tension; the last piece of tape is the only one applied under tension.

SKIN PREPARATION: With the patient sitting on an examination table, skin oils and other debris should be cleansed from the plantar aspect of the affected foot with alcohol. While the alcohol is allowed to dry, palpate the dorsalis pedis pulse. Document the presence or absence of the pulse.

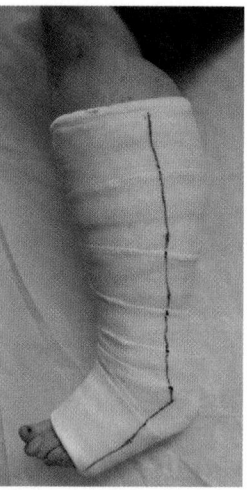

Fig. 175.11 When a cast is being removed, medial and lateral cuts are made posterior to the malleoli.

APPLICATION:

1. Place the foot in a neutral position (90 degrees), approximately the same position as if the patient were standing on it. From this position, it should be slightly inverted or "turned in" (sole of the foot facing slightly medially).

2. Apply skin tape (white tape) from the ball of the foot (Fig. 175.12A) to the middle of the heel (Fig. 175.12B). The upper edge of the tape will extend slightly up the medial side of the foot, but it should not be higher than one-third of the way up to the medial malleolus. In fact, keeping it low on the foot and simply taping around the posterior calcaneus may minimize any friction on the Achilles tendon. Smooth the wrinkles and bubbles; there should be no tension on the tape.

3. Locate the navicular bone. This is the bony projection about 1 inch anterior to the medial malleolus. Apply skin tape (white tape), under no tension, from the heel (Fig. 175.12C) up the medial aspect of the foot to end on top of the foot (Fig. 175.12D). This tape should cover and include the navicular bone and extend past the midline of the dorsum of the foot.

4. Apply tensile tape (brown tape) of the same length in the same location and manner as the first piece of skin tape, simply covering that skin tape. Smooth any wrinkles or bubbles, but do not apply any tension.

5. Apply a second piece of tensile tape (brown tape) over the second piece of skin tape. This tape should be applied under tension, but not enough tension to occlude the dorsalis pedis pulse.

6. When the patient stands, he or she should be almost symptom free because the tape bears the weight of the plantar fascia. For severe cases of plantar fasciitis, adding a slight degree of plantar flexion to the foot prior to taping, in addition to the slight inversion, will take the weight off the fascia even more.

7. Because it loses strength with weight bearing, the tape should be removed and reapplied daily for 4 to 6 weeks. Outlining the outside edges of the tape with a permanent marker may be helpful for patient education purposes. This outline may help them when reapplying the tape the next day. They may want to outline it each day or use a copy of Fig. 175.12 to remind them of how to reapply the tape. When the tape is being changed, the foot should be massaged and put through range-of-motion exercises. Using a commercial adhesive remover will help remove the debris from the prior day's skin tape.

8. For more severe cases, if the patient is symptomatic when bearing weight following taping, more degrees of plantar flexion should

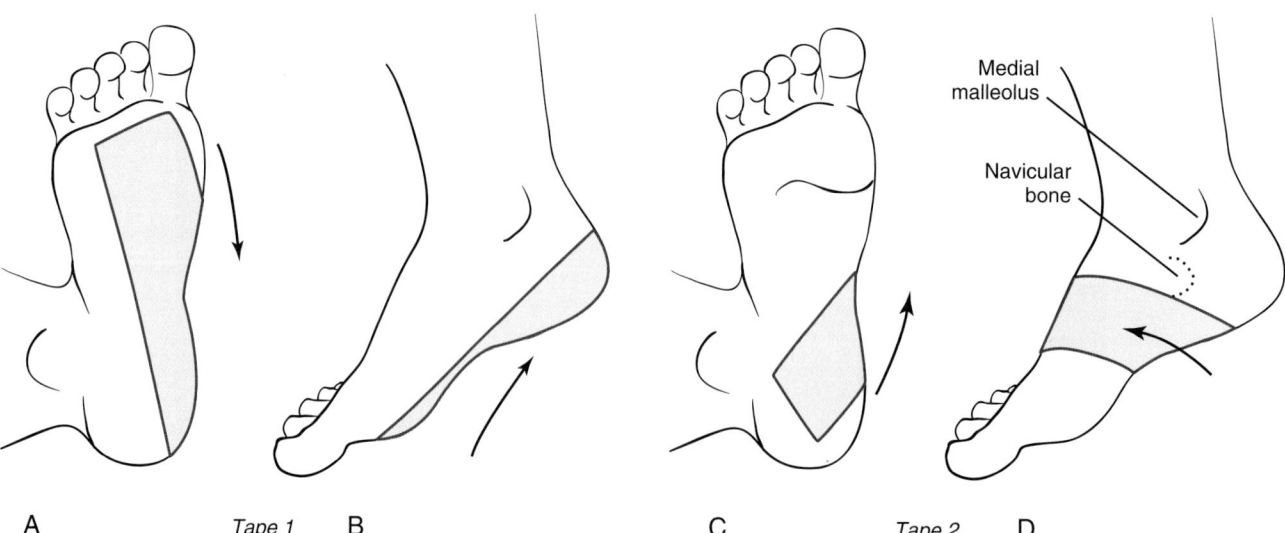

Fig. 175.12 Skin tape 1 (white tape) is applied from the ball of the foot (A) to the middle of the heel (B). Skin tape 2 (white tape) is applied from the heel (C) up the medial aspect of the foot to end on top of the foot (D). Tensile tape pieces 1 and 2 are applied in the same locations and directions. They should be the same lengths as the skin tape.

gradually be applied with each day of subsequent taping. The goal should be to bear weight with almost no symptoms for 4 to 6 weeks. This allows the fascia to heal.

9. Following resolution of symptoms and completion of the taping regimen, the foot should be rehabilitated aggressively with stretching and range-of-motion exercises.

NOTE: One of the success stories of the physical therapists who first used this technique was a woman who had plantar fasciitis for 7 years!

Ankle

SKIN PREPARATION: Ankle taping provides the greatest support when applied directly against the skin. However, daily application will likely cause skin irritation. The use of underwrap material can prevent this. Shave the foot and ankle. Apply a coating of skin preparation, usually benzoin, to protect the skin and provide better adhesion. Avoid the use of skin preparation in patients with a history of sensitivity or allergy to these products (underwrap is recommended in these patients [Fig. 175.13A]). Lubrication or padding may be applied to the skin at sites of potential friction or irritation (Fig. 175.13B).

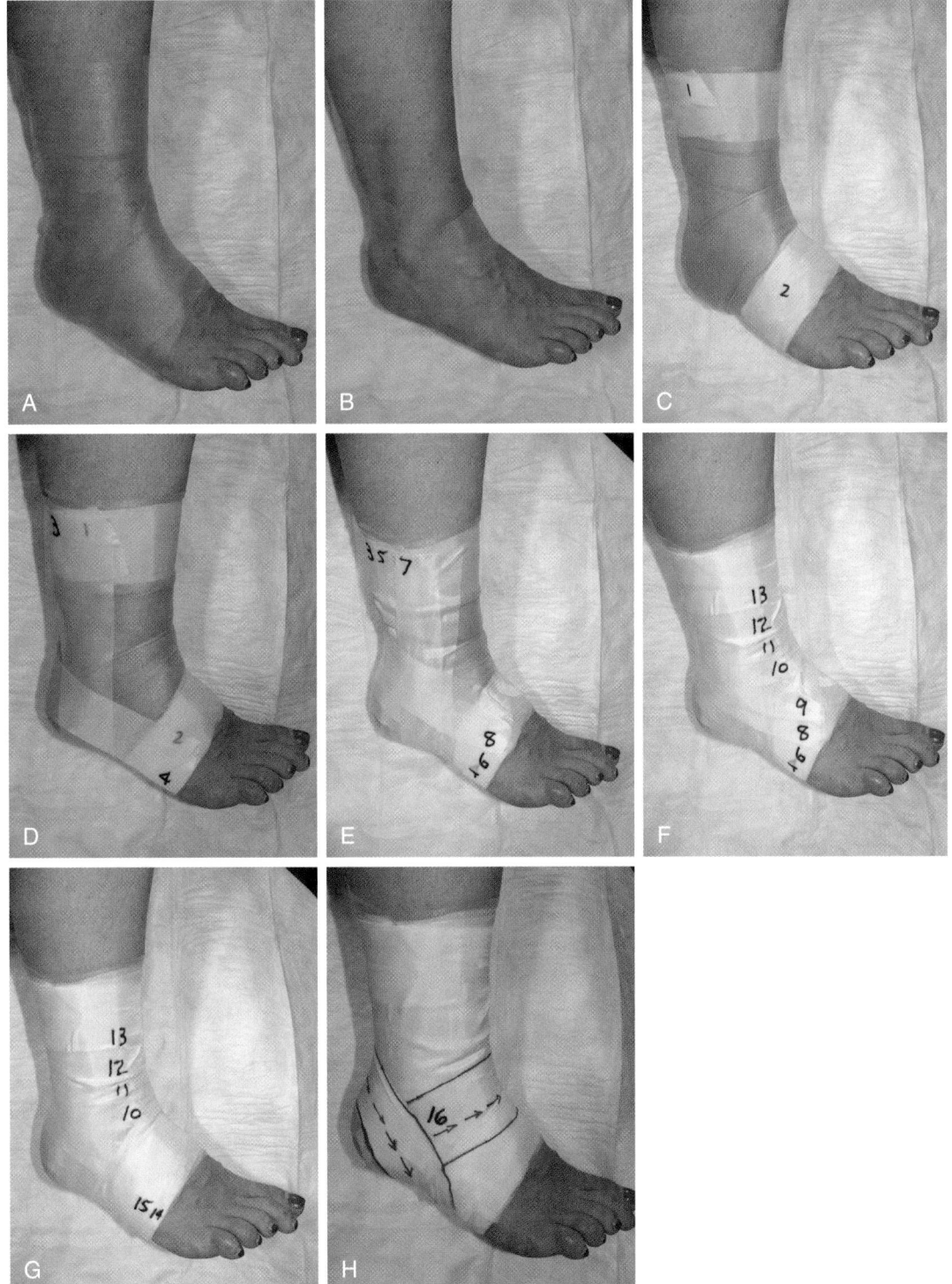

Fig. 175.13 Closed basket-weave (Gibney) technique. (A) Application of thin underwrap tape. (B) Application of padding at pressure points. (C) Anchor straps are placed either directly onto skin or over underwrap. (D) Application of first stirrup and Gibney strips. (E) Stirrup and Gibney strips are applied in an alternating fashion. (F) Gibney strips are continued up the ankle to the anchor strip. (G) Application of arch strips. (H) Heel locks are applied for additional support.

APPLICATION: Several methods can be used for taping the ankle. The most commonly used is the *closed basket-weave technique*, also known as the Gibney technique, which provides strong tape support (see Fig. 175.13). This extra support may be needed in either recently sprained or chronically weak ankles.

1. An anchor strip is placed around the ankle 5 to 6 inches above the malleoli (Fig. 175.13C).
2. A second anchor strip is placed around the instep.
3. A stirrup strip is placed posterior to the malleoli (Fig. 175.13D). For an inversion injury, hold the foot in *eversion* when applying the stirrup strips. Conversely, hold the foot in *inversion* for an eversion injury.
4. The first horizontal (Gibney) strip is placed under the malleoli, and attached to the foot anchor (Fig. 175.13D).
5. A second stirrup is placed overlapping the first by 50%, followed by a second Gibney strip, also overlapping the first by 50%. A third stirrup and Gibney are then placed in similar fashion (Fig. 175.13E).
6. Placement of the Gibney strips is then continued up the ankle to the anchor strip (Fig. 175.13F).
7. Two or three strips are placed around the arch for added support (Fig. 175.13G).
8. Lastly, heel locks are applied as a final support. Starting high on the instep, wrap the tape posteriorly across the Achilles tendon, downward, hooking the heel. It should then lead under the arch and up the opposite side to finish at the starting point. The heel lock is completed by repeating the wrap in the opposite direction (Fig. 175.13H).

An alternative method, the *open basket-weave technique*, allows for some degree of dorsiflexion and plantar flexion. This technique accommodates swelling and may be used after acute injury. The procedure for the open basket weave is the same as for the closed basket weave, with the notable exception of the Gibney strip placement. The Gibney strips are placed with a gap anteriorly. After the Gibney strips are placed, the gap is closed and the ends are locked by two to four strips running down the instep.

COMPLICATIONS

- *Nerve entrapment:* When casting, compression of the common peroneal nerve at the fibular head may lead to foot drop. Correct placement of the proximal end of the cast is essential.
- *Compartment syndrome:* This may be seen in patients with injuries due to high-velocity forces (e.g., motor vehicle accidents) or by applying the cast before swelling has reached its maximum. If the patient notes any pain caused by the cast, pain out of proportion to the injury, pain not controlled with oral analgesics, or progressively increasing pain, the cast should be bivalved or removed immediately to check compartment pressures (see Chapter 179, Compartment Syndrome Evaluation) and to evaluate for any neurovascular compromise. Treatment of the fracture or maintenance of reduction of the fracture is always a second priority to preserving the blood supply to the soft tissue and bone. **NOTE:** One of the earliest signs of an impending compartment syndrome is pain on resisted plantar flexion of the great toe. Have the patient dorsiflex his or her toe, and if pain radiates into the leg when the clinician attempts to plantarflex the toe, the cast should be bivalved or removed immediately.
- *Loosening of the cast:* Application of a cast when swelling is present may lead to cast looseness when the swelling abates. A loose cast will no longer provide adequate stability and immobilization.
- *Skin necrosis:* Skin necrosis may be caused by pressure over bony prominences. This is best prevented by placing extra padding at potential pressure points (Fig. 175.14). If necessary, a window may be cut in the cast to remove the source of irritation. A window should not be cut, however, in areas that

have acute swelling. In that case, a different form of immobilization should be employed.
- *Delayed union, nonunion, atrophic or hypertrophic union, or malunion:* All are possible complications of fractures. Inadequate assessment of the initial radiographs, improper management of the fracture (including incomplete reduction), poor patient adherence and compliance, increased age, medications, and presence of osteopenia or osteoporosis are all possible causes of these complications. Smoking or taking antiinflammatory medications delays the healing time and increases the risk for improper fracture healing, especially in weight-bearing bones such as the ankle, foot, or calcaneus. If the patient smokes, the fracture healing time in the ankle is doubled compared to a nonsmoker.
- *Joint stiffness:* Patients often suffer from joint stiffness as a result of immobilization. This is best prevented by not immobilizing joints any longer than what is needed for fracture healing.

POSTPROCEDURE PATIENT EDUCATION

In an acute injury, after immobilization, the patient should elevate the leg for 48 to 72 hours to prevent swelling. Ice can be used, in a sealed container, over the cast or splint to help alleviate pain. If a nonwaterproof cast or splint is used, every effort should be made to keep the cast or splint dry. Patients should remove or cover it when bathing. If a nonwaterproof cast or splint does become wet, patients may dry it with a hair dryer set on the cool setting.

Nothing should be inserted between a cast and the skin. This may cause abrasions and undetected infections. With a cast, patients should call immediately if they notice pain, fever, tightness or irritation, numbness, or discolored or cool toes.

CPT/BILLING CODES
Fracture Management
Fracture care CPT codes include initial management of fractures, along with initial splint or cast application. These codes include subsequent routine cast care and removal.

Codes for closed treatment without manipulation include the following:

27750 Tibial shaft fracture
27760 Medial malleolus fracture
27780 Proximal fibula or fibular shaft fracture
27786 Distal fibular (lateral malleolus) fracture

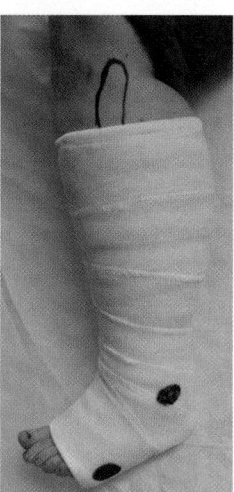

Fig. 175.14 Common locations for pressure sores are noted on the cast. Note the outline of the fibular head above the cast. This is the site of possible peroneal nerve entrapment.

Codes for closed treatment with manipulation include the following:

27752	Tibial shaft fracture
27762	Medial malleolus fracture
27781	Proximal fibula or fibular shaft fracture
27788	Distal fibular (lateral malleolus) fracture

Cast or Splint Application

The following codes can be used when not part of comprehensive fracture management, or when used for soft tissue injuries. If a cast needs replacement, these codes can also be used.

29405	Application of short-leg cast (below knee to toes)
29425	Walking or ambulatory type
29440	Adding walker to previously applied cast
29515	Application of short-leg splint (calf to foot)
29540	Strapping; ankle and/or foot
29700	Removal or bivalving of short-leg cast applied by another physician
29705	Removal or bivalving of full-leg cast applied by another physician
29730	Windowing of cast applied by another physician
29740	Wedging of cast applied by another physician
29799	Unlisted procedure, casting or strapping

SUPPLIES

A4565	Sling
A4570	Splint material
A4580	Plaster cast supplies
A4590	Special cast supplies (fiberglass)
99070	Miscellaneous supplies/materials provided over and above other services rendered

ICD-10-CM DIAGNOSTIC CODES

M72.2	Plantar fasciitis
M84.379a	Stress fracture unspecified toe(s) initial encounter
S82.109A	Tibial fracture unspecified, upper end closed
S82.839A	Fibular fracture unspecified, upper and lower end closed
S82.209A	Tibial shaft fracture unspecified, closed
S82.409A	Fibular shaft fracture unspecified, closed
S82.53XA	Medial malleolus fracture displaced, closed
S82.56XA	Medial Malleolus fracture nondisplaced, closed
S82.63XA	Lateral malleolus fracture displaced, closed
S82.66XA	Lateral malleolus fracture nondisplaced, closed
S82.843A	Bimalleolar fracture displaced, closed
S82.846A	Bimalleolar fracture nondisplaced closed
S82.853A	Trimalleolar fracture displaced, closed
S82.856A	Trimalleolar fracture nondisplaced, closed
S92.009A	Calcaneal fracture unspecified, closed
S92.109A	Talar fracture unspecified, closed
S92.253A	Navicular fracture of foot displaced, closed
S92.256A	Navicular fracture of foot nondisplaced closed
S92.213A	Cuboid fracture displaced, closed
S92.216A	Cuboid fracture nondisplaced closed

S92.226A	Cuneiform fracture undisplaced, closed
S92.223A	Cuneiform fracture displaced, closed
S92.309A	Metatarsal fracture unspecified, closed
S96.919A	Ankle sprain and strain

SUPPLIERS

Full contact information is available at www.expertconsult.com.

Braces
  Swede-O, Inc.
Casting and splinting materials
  Johnson & Johnson Professional, Inc. (extra-fast setting casting splints available)
  3M Health Care
Casting and splinting materials, accessories, braces
  M-Pact
Dressing retention sheet (skin tape)
  Hypafix
  Smith & Nephew, Inc.
High-tensile-strength adhesive tape
  FLA Orthopedics
  Jobst/BSN Medical
  Leukotape-P (specifically for use with McConnell taping)
Nocturnal splints
  AliMed, Inc.
  Freedom PF Night Splint II
Splints and braces
  Aircast, Inc., and DonJoy (owned by DJO)

RECOMMENDED READING

Batt ME, Tanji JL, Skattum N. Plantar fasciitis, a prospective randomized clinical trial of the tension night splint. *Clin J Sport Med.* 1996;6:158–162.

Bica D, Sprouse RA, Armen J. Diagnosis and management of common foot fractures. *Am Fam Physician.* 2016;93(3):183–191.

Boyd AS, Benjamin HJ, Asplund C. Principles of casting and splinting. *Am Fam Physician.* 2009;79:23–24. 16–22.

Eiff MP, Hatch RL. *Fracture Management for Primary Care.* 3rd ed. Philadelphia: Elsevier; 2012.

Goff JD, Crawford R. Diagnosis and treatment of plantar fasciitis. *Am Fam Physician.* 2011;15(6):676–682.

Reichman EF, Sloas HA. Casts and splints. In: Reichman EF, ed. *Emergency Medicine Procedures.* 2nd ed. New York: McGraw-Hill; 2013.

Mellion MB, Walsh WM, Madden C, et al. *The Team Physician's Handbook.* 3rd ed. Philadelphia: Hanley & Belfus; 2001.

Petrizzi MJ, Petrizzi MG, Miller A. A "three-way" ankle splint for acute ankle injury. *Phys Sportsmed.* 2000;28:99–100.

Petrizzi MJ, Petrizzi MG, Roos RJ. Making a tension night splint for plantar fasciitis. *Phys Sportsmed.* 1998;26:113–114.

Pfeffer G, Bacchetti P, Deland J, et al. Comparison of custom and prefabricated orthoses in the initial treatment of proximal plantar fasciitis. *Foot Ankle Int.* 1999;20:214–221.

Prentice W, Arnheim D. *Principles of Athletic Training.* 9th ed. Madison, WI: Brown & Benchmark; 1996.

Shahady E, ed. *Primary Care of Musculoskeletal Problems in the Outpatient Setting.* Cambridge: Blackwell Science; 2006.

Tiemstra JD. Update on acute ankle sprains. *Am Fam Physician.* 2012;85(12):1170–1176.

Cast Immobilization and Upper Extremity Splinting

Scott W. Eathorne • Todd M. Sheperd

Cast immobilization is a technique used to treat a variety of medical conditions encountered by the primary care clinician. Although newer technologies have led to an evolution in casting materials, the general principles of this valuable technique have stood the test of time. By having knowledge of the materials available and an understanding of the indications and fundamental precepts of cast immobilization as well as by developing the necessary manual dexterity skills, the primary care clinician can easily treat the patient who has an injury amenable to such therapy. Casting and splinting is a skill that requires some practice; cast application videos and simulators are emerging as educational techniques to augment casting skills (Mehrpour, 2013; Moktar, 2014).

The principle of casting a fracture is to apply three points of force. Two points of force should be applied at sites proximal and distal to the fracture on its concave side. The third point of force should be applied in the opposite direction over the convex side of the fracture site.

In the upper extremity, splints made from casting material (e.g., thumb spica, sugar tong) are occasionally used in place of circumferential casts. Some of these are covered in this chapter. Note that splinting and casting in the lower extremity are also discussed in Chapter 175, Ankle and Foot Splinting, Casting, and Taping.

History

The use of immobilization to treat acute fractures dates to the era of the Fifth Dynasty of Egypt (2498–2345 BC), when bark was used to splint fractures of the forearm. Gypsum, from which plaster of Paris is derived, was initially used around the 16th century in parts of the Ottoman Empire. With the development, in 1927, of the hard-coated plaster of Paris rolls, a binder was incorporated that improved adherence of the plaster to the cloth. Since then, various additives have been used to either accelerate (salicylic acid, zinc, or aluminum) or slow down (gums or glue) the setting process.

Currently fiberglass is the most common material used in casting. It has the advantages of being stronger and lighter (approximately two to three times stronger for any given thickness) than plaster, and it creates less heat during application. However, it is more difficult to mold. The cost of fiberglass continues to be more than that of plaster, but in recent years this difference has decreased significantly. Commercial splinting products are also now available from a variety of companies that incorporate layered fiberglass within prepadded water-repellent felt that allows easy one-step application. These products can be cut to length and then resealed to allow application for future patient needs. In addition to newer casting materials, the development of synthetic padding (i.e., similar to Gore-Tex) has allowed most casts to survive without damage after significant exposure to water.

Indications

- A variety of stable, acute fractures
- Dislocations that have been reduced
- Injuries to the soft tissues, including muscle, tendon, and ligament
- Congenital and acquired deformities (e.g., correction of talipes equinovarus, congenital clubfoot)
- For the stabilization and protection of vascular, tendon, and nerve injuries following surgical repair

The most common diagnosis for which the primary care clinician uses cast immobilization is the stable, nondisplaced, closed fracture of a long bone. The primary care clinician also often treats fractures involving the radius or ulna, phalanges, metacarpals, metatarsals, and malleoli (See Chapter 178, Fracture Care) with casting. Other treated conditions include certain grade III ligament sprains (e.g., ankle), Achilles tendon disruptions, and tendonitis refractory to other forms of therapy.

EDITOR'S NOTE: There are few indications to cast an acutely injured extremity. Most acute injuries should be initially stabilized with a splint.

Contraindications

There are no absolute contraindications to an upper extremity splint. Relative contraindications include soft tissue injuries or wounds that need regular care and evaluation.

For casting, it is a contraindication to cast an extremity that has the potential for significant swelling and edema, as this may lead to a compartment syndrome. Otherwise patients with significant soft tissue injuries or infections of the joint space, soft tissue, or skin should be not put in cast. Patients with soft tissue injuries or wounds that need regular care and evaluation should also not be put in a cast. A fracture that has not been adequately reduced should be not put in a cast. If there is concern for swelling, the cast should be univalved or bivalved; this is discussed in the Technique section.

Cast Application Equipment

- Rubber gloves
- Gown and shoe covers for the clinician
- Patient towels or drapes
- Stockinette (2-, 3-, and 4-inch widths)
- Felt padding, soft cotton (e.g., Webril), or synthetic (e.g., polyester) bandages (2-, 3-, 4-, and 6-inch widths). These should always be longer and wider than the plaster or synthetic casting materials
- Synthetic waterproof cast liner (e.g., Gore Procel, Scotchcast Wet or Dry, Delta-Dry, Waterpruf)
- Rubber heels (walking cast)

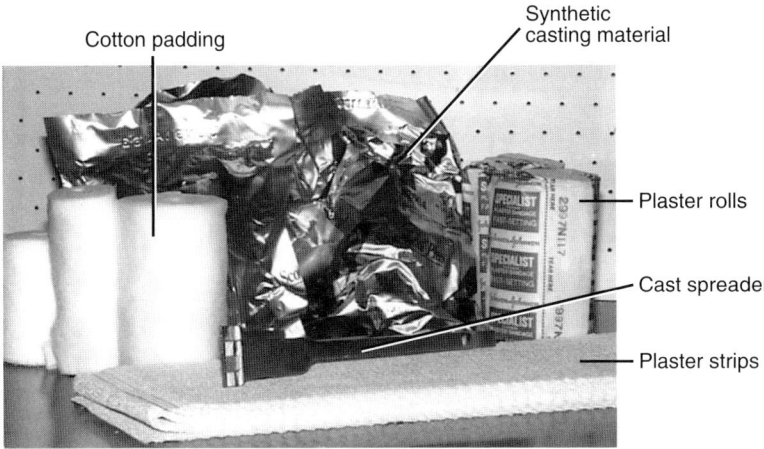

Cotton padding
Synthetic casting material
Plaster rolls
Cast spreader
Plaster strips

Fig. 176.1 Materials needed for casting: cotton padding, synthetic casting material or plaster rolls, cast spreader, cast cutter (not shown), and plaster strips.

- Cast removal protective strip (e.g., De-Flex) to eventually protect skin from the cast saw
- Casting material (Fig. 176.1), either plaster (e.g., plaster of Paris, avoid thicker than 10 ply, which can cause thermal injury to the patient, and if plaster is chosen, there should be traps in drains) or synthetic (e.g., fiberglass)
- Water source (water temperature <24°C/75°F)
- Elastic (e.g., Ace) bandages (2-, 3-, 4-, and 6-inch widths)
- Slings
- Scissors
- Chinese finger traps
- Leg stand

When water is added to the plaster, the water molecules are incorporated into the calcium sulfate hemihydrate (plaster of Paris) molecules with a resultant exothermic reaction. The powdery white substance is converted into a solid, semi-rock-hard material, and a significant amount of heat is generated. A curing process then follows over the next few days, characterized by continued water evaporation; this process is accelerated by low humidity, high ambient temperature, and increased air circulation.

Synthetic materials require immersion in water to activate the curing process, with generally less heat generated than with plaster. Attention to water temperature in this process is especially important, because water that is too warm (>24°C/75°F) can lead to rapid curing and significant difficulty in application. Water at higher temperatures than these or plaster of Paris thicker than 10 ply can also result in thermal injury to the patient.

Advantages of plaster casts over fiberglass include low cost, ease of molding, long shelf life, and low allergenicity. Synthetic cast material is more expensive, but this margin has narrowed in the years since fiberglass was introduced. Fiberglass has also improved in its ease of application and continues to be superior in strength, durability, weight, water resistance, and drying time. Both materials are available in multiple sizes, ranging from 2 to 5 inches in width for general, circumferential cast use.

EDITOR'S NOTE: Plaster should not be moved once it starts to set. This would cause fractures of crystals in the material and cause the plaster to lose strength. Conversely, careful lamination of the plaster using your hands while it is still wet enables the formation of longer, more durable crystals.

Ideally, a single room or area in the clinic, emergency department, or hospital should be dedicated to the application of casts and splints. This room should have a plaster trap in the sink, and all materials should be easily available. Rubber gloves, gowns, shoe covers, and towels or drapes should be available to protect both the clinician and patient from the inevitable exposure to casting materials. An easily cleaned examination table, stool, and leg stand can greatly facilitate the process of cast application.

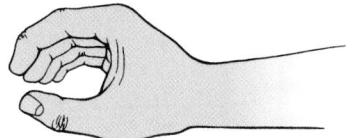

Fig. 176.2 Position of the wrist in the application of arm casts.

COMMON CAST TYPES

See Chapter 178, Fracture Care.

Short-Arm Casts

Short-arm casts are generally indicated in the treatment of stable sprains of the wrist as well as some stable fractures of the distal radius, ulna, carpal bones, and metacarpals. Clinicians performing cast immobilization should be aware of those fractures requiring orthopedic evaluation for possible open reduction and internal fixation. Materials required for short-arm cast applications include a 3-inch stockinette, two rolls of 3-inch cast padding (the waterproof liner replaces the need for both stockinette and padding), and two to four rolls of either 3- or 4-inch plaster bandage (or 2- or 3-inch fiberglass bandage). In general, adult males will require 4-inch plaster (3-inch fiberglass) and children will require 3-inch plaster (2-inch fiberglass). Adolescents and females may require either size depending on preference and size of the extremity. The patient should be supine or seated, with the arm abducted 90 degrees and the elbow flexed 90 degrees. The wrist should be slightly extended and in a position of function (Fig. 176.2). Chinese finger traps attached to the patient and suspended from above can support the arm and assist in maintaining the position of function. The cast extends from the proximal forearm (approximately 1 inch distal to the flexion crease of the elbow) distally to include the palm and dorsum of the hand, completely covering the forearm. The metacarpophalangeal joints are allowed complete motion, with the cast stopping just proximal to the distal palmar crease (Fig. 176.3). Extra padding should be applied over the ulnar styloid. Short-arm casts only partially immobilize the wrist joint and allow movement of the thumb, including opposition with the fifth digit. In addition, they allow for supination and pronation to occur because the elbow is not included. An adaptation of the short-arm cast is the short-arm thumb spica, in which the thumb is included to the level of the interphalangeal joint (Fig. 176.4). This type of cast may be used for injuries to the scaphoid, trapezium, first metacarpal, or any injury requiring wrist and thumb immobilization.

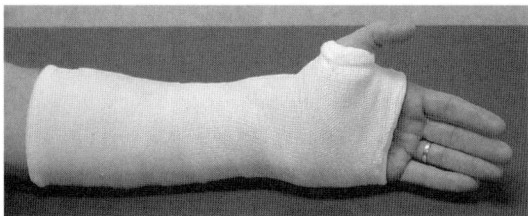

Fig. 176.3 Appearance of a completed short-arm cast. Note that the thumb and fingers are free to move.

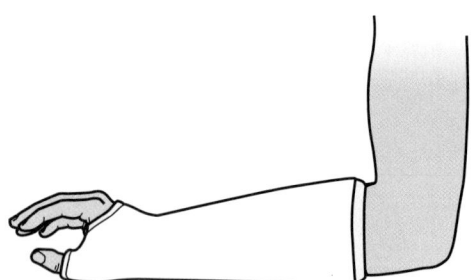

Fig. 176.4 Short-arm cast with thumb spica.

Long-Arm Casts

Long-arm casts can be fashioned by extending a short-arm cast proximally, with the elbow maintained in 90 degrees of flexion. The padding and plaster should be extended to the proximal humerus, ending two to three fingerbreadths below the axilla. Be careful to provide extra padding over the pressure point at the olecranon. Plenty of padding should also be placed over the proximal end of the cast or the patient will complain of the sharp edges.

Short-Leg Casts

Short-leg casts are indicated for certain stable ligamentous injuries to the ankle and stable fractures of the ankle, calcaneus, tarsals, and metatarsals. Materials include a 4-inch stockinette and three rolls of 4-inch cast padding (or waterproof liner). The use of fiberglass is generally preferred in these casts because of its increased durability; three rolls of 4-inch fiberglass bandage are generally needed. An extra reinforcing strip of heavy-duty fiberglass can also be used posteriorly along the bottom of the foot up the back of the leg. For plaster casts (used less often), materials vary widely based on personal preference, but they usually include two to three rolls of 6-inch plaster bandage and an adequate number of plaster splint strips (again for posterior and foot reinforcement), with size based on patient limb size. Application of the short-leg cast is achieved either in the sitting position, with the leg hanging over the table, or prone, with the knee flexed to 90 degrees to help relax the gastrocnemius muscle. The ankle is usually held at a 90-degree angle to the leg, but this angle may be altered depending on the type of injury. A foot stand or assistant can provide support to the foot. The cast extends from just below the knee joint, usually including the fibular head, and distally to the base of the toes, including the metatarsal heads (Fig. 176.5). Again, the ankle joint is only partially immobilized, since the cast does not involve areas both above and below the joint. For walking short-leg casts (Fig. 176.6), a posterior reinforcing strip is placed and molded after application of the second roll of fiberglass bandage and before placing the final roll. The walker can be applied the same day or at a later time. If applied initially, patients have a tendency to walk on it before the primary cast is dry enough, leading to breakdown of the cast.

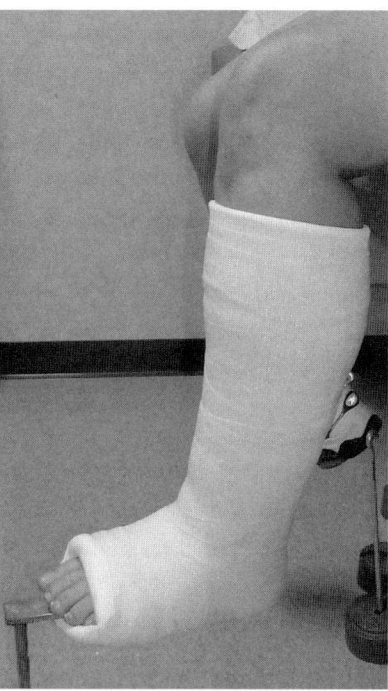

Fig. 176.5 Appearance of a completed short-leg cast. The cast should hold the ankle at 90 degrees. In addition, the proximal end of the cast should be far enough from the knee to eliminate the possibility of skin irritation with knee flexion.

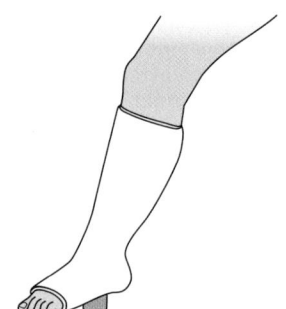

Fig. 176.6 Short-leg cast with walker.

Long-Leg Casts

Long-leg casts can be fashioned by extending a short-leg cast proximally up to the groin. The padding and plaster should be extended to the proximal femur, ending several fingerbreadths below the groin. The knee is in slight flexion and the foot is at 90 degrees. There should be no internal or external rotation of the foot. The knee should be supported in this slight flexion while the cast sets. To maintain strength, make sure there is adequate overlap of the casting material when extending it proximally from the knee. In addition, make sure that extra padding is provided over the pressure point at the anterior patella. Plenty of padding should also be placed over the proximal end of the cast or the patient will complain of the sharp edges.

Other Casts and Splints

Other types of common casts and splints are shown in Fig. 176.7. Even with splints, where casting materials do not totally surround the extremity, there is generally a layer of stockinette around the entire area followed by the padding, then the casting material. The casting material is held in place with an Ace wrap or similar material.

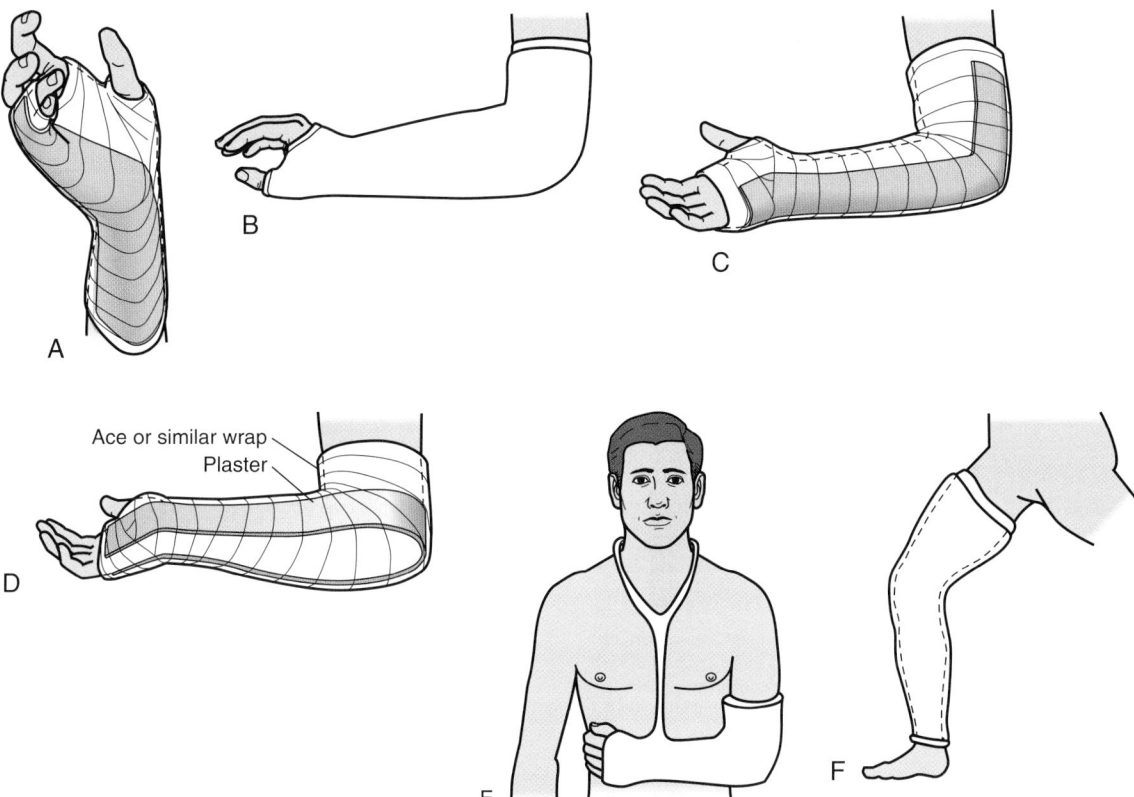

Fig. 176.7   Common casts and splints. (A) An ulnar gutter splint is used to immobilize fractures and serious soft tissue injuries of the ring and little fingers and fractures of the neck, shaft, and base of the fourth and fifth metacarpals. (B) Long-arm cast with thumb spica is used to treat navicular fractures, complicated Colles fractures, and nondisplaced radius and ulnar shaft fractures. (C) Long-arm posterior splint is used for severe lateral epicondylitis and elbow dislocation. (D) Sugar-tong splint is used for fractures of the distal radius and ulna. (E) Long-arm hanging cast. (F) Long-leg cast is used for fractures such as patellar, uncomplicated tibial plateau, and minimally displaced tibial/fibular shaft fractures as well as for medial collateral ligament or lateral collateral ligament avulsion and nondisplaced osteochondritis.

PREPROCEDURE PATIENT PREPARATION

After diagnosing an injury requiring cast immobilization and before application of the cast, the following issues should be discussed with the patient: the indications for casting, estimated duration of immobilization, potential complications, and potential impact on activities of daily living. Alternatives to casting, if available, should also be discussed. Discussion of common problems due to casting typically occur following application. Sample patient education handouts are available at www.expertconsult.com. If the cost of synthetic material may not be covered by the patient's insurance, this should be discussed prior to its use.

The patient should receive appropriate analgesia prior to manipulation of a fracture, especially if it is going to be reduced. Following a thorough examination and prior to any splinting or casting, make sure and document that the neurologic and vascular systems of the affected extremity are intact.

TECHNIQUE

Casts are generally applied to immobilize and protect an injured part of the body in a position that will facilitate healing. Three-point contact and stabilization are necessary to maintain most closed reductions. The following simple principles direct the fundamentals of cast immobilization. First, to best approach complete immobilization, a cast must conform precisely to the anatomy of the region being immobilized. Failure to accomplish this can lead to unacceptable movement of the injured area, leading to potential loss of reduction, malalignment of a reduced dislocation, or persistent inflammation in a refractory tendonitis. Second, effective immobilization is achieved only by including a sufficient amount of injured

area in the cast. Ideally, this is accomplished by including the joints above and below the area of injury. However, exceptions to this rule are made based on the nature of the injury. Achieving adequate immobilization requires attention to these fundamentals before application of the cast. If these goals cannot be met, the injury may best be served by another means of immobilization.

1. Before application of any casting materials, cleanse, dry, and thoroughly inspect the skin to be included in the cast for any lesions such as lacerations, abrasions, and ulcers. If present, they should be noted; if significant, they may contraindicate inclusion in the cast or may require special "window" techniques. Depending on the acuity of the injury and degree of soft tissue swelling, immobilization using circumferential casting may be contraindicated. In this situation, the injury may require the use of a splint for immobilization until the swelling has diminished or the contraindication has resolved.
2. After this assessment is completed, position the patient so that the injured area can be held most easily in the desired position throughout the application process. This positioning often requires the use of an assistant or assistive device (e.g., leg stand, finger traps).
   NOTE: Cast application is performed in a stepwise manner, and the use of a systematic approach will help ensure consistency and minimize the potential for error.
3. The first layer generally applied in casting is the stockinette. A poorly fitting stockinette can contribute to skin breakdown, so it must be applied carefully. Use a 3-inch-wide stockinette for adult arm casts and a 4-inch-wide one for legs, with exceptions based on the extremes of limb size. The material should go well past the toes or fingertips and 4 to 5 inches above the elbow

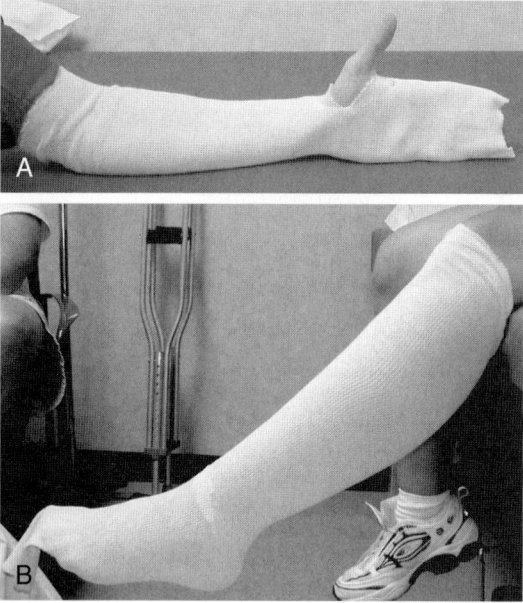

Fig. 176.8 (A) Demonstration of proper stockinette application for short-arm cast. Enough excess is present to allow a cuff to be created below the final layer of casting material. (B) Application of stockinette for a short-leg cast, demonstrating the technique to eliminate transverse wrinkle at ankle. Note the length of the stockinette for a short-leg cast.

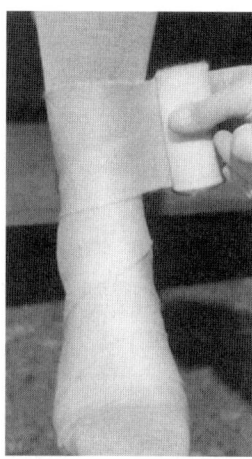

Fig. 176.9 Application of soft cast padding. Beginning at one end, cast padding is added while overlapping each turn by half.

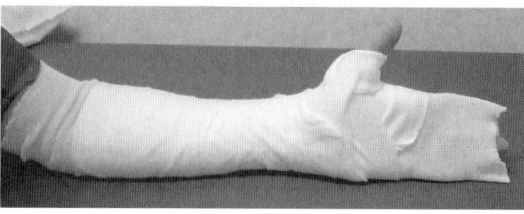

Fig. 176.10 Short-arm cast after application of cast padding and before addition of casting material.

or knee (Fig. 176.8A). (Cutting the stockinette too short is a common problem among those learning the procedure.) Some of this "extra" material is ultimately incorporated into the cast or, eventually, cut off.

4. Remove all transverse wrinkles; they become pressure points after cast application and can cause skin breakdown. This can be achieved by cutting the redundant material, which is usually at a joint. Fig. 176.8B shows a short-leg stockinette that has been cut and then overlaid at the anterior ankle to reduce wrinkles. Likewise, do not put tension on the stockinette by pulling it tightly.

5. After ensuring that the stockinette overlying the area is smooth and free of wrinkles, apply the second layer. The second layer consists of soft cast padding material (Webril), which comes in rolls and is applied in a circular manner. Start at one end (usually distal) and work toward the other; on the first turn around the extremity, roll the padding over itself to create an anchor. After this, each subsequent turn will overlap itself by 50% (Fig. 176.9). Two layers of cast padding can be applied, but care should be taken not to pad too much because this can lead to a loose cast. The goal with padding, as with the stockinette, is to avoid wrinkles, which may contribute to pressure points. Stretch or tear the advancing edge that is to encircle a larger portion of the extremity to avoid wrinkles. Keeping in mind the local anatomy, apply additional padding to bony prominences and likely areas of increased local pressure (e.g., flexion creases; fulcrum points such as the proximal anterior tibia where short-leg walking casts may rub; and common areas of nerve compression or pressure necrosis, such as over the proximal fibula). Felt pads appropriately fashioned can prevent common complications and improve comfort. Fig. 176.10 shows a short-arm cast after cast padding application and before application of cast material. Although padding is important, excess padding over bony prominences can also lead to excess pressure; therefore it should be avoided.

6. When waterproof cast liner is used, it is applied in the same manner as cast padding and eliminates the need for stockinette. By using this material, only two total layers of material are needed (cast liner and cast material). To apply, start unrolling onto the extremity from either the distal or proximal end. Remember to keep the adhesive side of the cast liner away from the patient's skin. The material is applied until the opposite end of the desired end point is reached, and it is extended 4 to 5 cm beyond the desired length of the cast. The excess will allow the ends to be folded back at the margins before the casting material is applied (Fig. 176.11A). Apply additional material to bony prominences to prevent pressure-related complications. Unlike traditional cast padding, the waterproof cast liner must be cut to achieve proper sizing because it does not tear (see Fig. 176.11B-C). In addition, because fewer layers of padding are used, waterproof cast liner requires the use of a protective strip below the cast material (see Fig. 176.11D) to protect the skin from the cast saw.

7. A protective strip can be placed under any cast to minimize the risk of thermal injury or damage to the skin with later use of the cast saw to remove the cast. Many experts will extend the strip an inch or so beyond the anticipated margin of the cast, far enough to enfold it into the end or cuff of the cast right over the stockinette. This simplifies locating and following the strip when the cast saw is later used, especially if the strip is extended into both the proximal and distal cuffs of the cast. The resistance of the strip to being cut by the saw is compromised over hard, bony surfaces; therefore its use over bony prominences should be avoided.

8. Apply the third layer (or second layer if cast liner was used), which consists of the cast material itself. The type of material used (plaster versus synthetic) dictates how the next step will be completed. Although application is quite similar, a few significant differences are worth noting. When plaster-impregnated rolls are being used, place each roll individually in water at room temperature and submerse until the bubbling stops. When the bubbling stops, the material is saturated, so it cannot absorb any more water. Cold water slows the setting process, whereas warmer water speeds it. (A faster-setting cast may be desirable when a recently reduced dislocation is being immobilized.)

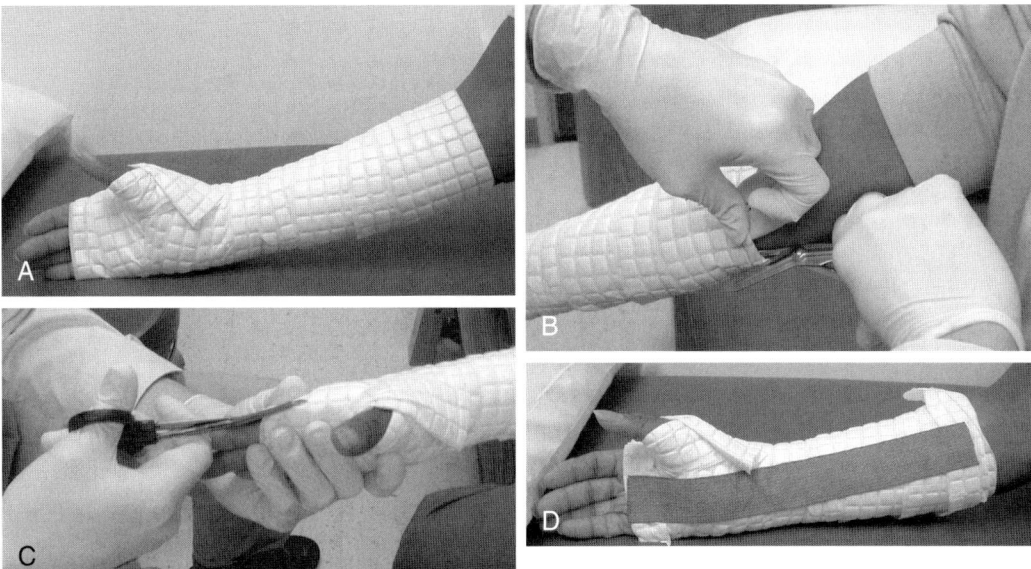

Fig. 176.11   Gore-Tex application. (A) Gore-Tex liner applied 4 to 5 cm beyond desired cast length. (B and C) Using scissors to cut material and allow liner to be folded. (D) Protective strip applied before application of cast materials. Extend the strip beyond the anticipated margin of the casting material.

After removing a roll from the water, gently squeeze it to eliminate excess water and begin the application (Fig. 176.12A). Do not twist the roll like a dish rag; it will cause loss of plaster into the sink or bucket. It is also not necessary to remove all the water, only the excess water. Placement of the plaster rolls should follow the direction of the cast padding and should be applied in a similar manner. The first turn has 100% overlap, and each additional turn overlaps approximately 50%. To avoid transverse wrinkles, plaster rolls can be tucked (folded over) at the edges when redundancy occurs and smoothed with the palm of the hand (see Fig. 176.12B-C). Avoid stretching and applying undue pressure with each turn. In a similar fashion, do not lift the roll off the extremity; instead, it should be rolled around the extremity while maintaining contact in a contiguous manner. Apply four to six layers of plaster evenly, with extra reinforcement in areas under increased stress. Apply each roll in a consistent manner, either distal to proximal or proximal to distal, with the length of the area to be immobilized covered with each layer. Covering only a portion of the extremity with one roll and overlapping with the next roll may lead to inherent weakness and future difficulties with the cast. Do not allow excessive time between successive applications of casting material; this may prevent lamination between layers and weaken the cast. Before placing the final layers, the ends of the stockinette should be folded over onto the initial layers. Reinforcing strips or cast cushions, if used, should be added now (depending on the type of cast being applied; see Fig. 176.12D).

9. Place the final layers of cast material and smooth the cast, using both hands. Make sure that it conforms to the contours of the local anatomy by using the palms to apply pressure to the cast (see Fig. 176.12E). Avoid using just the fingers to smooth the cast; if the fingers are used to conform (or mold) the cast, subtle pressure areas under the cast may be created. After the cast is applied, plaster should never touch the patient's skin directly. Positioning of the injured area while casting is critical. The ankle joint should be at 90 degrees and the hand and wrist in a position of function (slightly extended, relaxed). This position should be closely rechecked before hardening of the cast. See Fig. 176.2 for an example of the position of function used with short-arm casts. With certain fractures or tendon injuries, these positions may be altered to improve tissue healing. The provider should be aware of these needs before application of the cast.

Application of synthetic materials follows a similar course, with a few noteworthy exceptions. Water used to activate the curing process should be kept no warmer than room temperature to avoid too rapid setting. Normally, setting occurs in 2 to 3 minutes. Because of the flexibility of the synthetic bandage rolls, tucking of edges to avoid transverse creases is not necessary. However, care must still be taken to avoid pulling the cast material too tight. Molding should occur between each layer, with most synthetic casts requiring only two to three layers of cast material, depending on the area being immobilized (Fig. 176.13A–C). Strips of heavy-duty reinforcing material are available and frequently applied (e.g., to the posterior aspect of a short-leg walking cast) to increase durability (see Fig. 176.13D). After the final check of position, synthetic casts may require trimming of rough edges. If not trimmed, these edges may catch on clothing or injure the skin or soft tissue under the cast. Trimming can be done with a file, sandpaper, cast saw, or scissors; it is done with less difficulty when the cast is still soft (see Fig. 176.13E).

EDITOR'S NOTE: If there is concern for additional swelling after application of the cast, univalving or bivalving of the cast should be performed. Univalving is a complete cut through the cast for its full length. Bivalving is repeating this cut at a location 180 degrees from the first. Univalving results in a 30% drop in pressure, whereas bivalving results in a 60% drop. Ironically, univalving and bivalving cause a minimal drop in strength or support. In fact, some clinicians perform these maneuvers very frequently as a preventive measure; although a cast can always be replaced, the development of compartment syndrome may require a fasciotomy or result in loss of a limb.

POSTPROCEDURE PATIENT EDUCATION

After cast application, instruct the patient in proper cast care and advise him or her to be alert for signs and symptoms that require immediate attention. For plaster, advise avoidance of unnecessary forces to the cast, such as weight bearing for at least the first 24 to 48 hours, as the material will still be in the curing process. Synthetic casts usually develop sufficient durability to bear increased forces after 12 to 24 hours. Depending on the acuity of injury, elevation for the initial 48 to 72 hours may be recommended to reduce swelling.

Crutch walking is necessary for lower extremity injuries treated with casting until the cast has developed adequate strength to support weight bearing. Crutches that fit properly will be 1 to 1.5 inches below the axilla when placed vertically between the arm and body.

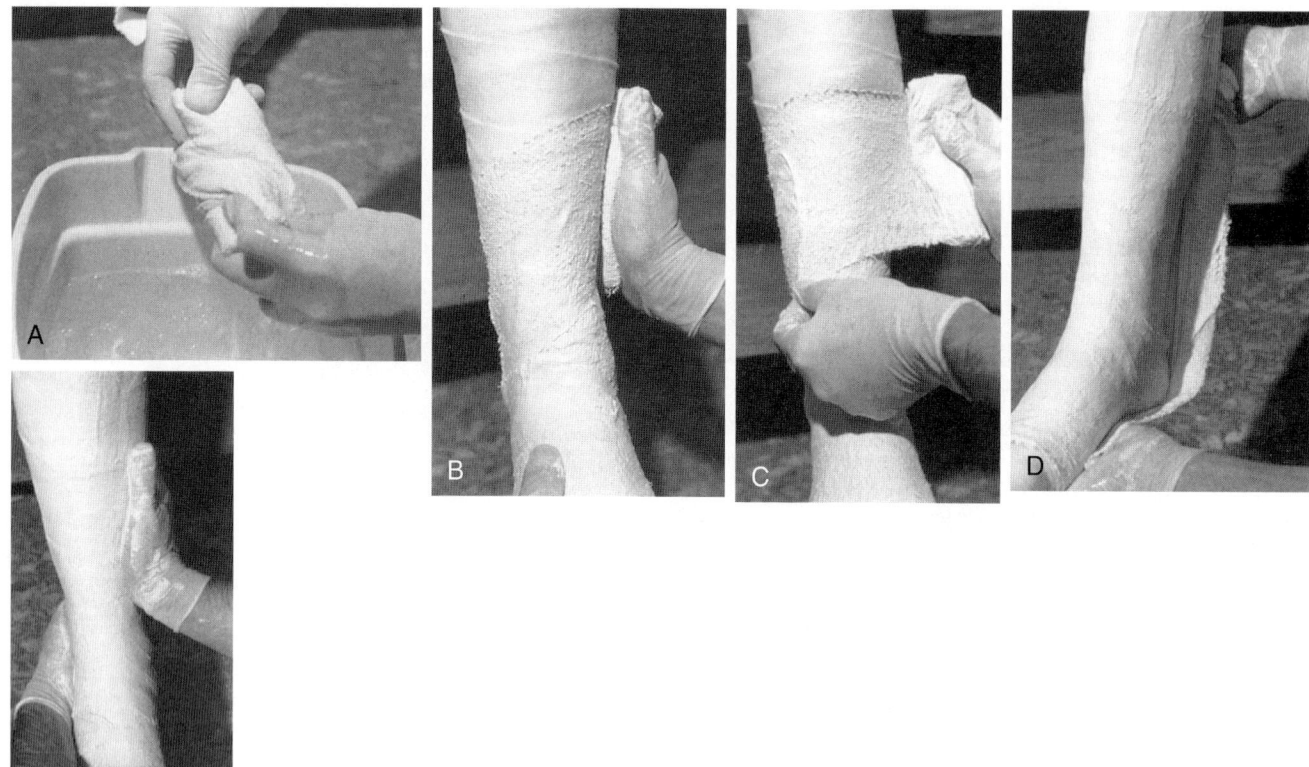

Fig. 176.12 Application of plaster cast material. (A) The plaster roll is removed from the water after the bubbling stops. The ends are pinched shut, and the roll is gently squeezed to expel excess water. Less water and excess wringing cause faster drying. (B) Beginning at one end, the plaster is pushed onto the extremity by using gentle pressure from the thenar eminence against the middle of the roll. The roll should remain in contact with the limb and is usually not lifted from it. Additional rolls are started where the previous one ends. The roll is applied so that the opening side faces the operator and not the extremity. (C) Tucks or pleats are taken as often as necessary to guide the roll and to accommodate any tapering of the limb. The stockinette is folded back and incorporated into the cast. (D) Reinforcing splints 5 to 10 layers thick applied to the sides or back add a great deal of strength without adding much weight. They are particularly useful at the ankle, where the cast is weakest and breakage is most common. (E) The cast is molded with the flat surface of the hands, if necessary, and trimmed, especially at the small toe.

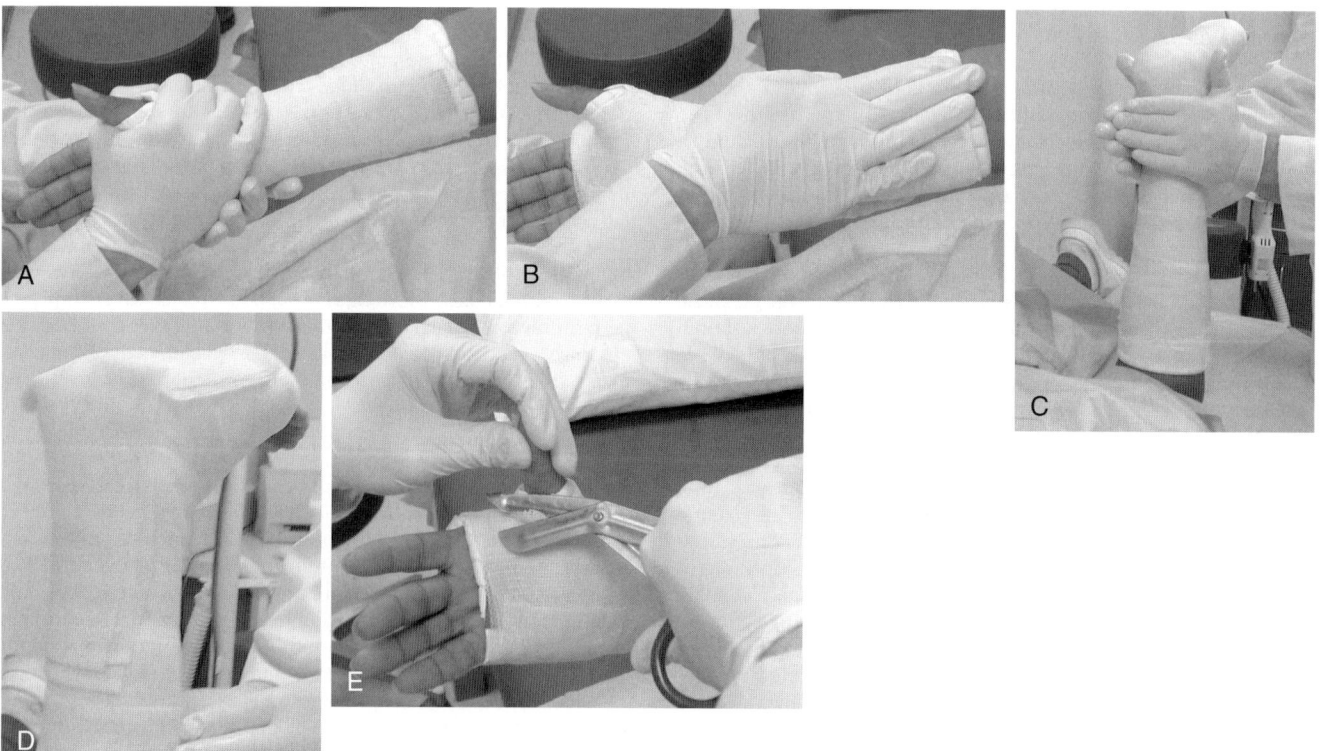

Fig. 176.13 Application of synthetic materials. (A) Molding short-arm cast at wrist. (B) Molding short-arm cast at forearm. (C) Molding short-leg walker at Achilles area. (D) Position of posterior reinforcement strip for short-leg walker. (E) Trimming excess cast material to avoid trauma to nearby skin.

The hand grips should be adjusted to allow the patient to have slightly flexed elbows during use. It is also important to remind patients that crutches are not intended to support the weight in the axilla, since this can lead to paresthesias in the arm. The weight of the body should be supported in the hands and the unaffected lower extremity (using a three-point gait). Prior to discharging the patient, it is also helpful to observe his or her gait with the use of crutches and to correct any problems that may occur.

Patients must take care to avoid getting the cast material wet and must be advised that submersion of even synthetic casts is unacceptable if routine stockinette and padding have been used. If the cast should get wet, the patient may try drying it with an electric blow dryer on the cool setting, being careful not to overheat the cast material. Soaked plaster casts and synthetic casts (with traditional stockinette and padding) in which the underlying cast padding is saturated require attention by a clinician and possible replacement. If the cast is not evaluated, the patient may suffer loss of immobilization, skin irritation, or maceration from the moisture under the cast material.

The patient must never introduce foreign objects (e.g., coat hangers) underneath the cast for any reason. Strategies for the patient with pruritus under the cast include using cool air from an electric blow dryer or talc or baby powder applied under the cast.

Patients using waterproof cast liner and fiberglass cast material may allow their cast to get wet. Bathing with mild soap is permitted. In general, a synthetic cast will require 1 to 4 hours to dry after submersion. Common sense should dictate the avoidance of swimming in areas that might allow the introduction of foreign bodies beneath the cast (e.g., fish, debris).

Cast wearers should contact their clinician if they develop increased pain in the immobilized region; numbness, tingling, or weakness in the affected area; a change in skin color distal to the cast; or persistent skin irritation.

CAST REMOVAL EQUIPMENT

* An electric, oscillating cast saw
* Cast spreaders
* Bandage/trauma scissors

PREPROCEDURE PATIENT PREPARATION

Patient counseling before starting the procedure, especially in the pediatric population, is likely to be the most effective means of minimizing fear and apprehension. Some practitioners solve this potential problem by allowing ancillary staff (nurses or other clinicians) to perform this function. In either case, it is good practice to describe the technique to the patient and include descriptions of any sensations (e.g., warmth, vibration) likely to be experienced. Actually turning the cast saw on and applying it briefly to one's own skin to show that it will not cut is sometimes used to demonstrate the safety of the procedure. The fear related to the noise generated by the cast saw can be reduced with the use of hearing protection. This may be especially helpful in the pediatric population. Once the patient is prepared, actual removal of the cast is fairly easy.

TECHNIQUE

Removal techniques differ based on the clinician's previous experience and training.

1. With the patient in a comfortable position and with a drape covering any clothing likely to be exposed to cast saw dust, stabilize the immobilized limb. Some patients will also appreciate being given a surgical mask to wear so as to reduce the inhalation of cast dust.
2. Determine the cut line before starting. If possible, avoid potentially sensitive areas. If a protective strip was utilized, the cut line is between where it appears on the cuffs at each end.
3. Hold the cast saw in one hand and, using the thumb and a finger (usually the index) of the other hand, stabilize the saw against the

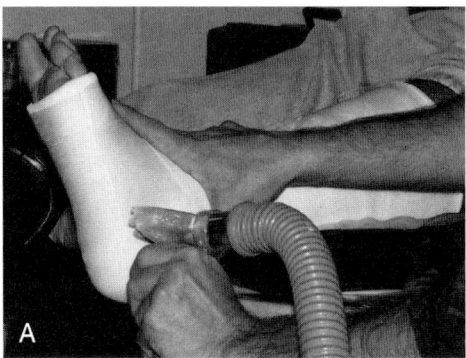

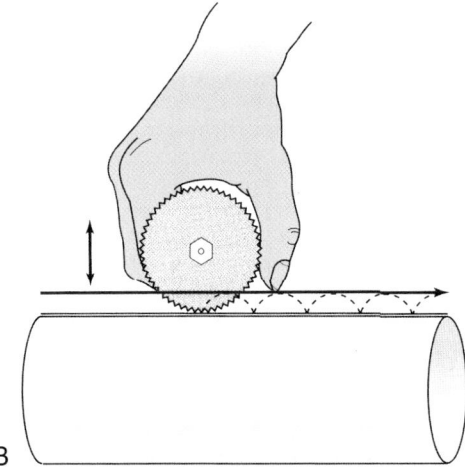

Fig. 176.14 Cast removal. (A) Hold the cast saw in one hand and use the thumb and another finger (usually the index) to stabilize the saw against the cast, which prevents the blade from injuring the underlying skin. (B) Cut down through both sides of the cast. Do not saw back and forth with the blade. Cut the cast at right angles to the material.

cast (Fig. 176.14). This technique allows control of the depth of cut. Constantly changing the area of the blade in contact with the cast and avoiding prolonged cutting in a single area should decrease the heat generated and limit the potential for saw-induced burns. Another technique to reduce the production of cast saw heat is to cut in a manner similar to a sewing machine needle. With this method the depth of the cast saw is constantly changing and exposes different areas of the saw blade to cast material. Depending on the cast material and the type of cast, either univalving or bivalving cuts along the entire length of the cast will be required.

4. After full-thickness cuts have been made through the casting material, use the cast spreaders to expose the underlying padding and stockinette (Fig. 176.15), which can then be cut with bandage/trauma scissors. If a protective strip is in place, the cast spreaders are frequently used to locate it and thereby maintain the cut line for the saw.
5. Once all material has been divided, remove the cast and allow the patient to cleanse the skin. Postprocedure cast care is injury specific and geared toward rehabilitation of the affected limb.

COMPLICATIONS

The best-known and most feared complication is the development of a compartment syndrome (see Chapter 179, Compartment Syndrome Evaluation). The process can occur with even a simple benign-appearing injury. If a snug circumferential cast is applied and tissue swelling continues after the initial injury, conditions are set for compromise of the microcirculation to the immobilized tissue. This may lead to ischemia of the affected area, producing muscle necrosis and further edema. If this process continues untreated and compartmental pressures reach a critical level, irreversible damage

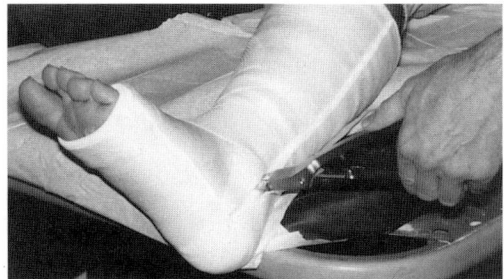

Fig. 176.15 Cast spreader or pliers separate the upper and lower portions of the cast, which has been cut on both sides.

to the involved tissues may ensue. Ultimately ischemic contractures (e.g., Volkmann) may occur, with loss of limb function.

Signs and symptoms of compartment syndrome include pain that is out of proportion to the injury or is elicited with pressure over the affected compartment or with stretching of involved muscle groups. Additional indications of impending compartment syndrome include paresthesias in the corresponding dermatome, the inability to generate a forceful muscle contraction, and normal pulses in the affected limb. Pulselessness and pallor are not characteristics of compartment syndrome because pressures will rarely rise high enough in a compartment to completely obstruct the major blood vessels in that area. All patients who receive a cast as part of their therapy should be counseled regarding the signs and symptoms of compartment syndrome. Should they occur, emphasis must be placed on the immediate need to contact the treating clinician or to seek care in an emergency department. Delayed diagnosis and treatment can lead to irreversible muscle and nerve damage.

Initial treatment in suspected cases of compartment syndrome is relief of the pressure generated by the cast, either through univalving, bivalving (as discussed in the section "Technique"), or complete removal. If univalving or bivalving is performed, the underlying cast padding must also be split. Splitting the plaster alone will not reduce the pressure adequately. Definitive diagnosis rests on characteristic signs, symptoms, and objective measurement of the compartmental pressure. Treatment of documented compartment syndrome may require surgical intervention in the form of fasciotomy.

Loss of reduction of the fracture is a possible complication. Therefore every effort should be made to maintain the reduction as the extremity is being cast. Likewise, every effort should be made to maintain the integrity of the cast, especially while it is setting and also afterward, when it is exposed to daily wear and the environment.

Various other skin conditions, nerve palsy, thermal injury, joint stiffness, disuse osteoporosis, and thromboembolic events may also complicate cast therapy. Of the skin conditions, cast dermatitis may be the most common, usually resulting in severe, bothersome pruritus from poor ventilation to the underlying skin. The use of absorbent powders (e.g., talc or baby powder) may help to limit the incidence of this condition. Two problems may result if patients introduce objects under the cast to relieve intense itching. First, the object may become trapped under the cast, producing a pressure point that can cause severe ulceration. Second, such instruments as coat hangers can easily lacerate the skin if used too aggressively, forming a nidus for infection or even requiring suture repair. Pressure necrosis or sores may result from poorly fitting casts that are insufficiently padded over bony prominences or inadequately molded to local anatomic contours (Fig. 176.16). As mentioned, transverse wrinkles in stockinette or cast padding or ridges in the cast material can lead to pressure necrosis. Pressure sores can occur as soon as 2 hours after the application of a cast. The patient who complains of persistent skin irritation characterized by burning or pain should be seen for evaluation and for possible opening of a window over the symptomatic area to facilitate direct examination. Additional skin damage may occur during cast removal as a result of heat generated by the cast saw. These burns are preventable with use of good technique, and their frequency may be reduced with the use of protective strips under the cast (e.g., De-Flex

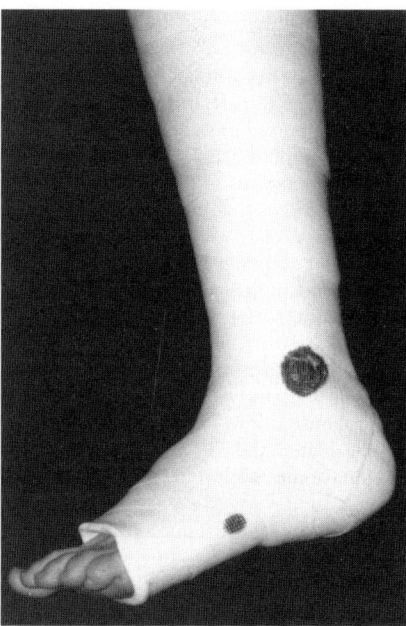

Fig. 176.16 Common locations of pressure sores (noted by ink on cast).

Strip). The use of a waterproof liner under the cast material increases the chance of burns during cast removal (this should be discussed with patients prior to cast application); however, the use of a protective strip under the cast material is highly recommended. Many providers have patients sign a consent form prior to using waterproof liner because of the increased risk of burns and because many insurance providers do not cover the additional cost of this material.

Any cast used to immobilize an anatomic region where superficial peripheral nerves lie in close proximity to underlying bone may lead to nerve palsy. Long-leg casts and those short-leg casts involving the head of the fibula can produce a common peroneal nerve palsy as the rigid cast compresses the nerve in its course over the fibular head (Fig. 176.17). Symptoms may include loss of sensation over the dorsolateral aspect of the involved foot, and "foot drop," or weakness in the ankle dorsiflexors. Other potential areas of involvement include the ulnar nerve as it passes through the cubital tunnel region, usually seen with long-arm casts, and the median nerve as it passes through the carpal tunnel (in both short- and long-arm casts). These neurologic injuries can be complete or incomplete, reversible or irreversible, and should be recognized and treated in a timely fashion.

Risk of thermal injury can be minimized by avoiding water that is too warm (>24°C/75°F) when using plaster of Paris and by avoiding casting that is thicker than 10 ply. A nearly universal complaint following cast immobilization is joint stiffness, which is directly related to duration of immobilization. This fact should be discussed with the patient at the time of cast application and should be taken into consideration when the length of treatment is being determined. In geriatric patients, the cast can likely be removed early to minimize the risk of contractures or loss of range of motion. Depending on the cause for initial treatment and response to therapy, the clinician can initiate fairly aggressive stretching exercises after cast removal to facilitate the return of normal joint function. Use of simple range-of-motion and other exercises involving nonimmobilized joints in the affected extremity (e.g., straight leg raising, finger or toe flexion/extension) can minimize the effects of prolonged disuse. Casting in the position of function also seems to minimize the effects of disuse.

Thromboembolic complications, such as deep venous thrombosis or pulmonary embolism, can occur with cast use (usually of the lower extremity) and must be considered when patients have suspicious symptoms. Diagnosis is difficult because of the presence of the original injury and limitations in examination. To exclude the diagnosis of venous thrombosis may require cast removal and ancillary testing (e.g., duplex ultrasound).

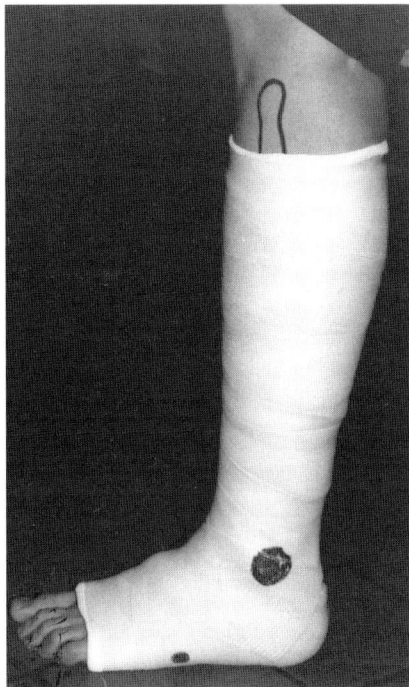

Fig. 176.17 Outline on the skin denotes the fibular head and indicates where the peroneal nerve is located. Excess pressure in this area can lead to paralysis and foot drop.

PATIENT EDUCATION GUIDES

See the sample patient education handouts available at www.exper tconsult.com.

CPT/BILLING CODES

The codes for fracture treatment include application of casts and splints. The clinician cannot use these codes for the initial application. Use the cast application codes listed here when any of the following occurs:

- Application of cast/splint is temporary and definitive treatment will be done later or by someone else (e.g., application performed in emergency room or office for patient comfort or to temporarily stabilize an injury).
- The cast must be replaced.
- The cast or splinting is performed as an initial service for treatment and no other procedure is planned (e.g., casting of a sprained ankle). Use a casting code in addition to an E/M code.

Casting and strapping codes include removal. Use removal codes only if the cast has been applied by another clinician.

If not listed here, see CPT codes 29000 to 29799 in the CPT code book.

Upper Extremity Casts

29065	Shoulder to hand (long arm)
29075	Elbow to finger (short arm)
29085	Hand and lower forearm (gauntlet)
29086	Finger (e.g., for contracture)

Upper Extremity Splints

29105	Application of long-arm splint (shoulder to hand)
29125	Application of short-arm splint (forearm to hand); static
29130	Application of finger splint; static

Lower Extremity Casts

29345	Application of long-leg cast (thigh to toes)
29355	Application of long-leg cast—walker or ambulatory type
29365	Application of cylinder cast (thigh to ankle)
29405	Application of short-leg cast (below knee to toes)
29425	Application of short-leg cast, walker or ambulatory type
29435	Application of patellar tendon bearing cast
29440	Adding walker to previously applied cast
29445	Application of rigid total contact leg cast

Lower Extremity Splints

29505	Application of long-leg splint (thigh to ankle or toes)
29515	Application of short-leg splint (calf to foot)

Lower Extremity Strapping

29530	Strapping, knee
29540	Strapping, ankle
29550	Strapping, toes
29580	Unna boot

Removal or Repair

Codes for cast removal should be used only for casts applied by another clinician.

29700	Removal or bivalving, gauntlet, boot, or body cast
29705	Removal or bivalving, full arm or full leg cast
29730	Windowing of cast
29740	Wedging of cast (except clubfoot casts)
29799	Unlisted procedure, casting or strapping

Also see Chapter 178, Fracture Care, for appropriate ICD-10 codes.

ONLINE RESOURCES

University of Ottawa: www.med.uottawa.ca/procedures/cast/

RECOMMENDED READING

Black WS, Becker JA. Common forearm fractures in adults. *Am Fam Physician.* 2009;80:1096–1102.
Boyd AS, Benjamin HJ, Asplund C. Principles of casting and splinting. *Am Fam Physician.* 2009;79:16–24.
Court-Brown CM, Heckman JD, eds. *Rockwood and Green's Fractures in Adults.* 8th ed. Philadelphia, Lippincott: Williams & Wilkins Wolters Kluwer; 2015.
Eiff MP, Hatch RL. *Fracture Management for Primary Care.* 3rd ed. Philadelphia: Elsevier Saunders; 2012.
Egol KA, Koval KJ, Zuckerman JD. *Handbook of Fractures.* 5th ed. Philadelphia, Lippincott: Williams & Wilkins Wolters Kluwer; 2015.
Mehrpour SR, Aghamirsalim M, Motamedi SM, Ardeshir Larijani F, Sorbi R. A supplemental video teaching tool enhances splinting skills. *Clin Orthop Relat Res.* 2013;471(2):649–654.
Moktar J, Popkin CA, Howard A, Murnaghan ML. Development of a cast application simulator and evaluation of objective measures of performance. *J Bone Joint Surg Am.* 2014;96(9):e76.
Reichman EF, Sloas HA. Casts and splints. In: Reichman EF, ed. *Emergency Medicine Procedures.* 2nd ed. New York: McGraw-Hill; 2013.

CHAPTER 177

KNEE BRACES

Scott A. Paluska

Traumatic, overuse, and degenerative knee injuries are common in the knee joint, which is the largest joint in the body. Strength, flexibility, and technique modification have traditionally been essential components in the treatment of knee pain. Improved surgical techniques, arthroscopic advances, and smaller incisions have also enhanced therapy for knee disorders over the last few decades. More recently, knee braces have been used in an attempt to prevent or treat several knee conditions.

Knee braces typically fall into one of several broad categories:

- *Prophylactic:* Braces designed to reduce the occurrence or facilitate the recovery of injury to the knee's medial collateral ligament (MCL) or lateral collateral ligament (LCL).
- *Functional:* Braces designed to restore normal knee kinematics, minimize tibial rotation, and reduce translation for anterior cruciate ligament (ACL)-deficient or ACL-reconstructed knees.
- *Patellofemoral:* Braces designed to keep the patella centered in the femoral trochlea and improve patellofemoral joint alignment.
- *Postoperative:* Braces designed to immobilize the knee or limit motion after surgery or an injury.
- *Osteoarthritic:* Braces designed to diminish painful forces exerted on an affected knee's tibial-femoral compartment (medial or lateral) for unicompartmental knee osteoarthritis.

Despite their popularity, the appropriate indications and true benefits of many knee braces have not been clearly defined or validated by rigorous research. In addition, brace manufacturers market several different knee braces to address conditions that may be nonspecific and diverse. As a result, confusion often exists regarding when and if knee braces should be used for the prevention or treatment of various knee abnormalities. At this point, it can be said that some knee braces may minimize knee injuries, but the efficacy of most braces has not been confirmed by well-controlled studies. In general, most individuals using knee braces express subjective symptomatic improvements that exceed objective findings. Clinicians must assess the costs and potential risks of knee braces when deciding to use them for individuals. Although knee braces appear relatively safe when used appropriately, they should be used only in conjunction with appropriate education, muscular rehabilitation, technique enhancement, and activity modification.

INDICATIONS

Prophylactic Knee Braces

- MCL or LCL injury protection during significant valgus or varus knee forces
- MCL or LCL stabilization during recovery following an MCL or LCL sprain
- Athletes or individuals at high risk for MCL or LCL injuries

Functional Knee Braces

- Mild-to-moderate ACL instability
- ACL-deficient knees treated nonsurgically

- Postoperative support following ACL reconstruction
- Support for mild-to-moderate posterior cruciate ligament (PCL) or MCL instability

Patellofemoral Knee Braces

- Patellar subluxation or dislocation
- Anterior knee pain syndromes
- Patellar tendonitis
- Osgood-Schlatter disease
- Compression of a knee effusion

Postoperative Knee Braces

- Stabilization following an acute knee injury or ligament sprain
- Postoperative immobilization
- Customized range-of-motion limitations for various knee conditions
- Stabilization following a femoral or tibial fracture
- Graft protection following knee ligament reconstruction

Osteoarthritis Knee Braces

- Unicompartmental, symptomatic tibial-femoral knee osteoarthritis
- Neutral or varus knee alignment (for a valgus-force brace)
- Neutral or valgus alignment (for a varus-force brace)

CONTRAINDICATIONS

General

- Unstable knees requiring prompt surgical management
- Body contours that preclude effective brace positioning
- Regional compartment syndrome that may be exacerbated by brace tension
- Open wounds, cellulitis, or lacerations that will be occluded by the brace

Prophylactic Knee Braces

Prophylactic knee braces should not be used for control of tibial translation or rotation in ACL-deficient knees.

Functional Knee Braces

Functional knee braces should not be used for complex knee injuries, such as posterolateral corner injuries.

Patellofemoral Knee Braces

- Knee disorders unrelated to the patellofemoral joint
- Moderate-to-severe patellofemoral osteoarthritis

Osteoarthritis Knee Braces

- Multicompartmental knee osteoarthritis
- Moderate-to-severe patellofemoral osteoarthritis
- Knee arthritis related to other conditions such as inflammatory, infectious, or autoimmune

EQUIPMENT AND SUPPLIES

General

- Tape measure
- Athletic tape (optional)
- Skin razor (optional)
- Prewrap on skin under brace to limit brace migration (optional, not beneficial for patellofemoral braces)
- Elastic wrap or brace cover (optional)

Prophylactic Knee Braces

- Custom or off-the-shelf (prefabricated) brace with unilateral or bilateral bars
- In addition to athletic tape, there may be manufacturer-supplied hook-and-pile fasteners

Functional Knee Braces

- Custom or off-the-shelf (prefabricated) brace
- In place of a tape measure, there may be specific measuring device supplied by the brace manufacturer

Patellofemoral Knee Braces

- Custom or off-the-shelf (prefabricated) brace
- Counterbalancing straps (optional)
- Patellar buttresses (optional)
- Inflation device for inflatable air pocket (optional)

Postoperative Knee Braces

An off-the-shelf (prefabricated) universally sized brace is used postoperatively.

Osteoarthritis Knee Braces

A custom or off-the-shelf (prefabricated) brace is used in cases of osteoarthritis.

PREPROCEDURE PATIENT EDUCATION

The clinician should identify the appropriate indication for using a knee brace and explain that the brace may or may not be helpful for a given individual. An appropriately sized prefabricated brace is generally sufficient for most individuals. Although custom braces may distribute weight and fit better and be made of materials more worthwhile for high-level athletes or individuals with abnormal limb contours, they are more expensive. If the individual is a minor, consent should be obtained from the parent or guardian. (See the sample patient consent form available at www.expertconsult.com.) The initial fitting and brace application should be scheduled with adequate time allowed for correct sizing and an explanation of recommended brace care and usage. (See the sample patient education form available at www.expertconsult.com.)

PROCEDURE

Prophylactic Knee Braces

Prophylactic knee braces are used to prevent injury to the MCL or LCL during contact sports or to provide stability during recovery

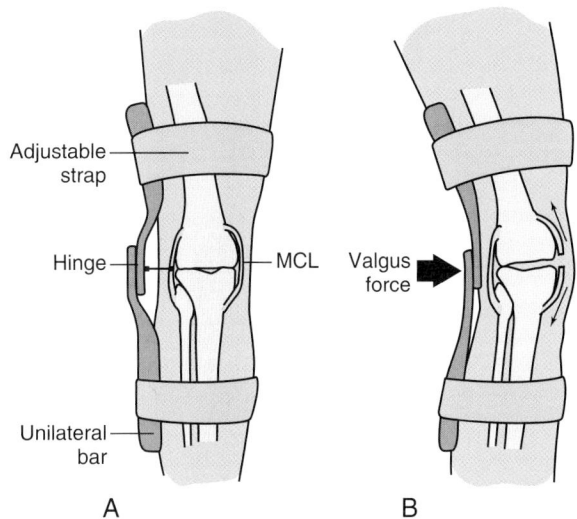

Fig. 177.1 Prophylactic knee brace. (A) Unilateral hinged bar prophylactic knee brace in a neutral position. (B) Valgus-applied force causing increased medial collateral ligament (MCL) tension and potential ligament rupture. Use of the brace would hopefully prevent the MCL tear seen here.

after an MCL or LCL sprain (Fig. 177.1). Although the routine use of prophylactic knee braces for collateral ligament injury prevention may be controversial, they do have a more well-defined role during MCL or LCL rehabilitation. Prophylactic knee braces are available as custom or off-the-shelf (prefabricated) models (Figs. 177.2 and 177.3). They have either a single lateral hinged support or bilateral supports with polycentric hinges that are connected by fabric and closures. Cost is greater for custom models, which appear to have greater efficacy during both knee flexion and extension. Although high-level athletes may profit from the weight distribution and fit characteristics of a custom brace, a prefabricated brace is sufficient for most individuals. At-risk athletes, such as football linemen, may particularly benefit from wearing well-fitting prophylactic knee braces on both knees during practices and games. However, it should be noted that prophylactic knee brace use may have a negative impact on an athlete's speed, agility, fatigability, and endurance.

1. Obtain the longest brace that the individual can wear comfortably (≥50 cm).
2. Select a brace with either unilateral or bilateral bars based on personal preference and cost. Bilateral bars may improve the brace's ability to transfer loads placed on the knee joint during impact.
3. Shave the skin under the brace, if desired, to maximize brace-to-skin contact.
4. Secure and adjust the athletic tape or brace enclosures to minimize brace movement.
5. Align the hinge(s) with the femoral condyles to minimize knee range-of-motion attenuation. Correct hinge placement relative to the knee joint is critical for optimal brace efficacy. The side bars may be bent if needed to accommodate the limb contours.
6. Cover the brace with the elastic wrap or brace cover, if desired, to minimize brace deterioration or injury to others during activities.
7. Tighten and adjust the brace regularly during prolonged athletic activities. It is common for the brace to migrate distally.
8. Hand wash and thoroughly dry the brace occasionally to prolong its life and reduce skin irritation.
9. Inspect the brace regularly for signs of deterioration or excessive wear.
10. Periodically apply a dry lubricant, such as Teflon spray, to the hinges.
11. Replace a broken or damaged brace.

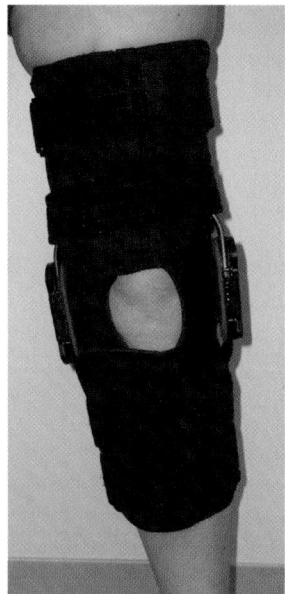

Fig. 177.2   Prophylactic knee brace with bilateral hinged bars seen from the front.

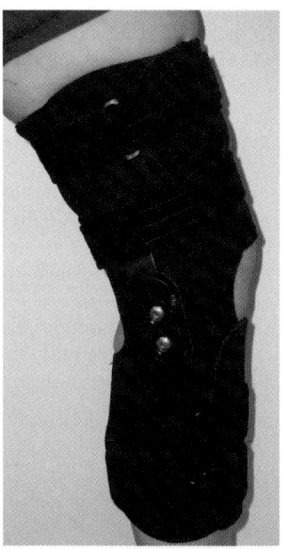

Fig. 177.3   Prophylactic knee brace with bilateral hinged bars seen from the side.

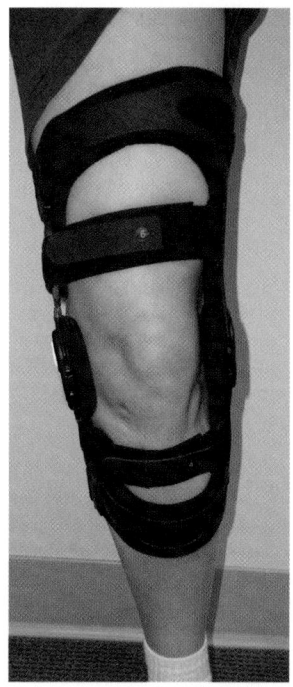

Fig. 177.4   Functional knee brace seen from the front.

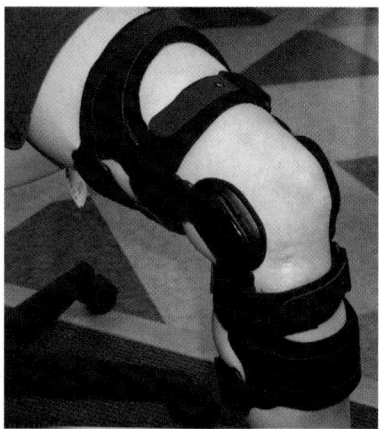

Fig. 177.5   Functional knee brace seen from the side.

Functional Knee Braces

The ACL is one of the knee's most important stabilizers for antero-lateral motion, and an ACL tear can cause significant knee dysfunction. Functional braces are designed to limit instability in ACL-deficient knees or to stabilize the surgical graft for ACL-reconstructed knees. They are often antirotational. The braces may also enhance proprioception and muscle-timing during activity. Even though most individuals report subjective improvements with brace wear, the braces' ability to limit knee laxity during high-load, in vivo conditions is clearly less than what has been observed in laboratory models. Theoretically, functional braces may also provide protection for an ACL graft by limiting strain during the initial surgical recovery period. However, functional bracing has not been definitively shown in long-term studies to improve subjective or objective outcomes after ACL reconstruction. As such, functional bracing may be superfluous following uncomplicated ACL surgery.

Functional knee braces are available as custom or off-the-shelf (prefabricated) models (Figs. 177.4 and 177.5). They have similar designs and use a "hinge-post-shell" or a "hinge-post-strap" design, which differ in the method of securing the brace around the user's thigh and calf. The "hinge-post-shell" braces provide better long-term durability and enhanced soft tissue contact. It is unclear whether the small mechanical and limb-contact advantages demonstrated in the laboratory for the more expensive custom models have clinically meaningful implications versus the less expensive off-the-shelf (prefabricated) knee braces. Custom braces may be more appropriate for individuals participating in high-level activities or having abnormal limb contours. Prefabricated braces are usually sufficient for most individuals. It is more important that the brace be secured snugly and aligned correctly on the affected leg to maximize its efficacy.

1. Measure the thigh circumference 6 inches above the mid-patella if using a prefabricated brace and select the corresponding brace size according to the manufacturer's instructions.
2. Measure the thigh, knee, and calf dimensions with the manu-facturer-specific instrument for custom braces. The submitted

measurements will be used to fabricate a brace that closely meets the affected individual's leg.

3. Choose the longest length brace that the individual can comfortably wear, generally mid-thigh to mid-calf. Longer braces may be more uncomfortable, so balanced brace length and comfort is important to improve compliance.
4. Set the bilateral hinge extension stops at 10 to 20 degrees of flexion to minimize potentially harmful knee hyperextension.
5. Center the condylar hinge pads over the medial and lateral joint lines to allow the brace's flexion axis to conform to the knee joint.
6. Fasten the brace securely around the individual's leg using the brace closures or straps.
7. Cover the brace with the elastic wrap or brace cover, if desired, to minimize brace deterioration or injury to others during activities.
8. Tighten and adjust the brace regularly during prolonged athletic activities. It is common for the brace to migrate distally.
9. Hand wash and thoroughly dry the brace occasionally to prolong its life and reduce skin irritation.
10. Inspect the brace regularly for signs of deterioration or excessive wear.
11. Periodically apply a dry lubricant, such as Teflon spray, to the hinges.
12. Replace a broken or damaged brace.

Patellofemoral Knee Braces

Patellofemoral knee braces are designed to treat a variety of highly prevalent anterior knee symptoms that occur during activities such as ascending or descending stairs, prolonged sitting, or frequent squatting. Although their mechanism of action is uncertain, patellofemoral braces may diminish pain via improved patellar tracking, lessened lateral patellar tilt, augmented sensory feedback, reduced patellofemoral joint stress, and enhanced joint contact between the undersurface of the patella and the femoral trochlea. Generally, the subjectively reported benefits exceed the objectively measured findings for patellofemoral knee braces.

Patellofemoral knee braces are available in many different styles, but most use an elastic sleeve, a patellar cut-out, and padding around the patella (Figs. 177.6 and 177.7). Some braces also include adjustable straps or moveable buttresses. Most individuals can use a prefabricated brace without the need for customization. No patellofemoral brace type or materials appear to be superior.

1. Measure the extended and relaxed leg circumference 6 inches above and 6 inches below the knee joint line or around the mid patella, depending on the manufacturer's instructions.
2. Obtain the corresponding brace size.
3. Pull the brace onto the individual's leg and center the patellar cut-out over the anterior knee.
4. Align the hinges, if present, with the medial and lateral femoral condyles.
5. Position the patellar buttress, if moveable, medial to the patella to apply laterally directed force (uncommon) or lateral to the patella to apply medially directed force (common).
6. Snugly secure the counterbalancing straps, if present, around the individual's thigh and calf. Moveable straps should be placed proximal to the patella for most individuals, except for those with patellar tendonitis who may benefit from a more distal placement.
7. Apply athletic tape to the top and bottom of the brace, if desired, to minimize brace migration during activities.
8. Hand wash and thoroughly dry the brace occasionally to prolong its life and reduce skin irritation.
9. Inspect the brace regularly for signs of deterioration or excessive wear.
10. Replace a broken or damaged brace.

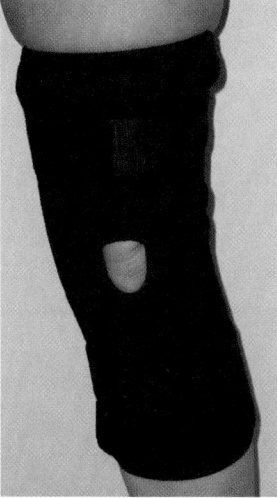

Fig. 177.6 Patellofemoral knee brace seen from the front.

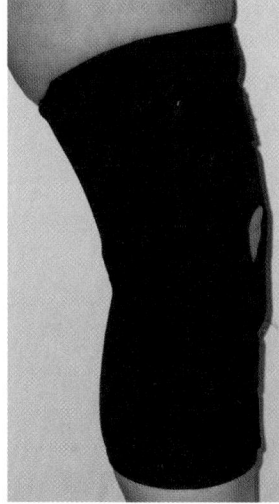

Fig. 177.7 Patellofemoral knee brace seen from the side.

Postoperative Knee Braces

Postoperative knee braces are designed to provide immobilization and protected range of motion following a knee ligament injury, fracture, or surgical procedure. The braces may be used to keep the knee fully extended or limited within any desired range of motion. During the course of treatment or recovery, the allowable motion is typically advanced gradually. Postoperative knee braces are not designed to be worn during athletic endeavors but may be used during full or partial weight-bearing ambulation.

Postoperative knee braces are primarily prefabricated and universally sized (Figs. 177.8 and 177.9). Some individuals with abnormal limb contours may need a custom brace. It is essential that the brace be correctly positioned and securely attached on the affected leg to stabilize the knee adequately.

1. Unfasten all of the buckles and loosen the strap enclosures.
2. Pull the brace onto the individual's leg and center the patellar cut-out over the anterior knee.
3. Wrap the foam thigh and calf inserts securely around the leg and attach the free ends together. The foam may be trimmed if necessary.
4. Adjust the brace length by pressing the medial and lateral release buttons, allowing the side bars to telescope to the desired

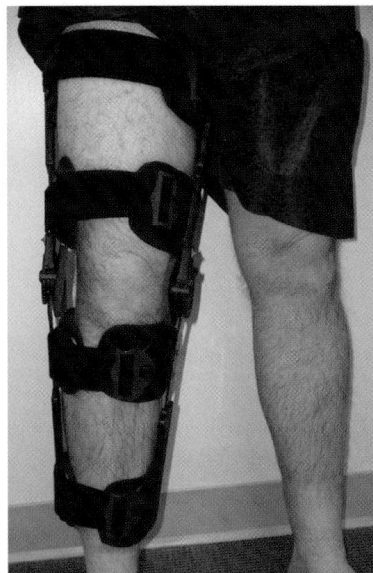

Fig. 177.8 Postoperative knee brace seen from the front.

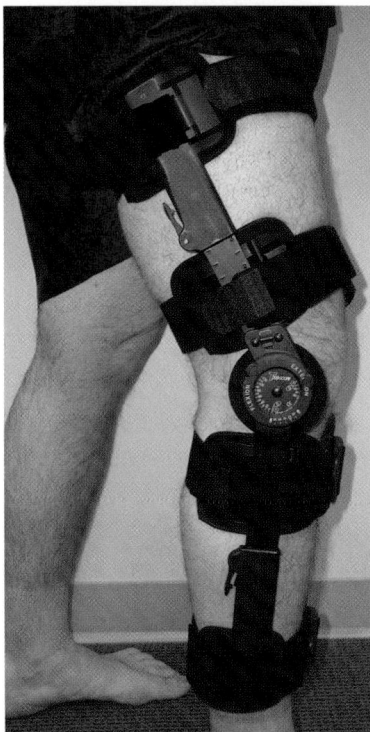

Fig. 177.9 Postoperative knee brace seen from the side.

length. If necessary, the bars may be fully extended from the upper thigh to the ankle. After finishing the adjustments, confirm that the release buttons have reengaged and that the side bars are equivalent in length.

5. Align the hinges with the patella and midline (anterior/posterior plane) of the affected leg. The lateral malleolus and greater trochanter may be used to verify midline placement. The hinge bars may be bent to fit varus or valgus knee alignments.
6. Confirm that the medial and lateral hinge heights are the same. Correct hinge placement is important for brace efficacy.
7. Adjust the brace's strap lengths and snap the buckles closed, starting with those closest to the patella.

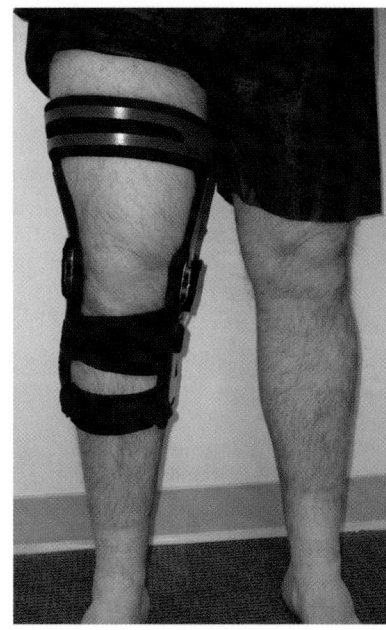

Fig. 177.10 Osteoarthritis knee brace seen from the front.

8. Open the bilateral hinge covers and set the desired limitations of flexion and extension by moving the adjustment pins.
9. Tighten and adjust the brace regularly during prolonged wear. It is common for the brace to loosen slightly or migrate distally.
10. Hand wash and thoroughly dry the brace to prolong its life and reduce skin irritation.
11. Inspect the brace regularly for signs of deterioration or excessive wear.
12. Periodically apply a dry lubricant, such as Teflon spray, to the hinges.
13. Replace a broken or damaged brace.

Osteoarthritis Knee Braces

Knee osteoarthritis is a widespread disorder, and osteoarthritis knee braces have gained prominence as nonsurgical adjuncts in the treatment of unicompartmental degenerative changes. Many studies have confirmed the braces' subjective and objective benefits among symptomatic individuals. Osteoarthritis knee braces (Figs. 177.10 and 177.11) play an important role in addition to standard treatments of pharmacotherapy, intraarticular injections, heel wedges, regional muscle strengthening, and lifestyle modifications. The brace applies three-point forces periarticularly to reduce load on one side of the tibial-femoral knee joint. A varus (force is laterally directed) knee brace provides distracting pressure on the knee to off-load symptomatic lateral tibial-femoral osteoarthritis, and a valgus (force is medially directed) knee brace provides distracting pressure on the knee to off-load symptomatic medial tibial-femoral degenerative changes.

Most individuals can use a prefabricated brace without the need for more expensive customized osteoarthritis knee braces. No brace type or materials have been shown to be superior for improving pain or function. Obese individuals or those with abnormal limb contours typically have less success with the use of osteoarthritis knee braces. Moreover, some individuals are unable to tolerate the forces created by osteoarthritis knee braces very well during daily activities.

1. Measure the thigh circumference 6 inches above the mid patella and select the corresponding brace size according to the manufacturer's instructions.
2. Some braces may also require measuring the calf circumference 6 inches below the mid patella or the circumference of the knee at the joint line.

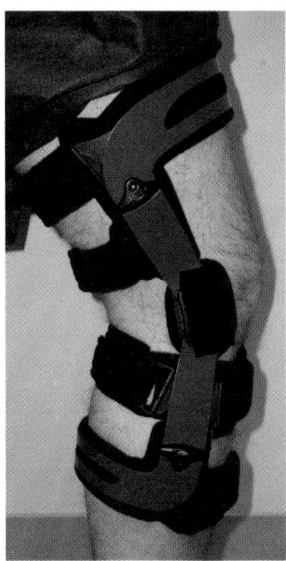

Fig. 177.11 Osteoarthritis knee brace seen from the side.

3. Loosely apply the brace to the leg without tightening the closure straps while the patient stands.
4. Adjust the varus and valgus alignment to fit the contours of the individual's leg. The side bars may be bent if needed.
5. Have the individual sit and flex the knee to 45 degrees. Position the side hinges 1 inch above the patella with the brace centered on the midline of the leg.
6. Secure the lower calf and the upper thigh straps snugly.
7. While the knee is still bent at 45 degrees, push both condylar hinges posteriorly to the midline of the leg. Hold the hinges in this position while securing the lower thigh strap.
8. While the knee is still bent at 45 degrees, pull both condylar hinges slightly forward but not anterior to the midline of the leg. Hold the hinges in place while securing the upper calf strap.
9. Confirm that both side hinges are centered just above the patella and slightly posterior to the leg's midline.
10. Tighten and adjust the straps after a few steps and then regularly during prolonged athletic activities. It is common for the brace to migrate distally or loosen slightly.
11. Trim the pads and straps as needed for comfort or to accommodate limb contours.
12. Cover the brace with the elastic wrap or a cover, if desired, to minimize brace deterioration or injury to others during activities.
13. Periodically apply a dry lubricant, such as Teflon spray, to the hinges.
14. Hand wash and thoroughly dry the brace occasionally to prolong its life and reduce skin irritation.
15. Inspect the brace regularly for signs of deterioration or excessive wear.
16. Periodically inspect and tighten the hinge screws as needed.
17. Replace a broken or damaged brace.

COMMON ERRORS AND COMPLICATIONS

In general, knee braces are associated with few complications when selected and worn appropriately. Careful brace sizing and maintenance may limit unwanted side effects. However, the following may occur:

- Skin breakdown or irritation may occur from brace-to-skin contact over bony prominences. Regular cleaning and air drying the brace will help protect the skin's integrity.
- Athletes or highly active individuals may note diminished endurance, performance, speed, and range of motion.

- Brace wear may require increased energy expenditure during vigorous activities.
- Premature muscle fatigue resulting from regional muscle ischemia and lactic acid accumulation may limit activities.
- While wearing a knee brace, an individual may harbor a false sense of security or invincibility regarding the brace's efficacy and subsequently sustain a more significant knee injury.
- Some knee braces may interfere with an individual's knee proprioception.
- Brace-related contact injuries to others may occur.
- Excessive preloading of the knee ligaments by some braces may potentiate the severity of a knee injury.
- Some braces may cause symptomatic regional ipsilateral or contralateral lower extremity discomfort due to altered knee kinematics and gait.

POSTPROCEDURE PATIENT EDUCATION

Give the individual a copy of any materials provided by the brace manufacturer. It is also important to remind him or her of the following:

- Routinely inspect the brace for any signs of wear or deterioration. It is common for braces that are used for extended periods of time to need new pads, foam inserts, or enclosure straps.
- Knee braces are only one part of a comprehensive knee rehabilitation program. More important components of knee injury prevention and treatment include muscular strengthening, flexibility enhancement, and technique modification.
- The patient should report any of the following in regard to the knee brace: poor fit, mechanical dysfunction, skin breakdown or irritation, new-onset knee pain, or concerns regarding proper brace usage.

PATIENT EDUCATION GUIDES

See the sample patient education and consent forms available at www.expertconsult.com.

CPT/BILLING CODES

For most fittings, E and M counseling codes will be used.

29530   Strapping, knee

HCPCS BRACE FITTING AND APPLICATION CODES

L1800   (Patella support) + L2795 (Patellar buttress) billed together for patellofemoral brace
L1815   (Hinged knee support) + L2425 (Additional hinge) billed together for a unilateral support prophylactic brace or L1815 + L2425 (×2) for a bilateral support prophylactic brace
L1832   Postoperative hinged knee
L1845   Prefabricated functional or osteoarthritis brace
L1858   Custom functional or osteoarthritis brace

ICD-10-CM DIAGNOSTIC CODES

M17.10   Osteoarthritis primary unilateral unspecified leg
M22.40   Chondromalacia of patella unspecified knee
M23.50   Old disruption of ACL unspecified knee
M25.469   Knee effusion unspecified knee
M76.50   Patellar tendonitis unspecified knee
M70.40   Prepatellar bursitis unspecified knee
M70.50   Infrapatellar or subpatellar knee bursitis unspecified knee

S82.109A	Tibial plateau fracture unspecified knee
S83.006A	Dislocation of patella, unspecified
S83.429A	LCL sprain unspecified knee
S83.419A	MCL sprain unspecified knee
S83.509A	Cruciate ligament of knee sprain unspecified knee

SUPPLIERS

(Full contact information is available at www.expertconsult.com.)

Functional Knee Braces

Bledsoe Ultimate CI (prefabricated)
  Bledsoe, Inc.
Breg Fusion (prefabricated or custom)
  Breg, Inc.
Donjoy Legend (prefabricated) or Defiance (custom)
  dj Orthopedics
Össur C.Ti.2 (prefabricated or custom)
  Össur
Townsend Design Rebel (prefabricated) or Premier (custom)
  Townsend Design

Osteoarthritis Knee Braces

Bledsoe Thruster 3
  Bledsoe, Inc.
Breg Fusion XT OA
  Breg, Inc.
DonJoy OA Adjuster
  dj Orthopedics
Össur GII Unloader
  Össur
Townsend Design Rebel Reliever
  Townsend Design
Patellofemoral Knee Braces
  BioSkin/Cropper Medical Q Lok
  BioSkin/Cropper Medical
Breg Lateral J
  Breg, Inc.
DonJoy Tru-Pull
  dj Orthopedics
Hely Weber Shields Brace
  Hely & Weber
Palumbo Patella Tracker
  Palumbo Orthopedics
Postoperative Knee Braces
  Bledsoe Merit OR
  Bledsoe, Inc.
Breg T-Scope
  Breg, Inc.
Donjoy TROM
  dj Orthopedics

Össur Innovator DLX
  Össur
Townsend Adjusta-ROM
  Townsend Design
Prophylactic Knee Braces
Bledsoe Sport Max (bilateral supports)
  Bledsoe, Inc.
Breg RoadRunner (bilateral supports)
  Breg, Inc.
DonJoy Playmaker (bilateral supports)
  dj Orthopedics
Hely Weber Velocity (bilateral supports)
  Hely & Weber
McDavid Protective Knee Guard (unilateral support) or Pro Stabilizer (bilateral supports)
  McDavid Sports Medical Products

RECOMMENDED READING

Arnold MJ, Moody AL. Common running injuries: evaluation and management. *Am Fam Physician.* 2018;97(8):510–516.

Dixit S, DiFiori JP, Burton M, Mines B. Management of patellofemoral pain syndrome. *Am Fam Physician.* 2007;75:194–202.

Duivenvoorden T, Brouwer RW, van Raaij TM, Verhagen AP, Verhaar JA, Bierma-Zeinstra SM. Braces and orthoses for treating osteoarthritis of the knee. *Cochrane Database Syst Rev.* 2015;3:CD004020.

Jones BQ, Cover CJ, Sineath MH. Nonsurgical management of knee pain in adults. *Am Fam Physician.* 2015;92(10):875–883.

Lowe WR, Warth RJ, Davis EP, Bailey L. Functional bracing after anterior cruciate ligament reconstruction: a systematic review. *J Am Acad Orthop Surg.* 2017;25(3):239–249.

Lun VMY, Wiley JP, Meeuwisse WH, et al. Effectiveness of patellar bracing for treatment of patellofemoral pain syndrome. *Clin J Sport Med.* 2005;15:235–240.

McDevitt ER, Taylor DC, Miller MD, et al. Functional bracing after anterior ligament reconstruction: a prospective, randomized, multicenter study. *Am J Sports Med.* 2004;32:1887–1892.

Miller MD, Thompson SR, eds. *DeLee and Drez's Orthopedic Sports Medicine.* 4th ed. Philadelphia: Saunders Elsevier; 2015.

Najibi SH, Albright JP. The use of knee braces, part 1: prophylactic knee braces in contact sports. *Am J Sports Med.* 2005;33:602–611.

Nadaud MC, Komistek RD, Mahfouz MR, et al. *In vivo* three-dimensional determination of the effectiveness of the osteoarthritic knee brace: a multiple brace analysis. *J Bone Joint Surg Am.* 2005;87A(suppl 2):114–119.

Pollo FE, Jackson RW. Knee bracing for unicompartmental osteoarthritis. *J Am Acad Orthop Surg.* 2006;14:5–11.

Powers CM, Ward SR, Chan LD, et al. The effect of bracing on patella alignment and patellofemoral joint contact area. *Med Sci Sports Exerc.* 2004;36:1226–1232.

Smith TO, Drew BT, Meek TH, Clark AB. Knee orthoses for treating patellofemoral pain syndrome. *Cochrane Database Syst Rev.* 2015;12:CD010513.

Soma CA, Cawley PW, Liu S, et al. Custom-fit versus premanufactured braces. *Orthopedics.* 2004;27:307–310.

Wright RW, Fetzer GB. Bracing after ACL construction: a systematic review. *Clin Orthop Relat Res.* 2007;455:162–168.

CHAPTER 178

FRACTURE CARE*

Robert L. Kalb • Grant C. Fowler

Primary care clinicians manage a wide range of fractures with good outcomes. However, to do this optimally, it is important to have adequate orthopedic training (perhaps on a rotation in residency) and supportive orthopedic backup. In fact, primary care clinicians so equipped can manage more complicated fractures, including about a third of fractures requiring reduction. A patient with multiple fractures or open, displaced, intraarticular, or epiphyseal plate fractures should generally be referred to an orthopedic surgeon. Adverse outcomes can be avoided by carefully choosing which fractures primary care clinicians manage, based on their level of training or appropriate consultation. This chapter provides guidelines for the office, urgent care, and emergency center management of fractures by the primary care clinician.

Decisions regarding whether to manage a displaced fracture are often influenced by the state's malpractice climate, insurance carriers, and premiums. Managing fractures requiring reduction often necessitates a higher level of malpractice coverage and higher premiums. Those clinicians treating fractures, especially fractures that require reduction, must have a good working relationship with an orthopedic surgeon willing to provide informal advice on management and on specific cases. It is ideal to have a relationship with an orthopedist who is able occasionally to examine a patient and return the patient to the referring clinician for follow-up care.

All the fractures discussed in this chapter can be treated by the primary care clinician, with or without local anesthesia. This chapter serves as a guide or a basic summary for primary care; it cannot possibly review the management of all fractures. Because the management of fractures in children often differs greatly from that of fractures in adults, children are considered separately.

With all fractures, healing starts when osteoclasts arrive at the fracture site, causing resorption of the dead, soon to be demineralized bone. This resorption results in the fracture line appearing larger in the follow-up radiograph (even in those fractures that are nondisplaced or initially have only hairline cracks). As the fracture heals further, callus forms and the pain and tenderness decrease. However, the radiograph will not show callus and healing until later, when it has mineralized, which may take 6 weeks or longer. It is only when mineralization has occurred that the x-ray beam no longer easily penetrates the callus, which results in the image of healing observed on the radiograph.

Box 178.1 lists types of casts. Chapter 175, Ankle and Foot Splinting, Casting, and Taping, and Chapter 176, Cast Immobilization and Upper Extremity Splinting, contain more details on casts than are discussed in this chapter.

EQUIPMENT

See the discussions of equipment in Chapter 175, Ankle and Foot Splinting, Casting, and Taping, and Chapter 176, Cast Immobilization and Upper Extremity Splinting.

TERMINOLOGY

Open fracture: This fracture communicates through a hole in the skin; therefore, by definition, an open fracture is contaminated and is more likely to become infected, especially if the hole is greater than 1 cm in diameter. Open fractures should almost always be referred to an orthopedic surgeon. (Previously, the term *compound fracture* was used to describe an open fracture.)

Closed fracture: This fracture is not openly communicating through a hole in the skin. The vast majority of fractures are closed, and the skin is unbroken.

Torus fracture: In this fracture, only one of the cortices is buckled.

Greenstick fracture: A greenstick fracture is a level worse than a torus fracture. It involves an actual crack or disruption of one cortex and buckling of the opposite cortex. This fracture is so named because the bony deformation is much like that seen after cracking a green tree twig in springtime: the tension side of the bent twig cracks, whereas the compression side (i.e., the concave side) merely buckles.

Comminuted fracture: In this fracture the bone is in more than two pieces. Often an additional piece, which is small and shaped like a butterfly and therefore named a *butterfly fragment,* is found at the fracture site.

Fracture dislocation: A joint is dislocated and associated with a bony fracture on one or both sides of the joint.

Intraarticular fracture: This fracture extends into the joint or articular surface. If an intraarticular fracture is displaced, the patient should be referred to an orthopedic surgeon.

Delayed union: Delayed union occurs when a fracture is not healed after a time interval that is twice the normal healing time. For example, a fracture of the radius would be considered a delayed union if it has not healed in 4 months because it has an expected healing time of 2 months.

Nonunion: The bone has not united after three times the normal healing time. For example, a distal radius fracture is expected to heal completely in 2 months. If it has not healed in three times that amount, or 6 months, it is considered a nonunion fracture.

Atrophic nonunion: A bone end near the fracture becomes pointed like a partially consumed peppermint stick or icicle without any sign of new bone formation.

Hypertrophic nonunion: The bone end forms new bone even though it is not united.

Malunion: A fracture has united with unacceptable angulation, rotation, or shortening.

FRACTURES IN ADULTS

Cervical Spine Fracture

The possibility of a cervical spine fracture being unstable with associated spinal cord complications should always be considered (in

---

* Also see Chapter 235, Principles of X-Ray Interpretation.

BOX 178.1 Types of Casts

Long-arm cast (see Fig. 176.7): Always begins at the level of the proximal palmar crease and ends at the upper two thirds of the humerus. It always holds the elbow in 90 degrees of flexion. It begins as a short-arm cast and is then extended in a second stage.

Short-arm cast (see Fig. 176.4): Always begins at the proximal palmar crease and ends just below the elbow crease.

Short-leg cast (see Fig. 176.5): Always begins at the tips of the toes with the ankle in a neutral position and extends up to just behind the knee, allowing the patient to bend the knee at least 90 degrees without pinching from the cast.

Long-leg cast (see Fig. 176.7F): Always extends from the tips of the toes up to the proximal thigh. A long-leg cast is always a combination of first applying the short-leg cast and then extending it into a long-leg cast as the second stage, just as for a long-arm cast application.

If the knee is in approximately 30 degrees of flexion, crutch walking is easier because the foot is out of the way on the non–weight-bearing side. The 30 degrees of flexion helps to control rotation of the tibia and ankle; it also prevents the patient from walking on the cast. Without 30 degrees of flexion, no rotational control is present.

See Chapter 176, Cast Immobilization and Upper Extremity Splinting.

fact, most are unstable). The exceptions would be a certain spinous process fracture (clay shoveler's fracture) or a simple anterior wedge fracture (defined as <25% loss of vertebral body height and no subluxation on dynamic flexion-extension radiographs of the cervical spine). The clay shoveler's fracture is an avulsion of the tip of the spinous process of C6 or C7 due to stress on the interspinous ligaments. These cervical fractures may require nothing more than a soft cervical collar and symptomatic management.

All patients with a suspected cervical spine fracture should have a three-view series of cervical spine radiographs: cross-table lateral, anteroposterior (AP), and open-mouth odontoid views. In most cases the lateral view should be taken first to rule out an occult fracture before the neck is moved. Overall, this view provides 90% of the information regarding the stability of the spine. The radiologist, neurosurgeon, or orthopedist can review the radiographs to exclude any associated problems. It should be noted that even minor fractures seen on plain radiographs (such as clay shoveler's and simple anterior wedge) may be associated with significant ligamentous injuries that render the cervical spine unstable; consultation with a neurosurgeon or orthopedist is helpful. Advanced imaging may include flexion-extension radiographs to assess for occult instability, computed tomography (CT), and/or magnetic resonance imaging (MRI). A systematic review (Holmes, 2005) found CT to be superior to plain radiographs for detecting cervical spine injuries in patients with blunt trauma. MRI can visualize soft tissue injuries, including ligamentous structures. These imaging strategies are optimally ordered in consultation with an appropriate specialist.

Thoracolumbar Spine Fractures

A thoracolumbar spine fracture can generally be treated with symptomatic management and brief (24 to 48 hours) bed rest with serial neurologic monitoring, followed by rehabilitative exercises with or without back support (thoracolumbosacral orthosis [TLSO]). A recent review (Giele et al., 2009) found no benefits from use of a brace; however, high-quality studies are lacking. Exceptions to conservative management include evidence of instability such as loss of greater than 50% of the anterior vertebral height (compared with posterior vertebral body height), presence of more than 20 degrees of angulation, an increased space between the spinous processes,

and disruption of the facet joints; these patients should generally be referred. Burst fractures or fractures associated with any sign of neurologic injury should also be referred for orthopedic or neurosurgical consultation to rule out instability (which may require surgical stabilization). Another exception to the use of a TLSO is a compression fracture occurring in an osteoporotic patient; in such cases, a TLSO is usually unnecessary and may impair return to function in the elderly.

Fractures of the upper thoracic spine (T1 to T9) tend to be more stable because of attachments of the rib cage, which in turn are further stabilized at the sternum. Fractures of L2 to L5 tend to be more stable because of the larger vertebral bodies; fractures of L5 and S1 tend to be unstable because of the high-energy forces required to cause injury at this level. Transverse process fractures, usually at L2, L3, or L4, and spinous process fractures are usually benign and do not affect spine stability. With a transverse or spinous process fracture in the general region of the kidneys, the possibility of a renal contusion should be considered. The significant forces required to fracture either a spinous or transverse process should also alert the clinician to consider other intraabdominal injuries.

For possible thoracolumbar spine fractures, radiographs should include AP, lateral, and oblique views of the entire thoracolumbar spine (patients often have fractures at more than one level). When managing a compression fracture, serial radiographs should be obtained at 3, 6, and 12 weeks to rule out a progressive kyphotic deformity (>20 degrees of angulation). CT scanning is particularly helpful in diagnosing multiple or occult fractures or bony impingement on the spinal canal. MRI is useful for evaluating soft tissue injury. Management of these fractures is bed rest for a few days and analgesics as needed. Patients may have symptoms for 4 to 6 weeks. Nonunion may occur, but rarely is it of any consequence. When managing these fractures, an accompanying ileus is fairly common. Osteoporotic fractures are managed the same as traumatic fractures except it may be even more important for early ambulation in the elderly to prevent complications from prolonged immobility. Always consider radiographs of the lumbar spine in a patient who has a calcaneal fracture because the axial loading associated with such an injury is often associated with a lumbar spine fracture.

Pelvic Fractures

Pelvic fractures managed by primary care clinicians tend to occur in osteoporotic older patients due to a fall. Otherwise, pelvic fractures are usually the result of significant trauma in a motor vehicle accident or a fall from a considerable height. Most fractures of the pelvis are diagnosed on the AP view. Additional views to assess the pelvis include inlet, outlet, and oblique views of the acetabulum. If there is concern for acetabular involvement, obturator (45 degrees of internal rotation) and iliac (45 degrees of external rotation) oblique views should be obtained; a radiologist or orthopedist will usually be able to determine from these views whether any question remains of acetabular involvement. If the acetabulum is involved, the patient should generally be referred to an orthopedist. If comminution is present, CT can be used for further delineation. Some experts recommend using CT to delineate extent of injury with all pelvic fractures. Orthopedic referral should also be considered if the pelvic ring is unstable. However, there must be two breaks in the pelvic ring, either from two fractures or a fracture plus a joint dislocation (usually the sacroiliac joint), for a pelvic fracture to be unstable. Fractures external to the pelvic ring are generally considered stable (Fig. 178.1).

If the pelvic fracture is considered stable, the patient can be treated with bed rest, analgesics, walking as tolerated, or full weight bearing with a walker. The pubic and ischial rami function only as tie rods for the anterior portions of the pelvis; they are not weight bearing. The typical older woman who falls and breaks her pelvis has a pubic or ischial ramus fracture only (see Fig. 178.1) and does

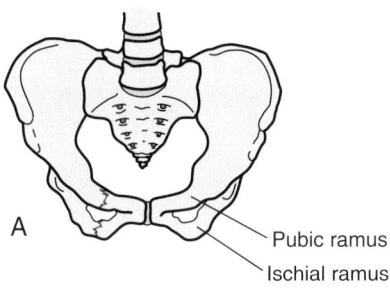

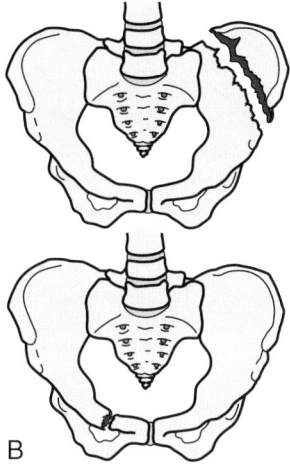

Fig. 178.1   Stable pelvic fractures. (A) Nondisplaced ramus fractures. (B) Fracture of the pelvis not involving the ring *(top)*. Stable, minimally displaced fracture of the ring *(bottom)*.

Pubic ramus
Ischial ramus

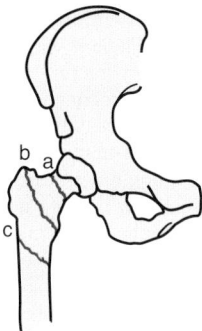

Fig. 178.2   Fractures of the proximal femur: Neck *(a)*; intertrochanteric *(b)*; subtrochanteric *(c)*.

not require either surgical intervention or bed rest. Otherwise, the length of bed rest is variable, usually from 2 to 4 weeks; the patient may sit as tolerated. During bed rest, gentle range of motion exercises of the lower extremities should be performed, especially in the elderly. Although walking may be uncomfortable, explain to the patient that it is not dangerous or harmful. Radiographs should be repeated after the patient has ambulated to make sure not displacement has occurred.

If the pelvic fracture occurs in an individual younger than 50 years or one involved in a motor vehicle accident, be prepared to resuscitate the patient, because hemorrhagic shock is the major cause of death. Consider the possibility of bladder, urethral, or external genitalia injury, especially with anterior pelvic fractures and especially in men. Always palpate the sacroiliac joint to ensure that it is nontender and therefore not involved in the injury.

Intertrochanteric Femur Fracture

The intertrochanteric femur fracture (Fig. 178.2) is the most common type of hip fracture. Occurring between the greater and lesser trochanter of the proximal femur, this fracture does not involve the hip joint itself; it is an extraarticular, extracapsular fracture. The patient typically presents with a markedly shortened and externally rotated leg, painful with any movement of the hip. An intertrochanteric fracture usually results from the patient tripping over a carpet, pet, or step or slipping and falling; the force of the direct fall onto the intertrochanteric area causes the fracture. This scenario is entirely different from the femoral neck stress fracture discussed next. Repair of the intertrochanteric fracture requires hip pinning with a compression screw. It may require open reduction with use of a bone plate device to achieve near-anatomic alignment. Without repair, the intertrochanteric fracture, even if nondisplaced, is at high risk for displacement with such minor activities as rolling over or moving

in bed. Therefore, if possible, these patients should be referred to an orthopedist for surgical repair. In the nonambulatory patient, such as the nursing home patient, nonoperative treatment may be a safer and less costly alternative. The patient should be managed symptomatically; Buck traction can be used intermittently to reduce pain. The patient should be mobilized to a sitting position within 2 to 3 days. Nonoperative treatment for the ambulatory patient is a rare possibility; it is beyond the scope of this chapter.

Femoral Neck Fracture

Fracture of the femoral neck (see Fig. 178.2) is the second most common type of hip fracture. For a younger person to sustain a femoral neck fracture from trauma takes significant force; therefore most of these fractures occur in older osteoporotic patients, often while just walking in the home. The hip suddenly gives way, and the patient falls to the floor; no history of tripping over a carpet, pet, or step is usually reported, and the patient does not know the reason for the fall. In most cases an osteoporotic femoral neck fracture is actually a stress fracture, which ultimately becomes complete. As the fracture completes itself, it results in the instability that causes the patient to fall. Most of these fractures are displaced; therefore appropriate treatment is prosthetic replacement (one-half of a total hip). Occasionally, these fractures are nondisplaced and can be treated with pinning. Because the femoral neck (most of it) is intracapsular, the greater the displacement, the greater the risk of vascular compromise. Because of this tenuous blood supply, all femoral neck fractures should be monitored for the development of avascular necrosis, even if a prosthesis is placed.

If a patient does not have a history of falling but complains of pain in the groin aggravated by walking and weight bearing, rule out hip osteoarthritis with a weight-bearing radiograph. Always be certain to order a true lateral radiograph of the hip because it will often show a fracture not visible on the plain AP or frog-leg AP view. If the hip joint is free of osteoarthritic findings, a diagnosis of impending stress fracture should be considered. In some patients the fracture is not visible on the radiograph but can be observed on limited MRI. MRI is now considered the standard of care because it is more sensitive and specific than either a bone or CT scan for diagnosing femoral neck stress fractures. Nonathletes with nondisplaced stress fractures in progress demonstrated by bone scan or MRI can be treated with a walker and no weight bearing on the involved side. This treatment often allows the fracture to heal completely and prevents surgery.

Femoral neck stress fractures can also occur in athletes, and inguinal or anterior groin pain is the most frequent symptom. If the diagnosis is delayed, night pain can occur. On physical examination, discomfort is noted at the extremes of internal and external rotation, especially internal rotation. Compression-type stress fractures occur on the inferior medial border of the femoral neck and are considered more stable; tension-type stress fractures occur on the superior lateral border, are less stable, are more prone to displacement, and subsequently require referral to an orthopedic surgeon to consider early operative intervention. Patients with a compression-type fracture with evidence of an overt fracture line should be referred to an orthopedist. Conservative treatment consists of modified bed rest followed by assisted crutch-walking as tolerated until healing is seen (usually 6 weeks); cross-training with cycling or swimming will be helpful for maintaining fitness. Serial radiographs should be obtained every 1 to 2 weeks for the first month or at any time the patient stops improving; if sclerosis extends through both cortices or a crack develops, the patient should be referred. If the patient fails to heal with non–weight bearing, he or she should be referred to an orthopedist. Otherwise, after 6 weeks, weight-bearing exercise can be resumed to preinjury levels over a span of 6 to 8 weeks; the patient should be able to walk a mile without pain before any running is allowed.

Femoral Shaft Fracture

Femoral shaft stress fractures can also occur in athletes. Lacking a history of trauma, the athlete often presents with vague thigh pain, diffuse tenderness, and a suspected quadriceps strain. These patients frequently wait 4 to 6 weeks following the onset of symptoms before seeking care; persistent, worsening symptoms finally bring them in. Fortunately, most femoral shaft stress fractures do not progress to complete fractures. Conservative care consists of relative rest with a switch to non–weight-bearing activities such as swimming or cycling for 6 to 8 weeks. Serial radiographs should be obtained and results managed as for a femoral neck stress fracture. Return to full activity can usually be anticipated after 3 to 4 months.

Other than stable stress fractures, femoral shaft fractures should always be referred for surgical stabilization. These fractures are at high risk for fat embolism and neurovascular problems. A distal femur fracture, which is often intraarticular (extending into the knee joint), should usually undergo surgery to stabilize the fracture, even if the fracture is nondisplaced.

Patellar Fractures

If the articular surface is smooth and the quadriceps mechanism intact, a nondisplaced patellar fracture (Fig. 178.3), whether comminuted or not, can be treated with a cylinder (from above malleoli to groin), full weight-bearing walking cast or with a knee immobilizer (in a reliable patient), crutches, and 10% partial weight-bearing activities. If a tense effusion is present, draining the hemarthrosis under aseptic conditions may provide some symptom relief. Consider referring severely comminuted fractures or fractures with more than 3-mm separation or more than 2-mm articular step-off to an orthopedist. Otherwise, a follow-up clinical examination is performed and AP and lateral radiographs assessed 2 weeks after initial treatment. If no displacement exists and tenderness with palpation is resolved, then gentle non–weight-bearing range of motion exercises can be started in an arc of 0 to 45 degrees. Another radiograph should be obtained 6 weeks after treatment; at this point, the fracture should be solidly healed and point tenderness over the patella resolved. Active and passive range of motion activities can now be initiated in therapy. During the healing phase, the patient should be encouraged to carry out quadriceps and hamstring isometric and straight-leg raising exercises to maintain muscle function and tone.

Marginal vertical fractures that are nondisplaced do not have to be immobilized. They can be treated with reduced activity for 4 to 6 weeks followed by progressive range of motion and strengthening exercises.

Tibial Plateau Fractures

The clinician should be certain that a tibial plateau fracture is not depressed or displaced, especially if it extends into the joint surface. Lateral, AP, and internal and external oblique radiographs

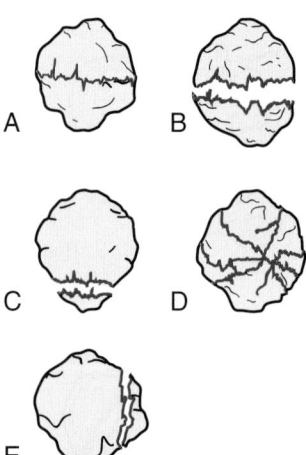

Fig. 178.3 Classification of patellar fractures. (A) Nondisplaced transverse. (B) Displaced transverse. (C) Upper or lower pole. (D) Comminuted. (E) Vertical.

should be obtained. A tunnel (notch) view is helpful for visualizing the intercondylar eminence. Tomograms are the only method to exclude displacement. CT will help to delineate the extent of articular involvement and fracture displacement; MRI also provides this information and can detect ligamentous and meniscal injuries. If any depression or displacement has occurred, the patient must be referred; fractures associated with ligamentous or meniscal injury should also be referred. These referrals should generally occur within 24 to 48 hours.

If the fracture is extraarticularly displaced (intraarticularly nondisplaced), it can be treated with crutches, non–weight-bearing activities for 3 months, and gentle range of motion activities. A hinged brace is excellent for this fracture, with gradual increased range of motion activities up to 90 degrees at 3 to 4 weeks. Otherwise, the patient should remain non–weight bearing for 4 to 6 weeks, until there is radiographic evidence of healing, and can then progress to partial weight bearing with crutches. Crutches should be used until solid union of the fracture is documented. These fractures need to be watched carefully with clinical examination and radiographs at 2-week intervals for the first month to be certain there is no displacement, which can occur with motion of the knee joint. Be certain to document the strength of the peroneal nerve.

Tibial Shaft Fractures

Tibial shaft fractures (Fig. 178.4) can be treated with a long-leg cast with the knee in 0 to 5 degrees of flexion and the ankle in neutral position (90 degrees). The patient can bear weight with this cast, and ambulation should be encouraged as soon as possible (as long as there is no risk for compartment syndrome [see Chapter 179, Compartment Syndrome Evaluation], which can occur at up to 10 days). As it turns out, most patients are not able to bear significant weight, due to discomfort, for 1 to 2 weeks.

Proximal shaft fractures are often due to high-energy forces, but distal fractures are usually the result of low-energy injuries; this concept is important to consider during management. There should be less than 5 mm of displacement in both the AP and mediolateral planes; otherwise, the patient should be referred. If any angulation of the tibial shaft fracture has occurred, a goniometer must be used to assess the amount. Angulation up to 10 degrees in the AP radiograph and up to 5 degrees in the mediolateral plane is acceptable. Angulation greater than these amounts requires correction by wedging the cast; these patients should be referred.

If less than 50% bone surface contact between fracture fragments is observed in the AP or lateral views, then the patient should be referred to an orthopedic surgeon. Degree of rotation should be

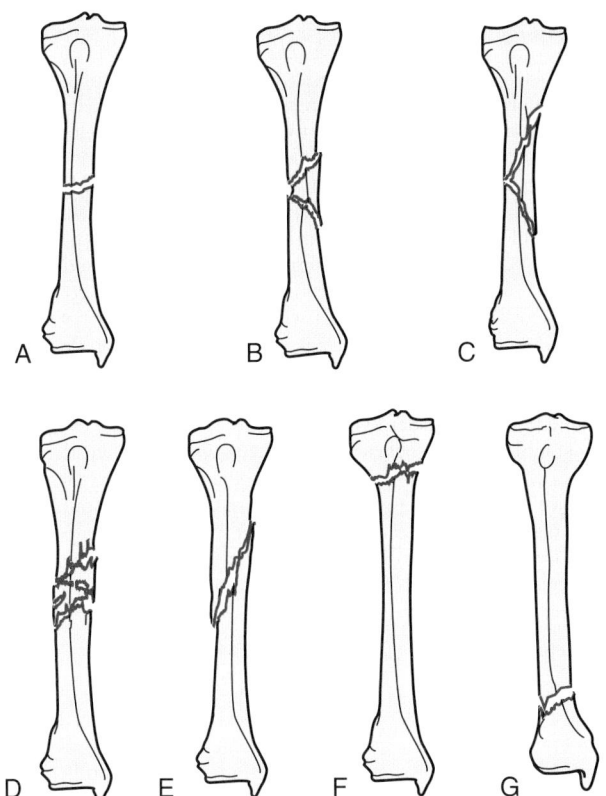

Fig. 178.4 Tibial shaft fractures. (A) Transverse or short oblique. (B) Small butterfly fragment. (C) Large butterfly fragment. (D) Segmental comminution. (E) Spiral. (F) Proximal one-fourth transverse or oblique. (G) Distal one-fourth transverse or oblique. The fracture in A is usually stable. The stability of the fractures shown in B and C is dependent on the size of the butterfly fragment. The fracture shown in D is usually unstable. The fractures shown in E to G are stable but difficult to control.

determined by the amount of discrepancy between transverse widths of the proximal and distal fragments; greater than 10 degrees of rotation should also be referred. Shortening greater than 2 cm is not acceptable and requires referral. If any doubt remains about the amount of overlap (which causes shortening), a bone length measurement radiograph can be obtained for the radiologist to compare the length of one tibia with the other.

For tibial fractures in which the fibula is not broken, very little chance exists of the tibia becoming unacceptably shortened because the fibula will splint the soft tissue at an appropriate length. If the fibula is broken in addition to the tibia, a higher incidence of shortening of the tibia exists as a result of unopposed muscle contraction. This is especially true in an oblique angle fracture; the oblique angle allows sliding of the fracture into a shortened position. If the fracture is transverse, then this sliding shortening cannot occur. Nevertheless, combined tibia-fibular fractures are frequently due to high-impact forces, are at high risk for compartment syndrome, and are rarely nondisplaced; these patients are frequently referred.

If the fracture is satisfactory in alignment and length, then a long-leg cast for a period of 4 to 6 weeks is appropriate. For the initial cast, plaster is usually easier to mold; fiberglass reinforcement can then be applied in a few days if this cast is left in place. The cast will usually need to be changed in 2 to 3 weeks because of loosening as the swelling decreases. Radiographs should be taken weekly for the first 3 or 4 weeks to verify fracture alignment, then every 2 to 4 weeks until healing confirmed. After 4 to 6 weeks, the cast can be cut down to a short-leg walking cast or a walking cast brace for an additional 10 to 14 weeks, until clinically healed. To verify clinical healing, there should be minimal tenderness over the fracture site and no motion or pain with bending stress in any direction.

Tibial fractures are notorious for developing compartment syndrome (see Chapter 179, Compartment Syndrome Evaluation) when any significant soft tissue trauma has occurred. If the tibial fracture is the result of a fall from a height greater than 6 feet or the result of a high-velocity injury such as in an automobile accident, be very cautious about the possibility of compartment syndrome. Be certain that the patient elevates the leg at home so that the calf is 2 feet higher than the heart at all times, except when going to the bathroom, for 1 week. Explain to the patient that the heart is the pump and that the fluid from the leg needs to drain toward the pump, which requires the fluid in the leg to be elevated higher than the pump. Seat cushions from the couch stacked three high under the calf can help to achieve this elevation. The patient's chest must be flat, although pillows can be placed under the head to facilitate reading and eating. However, sitting in a recliner does not provide adequate elevation because the chest is only at the level of the calf.

Patients at risk for compartment syndrome may use their crutches to go to the bathroom, placing no weight on the injured side. They should return to the bed, couch, or floor, lie down, and resume elevation of the leg as soon as possible. If there is loss of fine-touch sensation or two-point discrimination, distention and swelling of the calf, pain with passive motion of muscle groups (especially extension of the great toe), progressive pain, or pain not relieved by oral pain medication such as narcotics, then emergent testing should be performed or referral made to rule out compartment syndrome (see Chapter 179, Compartment Syndrome Evaluation). The peak time for compartment syndrome after a tibial fracture is on the third day after the injury.

Tibial stress fractures are one of the most common stress fractures in young athletes and military recruits. They occur more commonly at the junction of the middle and distal thirds of the tibia in runners, in the middle third in ballet dancers, and in the proximal third in military recruits. Symptoms are usually insidious in onset, increase with physical activity, and may become severe enough to persist for hours after activity or even at night. There is usually pain with palpation but minimal swelling at the site of tenderness. However, pain can often be elicited at the site by applying a tuning fork or by percussing the tibia away from the site. Radiographs are frequently negative for 2 to 4 weeks after the onset of symptoms; a triple-phase bone scan can be helpful if a stress fracture is strongly suspected. However, MRI has somewhat become the preferred imaging study for tibial stress fractures. MRI will remain positive for up to 12 months. Most tibial stress fractures are treated with elimination of impact activity for 4 to 6 weeks, cross-training, and crutches as needed for pain. Additional imaging is not necessary unless the patient fails to improve with treatment. In that situation, CT is the best study to detect extension of the fracture or nonunion.

Radiographs may demonstrate the dreaded "black line" fracture, which is an anterior midshaft tibial stress fracture associated with poor healing, a risk of nonunion, and risk of recurrence. These fractures typically take 6 to 12 months to heal; patients must refrain from impact loading activities until they are pain free and there is complete radiographic healing.

Fibular Shaft Fractures

Fibular shaft fractures require no immobilization or restriction of weight-bearing activities, other than for pain management, because the fibula supports only 15% of the weight in the lower extremity. In fact, the fibula can be used elsewhere as a bone graft without a problem. However, fibular fractures rarely occur alone. Always check for associated injury around the ankle, over the medial and lateral collateral ligaments, and the tibiofibular distal joint. It is common for a severe ankle-twisting injury to result in a small fracture around the ankle and an associated fracture somewhere along the fibula, including the proximal fibula (Maisonneuve fracture). Isolated fibular fractures can occur from a direct blow to the side of the calf. Again, these fractures require no immobilization or restriction of weight-bearing activities and almost always heal uneventfully within 6 to 8 weeks. Use of a stirrup splint, a short-leg walking cast, or a cast boot for 3 to 4 weeks may help to relieve moderate to severe pain. If a radiograph at 3 to 4 weeks documents some healing (e.g., some callus formation, filling in of fracture line), the splinting can be reduced to as needed and progressive rehabilitation initiated.

Always evaluate the function of the peroneal nerve when treating a fibular fracture by documenting the strength of active foot flexion and extension at the ankle, as well as eversion. If the peroneal nerve is affected, document this and consider referral to an orthopedist. Also consider referral for severely displaced or comminuted fractures, ligament instability, or painful nonunion after treatment.

Ankle Fractures

Point tenderness over the lateral malleolus (distal fibula) or medial malleolus (distal tibia) often indicates an ankle fracture as opposed to a sprain. The area of the posterior malleolus (distal tibia, immediately behind the medial malleolus) should also be palpated for tenderness. If no point tenderness is felt over the malleoli, then an x-ray is rarely necessary. This decision is supported by the Ottawa ankle rules, which indicate a radiograph is most predictive of fracture if the patient has pain over the malleolus and tenderness over the malleolus or the patient was unable to bear weight immediately at the time of injury and at the initial clinician visit. Point tenderness over the anterior and lateral ligaments (anterior talofibular and lateral calcaneofibular ligament) but not the fibula indicates an ankle sprain. A first-degree ankle sprain will have tenderness only over the anterior talofibular ligament, whereas a second- or third-degree ankle sprain has tenderness over the talofibular and calcaneofibular ligaments.

If ankle radiographs are indicated, obtain lateral, AP, and mortise (AP view with the foot in 15 degrees of adduction) views. The ankle mortise is the joint space between the top of the talus and the bottom of the tibia, as well as the medial and lateral malleoli. There should be symmetric spacing throughout the mortise; in other words, there should be less than 1 mm of displacement of the talus in any direction greater than elsewhere in the mortise. A nondisplaced fracture of the ankle is frequently seen in only one radiographic view of the ankle.

Small avulsion fractures, nondisplaced single malleolar fractures, and stable bimalleolar fractures can be treated nonoperatively. Small, nondisplaced avulsion fractures are treated with early mobilization and weight bearing, as tolerated, similar to an ankle sprain. A functional stirrup splint worn in a shoe may be adequate; functional rehabilitation exercises can be started as soon as symptoms allow. Isolated oblique lateral malleolar fractures at or below the ankle joint can be immobilized with a commercial walking fracture boot or short-leg walking cast for 4 to 6 weeks. Unstable fractures (e.g., malleolar fracture with ligament disruption on the opposite side), displaced single malleolar, large (>25% of articular surface) or displaced (>2 mm) posterior malleolar, or trimalleolar (bilateral plus posterior malleolar) fractures (or if clinician is unsure about the stability of the fracture) should be referred. Otherwise, medial and lateral malleolar fractures require a minimum of 4 weeks for clinical healing and possibly several months for radiographic healing. When following an ankle fracture with radiographs, the mortise view should always be examined for evidence of new instability or a shift.

If the patient smokes, the fracture healing time can be doubled; it can also be delayed in patients who are taking antiinflammatory medications. Patients should be informed that the incidence of complex regional pain syndrome (CRPS) (see the section on "Complications") after any injury in this area, including a fracture, is much higher when they smoke.

NOTE: A cast boot should be prescribed for any patient wearing a short-leg splint or cast or a long-leg splint or cast. The cast boot protects the toes and cast and prevents material from slipping through the end of the cast and up underneath the foot.

Medial and Posterior Malleolar (Distal Tibia) Fractures

If an isolated medial or small (<25% of the articular surface) posterior malleolar fracture is shown to be nondisplaced in the lateral, AP, and mortise views of the ankle, treatment with a short-leg weight-bearing cast (or walking fracture boot in a trusted, compliant patient) is appropriate. (Suspect Maisonneuve fracture in isolated posterior malleolar fracture.) Similar to isolated lateral malleolar fractures, the ankle should be immobilized in the neutral (90 degrees) position to minimize Achilles tendon shortening. The patient should be seen again in 2 weeks to assess the condition of the cast (or compliance with the walking boot) and at 4 weeks to repeat radiographs. If the initial fracture line is below (distal to) the level of the ankle mortise, immediate full weight-bearing activities may be allowed, as tolerated. If the fracture is at or above the ankle mortise and at 4 weeks is clinically healing (nontender over the fracture site and some evidence of radiographic healing such as callus formation), the patient may begin gradual weight bearing and ankle rehabilitation. If no radiographic evidence of healing is apparent at 4 weeks, the patient should remain in the cast another 2 weeks and return for repeat radiographs. At that point, if the patient is still not clinically healed, a fracture boot should be worn, and walking and ankle rehabilitation initiated.

Lateral Malleolar (Distal Fibula) Fractures

There are three types of fractures in the distal third of the fibula. Because these fractures can be associated with a medial ligament injury and subsequent instability, repeat radiographs should be obtained in 7 to 10 days to assess fracture alignment and the position of the mortise. A Weber A fracture occurs below the level of the ankle mortise and can be treated with an immediate weight-bearing short-leg cast or fracture boot for 6 to 8 weeks. A Weber B fracture occurs at the level of the ankle mortise. Again, if the lateral, AP, and mortise x-ray views show the fracture to be nondisplaced, it can be treated with a short-leg walking cast for 6 to 8 weeks. Because this fracture is at the level of the ankle mortise, weight bearing should not be allowed for the first 2 weeks. This restriction decreases stress at the ankle mortise, which could cause displacement at the fracture site. A Weber C distal fibular fracture occurs above the ankle mortise and has the greatest potential for displacement. This fracture disrupts a portion of the syndesmotic ligament area between the tibia and fibula distally, just above the ankle mortise. This fracture is also treated in a walking cast for 6 to 8 weeks with no weight bearing during the first 3 weeks.

Talar Fractures

Plain radiographs are frequently adequate for diagnosing talar fractures, although CT may be necessary to diagnose fractures of the talar head or stress fractures. Minor anterior and posterior avulsion fractures of the talus are occasionally seen in association with ankle injuries. Lateral avulsion fractures, just distal to the tip of the distal fibula, are occasionally seen in snowboarders (snowboarder's fracture) and can be large and comminuted. Small, or nondisplaced, anterior and posterior avulsion fractures are treated with a short-leg walking cast for 1 month followed by range of motion, stretching, and strengthening rehabilitation exercises. Anterior avulsion fractures should be cast with the ankle in the neutral position (90 degrees); posterior avulsion fractures benefit from being cast in 15 degrees of equinus (plantar flexion), which allows tiptoe weight bearing. Small (<2 mm), nondisplaced, noncomminuted lateral avulsion fractures are probably best managed in a short-leg, non–weight-bearing cast for 4 weeks followed by 2 weeks of progressive weight bearing in a walking cast or cast boot. If displacement has occurred for an avulsion fracture or the fragment is large or comminuted, the patient should be referred to an orthopedic surgeon. Small (<50% of talonavicular surface, <0.5 cm) talar head fractures are treated with immobilization for 6 to 8 weeks followed by a longitudinal arch support for 3 to 6 months. Nondisplaced fractures of the talar neck can be treated with 4 to 6 weeks short-leg non–weight-bearing cast followed by short-leg walking cast for 4 weeks. Nondisplaced talar body fractures can be treated with 6 to 8 weeks of short-leg non–weight-bearing cast.

Prolonged pain (several weeks to months) following an inversion injury of the ankle, often associated with point tenderness in the area, decreased range of motion, crepitus, and an effusion, should lead the clinician to suspect an osteochondral talar dome fracture. If plain films show no abnormality, a bone scan is highly effective for detecting these fractures. For positive bone scans, an MRI is effective at determining the exact location and stage. Symptomatic stage I (compressed, nondisplaced) and stage II (attached, nondisplaced) osteochondral talar dome fractures typically respond well to conservative treatment with immobilization for 6 to 8 weeks in a non–weight-bearing cast followed by rehabilitation; referral should be considered if symptoms persist after 4 to 6 months of conservative therapy. Stage III (detached, nondisplaced) and stage IV (displaced) talar dome fractures are best treated with early operative care (often just arthroscopy). Talar head fractures can be treated with a short-leg walking cast for 6 to 8 weeks followed by longitudinal arch support for several more weeks. Patients should be warned that this fracture may be complicated by persistent pain due to posttraumatic arthritis in the talonavicular joint.

The patient should be aware that despite perfect reduction, healing is often complicated by avascular necrosis in fractures of the talar neck and body. The nonunion rate may be as high as 50%, and there is an associated high incidence of osteoarthritis. Talar fractures are second only to scaphoid (navicular) fractures in the wrist as a site for chronic postfracture complications and pain. That said, nondisplaced talar neck fractures can be treated with a non–weight-bearing short-leg cast for 4 to 6 weeks followed by a short-leg walking cast for an additional 4 weeks. If there is no radiographic evidence of fracture union at 6 weeks, radiographs should be repeated every 2 to 3 weeks and the patient should remain in a walking cast until union is documented. CT scanning may be necessary to demonstrate fracture union. Nondisplaced talar body fractures should be immobilized in a short-leg non–weight-bearing cast for 6 to 8 weeks. All patients with a talar fracture should be instructed in range of motion, stretching, and strengthening rehabilitation exercises following cast removal. Patients should be seen 2 to 3 weeks into such a rehabilitation program and then followed until there is near-normal function.

Calcaneal Fractures

Obtain axial, lateral, and dorsoplantar radiographs of the calcaneus for suspected fractures. Comparison views of the opposite side may be helpful for diagnosing bilateral fractures (common) and for measuring anatomic angles. Oblique views may also be helpful. If radiographs are negative but there is high suspicion of fracture, obtain a CT. If any doubt remains about displacement, obtain a CT scan. A radiologist or orthopedist can offer suggestions about the need to obtain a CT scan after viewing the plain radiographs. Intraarticular (subtalar joint) fractures (approximately 70% of calcaneal fractures) or displaced extraarticular fractures should generally be referred to an orthopedist.

If the vertical forces were significant enough to cause a calcaneal fracture (e.g., a fall from a height), a radiograph of the thoracic and lumbar spine should also be obtained; there is a high incidence of associated axial fractures (e.g., thoracic and lumbar spine fractures). The clinician must also palpate the thoracic and lumbar spine for signs of tenderness in these patients.

For a nonarticular, nondisplaced fracture of the calcaneal body, pain management, treatment with a bulky compression soft wrap, and elevation are all that is needed. These fractures generally heal well regardless of treatment. Early, gentle, yet active range of motion exercises of the foot and ankle are appropriate to minimize the stiffness associated with these fractures. Maximal elevation is critical to minimize swelling and pain; swelling can be significant, even

causing blisters or skin loss with subsequent infection. Elevation with the patient lying down and the hip and knee both flexed to 90 degrees with couch cushions under the calf is the best management for the first week. Patients may be up on crutches only to go to the bathroom; otherwise, they should be supine with the leg elevated.

NOTE: If the patient is not instructed to keep the hip and knee bent 90 degrees with elevation, he or she may complain of sciatica. When pillows or blankets are placed underneath only the heel, the knee remains straight and can result in the sciatic nerve being stretched.

For extraarticular fractures of the anterior, medial, or lateral calcaneal processes, the patient should be placed in a short-leg walking cast for 4 weeks. Displaced fractures can usually be reduced with closed manipulation; otherwise, surgical reduction is necessary. Fractures of the tuberosity or sustentaculum tali should be managed with a short-leg non–weight-bearing cast for 6 to 8 weeks. Tuberosity fractures should be cast in 5 to 10 degrees of equinus (plantar flexion) and repeat radiographs obtained at 1 week to check for alignment. The patient should be seen every 2 to 4 weeks for management of all these fractures.

Midfoot Tarsal Bone (Cuneiforms, Cuboid, and Navicular) Fractures

Lateral, AP, and oblique radiographs should be obtained for suspected midfoot fractures. For nondisplaced fractures, apply a short-leg walking cast for weight-bearing activities as tolerated after the first week. For most, the cast should be in place for 4 to 6 weeks; fractures of the navicular body may benefit from casting for 8 weeks total. For nonunion of a navicular tuberosity fracture, 8 to 10 weeks of casting may be necessary. If fractures are displaced or severely comminuted, if there is nonunion of the navicular tuberosity after 10 weeks, or if there is a concomitant joint dislocation, refer the patient to an orthopedic surgeon.

Beware of a fracture or dislocation of the Lisfranc joint, which extends into the tarsometatarsal joint at the midfoot and occurs when an athlete falls forward on a plantar-flexed foot. To prevent future disability, it is critical to diagnose an unstable fracture of this area, so always obtain routine as well as weight-bearing lateral and AP radiographs for injuries to the bridge of the foot. Also suspect a Lisfranc injury when there is an avulsion "fleck" fracture of the lateral proximal first metatarsal or the medial proximal second metatarsal. The joint may appear nondislocated on the AP view; however, on the lateral view, anterior displacement may be observed. On the weight-bearing AP radiograph, widening may appear between the first and second metatarsals; on the weight-bearing lateral radiograph, a step-off (evidence of joint disruption) between the tarsal and proximal metatarsal may appear. A CT scan can be used to confirm the diagnosis. If any questions remain about an injury to the midfoot or about the radiographic views, ask a radiologist or orthopedic surgeon to review the films. These fractures are rare because of the rigidity of the midfoot.

Metatarsal Fractures

The most common metatarsal fracture is at the base of the proximal fifth metatarsal and represents an avulsion fracture of the styloid where the peroneus brevis tendon and plantar aponeurosis insert. With an inversion sprain-type injury to the forefoot and ankle, a small piece of bone can be pulled loose. The displacement is usually no greater than 3 mm; it is treated with a firm or wooden-soled fracture shoe with weight bearing as tolerated and ice and elevation for comfort. If the patient continues to experience significant discomfort at the first follow-up visit in 4 to 7 days, a short-leg walking cast (limited to 2 weeks) may help to reduce symptoms. The purpose of the wooden-soled shoe or cast is to prevent flexion at the midfoot when the patient walks, thereby preventing stress at the fracture site. The wooden-soled shoe is worn for 3 weeks or longer until the patient is comfortable without it and can return to wearing a regular shoe. However, impact sports should be avoided for a minimum of 2 months.

A metatarsal avulsion fracture must be differentiated from a Jones fracture, which is much less common and treated entirely differently. A Jones fracture occurs in nearly the same location; however, it extends (if not initially, eventually) across the entire shaft just distal to the base of the fifth metatarsal and into the joint between the bases of the fourth and fifth metatarsals. If the fracture is displaced, the patient should be referred to an orthopedic surgeon. If there are signs of stress fracture (e.g., widened fracture line, medullary sclerosis), referral should be considered to avoid prolonged immobilization or nonunion. If it appears acute and nondisplaced, it will usually heal well with a short-leg walking cast for 6 to 8 weeks and no weight bearing for the first 3 weeks. At this point, if neither clinical nor radiographic healing is apparent, a non–weight-bearing cast should be reapplied for 4 more weeks or the patient referred. This fracture is notorious for delayed union, especially in patients who smoke or take antiinflammatory medications. No impact sports should be allowed after this injury for a minimum of 3 months. This possible prolonged healing and delay in return to sport may cause some patients to request screw fixation, especially athletes.

A stress fracture of the fifth metatarsal can be confused with a Jones fracture, but it typically occurs in the proximal shaft. This fracture is also notoriously slow to heal. MRI has somewhat replaced bone scan for detecting early stress fractures because of increased sensitivity and specificity; it should be noted that specificity of MRI is not perfect, so clinical correlation is also important. Some experts recommend orthopedic consultation in every case because optimal conditions may require up to 20 weeks of immobilization and nonunion may still occur. With intramedullary screw fixation, the athlete may return to his or her sport much earlier. Stress fractures of the other metatarsal shafts are much more common and usually less severe. Symptoms may precede radiographic findings by 2 to 3 weeks. In most cases, these fractures can be managed without casting; merely eliminating impact (e.g., running, jumping) until clinical healing is documented is sufficient.

Nondisplaced fractures of metatarsal shafts can be treated with wooden-soled shoes for 4 to 6 weeks. If there is significant pain (e.g., first metatarsal, multiple fractures), the patient can be in a short-leg walking cast for 4 to 7 weeks and minimize weight bearing for the first 2 to 3 weeks. Most displaced fractures of the first metatarsal should be referred, even if the displacement appears mild. Patients with displaced fractures of multiple metatarsals, displaced fractures close to the metatarsal heads, and intraarticular fractures are probably best referred for pin fixation. Otherwise, fractures of the second through fourth metatarsals that are displaced only in the lateral or medial plane do not usually require reduction. Fractures of the second through fourth metatarsal shafts displaced more than 3 or 4 mm or angulated greater than 10 degrees in the dorsal or plantar plane should be reduced or referred. These fractures can often be reduced under local anesthesia hematoma block using Chinese finger (toe) traps and gravity or 2 to 5 lb of weight. After reduction, a short-leg walking cast can be used for 5 to 7 weeks with no weight bearing the first 2 to 3 weeks.

Although rare, clinicians must beware of compartment syndrome in the foot. This can occur with multiple fractures (e.g., three or more metatarsals) from a crushing-type injury and resultant extreme swelling.

Toe Fractures

For the great toe, displaced intraarticular fractures and fractures that spontaneously become displaced when traction is released after reduction may benefit from internal fixation, so these patients should generally be referred. For the other toes, fracture dislocations and intraarticular fractures that involve more than 25% of the joint surface may benefit from referral. Otherwise, rarely is a surgical

intervention required. Displaced fractures can be managed by reduction under digital block anesthesia followed by manual traction, pulling the toe into a corrected position. Many authorities recommend a short-leg walking cast with a toe platform for 2 to 3 weeks for fractures of the great toe followed by buddy taping and a wooden-soled shoe. For fractures of other toes, buddy taping to an adjacent toe for 3 to 6 weeks will stabilize the fracture. Use of wooden-soled shoes for 2 to 3 weeks, ice, and elevation may decrease pain. When taping digits together (fingers or toes), place dry cotton or gauze between them to prevent skin maceration from moisture. Patients can change this dressing after a shower and watch the alignment of the nail beds for development of a rotational deformity, which can be surgically repaired. Patients should be followed by the clinician every 2 to 4 weeks. Follow-up radiographs are generally not needed except for fractures of the great toe or intraarticular fractures.

Fractures in the distal phalanges of the fingers or toes sometimes involve injury to the nail bed or an open fracture caused by the bone pushing up through the nail bed. In these patients, the treatment should be digital block anesthesia followed by removal of the nail to irrigate the nail bed thoroughly at the site of the open fracture. The nail bed can be repaired with 5-0 absorbable suture, which will minimize nail deformity. Nail bed repair is usually more desirable for the fingers because many individuals will accept deformity of a nail plate in a toe but are concerned about a cosmetic deformity in a finger (see Chapter 24, Nail Bed Repair).

Clavicle Fractures

Because outcomes are basically the same, treatment for fractures of the clavicle is generally whatever best relieves the symptoms. Possibilities include a figure-of-eight brace or sling, both, or neither, depending on the patient's comfort level (see Fig. 178.8). Other considerations include whether the patient lives alone and can adjust a figure-eight; as opposed to a sling, use of a figure-eight also leaves the elbow and hand free for daily activities. If the fracture site produces pressure and tenting of the skin, refer the patient for possible surgery. Because nonunion of middle third (midshaft) fractures is rare (<1%), such fractures rarely require referral (usually only for fractures displaced more than 1 bone width, especially if associated comminution or significant shortening [>18 mm in men or >14 mm in women] or symptomatic nonunion after 12 to 16 weeks). These fractures comprise 69% of clavicular fractures. Inner third (proximal) clavicular fractures (rare, 3% of clavicular fractures) need to be referred only if there is significant displacement or an associated sternoclavicular dislocation. Distal third (lateral) clavicular fractures (28% of clavicular fractures) should be referred if the coracoclavicular ligament is torn and the proximal fragment displaced (type IIB, Fig. 178.5). Because distal third fractures that extend into the acromioclavicular joint can lead to future degenerative changes in that joint, some primary care clinicians also refer these fractures (type III, see Fig. 178.5). Otherwise, symptomatic therapy is indicated for most clavicular fractures.

Clavicular fractures require a minimum of 2 months for solid union (possibly a month longer in adults), and contact sports should be avoided for 8 to 10 weeks. (Do not be dismayed if the 1 month follow-up x-ray shows no sign of healing! In fact, this x-ray can be omitted if there are no new symptoms.) Patients should be seen every 2 to 3 weeks; radiographs are indicated only after clinical union (nontender locally and with full range of motion) has occurred or for late development of symptoms. Remember to adjust the figure-of-eight splint to ensure that it is tight enough to be supportive and keep the shoulders back ("position of attention") yet loose enough to avoid tingling and numbness from pressure on the brachial plexus where the splint wraps around the armpit. Instruct the patient to loosen or tighten the brace for more support, if needed, or to reduce restriction if tingling and numbness occur. It should be worn until there is no more tenderness or crepitus at the fracture site.

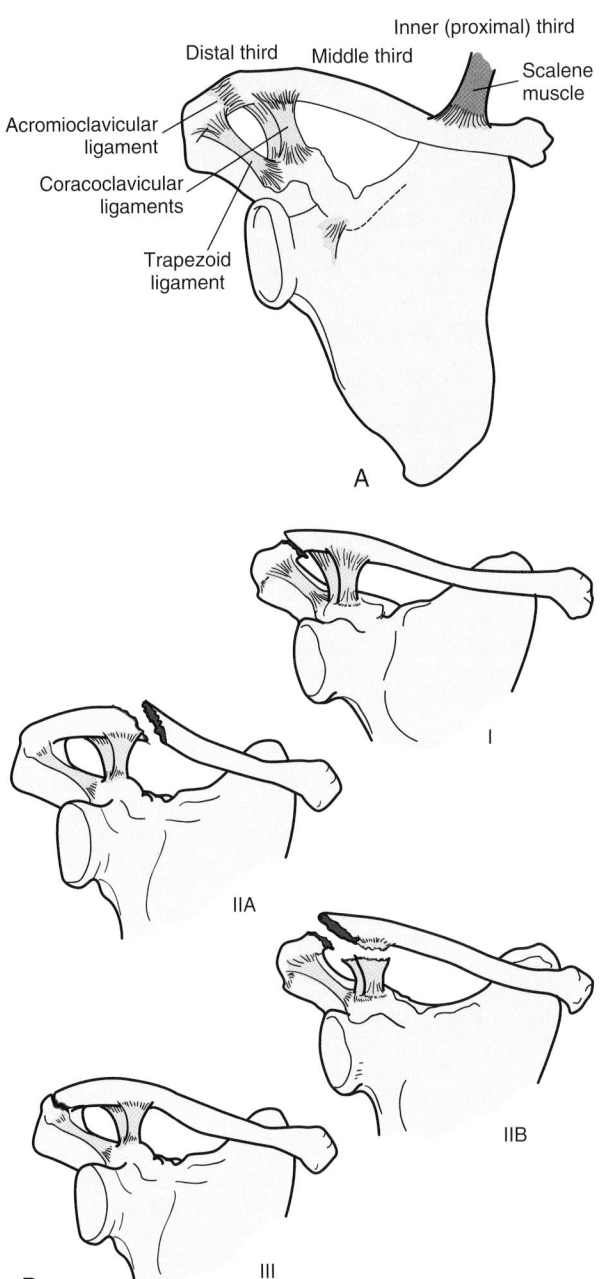

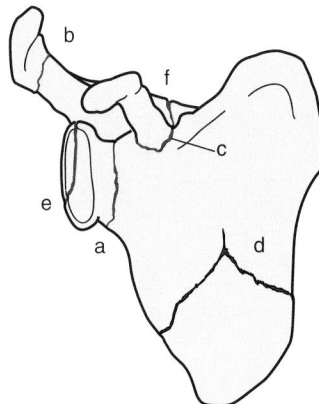

Fig. 178.6 Scapular fractures (anterior view): neck (*a*); acromion process (*b*); coracoid process (*c*); body (*d*); glenoid rim or articular cartilage (*e*); spinous process (*f*), which is posterior and only partially seen here.

Fig. 178.5 Clavicle fractures. (A) Fractures of the clavicle are classified by location into the distal (28%), middle (69%), and inner (proximal) (3%) thirds. Clavicle fractures can be nondisplaced, displaced, angulated, or non-angulated. (B) Classification of fractures of the distal third of the clavicle (Allman). Type I: minimal displacement with ligaments intact. Type IIA: proximal shaft is displaced with ligaments intact. Type IIB: clavicle displaced, coracoclavicular ligament ruptured but trapezoid ligament intact. Type III: fracture of the articular surface with no disruption of the ligaments.

For clavicular fractures, always listen to the chest to exclude a pneumothorax, especially for fractures due to motor vehicle accidents. A chest x-ray is also appropriate. Instruct the patient to report any shortness of breath immediately.

Scapular Fractures

The scapula is covered on all sides with muscle and has an excellent blood supply; therefore fractures of the scapula (Fig. 178.6) heal extremely well, even when displaced. Most fractures of the scapula need only a sling or shoulder immobilizer for comfort for 2 weeks. Even these measures may not be needed for fractures of the scapular spine, body, or coracoid. For suspected scapular fractures, always obtain a true AP of the glenohumeral (shoulder) joint, an axillary view, and a true lateral scapular Y view. These views will help to exclude any intraarticular extension into the glenoid shoulder socket. (A cephalic tilt view can help to evaluate the coracoid process.) If any questions remain about a fracture being intraarticular or displaced at the glenoid, a CT scan should be obtained. Significantly displaced coracoid fractures, especially if combined with a complete acromioclavicular separation, displaced acromion fractures, displaced glenoid neck fractures associated with a clavicular fracture or that exceed more than 1 cm displacement or more than 20 degrees inferior angulation, or glenoid fractures that involve more than 25% of the articular surface (or those with an associated subluxed humeral head) should be referred. Scapular body fractures that have separated the body and spine by more than 1 cm may require surgery. For all others, early range of motion activities should be encouraged, as tolerated. Patients should be seen every 2 to 4 weeks to ensure adequate progress in their rehabilitation program. Evidence of radiographic healing should be present before resistance exercises are initiated.

Proximal Humerus Fractures

After obtaining true AP and lateral scapular Y or axillary views, fractures of the proximal humerus can be classified by the Neer system (Fig. 178.7) and are considered a one-part fracture if they are displaced less than 1 cm or angulated less than 45 degrees. Patients with fractures displaced more than 1 cm (the minority of fractures) or associated with joint instability or a dislocation should generally be referred. Fractures involving the bicipital groove may interfere with function and therefore also probably warrant referral. Fractures involving the anatomic neck have a high risk of avascular necrosis, so these patients should probably be referred. Angulation up to 45 degrees is tolerated amazingly well by most individuals, so referral is necessary only for greater angulation; however, athletic or very active individuals may warrant consultation when angulation approaches 20 degrees. Most fractures in older patients are immediately below the tubercles, in the area of the surgical neck, which generally has a good blood supply (as opposed to the anatomic neck, immediately beneath the humeral head). As long as there is at least 50% overlap of fracture segments on the AP and scapular Y views, treatment with a sling or shoulder immobilizer for 2 weeks is appropriate, followed by gentle passive and active assistive range of motion exercises to minimize stiffness (Fig. 178.8). The sling should be discontinued 2 to 4 weeks after the injury. The shoulder immobilizer is most useful when angulation is greater

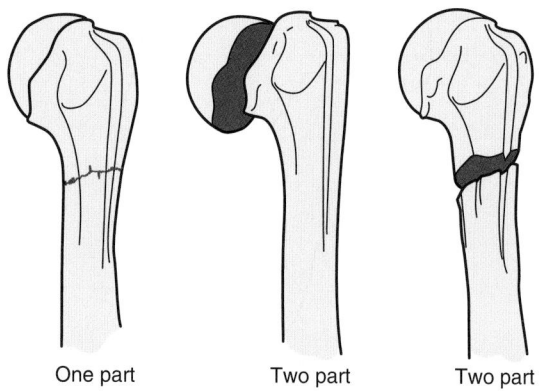

Fig. 178.7 Neer classification of proximal humerus fractures. One-part or minimally displaced fracture is defined as no segments displaced more than 1.0 cm or angulated more than 45 degrees. A two-part fracture is defined as one segment displaced more than 1.0 cm or angulated more than 45 degrees.

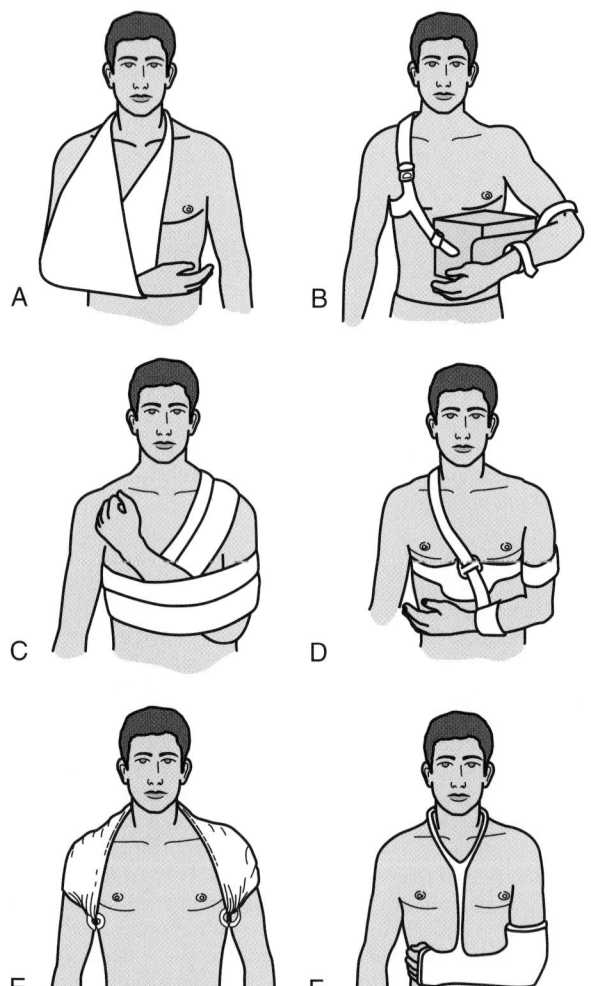

Fig. 178.8 Possible methods of immobilization of the shoulder. (A) Simple shoulder sling is used for humerus, clavicle, and radial head fractures. (B) Abduction pillow shoulder immobilizer is used for rotator cuff tendon tear after surgery. (C) Sling and swathe bandage is used for severe acromioclavicular separation and fractures of upper humerus. (D) Shoulder immobilizer is used for humeral neck fractures. (E) Figure-of-eight strap for fractures of the clavicle. (F) The hanging arm cast is used for humeral neck and humeral shaft fractures. It provides weight and traction to align the fracture pieces.

than 20 degrees and should be worn 24 hours a day, except when performing physical therapy or exercise. The shoulder immobilizer prevents displacement of the fracture at night while sleeping. Remind the patient not to use the arm for heavy activity during the day; however, activity of daily living should be encouraged after 2 weeks.

In all fractures, palpation for resolution of point tenderness at the fracture site is a very reliable clinical index of solid fracture union. This finding combined with radiographic union determines when patients can return to full activity without restriction.

Humeral Shaft Fractures

Humeral shaft fractures are unique in the amount of angulation (of a long bone) that can be allowed; they are also unique in their excellent healing rate (low incidence of nonunion) for long bone shaft fractures. These distinctions are due to the excellent blood supply provided, in part, by a large amount of surrounding muscle tissue. This surrounding muscle tissue can also shelter significant angulation with little resultant cosmetic defect.

For these reasons and because the shoulder and elbow have excellent motion, up to 30 degrees of mediolateral angulation, up to 20 degrees of AP angulation, and displacement of up to half the width of the humerus are acceptable when treating a humeral shaft fracture. Treatment consists of a hanging arm cast (see Fig. 178.8F) that extends from the humerus, around the elbow flexed at 90 degrees, and down to the wrist. This position is maintained until callus formation is detected and the fracture site is stable to manual stress, which can take from 8 to 14 weeks. Alternatively, if there is radiographic evidence of healing at 1 month and decreased tenderness at the fracture site, the hanging arm cast can be removed and a functional humerus cast brace (Fig. 178.9) applied. Such a brace is also preferred for transverse fractures which ironically have higher risk of nonunion than spiral fractures.

Made from polyethylene, functional humerus cast braces are available off the shelf at local brace supply shops. They wrap around the midshaft of the humerus and provide circumferential compression of the muscle belly, resulting in some hydraulic stabilization at the fracture site. The patient may move the shoulder and elbow in the brace and begin using the arm with such light activities as eating, brushing the teeth, and reading a newspaper. When immobilized, even for a short period, the elbow is notorious for becoming stiff with possible permanent limitation of motion. For this reason, any time the elbow is immobilized for treatment of a humeral fracture at the shaft or shoulder, encourage the patient to adjust the brace and allow the elbow to hang straight in full extension for 15 minutes each day.

When managing these fractures, weekly radiographs are recommended for the first 4 to 6 weeks, until it is clear that the fracture fragments are not moving appreciably. At that point, the patient can be seen and radiographs repeated every 2 weeks until a satisfactory functional result is obtained.

At the time of the fracture, patients with neurovascular deficits should be referred emergently; surgical exploration may be necessary. Although radial nerve exploration is not always indicated when radial nerve function is absent or weak (e.g., weakness in finger or wrist extension), many primary care clinicians will refer in this situation. (As it turns out, radial nerve function almost always returns during the 6 months following an injury, but neither the clinician nor the patient may be willing to wait.) If the patient's radial nerve function is initially normal but becomes impaired after splinting or casting, the splint or cast should be removed, a brace or shoulder immobilizer applied, and the patient referred to an orthopedist for evaluation and treatment. Other indications for referral at the time of the fracture include pathologic fractures, associated elbow injuries, and the presence of multiple injuries. Some primary care clinicians refer all transverse fractures due to their higher risk of nonunion.

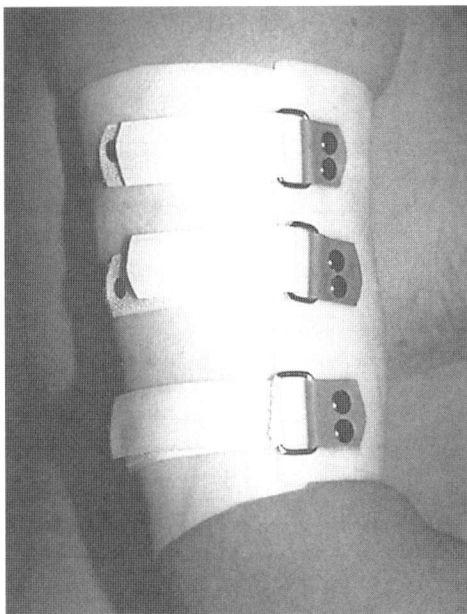

Fig. 178.9 Functional humerus cast or fracture brace. (Courtesy AliMed, Inc., Dedham, MA.)

Supracondylar and Transcondylar Humeral Fractures

Nondisplaced or minimally displaced (<20 degrees apex anterior angulation on lateral x-ray) supracondylar and transcondylar fractures (Fig. 178.10) can be treated with a posterior long-arm, fiberglass, one-step prepadded splint. The elbow should be held at 90 degrees of flexion and a shoulder immobilizer (see Fig. 178.8D) used. The distal pulses should be checked after splint application; if absent, the elbow should be extended until they return. True AP and lateral radiographs of the distal humerus should be obtained after immobilization to confirm that no displacement occurred during efforts to immobilize. During the first 7 to 10 days, frequent checks of neurovascular function are necessary. Follow-up radiographs should be reviewed weekly for the first 2 to 3 weeks and then every 2 weeks until callus formation is seen. When significant tenderness is no longer felt at the fracture site, the splint can be removed to allow gentle range of motion activities (usually at 2 weeks). The patient should be instructed to avoid any passive motion at the elbow because it will predispose the elbow to ectopic bone formation and permanent stiffness. The splint is used for protection until adequate callus forms (usually 6 to 8 weeks) but is removed for showers, bathing, and gentle exercise, usually starting 2 weeks after the injury.

Intercondylar Fractures

Displaced intercondylar fractures (see Fig. 178.10A) are unstable and should be referred to an orthopedic surgeon. By definition, intercondylar fractures are intraarticular. Nondisplaced fractures between the capitellum and trochlea can be managed the same as nondisplaced supracondylar or transcondylar fractures; however, the risk of neurovascular compromise is less, so the patient does not need as many follow-up visits in the first 7 to 10 days. Some experts recommend referral for all other intercondylar fractures.

Fractures of the Humeral Condyles

Type I fractures of the humeral (epi)condyles (Fig. 178.11) are treated with a splint in a manner similar to nondisplaced supracondylar and transcondylar fractures as previously discussed. The joint hemarthrosis should be aspirated and the elbow immobilized in a

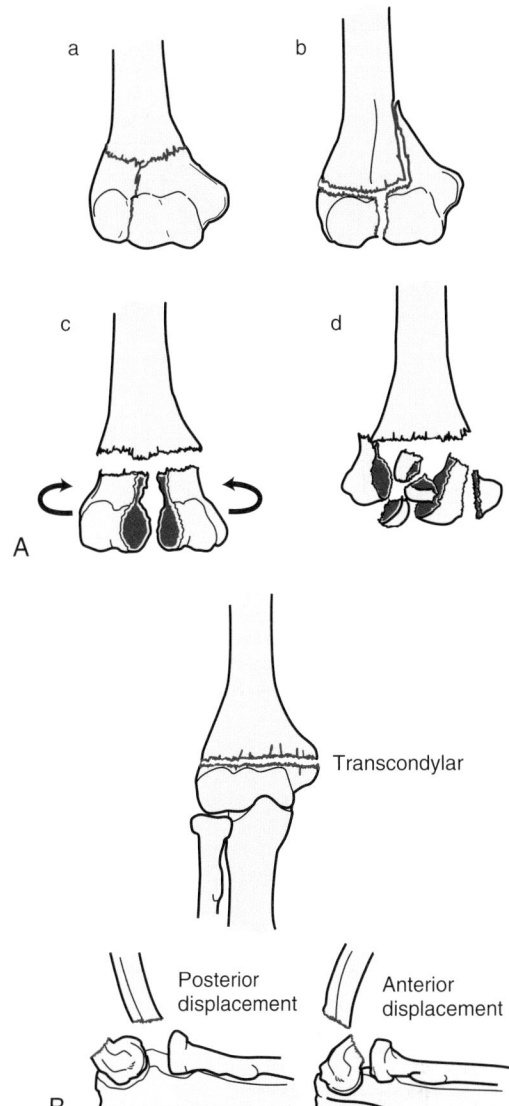

Fig. 178.10 (A) Intercondylar fractures of the humerus: No displacement of fragments (a); T-shaped fracture with the trochlear and capitellar fragments separated but not appreciably rotated in the frontal plane (b); T-shaped fracture with separation of the fragments and significant rotational deformity (c); T-shaped intercondylar fractures with severe comminution of the articular surface and wide separation of the humeral condyles (d). (B) Transcondylar fractures of humerus, demonstrating significant posterior (left) and anterior (right) displacement.

posterior splint with 90 degrees of flexion. For a medial condyle fracture, the forearm is placed in pronation and the wrist slightly flexed. For a lateral condyle fracture, the forearm is placed in supination and the wrist slightly extended. Radiographs should be obtained every 3 to 5 days for the first 2 weeks, then weekly thereafter to ensure no late displacement of the fragments. Patients with even slightly displaced type I and all type II fractures of the humeral (epi)condyles should be referred to an orthopedic surgeon.

Elbow Fractures

All displaced (>2 mm) olecranon fractures (Fig. 178.12) should be referred to an orthopedic surgeon. If the patient is unable to actively extend the elbow (i.e., loss of triceps function), an orthopedic surgeon should be consulted. Otherwise, the patient should be immobilized in 60 to 90 degrees of flexion and seen in follow-up in 5 to 7 days. Radiographs should be evaluated in that visit to ensure no

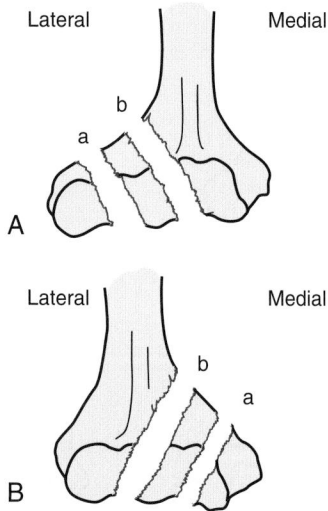

Fig. 178.11 Fractures of the humeral (epi)condyles. (A) Lateral humeral condyle: type I, simple fracture of the lateral condyle with lateral wall of trochlea attached to main mass of the humerus (a); type II fracture with lateral wall of trochlea attached to fractured lateral condylar fragment (b). (B) Medial humeral condyle: type I, simple fracture of medial condyle with medial wall of trochlea attached to main mass of the humerus (a); type II fracture with medial wall of trochlea attached to fractured medial condylar fragment (b).

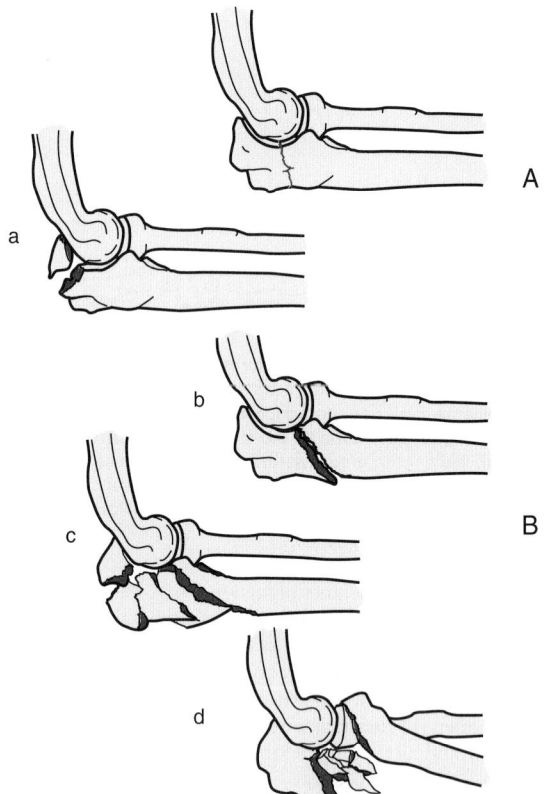

Fig. 178.12 Olecranon fractures. (A) Nondisplaced. (B) Displaced fractures: Avulsion fracture (a); oblique and transverse fracture (b); comminuted fractures (c); fracture dislocations (d).

displacement and at the 2- and 4-week visits. Range of motion activities should be started at 2 weeks with motion limited to 90 degrees of flexion until there is radiographic evidence of fracture healing.

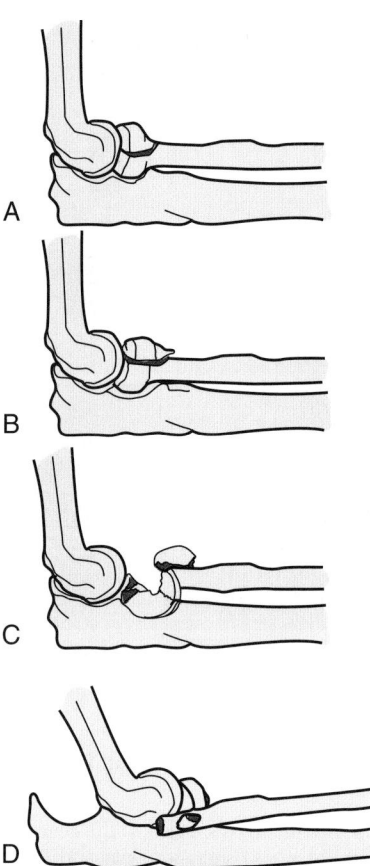

Fig. 178.13 Radial head fractures (Mason classification with Johnston modification). (A) Nondisplaced linear or transverse fractures. (B) Fractures with minimal displacement (or comminuted fractures without displacement [not shown]). (C) Comminuted fractures with marked displacement. (D) Radial head fracture with associated elbow dislocation.

Radial head fractures (Fig. 178.13) displaced more than 2 mm, involving more than a third of the articular surface, angulated more than 30 degrees, depressed more than 3 mm, severely comminuted, or with an associated dislocation should be referred to an orthopedic surgeon. Otherwise, treatment is range of motion activities such as pronation, supination, and elbow flexion and extension, as soon as pain permits, usually within 3 to 5 days. The patient should apply ice intermittently to the joint and keep it elevated for the first 48 hours. Significant pain relief can be provided by aspiration of blood from the joint followed by instillation of a local anesthetic. Immobilization is not required, but if the patient experiences too much pain without immobilization, a long-arm fiberglass one-step 90-degree splint and sling can be used. It should be removed as soon as possible to minimize stiffness. With radial head injuries, always check the wrist to ensure that there is no tenderness over the distal radius or ulna; associated injuries to the wrist often result in instability. If tenderness is present over the wrist, obtain true AP and lateral radiographs. For any displacement or dorsal subluxation of the ulna, with or without a fracture, the patient should be referred to an orthopedic surgeon.

Midforearm Fractures

An isolated fracture of the ulnar shaft (nightstick fracture) with no at least 50% apposition of fragments, less than 10 degrees angulation, and no fracture or dislocation of the radius can be treated with a long-arm splint and sling with the elbow in 90 degrees of flexion. The splint remains in place for protection for 6 to 8 weeks. Weekly radiographs should be obtained for the first 3 weeks to detect any displacement and then at 6 to 8 weeks to document union. The fracture of the ulna will become sticky, stable, and less painful after 3 weeks, allowing removal of the splint for gentle range of motion activities of the elbow, including pronation and supination of the forearm twice a day for 15 minutes to minimize stiffness. Alternatively, a functional forearm brace can be applied after the initial swelling goes down in 7 to 10 days and remain in place until union is documented radiographically.

A fracture of the radial shaft (Galeazzi fracture) requires surgery in all cases, so these patients should be referred to an orthopedic surgeon. Even if nondisplaced initially, the fracture will often become displaced, and the distal radioulnar joint is usually affected. Patients with both-bone shaft fractures (radial and ulnar shafts) should usually be referred to an orthopedic surgeon because these fractures usually require open reduction and internal fixation as a result of instability.

Distal Forearm Fractures

Colles Fracture

A Colles fracture involves the distal 2 cm of the radius, is angled dorsally (Fig. 178.14), and is the most common wrist fracture. If extraarticular and nondisplaced, it can be treated with a double sugar-tong splint (one splint from elbow to wrist, the other over initial splint and extending from elbow to axilla) for 3 to 5 days followed by a short-arm cast for 3 to 5 more weeks (if no reduction) or long-arm cast for 3 to 4 weeks followed by short-arm cast for total immobilization 6 to 8 weeks (if reduction was necessary). In the elderly, the length of time in long-arm cast can be reduced to 2 to 3 weeks followed by short-arm cast until healed. The fracture should be followed with radiographs at 1 (splint removed), 2, and 6 weeks to ensure no displacement and complete healing. At 6 weeks, the radiograph is taken after cast removal to assess fracture healing; if tenderness persists at the fracture site or there is incomplete union, an ulnar gutter splint should be applied. This splint can be removed to allow gentle range of motion activities but should then be reapplied each time until all tenderness resolves and a solid fracture union is noted on the radiograph.

Colles fractures require reduction if the lateral x-ray shows the distal radius articular surface to be tilted dorsally beyond the neutral position (determined by a line drawn straight through the distal radius, lunate, and capitate). After reduction, the distal articular surface should be perpendicular to the long axis of the forearm (neutral) or tilted volarly. If not reducible (more than 20-degree dorsal angulation), unstable, comminuted, displaced more than two-thirds the width of wrist, intraarticular, or with more than 5 mm radial shortening or ulnar angulation, these fractures are best treated by an orthopedic surgeon. Colles fractures in the dominant wrist of the high-demand (i.e., very active) patient are also more likely to require surgery for a satisfactory result.

On the AP view, if the radius is not equal to or longer than the length of the ulna, reduction is also indicated. Most patients have a radius that is longer than the ulna; this characteristic is referred to as negative ulnar variance as seen on the AP radiograph. (In a few patients, the radius and ulna are the same length; if any doubt remains, a comparison AP radiograph can be assessed). If there is displacement at the fracture site as defined by shortening of the radius on the AP view, reduction is indicated.

Reduction is simplified by injecting 10 mL of plain 1% lidocaine into the fracture site hematoma (hematoma block) for anesthesia. This injection should be performed slowly to minimize any pain associated with distention. The skin surface can be iced or sprayed with ethyl chloride to decrease the discomfort associated with the injection. Always clean the skin after applying the spray with an antiseptic preparation (e.g., povidone-iodine, chlorhexidine, alcohol) before injecting lidocaine. The patient should be supine during the entire procedure including the injection.

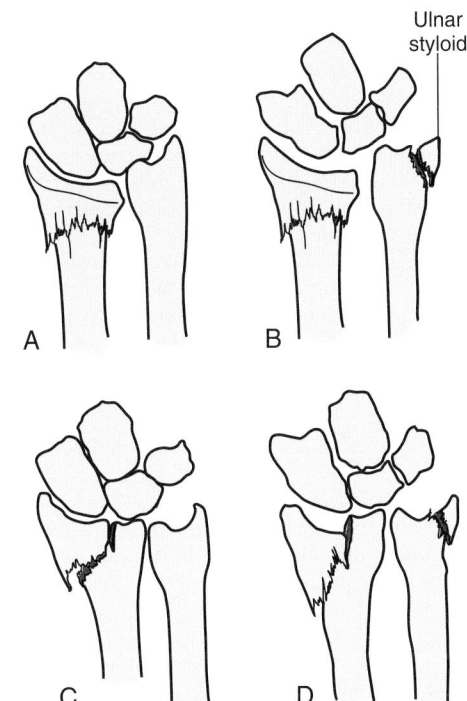

Fig. 178.14 Distal radius fractures. (A) Colles fracture. (B) Colles fracture is commonly associated with fracture of ulnar styloid. (C) Intraarticular fracture. (D) Intraarticular fracture of radius with associated fracture of ulnar styloid.

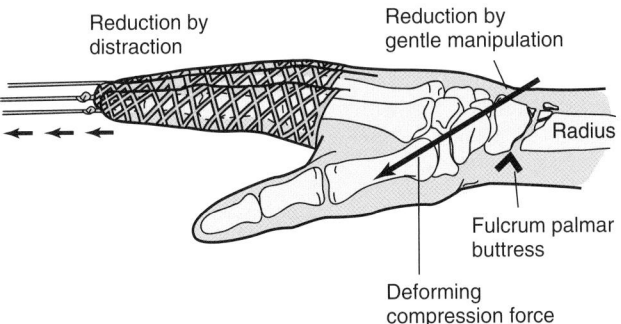

Fig. 178.15 Treatment of Colles fracture to effect reduction.

After the hematoma block has had time to take effect (10 minutes), hang the patient's hand in finger traps traction with the elbow flexed 90 degrees, and gradually add counterweights to a weight hanger, orthopedic felt sling, or stockinette draped over the humerus (Fig. 178.15). A weight of 5 to 10 lb is appropriate, and the patient should be in this suspended traction position for 15 to 20 minutes. At that point, reduction is usually achieved spontaneously by ligamentotaxis (the soft tissue attachments to the bone pull the bone into a reduced position in response to the traction). If any visible or palpable deformity remains after 15 to 20 minutes of traction, manual pressure can then be used to correct the deformity. Push from dorsal to volar over the distal radius, distal to the fracture site. Following reduction, with the arm still maintained in traction, as mentioned previously, the double sugar-tong splint should be applied. After 3 to 5 days, a long-arm, well-molded cast is applied (it is started as a short-arm cast and extended). Take great care to mold with your thenar cone at the base of the thumb, pressing into the patient's palm to prevent a gap in the volar portion of the cast at the palm. After the cast is hard, trim it back to the proximal palmar crease to allow full flexion of the metacarpophalangeal (MP) joints to prevent joint stiffness.

After the cast is hard and three-point molding is applied (pushing volarly distal to the fracture site, dorsally just proximal to the fracture site, and volarly against the elbow), the cast is extended to the long-arm level, which is at least 5 inches more proximal, above the elbow. Be careful to pad the cast margins well, proximally and distally, and to stop application of plaster or fiberglass at least 1 inch before reaching the padding margin.

True AP and lateral postreduction radiographs should then be obtained. If the dorsal tilt of the distal radius articular surface or shortening of the radius in relation to the ulna persists, then the reduction is unacceptable and referral should be made for repeat reduction under general anesthetic and the possible application of skeletal external frame traction.

Ulnar styloid fractures indicate a larger force of injury and a higher chance of eventual loss of reduction. However, surgical treatment is never required for an isolated displaced ulnar styloid fracture. These fractures often remain nonunited on follow-up radiographs, but this has no clinical significance. Although patients may look at the radiograph and think they have a loose piece of bone floating around the wrist, they should be reminded that this bone is attached to soft tissue, does not float freely, and will not move.

Smith Fracture

A Smith fracture is similar to a Colles fracture except that the angulation is volar (so it is sometimes called a reverse Colles). After reduction, this fracture is treated the same as a Colles fracture, with a double sugar-tong splint followed by a long-arm cast. If the fracture is intraarticular or the reduction is not anatomically correct, refer the patient to an orthopedic surgeon. This is an uncommon fracture and is often unstable; most should be referred.

Fractures of the Carpal Bones

Most chip and avulsion fractures of the carpal bones are treated with a gutter splint for comfort and protection for 4 to 6 weeks until symptoms resolve. The gutter splint can be removed for a shower. Hook of the hamate fractures should be referred to an orthopedist or hand specialist.

Scaphoid (Navicular) Fractures

When there is pain in the "snuff-box," always consider a scaphoid (navicular) injury (Fig. 178.16). Lateral, posteroanterior, and motion (flexion-extension, radial deviation–ulnar deviation) views may be helpful. If a fracture is seen, a scaphoid magnification view radiograph and consultation with a radiologist or orthopedist may help to confirm that the fracture is, in fact, nondisplaced. A limited CT or MRI scan may also be helpful. Because the best blood supply (and highest likelihood of healing) is distal, nondisplaced distal third fractures (see Fig. 178.16) can be treated with a short-arm thumb spica cast for 4 to 6 weeks. Middle or proximal third fractures (see Fig. 178.16) need a longer cast and treatment; a long-arm thumb spica cast is applied for 6 weeks, followed by a short-arm thumb spica cast for another 6 weeks. Some clinicians continue the short-arm thumb spica cast for up to 14 more weeks for proximal third fractures. A recent systematic review and metaanalysis demonstrated that early surgical management of nondisplaced and minimally displaced scaphoid fractures had better outcomes, in particular, early return to function, when compared with nonoperative therapy. Management of these potentially complex fractures should include a discussion of surgical options (Buijze et al., 2010).

A short-arm thumb spica cast is appropriate for any patient who has significant tenderness over the snuff-box (scaphoid), with follow-up radiograph and examination in 2 to 3 weeks without the cast. If at that time no tenderness is felt over the scaphoid and no fracture is visible, then there was no scaphoid fracture. Scaphoid fractures

are notorious for being difficult to diagnose radiographically in the acute setting. For this reason, always err on the side of immobilization when a scaphoid fracture is suspected. If after 2 to 3 weeks the cast is removed and no fracture line is visible but persistent tenderness is noted over the fracture site, immobilization for an additional 2 to 3 weeks is appropriate, followed by repeat radiographs. At that point, if no fracture line is visible, then there was no scaphoid fracture and gentle range of motion exercises can be initiated. A bone scan may also help to confirm a fracture.

Displaced scaphoid fractures should be referred to an orthopedic surgeon. Avascular necrosis, delayed union, nonunion, and arthritis are common complications of scaphoid fractures, even if managed appropriately; therefore the patient needs to be made aware of these risks at the start.

Metacarpal Fractures

Nondisplaced, noncomminuted metacarpal fractures, including those that are intraarticular (except thumb metacarpal), are treated with an ulnar or a radial gutter cast, depending on the fracture location. Nondisplaced, noncomminuted, nonarticular fractures of the thumb (first) metacarpal are treated with a thumb spica cast. An index (second) finger metacarpal fracture can be treated with a radial gutter cast with a hole cut out for the thumb to allow thumb function. Fractures of the middle (third), ring (fourth), and little (fifth) finger metacarpals are treated with an ulnar gutter splint. A gutter splint can be made using 6-inch wide one-step fiberglass prepadded splint material. Patients should be seen every 2 weeks.

Nondisplaced fractures of the metacarpal heads can be treated with a gutter splint for 2 to 3 weeks. Nondisplaced fractures of the second or third or mildly angulated fractures of the fourth (<30 degrees) or fifth metacarpal (<40 degrees) neck can be treated in the same manner for 3 to 4 weeks so long as there is no rotational deformity. If the fracture is in the midportion of the shaft and there is no rotational deformity, mildly angulated second or third metacarpal (<10 degrees) or fourth or fifth metacarpal (<20 degrees) fractures can be managed with gutter splinting for 3 to 4 weeks. For angulation greater than these parameters, reduction can be attempted. If reduction is unsuccessful or if there is a rotational deformity, the patient should be referred. Hematoma block reduction can be carried out with three-point pressure fixation in the splint, followed by postreduction radiographs. After 3 to 4 weeks, the gutter splint can be removed for range of motion exercises. When not performing range of motion movements, the metacarpal should remain protected in the splint for an additional 3 weeks.

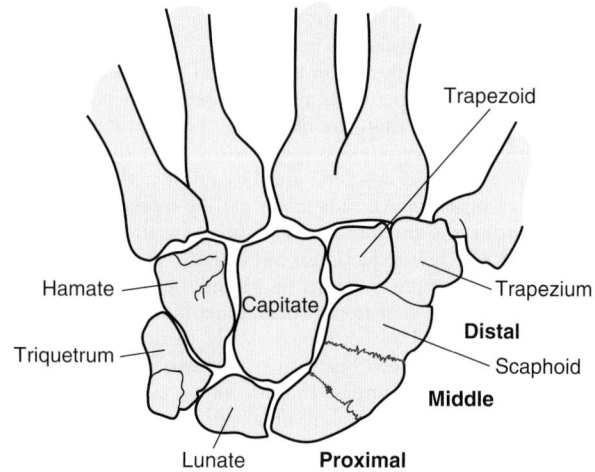

Fig. 178.16 Scaphoid (navicular) fractures.

Immobilize the metacarpals with 90-degree flexion at the MP joint and full extension of the interphalangeal and distal interphalangeal (DIP) joints of the fingers. Often referred to as the "intrinsic plus position," this position results in the MP joint lateral ligaments and those of the DIP and proximal interphalangeal (PIP) joints being in maximal stretch. This position prevents tightening during immobilization and secondary stiffness of the joint. The gutter cast should go from the tips of the fingers to the midforearm. Remember to place dry cotton ball padding between the fingers to prevent skin maceration from moisture accumulation.

Immobilizing all metacarpal fractures in an MP joint flexion 90-degree position minimizes the risk for future malrotation; the flexed finger at the MP joint serves to align the metacarpal in the correct direction with the adjacent metacarpals. This alignment acts as a reference angle because the protective fingers are also flexed 90 degrees. The exception to this rule is fractures of the metacarpal neck; to minimize loss of joint mobility, these may be placed in 70 to 90 degrees of flexion.

Patients with displaced intraarticular fractures (Bennett and Rolando fractures) should be referred to an orthopedic surgeon, especially those who have intraarticular fractures at the base of the thumb (Fig. 178.17). Even nondisplaced intraarticular fractures of the base of the thumb should probably be referred. Nondisplaced fractures of the thumb shaft with more than 30 degrees of angulation should be reduced under a Bier or hematoma block and managed with a thumb spica cast for 4 weeks.

Boxer fractures occur at the fifth metacarpal neck. As mentioned previously, angulation up to 40 degrees is acceptable for this fracture. However, the clinician must be certain not to confuse a boxer fracture (fifth metacarpal neck) with a fifth metacarpal shaft fracture (Fig. 178.18), because angulation of the shaft of the fifth metacarpal greater than 20 degrees is unacceptable. If the reduction is lost somewhat during healing of a fifth metacarpal neck, it will mainly result in a cosmetic, as opposed to a functional, deformity. In addition, explain to patients that with boxer fractures the bone will heal with abundant callus; consequently, they will have a bump over the dorsum of the hand because the callus is subcutaneous.

When treating boxer fractures, be cautious of any mark on the skin over the knuckle, which could suggest an open fracture or a human bite lesion that might become infected. If either is present, begin broad-spectrum antibiotics, possibly giving the first dose intravenously. The wound should be inspected again in 2 to 3 days to ensure no infection.

An isolated fracture involving one of the long or ring finger metacarpals can be treated without immobilization if the patient is comfortable and wishes to use the hand out of a cast. Approximately 3 to 5 mm of shortening of the finger may occur as the metacarpal overrides itself. However, no shortening will occur beyond this point because the fractured metacarpal is being suspended between the two intact metacarpals and associated interosseous ligaments that run between the metacarpals.

Phalangeal Fractures

Phalangeal fractures can be immobilized with aluminum foam splints, buddy taping, or stack splints (e.g., mallet finger fracture of distal phalanx). The splint should hold the DIP joint in extension for 3 to 4 weeks or until nonpainful to palpation. If there is any displacement of these fractures, closed reduction is unsuccessful, or reduction cannot be maintained, referral is appropriate. Volar plate avulsion fractures caused by hyperextension injuries at the PIP joint are best immobilized with a dorsal block splint holding the PIP joint in 45 degrees of flexion for 3 weeks.

Transverse or angulated fractures of the distal phalanx are often unstable and difficult to reduce because of interposition of soft tissue. Intraarticular fractures of one or more condyles of the middle or proximal phalanx at the level of the DIP or PIP joints, respectively, usually also need referral for internal fixation. Oblique or spiral proximal shaft fractures and large displaced avulsion fractures of the base of the proximal phalanx may also benefit from referral for operative repair. Conversely, mallet finger fractures should be treated with continuous slight hyperextension splinting for up to 8 weeks. Almost all other finger fractures can be treated with 3 or 4 weeks of buddy taping.

Always check the collateral ligaments by stress examination. Use a digital block if needed to perform the examination. If collateral ligaments are disrupted despite a negative x-ray, buddy taping is appropriate for protection for 1 month while allowing protected range of motion movement in the taped position.

In general, with metacarpal and phalangeal fractures, *malrotation* is the most common complication. To exclude malrotation with a metacarpal fracture, always hold the MP joints in 90 degrees of flexion to ensure perfect rotational alignment. For phalangeal fractures, always note the plane of the nail beds while looking at the fingers from the ends. Compare them with the opposite hand to ensure correct rotational alignment.

Any intraarticular fracture with displacement at the joint surface should be referred to an orthopedic surgeon for reduction and fixation. PIP joint fractures involving more than 40% of joint surface should be referred for probable internal fixation. Extraarticular and intraarticular fractures without displacement at the joint surface can be treated without referral. If any doubt remains as to whether displacement in the joint surface is present, consult a radiologist or orthopedist.

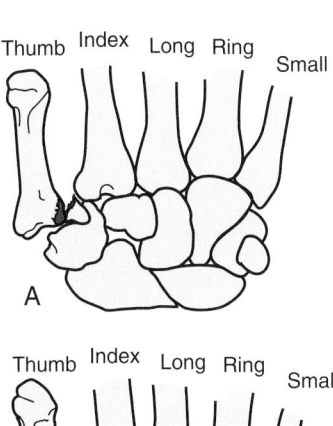

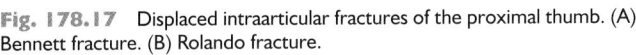

Fig. 178.17 Displaced intraarticular fractures of the proximal thumb. (A) Bennett fracture. (B) Rolando fracture.

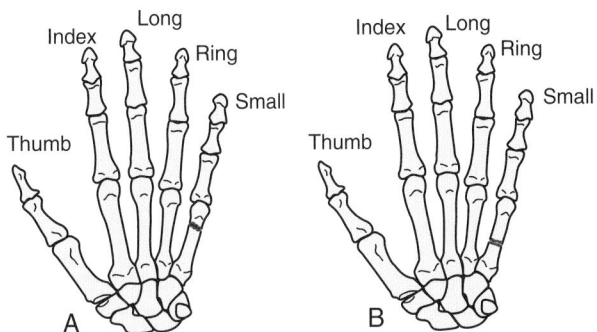

Fig. 178.18 (A) Boxer fracture. (B) Metacarpal shaft fracture.

CHILDREN'S FRACTURES

Children's bone tissue is elastic, similar to a plastic flyswatter handle. For this reason, their bones can deform and bow without cracking the cortex. This elastic deformation commonly occurs in the shaft of the radius or ulna and is referred to as a bone bow fracture. If concerned about the alignment of the forearm, remember that the ulna is always straight and that a small 10- to 20-degree bow is normally present in the radius. Assessment of a *comparison film* can determine what is normal for the patient. When viewing comparison films, always make sure the views are taken in exactly the same projection so that a true comparison can be made. Comparison films in children are also beneficial because the growth plates ossify at different ages.

Comparison radiographs in children are especially important when treating any elbow injury, because numerous ossification centers develop at various ages (from 3 to 12 years). Because of these various centers of ossification, if any sign or question of fracture is present, a radiologist should be consulted or referral to an orthopedist considered to review the films. Salter classification is commonly used for children's fractures involving the growth plate (Box 178.2 and Fig. 178.19).

It is appropriate to refer all fractures in children involving the spine or knee because fractures around the spine and knee are at high risk for growth plate arrest or neurologic injury.

Upper Extremity Fractures

Clavicle fractures do not generally require referral, reduction, or intervention unless tenting of the skin is observed with whiteness over the skin as a result of loss of blood supply. Exceptions include a clavicular fracture near the acromioclavicular joint that is displaced or in the proximal third of the clavicle displaced posteriorly; these should be referred to an orthopedic surgeon. However, the vast majority of fractures occur in the middle third of the clavicle or are nondisplaced and are treated with a figure-of-eight strap for immobilization and comfort. Remember, the figure-of-eight strap is applied only to increase comfort; children heal very rapidly (within weeks), and as soon as the child is comfortable without it, the strap is no longer required. In toddlers a figure-of-eight strap is unnecessary because healing occurs so quickly. In older children a sling may be more comfortable than a figure-of-eight strap. These straps and splints can be removed for bathing and then reapplied. To show patients how to put the straps back on and get the straps in the same position, instruct them to use a pen to make marks on the white straps at the level of the buckles. This "trick" will enable the patient to reapply the splint, sling, or brace in the same position with the same degree of tension as applied in the office.

Rib fractures, similar to those in adults, do not require treatment, immobilization, or bracing. Although patients may ask for any one of these treatments, remind them that splints or rib binders can cause atelectasis or pneumonia. Always auscultate the chest to exclude pneumothorax and respiratory compromise. Sometimes subcutaneous emphysema suggests lung puncture by a rib or clavicular fracture. This complication can be ruled out by palpating the skin around the area of the fracture to check for any crepitus.

Fractures around the shoulder usually involve only the surgical neck of the humerus. As long as there is 50% bone-on-bone contact and not too much angulation (<70 degrees before age 5, <40 degrees from age 5 to 16, <25 degrees after age 16), no reduction is necessary. As with adults, treatment is a hanging arm cast for 3 to 4 weeks until tenderness resolves on palpation and comfort is present. Humeral shaft fractures almost always heal well, and angulation up to 25 degrees on AP and lateral planes can be accepted. Always check for radial nerve dysfunction.

Distal humerus supracondylar fractures are best evaluated with comparison of true lateral radiographs. Remember that the distal humerus ordinarily has a tilt in an anterior direction. If the distal humerus is entirely straight, approximately 10 to 15 degrees of bending of the distal humerus has occurred in a posterior direction.

BOX 178.2 Salter Classification of Fractures

Salter type I fracture is diagnosed with a normal x-ray appearance and by point tenderness directly over the growth plate. No tenderness should be felt over the ligaments around the joint. This type of fracture is common in infants and young children. Treatment is always closed with cast immobilization.

Salter type II is a fracture through the growth plate and then through the metaphysis. This type of fracture is more common in older children. The prognosis for growth disturbance is very high when the fracture involves the distal femoral growth plate. Refer all patients with this type of fracture to an orthopedic surgeon if any displacement has occurred. Reduction is almost always performed with a general anesthetic to provide complete muscle relaxation. This relaxation allows the traction to decrease the force across the growth plate, which is required to set it. The less force required to set the fracture, the less recurrent injury to the growth plate itself (see Fig. 178.19).

Salter type III fracture involves the epiphysis extending into the epiphyseal plate. If any displacement has occurred, the patient should be referred to an orthopedic surgeon. These fractures are most common in the distal tibia and can be associated with growth arrest. Anatomic reduction is always required, and surgery may be required.

Salter type IV fracture extends from the joint surface through the epiphysis and on through the epiphyseal plate and out through the metaphysis. These fractures are often displaced and require open surgical treatment. This fracture most commonly occurs at the lateral humeral condyle at the elbow. These injuries extend into the joint. If the fracture appears nondisplaced and any question of displacement remains, it may be beneficial for a radiologist or an orthopedist to review the film and tomograms.

Salter type V injury is a crush injury of the epiphyseal plate and is uncommon. When this fracture occurs, it is usually at the knee or ankle and associated with growth arrest. The x-ray appearance may be normal as for a Salter type I fracture. For this reason, parents (and the child) should be cautioned that growth arrest can occur if there is tenderness over the growth plate, whether it is a Salter I or Salter V fracture (and often this is difficult to determine), because it may have extended into the growth plate. Osteoarthritis can occur as a result of any fracture that extends into the joint itself, whether this occurs in an adult or a child.

See Fig. 178.19.

However, this bending is acceptable as long as the humerus is not bent backward beyond the straight position. As it turns out, most supracondylar fractures in children are displaced and require referral. Nondisplaced fractures with good alignment can be treated with a long-arm cast for 3 weeks with the elbow at 90 degrees and the forearm in neutral rotation.

A supracondylar fracture or radial head or neck fracture can be identified with a posterior fat pad sign. The posterior fat pad sign is the result of intraarticular bleeding in the elbow joint with any fracture that is intraarticular. The blood goes into the olecranon fossa in the distal humerus and causes the fat pad that resides there to float posteriorly; therefore it is no longer hidden in the olecranon fossa. As it floats posteriorly, it is visible as a fat pad on the true lateral radiograph of the distal humerus. In the absence of any abnormality on the radiograph, a fat pad sign indicates bleeding into the joint and leads to a diagnosis of occult fracture most likely involving the radial head or neck. This involvement can be confirmed by point tenderness with palpation of the radial head and neck. Angulation

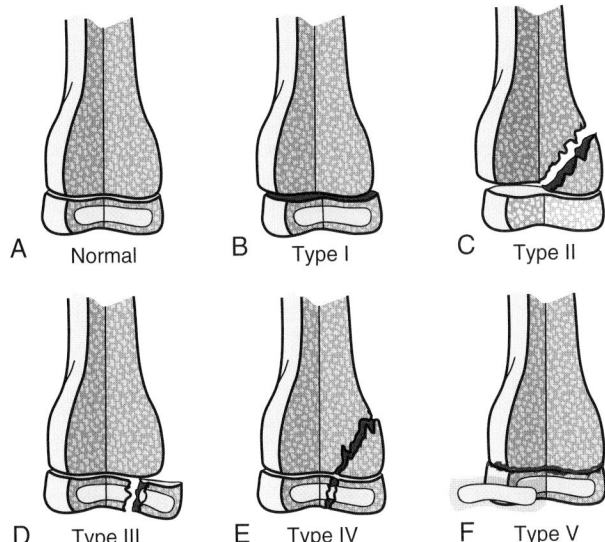

A Normal   B Type I   C Type II

D Type III   E Type IV   F Type V

Fig. 178.19 Illustrations of Salter classification for fractures in children (also see Box 178.2). (A) Normal. (B) Type I. (C) Type II. (D) Type III. (E) Type IV. (F) Type V.

up to 30 degrees and up to 4 mm translocation are acceptable in fractures of the radial head or neck; a child with greater angulation or translocation should be referred to an orthopedic surgeon for probable closed reduction.

Common fractures in the forearm include *torus fractures*. They are treated with a short-arm cast for 1 month until all tenderness resolves. *Greenstick fractures* are one level worse than torus fractures; these involve an actual crack or disruption of one cortex and often a buckling of the opposite cortex. These fractures are so named because they represent a deformation of the bone much like cracking a green twig on an apple tree in springtime. The tension side of the bent twig cracks, whereas the compression side (concave side) buckles and does not crack.

Any angulation in the radius greater than 10 degrees in children older than 8 (or >15 degrees in children younger than 8) requires reduction and should be referred. Significantly comminuted fractures or those associated with nerve injury should also be referred. With ulnar shaft fractures, angulation greater than 15 degrees should be reduced; if uncomfortable performing this reduction, the primary care clinician should refer the patient. For all other radial or ulnar shaft fractures (including both-bone fractures if nondisplaced or minimally displaced), a long-arm cast can be used for 6 to 8 weeks to prevent pronation and supination at the elbow. The cast is always applied with the elbow in at least 90 degrees of flexion, and the sling must always hold the arm in at least 90 degrees of flexion. If it does not do so or if the cast is applied in less than 90 degrees of flexion, the cast will continue to slip out of the sling.

Wrist and Hand Fractures

Fractures of the carpal bones are uncommon in children. Management of scaphoid fractures is very similar to that in adults. However, with a fall on the outstretched arm, the typical fracture is of the distal radius and ulna. These fractures can be reduced by hematoma block and finger traps traction, as in the adult. This technique should be reserved for the child who is 12 years or older and very cooperative and understanding. Younger children, who are uncooperative, anxious, or otherwise frightened of injections, should have a reduction under general anesthesia. This approach will provide a more comfortable, less frightening experience and allow maximum muscle relaxation for the least traumatic reduction potentially affecting later arm growth and length.

Metacarpal and phalangeal fractures that are nondisplaced are simply treated with ulnar or radial gutter splint immobilization. The position of immobilization and the angulation are the same as that used for treating adults. Remember, the fifth metacarpal neck can accept angulation up to 40 degrees, whereas the shaft angulation can be accepted only to 20 degrees. Phalangeal fractures, including mallet fingers, are treated the same for children and adults.

The so-called *octave fracture* is common in children and occurs at the base of the proximal phalanx of the little finger (fifth digit), where it is angulated ulnarly. It is so named because playing the piano requires children to stretch their fingers into wide abduction. Reduction is required and is easily done using a finger digital block anesthetic, followed by placement of a pen or pencil between the fourth and fifth fingers. The pen acts as a fulcrum between the two fingers. The little finger is then pulled back into place with traction and radial deviation until it is perfectly straight using the pen or pencil deep against the web space as a bolster or fulcrum. This technique works extremely well and should be followed by buddy taping and splint immobilization for a minimum of 3 weeks.

Again, a child with any displaced intraarticular fracture or displaced growth plate fracture should be referred to an orthopedic surgeon for reduction.

Lower Extremity Fractures

Fractures of the true pelvis are uncommon, except in automobile accidents or high-velocity trauma. Patients with these fractures should all be referred to rule out other associated injuries to the abdomen, genitourinary, and gynecologic systems. Apophyseal avulsion fractures are fairly common in young athletes. Those of the anterior inferior or superior iliac spine are usually minimally displaced; hamstring attachment avulsion fractures may result in a large displaced fragment. Conservative treatment consists of a brief period of rest followed by 2 to 3 weeks of crutch-assisted ambulation. Return to full function may take 6 to 12 weeks. Surgery is reserved for those with symptomatic nonunion.

Femur fractures are also uncommon and should be immediately referred to an orthopedic surgeon for further evaluation and treatment. Remember, a slipped capital femoral epiphysis or avascular necrosis of the femoral head in children (Perthes disease) can present with knee pain. The knee examination and radiograph may be entirely normal. The first clue to the diagnosis is limitation of hip internal rotation on the involved side. The Trendelenburg test often shows weakness in the gluteus medius on the involved side. If a child younger than 17 years of age complains of knee pain and the knee examination and radiographs are negative, always examine and carry out radiographs of the pelvis and hips. AP pelvic and true lateral radiographs of the hips are appropriate studies for this purpose.

Fractures of the distal femur that are nondisplaced and have normal radiographs are diagnosed by point tenderness over the distal femoral epiphysis, which is located 3 cm above the joint line. Treatment involves a cylinder cast for complete immobilization, crutches, and protective partial weight-bearing activities for 1 month. During the follow-up examination, a window can be placed in the cast through which the examiner's finger can palpate for tenderness. As long as tenderness is felt at the fracture site, the cast should remain in place. The tenderness should resolve within 8 weeks or sooner, depending on the child's age.

Patellar fractures are usually nondisplaced and are similarly treated with a knee immobilizer or cylinder cast. Immobilize the knee for 1 month until all tenderness resolves.

Beware of any intraarticular avulsion fractures along the lateral tibial plateau. This type of fracture indicates an anterior cruciate ligament avulsing a piece of bone. If there is any associated displacement, referral to an orthopedist should be carried out for surgical repair.

Proximal tibial fractures are treated the same as those of the distal femur and are diagnosed by point tenderness over the growth plate. Tibial shaft fractures can be treated in a long-leg cast without reduction if there is not more than 5 degrees angulation on the AP radiograph and not more than 10 degrees angulation on the lateral radiograph. If angulation exceeds these thresholds, referral to an orthopedic surgeon should be made for closed manipulation reduction.

Fibular fractures are of no concern and will heal uneventfully without treatment. However, if any angulation is present, an orthopedic surgeon should be consulted for probable closed manipulation reduction.

Foot and Ankle Fractures

Patients with any fracture around the ankle that is displaced should be referred to an orthopedist. Most fractures of the ankle should be managed by an orthopedist because most involve the growth plate. That said, fractures that are nondisplaced can be treated with a short-leg cast and no weight-bearing activity for 2 weeks, followed by advancing to weight-bearing activities for the remaining 3 to 4 weeks while in the cast.

Fracture of the talus, navicular, and cuneiform bones can be treated with a short-leg walking cast, provided there is no displacement. Fractures of the metatarsals are treated the same in children as for adults. Peroneus brevis avulsion fractures can be treated with a wooden-soled fracture shoe. Beware of the fracture of the proximal shaft of the fifth metatarsal (Jones fracture), which is different from a peroneus brevis avulsion fracture. For optimal healing, this type of fracture requires a short-leg fiberglass cast and no weight-bearing activities for 2 weeks, followed by weight-bearing activities for an additional 6 weeks.

Child Abuse

Any history or examination suspicious for child abuse should be assessed with long bone radiographs of the upper and lower extremities. This long bone study should be carefully reviewed for signs of fractures in various bones in different stages of healing, which would indicate a history of numerous injuries. A corner fracture is a typical radiographic finding, which is noted at the corner of the metaphysis of a long bone.

COMPLICATIONS (ADULT AND PEDIATRIC)

Compartment syndrome (see Chapter 179, Compartment Syndrome Evaluation) is the most devastating complication in fracture treatment and is caused by swelling and a tight cast leading to neurovascular compromise. This syndrome most frequently occurs in the calf and forearm. Any patient who requires more than the average dose of oral pain medication for fractures of the forearm or tibia (or any other fracture, for that matter) should be evaluated emergently. If the patient feels the cast is too tight, if there is excess pain beyond what would be reasonably expected, or if any swelling in the digits occurs, then the cast and padding should be immediately split (univalved or bivalved). Univalving results in a 30% drop in pressure, whereas bivalving results in a 60% drop. Ironically, univalving and bivalving do not cause a comparable drop in strength or support. In fact, very little strength or support is lost. If pain relief does not occur, the entire cast should be removed and the extremity inspected for signs of tenseness of the skin. If the skin is not tense and the calf is involved, perform a Doppler study to rule out phlebitis. Treatment of the fracture and maintenance of reduction of the fracture are always a second priority to preserving the blood supply to the soft tissue and bone. If any question of compartment syndrome remains, compartmental pressure measurements must be obtained and a fasciotomy performed if pressures are elevated.

The higher the velocity of the injury, the more comminuted the fracture, the higher the energy of the force, the more soft tissue trauma, and the higher the chance of swelling. For the upper extremity, always tell patients to carry the arm over the head in a "monkey-like" position for the first week. Children may go to school, but their arm should be propped up over the head or on a stack of books in front of them on their desk. At night, they should sleep with couch cushions elevating the arm. Parents should set their alarm clock for 3 AM and reposition the child's arm back up on the pillows because the child will have most likely wiggled the arm off the elevated position. Be certain that patients *do not* have slings to use for a long-arm cast for the first week. If they are given a sling, they will automatically carry the cast and arm down in front by their chest and it will be lower than the heart and promote swelling. The sling should not be used until after the first week.

Most open fractures should be referred to an orthopedist due to the increased risk of infection. The open fracture may be associated with only a small puncture wound in the skin, and this puncture may be located several inches from the fracture itself because of the forces of deformation at the time of the injury. Fractures of nail beds may become open fractures when the nail is removed; however, primary care clinicians can often repair these (see Chapter 24, Nail Bed Repair).

It is now known that CRPS involves, in fact, a shutdown of the capillary circulation system and results in arterial blood being shunted in a bypass fashion from arterioles to venules without adequate capillary profusion. This phenomenon has been demonstrated by sampling the oxygen content of venous blood in the involved extremity compared with the uninvolved extremity. The oxygen content in the venous blood in an extremity with CRPS is higher, which is due to the oxygen not being taken out by the tissues, as it would be if the blood were supplied normally to the capillary system.

The incidence of postfracture stiffness in a joint (especially at the elbow or where the fracture extends into the joint) is dramatically increased in patients who have diabetes and in those who smoke. Patients should understand that diabetes and smoking have similar effects on the capillary blood flow; they both diminish the flow.

Delayed union, nonunion, atrophic or hypertrophic union, and malunion are possible complications of fractures. Inadequate assessment of the initial radiographs, improper management of the fracture (including incomplete reduction), poor patient adherence and compliance, increased age, medications, and presence of osteopenia or osteoporosis are all possible causes of these complications. Smoking or taking antiinflammatory medications delays the healing time and increases the risk for improper fracture healing, especially in weight-bearing bones (e.g., ankle, foot, calcaneus). If the patient smokes, the fracture healing time in the ankle is doubled compared with the nonsmoker. Colles fracture healing may also be delayed in patients taking antiinflammatory medications or smoking.

Among other factors, risk of traumatic arthritis is increased by the proximity of the fracture to a joint (especially if intraarticular), the forces causing the fracture (risk of damage to cartilage), repetitive fractures, and fracture healing.

CPT/BILLING CODES

See Chapter 175, Ankle and Foot Splinting, Casting, and Taping, and Chapter 176, Cast Immobilization and Upper Extremity Splinting.

RECOMMENDED READING

Bica D, Sprouse RA, Armen J. Diagnosis and management of common foot fractures. *Am Fam Physician.* 2016;93(3):183–191.

Black WS, Becker JA. Common forearm fractures in adults. *Am Fam Physician.* 2009;80:1096–1102.

Boyd AS, Benjamin HJ, Asplund C. Principles of casting and splinting. *Am Fam Physician.* 2009;79:16–22, 23–24.

Court-Brown C, Heckman JD, McQueen MM, Ricci WM, Tornetta P, eds. *Rockwood and Green's Fractures in Adults.* 8th ed. Philadelphia, Lippincott: Williams & Wilkins; 2015.

Buijze GA, Doornberg JN, Ham JS, Ring D, Bhandari M, Poolman RW. Surgical compared with conservative treatment for acute nondisplaced or minimally displaced scaphoid fractures: a systematic review and metaanalysis of randomized controlled trials. *J Bone Joint Surg Am.* 2010;92(6):1534–1544.

Egol KA, Koval KJ, Zuckerman JD. *Handbook of Fractures.* 5th ed. Philadelphia, Lippincott: Williams & Wilkins Wolters Kluwer; 2015.

Eiff MP, Hatch RL. *Fracture Management for Primary Care.* 3rd ed. Philadelphia: Elsevier; 2012.

Ersoy H, Pomeranz SJ. Complex Regional Pain Syndrome. *J Surg Orthop Adv.* 2016;25(2):117–120.

Flynn JM, Skaggs DL, eds. *Rockwood & Wilkins' Fractures in Children.* 8th ed. Philadelphia: Lippincott; 2014.

Giele BM, Wiertsema SH, Beelen A, et al. No evidence for the effectiveness of bracing in patients with thoracolumbar fractures. *Acta Orthop.* 2009;80:226–232.

Herring JA. *Tachdjian's Pediatric Orthopedics from the Texas Scottish Rite Hospital for Children.* 3rd ed. Philadelphia: WB Saunders; 2002.

Holmes JF, Akkinepalli R. Computed tomography versus plain radiography to screen for cervical spine injury: a metaanalysis. *J Trauma.* 2005;58:902–905.

Salter RB. *Disorders and Injuries of the Musculoskeletal System.* Baltimore: Williams & Wilkins; 1970.

Salter RB, Harris WR. Injuries involving epiphysial plate. *J Bone Joint Surg.* 1963;45A:587.

Spinner M. Monteggia fractures in children with nerve palsies. *Clin Orthoped.* 1968;58:141.

Stiell IG, McKnight RD, Greenberg GH, et al. Implementation of the Ottawa ankle rules. JAMA. 1994;271:827–832.

CHAPTER 179

COMPARTMENT SYNDROME EVALUATION

Michelle E. Szczepanik • Francis G. O'Connor

Compartment syndrome occurs when the pressure inside a fascial compartment is higher than the perfusion pressure. This variance can be caused by an increase in the contents of a compartment (e.g., bleeding, muscle hypertrophy, edema due to increased capillary filtration or capillary pressure), a decrease in the volume of a compartment (e.g., closure of fascial defect following surgery, excessive traction on fracture, compression by cast, splint, dressing, or patient lying on limb), or externally applied pressure. In turn, this pressure imbalance can lead to compromise of the circulation to the soft tissues, especially the muscles and nerves, resulting in tissue ischemia and eventual necrosis. If the compartment syndrome is present for 8 hours or more, irreversible tissue damage is likely and can lead to subsequent fibrosis and contracture of the muscles and compartment tendons. The flexor tendons are involved most often and are usually the earliest to be affected because they are in the deepest compartments of the calf and forearm. To merely monitor distal pulses for the development of compartment syndrome is not adequate. An absent arterial pulse may indicate only damage to a single artery, congenital absence of an artery, or hypovolemia; conversely, normal pulses may be present despite dangerously elevated compartment pressures. Pain, pallor, and lack of pulse are end-stage compartment syndrome signs and symptoms; if these are relied on to make the diagnosis, it is usually too late. Surgical release using an incision through the fascial compartments (fasciotomy) is required to relieve the excessive pressure, hopefully before reaching the end stage.

Compartment syndrome can occur at any age but is much more common in adults than children. Be aware that the swelling may not peak for 24 to 72 hours after an injury; therefore, the clinician needs to consider the diagnosis, perform a careful examination, and continue measuring compartment pressures up to 3 days after severe injuries.

Compartment pressures can be measured once (as a spot check), periodically, or continuously with a needle being left in place. This chapter discusses the measurement of compartment pressures using a needle, which is the most common method these days; wick or slit catheters were designed to be used in a similar manner but are rarely used anymore.

CONDITIONS ASSOCIATED WITH COMPARTMENT SYNDROME

- Soft tissue injury only (without a fracture)
- Soft tissue injury with a fracture of the forearm, calf, hand, or foot (fractures of the forearm or tibia cause 58% of compartment syndrome cases seen in the Emergency Department)
- Supracondylar fracture of the elbow (Volkmann ischemia)
- Crush injury to hand, thigh, or foot
- Gluteal trauma
- Prolonged tourniquet application (>2 hours) and reperfusion after other causes of ischemia
- Nephrotic syndrome

- Infusion of fluids into forearm (e.g., leaking intravenous [IV] site, dialysis tubing, or intraosseous vascular access canula)
- Anticoagulated patient or patient with coagulopathy
- Arterial or venous thrombosis
- Bites (e.g., dog, shark, and snake) in susceptible areas
- Electrical injury, especially those involving muscle
- Burns, especially those involving muscle
- Obtunded patient
- Intensive use of muscles from severe exertion, seizures, eclampsia, tetany
- Exercise-induced compartment syndrome

It is important to understand that compartment syndrome can be the result of many different types of insults. Although it is more common in the calf or the forearm, compartment syndrome can also occur in the hand, foot, thigh, or buttocks. Rarely, it can occur in the lumbar region. When trauma is involved, the rule to be followed is the greater the amount of soft tissue trauma, the greater the chance of compartment syndrome. For this reason, any high-velocity injury should be treated with caution because the energy dissipated through the soft tissue can cause extreme swelling. Injuries commonly associated with compartment syndrome include automobile accidents and pedestrian trauma, especially bumper injuries to the buttocks, calf, or forearm. Gluteal compartment syndrome, which is frequently associated with an automobile accident or falling from a height, is due to the direct trauma and the associated swelling of the muscle compartment. Compartment syndrome can occur in the thigh because of a severe crush injury.

Compartment syndrome is a common result of trauma significant enough to cause a fracture. Volkmann ischemia is compartment syndrome in the forearm occurring after supracondylar fractures that cause a large amount of swelling around the elbow. Calcaneal fractures can also cause compartment syndrome, although this is rare. While a patient with a coagulopathy or on anticoagulation can develop spontaneous bleeding into a muscle compartment, leading to increased pressure, such a patient is even more likely to develop compartment syndrome if trauma is associated.

A chronic, low-grade form of compartment syndrome can occur with exertion, which usually increases as a training program progresses. Also known as exercise-induced compartment syndrome, chronic exertional compartment syndrome presents as a gradual development of pain with activity followed by a gradual resolution of symptoms with cessation of the activity. It is more common in runners, and usually involves the calf. It must be distinguished from other causes of chronic leg pain such as medial tibial stress syndrome, stress fracture, nerve or arterial entrapment, or muscle strain. A good history and postexercise examination are fundamental in differentiating between these varied causes of chronic leg pain.

Finally, some less common but certainly notable causes of compartment syndrome include nephrotic syndrome, a leaking IV site, dialysis tubing, or intraosseous vascular canula, large animal bites, snakebites, and infection. Prolonged application of a tourniquet (>2 hours) has been associated with the development of compartment syndrome when the tourniquet is released and reperfusion causes swelling and increased pressure. Reperfusion after other causes of ischemia can have similar results. Bites in an extremity from large animals, such as sharks or dogs, can cause crush injuries; snakebites are also associated with significant edema. Scratches, cuts, or bites from smaller animals or insects can result in infection that may cause a compartment syndrome, or may mask or restrict one. Patients who have electrical injuries, with or without a visible skin burn, can develop compartment syndrome. The mechanism is similar to that of a device available on the market to cook a hot dog, which is how the injury got its nickname "hot dogger." After a hot dog is punctured at both ends with a metal spike, an electrical current is delivered through the hot dog. This causes intense heat, thus cooking the hot dog. The same mechanism occurs with burn injuries with an entrance and exit point for the electrical energy. The "cooked" tissue inside swells, nearly to the point of bursting, but is restrained by the surrounding tissue. The extent of injury may not be visible on the patient's initial visit but can develop over the next 1 to 3 days. A clinician should always consider compartment syndrome when evaluating burns of any kind.

CONDITIONS THAT CAN CREATE, MASK, OR WORSEN COMPARTMENT SYNDROME

- Applying heat to injury
- Spinal cord injury or regional anesthetic block
- Intoxication, altered mental status, or changes in sensorium (e.g., head trauma and coma)
- Infection, burns, scarring, tight bandages, or being in a cast

An injury, with or without fracture, which is later subjected to warm water or any other intervention resulting in vasodilation, will have increased swelling and an increased chance of compartment syndrome. Patients with a severe bruise from a fall who then soak it in a hot tub of water can develop compartment syndrome. It can also happen when expansion of the soft tissue envelope (skin) is constricted by a cast, scarring, or infection. If any patient has pain out of proportion to objective findings, especially after trauma to an extremity or placement of a cast, the cast and padding should be removed entirely and the patient examined carefully for compartment syndrome. A cast, especially if applied too tightly, can be one of those things that applies constant external pressure which itself can cause compartment syndrome. If removal of the cast and padding does not bring immediate and complete relief of the intense pain, evaluation for compartment syndrome is indicated (with subsequent surgical treatment if present). Even without a cast, any feeling of tense, tight swelling in the forearm, hand, calf, or foot should lead to suspicion of compartment syndrome.

Another presentation for compartment syndrome is the intoxicated individual who falls and sustains an injury. Because of the intoxication (or any other reason for an altered sensorium), the pain is ignored. In addition, patients who have a spinal cord injury resulting from a motor vehicle accident will not have pain in the forearm or calf in spite of the swelling that may also occur as a result of the accident. Postoperative patients with a regional block may not have pain for the same reason. For the aforementioned reasons, immediate evaluation may be necessary and a fasciotomy considered in any such patient with a tense and swollen forearm, calf, hand, or foot.

In addition to the obtunded or unresponsive patient, consideration should be made to evaluate those patients who may not be able to reliably report pain, such as patients with multiple or distracting injuries, those with sensory neuropathy (which could be due to diabetes or fracture-associated nerve injury), uncooperative patients, or children.

INDICATIONS

A diagnosis of compartment syndrome made after the loss of pulses and the loss of capillary refill comes too late for optimal treatment. Therefore, the evaluation of compartment pressures in any of the conditions mentioned earlier that are associated with compartment syndrome or any of those conditions where compartment syndrome could be created, masked, or worsened, should be considered.

The most important and earliest symptom associated with compartment syndrome is *pain*. If pain after an injury is associated with swelling in an extremity and the pain is not relieved by medication (e.g., up to one or two Percocet tablets every 4 hours), compartment syndrome should be suspected, especially if the pain is progressive.

The earliest physical findings are (1) loss of fine touch, and (2) pain with extension of the great toe or the thumb. Compartment syndrome most commonly occurs first in the volar/dorsal compartment of the forearm, where the long flexor tendon of the thumb travels, and in the calf, where the long flexor tendon for the great toe is located. By passively extending the thumb or great toe, the muscle tendon unit in this deep compartment is stretched. If the muscle is ischemic because of early compartment syndrome, pain will be present and increased by extension of the thumb or toe. Two-point discrimination is also impaired early.

For chronic exertional compartment syndrome, certain symptoms help distinguish it from other causes of chronic leg pain. Typical symptoms are aching or cramping leg pain; gradual rather than immediate development of pain with activity; neurologic symptoms such as numbness or tingling; gradual resolution with cessation of activity; and shorter distances or intensities being required to produce the discomfort. Because routine physical examination is usually negative, a postexercise examination should be included to demonstrate tightness of the compartment involved, discomfort and tenderness with palpation, and involvement of the muscle mass rather than the muscle-tendon junction. The calf is most commonly involved, and approximately 80% of the time compartment syndrome occurs bilaterally.

Measurement of compartment pressures should be considered in any patient with a compatible history or a swollen and tense muscle group, and the following:

- Pain (the earliest and most sensitive symptom)
- Pain out of proportion to objective findings, especially if progressive
- Increasing pain not relieved by usual narcotic pain medication
- Loss of fine touch or two-point discrimination
- Pain with passive motion of the affected muscles (e.g., extension of great toe or thumb of affected limb)
- Increased discomfort when muscle trapped in the fascial compartment is moved (actively or passively), especially the flexor muscles
- Excessive constriction of the affected compartment
- Suspected chronic exertional compartment syndrome

CONTRAINDICATIONS TO MEASUREMENT

- When compartment syndrome is clinically obvious and measurement would delay definitive treatment
- Infection, cellulitis, or burn directly over the area to be measured (relative contraindication)
- Anticoagulation (relative contraindication)

PREPROCEDURE PATIENT PREPARATION

Indications, alternatives, risks, potential benefits, and expected results should be discussed with the patient or representative and signed informed consent should be obtained. The patient should expect some discomfort as needles are inserted. The procedure may need to be repeated at various locations and intermittently over time. Alternatively, a continuous monitor may be left in place (usually in a comatose patient). Let conscious patients know they will be warned before the insertion of a needle. It will also be important for them to remain very still during certain portions of the procedure. If moderate (conscious) sedation is to be used, IV access should be obtained and the patient should be monitored with pulse oximetry.

EQUIPMENT

- Gloves and other necessary equipment for the clinician to follow universal blood and body fluid precautions
- Povidone-iodine or chlorhexidine antiseptic solution
- Sterile drapes and towels
- 4 × 4 gauze squares
- Band-Aids to cover needle insertion sites
- Local anesthetic (1% lidocaine), syringe, and needles (optional)

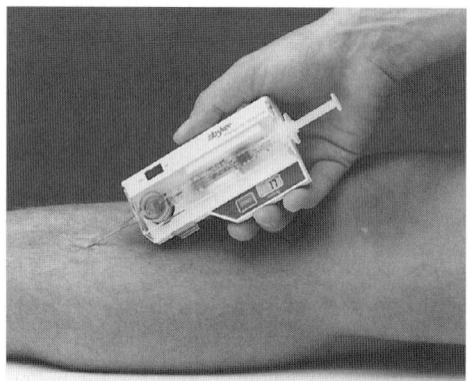

Fig. 179.1 Stryker intracompartmental pressure monitor system. (Courtesy Stryker Instruments, Kalamazoo, MI.)

STRYKER SYSTEM

- Prefilled syringe with saline
- Side-port needle
- Diaphragm chamber
- Hand-held pressure monitor
- Stryker quick-pressure monitor set (disposable pouch)

Needle–Manometer or Arterial-Line Type Transducer System

- Two 18-gauge needles (18-gauge spinal needle may be needed for deep measurements such as thigh or gluteal compartments)
- Two sets of extension tubing
- 20-mL syringe
- Three-way stopcock
- Sterile normal saline solution
- Manometer or pressure transducer, cable, monitor, and adjustable transducer stand

Clinicians primarily use one of two pressure measurement systems, either the Stryker intracompartmental pressure monitor system, which is a portable pen-like compartment pressure device made by the Stryker Company, or a needle–manometer or arterial-type transducer system. The Stryker (Fig. 179.1) is much like a tonometer for measuring glaucoma. All of these systems also can be converted to a continuous monitoring system.

TECHNIQUE

Each body "compartment" can become compromised. Various compartments are shown in Figs. 179.2 to 179.13. Suggested sites for placement of the needle are noted in Table 179.1. Most experts recommend multiple measurements at multiple sites with at least one being at the site of maximal tightness as determined by the examining clinician. A study by Whitesides and Heckman (1996) suggests

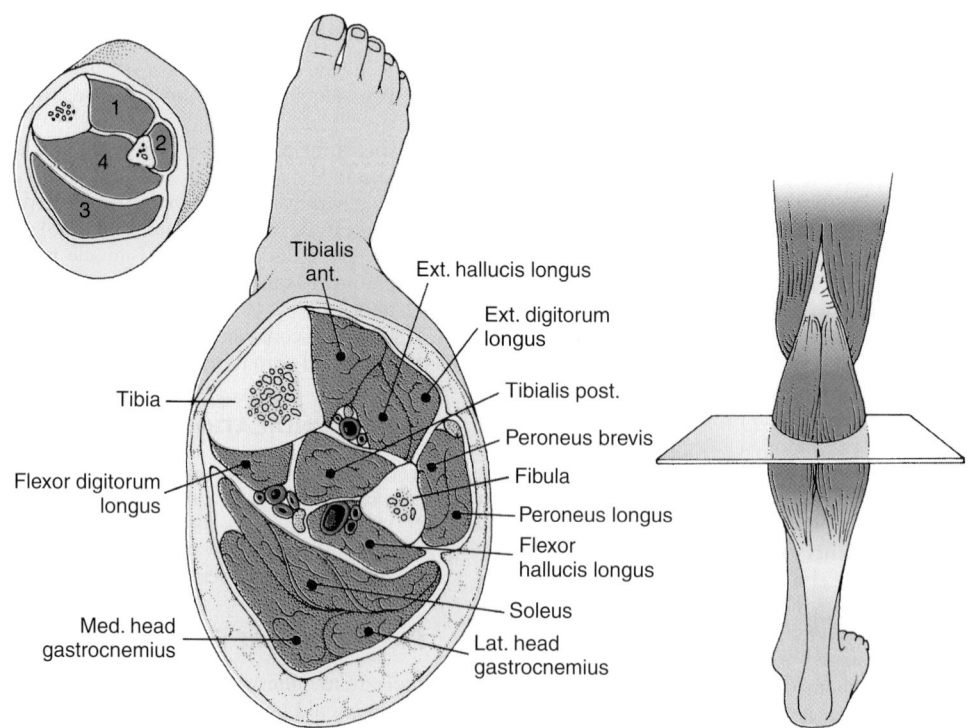

Fig. 179.2 Fascial compartments of the lower leg with enclosed muscle groups. *1*, Anterior; *2*, lateral; *3*, superficial posterior; and *4*, deep posterior compartments. (Modified from Roberts JR, Custalow CB, Thomsen TW, eds. *Roberts and Hedges Clinical Procedures in Emergency Medicine.* 6th ed. Philadelphia: Elsevier; 2014.)

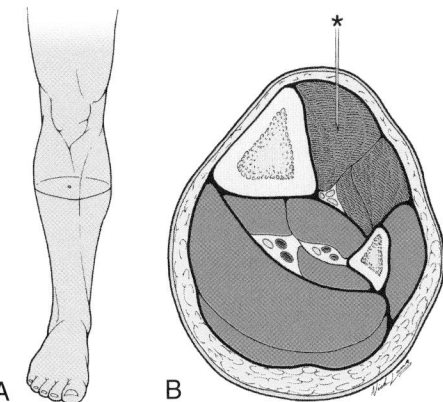

Fig. 179.3   Anterior compartment syndrome of the lower leg. (A) Suggested needle entry point is indicated by the small circle. (B) The needle should be inserted to a depth of 1 to 3 cm (asterisk). (Modified from Roberts JR, Custalow CB, Thomsen TW, eds. *Roberts and Hedges Clinical Procedures in Emergency Medicine*. 6th ed. Philadelphia: Elsevier; 2014.)

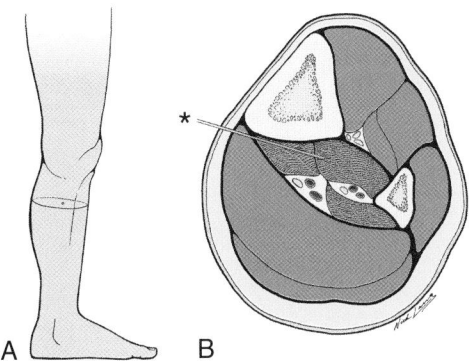

Fig. 179.4   Deep posterior compartment syndrome of the lower leg. (A) Suggested needle entry point indicated by the small circle. (B) The needle should be inserted to a depth of 2 to 4 cm (asterisk). (Modified from Roberts JR, Custalow CB, Thomsen TW, eds. *Roberts and Hedges Clinical Procedures in Emergency Medicine*. 6th ed. Philadelphia: Elsevier; 2014.)

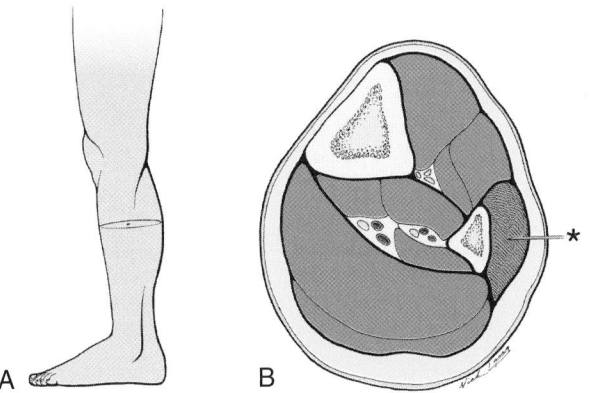

Fig. 179.5   Lateral compartment syndrome of the lower leg. (A) Suggested needle entry point indicated by the small circle. (B) The needle should be inserted to a depth of 1 to 1.5 cm (asterisk). (Modified from Roberts JR, Custalow CB, Thomsen TW, eds. Roberts and Hedges Clinical Procedures in Emergency Medicine. 6th ed. Philadelphia: Elsevier; 2014.)

that with fractures, measurements should be performed at the level of the fracture as well as locations proximal and distal to the zone of the fracture. They used a distance of 5 cm proximal and distal to the fracture site.

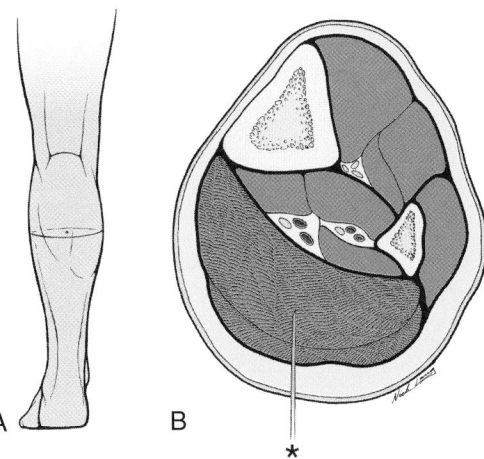

Fig. 179.6   Superficial posterior compartment syndrome of the lower leg. (A) Suggested needle entry point indicated by the small circle. (B) The needle should be inserted to a depth of 2 to 4 cm (asterisk). (Modified from Roberts JR, Custalow CB, Thomsen TW, eds. *Roberts and Hedges Clinical Procedures in Emergency Medicine*. 6th ed. Philadelphia: Elsevier; 2014.)

General

1. Obtain informed consent.
2. The compartment to be measured should be at the level of the patient's heart and positioned so the needle can enter perpendicular to the compartment.
3. Avoid any external pressures to the area; the region tested may need to be slightly elevated off the bed by an assistant. The patient must be cooperative and not move or contract the muscle group.
4. Prepare skin with antiseptic solution. Sterile technique should be maintained when setting up the equipment and inserting the needles. Sterile drapes should be used if more than one measurement is to be obtained.
5. A superficial local anesthetic can be given.
6. When taking pressure measurements, squeeze the involved area to see if pressure increases (or have the patient contract the affected muscle), which confirms that the unit is functioning.
7. Consider measuring opposite-side pressures as a control and if there is any question about proper readings on affected side.
8. When the needle is pulled between measurements, flush it to be sure it has not become plugged with blood or tissue. After measurements are obtained, needle insertion sites should be covered properly (e.g., with a Band-Aid).

Stryker Systems

9. Open the disposable Stryker 295 or 295-2 quick-pressure monitor setup (the 295 comes with the syringe barrel prefilled with saline and covered with a syringe cap. The plunger is separate. The 295-2 comes with the syringe prefilled with saline and the plunger in place).
10. Assemble the equipment (Fig. 179.14).

    For the Stryker 295:

11. Place the 18-gauge needle onto the diaphragm. Attach the prefilled syringe barrel on the other side. This is now the chamber diaphragm assembly. Open the cover of the monitor and insert the chamber into the device well with the block surface down. Be sure it is firmly in place. The chamber diaphragm assembly should all still be attached.
12. Gently snap the cover closed (do not force it). You should hear it snap closed.
13. Remove the syringe cap and insert the plunger.

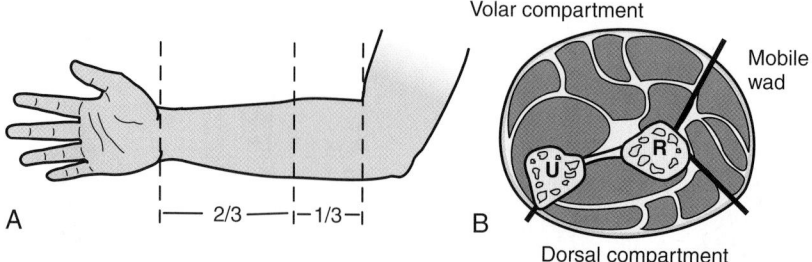

Fig. 179.7   (A) Level of needle insertion for the forearm. (B) Cross-section through the upper third of the forearm demonstrating the three forearm compartments (volar, dorsal, and mobile wad). *R*, Radius; *U*, ulna. (Modified from Roberts JR, Custalow CB, Thomsen TW, eds. *Roberts and Hedges Clinical Procedures in Emergency Medicine.* 6th ed. Philadelphia: Elsevier; 2014.)

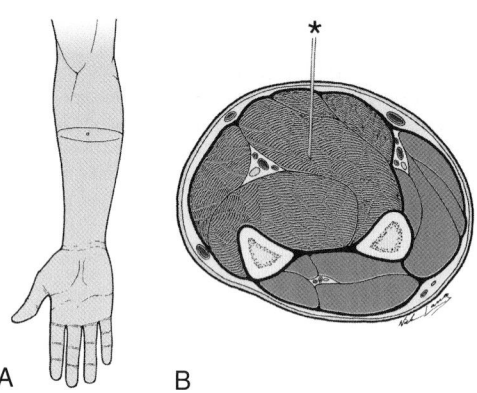

Fig. 179.8   Volar compartment syndrome of the forearm. (A) Suggested needle entry point indicated by the small circle. (B) The needle should be inserted to a depth of 1 to 2 cm (asterisk). (Modified from Roberts JR, Custalow CB, Thomsen TW, eds. *Roberts and Hedges Clinical Procedures in Emergency Medicine.* 6th ed. Philadelphia: Elsevier; 2014.)

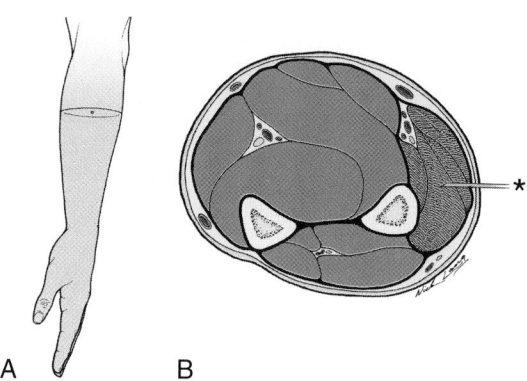

Fig. 179.10   Mobile wad compartment syndrome of the forearm. (A) Suggested needle entry point indicated by the small circle. (B) The needle should be inserted to a depth of 1 to 1.5 cm (asterisk). (Modified from Roberts JR, Custalow CB, Thomsen TW, eds. *Roberts and Hedges Clinical Procedures in Emergency Medicine.* 6th ed. Philadelphia: Elsevier; 2014.)

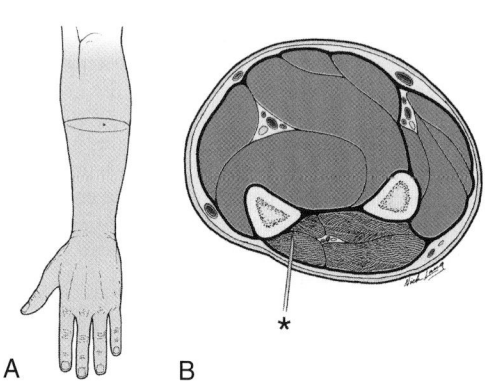

Fig. 179.9   Dorsal compartment syndrome of the forearm. (A) Suggested needle entry point indicated by the small circle. (B) The needle should be inserted to a depth of 1 to 2 cm (asterisk). (Modified from Roberts JR, Custalow CB, Thomsen TW, eds. *Roberts and Hedges Clinical Procedures in Emergency Medicine.* 6th ed. Philadelphia: Elsevier; 2014.)

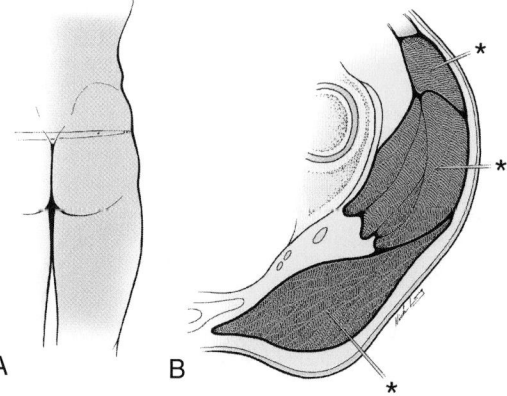

Fig. 179.11   Gluteal compartment syndrome. (A) Suggested needle entry point is indicated by the small circle. The needle should be inserted to a depth of 4 to 8 cm depending on which compartment is being measured. (B) Needle tips (asterisk) shown entering muscle compartments. (Modified from Roberts JR, Custalow CB, Thomsen TW, eds. *Roberts and Hedges Clinical Procedures in Emergency Medicine.* 6th ed. Philadelphia: Elsevier; 2014.)

For the Stryker 295-2:

11. Place the 18-gauge needle onto the tapered stem of the diaphragm chamber. Screw the prefilled syringe onto the other side of the diaphragm chamber. This is now the chamber diaphragm assembly.
12. Place the chamber diaphragm assembly into the pressure monitor, back side down. Gently push the chamber until it is well-seated in the device. The chamber diaphragm assembly should all still be attached. Snap the cover closed (do not force it). You should hear it snap into place.

For both systems:

14. Purge the system of air. Tilt the end of the needle up 45 degrees and slowly fill the system with saline. The saline must not roll back into the transducer well.
15. Turn on the unit. Readings should be between 0 and 9 mm Hg.
16. Simulate the angle of insertion and press the "zero" button. If the monitor does not read "00," there is a problem. Review the instructions supplied with the kit if necessary. A reading of "00" must be displayed or readings will be inaccurate.

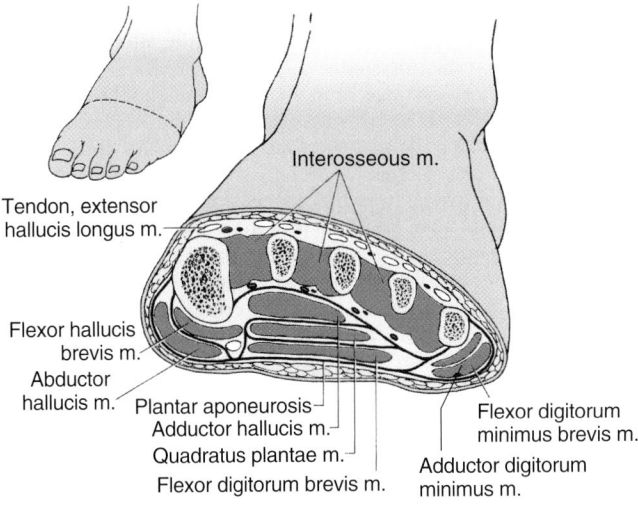

Fig. 179.12 Compartments of the foot. (Modified from Roberts JR, Custalow CB, Thomsen TW, eds. *Roberts and Hedges Clinical Procedures in Emergency Medicine.* 6th ed. Philadelphia: Elsevier; 2014.)

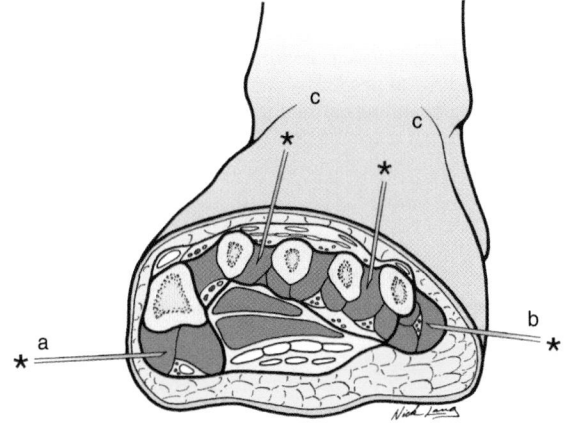

Fig. 179.13 Compartment syndromes of the foot. Suggested needle pathways (asterisk) to measure intracompartmental pressures are shown: Medial *(a)*; lateral *(b)*; and interosseous compartments *(c)*. The central compartment is located between these compartments. (Modified from Roberts JR, Custalow CB, Thomsen TW, eds. *Roberts and Hedges Clinical Procedures in Emergency Medicine.* 6th ed. Philadelphia: Elsevier; 2014.)

TABLE 179.1	**Landmarks for Suggested Needle Placement to Measure Compartment Pressures**				
Compartment	**Position**	**Location**	**Insert Needle***	**Depth (cm)**	**Confirm Proper Position by Pressure Variation**
Lower Leg					
Anterior	Supine	Junction of proximal and middle thirds of tibia anteriorly	1 cm lateral to anterior tibia (see Fig. 179.3)	1–3	Compression proximal or distal plantar flexion of foot Dorsiflexion of foot
Deep posterior	Supine	Junction of proximal and middle thirds of tibia anteriorly	Just posterior to medial border of tibia; direct at posterior border of fibula (see Fig. 179.4)	2–4	Toe extension Ankle inversion
Lateral	Supine	Junction of proximal and middle thirds, posterior border of fibula	Just anterior to posterior border of fibula; direct at fibula (see Fig. 179.5)	1–1.5	Compression inferior or superior to needle Inversion of foot and ankle
Superficial posterior	Prone	Junction of proximal and middle thirds of posterior leg	3–5 cm on either side of vertical line in middle of calf (see Fig. 179.6)	2–4	Compression inferior or superior to needle Foot dorsiflexion
Forearm					
Volar	Forearm in supination	Junction of proximal and middle thirds of forearm	Just medial to palmaris longus (midline of forearm); direct needle to palpated posterior border of ulna (see Fig. 179.7)	1–2	Compression proximal or distal to needle Extension of fingers or wrist
Dorsal	Forearm in supination	Junction of proximal and middle thirds of forearm, posterior aspect of ulna	1–2 cm lateral to posterior aspect of ulna (see Fig. 179.9)	1–2	Compression proximal or distal to needle Flex fingers or wrist
Mobile wad	Forearm in supination	Junction of proximal and middle thirds of forearm, most lateral portion of forearm	In muscle tissue lateral to radius	1–1.5	Compression proximal or distal to needle Ulnar deviation of wrist
Gluteal					
All three compartments	Prone	Point of maximal tenderness	Spinal needle	4–8	Compression of gluteal musculature
Foot					
Medial	Supine	Medial aspect of base of first metatarsal	Medial aspect of foot, inferior to base of first metatarsal into abductor hallucis	1–1.5	Compression of medial compartment
Central	Supine	Medial aspect of base of first metatarsal	Medial aspect foot inferior to base of first metatarsal, through abductor hallucis	3	Compression of central compartment
Lateral	Supine	Base of fifth metatarsal	Inferior to base of fifth metatarsal	1–1.5	Compression of lateral compartment
Interosseous	Supine	Dorsum, bases of second and fourth metatarsal	Dorsum of second and fourth web spaces	1	Compression of interosseous compartment

*Perpendicular to skin unless otherwise stated.

17. Insert needle into the tissue.
18. Inject up to 0.3 mL of saline.
19. Read the pressure once it stabilizes.
20. Repeat readings as needed by turning the unit off and withdrawing the needle and repeating the previous steps.

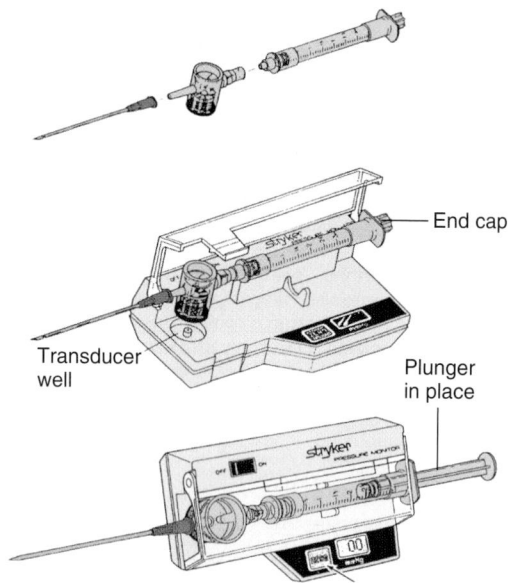

Fig. 179.14 Stryker 295 intracompartmental pressure monitor system assembly. (Courtesy Stryker Instruments, Kalamazoo, MI.)

Needle-Manometer System

Equipment for the needle-manometer technique is readily available and the least expensive, but it is also the least accurate.

9. Prepare setup (Fig. 179.15A). Use one 18-gauge needle to ventilate the sterile saline solution (i.e., ventilate by inserting the needle, which opens the bag or bottle to atmospheric pressure and breaks the vacuum in the bottle or bag). This needle should be left in place, ventilating the saline, during the next step, while the extension tubing is being partially filled with saline.

10. Attach the 20-mL syringe to the stopcock. Attach one extension tubing (with the other 18-gauge needle attached) to another port on the stopcock.
11. Using the 20-mL syringe, draw enough saline into the extension tubing to fill it about halfway. Then close the stopcock to the extension tubing. Be sure there are no air bubbles in the saline in the extension tubing.
12. Remove the syringe from the stopcock and fill it with approximately 15 mL of air. Reattach it to the stopcock.
13. Attach the other extension tubing to the stopcock. Attach the opposite end of this tubing to a manometer (see Fig. 179.15B).
14. With the stopcock still closed to the extension tubing with the needle attached, pull the needle out of the saline. Insert the needle into the desired compartment for pressure measurement (see Table 179.1). For deep measurements (thigh or gluteal compartments), an 18-gauge spinal needle may be needed.
15. *Slowly* depress the syringe plunger. This gives the manometer time to move. Watch the meniscus on the column of saline in the extension tubing. When it flattens, right before the saline starts moving in the tubing, the pressure in the syringe has matched the tissue pressure. Note the reading on the manometer, which is the compartment pressure.
16. Check a second recording by removing the needle and repeating as previously.

Arterial-Type Transducer System

Also see Chapter 225, Arterial Puncture and Percutaneous Arterial Line Placement.

Equipment for the arterial-type transducer system is also usually readily available. In the emergency department, the operating room, or the critical care unit, the nurse or respiratory therapist can often assist with flushing and hooking up the extension tubing, which is attached to a pressure transducer. The nurse or respiratory therapist also usually knows how to assemble and calibrate the rest of the equipment.

9. Connect the cable to the monitor.
10. Assemble the equipment (Fig. 179.16). Using one 18-gauge needle, fill the 20-mL syringe with sterile saline. One extension tubing will be used to connect the stopcock to the transducer; the other will have the other 18-gauge needle attached.
11. Attach the 20-mL syringe to the stopcock and fill the transducer, both sets of extension tubing, and the attached 18-gauge

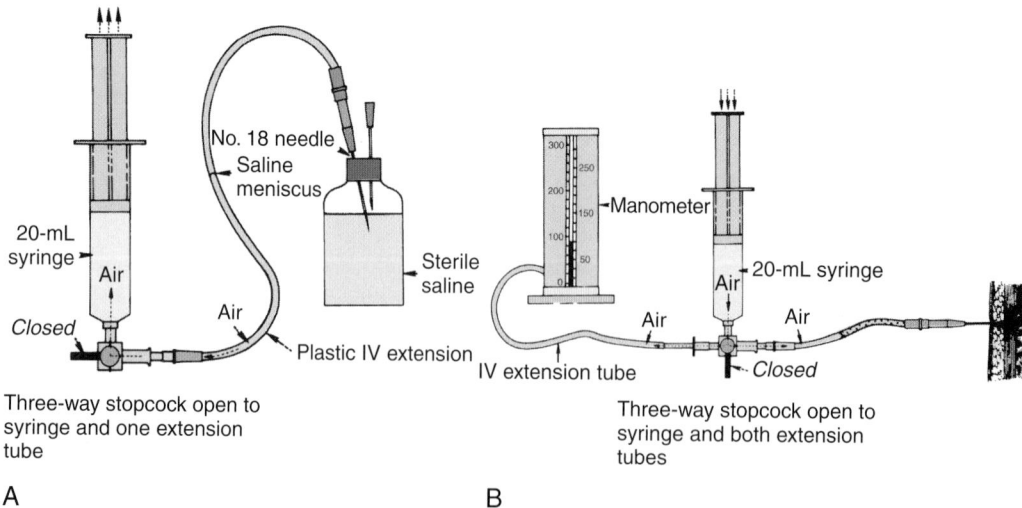

Fig. 179.15 Needle-manometer technique for compartment pressure monitoring. (A) Drawing up saline to partially fill tubing. (B) Completed system setup with needle inserted into compartment. *IV,* Intravenous. (From Whitesides TE Jr, Haney TC, Morimoto K, Harada K. Tissue pressure measurement as a determinant for the need of fasciotomy. *Clin Orthop.* 1975;113:43–51.)

needle with saline. Close the stopcock to the extension tubing attached to the 18-gauge needle.

12. Remove the 20-mL syringe and open the stopcock to air. Place the transducer at the level of the muscle compartment where pressures are being measured.

13. Calibrate to zero and close the stopcock.

14. Open the stopcock to the extension tubing with the 18-gauge needle attached (which will now be called the "arterial line" because the pressures will be measured and monitored like that of an artery) and insert the needle into the muscle compartment. Squeeze (or have the patient move) the muscles of the desired compartment. Pressures should elevate on the monitor. Allow the muscles to rest and measure the pressure.

15. Pull the needle and repeat the process for a second confirmatory measurement.

NOTE: Attempts should be made to minimize the injection of saline into the compartment being measured because it may elevate the pressure for subsequent measurements or worsen the compartment syndrome. Using a partially air-filled 20-mL syringe and a partially filled "arterial line" extension tubing, the technique described with the needle–manometer setup can also be used with the arterial-type transducer system. As the air-filled syringe is depressed, when the meniscus flattens and the saline starts moving toward the compartment, the measurement on the monitor will be equal to compartment pressure.

CRITERIA TO PERFORM FASCIOTOMY

- Compartment pressure reading over 30 mm Hg
- High clinical suspicion despite normal pressure readings (symptoms of pain out of proportion to objective findings, decreased sensation and pain with passive extension of the thumb or great toe, a tense compartment with clinical signs of compartment syndrome)

Although there is some debate, healthy compartment pressures generally range between 0 and 8 mm Hg. Normal pressures may be slightly higher in physically fit individuals. Readings in all compartments should be 30 mm Hg or below. Since the 1980s, this has been considered the pressure where fasciotomy is indicated. At a minimum, any reading above that level requires immediate consultation for possible surgical treatment of compartment syndrome. At this point, the consultant may interpret these results within the context of the clinical scenario; some individuals tolerate

these pressures without developing compartment syndrome. But the patient should be monitored closely. Compartment pressures 10 to 30 mm Hg below the patient's mean arterial pressure or the patient's diastolic pressure may also indicate the need for a fasciotomy. If multiple measurements are taken, some experts recommend using the highest measured pressures to make the decision for further intervention.

Do not rely solely on pressures to make clinical decisions. Fasciotomy may be indicated if the compartment is tense to palpation, if there is pain out of proportion to objective findings, or if there is decreased sensation and pain with passive extension of the thumb or great toe. If any of these findings are present, even in the face of what appears to be normal compartment pressures, consultation should be obtained immediately. Compartment pressure measurements can give false-normal readings at times. Therefore, such measurements are of value only when combined with the other information on physical examination and pain level.

CRITERIA FOR DIAGNOSIS OF CHRONIC EXERTIONAL COMPARTMENT SYNDROME

Once history and physical findings support the diagnosis, compartment pressures should be measured at rest followed by postexercise pressures after pain is reproduced. While there is considerable controversy over the most reliable protocol and criteria to diagnose chronic exertional compartment syndrome, the Pedowitz criteria (1990) are most commonly used to make a diagnosis. One of the following criteria must be met for the test to be positive in a symptomatic patient:

- A preexercise compartment pressure greater than 15 mm Hg
- One-minute postexercise compartment pressure greater than 30 mm Hg
- Five-minute postexercise compartment pressure greater than 20 mm Hg

COMPLICATIONS

- Bleeding
- Infection
- Increased pressure from extra fluid injected
- Pain
- Inaccurate, falsely reassuring readings

Each of the first three (bleeding, infection, and increased volume of fluid) could exacerbate compartment syndrome.

PATIENT EDUCATION GUIDES

See the sample patient education form available at www.expertconsult.com.

CPT/BILLING CODES

20950   Monitoring of interstitial fluid pressure (includes insertion of device, e.g., wick catheter technique, needle-manometer technique) in detection of muscle compartment syndrome

ICD-10-CM DIAGNOSTIC CODES

M79.A19   Nontraumatic compartment syndrome of unspecified upper extremity
M79.A29   Nontraumatic compartment syndrome of unspecified lower extremity
M79.A3   Nontraumatic compartment syndrome of abdomen
M79.A9   Nontraumatic compartment syndrome of other sites

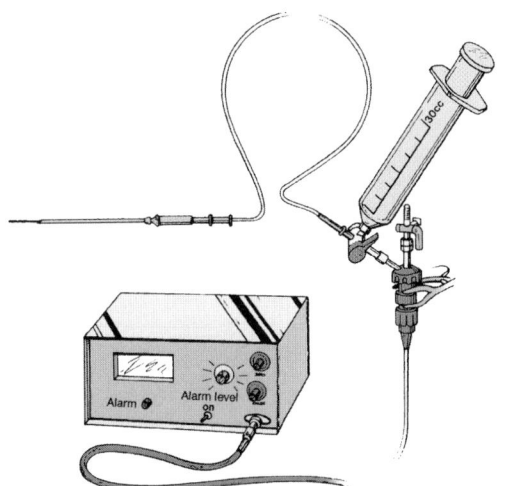

Fig. 179.16 Arterial-type transducer system for compartment pressure measurement. (From Rorabeck CH. Compartment syndromes. In: Browner BD, Jupiter JB, Levine AM, Trafton PG, eds. *Skeletal Trauma: Fractures, Dislocations, Ligamentous Injuries.* Vol 1, 2nd ed. Philadelphia: WB Saunders; 1992.)

S38.1XXA	Crushing injury of abdomen, lower back, pelvis initial encounter
S47.9XXA	Crushing injury of upper arm, shoulder unspecified arm, initial encounter
S57.80XA	Crushing injury of unspecified forearm initial encounter
S57.00XA	Crushing injury of unspecified elbow initial encounter
S77.10XA	Crushing injury of unspecified thigh initial encounter
S77.00XA	Crushing injury of unspecified hip initial encounter
S87.80XA	Crushing injury of unspecified lower leg initial encounter
S87.00XA	Crushing injury of unspecified knee initial encounter
T79.6XXA	Volkmann ischemic or posttraumatic muscle contracture initial encounter
T79.A0XA	Compartment syndrome, unspecified initial encounter
T79.A19A	Traumatic compartment syndrome of unspecified upper extremity initial encounter
T79.A29A	Traumatic compartment syndrome of unspecified lower extremity initial encounter
T79.A3XA	Traumatic compartment syndrome of abdomen initial encounter
T79.A9XA	Traumatic compartment syndrome of other sites initial encounter

SUPPLIERS

(See contact information available at www.expertconsult.com.)

Stryker Instruments

Acknowledgment

The editors recognize the contributions of Robert L. Kalb, MD, to this chapter in a previous edition of this text.

RECOMMENDED READING

Aweid O, Del Buono A, Malliaras P, Iqbal H, Morrissey D, Maffulli N, Padhiar N. Systematic review and recommendations for intracompartmental pressure monitoring in diagnosing chronic exertional compartment syndrome of the leg. *Clin J Sport Med.* 2012;22(4):356–370.

d'Amato TA, Kaplan IB, Britt LD. High-voltage electrical injury: a role for mandatory exploration of deep muscle compartments. *J Natl Med Assoc.* 1994;86:535–537.

Dellaero DT, Levin LS. Compartment syndrome of the hand: etiology, diagnosis, and treatment. *Am J Orthop.* 1996;25:404–408.

Gourgiotis S, Villias C, Germanos S, et al. Acute limb compartment syndrome: a review. *J Surg Educ.* 2007;64:178–186.

Griffiths D, Jones DH. Spontaneous compartment syndrome in a patient on long-term anticoagulation. *J Hand Surg Br.* 1993;18:41–42.

Hutchinson MR, Ireland ML. Common compartment syndromes in athletes: treatment and rehabilitation. *Sports Med.* 1994;17:200–208.

Kleinmaier M, Malik S. Compartment pressure measurement. In: Reichman EF, ed. *Emergency Medicine Procedures.* 2nd ed. New York: McGraw-Hill; 2013:473–490.

Laoteppitaks C. Compartment syndrome evaluation. In: Roberts JR, Custalow CB, Thomsen TW, eds. *Roberts and Hedges Clinical Procedures in Emergency Medicine and Acute Care.* 7th ed. Philadelphia: Elsevier; 2019:1125–1140.

Myerson M, Manoli A. Compartment syndromes of the foot after calcaneal fractures. *Clin Orthop.* 1993;290:142–150.

Olson SA, Glasgow RR. Acute compartment syndrome in lower extremity musculoskeletal trauma. *J Am Acad Orthop Surg.* 2005;13:436–444.

Pedowitz RA, Hargens AR, Mubarak SJ, Gershuni DH. Modified criteria for the objective diagnosis of chronic compartment syndrome of the leg. *Am J Sports Med.* 1990;18:35–40.

Peters CL, Scott SM. Compartment syndrome in the forearm following fractures of the radial head or neck in children. *J Bone Joint Surg Am.* 1995;77:1070–1074.

Schnall SB, Holtom PD, Silva E. Compartment syndrome associated with infection of the upper extremity. *Clin Orthop.* 1994;306:128–131.

Seybold EA, Busconi BD. Anterior thigh compartment syndrome following prolonged tourniquet application and lateral positioning. *Am J Orthop.* 1996;25:493–496.

Simpson NS, Jupiter JB. Delayed onset of forearm compartment syndrome: a complication of distal radius fracture in young adults. *J Orthop Trauma.* 1995;9:411–418.

Vidal P, Sykes PJ, O'Shaughnessy M, Craddock K. Compartment syndrome after use of an automatic arterial pressure monitoring device. *Br J Anaesth.* 1993;71:902–904.

Whitesides TE, Heckman MH. Acute compartment syndrome: update on diagnosis and treatment. *J Am Acad Orthop Surg.* 1996;4:209–218.

CHAPTER 180

JOINT AND SOFT TISSUE ASPIRATION AND INJECTION (ARTHROCENTESIS)

Thad J. Barkdull • Francis G. O'Connor • John M. McShane

Joint and soft tissue aspiration and injection are both clinically rewarding and relatively simple procedures for primary care clinicians to learn and perform. They are also very much appreciated by our patients. In the United States, 8% of ambulatory visits are for musculoskeletal conditions, and 13% of these patients have osteoarthritis (OA) as a comorbid condition. Steroid join injection fell into disfavor for many years because the procedure was overused and abused. When appropriate guidelines are followed, however, complications are extremely rare, and the injections can be very beneficial to the patient by reducing symptoms. The usual alternative to focal treatment with injection is systemic nonsteroidal antiinflammatory drugs (NSAIDs) which have significant toxicity and risk with prolonged use. In the United States, almost two-thirds of family physicians use corticosteroid injections as part of a treatment plan.

Primary care clinicians should master the technique of aspiration and injection for many reasons. If the clinician aspirates an inflamed joint, a diagnosis can often be made immediately. If a joint is distended, pain can be relieved rapidly by aspirating the fluid. Injecting an anesthetic, steroid, hyaluronic acid, prolotherapy, or other solution (e.g., botulinum toxin, intraarticular NSAIDs are being studied) can not only provide focal pain relief without the toxicity of the systemic medications, it can also provide valuable diagnostic information.

The clinician should not withhold the benefits of injection therapy because of incomplete familiarity with the exact anatomy involved. Basic knowledge of soft tissue and bony landmarks is enough to provide a reliable method for identification of needle insertion sites. The emerging role of musculoskeletal ultrasound in office-based practice offers additional opportunities to improve diagnostic and therapeutic techniques. The reader may want to refer to Chapter 171, Musculoskeletal Ultrasound, for related information. One joint that the process of injection is completely changed with ultrasound guidance is the knee. Instead of going very near cartilage, possibly bumping it when injecting blindly, without ultrasound, the suprapatellar pouch is localized with ultrasound. This is a pouch above the knee which communicates into the capsule. With ultrasound guidance, the pouch can be injected by directing the needle through the quadriceps muscle.

INDICATIONS

Diagnostic

* To evaluate synovial fluid and determine whether an effusion is from an infectious, rheumatic, traumatic, or crystal-induced origin
* To perform a therapeutic trial to differentiate between various conditions (e.g., costochondritis vs. coronary artery disease, trochanteric bursitis vs. deep hip disease, occipital trigger points vs. vertebral disease)
* To differentiate an intraarticular from extraarticular origin of pain symptoms

EDITOR'S NOTE: If you or your patient can localize the area of discomfort near a joint with one finger, a bursitis or tendonitis is much more likely the cause and it will likely benefit from an injection, especially if other therapies have failed.

Therapeutic

* To remove exudative fluid from a septic joint
* To relieve pain in a grossly swollen joint (e.g., traumatic effusion)
* To reduce pain and inflammation by injecting lidocaine, with or without corticosteroids, or saline for trigger points (see Chapter 181, Trigger-Point Injection), noninfectious inflammatory arthritis, tendinitis, bursitis, or neuritis
* To stimulate the body's inflammatory cascade in order to promote healing (i.e., prolotherapy, [Dagenais, 2007])

Indications for Corticosteroid Injections

Corticosteroids have a marked effect on inflammation. There are no good data to indicate that steroid injections decrease the long-term adverse effects of chronic degenerative OA, but there is no doubt that they result in acute symptomatic improvement, especially over the first 1 to 4 weeks. Several meta-analyses and systematic reviews support the use of the intraarticular corticosteroids in the treatment of adhesive capsulitis or impingement syndrome of the shoulder (Blanchard, 2010; Gaujoux-Viala, 2009; Griesser, 2011), osteoarthritis (OA) of the knee (Arroll, 2004; Cheng, 2012; Hepper, 2009) and tendon injections for lateral and medial epicondylitis of the elbow (Krogh, 2013; Coombes, 2010), carpal tunnel syndrome (Marshall, 2007), de Quervain tenosynovitis and trigger finger (Peters-Veluthamaningal, 2009). Randomized trial data also support steroid injection of the hip for OA (Qvistgaard, 2006). For trochanteric bursitis, now generally called greater trochanter pain, there is evidence supporting steroid injections (Brinks, 2011). Cochrane has recently found some systematic review evidence supporting steroid injections for plantar fasciitis (David, 2017).

Box 180.1 lists the conditions that are improved with local corticosteroid therapy. Localized pain that persists more than a few weeks after a trial of NSAIDs warrants an injection with steroids. Injections should be considered primarily when the potential toxicity or intolerance to NSAIDs outweighs the risk of local corticosteroids. Tramèr et al. (2001) noted in their metaanalysis that individuals chronically (≥2 months) using NSAIDs had a 1:1220 chance of dying from a gastrointestinal complication. Morbidity risks associated with prolonged NSAID use, including gastrointestinal bleeding, are even greater. In contrast, death occurring after intraarticular injections comes predominantly from septic arthritis, which occurs in anywhere from 1 in 3000 to 1 in 50,000 cases—with a mortality rate of about 15%.

Indications for Hyaluronic Acid Supplementation

Synovial fluid functions as a lubricant and a shock absorber in the joint. In OA, it retains very little of these intrinsic physical properties.

1221

At a critical load, normal synovial fluid changes its mechanical properties from viscous lubricant to elastic shock absorber. This change occurs between walking and running and is determined by the dynamic stress of both the frequency and the force of the load—a property which is diminished in OA. In addition, the concentration of hyaluronan in the synovial fluid in patients with OA is less than normal. Injected hylans and hyaluronans have properties similar to normal synovial fluid, and although they may only remain in the knee less than 2 weeks, the beneficial effects can persist up to a year (mean duration of 8.2 months). There is some evidence that they stimulate endogenous production of the synovial fluid. There is no evidence that viscosupplementation retards the progression of joint deterioration, but a Cochrane review (Bellamy, 2006) concluded that viscosupplementation showed beneficial effects on pain and patient function; this modality shows promise of postponing for years the need for total knee replacement. Studies are ongoing to assess its efficacy in other joints, because it is currently only Food and Drug Administration–approved for use in the knee. Certain

---

BOX 180.1   Conditions Improved With Local Corticosteroid Injection

Articular Conditions
Coccydynia
Crystal-induced arthritis
- Gout
- Pseudogout
Ganglions
Osteoarthritis
Rheumatoid arthritis
Seronegative spondyloarthropathies
- Ankylosing spondylitis
- Arthritis associated with inflammatory bowel disease
- Psoriasis
- Reiter syndrome

Nonarticular Conditions
Bursitis
- Anserine
- Olecranon
- Prepatellar
- Subacromial
- Trochanteric
Costochondritis
Fibrositis
- Localized (trigger points)
- Systemic
Morton neuroma
Neuritis
- Carpal tunnel syndrome
- Cubital tunnel syndrome
- Tarsal tunnel syndrome
Periarthritis
- Adhesive capsulitis
Tenosynovitis/tendonitis
- Bicipital tendonitis
- de Quervain disease
- Golfer's elbow (medial epicondylitis)
- Impingement syndrome
- Plantar fasciitis
- Rotator cuff
- Supraspinatus tendonitis
- Tennis elbow (lateral epicondylitis)
- Trigger finger
Tietze syndrome

Modified from Pfenninger JL. Injections of joints and soft tissue. Part I. General guidelines. *Am Fam Physician*. 1991;44:1196.

---

experts are already using it in other joints, although this is considered off-label and usually not covered by insurance. The materials injected (hylans and hyaluronans) are pharmacologically inert so the Food and Drug Administration classifies them as "devices," not "drugs."

- Approved for use in knee only
- May be used instead of, or after, intraarticular corticosteroid injections and before surgical intervention
- Effective in all stages of OA of the knee, although it wanes in the most advanced stages
- Is being studied for use in other joints

Indications for Prolotherapy

Prolotherapy is an alternative form of injection therapy, used by some clinicians to treat chronic musculoskeletal pain syndromes. *Prolo* is derived from proliferation, because the treatment causes the proliferation (growth and formation) of new connective tissue in areas that have become weak. The concept behind this technique is to stimulate the body's own inflammatory cascade to promote reabsorption of unhealthy tissue, such as degenerative fibroblasts in injured tendons, and the creation of new, healthy tissue. Inflammation-promoting agents (>10% dextrose solutions, phenol- or sodium-morrhuate–containing solutions, autologous blood, platelet-rich plasma) are injected into the area of injury, often with the aid of ultrasound to best localize the target.

Prolotherapy is most often described in use with tendinopathy, and there is some evidence to suggest that it is an effective therapy in treating the degenerative tissues identified. The treatment most likely achieves its maximal benefit when coupled with physical therapy focused on further stimulating growth of new tendinous tissue (Dagenais, 2007). As prolotherapy is an emerging technique that can be highly operator dependent, those interested in providing this service are encouraged to consult with a prolotherapist or complete a course of instruction prior to beginning prolotherapy injections in an office practice. As of 2014, a Cochrane review found insufficient evidence for use of platelet-rich plasma prolotherapy for treating musculoskeletal soft tissue injuries.

CONTRAINDICATIONS

- Cellulitis or broken skin over the intended entry site for the injection or aspiration
- Anticoagulant therapy that is not well controlled
- Severe primary coagulopathy
- Infected effusion of a bursa or a periarticular structure (for injection)
- More than three previous injections in a weight-bearing joint in the preceding 12-month period (relative—concern for theoretic joint destruction)
- Suspected bacteremia (Unless the joint itself is suspected as the source of the bacteremia, it should not be tapped. Doing so could inoculate the joint space and cause infection.)
- Unstable joints (for steroid injection)
- Inaccessible joints (For many primary care clinicians, this includes the hip joint, the sacroiliac joint, and the joints of the vertebral column.)
- Joint prostheses (If infection is suspected, consider a referral to the orthopedist that placed the prosthesis, if possible.)
- Pregnancy (relative)
- Lack of response to two or three prior injections (relative)

EQUIPMENT

In the past, joint injections were frequently performed without gloves with only an alcohol wipe. In contrast, some clinicians still use an extensive sterile draping procedure. Although the former is most likely inadequate, the latter is probably unnecessary unless the patient is immunosuppressed, diabetic, or at high risk of infection. Most injections are administered after an alcohol, chlorhexidine, or povidone–iodine wipe. Gloves (sterile or nonsterile) should be used. When a culture is anticipated, sterile gloves are more customary. Masks are unnecessary. Universal blood and body fluid precautions should be followed.

Required equipment includes the following:

- Chlorhexidine, povidone-iodine wipes, or alcohol wipes
- Sterile or nonsterile gloves
- Sterile drapes (optional)
- 22- to 27-gauge, 1.5-inch needle for injections
- 18- to 21-gauge, 1.5-inch needle for aspirations
- 30-gauge, 0.5-inch needle, if skin anesthesia is to be given (usually not needed)
- 1- to 10-mL syringe for injections (Luer-Lok is recommended)
- 3- to 50-mL syringe for aspirations
- Single-dose vials of 1% lidocaine

NOTE: There are two reasons to use single-dose vials. It is extremely rare to have an allergic reaction to lidocaine (an amide). Although rare, reactions do occur to the preservative (parabens) that is used in multidose vials. Local anesthetics with an ester base (e.g., procaine [Novocain]) can cause allergic reactions. So, using a single-dose vial of lidocaine makes it highly unlikely that there will be a reaction. Second, many steroids will precipitate when mixed with the parabens preservative. This leads to uneven distribution in the syringe as well as the injection of small crystals into the site, and these crystals themselves could cause an inflammatory process (Fig. 180.1). Theoretically, a homogeneous solution would be more efficacious, although no studies have looked at the issue and many feel it is a moot point and of little concern. Certain manufacturers, however, do not recommend injecting precipitated steroids.

Many practitioners will use a longer-acting local anesthetic such as bupivacaine (Marcaine). Although this addition in most cases will not have any untoward effects, it should be noted that there have been instances of myotoxicity associated with bupivacaine, and given that it is only intended to provide short- to medium-term relief of symptoms, one might question its regular use.

EDITOR'S NOTE: Although it is only one study (Karpie and Chi, 2007) and it only involved bovine cartilage, since reading this study, I have quit mixing any "caine" analgesic with injectable steroids for intraarticular injections. As it turns out, this allows me to give a slightly higher dose of steroid per injection and injected pure steroid preparations also seem to offer some immediate analgesic effect. When injecting a tendon or a bursa, I still mix the steroid with lidocaine; I want the steroid to diffuse over a large area.

- Hemostat (to be used if joint is to be aspirated then injected using different syringes but same needle)
- Tubes for culture or other laboratory studies (if aspiration is performed)
- Injectable corticosteroid preparation (Tables 180.1 and 180.2)

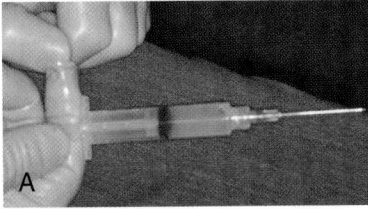
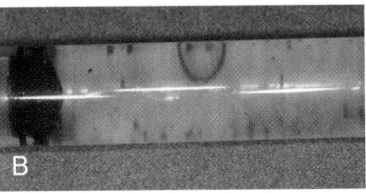

Fig. 180.1 (A) Example of precipitation of steroid (Celestone Soluspan) when mixed with lidocaine solution from a multidose vial. (B) Steroid in solution (Celestone Soluspan) when mixed with lidocaine from a single-dose vial. It is preferable to have the steroid in solution rather than in precipitated form. (Courtesy John L. Pfenninger, MD, The Medical Procedures Center, Midland, MI.)

TABLE 180.1   Relative Potency of Corticosteroids

Corticosteroid	Relative Anti-inflammatory Potency	Approximate Equivalent Dose (mg)
Short-Acting Preparations		
Cortisone	0.8	25
Hydrocortisone	1	20
Intermediate-Acting Preparations		
Prednisone	3.5	5
Prednisolone tebutate (Hydeltra-TBA)	4	5
Triamcinolone (Aristocort, Aristospan, Kenalog)	5	4
Methylprednisolone acetate (Depo-Medrol)	5	4
Long-Acting Preparations		
Dexamethasone (Decadron-LA)	25	0.6
Betamethasone (Celestone Soluspan)	25	0.6

Modified from Leversee JH. Aspiration of joints and soft tissue injections. *Prim Care* 1986;13:572.

TABLE 180.2   Common Corticosteroids and Recommended Dosages for Various Joint Injections

Corticosteroid	Concentration (mg/mL)	Large Joint* Dosage (mg)	Medium Joint† Dosage (mg)	Small Joint†,‡ Dosage (mg)	Ganglia (mg)	Tendon Sheath (mg)	Bursa (mg)
Hydrocortisone acetate	25, 50	40–100	20–40	8–20	20–40	20–50	40–90
Prednisolone tebutate (Hydeltra-TBA)	20	20–30	10–20	8–10	10–20	4–10	20
Prednisolone sodium phosphate	20	10–20	5–10	4–5	5–10	3–8	20
Triamcinolone hexacetonide (Aristospan)	5, 20	20–30	10–20	8–10	10–20	4–10	20
Triamcinolone diacetate (Aristocrat)	25, 40	20–40	10–20	8–10	10–20	4–10	20
Triamcinolone acetonide (Kenalog)	10, 40	20–40	10–20	8–10	10–20	4–10	20
Methylprednisolone acetate (Depo-Medrol)	20, 40, 80	20–40	10–40	8–10	4–20	4–10	20
Dexamethasone sodium phosphate (Decadron)	4	2–4	1–3	0.8–1	1–2	0.4–1	2–3
Dexamethasone acetate (Decadron-LA)	8	2–4	1–3	0.8–1	1–2	0.4–1	2–3
Betamethasone acetate/phosphate (Celestine Soluspan)	6	6–12	3–6	1.5–3	1–3	1.5–2	3–6

*Such as knee, shoulder, ankle.
†Such as elbow, wrist.
‡Such as metacarpophalangeal, interphalangeal, acromioclavicular, temporomandibular.

TABLE 180.3 Steroid Solubility	
Steroid	**Solubility (% wt/vol)**
Triamcinolone hexacetonide	0.0002
Triamcinolone acetate	0.004
Prednisolone tebutate	0.001
Methylprednisolone acetate	0.001
Hydrocortisone acetate	0.002

TABLE 180.4 Adverse Effects of Local Corticosteroid Therapy	
Complication	**Estimated Prevalence**
Postinjection flare	2%–5%
Steroid arthropathy	0.8%
Tendon rupture	<1%
Facial flushing	<1%
Skin atrophy, depigmentation	<1%
Iatrogenic infectious arthritis	0.01%
Transient paresis of injected extremity	Rare
Hypersensitivity reaction	Rare
Asymptomatic pericapsular calcification	43%
Acceleration of cartilage attrition	Unknown

From Gray RG, Gottlieb NL. Intraarticular corticosteroids: an updated assessment. *Clin Orthop Relat Res.* 1983;177:253.

A reasonable rule of thumb is that the greater the water solubility of the corticosteroid, the more rapid the onset of action, and the shorter the duration of effect. Thus steroids with a lower degree of water solubility would in general be more effective in a chronic disease process, such as OA, whereas an acute inflammatory process might be more responsive to a shorter-acting preparation (Table 180.3).

NOTE: It is best to pick out one or two preparations and learn them well. It is not necessary to be familiar with all the drugs listed. There is no consensus in the literature as to the "best" drug or the optimal dosages. Table 180.2 offers our recommendations for appropriate dosing. Instead of stocking them in a primary care clinic, which would be very expensive if allowed to expire, giving the patient a prescription to obtain the supplement at a pharmacy is usually an option.

- Ethyl chloride spray (optional)
- Hyaluronic acid preparation (if used)—sodium hyaluronate (Hyalgan, Supartz, Euflexxa, Orthovisc, Monovisc) and hylan G-F 20 (Synvisc and Synvisc-one); dosages, and estimated cost per treatment (note dynamic marketplace with marked variability) are as follows:
  - Hyalgan: five injections, 1 week apart ($990.00)
  - Supartz: five injections, 1 week apart ($1110.00)
  - Euflexxa: three injections, 1 week apart ($1110.00)
  - Orthovisc: three injections, 1 week apart ($1536.00)
  - Synvisc: three injections, 1 week apart ($1195.00)
  - Synvisc-one: one injection ($1195.00)
  - Monovisc: one injection ($1170)
- Adhesive bandage dressing
- Ultrasound (see later discussion for information regarding ultrasound-guided injections and Chapter 171, Musculoskeletal Ultrasound)

PREPROCEDURE PATIENT PREPARATION

Inform the patient of the risks, benefits, and possible complications of injection therapy. This information is especially important if steroids are used. Rarely is there ever a complication from the use of lidocaine alone. However, with steroids, and especially with repeated injections, there are some adverse consequences (see the Complications section and Table 180.4). There can be some pain or discomfort, and damage to nearby structures. Alternatives to injection should be discussed, if there are any. Warn the patient of a possible failure to obtain relief, and that a second or even a third injection may be needed. Whether or not steroids have significant adverse effects on the cartilage and bone itself when steroids are injected into the joint space, and the degree of this reaction, is controversial. However, the effects would appear to be minimal, especially when used appropriately. If they are diabetic, hyperglycemia can occur, so they may need to monitor their sugars more closely over the next few days. If a local anesthetic is going to be used in the skin, the patient should be warned. They should also be informed if ethyl chloride is available and will be used to numb the skin prior to injection.

EDITOR'S NOTE: Since I cannot always be sure I'll have ethyl chloride spray available, I have somewhat quit using it as an analgesic prior to musculoskeletal injections. If the patient has used it before, their patient satisfaction is generally much less if not available for the next injection. I have also quit using a subcutaneous local anesthetic injection or an injection along the anticipated needle track. Local anesthetic injections burn; there is also no way I can also guarantee where the steroid injection needle will track. For most intraarticular injections, I now use a 23-gauge needle, the same needle used for flu shots in our clinics. So I tell the patient we will be doing an injection very similar to a flu shot even though we are entering the joint. Almost all patients tolerate this very well.

TECHNIQUE

Before injection therapy, consider the differential diagnosis. If a tumor or fracture is possible, radiographs should be obtained. Many times, especially with trigger-point injection (see Chapter 181, Trigger-Point Injection), x-rays are unnecessary. Other diagnoses may also be fairly straightforward and not require a prior radiographic examination either. If the diagnosis is in question or if the patient is at risk for bone metastases (e.g., a history of breast or prostate cancer), the condition should be clarified before injection therapy.

Generally, the clinician injects a combination of lidocaine with the steroid of choice. Single-dose vials of lidocaine should be used to avoid the preservative/precipitation problems (see earlier comments and the "Complications" section). Using a rather large volume of lidocaine may be beneficial. Not only does it disperse the steroid in a less concentrated solution, the volume itself may have a therapeutic effect. In some instances, only a minimal amount of lidocaine can be used (e.g., ganglion cysts, trigger fingers). In other sites, larger amounts are recommended (e.g., lidocaine 5 to 10 mL in a shoulder or knee mixed with 0.5 to 1 mL of selected steroid). A good rule of thumb is to use more, not less, when it comes to lidocaine.

The recommended dosages of medications (Table 180.5) and the specific techniques for various injection sites (Figs. 180.2 to 180.24) are included in this chapter.

General

The general approach is as follows:

1. Identify the site of entry and mark it with a thumbnail, ballpoint pen, or indelible marker. Making a circular indentation at the designated site with the retracted end of a ballpoint pen is an excellent way to avoid losing your landmarks when cleaning the area.
2. Prep the area with an alcohol, chlorhexidine, or povidone-iodine wipe. (Note that alcohol often removes ink and skin marker solutions.)

TABLE 180.5	Needle Size and Drug Dosage for Injection Therapy		
Anatomic Structure	**Needle Gauge (Length)**	**Dose of 1% Lidocaine (mL)**	**Dose of Methylprednisolone Acetate (mg)**
Abductor tendon of thumb (de Quervain disease)	25 (1.5 inch)	3–4	10–20
Acromioclavicular joint	22–25 (1–1.5 inch)	2–4	4–10
Ankle	22 (1–1.5 inch)	3–5	20–40
Anserine bursa	22–25 (1.5 inch)	3–5	20–40
Biceps tendon	22 (1.5 inch)	5–10	10–20
Calcaneal bursa	22 (1.5 inch)	5	20–40
Carpal tunnel	25 (1.5 inch)	1	20–40
Elbow	25 (1.5 inch)	3–4	10–20
Radiohumeral joint	22 (1–1.5 inch)	3–5	20–30
Lateral or medial epicondyle ("tennis elbow," "golfer's elbow")	22–25 (1–1.5 inch)	3–5	10–30
Olecranon bursa	22 (1–1.5 inch)	2–3	10–20
Finger and toe joints (interphalangeal)	25 (1 inch)	0.5–1.0	4–10
Flexor tendon sheath (trigger finger)	25 (1 inch)	0.25–0.5	4–10
Ganglion of wrist, other	18–20 (1–1.5 inch)	0.25–0.5	4–10
Hip joint	20 (1.5–3 inch)	5	40–80
Knee intraarticular space	20 (1.5 inch)	5	20–80
Plantar fascia	22 (1.5 inch)	2–4	15–30
Prepatellar bursa	20–22 (1–1.5 inch)	3	20–40
Shoulder intraarticular space	20 (1.5 inch)	5–7	20–40
Shoulder rotator cuff tendon	18–20 (1.5 inch)	5	20–40
Shoulder subacromial bursa	22 (1.5–2 inch)	5–7	30–40
Tarsal tunnel	25 (1.5–1 inch)	1–2	10–20
Temporomandibular joint	25 (1.5–1 inch)	1–2	5–20
Trigger point	25 (1.5 inch)	3–5	10–30
Trochanteric bursa	22 (1.5–2 inch)	5–10	20–40
Wrist joint	22–25 (1–1.5 inch)	2–4	20–40

Modified from Pfenninger JL. Injections of joints and soft tissue. Part II. Guidelines for specific joints. *Am Fam Physician*. 1991;44:1690.

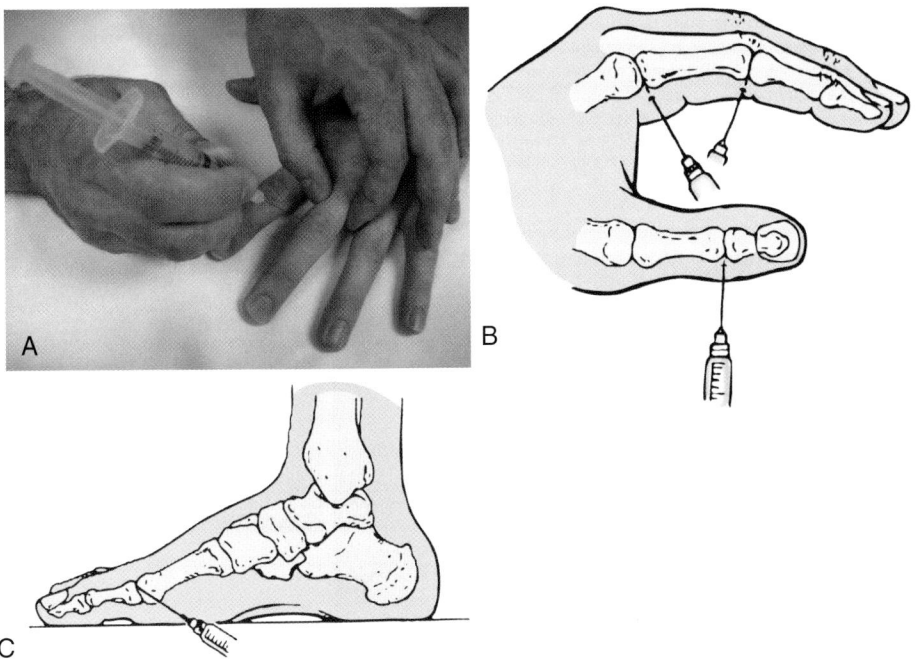

Fig. 180.2 Injecting finger and toe joints. (A) Appropriate technique for injecting a finger joint. Tendons run over the dorsum of the finger, whereas nerves and vessels run laterally. Open the joint slightly by flexing it and then inject between the ligaments and the vascular structures as noted. The needle enters at a 45-degree angle to the joint. Any of the finger (B) and toe (C) joints may be aspirated or injected in the lateral or medial aspect. Slightly flex the joint to open the joint space. Direct the needle to enter just medial or lateral to the extensor tendon, avoiding too lateral or medial an approach where the nerve and vascular structures run. Use a 25-gauge, 1-inch needle with 0.5 to 1.0 mL 1% lidocaine and 4 to 10 mg of methylprednisolone acetate or equivalent (see Tables 180.2 and 180.5).

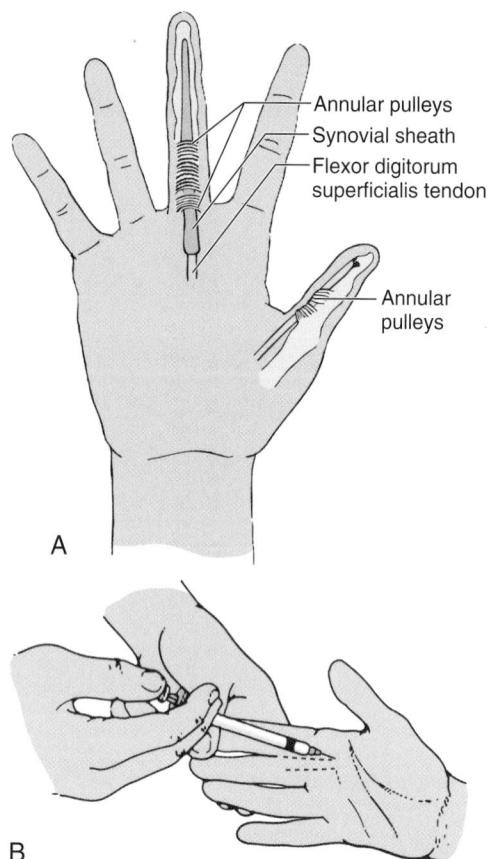

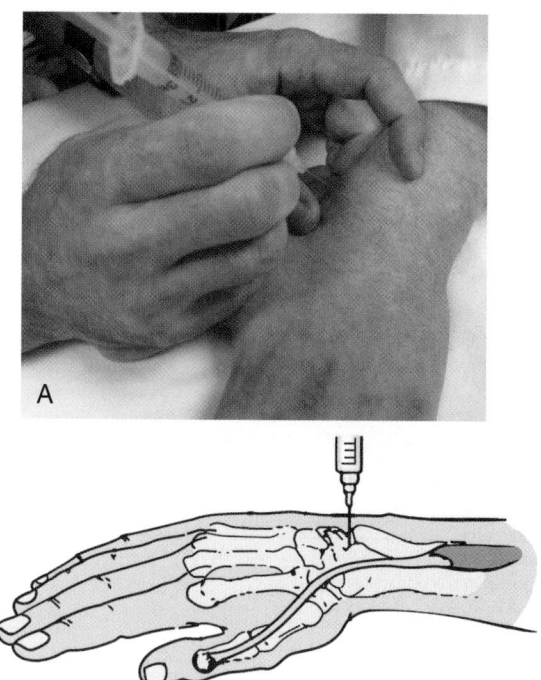

Fig. 180.3   Trigger finger. (A) The anatomy of a finger showing the annular pulleys, which maintain the flexor close to the bony structures. When the tendon becomes inflamed and enlarges, it catches on the pulleys, causing a snapping with extension or a "trigger finger." (B) Identify the flexor tendon involved. Insert the needle at the distal palmar crease. Attempt to position it peritendinously. When the needle is in position, the syringe will move with flexion of the finger. Use a 25-gauge, 1-inch needle with 0.25 to 0.5 mL 1% lidocaine and 4 to 10 mg of methylprednisolone acetate or equivalent (see Tables 180.2 and 180.5).

Fig. 180.4   Wrist joint. (A) Injection of the wrist joint. The hand is held in slight flexion, and the needle is inserted just distal to the radius in the "snuff box." (B) Flex the joint 20 degrees to open the joint spaces. The dorsal approach is generally used. Position the needle perpendicular to the skin surface. Enter at a site distal to the radial head and lateral to the extensor pollicis longus tendon (just ulnar to the anatomic "snuff box"). If the needle can be easily inserted to 1 or 2 cm, it is correctly positioned in the joint space. The intercarpal joints have interconnecting synovial spaces, and the contents of one correctly placed injection will disperse into the entire joint complex. Use an 18- to 20-gauge, 1- to 1.5-inch needle with 0.5 to 1.0 mL 1% lidocaine and 4 to 10 mg of methylprednisolone acetate or equivalent (see Tables 180.2 and 180.5).

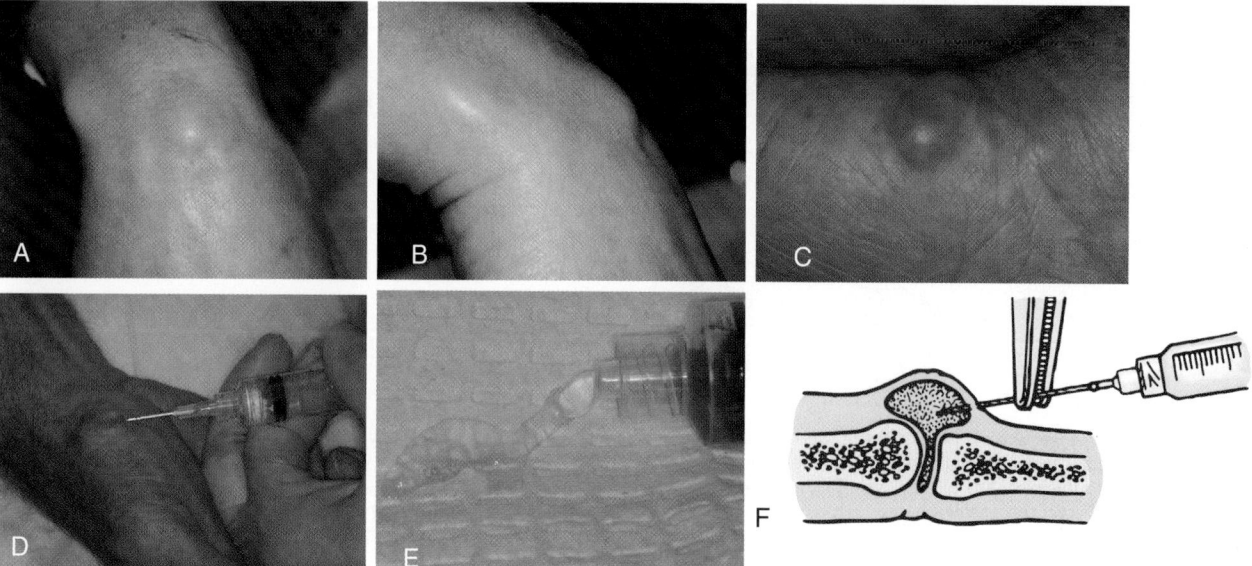

Fig. 180.5   A ganglion is a manifestation of joint inflammation. (A) Frontal view. (B) Side view. (C) Example of an unusual ganglion cyst on the thenar eminence. (D) Aspiration of the cyst. Hold the needle in position with the hemostat and remove the syringe. Attach the steroid-containing syringe and inject the contents. (Some have used fibrin sealants, hypertonic saline, and other irritants for attempts to "scar down" the cyst.) (E) The contents are often thick, and there may only be minimal return of a gel-like material. (F) Use an 18- to 20-gauge, 1- to 1.5-inch needle with 0.5 to 1.0 mL 1% lidocaine and 4 to 10 mg of methylprednisolone acetate or equivalent (see Tables 180.2 and 180.5). (A–E, Courtesy John L. Pfenninger, MD, The Medical Procedures Center, Midland, MI.)

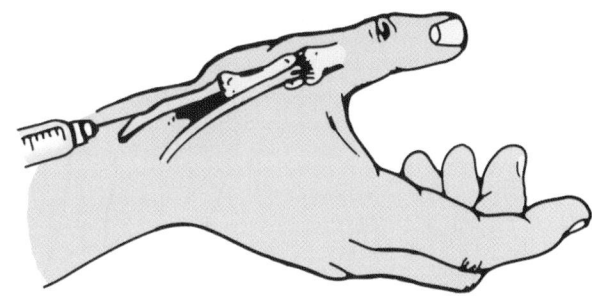

Fig. 180.6 De Quervain disease. Maximally abduct the thumb to accentuate and identify the tendon. Insert the needle parallel to (but not into) the tendon. Inject at the areas of greatest tenderness. Postinjection splinting may still be necessary. Use a 25-gauge, 1.5-inch needle with 3 to 4 mL 1% lidocaine and 10 to 20 mg of methyl-prednisolone acetate or equivalent (see Tables 180.2 and 180.5).

A

B

Median nerve
Palmaris aponeurosis
Flexor retinaculum
Palmaris longus tendon
Distal palmar crease

C

Distal crease
Flexor retinaculum
Radial artery
Flexor tendons
Median nerve   Palmaris   Ulnar artery   Flexor
aponeurosis   and nerve   tendons

D

E

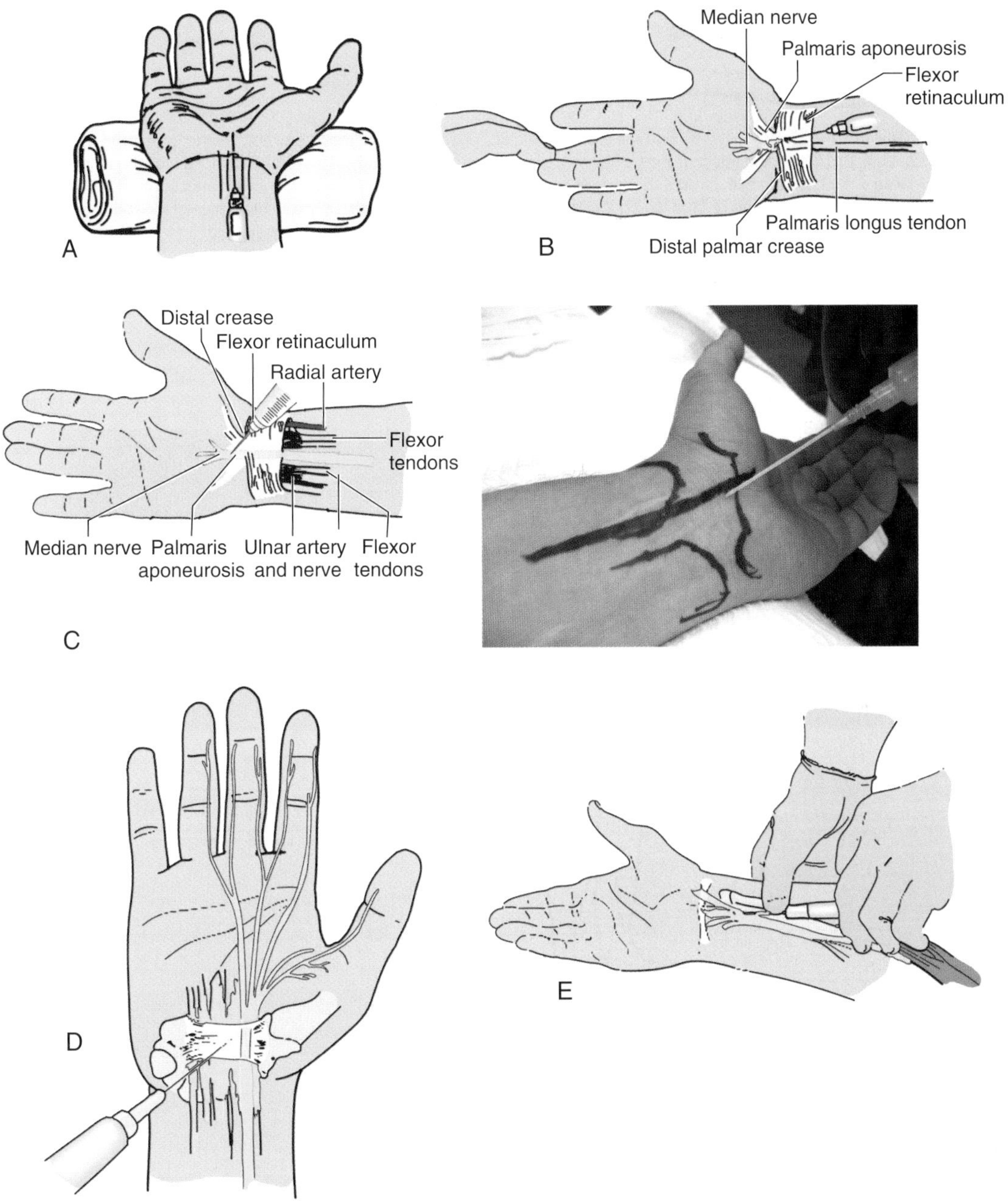

Fig. 180.7 Carpal tunnel syndrome. Four approaches to injection: (A) Traditional method. Dorsiflex the wrist 30 degrees or keep it flat and rest it on a rolled towel. Insert the needle at the distal crease of the wrist either lateral or medial to the palmaris longus tendon. (B) Find the tendon by having the patient flex the middle finger against resistance or abduct the thumb and little finger together. Angle the needle downward at a 45-degree angle toward the tip of the middle finger. If there is any discomfort in the fingers, withdraw and reposition the needle. Advance 1 to 2 cm until there is *no* resistance, and then inject the medication. (C) Alternative method. Insertion of the needle directly over the carpal tunnel. Use a perpendicular approach going directly through the flexor retinaculum into the median nerve space. (D) A third method of injecting the carpal tunnel. The needle is inserted just radial to the pisiform bone and directed toward the carpal tunnel just beneath the transverse carpal ligament. The needle goes dorsally and distally to terminate within the carpal tunnel just to the ulnar side and dorsal to the median nerve. (E) A more recent approach is to inject on the volar aspect of the forearm 4 cm proximal to the wrist crease between the palmaris longus tendon (see previous description) and the radial flexor tendon. The needle is inserted in a distal direction with the syringe lifted 10 to 20 degrees up from the parallel. This approach supposedly minimizes chances of trauma to the nerve. In all cases (A–E), the injection should be given with minimal pressure, slowly. If there is resistance or if the patient feels "pins and needles" in the fingers, stop immediately. If an intraneural injection occurs, there will be significant pain after injection and surgical decompression may be needed. Use a 25-gauge, 1.5-inch needle with 1 mL 1% lidocaine and 20 to 40 mg of methylprednisolone acetate or equivalent (see Tables 180.2 and 180.5).

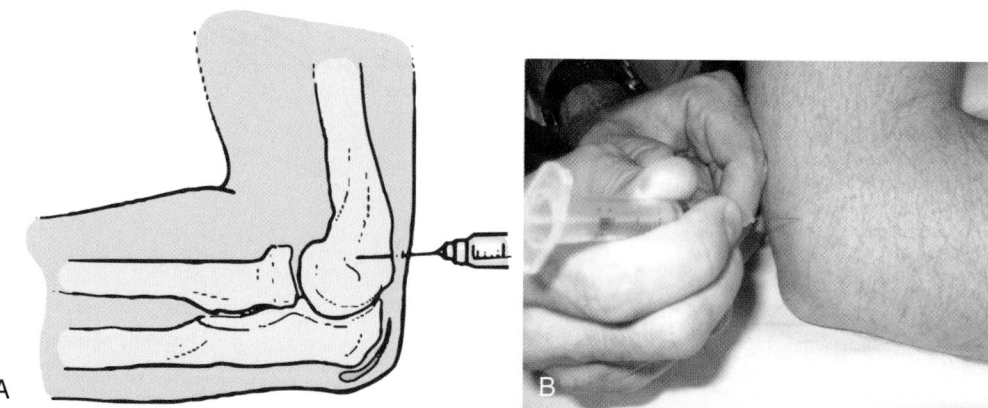

Fig. 180.8   Lateral epicondylitis (tennis elbow). (A–B) Find the area of greatest tenderness over the lateral epicondyle. Insert the needle perpendicularly until bone is felt. Withdraw the needle 1 to 2 mm and inject. It may be beneficial to fan out the injections in several directions into the extensor aponeurosis and the radial collateral ligament. Massage the injection site. If distal tenderness is still present after several minutes, another injection in a fanlike pattern may be necessary. Some experts recommend "fenestrating" the tendon by tapping it up to 20 times with the needle around the area of most discomfort. This may stimulate healing. Medial epicondylitis (golfer's elbow) is treated in a similar fashion. Use a 22- to 25-gauge, 1.5-inch needle with 3 to 5 mL 1% lidocaine and 10 to 30 mg of methylprednisolone acetate or equivalent (see Tables 180.2 and 180.5).

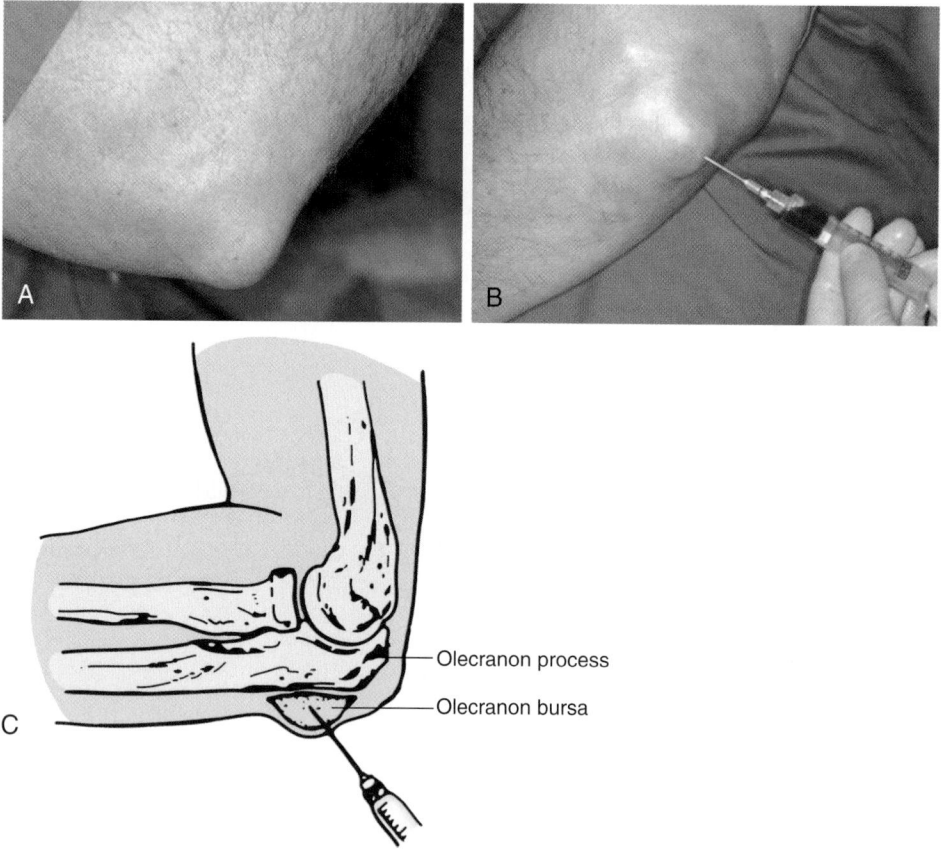

Olecranon process
Olecranon bursa

Fig. 180.9   Olecranon bursa, aspiration and injection. (A) An enlarged bursa secondary to bursitis. (B) Aspirating the olecranon bursa. This bursa is easily identified and entered. (C) Insert a large-bore needle directly into the bursa and aspirate until fluid is returned. Whether cloudy or not, the fluid should be submitted for culture and concurrent infection should be ruled out. Await the culture results before injecting with a steroid. It is next to impossible to tell whether the bursa is infected or not on a clinical basis. While waiting for the culture results, place the patient on nonsteroidal antiinflammatory drugs (NSAIDs) and wrap the area tightly. If infection is suspected, start an antibiotic to cover gram-positive pathogens while waiting for culture results. Once infection is ruled out, steroids can be used. In a double-blind study comparing focal steroid injection into the olecranon bursa with systemic NSAIDs, the most rapid benefit and most lasting effect came from steroid injections. Use an 18- to 21-gauge needle for aspiration. Use a 22-gauge, 1- to 1.5-inch needle with 2 to 3 mL 1% lidocaine and 10 to 20 mg of methylprednisolone acetate or equivalent for injection (see Tables 180.2 and 180.5). (Courtesy John L. Pfenninger, MD, The Medical Procedures Center, Midland, MI.)

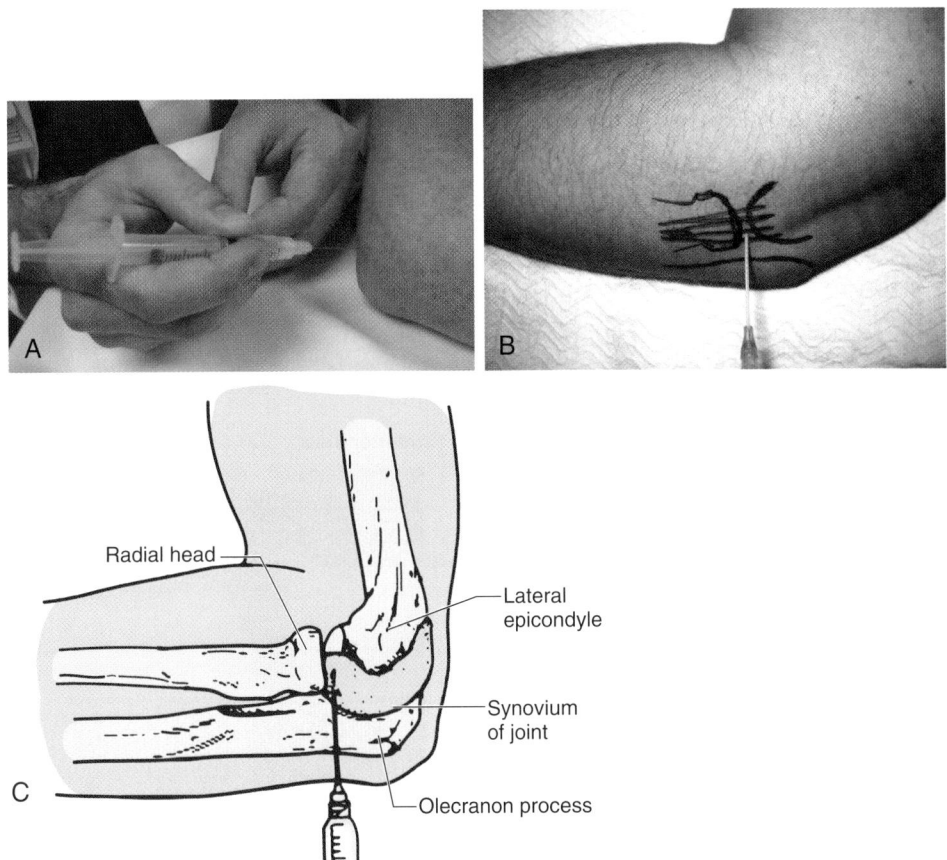

Fig. 180.10   Elbow joint. (A) Injection of the elbow joint. (B) Flex the elbow 45 degrees. Identify the lateral epicondyle. Inject into the joint space just distal to the lateral epicondyle and superior to the olecranon process of the ulna. A slight concavity can be felt just inferior to the radial head and helps identify the proper point of insertion. (C) Use a 22-gauge, 1- to 1.5-inch needle with 3 to 5 mL 1% lidocaine and 20 to 30 mg of methylprednisolone acetate or equivalent (see Tables 180.2 and 180.5).

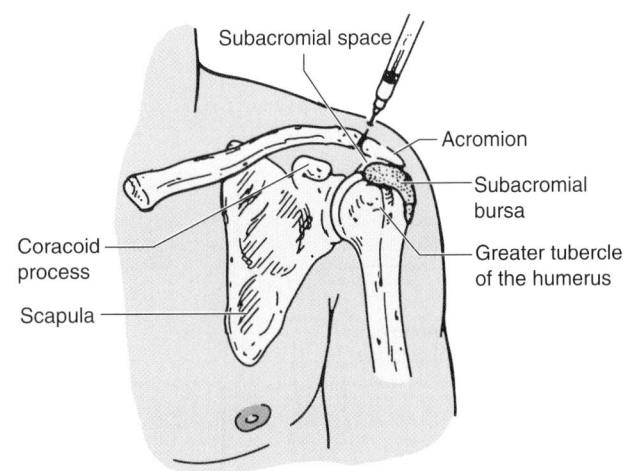

Fig. 180.11   Acromioclavicular joint. With the patient seated and arm at the side, palpate the clavicle, moving laterally until a prominence is felt. This is the acromioclavicular joint. It is about 1.5 to 2 cm inward from the lateral edge to the acromion. Insert the needle from an anterior or superior position into the joint and angle it medially, then inject. Use a 22-gauge, 1- to 1.5-inch needle with 5 to 7 mL 1% lidocaine and 30 to 40 mg of methylprednisolone acetate or equivalent (see Tables 180.2 and 180.5). Since there is limited space to inject, this is often a painful procedure and benefits from ultrasound guidance.

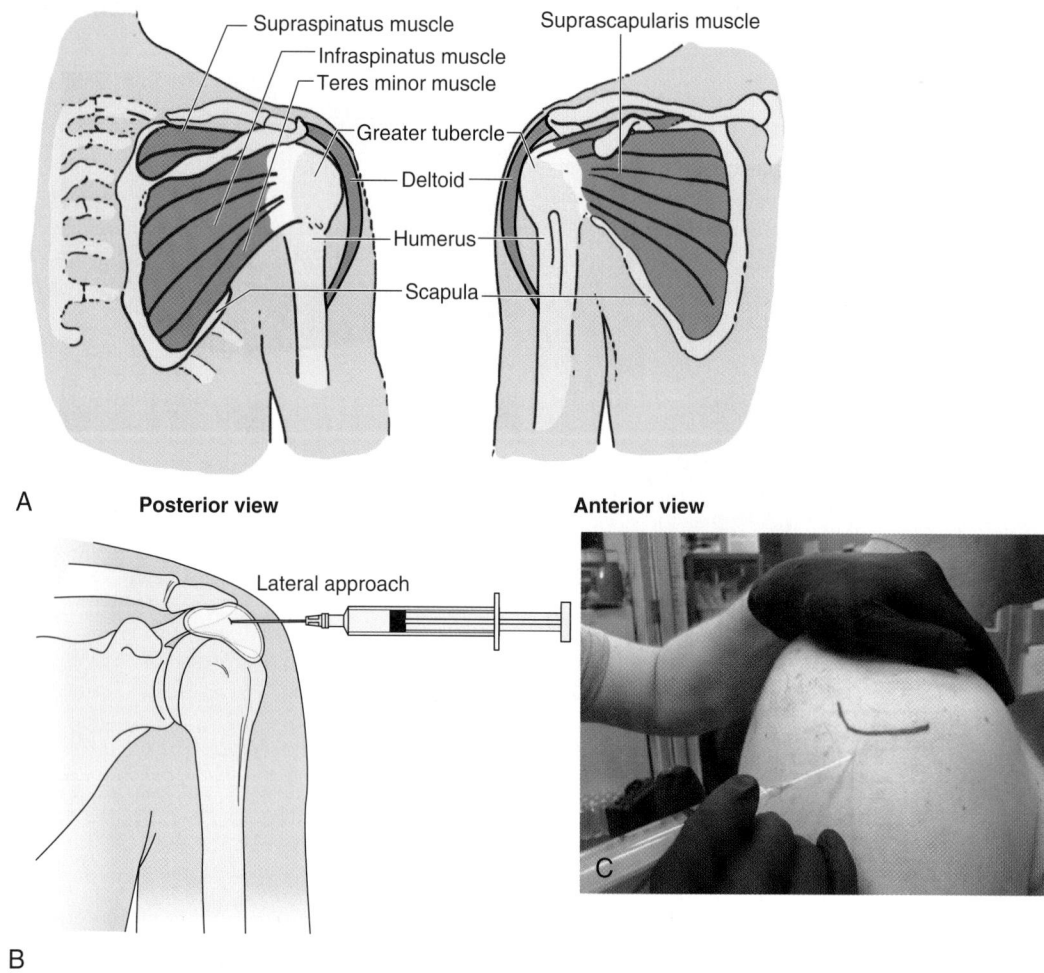

A   **Posterior view**   **Anterior view**

B

Fig. 180.12 Shoulder: Subacromial bursa. Most injection procedures involving the shoulder will include an injection into the subacromial bursa. Palpate the superior surface of the shoulder, progressing laterally until there is a slight drop-off. This is the lateral edge of the acromion. The now palpable soft spot above the humeral head is the location of the subacromial bursa. Direct the needle perpendicular to the surface and insert the needle through the deltoid muscle into the bursa. The needle should be free floating, since it is within a space, not in a muscle or tendon. The tendon of the supraspinatus, the muscle most commonly involved in a rotator cuff syndrome, is directly medial to this bursa and can be entered by directing the needle deeper. If the tendon is calcified as it is entered, a gritty sensation may be felt. Inject within the bursa, not within the tendon. (A) The muscles of the rotator cuff are demonstrated. They include the supraspinatus, the infraspinatus, teres minor, and the subscapularis. (B) The technique of a subacromial bursa injection, anterior view. (C) Injecting the subacromial bursa, posterior approach. Use a 22-gauge, 1- to 1.5-inch needle with 5 to 7 mL 1% lidocaine and 30 to 40 mg of methylprednisolone acetate or equivalent (see Tables 180.2 and 180.5). It can be reached from anterior, lateral, or posterior approach, but outcome studies suggest using lateral approach, especially in women who may have slightly smaller bursa.

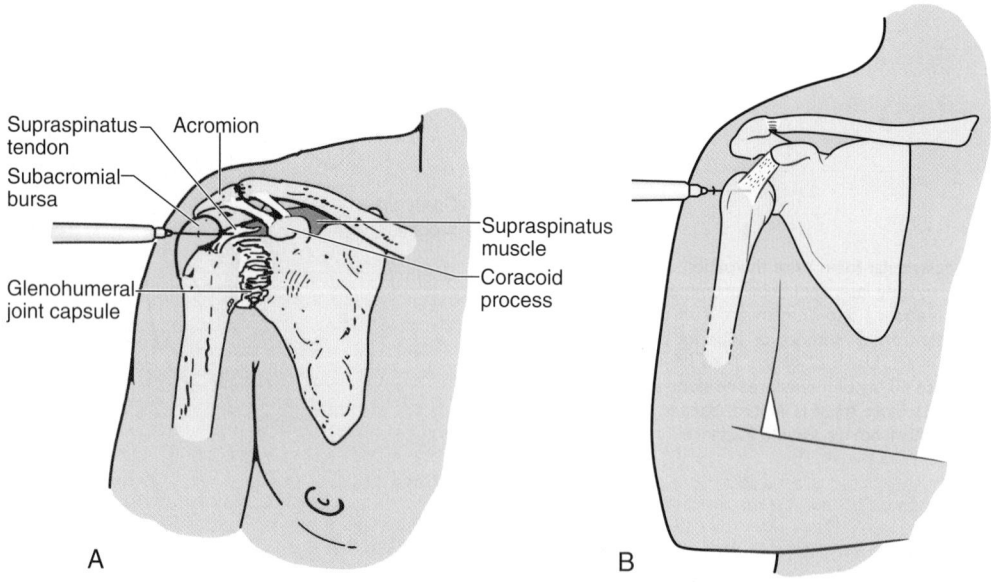

Fig. 180.13 Shoulder: Rotator cuff (supraspinatus tendinitis). (A) Use the same approach as that used for injecting the subacromial bursa (see Fig. 180.13). However, insert the needle deeper to reach the peritendinous area. (B) Alternatively, have the patient rotate the flexed arm behind the back. Palpate the inferior edge of the acromion. The greater tuberosity of the humerus lies just below it. The tendon lies in the hollow between these two bones. Use an 18- to 20-gauge, 1.5-inch needle with 5 mL 1% lidocaine and 20 to 40 mg of methylprednisolone acetate or equivalent (see Tables 180.2 and 180.5).

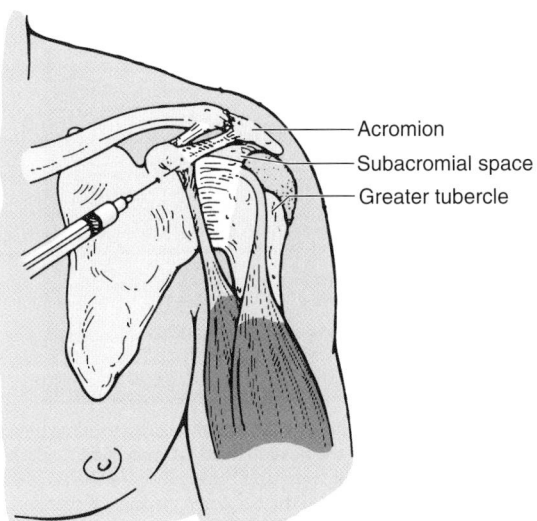

Acromion
Subacromial space
Greater tubercle

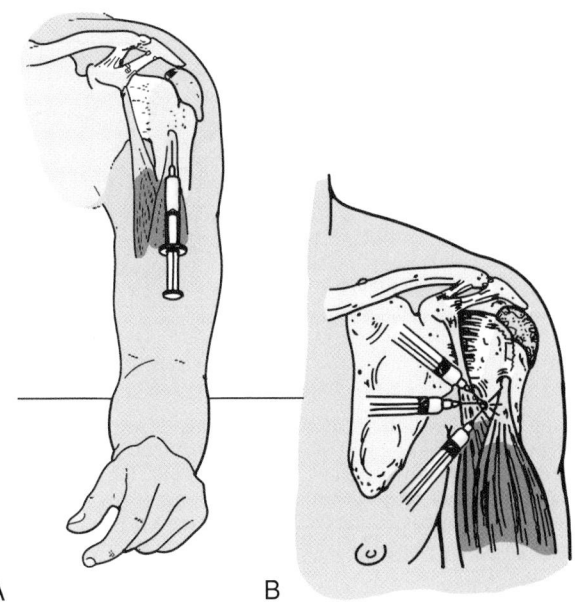

A   B

Fig. 180.14 Shoulder: Short head of the biceps. The short head of the biceps attaches to the coracoid process. This is the palpable bony prominence located inferior to the clavicle and medial to the humerus over the anterior portion of the shoulder. Rarely does this area have to be injected, but should a patient have pain and discomfort over the coracoid process, insert a needle directly into the point of maximal tenderness until it reaches the bone. Withdraw the needle 1 or 2 mm and inject. Only a small volume of steroid is needed along with relatively larger amounts of lidocaine. Additional steroid may be injected parallel to the tendon distally (if it is palpable). Use a 22-gauge, 1.5-inch needle with 5 to 10 mL 1% lidocaine and 10 to 20 mg of methylprednisolone acetate or equivalent (see Tables 180.2 and 180.5).

Fig. 180.15 Shoulder: Bicipital tendinitis (injection of the long head of the biceps tendon). (A) Have the patient seated with arm flexed 90 degrees. Identify the biceps tendon by placing your hand on the patient's shoulder with your fingers posteriorly and the thumb anteriorly over the proximal humerus. Internally and externally rotate the patient's arm. The bicipital groove is palpable anteriorly and the tendon "snap" can be felt under your thumb. Identify the most tender area of the tendon (usually in the bicipital groove on the humerus). Insert the needle into this groove and attempt to make a *peritendinous* injection of steroid and lidocaine. Often, a slip of the subacromial bursa surrounds the more proximal portion of the tendon. (B) If pain persists on palpation after the injection, further injection in a fanlike peritendinous pattern may be needed more distally. Use a 22-gauge, 1.5-inch needle with 5 to 10 mL 1% lidocaine and 10 to 20 mg of methylprednisolone acetate or equivalent (see Tables 180.2 and 180.5).

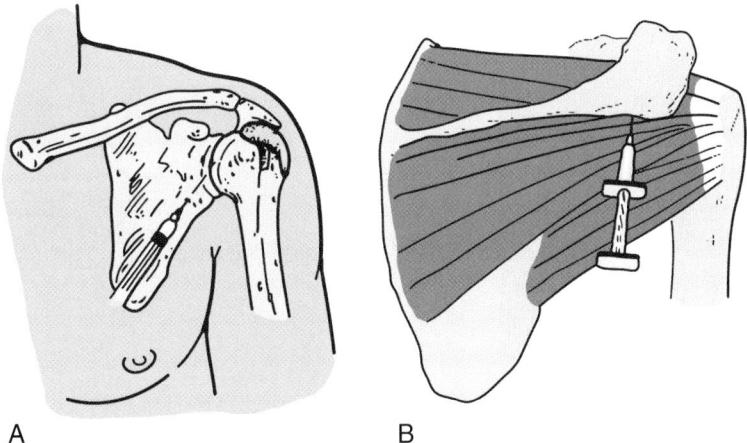

A   B

Fig. 180.16 Shoulder: Intraarticular shoulder joint injection. A posterior or an anterior approach can be used to inject into the space of the shoulder joint (scapulohumeral or glenohumeral joint). (A) In the anterior approach, externally rotate the shoulder. This movement opens the joint space. Identify the coracoid process. Insert the needle 1 cm inferior and 1 cm lateral to the coracoid process, and direct the needle perpendicularly, or slightly laterally, into the glenohumeral joint. The properly inserted needle should not contact bone. (B) With the posterior approach, the patient is again seated with the arm internally rotated across the waist. Palpate the inferoposterior aspect of the acromion with the thumb. Place the index finger on the coracoid process. Insert the needle just below the acromion and aim toward the coracoid. Insert 2 to 3 cm deep. Use a 20-gauge, 1.5-inch needle with 5 to 7 mL 1% lidocaine and 20 to 40 mg of methylprednisolone acetate or equivalent (see Tables 180.2 and 180.5).

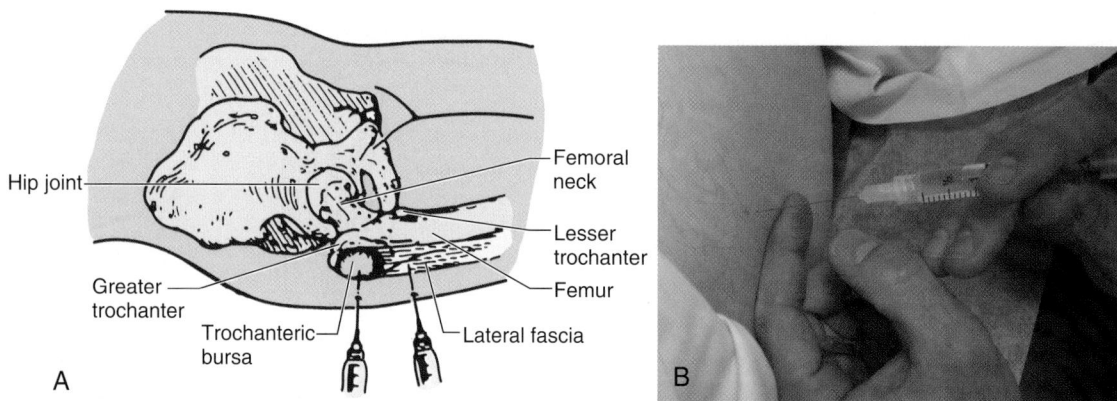

Fig. 180.17   Trochanteric bursa. (A) Trochanteric bursa is located at the most superior prominent portion of the femur. A bony prominence can be palpated. Tenderness in this area generally denotes trochanteric bursitis. Direct the needle perpendicular to the femur at the point of maximal tenderness, and insert until bone is felt. Withdraw the needle 2 to 3 mm and inject. Frequently the pain will radiate more distally (as it might with lateral epicondylitis in the arm) down the lateral portion of the femur along the fascia. If the patient is still experiencing discomfort 5 minutes after injection of the bursa and massage of the area, a more distal injection may be necessary at the areas of tenderness. (B) Injecting for trochanteric bursitis. Use a 22-gauge, 1.5- to 2-inch needle with 5 to 10 mL 1% lidocaine and 20 to 40 mg of methylprednisolone acetate or equivalent (see Tables 180.2 and 180.5).

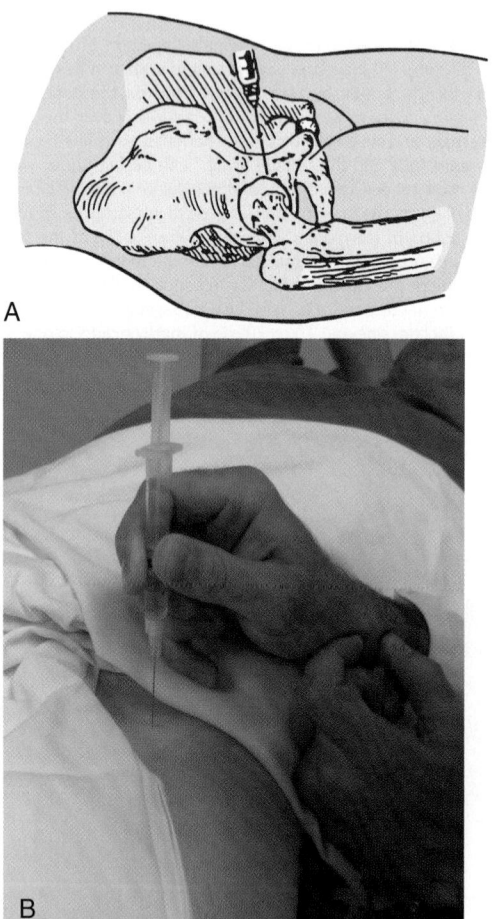

Fig. 180.18   Hip joint proper. (A) Experience is necessary to inject the hip joint itself. Even experienced practitioners often use fluoroscopy. An anterior or posterior approach can be taken. However, the anterior approach is most common. Great care must be taken to avoid entering any of the blood vessels or nerves coursing through the inguinal canal area. Position the hip so that the leg is maximally extended and internally rotated. Use a long needle to enter 2 to 3 cm below the anterior superior spine of the ilium and 2 to 3 cm lateral to the femoral pulse. The needle should point posteromedially at a 60-degree angle to the skin and then should course through the capsule ligaments until it reaches bone. Withdraw the needle slightly and aspirate for fluid. Injection may then be carried out, and there should be little resistance. (B) Injecting the hip. Use a 20-gauge, 1.5- to 3-inch needle with 5 mL 1% lidocaine and 40 to 80 mg of methylprednisolone acetate or equivalent (see Tables 180.2 and 180.5).

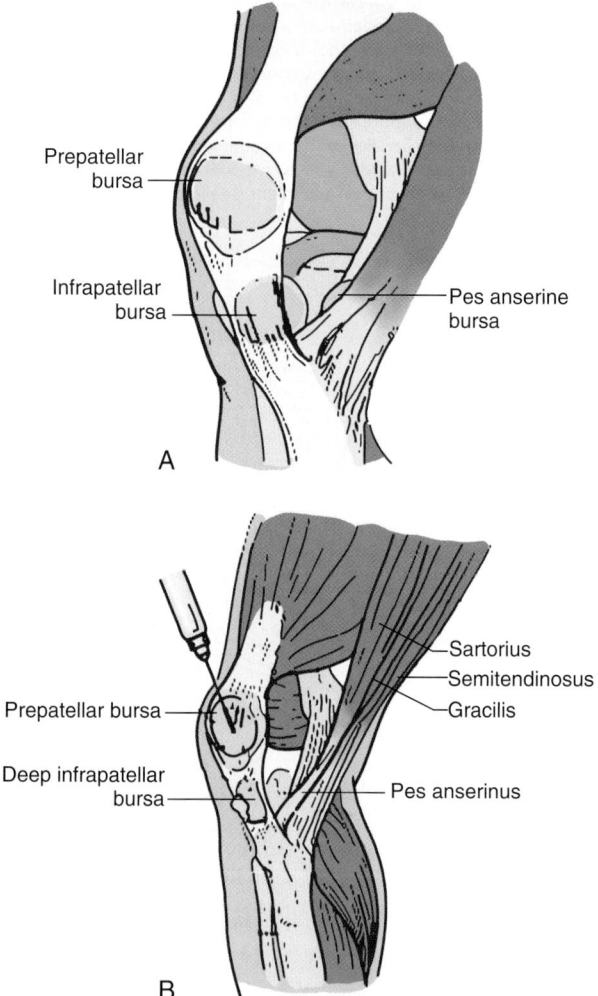

Fig. 180.19   Prepatellar bursa, one of nine bursa around the knee, but the one most frequently inflamed. (A) Identify the bursa, which is located between the skin and the patella. (B) Insert the needle just above the patella and at the lateral portion of the bursa, and direct it to the center of swelling. Aspirate fluid (for culture), switch syringes, and then inject. (Although the data are not as documented as for olecranon bursitis, the protocol for injecting this bursa can be the same.) Use a 20- to 22-gauge, 1- to 1.5-inch needle with 3 mL 1% lidocaine and 20 to 40 mg of methylprednisolone acetate or equivalent (see Tables 180.2 and 180.5).

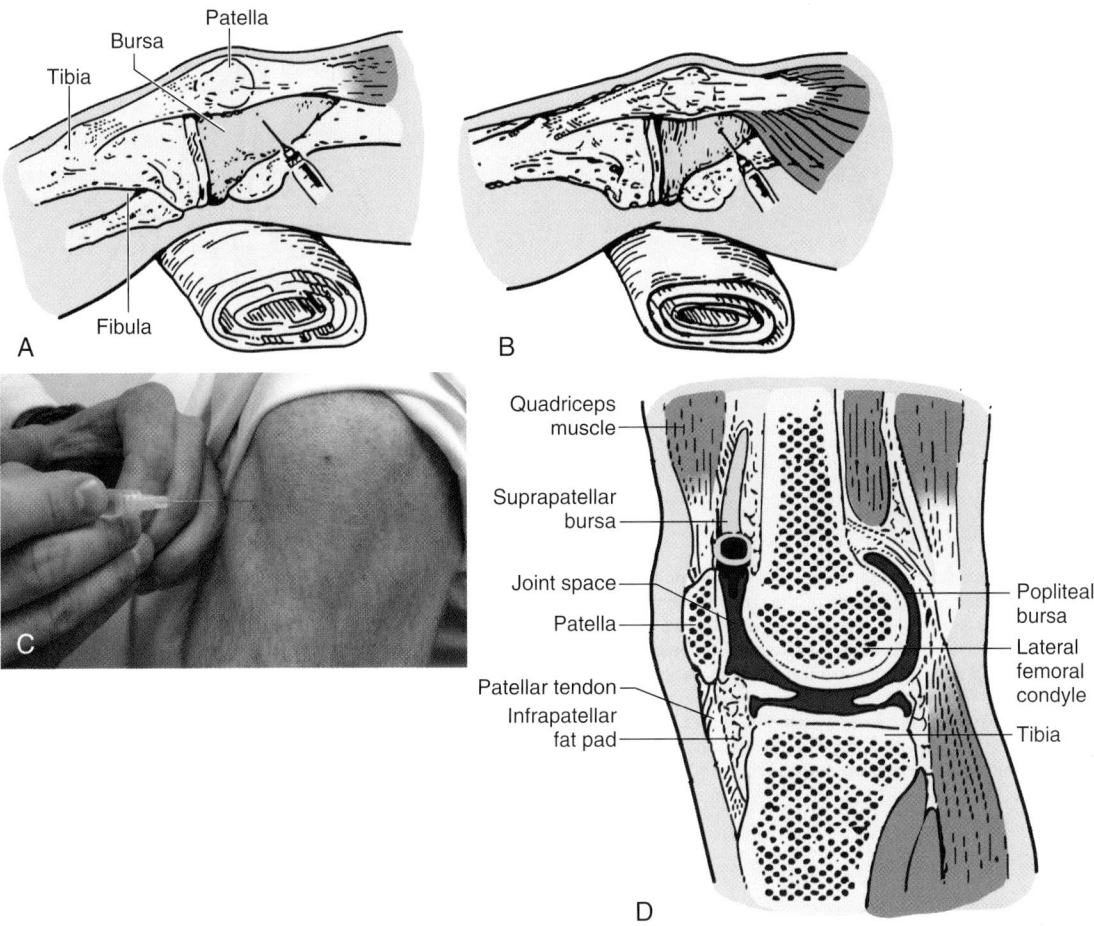

Fig. 180.20 Knee joint. The knee is one of the easiest joints to enter and one of the most common joints to aspirate and inject. Slightly flex the knee using a towel in the popliteal space with the patient lying on an examination table. Either a lateral (A) or medial (B) approach may be used. For the lateral approach, palpate the superior lateral aspect of the patella and insert the needle 1 cm superior and 1 cm lateral to this point. Apply gentle pressure on the contralateral side of the knee to encourage the fluid to pool in the area of aspiration. Direct the needle under the patella at a 45-degree angle to the midjoint area. Aspirate all fluid before injection. There should be no resistance. (C) Other approaches include entering medially or laterally directly above the joint line with the patient seated, or going directly through the patellar tendon just below the patella. Another option is to enter the joint capsule from either side of the patellar tendon just below the patella. This is an excellent location when there is little cartilage left; the knee is basically bone on bone so there is little room to maneuver the patella. (D) The knee joint space is large and is readily entered from multiple approaches. Use a 20-gauge, 1- to 1.5-inch needle with 5 mL 1% lidocaine and 20 to 80 mg of methylprednisolone acetate or equivalent (see Tables 180.2 and 180.5). A Baker cyst is a sac of synovial fluid that has leaked out of a hole in the posterior capsule of the knee. It generally indicates significant internal knee problems, and steroid injections are only a temporary relief frowned on by many clinicians. Insert the needle 3 cm medial to the midline and 3 cm below the popliteal crease. Take care to avoid the popliteal artery, vein, and nerve. Use a 20-gauge, 1- to 1.5-inch needle with 5 mL 1% lidocaine and 20 to 80 mg of methylprednisolone acetate or equivalent (see Table 180.2).

3. Draw up the proper amounts of steroid and anesthetic into a single syringe and mix well by tipping the syringe backward and forward.
4. Note that although using smaller caliber needles may provide the patient with less pain, it is more difficult to determine whether the appropriate space for injection has been entered. In contrast, larger bore needles will be more painful. Based on the site of injection, and the constitution of the patient, you may decide to inject a superficial anesthetic (e.g., lidocaine) or use ethyl chloride spray on the skin prior to the intraarticular injection to allow for the use of a larger needle.
5. Using appropriate syringes and needles, either aspirate or inject the site as indicated. After insertion but before injection, pull back the plunger to be sure the needle is not in a blood vessel. Universal blood and body fluid precautions should be followed.
6. If aspiration of an effusion is to be followed by injection, there are two choices: (1) have two needle/syringe setups and enter the area twice; or (2) enter once, aspirate, grasp the needle with a hemostat (being careful not to change the position of the needle tip), remove the syringe with the aspirate, then replace it with the lidocaine/steroid syringe, and finally inject the contents.

7. If lidocaine or steroid is to be injected, it is often necessary to inject in two or three slightly different areas at the site of tenderness. This is not necessary when the joint space itself has been entered, although some practitioners advocate repositioning within bursal spaces because of the potential presence of septations that may interfere with full dissolution within the desired area.
8. Although much has been written regarding laboratory evaluation of joint fluid aspirates, Schmerling (1990) reported that the white blood cell (WBC) count and polymorphonucleocyte percentage were the only helpful tests to determine the etiology of an exudate. Use lavender-topped Vacutainers for these studies. It is recommended that synovial fluid be examined within 1 hour after arthrocentesis. WBC counts of mildly inflammatory fluids can decrease to "noninflammatory range" within 5 to 6 hours. Glucose, protein, lactate dehydrogenase, complement fixation, electrolyte, uric acid levels, rheumatoid factor, and antinuclear antibodies are of little benefit. Fluids for chemistry testing if desired should be transported in green- or red-topped tubes and be analyzed within 4 hours.

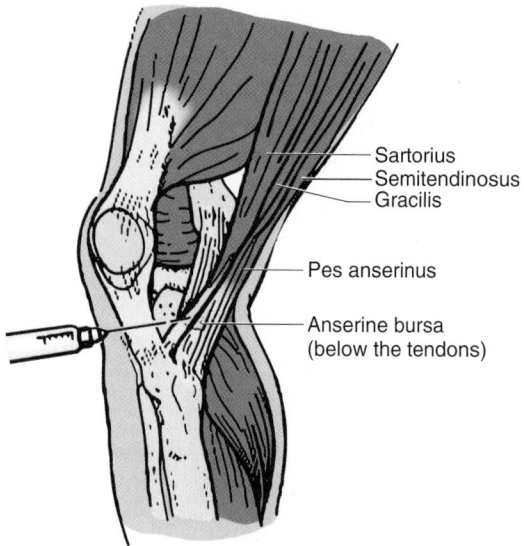

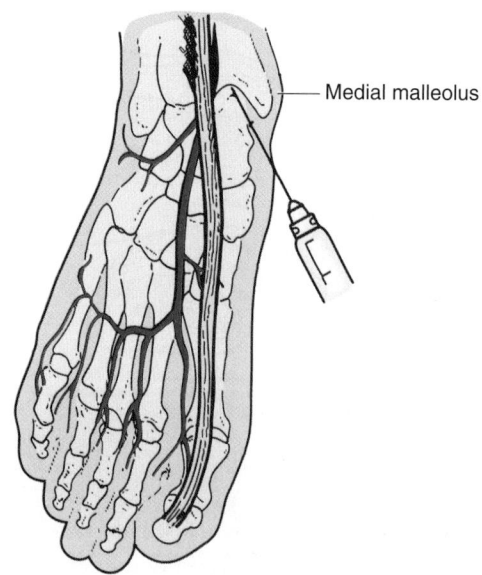

Fig. 180.21   Anserine bursa. The anserine bursa is located on the upper medial portion of the tibia under the insertion of the sartorius, semitendinosus, and gracilis tendons. This bursa frequently becomes inflamed in elderly, somewhat obese women; the symptoms are aggravated by going up and down stairs. Palpate and find the point of maximal tenderness, and insert the needle perpendicular to the tibia. When bony resistance is encountered, withdraw the needle 2 or 3 mm and inject several areas in a fanlike fashion. Use a 22- to 25-gauge, 1.5-inch needle with 3 to 5 mL 1% lidocaine and 20 to 40 mg of methylprednisolone acetate or equivalent (see Tables 180.2 and 180.5).

Fig. 180.22   Ankle joint. Anteromedial approach is the easiest. Have the patient maximally dorsiflex the toe, accentuating the extensor tendon. Identify the hollow between the anterior medial malleolus and the long extensor tendon. This is the spot for injection. The needle must be inserted approximately 3 cm and directed slightly lateral. Use a 22-gauge, 1- to 1.5-inch needle with 3 to 5 mL 1% lidocaine and 20 to 40 mg of methylprednisolone acetate or equivalent (see Tables 180.2 and 180.5).

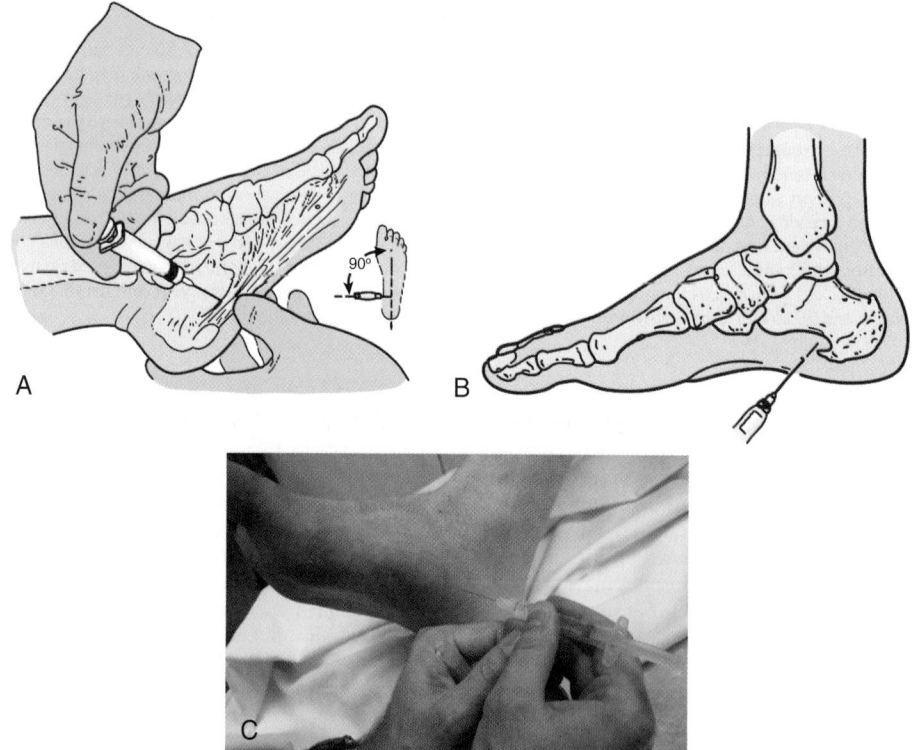

Fig. 180.23   Calcaneal spur/plantar fasciitis. Two approaches can be used. Many clinicians prefer to direct the needle from the lateral side of the foot (A) rather than from the inferior (plantar) side (B). The adipose tissue of the heel is uniquely segmented to provide cushion for the foot. If the plantar approach is used and steroid leaks out through the tract, atrophy could result, and thus the patient would have heel pain while walking. Nevertheless, many clinicians approach directly from the plantar position to inject steroid right over a calcaneal spur. Using the lateral approach, the clinician would direct the needle to enter just below the bony prominence of the calcaneus, and just anterior to the heel pad, and go to the midline until the point of maximal tenderness is reached (C). Use a 22-gauge, 1.5-inch needle with 2 to 4 mL 1% lidocaine and 15 to 30 mg of methylprednisolone acetate or equivalent (see Tables 180.2 and 180.5).

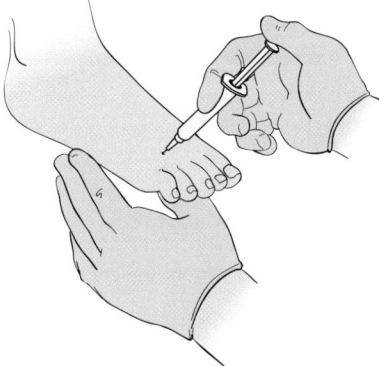

Fig. 180.24 Morton neuroma. Approach the foot from dorsal aspect. Insert needle 1 to 2 cm proximal to affected web space. Insert needle perpendicularly all the way to the plantar surface. Do not penetrate skin, but estimate depth by observing tenting of skin. Withdraw 1 cm and inject. Use a 25-gauge, 1.5-inch needle with 3 to 5 mL 1% lidocaine and 10 to 30 mg of methylprednisolone acetate or equivalent (see Table 180.2).

If the exudate is cloudy, the WBC count is elevated, or a septic joint is strongly suspected, do not inject the area, and a *culture* is also indicated. For cultures, submit as much fluid as possible. "Swabbed samples" may not be adequate. Large-volume specimens (over 2 mL) support viability of most microorganisms for up to 24 hours at room temperature. Nevertheless, transport to the laboratory ASAP. *Do not refrigerate!* Large samples may be sent in the syringe used to aspirate them or in a sterile 5- or 10-mL container that has no additives (i.e., a red-topped glass tube). For volumes less than 2 mL, consider using bottles with culture media (e.g., Port-A-Cul) inside. Test tube containers with anticoagulant additives (i.e., lavender- or green-topped containers) should not be used.

If there is any suspicion of gouty arthritis, examine the fluid for crystals under polarized light.

A peripheral smear may be helpful when a bloody tap is obtained after trauma. The presence of fat cells indicates a fracture.

The Pfenninger articles listed in the bibliography contain many tables of other characteristics of synovial fluid for differential diagnosis, although the benefit of additional studies is unproved.

Technique of Injection for Hyaluronic Acid "Devices"

- Must be intraarticular.
- More demanding than steroid intraarticular injections because it must be placed within the synovial space, not the surrounding soft tissue.
- Some experts use fluoroscopy or ultrasound to be certain of intraarticular injection.
- Do not mix with lidocaine or steroids.
- Drain all effusions before injection.
- Forced injections push material into the elasticity zone and then are very difficult to administer; slow injections must be given with a 22-gauge or larger needle (which again may necessitate the use of superficial anesthesia with lidocaine or ethyl chloride spray to allow for better tolerance by the patient).
- Patient should avoid strenuous activity for 48 hours.
- Derived from chicken or rooster combs, so an allergy to eggs or feathers would dictate caution.

Technique of Injection for Prolotherapy

A complete course of instruction prior to beginning prolotherapy injections in an office practice is recommended.

- Typically used in areas of degenerative tissue (i.e., tendinosis).
- Because of common usage with tendinous tissues, care must be taken to inject into the peritendinous areas rather than into the body of the tendon itself.
- Ultrasound can be considered to confirm placement of agent into the desired area.
- Because an inflammatory response is the desired outcome, educating the patient regarding anticipated pain over the next 24 to 48 hours is strongly encouraged. Some practitioners even advocate the use of opioid analgesics for pain control in the immediate postinjection period.
- There are no current recommendations for the ideal proinflammatory agent; availability (i.e., dextrose solutions) or desire to utilize the patient's own fluids (i.e., autologous blood, platelet-rich plasma) are two of the considerations made in determining the appropriate agent.
- Lidocaine should be injected to provide local anesthesia prior to using the other agents.
- Volume of agent should be based on the size of the area involved; most tendinous injections usually require no more than 5 mL of solution. Some areas will allow for a greater volume to be placed, but may cause more postinjection pain.
- Although there is no consensus as yet for the appropriate interval or total number of injections that should be administered, it is reasonable to wait at least 4 to 6 weeks between treatments. If more than five injections are necessary, consideration should be made for other therapies.

Ultrasound Guidance for Injections

Also see Chapter 171, Musculoskeletal Ultrasound.

Ultrasound is an extremely valuable modality that can allow the clinician to identify the structure to be injected and guide the needle to its precise location. This can be particularly beneficial in reducing the pain associated with "blind" localization of small joint spaces, making the patient more comfortable, and thus more compliant, during the procedure.

Ultrasound-guided injections also allow the clinician greater confidence in interpreting the results of an injection. For example, a missed injection into the acromioclavicular joint may suggest another etiology of a patient's shoulder pain, resulting in further erroneous testing and treatment regimens unless the error is identified on ultrasound. When the injection is performed with ultrasound, the clinician has objective evidence of appropriate placement of the medication and can therefore derive more accurate conclusions regarding the efficacy of the medication.

In order to perform ultrasound-guided injections, the clinician must have some training in the use of diagnostic ultrasound. The machine used should ideally have at least one multifrequency transducer in order to allow for visualization of both superficial and deeper structures. Power Doppler capability is also valuable because it allows the clinician to avoid vasculature and to better observe the flow of the medication in the actual space intended.

When performing ultrasound-guided injections, the following supplies are needed:

- Ultrasound gel
- Antiseptic, such as alcohol, chlorhexidine, or povidone-iodine
- Gauze pads and adhesive bandages
- Ethyl chloride spray (optional)
- Syringes (It is important to ensure that all air has been cleared out of both the needle and the syringes to be used, because air bubbles obscure ultrasound images.)
- Needles of appropriate length to reach the target
- A pair of forceps or a needle holder

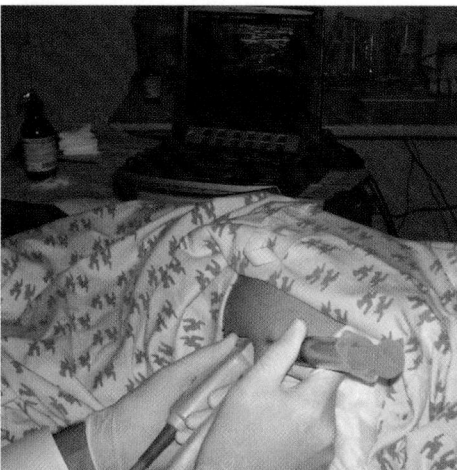

Fig. 180.25 Ultrasound-guided injection. Clinician demonstrates ultrasound guidance for injection of proximal hamstring tendinopathy. Note the needle is parallel to the longitudinal axis of the probe to facilitate visualization on the accompanying computer screen for identification. (Courtesy John M. McShane, MD.)

The standard technique for performing therapeutic injections under ultrasound guidance is as follows:

1. With the patient in a comfortable position, place some ultrasound gel over the area to be visualized and then use the ultrasound transducer to identify the structure to be injected.
2. Once the structure has been identified, place the transducer so that its long axis will be parallel to best line for the needle to take in order to reach its target (Fig. 180.25).
3. Use appropriate antiseptic solution to cleanse the skin at the end of the transducer where the needle will enter. Be sure not to move the transducer once the skin has been prepared.
4. If desired, use the ethyl chloride spray to superficially anesthetize the skin that will be punctured by the needle.
5. Take the needle and syringe containing the local anesthetic and hold it parallel to the ultrasound transducer with the tip of the needle aimed at the skin that has been cleansed. Keeping the needle constantly parallel to the transducer, enter the skin, and inject a small amount of anesthetic.
6. Using the ultrasound transducer, constantly keep the needle and the target to be injected in view. As the needle is advanced, repeatedly inject a small amount of anesthetic ahead of the tip. The fluid injected will be seen distending the tissue, and will help establish the location of the needle. If the needle is moved off target, slightly withdraw and redirect toward the target.
7. Once the structure to be injected is reached, if available, turn on the power Doppler and center it over the tip of the needle. Inject some anesthetic into the targeted area and watch for flow on the Doppler. If the needle is placed accurately, it will be confirmed by seeing flow on the Doppler in the desired location.
8. Once the location of the needle is confirmed, the needle is held in place by the forceps/needle holder and the syringe is removed. The syringe containing the fluid to be injected is then attached to the needle and the fluid is then injected.
9. The needle is withdrawn, pressure is placed over the puncture site, and an adhesive bandage is placed.

COMPLICATIONS

Box 180.2 lists the possible complications of intraarticular or soft tissue injections. Also see Table 180.4. Possible complications include the following:

- Injection into a vein or artery (This rarely causes a problem except that the therapeutic effect may not occur. Lidocaine

---

BOX 180.2   Possible Complications of Intraarticular or Soft Tissue Injections

Local Complications
- Bleeding
- Charcot-like arthropathy
- Fat necrosis
- Hemarthrosis
- Iatrogenic infection; septic arthritis
- Intraarticular calcification
- Nerve damage from inadvertent injection
- Osteonecrosis
- Pain
- Periarticular calcification
- Pneumothorax (thoracic trigger points)
- Postinjection flare
- Skin depigmentation
- Subcutaneous atrophy
- Tendon rupture
- Tenosynovitis

Systemic Complications
- Acne
- Adrenal suppression
- Allergic reactions or anaphylaxis from local or preservatives in multidose vials
- Avascular necrosis
- Flushing of the face
- Impaired glucose tolerance
- Menstrual irregularity; uterine bleeding
- Muscle wasting and myopathy
- Osteoporosis
- Pancreatitis
- Posterior subcapsular cataracts
- Psychological upset
- Steroid arthropathy
- Syncope

From McKeag D. Complication of joint aspiration/injection. *Clin Atlas Office Proc.* 2002;5:4.

---

and steroids are both given intravenously for other conditions.)
- Introduction of infection (usually Staphylococcus) into joint space (18 infections per 250,000 injections [0.072%])
- Trauma to articular cartilage
- Injury to nearby nerves (e.g., median nerve in carpal tunnel injection) or other nearby structures
- Pneumothorax (when injecting thoracic trigger points)
- Subcutaneous fatty or skin atrophy or hyperpigmentation/hypopigmentation (see Fig. 180.26)
- Adverse drug reaction (see Table 180.4)
- Allergic drug reaction (very rare)
- Injection of steroid into a septic joint (If there is any suspicion of infection, do not instill steroids until laboratory studies have ruled it out.)
- Osteoporosis and cartilage damage (This is rare; reported cases have usually occurred after 20 to 30 injections. For joints, especially weight-bearing joints, a limit of three steroid injections per year provides a wide margin of safety.)
- Inappropriate/missed diagnosis
- Tendon rupture (To reduce the possibility of tendon rupture, inject peritendinously instead of intratendinously. Ruptures usually occur after multiple injections and when the patient will not rest the area. Finger tendon ruptures have been reported after steroid injection. Gray and Gottlieb recommend setting a limit of five total injections per finger joint. Some experts recommend never injecting near the Achilles tendon.)

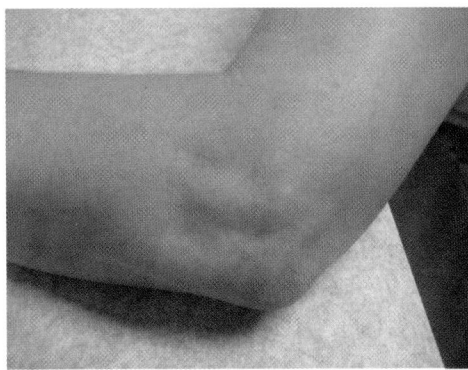

Fig. 180.26 Fatty atrophy. This patient received a steroid injection for lateral epicondylosis approximately 11 months before this photo was taken, showing an example of steroid fatty atrophy and hypopigmentation. Such changes may take up to a year to resolve, and some can be permanent changes.

- Reactions to anesthetic agent (True allergic reactions to lidocaine [an amide] itself is extremely rare. Allergic reactions have been reported to the esters more frequently [e.g., procaine/Novocain]; when reactions to lidocaine are suspected, the lidocaine has usually been drawn up from a multidose vial. These vials contain paraben preservatives, which can cause a reaction. So, if suspicions of a "caine" allergy arise, single-dose vials of lidocaine should be used. Another reason to use single-dose vials is to avoid precipitation of the steroid; see earlier discussion.)
- Steroid flare (Steroid flares occur rarely but are very painful. The patient actually experiences more discomfort after the injection. The flare is not associated with fever, occurs within 12 to 24 hours of the injection, and resolves spontaneously within 72 hours. It may be controlled with ice and nonsteroidal drugs.)
- Interference with glucose metabolism. Therefore glucose levels need to be followed more closely in diabetics in the first 24 hours.
- Problems with viscosupplementation injections
  - Injection site pain is more frequent.
  - Rash and itching, cramps, ankle edema, muscle pain, and tachyarrhythmia have been reported.
  - A local reaction can produce a massive effusion that resembles a septic joint; 69% with pain experience relief after effusion resolves.

POSTPROCEDURE PATIENT CARE AND EDUCATION

- An adhesive bandage dressing or other dressing should be left on for 8 to 12 hours.
- It is essential that the affected area be rested. Injection therapy is not a cure itself. It is used in conjunction with other modalities. Physical therapy, NSAIDs, and hot or cold compresses may all be indicated, depending on the specific problem. If a weight-bearing joint (such as the knee) is injected, rest is indicated for a longer period than that for a wrist ganglion cyst injection.
- The patient should report immediately if he or she develops fever, chills, or any sign of infection. If the discomfort from the injection does not resolve within 72 hours, the patient should be examined to rule out a septic joint.
- The patient may bathe normally.
- A short course of an NSAID is often beneficial at the time of injection; the two modalities combined may have a markedly beneficial effect.

CPT/BILLING CODES

Healthcare Common Procedure Coding System (HCPCS) Codes*

20526	Injection: therapeutic (e.g., local anesthetic, corticosteroid), carpal tunnel
20550†	Injection: tendon sheath, ligament, ganglion cyst
20551	Injection: therapeutic of tendon at its origin or insertion
20552	Injection: single or multiple trigger point(s), one or two muscle group(s)
20553	Injection: single or multiple trigger point(s), three or more muscle groups
20600	Arthrocentesis, aspiration and/or injection, small joint or bursa (e.g., fingers; toes); without ultrasound guidance, with permanent recording and reporting
20605	Arthrocentesis, aspiration and/or injection, intermediate joint or bursa (e.g., temporomandibular, acromioclavicular, wrist, elbow or ankle, olecranon bursa); without ultrasound guidance, with permanent recording and reporting
20610	Arthrocentesis, aspiration and/or injection, major joint or bursa (e.g., shoulder, hip, knee, subacromial bursa); without ultrasound guidance, with permanent recording and reporting
20604	Arthrocentesis, aspiration and/or injection, small joint or bursa (e.g., fingers; toes); with ultrasound guidance, with permanent recording and reporting
20606	Arthrocentesis, aspiration and/or injection, intermediate joint or bursa (e.g., temporomandibular, acromioclavicular, wrist, elbow or ankle, olecranon bursa); with ultrasound guidance, with permanent recording and reporting
20611	Arthrocentesis, aspiration and/or injection, major joint or bursa (e.g., shoulder, hip, knee, subacromial bursa); with ultrasound guidance, with permanent recording and reporting
M0076	Prolotherapy

*Can also charge for any injected medications using appropriate J code.
†Office visit can also be charged.

Steroids

J0702	Betamethasone acetate (Celestone Soluspan)
J0810	Cortisone
J1021	Methylprednisolone acetate
J1040	Depo-Medrol
J1095	Dexamethasone acetate
J1100	Dexamethasone sodium phosphate (Decadron)
J1690	Prednisolone tebutate (Hydeltra-TBA)
J1700	Hydrocortisone acetate
J2640	Prednisolone sodium phosphate
J3301	Triamcinolone acetonide (Kenalog)
J3302	Triamcinolone diacetate (Aristocort)
J3303	Triamcinolone hexacetonide (Aristospan)
J7506	Prednisone
J7321	Hyalgan or Supartz
J7323	Euflexxa
J7324	Orthovisc
J7235	Synvisc
J7327	Monovisc

ICD-10-CM Diagnostic Codes

M10.00	Gouty arthropathy site unspecified
G56.00	Carpal tunnel syndrome unspecified limb
G56.20	Lesion ulnar nerve unspecified limb
G57.50	Tarsal tunnel syndrome unspecified limb
G57.60	Morton's neuroma unspecified limb
L40.59	Psoriatic arthropathy other
M06.9	Rheumatoid arthritis unspecified
M19.019	Primary osteoarthritis unspecified shoulder
M19.029	Primary osteoarthritis unspecified elbow
M19.049	Primary osteoarthritis unspecified hand
M17.10	Unilateral primary osteoarthritis unspecified knee
M17.0	Bilateral primary osteoarthritis knee
M19.079	Primary osteoarthritis unspecified ankle and foot
M25.519	Pain unspecified shoulder
M25.529	Pain unspecified elbow
M25.539	Pain unspecified wrist
M25.549	Pain in joints of unspecified hand
M25.569	Pain unspecified knee
M25.579	Pain unspecified foot and ankle
M25.619	Stiffness unspecified shoulder
M25.669	Stiffness unspecified knee
M54.2	Neck pain
M54.5	Low back pain
M54.30	Sciatica unspecified site
M53.3	Coccydynia
M75.40	Impingement syndrome unspecified shoulder
M70.60	Trochanteric bursitis unspecified hip
M75.50	Bursitis unspecified shoulder
M75.100	Rotator cuff syndrome unspecified shoulder
M75.20	Tendinitis unspecified shoulder
M75.20	Bicipital tendinitis unspecified shoulder
M77.00	Medial epicondylitis (golfer's elbow) unspecified elbow
M77.10	Lateral epicondylitis (tennis elbow) unspecified elbow
M70.20	Olecranon bursitis unspecified elbow
M70.50	Pes anserine bursitis unspecified knee
M76.50	Patellar tendinitis unspecified knee
M70.40	Prepatellar tendinitis unspecified knee
M76.60	Achilles bursitis unspecified leg
M77.30	Heel spur unspecified foot
M65.30	Trigger finger unspecified finger
M65.4	de Quervain disease
M65.849	Tendinitis, unspecified hand/wrist
M65.879	Tendinitis, unspecified foot/ankle
M71.50	Bursitis unspecified site
M67.40	Ganglion, unspecified joint
M71.20	Baker cyst unspecified knee
M65.20	Calcific tendinitis unspecified site
M72.2	Plantar fasciitis
M79.7	Fibrositis
M72.9	Fasciitis
M79.629	Pain upper arm unspecified arm
M79.639	Pain forearm unspecified arm
M79.669	Pain lower leg unspecified leg
M79.659	Pain thigh unspecified leg
M79.676	Pain toe unspecified toe

Acknowledgment

The editors recognize the many contributions by John L. Pfenninger, MD, to this chapter in a previous edition of this text.

Learning Resource

National Procedures Institute: www.npinstitute.com (courses and DVDs on joint injection)

Online Resources

American Association of Orthopedic Medicine: http://aaomed.org/ Prolotherapy

Recommended Reading

Altman RD, Moskowitz R. Intraarticular sodium hyaluronate (Hyalgan) in the treatment of patients with osteoarthritis of the knee: a randomized clinical trial. J Rheumatol. 1998;25:2203.

Anderson B, Kaye S. Treatment of flexor tenosynovitis of the hand ("trigger finger") with corticosteroids: a prospective study of the response to local injection. Arch Intern Med. 1991;151:153.

Bellamy N, Campbell J, Welch V, Gee TL, Bourne R, et al. Viscosupplementation for the treatment of osteoarthritis of the knee. Cochrane Database Syst Rev. 2006;2:CD005321.

Blair B, Rokito AS, Cuomo F, et al. Efficacy of corticosteroids for subacromial impingement syndrome. J Bone Joint Surg. 1996;78-A:1685.

Blanchard V, Barr S, Cerisola FL. The effectiveness of corticosteroid injections compared with physiotherapeutic interventions for adhesive capsulitis: a systematic review. Physiotherapy. 2010;96(2):95–107.

Brinks A, van Rijn RM, Willemsen SP, et al. Corticosteroid injections for greater trochanteric pain syndrome: a randomized controlled trial in primary care. Ann Fam Med. 2011;9(3):226–234.

Carrabba M, Paresce E, Angelini M, et al. The safety and efficacy of different dose schedules of hyaluronic acid in the treatment of painful osteoarthritis of the knee with joint effusion. Eur J Rheumatol Inflamm. 1995;15:25.

Charalambous CP, Tryfonidis M, Sadiq S, et al. Septic arthritis following intraarticular steroid injection of the knee—A survey of current practice regarding antiseptic technique used during intraarticular steroid injection of the knee. Clin Rheumatol. 2003;22:386.

Cheng OT, Souzdalnitski D, Vrooman B, et al. Evidence-based knee injections for the management of arthritis. Pain Med. 2012;13(6):740–753.

Chumacher HR, Chen LX. Injectable corticosteroids in treatment of arthritis of the knee. Am J Med. 2005;118:1208.

Coombes BK, Bisset L, Vicenzino B. Efficacy and safety of corticosteroid injections and other injections for management of tendinopathy: a systematic review of randomised controlled trials. Lancet. 2010;376(9754):1751–1767.

Dagenais S, Yelland MJ, Del Mar C, Schoene ML. Prolotherapy injections for chronic low-back pain. Cochrane Database Syst Rev. 2007;(3):CD004059.

David JA, Sankarapandian V, Christopher PRH, Chatterjee A, Macaden AS. Injected corticosteroids for treating plantar heel pain in adults. Cochrane Database Syst Rev. 2107;(2):CD009348.

Dammers JW, Veering MM, Vermeulen M. Injection with methylprednisolone proximal to the carpal tunnel: randomised double blind trial. BMJ. 2000;321:884.

Divine JG, Zazulak BT, Hewett TE. Viscosupplementation for knee osteoarthritis: a systematic review. Clin Orthop Relat Res. 2007;455:113.

Fadale PD, Wiggins ME. Corticosteroid injections: their use and abuse. J Am Acad Orthop Surg. 1994;2:133.

Fitzgerald RH. Intrasynovial injection of steroids: uses and abuses. Mayo Clin Proc. 1976;51:655.

Foster ZJ, Voss TT, Hatch J, Frimodig A. Corticosteroid injections for common musculoskeletal conditions. Am Fam Physician. 2015;92(8):694–699.

Foster AH, Carlson BM. Myotoxicity of local anesthetics and regeneration of the damaged muscle fibers. Anesth Analg. 1980;59:727.

Gaujoux-Viala C, Dougados M, Gossec L. Efficacy and safety of steroid injections for shoulder and elbow tendonitis: a metaanalysis of randomised controlled trials. Ann Rheum Dis. 2009;68(12):1843–1849.

Gedda PO. Septic arthritis from cortisone. JAMA. 1954;155:597.

George E. Intraarticular hyaluronan treatment for osteoarthritis. Ann Rheum Dis. 1998;57:637.

Gowans JDC, Granieri PA. Septic arthritis: its relation to intraarticular injections of hydrocortisone acetate. N Engl J Med. 1959;261:502.

Griesser MJ, Harris JD, Campbell JE, et al. Adhesive capsulitis of the shoulder: a systematic review of the effectiveness of intraarticular corticosteroid injections. J Bone Joint Surg Am. 2011;93(18):1727–1733.

Gray RG, Gottlieb NL. Intraarticular corticosteroids: an updated assessment. Clin Orthop Relat Res. 1983;177:253.

Gray RG, Tenenbaum J, Gottlieb NL. Local corticosteroid injection therapy in rheumatic disorders. Semin Arthritis Rheum. 1981;10:231.

Hay EM, Paterson SM, Lewis M, et al. Pragmatic randomized controlled trial of local corticosteroid injection and naproxen for treatment of lateral epicondylitis of elbow in primary care. BMJ. 1999;319:964.

Hepper CT, Halvorson JJ, Duncan ST, et al. The efficacy and duration of intraarticular corticosteroid injection for knee osteoarthritis: a systematic review of level I studies. *J Am Acad Orthop Surg.* 2009;17(10):638–646.

Hernandez-Diaz S, Garcia-Rodriguez LA. Epidemiologic assessment of the safety of conventional nonsteroidal anti-inflammatory drugs. *Am J Med.* 2001;110(suppl 3A):20S.

Hollander JL. Intrasynovial corticosteroid therapy in arthritis. *Maryland State Med J.* 1970;19:62.

Jones A, Doherty M. Intraarticular corticosteroids are effective in osteoarthritis but there are no clinical predictors of response. *Ann Rheum Dis.* 1996;55:829.

Jones A, Regan M, Ledingham J, et al. Importance of placement of intraarticular steroid injections. *BMJ.* 1993;307:1329.

Juni P, Hari R, Rutjes AW, Fischer R, Silletta MG, et al. Intraarticular corticosteroid for knee osteoarthritis. *Cochrane Database Syst Rev.* 2015;3:CD005328.

Kamm GL, Hagmeyer KO. Allergic-type reactions to corticosteroids. *Ann Pharmacother.* 1999;33:451.

Karpie J, Chi C. Lidocaine exhibits dose and time dependent cytotoxic effects on bovine chondrocytes in vitro. *Am J Sports Med.* 2007;35:10.

Kendall H. Local corticosteroid injection therapy. *Ann Phys Med.* 1963;7:31.

Khohadee M. Common superficial bursitis. *Am Fam Physician.* 2017;95(4):224–231.

Kim SR, Stitik TP, Foye PM, et al. Critical review of prolotherapy for osteoarthritis, low back pain, and other musculoskeletal conditions: a physiatric perspective. *Am J Phys Med Rehabil.* 2004;83:379.

Kotz R, Kolarz G. Intraarticular hyaluronic acid: duration of effect and results of repeated treatment cycles. *Am J Orthop.* 1999;28:5.

Krogh TP, Bartels EM, Ellingsen T, et al. Comparative effectiveness of injection therapies in lateral epicondylitis: a systematic review and network metaanalysis of randomized controlled trials. *Am J Sports Med.* 2013;41(6):1435–1446.

Lavelle W. Intraarticular injections. *Med Clin North Am.* 2007;91:241.

Leversee JH. Aspiration of joints and soft tissue injections. *Prim Care.* 1986;13:572.

Marshall SC, Tardif G, Ashworth NL. Local corticosteroid injection for carpal tunnel syndrome. *Cochrane Database of Syst Rev.* 2007;2:CD001554.

McNabb JW. *A Practical Guide to Joint and Soft Tissue Injections.* 3rd ed. Philadelphia: Lippincott Williams & Wilkins Wolters Kluwer; 2014.

Moraes VY, Lenza M, Tamaoki M, Faloppa F, Belloti J. Platelet-rich therapies for musculoskeletal soft tissue injuries. *Cochrane Database of Syst Rev.* 2014;3:CD010071.

Nouette-Gaulain K, Sirvent P, Canal-Raffin M, et al. Effects of intermittent femoral nerve injections of bupivacaine, levobupivacaine, and ropivacaine on mitochondrial energy metabolism and intracellular calcium homeostasis in rat psoas muscle. *Anesthesiology.* 2007;106:1026.

Peters-Veluthamaningal C, van der Windt DA, Winters JC, Meyboom-de Jong B. Corticosteroid injection for de Quervain's tenosynovitis. *Cochrane Database Syst Rev.* 2009;2:CD005616.

Peters-Veluthamaningal C, van der Windt DAWM, Winters JC, Meyboom-de Jong B. Corticosteroid injection for trigger finger in adults. *Cochrane Database Syst Rev.* 2009;2:CD005617.

Pfenninger JL. Injections of joints and soft tissue. Part I. General guidelines. *Am Fam Physician.* 1991;44:1196.

Pfenninger JL. Injections of joints and soft tissue. Part II. Guidelines for specific joints. *Am Fam Physician.* 1991;44:1690.

Pfenninger JL, ed. Joint injection techniques. *Clin Atlas Office Proc.* 2002;5:4.

Qvistgaard E, Christensen R, Torp-Pedersen S, et al. Intraarticular treatment of hip osteoarthritis: a randomized trial of hyaluronic acid, corticosteroid, and isotonic saline. *Osteoarthritis Cartilage.* 2006;14(2):163–170.

Ryan M, Wong A, Taunton J, Wong J. A pilot investigation on a new treatment for chronic plantar fasciitis: ultrasound guided hyperosmolar dextrose injections. *Clin J Sport Med.* 2007;17:166.

Saunders S, Longsworth S. *Injection Techniques in Musculoskeletal Medicine: a Practical Manual for Clinicians in Primary and Secondary Care.* 4th ed. Philadelphia: Churchill Livingstone Elsevier; 2013.

Schmerling RH, Delbanco TL, Tosteson ANA, et al. Synovial fluid tests: what should be ordered? *JAMA.* 1990;264:1009.

Scott WA. Injection techniques and use in the treatment of sports injuries. *Sports Med.* 1996;22:406.

Sibbitt Jr WL, Peisajovich A, Michael AA, et al. Does sonographic needle guidance affect the clinical outcome of intraarticular injections? *J Rheumatol.* 2009;36:1892.

Slotkoff AT, Clauw DJ, Nashel DJ. Effects of soft tissue corticosteroid injection on glucose control in diabetics. *Arthritis Rheum.* 1994;37:S347.

Smith DL, McAfee JH, Lucas LM, et al. Treatment of nonseptic olecranon bursitis: a controlled, blinded prospective trial. *Arch Intern Med.* 1989;149:2527.

Stahl S, Kaufman T. The efficacy of an injection of steroids for medial epicondylitis. A prospective study of sixty elbows. *J Bone Joint Surg Am.* 1997;79(11):1648–1652.

Stefanich RJ. Intraarticular corticosteroids in treatment of osteoarthritis. *Orthop Rev.* 1986;15:65.

Stitik TP, Kumar A, Foye PM. Corticosteroid injections for osteoarthritis. *Am J Phys Med Rehabil.* 2006;85(suppl):S51.

Tramèr MR, Moore RA, Reynolds DJ, McQuay HJ. Quantitative estimation of rare adverse events which follow a biological progression: a new model applied to chronic NSAID use. *Pain.* 2001;91:401.

Troum OM. Office-based diagnostic needle arthroscopic lavage. In: Pfenninger JL, ed. *Joint Injection Techniques Clin Atlas Office Proc.* 2002;5:4.

Walker-Bone K, Javaid K, Arden N, et al. Medical management of osteoarthritis. *BMJ.* 2000;321:936.

Wen DY. Intraarticular hyaluronic acid injections for knee osteoarthritis. *Am Fam Physician.* 2000;62:565.

Wiggins ME, Fadale PD, Ehrlich MG, et al. Effects of corticosteroids on the healing of ligaments. *J Bone Joint Surg.* 1995;77-A:1682.

Wise CM. Arthrocentesis and injection of joints and soft tissue. In: Firestein GS, Budd RS, Harris ED, et al., eds. *Kelley's Textbook of Rheumatology.* 8th ed. Philadelphia: Saunders; 2008:721.

Young CC, Rutherford DS, Neidfeldt MW. Treatment of plantar fasciitis. *Am Fam Physician.* 2001;63:467.

Zink W, Missler G, Sinner B, et al. Differential effects of bupivacaine and ropivacaine enantiomers on intracellular Ca^{2+} regulation in murine skeletal muscle fibers. *Anesthesiology.* 2005;102:793.

Zuckerman JD, Meislin RJ, Rothberg M. Injections for joint and soft tissue disorders; when and how to use them. *Geriatrics.* 1990;45:45.

CHAPTER 181

TRIGGER-POINT INJECTION

Ashley Christiani

Myofascial pain is among the most common complaints for which patients seek care. In many cases, there is a defined, reproducible site of tenderness in the affected muscle, called a *trigger point*, that can be targeted for relief of pain and spasm. From 10% to 20% of the population are thought to be affected by trigger points, which may be effectively treated in the office through a trigger point injection. Understanding trigger point pathology and treatment can aid the clinician in addressing one of the most common and debilitating acute complaints encountered in the outpatient setting.

The term *trigger point* was coined by Dr. Janet Travell in 1942 to describe the clinical finding of a painful nodule in an indurated cord or "taut band" of muscle (Fig. 181.1). According to the American College of Rheumatology, trigger points should be painful to palpation with 4 kg of pressure, approximately the point at which the examiner's fingernail would begin to blanch. The taut band of muscle fibers may respond during palpation or needle activation with a local twitch response (LTR). Although the LTR phenomenon is not always visible, when present this response predicts an effective response to a trigger point injection.

It is thought that any one of the more than 600 striated muscles in the human body can develop trigger points, although not all can be accessed by direct palpation. Examples of the most common trigger points are shown in Fig. 181.2. Trigger points can form in response to an acute event such as a sudden strain placed on an already contracted muscle or in the context of insidious, repetitive strain. Trigger points are commonly classified as *active* or *latent*. Active trigger points (Box 181.1) are symptomatic, causing pain, stiffness, decreased range of motion, and referred symptoms such as paresthesias or a disturbance in motor or autonomic function. The pain experienced by patients may be well localized or diffuse, ranging in character from a dull ache to sharp, burning, and debilitating. Motor dysfunction includes muscle weakness and easy fatigability, as well as spasm of other muscles in the kinetic chain. Associated autonomic dysfunction can include abnormal sweating, lacrimation, salivation, pilomotor disturbance, mild edema, imbalance, dizziness, and tinnitus. Palpation of active trigger points typically reproduces the patient's symptoms. Latent trigger points may also cause stiffness and restriction of motion but are generally not noted by the patient to be painful until directly palpated by the examiner or when "unmasked" during the treatment of active trigger points.

Approximately 20% of patients with active trigger points also have fibromyalgia; it is important to differentiate this subset (Table 181.1) because patients with fibromyalgia usually have diffuse pain that may be better managed with systemic regimens and physical therapy as opposed to localized trigger point injections. Performing a trigger point injection in patients with fibromyalgia may actually worsen the pain. It should be noted that trigger points are frequently located near a bony prominence or moving part or where a muscle or tissue slides, whereas the tender points associated with fibromyalgia are often located in an area where the tissue is not subject to any local stress.

Trigger point injections may be performed quickly and effectively in the office setting to treat myofascial pain, producing immediate and often long-term results, especially when combined with complementary therapies such as physical therapy, transcutaneous electrical stimulation, therapeutic ultrasound, "spray and stretch," massage therapy, ischemic compression, or ergonomic retraining. (In fact, to avoid the patient becoming dependent upon the injections, some experts will not perform trigger point injections until the patient has tried these noninvasive therapies.) Trigger point injection is thought to work by causing a temporary relaxation of the taut muscle, allowing for improved local perfusion, replenishment of the adenosine triphosphate required to release actin-myosin chains, and clearance of noxious metabolites. In turn, this breaks the pain-tension cycle. Studies have demonstrated that it is the mechanical stimulation of the trigger point by the needle that releases the muscle spasm, whereas the substance injected provides only adjuvant therapy. A systematic review (Cummings) found that response rates are similar regardless of the substance injected; whether it is saline, a steroid, a local anesthetic, or a paralytic agent such as botulinum toxin injected, none has proven to be more effective than dry needling alone. However, the latter two substances may produce longer-lasting results because of caustic damage to the muscle. Injection of local anesthetic offers the additional benefit of significantly reducing postprocedure pain compared with saline or dry needling, without adding undue risk to the procedure. Most authorities recommend the use of 0.25% to 1% lidocaine without epinephrine or 2% procaine diluted to 0.5% for trigger point injections. We recommend against the use of steroids for trigger point injection.

INDICATION

Focal tender area identifiable by palpation without other identifiable neurologic or musculoskeletal findings or pathology is the indication for treatment. The tender area should be accessible by needle without significant risk.

CONTRAINDICATIONS

Absolute

- Trigger point not safely accessible by needle
- Cellulitis or other loss of skin integrity in area overlying trigger point

Relative

- Poorly controlled psychiatric disorder
- Resuscitation equipment not available
- Poorly controlled systemic illness that may compromise healing or predispose to infection
- Bleeding disorder, including anticoagulant use

- Severe fibromyalgia or presence of numerous trigger points
- History of keloid formation
- Highly anxious or needle-phobic patient

EDITOR'S NOTE: Some experts suggest that patients could become dependent upon injections for pain relief; therefore they reserve injection therapy for patients who have failed other therapies (e.g., physical therapy, transcutaneous electrical stimulation, therapeutic ultrasound, "spray and stretch," massage therapy, ischemic compression). Other experts do not perform trigger point injections in patients with fibromyalgia; they say it can worsen the pain.

PREPROCEDURE PATIENT PREPARATION AND EVALUATION

History and Physical Examination

Screening should include any history of trauma, fibromyalgia, collagen vascular disease, inflammatory condition, bleeding disorder, hypothyroidism, diabetes, hepatitis C (often associated with generalized myalgia), and any other systemic diseases or chronic conditions. The physical examination should include evaluation of the affected musculature and any associated musculature innervated by the same spinal segment to identify active and latent trigger points and to assess for other potential causes of pain. Significant muscle atrophy or sensory deficit is not commonly seen in isolated trigger point phenomena and should alert the clinician to other etiologies. Tender musculature should be palpated slowly and deliberately for taut bands and tender nodules with the muscle in a relaxed position. Trigger points are commonly found in the midbelly of the muscle where contraction is most acute, but the entire muscle from origin to insertion should be examined. Muscles that can be accessed in only one plane can be explored by flat palpation (Fig. 181.3), whereas those that can be partially enclosed in the fingers can be examined with the pincer grasp (Fig. 181.4). As discussed previously, palpation of an active trigger point generally elicits wincing or involuntary guarding by the patient and may generate an LTR. Ultrasound imaging can adjunctively assist

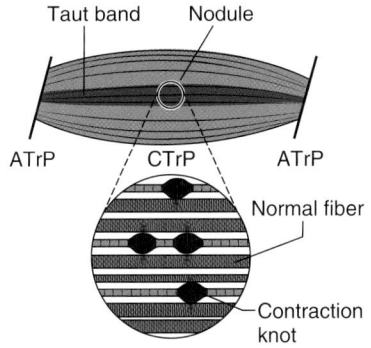

Fig. 181.1 Trigger point complex in muscle. *ATrP,* Attachment trigger point; *CTrP,* central trigger point. (From Simons DG, Travell JG, Simons LS. *Travell & Simons' Myofascial Pain and Dysfunction: The Trigger Point Manual.* 2nd ed. Philadelphia: Lippincott .Williams & Wilkins; 1999)

> **BOX 181.1 Diagnostic Criteria for Active Trigger Points**
>
> - Pain recognition (patient identifies pain at the trigger point as the pain he or she has been experiencing)
> - Presence of an exquisitely tender nodule in a palpable taut band
> - Referral of pain or symptoms in predictable pattern on palpation
> - Painful limitation of range of motion
>
> **Helpful If Present**
>
> - Local twitch response observed when trigger point is stimulated
> - Associated autonomic responses triggered with palpation of trigger point
> - Electromyographic demonstration of spontaneous electrical activity in region of tender nodule in the taut band

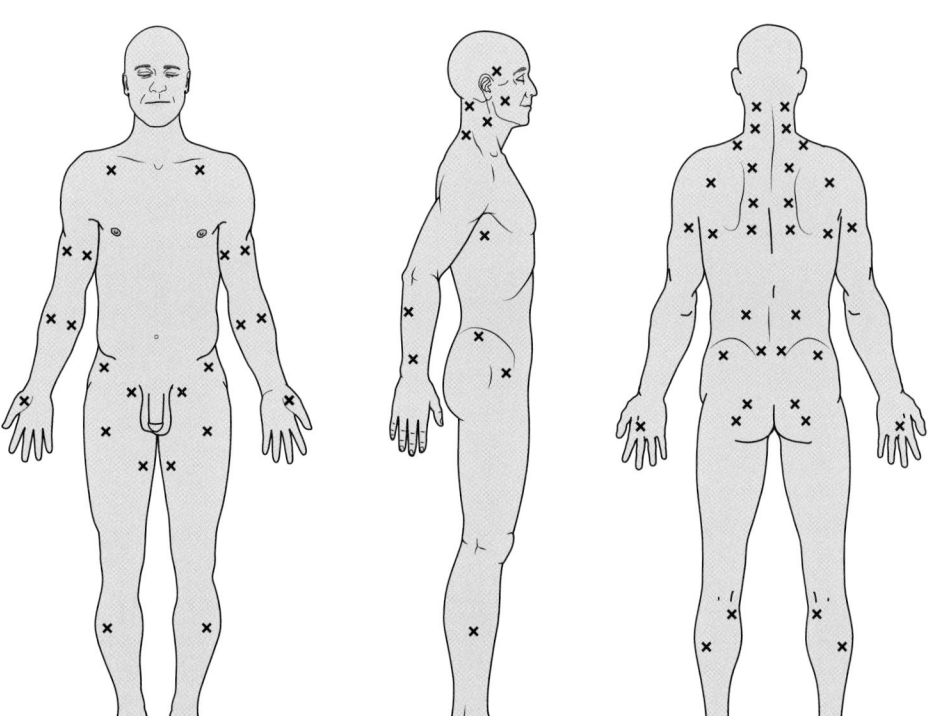

Fig. 181.2 Anterior, lateral, and posterior views of common trigger points. (From Simons DG, Travell JG, Simons LS. *Travell & Simons' Myofascial Pain and Dysfunction: The Trigger Point Manual.* 2nd ed. Philadelphia: Lippincott Williams & Wilkins; 1999.)

in manual palpation; this technology is evolving in the management of trigger points as both a diagnostic tool and to assist with ultrasound guidance (Kumbhare et al., 2016). The history and physical examination should also include investigation of mechanical etiologies and risk factors for development of recurrent trigger points such as leg length discrepancy, scoliosis, poor posture and body mechanics, or chronic trauma caused by carrying heavy items such as handbags, work equipment, or infants or young children. Behavior modification and physical therapy may help to prevent further injury in these cases.

Informed Consent

Provide the patient with a detailed explanation of the procedure and its potential risks, benefits, and alternatives (specific to the

TABLE 181.1	Myofascial Pain Due to Trigger Points Versus Fibromyalgia
Myofascial Pain Due to Trigger Points	**Fibromyalgia**
Male-female ratio 1:1	Male-female ratio ranges from 1:4 to 1:9
Local or regional pain and tenderness	Generalized or widespread pain* and tenderness
Taut muscle bands	Soft muscles
Muscle stiffness and decreased range of motion	Normal to hypermobile muscles and joints
"Trigger points"	11 of 18 "tender points"†
Immediate response to trigger point injection	Poor or delayed response to trigger point injection
Approximately 20% also have fibromyalgia	Approximately 70% also have active trigger points

*Widespread pain denotes pain that is bilateral and involving both the upper and lower body. Widespread pain must have been present for 3 months.
†Pain in at least 11 of the 18 specific tender points must be present. These tender points (bilateral) include the occiput (at suboccipital insertion), lower cervical spine (C5–C7 levels), trapezius (midpoint of upper border), supraspinatus (above scapular spine near medial border), second rib (at second costochondral junction), lateral epicondyle (2 cm distal to the epicondyle), gluteus (upper, outer quadrants of buttocks), greater trochanter (posterior to the trochanteric prominence), and knee (at the medial fat pad proximal to joint line).
Modified from Simons DG, Travell JG, Simons LS. *Travell & Simons' Myofascial Pain and Dysfunction: The Trigger Point Manual.* 2nd ed. Philadelphia: Lippincott Williams & Wilkins; 1999.

condition being treated), and obtain informed consent. If multiple trigger points are present on examination, they are generally best treated on the same visit unless they are too numerous (in which case other treatment modalities may be preferable). Explain to the patient that the relief resulting from the treatment can be followed by pain greater than the original pain, either in the same location or as an "unmasking" effect with pain in other untreated muscle groups, and that follow-up injections may be appropriate.

Patient Preparation

If not medically contraindicated, it may be advisable to discontinue aspirin or other anticoagulants at least 3 days before the procedure, to minimize bleeding. Patients who are anxious may benefit from pretreatment with a mild oral anxiolytic. In preparation for the procedure, the patient should generally be supine with pillows provided for rotational support, as needed, to minimize risk of vasovagal response.

EQUIPMENT

- Alcohol wipes.
- Gloves (nonsterile).
- Several gauze pads and simple adhesive bandages (e.g., Band-Aids).
- Ballpoint pen (with retracted nib) or skin marker.
- Lidocaine (0.25% to 1% without epinephrine), procaine (2% diluted to 0.5%), or bupivacaine (0.125% to 0.25%).
- Sodium bicarbonate 5% to 8.4% solution, for injection, available in 50-mL bottles with 50 mEq/50 mL, may be added as a buffer to local anesthetic. Add 1 mL per 10 mL of anesthetic.
- 25- to 27-gauge needle, depending on site to be injected. A 27-gauge, 1.5-inch needle is usually sufficient for the upper torso; a 25-gauge, 3.5-inch spinal needle may be required for large back or leg muscles.
- 3-, 5-, or 10-mL syringes.
- Resuscitation equipment (as with any injection).
- Pillows (optional).
- Vapocoolant spray such as ethyl chloride for topical anesthesia (optional).

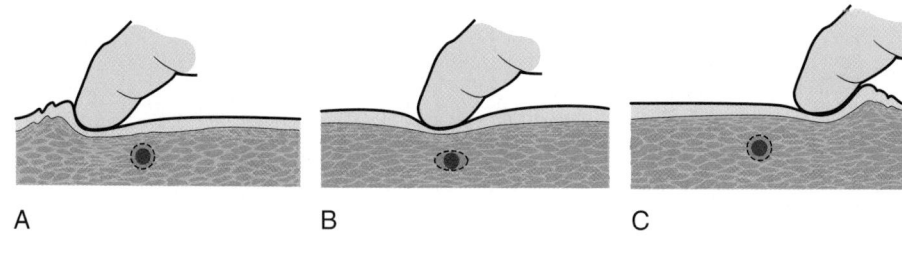

Fig. 181.3 Flat palpation technique. (A) Index finger pushes skin to one side. (B) Fingertip sweeps across the muscle to feel the taut band rolling beneath. (C) The skin is pushed to the other side, completing the movement. (From Simons DG, Travell JG, Simons LS. *Travell & Simons' Myofascial Pain and Dysfunction: The Trigger Point Manual.* 2nd ed. Philadelphia: Lippincott Williams & Wilkins; 1999.)

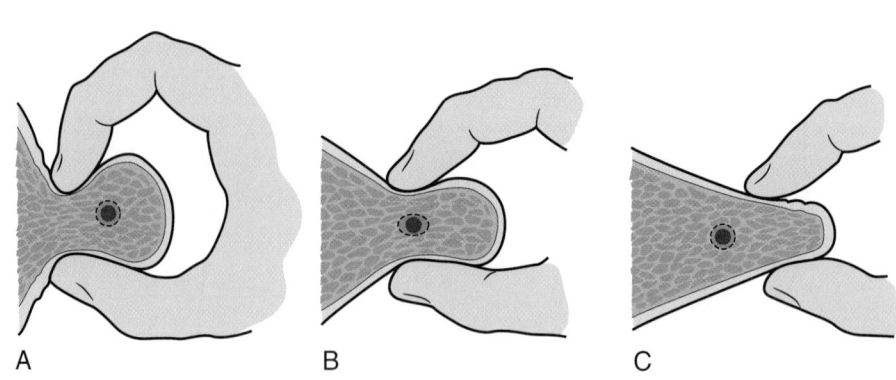

Fig. 18.4 Pincer grasp technique. (A) Muscles that are accessible from two sides may be gripped between the thumb and fingers. (B) The taut band may be felt as it is rolled between the digits. (C) The edge of the taut band is palpable as it rolls beneath the fingertips, often inciting a local twitch response. (From Simons DG, Travell JG, Simons LS. *Travell & Simons' Myofascial Pain and Dysfunction: The Trigger Point Manual.* 2nd ed. Philadelphia: Lippincott Williams & Wilkins; 1999.)

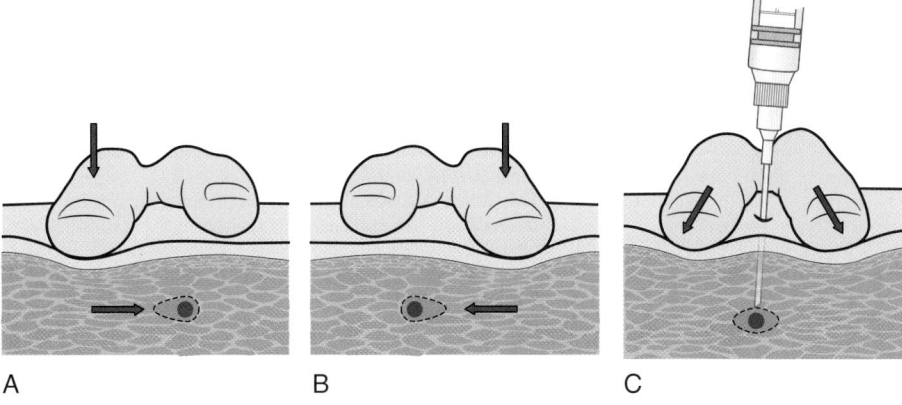

Fig. 181.5 Localizing and securing a trigger point for injection. (A–B) The use of alternating pressure helps to precisely localize the trigger point. (C) The trigger point is held in place with downward pressure and gentle traction to keep it from sliding away from the needle. (From Simons DG, Travell JG, Simons LS. *Travell & Simons' Myofascial Pain and Dysfunction: The Trigger Point Manual.* 2nd ed. Philadelphia: Lippincott Williams & Wilkins; 1999.)

TECHNIQUE

1. Place the patient in a comfortable or recumbent position (never standing) to protect them in the event of a vasovagal reaction.
2. Identify and mark the trigger point.
3. Using an 18-gauge needle, draw up 5 to 10 mL of 1% lidocaine, 0.5% procaine, or 0.125% to 0.25% bupivacaine into the syringe. If desired, sodium bicarbonate solution may be added in a 1:10 ratio by volume.
4. Replace the needle with a 25- to 27-gauge needle as appropriate for trigger point depth and muscle thickness.
5. Prepare the skin with an antiseptic solution or alcohol.
6. Reidentify the trigger point with gloved hands, observing aseptic technique. The trigger point should be stabilized between the fingers of the nondominant hand with downward pressure and slight tension on the skin surface (Fig. 181.5).
7. If superficial anesthesia is desired, 0.25 to 0.50 mL of local anesthetic may be injected into the skin to produce a wheal or a vapocoolant spray such as ethyl chloride may be applied to the site while maintaining stabilization of the trigger point.
8. Slowly advance the needle perpendicular to the skin toward the trigger point. Avoid infiltrating anesthetic until the needle is fully advanced into the target. A slight resistance should be felt on reaching the fascial plane of the muscle, at which point it is helpful to pause and inject 0.2 mL of solution. A gentle "pop" may be felt as the needle is advanced into the muscle itself. Once the needle is in the trigger point site, observe for LTRs and aspirate to confirm a nonvascular position.
9. Inject 0.1 to 0.2 mL of solution once the trigger point is located. Withdraw the needle slightly and reinject the site several times in a fanlike pattern, injecting as the needle is withdrawn (Fig. 181.6). No more than 2 mL should be injected into any particular muscle region. The patient will usually experience immediate relief if the injection is properly located.
   EDITOR'S NOTE: Dry needling is performed the same way, just without injecting any fluid or solution.
10. Remove the needle, and wipe the skin clean with a disinfectant.
11. After withdrawing the needle, place a simple adhesive bandage over the injection site, and massage the entire area to diffuse the anesthetic and check for pain relief. Put the affected muscle complex through full range of motion. If symptoms are still present, consider repeating the procedure with local anesthetic or dry needling.

COMPLICATIONS

- Vasovagal symptoms or syncope.
- Skin infection.
- Injury to nerves, vasculature, or other nearby structures.

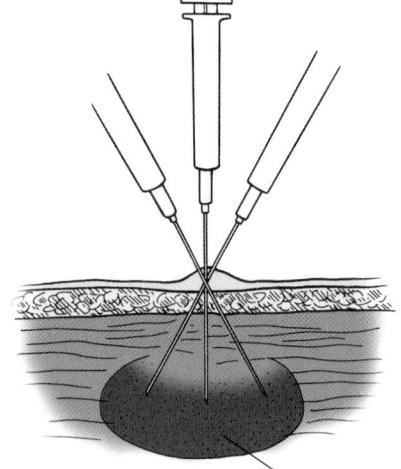

Area of identified tenderness

Fig. 181.6 Injection of a trigger point.

- Rebound pain.
- Reactions to the local anesthetic or steroid.
- Hematoma formation, bleeding, compartment syndrome.
- Pneumothorax (rare). Special care should be observed when injecting muscles of the thorax. Use pincer grasp when possible. Carefully select appropriate needle length. Use a tangential (instead of vertical) vector for the needle. It may be helpful to have the patient hold his or her breath during injection.

POSTPROCEDURE CARE

Active trigger points are generally treated with a series of injections over the course of days to weeks. Injections may be repeated as frequently as every 3 to 4 days. Temporary discomfort due to the injection itself may be treated with cold compresses or oral anti-inflammatory drugs. Patients should be instructed to report any redness, pus, streaking, increased pain, fever, chills, or other concerns. They should use the affected muscle through its full range of motion, but avoid strenuous activity for 1 to 3 days after the injection. Activity modification and ergonomic retraining may help to avoid reinjury.

PATIENT EDUCATION GUIDES

See the sample patient consent form available at www.expertconsult.com.

CPT/BILLING CODES

20552	Injection; single or multiple trigger point(s), one or two muscle(s)
20553	Injection; single or multiple trigger point(s), three or more muscles

NOTE: These codes are per session, not per injection.

ICD-10-CM DIAGNOSTIC CODES

723.1	Cervicalgia
723.9	Unspecified musculoskeletal disorders and symptoms referable to neck
724.1	Pain in thoracic spine
724.2	Lumbago
726.19	Other specified disorders (of rotator cuff syndrome of shoulder)
729.1	Myalgia and myositis, unspecified

Acknowledgment

The editors recognize the contributions by Gary Ruoff, MD, to this chapter in previous editions of this text.

RECOMMENDED READING

Alvarez DJ, Rockwell PG. Trigger points: diagnosis and management. *Am Fam Physician.* 2002;65(4):653–660.

Becker JP, Markowitz JE. Treatment of bursitis, tendonitis and trigger points. In: Roberts JR, Hedges JR, eds. *Clinical Procedures in Emergency Medicine.* Philadelphia: Elsevier; 2017.

Campagne D. Trigger point injections. In: Reichman EF, ed. *Emergency Medicine Procedures.* 2nd ed. New York: McGraw-Hill; 2013.

Christiani AK, Wallis D. Trigger point injection. In: Pfenninger JL, ed. *The Clinics Atlas of Office Procedures: Joint Injection Techniques.* Philadelphia: Saunders; 2002.

Crofford LJ. Fibromyalgia. In: Firestein GS, Budd RC, Gabriel SE, McInnes IB, Odell JR, eds. *Kelley and Firestein's Textbook of Rheumatology.* 10th ed. Philadelphia: Elsevier; 2016.

Cummings TM, White AR. Needling therapies in the management of myofascial trigger point pain: a systematic review. *Arch Phys Med Rehabil.* 2001;82:986–992.

Hong CZ, Hsueh TC. Difference in pain relief after trigger point injections in myofascial pain patients with and without fibromyalgia. *Arch Phys Med Rehabil.* 1996;77:1161–1166.

Kumbhare DA, Elzibak AH, Noseworthy MD. Assessment of Myofascial Trigger Points Using Ultrasound. *Am J Phys Med Rehabil.* 2016;95(1):72–80.

Simons DG, Travell JG, Simons LS. *Travell & Simons' Myofascial Pain and Dysfunction: The Trigger Point Manual.* 2nd ed. Philadelphia: Lippincott Williams & Wilkins; 1999.

Tough EA, White AR, Richards S, Campbell J. Variability of criteria used to diagnose myofascial trigger point pain syndrome: evidence from a review of the literature. *Clin J Pain.* 2007;23:278–286.

Wolfe F, Clauw DJ, Fitzcharles MA, et al. Fibromyalgia criteria and severity scales for clinical and epidemiological studies: a modification of the ACR Preliminary Diagnostic Criteria for Fibromyalgia. *J Rheumatol.* 2011;38(6):1113–1122.

CHAPTER 182

GANGLION TREATMENT

David T. Bortel

The most common tumor of the hand or wrist is the ganglion, which has a propensity for women. A ganglion can occur at almost any location adjacent to a joint or tendon sheath. The most common site is the dorsal wrist (Fig. 182.1), accounting for approximately 65% of ganglions; for this location, the scapholunate ligament and joint are usually the source or root of the pathology (Fig. 182.2). Volar cysts account for approximately 18% to 20% of ganglions and typically originate from the scaphotrapezial or trapeziometacarpal joints (Fig. 182.3). Another site of origin is the palmar fibro-osseous flexor tendon sheath, which accounts for approximately 10% of ganglions. A ganglion at this location normally presents as a hard, small or pea-sized, painful lesion at the proximal interphalangeal flexion crease (Fig. 182.4). Ganglion cysts can be seen at other body sites, with the foot and ankle being common locations (Figs. 182.5 and 182.6). Occasionally they can even be found intraosseously.

IDENTIFICATION AND CHARACTERISTICS

Patients usually present with an obvious mass and sometimes complain of pain and weakness. Ganglion cysts are usually easy to identify by their appearance. The most consistent characteristic is their location, as noted previously. The cyst is often rubbery, but it is sometimes firm. Occasionally a ganglion will allow fluid to be compressed from one septate area to another. The ganglion may transilluminate if it is of sufficient size. Seldom is it necessary to order additional studies to confirm the diagnosis; rather, confirmation is usually made by aspiration, which yields a viscous mucoid fluid (Fig. 182.7). A differential diagnosis includes extensor tenosynovitis, lipoma, sebaceous cyst, other hand tumors, or carpal or tarsal boss ("prominent bump" caused by bone spur). Musculoskeletal ultrasound can be useful for diagnosing occult ganglion cysts, as well as for guiding aspiration and injection (see Chapter 171, Musculoskeletal Ultrasound).

The ganglion cyst is a fibrous-walled, mucin-filled structure typically connected to the joint capsule or tendon sheath by a tortuous stalk. In fact, it is basically a herniation of the synovial lining of tendons, ligaments, or joints. A "one-way valve" probably predicates the formation of these nonmalignant, yet frequently painful, lesions. Use of the offending joint or tendon leads to increased production of the encapsulated mucin, thus magnifying the symptoms. The ganglion commonly is self-limiting (perhaps over several years) by rupture or resorption. These cysts may reflect an underlying ligamentous or arthritic pathology.

NOTE: A close cousin of the ganglion cyst is the mucous (or mucinous) cyst. Both are nearly identical histologically, but the mucous cyst often involves a more persistent if not ominous process. Mucous cysts often arise from an arthritic distal interphalangeal (DIP) joint (i.e., the cyst is a direct drainage conduit to the DIP joint; Fig. 182.8). Osteophytes are frequently noted in those undergoing surgery. Unfortunately, as these cysts enlarge with time, they will commonly erode into the germinal nail matrix, causing discomfort and nail distortion. (Nail distortion is a hallmark of this type cyst; it may precede cyst development by 6 months.) There is disagreement in the literature regarding optimal treatment

approaches. Dermatologists have reported success with conservative treatments such as needling, injection of sclerosing agents (Cordoba et al., 2008), aspiration, injection with a steroid, or curettage and electrocautery or cryotherapy of the base. Without treatment, the thinned local subcutaneous tissue may rupture spontaneously, leading to a septic joint or osteomyelitis. Lesions that recur more than a few times are particularly difficult to manage, even by skilled hand surgeons. Part of the disagreement regarding management may be due to the fact that hand surgeons are often referred the more refractory cases. During open surgery, they frequently remove osteophytes. Aspiration or injection, with curettage, cryotherapy, or electrocautery of the base of mucous cysts, can be attempted judiciously, but the risk of causing a septic joint must be discussed. If such treatment is implemented, the patient needs to be aware of the signs of infection.

EDITOR'S NOTE: Having seen at least one malignancy in a mucous cyst, if tissue is removed from the cyst, it should be sent for pathology.

PREPROCEDURE PATIENT PREPARATION

The patient should be informed that he or she will experience some discomfort similar to having a tooth numbed by a dentist. When the area is being anesthetized, a temporary burning sensation is felt. The local anesthetic typically lasts for 30 to 60 minutes. While anesthetized, the involved tissue could be prone to further unknown trauma until the anesthetic subsides. After the procedure, there will be a pressure-like sensation that may last for a few days. Typically, a pressure dressing will be necessary for several days over the ganglion site. Any steroid or sclerosant placed may produce a local reaction, which can be as simple as skin irritation or as dramatic as dermal atrophy, significant hypopigmentation, or subsequent cutaneous slough. Fortunately, the dramatic reactions are rare. Similarly, systemic manifestations to steroids are rare because dosages and volumes for these lesions are usually very small.

Ganglion cysts of the volar wrist near the distal radius are near the radial artery (Fig. 182.9). In fact, excision of a cyst in this region often requires dissecting scar tissue off the radial artery. Theoretically, incision and drainage of a ganglion in this area might predispose the patient to an arteriovenous malformation; however, a cyst that spontaneously ruptures in this area or is surgically removed may also predispose the patient to such a lesion.

Ganglion Cyst Excision

The patient should be informed of the alternative to either simple observation or aspiration and injection (with a 33% recurrence rate or higher), and that is surgical removal by a hand surgeon under regional or general anesthesia. Although the aspiration and injection procedure has a high recurrence rate, this must be weighed against the fact that it is a fairly simple procedure performed in the office and easily repeated, if necessary. Alternatively, two surgical approaches are available, with newer arthroscopic techniques demonstrating comparable recurrence rates as traditional open surgical

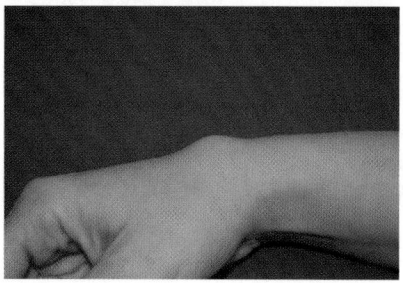

Fig. 182.1   Dorsal wrist ganglion. (Courtesy The Medical Procedures Center, Midland, MI.)

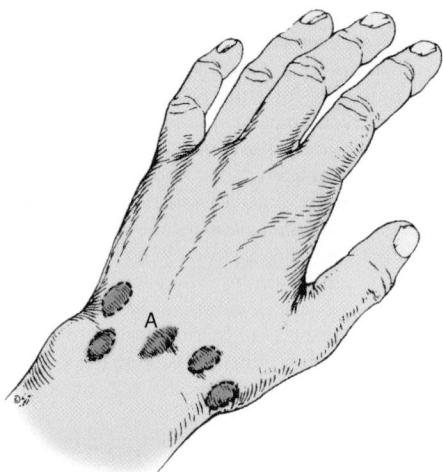

Fig. 182.2   A few of the many possible locations of dorsal wrist ganglions. The most common site (A) is directly over the scapholunate ligament. The others are typically connected to the scapholunate ligament through an elongated pedicle. (Modified from Athanasian EA. Bone and soft tissue tumors. In: Wolfe SW, Hotchkiss RN, Pederson WC, Kozin SH, Cohen MS, eds. *Green's Operative Hand Surgery*. 7th ed. Philadelphia: Elsevier; 2017:1987–2035.)

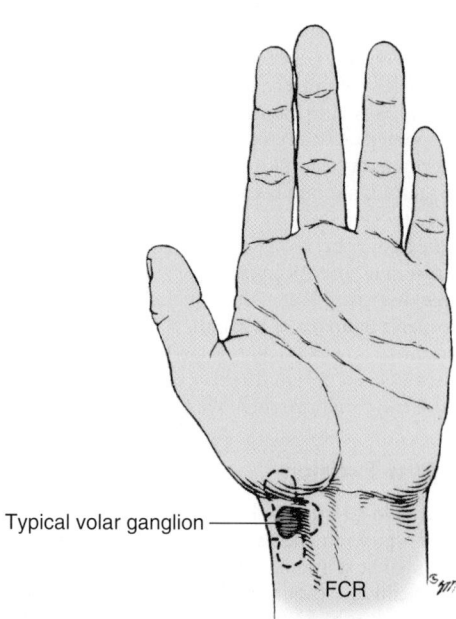

Fig. 182.3   Typical location of a volar wrist ganglion. Possible subcutaneous extensions (*dotted lines*) are often palpable. *FCR*, Flexor carpi radialis. (Modified from Athanasian EA. Bone and soft tissue tumors. In: Wolfe SW, Hotchkiss RN, Pederson WC, Kozin SH, Cohen MS, eds. *Green's Operative Hand Surgery*. 7th ed. Philadelphia: Elsevier; 2017:1987–2035.)

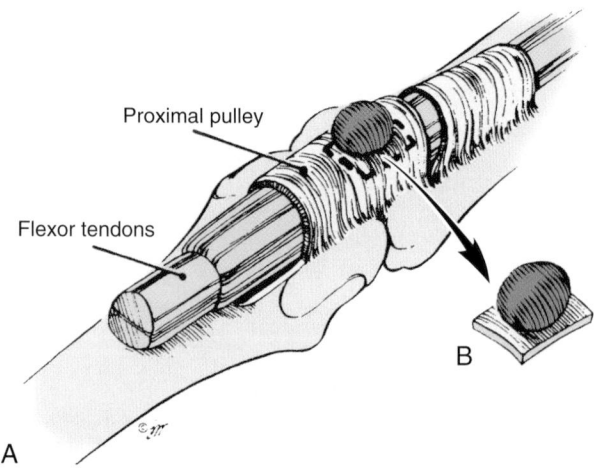

Fig. 182.4   (A) Volar retinacular ganglion in situ on the proximal annular ligament (A1 pulley) of the flexor tendon sheath. (B) Excised specimen with a surrounding margin of tendon sheath. (Modified from Athanasian EA. Bone and soft tissue tumors. In: Wolfe SW, Hotchkiss RN, Pederson WC, Kozin SH, Cohen MS, eds. *Green's Operative Hand Surgery*. 7th ed. Philadelphia: Elsevier; 2017:1987–2035.)

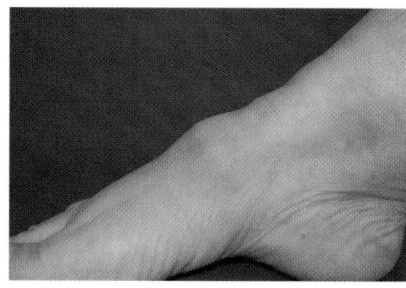

Fig. 182.5   Dorsal foot ganglion (differential includes tarsal boss, due to bone spur, which can be confirmed by x-ray).

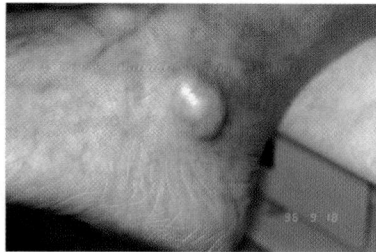

Fig. 182.6   Ganglion inferior to malleolus of ankle. (Courtesy The Medical Procedures Center, Midland, MI.)

techniques, or approximately a 25% recurrence rate. For surgery, typical anesthetic risks should be discussed, as well as the risks of surgery of this nature, including infection, neurovascular injury, rarely a venous thromboembolic event (much more common in the lower extremities), or recurrence of the ganglion. If the ganglion has resulted from a capsular or ligamentous defect, additional problems such as underlying joint destabilization and stiffness may occur.

INDICATIONS FOR ASPIRATION AND INJECTION

- Symptomatic ganglion cyst (e.g., pain, paresthesias, motion limiting)
- Patient desires aspiration and/or injection (may be due to cosmetic deformity)
- Diagnosis uncertain (although rare, malignant lesions can mimic ganglion cysts)

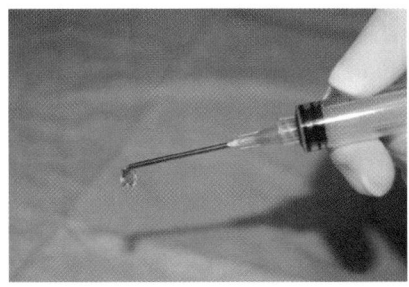

Fig. 182.7 Typical thick, honey-like consistency of ganglion mucin. (Courtesy The Medical Procedures Center, Midland, MI.)

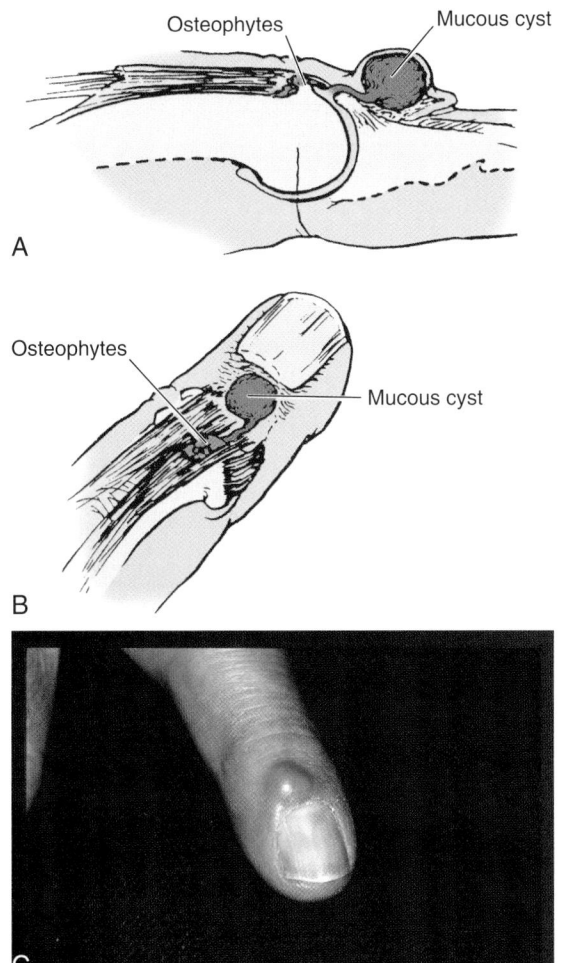

Fig. 182.8 (A) Relationship between mucous cyst and osteophyte of distal interphalangeal joint. Note that the cyst communicates with the joint. The osteophyte causes attrition of the extensor tendon, cyst formation, and decreased range of motion of the joint due to limited extension. (B) As seen from above. (C) Mucous cyst involving nailbed and distal interphalangeal joint. (A–B, Modified from Eaton RG, Dobranski AI, Littler JW. Marginal osteophyte excision in treatment of mucous cysts. *J Bone Joint Surg Am.* 1973;55:570–574. C, Courtesy The Medical Procedures Center, Midland, MI.)

CONTRAINDICATIONS TO ASPIRATION AND INJECTION

Be cautious and consider anatomic locations for critical neurovascular structures. The radial artery and dorsal sensory radial nerve are notable vulnerable structures and, as such, should be avoided.

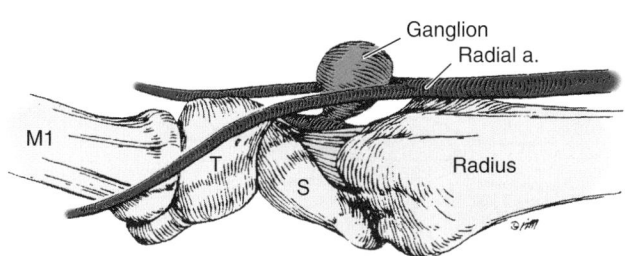

Fig. 182.9 Usual relationship of the ganglion to the radial artery and volar joint capsule. *M1*, First metacarpal; *S*, scaphoid; *T*, trapezium. (Modified from Athanasian EA. Bone and soft tissue tumors. In: Wolfe SW, Hotchkiss RN, Pederson WC, Kozin SH, Cohen MS, eds. *Green's Operative Hand Surgery.* 7th ed. Philadelphia: Elsevier; 2017:1987–2035.)

EQUIPMENT

- 25- or 27-gauge needle, 1 mL or less of lidocaine (1%), without epinephrine, in 1 or 3 mL syringe (it can be buffered with 0.1 mL of 7% to 10% sodium bicarbonate to minimize the stinging; see Chapter 5, Local Anesthesia)
- 18-gauge needle and 3- or 5-mL syringe for aspiration
- 1- or 3-mL syringe filled with steroid if injecting
- Small (2- to 4-inch) elastic bandage (e.g., Ace wrap) (optional)
  - Ultrasound guidance may be considered to guide ganglion aspiration.

Please refer to specified treatment techniques. Also see Chapter 180, Joint and Soft Tissue Aspiration and Injection (Arthrocentesis), as well as Chapter 171, Musculoskeletal Ultrasound.

TREATMENT OPTIONS

1. *Observation.* Unless the ganglion is symptomatic (unsightly, painful, or limits motion), no treatment is necessary. Aspiration is indicated if there is uncertainty with the diagnosis.
2. *Digital pressure or rupture with a mallet, large book (e.g., the Bible), or blade.* These have all been tried historically with minimal success. Simple incision and drainage or rupturing with a needle are variants of this method.
3. *Aspiration and injection.* Aspiration followed by a steroid injection remains a commonly used technique. Although recurrence rates are high (33% or higher), some consider it the initial treatment of choice.
4. *Surgery.* Excision may be simple or quite complex. It is generally performed with a sterile environment. Even though recurrence rate is low with surgery, it can be as high as 25% if the surgeon cannot remove the entire stalk and a portion of the joint capsule.

TECHNIQUE FOR ASPIRATION AND INJECTION

Steroids

1. Using a 25- or 27-gauge needle, 1 mL or less of local lidocaine (1%) without epinephrine is deposited in a wheal over the most superficial portion of the ganglion. If the cyst is small, avoid this step because it may obscure (i.e., make it difficult to palpate) the underlying lesion.
2. The clinician first stabilizes and localizes the ganglion by grasping it (or the area around it) between the thumb and index finger of the nondominant hand. Using the clinician's dominant hand, an 18-gauge needle attached to a 3- to 5-mL syringe is inserted centrally into the ganglion while aspirating. Entry into the cyst is confirmed by a flash (it may be a small amount) of gelatinous fluid into the syringe. All of the thick, gelatinous fluid is then aspirated (Fig. 182.10). Applying pressure on the cyst by squeezing it between the thumb and index finger of the nondominant hand may be helpful. (If no fluid is aspirated, yet the clinician is certain that the needle has entered the cyst, the needle has

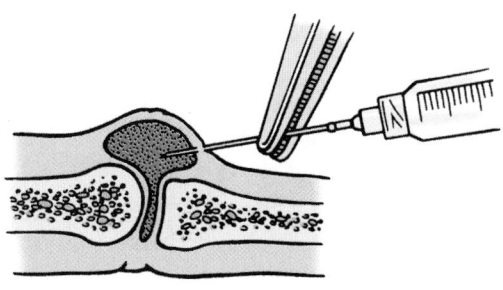

Fig. 182.10 Use an 18-gauge needle and a 1- to 3-mL syringe to enter the ganglion and aspirate its contents. The contents are often thick, and there may be only minimal return of a gel-like material. Hold the needle in position with the hemostat, and remove the syringe. Attach the steroid-containing syringe and inject the contents.

probably become obstructed with a skin plug or very viscous fluid. Withdraw and detach the needle, fill the syringe with air, and attempt to flush this air back through the needle with the needle directed into a biohazard bin. This may remove an obstruction caused by either a skin plug or clotted, viscous fluid. Reinsert the needle into the ganglion.) Optionally, ultrasound may be used for ganglion identification and needle guidance.
3. Secure this needle in place with a sterile hemostat (having verified that it is in the cyst) and remove the syringe filled with mucin.
4. Attach another syringe (1 or 3 mL) filled with a 50/50 mixture of 1% lidocaine and steroid of choice (e.g., betamethasone; see Chapter 192, Joint and Soft Tissue Aspiration and Injection [Arthrocentesis]), and inject into the confines of the cyst. Variable amounts are used depending on the size of the cyst (0.1 to 1 mL). To reduce local steroid complications, consider starting with even smaller amounts of steroid. After injection, withdraw the needle.
5. Pressure is held over the needle track with a sterile gauze pad; then some clinicians wrap the area with a small elastic bandage (e.g., Ace wrap) to maintain occlusion of the cyst walls.

Editor's Note: After successful aspiration, all efforts should be focused on keeping the tip of the needle in the cyst until it is injected. After the cyst has been aspirated, if at all possible, do not withdraw the needle and then attempt a second insertion to inject (unless the needle becomes obstructed and has to be withdrawn to remove the obstruction).

Sclerosants

1. Technique is as noted for aspiration/injection. Instead of using steroids, substitute 1 mL of 3% sodium tetradecyl sulfate or 1 mL of polidocanol. These are the same solutions used for sclerosing veins. Inject with approximately half the amount of the mucin withdrawn.
NOTE: This technique reportedly has an 80% resolution rate.
2. Maintain compression continuously for 2 weeks.

EDITOR'S NOTE: After successful aspiration, all efforts should be focused on keeping the tip of the needle in the cyst in the cyst until it is injected. After the cyst has been aspirated, do not withdraw the needle and then attempt a second insertion to inject.

POSTPROCEDURE PATIENT EDUCATION

The patient should be aware that if a steroid or sclerosing agent was reinjected into the cyst, the cyst may appear to be the same size. It may look and feel like nothing was done. However, unlike ganglion cyst fluid, this fluid will be rapidly reabsorbed. The patient should know to call the clinician's office or go to the emergency department

for bleeding from the site, a significant increase in pain or fever, or signs or symptoms of infection. If a pressure dressing is applied, he or she should be instructed how to care for it and when it should be removed.

COMPLICATIONS

Recurrence is the most common complication. That said, this procedure should not be taken lightly. Consideration of medical history and the location of the ganglion are of the utmost importance. The tissue overlying the ganglion commonly is thin with a poor blood supply and can slough because of bleeding, inadequate perfusion, or immune compromise. In addition, these cysts can be intertwined with neurovascular structures (see Fig. 182.9), and an intravascular or intraneural injection can have adverse results. Subcutaneous atrophy or depigmentation can occur if the steroid concentration is too high.

OPERATIVE TREATMENT

Surgical excision usually is 75% curative if the ganglion and stalk are removed with a small cuff of the adjacent joint capsule. The procedure should be approached with the same seriousness as any other hand surgery. A surgical suite with general or regional anesthesia is preferred. These operations should be performed by clinicians familiar with these lesions and the nearby anatomic structures. Even with surgical excision, the cysts can recur. The small, troublesome mucinous cyst on the dorsal DIP joint can actually require a fairly aggressive procedure to resolve.

CPT/BILLING CODES

10160	Puncture aspiration of abscess, hematoma, bulla, or cyst
20612	Aspiration and/or injection of ganglion cyst(s) any location
25110	Excision, lesion of tendon sheath, forearm and/or wrist
25111	Excision of ganglion, wrist (dorsal or volar); primary

NOTE: If the procedure is performed using ultrasound guidance, see Chapter 171 for appropriate coding additions and modifications.

ICD-10-CM DIAGNOSTIC CODES

| M67 | 40 Ganglion joint or tendon sheath unspecified site |

RECOMMENDED READING

Andrén L, Eiken O. Arthrographic studies of wrist ganglions. *J Bone Joint Surg Am.* 1971;53:299–302.
Athanasian EA. Bone and soft tissue tumors. In: Wolfe SW, Hotchkiss RN, Pederson WC, Kozin SH, Cohen MS, eds. *Green's Operative Hand Surgery.* 7th ed. Philadelphia: Elsevier; 2017:1987–2035.
Brown JS. *Minor Surgery: A Text and Atlas.* 4th ed. London: Oxford University Press; 2001.
Colio SW, Smith J, Pourcho AM. Ultrasound-Guided Interventional Procedures of the Wrist and Hand: anatomy, indications, and techniques. *Phys Med Rehabil Clin North Am.* 2016;27(3):589–605.
Cordoba S, Romero A, Hernandez-Nunez A, Borbujo JM. Treatment of digital mucous cysts with percutaneous sclerotherapy using polidocanol. *Dermatol Surg.* 2008;34(10):1387–1388.
Dias J, Buch K. Palmar wrist ganglion: does intervention improve outcome? A prospective study of the natural history and patient-reported treatment outcomes. *J Hand Surg Br.* 2003;28:172–176.
Head L1, Gencarelli JR1. Allen M1. Boyd KU2 Wrist ganglion treatment: systematic review and meta-analysis. *J Hand Surg Am.* 2015;40(3):546–553.

Holm PCA, Pandey SD. Treatment of ganglia of the hand and wrist with aspiration and injection of hydrocortisone. *Hand*. 1973;5:63–68.

Jayson MIV, Dickson ASJ. Valvular mechanism in juxta-articular cysts. *Ann Rheum Dis*. 1970;29:415–420.

Kleinert HE, Kutz JE, Fishman JH, McCraw LH. Etiology and treatment of the so-called mucous cyst of the finger. *J Bone Joint Surg Am*. 1972;54:1455–1458.

Loder RT, Robinson JH, Jackson WT, Allen DJ. A surface ultrastructure study of ganglia and digital mucous cysts. *J Hand Surg Am*. 1988;13:758–762.

Nelson CL, Sawmiller S, Phalen GS. Ganglions of the wrist and hand. *J Bone Joint Surg Am*. 1972;54:1459–1464.

Peimer CA. Surgery of the hand and wrist. In: Brunicardi FC, Andersen DK, Billiar TR, et al., eds. *Schwartz's Principles of Surgery*. 8th ed. New York: McGraw-Hill; 2005:1721–1787.

Peimer CA, Thompson JS. Tumors of the hand. In: Chapman MW, ed. *Operative Orthopaedics*. 3rd ed. Philadelphia: Lippincott Williams & Wilkins; 2001.

Richman JA, Gelberman RH, Engber WD, et al. Ganglions of the wrist and digits: Results of treatment by aspiration and cyst wall puncture. *J Hand Surg Am*. 1987;12:1041–1043.

Strenge KB, Mangan DB, Idusuyi OB. Postoperative toxic shock syndrome after excision of a ganglion cyst from the ankle. *J Foot Ankle Surg*. 2006;45:275–277.

Tallia AF, Cardone DA. Diagnostic and therapeutic injection of the wrist and hand region. *Am Fam Physician*. 2003;67:745–750.

CHAPTER 183

Transcutaneous Electrical Nerve Stimulation, Phonophoresis, and Iontophoresis

Russell D. White • Mary Beth Brown

The procedures described in this chapter—transcutaneous electrical nerve stimulation (TENS), phonophoresis, and iontophoresis—can be performed either by primary care clinicians in their office or by physical therapists when ordered by a clinician. The procedures are often used with other physical therapy modalities such as manual therapy, hot or cold therapy, or therapeutic exercise. The choice of procedure depends on the size (localized vs. diffuse) and depth (superficial vs. deep) of the proposed treatment area, as well as the specific pathologic process.

EQUIPMENT

- Scissors to trim hair
- Isopropyl alcohol 70% to cleanse skin
- For TENS: TENS unit with either disposable or reusable electrodes and gel
- For phonophoresis: therapeutic ultrasound unit, appropriate medication, and coupling gel
- For iontophoresis: direct-current generator with constant current output (calibrated in milliamperes), electrodes, and appropriate medications

PREPROCEDURE PATIENT PREPARATION

After discussing the patient's diagnosis, the risks and benefits of the selected treatment should be explained, along with any treatment options. Oral or written consent should be obtained from the patient. Patients should be aware that their skin will be cleansed and that their hair may be trimmed. The anticipated treatment plan and total number of treatments should also be discussed.

TRANSCUTANEOUS ELECTRICAL NERVE STIMULATION

TENS therapy uses low-voltage electrical pulses to stimulate the nervous system and is used for the treatment of pain syndromes. Skin surface electrodes are used to pass the electricity into the affected area. TENS units are class II, US Food and Drug Administration–approved devices and are typically selected for larger, generalized areas of pain, for acute or chronic joint pains, or for persistent myalgias. This procedure can be performed in the clinician's office and is reimbursable if performed by the clinician. However, TENS therapy is usually prescribed by a clinician and performed by the physical therapist. When prescribed for home use, the patient must be competent in operating a TENS unit. As it turns out, they are also now available over the counter.

TENS therapy is based on the gate theory of pain. According to this theory, nociperception (injury information) is transmitted through T cells that convey information to the higher brain centers. This information is presynaptically inhibited by interneurons in the substantia gelatinosa. TENS therapy bombards these interneurons, attempting to modulate or decrease the pain transmission by effectively blocking transmission of pain sensation. Other theories suggest that TENS therapy achieves its result by an acupuncture effect, by release of natural opiates, or by direct local vasodilation, which may reduce relative ischemia.

The goal of TENS therapy is to reduce or relieve pain and discomfort. This result may be either short-lived or prolonged. TENS therapy may slowly break the *pain-spasm-pain cycle* and reduce perceived discomfort. Unfortunately, TENS therapy is not effective for pain of central origin (e.g., headache). In fact, a systematic review (Khadilkar, 2005) found no benefit for chronic low back pain. In 2012, based on a review of evidence, the Centers for Medicare and Medicaid Services published a memorandum stating that "TENS is not reasonable and necessary for the treatment of chronic low back pain." A more recent Cochrane review (Johnson, 2015) found that TENS may reduce pain intensity when used as stand-alone therapy in acute pain. It has also been shown to be useful for diabetic neuropathic pain and for neuropathic pain from spinal cord injuries.

Treatment parameters are chosen based on several factors:

- *Intensity:* Small unmyelinated fibers require more current than large myelinated fibers. (Intensity is set according to patient comfort [strong but not painful] and can vary widely by body part undergoing treatment, by device used, and by individual sensation and tolerance.)
- *Pulse rate:* Small unmyelinated fibers respond better to a low-frequency rate (<100 Hz), whereas large myelinated fibers respond better to a high-frequency rate (>100 Hz).
- *Wave characteristics:* These characteristics are either monophasic (positive rectangular pattern) or biphasic (negative spike pattern).
- *Pulse width:* Small unmyelinated fibers respond to a long pulse (200 ms), whereas large myelinated fibers respond to a short pulse (50 ms).
- *Modulation:* Modulation allows gradual variation of the frequency or pulse width and retards accommodation of the nervous tissue.

Indications

- Chronic pain
- Acute pain
- Diabetic and spinal cord injury neuropathic pain

- Musculoskeletal pain
- Neurologic pain (e.g., herpes zoster)
- Phantom limb pain
- Before another procedure to elevate the pain threshold and to decrease patient discomfort after the procedure
- Postoperative pain
- Obstetric pain (after the first trimester)

Contraindications

- Patients with demand-type pacemakers (Newer pacemakers with improved shielding are not affected by TENS units. Check with a cardiologist or the manufacturer.)
- Patients in first-trimester pregnancy
- Patients with known cardiac dysrhythmias
- Mentally incompetent patients, uncooperative patients, those with paranoid disorders, or pediatric patients without adult supervision
- Undiagnosed pain syndromes without established etiology
- TENS therapy is also contraindicated over the following areas:
  - Carotid sinuses
  - Chest areas in patients with a cardiac history
  - Head or neck area of patients with an epileptic history
  - Laryngeal or pharyngeal muscles
  - Local areas of skin irritation or loss of skin integrity
  - Mucosal surfaces
  - Eyes

Technique

1. Before initiating therapy, organize the necessary materials (Fig. 183.1) and prepare the skin area to which the electrodes will be attached. Trimming hair and cleansing the skin with 70% isopropyl alcohol will promote the adhesion and conductivity of the electrodes.
2. Select the proper electrodes. For 24 hours or more of use, select either a carbon-impregnated rubber electrode with gel or a carbon-filled silicone electrode.
3. Attach electrodes to the selected treatment site, whether isolated trigger points, individual dermatomes or myotomes, or in the distribution of a specific nerve. Position the electrodes so that a paresthesia will be felt in the area of pain or dysfunction (Fig. 183.2). If the electrodes are secured poorly to the skin, they may cause a burning sensation instead of a paresthesia. In addition, electrodes should be placed at least 2 inches apart. Placing electrodes closer together can cause a burning sensation. The electrodes should also be placed so that the perimeter of the painful area is entirely surrounded by the electrodes.

4. Select the treatment parameters. Conventional settings use a high-frequency rate with a narrow pulse width. The intensity level is less than that which results in muscle stimulation.
5. With the amplitude control in the off position, attach wires to the TENS unit. Turn on the generator unit and increase the amplitude slowly, up to the patient's comfort level. Again, paresthesia should be felt by the patient before the threshold for motor stimulation.
6. If desired results (paresthesia with control of pain) are not achieved, change the stimulation sites or adjust the treatment settings.
7. Typically patients are treated once or twice daily for a duration of 30 to 60 minutes. Some patients may benefit from more frequent treatments and may require a home unit for therapy.
8. When the treatment is completed, turn off the unit, return the settings to zero, and remove the electrodes.

Complications

- Skin irritation from electrode placement
- Contact dermatitis resulting from electrode gels
- Pacemaker malfunction (typically an older pacemaker)
- Twitch response secondary to stimulation of a motor nerve or end plate in the treatment area by inappropriate current

PHONOPHORESIS

Phonophoresis uses therapeutic ultrasound to enhance the diffusion of medications across the skin and into body tissues. Commonly used medications include dexamethasone, hydrocortisone, topical nonsteroidal antiinflammatory cream, and lidocaine. Although phonophoresis is usually performed by the physical therapist, some clinicians provide this modality in the office setting. Clinicians can be reimbursed for phonophoresis, even if not performed by a physical therapist.

The dual action of phonophoresis—thermal and mechanical—counteracts the inflammatory response by a process called acoustic streaming, which increases cell membrane permeability. This effect also facilitates the passage of medications into body tissue. With *acute* inflammation, using pulse-mode ultrasound avoids an increase in tissue temperature. In addition to the alteration of tissue permeability, beneficial effects are obtained through nonthermal changes (e.g., stimulation of fibroblasts). With chronic inflammation, using continuous or nonpulsed ultrasound can produce thermal changes that counteract or prevent the chronic changes of scarring and tissue edema.

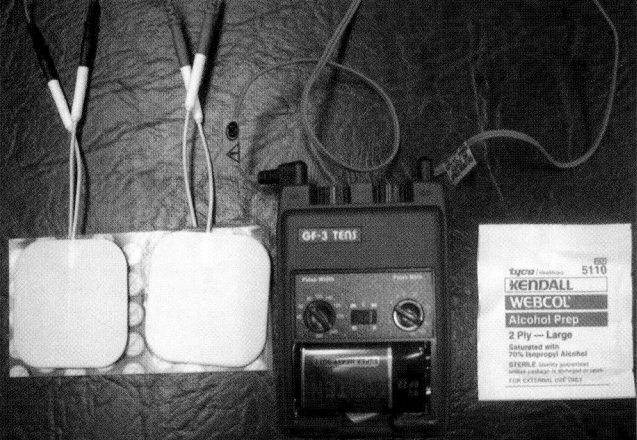

Fig. 183.1 Transcutaneous electrical nerve stimulation unit (generator) with supplies for skin preparation, electrodes, and electrode wires.

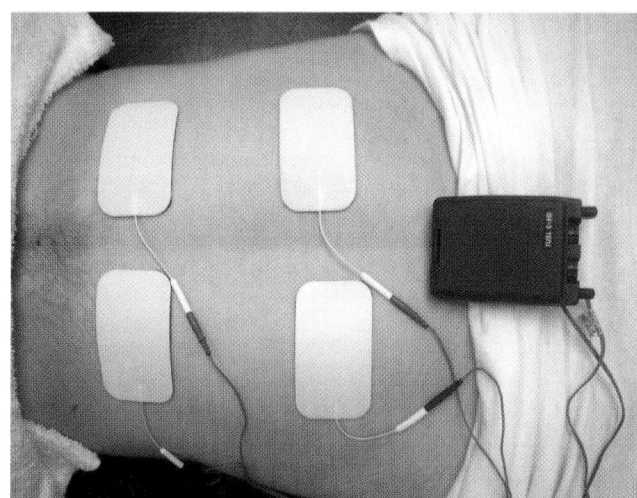

Fig. 183.2 Transcutaneous electrical nerve stimulation treatment.

Ultrasound dose is measured in intensity (intensity = W/cm^2), which is the acoustic energy delivered through the surface area of the head of the transducer. Areas of inflammation are usually treated with 1 to 2 W/cm^2 for 5 to 10 minutes. Results are measured by the improvement (either immediate or gradual) in pain or function of the treated area.

Indications

- Superficial periarticular disorders: bursitis, tendinitis, ligament sprains
- Contracture of joint capsules or adhesive scars
- Neuromas
- Reflex sympathetic dystrophy
- Plantar warts
- Muscular strains, fibrosis, spasm, myositis (limited evidence)
- Myofascial pain syndrome
- Carpal tunnel syndrome
- Epicondylitis
- Knee osteoarthritis
- Trigger point

Contraindications

- Allergy to medications being used
- Tumors or cancer
- Thrombophlebitis
- Pregnancy (therapeutic ultrasound is contraindicated over the abdomen and pelvis)
- Hemorrhagic or infected areas
- Cardiac disease (therapeutic ultrasound over the cervical ganglia, cardiac area, or an implanted pacemaker may produce a detrimental cardiac reflex)
- Unhealed fracture sites
- Phonophoresis should also be avoided over the following areas:
  - Epiphyseal plate in growing bones
  - Spinal cord or near laminectomy sites
  - Area of previous radiation therapy (wait 6 months before applying ultrasound)
  - Eyes
  - Near implant containing plastic

Technique

1. A clinician's prescription is required for the medications when phonophoresis is administered by a physical therapist.
2. Select an area of inflammation for treatment that is no greater than twice the surface area of the sound head.
3. Select the proper ultrasound equipment (Figs. 183.3 and 183.4).
4. Cleanse the general area to be treated. Inspect the skin for excessive dryness and trim excess hair. Skin areas may be pretreated with moist heat packs to facilitate drug absorption by dilating the hair follicles.
5. Because the chosen agent can affect ultrasound transmission, select only topical agents that transmit ultrasound. (Hydrocortisone 10% or ketoprofen 2.5 % in an aqueous base are commonly used medications for phonophoresis.) Apply the medication followed by the coupling gel or use coupling gels impregnated with medication.
6. Apply phonophoresis through the sound head in a moving pattern of overlapping strokes or circles (Fig. 183.5).
7. Recommended intensities of 1 to 2 W/cm^2 usually provide effective results. Use frequencies of 3 MHz for superficial tissues and 1 MHz for deeper tissues. Apply for 5 to 10 minutes. Treatment for greater than 10 minutes increases the risk of a negative effect (e.g., periosteal burn).
8. When finished, wipe away coupling gel but do not cleanse skin; there is some evidence that an occlusive dressing may further promote continued medication absorption.

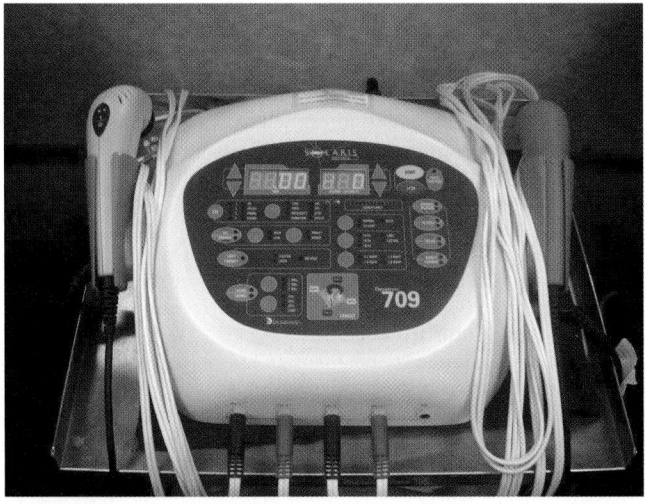

Fig. 183.3 Ultrasound–electrical stimulation combination unit used for phonophoresis and transcutaneous electrical nerve stimulation.

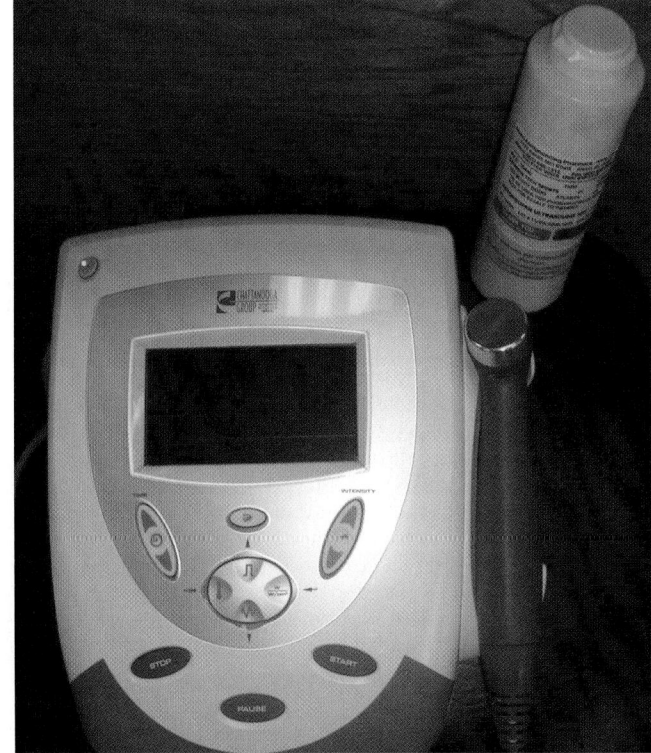

Fig. 183.4 Ultrasound unit.

Complications

- Previously unknown allergy or sensitivity to medication
- Systemic side effects from excessive absorption of applied medication
- Damage to susceptible areas (listed in "Contraindications" section)

IONTOPHORESIS

Iontophoresis uses direct electrical current to enhance the diffusion and absorption of charged medications across the skin and mucous membranes. With this technique, medicinal ions can penetrate tissue for 0.2 to 1.5 cm, depending on the drug used and the characteristics of the local tissue. This technique is based on repulsion of similarly charged ions; charged ions in solution are driven away from like-charged electrodes.

Iontophoresis works best when the pathologic process is superficial and localized. This treatment is usually performed in an outpatient rehabilitation setting or in the clinician's office. Primary care clinicians can be reimbursed for the procedure, even if it is not performed by a physical therapist.

The most common medications used are dexamethasone or lidocaine, and the amount depends on the size of the treatment area. The amount used also depends on the electrode size and the volume it takes to fill it. Electrode size varies from 1.5 to 3.5 cm³. Dexamethasone is the primary agent indicated for inflammatory lesions. Lidocaine is the agent typically used for preoperative topical anesthesia.

The electrical dose for administration is expressed in milliampere minutes (mA minutes) and is the product of the intensity (milliamperes) and duration (minutes). Most treatments last 10 to 20 minutes each and are repeated three to eight times (depending on patient response).

Indications

- Same indications as for a superficial injection of a therapeutic agent (superficial, because the medications penetrate only up to 1.5 cm with iontophoresis)
- Inflammation
  - Bursitis
  - Tendinitis
  - Fasciitis
  - Sprain
  - Strain
  - Trigger points

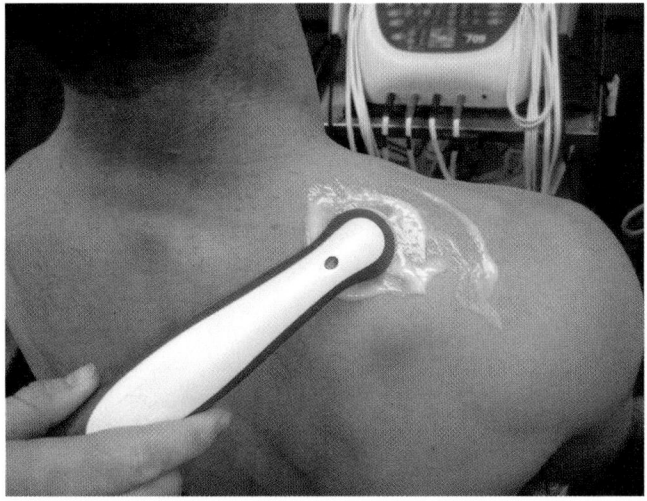

Fig. 183.5 Phonophoresis treatment.

- Carpal tunnel syndrome
- de Quervain disease
- Analgesia
  - Neuritis
  - Local anesthesia for invasive procedures, such as dermatologic procedures
- Other (limited case reports; Table 183.1)
  - Ganglion
  - Hyperhidrosis of feet or palms
  - Ischemic ulcer
  - Neuroma
  - Pain prophylaxis
  - Posttraumatic edema
  - Scar tissue
  - Tinea pedis
  - Turf toe
  - Warts
  - Wound healing

Contraindications

- Allergy or sensitivity to therapeutic agent
- Patients with pacemakers because electric current could interfere with sensitive implanted devices
- Iontophoresis should also be avoided over the following areas:
  - Areas of abnormal skin sensation (patients must be able to give feedback so that the intensity can be set correctly)
  - Superficial abrasions, cuts, and bruises
  - Areas of recent bleeding
  - Areas surrounding or superficial to an implanted or embedded wire, screws, staples, or other metallic objects
  - Recent scars or skin graft
  - Area over heart
  - Area over carotid sinus

Areas of abnormal sensation or a loss of skin integrity have decreased skin resistance; this raises the risk that an increased current dose may be given. Such a dose may lead to undesired skin reactions. Areas of increased vascularity or those near metal objects can also be subjected to enhanced current dosage.

Technique

1. A clinician's prescription is required for the medications administered by a physical therapist using iontophoresis.
2. Position the patient to obtain good exposure for the area to be treated. Inspect the skin of the treatment area for any recent injury or any contraindications previously listed.
3. Clip excessive hair but do not shave. Clean the skin treatment area with 70% isopropyl alcohol to remove surface oils and skin cells.
4. Before initiating therapy, the clinician should organize the equipment and select a direct-current generator (Fig. 183.6). Next, inject the premeasured medication into the electrode

Ion (Dose)	Polarity	Therapeutic Use
Acetic acid (3–4 mA × 10–20 min)	Negative	Calcified tendinitis, calcium deposit
Chloride, sodium (4 mA × 20–45 min)	Negative	Keloids, scar tissue
Copper sulfate (4 mA × 20–30 min)	Positive	Fungal infection
Dexamethasone (1–4 mA × 15–20 min)	Negative	Tendinitis, tenosynovitis, bursitis, arthritis
Hyaluronidase (1–2 mA × 20–40 min)	Positive	Edema, lymphedema, scleroderma
Iodine (2 mA × 1 min; then 4 mA × 5 min)	Negative	Fibrosis, scar tissue, trigger finger
Lidocaine 4% (4 mA × 20–30 min)	Positive	Skin anesthesia
Methylprednisolone (1–4 mA × 15–20 min)	Negative	Postherpetic neuralgia
Salicylate (4 mA × 45 min)	Negative	Analgesia, myalgia, plantar warts
Zinc (4 mA × 15 min)	Positive	Wound healing, ulcers

TABLE 183.1 Indications and Dosages for Common Iontophoresis Agents

reservoir according to the manufacturer's recommendations. (Properly filling electrodes to specified volumes decreases skin irritation.)

5. The active electrode (drug containment electrode) should be attached over the treatment area. It should have the same polarity as the medication to be used. Attach the larger dispersive electrode (indifferent electrode) over an area that is at least 3 inches distant (Fig. 183.7) from the active electrode.

6. Connect the electrode leads to the current generator. Current settings should range from 0.1 to 4 mA.

7. Determine the current dosage on the basis of the diagnosis and treatment. The recommended dosage for dexamethasone or lidocaine is listed in Table 183.1 and measured in mA × min (milliamperes [current] × minutes [time] = mA × min [dosage]).

8. Gradually increase the current until the patient barely feels it. Any sudden change in current may produce burning, stinging, or a twitch response. With most units, the treatment time is automatically set by the device once the intensity (current) and dosage are determined and entered.

9. During and after the procedure, ask the patient every 2 to 4 minutes if he or she is experiencing any adverse effects.

10. When the procedure is completed, remove the attached electrodes. Instruct the patient to report any delayed adverse effects. (Posttreatment erythema is common, resulting from either changes in skin pH or a histamine reaction.)

11. An alternative, recently developed technique is the use of a wearable, battery-powered iontophoresis patch. The patch is filled with medication by a physician or a physical therapist in the clinic and applied directly to prepared skin. Medication is iontophoretically delivered using a constant 0.06- to 0.45-mA current over 3 to 24 hours (varies by manufacturer) with automatic current shut-off when desired dosage is reached.

Complications

- Previously unknown drug allergy or sensitivity to medications
- Galvanic rash: hypersensitivity reaction to the direct current that develops within 5 minutes of initiating the electrical stimulation
- Twitch response secondary to stimulation of a nerve in the treatment area by inappropriate current
- "Negative electrode burn": skin burn resulting from a decrease in skin resistance and an alkaline reaction when the negative electrode (cathode) is the active electrode (newer electrodes stabilize the pH better and cause less skin irritation)
- Local immunologic inhibition from the steroid (dexamethasone is not detected in the bloodstream after treatment)

POSTPROCEDURE PATIENT CARE AND EDUCATION

The patient's results are evaluated by determining the decrease in pain or inflammation after treatment(s). Treatment(s) can be terminated when the patient has reached the desired clinical goal. The number or frequency of treatments can be increased to improve the results, as long as no adverse effects have been noted. On the contrary, after five treatments with any of these modalities, if there are no results, another type of therapy should be considered.

The patient should know to report any delayed adverse reactions to the clinician. He or she should also know when to make a follow-up appointment.

PATIENT EDUCATION GUIDES

See the patient education form available at www.expertconsult.com.

CPT/BILLING CODES

NOTE: Health Care Common Procedure Coding System codes are used for procedures and supplies when there is no CPT code. They are the alphanumeric codes listed here, and reimbursement is variable.

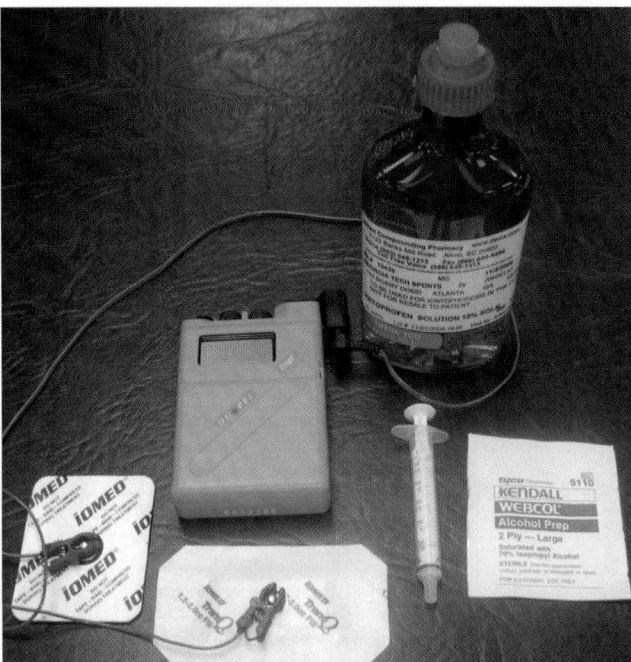

Fig. 183.6 Iontophoresis current generator with iontophoresis agent, measuring syringe, alcohol wipe for skin preparation, electrodes, and electrode leads.

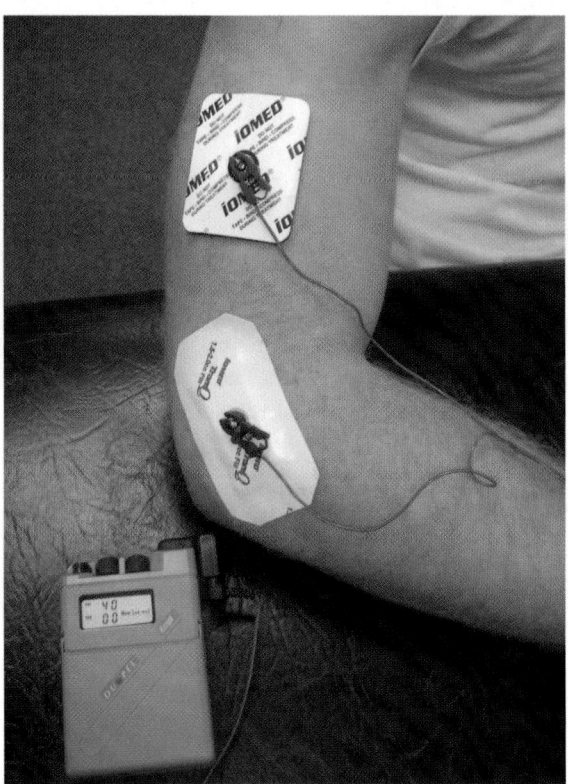

Fig. 183.7 Iontophoresis treatment.

Tens

64550   Application of surface transcutaneous neurostimulator (TENS)

Tens Unit

E0720   TENS, two lead localized stimulation*
E0730   TENS, four lead, larger/multiple nerve stimulation*

Phonophoresis

97035   Ultrasound therapy
A4558   Conductive paste or gel supplies

Iontophoresis

97033   Iontophoresis, each 15 minutes or application of each wearable patch

Medication and Supplies

A4556   Electrodes, per pair
J1100   Dexamethasone sodium phosphate, 4 mg/mL
J1020   Methylprednisolone acetate, 20 mg
J1030   Methylprednisolone acetate, 40 mg
J1040   Methylprednisolone acetate, 80 mg

ICD-10-CM DIAGNOSTIC CODES

B02.29   Other postherpetic nervous system involvement
B07.0   Plantar warts
B35.3   Tinea pedis
G90.50   Reflex sympathetic dystrophy unspecified
G50.9   Trigeminal neuralgia
G54.6   Phantom limb pain
G56.00   Carpal tunnel syndrome unspecified limb
G57.00   Lesion sciatic nerve, unspecified (Piriformis syndrome)
G57.60   Neuroma, Morton unspecified limb
I89.0   Lymphedema
M26.609   Temporomandibular syndrome
O99.89   Other diseases and conditions complicating pregnancy
L91.0   Keloids
L97.909   Nonpressure chronic ulcer, lower limbs unspecified w/unspecified severity
L90.5   Scar tissue
M15.0   Osteoarthrosis, general
M15.9   Osteoarthrosis, unspecified
M19.019   Osteoarthrosis, primary unspecified shoulder
M19.029   Osteoarthrosis, primary unspecified elbow
M19.039   Osteoarthrosis, primary unspecified wrist
M19.049   Osteoarthrosis, primary unspecified hand
M17.10   Osteoarthrosis, primary unspecified knee
M19.079   Osteoarthrosis, primary unspecified ankle/foot
M19.90   Osteoarthrosis, specified sites
M54.5   Low back pain
M75.00   Adhesive capsulitis of unspecified shoulder
M75.30   Tendinitis calcific unspecified shoulder
M70.70   Bursitis unspecified hip
M75.50   Bursitis unspecified shoulder

M77.00   Medial epicondylitis unspecified elbow
M77.10   Lateral epicondylitis unspecified elbow
M70.50   Bursitis unspecified knee
M76.899   Enthesopat, pes anserinus
M76.50   Tendonitis, patellar unspecified knee
M70.40   Bursitis, Prepatellar unspecified knee
M76.60   Tendinitis, Achilles unspecified leg
M77.9   Capsulitis, periarthritis, or tendinitis, NOS
M65.9   Tenosynovitis and synovitis, unspecified
M65.30   Trigger finger unspecified finger
M65.4   de Quervain disease
M67.40   Ganglion of joint or tendon sheath unspecified site
M65.20   Calcific tendonitis
M62.50   Muscle wasting and atrophy not elsewhere classified
M61.00   Myositis ossificans, traumatic
M72.2   Fasciitis, plantar
M62.40   Muscle spasm unspecified site
M60.9   Myositis, unspecified
M79.1   Myalgia
M79.2   Neuritis
R61   Hyperhidrosis
R20.9   Dermal pain
R60.9   Edema

NOTE: Injury diagnoses series need date of injury.

S93.409A   Ankle, sprains/strains, unspecified initial encounter
S93.429A   Ankle, sprain/strain, deltoid ligament initial encounter
S93.419A   Ankle sprain, calcaneofibular ligament initial encounter
S93.439A   Ankle sprain, tibiofibular ligament initial encounter
S986.019A   Ankle strain, Achilles tendon initial encounter
S93.609A   Foot, sprains/strains initial encounter
S93.529A   Sprain unspecified toe (turf toe) initial encounter
S40.019A   Contusion, shoulder initial encounter
S40.029A   Contusion, upper arm initial encounter
S50.10XA   Contusion, forearm initial encounter
S70.00XA   Contusion, hip initial encounter
S70.10XA   Contusion, thigh initial encounter
S80.10XA   Contusion, lower leg initial encounter
S80.00XA   Contusion, knee initial encounter
S79.80XA   Injury, shoulder and upper arm initial encounter
S89.80XA   Injury, knee, leg, ankle, and foot initial encounter

SUPPLIERS

(See contact information available at www.expertconsult.com.)

Iontophoresis
  Axelgaard
  IOMED
  Smith & Nephew
  Travanti Pharma for IontoPatch
  Trivarion
Phonophoresis
  AliMed, Inc.
  Chattanooga Group, Inc.
  Dynatronics
  DynaWave Corporation
  Sontra Medical
TENS units
  AliMed, Inc.
  Electro-Med Health Industries
  EMPI, Inc.
  RS Medical
  Thera-Tronics, Inc.

---

*Prior authorization is required by Medicare for this item.

RECOMMENDED READING

Abram SE. Advances in chronic pain management since gate control. *Reg Anesth.* 1993;18:66–81.

Anderson CR, Morris RL, Boeh SD, et al. Effects of iontophoresis current magnitude and duration on dexamethasone deposition and localized drug retention. *Phys Ther.* 2003;83:161–170.

Bakhtiary AH, Fatemi E, Emami M, Malek M. Phonophoresis of dexamethasone sodium phosphate may manage pain and symptoms of patients with carpal tunnel syndrome. *Clin J Pain.* 2013;29:348–353.

Bolin DJ. Transdermal approaches to pain in sports medicine management. *Curr Sports Med Rep.* 2003;2:303–309.

Cagnie B, Vinck E, Rimbaut S, Vanderstraeten G. Phonophoresis versus topical application of ketoprofen: comparison between tissue and plasma levels. *Phys Ther.* 2003;83:707–712.

Chen WS, Annaswamy TM, Yang W, Wang TG. Physical agent modalities. In: Cifu DX, Kaelin DL, Kowalske KJ, Lew HL, Miller MA, et al., eds. *Braddom's Physical Medicine and Rehabilitation.* 5th ed. Philadelphia: Elsevier; 2016:369–396.

Costello CT, Jeske AH. Iontophoresis: applications in transdermal medication delivery. *Phys Ther.* 1995;75:554–563.

DeSantana JM, Walsh DM, Vance C, et al. Effectiveness of transcutaneous electrical nerve stimulation for treatment of hyperalgesia and pain. *Curr Rheumatol Rep.* 2008;10:492–499.

Deyo RA, Walsh NE, Martin DC, et al. A controlled trial of transcutaneous electrical nerve stimulation (TENS) and exercise for low back pain. *N Engl J Med.* 1990;322:1627–1634.

Gudeman SC, Eisele SA, Heidt RS, et al. Treatment of plantar fasciitis by iontophoresis of 0.4% dexamethasone: a randomized, double-blind, placebo-controlled study. *Am J Sports Med.* 1997;25:312–316.

Guy RH, Kalia YN, Delgado-Charro MB, et al. Iontophoresis: repulsion and electroosmosis. *J Control Release.* 2000;64:129–132.

Johnson MI, Paley CA, Howe TE, Sluka KA. Transcutaneous electrical nerve stimulation for acute pain. *Cochrane Database Syst Rev.* 2015: CD006142. pub3.

Khadilkar A, Milne S, Brosseau L, et al. Transcutaneous electrical nerve stimulation for the treatment of chronic low back pain: a systematic review. *Spine.* 2005;30:2657–2666.

Klaiman MD, Shrader JA, Danoff JV, et al. Phonophoresis versus ultrasound in the treatment of common musculoskeletal conditions. *Med Sci Sports Exerc.* 1998;30:1349–1355.

Kuntz AR, Griffiths CM, Rankin JM, et al. Cortisol concentrations in human skeletal muscle tissue after phonophoresis with 10% hydrocortisone gel. *J Athl Train.* 2006;41:321–324.

Luksurapan W, Boonhong J. Effects of phonophoresis of piroxicam and ultrasound on symptomatic knee osteoarthritis. *Arch Phys Med Rehabil.* 2013;94:250–255.

Moll MJ. A new approach to pain: lidocaine and decadron with ultrasound. *USAF Med Serv Dig.* 1979;30:8–11.

Robinson AJ. Transcutaneous electrical nerve stimulation for the control of pain in musculoskeletal disorders. *J Orthop Sports Phys Ther.* 1996;24:208–226.

Rose JB, Galinkin JL, Jantzen EC, Chiavacci RM. A study of lidocaine iontophoresis for pediatric venipuncture. *Anesth Analg.* 2002;94:867–871.

Semalty A, Semalty M, Singh R, et al. Iontophoretic drug delivery system: a review. *Technol Health Care.* 2007;15:237–245.

Spielholz NI, Nolan MF. Conventional TENS and the phenomena of accommodation, adaptation, habituation, and electrode polarization. *J Clin Electrophysiol.* 1995;7:16–19.

Wang Y, Thakur R, Fan Q, Michniak B. Transdermal iontophoresis: combination strategies to improve transdermal iontophoretic drug delivery. *Eur J Pharm Biopharm.* 2005;60:179–191.

Wu PI, Meleger A, Witkower A, Mondale T, Borg-Stein J. Nonpharmacologic options for treating acute and chronic pain. *PM R.* 2015;7(suppl 11):S278–294.

Zempsky WT, Sullivan J, Paulson DM, Hoath SB. Evaluation of a low-dose lidocaine iontophoresis system for topical anesthesia in adults and children: a randomized, controlled trial. *Clin Ther.* 2004;26:1110–1119.

CHAPTER 184

ACUPUNCTURE

Victor S. Sierpina

The insertion of fine needles into the body at specific points, or "channels of energy flow" called *meridians*, has been used in the treatment of human and animal disease for thousands of years. The oldest reference to this traditional East Asian medical procedure dates to 2600 BC, when fine sharpened stone or bamboo needles are reported to have been used in the treatment and prevention of illness.

Contemporary use of acupuncture has become increasingly popular. It is offered not only by traditionally trained doctors of Oriental medicine but also by allopathic and osteopathic physicians and clinicians. Patients' interest and acceptance of acupuncture in the United States have resulted in its investigation and recognition by such bodies as the National Institutes of Health and the National Center for Complementary and Integrative Health (previously the Office of Alternative Medicine). Their advisory panel released a consensus statement in 2005 supporting the efficacy of acupuncture and acknowledging the potential benefit of acupuncture in a number of acute and chronic conditions. Furthermore, they recommended that the insurance industry consider wider coverage for this safe and effective technique. These statements have begun to change perceptions of this ancient medical art from that of a curiosity or an experimental treatment to that of an acceptable procedure within medical science. In 2009, the National Institute for Health and Care Excellence guidelines were released in the United Kingdom for the early management of low back pain in adults, endorsing the consideration of acupuncture among other modalities. However, this endorsement was revoked in the 2016 update of these guidelines. Most recently, the American College of Physicians endorsed acupuncture as an evidence-based nonpharmacologic therapy for acute, subacute, and chronic low back pain (Qaseem et al., 2017). At a minimum, acupuncture may be considered as an alternative for many pain syndromes, certainly as an alternative to the use of narcotics. Acupuncture has also been studied in the treatment of many addictive disorders; it may prove to be part of the solution to our current narcotic abuse pandemic.

Although the exact mechanism of its action is not known, acupuncture is the most widely studied alternative therapy, and many theories have been proposed in the effort to explain its effects. After having been used for many centuries, the traditional concept accepted by the Chinese and others to explain acupuncture is that it is a method of balancing *qi* (or *chi*), an invisible yet essential and ceaselessly flowing life energy that circulates silently and invisibly within the body. Because no scientist has ever measured or seen *qi*, only its effects can be observed. These effects are best demonstrated when the body is performing normally, an amalgam of all the physiologic, immunologic, and homeostatic functions of a living organism. Blockage of the flow of *qi*, an inadequate or waning supply of it, or its excessive amount can lead to conditions of pain, disease, and loss of homeostasis.

This quasi-mystical explanation is not always satisfying to the scientific mind. Thus attempts have been made over the years to derive a more robust explanation, one that would be understandable in terms of Western scientific tradition and terminology. The work of Pomeranz and others showed that some of the effects of acupuncture are achieved by activating the endorphin neuropeptide system, which can be blocked by the opiate receptor antagonist naloxone. Others have looked into the quantum physics realm and found parallels there in nonlocal effects, standing wave theory, and other quantum principles now used by physicists. Certain hybrid models apply Western medical and physiologic terminology to explain the effects of needling. These models discuss the ionic and electrical milieu of cells and tissues as well as the foreign-body effect and the pattern of injury currents induced by needling. Additional theories explain acupuncture results as being due to a "neurogate blocking phenomenon," various neural or endocrinologic events, effects on cytokine and prostaglandin inflammatory pathways, or electromagnetic field realignment. Given the sheer range and diversity of these explanations, it is likely that acupuncture works through a number of mechanisms and perhaps is not yet fully explicable by current scientific thought. However, its effects on humans and animals, its longevity as a healing art, and its resurgence in the Western medical community constitute inductive evidence of the value of acupuncture, whatever its mechanism of action.

Although there is considerable variability among training approaches for physicians and clinicians, the annual 300-hour course called Medical Acupuncture for Physicians, offered by the Helms Medical Institute (510-649-8488; www.hmieducation.com) and Stanford University (http://cme.stanford.edu/courses), is widely acknowledged as a benchmark minimum for those wanting to practice acupuncture. Classes are offered over several months, including distance learning by DVD and video, and are designed to give practical knowledge without requiring too much time away from a medical practice. The longer 3- to 4-year courses offered at Asian medical colleges are not usually required by states for the licensure for physicians and are often impractical for the practicing clinician to complete.

Laws governing physician acupuncture are listed on the American Academy of Medical Acupuncture's website, www.medicalacupuncture.org.

Blending this ancient medical art into a medical practice can be a source of satisfaction to both professionals and their patients. It can serve as a practice builder and provide new opportunities to attract patients. With the National Institutes of Health consensus panel's opinion on record, health care professionals have reason to anticipate better insurance coverage for acupuncture and a resulting increase in demand. In fact, some health maintenance organizations already reimburse for alternative therapies, including acupuncture.

INDICATIONS

Although acupuncture has been used to treat every imaginable human condition, to treat animals, and to prevent disease, most clinicians performing acupuncture find its greatest usefulness in the following conditions:

- Arthritis
- Asthma

- Back pain
- Carpal tunnel syndrome
- Dizziness
- Dysmenorrhea
- Gastrointestinal disorders
- Gynecologic problems
- Headache
- Irritable bowel syndrome
- Mental and mood disturbances
- Musculoskeletal pain
- Neuralgia
- Sciatica
- Sinusitis
- Skin disorders
- Substance addiction
- Tendonitis
- Tennis elbow
- Upper respiratory infections
- Urologic disease

EDITOR'S NOTE: The National Center for Complementary and Integrative Health has reviews of the evidence for many of these indications on its web page. Likewise, the Cochrane database has many systematic reviews available. Both organizations have called for more research in many areas.

CONTRAINDICATIONS

- Septic or extremely weakened patient.
- Local skin infection or loss of skin integrity (e.g., burns, cellulitis).
- Uncooperative patients or patients with delusions, hallucinations, or paranoia.
- Electroacupuncture should not be applied across the brain or heart.
- During pregnancy, a number of points are to be avoided (see acupuncture references for details) because some of these points may stimulate labor.
- The umbilicus, the nipple, points over major vessels and nerves, and an infant's fontanelle are points forbidden by both classic and contemporary practitioners.
- During menses (relative contraindication).
- Patient unable to lie down (relative contraindication; sitting or standing treatments should usually be avoided, especially for the first treatment).

EQUIPMENT

A variety of needles are available, ranging from very fine 34- or 36-gauge needles to 18-gauge needles used for veterinary acupuncture. The most commonly used needles are those from 0.5 to 3 inches in length and in the 30- to 34-gauge size. Acupuncture needles usually have solid stainless steel shafts and a copper, silver, or wound-steel-wire handle. The longer needles are used in thicker muscle groups, such as the back, buttocks, and legs, whereas the shorter, more delicate needles are used in the hands, face, and ears.

In addition to the needles, acupuncturists both in the United States and abroad, including China, now commonly use electrostimulation units (Fig. 184.1). These are small, handheld, battery-operated units, similar in design to the transcutaneous electrical nerve stimulation units used for pain control. Instead of the electrode pad used with the transcutaneous electrical nerve stimulation unit, a small alligator clip is placed on the shaft of an acupuncture needle to deliver the electrical current.

Other materials that may be used by an acupuncturist include embedded ear needles; metallic or magnetic beads; the herb moxa (*Artemisia vulgaris*), which is burned to heat the skin, needle, or acupuncture points; glass or bamboo cups used for a corollary procedure

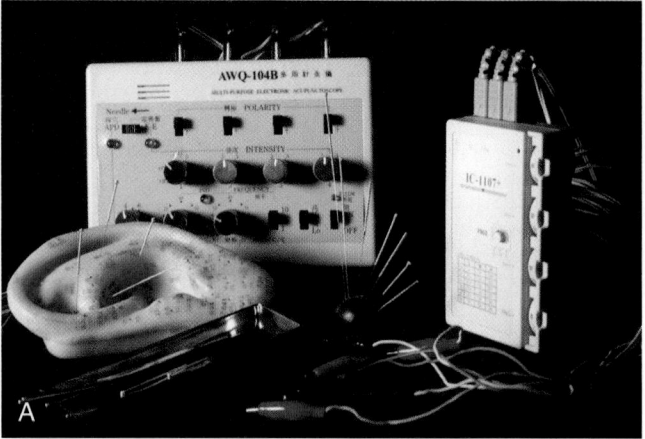

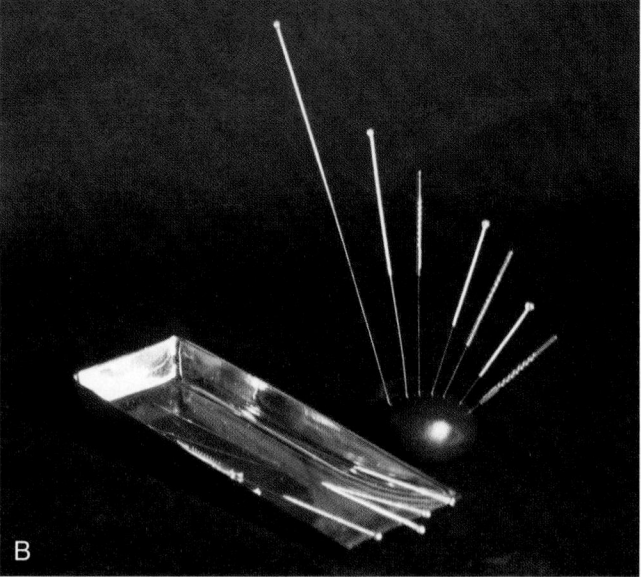

Fig. 184.1 An electroacupuncture stimulator (A) and acupuncture needles of various sizes (B).

called *cupping*; small hammers with several needles on the tip (plum blossom or seven-star needles); and electrical point locators, probes, or stimulators.

In general four sizes of needles and a few electrostimulator devices are all that is necessary for most medical acupuncture applications. The cost of these supplies varies, but a reasonable, complete set of equipment will usually cost less than $1000 (see the list of "Suppliers" at the end of this chapter).

PREPROCEDURE PATIENT PREPARATION

Although acupuncture is among the safest of invasive medical therapies, some precautions are needed. A thorough standard examination and diagnostic evaluation by a clinician are needed before acupuncture. Interestingly, performing these procedures often prepares the patient for acupuncture by giving him or her confidence through a known, established medical ritual—the routine physical. If the patient has never had acupuncture, the clinician should first show him or her the needles and stimulation devices. It is essential to assure the patient that the needles are sterile and disposed of after every treatment to allay fears of disease transmission. It is helpful to explain the risk of a needle reaction and the occasional endorphin rush, or "high," that follows some treatments.

As in the case of any other medical treatment or procedure, it is wise to discuss the pros and cons of treatment, any conventional therapy options that may not have been tried, the likelihood of success with acupuncture, its possible costs, and the expected number and length of treatments. Most conditions amenable to acupuncture will show a positive response within 4 to 10 treatments. With initial treatments, the patient may experience no response, a temporary worsening of the condition, or a gradual (or even sudden) improvement. For most chronic conditions, such as low back pain, a series of 4 to 10 treatments at $50 to $100 per treatment is often worth the investment for the patient seeking relief.

The topics just mentioned should be discussed with every patient before initiating a course of acupuncture treatments. The initial evaluation, review of records, discussion of options, and development of care plan usually occupy the entire first visit. Needle treatment is often deferred until the second visit. Usually no informed consent forms or releases are used in acupuncture therapy, although they may be useful in certain practice situations.

TECHNIQUE

Although the choice and location of points and the details of acupuncture therapeutics are beyond the scope of this chapter, the following text should give a general idea of how to interact with the patient and how a treatment session is staged and integrated into a medical practice.

1. After the patient and acupuncturist agree that a trial of acupuncture is appropriate and mutually acceptable, the patient is draped or gowned. Special efforts should be made to ensure patient comfort on the treatment table, using supports such as pillows, towels, and bolsters, because the patient will be lying down for a session lasting as long as 15 to 30 minutes or more. As noted earlier, sitting or standing treatments are avoided unless the patient is known to have tolerated them previously.
2. Acupuncture points are palpated on the body, extremities, ears, face, or scalp and the needle is inserted deftly with a slight twirling motion (Figs. 184.2–184.4). A sufficient depth of insertion has been reached when the patient feels a slight aching sensation, indicating that the *qi* has been reached (*de qi* sensation). Needle insertion should be painless other than the mild *de qi* sensation and a tiny prick the patient may feel as the needle penetrates the skin. Although some acupuncturists wipe the area of insertion with an alcohol swab, this is not necessary. However, cleansing before needling may be prudent in certain cases (e.g., patients who have an immune deficiency or diabetes or those who are concerned or worried).
3. A typical treatment may require 15 to 30 needles. After all the needles are in place, electroacupuncture electrodes are usually attached to several but not all of the needles. The electrostimulator is turned on and the current is gradually increased until the patient can feel a pulsing sensation. The current is then increased to the patient's maximal tolerance level and then backed off slightly (Fig. 184.5).
4. A timer is set, and a health care professional should remain within hailing distance to assist the patient if needed. The patient may be given a bell to ring if assistance is needed (e.g., if a needle falls out, the patient becomes uncomfortable or for some other reason may need the presence of another person).
5. At the end of the session, a nurse or medical assistant removes the wires and clips from the needles, removes the needles and disposes of them in a sharps container, and allows the patient to dress. The clinician or acupuncturist may return to evaluate the treatment or the patient may be discharged without further attention until the next visit. Usually the clinician is seeing or managing other patients while an acupuncture session is in progress. He or she may start another or even two more acupuncture sessions while the first is occurring, or the clinician may attend to other standard medical cases.

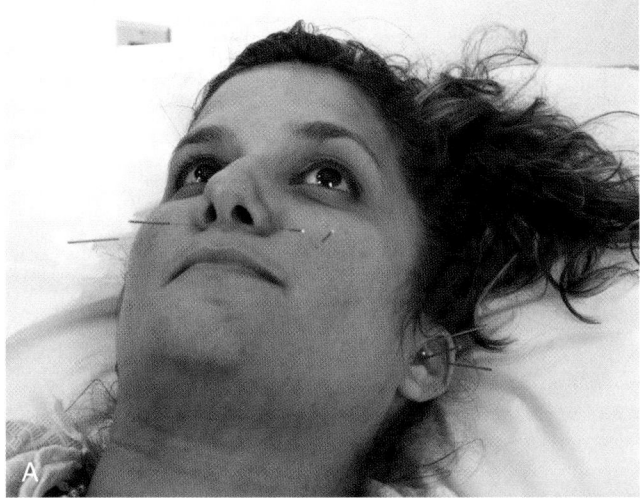
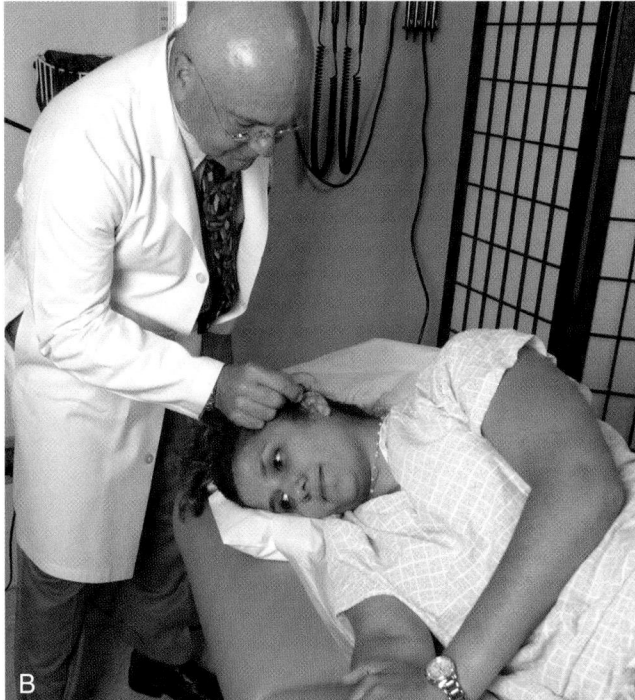

Fig. 184.2   (A) Treatment of facial and ear points. (B) Ear acupuncture.

6. Follow-up treatments are done at intervals of up to 2 weeks. During return visits, the acupuncturist interviews, examines, and reevaluates the patient and his or her progress. Treatment and needle location may be altered based on the patient's response, or the same or a similar pattern may be used. As the patient starts to improve, treatment intervals are spaced farther apart. Whereas some patients obtain permanent relief from acupuncture, others may require additional periodic treatments to sustain their improvement.
7. The patient's diagnosis, his or her vital signs, type of treatment, and needle application points used should be dictated into the medical record.

COMPLICATIONS

Complications are rare in acupuncture. Of those reported, the most common are local pain; swelling; hematoma formation; organ puncture; pneumothorax; metal allergy; needle reaction (fainting); a post-treatment period of euphoria; and local infections, such as

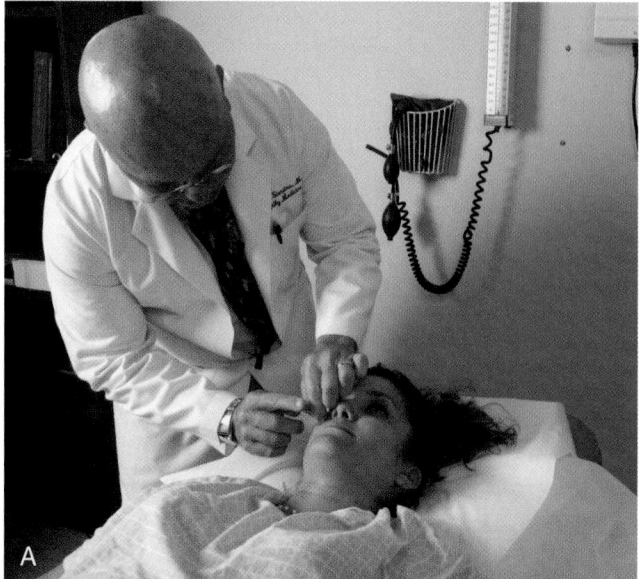

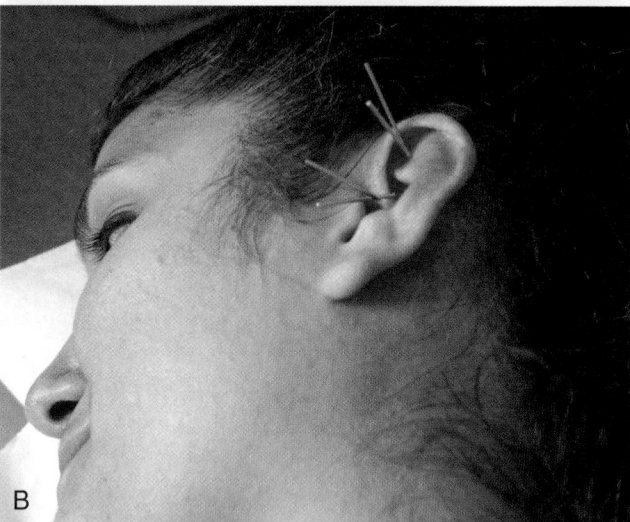

Fig. 184.3 (A) Facial points used for sinus problems. (B) Auricular points used for an addiction.

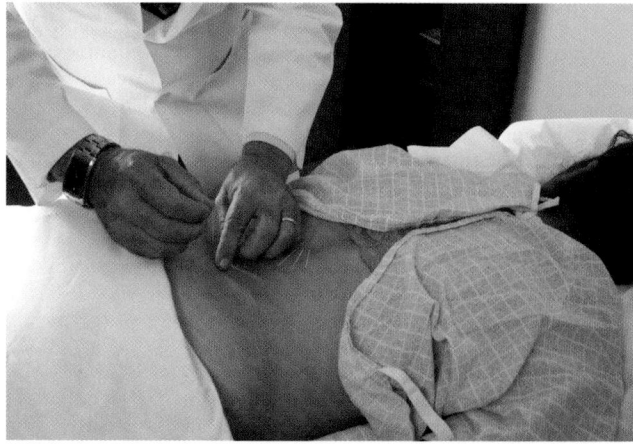

Fig. 184.4 Needle insertion in abdomen.

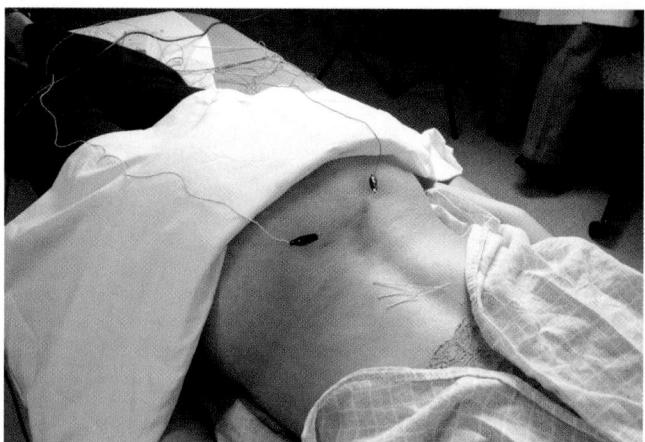

Fig. 184.5 Adjusting treatment settings (after checking pulse).

perichondritis, or even more serious infections, such as endocarditis. Systemic infections, such as hepatitis and acquired immunodeficiency syndrome, have been reported as transmitted by acupuncture needles. However, poorly qualified practitioners who reused needles and did not use sterile technique caused these infections.

POSTPROCEDURE PATIENT EDUCATION

Depending on the type of treatment, no special instructions are usually necessary. Band-Aids are not needed. Some patients, particularly at their first treatment, experience a euphoric spell thought to be related to endorphin release. The practitioner may instruct patients to drive carefully after a treatment or to have someone drive them home.

Some treatments are designed to increase general energy and vigor, especially in chronically weakened patients. Advice should be given to these patients to avoid heavy meals, alcoholic beverages, sexual relations, and intense exercise for about 8 hours after the treatment. This should enhance treatment benefits.

REFERRAL PROCESS

If you choose not to learn to use acupuncture in your practice, the clinical algorithm shown in Fig. 184.6 can be very useful in selecting proper cases for referral, assessing evidence, and managing follow-up for patients who are seen by an acupuncturist outside of your practice.

PATIENT EDUCATION GUIDES

See the sample patient education form available at www.expertconsult.com.

CPT/BILLING CODES

97810	Acupuncture, one or more needles; without electrical stimulation, initial 15 minutes of personal one-on-one contact with the patient
97811	Each additional 15 minutes of personal one-on-one contact with the patient, with reinsertion of needle(s) without electrical stimulation
97813	Acupuncture, one or more needles; with electrical stimulation, initial 15 minutes of personal one-on-one contact with the patient
97814	Each additional 15 minutes of personal one-on-one contact with the patient, with reinsertion of needle(s) with electrical stimulation

Need arises:

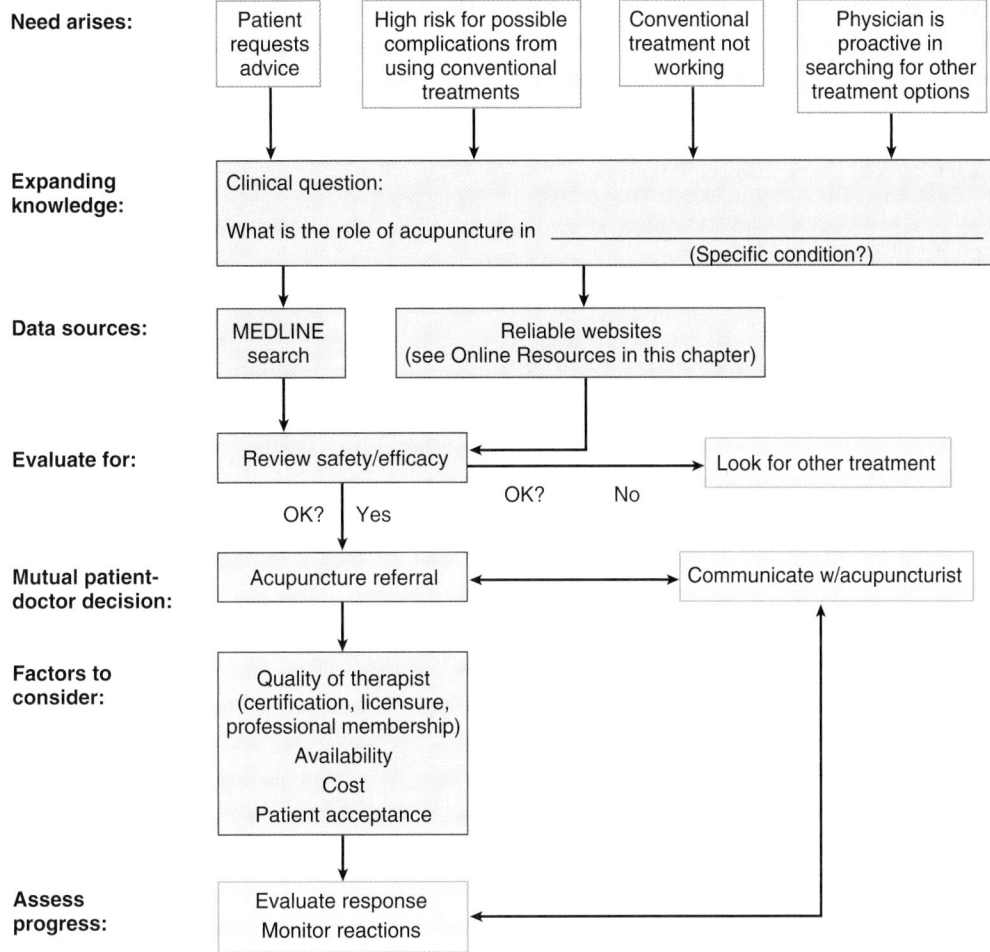

Fig. 184.6   Algorithm for integrating acupuncture into medical practice.

New codes are based on 15-minute increments; time must be documented in the chart for billing purposes. Most patients pay out of pocket, however, thus minimizing billing procedures.

Standardized fees depend on the client population, geography, and, increasingly, the rate of insurance reimbursement. However, treatments are billed in the range of $50 to $100 in most cases and locations.

ICD-10-CM DIAGNOSTIC CODES

F41.9	Anxiety
F10.20	Alcohol dependence syndrome, chronic, unspecified
F11.20	Drug dependence, opioid, unspecified
F13.20	Drug dependence, barbiturate, unspecified
F14.20	Drug dependence, cocaine, unspecified
F15.20	Drug dependence, amphetamine, unspecified
G44.209	Headache, tension
F43.21	Adjustment disorder with depressed mood
F32.9	Depressive disorder not otherwise classified
G43.109	Headache, classical migraine, not intractable
G43.009	Headache, common migraine, not intractable
G44.009	Headache, cluster, without intractable migraine
G56.00	Carpal tunnel syndrome unspecified limb
J32.9	Sinusitis, chronic
J45.20	Asthma mild intermittent uncomplicated
J98.8	Upper respiratory infection, chronic
K58.8	Irritable bowel syndrome

N30.10	Cystitis, chronic interstitial
N80.9	Endometriosis
N94.6	Dysmenorrhea
R10.2	Pelvic and perineal pain
L20.89	Dermatitis, atopic (eczema)
L40.8	Psoriasis
M06.9	Arthritis, rheumatoid, adult
M15.0	Arthrosis, osteoarthrosis, site unspecified or generalized
M54.30	Sciatica unspecified
M54.5	Back pain, low, or low back syndrome
M77.10	Lateral epicondylitis unspecified elbow
M77.9	Tendonitis, site not otherwise specified
M79.2	Neuralgia, unspecified
M79.609	Pain unspecified limb
M25.50	Pain unspecified joint
R42	Dizziness
R10.9	Abdominal pain, unspecified site

SUPPLIERS

(See contact information available at ww.expertconsult.com.)

Acupuncture needles and other equipment
   Lhasa OMS Medical, Inc.
Books and references on acupuncture
   Redwing Book Company

ONLINE RESOURCES

American Academy of Medical Acupuncture: www.medicalacupuncture.org. A physician-oriented site supported by the Medical Acupuncture Research Foundation to make available online the most comprehensive database of references on acupuncture in the English language.

British Acupuncture Council: https://www.acupuncture.org.uk/.

Helms Medical Institute: Medical Acupuncture for Physicians: www. hmieducation.com. Courses and physician education in acupuncture.

MedlinePlus: Acupuncture, MedlinePlus: Acupuncture: www.nlm.nih.gov/ medlineplus/acupuncture.html.

National Institute of Health (NIH) and NCCIH National Center for Complementary and Integrative Health (NCCIH): https://nccih.nih.gov/ health/acupuncture. Summary of indications and supporting evidence.

World Health Organization. Acupuncture Research. http://www.who.int/ traditional-complementary-integrative-medicine/publications/en/. Portal to traditional and complementary medicine.

RECOMMENDED READING

Allen JJ, Schnyer RN, Chambers AS, et al. Acupuncture for depression: a randomized controlled trial. *J Clin Psychiatry.* 2006;67:1665–1673.

Berman BM, Ezzo J, Hadhazy V, et al. Is acupuncture effective in the treatment of fibromyalgia? *J Fam Pract.* 1999;48:213–218.

Berman BM, Lao L, Langenberg P, et al. Effectiveness of acupuncture as adjunctive therapy in osteoarthritis of the knee: a randomized, controlled trial. *Ann Intern Med.* 2004;141:901–910.

Burke A, Upchurch D, Dye C, Chyu L. Acupuncture use in the United States: findings from the National Health Interview Survey. *J Altern Complement Med.* 2006;12:639–648.

Chou R, Deyo R, Friedly J, Skelly A, Hashimoto R, et al. *Noninvasive Treatments for Low Back Pain.* Agency for Healthcare Research and Quality (US) Report No.: 16-EHC004-EF; 2016.

Ernst E. Acupuncture: a critical analysis. *J Intern Med.* 2006;259:125–137.

Ezzo J, Hadhazy V, Birch S, et al. Acupuncture for osteoarthritis of the knee. *Arthritis Rheum.* 2001;44:819–825.

Filshie J, White A. *Medical Acupuncture: A Western Scientific Approach.* New York: Churchill Livingstone; 1998.

Helms J. *Acupuncture Energetics.* Berkeley, CA: Medical Acupuncture Publishers; 1996.

Helms J. An overview of medical acupuncture. *Altern Ther Health Med.* 1998;4:35–45.

MacPherson H, Hammerschlag R, Lewith G, Schnyer R. *Acupuncture Research: Strategies for Establishing an Evidence Base.* London: Churchill Livingstone; 2007.

Melchart D, Thormaehlen J, Hager S, et al. Acupuncture versus placebo versus sumatriptan for early treatment of migraine attacks: a randomized controlled trial. *J Intern Med.* 2003;253:181–188.

NICE guidelines. Low back pain and sciatica in over 16s: assessment and management. https://www.nice.org.uk/guidance/ng59/resources/low-back-pain-and-sciatica-in-over-16s-assessment-and-management-pdf-1837521693637; 2016.

National Institutes of Health: Acupuncture. *NIH Consensus Statement.* 1997;15(5). http://consensus.nih.gov/1997/1997Acupuncture107pdf.pdf.

Pomeranz B, Chiu D. Naloxone blockade of acupuncture analgesia: endorphin implicated. *Life Sci.* 1976;19:1757–1762.

Qaseem A, Wilt TJ, McLean RM, Forciea MA. Clinical guidelines committee of the American College of Physicians. Noninvasive treatments for acute, subacute, and chronic low back pain: a clinical practice guideline from the American College of Physicians. *Ann Intern Med.* 2017;166(7):514–530.

Richardson M, Freedman J. A model for acupuncture training in primary care. *Acupunct Med.* 2005;23:135–136.

Rubik B. Can Western science provide a foundation for acupuncture? *Altern Ther Health Med.* 1995;1:41–47.

Sierpina VS. *1000 Cures for 200 Ailments.* London: Collins Reference; 2007.

Sierpina V, Frenkel M. Acupuncture: a clinical review. *South Med J.* 2005;98:330–337.

White A, Tough E, Cummings M. A review of acupuncture clinical trials indexed during 2005. *Acupunct Med.* 2006;24:39–49.

CHAPTER 185

PODIATRIC PROCEDURES

Gary L. Snyder • Grant C. Fowler

ORTHOTICS

Orthotics are prescribed, in-shoe devices designed to protect and improve abnormal foot function. Orthotics are custom-made and, as such, may differ in the materials from which they are manufactured. Each prescription may have various modifications and additions, depending on the underlying diagnosis. The two most common types of orthotics are *functional* orthotics and *accommodative* orthotics. Both of these are made from precise casts, impressions, or scans of the patient's foot that have been placed in the position in which the practitioner wishes the foot to function. Although symptoms improve with conservative care in the majority of patients with plantar fasciitis in 3 to 6 months, no matter what the treatment, Cochrane evidence-based reviews found possible benefit with custom-made orthotics in patients with this disorder. Cochrane reviews also found possible benefit with custom orthotics in patients with painful pes cavus (high-arching foot), painful hallux valgus (bunion), rearfoot pain due to rheumatoid arthritis, and foot pain due to juvenile idiopathic arthritis (patients older than 5 years). Other reviews have found that 70% of patients improved with orthotics versus 30% with heel cups or injections. According to one study, after 1 year, most patients prefer custom orthotics to other devices (e.g., night splints) for preventing or managing foot pain.

EDITOR'S NOTE: Vendors with digital foot scanning systems have become more common and offer custom orthotics. It should be noted that such orthotics will not be able to provide the frequently needed accommodative pads or customized balance support. They also may not be as durable as custom orthotics and therefore need to be replaced more often.

Most (70%) patients are heel strikers, and in these patients, about 50% of the stress of weight bearing is borne or transferred through the calcaneus, whereas the other 50% is transferred to the first and fifth metatarsophalangeal (MTP) joints (about 35% to the first MTP). Although malalignment anywhere in the lower extremity can change this weight-bearing pattern, the normal pattern is therefore from the calcaneus, through the midfoot, and then off the first and fifth MTP joints. Orthotics can be useful for patients with abnormalities in their weight-bearing pattern. Corns and calluses may not only develop as a result of weight-bearing abnormalities, but their location may also help diagnose or confirm the abnormality. Exceptions to the normal weight-bearing pattern are patients with a very narrow heel and wide forefoot; they are likely forefoot strikers. Plantar warts, hammer (claw and mallet) toes, bunions, bunionettes, metatarsalgia, sesamoiditis, and hallux rigidus (stiff toe) can all be uncomfortable and have an impact on the weight-bearing pattern; significant relief is often provided by a simple podiatric adjustment or procedure.

Functional Orthotics

Functional orthotics are usually rigid or semirigid thermoplastic shells with built-in corrections or additions to change a foot's position or to control abnormal foot motion. Flexible deformities of the foot are most frequently treated with this type of orthotic.

Accommodative Orthotics

Accommodative orthotics are softer and more cushioned, designed to protect painful plantar lesions or bony deformities of the foot. A number of closed-cell and open-cell foam products—as well as cork, leather, rubber, and silicone—are used in the fabrication of accommodative orthotics. These designs are most frequently used with rigid foot deformities, arthritic foot changes, and certain diabetic conditions. In some cases, they may be useful early in a disease process that will later require surgery.

Indications

Rigid, Custom Orthotics

- Plantar fasciitis (with or without heel spur syndrome)
- Pes cavus (Although people with this high-arching foot [defined as >3 cm height from ground measured at navicular bone] may never have a problem, they have a sixfold increased risk of injury with sports, largely because of an inflexible foot that does not adjust well to uneven surfaces; they also have a higher risk of plantar fasciitis.)
- Pes planus (flat foot)
- Excessive pronation (Fig. 185.1) resulting in problems (e.g., tibialis posterior dysfunction or medial tibial stress syndrome, metatarsalgia, tarsal tunnel syndrome)

NOTE: Examination may reveal a long, narrow foot, usually resulting in the patient rolling the foot excessively (excessive pronation) with ambulation. Deviations from the normal leg-heel-forefoot alignment may also be noted. Direct observation or videotaping of training routines may also be necessary to diagnose biomechanical abnormalities that are not noticed on routine examination. Pes planus, tibia vara, tibial torsion, subtalar joint varus, and heel cord tightness are possible causes of malalignment.

- Painful corns and calluses (following treatment, to prevent recurrence)
- Hammer toes (flexible)
- Early bunion (hallux valgus) deformity
- Stiff toe (hallux rigidus)
- Morton neuroma
- Chronic lateral ankle instability

Soft, Accommodative Custom Orthotics

- Diabetic foot pathology such as Charcot changes or plantar ulcerations
- Patients with arthritis or arthrosis

Contraindications (Relative)

- Other than allergy to orthotic material, there are usually no contraindications.
- Care must be taken with the neuropathic (e.g., diabetic) foot to ensure an exact fit.

- Some difficulty exists in fitting prescription orthotics for women's and men's dress shoes, although specialty laboratories do manufacture these devices.
- When anticipating a functional rigid or semirigid orthotic, the patient's range of ankle dorsiflexion must be greater than 10 degrees with the knee extended.

Equipment

More than 100 different prescription orthotic laboratories are accredited throughout the United States. The choice of laboratory is left to the discretion of the practitioner. Langer Biomechanics, Inc., is an example of an excellent facility and can be a very helpful resource.

Impressions taken in the office can be performed with the following techniques:

- Johnson & Johnson Extra-Fast Setting plaster casting tape (available from Moore Medical Corporation)
- ScanCast 3D Optical Scanner (Fig. 185.2; Benefoot/Langer)
- Biofoam Impression Kit (Smithers Bio-Medical Systems)

Impression Techniques

Plaster Cast Technique

Four-inch-wide Johnson & Johnson Extra-Fast Setting casting splints can be used, usually two layers thick. The casting tape is wrapped around the foot to completely cover the heel, medial and lateral margins, plantar aspect, and toes (Fig. 185.3). The casting tape is then smoothed to ensure full contact with the foot, and the foot is immediately placed in the desired functional position. The procedure is repeated for the other foot. When the casting tape dries, the feet are easily released from these slipper casts.

Scan Cast Technique

Using ScanCast 3D (Benefoot/Langer), the foot is placed in the desired functional position in front of the ScanCast screen

(Fig. 185.4). Foot position is confirmed and visualized. The scan function is activated. Scanning takes approximately 1 second and is then repeated for the other foot. A digital image of the plantar surface of each foot is recorded. Orthotics are developed from these scans. (A positive model of each foot is constructed and the orthotic is molded onto this model.)

Biofoam Impression Technique

First, the patient's body should be aligned properly while they are seated. The hip, knee, and ankle should all be at 90 degrees (Fig. 185.5A). With one of the clinician's hands, the patient's ankle should be stabilized and held in a neutral position (neither pronated nor supinated; see Fig. 185.5B). Supporting the talus may help prevent pronation while the impression is being made. The patient's foot is then placed lightly over the foam in the impression kit, and the patient is instructed to avoid applying

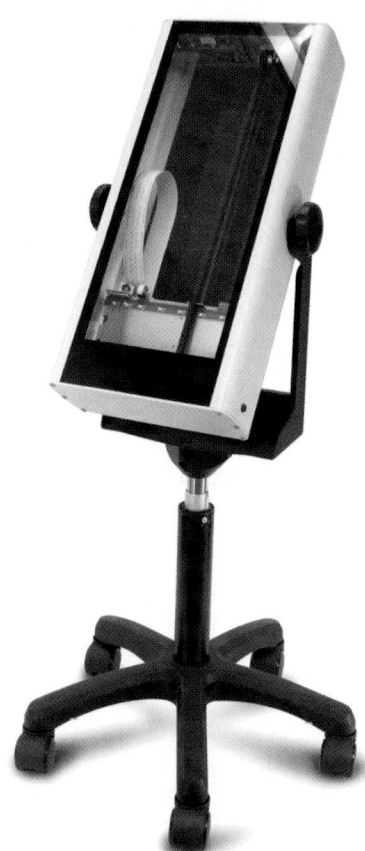

Fig. 185.2 ScanCast 3D is a portable, self-contained unit. (Courtesy Smithers Bio-Medical Systems, Kent, OH.)

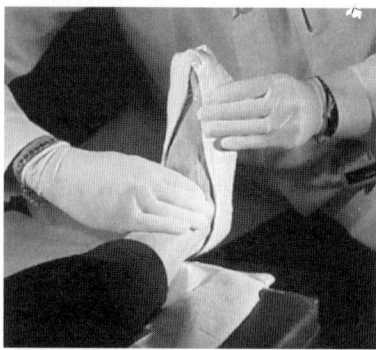

Fig. 185.3 Casting tape applied to foot. (Courtesy Benefoot/Langer Biomechanics, Ronkonkoma, NY.)

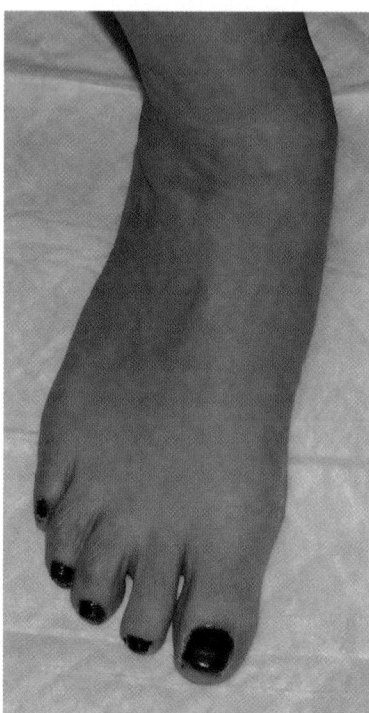

Fig. 185.1 Excessive, unchecked pronation demonstrated with weight bearing.

pressure. For additional stability, the clinician can quickly shift the stabilizing hand to the lateral aspect of the foot (see Fig. 185.5B), if not already there. Using the other hand, the clinician applies downward pressure on the patient's knee to make an impression of the foot in the foam. The foot should be pushed 1 to 1.5 inches into the foam while simultaneous, stabilizing pressure is applied to the lateral aspect of the foot. Finish the impression by using both hands to press the toes into the foam (see Fig. 185.5C). In this manner, weight-bearing flow is simulated, from heel to midfoot to toes, while the foot is maintained in the neutral position. Alternatively, with a good grasp on the lateral aspect of the foot, one hand can be used to both stabilize and push the foot into the foam and make the impression. Inspect each impression for defects, unevenness of the weight-bearing

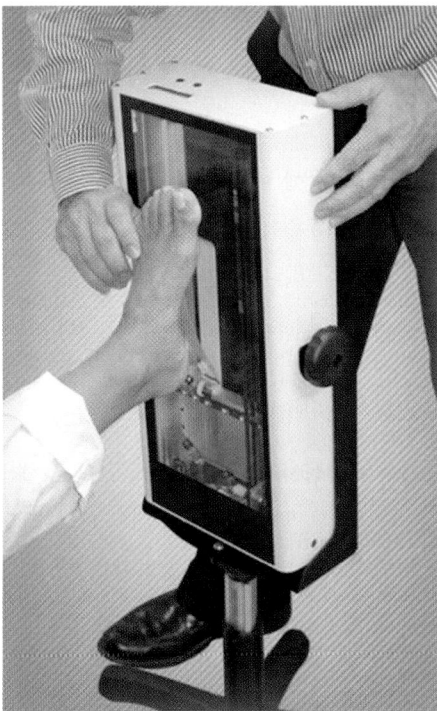

Fig. 185.4 Using the ScanCast 3D to scan the foot. (Courtesy Smithers Bio-Medical Systems, Kent, OH.)

surface, or abnormal plantar contour. Repeat the procedure with the patient's other foot.

Foot Position

There are four basic positions that may be used to obtain a cast of the foot for an orthotic:

1. Subtalar neutral position, non–weight bearing
2. Subtalar neutral position, partial weight bearing
3. Rectus position
4. Full weight bearing

NOTE: One of the authors (GLS) suspects it is of little consequence which position is used to obtain the cast, scan, or impression, as long as the midtarsal, subtalar, and ankle joints are in a neutral and locked position. His preference is to use the non–weight-bearing position for fitting custom orthotics, and he reserves a weight-bearing position for obtaining certain radiographs.

Subtalar Neutral Position, Non–Weight Bearing

This technique is used most frequently and captures the neutral position of the foot. The patient may be sitting, supine, or prone, with the feet hanging free over the end of the examination table. The ankle is kept at right angles to the leg. This technique can be used for the casting tape (see Fig. 185.3), ScanCast 3D Optical Scanner (see Fig. 185.4), or Biofoam Impression (see Fig. 185.5). First, get a feel for the neutral position of the foot by inverting and everting, pronating and supinating it while palpating the medial and lateral aspects of the head of the talus with the thumb and index finger (at the talonavicular joint) of one hand. Next, stabilize the talonavicular joint in a neutral, congruous position, midway between inversion and eversion, pronation and supination. Then, with the other hand, grasp the foot on the dorsal and plantar aspects of the fifth metatarsal head (at the MTP joint) and maximally pronate the midtarsal joint (see Fig. 185.4). (One author [GLS] grasps the great toe and gently pulls down and lateral so that the foot is in approximately 15 degrees of external rotation.) The foot is held in this position until the casting tape dries (see Fig. 185.3) or the scanning is completed, or while a Biofoam impression is made.

NOTE: This is useful when maximum biomechanical control of forefoot and rearfoot deformities is required (e.g., flexible pes planus [flat foot] deformity, tibialis posterior dysfunction or medial tibialis stress syndrome, most pediatric deformities). It is best for pes planus with greater than 10 degrees ankle dorsiflexion mobility, and most commonly used with sport orthotics.

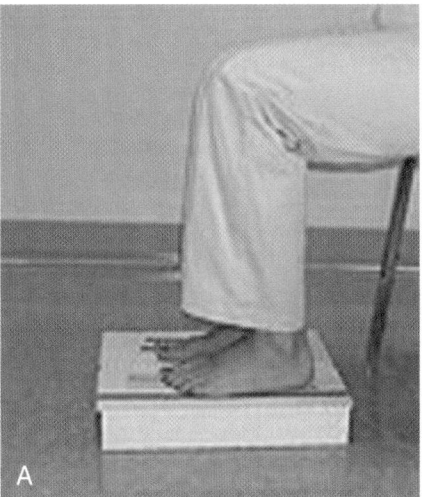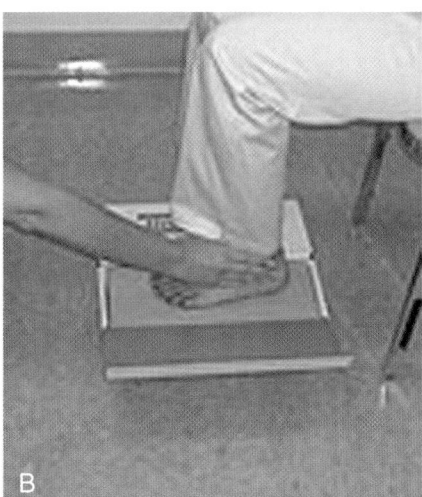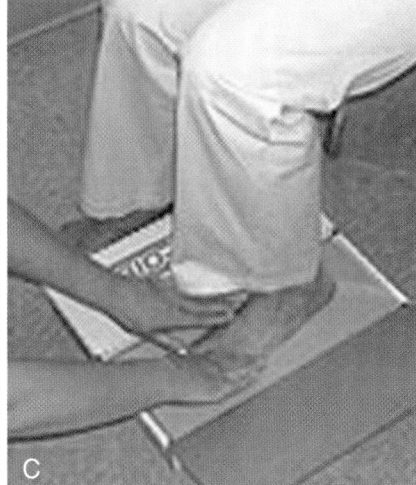

Fig. 185.5 Taking foam impressions. (A) With patient seated, hip, knee and ankle should be at 90 degrees. Foot should be in neutral position. (B) Make sure ankle is neither supinated nor pronated while applying lateral stability. (C) The foot should be pushed 1 to 1.5 inches into foam. Finish impression by pressing in toes with both hands. (Courtesy Smithers Bio-Medical Systems, Kent, OH.)

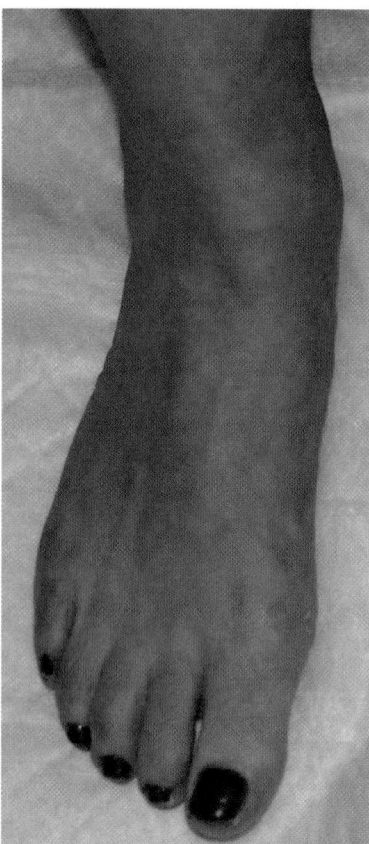

Fig. 185.6   Partial weight-bearing, neutral functional position.

Subtalar Neutral Position, Partial Weight Bearing

With this technique, the patient sits comfortably with the knee flexed at 90 degrees, the ankle at 90 degrees, and the center of the patella located directly over the second MTP joint. The foot is placed in the neutral position (Fig. 185.6), the position of function, and is then either wrapped in casting tape or placed over the Biofoam Impression Kit and carefully pressed into the foam (see Fig. 185.5). If casting tape is used, the patient is placed on a 2-inch-thick, plastic-wrapped foam pad until the casting tape dries. Care is taken to avoid inverting or everting the heel during the impression stage.

NOTE: This technique is indicated for most flexible foot deformities (e.g., pes cavus, pes planus, plantar fasciitis, heel spurs, bunions, painful corns, or calluses on the plantar aspect of the foot).

Rectus Position

This technique is similar to the non–weight-bearing neutral position, except that the forefoot is held parallel to the plantar aspect of the rearfoot during the time the plaster is drying or the foot is being scanned.

NOTE: This technique is indicated for childhood foot deformities (e.g., metatarsus adductus, pes cavus, pes planus, and calcaneal valgus).

Full Weight Bearing

The practitioner can choose plaster or a scanning system similar to the ScanCast Optical Scanner. The patient is instructed to stand in a normal angle and base-of-gait (with the foot held in the neutral position by the clinician while palpating the talonavicular joint; Fig. 185.7) while plaster is drying or the foot is being scanned.

NOTE: Full weight-bearing impressions are useful for rigid and arthritic foot deformities, where accommodative padding under pressure points will be beneficial.

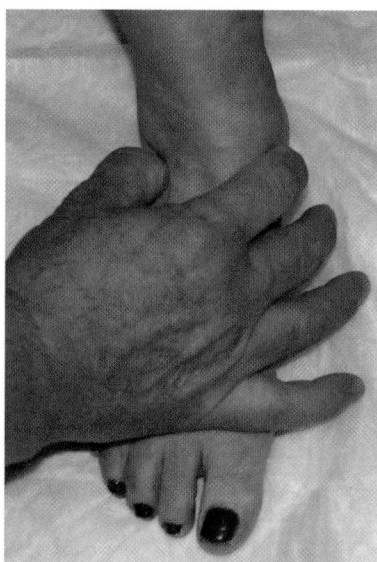

Fig. 185.7   Weight-bearing, neutral position, demonstrated by palpating the talonavicular junction.

Complications

Reported adverse effects include additional foot pain, ankle instability, and skin irritation. Many adjustments can be performed in the office to minimize these or other adverse effects, usually relating to thickness, width, or position of accommodation. Shoe fitting can be difficult with some dress shoes.

Postprocedure Patient Education

Patients are instructed to initially wear an oxford-style shoe, at least five eyelets per side, with a removable manufacturer's insole. They begin by wearing the orthotics approximately 1 hr/day; they can then increase the wearing time as tolerated. Average break-in period is between 4 and 12 weeks. If ankle equinus is present, the patient is instructed to continue with gastrocnemius-soleus stretching exercises. It usually takes 12 weeks to obtain the maximum benefit from orthotics.

CORNS (HELOMAS, CLAVI), CALLUSES (TYLOMAS), AND PLANTAR KERATOMAS

Corns are discrete, localized, well-circumscribed, round to oval hyperkeratotic lesions found on the toes, usually overlying bony prominences or digital deformities. They are usually painful and can be disabling. Corns involve the dermis and epidermis. *Soft corns* (heloma molle) are usually interdigital lesions resulting from abnormal pressure from deformed joints, bony prominences, or improper- or tight-fitting shoes (Fig. 185.8). Friction or structural deformities cause mechanical irritation between the toes. Soft corns are most commonly found between the fourth and fifth toes on the digital surface, but they can occur in any interdigital space or on the webspace. These lesions often become macerated (by absorbing moisture) and even secondarily infected. After paring or debridement, a small sinus tract can occasionally be identified and can be a source of underlying infection or inflammation. *Hard corns* (heloma durum) are usually found on the dorsum of an interphalangeal joint (second to fourth) or on the dorsolateral aspect of the fifth toe. These lesions result from structural deformities or bony prominences—pressure, shear forces, or friction from footgear over these prominences causes thickening and nucleation of the skin.

Corns are usually uniform in color and vary from whitish-gray to yellowish-gold. Subdermal hemorrhages can cause areas of discoloration that may appear dark red, brown, or black. Lesions are painful

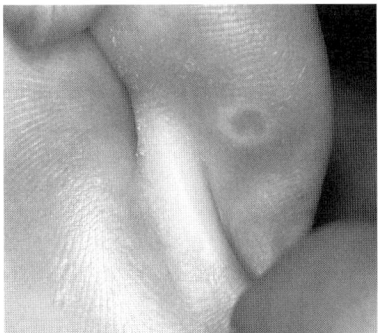

Fig. 185.8 Soft corn on lateral aspect of the toe. (Courtesy John L. Pfenninger, MD, The Medical Procedures Center, Midland, MI.)

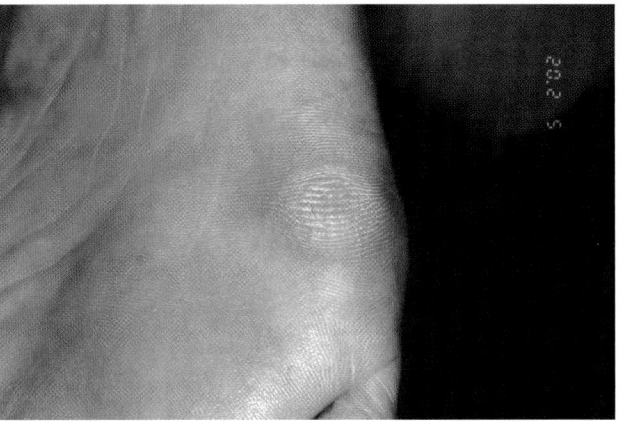

Fig. 185.9 Callus on foot. The differential includes a plantar wart. (Courtesy John L. Pfenninger, MD, The Medical Procedures Center, Midland, MI.)

BOX 185.1 Distinguishing Features of Warts and Plantar Corns

Wart
- Relatively rapid onset
- May or may not be under bony prominences
- Skin lines pass around lesion
- Maximum pain on squeezing side to side
- End arteries visible as red or black dots on paring
- Rapid recurrence after shaving and padding

Plantar Corn
- Develops over months or years
- Located under bony prominences
- Skin lines pass through lesion
- Maximum pain with direct pressure
- No end arteries visible on paring
- Slower recurrence after shaving

From Singh D, Bentley G, Trevino SG. Callosities, corns, and calluses. *BMJ.* 1996;312:1403–1406.

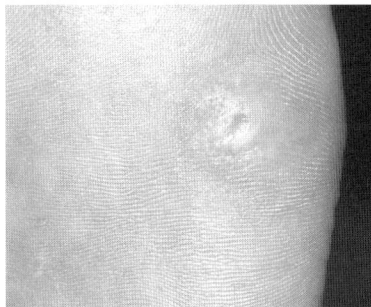

Fig. 185.10 Intractable plantar keratoma showing solid, smooth, hard central core. There are no pinpoint bleeders characteristic of a wart. (Courtesy John L. Pfenninger, MD, The Medical Procedures Center, Midland, MI.)

Fig. 185.11 Two molecules of cysteine are linked by disulfide bonds to form cystine, a major component of the underlying matrix in human keratin.

to direct and indirect pressure over the area. When debrided or pared down, a central, translucent, pearl-white core is usually found over the area of greatest pressure. Corns can be distinguished from warts by the lack of thrombosed tiny blood vessels on examination, as well as the lack of punctate bleeding when debrided. Skin lines pass through corns but around warts (Box 185.1). These skin lines are often more apparent after alcohol is used to cleanse the area.

Calluses are broad-based, poorly circumscribed, hyperkeratotic lesions commonly found on the plantar aspect of the foot at sites of friction or high pressure. They may be quite painful when located under the MTP joints. Calluses by definition involve primarily the epidermis and can occur diffusely around the heel or on the margins of the toes. Because most (70%) patients are heel strikers, and it is then normal to transfer weight through the midfoot and off the great (first) and fifth MTPs, calluses are common on the heels and under the first, second, and fifth MTP joints. (Calluses located between these areas often indicate abnormal foot structure or function.) A callus, differing from a corn, usually does not have a "nucleus" and instead consists of diffuse hyperkeratotic tissue (Fig. 185.9). The *intractable plantar keratoma* (Fig. 185.10) is a unique lesion consisting of an overlying callus with significant epidermal, dermal, and subdermal alterations, including fibrosis of the surrounding tissue. These are deep, nucleated plantar calluses found beneath an MTP joint and are often extremely painful with palpation and ambulation. They are usually circular, of smaller diameter than a tyloma, and exhibit a central plug or fibrous core on scalpel debridement. Intractable plantar keratomas are strong indicators of forefoot or rearfoot joint instability and therefore often benefit from rebalancing the weight-bearing surface with orthotics.

Etiology

Corns and calluses consist of multiple layers of flat sheets of α-keratin (β-keratin is found in reptile and fish scales), which has an underlying protein matrix consisting mostly of the amino acid cystine. Cystine, in turn, is formed by linking multiple molecules of the amino acid cysteine with disulfide bonds (Fig. 185.11). Clinicians are often familiar with the pungent sulfur odor released by these disulfide bonds when hair, skin, or a fingernail is cauterized or burned. Corns and calluses generally occur as a result of abnormally high pressure from a deformity, footgear, shear forces, or friction from ambulation. They can also be the result of permanently plantar flexed or hypermobile metatarsals, as well as instability of the joints of the forefoot and rearfoot. Fig. 185.12A shows normal metatarsal alignment; Fig. 185.12B and C show how to test for permanently inflexible joints or hypermobile joints by moving the second and third metatarsal heads through their full range of motion.

Differential Diagnosis

- Verrucae
- Digital bursa
- Dermal and epidermal malignancies
- Porokeratosis plantaris discreta (caused by keratin-plugged sweat duct)

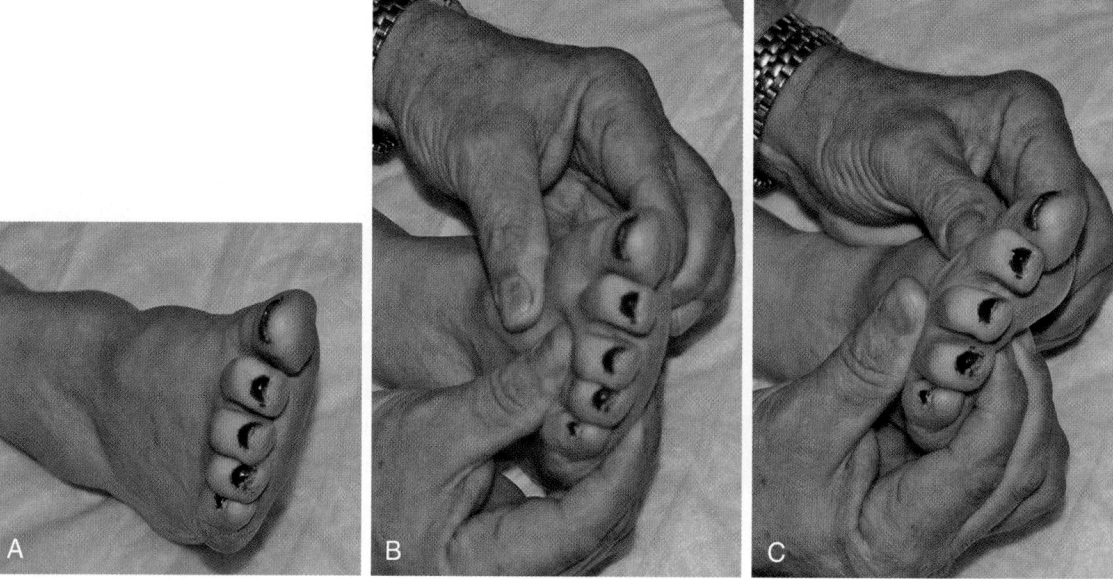

Fig. 185.12 (A) Normal metatarsal alignment. (B) Testing metatarsal head flexibility with excessive pronation. (C) Testing metatarsal head flexibility by hyperflexion.

Techniques

Treatment should not only provide symptomatic relief, but attempt to lessen or alleviate the underlying biomechanical cause(s) inciting the problem. Use of shoes with a wider toe box or thicker socks may remove some of the pressure (see the section on "Postprocedure Patient Education" for how to fit a shoe correctly using the Brannock device). Wearing a thin layer of cotton socks under a thicker layer of socks may reduce friction or shear forces on skin. Correcting or minimizing deformities with orthotics may prevent recurrence. Attempts should be made to correct bony angulation or flexibility defects with padding or orthotics, to see if they are beneficial, before performing corrective surgery.

Debridement

Debridement should be considered for hyperkeratotic lesions causing symptoms or showing signs of extreme dryness or intralesional cracking and fissuring. In the office, most clinicians use a No. 10 or No. 15 scalpel blade on a handle to remove hyperkeratotic tissue from corns or calluses. The scalpel is held parallel to the lesion and, using small, straight, or circular motions, the lesion is gradually shaved, debrided, or pared back. A thin layer is removed with each pass of the instrument. Because hyperkeratotic skin is devoid of innervation (has no sensation), the patient is usually able to tolerate debridement without a local anesthetic. To minimize discomfort, avoid placing pressure downward into the lesion; instead, pressure should be directed across the lesion with the scalpel. When most of the lesion has been removed, the clinician can usually visualize pink, viable skin just beneath it. This pink tissue has sensation, and as the clinician gets closer to shaving through it, the patient will usually sense or complain of some discomfort. This tissue also has a viable blood supply. In fact, the patient can guide and warn the clinician: as the sensation increases, the majority of the hyperkeratotic skin has been debrided, and this is the point where bleeding is likely to start.

Debridement can also be accomplished with various razor blade–containing devices, a pumice stone, electric drill, or keratolytic agents such as weak salicylic acid plasters. It is easier to use a pumice stone if the area has been soaked and softened. Of course, debridement is only a temporary cure, and the lesion will recur unless the primary cause for the excessive pressure is corrected. Use of aperture pads (Fig. 185.13) may decrease the likelihood of recurrence by taking pressure off the original site. Shoes must be evaluated and modified if necessary.

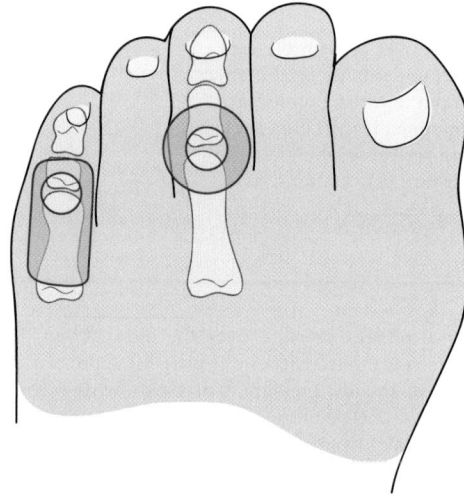

Fig. 185.13 Self-adherent aperture pads, usually placed over previously pared area to relieve pressure, often overlying a bony prominence. (Modified from Ehrlich M, Nemer JA. Management of select podiatric conditions. In: Reichman EF, Simon RR, eds. *Emergency Medicine Procedures.* New York: McGraw-Hill; 2004;1443.)

NOTE: If the clinician is untrained or uncomfortable performing debridement, he or she should consider referral, especially for those patients with compromised circulation or diabetes; options include a competent podiatrist.

Combined Approaches

Therapy for these disorders can also include mechanical supportive orthotics (either functional or accommodative), nonsteroidal anti-inflammatory drugs (NSAIDs), accommodative footgear, digital or metatarsal pads, and accommodations made of moleskin, Cushlin (Dr. Scholl/Schering-Plough Healthcare Products), or silicone (Silipos or Spenco; all available through Moore Medical Corp.).

Surgical Treatment

Surgical removal of bone exostosis, correction of digital deformities, osteotomies for elevation of depressed metatarsals, arthrodesis of midfoot, hindfoot, or ankle joint, or various joint-limiting procedures may be recommended when conservative therapies fail to provide lasting relief.

Complications

Secondary infections can occur with untreated corns or calluses. Ulcerations are a serious complication with diabetic neuropathy. Bursitis can occur with untreated lesions.

WARTS (VERRUCAE PLANTARIS)

Verrucae plantaris (plantar warts) are well-circumscribed, encapsulated, benign, tumorigenic, dermatotrophic lesions. The diagnosis is relatively simple, judging from appearance, the production of pain on lateral compression of the lesion, thrombosed tiny blood vessels, and pinpoint bleeding after debridement. Plantar verrucae appear different clinically from verrucae elsewhere because of being compressed and driven into the surrounding tissue.

Verrucae are encapsulated and well contained within the epidermis; the dermis is rarely involved. The lesion obliterates normal papillary skin lines. (This is an important diagnostic feature when treating warts. Often there is hyperkeratotic skin over the lesion. If this material is pared away after treatment and skin lines are then seen, the wart is considered resolved.) The appearance typically resembles grayish or brown papules with hypertrophic capillaries creating black or brown specks (end arteries, thrombosed capillaries) within the lesion. Plantar warts can occur singularly or in multiple clusters, which are referred to as *mosaic verrucae*. Smaller lesions surrounding the large centralized clusters are referred to as *satellite lesions*.

Etiology

Verrucae plantaris is caused by the human papillomavirus.

Differential Diagnosis

Warts are often confused with corns or deep calluses. Thrombosed tiny blood vessels and pinpoint bleeding after scalpel debridement are diagnostic hallmarks of verrucae plantaris. Other differential diagnoses include porokeratosis, epidermal malignancies (amelanotic melanoma), and various epidermal inflammatory conditions.

Treatment Options

There are a plethora of treatment methods, including chemical cautery with various acids, caustic chemotherapy such as 5-fluorouracil, cryotherapy, infrared coagulation, electrosurgery, immunotherapy (including imiquimod), injections (bleomycin, *Candida* antigen), CO_2 pulsed-dye laser, and surgical excision or curettage. Even duct tape has been reported to be beneficial, with an 85% cure rate. (Also see Chapter 30, Wart [Verruca] Treatment.)

Techniques

Chemocautery

Scalpel debridement of all hyperkeratotic tissue should be performed first. After debridement, the application of various acids, such as trichloracetic acid 85%, salicylic acid 60%, or pyrogallic acid 25%, can be used. Careful protection of the surrounding normal integument is paramount (some clinicians paint surrounding tissue with fingernail polish). The acids are usually followed by an occlusive, adhesive dressing. The patient is then instructed to keep the area dry and intact for approximately 2 to 7 days. This procedure is repeated until normal skin lines are visualized. Treatment response times vary greatly with individuals. If there is minimal improvement after a

reasonable number of treatments, another form of treatment, such as cryotherapy or other options as mentioned, should be considered.

Other Techniques

Specifics of treatment using other modalities are noted in the specific chapter dealing with each technique. (See Chapter 13, Approach to Various Skin Lesions; Chapter 14, Cryosurgery; Chapter 25, Radiofrequency Surgery [Modern Electrosurgery]; and Chapter 30, Wart [Verruca] Treatment.)

Complications

Posttreatment pain can be controlled with ice, NSAIDs, and acetaminophen. Chemical burns can create a sterile abscess site; fortunately, these rarely become infected. Painful plantar scarring should be avoided because walking on scars can feel like stepping on a pebble.

HAMMER (CLAW AND MALLET) TOES, BUNIONS (HALLUX VARUS AND VALGUS), AND BUNIONETTES (TAILOR BUNION)

Hammer, claw, and mallet toes are usually due to atrophy of the intrinsic muscles of the interphalangeal joints with subsequent loss of their stabilizing effect on the interphalangeal joints. As a result, the extrinsic muscles overpower the joints and pull them into permanent flexion or extension. Atrophy of the intrinsic muscles may be due to biomechanical faults, arthrosis, or constant pressure from tight shoes, resulting in toes being held in a constantly flexed or bent position; atrophy may also be due to other causes such as neuropathy from diabetes, alcoholism, or normal aging.

Hammer toes, like most nonacute foot deformities, are progressive. They start as flexible deformities where biomechanical control may be all that is necessary to prevent progression and even allow regression. A severe hammer toe deformity can indicate that there has been enough atrophy of the plantar capsule of the MTP joint to allow the metatarsal head to drop through the degenerated, torn capsule. Often this metatarsal head can be palpated as a hard bump on the bottom of the foot. It will also often result in the affected toes being splayed, and this can even be seen radiographically. Usually affecting the second toe, which is often the longest toe, this results in a permanently extended, dorsiflexed MTP joint. Subsequent pressure on the dorsum of the toe combined with an imbalance of muscles results in permanent plantar flexion at the proximal interphalangeal joint and the appearance of a hammer. This also often occurs in the third toe. If the distal interphalangeal (DIP) joint also becomes permanently plantar flexed, it results in a claw toe. Claw toes can affect all the toes with the exception of the great toe (which does not have a DIP joint). A mallet toe occurs when only the DIP joint is flexed, and although it can involve any of the toes, it frequently affects only the second toe because it is often the longest.

Such structural abnormalities and deformities often result in increased pressure on the overlying skin and development of hyperkeratotic lesions. The hammer toe frequently shows flexion of the proximal interphalangeal joint and extension of the DIP joint.

Bunions and bunionettes also result from the effects of biomechanical faults, footwear, osteoarthritis/osteoarthrosis, or various other anatomic, physiologic, and hereditary conditions. Just like the thumb, the MTP joint of the great toe is a common site for osteoarthritis. Bunions involve the first metatarsal head, resulting in lateral deviation of the great toe and medial deviation of the MTP joint (also known as *hallux abducto valgus*, the terms derived from movement related to the midsagittal plane of the foot); bunionettes affect the fifth metatarsal head, resulting in medial deviation of the fifth toe (adduction) and lateral deviation (abduction) of the fifth MTP joint (also known as a *tailor's bunion*).

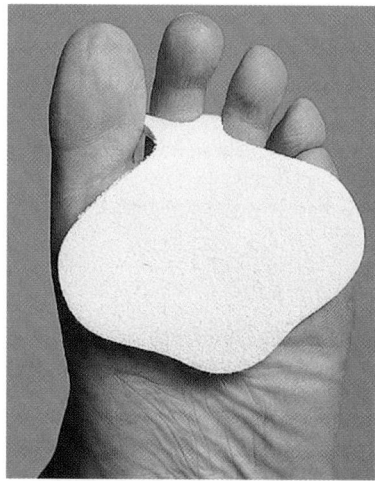

Fig. 185.14 Commercially available metatarsal pad; a similar pad can be cut from self-adherent felt.

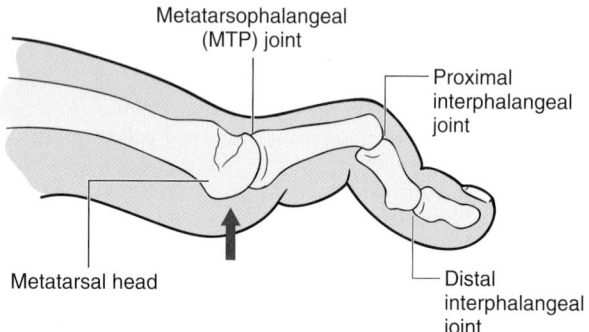

Fig. 185.15 Adding padding such as a metatarsal bar may correct the angle of dorsiflexion of the metatarsophalangeal joint by putting pressure on the plantar aspect of the joint.

Differential Diagnosis

Trauma and infectious or other inflammatory diseases are possible causes for painful or deformed joints at all of these sites. Radiographs may be helpful not only for determining the magnitude of the problem but also for excluding other causes. Laboratory analysis may be helpful for ruling out infectious or inflammatory arthritis. The differential diagnosis of a bunion also includes bursitis of the first MTP joint; it can occur on the medial aspect of the joint.

Techniques

The initial treatment of hammer, claw, and mallet toes and bunions or bunionettes is to consider changing footwear (see the section on "Postprocedure Patient Education" for how to fit a shoe correctly using the Brannock device). Shoes with a roomier toe box or use of thicker socks should minimize pressure against the inflamed, affected areas and allow them to heal. Hyperkeratotic lesions should be debrided or pared down. Padding and accommodative shields may help disperse local pressure and change balance. Precut metatarsal pads (Fig. 185.14) or bars are available or may be cut from 1-cm-thick felt (see the Suppliers section). For hammer or claw toes, decreasing the degree of plantar flexion of the MTP joint by using metatarsal pads (Fig. 185.15), placed just proximal to the metatarsal head, may decrease symptoms. This is partially accomplished by decreasing the pressure on the dorsum of the distal toe(s) from the inside top of the shoe. If a metatarsal pad is used early, it may even prevent the development of hammer or claw toes. Attempts should be made to correct bony angulation or flexibility defects with padding or orthotics, to see if they are beneficial, before performing corrective surgery.

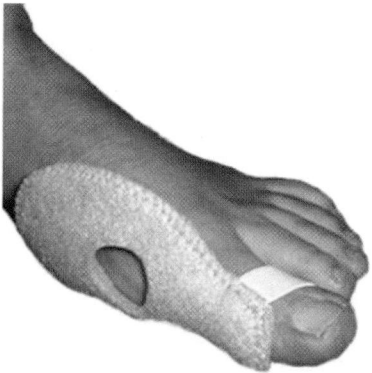

Fig. 185.16 Bunion shields are commercially available or can be cut from self-adherent felt.

Bunion shields (Fig. 185.16) are also available or may be cut from 1-cm felt. With a bunion shield in place, padding can be placed between the first and second toe to decrease the angle of lateral deviation of the bunion.

NSAIDs may help with pain and inflammation. The use of ice massage in the inflamed area after exercise may be helpful. An inflamed MTP bursa can be drained and reinjected with a steroid. Even if there is no bursitis, injection of corticosteroid into the area of inflammation may be helpful.

For those failing local care, surgical options include resection of the phalangeal head (arthroplasty), joint fusion (arthrodesis), removing tissue, or moving tendons in the toe joint. A fixed toe joint deformity usually requires surgery to relieve pain and correct the deformity.

METATARSALGIA, SESAMOIDITIS, AND STIFF TOE (HALLUX RIGIDUS)

Most commonly affecting the most distal portion of the metatarsal bone (i.e., the metatarsal head), metatarsalgia can affect the heads of any of the bones in the ball of the foot; however, it more commonly involves the second and third metatarsals. Frequently, a large callus is noted beneath the MTP joint. The ball of the foot is defined as the area between the arch of the foot and the toes.

Beneath the first metatarsal head are two sesamoid bones whose structure and function are similar to those of the patella. They may become painful as a result of overuse, a stress fracture, osteoarthritis, or chondromalacia. Because they are imbedded in the tendon, there is always an associated tendonitis. Plantar keratomas are frequently seen here, particularly with a plantar flexed first ray associated with high cavus foot deformity.

EDITOR'S NOTE: Anatomically, a "ray" is the digit plus the head and shaft of the respective metatarsal.

The great toe needs about 60 degrees of extension and 30 degrees of flexion for running and jumping sports; lack of flexibility causes discomfort. "Stiff toe," also known as *hallux rigidus*, is usually the result of a gradual process (over years) with a stiff, sore toe progressing to an inflexible first toe and pain even at rest. Although rheumatoid arthritis and gout can affect joint function, hallux rigidus is usually the result of a genetic predisposition combined with osteoarthritis. It can be a chronic, persistent cause of discomfort.

Differential Diagnosis

The location of hyperkeratotic lesions often helps differentiate between the possible causes of foot pain. Because of normal weight bearing, calluses are common under the first (and maybe second) and fifth MTPs; calluses between these locations may indicate other structural abnormalities of the foot or abnormal weight bearing, which may respond to orthotics or surgery.

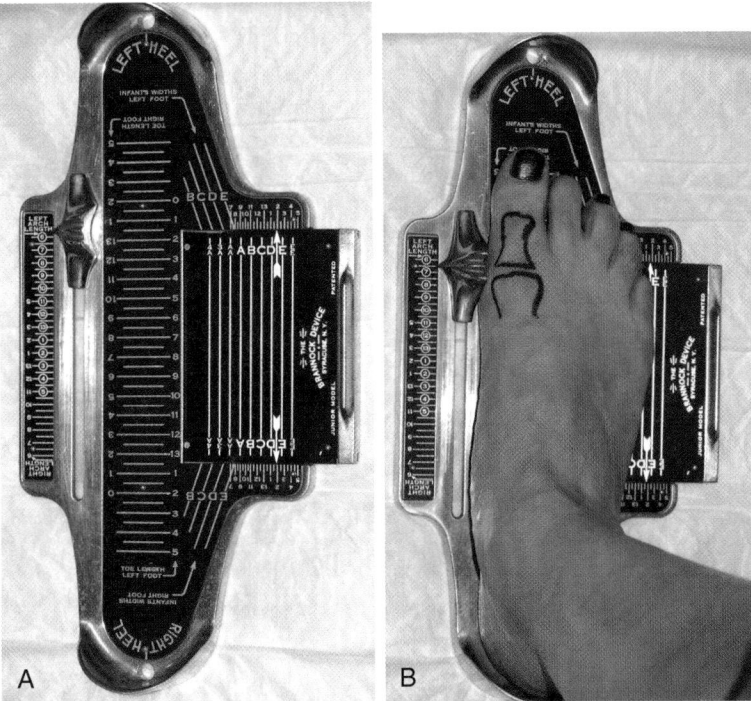

Fig. 185.17   (A) Brannock device for measuring shoe width and length. (B) Proper location to measure shoe width, just anterior to the first metatarsal head, between it and the first proximal phalanx, as drawn on this patient.

The patient can often point to the most painful area. Pain beneath the second or third metatarsal heads usually indicates metatarsalgia. Pain beneath the first metatarsal head suggests sesamoiditis. Pain with sesamoiditis is usually gradual in onset; pain due to a stress fracture is usually immediate. A bursa can also form in this area, between the skin and usually the medial sesamoid bone, and result in bursitis. A torn ligament or arthritis of an individual joint can cause similar pain. A radiograph can help distinguish between metatarsalgia and a metatarsal stress fracture, or sesamoiditis and a sesamoid stress fracture. On radiographs, the lateral sesamoid is often bipartite with smooth edges as opposed to jagged edges seen with a fracture. Radiographs of the metatarsal or sesamoid bones may initially be negative; however, serial radiographs taken 2 to 4 weeks later may reveal a fracture.

Techniques

Hyperkeratotic lesions should be debrided or pared. Use of a metatarsal pad placed just proximal to the second or third metatarsal head, under the diaphysis, should alleviate some of the symptoms of metatarsalgia; alternatively, the pad can be placed beneath the first metatarsal to force it to bear more weight (i.e., change the balance). Sesamoiditis also often responds to the use of metatarsal pads or a donut pad (a felt pad cut in the shape of a donut) to change the balance. Orthotics may prevent excessive pronation and decrease strain in the area. For a stiff first toe, early use of a metatarsal pad beneath the MTP joint may take off some of the stress and increase the leverage and range of motion of the first toe, not only decreasing but also possibly slowing the progression of symptoms. Attaching a pad to an ordinary insole of a shoe (or custom orthotic with first ray support, also known as *first ray post*) under the first MTP may also change balance, increase range of motion, and decrease symptoms. NSAIDs may help with pain and inflammation in all of these disorders. The use of ice massage in the inflamed area after exercise may be helpful. Injection of corticosteroid into the area of inflammation or intracapsular may also be helpful; caution should be observed in young athletes with such an injection to prevent fat pad atrophy and increased capsular laxity.

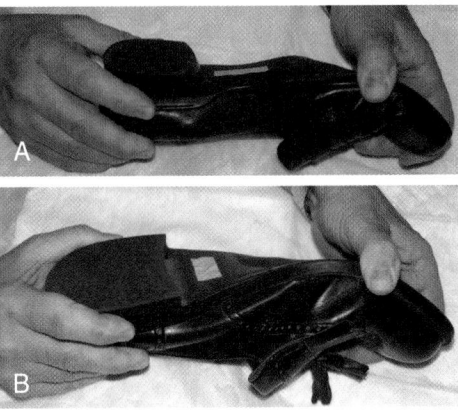

Fig. 185.18   (A) Determine shank stability by grasping counter (heel) and toe box and attempting to twist while observing the center of the shoe. (B) Ability to twist the shank indicates it will not offer much support.

POSTPROCEDURE PATIENT EDUCATION

Care should be taken to fit shoes properly. As a general rule, a proper-fitting shoe is longer and narrower than what most people wear. A Brannock device (Fig. 185.17A) is the most common instrument used for measuring shoe size. It comes in three sizes: men's, women's, and children's. The measurement for the widest part of the shoe should be made just anterior to the first metatarsal head (see Fig. 185.17B).

Shoes should also provide proper support, with steel shanks being preferable. It is simple to evaluate the effectiveness of any shank. Grasp the counter (heel) of the shoe with one hand and the toe box with the other hand (Fig. 185.18A), and attempt to twist the shoe. Observe the area of the shank, located between the center of the shoe and the heel; if that area deforms or twists (see Fig. 185.18B), it will offer little support. A steel shank in a well-made shoe will result in little or no deformation with twisting.

PATIENT EDUCATION GUIDE

See the sample patient education handout available at www.expertconsult.com.

CPT/BILLING CODES

Orthotics

A4580	Orthotic casting
L3030	Orthotics

Corns (Helomas)

L3030	Prescription orthotics
11055	Paring or cutting of benign hyperkeratotic lesion (e.g., corn or callus), single lesion
11056	Paring or cutting of benign hyperkeratotic lesions (e.g., corn or callus), two to four lesions
11057	Paring or cutting of benign hyperkeratotic lesions (e.g., corn or callus), more than four lesions

Warts (Verrucae Plantaris)

17000	Destruction (e.g., laser surgery, electrosurgery, cryosurgery, chemosurgery, surgical curettement), all benign or premalignant lesions, first lesion
17003	2 to 14 lesions (each)
17004	15 or more lesions (one set fee)

ICD-10-CM DIAGNOSTIC CODES

078.19	Verrucae (plana, plantaris, or plantar warts)
355.6	Morton neuroma
700	Corns and callosities (callus, heloma molle, heloma durum)
713.5	Charcot joint, neuropathic arthritis
715.17	Osteoarthrosis, localized, primary, ankle and foot
715.27	Osteoarthrosis, localized, secondary, ankle and foot
715.37	Osteoarthrosis, localized, not specified whether primary or secondary
716.17	Traumatic arthropathy, ankle and foot
719.47	Pain in joint, ankle and foot
726.73	Calcaneal (heel) spur
727.1	Bunion or bunionette
728.71	Plantar fasciitis
733.95	Stress fracture of other bone
733.99	Sesamoiditis
734	Pes planus (flat feet), acquired
735.0	Hallux valgus (similar to bunion)
735.1	Hallux varus
735.2	Hallux rigidus (inflexible or stiff big toe)
735.4	Hammer toes, acquired
736.73	Pes cavus
754.61	Pes planus, congenital (flat foot, rocker-bottom foot)

SUPPLIERS

(See contact information available at www.expertconsult.com.)

Corn, callus, hammer toe, and bunion supplies (also orthotics)
AliMed, Inc.
Feet Relief
Foot Smart
Moore Medical Corporation (subsidiary of McKesson Medical-Surgical, also supplies surgical instruments)
Myfootshop.com
Foam foot impression system
Smithers Bio-Medical Systems
Orthotics
Langer Benefoot Biomechanics, Inc.
Three Dimensional Systems, Inc.

Acknowledgment

The editors recognize the contributions of Joseph Ellis, DPM, and David Snider, DPM, to this chapter in previous editions of this text.

ONLINE RESOURCES

American College of Foot and Ankle Surgeons (patient information): www.footphysicians.com
American Orthopaedic Foot & Ankle Society, American Orthopaedic Foot & Ankle Society (patient information): www.aofas.org

RECOMMENDED READING

Banks AS, Downey MS, Martin DE, Miller SJ, eds. *McGlamry's Comprehensive Textbook of Foot and Ankle Surgery.* 3rd ed. Philadelphia: Lippincott Williams & Wilkins; 2001.

Bedinghaus JM, Niedfeldt MW. Over-the-counter foot remedies. *Am Fam Physician.* 2001;64:791–796.

Birrer RB, Dellacorte MP, Grisafi PJ. *Common Foot Problems in Primary Care.* Philadelphia: Hanley & Belfus; 1992.

Cole C, Seto C, Gazewood J. Plantar fasciitis: evidence-based review of diagnosis and therapy. *Am Fam Physician.* 2005;72:2237–2242.

DiPreta JA. Managing and treating common foot and ankle problems. *Med Clin North Am.* 2014;98(2):181–390.

Ehrlich M, Nemer JA. Management of select podiatric conditions. In: Reichman EF, Simon RR, eds. *Emergency Medicine Procedures.* New York: McGraw-Hill; 2004:1443.

Hawke F, Burns J, Radford JA, du Toit V. Custom-made foot orthoses for the treatment of foot pain. *Cochrane Database Syst Rev.* 2008;3:CD006801.

Jahss MH, ed. *Disorders of the Foot and Ankle.* 2nd ed. Philadelphia: WB Saunders; 1991.

Ringold S, Mendoza JA, Tarini BA, Sox C. Is duct tape occlusion therapy as effective as cryotherapy for the treatment of the common wart? *Arch Pediatr Adolesc Med.* 2002;156:975–977.

Samit MH, Dana AS. *Cutaneous Lesions of the Lower Extremities.* Philadelphia: JB Lippincott; 1971.

Singh D, Bentley G, Trevino SG. Callosities, corns, and calluses. *BMJ.* 1996;312:1403–1406.

Snoey ER, Miller S. Neuroma management. In: Reichman EF, ed. *Emergency Medicine Procedures.* 2nd ed. New York: McGraw-Hill; 2013:1177–1179.

Stadler TA, Johnson ED, Stephens MB. Clinical inquiries: what is the best treatment for plantar fasciitis? *J Fam Pract.* 2003;52:714–717.

CHAPTER 186

BODY FAT ANALYSIS

Russell D. White • Darrin Ashbrooks

Body fat analysis is a quantitative method for assessing obesity and lean body mass. Several methods of body fat analysis are listed in Table 186.1; each has its advantages and disadvantages. Body fat analysis is more accurate than using body mass index (BMI) to evaluate health and obesity.

Traditional methods such as densitometry and skin-fold measurements are based on the two-compartment model (fat and fat-free mass). Densitometry (underwater weighing) is cumbersome and not readily available. Infrared interactance is less accurate and assumes that the fat in the arm is proportionate to total body fat, which may not always be true. Alternative methods include dual-energy x-ray absorptiometry (DEXA) and total-body electrical conductivity (usually measured as somewhat the reciprocal of conductivity, which is resistance or impedance); these methods distinguish four compartments (water, protein, fat, and bone). Imaging techniques such as computed tomography (CT) scanning, magnetic resonance imaging (MRI), and ultrasound can also give estimates of subcutaneous and visceral fat. Although some of these methods are impractical and require expensive and bulky instruments, several methods can be performed quickly and easily in the office setting. These include skin-fold measurements, bioelectrical impedance, and infrared interactance.

INDICATIONS

- Assessment of conditioning or fitness level (often performed at a gym at the start of a fitness program)
- Assessment of nutritional status
- Obesity
- Risk stratification for disease states (e.g., hypertension, diabetes, coronary artery disease)

CONTRAINDICATIONS

- Patient refusal
- For MRI, patients with pacemakers, implantable defibrillators, spinal cord stimulators, or implantable pain pumps
- For bioelectrical impedance, caution in patients with implantable defibrillators or pacemakers

SKIN-FOLD MEASUREMENTS

In the outpatient setting the most widely used method is the measurement of skin-fold thickness in various predetermined sites.

Equipment

- Marking pen (optional)
- Measuring tape (optional)
- Skin-fold calipers (Fig. 186.1)

Technique

1. Although it matters little on which side of the body measurements are taken, by convention measurements are usually taken on the right side.
2. Measure exactly the same sites for serial comparisons.
3. Be familiar with the skin-fold site to be measured and pull the skin fold once or twice before the actual measurement.
4. Grasp the skin fold with the index finger and thumb of one hand and pull a fold away from the body with the sides approximately parallel. Asking the patient to contract the underlying muscle will help in grasping only skin and fat.
5. Place the caliper heads approximately 0.5 cm away from the fingers holding the skin fold. Place the caliper heads perpendicular to the skin fold and measure 4 to 5 seconds after releasing the lever arm of the calipers.
6. Maintain constant pressure with the thumb and index finger throughout the measurement.
7. To ensure consistency, take a minimum of two measurements 15 seconds apart at each site until consecutive measurements vary by no more than 1 mm.
8. Measuring obese subjects may require both hands to pull a skin fold away with parallel sides. In this case, an assistant will be needed to place the caliper heads on the skin fold.
9. Take measurements when the skin is dry and the subject is not overheated (e.g., after exercise). Vasodilation of the skin in these conditions will inflate normal skin-fold size.
10. Proficiency and accuracy require practice.

Measurements at seven common sites are described as follows (an alternate eighth site is also shown):

TABLE 186.1	Comparative Analysis of Methods for Body Fat Analysis		
Method	**Cost**	**Difficulty**	**Accuracy**
Skinfold measurements	1	2	3*
Bioelectrical impedance	3	1	3†
Near-infrared interactance (NIR)	3	1	3†
Underwater weighing (hydrostatic)	3	4	5
BOD POD (air displacement)	4	2	5
Magnetic resonance imaging	5	3	5
Computed tomography	4	3	5
Dual-energy x-ray absorptiometry (DEXA)	5	2	5
Total-body electrical conductivity	5	2	5

*Accuracy depends on the quality of the instrument and skills of the technician.
†Accuracy diminishes in very lean or very obese subjects.
Range: 1 is low; 5 is high.

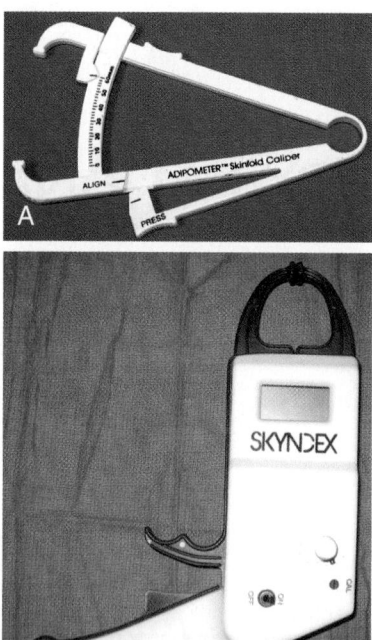

Fig. 186.1   Skin-fold calipers. (A) Manual readout. (B) Digital readout.

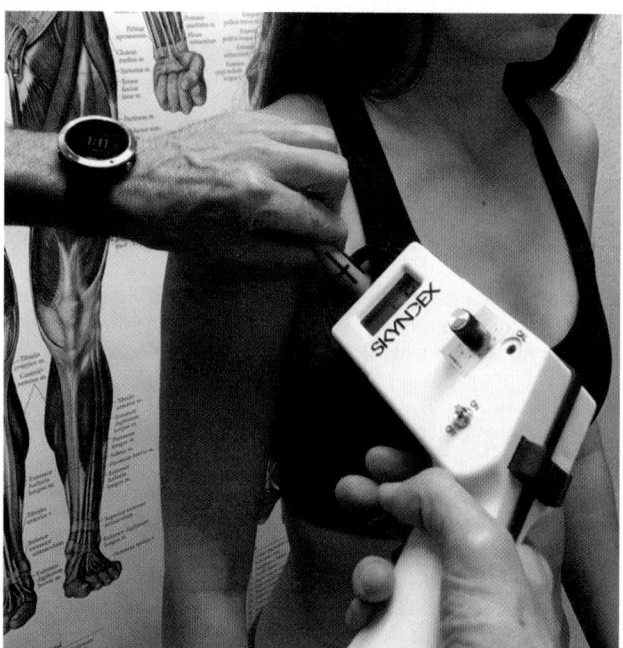

Fig. 186.2   Measurement of the chest or pectoral skin fold. (Courtesy Skyndex, LLC.)

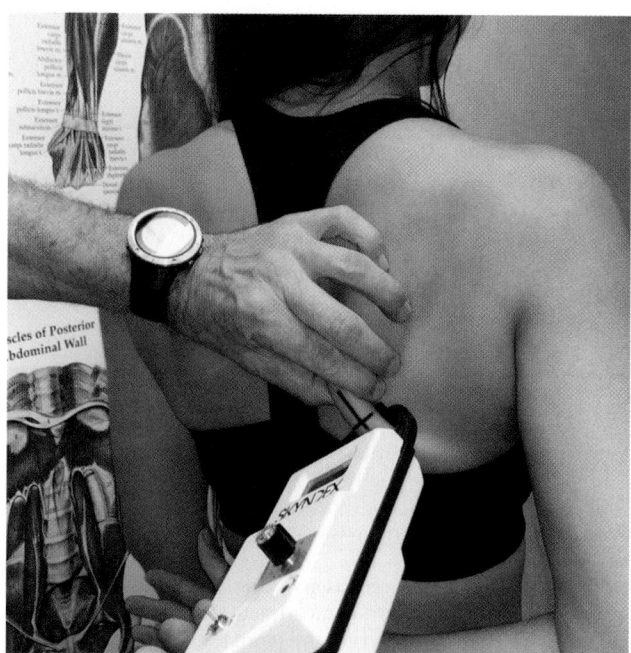

Fig. 186.3   Measurement of the subscapular skin fold. (Courtesy Skyndex, LLC.)

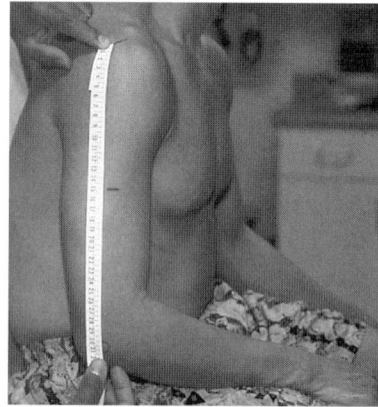

Fig. 186.4   Determining the midpoint between the lateral edge of the acromion and the inferior border of the olecranon.

1. *Chest:* Pick up the pectoral skin fold at the anterior axillary line with the long axis directed to the nipple. Place the skin-fold calipers approximately 2 cm anterior to the anterior axillary line (Fig. 186.2).
2. *Subscapular:* Lift a diagonal fold parallel to the medial border of the scapula at a point just below the inferior angle of the scapula (Fig. 186.3).
3. *Triceps:* Pick up a vertical fold on the posterior arm 1 cm above the midway point between the lateral edge of the acromion and the inferior border of the olecranon. A measuring tape may be helpful in determining the midpoint (Fig. 186.4). Measurements are taken with the arm hanging loosely at the side and the caliper heads placed precisely at the midpoint (Fig. 186.5).
4. *Abdomen:* Pick up a horizontal fold 3 cm lateral to and 1 cm below the navel (Fig. 186.6).
5. *Suprailiac:* Pick up a diagonal fold along the Langer lines above the iliac crest just posterior to the midaxillary line with the calipers placed approximately 1 cm anterior to the grasping fingers. The arm should hang naturally to the side but can be moved slightly to improve access (Fig. 186.7A). Some experts measure this anterior to the superior iliac crest and anterior to the midaxillary line (see Fig. 186.7B).
6. *Thigh:* Measure a vertical fold midway between the inguinal crease and the superior border of the patella. It may be helpful to use a measuring tape to determine the midpoint of the anterior thigh (Fig. 186.8). Pick up the skin fold 1 cm above this point. The subject should have his or her body weight shifted to the opposite side, with the measured leg in slight knee flexion and the foot flat on the floor (Fig. 186.9).
7. *Medial calf:* Measure a vertical fold at the level of the maximum calf circumference on the medial side of the calf. The measured leg should not bear weight and can be measured with the patient in either the standing or the seated position (Fig. 186.10).

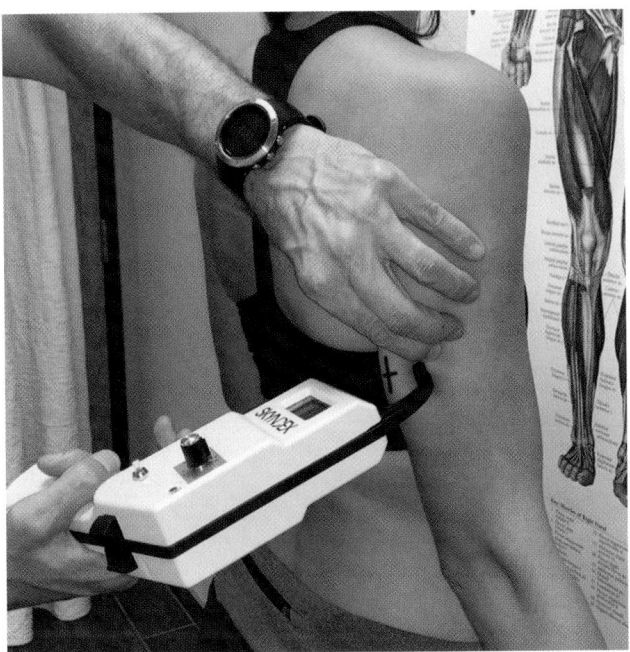

Fig. 186.5 Measurement of the triceps skin fold. (Courtesy Skyndex, LLC.)

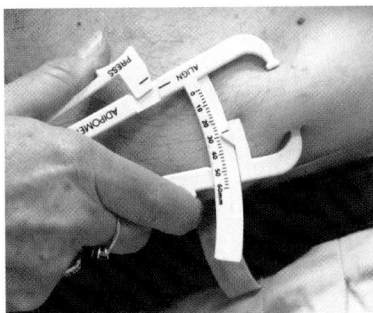

Fig. 186.6 Measurement of the abdominal skin fold.

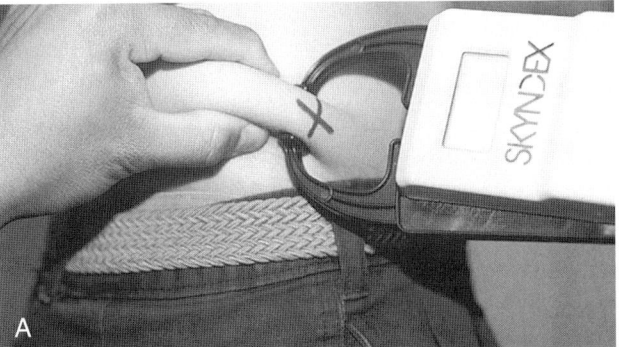

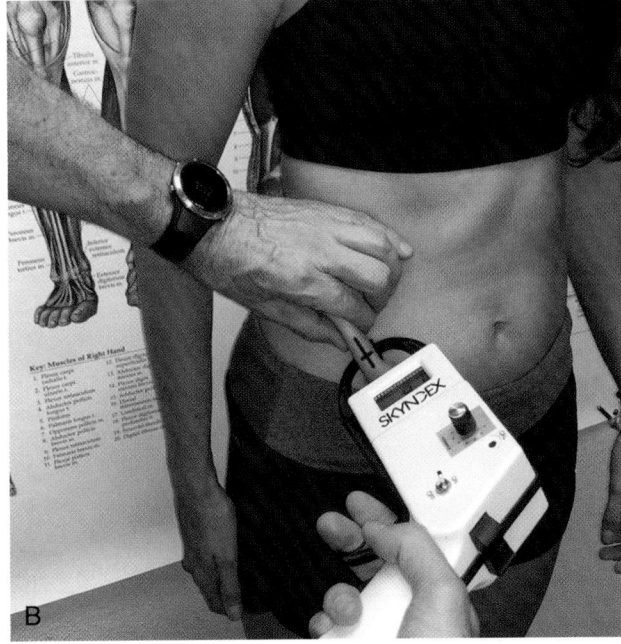

Fig. 186.7 Measurement of the suprailiac skin fold. (Courtesy Skyndex, LLC.)

8. *Biceps (optional):* Measure a vertical fold on the anterior arm midway between the antecubital fossa (proximal antecubital crease) and the insertion of the biceps tendon on the proximal humerus. This is usually over the largest portion of the belly of the biceps. Measurements are taken with the arm hanging loosely at the side and the caliper heads placed at this midpoint (Fig. 186.11).

Calculations

Numerous regression equations with various anthropometric measurements have been used to calculate body fat percentage. However, the following equations by the American Alliance for Health, Physical Education, Recreation, and Dance, used in children and youth (6 to 17 years of age), and those developed by Jackson and Pollock for adults are among the most widely used and accepted.

- For children and youth, a two-site skin-fold test is done, using the triceps and medial calf sites:
  - *Boys 6 to 17 years:* % body fat = (0.735 × sum of skin folds in mm) + 1.0
  - *Girls 6 to 17 years:* % body fat = (0.610 × sum of skin folds in mm) + 5.0
- For adults, the three-site equations developed by Jackson and Pollock are as follows:
  - Men: Body density = $1.1093800 - 0.0008267(x) + 0.0000016(x)^2 - 0.0002574(age)$
    where x = sum of chest, abdomen, and thigh skin folds in mm

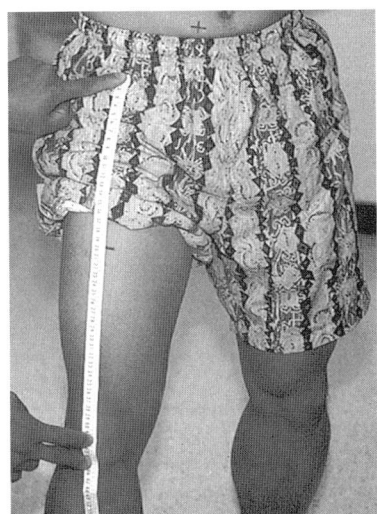

Fig. 186.8 Determining the midpoint of the anterior thigh between the inguinal crease and the superior border of the patella.

% body fat = (495/body density) − 450
or
% body fat = $0.39287(x) - 0.00105(x)^2 + 0.15772(age) - 5.18845$
where x = sum of abdomen, suprailiac, and triceps skin folds in millimeters

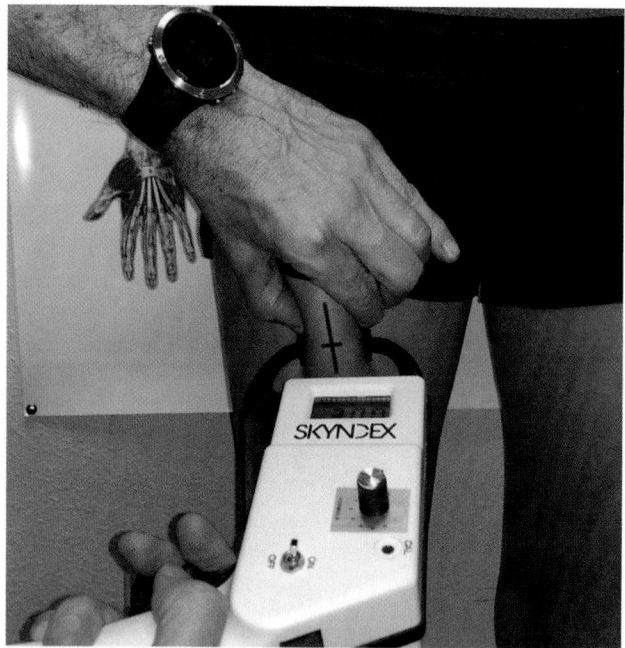

Fig. 186.9 Measurement of the thigh skin fold. (Courtesy Skyndex, LLC.)

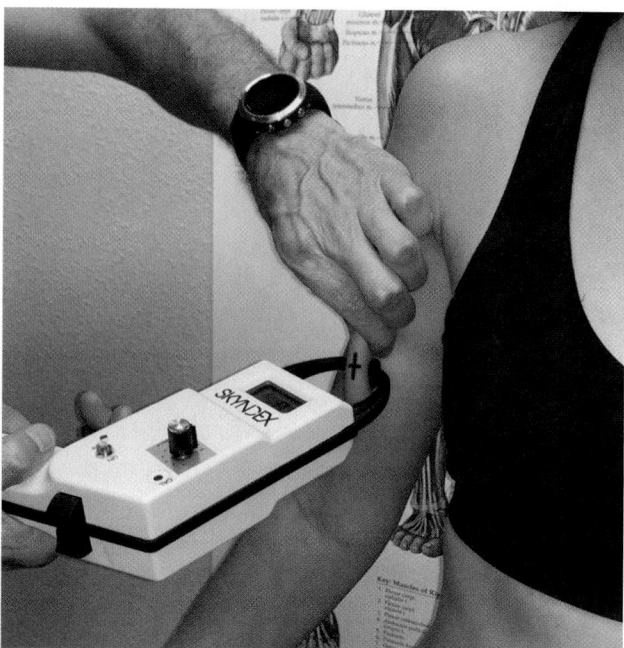

Fig. 186.11 Measurement of the biceps skin fold. (Courtesy Skyndex, LLC.)

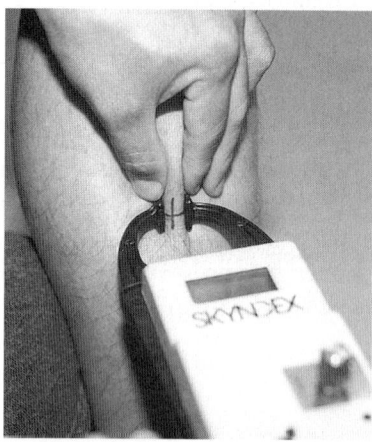

Fig. 186.10 Measurement of the medial calf skin fold. (Courtesy Skyndex, LLC.)

TABLE 186.2	Weight Classification (General Body Fat Percentage Categories)	
Classification	**Women (% of Fat)**	**Men (% of Fat)**
Essential fat	10–13	1–3
Athletes	14–20	6–13
Fitness	21–24	14–17
Acceptable	25–31	18–30
Obese	32+	31+

From American Council of Exercise: http://www.acefitness.org/blog/112/what-are-the-guidelines-for-percentage-of-body-fat/.

- *Women:* Body density = $1.0994921 - 0.0009929(x) + 0.0000023(x)^2 - 0.0001392$(age)
  where x = sum of triceps, suprailiac, and thigh skin folds in millimeters
  % body fat = (495/body density) − 450
  Or
  % body fat = $0.41563(x) - 0.00112(x)^2 + 0.03661$(age) + 4.03653
  where x = sum of triceps, abdomen, and suprailiac skin folds in millimeters

Other formulas have been used, such as those developed by Durnin and Womersley. Also, many clinicians have found the nomogram from American Alliance for Health, Physical Education, Recreation, and Dance useful for determining body fat percentage (Fig. 186.12). Table 186.2 shows weight classifications for men and women.

BIOELECTRICAL IMPEDANCE

Bioelectrical impedance is based on differences in electrical conductivity through tissue depending on the amount of fat-free mass. A greater percentage of fat-free mass increases electrical conductivity, which decreases impedance. Mass is measured by applying an electrode to one hand and one foot (Fig. 186.13C–D) or by having the patient stand on the foot plate of a special scale (see Fig. 186.13B). A variety of formulas have been developed to convert the impedance, which measures body water, into an estimate of body fat.

Equipment

- Bioelectrical impedance measuring device (see Fig. 186.13A)
- Foot plate of special scale (see Fig. 186.13B)
- Handheld unit

Technique A

See Fig. 186.13.

1. Subject should:
   - Be in a fasting state for at least 4 hours before the test.
   - Void completely before the test.
   - Avoid alcohol ingestion within 4 hours of the test.
   - Avoid diuretics within 24 hours of the test.
   - Avoid exercising for 12 hours before the test.
2. Have the subject lie flat on a table with the limbs not touching the body.

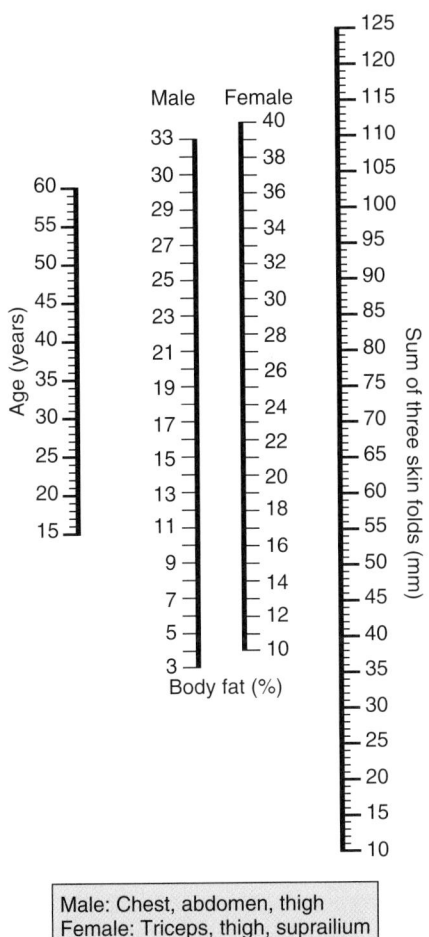

Male: Chest, abdomen, thigh
Female: Triceps, thigh, suprailium

Fig. 186.12 Nomogram for estimating body fat percentage by using the sum of three skin folds and age. (From Baun WB, Baun MR, Raven PB. A nomogram for the estimate of percent body fat from generalized equations. *Res Q Exerc Sport.* 1981;52:380–384.)

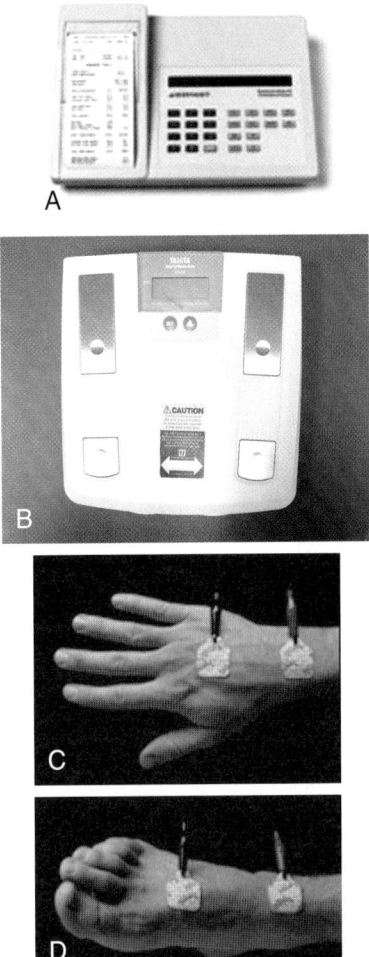

Fig. 186.13 (A) Bioelectrical impedance measuring device. (B) Foot plate of special scale. (C and D) Electrodes are placed on the right hand and right foot. (Courtesy Biodynamics Corp., Seattle, WA.)

3. Electrodes are placed on the right hand and right foot. A harmless, imperceptible 50-kHz current at 800 µA is generated and passes through the subject.
4. Electrical conductance (or impedance) is measured and percentage lean body mass is subsequently automatically calculated by the machine.

Technique B

1. Have the subject follow the guidelines given in step 1 of technique A.
2. Have the subject stand in limited clothing on the foot plate of a special scale (see Fig. 186.13B).
3. Electrical conductance (or impedance) is measured and percentage lean body mass is subsequently automatically calculated by the instrument.

Technique C

1. Have the subject follow the guidelines given in step 1 of technique A.
2. Have the subject stand in limited clothing with arms outstretched at 90 degrees in front holding a handheld device.
3. The analyzer automatically detects that it is being grasped with two hands and begins measurement. Within less than 10 seconds, body fat percentage and body fat mass are displayed on the digital panel.

Complications

Bioelectrical impedance should not be used in patients with implantable defibrillators or pacemakers.

NEAR-INFRARED INTERACTANCE

Near-infrared interactance is based on the principles of light absorption and reflection and uses near-infrared spectroscopy. The degree of infrared energy absorption is related to the composition of the substance through which the energy is passing and the particular wavelength of the energy. Hence lean body mass and fat can be distinguished from each other and a percentage calculated.

Equipment

A computerized, near-infrared spectrophotometer with fiberoptic probe, practical for office use (Fig. 186.14), is necessary.

Technique

The fiberoptic probe is commonly placed over the belly of the biceps muscle to gather the near-infrared data. Specific requirements, including anatomic location for probe placement, may differ depending on the individual spectrophotometer.

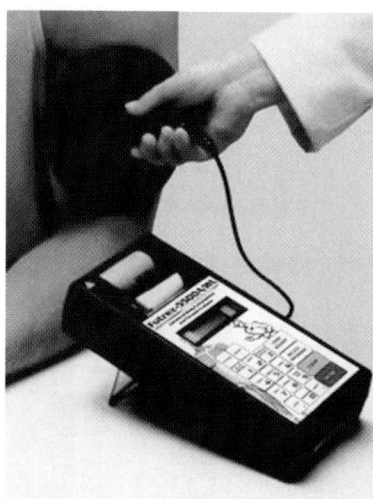

Fig. 186.14 Measurement using computed near-infrared spectrophotometer with fiberoptic probe. (Courtesy Futrex, Inc., Gaithersburg, MD.)

Complications

No complications are associated with near-infrared interactance.

DUAL-ENERGY X-RAY ABSORPTIOMETRY

Densitometry has been the gold standard for determining body fat. However, this technique has now been replaced by DEXA because of its ease of use.

NOTE: There have been questions regarding DEXA's accuracy in child and adolescent models. Compared with other methods, DEXA overestimated body fatness at lower values. It has been recommended that this method not be used to calibrate field methods in the pediatric population.

DEXA estimates lean mass, body fat, and bone mineral density by using the differential absorption of photon beams of two levels of intensity. DEXA relies on the principle that the intensity of a photon beam is altered by the thickness, density, and chemical composition of an object in its path. In children, the scan takes approximately 10 minutes. The average radiation dose is barely higher than normal background radiation and well below that of a chest radiograph.

Equipment

A DEXA scanner is required.

Complications

Although it is minimal, there is radiation exposure. DEXA is contraindicated in the first trimester of pregnancy and relatively contraindicated in the second and third trimesters.

MAGNETIC RESONANCE IMAGING, COMPUTED TOMOGRAPHY, AND ULTRASOUND

Regional body fat distribution can be determined reliably by either CT or MRI; ultrasound is an evolving modality for body fat analysis. CT uses x-radiation and computer analysis to determine the structure of internal organs. It is possible to obtain an accuracy within less than a 1% margin of error for body fat using a series of scans. With MRI the patient is placed in an electromagnetic field that creates tissue (body) images. Hydrogenated (^{1}H) atoms possess an unpaired proton and exhibit a spin that results in a magnet moment. ^{1}H atoms react to an external magnetic field when radio waves are pulsed to a patient at a specific frequency and are absorbed by the nuclei. Fatty tissue is high signal on T1-weighted images, whereas fluid (water)

is high signal on T2-weighted images. In addition, fat suppression techniques that cause fat to lose signal or become dark while fluid stays bright or high signal are available. The ratio of whole body fat/nonfat tissue can be determined because the human body is primarily fat and water. MRI takes longer to perform than CT and is considerably more expensive.

Although ultrasound has been used to measure adipose tissue for almost five decades, this technology is often disregarded by body composition clinicians and researchers. There is substantial literature that it is a reliable, reproducible, accurate, fast, and safe method to measure subcutaneous and visceral fat. Ultrasound machines are small, portable, and relatively inexpensive imaging devices that do not involve radiation, giving it many advantages over other imaging devices and laboratory body composition techniques. Additionally, the ability to assess regional composition provides another advantage over many other methods and allows for the unique assessments of some clinical populations. However, owing to the lack of standardized procedures and because results are highly dependent on the skill of the operator, ultrasound is currently not being widely used. New user-friendly devices with accompanying software designed specifically for body composition analysis may help to minimize these limitations, but they have yet to be adequately validated (Wagner, 2013).

Equipment

An MRI machine, CT scanner, or ultrasound device is necessary.

Technique

These scans are used mainly for analysis of body fat in a certain region, most commonly the abdomen. There are different methods of CT scanning, but the most common is to take a single cut through the L4 to L5 position and compute the regional body fat percentage from this cut. This method minimizes the patient's exposure to radiation. Likewise, MRI and ultrasound methods usually consist of scanning a region such as the abdomen and computing data from this region.

Complications

There is moderate radiation exposure with CT scans and they are relatively contraindicated in pregnancy. MRI is contraindicated in patients with pacemakers, implantable defibrillators, and intracranial metal clips (until 8 weeks after central nervous system surgery) or following documentation of material used in the procedure. After implantation, patients are issued a medical card indicating whether MRI is acceptable. Since 1995, new materials have been used for pacers and defibrillators, and many are now acceptable. As previously identified, MRI and ultrasound have the advantage of not utilizing ionizing radiation.

BOD POD

BOD POD (air displacement) is based on the same principle as underwater weighing and uses computerized sensors to measure how much air is displaced while a person sits for 20 seconds in a capsule. The BOD POD determines body mass and volume and from these two variables computes body density. From this calculation body fat is determined. The equipment is very expensive and limited in availability. Studies have shown that the results are comparable with underwater weighing. There has been some variance in outcomes (−3.0% to 1.7%) when air displacement is compared with other methods, such as DEXA scanning. These differences are likely due in part to differences in laboratory equipment, study design, and subject characteristics and, in some cases, to failure to follow the manufacturer's recommended protocol.

Equipment

The BOD POD capsule and associated computerized equipment are required.

Technique

1. The subject should avoid eating or exercising for at least 2 hours before testing.
2. The subject must remove clothing, jewelry, and eyeglasses and should wear form-fitting clothing (e.g., Spandex or Lycra swimsuit).
3. A swim cap is worn to compress air pockets from the hair.
4. The subject must avoid moving, talking, or laughing.
5. During the test, slight pressure changes occur, similar to what is experienced in a moving elevator.

CPT/BILLING CODES

76499   Unlisted diagnostic radiographic procedure: DEXA for Body Composition

There is no specific CPT code for body fat analysis. This unspecified code can be attempted or it is possible to code this in addition to using normal outpatient evaluation and management codes (e.g., 99202, 99203, 99213, 99214).

99354   Prolonged service in the office or other outpatient setting, requiring direct (face-to-face) patient contact beyond the usual service first hour*

99355   Each additional 30 minutes (list separately in addition to code for prolonged service)*

ICD-10-CM DIAGNOSTIC CODES

E66.9   Obesity unspecified
E66.2   Obesity, morbid
E66.3   Overweight

Use additional code to identify BMI:

Z68.20-Z68.29	BMI 20-29.9	Adult
Z68.30-Z68.39	BMI 30-39.9	Adult
Z68.40-Z68.45	BMI 40->70	Adult
Z68.51-Z68.54	BMI	Pediatric

Acknowledgment

The editors recognize the contributions of Arnold M. Ramirez, MD, to this chapter in a previous edition of this text.

SUPPLIERS

(See contact information available at www.expertconsult.com.)

Bioelectric impedance measuring device (approximate cost: $1500 to $2200)
Biodynamics Corporation
Near-infrared spectrophotometer (approximate cost: $3000 to $4000)
Futrex Inc.

Skin-fold calipers (approximate cost: $250 to $500)
Medco Supply Company
Micro Bio-Medics
Skyndex by Welltec-USA IDT International

RECOMMENDED READING

Baun WB, Baun MR, Raven PB. A nomogram for the estimate of percent body fat from generalized equations. *Res Q Exerc Sport.* 1981;52:380–384.

Boneva-Asiova Z, Boyanov MA. Body composition analysis by leg-to-leg bioelectrical impedance and dual-energy x-ray absorptiometry in non-obese and obese individuals. *Diabetes Obes Metab.* 2008;11:1012–1018.

Durnin JV, Wormersley J. Body fat assessment from total body density and its estimation from skinfold thickness. Measurements on 481 men and women aged 16–72 years. *Br J Nutr.* 1974;32:77.

Fields DA, Goran MI, McCrory MA. Body-composition assessment via aird-isplacement plethysmography in adults and children. A review. *Am J Clin Nutr.* 2002;75:453–467.

Fukuda DH, Wray ME, Kendall KL, Smith-Ryan AE, Stout JR. Validity of near-infrared interactance (FUTREX 6100/XL) for estimating body fat percentage in elite rowers. *Clin Physiol Funct Imaging.* 2017;37(4):456–458.

Goodpasture BH. Measuring body fat distribution and content in humans. *Curr Opin Clin Nutr Metab Care.* 2002;5:481–487.

Helba M, Blinkovitz LA. Pediatric body absorption analysis with dual-energy X-ray absorptiometry. *Pediatr Radiol.* 2009;39:647–656.

Horie LM, Barbosa-Silva MC, Torrinhas RS, et al. New body fat prediction equations for severely obese patients. *Clin Nutr.* 2008;27:350–356.

Kurniawan LB, Bahrun U, Hatta M, Arif M. Body mass, total body fat percentage, and visceral fat level predict insulin resistance better than waist circumference and body mass index in healthy young male adults in Indonesia. *J Clin Med.* 2018;1(5):7.

Kyle UG, Piccoli A, Pichard C. Body composition measurements. Interpretation finally made easy for clinical use. *Curr Opin Clin Nutr Metab Care.* 2003;6:387–393.

Lazzer S, Bedogni G, Agosti F, et al. Comparison of dual-energy x-ray absorptiometry, air displacement plethysmography and bioelectrical impedance analysis for the assessment of body composition in severely obese Caucasian children and adolescents. *Br J Nutr.* 2008;100:918–924.

Lee SY, Gallagher D. Assessment methods in human body composition. *Curr Opin Clin Nutr Metab Care.* 2008;11:566–572.

Lukaski HC. Methods for the assessment of human body composition. Traditional and new. *Am J Clin Nutr.* 1987;46:537–556.

Mattsson S, Thomas BJ. Development of methods for body composition studies. *Phys Med Biol.* 2006;51:R203–R228.

Pietrobelli A, Tato L. Body composition measurements. From the past to the future. *Acta Paediatr Suppl.* 2005;94:8–13.

Rao G. Office-based strategies for the management of obesity. *Am Fam Physician.* 2010;81(12):1449–1455.

Reilly JJ, Gerasimidis K, Paparacleous N, et al. Validation of dual-energy x-ray absorptiometry and foot-foot impedance against deuterium dilution measures of fatness in children. *Int J Pediatric Obes.* 2010;5:111–1115.

Ritz P, Salle A, Audran M. Comparison of different methods to assess body composition of weight loss in obese and diabetic patients. *Diabetes Res Clin Pract.* 2007;77:405–411.

Vescovi JD, Zimmerman SL, Miller WC, et al. Evaluation of the BOD POD for estimating percentage body fat in a heterogeneous group of adult humans. *Eur J Appl Physiol.* 2001;85:326–332.

Volgyi E, Tylavsky FA, Lyytikainen A, et al. Assessing body composition with DXA and bioimpedance. Effects of obesity, physical activity, and age. *Obesity.* 2008;16:700–705.

Wagner DR, Heywrd VH. Techniques of body composition assessment. A review of laboratory and field methods. *Res Q Exerc Sport.* 1999;70:135–149.

Wagner DR. Ultrasound as a tool to assess body fat. *J Obes.* 2013;280713.

Wells JC, Haroun D, Williams JE, et al. Evaluation of DXA against the four-component model of body composition in obese children and adolescents aged 5–21 years. *Int J Obes.* 2010;34:649–655.

CHAPTER 187

OFFICE NERVE CONDUCTION TESTING

Thomas A. Kintanar

The NC-stat System and ADVANCE NCS System (NeuroMetrix, Inc.) are designed to perform standard noninvasive nerve conduction studies. These systems have components that work together to accurately and rapidly evaluate peripheral nerve function. This enables clinicians to manage patient care more effectively and efficiently—all within the office or clinic setting. These diagnostic tools have the capability of approximating the results of more invasive electromyographic (EMG) testing, but with the purported advantage of patient comfort without sacrificing diagnostic accuracy. The neural waveform analysis provided is parallel to traditional EMG analysis without the pain conferred by traditional EMG. The units, connectors, and biosensors are all available from NeuroMetrix. Since this chapter was originally written, NeuroMetrix transitioned from the NC-stat system to the ADVANCE NCS System. Neither is being manufactured any longer; however, both systems continue to be supported by Neurometrix. Electrodes and supplies are still available. Neurometrix now produces DPNCheck, a fast, accurate, and quantitative nerve conduction test that is used to evaluate systemic neuropathies such as diabetic peripheral neuropathy (DPN). That said, this chapter details the functioning of the NC-stat system.

The NC-stat system is termed an automated system, which clearly delineates it from a standard EMG system, which is a manual system. There are some advantages, but also disadvantages, conferred by an automated system. The advantages include standardized methods and reference ranges; technical setup can be performed by staff with basic training; the process is rapid and consistent; support systems can aid the clinician with reports to assist in diagnosis; and the procedure is completely automated. The disadvantages of this system in deference to traditional needle EMG are that it is limited to nerves for which the system was specifically designed; is less flexible than other systems; is not suitable for children; and may not work well in anatomically challenged patients (e.g., amputees).

ANATOMY

Neurons serve as the primary functional unit of the nervous system. The basis of the evaluation is centered around the basic components of a neuron. The components consist of a *cell body* that contains a nucleus and axon (nerve fiber) and creates an electrochemical action potential to stimulate communication with other neurons or muscle fibers; a *dendrite* that receives input from other neurons and transmits the signal to the cell body for interpretation; and the *synapse*, which is the connecting point between a neuron and muscle fiber or two neurons.

Peripheral nerves are a collection of thousands of nerve fibers whose cell bodies are located in either the dorsal root ganglia (sensory neurons) or the anterior horn (motor neurons) of the spinal cord. Nerve fibers can be characterized by the amount of myelin surrounding each axon. Myelin is an insulator that enhances the speed of action potential propagation. Thus axons can be thinly myelinated (A-delta pain fibers), unmyelinated (temperature and pin prick), or thickly myelinated (motor or sensory fibers that carry vibration, light touch, and proprioception). Thin myelination is considered to be less than 0.5 mm, whereas thick myelination is greater than 1 mm.

INDICATIONS

Indications for NC-stat testing include the EMG diagnosis of the following:

- Polyneuropathies: diabetes, chronic inflammatory demyelinating polyneuropathy (toxic, metabolic, drug-induced polyneuropathy), acute demyelinating polyneuropathy (i.e., Guillain-Barré syndrome)
- Upper extremity neuropathies: carpal tunnel syndrome, cubital tunnel syndrome
- Spine and lower extremity disorders: tarsal tunnel syndrome, spinal stenosis, lumbosacral radiculopathy
- Generalized disorders: myopathy, motor neuron disease, disorders of neuromuscular transmission (e.g., myasthenia gravis)

CONTRAINDICATIONS

Relative

- Anticoagulation (for the needle examination).
- Check for medication administration (e.g., if patient has myasthenia gravis, medication may alter the validity of the examination).

Absolute

Other than placing a needle through an infected area, there are no absolute contraindications.

EQUIPMENT AND SUPPLIES

NC-Stat Biosensors

A biosensor is a preconfigured standard array of electrodes, eliminating the need for placement of multiple needles in very precise locations; multiple sites can be studied instead (Figs. 187.1 to 187.6). The NC-stat biosensor integrates flexible circuitry and a proprietary electrochemical gel with stimulus and sensing electrodes. An embedded chip monitors skin surface temperature, an important covariant for nerve conduction studies. A unique serial number is also embedded in the chip to conveniently link patients to their test results. Currently, biosensors are available for the median, ulnar, cubital, peroneal, sural, and tibial nerves.

NC-Stat Monitor

The NC-stat monitor houses sophisticated proprietary technology for conducting accurate nerve conduction studies. The monitor measures standard nerve conduction parameters—amplitude, latency, and conduction velocity—of the motor and sensory nerves. The NC-stat can record the smallest signals for early detection of disease.

A nerve conduction study is initiated with the press of a button. The monitor automatically stimulates the nerve, acquires all the response waveforms, and displays response parameters in real

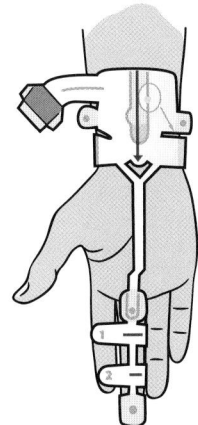

Fig. 187.1   Median nerve biosensor.

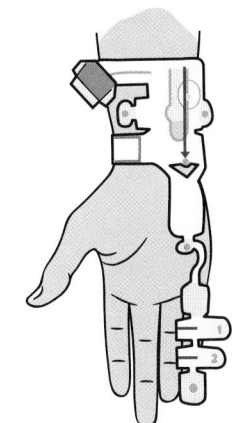

Fig. 187.2   Ulnar nerve biosensor.

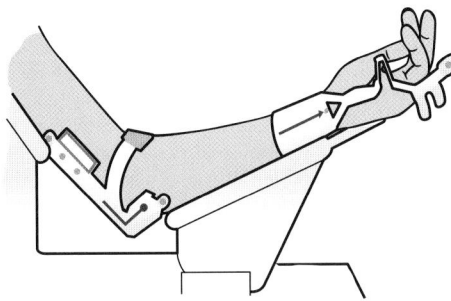

Fig. 187.3   Cubital nerve biosensor.

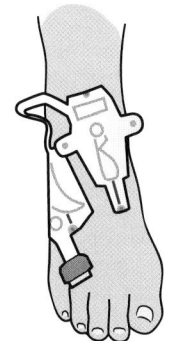

Fig. 187.4   Peroneal nerve biosensor.

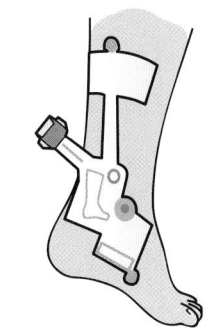

Fig. 187.5   Sural nerve biosensor.

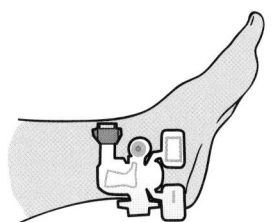

Fig. 187.6   Tibial nerve biosensor.

time on the liquid crystal display screen. Using advanced signal processing and control algorithms, the monitor determines stimulation intensity, waveform validity, real-time response parameters, noise artifacts, and appropriate NC-stat biosensor contact.

NC-Stat Docking Station

This component receives nerve conduction data and waveforms from the monitor and, at the clinician's direction, can automatically transmit the data to the On-Call Information System at NeuroMetrix through any available analog telephone line (such as those used by facsimile machines) in minutes. The monitor can also be remotely upgraded by the docking station, thus ensuring that the system is always up to date with the latest software (Fig. 187.7).

On-Call Information System

This component at NeuroMetrix receives data from the docking station and automatically generates a report in real time that is returned to the clinician within minutes by facsimile or email. The report includes nerve conduction data originally displayed by the monitor, response waveforms, comparison with reference data, and summary data. Nerve conduction data are archived for sequential testing and trending. Suggested interpretation and diagnostic considerations are provided.

Precautions

No general precautions are needed, except to remind the patient not to use lotions or oils, which may alter the quality of the signals evaluated. Alcohol wipes are sufficient to remove oils from contact points.

PREPROCEDURE PATIENT EDUCATION AND FORMS

Patient education forms and insurance/Medicare/Medicaid waiver forms are available at www.neurometrix.com.

PROCEDURE

The bulk of this procedure is performed by ancillary staff. The biosensors are placed by staff who are trained in the proper technique

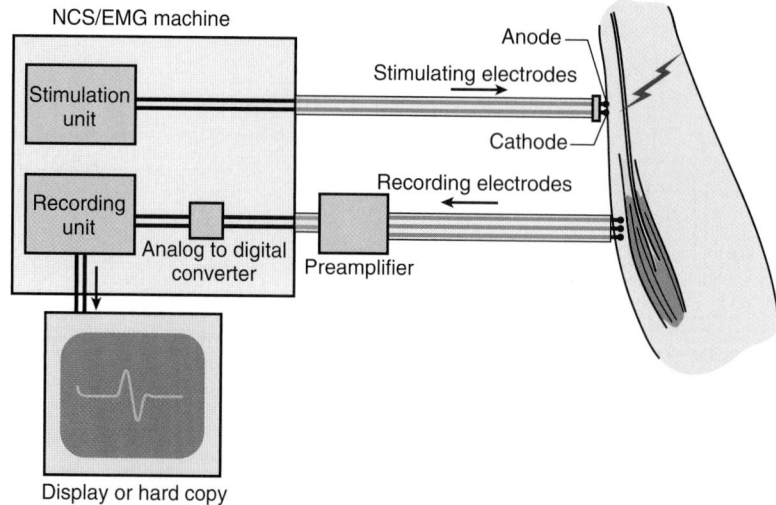

Fig. 187.7   The basic unit of operation in obtaining the recorded data. *EMG,* Electromyographic.

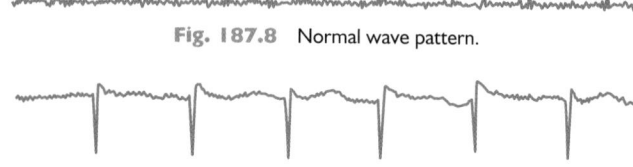

Fig. 187.8   Normal wave pattern.

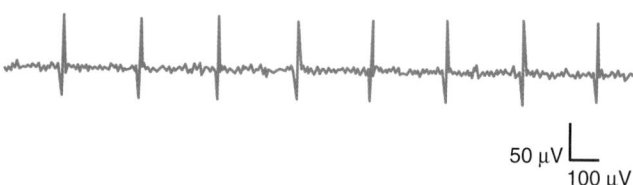

Fig. 187.9   Abnormal wave pattern demonstrating positive sharp wave.

50 μV ⌐
         100 μV

Fig. 187.10   Abnormal wave pattern demonstrating fibrillation potential.

or by the clinician. Proper placement of the biosensors is essential for accurate interpretation of the submitted data (see Figs. 187.1 to 187.6). Instructions for the accurate placement of the leads and operation of the NC-stat module are found at www.neurometrix.com. Proficiency in the use of the NC-stat system is easily attained. However, it is important to highlight the basic elements of interpretation of the traditional EMG, which correlate with the NC-stat system interpretation. The two major evaluative points of EMG or nerve conduction include (1) evaluation of spontaneous muscle activity performed while the muscle is at rest and (2) evaluation of voluntary activity performed when the patient is requested to contract the muscle. The oscilloscope findings may demonstrate the muscle electrical potential tracings shown in Figs. 187.8 to 187.10.

SAMPLE OPERATIVE REPORT

A sample operative report is available at www.neurometrix.com. The clinician uses the initial interpretation along with his or her cognitive knowledge of neural wave patterns and the clinical presentation of the patient to agree with or supplement the initial interpretation, or to synthesize another interpretation germane to the patient.

COMPLICATIONS

- For needle EMG: infection, bleeding, pain
- For NC-stat: none apparent except surface allergies to the biosensors

POSTPROCEDURE PATIENT EDUCATION

An appointment should be scheduled to review the results with the patient.

INTERPRETATION OF RESULTS

The basic electrophysiologic assessment of peripheral nerve conduction depends on the response of nerves to electrical stimulation. The study is objective and independent of patient input. It is also quantitative, providing numeric values that can be compared rigorously against reference ranges. The results of a nerve conduction study are reproducible and assess peripheral sensory neurons, motor neurons, and the neuromuscular junction. Nerve conduction studies also document the presence, nature, distribution, and severity of peripheral nerve impairment and have high diagnostic sensitivity and specificity for most types of peripheral nerve disorders.

There are no standard or normative reference ranges used for conduction studies. Each laboratory usually has its own reference range or uses published parameters determined using rigorous clinical study design. Reference values may depend on height, age, and sex. Only reference data that are demographically matched should be used for determining an abnormality. Obviating this detail may lead to poor sensitivity and specificity of resultant data. The basic components of a sensory nerve conduction study starting with baseline at 0 msec are shown in Fig. 187.11.

When stimulating the nerve, the stimulus should be strong enough to stimulate all axons in the nerve, which is termed supramaximal. A submaximal stimulus may lead to inaccurate data being recorded. This potential problem is minimized by the NC-stat technology.

Under the usual needle protocol, a strong, appropriate stimulus is achieved by slowly and gradually increasing the intensity and duration of the stimulus until maximal stimulus is achieved. The NC-stat technology performs this function through its biosensor units. In motor conduction studies, the nerve is stimulated at two or more points along its course while the electrical response of one of the muscles supplied is recorded. The muscle response is recorded by surface (biosensors) or subcutaneous needle electrodes, with the active electrode being placed over the end-plate region and the reference electrode over the muscle tendon. The response recorded is called the compound muscle action potential (CMAP), or M wave, and it represents the sum of the electrical activity of all the activated muscle fibers within the pickup region of the recording electrode. The shape, size, and latency of the response obtained by stimulating the nerve at different sites are measured. The conduction velocity can

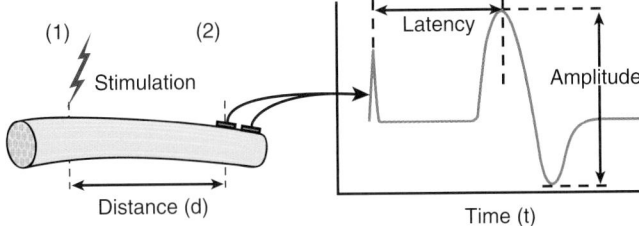

Fig. 187.11 Testing sequence. Components of a sensory nerve conduction study are defined as follows: Latency is the time (t) it takes the impulse to travel the distance (d) between the stimulator (1) and the detector (2), usually measured in milliseconds. Conduction velocity is the speed with which the impulse propagates, calculated as d/t, usually measured in meters per second. Amplitude is the height of the response and can be measured from the baseline to the peak or from peak to peak for sensory responses.

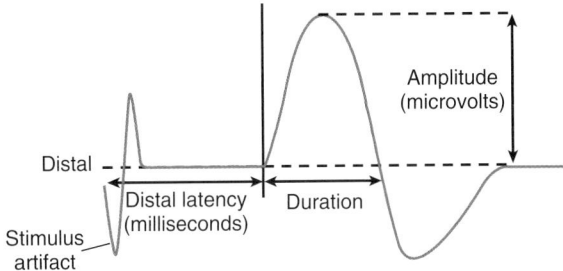

Fig. 187.12 Compound motor action potential.

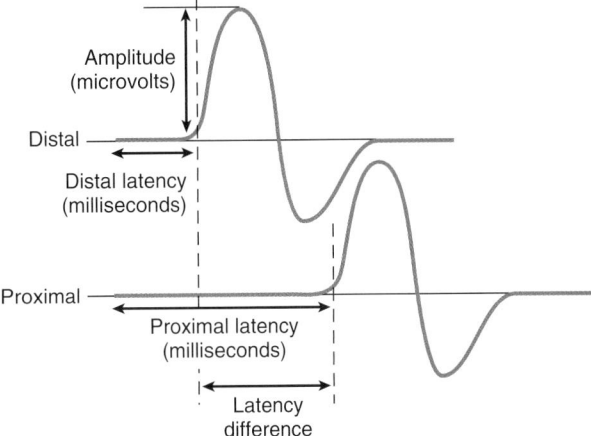

Fig. 187.13 Comparison of proximal and distal compound motor action potential responses.

then be determined by measuring the distance between stimulation sites and the time it takes to measure a response. This measurement can determine the fastest conducting fibers along the intervening segments of the nerve. The normal range of maximal motor conduction velocity is between 50 and 70 m/sec in the arms, and between 40 and 60 m/sec in the legs.

Sensory nerve conduction studies involve stimulating a sensory nerve and recording the response at another point along the course of the same nerve. Responses can also be recorded from a purely sensory nerve after stimulation of the parent nerve trunk from which it originates, or vice versa. This response is called the sensory nerve action potential (SNAP).

Nerve Conduction Study Components

The parameters for interpretation of the EMG/NC-stat are (1) the standard sensory nerve conduction study, (2) the standard motor nerve conduction study, and (3) an F-wave study.

Sensory Nerve Conduction Study

The components to evaluate this part of an EMG/NC-stat evaluation are as described earlier. The sensory response is termed the SNAP.

Standard Motor Nerve Conduction Study

The components to evaluate this part of an EMG/NC-stat include recording, reference, and stimulating electrodes, as noted previously. This portion of the study creates a characteristic waveform. The calculation for motor velocity conduction occurs at proximal and distal sites along the nerve and is called the CMAP (Figs. 187.12 and 187.13).

Differentiating Compound Muscle Action Potential (Motor) and Sensory Nerve Action Potential (Sensory) Responses

Several parameters differentiate CMAP and SNAP. The size of the signal involved is larger with CMAP. The signal is measured in millivolts rather than microvolts for SNAP. Although muscle can amplify the signal in CMAP, noise and other small artifacts can alter the quality of the reading with SNAP. CMAP can detect pathology in nerve and muscle, whereas SNAP can identify nerve changes only. The SNAP response is not affected by radiculopathies, whereas CMAP can be. The sensitivity of amplitude decrement to axonal loss is very high in SNAP because of the proportional relationship of amplitude to the number of axons in this study. This sensitivity is hard to overcome in CMAP because of vigorous muscle fiber reinnervation until advanced axonal loss occurs. As mentioned earlier,

CMAP requires stimulation at two locations to evaluate conduction velocity, whereas SNAP requires only one stimulation site.

F Wave

The F wave provides information on the integrity of the entire nerve, from the root to the muscle. Because its measurement requires evaluating signals from every nerve traversing the entire spine, its latency is considerably longer than for the CMAP. The minimum latency is the most frequently reported parameter in most traditional studies. Its limitation lies in its having the lowest sensitivity because a single normal nerve fiber can read as a normal minimum latency. Measurement of these parameters is the function of the biosensor system of NC-stat (Fig. 187.14).

There are several F-wave response parameters that help to generate optimal sensitivity and specificity. These include minimum F wave, which is the earliest latency among the ensemble of recorded F waves; chronodispersion, which is the time between the earliest and latest responses in the ensemble; and persistence, which is the percentage of stimuli that lead to a recordable F wave. Other factors that affect interpretation are the age, height, and temperature of the patient, as well as appropriate stimulation and placement of electrodes or biosensors. The sum of all of these parameters provide data to assist the clinician in coming to a meaningful clinical conclusion. By evaluating the nerve conduction data in their entirety, the clinician can assess how severe a nerve problem happens to be, the duration of the problem, and whether a nerve injury or muscle anomaly is generalized or involves specific nerves and muscles.

It is highly recommended that a clinician who wants to perform nerve conduction/EMG studies participate in a dedicated course in EMG waveform interpretation to understand the nuances of EMG interpretation. Suggested courses are found on the NeuroMetrix website. However, there is a distinct advantage conferred with the

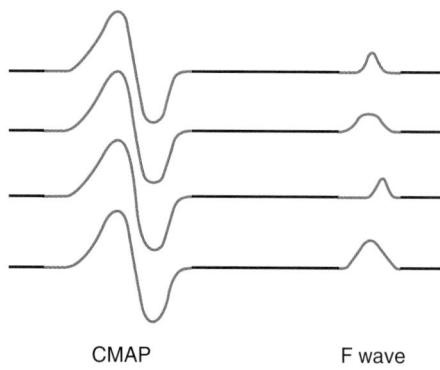

CMAP   F wave

Fig. 187.14   Illustration of a compound motor action potential (CMAP) and F wave.

TABLE 187.1	Sample Reimbursement Rates for Nerve Conduction Studies		
CPT Code	Global	−26 Modifier	TC Modifier
95900	$90.88	$32.38	$57.98
95903	$96.63	$46.48	$50.14
95904	$77.30	$26.64	$50.66

TC, Technical component.

NC-stat system in that the real-time automatic reports generated include very detailed waveform analysis and explanations that assist the clinician to correlate clinical findings with the most likely diagnosis without the patient experiencing the pain or discomfort of a needle prick. The report includes not only the waveforms and data but a preliminary diagnostic impression, which the clinician can confirm, refute, or include as additional commentary in the final diagnosis.

BILLING AND CODING

CPT/Billing Codes

95905   Motor and/or sensory nerve conduction, using preconfigured electrode arrays, amplitude and latency/velocity study, each limb, includes F-wave study when performed, with interpretation and report

95999   Some Medicare carriers require the use of 95999, unlisted neurologic or neuromuscular code

Coding Multiple Nerves

Units are used to indicate the number of nerves tested when coding nerve conduction studies. When performed with the NC-stat, a motor study with F wave of two separate nerves might be described as two units of 95907. Some payers have specific requirements for modifiers. For example, certain payers will require a specific local modifier to indicate billing for multiple nerves and, if not used, will reimburse for one nerve/unit of the procedure. Although nerve conduction CPT codes are designed to be billed per nerve by definition (no modifier needed), payers might not recognize this and reject this usage on a regular basis. A CMS 2000 OCI edit update suggested that the -59 modifier be used with CPT code to indicate it is a distinct procedural service being performed on a different area of the body (different nerve). It is good practice to regularly cross-reference units billed with reimbursement received.

Coding Components

Nerve conduction studies consist of a professional component, the amount paid for the clinician's interpretation of the results of the study and associated overhead, and a technical component (TC), the amount paid for all other services (including technician and equipment costs). The global charge describes both the professional and TCs. Most payers will process and reimburse for the global (entire) procedure when nerve conduction studies are billed without modifiers indicating the separate components (TC or -26 modifier). Note that some payers have specific requirements for modifiers. For example, certain payers require a local modifier to indicate billing

for the entire procedure and, if not used, will reimburse for one component of the procedure.

In essence, the real-time interpretation provided by NeuroMetrix is subject to the confirmation of the clinician providing direct service to the patient. Thus the eligible charges are credited to the primary provider of the service. NeuroMetrix is able to sustain its support to the medical community by the sale of its biosensors. An example of characteristic payment for the procedure is given in Table 187.1.

Nerve Conduction Policy

Medicare and other payers reimburse for medically appropriate nerve conduction studies. Most Medicare carriers have established lists of pertinent ICD-10 codes that indicate medical necessity for nerve conduction studies. Studies submitted with other diagnoses are considered not medically necessary and denied. Additional details for billing nerve conduction studies can be found in Medicare carrier Local Coverage Decisions (LCDs). The LCDs provide detailed conditions of coverage for nerve conduction procedures that address the following: type of procedures covered, number of nerves allowed, patients who are eligible to receive the procedure, requirements for providers of the procedure, the allowed testing frequency, and coding instruction.

Frequency of Testing

Electrodiagnostic testing frequency guidelines have been established according to the American Association of Neuromuscular and Electrodiagnostic Medicine (AANEM). Repeat electrodiagnostic testing should not be necessary in a 12-month period in most cases. Tests refer here to any area tested with a group or region of nerve distribution, not the number of nerves. These guidelines have been incorporated into many Medicare and other payer policies. These limits should not apply if the patient requires evaluation by more than one electrodiagnostic consultant (i.e., a second opinion or an expert opinion at a tertiary care center) in a given year or if the patient requires evaluation for a second diagnosis in a given year. Additional tests may be required or appropriate over and above these guidelines. In such situations, the reason for the repeat test should be included in the body of the report or in the patient's chart. Comparison with the previous test results should be documented.

Reimbursement

Medicare, workers' compensation carriers, and other payers reimburse medical providers for nerve conduction studies. Payment amounts and coverage policies for specific procedures vary by geographic location. To confirm reimbursement rates, consult with your local carrier or fiscal intermediary for specific procedure code reimbursement rates.

Location

Nerve conduction studies are reimbursed in hospital and office settings. The Medicare Diagnosis-Related Group (DRG) covers the TC of Medicare services for inpatients. When submitting bills to

Medicare, the clinician may submit and be reimbursed for only the professional component of these studies. Although the clinician cannot bill the carrier for the TC under the DRG system, he or she may either bill the institution or establish a separate contract to receive the appropriate reimbursement. This rule also applies to non-Medicare payers using DRG payment methods.

Technical Specifications

The NC-stat nerve conduction system meets or exceeds all the technical requirements for standard electrodiagnostic equipment. A detailed chart demonstrating each specification is available from NeuroMetrix on request.

Caveats

- When this technology was relatively new, a number of insurers considered this automated methodology experimental and did not pay for the procedures performed. New CPT codes that specifically reflected this procedure with commensurate charges were released in 2010.
- The biosensors are expensive, but their accuracy is impressive. Always make sure that lead placement is accurate and contact points are clean. If there seems to be a malfunctioning unit, always recheck electrical contact points to ensure power is adequate.
- In the unlikely event reports are not timely, one can usually contact NeuroMetrix for support.

- Do your due diligence to evaluate the payment policy in your practice arena. One size does not fit all. Take advantage of some of the patient handouts supplied by NeuroMetrix. These remind the patient this is not a needle procedure.

SUPPLIERS

(See contact information available at www.expertconsult.com.)

NeuroMetrix, Inc.

RECOMMENDED READING

Gozani SN, Fisher MA, Kong X, et al. Electrodiagnostic automation: principles and practice. *Phys Med Rehabil Clin North Am*. 2005;16:1015–1032.

Jabre JF, Salzsieder BT, Gnemi KE. Criterion validity of the NC-stat automated nerve conduction measurement instrument. *Physiol Meas*. 2007;28:95–104.

Kong X, Gozani SN, Hayes MT, Weinberg DH. NC-stat sensory nerve conduction studies in the median and ulnar nerves of symptomatic patients. *Clin Neurophysiol*. 2006;117:405–413.

Megerian JT, Kong X, Gozani SG. Utility of nerve conduction studies for carpal tunnel syndrome by family medicine, primary care, and internal medicine physicians. *J Am Board Fam Med*. 2007;20:60–64.

Morse J. *Technology assessment: NC-stat System, NeuroMetrix, Inc*. Office of the Medical Director, Washington State Department of Labor and Industries; 2006.

CHAPTER 188

MUSCLE BIOPSY

James R. Shepich

Many disorders of the motor unit can be identified by clinical presentation or electrodiagnostically, but occasionally a muscle biopsy is necessary for diagnosis. Muscle biopsy is a relatively straightforward procedure that may be performed under local anesthesia. However, many authorities contend that a better-quality specimen can be obtained under general anesthesia (e.g., propofol) because injudicious local infiltration can affect the histology. The site of biopsy and the type of biopsy (open vs. core needle) vary with the patient and disease.

The muscle of choice should show the effects of the disease process. For chronic disease, the most severely affected muscles should be avoided because the muscle mass may be replaced by scar tissue or fat, and an adequate pathologic diagnosis may not be possible. However, for acute disease, biopsies should be performed in those muscles with the most severe or at least moderate disease. Avoid muscles with recent trauma, including recent electromyography (EMG), injections, or infection (except when parasitic infection suspected). Muscle in areas of tendinous transition should not be sampled because the increased connective tissue may be mistaken for fibrosis during pathologic assessment. Some commonly biopsied muscles include the lateral aspect of quadriceps femoris, deltoid, biceps brachii, tibialis anterior, and gastrocnemius. In difficult cases, an MRI may help to locate the best pathologic muscle site to sample.

The biopsy method depends on clinical judgment. Core needle biopsy is less invasive and causes less pain and scarring than open biopsy. It is easier to perform, especially in children, and allows repeat biopsy of the same muscle if necessary. Open biopsy allows a larger specimen to be taken, which increases the chance of definitive diagnosis and allows multiple modalities of pathologic preparation of the specimen if needed, including electron microscopy. Open biopsy is also ideal if disease of the motor end plate is suspected. With either approach the muscle to be sampled should be placed in an extended, relaxed position.

INDICATIONS

A muscle biopsy is performed to identify syndromes of muscle weakness that do not present with classic findings. Several diseases, such as Duchenne muscular dystrophy, certain myotonias, Werdnig-Hoffmann disease, and myasthenia gravis, have classic presentations or electrodiagnostic findings, and therefore muscle biopsy is not necessary. Muscle biopsy can be used to distinguish between neurogenic and myopathic processes, identify congenital myopathies, and diagnose connective tissue disorders and muscle infections, such as trichinosis and toxoplasmosis. Muscle biopsy may help to diagnose certain conditions with silent manifestations in muscle such as amyloidosis, sarcoidosis, vasculitis, or microvasculopathies. Patients with abnormal lab tests (elevated creatine kinase) may benefit from muscle biopsy. Metabolic and symptomatic disorders of the muscle may also be diagnosed by biopsy. Biopsy may be useful for the identification and indexing of hereditary disorders.

CONTRAINDICATIONS

- Anticoagulation and bleeding disorders
- Recent trauma of the muscle, including EMG

- Clinical appearance of Duchenne muscular dystrophy (biopsy can cause scarring and contracture of muscle)
- Infection in region of proposed biopsy (unless suspected parasitic infection)
- Avoid biopsy for at least 1 month after an episode of rhabdomyolysis, if possible

EQUIPMENT

Open Biopsy

- Sterile drapes
- Povidone-iodine
- Local anesthesia (1% lidocaine without epinephrine)
- Scalpel with No. 11 or No. 15 blade
- Forceps, iris scissors, suture scissors
- 3-0 Vicryl or Monocryl sutures
- 4-0 Vicryl or Monocryl sutures
- Electrocautery or diathermy (not to be used until after biopsy sample is procured)
- 4 × 4 gauze sponges
- Tongue blade, cut into 6- to 7-cm lengths, with V-groove in ends, or 22-gauge needles to pin specimen
- 3-0 nylon suture
- Steri-Strips, Tegaderm, Op-Site, or dressing of choice

Core Needle Biopsy

- Sterile drape
- Povidone-iodine
- Local anesthesia
- Tru-Cut, Biopty, Conchotome, or equivalent needle
- Band-Aid

PREPROCEDURE PATIENT PREPARATION

The patient should be informed that the procedure is relatively painless but that the biopsy site may be sore for several days. Many patients experience a sensation of muscle bruising and occasionally a pulling sensation. Unless it is going to be performed under general anesthesia, the patient does not need to restrict food and fluids before the procedure. He or she should be instructed to wear loose-fitting clothes that readily allow access to the intended biopsy site. Little postprocedural disability or recovery time is expected, and the patient may return to usual activity immediately. Analgesic medication is rarely needed, and when it is necessary, it is usually only for 24 to 48 hours. Risks, benefits, and potential complications should be discussed with the patient before the procedure (see the sample patient education handout available at www.expertconsult.com).

TECHNIQUE

Open Biopsy

The patient should be prepared and draped, with the muscle in an extended, relaxed position. In the event of a vasovagal episode, the

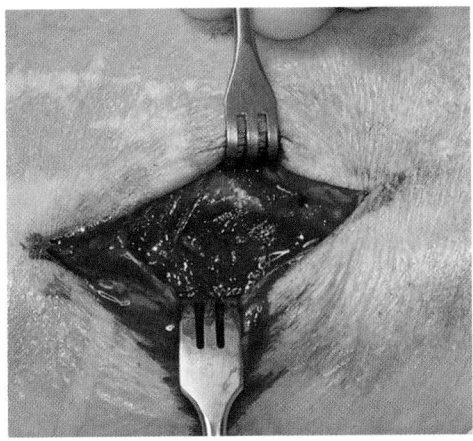

Fig. 188.1   Incision for biopsy of rectus femoris muscle.

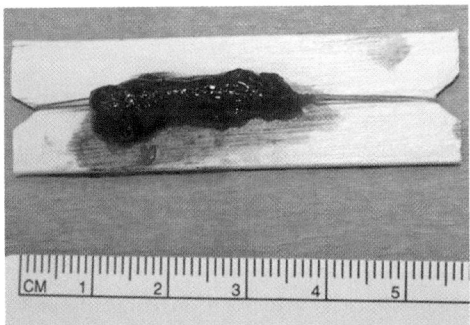

Fig. 188.2   Muscle portion approximately 1 × 1 × 2 cm stretched on a tongue blade.

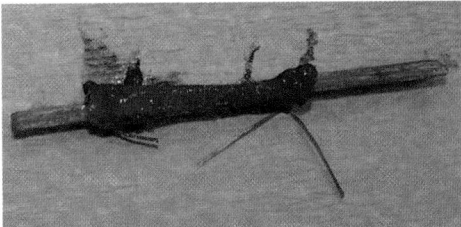

Fig. 188.3   Muscle fascicle tied in situ to splinter of tongue blade.

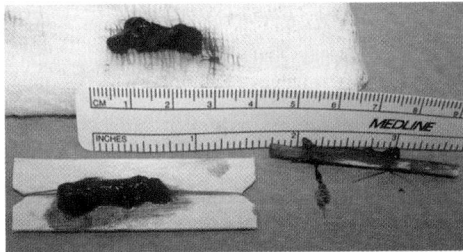

Fig. 188.4   Three specimens for histology, immunochemistry, and electron microscopy.

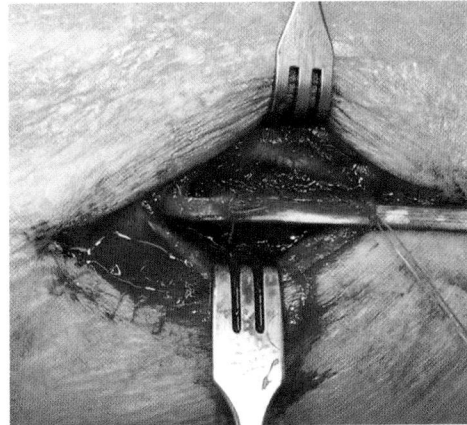

Fig. 188.5   Technique for in situ harvest of muscle fascicle.

patient should be lying down. The skin overlying the muscle to be sampled is infiltrated with local anesthesia. Care should be taken to avoid infiltration of the muscle itself. A 3- to 4-cm incision is made over the muscle belly, in an axial orientation to the muscle (Fig. 188.1). The skin and subcutaneous tissue are retracted and the fascia exposed. The fascia is opened sharply in a longitudinal fashion, and the muscle is exposed. Care should be taken to avoid injuring cutaneous nerve branches, which often lie on the fascia. A portion of muscle approximately 0.5 to 1 cm in diameter and 2 to 4 cm in length is excised after a nonabsorbable suture is placed at each end. The excisional sites are "outside" of the sutures. The specimen is maintained in an extended state and transferred to the tongue depressor, where the suture can be placed in a V-groove on either end or pinned to the surface with 22-gauge needles (Fig. 188.2). Hemostasis is achieved with diathermy or electrocautery.

Many pathologists require two specimens for a muscle biopsy. The first is a piece of muscle measuring 0.5 to 1 cm and 2 to 4 cm in length, and the second is an additional fascicle 2 to 3 cm in length and 5 mm in diameter that is tied to a splinter of tongue blade in situ, before it is excised (Figs. 188.3 to 188.5).

The fascia is then closed with 3-0 Vicryl sutures to prevent muscle herniation. The skin is closed with a running subcuticular stitch. Steri-Strips and a sterile dressing are applied. Dermabond or other skin adhesive may also be used.

Core Needle Biopsy

The patient is prepared, draped, and anesthetized as previously described for an open biopsy. A small nick is made in the skin with a No. 11 blade, and the bioptome is introduced. Care should be taken that the throw of the needle does not carry it into vital structures or bone. The bioptome is then activated. Multiple passes may be taken through the muscle in different areas, and usually three cores

of tissue are obtained. Pressure is held at the site for 2 to 3 minutes, and a Band-Aid is then applied.

COMPLICATIONS

Potential complications include bleeding, hematoma, or bruising at site of biopsy. The wound may become infected or be slow to heal, especially in patients with connective tissue disorders who have been on steroids. In some conditions, biopsy may lead to fibrosis and contracture of the muscle. Mild postprocedural discomfort is usual, and prolonged paresthesia can be experienced if a sensory nerve is injured. In addition, the biopsy may be nondiagnostic, requiring a repeat biopsy.

HANDLING OF TISSUE AND INTERPRETATION OF RESULTS

Note for the pathologist which muscle was sampled. (The deltoid muscle has an unusual connective tissue pattern that may be misinterpreted.) Other information supplied to the pathologist should include a clinical summary of symptoms and their distribution and duration. The results of EMG, nerve conduction velocity, and pertinent laboratory studies should also be included. Muscle biopsy should be performed in coordination with a pathologist because the specimen should never be placed in a fixative and should be processed within 30 minutes of its removal. (If this is not possible, discuss with the lab, a frozen specimen may be preferred.) A longer interval will cause specimen desiccation and architectural distortion. Wrap the specimen in gauze slightly moistened with normal saline. Do not immerse in saline, because that will also produce an artifact. Keep the specimen cool, but do not freeze unless the lab requests it prepared in that manner. Standard pathologic assessment includes sectioning after cryostat freezing of the specimen, electron microscopy, and immunohistochemical analysis. The pathologic diagnosis is based on the architecture of the muscle group, the characteristics of the individual fibers, and the presence of increased connective tissue or inflammatory cells. Electron microscopy will reveal abnormalities of the mitochondria and other cellular infrastructure. Special staining for oxidative, glycolytic, and hydrolytic enzymes will add information about enzyme deficiency, inflammation, and mitochondrial and lysosomal abnormalities. Stains with periodic acid–Schiff reagent and Oil Red O will help to diagnose glycogen and lipid storage disorders. Immunohistochemical assay will add information regarding dystrophin, major histocompatibility complex receptors, and autoimmune disorders.

POSTPROCEDURE PATIENT EDUCATION

The patient should be instructed to monitor the area of biopsy for signs or symptoms of infection, excessive bleeding, or hematoma formation. A small amount of serosanguineous fluid may accumulate beneath the dressing. The outer dressing should be maintained for at least 48 hours and then removed. The Steri-Strips may be removed between the fifth and seventh days after the biopsy (see the sample patient education handout available at www.expertconsult.com).

PATIENT EDUCATION GUIDES

See the sample patient education and consent forms available at www.expertconsult.com.

CPT/BILLING CODES

20200	Muscle biopsy, superficial
20205	Muscle biopsy, deep
20206	Muscle biopsy, percutaneous needle

ICD-10-CM DIAGNOSTIC CODES

G12.0	Werdnig-Hoffmann syndrome (muscular atrophy)
G72.89	Myopathy other specified
G71.8	Other primary disorders of muscles
M33.13	Dermatomyositis
M33.22	Polymyositis with myopathy
M62.50	Muscular atrophy not otherwise classified
M62.81	Muscle weakness (generalized)

In addition, see numerous specific conditions.

ONLINE RESOURCES

Neuromuscular: Muscle biopsy: http://neuromuscular.wustl.edu/lab/mbiopsy.htm

University of Iowa, Department of Pathology, Laboratory Services Handbook. Muscle biopsy: General instructions available at https://medicine.uiowa.edu/uidl/faculty-services/muscular-dystrophy-muscle-biopsy/muscle-biopsy-general-evaluation

RECOMMENDED READING

DuBowitz V, Sewry C, Oldfors A. *Muscle Biopsy: A Practical Approach.* 4th ed. Philadelphia: Elsevier; 2013.

Ekblom B. The muscle biopsy technique. Historical and methodological considerations. *Scand J Med Sci Sports.* 2016;26(12):1–4.

Keith J. Diagnostic skeletal muscle biopsy: quality assurance considerations for the anatomic pathology department. *Diagnostic Histopathology.* 2016;22(9):345–353.

SECTION 13

Urgent Care

Section Editor: THEODORE X. O'CONNELL

CHAPTER 189

Burn Treatment

Roberta E. Gebhard

Two million people sustain a burn-related injury every year in the United States; 450,000 receive medical evaluation and treatment, and 10% require hospitalization. Burn injuries can cause both severe psychological and physical disability. Patients sustaining burn injuries are predominantly male (70%), and nearly 80% are caused by flame, fire, or scalds. Early resuscitation and aggressive surgical intervention of burn injuries can reduce mortality and limit long-term morbidity.

BURN COMPLICATIONS REQUIRING RESUSCITATION

Inherent to burn injuries are a number of potential complications. Burn research has shown that the causes of early mortality are not the burns themselves but complications related to hypoxia, hypoventilation, and circulation disorders, including hypovolemia and hypothermia. Complications requiring early resuscitation are as follows:

- Airway injury (airway edema from thermal or chemical burns)
- Inhalation injury/hypoxia
  - Chemical fumes are the most common cause of pneumonitis/pulmonary edema.
  - Smoke or other particulate material causes pneumonitis.
  - Carbon monoxide (CO) poisoning is common with fires in enclosed spaces.
- Hypothermia from loss of skin integrity and evaporative losses
- Hypovolemia or shock resulting from intravascular-to-extravascular fluid shifts and pain vasoconstriction
- Cardiac asystole and arrhythmias (especially with high voltage burns)

RESUSCITATION FOR EARLY BURN COMPLICATIONS

Advanced burn life support (ABLS) courses are available both in traditional and online formats that help to focus resuscitation efforts to the most critical patient needs by using a simple-to-remember alphabetic mnemonic: A = airway, B = breathing, C = circulation, D = disability, E = exposure, F = fluids (see the "Online Resources" section at the end of the chapter).

A = Airway

Airway management is the crucial first step in resuscitating a severe burn victim. Early endotracheal intubation is recommended when an injured airway is first diagnosed. Although airway edema normally stays above the vocal cords, delayed intubation can be much more difficult or traumatic. The manifestations of airway injury are often subtle and may not appear for 24 hours. A history of the victim being confined in a burning building (or closed space) or of having impaired mentation is suggestive of acute inhalational injury. With this history, a search for clinical evidence of inhalation injury should be undertaken carefully. Clinical clues to acute inhalation injury include facial burns, singed eyebrow or nasal hairs, oropharyngeal carbon deposits, acute inflammation, and carbonaceous sputum. If hoarseness, a brassy

cough, or stridor develops, immediately intubate the patient. Intubation is also required before transport if transportation time will be prolonged. Airway injuries indicate major burn severity.

B = Breathing

Evaluate the patient for spontaneous respirations. Check for stridor, wheezing, or rales, and administer 100% O_2 as soon as it is available. Maintain oxygen saturation greater than 92%. CO poisoning should be assumed if the burn victim was trapped in an enclosed space.

C = Circulation

Rapid shifts in intravascular fluid occur in burns of greater than 20% to 25% total body surface area (TBSA). Hypovolemia resulting from capillary leak and evaporative losses should be anticipated and corrected (see "F = Fluids" section). High-voltage burns can cause cardiac arrest. Lower-voltage injuries may cause delayed arrhythmias. After removing the electrical source with a nonconducting piece of equipment or turning off the power source, begin basic life support in the pulseless victim. Advanced cardiac life support measures should be initiated as soon as appropriate equipment is available.

D = Disability

Remember to stabilize the cervical spine to prevent further disability. High-voltage injuries can cause tetanic muscle contractions severe enough to fracture the cervical spine, lumbar spine, or limbs. Jumps from burning buildings can also cause fractures.

E = Exposure

- Expose the patient by removing any nonadherent clothing, especially chemically contaminated or smoldering clothing, constricting clothing, and jewelry.
- Examine for associated injuries. Document these injuries and address them after the patient is stabilized.
- Brush away residual dry chemicals. Irrigate liquid residual chemicals copiously with water. Alkalis may require forceful irrigation (such as a shower) for up to an hour.
- Cover the patient with a clean, dry blanket to prevent hypothermia.

F = Fluids

Aggressive fluid resuscitation is required in patients with burns covering more than 20% TBSA in adults and 10% TBSA in children to prevent hypovolemia and shock resulting from capillary leak and evaporative losses.

Intravenous Access

Insert two large-bore intravenous (IV) lines, avoiding burned skin if possible. Central venous access may be needed.

Partial thickness (superficial)   Partial thickness (deep)   Full thickness

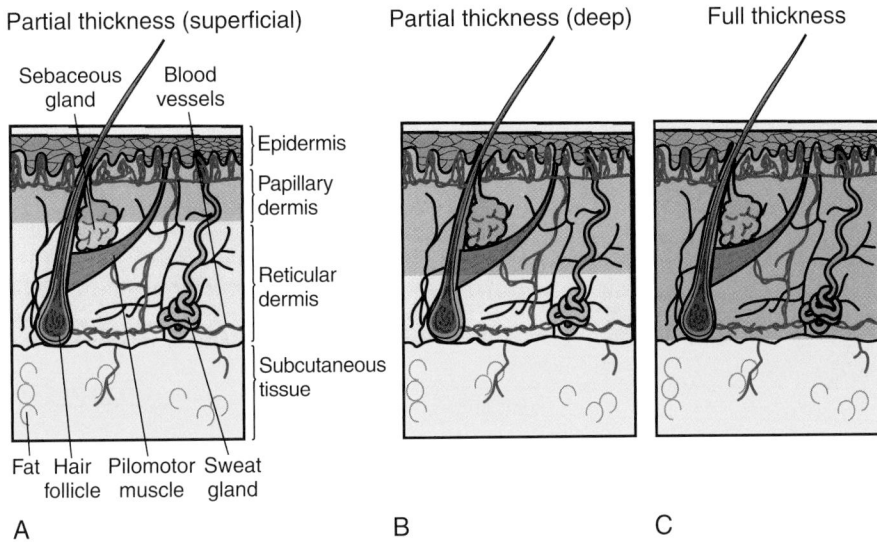

Sebaceous gland / Blood vessels

Epidermis
Papillary dermis
Reticular dermis
Subcutaneous tissue

Fat   Hair follicle   Pilomotor muscle   Sweat gland

A   B   C

Fig. 189.1 (A) Superficial partial-thickness burn. (B) Deep partial-thickness burn. (C) Full-thickness burn. *Coral background area* denotes depth of burn injuries. (From Edlich RF, Bailey TL, Bill TJ. Thermal burns. In: Marx JA, Walls R, Hockberger R, eds. *Rosen's Emergency Medicine: Concepts and Clinical Practice*, 5th ed. Philadelphia: Mosby; 2002:802–813.)

Parkland Formula

The most widely used formula for fluid resuscitation is the Parkland Formula, although there is some controversy that it may underestimate the initial need for fluid (see Holm and colleagues, 2004). The greatest intravascular-to-extravascular fluid shifts occur in the first 8 hours. Significant but slower fluid shifts continue for the next 16 hours. All fluid resuscitation formulas are designed to replace the intravascular volume as it is lost, most rapidly in the first 8 hours, then the next 16 hours.

- *First 24 hours:* lactated Ringer 4 mL/kg per percentage burn (first half given in first 8 hours, second half given in next 16 hours). Time is measured from the onset time of burn.
- *Second 24 hours:* colloid (5% albumin) 20% to 60% of plasma volume (approx. 40 mL/kg) + 2000 mL of 5% dextrose in water (given over second 24 hours). Increase dextrose volume to maintain urine output 0.5 to 1.0 mL/kg per hour in adults and 1.0 mL/kg per hour in children.
- *Example:* 70-kg adult with 50% TBSA partial- and full-thickness burns requires 14 L of lactated Ringer over the first 24 hours (4 mL × 70 kg × 50% burn = 14,000 mL/24 hr). Seven liters is given in the first 8 hours (875 mL/hr) and 7 L given in the next 16 hours (437.5 mL/hr). This is followed by 3000 mL albumin and 2000 mL D5W given over next 24 hours with D5W titrated to maintain adequate urine output.
- Evaluation of fluid resuscitation efforts is best gauged by urine output (see "Inpatient Management for the Primary Provider" section).

ESTIMATING BURN SEVERITY

Burn depth, size, and locations on the body must be assessed to determine the burn severity.

Burn Depth

Fig. 189.1 shows the skin in cross section with the layers involved with superficial partial-thickness, deep partial-thickness, and full-thickness burns.

Superficial burns are erythematous without blister formation and involve only the epidermis; pain is localized (Fig. 189.2). Superficial partial-thickness burns are painful, warm, and moist with blister formation; they involve the epidermis and superficial

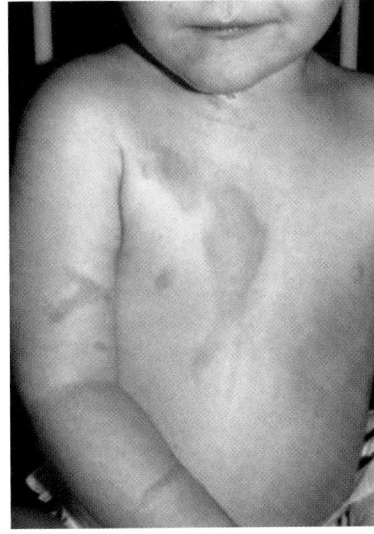

Fig. 189.2 Superficial burns are erythematous without blister formation, involve only the epidermis, and are characterized by localized pain.

papillary dermis (Fig. 189.3). With deep partial-thickness burns the skin is mottled, waxy, and white in appearance, with ruptured blisters. Pain sensation is absent, but pressure sensation is intact (Fig. 189.4). Full-thickness burns involve both the epidermis and dermis, have a white to gray, leathery appearance, and do not blanch with pressure. There is only sensation to deep pressure; there is no pain because pain receptors in the dermis are destroyed (Fig. 189.5).

Burn depth terminology no longer includes the use of "first-, second-, and third-degree burns." Note that superficial and superficial partial-thickness burns have minimal to no risk of scarring, are painful, and heal spontaneously by 3 weeks. Deep partial-thickness and full-thickness burns have a higher risk of scarring, decreased sensation, and delayed healing of greater than 3 weeks. Fourth-degree burn is the term still used to depict the most severe burns, extending through both the epidermis and the dermis and into the fascia and muscle. Fourth-degree burns are life-threatening and may never heal if they are present over more than 2% of TBSA (see later).

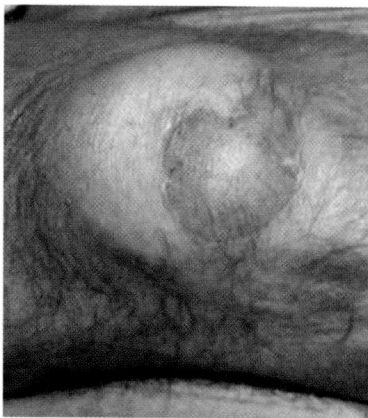

Fig. 189.3 Superficial partial-thickness burns are painful, warm, and moist with blister formation and involve the epidermis and superficial papillary dermis.

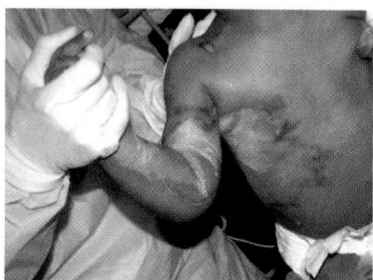

Fig. 189.4 With deep partial-thickness burns the skin is mottled, waxy, and white in appearance, with ruptured blisters.

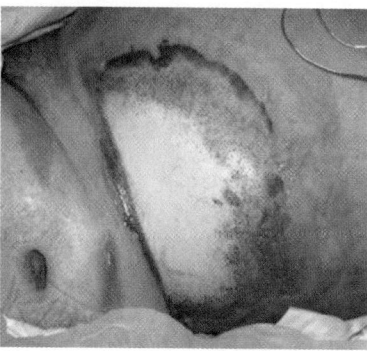

Fig. 189.5 Full-thickness burns involve both the epidermis and dermis, have a white to gray, leathery appearance, and do not blanch with pressure.

Initial estimates of the depth of the burn are crucial to timely triage. The final depth of injury cannot always be predicted at the initial evaluation; therefore sequential evaluations may be needed to revise the depth of the burn over the days and weeks after the injury. See Fig. 189.6 for treatment recommendations based on wound depth assessment.

Burn Size: Percentage of Total Body Surface Area

Burn size is an important determinant of burn healing. Healing occurs from fibroblasts migrating in from the burn margins and the oil glands and hair follicles (skin appendages). The skin appendages penetrate deep into the dermis and, except for full-thickness burns, are spared from destruction.

The adult body surface area can be divided into percentages of nine and multiples or fractions of nine: the "Rule of Nines" (Fig. 189.7). Infants have a greater proportion of TBSA on the head and

neck and less on the legs. The posterior torso, including buttocks, still equals 18%, with each buttock equaling 2.5%. Palms are 1.25%.

Burn Locations

The determination of whether a particular burn injury should be treated as an ambulatory case, a local hospital admission, or a direct admission to a regional burn center depends on burn involvement in some highly critical areas.

The American Burn Association (ABA) has set up criteria for referral to a burn center for treatment (Box 189.1). The ABA's grading system recommends disposition to a burn center for these critical conditions because of the significantly increased risk of morbidity.

Certain burn locations or other potential injuries lead to automatic classification as *moderate burn severity*. Fractures in association with burns increase the severity index.

Disposition of Patient Based on Burn Severity: American Burn Association Guidelines

The ABA guidelines for disposition of burn patients are based on burn severity, which is based on depth, size, and location of the burn (see Box 189.1).

- Minor burns: outpatient management
  - Involve less than 10% TBSA in adults, less than 5% TBSA in children and elderly
  - Less than 2% TBSA full-thickness burns
  - Do not involve face, hands, feet, genitalia, or respiratory tract
  - Are not circumferential
  - No associated injuries or comorbidities
- Moderate burns: hospitalization
- Major burns: burn center

COMPLICATIONS ENCOUNTERED DURING BURN MANAGEMENT

Additional complications are encountered during the treatment of burns, whether in the hospital or as an outpatient. Any life-threatening complications encountered during the resuscitation phase of burn care require continued attention after the patient is stabilized and disposition has been determined. Burn centers offer expertise in wound management and vigilance in late complications. Other complications that must be prevented if possible and addressed if they occur despite all preventive efforts include the following:

- Airway injury
  - Hypoxia
  - Airway edema
  - CO poisoning: PO_2 levels on blood gases may be normal even in the presence of CO poisoning. Carboxyhemoglobin (CO-Hgb) levels should be measured. The administration of 100% O_2 provides appropriate supplementation and reduces CO levels. (The half-time of CO-Hgb converting back to hemoglobin is reduced from 250 minutes on room air to 40 minutes on 100% O_2.) Severe cases of CO poisoning should receive hyperbaric oxygen therapy, which can be life-saving. See Fig. 189.8 for an algorithm on using the hyperbaric chamber for CO poisoning.
  - CO poisoning symptoms are related to the percentage of CO-Hgb; CO-Hgb levels less than 20% are usually asymptomatic. At CO-Hgb levels of 20% to 30%, headache and nausea occur. At CO-Hgb levels of 30% to 40%, confusion occurs, and coma ensues when CO-Hgb levels reach between 40% and 60%. Levels over 60% cause death.
- Cardiac arrhythmias: Can occur for up to 3 days after high-voltage injury
- Pain

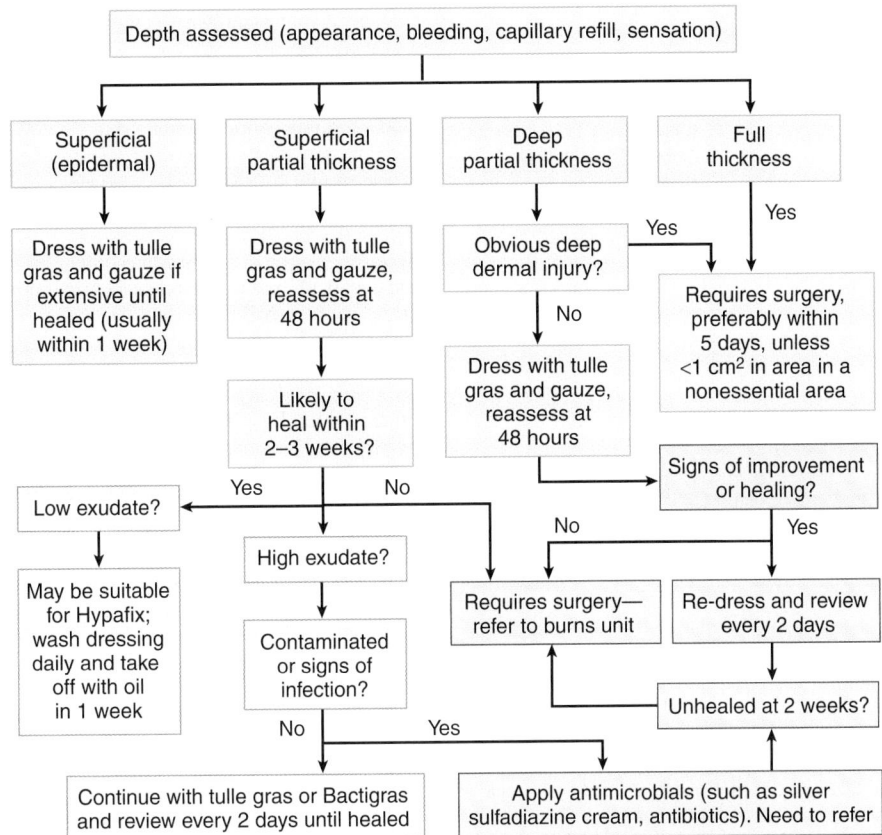

Fig. 189.6   Algorithm for assessing depth of burn wounds and suggested treatment.

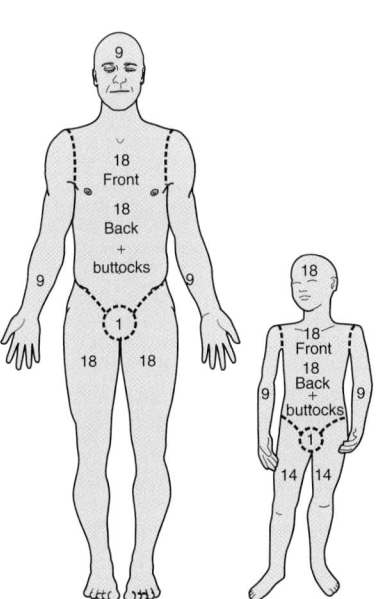

Fig. 189.7   Rule of nines. (Modified from Mazzeo AS, Price LA, Gerold KB. Burn care procedures. In: Roberts JR, Custalow CB, Thomsen TW, eds. *Roberts and Hedges Clinical Procedures in Emergency Medicine*, 6th ed. Philadelphia: Elsevier, 2014.)

BOX 189.1   Burn Center Referral Criteria

A Burn Center May Treat Adults, Children, or Both
Burn injuries that should be referred to a burn center include the following:

- Partial-thickness burns of greater than 10% of the TBSA.
- Burns that involve the face, hands, feet, genitalia, perineum, or major joints.
- Third-degree burns in any age group.
- Electrical burns, including lightning injury.
- Chemical burns.
- Inhalation injury.
- Burn injury in patients with preexisting medical disorders that could complicate management, prolong recovery, or affect mortality.
- Any patient with burns and concomitant trauma (such as fractures) in which the burn injury poses the greatest risk of morbidity or mortality. In such cases, if the trauma poses the greater immediate risk, the patient's condition may be stabilized initially in a trauma center before transfer to a burn center. Physician judgment will be necessary in such situations and should be in concert with the regional medical control plan and triage protocols.
- Burned children in hospitals without qualified personnel or equipment for the care of children.
- Burn injury in patients who will require special social, emotional, or rehabilitative intervention.

Modified from Committee on Trauma, American College of Surgeons. Guidelines for the operation of burn centers. In: *Resources for Optimal Care of the Injured Patient 2006*. Rockford, IL: American College of Surgeons, 2006:79–86.

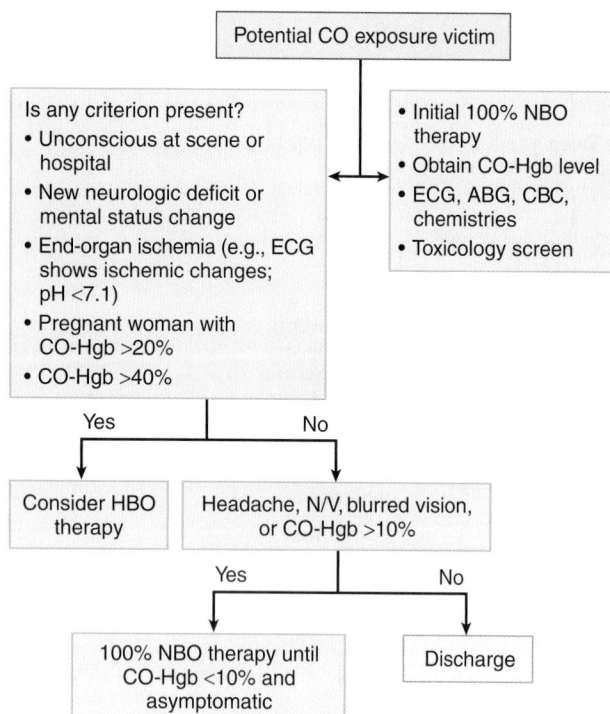

Fig. 189.8 Algorithm for using normobaric oxygen *(NBO)* and hyperbaric oxygen *(HBO)* after carbon monoxide exposure. *ABG,* Arterial blood gas; *CBC,* complete blood count; *CO-Hgb,* carboxyhemoglobin; *ECG,* electrocardiogram; *N/V,* nausea/vomiting. (Modified from O'Brien C, Manaker S. Carbon monoxide and smoke inhalation. In: Lanken PN, Hanson CW III, Manaker S, eds. *The Intensive Care Unit Manual.* Philadelphia: WB Saunders, 2001.)

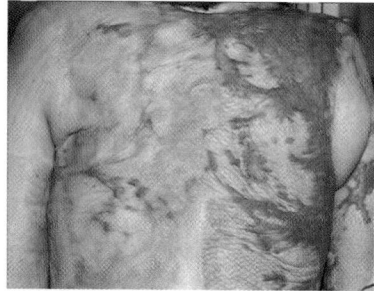

Fig. 189.9 Permanent disfigurement.

- Infection
  - Bacterial
  - Tetanus
  - Smoke inhalation/pneumonitis
  - Pneumonia
- Hypothermia
- Intravascular-to-extravascular fluid shifts
  - Hypovolemia/shock
  - Edema
  - Compartment syndrome
- Hypertrophic scars/contractures
  - Loss of function of hands, feet, eyes, joints, genitalia
  - Permanent disfigurement (Fig. 189.9)
- Pigmentary changes
  - Hypopigmentation for 6 to 24 months
  - Hyperpigmentation if not protected from ultraviolet damage
- Sensory dysfunction (sensory nerve damage)
  - Hyperesthesias
  - Pruritus

- Xerosis (damaged sweat glands)
- Psychological
  - Depression
  - Anxiety disorders
- Carcinoma (nonmelanoma skin cancers) in burn scars

INPATIENT MANAGEMENT FOR THE PRIMARY PROVIDER

According to the ABA's grading system for burn severity and disposition of patients, moderate and major burn injuries require hospitalization either locally or in a burn center. The primary provider may be the admitting provider for moderate and even severe burns if stabilization is needed before transfer to a burn center. The ABA's website (www.ameriburn.org) has search capability to assist in locating burn centers throughout the United States. Inpatient management of patients with moderate burn severity should include consideration of the following:

- History of burn injury
  - When? Initial time of burn important for fluid resuscitation.
  - How? Fire, steam, chemical, electrical, hot material?
  - Where? Enclosed space (inhalation injury)?
- Medical history
  - Medical problems: diabetes and chronic steroid use increase the risk of infection. Cardiopulmonary disease decreases physical reserves. Other medical problems will need to be addressed.
  - Medications: steroid use, blood thinners, diabetic medications, and so forth.
  - Allergies: sulfa allergy (use bacitracin ointment).
  - Last tetanus: boost if not received in last 12 months.
- Airway: suspected airway injury may need intubation if oropharyngeal edema develops during the 12 to 24 hours after injury. Observe for hoarseness, raspy cough, or stridor.
- Breathing: monitor for hypoxia.
  - CO poisoning: 100% O_2 or hyperbaric oxygen therapy (see Fig. 189.8).
  - Pneumonitis or pulmonary edema: ventilation with high O_2 and positive end-expiratory pressure may be needed.
  - Pneumonia: treat with appropriate systemic antibiotics.
- Circulation
  - Monitor urine output for adequate rehydration.
  - Monitor for cardiac arrhythmias with telemetry. Patients with high-voltage (>440 V) injuries can develop ventricular arrhythmias up to 3 days after the injury. The most common electrocardiographic (ECG) finding of cardiac injury after electrical burn is nonspecific ST segment–T-wave abnormalities. These patients should be admitted to the telemetry unit for cardiac monitoring until the ECG normalizes. Treat with appropriate antiarrhythmics.
  - Monitor for compartment syndrome for circumferential wounds or when significant rehydration is administered.
    - Clinical diagnostic signs: delayed capillary refill, distal anesthesia, increasing limb pain, and decreased or absent distal pulses. Clinical signs are only 60% sensitive (they miss 40% of true compartment syndromes).
    - Measure direct compartment pressures (see Chapter 179, Compartment Syndrome Evaluation).
    - Obtain surgical consultation for escharotomy of affected limb, including across joints. Rarely needed for circumferential burns of trunk.
    - Fasciotomy will be necessary if escharotomy is not effective.
- Disability: obtain an x-ray skeletal survey for high-voltage burn or other suspected bone injury. Tetanic convulsion can cause fracture of cervical spine, lumbar spine, or limbs. A cross-table lateral view of the cervical spine should be obtained before removal of full cervical spine precautions. Monitor the level of consciousness; mental alertness confirms adequate circulation.

- Exposure: Avoid hypothermia, which can increase peripheral vasoconstriction. Evaporative fluid loss and loss of barrier to infection result from partial- and full-thickness burns. Consider early excision of eschar and skin grafting or artificial covering.
- Fluids: Continue rehydration per urine output. For adults, adequate urine output is 0.5 mL/kg per hour; for children, 1.0 mL/kg per hour is needed. A Foley catheter is required. Excessive fluid administration can lead to increased edema, increased rate of compartment syndrome, and unnecessary fasciotomies. Higher urine output and osmotic diuretics are normally required for high-voltage burns to prevent acute renal failure from rhabdomyolysis.
- Requirements decrease as the capillary leakage decreases over 2 to 7 days.
  - Admission weight and daily patient weights are required. Increased insensible losses through open wounds make patient weight invaluable.
  - Inputs and outputs: hourly fluid input and output are required to monitor the massive amounts of fluid used for resuscitation.
- Give tetanus prophylaxis for burns deeper than superficial partial thickness (if time since last tetanus booster is >12 months).
- Early nutrition first 12 to 24 hours, enteral if possible. Burn injuries are associated with an increased metabolism of 1.3 to 2 times baseline. Enteral feedings decrease the risk of gastrointestinal ulceration. Parenteral feedings may be required but significantly increase the risk of sepsis at IV sites. Catheters should be replaced every 48 to 72 hours.
- Infection: Common sources of infection in burn patients include the burn wounds, pneumonia, IV line sepsis, and urinary tract sepsis from indwelling catheters. Burn wound infections usually require full-thickness biopsy and tissue culture to differentiate bacterial colonization from bacterial tissue invasion. Systemic antibiotics are required. Excision of infected burn tissue and grafting are often required. Culturing of central line catheter tips during replacement is recommended. Worsening pulmonary status should prompt a chest radiographic examination.
- Pain: Baseline pain medication with augmentation of pain relief by rescue medications is recommended. Some authorities recommend treatment of baseline pain with methadone and augmentation with morphine before dressing changes or activities such as physical therapy.

WOUND CARE

Burn Debridement

- Devitalized tissue removal is important to prevent bacterial colonization. Mild soaps such as chlorhexidine are recommended. Avoid povidone-iodine (Betadine), alcohol, and hydrogen peroxide and neomycin, which inhibit fibroblasts as well as bacteria, delaying the healing process.
- Remove ruptured blisters, blisters prone to rupture (e.g., over joints), and those with cloudy fluid that could be infected.
- Removal of small intact blisters is controversial. Some authorities recommend debridement of all blisters, whereas others recommend leaving them undisturbed as a natural sterile barrier to infection.
  NOTE: Delayed blister resolution longer than 2 weeks may indicate deep partial-thickness burn. Consider consultation for excision and skin grafting.
- Removal of adherent tar or clothing can be facilitated by application of petroleum jelly or bacitracin ointment for softening and removal during washing at dressing changes. Whirlpool baths are well tolerated for wound debridement.

Dressings

- Standard dressings are changed twice a day. After dressing removal, the wounds are washed, inspected for healing or onset of infection, patted dry, treated with topical antibiotics, and covered with Telfa (Smith & Nephew), a nonadherent dressing, and gauze or stockinet. Tulle gras dressings are gauze impregnated with paraffin, and Bactigras (Smith & Nephew) is a tulle gras with 0.5% chlorhexidine acetate. These, as well as Adaptic and Xeroform, are alternatives to Telfa. Hypafix (Smith & Nephew) is an adhesive retention tape that is air and moisture permeable and completely covers the entire dressing to reduce contamination. Next, cover and pad the wound with loose gauze fluffs. The entire dressing is then wrapped with an absorbent, slightly elastic material such as Kerlix.
- Consider Unna paste dressings. Advocates cite benefits such as decreased scarring, discomfort, and cost without increased infection rate. Dressings are changed every 3 to 7 days. Concerns include delayed detection of infection and overlooking early scarring or other complications because of infrequent wound observation.

Topical Antibiotics

Topical antibiotics are used to decrease bacterial colonization of open blisters and deep burns. Their use significantly decreases wound infections. No single agents can be used in all cases. Several choices include the following:

- *Silver sulfadiazine (Silvadene 1% cream).* Silver sulfadiazine is synthesized by combining silver nitrate with sodium sulfadiazine and has intermediate eschar penetration and a broad spectrum of antibacterial and anticandidal activity. It is clearly indicated for infected or heavily contaminated burns. It is easy to apply but should not be used on the face because of staining or in patients with sulfa allergy or glucose-6-phosphate dehydrogenase (G6PD) deficiency. Silver sulfadiazine should not be used in pregnant women, newborns, and breast-feeding women of children 2 months of age or younger owing to risk of sulfonamide kernicterus if it is absorbed through the skin. Silver sulfadiazine impedes reepithelialization and should be stopped when there is evidence of reepithelialization. A recent randomized trial (Genuino, 2014) found petrolatum gel alone to be slightly superior to silver sulfadiazine measured in time to healing for superficial partial thickness burns in adults. Results of a recent systematic review of 30 randomized trials (Wasiak, 2013) also have some experts questioning the value of silver sulfadiazine. Compared with biosynthetic dressings (skin substitute), silver-containing dressings, and silicon-coated dressings, silver sulfadiazine was associated with poorer outcomes. Therefore some experts no longer recommend silver sulfadiazine for most burns (other than infected or heavily contaminated burns).
- *Mafenide acetate (Sulfamylon 8.5% cream).* Mafenide acetate has excellent eschar penetration and has the best antibacterial spectrum. It can be used on ears for prevention of chondritis. Mafenide is painful after it is applied and is expensive. Sleep disturbance is fairly common after evening application. It is a carbonic anhydrase inhibitor; metabolic alkalosis may occur. With newer preparations available, mafenide is rarely used any more.
- *Bacitracin zinc ointment 1%.* Bacitracin is best used for facial burns, around mucous membranes, in patients with sulfa allergy, and for loosening adherent tar or clothing before removal. Advocates note that it is inexpensive, readily available without prescription, and often effective. Bacitracin does not have good eschar penetration, has a narrower spectrum of antibacterial action, and can cause topical sensitization. It has no activity against *Candida albicans*. Controlled trials are needed comparing bacitracin with silver sulfadiazine.
- *Aloe vera cream.* Commercially available in 50% or higher concentration with preservatives, it has been found to have antibacterial activity against at least four common burn wound pathogens. One study of 18 patients compared it with silver sulfadiazine and found it to have similar healing times in minor burns.

- *Honey.* Long advocated as inexpensive and effective, it may be superior to silver sulfadiazine for minor burn wound healing.
- *Alternatives to topical antibiotics.* Biologic dressings such as pigskin or allografts; biosynthetic dressings such as Integra (Integra Lifesciences), Alloderm (Allergan, Parsippany-Troy Hills), Epicel (Vericel), TransCyte and Biobrane (Smith & Nephew); and Xeroform (Smith & Nephew), a bismuth-impregnated petroleum gauze, produce faster healing and lower infection rates but need to be placed within 6 hours of injury. Their use is limited by lack of availability at the point of entry to the health care system, high cost, and difficulty of use.

Excision and Skin Grafting

- Benefits of excision of the eschar and skin grafting include prevention of hypertrophic scarring and contractures, as well as protection of deep tissues such as muscles and tendons (see Chapter 27, Skin Grafting). Decreases in evaporative fluid loss, pain, and susceptibility to infection are noted. Reduced time for rehabilitation and reduced time in the hospital are also significant.
- A negative aspect of early excision and grafting is significant blood loss in a critically ill patient. Decreased blood loss occurs if excision is performed one day and grafting the following day.
- Options for skin grafting with the patient's own skin (autograft) include full-thickness versus split-thickness grafts, as well as sheet grafts versus mesh grafts.
- Other grafting materials include allografts (cadaver), xenografts (usually porcine), cultured skin cells, and dermal substitutes such as collagen and bilayer substitutes (both dermal and epidermal components). See also the previous discussion of alternatives to topical antibiotics.

Prevention of Contractures and Hypertrophic Scarring

- Early consultation with a burn specialist or surgeon with burn experience is recommended. Hypertrophic scarring and contractures are best prevented and, once started, are more difficult to treat.
- Hypertrophic scarring can occur up to 2 years after the burn injury.
- There is an increased risk of contracture in deep partial-thickness burns and full-thickness burns, black patients, and at extremes of age range, both young and old.
- Late excision (after 2 weeks) of eschar and skin grafting for deep partial-thickness or full-thickness burns masked by blisters should be done. Nonresorption of blister by 2 weeks is a diagnostic clue.
- Early involvement with physical therapy and occupational therapy decreases contractures. Active range of motion (ROM) and stretching are superior to passive ROM in decreasing the risk of contracture. Avoid splinting of extremity burns if at all possible.
- Pressure dressings decrease hypertrophic scarring, even if initiated as late as 12 months after the burn injury, but early pressure dressing use is superior.
- Silicone sheeting such as ReJuveness or Scar Fx can reduce hypertrophic scarring if used up to 12 years after the injury.

AMBULATORY MANAGEMENT FOR THE PRIMARY PROVIDER

Management of the majority of the 450,000 burn patients per year in the United States occurs in an ambulatory setting. The primary provider is well equipped to manage the initial and follow-up burn care for minor burns. Minor burns involve less than 10% TBSA of adults, less than 5% TBSA of young and old patients, and less than 2% TBSA full-thickness burn; they do not involve the face, hands, feet, genitalia, or respiratory tract and are not circumferential. These patients do not have significant associated injuries or comorbidities that predispose to infection.

INITIAL AMBULATORY VISIT

- Evaluation of burn severity and inclusion of only minor burns.
- Tetanus prophylaxis, if indicated.
- Burn debridement. (Give field block or regional anesthesia for discomfort; remove devitalized tissue, ruptured blisters, and blisters likely to rupture.*)
- Wound washed with mild soap and warm water. (This is a clean but not sterile procedure.*) Skin disinfectants are no longer recommended because they are thought to delay wound healing.
- Wound dressing changes twice a day.* Teach the patient to keep extremities with burns elevated.
- Early referral for excision of eschar and skin grafting as outpatient, if indicated.†
- Pain control: nonsteroidal antiinflammatory drugs or acetaminophen recommended for baseline pain. (Prescribe oral narcotic pain relievers for before dressing changes, for breakthrough pain, and at bedtime for pain during sleep.)
- Avoidance of splinting and encouragement of active ROM and stretching.
- Full-thickness burns less than 3 cm in diameter in a nonfunctional, noncosmetic area with normal-thickness skin may be allowed to heal by contracture.
- Patient teaching guide (see the patient education form available at www.expertconsult.com).
- Follow-up appointment scheduled for the day after the burn injury.

Second Ambulatory Visit

- During the dressing change, reevaluation of burn severity (location, size, and depth), evaluation of pain control, and possible further wound debridement.
- Teaching wound care and dressing changes at this visit. Remind the patient to keep extremities with burns elevated.
- Teaching patient to observe for infection, scarring, or other complication.
- Patient referral to physical or occupational therapy for burns involving the hands, feet, or joints.

Subsequent Visits

- Follow-up weekly until the wound is epithelialized. Continue daily follow up if compliance of patient or communication with provider is not optimal.
- Epithelialized wounds no longer need antibiotic ointments or dressings, but they do need daily sunblock (SPF 15 or higher) for 6 to 24 months to prevent hyperpigmentation. Once repigmentation is complete and the wound no longer blanches from red-pink to white with pressure, additional sunblock is not needed.
- Subsequent follow-up for at least 6 months and reevaluation every 4 to 6 weeks to check for hypertrophic scarring, which can occur up to 2 years after the burn.
- Hypoallergenic, unscented moisturizing creams (cocoa butter, mineral oil, or Vaseline Intensive Care lotion) for pruritus and xerosis. Antihistamines such as diphenhydramine or hydroxyzine pamoate.
- Patient education handout for home care. (See the patient education form available at www.expertconsult.com.)

Considerations for Referral to Burn Specialist or Surgeon

- African-Americans, who have increased risk of hypertrophic scars (if not healed at 10 days)

---

*The "Inpatient Management for Primary Provider" section of this chapter includes more extensive discussion of this topic.
†See the "Considerations for Referral to Burn Specialist or Surgeon" section.

- Children and elderly (if not healed at 2 weeks)
- Adults (if not healed at 3 weeks)
- Wound infection
- Early hypertrophic scarring

PREVENTION

- Encourage installation of smoke detectors on each floor of domestic dwellings, particularly at prenatal visits or well-child visits.
- Encourage parents to teach their children about the proper fire safety precautions, fire escapes, and the hazards of matches and fireworks.
- Encourage families to know and practice fire escape routes. Purchase rope escape ladders for bedrooms on the second floor.
- Advise smokers to quit smoking and not to smoke in bed.

PATIENT EDUCATION GUIDES

See the patient education form available at www.expertconsult.com.

CPT/BILLING CODES

16000	Burns, initial, superficial, when no more than local treatment required
16020	Burns, dressings and/or debridement of partial thickness, initial or subsequent, small (<5% TBSA)
16025	Burns, dressings and/or debridement, medium (e.g., whole face, whole extremity, 5%–10% TBSA)
16030	Burns, dressings and/or debridement, large (e.g., more than one extremity, >10% TBSA)
16035	Burns, escharotomy, initial incision
16036	Burns, escharotomy, each additional incision

See Chapter 27, Skin Grafting, for procedural coding for skin grafts or skin substitutes.

ICD-10-CM DIAGNOSTIC CODES

T20.00X–T25.79X	Burns and corrosions external body surface specified by site

NOTE: Use additional code category T31 or T32 to identify extent of body surface involved.

Includes: first, second, and third degree.

The appropriate seventh character should be added: A = initial, D = subsequent, S = sequela.

T30.0–T31.99	Burns and corrosions of multiple and unspecified body regions

NOTE: T31.0 is primary if body site is unspecified.

SUPPLIERS

(See contact information available at www.expertconsult.com.)

Integra LifeSciences Corp.
Allergan Corporation
ReJuveness, LLC
ScarHeal Rejuvaskin, Inc.
Smith & Nephew, Inc.
Vericel, Inc.

Acknowledgment

The editors recognize the contributions of J. Fintan Copper, MD, and Timothy J. Downs, MD, FAAFP, to this chapter in a previous edition of this book.

ONLINE RESOURCES

Advanced Burn Life Support course online. www.aba.sitelms.org.
American Burn Association (listing regional burn centers by state). www.ameriburn.org.

RECOMMENDED READING

Cameron JL, Cameron AM, eds. *Current Surgical Therapy*. 12th ed. Philadelphia: Elsevier; 2016.
Genuino GA, Baluyut-Angeles KV, Espiritu AP, et al. Topical petrolatum gel alone versus topical silver sulfadiazine with standard gauze dressings for the treatment of superficial partial thickness burns in adults: a randomized controlled trial. *Burns*. 2014;40:1267–1273.
Holm C, Mayr M, Tegeler J, et al. A clinical randomized study on the effects of invasive monitoring on burn shock resuscitation. *Burns*. 2004;30:798–807.
Lloyd EO, Rodgers BC, Michener M, Williams MS. Outpatient burns: prevention and care. *Am Fam Physician*. 2012;85(1):25–32.
Mazzeo AS, Price LA, Gerold KB. Burn care procedures. In: Roberts JR, Custalow CB, Thomsen TW, eds. *Roberts and Hedges clinical procedures in emergency medicine*. 6th ed. Philadelphia: Elsevier; 2014:759–787.
Monafo WW. Initial management of burns. *N Engl J Med*. 1996;335:1581–1586.
Papini R. ABC of burns: management of burn injuries of various depths. *BMJ*. 2004;329:158–160.
Singer AJ, Lee CC. Thermal burns. In: walls RM, Hockberger RS, Gausche-Hill M, eds. *Rosen's Emergency Medicine*. 9th ed. Philadelphia: Elsevier; 2018:715–723.
Wasiak J, Cleland H, Campbell F. Dressings for superficial and partial thickness burns. *Cochrane Database Syst Rev*. 2013;3. CD002106.

CHAPTER 190

FISHHOOK REMOVAL

John Harlan Haynes III • Terrance S. Hines

Fishhook injuries are relatively common. Confidence in their management is important for successful outcomes. The method used to remove a fishhook depends on the anatomic location of the injury and the conditions under which the removal is to take place. The least harmful methods described are the *retrograde* and *string-yank* methods, which may be used without anesthesia by anglers on the water. These are best used on the more resilient skin surfaces with underlying bone and muscle. For more embedded hooks or for hooks in flaccid areas such as the earlobe, the needle cover *barb-sheath* or the *pull-through* technique may be more applicable. Local anesthesia with 1% lidocaine is usually appreciated by the anxious patient in an emergency setting. If the shank has already been clipped by a well-meaning first-aider, a strong needle driver or hemostat may be clamped over the exposed shank tip to facilitate removal. Unfortunately, if the shank has been cut too short and there is too little of the hook remaining to manipulate, it may complicate removal.

Occasionally, radiographs may help in determining the type of fishhook and depth of penetration. It may be helpful for the patient to draw the hook to determine what types of barbs to anticipate. Before a fishhook is removed, be sure to assess the proximity of the hook to underlying neurovascular or tendon structures and the potential for damage.

INDICATION

A fishhook embedded in subcutaneous tissue (most commonly, fingers and feet).

Contraindications

- Penetration into the eye with scleral perforation (necessitates ophthalmology referral)
- Deeply embedded hooks in or near the neck, genitalia, nerves, arteries, or the wrist (relative contraindications), or possible penetration of gastrointestinal mucosa

RETROGRADE TECHNIQUE
Equipment

- 2 to 3 mL of 1% lidocaine in syringe with a 30-gauge needle

Technique

1. Cleanse the skin with an iodinated soap or similar antiseptic solution.
2. Inject 2 to 3 mL of 1% local anesthetic around the hook.
3. Place the involved extremity on a flat surface to provide stabilization. Hold the extremity with your dominant hand for further stabilization. Grasp and depress the eye and shank of the hook toward and against the patient's skin with your nondominant free hand until either the barb disengages or

the shank meets resistance. Sometimes this alone is enough to disengage the barb. It may also require some slight wiggling of the hook or tilting of the shank to one side or the other to disengage the barb. If the barb disengages, it may be possible to back the fishhook out in a retrograde fashion with no other maneuvers required. Once the barb is disengaged, instead of using the string to yank as in (Fig. 190.1), merely using retrograde pressure from the nondominant hand may remove the hook. If resistance is encountered, another technique will be necessary. Although this is the simplest method for fishhook removal, it is also the least effective. If successful, it may also cause the least trauma, especially if the barb is not already protruding from the skin when the patient presents.

ANGLER'S STRING-YANK METHOD
Equipment

- Silk suture (0 or larger diameter), umbilical tape, or ordinary string, 2 to 3 feet in length
- 2 to 3 mL of 1% lidocaine in syringe with a 30-gauge needle
- Protective eyewear

Technique

1. Cleanse the skin with an iodinated soap or similar antiseptic solution.
2. Inject 2 to 3 mL of 1% local anesthetic around the hook.
3. Tie the midpoint of the string or suture around the curve of the fishhook. Securely wrap the other ends several times around your index and middle fingers of your dominant hand (Fig. 190.1A).
4. Place the involved extremity on a flat surface to provide stabilization. Grasp the eye and shank of the hook with your nondominant free hand and use your index finger to push them toward and against the patient's skin until it either disengages the hook or meets resistance. The clinician may be able to feel or sense the barb disengaging. It may also require some slight wiggling of the hook or tilting of the shank to one side or the other to disengage the barb. The shaft of the hook is then held approximately parallel to the underlying skin by continuing to grasp the eye with the thumb and middle fingers (Fig. 190.1B). These maneuvers should have disengaged the barb from the subcutaneous tissue, even if it was not felt or sensed.
5. With the shank depressed and the barb disengaged, with your dominant hand grasp the string 12 inches from the hook and firmly and quickly jerk the string, with follow-through, in one forceful move parallel to the shank (Fig. 190.1C). Sudden and forceful pulling on the suture is necessary to prevent failure of the technique. Bystanders should stand clear from the flight path, and protective eyewear should be worn. This method is effective and produces no additional wounds.

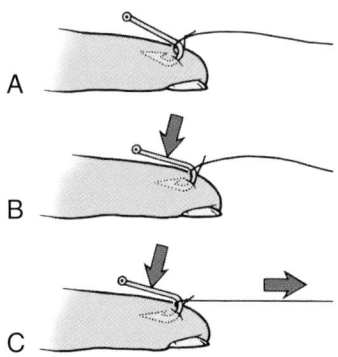

Fig. 190.1 (A–C) Angler's string-yank method of fishhook removal.

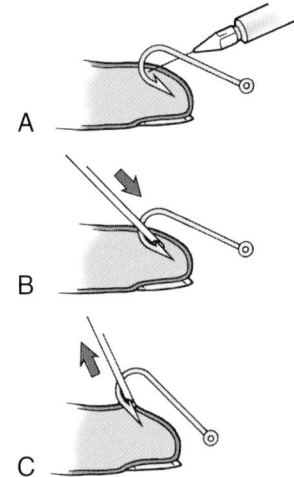

Fig. 190.2 (A–C) Removal of a fishhook with anesthetic when the hook is large and not too deep in the skin.

NEEDLE COVER OR BARB-SHEATH METHOD

Equipment

- 0.5 mL lidocaine 1% in a syringe with a 30-gauge needle
- 18-gauge needle
- Protective eyewear

Technique

1. After local anesthesia is injected, introduce the 18-gauge needle through the entrance track along the inside curvature of the hook, parallel to the shank, with the bevel toward the inside of the curve so that the needle opening can engage the barb (Fig. 190.2A–B).
2. Advance the hook slightly to dislodge the barb from the tissue. Gently pull and twist the hook so that the barb is firmly sheathed by the lumen of the 18-gauge needle.
3. Back the hook and needle out together as a unit (Fig. 190.2C).

TRADITIONAL PULL-THROUGH METHOD

Equipment

- 0.5 mL lidocaine 1% in syringe with a 27-gauge needle
- Wire clipper
- Protective eyewear

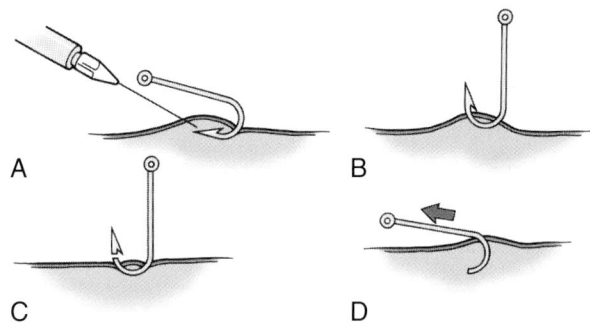

Fig. 190.3 (A–D) Traditional pull-through method for removing a small fishhook.

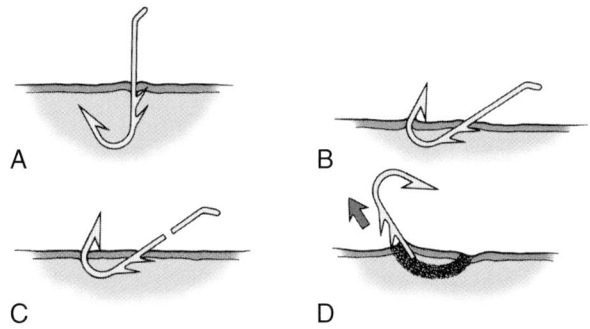

Fig. 190.4 Removal of a barbed fishhook. (A) The hook embedded in soft tissue. (B) Twist the hook forward until the sharp end is visible. (C) Cut off the eye of the hook. (D) Pull on the sharp end to remove.

Technique

1. Provide local anesthesia over the point of the hook (Fig. 190.3A).
2. Force the point through the anesthetized skin (see Fig. 190.3B).
3. When the barb tip is fully exposed, clip it off (see Fig. 190.3C).
4. Back the hook out along the direction of entry (see Fig. 190.3D).
5. Alternatively, if the shank has multiple barbs, clip off the eye of the hook and pull on the sharp end of the hook until the entire hook is removed (Fig. 190.4).

POSTPROCEDURE CARE

- Explore the wound for possible foreign bodies and debride it.
- Administer tetanus toxoid if more than 5 years has elapsed since its last administration.
- Prophylactic antibiotic therapy may be considered for persons who are immunosuppressed or have cancer, liver disease, diabetes, or peripheral vascular disease. Prophylactic antibiotics may also be used for deeper or contaminated wounds. Coverage should include normal skin flora (*Staphylococcus aureus* and *Staphylococcus pyogenes*) and potential water-borne pathogens (*Aeromonas* species, *Edwardsiella tarda*, *Erysipelothrix rhusiopathiae*, *Vibrio vulnificus*, and *Mycobacterium marinum*). Empiric coverage for soft tissue infections after water exposure includes either a first-generation cephalosporin *or* clindamycin *plus* levofloxacin *plus* either metronidazole (sewage- or soil-contaminated wound, not necessary if clindamycin given) *or* doxycycline (coverage of *Vibrio* species if seawater exposure).
- Dress the wound with a sterile adhesive bandage and antibiotic ointment.
- Wash the area well with soap and water four to six times a day for 2 days.
- Warn the patient of the possibility of infection.

CPT/BILLING CODES

10120	Removal of subcutaneous foreign body, simple
10121	Incisional removal, foreign body, complex

Removal of foreign body from the following:

20520	Muscle or tendon sheath, simple
23330	Shoulder subcutaneous
23333	Shoulder, deep (subfascial or intramuscular)
24200	Upper arm/elbow subcutaneous
27086	Pelvis/hip subcutaneous
28190	Foot subcutaneous
67938	Embedded, eyelid

ICD-10-CM DIAGNOSTIC CODES

H02.811–H02.819	Retained foreign body eyelid
M79.5	Residual soft tissue
L92.3	Foreign body granuloma of skin and subcutaneous
Z18.01–Z18.9	Use additional code to identify type of retained foreign body
S00.00XX–S00.97XX	Superficial wound head
S01.00XX–S01.95XX	Laceration with foreign body head
S40.01XX–S40.929X	Superficial wound shoulder and upper arm
S41.001X–S41.151X	Laceration with foreign body shoulder and upper arm
S70.00X–S70.929X	Superficial wound hip and thigh
S71.0001X–S71.159X	Laceration with foreign hip and thigh
S80.00X–S80.929X	Superficial knee and lower leg
S81.001X–S81.859X	Laceration with foreign body lower leg

Add appropriate seventh character: A = initial, D = subsequent, S = sequela.

RECOMMENDED READING

American Academy of Orthopedic Surgeons. Fishhook removal. In: Armstrong AD, Hubbard MC, eds. *Essentials of Musculoskeletal Care*. 5th ed. Rosemont, Ill: American Academy of Orthopedic Surgeons; 2015.

Baddour LM. Soft tissue infections following water exposure. https://www.uptodate.com/contents/soft-tissue-infections-following-water-exposure?search=soft%20tissue%20infections%20following%20water%20exposure&source=search_result&selectedTitle=1~150&usage_type=default&display_rank=1.

Gammons M, Jackson E. Fishhook removal. *Am Fam Physician*. 2001;63:2231–2236.

Halaas GW. Management of foreign bodies in the skin. *Am Fam Physician*. 2007;76:683–688.

Raveenthiran V. Soft palatal injury resulting from an unusual fishhook in a child. *J Trauma*. 2007;62:1060.

Reichman EF, Hamilton RC. Fishhook removal. In: Reichman EF, ed. *Emergency Medicine Procedures*. 2nd ed. New York: McGraw-Hill; 2013.

Stone DM, Scordino DJ. Foreign body removal. In: Roberts JR, Custalow CB, Thomsen TW, eds. *Roberts & Hedges' Clinical Procedures of Emergency Medicine*. 6th ed. Philadelphia: Elsevier; 2014.

CHAPTER 191

FOREIGN BODY REMOVAL FROM SKIN AND SOFT TISSUE

Grant C. Fowler

Patients frequently seek care from a primary care clinician for a foreign body in the skin or soft tissue. In fact, foreign bodies are present in 3% of wounds. In certain situations, removal may cause more trauma than leaving the object in place; hence the patient may require only information or reassurance. However, the presence of a foreign body increases the risk of infection in a wound, even if only slightly. A foreign body can also cause pain and discomfort. Fortunately removal is often accomplished with minimal trauma, usually leading the patient to express considerable appreciation.

A foreign body should be suspected whenever the skin is broken; many issues occur when one is not suspected. A foreign body should also be suspected in all wounds caused by a high-velocity missile or a sharp, fragile object. If a patient presents with an infected wound, a foreign body should be suspected. Objects that splinter, shatter, or break in the process of causing a wound often leave remnants behind. For example, a piece of glass that caused a wound by breaking on impact with the skin is more likely to leave shards in the wound than a piece of glass that was previously broken.

All wounds should be probed manually for the presence of a foreign body. Up to 38% of embedded objects are missed on the initial assessment; consequently the most common error in the management of soft tissue foreign bodies is the failure to detect their presence. Failure to diagnose soft tissue foreign bodies and manage them correctly is a common cause of malpractice litigation in both emergency and family medicine. With the techniques discussed in this chapter, attempts at removal may be simplified and the results optimized.

INDICATIONS

- Known foreign body in skin, subcutaneous, or soft tissue
- Pain or persistent inflammation from a foreign body
- Foreign body with toxic, infectious, or allergic potential
- Impairment of neurovascular or mechanical function due to a foreign body
- Foreign body near a fractured bone or open joint
- Foreign body causing a cosmetic deformity

NOTE: A general guideline is if one end of the foreign body can be palpated by hand or an instrument, it can be removed. Another is that removal may be more difficult than expected, even if the foreign body is large, palpable, and apparently superficial on radiographs; therefore adequate time should be set aside to evaluate, explore, plan, and pursue removal. However, some experts suggest spending no more than 15 to 30 minutes exploring; clinicians thereby avoid causing excessive damage by "looking too long for a needle in a haystack." Yet another guideline is that if a patient complains of a foreign-body sensation, the clinician should assume that there is

one, even if the radiographs are negative. One study found that such a foreign-body sensation was 43% sensitive and 83% specific for the presence of glass.

CONTRAINDICATIONS

- Lack of knowledge of anatomic structures surrounding the foreign body
- Proximity of the foreign body to a vital structure such as a nerve or artery
- An uncooperative patient who cannot be sedated (see Chapter 2, Pediatric Sedation and Analgesia) or anesthetized (see Chapter 5, Local Anesthesia)

NOTE: Consider referral for a foreign body in the soft tissues of the face or the deep spaces of the hands or feet, or for broken glass if there are multiple shards. Also, deeply imbedded objects, those in joints, and those impairing neurovascular or mechanical function may best be removed by a surgeon while the patient is under general anesthesia.

EQUIPMENT

- Blunt-tipped stiff (but bendable) sterile metal probe
- Small sharp-tipped dissecting scissors
- Sterile tweezers (splinter forceps are very helpful)
- Adson pickup forceps with teeth (an Allis clamp may also be helpful)
- Two mosquito hemostats
- Bright light that can be directed or focused (use of a head lamp allows both hands to be free for the procedure)
- Clear plastic tape
- Skin-marking pen or pencil
- Paper clips, BBs, or 27-gauge needles used for local anesthetic can be used as markers
- Scalpel (No. 11 or 15)
- Suture, if necessary for closure
- Local or topical anesthetic materials (see Chapter 5, Local Anesthesia, and Chapter 4, Topical Anesthesia)
- Irrigant, such as saline
- Syringes for irrigation (5 mL for small wounds, 10 to 30 mL for larger wounds) with optional 18-gauge needle
- Magnifying glass or loupes
- Antiseptic solutions such as chlorhexidine or povidone-iodine solution
- Powerful magnet for ferromagnetic objects
- Sterile adhesive bandage
- Liquid soap
- Blood pressure cuff to use as tourniquet and elastic (Ace) bandage (optional)

- Hair removal (depilatory) wax (optional)
- Skin hook (optional)
- 3-mm skin punch for biopsy (optional)
- 1-0 or 2-0 nylon suture, without needle, to use as probe (optional)
- Hemoclips, hemoclip applicator, and silk sutures (optional)
- Vinegar (5% acetic acid) and sharp edge (e.g., credit card) or shaving cream and razor (optional, for certain marine foreign bodies)

PREPROCEDURE PATIENT PREPARATION

Patients should be aware that in some situations removal may be too complicated, unsuccessful, or impossible. The clinician should also explain that it is safe for certain objects to be left in the skin permanently. For example, wounds containing a small metal fleck in a nonvital area will often heal with no problems. Even lead and other metal objects are sometimes safe to let "rest" in the skin indefinitely. Their removal, especially if deeply embedded, may cause more trauma than leaving them in place, especially if the patient is not experiencing symptoms and has no signs of infection. The only time extra effort should be made to remove lead is if it is bathed in synovial, pleural, peritoneal, or cerebrospinal fluid; in these situations, the lead may leach out over time and produce a significant elevation in blood lead levels. Otherwise the body tends to wall off nonporous materials and smooth objects such as bullets, glass, metal, and even shrapnel; if they are deeply embedded, therefore, they are often better left alone. However, heavily contaminated foreign bodies should be removed as soon as possible. Hair or marine foreign bodies, such as sea urchin spines, may cause granuloma formation, so they should usually be removed. Similarly, objects made of wood, vegetable fiber, or other organic materials—which are likely to cause an inflammatory reaction or infection—usually have to be removed. The same is true for any object with toxic or allergic potential.

Patients should also be aware that other foreign bodies may need to be left in the tissue until it forms a cyst or localizes (i.e., until edema subsides). Although it may take days, weeks, or even decades, certain objects will eventually work their way to the surface and can then be removed. If an infection develops, it will be treated with an antibiotic. If a small pocket of fluid develops, it may help with later removal. Inform the patient that if removal is attempted, certain techniques may be used to locate and remove the foreign body, including the taking of radiographs.

If removal is attempted, the patient should be informed that the object may not be removable or that it may be only partially removed. Even with what appears to be a simple extraction (e.g., of a splinter), the clinician may want to be cautious about telling the patient that it was removed entirely; perhaps a better explanation would be that all of the visible object was removed but that small fragments might still be present that are currently undetectable. With removal, there will be minor trauma and possibly scarring (from the original wound, an incision, or from sutures), and there is a possibility of damage to vital structures surrounding the object, such as a nerve, artery, vein, or tendon. Such trauma may be associated with discomfort during the procedure or some bleeding during or after the procedure. There is also a risk of infection after the procedure. In certain situations, minimal or no anesthesia will be used at first in order to localize or grasp the object. A patient's intact sensation is usually much more accurate than probing blindly under anesthetized skin when the clinician is attempting to locate an object, especially if the skin is distorted from an injection of local anesthetic. For small or difficult-to-locate objects, the patient's intact sensation may be the only way to find the object. As soon as the object is grasped, stabilized, or removed, the discomfort is usually decreased or eliminated. After the object is grasped, local anesthesia may then be used to minimize any discomfort.

The patient should be aware that glass objects, especially small ones, may be difficult to visualize on radiographs and that there may be multiple shards. For various reasons, glass objects are probably the most difficult to remove. If the clinician is not certain that all of the foreign object (or objects) has been removed, referral may be required.

If the decision is made to attempt to remove a foreign object, the patient should be aware that the procedure may be time consuming, although usually not more than 15 to 30 minutes will be spent exploring to keep tissue damage to a minimum. He or she should be in a comfortable position that can be maintained for this amount of time. The patient should also be aware of the importance of remaining immobile during the procedure.

TECHNIQUE

1. Before removal, obtain as much history as possible regarding the foreign body. Knowledge of the material and method of injury may help to determine which technique to use and whether a diagnostic study such as a radiograph would be helpful. Knowledge of the angle of entry (e.g., whether tangential or perpendicular to the skin surface) may be helpful for localization. Information regarding the speed and force of entry may also be helpful.
2. Most superficially embedded, visible objects can be magnified and removed from soft tissue with a sterile needle and tweezers. For very fine splinters in the skin surface (e.g., cactus spurs, glass slivers), it can be helpful to spread liquid soap lightly over the skin; this will often enhance visualization. Alternatively, such objects can be removed by applying clear plastic tape or hair removal wax to the skin and then peeling it off.
3. Good judgment should be used when foreign objects are being removed from cosmetically sensitive areas. For example, the risk of tattooing from an object left in place (e.g., graphite from pencil or asphalt, tar, or gravel from road) must be weighed against the risk of a scar from removal.
4. Toothpicks and splinters usually enter tangentially, and their tract can usually be envisioned based on the history. Occasionally, instead of using forceps or making an incision, a hypodermic needle can be inserted perpendicular to the splinter to "spear" it. The hypodermic is then used as a lever to ease the splinter out through the entry wound. Because wood splinters must be removed entirely to avoid local inflammation, one cannot just pull the splinter out; instead, many experts incise the entire tract of the splinter to remove it. They then irrigate the wound to ensure the removal of all fragments. Although this may seem excessive and creates a laceration where there was only a puncture wound, small pieces of the splinter may otherwise remain in the skin. This is especially important for splinters derived from cedar, cypress, or California redwood because of the pliable and reactive nature of the wood.
5. If the object is not visible because it is below the skin, consider the use of radiographs or other imaging techniques for localization and documentation.
   - *Radiographs* are 98% sensitive for detecting radiopaque materials such as metal, gravel, pencil graphite, or teeth. Sand, mammalian bone, and certain fish bones (e.g., haddock, cod, grey mullet, sole, red snapper) are also usually radiopaque. Some plastics produce at least a slight shadow on x-ray films. Painted wood can also sometimes be seen on radiographs. Although leaded glass is radiopaque, which improves its visibility on radiographs, most glass is nonleaded. However, in one cadaver study, radiographs were 90% sensitive for detecting nonleaded glass, with a false-positive rate of only 10%. (It should be noted that a diameter of less than 1.5 mm was associated with risk of failed detection.) Radiographs are also helpful, to make sure that there are not multiple shards, if

the glass shattered near the skin surface. Routine lateral and anteroposterior views may suffice. By ordering "soft tissue" x-rays, slightly underpenetrated films are provided, which can enhance visibility and localization efforts. (With digitized images, the contrast and brightness can be adjusted to produce the same effect.) If the object is positioned parallel to the central ray of the x-ray beam, the likelihood of detection is increased. Oblique and tangential views may also be helpful if the object is obscured by underlying bone.

EDITOR'S NOTE: in one study of malpractice cases for undetected foreign bodies, the failure to obtain a plain radiograph was a frequent factor in the final outcome.

- *High-frequency ultrasound* is available in most emergency departments as an alternative for localizing nonradiopaque objects (see Chapter 171, Musculoskeletal Ultrasound, and Chapter 214, Emergency Department, Hospitalist, and Office Ultrasound [POCUS]). Most authors have reported a greater than 90% sensitivity for the detection of objects larger than 4 to 5 mm. Although ultrasound has the benefit of avoiding radiation, it has the limitation of being operator dependent. Small objects perpendicular to the skin surface may also be difficult to visualize. The 7.5- to 10-MHz probe is better for shallow depths (<5 mm), whereas the 5-MHz probe should be used for deeper searching. Metal objects classically produce a comet-tail, "ring-down" shadow. Otherwise, solid objects are typically echogenic (white by convention), and cast sharp shadows behind or beneath them.
- *Xeroradiography* (the technology used in xeromammograms), although recommended in the past, has fallen out of favor because it has rarely been found to offer an advantage over plain radiographs. It also requires a much higher dose of radiation compared with plain radiographs and is not as readily available.
- *Fluoroscopy* has received more attention lately as a diagnostic and therapeutic tool in the emergency department. Compared with plain radiographs, bedside fluoroscopy usually requires less irradiation and is faster, more convenient, and less expensive. For objects that must be removed, needle localization under fluoroscopy may remain the final option.
- *Computed tomography* (CT) scanning is useful not only for further characterizing foreign objects seen on plain radiographs but also for diagnosing possible complications such as an abscess. CT is often useful for visualizing nonradiopaque objects made of plastic or wood. Consequently CT has evolved as the procedure of choice for excluding foreign objects if the plain radiograph is negative. With the development of spiral/helical CT scanning (i.e., real-time scanning) and its increased availability in emergency departments, the time required to visualize an image has been greatly reduced.
- *Magnetic resonance imaging* (MRI) in comparison studies was found to be the most accurate method of detecting foreign bodies such as thorns or those made of wood or plastic. MRI is also useful for detecting complications due to a foreign body, such as an abscess or the involvement of bone. However, MRI is limited when one is scanning gravel or ferrometallic foreign bodies because they produce streaking, which usually obscures visualization. And because CT scanning can also usually detect foreign bodies made of wood or plastic as well as abscesses, MRI is rarely used owing to the additional time it takes to obtain the images as well as the additional expense incurred.

6. Attempt to localize the object before incising the skin. Although the object may not be visible, there may be a discoloration beneath the skin. Any externally visible entry wound should be measured and its exact size and location recorded. Examine the wound entrance to determine the angle of penetration and possibly also the depth. Palpate the object, determine the exact orientation and approximate depth (Fig. 191.1A), and measure and record it. For larger metal objects, a powerful magnet may pull the object to the surface and tent the skin. If the skin tents, mark the outline of the object with the skin-marking pen. Glass is the most common foreign body, yet it is one of the more difficult substances to remove because it is transparent and slippery, and the sizes and outlines of the pieces are unpredictable. If glass is suspected, do not probe with your finger so as to avoid cutting yourself. An unknown number of shards may be involved, and if there is uncertainty about whether all of the shards have been removed, referral should be considered.

NOTE: Probing a wound with a gloved finger is not recommended for *any* possibly sharp foreign object because it may result in a puncture wound to the clinician and the spread of a body fluid- or blood-borne infection.

7. If the object is not visible at the entrance wound, after palpation for orientation and depth, prepare the skin with antiseptic solution and carefully use a sterile probe or mosquito hemostat to enter the wound. Gently follow the apparent tract of the wound to locate the nearest edge. Use small, light, deliberate probing motions, gradually fanning in all directions, until contact is made with the object. This may be felt or heard as a clicking sound when the probe contacts the foreign body. (For metallic objects, a magnetic probe can be used in the same manner, and the object will usually cause a click when it comes into contact with the magnet; it can then be pulled out of the wound.) Avoid excessive or unnecessary blind probing, which may conceal the foreign body further with blood and edema, or may push it deeper into the tissue. For small objects, before using local anesthetic, attempt to use the patient's sensation as a guide; it may be more accurate than using a probe. In this situation, avoidance of local anesthetic not only minimizes local skin distortion but limits the tissue destruction that may occur from cutting or exploring blindly under anesthesia. After the object has been removed, if the patient has not been anesthetized and the symptoms have completely resolved, this is somewhat reassuring that everything was removed. If the patient continues to have a foreign-body sensation, there may have been more than one foreign body, and exploration may have to be continued.

8. If the object is not palpable, an attempt can be made to follow the tract of the wound with a probe. However, because of the nature of the tissue, following the tract may be more difficult in muscle or fat. That said, the clinician must avoid probing only superficially because the subcutaneous tissue can reapproximate and give the appearance of a superficial wound. If necessary, the wound edges should be extended with a scalpel for direct visualization if there is concern regarding a retained foreign body. If the bottom of the wound is less than 5 mm deep and visible, there is a 96% chance that a foreign body has been ruled out. If the wound extends into subcutaneous fat, be aware that foreign bodies can migrate significantly in this layer. Repeated imaging may then be necessary. Probing in this layer may also displace the foreign body even further.

9. After the object has been located, fixate the probe in your nondominant hand. Rest this hand on a firm surface. Administer or inject local anesthetic with the dominant hand (see Fig. 191.1B). Occasionally the injection of anesthetic beyond the foreign body or on each side of the entry wound will force the foreign body out. Once the presence of a neurovascular bundle, tendon, or other important structure has been excluded and without moving the probe, cut down along the probe with a No. 11 or 15 scalpel blade until the foreign body is reached. Do not remove the probe. Reach into the incision and remove the foreign body with a pair of Adson forceps. Alternatively, if the entrance tract is

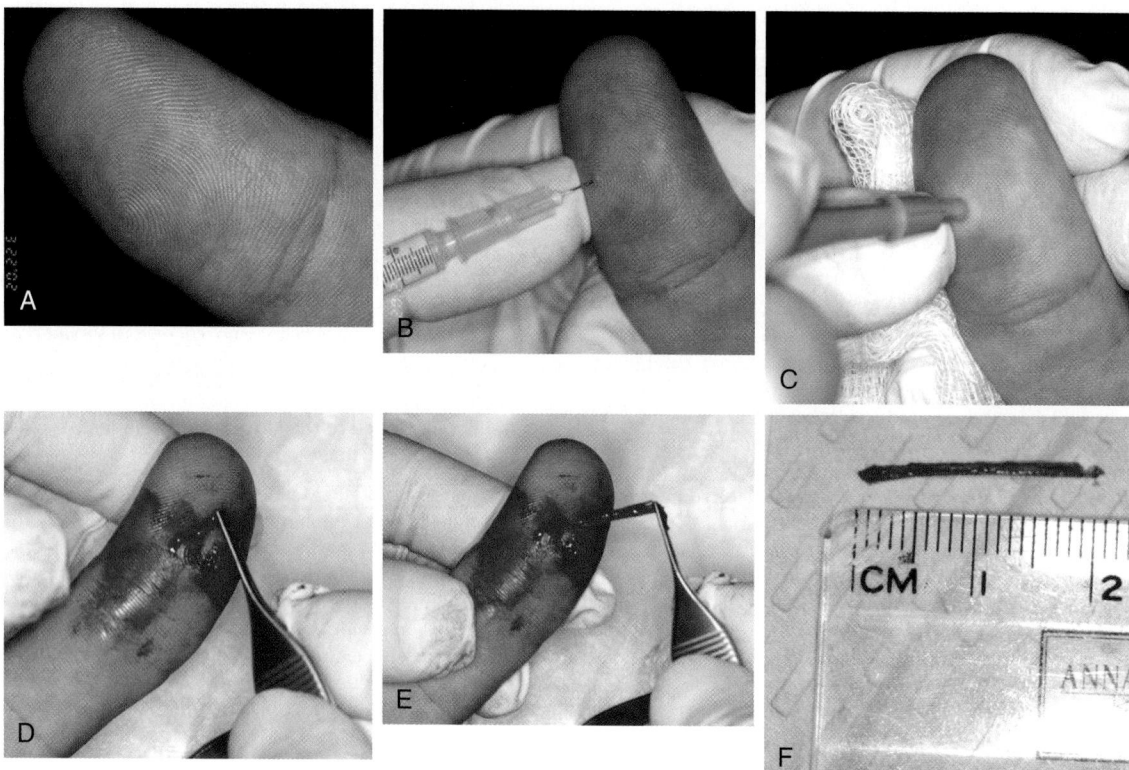

Fig. 191.1 Patient reports sensation of sliver in palmar surface of distal phalanx. (A) A fullness is palpable but no real foreign body is detected. (B) Lidocaine 2% 0.5 mL without epinephrine is injected. (C) A 3-mm disposable skin punch is used. It is inserted until a gritty sensation is appreciated. (D) Fine pickups without teeth are inserted and grasp the foreign body. (E) A long wooden sliver is removed. (F) The sliver.

fairly long and the foreign body is very superficial and easily palpable beneath the skin, it may be advantageous to simply cut down through the skin directly over the object to remove it without the use of a probe. The object should be stabilized between the fingers of your nondominant hand while the incision is being made.

NOTE: An inadequate incision is a common source of frustration when one is attempting to remove a foreign object, so the clinician should usually plan a slightly larger-than-necessary incision. Bleeding into the field, which may obscure the entrance wound or the object, can be another source of frustration. If the object is in the soft tissue of an extremity and the arterial circulation is otherwise intact, it is safe to inflate a proximal blood pressure cuff to greater than systolic arterial pressure for up to 2 hours to minimize bleeding. (Although this may cause some mild patient discomfort, patients usually tolerate it well.) The extremity can be elevated for a minute or an elastic (Ace) bandage can be wrapped tightly around the extremity, from distal to proximal, before inflating the blood pressure cuff to minimize venous backflow into the field. The elastic bandage can be removed as soon as the blood pressure cuff has been inflated.

10. For a wound less than 48 hours old, one technique that has been found to have a 92% success rate involves using nylon suture as a probe. The clinician grasps a 1-0 or 2-0 nylon suture (with no needle) between his or her thumb and index finger, then pushes it into the entrance wound while gently rotating it so that it follows the foreign body tract. Experienced clinicians report that the foreign body is easily felt when the suture contacts it. The suture is then left in the tract and the wound opened down to the foreign body by cutting alongside the suture with a scalpel.

11. If an edge of the object is somewhat superficial and easily located with a probe and the entrance wound is large, simply enlarging the entrance wound slightly with mosquito forceps may provide enough room for the clinician to grasp the object firmly with

forceps. The object can then be removed. If the object has been in place for long enough to form a cyst, the cyst wall will sometimes need to be incised. This may be performed by the use of very small, deliberate strokes with the scalpel while the object is held by one set of mosquito forceps. The other set of mosquito forceps can then be used to bluntly dissect down to the object by spreading anything that was incised with the scalpel. If the object is visible after incision of the cyst wall, it should be grasped through the incision with the second set of forceps. The first set of forceps can then be relaxed and the object removed. If the object is not visible, which is often the case when a foreign body has been in place for a long time, constant traction on the object with the first set of forceps may cause one end of the cyst to tent. Incise through this tent with the scalpel until the object is freed.

NOTE: Do not blindly grab something in a wound with a hemostat. Blind grasping can cause damage to a vital anatomic structure.

12. Another option for the not-yet-visible but readily palpable object is to perform a punch biopsy (see Fig. 191.1C through F; see Chapter 26, Skin Biopsy). As the punch biopsy is being performed, a hard "click" may reveal the position of the foreign body, thereby both localizing it and avoiding the need to make a larger incision. After the biopsy has been performed, tease apart the core of tissue removed and identify the foreign body. If the foreign body cannot be found in the tissue, probe the wound to make sure that the foreign body is not still beneath the biopsy site. If the punch biopsy missed the foreign body (because of an angled entry wound, it may be lateral to the biopsy site), undermine the subcutaneous fat all around the site using dissecting scissors. After undermining, if pressure is applied from various locations around the site toward the center of the biopsy site, the foreign body may be forced into the biopsy site. Foreign bodies located in subcutaneous fat are highly mobile, so lateral

pressure can move them a considerable distance. If the foreign body is beneath the biopsy site, the clinician must decide whether to deepen the site with the punch or to cut down with a No. 11 scalpel. Neither procedure should be performed if the object is located close to an underlying vital structure (e.g., nerve, artery, significant vein).

13. If a skin punch is not available, simple elliptical excision of a block of skin overlying the foreign body can be performed in the same manner. Limit the incision to just the skin, and while applying upward traction on the ellipse with forceps (or an Allis clamp) and with the subcutaneous fat still attached beneath, probe the subcutaneous fat lateral to and beneath the incision for the foreign object. If the object is not found with probing, use the dissecting scissors to undermine the subcutaneous fat in the same directions, attempting to come into contact with the object. If the object is not found with undermining, the probe can be used again under the ellipse or directed laterally. If the object is still not located, apply pressure to the skin lateral to the incision, attempting to force the object into view.

14. If the object is neither palpable through the skin nor located by probing through the entry wound (yet is visible on x-ray films), paper clips or BBs may be used for localization with a radiograph. Bend the paper clips into various shapes and tape them to the skin with clear plastic tape, or tape the BBs over the skin above and beside the approximate location of the object. With lateral and anteroposterior radiographs taken at precisely 90 degrees, the location of the foreign body can be predicted by measuring the distance from the paper clips or BBs on the film. Transfer this measurement to the skin with a marking pen. Next, remove the tape and clips, apply antiseptic solution and local anesthetic, incise the skin in the correct location to the depth measured on the x-ray film, and remove the object. A punch biopsy may also be used in this manner if the measurements from the x-ray film are very accurate; however, if there is any error in the measurement, an incision may be necessary to expand the search for the object.

NOTE: It is very important to have true lateral and anteroposterior views in order to use radiographic measurements for localization before incision; otherwise any variance in the angle of the x-ray beam to the film will cause significant distortion of the apparent location of the foreign body. This is especially true for small metal flakes.

15. For deeply embedded objects, after injecting local anesthetic, two 27-gauge needles can be inserted at a 45-degree angle to the skin and directed toward the object from either side. Radiographs can then be used for localization and an incision made down to the tip of the needle closest to the object. Needles used in such a manner are especially helpful when fluoroscopy is available; when the extremity is rotated under fluoroscopy, the needles provide a three-dimensional effect that can be useful for localizing, planning the overlying incision, and removing the object.

16. Localizing even a superficial foreign body can be difficult after the procedure has begun because of distortion by local anesthetic, edema, and tissue retraction. It can be especially difficult to localize deeply embedded foreign bodies owing to these conditions. One reported technique for localizing radiopaque foreign bodies uses hemoclips with silk sutures tied to them. After the clinician dissects down to where he or she thinks the foreign body is located, two or three hemoclips can be placed into the depths of the wound. On subsequent radiographs, the hemoclip located closest to the foreign body should be verified. It should then be left in place and the others removed. The incision and dissection pathway should then follow the silk suture down to the foreign body.

17. For marine venom-containing foreign bodies (nematocysts from Portuguese man-of-war, true jellyfish, fire coral, box jellyfish, or sea anemones), vinegar (5% acetic acid) is the decontaminat-

ing agent of choice because it will neutralize most (but not all) of these species. Apply it continuously for 30 minutes. Do not apply fresh water because it will activate all unfired nematocysts. After the wound has been decontaminated, remove all remaining visible tentacle fragments with forceps. The invisible remaining nematocysts can be removed by scraping the skin with a sharp-edged object such as a credit card or by applying shaving cream and shaving the area. For catfish spines, no antivenom exists. Immerse the affected body part for 30 minutes in hot water (>43°C/110°F). Infiltrate the area around the spine with bupivacaine and remove the spine and any remaining particles. The same treatment should be used for stingray spines, but irrigate with normal saline prior to soaking in hot water for a longer time period (30 to 90 minutes) before removal.

18. After removal of the foreign body, the wound should be irrigated with any remaining anesthetic. This irrigation should be followed by sterile saline pulsated from a syringe. Irrigation is helpful for removing any small remaining fragments or debris. A jetted irrigation can be performed by attaching an 18-gauge needle to the syringe.

19. If a significant incision was made or a punch biopsy performed, reapproximate the skin with suture. Cover the wound with a sterile adhesive bandage and give the patient postprocedure instructions.

20. For a splinter under a nail, a "V" can be cut in the distal nail to allow it to be reached and grasped or a portion or all of the nail can be removed under a local block (see Chapter 23, Nail Plate, Nail Bed, and Nail Matrix Biopsy, and Chapter 194, Ingrown Toenails, for similar situations). Alternatively, a 27-gauge needle can be bent at its tip to form a hook, inserted under the nail, and used to hook the splinter and drag it out. If the entire splinter cannot be removed, at least the part of the nail covering any possible splinter fragments should be removed to allow for irrigation. Otherwise, because the subungual area is very close to the distal phalanx, any remaining fragments may increase the risk of infection and subsequent rapid spread to osteomyelitis.

21. Tetanus prophylaxis should be provided if appropriate.

COMPLICATIONS

- Trauma to local vital structures, such as nerves, arteries, veins, or tendons.
- Infection or bleeding.
- Scarring from the original wound, or from the incision and sutures that were necessary to locate the object and close the wound.
- Failure to remove the object, partially or completely. Again, for those objects that must be removed, needle localization under fluoroscopy may remain the final option. The patient should be informed if there was failure to remove the object, and this should be documented along with any agreed-on plan for follow-up or removal.

POSTPROCEDURE PATIENT EDUCATION

After removal, a dull ache or stretching sensation in the area is normal for up to a day, especially if sutures were placed. Instruct the patient to watch for signs of infection. Itching is a normal sign of healing. The patient should follow up with the clinician in 2 days to check for infection (earlier if there are significant signs) and again in the appropriate number of days (7 days in most cases) for suture removal if sutures were placed. A topical antibiotic may be applied, and the dressing should remain over the wound for 48 hours. It should be changed if it gets wet during that time. After the first 48 hours, a dressing should be applied only if the wound continues to drain or if it could get dirty and the wound may be washed with soap and water.

CPT/BILLING CODES

NOTE: As with all coding, the reimbursement is usually greater if there is a more descriptive code that includes the location, depth, and complexity (e.g., 23330 is approximately twice the RVUs as 10120, whereas 28192 is approximately four times that of 10120).

10120	Incision and removal of foreign body, subcutaneous tissues; simple
10121	Incision and removal of foreign body, subcutaneous tissues; complicated

For codes 20100 through 20103, exploration is defined as exploration and enlargement of the wound; extension of dissection (to determine penetration); debridement; removal of foreign body or bodies; or ligation or coagulation of minor subcutaneous and/or muscular blood vessel(s) of the subcutaneous tissue, muscle fascia, and/or muscle not requiring thoracotomy or laparotomy.

20100	Exploration of penetrating wound (separate procedure); neck
20101	Exploration of penetrating wound (separate procedure); chest
20102	Exploration of penetrating wound (separate procedure); abdomen/flank/back
20103	Exploration of penetrating wound (separate procedure); extremity
20520	Removal of foreign body in muscle or tendon sheath; simple
20525	Removal of foreign body in muscle or tendon sheath; deep or complicated
23330	Removal of foreign body, shoulder, subcutaneous tissue
24200	Removal of foreign body, upper arm or elbow area; subcutaneous tissue
24201	Removal of foreign body, upper arm or elbow area; deep (subfascial or intramuscular)
27086	Removal of foreign body, pelvis or hip; subcutaneous tissue
28190	Removal of foreign body, foot; subcutaneous tissue
28192	Removal of foreign body, foot; deep
28193	Removal of foreign body, foot; complicated

ICD-10-CM DIAGNOSTIC CODES

L92.3	Foreign body granuloma of skin or subcutaneous tissue
M79.5	Residual foreign body in subcutaneous or soft tissue
S31.040A	Foreign body lower back through open wound
S31.122A	Foreign body abdominal wall unspecified quadrant through open wound
S41.129A	Foreign body arm (upper) through open wound unspecified arm
S61.429A	Foreign body hand through open wound unspecified hand
S81.029A	Foreign body calf, knee, leg through open wound
S00.95XA	Foreign body superficial unspecified part of head
S30.855A	Foreign body superficial external genital organs male
S30.856A	Foreign body superficial external genital organs female
S30.851A	Foreign body superficial abdominal wall
S30.850A	Foreign body superficial lower back and pelvis
S40.859A	Foreign body superficial unspecified arm
S50.859A	Foreign body superficial unspecified forearm
S60.559A	Foreign body superficial unspecified hand
S60.459A	Foreign body superficial unspecified finger
S70.259A	Foreign body superficial unspecified hip
S80.859A	Foreign body superficial unspecified lower leg
S80.359A	Foreign body superficial unspecified thigh
S90.859A	Foreign body superficial unspecified foot

RECOMMENDED READING

Buttaravoli P, Leffler SM. *Minor Emergencies. Splinters to Fractures.* 3rd ed. Philadelphia: Elsevier; 2012.

Chan C, Salam GA. Splinter removal. *Am Fam Physician.* 2003;67:2557–2562.

Gutman SJ, Secter MB. Subcutaneous foreign body identification and removal. In: Reichman EF, ed. *Emergency Medicine Procedures.* 2nd ed. New York: McGraw-Hill; 2013.

Lammers RL. Soft tissue foreign bodies. In: Tintinalli JE, Stapczynski JS, Ma OJ, et al., eds. *Tintinalli's Emergency Medicine. A Comprehensive Study Guide.* 8th ed. New York: McGraw-Hill; 2015.

Murtagh J. Removal of foreign bodies. In: Murtagh J, ed. *Practice Tips.* 7th ed. Sydney, Australia: McGraw-Hill; 2017.

Stone DM, Scordino DJ. Foreign body removal. In: Roberts JR, Custalow CB, Thomsen TW, eds. *Roberts and Hedges Clinical Procedures in Emergency Medicine and Acute Care.* 7th ed. Philadelphia: Elsevier; 2019:708–737.

Thomas SH, Goodloe JM. Foreign bodies. In: Marx JA, Hockberger RS, eds. *Rosen's Emergency Medicine. Concepts and Clinical Practice.* 8th ed. Philadelphia: Elsevier; 2014.

Wagstrom G. Management of foreign bodies in the skin. *Am Fam Physician.* 2007;76(5):683–690.

CHAPTER 192

INCISION AND DRAINAGE OF AN ABSCESS

Daniel J. Derksen

An abscess is a localized infection, a collection of pus surrounded by inflamed tissue. When an infected sweat gland or hair follicle forms an abscess, it is called a *furuncle* or *boil*. If multiple follicles are involved, it is referred to as a *carbuncle*. *Paronychia* is an abscess that involves the nail; a *felon* involves the tuft of soft tissue in the distal phalanx of the finger. A *hordeolum* is an abscess on the eyelid margin, whereas a *chalazion* is a chronic abscess of the eyelid itself in the meibomian glands beneath the tarsal plate (see Chapter 57, Chalazion and Hordeolum). *Hidradenitis suppurativa* is a chronic condition in the axilla and groin with recurrent abscesses. *Pilonidal abscesses* are discussed in Chapter 31, Pilonidal Cyst and Abscess: Current Management; *Perianal abscesses* in Chapter 86, Perianal Abscess Incision and Drainage; and *Bartholin's abscesses* in Chapter 118, Bartholin Cyst and Abscess: Word Catheter Insertion Marsupialization. For *olecranon* and *prepatellar* bursitis, see Chapter 180, Joint and Soft Tissue Aspiration and Injection (Arthrocentesis).

Most often, *Staphylococcus aureus* is the causative agent, but some abscesses are due to *Streptococcus* species or a combination of microorganisms, including gram-negative and anaerobic bacteria. Perianal abscesses are usually caused by a mix of aerobic and anaerobic enteric organisms. Abscesses can occur in any location, but they are commonly found on the extremities, buttocks, and breast or in hair follicles.

A small abscess may respond to warm compresses or antibiotics and drain spontaneously. If one enlarges, the inflammation, collection of pus, and walling off of the abscess cavity render such conservative treatments ineffective; the treatment of choice is incision and drainage (I&D), If this treatment is done properly, antibiotics are usually unnecessary. (See precautions for the facial triangle in "Contraindications," later.) In a nonlactating woman, a breast abscess that is not subareolar is rare. If one occurs anywhere other than the areola, it should prompt a biopsy, in addition to I&D, and raise the clinician's suspicion of a malignant tumor.

A patient with diabetes, debilitating disease, or compromised immunity should be observed closely after I&D of an abscess. Although usually not necessary, consider a culture obtained by aspiration or a swab of the cavity because it may have been caused by unusual organisms in an immunocompromised patient. The infection may also warrant the administration of antibiotics that cover *Staphylococcus* infection.

If an abscess recurs after I&D, methicillin-resistant *S. aureus* (MRSA) should be considered, a culture and sensitivity obtained, and the patient treated with appropriate antibiotics based on these results. Community-associated *S. aureus* is most often sensitive to clindamycin, trimethoprim/sulfamethoxazole, doxycycline, and linezolid. The frequency of MRSA skin and soft tissue infections has increased dramatically, and it is now the most common pathogen in abscesses in patients presenting to the emergency department.

Resistance changes rapidly and differs regionally. Initial treatment remains I&D, although some recommend treatment with one or more oral antibiotics based on culture and sensitivity.

INDICATIONS

A localized collection of pus that is tender and not resolving spontaneously. If the lesion is not "pointing" and localized, a trial of antibiotics may be indicated. However, antibiotics are usually inadequate once a collection of pus is present.

CONTRAINDICATIONS

Crepitus or gas seen on imaging suggests a more serious infection such as necrotizing fasciitis; emergent surgical referral is indicated. Be cautious with cysts involving the face; to minimize risk of scarring, aspiration and antibiotics may be best first option. Small, nonfluctuant facial furuncles without surrounding cellulitis should not be incised or drained if located within the triangle formed by the bridge of the nose and the corners of the mouth. These infections should be treated with antibiotics, with coverage for MRSA, and warm compresses because there is a risk of septic phlebitis with intracranial extension after I&D of a furuncle in this area. However, if the lesion is large and fluctuant, drainage is recommended, regardless of the site. In most instances, drainage alone is adequate, but in this area, antibiotics are also recommended.

EQUIPMENT

- Local anesthetic (1% to 2% lidocaine), sodium bicarbonate 7.5%, or diphenhydramine (Benadryl) 50 mg/mL
- Syringe with 25- to 30-gauge needle, usually 0.5 to 1 inch, because only the skin over the abscess is anesthetized
- Possibly a cryosurgery unit or ethyl chloride for anesthesia (to minimize the needle poke)
- Antiseptic solution (e.g., alcohol, povidone-iodine [Betadine] or chlorhexidine)
- 4 × 4–inch gauze
- No. 11 blade
- Curved hemostats
- Possibly iodoform gauze (0.25- to 0.5-inch width, and up to 24 inches long depending on abscess size)
- Culture materials
- Bandage scissors
- Dressing of choice
- Protective eyewear, gloves, and equipment necessary to observe universal blood and body fluid precautions

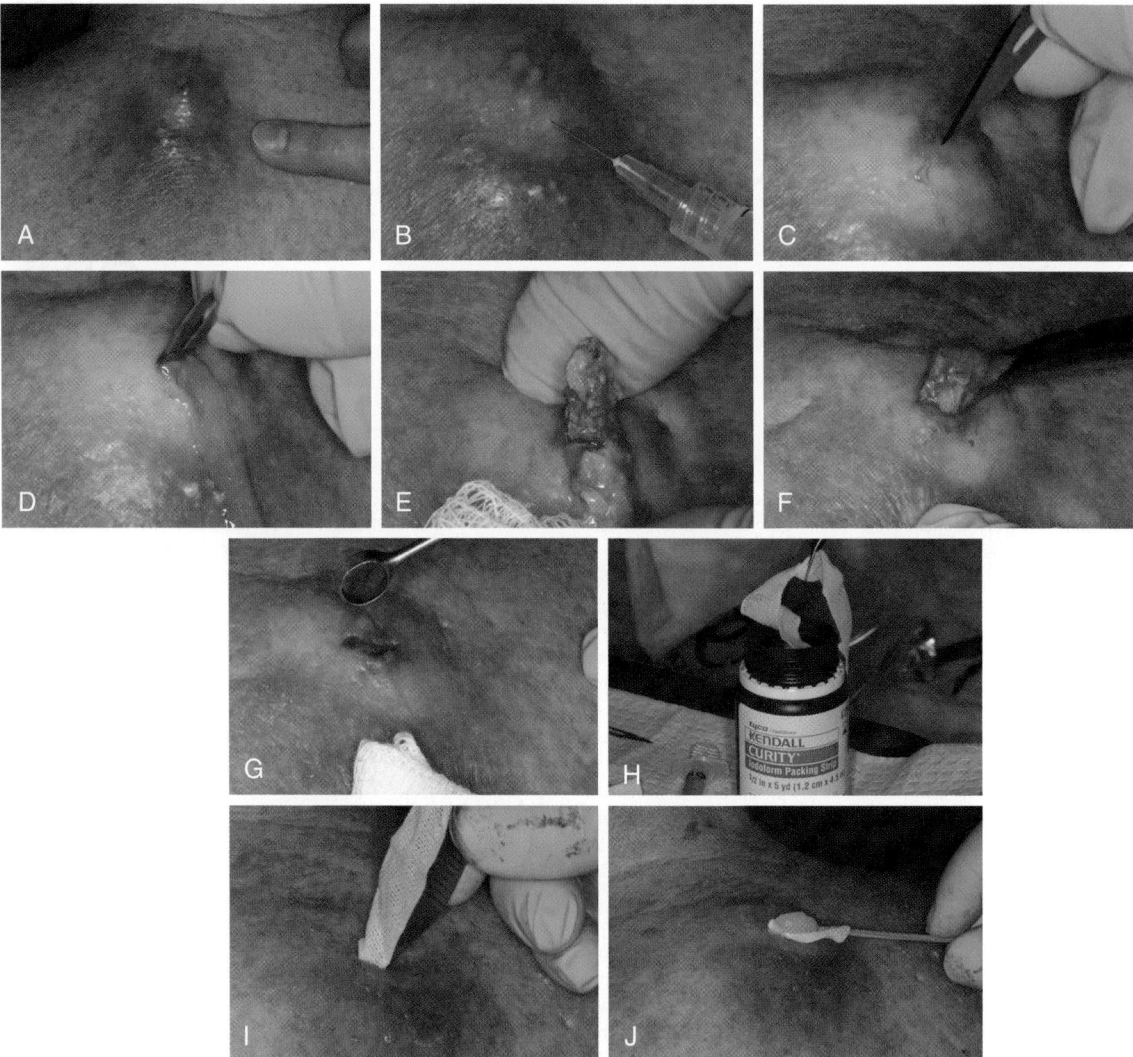

Fig. 192.1   (A) Large sebaceous cyst abscess of the back. (B) Injecting local anesthetic (2% lidocaine with epinephrine). May augment with field block if desired. (C) Incising abscess with No. 11 blade. (D) Purulent material is released from the lesion. (E) Apply digital pressure to evacuate contents of the infected cyst. (F) In the case of sebaceous cyst abscesses, the sac can often be grasped and removed using hemostats. It may be so necrotic in some lesions that it fragments, making removal more difficult. (G) In cases where total removal of the cyst sac is uncertain, a reusable dermal curette can be used to scrape the cavity and remove any residual sac. (H) Iodoform gauze (0.25 or 0.5 inch, depending on size of cavity) is used to pack the wound open. Premature closure will lead to recurrence of the abscess. Suturing the wound closed is contraindicated. (I) Insert the gauze using pickups without teeth. (J) Apply antibiotic ointment over the tail of the iodoform gauze to prevent the outer dressing from sticking to it.

TECHNIQUE

1. Prepare the abscess area with antiseptic solution (e.g., alcohol, povidone-iodine, or chlorhexidine). The clinician should observe universal blood and body fluid precautions including protective eyewear.
2. Administer local anesthetic; consider a field block (see Chapter 7, Peripheral Nerve Blocks and Field Blocks) or a ring block around the entire lesion to allow for an adequate incision to be made. Avoid infiltration of the abscess cavity; rather, concentrate on anesthetizing the perimeter of the tissue around the abscess. Injecting into the abscess cavity will not provide anesthesia, instead it will raise the pressure inside, possibly causing it to burst and spray or to spray when incised. More anesthetic than usual may be needed to relieve pain because local anesthetics usually work poorly in the acidic milieu of an abscess. Alternatively, diphenhydramine 10 to 25 mg can be injected into the area for anesthesia. Dilute a 50-mg (1-mL) vial in a syringe with 4 mL of normal saline (Fig. 192.1A–B). Cryocautery can also be used to chill or freeze the roof of the abscess. This can be performed

with a nitrous oxide unit, liquid nitrogen, or ethyl chloride. The incision is then made through the cooled skin, which is now anesthetized.

EDITOR'S NOTE: Lidocaine will nearly always be adequate, but larger volumes may be needed.

3. Make a sufficiently wide incision with a pointed No. 11 blade to allow drainage of the abscess cavity and to prevent premature closure of the incision. If a large abscess is present, a 1-cm incision is usually large enough. Make the incision in or following the skin lines. Recurrence of the abscess is most often due to an inadequate incision and premature closure of the incision (see Fig. 192.1C–D). Purulent material can squirt out, especially if digital pressure is applied. Protective glasses and other universal precautions such as a face shield are suggested.
4. If a culture is obtained, it should be from the abscess cavity and not from the superficial skin over the abscess. Alternatively, the abscess cavity can be aspirated with a large-bore (18-gauge) needle before the incision is made. The aspirated contents can then

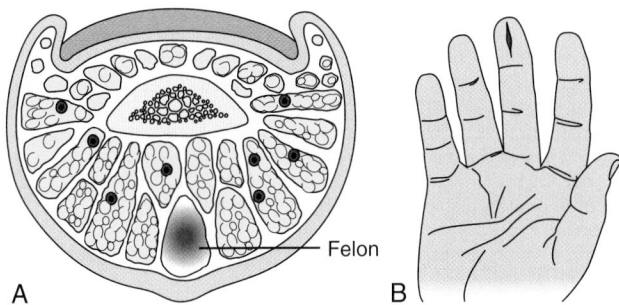

Fig. 192.2 (A) Anatomic cross section of the distal phalanx, showing the numerous fascial septa and a felon. (B) Incision of a felon. Incision should be in the longitudinal digital midline and should not cross a flexor crease.

be sent for the appropriate cultures in more complicated cases. This is rarely helpful in routine superficial abscesses.

5. Apply external pressure to express all pus (see Fig. 192.1E). The abscess cavity should also be thoroughly explored with a sterile cotton-tipped applicator or with hemostats. Attempts should be made to break down any walled-off pockets or possible septa (see Fig. 192.1F). If the lesion began as a cyst, a small reusable dermal curette can be used to curette the cavity in the hope of removing all of the sac (see Fig. 192.1G). (Disposable curettes are often too sharp and may cause excessive damage.) A residual sac can lead to a recurrent cyst. (See Chapter 13, Approach to Various Skin Lesions, for a minimally invasive technique for removing a sebaceous cyst.) The cavity can be packed with a Penrose drain or with packing material, preferably iodoform gauze. The length and width depend on abscess size. A small "tail" of gauze should be left protruding from the wound for drainage. Apply an ointment over the wound to prevent the gauze from sticking to the overlying dressing and being inadvertently removed when the dressing is changed (see Fig. 192.1H–J).

6. Depending on the location and the size of the abscess, the gauze can be removed slowly over several weeks. Slowly advancing the packing will ensure that the wound does not close off too soon; use of packing decreases the recurrence rate. The packing material can be changed daily, but it is painful and there is no real advantage to changing it. There may be some advantage to changing it after 5 to 7 days to reduce purulence and recheck the wound. For larger abscess cavities, leave the "wick" in for 4 weeks so that the abscess scars down from the inside. The patient can advance the drain every few days and cut off 2 inches at a time.

7. A sterile dressing can be applied over the area to collect discharge. This should be changed several times daily. Healing should progress from the inside out; that is, epithelialization of the abscess cavity should occur before healing of the incision site to minimize the chance of recurrence.

8. In patients with hidradenitis, I&D may traumatize the area and cause more long-term abscesses. However, the pain is usually so severe and acute with an abscess that I&D is necessary. Most patients with hidradenitis require long-term antibiotics, similar to patients with chronic acne. Some patients may require resection of all axillary or groin tissue involved.

9. A felon is an abscess in the distal tuft of the phalanx (Fig. 192.2A). A digital block serves best to anesthetize the area. Prepare with alcohol, povidone-iodine, or chlorhexidine. Incise the abscess in the midline parallel with the digit (see Fig. 192.2B). The large bilateral incisions of the past are now generally avoided. A small wick of iodoform gauze can be placed in the cavity for 24 hours. Many clinicians use antibiotics in patients with felons to cover for MRSA.

Usually I&D is sufficient to resolve an abscess. If cellulitis is present or the patient is at high risk for infection, an antibiotic can be used. It should cover MRSA.

COMPLICATIONS

If the packing is tight in the abscess cavity, the pain can be sufficient to warrant use of acetaminophen or nonsteroidal antiinflammatory drugs. Narcotics are rarely needed. I&D alone may provide sufficient pain relief from a tense abscess. Complications include the following:

- Recurrence
- Bleeding
- Scar or keloid
- Damage to adjacent structures
- Failure to resolve, causing cellulitis, or the progression to septicemia
- Formation of a fistula
- Osteomyelitis

An abscess in the palmar aspect of the hand can extend from superficial to deep tissue through the palmar fascia. Deep infection is suspected when the simple I&D fails to reduce the erythema, pain, pus, or swelling. More extensive surgical debridement, hospitalization, and intravenous antibiotics may be necessary in a patient with a deep palmar abscess, which is a surgical emergency.

A recurrent paronychia may require removal of the nail to resolve the infection (see Chapter 194, Ingrown Toenails, and Chapter 13, Approach to Various Skin Lesions). In addition, consider treatment for *Candida* infection in fingernail cases.

POSTPROCEDURE PATIENT PREPARATION

Some patients can be taught to change their own packing, replace the dressings, and advance the drain. Other patients may require a family member or home nurse visits or may have to return to the office to have this done. Patients should be instructed to watch for signs of recurrence of the abscess and for evidence of further infection such as cellulitis, and to notify the clinician immediately if any of the following occur:

- Re-collection of pus in the abscess
- Fever and chills
- Increased pain or redness
- Red streaks near the abscess
- Increased swelling in the area

In general, bathing and frequent changes of the overlying dressing are encouraged.

CPT/BILLING CODES

I&D CPT codes vary by complexity and site.

10040	Acne surgery
10060	I&D one abscess
10061	I&D multiple/complex abscess
10080	I&D pilonidal cyst, simple
10081	I&D complicated pilonidal cyst
10160	Aspirate abscess/cyst
10180	I&D complex/postoperative infection
19020	I&D deep, breast abscess
21501	I&D deep, neck or thorax
23030	I&D deep, shoulder
23930	I&D deep, arm/elbow
23931	I&D infected olecranon bursa
25028	I&D deep, forearm
26010	I&D simple, abscess finger
26011	I&D complex, finger (felon)
26990	I&D deep, hip area
26991	I&D infected bursa, hip area
27301	I&D deep abscess/bursa knee

27603	I&D deep, leg/ankle
28001	I&D bursa, foot
28002	I&D deep, foot
30000	I&D drainage abscess, nasal, internal approach
30020	I&D nasal septum abscess
40800	I&D vestibule mouth
40801	I&D complicated, mouth
41000	I&D lingual
41005	I&D sublingual (superficial)
41006	I&D sublingual, deep
41800	I&D gums
45005	I&D submucosal rectum abscess
46040	I&D perirectal abscess
46050	I&D superficial perianal abscess
54015	I&D deep, penis
54700	I&D epididymis
55000	Aspirate hydrocele
55100	I&D scrotal wall abscess
56405	I&D vulva
56420	I&D Bartholin abscess
67700	I&D eyelid abscess
69000	I&D abscess pinna
69005	I&D abscess, pinna, complicated
69020	I&D ear canal abscess

ICD-10-CM Diagnostic Codes

For ICD-10-CM diagnostic codes, look under "abscess" for specific site.

RECOMMENDED READING

Bobrow BJ, Pollack Jr CV, Gamble S, Seligson RA. Incision and drainage of cutaneous abscesses is not associated with bacteremia in afebrile adults. *Ann Emerg Med.* 1997;29:404–408.

Brooks I, Frazier EH. The aerobic and anaerobic bacteriology of perirectal abscesses. *J Clin Microbiol.* 1997;35:2974–2976.

Hankin A, Everett WW. Are antibiotics necessary after incision and drainage of a cutaneous abscess? *Ann Emerg Med.* 2007;50:49–51.

Moran GJ, Krishnadasan A, Gorwitz RJ, et al. Methicillin-resistant *S. aureus* infections among patients in the emergency department. *N Engl J Med.* 2006;355:666–674.

Nagle D, Rolandelli RH. Primary care office management of perianal and anal disease. *Prim Care.* 1996;23:609–620.

Ramakrishnan K, Salinas RC, Agudelo Higuita NI. Skin and soft tissue infections. *Am Fam Physician.* 2015;92(6):474–483.

Stulberg DL, Moran P. Incision and drainage. In: Usatine RP, Pfenninger JL, Stulberg DL, Small R, eds. *Dermatologic and Cosmetic Procedures in Office Practice.* Philadelphia: Elsevier; 2012:210–215.

Tuggy M, Garcia J. *Procedures Consult.* Incision and drainage of abscess. http://www.proceduresconsult.com/medical-procedures/incision-and-drainage-of-an-abscess-FM-006-procedure.aspx.

Usatine RP, Smith MA, Mayeaux EJ, et al., eds. *The Color Atlas of Family Medicine.* 2nd ed. New York: McGraw-Hill; 2013.

Yasuta M. Incision, draining and exteriorization techniques. In: Robinson JK, Hanke CW, Siegel DM, et al., eds. *Surgery of the Skin: Procedural Dermatology.* 3rd ed. Philadelphia: Elsevier; 2015.

CHAPTER 193

SUBUNGUAL HEMATOMA EVACUATION

Rebecca Beach

Injuries to the nail bed and fingertip are the most common injuries to the upper extremity. Most frequent among these is a subungual hematoma, which results from a direct blow to the fingernail or a squeezing-type injury to the distal finger, causing bleeding into the space between the nail bed and the fingernail itself. Intense throbbing pain can result from the pressure generated by such a hematoma. Evacuation of the hematoma by drilling (trephination) can produce significant relief from the pain and can be performed safely in the outpatient setting. Toenails can be treated in the same fashion. Evacuation of a hematoma may or may not prevent the eventual spontaneous avulsion of the nail that results from nail injury. Patients should be made aware of this possibility. Radiographs may be necessary, and, if a fracture is documented, antibiotics may be considered because this would then essentially be an open fracture. (In the two studies that evaluated this situation, no infections occurred, so an underlying fracture should not contraindicate trephination.)

INDICATION

A visible, painful hematoma beneath the involved nail (Fig. 193.1).

CONTRAINDICATIONS

- Crushed or fractured nail bed or angulated, displaced, unstable, or intraarticular phalanx fracture, or phalanx fracture that involves more than 30% of articular surface (these should be referred to a hand surgeon).
- Hematomas involving greater than 50% of the nail may indicate laceration of the underlying nail bed. (Removal of the nail and repair of the laceration are recommended by some experts to avoid a posttraumatic nail deformity. Others recommend leaving the nail in place as a splint, especially if the nail margins and nail are intact. The patient should be warned that the nail may be permanently deformed unless the nail bed is examined and treated. There is also the chance that even if the bed is examined and treated, it may be permanently deformed.)

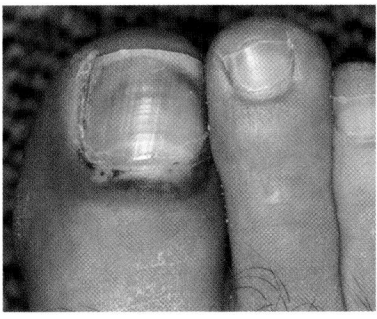

Fig. 193.1 Subungual hematoma.

EQUIPMENT

- Open flame (e.g., alcohol lamp, Bunsen burner, matches, cigarette lighter) or equivalent, metal paperclip, and forceps or hemostat
- *Or* battery-operated cautery unit
- *Or* 18-gauge needle or No. 11 scalpel
- *Or* automatic drill device (Dremel tool, dental burr, or Path-Former device)
- *Or* radiofrequency or electrocautery unit with needle or pointed electrode
- *Or* extra-fine 29-gauge insulin needles with syringes (work best for small hematomas or when the nails are very thick and difficult to penetrate)
- Equipment necessary to observe universal blood and body fluid precautions
- Antibacterial soap or sterile skin preparation (e.g., povidone-iodine, chlorhexidine) and sterile field, if available

TECHNIQUE

1. Wash the digit as thoroughly as possible with an antibacterial soap or use sterile skin preparation (if available) to decrease the possibility of contamination of the hematoma and subsequent infection. If available, the finger can then be placed in a sterile field.
2. Consider a digital or ring block with lidocaine without epinephrine because any pressure on the area can be painful (see Chapter 7, Peripheral Nerve Blocks and Field Blocks).
3. Create a hole in the nail directly over the center of the hematoma to allow decompression.
   - *Paperclip method.* Partially straighten a metal paperclip, grasp it with the forceps, and heat it over an open flame or equivalent. It should turn bright red or orange when hot enough. Place the heated clip firmly on the nail, allowing it to melt the tissue for a few seconds until the nail is completely perforated (Fig. 193.2). The clinician should feel the nail "give" as it is perforated; as soon as that happens, avoid going any deeper which might damage the nail bed. The clinician should be prepared to avoid any spray as the blood is expressed, sometimes it is under pressure.
   - *Cautery method.* In similar fashion, apply battery cautery tip to the nail and create a hole in the nail bed (Fig. 193.3). Some electrocautery units may work, but there is often too much keratin in the nail for it to be effective.
   - *Drill method.* Twist a large-bore needle or scalpel between your fingers gently in one place to create a 1- to 2-mm hole over the central area of the hematoma. A 2-mm, sharp, disposable punch biopsy unit can also be tried. Alternatively, a drill device (Dremel tool, dental burr, or PathFormer device) may be used. The only drawback to this method is that any pressure on the nail can cause pain, so proceed gently. It is also

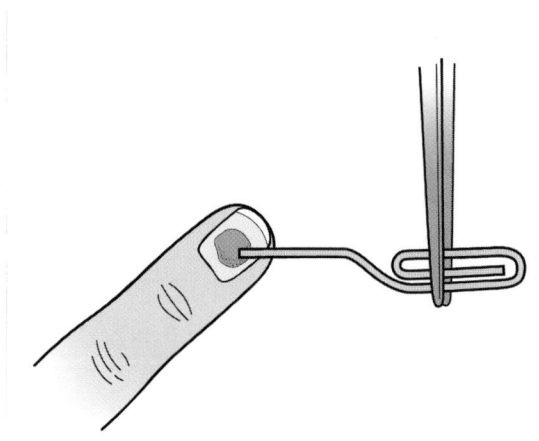

Fig. 193.2 Heated paperclip is placed directly over the hematoma to create a perforation of the nail.

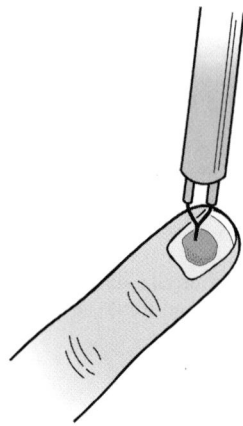

Fig. 193.3 Cautery unit may be used to perforate the nail and evacuate the subungual hematoma.

not as easy to feel the "give" of the nail as it is penetrated, so proceed slowly while observing for signs of blood being evacuated. The PathFormer device measures electrical resistance within the nail and can sense when penetration has occurred; it then stops and retracts.

4. The extra-fine 29-gauge insulin syringes method is an alternative to drilling a hole. After trimming the nail back as far as possible, instead of going through the nail, insert the needle beneath and parallel to the nail plate. Advance to the distal edge of the hematoma and aspirate or drain it.

5. The color of the nail usually returns to normal color almost immediately if the procedure has been successful. Multiple holes or attempts at drainage may be necessary to evacuate the hematoma completely. Blood usually remains liquid for 24 to 36 hours after a hematoma is formed, so it should be able to be expressed easily.

In the first two procedures mentioned, the heated tip is cooled by the hematoma on perforation of the nail, thereby preventing injury to the nail bed, especially if the clinician stops as soon as the nail "gives." This effect is maximal in the center of the hematoma, where the distance between nail and tissue is greatest. Similarly, with the drill technique, the tip of any drill/needle/scalpel will not touch sensitive tissue if it is placed in the center of the hematoma. The hole created in the nail should be of sufficient size so as not to close off within a few hours (adequate size is 1 to 2 mm). Elevation of the finger, cool compresses, and a simple dry bandage are recommended during the first 12 hours. Use of antibiotic ointment can serve dual purposes—to moisturize (minimizing blood clotting so that the hematoma will drain maximally and prevent blood from adhering to the bandage) and to minimize infection. Because patient anxiety can be severe, passing the needle through the fibers of a 4 × 4 gauze so that the patient cannot visualize it may make the drilling procedure more tolerable for a child.

COMPLICATIONS

- Recurrence (although a hot paper clip is easy to use, hematomas often recur and may need to be drained again)
- Infection of the remaining hematoma
- Pain
- Inadvertently lacerating the nail bed
- Not recognizing a fracture beneath the hematoma

CAUTIONS

- Neither the drill method nor the two heat methods by themselves should be painful, but the hematoma itself may be exquisitely tender, so the digit should be grasped gently, proximal to the injury.
- Either a local anesthetic or ethyl chloride may be used before these methods, if desired, to decrease pain. However, ethyl chloride is flammable and should not be used during or immediately before the cautery method or very close to the flame of the paperclip method. Holding the area in ice water is safer. Consider a digital block.
- Artificial acrylic nails may also be flammable.

CPT/BILLING CODES

11740	Subungual hematoma evacuation

ICD-10-CM DIAGNOSTIC CODES

S60.011X-S60.159X   Contusion finger(s) (nail) (subungual)

Add appropriate seventh character: A = initial, D = subsequent, S = sequela.

Acknowledgment

The editors recognize the contributions by James F. Peggs, MD, to this chapter in previous editions of this text.

SUPPLIERS

(See contact information available at www.expertconsult.com.)

Battery-operated cautery
Advanced Meditech International (AMI)

NOTE: Most medical suppliers also carry battery-operated cautery equipment.

Bovie Disposable Cautery
Delasco LLC
PathFormer
Path Scientific, LLC
Surgitron and Battery Unit
Ellman Cynosure

ONLINE RESOURCES

See patient education and patient consent forms available at www. expertconsult.com.

RECOMMENDED READING

Roberts JR, Custalow CB, Thomsen TW, eds. *Roberts and Hedges' Clinical Procedures in Emergency Medicine*. 6th ed. Philadelphia: Elsevier; 2014.

Salter SA, Ciocon DH, Gowrishankar TR, Kimball AB. Controlled nail trephination for subungual hematoma evacuation. *Am J Emerg Med.* 2006;24:875–877.

Simon RR, Wolgin M. Subungual hematoma: association with occult laceration requiring repair. *Am J Emerg Med.* 1986;5:302–304.

Usatine RP, Smith MA, Mayeaux EJ, et al., eds. *The Color Atlas of Family Medicine*. 2nd ed. New York: McGraw-Hill; 2013.

Van Beek AL, Kassan MA, Adson MH, Dale V. Management of acute fingernail injuries. *Hand Clin.* 1990;6:23–35.

Zook EG. Nail bed injuries. *Hand Clin.* 1985;1:701–716.

CHAPTER 194

INGROWN TOENAILS

Madelyn Pollock

Ingrown toenails usually present with pain, redness, swelling, and sometimes discharge. It is not uncommon for patients to have attempted self-remedies. Often, the irritation is long-standing enough to have caused granulation tissue to form. In essence, the nail acts as a foreign body, like a wooden splinter or thorn, and must be removed to allow for healing. The great toe is usually the only toe involved, and either the medial or lateral border of the nail may be affected.

Fig. 194.1 is an algorithm for the suggested treatment of an ingrown toenail.

Removal of the toenail, either partial or total, remains the definitive treatment for bothersome ingrown nails. For recurrent episodes, ablation of the germinal matrix tissue can be used to prevent regrowth of the nail. Permanent destruction can be performed by using chemicals or radiofrequency energy.

EDITOR'S NOTE: Repeated Cochrane reviews have concluded that surgical interventions are more effective than nonsurgical ones in preventing recurrence of an ingrowing nail. Application of phenol is probably more effective in the prevention of recurrence and regrowth. None of the postoperative treatments used, such as antibiotics or topical preparations, showed any significant difference when looking at infection rates, pain, or healing time.

ANATOMY

Fig. 194.2 illustrates the nail bed anatomy.

INDICATIONS

- Onychocryptosis (ingrown nail)
- Onychomycosis (fungal infection of the nail) with significant pain: medical therapy is necessary to prevent recurrence of the fungal infection
- Chronic recurrent paronychia (inflammation of the nail fold)
- Onychogryphosis (deformed, curved nail)

For a first occurrence, it is reasonable to remove only the offending portion of the nail and allow regrowth while educating the patient to correct all offending practices such as overtrimming nails and wearing tight-fitting shoes. If an ingrown nail recurs, consider permanent ablation of the portion of nail matrix causing the problem; some consider this to be indicated.

CONTRAINDICATIONS

- Allergy to local anesthetics (see Chapter 6, Local and Topical Anesthetic Complications).
- Bleeding diathesis.
- Diabetes mellitus and peripheral vascular disease are relative contraindications and should be considered on a case-by-case basis.
- Pregnant patients should not have phenol ablation.

EQUIPMENT AND SUPPLIES

- A 5- or 10-mL syringe with long (1.5-inch) needle (25 or 27 gauge).
- Nonsterile surgical gloves and equipment necessary to follow universal blood and body fluid precautions.
- Local anesthetic generally without epinephrine (e.g., 2% lidocaine with or without sodium bicarbonate buffer to decrease the sting; see Chapter 5, Local Anesthesia). Recent research does not confirm the previous concerns that epinephrine might cause excess vasoconstriction in the digits. However, with patients at high risk, such as those with long-standing diabetes or severe peripheral vascular disease, it may be best to avoid it.
- Narrow Locke periosteal elevator (nail elevator; Fig. 194.3).
- Sterile scissors with straight blades (or an English anvil nail splitter [Fig. 194.4] or miniblade with wedge tip).
- Wide rubber band, small Penrose drain, donut digital tourniquet (Ellman Corp.; Fig. 194.5), or a portable blood pressure cuff (tourniquets are optional but can be very helpful). A surgical glove can also be used to encircle the proximal toe and tied in a knot.
- Two straight hemostats.
- Silver nitrate sticks for cautery of granulation tissue (optional). Best to curette this tissue off with a reusable dermal curette.
- Alcohol swabs.
- Antiseptic solution (e.g., povidone-iodine, chlorhexidine).
- Monsel solution to control any possible bleeding after the tourniquet is removed.
- Sterile gauze and tubular gauze dressing.
- Antibiotic ointment (Polysporin or Bacitracin).
- Phenol solution (88%) and isopropyl alcohol for permanent ablation of the nail if desired.
- As an alternative to phenol, the Ellman Surgitron (radiofrequency unit) with specially designed, Teflon-insulated matrix ablation tips (less inflammation and excellent results; see Chapter 25, Radiofrequency Surgery [Modern Electrosurgery]).

PREPROCEDURE PATIENT EDUCATION AND CONSENT

See the patient education form available at www.expertconsult.com.

A *signed* consent is not mandatory but the patient must be well informed of the procedure and the intended outcome. A patient education handout that explains the nature of ingrown nails is helpful. The nail acts as a foreign body, like a wooden splinter or a thorn, and at least a portion of the nail must be removed to allow healing. Before beginning the procedure, be sure that the patient understands that the provision of anesthesia will be uncomfortable, but after that there should be minimal pain. With use of local anesthesia, inform the patient that if there is any residual pain, it is usually of a dull, achy nature as opposed to a sharp pain. There is no guarantee that removing the portion of ingrown nail will resolve the problem, but generally it will if the nails are cared for properly afterward. The major benefit to removing the toenail (or a portion of it) is pain relief, with the secondary benefit of allowing the body to heal the inflamed area.

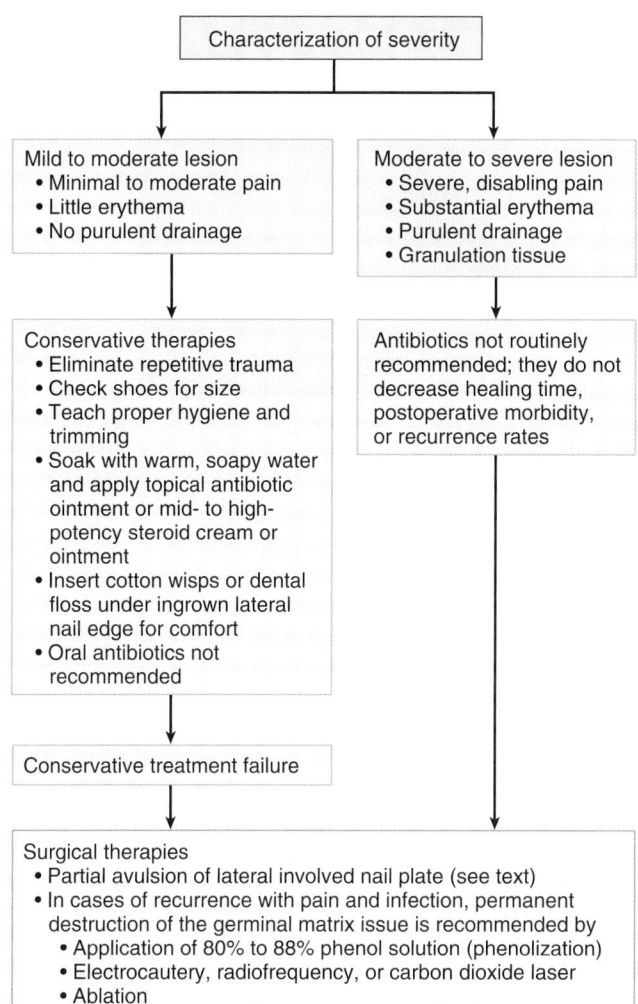

Fig. 194.1 refers to the algorithm below:

```
                    Characterization of severity
                              |
          _____
         |                                        |
  Mild to moderate lesion              Moderate to severe lesion
  • Minimal to moderate pain           • Severe, disabling pain
  • Little erythema                    • Substantial erythema
  • No purulent drainage               • Purulent drainage
         |                             • Granulation tissue
         |                                        |
  Conservative therapies               Antibiotics not routinely
  • Eliminate repetitive trauma        recommended; they do not
  • Check shoes for size               decrease healing time,
  • Teach proper hygiene and           postoperative morbidity,
    trimming                           or recurrence rates
  • Soak with warm, soapy water
    and apply topical antibiotic
    ointment or mid- to high-
    potency steroid cream or
    ointment
  • Insert cotton wisps or dental
    floss under ingrown lateral
    nail edge for comfort
  • Oral antibiotics not
    recommended
         |
  Conservative treatment failure
         |
  Surgical therapies
  • Partial avulsion of lateral involved nail plate (see text)
  • In cases of recurrence with pain and infection, permanent
    destruction of the germinal matrix issue is recommended by
    • Application of 80% to 88% phenol solution (phenolization)
    • Electrocautery, radiofrequency, or carbon dioxide laser
    • Ablation
```

Fig. 194.1 Algorithm for a suggested approach to the patient with an ingrown toenail. (Modified from Heidelbaugh JJ, Lee H. Management of the ingrown toenail. *Am Fam Physician*. 2009;79:303–308.)

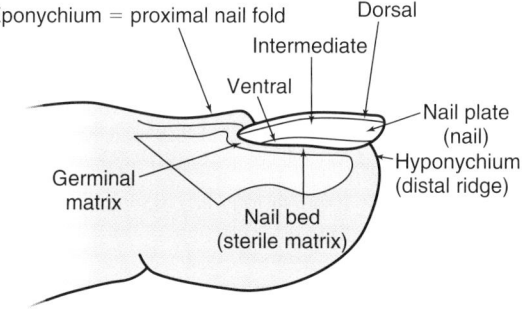

Fig. 194.2 Nail bed anatomy and terminology. Also see Chapter 24, Nail Bed Repair.

PROCEDURE

NOTE: Nonsterile gloves may be used in this procedure.

Removal of Partial or Full Nail

1. With the patient in the supine position, prepare the toe with antiseptic solution. If the patient has significant discomfort, anesthesia (step 2) can precede this step for patient comfort. (Almost everyone will benefit from anesthesia.)

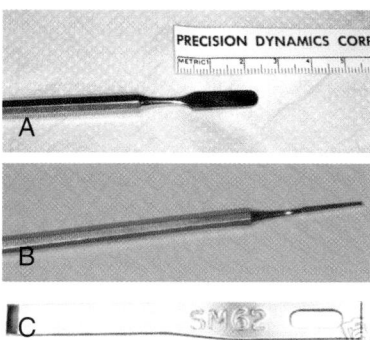

Fig. 194.3 Locke periosteal elevator. (A) Front view. (B) Side view. (C) Miniblade with wedge tip. (Courtesy John L. Pfenninger, MD, The Medical Procedures Center, Midland, MI.)

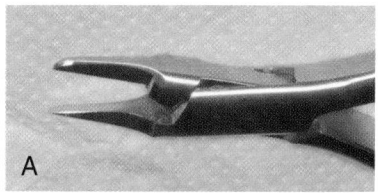

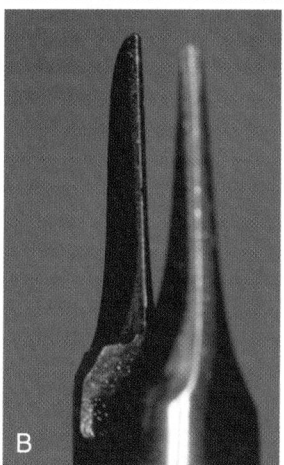

Fig. 194.4 Nail splitter. (A) Flat wedge-shaped jaw seen on bottom. (B) Beveled jaw on top. (Courtesy John L. Pfenninger, MD, The Medical Procedures Center, Midland, MI.)

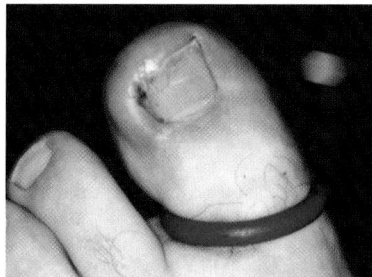

Fig. 194.5 The Ellman digital tourniquet. (Courtesy John L. Pfenninger, MD, The Medical Procedures Center, Midland, MI.)

2. Administer a digital block as described in Chapter 7, Peripheral Nerve Blocks and Field Blocks. During this and subsequent steps, universal blood and body fluid precautions should be followed. Adequate time must be allowed for anesthesia to take effect (5 to 10 minutes).

EDITOR'S NOTE: In a busy practice where many procedures are being performed, it may be worthwhile to see or interview

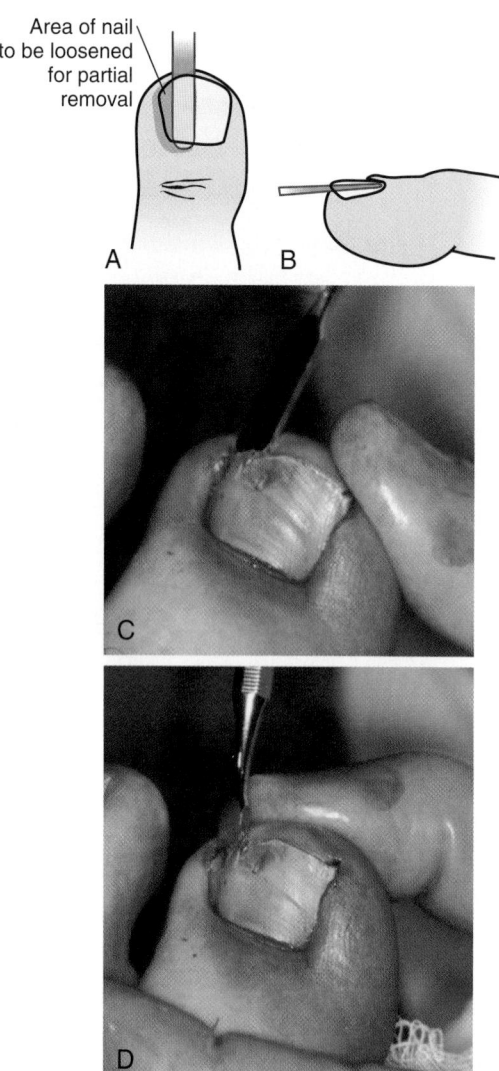

Area of nail to be loosened for partial removal

Fig. 194.6 (A) Periosteal elevator advanced all the way under the proximal nail fold. (B) Lateral view. The elevator is advanced with upward pressure on the nail and forward motion until more pressure is felt under the nail fold. (C) Inserting the elevator. (D) The instrument has been fully inserted, freeing up the lateral portion of the nail from the nail bed. (C–D, Courtesy John L. Pfenninger, MD, The Medical Procedures Center, Midland, MI.)

another patient while waiting for this anesthesia to take effect. In the absence of peripheral artery disease, a tourniquet can also be left in place for a few minutes without untoward effects.

3. Apply a tourniquet if desired. Options include the following:
   - Use a straight hemostat to firmly secure a wide rubber band or Penrose drain around the base of the toe.
   - Apply a blood pressure cuff at the calf so that it will not affect the operative field. To use this method, place the cuff around the calf, elevate the foot to about a 45-degree angle at the hip, and, after 1 to 2 minutes of elevation, raise the cuff pressure to above systolic, lock the cuff it so it stays inflated, and then lower the foot to the operative field. Maintain the pressure until the procedure is completed.
   - The Ellman donut tourniquets (see Fig. 194.5) are disposable and come in various sizes. After the procedure, simply cut them with scissors to remove them.
   - A surgical glove can also be stretched to encircle the proximal toe and tied in a knot.

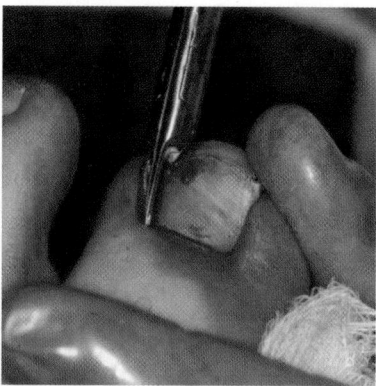

Fig. 194.7 Using the nail splitter to "cut" through the nail. Flat jaw is down, beveled side is up. (Courtesy John L. Pfenninger, MD, The Medical Procedures Center, Midland, MI.)

EDITOR'S NOTE: Tight application of the tourniquet may provide additional and significant anesthesia by placing pressure on the digital and surrounding nerves.

4. Identify the portion of the nail to be removed, which would be at least 20% to 25% of the nail.
5. When anesthesia has been achieved (5 to 10 minutes), loosen and lift the nail to be removed from the nail bed by using the flat, rounded blade of the scissors, a single jaw of a straight hemostat, or a narrow periosteal elevator. The elevator works best to decrease the likelihood of injury to the nail bed (see Fig. 194.3). Introduce and advance the instrument with continued upward pressure against the nail plate and away from the nail bed to minimize injury and bleeding (Fig. 194.6). It is important to completely free the proximal nail at its base under the nail fold to allow removal and to expose the germinal tissue of the nail bed. Push forward gently—the elevator moves easily when it is under the nail. Resistance will be felt when the proximal end of the nail plate has been loosened sufficiently. Elevate the entire nail plate in this fashion if the entire nail is to be removed. If an English nail splitter is used, slide the flat jaw that is wedge shaped under the nail. Since it has the shape of a wedge, it can be used to gently lift the nail itself, often without an elevator.
6. For partial nail removal, scissors or a nail splitter (see Fig. 194.4) should be used to completely split the nail 5 to 6 mm in from the lateral or medial margin in a longitudinal direction (Fig. 194.7). A miniblade with a wedge at the tip also works well. Include the base of the nail. This requires introducing your cutting instrument beneath the proximal nail fold. Take care to protect the nail fold from damage when you are making this part of the incision.

EDITOR'S NOTE: If no surrounding skin is damaged or cut, there will often be very little bleeding or oozing of blood, even after the tourniquet is removed.

7. Grasp the portion of the nail to be removed lengthwise with a straight hemostat and remove it, using a steady, strong pulling motion with a simultaneous upward twist of the hand away from the affected side (Fig. 194.8). This twisting action ensures that the offending nail spicule will be rolled out from beneath the affected nail margin instead of rolling over it. If the entire nail is to be removed, the nail may be removed in two halves or in its entirety after a thorough loosening and lifting of the nail. In removing the entire nail, the forceps should apply lift and distal traction on the nail as it separates from the nail bed. Indications for total removal include onychomycosis, which can cause painful pincer nails, or perhaps cases in which both the medial and lateral aspects of the nail are ingrown (Fig. 194.9).
8. Remove all granulation tissue by grasping with hemostats and pulling. Light curettage with a reusable dermal curette

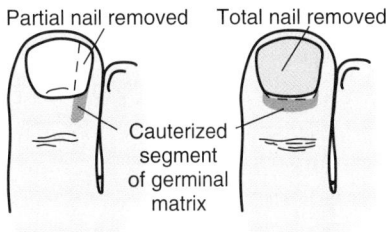

Fig. 194.11 Area of nail bed to be cauterized in partial *(left)* and total permanent nail removal (matrixectomy) *(right)*.

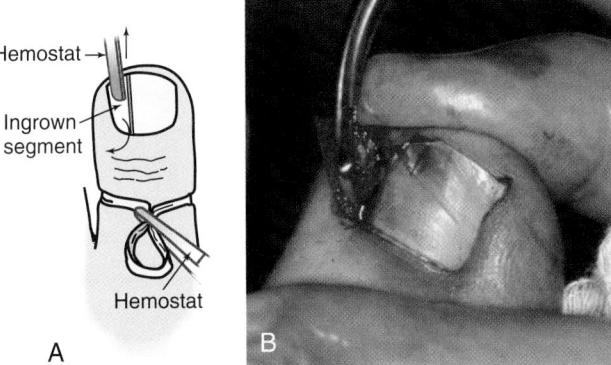

Fig. 194.8 Technique for nail removal after nail has been elevated and split. (A-B) Grasp that portion of the nail to be removed lengthwise with a straight hemostat and remove it using a steady pulling motion with a simultaneous upward twist of the hand away from the affected side. (B, Courtesy John L. Pfenninger, MD, The Medical Procedures Center, Midland, MI.)

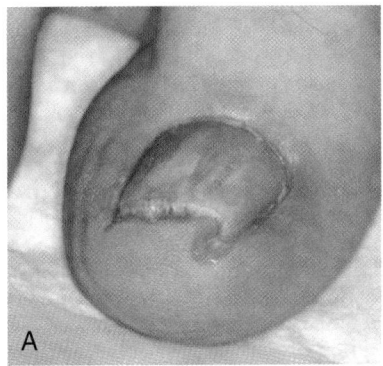

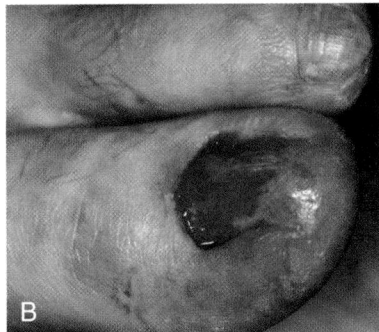

Fig. 194.9 Complete removal of the toenail. (A) Onychomycosis. (B) Appearance after the nail has been removed. (Courtesy John L. Pfenninger, MD, The Medical Procedures Center, Midland, MI.)

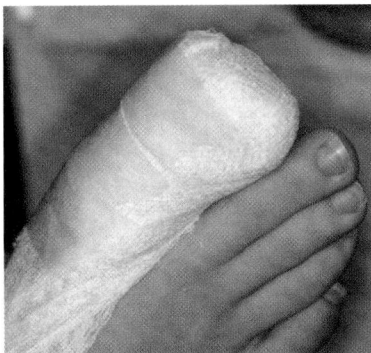

Fig. 194.10 A compression dressing is applied after most toenail procedures. (Courtesy John L. Pfenninger, MD, The Medical Procedures Center, Midland, MI.)

(not as sharp as the disposables) removes any residual tissue from the nail groove. Without a tourniquet there will be significant bleeding during this portion of the procedure, especially if there is significant granulation tissue. Application of silver nitrate or Monsel solution to the exposed nail bed will control bleeding and, with silver nitrate, discourage persistence of granulation tissue.

9. If ablation is to be performed, complete that portion at this step before the tourniquet is removed and the wound dressed (see later discussion).
10. Remove any tourniquet used.
11. Observe the area for hemostasis, using pressure as necessary. When hemostasis is obtained, dress with antibiotic ointment, nonadherent gauze pad, and tube gauze (Fig. 194.10).

Nail Bed Ablation (Matrixectomy)

If recurrent regrowth of the toenail with resulting pain or infection occurs, permanent ablation of the germinal tissue is recommended (matrixectomy).

Phenol Chemical Method

1. Remove total or partial nail as described previously. The area must be dry and not bleeding. Remove all granulation tissue.
2. Sponge the exposed nail bed dry with cotton swabs and then cauterize the germinal tissue, including that under the nail fold, by application of phenol on a cotton swab to the nail bed tissues (Fig. 194.11). It is important to achieve good hemostasis before this step so that the tissue is dry. Use caution to avoid phenol contact with normal skin. A skin hook can be helpful in elevating the skin fold from the nail matrix. Hold the phenol-dampened cotton swab in place for 3 minutes. Three separate 60-second applications with drying of the surface in between are also reported to be effective. The tissue will turn pale or gray at the area of application.
3. After 3 minutes, drip 70% isopropyl alcohol into the nail groove and swab the area to neutralize the phenol.

Radiofrequency Method

See Chapter 25, Radiofrequency Surgery (Modern Electrosurgery).

The radiofrequency method of ablation is quick and easy. Although formal studies have not been performed, it is thought that radiofrequency causes markedly less pain, swelling, and discharge than other methods. It is difficult to control liquid agents, and they tend to destroy more tissue than desired.

1. Remove whole or partial nail as described previously.
2. Place antenna lead under the heel of foot.
3. Turn unit to "Hemo-part rect" (hemostasis/coagulation setting) and set the power at 2 to 3.
4. Insert wide or narrow insulated matrixectomy tip over nail matrix, under the eponychium as far as it will go, with the insulated side up (Fig. 194.12). These electrodes are insulated with Teflon on one surface to prevent damage to the undersurface of

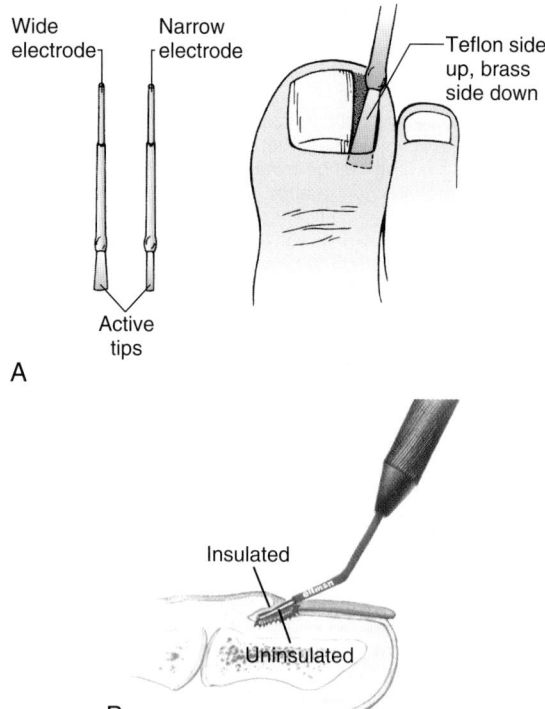

Wide electrode
Narrow electrode
Teflon side up, brass side down

Active tips

A

Insulated
Uninsulated

B

Fig. 194.12 Application of nail matrixectomy electrode with Teflon-coated side up: (A) top and (B) lateral views. The lateral 25% of the nail has been removed.

the proximal nail fold while ablating the nail matrix with the uninsulated surface beneath. A slight upward pressure should be exerted against the undersurface of the nail fold to ensure that no pressure is exerted on the underlying matrix. The field must be free of blood. For proper effect, there should be a slight gap between electrode and matrix.

5. Apply power and slowly withdraw the electrode, pulling distally. Contact should last for only 1 to 2 seconds, and a sizzling sound should be heard. This step can be repeated once or twice over the same area after a 15-second cooling period. If the entire nail matrix is to be ablated, multiple applications are necessary with side-to-side placements of the electrode; slight overlapping should not be a problem. Caution: two to three passes (maximum) over the same tissue area are sufficient. Avoid overtreatment. The matrix is very thin and bone lies immediately beneath it. Overtreatment can cause burns with prolonged healing times of up to 6 to 8 weeks. It is often easier to use the narrower electrode because the power level can be set lower and it affords better control. Side-by-side applications may then be needed even for partial nail removal.

Other Methods

Sodium hydroxide (10% solution) and CO$_2$ laser are also described in the literature for use in matrixectomy. Sodium hydroxide is applied similarly to phenol and is thought by some to decrease postoperative drainage and speed healing compared with the phenol method. It is not as commonly used in the United States as phenol. The CO$_2$ laser requires special equipment and training and is usually operated by dermatologists or podiatrists.

Once either partial or complete ablation has been accomplished, apply antibiotic ointment to the nail bed, cover with a sterile gauze pressure dressing, remove the tourniquet, and wrap with a tubular gauze dressing. Coban, CoFlex, and other similar self-adherent dressings provide a comfortable pressure wrap that holds the dressing in place.

SAMPLE OPERATIVE REPORT

Informed consent obtained: Yes_____ No_____
Site (circle one): Left Right Medial Lateral great toe
Anesthesia: Digital block _____% Lidocaine without epi ____mL
Tourniquet used: Yes_____ No_____
Nail removal (circle one): Complete Partial
Granulation tissue removed: Yes_____ No_____ Cautery Y Chem/elect N
Ablation performed: No_____ Yes_____ (Phenol radioablation [tip _____ wide _____ narrow, setting _____])
Other_____
Hemostasis was obtained.
The wound was dressed with antibiotic ointment and covered with a sterile dressing. The patient was given oral and written instructions in postoperative management. The patient tolerated the procedure without complications.

COMMON ERRORS

- Inadequate anesthesia resulting in patient discomfort. Ensure full anesthesia before starting procedure. Anesthetizing the toe generally requires 6 to 10 mL of lidocaine.
- Prolonged use of tourniquet resulting in ischemia. This can be avoided by foregoing use of the tourniquet in patients with possible decreased circulation and limiting the time under tourniquet pressure.
- Laceration of nail bed during lifting or splitting of the nail. This can result in difficult-to-control bleeding at the nail edge and scarring, leading to deformity of the nail when it grows back. Position any cutting instrument used such that the nail bed is protected during the incision. It can help to use the miniblade (also called a *Beaver* or *wedge blade*), which has no sharp edge on the portion of the blade facing the nail bed.
- Retained portion of nail results in persistent pain after procedure. Avoid this by careful examination of the nail fold and the removed portion of the nail after the procedure. A feathery edge of nail where it abuts the nail growth plate demonstrates that all the nail was removed. If necessary, explore the area and remove retained fragments.

COMPLICATIONS

- Infections (treat with soaking and appropriate antibiotics)
- Bleeding (generally controlled with pressure)
- Regrowth of nail and return of symptoms (regrowth rate after phenol cauterization is 4% to 25%; for radiofrequency, <5%)
- Excessive tissue destruction with radiofrequency unit, leading to prolonged healing time and possible osteomyelitis
- Ischemic damage to toe or loss of toe in patients with peripheral arterial disease if tourniquet is used or left in place too long

POSTPROCEDURE PATIENT EDUCATION AND MANAGEMENT

The foot should be rested and preferably elevated during the first 12 to 24 hours. Because phenol ablates the nerve endings of the nail plate, pain should be absent when phenol is used. There is minimal pain with the radiofrequency unit. Nonsteroidal antiinflammatory drugs or acetaminophen may be taken for discomfort.

The dressing should be changed in 12 to 24 hours, at which point ambulation can be encouraged; however, vigorous exercise should be avoided for 1 week. The toe should be washed with soap and water at least twice daily (depending on soiling) until healed. Topical antibiotic ointment should be applied and the area kept clean until healed. Tell the patient to expect a sterile exudate from the nail bed for several weeks. Explaining that the wound will "heal like a burn" can help patients understand that the exudate is not an indication of infection. Emphasize proper nail hygiene to prevent further recurrences (Fig. 194.13).

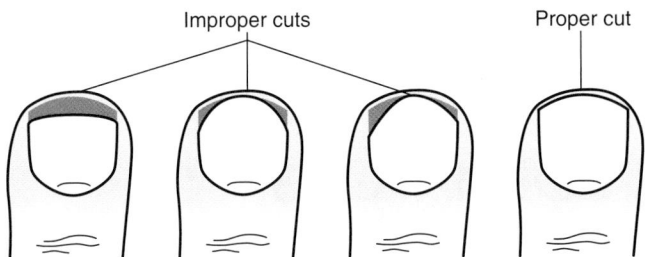

Fig. 194.13 Examples of improper and proper nail care. Trim the nail flat and straight across and not too short. (Modified from Heidelbaugh JJ, Lee H. Management of the ingrown toenail. *Am Fam Physician.* 2009;79:303–308.)

CPT/BILLING CODES

11730	Nail removal, partial or complete
11732	Avulsion, each additional nail
11750	Permanent nail removal (matrixectomy), partial or complete

ICD-10-CM DIAGNOSTIC CODES

B35.1	Onychomycosis
L60.0	Ingrown toenail
L60.2	Onychogryphosis

SUPPLIERS

(See contact information available at www.expertconsult.com.)

Toe tourniquets and Surgitron radiofrequency unit (see Chapter 25, Radiofrequency Surgery [Modern Electrosurgery])
Ellman

Other equipment can be obtained from most medical suppliers, such as Miltex and Delasco.

Acknowledgment

The editors recognize the contributions of James E. Peggs, MD, to this chapter in a previous edition of this text.

RECOMMENDED READING

Bos AMC, van Tilburg MW, van Sorge AA, Klinkenbijl JH. Randomized clinical trial of surgical technique and local antibiotics for ingrowing toenail. *Br J Surg.* 2007;94:292–296.

DeLauro NM, DeLauro TM. Onychocryptosis. *Clin Podiatr Med Surg.* 2004;21:616–630.

Denkler K. Dupuytren's fasciectomies in 60 consecutive digits using lidocaine with epinephrine and no tourniquet. *Plast Reconstr Surg.* 2005;115:802–810.

Eekhof JAH, Van Wijk B, Knuistingh Neven A, van der Wouden JC. Interventions for ingrowing toenails. *Cochrane Database Syst Rev.* 2012;(3):CD001541.

Freiberg A, Dougherty S. A review of management of ingrown toenails and onychogryposis. *Can Fam Physician.* 1988;34:2675–2681.

Heidelbaugh JJ, Hobart L. Management of ingrown toenail. *Am Fam Physician.* 2009;79:303–308.

Hettinger DF, Valinsky MS, Nuccio G, Lim R. Nail matrixectomies using radio wave technique. *J Am Podiatr Med Assoc.* 1991;81:317–321.

Ikard RW. Onychocryptosis. *J Am Coll Surg.* 1998;187:96–102.

Krunic AL, Wang LC, Soltani K, et al. Digital anesthesia with epinephrine: an old myth revisited. *J Am Acad Dermatol.* 2004;51:755–759.

McGee DL. Podiatric procedures. In: Roberts JR, Custalow CB, Thomsen TW, eds. *Roberts and Hedges' Clinical Procedures in Emergency Medicine and Acute Care.* 7th ed. Philadelphia: Elsevier; 2019:1057–1070.

Radovic P, Smith RG, Shumway D. Revisiting epinephrine in foot surgery. *J Am Podiatr Med Assoc.* 2003;93:157–160.

Reyzelman AM, Trombello KA, Vayser DJ, et al. Are antibiotics necessary in the treatment of locally infected ingrown toenails? *Arch Fam Med.* 2000;9:930–932.

Robb JE, Murray WR. Phenol cauterization in the management of ingrowing toenails. *Scott Med J.* 1982;27:236–239.

Thompson C, Lalonde D, Denkler K, Feicht A. A critical look at the evidence for and against elective epinephrine use in the finger. *Plast Reconstr Surg.* 2007;119:260–266.

Usatine R. Nail procedures. In: Usatine RP, Pfenninger JL, Stulberg DL, Small R, eds. *Dermatologic and Cosmetic Procedures in Office Practice.* Philadelphia: Elsevier; 2012:216–228.

Yang KC, Li YT. Treatment of recurrent ingrown great toenail associated with granulation tissue by partial nail avulsion followed by matricectomy with sharpulse carbon dioxide laser. *Dermatol Surg.* 2003;28:419–421.

Zuber T, Pfenninger J. Management of ingrown toenails. *Am Fam Physician.* 1995;52:181–190.

CHAPTER 195

RING REMOVAL FROM AN EDEMATOUS FINGER

John Harlan Haynes III • *Andrew Thomas Haynes* • *Terrance S. Hines*

Soft tissue swelling of a finger can occur with trauma, fluid retention, weight gain, arthritis, allergic reaction, infection, or iatrogenic infusion infiltration. When the finger is constricted by circumferential banding, such as with ring jewelry, venous outflow from the finger may be restricted, which can lead to a laceration, nerve damage, ischemia, and digital gangrene if the ring is not removed promptly.

The involved finger should be evaluated initially for any lacerations or neurovascular compromise. This can be accomplished by testing for sensory deficits with two-point discrimination to the distal fingertip and assessment of distal digital pulses with a Doppler flowmeter. In the absence of any signs of neurovascular compromise, ring-sparing techniques may be attempted initially; however, if signs of compromise are present, ring cutting is indicated. Embedded bands should be evaluated radiographically for bony involvement necessitating removal in the operating room.

If the ring is not yet constricting the finger, attempts should be made to remove the ring by applying distal traction and using a circular motion. Lubricate the finger first with a water-soluble lubricant (e.g., K-Y jelly).

Removal of a constricting ring is often described as a two-step process: (1) exsanguination of the finger and (2) removal of the ring. If a tourniquet is used to accomplish the first step, a maximum of 2 hours is recommended, although up to 4 hours has been reported. If ring removal is not accomplished by a trial of elevation, lubrication, application of ice for 5 minutes, application of a proximal blood pressure cuff, and circular traction, the clinician may try various techniques for intact removal of a constricting band (e.g., string-wrap method or glove method). Alternatively, division of a constricting ring may be necessary using a variety of tools (e.g., conventional hand-operated or motorized circular saw, circular-blade ring cutter Steinmann pin cutter, wire or bolt cutters, or other commercially available cutting device). However, the use of this equipment damages jewelry and could injure the patient. Care should be taken to avoid implantation of metal filings, which may lead to foreign body granuloma and synovitis if the ring is cut. Rings removed by cutting are often repairable by a jeweler. After ring removal by any of these methods, a neurovascular examination should be performed as mentioned earlier. If any deficits in sensation or vascular flow are noted, prompt consultation with a hand specialist is required.

INDICATIONS

Acute or chronic finger edema with proximal band constriction.

RELATIVE CONTRAINDICATIONS

- Open wound or fracture
- Deeply embedded ring erosion or laceration
- Lack of patient cooperation

STRING-WRAP METHOD

Equipment

- Between 2 and 3 yards of string, braided suture of 0 gauge or larger, or umbilical tape—preferably on a spool
- Adhesive tape
- Small hemostat
- 1.5 mL of 1% lidocaine without epinephrine (optional)
- 5-mL syringe with 27-gauge needle for digital nerve block (optional)
- Lubricating K-Y jelly, mineral oil, vegetable oil, or the like

Technique

1. Some patients may require a digital or metacarpal block (see Chapter 7, Peripheral Nerve Blocks and Field Blocks) in case the pain increases from the compression and unwinding. For a digital block, 0.5 to 0.75 mL of 1% lidocaine is infiltrated deep into the neurovascular bundle on the proximal volar aspect of the affected finger bilaterally.
2. Lightly lubricate the finger near the ring. Pass the hemostat from distal to proximal under the ring, grasp the end of the string, and thread it beneath the ring, pulling several inches of string through (Fig. 195.1A). Tape the proximal end to the hand (see Fig. 195.1B).
3. Wrap the string circumferentially around the finger, beginning just adjacent to the ring margin. Care should be taken to not wrap the string so tight as to obstruct arterial flow. Wind the string in a smooth single layer going distally, using moderate tension until it encompasses the point of greatest swelling (see Fig. 195.1C).
4. Untape the proximal end of the string and pull distally toward the fingertip. Maintain tension along the long axis of the finger, moving the ring distally as the string unwinds beneath it. Force the ring over that portion of the finger that has been compressed by the wrap (see Fig. 195.1D). Once past the area of largest diameter, usually the proximal interphalangeal joint, the ring will slide off easily.
5. The most difficult area to unwind is usually where the ring is over the largest diameter. If unsuccessful removing the ring with this method, it may be worth trying it again. Or it may be necessary to rewrap the ring if it was not done carefully the first time. It is not uncommon to produce skin trauma or abrasions using this technique.
6. Variations, including wrapping proximally to distally as well as vice versa, have been described. A number of devices have been used for this "sequential compression," including suture, thread, or floss; thicker umbilical tape, ribbon gauze, or tape; or more elastic items such as an intravenous tourniquet, rubber band, or Penrose drain.

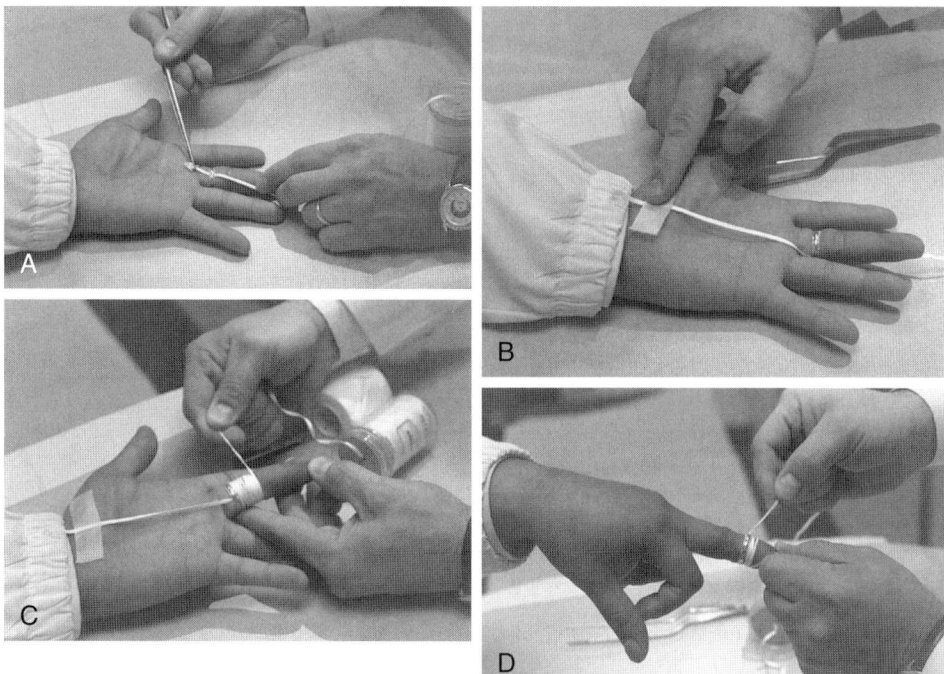

Fig. 195.1   String-wrap method of removing ring from a swollen finger.

CIRCULAR-BLADE OR STEINMANN PIN CUTTER METHOD

Equipment

- Hand-held circular-blade ring cutter (e.g., Beaver, Hawk, Mooney GEM) or Steinmann pin cutter with a McDonald elevator
- Large hemostats (e.g., Kelly clamps)
- 20-mL syringe filled with saline and 20-gauge Intracath sheath

Technique

1. Begin by draping the patient and providing eye protection to all persons in the work area. Slip the small hook of the ring cutter or elevator under the ring on the palmar surface to serve as a guide and barrier (Fig. 195.2). If elevation of this section is necessary for application of the ring cutter, the ring may be bent outward by using pliers with the jaws placed at 90 degrees from the cutting site.
2. Firmly grip the saw handle, and, using a 180-degree twisting motion, grind through the ring. Using the pin cutter, cut through the ring, over the elevator. This process generates heat and may be interrupted every 30 seconds to allow ring cooling to prevent further injury to the patient. Irrigation is helpful, but careful drying is necessary if electric tools are being used. Because sparks may be produced, flammable items (e.g., rubbing alcohol) must be removed.
3. The cut ends of the ring may be spread using large hemostats with steady opposing force. If the ring must be cut in two places, sharp edges should be protected with a gauze covering.
4. Rinse the area with high-pressure saline to ensure evacuation of all metal filings.
5. Alternatives include using a Dremel MultiPro cutting tool, fire department extrication tools, or carbide dental drills.
6. In cases of very hard titanium or tungsten alloy bands causing constriction, we recommend the use of a high-speed Dremel tool with an abrasive carbide cutting wheel. A variable-speed Dremel tool and 1-inch carbide cutting wheel are available at most hardware supply stores. The medial and lateral sides of the finger must be supported with malleable ribbons, and the finger should be protected by a stainless-steel ring support under the ring. A bulb syringe with sterile water is used to keep the ring as cool as possible while cutting.

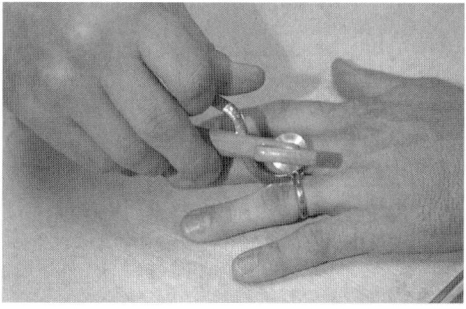

Fig. 195.2   Hook of the ring cutter serves as a guide and barrier.

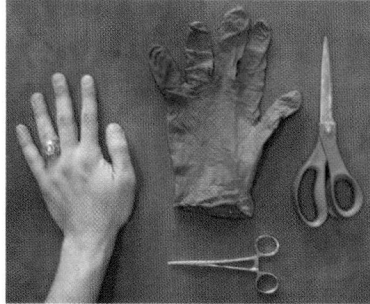

Fig. 195.3   Materials needed for ring removal from an edematous finger using the surgical glove method: surgical glove, hemostat, scissors. One finger is cut from the glove and the tip is removed to form a sleeve.

It may be necessary to consult a team member from maintenance or plant operations who is experienced in using a Dremel tool.
7. Alternatively, extremely hard rings, such as those made from tungsten alloy or ceramic can sometimes be cracked to remove them. Use standard locking pliers and adjust them to fit tightly and grasp the ring. Repetitively remove and readjust the pliers with increasing tension. Continue until the material cracks and falls apart. Some of these rings may be lined with a metal band which can then be removed as discussed previously.

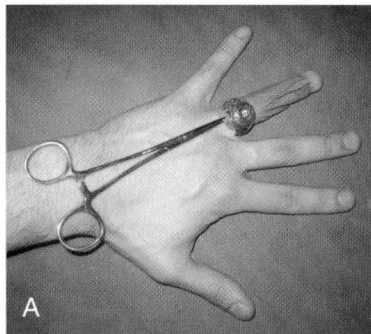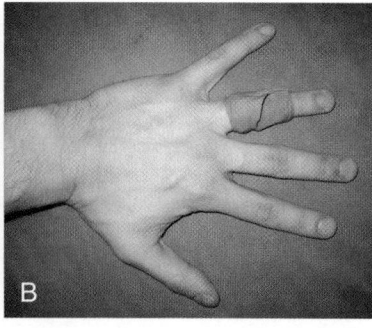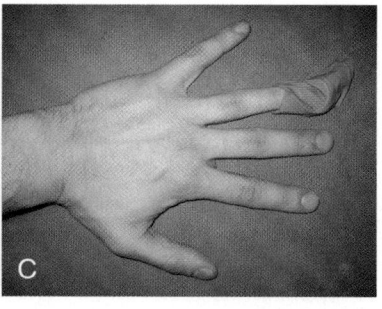

Fig. 195.4 (A) The rubber sleeve is pulled under the ring. (B and C) The sleeve is pulled over the ring, removing it from the finger.

SURGICAL GLOVE METHOD

Discussion

- Not universally recommended
- Can be used in the presence of fractures or soft tissue injury
- Causes minimal additional pain

Technique

1. Cut one finger from a surgical glove (Fig. 195.3).
2. Place on involved finger.
3. Slip proximal end under ring using hemostats (Fig. 195.4A).
4. K-Y Jelly may be used to lubricate.
5. Pull proximal end back over ring (see Fig. 195.4B).
6. Continue to pull and twist on the retroverted glove to advance ring distally (see Fig. 195.4C).
7. A variant of this technique involves using a Penrose drain. In the event of a failed removal, the drain may act as insulation against electrical burns should electrocautery be required during surgery.

POSTPROCEDURE PATIENT CARE

- Consider appropriate tetanus prophylaxis.
- Consider antibiotics in cases of contaminated wounds, patients with diabetes, patients with comorbidities, or the immunocompromised.

CPT/BILLING CODES

Ring removal is considered part of the standard evaluation and management (E&M) otherwise provided to the patient. However, if the ring removal were provided in the setting of a finger fracture, an appropriate CPT code (open, closed, manipulated) may be used if definitive treatment is provided. If definitive treatment is referred to another physician, coding for supplies and splinting may be used.

There is no specific code for removal of a ring. Use the appropriate E&M code.

RECOMMENDED READING

Belliappa PPL. A technique for removal of a tight ring. *J Hand Surg [Br]*. 1989;14:127.

Chiu TF, Chu SJ, Chen SG, et al. Use of a Penrose drain to remove an entrapped ring from a finger under emergent conditions. *Am J Emerg Med*. 2007;25:722–723.

Cresap C. Removal of a hardened steel ring from an extremely swollen finger. *Am J Emerg Med*. 1995;13:318–320.

Fasano Jr FJ, Hansen RH. Foreign body granuloma and synovitis of the finger: a hazard of ring removal by the sawing technique. *J Hand Surg [Am]*. 1987;12:621.

Fuchs SM. Ring removal. In: King C, Henretig FM, eds. *Textbook of Pediatric Emergency Procedures*. 2nd ed. Philadelphia: Wolters Kluwer; 2008.

Inoue S, Akazawa S, Fukuda H, Shimizu R. Another simple method for ring removal. *Anesthesiology*. 1995;83:1133.

McElfresh EC, Peterson-Elijah RC. Removal of a tight ring by the rubber band. *J Hand Surg [Br]*. 1991;16:225.

Mittiga MR, Ruddy RM. Procedures. In: Shaw KN, Bachur RG, eds. *Fleisher & Ludwig's Textbook of Pediatric Emergency Medicine*. 7th ed. Philadelphia: Wolters Kluwer; 2016.

Paterson P, Khanna A. A novel method of ring removal from a swollen finger [letter]. *Br J Plast Surg*. 2001;54:182.

Peckler B, Hsu C. Tourniquet syndrome: a review of constricting band removal. *J Emerg Med*. 2001;20:253–262.

Stone DM, Scordino DJ. Foreign body removal. In: Roberts JR, Custalow CB, Thomsen TW, eds. *Roberts & Hedges' Clinical Procedures of Emergency Medicine*. 6th ed. Philadelphia: Elsevier; 2014.

Thilagarajah M. An improved method of ring removal. *J Hand Surg [Br]*. 1999;24:118–119.

Tintinalli JE, Stapczynski JS, Ma OJ, et al., eds. *Tintinalli's Emergency Medicine: A Comprehensive Study Guide*. 8th ed. New York: McGraw-Hill; 2015.

CHAPTER 196

SKIN STAPLING

David James

In certain body areas, when performed with care, skin stapling provides a rapid and simple alternative to other methods of skin closure and wound repair. Clinical experience with stapling now spans decades, and improved equipment, such as absorbable staples, is being introduced on a regular basis. A variety of staplers with specific features for various purposes are now available. For example, staplers designed for small lacerations may hold only 5 fine staples, whereas staplers for general-purpose closure may hold up to 35 heavier-gauge staples.

ADVANTAGES

The final result of a stapled wound depends on its location, the condition of the wound being stapled, and operator experience. The best cosmetic results are seen in clean, uninfected linear wounds of the scalp, torso, and proximal extremities that have some degree of a subcutaneous fat "bed" and are not under tension. Poorer results occur when the wound is macerated, ragged, infected, or under tension or when the staples are placed directly over a bony prominence with thinner skin.

Numerous studies have supported stapling as an acceptable alternative to suture closure; in some studies a lower rate of infection has been found with stapling. Staples are generally well accepted by patients; in most cases it is a much faster procedure than suturing (three to four times faster, which may be very helpful in the uncooperative, agitated, or intoxicated patient). Well-placed staples evert the wound edges optimally and place less tension on wound edges than sutures. Surgical stainless steel staples are less reactive than sutures and potentially cause less postclosure inflammation and infection. Staple ends do not completely meet in the deeper tissues, thus resulting in less tissue constriction; this may also promote a lower infection rate.

DISADVANTAGES

Stapling has the potential to provide a result inferior to meticulous suturing, especially if the clinician is not familiar with stapling. Staples certainly do leave larger puncture scars proportional to the time they remain in the wound, and the cost-benefit ratio of using a stapling device in smaller wounds is not advantageous.

INDICATIONS

- To secure skin grafts or repair wounds whose edges are easily approximated and not under undue tension
- Long, linear wounds of the scalp, proximal extremities, or the torso where cosmesis is not a concern

CONTRAINDICATIONS

- Facial or neck tissue, or in areas where there is an inadequate subcutaneous base (where staples are difficult to place and can damage underlying structures)
- Over small mobile joints of the hand and foot, soles and palms, or any other location where the staples may interfere with the function of a body part
- In wounds that are macerated or infected, or over areas of large tissue loss unless the subcutaneous tissues can easily be approximated after undermining and buried deeper sutures are used to help approximate the skin edges
- In areas where magnetic resonance imaging may have to be performed

EQUIPMENT

- Skin hooks or two pairs of fine Adson forceps
- Skin stapler with appropriate-gauge staples (heavier gauge for longer wounds over thicker tissue, lighter gauge for smaller wounds; these are usually sterile, disposable, single-patient-use devices)
- Sterile surgical skin preparation solution (e.g., povidone-iodine, chlorhexidine), sterile drapes, gloves for the operators, equipment necessary to observe universal blood and body fluid precautions
- Local or topical anesthetic appropriate for the area to be repaired
- Suture kit with appropriate sutures on standby, in case deeper sutures need to be inserted to take tension off the skin edges
- Staple removers (again, these are usually sterile, disposable, single-patient-use devices; one can be given to patient if another practitioner will be removing the staples)

PREPROCEDURE PATIENT PREPARATION

Community standards or facility type will dictate the nature and extent of any consent forms involved. In all cases, the patient should be informed about the procedure to close the wound, the intent to use staples, the relative advantages and disadvantages of staple use in his or her particular wound, how to care for the repaired wound, and when to return for recheck and/or staple removal.

TECHNIQUE

1. The help of an assistant to hold the skin edges together for the stapler operator is often useful during the procedure (Fig. 196.1).
2. Prepare and drape the wound in the usual fashion.
3. Don sterile gloves. Observe universal blood and body fluid precautions.
4. Anesthetize the area to be repaired with injectable lidocaine 1% or 2% with or without epinephrine. Topical anesthetics (e.g., a solution of lidocaine, epinephrine, and tetracaine) may be used instead of injectable anesthetics.
5. If there is tissue loss or if the wound is gaping, undermine the edges of the wound and close the deeper layers with buried absorbable sutures. The skin edges should be well approximated and under no tension before stapling is performed.

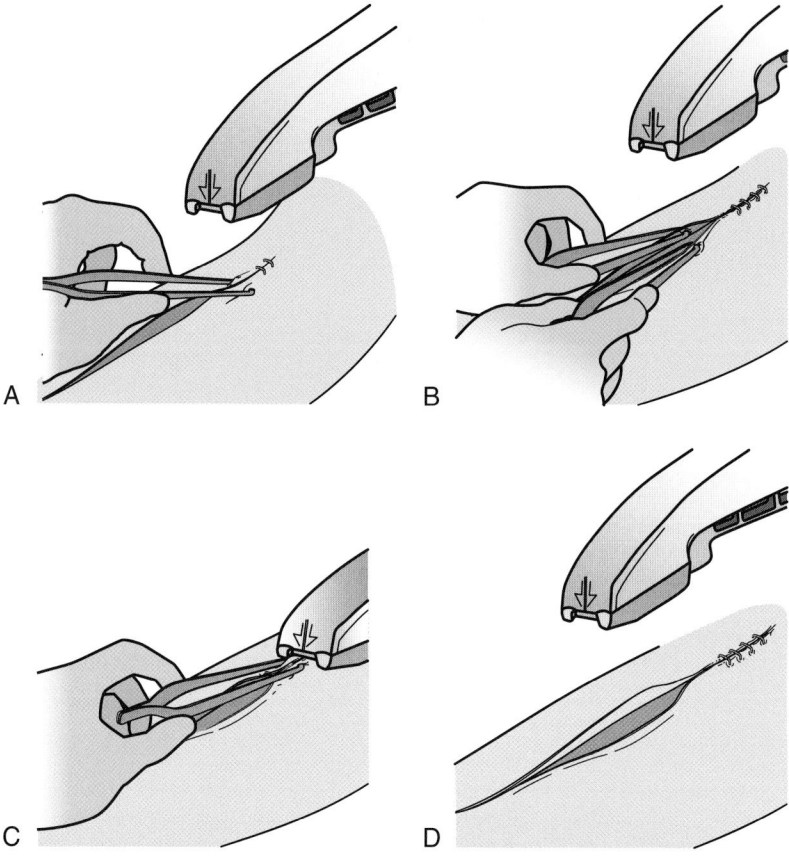

Fig. 196.1 Use of a skin stapler. Approximate skin edges so that they are slightly everted (A) with one forceps (B) or two forceps. (C) Position the instrument lightly over the everted skin edges, aligning the stapler arrow with the incision. Pressing down on the instrument too heavily may make staple removal difficult. (D) Squeeze the trigger quickly and firmly until the trigger motion is halted. Release the trigger and back the instrument off the staple.

6. Have assistant (if present) pick up the skin edges of the wound in front of the stapler with the skin hooks/forceps, and gently hold them together and slightly elevate or evert them (if the skin is held flat, the wound may have a gap or invert after stapling).
7. Start at one end of the wound, pointing the stapler toward the opposite end. Position the stapler guide (usually an arrow) over the laceration and press the stapler gently down onto the skin. (Do not indent the skin with the stapler, this will place the staple too deep.) Squeeze the trigger, placing one staple. Do not release the trigger yet, but pull up gently on the stapler. This will pull up the wound edges.
8. Release the stapler trigger and remove the stapler.
9. Place the stapler again over the laceration, and repeat step 6. A small gap should be located between the skin and each staple after it is placed; if a staple is flat against the skin surface, it is in too deep and should be removed.
10. Alternate step 7, followed by step 6, until the end of the wound is reached. If there is a "dog ear" of excess tissue, excise with forceps and iris scissors and place final staples.
11. The distance between staples depends on the operator and his or her experience, but the wound margins should be approximated without gaps when complete. This usually means placing staples every 3 to 5 mm.

    NOTE: Some clinicians prefer to start closing at the middle of a wound, lessening the chance of dog ears. They place a staple in the middle, then divide the distance on each side of the wound again and place an additional staple in each middle. They continue dividing the distance on each side and placing a staple in the middle until adequate closure is obtained.

12. A lone operator can approximate the skin edges with a single forceps by pulling the skin edges together before placing a staple or by placing the thumb and forefinger of the nonoperating hand along the edges of the skin to pull them together.

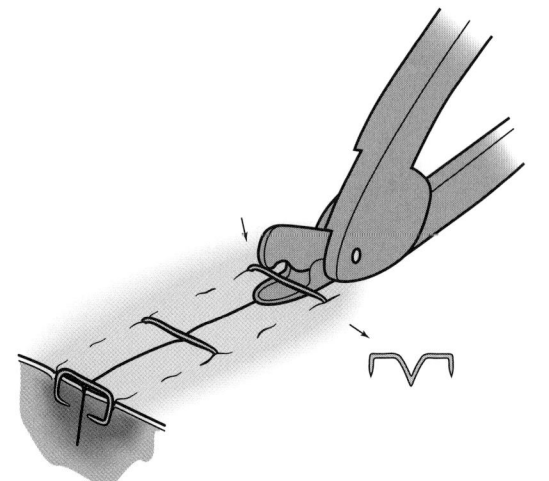

Fig. 196.2 Use of a staple remover.

13. After stapling is complete, reclean the wound and place an appropriate dressing.
14. Arrangements for follow-up and staple removal should be made. In general, staples should remain in place for 8 to 10 days. If necessary, stapled scalps may be washed after staple placement.
15. Removal of staples is best accomplished by a staple remover that bends the staple arms up and out of the skin (Fig. 196.2). These are also usually available in a single-patient-use disposable kit. If a kit is not available, two hemostats can be used to pry out each staple arm, but this should usually be done at the same time. Before doing this, careful attention should be paid to Fig. 196.2. Note that the end of each staple arm is bent 90 degrees to the downward direction of the staple, going under the skin and

parallel to the skin surface. Merely prying on one staple arm at a time causes the other arm to dig in and can be very painful; if attempts are made to remove staples with hemostats, both staple arms should probably be removed at once, attempting to mimic the maneuvers and directional forces made by the removal kit.

COMPLICATIONS

Complications, although rarely reported, include dehiscence, poor cosmesis, infection, and hematoma. These are similar to the complications seen with a sutured wound. There can also be complications with removal that can be difficult or uncomfortable, especially if the staples were placed incorrectly or left in place too long. If the patient is going to have the staples removed at another office, it may be prudent to give the patient a staple remover kit; many clinics do not routinely stock these.

POSTPROCEDURE PATIENT EDUCATION

See the sample patient education handout available at www.expert consult.com.

CPT/BILLING CODES

Coding is the same as for suture repairs; see Chapter 19, Laceration and Incision Repair, Table 19-4.

SUPPLIERS

(See contact information available at www.expertconsult.com.)

Minogue Medical
Most medical suppliers (e.g., Miltex, Delasco)
3M
Weck Closure Systems (Visistat and Skinstat skin staplers)

Acknowledgment

The editors recognize the contributions by J. Mark Wiedemann, MD, MS, to this chapter in a previous edition of this text.

RECOMMENDED READING

Brickman K, Lambert R. Evaluation of skin stapling for wound closure in the emergency department. *Ann Emerg Med.* 2009;18:1122–1125.

Dos Santos LR, Freitas CA, Hojaij FC, et al. Prospective study using skin staplers in head and neck surgery. *Am J Surg.* 1995;170:451–452.

James D. Repair of lacerations. In: James D, ed. *A Field Guide to Urgent and Ambulatory Procedures.* Philadelphia: Lippincott Williams & Wilkins; 2001:202–212.

Kanegaye JT, Vance CW, Chan L, Schonfeld N. Comparison of skin stapling devices and standard sutures for pediatric scalp lacerations: a randomized study of cost and time benefits. *J Pediatr.* 1997;130:808–813.

Lammers RL, Smith ZE. Methods of wound closure. In: Roberts JR, Custalow CB, Thomsen TW, eds. *Roberts and Hedges' Clinical Procedures in Emergency Medicine.* 6th ed. Philadelphia: Elsevier; 2014:649–652.

Orlinsky M, Goldberg RM, Chan L, et al. Cost analysis of stapling versus suturing for skin closures. *Am J Emerg Med.* 1995;13:77–81.

Reichman EF, Powell C. Basic wound closure. In: Reichman EF, ed. *Emergency Medicine Procedures.* 2nd ed. New York: McGraw-Hill; 2013:643–645.

CHAPTER 197

TICK REMOVAL AND PREVENTION OF INFECTION

David James

Persons frequenting outdoor areas may be exposed to ticks. Ticks often lurk in tall grasses or in overhead branches and will attach themselves to persons passing by them in search of a blood meal. Although most tick bites are harmless, ticks may be the vectors of several significant diseases. Because it is impossible to identify in the field whether a tick carries an infectious disease, it is good medical practice to promptly remove all ticks found on human skin. Ticks feed slowly, and several hours of attachment are thought to be required for transmission of tick-borne illnesses.

DISEASES TRANSMITTED BY TICKS

Ticks have eight legs and are members of the class *Arachnida*. Ticks belonging to the families *Argasidae* (soft ticks) and *Ixodidae* (hard ticks) are able to act as disease vectors to humans. The ixodid, hard ticks *Dermacentor* and *Ixodes* are most likely to be encountered by humans in North America, and they can transmit microorganisms hematogenously during all phases of their development. See Box 197.1 for a list of tick-borne diseases.

Ticks have powerful mouthparts to break the skin of their hosts and enable a blood meal. The saliva of the tick has anticoagulant properties to keep blood flowing. Pathogens in the gut of the tick migrate to the tick's salivary glands and thus are transmitted parenterally to the host during feeding. *In general, a tick must be attached for longer than 8 hours (possibly as long as 24 hours) for successful transmission of disease.*

Two of the tick-borne diseases bear special mention. *Tick-bite paralysis* is a serious illness that presents as an ascending neuromuscular paralysis, similar to Guillain-Barré syndrome. The paralysis is caused by envenomation of the host with a salivary neurotoxin secreted in the saliva of certain gravid *Dermacentor* ticks. Resolution of the paralysis occurs after removal of the often-overlooked tick.

Lyme disease is a fairly common illness affecting the cardiovascular, musculoskeletal, neurologic, and dermatologic systems. It is often seen in children and adults who spend time outdoors. Lyme disease is caused by the spirochete *Borrelia burgdorferi* and is transmitted to humans by the bite of the hard *Ixodes* tick. White-footed mice and white-tailed deer are the major reservoirs for *B. burgdorferi*. This disease is becoming prevalent throughout northeastern North America and is worth including in the differential diagnosis of unusual rashes, fevers, myalgias, and arthralgias. It is best diagnosed by enzyme-linked immunosorbent assay (ELISA) testing of serum for specific antibodies to *B. burgdorferi*. Treatment of Lyme disease is discussed in the section on Complications and Disease Prevention. See Table 197.1 for a synopsis of presenting features of other tick-borne diseases.

The lone star tick (*Amblyomma americanum*) has been associated with an erythema migrans–like rash in patients from the southeastern United States. This condition has been termed Southern tick–associated rash illness (STARI), although it also goes by several other names. In addition to a rash, symptoms can include headache, fatigue, fever, and muscle aches. Although these symptoms have resolved after a course of doxycycline, it is unknown whether the medication speeds recovery. The suspected causative agent of this disease, *Borrelia lonestari*, has never been isolated from a human with STARI, and numerous questions remain regarding the spectrum of clinical features and the pathophysiology of human illness following exposure to *B. lonestari*. Currently, STARI is considered a syndrome of unproven cause. Fortunately, it has not been linked to arthritis, neurologic disease, or chronic symptoms.

Hard ticks are best removed mechanically. Care must be taken to remove the tick's mouthparts, which will be firmly embedded in the host. The head and mouthparts may separate from the tick's body if not removed properly, thus increasing risk of disease transmission. An incision or punch biopsy of the tissue surrounding the mouthparts may then be necessary. *Home remedies*, such as the placement of oil on the tick to smother it or burning the tick with a hot match or cigarette *are not recommended*. Both techniques have the potential to cause the tick to regurgitate its blood meal and cause significant inoculation of disease pathogens.

INDICATIONS

- Any tick found attached to the skin, preferably within first 24 hours of attachment.

CONTRAINDICATIONS

- None

EQUIPMENT

- Blunt straight or curved forceps or tweezers or hemostat (if very small tick, having fine forceps or mosquito hemostat is helpful)
- Rubber gloves
- Antiseptic solution (e.g., povidone-iodine scrub or solution, chlorhexidine solution)

BOX 197.1 Tick-Borne Diseases
Babesiosis
Human granulocytic and monocytic ehrlichiosis
Lyme disease
Q fever
Rocky Mountain spotted fever
Tick fever
Tick-bite paralysis
Tularemia
Typhus

TABLE 197.1	Common Tick-Borne Diseases and Their Management			
	Lyme Disease	**Ehrlichiosis**	**Rocky Mountain Spotted Fever**	**Tularemia**
Pathogens	*Borrelia burgdorferi*	*Ehrlichia chaffeensis* *Ehrlichia ewingii*	*Rickettsia rickettsii*	*Francisella tularensis*
Geographic distribution in continental United States	Northeast and upper Midwest	South, Southeast, and Midwest	Southeast, Atlantic Coast states, Midwest	South and Midwest
Presenting symptoms	Erythema migrans, fatigue, myalgias, arthralgias, headache, fever, chills, neuropathies	Fever, chills, headache, myalgias	Macular rash, fever, myalgias, vomiting, fatigue, headache	Fever, chills, headache, cough, diarrhea, fatigue, vomiting, sore throat; contact with mice is a risk factor
Initial laboratory findings	Nonspecific; convalescent serology positive at 4–6 wk for antibodies to *Borrelia*	Leukopenia, thrombocytopenia, elevated liver aminotransferases; confirmatory convalescent serology at 1–2 wk	Leukopenia, thrombocytopenia, elevated liver aminotransferases, hyponatremia; confirmatory convalescent serology at 7–10 days	White blood cell count often normal, elevated erythrocyte sedimentation rate; confirmatory convalescent serology at 2 wk
Treatment	Doxycycline, amoxicillin, cefuroxime axetil	Doxycycline (preferred), chloramphenicol, rifampin	Doxycycline, chloramphenicol	Streptomycin, gentamicin, chloramphenicol, doxycycline (mild disease only), ciprofloxacin (mild disease only).

- Normal saline specimen container or culture medium *(optional)*
- Gauze and bandage
- In addition, for difficult removal or retained mouthparts:
  - Punch biopsy equipment for 3- to 6-mm punch as appropriate or #15 blade scalpel
  - Iris scissors
  - 1% Lidocaine 0.5 mL in syringe with 30-gauge needle
  - Aluminum chloride solution 6.25% on a cotton-tipped swab *(optional)*
  - 5-0 nylon suture and needle driver *(optional)*

TECHNIQUE

1. Gently paint the surrounding area with antiseptic solution.
2. With blunt forceps, tweezers, hemostat, or gloved fingers, grasp the tick as close to the skin surface as possible and pull axially or perpendicular to the skin with steady, even pressure (Fig. 197.1).
3. *Do not* twist or jerk the tick because this may break off mouthparts.
4. *Never squeeze*, crush, or puncture the body of the tick because its fluids may contain infectious agents.
5. The tick may be sent for microscopic analysis of the *Borrelia* spirochete or cultured for other organisms.
6. Disinfect the bite site with antiseptic solution or antibacterial soap. Inspect carefully for any signs of retained tick mouthparts.

In cases of a particularly tenacious tick, retained mouthparts, or high-risk endemic areas, perform the following technique:

1. Disinfect the area with antiseptic solution or antibacterial soap. Infiltrate the area beneath the bite with lidocaine.
2. Apply the punch biopsy instrument perpendicular to the skin so that it encompasses the tick or retained mouthparts. Stretch the skin on each side of the lesion. Advance the biopsy punch downward with moderate pressure, using a clockwise-counterclockwise twisting motion. Penetration through the epidermis and dermis is confirmed with a marked decrease in resistance (see Chapter 26, Skin Biopsy).
3. Remove the punch. Lift the biopsy specimen with forceps, and cut the pedicle with iris scissors. Submit the tissue for histologic study.
4. Disinfect the area again and apply pressure with gauze. If adequate hemostasis is not accomplished, cauterize with aluminum chloride solution or close with suture. Apply bandage.
5. As an alternative to punch biopsy, remove the tick or mouthparts and skin with a #15 scalpel blade.

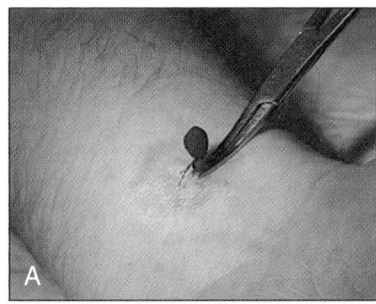
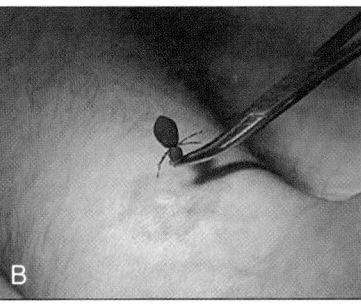

Fig. 197.1   Technique of tick removal. (A) Apply the instrument perpendicular to the skin, encompassing the tick. (B) Pull upward with a steady, even pressure.

COMPLICATIONS AND DISEASE PREVENTION

Local complications of tick removal may include transient *bleeding* or *cellulitis*. Bleeding is managed by locally applied pressure, whereas cellulitis is prevented by attention to area cleanliness and follow-up care.

The Infectious Disease Society of America (IDSA) recommends antibiotic prophylaxis with a single dose of doxycycline 200 mg orally only in patients who meet all of the following criteria:

1. Attached tick identified as an adult or nymphal *Ixodes scapularis* tick (deer tick)
2. Tick is estimated to have been attached for greater than or equal to 36 hours (by degree of engorgement or time of exposure
3. Prophylaxis is begun within 72 hours of tick removal

4. Local rate of infection of ticks with *B. burgdorferi* is greater than or equal to 20%, either where the patient lives or has recently traveled (these rates of infection have been shown to occur in parts of New England, parts of the mid-Atlantic States, and parts of Minnesota and Wisconsin; specifically in Connecticut, Delaware, Massachusetts, Maryland, Maine, Minnesota, New Hampshire, New Jersey, New York, Pennsylvania, Rhode Island, Virginia, Vermont, and Wisconsin)
5. Doxycycline is not contraindicated (i.e., the patient is not less than 8 years of age, pregnant, or lactating)

If the patient cannot take doxycycline, the IDSA does not recommend prophylaxis with an alternate antibiotic. Antibiotic treatment following a tick bite is not recommended to prevent anaplasmosis, babesiosis, ehrlichiosis, or Rocky Mountain spotted fever. There is no evidence this practice is effective, and it may simply delay onset of disease. The Centers for Disease Control and Prevention (CDC) reviewed these ISDA guidelines in 2017 and still recommends them.

PATIENT EDUCATION GUIDES

Following a tick bite or removal of a tick, patients should be alert for symptoms suggestive of tick-borne illness and consult a clinician if fever, rash, or other symptoms of concern develop. See patient education handouts available at www.expertconsult.com.

CPT/BILLING CODES

10120 Removal of superficial foreign body, skin
10121 Incisional removal of foreign body, complex

ICD-10-CM DIAGNOSTIC CODES

Injury, superficial, insect bite (nonvenomous) by site (see S00–S99)
Add appropriate seventh character: A = initial, D = subsequent, S = sequela.

Acknowledgment

The editors recognize the contributions of John Harlan Haynes III, MD, to this chapter in a previous edition of the text.

RECOMMENDED READING

Goodman JL. Ehrlichiosis: ticks, dogs, and doxycycline. *N Engl J Med.* 1999;341:195–197.
Hu L. Evaluation of a tick bite for possible Lyme disease. *UpToDate.* 2016.
James DM. Tick removal. In: James DM, ed. *Field Guide to Urgent and Ambulatory Care Procedures.* Philadelphia: Lippincott Williams & Wilkins; 2001:225–226.
Kassutto Z. Tick removal. In: Reichman EF, ed. *Emergency Medicine Procedures.* 2nd ed. New York: McGraw-Hill; 2013:679–681.
Needham G. Evaluation of five popular methods for tick removal. *Pediatrics.* 1985;75:997–1002.
Stone DB, Scordino DJ. Foreign body removal. In: Roberts JR, Custalow CB, Thomsen TW, eds. *Roberts and Hedges' Clinical Procedures in Emergency Medicine.* 6th ed. Philadelphia: Elsevier; 2014:709–713.
Tibbles C, Edlow J. Does this patient have erythema migrans? *JAMA.* 2007;297:2617–2627.
Wormser GP, Dattwyler RJ, Shapiro ED, et al. The clinical assessment, treatment, and prevention of Lyme disease, human granulocytic anaplasmosis, and babesiosis: clinical practice guidelines by the Infectious Diseases Society of America. *Clin Infect Dis.* 2006;42:1089.

CHAPTER 198

TISSUE GLUES

Rebecca Beach

The US Food and Drug Administration (FDA) approved cyano-acrylates for the repair of incisions and lacerations in 1998. The agents combine cyanoacrylates and formaldehyde. Some have added plasticizers for extra strength and flexibility. Dermabond (Ethicon) is available in different types of applicators; it forms a polymeric bond across apposed tissue edges on contact with moisture or air. Several other brands are available, including SurgiSeal (Pfizer) and LiquiBand (Advanced Medical Solutions). These are all versions of octyl cyanoacrylates with long side-chains that provide slightly more flexibility after drying, making them less brittle, less likely to fracture, and perhaps better for longer lacerations. Alternatives include Histoacryl (B Braun) and Indermil (Covidien Medtronics), which utilize butyl cyanoacrylates; these are probably best for short lacerations under no tension. Over-the-counter cyanoacrylates, such as Super Glue and Crazy Glue, are somewhat weaker and are not FDA approved for this indication, but they are used by many patients at home. The latter preparations have more difficulty binding to a moist surface. Cosmesis and final results with tissue glues is comparable or superior to sutures, and there is much greater acceptance, especially with children. The products have antimicrobial properties and negligible tissue toxicity and are easily applied. They may not require local anesthesia and significantly decrease wound repair time.

INDICATIONS

- Nonmucosal laceration or incision repairs
- Facial, scalp, neck, torso, or proximal extremity wounds
- After deep suture placement if skin tension is minimal
- Wounds less than 8 cm (gap <0.5 cm)
- Alternative to 5-0 or smaller suture
- Removal of foreign bodies in ear or nose (clinicians can apply a small drop of glue on the wooden end of cotton swab, touch the object for 30 seconds, and remove)
- Repair of lacerated nails or nail beds
- Because there is more scarring the longer the sutures are left in, consider removing any sutures a few days ahead of schedule after the wound has sealed over, and applying a tissue glue to keep the wound edges together
- Flap type lacerations or lacerations in thin skin where sutures may cause skin compromise

NOTE: Tissue glue is best with low-tension, short, small, straight-edged, and superficial wounds. However, long wounds can be divided into segments and each segment closed separately.

CONTRAINDICATIONS

- Mucosal lesions
- Significant wound margin tension
- Noncompliant patient
- Heavily contaminated wounds requiring debridement
- Wounds >6 to 12 hours old

- Human or animal bite or scratch wounds
- Puncture wounds
- Stellate, jagged, or crush wounds
- Wounds on axillae or perineum (moisture prevents adherence)
- Actively bleeding or oozing wound (moisture prevents adherence; attempts can be made to stop the bleeding with direct pressure or injection of local anesthetic with epinephrine)
- Hand or joint lacerations, feet (washing or repetitive and frequent movement can weaken bond)
- Allergy to formaldehyde or cyanoacetate

NOTE: While not a contraindication, great care should be taken if using glue near the eye; it can run and potentially seal the eyelids.

ADVANTAGES

- Faster than suturing or stapling
- Less painful
- Less need for painful injectable anesthetic
- As effective as suturing in appropriately selected patients
- A lower infection rate compared with staples and sutures (according to some studies)
- No need for suture removal
- Low cost
- Reduces risk of needle stick injury
- Hair apposition technique allows the treatment of scalp wounds without shaving, with less pain, and much more quickly than traditional techniques

DISADVANTAGES

- Bond not as strong as sutures at onset, but it reaches strength equivalent to sutures or naturally healed tissue at 7 days after repair
- Early dehiscence is the most common complaint. Again, wound strength on the first day is significantly less than with a suture
- Glue is very liquid, and inadvertent spillage or excessive application can cause adherence to gloves or other tissues as well as pain from heat of exothermic reaction
- Most bonding agents are available as single-use applicators that typically cost more than a single pack of nylon suture. However, the cost to the patient of sutures being placed is usually much higher

EQUIPMENT

- Dermabond single-use vials (Fig. 198.1) or alternative brands. Information on specific brands and their applicators are available at corporate websites: www.ethicon.com (Dermabond), www.liquiband.com (Liquiband), www.adhezion.com (Surgi-Seal), www.tissueseal.com (Histoacryl), www.connexiconmedical.com (Indermil)
- Gloves

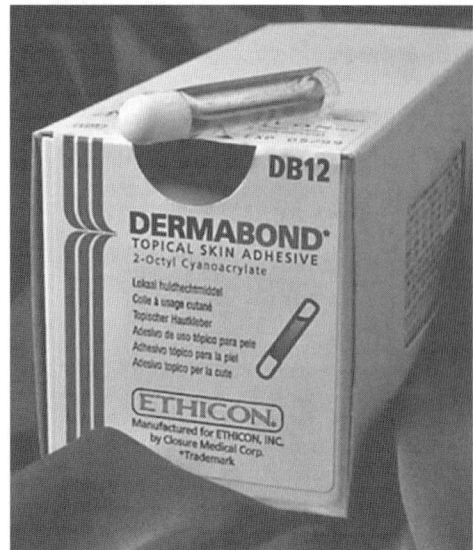

Fig. 198.1 Dermabond single-use vials.

- Wound cleaning and irrigation supplies
- Equipment necessary to follow universal blood and body fluid precautions
- Single-use tissue approximators (Bionix), gauze, or forceps (see Fig. 198.3A) (optional)
- Super Glue remover (optional). Acetone (nail polish remover) is the active ingredient
- Petrolatum jelly (optional). Might be used to remove glue, if needed, after the procedure. Might also be used to protect an area; however, avoid getting near the wound because it will make the wound edges too slippery to hold in apposition

PREPROCEDURE PATIENT PREPARATION

Obtain verbal informed consent for the procedure. Explain that the wound will be cleansed and prepared, possibly involving local anesthesia. Some children may need to be restrained. Explain the procedure and warn the patient there may be a slight sensation of heat or stinging.

TECHNIQUE

See Fig. 198.2.

1. Meticulous wound preparation is essential and may require topical or infiltrated anesthetics. Good hemostasis must be achieved before application. The clinician should follow universal blood and body fluid precautions.
2. The patient should be positioned so that the fluid glue does not run off the wound to other areas.
3. The edges of the laceration are manually apposed. Clean, not sterile, gloves are acceptable for use, provided the wound is not inadvertently contaminated. For better traction, gauze, forceps, or disposable plastic tissue approximators may be used (Fig. 198.3).
4. The vial is crushed to start the flow of glue, and the glue touched to the wound edges.
5. The glue is gently painted over the wound. Care should be taken to keep the glue from entering into the wound, which can impair healing and precipitate a foreign body reaction. If there is doubt that the tissue edges can be reapproximated completely and evenly, suturing or stapling should be considered.
6. Apply only a few drops at a time. Heat is produced proportionately to the amount of adhesive applied and can be painful. It can even cause a superficial burn if too much is applied too fast. By

the time the patient is feeling heat, it may be too late to wipe off the excess. Err on the side of caution.
7. The glue should be applied in an ovoid area (the wound being central) for best adhesive strength. A template can be cut from occlusive dressing and placed over the wound to delineate the oval pattern

   NOTE: Other experts use various patterns for application. Some paint a wide line down the wound, extending at least 5 to 10 mm outside the wound on both sides. Others paint strips of glue across the wound in a manner and pattern similar to where Steri-Strips would be placed.

8. While it is recommended to apply Dermabond in a single coat and SurgiSeal in one thick coat or two thinner coats, most experts apply several thin coats. If two or more coats are used, allow 30 to 60 seconds of drying time between coats. LiquiBand is also recommended to be applied as a single layer. The surface, when dry, looks slightly rougher and more undulant than when it is wet. Subsequent layers dry more rapidly. Excess adhesive must be wiped off within 10 seconds.
9. Remember to hold the wound edges apposed until the glue dries—for 60 seconds or longer in most cases. Steri-Strips, applied after drying, can help prevent wound dehiscence.
10. Hair apposition technique for scalp lesions:
    - After cleaning, prepping, and possibly anesthetizing the wound, twist together 5 to 15 hairs on each side of the scalp laceration. They should be twisted such as a "rope." Next, tie the two "ropes" together across the wound in order to close it and appose the edges.
    - Apply a few drops of glue to the laceration. Some also apply a few drops to the twisted hair.
    - Repeat every few millimeters along the laceration. Allow 60 to 90 seconds for the glue to dry and apply another coat if indicated. Complete this process until the wound is completely approximated.
    - Caution patient not to wash hair for 2 days or to vigorously brush or comb around the area of the laceration.

POSTPROCEDURE PATIENT EDUCATION

The adhesive is water resistant, and further dressing is not needed. The patient may wet the area but should pat it dry. Soaking is not recommended. Antibiotic ointment should be avoided because it will weaken the bond and dissolve the glue. A bandage may be appropriate for active people, children, or those inclined to pick or pull at the wound. The adhesive spontaneously sloughs in 5 to 14 days. Infections are unusual but can be detected early because the wound is visible and purulent exudate normally "unroofs" the adhesive. In these cases, the adhesive should be gently removed and standard wound infection treatment, possibly including systemic antibiotics, implemented. Reclosure with cyanoacrylate is not recommended.

COMPLICATIONS

- Early wound dehiscence.
- If the practitioner's instruments, gauze, or gloves accidentally adhere to the wound or patient, pressure is placed adjacent to the area and the object is "rolled off" in a way that does not place traction on the repair.
- Adhesive that inadvertently binds the eyelids should be covered with generous amounts of ophthalmic antibiotic ointment and not pried open. The bond usually weakens and separates—if not immediately, then in 1 or 2 days. Cyanoacrylates are not harmful to the eye and are used routinely in ophthalmologic practice. Appropriate placement of gauze during repairs can prevent spillage into the eyes.
- Petroleum jelly, antibiotic ointment, or a commercially available Super Glue remover can be used on dried runoff areas.
- Adhesive may insinuate itself between wound edges, resulting in unacceptable healing.

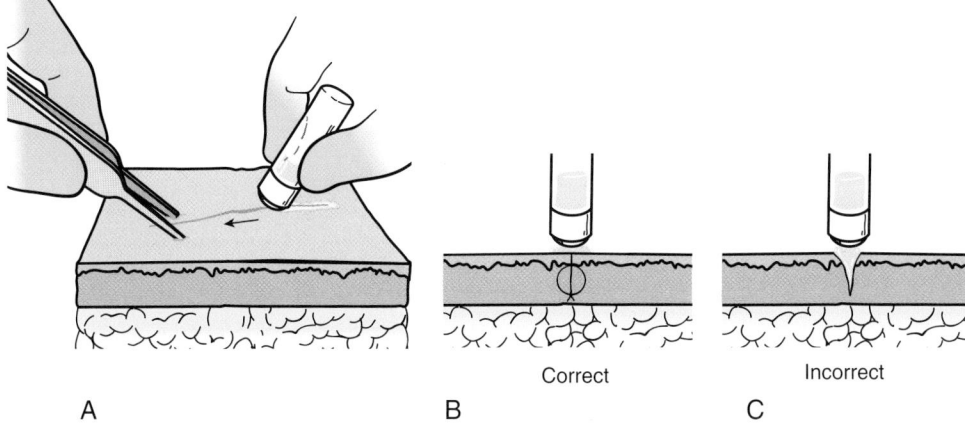

A   B   Correct   C   Incorrect

Fig. 198.2 (A) Approximate margins and apply glue. (B) Correct application. (C) Incorrect application into the wound itself.

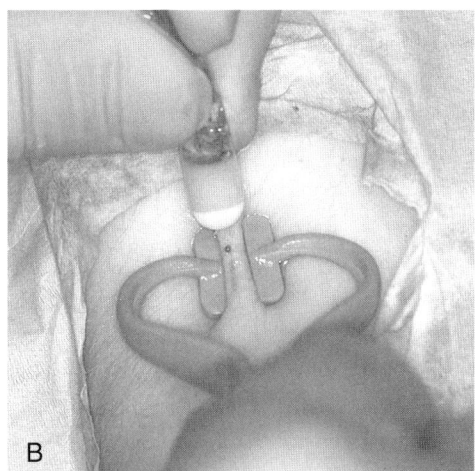

Fig. 198.3 (A) Plastic tissue approximators for the application of tissue glue. (B) Application of tissue glue with the aid of plastic approximators.

PATIENT EDUCATION GUIDES

See the sample patient education handout available at www.expert consult.com.

CPT/BILLING CODES

See Chapter 19, Laceration and Incision Repair, Table 19.4, for wound closure codes. The same codes are used whether the repair is performed with suture or with tissue glue.

ICD-10-CM DIAGNOSTIC CODES

ICD-10   Codes for wound or laceration vary by location, degree, depth, and tendon involvement. See also Chapter 19, Laceration and Incision Repair.

SUPPLIERS

(See contact information available at www.expertconsult.com.)

Octyl cyanoacrylates
   Dermabond, Ethicon, Inc.
   LiquiBand, Advanced Medical Solutions, Ltd.
   SurgiSeal, Pfizer, Inc.
Butyl cyanoacrylates
   Histoacryl, B Braun Corp.
   Indermil, Covidien Medtronic
Wound closure forceps
   Bionix Development Corp.

Acknowledgment

The editors recognize the contributions of J. Mark Wiedemanm, MD, and John L. Pfenninger, MD to this chapter in a previous edition of this text.

RECOMMENDED READING

Afarian HM. Tissue adhesives for wound repair. In: Reichman EF, ed. *Emergency Medicine Procedures.* 2nd ed. New York: McGraw-Hill; 2013:647–649.

Hock MO, Ooi SB, Saw SM, Lim SH. A randomized controlled trial comparing the hair apposition technique with tissue glue to standard suturing in scalp lacerations (HAT Study). *Ann Emerg Med.* 2002;40:19–26.

Lammers RL, Smith ZE. Methods of wound closure. In: Roberts JR, Custalow CB, Thomsen TW, eds. *Roberts and Hedges' Clinical Procedures in Emergency Medicine.* 6th ed. Philadelphia: Elsevier; 2014:646–649.

Pfenninger JL. Use of tissue glues (cyanoacrylate tissue adhesives). In: Rakel R, ed. *Saunders Manual of Medical Practice.* Philadelphia: WB Saunders; 2000.

Quinn J, Wells G, Sutcliffe T, et al. A randomized trial comparing octyl-cyanoacrylate tissue adhesive and sutures in the management of lacerations. *JAMA.* 1997;277:1527–1530.

Simon HK, McLario DJ, Bruns TB, et al. Long-term appearance of lacerations repaired using a tissue adhesive. *Pediatrics.* 1997;99:193–195.

Singer AJ, Hollander JE, Valentine SM, et al. Prospective, randomized, controlled trial of tissue adhesive (2-octylcyanoacrylate) vs. standard wound closure techniques for laceration repair. Stony Brook Octylcyanoacrylate Study Group. *Acad Emerg Med.* 1998;5:94–99.

CHAPTER 199

TOPICAL HEMOSTATIC AGENTS

Dale A. Patterson • Matt D. Roth

In medical training, there is a cynical phrase quoted to novice medical students on a surgery rotation: "All bleeding stops eventually." Although this is true, the lesson to learn is that usually the best amount of bleeding is the least amount. Effective, rapid hemostasis is the goal of clinicians performing cutaneous surgery. This chapter covers the most useful methods of achieving topical hemostasis (Table 199.1).

The various methods range from physical techniques, such as simple pressure with an index finger and gauze pad, to chemical, electrical, and even laser techniques. The method used depends on the specifics of the surgery being performed, the experience of the office surgeon, and the availability of the agents or equipment.

Each method has its own benefits and drawbacks, and the astute clinician will match the method that best fits the needs of the particular situation and patient. The older chemical agents (so-called vasoconstrictive, vaso-occlusive, or denaturing agents) produce an eschar and actually cause some tissue damage. Newer, so-called physiologic, agents facilitate the clotting mechanism but can be exorbitantly expensive (e.g., $30 or more for a single pack of Gelfoam). It is therefore important for the clinician to be familiar with multiple methods and competent in their use to ensure the most positive outcome.

INDICATIONS

- For the treatment of:
  - Bleeding after cutaneous surgery, such as a shave biopsy
  - Abrasions or denuded skin
  - The nail bed after either partial or full removal of a nail
  - Cuts or open wounds that cannot or will not be primarily closed
- To cauterize excess granulation tissue

CONTRAINDICATIONS

Absolute

- Profuse bleeding. Topical agents will not control briskly bleeding vessels.
- Allergy to the hemostatic agent used.

Relative

- Large, deep wounds that require primary surgical closure with suture (use mechanical methods only).
- A cardiac pacemaker may preclude the use of electrosurgery (e.g., Bovie, Hyfrecator).

NOTE: *Cautery* technically refers to a hot wire (most often in a battery-powered unit). This method is generally safe for patients with a pacemaker. On the other hand, *electrocautery* (e.g., Bovie, Hyfrecator, Ellman Surgitron) produces a low-amperage current (causing electrofulguration, electrodesiccation, or electrocoagulation) that may pose a risk to pacemaker users. Most new pacemakers are shielded. Use of these electrosurgical units should not be a problem, but other safe alternatives exist. See Chapter 25, Radiofrequency Surgery (Modern Electrosurgery) for details of electrosurgical principles.

EQUIPMENT AND SUPPLIES

Hemostatic Agents

See Fig. 199.1 for a depiction of several common hemostatic agents.

Vaso-occlusive Denaturing Agents

Most commonly used

- Ferric subsulfate solution (20%; Monsel solution)
- Aluminum chloride (30% solution; Drysol)
- Silver nitrate sticks or 20% to 50% solution
- Hydrophilic polymer and potassium salt (QR powder)

Not recommended

- Trichloroacetic acid (50% to 85% solution)
- Zinc chloride paste
- Phenol 50% solution
- Hydrogen peroxide 3% solution

Agents Producing a Physical Meshwork

- Absorbable gelatin sponge (Gelfoam)
- Oxidized cellulose (Surgicel)
- Microfibrillar collagen (Avitene)
- Cyanoacrylates (Dermabond, IsoDent; see Chapter 198, Tissue Glues)

Physiologic Hemostatic Agents

- Epinephrine or lidocaine with epinephrine
- Thrombin (Thrombostat)
- Fibrin sealant
- Cocaine hydrochloride solution

Combination Products

- Flowable bovine collagen and bovine platelets (CoStasis)
- Flowable bovine gelatin matrix and bovine thrombin (FloSeal)

Agents for Traumatic Injuries

- QuikClot (granular zeolite powder)
- HemCon (Chitosan dressing)
- ChitoFlex (Chitosan dressing)

Mechanical Methods

- Electrocautery (hot wire, battery-operated unit)
- Electrosurgery (e.g., Bovie, Hyfrecator, Ellman Surgitron)
- Laser (carbon dioxide)
- Shaw scalpel (a Teflon-coated scalpel blade with a heating element)

TABLE 199.1 Topical Hemostatic Agents					
Generic/Product Name	Effectiveness	Difficulty of Preparation/ Application	Undesired Tissue Destruction	Chance of Pigment Stain (Usually Temporary)	Cost
Vaso-occlusive/Denaturing Agents					
Recommended					
Ferric subsulfate solution (20%; Monsel solution)	+++	++	+	++	$$
QR powder	+++	+	−	−	$$
Aluminum chloride (30%)	++	++	+	−	$$
Silver nitrate sticks	+++	+	++	++++	$$
Not recommended					
Trichloroacetic acid (50%–85%)	++	+++	+++	−	$$
Zinc chloride paste	++	++	+	−	$$
Phenol 50%	++	++	+++	−	$$
Hydrogen peroxide	+	+	+	−	$
Agents Producing a Physical Meshwork					
Absorbable gelatin sponge (Gelfoam, Surgifoam)	+++	++	−	−	$$$$
Oxidized cellulose (Surgicel)	++++	+++	−	−	$$$$
Microfibrillar collagen (Avitene)	+++++	+++++	−	−	$$$$$
Physiologic Hemostatic Agents					
Cocaine hydrochloride	+++	++++	−	−	$$$
Epinephrine	+++	+	−	−	$
Thrombin (Thrombostat)	+++++	++++	−	−	$$$$$
Fibrin sealant	+++++	++++	−	−	$$$$
Combination Agents					
CoStasis, FloSeal	+++++	+++++	−	−	$$$$$

Agents rated from mildly effective (+) to highly effective (+++++), easy to prepare/apply (+) to difficult to prepare/apply (+++++), minimal damage (+) to significant destruction (+++++), low pigment stain (+) to high chance of pigment stain (+++++), and low cost ($) to high cost ($$$$$).
−, No effect.

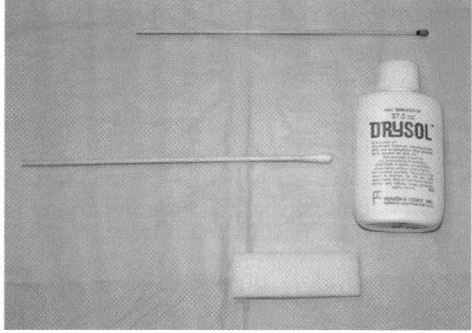

Fig. 199.1 Common hemostatic agents. *Top to bottom,* silver nitrate stick, aluminum hydroxide with applicator, absorbable Gelfoam.

- Application of ice
- Pressure dressings
- Blood pressure cuff inflated proximally

PREPROCEDURE PATIENT EDUCATION

Discuss the procedure, including the rare but possible risks of pain, further bleeding, infection, nerve or other nearby structural damage, and scarring. Determine if the patient is known to be allergic to any of the agents. If using silver nitrate or Monsel solution, inform the patient of the possibility of pigmentary change ("tattooing"), which is usually temporary but still requires discretion when it is being used in exposed areas such as the face.

PROCEDURE

See the corresponding chapter for the initial procedure being performed. Topical hemostatic agents are not a substitute for meticulous surgical technique and many cannot be used inside a wound to be sutured. When topical hemostatic agents are required, make sure that the patient is positioned on the examination or procedure table in a way that provides adequate access to the wound. Inflating a blood pressure cuff proximally may help to start with a dry field, thus enhancing chemical or electrical cautery.

Vaso-occlusive Denaturing Agents

These agents are applied topically and are not used if a wound is to be closed surgically. To maximize the coagulation effect, these agents should be applied as close to the source of bleeding as possible and the wound should be sponged free of excess blood just before their application.

Ferric Subsulfate Solution (20%; Monsel Solution)

First described by Leon Monsel in 1856, this liquid is perhaps the most commonly used topical hemostatic agent (Fig. 199.2). The solution is dark brown, almost black. If the bottle is left open, evaporation results in a pasty solution that, because it is more concentrated, is more effective. Do not let it become too thick, however. If it crystallizes, it can be reconstituted with water. Keep the container covered once the desired consistency has been obtained. Hemostasis is effective with only rare staining, which can last up to 3 months. The application of Monsel solution to a relatively dry wound bed (achieved by stretching and blotting the skin) controls oozing effectively.

Monsel solution is applied with a cotton-tipped swab after drying and stretching the skin with the other hand. The swab is applied with light pressure. The low pH and subsulfate group denature protein and occlude blood vessels. The practitioner cannot use too much, meaning, there is not a limit to the amount used. Once in contact with blood, the black, coagulated mixture can be wiped away. Monsel solution works particularly well after cervical biopsies, loop electrosurgical excision procedures, and anorectal biopsies. It is also commonly used after shave excision and punch biopsies except in very fair-skinned individuals.

Monsel solution is inexpensive, easily applied, easily stored, and readily available. However, there is a rare risk of "tattooing," so some

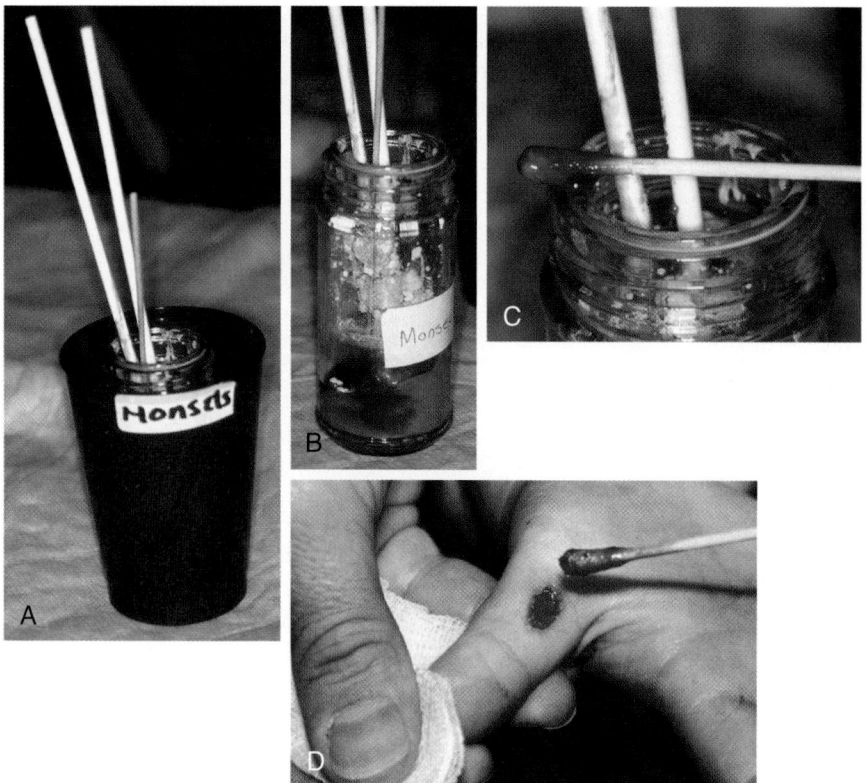

Fig. 199.2 Topical astringent. (A) Monsel solution in open bottle, which allows it to thicken. (B) Inner bottle. (C) Cotton-tipped applicator used to apply thickened solution (do not reinsert into bottle/container). (D) Applying Monsel with cotton-tipped applicator.

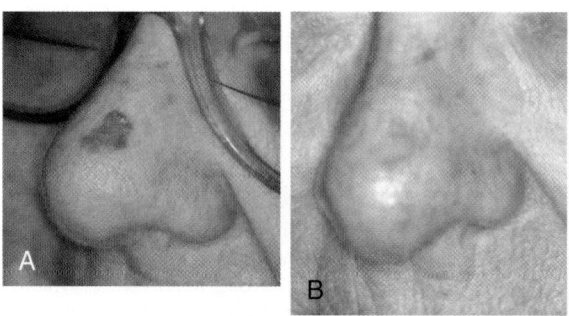

Fig. 199.3 Monsel staining. (A) Three weeks after initial use. (B) Spontaneous resolution after 6 to 8 weeks.

clinicians do not recommend it for the face, especially on light skin (Fig. 199.3). In clinical practice there is often a compromise in which Monsel solution, given its superior hemostatic properties, is still used for the face and on patients with a very light complexion. (Aluminum chloride is nonstaining and should be tried first in these cases.) The tattooing can last for several months. Monsel solution may also cause temporary artifactual changes in skin and cervical biopsies, confounding the histologic evaluation of reexcisions for a few weeks thereafter. It also stains clothing. Stains on laboratory coats can be removed with dilute hydrochloric acid, such as that often found in toilet bowl cleaners, or by using Iron-Out. Monsel solution stains must be treated before washing in hot water or drying with heat because each maneuver seems to set the stain permanently.

Aluminum Chloride (30%)

Aluminum chloride is usually applied topically to a wound as a 30% solution (e.g., Drysol, Lumicain) on a swab with light pressure (Fig. 199.4). It is colorless and forms a thin coagulum over the wound.

Although not as effective as Monsel solution, it does not cause tattooing. This solution is commonly used after surgical shave biopsies.

Silver Nitrate

Silver nitrate is available as a 20% to 50% solution and as a solid on a wooden stick. The sticks are more convenient and consequently more popular. The silver nitrate on the end is activated when the tip is placed on a moist wound bed. Silver ions cause proteins to denature and precipitate, which occludes blood vessels. The eschar that forms in the wound bed prevents deeper tissue penetration by the hemostatic agent. Silver salts stain the tissue black because of the deposition of reduced silver. Although most of the stain disappears spontaneously within a few weeks, there is a modest possibility of permanently tattooing the treated site. Care must be used with silver nitrate to avoid damaging normal tissue surrounding a wound. Because of these concerns, silver nitrate is most often restricted to cauterization of excess granulation tissue or for use in nonvisible areas (e.g., cervix, rectum). Fig. 199.5 shows silver nitrate hemostasis of a shave biopsy. Without anesthesia it can be uncomfortable, so the patient should be warned.

Trichloroacetic Acid (50% to 85%)

Trichloroacetic acid is a topically applied agent that also forms an eschar at the wound bed. When it touches the tissue, the acid also causes superficial tissue destruction; it is therefore rarely used for hemostatic purposes and is not recommended. Without anesthesia it can be painful, so application should be precise and rapid.

QR Powder (Hydrophilic Polymers and Potassium Salt)

This product is available over the counter and for professionals (Fig. 199.6). Blood must be present for it to work. The product is supplied in an individual-use packet at a cost of about $2 per packet. A thin coating of the powder is applied to the wound and pressure held for 15 to 60 seconds. Pressure is applied until bleeding stops (see Fig. 199.6D and E). If bleeding recurs, another application of the product can be made, even by the patient at home. The eschar should be left in place until it naturally falls off. It is safe to wash and bathe the area 1 hour after application of the product. QR powder is not biologically derived and is not known to cause allergic reactions, tattooing, or discoloration of the skin. It can be used on any wound

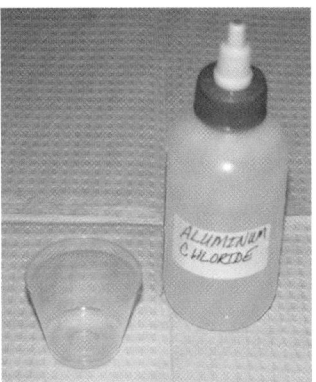

Fig. 199.4   Aluminum chloride (clear solution).

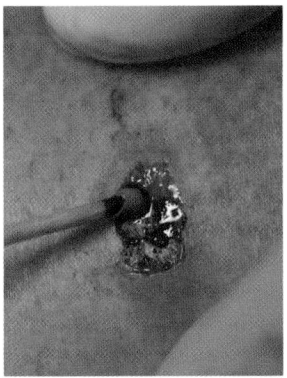

Fig. 199.5   Shave biopsy partially cauterized by silver nitrate stick.

left to heal by secondary intention and has been successfully used to stop bleeding from the nose, abrasions, punctures, and minor surgical procedures. It should not be used below the surface of the skin on sutured wounds and is for topical/external use only. It does not cause pain or any pigment changes.

Other Agents

Zinc chloride paste is an effective hemostatic agent that was used in the original fixed-tissue Mohs micrographic surgery, and it is still occasionally used today. *Phenol 50%* is effective, but the severe caustic effects on normal tissue may enlarge a wound. For this reason, it may be useful in nail removal for achieving hemostasis while providing destruction of the nail matrix. *Hydrogen peroxide* is readily available and is a weak hemostatic agent. It has obvious germicidal action, is inexpensive, and is easy to apply. Hydrogen peroxide is commonly applied directly to the wound in saturated gauze with direct pressure. It too causes some degree of tissue destruction and is rarely used for hemostasis alone.

Agents Producing a Physical Meshwork

Surgical wound closure is acceptable after use of most of the following agents.

Absorbable Gelatin Sponge (Gelfoam, Surgifoam)

Gelatin powder is applied dry to the wound bed with light pressure. Absorbable gelatin sponges are manufactured in various forms from purified gelatin solution. Gelatin sponges can be applied dry or moistened with saline or thrombin. Absorbable gelatin holds blood and provides a matrix for clot formation and granulation tissue to form. The sponges are costly for a private office but are convenient and easy to handle. The gelatin powder can be difficult to handle and may be less effective than other meshwork agents. Following application, the wound can often be covered with a pressure dressing. After a few minutes, the resultant dry field can often be approximated with sutures.

Potential side effects include excessive granuloma formation and fibrosis. Care should be taken if these sponges are used near tendons because they have been known to cause excessive fibrosis, especially in these areas.

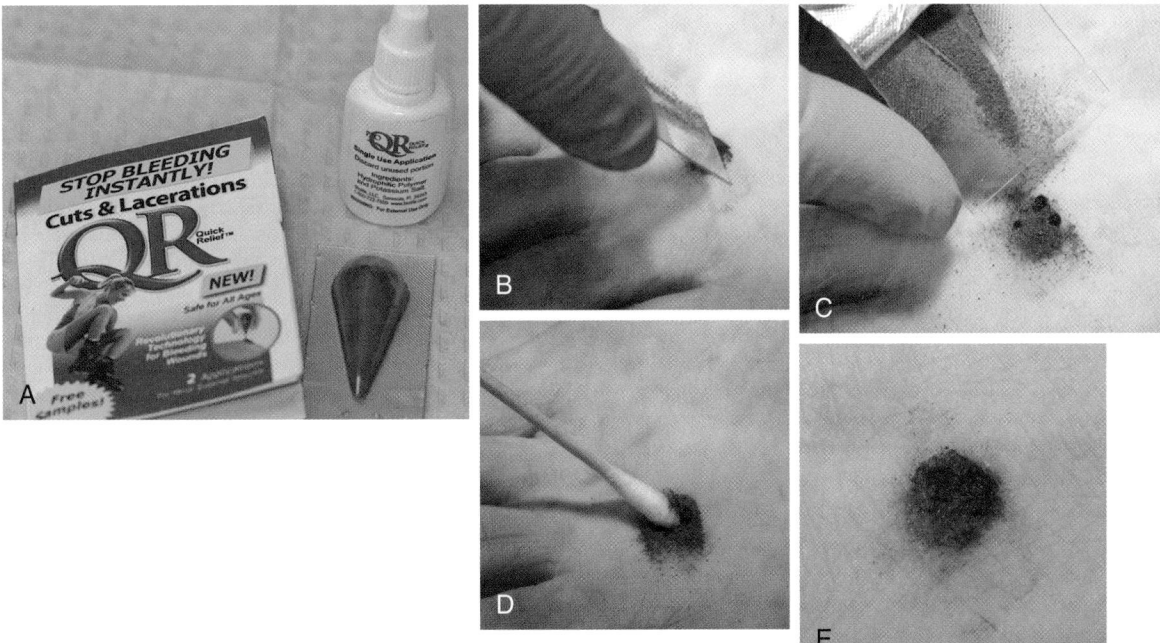

Fig. 199.6   QR (Quick Release) powder. (A) Available in packets *(lower right)* or bottle dispensers. (B) QR in use: applying from packet to shave excision. (C) Appearance on wound before applying pressure. (D) Applying pressure with a cotton-tipped applicator. (E) Final appearance; hemostasis is obtained. A dressing is applied without antibiotic ointment.

Oxidized Cellulose (Surgicel)

Oxidized cellulose consists of absorbable fibers prepared from cellulose. Woven strips or sheets of cellulose can be cut and held with firm pressure on the wound bed. Oxidized cellulose provides a meshwork for coagulation and causes local vasoconstriction. This preparation is moderately priced, easy to handle, and mildly bactericidal.

Foreign-body reaction is possible if excessive amounts of cellulose are left in a wound. Cellulose should not be used under grafts or flaps because it separates the graft from the blood supply. Some experts believe that the removal of oxidized cellulose after obtaining hemostasis frequently produces rebleeding.

Microfibrillar Collagen (Avitene)

Microfibrillar collagen is prepared by mechanically breaking down bovine collagen into fibrils. It is available in a fibrous (granular) form or a web form. The fibrous form is applied directly to the wound and held in place. The highly effective collagen products aggregate platelets on their surface. Collagen matrix applied to skin biopsy sites produces fewer infections, faster healing, and better cosmetic results than Monsel solution.

Microfibrillar collagen adheres to wet gloves or surfaces, and it must be applied with dry instruments. Although the collagen is eventually absorbed, it cannot be used at skin closure sites because it impedes the healing of wound edges. Its high cost and difficulty in handling make this agent impractical for most office dermatologic surgery.

Cyanoacrylates (Dermabond, IsoDent)

Tissue glues can seal wound edges and halt bleeding. See Chapter 198, Tissue Glues.

Physiologic Hemostatic Agents

Epinephrine

Epinephrine is a potent activator of adrenergic receptors, and the activation of α-adrenergic receptors produces vasoconstriction in the skin. Epinephrine is available in local anesthetics such as lidocaine with epinephrine or as adrenaline chloride solutions. Epinephrine is inexpensive and readily available, and it does not harm normal tissue at the base of the wound. It can be applied topically to control bleeding (e.g., from the nose) or injected into a bleeding site (e.g., cervical biopsy). Effects are temporary (about 2 hours). Control of the bleeding, however, allows electrocoagulation or the application of other topical agents if necessary. Use caution and aspirate prior to injection to make sure that the epinephrine is not being injected intravascularly. Attention should be paid to the total dose, even when applied topically, to avoid systemic side effects such as hypertension, tachycardia, and seizure.

Complications are quite rare. The precaution is always to avoid its use in end-arterial areas (i.e., finger, nose, penis, toes) for fear of causing distal necrosis. This rarely occurs. However, caution is advised in the vascular-compromised patient. Rebound vasodilation can potentially cause delayed bleeding. Cardiac arrhythmias and neurologic symptoms have been reported with the use of epinephrine in dermatologic procedures.

Thrombin (Thrombostat)

Thrombin is a potent physiologic clotting agent produced by the activation of bovine prothrombin. This freeze-dried powder can either be mixed with isotonic saline and sponged or sprayed on the wound bed, or it can be applied directly as powder. The wound should be sponged free of excess blood before thrombin is applied. For superficial surgery or plastic surgery involving flaps, dilute solutions of 100 U/mL may be effective.

Thrombin does not injure tissue or produce residue on the tissue bed. Once the solution has been prepared, it must be used within 6 hours. Thrombin is expensive, prohibiting the routine use of this agent for office procedures.

Fibrin Sealant

Fibrin sealant is produced by making two components of human clotting factors immediately before application. Fibrin clot forms in about 30 seconds; the sealant can be applied with a special spraying device that mixes the components as they are delivered into the wound. Fibrin glue is one of the most effective agents available for hemostasis. The cost, the risk associated with the use of human blood products, and the cumbersome method of administration make this therapy undesirable for routine dermatologic surgery.

Cocaine Hydrochloride

Cocaine hydrochloride is useful as a powerful vasoconstrictor, but the potential for abuse, the cost, and the need for locked storage make its use problematic.

Combination Products

Combination products, such as CoStasis and FloSeal, use both meshwork and hemostatic agents in surgical procedures when conventional methods of hemostasis have been unsuccessful. They are impractical for office procedures owing to their cost (e.g., up to $500 per use for Floseal) and limited applicability in routine procedures. PRO QR powder, a combination of a hydrophilic polymer and a potassium iron oxyacid salt, has more recently become available and is gaining popularity in office and emergency department settings.

Agents for Traumatic Injuries

QuikClot (Granular Zeolite Powder)

QuikClot has been approved by the US Food and Drug Administration for the treatment of external hemorrhage. Much of the experience in the use of QuikClot has been in military applications. When applied to a wound, the granular zeolite powder attracts water and dries the wound in an exothermic reaction. This drying effect increases the rate at which red blood cells aggregate and decreases blood loss. The product has been shown to reduce hemorrhage from major traumatic wounds and has been used by the military in Iraq and Afghanistan. QuikClot is supplied in various forms, including sponges, bandages, granular packets, and nasal applicators. Each of these forms is applied directly to an external bleeding wound and combined with pressure to stop hemorrhage. The original product caused a significant temperature elevation in the surrounding tissue, but a reformulated product has been released that decreases the amount of heat released during application.

HemCon and ChitoFlex (Chitosan Dressings)

Chitosan is a mucoadhesive, biodegradable polysaccharide derived from shellfish. HemCon and ChitoFlex supply chitosan in ready-to-apply bandages. When exposed to blood, the bandages become extremely adherent and facilitate clotting. The molecule is also positively charged and may attract negatively charged erythrocytes, further enhancing clot formation. HemCon bandages are larger and supplied in various sizes to treat external wounds. ChitoFlex bandages are more flexible and compact, facilitating the treatment of penetrating trauma tracts. Both are latex-free and have no known complications or contraindications. They can be left in place for up to 48 hours and should be removed with water or saline for definitive wound treatment. Traumadex is another polysaccharide-derived powder and sponge that dehydrates the blood, concentrates blood constituents, and promotes clot formation. In a swine model of lethal hemorrhage, it did not perform quite as well as HemCon or QuikClot.

Mechanical Methods

- *Cautery (electrosurgical or battery-operated unit):* For hemostasis, use the coagulation or fulguration settings and set at a very low power. Gently "tap" the area, being careful to avoid excessive tissue damage. Larger vessels (>2 to 3 mm) should be tied off rather than coagulated.
- *Laser (carbon dioxide):* Rarely used for this purpose.
- *Shaw scalpel* (a Teflon-coated scalpel blade with a heating element).
- *Ice packs:* Cause vasoconstriction and reduce bleeding and swelling.
- *Pressure dressings* (see Chapter 26, Skin Biopsy, Fig. 26.8).

COMMON ERRORS

- Using agents capable of producing "tattooing" (Monsel solution or silver nitrate) in a visible area on a light-skinned person. Choose an agent that does not pose this risk.
- Overcauterizing an area of bleeding, leading to more tissue destruction than necessary. Use only the minimal amount of chemical, electric, or thermal cautery to stop the active bleeding.
- Using ferric subsulfate, aluminum chloride, or silver nitrate inside a wound that must be sutured closed.

COMPLICATIONS

- Rebound bleeding
- Infection
- Nerve damage
- Scarring or tattooing
- Swelling
- Excessive tissue damage

POSTPROCEDURE PATIENT INFORMATION

Instruct the patient on the following:

- Keep the area clean and moist but avoid maceration. Any ointment, including those with antibiotics (except Neosporin), will aid healing. For dermatologic applications, petrolatum jelly has been found to be as effective as antibiotic ointments.
- Change the dressing at least two to three times a day (preferably four) and wash gently with soap and water.
- Follow up as directed; do so sooner if there is an increase in redness, swelling or if the patient reports pain, fever, night sweats or chills or other signs of infection such as purulent drainage.
- Avoid cleansing with hydrogen peroxide because it kills fibroblasts.

CONCLUSION

Hemostatic agents are useful during cutaneous surgery or when the clinician is faced with an open wound that cannot be primarily closed with sutures. Topical hemostatic agents are not a substitute for meticulous surgical technique, and many cannot be used inside a wound to be sutured. Physical measures such as direct pressure, cold application, or suture ligatures should also be considered when one is trying to control bleeding. The various agents have benefits and limitations. It is important to become familiar with several, such as Monsel solution, aluminum chloride, absorbable gelatin sponge (Gelfoam), and oxidized cellulose (Surgicel).

BILLING AND CODING

Application of topical hemostatics is included in the wound care charge and should not be unbundled. If a patient presents with a condition requiring topical hemostasis, the appropriate level of service should be billed. ICD-10-CM codes are indicated for the particular lesion or presenting concern being addressed.

SUPPLIERS

(See contact information available at www.expertconsult.com.)

Nearly every medical supplier (such as Delasco) can provide the routine and common hemostatic agents. For the newer agents, consult the following:

HemCon by Tricol Biomedical Technologies, Inc.
Z-Medica Corporation

RECOMMENDED READING

Freeman C, Reichman EF. Hemorrhage control. In: Reichman EF, ed. *Emergency Medicine Procedures.* 2nd ed. New York: McGraw-Hill; 2013:731–738.

Gabay M. Absorbable hemostatic agents. *Am J Health Syst Pharm.* 2006;63:1244–1253.

Guttman C, Susan H, Weinkle MD. Pearls of wisdom: dermatologist. *Dermatol Surg.* 2008;34:96.

Ho J, Hruza G. Hydrophilic polymers with potassium salt and microporous polysaccharides for use as hemostatic agents. *Dermatol Surg.* 2007;33:1430–1433.

Kircik L. *Comparative Efficacy of Topical Hemostatic Powder vs. Foam Sterile Compressed Sponge in Second Intention Healing After Mohs Micrographic Surgery: Pilot Study.* Presented at the American College of Mohs Surgery Annual Meeting, Vancouver, British Columbia, Canada; May 3, 2008.

Lammers RL, Smith ZE. Principles of wound management. In: Roberts JR, Custalow CB, Thomsen TW, eds. *Roberts and Hedges' Clinical Procedures in Emergency Medicine.* 6th ed. Philadelphia: Elsevier; 2014:611–643.

Kuwahara RT, Ammonette RA. A novel method to remove Monsel's stain. *Dermatol Surg.* 2000;26:507.

Mabry R, McManus JG. Prehospital advances in the management of severe penetrating trauma. *Crit Care Med.* 2008;36(suppl):S258–S266.

Palm MD, Altman JS. Topical hemostatic agents: a review. *Dermatol Surg.* 2008;34:431–445.

Spitzer M, Chernys AE. Monsel's solution-induced artifact in the uterine cervix. *Am J Obstet Gynecol.* 1996;175:1204–1207.

Take 5 Pearls Surgical. QR powder to control bleeding. *Pract Dermatol.* 2008;5:64.

Wang DS, Chu LF, Olson SE, et al. Comparative evaluation of noninvasive compression adjuncts for hemostasis in percutaneous arterial, venous and arteriovenous dialysis access procedures. *J Vasc Interv Radiol.* 2008;19:72–79.

CHAPTER 200

CORNEAL ABRASIONS AND REMOVAL OF CORNEAL OR CONJUNCTIVAL FOREIGN BODIES

Grant C. Fowler

Patients with "something in the eye," a foreign body, or corneal or conjunctival abrasion, are common for primary care clinicians. In most cases, the management is uncomplicated and can be completed in the clinician's office; however, knowledge of certain principles should help to avoid impaired vision or blindness.

A detailed history is important, especially knowing what the patient was doing when they first noticed a problem. For instance, was the patient wearing eye protection? Was he or she around hammered metal? Did he or she come into contact with a high-velocity foreign body?

NOTE: In the past, corneal abrasions were treated with eye patching and mydriatics; however, there is little evidence to support eye patching, which may even impair healing. Consequently, most clinicians now use ophthalmic nonsteroidal antiinflammatory drugs (NSAIDs) and an ophthalmic antibiotic for treatment. Some of the evidence supporting this approach is discussed further in the "Technique" section. Also, if a slit lamp is available, a more thorough evaluation of the eye may be performed for a corneal abrasion or foreign body (see Chapter 201, Slit-Lamp Examination). In the absence of a slit lamp, this chapter indicates when a slit-lamp referral is required.

FLUORESCEIN EXAMINATION OF THE CORNEA AND CONJUNCTIVA

Indications

- Unilateral foreign body sensation, hypersensitivity to light, excess tearing, or pain—especially on opening or closing the eye
- Red eye
- Eye trauma
- After airbag deployment in automobile accidents
- Unilateral, persistent eye irritation in a contact lens wearer
- History of exposure to ultraviolet light from such sources as a welding torch, sunlight, or a tanning bed (ultraviolet light can penetrate the cornea even when the patient's eyes are closed if protective lenses are not worn)
- Mild chemical exposure to eye
- Neonates or infants with persistent crying, unilateral tearing, hypersensitivity to light, or conjunctival inflammation
- Eye discharge in a mask-ventilated newborn or a heavily sedated or paralyzed adult on a ventilator

NOTE: Hypersensitivity to light, excess tearing, and painful or red eye are also signs and symptoms of glaucoma (see Chapter 58, Tonometry). If there is no foreign body sensation, the patient should be evaluated for acute glaucoma.

Contraindications

Patients with the following symptoms should be referred to an ophthalmologist after they have been provided initial urgent care:

- Suspected high-velocity injury to the eye (e.g., patients exposed to metal hammering or heavy machinery). High-speed metallic or nonmetallic fragments can penetrate the globe while only causing minimal symptoms and damage to the cornea. As a result, significant internal damage must be excluded. If penetration of the globe is apparent, fluorescein staining is usually avoided because it may make further evaluation or surgery more difficult.
- A hyphema, lens opacification, scleral tear, abnormal anterior chamber examination, or irregularity of the pupil. These findings suggest that the globe has been penetrated, and an ophthalmologist needs to be involved. Orbital x-ray films may confirm a metal foreign body. A spiral computed tomography scan or ultrasonography may also confirm a metal foreign body; magnetic resonance imaging is contraindicated if there is a possible ferromagnetic object.
- Long-standing (>24 hours) inflammation as evidenced by iritis, photophobia, or ciliary blush. These findings suggest the presence of an intraocular foreign body or a more serious injury and require slit-lamp examination and evaluation by an ophthalmologist.

NOTE: A pressure patch is contraindicated in a penetration injury of the globe or a complex lid laceration. For such injuries, a nonpressure protective eye shield should be applied before referral. Metal shields are manufactured for this purpose, or a nonpressure shield can be fashioned from a paper cup (Fig. 200.1). All patches and shields should be taped in the same direction, from the medial forehead across the eye and toward the ear.

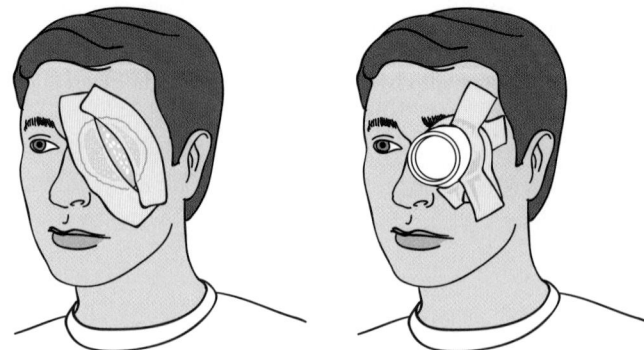

Fig. 200.1 Nonpressure patch to protect ruptured globe. A metal shield or a paper cup can be used.

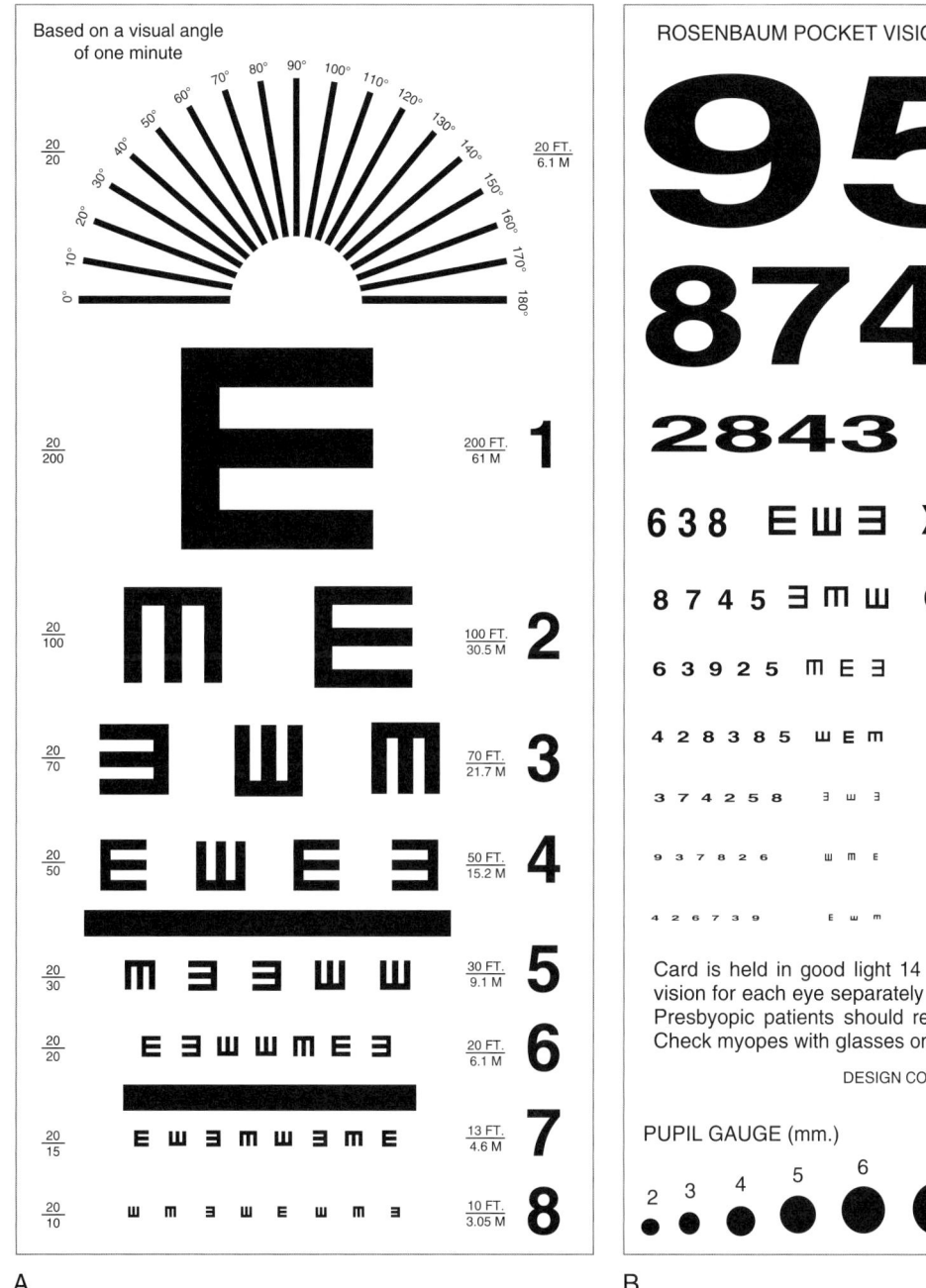

Fig. 200.2 (A) Illiterate E chart. (B) Near-vision chart.

- Exposure to caustic or acidic media. Immediate management includes copious irrigation for at least 15 minutes. (It can begin at home with tap water from a shower or hose.)
- Mild chemical exposure. If the clinician is not knowledgeable about or comfortable with managing the case after contacting a Poison Control Center, the patient should be referred.
- Ruptured globe.
- Uncooperative patient. (Infants may have to be sedated; see Chapter 2, Pediatric Sedation and Analgesia.)

Equipment

- Snellen chart at 6 m (20 ft), or an equivalent visual acuity chart (Fig. 200.2). If a chart is unavailable, ask the patient to read a magazine at arm's length. If the patient cannot do so, measure and record the distance at which the patient can count fingers.

- Topical ophthalmic anesthetic such as 0.5% proparacaine (e.g., Alcaine, Kainair, Ophthaine, Ophthetic, Paracaine, Proparacaine), unless contraindicated (e.g., ruptured globe or allergy to local anesthetics). Benoxinate 0.4% is compatible with fluorescein in solution.

  NOTE: Proparacaine has been proven to cause less discomfort than tetracaine 0.5% to 1.0% (Pontocaine).

- Sterile fluorescein sodium strips. (Because fluorescein is incompatible with preservatives effective against *Pseudomonas* and *Proteus*, multidose dropper bottles of fluorescein solution should not be used. Inoculating abraded corneal epithelium with bacteria could cause infection, permanent scarring, or blindness.)
- Bright white light source (a single-point source such as a penlight is preferable).
- Cobalt-blue light source (Wood's lamp is adequate).

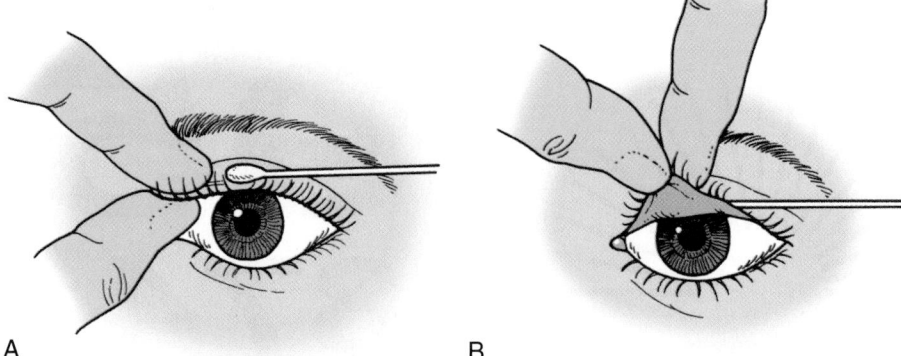

Fig. 200.3 (A) Grasp the upper eyelashes between the thumb and index finger. With the tip of the other index finger or a cotton-tipped applicator, press down gently on the skin of the upper lid. (B) Pull outward on the lashes and rotate the tarsal plate upward until it forms a right angle with the eyeball. A gentle tug upward should flip the plate into eversion, clearly exposing the conjunctival surface of the upper lid.

- An 8- to 10-power magnification lens (loupes, a magnifying glass, a colposcope, or an ophthalmoscope on the +20 to +40 diopter setting).
- Sterile cotton-tipped applicators.
- Isotonic ophthalmic irrigant (e.g., Dacriose, Ringer lactate, normal saline).
- Facial tissues (e.g., Kleenex).

Preprocedure Patient Preparation

The indications for the examination should be explained to the patient as well as any risks or alternatives. The patient needs to know what will occur during the examination and that they may be asked to direct their vision to certain locations. Eyedrops and dye will probably be necessary to enhance the examination. Contact lenses should be removed before the eye is stained (fluorescein can stain them permanently). Before instilling fluorescein, the patient should be warned that objects in his or her vision may temporarily appear yellow. Tears may also remain yellow for a short time after the examination and might stain skin or clothing, at least temporarily, so the patient should avoid rubbing his or her eyes or drying tears on something that might stain.

Patients should be instructed to breathe normally and, especially children, may be asked at certain times to remain as still as possible. Children may need assistance with holding still. Patients should know to blink normally unless their eye is being held open by the examiner or they are asked to hold their eye open. They should be aware of the need for the examiner to touch their face and even to pull on their eyelids. Before instilling the topical anesthetic, tell the patient that it may cause a burning sensation until the eye becomes numb. Because patients with a corneal abrasion are usually hypersensitive to light, let them know when you are going to need a bright white light for only a short while, and that the room will otherwise be darkened. The remainder of the examination is done with a blue light, which should be more comfortable. Reassurance that this bright light will not cause permanent visual damage is usually appreciated. In fact, patients should be told that the reason for using this bright light (in most cases) is to *prevent* permanent damage to their vision. After the clinician has located the necessary equipment, the lights in the room can be dimmed during the remainder of the examination.

If an abrasion is diagnosed, emphasize the need for the patient to follow up daily with the clinician until it is completely healed. This will detect early complications such as infection. Instruct the patient to call the office if persistent or recurrent symptoms occur. Patients should also be instructed not to drive if the abrasion impairs their vision or depth perception.

Technique

1. Check and document visual acuity in both eyes before instilling topical anesthetic. Documentation of baseline visual acuity before the topical anesthetic is applied is important because initial discomfort due to the anesthetic (e.g., burning, stinging) may be suspected later by the patient as having caused impaired vision. If the patient normally wears corrective lenses (e.g., glasses) for refractive error, check visual acuity with refraction. After the acuity check, the patient will probably be most comfortable in the supine position for the remainder of the examination.

   NOTE: If the patient's corrective lenses are not available, a pinhole myopia corrector can be used. These are commercially available, but they are also easy to make. With an 18-gauge needle, punch 8 to 10 holes within a 5-cm (2-inch) circle on an index card. Have the patient select the hole that provides the best vision when viewing the Snellen chart. This effectively corrects the patient's vision.

2. Hand the patient a tissue and instill one to two drops of topical anesthetic into his or her affected eye. (This is not mandatory but does facilitate patient cooperation and comfort.)

3. Inspect the affected eye, briefly but thoroughly, with a bright white light source, and compare it with the opposite eye. The sclera should be intact. The anterior chamber should be free of pus or blood. The iris should be normal in size and shape. The pupil should be normal in size, shape, and reactivity, and it should be symmetric with the other pupil unless there is a history of asymmetry (anisocoria). If all of these conditions are not met, the patient should be referred to an ophthalmologist.

4. Eversion of the upper lid is usually necessary to examine the entire conjunctiva (Fig. 200.3). After grasping the lower lid and applying traction, examine the conjunctiva beneath it as well. Inspect the entire bulbar and palpebral conjunctiva for trauma, foreign body, or other sources of symptoms, such as a hordeolum or an ingrown or inverted eyelash. Examine carefully the groove about 2 mm from the lash margin of the everted lid. Tiny objects frequently lodge here and may not be immediately visible. Use magnification if necessary. For a foreign body, refer to the "Corneal or Conjunctival Foreign Body Removal" section later in this chapter. Older patients often have ingrown hairs (trichiasis) that can cause a foreign body sensation (see Chapter 46, Epilation of Isolated Hairs [Including Trichiasis]). Trichiasis most frequently involves the lower lid, and if there are only a few hairs, they can be plucked out with fine forceps. The patient with many hairs should be referred for electrolysis of the roots.

5. Instill fluorescein dye by moistening a sterile fluorescein strip with one or two drops of sterile saline or topical anesthetic, asking the

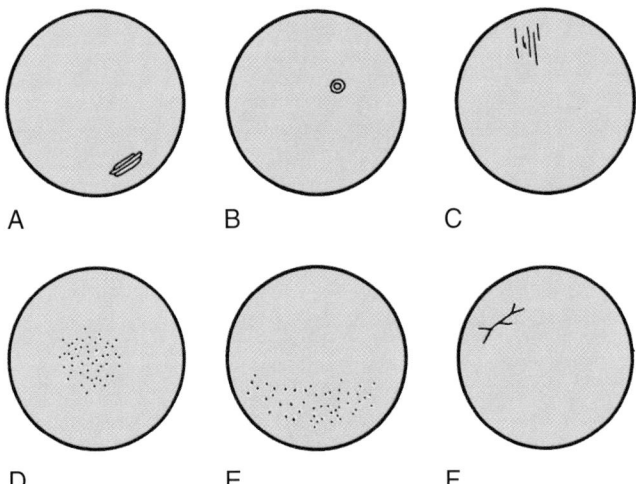

Fig. 200.4 Corneal defect staining patterns for specific injuries. (A) Typical abrasion. (B) Abrasion around a corneal foreign body. (C) Abrasion from a conjunctival foreign body under the upper lid. (D) Abrasion from excessive wearing of a contact lens. (E) Ultraviolet exposure (resulting from sunlamp exposure, welding, or snow blindness). (F) Herpetic dendritic keratitis.

patient to look up, and gently touching the lower conjunctival sac for 3 to 5 seconds. Use a minimal amount of solution when wetting the strip. This usually helps visualize the defect by staining only the defect as opposed to staining the entire eye. Try not to touch the cornea directly with the strip because this may cause iatrogenic staining. After instilling the fluorescein, have the patient blink a few times to remove excess tears, and blot them with the tissue. This is helpful to distinguish true staining from fluorescein saturation of the tear film.

6. Inspect the cornea with magnification under a cobalt-blue light source. If the entire cornea is stained, irrigate the eye again and re-examine. Abraded areas of the cornea should remain highlighted with fluorescein.

   NOTE: Rivulets of fluorescein (Seidel sign) tracking from a puncture site indicate an unsuspected penetration of the globe and require ophthalmologic consultation.

7. Make a drawing of the cornea for later reference, detailing the area(s) of abnormality.
8. If no cause of symptoms is found or if vertical streaking is found on the cornea, suspect an embedded conjunctival foreign body in the eyelid and examine the entire conjunctiva under cobalt-blue light. Keep in mind that fluorescein is taken up by mucus on the conjunctiva; therefore fluorescein staining with a conjunctival injury is less specific than with a corneal injury.
9. At this point, if no cause for the symptoms can be found, the eye should be examined under a slit lamp (see Chapter 201, Slit-Lamp Examination). A slit lamp is helpful when a plain fluorescein examination is nondiagnostic. For deep, dendritic, or central ulcerations or for ulcerations in which infection is suspected (i.e., if there is clouding of the cornea or a purulent discharge), the patient should be referred to an ophthalmologist (Fig. 200.4).

TREATMENT OF UNCOMPLICATED CORNEAL ABRASIONS

Considerations

Some clinicians working in the emergency department refer all corneal abrasions to ophthalmologists for follow-up. Others rely on their knowledge, skills, and experience to make decisions regarding referral. Knowing that the risk for permanent visual impairment is affected by several factors associated with the abrasion (e.g.,

depth, size, location, susceptibility to infection) can be helpful for clinicians when making their decision. Lacking the magnification available with a slit lamp, the depth of the abrasion is often difficult to assess, so referral should be considered. Referral should also be considered for suspected deep or large lesions or for those located centrally in the line of vision. One way to assess a borderline case is to wait until the follow-up examination the next day. The corneal epithelium is one of the fastest-healing areas of the body, and if considerable progress toward healing has not been made by the next day or if there are signs of infection (cloudiness of the cornea or pus), the patient should be referred immediately.

Equipment

- Topical ophthalmic anesthetic.
- Isotonic irrigant (Dacriose, Ringer lactate, sterile saline).
- Ophthalmic antibiotics (ointment is better lubricating and less expensive than drops): erythromycin ointment, trimethoprim-polymyxin B drops, sulfacetamide ointment, fluoroquinolone drops, or azithromycin drops. Fluoroquinolones are not first-line therapy for routine cases of bacterial conjunctivitis because of concerns regarding emerging resistance and cost, except in contact lens wearers (see below). Sulfacetamide ophthalmic drops are available but are not a first-line option because of the potential for rare but serious allergic events. Aminoglycoside drops and ointments are poor choices because they are toxic to the corneal epithelium and can cause a reactive keratoconjunctivitis after a few days of use. Interestingly, although commonly used, there is no standard of care supported by evidence regarding the use of ophthalmic antibiotics after the removal of a foreign body.
- Contact lens wearers have a high risk of pseudomonal keratitis, especially with the use of extended-wear lenses. In contact lens wearers, the presence of keratitis should be ruled out prior to presuming and treating for conjunctivitis. Once keratitis has been ruled out, cover for *Pseudomonas* with a topical fluoroquinolone antibiotic.
- (Optional) Cycloplegic, mydriatic drops, such as tropicamide 0.5% or 1% (Tropicacyl, Mydriacyl) or 0.5%, 1%, or 2% cyclopentolate (Cyclogyl, Pentolair), or 5% homatropine may be useful for pain control. Their duration of action ranges from hours to a day.
- (Optional) Sterile "bandage" contact lens or eyepatches and 1-inch (preferably nonallergenic) paper tape.

NOTE: Topical steroids have no place for routine use in a traumatic corneal abrasion.

Technique

1. With the patient in the supine position, irrigate the eye copiously with ophthalmic irrigant, with the patient's head turned laterally toward the affected side.
2. Instill one to two additional drops of local anesthetic.
3. Apply an antibiotic ointment or drops. For patients who wear contact lenses, keratitis should be ruled out and antipseudomonal antibiotic drops should be chosen (see above for details). Even under the best of conditions, infection is a possibility because of the avascular nature of the cornea. Prophylaxis with antibiotic ointment or drops is important.

   NOTE: In the past, eye patching was thought to decrease pain from a corneal abrasion by decreasing blinking and reducing eyelid-induced trauma. By being a physical barrier, it was also thought to reduce the risk of infection and prevented the patient rubbing their eye when asleep. However, at least one meta-analysis and several subsequent randomized clinical trials have found no benefit to patching regarding either pain or healing. In fact, eye patching was the source of pain in 48% of patients in one study! Furthermore, eye patching decreases oxygen delivery, increases heat and moisture, and may increase the risk of infection. In various trials, ophthalmic topical NSAIDs provided pain relief that was superior to patching.

As a result of this evidence, many clinicians no longer use eye patching. However, the technique for patching remains in this chapter as an option. The evidence is somewhat lacking for lesions greater than 10 mm in diameter. Another option that is being used, but needs more study in the hands of primary care clinicians, is a soft contact "bandage" lens as a protective barrier. This is an excellent option for the busy patient who must have continuous use of both eyes. As long as the cause of the abrasion was not a contact lens, the use of a soft contact lens usually provides comfort and protection and should not impair healing. However, if a soft contact lens is used, the patient should be followed closely and warned about signs of infection.

4. Pain medication should be prescribed in an amount appropriate to the symptoms. However, additional local anesthetic should not be prescribed because it may retard corneal healing and cause corneal scarring. Topical ophthalmic NSAIDs such as ketorolac (Acular) or diclofenac (Voltaren) have been found to reduce pain by about 14% compared with placebo. A systematic review of the literature found that patients using ophthalmic NSAIDs may take fewer oral analgesics, return to work earlier, and take fewer narcotics.

5. In the past, mydriatics were thought to relieve the pain related to ciliary muscle spasm associated with any corneal abrasion. Although there is minimal evidence supporting this practice, it may be reasonable to use a mydriatic when there is obvious spasm, iritis, or irregularity of the pupil (these patients should also be referred to an ophthalmologist). It may also be reasonable to use a mydriatic when the patient presents with photophobia or significant eye discomfort.

6. Re-examine the eye in 24 hours using fluorescein and magnification. If the abrasion has healed, antibiotic ointment or drops should be used for an additional 3 days. If the defect is smaller, instill antibiotic ointment and examine again in 24 hours. If at any time during the follow-up corneal cloudiness or suppuration is seen, refer the patient to an ophthalmologist.

7. The visual acuity test should be repeated and documented just before the patient is discharged from care.

8. Tetanus prophylaxis should be verified or provided.

NOTE: Abrasions resulting from fingernails or plant matter are notoriously slow to heal. Their progress should be followed patiently, just like any other abrasion, while observing for any signs of early infection.

9. (Optional) A double patch (pressure patch) can be used. Before patching, an ophthalmic ointment (as opposed to solution) should be applied. The first patch is then folded and the fold placed immediately under the upper brow (this adds padding and prevents opening of the eye). This patch is covered with the second patch. With three to five strips of paper tape, secure the patches by taping from the middle of the forehead, across the eye, and toward the ear (Fig. 200.5)

NOTE: If infection is suspected, an eyepatch is contraindicated. Also, abrasions from organic material have fungal potential, so they should not be patched. Abrasions due to contact lenses increase the risk of infection with *Pseudomonas* so they should not be patched. Do not use eyepatches on young children. There is the theoretical risk of permanently affecting the use of one eye or of making amblyopia worse. Very young children typically remove a patch anyway.

Complications

- Infection.
- Scarring (the highest morbidity occurs when the abrasion is near the central line of vision).
- Permanent visual impairment.

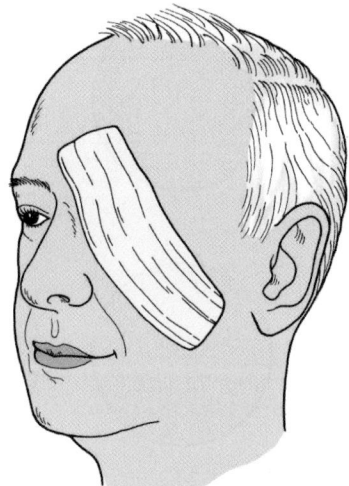

Fig. 200.5 Pressure eyepatch.

- Recurrent corneal erosion (symptoms include foreign body pain, ocular pain, decreased vision, photophobia, increased lacrimation on wakening, and blepharospasm). Although the symptoms may be annoying, they do not interfere with activities in most patients.

Postprocedure Patient Education

Instruct the patient not to rub his or her eyes, especially upon wakening in the morning. Rubbing the eye may disrupt new layers of epithelializing cornea. Re-epithelialization can take weeks to complete. Inform the patient that the local anesthetic used during the examination will wear off in a few minutes to hours and that they may feel the foreign body sensation again. Additional pain medication may be necessary. Topical ophthalmic NSAIDs have been found to be safe and somewhat effective. Moist compresses may be applied for some relief if the patient's eye has not been patched. Instruct the patient to return to the office daily until healed or if persistent or recurrent symptoms develop. If a mydriatic was used, inform the patient which one. Also inform the patient to tell any other clinician involved that a mydriatic was used, and which one, if he or she will be seen in another center or referred so that the clinician can know how long to expect the pupil to remain dilated. Instruct the patient not to overuse the affected eye, such as by watching television or reading for prolonged periods. This is especially true for children or anyone with a history of amblyopia. Although there is not a lot of evidence supporting such an intervention, if the abrasion is due to a contact lens, the patient probably should avoid contact lenses until the abrasion is completely healed. It is important to document the degree of healing observed during the discharge examination. Safety goggles or protective glasses should be emphasized if the abrasion was an occupational, exposure, or sports injury. If the eye is patched, the patient should not drive owing to the loss of depth perception. Even if the eye is not patched, the patient should not drive until the injury heals if there is loss of vision or depth perception.

CORNEAL OR CONJUNCTIVAL FOREIGN BODY REMOVAL

Indications

Noninfected, small, recent corneal or conjunctival foreign body.

Contraindications

The contraindications (those that should be referred to ophthalmology) are the same as those for "Fluorescein Examination of the Cornea and Conjunctiva," as well as the following:

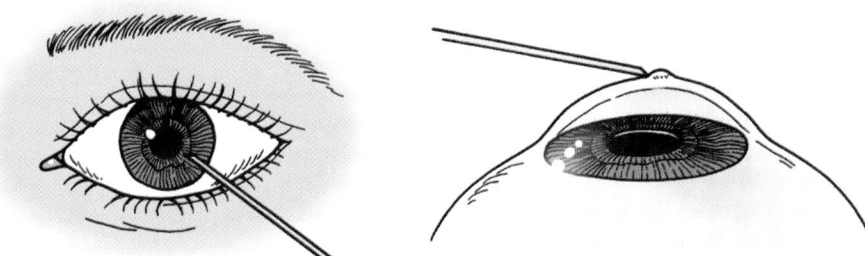

Fig. 200.6   Removal of a superficial corneal foreign body. Side view illustrates the thickness of the cornea relative to the beveled needle edge. The needle or eye spud should be held tangential to the cornea, and the object should be gently lifted off of the cornea.

- Signs or symptoms that suggest infection, such as edema and clouding of the cornea surrounding the foreign body, ulceration exceeding the size of the foreign body, or purulent discharge
- Large metal foreign body or foreign body with potential to cause a large rust ring (e.g., embedded in the cornea for longer than 24 hours)
- Deeply or centrally embedded foreign body or one that has healed and is covered by epithelium

Equipment

- Topical ophthalmic anesthetic
- Sterile cotton-tipped applicators
- Bright white and cobalt-blue light sources
- Magnification as previously listed (it may be necessary to have an assistant hold the magnifier to allow the operator to use both hands)
- Isotonic ophthalmic irrigant, such as Dacriose, Ringer lactate, or sterile saline
- Snellen chart or equivalent visual acuity chart
- Sterile 18-gauge needle with small syringe
- Sterile dental burr or cornea drill (optional)

NOTE: Instead of an 18-gauge needle, a tuberculin syringe with a 26-gauge needle, a sterile eye, or a small, sterile chalazion curette may be substituted, depending on user experience.

Preprocedure Patient Preparation

Instruct the patient that it will be important to fix their gaze on a distant object, maintain that gaze, and hold the head motionless, regardless of what is seen or experienced. The patient will have the urge to blink, but it will be important to keep the eye open. Inform the patient that the eye will be numb from the local anesthetic, but that he or she may feel pressure during the procedure. The patient should know that you will need to touch him or her.

Advise the patient of possible complications and that referral may be necessary regardless of outcome. Some clinicians obtain signed informed consent.

Technique

Controversy exists about the use of a swab or a spud to remove a corneal foreign body and whether this causes more damage. Only experienced users should consider a swab or spud, and they should use them only for a small foreign body. The swab will be more successful with a very recent, superficial foreign body. Irrigation alone is not usually successful unless the foreign object is very recent, consists of carbon, or is water soluble. The patient's tears would normally have already washed away anything that irrigation would remove.

NOTE: Some experts no longer recommend the use of swabs, saying they are never successful and can cause more harm than good. Also, if multiple foreign bodies are present, such as from an explosion, ophthalmologists may simply denude the epithelium, so a referral may be indicated. It may take years for deep foreign bodies to work their way to the surface. Likewise, it may be prudent to avoid significant corneal procedures in patients with a prior history of a laser-assisted in situ keratomileusis procedure for nearsightedness because there may be increased risk of damaging the cornea. Clinicians should also examine patients who have undergone radial keratotomy very closely under magnification. The corneal incisions in these patients have been known to gape for 6 years postprocedure, and these can entrap a foreign body.

1. Record the patient's visual acuity.
2. With the patient supine, hold the eyelids apart with your thumb and index finger, and position the patient's head so that the foreign object is at the highest point on the eyeball. The patient should fix his or her gaze. For a conjunctival foreign body, the head should be positioned for maximal access.
3. Attempt to dislodge the object. Noting the controversy regarding swab or spud use, try to lift the object by lightly touching it with a cotton swab moistened with local anesthetic. This occasionally dislodges the particle. Never use any force to rub the cornea because this will dislodge the epithelium and cause a larger abrasion. The same maneuver can be attempted for a conjunctival foreign body.
4. To use a sterile needle, approach the object from a direction tangential to the eyeball, with the needle bevel upwards and the syringe held with a pencil grip (Fig. 200.6). Rest your hand on the patient's zygoma so that if the patient moves, your hand will move with the patient. Use the needle tip to lift the object gently from its bed. Several attempts may have to be made, but the use of a slit lamp (see Chapter 201, Slit-Lamp Examination) or referral should be considered if further corneal damage is anticipated. If several attempts with a needle are unsuccessful, a spud or chalazion curette may be considered (again, noting the controversy discussed previously). For a conjunctival foreign body, the technique is the same; attempt to lift it from its bed with the same instruments. More vigorous force, if controlled, may be used on the conjunctiva.
5. A rust ring can develop within hours. After removal of the foreign body, if a residual rust ring is found, it can occasionally be removed with the sterile needle alone. A cornea drill may also be considered. It should have a pressure-sensitive automatic shut-off to minimize corneal damage. Another published technique involves the use of a sterile dental burr held between the thumb and forefinger to approach the rust ring vertically (Fig. 200.7). After the burr has made one gentle rotation, re-examine the eye under magnification to verify complete removal of the ring.

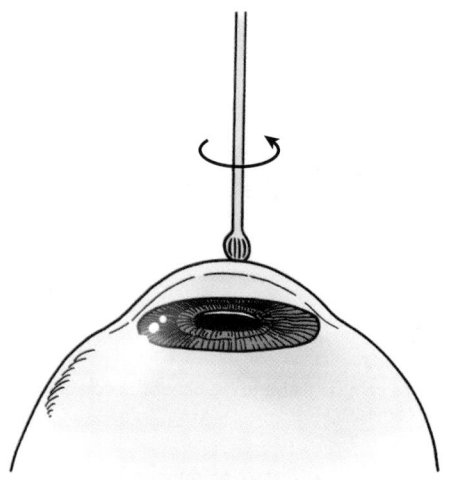

Fig. 200.7 Dental burr rotated once to remove corneal rust ring. Note the vertical approach.

Another approach to a rust ring is to re-examine the patient in 24 to 48 hours (preferably 24 hours). Rust is toxic to corneal epithelium and prevents healing; therefore, given a day or two, the tissue around the rust ring will soften, and often it will come out with one solid plug. If attempts to remove the rust ring are unsuccessful or if they will cause significant damage to corneal epithelium, referral should be made for management under slit-lamp magnification. A rust ring should not be left in place more than 48 hours as it can cause significant damage to the cornea. Remaining rust rings may also cause night-time visual defects.

NOTE: Some experts suggest that the use of a corneal drill or dental burr is contraindicated when the foreign body or rust ring is in the central line of vision. Instead, they recommend referral.

6. Retest and record the patient's visual acuity. The corneal defect that is present after removal of the foreign body should now be managed the same as a corneal abrasion.

NOTE: As mentioned previously, topical steroids have no place for routine use in a traumatic corneal abrasion.

Postprocedure Patient Education

Follow the treatment previously mentioned for an uncomplicated corneal abrasion. If the object cannot be removed, the resultant rust ring is too large, or the patient is referred to an ophthalmologist for any other reason, the ophthalmologist should provide further patient education.

Complications

- Same as the complications associated with treatment of a routine corneal abrasion, except the risk of corneal scarring is higher
- Perforation of the cornea or globe
- Incomplete removal of a foreign body
- Failure to heal because of a retained rust ring, infection, or other causes

CPT/BILLING CODES

65205   Removal of foreign body, external eye; conjunctival superficial
65210   Removal of foreign body, external eye; conjunctival embedded (includes concretions), subconjunctival, or scleral nonperforating
65220   Removal of foreign body, external eye; corneal without slit lamp

99070   Eye tray: supplies and materials (except spectacles) provided by physician over and above those that are usually included with the office visit or other services rendered (list drugs, trays, supplies, or materials provided)
99173   Screening test of visual acuity, quantitative, bilateral (e.g., Snellen chart)

NOTE: Some insurers will deny 99070 as not being specific enough; HCPCS codes are more specific and are often covered.

ICD-10-CM DIAGNOSTIC CODES

H44.701-H44.799   Intraocular foreign body, unspecified nonmagnetic retained
H44.601-H44.699   Intraocular foreign body, unspecified magnetic retained
H33.001-H33.43   Retinal detachment and breaks
H20.011-H20.9   Acute and subacute iritis
H21.501-H21.509   Adhesions of iris, unspecified
H16.101-H16.109   Superficial corneal keratitis without conjunctivitis
H16.131-H16.139   Photokeratitis
H18.821-H18.829   Corneal injury due to contact lens
S05.00X-S05.02X   Superficial injury of conjunctiva and corneal abrasion
T15.00X-T15.02X   Corneal foreign body
T15.10X-T15.12X   Foreign body in conjunctival sac

Add appropriate seventh character: A = initial, D = subsequent, S = sequela.

SUPPLIERS

(See contact information available at www.expertconsult.com.)

Sterile fluorescein sodium strips
Fluor-I-Strip and Fluorets: Bausch and Lomb
Ful Glo: Akorn Pharmaceuticals

RECOMMENDED READING

Arbour JD, Brunette I, Boisjoly HM, et al. Should we patch corneal erosions? *Arch Ophthalmol.* 1997;115:313–317.
Brunette DD. Ophthalmology. In: Marx JA, Hockberger RS, eds. *Rosen's Emergency Medicine: Concepts and Clinical Practice.* 8th ed. Philadelphia: Elsevier; 2015.
Buttaravoli P, Keller R. Foreign body, corneal. In: Buttaravoli P, Leffler SM, eds. *Minor Emergencies: Splinters to Fractures.* 3rd ed. Philadelphia: Elsevier; 2012.
Cheng KH, Leung SL, Hoekman HW, et al. Incidence of contact-lens-associated microbial keratitis and its related morbidity. *Lancet.* 1999;354:181.
Flynn CA, D'Amico F, Smith G. Should we patch corneal abrasions? A meta-analysis. *J Fam Pract.* 1998;47:264–270.
Knoop KJ, Dennis WR. Ophthalmologic procedures. In: Roberts JR, Custalow CB, Thomsen TW, eds. *Roberts and Hedges' Clinical Procedures in Emergency Medicine.* 6th ed. Philadelphia: Elsevier; 2014:1259–1277.
Parmar P, Salman A, Kalavathy CM, et al. Comparison of topical gatifloxacin 0.3% and ciprofloxacin 0.3% for the treatment of bacterial keratitis. *Am J Ophthalmol.* 2006;141:282.
Reichman EF. Corneal foreign body removal/corneal rust ring removal. In: Reichman EF, ed. *Emergency Medicine Procedures.* 2nd ed. New York: McGraw-Hill; 2013:1043–1050.
Tabbara KF, El-Sheikh HF, Aabed B. Extended wear contact lens related bacterial keratitis. *Br J Ophthalmol.* 2000;84:327.
Thomas SH, Brown DFM. Foreign bodies. In: Marx JA, Hockberger RS, Walls RM, eds. *Rosen's Emergency Medicine: Concepts and Clinical Practice.* 6th ed. St. Louis: Mosby; 2006:859–861.
Usatine RP, Smith MA, Mayeaux EJ, et al., eds. *The Color Atlas of Family Medicine.* 2nd ed. New York: McGraw-Hill; 2013.
Walker RA, Adhikari S. Eye emergencies. In: Tintinalli JE, Stapczynski JS, Ma OJ, et al., eds. *Tintinalli's Emergency Medicine: A Comprehensive Study Guide.* 8th ed. New York: McGraw-Hill; 2015.

CHAPTER 201

SLIT-LAMP EXAMINATION

Christopher J. Bigelow

The slit-lamp biomicroscope is used for a thorough evaluation of the eye as well as for the diagnosis of various eye conditions. In short, the eyes remain in a fixed position while the light and microscope are independently moved and adjusted. As with any instrument, repeated use facilitates clinician comfort with the scope as well as his or her ability to obtain the desired or necessary information. With its many levers and knobs (Fig. 201.1), the slit lamp can be somewhat intimidating at first. However, after learning a few simple techniques, even the infrequent user should feel comfortable. Granted, not every primary care clinician's office has a slit lamp. However, if one is available, it can offer invaluable diagnostic opportunities that should not be missed because of lack of experience. Clinicians working in an urgent care center or emergency department can also benefit from knowing how to use a slit lamp. The goal of this chapter is to provide even the novice user with guidance for performing a useful and reproducible slit-lamp examination.

A slit lamp consists of both an illumination and an observation system (see Fig. 201.1). The light source is an incandescent lamp contained in the body of the instrument. Light from the lamp passes through a condenser, the slit mechanism, and an objective lens and is then reflected by an inclined mirror onto the patient's eye. When projected onto the globe, the slit beam of incandescent light creates an optical cross section of the eye. The height and width of the beam (Fig. 201.2) can be adjusted with controls (often different on each slit lamp). The beam can be changed from a small pinpoint spot to a slit beam or made even wider for broad illumination. As the beam is narrowed, the scattered light from adjacent tissue is minimized, allowing greater detail to be seen in the cross section. Beam sizes, their widths, and their usefulness are discussed in the "Technique" section. Light intensity can also be adjusted. In general brighter illumination settings are better tolerated (i.e., less photophobia) with a short, narrow beam, whereas a long, wide beam is usually better tolerated with a lower-power illumination setting. The observation system is a microscope with a long working distance. Most slit lamps offer a choice of magnification between 5× and 50×. The necessary degree of magnification depends on the tissue being examined.

Use of the slit lamp is indicated in any situation where brighter illumination and increased magnification of the lids, conjunctiva, or anterior segment structures (e.g., cornea, iris, lens) would be helpful. If desired, the clinician can use a slit lamp for most examinations of the eye. With increased magnification, oblique illumination, and a stereoscopic view, a much better evaluation of lesions can be obtained, especially their depth. Attachments are also available to perform applanation (Goldmann) tonometry (see Chapter 58, Tonometry), which is considered the most accurate form of tonometry. In addition, high-powered lenses are available for most slit lamps to allow visualization of the posterior structures (e.g., retina, optic nerve).

INDICATIONS

- Need for bright illumination or magnification of lids, conjunctiva, or anterior segment structures (e.g., chronic blepharitis, keratitis, iritis).

- Same indications as for routine fluorescein examination or for foreign body removal (see Chapter 200, Corneal Abrasions and Removal of Corneal or Conjunctival Foreign Bodies). If a slit lamp is available, it will enhance the techniques found in that chapter.
- Patient with a foreign body sensation when routine fluorescein examination is negative, or when the routine fluorescein examination is inconclusive or unsuccessful.

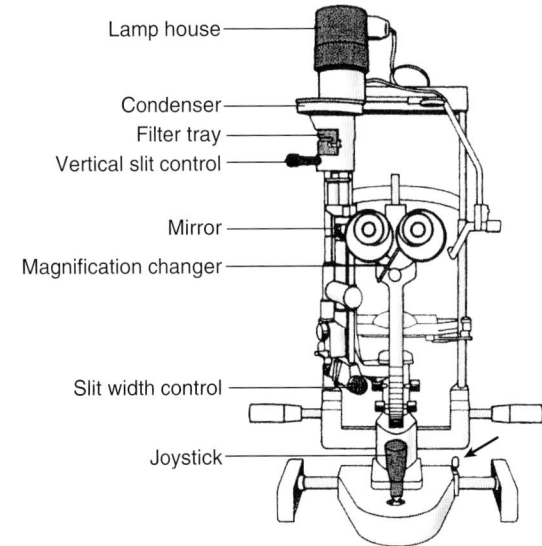

Fig. 201.1 Slit lamp and its optics. (From Solley WA, Broocker G. General eye exam. In: Palay DA, Krachmer JH, ed. *Ophthalmology for the Primary Care Physician*. St. Louis: Mosby; 1997:1–22.)

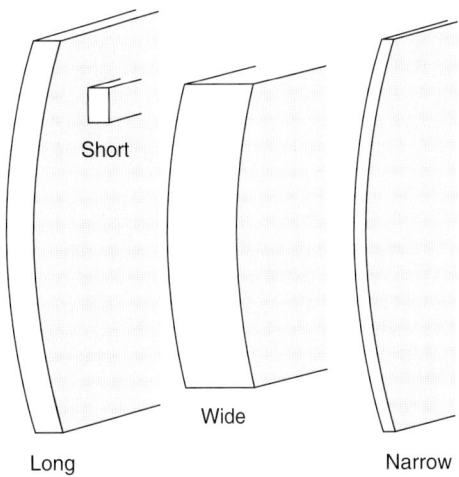

Fig. 201.2 Different dimensions of the slit-lamp beam.

- Suspected deep or large abrasions or those centrally located in the line of vision on fluorescein examination. Such lesions increase the risk of vision loss and should be evaluated thoroughly and followed clinically with a slit lamp.
- After several unsuccessful attempts at removing a corneal foreign body in the standard fashion and before additional trauma is inflicted on the cornea, the foreign body and cornea should be evaluated under a slit lamp. It may also be necessary to remove the foreign body with slit-lamp guidance.
- When routine fluorescein examination is relatively contraindicated (e.g., when there is long-standing [>24 hours] inflammation, and/or possible perforation). The presence of iritis, photophobia, or ciliary blush may indicate long-standing inflammation, or it may be the result of an intraocular foreign body or a more serious injury. If the etiology is not evident with a slit-lamp examination, the patient should be referred to an ophthalmologist.
- Recent eye trauma (e.g., to exclude perforation).

CONTRAINDICATIONS

After urgent care has been provided, patients with the following symptoms should be referred to an ophthalmologist:

- Suspected high-velocity injury to the eye (e.g., patients exposed to metal hammering or heavy machinery). Although a slit lamp may diagnose a perforation, it is possible for high-speed metallic or nonmetallic fragments to penetrate the globe with unnoticeable damage to the cornea. Although there may be minimal symptoms, significant internal damage may have occurred. A hyphema, lens opacification, an abnormal anterior chamber examination, or an irregularity of the pupil may suggest that the globe has been penetrated. Orbital radiographs may confirm a metal foreign body.
  NOTE: A pressure patch is contraindicated in a penetration injury of the globe. Also, for complex lid lacerations, a nonpressure protective eye shield should be applied before referral (see Chapter 200, Corneal Abrasions and Removal of Corneal or Conjunctival Foreign Bodies, Fig. 200.1).
- Exposure to caustic or acidic media: urgent management includes copious irrigation, which should continue for at least 15 minutes. (It can begin at home with tap water from a shower or hose.)
- Other chemical exposure if the clinician is not knowledgeable about its management after contacting a Poison Control Center.
- Ruptured globe.
- An uncooperative patient. (Mild sedation for infants may be helpful; see Chapter 2, Pediatric Sedation and Analgesia.)
- Foreign body removal if there are signs or symptoms that suggest infection (e.g., edema and clouding of the cornea surrounding the foreign body, ulceration exceeding the size of the foreign body, or purulent discharge). If infection is suspected, patching is contraindicated and referral is necessary.
- Large metal foreign bodies or those with potential to cause a large rust ring (i.e., those that have been embedded in the cornea for longer than 24 to 48 hours).
- Apparently deeply or centrally embedded foreign bodies.

NOTE: For these contraindications, although the slit lamp may be helpful to a primary care clinician, management by an ophthalmologist is the usual care.

EQUIPMENT

- Topical ophthalmic anesthetic, such as 0.5% proparacaine (Alcaine or Ophthaine) or 0.5% tetracaine (Pontocaine) unless contraindicated (e.g., ruptured globe or allergy to local anesthetics).

NOTE: The use of proparacaine has been found to cause less discomfort than tetracaine.
- Sterile fluorescein sodium strips. (Because fluorescein is incompatible with preservatives effective against *Pseudomonas* or *Proteus*, multidose dropper bottles of fluorescein solution should not be used. Inoculation of abraded corneal epithelium with either of these bacteria could cause infection, scarring, or permanent blindness.)
- Sterile cotton-tipped applicators.
- Isopropyl alcohol swab.
- Isotonic ophthalmic irrigant (e.g., sterile saline, Dacriose).
- Slit lamp: the two most common slit lamps in use are manufactured by Haag-Streit and Zeiss (see "Suppliers" section).

PREPROCEDURE PATIENT PREPARATION

Patients should be informed about the indication(s) for and alternatives to the slit-lamp examination. Once a patient's chin has been placed on the scope, he or she should be asked to get into a comfortable position that can be maintained for a while. Patients should be instructed to breathe normally and, especially children, asked to remain as still as possible. Children may need assistance with holding still. Patients should know to blink normally unless their eyes are being held open by the examiner or they are asked to hold their eyes open. They should be aware of the need for the examiner to touch their faces and even to pull on their eyelids. It should be explained that the room is going to be darkened and that a bright light can be expected, especially if the pupil is dilated. Reassurance that this bright light will not cause permanent vision damage is usually appreciated. In fact, patients should be told that the reason for using this bright light (in most cases) is to *prevent* permanent damage to their vision.

Patients need to know that they will be asked to direct their vision to certain locations and that eyedrops or dye may have to be used to enhance the examination. Before fluorescein is instilled, the patient should remove contact lenses (if present) and warned that objects in his or her line of vision may temporarily appear yellow. Tears may also remain yellow for a short time after the examination and might stain skin or clothing, at least temporarily, so patients should avoid rubbing their eyes or drying their tears on something that might stain. Before topical anesthetic is instilled, the patient should be warned that it may cause a burning sensation until the eye becomes numb.

TECHNIQUE

1. Clinicians should be familiar with the anatomy of the external eye before evaluation with a slit lamp (Fig. 201.3). For the novice or infrequent user of a slit lamp, it may also be helpful to get comfortable with the instrument before the patient is in the room. Learn to locate and loosen the locking nut for the mechanical assembly. Practice with the joystick, turn the knobs, and watch the results. The clinician may then benefit from focusing the slit lamp on an object or his or her skin to gain some sense of perspective. In an urgent care center or emergency department, practicing before the patient is in the room may be important because the slit lamp is often left in complete disarray by others.
2. Proper patient positioning is absolutely essential for a satisfactory examination. Both the patient and the examiner should be comfortable. An improperly positioned patient is more likely to move backward and out of focus. He or she is also less likely to maintain positioning for extended periods of time. The patient is seated during the examination. Clean the chin rest with an alcohol swab. The height of the examination chair should be such that the patient can easily place his or her chin on the adjustable chin rest with the forehead against the headrest. Some slit lamps have an eye-level marker to assist in gauging head po-

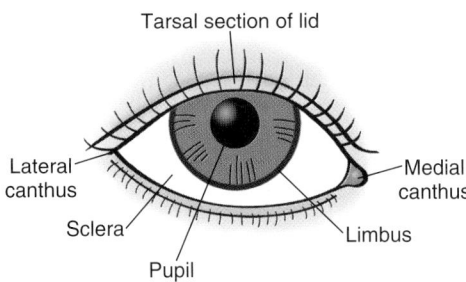

Fig. 201.3 External anatomy of the eye.

sitioning. If the patient is unable to place the forehead against the headrest, either elevate the chair or lower the chin rest. If the patient is not positioned against the headrest, it will be difficult to focus on deeper ocular structures. This common mistake often causes a great deal of frustration for the novice slit-lamp user. After the patient is positioned, loss of focus may indicate that he or she has moved his or her head backward. It should then be repositioned. Small children should sit in the chair on their knees, stand up on the footrest, or sit in a parent's lap.

3. Examiner positioning is also important. The clinician should be able to reach the patient's eye comfortably and easily rest an elbow on the slit-lamp table. Such a position is important if the eyelids need to be manipulated or for holding instruments used in foreign body removal. The examiner should also be seated comfortably in the chair so that his or her eyes easily reach the eyepiece without leaning forward. This description may seem overly simplistic, but many a novice slit-lamp examiner looks like a baseball catcher coming up from a crouch. This is not a position that can be maintained for very long.

4. Turn on the power to the lamp (the switch is usually located on the left lower side, just under the table base), and select the degree of illumination anywhere from low power (preserves bulb life the longest) to the next-to-highest power. The illumination power setting rheostat is usually part of the power switch or located nearby. The eyepieces can then be adjusted to correct the clinician's refractive error, although it is often simpler for the clinician to set the eyepieces at zero (1×) and wear his or her spectacles or contact lenses. Once the eyepieces are adjusted, the interpupillary distance is set. After this adjustment, no further manipulation of the eyepieces should be necessary. Magnification can be changed with a knob found anterior to the eyepieces on some slit lamps or by shifting a lever found below the eyepieces on other models.

5. After positioning and eyepiece adjustment, darken the examination room as much as possible. The eyepieces (and thus the examiner) should remain perpendicular to the chin rest throughout the examination. The light source, not the oculars, should be moved to facilitate viewing. Move the light source vertically by using the control lever located at the base of the slit lamp. Horizontal movement is accomplished by moving the swing arm with the examiner's other hand. Position the slit beam at an oblique angle, starting at the temporal side of each eye and moving the light nasally. Beware when moving the light source from the temporal side; from this position, if the examiner is not careful, the patient's nose may be struck by the mirror or light source. To view the nasal portion of an eye, have the patient gaze temporally on that side, which should bring the desired area into focus.

6. The depth of focus is adjusted by moving the slit lamp backward and forward. Focusing is typically accomplished at the same time as vertical positioning with the joystick. Remember to examine both eyes, even if the symptoms are monocular. The "normal" eye can be used for comparison with any pathology in the other eye.

7. At the start of the examination, the patient should be instructed to look toward the examiner's ear opposite to the eye being examined (i.e., the patient looks at the examiner's left ear while his or her right eye is being examined). Some slit lamps have a fixation light to direct the patient's gaze, but it is often simpler to instruct the patient to focus on a larger, nonmoving object such as the examiner's ear.

8. Evaluation of the ocular structures has already begun with a focused history, the measurement of visual acuity in both eyes, and a gross hand-light examination of the eyelid skin and surrounding structures. The slit-lamp examination should then proceed in a systematic manner from external (lids and lashes) to internal (vitreous). Failure to be systematic can cause the examiner to get caught up in the fine detail that the slit lamp provides. As a result, the examiner may "miss the forest for the trees."

9. Choose the white light beam filter lens. A long, wide beam is useful for scanning tissues such as the lids and lashes. For these structures, a low-power magnification (e.g., 10× to 16×) should be adequate.

   NOTE: Avoid focusing the light into the pupil for an extended period. This can be very uncomfortable for the patient and may result in injury.

   • Observe the general appearance of the lid margin; the lid's color, position, and vascularity; and any meibomian gland openings. Thickening, crusting, and erythema of the eyelid margins are consistent with blepharitis. Examine the lashes and eyebrows for the presence of inflammation, scaling, or elevated or ulcerated lesions. Also examine the lashes for evidence of lid debris and for missing or additional lashes. Scan for the misdirection of lashes (trichiasis), which can cause a severe foreign body sensation in an otherwise normally positioned lid. If there are only a few misdirected eyelashes, pluck them with fine forceps. If there are many, the patient should be referred for electrolysis (see Chapter 46, Epilation of Isolated Hairs [Including Trichiasis]) of the roots. Also evaluate lid position for being turned in (entropion) or out (ectropion). Note discrete changes in lid pigmentation.

   • Examination of the lower lid is aided by having the patient look up while you are pulling the lower lid down with your index finger. This exposure provides a good view of the posterior lid margin and the lower palpebral conjunctiva. Eversion of the upper lid is necessary to properly examine the upper palpebral conjunctiva (e.g., to exclude foreign bodies). Lid eversion can be performed by having the patient close his or her eyes and look down (see Chapter 200, Corneal Abrasions and Removal of Corneal or Conjunctival Foreign Bodies, Fig. 200.3). Grasp the upper lid margin gently between your thumb and index finger. Then place a cotton-tipped swab about 15 mm from the lid margin. The lid is then moved out, up, and over the cotton-tipped swab. A drop of local anesthetic often enhances patient comfort with this procedure. Carefully examine the few millimeters proximal to the lid margin. This is a common location for small foreign bodies missed on the routine examination.

10. A long, wide beam is also used to examine the conjunctiva. Low-power magnification (e.g., 10× to 16×) should be adequate. The examiner gently separates the eyelids with the opposite hand while the patient is asked to look in all directions of gaze. The conjunctiva is normally a transparent tissue with the white sclera visible beneath. Occasionally, there are slightly elevated yellow lesions at the 3- and 9-o'clock positions at the limbus (edge of cornea), called *pinguecula*. These benign lesions are more common with advancing age. Areas of pigmentation of the conjunctiva can also be seen. These are commonly benign nevi, most often translucent and flat. For irregularly shaped or pigmented lesions suspicious for melanoma, the patient should be referred to an ophthalmologist.

11. A long narrow beam, which produces an optical cross section, is usually best for examining the cornea. Higher-power magnification (e.g., more than 20×) may be useful when the cornea is being examined in minute detail. Within this cross section, the epithelium or tear film is seen as the most anterior band. The stroma can be seen as the large middle layer, and the posterior band represents the endothelium (Fig. 201.4). The examiner brings the slit-lamp beam across the cornea from the temporal to the nasal limbus while paying attention to the regularity of the corneal surface. Any disruption of the corneal surface such as an abrasion should be easily noted as an irregular, distorted, or dulled light reflex. When the light is shone from a lateral position, it produces greater shadows; this, in turn, enhances the ability to determine the depth and texture of corneal lesions.

    - One way of screening for a corneal lesion or foreign object is to use limbal scatter. To do this, light is directed from the laterally placed scope to the closest portion of the limbus. The cornea then simulates a fiberoptic element, and light is transmitted through the cornea medially to the limbus on the other side. A lesion or foreign body in the cornea should cause light to backscatter; consequently the lesion should be seen clearly against the dark pupillary background.
    - Deeper focus allows examination of the corneal stroma, which makes up 90% of the corneal tissue. A narrow slit beam allows for accurate determination of the depth of either a foreign body or a penetrating injury involving this area. Opacities or haze may be noted, both of which are indicative of previous trauma, infection, or inflammation. Old lesions tend to be more circumscribed, whereas an active keratitis usually produces a diffuse pattern of corneal haze.
    - The endothelium is visible as the posterior line in the optical section. Abnormalities may present either as folds in the endothelium or as changes that resemble the surface of a golf ball, called *corneal guttae*. Both of these changes may be indicative of endothelial cell loss.

12. The anterior chamber is the space between the corneal endothelium and the iris. Continuing to use a narrow beam, gauge the anterior chamber depth by estimating the distance between the corneal endothelium and the front surface of the iris. This distance is normally 3 mm or more. When the light is shining from the temporal to the nasal side, a normal anterior chamber will allow this narrow beam to project evenly from side to side. A narrowed anterior chamber will have a lighted temporal side and a narrowed nasal side.

13. The aqueous humor is normally clear, so that the light passes through it without change. To examine the aqueous humor for the presence of cells or flare, a short (3- or 4-mm) narrow beam with bright illumination and high magnification (e.g., 20× to 30× or more) should be used. The presence of cells in the aqueous humor may indicate inflammation (iritis) or hemorrhage (hyphema). While keeping the beam centered on the pupil, any white (i.e., white blood cells, indicating iritis) or red (i.e., red blood cells, indicating a hyphema) specks will be highlighted against the dark pupillary background. Protein in the aqueous humor (i.e., intraocular inflammation) causes a visible flare (Tyndall effect). This effect is similar to that seen when one is shining a flashlight through smoke (Fig. 201.5). Take care to examine the lower aspect of the anterior chamber, because cells and inflammatory products tend to settle in this part of the eye and may form a meniscus when the patient is seated upright.

14. The iris has numerous crypts that should be plainly visible with the slit lamp. Nevi, surgical openings, neovascularization, atrophy, tears, or abnormally pigmented lesions may be seen with magnification. If the iris is scarred to the lens (posterior synechiae) or cornea (anterior synechiae), it should be noted. Of interest in those patients who have undergone cataract extraction, a tremulousness of the iris called *iridodonesis* is often seen. It is caused by removal of the support usually provided by the lens.

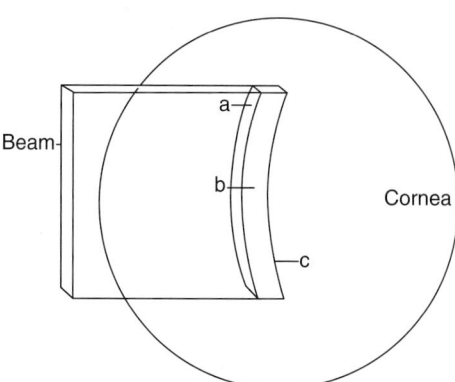

Fig. 201.4 Optical cross section of the cornea. *a,* Corneal epithelium; *b,* corneal stroma; *c,* corneal endothelium.

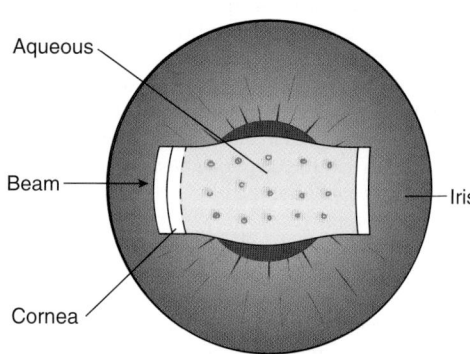

Fig. 201.5 Optical cross section of the anterior chamber showing cell and flare.

15. Next, use a long, narrow slit beam to examine the layers of the lens. Dilating the pupil allows for the most thorough evaluation of the lens. Any opacity in the crystalline lens is called a *cataract.* The slit beam passes through multiple layers from anterior to posterior: anterior capsule, anterior cortex, nucleus, posterior cortex, and posterior capsule (Fig. 201.6). Cortical cataracts resemble spokes radiating from the lens equator. Nuclear cataracts are central and are often seen as a yellow or amber hue discoloring the normally clear lens. Posterior subcapsular cataracts often appear as clustered punctate vacuoles. These can be seen either directly or with retroillumination.

    - Retroillumination uses the red reflex and will often provide a striking view of a lens opacity, especially through a dilated pupil. The slit beam is directed parallel to the visual axis to either the nasal or temporal side of the lens. The examiner then views the red reflex, which is the light reflected off the retina and back through the lens. Lens opacities such as capsular cataracts are prominently displayed against this red background.

16. After examining the posterior lens capsule, examine the anterior vitreous humor. Normally, the vitreous humor is a relatively clear fluid with minimal cellular material. If cellular material is noted, refer the patient to an ophthalmologist. Gross vitreous opacities, such as floaters, can also be seen with the slit beam.

17. At this point, if a corneal abrasion is suspected but not yet seen, a fluorescein strip should be used. It will stain areas of absent epithelium bright green when viewed with a cobalt-blue light filter. A wider slit beam is better tolerated by patients (i.e., causes less photophobia) if it is blue. (For instilling fluorescein, see Chapter 200, Corneal Abrasions and Removal of Corneal or Conjunctival Foreign Bodies.) Be careful to use minimal amounts of fluorescein to avoid flooding the eye and obscur-

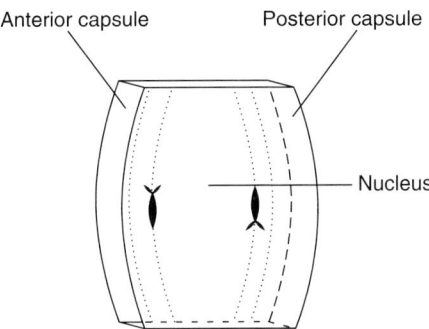

Anterior capsule Posterior capsule

Nucleus

Fig. 201.6 Optical cross section of the lens.

ing the abnormal epithelium. (Also, avoid staining the patient's skin and clothing with fluorescein!) Avoid touching the cornea directly with a fluorescein strip because this may result in an iatrogenically stained cornea. If either of these occurs, have the patient blink, blot the excess fluorescein away, and then reexamine. If the eye is still flooded, flush it with ophthalmic saline and again have the patient blot away the excess. The fluorescein examination is usually performed after the remainder of the eye has been examined with the slit lamp to avoid any light scatter that could be caused by fluorescein adsorbed by a corneal abrasion.

18. Using special lenses, often through a dilated pupil, the vitreous body, retina, and optic nerve can also be viewed with a slit lamp. For example, a Hruby lens can be attached by inserting the lens spindle into the groove of the lens guide plate on the slit lamp. A handheld lens positioned in front of the patient's eye can be used in the same manner. When a lens is being used, the slit beam is positioned parallel to the visual axis. (Distracting light reflections off the lenses can often be resolved by tilting the lens slightly.) The posterior structures of the eye can then be examined. This part of the examination should probably not be performed if the patient has an iritis or a corneal abrasion because of the associated severe photophobia.

POSTPROCEDURE PATIENT EDUCATION

The findings, as well as any needed postprocedure care, should be discussed with the patient. Any necessary referrals should be made. For corneal foreign bodies or abrasions, see Chapter 200, Corneal Abrasions and Removal of Corneal or Conjunctival Foreign Bodies, for management and postprocedure patient information.

CPT/BILLING CODES

65222	Removal of foreign body, external eye; corneal with slit lamp
92002	Ophthalmologic services: medical examination and evaluation with initiation of diagnostic and treatment program; intermediate, new patient
92012	Intermediate, established patient

NOTE: Intermediate examination includes biomicroscopy.

99070	Eye tray: supplies and materials (except spectacles) provided by physician over and above those that are usually included with the office visit or other services rendered (list drugs, trays, supplies, or materials provided)

ICD-10-CM DIAGNOSTIC CODES

H20.00	Acute or subacute iritis
H20.011–H20.019	Acute, primary iritis
H20.021–H20.029	Acute, primary recurrent
H20.031–H20.039	Iritis, secondary, infectious
H20.041–H20.049	Iritis, secondary noninfectious
H20.10–H20.13	Iritis, chronic
H21.50–H21.509	Adhesions of iris, unspecified
S05.00XX–S05.02XX	Corneal abrasion and injury of conjunctiva
T15.10XX–T15.12XX	Foreign body in conjunctival sac
T15.00XX–T15.02XX	Corneal foreign body

Use appropriate 7th character: A = initial, D = subsequent, S = sequela.

H16.101–H16.109	Superficial or unspecified keratitis w/o conjunctivitis
H16.131–H16.139	Welder's or photokeratitis
H16.201–H16.209	Superficial corneal keratitis with conjunctivitis
H18.821–H18.829	Corneal injury due to contact lens
H33.001–H33.009	Retinal detachment with retinal defect, unspecified
H44.601–H44.699	Intraocular foreign body magnetic
H44.701–H44.799	Intraocular foreign body nonmagnetic

Use additional code to identify foreign body: Z18.11, Z18.01–Z18.9

SUPPLIERS

(See contact information available at www.expertconsult.com.)

Sterile fluorescein sodium strips
  Haag-Streit
  Zeiss
  HUB Pharmaceuticals

RECOMMENDED READING

Albert DA, Miller JW, Azar DT, et al., eds. *Albert & Jakobiec's Principles and Practice of Ophthalmology.* 3rd ed. Philadelphia: Elsevier; 2008.

James D. Use of the slit lamp. In: James DM, ed. *Field Guide to Urgent and Ambulatory Care Procedures.* Philadelphia: Lippincott Williams & Wilkins; 2001:1–3.

Knoop KJ, Dennis WR. Ophthalmologic procedures. In: Roberts JR, Custalow CB, Thomsen TW, eds. *Roberts & Hedges' Clinical Procedures in Emergency Medicine.* 6th ed. Philadelphia: Elsevier; 2014:1259–1297.

Reichman EF. Corneal foreign body removal/ corneal rust ring removal. In: Reichman EF, ed. *Emergency Medicine Procedures.* 2nd ed. New York: McGraw-Hill; 2013:1043–1050.

Schabowski S. Eye examination. In: Reichman EF, ed. *Emergency Medicine Procedures.* 2nd ed. New York: McGraw-Hill; 2013:1007–1022.

CHAPTER 202

AURICULAR HEMATOMA EVACUATION

George D. Harris

The external ear is subject to a wide variety of injuries. Traumatic injury to the ear is commonly seen in athletes, particularly wrestlers, boxers, and rugby players. Such trauma can also be the result of motor vehicle accidents, assaults, fights, and falls. Although the cushion of subcutaneous fat on the medial surface of the auricle can dissipate a direct force, allowing the skin to slide over the underlying cartilage, the lateral surface lacks this layer of fat. Consequently, blunt trauma over the lateral surface causes shearing forces between the perichondrium and the underlying cartilage, resulting in torn blood vessels in the perichondrium and the formation of a hematoma. The location of the hematoma has classically been described as between the perichondrium and cartilage; however, the hematoma can arise within the cartilage itself.

Untreated hematomas affecting the external ear (pinna) can lead to overt disfigurement (cauliflower or wrestler's ear), especially if there is a delay in diagnosis and management.

With trauma, swelling can occur immediately or up to several hours later. Auricular hematomas can also occur spontaneously in older patients and in patients with a blood dyscrasia. A hematoma between the auricular cartilage and the perichondrium deprives the cartilage of its nutrient supply. If left untreated, a hematoma is at risk for secondary infection, causing perichondritis, cartilage necrosis, contracture, and neocartilage formation. The goals of treatment are to evacuate the hematoma, provide compression in the area, prevent the reaccumulation of fluid, prevent infection, and maintain the cartilage contour. Early treatment helps prevent aseptic necrosis and the loss of cartilage, and, it is hoped, avoids the permanent cosmetic ear deformity (cauliflower ear) from clot organization with fibrin deposition.

This chapter gives primary care clinicians, especially those involved in sports medicine, the information necessary to become familiar with the clinical presentation, appropriate treatment, and complications encountered when faced with an auricular hematoma.

NOTE: Patients presenting more than 7 days after the time of injury typically need extensive management. By this time, the clot has organized and there is newly formed cartilage and perichondrium; treatment of these patients is beyond the scope of this chapter.

INDICATIONS

Auricular hematoma: red, reddish-purple, or bluish fluctuant swelling, usually involving the entire lateral auricle. It is also usually quite tender.

CONTRAINDICATIONS

- Hematoma more than 7 days after injury or accompanied by auricular laceration, cellulitis, perichondritis
- Injury beyond the abilities of the clinician

EQUIPMENT

- Topical antiseptic, such as povidone–iodine (Betadine) or chlorhexidine
- For aspiration, 18- or 20-gauge needle and syringe
- Adhesive plastic ear drape or fenestrated drape
- Kidney or ear basin
- Sterile gloves
- No. 15 scalpel blade and holder
- Curved hemostat
- Forceps
- For anesthesia, 30-gauge needle and syringe
- Local anesthetic such as lidocaine 1% (optional, mixed with 1:100,000 epinephrine)
- Small suction catheter or curette
- 18-gauge intravenous catheter (needle removed), syringe, and normal saline for irrigation
- Penrose drain or sterile rubber band and scissors
- Gauze dressing
- Petrolatum gauze, or cotton balls soaked with petroleum jelly or mineral oil
- For alternative compression techniques: (1) cotton dental roll, tightly folded gauze or thermoplastic splinting material and monofilament nylon suture (3-0 or 4-0) with needle and a needle holder; (2) otolaryngologist's (ear, nose and throat [ENT]) silicone putty or dental impression material (Exaflex type O putty [GC America, Inc.]), (3) 3-0-4-0 nylon, Vicryl, or chromic catgut suture
- Topical antibiotic ointment (bacitracin/polymyxin or mupirocin)
- Eye protection and equipment necessary to follow universal blood and body fluid precautions

PREPROCEDURE PATIENT PREPARATION

Explain the indications for, alternatives to, and possible complications of the procedure, as well as the possible complications from not performing the procedure. Obtain informed consent, if possible. Also explain the discomfort of injected local anesthetic and the necessity for the patient to remain very still during the procedure. The patient should be prepared for some mild discomfort during hematoma removal, even with use of the local anesthetic.

TECHNIQUE

Treatment requires the complete drainage of the hematoma to prevent deformity. This can be done in multiple ways, but the predominant methods are needle aspiration and incision and evacuation. Both should be followed by some type of compression dressing to prevent reaccumulation. There is controversy about which method of drainage is superior. In addition, there are no randomized trials, case-controlled trials, or cohort studies to support one treatment over another regarding the best cosmetic result with the least permanent deformity. Because of the difficulty in removing the entire hematoma, the difficulty in eliminating the dead space, the consequent high risk of recurrence, and the frequent need for a second procedure after needle aspiration, many experts prefer the incision and evacuation technique.

1. Position the patient comfortably in the supine position with the injured ear accessible. Universal blood and body fluid precautions should be followed.
2. Cleanse the helix with antiseptic solution. Examine for associated lacerations. Anesthesia is achieved by performing a regional block (see Chapter 7, Peripheral Nerve Blocks and Field Blocks) or by placing a skin wheal of local anesthetic over the hematoma. Many clinicians prefer a regional block because it is very difficult to inject local anesthetic at the site. (There is no subcutaneous layer of fat below the skin; consequently, the skin is tightly adherent to perichondrium.) The hematoma should not be injected because the anesthetic will only cause the hematoma to expand and increase the damage.
3. Attempt aspiration of the most fluctuant area of the hematoma using an 18- or 20-gauge needle (Fig. 202.1). To ensure complete evacuation of the hematoma, it may be helpful to express or "milk" the hematoma between the thumb and index finger of the opposite hand while aspirating. After evacuation, hold pressure over the area for at least 3 to 5 minutes to make sure the hematoma does not recur and that all was removed. If there has been recurrence or an incomplete evacuation, aspirate again. If successful, this technique may be all that is necessary to evacuate the hematoma, especially if the injury is quite recent and the hematoma is small. Place antibiotic ointment over the aspiration site; proceed to step 10 or the "Alternative Compression Techniques" sections. **NOTE:** Using a simple aspiration technique is not adequate for preventing recurrence; consequently one must also use a compression bandage of some sort. If the hematoma has been present for 6 to 8 hours, it is likely an organized clot. This will be difficult to aspirate, and incision and drainage will probably be required. However, if the patient presents slightly less than 1 week postinjury, sometimes the clot will have broken down (liquefied) and aspiration can be attempted. Larger hematomas may require an open approach or the placement of a drain.
4. If aspiration does not completely evacuate the hematoma, incision and evacuation will need to be performed. While maintaining a sterile field, if not performed previously, a regional block should be performed. (A regional block is necessary for reasons previously mentioned, including the lack of a subcutaneous layer of fat.)
5. While waiting 10 to 15 minutes for the anesthetic to take effect, if not previously performed, drape the patient in a manner that keeps his or her hair away from the involved area.
6. Note the anatomy of the external ear (Fig. 202.2). With the No. 15 scalpel, make a curvilinear incision over the hematoma, usually 4 to 5 mm in length (no longer than 1 cm). For the best cosmetic result, the incision should follow the natural recessions of the ear between the helix and antihelix, or the antihelix and the concha (Fig. 202.3). Multiple incisions may be needed. The hematoma may then be expressed or removed using the forceps, gentle suctioning, or curettage.
7. Probe the cavity with the hemostat to ensure complete evacuation. Additional manipulation can be performed, if necessary, with digital pressure applied to assist with complete evacuation. Apply pressure until hemostasis is obtained, for at least 3 to 5 minutes. After hemostasis is obtained, some clinicians will irrigate the cavity with normal saline, pulsed in from a soft intravenous catheter and collected in a basin.
8. If necessary, insert a piece of the sterile Penrose drain or rubber band into the incision. (This should be removed within 48 hours to minimize the risk of infection.)

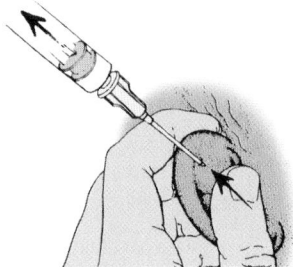

Fig. 202.1 While stabilizing the pinna with the thumb and fingers, puncture the most fluctuant part of the hematoma. Use the thumb and index finger to express or "milk" the hematoma into the syringe.

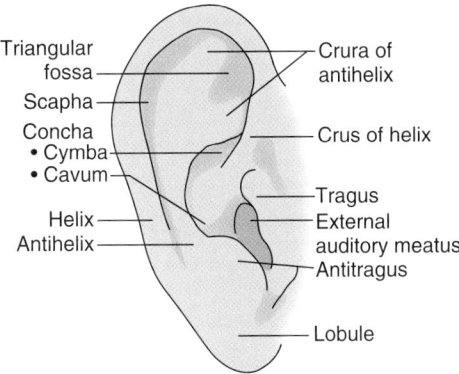

Fig. 202.2 Anatomy of the external ear. (From Bisaccia E, Lugo A, Johnson B, Scarborough D. The surgical correction of protuberant ears. *Skin Therapy Lett.* 2005;10:7–9.)

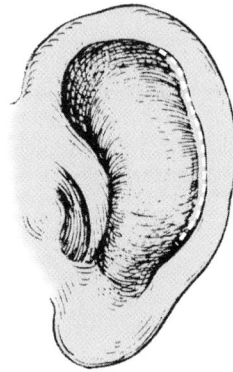

Fig. 202.3 A 3- to 5-mm curvilinear incision is made along this line near area of greatest fluctuance. It can be made larger, but should not exceed 1 cm.

9. Apply antibiotic ointment to the area of the aspiration or incision.
10. Place a piece of sterile dry cotton in the external auditory canal.
11. Fit petroleum jelly–treated gauze or petroleum jelly– or mineral oil–soaked cotton balls externally onto the contours of the ear. They should be placed in layers until level with the lateral helical rim. Trimmed gauze squares should then be placed between the ear and the head. Finally, over these layers of gauze or cotton, apply an elastic gauze compression dressing to the ear (Fig. 202.4).
12. Prescribe prophylactic oral antibiotics for 5 days and appropriate analgesia. Antibiotics are important if the hematoma has been present for more than 24 hours, if the hematoma recurs and requires repeated incision and drainage, or if there are signs

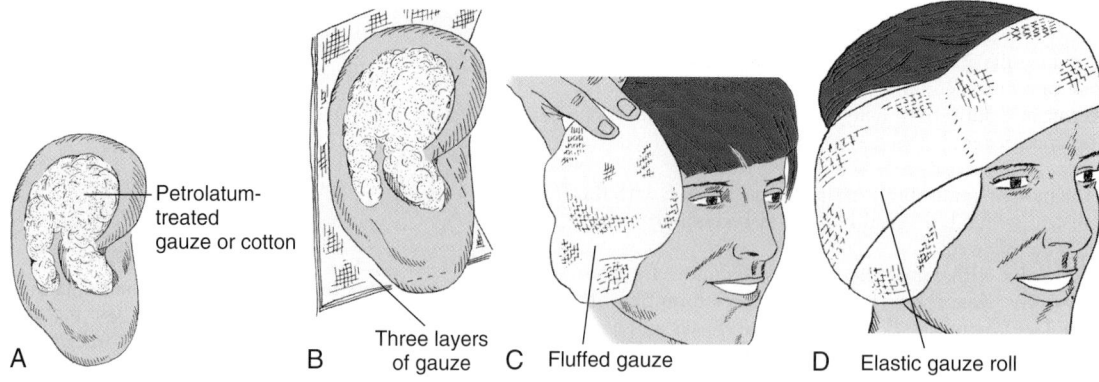

Fig. 202.4 External gauze compression dressing. (A) Dry cotton is first placed into the ear canal. A conforming material is then carefully molded into all the convolutions of the auricle. (B) When the convolutions are fully packed, a medial gauze pack is placed behind the ear. A V-shaped section has been cut from the gauze to allow it to easily fit behind the ear. (C) Multiple layers of fluffed gauze are placed over the packed ear. (D) The entire dressing is held in place with Kling or an elastic gauze roll. The ear is thus compressed between two layers of gauze, and the packing ensures even distribution of pressure to all parts of the auricle.

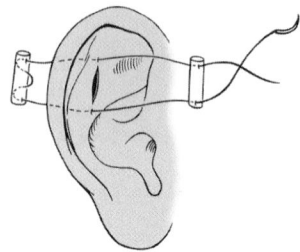

Fig. 202.5 Alternative technique using cotton dental roll for compression. Cut pieces of softened thermoplastic splinting material can be used in same manner.

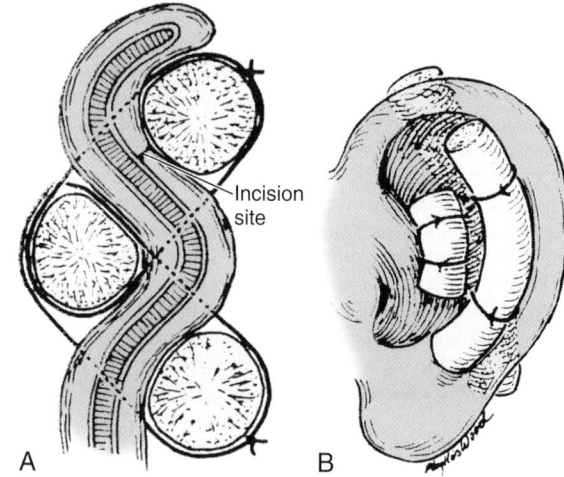

Fig. 202.6 Multiple dental rolls used for compression after evacuation of a large hematoma. (A) Medial auricular. (B) Lateral auricular. (From Cummings CW, ed. *Otolaryngology: Head and Neck Surgery*. 2nd ed. St. Louis; Mosby; 1993.)

of cellulitis. They should cover skin flora and *Pseudomonas aeruginosa* (amoxicillin-clavulanic acid in children; levofloxacin in adults).

13. Instruct the patient to remove the elastic gauze bandage daily to evaluate the auricle. He or she should return in 24 to 48 hours for complete dressing removal and reevaluation. Redrain the ear or reapply the dressing as needed to maintain ear compression for 1 week.

ALTERNATIVE COMPRESSION TECHNIQUES

Cotton Dental Rolls

This alternative compression technique uses cotton dental rolls or cut pieces of thermoplastic splinting material for compression *after* evacuation. First, follow steps 1 through 10, as described previously.

11. Next, cut a dental roll or piece of thermoplastic splinting material to fit over most of the hematoma. The smaller remnant of the cut roll or a smaller piece of thermoplastic splint will be stitched medially. Soften the splint in water before applying it. (Two tightly packed pieces of gauze can be stitched in a similar manner, with similar effects.)
12. After slightly straightening the suture needle, pass it through one end of the cut dental roll or thermoplastic splint.
13. Pass the needle through the most cephalic end of the hematoma from lateral to medial. To use the smaller remaining piece of dental roll or thermoplastic splint as medial compression, pass the needle back and forth through the smaller roll or splint (Fig. 202.5).
14. Next, pass the needle through the inferior portion of the hematoma from medial to lateral and then through the other end of the lateral dental roll or splint. If necessary, multiple rolls or

pieces of splint can be used (Fig. 202.6).
15. Tie the suture securely. This creates both lateral and medial compression of the hematoma.
16. Apply antibacterial ointment liberally over the dental rolls and the ear. Next, apply an elastic gauze dressing. Oral antibiotics are given as in preceding step 12.
17. Ask the patient to return in 24 hours, at which time the elastic gauze dressing is removed. Instruct the patient to continue applying antibacterial ointment until the dental roll or splint dressing is removed in 2 weeks.

NOTE: This technique requires an aseptic procedure, anesthesia, and frequent daily dressings. Patients frequently complain of auricular pain for several days after a stitched compressed dressing is applied. The stitched compressed dressing can sometimes lead to pressure necrosis of the auricle.

Ear, Nose, and Throat Silicone Putty or Dental Impression Material

The technique using ENT silicone putty or dental impression material first follows steps 1 through 10, described previously.

11. Next, mold ENT silicone putty to fit the lateral ear just lateral to the external auditory meatus. Wrap the putty medially to

match the pinna (Fig. 202.7). The putty contains a hardener, causing it to solidify in a few minutes. Dental impression material can be mixed and used in the same manner (Fig. 202.8).

12. An elastic gauze head bandage is then applied for 2 days, after which it can be removed. The ENT putty or hardened dental impression material mold should be left in place for a week. Use oral antibiotics as described previously. Instruct the patient to return in 48 hours for reevaluation.

Oversewing Technique

Dental or ENT putty, dental rolls, or even thermoplastic splints are not always available in an emergency department or urgent care center. They are even less likely to be available in a primary care office. Since the goal of this procedure is to drain the hematoma and prevent it from coming back by closing the dead space, after draining the hematoma (following steps 1 through 10), the dead space can be

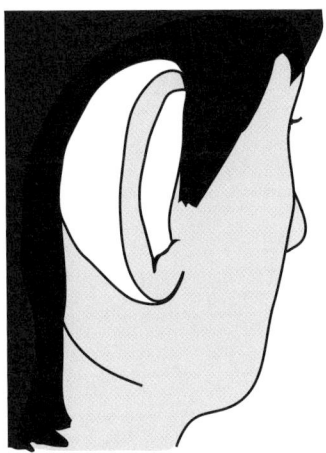

Fig. 202.7 Ear, nose and throat putty used for compression. The putty is molded to fit the ear, and an external compression dressing is used for 2 days. By then the putty is hardened and can be left open to air.

closed by merely oversewing the pinna using a continuous horizontal mattress stitch. The needle should be passed back and forth through the pinna. This will require a sturdy, 3-0 to 5-0 nylon, Vicryl, or chromic cat gut stitch. The patient should be seen in follow-up in 24 to 48 hours to reassure a hematoma has not recurred.

POSTPROCEDURE PATIENT EDUCATION

The patient should be aware of the importance of follow-up with the clinician and maintaining compression for at least a week. He or she should understand the risk of complications, regardless of management, and should see a clinician if there are signs of infection (e.g., increasing redness, drainage, tenderness, warmth, pain at the site). If an external elastic gauze is used to cover the site (see Fig. 202.4), it should be removed daily to check for signs of infection or complications and then reapplied. Oral antibiotics are indicated for 5 days with any puncture, incision, or laceration of the auricle, so patients should know how to take them and the importance of taking them. The patient should know when to return to the clinician's office and what possible complications to report.

COMPLICATIONS

- Bleeding or recurrence of hematoma
- Scar at the site of the incision
- Infection including perichondritis (risk minimized by prophylactic oral antibiotics)
- Auricular deformity, either in spite of appropriate treatment, or because the treatment is inadequate

CPT/BILLING CODES

69000	Drainage external ear, abscess or hematoma; simple
69005	Complicated

ICD-10-CM DIAGNOSTIC CODES

H61.121-H61.129   Auricular hematoma

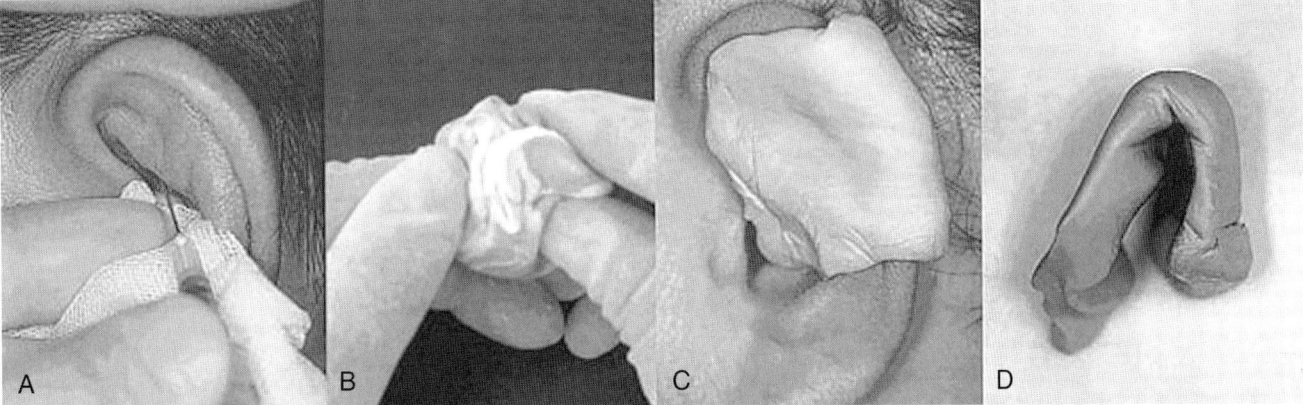

Fig. 202.8 Technique for treatment of auricular hematoma using dental impression material. (A) Follow steps 1 through 9 of the procedure. (B) The impression material is prepared using equal parts (one scoop) of base and catalyst of Exaflex type O putty (GC America, Inc.), which is composed of vinyl polysiloxane and spontaneously cures after base and catalyst are mixed. The materials are kneaded in the hands for 1 minute or until uniform in color. (C) The mixed impression material is placed on both the lateral and medial surfaces of the auricle. Make sure the lateral surface of the auricle is adequately covered, including the cavum concha area, to maintain the normal contour of the auricle. It takes about 3 to 5 minutes for the Exaflex mixture to cure spontaneously. (D) The dental impression material is contoured into the shape of an inverted "U," which acts to stabilize the frame. The cured dental frame is fixed and stabilized with paper tape and then dressed simply with gauze. The patient is checked again 3 days after the procedure, and then on day 7. At that time, the impression material is removed. (From Choung YH, Park K, Choung PH, Oh JH. Simple compressive method for treatment of auricular haematoma using dental silicone material. *J Laryngol Otol.* 2005;119:27–31.)

RECOMMENDED READING

Ghanem T, Rasamny JK, Park SS. Rethinking auricular trauma. *Laryngoscope*. 2005;115:1251–1255.

James DM. Management of auricular hematoma. In: James DM, ed. *Field Guide to Urgent and Ambulatory Care Procedures*. Philadelphia: Lippincott Williams & Wilkins; 2001:33–35.

Jones SE, Mahendran S. Interventions for acute auricular hematoma. *Cochrane Database Syst Rev*. 2004;2:CD004166.

Lee D, Sperling N. Initial management of auricular trauma. *Am Fam Physician*. 1996;53:2339–2344.

Reichman EF. Auricular hematoma evacuation. In: Reichman EF, ed. *Emergency Medicine Procedures*. 2nd ed. New York: McGraw-Hill; 2013:1078–1084.

Riviello RJ. Otolaryngologic procedures. In: Roberts JR, Custalow CB, Thomsen TW, eds. *Roberts & Hedges' Clinical Procedures in Emergency Medicine*. 6th ed. Philadelphia: Elsevier; 2014:1317–1320.

Schuller DE, Dankle SD, Strauss RH. A technique to treat wrestlers' auricular hematoma without interrupting training or competition. *Arch Otolaryngol Head Neck Surg*. 1989;115:202–206.

CHAPTER 203

REDUCTION OF DISLOCATED TEMPOROMANDIBULAR JOINT (WITH TEMPOROMANDIBULAR JOINT SYNDROME EXERCISES)

Robert S. Tan • Grant C. Fowler

Although dislocation of the temporomandibular joint (TMJ) can happen to anyone, it occurs more commonly in older patients. Associated conditions and situations include rheumatoid arthritis, osteoarthritis, excessive laughter, or yawning. Trauma can cause a TMJ dislocation; the history often reveals a blow to the chin while the mouth is slightly open. Dystonic reactions to medications can also cause dislocation. Patients who have had one dislocation are prone to further dislocations.

Anterior dislocation occurs when the muscles and ligaments supporting the mandible are relaxed enough to allow the condyle to jump anteriorly over the articular eminence of the fossa. Posterior dislocation is rare and usually the result of a direct blow to the chin that does not break the condylar neck. Once any dislocation occurs, trismus and muscle spasms prevent the joint from returning to its natural position. Consequently, the patient presents to the clinician with an open mouth that cannot be closed and difficulty swallowing and talking. For anterior dislocation, pain is usually localized anterior to the tragus. There will be a visible and palpable preauricular depression from the displacement of the mandibular condyle. Although unilateral dislocation causes a deviation away from the affected side, the more common bilateral dislocation prevents the mouth from being closed.

For clicking or tender TMJs, splinting by a dentist or oral surgeon is a common treatment. In the "Postprocedure Patient Education" section, three published alternatives to splint therapy are described as well as a TMJ "rest" program. For an acutely painful TMJ, as described in the "Passive Reduction" section, the joint can also be injected with a lidocaine/corticosteroid mixture.

INDICATIONS

Unilateral or bilateral TMJ dislocation(s) without fractures (the dislocation should be confirmed with a radiograph, which also rules out a fracture).

CONTRAINDICATIONS

Fractured condyle(s) (patient should be referred to a maxillofacial surgeon)

EQUIPMENT

- Gloves, mask, goggles, and equipment necessary to maintain universal blood and body fluid precautions

- Gauze and tongue blade to protect the clinician's thumbs
- Parenteral muscle relaxant may be helpful (e.g., diazepam, lorazepam, midazolam).
- Examination chair with firm neck rest
- 5 mL of 2% lidocaine in a 10-mL syringe with a 25-gauge needle, 4 × 4 inches gauze sponges, skin antiseptic solution such as povidone-iodine or chlorhexidine (optional)
- Injectable corticosteroid (optional)

PREPROCEDURE PATIENT PREPARATION

Inform the patient which technique(s) will be attempted, whether passive or active, and the indications for, risks of, and alternatives to these techniques. If the passive technique is to be attempted, explain how muscle spasm is inhibiting reduction of the dislocated TMJ, and that an intravenous muscle relaxant may be all that is necessary.

Alternatively, an injection of local anesthetic into the TMJ may allow patients to reduce the dislocation themselves. If the active technique is necessary, patients should know that while the joint is being reduced, they may experience considerable pressure on the molars. They may also experience some referred pain to the neck, face, or ear, as well as mild, aching TMJ arthralgia after the reduction. It will be important for them to remain relaxed and immobile while the joint is being reduced.

NOTE: If an intravenous muscle relaxant is used, the patient should be accompanied by someone and not be allowed to drive that day. The patient should also be aware that his or her urine would test positive for benzodiazepines should drug testing be done.

TECHNIQUE

Passive Reduction

One theory suggests that muscle spasm is all that is inhibiting reduction; therefore, an intravenous muscle relaxant should suffice. However, another theory suggests that painful stimuli arising from the capsule cause the muscle spasm. Consequently, injection of lidocaine into the joint would be needed to overcome these painful stimuli and allow for passive reduction. The choice of technique may be determined by patient desire or by what is available in the clinic setting. Universal blood and body fluid precautions should be followed when performing this procedure.

1. If *intravenous muscle relaxation* is chosen, administer titrating doses of a muscle relaxant (e.g., diazepam, lorazepam, midazolam). Often, as the medication is titrated, the joint reduction occurs spontaneously.

    NOTE: When benzodiazepines are administered intravenously, appropriate airway and hemodynamic monitoring is required. Moderate (conscious) procedural sedation privileges may also be required (see Chapter 1, Procedural Sedation and Analgesia).

2. If *TMJ injection* is chosen, have the patient open their mouth at least 4 cm. Palpate the joint line anterior to the tragus of the ear and the condyle of the mandible located immediately beneath the zygomatic arch. These landmarks are further confirmed by having the patient open and close the jaw while the clinician is palpating the joint line. After preparing the site with antiseptic solution, 3 to 5 mL of lidocaine should be injected into the joint. The needle should be inserted just below the zygomatic arch, one fingerbreadth anterior to the tragus, and directed inward and slightly upward. It will move freely when the tip is in the joint cavity.

    NOTE: For an acutely painful TMJ, injection with a combination of 0.5 mL corticosteroid and 0.5 mL local anesthetic may be helpful. Joint rest, as described in the "Postprocedure Patient Education" section, may also be helpful.

3. The injection of lidocaine alone may allow for spontaneous reduction (Fig. 203.1). Otherwise, a few minutes after the injection, even with bilateral dislocation, the patient might be able to close his or her mouth and retract the mandible into its normal position.

4. If passive reduction by muscle relaxation or TMJ injection is unsuccessful, active reduction may be necessary.

Active Reduction

This technique can be used for unilateral or bilateral dislocation.

1. The patient's head should be placed against a wall or high headrest to prevent backward movement. To allow for adequate leverage, the level of the patient's mandible should not be higher than the clinician's elbow. Take care to protect your thumbs because the mandible usually snaps sharply back into place with tremendous pressure, and this is an involuntary reflex. At a minimum, gauze should be wrapped over the gloved thumbs to protect them. Fortifying the gauze with two pieces of tongue blade is a good idea.

2. While standing in front of the patient (or behind), have the patient open his or her mouth slightly and place your thumbs on the occlusal surfaces of his or her posterior lower teeth.

3. Firmly grasp the mandible on the outside with your fingertips. Exert downward force on the molars (Fig. 203.2) in a slow and firm manner.

4. For anterior dislocation, after 30 to 60 seconds of downward pressure, apply very light pressure in a posterior direction and elevate the chin. (Pressure should be exerted in the opposite direction for a posterior dislocation.) This light posterior pressure and chin elevation can be accomplished by rotating the posterior or inferior mandible with your fingertips. At this point, the condyles should clear the articular eminence and allow the mandible to slide into its normally closed position (Fig. 203.3). If unsuccessful, this step may be repeated once or twice. With posterior dislocation, because the condyle may have prolapsed into the external auditory canal, baseline hearing should be documented (see Chapter 59, Audiometry).

5. Should these procedures fail, attempt to reduce the TMJ under more aggressive procedural sedation (see Chapter 1, Procedural Sedation and Analgesia). Should this also fail, consultation should be considered because reduction may need to be done under general anesthesia.

6. If the patient can swing his or her jaw from side to side, the reduction has been successful. Postprocedure radiographs are not re-

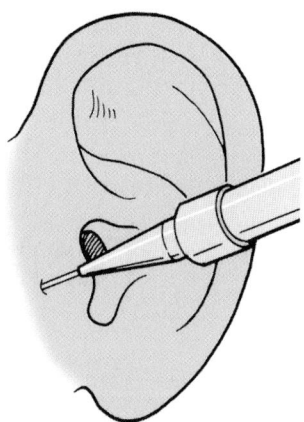

Fig. 203.1 Injection of lidocaine into the joint.

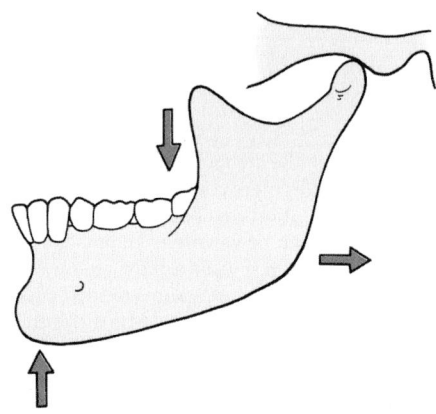

Fig. 203.2 Direction of combined forces necessary for reduction.

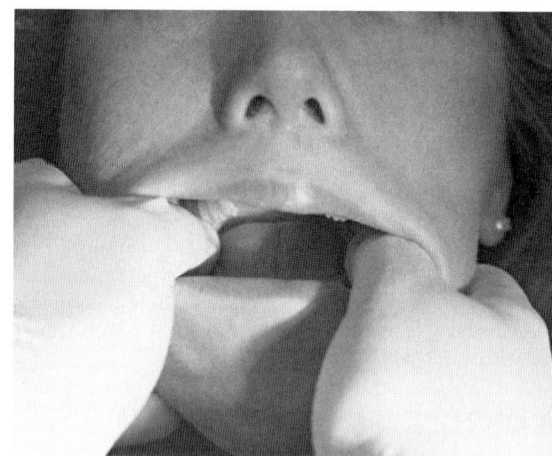

Fig. 203.3 Reduction of a dislocated mandible from a position in front of the patient.

quired unless the procedure was difficult or traumatic, or there is significant postreduction pain. If the jaw immediately dislocates after successful reduction, a Kerlix-type gauze or a Barton bandage (elastic fabricated bandage) should be wrapped around the jaw and over the top of the head, producing a pressure-type dressing to keep the jaw closed. In this situation, the patient should also be referred to a dentist or an oral or maxillofacial surgeon.

7. A recently technique published uses a 5- to 10-mL syringe for a hands-free reduction of nontraumatic dislocation. The syringe is placed between the upper and lower posterior molars (or gums if edentulous) on the affected side. Ask the patient to gently bite down on the syringe and roll it back and forth. In so doing, the syringe acts as a rolling fulcrum to help the anteriorly displaced condyle slip back into the normal position.

NOTE: For recurrent dislocations, search for possible causes (e.g., occlusal disharmony causing muscle spasm, medication-induced trismus, rheumatoid arthritis).

COMPLICATIONS

All of the following complications occur only rarely.

* Posterior dislocation of the TMJ from reduction of anterior dislocation, and vice versa
* Iatrogenic fracture or avulsion of the articular cartilage
* Anesthesia complications (e.g., allergic reaction to lidocaine)
* Nerve damage
* Permanent TMJ arthritis related to an improperly managed or undiagnosed condylar fracture; this is particularly a risk if the fracture extends into the articular surface. Prolonged disarticulation (several days) or recurrent disarticulation is also associated with TMJ arthritis.

POSTPROCEDURE PATIENT EDUCATION

Patients should be instructed to avoid opening their mouth more than 2 cm (the width of their thumb) for 2 weeks, and they should not yawn widely, take large bites of food, or laugh excessively for 4 to 6 weeks. They should also be placed on a soft diet for 2 weeks, and acetaminophen or nonsteroidal analgesics may be helpful for any discomfort. Patients should be taught to support the mandible with a hand when they yawn. In some instances, immobilization of the jaw is needed after reduction; consider referral to a dentist. Some dentists immobilize the jaw for up to 2 weeks to give the stretched muscles and ligaments an opportunity to heal. This also allows the edema to subside. Inadequate immobilization may lead to the recurrence of dislocation. If the dislocation was not traumatic, inform the patient that repeating the action that caused it will again cause dislocation. This is particularly true in the 4 to 6 weeks after reduction when the ligaments are not fully healed. Also warn the patient that recurrent dislocations may lead to permanent TMJ arthritis. In recurrent TMJ dislocation, the patient should be referred and the jaw immobilized for 4 to 6 weeks.

Three Alternatives to Splint Therapy for a Tender or Clicking Temporomandibular Joint

Patients with a tender or clicking TMJ are frequently referred to a dentist or oral surgeon for internal splinting or splint therapy. A custom splint is made to be inserted between the upper and lower molars and provide constant tension on the TMJ by separating the molars. Such constant tension and immobilization of the TMJ hopefully allows it to heal. Some primary care clinicians use a "boil and bite" mouthpiece (which can be bought in most sporting goods stores to protect teeth during contact sports) in the same manner. The following exercises have been published as alternatives to splinting in the patient with no obvious malocclusion or organic disease such as rheumatoid arthritis. These exercises often alleviate symptoms in about 2 weeks. If they fail, rest therapy (as noted in the section the follows) may be an option.

Method A

1. Have the patient obtain a soft wooden or plastic rod, approximately 15 cm long and 1.5 cm in diameter (e.g., a wooden dowel).
2. At least three times a day, the patient should thrust the mandible forward and grasp the rod with his or her back molars.

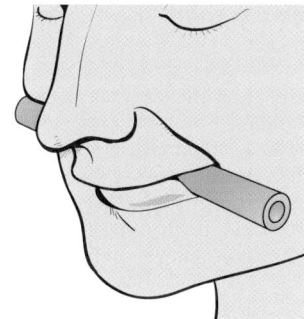

Fig. 203.4   Wooden rod chewing exercise.

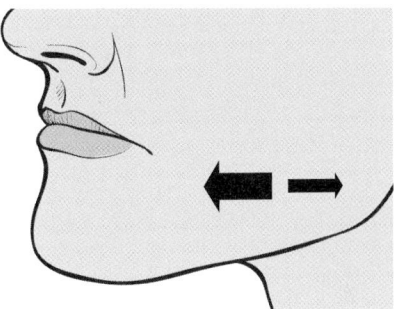

Fig. 203.5   Lower jaw thrust exercise.

3. For 2 to 3 minutes, the patient then rhythmically bites on the rod with a grinding movement (Fig. 203.4).

Method B

1. Although it may be initially uncomfortable, this exercise should eventually lead to some relief in uncomplicated TMJ syndrome.
2. At least four to five times a day, for 15 repetitions, the patient should rhythmically thrust the lower jaw forward and backward, in an anterior-posterior direction. The mouth should be slightly open, and when the exercise is performed correctly, the patient will look like a pouting child exposing the bottom lip (Fig. 203.5).

Method C

This method consists of six exercises to be repeated six times each, six times per day (6 × 6).

NOTE: These exercises were recommended by an oral surgeon and should not cause pain while being performed. If performance causes discomfort, the intensity, rather than the number and frequency of the repetitions, should be reduced.

1. Have the patient hold the front third of his or her tongue to the roof of the mouth and take six deep breaths.
2. Next, have the patient hold his or her tongue to the roof of the mouth and open the mouth six times. The jaw should not click.
3. Have the patient hold the chin with both hands, keeping the chin still. Without actually letting it move, the patient should attempt to move his or her chin up, down, and to each side.
4. Next, with the chin between the heels of both hands, and the fingertips behind the neck, have the patient pull his or her chin toward the neck. Hold for 6 seconds.
5. Next, have the patient push his or her upper lip back as if to push the head straight back while using the neck muscles to prevent the head from being pushed back. Hold for 6 seconds.
6. To finish the exercises, have the patient pull the shoulders back, as if to touch the shoulder blades together, and hold for 6 seconds.

Temporomandibular Joint "Rest" Program

The following instructions may be given to patients:

1. Avoid biting any food with your front teeth—use small, bite-size pieces.
2. Food should be in small enough pieces to avoid opening your mouth wider than the thickness of your thumb.
3. Avoid eating food that requires prolonged chewing (e.g., raw vegetables, tough meat, hard crusts of bread).
4. Avoid protruding your jaw (e.g., talking, applying lipstick) or your tongue.
5. Try to breathe through your nose at all times.
6. Do not sleep on your jaw; attempt to always sleep on your back.
7. Avoid clenching your teeth—keep your lips together and your teeth apart.
8. Avoid chewing gum.
9. Always try to open your mouth in a hinge or arc motion.
10. Practice a relaxed lifestyle so that your jaws and face muscles feel relaxed.

CPT/Billing Codes

21480   Closed uncomplicated treatment of temporomandibular dislocation, initial or subsequent

21485   Closed complicated treatment of temporomandibular dislocation (e.g., recurrent requiring intermaxillary fixation or splinting), initial or subsequent

ICD-10-CM Diagnostic Codes

M26.601-M26.609	Temporomandibular joint-pain-dysfunction syndrome
M26.621-M26.629	Temporomandibular joint arthralgia
M26.69	Temporomandibular joint sounds on opening/closing the jaw
S03.00XX-S03.03XX	Dislocation of temporomandibular joint, recurrent or closed

Add appropriate seventh character: A = initial, D = subsequent, S = sequela.

RECOMMENDED READING

Pedigo RA, Amsterdam JT. Oral medicine. In: Walls RM, Hockberger RS, Gausche-Hill M, eds. *Rosen's Emergency Medicine*. 9th ed. Philadelphia: Elsevier; 2018:771–789.

James DM. Reduction of a dislocated mandible. In: James DM, ed. *Field Guide to Urgent and Ambulatory Care Procedures*. Philadelphia: Lippincott Williams & Wilkins; 2001:44–47.

Lareau SA, Heitz CR. Face and jaw emergencies. In: Tintinalli JE, Stapczynski JS, Ma OJ, et al., eds. *Tintinalli's Emergency Medicine: A Comprehensive Study Guide*. 8th ed. New York: McGraw-Hill; 2015.

Murtagh J. *Musculoskeletal medicine*. In: Murtagh J. *Practice Tips*. 7th ed. Sydney, Australia: McGraw-Hill; 2017:129–130.

CHAPTER 204

REMOVAL OF FOREIGN BODIES FROM THE EAR AND NOSE

John Harlan Haynes III • Michael Zeringue

The nasal orifice and external auditory canal occasionally collect small objects such as beads, insects, peanuts, pebbles, or beans. Foreign bodies in this area are especially common in pediatric and mentally impaired individuals. Living insects are the most common foreign bodies in the ears of adults. Knowledge of the type of foreign body and how long it has been lodged is very helpful. If an expandable material is suspected (e.g., organic materials, beans, seeds), irrigation with water or saline may be contraindicated because it could cause additional expansion of the object. Timeliness is a priority because the object could become more firmly lodged in place as the mucosa swells. Reactive debris may accumulate as a local response to the irritation. Manual removal or suction may be required to remove these objects and the accompanying debris.

Various techniques are available for removing foreign bodies with instruments; however, simple attempts at removal should generally be pursued before instrumentation. In children with a nasal foreign body, a nebulized decongestant may assist expulsion with simple nose blowing. A positive-pressure technique (as in mouth-to-mouth resuscitation) using an appropriately sized bag-valve-mask (Ambu bag) may be all that is needed in infants, young children, and impaired adults. While not exceeding recommended maximal pressure with the bag-valve-mask (by cardiopulmonary resuscitation guidelines), block the unaffected nostril to force air briskly through the oropharynx and affected nostril. This will often dislodge the object. In older children and adults, vasoconstrictive nasal solutions (e.g., phenylephrine, epinephrine, oxymetazoline) may be used to reduce mucosal edema. Wait 10 minutes after application, then have the patient obstruct one nostril and blow forcefully through the other. Even if the object does not come out, the relaxed and decongested mucosa will give the clinician more room to work.

EDITOR'S NOTE: A "parent's kiss" technique has also been described; studies have found it to be very effective. With the child supine, have the parent occlude the opposite nostril with a thumb. Next, as in mouth-to-mouth resuscitation, have the parent make a seal with their mouth over the child's open mouth and give a short, sharp puff of air briskly into the child's mouth. Even if the object does not pop out of the nose, it may move it into a position that makes it easier for the clinician to retrieve. This may be repeated, if necessary. A modification of this technique uses a large straw. With the parent holding the child's opposite nostril closed, ask the child to make a tight seal on the straw, as if they were going to sip a liquid. The parent can then give a sharp puff on the straw.

In the external ear canal, pulsed saline irrigation through an 18-gauge plastic catheter directed posteriorly may dislodge the impacted object. However, irrigation is contraindicated if tympanic membrane perforation is suspected.

The use of strong acrylic glue (cyanoacrylate) has been advocated for removing beads from the nose or external canal, but the patient must be able to remain very still. The ultimate goal when removing a foreign body with this technique, as well as with all other techniques, is to remove the object with as little trauma as possible while avoiding pushing it further into the orifice. If this technique is used, make sure acetone is available to remove any misplaced cyanoacrylate (see section on "Alternate Technique: Glue").

Having acetone available may also be helpful if the foreign body turns out to be chewing gum or polystyrene foam (e.g., Styrofoam) or beads. In addition to dissolving cyanoacrylate glue, acetone has been reported in the literature to dissolve or soften polystyrene; it also reduces the adherence of particles consisting of these substances or gum. Ethyl chloride has been used in the same manner. It should be noted that there have been no studies regarding any possible toxicity from acetone, dissolved polystyrene, or ethyl chloride in contact with a mucous membrane. Therefore, only a few drops of the acetone or ethyl chloride should be dripped directly onto the foreign body under guidance with an otoscope. After being left in place for 5 minutes or less, the resulting combination should be removed with forceps, suction, or irrigation. Ultimately, the ear should be irrigated to remove any residual chemicals after the object is removed. Again, if there is a possibility of a perforated tympanic membrane, this process is contraindicated.

Both reassurance and immobilization are important when removing nasal or external canal foreign bodies. Availability of the proper tools and an adequate light source are also critical. To minimize the risk of lacerations or abrasions, all attempts to remove foreign bodies should be made under direct visualization with magnification if possible. The clinician should set realistic limits on the amount of time to be spent and number of attempts to be made. Referral to an ear, nose, and throat specialist may be prudent (1) if the examiner is dealing with an expandable material (unless there is a high probability of successful removal); (2) when the nasal passage or external ear canal is completely occluded and surrounded by marked edema and inflammation; (3) if the object is adherent or adjacent to the tympanic membrane; or (4) if attempts to remove the object have been unsuccessful or will worsen the scenario. For such difficult removals, local anesthesia, conscious sedation, or even general anesthesia may be necessary. If an ear, nose, and throat specialist agrees, and if the patient is in considerable pain, instillation of topical anesthetic drops before transportation may be appreciated.

NOTE: Miniature button or disk batteries are commonly used in watches, calculators, cameras, hearing aids, and even greeting cards that play music. Consequently, they are frequent foreign objects in noses and ears. Removal is a high priority because permanent damage can result (usually localized electrical burns, but bone and cartilage can be destroyed) if allowed to remain for more than a short time. Although miniature batteries contain toxic heavy metals, such as mercury, their greater danger lies in the fact that they can produce electrochemical current. They should be removed promptly; irrigation, nose drops, or eardrops are strictly contraindicated.

NOTE: If a recently acquired foreign body turns out to be a moth, take the patient into a dark room and shine a flashlight into the ear or nose. The moth may fly out toward the light!

INDICATION

A known foreign body is the indication for treatment.

NOTE: A general rule for foreign bodies in the ear is that if the object is in the outer two-thirds of the canal and is easily accessible, it can usually be removed. If it is closer to the eardrum and cannot be removed by irrigation, referral should be considered.

CONTRAINDICATIONS

Consider referral if any of the following contraindications apply.

- Lack of knowledge of normal anatomy of nasal passage or external ear canal.
- Nasal passage or external ear canal is obscured because of trauma. With a foreign body that has perforated the tympanic membrane, removal may cause further damage to the tympanic membrane, damage to middle ear ossicles, and loss of hearing.
- The airway is in danger from a nasal foreign body.
- A large foreign body is impaled in the external ear canal.
- The patient is uncooperative and cannot be sedated (see Chapter 2, Pediatric Sedation and Analgesia) or anesthetized (see the section on "Anesthesia for Auditory Canal" and Chapter 5, Local Anesthesia; Chapter 8, Oral and Facial Anesthesia; Chapter 4, Topical Anesthesia).
- For a miniature battery, do not use nose or ear drops.
- For organic or expandable materials, unless the clinician is fairly certain of a successful removal, flushing with saline or water is contraindicated. Flushing can hasten or enhance the swelling.
- Irrigation is contraindicated with an acute or chronic ruptured tympanic membrane.
- For other contraindications to removal from ear, see Chapter 62, Cerumen Impaction Removal.

EQUIPMENT

- Traditional foreign body extraction tools such as a Frazier suction tip; ear curette (Fig. 204.1) or wire loop curette; nasal bayonet (see Fig. 204.1), alligator (Fig. 204.2; see Fig. 204.1), or Hartmann forceps; fine tissue or Adson forceps; right-angle hook (can be made from 21-gauge needle; Fig. 204.3) or ball-tipped right-angle hook.
- Cotton-tipped swabs.
- Nasal or ear speculum (select the largest that will fit the orifice or canal; visibility and room for instrumentation is better with a speculum than with an otoscope).
- Magnification, in the form of either an otoscope with an operating head or a loupe.

- Bright light that can be directed or focused. If a headlamp is available, both hands will be free to perform the procedure.
- Topical anesthetic such as 2% to 5% lidocaine (see the section on "Anesthesia for Auditory Canal" and see Chapter 4, Topical Anesthesia). Benzocaine spray (14%, Cetacaine) can be used for nasal anesthesia; 20% benzocaine solution can be used for the external ear canal.
- For a local field ear block, use a 27-gauge, 1.5-inch needle. An anesthetic such as 1% to 2% lidocaine with epinephrine or 0.25% bupivacaine with epinephrine can be used on the external canal. For subcutaneous injections deeper inside the canal, plain 2% lidocaine may be useful (see also Chapter 5, Local Anesthesia, and Chapter 8, Oral and Facial Anesthesia). Adding a 1:10 mixture of 8.4% sodium bicarbonate to lidocaine helps reduce the pain of injection.
- Nasal decongestant such as phenylephrine (0.25% to 2%; Neo-Synephrine, Vicks), epinephrine (1:50,000; Adrenalin), or oxymetazoline hydrochloride (0.05%; Afrin, Neo-Synephrine 12 hour) spray. An atomizer is helpful if available.
- Irrigant such as saline.
- Irrigation equipment (e.g., surgical Chux, kidney basin) as noted in Chapter 62, Cerumen Impaction Removal.
- Wall or portable suction unit.
- Equipment necessary for the clinician to follow universal blood and body fluid precautions, especially when working near mucous membranes.

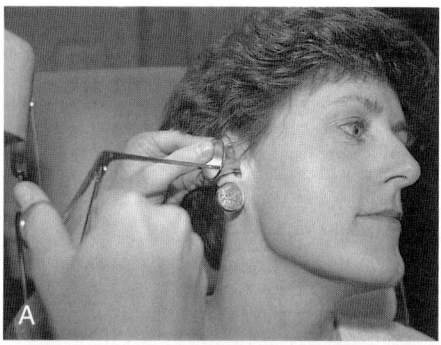
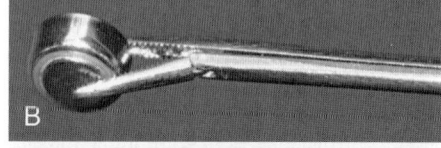
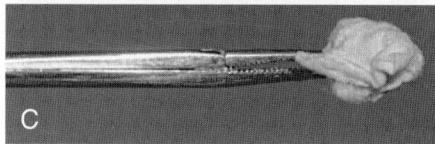

Fig. 204.2 Alligator forceps (A) for retrieving small batteries (B) and paper balls (C) from auditory canal.

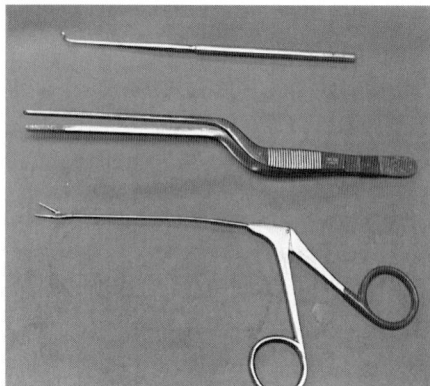

Fig. 204.1 Traditional instruments used for foreign-body extraction: Ear curette (top), nasal (bayonet) forceps (middle), and alligator forceps (bottom).

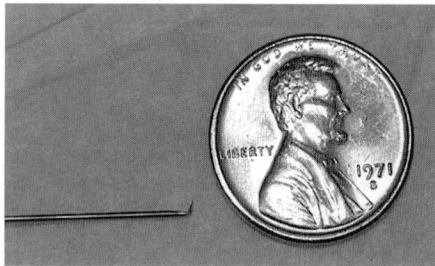

Fig. 204.3 Precise right-angle hook made from bending a 1.5-inch, 21-gauge needle tip at a right angle is an excellent tool for removing smooth objects such as beans and corn kernels.

- Strong magnet and magnetizable nail for retrieving metal foreign bodies.
- Optional: 2- to 6-Fr diameter Fogarty (biliary or cardiovascular), Foley, Swan-Ganz or Schuknecht FB catheter, or Katz otorhinologic foreign body remover (single-use balloon-tipped catheter attached to syringe). The balloons on the Fogarty, Foley, or Swan-Ganz catheters will need to be inflated with a 2-mL syringe.
- Optional: Commercially available, single-use, disposable, Hognose (4-, 5-, or 6-mm) or Gatornose (small or large) otoscope tip.
- Alternate technique, suction: 30-inch plastic intravenous extension tubing or 10-Fr suction catheter, heat source (e.g., burner, alcohol lamp, lighter), blunt end of metal ear curette handle or atomizer tip, and hemostat.
- Alternate technique, glue: Dacron-tipped applicator, thin paintbrush, plastic ear curette, straightened paperclip, toothpick, or the wooden end of cotton-tipped swab and strong acrylic glue (cyanoacrylate; Dermabond or Superglue), with acetone to remove the glue if necessary.

PREPROCEDURE PATIENT PREPARATION

- Stress the importance of remaining still during the procedure.
- For otic body removal, warn the patient that they may hear some loud noises since work will be ongoing in the ear canal
- For nasal or otic foreign body removal, discuss the chance of minor trauma. This may be associated with discomfort during the procedure or some bleeding after the procedure.
- For nasal foreign bodies, the risk of aspiration should be discussed.
- For ear irrigation or instrument removal, discuss the risk of perforation and dizziness.
- Alternatives, risks, and benefits should be explained and informed consent obtained.
- If instrumentation is to be performed, after the topical anesthetic is applied, touch the mucosa with the instrument slightly inside the orifice so that the patient knows what to expect and to avoid being startled.

TECHNIQUE: NASAL FOREIGN BODY

1. Topical anesthesia and vasoconstriction can be applied as a spray or with drops (e.g., a mixture of 2% to 5% lidocaine and 0.25% to 2% phenylephrine hydrochloride or 0.5% oxymetazoline hydrochloride). After waiting a few minutes for the mixture to work, carefully examine the nostril and determine the best instrument or technique. Alternatively, the decongestant can be sprayed first; after waiting a few minutes for the decongestant to work, if the topical anesthetic is then sprayed, it may last longer. The disadvantage of spraying the decongestant and topical anesthetic separately is that the clinician then has to wait a few more minutes for the topical anesthetic to work.
2. The patient may be sitting or lying. Extend the patient's head. Apply pressure on the tip of the nose in a superior and posterior direction to help visualize the nasal canal. Irrigation should not be used in the nasal cavity because it may push the object into the oropharynx or larynx, causing aspiration.
3. Smooth, round objects can be removed using suction or right-angle hooks. For the right-angle hook, slide it past the object with the tip parallel to the nasal sidewall. Once it has passed the object, rotate it 90 degrees so that the tip is behind the object, and then gently pull the object out.
4. Alligator or bayonet forceps may be used to grasp an object that has a small leading edge.
5. A lubricated, small Fogarty, Foley, Swan-Ganz, or Schuknecht FB catheter, or a Katz otorhinologic foreign body catheter can be passed beyond the foreign body. After inflating the balloon or opening the umbrella, gentle traction will either facilitate

removal or stabilize the foreign body to prevent oropharyngeal aspiration. This technique may slightly increase the risk of trauma and epistaxis; it is rare to visualize much of the catheter tip during insertion.
6. In all cases, instruments introduced into the nasal passage require a steady hand resting on the patient's head in case of sudden movements, which can be involuntary if pain is elicited.
7. After removal, examine the orifice closely to make sure that another foreign body was not behind the first and that all debris has been removed. Any particles left behind can lead to irritation, inflammation, drainage, or chronic granulation. Also check the unaffected nasal and ear orifices for any other surprises.

TECHNIQUE: OTIC FOREIGN BODY

1. Many clinicians perform hearing testing (see Chapter 59, Audiometry) to determine the baseline before inserting instruments. Some also perform tonometry (see Chapter 58, Tonometry) to attempt to determine if the tympanic membrane has been perforated.
2. Small children may need to be sedated (see Chapter 2, Pediatric Sedation and Analgesia). If an attempt is to be made without sedation, they may want to sit on the lap of a parent or attendant with the ear facing the clinician. Adults usually want to remain seated with the affected ear facing the clinician. The patient also may be comfortable lying down with the affected ear facing upward.
3. With the ear turned upward, instill a topical anesthetic. After several minutes, use suction to remove pus, topical anesthetics, or blood as necessary to visualize the object. The patient should be warned that suction can be very loud.
4. With adults, visualization of the external ear canal is aided by pulling the auricle upward and backward to straighten the canal. In small children, the auricle is pulled downward. If an instrument is to be used, it should be used only under direct visualization. Insert it slightly inside the auricle, at first, to help the patient accommodate to the noise and sensation of instrumentation. Compared with the internal canal, the external third of the canal has a thicker layer of skin and subcutaneous tissue that covers cartilage; the internal two-thirds has a thinner, more fragile layer of skin covering only bone.
5. The depth and surface qualities of the object usually suggest which tool(s) to use. Grasp fibrous objects (e.g., cotton, plant matter) with the alligator forceps (see Fig. 204.2). Smooth objects (e.g., beans, seeds, popcorn kernels) that are blocking no more than half the diameter of the canal might be dragged out by passing an ear curette or wire loop beyond the object and gently withdrawing it. Larger, smooth, and hard items, such as small batteries and BBs, may be teased out with a fine, 1-mm, right-angle hook (see Fig. 204.3) or a ball-tipped right-angle hook. Slide the right-angle hook past the object with the tip parallel to the canal sidewall. Once it has passed the object, rotate it 90 degrees so that the tip is now behind the object, and gently pull the object out. Objects with sharp projections, such as earrings and screws, may need to be grasped with forceps to avoid laceration of sensitive membranes.
6. Irrigation may move a foreign body far enough away from the eardrum to increase the chance of extraction.
7. Occasionally, iron-containing items, such as a BB, can be removed with a small magnet probe. A probe can be fashioned from a nail that has been blunted and magnetized by drawing it across any strong permanent magnet. Permanent magnets are available in hardware stores or can be found in the rear of stereo speaker cones.
8. Irrigation may be useful in certain instances after object removal, such as when small fragments of debris remain.
9. Insects in the auditory canal should be drowned or smothered by instilling lidocaine or a benzocaine solution or mineral oil. The

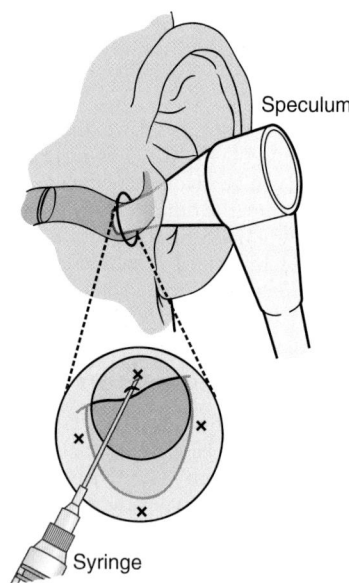

Fig. 204.4 Four-quadrant field block anesthesia of the external auditory canal. Local anesthetic is injected subcutaneously in the four quadrants of the lateral portion of the ear canal. The largest speculum that will fit is used to guide the injections. The speculum is withdrawn slightly, tilted toward each of the four quadrants, and the needle is inserted subcutaneously (*x*). A very small amount of anesthetic (0.25 to 0.5 mL) is injected to produce a slight bulge in the soft tissue. A total of 1.5 to 2 mL of anesthetic is usually sufficient to anesthetize the ear canal and permit painless removal of a foreign body. (From Riviello RJ. Otolaryngologic procedures. In: Roberts JR, Custalow CB, Thomsen TW, eds. *Roberts & Hedges' Clinical Procedures in Emergency Medicine*. 6th ed. Philadelphia: Elsevier; 2014.)

liquid kills the insects, which halts their disturbing and painful movements. An alligator forceps can then be used to grasp and remove the insect. Suction can also be used to remove both the insect and the liquid. Some clinicians suggest that mineral oil immobilizes insects faster; however, mineral oil does not provide anesthesia for the patient, and other clinicians say mineral oil is more likely to cause the insects to break into fragments during attempts to remove them.

10. In all situations, instruments introduced into the auditory canal require a steady hand resting on the patient's head in case of sudden movements, which can be involuntary if pain is elicited.

11. Light, moderate (e.g., intramuscular or intravenous), or general anesthesia may be needed to remove foreign bodies in individuals who cannot tolerate instrumentation with or without local agents. Field block anesthesia of the external auditory canal may be helpful, if tolerated (Fig. 204.4).

12. After removal, make sure that another foreign body is not behind the first and that all debris has been removed. Any particles left behind can lead to irritation, inflammation, drainage, or chronic granulation. Some clinicians repeat hearing tests after removing a foreign body to compare with baseline. Also check the unaffected nasal and ear orifices for any other surprises.

ALTERNATE TECHNIQUE: SUCTION

Suction is especially useful for removing round foreign bodies from the ear or nasal cavity.

1. Cut off the tip of the tubing or suction catheter (Fig. 204.5A). Heat the end of the curette handle or metal atomizer tip (see Fig. 204.5B). Flange the cut tube end with the preheated handle or tip so that it molds to the blunt, rounded metal (see Fig. 204.5C–D). An alternative to this self-made catheter is the commercially available Hognose otoscope tip.

2. Clamp the tubing with a hemostat and attach the opposite end to the suction unit (see Fig. 204.5E). Alternatively, apply low to medium suction to the Hognose suction line.

3. Gently insert the flanged end into the orifice containing the foreign body under direct visualization and advance it to the object.

4. When the flange is in contact with the object, quickly unclamp the suction catheter tubing (see Fig. 204.5F) and apply full suction immediately through the suction cup onto the foreign object. Alternatively, using the Hognose otoscope tip, apply suction when the soft tip is in contact with the object.

5. While suctioning, gently extract the tubing and the suction-attached foreign body (see Fig. 204.5G).

ALTERNATE TECHNIQUE: GLUE

This technique is especially useful for removing smooth, round objects that are difficult to grasp (e.g., plastic beads) from the nasal cavity or ear. It may be more useful in adults because cooperation is required.

1. Place a small drop of acrylic glue (cyanoacrylate such as Dermabond or Superglue) on the blunt end of an applicator (e.g., Dacron-tipped applicator, thin paintbrush, curette, straightened paper clip, toothpick, or the wooden end of a cotton-tipped swab). Allow the glue to become tacky.

2. Quickly, but carefully, touch the glue on the end of the applicator to the foreign body. Establish and maintain contact. Avoid contacting the mucosa en route or pushing the object any farther inward. Hold the applicator still and maintain contact for 30 seconds until the glue hardens.

3. Gently pull the applicator out of the orifice with the foreign body stuck to it.

ANESTHESIA FOR AUDITORY CANAL

For local anesthesia, instill five drops of 2% to 5% lidocaine or 20% benzocaine solution into the canal and allow it to remain for 5 to 10 minutes. Suction to remove fluid and canal debris before injection of a local anesthetic (if needed) under direct visualization. If tympanic membrane rupture is suspected, eardrops and irrigation are contraindicated.

For local field anesthesia of the external half of the auditory canal, inject small amounts (usually <2 mL total) of 1% lidocaine with epinephrine at three or four sites equally spaced along the exterior verge of the canal (see Fig. 204.4). For deeper canal anesthesia (much more sensitive area), subcutaneous injections (0.5 to 1 mL) of plain 2% lidocaine may be considered; however, this is not recommended because the need for multiple injections is usually much more traumatic than the actual foreign body removal. This is especially true for the pediatric population, where, in many instances, it is more appropriate to use sedation. If subcutaneous injections are used, they are placed in the canal just external to the junction of the cartilaginous and bony canal (approximately one-third of the way into the canal). Beginning at the posterior and superior aspect of the canal, use a 27-gauge, 1.5-inch needle to slowly infiltrate lidocaine. Repeat this at two or three spots equally spaced around the canal. Allow the lidocaine to dissect down, "blanching" the ear canal and drum, if visible. Topical lidocaine or benzocaine applied to the auditory canal before an injection is often useful. Wait 5 to 10 minutes before instrumentation.

COMPLICATIONS

- Trauma to mucous membranes (e.g., excoriation, laceration) with the possibility of trauma-related infection or bleeding.
- Injury to a nasal passage, external canal, tympanic membrane, or middle ear.

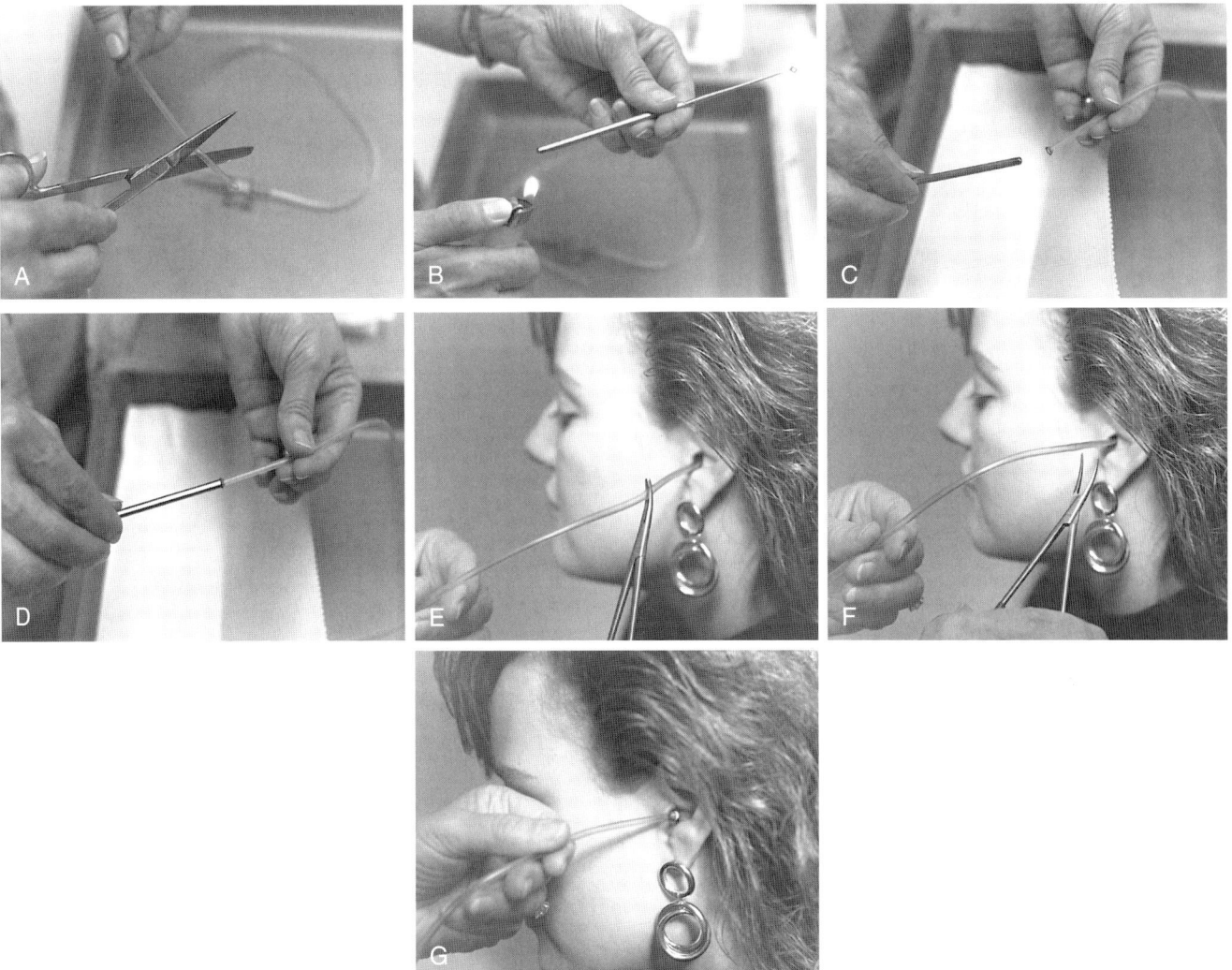

Fig. 204.5 **Technique for removing spherical foreign bodies from the ear. (A) Cut tip off tubing or suction catheter. (B) Heat end of instrument to be used to flare tubing. (C) Press cut end of tubing against heated instrument. (D) With end of tubing softened from heat, use slight pressure against instrument to form a flare on cut end. (E) Clamp tubing with hemostat, attach opposite end to suction. (F) Press flared end of tubing against foreign body. Release the hemostat, apply suction to foreign body. (G) Gently remove the foreign body.**

- Deeper progression of the object leading to the inability to extract in the office.
- Aspiration (nasal passage foreign bodies).
- With delayed or incomplete removal of nasal foreign bodies, the patient may be at risk of obstructive sinusitis and even meningitis from local extension of the sinusitis.
- With foreign bodies of the ear, acute otitis externa is common and may result from injury caused by the foreign body itself or by its removal. Also, when instruments are placed in the ear, the patient may experience bradycardia, or nausea or vomiting (or both).
- Complications of using cyanoacrylate glue include abrading or excoriating the mucosa with the applicator, dripping or spilling the glue on the mucosa, or gluing the applicator to the mucosa. Acetone can be used to remove the glue.

POSTPROCEDURE PATIENT EDUCATION

Inform the patient to watch for signs of infection (see Chapter 62, Cerumen Impaction Removal). The patient should follow up with the clinician in 1 to 2 days. He or she should report a headache, fever, or drainage after removal of a foreign body. These symptoms could indicate sinusitis or meningitis or other serious

infection. After removal of nasal foreign bodies, the patient should use saline irrigation, two to three times a day for 2 or 3 days. Many clinicians prescribe several days of antibiotic otic drops to prevent external otitis after the mucosa has been possibly abraded, excoriated, or lacerated with irrigation or the removal of a foreign body.

PATIENT EDUCATION GUIDES

See the sample patient education and consent forms available at www.expertconsult.com.

CPT/BILLING CODES

30300	Removal foreign body, intranasal; office type procedure
30310	Removal foreign body, intranasal; requiring general anesthesia
69200	Removal foreign body from external auditory canal; without general anesthesia
69205	Removal foreign body from external auditory canal; with general anesthesia

ICD-10-CM Diagnostic Codes

T16.1XXX	T16.9XXX Foreign body in ear, auditory canal or auricle
T17.0XXX	T17.1XXX Foreign body in nose, nasal sinus or nostril

Add appropriate seventh character: A = initial, D = subsequent, S = sequela

Suppliers

(See contact information available at www.expertconsult.com.)

Hognose and Gatornose otoscope attachments/specula
IQDr., Inc.
Katz Extractor Oto-rhino Foreign Body Remover
Inhealth Industries

Acknowledgment

The editors recognize the many contributions of Gary Newkirk, MD, to this chapter in a previous edition of this text.

RECOMMENDED READING

Backlin SA. Positive-pressure technique for nasal foreign body removal in children. *Ann Emerg Med.* 1995;25:554–555.

Douglas AR. Use of nebulized adrenaline to aid expulsion of intra-nasal foreign bodies in children. *J Laryngol Otol.* 1996;110:559–560.

Finkelstein JA. Oral Ambu-bag insufflation to remove unilateral nasal foreign bodies. *Am J Emerg Med.* 1996;14:57–58.

Hanson RM, Stephens M. Cyanoacrylate-assisted foreign body removal from the ear and nose in children. *J Paediatr Child Health.* 1994;30:77–78.

Jensen JH. Technique for removing a spherical foreign body from the nose or ear. *Ear Nose Throat J.* 1976;55:270–271.

Kadish H. Ear and nose foreign bodies: it is all about the tools. *Clin Pediatr (Phila).* 2005;44:665–670.

Kadish HA, Corneli HM. Removal of nasal foreign bodies in the pediatric population. *Am J Emerg Med.* 1997;15:54–56.

Paredes Luck R. Nasal foreign body removal. In: Reichman EF, ed. *Emergency Medicine Procedures.* 2nd ed. New York: McGraw-Hill; 2013:1084–1092.

Riviello RJ. Otolaryngologic procedures. In: Roberts JR, Custalow CB, Thomsen TW, eds. *Roberts & Hedges' Clinical Procedures in Emergency Medicine.* 6th ed. Philadelphia: Elsevier; 2014:1298–1341.

CHAPTER 205

MANAGEMENT OF EPISTAXIS

Scott Savage

Nosebleed is a common complaint with an incidence of approximately 1 per 1000 patients annually in the United States. Ninety percent of nosebleeds resolve either spontaneously or by pinching the outer soft tissue of the nose (Fig. 205.1) or by applying an ice pack to the bridge (Fig. 205.2). Management of the other 10% is the topic of this chapter.

The most common cause of a minor nosebleed is dry nasal mucosa (i.e., low-humidity environment such as in the desert or in a cold climate where heating is used). A moderate nosebleed is usually caused by nasal trauma; a severe nosebleed is often a complication of a cancer or medical condition such as a coagulopathy caused by medications, cancer, or cirrhosis. Although hypertension is often seen in patients with nosebleeds, studies have been unable to confirm this as a cause. Rather, it appears that nosebleeds can cause stress and anxiety, and this stress and anxiety leads to hypertension. Localized causes of nosebleeds also include inflammation from colds and allergies, foreign bodies, nasal septum deformities, chronic use of nasal steroid sprays, and sinonasal neoplasms. Systemic causes include coagulopathies, Osler-Weber-Rendu disease (hereditary hemorrhagic telangiectasia), and use of nonsteroidal antiinflammatory drugs or anticoagulants. Osler-Weber-Rendu disease is an autosomal dominant condition in which the vascular walls lack contractile elements; consequently, prolonged and heavy bleeding can occur despite a normal coagulation profile. The diagnosis can be suspected when there is a family history compatible with the disease.

Nosebleeds can be divided into three groups: anterior, posterior, and mixed. Anterior bleeds account for approximately 90% of epistaxis. Posterior and mixed bleeds can be clinically suspected in patients who have brisk, bilateral, nontraumatic bleeding that does not abate with anterior packing. Posterior bleeding can be life-threatening and is more common in patients older than 40 years. Usually the patient can tell you which side of the nose started bleeding. With posterior bleeding, blood also usually runs down the back of the throat.

Understanding the anatomy of the nasal cavity is important for obtaining control of bleeding. The blood supply for the nasal septum arises from both the internal and external carotid arteries. A primary source for the posteroinferior septum is the sphenopalatine artery, a branch of the internal maxillary artery, which in turn is a branch of the external carotid system. The uppermost part of the nasal septum is supplied by the anterior and posterior ethmoid arteries, which arise indirectly from the internal carotid system. The blood supply for the anterior nasal septum is the superior labial artery, which is also indirectly a branch of the internal carotid system. All these arteries anastomose in the anterior central portion of the nasal septum, an area known as *Kiesselbach plexus* (Fig. 205.3). It is estimated that 95% of anterior nasal bleeds occur there. An occasional source of anterior bleeding is an exposed edge from a perforated nasal septum. Anterior bleeding from the lateral nasal cavity is rare, although telangiectases from Osler–Weber-Rendu disease can be seen here. Trauma can also result in lateral bleeding.

The clinician treating epistaxis must also understand the anatomy of the nose and nasal septum, and its appropriate midline position.

He or she should be able to identify the inferior and middle turbinates. With an understanding of normal anatomy, when a patient has a nosebleed, the examiner should quickly notice any anatomic abnormalities (e.g., deviated nasal septum, a nasal polyp, a mass). Bleeding is not unusual on either side of a deviated nasal septum.

INDICATIONS

- Nosebleed lasting longer than 10 minutes despite pinching outer nasal tissue or application of ice
- Recurrent nosebleeds despite treatment
- Traumatic nosebleed with suspected nasal fracture
- Nosebleed associated with a septal perforation or other nasal abnormality
- Nosebleed in patient with a high-risk medical condition
- Nosebleed in a frail patient

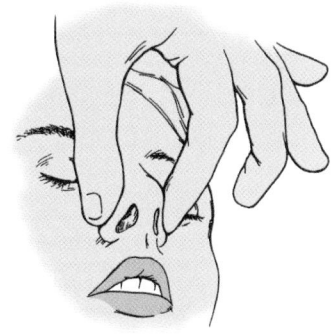

Fig. 205.1   Apply pressure by pinching the nose to stop the bleeding.

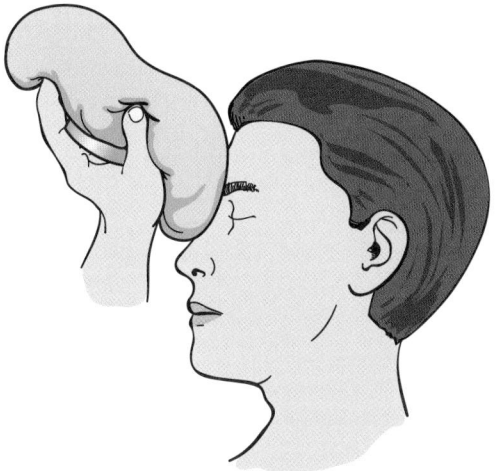

Fig. 205.2   An ice pack can be applied to the bridge of the nose.

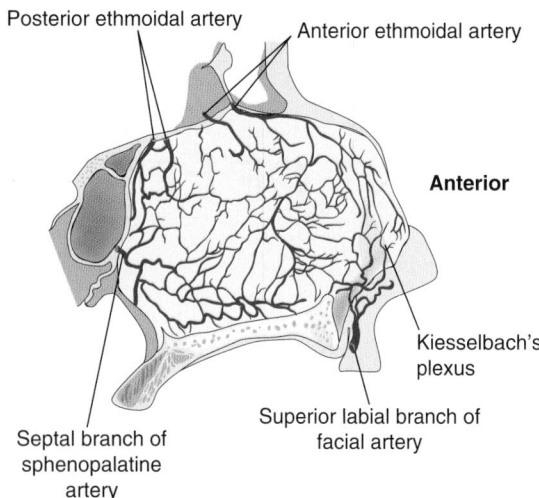

Fig. 205.3   Anatomy of the septal blood supply.

CONTRAINDICATIONS (RELATIVE)

- Patients with advanced chronic obstructive pulmonary disease or other advanced cardiac or pulmonary conditions (nasal packing can induce the nasopulmonary reflex, causing the arterial oxygen pressure to drop by as much as 15 mm Hg).
- Untreated coagulopathy, a displaced fracture, or Osler-Weber-Rendu disease (nasal packing, especially posterior packing, can disrupt friable tissue and should be done with caution in these patients; attempts should be made to normalize clotting factors, if possible, before instrumentation).
- Massive facial trauma with possible basilar skull fracture (balloon or packing may travel into the skull cavity).
- Other critical conditions, such as a threatened airway or other problem that should be managed first, may mandate a delay in managing a nosebleed.

EQUIPMENT

Preparing a "nosebleed tray" in advance is useful.

- Headlight
- Tongue depressor
- Yankauer suction catheter
- Frazier suction catheters, No. 5 and No. 7
- Nasal speculums, short and medium length
- Bayonet or offset forceps (see Chapter 204, Removal of Foreign Bodies from the Ear and Nose, Fig. 204.1)
- Fine Adson forceps
- Emesis (kidney) basin
- Cotton balls
- Cotton-tipped swabs (wooden handle preferred if applying Gelfoam or Surgicel)
- Gelfoam or Surgicel (Surgicel may be better for coagulation but may delay healing, so it is often reserved for when Gelfoam is not effective or available)
- 4 × 4 gauze sponges
- Silver nitrate sticks
- Petroleum impregnated gauze, ½-inch wide, up to 72 inches long
- Nasal sponges/tampons (Fig. 205.4), Rapid Rhino (Fig. 205.5) or Rhino Rocket (Fig. 205.6)
- Nasal balloon devices (Fig. 205.7)
- 12- to 14-Fr Foley (pediatric) catheter with 30-mL balloon, umbilical clamp, and padding
- Red rubber (in and out or Robinson) soft catheter(s)
- Bite block
- 3-inch dental gauze roll

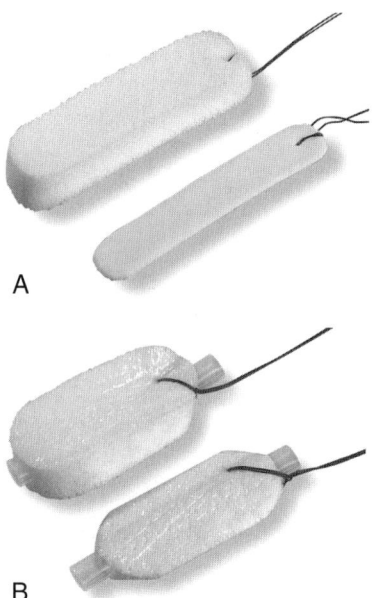

Fig. 205.4   Nasal sponges. (A) Pope pack. (B) Nasal sponge with airway (Merocel 2000 4.5 cm, also Merocel Doyle). (A and B, Courtesy Medtronic Xomed ENT, Inc., Jacksonville, FL.)

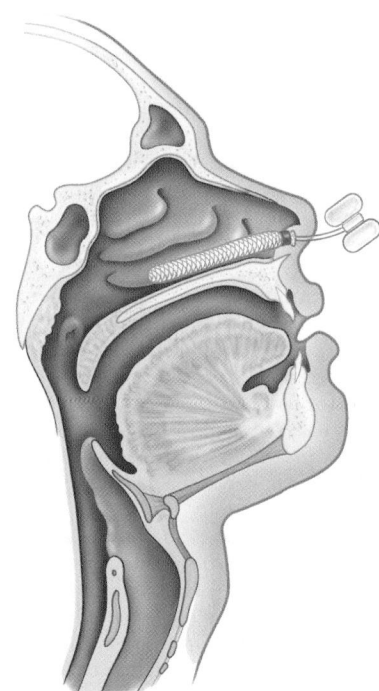

Fig. 205.5   Rapid Rhino nasal system, a hydrocolloid fabric covered balloon. (Copyright 2018 Smith & Nephew.)

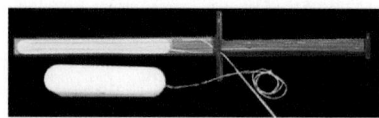

Fig. 205.6   Rhino Rocket nasal sponge system. (Courtesy Shippert Medical Technologies, Centennial, CO.)

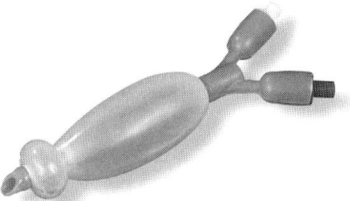

Fig. 205.7 Nasal balloon device. The Medtronic Xomed EpiStat I (pictured) is a double (anterior and posterior) balloon catheter. The EpiStat II is a posterior balloon catheter with anterior soft packing attached. It also contains an airway and can be used for bleeding from an indeterminate site, whether posterior, anterior, or both. If posterior bleeding stops, the balloon catheter and airway can be removed, leaving the anterior packing in place. (Courtesy Medtronic Xomed ENT, Inc., Jacksonville, FL.)

- Umbilical tape or heavy silk (nonabsorbable) sutures, two pieces at least 18 inches long each
- Petroleum jelly (Vaseline) or other lubricant
- Phenylephrine 2% or oxymetazoline 0.05%
- Epinephrine 1:1000
- Local anesthetic such as lidocaine 2% to 5%, benzocaine 14% spray or 20% solution, or tetracaine 2%
- Tuberculin syringe and needle with 2% lidocaine and epinephrine (optional, if bleeding site is easily visible)
- Gowns, gloves, and face shield as necessary for clinician to follow universal blood and body fluid precautions
- Chux or towels
- Antibiotic ointment
- Tranexamic acid (optional, usually as last resort)
- Pulse oximetry (optional, consider for severe epistaxis, medically compromised patients)

PREPROCEDURE PATIENT EDUCATION

Nasal bleeding can be very frightening, so reassurance is important; explain that most bleeding can be easily stopped with minimal discomfort. That said, the patient or guardian should also know about the risks (as listed in the section on "Complications"), benefits, and any options for the procedure as well as the procedure itself. Obtain written informed consent if the patient's condition allows (see consent form available at www.expertconsult.com). Warn the patient that the procedure may be uncomfortable, especially initially, but that everything possible will be done to minimize the discomfort. If the patient is stable, a mild narcotic or sedative may be helpful, especially for posterior packing (see Chapter 1, Procedural Sedation and Analgesia, Chapter 2, Pediatric Sedation).

TECHNIQUE

Patient and Clinician Preparation

1. Obtain vital signs and address any significant vital sign abnormalities. Consider pulse oximetry (vasoactive drugs will be used; packing can provoke the nasopulmonary reflex with subsequent decreases in oxygen saturation).
2. Have the patient sit back on a procedural chair or gurney with the head elevated approximately 45 degrees. Gown and drape the patient appropriately to protect their clothing; the patient also can be given an emesis basin. While getting the patient positioned, ask which side started bleeding first and which side is currently bleeding the most. Have the patient continue to apply ice or pressure while the equipment is being assembled.
3. Connect the suction tubing and catheters to wall suction. Don the headlamp. Good lighting is critical to the procedure. Universal blood and body fluid precautions should be observed while performing this procedure.

4. Inspect the oropharynx for trauma, or any other abnormality. Plan to inspect the nasal cavity that is not actively bleeding first. If both are bleeding, and the patient cannot state which side started bleeding first, inspect the nostril on the same side as the patient's dominant hand. Many nosebleeds are caused by nose-picking, and people are less clumsy with their dominant hands. This side will generally be easier to examine.
5. Have the patient blow his or her nose gently to remove any loose clots that may obstruct the examination. While this may increase the bleeding slightly at first, it is necessary to identify the bleeding source. Insert the short nasal speculum and open it vertically. Suction any blood or clots and inspect the nasal cavity, specifically looking at the floor, vestibule, turbinates, and septum. Forceps may be helpful for manual removal of large clots.
   NOTE: If you are able to get behind the source of the bleeding with the suction tip, the condition can be managed in the office. If the source of bleeding can be seen, submucosal injection of a small amount of 2% lidocaine with epinephrine using a tuberculin syringe may help decrease or stop the bleeding.
6. Vasoconstrict and anesthetize the nasal mucosa using appropriate agents. If using separate agents for these purposes, apply the anesthetic first unless bleeding is so rapid that the anesthetic is likely to be washed out before being effective. Having the patient sniff an aerosolized solution is the easiest way. If time allows, best results are obtained if the anesthetic has been in place for at least 15 minutes. After or while the anesthetic solution is being applied, also apply the vasoconstrictive solution.
7. Alternatively, pledgets soaked with an agent can be applied. Monitor the patient's vital signs when using vasoconstrictive agents.

NOTE: The offset forceps can be used to make a pledget. First, flatten and grasp with the forceps most of the length of an appropriate amount of cotton pulled from a cotton ball. Next, grasp the opposite end of the cotton with the other hand, and while holding this end, twirl the forceps to twist the cotton in and around the long blades. Finally, relax the forceps and slip the pledget off the end. It is now ready to be soaked and inserted.

Absorbable Dressings

Although several types of absorbable dressings are available, the two most commonly used are still Gelfoam and Surgicel. These dressings form a scaffold for the formation of a blood clot. Although Surgicel may be better for stimulating coagulation, it is more expensive and may delay healing; therefore, Gelfoam is usually preferred. Surgicel is often reserved for when Gelfoam is not effective or available. These dressings may be used as a primary technique for discrete bleeding, as a bandage over a previously cauterized site, or as a mucosal sheet over an area of diffuse bleeding (e.g., coagulopathy) before packing is applied. If these are in place before packing is removed, it may prevent the clot from being dislodged.

1. When applying these dressings, it is helpful to use forceps and a cotton-tipped swab stick with a wooden handle to manipulate the dressing, to press it onto the bleeding site, and especially to hold it down when releasing the forceps so the dressing does not dislodge.
2. Before using the swab stick, remove about half of the cotton to make it small enough to be useful, and moisten the tip with saline or tap water to prevent the dressing from sticking to it.

Cauterization

Cauterization is suitable for discrete areas of bleeding in the anterior nares. The preferred method is to use silver nitrate sticks, which are especially useful in children. Do not perform cautery at the same location on both sides of the septum because it may interrupt the entire blood supply to the septum, resulting in permanent damage or necrosis. Electrocautery should be done only by an experienced operator because damage to the septal cartilage may occur.

1. Suction the nares and keep a small Frazier suction catheter ready to suction excessive blood. Attempt to dry the surrounding mucosa with a dry cotton swab; silver nitrate needs to be applied to a dry area to be effective. Drying the area will also minimize spread of silver nitrate beyond the area. As mentioned earlier, a submucosal injection of a small amount of 2% lidocaine with epinephrine using a tuberculin syringe near, surrounding or under the area of bleeding may help blanch and keep the area dry.

2. Apply the silver nitrate stick with gentle pressure for 3 to 10 seconds. Do not use the stick for more than 10 seconds in any area, or septal cartilage may be damaged. Do not cauterize an area greater than 1 cm in diameter, which is equivalent to about four dabs of the stick if only the bulb portion is used. As mentioned previously, do not cauterize both sides of the septum at the same location. Silver nitrate causes a burning sensation, so the patient will appreciate having the anesthetic in place for at least 15 minutes. Most patients sneeze after the application of silver nitrate. Some authors apply the silver nitrate peripherally (approximately 0.5 cm from site) and in a circular motion around the offending area or vessel. They then gradually move toward the center of the site until the bleeding stops. Electrocautery should be applied in the same manner. Some clinicians apply electrocautery directly down the Frazier suction tip by touching it with the cautery unit.

3. After hemostasis is obtained, use Gelfoam, Surgicel, or an equivalent specialized dressing to protect the cauterization site. If these are not available, use a small amount of antibiotic ointment or petroleum jelly and gently place it on the cautery site. One study (Loughran et al., 2004) found antibiotic ointment to be superior to petroleum jelly for preventing recurrence.

4. Antibiotic therapy is considered optional in these cases. If cauterization fails or bleeding recurs within 72 hours, consider the use of packing or a balloon device.

Expandable Nasal Sponge and Tampon Packing

This technique is generally easy and effective in mild to moderate anterior bleeding. The sponges/tampons come in a variety of sizes and shapes, and the 4- to 6-cm sizes are usually ideal (see Fig. 205.4). They are initially rigid but soften when saline or tap water is applied or blood is absorbed.

1. Prepare the sponge/tampon by opening the package and removing the string (the string is not necessary and is usually irritating to the patient). If necessary, trim the sponge to a size and shape that appears consistent with the patient's nasal opening, usually about 4 to 6 cm in length. An exact fit is not required, but using a wide, 10-cm-long sponge in a small patient is uncomfortable, unnecessary, and more difficult to remove. Likewise, if only a small sponge is available, and the patient has a large nasal opening, then consider using two sponges side by side. When cutting the sponge, make sure to avoid leaving any corners or other sharp edges.

2. Coat all but the distal tip of the sponge in petroleum jelly to avoid premature softening of the sponge. The use of an antibiotic ointment may decrease the risk of epistaxis recurrence (Loughran et al., 2004). The Rapid Rhino (see Fig. 205.5) is an air-inflatable balloon coated with a hydrocolloid fabric, which eases insertion and removal. If using the Rhino Rocket (see Fig. 205.6), remove the sponge from the syringe-like device before inserting it. The syringe can generate enough force to damage the nasal mucosa, septum, or other structures. It should be soaked in sterile water first, for 30 seconds; saline should not be used because it can affect its gelling properties.

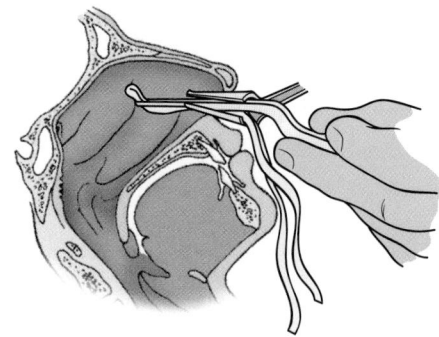

Fig. 205.8 Insert anterior pack with the folded end inserted first.

EDITOR'S NOTE: One study (Singer et al., 2005) comparing Rapid Rhino with Rhino Rocket found equal efficacy in stopping nosebleeds but better patient comfort and ease of removal with Rapid Rhino. Another study (Moumoulidis et al., 2006) found less discomfort with insertion and removal of Rapid Rhino than with Merocel.

3. Insert the sponge in a smooth motion, entering in a near vertical direction, and then rotating it to a horizontal direction. Continue passing the sponge along the inferior nasal floor until it is completely inside the nasal passage. When in place, the trailing tip of the sponge should be visible inside the nostril but not protruding from it.

4. Slowly drip about 2 mL of saline or tap water onto the tip to help the sponge expand more quickly (use only sterile water for the Rhino Rocket).

5. Closely monitor the patient for 3 to 5 minutes for complications and to see if the technique was adequate to abate the bleeding. Keep the patient in observation status for approximately 30 minutes after completing the packing.

6. If successful, packing should be left in place for 48 hours. The routine use of antibiotics with the treatment of anterior bleeding is controversial, so the decision regarding prescribing antibiotics should be individualized to the patient. Persistent bleeding may be due to a bowed septum; inserting the same size sponge on the contralateral side may halt bleeding. If bleeding persists, choices include removing the sponge to insert a larger sponge or two smaller sponges, or proceeding to anterior packing or insertion of a nasal balloon (see Fig. 205.7).

Anterior Packing

Packing is a time-consuming process but is a viable alternative where there is diffuse bleeding but a nasal sponge/tampon is either unavailable or insufficient. One study (Corbridge et al., 1995) found no difference between efficacy, patient tolerance, and complications when comparing traditional anterior nasal packing with commercial products.

1. Because of the increased time it takes for this technique, it is generally advisable to give the patient a narcotic or sedative medication, or both (see Chapter 1, Procedural Sedation and Analgesia, Chapter 2, Pediatric Sedation), unless a contraindication exists. If using a combination analgesic, take caution to use one that does not increase bleeding.

2. Fold a ½- by 72-inch piece of petrolatum gauze in half. Using bayonet forceps, place the center-folded end (not the free end) into the nostril (Fig. 205.8). Make sure the gauze is placed back all the way to the posterior soft tissue.

3. Pat down the gauze, and continue to layer it in an accordion fashion, patting down each layer. Gauze should be layered from nasal floor to turbinates (Fig. 205.9). Approximately 4 to 5 feet of gauze will be required.

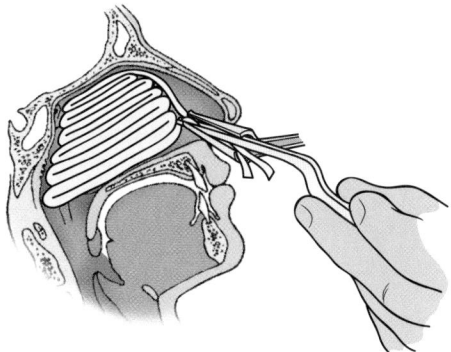

Fig. 205.9 Pack folded gauze in layers, from nasal floor to turbinates.

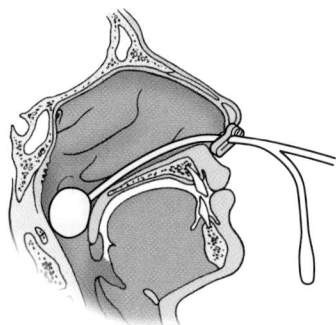

Fig. 205.10 Foley catheter as posterior pack.

4. Leave at least an inch of gauze protruding from the nostril. This should be taped to the patient's cheek to avoid inadvertent removal.
5. If successful, leave the packing in place for 48 hours. Again, the routine use of antibiotics with anterior packing is controversial. If this incompletely stops the bleeding, then packing the contralateral nostril in a similar fashion may buttress the original dressing by preventing bowing of the septum. If bleeding persists, choices include removing the packing to insert an anterior nasal balloon, a posterior balloon, or posterior packing.

Balloon Tamponade

These devices are fast and easy to place. They come in several sizes, shapes, and configurations (e.g., single-balloon, dual-balloon). The most versatile device is the dual-balloon (see Fig. 205.7); it can be used for both anterior and posterior bleeding. Although nasal balloon devices are more expensive than sponges or gauze, they often save the clinician time. Regardless of mechanism, one benefit of placing a posterior pack is that it puts pressure on the sphenopalatine artery.

1. Place the balloon in a basin of water, inflate it with air according to manufacturer specifications, and observe for air leaks. Then deflate the balloon and coat the tip of the device with petroleum jelly or other lubricant.
2. Insert the catheter with the longer portion of the bevel toward the nasal septum to prevent damage to the turbinates or mucosa.
3. Inflate the anterior balloon with air according to manufacturer specifications. Do not use saline or tap water. (If the balloon were fluid-filled and it leaked, the patient might aspirate the contents.) If the patient complains of pain at a pressure lower than manufacturer specifications, the balloon may be larger than the nasal cavity. Deflate the balloon until the pain subsides. Do not inflate the posterior balloon at this time unless the patient has such significant bleeding that there is a risk of aspiration or exsanguination.
4. Observe the patient for further bleeding. The routine use of antibiotics is controversial. These devices are uncomfortable, so analgesics and even sedative medications are generally indicated. If bleeding persists, it is likely due to an area high in the nasal cavity, where the balloon does not reach. One solution is to deflate the balloon, leave it in place, and use anterior petroleum gauze packing on top of it. The balloon can then be reinflated to seal the packing in the upper portion of the anterior nasal cavity. Persistent bleeding may also be due to a bowed septum; packing the contralateral side may halt bleeding by correcting the bowing. If these maneuvers fail to relieve the bleeding, then it is likely the patient has a posterior bleed. At this time, inflate the posterior balloon.
5. It is important to document the procedure, notify the follow-up clinician if there is additional packing, and tell the patient that

this second packing is present so that it is not left behind when the balloon is removed.

Foley Catheter

If posterior bleeding is suspected, this technique may be used. It also may be used to provide a posterior buttress for anterior packing. Use a catheter with a 30-mL balloon.

1. Prepare the catheter by cutting off the portion of the catheter that is distal to the balloon. Test the balloon by inflating with air and checking for leaks. Deflate the balloon and lubricate the distal catheter with petroleum jelly or equivalent.
2. If present, remove the anterior packing.
3. Have the patient open his or her mouth widely. Pass the catheter along the floor of the nasal cavity until a small portion of the balloon is visible in the mouth. Inflate the balloon with 7 to 10 mL of air.
4. Retract the balloon until it gently lodges against the soft tissue of the choanal arch. If it withdraws into the nasal cavity, advance it back into the nasopharynx and add an additional 3 to 5 mL of air. Keep adding air in 3- to 5-mL aliquots until the balloon lodges upon withdrawal. The balloon is overinflated if the soft palate bulges or the patient complains of pain.
5. While an assistant maintains gentle traction on the catheter, place or replace anterior packing with a sponge or gauze as clinically indicated. Place an umbilical clamp on the catheter just outside the nares to secure the device (Fig. 205.10). Pad the umbilical clamp to prevent pressure necrosis.
6. Secure the proximal portion of the catheter by taping it to the side of the face. Do not tape it to the neck; if the patient were to turn his or her head, the device might be dislodged. Avoid cutting the proximal catheter; this may cause the balloon to deflate.
7. This procedure can be repeated on the opposite side if necessary. Use analgesics as indicated. The routine use of antibiotics is controversial.

Posterior Packing

Although posterior packing is described in many textbooks, in practice it is a technically difficult procedure and is very time consuming. I believe it is best left to the otolaryngologist. A simpler technique is to use either a commercially available dual-balloon tamponade device or, failing that, the Foley catheter technique previously described. Balloon tamponade devices are available with channels for the patient to breathe through, making them a more acceptable alternative. A long, expandable sponge also may be attempted, but these have limited success. Posterior packing is included in this chapter for the sake of completeness, or for when the otolaryngologist is not available.

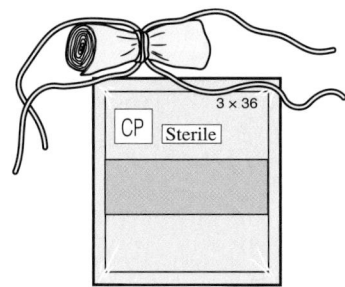

Fig. 205.11 Prepare posterior pack.

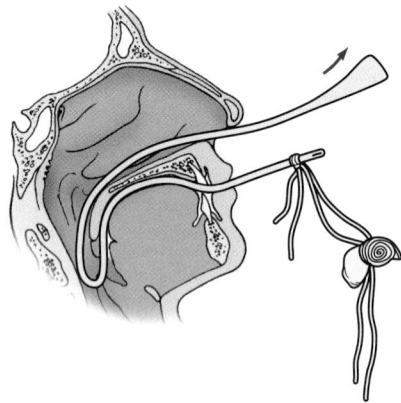

Fig. 205.12 Tie or suture posterior pack to catheter.

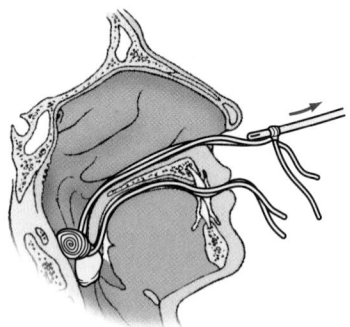

Fig. 205.13 Pull pack into position.

1. A posterior pack can be made from a 3 × 36-inch piece of petrolatum gauze rolled into a tight, cylindrical, 3-inch long pack. Two 18-inch pieces of umbilical tape (or heavy nonabsorbable suture) should be tied around the middle of the pack (Fig. 205.11).
2. Before inserting the pack, spray the posterior pharynx with anesthetic (e.g., benzocaine spray).
3. Next, insert a soft red rubber catheter through the bleeding nostril. Visualize the catheter tip through the patient's open mouth as it passes behind the palate. Pull the tip from the pharynx and out of the patient's mouth with forceps. Tie both ends of umbilical tape around the catheter (Fig. 205.12). Pull the catheter back through the nose and snug the roll of gauze against the posterior aspect of the choanal arch (Fig. 205.13). While using something to protect yourself from being bitten (e.g., a bite block), guide the pack into this location after pushing it around the soft palate with your finger. Leave the second piece of umbilical tape hanging from the mouth for pack removal in the future.

NOTE: Some clinicians use two soft red rubber catheters to perform posterior packing, inserting one through each nostril and then tying the umbilical tape from each side of the posterior pack to the respective red rubber catheter.

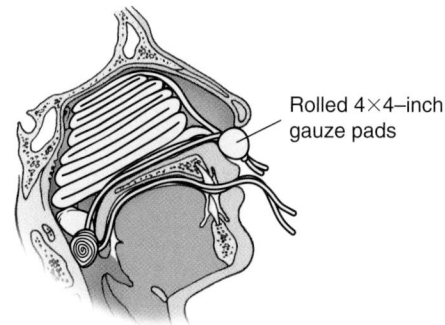

Rolled 4×4–inch gauze pads

Fig. 205.14 Securing posterior pack after placing anterior pack.

4. Secure the posterior pack by tying the piece of umbilical tape that is in the patient's nose around rolled 4 × 4 gauze pads. These rolls should be fitted flush, but not too firmly, against the nares (Fig. 205.14).
5. If bleeding slows but does not subside, it will be necessary to also place an anterior nasal sponge/tampon or gauze packing.

NOTE: Nasal packing fails to stop epistaxis in up to 25% of cases. If bleeding does not subside with these techniques, otolaryngology consult is indicated; if available, tranexamic acid can be considered (see below). Sinus endoscopes can be used to locate the site of bleeding and to cauterize it. Septoplasty or ligation of the anterior or posterior ethmoid, internal maxillary, sphenopalatine, or external carotid artery may be necessary. Arterial embolization is another option.

Tranexamic Acid

In the United States, tranexamic acid is approved by the US Food and Drug Administration for short-term use in hemophiliacs to prevent hemorrhage and to decrease the need for factor replacement following dental extraction and for heavy menstrual bleeding. Two studies (Zahed et al., 2013; Utkewicz et al., 2015) have found benefit from topical application of injectable tranexamic acid to the nares for epistaxis. One used soaked cotton pledgets, the other used a compounded topical gel.

Removing Packing

Posterior packing should be removed by a specialist. Anterior packing may be removed in the medical office if the patient is medically stable and healthy, does not take anticoagulant medications or have an uncontrolled coagulopathy, and has not had significant complications of therapy. Have an epistaxis tray in the room in case the nosebleed recurs. Having good lighting is critical to the procedure.

1. Soften and rehydrate the dressing with saline, taking care not to use so much as to cause the patient to aspirate. Usually, 3 to 5 mL of saline is sufficient. Give the fluid a few minutes to diffuse through the material. To remove the Rapid Rhino, first deflate the balloon.
2. Follow universal precautions and protect the patient, furniture, and flooring from potential blood spills. Have the patient sit up and lean forward, bracing himself or herself with arms grasping a supporting surface—the mattress of the examination table, or the arm of the chair. Instruct the patient to mouth breathe, to remain still, to not blow his or her nose or snort.
3. With a basin in one hand, and bayonet forceps in the other, gently and smoothly remove the packing.
4. Inspect the nasal mucosa for residual bleeding and retained packing. If present, treat appropriately. Often there will be some mild drainage that is nasal mucus mixed with old blood. This drainage rapidly subsides and does not require further treatment.

COMPLICATIONS

- Hypoxia, causing cardiac or respiratory distress
- Hypercapnia
- Posterior migration, local abrasions, premature dislodgment (anterior packing)
- Cardiac dysrhythmias, myocardial infarction, death (posterior packing)
- Pressure necrosis of soft tissue
- Sinusitis
- Nasal septal perforation
- Rebleeding
- Otitis media
- Toxic shock syndrome
- Aspiration
- Bacteremia
- Allergic reaction to materials or anesthetics

POSTPROCEDURE CARE

Acetaminophen or narcotics can be used for pain; the use of aspirin and other nonsteroidal antiinflammatories should be minimized for the next 4 days because they may encourage bleeding. Patients should be cautioned against nose picking, straining, and bending over. Children's nails should be trimmed short to avoid trauma (parents may want them to wear mittens or socks over their hands at night to protect the nose during sleep). If patients feel that sneezing is imminent, instruct them to keep their mouth open. Patients treated with cautery alone should keep the nasal mucosa moist with antibiotic ointment, petroleum jelly, or A&D ointment three times daily for a week. The routine use of antibiotics in patients with packing is controversial and should be individualized to the patient. It may be reasonable to prescribe antibiotics to patients at greater risk of infection such as those with diabetes, immunosuppression, or advanced age. If an antibiotic is prescribed, amoxicillin-clavulanate is a reasonable choice. All patients should be instructed to notify health care providers if there is increasing pain, if rebleeding is not controlled with 15 minutes of nose pinching/ice application, or if fever occurs. Patients should also receive instructions on how to keep the packing moist with a humidifier at home and frequent applications of nasal saline drops. Patients with anterior packing should have the packing removed by an experienced health care provider in 48 to 72 hours. If the patient is medically frail, had significant bleeding, or if posterior packing was performed, hospital admission may be indicated. Patients needing posterior packing or insertion of a Foley catheter or posterior balloon device generally require admission to an intensive care unit and specialist consultation. Nearly 40% of these patients will eventually require intubation.

PATIENT EDUCATION GUIDES

See the sample patient education and consent forms available at www.expertconsult.com.

CPT/BILLING CODES

30901	Control nasal hemorrhage, anterior, simple (limited cautery and/or packing), any method
30901-50	(use modifier "-50" for bilateral)
30903	Control nasal hemorrhage, anterior, complex (extensive cautery and/or packing), any method
30903-50	Bilateral
30905	Control nasal hemorrhage, posterior, with posterior nasal packs and/or cautery, any method, initial
30906	Subsequent

ICD-10-CM DIAGNOSTIC CODES

J34.89	Other diseases of nasal cavity and sinuses (necrosis of nose [septum], ulcer of nose [septum], nasal septal perforation [nontraumatic])
R04.0	Epistaxis (acute)

Acknowledgment

The editors recognize the contributions of Nancy Schantz, MD, Robert Beck, MD, and Jerry Hizon, MD, to this chapter in previous editions of this text.

SUPPLIERS

(See contact information available at www.expertconsult.com.)

Boston Medical Products
  Epistaxis catheters
Rhino Rocket and Epistax Balloon
  Shippert Medical Technologies
Rapid Rhino
  Smith & Nephew Arthrocare
Xomed EpiStat and Merocel
  Medtronic Xomed Surgical Products, Inc.

RECOMMENDED READING

Buttaravoli P, Leffler SM. *Minor Emergencies*. 3rd ed. Philadelphia: Elsevier; 2012.

Corbridge RJ, Djazaeri B, Hellier WPL, et al. A prospective randomized controlled trial comparing the use of Merocel nasal tampons and BIPP in the control of acute epistaxis. *Clin Otolaryngol*. 1995;20:305–307.

Kelanic SM, Caldarelli DD, Reichman EF. Epistaxis management. In: Reichman EF, ed. *Emergency Medicine Procedures*. 2nd ed. New York: McGraw-Hill; 2013.

Loughran S, Spinou E, Clement WA, et al. A prospective, single-blind, randomized controlled trial of petroleum jelly/Vaseline for recurrent paediatric epistaxis. *Clin Otolaryngol*. 2004;29:266–269.

Marx JA, Hockberger RS, eds. *Rosen's Emergency Medicine: Concepts and Clinical Practice*. 8th ed. Philadelphia: Elsevier; 2014.

Moumoulidis I, Draper M, Patel H, Piyush J, Price T. A prospective randomized controlled trial comparing Merocel and Rapid Rhino nasal tampons in the treatment of epistaxis. *Eur Arch Otorhinolaryngol*. 2006;263:719–722.

Riviello RJ. Otolaryngologic procedures. In: Roberts JR, Custalow CB, Thomsen TW, eds. *Roberts & Hedges' Clinical Procedures in Emergency Medicine*. 7th ed. Philadelphia: Elsevier; 2019.

Singer AJ, Blanda M, Cronin K, et al. Comparison of nasal tampons for the treatment of epistaxis in the emergency department: a randomized controlled trial. *Ann Emerg Med*. 2005;45:134–139.

Tintinalli JE, Stapczynski JS, Ma OJ, eds. *Tintinalli's Emergency Medicine: a Comprehensive Study Guide*. 8th ed. New York: McGraw-Hill; 2015.

Utkewicz MD, Brunetti L, Awad NI. Epistaxis complicated by rivaroxaban managed with topical tranexamic acid. *Am J Emerg Med*. 2015;33:1329. e5–1329.e7.

Wurman LH, Sack JG, Flannery JV, Lipsman RA. The management of epistaxis. *Am J Otolaryngol*. 1992;13:193–209.

Zahed R, Moharamzadeh P, AlizadeArasi S, et al. A new and rapid method for epistaxis treatment using injectable form or tranexamic acid topically: a randomized controlled trial. *Am J Emerg Med*. 2013;31:1389–1392.

CHAPTER 206

PERITONSILLAR ABSCESS DRAINAGE

Roger K. Waage

Peritonsillar abscess, also known as quinsy, is an infection in the space between the palatine tonsil and the pharyngeal constrictors; it is the most common deep infection or abscess of the head and neck. Approximately 45,000 cases occur annually in the United States, usually in patients in their second or third decade of life; it rarely occurs in immunocompetent children younger than 6 years. The patient usually has symptoms for about 4 days; these can include fever, malaise, severe sore throat, trismus, odynophagia, and dysphagia with drooling. he or she may be dehydrated from a lack of oral intake. Pain is often referred to the ear, and the patient's voice may have a muffled resonance known as a "hot potato" voice. Signs of peritonsillar abscess include nonexudative pharyngitis in the majority of cases, marked edema of the soft palate, and a fluctuant fullness of the tonsil, which is covered superiorly by a shiny membrane. There is often inferior and medial displacement of the affected tonsil. The classic sign is deflection of the swollen uvula to the opposite side (Fig. 206.1). Bilateral peritonsillar abscesses are rare. Tender cervical adenopathy is usually present.

The local anatomy must be understood before attempting to aspirate or drain a peritonsillar abscess. The palatine tonsils lie between the palatoglossal and palatopharyngeal arches. These two pillars form the anterior and posterior borders of the tonsil. The surface of each tonsil has a covering of mucosa with an irregular number of indentations known as *tonsillar crypts*. Beneath the mucosa, each tonsil is surrounded by a fibrous capsule. A peritonsillar abscess is a collection of pus between the fibrous capsule of the tonsil and the superior constrictor muscle of the pharynx, which forms a lateral wall near the tonsil. Progression of pus formation and lateral extension of cellulitis irritate the surrounding musculature, particularly the internal pterygoids, resulting in spasm and trismus. It is also important to note for this procedure that the internal carotid artery lies approximately 2.5 cm posterolateral to the tonsil, whereas the facial artery lies lateral to the tonsil.

Historically it was thought that a peritonsillar abscess developed as the progression of an acute exudative tonsillitis. Currently a peritonsillar abscess is thought to originate in the Weber salivary glands, which are found in a space just above the tonsil known as the *supratonsillar fossa*. These salivary glands are a group of about 20 mucous salivary glands that assist with the digestion of food particles trapped in the tonsillar crypts. They are connected to the palatine tonsil by a duct that extends to the surface of the tonsil. Supporting the theory that the Weber glands are involved in the pathogenesis of peritonsillar abscess are the facts that a peritonsillar abscess can occur after tonsillectomy, even while the patient is on appropriate antibiotics and that the majority of abscesses are found in the superior pole of the palatine tonsil. Only 20% of abscesses are found in the midtonsil, and only 10% occupy the lower pole.

A peritonsillar abscess is usually polymicrobial. The most common aerobic organisms are *Streptococcus pyogenes* (group A β-hemolytic *Streptococcus*) and *Staphylococcus aureus*. The most common anaerobes are *Bacteroides* and *Fusobacterium*; other anaerobes include *Peptostreptococcus* and *Prevotella*. Throat cultures are of

no benefit, and cultures from the aspirate have rarely been found to be helpful for the selection of antibiotics.

The differential diagnosis of peritonsillar abscess includes unilateral tonsillitis, peritonsillar cellulitis, intratonsillar abscess, neoplasm, retropharyngeal abscess, leukemia, herpes simplex tonsillitis, infectious mononucleosis, foreign body aspiration, aneurysm of the internal carotid artery, and retromolar abscess. The most common entity that is confused with peritonsillar abscess is peritonsillar cellulitis. This condition has the same symptoms and perhaps similar physical findings, but because there is no pus between the tonsil and the lateral muscles, there is no fluctuance in the peritonsillar area.

If visualization is inadequate, placing a gloved index finger into the mouth to feel for hardness versus fluctuance in the peritonsillar region may be helpful.

Intraoral ultrasound and ultrasound-directed aspiration of peritonsillar abscess has been described in the emergency medicine literature since 2003. It is very helpful for distinguishing between cellulitis and abscess noninvasively; however, the examination may also be limited by trismus. Intraoral ultrasound is probably most useful for locating the abscess when aspiration or incision and drainage is unsuccessful. Transcutaneous ultrasound can also be performed by placing the transducer over the submandibular gland and scanning the tonsillar area. But there is a loss in the resolution of the image because of the distance from the transducer, so this is rarely used. Computed tomography (CT) is occasionally helpful. The CT should be done with contrast and may be helpful for ruling out an extension of the abscess.

The initial treatment of all patients with peritonsillar abscess should include adequate pain relief, hydration, and antibiotics. Antibiotics should cover group A streptococcus, *S. aureus*, and respiratory anaerobes. β-Lactamase–producing organisms are increasingly prevalent. Reasonable empiric regimens include amoxicillin-clavulanate or clindamycin. Consideration should be given to covering for methicillin-resistant *S. aureus* (MRSA) based on the severity of the patient's illness, the prevalence of MRSA in the community, and whether the patient is likely to be colonized with MRSA. If MRSA coverage is desired, clindamycin or linezolid are reasonable choices. The evidence regarding the use of glucocorticoids in the treatment of peritonsillar abscess is inconsistent; additional studies are needed before the use of glucocorticoids should be recommended.

Historically the surgical treatment of peritonsillar abscess has been either abscess tonsillectomy or incision and drainage. If untreated, the abscess can rupture, possibly resulting in laryngeal aspiration, pneumonia, sepsis, or death. An untreated abscess can also spread locally or hematogenously, causing extensive local infection or even meningitis. Patients with a peritonsillar abscess and a history of three episodes of tonsillitis in the past year should probably be sent for an abscess tonsillectomy. However, for those without recurrent tonsillitis, there is growing evidence that needle aspiration is the treatment of choice. It has been shown to have an 85% to 100% success rate. Of those patients who respond initially, only 4% to 10% will have a recurrence. A second needle aspiration also has a high success rate. Patients who fail a second or third needle aspiration should probably have an abscess tonsillectomy. (Even those patients who respond to a third aspiration should probably have a tonsillectomy, especially if this is the third infection in a year; see Chapter 66, Tonsillectomy and Adenoidectomy). The small percentage of patients whose abscess fails to resolve with a needle aspiration should probably have an incision and drainage procedure or be referred to an otolaryngologist to rule out a possible abscess of the pterygomaxillary space. An algorithm for the management of peritonsillar abscess is shown in Fig. 206.2. Considering that the incision and drainage technique is now typically reserved for more difficult cases, it is not

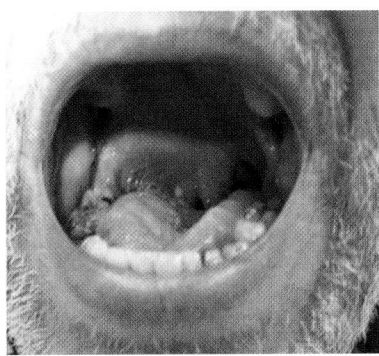

Fig. 206.1 Peritonsillar abscess on patient's right side. Note fluctuance, lack of exudate on tonsil, soft palate edema, and deviation of uvula to the opposite side.

surprising that the recurrence rate is slightly higher than in the past, ranging from 6% to 24%. However, overall, the recurrence rate of incision and drainage is slightly less than that of needle aspiration.

Needle aspiration does have some drawbacks. It is painful, invasive, and—unless ultrasound-directed—is performed somewhat blindly. A series of 12 patients evaluated by Haeggstrom and associates demonstrated that abscesses were located within 4 to 25 mm from the carotid artery. In addition, needle aspiration samples only one area in the tonsillar fossa and may require repeated attempts. From 12% to 24% of abscesses are missed on the first aspiration attempt. However, it is relatively simple to perform (even by those with little experience and who are not ear, nose, and throat specialists), and it does not require expensive or specialized equipment. Successful aspiration or incision and drainage may also help the patient avoid a hospitalization.

INDICATIONS

Peritonsillar abscess in a patient who is not indicated for abscess tonsillectomy

CONTRAINDICATIONS (ABSOLUTE AND RELATIVE)

- Septic shock or impending respiratory compromise (patient should first be stabilized)
- Uncooperative patient or one that is unable to sit upright
- Operator unfamiliar with the anatomy

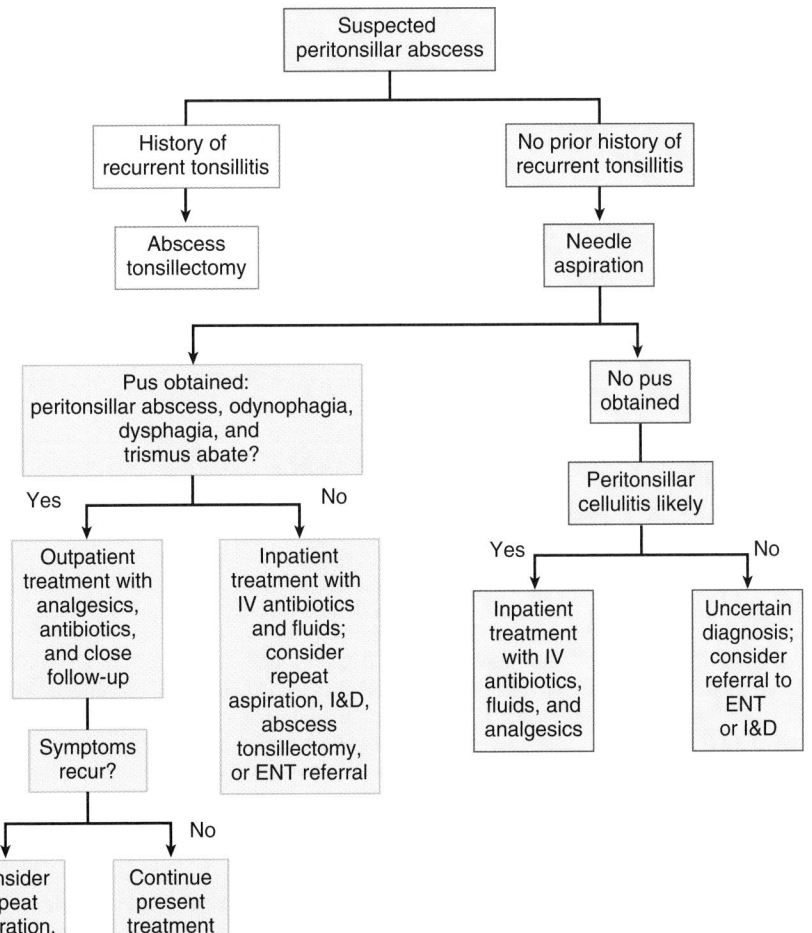

Fig. 206.2 Algorithm for the management of peritonsillar abscess. *ENT*, Ear, nose, and throat; *I&D*, incision and drainage.

- Anticoagulated patient or patient with coagulopathy (either the anticoagulation/coagulopathy should be reversed or otolaryngology consulted)
- Inadequate equipment

EQUIPMENT

Needle Aspiration

- Topical anesthetic—lidocaine, tetracaine, or benzocaine (Cetacaine) spray or 4% cocaine
- 2% lidocaine with epinephrine 1:100,000 in a 3- to 5-mL syringe with a 25- or 27-gauge 1.5-inch needle or tonsil needle
- 18-gauge 1.5-inch or longer needle or spinal needle
- 10-mL syringe

    NOTE: As a guide to keep from going too deep, place a piece of tape or 8-mm Steri-Strip proximal to the needle tip or cut 1 cm off the end of the needle cover and put it back on the needle, leaving 1 cm of needle exposed.

- Suction: tonsillar, No. 8 Frazier or Yankauer
- Good lighting: headlight or head mirror with gooseneck lamp
- Kidney basin
- Tongue depressor
- Bite block or heaped gauze (as thick as the clinician's finger) folded over the patient's incisor teeth to help the clinician avoid being bitten when palpating the area
- Surgical assistant to help with the equipment and procedure
- Culturettes or culture bottles
- Gloves, gown, and face shield for the clinician to observe universal blood and body fluid precautions
- For ultrasound-guided: ultrasound machine, high-frequency, endocavitary probe, sterile ultrasound gel, ultrasound probe cover

Incision and Drainage

All of the aforementioned plus a curved Kelly, hemostat or tonsillar clamp and a No. 15 scalpel blade marked with tape or Steri-Strip 1 cm from the tip. The patient will need something to rinse the mouth afterward, such as water, normal saline, half-strength peroxide, or chlorhexidine (Peridex) solution.

PREPROCEDURE PATIENT EDUCATION

The procedure of choice for most patients is needle aspiration, and this procedure should be explained, as well as the risks and any alternatives. Advise the patient that he or she may experience some discomfort while attempting to hold the mouth (or as it is held) open and when the local anesthetic is injected (even though the pharynx will be sprayed first with a topical anesthetic). The patient may also experience some discomfort when the abscess is aspirated or incised and drained. However, after a successful procedure, the patient's symptoms should improve dramatically; even the trismus should resolve. If the procedure is ultrasound-directed, the patient should know than a transducer with a sterile cover will be placed in his or her mouth. If aspiration fails, the procedure may shift to incision and drainage, and the patient should know the difference. He or she may gag or experience fluid running down the throat. Fortunately the pus can usually be aspirated or incised and drained successfully; if so, the symptoms will improve dramatically and the patient can then be treated with oral antibiotics and analgesics. Hospitalization can usually be avoided. If the abscess is not successfully drained or the symptoms do not resolve, further treatment and hospitalization may be required. The patient should also be told that there is a 10% chance of recurrence after aspiration and a 6% to 24% chance of recurrence after incision and drainage. If the abscess recurs after successful aspiration, there is a high success rate for merely repeating the aspiration. However, even if aspiration is successful three times,

the patient would probably benefit from tonsillectomy, especially if three infections have occurred in the same year. Fortunately new methods for tonsillectomy and adenoidectomy are available (see Chapter 66, Tonsillectomy and Adenoidectomy) that can usually be performed in the outpatient setting and that minimize postoperative pain and recovery time. Obtain a signed informed consent from the patient or his or her representative for all of these procedures.

TECHNIQUE

Precautions

One potential disaster to avoid is aspiration or incision of the carotid or facial arteries or an undiagnosed carotid artery aneurysm. (Fortunately there are no recent reports in the literature of this occurring, so it is extremely rare.) Another potential disaster to avoid is patient aspiration of purulent material into his or her lungs. The risk of the first can be minimized by directing the needle or scalpel only posteriorly when performing the procedure (the major vessels are located laterally) and never inserting it more than 1 cm. The risk of such aspiration can be minimized by ensuring the availability of adequate operative wall suction at the time of incision and drainage.

Procedure

1. Seat the patient leaning slightly forward, in the sniffing position, at eye level with the operator. His or her neck should be supported posteriorly to prevent any abrupt moves. A kidney basin should be available for the patient to expectorate. Suction must be readily available with either a tonsillar, No. 8 Frazier, or Yankauer tip. Good lighting is necessary, provided by either a headlight or a head mirror with a bright light source behind the patient.
2. Have the patient open his or her mouth as wide as possible. If trismus restricts jaw motion, the patient may need some encouragement to open more widely. Mild pressure on the lower jaw may also be necessary to help open the mouth. The cheek may be retracted laterally to improve visualization. Your assistant can help provide exposure by placing mild pressure on the jaw and lateral traction on the cheek. For moderate to severe trismus, sedation may be beneficial (see Chapter 1, Procedural Sedation and Analgesia). Palpate the soft palate and tonsil to localize the fluctuant area, and administer topical anesthetic to the affected side. A bite block or some heaped gauze folded over the patient's incisor teeth may help the clinician to avoid being bitten. Be prepared to avoid a bite when palpating the area because the patient may not be able to hold his or her mouth open for very long. The patient may also gag when the area is palpated. When the topical anesthetic has taken effect, inject 2% lidocaine with epinephrine (using a 25- to 27-gauge 1.5-inch needle, or tonsil needle on a smaller syringe) into the mucosa, just above and lateral to the tonsil. Avoid injecting into the abscess.

    NOTE: Novel techniques to visualize the area and assist in the drainage procedure have recently been described in the literature. One describes the use of a laryngoscope with a shiny curved blade. This blade not only helps keep the tongue out of the way but also provides additional light to the area of the tonsil. Another technique describes using half of a disassembled disposable vaginal speculum combined with a fiberoptic light source. What is nice about both of these methods is that an assistant can help without getting in the way of the clinician while allowing him or her to focus on the procedure. Finally, a group has described performing the procedure with the patient in the Trendelenburg position and the operator seated behind the patient's head. This may provide superior comfort for both patient and clinician.
3. After a few minutes, attempt aspiration. Hold the tongue depressor in your nondominant hand and the aspirating syringe in your dominant hand. (Some clinicians find that using an index finger to hold the tongue out of the way allows for better visualization

using a tongue depressor.) You may need to ask your assistant to create suction with the syringe. Insert the 18-gauge long or spinal needle on a 10-mL syringe toward the area of maximal fluctuance, usually in the upper pole of the tonsil. Direct the needle parallel to the floor and straight posteriorly (a smaller-gauge needle will not allow thick pus to be aspirated). When the needle has been inserted, attempt aspiration (Fig. 206.3). The needle should not be inserted more than 1 cm. If you aspirate pus, continue until no more pus returns. Evidence suggests there is no reason to culture the aspirated fluid, which is usually between 2 and 14 mL of pus.

4. If you do not aspirate any pus, withdraw the needle slightly and redirect it inferiorly, into the middle pole of the tonsil. When performing this procedure, again be aware that the carotid artery lies approximately 2.5 cm posterior and lateral to the tonsillar pillars. In addition, the more the needle is directed toward the lower pole of the tonsil, the more likely it is to enter the carotid artery. Therefore make sure that it is directed only posteriorly. Never aspirate lateral to the molar. If no pus is obtained on the second aspiration attempt, redirect the needle inferiorly into the inferior pole. If blood returns on aspiration, the procedure should be stopped, the needle removed, and direct pressure applied to the puncture site. An otolaryngologist should be consulted immediately.

5. It is recommended that aspiration be performed prior to incision and drainage so as to localize the pus and enable a more accurate incision and drainage. However, if the third aspiration is unsuccessful and the diagnosis of peritonsillar abscess is certain (i.e., confirmed by palpation or imaging), immediate incision and drainage can be performed. To do this, direct a No. 15 scalpel blade posteriorly and make a horizontal stab incision just through the mucosa in the upper pole of the tonsil at the point of maximum fluctuance or prominence (Fig. 206.4). This point is usually

seen as a shiny membrane over the abscess. Avoid inserting the scalpel blade more than 1 cm into it. After an incision through this membrane has been made, there is often a prompt expression of pus. Immediate and aggressive suction is now required. Having the surgical assistant ready with the suction placed at the incision site, before the incision is made, often reassures the patient and keeps him or her comfortable. This may also help the patient to avoid any gagging or the drowning sensation that can occur when pus is released into the pharynx.

NOTE: If the third aspiration is unsuccessful and ultrasound is not available, the performance of incision and drainage is contraindicated. The diagnosis is then probably tonsillar cellulitis or it may be too early for the abscess to have formed.

6. Sometimes the incision must be widened with a curved Kelly, hemostat, or tonsillar clamp. Any loculations that are apparent should be opened. Loculations are especially common inferiorly. Any remaining pus or blood should be suctioned before the procedure is completed. The patient can then rinse his or her mouth with tap water, normal saline, half-strength peroxide, or chlorhexidine solution. The patient should be observed directly for a few minutes after incision and drainage for any persistent drainage. If drainage persists, the patient should be admitted for intravenous antibiotics. The patient should also be observed for at least an hour before discharge to ensure stable vital signs and absence of bleeding.

7. All patients successfully treated by needle aspiration or incision and drainage may be sent home with antibiotics such as amoxicillin-clavulanate or clindamycin. Liquid elixirs are much easier for the patient to swallow. If MRSA is a consideration, clindamycin or linezolid are good empiric choices. The patient should be seen in follow-up the next day.

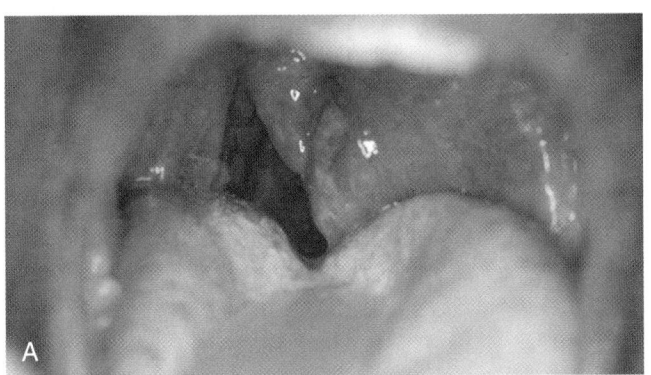

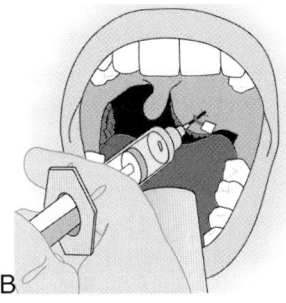

Fig. 206.3 Aspiration of peritonsillar abscess. (A) Abscess. (B) The abscess should be anesthetized topically and locally and then aspirated with an 18-gauge long needle or spinal needle at the point of maximal fluctuance (prominence). The needle is directed straight back and parallel to floor of the mouth.

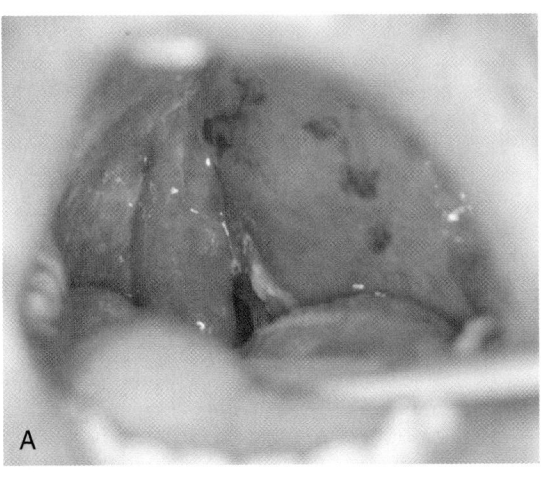

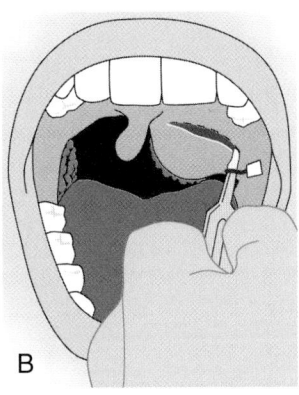

Fig. 206.4 Incision and drainage of peritonsillar abscess. (A) Abscess. (B) After topical and local anesthesia, the incision should be made in the upper pole of the tonsil at the point of maximal fluctuance (prominence). The incision may have to be probed or widened with a curved Kelly, hemostat, or tonsillar clamp.

Ultrasound-Directed Procedure

1. Seat the patient, set up the equipment, and anesthetize the area as previously described. Apply the sterile ultrasound gel onto the probe and cover the probe; attempt to avoid trapping bubbles between the probe and cover. Next apply sterile gel over the covered ultrasound probe.
2. Insert the probe until it rests on the patient's posterior pharynx. To maximize visualization of the posterior pharynx, the probe is usually maintained in a transverse orientation (marker dot to the patient's right side: see Chapter 214, Emergency Department, Hospitalist, and Office Ultrasonography [POCUS]).
3. Note the palantine tonsil (a small oval structure with low-level echoes) and the pulsating internal carotid arteries. An abscess is usually cystic and adjacent to the tonsils; it can have heterogeneous tissue in it as well as around it. Note the depth, angle, location of the maximal area of the abscess as well as where it lies relative to the carotid artery. Color Doppler can be used to distinguish the carotid if not already clearly visible. The ultrasound probe can then be laid down and the aspiration needle advanced at the same angle and depth to the area of maximal abscess diameter seen on imaging (two-handed unassisted technique). Or the needle can be advanced under the probe to visualize the aspiration, using a one- or two-person technique (see Chapter 214, Emergency Department, Hospitalist, and Office Ultrasonography [POCUS] and Chapter 171, Musculoskeletal Ultrasound).

COMPLICATIONS

- Hemorrhage
- Tracheal aspiration of purulent material
- Respiratory distress
- Pneumonia
- Failed aspiration or incision and drainage, persistent cellulitis
- Recurrence

SAMPLE OPERATIVE REPORTS

See sample operative reports available at www.expertconsult.com.

POSTPROCEDURE PATIENT EDUCATION

All patients who have been treated for a peritonsillar abscess need adequate antibiotics and analgesia, preferably in liquid form. Warm gargles may help to keep the area clean and provide mild analgesia. Patients will want to maintain a liquid or soft diet until the discomfort has resolved. They should be instructed to return if they experience a recurrence of symptoms, fever greater than 101°F, severe pain, significant bleeding, or trouble breathing or swallowing. A follow-up appointment within 48 hours should be scheduled.

CPT/BILLING CODES

42700   Incision and drainage of peritonsillar abscess
88170   Needle aspiration (location needs to be recorded for insurance billing)
76942   Ultrasonic guidance for needle placement (e.g., biopsy, aspiration, injection, localization device), imaging supervision and interpretation

ICD-10-CM DIAGNOSTIC CODES

J36   Peritonsillar abscess, quinsy, peritonsillar cellulitis

ONLINE RESOURCES

Medline Plus: Peritonsillar abscess: www.nlm.nih.gov/medlineplus/ency/article/000986.htm.

RECOMMENDED READING

Chau JK, Seikaly HR, Harris JR, et al. Corticosteroids in peritonsillar abscess treatment: a blinded placebo-controlled clinical trial. *Laryngoscope.* 2014;124:97.
Epperly T, Wood T. New trends in the management of peritonsillar abscess. *Am Fam Physician.* 1990;42:102–112.
Galioto NJ. Peritonsillar abscess. *Am Fam Physician.* 2008;77:199–202.
Haeggstrom A, Gustafsson O, Engquist S, et al. Intraoral ultrasonography in the diagnosis of peritonsillar abscess. *Otolaryngol Head Neck Surg.* 1993;108:243–247.
Herzon FS, Martin AD. Medical and surgical treatment of peritonsillar, retropharyngeal, and parapharyngeal abscesses. *Curr Infect Dis Rep.* 2006;8:196.
Herzon F, Aldridge J. Peritonsillar abscess: needle aspiration. *Otolaryngol Head Neck Surg.* 1980;89:910–911.
Lamkin RH, Portt J. An outpatient medical treatment protocol for peritonsillar abscess. *Ear Nose Throat J.* 2006;85:658–660.
Ozbek C, Aygenc E, Tuna EU, et al. Use of steroids in the treatment of peritonsillar abscess. *J Laryngol Otol.* 2004;118:439.
Reichmann EF, Hughes KD, Meer J. Peritonsillar abscess incision and drainage. In: Reichman EF, ed. *Emergency Medicine Procedures.* 2nd ed. New York: McGraw-Hill; 2013.
Riviello RJ. Otolaryngologic procedures. In: Roberts JR, Custalow CB, Thomsen TW, eds. *Roberts & Hedges' Clinical Procedures in Emergency Medicine.* 6th ed. Philadelphia: Elsevier; 2014.
Steyer T. Peritonsillar abscess: diagnosis and treatment. *Am Fam Physician.* 2002;65:93–96.
Wald ER. Peritonsillar abscess and cellulitis. *UpToDate.* https://www.uptodate.com/contents/peritonsillar-cellulitis-and-abscess?search=peritonsillar%20abscess&source=search_result&selectedTitle=1~53&usage_type=default&display_rank=1. 2017.

CHAPTER 207

MANAGEMENT OF DENTAL INJURIES AND REIMPLANTATION OF AN AVULSED TOOTH

Grant C. Fowler

Dental trauma, ranging from a slight chip of the enamel to avulsion of a tooth, encompasses some of the most common injuries to the face. An occlusive misadventure (e.g., biting a hard object, a seizure) or a blow to the face can cause dental trauma. Up to 10% of emergency department visits are due to dental trauma. Injuries to the maxillary central incisors account for 70% of dental injuries, subluxations account for about 50% of injuries to the teeth, and up to 5 million avulsions occur annually in the United States. It is estimated that 50% of children will experience dental injuries, and the majority of these will involve the permanent teeth. Management depends on the age of the patient and the nature of the injury. Often, the primary care clinician is the first to evaluate such an injury. Occasionally the clinician will receive a phone call from a patient requesting guidance after a fracture, subluxation, luxation, or avulsion. Proper management of dental trauma may minimize pain and disfigurement. For example, knowledge of proper storage and treatment of an avulsed tooth is crucial to optimize the chances of successful reimplantation.

NOTE: If a tooth or portion of a tooth is missing and it cannot be unequivocally located by history or physical examination, attempts should be made to locate it with radiographs. Facial films may find it in a maxillary sinus (which may necessitate surgery), a chest radiograph may document that it has been aspirated (requiring bronchoscopic retrieval), or abdominal films may document that it has been swallowed. Also, with a luxation or avulsion, care should be taken to determine whether a tooth in a child is primary (i.e., deciduous, milk, and temporary) or permanent because it may change the management (Fig. 207.1). This determination may be tricky in children between the ages of 6 and 12 years who may have "mixed" dentition. The patient's should also be aware that it may not always be possible to detect the presence or extent of a dental fracture with the initial examination and radiographs. Root fractures (although rare), which may require extensive dental care, are notorious for avoiding detection by radiography; they may be diagnosed only later by radiography as they are healing.

Management of a dental fracture is based on the extent of the fracture (Fig. 207.2) and the age of the patient. Ellis I fractures involve only the enamel of the tooth. Such a fracture may be only a chip off of the tooth. Management is necessary only if a resultant sharp edge is disturbing the adjacent soft tissues. In that case, a nail file (emery board) can be used to file down the edge. (Be careful not to be overzealous with the emery board and thus convert an Ellis I into Ellis II.) Referral can be made to a general dentist for cosmetic restoration. Patients or parents may appreciate being reassured that the tooth can usually be restored to its natural appearance with the use of enamel-bonding plastic materials.

Ellis II fractures, which account for 70% of tooth fractures, not only involve the enamel but also expose the dentin layer, which has a creamy or ivory-yellow color compared with the white enamel. Beneath the dentin lies the pulp, which continually lays down dentin for the life of the tooth; the goal of emergency management of Ellis II fractures is to maintain the vitality of this pulp. Patients usually complain of sensitivity to heat, cold, or even air passing over the exposed surface as they breathe. They should be warned that this type of trauma to the tooth may lead to pulpal necrosis or tooth resorption regardless of management and that dental referral is required within 24 hours. Patients below 12 years of age have less dentin, so there is usually less discomfort. However, because dentin is a microtubular structure that can allow bacteria to penetrate the pulp, tooth fractures in children and adolescents involving the dentin are more serious because the pulp is more likely to be contaminated. Fortunately this age group also has much greater pulpal regenerative ability. Early treatment may prevent contamination of the pulp and the need for subsequent root canal, so a pediatric or general dentist should be notified right away. For patients above 12 years of age, because they have more dentin and less pulp, referral can be made for the next working day. Regardless of age, warming the sterile saline before flushing may decrease temperature sensitivity. A thin layer of protective dressing that is also a sedative to the pulp (e.g., calcium hydroxide paste or zinc oxide with eugenol; see Suppliers section) or even toothpaste should be applied with a small applicator. The exposed dentin should be covered and then the paste covered with dry gauze. The fractured tooth must be dry for the calcium hydroxide paste to adhere, so having the patient gently bite on a piece of dry gauze prior to application may be helpful. Several dry, sterile cotton-tipped applicators may be used for same purpose. To maintain a dry field while working, cotton gauze or rolls can be placed on either side of the tooth. Patients above 12 years of age should then be advised to avoid extremes of intraoral temperatures. A piece of dental foil or aluminum foil placed over the paste-covering gauze may provide additional protection from discomfort associated with temperature extremes until the dentist can see the patient. If available, instead of gauze, three to four coats of dental varnish (see Suppliers section) or clear nail polish can be painted over the paste. Allow time to dry between coats; this may help to protect against temperature extremes. If applied with care, such a dressing should last 3 to 4 days. The patient should minimize chewing until seen by a dentist; therefore he or she should eat only soft or liquid foods.

Ellis III fractures expose the pulp of the tooth. Again, because there is more pulp relative to dentin in children, fractures involving the pulp are more common in children. Pulp can easily be distinguished from dentin because exposed pulp produces a red blush or a drop of blood when brushed with sterile gauze. These fractures are dental emergencies, and the usual treatment is removal of the

Primary dentition
Age of primary tooth
eruption (months)

Adult (permanent) dentition
Age of permanent tooth
eruption (years)

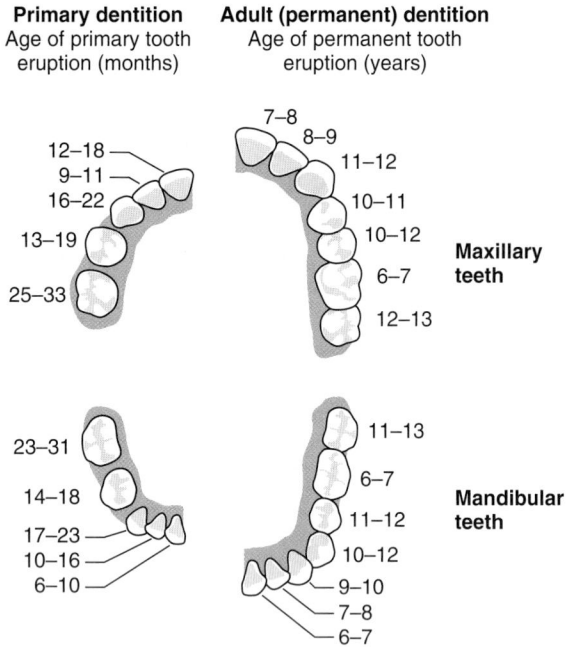

**Maxillary
teeth**

**Mandibular
teeth**

Fig. 207.1 Normal eruptive patterns of primary and permanent teeth. Extra or fewer teeth are common in both types of teeth. (Modified from Ross DJ. Fractured tooth management. In: Reichman EF, ed. *Emergency Medicine Procedures*, 2nd ed. New York: McGraw-Hill; 2013.)

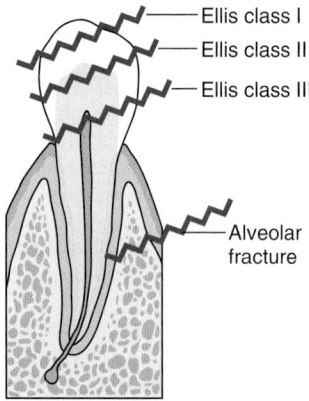

Ellis class I
Ellis class II
Ellis class III

Alveolar
fracture

Fig. 207.2 Ellis classification for fractures of anterior teeth. (From James DM. Immediate management of tooth fracture and avulsion. In: James DM, ed. *Field Guide to Urgent and Ambulatory Care Procedures*. Philadelphia: Lippincott Williams & Wilkins; 2001.)

diseased pulp (pulpotomy, a partial root canal) or root canal. Significant delay in care can lead to long-term pain and abscess formation. The clinician should not attempt to probe the pulp or remove any material; instead, the affected area should be covered with aluminum foil, adequate analgesia provided, and oral antibiotics effective for mouth flora prescribed. Such a fracture can cause considerable pain, so a dental anesthetic nerve block may be appreciated. The patient should consult a dentist immediately because definitive treatment for all but the smallest pulpal exposures is endodontic or root canal therapy. If a dentist will not be available, bleeding can be stopped by dripping dilute epinephrine (or lidocaine with epinephrine) over the site. Injection of lidocaine with epinephrine around the tooth also often provides hemostasis. If this is unsuccessful, pressure can be applied with a saline- or lidocaine-moistened sterile cotton-tipped applicator. It may take 3 to 5 minutes for hemostasis to occur. A thick coat of calcium hydroxide or zinc oxide with eugenol paste can then be applied to the tooth and an adjacent tooth (for stability),

making sure that it is not so thick as to interfere with occlusion. If a dentist is not available, a minimal Ellis III fracture (<1 to 2 mm of pulp exposure) can be treated as an Ellis II fracture and followed up by a dentist within 24 hours, although this alternative is less than ideal.

Teeth are held in place by surrounding periodontal membrane fibers and ligaments, a fragile cell layer lining the root known as the *cementum*, and alveolar bone (Fig. 207.3). These structures combined are known as the *attachment apparatus*. The crown is the hard enamel portion of the tooth located above the gum line. With trauma, periodontal fibers and the attachment apparatus may be concussed (Fig. 207.4); a tooth may be subluxed (ligaments damaged) or luxated (dislocated) extrusively, intrusively, or laterally; or an entire tooth may be avulsed (Fig. 207.5). Concussion is defined as injury to the tooth, and although the tooth will be tender to palpation, there is no increased mobility. The radiograph will be negative. If examination of the surrounding gingiva reveals blood, there has also usually been ligamentous damage, which is confirmed if the tooth can be wiggled. Ligamentous damage can be caused by subluxation or luxation, with subluxation resulting in a loose tooth that may or may not be sensitive to touch. Extrusive luxation results in a misaligned loose tooth that is often elevated above those bordering it. The patient frequently complains of malocclusion because this tooth contacts the opposing teeth early when chewing. Intrusive luxation is a more severe form of luxation in which the tooth is driven into the alveolar bone. With primary teeth, this process can cause damage to the permanent tooth bud. Depending on the force involved, the tooth can even be driven into the maxillary sinus and appear avulsed. If intrusive luxation is suspected and the tooth is not visible, a radiograph may be needed to locate the tooth. Although an extrusive luxation is the result of a partial avulsion or dislodgment of the tooth, there is no fracture, so the radiograph will be negative. Lateral luxation is the result of an alveolar bone fracture with lateral displacement of the tooth in the mesial, distal, buccal, or lingual direction. A radiograph should confirm the fracture.

Treatment of a concussed tooth is directed by the severity of the discomfort. Nonsteroidal antiinflammatory drugs (NSAIDs) and a soft diet may be all that is necessary to manage the pain. For subluxation, a minimally mobile tooth will usually "firm up" over a week or two, and splinting is usually not required. Severely subluxed primary teeth should be extracted; otherwise concussed and subluxed primary teeth are treated in the same manner as permanent teeth. For subluxed permanent teeth, the patient should maintain a soft diet and avoid undue pressure on the affected tooth during that time; he or she may benefit from NSAIDs for pain control. For either concussion or subluxation, referral to a dentist may be prudent, not only to confirm the diagnosis but also to exclude more serious injury.

An extrusively luxated primary tooth should be removed; conversely, an extrusively luxated permanent tooth should be repositioned. Firm, gentle pressure will usually realign the tooth to its original position, and this maneuver may be better tolerated if a local anesthetic is injected. Avoid excessive pressure when attempting this maneuver; a hematoma may be blocking repositioning and require more definitive care by a dentist. If repositioning is successful, splinting should be provided to stabilize the tooth for 1 to 2 weeks during healing, either by a dentist with flexible wire splinting or by a primary care clinician using a cold-curing periodontal pack (see Suppliers section) or dressing until a dentist, oral surgeon, or maxillofacial surgeon can provide definitive care (ideally within 24 hours). To use a cold-curing periodontal pack, thoroughly mix equal portions of the epoxy and catalyst on an uncontaminated surface until it has the consistency of putty. It should be allowed to dry slightly for a few minutes and then be applied by molding it to the exterior buccal surface of the tooth and adjacent teeth on either side. Avoid covering any of the occlusal surface. The patient should remain in the clinic until the splinting material has completely hardened; reexamination ensures the absence of impingement of an occlusal surface or soft tissue sufficient to cause local irritation.

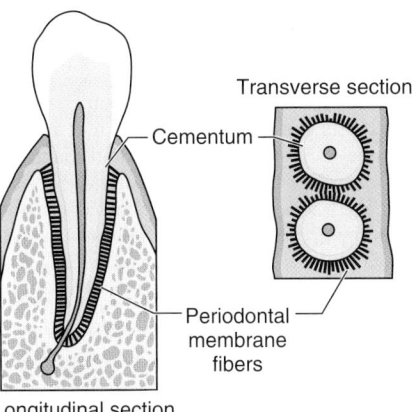

Fig. 207.3 Arrangement of periodontal fibers. The cementum is a thin cell layer lining the root between the root and the periodontal fibers. Together, the cementum, periodontal fibers, and alveolar bone form the attachment apparatus.

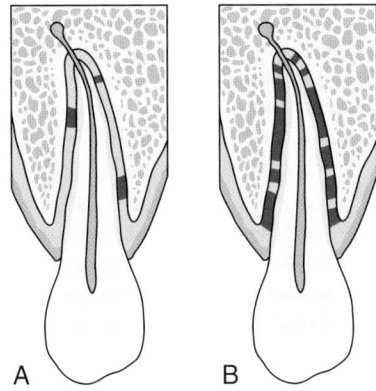

Fig. 207.4 Slightly (A) and moderately (B) concussed teeth.

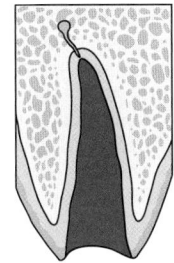

Fig. 207.5 Avulsed tooth.

Dental utility wax or beeswax may be used in the same fashion if a cold-curing periodontal pack is not available.

Intrusive luxation is a more serious injury, resulting in alveolar fracture. Management consists of defining the extent of injury (e.g., is a sinus involved?), locating the tooth, providing analgesics, and referral. Laterally luxated primary teeth should be extracted. With permanent teeth, because lateral luxation causes a fracture, repositioning the tooth may be more difficult. However, by grasping the tooth firmly between thumb and forefinger, the clinician will usually be able to realign the tooth. After referral, stabilizing with a splint is necessary for a minimum of 2 weeks.

In the event of avulsion, the neurovascular supply is disrupted. Primary teeth are usually not reimplanted (to avoid damaging the developing permanent teeth); however, the more rapidly a permanent tooth is reimplanted, the more likely it is that the tooth will remain viable. If the tooth can be replanted within 5 minutes, there is a greater than 80% chance that it will remain vital. Given this urgency, bystanders or clinicians should not be overly concerned about cleaning or flushing the socket or tooth before reimplanting. When the tooth is being prepared for reimplantation, only the crown should be touched; touching the root can devitalize it. Significant debris and large clots can merely be brushed off; small clots or dirt can be removed by the patient by placing the tooth under his or her tongue for a few seconds. If it is going to be reimplanted immediately, the tooth can be flushed with saline or tap water. Reimplantation should then be performed, with follow-up by a dentist.

For the tooth that is not immediately reimplanted, proper storage is crucial. Prognosis for later reimplantation deteriorates rapidly—within minutes—if the tooth dries out, causing pulpal and periodontal damage. Storage media available to prevent drying, in order from most to least successful, are cell culture medium (e.g., Viaspan [a special cell culture medium, or SCCM, used for the preservation of transplant donor tissue], Hanks balanced salt solution [a pH-balanced cell culture medium]), milk, physiologic (normal) saline, and saliva. There may be slight benefit of SCCM over Hanks balanced salt solution. An egg white may also be used. These fluids have an osmotic pressure similar to those of the pulp and periodontal tissues and therefore help preserve these structures. Tap water is not an appropriate storage medium because of its hypotonicity.

Although cell culture medium and milk are superior to saliva as storage media, the prevention of desiccation is much more important than waiting until SCCM, Hanks balanced salt solution, or milk is available. If none of these is immediately available, the tooth can be stored in saliva. Perhaps the most readily available preservative other than saliva is fresh whole milk on ice (between 4°C and 20°C); however, parents, schools, teams, and facilities that sponsor sporting events now often have cell culture medium (e.g., SCCM, Hanks solution) in a kit. These solutions have been shown to keep periodontal ligaments alive for 4 to 6 hours. Successful results have been reported with teeth suspended in Hanks solution for up to 96 hours. It has also been found to restore cell viability in a tooth that has been avulsed for longer than 60 minutes. These kits contain a basket and net or a similar system to suspend, clean, and store the tooth in preservative solution while it is being transported for reimplantation (see Suppliers section). A basket allows the clinician to remove the tooth from the solution without touching it with fingers or forceps.

INDICATIONS

- Avulsed permanent tooth with minimal pulpal and periodontal damage, especially a tooth from the front of the mouth
- Tooth out of its socket for only a short time
- Tooth stored in the proper physiologic medium

NOTE: One readily available source of saliva is the patient's mouth, and the tooth can be stored under the tongue. Another option is the mouth of a relative if the patient is unconscious or uncooperative. If the tooth is stored in the patient's mouth, he or she must concentrate on not swallowing the tooth! Universal blood and body fluid precautions should be remembered if the tooth is to be stored in someone else's mouth.

CONTRAINDICATIONS

- Primary (i.e., deciduous, milk, temporary) teeth should not be reimplanted. (Reimplanting these teeth may result in their fusion to the supporting bone and possible facial deformity. It may also damage or interfere with the development of the permanent teeth.)
- Avulsed teeth with gross caries or fractures should not be reimplanted.
- Patients with significant loss of periodontal support (periodontitis) should not have teeth reimplanted.

EQUIPMENT

- Adequate light
- Equipment necessary to follow universal blood and body fluid precautions (gloves, eye protection, and mask)
- Sterile normal saline
- Irrigation syringe
- Local anesthetic (lidocaine with epinephrine), syringe (dental aspirating type or 3 mL), and 2-inch 25- to 27-gauge needle
- Sterile 2- × 2-inch cotton gauze squares or cotton rolls
- Nail file or emery board for tooth fracture, dental drill if available
- Tooth forceps
- Fraser suction catheter, suction source, and tubing
- Calcium hydroxide or zinc oxide and eugenol paste (protective and sedative for pulp; see Suppliers section) or toothpaste
- Dental dry foil or aluminum foil
- Small brush and cavity varnish (see Suppliers section) or clear nail polish
- Cold-curing periodontal pack (i.e., elastic quick-setting dressing), dental utility wax, or beeswax (see Suppliers section)
- Applicator sticks (e.g., tongue depressor, wooden ends of cotton swabs)
- Dental radiography equipment and supplies
- Penicillin V potassium (penicillin VK) 500-mg tablets (18 to 26 tablets) or clindamycin (parenteral antibiotics for those at risk; see Chapter 69, Antibiotic Prophylaxis)
- Cell culture medium (e.g., SCCM, Hanks balanced salt solution)
- Tooth-saving system (contains cell culture medium; see Suppliers section)
- Citric acid, 2% stannous fluoride, doxycycline syrup or suspension (*optional,* especially useful if a dentist is not available and tooth has dried more than an hour)
- Cyanoacrylate glue (optional, especially useful if a dentist is not available)
- Paper clip (optional, especially useful if a dentist is not available)

PREPROCEDURE PATIENT PREPARATION

Explain to the patient the procedure, possible complications, benefits, and the need for follow-up. The patient will have to remain still during the procedure, but discomfort should be minimal. Informed consent should be obtained.

NOTE: Immediate reimplantation (within 5 minutes) is one of the most critical factors related to periodontal healing. If the tooth is not stored in a proper medium and the interval is more than 30 minutes before reimplantation, the success rate falls to less than 20% and the tooth will inevitably require endodontic therapy. If the patient or family member calls and is more than 5 minutes away from clinical care, an immediate attempt to reimplant the tooth will provide the best outcome. Have the patient rinse the tooth under cold water or place it under his or her tongue for a few seconds and then reimplant it at once. Instructions or words of encouragement may be needed. However, accident-associated factors such as the person's emotional state, a lack of knowledge of proper first aid, a lack of confidence on the part of bystanders, or informed consent issues are often obstacles at the accident site. If these obstacles cannot be overcome, the only choice may be to store the tooth in the best medium available and to transport it and the patient to the clinic. There are isolated cases of teeth remaining viable for many hours or even days, so the clinician may consider replantation; however, the patient should understand that the chances usually decrease dramatically the longer a tooth is out of the socket. Attempting to contact a dental professional for guidance is also very worthwhile.

TECHNIQUE

1. If the tooth is stored in a cell culture medium or milk on arrival, leave it in the medium. If it is stored in saliva or no medium, place the avulsed tooth in cell culture medium or normal saline as soon as possible. If the tooth has been dry for 20 to 60 minutes, it should be soaked in cell culture medium for 30 minutes. If it has been dry for more than an hour, the periodontal cells will be dead and the goal will be to reduce root resorption. In that situation, dentists often recommend soaking the tooth for 5 minutes in each of three different solutions before reimplantation: citric acid, followed by 2% stannous fluoride, and finally doxycycline syrup or suspension. The tooth should never be merely discarded; attempts should be made to contact a dental professional for guidance.

2. If the patient is at risk for bacteremia, administer parenteral antibiotics.

3. Conduct a rapid medical history and systematic evaluation of the traumatized individual:
   - Where, how, and when did the trauma occur? Are there fractures?
   - Is there any neurologic damage? Unconsciousness? Amnesia? Headache? Nausea?
   - Are there any underlying medical conditions? Immunocompromise? Diabetes? Prostheses? Cardiac conditions for which antibiotic prophylaxis is recommended? See Chapter 69, Antibiotic Prophylaxis. If any of these are life- or limb-threatening, they should be managed first. If not, make mental notes of other problems while rapidly preparing to reimplant the tooth.

4. When the patient is stable, administer local anesthetic to the socket area if necessary. The clinician should follow universal blood and body fluid precautions.

5. Perform a brief clinical examination:
   - Are there any other intraoral lacerations or disturbances?
   - Is the bite disturbed by other displaced teeth?
   - Make mental notes of these findings while rapidly preparing to reimplant the tooth.

6. Examine the tooth socket and flush with normal saline. Remove all clot material.
   NOTE: Although flushing the socket is commonly suggested in practice guidelines, there is little scientific evidence to support this activity; thus the socket should be manipulated as little as possible. (That is why reimplanting the tooth at the scene of the accident, if it can be accomplished within 5 to 10 minutes, is much more important than waiting to flush the socket or tooth.)

7. Remove the tooth from its soaking medium and, while holding the crown with gauze or tooth forceps, reimplant it as close as possible to its normal position, using finger pressure. *Do not touch the root.* The patient can assist the reimplantation by gently biting on gauze; this maneuver can also be used to help stabilize the tooth after reimplantation until more permanent stabilization can be arranged. Make sure the alignment is anatomic (remember that the curved side faces the tongue!). Observe the patient for malocclusion. If the tooth contacts another tooth with occlusion, it may be better to transport the tooth in preservation medium to a dental professional for definitive reimplantation.

8. Take a radiograph of the area if possible.

9. Refer to a dentist for semirigid splinting and follow-up. If a dentist is unavailable, a cold-curing periodontal pack, aluminum foil wrapped over the tooth and the neighboring teeth, or dental wax or beeswax can act as a splint. For a more rigid splint, a small paper clip bent to conform to the buccal side of the neighboring teeth can be glued to the reimplanted tooth as well as two or three neighboring teeth with cyanoacrylate glue. The dentist can later remove the glue with a dental pick.

10. Immediately administer penicillin VK 1 g orally (for those not already given parenteral dose), then 500 mg orally four times a day for 4 to 6 days (clindamycin for those allergic to penicillin).

11. Administer tetanus toxoid if the patient has not had a booster within 5 years.

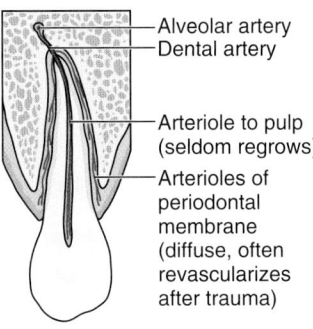

- Alveolar artery
- Dental artery
- Arteriole to pulp (seldom regrows)
- Arterioles of periodontal membrane (diffuse, often revascularizes after trauma)

Fig. 207.6 Blood supply to tooth.

POSTPROCEDURE PATIENT EDUCATION

NSAIDs and occasionally a narcotic analgesic may be all that is necessary to manage the pain. The patient should avoid chewing in the area of the tooth; he or she should follow a soft diet and avoid extremes of temperature. Patients should be warned that any trauma to the tooth may cause pulpal necrosis or tooth resorption regardless of management. For an avulsed tooth, inform the patient that the prognosis depends on the length of time the tooth was out of the socket and the medium in which it was stored. Fortunately a tooth has two sources of blood supply (Fig. 207.6). However, pulpal revascularization through the pulpal arterioles is almost nonexistent in teeth after complete root development (adult teeth). It is unusual even with immature root development. Periodontal ligament preservation is also infrequent, depending on the length of drying time to which the tooth was exposed. Fortunately the periodontal ligament has a more diffuse blood supply and revascularizes more readily than the pulp. However, the importance of consulting a dentist for the appropriate follow-up care should be stressed, especially if further splinting will be necessary.

COMPLICATIONS

- Necrosis of the pulp or periodontal ligament or complete loss of the tooth can occur. (Necrotic pulp tissue necessitates subsequent endodontic work.)
- An inadequately splinted tooth can remain loose, cause further damage to the attachment apparatus, and decrease the chance of tooth viability. If the tooth becomes dislodged, it could result in aspiration.
- With a nonvital periodontal ligament, ankylosis or osteoclastic root resorption can occur, which requires a root canal.
- Localized infection or bacteremia can occur, but it is very rare.
- If avulsed teeth are unaccounted for, the possibility of aspiration or entrapment in soft tissues should be considered.

CPT/BILLING CODES

D7270   Tooth reimplantation and/or stabilization of accidentally avulsed or displaced tooth (HCPCS Code)

ICD-10-CM DIAGNOSTIC CODES

K03.81	Cracked tooth
K08-111–K08.119	Loss of teeth due to trauma complete
K08.411–K08.419	Loss of teeth partial due to trauma
S02.5XXX	Tooth broken or fractured due to trauma

Add appropriate 7th character: A = initial; D = subsequent; S = sequela.

SUPPLIERS

(See contact information available at www.expertconsult.com.)

Calcium hydroxide or zinc-oxide eugenol paste
   Dycal (calcium hydroxide) by Dentsply Caulk
   IRM (intermediate restorative material, zinc-oxide eugenol) by Dentsply Caulk
   UltraCal XS (calcium hydroxide) by Ultradent Products, Inc.
Cavity varnish or sealant
   Copalite by Temrex (formerly by Cooley and Cooley)
Cold-curing periodontal packs
   Coe-Pak Automix by GC America, Inc.
   Periocare Periodontal Dressing by Pulpdent Corporation
Special Cell Culture Medium (SCCM)
   Viaspan (SCCM) by Barr Teva Pharmaceuticals
Tooth-saving systems
   Dentosafe (SCCM) by Medice
   EMT Tooth Saver Bottle (SCCM) by Smart Practice
   Save-A-Tooth System (Hanks balanced salt solution) by Phoenix-Lazerus

RECOMMENDED READING

Benko KR. Emergency dental procedures. In: Roberts JR, Custalow CB, Thomsen TW, eds. *Roberts and Hedges' Clinical Procedures in Emergency Medicine*. 6th ed. Philadelphia: Elsevier; 2014:1342–1351.

James DM. Immediate management of tooth fracture and avulsion. In: James DM, ed. *Field Guide to Urgent and Ambulatory Care Procedures*. Philadelphia: Lippincott Williams & Wilkins; 2001:36–39.

Ross DJ. Fractured tooth management. In: Reichman EF, ed. *Emergency Medicine Procedures*. 2nd ed. New York: McGraw-Hill; 2013:1161–1164.

Ross DJ. Subluxed and avulsed tooth management. In: Reichman EF, ed. *Emergency Medicine Procedures*. 2nd ed. New York: McGraw-Hill; 2013:1154–1161.

CHAPTER 208

MANAGEMENT OF FECAL IMPACTION

George G. Zainea

Fecal impaction is a common condition that typically occurs in the bedridden or nursing home patient. Individuals who suffered a cerebrovascular accident are at particular risk. Fecal impaction is the most common gastrointestinal disorder occurring in patients with a spinal cord injury. Medications such as narcotics predispose to this problem, and there are now medications available (e.g., Naloxegol) to offset this effect, but they are expensive. Fecal impaction is also a common complication of anorectal procedures as a result of reflex spasm of the anal sphincter. Painful anal fissures may cause the same problem.

DIAGNOSIS

Fecal impaction should be suspected when a patient has unexplained constipation or diarrhea. Diarrhea occurs as liquid stool passes around the hard fecal bolus. Rectal distention from the fecaloma causes reflex relaxation of the internal anal sphincter. The patient may have acute or chronic large bowel obstruction, both clinically and by radiographic examination. The chronic obstruction will increase mucosal water and electrolyte secretion, leading to frequent, loose, watery stools that pass around the bolus. The patient with spinal cord injury may demonstrate autonomic hyperreflexia with pain, fever, tachycardia, and abdominal distention.

Digital rectal examination reveals palpable impacted feces in the rectum. It is important to assess for size and consistency of the bolus, as well as for the presence of blood. In the normal situation, the rectal ampulla remains empty. A fecal bolus does not pass beyond the rectosigmoid junction until the act of defecation commences.

Complications of fecal impaction can include acute or chronic bowel obstruction, mucosal ulceration, and hemorrhage.

After disimpaction, particularly in the recurrent setting, it is important to rule out an anatomic cause of obstruction. This may require colonoscopy, sigmoidoscopy, or a water-soluble contrast radiographic examination. Impaction may be associated with an anal or rectal stricture. The practitioner must assess for the presence of a tumor. Last, a deep mucosal ulcer may cause bleeding or infection as a result of fecal impaction. This is known as a *stercoral ulceration*.

TECHNIQUE

An attempt at medical therapy in an otherwise ambulatory patient is a reasonable first step. Careful administration of one or two warm water (3 to 6 ounces) or Fleet (sodium phosphates) enemas into the bolus to soften and hydrate the stool should be followed in 1 hour by the administration of a mineral oil enema to assist in passage of the softened stool. Soapsuds or hydrogen peroxide enemas are discouraged because they may irritate the mucosa and result in bleeding. An alternative is an attempt at antegrade cleansing with either polyethylene glycol (PEG) solution or mineral oil. The dose of PEG solution is 20 mL/kg daily for 2 consecutive days. The dose of mineral oil is 30 mL/10 kg orally in two divided doses for 2 consecutive days.

NOTE: Sodium phosphate enemas have been found in one study (Ori, 2012; mean age, 80 years) to cause multiple complications (e.g., hypotension, volume depletion, hyperphosphatemia, hypokalemia and hyperkalemia, hypercalcemia, renal failure, metabolic acidosis, prolonged QT interval) in the elderly. The American Geriatrics Society also recommends against use of oral mineral oil in the elderly due to risk of aspiration and other complications, partly because there are alternatives available (PEG).

Manual disimpaction is required in most patients. This is best performed after a circumanal block of the anal musculature with local anesthetic. A four-quadrant field block allows for complete muscle relaxation and a painless disimpaction. Use 0.5% lidocaine drawn up in a 10-mL syringe. A 22-gauge, 0.5-inch needle is used. Insert the needle all the way to the hub in each of the right, left, anterior, and posterior positions 1 cm away from the anal verge (Fig. 208.1). Fan it out in three directions at each of the injection sites, depositing a total of 2 to 3 mL of local anesthetic in each of the four sites as the needle is slowly withdrawn. The left decubitus position with hips and knees flexed to the chest is the most comfortable for the patient.

Gentle digital dilation of the sphincter is then performed as the fecal bolus is fragmented and extracted. If a large amount of stool is removed but there is stool remaining above the finger, one option is to restart daily administration of enemas for up to 3 days. Or, a large, rigid proctoscope may be necessary to soften and break up stool residing higher in the rectum. After passing the rigid scope up to the fecal bolus, warm water or phosphate enema solution is passed through the scope to soften the stool. A long rigid aspirator is then passed through the scope to break up the softened stool and allow for evacuation. This process is repeated as many times as necessary to empty the bowel of stool.

Manual disimpaction may be facilitated by intravenous or intramuscular administration of a narcotic or anxiolytic. Early

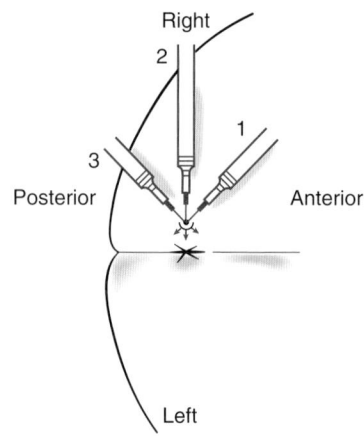

Fig. 208.1 Circumanal block with local anesthetic. Patient is in the left lateral decubitus position. Repeat the injection as shown, 1 cm from the anal verge, in all four quadrants (right, left, posterior, and anterior).

posthemorrhoidectomy impaction may be managed best in the operating room under general or regional anesthesia.

After disimpaction, it is prudent to institute a bowel habit program that should produce a stool at least every other day; sorbitol, lactulose, PEG solution, or a combination may be effective. Bisacodyl or glycerin suppositories should be used if there is no defecation after 2 days. Toileting should be scheduled after meals to take advantage of meal-stimulated increases in motility. Fiber intake should be gradually increased over weeks and should be matched with adequate fluid intake. Stimulant laxatives may be necessary, but long-term use of magnesium containing compounds should be avoided due to potential toxicity. For bedridden or demented patients, a fiber restricted diet combined with cleansing enemas once or twice a week will assist nursing management of bowel function.

CPT/BILLING CODES

45300   Rigid proctosigmoidoscopy
45915   Removal of fecal impaction or foreign body under
         anesthesia
45999   Procedure rectum (unspecified)

ICD-10-CM DIAGNOSTIC CODES

K56.41   Fecal impaction

RECOMMENDED READING

Araghizadeh F. Fecal impaction. In: *Clinics in Colon and Rectal Surgery*. Vol 18. New York: Thieme; 2005:116–119.
Mounsey A, Raleigh M, Wilson A. Management of constipation in older adults. *Am Fam Physician*. 2015;92(6):500–504.
Ori Y, Rozen-Zvi B, Chagnac A, Herman M, Zingerman B, et al. Fatalities and metabolic disorders associated with use of sodium phosphate enema. *Arch Int Med*. 2012;172(3):263.

CHAPTER 209

GASTROINTESTINAL DECONTAMINATION

Theodore X. O'Connell • Grant C. Fowler

The overall mortality from acute poisoning is less than 1%; therefore the challenge to clinicians is to determine which patients face serious complications from poisoning if not treated. If the decision is made to treat, activated charcoal is the first-line treatment for most ingested toxins, especially for ingestion of a small or moderate amount. Multiple doses of charcoal may be indicated in some situations such as ingestions of toxins recycled in the enterohepatic circulation or those with long half-lives. However, evidence for multidose activated charcoal is limited and opinions among toxicologists vary. Even use of single dose activated charcoal has decreased markedly since its introduction; it was recommended in less than 1% of cases in children in 2015. The American Academy of Clinical Toxicology (AACT) or the European Association of Poisons Centres and Clinical Toxicologists (EAPCCT) does not recommend it for routine use. Whole-bowel irrigation is the administration of polyethylene glycol (PEG) electrolyte solution to induce liquid stool and mechanically flush pills, tablets, or drug packets from the gastrointestinal tract. Gastric lavage is also rarely used due to unclear benefit and the risk of serious complications such as aspiration. However, poison control centers may still recommend its use in certain situations. Syrup of Ipecac is also no longer recommended for routine use by the AACT or the EAPCCT. The American Academy of Pediatrics recommends that it be removed from the home. It is no longer manufactured and is difficult to obtain (even though it remains active many years beyond the expiration date). That said, it was recommended 29 times by poison control centers in the United States in 2015. Cathartics such as magnesium citrate, magnesium sulfate, sorbitol, and mannitol are intended to decrease poison absorption by increasing rectal evacuation of the toxin. The AACT and EAPCCT advise against using cathartics as single agent therapy. Consultation with a medical toxicologist or regional poison control center (800-222-1222) may help guide the choice of intervention.

MECHANISMS OF ACTION AND EVIDENCE

Charcoal is activated by the manufacturer by heating it to approximately 900°C and washing it in a stream of carbon dioxide gas or steam. This increases the surface area from 2 m^2/g to greater than 2000 m^2/g; consequently, a 50-g dose has the surface area of 10 football fields. When ingested, there is no modification of charcoal's structure by digestive enzymes as it passes through the stomach and intestines, nor is it absorbed across the intestinal wall. Activated charcoal binds with toxins and then passes through the gastrointestinal tract to be eliminated in the stool as a sticky black substance. As the charcoal absorbs the toxin in the intestine and passes distally, it creates a diffusion gradient. This in turn causes already absorbed toxins to diffuse back across the intestinal membrane and into the lumen; it somewhat dialyzes the intestinal blood. Thus charcoal decreases systemic absorption of toxins by both its absorptive mechanism and its ability to form a diffusion gradient.

Charcoal has an excellent safety profile; it is even considered safe during pregnancy, in lactating women, and in the pediatric population. Although studies show a better safety profile and a more effective decrease in toxin absorption compared with lavage or ipecac-induced emesis, no significant decrease in mortality, length of hospital stay, or likelihood of clinical deterioration has been demonstrated with the use of activated charcoal. In studies using a single dose of at least 50 g of activated charcoal, there was a 47% to 21% reduction in toxin absorption when administered 30 to 180 minutes after toxin ingestion, respectively. According to the AACT (Position Statement 2004), the administration of activated charcoal may be considered if a patient has ingested a potentially toxic amount of a poison up to 1 hour following ingestion. Activated charcoal may be considered more than 1 hour after ingestion, but there are insufficient data to support or exclude its use.

Similarly, although studies have shown statistical significance for multidose charcoal's effectiveness in removing toxins, it has not been shown to reduce morbidity or mortality. Therefore multidosing is usually not recommended except for a select list of drugs (see section on "Indications"). Although there is no evidence supporting their use, cathartics are added to activated charcoal by some experts to hasten elimination. This may be helpful when large doses of charcoal have been administered, which can be constipating. Sorbitol, which is used as a preservative and to decrease the grittiness of charcoal, also enhances the flavor of charcoal by making it slightly sweet. It is not absorbed and therefore encourages water secretion into the lumen, which in turn stimulates bowel peristalsis. However, it can cause severe cramping, hypotension, and vomiting and increase the risk of pulmonary aspiration. Sorbitol with activated charcoal may cause electrolyte imbalances and is not recommended in children. Magnesium, another cathartic, is contraindicated in patients with hypermagnesemia, myasthenia gravis, renal insufficiency, or cardiac arrhythmias. Sodium-based cathartics should be avoided in patients with severe hypertension, renal failure, or congestive heart failure. Mineral oil or other oil-based cathartics should not be used because of risk of aspiration. The concurrent use of a cathartic is not recommended with multidose activated charcoal due to the risk of diarrhea leading to fluid shifts and electrolyte imbalances.

Whole-bowel irrigation uses the infusion of PEG electrolyte solution (the same as used for preparation for colonoscopy) at a rate faster than normal for a bowel preparation. PEG infusion works by decreasing enteric transit time, thereby reducing toxin contact time with the intestinal wall and decreasing absorption. Whole-bowel irrigation does not cause electrolyte disturbances because it does not create an osmotic differential across the intestinal membrane. Whole-bowel irrigation is especially useful for ingestions of toxins not absorbed by charcoal (e.g., iron, lithium, heavy metals), sustained-release or enteric-coated pills (if multidosing charcoal is not indicated), or illegal drug packets. Studies have found whole-bowel irrigation to decrease toxin bioavailability by up to two thirds.

Gastric lavage used to be the chosen method to decontaminate the intestinal tract. However, the American Association of Poison Centers and the EAPCCT have issued a joint statement that gastric lavage should not be used routinely, if ever, in the management of poisoned patients. There are rare cases, such as a recent and potentially lethal ingestion or when other supportive modalities are inadequate or unavailable, in which gastric lavage may be considered after carefully weighing the risks and benefits, preferably in consultation with a poison control center.

As mentioned previously, Syrup of Ipecac is no longer recommended for routine use by the AACT or the EAPCCT. The recommends it be removed from the home. Studies have demonstrated that Syrup of Ipecac is less effective at decreasing systemic absorption than activated charcoal, yields inconsistent results, and has a higher risk of aspiration and other adverse effects as more effective decontamination measures.

INDICATIONS

Activated Charcoal

- Most toxic substances
- Toxins metabolized by the liver and secreted into the bile
- Toxins that are recycled in the enterohepatic circulation and have long half-lives

Multidose Activated Charcoal

- Toxins that are recycled in the enterohepatic circulation and have long half-lives, including some sustained-release or enteric-coated preparations.
- Specific medications include amitriptyline, carbamazepine, dapsone, diazepam, digoxin, doxepin, phenobarbital, phenytoin, piroxicam, quinine, salicylates, tricyclic antidepressants, theophylline.

Whole-Bowel Irrigation

- Life-threatening or serious ingestion not effectively removed by activated charcoal
- Medications with delayed absorption or sustained-release or enteric coatings
- Ingested packets of illicit drugs
- Iron (often seen on flat-plate radiograph)
- Lithium
- Heavy metals
- Activated charcoal not indicated or available

Gastric Lavage

- Gastric lavage should not be routinely used in the management of poisoned patients. Only used in rare cases and after consultation with a toxicologist or poison control center.
- Oral activated charcoal alone is considered superior to gastric lavage if a drug is absorbed by charcoal. Whole bowel irrigation should also be considered prior to lavage.
- Patients who have ingested a potentially life-threatening amount of poison in whom the procedures can be performed within 60 minutes of ingestion are candidates for gastric lavage.
- Substances able to be neutralized (after consultation with toxicologist or poison control center): fluoride, formaldehyde, iodine, oxalic acid.
- Substances with high risk of morbidity or mortality: β-blockers, calcium channel blockers, chloroquine, colchicine, cyanide, heterocyclic antidepressants, paraquat, selenious acid.
- Substances poorly absorbed by activated charcoal: iron, lithium, heavy metals, toxic levels of alcohol.

- Substances that form concretions (with evidence of concretions forming): sustained-release or enteric-coated preparations, phenothiazines, salicylates.

Induced Emesis (Syrup of Ipecac)

- Activated charcoal, whole-bowel irrigation, gastric lavage are not indicated or available.
- Conscious, alert patient
- Potentially toxic dose of poison ingested within 60 minutes

CONTRAINDICATIONS

Activated Charcoal

- Unprotected airway
- Comatose or convulsing patient (unless the airway can be protected)
- Recent gastrointestinal surgery
- Ingestion of corrosive agent and endoscopy is planned.
- Bowel obstruction or ileus
- Recent use of anticholinergic or antiperistaltic drugs
- Substances not absorbed by activated charcoal such as iron, lithium, potassium, inorganic salts, lead, and other heavy metals, cyanide, acids, alkalis, alcohol, boric acid, petroleum distillates (hydrocarbons), pesticides

Use of Cathartic with Activated Charcoal

- Ingestion of a toxin that already causes diarrhea
- Electrolyte abnormality
- Debilitated or elderly patient who may not tolerate
- Children younger than 5 years
- Intestinal obstruction
- Severe dehydration
- Mineral oil or other oil-based cathartics

Use of Sodium-Based Cathartics

- Severe hypertension
- Renal failure
- Congestive heart failure

Use of Magnesium-Based Cathartics

- Hypermagnesemia
- Myasthenia gravis
- Renal failure
- Abnormally slow heart rate

Whole-Bowel Irrigation

- Unprotected airway
- Abnormal gastrointestinal anatomy (e.g., strictures, anomaly) or recent gastrointestinal surgery
- Bowel perforation, obstruction, or ileus
- Ingestions of substances that cause an ileus (e.g., anticholinergics, antiperistaltics, opioids)
- Gastrointestinal bleed
- Vomiting
- Patient unable to remain sitting on toilet (relative contraindication)

Gastric Lavage

- Depressed mental status or inactive or diminished airway reflexes (unless airway can be protected)
- Combative or uncooperative patient
- Ingestion of corrosive agents (acids or alkalis) or hydrocarbons (unless they contain highly toxic substances such as pesticides)

- Known esophageal strictures, gastric bypass surgery, or other abnormal or absent pharyngeal or upper gastrointestinal anatomy
- Active or substantial antecedent vomiting
- Coagulopathy
- Large pills or particles (e.g., mushrooms)
- Large or sharp foreign body
- Nontoxic or minimally toxic ingestion
- Significant risk if aspirated (e.g., low-viscosity hydrocarbon or petroleum distillates)
- More than 60 minutes after ingestion
- Infants and neonates (problematic but not an absolute contraindication)

EQUIPMENT

- Equipment necessary for the clinician to follow universal blood and body fluid precautions (e.g., eye protection, mask, gloves, gown).
- Nasogastric tube. (Optional for administration of activated charcoal [i.e., for the patient who refuses to swallow charcoal], but use at least a 16-Fr diameter in adults for activated charcoal. A 10- to 12-Fr tube can be used for whole-bowel irrigation in anyone older than 1 year; infants can usually tolerate an 8-Fr tube.) An orogastric or nasogastric tube may be used for gastric lavage.
- 2% viscous lidocaine gel, or benzocaine; phenylephrine decongestant nasal spray for nasogastric tube insertion.
- 50-mL tube syringe (Toomey).
- Towel or surgical Chux for covering patient's clothing.
- Paper tissues.
- Emesis basin.
- Suction tube with vacuum generator.
- Endotracheal tube with cuff for obtunded patients or those with an altered mental status or at risk of altered mental status or convulsions because of what they have ingested. Intubation should also be considered to protect the airway in patients who have ingested hydrocarbons.
- Intravenous (IV) antiemetics (e.g., promethazine); optional, but must avoid sedating dose.

Activated Charcoal

Activated charcoal (1 g/kg): Available in doses ranging from 15 to 500 g that must be mixed with water. Premixed suspensions are available; it is also available in capsules or tablets. Flavored versions (e.g., cherry) are available. Preparations are also available containing sorbitol, which is an artificial sweetener and may make the charcoal slurry or solution seem less gritty and more palatable; however, sorbitol is also a laxative.

Whole-Bowel Irrigation

Use 4 to 8 L of balanced PEG electrolyte solution (e.g., Colyte, GoLYTELY, MoviPrep) at body temperature for whole-bowel irrigation.

Gastric Lavage

Use 3 L of normal saline at body temperature for gastric lavage.

- 36- to 40-Fr orogastric tube for adults or a 24- to 28-Fr orogastric tube for children (to be passed through the mouth only).
- Bite block.
- Cetacaine or benzocaine spray for alert patient.
- Oral airway.
- Alternatively, an 18-Fr nasogastric Salem sump tube may be used (may be passed through the nose or the mouth).
- 50-mL syringe.

- Gastric lavage system.
- Large, rigid suction catheter (e.g., Yankauer) attached to wall suction.
- Pulse oximeter, cardiac monitor, noninvasive blood pressure monitor.

PREPROCEDURE PATIENT PREPARATION

The patient or representative should know what to expect when activated charcoal is administered, especially if multiple doses will be needed or a cathartic will be used. The patient should be aware that if he or she is unwilling or refuses to swallow the charcoal, a nasogastric tube will be inserted. Likewise, a nasogastric tube will be inserted for whole-bowel irrigation, and a larger nasogastric or orogastric tube inserted for gastric lavage. The patient or representative should also know what to expect if whole-bowel irrigation or gastric lavage will be performed. IV antiemetics may be used to minimize nausea when any of these procedures are performed (except, of course, induced emesis, unless vomiting is prolonged). Although administration of activated charcoal, whole-bowel irrigation, or gastric lavage is typically performed as an urgent or emergent procedure and most hospitals do not require written informed consent, the risks, benefits, indications, and any possible alternatives should be explained to the patient or representative.

Insertion of a nasogastric or orogastric tube can be very distressing for the conscious patient (see "Preprocedure Patient Preparation" section in Chapter 217, Nasogastric and Nasoenteric Tube Insertion, for additional information).

Airway protection with a cuffed endotracheal tube (see "Preprocedure Patient Preparation" section in Chapter 222, Tracheal Intubation) is very important for a patient whose level of consciousness is depressed, whose airway-protective reflexes are diminished, or who is otherwise in danger of aspiration (e.g., altered mental status, obtunded, unconscious, convulsing). For activated charcoal or whole-bowel irrigation, the patient should be upright or semiupright. For whole-bowel irrigation, the patient should optimally be capable of sitting on the toilet for a few hours. For gastric lavage, the patient should be positioned in the left lateral decubitus position with the head lowered approximately 20 degrees (Trendelenburg position). These positions decrease the risk of aspiration should vomiting occur.

TECHNIQUE

Activated Charcoal

1. If the patient is unable, unwilling, or refuses to swallow the charcoal, place at least a 16-Fr nasogastric tube in adults and confirm its placement before administration of any fluids (see Chapter 217, Nasogastric and Nasoenteric Tube Insertion). Aspirated gastric contents can be saved or sent for analysis if the toxin is unknown. If the patient is unable to protect his or her airway, endotracheal intubation should be considered (see Chapter 222, Tracheal Intubation). (The absence of blinking after touching the eyelashes is strong evidence of inability to protect the airway from vomitus.) Intubation should also be considered in any patient who has ingested a central nervous system depressant or any substance that can cause altered mental status or seizures. The patient should not undergo endotracheal extubation until 4 hours after the last dose of charcoal is administered.
2. Charcoal can be ordered as capsules, tablets, powder, or oral suspension/solution. However, with an acute toxin ingestion, only powder mixed with water or a premixed oral suspension or solution, with or without a cathartic, is recommended. Older-style preparations or suspensions were gritty and, although they had no taste, were unpleasant to swallow. Newer-style preparations dissolve completely when added to water and form a solution.

3. Optimally, administration of charcoal should occur within the first hour of ingestion.
4. Mix the powder in water to achieve a slurry.
5. It has become standard practice to administer 50 to 100 g of charcoal for an adult and 1 g/kg (maximum 50 g) for a child.
6. An IV antiemetic can be administered to decrease vomiting/nausea. Avoid a sedating dose.
7. In adults, activated charcoal can be mixed with 70% sorbitol (1 g/kg) or 10% solution of magnesium citrate (typically given as 250 mL for adults).
8. For multidose charcoal treatment, follow the initial dose of 50 to 100 g with 25 to 50 g every 4 hours, possibly alternating with and without a cathartic. (A cathartic is not used with each dose to avoid side effects such as very large stools, dehydration, and electrolyte abnormalities.) Monitor the patient between doses to verify the presence of bowel sounds and to confirm the absence of distention or an ileus.
9. The nasogastric tube should be removed at least before extubation to avoid aspiration of charcoal as the nasogastric tube is being removed.

Whole-Bowel Irrigation

1. Place the nasogastric tube and confirm its placement before administration of any fluids (see Chapter 217, Nasogastric and Nasoenteric Tube Insertion). Consider endotracheal intubation in the patient who may become obtunded or sedated or may convulse. A 10- to 12-Fr tube can be used for whole-bowel irrigation in anyone older than 1 year; infants can usually tolerate an 8-Fr tube.
2. Introduce PEG electrolyte into the nasogastric tube at an initial rate at 25 mL/kg per hour. Increase the rate, depending on patient tolerance, while also trying to avoid vomiting and abdominal distention. Adults often tolerate greater than 3 L of PEG per hour.
3. Continue treatment until the patient passes the ingestant or clear rectal fluid.
4. The patient should be continually assessed for any signs of airway compromise, ileus, or abdominal distention. If significant abdominal distention occurs or there is a loss of bowel sounds, irrigation should be held for 30 to 90 minutes and the patient reassessed. If bowel sounds have returned, irrigation can be resumed at a reduced rate. If the patient tolerates irrigation at the reduced rate, and the clinical status improves, it can be continued at this rate or possibly increased gradually as tolerated.

Gastric Lavage

1. Before lavage, obtain IV access and begin continuous cardiac monitoring and pulse oximetry.
2. If the patient is highly anxious, consider giving a small dose of benzodiazepine (e.g., 1–2 mg midazolam IV).
3. Consider rapid-sequence induction and intubation, with a cuffed endotracheal tube if the patient has a depressed level of consciousness, questionable airway, or if airway compromise may occur during the procedures.
4. Premeasure and mark the length of the tube needed by estimating the distance from the nose, around the ear, and down to the midepigastrium.
5. Position the patient the left lateral decubitus position with the head lowered approximately 20 degrees (Trendelenburg position) to reduce the risk of aspiration of gastric contents if vomiting occurs.
6. Restrain the hands of an uncooperative patient to prevent removal of the gastric or endotracheal tube.
7. A bite block or an oral airway may prevent the patient from biting on the orogastric tube or biting the fingers of the inserter.

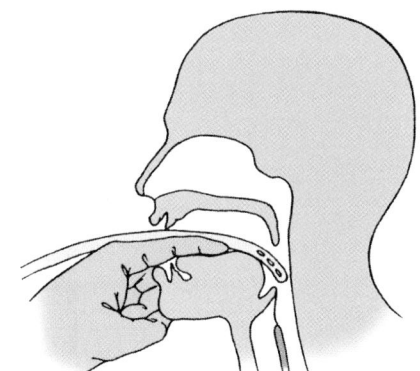

Fig. 209.1 Orogastric tube insertion.

8. If using a nasogastric tube for nasal insertion, see the procedure for nasogastric tube insertion in Chapter 217, Nasogastric and Nasoenteric Tube Insertion.
9. For orogastric tube insertion, if the patient is alert, spray the posterior pharynx with topical benzocaine or Cetacaine spray. Position the patient's head so that it is flexed as far forward as possible, and while ensuring against being bitten (bite block in place), insert your gloved finger and middle finger over the base of the patient's tongue. Guide the lubricated gastric tube over the dorsum of your fingers as the patient swallows (Fig. 209.1). Pass it gently to avoid damage to the posterior pharynx. Never use force to pass the tube. If the patient gags, advance the tube immediately after gagging. When the pharynx has been entered, put the patient's chin on the chest to facilitate passage of the tube into the esophagus. Cough, stridor, or cyanosis indicates tracheal intubation; withdraw the tube immediately and reattempt passage.
10. Confirm intragastric tube placement initially by auscultating the stomach while introducing air with a 50-mL syringe. In an intubated or obtunded patient or a young child, confirm tube position radiographically before lavaging, although this is not routinely performed. Verify the final placement by aspirating and confirming gastric contents. *It is critical to avoid infusion of fluids until tube placement is confirmed.*
11. Before beginning gastric irrigation, remove the gastric contents by careful aspiration with repeated repositioning of the tip of the tube.

Open-System Procedure (Fig. 209.2)

12. With the Y-connector closed system, perform lavage by clamping the drain arm of the Y-adapter and infusing aliquots of fluid (2–3 mL/kg per cycle) into the stomach from a reservoir. Clamp the reservoir arm of the Y; then open the drainage arm to permit drainage of the stomach contents via gravity. Repeat this procedure. Some resistance is produced by the Y-connector and tubing. Apply suction intermittently to the drainage tubing to enhance emptying of the stomach. With an active system, use a syringe or vacuum suction equipment, instead of gravity, to evacuate the gastric contents.
13. Prewarmed normal saline at body temperature is generally preferred, particularly in children due to the risk of electrolyte disturbances with the use of tap water. Alternatively, tap water can be used to perform gastric lavage in adults.
14. Repeatedly introduce small aliquots of lavage solution (200–300 mL) and remove them. Continue irrigation until you have used at least 3 L of lavage for adults and the return is clear on visual inspection.
15. Alert patients should take oral activated charcoal as necessary. For the nonalert patient, a slurry of activated charcoal can be administered through the same system.
16. If an awake patient begins to vomit during lavage, remove the tube immediately to allow the patient to protect the airway.

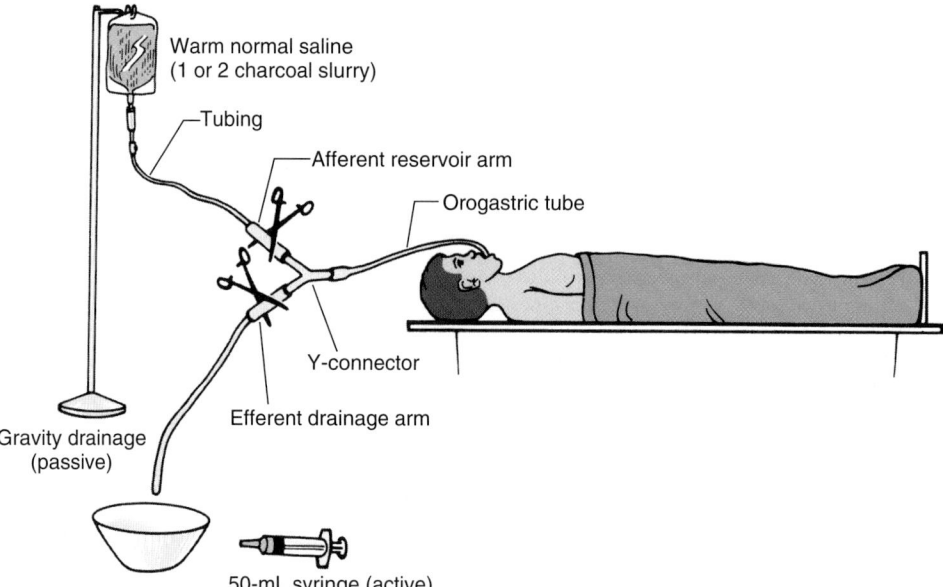

Fig. 209.2   Open gastric lavage system assembly with components.

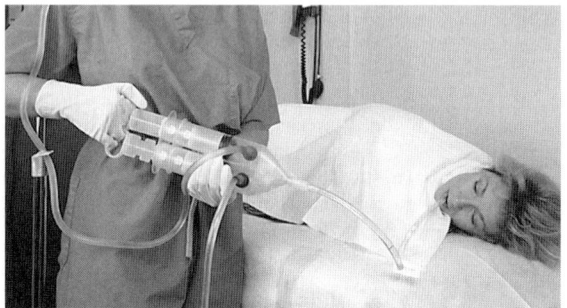

Fig. 209.3   Gastric lavage system assembly with components.

17. When the procedure is completed, clamp or pinch the gastric tube during removal to prevent contaminating the lung with gastric contents or charcoal. If repeated doses of charcoal are deemed necessary, the large tube maybe replaced with a standard, smaller nasogastric tube. In the obtunded, intubated patient, leave the endotracheal tube in place for at least 15 minutes after gastric tube removal to prevent aspiration. Confirm adequate spontaneous respirations and oxygenation by pulse oximetry before removing the endotracheal tube.

Closed-System Procedure (Fig. 209.3)

18. With a waste bag hanging from the bed, close the fluid bag clamp and fill the fluid bag. Hang the fluid bag from an IV pole. The position of the gastric tube should have been previously confirmed. Advance both syringe plungers to the fully forward position.
19. Open the fluid bag clamp, and pull both plungers back. This should fill one syringe with fluid from the IV bag, and the other with gastric contents. Then again advance both plungers to the fully forward position. This should empty the gastric contents into the drainage bag while instilling additional fluid into the stomach.
20. Repeatedly introduce small syringes full of lavage solution and removing them until you have used at least 3 L of lavage for adults and the return is clear on visual inspection. Next, follow steps 15 through 17 from the Open Drainage System procedure.

COMPLICATIONS

The main complications of activated charcoal administration are aspiration, intestinal obstruction, and electrolyte imbalances or dehydration from cathartic use. Aspiration is prevented by following the patient's alertness and gag reflexes as he or she is ingesting the activated charcoal, or by endotracheal intubation. Anticholinergic and antiperistaltic drugs should not be administered around the time of activated charcoal administration because they slow down gastrointestinal transit time and increase the risk of bezoar formation.

Caution should be taken when giving a cathartic with activated charcoal. Cathartics should be withheld in any patient who has ingested a toxin that may itself already cause diarrhea. Also, they should not be given to children younger than 5 years. Cathartic-induced hypernatremia is a serious side effect that has been reported in young children. Magnesium should not be administered in patients with hypermagnesemia, myasthenia gravis, an abnormally slow heart rate, intestinal obstruction, or kidney failure. Finally, cathartics are not recommended with every dose of multidose charcoal.

Pulmonary aspiration with subsequent chemical pneumonitis can be a devastating complication of gastric lavage. It is less likely with whole-bowel irrigation. Such risk can be minimized by proper patient positioning and observing the patient closely. Laryngospasm and resultant hypoxia are possible complications of any aspiration. Risks versus benefits must be considered when performing any of these procedures.

Mucosal injury or perforation of the upper gastrointestinal tract is also a possible complication of nasogastric or orogastric intubation or gastric lavage. Up to 50% of patients will complain of nausea, gassiness, mild discomfort, or distention with whole-bowel irrigation; however, these symptoms do not mandate discontinuation of the procedure.

Fluid and electrolyte disturbances are possible with gastric lavage; these are more common when tap water is used instead of saline. The risk of hypothermia can be minimized by using body-temperature PEG or saline. Cardiac dysrhythmias, due to aspiration or otherwise, are possible complications of gastric lavage. Other possible complications are the same as for nasogastric tube insertion (see Chapter 217, Nasogastric and Nasoenteric Tube Insertion).

PATIENT EDUCATION GUIDES

See the sample patient education form available at www.expertconsult.com.

CPT/Billing Codes

43754   Gastric intubation and aspiration(s) therapeutic, necessitating physician's skill (e.g., for gastrointestinal hemorrhage), including lavage if performed

ICD-10-CM Diagnostic Codes

NOTE: Most of these codes need a specific fourth digit.

T36.94XX	Poisoning by antibiotics
T37.8X4X	Poisoning by other anti-infectives
T38.804X	Poisoning by hormones and synthetic substitutes
T45.94XX	Poisoning by primarily systemic agents
T37.2X4X	Poisoning by agents primarily affecting blood constituents
T39.8X4X	Poisoning by analgesics, antipyretics, and antirheumatics
T42.8X4X	Poisoning by anticonvulsants and antiparkinsonian drugs
T42.74XX	Poisoning by sedatives and hypnotics
T41.204X	Poisoning by other central nervous system depressants and anesthetics
T43.8X1X	Poisoning by psychotropic agents
T43.604X	Poisoning by central nervous system stimulants
T44.904X	Poisoning by drugs primarily affecting the autonomic nervous system
T46.904X	Poisoning by drugs primarily affecting the cardiovascular system
T47.8X4X	Poisoning by drugs primarily affecting the gastrointestinal system
T50.4X4X	Poisoning by water, mineral, and uric acid metabolism drugs
T48.204X	Poisoning by agents primarily on muscles
T51.94XX	Toxic effect of alcohol
T52.0X4X	Toxic effect of petroleum products
T54.1X4X	Toxic effect of corrosive aromatics, acids, and caustic alkalis
T56.0X4X	Toxic effect of lead and its compounds

Add appropriate seventh character: A = initial, D = subsequent, S = sequela.

Suppliers

(See contact information available at www.expertconsult.com)

Activated charcoal
Paddock Laboratories
Vista Pharmaceuticals
Gastric lavage: closed system
Evacu-Stat
Mason Tayler Medical Products
TUM-E-VAC (available with activated charcoal systems)
Ethox Corp.
Gastric lavage open system: Argyle Edlich gastric lavage tray
Cardinal Health
Kendall Company (Covidien)
PEG solution
Braintree Laboratories

Acknowledgment

The editors recognize the contributions of John Harlan Haynes III, MD, Andrew Thomas Haynes, MD, and Michael Zeringue to this chapter in previous editions of this text.

RECOMMENDED READING

Aks SE, Gummin DD. Whole bowel irrigation. In: Reichman E, ed. *Emergency Medicine Procedures.* 2nd ed. New York: McGraw-Hill; 2013.

American Academy of Pediatrics Committee on Injury. Violence, and Poison Prevention. Poison treatment in the home. American Academy of Pediatrics Committee on Injury, Violence, and Poison Prevention. *Pediatrics.* 2003;112:1182.

Bond G. The role of activated charcoal and gastric emptying in gastrointestinal decontamination: a state-of-the-art review. *Ann Emerg Med.* 2002;39:273–286.

Haynes JH. Gastric lavage for serious poisonings. *Fam Pract Recert.* 1992;14:45.

Hendrickson RG, Kusin S. *Gastrointestinal Decontamination of the Poisoned Patient;* 2017. www.uptodate.com.

Holstege CP, Borek HA. Decontamination of the poisoned patient. In: Roberts JR, Custalow CB, Thomsen TW, eds. *Roberts & Hedges' Clinical Procedures in Emergency Medicine.* 6th ed. Philadelphia: Elsevier; 2014.

Lu JJ. Gastric lavage. In: Reichman E, ed. *Emergency Medicine Procedures.* 2nd ed. New York: McGraw-Hill; 2013.

Lu JJ. Activated charcoal administration. In: Reichman E, ed. *Emergency Medicine Procedures.* 2nd ed. New York: McGraw-Hill; 2013.

Marx JA, Hockberger RS, eds. *Rosen's Emergency Medicine: Concepts and Clinical Practice.* 8th ed. Philadelphia: Elsevier; 2014.

Mowry JB, Spyker DA, Brooks DE, Zimmerman A, Schauben JL. 2015 annual report of the American Association of Poison Control Centers' National Poison Data System (NPDS): 33rd annual report. *Clin Toxicol.* 2016;54(10):924–1109.

Olson KR. Poisoning. In: McPhee SJ, Papadakis MA, eds. *Current Medical Diagnosis and Treatment.* 48th ed. New York: McGraw-Hill; 2009:1388–1416.

Position statement and practice guidelines on the use of multi-dose activated charcoal in the treatment of acute poisoning. American Academy of Clinical Toxicology; European Association of Poisons Centres and Clinical Toxicologists. *J Toxicol Clin Toxicol.* 1999;37:731.

Position paper. Whole bowel irrigation. *J Toxicol Clin Toxicol.* 2004;42:843.

Position paper. Ipecac syrup. *J Toxicol Clin Toxicol.* 2004;42:133.

Position paper. Cathartics. *J Toxicol Clin Toxicol.* 2004;42:243.

Position paper. Single-dose activated charcoal in the treatment of acute poisoning. American Academy of Clinical Toxicology and European Association of Poisons Centres and Clinical Toxicologists. *Clin Toxicol.* 2005;43:61–87.

Smith SW, Ling LJ, Halstenson CE. Whole bowel irrigation as a treatment for lithium overdose. *Ann Emerg Med.* 1991;20:536–539.

Tenenbein M. Whole bowel irrigation. In: King C, Kenretig FM, eds. *Textbook of Pediatric Emergency Procedures.* 2nd ed. Philadelphia: Wolters Kluwer; 2008.

Tintinalli JE, Stapczynski JS, Ma OJ, et al., eds. *Tintinalli's Emergency Medicine: A Comprehensive Study Guide.* 8th ed. New York: McGraw-Hill; 2015.

Vale JA, Kulig K. American Academy of Clinical Toxicology, European Association of Poisons Centres and Clinical Toxicologists. Position paper: gastric lavage. *J Toxicol Clin Toxicol.* 2004;42:933.

CHAPTER 210

DIAGNOSTIC PERITONEAL LAVAGE

Eric Skye

Diagnostic peritoneal lavage (DPL) is a procedure that consists of two components. The first involves attempting to aspirate any free blood in the peritoneal cavity. If this initial portion of the procedure is positive (i.e., reveals hemoperitoneum), the remainder of the procedure is aborted. Hemoperitoneum in this circumstance is highly predictive of intraperitoneal injury and warrants a laparotomy.

If there is no free blood during the initial aspiration, the second portion of the procedure is performed. This involves infusion of normal saline or lactated Ringer solution into the peritoneal cavity. The fluid is then drained and analyzed; results may not only confirm an injury but also suggest the nature of the intra-abdominal pathology.

Physical examination can be misleading in up to 45% of patients with blunt abdominal trauma. Spiral (helical/real-time) abdominal computed tomography and focused abdominal sonography for trauma (often performed at the bedside; see Chapter 214, Emergency Department, Hospitalist, and Office Ultrasound [Clinical Ultrasound]) are generally the preferred initial diagnostic tests for these patients. However, DPL continues to be an important test in patients who are hemodynamically unstable (i.e., cannot be safely transported to radiology) or for whom bedside ultrasound is not available. While DPL is invasive, it is the most sensitive of these three tests for mesenteric and hollow viscous injuries. DPL also serves as an adjunct in the evaluation of the patient with penetrating trauma. While it is beyond the scope of this chapter, peritoneal lavage can also be used to warm the hypothermic patient by infusion of large volumes of warmed fluid.

ANATOMY

DPL is traditionally performed in the midline, 1 to 2 cm below the umbilicus, which allows entry into the peritoneal cavity through the linea alba (the fibrous structure separating the rectus abdominis muscles). This fibrous band is relatively avascular and provides safe access for both the open and closed techniques. If DPL is performed above the umbilicus, the omentum frequently interferes. When performed below the umbilicus, it is also usually easier to advance the catheter into a dependent location such as the pelvis.

INDICATIONS

- Blunt abdominal trauma in a patient who is either hemodynamically unstable or has an altered mental status or abnormal sensation (e.g., spinal cord injury).
- Penetrating injuries (e.g., stab wound or gunshot wound) to the abdomen, flank, back, or lower chest. (Gunshot wounds that penetrate the peritoneum result in intraperitoneal injury in 98% of cases, so they warrant laparotomy. DPL should only be used for tangential gunshot wounds to the abdomen. Likewise, penetration into the peritoneum from a thoracoabdominal wound results in a diaphragmatic injury that, by definition, needs to be repaired; they warrant going straight to surgery. Penetration through the retroperitoneum from the back or flank will cause a significant injury in 73% of cases; DPL may help determine whether the retroperitoneum has been traversed. Only two thirds of stab wounds to the anterior abdomen will penetrate the peritoneum, and of these, only 50% will require repair. Use of DPL in these cases may reduce the need for laparotomy.)
- Penetrating injuries to the abdomen, flank, back, or lower chest or blunt abdominal trauma in a patient who has an unreliable physical examination or in whom serial physical examinations are not practical (e.g., patient under anesthesia for orthopedic or neurosurgical procedure or taking postoperative analgesics).
- Patient in shock after trauma who has other potential sources of hemorrhage (e.g., thoracic, retroperitoneal) to determine whether intraperitoneal hemorrhage is contributing to shock. DPL can frequently be performed while the patient is undergoing resuscitative efforts.

CONTRAINDICATIONS
Absolute

Acute abdomen requiring immediate surgery is the only absolute contraindication.

Relative

If DPL is performed, use the open technique.

- Previous abdominal surgery (bowel may be adherent to midline; although DPL may be performed in area away from scar, compartmentalization of abdomen may have occurred, preventing blood circulation and causing false-negative DPL result).
- Coagulopathy.
- Pregnancy (DPL should be performed above the level of the uterine fundus; possibly below umbilicus in early-stage pregnancy).
- Morbid obesity (the locator needle may not be long enough to pierce abdominal wall).
- Pelvic fracture (use open technique above the umbilicus; closed technique may result in penetration of a retroperitoneal hematoma, a false-positive result, and decompression of the hematoma).
- Abdominal wall infections.
- Inability to insert Foley catheter to decompress bladder (e.g., urethral injury or stricture).
- Clinician with lack of training or familiarity with DPL.

EQUIPMENT

Commercially prepared kit or the following equipment:

- Skin-cleansing solution (povidone-iodine or chlorhexidine).
- Sterile gloves, mask, and equipment to maintain universal blood and body fluid precautions.
- Sterile marking pen (if area has not been marked indelibly before skin preparation).
- Sterile drapes.
- 4 × 4 gauze squares.

- 1% or 2% lidocaine with epinephrine.
- No. 11 scalpel.
- 9- to 18-Fr peritoneal catheter (kit equipped with catheter-over-wire system for closed or Seldinger technique).
- 10-mL syringe for anesthetic in the alert patient.
- 10-mL syringe for diagnostic tap.
- 50-mL syringe, if using stopcock technique.
- 18-gauge, 1.5- to 3-inch locator needle; alternatively, an 18- or 20-gauge, 1.5- to 3-inch spinal needle may be substituted.
- 25- or 27-gauge, 1.5-inch needle.
- Purple-topped blood collection tube.
- Sterile intravenous (IV) fluid (1 L warmed lactated Ringer solution or normal saline, as opposed to fluid at room temperature, is preferred) and tubing.
- Foley catheter.
- Nasogastric tube.
- Three-way stopcock (for use with 50-mL syringe) (optional).

Additional equipment for open technique:

- Razor
- No. 15 blade
- Instruments for retraction such as Army-Navy retractors
- Two tissue forceps
- Two Allis clamps
- Four hemostats
- Needle holder
- Nylon skin suture (4-0 or 5-0) on cutting needle
- Absorbable sutures (2-0 Vicryl) for peritoneum and fascia

PRECAUTIONS

- An open technique should be considered if the patient has a relative contraindication such as coagulopathy, pregnancy, previous abdominal surgery, pelvic fracture, or morbid obesity.
- A surgical assistant is recommended for open DPL.
- DPL will not diagnose retroperitoneal hemorrhage.

PREPROCEDURE PATIENT PREPARATION

- Explain the procedure and its risks and benefits to the patient as well as any alternatives if possible (see the section on "Complications").
- Obtain verbal or written informed consent if possible.
- Place patient in the supine position.
- If necessary, use wrist restraints, especially for patients with altered mental status, to prevent contamination of the sterile field or self-injury.
- Consider procedural sedation (see Chapter 1, Procedural Sedation and Analgesia), especially if performing an open DPL.

EDITOR'S NOTE: Reviewing Chapter 219, Abdominal Paracentesis, may also be helpful.

TECHNIQUE

Procedural setup and fluid removal are identical for the open and closed techniques.

1. Use a nasogastric tube and Foley catheter for decompression of the bladder and stomach, respectively. (See Chapter 217, Nasogastric and Nasoenteric Tube Insertion, and Chapter 96, Bladder Catheterization [and Urethral Dilation].)
2. Prepare the abdominal skin at the puncture site with standard preparation solutions such as povidone–iodine or chlorhexidine, and apply sterile drapes as appropriate. The ideal site is immediately inferior to the umbilicus (Fig. 210.1). Again, the supraumbilical approach may be used in second- or third-trimester pregnant patients, patients with prior lower abdominal surgery, or patients with pelvic fractures.

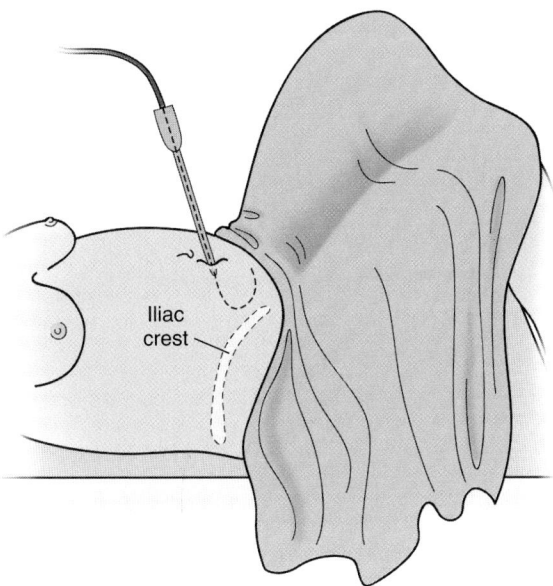

Fig. 210.1   Insertion of the needle into the peritoneal cavity in the midline, immediately inferior to the umbilicus.

3. Infiltrate the skin, subcutaneous tissues, and fascia with lidocaine with epinephrine.

Closed (Seldinger) Technique

This is the preferred technique, if not contraindicated.

4a. Attach an 18-gauge locator needle to the syringe and insert it into the midline, 1 to 2 cm inferior to the umbilicus, directed at a 45-degree angle to the skin and toward the pelvis. Applying negative pressure on the syringe, insert the needle through the skin and directly into the peritoneal space. Three "pops" are felt as the needle penetrates the skin, the fascia, and the peritoneum. If blood is aspirated during this step, it is considered a positive result. If not, proceed to step 5.
5a. The guidewire is introduced through the 18-gauge needle until only 7 to 10 cm of the guidewire remains outside the needle. You may then safely remove the needle, although there must be continuous control of the wire to prevent inward migration and injury to peritoneal structures. If there is difficulty inserting the guidewire or the patient complains of pain, both the needle and guidewire should be removed as a unit. To avoid shearing it off, do not withdraw the guidewire through the needle.
6a. Slide the peritoneal catheter over the wire using gentle twisting motions. With the closed technique, it may be necessary to make a small skin nick at the entry site with the scalpel to allow for passage of the lavage catheter.
7a. Remove the wire after the catheter is in the peritoneum. Proceed to step 8.

Open Technique

4b. The skin should be shaved before preparation. Using the No. 11 blade, create a 4- to 6-cm vertical skin incision in the midline.
5b. By blunt dissection, proceed down to the rectus fascia. Clamp and ligate any bleeders with absorbable suture before opening the fascia to prevent a false-positive test result. Open the rectus fascia using the No. 15 blade. Proceed down to the peritoneum by sharp and blunt dissection.
6b. A 2- to 3-mm opening of the fascia is adequate for a semiopen technique. This technique provides room for the catheter to be inserted directly into the peritoneal space, even though visualization of the structures is not possible.

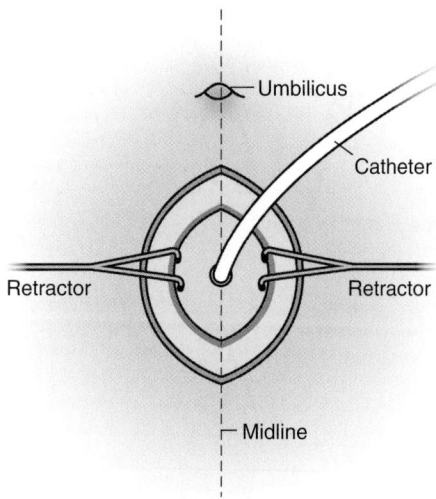

Fig. 210.2 Open technique, view from above. Superficial layers have been opened and are retracted away from the field of view. Catheter is inserted through the opened peritoneum directly into the peritoneal space.

7b. A slightly longer incision of the fascia is required for the open technique. The longer incision allows for the peritoneal space to be opened and visualized. The catheter can then be inserted into the peritoneal space under direct visualization (Fig. 210.2). Proceed to step 8.

Both Techniques

8. Attach the syringe to the catheter and attempt to withdraw fluid. If more than 10 mL of blood is obtained, the patient should be prepared for emergent laparotomy. If the tap is dry, proceed to peritoneal lavage.
9. Connect the IV tubing and infuse lactated Ringer solution or normal saline. The amount infused is 1 L for adults and 15 mL/kg for children.
10. The infused fluid is then removed by placing the IV bag on the floor and allowing the fluid to return by gravity. Alternatively, the IV tubing may be connected to a 1-L vacuum jar. The fluid should return at a steady rate of flow. If this flow is interrupted, it is probably due to omentum blocking the holes in the catheter. Placing pressure on the patient's abdomen may increase the flow; alternatively, the catheter may need to be withdrawn slightly and reinserted. If these maneuvers do not increase the return flow, a second liter of IV fluid may be infused.
11. At least 200 to 300 mL of lavage fluid should be returned for a valid test. After the maneuvers described previously have been performed, if less than 200 to 250 mL of return flow is obtained, a second catheter should be inserted. This should be inserted 1 cm below the first in the same manner as the first, in the midline. A second IV bag should then be attached and lowered to collect fluid via gravity drainage. After the fluid is removed, gently remove the catheter and apply pressure to the wound. When the open technique is used, close the peritoneum and rectus fascia with absorbable suture. The skin is then closed with nylon suture. If the closed technique was used, placement of a pressure dressing alone may suffice, although a single nylon skin suture may be necessary in some patients. A small amount of fluid should be transferred to the purple-topped tube for laboratory analysis.

SAMPLE OPERATIVE REPORT

See the Sample Operative Report online at www.expertconsult.com.

COMPLICATIONS

Complication rates range from 0.6% to 2.3% of all DPLs. There is no difference in complication rates among the techniques discussed.

- Bladder perforation
- Bowel perforation
- Laceration of a major vessel
- Abdominal wall hematoma
- Abdominal wall dehiscence after open technique
- Infection (local, intraperitoneal, or systemic)
- False-positive result (vessel laceration during procedure) or false-negative result (poor catheter placement or loss of fluid into the thoracic cavity)

POSTPROCEDURE PATIENT EDUCATION

If the DPL result is positive, the patient should be informed of the need for emergent surgery. The patient with a negative DPL should be observed in the hospital for up to 24 hours. He or she should remain NPO during the initial observation period and receive analgesics as needed. Before discharge, it is useful to determine whether the patient can tolerate a regular diet. Also before discharge, educate the patient about the signs and symptoms of a complication such as bleeding, pain, vomiting, or infection. The patient should be given instructions regarding wound care.

INTERPRETATION OF RESULTS

The aspiration of greater than 10 mL of gross blood on entering the peritoneal cavity or through the locator needle is considered a positive finding. If not grossly bloody, fluid aspirated through the catheter should be sent for a red blood cell (RBC) count, a white blood cell count, and possibly to check for amylase. A finding of more than 100,000 RBCs/mm^3 is also considered positive (half these numbers if 2 L of fluid were infused). Finding 20,000/mm^3 to 100,000/mm^3 RBCs should be considered equivocal. In these patients, an observation period of 12 to 24 hours should be considered. Two situations provide exceptions to these general rules: (1) stab wounds to the lower chest where diaphragmatic injury is suspected (the diaphragm does not bleed as readily as other abdominal organs), and (2) gunshot wounds. The threshold for a positive RBC count should be 5000 RBC/mm^3 in these situations. Always be mindful of the hemodynamic stability of the patient when interpreting these results.

A white blood cell count greater 500 cells/mm^3 is also considered a positive test and warrants laparotomy. Amylase may be elevated when there is injury to the gastrointestinal tract; however, a positive amylase test is neither sensitive nor specific. Confusion sometimes exists when a small amount of gross blood (<10 mL) is aspirated directly from the catheter (as opposed to the locator needle). This may have been the only blood located in a dependent portion of the abdomen and may not indicate the patient is unstable. The patient does not need a laparotomy if the subsequent lavage is negative.

CPT/BILLING CODES

49084   Peritoneal lavage, including imaging guidance, when performed

ICD-10-CM DIAGNOSTIC CODES

K66.1   Hemoperitoneum (nontraumatic)
S21.309X   Injury, diaphragm, with open wound into cavity
S36.39XX   Injury to stomach
S36.119X   Injury to liver
S36.09XX   Injury to spleen
S37.009X   Injury to kidney
S37.99XX   Injury to pelvic organs

| S36.899X | Injury, other intra-abdominal organs, without mention of open wound into cavity |
| S36.81XX | Injury, peritoneum, without mention of open wound into cavity |

SUPPLIERS

(See contact information available at www.expertconsult.com.)

PERITONEAL LAVAGE KIT

Teleflex Inc.

Acknowledgment

The editors recognize the contributions of Michael Brown, MD, Brett White, MD, and Kenneth Hu, MD, to this chapter in previous editions of this text.

RECOMMENDED READING

Diercks DB, Mehrotra A, Nazarian DJ, Promes SB, Decker WW, Fesmire FM. American College of Emergency Physicians. Clinical policy: critical issues in the evaluation of adult patients presenting to the emergency department with acute blunt abdominal trauma. *Ann Emerg Med.* 2011;57(4):387–404.

Johar S, Lakshmanadoss U. Diagnostic peritoneal lavage. In: Reichman EF, ed. *Emergency Medicine Procedures.* 2nd ed. New York: McGraw-Hill; 2013.

Puskarich MA, Marx JA. Abdominal trauma. In: Marx JA, Hockberger JS, eds. *Rosen's Emergency Medicine: Concepts and Clinical Practice.* 8th ed. Philadelphia: Elsevier; 2014.

Runyon MS, Marx JA. Peritoneal procedures. In: Roberts JR, Custalow CB, Thomsen TW, eds. *Roberts & Hedges' Clinical Procedures in Emergency Medicine.* 6th ed. Philadelphia: Elsevier; 2014.

CHAPTER 211

TUBE THORACOSTOMY AND EMERGENCY NEEDLE DECOMPRESSION OF TENSION PNEUMOTHORAX

Scott Savage

Tube thoracostomy, or chest tube insertion, is performed to evacuate air or fluid from the pleural space. A related procedure, emergency needle decompression, is performed to relieve a tension pneumothorax, is a life-threatening condition. Air progressively accumulates in the pleural space, eventually compressing the lung and the mediastinum; this causes decreased blood flow in the great vessels and subsequent death. Patients with tension pneumothorax present with dyspnea, tachycardia, and hypoxia. Jugular venous distention and midline tracheal shift are classically described but rarely present. Hypotension is an ominous sign that signifies obstructive shock.

The radiographic features of a tension pneumothorax are a 100% pneumothorax with a midline shift away from the collapsed lung. However, if this condition is clinically suspected, an emergency needle decompression should be performed; to wait for a confirming chest radiograph is unnecessary. A preprocedural chest radiograph should be obtained only in stable patients in whom the diagnosis is in question.

It may be difficult to diagnose a tension pneumothorax in an infant because lobar emphysema can mimic a pneumothorax. Making the correct diagnosis is essential because chest tube insertion in the presence of lobar emphysema can make the infant worse. If the infant is hemodynamically stable, it is advisable to get three radiographic views of the chest—lateral, anteroposterior, and lateral decubitus—with the affected side inferior. A specialist in radiology, pediatrics, or pediatric emergency medicine should be consulted to help with film interpretation.

EMERGENCY NEEDLE DECOMPRESSION

Indication

Tension pneumothorax indicates the need for emergency needle decompression.

Contraindication

Lobar emphysema in infants is a relative contraindication. In the patient with a coagulopathy, it is very important to make sure that anatomic landmarks are correct and the procedure is performed correctly.

Equipment

- Antiseptic solution (e.g., povidone-iodine, chlorhexidine)
- Sterile hemostat
- 10-mL syringe half-filled with 2% lidocaine with epinephrine (or

equivalent) attached to a large-bore (18-gauge or larger), 2-inch catheter-over-needle (angiocatheter). A 20- or 22-gauge 1-inch catheter-over-needle should be used in preterm infants, neonates, and children up to 1 to 2 years of age. An 18- or 20-gauge 1.5-inch catheter-over-needle should be used for children 1 to 6 years of age. (Increase needle size and length in older children based on body habitus compared with adults.) Some clinicians prefer using a butterfly needle with attached tubing in preterm children, neonates, and infants up to 1 year of age. The tip of the attached tubing should be submerged in sterile water or saline in a specimen container.
- Supplemental oxygen (100% face mask oxygen), continuous cardiac monitoring, pulse oximetry, and blood pressure monitoring, if available.
- Equipment necessary to follow universal blood and body fluid precautions.
- Ultrasound machine (optional) with low-frequency (2.5–5 MHz) probe and sterile ultrasound gel.

Technique

1. Place the patient in the semiupright position (head of bed elevated to 30 to 60 degrees).
2. Provide supplemental oxygen. If available, continuous cardiac monitoring, pulse oximetry, and blood pressure monitoring is helpful. Intravenous access is desirable if available.
3. Obtain rapid verbal consent with a witness present if possible.
4. Apply antiseptic solution to a generous area of the second intercostal space where a line drawn laterally from the level of the sternomanubrial junction (Lewis line) would intersect a line drawn down from the midclavicle (midclavicular line).
5. Locate the upper border of the third rib at this intersection.
6. Insert the catheter-over-needle perpendicular to the skin just above the upper border of the third rib (Fig. 211.1). (Remember that the neurovascular bundle runs below the ribs.) Universal blood and body fluid precautions should be followed. Once through the skin, infiltrate the tissue with half of the anesthetic solution.
7. Before proceeding further, attempt aspiration. If air is obtained, then the catheter-over-needle is not secured to the syringe tightly enough. Use the hemostat to tighten the catheter hub on the syringe before advancing the catheter-over-needle any farther.
8. After creating the skin wheal and testing the seal, advance the catheter-over-needle at a moderate rate with continuous aspiration until air is obtained—this will be noted by bubbles in the syringe and easy aspiration. There may also be a rush of air, with or without blood, into the syringe.

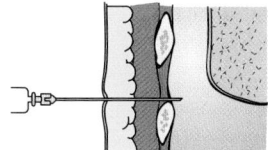

Fig. 211.1 Placement of a catheter within a needle. The needle is inserted slightly above the rib, and air should return or express itself through the needle.

9. Advance the catheter-over-needle an additional half centimeter to prevent accidental dislodgement.
10. Using the hemostat, unscrew the syringe to allow free passage of air. Do not hook the needle up to suction. The air in the thoracic cavity is under pressure (under tension) and will exit the needle spontaneously; it should gush out. Intrathoracic pressure will equilibrate with room air, which is acceptable until a tube thoracostomy is placed.
11. Do not remove the needle at this point. In older texts, it was advised to remove the needle because the plastics in older catheters were much harder than the soft Silastic catheters now used. Unlike the older catheters, the new catheters are too soft to endure the tissue pressure of the intercostal muscles and will rapidly collapse, causing reaccumulation of the tension pneumothorax. Concerns that the reexpanding lung will be impaled on and lacerated by the needle (pulmonary laceration) are generally unfounded. In the presence of a 100% pneumothorax, it is unlikely that lung tissue will be near the needle tip as long as suction is not used. The purpose of this procedure is to relieve excessive intrathoracic pressure and allow blood to circulate. Subsequent tube thoracostomy, hopefully performed very soon after emergency needle decompression, will provide full lung reexpansion. The time to remove the catheter-over-needle (angiocatheter) is just prior to applying suction to the chest tube.
12. If the first attempt fails to decompress the pleural space, ultrasound can be used to measure the chest wall's thickness and thus to determine appropriate needle length.

NOTE: In one ultrasound study (Ball and collegues, 2010), a catheter-over-needle 1.25-inch long failed to reach the pleural space in 65% of adults; however, a 1.75-inch catheter-over needle should reach the pleural space in 96% of adults.

TUBE THORACOSTOMY

Indications

- Pneumothorax
- After needle decompression of a tension pneumothorax
- Chylothorax
- Hydrothorax
- Empyema.
- Hemothorax
- Malignant pleural effusion
- Pleurodesis
- Recurrent pleural effusion
- Prevention of a hydrothorax after thoracotomy (cardiothoracic or lung resection surgery)
- Tube thoracostomy is often needed following blunt or penetrating trauma to the chest. The tube may be placed prophylactically in patients with penetrating injuries to the chest who are about to undergo endotracheal intubation and general anesthesia.

Contraindications

- No contraindications if the procedure is emergent.
- Bleeding dyscrasia.

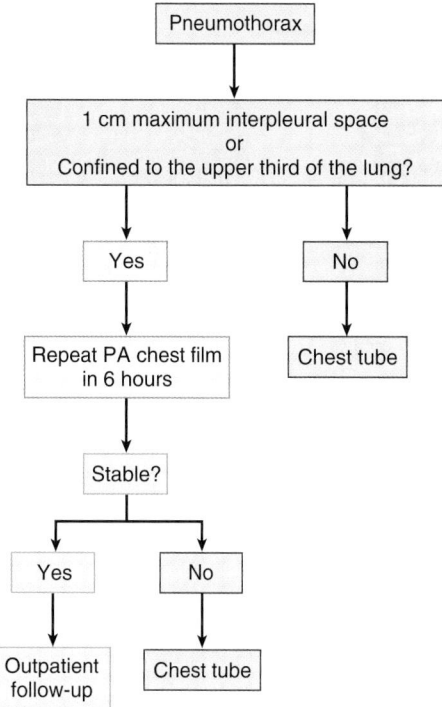

Fig. 211.2 Algorithm used for deciding on the necessity for thoracostomy. *PA,* Posteroanterior.

- Severe thrombocytopenia (platelet count <50,000/mL relative contraindication).
- Large pulmonary blebs or bullae (relative contraindication).
- Conditions causing pleural scarring in the area of planned insertion.
- Empyema with acid-fast organisms.
- History of pleurodesis.
- Use caution if loculated fluid collections are present.
- Pneumothorax of less than 20% that is stable for 6 hours (Fig. 211.2). Also if there is no associated hemothorax following trauma.
- Known or suspected mesothelioma.
- Patients requiring open thoracotomy.
- Skin infection over insertion site.

There are many methods to determine whether or not a pneumothorax is greater than 20%. One method is to use the "1 cm and one-third rule": if a pneumothorax creates no more than 1 cm distance between the pleural line and the inner chest wall and is also confined to the upper third of the chest on an anteroposterior upright radiograph, the pneumothorax is less than 20%. This may resolve without any intervention (see Fig. 211.2). Stability is gauged by comparing a chest radiograph taken initially to one obtained 6 hours later. Although it may require thoracostomy, a simple pneumothorax is the accumulation of air that is not under pressure within the pleural space.

Results from some studies suggest that mere aspiration of a simple pneumothorax can be performed without placing a chest tube. However, this method is still controversial because other studies indicate little better than a 50% success rate. The success rate may be higher in carefully selected patients.

Equipment

- Adhesive tape (Tensoplast or Elastoplast preferred)
- Antiseptic solution (e.g., povidone-iodine, chlorhexidine)
- Chest tube (alternatives are Seldinger guidewire kit or catheter-over-needle kit; Heimlich valve can be attached)
- Connector (5-in-1, also known as Christmas tree connector)

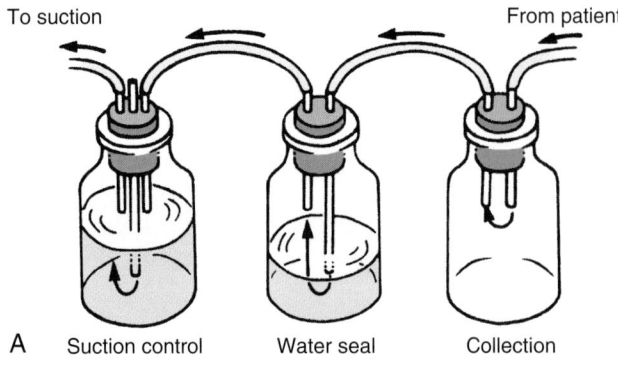

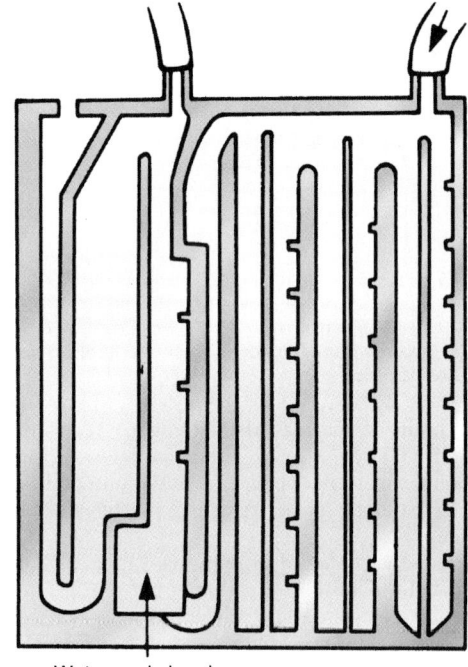

Fig. 211.3 (A) Three-bottle system: the first bottle *(right)* is the collection chamber; the second bottle *(center)* is the water seal; and the third bottle *(left),* closest to the wall suction, is the suction control chamber. (B) Disposable suction unit.

- Local anesthetic
- Petroleum-impregnated gauze
- Sterile drapes
- Sterile gown and gloves
- Suction-drainage system (Fig. 211.3)
- Surgical mask, cap, and goggles; equipment necessary to follow universal blood and body fluid precautions
- Wall suction unit
- Supplemental oxygen, pulse oximetry, continuous cardiac and blood pressure monitoring
- Thoracostomy tray
  - 4 sterile towels
  - 1 package 4 × 4 inches sterile gauze pads
  - 4 towel clips (optional)
  - 1 large straight scissors
  - 1 large curved (Mayo) scissors
  - 2 large curved (Kelly) clamps
  - 2 medium-sized clamps
  - 1 needle holder
  - 1 package of 2-0 to 4-0 nonabsorbable suture (e.g., silk, nylon)
  - 1 No. 11 or No. 10 scalpel mounted on a holder
  - Sterile water or saline

NOTE: Trocars have a high complication rate and should not be used.

Adult tube size selection
- Primary spontaneous pneumothorax: 7 to 14 Fr
- Secondary spontaneous pneumothorax: 20 to 28 Fr
- Trauma, mechanical ventilation, or detectable pleural fluid: 28 to 40 Fr

Secondary spontaneous pneumothoraces are associated with underlying lung diseases such as chronic obstructive pulmonary disease, asthma, cystic fibrosis, infection, interstitial lung disease, neoplasms, connective tissue disease, pulmonary infarction, and endometriosis.

PROCEDURES

Initial Preparation (for All Techniques)

1. Obtain written informed consent if possible. Patient should be aware of the indications, risks, and complications of the procedure and know whether any alternatives exist.
2. Because the procedure can be rather painful, the patient should be warned and prepared, even if a local anesthetic is used. Procedural sedation is recommended (see Chapter 1, Procedural Sedation and Analgesia). If time allows, obtain a partial thromboplastin time, international normalized ratio, and platelet count.
3. Place the patient on 100% oxygen. (Use of oxygen increases the resorption rate of pneumothorax fourfold.)
4. Monitor the patient with pulse oximetry and continuous cardiac and blood pressure monitoring.
5. An ultrasound (see Chapter 214, Emergency Department, Hospitalist, and Office Ultrasound [POCUS]) may be helpful for localizing the air or fluid levels and for possibly excluding any anatomic variants that could place the patient at risk. It can also be used to measure chest wall thickness to determine how far to penetrate.
6. Assemble the suction-drainage system according to the manufacturer's recommendations.
7. Connect the suction-drainage system to suction.
8. Create a sterile field for the equipment.
9. Measure the length of tube to be inserted from the midaxillary line at the fifth intercostal space to the inferior tip of the scapula. A piece of suture with the needle removed is often used to make this measurement.
10. In a sterile manner, open the package containing the tube and occlude the distal end at the properly measured distance with a large sterile clamp.
11. The distal end (usually beveled) of the tube can be cut so that it is "squared off," if needed, to ensure a firm connection.
12. Place the patient in the semiupright position (elevate head of bed 30 to 60 degrees if possible) with the ipsilateral arm placed overhead and the wrist secured with a soft restraint. Use standard restraint monitoring.
13. Maintain sterile technique, including use of face mask, gown, and sterile gloves, and observe universal blood and body fluid precautions.
14. Mark the fifth intercostal space just slightly anterior to the midaxillary line. In males, this is generally one space below the nipple line. In females, it is generally two fingerbreadths above the base (not the tip) of the xiphoid. Although an anterior approach was used in the past for pure pneumothoraces, it has fallen out of favor. (Studies have failed to demonstrate a significant clinical advantage, and this approach leads to worse cosmetic results.) The posterior approach is generally reserved for thoracentesis.
15. Prepare the incision site with antiseptic solution and drape the patient to create an adequate sterile field.

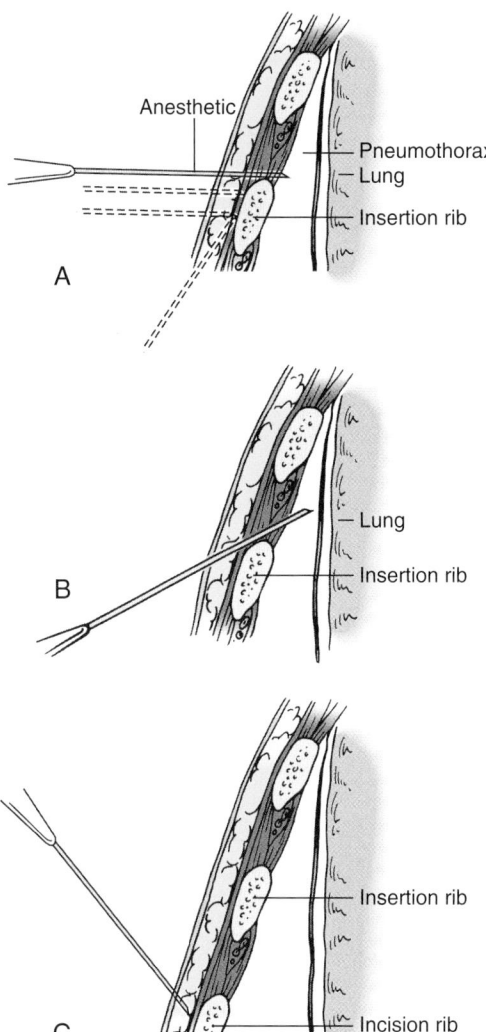

5. Once air, blood, or fluid has been obtained, feed the guidewire posteriorly and superiorly toward the scapula in adults or anteriorly and superiorly toward the manubrium or sternal notch in small children.
6. Maintaining manual control of the guidewire at all times, remove the locator needle and nick the skin in a direction parallel to the rib with a No. 11-blade scalpel to about one third the depth of the scalpel blade.
7. Feed the smallest dilator over the guidewire with a twisting motion, and once through the skin, aim toward the tip of the scapula in adults and the sternal notch in small children.
8. If progressive dilators are available, use these to gradually widen the insertion track.
9. Remove the dilators and insert the chest tube over the guidewire to the premeasured length.
10. Remove the guidewire.
11. Attach the chest tube to the suction-drainage system. Be careful when removing the distal clamp, as blood or fluid may flow forcefully from the tube.
12. Have the patient cough, and check for bubbles in the water seal, which indicates good flow. (A Heimlich valve may then be used for a simple pneumothorax with no recurrent leaking.)
13. Secure the tube with tape (Tensoplast or Elastoplast tape is preferred; avoid taping the nipple), and obtain a chest radiograph. Suturing is not absolutely necessary, although it is recommended to ensure that the tube does not get dislodged. Likewise, petroleum gauze is not absolutely required unless an air leak is identified.
14. If no adjustment is needed, tape the suction connector to the tube.
15. Consider the use of prophylactic antibiotics. Guidelines from the Eastern Association of Surgeons of Trauma recommend the use of first-generation cephalosporins (e.g., cephalexin) during the first 24 hours for patients undergoing chest tube drainage for hemothorax (Luchette et al., 2000).

Using Pneumothorax Evacuation Kits (Catheter-Over-Needle, Heimlich Valve)

1. Special kits containing a single catheter-over-needle device, a connector, and a Heimlich valve are available. They are used only with simple pneumothoraces but are very convenient and effective for that purpose.
2. Prepare as directed under "Initial Preparation," Enter the interspace using the locator needle. Remove the needle.
3. Insert the catheter-over-needle tip just above the top of the rib in the anesthetized area, slowly advance the needle perpendicular to the thorax, and enter the pleural cavity while aspirating for air (similar to Fig. 211.1).
4. Once air is obtained, the catheter is advanced, the needle removed, and the Heimlich valve connected.
5. The Heimlich valve is taped to the anterior chest wall. This reduces the chance of the patient accidentally dislodging it with his or her elbow.
6. A postprocedural radiograph is required.
7. Although clinical judgment is required, it has been suggested that many patients receiving these types of devices may be discharged for next-day follow-up.

Traditional (Open) Technique

1. Prepare as directed under "Initial Preparation."
2. At the fifth intercostal space in the midaxillary line where the lower skin wheal was anesthetized, create a 2- to 5-cm skin incision (approximately two fingerbreadths) that follows the rib (Fig. 211.5).
3. Using a curved Kelly clamp, bluntly dissect until bone or muscle fascia is reached.
4. From this position, change the direction of the dissection superiorly, with the tips of the clamp directed upward, until the upper border of the next rib is reached (Fig. 211.6). This should be at the level of the second anesthetic wheal.

Fig. 211.4 Infiltration of the skin, subcutaneous muscle, and periosteum of the rib (A), the pleura (B), and skin incision site (C) with local anesthetic.

16. In a sterile fashion, infiltrate the skin with 2 to 4 mL of lidocaine 2% with epinephrine or equivalent local anesthesia at the incision site. Be careful to insert the needle just above the upper border of the rib. This avoids damage to the neurovascular bundle, which lies in a groove at the lower border of the ribs. Then use up to 6.5 mg/kg lidocaine with epinephrine (1 mL of 2% lidocaine contains 20 mg of lidocaine) to anesthetize the deeper structures along the tract that the chest tube will traverse and enter the pleural space (Fig. 211.4 shows a Z-tract technique).

Seldinger Guidewire Technique

1. Prepare as directed under "Initial Preparation."
2. The Seldinger guidewire technique requires use of a prepackaged kit but it is generally preferred to the traditional open technique. For most operators, it is simpler, faster, and safer than the open technique. A Z-tract technique is unnecessary.
3. Open the kit and check the inventory to make sure that all necessary materials are present and double check that the items listed on the package cover have been properly packaged. (Note that some kits do not include the ancillaries [cleaning swabs, tape, lidocaine for anesthetic].)
4. Using the locator needle, insert the tip just above the top of the rib in the anesthetized area, slowly advance the needle perpendicular to the thorax, and enter the pleural cavity while aspirating for air, blood, or other fluid (similar to Fig. 211.1).

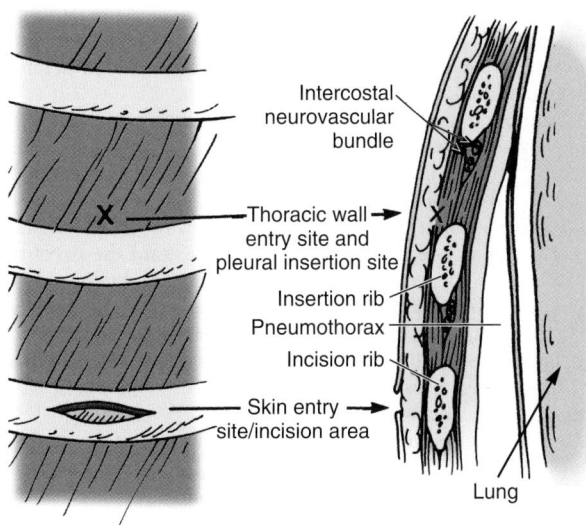

Fig. 211.5 A skin incision is made one rib below the rib over which the tube will pass. Location of the intercostal neurovascular bundle is shown.

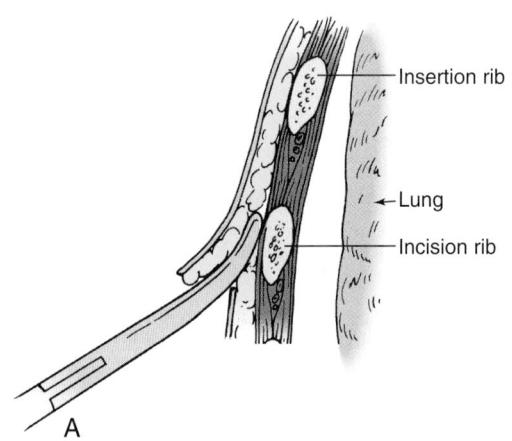

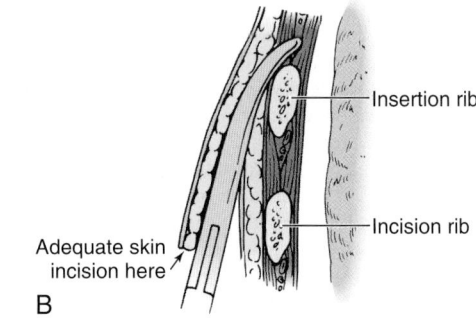

Fig. 211.6 Tunneling procedure for forming a Z-tract.

5. From that position, rotate the tip of the curved clamp inward and use it to push through the intercostal muscle and parietal pleura. A popping sensation is often felt. (Do not push the clamp too far into the pleural space, where it could cause damage to the great vessels, heart, diaphragm, or lungs.)

6. Once inside the pleural space, open the clamp and withdraw partially to widen the space. Be careful not to withdraw completely, as you may then lose the opening and therefore have to begin again.

7. Using the other hand, place a gloved finger in the pleural space (Fig. 211.7) as you withdraw the open curved clamp completely. The idea is to keep either the clamp or your finger in the hole at all times to prevent losing the opening.

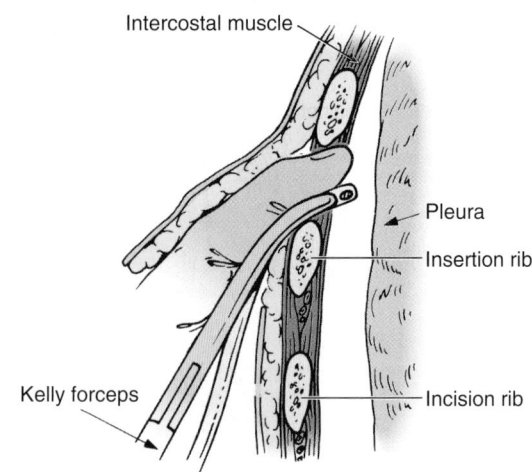

Fig. 211.7 Tip placement in the pleural cavity using the finger as a guide.

8. Sweep the finger to confirm proper placement (you should not feel the diaphragm) and to detect and break up any adhesions.

9. Estimate the distance from the skin incision to the apex of the lung by laying the chest tube over the patient. The apex of the lung is at about the level of the clavicle. Apply a clamp onto the chest tube at the estimated site at which the tube is to exit the skin incision. Using the other curved clamp, grasp the proximal end of the tube (fenestrated end) and guide the tube into the pleural space. Release the lead clamp and withdraw your finger as you advance the tube into the pleural space. Again, the idea is to keep either your finger or the tube in the hole at all times to avoid losing the opening. Advance until the fenestrations are no longer visible and the marking clamp is at the skin incision. The marking clamp can then be removed. To confirm placement in the pleural cavity, you can slide a finger along the tube to verify that it is in the proper location. Condensation is often seen inside the tube and air movement should be audible during respirations. The tube should rotate freely in your hand. A chest radiograph is eventually taken to verify placement.

10. Connect the tube to the suction-drainage system. Be careful when opening the distal clamp, as blood or fluid may flow forcefully from the tube.

11. Attach the suction-drainage system to suction.

12. Have the patient cough, and check for bubbles in the water seal; this indicates a patent system.

13. Suture the tube in place, taking care not to puncture the tubing. A variety of techniques are acceptable. A common one is to use a single horizontal mattress suture to close the incision around the tube. After tying a knot and before cutting the suture ends, wind one end around the tube several times and back to tie to the other end (Fig. 211.8). Alternatively, a second suture can be placed through the skin; it is then wound around the tube several times and secured with a knot. Centurion Medical Products manufactures chest tube trays as well as a Centurion Chest Tube Anchor (Centureon Medical Products).

14. Wrap the tube with petroleum gauze and secure the tube with tape (avoid taping the nipple).

15. Obtain a chest radiograph. If the chest tube is kinked, bent, in the fissure of the lung, or in the subcutaneous tissues, remove it and insert a new one.

16. If no adjustment is needed, then tape the suction connector to the tube and the tube to the patient's side. (Tensoplast or Elastoplast tape is preferred.)

17. Consider the use of prophylactic antibiotics. Guidelines from the Eastern Association of Surgeons of Trauma recommend the use of first-generation cephalosporins (e.g., cephalexin) during the first 24 hours for patients undergoing chest tube drainage for hemothorax (Luchette et al., 2000).

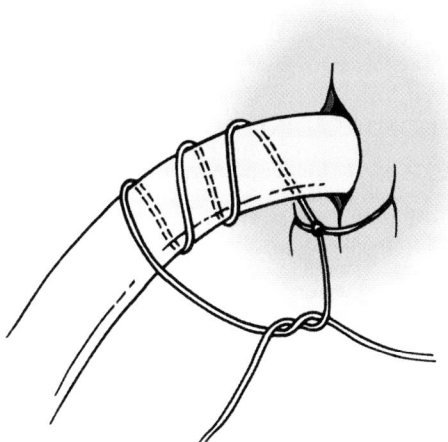

Fig. 211.8   Chest tube fastened with a stay suture.

MANAGEMENT

After the chest tube has been inserted, it should be connected to the suction-drainage system. Suction should be maintained until there is no air leak. Although many different protocols exist as to when to consider removing the tube, the most prudent method is to turn off the suction after the patient's lung reexpands and allow the patient to remain on water seal for 6 to 12 hours to detect occult air leaks. Chest tube dressings should be changed every 24 hours, or sooner if the dressing becomes saturated.

A chest radiograph taken 4 to 6 hours after chest tube insertion should show improvement in the pulmonary condition. If the patient's condition is not improved, check for persistent bubbling in the system. If bubbling is present, check the connections between the chest tube, connectors, and hosing throughout the system. If the air leak continues, place cloth tape over all the connections. Examine a chest radiograph to confirm that all fenestrations are within the thoracic cavity. If not, replace the tube (merely advancing the current chest tube may track infectious material into the pleural cavity). If the air leak persists, check the tubing for holes or cracks and replace any damaged tubing. If the air leak continues, place a second chest tube and prepare the patient for thoracoscopy, bronchoscopy, or esophagoscopy to diagnose the etiology of the leak.

Pain can be managed with parenteral analgesics and sedation. If the source of the pain is thought to be the chest tube, it may respond to intrapleural administration of bupivacaine. Administer 20 to 40 mL of 0.25% bupivacaine through the chest tube and into the pleural cavity. Clamp the chest tube for up to 10 minutes to allow the bupivacaine to coat the pleural cavity. Monitor and observe the patient for tension pneumothorax while the tube is clamped. Unclamp the chest tube and allow excess anesthetic to drain into the collecting system.

CHEST TUBE REMOVAL

Indications

* No air drainage for 24 hours
* Less than 150 mL fluid drainage in 24 hours

Contraindication

A persistent need for a chest tube contraindicates its removal.

Equipment

* Suture scissors
* Petroleum gauze

* Several sterile 4 × 4 inches gauze sponges
* Tape (Tensoplast or Elastoplast preferred)
* Equipment necessary to follow universal blood and body fluid precautions
* Equipment necessary to replace chest tube if required (patient may require urgent replacement)

Removal Technique

1. If sutures were used to secure the tube during placement, cut the sutures. Observe universal blood and body fluid precautions.
2. Disconnect the tube from the suction-drainage system.
3. If the patient is awake and cooperative, have the patient exhale and hold his or her breath. (This prevents ambient air being drawn in.) If the patient is nonalert and artificially ventilated, pause the ventilator in exhalation.
4. Swiftly and smoothly remove the tube.
5. Apply petroleum gauze covered by sterile 4 × 4 inches gauze sponges.
6. Apply a pressure dressing with tape (Tensoplast or Elastoplast preferred).
7. Repeat the chest radiograph in 6 to 12 hours.
8. Observe for complications.
9. After 48 hours, the dressing may be removed. The patient should follow routine wound care instructions.

COMPLICATIONS

* Injury to the heart, great vessels, lung, diaphragm, liver, spleen, or even the intestines
* Subdiaphragmatic placement of tube
* Open pneumothorax
* Tension pneumothorax
* Dislodgement of the tube
* Subcutaneous emphysema
* Reexpansion pulmonary edema
* Unexplained or persistent air leakage
* Hemorrhage from an injured intercostal artery
* Local or more generalized infection

CPT/BILLING CODES

32550	Insertion of indwelling tunneled pleural catheter with cuff
32551	Tube thoracostomy, includes connection to drainage system (e.g., water seal), when performed, open
32552	Removal of indwelling tunneled pleural catheter with cuff
32554	Thoracentesis, needle or catheter, aspiration of the pleural space; without imaging guidance
32555	With imaging guidance
32556	Pleural drainage, percutaneous, with insertion of indwelling catheter; without imaging guidance
32557	With imaging guidance

ICD-10-CM DIAGNOSTIC CODES

A15.0	Pneumothorax, tuberculous
A15.6	Empyema, tuberculous
C78.2	Pleura malignant or pleural effusion, malignant
J94.8	Chylous hydrothorax
J86.9	Empyema, without mention of fistula (use additional code to identify infectious organism [B95–B97])
J90	Pleurisy with effusion, bacterial, nontuberculous
J94.2	Hemothorax or hemopneumothorax
J91.8	Pleural effusion, unspecified
J93.0	Pneumothorax, tension, spontaneous

J95.811	Pneumothorax, due to operative injury of chest wall or lung
512.8	Pneumothorax, spontaneous
P28.9	Hemothorax, newborn
S27.0XXA	Pneumothorax, traumatic, without mention of open wound into thorax
S27.1XXA	Hemothorax, traumatic, without mention of open wound into thorax
S27.2XXA	Pneumohemothorax, traumatic, without mention of open wound into thorax

Acknowledgment

The editors recognize the contributions of Nelly Otero, MD, and José Ramón García, MD, to this chapter in previous editions of this text.

SUPPLIERS

(Full contact information is available at www.expertconsult.com.)
Atrium Ocean wet suction water seal chest drain system and thoracostomy tubes
   Atrium Maquet Getinge Group
Emergency pneumothorax kits
   Cook Medical, Inc.
Pleur-Evac water seal chest drain system and thoracostomy tubes
   Teleflex Medical
Thoracentesis tray with catheter-over-needle
   Cardinal Healthcare Company
Water seal chest drain systems, thoracostomy tubes, thoracentesis trays, and pneumothorax tray with 8-F catheter; Argyle Aqua-Seal Systems; Argyle Turkel Safety thoracentesis and pneumothorax tray
   Medtronic

ONLINE RESOURCES

Merck Manual: How to Do a Needle Thoracostomy: http://www.merckmanuals.com/professional/pulmonary-disorders/diagnostic-and-therapeutic-pulmonary-procedures/how-to-do-needle-thoracostomy

RECOMMENDED READING

Ball CG, Wyrzykowski AD, Kirkpatrick AW, et al. Thoracic needle decompression for tension pneumothorax: clinical correlation with catheter length. *Can J Surg.* 2010;53:184–188.

Cline DM, Ma OJ, Cydulka RK, eds. *Emergency Medicine: Just the Facts.* 3rd ed. New York: McGraw-Hill; 2013.

Luchette FA, Barrie PS, Oswanski MF, et al. Practice management guidelines for prophylactic antibiotic use in tube thoracostomy for traumatic hemopneumothorax: the EAST practice management guidelines work group. *J Trauma.* 2000;48:753–757.

Marx JA, Hockberger R, eds. *Rosen's Emergency Medicine.* 8th ed. Philadelphia: Elsevier; 2014.

Reichmann EF, ed. *Emergency Medicine Procedures.* 2nd ed. New York: McGraw-Hill; 2013.

Roberts JR, Custalow CB, Thomsen TW, eds. *Roberts and Hedges Clinical Procedures in Emergency Medicine and Acute Care.* 7th ed. Philadelphia: Elsevier; 2019.

Sun J, Xu Z. The role of prophylactic antibiotics in thoracostomy. *Aust N Z J Surg.* 2010;80:127–128.

Tintinelli JE, Stapczynski JS, Ma OJ, eds. *Tintinalli's Emergency Medicine: A Comprehensive Study Guide.* 8th ed. New York: McGraw-Hill; 2015.

CHAPTER 212

ANAPHYLAXIS

Daniel J. Derksen

Anaphylaxis is an acute and serious allergic reaction in response to antigen exposure in a previously sensitized patient. It can be encountered after administration of intramuscular (IM) antibiotics; vaccines; contrast material, such as intravenous (IV) pyelography or computed tomography contrast; local anesthetics; allergy injection in the office setting; or exposure to latex. Patients may also report to a clinician's office with a clinical picture of anaphylaxis after being bitten by an insect (Fig. 212.1) or snake or exposed to some other allergen (e.g., pollen, latex, certain food products). The source of the allergic reaction may be unknown to the patient. The exact incidence of anaphylaxis is unknown, but it is estimated that there are 1500 fatal cases per year in the United States and the incidence is increasing. Although previously the term "anaphylactoid" was used to distinguish non–immunoglobulin E-mediated events from immunoglobulin E-mediated "anaphylaxis," because the clinical presentation and treatment are identical, the current World Allergy Organization guidelines (2013) no longer use the term anaphylactoid.

Medical procedures frequently require injections or use of foreign materials. The clinician must be prepared to treat the rare but serious complication of anaphylaxis.

DIAGNOSIS

Depending on the severity of reaction, patients may have a variety of symptoms, including swelling, rash, urticaria, pruritus, dyspnea, abdominal pain, vomiting, and decreased blood pressure from baseline (Figs. 212.2 and 212.3). As the anaphylaxis proceeds, respiratory compromise may occur with laryngeal edema, bronchospasm, and hypoxia. The patient may progress into shock as manifested by hypotension, tachycardia, peripheral vasodilation, and mental status changes. If the clinician does not take immediate steps to reverse the anaphylactic reaction in the final stages, vascular collapse and death can occur within minutes.

Vasovagal reactions (e.g., fainting and seizure-like activity) and injection of intravascular anesthetic that can cause lightheadedness and ringing in the ears may be confused with an anaphylactic response. However, vasovagal reactions are usually associated with bradycardia, hypotension, and pallor as opposed to the tachycardia, urticaria, and respiratory distress associated with anaphylaxis.

EQUIPMENT

Clinicians should be prepared to treat anaphylaxis in the office, especially if any injections are given. A collection of medications and equipment, the "crash cart," can be gathered and placed in one area. Alternatively, a fishing tackle box or medical emergency kit can be made. The simplest and best-organized method is to use commercially available Banyan kits (Fig. 212.4). These kits, similar to suitcases, are stocked with various medications. They vary in size, contents, and cost ($800 to $1000). The Banyan Stat Kit 750 (approximately $1795 to $1995) is essentially a portable crash cart, lacking only a defibrillator. The specifics on medications and

equipment needed are too extensive to detail in this chapter. The Banyan Stat Kit 750 includes Banyan's KMCA Refill System, which monitors and automatically replaces expiring medications.

Whether the commercially available kits are used or a do-it-yourself collection is assembled, the entire office staff must know where the kit is stored. One person must be in charge of keeping the medications current. Drugs cannot be borrowed from this kit for other purposes. It may be worth using a cable tie to keep the box sealed with an expiration date on it to prevent inadvertent use.

The clinician in charge of office procedures must be prepared for emergencies. Assembling a crash cart or obtaining a Banyan kit may appear expensive, but it is a good practice to have one available and is an inexpensive form of malpractice coverage in the event of an emergency.

TECHNIQUE

Patients who exhibit signs and symptoms of anaphylaxis should be treated immediately. Any triggering agent (e.g., insect stinger, infusion of medication) should be removed. The patient should be placed in the supine position, IV access established, and supplemental oxygen provided, as well as continuous cardiac and blood pressure monitoring and pulse oximetry. In the earliest stages, anxiety, swelling, urticaria, pruritus, and mild dyspnea respond quickly to epinephrine. The dose can be 0.3 to 0.5 mL of a 1:1000 solution (pediatric 0.1 mg/kg), given subcutaneously or IM (anterolateral thigh) every 5 to 10 minutes as needed (to a maximum of three doses). In the milder reactions, antihistamines such as diphenhydramine hydrochloride (Benadryl), 25 to 50 mg (pediatric 1 mg/kg) by the IV, IM, or oral route every 6 hours, can be given. Some suggest that using both histamine type 1 and 2 receptor antagonists (H_1 and H_2 blockers; e.g., 50 mg diphenhydramine and 150 mg ranitidine [pediatric 1 mg/kg] oral or IV) may be more effective than diphenhydramine alone

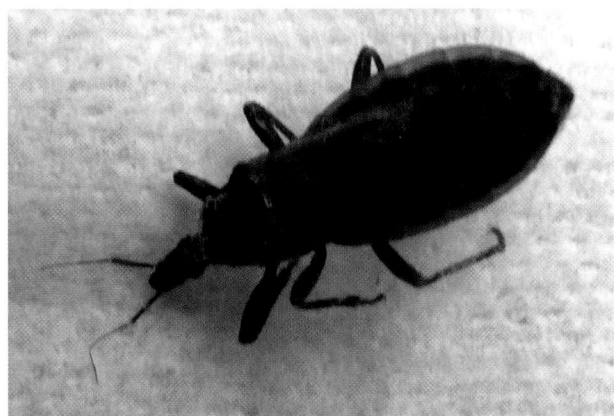

Fig. 212.1 Insect bites, such as those caused by kissing bugs (Reduviidae kissing bugs), can cause anaphylactic reactions in a small percentage of the population. The reaction may start as urticaria (hives) at the site of the bite.

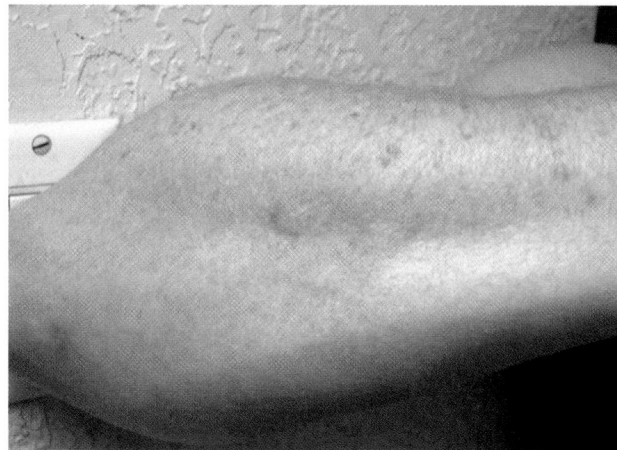

Fig. 212.2 Urticaria. Without prompt treatment, urticaria can quickly progress to angioedema.

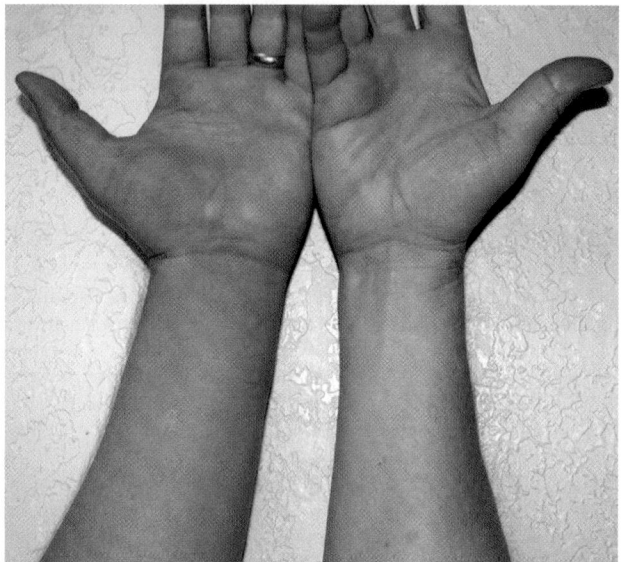

Fig. 212.3 Angioedema of the left arm and generalized anaphylaxis.

(despite little evidence supporting this combination). Although not helpful in the acute situation, systemic steroids can be given as a prednisone taper, beginning with 30 to 60 mg (pediatric 1 mg/kg) the first day and gradually tapering to nothing over a 2-week period.

In truly emergent situations, 5 mL (pediatric 0.1 to 0.25 mL/kg) of a 1:10,000 solution of epinephrine should be given IV over 10 minutes and repeated every 5 minutes as needed. Consider an IV continuous epinephrine drip or other pressors (e.g., dopamine, norepinephrine, phenylephrine, vasopressin). Although not helpful in the acute situation, 125 to 250 mg methylprednisolone (Solu-Medrol; pediatric 1 to 2 mg/kg) IV can be given. Infusion of 1 to 2 liters (pediatric 20 mL/kg) of normal saline through large-bore IV lines may be supportive.

If bronchospasm occurs, aerosolized albuterol 2.5 mg diluted to 3 mL of normal saline can be given continuously to both adults and children. Ipratropium 0.5 mg (pediatric 0.25 mg) in 3 mL normal saline can be given and repeated as necessary. In addition, consider summoning an ambulance. Patients on β-blockers may exhibit more severe anaphylactic symptoms and be refractory to epinephrine. Administration of glucagon (1-mg ampule), atropine (1 mg IV), or isoproterenol (0.1 mg/kg initially) may be necessary to stabilize patients on β-blockers who do not respond to epinephrine.

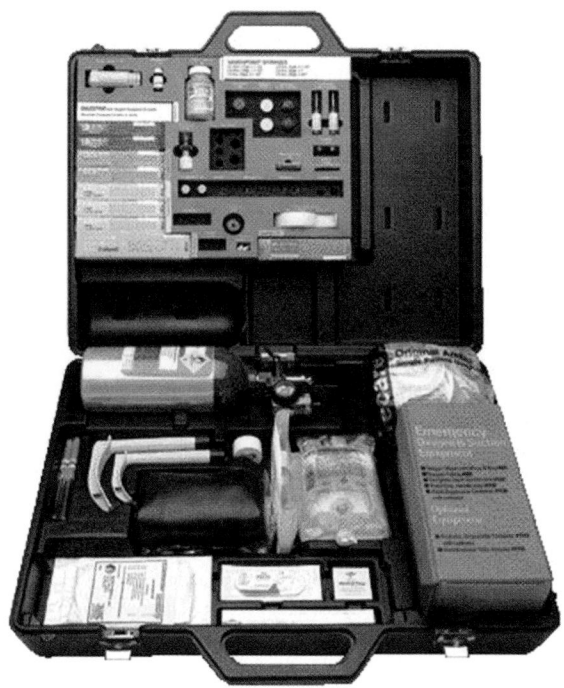

Fig. 212.4 **Banyan kit.** (Courtesy Banyan International Corporation, Mukilteo, WA.)

Clinicians should consider basic life support and advanced cardiac life support training and certification as appropriate if administering medications or therapies that might cause anaphylactic reactions. If the patient responds rapidly to epinephrine and has no further symptoms, a shorter monitoring period may be possible. For those patients refractory to treatment, or those requiring multiple doses, it may be necessary to be more aggressive, including summoning an ambulance and following basic life support and advanced cardiac life support protocols until the patient is safely transported.

Patients with anaphylactic reactions must be observed for an appropriate period after treatment to ensure there is no recurrence. Up to 20% of patients may have a biphasic reaction which is recurrence of symptoms without reexposure to the triggering agent. Most occur within 8 hours, but it can happen as far out as 72 hours. Patients who presented with wheezing, laryngeal edema, or gastrointestinal symptoms or those with asthma or who ingested the allergen are more likely to have a biphasic reaction. Guidelines suggest an observation period of 4 to 8 hours if they have complete resolution of symptoms. Consider hospitalization for patients with protracted anaphylaxis, airway involvement, or hypotension, those that required more than two doses of subcutaneous or IM epinephrine or IV epinephrine, or those with poor social support.

NOTE: A quick way to administer epinephrine is to have a preloaded syringe system of epinephrine (e.g., EpiPen Epinephrine 0.3 mg, Adrenaclick 0.3 mg, or Auvi-Q 0.3 mg Auto-Injectors for those weighing more than 30 kg [66 lb] or EpiPen Jr. 0.15 mg, Adrenaclick 0.15 mg, or Auvi-Q 0.15 mg Auto-Injectors for those weighing 15–30 kg [33–66 lb]). These systems eliminate the delay involved in drawing up epinephrine in a syringe before administration. Appropriate examination and treatment rooms should have one of these injection systems taped to a cabinet door for easy accessibility.

PREVENTION WITH PREVIOUS HISTORY

Some patients may require tests that necessitate the use of known allergens. For example, patients may require a computed tomography scan with contrast material that previously caused urticaria, dyspnea, or other signs of early anaphylaxis. If an alternative contrast agent cannot be used and the test is critical to the diagnostic work-up, the patient can be counseled about the risks, asked to sign an informed consent form, and premedicated with diphenhydramine and steroids to minimize the risk of an anaphylactic reaction. This premedication can be done with 50 to 100 mg of diphenhydramine orally and 100 mg of hydrocortisone or 50 mg of methylprednisolone (Solu-Medrol) intravenously; both the oral and IV forms of premedication are given 1 hour before the procedure. The clinician can also consider ephedrine 25 mg by mouth an hour before the procedure. In addition, ranitidine 150 mg can be given by mouth 3 hours prior to the procedure. An alternate oral steroid dose is 50 mg prednisone given 13 hours, 7 hours, and 1 hour prior to the procedure. The patient should be observed carefully for at least 6 hours after the procedure.

For patients with a history of allergies to local anesthetics, a few simple steps need to be followed. Allergies have been reported to ester drugs (e.g., procaine [Novocain]) but are very rare with amide derivatives (e.g., lidocaine [Xylocaine]). If someone is suspected of having an allergy to a local anesthetic, the clinician should use an amide drug from a single-dose vial. Single-dose vials do not contain any preservatives (parabens), which is often the source of allergy. As such, allergic reaction to amide local anesthetics from single-dose vials is very rare. However, it is still judicious to observe the reaction to a small wheal of injected solution (0.05 mL) for 10 to 15 minutes before injecting a larger volume.

PRECAUTIONS

Procedures and medications that could result in anaphylaxis should not be administered unless the office is equipped to deal with this complication. At a minimum, the office should be able to administer subcutaneous epinephrine, supply supplemental oxygen, and provide ventilation to the patient until emergency services can arrive. In general, procedures and medications that carry a high risk of anaphylaxis should be followed by an appropriate observation period after the procedure to watch for signs and symptoms.

POSTPROCEDURE PATIENT EDUCATION

Sensitized patients should receive detailed patient education. Such patients should be encouraged to wear a medical identification bracelet that identifies the agent that could cause anaphylaxis (e.g., penicillin, bee sting, IV pyelography contrast). Some patients with recurrent, severe anaphylactic reactions should carry a kit with them (containing 1:1000 epinephrine that can be injected) so that initial treatment can begin without delay. For example, a beekeeper with a known sensitivity to bee stings and who refuses to explore a new profession should be encouraged to carry a kit. Patients with previous anaphylaxis should be instructed to seek prompt medical attention for the following symptoms:

- Shortness of breath
- Swelling of eyes, legs, or hands
- Dizziness
- Sensation of swelling in the throat
- Raised, red rashes (urticaria)
- Change in mental status

ICD-10-CM DIAGNOSTIC CODES

D69.0	Purpura
T50.90-T50.901	Overdose or wrong substance given or taken
T63.30X-T63.484X	Toxic effect venom

T88.6XXX	Anaphylactic reaction (correct substance properly administered)
T78.00XX	Anaphylactic reaction due to unspecified food
T78.01XX	Anaphylactic reaction; peanuts
T78.02XX	Crustaceans
T78.04XX	Fruits; vegetables
T78.05XX	Nuts (including tree nuts); seeds
T78.03XX	Fish
T78.06XX	Additives
T78.07XX	Milk and dairy products
T78.08XX	Eggs
T78.1XXX	Specified NEC
T80.51-T80.59	Immunization; serum

Add appropriate seventh character: A = initial, D = subsequent, S = sequela.

Specified drug (see Table of Drugs and Chemicals)

SUPPLIERS

(See contact information available at www.expertconsult.com.)

Banyan kits
Banyan International Corporation
EpiPen
Mylan Specialty, LP

RECOMMENDED READING

Barksdale AN, Muelleman RL. Allergy, hypersensitivity, and anaphylaxis. In: Walls RM, Hockberger RS, Gausche-Hill M, eds. *Rosen's Emergency Medicine*. 9th ed. Philadelphia: Elsevier; 2018:1418–1429.

Fader DJ, Johnson TM. Medical issues and emergencies in the dermatology office. *J Am Acad Dermatol*. 1997;36:1–16.

Hash RB. Intravascular radiographic contrast media: issues for family physicians. *J Am Board Fam Pract*. 1999;12:32–42.

Joint Task Force on Practice Parameters. American Academy of Allergy, Asthma, and Immunology; American College of Allergy, Asthma, and Immunology; Joint Council of Allergy, Asthma, and Immunology: Anaphylaxis—a practice parameter update 2014. *Ann Allergy Asthma Immunol*. 2015;115:341–384.

Joint Task Force on Practice Parameters. American Academy of Allergy, Asthma, and Immunology; American College of Allergy, Asthma, and Immunology; Joint Council of Allergy, Asthma, and Immunology: Emergency department diagnosis and treatment of anaphylaxis: a practice parameter. *Ann Allergy Asthma Immunol*. 2014;113:599–608.

Kemp SF, Lockey RF, Simons FE, Epinephrine. The drug of choice for anaphylaxis. A statement of the World Allergy Organization. *Allergy*. 2008;63:1061–1070.

Kemp SF, Lockey RF, Wolf BL, Lieberman P. Anaphylaxis: a review of 266 cases. *Arch Intern Med*. 1995;155:1749–1754.

Lieberman P. Epidemiology of anaphylaxis. *Curr Opin Allergy Clin Immunol*. 2008;8:316–320.

Lin RY, Curry A, Pesola GR, et al. Improved outcomes in patients with acute allergic syndromes who are treated with combined H_1 and H2 antagonists. *Ann Emerg Med*. 2000;36:462–468.

Sampson HA, Munoz-Furlong A, Campbell RL, et al. Second symposium on the definition and management of anaphylaxis: summary report—Second National Institute of Allergy and Infectious Disease/Food Allergy and Anaphylaxis Network Symposium. *Ann Emerg Med*. 2006;47:373–380.

CHAPTER 213

PREVENTION AND TREATMENT OF WOUND INFECTIONS

Madelyn Pollock • Farin W. Smith

Infection is one of the possible adverse outcomes of many procedures. In general, infection rates in the controlled environment of an office procedure are low, and prophylactic antibiotic use is usually not indicated. The rate of infection in traumatic wounds is somewhat higher. Clinicians must decide whether to use prophylactic antibiotics in managing surgical or traumatic wounds. Making the right choice involves evaluating the wound, the patient, and the risk-benefit balance. Much of the information available in making that choice is based on opinion, with little being evidence based.

(See Chapter 69, Antibiotic Prophylaxis for a discussion of antibiotic prophylaxis to prevent surgical site infections, as well as for guidelines for antibiotic prophylaxis for certain gastrointestinal, genitourinary, gynecologic, and obstetric procedures.)

INITIAL WOUND MANAGEMENT

After ensuring that the patient is medically stable, treatment of any wound should begin with hemostasis and a thorough physical examination, with particular attention to motor, sensory, and vascular components. The wound should be anesthetized (local and/or regional) and copiously irrigated, and any devitalized tissue should be debrided. Use a 30-mL syringe with a large-bore needle (16 to 18 gauge), with a steady, firm force, and at least 250 mL of fluid. Warmed irrigant is generally more comfortable for patients. For large wounds, use at least 500 mL of fluid. Irrigation should continue until all visible, loose particulate matter has been removed. A quick method is to hook up a three-way stopcock to a bag of saline. Clean wounds do not need irrigation. However, if there is significant manipulation of a wound (e.g., difficult removal of a deep lesion) or if a cyst has been ruptured during removal, irrigation will help to remove small pieces of adipose tissue or cystic contents. In the Cochrane Review "Water for Wound Cleansing" (Fernandez and Griffiths, 2008, 2012), tap water was determined to be as safe as sterile water or saline for this irrigation. If the possibility of a retained foreign body exists, a radiograph should be considered (see Chapter 19, Laceration and Incision Repair, for more details). Most wounds can be closed safely up to 6 to 8 or even 12 hours after the time of injury if it can be adequately cleaned. However, clinical judgment may allow the time in the lowest-risk wounds to extend much longer. For instance, the highly vascular face and scalp can be safely closed for up to 24 hours or longer in healthy patients. Grossly contaminated wounds and most wounds older than 12 hours should be allowed to heal by secondary intention or undergo delayed closure in 4 to 5 days. Puncture wounds should not be closed unless by delayed closure. Buried absorbable subcutaneous sutures increase the infection rate in irrigated contaminated wounds and should be avoided. Shaving hair from wound sites should be avoided if possible because it increases the likelihood of infection.

DELAYED CLOSURE

There is a common misconception that all wounds must be closed within a few hours or left open to heal slowly by secondary intention. Unfortunately, healing by secondary intention results in much more inflammation, fibroplasia, and contraction and can result in an unsightly, larger than necessary scar and other complications such as contractures. As it turns out, in the short-term, wounds cleaned and left unsutured appear to have higher resistance to infection than closed wounds. Therefore reinspecting the wound after 3 to 5 days may allow for delayed closure. This delay actually allows the wound to gain resistance to infection. Despite its effectiveness, delayed closure remains largely unappreciated and probably underused by clinicians.

For delayed closure, the wound should have been initially cleaned and debrided carefully as soon as possible after the primary injury. The wound should then be packed with sterile, saline-moistened, fine mesh gauze. In turn, this packing should be covered with a thick, absorbent sterile dressing. Depending on the nature of the wound and the ability of the patient to provide care, this packing may be changed daily at home or in the clinician's office, or even left undisturbed for several days. Although there is no evidence supporting the use of prophylactic antibiotics, some clinicians prescribe them. On the fourth or fifth postoperative day, the clinician reevaluates the wound, and if there is no evidence of infection, it can be closed (delayed primary closure). Additional debridement may be necessary. Another option is to excise the wound and then close it (secondary closure). Because the wound is closed before the proliferative phase of healing, there is no delay in final healing. The results are often indistinguishable from those of initial primary closure.

Certain wounds should almost always be managed with delayed closure, if closed at all. Wounds heavily contaminated by soil, organic matter, or feces or that are already infected often respond well to delayed closure. Wounds associated with extensive tissue damage such as those caused by bites (except human bites), explosions, crush injuries, or high-velocity missiles are often managed in this manner. Even deep puncture wounds can be managed in this manner. An additional benefit of delayed closure is that it allows the clinician to determine which tissue is viable, thereby minimizing debridement.

PATIENT FACTORS

Certain patient or wound characteristics are associated with a possible increase in wound infection. When these higher-risk situations apply, there is little evidence to guide the practitioner's decision to use or not use prophylaxis. Conditions to consider are listed in Box 213.1. All of these conditions or characteristics can increase the risk of infection. These should be weighed against the facts that antibiotic use carries the risks of allergic reaction, development of resistant organisms, antibiotic-associated colitis, fungal superinfections, and increased costs to the medical system. A careful assessment of potential risks and benefits should be made before making the choice.

<table>
<tr><td colspan="2">

BOX 213.1 Factors That Increase the Risk of Wound Infection When to Consider Antibiotic Prophylaxis for Surgical and Traumatic Wounds

</td></tr>
</table>

Comorbid Conditions
- Diabetes mellitus
- Peripheral vascular disease (if wound on extremity involved)
- Elderly
- Immunocompromised
- History of radiation to site of wound
- Malnutrition (e.g., alcoholic, chemotherapy, chronic debility)
- History of previous wound infection or slow healing
- Chronic steroid use
- Obesity
- Pedal edema with leg wounds
- History of poor healing
- Collagen vascular diseases
- Coexisting infection at a distant site
- Colonization with a pathologic organism

Wound Locations and Characteristics
- Increased bacteria: axilla, inguinal fold, mouth, anogenital area
- Over joint spaces where invasion of space possible (finger and toe joints in particular)
- Residual devitalized tissue (should be rare)
- Penetrating injury, particularly if mucous membrane perforation possible
- Stellate wounds
- Wounds deeper than the subcutaneous tissue

Contamination
- Dirty wounds, particularly if contaminated with feces, meat, seawater
- Break in sterile technique
- Deep puncture wounds
- Bites (human and cat; <5% of dog bites result in infection)
- Presence of residual foreign body

WOUND FACTORS

Prophylaxis in Clean Surgical Wounds

The use of prophylactic antimicrobials is not indicated in the vast majority of dermatologic procedures. In certain patient types and in some wound locations, antimicrobial prophylaxis may be considered if the clinician feels that the risk of infection is high, although there is little evidence for doing this (see Box 213.1). If an antibiotic is to be administered, the most common regimen for adults is a first-generation cephalosporin such as cephalexin. The dose should be given at least 30 minutes but not longer than 1 hour before the incision in clean, scheduled cases. This timing is important. Efficacy decreases with doses given earlier or later.

Topical application of antibiotic ointment has not been shown to decrease wound infections better than petrolatum alone. Mupirocin ointment applied after clean procedures is not more effective than commonly available triple-antibiotic ointment in preventing infection and is much more expensive. Because of the risk of hypersensitivity, topical neomycin should be avoided if possible. Neomycin is present in most generic triple-antibiotic formulations and in Neosporin; it is not present in Polysporin or Bacitracin. If a patient complains of redness and itching and is using a neomycin product (or some other topical antibiotic), the clinician should suspect allergy rather than infection.

Prophylaxis in Traumatic Wounds

Prophylactic antimicrobials in traumatic wounds are those used within 24 hours of the event and before there is evidence of infection. Their use is not indicated in the vast majority of traumatic wounds in healthy patients. Copious and thorough wound irrigation (and careful debridement where necessary) is the most important intervention to prevent infection. When risks are particularly high, either because of patient factors or wound characteristics, prophylactic antibiotics may be considered. First-generation cephalosporins are the drugs of choice, although coverage for methicillin-resistant *Staphylococcus aureus* (MRSA) as previously discussed may be considered. Injuries associated with contamination from saliva, blood, feces, meat, and seawater are more likely to become infected. However, there is no clear indication for antibiotics versus copious irrigation and early treatment if infection develops (Table 213.1).

TABLE 213.1	Choice of Antibiotic Prophylaxis When Indicated	
Setting	**Recommendation**	**Comments**
Adult human bites (or child >40 kg) with wound from human mouth contact (bite or punch)	Amoxicillin-clavulanate 875/125 mg PO every 12 hr for 3–5 days. For high-risk wounds (on the hands, genitalia, face, or in close proximity to a bone or joint) or bite wounds in immunocompromised hosts, consider an initial dose parenterally.	Prophylaxis should be provided for human bites through the dermis, especially wounds to the hand. Also consider viral prophylaxis. Any unvaccinated patient or individual negative for anti-HBs antibodies who is bitten by an individual positive for HBsAg should receive both hepatitis B immune globulin and hepatitis B vaccine. If the source is unknown or not available for testing, initiate the hepatitis B vaccine. The risk of HIV or hepatitis C infection through saliva is very low, but counseling regarding postexposure HIV prophylaxis is appropriate.
Dog bites, low risk (superficial injury, not a puncture wound)	No antibiotics in healthy patients	Infection rate <5% if wound is irrigated well. Consider tetanus and rabies prophylaxis, as appropriate.
High-risk dog bites and all cat bites	Amoxicillin-clavulanate 875/125 mg PO every 12 hr for 3–5 days. Consider initial dose of parenteral antibiotics in high-risk wounds, as noted in the text.	High-risk dog bites include hand bites, deep punctures. Consider tetanus and rabies prophylaxis, as appropriate.
Wounds sustained in seawater or in wet/dirty environments (e.g., plumber)	Tetracycline or fluoroquinolone	*Vibrio* species often the organism; treat based on culture when possible.
Intraoral wounds, full thickness or "through-and-through" in adults	Penicillin, amoxicillin, or cephalexin for 5 days. Clindamycin may be used in penicillin-allergic patients.	Increased rate of infection if sutures used.
Most surgical wounds, clean	Prophylactic antibiotics not indicated	Copious irrigation recommended for most traumatic wounds.
Surgical wounds when risk of infection is high. (see Box 213.1)	Prophylactic antibiotics generally not indicated, but first-generation cephalosporin could be considered if risk of infection is felt to be sufficiently high.	If penicillin allergic, clindamycin 300 mg PO.

HB, Hepatitis B; *HBsAg,* hepatitis B surface antigen; *IV,* Intravenous; *PO,* oral.

Rabies Prophylaxis in Animal Bites

The Cochrane Database (Medeiros and Saconato, 2001) reports that there is good evidence to support routine use of prophylactic antibiotics in wounds from cat and human bites because these are likely to get infected even when copiously irrigated (see Table 213.1). Blunt trauma resulting from contact with the human mouth (e.g., a punch to the face) should be treated as a human bite if the skin is broken. Dog bites become infected less than 5% of the time. Amoxicillin-clavulanate is the recommended antibiotic for prophylaxis in bite wounds. Rabies should always be a consideration when treating patients with animal bites. The animal's location and rabies vaccination status should be assessed, and the local public health department should be contacted. Decisions regarding postexposure rabies prophylaxis are complex and depend on the animal involved, the degree of contact, local epidemiology, and the results of testing, when available. In most states a period of observation is required and rabies prophylaxis can be delayed unless and until the offending animal exhibits clinical signs of infection.

TREATMENT OF WOUND INFECTIONS

Patients should always be educated about the signs and symptoms of wound infection after a procedure and asked to return for early evaluation should the classic signs of redness, swelling, warmth, increased pain, or purulent drainage develop. An early postoperative evaluation of the wound at 48 to 72 hours might be useful in patients at high risk of infection. If infection is detected, extraction of some or all suture material with irrigation and exploration of the wound may be indicated if there is no marked improvement in 24 hours with antibiotics. Devitalized or obviously infected tissue should be debrided. A Gram stain and culture of the wound should guide the choice of antibiotic therapy.

The most common organisms present are staphylococci or streptococci. As the prevalence of MRSA has increased, it has become important to consider coverage for this organism if the infection is purulent, if the patient has a history of MRSA, or if there are high rates of MRSA in the community. Trimethoprim/sulfamethoxazole preparations provide good coverage for MRSA; other options include doxycycline, clindamycin, or linezolid. In the specific setting of bite wounds, amoxicillin-clavulanate is recommended as first-line therapy if not used as a prophylactic antibiotic. For cat bites, the most common cause of infection is *Pasteurella multocida*, which should be treated with amoxicillin-clavulanate. Deep or severe bite wounds from dogs or cats should be treated with intravenous antibiotics. In wounds close to bony structures, osteomyelitis should be considered when the response is not prompt.

Seawater Wounds

For the special circumstances of wounds associated with exposure to seawater, and the possibility of infection with *Vibrio* species, tetracycline or a fluoroquinolone is the drugs of choice. Treatment should be based on culture when possible.

TETANUS PROPHYLAXIS

An important, and too often overlooked, aspect of wound management is tetanus prophylaxis. It is easy to overlook in atypical wounds, such as foreign bodies in the eye or superficial burns. All wounds that penetrate the superficial skin should be considered for tetanus prophylaxis based on immunization history and type of wound. The recent release of the tetanus toxoid, reduced diphtheria toxoid, and acellular pertussis (Tdap) vaccines Boostrix and Adacel has changed the Centers for Disease Control and Prevention recommendations for use of tetanus in adults and adolescents (Table 213.2). Of note,

TABLE 213.2 Guide to Wound Management and Tetanus Prophylaxis in Routine Wound Management among Adults and Adolescents Aged 11 to 64 Years

Previous Doses of Tetanus Toxoid[†]	Clean, Minor Wound		All Other Wounds*	
	Tetanus Toxoid–Containing Vaccine[‡]	Human Tetanus Immune globulin	Tetanus Toxoid–Containing Vaccine[‡]	Human Tetanus Immune globulin
Unknown or <3 doses	Yes	No	Yes[§]	Yes[¶]
≥3 doses	Only if last dose given ≥10 yr ago	No	Only if last dose given ≥5 yr ago[¶]	No

*Such as, but not limited to, wounds contaminated with dirt, feces, soil, and saliva; puncture wounds; avulsions; and wounds resulting from missiles, crushing, burns, and frostbite.

[†]Tetanus toxoid may have been administered as diphtheria-tetanus toxoids adsorbed (DT), diphtheria-tetanus-whole cell pertussis (DTP, DTwP; no longer available in the United States), diphtheria-tetanus-acellular pertussis (DTaP), tetanus-diphtheria toxoids adsorbed (Td), booster tetanus toxoid-reduced diphtheria toxoid-acellular pertussis (Tdap), or tetanus toxoid (TT). *Td*, tetanus and diphtheria toxoids vaccine; *Tdap*, tetanus toxoid, reduced diphtheria toxoid, and acellular pertussis vaccine; *TIG*, tetanus immunoglobulin; *TT*, tetanus toxoid.

[‡]Tdap is preferred to Td for adults or adolescents who have never received Tdap. Td is preferred to TT for adults or adolescents who received Tdap previously or when Tdap is not available. If TT and TIG are both used, tetanus toxoid adsorbed rather than tetanus toxoid for booster use only (fluid vaccine) should be used. The preferred vaccine preparation depends upon the age and vaccination history of the patient:

* <7 years: DTaP.
* Underimmunized children ≥7 and <11 years who have not received Tdap previously: Tdap. Children who receive Tdap between 7 and 11 years do not require revaccination at age 11 years.
* ≥11 years: a single dose of Tdap is preferred to Td for all individuals in this age group who have not previously received Tdap. Pregnant women should receive Tdap during each pregnancy.
* Td is preferred to TT for those who received Tdap previously and when Tdap is not available.

[§]The vaccine series should be continued through completion as necessary.

[¶]250 units intramuscularly at a different site than tetanus toxoid; intravenous immune globulin should be administered if human tetanus immune globulin is not available.

[¶]Booster doses given more frequently than every 5 years are not needed and can increase adverse effects. Yes, if ≥5 years since the last tetanus toxoid–containing vaccine dose.

Data from: (1) Advisory Committee on Immunization Practices. Recommended adult immunization schedule: United States, 2012. *Ann Intern Med.* 2012;156:211. (2) Centers for Disease Control and Prevention (CDC). Updated recommendations for use of tetanus toxoid, reduced diphtheria toxoid and acellular pertussis (Tdap) vaccine from the Advisory Committee on Immunization Practices. *MMWR Morb Mortal Wkly Rep.* 2011;60:13. (3) Centers for Disease Control and Prevention. Updated recommendations for use of tetanus toxoid, reduced diphtheria toxoid, and acellular pertussis (Tdap) vaccine in adults aged 65 years and older—Advisory Committee on Immunization Practices (ACIP), 2012. *MMWR Morb Mortal Wkly Rep.* 2012;61(25):468–470. (4) Centers for Disease Control and Prevention (CDC). Updated recommendations for use of tetanus toxoid, reduced diphtheria toxoid, and acellular pertussis vaccine (Tdap) in pregnant women—Advisory Committee on Immunization Practices (ACIP), 2012. *MMWR Morb Mortal Wkly Rep.* 2013;62(7):131–135. Modified from American Academy of Pediatrics. Tetanus (lockjaw). In: Kimberlin DW, Brady MT, Jackson MA, Long SS, eds. *Red Book: 2015 Report on the Committee on Infectious Diseases.* 30th ed. Elk Grove Village, IL: American Academy of Pediatrics, 2015 and from Hibberd PL. Tetanus-diphtheria toxoid vaccination in adults. In: UpToDate.com, 2017.

for individuals with an unknown number or fewer than three tetanus-containing immunizations before the injury, the Centers for Disease Control and Prevention recommends use of tetanus immunoglobulin for all but "clean, small" wounds. These guidelines do not use age of wound, mechanism of injury, or presence of devitalized tissue to distinguish between wounds that might be an indication for tetanus immunoglobulin and those that are not.

CPT/BILLING CODES

The postoperative management of wound infections usually will be included in the initial charge for the wound management or operative procedure if it occurs within 10 days ("10-day global period"). If the treatment of the infection is complex, the following code can be used:

10180	Incision and drainage of complex postoperative wound infection
Other	codes that may be useful in certain situations include the following:
12020	Treatment of superficial wound dehiscence, simple closure
12021	Treatment of superficial wound dehiscence with packing
13160	Secondary closure of surgical wound or dehiscence, extensive or complicated

ICD-10-CM DIAGNOSTIC CODES

NOTE: Always include date of injury and measurement of wound.

A28.0	Infection by *Pasteurella multocida* including septic infection (cat or dog bite)
T81.33XX	Posttraumatic wound infection, not elsewhere classified
T81.30XX	Disruption, dehiscence, or rupture of operation wound
T81.31XX– T81.62XX	Postoperative infection

Add appropriate seventh character: A = initial, D = subsequent, S = sequela.

Excludes: infection due to implanted device or postoperative obstetric wound

RECOMMENDED READING

Bratzler DW, Dellinger EP, Olsen KM, Perl TM, Auwaerter PG, et al. Clinical practice guidelines for antimicrobial prophylaxis in surgery. *Surg Infect.* 2013;14:73.

Fernandez R, Griffiths R. Water for wound cleansing. *Cochrane Database Syst Rev.* 2012;1:CD003861. pub3.

Harper M. *Clinical manifestations and initial management of animal and human bites.* UpToDate.com, February 2017;13.

Lammers RL, Smith ZE. Principles of wound management. In: Roberts JR, Custalow CB, Thomsen TW, eds. *Roberts and Hedges Clinical Procedures in Emergency Medicine.* 6th ed. Philadelphia: Elsevier; 2014:611–643.

Lohiya GS, Tan-Figueroa L, Lohiya S, Lohiya S. Human bites: bloodborne pathogen risk and postexposure follow-up algorithm. *J Natl Med Assoc.* 2013;105:92.

Emergency department wound management. Mcmanus J, Wedmore I, Schwartz RB, eds. *Emerg Med Clin North Am.* 2007;25:1–248.

Medeiros I, Saconato H. Antibiotic prophylaxis for mammalian bites. *Cochrane Database Syst Rev.* 2001;2:CD001738.

Mehta PH, Dunn KA, Bradfield JF, Austin PE. Contaminated wounds: infection rates with subcutaneous sutures. *Ann Emerg Med.* 1996;27:43–48.

Morris JRJG. *Vibrio vulnificus infections.* UpToDate.com; 2017.

Stevens DL, Bisno AL, Chambers HF, Dellinger EP, Goldstein EJC, et al. Practice guidelines for the diagnosis and management of skin and soft tissue infections: 2014 update by the Infectious Diseases Society of America. *Clin Infect Dis.* 2014;50(2):e10–e52.

CHAPTER 214

Emergency Department, Hospitalist, and Office Ultrasound (POCUS)

Grant C. Fowler • Nicholas Lefevre

For many reasons—including improvements in image quality, portability (probes are now available for use with smart phones), and affordability—real-time, point-of-care ultrasound (POCUS) has become a valuable tool for primary care clinicians. Results from high-quality research and more widely available educational programs have also supported the use of POCUS by primary care clinicians. In many settings, patient care quality has been improved and lives have been saved with immediately available POCUS.

Studies continue to demonstrate the safety and efficacy of ultrasound in the hands of nonradiologists, as well as to clarify its indications. How did we get here? In 1991, the American College of Emergency Physicians (ACEP) Board of Directors first adopted a policy recognizing the need for emergency ultrasound imaging on a 24-hour basis and encouraged emergency physicians to perform such examinations. This policy was soon endorsed by the Society for Academic Emergency Medicine, and they rapidly encouraged residency programs to offer ultrasound training. All emergency medicine residency programs now provide POCUS training; it is required by the American College of Graduate Medical Education for that specialty. ACEP now considers POCUS to be within the scope of practicing emergency clinicians in 12 core areas: cardiac/hemodynamic assessment, pregnancy/gynecology, abdominal/bowel, biliary tract, urinary tract, aorta, thoracic/airway, trauma, ocular, venous thrombosis, musculoskeletal/soft tissue, and ultrasound-guided procedures (an excellent reference is the *ACEP Ultrasound Guidelines: Emergency, Point-of-Care and Clinical Ultrasound Guidelines in Medicine*, 2017). Advanced applications continue to be developed. The American College of Chest Physicians now offers courses in critical care ultrasound. The American College of Surgeons has offered courses and videos on ultrasound since 1998. The 3rd edition (2017) of *Ultrasound for Surgeons: The Basic Course* is available online. Many medical schools are now teaching ultrasound as a part of their anatomy course. Training opportunities in other specialties including primary care internal medicine and family medicine are also rapidly expanding.

Although many of the applications in emergency medicine are useful for hospitalists and in the offices of primary care clinicians, ultrasound in those settings has not been studied as extensively. That said, since the first edition of this text (1994), which contained a chapter on ultrasound, it has found its way into the armamentarium of primary care clinicians. Since the 1990s, the American Academy of Family Physicians (AAFP) has sponsored various task forces on ultrasound; in 2016, the AAFP formed an interest group on POCUS. As a result of their work, the Recommended Curriculum for Family Medicine residents on POCUS (AAFP Reprint #290-D) was developed. This recommended curriculum defines 12 core indications for POCUS that are very similar to those from ACEP. Most of these indications will be covered in this chapter, as well as many indications for POCUS.

Because ultrasound enhances physical examination skills, its use is also anticipated to enhance periodic health evaluations. In so doing, cancer, carotid atherosclerosis, urinary retention, hydronephrosis, abdominal aortic aneurysms (AAAs), and other disease processes might be diagnosed earlier. One study (Siepel, 2000) of ultrasound-enhanced periodic health evaluations in the elderly found a new diagnosis in 31% of patients who had already undergone a conventional physical examination. Seven percent of the patients required prompt treatment for a serious, unsuspected condition. Musculoskeletal ultrasound has also evolved as an adjunct to the history and physical examination and to guide procedures for primary care clinicians providing musculoskeletal care, especially those in sports medicine (see Chapter 171, Musculoskeletal Ultrasound). All primary care sports medicine fellowships are required to have a curriculum in musculoskeletal ultrasound, and fellows are encouraged to obtain 150 scans during their fellowship. Both screening for atherosclerosis with ultrasound and musculoskeletal ultrasound have been endorsed by the American Institute for Ultrasound in Medicine, and guidelines and videos have been developed. Ultrasound has also been used by primary care clinicians to direct prostate biopsy (see Chapter 106, Prostate and Seminal Vesicle Ultrasonography and Biopsy).

Primary care clinicians already performing obstetric ultrasound (see Chapter 142, Obstetric Ultrasound) are often comfortable with the principles of ultrasound and capable of extending its use beyond obstetrics with little additional training. Primary care clinicians who use ultrasound when covering emergency departments or urgent care centers often extend its use into their hospital and office practices. Even primary care clinicians not comfortable using ultrasound for diagnostic purposes may find it useful for directing procedures (e.g., insertion of central lines; guiding aspiration of bladder, breast or thyroid cysts, abscesses, or pericardial, pleural, peritoneal, or joint fluid), especially invasive procedures. Such use may help identify relative anatomy and pathology to minimize the number of attempts necessary when performing a procedure, thereby increasing patient safety. Having ultrasound available may also increase clinician confidence when performing procedures. Gastroenterologists and nephrologists now use ultrasound to direct liver and renal biopsies. The subspecialty of interventional radiology has grown very rapidly, and clinicians (e.g., physicians, physician assistants) in this field frequently use ultrasound to guide procedures formerly performed "blindly" or "landmark-based" by primary care and other clinicians. The use of ultrasound for certain procedures such as central venous line placement is now considered a core safety measure by certain national academies (e.g., Institute of Medicine). Clinicians accustomed to performing "landmark-based" procedures can quickly adapt to the addition of ultrasound guidance.

When first getting started, it is important to ask what clinical question(s) can be answered while scanning. Perhaps the answer in the emergency department can be provided with a limited scan rather than a standard or complete ultrasound survey. Sonographers and radiologists are trained for formal, complete ultrasound surveys. Applications for ultrasound in the emergency department are also defined as either *primary*, which have been evaluated and defined in the medical literature, or *extended*, which generally require more training or experience. Primary scans are often brief and goal-oriented to answer specific questions raised by the clinical presentation. If a definitive clinical answer cannot be obtained with portable scanning, comprehensive ultrasound performed by radiology can be ordered.

POCUS was defined by Kendall in 2007 and has six principles: the exam is well-defined, its purpose is to improve patient outcome, it is focused and goal-oriented, its findings are easily recognizable, it is easily learned, and it is quickly performed at bedside. POCUS is used as a component of the overall clinical evaluation of the patient. It is used in conjunction with history, physical, and laboratory information, and provides additional data for decision making and guiding procedures. POCUS usually answers specific questions about a particular patient's condition or anatomy. Although other imaging tests may provide more information in more detail, have greater anatomic specificity, or identify alternative diagnoses, POCUS has the advantages of being noninvasive, rapidly deployed, and not requiring the patient to visit another unit or facility. Furthermore, use of POCUS avoids or minimizes the delays, costs, use of specialized technical personnel, and administration of contrast agents or exposure to biohazards (e.g., radiation). These advantages make POCUS a valuable addition to available diagnostic and procedural resources. It is particular useful in time-sensitive or emergent situations.

PRINCIPLES OF ULTRASOUND

Similar to sonar used by submarines and fishing boats, ultrasound technology analyzes echoes from pulsed sound waves to generate images. Real-time ultrasound provides continuously updated or "live" images while the patient is being scanned. Live images often allow the clinician to immediately exclude certain diagnoses and to redirect clinical suspicions elsewhere. Live images may also improve the clinician's understanding of a particular patient's underlying anatomy. In addition, the best images are often obtained when scanning "live" because the clinician can immediately reposition the patient, if needed.

One general principle of ultrasound is that the higher the frequency, the sharper the resolution of the image. However, the higher the frequency, the less depth of tissue penetration (Fig. 214.1). With these principles in mind, the clinician chooses the probe, or *transducer*, that best matches his or her needs. Although recently developed probes can vary the frequencies, most probes are dedicated to one frequency range—a *high-* (7.5 to 10 MHz), an *intermediate-* (5 to 7.5 MHz), or a *low-* (3.5 to 5 MHz) frequency probe. High-frequency probes are useful for scanning tissue close to the skin surface, such as breast or thyroid lumps, testicles, arteries, veins, or foreign bodies in the skin. Low-frequency probes are useful for scanning deep internal structures such as those of the abdomen, pelvis, and chest. (Even lower-frequency probes [2 to 2.25 MHz] are being used to scan obese patients.) Intermediate-frequency probes may be useful for scanning children. *Linear* probes are elongated and use parallel sound waves to produce a square or rectangular image (Fig. 214.2A). They require more surface contact, basically throughout the length of the probe, than *sector* probes. With sector probes, sound waves originate from one point source and are directed through a field to produce a pie-shaped image (see Fig. 214.2B). *Curvilinear* probes are basically linear probes with a curved surface, also requiring less surface contact (see Fig. 214.2C) and making it easier to scan areas where it is difficult to maintain good surface contact with a linear probe (e.g., between ribs).

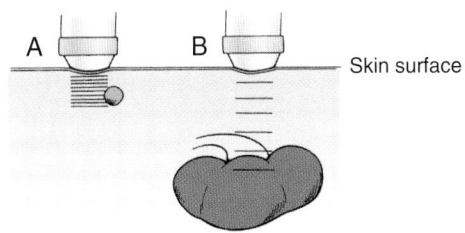

Fig. 214.1 (A) High-frequency probe (7.5 to 10 MHz) provides higher-resolution images but cannot be used to scan deep organs. This probe is especially useful for organs or structures near the skin surface such as breast or thyroid tissue, veins, or arteries. (B) Low-frequency probe (3.5 to 5 MHz) for deeper tissue such as abdominal or pelvic organs.

Another principle of ultrasound is that sound waves travel more readily and rapidly through solids and liquids than through air. Attempts at imaging through structures filled with air or gas may limit visualization, particularly in abdominal studies where bowel gas can be obstructive. (However, even the artifacts produced by air are being interpreted clinically as is the case with lung sonography.) In contrast, the liver, spleen, heart, bladder, and uterus (during pregnancy) are predominantly fluid-filled and therefore provide their own excellent "windows" for imaging. They also provide windows to view surrounding organs or structures. A "window" is an area or organ near the body surface through which sound waves can easily be transmitted to obtain images. For tissue very close to the skin surface, such as thyroid, breast, and femoral veins, there is little tissue to be used for a window. In other words, there is little fluid between the probe and the organ. As a result, high-frequency probes often have their own built-in windows. Because ultrasound is best transmitted through solids and liquids, ample acoustic gel must also be applied between the body surface and any probe to form a good interface. Nevertheless, even with ample gel applied and excellent equipment, there will sometimes be difficulty obtaining images of certain organs for various reasons (e.g., inadequate window, organ obscured by bowel gas, body habitus, local trauma). In that situation, the reasons for being unable to scan an area or an organ should be documented and other imaging modalities considered.

NOTE: An after-market standoff or water path can usually be purchased and attached to a low-frequency probe so that, in addition to scanning deep organs, the same probe can be used for scanning near the body surface. If the clinician is not concerned about seeing bubbles, a bag of intravenous (IV) fluid can be used in the same manner, even if it is sometimes awkward to scan through it. A hand or foot can be submerged in a water bath and the probe placed underwater to provide better views of these difficult-to-image areas. Although a higher-frequency probe would certainly produce better images in this situation, for beginners, using a standoff with a low-frequency probe can save the cost of a high-frequency probe. This allows the primary care clinician to become very proficient with his or her "workhorse" or primary probe, usually a low-frequency 3.5-MHz probe.

Fluid such as amniotic fluid, urine, pus, or blood in the aorta or inferior vena cava (IVC) appears dark by convention on an ultrasound image and is *sonolucent* (sound waves pass through it). Predominantly fluid-filled organs such as the liver, spleen, or renal cortex appear dark or gray on the screen with intermittent bright echoes within their structure. Solid objects such as polyps, bones, or gallstones are white or *echogenic* (i.e., produce a lot of echoes). If a solid object (calcified or hardened such as a gallstone) is larger than 3 mm, it should cast a well-defined shadow. This type of well-demarcated or "sharp" shadow can be differentiated from shadows cast by air, such as air in the gut. Artifact and shadows produced by

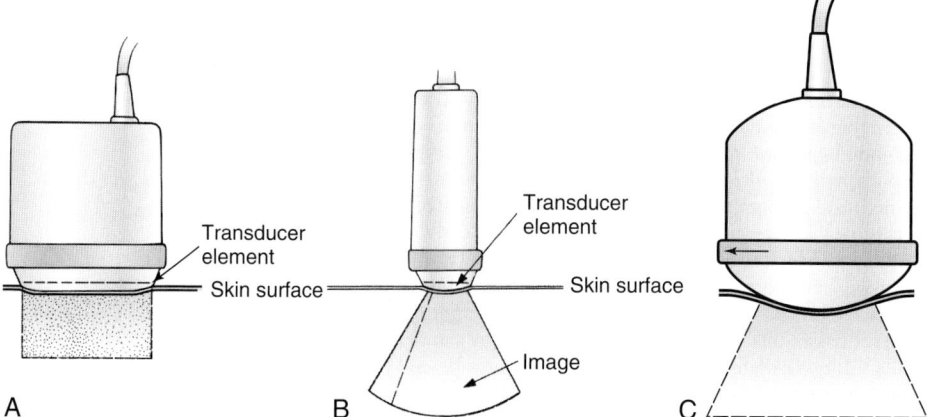

Fig. 214.2 (A) Linear probe produces a rectangular image and works especially well for obstetric scans. (B) Wedge-shaped image produced by sector scanning probe may be adequate for most applications, depending on width of image. (C) Curvilinear probe may be easier to maneuver between ribs. Note wedge-shaped image with curved anterior edge.

air are often diffuse or "soft" and change considerably with changes in the placement, angle, or pressure of the probe, or with peristalsis. Shadows produced by air are typically gray and are sometimes referred to as "dirty," whereas shadows produced by calcified objects are black.

From an ultrasound perspective, a cyst is any fluid-filled structure with smooth walls. Examples include cysts in the ovary, liver, or kidney, but also a full gallbladder, uterus during pregnancy, or full urinary bladder. In some ways, the IVC and abdominal aorta demonstrate cystic properties, such as the following:

- Cysts have smooth walls.
- No echoes or shadows are normally found in simple cysts.
- There is enhanced visualization of structures or tissue posterior to cysts (an artifact referred to as "posterior acoustic enhancement").
- Cysts demonstrate a penumbra effect.

Because of the third property, cystic structures often serve as excellent windows for tissue being scanned behind or around them. The fourth property manifests as "semishadows," or what appear to be shadows, often seen below both sides of a cyst and spreading outward (i.e., the penumbra effect, sometimes called "edge artifact"). Combined, the appearance of all four acoustic properties may help confirm that whatever is being scanned is a cystic structure. These phenomena may be important after localizing a palpable mass, especially when trying to determine whether it is truly a cyst and might benefit from draining, or whether it is an adenoma.

QUALITY ASSURANCE

Clinicians should follow local and national standards for the performance of POCUS, archiving of images, and documentation in the medical record. Limited or focused studies can be used to answer a particular clinical question, to improve patient care, or as a follow-up to streamline patient care. Similar to interpreting plain radiographs, the clinician at the bedside knows exactly where the patient is experiencing pain. This information is helpful when interpreting limited scans, especially when there are abnormalities. In complex cases or in cases in which portable ultrasound is inconclusive, if the patient is stable, referral to a radiology department can be considered. If the clinical question cannot be answered with certainty, referral or consultation should be considered, especially if it might change the management. If these principles are followed, perhaps the rare yet most dreaded error of failure to diagnose can be avoided. Clinicians performing POCUS should make clear in their documentation and communication with consultants what focused question the study is intended to answer, such that comprehensive imaging is still performed when indicated.

A quality assurance program should be implemented. This could consist of some method of tracking outcomes or comparing results. One method of comparing outcomes while the clinician is learning is to not charge for "beginner" or "learner" scans and to follow up every scan with a formal scan in the radiology department. Log sheets should be created and used to compare results with consultative scans. Results should continue to be compared until an acceptable level of clinical accuracy is achieved. Although formal interpretations may differ slightly from "beginner" or "learner" interpretations, the evaluation standard is whether the formal interpretation will lead to a change in clinical management. Having a radiologist or trained ultrasound program director overread every scan is another method of ensuring quality; standard images could be obtained with each scan and then reviewed by a radiologist. Internet overreading services by a radiologist are now continuously available (see the Suppliers section). Quality assurance programs are also established in most academic emergency departments, and emergency medicine ultrasound directors may be willing to work with primary care colleagues in image review. With either method of quality assurance, proof of high-quality clinical data can be maintained and liability minimized, especially the liability of failure to diagnose. With these methods of quality assurance, the process of verifying and documenting clinician competence can be customized for each individual clinician. The ACEP ultrasound guidelines, and other specialty guidelines, such as the residency curriculum guidelines by the AAFP, offer a pathway for both residents and practicing clinicians to obtain ultrasound credentialing. These standards have been used by hospital credentialing committees to develop such credentialing.

For procedural purposes, there has been speculation that national hospital accrediting organizations will someday require certain emergency department and hospital procedures to be ultrasound-guided. At the time of this publication, the author informally surveyed hospitalists and emergency medicine experts, and few saw the need for such guidelines. Although there is individual variation, the literature suggests that the vast majority (>80%) of hospital and emergency medicine procedures are not currently ultrasound-guided. The majority of clinicians use ultrasound guidance only in those patients with a challenging body habitus or when there has been difficulty performing a procedure.

As with many procedures in primary care, beginners should develop a relationship with a consultant, either a radiologist or a clinician competent with ultrasound (sonologist). Ultrasound technicians (sonographers) often have extensive skill in multiple areas and can be helpful consultants, especially in rural areas. As the clinician begins performing ultrasound scanning, cases should be discussed and consultation or supervision should be available.

CREDENTIALING

For departments implementing ultrasound as a procedure, in addition to quality assurance, policies should be in place regarding credentialing. Such policies should identify eligible providers, specify training or experience requirements, and specify ultrasound privileges. For certain clinicians, scanning with ultrasound can seem quite simplistic, and it can even be seductive; operators may become overconfident. Without credentialing, the liability of failing to diagnose may increase with potentially catastrophic outcomes, especially in urgent care centers or emergency departments. The author knows of cases in which watchful waiting (e.g., leaking AAA, ectopic pregnancy) was inappropriate management. These near-catastrophes could have been avoided with appropriate departmental policies, credentialing, or a supervision process.

ACEP guidelines for credentialing nonradiologists in an emergency department require a minimum of 150 to 300 recorded scans for general emergency ultrasound privileges and 25 scans per primary indication. For procedural ultrasound, the clinician should demonstrate competence with basic ultrasound scanning by being credentialed for at least one primary indication. ACEP (and the literature) supports these numbers and notes that the range needed to document proficiency is between 25 and 50 scans per primary indication. These scans should be followed up with consultative scans, overreading, or by tracking clinical outcomes to document and demonstrate accuracy. When competence for primary scans has been documented, scanning for other diagnoses (extended scans) can be managed on a case-by-case basis. Although there is much more to using ultrasound than can be learned by performing a certain number of scans, using these numbers as guidelines is helpful when attempting to decide whether a clinician is ready to demonstrate competence. A certification in various POCUS applications has been designed for clinicians by the Alliance for Physician Certification and Advancement, a branch of the organization that certifies sonographers (American Registry for Diagnostic Medical Sonography). Certification is voluntary. The AAFP does not have a credentialing guideline, but as previously mentioned, it did endorse the residency curriculum guidelines on ultrasound that suggest a similar number and training structures to that designed by ACEP. It should be noted that the AAFP does not endorse using a particular number of procedures performed (or documented) to credential for most procedures.

LIABILITY

When deciding whether using POCUS will raise a clinician's liability, the risk of not having POCUS immediately available should be weighed against making an incorrect diagnosis using ultrasound as a nonradiologist. For example, if certain diagnoses are not made urgently (e.g., pericardial tamponade, ectopic pregnancy, leaking aortic aneurysm, hemoperitoneum), patients may be endangered and liability may increase. In fact, failure to diagnose ectopic pregnancy is the second leading cause (in total dollar amounts) of malpractice awards against emergency physicians; POCUS is the initial procedure of choice to exclude ectopic pregnancy. For these and many other reasons, emergency clinicians now perform POCUS in most large emergency departments. Since POCUS training became routine for residents in emergency medicine, the standard of care also changed to that of a prudent emergency department physician, not a radiologist. Unfortunately, the standards of care for hospitalists and other primary care clinicians are not as well defined; therefore documentation of competence, absolute certainty of interpretation, and having images overread may be important.

DOCUMENTATION

In many cases, ultrasound images are interpreted by the primary care clinician as they are being obtained. These interpretations often guide

---

> **BOX 214.1 Probe Frequencies and Potential Applications (From Low to High Frequency)**
>
> **3.5 MHz**
> Abdominal
> Cardiac
> Lumbar puncture in morbidly obese
> Pelvic and obstetric
> Pleural effusion
>
> **5 MHz**
> Pediatric, including bladder
> Transvaginal
>
> **7.5–10 MHz**
> Breast mass or cyst
> Carotid arteries
> Pediatric bladder
> Testicular mass or torsion
> Thyroid mass or cyst
> Transvaginal
> Venous vessels in neck and extremities

---

contemporaneous clinical decisions; however, a report needs to be placed on the patient's chart. It can be a handwritten, dictated, or templated note, and should include the indication for ultrasound (e.g., preliminary diagnosis), what organs or structures were imaged, a copy of recorded images, appropriate measurements, and the final interpretation. Printed images or images uploaded to a picture archiving and communication system are usually necessary for liability and billing purposes. If bowel gas or other technical factors prevent a thorough scan, these limitations should be identified and documented. Whenever feasible, images should be stored as part of the medical record and done so in accordance with facility policy requirements. Documentation is especially important if the clinician will be billing for ultrasound imaging or directed procedures; however, given the possible emergent use of POCUS by primary care clinicians, the timely delivery of care should not be delayed to archive images.

EQUIPMENT

- Acoustic gel (High-level disinfection is also required by regulatory agencies.)
- For cardiac and abdominal scanning, a 2.5- to 5-MHz sector or curvilinear transducer and scanner is needed. These scanners, or a linear scanner of the same frequency, can also be used for transabdominal obstetric–gynecologic scanning.
- For transvaginal scanning, a 3.5-, 5-, or 7.5-MHz sector, linear, or curvilinear transducer can be used. Special transvaginal probes are manufactured at those frequencies. Again, the higher the frequency, the higher the resolution and the sharper the image. However, the depth of scanning is decreased with a high-frequency probe, so the transvaginal probe must be applied directly to the cervix or in the nearby vicinity. For transvaginal scanning, a probe cover, plain-tipped condom, or examination glove is necessary to place over the probe.
- For pediatric or vascular scans, a 5- to 10-MHz sector, curvilinear, or linear scanner can be used.
- For scanning tissue close to the body surface (e.g., thyroid, testicular, breast)—also known as "small-parts scanning"—a high-frequency, 7.5- to 10-MHz sector, curvilinear, or linear scanner can be used (Box 214.1).

BEGINNER SCANNING

Most clinicians learn human anatomy in three dimensions by dissection. Interpreting ultrasound images requires an ability to

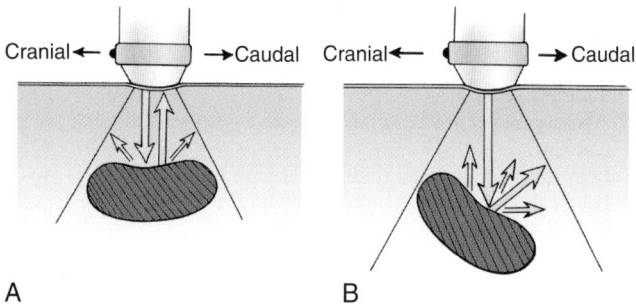

Fig. 214.3 (A) Best image is produced when the ultrasound beam is perpendicular to the organ interface. (B) When the ultrasound beam is not perpendicular to the organ interface, scatter is seen, which may cause artifacts.

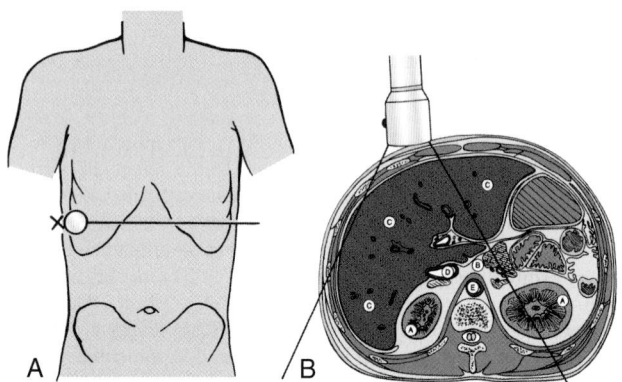

Fig. 214.4 (A) Marker dot toward the patient's right side produces a transverse image of the abdomen. (B) Transverse image: kidneys *(A)*, pancreas *(B)*, liver *(C)*, inferior vena cava *(D)*, and aorta *(E)*.

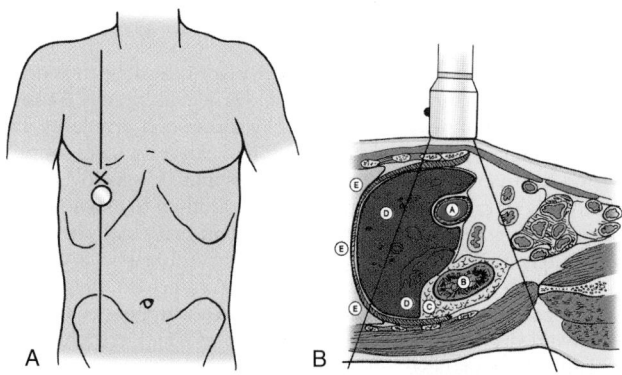

Fig. 214.5 (A) Marker dot toward the patient's head produces a longitudinal image of the abdomen. (B) Longitudinal image: gallbladder *(A)*, right kidney *(B)*, perirenal fat *(C)*, liver *(D)*, and diaphragm *(E)*.

translate that knowledge into two dimensions. For proper probe placement and angulations, beginners should know that the best image is generated when the probe is perpendicular to the tissue being studied (Fig. 214.3). It may be helpful for beginners to minimize the planes of anatomy needed to learn by limiting their initial scanning to transverse and longitudinal planes. In other words, beginners should consider placing the transducer marker dot only toward the patient's right side (transverse) or head (longitudinal), while holding the probe perpendicular to the organ or tissue being scanned. If the probe can be held perpendicular to the skin surface, it is also usually easier to scan. Even for experienced sonographers, using these techniques may be helpful when getting oriented to a patient's anatomy at the beginning of a scan.

By convention, when the marker dot is to the patient's right side, it produces a transverse image similar to computed tomography (CT) orientation (Fig. 214.4). The patient's right side will be to the left of the image on the screen. With the marker dot toward the patient's head, the image is what the clinician would see if the patient were dissected longitudinally and viewed looking into the body from the right side with the patient's head to the left of the screen (Fig. 214.5). A good impression of all of the anatomy and images of most organs can be obtained with longitudinal scanning, alone, at first.

NOTE: Some European manufacturers reverse the orientation so that the marker dot is found on the right side of the image. Cardiac packages also often reverse the screen orientation.

INDICATIONS

Diagnostic Ultrasound

Cardiac Indications

- Electromechanical dissociation (EMD): narrow electrical complexes on electrocardiogram (ECG) without measurable blood pressure or clinical evidence of perfusion*
- Evaluation of gross cardiac activity in setting of cardiopulmonary resuscitation*
- Suspected pericardial effusion (enlarged cardiac silhouette on chest x-ray, electrical alternans or decreased voltage on ECG)*
- Suspected pericardial tamponade (unexplained hypotension, prominent jugular venous distention, pulsus paradoxus, or EMD)*
- Penetrating wounds to the chest (to exclude hemopericardium*; see also the discussion of the focused assessment with sonography for trauma [FAST] examination, in the Trauma section)
- Evaluation of global left ventricular function*
- Gross estimation of intravascular volume status and cardiac preload
- Identification of acute right ventricular dysfunction or acute pulmonary hypertension in the setting of acute or unexplained chest pain, dyspnea, or hemodynamic instability
- Identification of proximal aortic dissection or thoracic aortic aneurysm

Pregnancy/Gynecologic Indications

- First-trimester vaginal bleeding/threatened abortion*
- Suspected ectopic pregnancy*
- Identification of uterine pregnancy*
- Evaluation of fetal viability (e.g., maternal demise, maternal trauma, inability to auscultate fetal heart tones by Doppler)*
- Misplaced intrauterine device
- Suspected ovarian cyst, tubo-ovarian abscess, or adnexal/ovarian torsion
- Uterine fibroid

Biliary Indications

- Right upper quadrant (RUQ) pain
- Symptoms suggestive of biliary tract disease*
- Suspected acute cholecystitis*

---

*These indications have been evaluated and defined in the medical literature and are considered primary applications in emergency medicine. The remaining indications listed for scanning by nonradiologists have also been published, and in many cases studied extensively.

Urinary Tract Indications

- Obstructive uropathy and renal colic*
- Hematuria
- Suspected renal abscess
- Incontinence or urinary retention
- Ultrasound evaluation of the bladder before suprapubic aspiration (SPA) or cannulation in infants or adults, or for documentation of postvoid residual (PVR)

Aorta or Abdominal Indications

- Pulsatile abdominal mass or suspected AAA*
- Screening for AAA* (US Preventive Services Task Force and Medicare guidelines)
- Pneumoperitoneum (in some countries, ultrasound is used first line for diagnosing diverticulitis)
- Small bowel obstruction and ileus (more sensitive and specific than plain x-rays)
- Appendicitis (60% to 90% sensitivity and specificity in ED, so CT is still the gold standard)

Thoracic and Airway Applications

- Shortness of breath
- Suspected pneumothorax*
- Suspected pulmonary edema or pleural effusion
- Suspected pneumonia
- Airway-Confirmation of Endotracheal Tube Placement (see Miscellaneous section)

Trauma

- Suspected hemoperitoneum or hemopericardium (e.g., FAST examination),* especially when real-time spiral (helical) CT is not available or the patient is not stable enough for CT (hemoperitoneum and hemopericardium need to be excluded in a patient with a history of blunt or penetrating trauma to the chest or abdomen or with an altered mental status and an acute abdomen)

Ocular

- Vision loss or changes (detached retina*, vitreous detachment*, vitreous hemorrhage*, intraocular foreign body)
- Suspected increased intracranial pressure (papilledema)

Venous Thromboembolic Disease

- Suspected proximal, lower extremity deep venous thrombosis*

Musculoskeletal/Soft Tissue

- Subcutaneous foreign body
- Superficial fracture evaluation (e.g., finger, rib; see also Chapter 171, Musculoskeletal Ultrasound)
- Distinguishing cellulitis from abscess (see Chapter 171, Musculoskeletal Ultrasound)
- Evaluation for tenosynovitis (i.e., fluid around a tendon; see Chapter 171, Musculoskeletal Ultrasound)

Other Advanced Indications

- Testicular pain or mass

Combined Diagnostic–Procedural Ultrasound

- Insertion of central lines*
- Arterial puncture and cannulation

---

*These indications have been evaluated and defined in the medical literature and are considered primary applications in emergency medicine. The remaining indications listed for scanning by nonradiologists have also been published, and in many cases studied extensively.

- Lumbar puncture or other spinal procedures in a morbidly obese individual (increasingly used by anesthesiologists, at least for localization of puncture site; see Chapter 221, Lumbar Puncture)
- Thyroid or breast mass or cyst, diagnosis, or aspiration
- Pericardial effusion and ultrasound-guided pericardiocentesis (see Chapter 230, Pericardiocentesis)
- Pleural effusion and ultrasound-guided thoracentesis (see Chapter 218, Thoracentesis)
- Ascites and ultrasound-guided paracentesis (see Chapter 219, Abdominal Paracentesis)
- Soft tissue abscess and ultrasound-guided drainage (see Chapter 171, Musculoskeletal Ultrasound)
- Joint effusion and arthrocentesis (see Chapter 171, Musculoskeletal Ultrasound)
- Fracture, long bone, and fracture reduction (see Chapter 171, Musculoskeletal Ultrasound)
- Endotracheal tube placement confirmation (see Chapter 222, Tracheal Intubation)
- Transvenous and transthoracic pacemaker placement (for localization of insertion site and when having difficulty with capture; see Chapter 232, Temporary Pacing)

CARDIAC ULTRASOUND (ECHOCARDIOGRAPHY)

In the unstable hypotensive patient or the patient in shock, narrow QRS complexes on the ECG confirm the diagnosis is EMD. The possible etiologies include anything that could cause abrupt cessation of venous return to the heart (including massive pulmonary embolism, tension pneumothorax, cardiac tamponade), acute malfunction of a prosthetic valve, and exsanguination. During resuscitative measures, exclusion of reversible causes is imperative, especially tamponade. Cardiac ultrasound (echocardiography) is the diagnostic procedure of choice for excluding reversible causes of EMD.

A patient with a large pericardial effusion can be completely asymptomatic, or deteriorate rapidly as a result of tamponade, or be in between. Several scenarios may lead the clinician to suspect a pericardial effusion (e.g., an enlarged cardiac silhouette on the chest radiograph, electrical alternans or decreased voltage on an ECG), especially in a patient at risk of an effusion. Pericardial tamponade may also result from a penetrating wound to the chest or be the cause of unexplained hypotension, prominent jugular venous distention, or a pulsus paradoxus on physical examination. Echocardiography is also the diagnostic procedure of choice for identifying and quantifying a pericardial effusion. Because rapid intervention is often a necessity in tamponade, ultrasound-directed aspiration of the effusion has become the treatment of choice.

Many emergency department clinicians, hospitalists, and cardiologists now also include a quick portable ultrasound of the heart when evaluating patients with chest pain. (See also Chapter 75, Echocardiography.) During this evaluation, gross cardiac activity can be assessed, including left ventricular function. Wall motion abnormalities (suggesting ischemia or scar) or severe valvular dysfunction may be noted, often early in the evaluation. Intravascular volume status can often be estimated, and right ventricular dysfunction or acute pulmonary hypertension identified (possibly indicating a pulmonary embolism). In the setting of chest pain, occasionally the diagnosis of proximal aortic dissection or a thoracic aortic aneurysm can be made.

Preprocedure Patient Preparation

Indications for the study and possible findings should be explained to the patient. The patient should be prepared to change positions, if possible, during scanning. He or she may experience some pressure from the probe as images are being obtained. Adequate gel should

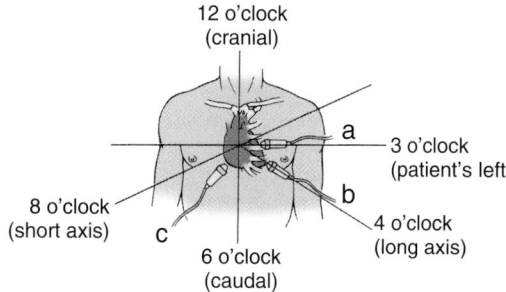

Fig. 214.6 Typical probe positions (placement) for emergency department echocardiography: *a*, parasternal position of probe; *b*, apical position of probe; and *c*, probe in subxiphoid position.

be applied to the parasternal, apical, and possibly subxiphoid areas of the chest wall. The patient should be in the supine or left lateral decubitus position when scanning is initiated.

Technique

While viewing the front of the chest—if the 12 o'clock position is considered cephalic and the 6 o'clock direction caudal—note that the axis of the heart is directed toward the 4 o'clock position. Placing the marker dot of the transducer at about the 4 o'clock position in the second, third, or fourth intercostal space on the left produces the parasternal long-axis view of the heart. The parasternal long-axis view is essentially the "longitudinal" view of the heart, if described in the conventional ultrasound terminology for the remainder of the body. Rotating the marker dot almost 90 degrees to the 8 o'clock position produces the parasternal short-axis view of the heart, which is basically a "transverse" view of the heart (Fig. 214.6). For unresponsive patients, those who cannot be moved, or patients with pulmonary hyperinflation (e.g., chronic obstructive pulmonary disease, intubated), a subxiphoid view may be useful. However, a subxiphoid view may not be possible in patients with abdominal distention or pain, so the clinician should be comfortable using several cardiac windows.

1. With the patient in the supine position, place the low-frequency transducer in the parasternal (third to fourth or fifth intercostal space) or apical (inferolateral to the left nipple at the point of palpated maximal cardiac impulse) location. These are the same two traditional locations used for auscultation with a stethoscope.
2. In the parasternal space, the probe or marker dot will be rotated to either the 4 o'clock (long-axis) or 8 o'clock (short-axis) position.
3. The short-axis view at the level of the mitral valve is often used to assess the adequacy of the window because the mitral valve is usually prominent and easy to locate. In this view, with the probe directed almost straight posteriorly, nearly perpendicular to the hospital bed, the mitral valve produces the characteristic "fishmouth" image (Fig. 214.7), especially if there is any degree of stenosis. This is basically a "transverse" view of the mitral valve. After this transverse view is obtained, if the probe is directed or angled superiorly, toward the patient's right scapula, the aortic valve can often be seen in cross-section. (This is more of an extended scan, so see also Chapter 75, Echocardiography, and Fig. 75.4.) Conversely, from the transverse view of the mitral valve, if the probe is directed or angled inferiorly, toward the patient's left hip, the papillary muscles of the mitral valve can be seen in cross-section (see Chapter 75, Echocardiography, Fig. 75.5). They are echogenic (bright white) structures, surrounded by fluid in the heart (dark), which in turn is enclosed by the echogenic left ventricular walls seen in cross-section.

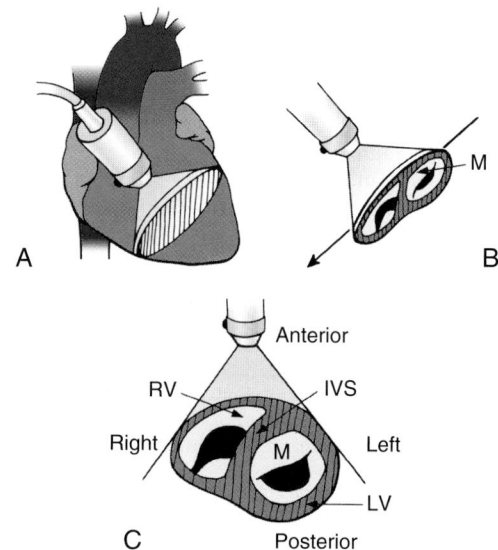

Fig. 214.7 Short-axis view at mitral valve level. Probe is in parasternal position with marker dot at the 8 o'clock position. (A) Ultrasound plane transects the short axis of the heart at the level of the mitral valve. (B) Actual endocardiac structures viewed with probe in this position. (C) Short-axis view as it appears on the ultrasound screen. The image is displayed as if it is being viewed from the apex of the heart looking up toward the base. Note "fish mouth" appearance of mitral valve *(M)* as seen from this view. *IVS,* Interventricular septum; *LV,* left ventricle; *M,* mitral valve; *RV,* right ventricle.

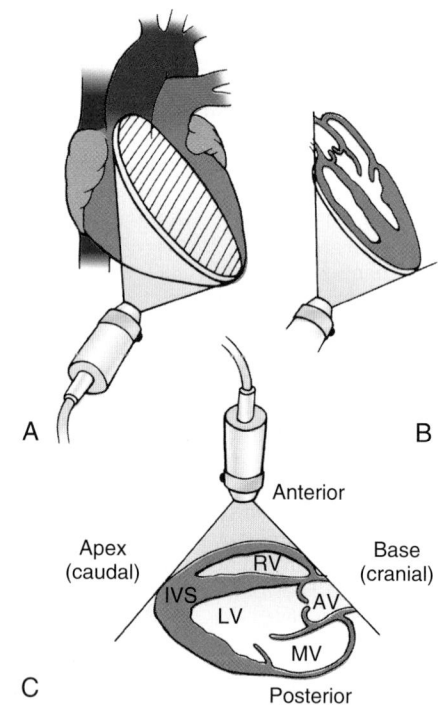

Fig. 214.8 Parasternal long-axis view of the heart. Probe is in parasternal position with the marker dot at the 4 o'clock position. (A) Ultrasound plane transects heart through the long axis. (B) Actual endocardiac structures viewed. (C) Image as it appears on ultrasound screen. *AV,* Aortic valve; *IVS,* interventricular septum; *LV,* left ventricle; *MV,* mitral valve; *RV,* right ventricle.

4. Directing the probe straight posteriorly, again perpendicular to the hospital bed, the parasternal long-axis view can be obtained from the short-axis view by simply rotating the probe about 90 degrees counterclockwise (i.e., marker dot directed toward the 4 o'clock position; Fig. 214.8A and B). This is basically a "longitudinal"

view of the mitral valve, with the echogenic ventricular septum located above the mitral valve on the image and the posterior wall located below it. The dark, fluid-filled right ventricle is located above the septum, and the left ventricle below it (see Fig. 214.8C). To the right side of the image will be the aortic root, located to the right of the aortic valve and above the left atrium (see Fig. 214.8C). The left atrium in this view is located to the right of the mitral valve. The aortic valve cusps will also be seen opening and closing in a longitudinal view.

5. If the patient's position can be changed easily, place the patient on his or her left side. This allows the lingula of the lung to fall away from the heart and often provides a better window for all cardiac imaging.

   NOTE: Some ultrasound equipment places the marker dot 180 degrees away from this standard orientation (i.e., the 6 o'clock position for some is the 12 o'clock position for others). To allow the user to determine the orientation of the probe, the marker on the image should be found. It corresponds with the marker dot on the probe.

6. In the apical location (again, a more extended scan, so see also Chapter 75, Echocardiography), the majority of scanning can be performed with the marker dot rotated toward the patient's right side or at the 8 o'clock position. The probe is then directed toward the patient's right shoulder. The apex of the heart will be in the center at the top of the image, with the septum also in the center and coursing vertically downward. The left ventricle and atrium will be on the right side of the image, and the right ventricle and atrium on the left, so it is called the *apical four-chamber view* (see Chapter 75, Echocardiography, Fig. 75.7).

7. A subxiphoid view may be needed to obtain a good window. Place the transducer directly below the xiphoid with the marker dot toward the patient's right side and angle it toward the patient's left scapula or even higher on the back. In fact, because the heart lies immediately beneath the sternum, the angle or plane of the probe will be almost horizontal or parallel to the patient's bed. A portion of liver will typically be seen at the top of the image (Fig. 214.9). Firm downward pressure may need to be applied with the probe, especially if the patient has a protuberant abdomen. Cardiac structures from this window will appear similar, but in a mirror image (rotated 180 degrees), to the parasternal long-axis view.

8. Search for fluid posterior to the heart. If present, it will usually appear at the bottom of the image. If found, quantify the amount of fluid (Fig. 214.10). For various reasons (including body habitus), up to 10% of patients cannot be scanned adequately for a complete echocardiogram with portable equipment, even under optimal conditions. However, almost all patients with a clinically significant effusion can be diagnosed, so scan patiently and methodically. With a significant effusion, almost any view is acceptable. If an effusion is not readily apparent, vary the probe angles and amount of pressure applied on the probe for 5 to 10 minutes, if necessary, to find a window. Changing the patient's position may be helpful. All of these maneuvers may be necessary when there is a challenging body habitus or too much air in the lungs obscuring the image. If a good window is found with the parasternal short-axis view, many experts suggest using the parasternal long-axis view to exclude an effusion (see Fig. 214.8) because it provides a lengthwise image of the gravity-dependent portion of the heart (the posterior wall) when the patient is lying down. This is where a nonloculated effusion is most likely to settle.

NOTE: Even large effusions may develop gradually and not cause EMD or tamponade.

Interpretation

Pulseless Electrical Activity (Electromechanical Dissociation)

For patients undergoing cardiopulmonary resuscitation or with EMD, a subjective estimate of the organized cardiac activity can be made. Terminal cardiac dysfunction typically progresses from global ventricular hypokinesis with incomplete valve closure, to absence of ventricular wall and valve motion, to eventual cardiac standstill. This information, combined with the clinical scenario, may be helpful for determining futility during resuscitative efforts. Patients with poorly organized or absent cardiac activity on ultrasound have a prognosis similar to that of patients with the ECG pattern of asystole (very poor). Patients with no obtainable blood pressure yet good cardiac contractility appear to carry a better prognosis, so an aggressive search for reversible causes of EMD should be pursued. If the EMD is due to pericardial tamponade, at least one chamber of the heart should collapse during diastole, and there will usually be a moderate to large pericardial effusion. However, even without identified collapse of a chamber, hemodynamic instability associated with a moderate to large pericardial effusion is suspect for tamponade. A plethoric, noncollapsing IVC is further support for tamponade in these cases, and a collapsing IVC is highly predictive for the absence of clinically significant tamponade. The cardiac activity is often well organized, with the rhythm regular and the rate tachycardic. Pericardiocentesis may be life-saving. After the patient has been stabilized the findings should be recorded, including the size of the effusion.

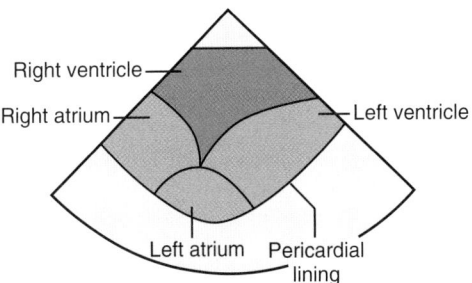

Fig. 214.9 Subxiphoid (subcostal) view of heart.

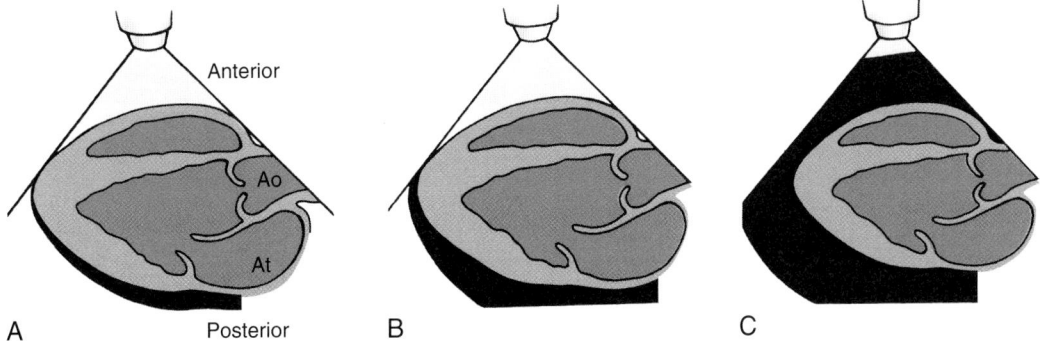

Fig. 214.10 Effusions using a parasternal long-axis view. (A) Small (may be physiologic). (B) Moderate. (C) Large. *Ao,* Aortic root; *At,* left atrium.

Effusions

A small amount of pericardial fluid may be physiologic. If an effusion is diagnosed, it should be quantified (small, moderate, large, or very large) and recorded (see Fig. 214.10). Any hemodynamic compromise should also be noted.

- *Small:* With the patient in the supine position, pericardial fluid is confined posteriorly without anterior, lateral, or apical spread. It will be less than 10 mm width in diastole.
- *Moderate:* Effusion more evenly distributed anteriorly, laterally, and apically, no part greater than 10 mm width in diastole.
- *Large:* Effusion extends entirely around the heart, 10 to 20 mm width in diastole.
- *Very large:* Greater than 20 mm width as well as evidence of tamponade.

Epicardial fat pads can occasionally be mistaken for a pericardial effusion. However, epicardial fat pads usually have some internal echoes and are not distributed evenly around the heart. The descending aorta can also be mistaken for a pericardial effusion, but rotating the probe into a transverse plane will often help distinguish that structure. See Chapter 230, Pericardiocentesis, for treatment of a pericardial effusion. Pleural effusion may also be mistaken for pericardial effusion. The peristernal long-axis view can be helpful in distinguishing the two, as a pericardial effusion will track between the descending aorta and the heart and a pleural effusion will not extend past the descending aorta.

Global Left Ventricular Systolic Function

Published reports indicate clinicians can accurately estimate left ventricular ejection fraction (EF) as normal (EF >50%), moderately impaired (EF 30% to 50%), or severely impaired (EF <30%) with little training and experience.

Dilated Left Atrium or Aortic Root

The diameter of the left atrium should be approximately the same as that of the aortic root on the parasternal long-axis view (see Fig. 214.10), and normal for both is about 2 cm. Disparities may suggest the need for a formal echocardiogram. A dilated aortic root may be suggestive of a thoracic aortic aneurysm, whereas an enlarged atrium increases the risk for atrial fibrillation and may indicate valvular or left ventricular dysfunction.

Right Ventricular Function, Intravascular Volume, and Preload Assessment

Using the subxiphoid view (or during abdominal scanning), the IVC can be located. Comparing the maximal diameter of the IVC during exhalation with the minimal diameter during inhalation may provide a quantitative estimate of preload. Collapse of 50% to 99% is normal, complete collapse may indicate volume depletion, and less than 50% collapse may indicate volume overload, pericardial tamponade, or right ventricular strain or failure. However, it can also indicate acute right ventricular infarct, pulmonic stenosis, and chronic pulmonary hypertension. An estimate of preload can also be made by measuring the height of the meniscus sonographically in the internal jugular from the sternal notch and adding 5 cm.

NOTE: Lack of right ventricular strain on ultrasound does not exclude pulmonary embolism.

Mitral Valve Function

The parasternal long-axis view (because it cuts the mitral valve lengthwise) can be used to assess the mitral valve quantitatively (M-mode) and qualitatively. The anterior leaflet is seen on the superior aspect of the image, and the posterior leaflet is located inferiorly (see Fig. 214.8). With real-time scanning, leaflets can be observed opening and closing. In systole, the leaflets should close to about a 90-degree angle from the septal and posterior walls and lie flat against the plane of the annulus. If the leaflets close and then billow beyond the 90-degree angle or the plane of the annulus, they are prolapsing, and a formal echocardiogram may be helpful to confirm the diagnosis. Severe prolapse can be the result of papillary muscle dysfunction or disruption due to an acute myocardial infarction. The apical four-chamber view (see Chapter 75, Echocardiography, Fig. 75.7) is also helpful for assessing mitral valve function.

OBSTETRIC-GYNECOLOGIC ULTRASOUND

With the advent of transvaginal probes, an alternative to transabdominal scanning became available for evaluating the female pelvis. Advantages of transvaginal over transabdominal scanning include the use of a higher-frequency probe with higher resolution, fewer tissue layers through which to scan (nine layers on transabdominal), resulting in less artifact, and less patient preparation required, especially regarding the bladder. These advantages allow an intrauterine pregnancy to be diagnosed by about 5 weeks after the first day of the patient's last menstrual period. Fetal cardiac activity can frequently be seen by 6 weeks. With transvaginal scanning, there is also a greater likelihood of visualizing an ectopic pregnancy in a tube or the adnexa. Disadvantages to transvaginal scanning include the necessities of an extra probe, a sheath, and additional training. Interpretation is slightly more confusing, and the field of imaging is slightly narrower. Patients are becoming more familiar with and accepting of this technology, but transvaginal scanning is also slightly more invasive.

Transabdominal Scanning

Preprocedure Patient Preparation

The patient is scanned in the supine position. For an adequate window, the patient's bladder must be full, occasionally to the point of discomfort. For best scanning, the bladder should be so full that the dome extends 1 or 2 cm above the fundus. If scanning above the pubis does not immediately provide an adequate view, the patient's clinical stability should be evaluated. If she is stable, either a Foley catheter infusion of fluid (300 to 500 mL) or oral or IV hydration can be used to fill the bladder. If a Foley catheter is used to infuse fluid, the clinician should try to avoid instilling air bubbles into the bladder, which can cause echoes and produce a confusing image.

Technique

1. Scanning the bladder first with a low-frequency probe and the marker dot at the patient's right side may help determine the shape and orientation of the uterus behind the bladder (Fig. 214.11). Because the bladder is rarely full of floating debris, the gain should be lowered until a minimal number of echoes are demonstrated in the bladder. This will decrease artifact. Confirm that the bladder, as opposed to a large ovarian cyst, is being used as a window. A large ovarian cyst is usually irregularly shaped, is oval or round, and often contains complex or echogenic contents. The bladder is basically square in a transverse view.

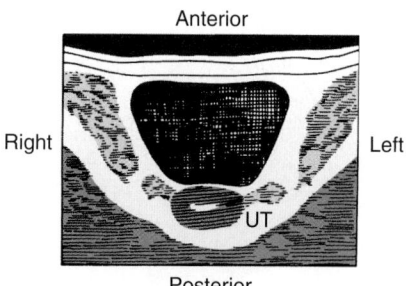

Fig. 214.11 Transverse view of the bladder. Note uterus (*UT*), viewed transversely, is found posterior to the bladder.

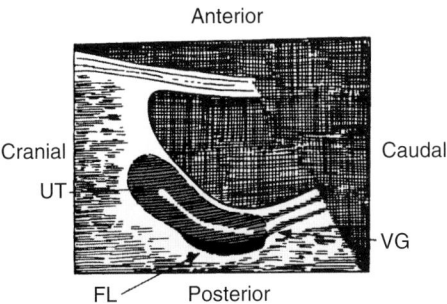

Fig. 214.12 Longitudinal view of the bladder. Note uterus (*UT*), viewed longitudinally, behind the bladder. Fluid in the cul de sac (*FL*) is found posterior to the uterus. *VG*, Vagina.

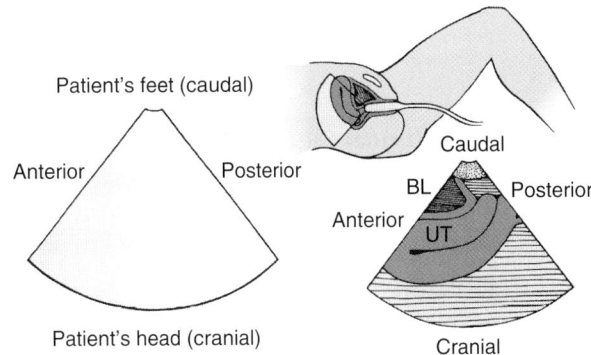

Fig. 214.13 Longitudinal orientation with transvaginal scanning. *BL*, Bladder; *UT*, uterus.

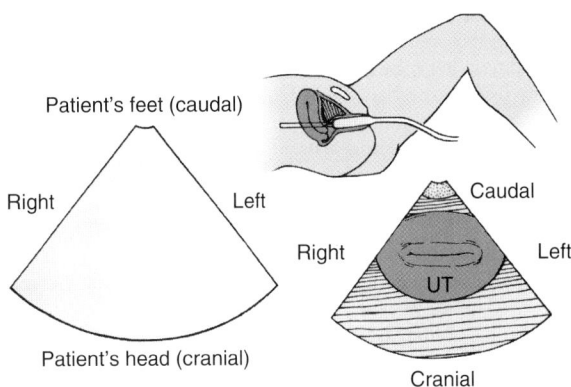

Fig. 214.14 Transverse orientation with transvaginal scanning. *UT*, Uterus.

2. Turn the marker dot cephalad for a longitudinal view (Fig. 214.12). Often the uterus is not quite in the midline, as will have been demonstrated on the transverse view, so the probe may need to be rotated slightly out of the midline for a longitudinal image of the uterus. An echogenic line in the midline of the uterus is normal and represents the interface between the anterior and posterior endometria. A pair of dark fluid lines anterior and posterior to the central echogenic line represents endometrium during the proliferative phase. During the secretory phase, the endometrium becomes progressively thicker and echogenic. Scan the uterus from fundus to cervix. Occasionally an echogenic line known as the *vaginal stripe* may be visualized in the vagina, distal to the cervix. It represents another interface.

3. Photograph and document any object or fluid accumulation within the uterus or posterior to it in the cul de sac (pouch of Douglas).

4. Scan the adnexa and note any fluid accumulations or abnormalities. Adnexa are usually located by first finding the midline of the uterus and then rotating the probe slightly. More specifically, with the probe producing a longitudinal view of the uterus, rotate it slightly clockwise (left adnexa) or counterclockwise (right adnexa) so that the marker dot is somewhat oblique to the uterus. If the adnexa cannot be located with this maneuver, move the probe laterally off of the midline and, while maintaining a longitudinal orientation, scan across and through the bladder to the opposite adnexa. In other words, angle the probe about 15 degrees off of the vertical to scan from the patient's left paramedian position. Scan across the midline through the bladder to visualize the patient's right adnexa, and vice versa for the left. The ovary often indents the wall of the bladder. Ovaries are oval structures of medium echogenicity and lie immediately anterior and medial to the internal iliac arteries, which are pulsatile and have echogenic walls. The iliac veins are also nearby. In women of reproductive age, demonstration of internal follicles often distinguishes ovaries from surrounding structures. Normal ovaries are 2.5 to 5 cm long, 1.5 to 3 cm wide, and 0.6 to 1.5 cm thick. Evidence of peristalsis on the patient's left side confirms that the colon is being scanned instead of the ovary.

Transvaginal Scanning

Preprocedure Patient Preparation

The patient is scanned in the supine or lithotomy position. Transvaginal scanning is usually preceded by transabdominal scanning with a full bladder, perhaps allowing the clinician to make the diagnosis and, if not, to assess the overall anatomy. The bladder can then be emptied; however, some residual urine can serve as a useful marker for locating the bladder with transvaginal scanning.

Technique

1. Prepare the probe by covering it with a probe sheath, a plainended latex condom, or an examination glove. Adequate gel should be placed on the tip of the transducer before covering it. Any bubbles between the cover and transducer should be smoothed out before scanning.

2. Perform a preliminary pelvic examination to relax the vagina as well as to evaluate for palpable masses. Determine the size, shape, and position of the uterus, and define any areas of tenderness. Any tampons should be removed. Counsel the patient about the transvaginal ultrasound examination and obtain verbal consent. A chaperone should be present.

3. While continuing to wear examination gloves, apply more gel to the transducer cover and gently insert the probe with posterior vaginal pressure to a position anterior to the cervix.

4. Scanning starts as soon as the transducer is inserted; avoid inserting the transducer too far, which can cause the clinician to miss the cervix and lower uterine segment. With the marker dot anterior, locate the midline of the uterus in the image.

5. Obtain both longitudinal and coronal scans of the uterus and adnexa by turning the marker dot anterior to the patient or toward her right side. For longitudinal scanning, the image orientation changes slightly (Fig. 214.13) compared with transabdominal scanning. Because the marker dot is pointed toward the anterior abdominal wall of the patient, the left side of the resultant image is actually anterior instead of cranial. Transverse orientation also changes slightly because true anteroposterior (AP) images of the uterus cannot be obtained by scanning from below. However, various coronal images are obtained that are similar to transverse images. The patient's right side remains on the left side of the image because the marker dot is turned to the patient's right side (Fig. 214.14).

6. Scan the uterus by performing a series of longitudinal, coronal, and oblique scans with the transducer at varying depths of penetration. Oblique views are obtained by rotating the probe with the marker dot in the longitudinal position to either the right or left side of the patient. Oblique views are used to scan the adnexa.

7. Note any evidence of a fetus or fluid accumulations. Any areas of tenderness should be documented, along with any other important findings.

First-Trimester Vaginal Bleeding

Approximately 25% of all pregnancies experience bleeding during the first half (see Chapter 142, Obstetric Ultrasound, for differential). Abdominal pain is also common during pregnancy. Ultrasound is recommended as the first test in patients experiencing bleeding or pain beyond 5 to 7 weeks after their last menstrual period. Two frequent causes of first-trimester vaginal bleeding are ectopic pregnancy and threatened abortion.

NOTE: If a fetal heart beat is demonstrated by the less-expensive hand-held Doppler, pregnancy loss has effectively been ruled out and ectopic pregnancy is much less likely. Doppler heart beats are not heard until 9 or 10 weeks, and most ectopic pregnancies become symptomatic before that time. With a threatened abortion, demonstration of fetal heart beats decreases the likelihood of miscarriage to less than 10%. If the hand-held Doppler is used during a bimanual pelvic examination and aimed directly at the uterine fundus as it is elevated by the examiner's hand, the likelihood of hearing fetal heart beats is much improved.

Suspected Ectopic Pregnancy

Ectopic pregnancies vary in prevalence from 1 in 28 to 1 in 200 pregnancies. They account for the majority of first-trimester maternal deaths. The incidence has quadrupled since 1970, and there has been a sevenfold increase in maternal mortality. More than 40% of ectopic pregnancies are misdiagnosed on first presentation to the health care provider.

POCUS coupled with immediately available sensitive radioimmunoassay for human chorionic gonadotropin (hCG) and the doubling time has decreased the morbidity and mortality of ectopic pregnancies.

RISK FACTORS FOR ECTOPIC PREGNANCY (IN DESCENDING ORDER OF SIGNIFICANCE) AND SYMPTOMS:

- Intrauterine device currently in place or recently used
- Previous tubal, abdominal, or pelvic surgery
- Prior ectopic pregnancy
- Prior sexually transmitted infection, especially pelvic inflammatory disease
- Infertility
- Recent therapeutic abortion

In several large studies, pain (97% to 100% of patients) and amenorrhea (74% to 84%) were more common complaints than vaginal bleeding, although bleeding occurred in the majority of ectopic pregnancies.

INTERPRETATION: TRANSABDOMINAL SCANNING: One technique for excluding or ruling out an ectopic pregnancy is to confirm or rule in an intrauterine pregnancy. With transabdominal scanning, to diagnose an ectopic pregnancy by actually visualizing the fetus in a tube or the adnexa is rare (<10% of ectopic pregnancies). Even with higher-resolution transvaginal scanning, only occasionally will the ectopic pregnancy be visualized (<25% of ectopic pregnancies).

To confirm an intrauterine pregnancy, a gestational sac with a fetus or fetal pole or yolk sac should be noted. A gestational sac appears as an anechoic (dark) structure within the uterus with highly echogenic borders. The first small echogenic structure seen in the gestational sac is the yolk sac at about 5.5 weeks. About a week later, a small collection of echoes may be seen; they constitute the fetal pole. The presence of a gestational sac with a fetal pole in the uterus reduces the chance of an ectopic pregnancy to about 1 in 10,000 cases. This figure represents the likelihood of a concomitant ectopic during an intrauterine pregnancy, the so-called combination

TABLE 214.1	Dates From Last Menstrual Period Correlated to Findings by Transabdominal Imaging
Finding	**Weeks**
Gestational sac	5–6
Yolk sac	5–6
Fetal pole	6–7
Cardiac activity	7–8
Placenta	8–9
Somatic activity	9–10

Transvaginal imaging can usually locate the same finding 1 wk earlier.

or heterotopic pregnancy. Exceptions to this statistic are found in patients undergoing assisted reproduction in which the risk of heterotopic pregnancy may be as high as 1 in 7000, or in patients taking ovulation-stimulating fertility drugs (e.g., clomiphene), in which the incidence may be as high as 1 in 100. If no fetal pole or yolk sac is seen within what appears to be a gestational sac, the clinician must consider that 10% to 20% of ectopic pregnancies produce pseudogestational sacs in the uterus and that the possibility of an ectopic pregnancy cannot be completely dismissed.

The gold standard for diagnosing an intrauterine pregnancy is the visualization of embryonic cardiac activity. This may be seen as early as 7 weeks after the first day of the patient's last menstrual period or when the mean sac diameter is 12 to 16 mm, depending on the resolution of the equipment and the skill of the examiner. *Mean sac diameter* is determined by measuring a single diameter if the sac is round. It is the average of the three largest diameters (transverse, longitudinal, and AP) if the sac is oval. If a fetus is seen, gestational age can also be determined from what else is visualized (Table 214.1). When a gestational sac with a mean diameter greater than 25 mm (17 mm for transvaginal scanning) lacks an embryo or when the gestational sac is grossly distorted, abnormal pregnancy is almost certain. Using these criteria, 76% of abnormal pregnancies and 93% of normal pregnancies will be correctly classified by only one ultrasound scan. The most accurate estimate of gestational age is at 9 to 11 weeks, using the crown-rump length.

If the patient is obese or her bladder is empty, transabdominal ultrasound findings may be limited; transvaginal scanning may be the only option. In all cases, failure to define an intrauterine pregnancy is interpreted in the proper clinical setting as an ectopic pregnancy until proven otherwise. Eight options exist when an intrauterine pregnancy is not demonstrated by POCUS (Table 214.2). Correlation with hCG titers may be necessary to complete the interpretation. With a healthy intrauterine pregnancy, hCG values rise predictably, doubling every 2 to 3 days for the first 8 weeks. In contrast, the hCG titer tends to rise at a slower rate in a patient with an ectopic pregnancy.

Even if an ectopic pregnancy is not demonstrated with POCUS, there are associated sonographic findings (Table 214.3) that, if seen, significantly increase the likelihood of ectopic pregnancy. In the case of a ruptured ectopic, scanning the upper abdomen may reveal free fluid representing intra-abdominal hemorrhage. Although a moderate to large amount of fluid is highly correlated with an ectopic pregnancy, any free fluid is significant in the proper clinical situation. A demonstrated echogenic pelvic mass also significantly increases the likelihood of ectopic pregnancy.

If a normal intrauterine pregnancy is demonstrated, the search for other causes of the patient's symptoms might be facilitated with ultrasound. The clinician should scan for evidence of urolithiasis, intact or ruptured ovarian or corpus luteum cyst, adnexal/ovarian torsion, tubo-ovarian abscess (dilated fallopian tubes/hydrosalpinx, usually bilateral, indicate pelvic inflammatory disease), or appendiceal abscess (appendicitis). Although a thorough description of the ultrasound findings for most of these situations is beyond the scope of this chapter, a ruptured ovarian cyst frequently is noted as

TABLE 214.2	Possible Diagnoses If an Intrauterine Pregnancy Is Not Demonstrated by Transabdominal Ultrasound	
Diagnosis	**Finding**	**Management**
Confirmed ectopic pregnancy	Empty uterus and ectopic fetal heart activity	Surgery or emergent consultation
Highly likely ectopic pregnancy	Empty uterus and echogenic pelvic mass or free pelvic fluid or hemoperitoneum	Surgery, culdocentesis, or emergent consultation
Very early normal pregnancy		Repeat quantitative hCG in 48–72 hr
Occult unruptured ectopic pregnancy	Empty uterus or may see pseudogestational sac in uterus (seen in 10%–20% of ectopic pregnancies)	Surgery, consultation, or repeat quantitative hCG in 48–72 hr if stable
Complete or incomplete spontaneous abortion	Empty uterus or atypical echogenic or sonolucent findings in uterus such as a misshapen sac, located low in the uterus, or debris in the sac	D&C to treat or confirm, consultation, or repeat quantitative hCG; emergency treatment necessary if cannot exclude ectopic pregnancy, if patient is unstable, or for heavy bleeding
Dead embryo	Crown–rump length >5 mm and no cardiac motion after continuous observation	Serial quantitative hCGs or repeat ultrasound in a few days; emergency treatment necessary only for heavy bleeding
Embryonic resorption/blighted ovum	Mean sac diameter of >2.5 cm and no fetal pole or >2.0 cm and no yolk sac (see text for calculating mean sac diameter); also, a misshapen empty sac, located low in uterus, or debris in the sac	Emergency treatment necessary only for heavy bleeding
Hydatidiform mole or trophoblastic disease	Snowstorm appearance of uterine contents	Consultation or D&C

D&C, Dilation and curettage; *hCG*, human chorionic gonadotropin; *IRP*, International Reference Preparation.

TABLE 214.3	Using Transabdominal Ultrasound to Determine Risk of Ectopic Pregnancy in Patients with Positive Human Chorionic Gonadotropin and Empty Uterus
Ancillary Findings	**Risk of Ectopic Pregnancy (%)**
Any free fluid	20
Echogenic mass	71
Moderate to large amount of fluid	95
Echogenic mass with fluid	100
No ancillary findings	20

an irregular adnexal mass, accompanied by fluid in the cul de sac. Evidence of clotting blood seen as an echogenic mass difficult to separate from the uterus. The appearance will be the same with a ruptured corpus luteum cyst; however, the ovary will be noted in the middle of the irregular adnexal mass. If color Doppler is available, it may diagnose probable adnexal/ovarian torsion by demonstrating an enlarged ovary with absent blood flow compared with the opposite adnexa. However, two arterial sources supply the ovary, the ovarian and the uterine arteries, so normal blood flow does not exclude ovarian torsion. A torsioned cyst is often associated with a torsioned ovary, and may have a fluid-fluid level and a thickened rim of tissue, and be tender with palpation with the transvaginal probe. Urolithiasis is discussed in a separate section of this chapter. However, it should be noted that diagnosing ovarian torsion is one of the pitfalls of POCUS; it is technically very challenging.

INTERPRETATION: TRANSVAGINAL SCANNING: The interpretation for transvaginal scanning is the same as for transabdominal scanning, except that with a fetus everything is visualized approximately 1 week earlier than with transabdominal scanning (see Table 214.1).

Threatened Abortion

Management of a threatened abortion consists of ruling out possible causes (or treating them), assessing the amount of bleeding, and predicting the prognosis for the pregnancy. If bleeding is minimal and no specific cause is identified, such as infection (e.g., urinary tract or cervix) or anemia, the patient is discharged in most cases with instructions for bed rest, to minimize stress, and to increase hydration. If the evaluation can be completed entirely in the emergency department or the office, treatment goals are more readily accomplished than if the patient must undergo a stressful evaluation in another department. Using specific sonographic criteria, the clinician may determine which patients need additional

ultrasound studies as well as reasonably estimate the prognosis of the early pregnancy. Without POCUS, the only prediction the clinician can make is that 50% of threatened abortions will progress to miscarriage.

INTERPRETATION: Frequently, the diagnosis of threatened abortion is made after ruling out ectopic pregnancy. The presence of fetal cardiac activity is an encouraging finding in an early pregnancy because the risk of spontaneous abortion is less than 2% to 4% if fetal cardiac activity is seen after 12 weeks. The risk of miscarriage is less than 16% if cardiac activity is noted at less than 8 postmenstrual weeks, which is much lower than the 50% predicted if POCUS is not available or performed.

With earlier pregnancies (even before the embryo is visible), major and minor criteria are available for evaluating gestational sacs (see Chapter 142, Obstetric Ultrasound). Again, patients with gestational sacs meeting most or all of these criteria by ultrasound scanning are much less likely to miscarry than the 50% rate predicted if the patients are evaluated by clinical means alone.

Failure to meet at least one major criterion is 100% specific in predicting spontaneous abortion. Fifty-three percent of abnormal pregnancies are identified by the same criteria. If there is a question about an abnormal sac, the patient should be scanned 7 to 10 days later. As an additional criterion during that time, the mean sac diameter in normal pregnancies should increase by about 1 mm/day.

Examples of abnormalities include low-lying gestational sacs (sacs in the cervical region) and abnormally shaped sacs. Both of these are worrisome findings and should be followed with a scan 1 week later. Frequently, low-lying sacs lead to spontaneous abortions, whereas abnormally shaped sacs lead to abnormal pregnancies. Worrisome findings also include failure of the sac to gain 1 cm in mean diameter in 1 week or the inability to visualize an embryo when the sac reaches 2.5 cm in mean sac diameter. These findings may assist the clinician in preparing the patient for the possibility of an abnormal pregnancy, such as one resulting in a spontaneous miscarriage.

Fibroids are present in 40% of women older than 40 years, have an echogenicity similar to the uterus (although the tissue is frequently organized in whorls), and can calcify. They are an overgrowth of uterine tissue and may be intracavitary, submucosal, intramural, subserosal, or pedunculated. Intracavitary fibroids almost always cause cramping and bleeding. Subserosal fibroids lie on the edge of the uterus and may indent the bladder, submucosal fibroids border lie on the endometrial lining, and intramural fibroids lie entirely within the myometrium. Pedunculated fibroids are connected by a neck to the body of the uterus and may be confused with adnexal masses.

Evaluation of Fetal Viability

Detection of fetal heart activity by the second and third trimester of pregnancy should be reliable by transabdominal scanning (see Chapter 142, Obstetric Ultrasound). Earlier detection may require transvaginal scanning.

Interpretation

The absence of fetal cardiac activity and fetal movement after scanning for a 5-minute interval in a pregnancy of more than 20 weeks' gestation is said to be 100% reliable for diagnosing a fetal demise. For a first-trimester pregnancy, if uncertainty exists about fetal heart activity, rescanning should be performed in 1 to 2 weeks.

Secondary criteria for fetal demise using POCUS include fetal anomalies such as hydrops, ascites, and pleural or pericardial effusions. Echogenic gas in the fetal heart and vessels may be early findings. Late findings include morphologic changes such as skeletal anomalies and unusual fetal positioning.

Reaction to external stimulation or uterine manipulation should cause brisk reflexes in viable fetuses, as opposed to the passive motions seen with a fetal demise. Avoid misinterpreting the passive motions from uterine contractions around a dead fetus as fetal activity.

Because abruptio placentae cannot always be diagnosed with ultrasound (i.e., it is a clinical diagnosis), ultrasound studies should be used in conjunction with maternal–fetal monitoring in the pregnant patient with significant abdominal trauma. A 4-hour monitoring period should be sufficient to identify fetal distress.

Misplaced Intrauterine Device

Intrauterine contraceptive devices (IUDs) are approved for 3 to 10 years of continuous use. This length of time offers many opportunities to lose the string. The manufacturers now recommend cutting the strings shorter; this also increases the risk of a missing string. When a string is not visible or palpable on an IUD, possible causes include a properly positioned IUD in the uterus that has lost its string, strings located in the cervix, an extruded IUD, or an IUD that has perforated the uterus and may even be lying in the abdomen. IUD users who have not lost the string also warrant further evaluation if they are experiencing cramping, pain, or abnormal bleeding. A flat-plate radiograph may document the presence of the IUD, but it will not help determine whether the IUD is in the uterus. Gynecologic instrumentation is another option, but instrumentation places the patient at risk of infection. In most cases, it should be reserved for removal of the IUD after the location is documented. Ultrasound is usually the diagnostic procedure of choice to determine the location of an IUD. However, the diameter of most IUDs is less than 3 mm; therefore scanning for IUDs in some cases is more difficult than expected.

Interpretation

An IUD on ultrasound produces a very straight, sharp-edged, echogenic image. Document the location of the IUD in both longitudinal (Fig. 214.15A) and transverse or coronal views (see Fig. 214.15B). It may be accompanied by a small "ball" of echoes in the cervix—the string coiled up, which can often be retrieved with a cervical brush used for Papanicolaou smears (see Chapter 135, Intrauterine Device Insertion and Removal). If an IUD is not demonstrated and the posterior wall of the uterus is not easily identified, formal scanning may be necessary. IUDs may be difficult to locate when the uterus is retroverted.

Decidual reaction may mimic an IUD. To differentiate, an IUD should produce shadowing in at least one plane. Echoes from an IUD are typically straighter and sharper-edged than those from a decidual reaction.

A perforation should be recorded as either complete or incomplete. For an incomplete perforation, a portion of the IUD can be

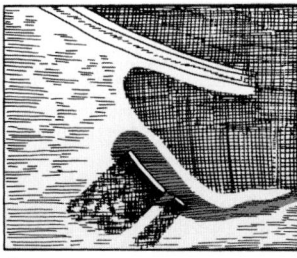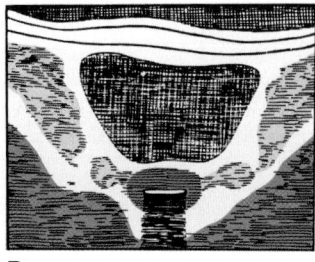

Fig. 214.15   Intrauterine device in longitudinal (A) and transverse (B) views.

demonstrated within the uterine wall. A flat-plate x-ray film may be necessary to document a complete perforation if it is not visible by ultrasound.

ABDOMINAL ULTRASOUND

Various tests can be used when deciding whether conditions are good enough to perform a complete abdominal survey, especially if using portable equipment. The gain can also be set when performing these tests. First, if the bladder is full, an attempt should be made to scan it; if a full bladder cannot be scanned, the body habitus or conditions are probably not conducive for obtaining a complete abdominal survey. If the bladder can be scanned, the gain on the machine should be set low enough to eliminate echoes from a normally nonechogenic organ. Next, the clinician should attempt to scan the aorta lengthwise. Repositioning may be required, and the liver may be needed as a window. If the aorta is located, the gain should be set to minimize internal echoes because this organ normally has no echoes. (This gain setting can then generally be used to scan the majority of the abdomen.) If the clinician is unable to locate the aorta after several attempts and several minutes of scanning, body habitus or conditions may preclude a complete abdominal survey or scan. The clinician may be restricted to a focused or limited scan. The pelvis with a full bladder and the liver, right kidney, and RUQ structures will probably be easiest to scan. A referral may be necessary for a formal, complete scan for other abdominal structures.

Biliary Tract Disease

Acute cholecystitis in the ambulatory setting in the United States results from obstruction of the cystic duct by gallstones in approximately 95% of cases. Unfortunately, the diagnosis of acute cholecystitis by purely clinical means (without ultrasound) has an accuracy of only 50%, even with a positive Murphy sign (pain over the gallbladder with palpation during inspiration). Therefore ultrasound is the preferred diagnostic test for acute cholecystitis, and POCUS can be used. A "sonographic Murphy sign" combined with the presence of gallstones increases the diagnostic accuracy for acute cholecystitis to more than 90%. A sonographic Murphy sign is described as pain elicited with probe compression over the gallbladder, especially if stones are present. Because early surgical management is now the treatment of choice for acute cholecystitis, early diagnosis is also important. POCUS is useful in diagnosing most cases of cholelithiasis and acute cholecystitis; however, obscure cases may require additional studies.

Preprocedure Patient Preparation

If possible, the patient should have been in the fasting state for at least 8 hours; this ensures that the gallbladder is fully distended. Early-morning scanning may minimize bowel gas interference.

Technique

1. Scan the patient in the supine or left-lateral position, longitudinally, with a low-frequency probe until you locate the gallbladder.

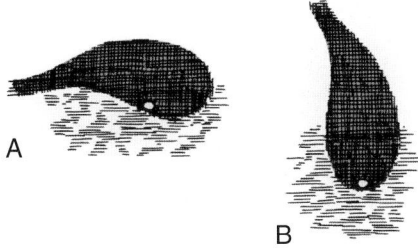

Fig. 214.16 (A) Gallstone is small and shadowing is not seen. (B) However, it moves when the patient is repositioned.

It is usually located in about the midclavicular line, just above the inferior edge of the liver; however, it can be located anywhere between the midline and the anterior axillary line. A combination of subcostal and intercostal windows may be needed. Sustained inspiration by the patient may move the liver below the ribs and improve the subcostal window. The normal gallbladder is a cystic structure; when distended, it demonstrates the sonographic properties of cysts elsewhere in the body. The walls are smooth, usually no echogenic matter exists between them, and tissue behind the posterior wall is more clearly defined.

Other cystic structures located nearby that can be confused with the gallbladder include hepatic cysts, hepatic veins, the portal vein, renal cysts, the duodenum, the IVC, and the abdominal aorta. Hepatic cysts have very thin walls and are usually located much deeper in the hepatic parenchyma than the gallbladder. Hepatic veins usually run vertically within the liver when the patient is supine. They also have very thin walls that are compressible with probe pressure. Veins also collapse with inspiration and expand with a Valsalva maneuver. If followed posteriorly, the location just below the diaphragm where the hepatic veins empty into the IVC can usually be seen. Although the portal vein has echogenic sidewalls similar to the gallbladder, it can usually be viewed coursing horizontally through the liver. Often, tributaries to the portal vein, such as the splenic vein, can be traced from their origin to where they join to form the portal vein near the liver. Renal cysts can usually be demonstrated as very thin-walled and contiguous with renal tissue (Fig. 214.16). They are located much further lateral and posterior than the gallbladder. Although the abdominal aorta has echogenic walls, it demonstrates pulsations and can be followed distally. Color Doppler can also help distinguish vascular structures; the gallbladder has no internal flow. Pulsations transmitted from the aorta may also be noted in the IVC. Having the patient take in a large breath should collapse the vena cava; a Valsalva maneuver should cause significant dilation. The duodenum can usually be distinguished from the gallbladder because peristalsis is observed. Having the patient drink water can also stimulate and demonstrate peristalsis in the duodenum. Air in the duodenum usually casts confusing, irregular shadows as opposed to the sharp shadows of gallstones.

2. Compared with other abdominal organs, the gallbladder usually has a rather superficial location on the inferior edge of the liver. After locating the gallbladder with the probe in the longitudinal position, obtain a long-axis view by rotating the probe out of the longitudinal plane of the body until the maximal length of the gallbladder is visualized and an image recorded. The maximal transverse diameter of the gallbladder should also be measured and recorded.

3. Obtain additional views of the gallbladder by moving the patient into one other position: the decubitus (right side up) position or the erect position. Repositioning the patient helps avoid missing stones that may have rolled into a dependent position out of view.

4. Attempt to identify the source of any local tenderness and scan that area. The porta hepatis, which consists of the common bile duct, the hepatic artery, and the portal vein, can often be located by following the portal vein from the confluence of the splenic

vein and the superior mesenteric vein. Conversely, the portal vessels in the liver can be followed horizontally until they coalesce as the portal vein at the hepatic hilum. The porta hepatis also can be located by tracking the hepatic artery from the celiac axis. Color Doppler can help distinguish the common bile duct from the hepatic artery.

Interpretation

An echogenic structure within the gallbladder is a gallstone if it shows prominent posterior shadowing, has circumferential bile visible in at least one view, and has demonstrated mobility when the patient is placed in various positions (Fig. 214.17). When coupled with a positive sonographic Murphy sign, this is diagnostic of acute cholecystitis. Otherwise, gallstones can have several variations when viewed sonographically:

- *Nonshadowing:* Gallstones less than 2 to 3 mm in size often do not cast a shadow. In that situation, the differential also includes echogenic structures such as polyps or folds in the gallbladder. In fact, echogenic structures in the gallbladder that are nonshadowing are calculi in only 50% of cases. If, however, an echogenic structure is noted to have gravity-dependent motion, it is usually a stone (Fig. 214.18).
- *Intermittent shadowing:* Multiple small stones may form an irregular layer in the most dependent portion of the gallbladder. They may also cast a variable or intermittent shadow. This may be highly suspect for cholelithiasis, but further studies are necessary if there is no well-defined shadowing.
- *Filled gallbladder:* If the gallbladder is entirely filled with stones, bile may not be noted circumferentially around any one stone. Shadowing may be less prominent or hazy. Because a gas-filled duodenum can have the same appearance, it must be carefully eliminated from the differential by studying for other characteristics (e.g., peristalsis).
- *Adherent stones:* These can appear as echogenic structures that are not gravity dependent. If no shadowing is seen, further studies may be necessary to exclude a polyp, tumor, or fold, which can also be echogenic.
- *Floating stones:* Either one stone or a collection of stones may float and appear as an echogenic structure or a line of echoes in a nondependent portion of the gallbladder. If they do not cast a shadow, further studies may be necessary.
- *Absent gallbladder:* This sonographic finding (absence) may also be noted in a nonfasting patient or in one with chronic cholecystitis and severe scarring preventing expansion of the gallbladder. A patient with a completely stone-filled gallbladder, with a previous cholecystectomy, or with congenital absence of a gallbladder may also have a nonvisible gallbladder. If the gallbladder is not readily imaged and the patient is clinically stable, additional scanning should be performed several hours later with the patient fasting.

Additional echogenic structures that can be noted in the gallbladder include folds and septations (very common, the so-called phrygian cap) or polyps (less common). These are immobile and do not cast shadows. Other possible findings within and around the gallbladder include the following:

- *Increased diameter:* A gallbladder diameter greater than 5 cm may be evidence of cholecystitis.
- *Sludge:* Low-level to mixed echogenic material that is slow to layer out after the patient changes positions may be gallbladder sludge. It most commonly represents biliary stasis and may occur in various conditions (e.g., obstructive jaundice, liver disease, sepsis) or in patients receiving hyperalimentation or certain other medications. It may also precede the formation of gallstones by a few years.
- *Edema/pericolic fluid:* A thin, dark line of fluid around the gallbladder wall may represent gallbladder edema, which can be

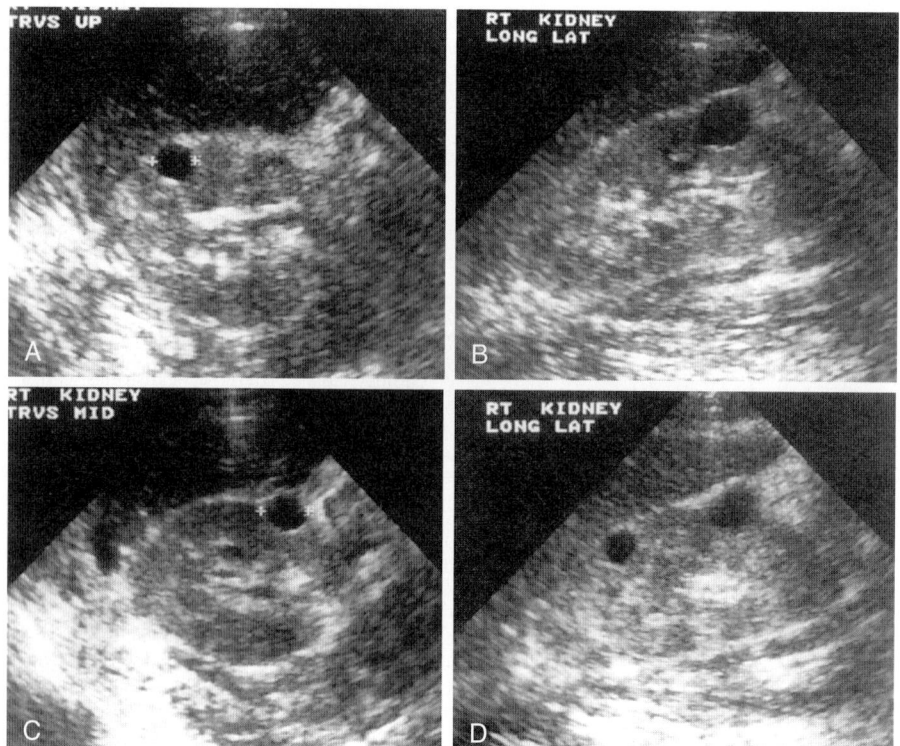

Fig. 214.17 Transverse (A and C) and longitudinal (B and D) scans of two small renal cysts along the lateral wall of the kidney. Borders are smooth and well defined. No echoes are present.

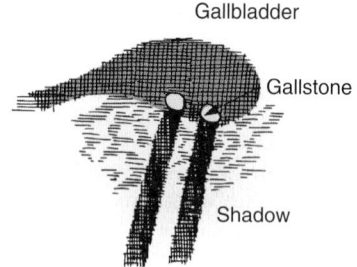

Fig. 214.18 Acoustic shadowing behind two gallstones. Note the "sharpness" of the shadow.

found in acute cholecystitis or other conditions such as hypoalbuminemia, hepatitis, and ascites. In the situation where the patient has a sonographic Murphy sign, discrete pockets of fluid may represent small abscesses. These abscesses are often near the fundus and are definitive evidence of acute cholecystitis.

- *Thickening:* Wall thickening is not specific for acute cholecystitis. The anterior wall is usually the easiest to measure. A rim of diffuse echogenicity greater than 3 mm thick may represent contraction after a recent meal, hepatic dysfunction, congestive heart failure, renal disease, ascites, sepsis, or neoplasms elsewhere (decreased osmotic pressure or elevated portal venous pressure). Patients with acquired immunodeficiency syndrome may also have diffuse thickening. Irregular wall thickening is also common with both acute and chronic cholecystitis. If no stone is present yet the patient has a positive sonographic Murphy sign, acalculous cholecystitis is a possibility.

- *Dilated common bile duct:* The normal common bile duct is less than 5 mm in diameter, but it can increase with age by 1 mm per decade after age 50 without indicating a pathologic process. A diameter greater than 1 cm is likely pathologic no matter what the age.

Other entities, including hepatic tumors and abnormalities of the pancreas or portal system, would not usually be identified by a limited or focused examination. However, hepatic cysts are common (although not as common as renal cysts), are usually smooth walled, and demonstrate properties of cysts elsewhere. Hepatic malignancies usually demonstrate a variation in density from the normal surrounding tissue, but this can be very subtle.

Urinary Tract (Obstructive Uropathy, Renal Colic, Hematuria, Renal Abscess, Evaluation of Bladder)

Obstruction of the collecting ducts of the kidney may be acute or chronic and unilateral or bilateral. Renal failure due to obstruction may be relatively asymptomatic, so an ultrasound study may be helpful, especially in those at risk (e.g., older man with benign prostatic hyperplasia). Up to 15% of American men will experience an episode of renal colic severe enough to require emergent medical attention. With flank pain and hematuria being the hallmark signs and symptoms for a stone, if a small stone is identified and the patient responds to analgesics, expectant management may be adequate. If available, real-time helical/spiral CT scanning using a stone protocol has somewhat become the diagnostic procedure of choice for identifying stones. Though CT is the gold standard in the diagnostic evaluation of renal colic, a strategy of ultrasound-first is safe and effective. If a spiral CT and ultrasound are not available, studies have found that plain radiographs (KUB: kidney, ureter, and bladder) rarely change the clinician's management of renal colic. Intravenous pyelograms (IVPs) can be used when direct imaging of the urinary tract is necessary. Studies comparing sensitivity of ultrasound and IVP have found them to be relatively comparable. However, most studies have found IVP to be somewhat more specific. Nonetheless, in certain situations, ultrasound may be preferred over IVP (Box 214.2). Even if ultrasound does not reveal the diagnosis, at least it is noninvasive and certainly can be followed up with an IVP.

Evaluation of hematuria in the asymptomatic person probably warrants cystoscopy (see Chapter 97, Diagnostic Cystourethroscopy);

however, it may warrant an ultrasound scan, even though evaluating all of the possible sources requires considerable scanning experience. The patient with a possible renal abscess (e.g., fever from pyelonephritis defervesced on IV antibiotics for a few days and then spiked again) may also benefit from use of ultrasound, especially in the area of the original flank pain. Scanning the patient for possible renal trauma is discussed with the FAST examination.

NOTE: A leaking or dissecting AAA may produce signs and symptoms similar to left-sided renal colic, including hematuria. In fact, left-sided renal colic is the most common misdiagnosis in elderly patients with a symptomatic AAA. In patients older than 55 years with left-sided renal colic, CT or ultrasound should be considered to exclude this potentially fatal diagnosis.

Preprocedure Patient Preparation

Under optimal conditions, the patient should have been in the fasting state for at least 8 hours to minimize bowel gas. Early-morning scanning may be preferable; bowel gas is usually minimal. Understanding that patients do not always come to the hospital or the office under these conditions, the clinician may need to hydrate the patient to increase hydronephrosis and enhance the acoustic window. Therefore, administering IV fluids may be not only therapeutic but helpful for making the diagnosis.

Technique

1. Scan the patient in the supine position, longitudinally, with a low-frequency probe until the kidney is located. Kidneys are football shaped with a white stripe (echogenic renal sinus) down the middle. The renal sinus is surrounded by the echolucent renal cortex, which in turn is surrounded by the echogenic renal capsule (Fig. 214.19A). Compared with other abdominal organs, the kidneys are very posterior and lateral organs. On the right, the kidney is located at the posterior inferior edge of the liver, far lateral to the midclavicular line. Prolonged deep inspiration by the patient should bring the liver edge down from under the subcostal margin to improve the window and facilitate locating the kidney. Scanning between the ribs may also be necessary to obtain a good window through the liver.

2. The left kidney is located slightly higher than the right. On the left, the same maneuvers may enhance the use of the spleen as an acoustic window. Having the patient turn completely onto his or her right side to facilitate scanning in the coronal and transverse planes may also be helpful. Even scanning between the ribs from the back may be useful. Occasionally, having the patient sit in the erect position will bring the kidney into view. If no kidney is found on the left side, attempt to locate the kidney by scanning the pelvis for a pelvic kidney or the midline for a horseshoe kidney.

3. After locating each kidney, with the probe in the longitudinal position, obtain a long-axis view. Rotate the probe out of the longitudinal plane of the body until the maximal length of the organ is visualized.

4. Attempt to assess for the presence or absence of hydronephrosis or hydroureter in both kidneys. Also attempt to locate any other intrarenal or extrarenal fluid collections, masses, or calcifications. The bladder should be scanned (see the section Ultrasound Evaluation of the Bladder), especially if there is hydronephrosis or hydroureter.

BOX 214.2   Conditions in Which Ultrasound May Be Preferable to Intravenous Pyelography

Dehydration
Contrast allergy
Diabetes mellitus
Differential diagnosis includes dissecting aortic aneurysm or acute cholecystitis
Inadequate abdominal preparation for intravenous pyelography
Poor venous access
Pregnancy
Renal failure or proteinuria
Time constraints

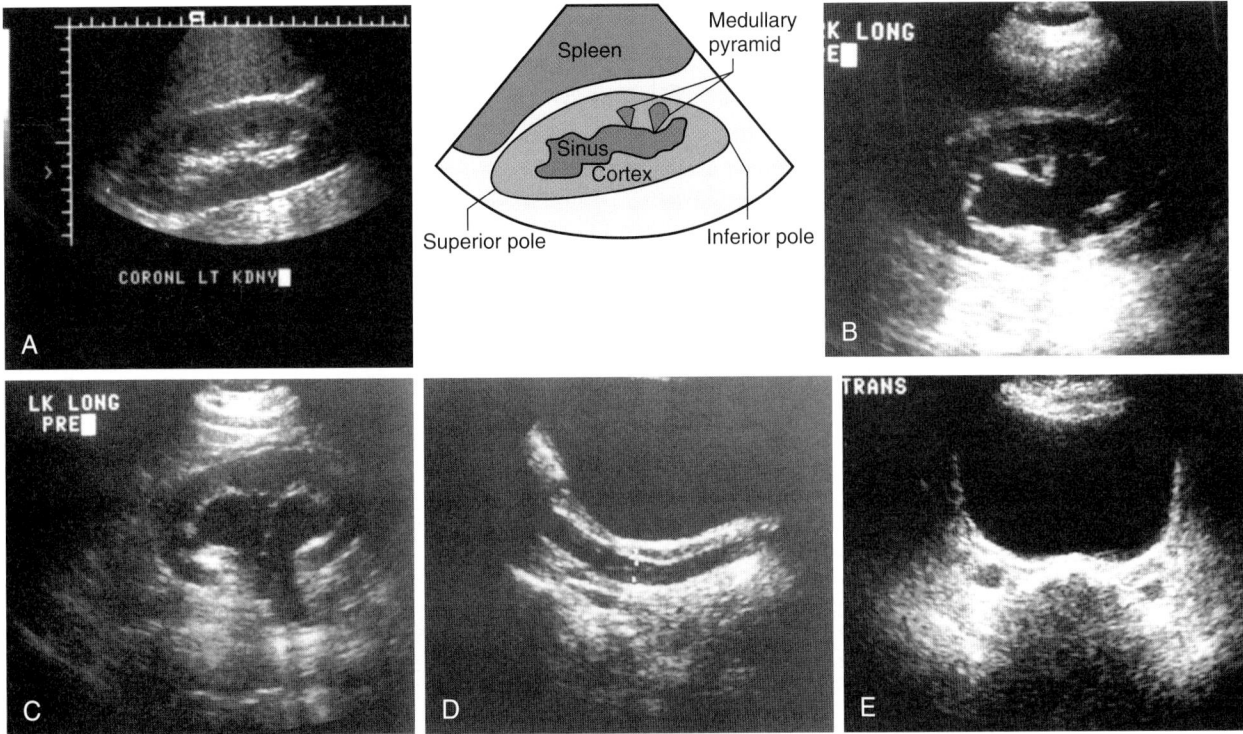

Fig. 214.19 Longitudinal view of the left kidney (A), including inferior and superior poles. Pseudohydronephrosis of both kidneys (B and C) and ureters (D) associated with a full bladder (E).

Interpretation

Because most episodes of renal colic are caused by small stones (2 to 4 mm), visualizing the stone is not common. The confirmation of renal colic is usually made by demonstrating hydronephrosis or hydroureter in the correct clinical setting (flank pain, hematuria). Associated intrarenal calcifications further support the diagnosis. However, absence of hydronephrosis does not exclude the possibility of a stone; it may be small or have already passed.

The normal ureter is rarely visualized with the POCUS, so demonstration of a dark, fluid-filled ureter (hydroureter) is usually abnormal. With accumulation of additional fluid, as seen in hydronephrosis, the normal echogenic renal sinus stripe may actually be split by fluid, appearing as an intervening dark stripe. Along with this intervening stripe, the full appearance of hydronephrosis is characterized by increased fluid throughout the kidney, often contiguous with the hydroureter. Make sure the patient has voided before the ultrasound examination because a very full or overdistended bladder can cause pseudohydronephrosis, which appears identical to mild or moderate hydronephrosis (see Fig. 214.19B and C). Dehydration may also mask hydronephrosis, so IV hydration may be necessary before the scan.

When hydronephrosis is noted, an attempt should be made to follow the hydroureter(s) distally to the source of the obstruction. When associated with hydronephrosis, an echogenic structure found as the source of an obstruction, with or without prominent posterior shadowing, is diagnostic of urolithiasis. A stone larger than 3 mm should be highly echogenic and cast a well-defined shadow. With a good acoustic window and minimal bowel gas, the ureterovesical junction may be visualized and is a common place to find stones; stones frequently lodge at this level. Occasionally a stone will have passed this junction and be found in the bladder. Even if a stone cannot be located distally, scanning the kidney may reveal intrarenal calcifications. As mentioned previously, intrarenal calcifications associated with hydroureter support the diagnosis of renal colic due to a stone.

With moderate chronic hydronephrosis, there is thinning of the renal medulla (Fig. 214.20A). With severe, long-standing, chronic hydronephrosis, there may also be thinning of the renal cortex (see Fig. 214.20B and C). If bilateral obstructions are found, they are more likely due to an obstruction at the bladder outlet. In this situation, the bladder will be distended, should be easily scanned, and should be scanned carefully for the source of obstruction. One system grades hydronephrosis as mild or grade I (any hydronephrosis up to grade II), moderate/grade II (renal sinus is split and confluent with calyces), or severe/grade III (causing effacement of renal parenchyma).

Hydronephrosis can be a normal finding in pregnancy, especially on the right side. Renal cysts may also mimic hydronephrosis. With POCUS, simple renal cysts appear like cysts elsewhere in the body. They have smooth borders and no echogenic material within them. Renal cysts are common, occurring in 50% of individuals older than 50 years. As opposed to hydronephrosis, renal cysts are well-circumscribed and do not communicate with fluid outside the kidney (see Fig. 214.18). Renal cell carcinoma, which may appear as an echogenic mass in the kidney, can also cause hematuria. Transitional cell carcinoma can be seen as a mass anywhere along the length of a ureter or in the bladder. Fluid around the capsule, which appears as a dark stripe and can be irregular, may represent a perinephric abscess or, in the trauma patient, hemoperitoneum or a hematoma; hence clinical correlation will be important.

Ultrasound Evaluation of the Bladder

Up to 8% of infants younger than 8 weeks in the emergency department with a temperature of 100.6°F or higher have a urinary tract infection (UTI). As much as 5% of infants younger than 2 years with unexplained fever have UTIs. The rate is 8% in girls and uncircumcised boys but less than 1% in circumcised boys. White girls have a much higher rate (up to 15%) than black girls. Boys are at the highest risk during the first 3 to 6 months of life.

Using an evidence-based approach, in those infants or children sufficiently ill to warrant immediate antibiotic therapy, the practice parameter of the American Academy of Pediatrics recommends a SPA or transurethral catheterization to obtain a urine specimen and then treating with antibiotics. In those not sufficiently ill to require immediate antibiotics, the same diagnostic approach can be used; however, a bag collection is another option. If a urinalysis obtained by the most convenient means indicates a UTI, a sterile urine specimen should then be obtained in the same manner as listed earlier. These recommendations are based on a summary of the evidence and good clinical judgment; however, although a negative culture from a bagged specimen effectively rules out UTI, culture results are not available immediately. Bagged specimen cultures are also rarely negative, and unfortunately culture results cannot be predicted from urinalysis in most cases. Therefore many clinicians opt for SPA or catheterization.

Although catheterization is less invasive than SPA, the process of catheterization may actually cause a UTI. SPA is inherently invasive, yet few serious complications have been reported, and numerous studies have demonstrated the superiority of SPA over alternative techniques. Limiting SPA to patients with proven full bladders further minimizes the risk to the infant (see Chapter 168, Pediatric Suprapubic Bladder Aspiration). One change to the most recent American Academy of Pediatrics guidelines is that a voiding cystourethrogram is no longer recommended after the first documented UTI; however, ultrasound imaging of the kidneys and bladder is still recommended.

In adults, there are indications in the emergency department, hospital, and the office for SPA or suprapubic cannulation (SPC). SPA can be useful for obtaining a urine culture whenever a urethral catheter cannot be placed (or is contraindicated) or may be particularly useful in critically ill, potentially septic, or unresponsive adults. SPC is indicated whenever a urethral catheter is indicated yet cannot or should not be placed (e.g., trauma patients who have serious injury to the urethra, patients who recently underwent bladder or gynecologic surgery, or when a sufficiently wide catheter is unable to be passed through the urethra for diagnostic cystometry; see also Chapter 99, Suprapubic Catheter Insertion and/or Change, and Chapter 100, Suprapubic Tap or Aspiration).

Ultrasound may also be used in adults to estimate PVR to evaluate the significance or status of urethral obstruction (e.g., significant prostatic hyperplasia) or a neurogenic bladder. PVR can be measured more precisely, albeit more invasively, by inserting a catheter; however, ultrasound provides reasonable estimates of PVR in a much more comfortable manner with less risk of inducing an infection.

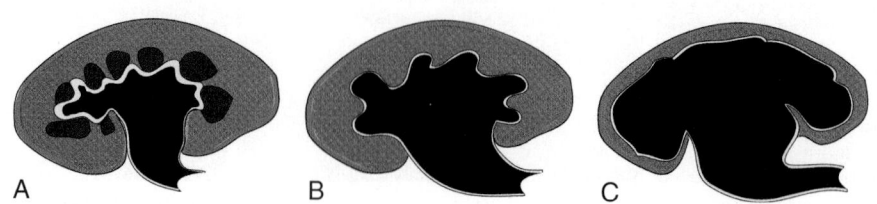

Fig. 214.20 (A) Mild hydronephrosis. Note hydroureters. (B) Moderate hydronephrosis. (C) Severe hydronephrosis.

Given the fact that recent studies have failed to document an exact level of PVR that would benefit from transurethral resection of the prostate (TURP) as opposed to watchful waiting, PVR estimates from ultrasound may be more than adequate in that situation (considering TURP).

Preprocedure Patient Preparation

The patient (or his or her parents or caregiver) should be informed about the indication for the study. If a suprapubic tap or cannulation is to be performed, counseling should be given for informed consent.

Technique

1. Infants should be placed in the supine, frog-leg position; adults should be supine. Perform the scanning in a transverse manner with a high-frequency transducer in infants. The marker dot should be directed toward the infant's right side, with the transducer placed slightly above the symphysis pubis. The transducer should be directed posteriorly or slightly caudad to locate the bladder. In adults, a low-frequency probe is used with the transducer and marker dot in the same location. The transducer should be angled in more of a caudal direction.

   NOTE: In infants younger than 2 years, the bladder is an abdominal organ. As the pelvis grows, the bladder moves into the pelvis; therefore the transducer should be angled more caudad.

2. Move and angle the probe to locate the maximal transverse diameter of the bladder. In infants, this is the probe location and angle to take measurements for determining whether the bladder is full. Take measurements in both the AP and transverse diameters.

3. For aspiration or cannulation, note the angulation of the probe necessary to locate the maximal transverse diameter of the bladder. Note the depth necessary to penetrate the bladder. The same angulation and depth should be used when directing the aspiration needle or trocar.

4. To estimate bladder volume in an adult, including PVR, three diameters should be determined. First, measure and record the greatest transverse measurement (w in Fig. 214.21A). Next, turn the marker dot cephalad and find the longest longitudinal plane. Measure and record the maximal superoinferior measurement (h in Fig. 214.21B) in this plane. In the same plane, with that same image, measure and record the maximal AP measurement (Fig. 214.22; see d in Fig. 214.21B).

Interpretation and Results

In infants, a pocket of fluid larger than 2 × 2 cm in the retropubic area measured in the AP and maximal transverse diameters defines a "full" bladder (see Fig. 214.22). In adults, the pocket should be much larger to reach it with a needle or trocar. Again, SPA or SPC should be attempted at the same angle with which the maximal transverse bladder diameter was measured (Fig. 214.23). One study resulted in obtaining urine in 79% of children meeting these criteria and undergoing aspiration. If the bladder is found to be empty and the patient is clinically stable, repeat scanning to search for a full bladder should be performed 30 minutes to 1 hour after the initial scan. If a full bladder cannot be found on the repeat scan, bladder catheterization should be considered.

In adults, bladder volume can be calculated with this formula, which accommodates for the irregular shape of the bladder:

$$0.7 \times h \times d \times w$$

This yields a standard error of approximately 21%. Although 21% may seem like a large error, as mentioned earlier, it is now known that no certain PVR threshold exists where surgery (TURP) ensures success and avoids future morbidity. For that reason, this crude measurement may be more than adequate. If more precise volumes are needed, more sophisticated formulas are available with correction factors, depending on the degree of distension of the bladder. In addition, software packages are available for more precise estimates

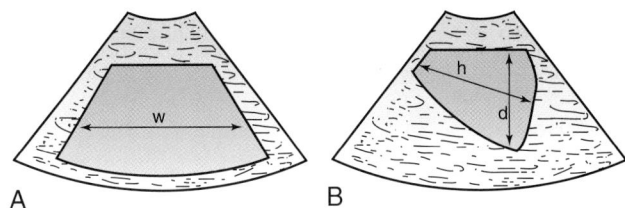

Fig. 214.21 (A) Greatest transverse diameter of bladder is shown by w. (B) Maximal superoinferior measurement is shown by h; the maximal anteroposterior measurement is shown by d.

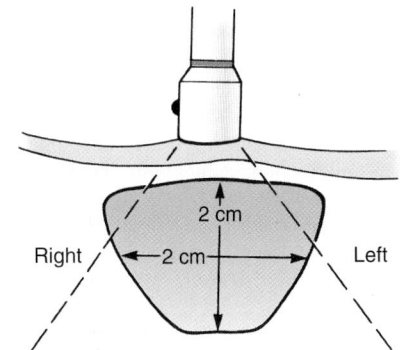

Fig. 214.22 Transverse view of a full infant bladder.

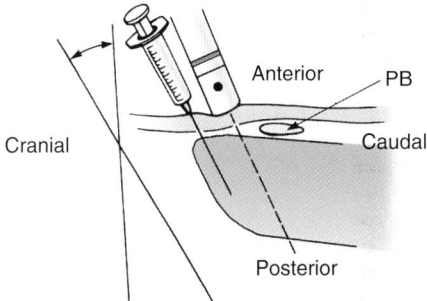

Fig. 214.23 Needle should be inserted next to the probe and parallel to whatever angle demonstrated the greatest diameter of the bladder. *PB*, Pubic bone.

using large machines that can take more precise measurements. Portable ultrasound equipment is also available that is used solely for making urologic measurements. Such equipment has been studied extensively, and its accuracy has been documented.

Aorta

Unlike coronary artery disease and cerebrovascular disease, the incidence and associated mortality rate of AAAs continue to increase. Men are affected three to four times more frequently than women. The prevalence of AAA has climbed to 10% in people older than 65 years, and ruptured AAA has also become the 10th leading cause of death in men older than 55 years. Consequently, the United States Preventive Services Task Force recommends screening for AAA and Medicare will reimburse for a screen in men aged 65 to 75 who have smoked at least 100 cigarettes or men and women at age 65 who have a family history of AAA.

The natural history of an AAA is to expand at a rate of 0.21 to 0.4 cm/yr. Over 5 years, a 4-cm AAA has a 10% chance of rupture, a 5-cm aneurysm an 18% chance, and a 6-cm aneurysm a 30% or greater likelihood of rupturing. Controlling blood pressure and cessation of smoking may diminish the risk of rupture. At all comparable sizes, women may have a higher risk of rupture. Elective repair in most large centers has a mortality risk of less than 5%, compared with up to 80% in those patients who live long enough to reach the operating room after rupture. Therefore stenting or elective resection is indicated for low- to moderate-risk patients with aneurysms that measure more than 5 cm in diameter.

Risk Factors

- Male sex
- 50 years of age or older
- Use of tobacco
- Hypertension
- Family history of AAA*
- Other atherosclerotic risk factors may also be AAA risk factors.

The classic triad of ruptured AAA is pulsatile abdominal mass; low back, flank, or abdominal pain; and hypotension. Less than 50% of victims, however, possess this triad, and less than 25% are hypotensive on admission. Unfortunately, low back, flank, or abdominal pain is a frequent complaint for patients in the age group at risk for AAA. Patients with a leaking AAA may have many other signs and symptoms as well, including chest pain, ecchymoses, or a scrotal mass. The most common incorrect diagnosis in an elderly patient with a symptomatic AAA is left-sided renal colic. A leaking AAA may even be associated with hematuria; therefore any elderly patient with left-sided renal colic should be considered to have an AAA until proven otherwise.

Most aortic aneurysms are found in the mid-abdomen, just above the iliac bifurcation (about the level of the umbilicus). Physical examination is extremely inaccurate for diagnosing AAA. Aortography may underestimate the size of an aneurysm if it is filled with thrombus or is dissecting, and lateral radiographs overestimate the possibility and size. Ultrasound has been shown to be accurate in identifying both aneurysmal and normal aortas, especially infrarenally. For screening, ultrasound is comparable with CT scanning, which is the gold standard for both diagnosis and estimation of size. However, ultrasound may be a difficult study if there is a large amount of bowel gas, retained barium, or marked obesity. In addition, CT scanning is better than ultrasound for identifying a leaking aneurysm, although POCUS may be useful when there is not enough time to perform a CT scan (emergent situation).

Preprocedure Patient Preparation

Under optimal conditions, the patient should have fasted for at least 8 hours to minimize bowel gas. Early-morning scanning may also be preferable because bowel gas is usually minimal. Patients do not always present to the primary care clinician under these conditions; however, if a pulsatile mass is palpable through the anterior abdominal wall, it should be readily scannable. The patient should be informed of possible diagnoses and the indication for scanning.

Technique

1. With a low-frequency probe and the patient in the supine position, attempt to define the general outline of the aorta with longitudinal scanning (Fig. 214.24). It is thick walled and pulsating. The IVC runs parallel and may be transmitting pulsations but will be thin walled and will collapse with inspiration and distend with a Valsalva maneuver. If a pulsatile mass is palpated, it should not be difficult to determine whether it is contiguous with the abdominal aorta. If the aorta cannot be identified with longitudinal scanning, rotate the probe for a transverse scan and the aorta will often be revealed slightly anterior and to the left of the patient's vertebral body. A transverse view of the IVC will be noted to the patient's right (to the left of the image).

2. After defining the general outline, measurements should be taken of the largest AP diameter on transverse scanning at 1 to 2 cm increments from immediately below the diaphragm (at level

*Family history is most significant when a female relative has been diagnosed. Elastinolytic enzymes, decreased type III collagen, decreased elastin, and other biochemical variants are being studied to determine what is probably a multifactorially inherited etiology.

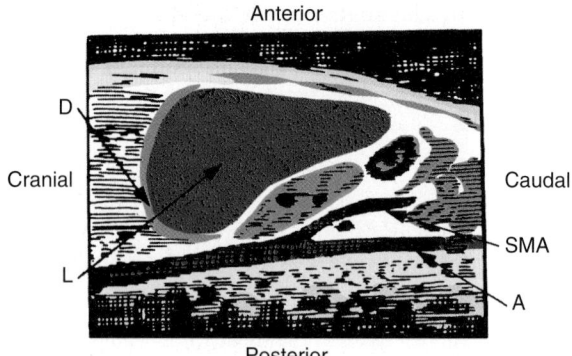

Fig. 214.24 Longitudinal scan slightly to the left of the midline showing normal structures and orientation. *A*, Aorta; *D*, diaphragm; *L*, liver; *SMA*, superior mesenteric artery.

of xiphoid) to a level 3 cm below the umbilicus. Measurements are taken from the outside wall to the opposite outside wall. Be aware that the transverse diameter of the aorta on a transverse scan may be exaggerated if the aorta is tangentially imaged when it makes a lateral turn. In addition, avoid applying too much probe pressure, which can also distort AP measurements. That being said, both AP and lateral transverse diameters should be measured because the lateral diameter of an AAA is often larger than the AP diameter. The lateral diameter may be slightly more difficult to obtain because the AP walls and diameter are usually more sharply demarcated. Longitudinal measurements should never be taken, as the diameter will be underestimated if taken slightly off midline.

3. If there is considerable truncal obesity or overlying bowel gas, increased surface pressure with the probe may enhance visualization. Immediately below the xiphoid, the liver can often be used as a window, especially if the patient suspends breathing briefly after a deep inspiration. Despite these maneuvers, bowel gas frequently obscures a 4- or 5-cm segment between the xiphoid and umbilicus. Using a rocking motion with the probe and scanning from above and below this segment may allow for a complete, systematic evaluation of the entire abdominal aorta. Turning the patient to the right or left lateral decubitus position may enhance scanning the aorta in the area of the kidneys, although the iliac bifurcation may not be visible unless the liver or spleen is enlarged. With the patient in the left lateral decubitus position (left side down), scanning intercostally from the right midaxillary line may reveal the aorta lying "deep" to the IVC. Alternatively, placing the probe in the left paraumbilical region may allow evaluation of the distal aorta.

Interpretation

With normal anatomy, mean abdominal aortic diameters are approximately equal in males and females during the second decade of life: 12.2 mm and 12.3 mm, respectively. By the eighth decade, the mean diameter increases to 22.8 mm in men and 16.9 mm in women. An AAA is defined by an aortic diameter of greater than 3 cm in a man and greater than 2.5 cm in a woman, or an enlargement of greater than 0.5 cm throughout the length of the aorta (the normal aorta tapers and decreases in diameter as it descends to its bifurcation). Surgery should be considered for any patient with symptoms compatible with an acute AAA and meeting these definitions because he or she is at risk for rupture.

If an AAA is found (Fig. 214.25) and the patient is hemodynamically stable, the clinician should attempt to determine whether branching vessels are involved and whether there is free intraperitoneal (in the manner of the FAST examination; see the Trauma section) or retroperitoneal fluid (although ultrasound is not always reliable for diagnosing retroperitoneal hemorrhage). Usually located along the left side of the spine or anterior to a

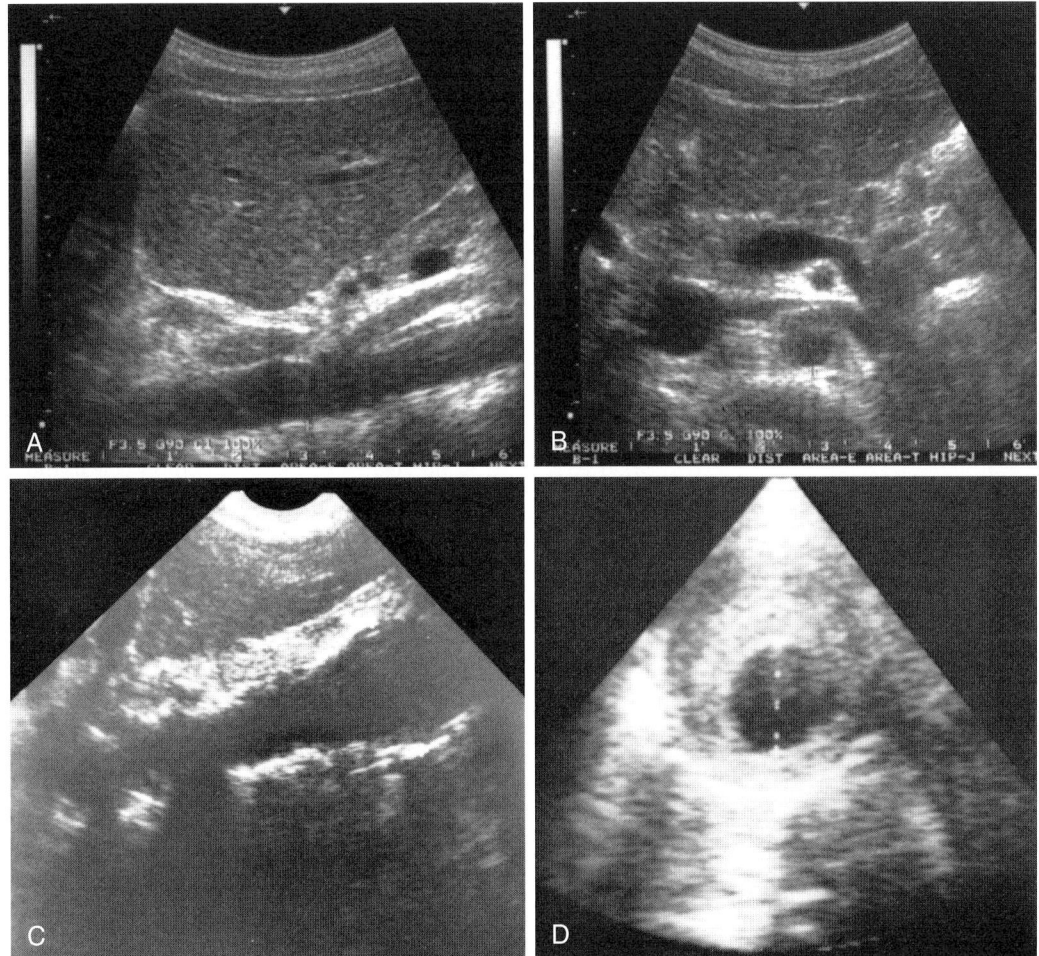

Fig. 214.25   (A) Longitudinal view of an abdominal aortic aneurysm (AAA). (B) Transverse view of an AAA. (C) Longitudinal view of intrarenal AAA. (D) Transverse view of a rupturing AAA with thrombus.

kidney, the presence of fluid may indicate a ruptured or leaking aneurysm; surgical consultation should be obtained immediately. It should be noted that the lack of free intraperitoneal fluid does not rule out an acute AAA because the majority of acute AAAs present without free intraperitoneal fluid. If no fluid is visualized and the patient is hemodynamically stable, a CT scan may be useful to check for retroperitoneal hemorrhage. CT angiography and magnetic resonance angiography are best for delineating whether other arteries are involved. Again, surgery should be considered in any patient with persistent abdominal pain and a known AAA. At the same time, because AAAs are common in older patients, just because a patient has a new or known AAA does not guarantee it is the source of symptoms. Endovascular aneurysm repair (endovascular stents) are now offered as an alternative (and probably safer choice) for patients with asymptomatic AAAs, especially those greater than 5 cm.

Most AAAs are fusiform and extend over a segment of the aorta; however, saccular aneurysms are often confined to a short segment. Therefore, to avoid overlooking an AAA, all segments of the aorta should be scanned methodically and systematically.

Echogenic material in the lumen may represent a thrombus or dissection. Alternatively, the clinician should check the gain setting elsewhere on the aorta to make sure it is not artifact. Large para-aortic lymph nodes (usually anterior but may be posterior and even displace the aorta away from the vertebrae) may be confused with the aorta or an AAA. However, compared with the aorta, nodes are usually irregular and nodular; color Doppler will demonstrate an absence of blood flow.

THORACIC (SEE MISCELLANEOUS FOR AIRWAY SCANNING)

A pneumothorax may also be detected by scanning the rib interspaces anteriorly and longitudinally in the midclavicular line using a high-frequency probe. In the normal lung, pleural sliding should be noted in the somewhat superficial visceral–parietal pleural interface during respiration. Absence of normal pleural sliding suggests separation of the visceral and parietal pleura due to pneumothorax. When compared with CT or other techniques, POCUS demonstrated better than 92% sensitivity, specificity, positive predictive accuracy, and negative predictive accuracy (Blaivas, 2005) for diagnosing pneumothorax.

See the Combined Diagnostic: Procedural for Pleural Effusions and Ultrasound-Guided Thoracentesis section.

TRAUMA

Studies indicate that physical examination fails to reveal significant injuries in 25% to 40% of trauma patients. Although a spiral CT scan may detect damage to abdominal organs, free fluid released from injured organs has long been used as a marker for significant injury. For many years in the United States, diagnosis of intraperitoneal blood was made almost exclusively with diagnostic peritoneal lavage (DPL; see Chapter 210, Diagnostic Peritoneal Lavage). However, after dozens of prospective, controlled studies demonstrated the accuracy of POCUS for detection of hemoperitoneum, diagnostic techniques changed, first in

Europe and Japan, and then in the United States. Investigators demonstrated that in the hands of capable, properly trained personnel, the sensitivity of ultrasound for diagnosing hemoperitoneum was at least as great as that of DPL. In recent years, the FAST examination was developed, which also includes a quick scan of the heart and pleural space. (See also the Miscellaneous section for a brief discussion of scanning for rib fractures or pneumothorax.) The indications for the FAST examination include but are not limited to traumatic injury to the torso. Not only is such rapidly available diagnostic information very valuable in the emergency department; it may be very useful for triage in the setting of mass casualties or on the battlefield. There are no absolute contraindications to the FAST examination, and the only relative contraindications include morbid obesity, massive subcutaneous emphysema, and extensive abdominal or chest wall trauma because these patients may be difficult to scan. Patients with intraabdominal fluid due to ascites, peritoneal dialysis, a ventriculoperitoneal shunt, a prior DPL, a ruptured ovarian cyst, or other pelvic inflammatory processes may also be difficult to evaluate. It may also be difficult to detect free fluid in some children and patients with isolated penetrating injury to the torso. The emergent need for laparotomy may be a relative contraindication; however, it may be important to make the diagnosis of pericardial tamponade or hematothorax with the FAST examination before taking such a patient to surgery.

NOTE: Unfortunately, individuals who already have free fluid in the abdomen (e.g., ascites due to alcoholic cirrhosis) are often prone to abdominal trauma, and yet they frequently are not the best candidates for DPL or surgery. Serial ultrasound scans can be used in such patients to document rapidly increasing fluid; the decision can then be made whether this is likely due to bleeding and thereby justifies surgery.

Preprocedure Patient Preparation

If the patient is hemodynamically compromised, attempts should be made to stabilize him or her before scanning. A full bladder may enhance scanning. The patient may experience some discomfort when scanning is performed over a contusion. The patient may also be asked to change positions.

Technique

1. If the bladder is about to be emptied, consider proceeding to step 5. The location of initial scanning may also be determined by a history of or evidence of trauma over a particular area. Otherwise, most clinicians scan the RUQ first. This is the most important and easiest region to visualize and is usually the earliest and most accurate for detecting blood. Factors that may affect the sensitivity include the positioning of the patient and a history of prior abdominal surgery or intraabdominal adhesions. If no fluid is seen in the supine position, Trendelenburg positioning may increase the sensitivity. Scan the patient's RUQ longitudinally with a low-frequency probe until you locate the right kidney. It is quite lateral and behind the organ used as a window, the liver. If the kidney is not immediately visible and the patient is conscious, have him or her inspire and briefly suspend breathing to bring the liver down. This often provides a better window and pushes bowel gas out of the way. If not, it may be necessary to scan between the ribs. The probe may need to be turned counterclockwise out of the longitudinal orientation to scan between the ribs. The probe may also need to be moved as far posterior as the posterior axillary line if bowel gas is interfering. The potential space located between the liver and the kidney is the Morison pouch (Fig. 214.26), also known as the *hepatorenal space*. This area, as well as the other spaces, should be scanned meticulously and in at least two perpendicular planes to rule out even a small collection of fluid.

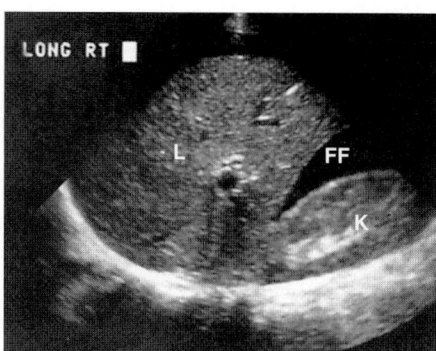

Fig. 214.26 Fluid in Morison's pouch or hemoperitoneum. *FF*, Free fluid; *K*, right kidney; *L*, liver.

2. If no fluid is seen in the Morison pouch, three additional potential spaces should be scanned in the RUQ. By angling the probe cephalad and using a gentle rocking motion, the pleural space above the echogenic diaphragm can usually be seen. The diaphragm will be moving with inspiration and expiration. Fluid above the diaphragm indicates either a hemothorax or a preexisting fluid collection (e.g., pleural effusion, empyema); fluid below it, in the subphrenic space, indicates intra-abdominal fluid. The potential space immediately below the kidney should also be scanned; it is an extension of the Morison pouch from above and the right paracolic gutter below.

3. Next, with the marker dot turned to the patient's right side, the probe should be moved to the midline and angled upward for a subxiphoid (subcostal) view of the heart and pericardium. The probe should be angled toward the patient's left scapula or even higher on the back, almost horizontal or parallel to the patient's bed. Again, the liver is usually used as a window. The area around the heart should be searched for fluid (usually located posteriorly, and possibly extending laterally) or evidence of tamponade. Avoid confusing a dark stripe due to pericardial fat pads, a pericardial cyst, or the descending thoracic aorta with a pericardial effusion. Scanning in more than one plane will usually help define the aorta. (See the section on Cardiac Ultrasound for a discussion of subxiphoid scanning as well as alternative windows to use, such as the parasternal and apical windows, in case the subxiphoid view cannot be used owing to local trauma or body habitus.) Also, if pericardial fluid is noted, an attempt should be made to determine whether the patient has a diagnosis that could be associated with a preexisting effusion.

4. The probe should then be moved to the left upper quadrant (LUQ). Scan it longitudinally and survey the same four potential spaces that were scanned around the right kidney. The area should be scanned meticulously and the probe rotated to scan in at least two perpendicular planes to rule out small pockets of fluid. Scan the areas around the left kidney and spleen, the space between the kidney and spleen (splenorenal space), the pleural space above the diaphragm, the subphrenic space, and the space below the left kidney. The splenorenal ligament on the left side may prevent accumulation of fluid in the splenorenal space, so scanning the other areas around the spleen becomes more important. Similar to the right side, the space below the left kidney is an extension of the splenorenal space from above and the paracolic gutter below. Realizing that the spleen is smaller than the liver and often more difficult to locate, use modest inspiration to bring it down to facilitate a window. If subcostal scanning does not provide an adequate window, intercostal scanning may be necessary. Rotate the probe counterclockwise to fit between the ribs. Because it is even more likely that bowel gas will interfere when scanning the LUQ, the clinician needs to be very patient when scanning, rocking the probe gently. The probe may need to be moved even more laterally than on the patient's right side, beyond the posterior axillary line to the flank or the back.

NOTE: Scanning the paracolic gutters requires considerable sonographic experience. When scanning immediately beneath the kidneys, windows from above are usually available; however, when attempting to scan inferiorly, windows next to the iliac crests may be more difficult to locate. Large amounts of fluid surrounding the bowel may facilitate scanning; however, it usually requires more experience to be comfortable with declaring an absence of fluid. Although studies indicate that scanning this area only minimally improves the sensitivity, such scanning significantly increases the time required. Clinicians should also be aware that scanning these areas increases the number of false-positive findings because of confusion of soft tissue for fluid.

5. If the preceding scans are negative and the patient remains stable, the region of the pelvic cul de sac can be scanned after placing the patient in the reverse Trendelenburg or sitting position. Scan transversely by placing the probe immediately above the suprapubic bone, turning the marker dot toward the patient's right side, and angling the probe downward into the pelvis. Rock it gently and scan meticulously all planes of tissue from the dome of the bladder to the inferior aspect of the cul de sac. The marker dot can then be turned cephalad for a longitudinal scan, which sometimes allows a better appreciation of the pelvic anatomy. If time allows, a full bladder increases the sensitivity of scanning in this area; however, adequate views can often be obtained with a partly full bladder, especially if there are large amounts of blood. Conversely, if the bladder is empty, small amounts of blood in the cul de sac may be missed. In women, transvaginal scanning replaces the need for a full bladder and is exquisitely sensitive for free fluid (capable of visualizing as little as 5 mL).

6. If the patient remains stable, serial scans may be helpful for the detection of newly accumulating fluid. Conversely, if the patient suddenly becomes unstable, another scan may locate the cause.

Interpretation

The entire examination can be performed very rapidly, with all four areas being scanned in less than 5 minutes. Intraperitoneal blood in small amounts usually first accumulates lateral to the right kidney. Fresh, unclotted blood has the same appearance as any free fluid in the abdomen. In the setting of a patient with a possible hemoperitoneum, the appearance of free fluid as a dark stripe is diagnostic (Fig. 214.27, and see Fig. 214.26) or a positive examination. As little as 10 mL has been diagnosed in the upper abdomen with transabdominal scanning; however, studies indicate the usual threshold for diagnosing hemoperitoneum is 500 mL. Therefore a negative FAST examination does not preclude early or slowly bleeding injuries. A 1-cm fluid stripe roughly corresponds to 1 L of intra-abdominal fluid. Again, the Morison pouch in the RUQ is one of the most sensitive areas to find fluid.

In the setting of trauma, the spleen is the most commonly injured abdominal organ. In the LUQ, fluid does not always accumulate between the spleen and the kidney; it can be located between the spleen and the abdominal wall. Conversely, it may completely surround the spleen (see Fig. 214.27). Spontaneous rupture of the spleen occurs occasionally, such as in teenagers or individuals in their early twenties after an Epstein-Barr virus infection (mononucleosis). In that situation, fluid will usually be found surrounding the spleen.

Free fluid in the abdomen may also be due to urine or bile and denote injury to the urinary or biliary tract, respectively. With large amounts of blood, fluid may be visible from almost anywhere in the abdomen or pelvis. It may accumulate as fluid in the cul de sac (see Fig. 214.12). As soon as the clotting process begins, blood may produce variable echoes as the fibrin and degenerating cells become more prominent. As clotting progresses further, which can occur rapidly, the fluid may develop the sonographic qualities of soft tissue; however, such an accumulation of soft tissue is unusual in dependent areas such as the cul de sac.

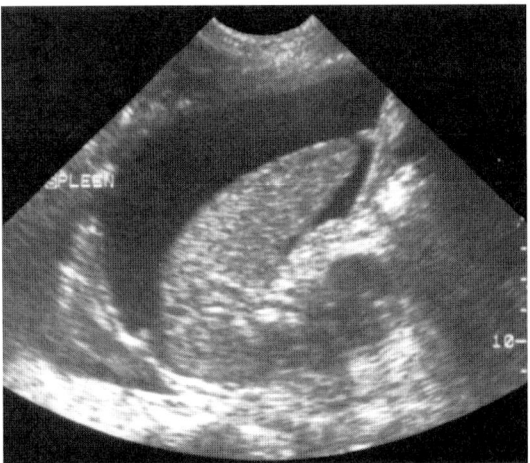

Fig. 214.27 Free fluid in the left upper quadrant.

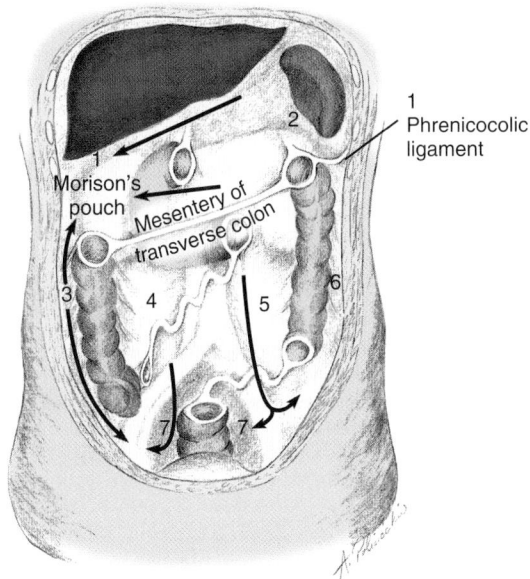

Fig. 214.28 Posterior peritoneum and reflections, indicating potential sites of intra-abdominal fluid localization and spread. *1* and *2*, Right and left supramesocolic regions—above the transverse mesocolon and separated by the ridge of the lumbar spine; *3*, right paracolic gutter; *4*, right inframesocolic gutter; *5*, left inframesocolic gutter; *6*, left paracolic gutter; *7*, pelvic cul de sac. *Arrows* indicate movement of free fluid (hemorrhage).

Avoid confusing fluid in the stomach or bowels as free fluid; search for the peristalsis associated with this fluid. Likewise, avoid confusing a dark stripe due to perinephric fat with free fluid. Obese patients may have a significant amount of such hypoechoic perinephric fat. However, fat tends to accumulate along the upper and lateral aspect of the kidney, whereas fluid often completely surrounds the kidney. Comparison with the opposite kidney may demonstrate a similar accumulation of fat, confirming the false-positive result. Patients with multiple abdominal surgical scars and adhesions may accumulate fluid in different patterns and locations because the normal flow of fluid in the abdomen (Fig. 214.28) is disrupted. Likewise, adhesions in the chest may result in fluid accumulating in areas other than a dependent location.

After examining all four areas for free fluid, the liver, spleen, and kidney capsules and the parenchyma should be reexamined for disruption or hematoma. After a recent hepatic, renal, or splenic contusion, if an intracapsular hematoma accumulates, it will usually appear cystic with irregular borders. A renal or splenic contusion with a ruptured capsule often appears as fluid surrounding either the kidney or spleen. Keep in mind, it is more difficult to evaluate the spleen for such injuries because the spleen is normally hypoechoic in texture. Consequently, large intraparenchymal and subcapsular splenic injuries can be missed. To avoid missing clinically significant splenic injuries, the ultrasound, along with a hematocrit, should be repeated in 2 to 3 hours or if there is a change in vital signs. As it turns out, a negative FAST examination does not exclude most solid organ, mesenteric vascular, hollow viscus, or diaphragmatic injuries. Major disruptions of the capsules of all of these organs can be missed by ultrasound; spiral CT scanning is more likely to diagnose such injuries.

OCULAR

Since 2002, a number of studies have indicated that emergency clinicians can accurately diagnose ocular pathology using high-frequency ultrasound. Since the eye is predominantly fluid-filled, it provides an excellent window for ultrasound scanning.

Technique

1. With the patient in the supine position, and eyes closed, place a liberal amount of ultrasound gel over the eyelid. A biooclusive dressing can be used to shield the eye from the gel.
2. With the marker dot directed toward the patient's right side, obtain a transverse image of the globe by applying gentle pressure with the transducer over the gel on the patient's eyelid. Make sure to scan the entire eye to avoid missing a small retinal detachment in the periphery of the eye. It may be necessary to have the patient gaze upward and downward while tilting the transducer accordingly to scan the entire retina.
3. When scanning, the echogenic structures in the anterior portion of the eye are the lens and supporting structures. The vitreous is normally dark or fluid-filled. The optic nerve is seen as a less echogenic streak leading from the posterior aspect of the eye. To measure optic nerve sheath diameter, the lateral diameter of the optic nerve is measured 3 mm posterior to the globe (Fig. 214.29).

Interpretation

The normal retina is not visible; it should be contiguous with the other posterior elements of the eye. A retinal detachment will appear as a thick, hyperechoic, undulating septum or membrane in the posterior aspect of the eye. While a vitreous detachment can look very similar, the retina is typically a thicker membrane that does not move if the patient changes their gaze. In contrast, the membrane seen with a vitreous detachment usually appears more mobile. If there is concern about normal versus abnormal pathology, the opposite eye can be scanned for comparison. However, it should be kept in mind that there is a 3% to 33% chance the patient is developing a retinal detachment in the other eye at the same time. If shadowing or reverberation artifact noted, this more likely indicates a foreign body of vitreous hemorrhage.

The optic nerve sheath diameter is measured 3 mm posterior to the globe, where demarcation is most easily seen. Normal optic sheath diameter in an adult is less than 5 mm; in children older than 1 year, it is less than 4.5 mm; in infants younger than 1 year, it is less than 4 mm. With papilledema, occasionally a bulb will be noted over the optic nerve as it exits the posterior aspect of the eye. This bulge is due to increased intracranial pressure.

Suspected Deep Venous Thrombosis

See Chapter 77, Noninvasive Venous and Arterial Studies of the Lower Extremities. Even when duplex equipment is available, compression ultrasound scanning using the high-frequency probe should be the initial study performed in most cases.

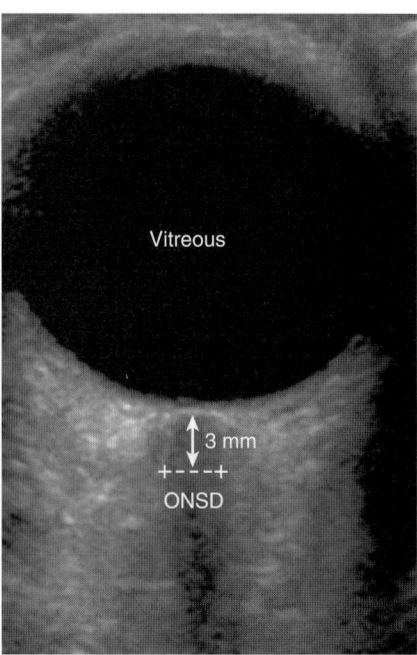

Fig. 214.29 Ocular scan. Measure the ophthalmic nerve sheath diameter *(ONSD)* 3 mm posterior to the retina.

MUSCULOSKELETAL/SOFT TISSUE

There are many applications for musculoskeletal ultrasound that are covered in Chapter 171, Musculoskeletal Ultrasound. For example, one published study found that rib fractures can be accurately diagnosed with ultrasound. The entire outline of the affected ribs was scanned with high-frequency ultrasound, searching for breaks in the normal smooth cortex which is diagnostic of a fracture. Accuracy, in certain situations, was better than that found with radiographs. Use of ultrasound also spared the patient from radiation exposure. This technique can also be used for diagnosing finger fractures.

Subcutaneous Foreign Bodies

Missed foreign bodies are the second most frequent cause of lawsuits against emergency medicine clinicians. Objects composed of wood, plastic, glass, and vegetable material may not be radiopaque or visible with standard x-ray examinations. Modern military armor is also an example. Most is now fiberglass or cloth, and therefore shrapnel is not often visible on routine radiographs. Although fine needles and splinters may be missed, high-frequency ultrasound is usually helpful not only for confirming the presence of a foreign body but for localization before removal. (See also Chapter 191, Foreign Body Removal from Skin and Soft Tissue, and Chapter 171, Musculoskeletal Ultrasound.)

Preprocedure Patient Preparation

The patient should be informed about the indication for the study and should understand that not all foreign bodies are visible with either ultrasound or standard x-ray examinations. If a foreign body is located, the patient should decide whether he or she wants it removed. The patient needs an understanding of the possible complications of removing the object as opposed to not removing the object. (See Chapter 191, Foreign Body Removal From Skin and Soft Tissue.)

Technique

1. In most cases, a high-frequency probe is preferred. For objects very near the skin surface, a standoff pad may be needed to raise the probe several millimeters off the skin. Such a device can either be purchased commercially or created using a latex glove filled with water or acoustic gel. Place the glove or pad on the

skin and scan through it with the transducer. Alternatively, the body part can also be submersed in a water bath.

2. Understanding that layers of normal subcutaneous tissue are not always uniform, scan in the area of the possible foreign body. Scan the contralateral "normal" side if unsure of the finding. Scan both longitudinally and transversely, and attempt to clarify the largest dimensions when located.

Interpretation and Results

Foreign bodies may appear as hyperechoic in contrast to the surrounding tissue. If the resolution of the probe is great enough and the foreign body thick enough, an acoustic shadow may also be seen. Metal and glass are more echoic than plastic or wood. Foreign bodies may also be surrounded by a hypoechoic halo representing fluid or inflammation. The exact location of the foreign body should be marked; if it is not round, the predominant direction in which it is lying should be noted. The depth of the object, especially if it is to be removed, should also be noted.

MISCELLANEOUS

There are many applications being used and further studied for POCUS in the emergency department, hospitalist, and office settings. The following sections discuss some of the newer indications in the emergency department, hospital, or office for which an ultrasound application has been either studied or published.

Airway Confirmation of Endotracheal Tube Placement

Technique

1. Gently place a high-frequency linear probe transversely at the level of the suprasternal notch.
2. The trachea will appear as an echogenic, curvilinear structure with shadowing (Fig. 214.30A). Deep or posterior to the trachea, the shadowing will be a mixture of reverberation artifact or "comet tails" because of the air in the trachea. However, if an endotracheal tube is properly placed, it will appear as a second curvilinear structure posterior to the somewhat superficial trachea (see Fig. 214.30B). If instead the endotracheal tube is in the esophagus, it will appear as two tracheas, with one to the patient's left (to the right side of the image) and more posterior (see Fig. 214.30C).

Testicular Mass or Possible Torsion

High-frequency ultrasound is helpful in diagnosing testicular cancer as well as for differentiating the four most common causes for a scrotal mass: spermatocele, hydrocele, varicocele, and tumor. Transillumination with a bright penlight can often differentiate a spermatocele or hydrocele from other possible causes of a scrotal mass. When there is still a question after transillumination, ultrasound is the procedure of choice.

Although radioisotope scans have been the procedure of choice for diagnosing a torsioned testicle, they often take hours to obtain, and time is of the essence when making this diagnosis. Because it can be performed fairly rapidly, color and pulsed wave Doppler ultrasound is becoming the diagnostic procedure of choice for testicular torsion (see Chapter 112, Manual Testicular Detorsion).

Preprocedure Patient Preparation

The patient should be informed about the indication for the study. Using a towel, the patient can retract the penis. The testicle and the scrotum are supported by the clinician's hand or by a towel under the scrotum. Either a very cooperative patient or an assistant may be needed to allow the clinician to use both hands for the ultrasound equipment.

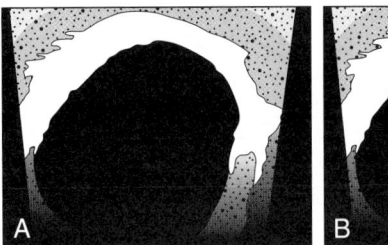
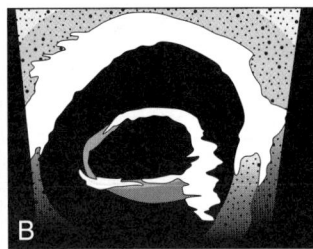
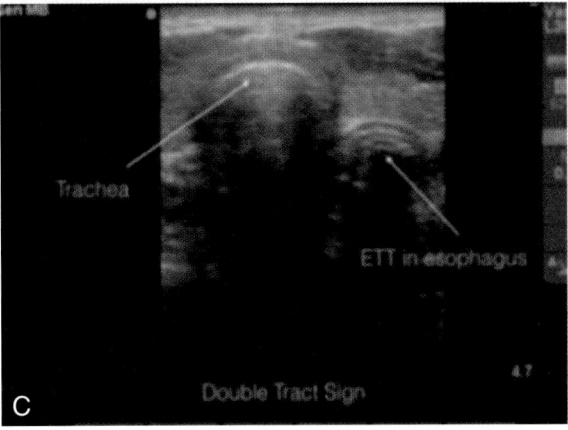

Fig. 214.30 (A) Normal trachea with echogenic curvilinear structure anteriorly, shadowing from air posterior to it. (B) Properly placed endotracheal tube has two echogenic curvilinear structures, one inside the other. (C) Endotracheal tube placed improperly in the esophageal appears like two trachea, side by side, with one located more posteriorly in the esophagus.

Technique

1. Using the same orientation as for the rest of the body, first turn the marker dot toward the patient's head for a longitudinal scan. Parallel longitudinal scans should be made with the high-frequency probe about every 5 mm.
2. Next, turn the marker dot toward the patient's right side for a transverse scan. Transverse scans should also be made approximately every 5 mm.
3. The opposite testicle should be scanned, if indicated, or for a comparison for questionable areas. Any palpable abnormalities should be scanned.

Interpretation and Results

Testicles are normally symmetric in size. A small amount of fluid in the scrotal sac is normal. A normal sonographic finding known as the *mediastinum testis* is seen as an echogenic longitudinal central line within the testicle (Fig. 214.31A). The epididymis usually appears as a slightly sonolucent structure posterior to the testes.

A small mass within the testicle is cancer until proven otherwise, especially in a patient younger than 40 years (see Fig. 214.31B). A seminoma, the most common testicular tumor, usually appears as a hypoechoic mass within the testicle. Teratomas and embryonal cell cancers are usually irregularly echogenic.

Hydroceles, spermatoceles, and varicoceles should all be extratesticular. Spermatoceles are usually found superior to the testicle and attached to the vas deferens. Hydroceles may surround the testicle and are predominantly fluid filled. Varicoceles are usually found in the region of the epididymis, extending superiorly. They will often increase considerably in size with a Valsalva maneuver.

A torsioned testicle often appears enlarged, less dense, and less echogenic compared with the normal testicle (see Fig. 214.31C and D). The texture of the ischemic testicle is often blurry, and even sharp intratesticular markings (mediastinum testis) may be diminished. If available, color Doppler (especially spectral Doppler) usually reveals decreased blood flow on the torsioned side.

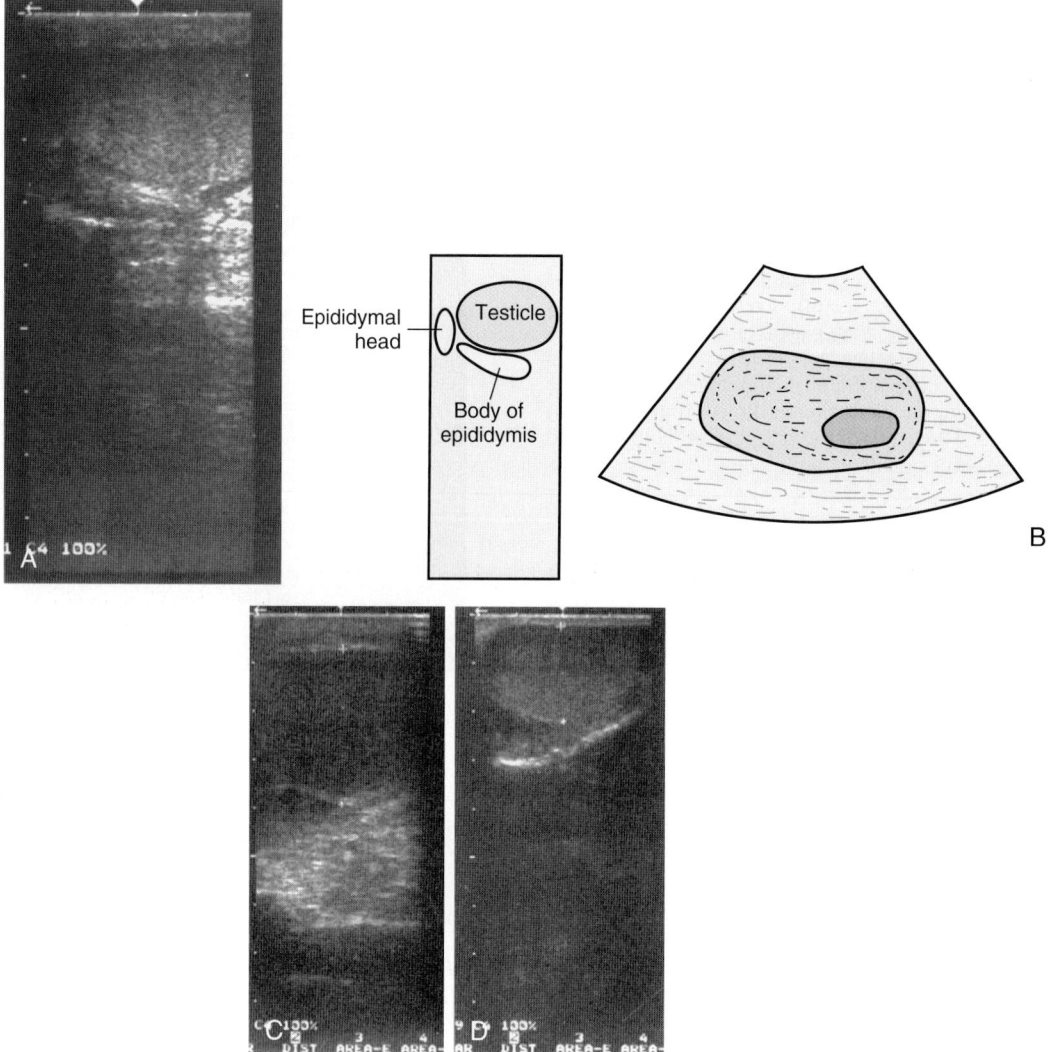

Fig. 214.31 (A) Normal testicular tissue with mediastinum testis. (B) Testicular mass suspect for cancer. (C) Torsion of right testicle demonstrated by an enlarged, hypoechoic testicle. (D) Normal left testicle.

However, flow cannot always be established by certainty with Doppler; if flow cannot be demonstrated in the opposite testicle, a radioisotope scan may be necessary to exclude torsion. If bilateral blood flow is documented and symmetric, the intratesticular markings are sharp and symmetric, and there is a difference in appearance between epididymides, epididymitis on the tender side is the likely diagnosis.

COMBINED DIAGNOSTIC-PROCEDURAL ULTRASOUND

Procedures can be guided either statically with ultrasound or in real time. For the static technique, anatomic structures, the insertion site, and the angle and depth of insertion are first identified with ultrasound, and then the probe is laid aside. If a fluid collection is to be aspirated, the amount can also be estimated (e.g., 1 cm^3 equates to approximately 1 mL of fluid). The key portions of the procedure are then performed without ultrasound imaging. For the real-time technique, a sterile probe cover is used and the key components of the procedure are performed with simultaneous ultrasound imaging. A needle guide for the probe is

helpful for real-time guidance; either a one-person or two-person technique can be used.

Insertion of Central Lines

Several studies indicate that the use of ultrasound as an adjunct for inserting central venous catheters not only decreases the failure rate; it decreases the overall incidence of complications, as well as the number of attempts necessary. Consequently, the Institute of Medicine, the Agency for Healthcare Research and Quality, and the National Institute for Health and Clinical Excellence now recommend this technique. Patient satisfaction should also be improved. A real-time, two-person technique for internal jugular cannulation is described here. Similar techniques can be used for other sites (e.g., external jugular, subclavian, femoral). With the advent of tunneled catheters, such techniques can also be used to cannulate the brachial and cephalic veins for central venous access. Equipment is now available in many large intensive care units and other areas of the hospital that is portable and dedicated to the insertion of central lines. Such equipment may facilitate a one-person technique. It also frequently has a needle guide that attaches to or is built into the probe.

Preprocedure Patient Preparation

See Chapter 228, Central Venous Catheter Insertion.

Technique

1. For internal jugular cannulation, the patient is positioned supine, in 15 degrees of Trendelenburg, with the head turned slightly to the opposite side. (See Chapter 228, Central Venous Catheter Insertion, for techniques in locations other than the internal jugular.)
2. Perform a preliminary transverse scan with the high-frequency probe just above the clavicle near the insertion of the two heads of the sternocleidomastoid muscle. The pulsatile internal carotid artery should appear in cross-sectional view beside and medial to the larger internal jugular vein. With a Valsalva maneuver, the internal jugular will increase in diameter, significantly. Avoid applying too much pressure with the probe initially, which may temporarily collapse the vein and make it hard to locate. After it is identified, apply pressure to demonstrate that it is indeed collapsible as opposed to the noncollapsible carotid artery.
3. Cover the probe with a sterile cover (e.g., a sterile glove). A ribbon of acoustic gel should have been placed on the probe before covering; pay special attention to eliminating all bubbles between the cover and the head of the transducer. Prepare and drape the patient in the usual sterile fashion.
4. A small amount of sterile acoustic gel is placed over the site to be scanned. The sterilely gowned and gloved ultrasound operator should be located next to the clinician (similarly gowned and gloved) performing the cannulation. The ultrasound probe should be operated beneath the drape to avoid interfering with the cannulation.
5. Position the probe so that the internal jugular vein is centered under the probe, which also means centered in the monitor screen. The person performing the cannulation should aim the needle toward the center of the probe. Unless there is a needle guide, the needle will not always be visualized; if it is, it will appear as a linear, echogenic structure with shadowing. The needle will typically cause slight tenting of the vessel as it enters. The flash of blood in the syringe is often anticipated by the sonographer when he or she sees tenting of the vein immediately before the needle enters. After the flash of blood and confirmation of needle placement, if a guidewire is used it can often be visualized as it passes into the vein.

EDITOR'S NOTE: In recent years, with more experience performing these procedures and with better equipment, the needle is observed during a "dynamic" ultrasound-guided procedure instead of the "static" one described here.

Arterial Puncture and Cannulation

Techniques are described using a hand-held Doppler to assess collateral flow before arterial puncture and to facilitate arterial cannulation in Chapter 225, Arterial Puncture and Percutaneous Arterial Line Placement. The technique just described for ultrasound-guided central venous catheter insertion can also be used to localize the vessel and then for arterial puncture and cannulation.

Lumbar Puncture in the Morbidly Obese Individual

In morbidly obese individuals, lumbar puncture is often complicated by the inability to palpate the spinous processes. The goal of ultrasound is to locate the midline of the spine. (Using ultrasound to localize the spine is also helpful for performing other spinal procedures and is being used more frequently by anesthesiologists.)

Preprocedure Patient Preparation

See Chapter 221, Lumbar Puncture.

Technique

1. Ultrasound scanning can be performed either under nonsterile conditions, to mark the midline, or under sterile conditions for

ultrasound guidance of the needle. A low-frequency probe is usually preferred.
2. With the patient in either the lateral recumbent or sitting position, apply adequate acoustic gel over the midline of the spine. Scan initially in transverse dimensions to locate a vertebra. The L4 spinous process should be noted below a line drawn between the iliac crests. When this vertebra is noted, maneuver the transducer so that the spinous process is centered on the monitor. Next, rotate the probe 90 degrees to scan longitudinally and locate several spinous processes. Mark the location and note the angle necessary to penetrate between the L3 and L4 spinous processes. After local anesthetic is given, insert the spinal needle and follow the remaining technique as described in Chapter 221, Lumbar Puncture.
3. To perform the scan under sterile conditions, cover the probe with a sterile barrier (sterile glove) as noted previously for central line insertion. When performing the lumbar puncture, use the same technique as for central line insertion and observe the needle passing over the L4 spinous process.

Interpretation and Results

The spinous process should appear hyperechoic in contrast to surrounding tissue. The vertebral bodies should also be hyperechoic and cast shadows. Spinal fluid is rarely imaged between the spinous processes in adults, but the angles and depths to the vertebral bodes can usually be more clearly defined.

Thyroid Mass

Palpable thyroid nodules occur in 3% to 4% of the population. One important goal when scanning a thyroid nodule is to determine whether there is more than one nodule. If multiple nodules are present (40% possibility), the risk of malignancy is very low (1% to 6%), with the exception of those that have been exposed to low-dose radiation therapy. In the past, this was usually done for children with croup or acne; however, these treatments were stopped so many years ago that patients have likely outlived their risk (i.e., they would have already developed their malignancies). More recently, patients exposed to nuclear accidents such as Chernobyl or those exposed to a terrorist "dirty bomb" may be at risk. These patients have a 30% to 40% lifetime risk of malignancy.

The next goal of scanning a thyroid nodule is to determine whether it is cystic (Fig. 214.32A), solid (see Fig. 214.32B), or both (complex). Cold nodules on nuclear studies can be cystic with low risk of malignancy (20%), malignant (20%), or benign (60%).

If the nodule is cystic, aspiration may be an option and the fluid may be sent for cytologic analysis. Fine-needle aspiration is also an option for solid lesions.

Preprocedure Patient Preparation

The patient should be informed about the indication for the study. If an aspiration is to be performed, the patient should be counseled for informed consent.

Technique

1. With the patient in the supine position and the neck slightly hyperextended, apply an adequate amount of acoustic gel. Using a high-frequency probe, scan transversely (marker dot to the patient's right side) in a lateral-to-medial fashion on one side. Next, scan the opposite side at the same level from lateral to medial. Apply minimal pressure at the midline to avoid obscuring the texture of the isthmus. Proceed in 5-mm increments throughout the entire gland.
2. Next, scan with longitudinal planes at 5-mm intervals. Observe each plane and then move medially from the carotid artery. Good surface contact is usually obtained at a 10- or 20-degree angle from the vertical. Scan the opposite side in the same manner.
3. For aspiration, see the next section Breast Mass. If aspiration is to be attempted, mark the location. Note the angle and depth of any nearby structures that need to be avoided.

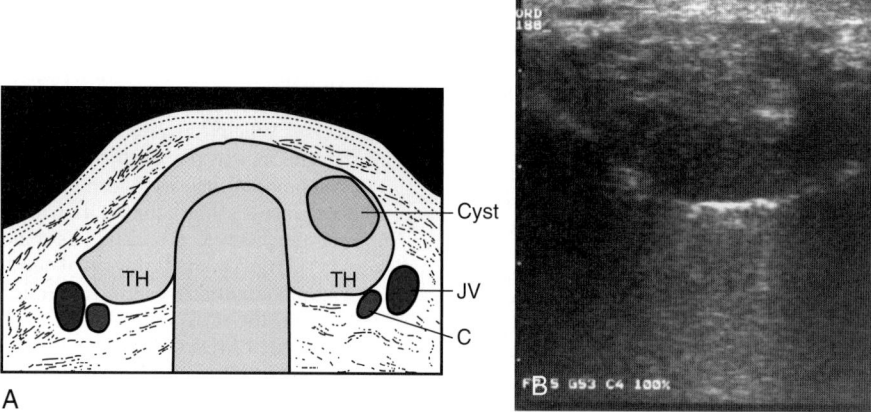

Fig. 214.32 (A) Thyroid cyst. *C,* Carotid artery; *JV,* internal jugular vein; *TH,* thyroid. (B) Thyroid mass (adenoma).

Interpretation and Results

Carcinomas of the thyroid are usually single nodules with irregular borders, and most are hypoechoic. They can be cystic, solid, or both (complex), and they are frequently accompanied by adenopathy. However, there is no pathognomonic feature of cancer of the thyroid. If unsure, the clinician should consider fine-needle aspiration or surgical removal, especially for solitary nodules.

The most common thyroid masses are adenomas. Adenomas almost invariably occur as multiple lesions. They can appear with a halo of hypoechoic tissue surrounding a more echogenic mass, as a solid homogeneous mass with few internal echoes, or as a densely echogenic mass. Goiters appear as a diffuse, asymmetric expansion of the thyroid with a coarse texture. Multiple nodules are often present. Thyroiditis usually appears as a diffuse enlargement of the thyroid with multiple nodules. Parathyroid glands are rarely seen and usually appear on the posterior aspect of the thyroid near the carotid artery. They are relatively sonolucent; if larger than 5 mm, they are abnormal.

Breast Mass

Ultrasound is very helpful for evaluating breast masses, whether confirming the presence of a palpable mass or locating a nonpalpable mass seen on mammography, evaluating young fibroglandular breasts where mammography is less helpful, or differentiating solid from cystic lesions.

Preprocedure Patient Preparation

The patient should be informed about the indication for the study. The patient should be aware that this procedure is being used only to evaluate palpable lesions (or lesions noted on mammograms), to localize them, or to determine whether they are cystic or solid. It is not being used solely to exclude cancer. Portable ultrasound may also be used to assist with aspiration of a breast cyst or with fine-needle aspiration of a suspected adenoma. Informed consent should be obtained if aspiration will be attempted.

Technique

1. Place the patient in the supine position. After application of acoustic gel, scan palpable lesions with a high-frequency probe. To locate nonpalpable lesions noted on a mammogram, scan longitudinally in 5-mm parallel increments in the appropriate quadrant. If the lesion is not located, scan in transverse increments through the same quadrant.
2. For cyst aspiration, either a one- or two-person technique can be used. The one-person technique may be adequate for large cysts, especially if they are readily palpable. The ultrasound scanning

can be performed under nonsterile conditions. The goal of the ultrasound study is to locate the cyst, note the surrounding structures (especially those that should be avoided), determine the necessary depth for puncture, and mark the puncture site. The transducer can then be set aside and the procedure performed under sterile conditions, as noted elsewhere (e.g., SPA, thoracentesis).

3. For smaller or deeper cysts that are difficult to localize, use the two-person technique. Just as with insertion of central lines, one person localizes the cyst with a high-frequency probe and keeps it in the center of the image while maintaining sterile conditions. The second clinician then punctures the cyst, also under aseptic conditions. Occasionally the needle can be visualized on the screen as it enters the cyst. The needle usually indents the cyst wall before it punctures.
4. After aspiration, the contents should be sent for cytology. A sample can also be prepared as a smear between two microscope slides that are then pulled apart, sprayed with the same fixative used for Pap smears, allowed to air dry, and sent for cytology.

Interpretation and Results

Breast cysts have the sonographic appearance of cysts elsewhere in the body and are the most common breast masses in women between 35 and 50 years of age. They normally have smooth walls and an absence of internal echoes; therefore they are uniformly hypoechoic. Tissue behind the posterior wall of the cyst is usually more sharply defined than tissue anterior to the cyst. The penumbra effect may be seen.

The cyst should be measured in three dimensions: AP, longitudinal, and transverse. If aspiration is to be attempted, the depth necessary for penetration should be recorded. Nearby structures should also be noted.

Adenomas are usually ovoid, with lateral diameters larger than AP diameters. They usually have uniform and regular borders. If the gain is set improperly (too low) and no internal echoes are noted, adenomas may also appear cystic.

In contrast, ductal carcinomas usually have irregular borders and may be dense enough to cast acoustic shadows. Their AP diameter may be as great or greater than the lateral diameter. If they are blocking ducts, the ducts can often be traced to the site of the mass. Medullary carcinoma may be difficult to differentiate from adenomas, with the only differences being a more irregular border and more internal echoes. For this reason, solid solitary breast lesions should undergo either fine-needle aspiration or surgical removal.

Papillary carcinoma is fairly rare, but it can appear as finger-like projections protruding from a cyst wall. After cyst aspiration, if any tissue remains palpable, it should probably be surgically removed to exclude the possibility of papillary carcinoma. Also after aspiration, air can be reinjected into the cyst and a repeat mammogram performed. The location of the cyst will be marked by the air when the mammogram is repeated. In this manner, a mammogram can be used to help exclude papillary carcinoma.

Pericardial Effusion and Ultrasound-Guided Pericardiocentesis

See Chapter 230, Pericardiocentesis. Even when duplex equipment is available, plain ultrasound scanning using the low-frequency probe should be the initial study performed in most cases.

Pleural Effusion and Ultrasound-Guided Thoracentesis

POCUS is an alternative to the use of decubitus x-ray films for confirmation of an effusion (e.g., patient with blunting of costovertebral angles on radiography). Once the effusion is confirmed, not only can the amount of fluid be quantified, but the best angle and the depth necessary for inserting the needle can be determined. In patients with a small amount of pleural fluid or a loculated effusion, routine thoracentesis is often unsuccessful and possibly dangerous. Ultrasound-directed thoracentesis should minimize the danger while maximizing the results.

Preprocedure Patient Preparation

The patient should be informed about the indications for the procedure as well as the risks and possible complications. The usual risks of pneumothorax, solid organ puncture, and procedural failure are reduced when thoracentesis is ultrasound-guided. Signed, informal consent should be obtained for thoracentesis. (See Chapter 218, Thoracentesis.)

Technique

1. With the patient in the proper position (usually sitting and leaning forward, but can be supine or lateral decubitus), use a low-frequency probe to scan the back intercostally on the appropriate side, just above the liver or spleen. It may be helpful to actually scan the liver or spleen first, and to then move the probe in a cranial direction to locate the effusion. With the patient in the sitting position and the marker dot located cephalad, scan the entire thorax in longitudinal planes. After scanning near the midline, move the transducer laterally and map the dimensions of the effusion from superior to inferior, medial to lateral. Then turn the marker dot counterclockwise to fit between the ribs, and again scan to note the lateral dimensions of the effusion.
2. Mark the location of the largest collection of effusion that is safely accessible with the needle. The diaphragm will appear echogenic and moving with respiration; also note the location of the spleen or liver, and avoid inserting the needle in those locations. If the procedure will be performed with the patient in the supine or lateral decubitus position, be sure to demarcate the extent of the effusion relative to the hemithorax that will be accessible. Effusions may move with respiration, so note where to direct the needle relative to each phase of respiration. Plan to perform the insertion during the optimal phase. Note the depth necessary to reach fluid, especially for large or obese patients; an extra-long needle may be necessary for these patients. A needle stop, set to the appropriate depth, may be helpful for preventing penetration of lung tissue and causing a pneumothorax.
3. For smaller or loculated effusions, the thoracentesis is best performed with ultrasound guidance. Cover the probe with a sterile barrier (e.g., sterile glove) as noted previously for central line insertion. This procedure may also require two persons: one to hold the transducer while the other performs the aspiration. When performing ultrasound-guided thoracentesis, use the same technique as for central line insertion. With the probe held scanning longitudinally, the top of the rib over which the thoracentesis is to be

performed should be highlighted by the transducer. If a curvilinear or sector scanner is being used, the transducer should be held at the same optimal angle as that needed to reach the effusion. The thoracentesis needle should then be advanced to the appropriate depth at the same angle as the transducer. Again, a properly set needle stop may prevent penetrating lung tissue and causing a pneumothorax. Occasionally the echogenic needle will be observed passing over the rib. Once fluid is obtained, complete the procedure in the same manner as if it were not ultrasound-guided.

Interpretation and Results

Pleural effusions that are predominantly fluid appear dark or hypoechoic with ultrasound imaging. They are located above the echogenic diaphragm, which moves with respiration (Fig. 214.33). An empyema may demonstrate echogenic objects in the fluid. Loculations and the diaphragm appear as echogenic borders to the fluid. Fluid located below the diaphragm (and not within an organ) is ascites.

Ascites and Ultrasound-Guided Paracentesis

As discussed in the Trauma section, the presence of abdominal fluid is not always obvious on physical examination. Ultrasound can be used to confirm the presence of ascites and to determine the best location for diagnostic paracentesis. Although routine paracentesis may be contraindicated in certain situations (e.g., in patients with adhesions from prior abdominal surgery), ultrasound-directed paracentesis may remain an option for those patients. Similar to the FAST examination, ascites is usually diagnosed earliest (even small amounts) in the Morison (hepatorenal) pouch.

Preprocedure Patient Preparation

The patient should be informed about the indications for the procedure as well as the risks and possible complications. The usual risks for paracentesis of solid organ perforation, vascular injury, bowel perforation, and procedural failure are decreased when ultrasonographic guidance is used. If there is a relative contraindication, the patient should be informed of the increased risk. (See Chapter 219, Abdominal Paracentesis.)

Technique

1. With the patient in the supine or sitting upright position, use a low-frequency probe to scan the usual location for performing paracentesis (in the midline, approximately one-third the distance from the umbilicus to the pubic symphysis, or in a lower quadrant [left usually preferred], about one-third the distance from the umbilicus to the anterior iliac crest). Note the location of any solid organs to avoid. Next, locate the largest, safest collection of fluid for a successful paracentesis. Also, confirm absence of bowel (would be floating in fluid; air in bowel usually causes scatter artifact) and whether the bladder has been emptied adequately. Color Doppler can also be used to avoid the area of the epigastric arteries. If these conditions are met, perform the procedure in the usual manner.

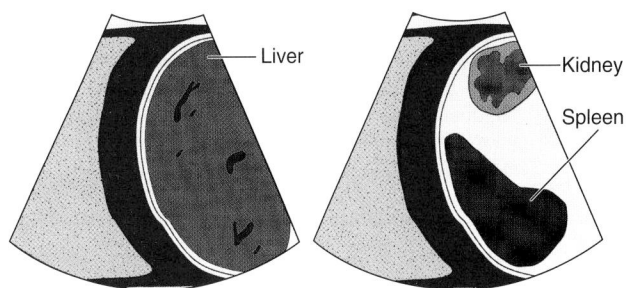

Fig. 214.33 Pleural effusion. Note the fluid is above the diaphragm.

2. For small amounts of fluid, or if there is need for stereotactic paracentesis, perform it under ultrasound guidance. Cover the probe with a sterile barrier (e.g., sterile glove) as noted previously for central line insertion. When performing the paracentesis, use the same technique for ultrasound guidance as for central line insertion or thoracentesis. In some cases, the echogenic needle may be observed passing into the fluid.

Interpretation and Results

Peritoneal fluid appears dark or hypoechoic on ultrasound images. Bowel or bladder wall is relatively echogenic. With peritonitis, echogenic objects will occasionally be seen floating in the fluid.

OVERREADING SERVICES

Overreading services are available through the following website: www.nighthawkradiologyservices.com.

NOTE: These require T1 internet access; DSL is not compliant with the Health Insurance Portability and Accountability Act Privacy Rule.

PATIENT EDUCATION GUIDES

See the sample patient consent form available at www.expertconsult.com.

CPT/BILLING CODES

NOTE: Only one limited scan can be billed per body part or region per patient encounter.

Cardiac

93307	Echocardiography, transthoracic, real time with image documentation (2D) with or without M-mode recording; complete, with spectral flow Doppler and with color flow Doppler
93308	Echocardiography, follow-up or limited study

Obstetric-Gynecologic

See also Chapter 142, Obstetric Ultrasound.

76801	Ultrasound, pregnant uterus, real-time with image documentation, <14 wk, transabdominal, single or first gestation
76802	Ultrasound, pregnant uterus, transabdominal, each additional gestation
76805	Ultrasound, pregnant uterus, >14 wk, transabdominal, single or first gestation
76810	Ultrasound, pregnant uterus, >14 wk, transabdominal, each additional gestation
76815	Ultrasound, pregnant uterus, real-time with image documentation, limited (e.g., fetal heartbeat, placental location, fetal position and/or qualitative amniotic fluid volume), one or more fetuses
76816	Ultrasound, pregnant uterus, real-time with image documentation, follow-up (e.g., reevaluation of fetal size, reevaluation of organ system[s] suspected or documented to be abnormal on previous scan), transabdominal approach
76817	Ultrasound, pregnant uterus, real-time with image documentation, transvaginal

Gynecologic

76830	Ultrasound, transvaginal
76856	Ultrasound, pelvic (nonobstetric), real-time with image documentation; complete
76857	Ultrasound, pelvic (nonobstetric), limited or follow-up study (e.g., for follicles)

Abdominal and Trauma

76700	Ultrasound, abdominal, real-time with image documentation; complete
76705	Ultrasound, abdominal, limited (e.g., single organ, quadrant, follow-up)
76770	Ultrasound, retroperitoneal (e.g., renal, aorta, nodes), real-time with image documentation; complete
76775	Ultrasound, retroperitoneal, limited study

Miscellaneous

See also Chapter 77, Noninvasive Venous and Arterial Studies of the Lower Extremities.

76604	Ultrasound, chest (includes mediastinum), real-time with image documentation
76870	Ultrasound, scrotum and contents

Combined Diagnostic–Procedural

76510	Ophthalmic ultrasound, diagnostic; B-scan
76536	Ultrasound, soft tissue of head and neck (e.g., thyroid, parathyroid, parotid), real-time with image documentation
76645	Ultrasound, breast(s) (unilateral or bilateral), real-time with image documentation
76930	Ultrasonic guidance for pericardiocentesis, imaging supervision and interpretation
76937	Ultrasonic guidance for vascular access requiring ultrasound evaluation of potential access sites, documentation of selected vessel patency, concurrent real-time ultrasound visualization of vascular needle entry, with permanent recording and reporting (list separately in addition to code for primary procedure)
76942	Ultrasonic guidance for needle placement (e.g., biopsy, aspiration, injection, localization device), imaging, supervision and interpretation

ICD-10-CM DIAGNOSTIC CODES

Cardiac

I30.9	Pericardial effusion, acute
I30.0	Pericarditis, acute, idiopathic
I30.8	Pericarditis, acute purulent
I31.4	Cardiac tamponade
I31.9	Pericardial effusion (chronic), or unspecified disease of pericardium
I46.9	Asystole

Obstetric-Gynecologic

See also Chapter 142, Obstetric Ultrasound, for additional coding on gravid uterus.

Z30.431	Intrauterine device, checking, reinsertion, or removal
D25.9	Uterine fibroid, unspecified
N70.93	Tubo-ovarian, ovarian, or fallopian tube abscess, salpingitis, or oophoritis, acute or chronic
N83.10	Ovarian cyst, corpus luteum
N83.209	Ovarian cyst, unspecified
N83.53	Torsioned ovary, ovarian pedicle or fallopian tube
N89.8	Vaginal bleeding
O01.9	Hydatidiform mole
O02.81	Blighted ovum
O02.1	Missed abortion
O00.00	Abdominal pregnancy
O00.109	Tubal pregnancy
O00.90	Ectopic pregnancy, unspecified
O03.9	Abortion or miscarriage, complete, without complication
O02.0	Threatened abortion, antepartum
O36.8190	Decreased fetal movements, antepartum
O36.4XX0	Intrauterine fetal death, late (after 22 weeks' gestation)

Abdominal

I71.02	Abdominal aortic aneurysm, dissecting
I71.3	Abdominal aortic aneurysm, ruptured
I71.4	Abdominal aortic aneurysm, without mention of rupture
K80.20	Cholelithiasis, without obstruction, without mention of cholecystitis
K80.21	Cholelithiasis, with obstruction, without mention of cholecystitis
K80.62	Calculus of gallbladder and bile duct with acute cholecystitis, without mention of obstruction
K82.0	Obstruction of gallbladder
K82.9	Pain, gallbladder
K81.9	Cholecystitis, unspecified
K81.1	Cholecystitis chronic
K81.2	Cholecystitis, acute and chronic
K83.8	Cholestasis
K83.9	Pain, bile duct
N15.1	Renal abscess
N13.30	Hydronephrosis
N20.0	Calculus of kidney
N20.1	Calculus of ureter
N13.4	Hydroureter
N21.0	Urinary bladder stone
R31.9	Hematuria
N23	Renal colic
R10.11	Pain, abdominal, right upper quadrant
R19.00	Abdominal mass

Trauma

See also Chapter 210, Diagnostic Peritoneal Lavage, and Chapter 230, Pericardiocentesis.

I31.2	Hemopericardium
R58	Hemorrhage, unspecified
K66.1	Hemoperitoneum
S36.112A	Hematoma, traumatic liver, subcapsular
S26.99XA	Injury to heart, without mention of open wound into thorax
S21.309A	Injury to heart, with open wound into thorax
S27.309A	Injury to lung, without mention of open wound into thorax
S21.309A	Injury to lung, with open wound into thorax
S27.899A	Traumatic pleural effusion
S36.112A	Injury to liver, without mention of open wound, hematoma without rupture of capsule
S36.029A	Injury to spleen, without mention of open wound, hematoma without rupture of capsule
S37.029A	Injury to kidney, without mention of open wound, hematoma without rupture of capsule

Miscellaneous

See also Chapter 191, Foreign Body Removal from Skin and Soft Tissue, Chapter 77, Noninvasive Venous and Arterial Studies of the Lower Extremities, Chapter 100, Suprapubic Tap or Aspiration, and Chapter 168, Pediatric Suprapubic Bladder Aspiration.

C62.90	Primary neoplasm of testicle
J93.9	Pneumothorax, spontaneous, acute, or chronic
N30.00	Cystitis, acute
N39.0	Urinary tract infection, site not specified
N50.89	Testicular mass
R33.9	Urinary retention, NEC
R39.14	Urinary retention, bladder incomplete emptying
M79.5	Residual foreign body in soft tissue
S22.39XA	Rib fracture, closed, unspecified number of ribs
S22.39XA	Rib facture, closed, one rib

Combined Diagnostic-Procedural

See also Chapter 171, Musculoskeletal Ultrasound, Chapter 221, Lumbar Puncture, and Chapter 228, Central Venous Catheter Insertion.

A15.6	Tuberculous pleurisy, pleural effusion, empyema, or hydrothorax
A87.9	Unspecified viral meningitis, or abacterial or aseptic meningitis
C50.819	Primary breast neoplasm, upper or lower
C73	Malignant neoplasm of thyroid gland
C78.2	Secondary malignant neoplasm pleura
D34	Benign neoplasm of thyroid
E04.2	Nontoxic multinodular goiter
E05.20	Toxic multinodular goiter
E04.1	Cyst of thyroid
G00.9	Meningitis due to unspecified bacterium
J90	Bacterial, nontuberculous pleural effusion
J91.8	Pleural effusion
K65.0	Suppurative peritonitis
N60.09	Solitary cyst of breast
N60.19	(Fibro) Cystic breast
N63.0	Lump or mass in breast
L03.90	Other cellulitis and abscess, unspecified site
R18.8	Ascites
T81.69XA	Chemical peritonitis

SUPPLIERS

See Suppliers sections in Chapter 142, Obstetric Ultrasound, and Chapter 171, Musculoskeletal Ultrasound.

ONLINE RESOURCES

Alliance for Physician Certification and Advancement: www.apca.org (branch of ARDMS, the certifying agency for sonographers)

American College of Chest Physicians: www.chestnet.org/Education/Advanced-Clinical-Training/Certificate-of-Completion-Program/Critical-Care-Ultrasonography (critical care ultrasound courses)

American College of Surgeons: www.facs.org/about-acs/statements/31-ultrasound-exam and www.learning.facs.org/content/ultrasound-surgeons-basic-course-3rd-edition-online-course.

American Institute of Ultrasound in Medicine (AIUM): www.aium.org., DVDs and videos available for many areas of scanning [e.g., abdominal aorta, abdominal/retroperitoneal scanning, FAST exam, musculoskeletal system, pelvis, ultrasound-guided procedures, scrotum]

American Registry for Diagnostic Medical Sonographers (ARDMS): www.ardms.org

Challenger Fundamentals. EM Ultrasound: www.onlinelibrary.wiley.com/doi/full/10.1111/j.1553-2712.2011.01263.x (course designed to teach the basic techniques of emergency ultrasonography; contains a combination of still and video segments as well as diagrams, three-dimensional animations, and interactive multimedia that describe the key concepts of ultrasonography)

Society for Academic Emergency Medicine: www.saem.org (Online teaching and narrated slides, including ultrasound images, for various emergency medicine topics)

Sonosite: www.sonosite.com (video series for learning ultrasound, from bedside invasive procedures, to emergency medicine, critical care medicine, and anesthesiology procedures)

RECOMMENDED READING

American College of Emergency Physicians. *ACEP Policy Statement: Emergency Ultrasound Imaging Criteria Compendium.* Board of Directors; 2014. https://www.acep.org/globalassets/uploads/uploaded-files/acep/by-medical-focus/ultrasound/emergency-ultrasound-imaging-criteria-compendium.pdf.

American College of Emergency Physicians. ACEP policy statement: ultrasound guidelines: emergency, point-of-care and clinical ultrasound guidelines in medicine. *Ann Emerg Med.* 2017;69:e27–e54.

American Institute of Ultrasound in Medicine. AIUM practice parameter for documentation of an ultrasound examination. 2014. www.aium.org/resources/guidelines/documentation.pdf.

American Institute of Ultrasound in Medicine. AIUM practice parameter for the performance of the focused assessment with sonography for trauma (FAST) examination. 2014. www.aium.org/resources/guidelines/fast.pdf.

American Institute of Ultrasound in Medicine. AIUM practice parameter for the performance of scrotal ultrasound examinations. 2015. www.aium.org/resources/guidelines/scrotal.pdf.

American Institute of Ultrasound in Medicine. AIUM practice parameter for the performance of selected ultrasound-guided procedures. 2014. www.aium.org/resources/guidelines/usGuidedProcedures.pdf.

American Institute of Ultrasound in Medicine. AIUM practice parameter for the performance of an ultrasound of the abdomen and/ or retroperitoneum. 2017. www.aium.org/resources/guidelines/abdominal.pdf.

American Institute of Ultrasound in Medicine. AIUM practice parameter for the performance of ultrasound of the female pelvis. 2014. www.aium.org/resources/guidelines/femalePelvis.pdf.

Blaivas M, Lyon M, Duggal S. A prospective comparison of supine chest radiography and bedside ultrasound for the diagnosis of traumatic pneumothorax. *Acad Emerg Med.* 2005;12:844–849.

Bornemann P, ed. *Ultrasound in Primary Care.* Philadelphia: Wolters Kluwer; 2018.

Daniels JM, Hoppmann RA, eds. *Practical Point-of-Care Medical Ultrasound.* Switzerland: Springer International Publishing; 2016.

Deutchman M. The problematic first-trimester pregnancy. *Am Fam Physician.* 1989;39:185–198.

Gochman RF, Karasic RB, Heller MB. Use of portable ultrasound to assist urine collection by suprapubic aspiration. *Ann Emerg Med.* 1991;20:631–635.

Heller M, Jehle D, eds. *Ultrasound in Emergency Medicine.* Philadelphia: WB Saunders; 1995.

Jehle D, Davis E, Evans T, et al. Emergency department sonography by emergency physicians. *Am J Emerg Med.* 1989;7:605–611.

Kendall JL, Hoffenberg SR, Smith RS. History of emergency and critical care ultrasound: the evolution of a new imaging paradigm. *Crit Care Med.* 2007;35(suppl 5):S126–S130.

Mortality results for randomized controlled trial of early elective surgery or ultrasonographic surveillance for small abdominal aortic aneurysms: the UK Small Aneurysm Trial Participants. *Lancet.* 1998;352:1649–1655.

Roberts KB. Revised AAP guideline on UTI in febrile infants and young children. *Am Fam Physician.* 2012;86(10):940–946.

Rodney JR, ed. *Family Medicine: Obstetrical Ultrasound.* Indianapolis: Dog Ear Publishing; 2014.

Sanders RC, Hall-Terracciano B, eds. *Clinical Sonography: A Practical Guide.* 5th ed. Philadelphia: Wolters Kluwer; 2016.

Schlager D, Lazzareschi G, Whitten D, et al. A prospective study of ultrasonography in the ED by emergency physicians. *Am J Emerg Med.* 1994;12:185–189.

Siepel T, Clifford DS, James PA, Cowan TM. The ultrasound-assisted physical examination in the periodic health evaluation of the elderly. *J Fam Pract.* 2000;49:628–632.

Simon B, Snoey E, eds. *Ultrasound in Emergency and Ambulatory Medicine.* St. Louis: Mosby; 1997.

Soni NJ, Artnfield R, Kory P, eds. *Point-of-Care Ultrasound.* Philadelphia: Elsevier; 2015.

CHAPTER 215

HEIMLICH MANEUVER

Raymond F. Jarris Jr

Each year in the United States, 3000 people die from swallowing or aspirating objects. When a patient displays the distress signal for choking (i.e., clutching the neck) or becomes cyanotic, unconscious, or unable to cough or breathe effectively (suggesting complete obstruction), efforts to clear the obstruction are warranted. The Heimlich maneuver (abdominal thrusts) causes a sudden increase in intrathoracic pressure, forcing an obstructing object from the glottis (Fig. 215.1). The 2010 International Consensus Conference on Cardiopulmonary Resuscitation and Emergency Cardiopulmonary Care found good evidence for the use of abdominal thrusts, chest thrusts, and back blows or slaps for clearing the airway of a foreign body obstruction. There was insufficient evidence to determine which technique is best or which should be used first. There was some evidence that chest thrusts may generate higher peak airway pressure than the Heimlich maneuver. Chest thrusts are usually performed in the child younger than 1 year, in patients in whom the Heimlich is contraindicated, or in an older patient after he or she has collapsed to the floor. They are performed in the same manner and at the same rate as chest compressions used with cardiopulmonary resuscitation (CPR). In fact, more than one technique may be needed to clear an obstruction; if so, they should be alternated rapidly until the airway is cleared.

NOTE: In the event of partial foreign body aspiration, if the patient is able to move air or speak, the Heimlich maneuver and probing of the oropharynx should be avoided and the patient be transported to a source of emergency medical care.

INDICATION

Asphyxiation from a foreign body obstruction of the upper airway indicates the need for emergent intervention. If forceful coughing is occurring, do not interfere with the coughing. However, the Heimlich maneuver is indicated if the cough becomes silent, respiratory difficulty increases and is accompanied by stridor, or the victim becomes unresponsive. The Heimlich is most effective when a solid food bolus is obstructing the larynx. In the unresponsive patient, a "finger sweep" of the posterior oropharynx should be used only when the provider can see solid material obstructing the airway.

CONTRAINDICATIONS

The Heimlich maneuver is relatively contraindicated in infants, small children, pregnant women, and individuals with a protuberant abdomen (abdominal thrusts inappropriate). It may also be difficult to accomplish in obese patients if the clinician is unable to encircle the victim's abdomen. In infants, abdominal thrusts are not recommended because infants may be at higher risk for iatrogenic injuries. In infants, pregnant women, individuals with a protuberant abdomen, and obese patients, chest thrusts may be appropriate.

TECHNIQUE

Adults and Children Older Than 1 Year

Sitting or Standing

1. Stand behind the patient with arms wrapped around the patient's waist.
2. Grasp the fist or wrist of one hand with the other, place the hands against the patient's abdomen between the navel and rib cage, and press the fist into the patient's abdomen. Deliver a quick thrust inward and upward, aiming toward the diaphragm while avoiding the ribs (Fig. 215.2A).
3. Apply three to five abdominal or chest thrusts. These thrusts lift the diaphragm and/or force enough air from the lungs to create an artificial cough to move and expel an obstructing foreign body in an airway.

Lying

1. If the patient has collapsed or is unable to be lifted, place him or her in the supine position. The clinician should kneel beside the patient's abdomen or straddle it.
2. Place one hand on top of the other, with the heel of the bottom hand positioned in the midline of the patient, between the umbilicus and the xiphoid.
3. Lean forward with shoulders over the patient's abdomen and quickly press inward and upward toward the diaphragm three to

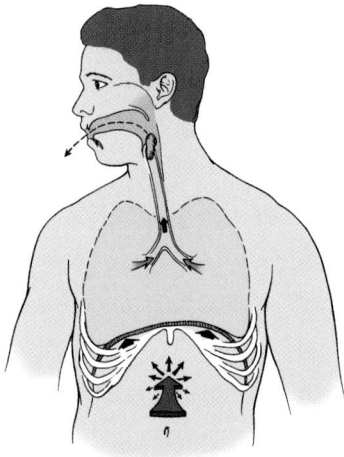

Fig. 215.1 The Heimlich maneuver causes a sudden increase in intrathoracic pressure, forcing an obstructing object from the glottis. If the patient is sitting or standing, the clinician should stand behind the patient and wrap his or her arms around the patient's waist. The clinician's fist should be placed with the thumb side against the patient's abdomen, above the umbilicus but below the rib cage.

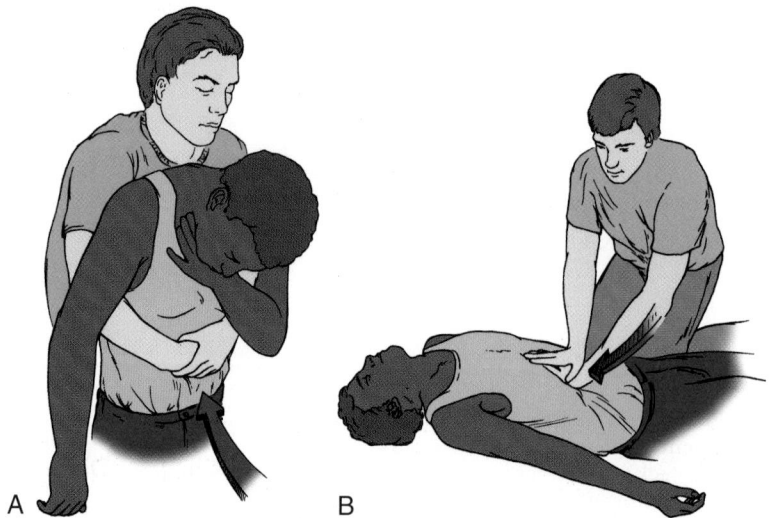

Fig. 215.2 Abdominal thrusts. (A) Patient sitting or standing, (B) Patient collapsed or lying down.

five times (see Fig. 215.2B). The clinician should not press to the right or left of the midline.

4. In a patient who has lost consciousness or in pregnant or obese patients or those with a protuberant abdomen, use chest thrusts delivered in the same fashion as in step 3 but place your hands over the sternum. After 30 seconds of chest compressions in the unconscious patient, remove the obstructing object if you see it, attempt two breaths, and continue CPR.

5. Clear visible material from the oropharynx with a finger sweep or Magill forceps.

Infants to 1 Year of Age (or Those Small Enough to Be Held in the Head-Down Position)

1. Place the child face down on your arm with the head directed downward, supporting the head and neck with a knee and one hand (Fig. 215.3).
2. Deliver three to five gentle back blows between the scapulae with the palm of your hand.
3. If obstruction is still present, roll the child over, lower his or her head, and deliver chest thrusts gently with two to three fingers as in CPR.
4. Repeat steps 2 and 3 until the object is cleared or surgical intervention is required (see Chapter 223, Cricothyroid Catheter Insertion, Crycothyroidotomy, and Tracheostomy).

COMPLICATIONS

- Abdominal aortic aneurysm thrombosis
- Internal carotid artery dissection
- Esophageal rupture
- Gastric rupture
- Mesenteric laceration
- Jejunal rupture
- Liver, spleen, or pancreas injury
- Pneumomediastinum and pneumothorax
- Punctured lung
- Regurgitation
- Retinal detachment
- Rib fracture

The Heimlich maneuver is usually performed outside of medical facilities. Although complications are rare, most of the complications are severe and can be life-threatening. For example, gastric rupture has a high mortality rate. A clinician should evaluate all persons who have been subjected to the Heimlich maneuver. Focused evaluation by the clinician should include history and physical

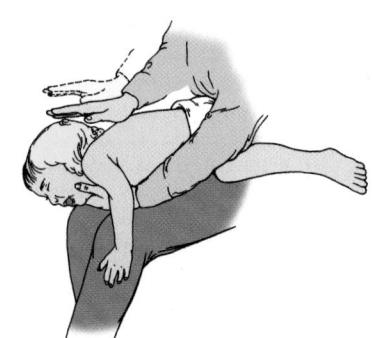

Fig. 215.3 Back blows for infants and small children.

examination of the respiratory and gastrointestinal system. Early intervention may reduce the morbidity and mortality associated with these complications.

RECOMMENDED READING

2015. American Heart Association Guidelines Update for Cardiopulmonary Resuscitation and Emergency Cardiovascular Care. *Circulation.* 2015;132:S313–S314.

Bradley RN, Lerakis S. American Red Cross SAC Advisory on Obstructed Airway-Adults. *American Red Cross Scientific Advisory Council.* 2015;24. January.

Bintz M, Cogbill TH. Gastric rupture after the Heimlich maneuver. *J Trauma.* 1996;40:159–160.

Espinoza T, Menon S, Bailitz J. Relief of choking and upper airway foreign body removal. In: Reichman EF, ed. *Emergency Medicine Procedures.* 2nd ed. New York: McGraw-Hill; 2013:1181–1184.

Haynes DE, Haynes BE, Yong YV. Esophageal rupture complicating Heimlich maneuver. *Am J Emerg Med.* 1984;2:507–509.

Kirschner RL, Green RM. Acute thrombosis of abdominal aortic aneurysm subsequent to Heimlich maneuver: a case report. *J Vasc Surg.* 1985;2:594–596.

Majumdar A, Sedman PC. Gastric rupture secondary to successful Heimlich maneuver. *Postgrad Med J.* 1998;74:609–610.

Otero Palleiro MM, Barbagelata López C, Fernández Pretel MC, Salgado Fernández J. Hepatic rupture after Heimlich maneuver. *Ann Emerg Med.* 2007;49:825–826.

Razaboni RM, Brathwaite CE, Dwyer Jr WA. Ruptured jejunum following Heimlich maneuver. *J Emerg Med.* 1986;4:95–98.

Reardon RE, Mason PE, Clinton JE. Basic airway management and decision making. In: Roberts JR, Custalow CB, Thomsen TW, eds. *Roberts and Hedges Clinical Procedures in Emergency Medicine.* 6th ed. Philadelphia: Elsevier; 2014:41–42.

CHAPTER 216

ZIPPER INJURY MANAGEMENT

Grant C. Fowler • Michael A. Hansen

Zipper injuries happen. Sometimes alcohol or another form of intoxication is involved. Such injuries are most common in uncircumcised young boys, but can occur in adults, especially those with cognitive or physical impairment and in a hurry. In one pediatric emergency department study (Wyatt), 60% of males were wearing underwear at the time of injury, 84% of injuries were self-inflicted, and 92% occurred as the zipper was being pulled up. Zipper injuries accounted for 1 in 4000 pediatric emergency room visits.

ANATOMY

A zipper consists of a sliding piece or fastener that moves in two directions along a row of teeth. It can be composed of metal, plastic, or other materials such as nylon. The fastener has a front and back plate connected by the median bar. A finger grip is usually attached to the front plate, and is used to place traction on the sliding piece.

The anatomic parts most likely to be entrapped by a zipper are the foreskin, the penis, or the scrotum. Occasionally, other body parts are entrapped.

INDICATIONS

Skin entrapped in a zipper. The skin should be released as soon as possible to minimize edema and risk of skin necrosis.

CONTRAINDICATIONS

Patient refusal.

EQUIPMENT AND SUPPLIES

* Heavy duty wire cutter (consider borrowing from maintenance department, preferably long, and narrow-nosed cutter for better maneuverability) or bone cutter
* Miniature hacksaw or large flathead screwdriver (if wire cutter or bone cutter not available)
* Povidone iodine or chlorhexidine
* Heavy scissors, bandage or Mayo
* Light scissors, small or iris
* Topical anesthetic (e.g., lisosomal lidocaine [LMA], lidocaine-prilocaine cream [EMLA])
* Local anesthetic solution without epinephrine
* Mineral oil
* 27-gauge needle
* 5 mL syringe

PREPROCEDURE PATIENT PREPARATION

The procedure should be explained to the patient or their representative in a gentle and reassuring manner. Informed consent should be obtained if damage to skin is anticipated. In most cases, the patient will be anxious and probably embarrassed because of the tissue entrapped. Reassure the patient that everything possible will be done to keep them comfortable and to minimize damage to whatever is entrapped. In most cases, this will be a fairly quick procedure, but it will be important for the patient to remain as still as possible while it is being performed. If tissue is entrapped by the zipper fastener, this procedure is usually more difficult than when the entrapment is just in the zipper teeth. Topical anesthesia such as LMX or EMLA can be applied (see Chapter 4, Topical Anesthesia), but this may result in significant delay while waiting for the anesthetic to take effect. If the patient is in significant pain, local anesthetic can be infiltrated around the entrapped skin or a penile block can be performed (see Chapter 166, Dorsal Penile and Subcutaneous Ring Block for Newborn Circumcision). In rare cases, parenteral analgesia or procedural sedation may be required.

TECHNIQUE

Manual Removal

1. Place the patient in a comfortable position and in a position where the clinician can apply significant traction on the finger grip, usually with the patient lying down. Apply mineral oil liberally to the zipper and entrapped skin, and allow to soak for 10 to 15 minutes. Patients are usually very anxious, especially young males, so approaching the patient in a firm, reassuring, and confident manner can sometimes allay anxiety.
2. Wipe any oil off the zipper finger grip. If tissue is entrapped by the zipper fastener, while attempting to avoid further injury, apply gentle and steady traction on the finger grip directed away from the entrapped tissue. If tissue is entrapped by the zipper teeth, the zipper may need to be pulled back over the entrapped tissue. As an alternative, significant lateral traction on either side of the zipped teeth will sometimes merely pull the zipper apart; this will free the entrapped tissue. This especially works well with nylon zippers.
3. Avoid use of excessive force on the finger grip, which can result in avulsion of tissue or a laceration. If this technique fails, consider the techniques described later.

Cutting of the Median Bar

1. This is the preferred technique. If the wire cutter is borrowed from maintenance, it might be prudent to coat the wire cutter and prepare the skin with povidone-iodine or chlorhexidine. Avulsions, bruising, and lacerations can happen with this technique.
2. Maneuver the cutter from above the zipper fastener to cut the median bar (Fig. 216.1). The front and back plates of the fastener should separate. If skin is entrapped by the zipper fastener, it should be released. If skin is trapped between zipper teeth, after the median bar is cut, the clinician should be able to manually pull the rows of teeth below the fastener apart to free the entrapped tissue.

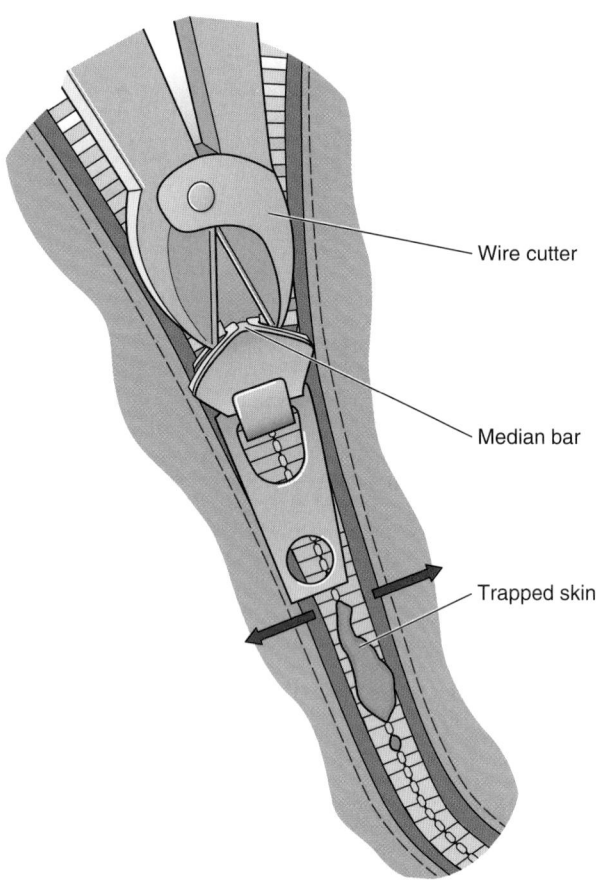

Fig. 216.1 Cut the median bar to remove the zipper. If the skin is entrapped between the zipper fastener and the teeth, this should release the entrapped skin. If the skin is entrapped in the zipper teeth, below the zipper fastener, it may be necessary to manually separate the two rows of zipper teeth (*arrows*).

Cutting the Cloth Surrounding Zipper Teeth

1. If a wire cutter or bone cutter is not available, this technique is an option, especially if the skin is trapped between the zipper teeth.
2. Using heavy scissors, and being careful to avoid any tissue beneath, two cuts should be made along a line parallel to the zipper on either side (Fig. 216.2). In this manner, cut the cloth portion of the zipper.
3. Using light scissors, cuts should now be made across the zipper, between the teeth, carefully avoiding any tissue beneath the teeth. This should free the entrapped tissue.

Cutting Between the Zipper Teeth

1. Using heavy scissors, above or below the entrapped tissue, the clinician can cut across the zipper, between the teeth. This allows the zipper teeth to be manually separated above or below the cut to free the entrapped tissue. This method is faster than cutting the median bar if tissue is only trapped in the zipper teeth.

Alternative Techniques

If the listed equipment is not available or the previous techniques are unsuccessful, alternative techniques have been published. One option is to excise the entrapped skin, but only if the tissue is readily accessible and superficial or redundant. Local anesthetic should

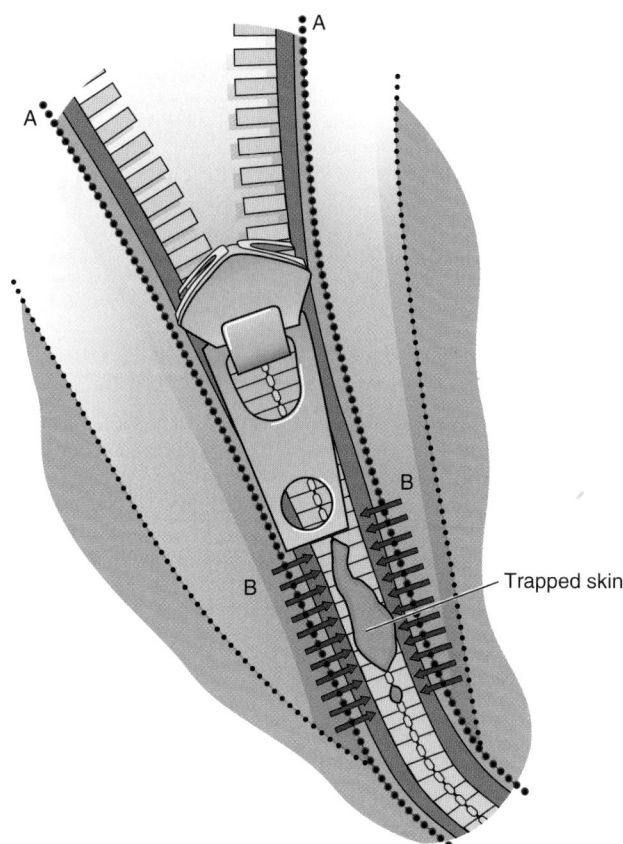

Fig. 216.2 (A) With heavy scissors, cut the cloth holding the zipper to the pants (*along the heavy dashed lines*). (B) Next, with light scissors, cut the cloth between the teeth (*along the dotted lines with directional arrows*).

be used, if possible. A miniature hacksaw can be used as a second option. However, this technique carries the risk of significant injury to nearby skin and soft tissue. Use the hacksaw to cut the median bar, paying careful attention to avoid damaging surrounding tissue. A third published technique uses a large flathead screwdriver. The flat blade of the screwdriver should be gradually and gently inserted between the inner and outer faceplates on one side of the zipper. It should then be turned or twisted clockwise and counterclockwise to pry open the zipper, free the zipper teeth, and release the entrapped skin.

COMPLICATIONS

- Superficial abrasions and lacerations, bruising, and pain are possible.
- Deep lacerations are possible, usually due to improper positioning of the wire cutter or scissors.
- Damage to the urethra or other genitourinary structures. The urethra should be carefully inspected following this procedure. Follow-up with a urologist may be necessary if there is suspicion of urethral damage.

POSTPROCEDURE PATIENT EDUCATION

Tetanus immune status should be verified if there was a break in the skin. Likewise, the patient should be instructed in local wound care and how to monitor for signs of infection. Pain with urination should be expected for 1 to 2 days after the procedure. If dysuria persists beyond this time, the patient should be seen in follow-up or consult a urologist. Medical care should be sought if the patient is unable to avoid or has fever or hematuria.

CPT/Billing Codes

10120   Incision and removal of foreign body, subcutaneous tissues; simple

Or an appropriate E&M code can be used. If definitive treatment is referred to another physician, coding for supplies and splinting may be used.

RECOMMENDED READING

Kassutto Z. Zipper injury management. In: Reichman EF, ed. *Emergency Medicine Procedures*. 2nd ed. New York: McGraw-Hill; 2013:1004–1006.

Kanegaye JT, Schonfeld N. Penile zipper entrapment: a simple and less threatening approach using mineral oil. *Pediatr Emerg Care*. 1993;9(2):90–91.

Stone DM, Scordino DJ. Foreign body removal. In: Roberts JR, Custalow CB, Thomsen TW, eds. *Roberts & Hedges' Clinical Procedures of Emergency Medicine*. 6th ed. Philadelphia: Elsevier; 2014:712–714.

Wyatt JP, Scobie WG. The management of penile zip entrapment in children. *Injury*. 1994;29(1):59.

SECTION 14

Hospitalist

Section Editor: GRAHAM V. SEGAL

CHAPTER 217

NASOGASTRIC AND NASOENTERIC TUBE INSERTION AND REMOVAL

Yong Sik Kim

Nasogastric tube insertion is a common procedure performed in the hospital and emergency department; it is also occasionally performed in the office setting. The nasogastric tube was initially developed for gastric feeding in 1760. The indications were expanded to gastric lavage in the case of poisoning in the early 1800s. One current design, by Dr. Levin, became available in 1921, and soon became popular for preventing intraoperative and postoperative gastric distention. In the 1960s, improved technology allowed the manufacture of a double-lumen tube; later developments include special soft tubes made of polyurethane and silicone. These later tubes are also very thin and have a noncomplicated, smooth surface—useful characteristics for prolonged nasoenteric feeding.

A nasogastric tube can be used for either diagnostic or therapeutic purposes. The Levin nasogastric tube is a firm, straight, single-lumen tube with multiple distal side ports, and is used predominantly for diagnostic aspiration or to instill materials into the stomach. Unfortunately, even when low–flow-rate suction is applied to a Levin tube, or if it is applied for a very long time, the lumen frequently becomes occluded with gastric mucosa. This can damage the gastric mucosa. In contrast, the Salem nasogastric sump tube is a double-lumen tube. The second lumen, or vent lumen, is smaller than the main suction lumen and runs alongside the larger lumen, providing a low level of continuous airflow to the stomach. This airflow prevents the main lumen from becoming occluded by gastric mucosa, thereby minimizing the risk of damage (Fig. 217.1). The blue "pigtail" on the Salem sump is an extension of this vent lumen (Fig. 217.2). Similar to the Levin tube, the Salem sump has multiple distal side ports. Antireflux valves are available to prevent gastric contents from leaking out of the vent lumen. Multiport adapters are available for the proximal end so that the same tube can be used for feeding, irrigating, suctioning, or medicating. Even though the Levin tube is still manufactured and available, hospitals predominantly stock the Salem sump tube because it can be used for most applications, is more effective, and is safer.

Salem sump tubes are usually clear, yet radiopaque, and made of polypropylene or silicone, whereas Levin tubes are available in various versions, including red rubber and clear polypropylene. Levin tubes can be either radiopaque or radiolucent. Although both can be used for short-term (up to 4 weeks) gastric or nasoenteric feeding, polypropylene is too rigid for long-term use, so most facilities now have the longer and smaller-diameter polyurethane tubes specially designed for this purpose (Fig. 217.3). These softer tubes (especially softer at body temperatures) usually have a tungsten-weighted tip or balloon near the tip to facilitate passage beyond the pylorus. They may also have a stiffening wire or stylet available for use during insertion; many have been designed to resist collapse when checking the gastric residual. Other styles of tubes include those equipped with a large esophageal balloon that can be used to tamponade a bleeding esophageal lesion (e.g., esophageal varices). Larger gastric tubes are also available for gastric lavage (see Chapter 209, Gastrointestinal Decontamination).

ANATOMY

The nasal cavity is lined by highly vascularized and innervated mucosa and continues posteriorly as the nasopharynx. Within the nasal cavity are the superior, inferior, and middle nasal conchae (turbinates), which divide the cavity into four passages (Fig. 217.4), the meatuses. Traditionally, the nasogastric tube is inserted blindly through the middle or inferior meatus. Beyond the nasal cavity, the pharynx extends from the base of the skull to the inferior border of the cricoid cartilage. It is divided into three parts: the nasopharynx, oropharynx, and laryngopharynx (hypopharynx). The nasopharynx gives rise to the oropharynx at the level of the soft palate, which then gives rise to the laryngopharynx (hypopharynx) at the superior border of the epiglottis (see also Chapter 64, Nasolaryngoscopy, Fig. 64.6). The laryngopharynx becomes continuous with the esophagus at the inferior border of the cricoid cartilage. The posterior part of the upper nasopharynx is surrounded by the cribriform plate and the body of the ethmoid and sphenoid bones, which can easily be broken by a traumatic blow to the midface, resulting in a maxillofacial

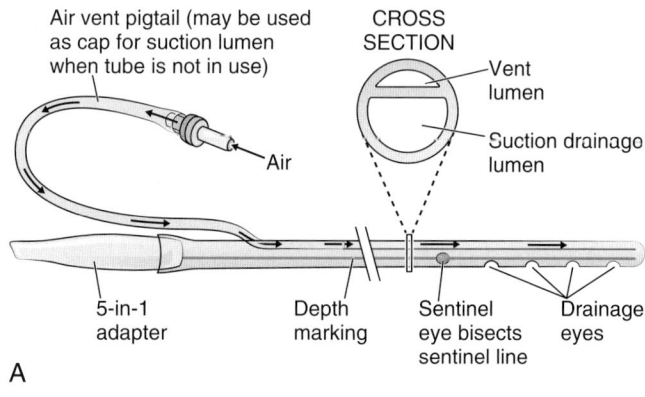

A

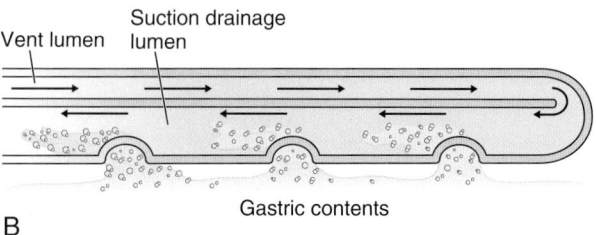

B

Fig. 217.1 Diagram of the Salem sump tube. (A) General design. (B) Diagram of the double lumen principle for suction. (Courtesy Covidien Medtronic, Dublin, Ireland.)

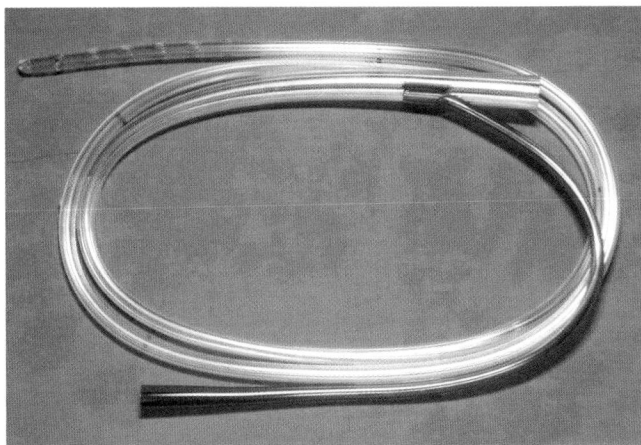

Fig. 217.2 Sump suction (Salem) tube. (Courtesy Covidien Medtronic, Dublin, Ireland.)

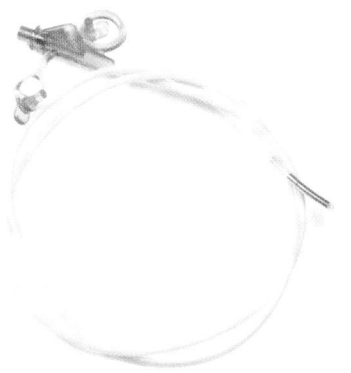

Fig. 217.3 Feeding nasogastrostomy tube with weighted, radiopaque tip. (COMPAT Nasogastric Tube, courtesy Nestlé Nutrition, Minnetonka, MN.)

or basilar skull fracture. Such fractures can create a route into the cranial vault, which is a prerequisite for one of the most disastrous complications of inserting a nasogastric tube, intracranial intubation. This can result in brain damage or death. Therefore, placement of a nasogastric or nasoenteric tube in a patient with a possible skull or maxillofacial fracture should be avoided, if possible (an orogastric route may be a better option).

Beyond the laryngopharynx and the larynx, the trachea lies anterior to the esophagus at the level of the cricoid bone and is supported by fibrocartilaginous tracheal rings. The superior aperture is covered by the epiglottis of the larynx during swallowing.

EDITOR'S NOTE: Knowing whether the patient has had bariatric surgery is important, because the anatomy may have been changed. Normally the stomach wall is thick and there is plenty of room to accommodate even an extra loop of nasogastric tube. However, the gastric pouch may have been significantly reduced; the intestinal wall is also very thin. (Van Dinter reported a case of late intestinal perforation [9 years] after a Roux-en-Y gastric bypass.) So, preferably, the clinician will know what type of bariatric procedure was performed. At a minimum, the clinician should proceed with caution. If a band is in place, more resistance may be encountered with nasogastric tube insertion. If the surgery is recent, consultation with the surgeon should be considered.

Knowing the anatomy also confers the ability to estimate the length of tube that should be inserted. Because the median distance from the anterior aspect of the nasal septum to the cricopharyngeus muscle (tracheoesophageal junction) is about 8 inches and the esophagus is on average about 10 inches long, and given that the tip of a nasogastric tube should lie 4 inches below the gastroesophageal junction when in place, the nasogastric tube should ideally be secured at the 20- to 24-inch mark at the nasal vestibule. Alternatively, the distance can be approximated by holding the tube up to the patient's ear and across to the nose, and then extending it to the xiphoid process and adding 6 inches (adding 8 to 10 inches for a nasoenteric tube; described later in the "Technique" section).

The anatomy of children regarding the insertion of a nasogastric tube warrants a special note. Children have larger tonsils and adenoids, and their tongues are large compared with adults and may push into the oropharynx; all of this can hamper the insertion of

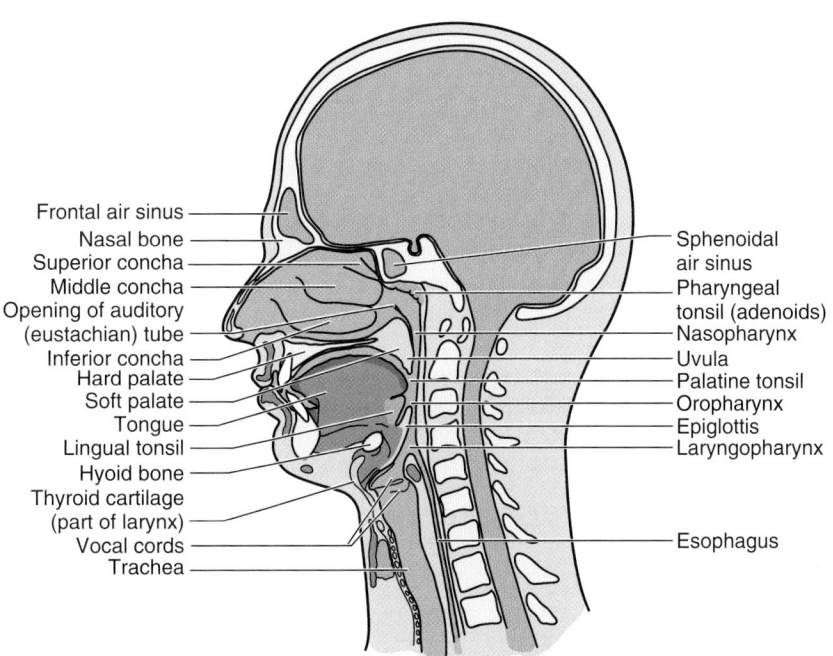

Fig. 217.4 Pharyngeal anatomy: sagittal section of the head and neck. (From Thibodeau C, Patton KT. *Structure and Function of the Body*. 11th ed. St. Louis: Mosby; 2000.)

a tube. At the same time, these tissues are soft and easily injured, thereby increasing the risk of bleeding with nasogastric intubation. Limiting the size of the tube to the smaller sizes of the nostrils and nasal cavity in children usually minimizes the difficulty with insertion, as well as tissue damage, despite these anatomic differences. See the "Equipment" section to estimate size for nasogastric tubes in children.

INDICATIONS

Therapeutic

- Drainage of gastric contents/gastric decompression. Examples include small bowel or gastric outlet obstruction, paralytic ileus, upper gastrointestinal bleeding, refractory vomiting, severe pancreatitis with obstruction, gastric lavage (for drug overdose), prevention of aspiration, or before diagnostic peritoneal lavage or pericardiocentesis.
- Instillation of feedings or medications for patients unable to take by mouth (e.g., nutritional supplements, activated charcoal for drug overdoses).

NOTE: In patients with upper gastrointestinal hemorrhage, extended irrigation of the stomach with water can result in hypokalemia; animal studies suggest that cold water lavage can cause rather than control the bleeding.

Diagnostic

- Sampling gastric contents (e.g., gastrointestinal bleeding, mycobacterial infection)
- Instillation of diagnostic agents (e.g., radiopaque contrast media for delineation of a transdiaphragmatic hernia, air inserted to assess for an intraperitoneal perforation)

NOTE: The fecal Hemoccult should not be used to test for occult blood in gastric contents; instead, the Gastroccult card uses a developer that neutralizes pH, rendering it able to detect hemoglobin.

CONTRAINDICATIONS

All the following contraindications are relative:

- Facial fractures, especially midface, or basilar skull fractures with possible cribriform plate injuries (may result in intracranial intubation; orogastric intubation may be a better option)
- Esophageal obstruction, strictures, or a history of alkali ingestion (increases the possibility of esophageal perforation)
- Esophageal varices (may lead to rupture and uncontrollable hemorrhage)
- Comatose patients without protected airways (increases the risk of aspiration)
- Penetrating neck wounds in the awake trauma victim (gagging might stimulate increased bleeding from the wound)
- Choanal atresia
- Recent oropharyngeal, nasal, or gastric surgery (especially bariatric surgery, consider consultation with the surgeon)
- Zenker diverticulum
- Percutaneous endoscopic gastrostomy tube indicated (see Chapter 92, "Percutaneous Endoscopic Gastrostomy Placement and Replacement")
- Severe coagulopathy (orogastric intubation may be a better option)
- Tube feeding in patients with advanced dementia (there is little evidence that the outcome will be improved)

Previous bariatric surgery is not a contraindication; however, it may be helpful to know the type of bariatric surgery performed. Clinicians inserting a nasogastric tube should be somewhat familiar with the resultant anatomy and proceed with caution.

EQUIPMENT AND SUPPLIES

- Gloves, mask, goggles, and an impervious gown
- Towel or surgical Chux for covering patient's clothing
- Paper tissues
- Emesis basin
- Tongue depressor
- Nasogastric tube (For adults, use a 16- or 18-Fr Salem sump [with antireflux valve, if possible] or Levin tube. Use 10- to 12-Fr tube for smaller children, 12- to 14-Fr for larger children, or use formula [age in years+16]/2.)
- For nasoenteric feeding tubes (5 to 12 Fr). Larger tubes (12 Fr) should be used for shorter periods because they are less comfortable and more likely to become occluded than smaller tubes (5 to 8 Fr).
- Tincture of benzoin
- Hypoallergenic tape (e.g., Hy-Tape), NG Secure, or NG Strip
- Stethoscope
- Large (60-mL) syringe with catheter tip (Toomey)
- Suction equipment
- Cup of water with drinking straw
- Decongestant such as phenylephrine (0.25% to 2%) spray (Neo-Synephrine, Vicks), oxymetazoline hydrochloride 0.05% spray (Afrin, Neo-Synephrine 12 hour), or ephedrine 3%
- Water-soluble lubricant gel (Surgilube) or 2% lidocaine gel (Xylocaine Jelly)
- Topical anesthetic spray such as benzocaine (Hurricaine) or tetracaine hydrochloride (Cetacaine), or both. Topical cocaine is an option, and it works as both a decongestant and anesthetic. However, its use may be a problem if the patient must undergo drug testing. In addition, purchase and storage by clinician or hospital requires significant record-keeping and may increase the risk of theft.
- Laryngoscope for difficult insertions
- pH indicator strips with 0.5 gradations or paper with a range of 0 to 6 or 1 to 11
- Soft nasal trumpet airway (optional)

PREPROCEDURE PATIENT PREPARATION

Although the insertion of a nasogastric tube is a common and fairly simple procedure, serious complications can occur. The risk for complications can be minimized by taking a few precautions: obtaining the full cooperation of the patient, informing the patient carefully at each step of the process, using a decongestant and local anesthesia for the nasal and retropharyngeal mucosa, premeasuring and marking the length of the tube needed for insertion, using gentle technique during insertion, and carefully confirming that the tube is in the proper position before use.

To have a nasogastric tube inserted into them is considered by many patients to be one of the most uncomfortable and distressful procedures they have ever experienced. Although most hospitals do not require written informed consent, the risks, benefits, indications, and any possible alternatives should be explained to patients. Even with the use of decongestants and anesthetics, patients should be prepared for some discomfort. The unpleasant nature of the procedure should not be minimized.

Patients should know that their eyes may water and they may have some tearing. They may have an intense tickling sensation or an urge to sneeze. During insertion, they may experience a gagging sensation. (Some clinicians premedicate with ondansetron 4 mg or metoclopramide 10 mg intravenously 5 minutes before the procedure, although there is scant evidence supporting this intervention.) Swallowing rapidly will minimize this response and shorten the total length of the procedure. At some point during the procedure, they will probably be asked to assist by sniffing or later by swallowing. To help them swallow, give them a glass of water and a straw. If they are not able to swallow, mimicking swallowing or saying "eeee" may help. Patients should be reassured that after the tube has been placed, they will usually adapt to it very soon and no longer notice it.

Before nasogastric tube removal, the patient should be informed of the procedure and what to expect. Towels, surgical Chux, or other drapes should be placed around the patient's neck and chest. He or she should be handed an emesis basin and tissues.

TECHNIQUE

Observe universal blood and body fluid precautions during the procedure. Wear gloves, goggles, a face mask, and an impervious gown.

1. Elevate the head of the bed into a high Fowler (sitting) or semi-Fowler position. Rest the back of the patient's head on a pillow or directly on the bed for support. The patient's clothing needs to be protected with a towel or surgical Chux. An emesis basin should be available on the patient's lap.
2. Check for a clear nasal passage. Various conditions may cause asymmetric nostril openings—for example, septal deviation, nasal polyps, septal spurs. So examine both nostrils to determine which is the largest and most open. You can also watch the patient inhaling through his or her nose to determine which nostril is more open.
3. After the application of a nasal decongestant such as phenylephrine, oxymetazoline, or ephedrine, adding a topical anesthetic usually increases the patient's comfort. Although this procedure is usually brief, application of the decongestant before the anesthesia usually results in the anesthesia lasting longer. The decongestant may also minimize damage to the nasal mucosa and decrease the incidence of epistaxis.

   NOTE: A randomized, controlled trial (Singer and Konia, 1999) showed improved comfort when a decongestant/anesthetic was used, compared with plain lubrication for nasogastric tube insertion. In the study, topical anesthesia was applied (after the decongestant) by injecting 5 mL of 2% lidocaine gel (Xylocaine Jelly) into the nostril before insertion. The pharynx was then sprayed with both benzocaine (Hurricaine) and tetracaine hydrochloride (Cetacaine) to minimize the gag reflex. If possible, allow a few minutes for the decongestants and anesthetics to take effect before inserting the tube. Topical cocaine solution can also be used, but it often causes a strong burning sensation on application (see the "Equipment" section for other warnings). Application of topical anesthesia should be considered the standard of care, except in emergency situations where adequate lubrication alone may be acceptable.
4. An alternative option is to lubricate a soft nasal airway with 2% lidocaine gel and allow the patient to insert the lubricated airway into his or her nares. The nasogastric tube can then be inserted through the soft airway. As the patient swallows the gel, it will anesthetize the pharynx. A soft airway not only minimizes patient discomfort; it can also decrease the risk of severe epistaxis, intracranial intubation, and kinking of the nasogastric tube into the mouth.
5. While waiting for the anesthetic to take effect, choose an optimal tube for the patient. A large-bore nasogastric tube (16 or 18 Fr), Salem sump (with antireflux valve, if available), or Levin tube should be used for adults. Select the largest tube possible for the patient's nostril size. The Salem sump tube has marks at 18, 22, 26, and 30 inches from the distal end. Measure the tube to fit the patient by holding the nasogastric tube above the patient with the distal end at the xiphoid process. After looping the midportion over the patient's earlobe, extend the proximal end to the nose, and then add 6 inches for a nasogastric tube (add 8 to 10 inches for a nasoenteric tube). Note the tube marks based on these measurements or mark the tube with a piece of tape to avoid inserting the tube too far (Fig. 217.5). The nasogastric tube should generally be secured with the 20- to 24-inch mark at the nasal vestibule.

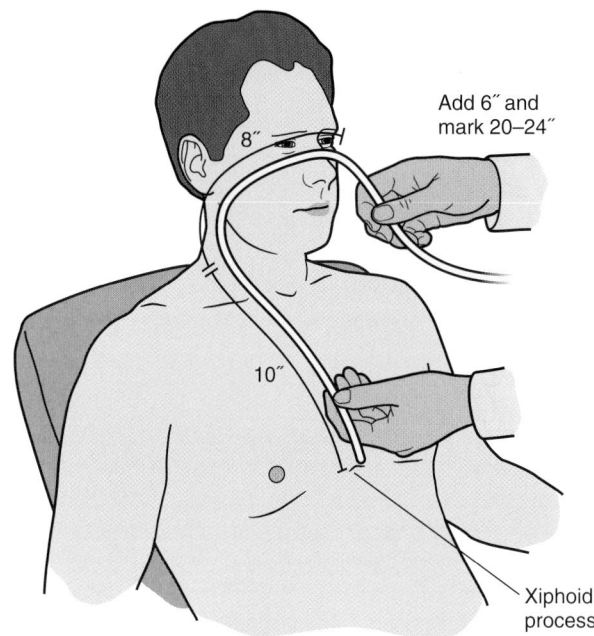

Fig. 217.5 Measuring the length of nasogastric tube for placement into stomach.

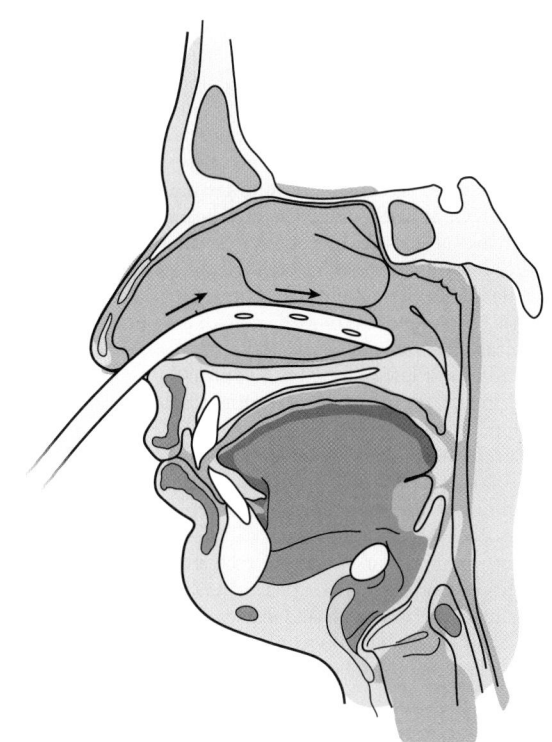

Fig. 217.6 Horizontal insertion of nasogastric tube into nasopharynx.

6. Lubricate the tip of the tube with additional anesthetic jelly or a water-soluble lubricant. Curl the tube by rolling 18 to 20 inches of the distal tube clockwise onto the first three fingers of your nondominant hand.
7. Introduce the lubricated tube tip into the nostril, pointing straight to the back of the nasal cavity and toward the base of the skull (Fig. 217.6). Recalling the anatomy, it should be inserted horizontally, along the floor of the nasal passage, and directed straight back, not upward. Feed the tube slowly with the dominant hand into the

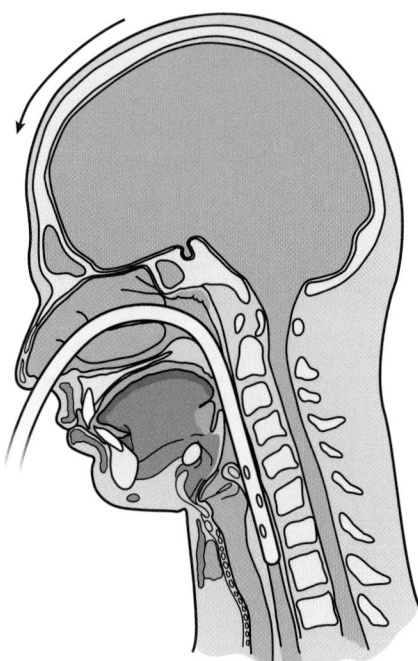

Fig. 217.7 Have the patient flex his or her head. Next, gently advance the tube while asking the patient to swallow.

nostril using continuous movement while unrolling the curled tube with the nondominant hand. The patient can sniff to assist the insertion. Never force a tube against resistance; however, spinning or twisting the tube slightly may help overcome resistance.

8. Have the patient flex his or her neck slightly forward to narrow the pharyngeal airway. When the tip of the tube reaches the pharynx, a slight increase in resistance will be noted (Fig. 217.7). Continue to advance the tube, and when the resistance decreases again, ask the patient to swallow or drink some water with a straw. Continue to push the tube with the same motion while asking the patient to continue swallowing. If the patient starts coughing or becomes distressed, or fog is seen in the tube, the tube has probably entered the trachea. The tube should be withdrawn a few inches, but not entirely, twisted slightly, and the process started again. If a patient cannot swallow, it is also helpful to mimic swallowing or say "eeee."

9. Continue to push the tube until the desired mark is reached if the patient is not coughing. In adults, this is slightly past the 22-inch mark—the second mark—on a Salem sump tube. The gastroesophageal junction is usually about 16 to 18 inches from the nose—the first mark—and the tube should be inserted about 4 inches beyond the gastroesophageal junction. If the stomach is full, an immediate return of fluid may occur. Use the emesis basin to collect this. If there is no return of fluid, open the patient's mouth to confirm that the tube is not curled in the mouth or pharynx.

NOTE: If significant resistance, respiratory distress, or a nasal hemorrhage occurs, or the patient suddenly becomes unable to speak, the tube should be withdrawn.

10a. Extra steps to facilitate placement of a *nasoenteric feeding tube* include the following:
   - Having placed the tube into the stomach, leave some extra tubing or slack to facilitate passage of the tip into the duodenum.
   - Place the patient in a right lateral decubitus (right side down) position.
   - A 60-mL syringe (Toomey) can be used to inject 400 mL of air to distend the stomach. This may allow a feeding tube coiled in the fundus of the stomach to uncoil and pass more freely into the duodenum.

   - In refractory cases, metoclopramide 10 mg may be given intravenously, with or without erythromycin 250 mg intravenously, to increase gastric motility.

10b. Extra steps to facilitate *any tube placement* include the following:
   - If the tube persistently kinks or coils into the mouth, cooling the tube in ice chips or a refrigerator for 5 minutes may stiffen it to prevent coiling. A larger-bore tube is also less likely to coil.
   - Applying external and medially directed pressure on the ipsilateral neck at the level of the thyrohyoid membrane may increase the success rate in difficult insertions. This maneuver collapses the piriform sinus and further clears the way for the nasogastric tube. If the tube passes to the level of the hypopharynx but then meets resistance, grasping the thyroid cartilage and lifting it anteriorly and upward may facilitate passage into the upper esophagus. Simply elevating the jaw or having the patient flex their neck slightly more, into the "sniffing" position, may also assist with passage.
   - Orotracheally intubated patients often present the most difficult challenge for inserting a nasogastric tube. If nasogastric insertion is deemed impossible, a second endotracheal tube may facilitate orogastric tube placement. Remove the respiratory adapter from the proximal end of the second endotracheal tube, lubricate it liberally, and insert it through the patient's mouth and into the esophagus. A well-lubricated nasogastric tube can then be inserted through the second endotracheal tube, which can then be removed over the proximal end of the nasogastric tube. Some clinicians use scissors to cut down the entire length of one side of the endotracheal tube to facilitate later removal; even when one side is cut, it maintains most of its rigidity.
   - Nasogastric placement may be facilitated manually through the oropharynx with three fingers, if necessary. However, unless the patient is unconscious or paralyzed, a bite block should be in place for this maneuver to prevent the clinician from being bitten.
   - In difficult cases, a laryngoscope may be helpful for guiding or confirming proper placement.
   - Fluoroscopic or endoscopic assistance may also be necessary.

11. Confirm the location of the tip as soon as possible after the tube is passed. Ask the patient to speak after placement. If he or she is unable to speak, the tube is in the trachea and should be withdrawn. (Be aware that cases have been reported in which the patient could talk despite tracheal placement of a small-bore feeding tube.) Otherwise, the position of the tip should be confirmed by a chest radiograph (the most accurate method of confirming placement). In addition, there are two traditional methods for confirming proper nasogastric placement: checking for absence of rhythmic airflow and auscultating for gastric bubbling when air is injected into the stomach. As it turns out, both of these techniques have been found to be inaccurate, and therefore they are not recommended. Even if the tip of the tube is located in the esophagus, duodenum, jejunum, pleural space, or respiratory tract, a bubbling sound may be heard. If proper location is misdiagnosed, the instillation of feeds or air has been reported to result in a pneumonia or pneumothorax with a high chance of an adverse outcome. Fortunately, placement can also be confirmed by aspiration (to check for gastric contents) and by ultrasonography.

NOTE: If gastric juices are aspirated, correct placement has been demonstrated. To confirm gastric juices, we recommend pH indicator strips with 0.5 gradations or paper with a range of 0 to 6 or 1 to 11. It is important that the resulting color change on any indicator strip or paper is easily distinguishable, particularly between the pH 5 and 6 range. The old type of litmus paper should not be used. Rakel and colleagues (1994) reviewed several studies and found that gastric fluid should have a pH of 0 to 4. If the pH is less than 4, there is a 95% chance the tube is in the stomach and nonrespiratory placement is almost guaranteed. If the patient is

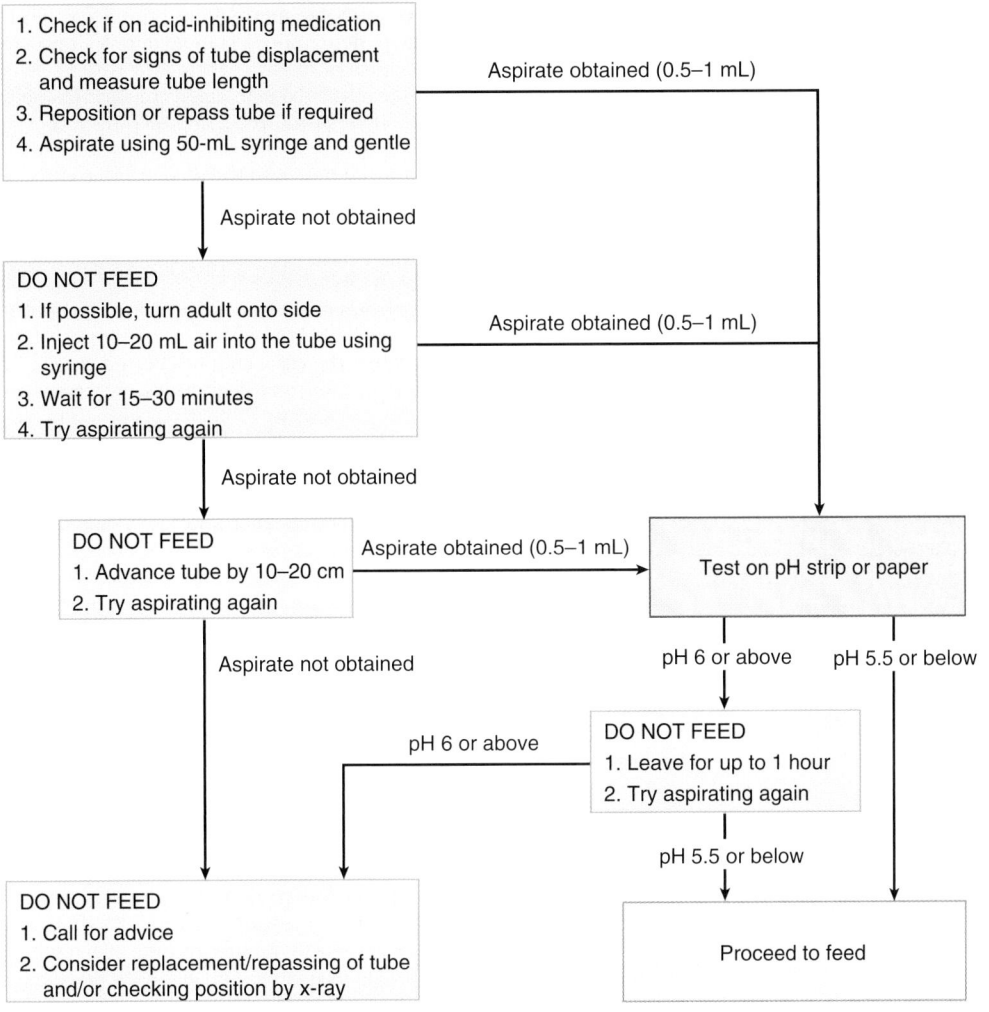

1. Check if on acid-inhibiting medication
2. Check for signs of tube displacement and measure tube length
3. Reposition or repass tube if required
4. Aspirate using 50-mL syringe and gentle

Aspirate obtained (0.5–1 mL)

Aspirate not obtained

DO NOT FEED
1. If possible, turn adult onto side
2. Inject 10–20 mL air into the tube using syringe
3. Wait for 15–30 minutes
4. Try aspirating again

Aspirate obtained (0.5–1 mL)

Aspirate not obtained

DO NOT FEED
1. Advance tube by 10–20 cm
2. Try aspirating again

Aspirate obtained (0.5–1 mL)

Test on pH strip or paper

Aspirate not obtained

pH 6 or above   pH 5.5 or below

pH 6 or above

DO NOT FEED
1. Leave for up to 1 hour
2. Try aspirating again

pH 5.5 or below

DO NOT FEED
1. Call for advice
2. Consider replacement/repassing of tube and/or checking position by x-ray

Proceed to feed

CAUTION: If there is ANY query about position and/or the clarity of the color change on the pH strip, particularly between ranges 5 and 6, then feeding should not commence.

Fig. 217.8 Algorithm to confirm the correct position of nasogastric feeding tubes in adults. (From the National Patient Safety Agency [NPSA]. Reducing the harm caused by misplaced nasogastric feeding tubes: Interim advice for healthcare staff—February 2005: How to confirm the correct position of nasogastric feeding tubes in infants, children and adults. www.nrls.npsa.nhs.uk/resources/?EntryId45=59794.)

on antacids, histamine type 2 inhibitors, or proton pump inhibitors, the pH is between 0 and 6 approximately 70% to 80% of the time. Fluid aspirated from the duodenum averaged a pH of 6.5. Fluid aspirated from tracheobronchial secretions ranged from pH 6.74 to 8.79. In other words, suspect that fluid from the respiratory tract has been aspirated when the pH is greater than 6.

Neumann and colleagues (1995) concluded that when the pH of the nasogastric tube aspirate is less than 4.0, radiographs are not needed to confirm tube placement. In 2005, the National Patient Safety Agency in the United Kingdom recommended the use of a pH value of less than 5.5 for tube placement confirmation; they concluded a pH value of less than 4.0 (as recommended by Neumann and associates) is too low to evaluate patients practically. If the pH is greater than 5.5, a chest radiograph, still the gold standard, is required to confirm tube placement (Fig. 217.8). However, chest radiography adds cost and prolongs waiting time before use (it can take up to 8 hours to receive notification from the radiologist). It also increases radiation exposure. There are also case reports of inaccurate confirmations by radiographs, with the tube located in the midline after perforating the esophagus, subclavian vein, or atrium of the heart.

Recently, bedside sonographic examination performed by experienced clinicians has been reported to be a sensitive method for confirming position. It is faster than conventional radiography and can easily be taught to nonradiologists. Regardless of how, confirmation must be done on all nasogastric or nasoenteric tubes used for instillation or feeding purposes before starting to avoid massive aspiration. The distal tips of feeding tubes should be allowed to migrate to the duodenum before enteral feeding is initiated.

12. Secure the tube to the patient's nose after confirmation of proper placement. First, apply alcohol to the dorsum of the nose. If available, tincture of benzoin may then be applied after the alcohol dries. Next, obtain a 5-inch piece of 1-inch-wide hypoallergenic tape. Make a 3-inch cut lengthwise in the middle, thereby forming two narrow strips of tape at one end of the 5-inch piece (Fig. 217.9). The two narrow strips of tape should be applied in a spiral down and around the nasogastric tube, going away from the patient's nose. Attempt to tape the tube so that it will rest in the middle of the nostril to minimize direct contact of the tube with the skin of the nose and avoid pressure necrosis. Recently, several commercial products (e.g., NG Secure, NG Strip) have been developed for this special purpose.

13. Also secure the nasogastric tube to the patient's gown. Place a slipknot over the tube with a rubber band, and then pin it to the patient's gown. This should reduce the risk of the nasogastric tube being tugged out of position. The Salem sump tube vent, or blue pigtail, must remain above the patient's waistline at all times to prevent gravity from siphoning fluid. Inadvertent siphoning of gastric contents could block the sump vent. When suction is discontinued during ambulation, the pigtail should be attached to the connector of the main lumen to close the system and avoid the spillage of gastric fluids.

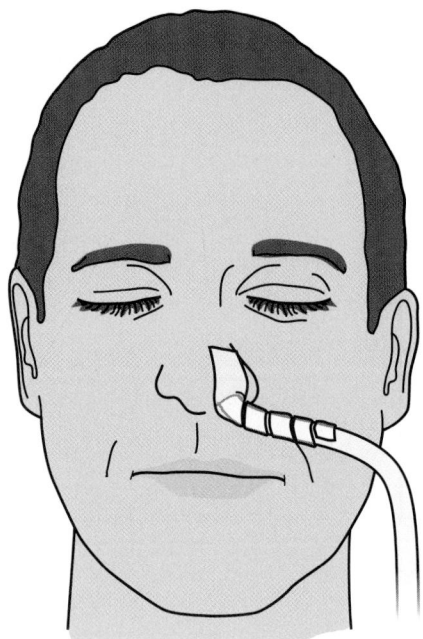

Fig. 217.9 Secure the tube with a 5-inch piece of 1-inch-wide hypoallergenic tape, partially cut lengthwise. Apply to the dorsum of the nose and spiral the cut portions down the tube away from the nose.

14. For removal, again place the patient in the sitting (Fowler or semi-Fowler) position and cover his or her neck and chest with towels, surgical Chux, or other drapes. Disconnect the nasogastric tube from the patient, from his or her nose, and from suction. Hand the patient an emesis basin and some tissues. Fold over the proximal end of the tube to prevent leakage and hold it tightly. Ask the patient to flex the neck, breathe in, and hold his or her breath. Place a drape around the tube and withdraw the tube from the patient's nose through the drape. The patient can then resume breathing. Discard the tube and the drape.

COMPLICATIONS

The most common complication is discomfort for the patient. The traumatic insertion of a nasogastric tube can cause epistaxis, but this is often avoided by using careful technique and a decongestant. Epistaxis can be massive and require packing. It can even compromise the airway. Gagging can occur with insertion and induce vomiting with aspiration of gastric contents. This can cause an aspiration pneumonitis or pneumonia with a mortality rate as high as 30%. Patients with an altered mental status from severe trauma or other causes should have their airway secured with an endotracheal tube before placement of a nasogastric tube. Long-term use of a nasogastric tube also predisposes patients to aspiration because of tube-induced hypersalivation, depressed cough reflex, or physiologic or mechanical impairment of the glottis. Aspiration is also quite common with nasoenteric feedings in debilitated patients for the same reasons, hence the value of gastrostomy tubes (see Chapter 92, "Percutaneous Endoscopic Gastrostomy Placement and Replacement").

Another common complication is misplacement into the respiratory tree, which is estimated to occur in 15% of cases. This should be recognized rapidly in the conscious patient when it causes him or her to cough, choke, or develop respiratory distress or an inability to talk. The vocal cords may also be traumatized. In a patient with decreased consciousness, tracheal intubation can go undetected, creating multiple complications such as atelectasis, pulmonary edema, pneumonia, or lung abscess.

Nasogastric tube syndrome is a reported life-threatening complication with laryngeal and upper airway obstruction and vocal cord abduction paralysis. This syndrome results from postcricoid ulceration and its effect on the posterior cricoarytenoid muscles, and can be prevented by early recognition and by checking the patient every day when making rounds. It is treated with emergent tracheostomy, immediate removal of the nasogastric tube, and administration of systemic antibiotics.

Penetration of a nasogastric tube into the pleural space is a rare but reported complication, with further possible complications including lung abscess, pneumothorax, isocalothorax, empyema, and sepsis. Intravascular penetration of the internal jugular and subclavian vessels has also been reported.

Perforation of the esophagus is a very serious reported complication that often results in mediastinitis, with a mortality rate of up to 30%. This may occur when the esophagus has been damaged by chemical burns or esophageal cancer, or if strictures are present, or with insertion after esophageal surgery. Prompt recognition of this complication, surgical repair, and parenteral antibiotics can significantly reduce the mortality rate. Bleeding from esophageal varices is not usually caused by nasogastric intubation. Duodenal perforation is very rare but has also been reported. Tube knotting, coiling, kinking, obstruction, and rupture can occur.

With long-term use, sinusitis, erosion of nasal tissue, or even a tracheoesophageal fistula can occur. Tracheoesophageal fistulas are usually associated with simultaneous use of an endotracheal tube. Sinusitis can cause a fever of unknown origin in patients.

If the tube is forced against resistance, cribriform plate fracture may result, with subsequent intracranial intubation. Individuals with midfacial or maxillofacial trauma or a basilar skull fracture have a significantly increased risk of inadvertent intracranial intubation. The risk of this complication can be reduced by using the orogastric route or by initially introducing a nasotracheal tube or a soft rubber nasal airway, through which a smaller-diameter nasogastric tube can then be passed. This technique decreases the danger of penetrating the cranium, reduces discomfort during insertion, decreases epistaxis, and decreases the frequency of the nasogastric tube kinking into the mouth. The long-term use of nasoenteric tube feeding may result in diarrhea, infection, electrolyte imbalance, and malnutrition.

POSTPROCEDURE MANAGEMENT

The nares should be assessed for skin irritation, erosion, or necrosis by health providers at regular intervals. The patient should be asked if he or she has any pain or pressure in the nose, throat, or sinuses. Any old or detached tape should be replaced after cleaning the skin of the nose with alcohol and applying tincture of benzoin. On a regular basis, the nursing team should record the patency of the tube, the level of graduated marks on the tube, any symptoms or patient complaints, the volume and nature of anything infused, and any residual volume. If it becomes difficult to aspirate from the tube, it should be flushed with 30 mL water. If patency is still uncertain, it should be repositioned by advancing 1 inch or withdrawing 1 inch. The same maneuver should then be tried again to confirm patency. Because the use of acidic substances for flushing can cause whole-protein formulas to coagulate and clog the tube, this practice should be discouraged. The tube should be flushed before and after each intermittent feeding, after medication administration, or every 4 to 6 hours in case of continuous infusion. When the volume of residual is higher than 300 to 400 mL or there is significant gastric distention, the clinician should be notified and any infusions held. Infusions should be held for several hours and the residual rechecked before restarting. For the infusion of medications, liquid forms should be used if possible. If pills are used, they should be crushed to a fine powder and mixed with water. If the result is sticky or highly concentrated, dilute it further with water. When the tube is clogged, it can be irrigated with warm water or, if unsuccessful, a pancreatic enzyme solution injected. Reinsertion of a device, for example a stylet or guidewire, into a nasoenteric tube should never be tried because it can result in gastrointestinal tract injury. If there are unusual gastrointestinal symptoms like nausea, cramping, abdominal distention, or severe diarrhea, the infusion should be stopped and the clinician notified immediately. The clinician must assess the patient and the tube at this point.

When the nasogastric tube is used for gastric decompression or postoperative drainage, clinicians should understand the mechanics of nasogastric suction. Suction strength is inversely proportional to flow; therefore, the lower the flow rate through the suction lumen, the higher the suction strength. In addition, a suction force of more than 25 mm Hg causes tissue capillary fragility and may damage the gastric mucosa. One advantage of the double-lumen Salem sump tube over the Levin tube is that it allows constant airflow through the secondary lumen, keeping the necessary suction in the main lumen at a minimum. Therefore the vent lumen must not be clamped or plugged. When the Levin tube is used, an intermittent suction pump should be connected to prevent injury of the gastrointestinal mucosa. The length of time the tube can be used depends on the patient's condition, feeding needs, and the tube design. With proper care and maintenance, most nasogastric tubes can be used for up to 30 days. For longer use, a percutaneous endoscopic gastrostomy tube should be considered (see Chapter 92, "Percutaneous Endoscopic Gastrostomy Placement and Replacement").

CPT/BILLING CODES

44500	Introduction of long gastrointestinal tube (e.g., Miller-Abbott)
42753	Gastric intubation and aspiration(s) therapeutic, necessitating physician's skill (e.g., for gastrointestinal hemorrhage), including lavage if performed
43754	Gastric intubation and aspiration, diagnostic, single specimen, for chemical analysis or cytopathology
43755	Gastric intubation and aspiration(s), collection of multiple fractional specimens with gastric stimulation, single or double lumen tube
43756	Duodenal intubation and aspiration; diagnostic, includes image guidance, single
43761	Repositioning of a nasogastric or orogastric feeding tube, through the duodenum for enteric nutrition

ICD-10-CM DIAGNOSTIC CODES

A18.32	Tuberculosis, gastrocolic, labs pending
E43	Calorie deficiency, severe
E46	Malnutrition, protein-calorie
R11.2	Vomiting, persistent, unspecified
K31.1	Gastric outlet obstruction, acquired or adult
K56.0	Ileus, paralytic
K56.50	Small intestine obstruction, due to adhesions
K85.90-K85.92	Pancreatitis, NOS or acute
K86.1	Pancreatitis, chronic
K92.0	Hematemesis or gastrointestinal hemorrhage
K92.1	Hematochezia
K92.2	Gastrointestinal bleeding, unspecified
R11.2	Vomiting, NOS with nausea
R11.10	Vomiting, NOS
T36-T50	Poisoning by, adverse effect of and underdosing of drugs or medicaments and biological substances

Code first for adverse effects, nature of adverse effect; use additional codes to specify manifestations of poisoning.

SUPPLIERS

(See contact information available at www.expertconsult.com.)

Feeding tubes
  Bard Medical
  Cook Incorporated
  CORPAK MedSystems
  Covidien Kendall Medtronic (Dobhoff)
  NeoDevices
  Nestle Health Science
Latex-free, zinc oxide tape
  Hy-Tape International
Levin, Salem sump, and feeding tubes
  Bard Medical
  Covidien Kendall Medtronic
Nasogastric tube guard
  NG Secure (M.C. Johnson)
  NG Strip (Derma Sciences)
Topical anesthetic
  Cetacaine, Cetylite Industries, Inc.
  Hurricane Spray, Beutlich Pharmaceuticals

Acknowledgment

The editors recognize the contributions of Julie Graves Moy, MD, and Ramiro Sanchez, MD, to this chapter in previous editions of this text.

ONLINE RESOURCES

National Patient Safety Agency (NPSA) UK. *Reducing the harm caused by misplaced nasogastric feeding tubes: Interim advice for healthcare staff—February*; 2005. www.npsa.nhs.uk/advice.

Thomsen TW, Shaffer RW, Setnik GS. Nasogastric intubation. Videos in Clinical Medicine. *N Engl J Med.* 2006. http://content.nejm.org/cgi/video/354/17/e16/ or www.youtube.com/watch?v=ARHfqRB3t4M.

RECOMMENDED READING

Fisman DN, Ward ME. Intrapleural placement of a nasogastric tube: an unusual complication of nasotracheal intubation. *Can J Anaesth.* 1996;43:1252–1256.

Grossheim LF. Nasogastric intubation. In: Reichman EF, ed. *Emergency Medicine Procedures.* 2nd ed. New York: McGraw-Hill; 2013:387–391.

Marcus EL, Caine Y, Hamdan K, et al. Nasogastric tube syndrome: a life-threatening laryngeal obstruction in a 72-year-old patient. *Age Ageing.* 2006;35:538–539.

Neumann MJ, Meyer CT, Dutton JL, et al. Hold that x-ray: aspirate pH and auscultation prove enteral tube placement. *J Clin Gastroenterol.* 1995;20:293–295.

Pillai JB, Vegas A, Brister S. Thoracic complications of nasogastric tube: review of safe practice. *Interact Cardiovasc Thorac Surg.* 2005;4:429–433.

Rakel BA, Titler M, Goode C, et al. Nasogastric and nasointestinal feeding tube placement: an integrative review of research. *AACN Clin Issues Crit Care Nurs.* 1994;5:194–206. quiz 218–219.

Samuels LE. Nasogastric and feeding tube placement. In: Roberts JR, Custalow CB, Thomsen TW, eds. *Roberts and Hedges' Clinical Procedures in Emergency Medicine.* 6th ed. Philadelphia: Elsevier; 2014:804–830.

Singer AJ, Konia N. Comparison of topical anesthetics and vasoconstrictors vs lubricants prior to nasogastric intubation: a randomized, controlled trial. *Acad Emerg Med.* 1999;6:184–190.

Van Dinter TG, John L, Guileyardo JM, Fordtran JS. Intestinal perforation caused by insertion of nasogastric tube late after gastric bypass. *Proc (Baylor Univ Med Cent).* 2013;26(1):11–15.

Vigneau C, Baudel JL, Guidet B, et al. Sonography as an alternative to radiography for nasogastric feeding tube location. *Intensive Care Med.* 2005;31:1570–1572.

CHAPTER 218

THORACENTESIS

Terry S. Ruhl • Jennifer L. Good

Pleural effusions are common in primary care. Sampling the fluid may not only yield information important for treatment decisions but may also improve patient symptoms. Similar techniques can also be used to treat certain pneumothoraces.

ANATOMY

The pleural "space" is a potential space between the visceral pleura, which is adherent to the lung, and the parietal pleura, which is adherent to the chest wall. Normally it contains only a thin film of lubricating fluid. When this space becomes filled with air or extra fluid, it may become painful or increase the work of breathing.

When performing thoracentesis, the lower border of the ribs should be avoided. This is where the neurovascular bundle (intercostal vessels and nerve) is located.

INDICATIONS

- Any significant (>10 mm on lateral decubitus radiograph) pleural effusion of unknown etiology (effusions with an easily explained cause, such as congestive heart failure, may be observed for 3 days for response to therapy).
- Large symptomatic effusion.
- Spontaneous pneumothorax (a minimally symptomatic, spontaneous pneumothorax of less than 20% may be merely observed if the patient has no significant underlying lung disease).

CONTRAINDICATIONS

Absolute

- Patient refuses the procedure, refuses to give informed consent, or is uncooperative. Uncooperative patients or those with an altered level of consciousness may need procedural sedation or anesthesia.
- When chest tube placement is planned and would be more appropriate.
- Known or suspected hemothorax.
- Empyema or complicated parapneumonic effusion.
- Large spontaneous pneumothorax.
- Spontaneous pneumothorax in a patient with underlying lung disease.

Relative

- Coagulopathy or patient undergoing anticoagulant therapy (international normalized ratio >1.5; consider reversing the coagulopathy or anticoagulant before performing thoracentesis).
- Thrombocytopenia (platelet count <50,000/μL).
- Very small pleural effusions (<10 mm thick on lateral decubitus chest radiograph), unless aided by real-time ultrasound.
- Local skin compromise (e.g., cellulitis, burn, pyoderma, herpes zoster infection).

- Unstable medical condition.
- Positive-pressure ventilation (e.g., mechanical ventilator, bilevel positive airway pressure, continuous positive airway pressure, although one study has found thoracentesis to be as safe in ventilator-dependent patients as in patients not being mechanically ventilated).
- Radiographic evidence of loculated pleural effusions making localization of fluid uncertain unless aided by real-time ultrasound.
- Patients with chronic obstructive pulmonary disease are at increased risk for complications.
- Unsupervised clinicians with little or no experience should not perform this procedure, as the risk of complications is increased (Gordon).

EQUIPMENT AND SUPPLIES

Commercial thoracentesis trays are available (e.g., Safe-T-Centesis). These now have one-way valves to prevent entry of air into the catheter when the needle is being removed. A blunt, spring-loaded safety cannula extends beyond the sharp tip to prevent lung puncture or laceration after the pleura is entered. Built in side-ports are available for drainage of fluid, so three-way stopcocks are no longer needed. If a commercial tray is used, the manufacturer's instructions *must* be reviewed because equipment varies. Alternatively, the equipment described in the following sections can be assembled. Equipment to follow universal blood and body fluid precautions should be available (e.g., face mask with face shield or goggles).

Preparation and Anesthesia

- Povidone-iodine solution or chlorhexidine and applicators
- Fenestrated drape or sterile towels
- 10-mL syringe (having Luer-Lok is very helpful)
- 25-gauge or smaller needle
- 1.5- to 2-inch, 22-gauge needle
- Lidocaine 1% to 2% with epinephrine

Insertion

- Sterile gloves
- 50- to 60-mL syringe (having Luer-Lok is very helpful), three-way stopcock
- 2.5-inch, 18-gauge needle (for air), 2.5-inch, 15- to 20-gauge needle (for fluid), or 16- to 20-gauge catheter over needle (can decrease risk of pneumothorax, but kinks can increase the "dry tap" rate)

NOTE: Obese people may require longer needles. If only small volumes of fluid are needed for diagnostic purposes, the needle technique may be preferred. For larger volume, therapeutic procedures, the catheter over needle may be preferred to avoid prolonged insertion of a needle in the pleural space while large volumes of fluid are being removed.

- Specimen tubes: one red top, one lavender top, culture tubes (aerobic and anaerobic), 10- to 50-mL red top for cytology, possibly 1 green top, ice for pH

Optional

- Sterile plastic tubing
- Curved clamp for marking insertion depth on needle
- 500- or 1000-mL vacuum bottles
- Telemetry, oximetry, blood pressure monitoring, and supplemental oxygen

Dressing

Use sterile gauze pads and adhesive tape or adhesive bandage with antibiotic ointment.

PRECAUTIONS

The use of real-time ultrasound guidance is helpful in situations where there is a small effusion (<10 mm free-flowing pleural fluid on lateral decubitus radiograph), there is presence of a loculated pleural effusion, the patient is receiving positive-pressure mechanical ventilation, or in other high-risk situations such as malignant effusions. "Marking" the location for later drainage is unhelpful because fluid shifts, but marking at the time of aspiration may be helpful. Use of ultrasound may also help determine needle depth and the angle at which the needle should be directed. Interestingly, a recent systematic review (Wilcox et al., 2014) found no benefit of decreased pneumothoraces if a radiologist marks the skin prior to thoracentesis or if it was ultrasound-guided. This differs from multiple prior studies showing reduced risk of pneumothorax when thoracentesis is ultrasound-directed (e.g., Cavanna, Patel). Removal of large amounts of fluid may increase the incidence of postprocedure complications, although some advocate "draining it dry." Most experts recommend removing no more than a maximum of 1500 mL of fluid; removing more has been associated with symptomatic hypovolemia and the potentially fatal complication of reexpansion pulmonary edema.

TECHNIQUE

Patient Positioning and Insertion Site

1. Seat the patient comfortably (Fig. 218.1) with arms supported on a table. The lower back should be kept as vertical as possible so that the most dependent portion of the hemithorax is posterior, thereby keeping free-flowing fluid in a posterior location.
   NOTE: Debilitated patients can be placed in the lateral decubitus position, lying on the side of the effusion with their back near the edge of the bed. The procedure would then be performed in the midscapular line or the posterior axillary line.
2. Confirm the location and extent of fluid or air by percussion, tactile fremitus, auscultation, and study of posteroanterior, lateral, and lateral decubitus (fluid-affected side down) chest radiographs.
   NOTE: If available, ultrasound may be very helpful for completing this step (see Chapter 214, Emergency Department, Hospitalist, and Office Ultrasonography [Clinical Ultrasonography]).
3. Select the needle insertion site. Use an area one or two interspaces below the fluid level and 5 to 10 cm lateral to the spine. Do not insert below the eighth intercostal space.
4. Mark insertion site with marker or by applying pressure from the hub of a needle or pen.

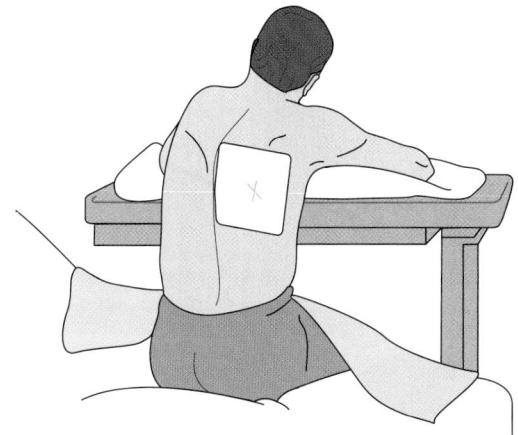

Fig. 218.1   Position for fluid removal.

5. Verify the patient's identity, ensure the insertion site is correctly marked, and take a "time-out" to verify this with everyone present.

Preparation and Anesthesia

1. Prepare the skin with povidone–iodine or chlorhexidine. Use sterile technique and follow universal blood and body fluid precautions. Drape with sterile towels or fenestrated drape. Some experts monitor all patients with telemetry, oximetry, and automatic blood pressure equipment and have supplemental oxygen available during this procedure, especially if the patient has underlying pulmonary disease.
2. Observing universal blood and body fluid precautions, raise a skin wheal using lidocaine with epinephrine and a 25-gauge or smaller needle attached to a 10-mL syringe.
3. Angle a 1.5- to 2-inch 22-gauge needle slightly downward, and insert it through the skin wheal so that the needle tip touches the superior border of a rib, alternately aspirating and injecting as you advance. "Walk" the needle over the superior margin of the rib and deeper into the interspace, anesthetizing the intercostal muscle layers (Fig. 218.2A).
4. To confirm the presence of fluid or air with the small anesthesia needle, continue advancing the needle while aspirating and injecting until the parietal pleura has been penetrated. (A "pop" may be felt, or fluid/air aspirated.) Warn the patient that there may be a twinge of pain as you go through the pleura. After entering the pleura, inject more lidocaine. Note the depth. Consider placing a clamp on the needle at the skin level to mark the depth (see Fig. 218.2B). Withdraw the needle. If no fluid is obtained, ultrasound guidance is recommended. If air is unexpectedly obtained, try a lower intercostal space.

Aspiration Option 1 (If No Kit Available): Needle-Only Insertion Technique

1. Prepare the equipment. Attach a 15- to 20-gauge needle to a 50-mL syringe with a three-way stopcock. Mark the previously measured depth on this needle with a clamp. Test the equipment to be sure you are well acquainted with the use of the stopcock. Open the stopcock to the syringe.
2. Insert the thoracentesis needle in the same track as the anesthesia needle, and advance it to the level of the clamp. ("Walk" over the rib, not under it, to avoid damaging vessels and nerves.) Aspirate to confirm placement. Keep the clamp attached to prevent penetrating too deeply.

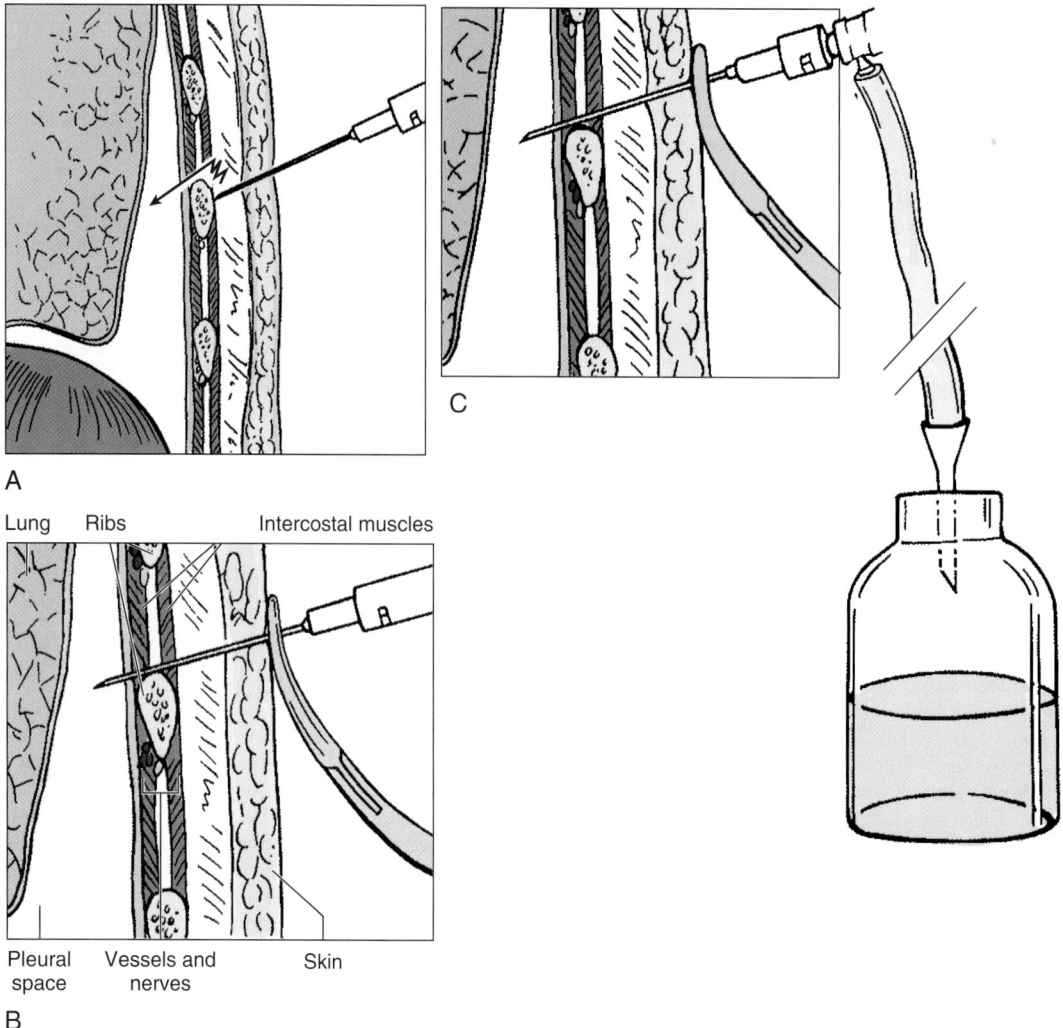

Lung   Ribs   Intercostal muscles

Pleural   Vessels and   Skin
space   nerves

Fig. 218.2 (A) Anesthetizing the intercostal muscle layers. Needle is "walked" over the rib. (B) Clamp is placed to mark the depth to the effusion. (C) Needle in pleural space with fluid draining into evacuated bottle.

Aspiration Option 2: Catheter-Over-Needle Insertion Technique

(If using a commercially prepared thoracentesis tray, read the manufacturer's instructions carefully.)

1. Prepare the equipment. Familiarize yourself with the stopcock. Visualize the measured insertion depth on the needle.
2. Insert the thoracentesis needle in the same track as the anesthesia needle, aspirating with the syringe until fluid is obtained. As soon as fluid is obtained, stop insertion and insert the catheter over the needle.
3. Making sure the stopcock is turned off to the environment, completely withdraw the needle, leaving the catheter in the pleural space. As the needle is removed, quickly turn the stopcock to close the catheter to the environment. Alternatively, a gloved finger can be used to quickly cover the catheter hub after the needle is removed to prevent air from entering the pleural cavity.

Completing the Procedure

1. For stopcock and evacuated container: Attach one end of the tube to the stopcock and the other end to a second 15- to 18-gauge needle. Insert the needle through the seal of an evacuated container, and open the stopcock to the evacuated container (see Fig. 218.2C). For stopcock and open container: Pull the fluid into the syringe. Turn the stopcock off to the needle, being careful not to open the needle to the environment. Push the fluid out of the syringe into the container. Alternate aspiration into the syringe and emptying into the container.
2. After withdrawal of the necessary amount of fluid, remove the needle while the patient is exhaling. For diagnostic thoracentesis, 50 to 100 mL of fluid should be adequate. For therapeutic thoracentesis, most experts recommend a maximum of 1500 mL (see section on "Precautions").
3. Dress the site with an occlusive, sterile dressing.
4. Send the fluid for analysis (see section on "Interpretation of Results" for details).
5. Consider an end-expiratory chest radiograph to check for a pneumothorax. Some experts repeat this radiograph in 4 to 6 hours to look for delayed pneumothorax. Some institutions do this routinely, although the yield is usually very low. Studies suggest no benefit from routine chest radiograph unless multiple passes of the needle were necessary, air was aspirated (which suggests the visceral pleura was penetrated), the patient is mechanically ventilated or critically ill and would not tolerate pneumothorax, or develops symptoms (Gordon, Aleman).

Thoracentesis for Aspiration of a Simple Spontaneous Pneumothorax

1. Position the patient supine with the head of the bed elevated at a 30- to 45-degree angle and infiltrate local anesthetic into the second or third intercostal space in the midclavicular line (Fig. 218.3). (Alternatively, the patient can be placed in the lateral decubitus position and the fourth or fifth intercostal space in the midclavicular line can be used.)
2. Observe sterile technique and follow universal blood and body fluid precautions. The catheter over a needle should be at least 16 Fr and 2 inches long. As described earlier, "walk" the catheter/needle over the cephalic surface of the rib.
3. When the pleural space is entered, remove the needle from the catheter during exhalation and attach a three-way stopcock and 50- to 60-mL syringe (preferably Luer-Lok) to the catheter. Be sure to occlude the hub of the catheter during this maneuver to prevent air entry into the pleural space.
4. Using the three-way stopcock, manually aspirate air into the 60-mL syringe. Stop when resistance to aspiration is felt, the patient coughs excessively or experiences chest pain or dyspnea, or more than 2 L of air is removed (this suggests the need for a chest tube). Remove the catheter.
5. Obtain a chest radiograph. If the pneumothorax is very small or has resolved, the procedure has been successful. Monitor for another 4 to 6 hours and discharge if a subsequent chest radiograph shows no recurrence of the pneumothorax.

SAMPLE OPERATIVE REPORT

See a sample operative report available at www.expertconsult.com.

COMMON ERRORS

- Stopcock confusion—mistakenly opening the needle or catheter to the environment
- Missing the effusion—by shifting patient position or not using ultrasound for small effusions
- Wrong side procedure—may occur if radiographs are malpositioned, mislabeled, or not confirmed by physical examination
- Kit changes—being given an unfamiliar kit without reviewing the instructions

COMPLICATIONS

- Pneumothorax may result if air is introduced through the needle or catheter, or if the visceral pleura is punctured. Between 3% and 20% of procedures produce a pneumothorax, which requires treatment with a chest tube about 20% of the time. Despite one recent systematic review finding differently (Wilcox et al., 2014), the editors believe pneumothorax incidence may be reduced with ultrasound-guided thoracentesis (e.g., Cavanna, Patel). Insert the needle only as far as needed to obtain fluid. Get comfortable with the equipment, especially the stopcock, before insertion. Use of smaller needles and short bevels, and removal of less fluid, may also decrease the risk of pneumothorax.
- Hemothorax may result from laceration of intercostal vessels or internal mammary vessels, but is rare. To reduce the risk of hemothorax, insert the needle just above the rib, avoiding the neurovascular bundle that runs below each rib. Never puncture medial to the midclavicular line.
- The spleen, liver, or diaphragm may be lacerated. To avoid lacerations to these organs, do not insert the needle lower than the eighth intercostal space posteriorly.
- Risk of hypovolemia and reexpansion pulmonary edema can be minimized by removing less than 1500 mL of fluid at a time (although some experts advocate draining the effusion dry). Remove fluid slowly and stop if the patient develops a cough, dyspnea, or chest pain.

- A catheter fragment may be left in the pleural space. To avoid this possibility, *never* withdraw a catheter over the needle.
- Failure to obtain fluid can occur. For improved success rates, pay close attention to landmarks obtained by auscultation, percussion, and radiographic examination. Consider ultrasound guidance.
- Infection can occur. To minimize this possibility, use sterile technique and avoid inserting through infected skin.
- Pain is associated with thoracentesis. Use adequate local anesthesia, especially at the pleura.
- Hypoproteinemia is a possibility. To reduce the risk of this problem, avoid repeated thoracenteses.

POSTPROCEDURE MANAGEMENT

Because the risk of complications is low, a postthoracentesis chest radiograph is necessary only if air was obtained during the thoracentesis, or if the patient is mechanically ventilated or critically ill and would not tolerate a pneumothorax or develops cough, chest pain, hypoxia, or dyspnea during or after the procedure (Gordon, Aleman). If multiple passes with the needle were necessary to obtain fluid, it may be prudent to obtain a radiograph. If a thoracentesis is performed for the management of a small, primary spontaneous pneumothorax, a chest radiograph should be obtained and the patient should be observed for recurrent pneumothorax for at least 6 hours.

Hypoxemia is very common after thoracentesis and occurs because of ventilation–perfusion mismatching in the newly expanded lung. Oxygenation should be checked periodically by pulse oximetry after thoracentesis and supplemental oxygen provided if necessary.

POSTPROCEDURE PATIENT EDUCATION

The dressing should stay on for 24 hours. The patient should inform someone if shortness of breath increases, there is fever, or there is redness at the puncture site.

INTERPRETATION OF RESULTS

First take a look at the fluid (Table 218.1). Food particles in the fluid suggests an esophageal perforation; black fluid suggests an *Aspergillus* infection. Milky fluid indicates a chylothorax or pseudochylothorax, whereas bile-staining suggests a biliary fistula (cholothorax). Anchovy paste suggests an amoebic abscess; a putrid odor suggests anaerobic empyema.

If etiology is not determined by the appearance of the fluid, the next important distinction is whether the fluid is a transudate (unbalanced hydrostatic forces) or an exudate ("leaks in the system or a damaged system"). If the lactate dehydrogenase (LDH) levels in

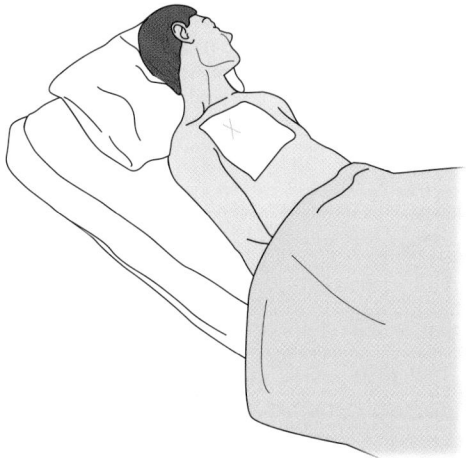

Fig. 218.3 Position for air removal.

the fluid and the pleural fluid/serum ratios for LDH and protein are all normal (these are the Light criteria; see Table 218.2), the fluid is a transudate and further studies are unlikely to give useful information. Light criteria are 99.5% sensitive for diagnosing exudative effusion; they differentiate exudative from transudative effusions in 93 to 96% of cases. In the absence of known serum levels, simply knowing pleural fluid protein (≥30g/L) and LDH levels (>0.45 of upper limit of normal serum level) is useful. These values have a 92% concordance with the Light criteria (Murphy). A recent systematic review found that a pleural cholesterol level greater than 55 mg/dL, a pleural to serum cholesterol ratio greater than 0.3, or a pleural LDH level greater than 200 IU or U/L were among the most specific findings for diagnosing exudate (Wilcox et al., 2014).

Most transudates are from congestive heart failure, with the rest associated with hypoalbuminemia, hepatic hydrothorax, hydronephrosis, pulmonary embolism, peritoneal dialysis, or trapped lung. Occasionally, pleural effusions that appear to be due to congestive heart failure may be classified as an exudate using traditional measures of LDH and total protein, particularly if the patient has been treated with diuretics. In this case, the use of a serum–pleural effusion albumin gradient (SEAG) can be useful. A serum–pleural effusion albumin gradient of greater than 1.2 g/dL will classify the pleural effusion as transudative, and less than 1.2 g/dL as exudative (Roth and colleagues, 1990). One diagnostic approach is to send some of the fluid for protein, pH, LDH measurement, and possibly aerobic and anaerobic culture and sensitivities while storing the remaining fluid for the other tests if the fluid proves to be an exudate (Fig. 218.4). Causes of exudates include cancer, pneumonia, trauma, tuberculosis, pulmonary embolism, pancreatitis, rheumatoid arthritis, and systemic lupus erythematosus. Up to 50% of patients with a pulmonary malignancy will have neoplastic cells in the pleural fluid, so sending exudates for cytology is important. Low pH (<7.2) can indicate a complicated parapneumonic effusion, which may require chest tube drainage. See Table 218.2 for potentially useful tests and their significance.

CPT/BILLING CODES

32554	Thoracentesis, needle or catheter, aspiration of the pleural space, without imaging guidance
32555	Thoracentesis, needle or catheter, aspiration of the pleural space, with imaging guidance
99070	Surgical tray (when performed in a clinician's office)

ICD-10-CM DIAGNOSTIC CODES

A15.6	Pleural effusion, tuberculous, unspecified
J91.0	Pleural effusion, malignant; code first underlying neoplasm
J91.8	Pleural effusion, bacterial; code first underlying disease
J90	Pleural effusion, unspecified
J93.0	Pneumothorax, tension
J95.811	Pneumothorax, iatrogenic or postoperative
J93.0	Pneumothorax, spontaneous, acute, or chronic
S27.2XXX	Pneumothorax, tension, traumatic

Add appropriate seventh character: A = initial, D = subsequent, S = sequela.

SUPPLIERS

(See contact information available at www.expertconsult.com.)

Thoracentesis trays
  Arrow International (Teleflex)
  Becton, Dickinson, and Company (Safe-T-Centesis)
  CardinalHealth
  Kendall Healthcare Products Covidien

ONLINE RESOURCES

Kaufmann DA: Thoracentesis. Medline Plus Medical Encyclopedia http://www.nlm.nih.gov/medlineplus/ency/article/003420.htm. Patient education handout linked to other information.

TABLE 218.1	Gross Pleural Fluid Findings and Potential Etiologies
Finding	**Potential Etiology**
Anchovy brown	Amoebic abscess
Bile staining	Cholothorax (e.g., biliary fistula)
Black fluid	*Aspergillus* infection
Food particles	Esophageal perforation
Milky fluid	Chylothorax or pseudochylothorax
Putrid odor	Anaerobic empyema

Modified from Hooper C, Lee YC, Maskell N; BTS Pleural Guideline Group. Investigation of a unilateral pleural effusion in adults: British Thoracic Society Pleural Disease Guideline 2010. *Thorax*. 2010;65(suppl 2):ii4–17, with additional information from McGraph.

TABLE 218.2	Potentially Useful Tests in the Evaluation of Pleural Effusions	
Pleural Fluid Test	**Abnormal Values**	**Frequently Associated Condition**
*Protein (PF/S)	>0.5	Exudate
*LDH (PF/S)	>0.6	Exudate
*LDH (IU)	>2/3 upper limit of normal for serum	Exudate
Red blood cells (per mm³)	>100,000	Malignancy, trauma, pulmonary embolism, tuberculosis
White blood cells (per mm³)	>10,000	Pyogenic infection
Neutrophils (%)	>50	Acute pleuritic
Lymphocytes (%)	>90	Tuberculosis, malignancy, sarcoidosis, fungal infection
Eosinophilia (%)	>10	Asbestos effusion, pneumothorax, resolving infection
Mesothelial cells	Absent	Tuberculosis
Glucose (mg/dL)	<60	Empyema, tuberculosis, malignancy, RA, SLE
pH	<7.20	Complicated parapneumonic process (needs chest tube), empyema, esophageal rupture, tuberculosis, malignancy, urinothorax, SLE
Amylase (PF/S)	>1	Pancreatitis
Bacteria	Positive	Infection
Cytology	Positive	Malignancy

*Light criteria. *IU*, Concentration in international units; *LDH*, lactate dehydrogenase; *PF/S*, pleural fluid/serum ratio; *RA*, rheumatoid arthritis; *SLE*, systemic lupus erythematosus.

  Modified from Kinasewitz GT. Pleural fluid dynamics and effusions. In: Fishman AP, ed. *Fishman's Pulmonary Diseases and Disorders*. 5th ed, vol 1. New York: McGraw-Hill; 2015.

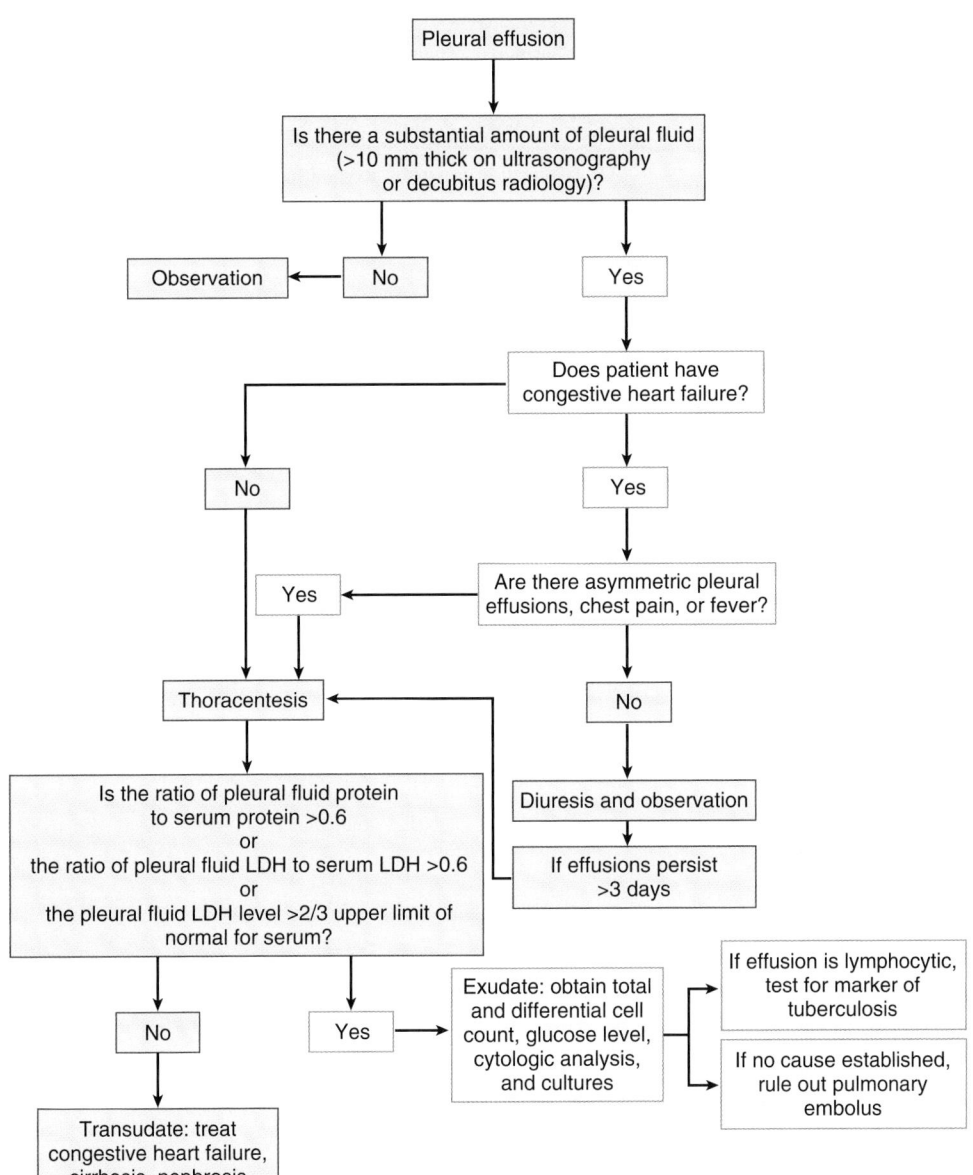

Fig. 218.4 Diagnostic scheme for pleural effusion. *LDH,* Lactate dehydrogenase. (From Light RW. Clinical practice. Pleural effusion. N Engl J Med. 2002;346:1971–1977.)

Sonosite. Teaching videos for ultrasonically directed thoracentesis. www.sonosite.com.

Thomsen TW, DeLaPena J, Setnik GS. *Thoracentesis. N Engl J Med Videos in Clinical Medicine*; 2016. https://www.youtube.com/watch?v=ivTyH09BcHg.

Tuggy M, Garcia J, Gaufberg SV. Procedures Consult: Thoracentesis. http://www.proceduresconsult.com/medical-procedures/thoracentesis-FM-042-procedure.aspx.

ADDITIONAL RESOURCES

See patient education and patient consent forms available at www.expertconsult.com.

RECOMMENDED READING

Adler EH, Block BK. Thoracentesis. In: Roberts JR, Custalow CB, Thomsen TW, eds. *Roberts and Hedges Clinical Procedures in Emergency Medicine.* 6th ed. Philadelphia: Elsevier; 2014:173–188.

Alemán C, Alegre J, Armadans L, Andreu J, Falco V, et al. The value of chest roentgenography in the diagnosis of pneumothorax after thoracentesis. *Am J Med.* 1999;107(4):340–343.

Cavanna L, Mordenti P, Berte R, Palladino MA, Biasini C, et al. Ultrasound guidance reduces pneumothorax rate and improves safety of thoracentesis in malignant pleural effusion: report of 445 consecutive patients with advanced cancer. *World J Surg Oncol.* 2014;12:139.

Ferrer JS, Muñoz XG, Orriols RM, et al. Evolution of idiopathic pleural effusion: a prospective, long-term follow-up study. *Chest.* 1996;109:1508–1513.

5th ed. Fishman AP, ed. *Fishman's Pulmonary Diseases and Disorders.* Vol 1. New York: McGraw-Hill; 2015.

Gordon CE, Feller-Kopman D, Balk EM, Smetana GM. Pneumothorax following thoracentesis: a systematic review and meta-analysis. *Arch Intern Med.* 2010;170(4):332–339.

Light RW. Pleural effusion. *N Engl J Med.* 2002;346:1971–1977.

McCartney JP, Adams JW, Hazard PB. Safety of thoracentesis in mechanically ventilated patients. *Chest.* 1993;103:1920–1921.

McGrath EE, Anderson PB. Diagnosis of pleural effusion: a systematic approach. *Am J Crit Care.* 2011;20(2):119–127.

Miller AC, Harvey JE. Guidelines for the management of spontaneous pneumothorax. *BMJ.* 1993;307:114–116.

Murphy MJ, Jenkinson F. Categorisation of pleural fluids in routine clinical practice: analysis of pleural fluid protein and lactate dehydrogenase alone compared with modified Light criteria. *J Clin Pathol.* 2008;61(5):68–685.

Patel PA, Ernst FR, Gunnarsson CL. Ultrasonography guidance reduces complications and costs associated with thoracentesis procedures. *J Clin Ultrasound.* 2012;40(3):135–141.

Peterson WG, Zimmerman R. Limited utility of chest radiograph after thoracentesis. *Chest.* 2000;117:1038–1042.

Reichman EF, Cristia CR, Meer J. Thoracentesis. In: Reichman EF, ed. *Emergency Medicine Procedures.* 2nd ed. New York: McGraw-Hill; 2013:250–263.

Roth BJ, O'Meara TF, Cragun WH. The serum-effusion albumin gradient in the evaluation of pleural effusions. *Chest.* 1990;98:546–549.

Saguil A, Wyrick K, Hallgren J. Diagnostic approach to pleural effusion. *Am Fam Physician.* 2014;90(2):99–104.

Wilcox ME, Chong CA, Stanbrook MB, Tricco AC, Wong C, Straus AC. Does this patient have an exudative pleural effusion? The rational clinical examination systematic review. JAMA. 2014;311(23):2422–2431.

CHAPTER 219

ABDOMINAL PARACENTESIS

Eric Skye

Paracentesis, or an *abdominal tap,* is an important clinical procedure for primary care clinicians. With the advent of new radiologic and minimally invasive techniques, diagnosis of intra-abdominal pathology has generally become less invasive. Nevertheless, paracentesis is the diagnostic test of choice in patients who have new-onset ascites, in patients with suspected malignant ascites, and in patients with preexisting ascites where infection needs to be ruled out. Therapeutic large-volume paracentesis (>5 L) also remains an important treatment option for many hemodynamically stable patients, particularly those with chronic tense or diuretic-resistant ascites. If ultrasound is available for guidance, it simplifies this procedure and decreases the risk of complications, especially in the overweight patient (see Chapter 214, Emergency Department, Hospitalist, and Office Ultrasonography [Clinical Ultrasonography]). In fact, Medicare carriers may refuse to reimburse for complications of paracentesis that was not ultrasound-directed.

ANATOMY

Abdominal anatomy must be considered when performing paracentesis. Large volumes of ascitic fluid tend to float the air-filled bowel anteriorly and toward the midline when the patient is in the supine position. Other pelvic organs that must be considered include an overly distended bladder and a gravid uterus. In addition, the cecum is relatively fixed and less mobile than the sigmoid colon; thus bowel perforation is more likely to occur in the right lower quadrant than in the left. Traditionally, the procedure has been performed through the linea alba using a midline insertion 2 cm below the umbilicus with the patient in a semiupright position (Fig. 219.1). Increasingly, a lateral approach has been advocated, with access obtained 3 to 5 cm medial and cephalad to the anterior superior iliac spine (Fig. 219.2). Using this approach, one must remain lateral to the rectus sheath to avoid the inferior epigastric artery. So either a supine or lateral decubitus position (or slight variants of these) can be used, which "floats" the bowel away from the insertion site and possibly provides access to a deeper ascitic pool.

INDICATIONS

Diagnostic

- New-onset ascites
- Suspected malignant ascites
- Rule out infection (consider for all hospitalized patients with known ascites)

EDITOR'S NOTE: It is unusual to have ascites without pedal edema. In diagnostically uncertain cases, transabdominal ultrasound (low-frequency probe) can detect as little as 100 mL of intra-abdominal fluid. Endoscopically guided ultrasound (high-frequency probe) can detect as little as 10 mL of fluid, which is more sensitive than computed tomographic scanning.

Therapeutic

- Temporary relief of tense ascites (causing gastrointestinal or cardiorespiratory symptoms such as pain, early satiety, or dyspnea)
- Symptom relief in patients with chronic tense or diuretic-resistant ascites

CONTRAINDICATIONS

Absolute

- Acute abdomen requiring immediate surgery (and even in this situation, paracentesis may be performed by the surgeon at the time of surgery)
- Coagulopathy when there is evidence of disseminated intravascular coagulation (DIC) or fibrinolysis

Relative

- Current bowel obstruction or severe bowel distention (Consider ultrasound-guided; see Chapter 214, Emergency Department, Hospitalist, and Office Ultrasonography [Clinical Ultrasonography].)
- Previous abdominal surgery (Bowel may be adherent to abdominal wall, so perform in an area away from prior incision or, even better, consider ultrasound-guided, especially in the overweight patient. Pockets of fluid may have formed and the ultrasound may be needed to locate them.)
- Anticoagulated patient or patient with coagulopathy without evidence of DIC or fibrinolysis. (Consideration should be taken to reverse the process, if possible, before paracentesis [see also the section on "Precautions"].)
  NOTE: Many patients undergoing paracentesis will have baseline coagulopathies or thrombocytopenia; however, the incident of clinically significant bleeding is extremely low. Therefore routine use of fresh frozen plasma or platelets is not recommended.
- Pregnancy (ultrasound-guided paracentesis is recommended after the first trimester)
- Distended bladder that cannot be emptied with a urinary catheter (consider ultrasound guided)
- Obvious infection at the intended site of needle insertion (cellulitis or abscess)

EQUIPMENT AND SUPPLIES

Commercially prepared kit or the following equipment:

- Skin cleansing solution (povidone-iodine or chlorhexidine)
- Sterile gloves and equipment necessary to follow universal blood and body fluid precautions
- Sterile marking pen (if area has not been marked indelibly before skin preparation)

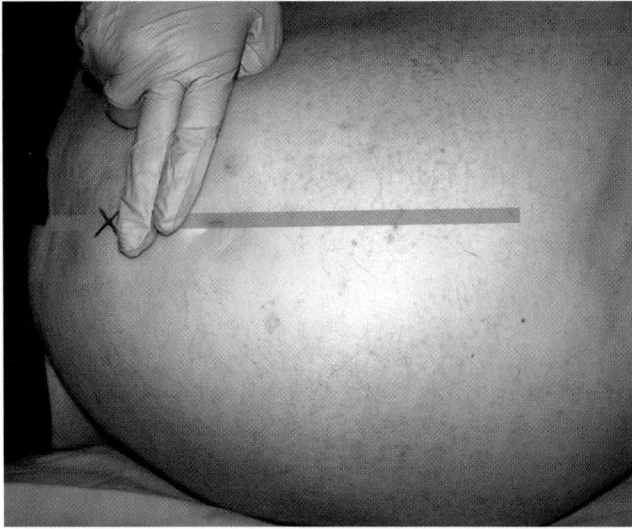

Fig. 219.1   View of the midline approach with anatomic landmarks.

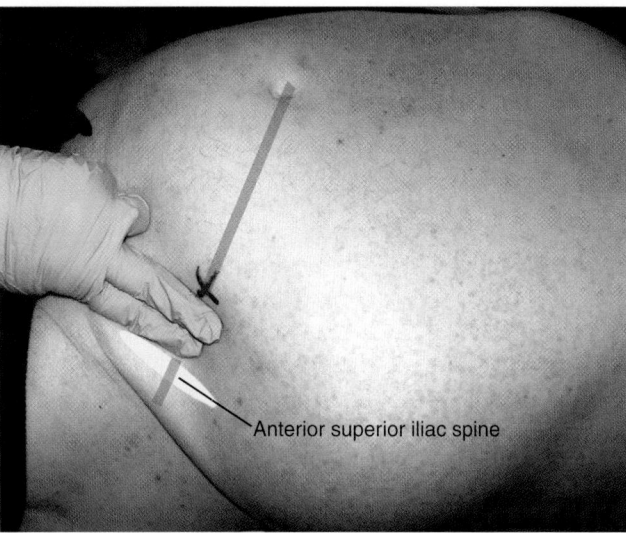

Anterior superior iliac spine

Fig. 219.2   View of the lateral approach with anatomic landmarks.

- Sterile drapes (sterile gown optional)
- 4 × 4 gauze squares and tape or material necessary for sterile occlusive dressing
- 1% or 2% lidocaine, 5 to 10 mL, with or without epinephrine
- 5-mL syringe for anesthetic
- 20-mL syringe for diagnostic paracentesis (also purple-topped blood collection tube for cell count, red-topped tubes for chemistries, blood culture bottles if infection suspected)
- 25- or 27-gauge, 1.5-inch needle for local anesthesia
- 18-gauge, 1.5- to 3-inch needle

Alternative devices: 18- or 20-gauge spinal needle, 18- or 20-gauge, 1.5- to 3-inch angiocatheter needle, 3.5-inch Caldwell needle (needle/cannula system designed for therapeutic large-volume paracentesis; studies have suggested this is the most expedient technique), or catheter-over-wire system (Seldinger technique). Paracentesis specific needle catheter assemblies are also available with a blunt obturator that is deployed after penetration of the abdominal wall to avoid organ damage (Safe-T-Centesis, Becton-Dickinson; see the section on "Online Resources").

- No. 11 blade scalpel if large catheter to be inserted
- Sterile intravenous (IV) tubing

- 1-L vacuum bottles, a sufficient number if large-volume paracentesis is needed
- Equipment to monitor blood pressure and heart rate if large-volume paracentesis will be performed
- Foley catheter (if bladder decompression needed)
- Nasogastric tube (if gastric decompression needed)
- Albumin for IV infusion if the patient is hypoalbuminemic and >5 L large-volume paracentesis will be performed (optional)
- Three-way stopcock (for use with 50-mL syringe) (optional)
- 50-mL syringe, if using stopcock technique (optional)

PRECAUTIONS

Careful attention to site selection, as discussed in the section on Anatomy, will minimize the risk of bleeding, infection, and injury to the bowel. Sites should be avoided where there is local skin breakdown, cellulitis, abdominal wall hematoma, or large engorged subcutaneous veins. In addition, entry near prior surgical scars should be avoided because there is a risk of adherent bowel loops near surgical scars. Blood pressure and heart rate should be monitored during large-volume paracentesis. The slow introduction of the needle through the abdominal wall minimizes the risk of bowel injury because the needle can push mobile bowel away rather than injure it. The application of intermittent negative pressure (aspiration) with the syringe while introducing the needle is generally preferred to constant negative pressure because the latter can quickly attract bowel or omentum on entry to the peritoneal cavity and occlude the needle. Needle occlusion can mask your entry into the peritoneal cavity and increase the risk of bowel injury, as well as lead to a false sense of a "dry tap." For patients taking warfarin or who have any coagulopathy other than DIC or fibrinolysis, some experts recommend the process being reversed before paracentesis. If possible, antiplatelet medications should be held for 5 to 7 days. Warfarin can be held for 5 to 7 days (until the international normalized ratio [INR] normalizes) and the patient converted to low-molecular-weight heparin during this time, with the dose being held the day of the procedure. Alternatively, the INR can be reversed the day of the procedure with fresh-frozen plasma. These experts suggest that patients with thrombocytopenia or an abnormal INR (for reasons other than taking warfarin) be given platelets or the INR reversed with factor replacement; however, this process is considered controversial and there are no data to support it. The only prospective study (Runyon, 1986) of bleeding complications determined that transfusion requiring abdominal hematomas occurred in less than 1% of cases despite 71% of patients having an abnormal prothrombin time (coagulopathy). In another prospective study (Grabau et al., 2004) of 1100 large-volume paracenteses, there were no bleeding complications with no pre- or postprocedure transfusions despite INRs as high as 8.7 and platelet counts as low as 19,000/mL. Consequently, the routine use of routine use of fresh frozen plasma or platelets is neither considered standard nor mandated, and imposes additional cost and risk of posttransfusion complications with little gain.

PREPROCEDURE PATIENT EDUCATION

Explain the procedure to the patient outlining the indications relevant to his or her medical situation and the anticipated benefits (diagnosis, ruling out infection, or decreased symptoms from therapeutic paracentesis). Risks of the procedure, as noted in section "Complications," should also be explained and informed consent obtained. Discuss anticipated patient positioning and ensure the patient is able to maintain the desired position. The patient should be aware that the local anesthetic may cause some discomfort, as well as the needle (or catheter) used to perform paracentesis.

TECHNIQUE

1. Examine the abdomen, delineate areas of shifting dullness, and find landmarks. Mark if necessary. Avoid sites where there is skin breakdown, cellulitis, abdominal wall hematoma, or large engorged subcutaneous veins. If clinical uncertainty exists about the presence of ascites, then ultrasound examination is recommended (see Chapter 214, Emergency Department, Hospitalist, and Office Ultrasonography [Clinical Ultrasonography]).

2. Assess for bowel and bladder distention and use a Foley catheter or nasogastric tube, if necessary, to decompress the bladder or stomach (see Chapter 96, Bladder Catheterization [and Urethral Dilation], and Chapter 217, Nasogastric and Nasoenteric Tube Insertion). Consider ultrasound guidance if needed.

3. Position the patient in the semiupright or lateral position, as tolerated, if the infraumbilical approach is used (see Fig. 219.1). Place the patient in the supine position if the lateral approach is taken (patient may be tilted slightly to the side of collection for improved fluid collection; see Fig. 219.2).

4. Prepare the abdominal skin at the puncture site with povidone–iodine or chlorhexidine solution.

5. Apply sterile drapes while confirming anatomic landmarks. The clinician should observe universal blood and body fluid precautions.
   - *Midline approach:* Insert the needle in the midline 2 to 3 cm below the umbilicus (two fingerbreadths). Patient is preferentially positioned in the semiupright or lateral position (see Fig. 219.1). Three "pops" will usually be felt as the needle penetrates the skin, the fascia, and the peritoneum.
   - *Lateral approach:* Enter 3 to 5 cm medial and cephalad to the anterior superior iliac spine. Patient may be in the supine position or tilted slightly to the side of collection (see Fig. 219.2). At least two pops will be felt as the needle penetrates the skin and the peritoneum (fluid returns). One or two additional pops may be felt in between these two as the needle penetrates fascia before penetrating the peritoneum.

6. Infiltrate the skin, subcutaneous, and other tissues down to the peritoneum with lidocaine (with or without epinephrine). Attempt to locate the very sensitive peritoneum and infiltrate 5 to 10 mL lidocaine across the peritoneum. Again, resistance is generally felt (a pop) as the needle perforates the peritoneum.

7. Direct the 18-gauge needle (or a catheter system) either perpendicular to the skin at the selected site when using a Z-tract or at a 45-degree angle to the skin and caudally. (A 20- or 22-gauge needle may be preferred for diagnostic paracentesis to minimize subsequent leakage of ascitic fluid.) A Z-tract technique should be used (Fig. 219.3) if there are tense ascites. Two alternate Z-tract techniques are described: (a) the needle is inserted just through the skin, and the skin is then pulled taut from a cranial or caudal direction, moving the needle 1 or 2 cm, before the needle is advanced through deeper abdominal structures down to the peritoneum; or (b) the needle is inserted in a caudal direction at a 45-degree angle, just through skin and subcutaneous tissue. The skin is then pulled taut in a caudal direction, pulling the needle toward a more perpendicular position. It is then inserted down into the peritoneal cavity. The theoretical advantage of these techniques is the self-sealing of the needle tract when the tension on the skin is released after the procedure is completed, thus minimizing leaking of peritoneal fluid. With either method it is important to apply suction only intermittently as the needle is inserted through the deeper structures. Applying continuous suction after the needle has penetrated the peritoneum may attract bowel loops or omentum, occlude flow, and create the appearance of an unsuccessful tap, all of which increase the likelihood of bowel perforation. Insert the needle until fluid returns in the syringe. The needle can be rotated 180 degrees if peritoneal tenting is suspected because this helps enter the peritoneal cavity. If no fluid returns from an area of shifting dullness after rotating the needle, withdraw the needle to just below the skin and then redi-

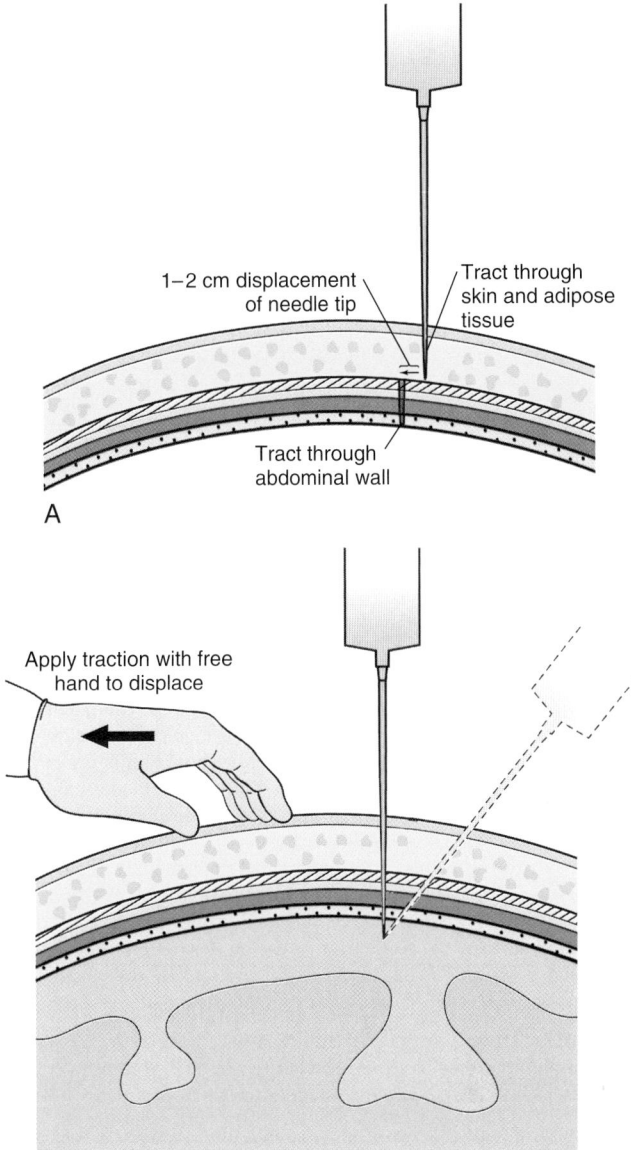

Fig. 219.3 The Z-tract technique. (A) Transverse view through the abdominal wall demonstrating the Z-tract. (B) The needle is inserted perpendicular to the skin on the abdominal wall, which is then pulled taut or retracted a few centimeters caudad (or cephalad) by the non–needle-bearing hand *(arrow)*. The needle is then advanced through the subcutaneous and deeper structures until it pierces the peritoneum and fluid is obtained. (As an alternative, the needle can be inserted into just the skin and subcutaneous tissue at a 45-degree angle, directed caudally. When traction is placed on the skin or the skin is pulled taut in a caudal direction, the needle will be pulled more upright, toward a position more perpendicular to the skin. The needle is then advanced downward until fluid is obtained.) When the procedure is finished, the needle is withdrawn, traction is released, and the abdominal wall layers will shift back to their natural positions to facilitate closure of the needle tract.

rect the needle in an area just inferior (midline approach) or just lateral (lateral approach) to the previous attempt. If still no fluid returns, another attempt can be made using a different location. If the initial attempt was made in the midline, consider another attempt in the lateral location (if not contraindicated) or in the midline 1 cm below the prior attempt. If the initial attempt was in the lateral location, consider another attempt in the midline (if not contraindicated) or 1 cm lateral to the prior attempt. If these attempts are unsuccessful, ultrasound should be used to guide the paracentesis. Ultrasound can be used to quantify the amount of fluid expected (1 cm³ of fluid equals 1 mL) as well as to determine the direction necessary to obtain this fluid. It can also be used to make sure no vital organs are in the pathway chosen for aspiration (see Chapter 214, Emergency Department, Hospitalist, and Office Ultrasonography [Clinical Ultrasonography]).

If a catheter-over-needle system is used, advance the needle 1 to 2 mm after the flash of ascitic fluid is seen. Occlude the needle hub temporarily with a sterile gloved finger. Using the No. 11 blade scalpel, a small nick in the skin near the catheter (taking care not to cut the catheter) may facilitate passage of the catheter. Directing the needle toward a fluid-dependent position, advance the catheter over the needle, using a twisting motion, until the hub is against the skin. Gently withdraw the needle while holding the hub securely against the skin. Attach a syringe, if fluid is needed for diagnostic reasons, or the sterile IV tubing for therapeutic paracentesis.

For the Seldinger technique (catheter-over-wire system such as that used for central venous catheter insertion), advance the needle 1 to 2 mm after a flash of ascitic fluid is seen. (These are special needles tapered at the hub to facilitate advancement of the guidewire; standard hypodermics will generally not allow passage of a guidewire.) Occlude the needle hub temporarily with a sterile gloved finger, and then insert the guidewire through the hub. Insert the guidewire to the desired depth, always making sure at least several centimeters remains outside the beveled end of the hub. Holding the guidewire securely on the proximal end, remove the needle over the guidewire. After the needle tip has been removed from the skin, grasp the guidewire below the needle with sterile gloved fingers to prevent it from being pulled out of the peritoneal cavity. Using the No. 11 blade scalpel, a small nick in the skin near the guidewire (taking care not to cut the guidewire) may facilitate passage of the dilator/sheath unit through the skin. Place the dilator through the sheath to form a unit, and then advance the dilator/sheath unit over the guidewire, using a twisting motion, up to the hub. Holding the hub securely against the skin, remove the guidewire and dilator, and attach a syringe to the hub, if fluid is needed for diagnostic reasons, or the sterile IV tubing for therapeutic paracentesis.

NOTE: When using a catheter-over-wire system, never let go completely of the proximal end of the wire. This precaution is to prevent loss of the wire into the peritoneal cavity.

8. After entry into the peritoneal cavity, fluid (usually 20–50 mL) should be withdrawn and collected for analysis (see the section on "Interpretation of Results"). Note the color and clarity of the fluid; normal ascitic fluid is clear and straw colored. If a therapeutic large-volume paracentesis is indicated, the needle may be attached to sterile IV tubing. This is then connected to vacuum bottles, if available, or a stopcock can be used with sequential aspiration using a 50-mL syringe. Blood pressure and heart rate should be monitored during large-volume paracentesis. The needle may need to be repositioned to allow for continuous flow (omentum or a loop of bowel may have occluded the flow).

NOTE: Never reposition the needle while the tip is within the peritoneal cavity; doing so may lacerate the bowel, the omentum, or a blood vessel. Instead, withdraw the needle into the subcutaneous tissue, redirect the needle, and then readvance it into the peritoneal cavity. Alternatively, the patient may need to be repositioned slightly or slight pressure applied to the abdomen.

There is controversy regarding hypotension caused by a large-volume paracentesis (>5 L). Some clinicians give colloid replacement (e.g., albumin, 6–8 g IV per liter of ascetic fluid removed) after paracentesis, especially in patients with cirrhosis and hypoalbuminemia; however, there is no evidence that this practice should be adopted universally and it is rarely recommended for procedures removing less than 5 L of ascitic fluid. After a large-volume paracentesis, there tends to be initial improvement in circulatory function; however, total paracentesis in patients with cirrhosis may cause delayed (>12–24 hours after the procedure) hypotension due to effective hypovolemia, so consider monitoring blood pressure and heart rate or colloid infusion. Although the literature suggests this hypovolemia may be avoided by prophylactic colloid infusion, it is difficult to obtain albumin in the outpatient setting; therefore, these infusions typically have to be done in the hospital.

9. After the fluid is removed, gently remove the needle (or catheter), cover the entry site with 4 × 4 gauze pads, and apply pressure. If the wound is still leaking fluid after 5 minutes of direct pressure, consider suturing the puncture site using a mattress suture or apply a pressure dressing.

COMPLICATIONS

Complications are rare during paracentesis but include the risk of the following:

- Perforation of viscus organ (e.g., stomach, small bowel, colon; rare, and tend to be self-healing).
- Lacerations of major vessels with subsequent hemorrhage.
- Abdominal wall hematoma (most common).
- Infection (local or intraperitoneal).
- Persistent ascitic fluid leak.
- Hypotension (e.g., vasovagal reaction, hemorrhage, reaccumulation of fluid).
- Postparacentesis circulatory dysfunction may lead to hypotension, renal failure, hyponatremia, and shortened survival. While controversial, these may be minimized or avoided by albumin infusion, especially if greater than 5 L fluid was removed with paracentesis.
- Bladder perforation.
- Hepatic encephalopathy.

POSTPROCEDURE PATIENT MANAGEMENT AND EDUCATION

Complications of the procedure are rare, and patients are usually able to return to their normal activities after this procedure. A brief observation period of 1 hour while monitoring vital signs is appropriate. Educate the patient about signs and symptoms of complications such as those listed (e.g., hypotension, bleeding, fever, abdominal pain or distention, nausea, vomiting), and instruct him or her to call or return to the clinician's office or the emergency department if these occur. If the site continues to ooze (e.g., tense ascites), the patient should be instructed about how to change the dressings regularly. When paracentesis is performed as an outpatient procedure, plans should be made to discuss with the patient the results of any tests performed.

INTERPRETATION OF RESULTS

Although numerous tests are possible for ascitic fluid, the key questions of whether the fluid is infected and whether portal hypertension exists can usually be answered by obtaining the following:

- Cell count and differential (usually a purple-topped or EDTA tube)
- Bacterial culture (sensitivity and yield are increased by inoculating culture bottles at the bedside; the same bottles used for blood cultures may be used.)
- Concurrent serum and ascitic fluid albumin and protein (usually a red-topped tube) to calculate serum–ascites albumin gradient (Table 219.1), which is approximately 97% accurate for diagnosing portal hypertension

To determine if preexisting ascites has become infected, some authors suggest using the cell count as the initial screen; if values are normal (<250/mm³), the likelihood of infection is low. If the cell count is elevated, a confirmatory culture is required, but the patient should be admitted for empiric treatment with IV antibiotics

	TABLE 219.1 Ascitic Fluid Analysis		
Laboratory Test		**Suggests Cirrhosis or Portal Hypertension***	**Suggests Inflammatory Process†**
White blood cell count (mm³)		<250	>250 (often >500 with >50% polymorphonuclear leukocytes)
SAAG (g/dL)‡		≥1.1 suggests portal hypertension	<1.1
Protein (g/dL)		<3	>3
Lactate dehydrogenase (fluid/serum ratio)		<0.6	≥0.6

*Some causes of portal hypertension: Cirrhosis, congestive heart failure (cardiac ascites), inferior vena caval obstruction or other veno-occlusive disease, Budd-Chiari syndrome (hepatic vein or inferior vena caval thrombosis), portal vein thrombosis, sarcoidosis, fulminant hepatic failure, alcoholic hepatitis, massive liver metastases, myxedema, mixed ascites.
†Some causes of inflammatory processes: Spontaneous bacterial peritonitis, malignancy, tuberculosis, pancreatitis, connective tissue disease. Nephrotic syndrome can cause ascites without an inflammatory process and serum–ascites albumin gradient.
‡Serum–ascites albumin gradient = [Serum albumin] − [Ascitic fluid albumin] alone is approximately 97% accurate in diagnosing portal hypertension. Increased red blood cell count can be seen in malignancy, tuberculosis, endometriosis, mesenteric thrombosis, pancreatitis, abdominal trauma, and perforated viscus.

(typically a third-generation cephalosporin, such as cefotaxime, which covers 98% of the causative agents for this disorder [*Escherichia coli* and streptococcal species; ampicillin should be added if *Enterococcus* is suspected]). It is also acceptable to culture all samples but treat empirically only when cell counts are abnormal. For the evaluation of new-onset ascites, the initial evaluation often centers around whether the etiology is portal hypertension (often due to cirrhosis) or other factors. An increased red blood cell count can also be seen in malignancy, tuberculosis, endometriosis, mesenteric thrombosis, pancreatitis, abdominal trauma, and perforated viscus.

Additional studies on ascitic fluid to determine the etiology of new-onset ascites might include Gram stain (usually not helpful because bacterial concentrations are very low unless bowel is ruptured or perforated), triglyceride level (particularly if "milky" appearance, e.g., pancreatitis), smear for acid-fast bacteria (AFB), or assay for AFB by RNA polymerase chain reaction and AFB culture. (Suspect AFB in immunocompromised patients or those who have immigrated from areas where mycobacterial diseases are endemic; AFB culture has a sensitivity of about 50%.) Chemistries that might be obtained on both serum and ascitic fluid include glucose, lactate dehydrogenase, and amylase. Table 219.1 lists some common values to assist in laboratory interpretation.

Peritoneal carcinomatosis is possible in patients with a prior history of colon, breast, gastric, pancreatic, hepatobiliary, hepatocellular, ovarian, or other cancers. Ascitic fluid should be sent for cytologic study in these patients or anyone suspected of having a malignancy.

CPT/BILLING CODES

49082* Peritoneocentesis, abdominal paracentesis, or peritoneal lavage (therapeutic or diagnostic); initial
49083* Peritoneocentesis, abdominal paracentesis, or peritoneal lavage; subsequent
99070* Supplies and materials (except spectacles), provided by the physician over and above those usually included with the office visit or other services rendered (list drugs, trays, supplies, or materials provided)

*Health Care Financing Administration (HCFA, for Medicare) allows additional payment for a tray for this procedure when performed in a physician's office.

ICD-10-CM DIAGNOSTIC CODES

A18.31 Ascites, tuberculous
C78.6 Ascites, malignant (secondary malignant neoplasm of respiratory and digestive system, retroperitoneum and peritoneum)
I50.810 Ascites, cardiac
I89.8 Ascites, chylous
K65.2 Spontaneous bacterial peritonitis
K70.31 Alcoholic cirrhosis of liver with ascites
R18.8 Ascites, unspecified site

SUPPLIERS

(See contact information available at www.expertconsult.com.)

Abdominal paracentesis kit
Safe-T-Centis (Becton-Dickinson and Company)
Arrow International (Teleflex Medical)

Acknowledgment

The editors recognize the contributions of Michael Brown, MD, Brett White, MD, and Kenneth Hu, MD, to this chapter in previous editions of this text.

ONLINE RESOURCES

Thompsen TW, Shaffer RW, White B, Setnik GS. Paracentesis. Videos in Clinical Medicine: Safe-T-Centesis system. *N Engl J Med*. www.youtube.com/watch?v=KVpwXK7cvzQ.
Perera P. Ultrasound directed paracentesis. www.youtube.com/watch?v=bWxv_a9CkBs.
Sonosite Inc: multiple videos for ultrasound-directed procedures: www.sonosite.com/education

RECOMMENDED READING

European Association for the Study of the Liver. EASL clinical practice guidelines on the management of ascites, spontaneous bacterial peritonitis, and hepatorenal syndrome in cirrhosis. *J Hepatol*. 2010;53(3):397–417.
Grabau CM, Crago SF, Hoff LK, et al. Performance standards for therapeutic abdominal paracentesis. *Hepatology*. 2004;40(2):484.
Ong JP. Paracentesis. *Am J Gastroenterol*. 2006;101:1954–1955.
Promes SB, Datner EM, Hsu S. Paracentesis. In: Reichman EF, ed. *Emergency Medicine Procedures*. 2nd ed. New York: McGraw-Hill; 2013:421–430.
Runyon BA. Paracentesis of ascitic fluid: a safe procedure. *Arch Int Med*. 1986;146:2259–2261.
Runyon BA. American Association for Study of Liver Diseases. Management of adult patients with ascites due to cirrhosis: update 2012. *Hepatology*. 2013;57(4):1651–1653.
Runyon BA. Ascites and spontaneous bacterial peritonitis. In: Feldman M, Friedman LS, Brandt LJ, eds. *Sleisenger and Fordtran's Gastrointestinal and Liver Disease*. 10th ed. Philadelphia: Elsevier; 2016.
Runyan MS, Marx JA. Peritoneal procedures. In: Roberts JR, Hedges JR, eds. *Roberts and Hedges' Clinical Procedures in Emergency Medicine*. 6th ed. Philadelphia: Elsevier; 2014:862–872.

CHAPTER 220

BONE MARROW ASPIRATION AND BIOPSY

Beth A. Choby

Bone marrow examination is a useful adjunct in the evaluation of various diseases, both hematologic and nonhematologic in origin. Bone marrow aspiration and biopsy supply additional clinical information when peripheral blood smears or other routine laboratory tests are inconclusive. Certain patients require this procedure for cytogenetic analysis, molecular studies, flow cytometry, or microbiologic cultures. The two procedures are usually performed sequentially and supply complementary information. Bone marrow aspiration allows visualization of cell morphology and a count of marrow cellular elements, whereas bone marrow (trephine) biopsy evaluates marrow cellularity and detects focal lesions such as metastatic cancer, lymphoma, or granulomas.

Bone marrow aspiration and biopsy are performed through one skin incision but sample separate areas of bone about 5 mm apart. The aspirate is usually collected first. A drawback of this approach is aspiration artifact—the artifactual hypocellularity and contamination with sinusoidal blood seen on the subsequent marrow biopsy specimen. Although the bone marrow biopsy can be done first, thromboplastic substances are released, making an adequate aspirate less likely.

ANATOMY

Site selection for bone marrow aspiration depends on the patient's age and the clinician's experience. The posterior iliac crest is the most common site for bone marrow aspiration; bone marrow biopsy is almost exclusively performed at this site (Fig. 220.1A). The sternum can be used for aspiration in adults, but it is never appropriate for biopsy (see Fig. 220.1B); cardiac tamponade is a possibility if the posterior sternum were to be inadvertently penetrated. Fig. 220.2 shows the Illinois needle, designed specifically for sternal bone marrow aspiration. The anterior iliac crest is an option for both bone marrow aspiration and biopsy, although the harder, thicker cortical layer of bone at this location makes this approach more technically challenging. The anterior iliac crest is most often used when biopsy of the posterior iliac crest is contraindicated (e.g., significant obesity, physical disability, or presence of a cast). The anterior tibia is an option for marrow aspiration in infants younger than 18 months.

Aspiration and biopsy techniques for the posterior iliac crest are described in this chapter. Aspiration and biopsy are both easily implemented at this site and safe when performed properly.

UNILATERAL VERSUS BILATERAL

Unilateral iliac sampling was previously considered adequate in patients with multiple myeloma, chronic myeloproliferative disorders, and myelodysplastic syndromes. Bilateral iliac sampling has been shown to increase the likelihood of confirming bone malignancy in patients with Hodgkin disease, sarcomas, carcinomas,

and non-Hodgkin lymphoma. However, at present, with the use of positron emission scanning to stage lymphomas and confirm bone involvement, bilateral bone marrow biopsies are rarely done.

INDICATIONS

- Evaluation of anemia or iron metabolism
- Thrombocytopenia
- Leukopenia or leukocytosis
- Pancytopenia
- Unexplained splenomegaly

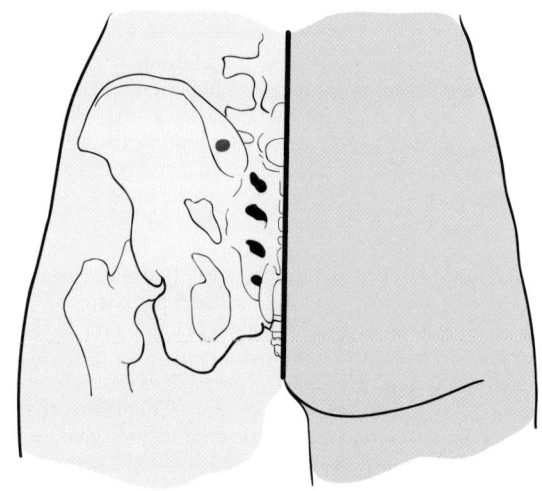

A

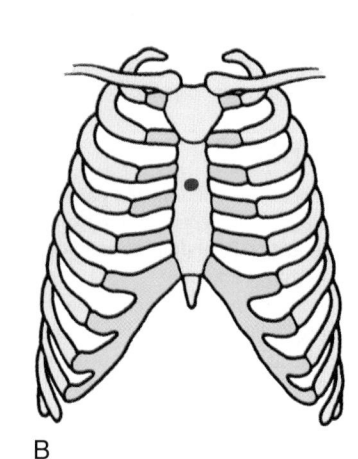

B

Fig. 220.1 (A) Posterior iliac sampling site. (B) Sternal sampling site.

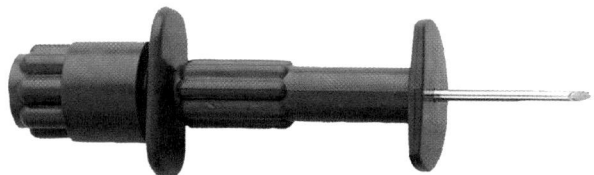

Fig. 220.2 Illinois needle for sternal bone marrow aspiration. (Courtesy Cardinal Health, Dublin, OH.)

- Workup for fever of unknown origin
- Diagnosis and staging of leukemia and lymphoma
- Multiple myeloma, myelodysplastic syndrome, myeloproliferative disorders
- Metastatic carcinoma
- Granulomatous diseases such as sarcoid
- Workup for bone marrow transplantation
- Staging of nonhematologic cancers such as neuroblastoma
- Monitoring of chemotherapy- and radiation-induced damage from cancer treatment
- To obtain samples for chromosomal studies
- Workup of dysproteinemia or lysosomal storage diseases
- Diagnosis of opportunistic infection in patients with human immunodeficiency virus infection/acquired immunodeficiency syndrome (e.g., *Mycobacterium avium intracellulare*)
- Unusual infections (e.g., tuberculosis, fungal infections, leishmaniasis)

CONTRAINDICATIONS

Absolute

- Hemophilia and related bleeding disorders
- Uncooperative patient
- Skin infection or osteomyelitis at the proposed biopsy site

Relative

- Significant obesity
- Severe osteoporosis (risk of bone perforation and injury to underlying tissues)
- Previous radiation therapy at the biopsy site

NOTE: Isolated thrombocytopenia is not a contraindication to bone marrow aspiration or biopsy. When a patient requires anticoagulation therapy, it does not need to be reversed or held before the procedure. Patients taking anticoagulants should have an activated partial thromboplastin time and prothrombin time/international normalized ratio within the therapeutic range for heparin or warfarin before the procedure (i.e., not be excessively anticoagulated, such as an international normalized ratio >5).

EQUIPMENT

Necessary equipment is available in sterile, disposable, prepackaged kits (Fig. 220.3).

- Antiseptic solution (e.g., povidone-iodine or chlorhexidine)
- Sterile fenestrated drape
- 1% lidocaine
- 5- and 10-mL syringes
- 22-gauge (1.5-inch) and 25-gauge (1.5-inch) needles
- No. 11 scalpel
- Bone marrow aspiration needle (Fig. 220.4)
- 11-gauge Jamshidi bone marrow biopsy needle (Fig. 220.5)
- 10-mL syringe rinsed with ethylenediamine tetra-acetic acid (EDTA)

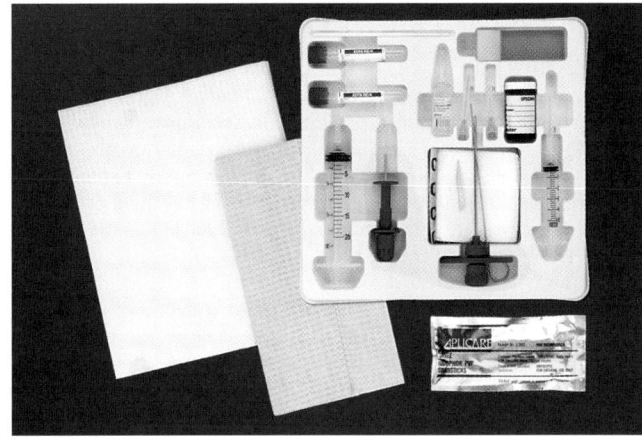

Fig. 220.3 Prepackaged sterile Jamshidi bone marrow biopsy kit. (Courtesy Cardinal Health, Dublin, OH.)

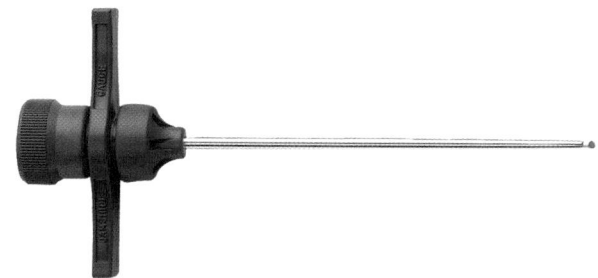

Fig. 220.4 Bone marrow aspiration needle. (Courtesy Cardinal Health, Dublin, OH.)

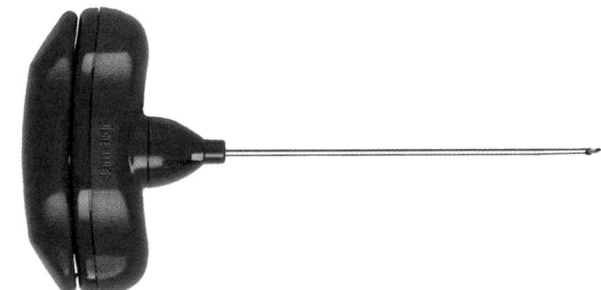

Fig. 220.5 Jamshidi bone marrow biopsy needle. (Courtesy Cardinal Health, Dublin, OH.)

- EDTA (purple-topped) tube
- Glass slides (10)
- Bottle or tube with fixative (formalin)
- 4 × 4 gauze
- Pressure dressing and tape

PRECAUTIONS

Review the patient history and indications for bone marrow sampling. Question the patient about recent use of medications that might depress bone marrow function or stimulate blood formation (e.g., cytokines). The results of a complete blood count and peripheral blood smear should be reviewed before considering bone marrow aspiration and biopsy.

PREPROCEDURE PATIENT EDUCATION

A cooperative patient is essential. Discuss indications for the procedure, as well as risks and benefits. Obtain a signed informed consent (see the sample patient consent form available at www.expertconsult.com). Inquire about any coagulation abnormalities or allergies (e.g., povidone-iodine or lidocaine). Explain that numbing the skin and periosteum, penetrating the iliac crest, and aspirating marrow is sometimes uncomfortable. Have the patient empty his or her bladder before the procedure. In overly apprehensive patients, premedication with a mild anxiolytic or analgesic is appropriate. Oral lorazepam (1–2 mg) and hydromorphone (1–2 mg) or equivalent given 60 to 90 minutes before the biopsy will lessen pain and induce varying degrees of amnesia. General anesthesia may be needed in infants and pediatric patients, especially if the anterior tibial location is utilized.

TECHNIQUE

Optimal bone marrow evaluation requires examination of both the marrow aspirate and a biopsy specimen (smear preparations and sections). Obtaining both samples simultaneously is better in terms of cost, patient comfort, and diagnostic information gleaned. The aspirate is usually performed first. The following instructions describe bone marrow aspiration and biopsy using the posterior iliac approach.

Bone Marrow Aspiration

1. Have the patient lie either in the lateral decubitus position with knees flexed at the hip or in the prone position. Identify each iliac crest and follow it to its posterosuperior spine (see Fig. 220.1). Mark this location using ink or pressure from a needle cap.
2. Put on sterile gloves and prepare the biopsy area with 10% povidone-iodine antiseptic in a circular pattern. Drape the site with the fenestrated sterile drape. Position the fenestration over the center of the intended biopsy site.
3. Using the 25-gauge needle and 5-mL syringe, make a skin wheal with 1% lidocaine. Switch to the 22-gauge needle/5-mL syringe to anesthetize deeper structures. Introduce the needle until the periosteum is encountered. Infiltrating the periosteum with 1 mL of lidocaine is important because most of the bone pain fibers are located here. Inject 2 to 3 mL of lidocaine along the outgoing tract as the needle is removed.
4. Make a 2- to 3-mm skin incision (basically nick the skin) with the scalpel to enhance insertion of the aspiration needle.
5. Insert the aspiration needle perpendicularly to the bone, making sure that the stylet is locked in place. Insert the needle until it rests against the anesthetized periosteum. Rotate the needle clockwise and counterclockwise using enough force to penetrate the bony cortex. "Give" is felt when the marrow cavity is entered. Stop pushing and check that the needle remains stationary without support.
6. Remove the stylet and attach a 10-mL EDTA-rinsed syringe. Warn the patient that he or she will experience pain as the marrow is aspirated. Pull the plunger and rapidly aspirate 0.2 to 2 mL of marrow for slide preparation (higher volumes dilute the specimen with blood). If more material is needed for other studies, an additional 5 mL of aspirate may be withdrawn.
7. Give the aspirated material to an assistant for slide preparation. Aspirate quality is assessed by the presence of grossly visible marrow spicules. Thin films should be prepared quickly with minimal specimen manipulation. Several drops of aspirate are placed on the edge of a glass slide while the edge of another slide is used to thinly spread the aspirate across the first slide. Four slides are prepared and allowed to air dry. Slides are stained with either Wright or May-Grünwald-Giemsa stain.

8. Place the remaining aspirate in a tube with EDTA, mix well, and allow it to clot for later fixation and processing by the histologist. If extra material is needed for flow cytometry, culture, cytogenetics, or other special studies, use another sterile syringe to withdraw more aspirate from the aspirate needle.
9. If a dry tap is encountered (no aspirate despite seemingly good needle placement), replace the stylet and advance the needle 1 to 2 mm. If still no aspirate is obtained, remove the needle and reinsert it at another part of anesthetized periosteum near the original site.
10. Once the aspirate sample has been judged adequate, replace the stylet and remove the entire needle using a twisting motion.
11. Place dry gauze over the site and apply pressure until the bleeding stops. Cover the area with an adhesive bandage unless proceeding with a bone marrow biopsy.

Bone Marrow Biopsy

Bone marrow biopsy is performed immediately after aspiration. Some kits allow use of the same needle for both aspiration and biopsy, but the clinician must remember to redirect the needle to a different location for biopsy. Otherwise, once the bone marrow aspiration needle has been removed, the following steps are taken:

1. Confirm that the stylet of the Jamshidi biopsy needle is locked into place with the cap secured (see Fig. 220.5). Place the capped end in the palm of your hand so that the shaft lies between the index and middle fingers. Introduce the needle into the skin incision and push past the soft tissue until the periosteum of the posterior iliac spine is reached. Position the needle at least 5 mm away from the periosteal entry point used for the aspirate collection (to avoid aspiration artifact). Using clockwise and counterclockwise rotation with considerable downward pressure, pierce the bony cortex and enter the marrow. The cortex is usually about 1 cm thick and entrance into the marrow cavity is detected by decreased resistance (Fig. 220.6).
2. Unlock the cap and remove the stylet.
3. Slowly and gently advance the needle millimeter by millimeter to a total of 1.5 to 2 cm while alternating a clockwise-counterclockwise motion to obtain an adequate specimen.
4. Pull the needle back 2 to 3 mm and redirect the tip approximately 15 degrees. Advance the needle 2 to 3 mm forward in this new position while rotating it. This will break off the specimen.
5. Rotate the biopsy needle 360 degrees four times to the right and then four times to the left.
6. Remove the needle from the patient using rotational movements. The sample should stay in the Jamshidi needle.
7. Remove the biopsy specimen by inserting the blunt probe into the needle tip, pushing the specimen toward the hub/handle and out onto sterile gauze. Take care not to injure yourself on the sharp cutting edge (see Fig. 220.6D) of the needle tip.
8. Prepare the specimens or give the sample to the technician for preparation. Touch preparations (five) are made by gently pressing five glass slides against the biopsy specimen. The slides are usually stained with Wright or Giemsa stain. The remaining biopsy sample is placed into a container with formalin and sent for sectioning and staining (Fig. 220.7).
9. Cover the biopsy site with gauze and apply firm pressure until the bleeding stops. Cover the area with gauze and an adhesive bandage to form a pressure dressing. If there is no bleeding at the site after 5 minutes of observation, the patient can be mobilized. If there is bleeding, the patient should lie on the biopsy site for a minimum of 30 minutes.

SAMPLE OPERATIVE REPORT

See the Sample Operative Report available at www.expertconsult.com.

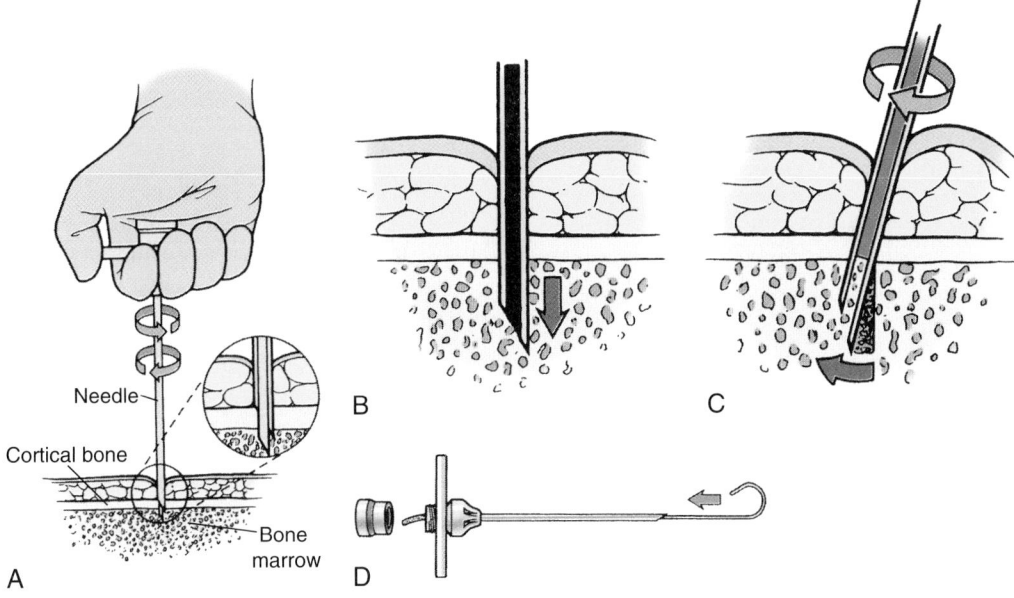

Fig. 220.6 Technique for obtaining a bone marrow biopsy specimen. (A) The needle is advanced through the cortical bone. (B) The stylet is removed and the needle advanced an additional 1.5 to 2 cm using a downward rotational force. (C) The needle tip is withdrawn 2 to 3 mm, then readvanced 2 to 3 mm after being redirected 15 degrees. When the needle is now rotated, the specimen should be broken off. (D) After withdrawing the needle completely, the probe is used to push the specimen onto gauze. It is threaded through the needle tip toward the biopsy needle's handle.

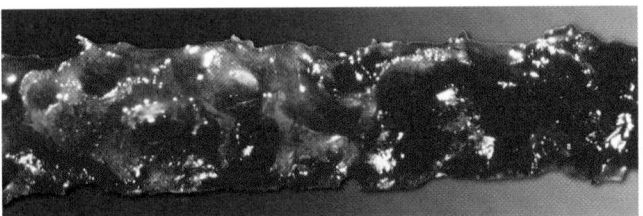

Fig. 220.7 Biopsy specimen from bone marrow biopsy with Jamshidi needle. (Courtesy Cardinal Health, Dublin, OH.)

COMMON ERRORS

- *Failure to adequately anesthetize the periosteum.* Most of the bone pain fibers are located in this layer. The periosteum should be gently probed or tested with the sharp point of the 22-gauge needle before aspiration or biopsy. If the patient experiences sharp pain, an additional 1 to 2 mL of lidocaine should be injected.
- *Failure to locate the posterosuperior iliac crest.* This occurs more commonly in obese patients. Having the patient locate his or her hip may help to identify the pelvic rim. It is not uncommon for the clinician to mistake the lateral sacral crest for the posterosuperior iliac crest and biopsy at this location can result in a dry tap.
- *Inadequate specimen length obtained on the bone marrow biopsy.* The ideal length of an adequate bone marrow biopsy is not well defined. Specimen lengths ranging from 1.6 to 3 cm have been recommended by various authorities. Because the core biopsy shrinks by up to 25% during processing, obtaining an adequate biopsy is important.
- *Dry tap.* A dry tap is the failure to aspirate fluid or find bone marrow particles during bone marrow aspiration. The most common cause is faulty positioning of the aspiration needle into the marrow cavity. The stylet can be replaced and the aspiration needle advanced to attempt a second aspirate. Dry taps occur in 4% to 7% of cases. A repeat dry tap is suggestive of myelofibrosis, hairy cell leukemia, aplastic anemia, myeloma, lymphoma, or leukemia. A bone marrow biopsy is then required to obtain touch imprints that "substitute" for the aspirate.
- *Preparation of low-quality aspirate smears.* Bone marrow clots quickly, so aspirate slides are usually prepared at the bedside by the provider or a trained technician. The simplest preparation is a wedge technique similar to that used for peripheral blood smears. A drop of marrow is placed at one end of a glass slide while a second slide held at a 30-degree angle is used to feather the aspirate across the first slide. Particle crush methods and coverslip preparations are more challenging to prepare.
- *Dilution by peripheral blood.* This happens when a large volume of bone marrow is aspirated.

COMPLICATIONS

Complications of bone marrow aspiration and biopsy are exceedingly rare. Major adverse events occur 0.05% to 0.07% of the time. Adverse outcomes include the following:

- Retroperitoneal hemorrhage or bowel damage from perforation of the iliac bone in osteoporotic patients
- Hemorrhage at the biopsy site
- Infection at the biopsy site (unusual if sterile technique is followed)
- Perforation of the lower sternal plate, resulting in cardiac tamponade and sudden death
- Breakage of the bone marrow needle or handle separation during insertion into the bone (rare)
- Unilateral lower extremity weakness or numbness due to irritation of the sacral nerve plexus (rare and transient)
- Pain (usually resolves within a day)

POSTPROCEDURE MANAGEMENT

The patient lies on the bandaged biopsy site for 1 hour while being monitored. If the patient was thrombocytopenic before the procedure, a pressure bandage is applied and the site checked frequently for excessive bleeding.

POSTPROCEDURE PATIENT EDUCATION

Emergency contact numbers are provided and the patient instructed to call in case of bleeding, pain, fever, or erythema at the biopsy site. The pressure dressing is removed after 12 to 24 hours. Pain medication should be provided as needed.

INTERPRETATION OF RESULTS

The bone marrow aspirate and biopsy specimens are examined by a trained histopathologist who interprets the results. A written report is generated and sent to the clinician who performed the tests. Providing adequate clinical information aids the pathologist in reaching an accurate diagnosis.

PATIENT EDUCATION GUIDES

See patient education and patient consent forms available at www.expertconsult.com.

CPT/BILLING CODES

38220	Bone marrow aspiration
38221	Bone marrow biopsy
85060	Peripheral blood smear interpretation with written report
85097	Bone marrow smear with interpretation

ICD-10-CM DIAGNOSTIC CODES

A19.9	Tuberculosis, disseminated, not otherwise specified
C85.89	Non-Hodgkin lymphoma, not otherwise specified, unspecified site
C90.00	Multiple myeloma, without mention of remission
C90.01	Multiple myeloma, in remission
C95.00	Leukemia, acute, without mention of remission
C95.10	Leukemia, chronic, without mention of remission
C95.11	Leukemia, chronic, in remission
D50.8	Anemia, iron deficiency, due to inadequate iron intake
D16.818	Pancytopenia, acquired
D69.6	Thrombocytopenia, not otherwise specified
D72.819	Leukopenia, not otherwise specified
D72.829	Leukocytosis
R50.9	Fever of unknown origin
R16.1	Splenomegaly, unspecified or unknown etiology

Acknowledgment

The editors recognize the many contributions by John M. O'Brien, MD, to this chapter in a previous edition of this text.

SUPPLIERS

(See contact information available at www.expertconsult.com.)

Goldenberg Snarecoil bone marrow aspiration and biopsy tray (Covidien)
Jamshidi bone marrow biopsy/aspiration needle (Cardinal Health)

RECOMMENDED READING

Bain B. Bone marrow aspiration. *J Clin Pathol*. 2001;54:657–663.
Bain B. Bone marrow trephine biopsy. *J Clin Pathol*. 2001;54:737–742.
Islam A. Bone marrow aspiration before bone marrow core biopsy using the same bone marrow biopsy needle: a good or bad practice? *J Clin Pathol*. 2007;60:212–215.
Riley R, Hogan T, Pavot D, et al. A pathologist's perspective on bone marrow aspiration and biopsy: I. Performing a bone marrow examination. *J Clin Lab Anal*. 2004;18:70–90.
Wilkins BS. Pitfalls in bone marrow pathology: avoiding errors in bone marrow trephine biopsy diagnosis. *J Clin Pathol*. 2011;64(5):380–386.

CHAPTER 221

LUMBAR PUNCTURE

Jeffrey A. German • John O'Brien

Lumbar puncture is performed to obtain cerebrospinal fluid (CSF) and is vital for making many neurologic diagnoses. In ordinary circumstances, the adult brain floats in about 150 mL of CSF and is capable of manufacturing about 500 mL/day. Examination of the CSF remains the most direct and accurate method of determining if there is a central nervous system infection. Lumbar puncture should be a routine procedure in febrile adults with an altered mental status and no other source of fever and in febrile children who appear toxic, regardless of age. Whereas computed tomography (CT) and magnetic resonance imaging have somewhat superseded lumbar puncture for making various neurologic diagnoses, they have also increased the safety of performing a lumbar puncture. Although the sensitivity of CT for making the diagnosis of subarachnoid hemorrhage (SAH) can range from 92% to 98% when performed within 24 hours of the onset of symptoms, it decreases to 75% when performed at 48 to 72 hours. It is often negative in patients with a sentinel bleed, which occur in 20% to 50% of patients, hours, days, weeks, or months before a major SAH. Xanthochromia, when measured by spectrophotometry, has a sensitivity approaching 100% when performed between 12 hours and 2 weeks after SAH; therefore, a lumbar puncture must be performed if SAH is still suspected after a negative CT. If adequate time has elapsed (>2 hours), xanthochromia and red blood cells (RBCs) should be seen. If there has not been adequate time for RBCs to migrate to the lumbar spine area, a cerebral angiogram or repeat lumbar puncture in 12 to 18 hours should be performed. Although lumbar puncture is generally a diagnostic procedure, it can also have therapeutic applications (e.g., pseudotumor cerebri, elevated CSF pressure, normal pressure hydrocephalus).

INDICATIONS

- Suspected central nervous system infection (e.g., meningitis, encephalitis)
- Suspected SAH (If available, a CT scan should be done first. It will exclude certain causes for increased intracranial pressure. However, CT has a false-negative rate of up to 25% for blood. With a bleed, xanthochromic color of CSF [visible >2 hours after the bleed] and an abnormal RBC count [>1000/mm^3] should be seen.)
- Pseudotumor cerebri (now known as *idiopathic intracranial hypertension*; lumbar puncture can be diagnostic or therapeutic) or normal-pressure hydrocephalus (diagnostic)
- New onset seizures
- Guillain-Barré syndrome (very high CSF protein level [>200 mg/dL])
- Multiple sclerosis (Usually the immunoglobulin G [IgG] level is elevated and oligoclonal banding is present on electrophoresis.)
- Spinal analgesia
- Lupus cerebritis (CSF may be normal, but some reports have noted elevated levels of anti-DNA antibodies, IgG, oligoclonal banding, immune complexes, interleukin-6, and the chemokine CXCL10.)

- Acute demyelinating disorders (e.g., encephalomyelitis, transverse myelitis)
- Dementia (if normal-pressure hydrocephalus, syphilis or other chronic infection, or vasculitis is suspected as a cause)
- Meningeal carcinomatosis
- Unexplained neurologic disorders if CT is negative (e.g., altered level of consciousness, polyneuropathy)
- Intrathecal antibiotics or chemotherapeutics
- Imaging procedures (e.g., myelography, cisternography)

CONTRAINDICATIONS

- Local skin infection (absolute contraindication)
- Raised intracranial pressure (suggested by the presence of papilledema, suspected SAH, or clinical risk factor[s] for intracranial pathology [Box 221.1] unless the CT scan is negative)
  NOTE: The absence of papilledema is not always a reliable sign of normal intracranial pressure because it often takes more than 48 hours for papilledema to develop. Papilledema will be absent in up to 15% of adults and 50% of children with early increased intracranial pressure.
- Supratentorial mass lesions (should be evaluated by CT scan first)
  NOTE: Certain CT findings indicate a predisposition to herniation if a lumbar puncture is performed: (1) a midline shift, (2) a loss of the suprachiasmatic and basilar cisterns, or (3) any evidence of a posterior fossa mass or obliteration of the superior cerebellar cistern or the quadrigeminal plate cistern caudal to the midbrain. Brain abscesses seem to be particularly predisposing to herniation.

BOX 221.1 Clinical Findings Associated With Increased Risk of Intracranial Pathology

Abnormal language
Age 60 yr or older
Altered level of consciousness
Arm drift
Facial palsy
Gaze palsy
History of central nervous system disease
Immunocompromised state
Inability to correctly answer two questions
Inability to follow two consecutive commands
Leg drift
Seizure within 1 wk of presentation
Visual field abnormality

From Straus SE, Thorpe KE, Holroyd-Leduc J. How do I perform a lumbar puncture and analyze the results to diagnose bacterial meningitis? JAMA. 2006;296:2012–2022.

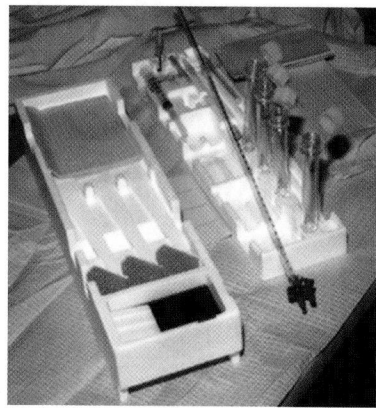

Fig. 221.1 Lumbar puncture equipment tray.

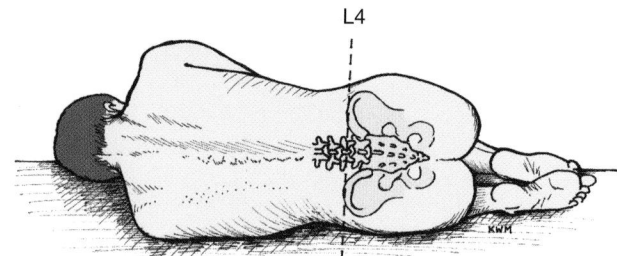

Fig. 221.2 Location of anatomic landmarks.

- Severe bleeding diathesis or coagulopathy (e.g., platelet count dropping rapidly or <20,000/mm³ [platelets should be transfused]), or anticoagulated patient (international normalized ratio >1.4) (relative contraindications; however, the most experienced clinician should perform the procedure using the smallest-gauge needle available)
- Unstable patient (If patient has hypotension, shock, status asthmaticus, or unstable airway, lumbar puncture should be delayed until patient is stable.)
  NOTE: Meningitis itself can cause increased intracranial pressure. Consequently, patients with decorticate or decerebrate posturing, focal neurologic signs, or no response to pain should receive antibiotics without lumbar puncture even if the CT scan is negative.
- Uncooperative adult patient (Sedation may need to be considered.)
- Prior lumbar fusion or laminectomy (It is technically difficult to enter subarachnoid space in the presence of significant postoperative changes.)

PREPROCEDURE PATIENT PREPARATION

Indications, alternatives, risks, potential benefits, and expected results should be discussed with the patient or representative, and he or she should sign an informed consent form (see the sample patient education and consent forms available at www.expertconsult.com). The patient should expect some discomfort with injection of the local anesthetic and as the spinal needle is inserted. It will be important for him or her to remain very still during certain portions of the procedure. If the patient is a child or minor, the parents or caregiver can be asked if they would like to be present during the procedure.

EQUIPMENT

Spinal tray (Fig. 221.1) containing the following:

- Skin antiseptic swabs such as those with povidone–iodine or chlorhexidine
- Alcohol swab
- Fenestrated drape and sterile gloves
- Manometer, three-way stopcock
- 1% lidocaine
- 3-mL syringe with 20- to 23-gauge needle (for drawing up anesthetic)
- 25- to 27-gauge skin needle
- 20- to 22-gauge spinal needle plus a spare (Traditional is Quincke spinal needle with sharp, beveled end, which is a cutting needle; options include Sprotte or Whitacre, which are noncutting or pencil point. However, passage of a thin atraumatic needle may be difficult in a thick-skinned individual; initiating the proce-

dure with a Quincke, down to level of interspinal ligament, and finishing with an atraumatic needle may be helpful.)*
- Four numbered, capped test tubes
- Sterile dressing (Band-Aid)
- Pulse oximetry (optional, may be especially helpful for children)
- Lidocaine-prilocaine (eutectic mixture of local anesthetic or EMLA) cream (optional; although shown to be more effective in adults than lidocaine infiltration alone, it must be applied 30 to 60 minutes before the procedure and local anesthetic should still be injected)
- 1-mL syringe (optional, but may be helpful if CSF not flowing)
- 21- to 25-gauge butterfly needle (optional)
- Ultrasound machine, high frequency probe (5 to 10 MHz), ultrasound gel, pen, or surgical skin marker (Technique can be used when landmark-guided approach has failed or when spinal landmarks are difficult to palpate.)

NOTE: Some experts advocate the use of a butterfly needle in children; the tubing is then used to estimate opening pressure. However, epidermoid tumors due to implanted dermal cells have been associated with use of a spinal needle without a stylet.

TECHNIQUE

1. In patients with focal neurologic findings, altered mentation, immunocompromise, suspected SAH, or papilledema (see Box 221.1), consider CT scan first.
   NOTE: If meningitis is suspected, the initiation of antibiotics should not be delayed while awaiting the CT scan results.
2. Position the patient near the edge of the bed (or the examination table) in the lateral decubitus or sitting position. Slightly flex the neck anteriorly. If the patient is lying down, give the patient a pillow to keep the head in line with the vertebral axis, and ask him or her to "curl up into a ball" with the knees drawn up to the abdomen (Fig. 221.2). The shoulders and pelvis should be aligned vertically without forward or backward tilt. If the patient is lying down, his or her shoulders, back, and hips should be exactly perpendicular to the bed. Identify the L3-L4 interspace (a line drawn between the superior aspect of the iliac crests intersects the body of L4). If necessary, the L2-L3, L4-L5, or L5-S1 interspaces can be used (Fig. 221.3). Some clinicians mark the site with a pen or make a small indention with the hub of a needle. In infants, the cord can reach the L3 vertebrae, so the needle should be place at the L4-L5, or L5-S1 interspace.
   NOTE: Although the lying position may be more comfortable for the patient, the sitting position is most commonly used in adults. With the patient sitting, it is usually easier to identify the midline and palpate the spinous processes, particularly when the patient is obese. The sitting position may also increase hydrostatic pressure in a dehydrated patient, but the clinician should be cautious for orthostatic changes in blood pressure. Flexing the patient's hips when sitting by using a stool to support the patient's feet will increase lumbar interspinous width.

---

*Atraumatic spinal needles have been shown to reduce the complication of spinal headache (i.e., less risk of a CSF leak).

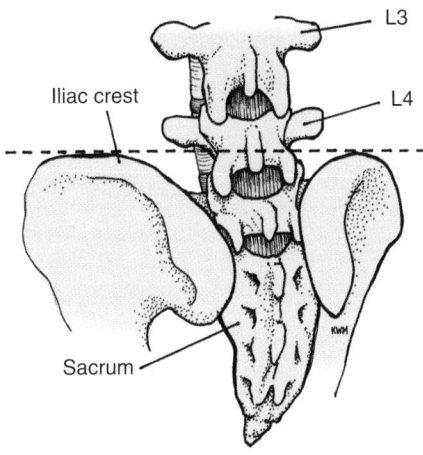

Fig. 221.3 Line across the iliac crests intersects the body of L4.

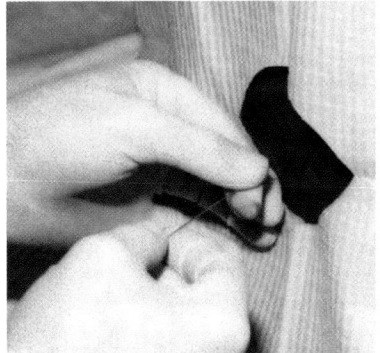

Fig. 221.4 Proper angle for entering spinal canal (with patient seated). Needle is directed cephalad.

3. Open the spinal tray in a sterile manner. Put on sterile gloves. Prepare the patient's skin at the selected interspace, plus the one above and below, with an antiseptic solution such as povidone–iodine or chlorhexidine. The prepared area is usually at least 10 cm in diameter; cover the area with a fenestrated drape. If lidocaine–prilocaine (EMLA) cream is used, it must be applied at least 30 to 60 minutes before beginning the procedure, and it only anesthetizes the skin and subcutaneous tissue, so a local anesthetic will still need to be injected.
4. Draw 3 mL of 1% lidocaine into the syringe with the 20- to 23-gauge needle. Administer local anesthetic with the skin needle and raise a wheal over the L3-L4 interspace in the midline. Inject a small amount deeper into the posterior spinous region, in the direction that the spinal needle will follow. (Some experts perform a field block for anesthesia. Sensation to the interspinous ligaments and the periosteum is supplied by the recurrent spinal nerves, which branch off the nerve roots exiting the spinal canal at the same level. A field block is performed by first injecting a small amount of local anesthetic into the interspinous ligaments in the midline, and then above and below the intended location of the lumbar puncture. The block is completed by redirecting the needle laterally, to both sides of the intended lumbar puncture site, and injecting a small amount of anesthetic.)
5. Preassemble the manometer while waiting for the anesthetic to take effect. It is usually in two pieces that slide together. Insert the manometer into the vertical port of the three-way stopcock and set this assembly to the side on the sterile field. Next, open the numbered test tubes. Place them upright, in order, in the slots provided in the plastic tray.
6. Palpate the posterior spinous process. Using this and the umbilicus as landmarks, insert a 20- or 22-gauge spinal needle through the skin in the midline. The needle can be held with both index fingers and advanced with the thumb(s), or it can be guided with a thumb and forefinger near the puncture site while the other hand advances the needle by putting pressure on the hub. Angle the needle about 15 degrees cephalad, toward the umbilicus, keeping it level with the sagittal midplane of the body (Figs. 221.4 and 221.5). Keep the bevel of the needle parallel to the longitudinal axis of the spine (point turned upward or downward with the patient in the lateral decubitus position, or to one side if the patient is sitting) as the needle is advanced. If bone is encountered, withdraw the needle slightly and change its angle, usually more cephalad. Depending on the size of the patient, after the needle has advanced about 3 to 4 cm, stop, withdraw the stylus, and check the hub for fluid. If there is no fluid, replace the stylus and advance another fraction before repeating this again. In obese patients, the

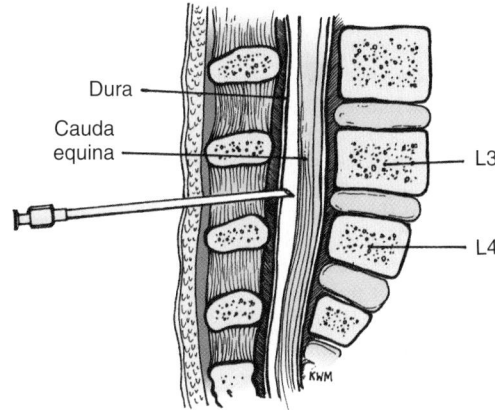

Fig. 221.5 Drop in resistance will be felt as the needle penetrates the dura.

needle may need to be advanced to the hub. Usually a slight "pop" is felt as the spinal needle penetrates the dura; however, this may not be felt using a Quincke needle. Advance the needle 1 to 2 mm farther and withdraw the stylus. Rotating the needle 90 to 180 degrees is sometimes helpful if no fluid returns. If the patient experiences pain radiating down one leg or the tap is "dry," remove the needle completely and make an attempt at a different interspace. A dry tap is more often due to a poorly positioned patient or an improperly placed needle than to an obliterated subarachnoid space; often the needle tip has migrated laterally out of the midline. For repeated dry taps, reposition the patient from lying to sitting, or vice versa, and attempt puncture again while making sure the needle is directed toward the midline. Approach from a lateral site is also described later. CSF may fail to flow in certain low intracranial pressure situations (e.g., dehydrated patient), so gentle suction with a 1-mL syringe may be helpful.

NOTE: For very large or obese patients, it may be impossible to palpate the spinous process for use as a landmark. Ultrasound may help locate the bone in the spinous process and the technique is described later (see also Chapter 214, "Emergency Department, Hospitalist, and Office Ultrasound [Clinical Ultrasound]").

7. Once fluid is obtained, the needle hub should be "anchored," or held firmly between the thumb and index finger of one hand that is braced against the patient's back. Whenever anything is attached or removed from the needle, use the other hand. Next, place the end of the stopcock with the attached manometer onto the hub of the needle. Have the patient straighten the legs and relax his or her position so that the opening pressure is not artificially elevated. The CSF should rise in the manometer to the level of the opening pressure. The pressure

TABLE 221.1	Normal Cerebrospinal Fluid Values		
Value	**Term Infant**	**Child**	**Adult**
Opening pressure (mm H₂O)	50–80	50–80	70–200 (up to 250 in obese)
WBC count (WBC/mm³)	9 (range, 0–22, 19 for infants 28 days or younger)	<7	<5
Neutrophils	61%	None	None
Glucose (ratio of blood/CSF glucose and CSF level [mg/dL])	60%–128% (34–119)	50% (40–80)	60%–70% (50–80)
Protein level (mg/dL)	20–170 (mean 90)	5–40	15–45

CSF, Cerebrospinal fluid; *WBC,* white blood cell.

TABLE 221.2	Recommended Cerebrospinal Fluid Tests		
Tube 1: Bacteriology	**Tube 2: Biochemistry**	**Tube 3: Hematology**	**Tube 4: Optional**
Gram stain	Glucose	Cell count	VDRL*
Acid-fast stain*	Protein	Differential	India ink*
Culture	Protein		Cryptococcal antigen*
Bacteria	electropho-		Cytology*
Fungal*	resis* (need		Oligoclonal bands*
Tuberculosis*	concurrent		Myelin basic protein*
Viral*	serum study)		Countercurrent immunoelectro-phoresis*
			Serologic, PCR and genetic tests for other microor-ganisms*
			Anti-DNA antibod-ies, immune complexes, interleukin-6, chemokine, and CXCL10 levels*

*If clinically indicated.
CXCL10, chemokine (C-X-C motif) ligand 10; *PCR,* Polymerase chain reaction; *VDRL,* Venereal Disease Research Laboratory.

is accurate only if the patient is lying on his or her side in a relaxed position. If tubing is in between the needle and manometer, the base of the manometer should still be held at the level of the needle hub for accurate readings. Note the color of the fluid and the opening pressure. CSF pressure should oscillate slightly with respiration (and sometimes with the pulse).

8. In case the fluid is bloody and does not clear after the first few drops of fluid (bloody tap), replace the stylus and remove the spinal needle. Select an alternative lumbar interspace above or below the current level and reattempt lumbar puncture as described in steps 4 through 7.

   NOTE: Bloody CSF due to SAH will not clot. Also, after spinning in a centrifuge, the supernatant is xanthochromic.

9. Turn the stopcock to allow the CSF to flow into the test tubes. Keep track of the order in which they are filled. Fill at least three test tubes with 2 to 3 mL of CSF each (at least 2 mL is necessary for cytology or antigen testing). Label each tube in the order it was collected. A fourth tube can be filled and frozen in case further studies are needed. Table 221.1 shows normal CSF values, and Table 221.2 lists recommended CSF tests. Tube 1 is most likely to be contaminated with blood from the needle insertion; therefore tube 3 should be tested for the cell count and differential. Minor blood contamination usually clears by the third tube.

10. Once you have obtained enough CSF, replace the stylus and withdraw the needle.

11. Cover the puncture site with a sterile dressing.

12. For a therapeutic lumbar puncture (i.e., for pseudotumor cerebri), remove enough CSF to reduce the closing pressure to 100 mm H₂O or less (usually 25 to 35 mL of CSF). For a diagnostic tap, removal of 35 to 50 mL may result in transient improvement in gait or cognition for suspected normal-pressure hydrocephalus.

Technique for Lateral Approach

The lateral approach technique may be preferred in elderly patients with calcified supraspinous and intraspinous ligaments. It may also be used if the midline approach has failed. The patient may be in either the sitting or the lateral decubitus position, and should be prepared and draped in the same interspaces as described previously. Anesthesia should be applied/injected in a location 1.5 to 2 cm lateral to the midline, on either side if the patient is in the sitting position or on the lower side if the patient is in the lateral decubitus position. Local anesthetic should be injected in the location and direction that the spinal needle will follow. The spinal needle should be directed approximately 15 degrees cephalad and 20 degrees to the midline (Fig. 221.6). From this location, the needle usually bypasses the supraspinous and infraspinous ligaments, and instead penetrates the erector spinae muscles and the paraspinous ligaments, and then the ligamentum flavum, dura, and

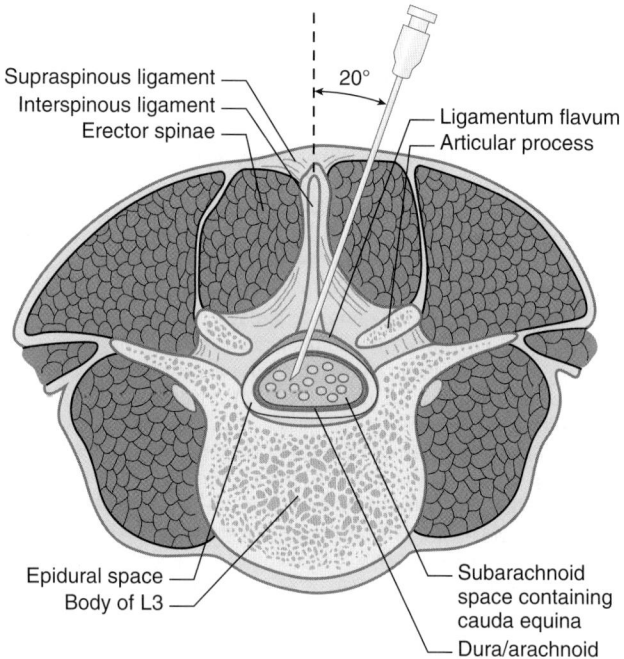

Fig. 221.6 Using the lateral approach, the needle is inserted 1.5–2 cm lateral to the midline and is directed approximately 20 degrees toward the midline and 15 degrees cephalad. (From Reichman EF, ed. *Emergency Medicine Procedures,* 2nd ed. New York: McGraw-Hill; 2013.)

subarachnoid space. If bone is encountered, the needle should be withdrawn slightly and redirected in the same angle toward the midline but slightly more cephalad. The remainder of the procedure is as described previously.

Technique for Pediatric Patients

The preferred position for infants (especially premature infants and neonates) is with the infant seated with the head only slightly flexed.

Overflexion of the head can lead to hypoxia and respiratory arrest in young infants. Likewise, increased intra-abdominal pressure caused by flexing the knees into the abdomen may lead to compression of the diaphragm and hypoxia. Consequently, the child should be monitored visually and possibly with pulse oximetry during the procedure. Proper positioning is usually best accomplished by an assistant who can also monitor the airway and oxygenation. If the infant suddenly stops crying, check the airway immediately. Preoxygenation with 100% oxygen by face mask for 2 to 5 minutes before the procedure may prevent hypoxia. If the procedure is performed with the child lying, a modified lateral decubitus position should be used (i.e., hips flexed only to 90 degrees). Draping should be done conservatively to avoid interfering with any infant monitors. The skin can be anesthetized initially with a patch containing EMLA cream, if it is available, followed 30 to 60 minutes later by an injection with lidocaine. The spinal needle is directed slightly cephalad. In young infants a "pop" or change in resistance may not be felt as the needle penetrates the dura. Use a 20- to 22-gauge, 1½-inch needle for infants. A 3.5-inch spinal needle can be used in children older than 12 years.

NOTE: Local anesthetic should be used in all children. There is evidence that pain perception is present even in premature neonates.

Technique for Ultrasound-Guided Lumbar Puncture

Anesthesiologists and interventional radiologists have been using ultrasound to guide spinal procedures such as lumbar puncture for many years. This technique is most helpful when the landmark-guided approach has failed or when spinal landmarks are difficult to palpate such as in an obese patient. While a high frequency probe (5 to 10 MHz) will generally be useful, it may result in an image that is too superficial to see a spinous process. Therefore, a lower frequency probe, such as a curvilinear 3.5 to 5 MHz probe, may be needed in the obese patient.

With this technique, ultrasound is basically used to define and mark the site for lumbar puncture using the vertebral spinous processes as landmarks. In so doing, longitudinal and transverse views are utilized. For a longitudinal scan, orient the probe so that the marker dot is toward the patient's head (cephalad); for a transverse scan, turn the marker dot to the patient's right side (see also Chapter 214, "Emergency Department, Hospitalist and Office Ultrasound [Clinical Ultrasound]"). Ultrasound will not penetrate bone, so the spinous processes appear as echogenic, dense white structures curving away from the probe with shadows cast below them. From the longitudinal view, two spinous processes should be located in the midline. Using the marker pen, place a mark or dot beside the probe at the midway point between these two spinous processes at the appropriate level (slightly above or below the level of the iliac crest). Next, rotate the probe 90 degrees for a transverse view (marker dot to the patient's right side). Center the probe over the spinous process above and below the previous mark, and mark the midline of the spine with a dot beside the probe above each spinous process. A line connecting these two dots should cross the point determined as midway from the longitudinal scan. This is the site for lumbar puncture to be performed in the same manner as described previously.

COMPLICATIONS

- *Post–lumbar (post–dural) puncture headache* occurs in 10% to 25% of patients and is usually self-limited. The headache usually lasts for only a few days, but may last longer than a week and can be debilitating. Cases lasting months have been described. Ninety percent of spinal headaches occur within 48 hours after dural puncture, but may occur up to 14 days later. While the headache is postural, or exacerbated by sitting upright and is relieved by lying down, there appears to be no benefit from enforcing bed rest following lumbar puncture for preventing the headaches. The incidence increases with repeat lumbar punctures in a patient;

it is also age dependent, with the highest incidence in 18- to 30-year-olds, and a decreased incidence after age 60 for reasons unknown. It is also more common in women and in individuals with a history of headache. The incidence is reduced by using a higher-gauge (24- to 27-gauge) or atraumatic needle, but these smaller needles have a higher failure rate and take longer to obtain samples, and opening pressures cannot be measured; therefore, in practice, a 22-gauge needle is typically used. The incidence of headache was thought to be reduced by keeping the bevel of the needle oriented parallel to the long axis of the patient's spine, thereby spreading rather than cutting the fibers of the ligamenta flava and dura. However, it is now known that the orientation of the dural fibers are random and not longitudinal; nevertheless, using a longitudinal orientation of the needle has been found to cause fewer headaches. Replacement of the stylet before removing the spinal needle has also been shown to decrease the risk of spinal headaches. Oral caffeine, 300 mg, or theophylline, 200 mg, if not contraindicated, may provide relief in adults. Intravenous caffeine benzoate, 500 mg given over a few minutes, or aminophylline, 5 to 6 mg/kg, can also be used to treat refractory spinal headaches in adults. A repeat dose of caffeine can be given in 1 hour for an 85% chance of alleviation of symptoms. Other medications that have been advocated include barbiturates, codeine, neostigmine, ergots, diphenhydramine, amphetamines, ephedrine, intravenous fluids, magnesium sulfate, and vitamins, but benefits are largely unproven. Bed rest with the head in the horizontal position and avoiding dehydration seems like reasonable management for the first 24 hours. An occipital nerve block may also resolve the headache.

- Twenty-four hours after lumbar puncture, if there has been no relief from caffeine, an epidural blood patch can be performed. This usually provides relief in up to 85% of patients; after a second patch is performed, if necessary, 98% of patients experience relief. Perform the blood patch by injecting 15 mL of autologous blood into the dural space at the level of the previous lumbar puncture. Slow or discontinue the injection if back pain or paresthesias develop. Keep the patient supine for an hour while administering intravenous fluids; relief usually occurs within 20 to 30 minutes. The mechanism of action appears to be from forming a gelatinous tamponade to stop the dural leak; however, it is less likely to be effective if symptoms have been present for 2 weeks. Because the patient already has a spinal headache, the most experienced clinician available, such as an anesthesiologist, should probably perform the blood patch(es). Transient complications of the blood patch include back pain, paresthesias, radiculopathies, and weakness; rarely, spinal subdural hematoma has been reported. Before repeating a blood patch, some clinicians recommend consultation with a neurologist.

- *Epidermoid tumors* have been associated with lumbar punctures performed in the neonatal period, especially when needles are used without a stylus.

- *Seizures* have been reported in a small percentage of patients with post–dural puncture headaches.

- A *traumatic or "bloody" tap* from inadvertent puncture of the spinal venous plexuses is possible. This is self-limiting in the majority of patients but could lead to a spinal hematoma in patients with bleeding disorders. Some authorities recommend sending the first and fourth tubes for cell count (RBCs and WBCs with a differential) if a traumatic tap is suspected. The RBC count will decrease from tube 1 to tube 4 in the case of a traumatic tap. A correction can be made for CSF leukocytes and CSF protein if the tap is traumatic. For every 700 RBCs, CSF leukocytes increase by 1 and CSF protein rises 1 mg/dL.

- *Brain herniation* from a supratentorial mass or increased intracranial pressure is another complication. Always check the fundi for papilledema before performing lumbar puncture. If a tumor, intracranial bleed, intracranial pathology (see Box 221.1), or marked increased pressure is suspected, an emergency CT scan should be obtained before a lumbar puncture is done, to reduce the chance of herniation.

- *Intracranial subdural hematoma* is a rare complication and is due to the same mechanism that causes post–lumbar puncture headache (especially with persistent CSF leakage) or brain herniation—that is, downward displacement of the brain. Such displacement can result in tearing of the bridging veins and lead to bilateral or unilateral subdural hematoma.
- *Spinal epidural or subdural hematoma* can present with paraplegia, lower extremity weakness, sensory deficits, or incontinence. Anticoagulated patients or those with a coagulopathy should be monitored closely for this complication.
- *Paresthesias* in the lower extremities are common and usually transient, but in rare cases can last for more than a year.
- *Local pain* in the back may be due to injury of the local tissue, the periosteum, or the spinal ligaments. Mild, transient pain is common.
- *Disk herniation* is a very rare complication and is caused by a needle passing through the entire subarachnoid space and into the annulus fibrosus. It can also result in diskitis or vertebral collapse.
- *Cranial nerve palsies* involving cranial nerves III, IV, V, VI, VII, and VIII have been reported. These are usually transient, present with visual and auditory symptoms, and are caused by traction on the nerve due to low intracranial pressure after lumbar puncture.
- *Nerve root aspiration* is a possible complication. Replacing the stylus before withdrawing the needle may prevent aspiration of nerve roots. Very rarely, nerve root diverticula can rupture as a result of lumbar puncture, causing a brief CSF leak and a spinal headache.
- *Meningitis* resulting from the procedure is a theoretical complication. Bacteremia is not a contraindication to lumbar puncture.

PATIENT EDUCATION GUIDES

See the sample patient education and consent forms available at www.expertconsult.com. A video of ultrasonically directed lumbar puncture can be purchased at www.Sonosite.com.

CPT/BILLING CODES

- 62270   Spinal puncture, lumbar, diagnostic
- 62272   Spinal puncture, therapeutic, for drainage of cerebrospinal fluid
- 62273   Injection, epidural, of blood or clot patch
- 62311   Injection, single, of diagnostic or therapeutic substances; (including anesthetic, antispasmodic, opioid, steroid, other solution), lumbar, sacral
- 76942   Ultrasonic guidance for needle placement (e.g., biopsy, aspiration, injection, localization device), imaging, supervision and interpretation

ICD-10-CM DIAGNOSTIC CODES

D49.7	Meningeal carcinoma or neoplasm
F02.80	Dementia in conditions classified elsewhere
G00.0	Meningitis due to hemophilus meningitis
G00.1	Pneumococcal meningitis
G00.2	Streptococcal meningitis. *Use additional code to identify organism*
G00.3	Staphylococcal meningitis. *Use additional code to identify organism*
G00.9	Meningitis due to unspecified bacterium
G03.0	Nonpyogenic meningitis
G03.9	Meningitis, unspecified
G04.89	Encephalitis, myelitis, and encephalomyelitis, unspecified cause
G35	Multiple sclerosis
G93.2	Pseudotumor cerebri
G61.0	Guillain-Barré syndrome
I60.9	Subarachnoid hemorrhage, nontraumatic
M32.9	Systemic lupus erythematosus
S06.6X0X	Subarachnoid hemorrhage after injury without open intracranial wound, unspecified state of consciousness

Use additional seventh character: A=initial, D=subsequent, S=sequela.

RECOMMENDED READING

Behrman RE, Kliegman RM, Jenson HB, eds. *Nelson Textbook of Pediatrics.* 20th ed. Philadelphia: Saunders; 2016.

Eng RH, Seligman SJ. Lumbar puncture-induced meningitis. *JAMA.* 1981;245:1456–1459.

Euerle BD. Spinal puncture and cerebrospinal fluid examination. In: Roberts JR, Custalow CB, Thomsen TW, eds. *Roberts and Hedges Clinical Procedures in Emergency Medicine.* 6th ed. Philadelphia: Elsevier; 2014:1218–1242.

Reichman EF, Polglaze K, Eurle B. Lumbar puncture. In: Reichman EF, ed. *Emergency Medicine Procedures.* 2nd ed. New York: McGraw-Hill; 2013:747–761.

Johnson KS, Sexton DJ. Lumbar puncture: technique; indications; contraindications; and complications in adults. In: Rose BD, ed. *UpToDate.* 2005. www.uptodate.com.

Siberry GK, Iannone R. *The Harriet Lane Handbook.* 21st ed. St. Louis: Mosby; 2017.

Straus SE, Thorpe KE, Holroyd-Leduc J. How do I perform a lumbar puncture and analyze the results to diagnose bacterial meningitis? *JAMA.* 2006;296:2012–2022.

Thomas SR, Jamieson DR, Muir KW. Randomized controlled trial of atraumatic versus standard needles for diagnostic lumbar puncture. *BMJ.* 2000;321:986–990.

CHAPTER 222

TRACHEAL INTUBATION

Dan F. Casey

Airway emergencies can be some of the most daunting situations a practitioner encounters. Radical advances in airway management have been made and are reviewed in this chapter.

INDICATIONS

- Hypoxia
- Respiratory distress
- Protection of the airway
- Cardiopulmonary arrest
- Need to maintain hyperventilation (e.g., with traumatic brain injury)

CONTRAINDICATIONS

- Need for emergent surgical airway
- Severe facial or neck trauma (consider needle or surgical cricothyroidotomy; see Chapter 223, Cricothyroid Catheter Insertion, Cricothyroidotomy, and Tracheostomy)
- Intact tracheostomy or stoma (replace tracheostomy tube)
- Cervical spine injury (may use video and optical laryngoscopes, fiberoptic laryngoscope, or digital [tactile] technique)
- Cervical spine severely immobilized due to arthritis (may use video and optical laryngoscopes, fiberoptic laryngoscope, or digital [tactile] technique)
- Expanding neck hematoma (relative, must use caution but may require surgical airway)
- Uncontrolled oropharyngeal hemorrhage (relative, may require surgical airway)
- Combative patient (consider rapid-sequence intubation [RSI])
- Trismus (consider RSI or nasotracheal intubation)
- When a less invasive technique may be adequate in a patient whose medical conditions are likely to respond quickly to medical interventions (e.g., cardiogenic pulmonary edema or pneumonitis may respond to diuresis and continuous positive airway pressure [CPAP] or bilateral positive airways pressure [BIPAP] if they have a normal mental status and are breathing spontaneously)

EQUIPMENT

See Fig. 222.1.

- Laryngoscope (and fresh batteries)
- Laryngoscope blades (at least two different types)
  - Size 1 for infants age 1 month to 2 years, size 2 for children 3 to 6 years, size 2 or 3 for children between 6 and 12 years, size 3 for adolescents, women, and average-sized males, size 4 for large males. To estimate size, place base of blade, excluding the insertion block, at the level of the patient's upper incisor teeth. The tip of blade should be 1 cm proximal or distal to angle of mandible.
- Endotracheal tubes
  - Adult men sizes 7 to 9
  - Adult women sizes 6 to 8
  - Nasotracheal intubation sizes 5 to7

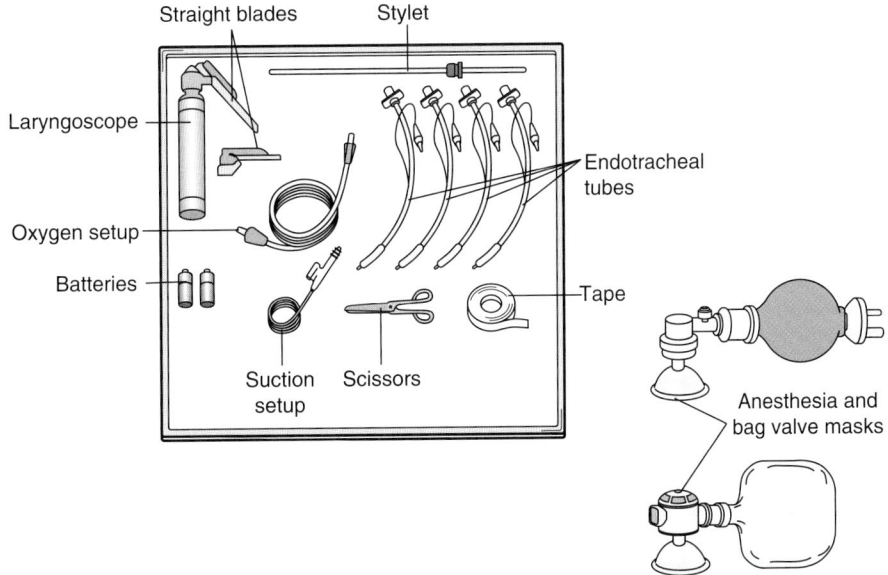

Fig. 222.1 Suggested intubation equipment.

- Pediatrics—Consult Broselow tape or use the size equal to the width of the fingernail of the little finger. Use uncuffed tubes in infants and small children up to 8 years of age.
- Stylet (optional, but most useful when bent to 35 degrees in hockey stick configuration) or esophageal bougienage (bougie with coudé tip, which has hockey stick configuration)
- Water-soluble lubricant
- 10-mL syringe
- Umbilical tape or endotracheal tube holding device
- Scissors
- Bag-valve-mask device (Ambu-bag) with 100% oxygen delivery system
- Suction system with dental or Yankauer tip
- Stethoscope
- Pulse oximeter
- Capnograph, carbon dioxide detector, esophageal detector, or other device to confirm tube placement
- Cardiac monitor and defibrillator
- Blood pressure monitor
- Gloves
- Face mask, goggles, or eye shield, and any other equipment necessary to follow universal blood and body fluid precautions
- Intravenous line (if possible)
- Ventilator
- Cricothyroidotomy kit
- Sedative medication to use for chemical restraint (e.g., Propofol, benzodiazepines)
- For rapid sequence intubation, paralytic agent (e.g., succinylcholine, rocuronium, vecuronium, atracurium, mivacurium), sedative agent (e.g., etomidate, ketamine, midazolam, thiopental), and adjuncts (e.g., lidocaine, atropine)
- Glidescope or equivalent for video-assisted intubation (see Fig. 222.9)

EDITOR'S NOTE: The ET tube and cuff should be examined for defects before use. No matter which hand is dominant for the physician, laryngoscopes are designed to be used in the left hand. The two basic laryngoscope blades are the Macintosh (curved; the tip fits into the vallecula) and the Miller (straight; the tip fits directly under the epiglottis to lift it), with the Macintosh being the most commonly used. Blade size is very important; correct size allows for approximately 90% of first attempt intubations to be successful versus 57% if the blade is too small.

CRICOID PRESSURE (SELLICK MANEUVER)

Providing or performing cricoid pressure may help protect against regurgitation of gastric contents; it also increases visibility by moving the trachea into the visual field of the person intubating. To perform cricoid pressure (Sellick maneuver), first find the thyroid cartilage (Adam's apple), and then the small indentation beneath it (cricothyroid membrane). The cartilage beneath this small indentation is the cricoid bone. Cricoid pressure is performed by pinching the extended thumb, index, and middle finger together into a double "V," or tripod. This is then placed on the cricoid bone and pressed down with enough pressure to occlude the esophagus (Fig. 222.2). The pressure should be applied toward the patient's back and the head somewhat. Cricoid pressure should not be released until intubation is completed and confirmed and the cuff inflated.

NOTE: The effectiveness of the Sellick maneuver has been questioned. Because of the wide variation in pressure applied by operators, cricoid pressure should be removed if there is difficulty in visualizing the airway. Another technique known as optimal external laryngeal manipulation (OLEM) can be tried. For OLEM, the intubator uses their right hand to manipulate the larynx into optimal position while simultaneously viewing the patient's airway and controlling the laryngoscope with their left hand. One study found

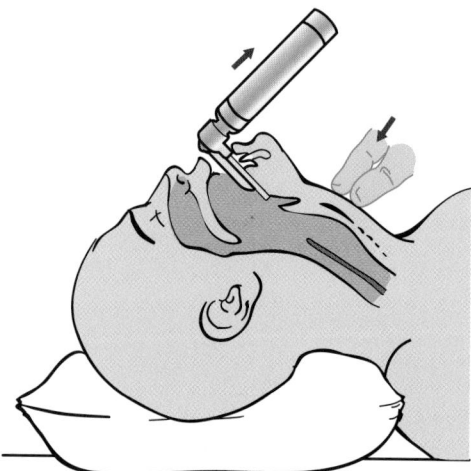
Fig. 222.2   Sellick maneuver. Either the practitioner or assistant uses the thumb and index and middle fingers pinched into a double "V" or tripod. Posterior pressure is then applied to the cricoid to avoid aspiration and bring the larynx into view. Note the upward and forward direction of forces applied in a nonfulcrum manner by the laryngoscope.

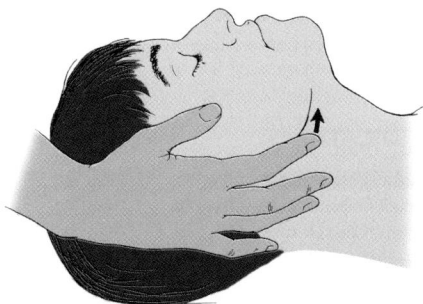
Fig. 222.3   Jaw thrust. Rotate mandible forward with index fingers. Arrow indicates motion to bring soft tissues forward to relieve airway obstruction.

that applying pressure to the thyroid cartilage was helpful in 88% of cases, while applying pressure on cricoid cartilage was only helpful in 11% (Benumof and Cooper, 1996). Once the best position is found, an assistant assumes control of the larynx by applying similar pressure in the same location and direction.

AIRWAY ASSESSMENT

Begin with the patient on 100% nonrebreather mask if spontaneously breathing. Remember that 5 minutes of preoxygenation provides 5 minutes of protection. The jaw thrust maneuver can be used to keep the airway open (Fig. 222.3), or begin bag-valve-mask breathing with a second assistant providing cricoid pressure (Sellick maneuver). Nasopharyngeal oxygen insufflation, even during apnea, has been found to be beneficial. Morbidly obese patients are best preoxygenated in a 25-degree head up position. The practitioner should be familiar with the anatomic landmarks (Fig. 222.4). Many airway management failures can be traced to lack of airway assessment. Patients can be classified into three groups (shades) based on two criteria: anticipated difficulty in intubation and ability to maintain oxygen saturation greater than 90% by bag-valve-mask ventilation. Airway assessment is critical. An experienced person can assess an airway in less than 4 seconds, and an inexperienced person should be able to do so in less than 8 seconds.

The mnemonic for assessing difficulty in intubation is 332-NUTS:

- 3—fingerbreadths, mouth opening
- 3—fingerbreadths, mentum (distance from the tip of the chin to the anterior soft tissue of the neck)

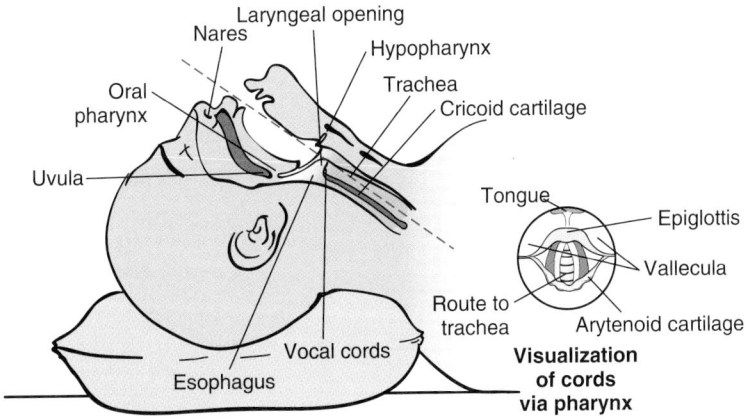

Fig. 222.4 Anatomic landmarks of the head and neck.

- **2**—fingerbreadths, thyromental distance (distance from the top of the thyroid cartilage to the upper soft tissue angle of the neck)
- **N**—normal neck flexion
- **U**—uvula visible when opening the mouth
- **T**—no tension pneumothorax
- **S**—no "soup" (foreign body in the airway)

Meeting all these criteria indicates a low-risk intubation; conversely, the fewer the criteria present, the higher the risk. Although the last two categories, tension pneumothorax and foreign body, do not strictly determine the anatomic difficulty of intubation, establishing their absence is a vital part of early airway assessment. The Mallampati system has previously been used to assess the uvular portion of the mnemonic; however, it is important to note that this classification was designed to assess a patient sitting upright with voluntary mouth opening—a condition rarely encountered in clinical practice outside anesthesiology. A simpler method is to open the mouth with the thumb while standing to either side of the patient's head. (Standing at the head of the patient changes the angle of view and may produce a false result.) If any portion of the uvula can be seen, then intubation will likely be unimpeded by this factor. The three risk groups (shades) are as follows:

- **Pink**—Able to keep the oxygen saturation greater than 90%; anticipate easy intubation and use standard technique.
- **Purple**—Able to keep the oxygen saturation greater than 90% but anticipate difficult intubation. Attempt awake laryngoscopy. If successful, perform an assisted intubation with a gum elastic bougie, lighted stylet, intubating, fiberoptic or video laryngoscope, or similar device. If not, use an intermediate airway (laryngeal mask airway [LMA] or King LTS-D) if possible, and obtain expert assistance for further management.
- **Blue**—Unable to keep the oxygen saturation greater than 90%. If possible, perform a single attempt at an intermediate airway (LMA or King LTS-D). If successful and easy intubation is anticipated, attempt assisted intubation as in the purple patient. If difficulty is anticipated, obtain expert assistance for further management if time permits. If not, needle or surgical cricothyroidotomy may be needed.

STANDARD OROTRACHEAL INTUBATION

Preparation

Lack of proper preparation is another common reason for failure to intubate. If the airway risk is purple or blue, auxiliary techniques should be strongly considered. However, if the patient is classified in the pink group, attempt standard orotracheal intubation. Prepare for intubation using the mnemonic "airway START." The airway prefix distinguishes it from a similar mnemonic used for triage in mass disasters.

- **S**—shade (classify the patient as pink, purple, or blue and select the proper technique)
- **T**—technicians (respiratory technician and cricoid pressure technician)
- **A**—assemble (ensure all the equipment and drugs are prepared)
- **R**—respiration (preoxygenate with at least eight vital capacity breaths. If time permits, and the patient is breathing spontaneously, 5 minutes of preoxygenation provides 5 minutes of protection.)
- **T**—tilt (ensure both the patient and the practitioner are properly positioned)

Technique

The cricoid pressure technician should initiate cricoid pressure using the Sellick maneuver as soon as the respiratory therapist begins bagging. This will reduce stomach insufflation and the risk for vomiting. The cricoid pressure technician also watches the oxygen saturation of the patient and announces saturations below 90% to the practitioner. In addition, this technician holds the endotracheal tube and passes it to the practitioner so the practitioner can focus uninterrupted on the intubating view.

"Tilt" or position of the patient and the practitioner is often overlooked, but this is probably the most critical component of successful intubation. If the patient is not suspected of having neck problems that could be worsened by movement, place the patient in the "sniffing" position with the neck flexed and the head extended backward (Fig. 222.5). The neck may be flexed by raising the head several inches using a folded towel or firm pillow. It is important to remember that the padding should be placed under the head and not between the shoulders (see Fig. 222.4).

The position of the practitioner is even more important. The most common problem is having an angle of view that is too high to visualize the anatomy, which is caused by being both too close to and too high above the patient. Crowded conditions at the head of the bed in most care settings compound this problem. Unfortunately, the practitioner usually reacts by bending forward at the waist, which serves only to worsen the angle of view. Raise the bed and move it a full 2 feet or more forward if possible. If a lower angle of view is needed, the practitioner should bend at the knees and not at the waist.

Intubation

The paraglossal technique has supplanted older methods of intubation. It is easier to learn, has a higher success rate, and uses the same technique regardless of whether a curved or straight blade is

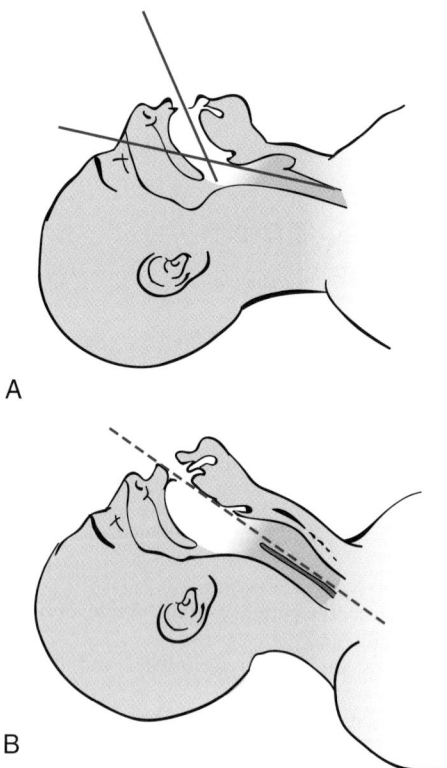

Fig. 222.5 Proper head position is important for successful endotracheal intubation. Axes of the mouth, pharynx, and larynx need to be aligned. (A) Divergent axes. (B) Axes in line, or "sniffing position."

used. Dr. Scott Savage, a previous author, nicknamed the method the "Diamond Technique," based on the four "Ds" of the steps used to intubate:

- **Dental**—Always hold the laryngoscope in the left hand. Place the flange of the blade against the right molars with no tongue intervening.
- **Deep**—Sweep the tongue centrally and insert the blade to the hilt or until resistance is met in the esophagus. If the patient is in the sniffing position, this is usually easy. If the patient cannot be moved safely into the sniffing position, follow the contour of the base of the tongue to reach the esophagus. Place the blade deeply and in the esophagus on purpose. In this position, the location of the tip of the blade is known and, more important, so is the location of the airway: shallow and superior to the blade tip.
- **Direct**—Once the blade is in the esophagus, lift the handle upward and forward (see Fig. 222.2), using the same technique as in the older methods of intubation.
- **Depart**—From this position, withdraw the blade while monitoring the view. Most of the time, there will be a slight sensation of "give" when the blade clears the esophagus, and a good intubating view is obtained.

From this position, the practitioner requests the tube from the cricoid pressure technician. Once received, the practitioner inserts it with the right hand guiding the tip down against the right buccal mucosa to avoid obstructing the intubating view (Fig. 222.6). A common mistake is to try to slide the tube straight down the center. This obstructs the view and increases the probability of accidental esophageal intubation. The endotracheal tube is advanced until the tip is at least 2 to 3 cm beyond the vocal cords.

Rarely, the tip of the epiglottis is encountered. If this is the case, lift the epiglottis with the blade tip. Using the right hand, after handing the tube back to the technician, replace the pressure on the cricoid cartilage that is being applied by the pressure technician. Consider

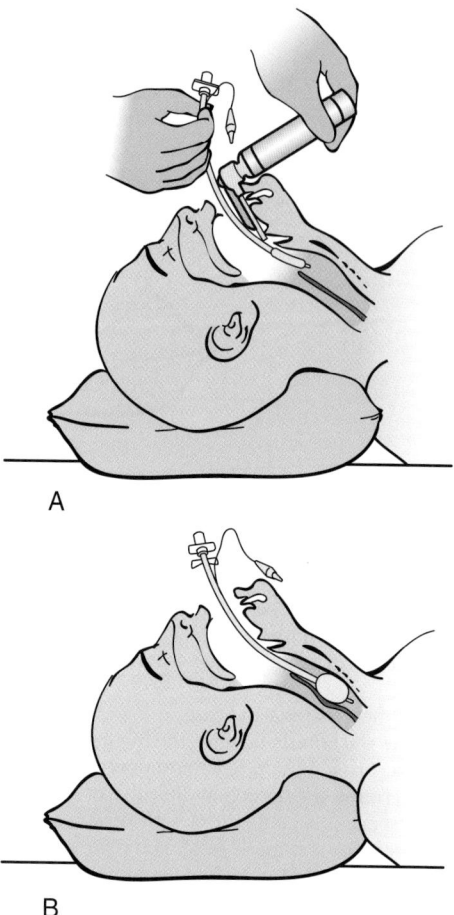

Fig. 222.6 Insertion of tube with laryngoscope in place. (A) Insert the tube with the tip initially against the right buccal mucosa so that a clear view of the vocal cords can be maintained at all times. As it advances, watch the tube pass through the cords. (B) The tube is correctly placed when the tip is 2 to 3 cm beyond the vocal cords.

OLEM to manipulate the trachea to obtain a good view (commonly, the cricoid pressure technician will use too much pressure). When a good view is obtained, have the cricoid pressure technician replace the same amount of pressure to maintain a constant view. The technician then hands the endotracheal tube back to the practitioner, who intubates the trachea as described previously. The tip and cuff of the ET tube must be visualized passing through the vocal cords to ensure proper placement. The tube insertion depth can be approximated by the Chula formula: 4 cm + (patient height in inches/4). In most patients, this will be between 21 and 23 cm. Inflate the balloon according to manufacturer directions. Most balloons take 10 mL of air.

Confirm Placement

Listen at the stomach to assess for an esophageal intubation, and then listen in each axilla to assess for equal breath sounds. Listening over the anterior chest is not as accurate as listening in the axillae for determining proper tube placement (Fig. 222.7). Asymmetric breath sounds suggest that the mainstem bronchus was intubated—typically, the right mainstem bronchus because it is more vertical than the left mainstem bronchus.

Next, use a secondary device to ensure proper placement. The devices available include bulb-type and syringe-type esophageal detector devices or carbon dioxide colorimetric devices. These devices are attached to the endotracheal tube after intubation. The bulb device is squeezed shut before being placed on the tube. If the bulb reinflates, the tube is in the proper location. One way to remember this is "reinflate means you're great." If a syringe device is used,

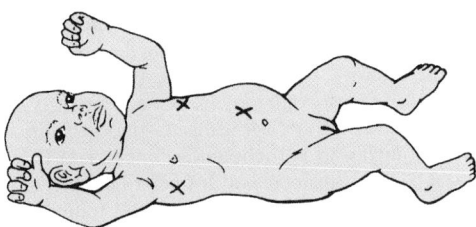

Fig. 222.7 Auscultation points for confirmation of placement are over the stomach (should be lack of sound) and the axillae. The same locations should be used to auscultate in the adult.

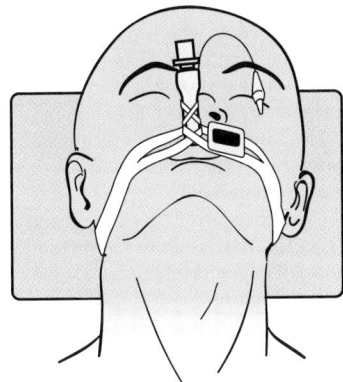

Fig. 222.8 Secure the tube to minimize patient discomfort while maintaining correct positioning. Consider a bite block.

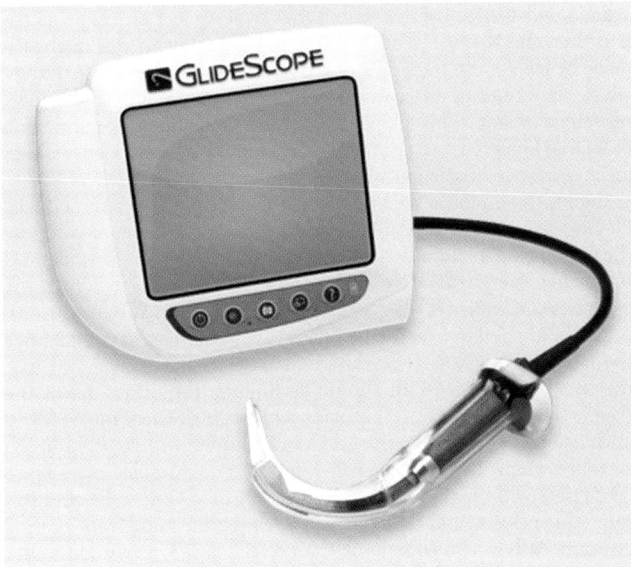

Fig. 222.9 Video-assisted laryngoscope (GlideScope). (Courtesy Verathon Inc.)

aspiration of more than 30 mL of air indicates proper tube placement. Colorimetric devices, which change from yellow to purple with an elevated carbon dioxide level, are also useful. These end-tidal carbon dioxide detectors are placed between the tube and the bag-valve device after intubation: the detectors will change from purple to yellow if the tube is in the proper location. An easy way to remember the colors is "yellow, yellow in the bellow." Carbon dioxide capnographic devices should show adequate respiratory waveforms. These forms are characterized by three phases: baseline, rapid upstroke, and long alveolar plateau, similar to a small "r" written in longhand.

Secure

Secure the tube with umbilical tape or a commercial device made for that purpose (Fig. 222.8). Avoid using tape or tincture of benzoin on the face because facial irritation can cause at least temporary skin changes. Consider inserting a bite block if the patient might bite the tube. Insert a nasogastric or orogastric tube. Use chemical restraints with appropriate monitoring to prevent tube removal. Finally, take a chest radiograph to ensure proper depth and placement. The ideal location is to have the tube 2 to 3 cm above the carina.

VIDEO-ASSISTED INTUBATION (GLIDESCOPE)

Video-assisted intubation is indicated for both routine and difficult intubations and is very useful in the patient with an immobilized cervical spine. The GlideScope was the first to market of the newer generation video-assisted laryngoscopes (Fig. 222.9); it is likely the most studied. In the patient with tongue edema, GlideScope has been shown to have an advantage over the Macintosh blade. It can be used in pediatric patients that weigh as little as 1.8 kg. There are no contraindications for using this device.

Preparation

Attach the GlideScope blade to the monitor using the video cable. If a single-use STAT blade is to be used, insert the baton into the

STAT blade. A click will be heard when the baton is in place. Turn on the device, and it is ready to use. Next, prepare the ET tube by inserting the GlideRite malleable stylet. The curve or angle of the stylet should somewhat match the hockey stick shape of the GlideScope blade, usually about 35 degrees. While use of a stylet generally facilitates manipulation of the ET tube, it is not required.

Technique

Similar to traditional intubation, open the patient's mouth and insert the blade into the midline of the oral cavity. Avoid any sweeping of the tongue; instead insert under direct visualization down the midline of the tongue, and finally over the tongue at the base. Next, turn your attention to the monitor and observe while advancing the blade through the pharynx. Continue to advance until the epiglottis is observed. Lift the blade, if necessary, to elevate the epiglottis and observe the vocal cords. The tip of the blade can be inserted gently into the vallecula, if needed. If the glottis is not well visualized, tilt the handle back slightly.

Next, advance the ET tube under direct visualization, past the tip of the GlideScope and toward the vocal cords. Before inserting the ET tube through the vocal cords, withdraw the GlideRite stylet approximately 2 cm. Turn your attention back to the monitor and advance the ET tube through the vocal cords. Advance until the marker line reaches the glottis. Inflate the ET tube cuff and finish withdrawing the stylet. Confirm proper placement of the ET tube using the previously described methods.

EDITOR'S NOTE: Novice operators should probably practice use of the GlideScope on mannequin models and for routine intubations before having to use it as a rescue device for a difficult intubation. Otherwise, the time to intubation may actually be longer than with direct laryngoscopy.

BOUGIENAGE-ASSISTED (BOUGIE) INTUBATION

Many critical care clinicians carry a bougie with them in their coat pocket in case there is need for emergency intubation in a difficult airway. Similar to traditional intubation, open the patient's mouth and insert the laryngoscope blade into the midline of the oral cavity. Using the laryngoscope in the usual manner, attempt to find the epiglottis. If you can find the epiglottis, you will be able to intubate the patient. Find the best view of epiglottis possible and insert the bougie with the distal coudé tip (hockey stick configuration) turned upward against the epiglottis. Riding the epiglottis inward (bougie tip pressed upward against undersurface of epiglottis), the distal tip will enter the glottis and then the trachea. Confirmation of placement in the trachea is made by feeling the tracheal rings. If unable to feel the tracheal rings, when you continue to advance the tip, at some point it will meet resistance or stop. This happens when the tip reaches the carina or a bronchial branch. Conversely, if in the esophagus, the bougie will not meet resistance; instead, it will continue to advance.

Next, the endotracheal tube must be advanced over the bougie. Having an assistant available is very helpful for this step. Make sure there is adequate lubrication on the outside of the endotracheal tube; have the assistant get the endotracheal tube started down the bougie and advance it until you can take it further. While continuing to hold the laryngoscope in place with your left hand, advance the endotracheal tube down the remainder of the bougie and into the trachea. The assistant should be holding the other end of the bougie steady and prevent it moving while you advance the endotracheal tube. Occasionally, the endotracheal tube will get held up on cartilage when advancing; gently rotating it counterclockwise up to 90 degrees will usually ease it into place. It may need to be counter-rotated gently several times as you advance the tube into its final position. When the tube is in the correct position, withdraw the bougie, remove the laryngoscope, and confirm proper placement.

Rapid-Sequence Intubation

RSI is an important technique to assist intubation in patients who are combative. It prevents laryngospasm and can have other therapeutic benefits. The prime candidate has been the "can't intubate, can't ventilate patient," but in actual practice this is rare. Airway assessment before the procedure should detect patients at risk for this problem, and often alternative methods can be used. Rarely, this may occur without warning, so an intermediate airway, such as an LMA or Combitube, as well as a cricothyroidotomy kit, needs to be readily available. There are many medications from which to choose, and the topic can be complex. Here, only the most common technique is explained, and this will be suitable for patients without suspected bronchospasm or increased intracranial pressure.

- Choose the paralytic agent. Succinylcholine 1.5 mg/kg is the first choice unless contraindicated. The vagal stimulatory effects of succinylcholine can cause bradycardia, hypotension, and other muscarinic effects. Contraindications are conditions in which hyperkalemia may be worsened, where there is concern that increased intracranial pressure or intraocular pressure may worsen the patient's condition, or there is a risk of malignant hyperthermia such as the following:
  - End-stage renal disease with missed dialysis
  - Rhabdomyolysis (e.g., patients found down for a long time)
  - Muscular dystrophy of any type
  - History of spinal cord injuries
  - Open globe injury (of controversial significance)
  - Conditions under which there may be increased intracranial pressure
  - History of a recent cerebrovascular accident
  - Burns of greater than 10% body surface area more than 24 hours old but incompletely healed
  - Patients with crush injuries more than 24 hours old
  - Family history of an anesthetic reaction
- If succinylcholine is indicated, then a standard dose is 2 mg/kg intravenously. It should not be given until other preparations are made.
- If succinylcholine is contraindicated, rocuronium 0.6 to 1 mg/kg is considered by many to be the best alternative. It has a rapid onset of action, but paralysis lasts an average of 50 minutes (possibly longer in geriatric patients), placing it second to succinylcholine. Vecuronium and atracurium are intermediate-acting agents with an onset of action of approximately 3 minutes and a duration of action of 30 minutes. Mivacurium has an onset of action of 2 to 3 minutes and a duration of action of 15 to 20 minutes. Fortunate-

ly, these drugs have minimal cardiovascular effects and, with the exception of mivacuronium, cause minimal release of histamines.
- Choose the sedative agent. Etomidate (0.3 mg/kg intravenous perfusion) is the most common choice because of its lack of cardiovascular depression and versatility. Other agents include ketamine 1 to 2 mg/kg in bronchospasm, midazolam 0.2 mg/kg, or thiopental 3 mg/kg in increased intracranial pressure. Each has its benefits and drawbacks, which should be studied before use.
- Choose the adjuncts. Although not indicated in all cases, lidocaine 1.5 mg/kg is considered useful in patients with bronchospasm or concerns for increased intracranial pressure. Atropine should be administered to children younger than 10 years at 0.02 mg/kg (minimum 0.1 mg, maximum 1 mg) to inhibit reflex bradycardia before the use of succinylcholine. Atropine should be considered for any adult who is receiving either ketamine or a second dose of succinylcholine during the intubation or reintubation procedure to reduce complications.
- Three minutes before intubation, give adjuncts.
- Two minutes before intubation, give a priming dose (10% of the dose drawn up in the syringe) of succinylcholine (if this medication is to be used for paralysis).
- One minute before intubation, give the paralytic agent (succinylcholine or rocuronium), followed immediately by the sedative (etomidate, midazolam, or thiopental). Begin giving the patient eight vital capacity breaths.
- Assess for adequate paralysis by gently stroking the eyelashes. If there is no response, proceed with intubation as described in previous sections.

NASOTRACHEAL INTUBATION

Nasotracheal intubation generally requires the patient to be breathing spontaneously and has the complications of nasal bleeding and sinusitis. It is of limited usefulness, except in cases where awake intubation is required. This technique is relatively contraindicated in the combative patient and in those patients with a coagulopathy or bleeding diathesis. It is important to examine the facial anatomy and nares for distortion, trauma, or other contraindications. If no contraindications are noted, use the side with the larger passage. If they are equal, use the right side because this helps reduce trauma from the tube bevel. Use a 6.5-mm tube or smaller, if anatomically indicated.

Preparation

Most nasotracheal intubation failures are the result of inadequate preparation.

- Get an assistant.
- Explain the procedure to the patient. This is the most important step.
- Place the patient in the standard "sniffing" position, as described previously.
- Determine if nasal vasoconstriction is safe. If the patient appears to be at risk for limited perfusion to the nasal area from either local or systemic disease, avoid the use of a vasoconstrictor.
- Prepare the nasopharyngeal path. Place 15 mL of 2% lidocaine with epinephrine (or plain lidocaine, if vasoconstriction is contraindicated) in a Toomey syringe.
- Have one assistant keep the syringe upright to prevent spillage and connect the Toomey syringe to a small Foley catheter. A red Robinson catheter is preferred.
- While an assistant continues to hold the catheter upright, lubricate the distal catheter with a water-soluble lubricant.
- With the free hand, apply cricoid pressure. This facilitates entry of the catheter into the airway. Insert the catheter through the nose to the level of the vocal cords. This is approximately twice the distance from the front of the lips to the tragus of the ear. Ideally, the patient will cough, indicating vocal cord stimulation.

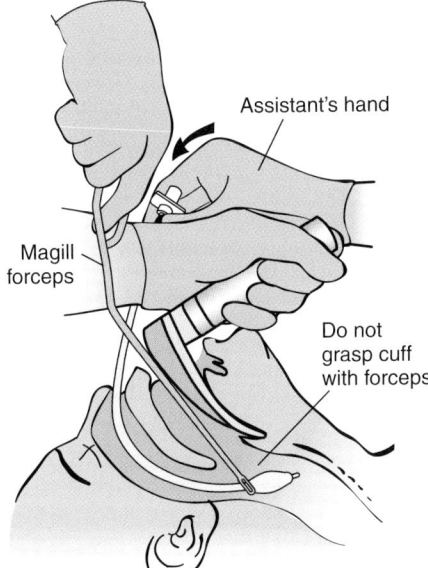

Fig. 222.10 Nasotracheal intubation using a laryngoscope and Magill forceps. The forceps are not used to pull the tube; rather, they serve to guide the tip of the tube through the vocal cords while an assistant advances the tube. The cuff is frequently damaged if it is grasped.

- Have the assistant turn the syringe upright and administer about 5 mL of the solution while the patient coughs, which helps disperse the solution.
- Withdraw the catheter, administering another 5 mL of the solution as the catheter is removed.
- Administer the last 5 mL at the Kiesselbach plexus in the anterior nasal passage of the septum. Allow the solution to work while lubricating the endotracheal tube and checking the balloon.

Two-Handed Nasotracheal Intubation Technique

- Standing at the side of the patient, insert the tube so the leading edge of the bevel is away from the septum. If the left nostril is used, the tube will be initially inserted with most of it positioned above the face and scalp, and then rotated 180 degrees once the turbinates are passed.
- Once the tube is about halfway in, apply cricoid pressure with the nondominant hand. Remember that unlike in training models, the trachea is a mobile structure. Use this advantage to move the trachea to assist placing the tube.
- Lean forward and listen for breath sounds through the end of the tube, adjusting both the tube and the trachea to create maximum breath sounds. Once resistance is felt at the vocal cord opening, await inspiration and then guide the tube past the vocal cords. This is often easily felt with the hand manipulating the trachea.
- Pass the tube 26 to 28 cm in an adult, depending on the size of the patient.
- Check and secure the tube in the standard fashion (see Fig. 222.8).
- Direct visualization can also be used for nasotracheal intubation. With the patient supine, use the laryngoscope in the same manner as for standard intubation. While visualizing the cords, use the Magill forceps to grasp the tube already inserted through the nasopharynx and pass it through the cords (Fig. 222.10). Avoid tearing the cuff when grasping the tube with forceps.

POSTPROCEDURE PATIENT CARE

- Order daily chest radiographs to verify tube placement.
- The respiratory services department of the hospital usually supplies the ventilator, tape, and other equipment as well as providing care; however, the clinician is ultimately responsible.

- Check the patient and the respiratory setup frequently. Carbon dioxide detectors and whistles can be used to confirm expiratory efforts.

COMPLICATIONS

- Short-term laryngeal edema: Sore throat occurs in almost every patient after extubation (repeated attempts at intubation by unskilled personnel may cause enough edema to preclude intubation by highly skilled clinicians).
- Trauma
  - Broken teeth
  - Oral lacerations or ulcerations (lip, tongue, pharynx, esophagus, or trachea)
  - Bleeding, hematoma, or abscess formation as a result of trauma
  - Avulsion of arytenoid cartilage
- Hypoxia resulting from
  - Long duration of procedure
  - Esophageal intubation (most commonly results from not visualizing the vocal cords)
  - Intubation of a bronchus
  - Failure to recognize esophageal or bronchial intubation
  - Pneumothorax
  - Failure to secure the placement
  - Failure to recognize misplacement of the tube
  - Aspiration of vomited material, especially in unconscious or semiconscious patient
  - Laryngospasm
- Hypertension/hypotension
- Bradycardia
- Tachycardia with or without arrhythmias
- Sequelae of long-term endotracheal tube placement
  - Nosocomial infection
  - Pneumothorax
  - Corneal abrasions
  - Epistaxis
  - Sinusitis
  - Vocal cord damage or paralysis (left cord more frequently involved than right)
  - Tracheomalacia and stenosis (occur more frequently in men; are more common with older tubes that use higher cuff pressures)
  - Tracheoesophageal fistula
  - Innominate artery erosion by endotracheal cuff

NOTE: Rarely are teeth broken with nasotracheal intubation. However, acute epistaxis and nasal trauma can result. Pulmonary infection can also be caused by nasal flora introduced through the nasotracheal tube.

CPT/BILLING CODES

31500   Intubation, endotracheal, emergency procedure

ICD-10-CM DIAGNOSTIC CODES

E87.2	Acidosis
E87.3	Alkalosis
E87.4	Acid-base mixed disorder
I46.9	Cardiac or cardiorespiratory arrest unspecified
I50.1	Pulmonary edema (left heart failure)
J44.9	Chronic obstructive bronchitis, unspecified
J44.1	Chronic obstructive bronchitis, with (acute) exacerbation
J43.9	Emphysema, not otherwise specified
J45.22	Asthma, extrinsic with status asthmaticus
J45.902	Asthma, unspecified with status asthmaticus
J95.2	Pulmonary insufficiency following nonthoracic surgery

J96.00	Respiratory failure, not otherwise specified
J80	Respiratory distress, insufficiency, or syndrome; acute
J96.10	Respiratory failure, chronic
R40.20	Coma, unspecified
R57.9	Shock, unspecified
R57.0	Shock, cardiogenic
R65.21	Shock, septic
R57.1	Shock, hypovolemic or other
R06.03	Respiratory distress or insufficiency, other, including hypercapnia
R09.02	Hypoxemia
R09.2	Respiratory arrest or cardiorespiratory failure

SUPPLIERS

(See contact information available at www.expertconsult.com.)

Cook Medical
Mallinckrodt, Inc.
Rusch
Sims Portex, Inc.

Acknowledgment

The editors recognize the contributions of Len Scarpinato, DO, and Scott Savage, DO, to this chapter in previous editions of this text.

RECOMMENDED READING

Ambrosio A, Pfannenstiel T, Bach K, Cornelissen C, Gaconnet C, Brigger MT. Difficult airway management for novice physicians. A randomized trial comparing direct and video-assisted laryngoscopy. *Otolaryngol Head Neck Surg.* 2014;150(5):775–778.

American Heart Association. *Advanced Cardiovascular Life Support Provider Manual.* Dallas: American Heart Association; 2015.

Benumof JL, Cooper SD. Quantitative improvement in laryngoscopic view by optimal external laryngeal manipulation. *J Clin Anesth.* 1996;8:136.

Butler J, Sen A. Best evidence topic report. Cricoid pressure in emergency rapid sequence intubation. *Emerg Med J.* 2005;22:815–816.

Ellis DY, Harris T, Zideman D. Cricoid pressure in emergency department rapid sequence tracheal intubations. A risk-benefit analysis. *Ann Emerg Med.* 2007;50:653–665.

Hagberg CA, Artime CA, Aziz MF, eds. *Hagberg and Benumof's Airway Management.* 4th ed. Philadelphia: Churchill Livingstone Elsevier; 2017.

Kopman AF, Zhaku B, Lai KS. The "intubating dose" of succinylcholine. The effect of decreasing doses on recovery time. *Anesthesiology.* 2003;99:1050–1054.

Marx JA, Hockberger RS, Walls RM, eds. *Rosen's Emergency Medicine. Concepts and Clinical Practice.* 9th ed. Philadelphia: Mosby; 2017.

Naguib M, Samarkandi AH, El-Din ME, et al. The dose of succinylcholine required for excellent endotracheal intubating conditions. *Anesth Analg.* 2006;102:151–155.

Reichman EF, ed. *Emergency Medicine Procedures.* 2nd ed. New York: McGraw-Hill; 2013.

Roberts JR, Custalow CB, Thomsen TW, eds. *Roberts and Hedges' Clinical Procedures in Emergency Medicine and Acute Care.* 7th ed. Philadelphia: Elsevier; 2019.

Tintinalli JE, Kelen GD, Stapczynski JS, eds. *Emergency Medicine. A Comprehensive Study Guide.* 8th ed. New York: McGraw-Hill; 2016.

Walls RM, Murphy MF, Luten RC, Schneider RE, eds. *Manual of Emergency Airway Management.* 4th ed. Philadelphia: Lippincott Williams & Wilkins; 2012.

CHAPTER 223

CRICOTHYROID CATHETER INSERTION, CRICOTHYROIDOTOMY, AND TRACHEOSTOMY

David Roden

Establishing an airway is crucial to a patient's survival and is of paramount importance in an emergency. If endotracheal or nasotracheal intubation is impossible, or it must be prolonged, several techniques can be used to establish a surgical airway. Cricothyroid catheter insertion (also known as percutaneous transtracheal jet ventilation) and cricothyroidotomy are usually performed in emergencies, whereas tracheostomy is usually performed under controlled conditions. Once a cricothyroid catheter has been inserted, kits are available to convert it to a cricothyroidotomy using a guidewire and the Seldinger technique. Retrograde intubation can also be achieved using the Seldinger technique through a cricothyroid catheter.

Cricothyroid catheter insertion is the least invasive procedure, requires the least surgical skill, does not require an assistant, and is the quickest technique. It also has the lowest risk of complications, such as bleeding, glottic stenosis, subglottic stenosis, or tracheal ulceration. This technique provides a temporary airway to preserve oxygenation until a larger airway can be established. (If used with intermittent jet of pressurized 100% oxygen at 50 lb/in², adequate ventilation is also provided; exhalation occurs passively due to secondary recoil of the lungs and chest wall.) Emergency personnel also use cricothyroidotomy as a lifesaving maneuver. One advantage of cricothyroid catheter insertion and cricothyroidotomy is the speed with which they can be performed. They also do not require a lot of equipment and result in less scarring than tracheosotomy. Because the airway is most superficial at the level of the cricothyroid membrane and anatomic landmarks are easily identifiable, this location is ideal for rapid access. Serious bleeding and perforation of other structures can also usually be avoided at this site.

Tracheostomy is the most complicated surgical airway procedure and requires the most equipment. It is performed at a level two tracheal rings below the cricothyroid membrane. This site is farther away from the larynx, so the incidence of laryngeal injury is much lower, especially if the opening is maintained for a prolonged time. Dissection is more complicated because the trachea is located deeper than the cricothyroid membrane, so the clinician must be familiar with local anatomy to minimize risk. Tracheostomy is associated with two to five times the complication rate when performed as an emergency procedure; therefore it is rarely performed except under controlled circumstances in the operating room. In addition, the complete procedure usually takes too long to be useful for emergency airway management and can be difficult for the untrained clinician to perform. The only situation in which emergency tracheostomy is preferred is when the specific location of the injury or disease (e.g., subglottic tumor, thyroid cartilage fracture) precludes alternatives.

CRICOTHYROID CATHETER INSERTION

Indications

- Temporary need for an airway, especially if patient cannot be ventilated with a bag-valve mask (Ambu), laryngeal mask airway, endotracheal tube, or otherwise
- Upper airway obstruction, usually resulting from foreign body, infection, neoplasm, edema, or trauma
- Preferred technique for establishing emergency airway in pediatric age group if endotracheal intubation fails
- Elective procedure for surgery involving the larynx and subglottic areas
- Alternative to cricothyroidotomy

Contraindications

- There is an intact nonsurgical airway or the possibility that one can be established.
- Subglottic obstruction exists.
- Thyroid cartilage fracture or damage to larynx or cricoid cartilage: anterior neck trauma may be a contraindication if these structures are possibly damaged. In these situations, tracheostomy is preferred.
- Lower tracheal or proximal bronchial tree disruption can result in an increased risk of pneumothorax or pneumomediastinum with high-pressure ventilation.
- Complete airway obstruction is a contraindication for jet ventilation (results in barotrauma or auto-positive end-expiratory pressure; a patent airway is needed for outflow of gas with expiration).

Equipment

- Goggles or eye protection
- Mask, cap, gown, and sterile gloves
- Commercially available kit (Instrumentation Industries, Bethel Park, PA; VMM Medizintechnik, West Germany), or assembled equipment including 12-, 14-, or 16-gauge, 2- to 3-inch over-the-needle catheter (angiocatheter); 5- or 10-mL syringe containing 3 to 5 mL of sterile saline
- Lidocaine 1% or 2% with epinephrine in 10-mL syringe with 22-gauge, 0.5-inch needle
- Skin-sterilizing supplies such as povidone-iodine (if time allows)
- Adhesive tape
- Umbilical tape, 2-0 monofilament nylon suture, and needle holder or commercially available endotracheal tube connecter
- High-pressure oxygen tubing

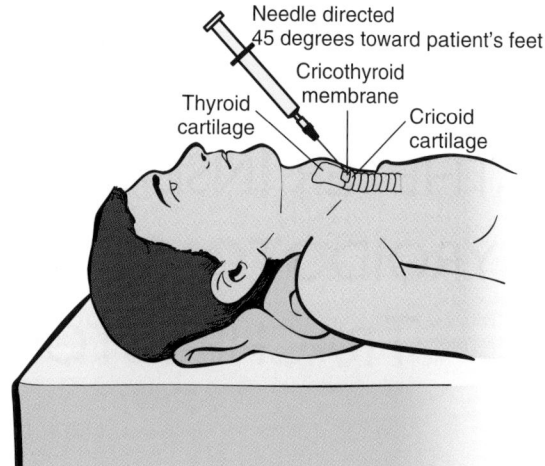

Fig. 223.1 Over-the-needle catheter is inserted through cricothyroid membrane with syringe attached. The clinician should aspirate while inserting the needle.

- High-pressure oxygen supply (30 to 60 pounds per square inch) with a pressure gauge and a pressure-regulating valve (if high-pressure oxygen is not available, a 3-mL syringe barrel [without a plunger] can be attached to the catheter; a standard endotracheal tube connector can then be used to attach the catheter to a bag-mask-valve device)
- Hand-operated valve connected inline to tubing and catheter
- Alternate: an oxygen regulator and manual trigger (ENK modulator set, Cook Critical Care)
- Cardiac monitor
- Pulse oximeter
- End-tidal CO_2 monitor (capnography)

PREPROCEDURE PATIENT PREPARATION

No patient education is needed in the emergency setting. Documentation should be made in the patient's chart that informed consent was obtained if time allows. If time does not allow, an explanation of the emergent need for this procedure should be documented.

Procedure

1. Position the patient in the supine position with the chin directly midline and maximally extended (if no cervical spine trauma). If a cervical fracture is suspected, the neck should remain immobilized in a neutral position.
2. Clean the neck with povidone–iodine or other antiseptic solution.
3. Observe universal blood and body fluid precautions. Observe sterile technique (cap, gloves, mask, gown, and drapes).
4. Use the nondominant hand to palpate and identify the cricothyroid membrane, which is located immediately caudal to the prominent thyroid cartilage (Adam's apple). It is the first small depression or indentation inferior to the hard thyroid cartilage, between the cricoid and thyroid cartilages. It should be easily palpable, even in obese individuals.
5. If the patient is awake, and time allows, infiltrate lidocaine as a wheal and then down to the membrane in the desired location using a 10-mL syringe with a 22-gauge needle.
6. With the nondominant hand, immobilize the thyroid cartilage and hold the skin taut over the cricothyroid membrane.
7. Direct the catheter-over-needle attached to the syringe partially filled with sterile saline downward in the midline and caudally at an angle of 45 degrees (Fig. 223.1). Inserting the catheter-over-needle in the inferior aspect of the cricothyroid membrane minimizes risk of injury to the cricothyroid arteries. Aspirate

with the syringe during insertion. When air bubbles appear in the syringe, the needle has entered the trachea.
8. Avoid injection of any of the saline while advancing the catheter over the needle. Advance the catheter until the hub is against the skin. Withdraw the needle and syringe and attach the syringe again to the hub. Aspirate again to confirm placement. Attach the distal end of the high-pressure oxygen tubing to the catheter.
9. Open the hand-operated release valve to deliver pressurized oxygen to the trachea. As soon as the chest rises, assume that the patient has been oxygenated; the valve should then be closed. Open the valve, watch the chest rise, and close the valve—in a rhythmic pattern—to approximate actual breathing. Adjust the overall pressure level to allow adequate lung expansion.
10. Most upper airway obstructions are incomplete and allow some ventilation to occur with forced exhalations. (If the chest remains inflated during the exhalation phase, a complete proximal airway obstruction may be present. In this case, a second large-bore over-the-needle catheter can be inserted next to the original catheter. If the chest remains distended, cricothyroidotomy should be performed.)
11. The oxygen line should be taped to the catheter. Next, secure the catheter and oxygen tubing by placing a stitch through the skin near the catheter (after infiltration of lidocaine in the conscious patient), wrapping one end of the suture around the catheter several times and tying it to the base of the other end of the suture near the skin. The other end of the suture can then be wrapped several times around the oxygen tubing and tied to the original end of the suture near the skin. Alternatively, a piece of umbilical tape or adhesive tape can be wrapped around the patient's neck, the catheter hub, and the oxygen tubing. As another option, a commercially available endotracheal tube holder can be wrapped around the patient's neck and connected to the oxygen tubing; the catheter will still have to be secured with suture or by being taped to the tubing and skin.
12. Obtain an arterial blood gas. Pulse oximetry, blood pressure, and telemetry should be monitored. Capnography can be used to assure adequate ventilation.
13. Monitor regularly for signs of crepitus in the neck or torso. If crepitus is present, the catheter tip is likely located directly against or directed toward the posterior mucosa of the tracheal wall. It should be removed and a new one inserted.

Complications

- Inadequate ventilation or hypoxia (often due to catheter kinking as it travels through the tissue; use of commercially available kink-resistant catheters minimizes this risk)
- Barotrauma (can cause pneumothorax, pneumomediastinum, or pneumopericardium; auto-positive end-expiratory pressure can result in decreased mean arterial pressure)
- Subcutaneous emphysema
- Aspiration (pressurized airflow may minimize risk of aspiration; however, make sure to suction upper airway before discontinuing cricothyroid catheter)

NOTE: Cricothyroid catheter insertion through the cricothyroid membrane may maintain spontaneous respirations for a few minutes. This is the procedure of choice for children under 12 years old because the cricothyroid membrane is small. If this maneuver is inadequate, formal tracheostomy is indicated.
ADDITIONAL NOTE: There are kits available (Melker, Cook Inc.) that use the Seldinger technique to convert a transcutaneous cricothyroid catheter into a cricothyroidotomy. Similarly, kits are available (Cook Retrograde Intubation Set, Cook Inc.) for retrograde intubation. Instead of directing it caudally, a cricothyroid catheter is directed cephalad to insert a guidewire up through the vocal cords and out through the mouth. The endotracheal tube is then advanced down the firmly held guidewire until it meets resistance

which means the tip should be at the cricothyroid membrane. The guidewire and catheter are then removed and the endotracheal tube advanced further into the proper position above the carina.

CRICOTHYROIDOTOMY

Indications

- Upper airway obstruction, usually resulting from foreign body, infection, neoplasm, edema, or trauma
- When endotracheal or nasotracheal intubation has failed, is contraindicated, or is unavailable
- Patient with a cervical spine fracture who cannot extend neck for intubation
- Prior cricothyroidotomy catheter insertion complicated by carbon dioxide retention or air entrapment

Contraindications

- Intact nonsurgical airway
- Subglottic obstruction
- Thyroid cartilage fracture or damage to larynx or cricoid cartilage (anterior neck trauma may be contraindication if these structures are possibly damaged); in these situations, tracheostomy preferred
- Patient younger than 8 years old (cricothyroid catheter insertion or needle cricothyroidotomy is the preferred procedure for this age group)
- Relative contraindications: a coagulopathy, massive neck swelling or hematoma, or previously prolonged endotracheal intubation (tracheostomy or conversion to tracheostomy may be preferred)

Equipment

- Goggles or eye protection
- No. 15 scalpel blade with handle
- Size 4 to 6 endotracheal tubes or size 4 to 6 Shiley cuffed tracheostomy tubes
- Adhesive tape
- Umbilical tape and 2-0 monofilament nylon suture and needle holder (if a tracheostomy tube is used)
- Sterile 4 × 4-inch gauze sponges
- Self-refilling bag-valve-mask unit (Ambu bag) with tubing and oxygen source
- Suction and suction catheters

If time allows:

- Povidone-iodine (Betadine) or other antiseptic skin preparation
- Mask, cap, gown, and sterile gloves
- Sterile fenestrated drape
- Lidocaine 1% or 2% with epinephrine in 10-mL syringe with 22-gauge, 0.625-inch needle

If a tracheostomy tray is available:

- Hemostat clamps (2)
- Kelly clamps (2)
- Tracheal dilator (Trousseau)
- Tracheal hook
- Curved scissors
- Cardiac monitor
- Pulse oximeter
- End-tidal CO_2 monitor

Preprocedure Patient Preparation

No patient education is needed in the emergency setting. Documentation should be made in the patient's chart that informed consent was obtained, if time allows. If time does not allow, an explanation of the emergent need for this procedure should be documented.

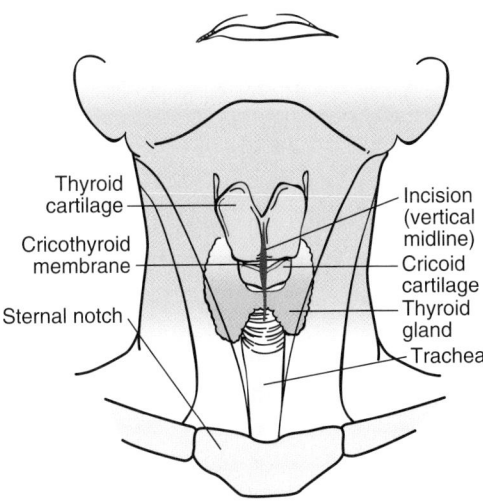

Fig. 223.2 Neck extended, with cricothyroid membrane identified.

Technique

NOTE: In extremely urgent situations, the goal is to save a life, so some concerns about sterile technique should be postponed.

1. Position the patient in the supine position with the chin directly midline and maximally extended (if no cervical spine trauma). If a cervical fracture is suspected, the neck should remain immobilized in a neutral position.
2. Clean the neck with povidone-iodine or other antiseptic solution.
3. Observe universal blood and body fluid precautions. Observe sterile technique (cap, gloves, gown, mask, and drapes). If right-hand dominant, stand on the patient's right side.
4. Use the nondominant hand to palpate and identify the cricothyroid membrane, which is located immediately caudal to the prominent thyroid cartilage (Adam's apple). It is the first small depression or indentation inferior to the hard thyroid cartilage, between the cricoid and thyroid cartilages. It should be easily palpable, even in obese individuals.
   NOTE: The cricothyroid membrane averages 9 mm in the cephalad-caudad dimension and 30 mm in the left-to-right dimension in adults. It should be easily palpable and accessible.
5. If the patient is awake, and time allows, use the 10-mL syringe with the 22-gauge needle to infiltrate lidocaine in a large subcutaneous wheal encompassing the future vertical skin incision. Next, infuse lidocaine in a transverse line across the membrane.
6. With the nondominant hand, immobilize the thyroid cartilage and hold the skin taut over the cricothyroid membrane. Using the no. 15 blade, make a 3-cm vertical (longitudinal) skin incision centered over the cricothyroid membrane (Fig. 223.2).
   NOTE: Certain authorities recommend a transverse skin incision. Making a longitudinal incision slows down the procedure and requires repositioning after the skin incision; however, if the transverse skin incision is accidentally extended too far laterally (e.g., when the procedure is performed under duress), the anterior jugular veins may be injured. If a patient has a suspected laryngeal injury, the longitudinal incision is indicated in the event it needs to be extended inferiorly to perform an emergency high tracheostomy.
   In a dire emergency, certain experts make the initial skin incision in the transverse direction and carry the initial incision all the way through the skin, subcutaneous tissue, and cricothyroid membrane. A tracheal hook can then be used to apply

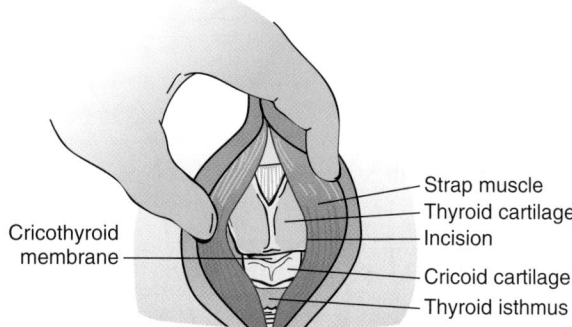

Fig. 223.3 After a vertical skin incision, soft tissue structures are retracted laterally with the nondominant hand.

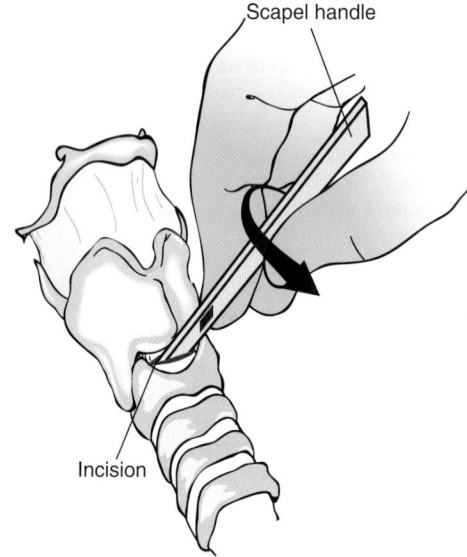

Fig. 223.4 Scalpel handle inserted into incision and twisted vertically to open it.

traction in the caudal direction, stabilizing the trachea, while a tracheostomy or endotracheal tube is inserted through the opening.

7. Use the finger and thumb of the nondominant hand to retract the incision edges laterally (Fig. 223.3).

8. Divide the neck fascia and strap muscles vertically in the midline with the scalpel until the thyroid and cricoid cartilages are encountered. In general, cartilage provides considerable resistance to the scalpel, so these structures are not easily injured.

9. Retracting soft tissue structures laterally, locate the cricothyroid membrane by palpation with the dominant hand and use the scalpel to create a 1- to 2-cm transverse incision centered in the midline, immediately above the cricoid cartilage. Be aware that at this point any respiratory effort by the patient will expel sputum, blood, and air into the wound. A low incision should avoid vocal cord injury and the cricothyroid arteries. The posterior aspect of the cricoid cartilage should be avoided, but even if the knife goes too deep, the cricoid cartilage should stop the progression of the knife.

10a. While keeping the cricothyroidotomy incision open with the nondominant index finger or an instrument, reverse the scalpel, placing the handle into the incision horizontally. Rotate the handle 90 degrees to open the incision (Fig. 223.4). If a tracheostomy tray is available, an alternative to Step 10 is as follows:

10b. After using the scalpel to make a transverse midline incision in the cricothyroid membrane, insert a hemostat or Kelly clamp with the points downward into the trachea and spread laterally.

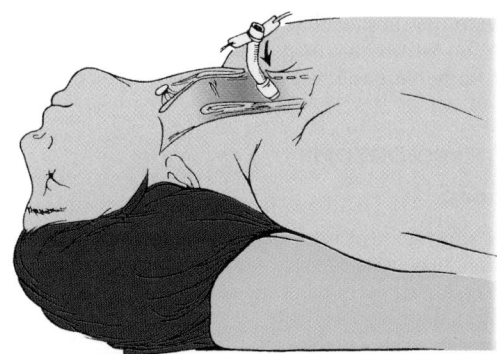

Fig. 223.5 Tube is inserted into the incision. Scalpel handle is still in cricothyroid membrane (not shown for clarity).

A rush of air indicates patency of the airway. Alternatively, a tracheal dilator can extend the cricothyroid membrane incision laterally approximately 1 cm on each side of the midline. Usually the dilator is inserted to extend the cricothyroid incision vertically, at first, and then the handles are rotated 90 degrees to extend the incision laterally. From here, continue with the remainder of the steps in the technique.

11. If available, place a tracheal hook into the incision and grasp the inferior border of the thyroid cartilage. Use the nondominant hand or an assistant to maintain traction in an upward or cephalad direction. With the dominant hand, place the largest possible endotracheal tube or, preferably, tracheostomy tube into the incision. The scalpel handle can be also be used as both a retractor and a guide. Direct the tube tip toward the patient's feet and attempt to visualize its insertion into the trachea (Fig. 223.5). Remove the tracheal hook or Trousseau dilator. Be very careful not to puncture the cuff when removing the hook. Do not release the hold on the tracheostomy or endotracheal tube until it is secured.

12. Connect the bag-valve-mask unit to the tube and ventilate with 100% oxygen. Check for bilateral breath sounds to ensure that the tube is properly placed above the carina.

13. Inflate the cuff with enough air to stop any audible air leaks.

14. Secure the tube and then apply a dressing. If an endotracheal tube is being used, secure the tube in place using tape. If a tracheostomy tube is being used, secure the tube with umbilical tape around the patient's neck. Place four interrupted sutures with 2-0 nylon through the tube's flange to secure it to the skin.

15. Suction the trachea.

16. Obtain an arterial blood gas and a chest radiograph. The radiograph should demonstrate tube position above the carina and should ensure the absence of an iatrogenic pneumothorax.

Complications

- Intraoperative and postoperative bleeding (direct pressure will usually stop bleeding after the airway is established)
- Improper tube placement with asphyxia
- Tube displacement or obstruction with subsequent hypoxia or death
- Subcutaneous or mediastinal emphysema
- Laryngeal or vocal cord injury (especially if tracheostomy tube is larger than cricothyroid membrane)
- Voice changes (e.g., hoarseness)
- Infection
- Persistent stoma
- Subglottic stenosis
- Perforated esophagus

If the opening of the cricothyroid membrane is not stabilized during insertion of the tube, the tube can be inadvertently placed in subcutaneous tissue. This will result in subcutaneous emphysema when first trying to ventilate the patient. Another cause of subcutaneous or mediastinal emphysema or infection is closing the skin incision around the tube; this should be avoided. If the cricothyroidotomy is only necessary for 48 to 72 hours (e.g., resolving infection, angioedema of tongue), the patient can be decannulated without converting to a tracheostomy. If a longer period of intubation is required (see the Tracheostomy section for a discussion of the controversies of timing), the procedure should be revised to a tracheostomy to prevent subglottic stenosis.

Postprocedure Patient Education

If prolonged airway management is needed, convert the cricothyroidotomy to a tracheostomy and provide the appropriate patient education. If the cricothyroidotomy can be removed within 48 to 72 hours, give the patient instructions for the routine care of a skin laceration. The patient should be aware that the fistula will close spontaneously. He or she should have a follow-up appointment within a week and should call or go to the emergency room for signs of hemorrhage, infection, airway distress, or subcutaneous emphysema.

TRACHEOSTOMY

Indications

- Chronic ventilatory failure (most common indication)
- Upper airway obstruction usually resulting from congenital anomaly, infection, neoplasm, edema, or trauma; also obstructive sleep apnea or bilateral vocal cord paralysis
- Anticipated prolonged endotracheal intubation
- Facial, tracheal, or other head and neck trauma or surgery with compromised airway
- Fractured larynx or subglottic obstruction (cricothyroidotomy contraindicated)
- Laryngospasm or angioedema
- Chronic impaired pulmonary toilet
- Management of chronic aspiration
- Unstable cervical spine
- Inability to intubate by other measures

NOTE: Management of bronchial secretions is much easier with a tracheostomy tube than with an endotracheal tube. Risk of endotracheal tube complications (e.g., tube displacement, sinusitis, tube kinking) is also reduced with conversion to a tracheostomy. However, the recommended timing for conversion has been debated extensively. Supporters for early conversion (7 days) suggest that laryngeal complication rates and patient comfort are improved with early conversion. Advocates for delayed placement of tracheostomy (14 to 21 days) state that unnecessary procedures will be avoided, reducing local wound and other surgical complications. Most experts have adopted an intermediate approach that is individualized to the patient. If the patient is expected to be intubated for considerably longer than 7 days, a tracheostomy is placed early. However, if the patient's course cannot be predicted, the conversion can be delayed until prolonged need becomes evident.

Contraindications

- Other methods can be used to secure an airway
- Lack of familiarity with the procedure
- Known preexisting severe tracheal disease or trauma
- Uncontrolled coagulopathy

EDITOR'S NOTE: Cricothyroidotomy is the procedure of choice when an invasive approach to the airway is needed.

Equipment

- Povidone–iodine or other antiseptic solution
- 1 package of 4 × 4-inch sterile gauze sponges

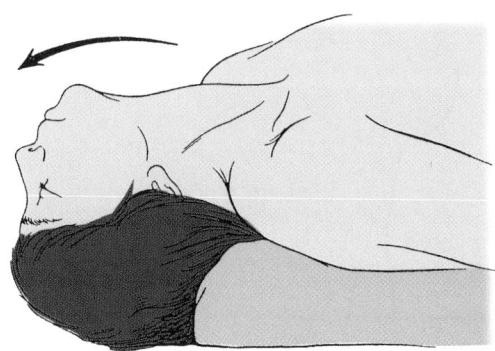

Fig. 223.6 Patient is positioned for tracheostomy.

- Sterile gown and gloves
- Sterile fenestrated drape
- Cap, mask, and eye protection
- Electrocautery machine
- 10- and 50-mL syringes
- 22- and 25-gauge, 0.625-inch needles
- Lidocaine 1% or 2% with epinephrine in 10-mL syringe with 22-gauge, 0.625-inch needle (if patient awake)
- No. 15 scalpel blade with handle
- Mosquito hemostats (4)
- Skin forceps
- Kelly clamps (2)
- Subcutaneous or Army-Navy retractors (2)
- Trousseau (tracheal) dilator
- Allis clamps (2)
- Tracheal hooks (2)
- Sizes 4, 6, and 8 cuffed Shiley tracheotomy tubes
- Needle holder
- Umbilical tape and 2-0 monofilament nylon suture
- Suction apparatus, tubing, and catheters
- Cardiac monitor
- Pulse oximeter
- End-tidal CO_2 monitor
- Ventilation equipment: bag-valve-mask unit (Ambu bag) with tubing and 100% oxygen available
- 3-0 Dexon or chromic absorbable suture on a cutting needle

Preprocedure Patient Preparation

Education of the patient and family should include the indication for tracheostomy and possible complications. Benefits of the procedure, as well as the risks of not performing it, should be explained to the patient and family. If there are alternatives to this procedure, they should be explained. Informed consent should be obtained in nonemergent situations.

Technique

1. Tracheostomy can be performed under local anesthesia on a spontaneously breathing patient, or under general anesthesia on an intubated patient. Exercise caution in administering sedation to a nonintubated patient with a compromised airway. The patient should be monitored continuously by pulse oximetry and telemetry while the procedure is being performed.
2. Position the patient in the supine position with a roll under the shoulders and, if there is no cervical spine trauma, with the neck maximally extended (Fig. 223.6). Placement of an endotracheal tube before elective tracheostomy (or leaving an existing tube) allows for better airway control and minimizes complications, especially in children. The anesthetist should stand above the patient's head for better access to the endotracheal tube, if present.

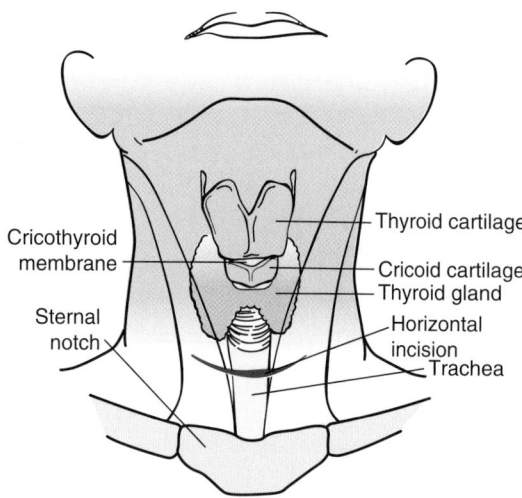

Fig. 223.7   Horizontal incision is made through the skin.

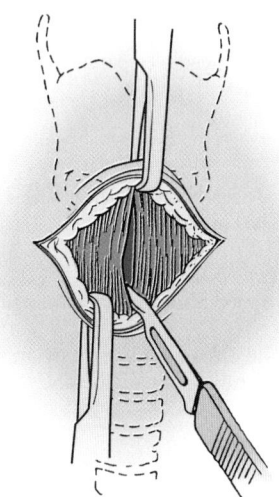

Fig. 223.8   Fascia and strap muscles are divided in the midline.

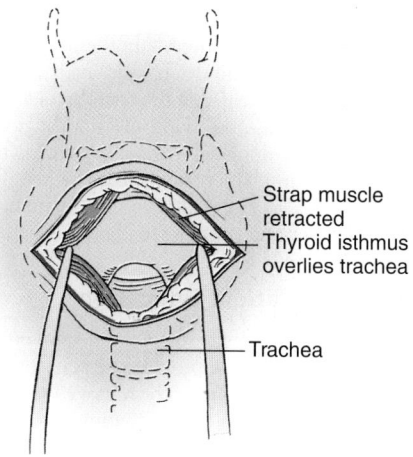

Fig. 223.9   Strap muscles are retracted laterally to expose the thyroid isthmus.

3. Prep the neck with povidone–iodine or other antiseptic solution from sternum to chin, and laterally to the sternocleidomastoid muscles. Apply the fenestrated drape.
4. Check the tracheostomy tube cuff for leaks prior to making the incision. A second tube should be tested and available, if possible.
5. Palpate landmarks: the sternal notch, cricoid cartilage, and inferior border of the thyroid cartilage. Outline a horizontal incision two fingerbreadths above the sternal notch, centered in the midline over the trachea.
6. For conscious patients, inject lidocaine subcutaneously around the intended incision site. Lidocaine can then be injected down to the anterior tracheal wall beneath the incision.
7. Using the scalpel, make a horizontal incision through skin and subcutaneous tissue down to the strap muscles (Fig. 223.7). Alternatively, once the skin has been incised, electrocautery can be used to divide the subcutaneous tissue horizontally, deepening the incision until the strap muscles are encountered.
8. Clamp the subcutaneous tissue with Allis clamps and retract superiorly and inferiorly. Next, incise the fascia vertically in the midline, in the raphe between the strap muscles. Incise down to the pretracheal fascia (Fig. 223.8).
   NOTE: Often the strap muscles are fused in the midline and covered by a network of troublesome veins. Attempts should be made to cauterize or ligate these veins.

9. Place retractor(s) beneath the strap muscles and apply traction laterally. Incise the pretracheal fascia to expose the thyroid isthmus and tracheal rings (Fig. 223.9).
10. Retract the thyroid isthmus superiorly, if possible, to increase visibility. If exposure is inadequate, horizontally incise the fascia immediately caudal to the lower border of the cricoid cartilage but do not enter the trachea. Insert a hemostat through this incision pointed toward the patient's feet, parallel to the trachea. Bluntly dissect the thyroid isthmus off the anterior wall of the trachea. After an additional attempt at superior or inferior retraction, if visibility is still inadequate, it may be necessary to divide the thyroid isthmus with clamps and suture the ligated edges (Fig. 223.10). A 3-0 chromic suture is used to oversew each edge for hemostasis.
    NOTE: It is important to remain in the midline with this procedure to minimize complications, especially in children.
11. If unsure that the object visualized is the trachea, aspirate for air with a small-bore needle into a syringe partly filled with sterile saline to confirm (bubbles should be seen) before proceeding. Next, place a tracheal hook beneath the cricoid cartilage and elevate it toward the surgeon and toward the patient's head. If using local anesthesia, 1 to 2 mL should be injected beneath the second tracheal ring into the tracheal lumen. This should stimulate the nonanesthetized patient to cough.
12. Make a transverse incision between the second and third rings (Fig. 223.11). Be prepared for a spurt of blood, air, or sputum, and have suction ready. Do not use electrocautery to incise the trachea because there is the risk of airway fire. Take care not to puncture the endotracheal tube cuff if present or the posterior wall of the trachea. (Alternatively, some clinicians make an inverted U-shaped incision. Others make a square "window" incision and remove the anterior portion of the second and third tracheal rings. A midline vertical incision through the second, third, and fourth tracheal rings is the incision of choice for an emergency tracheostomy.)
13. Insert a Trousseau dilator into the trachea and dilate laterally (Fig. 223.12).
14. Withdraw the endotracheal tube (if one is in place) until the tip is just above the tracheostomy. Under direct visualization, insert the appropriately sized tracheostomy tube through the dilated incision, with the tube tip directed downward (Fig. 223.13). Most adults will fit a size 8 Shiley tube. Inflate the tracheostomy tube cuff. Suction through the tube with a flexible suction catheter. Bronchoscopy can be performed at this point to confirm proper tracheostomy tube placement.
15. Attach the tube to the bag-valve-mask device and check for bilateral breath sounds with ventilation.

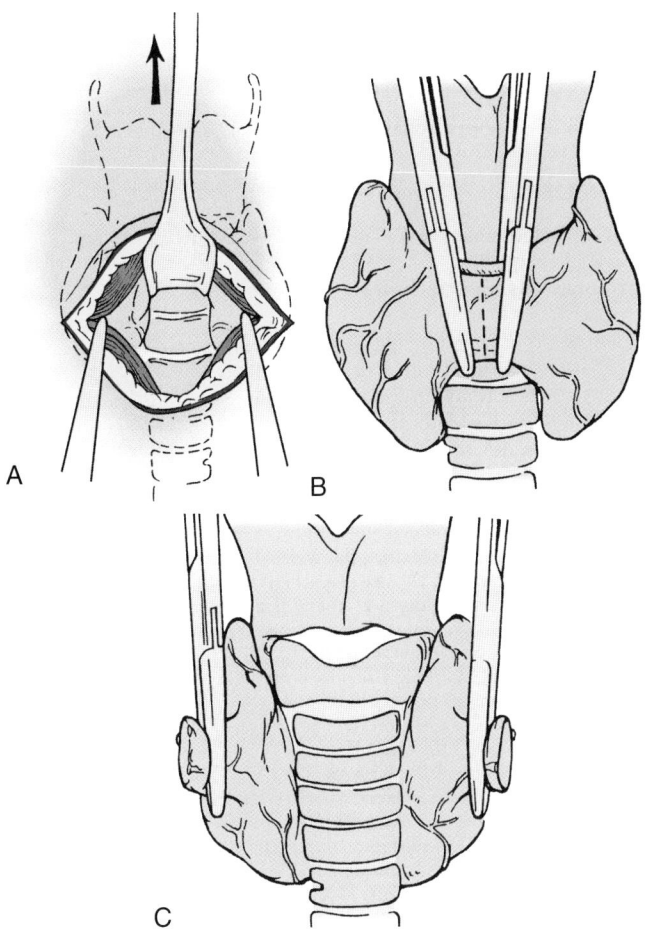

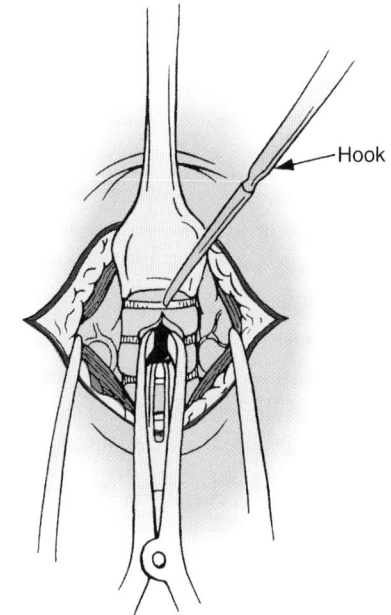

Fig. 223.12   Insert the dilator into the trachea.

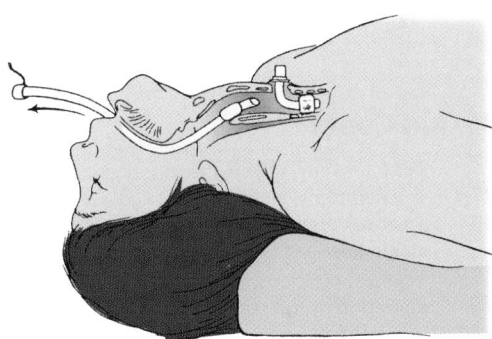

Fig. 223.10   (A) Thyroid isthmus is retracted upward or in cephalad direction. If exposure is inadequate, the thyroid isthmus should be clamped (B) and divided (C).

Fig. 223.13   Remove the endotracheal tube after inserting the tracheostomy tube.

17. Apply a sterile dressing around the tube.
18. A chest radiograph should be considered to assess tube placement above the carina and to ensure the absence of an iatrogenic pneumothorax.

To prevent infection, pneumomediastinum, or subcutaneous emphysema, do not close the skin incision around the tracheostomy tube. A tracheostomy tube provides access to the trachea for an unlimited amount of time. Once the indication for the tube has resolved, it is removed to allow the tracheocutaneous fistula to close spontaneously.

Complications

- Bleeding
- False passage
- Subcutaneous emphysema
- Wound infection
- Pneumomediastinum
- Pneumothorax
- Tracheoesophageal fistula
- Tracheoinnominate artery fistula
- Recurrent laryngeal nerve damage
- Carotid artery or jugular vein damage
- Aspiration

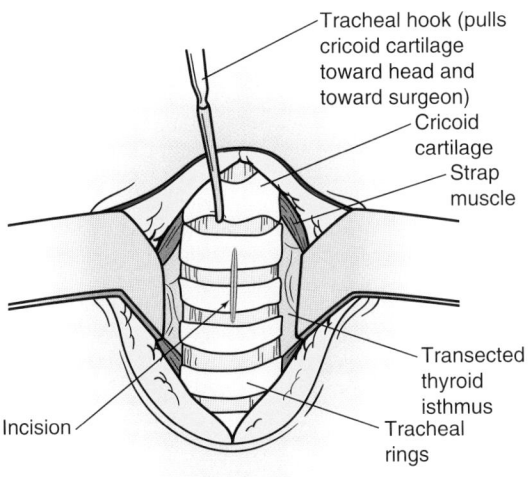

Fig. 223.11   Tracheal hook is placed in the cricoid cartilage and elevated anteriorly. The incision is made between the second and third rings.

16. Remove the retractors and the cricoid hook when the tube is adequately positioned. Secure the tracheostomy tube around the neck with umbilical tape. Secure the flange to the patient's skin with four interrupted 2-0 nylon sutures.

- Tube obstruction
- Malpositioned or displaced tube with subsequent hypoxia or death
- Tracheal stenosis
- Persistent stoma
- Dysphagia
- Sepsis, pneumonia, tracheitis, mediastinitis

NOTE: Placement of tracheostomies can be technically difficult, especially in children, obese patients, and patients with deformed or fixed cervical spines. Complication rates are higher in children. For these individuals, tracheostomies should definitely be avoided in emergency situations and performed under controlled circumstances.

Postprocedure Patient Education

Initially, the patient will be cared for in the hospital. Postprocedure education includes cleaning of the appliance and suctioning. If the patient is discharged with a tracheostomy, caretakers will need to continue this care at home. Patients will not be able to speak if the tube balloon is inflated. If the balloon is deflated, patients can eat normally and can speak if the tube lumen is occluded with the patient's finger during exhalation. A speaking valve can also be fitted to passively close the lumen during exhalation.

PATIENT EDUCATION GUIDES

See the sample patient education and consent forms available at www.expertconsult.com.

CPT/BILLING CODES

31600	Tracheostomy, planned (separate procedure)
31603	Tracheostomy, emergency procedure; transtracheal
31605	Tracheostomy, emergency procedure; cricothyroid membrane
31612	Tracheal puncture, percutaneous with transtracheal aspiration or injection

ICD-10-CM DIAGNOSTIC CODES

J38.7	Unspecified diseases of larynx, not elsewhere classified (abscess, obstruction, necrosis)
J95.89	Pulmonary insufficiency following trauma or surgery
J96.00– J96.02	Acute respiratory failure
J96.10– J96.12	Chronic respiratory failure
S12.8XXX	Fracture, larynx and trachea, closed

Use additional seventh character: A, initial; D, subsequent; S, sequela.

SUPPLIERS

Full contact information is available at www.expertconsult.com.

Percutaneous transtracheal jet ventilation kits
 Instrumentation Industries
 Life Assist Emergency Medical Supplies
 VMM Medizintechnik, West Germany
Shiley tracheostomy products
 Bivona/Smith's Medical
 Mallinckrodt/Covidien

RECOMMENDED READING

Boon JM, Abrahams PH, Meiring JH, Welch T. Cricothyroidotomy. A clinical anatomy review. *Clin Anat.* 2004;17:478–486.
Griffiths J, Barber VS, Morgan L, Young JD. Systematic review and meta-analysis of studies of the timing of tracheostomy in adult patients undergoing artificial ventilation. *BMJ.* 2005;330:1243.
Hebert RB, Bose S, Mace SE. Cricothyrotomy and percutaneous translaryngeal ventilation. In: Roberts JR, Custalow CB, Thomsen TW, eds. *Roberts and Hedges Clinical Procedures in Emergency Medicine.* 6th ed. Philadelphia: Elsevier; 2014:120–133.
Jackson C. Tracheotomy. *Laryngoscope.* 1909;19:285–290.
Reichman EF, Brown A. Percutaneous transtracheal jet ventilation. In: Reichman EF, ed. *Emergency Medicine Procedures.* 2nd ed. New York: McGraw-Hill; 2013:143–148.
Reichman EF. Cricothyroidotomy. In: Reichman EF, ed. *Emergency Medicine Procedures.* 2nd ed. New York: McGraw-Hill; 2013:148–161.
Romano TM, Haines CJ. Tracheostomy. In: Reichman EF, ed. *Emergency Medicine Procedures.* 2nd ed. New York: McGraw-Hill; 2013:161–170.
Weissler M. Tracheotomy and intubation. In: Bailey B. *Head and Neck Surgery: Otolaryngology.* 5th ed. Philadelphia: Lippincott Williams & Wilkins; 2014.

CHAPTER 224

MECHANICAL VENTILATION

Joe Esherick

Modern mechanical ventilation was developed out of necessity during the polio epidemic of the 1930s. The original machines were negative-pressure ventilators, known as "iron lungs." These devices soon became obsolete with the development of positive-pressure ventilators during the 1950s. The advent of positive-pressure ventilation ushered in the era of modern-day surgery, anesthesia, and critical care medicine.

Mechanical ventilators assist in patients' oxygenation and ventilation. Ventilators improve pulmonary gas exchange and aim to reverse hypoxemia and acute respiratory acidosis. Mechanical ventilation also unloads the respiratory muscles and therefore significantly decreases the body's oxygen consumption in both shock and respiratory failure. Although positive-pressure ventilation can aid in pulmonary mechanics, it can also lead to ventilator-induced lung injury if improperly applied.

CLASSIFICATION OF MECHANICAL VENTILATION

All modern ventilators use positive-pressure ventilation; it can be administered noninvasively (e.g., using bilevel positive airway pressure or continuous positive airway pressure [CPAP] machines). However, this chapter focuses on positive-pressure ventilation delivered by an endotracheal or tracheostomy tube.

INDICATIONS

- Inability to protect the airway
- Hypoxic respiratory failure
- Hypercapnic respiratory failure
- Increased work of breathing or inspiratory muscle weakness
- Cardiac arrest or acute decompensated congestive heart failure

CONTRAINDICATIONS

- Advanced directives specifying no intubation or resuscitation

EQUIPMENT AND SUPPLIES

- Ventilator
- Ballard suction catheter
- Suction canister and suction tubing
- Yankauer suction tip
- Bite block or oral airway
- Heat and moisture exchanger
- Ventilator circuit tubing
- Metered-dose inhaler adapter
- Bag-valve-mask device
- Continuous arterial blood pressure and pulse oximetry monitoring; end-tidal capnography and ventilator waveform monitoring may be considered

PRECAUTIONS

- Inadequate sedation may lead to patient-ventilator dyssynchrony.
- High plateau pressures (PPLAT; >30 cm H_2O) lead to increased risk of barotrauma (e.g., pneumothorax, pneumomediastinum, and pneumopericardium).
- Inadequate head elevation predisposes to ventilator-associated pneumonia.
- High (e.g., >8–10 cm H_2O) positive end-expiratory pressure (PEEP) levels can decrease cardiac output, leading to hypotension, and can increase intracranial pressure.
- High-tidal-volume (VT > 10 mL/kg predicted body weight [PBW]) ventilation may cause ventilator-induced lung injury and acute renal failure.
- Prolonged mechanical ventilation predisposes to:
  - Stress gastric ulcers
  - Subglottic stenosis and tracheomalacia
  - Sinusitis
  - Decubitus pressure ulcers
  - Intensive care unit psychosis

TECHNIQUE

Modes of Ventilation

There are four main modes of ventilation: controlled mode, assist-control (AC) mode, synchronized intermittent mandatory ventilation (SIMV) mode, and support mode (Table 224.1). Each of these modes is subclassified into volume-cycled or pressure-cycled methods of ventilation. There are very few data showing definitive improvement in clinically relevant outcomes when one mode is compared with another; therefore clinician familiarity, unit, and institutional practice patterns largely determine which mode is used.

Controlled Mode

Controlled ventilation (or intermittent mandatory ventilation) is restricted to use in heavily sedated or paralyzed patients. It is the principal mode of ventilation used for general anesthesia in the operating room. This mode will deliver a preset VT at a specified rate independent of patient effort. The advantage to its use is that the clinician controls the patient's minute ventilation with absolute certainty. However, the disadvantage is that heavy sedation is required to prevent the development of patient-ventilator dyssynchrony.

Assist-Control Mode

AC ventilation is capable of both *assisted* ventilation and *controlled* ventilation. If patients are breathing spontaneously, the ventilator will synchronize with a patient-initiated breath and thereby assist ventilation. If the patient fails to initiate a breath within a given

TABLE 224.1   Modes of Ventilation

Controlled	Assist-Control	Synchronized Intermittent Mandatory Ventilation	Support
Pressure of volume preset	Pressure of volume is preset	Volume is usually preset	Pressure is usually preset
Used in paralyzed patient	Used as an initial ventilatory mode	Used in spontaneously breathing patient	Used only in spontaneously breathing patient with adequate respiratory drive
Patient receives mandatory preset ventilator rate	Patient receives mandatory preset ventilator rate	Patient receives mandatory preset ventilator rate	Patient receives no mandatory preset ventilator rate
All breaths are ventilator-initiated	All spontaneous breaths are ventilator-assisted	Spontaneous breaths are not ventilator-assisted	All spontaneous breaths are ventilator-assisted
No spontaneous breathing problems	Can be used as a weaning mode	Can be used as a weaning mode	

From Lapinsky SE, Slutsky AS. Ventilator management. In: Wachter RM, ed. *Hospital Medicine*. 2nd ed. Philadelphia: Lippincott Williams & Wilkins; 2005:173–182.

time (as determined by the preset ventilator rate), the machine will provide a controlled breath. AC mode can be volume-cycled (volume control [VC]), pressure-cycled (pressure control [PC]), or a hybrid of the two (pressure-regulated volume control [PRVC]).

With VC ventilation, each AC breath delivers a preset V_T. In other words, both *assisted* breaths and *controlled* breaths receive a preset V_T regardless of the pressure required. The machine ensures that the patient will receive a minimal number of breaths per minute based on the set ventilator rate, even in the absence of patient effort. An advantage is that this mode requires less patient sedation. However, AC cannot limit the respiratory rate of patients who have a high spontaneous respiratory rate. Patients with obstructive lung disease (e.g., chronic obstructive pulmonary disease, status asthmaticus) and a rapid respiratory rate may develop air trapping. Air trapping can cause auto-PEEP and potentially barotrauma.

With PC ventilation, the ventilator delivers gas at a flow rate necessary to achieve a preset peak pressure. As in VC, the ventilator synchronizes with patient effort, when present, and ensures a minimum ventilatory rate. In PC ventilation the peak inspiratory pressure (PIP) remains constant, but its major disadvantage is that the V_T varies from breath to breath depending on the dynamic lung compliance; therefore the V_T can fall to very low levels if the lungs are stiff, which can compromise the minute ventilation.

PRVC is a hybrid between VC and PC. PRVC is essentially a volume-cycled mode of ventilation with gas flow characteristics similar to those of PC ventilation. The ventilator will deliver a preset tidal volume with each breath using a decelerating flow curve. PRVC allows the delivery of a preset V_T at lower peak and mean airway pressures compared with VC.

The primary disadvantage of all modes of AC ventilation is the potential for developing auto-PEEP. At the same minute ventilation, auto-PEEP occurs with fairly equal frequency in VC, PC, and PRVC. See the later discussion of auto-PEEP for more details.

Synchronized Intermittent Mandatory Ventilation Mode

SIMV is a mode of ventilation that ensures a preset minimal number of "machine breaths" while allowing spontaneous patient breaths in between. The ventilator waits for a preset time, allowing the patient to breathe spontaneously, and then delivers a "machine breath" synchronized with the patient's inspiratory effort. The main difference between the AC and SIMV modes is that every breath in the AC mode is ventilator-assisted, whereas only a minimum number of breaths per minute are ventilator-assisted in SIMV. SIMV can be administered in VC, PC, or PRVC mode; therefore the ventilator mode can be set as SIMV/VC, SIMV/PC, or SIMV/PRVC. If necessary, pressure support (PS) or PEEP can be added to assist spontaneous breathing in the SIMV mode.

Pressure Support Mode

The PS mode is used solely for spontaneously breathing patients. All breaths in this mode are patient-initiated breaths and can be augmented by varying degrees of PS. The least amount of PS that should be added is 6 to 10 cm H_2O to overcome the resistance of the endotracheal or tracheostomy tube. Higher PS levels may be applied to aid respiratory mechanics and achieve an adequate V_T.

Ventilator Settings and Terminology

- *Inspiratory time:* The inspiratory time (I_T) can be adjusted to change the inspiratory–expiratory (I:E) time ratio. The normal I:E ratio in nonintubated, spontaneously breathing patient is 1:4, common for the intubated patient it is 1:2. A decreased I_T is often helpful for conditions requiring a prolonged expiratory time, such as severe bronchospasm (e.g., chronic obstructive pulmonary disease, asthma exacerbations). An increased I_T may be indicated for severe hypoxia refractory to high PEEP levels. A significantly prolonged I_T is usually very uncomfortable, typically requires heavy sedation, and may lead to auto-PEEP.
- *Triggering sensitivity:* The triggering sensitivity is the amount of negative pressure/flow needed to trigger a ventilator-assisted breath. This is set in all ventilator modes while watching patient effort. The aim is to achieve optimal patient comfort.
- *Positive end-expiratory pressure:* PEEP is applied by regulating the pressure in the expiratory limb of the ventilator circuit. The goal of PEEP is to keep the alveoli open after expiration to increase the surface area available for gas exchange. Specifically, the longer the alveoli are open, the more oxygen can be exchanged; carbon dioxide clearance is rather efficient even in hypoxic conditions. In addition, PEEP can recruit lung volume by opening closed alveoli; however, it also raises intrathoracic pressure, which can decrease cardiac preload. High levels of PEEP (>8–10 cm H_2O) can improve oxygenation so that lower levels of inspired oxygen (FIO_2) can be administered. Furthermore, a high level of PEEP is often needed during lung-protective ventilation in patients ventilated for either acute respiratory distress syndrome (ARDS) or acute lung injury. PEEP must be used with extreme caution in shock states or if there is any evidence of increased intracranial pressure because high levels of PEEP can worsen both of these conditions.
- *Auto-PEEP:* Auto-PEEP occurs when there is inadequate time for expiration. It causes an increase in the functional residual capacity and raises intrathoracic pressure, increasing the risk of barotrauma. Volume-cycled AC modes have a higher risk of auto-PEEP compared with the SIMV modes of ventilation. Additional risk factors include severe bronchospasm, high respiratory rates, and a high I:E time ratio.
- *Tidal volume:* A preset V_T is used for all volume-cycled modes of ventilation (VC or PRVC). The ventilator displays both an inspiratory V_T and an expiratory V_T, which should be the same unless the circuit is occluded or has a leak. V_T should be monitored closely when ventilating in PS mode.
- *Peak inspiratory pressure:* The PIP is the maximal airway pressure experienced by the patient. The PIP is a measure of dynamic lung

compliance and is a pressure preset in PC mode. The PIP levels vary in volume-cycled ventilation depending on the breath-to-breath changes in dynamic lung compliance. Causes of a high PIP are described later in the discussion of high airway pressures in the section "Ventilator Complications."

- *Plateau pressure:* The PPLAT is the airway pressure measured after an end-inspiratory hold. This pressure reflects the static lung compliance and is a barometer for the risk of barotrauma. Every effort should be made to keep the PPLAT 30 cm H_2O or less. A patient with a high PPLAT may require a lower VT (in the case of ARDS), increased sedation (if there is patient-ventilator dyssynchrony), loop diuretics (if there is congestive heart failure), or an investigation for abdominal compartment syndrome or pneumothorax.
- *Fraction of inspired oxygen:* The FIO_2 can vary from 0.21 (room air) to 1.0. The initial ventilator settings typically start with an FIO_2 between 0.8 and 1.0 until adequate oxygenation has been ensured. Prolonged administration of an FIO_2 greater than 0.6 can lead to oxygen toxicity through the formation of oxygen free radicals; therefore every effort must be made to wean the FIO_2 level down to at least 0.6 as quickly as possible.
- *Flow rate:* The flow rate is typically set at 60 L/min. This is found in volume-targeted modes but not pressure-targeted modes. The flow rate can be increased to deliver the set volume faster and shorten the I_T with its subsequent effect on inspiratory-expiratory (I:E) time ratio.

Initiating Mechanical Ventilation

The steps involved in the initiation of mechanical ventilation and required monitoring are outlined in Box 224.1. The initial mode of ventilation is often the AC mode. Keep in mind that the primary goals of ventilatory support are adequate oxygenation/ventilation, reduced work of breathing, synchrony between the patient and ventilator, and avoidance of high end-inspiratory alveolar pressures.

Rules of Thumb for Mechanical Ventilation

- Adjust ventilation by changing minute volume, to modify the pH (preferably) but also the partial pressure of arterial carbon dioxide ($PaCO_2$):
  - Minute volume = respiratory rate × tidal volume (in liters)
- Methods to improve oxygenation are as follows:
  - Increase FIO_2 or PEEP first.
  - Increase the I_T for refractory hypoxia.
- Keep PPLAT no greater than 30 cm H_2O.
- Avoid ventilating with VT greater than 10 to 12 mL/kg (PBW).
  - Typical VT is 6 to 8 mL/kg PBW initial can be 8 to 10 mL/kg.
  - PBW for men (kg) = 50 + (2.3 × [height in inches − 60]).
  - PBW for women (kg) = 45.5 + (2.3 × [height in inches − 60]).
- Avoid paralytics (if possible) because of concerns regarding critical illness polyneuropathy.
- Sedation during mechanical ventilation should include agents that provide anxiolysis, analgesia, and, ideally, amnesia. Sedation should be titrated to an accepted sedation scale (e.g., the Ramsey scale) and continuous sedation should be interrupted on a daily basis.
  - Opiate and benzodiazepine combination
  - Opiate and Propofol combination
  - Ketamine and benzodiazepine combination
- Scheduled and routine suctioning of patient secretions should be avoided (because of insufficient data and complications); however, removal of oral and bronchotracheal secretions is commonplace and standard of care for mechanically ventilated patients. Data are conflicting regarding the benefit of closed- versus to open-circuit catheters. Caregivers performing suctioning should be aware of potential complications such as hypoxia, cardiac arrhythmias, and airway trauma.

BOX 224.1 Initiating Mechanical Ventilation

1. Choose the mode of ventilation
   - AC if very limited patient effort or with heavy sedation (VC or PRVC)
   - SIMV if some respiratory effort or patient-ventilator dyssynchrony on AC
2. Choose the settings for oxygenation
   - Initial FIO_2 0.8–1.0, adjust according to SaO_2
   - Initial PEEP 5 cm H_2O, adjust according to FIO_2
   - Aim for SaO_2 ≥90%, PaO_2 ≥60 mm Hg
   - Aim to titrate FIO_2 ≤0.6
3. Settings for ventilation
   - Tidal volume: 6–10* mL/kg predicted body weight
   - Ventilator rate: 10–16/min, adjust based on pH, not $PaCO_2$ (consider initial rate of 20–24 in ARDS)
   - Keep plateau pressure at ≤30 cm H_2O
4. Additional ventilator settings
   - Triggering sensitivity: adjust to minimize patient effort, usually set at −1 to −2 cm H_2O
   - I:E ratio: initially 1:2, decrease inspiratory time for severe bronchospasm and can increase inspiratory time for refractory hypoxia
   - Pressure support: if SIMV mode, can adjust between 6 and 20 cm H_2O titrated to patient comfort
5. Monitoring
   - Continuous cardiopulmonary monitor
   - Ventilator: tidal volume, minute volume, airway pressures, serial arterial blood gases
   - $ETCO_2$ monitors desirable for ventilator weaning

AC, Assist-control; *ARDS,* acute respiratory distress syndrome; $ETCO_2$, end-tidal carbon dioxide; FIO_2, fraction of inspired oxygen; *I:E,* inspiratory-expiratory time ratio; $PaCO_2$, partial pressure arterial carbon dioxide; PaO_2, partial pressure arterial oxygen; *PEEP,* positive end-expiratory pressure; SaO_2, arterial oxygen saturation; *SIMV,* synchronized intermittent mandatory ventilation; *VC,* volume control; *PRVC,* pressure-regulated volume control.

Weaning from Mechanical Ventilation

Weaning from mechanical ventilation involves the transition from full ventilatory support to spontaneous breathing and then to eventual extubation (Fig. 224.1). There have been numerous approaches to ventilator weaning but none as successful as daily spontaneous breathing trials (SBT). Patients who pass an SBT can be successfully extubated 85% of the time.

Patients should be assessed on a daily basis as to whether they are ready for an SBT; in part, this consists of clinicians interrupting continuous sedation on a daily basis. Patients should meet the following criteria to be ready for an SBT: (1) awake, cooperative, and able to follow commands; (2) clinically stable and preferably off vasopressor medications; (3) the underlying disease leading to intubation has sufficiently resolved; (4) good gag reflex and strong cough; (5) minimal pulmonary secretions; (6) spontaneous respirations with a PEEP less than 5 to 8 cm H_2O; (7) a partial pressure of arterial oxygen (PaO_2)/FIO_2 ratio of at least 150 to 200; (8) a pH of at least 7.25; and (9) a rapid shallow breathing index (RSBI) of less than 105. The RSBI is checked by placing

---

*Desired tidal volume is 6 to 8 mL/kg predicted body weight; however, patients with acute respiratory failure due to neuromuscular disease often require a tidal volume of 10 to 12 mL/kg to satisfy air hunger. In patients with ARDS it is recommended to use a tidal volume of 6 mL/kg and to keep inspiratory plateau pressure at 30 cm H_2O or less.

the patient on CPAP of 5 cm H_2O with a PS of 0 cm H_2O for 3 minutes and determining the average respiratory rate divided by the V_T (in liters). Patients who have an RSBI greater than 105 fail an SBT 95% of the time.

If the aforementioned criteria are met, an SBT should be performed daily. An SBT can be performed with the patient either on a CPAP level of 5 cm H_2O and PS of 6 to 8 cm H_2O or on a T-piece with an FIO_2 no greater than 0.4 to 0.5. Watch the patient for 30 to 120 minutes and terminate the SBT if the patient develops any of the following signs of intolerance: respiratory rate greater than 35 minutes, arterial oxygen saturation less than 90%, PaO_2 less than 60 mm Hg, heart rate greater than 140 minutes, systolic blood pressure greater than 180 mm Hg or less than 90 mm Hg, agitation, diaphoresis, increased work of breathing, or a V_T less than 325 mL (or less than 4 mL/kg PBW). After 30 to 120 minutes, an arterial blood gas can be drawn to ensure adequate oxygenation and ventilation. A $PaCO_2$ greater than 50 mm Hg (or an increase of >10 mm Hg) or a PaO_2 less than 55 mm Hg (on $FIO_2 = 0.4$) would be additional reasons to continue mechanical ventilation.

If an SBT fails, reasons should be sought. Possibilities include left ventricular dysfunction, respiratory muscle fatigue, sedation, weakness, or delirium.

VENTILATOR COMPLICATIONS

- *High airway pressures:* A high airway pressure can be divided into conditions associated with a high PIP or with a high PPLAT. The conditions associated with a high PIP but an unchanged PPLAT include aspiration, bronchospasm, or endotracheal tube obstruction (kinking or secretions). Conditions that involve elevations in both the PIP and PPLAT include "bucking the ventilator," pulmonary edema, pneumothorax, auto-PEEP, severe abdominal distention, ARDS, or chest wall noncompliance. "Bucking the ventilator" may be caused by inadequate sedation, paroxysms of coughing, or patient-ventilator dyssynchrony.
- *Barotrauma:* Barotrauma is defined as lung injury due to high mean airway pressures. It occurs when there is an alveolar leak causing one of the following clinical conditions: pneumomediastinum, pneumopericardium, pneumothorax, or subcutaneous emphysema. Those at highest risk for barotrauma have one of the following conditions: very stiff lungs (e.g., in ARDS), severe bronchospasm, PPLAT greater than 30 cm H_2O, use of a high I_T, the development of auto-PEEP, and V_T greater than 10 mL/kg PBW.

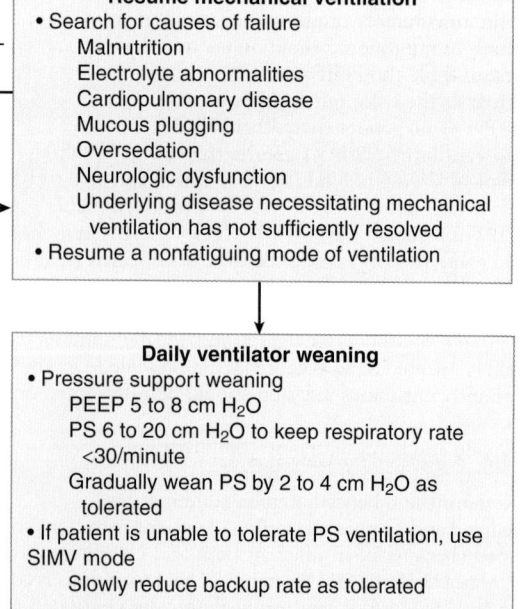

Patient is ready for a spontaneous breathing trial if the following criteria are met:
- Awake, cooperative, and follows commands
- Good gag reflex
- Strong cough
- Minimal secretions
- Hemodynamically stable off vasopressors
- The underlying disease leading to intubation has resolved
- Hemoglobin ≥8 g/dL
- Spontaneously breathing on PEEP <5 to 8
- PaO_2/FIO_2 ratio ≥150–200 (or SaO_2 ≥90% with FIO_2 ≤0.4)
- Systemic pH ≥7.25
- Minute ventilation <15 L/minute
- Rapid shallow breath index <105

↓

Spontaneous breathing trial (SBT)
- Settings: T-piece or PEEP 5 cm H_2O and PS 6 to 8 cm H_2O
- Duration: 30 to 120 minutes
- Patient passes SBT if
  RR ≤35
  HR <120 to 140/minute
  SBP >90 and <180 mm Hg
  SaO_2 ≥90% or PaO_2 ≥55 mm Hg on FIO_2 ≤0.4
  V_T ≥4 mL/kg predicted body weight or ≥325 mL (in adults)
  $PaCO_2$ increase <10 mm Hg
  Absence of agitation, diaphoresis, or increased work of breathing

↓ Daily SBT trials / Fails SBT →

Resume mechanical ventilation
- Search for causes of failure
  Malnutrition
  Electrolyte abnormalities
  Cardiopulmonary disease
  Mucous plugging
  Oversedation
  Neurologic dysfunction
  Underlying disease necessitating mechanical ventilation has not sufficiently resolved
- Resume a nonfatiguing mode of ventilation

↓

Extubate if successful SBT

Daily ventilator weaning
- Pressure support weaning
  PEEP 5 to 8 cm H_2O
  PS 6 to 20 cm H_2O to keep respiratory rate <30/minute
  Gradually wean PS by 2 to 4 cm H_2O as tolerated
- If patient is unable to tolerate PS ventilation, use SIMV mode
  Slowly reduce backup rate as tolerated

Fig. 224.1 Weaning and liberation from mechanical ventilators. *FIO_2*, Fraction of inspired oxygen; *HR*, heart rate; *PaCO_2*, partial pressure of arterial carbon dioxide; *PaO_2*, partial pressure of arterial oxygen; *PEEP*, positive end-expiratory pressure; *PS*, pressure support; *RR*, respiratory rate; *SaO_2*, arterial oxygen saturation; *SBP*, systolic blood pressure; *SIMV*, synchronized intermittent mandatory ventilation; *VT*, tidal volume. (Modified from MacIntyre NR, Cook DJ, Ely EW Jr, et al. Evidence-based guidelines for weaning and discontinuing ventilatory support. *Chest.* 2001;120[6 Suppl]:375S–395S.)

- *Low airway pressures:* A low airway pressure usually means a leak in the ventilator circuit. This can be caused by the patient becoming disconnected from the ventilator, a loose tubing connection, or a large cuff leak.
- *Hypotension:* The causes of hypotension in a ventilated patient can be divided into ventilator-related causes, patient-related causes, and medication-induced hypotension. The ventilator-related causes include high PEEP levels, the development of auto-PEEP, or a tension pneumothorax. Patient-related causes include hypovolemia, a worsening shock state (e.g., septic, cardiogenic, and anaphylactic), abdominal compartment syndrome, a massive pulmonary embolus, unstable arrhythmia, or a massive myocardial infarction. Finally, medication-induced hypotension may be caused by excessive sedation (e.g., opiates, propofol, and benzodiazepines), medication hypersensitivity response, or the excessive use of antihypertensives.
- *Reversible causes of hypoxia:* The reversible causes of hypoxia in a ventilated patient can be remembered by the mnemonic CD-SPIES (Box 224.2). Causes of *chronic* hypoxia are not included as etiologies. Splinting applies only to spontaneous breathing in a support mode when the V_T is limited by pain.
- *High respiratory rates:* The most common causes of a high respiratory rate in a ventilated patient are inadequate sedation, hypoxia, and anxiety. Other causes include a profound metabolic acidosis with a compensatory stimulus to hyperventilate, neurogenic hyperventilation, a pulmonary embolus, and toxic overdoses that stimulate the medullary respiratory center (e.g., salicylate overdose).
- *Apnea:* The most common cause of apnea in a ventilated patient is oversedation or the use of paralytics. Other potential causes include a central nervous system catastrophe or central sleep apnea.
- *Ventilator-induced lung injury:* Ventilator-induced lung injury results either from shear stress or overdistention injury. Shear stress is caused by the repetitive opening and collapsing of alveoli. Overdistention injury results from the prolonged application of high-V_T ventilation (V_T >10 mL/kg PBW). Overdistention injury is especially common if there are areas of normal and diseased lung; the normal lung will be preferentially ventilated and therefore is at risk of overinflation. Conditions associated with poor lung compliance, such as ARDS, are at highest risk for ventilator-induced lung injury and therefore are indications for the use of lung-protective ventilation (Table 224.2).
- *Self-extubation:* Self-extubation can occur for several reasons. First, it can be the inadvertent consequence of moving the patient without adequate attention to the airway. It can also occur as a result of inadequate sedation or loose restraints in an agitated patient.
- *Decubitus pressure ulcers:* Patients who have been mechanically ventilated for a prolonged period are at risk for the development of pressure ulcers of the occiput, sacrum, and heels. Frequent turning is imperative.
- *Venous thromboembolism:* Mechanical ventilation is a risk factor for venous thromboembolism. All ventilated patients should receive prophylactic heparin or sequential compression stockings to minimize the risk of a deep venous thrombosis.
- *Stress gastric ulcers:* Mechanical ventilation for longer than 48 hours places patients at risk for a stress ulcer. Therefore, histamine type 2 blockers or proton pump inhibitors should be administered as prophylaxis against the development of a stress gastric ulcer.
- *Ventilator-associated pneumonia:* Patients who have required mechanical ventilation for longer than 48 hours are at risk for a ventilator-associated pneumonia. The risk of ventilator-associated pneumonia can be decreased by performing the following interventions: raise the head of the bed to 45 degrees, avoid gastric overdistention, minimize ventilator circuit changes/manipulation, drain ventilator circuit condensate on a regular basis, use appropriate hand disinfection before patient care, consider kinetic bed therapy for prolonged mechanical ventilation, and administer twice-daily oral care with chlorhexidine rinses. Selective gut decontamination has a role in trauma patients. Other promising interventions include endotracheal tubes with either low-volume/high-compliance cuffs or those that allow for con-

---

BOX 224.2 Reversible Causes of Hypoxia in Ventilated Patients

C: Congestive heart failure
D: Drugs (oversedation leading to hypoventilation in spontaneously breathing patients)
S: Secretions or splinting (leading to atelectasis in spontaneously breathing patients)
P: Pneumothorax
I: Infection (ventilator-associated pneumonia)
E: Embolism (pulmonary embolism)
S: Spasm (bronchospasm)

TABLE 224.2 Protocol for Lung-Protective Ventilation

1. Assist-control mode with FiO_2 = 100%
2. V_T = 8 mL/kg predicted body weight (PBW)
   PBW for men (kg) = 50 + [2.3 × (height in inches − 60)]
   PBW for women (kg) = 45.5 + [2.3 × (height in inches − 60)]
   Decrease V_T 1 mL/kg PBW every 1–2 h until V_T = 6 mL/kg PBW
3. Initial respiratory rate typically 12–16/min, but can increase up to 35/min
4. Initial PEEP 5–8 cm H_2O, and adjust based on PEEP-FiO_2 algorithm (see below)
5. Adjust PEEP and FiO_2 to keep PaO_2 > 55 mm Hg or SaO_2 > 88%
6. Decrease V_T as low as 4 mL/kg PBW if P_{PLAT} >30 cm H_2O despite adequate suctioning and sedation
7. Allow permissive hypercapnia and may use sodium bicarbonate to keep pH >7.15

PEEP-FiO_2 Algorithm for Lung-Protective Ventilation

FiO_2	0.3	0.4	0.4	0.5	0.5	0.6	0.7	0.7	0.7	0.8	0.9	0.9	0.9	1.0	1.0	1.0	1.0
PEEP*	5	5	8	8	10	10	10	12	14	14	14	16	18	18	20	22	24

*PEEP measured in cm H_2O.
FiO_2, Fraction of inspired oxygen; PaO_2, partial pressure of arterial oxygen; *PEEP*, positive end-expiratory pressure; P_{PLAT}, plateau pressure; SaO_2, arterial oxygen saturation; V_T, tidal volume.
Adapted from Brower RG, Lanken PN, MacIntyre N, et al. for the ARDS Clinical Trials Network: Higher versus lower positive end-expiratory pressures in patients with the acute respiratory distress syndrome. *N Engl J Med.* 2004;351:327–336; and Brower RG, Matthay MA, Morris A, et al., for the ARDS Clinical Trials Network: Ventilation with lower tidal volumes as compared with traditional tidal volumes for acute lung injury and acute respiratory distress syndrome. *N Engl J Med.* 2000;342:1301–1308.

tinuous subglottic suctioning. Most hospitals now have "ventilator bundle checklists" and the frequency of implementation and compliance is monitored to minimize risk of ventilator-acquired pneumonia.

Postprocedure Management

- Check a daily chest radiograph in all endotracheally intubated patients.
- Assess ventilator settings frequently and adjust accordingly.
- Make sure that the patient is receiving interventions to prevent decubitus ulcers, gastric ulcers, a ventilator-associated pneumonia, or a deep venous thrombosis and assess daily for vent complications.
- Assess patients daily for potential to wean or discontinue ventilatory support.

CPT/BILLING CODES

94002	Ventilation assist and management; hospital inpatient/observation, initial day
94003	Ventilation assist and management; hospital inpatient/observation, each subsequent day
94004	Ventilation assist and management; nursing home, per day

(94002 to 94004 not to be reported with E/M services 99201–99499)

94005	Home ventilator management care plan oversight; in home or assisted living, within a calendar month, ≥30 minutes

(94005 code not to be reported with 99339–99340 or 99374–99378)

ICD-10-CM DIAGNOSTIC CODES

E87.2	Acidosis
E87.3	Alkalosis
E87.4	Acid-base mixed disorder
I46.9	Cardiac or cardiorespiratory arrest cause unspecified
I50.1	Left ventricular failure, unspecified
J44.9	Chronic obstructive pulmonary disease unspecified
J44.1	Chronic obstructive bronchitis, with or without emphysema, with acute exacerbation
J43.9	Emphysema, NOS
J45.22	Asthma, mild with status asthmaticus
J45.909	Asthma, unspecified uncomplicated
J95.3	Pulmonary insufficiency following surgery
J96.00	Acute respiratory failure, NOS
R06.03	Respiratory distress, acute
J96.10	Respiratory failure, chronic
R40.20	Coma
R57.9	Shock, unspecified, without mention of trauma
R57.0	Shock, cardiogenic
R65.21	Shock, septic
R57.1	Shock, other (hypovolemic, anaphylactic)
R06.89	Other abnormalities of breathing (hypercapnia)
R09.02	Hypoxia
R09.2	Respiratory arrest

SUPPLIERS

(See contact information available at www.expertconsult.com.)

Maquet Getinge Critical Care AB
Puritan Bennett
Siemens

RECOMMENDED READING

Brower RG, Matthay MA, Morris A, et al, for the ARDS clinical trials network. Ventilation with lower tidal volumes as compared with traditional tidal volumes for acute lung injury and acute respiratory distress syndrome. *N Engl J Med.* 2000;342:1301–1308.

Fuller BM, Cinel I, Dellinger RP. General principles of mechanical ventilation. In: Parrillo JE, Dellinger RP, eds. *Critical Care Medicine: Principles of Diagnosis and Management in the Adult.* 4th ed. Philadelphia: Elsevier; 2016:138–152.

Lapinsky SE, Slutsky AS. Ventilator management. In: Wachter RM, ed. *Hospital Medicine.* 2nd ed. Philadelphia: Lippincott Williams & Wilkins; 2005:173–182.

MacIntyre NR. Assist-control mechanical ventilation. In: Fink MP, Abraham E, Vincent J-L, Kochanek P, eds. *Textbook of Critical Care.* 5th ed. Philadelphia: Saunders; 2005:497–518.

MacIntyre NR, Cook DJ, Ely EW, et al. Evidence-based guidelines for weaning and discontinuing ventilatory support. *Chest.* 2001;120(suppl 6):375S–395S.

Markowitz DH, Irwin RI. Mechanical ventilation: initiation and discontinuation. In: Irwin RI, Rippe JM, eds. *Manual of Intensive Care Medicine.* 5th ed. Philadelphia: Lippincott Williams & Wilkins; 2010.

Santanilla JI. Mechanical ventilation. In: Roberts JR, Custalow CB, Thomsen TW, eds. *Roberts and Hedges Clinical Procedures in Emergency Medicine and Acute Care.* 7th ed. Philadelphia: Elsevier; 2019:160–180.

ARTERIAL PUNCTURE AND PERCUTANEOUS ARTERIAL LINE PLACEMENT

Grant C. Fowler • Donna A. Landen

ARTERIAL PUNCTURE

An arterial puncture can provide useful information for various urgent, acute, or chronic conditions or whenever an arterial blood sample is needed. If frequent sampling or (intra)arterial blood pressure monitoring is necessary, placement of an arterial line should be considered instead. With proper technique and equipment, an arterial puncture is a safe and simple procedure. That said, advancements in technology for noninvasive monitoring such as pulse oximetry (arterial oxygen saturation) and end-tidal CO_2 are decreasing the need for arterial puncture. In most cases, an arterial puncture is used currently only to assess and confirm hypoxia or hypercapnia when indicated by noninvasive monitoring. Although venous sampling may occasionally be used to monitor pH (e.g., diabetic ketoacidosis), venous blood pH is much less reliable as a surrogate marker for arterial pH in patients with shock and other critical illnesses; therefore arterial puncture is still necessary in these patients.

Indications

- To confirm a clinically suspected acute problem with carbon dioxide or oxygen exchange, or with acid-base balance, such as patients with shock, asthma or chronic obstructive pulmonary disease (COPD) exacerbation, pulmonary thromboembolism, diabetic ketoacidosis, or refractory cardiac dysrhythmias, or for patients who are newly comatose or have a depressed level of consciousness.
- To confirm the clinical status in a patient with a chronic condition that affects gas exchange or acid-base balance, such as chronic COPD. Long-term continuous oxygen therapy has proven beneficial (e.g., decreased mortality and hospitalizations) in patients with COPD with a partial pressure of arterial oxygen (PaO_2) less than 59 mm Hg (especially with comorbid disease, e.g., cor pulmonale, pulmonary hypertension), and even more if the PaO_2 is less than 55 mm Hg.
- To confirm hypoxia when pulse oximetry may not be reliable or is not available or obtainable (e.g., patient with severe hypoxia or severe hypotension).
- To confirm hypoxia, when pulse oximetry suggests this diagnosis.
- To confirm hypercapnia when end-tidal CO_2 monitoring may underestimate (e.g., patient with large dead space ventilation or low cardiac output).
- To confirm the need for oxygen therapy at home. Medicare has requirements for home oxygen therapy, and usually either pulse oximetry or arterial blood gas sampling can be used to determine if the patient qualifies. The company providing the oxygen cannot be the same company that does the testing in the home or hospital.

- To obtain arterial blood for certain laboratory tests (lactic acid, ammonia, carboxyhemoglobin, methemoglobin, or carbon monoxide levels, although some laboratories can use venous blood).
- To obtain a blood sample in an emergent situation when phlebotomy cannot be performed or when there are no venous sites.

Contraindications

- When a functional arterial line is present.
- Overlying skin compromised by trauma, burns, infection, severe dermatitis (relative contraindication in life-threatening situation).
- Known or suspected severe arterial disease of aneurysmal, atherosclerotic, inflammatory, or vasospastic nature (relative contraindication in life-threatening situation).
- Previous surgery in the area that may have caused scarring, thereby complicating the procedure (relative contraindication, can always use hand-held Doppler technique).
- Poor collateral perfusion from the ulnar or posterior tibial artery when the radial or dorsalis pedis artery, respectively, is the intended puncture site (may be relative contraindication).
- Inability to palpate arterial pulsation (relative contraindication, can always use hand-held Doppler technique).
- Synthetic vascular graft (relative contraindication).
- Additional relative contraindications: bleeding dyscrasias, anticoagulant therapy, or possible later thrombolytic or fibrinolytic therapy. These patients should be monitored carefully after arterial puncture to prevent complications.

NOTE: If drawing of frequent arterial specimens or continuous pressure monitoring is necessary, placement of an arterial line should be considered.

Equipment

- 3- to 5-mL sterile plastic or glass syringe with a freely movable plunger. (Kits are made in which the preheparinized syringe plunger should not be moved. A lyophilized heparin pellet may be in the syringe which means use of additional heparin is not necessary. These kits also contain the needle and rubber stopper or syringe plug.)
- 22- to 25-gauge, 0.625-inch (1.6 cm) to 1.5-inch (3.8 cm) needle for radial, brachial or dorsalis pedis puncture. For femoral puncture, a 20- to 22-gauge, 2.5-inch (6.4 cm) needle may be helpful, especially in obese patients.
- 1 or 2 mL heparin (1000 U/mL) if not using kit with preheparinized syringe
- Plug for syringe or rubber stopper for end of needle

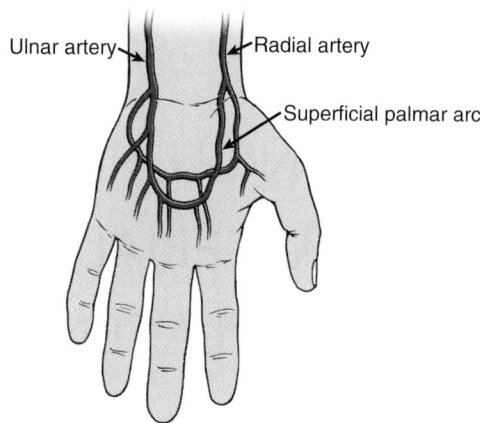

Fig. 225.1   Anatomy of radial and ulnar arteries at wrist and superficial palmar arch.

- Antiseptic skin preparation, such as povidone-iodine, chlorhexidine, or 70% isopropyl alcohol
- Sterile 4 × 4 gauze pads
- Hypoallergenic adhesive tape
- Container with 2 to 3 inches of crushed ice for sample transport (e.g., plastic bag, emesis basin, cup)
- Sterile gloves
- Equipment for the clinician to observe universal blood and body fluid precautions
- In the alert patient (optional), 1% or 2% lidocaine without epinephrine and a 1- or 3-mL syringe with 25- or 27-gauge, 0.625-inch (1.6 cm) needle
- Hand-held Doppler (same as used for obtaining fetal heart tones) or pulse oximeter (optional)
- Ultrasound machine, high frequency probe (5 to 10 MHz), sterile ultrasound gel, sterile ultrasound probe cover (optional technique, see "Percutaneous Arterial Line Placement" section for details)

Arterial Site Selection

Each site for arterial puncture has its own risks and benefits. Because of its proximity to the skin surface, the radial artery in the patient's nondominant hand is the preferred site. It is an excellent location if there is adequate ulnar artery collateral circulation (see the following section) and if the clinical situation is stable. In severely hypotensive patients or during cardiopulmonary resuscitation, the femoral artery is usually the most readily palpable and most conveniently located artery, in spite of its higher risk of complications with puncture. Alternative sites, in decreasing order of preference, include the brachial, dorsalis pedis, and superficial temporal arteries. The brachial artery should be reserved for use when radial artery puncture cannot be performed or is contraindicated. Although the dorsalis pedis artery is absent, usually bilaterally, in 12% of the population, it is another option for puncture. Before dorsalis pedis artery puncture is performed, collateral flow should be demonstrated in a manner similar to the Allen test (see the following section). Superficial temporal artery puncture will not be discussed. Ultimately, clinician experience and local anatomy are the deciding factors in choice of site. If possible, the clinician should avoid an artery where the overlying cutaneous defenses are disrupted because of infection, burn, severe dermatitis, or other skin damage.

Assessment of Ulnar Collateral Circulation

Radial artery puncture can lead to thrombosis of the distal artery. Because 12% of hands have inadequate collateral flow because of an incomplete palmar arch (Fig. 225.1), to minimize the risk of permanent ischemic damage to the hand, many experts suggest confirming adequate collateral circulation before puncture. Even if there is excellent collateral flow, the nondominant hand should be used, if possible. However, other experts have questioned the value of testing for collateral

circulation. At least one large case series of patients demonstrated the safety of radial artery cannulation without testing for collateral circulation with the modified Allen test in patients without major peripheral arterial disease (Slogoff et al., 1983). Thus it is recommended, but not required, to use another site if the modified Allen test is abnormal.

Modified Allen Test

The Allen test, used to evaluate ulnar collateral flow, was first described in 1929. To minimize falsely abnormal results, the modified Allen test can be used:

1. The hand should be at least room temperature (>70°F). It can be warmed in water, if necessary. The patient should hold his or her arm above heart level and then open and close the hand several times to exsanguinate it. Next, the patient should clench the fist tightly. The clinician then compresses both the radial and ulnar arteries (Fig. 225.2A). (In a comatose or anesthetized patient, the hand can be elevated and clenched passively by an assistant.)
2. After a minute is allowed for blood to drain from the hand, the fist should be lowered below the level of the heart and unclenched (see Fig. 225.2B), and pressure on the ulnar artery (see Fig. 225.2C) should be released. Care should be taken to avoid hyperextension of the wrist or fingers, which can lead to a falsely abnormal test result. When the pressure on the ulnar artery is released, the cadaveric color of the entire hand should return to its normal color within 6 seconds (see Fig. 225.2D). Color usually returns to the palm first, and then to the entire hand. If any area of the hand does not rapidly (within 6 seconds) return to normal color, this is a positive modified Allen test. The thumb, index finger, and thenar eminence are the areas most commonly involved in a positive test. These areas often have inadequate collateral blood flow and may be entirely dependent on the radial artery for perfusion.

An abnormal or equivocal modified Allen test result, although it may not preclude arterial puncture or cannulation, should alert the clinician to potential complications, a need for caution when performing the procedure, and a need to monitor the patient closely postprocedure. Various types of noninvasive studies are also useful for further patient evaluation. Hand-held Doppler or pulse oximetry can be used to rapidly assess perfusion with techniques more sensitive and specific than the modified Allen test. If time allows, formal arterial Doppler ultrasound, either portable or in the radiology department, can be used to further evaluate the collateral circulation or direct the puncture.

Hand-Held Doppler Evaluation

1. After placing the probe between the heads of the third and fourth metacarpals on the palm, angulate the probe and advance it proximally until maximal auditory signal is obtained (Fig. 225.3).
2. With the palmar arch identified and maximal signal obtained, compression of the radial artery should not cause a change of the signal if the palmar arch is complete and supplied by collateral ulnar circulation. A decrease in signal indicates poor collateral flow. This is a much more sensitive and specific test than the modified Allen test.

Pulse Oximetry Evaluation

This is especially useful in the unconscious patient.

1. Place the sensor of a pulse oximeter with a visual pulse waveform display on the patient's thumb.
2. While examining the waveform on the monitor, occlude the radial artery. If the waveform remains unchanged after radial artery occlusion, the patient has adequate collateral circulation, probably from the ulnar artery.

Assessment of Dorsalis Pedis Collateral Circulation

To minimize the risk of permanent ischemic damage to the distal foot, some experts suggest confirming adequate collateral circulation before dorsalis pedis artery puncture is attempted.

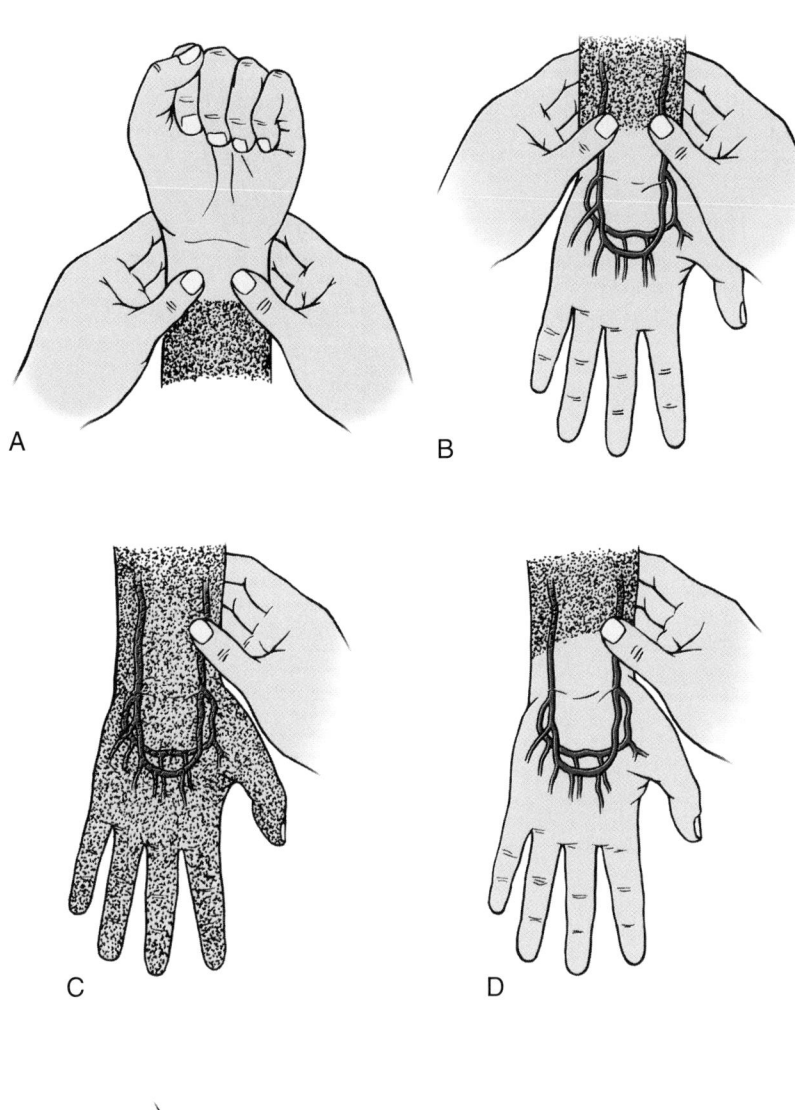

Fig. 225.2 Modified Allen test. (A) Hand is elevated and fist clenched while radial and ulnar arteries are occluded for 1 minute. (B) Hand is lowered and fist is unclenched. Hand is cadaveric. (C) Ulnar artery compression is released while radial artery compression is continued. In a negative test, the entire hand regains color within 6 seconds. (D) Positive test. With inadequate collateral perfusion from the ulnar artery, the hand remains cadaveric as long as radial artery compression is maintained. When inadequate collateral perfusion is demonstrated, another puncture or cannulation site should be considered.

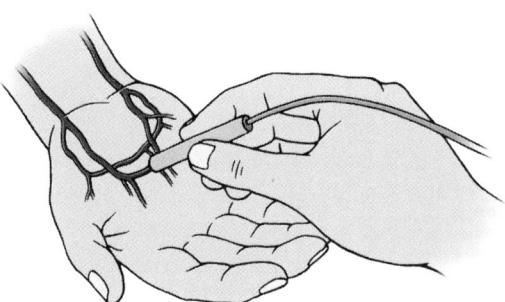

Fig. 225.3 Assessment of the superficial palmar arch with hand-held Doppler ultrasound.

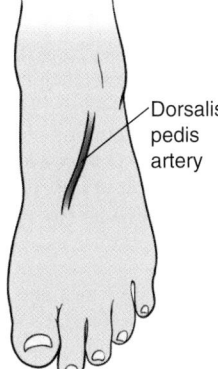

Dorsalis pedis artery

Fig. 225.4 **Location of the dorsalis pedis artery.**

1. The foot should be at least room temperature (>70°F). It can be warmed in water, if necessary.
2. After locating and palpating the dorsalis pedis artery (Fig. 225.4), occlude it with compression.
3. Blanch the great toenail by compressing for several minutes.
4. Release pressure on the nail and observe for flushing. A rapid return of color indicates adequate collateral flow.

NOTE: In most persons, collateral circulation of the foot is provided by a branch of the posterior tibial artery. Hand-held Doppler can be used to assess collateral flow between the dorsalis pedis and posterior tibial arteries in a manner similar to that used in the palmar arch.

Preprocedure Patient Preparation

The clinician and patient should be in a comfortable position that can be maintained for 10 to 15 minutes. The procedure, its necessity, alternatives (if there are any), and possible complications should be explained to the alert patient. In nonemergent situations, informed consent should be obtained (see the sample patient consent form available at www.expertconsult.com). The patient should be prepared for some discomfort.

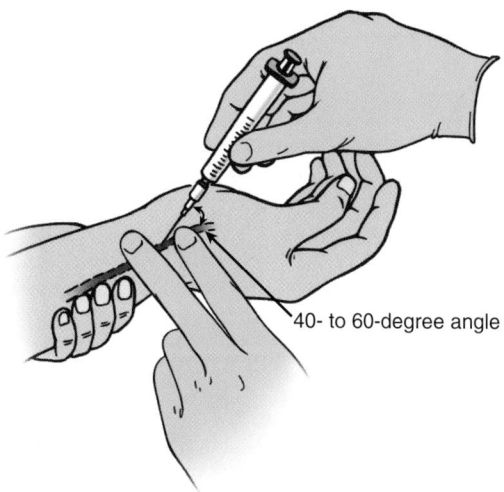

40- to 60-degree angle

Fig. 225.5   This patient is left-hand dominant. Palpate the patient's radial pulse with your left hand. While holding the heparinized syringe with your right hand (reverse hands if left-handed), puncture the skin at approximately a 60-degree angle to the skin, directing the needle toward the radial pulsation.

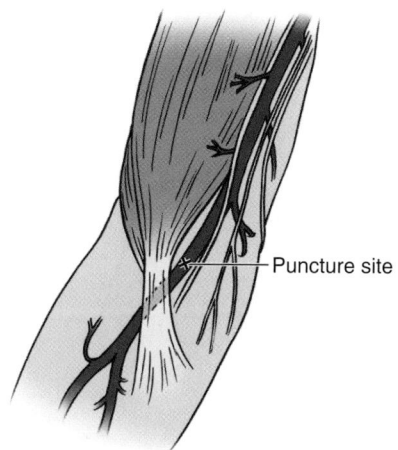

Puncture site

Fig. 225.6   Right brachial artery and its branches, and the anatomic site for brachial artery puncture.

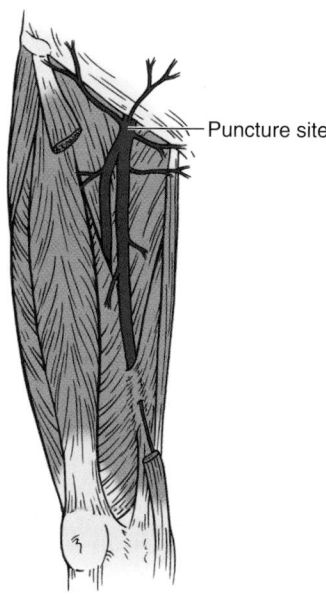

Puncture site

Fig. 225.7   Right femoral artery and its branches, and the anatomic site for femoral artery puncture.

Technique

1. Rinse the syringe with a small amount (1 or 2 mL) of heparin, and then empty it through the needle. For glass syringes, this step not only coats the syringe with heparin, it eliminates the dead space in the syringe and needle. Although heparin does not adhere to plastic syringes, performing this step with plastic syringes will displace any air and fill the dead space.
   NOTE: Certain kits contain syringes that are already heparinized (often containing a pellet of lyophilized heparin which means use of additional heparin is not necessary) and the plunger should not be moved.
2. Following universal blood and body fluid precautions, prepare the skin in an aseptic manner and put on sterile gloves.
3. The clinician should use his or her nondominant hand to palpate the selected artery with the balls of two or three fingers and immobilize it with these fingers along its course.
4. Optional: Local anesthetic (lidocaine) can be injected for a particularly anxious patient to minimize hyperventilation artifact. However, use minimal amounts to avoid anatomic distortion, which could make it difficult to palpate and puncture the pulse.
5. Holding the barrel of the syringe like a pencil in the dominant hand, keep the needle bevel up.
6. Depending on the site selected, perform the puncture.
   - *Radial artery puncture:* Dorsiflex the supine wrist (approximately 30 degrees) of the patient's nondominant hand and rotate it outward (externally), slightly. The wrist should be supported by a firm surface, such as an assistant's hand, a rolled towel or washcloth, or a 500-mL intravenous (IV) fluid bag. Insert the needle where the pulse is most prominent—0.5 to 1 inch proximal to the wrist crease—at a 40- to 60-degree angle to the skin (some experts advocate a 30- to 45-degree angle, similar to that used for cannulation). Direct it slowly in the long axis of the artery toward the pulsation (Fig. 225.5).
     NOTE: Avoid "spearing" (going through) the artery. Osteomyelitis and large hematomas can result from "spearing" the artery.
   - *Brachial artery puncture:* Place the patient's elbow on a rolled towel or washcloth. With the elbow fully extended, the arm should be supinated (palm up) and the patient's wrist in the anatomic position but rotated slightly outward. The brachial artery pulsation should be palpable in the medial aspect of

the antecubital fossa (Fig. 225.6), lateral to the medial epicondyle, but medial to the biceps tendon. Insert the needle at approximately a 45- to 60-degree angle, slightly above the elbow crease, in the antecubital fossa or slightly proximal to it. Aim along the long axis of the artery toward the pulsation.
   - *Femoral artery puncture* (Fig. 225.7): With the patient in a supine position and legs straight, rotated slightly outward, insert the needle 1 to 1.5 inches distal to the inguinal ligament at about the inguinal crease. It should be at a 60- to 90- degree angle to the distal skin and aimed toward the pulsation (Fig. 225.8). Avoid puncturing lateral to the pulsation because the femoral nerve could be damaged.
   - *Dorsalis pedis artery puncture* (Fig. 225.9): With the patient in a supine position, insert the needle where the pulse is most prominent, at a 20- to 30- degree angle to the skin (it is a fairly superficial artery). Aim toward the pulsation. Avoid plantar flexing the foot more than 45 degrees which can occlude the artery.

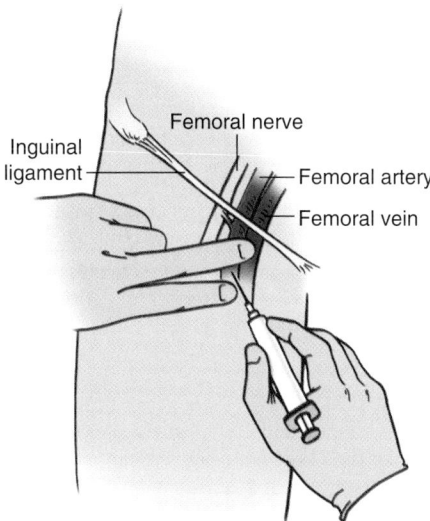

Fig. 225.8 Technique of femoral artery puncture. The first two fingers of the free hand are used to palpate the femoral artery.

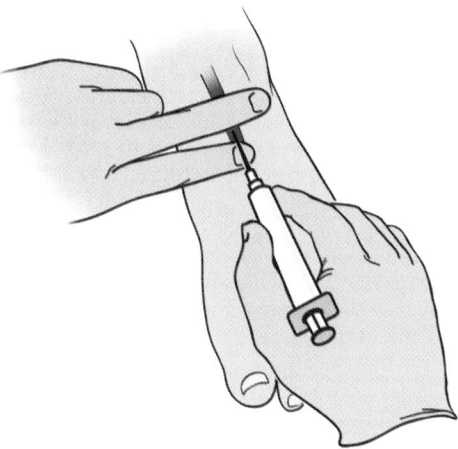

Fig. 225.9 Technique of dorsalis pedis artery puncture.

7. Although penetration into the artery can occasionally be sensed, puncture is usually detected when blood enters the syringe. It should enter the syringe spontaneously without withdrawing the plunger if the syringe is specifically designed for arterial puncture. With plastic syringes or in severely hypotensive patients, slight aspiration may be necessary. Otherwise, attempt to avoid aspiration to decrease the chance of obtaining venous blood. If blood is not obtained during the insertion, slowly withdraw the needle and stop when blood appears.

8. If no blood appears, withdraw the needle completely and start again. For additional attempts, advance the needle without changing the angle of approach but with the needle directed 0.125 inch to either side of the previous attempt.

9. When blood appears, collect 3 mL of blood, and remove the needle from the artery with a smooth, swift motion while applying pressure to the site. Steady pressure should be maintained for at least 5 minutes (longer in hypertensive or anticoagulated patients).

10. While applying pressure at the site with one hand, use the other hand to hold the syringe with the needle tip upright and expel any air bubbles. Tapping the syringe may help to expel bubbles clinging to the sides.

11. Secure the needle tip by impaling it on a rubber stopper or re-

move the needle and cap the syringe securely. (Special rubber caps are available for this purpose.) Do not allow any room air to get into the syringe or any air bubbles to remain.

12. Roll the syringe between the palms of the hands 4 or 5 times to mix the blood uniformly with the heparin.

13. Label the syringe appropriately with the patient's name and number(s) and place the syringe on ice. Immediately transport the syringe to the laboratory.

14. Return in 10 to 15 minutes and check the puncture site for hematoma formation and for adequate distal perfusion.

Complications

- Repeated punctures at the same site increase the risk of complications.
- Hemorrhage or hematoma is the most common complication. Risk can be minimized by prompt, continuous application (for 5 to 10 minutes) of pressure after the procedure, and by using a small-gauge (22- to 25-gauge) needle, if possible.
- Thrombosis is a possible complication of any arterial puncture. It more commonly results from puncture of the radial artery or any artery with occlusive disease. The risk increases with repeated punctures. For a diminished pulse after puncture, prompt vascular surgical consultation should be obtained. Ischemia and resulting gangrene are additional possible complications.
- Nerve damage can occur, either from direct needle insertion into the nerve or from the pressure of a resultant hematoma. This is more common with brachial and femoral artery punctures.
- Infection, including septic arthritis from a femoral artery puncture, is a possible complication. Try to avoid puncturing down to the bone with a femoral artery puncture (or any other puncture).
- Pseudoaneurysms have been reported, especially with femoral artery puncture. A pseudoaneurysm appears as a "pulsating tumor," anterior to the artery, often associated with a bruit. These occur more often after resolution of a large hematoma. Treatment is surgical removal of the pseudoaneurysm by a vascular surgeon.
- An arteriovenous fistula may form after femoral puncture. This is partly why the radial artery is a preferred site because there is no accompanying large vein.
- Spurious laboratory results are most often the consequence of mixing venous blood with the arterial sample, but they can also be due to an excessive quantity of heparin in the syringe. Heparin has a very low pH; therefore using too much can cause not only a falsely low partial pressure of arterial carbon dioxide ($PaCO_2$) but also a low pH. Delay in analyzing the specimen or improper chilling can cause the blood to metabolize the oxygen or the oxygen to dissociate from hemoglobin. This will falsely lower the oxygen and pH and falsely elevate the $PaCO_2$. Air in the syringe may markedly lower the $PaCO_2$ because room air contains little carbon dioxide. Depending on whether the initial partial PaO_2 was greater or less than room air, mixing the sample with air may either falsely lower or elevate the PaO_2. Vacutainers should not be used to draw arterial blood; even though they are filled with nitrogen, they contain measurable amounts of oxygen. Even this small amount of oxygen will significantly alter the PaO_2.

Postprocedure Patient Education

The patient should be instructed to avoid rubbing the site. He or she should report any bleeding, pain, swelling, numbness, or tingling after the arterial puncture. If the extremity turns cold or blue, the patient should inform the nurse or clinician. If the patient is awake and alert, he or she can help to hold pressure on the site while the clinician is delivering the specimen to the laboratory.

PERCUTANEOUS ARTERIAL LINE PLACEMENT

Intraarterial procedures are now common, with arterial dye studies and angioplasty even being performed by noncardiologists and nonsurgeons (e.g., interventional radiologists). The most common intraarterial procedures performed are arterial puncture and arterial cannulation. If arterial cannulation is to be performed, support staff and facilities must be properly trained and prepared to deal with setup and possible complications, which can be more frequent and severe than with IV cannulation or arterial puncture. The site (radial, femoral, or dorsalis pedis artery) should be chosen according to the same risks and priorities established in the Arterial Puncture section. Benefits of arterial cannulation include accurate arterial pressure measurements, less discomfort and injury than with frequent arterial punctures, and the ability to obtain arterial samples without disturbing the steady state (e.g., pain induced with arterial puncture can cause hyperventilation, resulting in falsely low $PaCO_2$ measurements).

NOTE: For noninvasive monitoring of arterial pressure, Korotkoff sounds are commonly used. With increased wall tension (e.g., in vasoconstricted patients, such as those with increased systemic vascular resistance from shock), the ability of the arterial walls to produce the Korotkoff sounds may be altered. Therefore, in these patients, low cuff pressure does not necessarily indicate hypotension. Relying on Korotkoff sounds alone in such patients can result in dangerous errors in therapy. Stiff walls from atherosclerosis can also alter Korotkoff sounds.

Indications

- When there is difficulty obtaining or risk of inaccuracy of cuff blood pressure in a critically ill patient
- When continuous monitoring of arterial blood pressure is needed, especially in patients with shock, patients with resultant increased systemic vascular resistance, patients who have the potential to become hemodynamically unstable, and during major surgery or administration of parenteral vasopressor or dilator medications
- With labile or accelerated hypertension and evidence of progressive vascular damage (mean arterial pressure [MAP] is a much more consistent parameter for accelerated hypertension than the systolic or diastolic pressure alone)
- To monitor MAP in patients in whom it is necessary to maintain MAP at a certain level (e.g., to maintain cerebral perfusion pressure in a patient poststroke)
- When continuous access to arterial blood is needed (to avoid repeated arterial punctures)
- To measure cardiac output by the dye dilution method
- To perform an angiogram

Contraindications

Absolute

- Inadequate collateral blood flow distal to where the arterial line will be placed (e.g., abnormal modified Allen test or dorsalis pedis collateral flow test result, or hand-held Doppler or pulse oximetry reveals inadequate collateral arterial circulation; see the controversy in the Arterial Puncture section)
- Patients with a significant injury to the same extremity, especially if it may compromise distal perfusion
- Hypercoagulable states

Relative

The following are relative contraindications; in life-threatening or certain other situations, the benefits of arterial cannulation may outweigh the risks. In some patients, arterial cannulation will decrease the risks of bleeding from multiple punctures.

- Severe atherosclerotic or vasospastic arterial disease
- Local skin compromise, such as with trauma, infection, burn, or severe dermatitis

- Anticoagulation from bleeding disorders, anticoagulant therapy, or potential future thrombolytic therapy
- Synthetic vascular graft
- Artery not palpable

NOTE: In general, it is a bad idea to attempt arterial puncture or cannulation if the artery is not palpable. Such attempts are usually fruitless and sometimes hazardous. Instead, consider ultrasound-guided puncture or cannulation. In addition, although certain experts no longer recommend cannulation of the brachial artery because of the increased potential for thrombosis and ischemia of the lower arm and hand, others prefer brachial artery cannulation to radial or dorsalis pedis artery cannulation in certain patients (e.g., the patient with anasarca).

Equipment

- Sterile gloves, drapes, and 4 × 4 gauze sponges
- Equipment for the clinician to observe universal blood and body fluid precautions
- Antiseptic skin preparation, such as povidone-iodine or chlorhexidine solution
- In the alert patient (optional), 1% or 2% lidocaine without epinephrine and a 3-mL syringe with 25- or 27-gauge, 0.625-inch (1.6-cm) needle
- Short arm board/wrist extensor splint and a rolled gauze, towel, or washcloth, approximately 3 inches in diameter, for radial artery cannulation; arm board and the same rolled gauze, towel, or washcloth for brachial artery cannulation
- For radial, dorsalis pedis, or brachial artery cannulation, a 20-gauge, 1.25- to 2-inch (3.2- to 5.1-cm) Teflon catheter-over-needle with a nontapered shaft
- For femoral artery cannulation, a 19- or 20-gauge or 4-Fr, 6-inch (15- to 16-cm) single-lumen cannula
- For the Seldinger or wire-guided technique, a flexible guidewire small enough to pass through the catheter and needle
- Fluid-filled connector tubing attached to sterile three-way stopcock and transducer (using a stiff, low-capacitance tubing will minimize the artifact; in addition, attempt to minimize the length of tubing); transducers are available with needleless sampling ports
- Antibiotic ointment, such as povidone-iodine ointment
- Nylon 3-0 or 4-0 suture, preferably on a skin needle
- Hypoallergenic adhesive tape
- Suture scissors
- Bag of sterile dextrose 5% in water (D_5W) IV fluid mixed with heparin to make a 1-U/mL solution for flushing (this should be in-line with the connector tubing)
- Scissors for clipping hair for femoral insertion
- Hand-held Doppler (same as used for obtaining fetal heart tones, optional technique)
- Ultrasound machine, high frequency probe (5 to 10 MHz), sterile ultrasound gel, sterile ultrasound probe cover (optional technique)
- No. 11 or No. 15 blade scalpel, mosquito hemostat, and nylon 3-0 suture for cutdown (optional technique)

Preprocedure Patient Preparation

Explain the indications, complications, and necessity of the procedure to the patient if he or she is alert and awake. If the patient is unconscious, explain this to the next of kin. If there are alternatives available, discuss them as along with the benefits of this procedure. Discuss the importance of immobilization while the procedure is being performed, and warn the patient of the discomfort that will be felt with the insertion of the catheter. Inform the patient that this catheter is more dangerous than an IV catheter and that care must be taken with the catheter after insertion. Obtain written consent for the procedure or document implied consent in the chart if the patient is unconscious.

Technique

1. The clinician and the patient should be in a comfortable position that can be maintained as long as necessary to complete the procedure. When using nonclosed systems, observe universal blood and body fluid precautions.
2. The clinician should palpate the artery selected and immobilize it along its course with two or three fingers of his or her nondominant hand.
3. Prepare the skin in an aseptic manner. For femoral cannulation, use scissors to clip any long hairs near the cannulation.
4. Local anesthetic (lidocaine) can be injected for a particularly anxious patient. It may also prevent arterial spasm when the artery is punctured. Use minimal amounts to prevent anatomic distortion, which may make it difficult to palpate the pulse. If the anatomy does get distorted from the anesthetic injection, attempt to massage it into the surrounding skin and soft tissue.
5. Drape the area with sterile towels.
6. Wearing sterile gloves, the clinician should hold the catheter needle hub like a pencil in his or her dominant hand with the needle bevel up. The clinician should be positioned to avoid any arterial spray that could occur after cannulation.
7. Depending on the site selected, perform the cannulation.
   - *Radial artery cannulation:* On the patient's selected hand (preferably the nondominant hand), slightly dorsiflex (approximately 30 degrees), slightly rotate outward, and immobilize the wrist by taping a gauze roll between the supinated wrist and the dorsally applied arm board (Fig. 225.10A). The 3-inch roll should be between the arm and the board. Apply tape over the proximal interphalangeal joints (excluding the thumb) and around the arm board. Also apply tape more proximally, securing the forearm to the arm board. Insert the needle 0.5 to 1 inch proximal to the wrist crease, at approximately a 30-degree angle to the distal skin. Direct it slowly down the long axis of the artery toward the pulsation (see Fig. 225.10B).
   - *Femoral artery cannulation:* With the patient in the supine position and legs straight, rotated slightly outward, insert the needle at a 45-degree angle to the skin and direct it toward the patient's head. In addition, direct it toward the femoral artery pulsation, 2 to 5 cm distal to the inguinal ligament at the inguinal crease. After the flash of blood, the angle can be lowered to 20 or 30 degrees relative to the distal skin.
   NOTE: Large hematomas are not uncommon in this area because of the amount of surrounding soft tissue. Femoral artery cannulation also carries the risk of more serious complications. Avoid puncturing proximal to the inguinal ligament, which could cause a retroperitoneal hematoma. The proximity of this location to the groin may increase the risk of infection. This location is also less popular for patients if they are awake; they should not ambulate with a femoral artery cannulation in place (see Fig. 225.7).
   - *Dorsalis pedis artery cannulation:* With the patient in the supine position and the foot slightly plantar flexed (not beyond 45-degrees) and stabilized on a firm surface, such as the bed, the dorsalis pedis artery should be palpated. Use two fingers of the nondominant hand to further localize and stabilize the artery. Following sterile technique (Fig. 225.11), direct the needle tip and catheter slowly along the axis of the artery, aimed toward the arterial pulsation, at a 20- to 30-degree angle to the distal skin.
   NOTE: Because collateral circulation in the foot is usually good, dorsalis pedis arterial cannulation should be considered when radial artery cannulation is not a good option. In patients with good cardiac output and palpable dorsalis pedis and posterior tibial pulses, dorsalis pedis arterial cannulation by experienced personnel has been demonstrated to have minimal risk of adverse events such as ischemia and thrombosis. It also allows the patient a little more mobility than with femoral artery cannulation.
   - *Brachial artery cannulation:* With the patient's elbow on a rolled towel or washcloth, fully extend the elbow and supinate the patient's nondominant arm so the patient's wrist lies in the anatomic position but rotated slightly outward. Immobilize the arm with tape and an arm board, preventing flexion at the elbow. The brachial artery lies lateral to the medial epicondyle but medial to the biceps tendon and courses through the antecubital fossa. Palpate and stabilize the artery using sterile technique. Direct the needle tip and catheter slowly along the axis of the artery, aimed toward the arterial pulsation, at a 20- to 30- degree angle to the distal skin (Fig. 225.12).

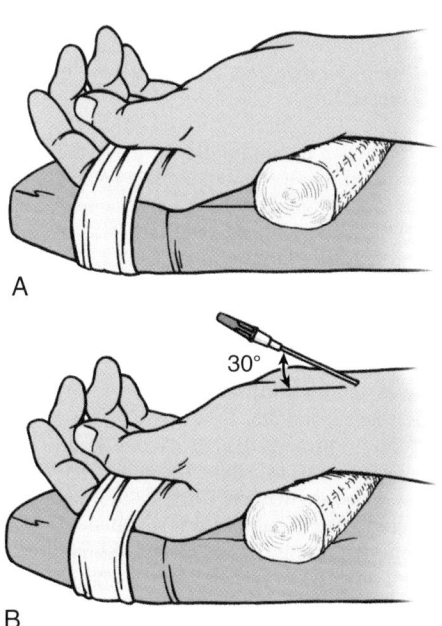

Fig. 225.10 (A) Position for radial artery cannulation. (B) Catheter is directed along the long axis of the artery.

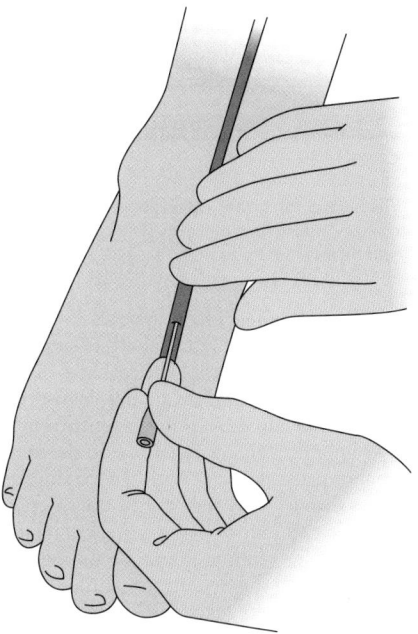

Fig. 225.11 Dorsalis pedis artery cannulation. (Modified from American Heart Association. *Textbook of Advanced Cardiac Life Support.* Dallas: American Heart Association; 1997.)

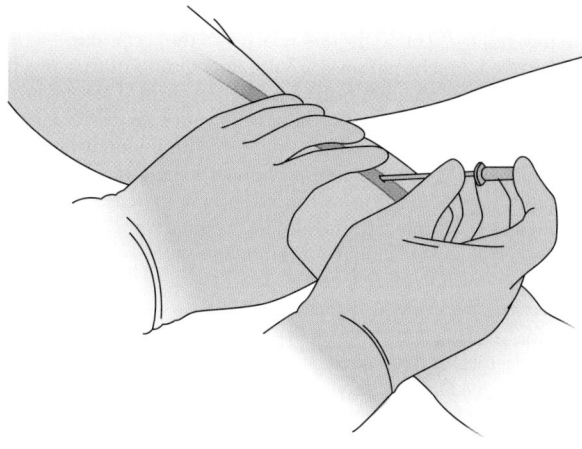

Fig. 225.12 Brachial artery cannulation. (Modified from American Heart Association. *Textbook of Advanced Cardiac Life Support*. Dallas: American Heart Association; 1997.)

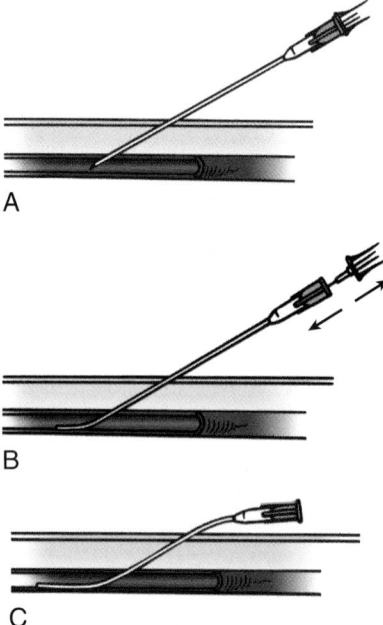

Fig. 225.13 Technique for artery cannulation. (A) Insert angiocatheter through skin, into artery, noting flash of blood. (B) Advance catheter carefully. (C) Catheter should be inserted up to hub.

8. Puncture is detected when blood appears in the needle hub. For radial, dorsalis pedis, and brachial artery cannulation, while holding the needle fixed, advance the catheter-over-needle into the artery (Fig. 225.13). Avoid advancing against resistance; the cannula may advance more easily if it is gently rotated while advancing. For femoral artery cannulation, do the same unless the Seldinger technique is desired. With the Seldinger technique, insert the wire through the needle into the artery, remove the needle, insert the catheter over the wire, and remove the wire. A modified Seldinger technique can be used for radial artery cannulation. Although the Seldinger technique is useful, an ordinary cannula is usually quicker and easier.
   NOTE: The wire-guided technique may be more successful for arterial cannulation when the pulse is either weak or absent, especially in female patients.

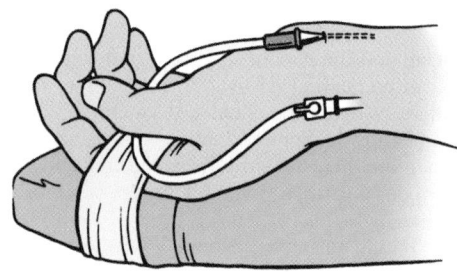

Fig. 225.14 Attach connector tubing to the catheter and fix in position.

9. If the artery cannot be cannulated after the flash of blood has appeared, the posterior artery wall has probably been penetrated. Remove the needle entirely, slowly withdraw the catheter until blood flows into it, and readvance the catheter. Advancing the catheter with a rotating motion may be helpful, especially if resistance is encountered.
10. For the Seldinger technique, to minimize the chance of intramural insertion or dissection, make sure the wire passes without *any* resistance.
11. If after three attempts the artery has not been entered, discontinue the procedure on that side and attempt on the other side or at another site. Pressure should be applied to the unsuccessful site for at least 10 minutes, followed by a pressure dressing. A cutdown might also be considered, with the technique described in a later section being similar to that used for venous cutdown (see Chapter 227, Venous Cutdown).
12. After insertion, advance the catheter until the hub is in contact with the skin and attach it to the connector tubing (Fig. 225.14). Flush the catheter and zero the transducer system by opening the three-way stopcock to atmosphere and pushing the "zero" button on the pressure monitor. Return the three-way stopcock to the patient position and observe the arterial tracing. It should be sharp and clean. If it is not, reposition the catheter. If successful, stitch the catheter into position, apply antibiotic ointment, and cover with a sterile dressing. For radial or brachial artery cannulation, remove the 3-inch roll.
13. Staff should check the extremity every 4 hours for perfusion and the site for signs of a hematoma or early cellulitis. The dressing should be changed daily, along with regular flushing of the line as long as it remains cannulated. After catheter removal, observe the patient for bleeding, extremity pain, numbness, swelling, or discoloration.

NOTE: If the Seldinger technique is not used, the "liquid stylet" method may be useful. If a flash of blood is seen in the hub and the artery cannot be cannulated, fill a 10-mL syringe with 5 mL of sterile normal saline. Attach the syringe to the catheter hub and aspirate 1 to 2 mL of blood to verify intraluminal position. The blood should be very easy to aspirate. Slowly inject fluid from the syringe and advance the catheter behind the fluid wave.

Alternate Method: Hand-Held Doppler Guided

1. Position the extremity in the position previously described, and prepare, anesthetize, and drape the area.
2. Using antiseptic ointment (e.g., povidone-iodine) as transmission gel, have an assistant align the hand-held Doppler with the artery, at a site slightly proximal to the puncture site. The assistant should pass it back and forth medial to lateral over the artery and determine the point of maximal flow. He or she should then hold the Doppler in place at the point of maximal volume.
3. Insert and advance the catheter-over-needle slowly and with constant pressure, at a 45-degree angle to the skin and directed toward the point of maximal flow (Fig. 225.15A and B).

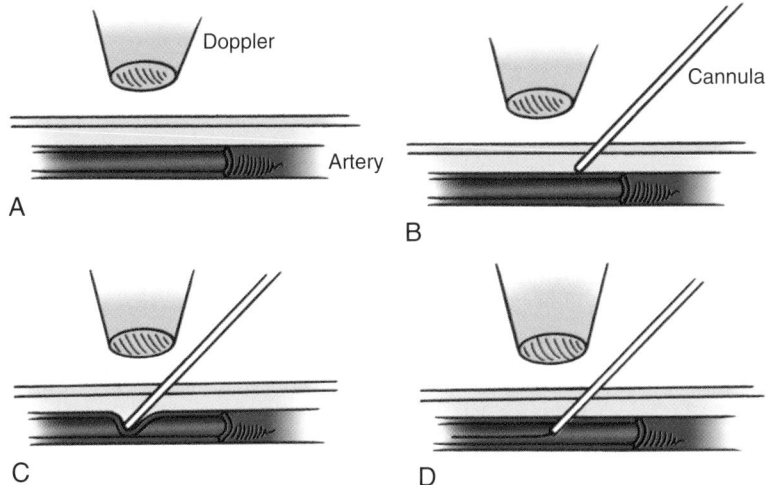

Fig. 225.15 Radial artery cannulation guided by hand-held Doppler. (A) Doppler is used to find maximal flow with loudest pulse. (B) Catheter inserted down to artery. (C) Pulse decreases or is temporarily inaudible when catheter enters artery. (D) The catheter then punctures the arterial wall (blood flashes in catheter), after which it is advanced intraluminally.

4. Contact with the artery is discerned by a slight decrease in arterial flow sound.
5. As the needle compresses the artery before puncture, the flow sound may transiently decrease or cease (see Fig. 225.15C and D).
6. The characteristic sound of arterial blood flow should resume as the artery is punctured and a flash of bright red blood is seen in the needle hub.
7. Advance the cannula, and secure and calibrate it as described previously.

NOTE: Use of hand-held Doppler or ultrasound may help to decrease the number of attempts necessary, the time spent gaining access, and complications such as hematoma and arterial laceration.

Alternate Method: Ultrasound-Guided (See Also Chapter 214 Emergency Department, Hospitalist, and Office Ultrasound [Clinical Ultrasound], Especially Section on Ultrasound-Guided Central Venous Catheter Insertion)

1. Position the extremity as previously described. Clean and prep the area over the artery, consider local anesthesia, and apply some ultrasound gel on the probe before inserting it into a sterile probe cover. Apply sterile ultrasound gel over the artery.
2. Orient the probe so that the marker dot is cephalad for a longitudinal scan or to the patient's right side for transverse scan. The artery should appear on a longitudinal scan as a pulsatile, thick-walled, noncompressible vessel. On transverse scan, it should be round and pulsatile. If color Doppler is available, it can be used to localize even very small arteries.
3. Move the probe proximally and distally to approximate the course of the artery which may not be perfectly longitudinal to the extremity. The probe can then be turned to either yield a transverse view of the artery or a longitudinal view, depending on the clinician's preference for guiding insertion.
4. If using a transverse view, center the artery in the image. Holding the probe in the clinician's nondominant hand (or having an assistant hold the probe), insert the needle 1 to 2 cm distal to the probe. When the needle is in subcutaneous tissue, rock the needle back and forth until it is identified in the image. This in turn will help to identify the location of the needle relative to the artery. If using a longitudinal view, attempt to localize and view as much of the artery in the image as possible. The longitudinal view is often reserved for ultrasound equipment with a needle guide so that the needle is seen in the plane of the image.
5. Carefully and slowly advance the needle toward the artery. Although the needle tip itself may not be identified, the motion through the tissue can infer the site and depth of the tip

and how close it is to the artery. When the needle reaches the artery, it will dimple the wall of the artery. Advance the needle further while watching for a flash of blood in the hub. Proceed at this point with cannulation as with the other techniques.
6. If the clinician "loses" the artery, or is having difficulty distinguishing it from surrounding tissue, turning on color Doppler will often verify the location of the artery.

Alternate Method for Radial or Brachial Artery Cannulation: Cutdown

1. Position the wrist or arm in the previously described position and prepare, anesthetize, and drape the area.
2. Wearing sterile gloves and maintaining sterile technique, make a 1.5- to 2-cm transverse skin incision perpendicular to the artery yet centered over it. Limit the depth of the incision to the skin; avoid cutting into the subcutaneous tissue to avoid damaging the nerve, artery, vein, lymphatics, tendons, or other nearby or deeper structures.
3. Using a mosquito hemostat, spread the subcutaneous tissue in a direction perpendicular to the incision, but along and above the artery. Expose approximately a 1-cm length of the artery.
4. Pass a nylon suture under the artery (internal suture) and prepare to elevate the artery to assist with cannulation.
5. Insert a catheter-over-needle through the skin, distal to the incision, and tunnel it under the skin and into the visible area of the incision.
6. While the clinician directly observes and controls the artery with two fingers of his or her nondominant hand or the suture, advance the catheter-over-needle into the artery. For the clinician to avoid being sprayed with arterial blood, the suture can be tied (lightly, without cutting the suture) proximal to where the catheter-over-needle will be inserted into the artery. After puncturing the artery with the catheter-over-needle, the knot in the suture can then be loosened (or released), as needed, to advance the catheter-over-needle further into the artery.
7. Advance the cannula, release the internal suture completely, and externally secure the arterial line and calibrate it as described previously. After the arterial line is secured externally and calibration confirmed, suture will also be needed to close the incision.

NOTE: Unlike venous cutdown (a procedure in which the internal suture is often tied, cut, and left within the incision), when an arterial cutdown is performed for arterial line insertion, the internal suture is only used temporarily to provide control while the artery is being cannulated.

Troubleshooting for a Variance between Cuff and Intraarterial Pressure and Preventive Maintenance for Accurate Readings

A variance or disparity of 5 to 20 mm Hg between measured cuff (indirect) and intraarterial (direct) pressures is normal and expected. If the intraarterial pressure is higher than cuff pressure, possible causes include improper cuff size or placement and improper calibration or zeroing of the transducer.

If cuff pressure is recorded as higher than intraarterial pressure, either improper cuff size, equipment malfunction, or technical error is likely. Damping of the arterial waveform suggests a problem with the intraarterial measurement. Air bubbles or blood in the line or transducer dome, a clot at the catheter tip, mechanical occlusion of the catheter or tubing, and loose or open connections are all possibilities. If the arterial waveform is not dampened and the cuff size and placement are correct, other possible causes include failure to calibrate the sphygmomanometer or the transducer, or an error in electrically or mechanically zeroing the transducer.

The variance of 5 to 20 mm Hg may be physiologic because the arterial pulse wave is transformed as it travels peripherally. As a result, the systolic pressure may become higher and the diastolic pressure lower. However, MAP is unchanged.

If the disparity is 20 to 30 mm Hg, severe vasoconstriction (e.g., patient with shock or hypothermia) may be the cause, and inevitably the auscultated cuff pressure is lower. With occlusive atherosclerotic peripheral disease, if the radial or dorsalis pedis artery has been cannulated, cuff pressures are frequently higher than the directly measured pressures because of the more distal location of cannulation.

If the disparity is greater than 30 mm Hg, the most common cause is resonance in the catheter system. This can be minimized by using stiff tubing that is kept as short as possible. Directly measured pressure may be significantly higher than cuff pressure when a single–end-hole catheter is used in a narrow artery with high flow. If the hole faces the flow, the direct blood pressure may be falsely elevated.

To minimize disparities and to maximize accurate readings, the following preventive steps should be followed or considered:

1. Allow the transducer and the amplifier to warm up for at least 10 minutes before zeroing and calibrating the system.
2. Purge all air from the pressure system; always observe for bubbles in the line and attempt to remove them if seen.
3. Use stiff, noncompliant extension tubing of the shortest possible length. Avoid the use of more than one stopcock between the catheter and the transducer. Place the extension tube near the patient to prevent a pulsating line.
4. Electrically zero and calibrate the system with an accurate manometer or a water column.
5. Mechanically zero the transducer.
6. At least once a shift, staff should check all fittings for tightness, check the zero setting (both electrically and mechanically), and check the calibration.
7. Avoid draining blood samples from the full length of the plumbing system.
8. Maintain a continuous low-flow flushing system (3 to 4 mL/hr) to avoid clotting. Traditionally, heparinized saline was used for flushing. Interestingly, the use of heparinized saline has not been shown to prevent thrombosis, increase the duration of catheter patency, or improve functionality of arterial cannulation. Therefore saline alone is adequate for flushing, and its use may reduce the risk of heparin-induced thrombocytopenia.
9. When the level of the patient is changed, recheck the mechanical and electrical zero positions and recalibrate the system if necessary.
10. Avoid making adjustments to the amplifier except at the time of calibration.

Complications

- *Significant blood loss* can occur if the tubing becomes disconnected.
- *Arterial thrombosis* (risk minimized by reducing the duration of cannulation, by choosing larger arteries, and by flushing properly). The risk of thrombosis increases if the cannula is left in place for longer than 72 hours.
- *Embolism*, usually distal. Retrograde arterial embolism can also occur from retrograde flushing of the cannula and may enter the cerebral circulation. This danger is greater with smaller patients. For all patients (and especially for smaller patients), make sure to either maintain a slow continuous flushing system or to use volumes of heparinized solution smaller than 3 mL to avoid dislodging thrombi.
- *Arterial occlusion.* With the Seldinger technique, it is possible to cause a small dissection and arterial occlusion by passing the guidewire between the intima and the media. With any technique, the result can be stenosis or permanent occlusion.
- *Ischemia or necrosis* distal to the site of arterial thrombosis, embolism, stenosis, or occlusion. Risk of amputation from necrosis is less than 1 in 2000 catheterizations.
- *Hemorrhage or local hematoma.*
- *Aneurysm or pseudoaneurysm.* The patient will present with a pulsatile mass. Management is surgical removal.
- *Local infection or sepsis*, usually related to length of time the catheter is in place, particularly after approximately 4 days. The infection rate for femoral and radial sites are similar.
- *Arteriovenous fistula.* This is more common with femoral artery cannulation because of the proximity of the large vein.
- *Neurologic complications*, same as with arterial puncture.
- *Vasovagal reactions.*

NOTE: A vascular surgeon should be consulted immediately if arterial flow is compromised in any way.

Postprocedure Patient Education

Explain to the alert patient and family the greater danger of a disconnected arterial line compared with a normal IV line. Instruct the patient not to rub or manipulate the site, line, or connectors. The patient should report any local pain, swelling, discoloration, or numbness at the site or any bubbles in the line. He or she should also report any blood or dampness near the site. After catheter removal, the patient should report any bleeding, extremity pain, numbness, swelling, or discoloration.

PATIENT EDUCATION GUIDES

See patient education and consent forms available at www.expertconsult.com.

CPT/BILLING CODES

36600	Arterial puncture; withdrawal of blood for diagnosis
36620	Arterial catheterization or cannulation for sampling, monitoring, or transfusion (separate procedure); percutaneous
36625	Arterial cutdown
76942	Ultrasonic guidance for needle placement (e.g., biopsy, aspiration, injection, localization device), imaging, supervision and interpretation
76937	Ultrasonic guidance for vascular access requiring ultrasound evaluation of potential access sites, documentation of selected vessel patency, concurrent real-time ultrasound visualization of vascular needle entry, with permanent recording and reporting (list separately in addition to code for primary procedure)

ICD-10-CM Diagnostic Codes

Arterial Puncture

E11.10	Diabetic ketoacidosis, without mention of coma
E87.2	Acidosis, lactic, metabolic or respiratory
E87.3	Alkalosis, metabolic or respiratory
E87.4	Acid-base mixed disorder
I26.09	Pulmonary embolism and infarction
I46.9	Cardiac or cardiorespiratory arrest
I50.1	Left heart failure, with pulmonary edema or cardiac dyspnea (cardiac asthma)
J44.9	Chronic obstructive bronchitis, with emphysema, without exacerbation
J44.1	Chronic obstructive bronchitis (COPD), with acute exacerbation
J43.9	Emphysema, NOS
J45.20	Asthma, extrinsic, unspecified
J45.22	Asthma, extrinsic with status asthmaticus
J45.21	Asthma, extrinsic, with acute exacerbation
J95.89	Pulmonary insufficiency following shock, trauma, or surgery
J96.00–J96.02	Respiratory failure, acute, NOS
J96.90	Respiratory distress or other pulmonary insufficiency, acute, not elsewhere classified
J96.10–J96.12	Respiratory failure, chronic
J96.20–J96.22	Respiratory failure, acute and chronic
R40.20	Coma
R57.9	Shock, unspecified, without mention of trauma
R57.0	Shock, cardiogenic
R65.21	Shock, septic
R57.1	Shock, other (hypovolemic, septic)
R06.02	Shortness of breath
R06.03	Respiratory distress or insufficiency, NOS
R09.01	Asphyxia
R09.02	Hypoxia
R09.2	Respiratory arrest
T58.01XX–T58.94XX	Carbon monoxide, toxic effect

Use additional seventh character: A, initial; D, subsequent; S, sequela.

Percutaneous Arterial Line Placement

In addition to ICD-9-CM diagnostic codes used for arterial puncture, the following are commonly used for arterial lines:

V42	Organ or tissue replaced by transplant
V43	Organ or tissue replaced by other means
V45	Postprocedure states
V45.81	Postprocedure status, aortocoronary bypass
V46.1	Dependence on machines, respirator (ventilator)
401.0	Hypertension, accelerated, malignant
410.9	Myocardial infarction, acute, NOS or unspecified site
411.1	Angina, unstable
434.9	Cerebral artery occlusion, unspecified

SUPPLIERS

(See contact information available at www.expertconsult.com.)

Arrow International (Teleflex Medical)
Becton, Dickinson and Co.
Cook Medical
Edwards Life Sciences Corp. (formerly a division of Baxter), closed needleless sampling systems

RECOMMENDED READING

Allen EV. Thromboangiitis obliterans: methods of diagnosis of chronic occlusive arterial lesions distal to the wrist with illustrative cases. *Am J Med Sci.* 1929;178:237–244.

Foyd Z, Stroud S. Arterial puncture and cannulation. In: Reichman EF, ed. *Emergency Medicine Procedures.* 2nd ed. New York: McGraw-Hill; 2013:376–385.

Gerber DR, Zeifman CW, Khouli HI, et al. Comparison of wire-guided and non-wire-guided radial artery catheters. *Chest.* 1996;109:761–764.

Kamienski RW, Barnes RW. Critique of the Allen test for continuity of the palmar arch assessed by Doppler ultrasound. *Surg Gynecol Obstet.* 1976;142:861–864.

Lau J, Chew PW, Wang C, White AC. *Long Term Oxygen Therapy for Severe COPD.* Rockville, MD: Agency for Health Care Research and Quality (AHRQ) Technology Assessment Program, U.S. Department of Health and Human Services, Public Health Services; 2004.

Maher JJ, Dougherty JM. Radial artery cannulation guided by Doppler ultrasound. *Am J Emerg Med.* 1989;7:260–262.

Mangar D, Thrush DN, Connell GR, Downs JB. Direct or modified Seldinger guide wire-directed technique for arterial catheter insertion. *Anesth Analg.* 1993;76:714–717.

Milzma D, Jaudan T. Arterial puncture and cannulation. In: Roberts JR, Hedges JR, eds. *Clinical Procedures in Emergency Medicine.* 6th ed. Philadelphia: Saunders; 2014:368–384.

Slogoff S, Keats A, Arlund C. On the safety of radial artery cannulation. *Anesthesiology.* 1983;59:42–47.

CHAPTER 226

INTRAOSSEOUS VASCULAR ACCESS

Raymond F. Jarris Jr. • *Grant C. Fowler*

One of the most frustrating and difficult challenges faced by a clinician is the establishment of vascular access in the critically ill patient. Establishment of peripheral intravenous (IV) access is often difficult in the severely dehydrated patient, the burn patient, the trauma patient, or the patient who is in shock or cardiac arrest—especially the obese patient. It is notoriously difficult in the small pediatric patient. For children younger than 5 years, thin bones and a vascular marrow make intraosseous vascular access (IOVA) a fairly simple alternative. For years, plain hypodermic needles, spinal needles, or bone marrow aspiration needles (e.g., Jamshidi) were used for IOVA. Now that special IOVA needles and kits are available, hypodermic needles and spinal needles are rarely used due to their propensity to bend and their frequent failure to reach the bone cortex. While bone marrow aspiration needles are still acceptable, later IOVA models have flanges, making them easier to secure to the patient with tape after insertion. Kits also combine IOVA needles with either a small, portable, battery-powered drill, a hand-powered drill, an impact-driven device, or a spring-loaded disposable needle gun, resulting in increased use in adults. In fact, many first responders and the military now use IOVA in adults more often than in children. Using IOVA, after the needle traverses the cortex, the venous plexus in the marrow cavity (Fig. 226.1) functions as a rigid "vein" or conduit for fluid; it does not collapse with hypovolemia or even shock. This procedure has been so successful that many national and international organizations recommend its use as the primary or secondary method of obtaining and maintaining vascular access in the critically ill patient. The use of IOVA is also increasingly common and accepted as an alternative to a central line for short-term infusions in nonemergent situations.

IOVA was originally described in the 1920s. However, with the introduction of plastic catheters and improved peripheral IV access procedures (e.g., cutdown) and skills, the need and interest for IOVA diminished. In the 1980s, IOVA saw a resurgence in pediatric shock emergencies. IOVA has now been studied and proven to be a safe, reliable, and rapid temporary method for vascular access in adult shock emergencies, especially when compared with percutaneous IV access. The American Heart Association, the American Academy of Pediatrics, and the American College of Surgeons recommend vascular access by IOVA in emergency situations when venous access is not immediately possible. Since 2010, the American Heart Association no longer recommends endotracheal administration of resuscitation drugs unless IV or intraosseous access is not obtainable. As mentioned previously, the military has also had excellent results with IOVA.

Any medication or fluid that can be given IV can also be administered by IOVA. After a 5- to 10-mL flush with normal saline, medications are immediately absorbed into the systemic circulation; drug concentrations and onset of action match those given through a central venous line during cardiopulmonary resuscitation (CPR). In addition to serving as a route for fluid administration, the IOVA needle may be used for obtaining blood type, cross-matching labs, blood cultures, and blood chemistries from the marrow cavity. Serum electrolyte, blood urea nitrogen, creatinine, glucose, and calcium levels are very similar to those in samples obtained from an IOVA aspirate.

One disadvantage of IOVA is the temporary nature of the procedure (it should not be used for more than 24 to 48 hours). Another, disadvantage is that infusion rates may be limited; however, rates can also reach more than 150 mL/min with a 16-gauge IOVA needle and a pressure infusor bag (blood pressure cuff inflated to 300 mm Hg around the IV fluid bag), an infusion pump, or with forceful manual pressure. The rate-limiting factor is usually the size of the marrow cavity. Infusion through IOVA can also be uncomfortable. IOVA also is not universally successful; however, success rates have improved since the development of kits specially designed for this procedure.

One retrospective study of pediatric cardiopulmonary arrest patients revealed that, although the time to obtain peripheral IV was occasionally minimal, the average time was a disappointing 7.9 ± 4.2 minutes. The overall peripheral IV success rate was only 17%. Of all techniques used, the success rate was highest with IOVA (83%); the next most successful was surgical cutdown (81%); and central venous line placement (77%) came in third. The average time required to establish vascular access was 4.7 minutes for IOVA (using older equipment not specially designed for this procedure), 8.4 minutes for central venous line placement, and 12.7 minutes for venous cutdown. Using newer kits specially designed for IOVA, the access time has been reduced to as little as 10 seconds, and the success rate has significantly improved over the prior 83%.

In the cardiopulmonary arrest situation, it is reasonable to use IOVA as the initial approach for vascular access because of the high success rate and the rapidity of the procedure. In fact, all providers of emergency care (including hospitalists) should be familiar with IOVA because in certain situations it may be the only available means of obtaining vascular access.

To learn the procedure or to maintain skills for IOVA, clinicians can practice on cadavers, raw chicken drumsticks, swine ribs, or piglet tibias. Mannequins are also available for practice from the manufacturers of the special IOVA kits.

The proximal tibia (Fig. 226.2), just below the growth plate, is the preferred site for IOVA in children younger than 6 years. At this

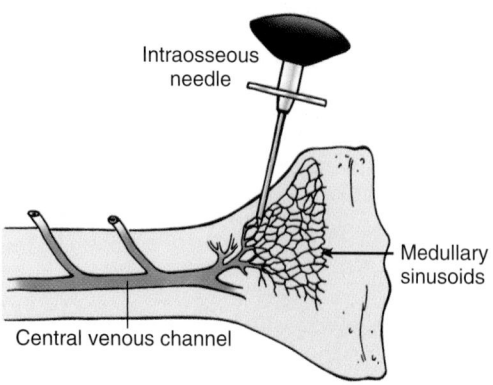

Fig. 226.1 Intramedullary venous system. With intraosseous venous access, the marrow cavity functions as a "vein" that will not collapse.

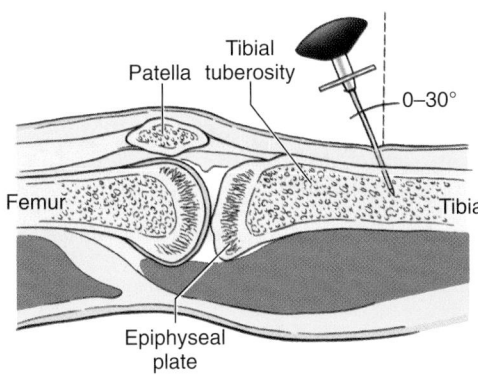

Fig. 226.2   Proximal tibial needle insertion.

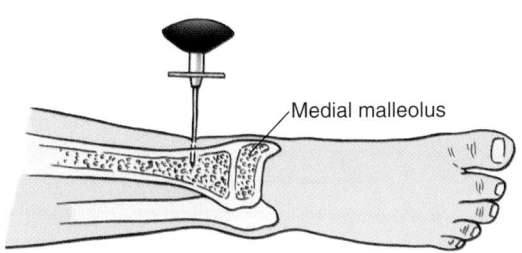

Fig. 226.3   Distal tibial needle insertion.

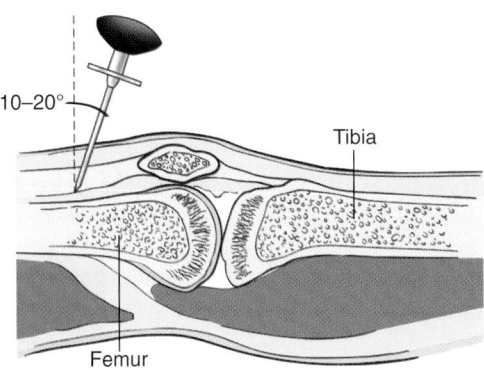

Fig. 226.4   Distal femoral needle insertion.

level, the tibial tuberosity is a broad, flat surface close to the skin, and there are few intervening muscles, nerves, and blood vessels; therefore bony landmarks are easily recognized.

Since an IOVA kit has been developed specifically for the adult sternum (FAST-1, Teleflex Inc.), it has been noted that the tibia may be a less desirable location for IOVA in adults because the red marrow has been replaced by yellow marrow. In contrast, the sternum has been advocated as a better site because it has red marrow, is large and flat, and can be readily located, even in obese individuals. In addition, the sternum's cortical bone is thin (1 to 2 mm) and the marrow space relatively uniform (6 to 11 mm). Also, it can be used during CPR because the site on the sternum for IOVA is different from that where chest compressions are recommended.

IOVA kits with a battery-powered drill (EZ-IO; Teleflex Inc.), a hand-powered drill (NIO; PerSys), or a spring-loaded disposable needle gun (Bone Injection Gun [BIG]; WaisMed PerSys) have been demonstrated to be effective for use in the proximal humerus; having vascular access above the diaphragm during CPR is considered important by many clinicians. The distal tibia (Fig. 226.3), just above the medial malleolus, the lateral or medial malleolus, the distal radius, ulna, or femur (Fig. 226.4) and the anterior-superior iliac spine are alternate sites for IOVA. Whereas the distal tibia is a good choice because the bone and tissues are thin, the distal femur is covered with muscles and fat, often making palpation of bony landmarks difficult. The distal femur should probably be reserved for those cases in which other sites cannot be used. The sternum and iliac crest are seldom used in children because the width of the marrow space is inadequate if the child is younger than 3 years, and insertion may be technically difficult and dangerous; the sternal site carries a risk of mediastinal puncture. The clavicle and calcaneus also may be used, but these sites are rarely necessary. Note that sites are device specific and should follow the manufacturer's indications and instructions for use.

INDICATIONS

- As an alternative to a central line for short-term infusions
- Any emergency condition that requires immediate vascular access (IOVA can often be achieved in 10 to 60 seconds)
- When IV access cannot be achieved (e.g., small veins, venofibrosis, edema, obesity; also, for regional anesthesia when the distal extremity is injured)
  NOTE: When a large-volume infusion is needed very rapidly, bilateral IOVA may be necessary as well as the use of a pressure infusor bag, an infusion pump, a large syringe, or forceful manual pressure.
- IOVA is preferred over the endotracheal route for medication administration (certain fluids or medications can be given only by IV or IOVA route, and *not* through an endotracheal tube; e.g., blood, sodium bicarbonate, dextrose)
- Newborns in whom conventional IV access failed (in one study of simulated resuscitation, IOVA was faster than umbilical vein catheterization for individuals that do not perform neonatal resuscitation frequently)

CONTRAINDICATIONS

Contraindications to IOVA are few and are all relative, especially since this is a very temporary and often life-saving procedure. That said, the risks and benefits of the procedure should be considered.

- Ipsilateral fracture or crush injury of an extremity (increases the risk of subcutaneous extravasation, compartment syndrome and nonunion of the fractures, so another extremity should be used)
- Previous orthopedic procedure near the selected insertion site
- Previous IOVA attempts in the same bone (even if IOVA was obtained, fluid would leak out of the previously attempted site)
- Infection or burn at the selected insertion site
- Inability to locate landmarks (e.g., obesity or excessive tissue over the insertion site; these may also prevent the device from reaching the medullary cavity)
- Brittle bones (e.g., osteogenesis imperfecta or anything increasing risk of fracture)
- Patients with right-to-left intracardiac shunts may be at higher risk for fat or bone marrow embolization complications
- Sternal IOVA in the patient weighing less than 50 kg, or in those patients with a small sternum, a congenital sternal malformation, blunt trauma with a sternal fracture or soft tissue injury over the sternum, or prior sternotomy. The exception to these in the smaller patient is the FAST-1 device, which has US Food and Drug Administration approval for age 12 and older.
- Disposable intraosseous needle, 16- to 20-gauge, preferably with stylet. Options include kits with a small, portable battery-powered drill, intraosseous needle, and integrated stylet that doubles as a battery-powered driver (15-gauge needle sets are available in three lengths with weight-based guidelines; Fig. 226.5A), a manual drilling device (NIO; see Fig. 226.5B), an impact-driven device designed for sternal placement (FAST-1; see Fig. 226.5C), a spring-loaded bone injection gun (BIG Adult or BIG Pedi; see Fig. 226.5D), or an IOVA needle with a built-in handle (see Fig. 226.5E). Aspects of all of these are disposable. If none of these

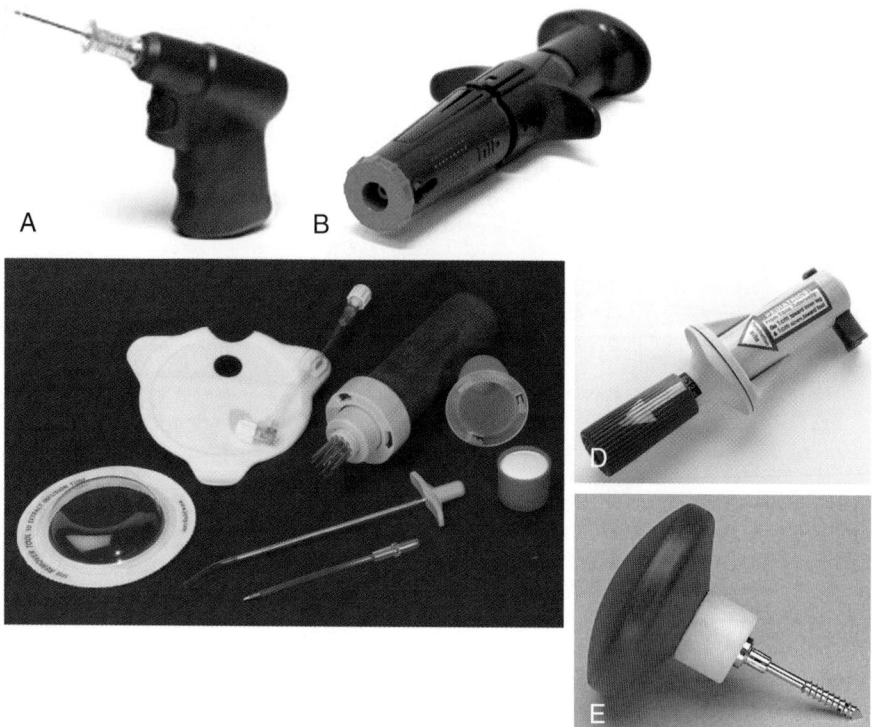

Fig. 226.5 (A) Intraosseous needle, battery-powered driver stylet, battery-operated drill (EZ-IO). (B) A manually driven device (NIO). (C) Impact-driven FAST-1. (D) Spring-loaded needle gun (Bone Injection Gun [BIG]). (E) Intraosseous vascular access needle with handle. (A, Courtesy Teleflex Inc., Morrisville, NC.B, Courtesy PerSys Medical, Houston, TX. C, Courtesy Teleflex Inc., Morrisville, NC. D, Courtesy WaisMed PerSys Medical, Houston, TX. E, Courtesy Cook Critical Care, Bloomington, IN.)

are available, bone marrow aspiration needles (e.g., Jamshidi) have been used to perform this procedure in children for years. **EDITOR'S NOTE:** Specific supplies and procedures should be followed based on device manufacturer recommendations.
- Sterile latex gloves.
- Goggles and equipment necessary to follow universal blood and body fluid precautions.
- Sterile drapes.
- Antiseptic solution (povidone–iodine, chlorhexidine, or alcohol).
- Two 10-mL syringes for aspirating medullary contents and flushing with normal saline.
- 2 × 2 gauze pads.
- 4 × 4 gauze pads.
- Tape.
- IV solution (isotonic crystalloid or colloid), tubing, and pressure infusor bag (can use a blood pressure cuff) or infusion pump (large syringes can also be used for boluses).
- Extremity or torso restraints for the uncooperative patient.
- Plastic or Styrofoam cup.
- In the alert patient, 2% lidocaine without preservatives (cardiac lidocaine) and without epinephrine and a 10-mL syringe

PREPROCEDURE PATIENT EDUCATION

In most cases, IOVA is performed emergently. When time allows, the indications should be documented and explained to the parent or other relative, if present. If performed electively, the indications, alternatives, benefits, and risks should be explained to the patient or parent, and signed informed consent should be obtained. The alert patient should be aware of the possibility of some dull pain with rapid infusion.

TECHNIQUE

NOTE: The following techniques and angles are for the standard IOVA needle. For the kits, the FAST-1 utilizes the sternal site; the others are used most often at the proximal tibial site in children and at the proximal humeral site in adults or the distal tibial site.

The instruments should be held perpendicular to the bone during insertion of the needle. The operator should be familiar with the particular device available for IOVA and review the device-specific protocol prior to use because the application of each device may vary slightly. (For these instructions, a manual needle is being used.)

1. If an extremity is the chosen site, place a small sandbag or pillows beneath it. An assistant or restraint may be useful for an infant or a confused patient. If an extremity is the desired site, everyone should avoid placing a hand behind the extremity in case of through-and-through bone penetration.
2. Prepare the skin with antiseptic solution and drape the area. Follow universal blood and body fluid precautions.
3. Administer local anesthetic down to the periosteum (this is optional, if time allows in the critically-ill patient; it may not be necessary for patients with an altered mental status).
4. To avoid through-and-through bony penetration, hold your index finger approximately 1 cm from the needle tip and avoid pushing past this mark. This step is not necessary if using a kit.
5. Perform the procedure according to the selected insertion site:
   - Proximal tibia
     Palpate the tibial tuberosity with your finger (it is the most prominent point on the tibia, noted immediately distal to the patella). In children, select a site approximately one or two fingerbreadths (1 to 2 cm) below the tibial tuberosity and one or two fingerbreadths medial to it. This should place the IOVA on the flat surface of the proximal, anteromedial tibia. In adults, the IOVA site can be found by first moving one or two fingerbreadths medial to the tibial tuberosity, and then moving one or two fingerbreadths above or below this location.
   Grasp the medial aspect of the tibia with the thumb and fingers of your nondominant hand to secure it.
   Using your dominant hand, with the stylet in place, insert the IOVA needle with a gentle, but firm, boring or screwing motion at an angle of 60 to 80 degrees to the proximal skin (which is a 10- to 30-degree angle to vertical; see Fig. 226.2). *To avoid bending the needle, twist it*

rather than pushing it. If the needle is threaded, it should be twisted clockwise to screw it into the bone. The needle should be pointed caudad, in the direction of the long axis of the bone, away from the epiphysis. The IOVA needle from a kit can be used in the same location, but should be held perpendicular to the bone. Again, every effort should be made to avoid the epiphysis.
- Head of humerus
  Palpate the anterior aspect of the head of humerus.
  Grasp the humerus in the nondominant hand to secure it. Make sure your nondominant hand is well below the insertion site in case there is through-and-through needle penetration of the bone.
  Using your dominant hand, the IOVA needle from a kit should be held perpendicular to the bone.
  The needle should then be inserted. Care should be taken when disconnecting the needle from the insertion instrument provided by a kit to avoid dislodging the needle.
- Distal tibia
  Insert the IOVA needle into the distal medial tibia at the broad, flat area proximal to the medial malleolus and posterior to the saphenous vein. It should be inserted at an angle perpendicular to the skin (see Fig. 226.3). Again, the IOVA needle from a kit can be used at this location and directed at the same angle.
- Distal femur (EZ-IO not indicated in this location)
  Insert the needle 2 to 3 cm above the epicondyles in the anterior midline.
  Direct the needle cephalad at an angle of 70 to 80 degrees to distal skin (10 to 20 degrees from the vertical; see Fig. 226.4).
6. Placement in the marrow space is confirmed by the following:
   - There is a decrease in resistance (it "gives") as the needle passes through the cortex into the softer medulla. The skin-to-cortex distance is rarely more than 1 cm in infants and children.
   - The needle should stand upright without support when the stylet is removed.
   - Marrow should be easily aspirated into a syringe, followed by blood (*note:* marrow or blood may not be aspirated in every case).
   - Fluids should infuse easily without extravasation.
7. Radiographs can be used to confirm needle position if time and the clinical situation permits (optional).
8. Flush the needle with saline solution (heparin is optional). Check for swelling (extravasation of fluid) around the needle or behind the extremity. If the test injection is unsuccessful (i.e., extravasation is noted), the IOVA should be removed and another site chosen. If an extremity is to be used, it should be another one. If the same extremity is used, fluid will leak through the prior hole in the cortex, possibly causing damage by extravasation
   NOTE: Common reasons for inadequate flow are over- or underpenetration of the cortex. This can occur despite the needle appearing to be in the marrow cavity. Underpenetration usually also causes extravasation; in this situation, replace the stylet and advance the needle until bone marrow contents are aspirated and fluid flows freely. Overpenetration results in penetrating the opposite cortex; if this is suspected, withdrawing the needle 1 to 2 mm may result in fluid flowing freely.
9. For the alert patient, 2% lidocaine without preservatives and without epinephrine (i.e., cardiac lidocaine, observing same contraindications and precautions as cardiac lidocaine; up to 5 mL in adults, less for children, adjusted for weight) can be infused very slowly (slow enough to prevent it being sent directly into the central circulation) to decrease the discomfort associated with later infusions. Lidocaine infused in this manner goes directly into the marrow to provide analgesia, prior to the saline flush.
10. If the IOVA has a flange, it should be taped down. A sterile

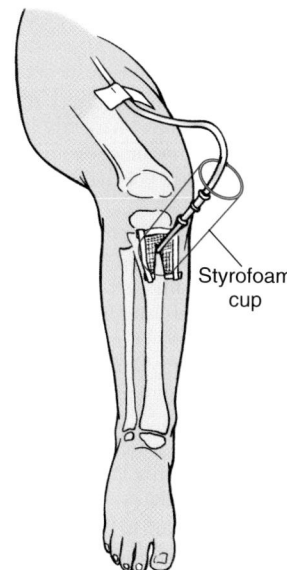

Fig. 226.6 Completed intraosseous vascular access with cup protector.

2 × 2 gauze pad cut to fit around the needle should also be taped down as a dressing. Next, place a cup (Styrofoam or plastic, with the bottom removed) over the IOVA site and firmly secure it with tape (Fig. 226.6)
NOTE: The cup offers additional protection for the IOVA in the case of inadvertent extremity movement.
11. Attach the pressure bag infusor or an infusion pump to the IV bag, and tape the IV tubing in place. The tubing should be taped both to the patient (to avoid putting tension on the IOVA) and to the IV line (to avoid it being disconnected). Pressure bag infusors, infusion pumps, or forceful manual pressure can be used to administer large volumes. Large fluid boluses can also be given with a large syringe, either through a medication port in the IV line or through a saline lock attached to the IOVA. When giving large volumes under pressure, care should be taken to avoid air embolism. Unfortunately, giving large volumes under pressure in places other than the sternum may result in considerable discomfort if lidocaine has not been infused.
12. Restrain the limb with soft restraints to avoid inadvertent movement.
13. Monitor the infusion site for evidence of needle displacement or extravasation. Needle displacement can result in severe complications from extravasation (e.g., compartment syndrome, tissue necrosis). Establish peripheral IV access within 24 to 48 hours after IOVA placement, and then remove the IOVA.

Removal

1. Rotate the needle slightly to loosen its seal. (If threaded, such as that inserted by portable, battery-powered or hand-powered drilling, rotate the needle clockwise.) Withdraw the needle with a firm, quick motion.
2. Place a sterile pressure pad over the puncture site; apply firm pressure for 5 minutes to prevent hematoma formation. Next, apply a sterile dressing to the extremity. Do not constrict the extremity with the dressing.

POSTPROCEDURE MANAGEMENT

After IOVA removal, the dressing must be changed daily. Dressings may be discontinued after 48 hours. The patient, his or her family, and the nursing staff, should be taught to monitor for signs of infection and other possible complications.

COMPLICATIONS

- The most common complication is unsuccessful placement. This was previously often due to the technical difficulty of the procedure; however, IOVA kits have markedly increased the success rate. Technical failure is now most commonly due to a lack of familiarity with the equipment or the landmarks, or an improper technique.
- Clotting of marrow in the needle or displacement of the needle may lead to loss of vascular access.
- Subcutaneous, or occasionally subperiosteal, infiltration of fluid or leakage from the puncture site is common. This is especially common with the use of pressure infusor bags, infusion pumps, or manual pressure, or with long-term use of IO infusion. Extravasated crystalloid is usually not a problem, but solutions containing calcium chloride, epinephrine, or sodium bicarbonate (or other potentially cytotoxic agents) should be stopped or slowed to minimize extravasation. Muscle or tendon compartment syndromes from excessive fluid extravasation are a possibility.
- Slow infusion rates may be due to underpenetration or overpenetration (see above), or a small, fibrotic marrow cavity (rare). Initially, flow rates may be slow because the needle is plugged by marrow contents. Flushing the needle with 5 to 10 mL of saline often clears the needle.
- No lasting effects have been noted in bone, growth plate, or marrow elements after IOVA. The needle is directed away from the growth plate, or the insertion site is distal enough to avoid inadvertent injury to this structure. After successful placement, a small defect is created in the cortex that is visible as a small radiolucent area on radiographs. It should resolve in 30 to 40 days. In one case report, tibial fractures were seen after unsuccessful IOVA attempts, but these are very rare.
- Localized cellulitis or a subcutaneous abscess may be observed in less than 1% of cases. In most studies, the incidence of osteomyelitis was less than 1%. Infections were usually associated with prolonged catheter placement, placement in bacteremic patients, or use of hypertonic infusions.
- Hematomas are most likely caused by local trauma from needle insertion.
- Pain is possible with insertion and when intramedullary pressure is increased during infusion. It is generally not a problem with slow infusions or in the unconscious patient. Slowing the infusion rate in the conscious patient may relieve symptoms.
- A theoretical complication is creation of a bone embolus when a needle without a stylet is used. No documented cases of a bone embolism have been reported. A fat embolism has been reported from tibial infusion in adults but not in children, probably because the marrow in children is relatively fat free.
- Bone marrow elements (immature blood cells, including blasts) have been observed in venous blood sampled proximal to IOVA infusion sites. Before more invasive diagnostic measures are undertaken, a repeat complete blood count with differential should be performed, preferably from the more permanent replacement IV site on another extremity.
- With sternal puncture with a plain needle, death has occurred from mediastinitis, hydrothorax, or injury to the heart or great vessels. This is avoidable if the FAST-1 system is used or sites other than the sternum are chosen.
- Through-and-through placement of the needle can occur. Placing your index finger approximately 1 cm from the needle tip can prevent advancement of the needle through the opposite side of the bone. Your finger will prevent pushing too deep. (Some intraosseous needles have a preset depth indicator on the shaft.)

PATIENT EDUCATION GUIDES

See patient education and patient consent forms available at www.expertconsult.com.

CPT/BILLING CODES

| 36680 | Placement of needle for intraosseous infusion |

ICD-10-CM DIAGNOSTIC CODES

E86.0	Volume depletion, dehydration
G40.311	Status epilepticus
I46.9	Cardiorespiratory arrest
P54.9	Hemorrhage, unspecified in newborn (NOS)
R57.9	Shock (without trauma), unspecified
R65.21	Shock, septic, endotoxic
R57.1	Hypovolemic shock (NEC)
R09.2	Respiratory arrest
T79.4XXX	Hemorrhagic shock or shock syndrome due to trauma
T78.2XXX	Shock, anaphylactic

Use additional seventh character: A, initial; D, subsequent; S, sequela

SUPPLIERS

(See contact information available at www.expertconsult.com.)

Cook Medical: IOVA needles with handles, with or without flanges
PYNG Teleflex Medical: Fast1 impact driven sternal IO device
Vidacare Teleflex Medical: EZ-IO AD for adults, EZ-IO PD for children; includes small, portable, battery-powered drill
WaisMed PerSys Medical: NIO Adult and NIO Pediatric, hand-powered drill; BIG Adult and BIG Pediatric, spring-loaded devices
Training videos and practice equipment are available from all these companies.

Acknowledgment

The editors recognize the contributions of Kelly T. Locke, MD, and Rafael F. Cruz, MD, to this chapter in previous editions of this text.

RECOMMENDED READING

American Heart Association. *Advanced Cardiac Life Support (ACLS) Provider Manual*. Dallas: American Heart Association; 2011.

American Heart Association. *Pediatric Advanced Life Support (PALS) Provider Manual*. Dallas: American Heart Association; 2011.

Deitch K. Intraosseous infusion. In: Roberts JR, Custalow CB, Thomsen TW, eds. *Roberts and Hedges' Clinical Procedures in Emergency Medicine*. 6th ed. Philadelphia: Elsevier; 2014:455–468.

Glaeser P, Hellmich T, Szewczuga D, et al. Five-year experience in prehospital intraosseous infusions in children and adults. *Ann Emerg Med*. 1993;22:1119–1124.

Munk A, Ma J. Intraosseous infusion. In: Reichman EF, ed. *Emergency Medicine Procedures*. 2nd ed. New York: McGraw-Hill; 2013:361–369.

Orlowski JP, Porembka DT, Gallagher JM, Van Lente F. The bone marrow as a source of laboratory studies. *Ann Emerg Med*. 1989;18:1348–1351.

CHAPTER 227

VENOUS CUTDOWN

Wm. MacMillan Rodney • J.R. MacMillan Rodney

Obtaining vascular access is a life-saving procedure for critically ill patients in a variety of situations, but hypovolemic shock and cardiac arrest are the most common vascular access emergencies. Venous cutdowns were first described in World War II. With the advent of intensive care units in the 1960s, surgical cutdowns were frequently replaced by percutaneous approaches to the subclavian and internal jugular veins. In the 1970s, placement of these "central lines" became core curriculum in the newly established course known as advanced cardiac life support. This course was usually taught by demonstration and did not require the traditional surgical skills of dissection and suture.

By 1980 the American College of Surgeons implemented the advanced trauma life support (ATLS) course, which required live tissue to demonstrate vascular access techniques. (For ATLS, plastic simulators do not realistically reproduce the in vivo experience.) These included "venous cutdowns," but since then, percutaneous techniques have replaced most of the cutdowns. This was at least partly due to a multicenter, prospective randomized trial in 1994 (Westfall), which showed that the time needed to obtain percutaneous femoral venous access and start an infusion was significantly less compared with venous cutdown. In recent years, venous cutdowns have become an optional part of the ATLS curriculum, offered at the discretion of the instructor. More recently, use of ultrasound has dramatically improved the ability to visualize central and peripheral veins, often directing cannulation (e.g., percutaneous inserted central catheter).

In situations where ongoing chest compressions, burns, or trauma make central line placement difficult, the intraosseous route (see Chapter 226, Intraosseous Vascular Access) is quickest and most reliable for clinicians with limited surgical experience. However, intraosseous needles and central line kits are not as universally available as scalpels, hemostats, and suture. In developing countries and most locations more than 1 mile from an academic medical center, venous cutdown may be the most readily available method for rapid vascular access. Ironically, clinicians in these locations are often less likely to have any experience or training with venous cutdown.

This chapter describes cutdowns of the distal great saphenous vein near the ankle and the proximal great saphenous vein beneath the inguinal crease. Brachial or basilic vein cutdowns in the antecubital fossa are rarely a first choice, because of the time required for dissection, but are also discussed. In cases where the patient is undergoing chest compressions, space around the patient can be limited, and choosing a more distal location is usually better.

INDICATIONS

- Multiple failed attempts at percutaneous insertion in a critically ill or injured patient
- Hypotensive shock
- Patient requiring immediate administration of intravenous (IV) fluids or drugs
- Cardiac or respiratory arrest
- Burns, trauma, or ongoing resuscitation preventing timely insertion of percutaneous central lines

- Intraosseous vascular access contraindicated (see Chapter 226, Intraosseous Vascular Access) or equipment not available
- Surgical consultation not available (e.g., because of time or distance limitation)
- Lack of percutaneously accessible vein (e.g., obesity, unusually small or fragile veins [as in some adults and most infants], or venous sclerosis from aging, IV drug abuse, or previous multiple venipunctures)

CONTRAINDICATIONS

- When less-invasive and adequate alternatives (e.g., intraosseous vascular access, percutaneous central or peripheral lines) are immediately available
- Long bone fracture present proximally in extremity
- Evidence of severe peripheral vascular disease such as thrombophlebitis, vascular insufficiency, history of vein stripping, or history of vein sclerosis (clinician should consider different site)
- Lack of equipment
- Local infection, burns, or trauma in the area of the cutdown (relative)
- Prolonged use for administration of hypertonic fluids (relative)
- Inadequate local arterial supply (relative, arterial supply is important for postprocedural healing, so consider a different site)
- Bleeding disorder (relative)

EQUIPMENT

- Tourniquet and tape
- Sterile gloves, goggles, equipment to follow universal blood and body fluid precautions
- Sterile gauze sponges, gauze pads, and drapes
- Antiseptic skin preparation (if time permits), such as povidone-iodine or chlorhexidine soap or solution (alcohol is not preferred)
- A 3- to 5-mL syringe of local anesthetic (any kind of lidocaine; epinephrine is not necessary but is not harmful)
- Basic surgical equipment (e.g., scalpel [No. 10 or No. 15 blade for skin, No. 11 blade for minivenotomy], hemostats [large and mosquito, curved and straight], thumb forceps [pickups] with and without teeth, suture scissors, tissue dissection scissors [Metzenbaum], and a needle holder)
- Although silk ligatures (4-0) for the vein and nonabsorbable skin suture (4-0) have been recommended for the skin, this is an emergency and any suture will work. In general, braided or monofilament absorbable sutures varying from 0 to 4-0 work fine. Concerns about infection risk with braided suture are more theoretical than real. Silk is the most reactive of all sutures in the skin and is not the first choice.
- IV fluids and setup. Cannulation is possible using a wide variety of tubes and catheters. Using the IV tubing itself (hub cut off) to cannulate permits the most rapid infusion but usually requires a vein as large as the proximal saphenous, and a backup IV catheter should be available. Ten- to 14-gauge plain peripheral IV

catheters are almost as good for infusion of large amounts of fluid, but anything will work if cardioactive drugs are needed.

- Ultrasound machine with high-frequency probe (5 to 10 MHz) and ultrasound gel to visualize or define the venous anatomy at the groin or antecubital fossa (optional; if time and the urgency of the situation allow)

PATIENT PREPARATION AND GENERAL CONSIDERATIONS: ANATOMY

1. The clinician should be familiar with the basic anatomy of the area (Fig. 227.1).
2. If the patient is alert, explain the need for IV access and the procedure. If time and the urgency of the situation allow, obtain informed consent.
3. For distal saphenous or basilic vein cutdowns, have an assistant apply a tourniquet proximal to the incision site and control it. This will enable the clinician to more easily visualize and palpate the vein. A tourniquet applied high on the thigh may help with locating the proximal saphenous vein. To minimize bleeding, tourniquets should be released at the time of venipuncture. Observe universal blood and body fluid precautions.
4. Cleanse the skin in the area around the vein and incision site thoroughly with antiseptic soap or solution.
5. To provide ample working space, if time and the urgency of the situation allow, extend a wide sterile field 8 to 10 cm proximally and distally and apply sterile drapes.
6. Regardless of which cutdown site is chosen, incisions can be made horizontally (i.e., laterally), which is also transversely. When subcutaneous fat protrudes from the incision, use blunt dissection and spread the tissue longitudinally along the axis of the vein. All these veins are in superficial fat layers, so with a proximal saphenous or basilic vein cutdown, if the incision exposes muscle fascia, it is too deep.

7. The vein should appear pulseless and thin-walled, and it should blanch with the application of distal traction. If a vein is not readily identified, have an assistant tighten the tourniquet, which may make it more apparent or palpable.
8. With all cutdowns, the vein should be dissected free and isolated for 2 to 4 cm along its axis.

CUTDOWN
Distal Saphenous Vein (Ankle)
Advantages

- No interference or disruption of other resuscitative procedures (e.g., obtaining blood gases in same area, cardiopulmonary resuscitation [CPR], or endotracheal intubation)
- IV access on inferior side of diaphragm
- Minimal training needed and low risk of complications compared with central access
- No valves at this level of the vein because of the minimal volume and pressure
- Most consistent vein of the lower extremity, especially in its location anterior to the medial malleolus

Disadvantages

- Phlebitis and infection are common complications of the lower extremity cutdown
- Less than ideal route for cardiac drug administration (especially during CPR)
- Not good for hypertonic solutions (risk of sclerosis)
- May be absent if the patient has had vein stripping or harvest (e.g., used for a coronary artery bypass graft) or nonfunctional due to prior cutdown
- Older patients may have vein narrowing
- May not be useful in the patient with unstable pelvic fracture or major knee trauma because of iliofemoral venous interruption

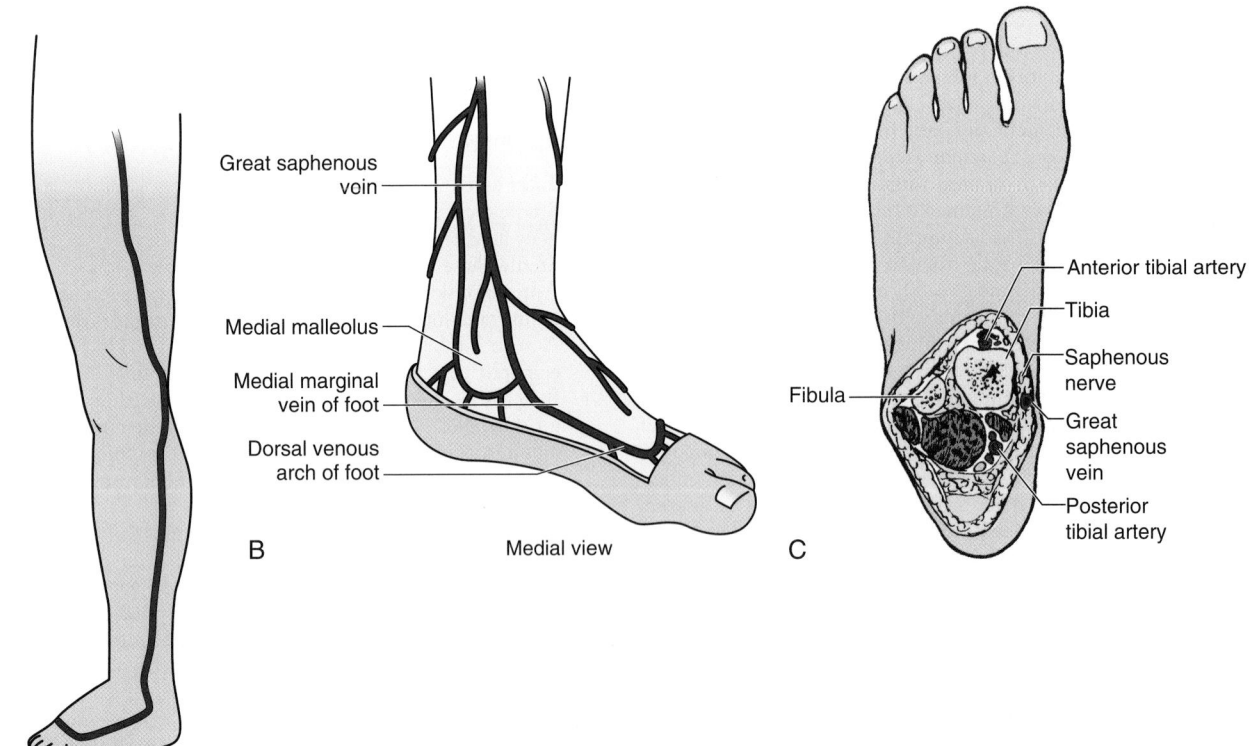

Fig. 227.1 (A) Anatomy of great saphenous vein of the lower extremity. (B) Superficial veins of the leg and foot (great saphenous vein at the ankle). (C) Cross-sectional view; the great saphenous vein may be isolated easily and safely at the ankle. Only the minor saphenous nerve lies nearby.

Technique

1. With the tourniquet in place, palpate the distal saphenous vein just anterior to the medial malleolus (see Fig. 227.1B).
2. Incise skin above the medial malleolus, starting at the proximal anterior border of the tibia and extending to the posterior border of the tibia (Fig. 227.2).
3. Using a closed, curved hemostat, with the point downward and adjacent to the tibia, advance the instrument in the line of the incision to lift the superficial tissue (Fig. 227.3).
4. Rotate the point upward, still holding the tissue. Spread to reveal the distal saphenous vein and nerve.
5. Proceed to cannulation as described in that section.
6. Apply dressing (Fig. 227.4).

Proximal Saphenous Vein (Groin)

Advantages

- IV access on inferior side of the diaphragm
- Minimal training and risk compared with central access
- Larger vein caliber facilitates cannulation and bolus infusion in profoundly hypovolemic patients

Disadvantages

- Phlebitis and infection are common complications in the groin
- Less than ideal route for cardiac drug administration (especially during CPR)

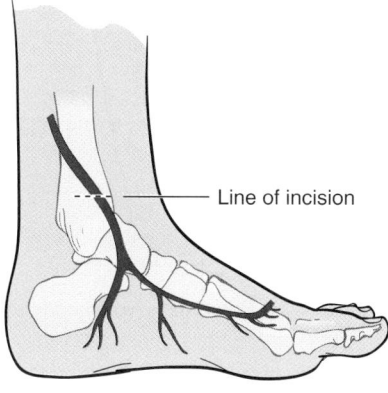

Fig. 227.2 Anatomic relationship of the saphenous vein and the line of incision.

- Not good for hypertonic solutions (risk of sclerosis)
- Proximity of femoral neurovascular bundle and other structures may introduce greater risk for complications
- May not be useful in patient with unstable pelvic fracture or major knee trauma because of iliofemoral venous interruption

Technique

1. If time and the urgency of the situation allow, identifying and visualizing the anatomy with high-frequency (5 to 10 MHz) ultrasound is very helpful (Fig. 227.5). (Also see Chapter 214, Emergency Department, Hospitalist, and Office Ultrasonography [Clinical Ultrasonography].) The high-frequency probe (even the transvaginal probe is a high-frequency probe) can be applied directly to ultrasound jelly on the skin to obtain images.
2. Incise laterally starting at the junction of the scrotal/labial fold and the medial thigh (Fig. 227.6). Extend the incision to the outer portion of the mons pubis. Visible muscle fascia means the incision is too deep.
3. The proximal saphenous vein lies in the superficial fat layer where a vertical, imaginary line starting from the pubic tubercle crosses the incision (see Fig. 227.6). Cannulate as noted in that section.

Basilic Vein (Antecubital Fossa)

Advantages

- IV access on superior side of the diaphragm
- Minimal training and risk compared with central access
- Larger vein caliber facilitates cannulation and bolus infusion in profoundly hypovolemic patients
- Less risk of phlebitis than with lower extremity cutdowns

Disadvantages

- With ongoing CPR, cannulation can be difficult at this site.
- Compared with the groin, the smaller diameter of the basilic vein theoretically limits rapid infusions of large volume. However, the cannulas are the same size in all sites; therefore the basilic vein diameter is unlikely to be a negative factor.
- Deep dissection in the antecubital fossa can damage other structures.

Technique

1. Take the distance between the olecranon and the acromion, and divide it into thirds. With the tourniquet applied proximally, palpate the vein on the medial aspect of the arm where it lies in the

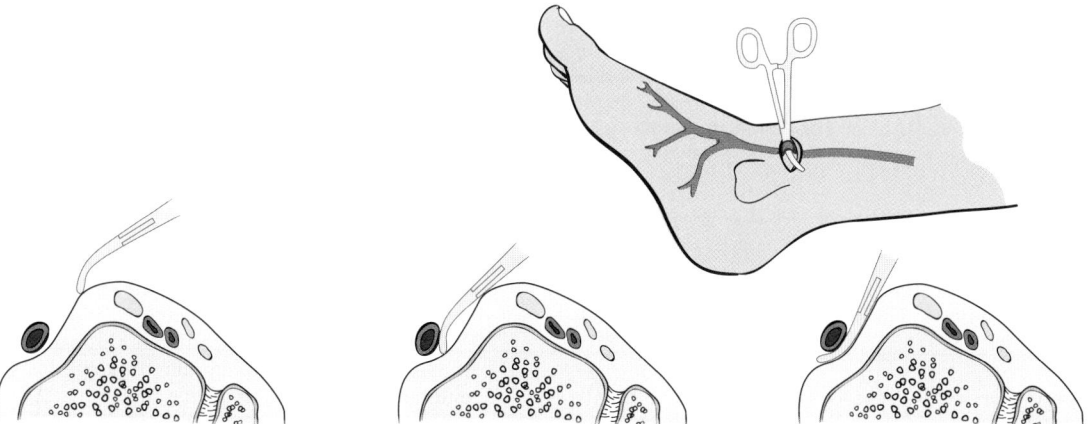

Fig. 227.3 Curved mosquito clamp is inserted into the edge of the incision and the tip turned downward and placed adjacent to the tibia. It is then advanced under the saphenous vein and swept across the tibia. Then the clamp is turned over so that the tips are pointed upward. The tips are spread to reveal the saphenous vein and nerve.

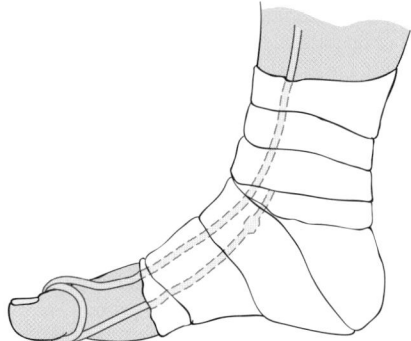

Fig. 227.4 Dressing to prevent decannulation.

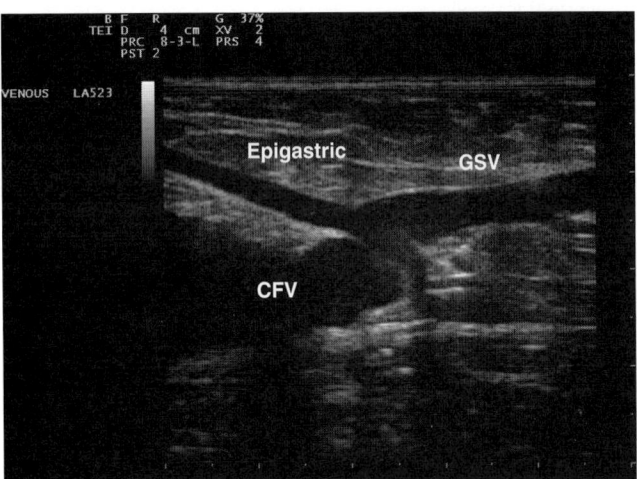

Fig. 227.5 High-frequency (5–10 MHz) ultrasound image of the groin, defining bifurcation of great saphenous vein (*GSV*) from common femoral vein (*CFV*).

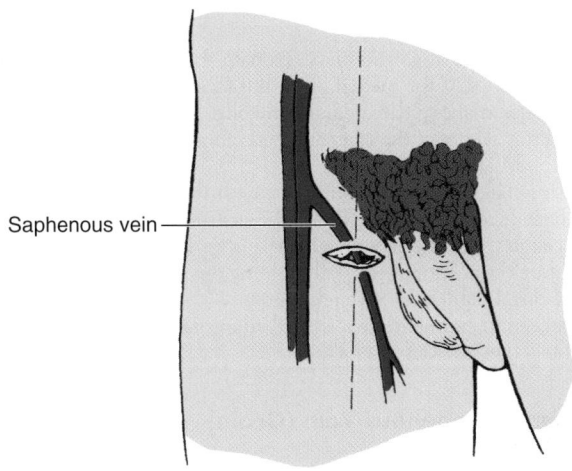

Fig. 227.6 Cutdown location for great saphenous vein at the groin.

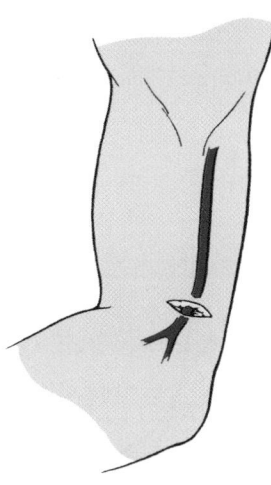

Fig. 227.7 Incision is made between the biceps and triceps for basilic vein cutdown (right arm).

groove between the triceps and biceps muscles. On the medial arm, the vein follows a course slightly anterior and superficial to the brachial artery.
2. Make a horizontal, superficial incision from the biceps across the groove to the triceps (Fig. 227.7).
3. Locate the basilic vein by dissecting the superficial fat layer. Visible muscle fascia or the brachial artery means the incision is too deep.
4. If time and the urgency of the situation allow it, identifying and visualizing the anatomy with high-frequency (10 MHz) ultrasound is very helpful (see Fig. 227.5; also see Chapter 214, Emergency Department, Hospitalist, and Office Ultrasonography [Clinical Ultrasonography]). The basilic vein will best be visualized with the tourniquet in place.
5. Proceed to cannulation.

CANNULATION

1. Isolate 3 to 4 cm of the chosen vein, dissecting aside loose adipose or adventitial tissue. The scissors can be spread longitudinally along the length of the vein to improve access and help to visualize it.
2. Pass suture ties under the vein, both proximally and distally. Pass the distal suture as far distal as possible; use this as a retractor to bring the vein into the incision.
3. If the distal vein is to be sacrificed, the distal ligature should be tied and left long to help control and manipulate the vein.

Clamp the ends of the ligature with a hemostat, and use its weight to maintain tension on the ligature.
4. Place traction on the proximal suture to minimize rebleeding; it should not be tied at this point.
5. Loosen the tourniquet if one has been applied.
6. Select a site near the distal ligature for venotomy. If the vein is large enough, it can be catheterized directly. Otherwise, incise one-third of the vein's diameter at a 45-degree angle to the skin in distal-to-proximal fashion (Fig. 227.8A). The result should be a V-shaped incision (see Fig. 227.8B). While maintaining proximal ligature traction, expand the lumen with a mosquito hemostat (see Fig. 227.8C).
   EDITOR'S NOTE: Avoid cutting the entire vein with the scissors or scalpel, which could cause excessive bleeding; it may also result in retraction of the vein from the incision, thereby increasing the difficulty of the procedure.
7. Once the skin has been entered through a separate stab wound, introduce the cannula through the vein incision, maintaining the same 45-degree angle (Fig. 227.9). This is the most difficult portion of the procedure. Use caution in great saphenous vein cannulations, making sure not to occlude the femoral vein with the cannula (avoid advancing the cannula too far).

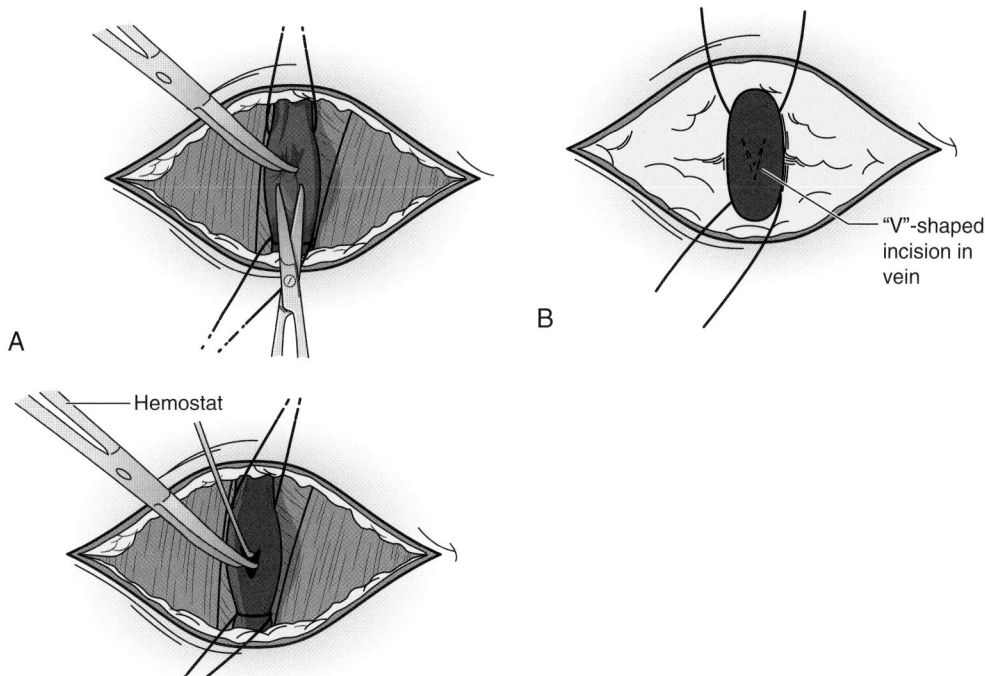

A

B

—"V"-shaped
incision in
vein

—Hemostat

C

Fig. 227.8   (A) Angled wedge cut
is made in the anterior wall of the
vein. Traction should be maintained
on the vein with proximal and distal
ligatures. If sacrificed, the distal vein
ligature can be tied. (B) Resultant V-
shaped incision in vein. (C) The vein
is dilated with a hemostat.

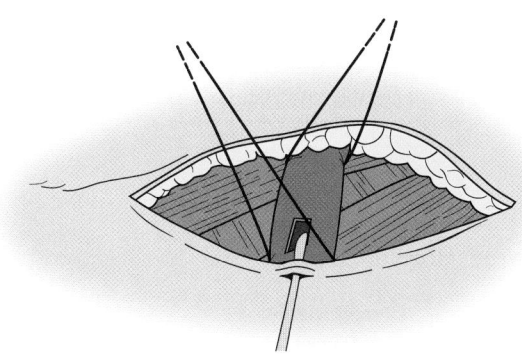

Fig. 227.9   Catheter is threaded through a separate skin stab wound and
then into vein.

8. Aspirate air from the cannula; tie the proximal ligature around
   the cannula and vein wall.
9. Cut both ligatures and close the wound (Fig. 227.10).
10. Remove the tourniquet and observe for incision leakage of
    blood or fluid.
11. Secure the catheter hub to the skin with an additional stitch.
    Apply sterile dressing.

MINICUTDOWN WITH ANGIMOCATHETER OR SELDINGER WIRE

The minicutdown is the fastest technique when an angiocatheter
needle (standard catheter-over-needle) of adequate size (16 to 18
gauge) or a Seldinger wire introducer or modified Seldinger wire
kit is available. The vein is located and isolated surgically as previously described, but the incision can be much smaller ("mini,"
or just large enough to locate the vein). Then the angiocatheter
unit is placed through the skin, approximately 1 cm distal to the

incision. The angiocatheter is threaded into the vein in the same
manner as with percutaneous catheterization. An optional suture
through the skin proximal to the incision, around the catheter
and vein, and then tied loosely can stabilize the catheter in the
vein. However, inserting the angiocatheter through skin distally
usually stabilizes it. Closure of the wound provides further stabilization. The hub should also be stabilized with an additional skin
suture. In 1 to 2 days, after the patient is stable and has routine
peripheral IV access, the hub (and optional catheter) sutures can
be removed and the Teflon catheter withdrawn without reopening
the incision.

To ease cannulation of the vein, a straight hemostat can be
inserted beneath the vein and spread open. The scalpel can then be
used to make a 1- to 2-mm venotomy (Fig. 227.11) and the angiocatheter inserted through the venotomy.

The Seldinger technique for venous cutdown can also use a small,
1- to 2-mm, venotomy (see Fig. 227.11) and a Seldinger wire-guided
catheter (found in prepackaged central line set). The Seldinger unit
comes assembled with dilator and catheter. The catheter-over-needle
is advanced through the skin, 1 cm distal to the incision and then
through the venotomy. The needle is removed and the wire advanced
into the vein through the catheter. The catheter is then removed
while the guidewire stays in place. Next, place the dilator through the
introducer sheath and thread the combined dilator-introducer sheath
down the guidewire. Holding the free end of the guidewire to prevent
it from advancing, and using a twisting motion, advance the dilator
and introducer sheath further down the guidewire and into the venotomy. This effort also dilates the vein. Most of the time, this technique
eliminates the need for tying off the distal vein. When the hub of the
introducer sheath reaches the skin level, remove the guidewire and
dilator as a unit, leaving the introducer sheath in place. Securing the
introducer in the vein with a suture around them both is usually not
necessary.

The modified Seldinger wire-guided technique for venous
cutdown is even easier to learn and has been shown to be 22%
faster than the classic technique. Assemble the unit (Fig. 227.12)

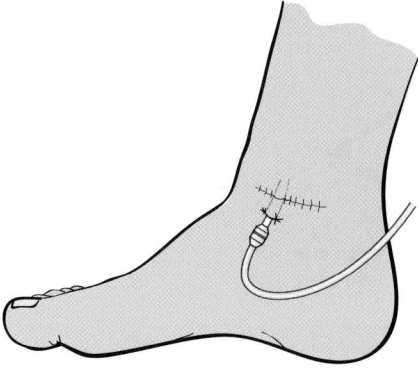

Fig. 227.10 Incision is closed to minimize risk of infection and catheter is then sutured in place.

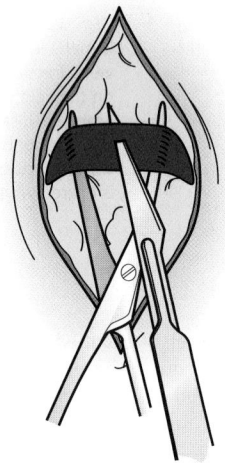

Fig. 227.11 A spread straight hemostat and No. 11 blade used to make 2-mm minivenotomy incision. (From Klofas E. A quicker saphenous vein cutdown and a better way to teach it. *J Trauma*. 1997;43:985–987.)

by placing the dilator through the sheath and then inserting the guidewire through the dilator. The guidewire should protrude 3 to 4 mm beyond the tip of the dilator. This guidewire is then inserted through a 1- to 2-mm venotomy and advanced. With a twisting motion, the entire unit is then inserted over the guidewire, up to the hub.

The skin incision can then be closed with sutures and the catheter hub sutured in place. Even when pressure infusion techniques are used, additional sutures may not be necessary.

COMPLICATIONS

Possible complications include hematoma, embolism, bacteremia, and sepsis. These are rare, especially if the catheter is removed within 12 hours of placement. There has been no value to using prophylactic antibiotics to prevent infection. Use of a daily topical antibiotic ointment decreases the risk of colonization. There is always the possibility of injury to nearby structures, especially using the basilic vein technique, which is the most difficult approach. The second most difficult approach uses the proximal saphenous vein. The distal saphenous vein is least likely to result in damage to other structures. In the unstable emergency patient, there is the possibility of taking too much time during an attempt to perform venous cutdown, leading to a worsening of the clinical situation.

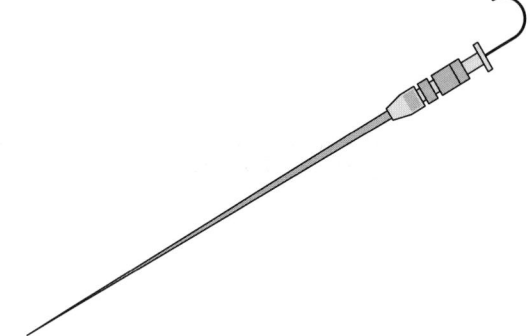

Fig. 227.12 The wire-guided catheter, already mounted on the wire and dilator. (From Klofas E. A quicker saphenous vein cutdown and a better way to teach it. *J Trauma*. 1997;43:985–987.)

CPT/BILLING CODES

36410   Venipuncture, child over 3 years or adult, necessitating physician's skill for diagnostic or therapeutic purposes (not to be used for routine venipuncture)
36425   Venipuncture, cutdown; aged 1 year or older
76937   Ultrasound guidance for vascular access

ICD-10-CM DIAGNOSTIC CODES

E86.0   Volume depletion, dehydration
E86.1   Volume depletion, hypovolemia
I46.9   Cardiopulmonary arrest
R58   Hemorrhage, nonspecific
I99.8   Venofibrosis
P54.9   Hemorrhage, unspecified in newborn (not otherwise specified)
R57.9   Shock (without trauma), unspecified
R65.21   Shock, septic or endotoxic
R57.1   Hypovolemic shock not elsewhere categorized
R09.2   Respiratory arrest
T79.4XXX   Hemorrhagic shock or shock syndrome due to trauma
T78.2XXX   Shock, anaphylactic

Use additional seventh character: A, initial; D, subsequent; S, sequela.

Acknowledgment

The editors recognize the contributions of Pauline Aham-Neze, MD, and Grant C. Fowler, MD, to this chapter in previous editions of this text.

RECOMMENDED READING

American College of Surgeons. Shock. In: *Advanced Trauma Life Support Student Course Manual*. 6th ed. Chicago: American College of Surgeons; 1997:87–125.

Keenan SP. Use of ultrasound to place central lines. *J Crit Care*. 2002;17:126–137.

Klofas E. A quicker saphenous vein cutdown and a better way to teach it. *J Trauma*. 1997;39:985–987.

Nobay F. Peripheral venous cutdown. In: Reichman EF, ed. *Emergency Medicine Procedures*. 2nd ed. New York: McGraw-Hill; 2013:350–361.

Shockley LW, Butzier DJ. A modified wire-guided technique for venous cutdown access. *Ann Emerg Med*. 1990;19:393–395.

Westfall MD, Price KR, Lambert M, et al. Intravenous access in the critically ill trauma patient: a multicentered, prospective, randomized trial of saphenous cutdown and percutaneous femoral access. *Ann Emerg Med*. 1994;23(3):541–545.

CHAPTER 228

CENTRAL VENOUS CATHETER INSERTION

David James

Over the past several decades, the use of central venous catheters increased to keep pace with other medical and technological advances. While the use of peripherally inserted central catheters has decreased the need somewhat, emergency resuscitation protocols, specialized cardiovascular monitoring techniques, and transvenous pacer insertion all demand access to a large central vein.

Expeditious placement of a large central venous catheter presents a challenge to the clinician, because the central veins are neither readily visible to the eye nor distinctly palpable. If the patient is critically ill or hypovolemic, the challenge is magnified. Fortunately, the larger central veins have predictable and constant relationships to readily identifiable anatomic landmarks.

In recent years, increasing emphasis has been placed on using ultrasound to guide placement of central venous catheters (see Chapter 214, Emergency Department, Hospitalist, and Office Ultrasonography [Clinical Ultrasonography]). Ultrasound guidance can assist not only with excluding thrombosis in the chosen vein but also with defining local anatomy; it has been shown to increase success rate and decrease procedure time and complication rates. Although ultrasound guidance was not considered the standard of care in a recent informal survey of hospitalists, Medicare guidelines suggest monitoring very closely for iatrogenic puncture wounds of vital organs in hospitalized patients. Consequently, many hospitals now require the use of ultrasound guidance for the placement of all non-emergent central venous catheters. Meanwhile, it has been shown that compliance with a central line bundling policy can reduce central line-associated bloodstream infections.

NOTE: Remember that a short, large-diameter IV catheter (e.g., 14-, 16-, or 18-gauge peripheral catheter) has less resistance to flow than a long, skinny central catheter! Rapid, large-volume infusion is faster with a peripheral, large-bore catheter and is preferred in an emergent situation. Depending on local availability and expertise, kits are available to rapidly and dependably obtain intraosseous vascular access (IOVA; see Chapter 226, Intraosseous Vascular Access). In some facilities, this has become the preferred temporary backup or alternative to obtaining central or peripheral venous access, especially in children (see Chapter 164, Pediatric Arterial Puncture and Venous Minicutdown).

INDICATIONS

- Venous access in those patients who are either so obese or so debilitated that their peripheral veins are not accessible for intravenous (IV) cannulation
- Emergency venous access after a cardiac arrest
- Administration of cardiac medications during cardiopulmonary resuscitation (CPR)
- Large-volume parenteral fluid administration needed when peripheral IV cannulation is not readily obtainable

- Central venous pressure monitoring
- Administration of certain chemotherapeutic agents
- Administration of vasopressor medications
- Administration of hyperosmolar or other irritating solutions (e.g., total parenteral nutrition) that have the potential to cause thrombophlebitis or to cause soft tissue necrosis if extravasation occurs
- Patients with significant burns on peripheral areas that may prevent placement of a peripheral catheter
- Placement of a pulmonary artery (Swan-Ganz) catheter (see Chapter 229, Swan Ganz [Pulmonary Artery] Catheterization)
- Placement of a temporary transvenous pacemaker wire (see Chapter 232, Temporary Pacing)
- Performance of right cardiac catheterization and pulmonary angiography
- Performance of hemodialysis or plasmapheresis

CONTRAINDICATIONS

Absolute

- Dependent on the patient's overall condition, urgency of need, and alternatives available
- Patient refusal
- Combative or agitated patient (may require procedural sedation, see Chapter 1, Procedural Sedation and Analgesia)
- Distortion of local anatomy or landmarks unless ultrasound guidance available (e.g., prior surgery, trauma, radiation therapy, orthopedic conditions, masses)
- Superior vena cava syndrome
- Cellulitis over the proposed insertion site
- Pneumothorax or hemothorax on the contralateral side, or inability to tolerate a pneumothorax on the ipsilateral side (for subclavian and internal jugular locations; generally the central line is placed on the side of the chest injury as long as the vein is not known to be injured)
- Trauma to the proposed insertion site
- Venous thrombosis of the proposed vein
- Avoid internal jugular location if cervical spine fracture, penetrating neck injury or C-collar in place.
- Avoid femoral vein if known or suspected intraabdominal hemorrhage.
- Allergy to any component of the catheter such as latex or to the medication in impregnated catheters
- Cardiac-paced patient (for Seldinger wire technique, whether pacer temporary, internal, or permanent)
- Highly unstable arrhythmias (for Seldinger wire technique, especially ventricular arrhythmias)
- Right-sided endocarditis or mural thrombus

Relative

- Suspected injury to proposed vein (may then use vein on contralateral side, if no associated hemothorax or pneumothorax, when using subclavian or internal jugular)
- Morbid obesity (ultrasound guided internal jugular probably best route)
- Marked cachexia
- Full-thickness burn (no increased risk of infection for 3 days, time it takes for burn to colonize with bacteria)
- Vasculitis that predisposes to sclerosis or thrombosis of veins
- Prior injection of a sclerosing agent into the proposed vein
- Previous long-term central catheterization or recently discontinued central catheter in proposed vein
- Proposed mastectomy on same side of subclavian vein access
- Patients receiving ventilatory support with high end-expiratory pressures (if possible, for subclavian or internal jugular, ventilation should briefly be interrupted while central vein is cannulated with needle)
- Patients undergoing CPR (should use femoral or internal jugular vein locations)
- Children younger than 2 years old (for whom the internal jugular vein is preferred location; however, if clinician is experienced with subclavian insertion, has been proven safe)
- Severe hypovolemia (try large bore peripheral IV or IOVA first)
- Bleeding diathesis or excessive anticoagulation and a noncompressible vessel (ultrasound guidance of internal jugular [compressible] preferred, see Editor's Note below)
- Prosthetic right heart valve (Seldinger wire technique contraindicated)
- Avoid internal jugular or subclavian vein locations if patient unable to lie in the Trendelenburg position.
- Left bundle branch block (use of Seldinger wire can cause complete heart block)
- Avoid internal jugular location if known severe carotid artery stenosis or atherosclerosis on the desired side (accidental artery puncture may result in plaque rupture and stroke).
- Personnel capable of handling complications not immediately available

EDITOR'S NOTE: One study (Mumtaz) found only a 3% risk of bleeding complications, usually limited to the insertion site and controlled by sutures, in patients with thrombocytopenia (platelet count <50 × 10^9/L). A 2005 review (Segal) found that if good technique is used, correction of coagulopathy is not necessary.

EQUIPMENT

Many commercially prepared central venous catheter kits are available. Most institutions have a relationship with a hospital supplier that provides a catheter kit. These kits, often from a company such as Baxter or Cook, have all the components needed to insert a central venous catheter. These kits often utilize a Seldinger wire technique (most common method) to place the catheter: a needle enters the vein, a guidewire is threaded through the needle into the vein lumen, and the cannulating needle is removed. A larger, flexible catheter is then passed over the guidewire into the vein, and the guidewire is removed. While almost any needle can be used to introduce a guidewire, a Seldinger needle has a funnel-shaped, tapered lumen that allows easy entry of the guidewire.

- IV solution and connector tubing, flushed and ready
- Towel
- Pressure transducer and monitor, if monitoring central venous pressure
- Supplemental oxygen
- Continuous pulse oximetry and cardiac and blood pressure monitoring

- Fully stocked code cart and defibrillator nearby
- Surgeon's cap
- Sterile gloves and gown
- Sterile drapes
- Bio-occlusive dressing (e.g., Tegaderm, Opsite) to cover insertion site, especially useful if clear so the wound can be more easily inspected
- Goggles or eye protection and other equipment necessary to follow universal blood and body fluid precautions

If a commercially prepared kit is unavailable, the following equipment list will supply what is needed:

- Sterile prep solution (chlorhexidine antiseptic preferred over povidone-iodine solution) and swabs
- Prep razor
- Sterile 4 × 4 inch gauze pads
- Lidocaine 1% to 2% with or without epinephrine for local anesthesia
- 3-mL syringe with 25-gauge needle for anesthetic injection
- 5-mL syringe with 22-gauge 1.5- to 2.5-inch seeker needle to find the vein
- 10-mL syringe with 2.5-inch 18-gauge needle to introduce guidewire
- No. 11 scalpel blade and holder
- Guidewire or J-wire (flexible wire 45 cm long, 0.064 to 0.089 cm diameter, 3 mm radius of curvature; J-wires possibly better for tortuous vessels, straight wires for vessels with linear configuration)
- Central venous catheter
- 3-0 silk suture on straight needle to suture catheter into place
- Suture scissors
- Topical antimicrobial ointment
- Saline flushes

PREPROCEDURE PATIENT EDUCATION

If the clinical situation permits, informed consent must be obtained prior to the procedure. Inform the patient (or family) why this procedure is necessary and of potential major complications and their management, which could require chest tube insertion, surgery, or cardioversion. Alternatives, if available, should be discussed. To minimize patient anxiety during procedure, explain the major steps of the procedure, the possible necessity of remaining in a head down (Trendelenburg) position during placement, and the near impossibility of a completely painless procedure.

TECHNIQUES

Several distinct options should be discussed for placement of a central venous catheter. These approaches include cannulation of the subclavian vein (using either the supra- or infraclavicular routes), the internal jugular vein, or the femoral vein.

In general, the preferred veins are on the right side of the patient. This preference is because the right-sided veins have a more direct course to the right atrium, and thus can be utilized for placement of a pacemaker wire or Swan-Ganz catheter with greater ease than the left-sided veins. The left-sided veins tend to have a more tortuous course and are in closer proximity to the thoracic duct and dome of the lung pleura.

The internal jugular vein is accessible without terminating CPR, although chest compressions and the lack of a carotid pulse may make access more difficult. However, having an internal jugular line requires limiting patient neck mobility, which can be uncomfortable, so the subclavian route may be preferable for long-term lines. Likewise, a femoral line limits ambulation, so the subclavian route may be preferable. Ongoing or impending thrombolytic or fibrinolytic therapy is a contraindication to internal jugular puncture. Femoral vein access may be the easiest to obtain and may be preferable in emergencies or during CPR. It may also be preferred for patients with respiratory distress or pulmonary edema because the patient

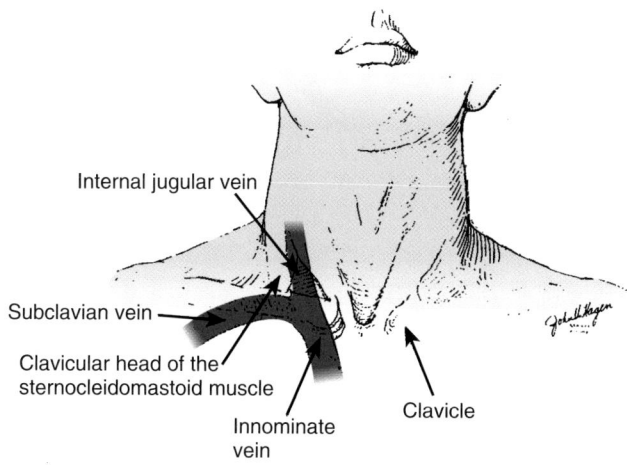

Fig. 228.1   Relationship of great vessels in and about the right neck.

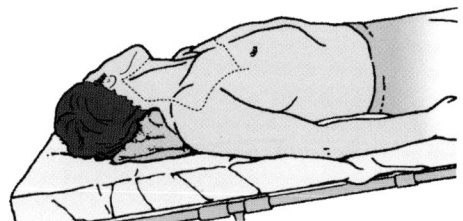

Fig. 228.2   Moderate Trendelenburg position for subclavian central vein catheter insertion.

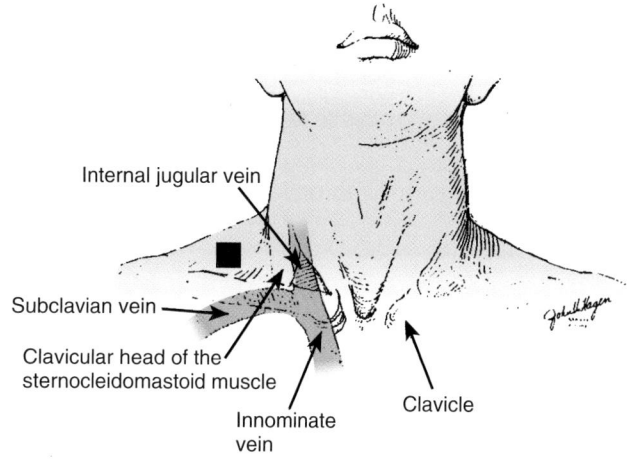

Fig. 228.3   Supraclavicular approach: *black box* represents entry point 1 cm lateral to the clavicular head of the sternocleidomastoid muscle, and 1 cm above the superior border of the clavicle.

should not be placed in the Trendelenburg position. Supplemental oxygen should be provided and the patient monitored continuously during this procedure. Passage of a guidewire into the right side of the heart can induce arrhythmias and complete heart block; the clinician should be prepared to treat these problems accordingly.

EDITOR'S NOTE: Cannulation may not succeed on the first attempt. It is reasonable to try again, but after three or four unsuccessful attempts, it is wise to move to a different anatomic approach or to allow a colleague to attempt the procedure. Even if the attempts were unsuccessful, it is advisable to obtain radiographs of the chest.

Subclavian Venipuncture

The subclavian vein begins as a continuation of the axillary vein at the lateral border of the first rib, and it joins the internal jugular vein to form the innominate vein (Fig. 228.1). As it crosses behind the first rib, the subclavian vein lies posterior to the medial third of the clavicle. It is only in this "middle region" that an intimate relationship exists between the subclavian vein and the clavicle. The subclavian vein contains no valves and is between 1 and 2 cm in diameter for most people. The subclavian artery is superior and posterior to the vein, and is separated from the vein by the anterior scalene muscle. Other important structures nearby include the phrenic nerve, the thoracic duct (left side), lymphatic duct (on the right side, it joins the subclavian vein near its merger with the internal jugular vein), and the dome of the pleura of the lung. The dome of the pleura may extend above the first rib on the left side but is rarely found this far cephalad on the right.

Patient Position

Proper positioning of the patient increases chances of a successful cannulation and reduces risk of complications of this procedure. Place the patient in Trendelenburg position at an angle of 15 to 20 degrees (Fig. 228.2). This position fills these low-pressure great veins by gravity, thus making them swell in diameter and increasing your chances of finding them. It also reduces the risk of air embolism.

- Have the patient turn his or her head contralaterally. (Have an assistant turn the head if the patient is unable to do so.) This gives a wider field of operation.
- Consider placing a rolled-up towel vertically between the patient's shoulder blades. This may cause the shoulders to fall back from the clavicles, which could help define the relevant anatomy and improve access to the subclavian vein. However, it should be noted that certain experts avoid placing a towel between the shoulder blades because it can decrease the distance between the clavicle and first rib, thereby compressing the subclavian vein and making it more difficult to cannulate.

Supraclavicular Approach to the Subclavian Vein

This approach may sound complicated, but the author believes it to be the least complicated and most efficient technique. It is rapid, stays away from other vital structures, and is easily performed in patients undergoing CPR. In addition, it is easily and reliably performed in an obese patient.

1. With the patient in the previously described position, locate the insertion area: a spot 1 cm lateral to the lateral head of the sternocleidomastoid muscle and 1 cm superior to the clavicular border (Fig. 228.3).
2. Review Fig. 228.4 for an overview of the catheter-over-wire (Seldinger) technique described here.
3. Assemble equipment on a work surface of convenient height, and within your reach. Wash your hands and put on mask, cap, eye protection, sterile gown, and gloves. A strict sterile technique should be observed from this point onward. Cleanse the area with skin prep solution (some kits will have a chlorhexidine or povidone–iodine prep swab enclosed), and drape to define a sterile field. Optimally, the entire neck and clavicular area are prepped. That way, in case of unsuccessful cannulation, another site can be attempted without having to repeat the prep. Drape as large of an area as possible, including the majority of the patient and the bed. A three-quarter sheet works well for this purpose. Follow universal blood and body fluid precautions.
4. Draw up 2 mL of 1% lidocaine into the 3-mL syringe, and raise a skin wheal at the site of the proposed insertion; infiltrate the deeper tissues with the remainder of the lidocaine.
5. With the 22-gauge needle on a 5-mL syringe, seek the subclavian vein; insert the needle at the entry point diagrammed in Fig. 228.3. Aim just under the clavicle, angled toward the contralateral nipple. Usually, in people of normal weight and habitus, the vein is quite shallowly located. In an obese patient, or

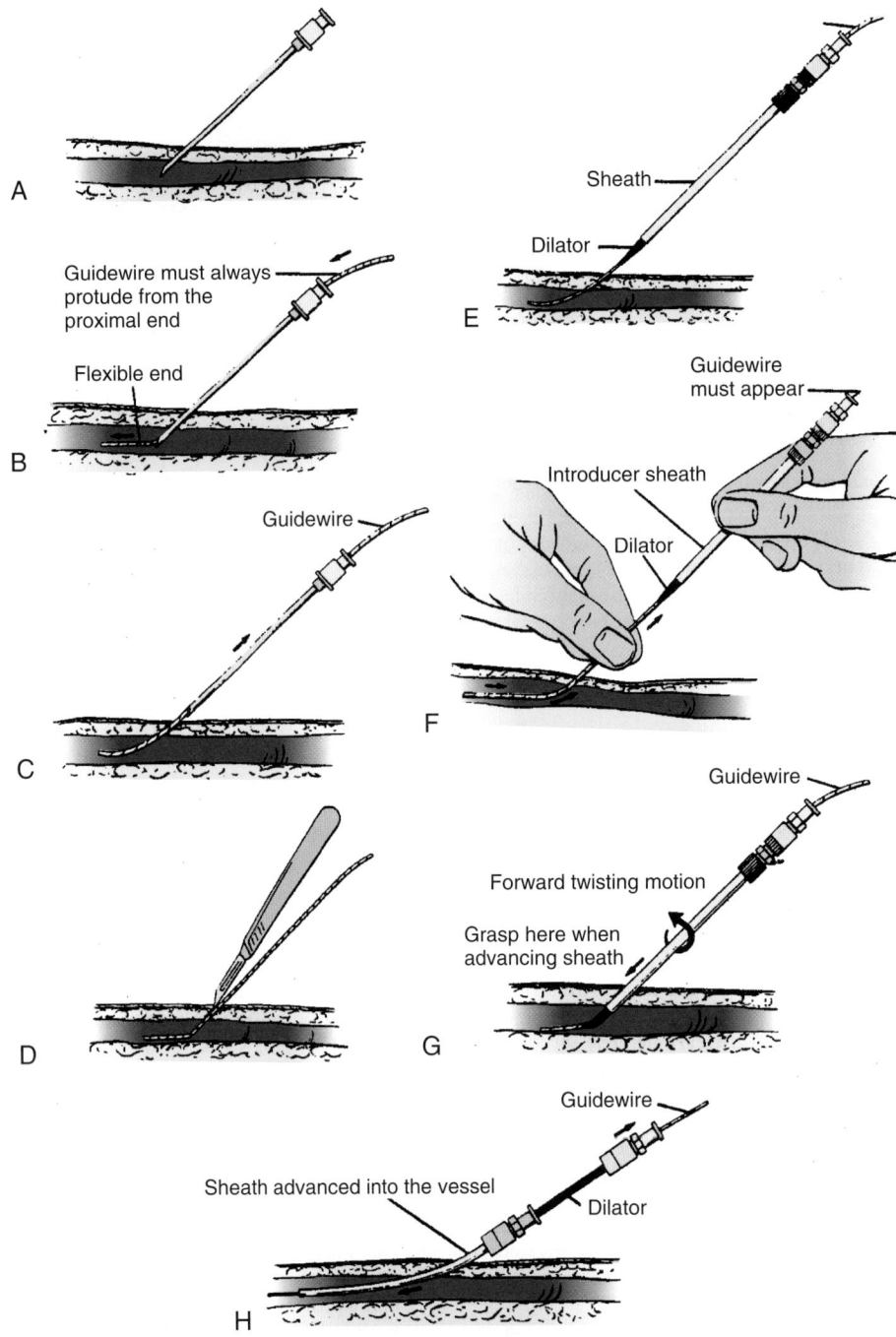

Fig. 228.4 Placement of Seldinger-type guidewire and catheter. (A) Introducing needle with tip in lumen. (B) Advance guidewire into vein. (C) Remove introducing needle over guidewire. (D) Make small skin incision. (E) Advance dilator and sheath until tip is near skin. (F) If guidewire tip cannot be grasped, withdraw it slightly from the vein by grasping below the dilator tip. (G) Advance dilator and sheath along guidewire and into vein. (H) After sheath is fully advanced, slowly withdraw dilator and then guidewire. Immediately cover catheter hub with finger and attach to intravenous tubing. (Modified from Roberts JR, Hedges JR, eds. *Clinical Procedures in Emergency Medicine*, 3rd ed. Philadelphia, WB Saunders; 1998.)

those with chest hyperinflation from chronic obstructive pulmonary disease, the vein is deeper. Maintain suction on the syringe until dark red blood flows easily into the syringe.

6. Insert the 18-gauge 1½-inch needle mounted on a 5- or 10-mL syringe parallel to the seeker needle to enter the subclavian vein. The position of this needle should be identical to that of the seeker needle (i.e., the same direction, depth, and angle of penetration). Insert while aspirating with the syringe plunger. Placement within the vein is confirmed by easy return of dark red blood. Rotate the syringe/needle unit until the bevel of the needle faces caudally.

7. In many central line kits, a Raulerson syringe (Teleflex Arrow), which has an 18-gauge port that runs through the plunger and right out through the needle, is provided. This syringe allows guidewire insertion directly into the vein from the syringe plunger and allows the needle/syringe unit to be left in place where the subclavian vein was entered, thus minimizing the risk of unintentional movement of the needle out of the vein. If you do not have a kit with the plunger port, you will need to remove the syringe from the 18-gauge 2.5-inch needle hub, making sure the needle does not move from its position. Occlude the needle hub with your nondominant thumb.

EDITOR'S NOTE: An intended benefit of use of a blue Raulerson syringe is the ability to differentiate arterial from venous blood by its color in the syringe. However, in patients with certain conditions (e.g., severe hypoxia, shock), arterial blood can be dark and mimic venous blood with adverse consequences. By disconnecting the introducer needle from the syringe, the clinician can determine whether the blood is pulsatile (arterial) or not. If there is any question, a sterile arterial blood gas syringe can be dropped into the field and a sample sent immediately for blood gas analysis. Make sure to cap the introducer needle hub while waiting for the result.

8. Insert the guidewire through the needle hub or plunger port. Most guidewires have a J loop at the end; straighten the loop by withdrawing the wire into its sheath. Then, once the straightened end of the wire is inserted into the needle, advance the guidewire approximately half of its length into the subclavian vein.

9. Withdraw, over the wire, the introducer needle/syringe unit. Make sure the wire stays steady and does not advance inadvertently its entire length into the vein, where it could embolize.

10. Using the no. 11 scalpel blade, make a small nick in the skin where the guidewire enters; this makes room for the dilator and introducer sheath. It is often easiest to just slide the blade on top of the wire. Slide the dilator over the wire, and insert/withdraw the dilator several times to dilate the entry site tissues. Using a twisting motion while inserting the dilator may facilitate its advance. Withdraw the dilator over the guidewire and set it aside.

11. If color-coded, remove the brown hub (most distal port) from the central venous catheter. In some kits, the catheter is stiff enough to be inserted alone, directly over the guidewire. Otherwise, insert the dilator into the catheter (or some kits have a smaller diameter introducer that fits into the catheter to stiffen it). Slide the catheter (and dilator/introducer if needed, as a unit) over the wire, and advance the guidewire up into the catheter until it just pokes out of the open port. Holding the end of the wire, slide the catheter (and dilator/introducer if needed) down over the wire to the desired depth of insertion. Using a twisting motion when advancing the catheter may facilitate its advance.

12. Remove the dilator/introducer over the guidewire and then remove the guidewire and set it aside. This leaves the catheter in place. Secure the catheter to the skin with a suture (most kits have a plastic hub that fits over the catheter and has preformed suture holes for securing to the skin). The insertion area and exposed catheter should be covered with a sterile dressing. (A clear bio-occlusive dressing such as Tegaderm or Opsite provides added security.)

13. Reattach the brown hub, or the required clave-type hub, to the catheter port, and aspirate each port to ensure easy blood return. Flush all ports with saline. You may hook up any IV tubing/fluids at this time.

14. Obtain a postinsertion chest radiograph to ensure that there is no iatrogenic pneumothorax and to check the catheter tip location.

15. If the catheter tip lies within the right atrium or ventricle, the catheter should be withdrawn so that the tip resides within the superior vena cava. The right atrium is very thin-walled and easy to perforate; to prevent this, the tip needs to reside in the vena cava.

Infraclavicular Approach to the Subclavian Vein

This approach is very familiar because of the easily identified anatomic landmarks.

1. Position the patient in a moderate Trendelenburg position, as illustrated in Fig. 228.2.

2. Orient yourself regarding landmarks, and establish an insertion site (Fig. 228.5). Place the thumb of your nondominant hand on the distal end of the clavicle and the middle finger of the same

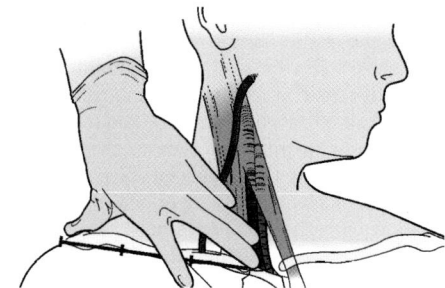

Fig. 228.5 Orientation for subclavian catheter insertion, infraclavicular approach. Thumb of nondominant hand is on distal clavicle, middle finger on sternoclavicular joint.

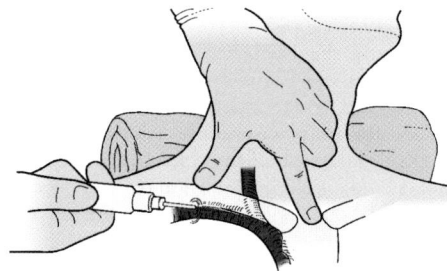

Fig. 228.6 Inserting the seeker needle.

hand on the sternoclavicular joint. Let the index finger extend comfortably. The site for insertion will be immediately under the index finger, where it crosses the clavicle. Mark this site with your fingernail or a marker pen.

3. Open the central line catheter kit, wash your hands, don personal gear (mask, cap, eye protection, sterile gown, and gloves), and prep and drape the area in the usual fashion. Observe universal blood and body fluid precautions.

4. Using a 3-mL syringe with a 25-gauge needle attached, draw up 2 mL of 1% plain lidocaine and use this to anesthetize the insertion area. Infiltrate anesthesia into the deeper tissues under the clavicle as well.

5. Have patient turn his or her head contralaterally, or have an assistant hold the head rotated contralaterally.

6. Use the 3-mL syringe with the 22-gauge needle as a "seeker" needle. Position the thumb of your nondominant hand over your mark and place the index finger of the same hand between the two clavicular heads in the suprasternal notch. Insert the seeker needle 1 to 2 cm inferior to the clavicle. Aim for the suprasternal notch (Fig. 228.6). Keep the shaft of the seeker needle in contact with the inferior border of the clavicle as you work it under the clavicle. Aspirate as you go; entry into the subclavian vein is confirmed by the easy return of dark venous blood into the syringe. If the first attempt is unsuccessful, withdraw the seeker needle, flush it, confirm landmarks, and reinsert it under the clavicle, directing the needle somewhat cephalad and deeper. At times, the 1.5-inch "seeker" needle will be too short to enter the subclavian vein with the infraclavicular approach.

7. Once the subclavian vein has been located, remove the seeker needle. Using the 18-gauge 2.5-inch needle on a 5-mL syringe, insert it along the track of the seeker needle (i.e., the same direction, angle, and depth of penetration) to enter the subclavian vein. Entry is confirmed by the easy return of dark red blood into the syringe. Once in the vein, roll the syringe, so that the bevel of the needle is directed inferiorly.

8. If the 5-mL syringe has a plunger entry port, insert the guidewire through the port and into the vein. Leave one third of the wire's length free, and maintain control of this end with your

dominant hand. If the 5-mL syringe does not have a plunger entry port, remove the syringe from the needle hub, and occlude the needle hub with your nondominant thumb until you insert the guidewire. If you do not have to traverse the syringe's length, leave half of the guidewire free and secured.

9. Using your nondominant hand, remove the syringe/needle assembly, gliding it along the guidewire. Be sure to maintain the position of the guidewire in the superior vena cava.
10. Nick the skin with the no. 11 scalpel blade by following the guidewire as it courses into the deeper tissues. Slide the dilator over the guidewire, and run it along the guidewire into the subclavian vein up to the hub. Using a twisting motion while inserting the dilator may facilitate its advance. Continue to maintain control of the guidewire. Remove the dilator by sliding it out of the vein and off the guidewire.

Follow steps 11 through 15 above.

NOTE: Occasionally, the subclavian artery may be entered during placement of the catheter. This is marked by a rush of bright red arterial blood into the syringe or out of the needle hub. If this occurs, withdraw all needles, and place pressure over the site for 10 minutes. Obtain an urgent radiograph of the chest to check for pneumothorax/hemothorax, and check the distal arm pulse frequently. Recheck the hematocrit in 1 hour, and choose another site for venous access. If the catheter is seen to loop *up* the ipsilateral jugular vein, contralateral innominate vein, or contralateral subclavian vein on postplacement radiograph, the catheter will need repositioning. Because the sterile field has been removed, repositioning the catheter will involve a rewiring procedure. This procedure involves withdrawing the catheter until the tip lies just outside the ipsilateral jugular or innominate vein and then threading a sterile wire through the brown port of the preexisting catheter. The preexisting catheter is then removed, leaving the wire in place, and a new sterile catheter is introduced over wire using the Seldinger technique. Care must be taken to keep the wire sterile while discontinuing the "old" catheter.

Internal Jugular Vein Catheterization

Advantages of the internal jugular technique include the ability to cannulate the vessel during ongoing CPR and a relatively low iatrogenic complication rate. Bleeding complications are easily controlled by direct compression; hence this is the preferred approach for those patients who have a concurrent coagulopathy. Disadvantages include limited neck motion of the patient after insertion and injuries to the recurrent laryngeal nerve, phrenic nerve, and brachial plexus during insertion. A rare complication is ipsilateral pneumothorax. The central approach to internal jugular vein catheterization is as follows:

1. Prepare the central catheter kit for use.
2. Position the patient as in Fig. 228.2. Review the relevant anatomy, remembering that the internal jugular vein appears just under the triangular apex formed by the sternocleidomastoid muscle as it splits into sternal and clavicular heads. The vein then runs closely along the anterior border of the clavicular head of the sternocleidomastoid muscle and is lateral to the carotid artery.
3. Prep and drape the area to define a sterile field, and don mask, cap, eye protection, sterile gloves, and gown. Maintain strict sterile technique from here onward. Observe universal blood and body fluid precautions.
4. Anesthetize with 1% lidocaine a 1- to 2-cm diameter area just caudal to the apex of the sternocleidomastoid muscle. Attach the 22-gauge seeker needle to the 3-mL syringe.
5. The insertion site is located just at, or slightly caudal to, the apex of the sternocleidomastoid triangle, in the anesthetized field. Insert the seeker needle; aim toward the ipsilateral nipple at a 30-degree angle. Entry to the vein is marked by the easy

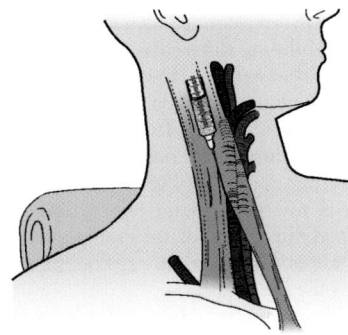

Fig. 228.7   Needle approach to the internal jugular vein.

return of dark red blood into the syringe. Fig. 228.7 shows the needle's approach to the vein. Having the patient perform a Valsalva maneuver or hum increases the size of the vessel by 30% to 40% and possibly enhances the likelihood of successful cannulation.

6. Once the internal jugular vein has been located, remove the seeker needle. Using the 18-gauge 2.5-inch needle on a 5-mL syringe, insert it along the track of the seeker needle (i.e., the same direction, angle, and depth of penetration) to enter the internal jugular vein. Entry is confirmed by the easy return of dark red blood into the syringe.
7. If the 5-mL syringe has a plunger entry port, insert the guidewire through the port and into the vein. Leave one-third of the wire's length free, and maintain control of this end with your dominant hand. If the 5-mL syringe does not have a plunger entry port, remove the syringe from the needle hub, and occlude the needle hub with your nondominant thumb until you insert the guidewire. If you do not have to traverse the syringe's length, leave half of the guidewire free and secured.
8. Using your nondominant hand, remove the syringe/needle assembly, gliding it along the guidewire. Be sure to maintain the position of the guidewire in the internal jugular vein.
9. Nick the skin with the No. 11 scalpel blade by following the guidewire as it courses into the deeper tissues.
10. Slide the dilator over the guidewire, and run it along the guidewire into the internal jugular vein up to the hub. Using a twisting motion while inserting the dilator may facilitate its advance. Continue to maintain control of the guidewire. Remove the dilator by sliding it out of the body and off the guidewire.

Follow Steps 11 through 15 provided.

Femoral Vein Catheterization

Femoral vein catheterization is an alternative route to access the central venous system. Like the methods discussed previously, femoral vein catheterization may be used to deliver large volumes of fluid, chemotherapeutic agents, or total parenteral nutrition. By converting a femoral venous catheter to a percutaneous sheath introducer, a transvenous pacing wire or a Swan-Ganz catheter may be inserted. The femoral vein is easier to cannulate than the internal jugular or subclavian veins, and is readily accessible during CPR or other resuscitation. The few disadvantages to a femoral approach include the difficulty in sterilizing the groin insertion site, difficulty keeping it clean once the line is inserted, the increased risk of catheter-related venous thrombosis, and the fact that it limits patient mobility if the patient is ambulatory.

Contraindications to femoral line insertion include ipsilateral groin surgery or cellulitis over the proposed insertion site; a prosthetic vascular graft on the side of the proposed insertion, venoocclusive diseases of the extremities or femoral venous thrombosis, and any uncontrolled bleeding diathesis. Because of the relatively

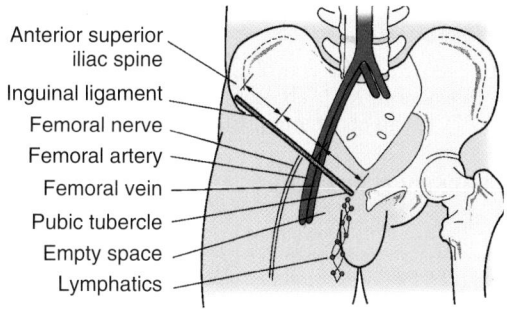

Anterior superior iliac spine
Inguinal ligament
Femoral nerve
Femoral artery
Femoral vein
Pubic tubercle
Empty space
Lymphatics

Fig. 228.8 Relevant anatomy of groin showing relationship of femoral vein to surrounding structures.

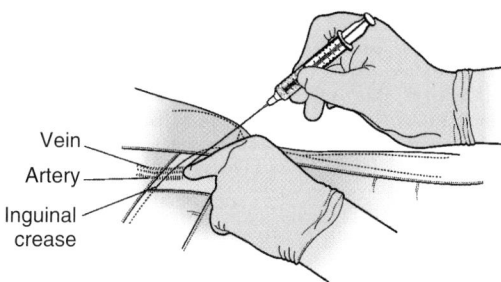

Vein
Artery
Inguinal crease

Fig. 228.9 Approach to femoral vein cannulation.

superficial location of the femoral vein, direct pressure may be readily applied if required, and this author recommends this approach for those patients who are anticoagulated and require rapid central venous access.

Review the relevant anatomy in Fig. 228.8. Note the neurovascular structures run in the following sequence from lateral to medial: nerve, artery, vein, "empty space," and lymphatics. The insertion site for femoral vein catheterization is just inferior to the femoral ligament, and 1 to 1.5 cm medial to the femoral artery, whose palpable pulse forms an important landmark for this procedure.

1. The patient should be flat in the supine position or in slight reverse Trendelenburg position. (The Trendelenburg position is contraindicated for this route of access due to the risk of venous air embolism.)
2. Set up the central venous catheter kit.
3. Wash hands and don mask, cap, eye protection, sterile gown, and gloves. Observe universal blood and body fluid precautions.
4. Prep and drape the groin area to obtain a sterile field. In obese persons, you may need an assistant to hold back any redundant pannus from the groin area to gain access to the femoral vein.
5. Locate the femoral pulse with fingers of your nondominant hand.
6. Using the 25-gauge needle on a 3-mL syringe, draw up 3 mL of lidocaine and anesthetize the area just medial to the femoral artery.
7. You may use the 22-gauge needle on a 3-mL syringe as a seeker, or proceed directly with the 2.5-inch 18-gauge needle on the 5-mL syringe with plunger port to find the femoral vein. Refer to Fig. 228.9 for the approach to cannulation. With bevel down, angle the needle at 30 degrees to the skin, and aim at the ipsilateral nipple. Aspirate as you insert the needle. Entry into the femoral vein is marked by the easy return of dark red blood into the syringe. Once a free flow of blood is verified, stop advancing the needle.
8. Stabilize the 2.5-inch needle and syringe assembly with your nondominant hand. If the syringe has a plunger port, pass the guidewire down this port, feeding approximately half of the wire into the femoral vein. If there is no plunger port, carefully rotate

the syringe off the needle hub, and advance the guidewire into the vein.
9. Maintain control of the distal end of the guidewire with your dominant hand, and remove the 2.5-inch needle/syringe assembly over the wire with your nondominant hand.
10. Nick the skin at the entry site of the guidewire with the No. 11 scalpel blade. Thread the dilator over the guidewire, and run it into the groin several times to create a passage for the central venous catheter assembly. Maintain control of the distal end of the guidewire at all times. Remove the dilator over the guidewire.

Follow steps 11 through 15 provided.

16. Some practitioners may elect to perform an abdominal flat plate radiograph at this time to ensure placement of the catheter in the common iliac vein.
17. Lastly, some practitioners elect to give a dose of a broad-spectrum antibiotic at this time (although there is no evidence to support this practice).

COMPLICATIONS

- Thrombosis of the vein
- Hemorrhage or hematoma at the insertion site
- Local, systemic, or catheter-related infection (often from poor sterile technique, but not always)
- Hydrothorax from infusion of IV fluids into the chest cavity from erroneous placement of a catheter using subclavian or internal jugular approach
- Tracheal perforation
- Perforation of an endotracheal tube cuff
- Air embolus (usually with subclavian or internal jugular vein catheter insertion if patient was not placed in Trendelenburg position prior to vein cannulation)
- Guidewire fragment embolus (results from shear of guidewire when it is pulled back out of insertion needle)
- Lost guidewire
- Laceration of a lymphatic duct
- Arteriovenous fistula
- Superior vena caval obstruction
- Pericardial tamponade
- Injury to local nerve structures
- Catheter malposition (a catheter inserted into the subclavian or internal jugular vein may thread itself back up into the neck or the arm)
- Catheter kinking
- Cardiac dysrhythmias

CPT/BILLING CODES

36555   Insertion of nontunneled centrally inserted (includes femoral vein) catheter into central vein, younger than 5 years
36556   Insertion of nontunneled centrally inserted (includes femoral vein) catheter into central vein, age 5 years or older
76937   Ultrasound guidance for vascular access

ICD-10-CM DIAGNOSTIC CODES

See also ICD-9-CM codes for Chapter 229, Swan-Ganz (Pulmonary Artery) Catheterization, and Chapter 232, Temporary Pacing.

E46   Protein calorie malnutrition unspecified
E43   Severe calorie deficiency unspecified
E86.0   Dehydration

E86.1	Hypovolemia
E87.70	Fluid overload or fluid retention unspecified
I10	Accelerated or malignant essential hypertension
I21.09	ST Myocardial infarction, anterior wall
I21.3	Myocardial infarction, acute, unspecified, 415.0 Cor pulmonale, acute
I31.4	Cardiac tamponade
I31.9	Pericardial effusion or unspecified disease of pericardium
I47.2	Paroxysmal ventricular tachycardia
I46.9	Cardiac or cardiorespiratory arrest
I50.814	Right-sided heart failure, secondary to left or heart failure, congestive, unspecified
I50.1	Pulmonary edema (left-sided heart failure)
N17.9	Acute renal failure, unspecified
N18.9	Chronic renal failure
O75.1	Shock, obstetric
R57.9	Shock, unspecified
R57.0	Shock, cardiogenic
R65.21	Shock, septic
R57.1	Shock, other (hypovolemic)
T79.4XXA	Traumatic shock initial encounter
T88.2XXA	Shock, anaphylactic
T81.10XA	Surgical or postoperative shock

Acknowledgment

The editors recognize the contributions of John F. Donnelly, MD, John M. Passmore Jr, MD, Thomas A. Bzoskie, MD, and Brian D. Madden, MD, to this chapter in previous editions of this text.

RECOMMENDED READING

Kumar A, Chuan A. Ultrasound guided vascular access: efficacy and safety. *Best Pract Res Clin Anaesthesiol.* 2009;23:299–311.

Leung J, Duffy M, Finckh A. Real-time ultrasonographically-guided internal jugular vein catheterization in the emergency department increases success rates and reduces complications: a randomized, prospective study. *Ann Emerg Med.* 2006;48:540–547.

Mumtaz H, Williams V, Hauer-Jensen M, et al. Central venous catheter placement in patients with disorders of hemostasis. *Am J Surg.* 2000;180:503–505.

Nagdev A, Sisson C. Central venous access. In: Reichman EF, ed. *Emergency Medicine Procedures.* 2nd ed. New York: McGraw-Hill; 2013:308–327.

Rezaie SR, Coffey EC, McNeil CR. Central venous catheterization and central venous pressure monitoring. In: Roberts JR, Custalow CB, Thomsen TW, eds. *Roberts and Hedges' Clinical Procedures in Emergency Medicine and Acute Care.* 7th ed. Philadelphia: Elsevier; 2019:405–438.

Segal JB, Dzik WH. Paucity of studies to support that abnormal coagulation test results predict bleeding in the setting of invasive procedures: an evidence-based review. *Transfusion.* 2005;45:1413–1425.

CHAPTER 229

Swan-Ganz (Pulmonary Artery) Catheterization

Stuart Forman

For more than 25 years the use of the balloon-flotation, flow-directed pulmonary artery (PA) thermodilution (Swan-Ganz) catheter symbolized modern care of the critically ill patient. However, since the 1990s, several studies found that the PA catheter did not reduce morbidity or mortality, despite its invasive nature. These studies were first summarized in a Cochrane review that stated "even though the trials measured numbers of deaths in each group at different points of time, all reported that there were no differences between patients who did and did not have a PA catheter inserted" (Harvey, 2006). Another meta-analysis in the *Journal of the American Medical Association* similarly showed that "the use of PA catheter neither increased overall mortality in the hospital nor conferred benefit" (Shah, 2005). A more recent Cochrane review (Rajaram, 2013) found no benefit with use of PA catheter from perspective of hospital or intensive care unit length of stay or cost. As a result, most intensive care units have decreased the use of PA catheters; and instead often use less invasive methods such as central lines for central venous pressure (CVP) monitoring and echocardiograms to evaluate cardiac function (see Chapter 75, Echocardiography, and Chapter 214, Emergency Department, Hospitalist, and Office Ultrasonography [Clinical Ultrasonography]).

As an alternative to PA catheterization, early goal-directed therapy (EGDT) was developed, which uses a regular central line and monitors central venous pressure and central venous oxygen saturation [S_{CVO_2}]) in patients with septic shock. EGDT demonstrated impressive survival rates in a landmark study in 2001 (Rivers, 2001). The standard therapy group had an in-hospital mortality rate of 46.5%, compared with 30.5% for those assigned to EGDT. Protocol patients were resuscitated to a CVP of 8 to 12 mm Hg and a mean arterial pressure of 65 mm Hg. If at this point their S_{CVO_2} was below 70%, packed red cells were transfused to a hematocrit of 30% and dobutamine added, if necessary, until their S_{CVO_2} normalized to 70%. If still not there, mean arterial pressure was titrated to 65 mm Hg with either norepinephrine or dopamine (Rivers, 2001). Subsequent trials have validated these results with similar or better findings (Otero, 2006). There is also technology available that provides continuous measurement of cardiac output using just a radial arterial line.

That said, PA catheters still have a major role in critical care. It should be realized that they are not a therapeutic intervention, but rather a monitoring device; hence improved outcomes might not be the best measure for usefulness. There is a core of accurate and reliable hemodynamic data obtainable from PA catheterization that is not readily available using any other device. In fact, newer, less invasive methods of monitoring hemodynamic data need to be validated against PA catheterization prior to use in critically ill patients. Pinsky (2005) proposed an algorithm for use of PA catheters (Fig. 229.1) that is still somewhat useful; their criteria for initiation of the protocol "would be ongoing circulatory shock despite initial fluid resuscitation efforts or, in the setting of normotension, persistent tachycardia, metabolic acidosis, lactic acidosis, altered mental status, or decreased

urine output, since all these are signs or indirect markers of inadequate tissue perfusion." Further study is needed to compare PA catheter-derived outcomes with those using a mere central line. As of this writing, PA catheters still remain an important, although less frequently used, assessment tool in critical care.

This chapter was written for the primary care clinician preparing to insert a PA catheter. All PA catheters generate data such as cardiac output, PA wedge pressure, systemic vascular resistance, and stroke work index; therefore, clinicians using PA catheters should be capable of interpreting and acting on these and other results. Many PA catheters are capable of continuously monitoring cardiac output and mixed venous oxygen saturation (S_{VO_2}). Further specialized catheters often provide a port or built-in electrode for pacing, four lumens, or the ability to gather specific data regarding right ventricular function. These specialized catheters are beyond the scope of this chapter.

Although many clinicians are proficient with similar procedures and may have crossover skills, beginners should first observe PA catheter placement several times. Attempts to place the first few catheters should be supervised by a trained, skilled, and experienced clinician. After the clinician gains mastery of the skill of insertion, further study and use of the catheter should increase his or her skills, interest, knowledge, and abilities in the maintenance of a PA catheter as well as in obtaining data. Attending courses devoted to the technology will further enhance proficiency, especially for the subtler applications.

INDICATIONS

- Refractory acute respiratory distress syndrome (ARDS) or pulmonary edema, especially in patients with renal failure
- Severe hypoxemia requiring high levels (>10 cm) of positive end-expiratory pressure (PEEP)
- Presence of hemodynamic deterioration due to a mechanical complication (e.g., differentiate between mitral regurgitation and acute ventricular septal defect)
- Evaluation of left ventricular function if echocardiogram not available (e.g., inadequate echo windows)
- Diagnose/manage cardiac tamponade
- Suspected right ventricular dysfunction or infarction
- Oxygen delivery and consumption assessment
- The evaluation of and drug titration for severe pulmonary hypertension
- Unable to transport patient for further diagnostic testing (e.g., computed tomography [CT] angiogram)

MONITORING

- In setting of sepsis, trauma, burns, multiple organ failure, pulmonary embolus, drug overdose
- Titration of drugs or other interventions in a highly unstable patient (e.g., vasodilators, inotropes, pacemaker)

Resuscitate to a mean arterial pressure of >65 mm Hg

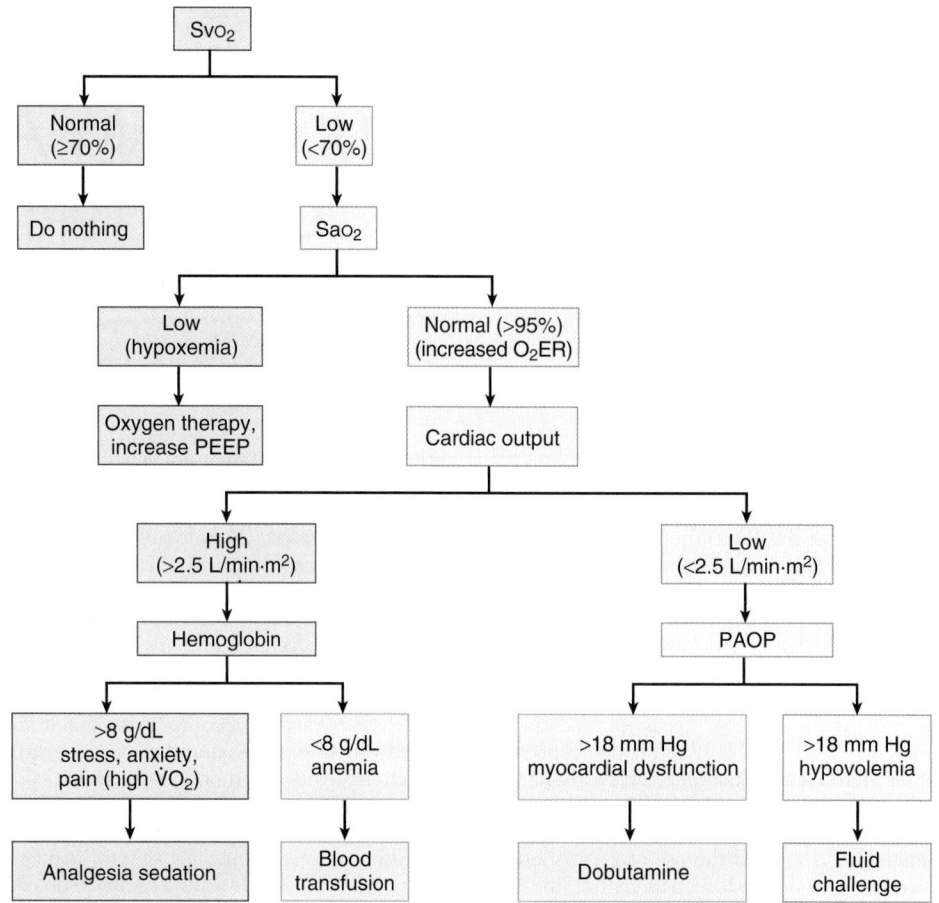

Fig. 229.1 Sample diagnostic and therapeutic algorithm based on mixed venous oxygen saturation (SvO_2) measurements: therapeutic options to be considered are presented in the rectangles. SaO_2, Arterial oxygen saturation; O_2ER, oxygen extraction ratio; *PEEP*, positive end-expiratory pressure; *PAOP*, pulmonary artery occlusion pressure; VO_2, oxygen consumption. (From Pinsky MR, Vincent JL. Let us use the pulmonary artery catheter correctly and only when we need it. *Crit Care Med.* 2005;33:1119–1122.)

- Refractory heart failure
- Hemodynamically unstable patient unresponsive to conventional therapy
- Unstable myocardial infarction with severely decompensated heart failure
- Right-sided heart failure resulting from severe obstructive lung disease, ARDS, or pulmonary embolism
- Refractory sepsis
- Fluid management in certain complex situations (e.g., shock, postoperative state, ARDS, acute renal failure, intraoperative)

Preoperative (Optimization of Extremely High-Risk Surgical Patients)

- High-risk cardiac surgery (e.g., multiple valve replacement, ventricular aneurysm resection, CABG in frail elderly patients or patient with multiple comorbidities)
- Complicated vascular surgery (e.g., dissecting aneurysm, resection of thoracic or abdominal aneurysm)
- Other surgical patients with multiple risk factors
- Myocardial infarction within 6 months
- Poor left ventricular function
- Elevated American Society of Anesthesiologists score

Therapeutic

- Pacing
- Aspiration of air emboli during seated neurosurgery

CONTRAINDICATIONS

Contraindications are the same as those for central venous catheterization (see Chapter 228, Central Venous Catheter Insertion), plus the following relative contraindications:

- Diagnostic information could be provided by less invasive means (e.g., echocardiography, a therapeutic trial of fluid administration in the hypovolemic patient)
- Prosthetic right heart valve
- Cardiac-paced patient (temporary, internal, or permanent)*
- Severe hypotension
- Known pulmonary hypertension
- Highly unstable arrhythmias (especially ventricular)
- Right-sided endocarditis or mural thrombus
- Highly unstable respiratory status
- Lack of nursing staff or clinicians trained in use of PA catheters
- Lack of a compatible pressure monitoring apparatus
- Allergy to any component of the catheter (e.g., latex)

---

*Left bundle branch block (LBBB) was previously a contraindication because of the frequent occurrence of natural or induced right bundle branch block (RBBB) during passage of a PA catheter. This could cause complete heart block (i.e., RBBB + LBBB = complete heart block). A chronic indwelling catheter may also increase the risk of RBBB. Evidence suggests that the risk of complete bundle branch block is low; however, it may be prudent to use fluoroscopy when placing a PA catheter in a patient with an LBBB. A transvenous or transcutaneous pacer or a PA catheter with pacing capabilities should be available.

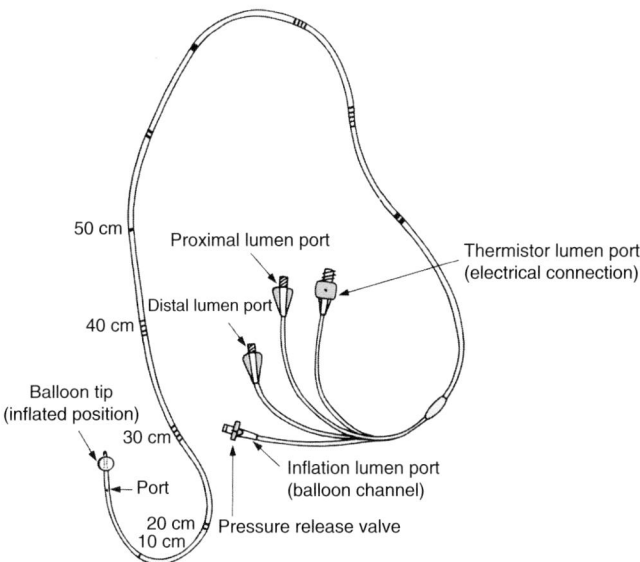

Fig. 229.2   Balloon-tipped thermodilution catheter.

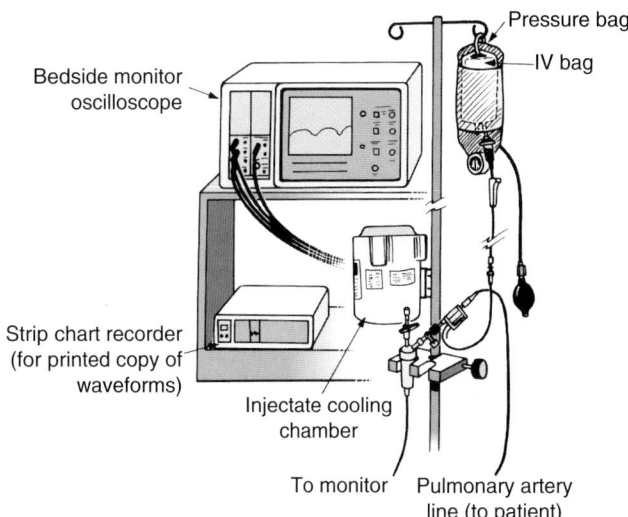

Fig. 229.3   Pulmonary artery catheter setup.

NOTE: If the underlying relative contraindication can be altered, catheterization may be worth the risk if there are no alternatives.

EQUIPMENT

- Central venous access with an 8.5-Fr percutaneous sheath introducer kit (see Chapter 228, Central Venous Catheter Insertion)
- Radiopaque PA catheter (7 to 7.5 Fr for adults; Fig. 229.2) with syringe for balloon inflation, occlusive caps for each port, and catheter protective shield
NOTE: Standard thermodilation catheters now usually have four lumens. The distal lumen at the tip measures PA and PA occlusion pressures and is used for blood sampling. A more proximal lumen (injectate) is used for injecting a thermal bolus for cardiac output measurement (if your Swan-Ganz catheter does not have continuous cardiac output capability). The third lumen is a proximal infusion port for medications; this port may also be used for a thermistor (electrical connection). A fourth lumen is used to inflate the balloon. There may be additional proximal lumens with ports. Catheters coated with chlorhexidine or heparin are also available to reduce the risk of infection and thrombosis, respectively.

- Pressure transducer and monitor (Fig. 229.3)
- High-pressure tubing, connectors, and two three-way stopcocks
- Heparinized saline flush system
- Povidone-iodine solution
- Sterile gowns, drapes, gloves, masks, and goggles
- Surgeon's cap
- Guidewire if changing central line to an introducer sheath (make sure it is the correct diameter and long enough to properly fit through both catheters)
- Suture and sterile dressing for site
- Supplemental oxygen
- Continuous pulse oximetry, cardiac, and blood pressure monitoring
- Fully stocked code cart and defibrillator nearby

PREPROCEDURE PATIENT PREPARATION

Because PA catheterization is usually an emergency procedure, written informed consent cannot always be obtained. However, explain the indications, risks, benefits, and any available alternatives to the patient and the family, if possible. If the consent is implied, it should be documented. If time allows, the patient or family should sign for informed consent. Venous access may be established by the procedure

outlined in Chapter 228, Central Venous Catheter Insertion. As delineated in Chapter 232, Temporary Pacing, catheterization of the right internal jugular vein provides the most direct access to the right atrium and ventricle, but its use may restrict patient mobility. The broad curve of the left subclavian vein may make it more difficult to traverse than the right internal jugular, but it is a reasonable second choice. The left internal jugular and right subclavian veins are acceptable alternatives. The femoral vein is another option, but it is infrequently used and often necessitates the use of fluoroscopy to properly advance the catheter. The external jugular, axillary, and basilic veins are additional options, but are also often difficult to traverse.

TECHNIQUE

Before Insertion and General Guidelines

1. Supplemental oxygen should be supplied. If the patient is on a ventilator, the ventilatory settings and alarms should be checked. The endotracheal tube should be secured and suctioned.
2. Before the heart undergoes invasive monitoring or an area of the heart is traversed for any reason, record a baseline electrocardiogram (ECG).
3. A "time out" should be taken before this (and any) procedure to make sure you have the right procedure, site, and patient.
4. Because this procedure may induce arrhythmias, an additional, separate intravenous access site should be available. The introducer sheath has a separate intravenous access site if no other access is available.
5. To prevent the loss of a guidewire in a patient, never let go of the guidewire during catheter manipulation.
6. Observe strict sterile technique. Scrub after donning hair cover, goggles or eye protection, mask, and gown; wear sterile gloves and maintain sterile technique throughout the procedure. Optimally, the entire neck and clavicular area are prepared with povidone-iodine if the internal jugular or subclavian routes are to be used; a similarly sized area should be prepared if another route is to be used. Drape as large of an area as possible, including the majority of the patient and the bed. A three-quarter sheet works well for this purpose. Follow universal blood and body fluid precautions.

Conversion to a Sheath or an Introducer

If the venous catheter in place is a multilumen catheter, or the single-lumen sheath is not large enough to accept the PA catheter, it must be converted. Use an 8.5-Fr introducer sheath for a 7- or 7.5-Fr PA catheter.

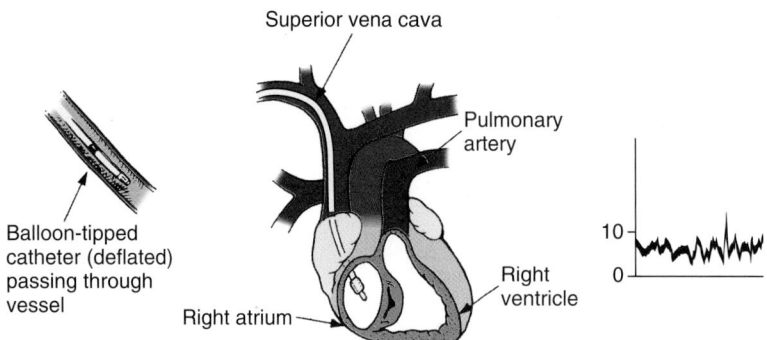

Fig. 229.4   Balloon-tipped catheter passing through vessel to the 10- to 15-cm mark. If passed through internal jugular or subclavian vein, it enters right atrium at 15- to 20-cm mark. Note pressure.

1. Insert a guidewire of proper diameter and sufficient length through the existing venous access line. Always maintain control of the guidewire. (Letting go could allow it to slip into the vein and embolize.) Carefully remove the existing venous access line (catheter or sheath) over the guidewire.

2. Leaving the guidewire in place, advance the dilator over the guidewire and into the vein to enlarge the lumen. A nick at the skin may be needed to advance the dilator; using a twisting motion when advancing may also be helpful.

3. Leaving the guidewire in place, remove the dilator.

4. Now place the dilator through the PA catheter introducer sheath and pass them both, as a unit, over the guidewire and into the patient's central circulation. Again, using a twisting motion while advancing the unit may facilitate this part of the procedure.

5. Remove the guidewire and the dilator, leaving the introducer sheath in place, and cap the sheath with the special cap that allows for PA catheter placement (usually a diaphragm on it).

Insertion of the Pulmonary Artery Catheter

1. Have an assistant set up, check, calibrate, and zero the electrical equipment. He or she should also level the transducer (see Fig. 229.3).

2. Remove the PA catheter from its sterile packaging. If used, thread the catheter protective sleeve (contamination shield) over the distal end of the catheter. Make sure that the docking mechanism is facing the correct direction. It should be able to be connected to the introducer sheath that was inserted earlier. Slide the protective sleeve up the PA catheter, far away from the tip, to keep it out of the way of the tip. Flush the catheter by injecting sterile heparinized saline into the three open ports of the catheter. Make sure that all ports are patent.

3. Next, test the balloon before insertion. Attach the smaller syringe to the balloon port and fill the balloon with air. A built-in safety mechanism in the syringe prevents overdistention of the balloon. Allow the balloon to deflate. (Never forcibly deflate the balloon.)

4. Hand the proximal end of the catheter to the assistant. Three-way stopcocks should be attached to the three lumens. Have the assistant connect the PA catheter to pressure tubing after internally flushing it with sterile saline.

5. Hook up the distal port to the PA transducer and jiggle the end of the catheter. You should see corresponding jiggling on the computer screen. If you do not, have your assistant check the connections.

6. Mark the patient's lateral midchest with an indelible ink spot so that the equipment can be lined up horizontally; this spot is considered the zero point. Record this height and the height of the bed mattress from the floor. The strict recording of heights is necessary because a change in height of 1 inch corresponds to a 1.8 mm Hg change in monitored pressure. An assistant or nurse will usually do this.

7. If using the right internal jugular approach, direct the catheter toward the superior vena cava. If using the right subclavian approach, aim the curve of the catheter so that it is pointing down clockwise toward the superior vena cava.
   EDITOR'S NOTE: The distance from the right internal jugular vein to the corresponding landmarks is about 5 cm more than when using the right subclavian vein approach.

8. ECG monitoring should be continuous throughout the procedure. Pass the deflated balloon-tipped catheter through diaphragm on the protective sleeve and then the sheath to the 20-cm mark; it is marked in 10-cm increments. Watch these distance markings carefully.

9. Watch the waveform monitor for a characteristic central venous tracing or a right atrial tracing. The normal range of pressure for the right atrium should be from 0 to 10 mm Hg and the monitor should show respiratory variation. An assistant should monitor the heart rhythm and record these pressures (Fig. 229.4). Three positive deflections can be seen if the scale is enlarged enough on the monitor: the a, c, and v waves.

10. Verify that the appropriate scale was picked on the monitor. If the patient is asked to cough, there should be an abrupt increase in the pressure tracing correlating with the abrupt increase in intrathoracic pressure.

11. After passing to 20 cm (out of the introducer sheath), rotate the entire catheter 180 degrees so the catheter tip is now pointing up (although you cannot see it) and counterclockwise, matching the curve of the passage through the heart (see Fig. 229.4).

12. Using the syringe provided with the kit, inflate the balloon with air to the recommended full volume as indicated on the package or the syringe (0.8 to 1.5 mL of air). To avoid vessel damage, never advance the catheter beyond this point without an inflated balloon. The provided syringe is designed to prevent the entry of undesired air. As long as it is not overdistended, the balloon will typically provide a buffer around the distal hard tip of the catheter. Avoid overfilling the balloon! It can burst with dire consequences. Never force air into a PA catheter (Fig. 229.5).
   EDITOR'S NOTE: Once out of the introducer sheath, never advance the PA catheter without the balloon being inflated. Never withdraw the PA catheter without the balloon being deflated.

13. Pass the catheter to the 30- or 40-cm mark in a quick but not too rapid fashion. While passing the catheter, watch the pressure monitor for the characteristic right ventricular tracing. This tracing looks like a large square root sign without a dicrotic notch. A dramatic rise in the systolic pressure should occur during this manipulation (Fig. 229.6A). Record the right ventricular pressures. Also watch the ECG monitor for any ectopy at this stage.

14. After confirming its presence in the right ventricle, pass the catheter without delay to the 40- to 50-cm mark, into the PA. The PA will have the same systolic pressures as the right ventricle, but the diastolic pressures will be higher. You will see a

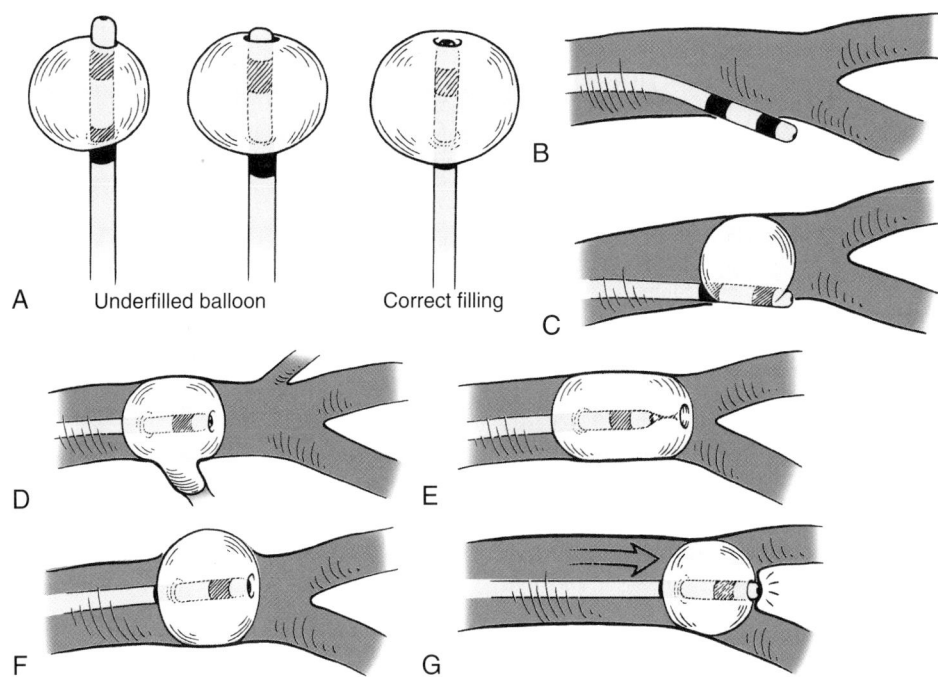

Fig. 229.5 Correct filling of the balloon and possible complications. (A) Underfilled and correct filling. (B) Tip perforates wall of vessel when balloon is not inflated. (C) Eccentric balloon (inaccurate wedge) with risk of wall rupture. (D) Overfilled balloon inadvertently distending down side vessel. (E) Inaccurate and overdistention of balloon can cause catheter tip occlusion. (F) Overwedge (see Troubleshooting section). (G) Underinflated catheter with protruding tip.

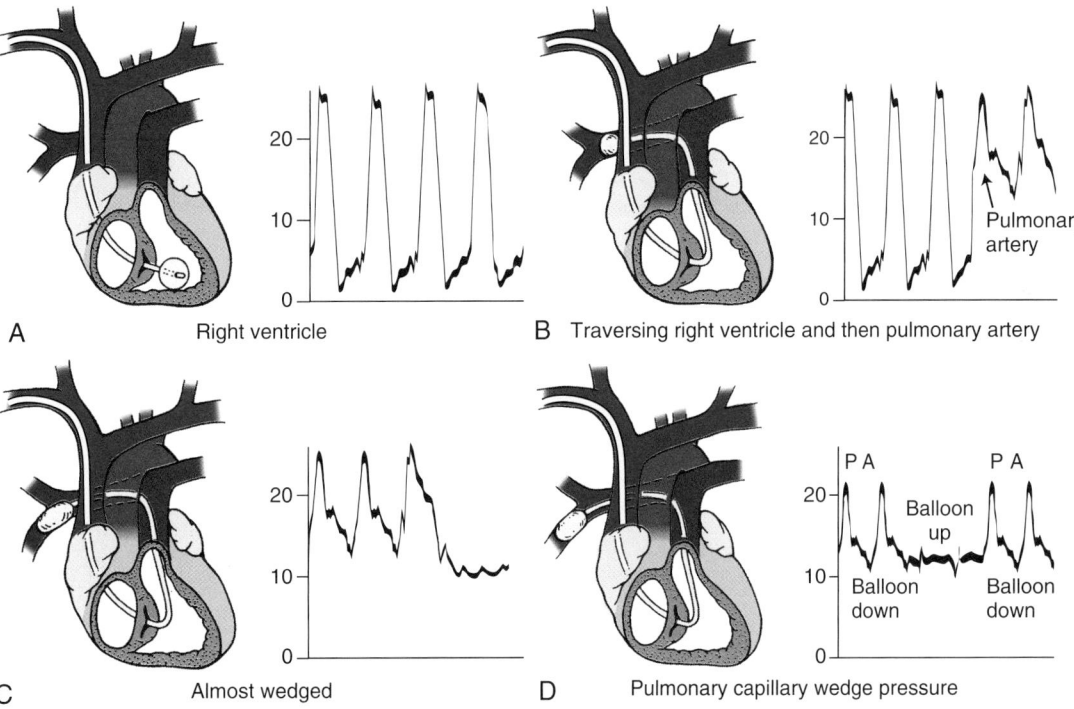

Fig. 229.6 Tracings recorded through the catheter as it traverses the right ventricle and pulmonary artery and is wedged: the right ventricle (A), the pulmonary artery (B), almost wedged (C), and, finally, the wedged position (D).

dicrotic notch on the downhill distal side of the triangles (see Fig. 229.6B). Record the pressures. Normal PA pressures are 15 to 25 mm Hg systolic and 8 to 16 mm Hg diastolic, with a mean of 10 to 20 mm Hg.

15. Once in the PA, continue passing the catheter at a much slower pace, watching for the characteristic pulmonary capillary wedge pressure (PCWP) tracing at about the 50-cm mark on the catheter (see Fig. 229.6C). With PCWP tracings, the systolic pressure is lost and you are left with the "wedge pressure." In fact, the PA diastolic pressure is a good estimate of the wedge pressure if for some reason you cannot get a wedge pressure. This is the place where the vessel has become occluded and the catheter no longer reads PA pressures; rather, it reads pressure reflected back from the left atrium through the capillaries. If the patient has a normal mitral valve, the PCWP approximates the left ventricular diastolic pressure (see Fig. 229.6D). In the absence

of elevated end-expiratory pressures or obstruction of the pulmonary veins, PCWP approximates left atrial mean pressure to within 2 mm Hg. If desired, using the Starling pressure–volume relationships, left ventricular end-diastolic volume can also be estimated.

16. Once the balloon is wedged, allow it to passively deflate and watch for the phasic PA tracing. Do not aspirate to deflate the balloon; active deflation may cause rupture.

17. Inflate the balloon again and allow it to deflate to observe the two different tracings. If the syringe and balloon were designed to hold 1.5 mL, this should be the amount required to wedge the catheter safely. If any less accomplishes it, the catheter's location is too distal; withdraw it until 1.5 mL wedges it. If 1.5 mL does not wedge the balloon, pass the catheter further. Although the PCWP is called an occlusion pressure, the inflated balloon actually floats distally and then occludes the vessel. The vessel is not occluded from inflation at a fixed location. The catheter should be placed at the most proximal point where a wedge pressure is observed. If you deflate the balloon and do not see the PA pressures, either the balloon did not truly deflate, or you have a "permanent wedge." If the latter is the case, you must withdraw the catheter until you see PA pressures again and then refloat the catheter.

18. The wedge pressure should be read at end expiration and recorded.

19. Extend the catheter protective sleeve, if used, and attach it to the sheath with the docking mechanism.

20. Secure the entire assembly with suture and adequate tape. Apply a sterile dressing.

21. Order a chest radiograph and auscultate the chest bilaterally to exclude a pneumothorax.

22. Begin infusion of necessary fluids or medications.

23. If the patient was moved, the assistant should reset the equipment to zero.

24. Document the procedure in the chart, including the tracings, and record end-expiratory values. Additional documented values should include the PA pressure, the PCWP, and the cardiac output (performed by the assistant and not detailed here).

Confirmation of Proper Placement

1. Obstruction is excluded by the ability to flush the catheter before inflating the balloon.

2. When the balloon is inflated, the typical PA tracing disappears. It reappears promptly after the balloon deflates.

3. PCWP is lower than or equal to PA diastolic pressure.

4. A chest x-ray should be obtained to confirm placement and view the course of the tip. If the tip is nearer the periphery of the lung, for example, beyond the midclavicular line, it is probably overinserted and needs to be checked or pulled back.

TROUBLESHOOTING

It is common to get salvos of premature ventricular contractions as the catheter passes through the right ventricle. Usually this problem will resolve with passage of the catheter to the PA. If the ectopy does not resolve, the balloon must be deflated and the catheter brought back to the superior vena cava. The catheter may also be coiling in the right ventricle. If further attempts to pass it are unsuccessful, administer an intravenous bolus of lidocaine (75 to 100 mg) and attempt passage under fluoroscopy.

If a PA or PCWP tracing cannot be obtained, keep the balloon deflated, pull the catheter back to 20 cm, and try inserting again. Consider inserting the catheter using a clockwise twisting action. If this fails, try counterclockwise reinsertion. Having the patient take some deep breaths may also help pass the catheter. Occasionally the tip of the PA catheter gets malpositioned in the chest. If the tip lies above the level of the left atrium (with the patient lying down,

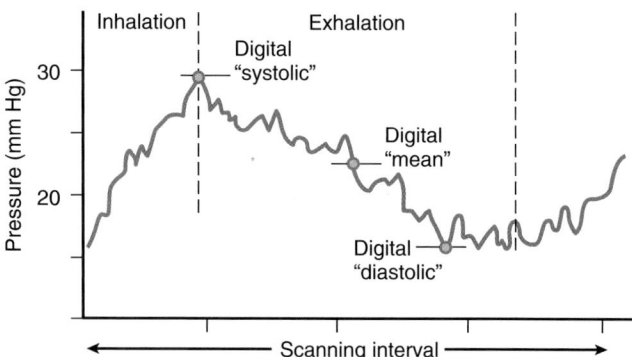

Fig. 229.7 Respiratory variation of the pulmonary artery catheter tracing. (From Wiedemann HP, Matthay MA, Matthay RA. Cardiovascular-pulmonary monitoring in the intensive care unit: Part I. *Chest* 1984;85:537–549.)

this would be anterior), the alveolar pressure may be greater than the pulmonary capillary pressures and you will get an errant reading. Again, fluoroscopy may be helpful here.

Some clinicians recommend injecting cold, sterile saline solution to enhance passage; this may stiffen the catheter, which may have softened because of the warmth of the body. Occasionally, a guidewire and fluoroscopy are necessary to advance the catheter. Repositioning the patient may help.

In patients with a very low ejection fraction, an inotrope may have to be administered to facilitate passage. It may also be difficult to pass a PA catheter in patients with tricuspid regurgitation or pulmonary hypertension. Again, having the patient take deep breaths may facilitate passage in all of these situations.

For a normal-sized adult, from the subclavian or internal jugular site, insertion beyond 50 cm (or 15 cm after entering the right ventricle) predisposes the catheter to coiling, which can lead to knotting.

When a catheter's location is too distal in the vessel, a tracing called an *overwedge* may be seen. This is likely to occur when the balloon is not filled with enough air. After allowing the balloon to deflate, withdraw the catheter and attempt to wedge it again, this time with the balloon fully inflated to its correct volume (see Fig. 229.5). Persistent underinflation of the balloon when wedging can damage the pulmonary vessels or the endocardium and may cause arrhythmias, especially if the catheter tip is exposed (see Fig. 229.5A and G). There are several possible mechanisms, such as overinflation or underinflation of the balloon (see Fig. 229.5), that could cause rupture of the PA; fortunately, these are unlikely.

When air is present in the catheter damping can occur, which has an opposite effect to that of overwedging. It appears like a regular tracing, but the variations are damped. Air bubbles should be removed from the connecting tubes by aspirating and flushing the catheter. If blood cannot be aspirated, yet the catheter flushes easily, suspect a ball-valve thrombus at the catheter tip. Inject 5000 U of heparin into the lumen and allow 15 to 30 minutes for it to take effect. Initiate a continuous drip of heparin (not to exceed 20,000 U for 24 hours). If still unsuccessful, withdraw the catheter gradually 5 cm at a time, watching for waveforms.

The most accurate readings obtained are the continuous systolic and diastolic PA pressures; the least accurate is the PA occlusion (wedge) pressure. Lesions obstructing the mitral valve, such as mitral stenosis, can interfere with the accuracy of the PCWP as an estimate of left ventricular diastolic pressure. Respirations can also cause significant variations in the pressure readings for the PA catheter. Make calibrated strip chart recordings for all measurements derived from the catheter and then measure again at end expiration (Fig. 229.7). Turning off sequential compression devices and holding fluid infusions (through the introducer) increases accuracy when measuring cardiac output using the thermodilution catheter.

Finally, high PEEP settings on a ventilator can falsely elevate wedge pressures.

COMPLICATIONS

Possible complications are the same as for central venous catheterization (see Chapter 228, Central Venous Catheter Insertion), *plus* those discussed in the following sections.

During Pulmonary Artery Catheter Placement

- *Pulmonary infarction:* Can result from leaving the balloon inflated too long
- *Atrial and ventricular ectopy or conduction changes:* Advancement into the PA may decrease ectopy. However, withdrawal of the catheter may be necessary. Usually the ectopy is transitory, but if an unstable rhythm persists, medical treatment or electrical conversion may be necessary.
- *Knotting of the catheter* can occur inside or outside of the heart (more likely with smaller-bore catheters [e.g., 5 Fr]) and, rarely, cause injury to intracardiac structures. Inflating the balloon while in the subclavian vein or superior vena cava may minimize the risk of knotting. On the contrary, to avoid injury to the pulmonic or tricuspid valve, do not withdraw the catheter with the balloon inflated. Also, if resistance is noted with attempted withdrawal, obtain a chest radiograph to exclude the possibility of knotting or entanglement in the heart. The catheter rarely can get looped around the papillary muscle of the tricuspid valve so that removal is impossible.
- *Malposition:* The most common malposition occurs when the PA catheter turns up the internal jugular instead of down into the superior vena cava. If, while advancing, you feel resistance, deflate the balloon, do not advance any further, and get a radiograph. If the PA catheter is malpositioned, try to carefully reposition it or use fluoroscopy. Rarely, vessel wall puncture and insertion into undesirable places (e.g., subclavian artery, pleural space) may occur.
- *Cardiac perforation and tamponade* (extremely rare)
- *Valvular damage* can occur during insertion with continued presence.

With Continued Presence of the Pulmonary Artery Catheter in the Central Circulation

- *Pulmonary infarction:* Leaving the balloon inflated too long or downstream displacement of the deflated balloon (causing "permanent wedge"—described earlier) can block an artery and cause infarction. Infarction can also result from thrombosis.
- *Pulmonary hemorrhage:* More common in the presence of pulmonary hypertension, possibly associated with the higher pressures forcing the tip through the vessel wall. Cautiously obtain PCWP in patients with pulmonary hypertension. Hemorrhage can also result from pulmonary infarction.
- *Mural (or elsewhere) thrombus formation:* Thrombosis may develop anywhere throughout the course of the catheter. It can occlude any of the veins through which the catheter has passed (or elsewhere).
- *Balloon rupture or catheter fracture:* If balloon rupture is suspected, aspirate into the syringe the same gas volume used for inflation, disconnect the syringe, and leave the stopcock open to vent the balloon. Remove the catheter immediately to prevent latex fragments from embolizing.
- *A right bundle branch (RBBB) or complete heart block.*
- *Endocarditis:* Aseptic vegetations are found on autopsy in approximately 30% of patients who have had a PA catheter. Both aseptic and septic vegetations may be more common in burn patients.
- *Sepsis:* Frequent manipulations of the catheter, as well as leaving the catheter in place more than 3 days, increase the risk of positive blood cultures. After 24 to 48 hours, if the catheter has become partially withdrawn, advancing the catheter may introduce bacteria from the skin insertion site or the catheter itself. No data show that aseptic protective sleeves prevent this from happening. PA catheters, like any other catheters, should be left in place only as long as necessary.
- *Hemoptysis:* Can be caused by flushing the catheter when it is in the wedged position.
- *Embolism* (air or thrombotic).
- *PA rupture.*
- *Pseudoaneurysm.*
- *Inaccurate diagnosis* because of malfunctioning or malpositioned catheter.

POSTPROCEDURE CATHETER CARE

- Flush the catheter with heparinized saline every 30 minutes.
- Inflate the balloon only when measuring the PCWP. To avoid pulmonary infarction, leave it inflated for a maximum of 60 seconds only. To exclude the possibility of catheter obstruction before inflation, flush the catheter each time before inflating the balloon. If the catheter is occluded, there is no point in inflating the balloon.
- For obstruction, attempt to reposition the catheter. If a thrombus is suspected, use the same technique as used for clearing a ball-valve thrombus.
- Adjust the position of the catheter as necessary. Otherwise, the catheter may soften and migrate to a more distal site, predisposing to distal or branch vessel occlusion. If the PA pressure tracing shows a loss in phasicity and begins to resemble the PCWP tracing (without balloon inflation), withdraw the catheter until the typical phasic PA tracing reappears. Always deflate when withdrawing to avoid damage to intracardiac structures.
- Remove, inspect, and replace the sterile dressing daily.
- Obtain daily chest radiographs to check for catheter migration and to exclude pulmonary infarction.

PATIENT EDUCATION GUIDES

See the sample patient education handout available at www.expertconsult.com.

CPT/BILLING CODES

93503   Insertion and placement of flow-directed catheter (e.g., Swan-Ganz) for monitoring purposes

ICD-10-CM DIAGNOSTIC CODES

I10	Accelerated or malignant essential hypertension
I21.09	Myocardial infarction, initial episode, anterior wall (can include damage such as ruptured myocardium)
I21.3	Myocardial infarction, acute, unspecified, initial episode (can include damage such as ruptured myocardium)
I20.0	Angina, unstable
I26.09	Cor pulmonale, acute
T81.718A	Pulmonary embolism or infarct, postoperative or iatrogenic
I26.99	Pulmonary embolism or infarct, unspecified
I27.0	Pulmonary hypertension, chronic primary
I27.29	Pulmonary hypertension, chronic secondary
I31.2	Hemopericardium
I31.4	Cardiac tamponade
I31.9	Pericardial effusion or unspecified disease of pericardium
I34.8	Mitral valve disorders
I35.8	Aortic valve disorders
I36.8	Tricuspid valve disorders

I37.8	Pulmonic valve disorders
I47.2	Paroxysmal ventricular tachycardia
I50.814	Right heart failure, secondary to left
I50.9	Heart failure, congestive, unspecified
I50.1	Pulmonary edema (left heart failure)
J95.3	Pulmonary insufficiency after trauma and surgery
R57.9	Shock, unspecified
R57.0	Shock, cardiogenic
R65.21	Shock, septic
R57.1	Shock, other (hypovolemic)

SUPPLIERS

(See contact information available at www.expertconsult.com.)

Arrow Teleflex
Edwards Lifesciences Corp (formerly a division of Baxter)

Acknowledgment

The editors recognize the contributions of Len Scarpinato, DO, to this chapter in previous editions of this text.

ONLINE RESOURCES

American College of Cardiology. Policy guidelines for cardiac catheterization, pulmonary artery catheterization, and the consensus statement on right heart catheterization. https://www.ncbi.nlm.nih.gov/pubmed/14508336

American Society of Anesthesiologists. Practice guidelines for pulmonary artery catheterization: An updated report by the American Society of Anesthesiologists Task Force on Pulmonary Artery Catheterization. www.asahq.org/publicationsAndServices/pulm_artery.pdf

Manbit Technologies: www.manbit.com (PA catheter insertion simulators and description of the procedure)

Pulmonary Artery Catheter Education Project: www.pacep.org (educational resources on how to use the PA catheter)

RECOMMENDED READING

American Heart Association. *Textbook of Advanced Cardiac Life Support.* Dallas: American Heart Association; 1997.

Bernard GR, Sopko G, Cerra F, et al. Pulmonary artery catheterization and clinical outcomes: National Heart, Lung, and Blood Institute and Food and Drug Administration workshop report consensus statement. JAMA. 2000;283:2568–2572.

Connors AF, Speroff T, Dawson NV, et al. The effectiveness of right heart catheterization in the initial care of critically ill patients: SUPPORT investigators. JAMA. 1996;276:889–897.

Hall JB. Use of the pulmonary artery catheter in critically ill patients: was invention the mother of necessity? JAMA. 2000;283:2577–2578.

Harvey S, Young D, Brampton W, et al. Pulmonary artery catheters for adult patients in intensive care. *Cochrane Database Syst Rev.* 2006;3:CD003408.

Doshi P. Pulmonary artery (Swan-Ganz) catheterization. In: Reichman EF, ed. *Emergency Medicine Procedures.* 2nd ed. New York: McGraw-Hill; 2013:344–350.

Leibowitz AB, Oropello JM. The pulmonary artery catheter in anesthesia practice in 2007: an historical overview with emphasis on the past 6 years. *Semin Cardiothorac Vasc Anesth.* 2007;11(3):162–176.

Mueller HS, Chatterjee K, Davis KB, et al. ACC expert consensus document: Present use of bedside right heart catheterization in patients with cardiac disease. American College of Cardiology. *J Am Coll Cardiol.* 1998;32:840–864.

Otero RM, Nguyen HB, Huang DT, et al. Early goal-directed therapy in severe sepsis and septic shock revisited: concepts, controversies, and contemporary findings. *Chest.* 2006;130:1579–1595.

Pinsky MR, Vincent JL. Let us use the pulmonary artery catheter correctly and only when we need it. *Crit Care Med.* 2005;33:1119–1122.

Rajaram SS, Desai NK, Kalra A, et al. Pulmonary artery catheters for adult patients in intensive care. *Cochrane Database Syst Rev.* 2003;(3):CD003408.

Rivers E, Nguyen B, Havstad S, et al. Early goal-directed therapy in the treatment of severe sepsis and septic shock. *N Engl J Med.* 2001;345:1368–1377.

Shah MR, Hasselblad V, Stevenson LW, et al. Impact of the pulmonary artery catheter in critically ill patients: meta-analysis of randomized clinical trials. JAMA. 2005;294:1664–1670.

Yunen RA, Oropella JM. Pulmonary artery catheterization. In: Oropella JM, Pastores SM, Kvetan V, eds. *Critical Care.* New York: McGraw-Hill; 2016. Chapter 107.

CHAPTER 230

PERICARDIOCENTESIS

David James

The normal pericardial space contains 10 to 50 mL of serous fluid, which serves to reduce friction between the surfaces of the visceral and parietal pericardium as the heart moves through the cardiac cycle. An increased amount of fluid in this space may result from a variety of disease processes or trauma. Because the pericardial sac is relatively nondistensible, an increased amount of pericardial fluid may exert pressure on the more compressible myocardium. This in turn may compromise cardiac performance and result in cardiac tamponade. Clinically, this is demonstrated with markedly elevated jugular venous pressure (i.e., jugular venous distention), hypotension, and distant heart sounds. Although less than 40% of patients will have all three of these clinical findings, almost all will have at least one unless they are hypovolemic. The patient may also exhibit restlessness, fatigue, and tachycardia; pulmonary edema may be present with corresponding tachypnea. Estimates of the volume of fluid required to accumulate acutely to produce tamponade range from 60 to 200 mL. A chest radiograph may show a dilated heart, classically in a "water bottle" shape. Electrocardiographically, pericardial effusions are identified by low voltage in all leads or electrical alternans (i.e., the QRS amplitude or morphology changes on the electrocardiogram [ECG] as the heart swings to and fro within the pericardial fluid). However, electrocardiographic and radiographic signs of cardiac tamponade are often absent. If ultrasound is available, a dark fluid echo will be present in the pericardial space. Further ultrasonic confirmation of tamponade when using two-dimensional (2D) echocardiography (see Chapter 214, Emergency Department, Hospitalist, and Office Ultrasonography [Clinical Ultrasonography]) includes dilation of the inferior vena cava and collapse of the right and left atrial and ventricular chambers. Further confirmatory findings can often be seen with M-mode and Doppler echocardiography (Table 230.1).

Additional findings with tamponade on physical examination include a paradoxic increase in jugular venous distention during inspiration and pulsus paradoxus (a drop in systolic pressure of >10 mm Hg during inspiration). To measure pulsus paradoxus, inflate the blood pressure cuff to greater than systolic pressure. Slowly release the cuff pressure until beats are heard only during expiration, and record this pressure. Keep deflating the cuff pressure until beats are heard continuously during expiration and inspiration, and record this pressure. The difference between these recorded pressures is pulsus paradoxus, as noted by Kussmaul, and is increased because the right ventricle and interventricular septum are forced into the left ventricle by tamponade.

Cardiac tamponade should always be considered as a possible cause in a medical patient in shock. This includes patients taking oral or parenteral anticoagulants or high-dose steroids, otherwise immunocompromised, having known cancer or pericardial disease, suspected of having an aortic dissection, or having had a recent myocardial infarction (e.g., ruptured myocardium). In the trauma patient, cardiac tamponade is the most common presentation for a penetrating cardiac injury. It occurs in 80% to 90% of stab wounds and in 20% of gunshot wounds near the heart. Tamponade can also be due to iatrogenic causes such as central venous line placement, temporary pacing (transthoracic or transvenous), and cardiopulmonary resuscitation. The causes of effusions, in order of frequency from most to least, include cancer, idiopathic, infectious (including human immunodeficiency virus), postpericardiotomy syndrome, connective tissue disease, radiation therapy, trauma, and uremia.

Pericardial effusions may be asymptomatic or associated with life-threatening cardiac compromise. The aspiration of pericardial fluid (pericardiocentesis) has diagnostic and possibly therapeutic applications. Pericardiocentesis is an infrequently performed procedure that has the potential for significant patient morbidity and mortality. Optimally, the procedure should be performed in the cardiac catheterization laboratory or intensive care unit, where complete cardiac monitoring and trained support personnel are available. Ideally, the procedure should be performed under real-time guidance using ultrasound or fluoroscopy to continuously visualize the pericardial fluid. With ultrasonic or fluoroscopic experience, the clinician should be able to estimate the amount of fluid that can be aspirated and the depth and angle of penetration necessary for pericardiocentesis (see Chapter 214, Emergency Department, Hospitalist, and Office Ultrasonography [Clinical Ultrasonography]). If using 2D echocardiography, clinicians should be aware of other conditions or even normal anatomy that may mimic a pericardial effusion [Box 230.1]).

However, pericardiocentesis may be required in urgent or emergent situations and in a suboptimal clinical setting if a patient presents with hemodynamic compromise from pericardial tamponade. Patients in whom urgent/emergent pericardiocentesis is contemplated should have intravenous (IV) access and continuous cardiac monitoring. Continuous oximetry, blood pressure monitoring, and supplemental oxygen may also be helpful. If the clinical situation permits, a 12-lead ECG and a chest radiograph should be obtained for review before the procedure (assess for mediastinal shift). Full resuscitation equipment should be readily available.

If time allows, the European Society of Cardiology Working Group has provided guidelines with a scoring system to help determine whether pericardiocentesis should be performed emergently or the patient referred. First, the etiology of the effusion is scored, with malignancy and tuberculosis each receiving two points. Next, the clinical presentation is scored, with orthopnea in the absence of rales scoring three points and pulsus paradoxus greater than 10 mm Hg and rapid worsening of symptoms each scoring two points. Finally, the results from imaging are scored, with circumferential pericardial effusion greater than 2 cm thick scoring three points and left atrial collapse scoring 2 points. When the score is 6 or greater, urgent pericardiocentesis is indicated (see Table 230.2 for the complete scoring system).

Before performing pericardiocentesis, the clinician should review the relevant anatomy of the heart, pericardium, and rib cage (Fig. 230.1). It may also be useful to insert a nasogastric tube to decompress the stomach (see Chapter 217, Nasogastric and Nasoenteric Tube Insertion). If time allows, efforts to stabilize the patient with cardiac tamponade include aggressive treatment with IV fluids and parenteral inotropic agents to increase ventricular filling pressures. Preload-reducing agents such as nitrates or diuretics may worsen the patient's condition or even be fatal.

TABLE 230.1   Ultrasound Findings of Cardiac Tamponade

Ultrasound Mode	Finding
Doppler	Mitral flow decreases during inspiration/increases during expiration
	Tricuspid flow increases during inspiration/decreases during expiration
	Peripheral flow decreases in expiration
M-mode color Doppler	Mitral flow decreases during inspiration/increases during expiration
	Tricuspid flow increases during inspiration/decreases during expiration
M-mode/two dimensional	Diastolic collapse of the right ventricular free wall (less sensitive than right atrial collapse, but specific sign for tamponade)
	Inferior vena cava dilation and does not collapse on inspiration
	Increase left ventricular wall thickness in diastole
	Left atrial (a very specific sign for tamponade), left ventricular, right atrial collapse (highly specific and sensitive sign for tamponade)
	Swinging heart to and fro

Modified from Seferovic PM, Ristic AD, Imazio M, et al. Management strategies in pericardial emergencies. *Herz* 2006;31(9):891–900.

BOX 230.1   Conditions Possibly Mimicking Pericardial Effusion on Two-Dimensional Echocardiography

Large left pleural effusion
Any tumor surrounding the heart
Pericardial fat
Normal descending thoracic aorta
Catheter in the right ventricle
Enlarged left atrium
Annular subvalvular LV aneurysm
Bronchogenic cyst
Mitral annular calcification

Modified from Yarlagadda C. Cardiac tamponade workup. *Medscape.* https://emedicine.medscape.com/article/152083-workup.

INDICATIONS

Diagnostic

Determination of the etiology or confirmation of the presence of an effusion.

Therapeutic

The relief of cardiac tamponade (should be performed emergently only if bedside ultrasound confirms, or diagnosis is consistent with known prior disease or mechanism of injury, or in a resuscitation patient when other causes of pulseless electrical activity [electromechanical dissociation] have been excluded [e.g., hypovolemia excluded by aggressive fluid replacement, tension pneumothorax excluded by needle thoracostomy]).

CONTRAINDICATIONS

* Anticoagulated patient or patient with uncontrolled coagulopathy (relative contraindication in life-threatening situation, absolute contraindication in stable patient).

TABLE 230.2   Severity Scoring System for Pericardial Effusion

Score the etiology
Malignant disease	2
Tuberculosis	2
Recent radiation therapy	1
Recent viral infection	1
Recurrent pericardial effusion/recent pericardiocentesis	1
Chronic terminal renal failure	1
Immunodeficiency or immunosuppression	1
Hypothyroidism or hyperthyroidism	−1
Systemic autoimmune disorder	−1

Score the clinical presentation
Dyspnea/tachypnea	1
Orthopnea (no rales on lung auscultation)	3
Hypotension (SBP <95 mm Hg)	0.5
Progressive sinus tachycardia (in the absence of medications affecting heart rate, hyperthyroidism and uremia)	1
Oliguria	1
Pulsus paradoxus >10 mm Hg	2
Pericardial chest pain	0.5
Pericardial friction rub	0.5
Rapid worsening of symptoms	2
Slow evolution of the disease	−1

Score the imaging
Cardiomegaly on chest x-ray	1
Electrical alternans on ECG	0.5
Microvoltage in ECG	1
Circumferential pericardial effusion (>2 cm in diastole)	3
Moderate pericardial effusion (1–2 cm thick in diastole)	1
Small pericardial effusion (<1 cm in diastole), no trauma	−1
Right atrial collapse more than one-third of cardiac cycle	1
Inferior vena cava >2.5 cm, collapse <50% on inspiration	1.5
Right ventricular collapse	1.5
Left atrial collapse	2
Mitral/ tricuspid respiratory flow variations	1
Swinging heart	1

Note: Urgent pericardiocentesis indicated when score ≥6.
ECG, Electrocardiogram.
From Ristic AD, Imazio M, Adler Y, et al. Triage strategy for urgent management of cardiac tamponade: a position statement of the European Society of Cardiology Working Group on Myocardial and Pericardial Diseases. *Eur Heart J.* 2014;35(34):2279–2284.

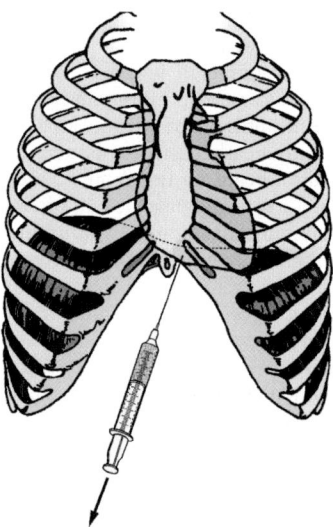

Fig. 230.1 Anatomic relationships of the heart, pericardium, and rib cage. Note the inferior border of the pericardium in relation to the xiphoid process and the angle the aspirating syringe takes as it enters under the rib cage.

- Presence of prosthetic heart valve, pacemaker, or cardiac device (relative contraindication in life-threatening situation, absolute contraindication in stable patient).
- Previous thoracoabdominal surgery (relative contraindication in life-threatening situation, absolute contraindication in stable patient).
- Because of the risk of complications, pericardiocentesis should not be performed if a safer alternative exists (e.g., medical management of an effusion).
- In a stable patient, pericardiocentesis should not be performed without ultrasonic or fluoroscopic demonstration of an effusion.
- In a stable patient, diagnostic pericardiocentesis should be guided by ultrasound or fluoroscopy in a cardiac catheterization laboratory or intensive care unit.
- In a stable patient, pericardiocentesis should not be performed for small, loculated, or posteriorly located effusions.
- Cardiac tamponade associated with an aortic dissection.
- In trauma patients, some experts argue that prompt sternotomy should be performed instead of pericardiocentesis; in patients too unstable to make it to the operating room, they argue for an emergency thoracotomy.
- Aggressive fluid resuscitation, as well as needle thoracostomy (to rule out tension pneumothorax), should also be considered prior to pericardiocentesis in the trauma patient.

EQUIPMENT

- Pericardiocentesis needle (18-gauge, 4-inch spinal needle with stylet)
- Two 10-mL syringes (preferably Luer type), one with 25-gauge, 2-inch needle
- 50-mL syringe (preferably Luer type)
- 10 mL local anesthetic (e.g., 1% lidocaine)
- ECG machine
- Wire connector with alligator clips (to connect pericardiocentesis needle to ECG lead)
- Basin
- Skin preparation solution (e.g., povidone-iodine, chlorhexidine)
- Sterile towels
- Mask, sterile gloves, eye protection, possibly sterile gown
- Kelly clamp
- Cardiac monitoring equipment, pulse oximetry, supplemental oxygen, automatic blood pressure cuff
- Nasogastric tube
- Access to chest radiography
- Bedside ultrasound machine or fluoroscopy (in emergent situations, optional but desirable)
- Cook 8-Fr Fuhrman pericardiocentesis catheter kit (usually a soft, multihole catheter; in an emergency, a single-lumen, 6- to 10-Fr central venous catheter can be used), No. 11 blade scalpel, nylon suture (if inserting a catheter for continuous drainage)

NOTE: Complete kits are available (see Supplier section later). In an emergent situation, a large central venous line access kit could be substituted.

PREPROCEDURE PATIENT EDUCATION

If the clinical situation allows, describe the procedure to the patient or representative and obtain informed consent. Signed informed consent is not necessary in an emergent situation. Explain that there will be some discomfort involved but that removal of even a small amount of pericardial fluid may make an enormous improvement in the patient's clinical status. The alert patient should attempt to remain as still as possible because the needle will be inserted near moving vital organs. If time allows, conscious sedation should be considered.

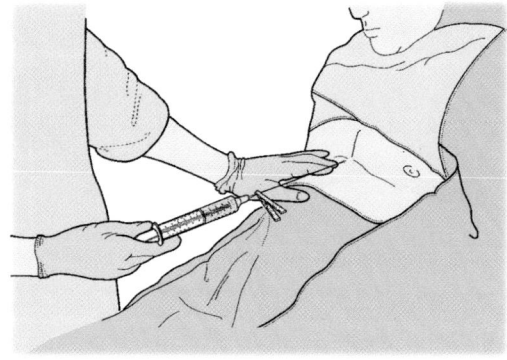

Fig. 230.2   Patient lying in semirecumbent position.

TECHNIQUE

1. Assemble and connect supplemental oxygen and all cardiac, blood pressure, and oximetry monitoring equipment, and have IV access in place and resuscitation equipment nearby. Some clinicians insert an arterial line for monitoring. Consider insertion of a nasogastric tube to decompress the stomach and decrease the risk of perforation of the stomach.
2. Place patient in a semirecumbent position (Fig. 230.2) at approximately 30 to 45 degrees. This position allows the myocardium to "fall back" slightly within the pericardial sac and lessens the likelihood of puncturing the myocardium. The supine position is an acceptable alternative.
3. Hook up limb leads of ECG machine and attach one end of connector to lead V_1 (or any precordial V lead).
4. Prepare skin of epigastrium, xiphoid area, and lower chest. Drape with towels to define a sterile field. If time allows, consider using a sterile gown. The clinician should follow universal blood and body fluid precautions when performing this procedure.
5. If the patient is awake, anesthetize the subxiphoid area skin with 1% lidocaine solution. (Alternatively, the right or left sternocostal margin near the xiphoid can be used. These sites are chosen because they are outside the pleura and should decrease the risk for pneumothorax.) Anesthetize the deeper tissue with the 25-gauge, 2-inch needle. Direct the needle under the xiphoid or costal margin toward the left shoulder (alternatively, the suprasternal notch or right or left midclavicle), aspirating continuously. Some advocate directing the needle at 45-degree angle to the abdominal wall and at a 45-degree angle to the midsagittal plane. If blood or pericardial fluid returns, withdraw the needle slightly.
6. Turn the ECG machine on.
7. Insert the pericardiocentesis needle through the anesthetized skin, advancing in the same direction that anesthesia was distributed, toward the left shoulder (alternatively, toward the suprasternal notch or right or left midclavicle). Remove the stylet and attach the 10-mL syringe. Attach the other end of the ECG connector to the pericardiocentesis needle (Fig. 230.3), close to the hub and advance the needle 4 to 5 cm while applying negative pressure to the syringe. This may be guided by ultrasound or fluoroscopy, if equipment is available (see later). Continue advancing the pericardiocentesis needle until blood or pericardial fluid is aspirated, cardiac pulsations are felt, or the ECG shows (a) increased P-wave amplitude, (b) ST segment elevation (i.e., current of injury), or (c) ectopic beats. All of these ECG findings are suggestive of penetration of the epicardium and require withdrawal of the needle slightly, in 1- to 2-mm increments, until the findings disappear.

   NOTE: To minimize the risk of damaging vital organs, never rock or redirect the pericardiocentesis needle without withdrawing it almost completely (to just below the skin).

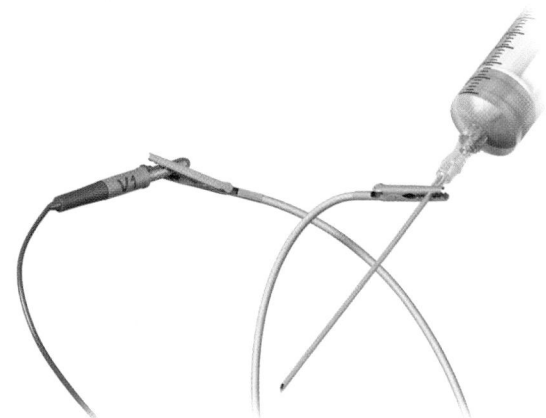

Fig. 230.3 Spinal needle attached to electrocardiogram lead V₁ (or any precordial lead V). (From *Roberts and Hedges' Clinical Procedures in Emergency Medicine and Acute Care*, Philadelphia: Elsevier; 2019.)

8. The clinician will often feel the needle give or a "pop" as it enters the pericardium. (The awake patient often complains of chest pain when the pericardium is entered.) Once blood or pericardial fluid begins to flow into the syringe, attach the Kelly clamp to the needle where it penetrates the skin. This will limit any further unwanted travel of the needle.

9. Remove the 10-mL syringe, attach the 50-mL syringe to the needle hub, and aspirate the desired amount of fluid. The fluid may be discarded into the basin or sterile containers if laboratory analysis is required. If the blood or pericardial fluid withdrawn clots, it is probably fresh blood from a cardiac chamber. Withdraw the needle slightly and aspirate again. Pericardial fluid may be bloody, but it should not clot.

Ultrasound-Guided Technique

1. Many experts believe that ultrasound-guided pericardiocentesis is now the standard of care. If this technique is used, the 12-lead ECG lead does not need to be attached to the spinal needle. However, the patient should be monitored continuously with either telemetry or a 12-lead ECG machine running continuously with the leads placed in the standard locations.

2. Follow previous steps 1 through 6 as much as possible (except the V₁ ECG lead does not need to be attached to the needle and the best location for puncture as determined by ultrasound scanning should be prepped and anesthetized). The patient should be scanned in the semierect or the left lateral decubitus position if there are no contraindications to this position. Apply ultrasound gel and scan using a low-frequency (3.5 to 5 MHz) probe, and attempt to locate the largest and most superficial pocket of fluid. The ideal puncture site and pathway should be near the largest and most superficial accumulation of fluid. This will usually be with the probe in either the left parasternal or apical location (see Chapter 214, Emergency Department, Hospitalist, and Office Ultrasonography [Clinical Ultrasonography]). The ideal path should also avoid other organs (e.g., lung, liver); the subxiphoid position should therefore usually not be used with an ultrasound-guided procedure because a portion of liver is usually included in the puncture path.

3. Pericardial fluid is dark by convention on the image and located in a dependent location which is usually in the lower portion of the image. Note on the image the amount of fluid, the distance from the probe to the fluid, and the angle of insertion; the needle should usually be inserted either parallel to the probe or in the middle of the probe where it can be visualized. The skin should then be prepped in a sterile manner over this area and anesthetized. Next, insert a sterile probe cover over the ultra-

sound probe. Sterile ultrasound gel should be applied generously between the probe cover and the patient's skin.

4. Insert the pericardiocentesis needle through the anesthetized skin, advancing at the same angle as the probe and toward the largest pocket, aspirating continuously. Some experts advocate direct visualization of the needle with ultrasound as it is advanced. If inserting near a rib, insert the needle over the superior aspect to avoid the neurovascular bundle located under the inferior portion of rib. Advance the spinal needle until blood or pericardial fluid is aspirated or cardiac pulsations are felt.

NOTE: In theory, the coronary arteries near the apical location are smallest and therefore less likely to be lacerated by the needle. However, the lingua and left pleural interspace are located nearby increasing the risk of pneumothorax. If using the parasternal location, avoid the intramammary artery which lies approximately 3 to 5 mm medial to the parasternal border.

Blind Insertion Technique

1. In an emergency, pericardiocentesis may have to be performed blindly (usually because neither connectors to attach the ECG lead to the pericardiocentesis needle nor an ultrasound machine is available). In that situation, a 12-lead ECG machine should still be running continuously with the leads placed in the standard locations.

2. Follow previous steps 1 through 6 as much as possible. Next, insert the pericardiocentesis needle through the subxiphoid skin, advancing toward the left shoulder (alternatively, directed toward the suprasternal notch or right or left midclavicle), aspirating continuously. Advance the spinal needle until blood or pericardial fluid is aspirated, cardiac pulsations are felt, or the 12-lead ECG shows (a) ST segment elevation (i.e., current of injury) or (b) ectopic beats. Again, these ECG findings are suggestive of penetration of the epicardium and require withdrawal of the needle slightly, in 1- to 2-mm increments, until the findings disappear.

Placing a Fuhrman Pericardial Drainage Catheter (Seldinger Technique)

Recurrence of an effusion is common; placing a pericardial catheter can minimize the risk of recurrence and decrease the risk of complications with repeat needlesticks.

1. Follow previous steps 1 through 8. Then remove the 10-mL syringe from needle hub, grasp the needle firmly, and pass the guidewire through the needle into the pericardial space (Fig. 230.4). Advance the guidewire until approximately one-third of its length is within the patient.

2. Stabilize the guidewire with one hand, and remove the needle while leaving the guidewire in place. Nick the skin, with a No. 11 blade, where the guidewire enters.

3. Slide the dilator over the guidewire, and dilate the skin tract. Several passes will be necessary. Slide the dilator off the guidewire, and set it aside.
   NOTE: The clinician must obtain some assurance that the guidewire is not located in the myocardium; dilating a tract through the myocardium will result in cardiac tamponade or hemorrhage.

4. Again, stabilize the guidewire with one hand, and with the other thread the 8-Fr pigtail (Fuhrman) catheter over the guidewire. Pass the catheter up through the dilated subcutaneous tract into the pericardium. Advance the entire catheter into the body except for the last 1 inch before the hub. Remove the guidewire, and set it aside.

5. Suture the pigtail catheter onto the skin, wrapping suture around the catheter between the hub and where it enters the skin.

6. Attach and secure the suction device.

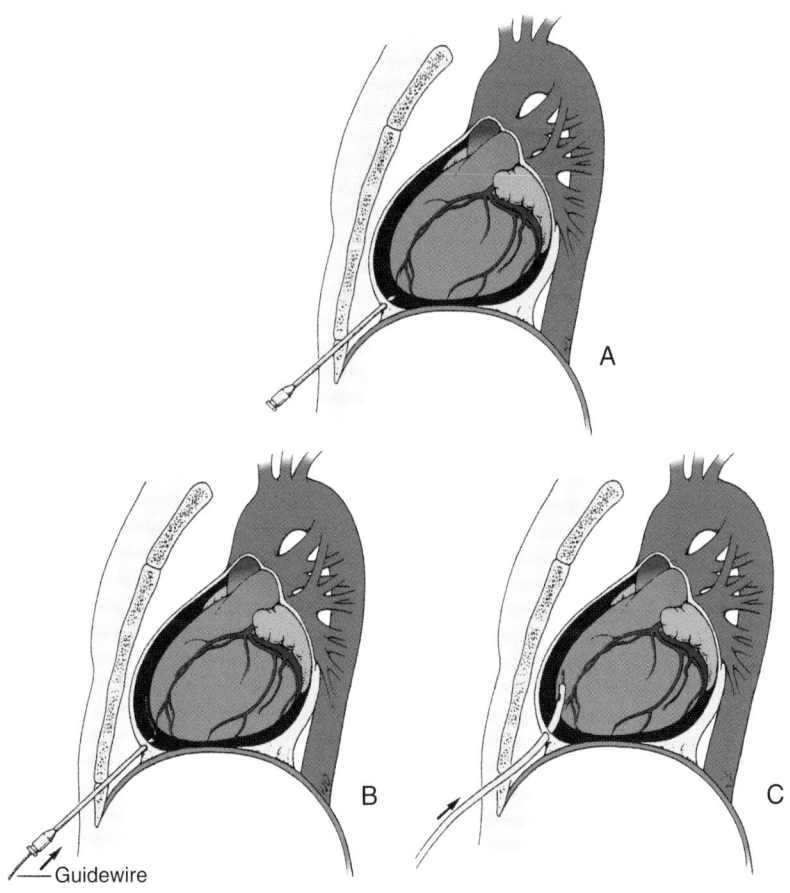

Fig. 230.4   (A) The needle is first advanced into the pericardial space. (B) The syringe is then disconnected from the needle and the flexible guidewire advanced carefully into the pericardial space (best performed under fluoroscopic guidance). (C) The needle is withdrawn over the guidewire, the needle tract dilated, and a multihole, soft pigtail catheter advanced into the pericardial space. (From Spodick DH. The technique of pericardiocentesis. *J Crit Illn.* 1987;2:91–96.)

POSTPROCEDURE PATIENT CARE

1. If just a simple aspiration was performed, remove the needle after aspiration is complete and dress the puncture site.
2. If a Fuhrman catheter is to be left in place, make sure both the catheter and drainage apparatus are secured. They tend to migrate out of the patient if they are not secured.
3. Obtain a postprocedure ECG to look for cardiac injury, and a chest radiograph, looking for pneumothorax. A repeat ultrasound scan is advised to see if fluid remains. An additional ultrasound scan the next day may diagnose a reaccumulation.

Tamponade should be promptly relieved even with a small amount of fluid removed because of the steep pressure-volume relationship of the pericardium. False-negative aspiration rates as high as 80% have been reported with blind or ECG-directed pericardiocentesis. This false-negative aspiration result is often due to clotted blood in the pericardial space that cannot be aspirated or failure to transverse the pericardium. If fluid is removed and relief of tamponade with improvement in hemodynamic status does not occur, consider another diagnosis and arrange transfer of care to the appropriate consultant. Continue to monitor the hemodynamic status in the meantime. Other diagnoses may include constrictive pericarditis, lung disease with left ventricular failure, right ventricular infarction, or biventricular failure. Consult a cardiothoracic surgeon if purulent material is expressed with pericardiocentesis.

After diagnostic pericardiocentesis, fluid should be sent for studies similar to those for pleural fluid (e.g., chemical, cytologic, microbiologic analyses). It can be sent for a cell count and differential, glucose, total protein (body fluid/serum ratio), lactate dehydrogenase, pH, appearance (e.g., clear, cloudy), Gram stain and culture, acid-fast bacillus stain and culture, fungal culture, and cytology.

COMPLICATIONS

Complication rates vary from 4% to 40% including myocardial puncture with hemopericardium, laceration of the coronary vessels, bradyarrhythmias and tachyarrhythmias, pneumothorax, hemothorax, air embolism, liver laceration, hemorrhage, hypovolemic hypotension from removing large volumes of fluid (e.g., patients with >1 L pericardial effusions), infection, recurrence (up to 70% using blind technique; reduced to 25% if Fuhrman catheter placed), cardiac arrest, and even death. Death usually occurs as the result of recurrence or occurrence of tamponade, hemorrhage, or dysrhythmias. Few if any deaths have been associated with ultrasound-guided pericardiocentesis. Overall, the complication rate of ultrasound-guided pericardiocentesis has been reported to be less than 5%. A less serious complication is vasovagal reaction in the alert patient.

CPT/BILLING CODES

33010	Pericardiocentesis, initial
33011	Pericardiocentesis, subsequent
33015	Tube pericardiostomy
76930	Ultrasound guidance for pericardiocentesis, imaging supervision and interpretation

ICD-10-CM Diagnostic Codes

A18.84	Pericarditis, tuberculous
I01.0	Acute rheumatic fever with pericarditis (can include effusion)
I32	Acute pericarditis in diseases classified elsewhere (first code the underlying disease)
I30.9	Acute pericarditis, unspecified
I30.8	Effusion, pericardial (acute)
I30.8	Pericarditis (acute), pneumococcal, purulent, staphylococcal, streptococcal, suppurative, or pyopericardium
I31.2	Hemopericardium
I31.4	Cardiac tamponade (first, code the underlying cause)
I31.9	Effusion, pericardial

Suppliers

Pericardiocentesis kits
Boston Scientific
Cook Medical
Merit Medical

RECOMMENDED READING

James D. Pericardiocentesis. In: James D, ed. *A Field Guide to Urgent and Ambulatory Procedures*. Philadelphia: Lippincott Williams & Wilkins; 2001:125–129.

Mallernat HA, Tewelde SZ. Pericardiocentesis. In: Roberts JR, Custalow CB, Thomsen TW, eds. *Roberts and Hedges' Clinical Procedures in Emergency Medicine*. 6th ed. Philadelphia: Elsevier; 2014:298–318.

Reichman E, Kang E, Meer J. Pericardiocentesis. In: Reichman EF, ed. *Emergency Medicine Procedures*. 2nd ed. New York: McGraw-Hill; 2013:225–236.

Seferovic PM, Ristic AD, Imazio M, et al. Management strategies in pericardial emergencies. *Herz*. 2006;31(9):891–900.

Ristic AD, Imazio M, Adler Y, et al. Triage strategy for urgent management of cardiac tamponade: a position statement of the European Society of Cardiology Working Group on Myocardial and Pericardial Diseases. *Eur Heart J*. 2014;35(34):2279–2284.

Spodick DH. The technique of pericardiocentesis. *J Crit Illn*. 1987;2:91–96.

Yarlagadda C. Cardiac tamponade workup. *Medscape*. 2016. Accessed September 4, 2017.

CHAPTER 231

ELECTRICAL CARDIOVERSION

Jeremy Fish

Transthoracic direct-current electrical shock, or electrical cardioversion, is a safe and effective procedure for terminating most sustained tachyarrhythmias. It is useful for converting acute arrhythmias that are causing clinical deterioration of the patient's condition, and for chronic arrhythmias that are symptomatic, carry a poor prognosis, or are unresponsive to drug therapy. Cardiac arrhythmias often can be converted to sinus rhythm with medications (chemical cardioversion), but electrical cardioversion refers to the direct application of electrical current.

CARDIOVERSION VERSUS DEFIBRILLATION

Cardioversion differs from defibrillation in that, with electrical cardioversion, the electrical discharge is synchronized with the R wave of ventricular depolarization to minimize the risk of triggering ventricular fibrillation (VF). External paddles or patches are used to apply the electrical current, which causes total depolarization of the atria and ventricles. This depolarization frequently causes the instantaneous conversion of an arrhythmia to sinus rhythm.

Electrical defibrillation is a procedure in which nonsynchronized electrical current is applied to convert chaotic fibrillation or pulseless ventricular tachycardia (VT) to a normal sinus rhythm. Defibrillation is warranted in an unconscious, pulseless, and apneic patient once VF or pulseless VT is identified. Patients in VF or pulseless VT should receive immediate defibrillation at 360 joules (J) if using a monophasic device or 200 J if using a biphasic device. Defibrillation should be repeated at 360 J (monophasic energy) or 200 J (biphasic energy) if the rhythm does not convert. Defibrillation is an emergency procedure. One of the most generally accepted protocols for defibrillation is available through advanced cardiac life support (ACLS) courses given by many local hospitals and registered through the American Heart Association (AHA).

INDICATIONS

- Atrial fibrillation (AF)
- Atrial flutter
- Hemodynamically stable VT unresponsive to pharmacologic therapy
- Hemodynamically unstable VT with a pulse
- Hemodynamically unstable supraventricular tachycardic (SVT) arrhythmias
- Certain SVT arrhythmias unresponsive to pharmacologic therapy, including reentrant bypass tract SVT (e.g., Wolff-Parkinson-White syndrome)

CONTRAINDICATIONS

Absolute

- Absent pulse (patient needs AHA basic life support measures or defibrillation)
- Severely unstable patient (patient needs resuscitation)

- Severe electrolyte disturbances
- Digitalis toxicity
- Left atrial or atrial appendage thrombus (for elective cardioversion, consult cardiology)
- Left ventricular mural thrombus (for elective cardioversion, consult cardiology)

Relative

- Large left atrial diameter (>4.5 cm) in patients with AF (unlikely to remain converted)
- Sick sinus syndrome (can result in worse postshock rhythm, consult cardiology)
- Ectopic or multifocal atrial tachycardia (can result in worse postshock rhythm, consult cardiology)
- Junctional or sinus tachycardia (can result in worse postshock rhythm, consult cardiology)
- Minimal hemodynamic or clinical improvement while in sinus rhythm
- AF duration greater than 6 months
- Inadequate anticoagulation and more than 48 hours' duration of AF (unless transesophageal echocardiography [TEE] negative)

A left atrial diameter greater than 4.5 cm or AF duration greater than 6 months is associated with a low likelihood of maintaining sinus rhythm. Patients with sick sinus syndrome or sinoatrial node block should not undergo cardioversion until a pacemaker has been placed. Ectopic or multifocal atrial, junctional, and sinus tachycardias do not normally respond to cardioversion. These rhythms have an automatic focus arising from cells that are depolarizing at a rapid rate; delivery of a shock may actually increase the rate of the tachyarrhythmia. Patients with a history of minimal hemodynamic or symptomatic improvement while in sinus rhythm should not undergo cardioversion because of an increased risk-to-benefit ratio. Inadequately anticoagulated patients with AF of longer than 48 hours' duration have an increased risk of thromboembolic stroke or arterial embolization after cardioversion (5% risk in the first 2 weeks).

EQUIPMENT

- Hand-held paddle electrodes, or 8- to 12-cm diameter, self-adherent pad electrodes or posterior paddle adapter
- Electrode gel or patches
- ACLS equipment
  - Oxygen source, nasal cannula or face mask
  - Pulse oximeter
  - Airway and intubation equipment
  - Ambu bag
  - Suction equipment, tubing, and catheter
  - Emergency drug kit, including IV
  - Medications needed to follow ACLS protocols
- Electrocardiography (ECG) electrodes and ECG monitoring capabilities

- Blood pressure monitoring equipment
- Direct-current defibrillator–cardioversion unit, with synchronization capabilities and optional "quick-look" paddles
- Sedatives for procedural sedation for elective cardioversion (see Chapter 1, Procedural Sedation and Analgesia)

Choice of Cardioversion Unit: Biphasic Versus Monophasic

Biphasic waveform automated external defibrillators and cardioversion units were developed in the late 1990s and have been shown to provide superior AF conversion rates with lower-energy shocks compared with traditional monophasic units currently in use—86% of patients with AF returned to sinus rhythm after a single biphasic shock, versus 51% with the first monophasic shock. Biphasic equipment usually weighs less; therefore most commercially available automated external defibrillators in the United States use biphasic waveforms, whereas most cardioversion units in hospitals and emergency departments continue to provide monophasic waveform shock. Cost and retraining of medical staff are likely barriers to wider use of biphasic cardioversion units.

Electrical Versus Chemical Cardioversion

Given the procedural sedation (see Chapter 1, Procedural Sedation and Analgesia) required for nonemergent electrical cardioversion, much effort has been exerted to find an ideal antiarrhythmic medication for chemical cardioversion. Two classes of agents are currently used, sodium and potassium channel blockers. Sodium channel blockers such as flecainide, propafenone and quinidine work by slowing down the heart's ability to conduct electricity. Potassium blockers such as amiodarone, sotalol and dofetilide work by slowing down the electrical signals that cause AF. Ibutilide is another available agent. Unfortunately, each of these agents has also been shown to be proarrhythmic—especially in the setting of decreased left ventricular ejection fraction (a relatively common finding in patients with AF). Amiodarone, although a slightly less effective agent that has delayed cardioversion effects in AF, has been shown to be safer in patients with a low ejection fraction. That said, some experts still recommend treating hemodynamically stable VT with amiodarone, 150 mg intravenously, and repeated as needed up to 2.2 g/24 hr. Most paroxysmal atrial tachycardia will respond to intravenous adenosine. If unsuccessful in these cases, or the patient becomes unstable, cardioversion can be performed.

The advantage of chemical cardioversion is primarily related to the avoidance of procedural sedation in patients at high risk for airway compromise during procedural sedation (e.g., obstructive sleep apnea, known tracheal stenosis, prior tracheostomy, macroglossia). Like electrical cardioversion, chemical cardioversion in a nonurgent setting requires full anticoagulation for 3 weeks to avoid thromboembolic complications.

Rhythm Control Versus Rate Control, Combined With Anticoagulation, in Persistent Atrial Fibrillation

Multiple studies over the years have demonstrated little difference in clinical outcome between rate and rhythm control strategies for patients with AF. In fact, rate control strategy is associated with fewer hospitalizations and less adverse drug effects when compared with rhythm control. Based on this evidence, most guidelines now strongly recommend rate control and anticoagulation as primary therapy for persistent AF. The latest American Academy of Family Physicians guidelines on newly detected AF (2017) recommend rate control with chronic anticoagulation for most patients. Drugs recommended for rate control are β-blockers (e.g., metoprolol, carvedilol, atenolol) and nondihydropyridine calcium channel blockers (e.g., diltiazem, verapamil) and digoxin. β-Blockers and calcium channel blockers consistently outperform digoxin for rate

control, so digoxin is not recommended as first-line management. Rhythm control may be considered for certain patients based on symptoms, exercise tolerance, and patient preference. Anticoagulation should be decided based upon risk of stroke versus bleeding; standardized risk calculators are available for both. Clinicians should consider using the continuous CHADS2 or continuous CHA2DS2-VASc for prediction for risk of stroke and HAS-BLED for prediction of risk for bleeding.

PREPROCEDURE PATIENT PREPARATION

Urgent cardioversion is indicated when the patient is unstable. Examples include symptomatic hypotension with central nervous system changes or syncope resulting from decreased perfusion. If the patient is alert, briefly explain the procedure while connecting the equipment. Informed consent is unnecessary for a life-threatening situation. Document the indications and risks to the patient as time permits. The following preparation for elective cardioversion is not required for urgent cardioversion (i.e., if the clinical status of the patient is so tenuous that he or she would not survive).

Echocardiography

TEE is helpful before elective cardioversion to estimate left atrial diameter (see Chapter 75, Echocardiography). TEE can identify small atrial thrombi, especially in the left auricular appendage, that are not visible with transthoracic echocardiography in patients for whom anticoagulation with warfarin poses high risk.

Anticoagulation and Antiarrhythmics

All patients with AF for more than 48 hours should be anticoagulated adequately for 3 weeks before elective cardioversion because of the risk of embolizing intra-atrial thrombi when sinus rhythm (and atrial contractions) are reestablished. The incidence of emboli may be up to 5% for the first 2 weeks after cardioversion in nonanticoagulated patients. Recent trials indicate the benefits of anticoagulation in all patients with chronic AF. If warfarin is used, the international normalized ratio should be maintained between 2 and 3 for at least 3 weeks before and 4 weeks after the cardioversion. The routine use of anticoagulation in arrhythmias other than AF is controversial.

EDITOR'S NOTE: A TEE is much more sensitive than a transthoracic echocardiogram for detecting thrombi, especially in the atrial appendage. Although the absence of a detectable thrombus does not preclude thromboembolism after cardioversion, a TEE-guided strategy (Klein, 2000) for elective cardioversion of AF has long resulted in outcomes comparable with those obtained using a conventional anticoagulation strategy.

There is some evidence suggesting that having the patient already on antiarrhythmic therapy before cardioversion may prevent recurrence. In the event the patient might chemically convert, he or she should have been adequately anticoagulated or have a TEE negative for thrombus before starting antiarrhythmics.

Fasting and Informed Consent

Instruct the patient to fast after midnight or for at least 4 to 6 hours before the procedure. Explain the indications for the procedure and the risk of complications. Explain that sedation will be used but that the patient may experience some achy discomfort in the arms and chest after the procedure. ECG monitoring for at least several hours will be necessary because of the risk of a recurrent or new arrhythmia. In addition, a minor skin irritation or burn may occur. Document the informed consent discussion, and obtain the patient's signature on the consent form (see the sample patient consent form available at www.expertconsult.com).

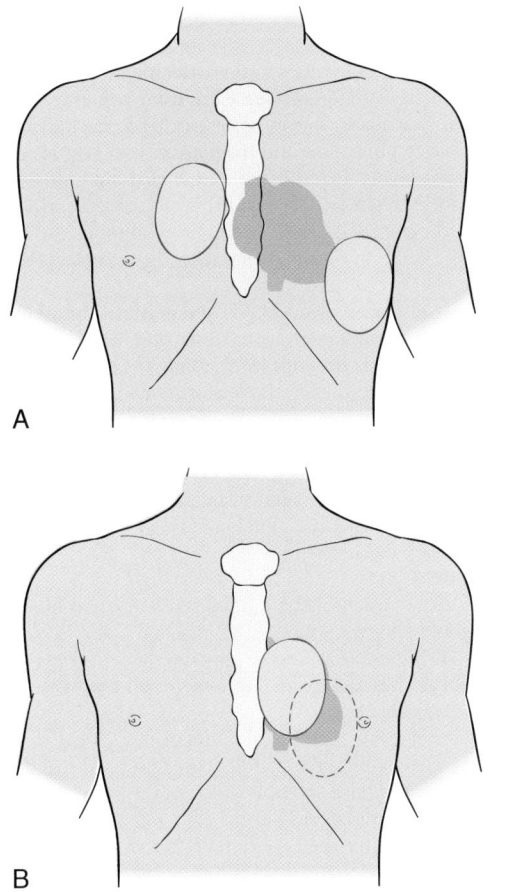

Fig. 231.1 (A) Standard electrode position. (B) Alternative (anteroposterior) electrode position.

TECHNICAL CONSIDERATIONS FOR ELECTIVE CARDIOVERSION

Paddle and Electrode Selection and Placement

Apply the electrodes in either the standard paddle position (right upper parasternal [second or third interspace, just below the clavicle] and left apical [fourth, fifth or sixth interspace, left midaxillary line]; Fig. 231.1A) or the anteroposterior paddle position. For anteroposterior placement, the anterior electrode is centered over the sternum and the posterior electrode is placed between the scapulae, or both can be placed slightly to the patient's left, on the left side of the sternum and beneath the left scapula (see Fig. 231.1B). Hand-held paddle electrodes or self-adherent pad electrodes 8 to 12 cm in diameter deliver adequate energy for cardioversion. To maximize the current flow to the heart, correct paddle or electrode placement is crucial. Either positioning technique is acceptable, but anteroposterior positioning may reduce energy requirements for cardioversion (through reduced electrical resistance) by up to 50%. In a large patient, this may increase cardioversion success. Anteroposterior placement is often used with disposable patches rather than paddles. Either paddles or electrodes must be positioned far enough apart so that electrical current travels through the heart. Gel or paste must be placed between the paddle or electrode and the chest wall to minimize resistance. However, avoid paste or gel smeared on the skin between electrodes, which might allow the current to travel along the external chest wall. Electrodes should also be placed far enough away from a pacemaker generator to prevent damage to its electrical components.

Electrocardiographic Monitoring

A set of ECG electrodes connected to the defibrillator should be placed on the patient so that the shock can be synchronized. An additional set of ECG electrodes can be connected to a telemetry monitor.

Synchronization

Synchronization refers to the delivery of electrical current to the myocardium during a nonrefractory period (e.g., not when repolarization of the entire myocardium is occurring). Shocking the myocardium during the relative refractory period (the T wave) can simulate the R-on-T phenomenon and induce VF. In synchronized mode, the energy is delivered at the peak of the QRS complex, the R wave. Synchronized administration reduces the energy requirements and complication rates of elective cardioversion.

Most defibrillators indicate when active synchronization is selected by highlighting the QRS peak (R wave). The practitioner can simply select and press the synchronization button for most cases of elective cardioversion. In cases with rapid ventricular response, the defibrillator in a synchronized mode may not be able to distinguish between the peak of the QRS complex and the peak of a T wave. As a safety feature, the defibrillator will not discharge if QRS complex and T waves cannot be distinguished. In this case, the provider should switch off the synchronization switch and perform unsynchronized defibrillation, realizing the increased risk of precipitating VT or VF. Alternatively, medications may be added to reduce the rapid ventricular response.

Energy Selection

Cardioversion is accomplished by passing an electrical current of sufficient magnitude through the heart to depolarize the myocardial tissues. Current flow is determined by the energy flow as measured in joules and by the resistance of the thoracic wall tissues as measured in ohms. The transthoracic resistance in an average adult is 70 to 80 ohms. If the transthoracic resistance is too high, the energy may fail to accomplish cardiac depolarization.

Some SVT arrhythmias are very sensitive to electrical current. Low energy settings may depolarize the myocardium in atrial flutter and allow the heart to resume a sinus rhythm. Recommended initial energy settings for cardioversion of various arrhythmias are listed in Table 231.1. For AF, the usual recommended initial energy setting is 100 J. However, recent evidence suggests that higher initial energy settings are more effective at achieving cardioversion, and some authors currently recommend an initial energy setting of 360 J. From there, some will increase the energy setting even further; one study found a good response to 720 J for the treatment of refractory VF.

Cardioversion energy for VT depends on the rate and morphologic features of the electrical activity. Monomorphic VT presents with a regular ECG form (wide-complex) and rate, and it is generally responsive to cardioversion beginning at energies of 100 J. Polymorphic VT has an irregular form and rate and is less responsive to electroshock therapy. Polymorphic VT behaves like VF, and the initial defibrillator shock energy should be 200 J (unsynchronized).

If the first shock fails to cardiovert any arrhythmia, repeated attempts should be undertaken with stepwise energy increases. The transthoracic resistance increases after each shock, so the energy must be increased to overcome that resistance. The standard sequence for synchronized cardioversion is 100, 200, 300, and 360 J; the energies used depend on the initial energy selected. For example, after starting with 200 J, the second attempt to convert polymorphic VT should be with an energy of 300 J. Patients with large thoraces,

TABLE 231.1	Recommended Initial Energy Settings for Electrical Cardioversion		
		Initial Energy Settings (J)	
		Monophasic	Biphasic
Adults			
Atrial flutter		50	50*
Atrial fibrillation		200	100*
Paroxysmal supraventricular tachycardia		50	50*
Monomorphic ventricular tachycardia		100	50*
Polymorphic ventricular tachycardia		200	100*
Children			
Supraventricular tachycardia		0.5 J/kg	0.5 J/kg*
Ventricular tach and defibrillation		2 J/kg	2 J/kg*

*Standards for biphasic cardioversion have not been established.

chest wall deformities, or large amounts of adipose tissue may require higher initial settings.

Energy levels differ between monophasic and biphasic cardioversion units. They can also differ between biphasic units (biphasic rectilinear waveform versus biphasic truncated exponential waveform); if possible, the clinician should be familiar with the recommended energy settings for a particular unit. In general, the energy requirements for biphasic cardioversion units are approximately half those for monophasic units. For example, patients with chronic AF often require 200 to 360 J of monophasic countershock; however, only 100 to 150 J of biphasic countershock is usually required (see Table 231.1).

Environment and Personnel

Elective cardioversion should be performed in a prepared environment, usually in a cardiac care unit with telemetry capabilities. The American College of Cardiology/AHA guidelines review the cognitive and technical skills necessary to perform external direct-current cardioversion and suggest a minimum requirement of eight prior supervised electrical cardioversions. Sedation or anesthesia is typically used with elective cardioversion, requiring appropriate personnel and monitoring.

Choice of Sedation Agents

Many factors play into the decision for procedural sedation during elective cardioversion, including anticipated energy levels for cardioversion, patient factors (e.g., airway, obesity, hepatic and renal disorders), and desired length of sedation. In general, the extent of sedation needed depends on the amount of energy to be used:

- 50 to 100 J: mild sedation
- More than 100 to 150 J: moderate to deep sedation

Mild sedation usually requires only short-acting benzodiazepines, such as midazolam or lorazepam, and fentanyl, a narcotic with fewer hemodynamic effects than morphine.

Moderate to deep sedation agents often used for cardioversion include the following:

- Etomidate: advantage, little hemodynamic compromise; caution in liver disease
- Propofol: advantage, rapid on, rapid off; caution, may cause hypotension
- Barbiturates, primarily thiopental: losing favor because of long recovery

See Chapter 1, Procedural Sedation and Analgesia.

TECHNIQUE

1. Review laboratory values and echocardiography results or obtain an echocardiogram (see Chapter 75, Echocardiography). Confirm adequate anticoagulation and normal electrolyte (particularly potassium and magnesium) and serum digoxin (if indicated) levels. If indicated, patients should already be on a therapeutic regimen of antiarrhythmic medication. Review echocardiogram findings, noting the absence of intra-atrial thrombi (if appropriate) and an atrial diameter less than 4.5 cm.
2. Ensure that the patient has fasted.
3. Obtain a resting 12-lead ECG, and confirm the persistence of the rhythm disturbance.
4. Obtain informed consent (see the sample patient consent form, "Cardiac Procedure—Cardioversion," available at www.expertconsult.com).
5. Premedicate the patient with a sedative. Many experts recommend anesthesia standby if this service is available. Administration of a sedative (e.g., diazepam, midazolam) or a barbiturate can be combined with an analgesic (e.g., meperidine, fentanyl) to improve patient comfort.
6. The patient should be lying on a flat, dry surface.
7. Monitor the patient's ECG, pulse oximetry, and blood pressure throughout the procedure.
8. Initiate intravenous access. Apply supplemental oxygen.
9. Have suction, resuscitation equipment, and support staff immediately available.
10. Apply conductive material and electrodes. (If gel is applied directly to the paddles, the paddles can be rubbed together to coat the electrode surfaces completely.)
11. Turn on the cardioversion unit.
12. Select the appropriate energy level for the dysrhythmia, body habitus, and electrode positioning.
13. Turn on the synchronizer circuit. Look for markers on the R wave indicating synchronization mode. Adjust monitor gain, if necessary, until synchronization markers occur with each R wave.
14. Charge the capacitors to the preselected energy level.
15. Position the paddles or electrodes. Apply the pads firmly to the torso. (The paddles should be separated from each other by at least 2 to 3 cm to prevent arcing.)
16. Call "All clear!" to indicate all personnel should move away from the patient's bed to avoid receiving a shock. Double-check by visually confirming all personnel (including yourself) have moved back and have no physical contact with the patient or the bed.
17. Deliver electrical energy by depressing appropriate discharge buttons on both paddles. (There is often a brief delay. Keep buttons depressed until the shock is delivered.)
18. Assess the cardiac rhythm on the monitor.
19. Assess the patient, and administer more sedation if needed.
20. If necessary, repeat cardioversion process (steps 12 through 17) at a higher energy setting.
21. Remember to reset the synchronization switch, if necessary. Some defibrillators reset the switch to the "off" position after a shock is delivered.
22. If cardioversion is unsuccessful after a shock at 360 J, consider aborting the procedure and using additional antiarrhythmic medications.

COMPLICATIONS

- Unsuccessful cardioversion
- Transient mild arrhythmias
- Conversion to VT or VF
- Bradycardia, heart block
- Elevated cardiac enzymes (up to three times normal values)
- Localized cutaneous burns

- Accidental shock to attending personnel because of contact with the patient or bed
- Damage to electrical equipment in contact with the patient or bed
- Thromboembolic events
- Recurrence of original arrhythmia

If the original arrhythmia persists after more than three shocks and up to 360 J, the cardioversion is generally considered unsuccessful. In this case the procedure should be aborted. Allow the patient to waken. Explain that the cardioversion was unsuccessful despite maximal safe efforts, and list the various options available to the patient and anyone else present. Options include internal cardioversion, antiarrhythmic medications, devices such as pacemakers, and no further treatment. Catheter ablation techniques are also sometimes available. In a significant number of patients with unresponsive AF, internal cardioversion with intracardiac electrode catheters has been successful. In this case, anticoagulation needs to be withheld temporarily because of the risk of bleeding at the catheter site. Alternatively, additional, more specific antiarrhythmic medications could be considered. The cardioversion may be reattempted after therapeutic blood levels are achieved (usually a few days). The patient may decide that further attempts are not worth the perceived risks.

Other complications after cardioversion are uncommon in the absence of digitalis toxicity or hypokalemia and with a properly delivered shock. Bradycardia is sometimes noted immediately after cardioversion in patients with a history of inferior myocardial infarction. If the bradycardia is symptomatic, atropine may be used. Transient mild arrhythmias or creatine kinase elevations of less than three times normal may be noted, but they are generally inconsequential.

With any cardioversion, especially with rapid heart rates, there is a risk of producing a worse rhythm, such as VT or VF. Any attempted cardioversion that results in VF should be defibrillated (synchronization off) immediately, starting with 200 J of energy. On some defibrillators, the synchronization must be shut off manually to administer a nonsynchronized shock.

Application of adequate amounts of electrode paste to the paddles can minimize cutaneous burns. Electrical shock is a possibility for anyone in contact with the patient or the patient's bed. Any attached electrical equipment can be damaged. Systemic emboli may develop if the patient is not adequately anticoagulated, causing neurologic deficit or occlusion of a peripheral artery. The original arrhythmia may recur despite successful cardioversion.

POSTPROCEDURE MONITORING

Monitor the patient for 2 to 4 hours. An example of monitoring orders includes vital signs with neurologic checks every 15 minutes for 1 hour, then every hour for 2 hours. Provide continuous ECG telemetry during this time. Atrial or ventricular ectopy and bradycardia are not uncommon in the first 15 to 30 minutes after cardioversion.

CPT/BILLING CODES

92950   Cardiopulmonary resuscitation
92960   Cardioversion, elective; electrical conversion of arrhythmia, external

SUPPLIERS

Most hospitals have cardioversion equipment. Familiarize yourself with the equipment available in your particular setting.

Acknowledgment

The editors recognize the contributions of Thomas J. Zuber, MD, John L. Pfenninger, MD, Les B. Forgosh, MD, FACC, FACP, and David V. Power, MD, MPH, to this chapter in previous editions of this text.

RECOMMENDED READING

American Heart Association. *Advanced Cardiovascular Life Support Provider Manual.* Dallas: American Heart Association; 2015.

Boos CJ, Carlsson J, More RS. Rate or rhythm control in persistent atrial fibrillation? *Q J Med.* 2003;96:881–902.

Catherwood E, Fitzpatrick WD, Greenberg ML, et al. Cost-effectiveness of cardioversion and antiarrhythmic therapy in nonvalvular atrial fibrillation [see comments]. *Ann Intern Med.* 1999;130:625–636.

Frost JL, Campos-Outcalt D, Hoelting D, et al. *Pharmacologic Management of Newly Detected Atrial Fibrillation: Updated American Academy of Family Physicians Clinical Practice Guideline;* June 2017.

Joglar JA, Hamdan MH, Ramaswamy K, et al. Initial energy for elective external cardioversion of persistent atrial fibrillation. *Am J Cardiol.* 2000;86:348–350.

Klein EA. Assessment of cardioversion using transesophageal echocardiography (TEE) multicenter study (ACUTE I): clinical outcomes at eight weeks. *J Am Coll Cardiol.* 2000;36:324.

Mathew TP, Moore A, McIntyre M, et al. Randomised comparison of electrode positions for cardioversion of atrial fibrillation. *Heart.* 1999;81:576–579.

Minczak BM. In: Roberts JR, Custalow CB, Thomsen TW, eds. *Roberts and Hedges' Clinical Procedures in Emergency Medicine.* 6th ed. Philadelphia: Elsevier; 2014:228–247.

Page RL, Kerber RE, Russell JK, et al. For the Bicard Investigators: biphasic versus monophasic shock waveform for conversion of atrial fibrillation: the results of an international randomized, double-blind multicenter trial. *J Am Coll Cardiol.* 2002;39:1956–1963.

Sattar P. Cardioversion and defibrillation. In: Reichman EF, ed. *Emergency Medicine Procedures.* 2nd ed. New York: McGraw-Hill; 2013:193–197.

Stroke Prevention in Atrial Fibrillation Investigators. Stroke prevention in atrial fibrillation study: final results. *Circulation.* 1991;84:527–539.

CHAPTER 232

TEMPORARY PACING

William Ellert

For various reasons, primary care clinicians may need to perform temporary cardiac pacing. Several types of pacing are available, with the primary purpose being to maintain circulatory stability until either the situation resolves or a permanent pacemaker can be installed. This chapter covers external (transcutaneous) and internal (transvenous) emergency ventricular pacing. Transesophageal pacing, usually limited to atrial pacing, and transmyocardial transthoracic pacing are beyond the scope of this chapter.

The basic uses for temporary cardiac pacing are if complete heart block occurs, as a standby should the patient become symptomatic, or as a way to increase heart rate during periods of symptomatic bradycardia. In addition, overdrive pacing may be used to terminate arrhythmias (e.g., sustained supraventricular or ventricular tachycardia); atrioventricular (AV) sequential pacing may be used to prevent arrhythmias. "Medicinal" pacing (e.g., atropine, isoproterenol) is also available, with advanced cardiac life support (ACLS) guidelines being helpful to guide its use. Overall, the indications for temporary pacing can be divided into therapeutic, prophylactic, and diagnostic categories. For the purposes of this chapter, only therapeutic and prophylactic pacing are covered.

EXTERNAL (TRANSCUTANEOUS) PACING

Most defibrillator/cardioversion units are now capable of performing external transcutaneous pacing. Modern transcutaneous pacing units represent a major improvement over the units first developed in the 1950s. Those units frequently inflicted severe chest and back muscle stimulation and discomfort, and they often left burns on the skin. At least one suicide was recorded of a pacer-dependent patient who removed the leads to "end the pain." In the 1960s, transcutaneous pacing was largely replaced with the newly available transvenous pacing.

Subsequent discoveries rejuvenated transcutaneous pacing, especially since the 1980s. Researchers found that increasing the pulse duration from 2 to 20 ms not only increased the safety of transcutaneous pacing (reduced the risk of ventricular fibrillation), but also reduced the required current. Reduced current meant less pain and fewer burns. The development of electrodes with a larger surface area also decreased the pain and risk of tissue burn. Use of larger electrodes allows for a reduction in the current density, or the amount of current penetrating per square unit of skin. These developments have resulted in more frequent use of transcutaneous pacing, especially on a standby basis, and consequently decreased the use of transvenous pacing.

One of the shortfalls of external pacing, even with today's sophisticated equipment, is difficulty achieving capture in about one-fifth of patients. The reasons for difficult or ineffective external pacing include increased intrathoracic air (such as barrel chests or chronic obstructive pulmonary disease), a large pericardial effusion or tamponade, recent thoracic surgery, obesity, and the improper placement of electrodes. Increased output for capture may be required in these individuals. Another shortfall is that it is rare for patients not to complain of some pectoral muscle stimulation. Although most patients rate the discomfort as mild or moderate and easily tolerable, approximately one-third of patients rate the pain as severe or intolerable. Therefore, analgesics, narcotics, or sedatives should be considered when using external pacing, especially if the required mean current for capture is 50 mA or more (a common threshold).

Because the high voltages required for external pacing produce significant muscle twitching, conventional electrocardiographic (ECG) monitors and recorders are useless. To provide decent tracings despite the large pacer spikes and their aftermath, routine ECG monitors must be equipped with an output adapter. Fortunately, most external pacer units come equipped with a monitor capable of filtering the spikes. Without an adequate ECG monitor, treatable ventricular fibrillation could be masked by the large pacing spikes, with disastrous results. This is one of the grave risks of transcutaneous pacing.

Indications

- Short-term pacing until transvenous pacing can be initiated or underlying conditions are corrected (e.g., drug overdose, hyperkalemia)
- When medical therapy is not immediately available, or when significant bradyarrhythmias have not responded to medical therapy (e.g., atropine, isoproterenol)
- Symptomatic patients (e.g., syncope, presyncope, dizziness, fatigue) with type I or type II second-degree AV block, third-degree or complete AV block, asystolic pauses exceeding 3 seconds, or an escape pacemaker rate less than 40 beats/min; also for patients who become symptomatic because of a bifascicular block or sinus node dysfunction
- Overdrive pacing may be used to terminate arrhythmias (e.g., sustained supraventricular or ventricular tachycardia)
- As a standby or prophylaxis in conscious patients with hemodynamically stable bradycardia
- As a standby or prophylaxis before surgery in patients with a pre-existing cardiac conduction block (anesthesia can exacerbate the block); also before cardiac diagnostic studies
- As a standby or prophylaxis in conscious patients with an expected bradyarrhythmia or a new type II second-degree, third-degree, or complete AV heart block in the setting of ischemia or infarction (frequently seen with acute anterior or inferior wall myocardial infarctions or digoxin overdose)

  NOTE: Preliminary trial of pacing should be performed to ensure that capture is achievable and that pacing is tolerated by the patient.

- In children with primary bradycardia from congenital defects or after open-heart surgery
- To be considered when fluoroscopy (the preferred technique) is not available for transvenous pacer insertion

Contraindications

All of the contraindications are *relative*.

- Bradycardia in a patient with significant hypothermia; as the core temperature drops, the ventricles become more irritable and prone to fibrillation that is resistant to defibrillation. In addition, bradycardia may be physiologic due to a decreased metabolic rate in these individuals.

- Bradycardia in children: usually due to hypoxia or hypoventilation, the best intervention is to provide an adequate airway as opposed to pacing (exceptions as mentioned in the Indications section).
- Overdrive pacing in tachyarrhythmias with rates greater than 180 beats/min because that is the maximal rate of most external pacers.
- Bradyasystolic or asystolic arrest of more than 20 minutes' duration because of the well-documented poor resuscitation rates.
- Patient is unable to cooperate or tolerate the procedure (in a life-threatening situation, provide sedation).
- Lack of therapeutic benefit because of advanced disease or terminal illness.

Equipment

- Two 13 by 15 cm^2 electrodes for adults (two 6 by 7 cm^2 electrodes for infants and small children). These are usually round or rectangular and packaged in pairs. The negative electrode may also be labeled "front," "apex," or "anterior"; the positive electrode may be labeled "back" or "posterior."
- Razor or scissors to remove body hair from the area of electrode placement.
- Pacing unit (contains pulse generator and monitor) with pacing cable. The best units allow either fixed-rate or demand mode. Most allow a range from 30 to 180 beats/min, with current output from 0 to 200 mA. Pulse durations vary from 20 to 40 ms and are not adjustable by the operator. To protect health care providers, some pacers shut off when an electrode falls off the chest.

NOTE: Most defibrillator/cardioversion units contain a transcutaneous pacing unit as an integral part of the system.

- ECG leads and electrodes capable of monitoring during transcutaneous pacing. If not purchased as part of the pacing or defibrillator/cardioversion system, an output adapter to a separate ECG monitor is required to "blank" or neutralize the large electrical spikes from the pacer.
- Sedative and analgesic medications

Preprocedure Patient Preparation

If time allows, explain the purpose and benefits of the procedure as well as the risks of not performing the procedure to the patient or representative. The patient should know what to expect, the sensations he or she may experience (e.g., muscle contractions, a slight tingling, burning or shocking sensation), and that although this may be uncomfortable, the majority of patients tolerate it well. Explain what will be done to minimize the discomfort (e.g., sedative, analgesic). A signed consent is not required in emergent situations, but is preferred if time allows; at a minimum, implied consent should be documented in the medical record (e.g., "the risks and benefits have been explained to the patient, who agrees with having the procedure").

Any dirt or debris should be cleaned from the skin; however, avoid using any flammable liquids such as alcohol. Patients with significant body hair may need to be shaved (unconscious patients) or the hair clipped or trimmed (conscious) to ensure good skin–electrode contact. Shaving should be avoided, if possible, in the conscious patient because any nicks or lacerations can increase the discomfort and skin irritation during pacing.

Technique

1. Attach the exposed adhesive surfaces of two large electrode patches to the anterior and posterior chest walls (Fig. 232.1). The negative (anterior) electrode should be placed over the apex

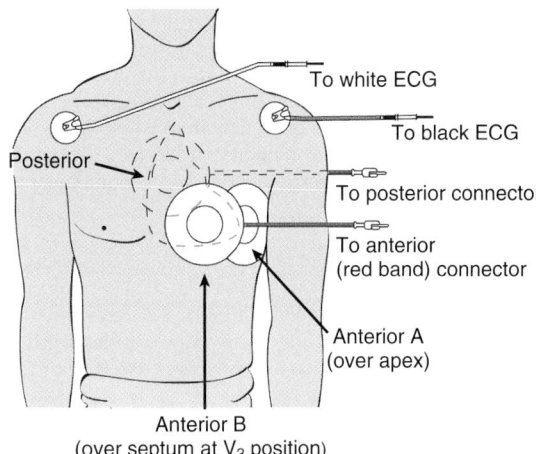

Fig. 232.1 External (transcutaneous) pacing. The anterior electrode is placed at the apex (A), which is to the left of the sternum over the point of maximal impulse, or over the septum (B), which is the V$_3$ position. The posterior electrode is placed to the left of the spinal column on the back, directly behind the anterior electrode. (Modified from Dahlberg ST, Benotti JR. Temporary cardiac pacing. In: Rippe JM, Irwin RS, Alpert JS, Fink MP, eds. *Intensive Care Medicine.* 2nd ed. Boston: Little, Brown; 1991.)

(at the point of maximal impulse) or the septum of the heart (the lead V$_3$ position), and the positive (posterior) electrode directly behind the anterior electrode, to the left of the thoracic spine, between the spine and the left scapula. Alternatively, the positive electrode can be placed on the right upper chest (immediately below the clavicle in a parasternal location) with the negative electrode over the apex of the heart. Avoid trapping any air between the skin and the electrodes.

2. If time allows, prepare the patient with analgesia such as a narcotic or sedation with a benzodiazepine (especially helpful if the required mean current for capture is ≥50 mA).

3. Turn on the pacing unit. Set the heart rate (e.g., 80 beats/min) to demand pacing. Set the current output (mA) dial as low as possible and sensing thresholds at levels similar to those used for internal pacing. Keep in mind that for demand pacing, external units often do not have sensing thresholds. The final current output setting is usually 1.25 times the initial capture threshold. Patients with conditions that cause difficult or ineffective pacing may require higher outputs for capture. At these higher outputs, the resultant muscle twitches may be too severe for external pacing to be used.

4. Apply the electrical stimulation to the electrodes. For conscious patients, slowly increase the output from the minimal setting, at 5- to 10-mA increments, until capture is achieved. Electrical capture is usually indicated by a widening of the QRS complex and especially by a broad T wave. The output required to obtain capture is defined as the pacing threshold. For near arrest, asystolic or unconscious patients, begin at full output (200 mA) and decrease until capture is achieved, which defines the pacing threshold. The final current output should be set at the pacing threshold or 5 to 10 mA above it. When transcutaneous pacing is used as a standby technique, most clinicians document capture by initiating a brief period of pacing at a rate slightly higher than the patient's intrinsic rate. The pacing output threshold is then recorded and the pacing unit is returned to standby mode.

5. When successful pacing is achieved, prophylactic intravenous access (central venous catheter) through the right internal jugular vein may be helpful in case an internal pacer is needed urgently. Because external pacers have up to a 20% failure rate, having central venous access available minimizes the risk of having to obtain it during a "code" situation.

6. Monitor continuously for capture, potential complications (e.g., treatable ventricular fibrillation, burns), and patient comfort. The only sure sign of electrical capture is the presence of a consistent ST segment and T wave after each pacer spike. Palpation of the carotid to confirm a pulse may not be helpful because the muscle stimulation and contractions produced by the pacer simulate a carotid pulse; therefore palpation of a femoral pulse may be necessary.

NOTE: The increased use of external pacers has surely reduced the number of prophylactic internal pacers placed. However, in nontransient situations, external pacing is always a temporary measure until an internal pacer (probably transvenous, as described in the next section) can be placed.

INTERNAL (TRANSVENOUS) PACING

Clinicians who may need to insert a transvenous pacemaker should be familiar with the equipment and its use before needing it in an emergent situation. There are usually two lights, a sense indicator light, which is illuminated when a cardiac impulse is sensed, and a pace indicator light, which is illuminated whenever a pacing stimulus is generated. There is also usually a button to test the battery to ensure adequate voltage to operate the pacemaker generator. Although newer models have digital displays and more sophisticated pacing options, they function basically the same as older models.

Indications

Therapeutic

- Symptomatic, hemodynamically compromising or life-threatening bradyarrhythmias unresponsive to pharmacologic therapy (e.g., systolic blood pressure <80 mm Hg, change in mental status, angina, pulmonary edema), including sick sinus syndrome, atrial fibrillation with a slow ventricular response rate
- Overdrive pacing may be used to terminate arrhythmias (e.g., sustained supraventricular or ventricular tachycardia)
- Bradycardia with ventricular escape rhythm unresponsive to pharmacologic therapy

NOTE: For tachyarrhythmias of less than 150 beats/min, neither immediate cardioversion nor an immediate pacer is necessary.

Prophylactic (in Setting of Acute Myocardial Infarction)

- Symptomatic sinus node dysfunction or Mobitz type I second-degree AV heart block that is not responsive to atropine therapy
- Second-degree Mobitz type II, third-degree, or complete AV heart block*
- Newly acquired bundle branch block with first-degree AV block
- Bilateral or alternating bundle branch blocks
- An old right bundle branch block with first-degree AV block and a new fascicular block

Contraindications

Contraindications include those listed in Chapter 228, Central Venous Catheter Insertion, and those listed previously for external pacing. Other contraindications include the following:

- A situation in which the bradycardia is well tolerated and the symptoms are intermittent, mild, or rare.*

---

*In patients with an inferior myocardial infarction, relatively asymptomatic second- or third-degree heart block can occur. Pacing in such patients should be reserved for symptoms or the presence of a deteriorating bradycardia. If not paced, patients should be monitored closely with a pacer nearby or on standby. It should have been tested for capture and patient tolerance.

- Bradycardia in patients with significant hypothermia; as the core temperature drops, the ventricles become more irritable and prone to fibrillation (especially if the pacing wire contacts the heart muscle) that is resistant to defibrillation. In addition, bradycardia may be physiologic because of a decreased metabolic rate in these individuals (relative contraindication).
- Digoxin toxicity and other drug ingestions that may increase the irritability of the myocardium (relative contraindication in life-threatening situation).
- Presence of a prosthetic tricuspid valve (relative contraindication in life-threatening situation).
- Depending on access site, planned neck or clavicle surgical procedures (relative contraindication, may affect choice of site).
- Distortion of local anatomy or landmarks; for insertion from subclavian, moderate to severe chest wall deformities that distort local anatomy (relative contraindication, may affect choice of site).
- Suspected injury to the superior vena cava (relative contraindication, may affect choice of site; e.g., superior vena cava syndrome, in which insertion from below the diaphragm is preferable).
- Bleeding diathesis, anticoagulation therapy, or concurrent thrombolysis or fibrinolysis (unless emergent pacing is required, and then antecubital venous cutdown access is preferred).
- Full-thickness burn, cellulitis, or other infection over the anticipated insertion site (relative contraindication, may affect choice of site).
- The absence of informed consent (relative contraindication in life-threatening situation).
- Patient is unable to cooperate or tolerate the procedure (relative contraindication in life-threatening situation, provide sedation).
- Bradyasystolic and asystolic arrest of more than 20 minutes' duration because of the well-documented poor resuscitation rates (relative contraindication).
- Lack of therapeutic benefit because of advanced disease or terminal illness (relative contraindication).
- Contraindications specific to internal jugular vein access include significant carotid artery disease, distorted cervical anatomy, and recent, unsuccessful contralateral cannulation (to prevent bilateral neck hematomas, which could compromise the patient's airway).
- Subclavian insertion during cardiopulmonary resuscitation (CPR). (If CPR can be halted briefly, this may be beneficial; jugular access usually can be obtained without stopping CPR. Otherwise, peripheral access may be preferable.)
- Children (relative contraindication and rarely needed; better intervention is to treat the cause [e.g., hypoxia]. If pacing is needed, the internal jugular vein is probably the best access route. However, the femoral vein is often used in infants and younger children and often requires fluoroscopy.)
- Patients with morbid obesity, marked cachexia, or severe hypovolemia may be better served by using common femoral or peripheral vein access.
- Severe hypovolemia (relative contraindication due to difficulty in insertion).

Equipment

- Bipolar transvenous pacing catheters (Fig. 232.2), 4 to 6 Fr for adults (3 or 4 Fr for infants and children), may be soft and pliable and made from extruded plastic or firm, relatively nonpliable, and made from woven Dacron. Some practitioners prefer soft, flexible, semifloating catheters; however, these are more difficult to maneuver and less stable once positioned. Flow-directed, flexible, balloon-tipped pacing catheters are also available. They are similar to balloon-tipped pulmonary artery catheters, but without an open lumen (see Fig. 232.2). Stiffer catheters are usually easier to maneuver than balloon-tipped catheters; however, balloon-tipped cathe-

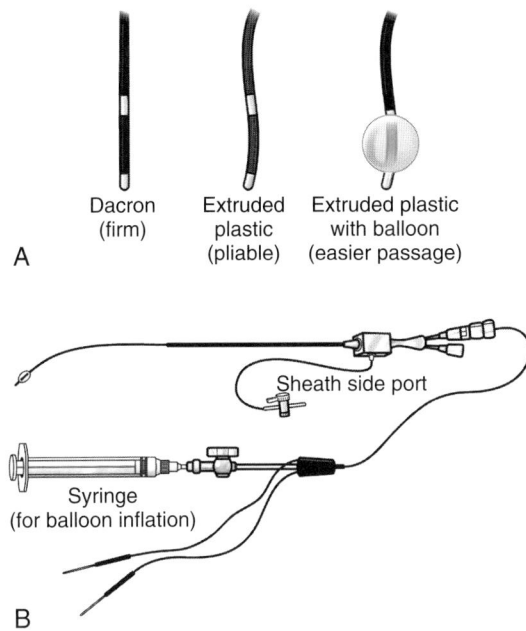

A

Dacron   Extruded   Extruded plastic
(firm)   plastic   with balloon
               (pliable)   (easier passage)

Sheath side port

Syringe
(for balloon inflation)

B

Fig. 232.2 **(A)** Distal tips of transvenous pacers. (B) Transvenous balloon-tipped temporary pacer.

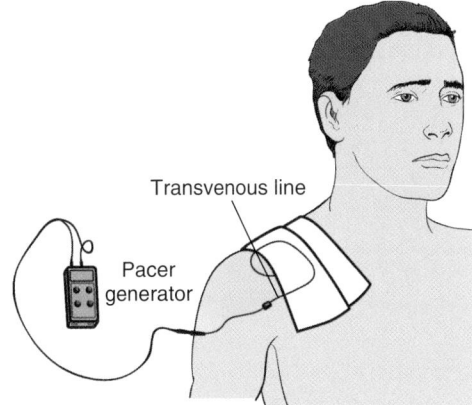

Transvenous line

Pacer
generator

Fig. 232.3 Transvenous line and pacer in place.

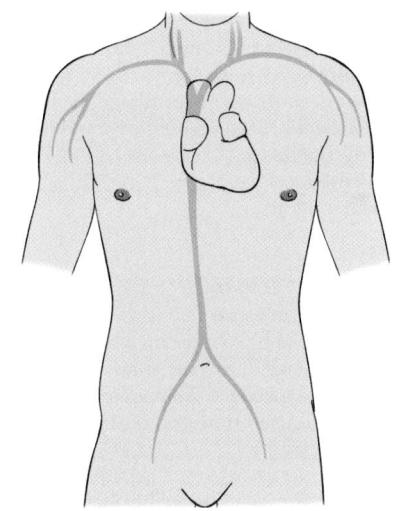

Fig. 232.4 Temporary pacer in right internal jugular vein.

ters are easier to insert without fluoroscopy. There is also always the option of using a balloon-tipped, pacer-equipped pulmonary artery catheter (Swan-Ganz). One prospective, randomized trial (Ferguson and colleagues, 1997) demonstrated that balloon-flotation pacing wires are easier to insert, quicker to position, and more likely to be optimally positioned than semirigid electrode wires.

- Unipolar electrode catheters are available; however, unipolar catheters must rely on a second, external electrode to be placed on the skin. This electrode is very susceptible to any external electrical interference; therefore, bipolar catheters are preferred.
- A flexible J-shaped catheter is available specifically for temporary atrial pacing.
- Availability of fluoroscopy is ideal.
- Pacer pulse generator (Fig. 232.3) with a new or spare battery.
- Extension cable with alligator clips on either end to connect pacer to ECG lead.
- ECG monitoring capability during insertion.
- Venous insertion site.
- Povidone iodine or chlorhexidine.
- Equipment for clinician to follow universal blood and body fluid precautions.
- Gauze squares.
- 3-0 nylon suture.
- ACLS equipment (defibrillator, airway management equipment, resuscitative drugs).

Preprocedure Patient Preparation

See Chapter 228, Central Venous Catheter Insertion.

If possible, obtain written informed consent. The conscious patient should know what to expect, the sensations he or she may experience (e.g., possibly being covered by a drape, needlesticks while obtaining central access), and that although this may be uncomfortable, everything possible will be done to minimize the discomfort (e.g., local anesthetic). In many cases, pacing is an emergency procedure and written informed consent cannot be obtained. However, after the patient is stabilized, the situation, risks, and benefits should be explained to the patient or representative. Implied consent should be documented in the medical record (e.g., in the conscious patient: "the risks and benefits have been explained to the

patient, who agrees with having the procedure"). Always outline the complications of either performing or withholding the procedure.

Technique

All steps should be performed using an aseptic technique and following universal blood and body fluid precautions. Venous access is established by the procedure outlined in Chapter 228, Central Venous Catheter Insertion. Inspect the leads on the pacing catheter for any breaks or manufacturing defects.

Access Route

The most direct route for internal pacemaker insertion is through a central venous catheter in the right internal jugular (even then, there is a failure rate of up to 8%). The subclavian vein (left preferred over right, with up to 17% failure rate on left) also can be used, especially for relatively long-term use, but this route of insertion may be more difficult because of the turns the electrode has to negotiate (Fig. 232.4). Brachial and femoral approaches are discouraged (except the femoral approach is preferred in infants and small children and usually requires fluoroscopy). The brachial approach has an increased risk of cardiac puncture and the femoral approach has an increased risk of deep venous thrombosis and infection.

Catheter Conversion

If necessary, insert a larger catheter into the established venous access site.

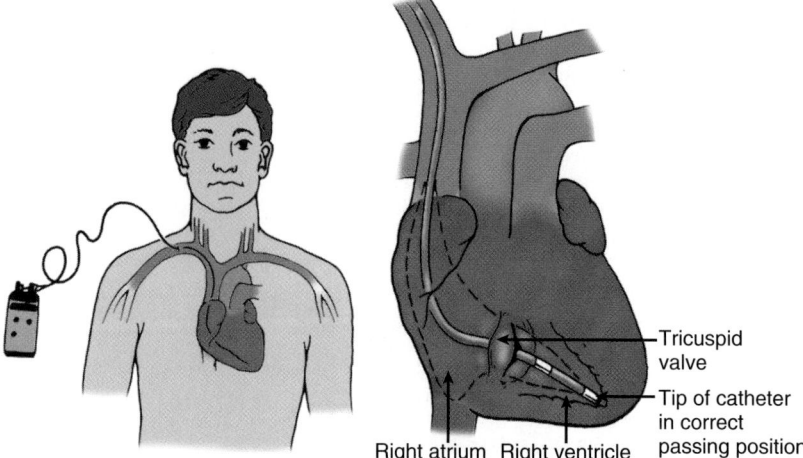

Fig. 232.5 Correct positioning of pacer catheter. When the tip reaches the apex, it stops moving under fluoroscopy.

1. Place a guidewire down the central venous access line.
2. Remove the catheter.
3. Use an obturator over the wire to enlarge the lumen.
4. Pass an introducer with catheter (e.g., Swan-Ganz or Cordis) assembly over the guidewire.
5. Remove the introducer.
6. Check for venous return.

Pacer Placement

FLUOROSCOPY-GUIDED TECHNIQUE: By far, the best method of temporary pacer placement involves fluoroscopic guidance of the semifloating or balloon-tipped bipolar pacing leads. Many intensive care units and some emergency departments have beds that will accommodate C-arms for fluoroscopy. If C-arms cannot be accommodated, and if time and clinical conditions permit, the patient might also be moved to the radiology suite.

1. Pass the catheter through the rubber diaphragm of the introducer sheath and to the 10- to 12-cm mark (10-cm segments are marked on the catheter).
2. If the balloon is used, blow it up and advance the catheter; it should move easily into the right atrium (RA).
3. Pass the tip across the tricuspid valve and advance it to the apex of the right ventricle (RV). Ask the patient to take deep breaths or to cough; this will facilitate passage across the valve. Under fluoroscopy, once the radiopaque tip is at the apex, the last 2 to 3 cm of the lead should show minimal or no longitudinal motion if an attempt is made to advance the catheter farther. The remainder of the catheter may have horizontal and longitudinal motion (Fig. 232.5), but not the tip. If a balloon is used, deflate it as soon as it passes across the tricuspid valve and washes to the ventricular wall. If the catheter tip curls up against the atrial wall, advance it 1 to 2 cm to create a partial loop. Next, rotate it clockwise and watch it straighten as it enters the plane of the tricuspid valve.
4. The best final position for the catheter tip is at the right ventricular apex. Electrodes residing in the pulmonary outflow tract or along the free wall are less stable and more likely to cause perforation.
5. If a balloon is used, it must be deflated before withdrawal for repositioning.
6. Coiling the proximal electrode catheter around the insertion site and firmly suturing and taping it to the skin prevents inadvertent dislodgement of the distal electrode. Using the extension cable, connect the pacer electrodes to the pacer unit.

ECG-GUIDED TECHNIQUE (WITHOUT FLUOROSCOPY): A flexible, semifloating or balloon-tipped catheter can be advanced and positioned much like a pulmonary artery catheter (see Chapter 229,

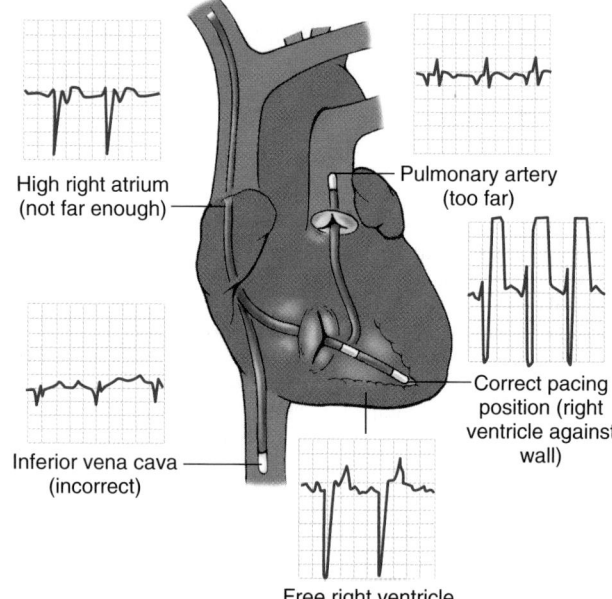

Fig. 232.6 Pattern of recorded electrocardiogram from intracardiac pacemaker electrodes at various locations in the venous circulation.

Swan-Ganz [Pulmonary Artery] Catheterization), except that the negative catheter electrode is attached to an ECG machine (usually the V_1 lead, a unipolar lead) using a connector with alligator clips.

1. Connect the limb leads of an ECG machine to the patient.
2. Turn on the ECG machine and set it to the appropriate lead to monitor insertion (again, usually the V_1 lead). Use an extension cable with alligator clip on each end to attach the ECG lead to the negative pacing catheter electrode. Next, touch the ECG lead to the ECG monitor to confirm that the ECG is obtaining a signal. A large wave should be seen on the monitor when the ECG lead touches the monitor.
3. Insert the pacemaker catheter through the rubber diaphragm of the introducer sheath and to the 10-cm mark. If the balloon is used, inflate it and advance the catheter; it should move easily into the RA.
4. The change in the recorded QRS complex allows the practitioner to approximate the tip location (Fig. 232.6). Follow the same passage route: into the veins and then RA, across the tricuspid valve, and to the apex of the RV. In the internal jugular or sub-

clavian vein, the P wave and the QRS complex are both small in amplitude and inverted. In the superior vena cava, the P wave increases in amplitude while the QRS complex is unchanged. As the electrode enters the RA, the P wave appears quite large but remains inverted until it reaches the lower RA, where it turns upright. As it passes the tricuspid valve, the QRS amplitude increases. When the electrode is freely floating in the RV, the QRS amplitude appears large and normal (inverted in V$_1$ lead). The balloon should be deflated. Advance the catheter until a large, elevated ST segment is observed. This indicates that the catheter is abutting the RV wall and is in the correct location.

5. If the catheter does not advance across the tricuspid valve, rotate it clockwise while advancing it 1 cm to flip the tip across the valve. If the catheter exits the RA and enters the inferior vena cava, the amplitudes of the P wave and QRS complex will decrease. Withdraw the catheter until the largest P wave is noted and then readvance the catheter. If the catheter exits the RA and enters the pulmonary artery, the P wave will become negative and the QRS will decrease. Withdraw the catheter until the normal right ventricular P wave and QRS complex are seen and then readvance the catheter.

6. Disconnect the negative pacemaker catheter lead from the extension cable and attach the positive and negative leads to the positive and negative terminals of the pacemaker generator, respectively.

ULTRASOUND-GUIDED TECHNIQUE: A pacing electrode is usually visible on ultrasound; therefore ultrasound cannot only be helpful for guiding insertion but also for confirming the final position. Generally, a low-frequency curvilinear probe (3.5 to 5 MHz) is preferred for cardiac ultrasound. Using the subxiphoid view, obtained with the patient in the supine position, the RA and RV are usually visible. By scanning through the liver (i.e., using the liver as a window), the catheter appears as a white, echogenic linear structure passing through the RV to the apex. Take care not to confuse the ventricular wall or septum for the electrode. While the ventricular wall and septum will be mobile and more echogenic than the fluid in the atrial and ventricular cavities, the catheter is usually thinner and more echogenic. Unfortunately, body habitus (e.g., obesity, chronic obstructive pulmonary disease) can limit the ability to visualize the heart with ultrasound in approximately 10% of individuals; however, ultrasound can often be combined with the ECG-guided technique to increase the likelihood of proper pacemaker placement (see also Chapter 214, Emergency Department, Hospitalist, and Office Ultrasound [Clinical Ultrasound]).

EMERGENCY TECHNIQUE: Unfortunately, situations frequently require placement of a temporary pacer under emergent or extreme conditions, without fluoroscopic or ECG guidance, such as during a code with the patient lying in a hospital bed (often this is necessary because the alligator clips and connector are not available for ECG guidance).

1. A flexible catheter should be used, and it may be inserted blindly to about 12 cm. The catheter is then attached to the pacemaker and the pacemaker turned on.

2. Set the rate higher than the patient's highest native heart rate (usually 80 to 120 beats/min), the amperage (ventricular output current) at 5 mA, and the mode at asynchronous (sensitivity off).

3. A surface or conventional ECG or rhythm strip should be running while the catheter is being passed. Capture is noted by an obviously paced rhythm seen on the surface ECG. Do not advance the catheter against resistance or more than 12 cm beyond the point at which the pacemaker was turned on. If capture does not occur at this point, withdraw the catheter and rotate it 90 degrees and readvance. Multiple attempts at passage may be necessary. When capture occurs, decrease the ventricular rate to 70 or 80 beats/min.

4. Alternatively, the sensing indicator on the pacemaker can be used to guide placement. Advance the flexible catheter to about 12 cm, inflate the balloon, attach and turn on the pacemaker, and set it on demand mode with a rate twice the patient's highest native heart rate (again, usually 80 to 120 beats/min) and the amperage at 1.5 to 2 mA. Advance the catheter, and when it enters the RV, the sens-

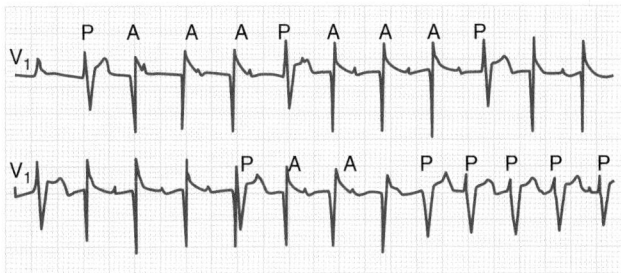

Fig. 232.7 Pacing with intermittent capture. *A*, pacer artifact without capture; *P*, paced beats. (From Dahlberg ST, Benotti JR. Temporary cardiac pacing. In: Rippe JM, Irwin RS, Alpert JS, Fink MP, eds. *Intensive Care Medicine*. 2nd ed. Boston: Little, Brown; 1991.)

ing indicator will illuminate with every other heart beat (because the pacemaker rate was set at twice the native heart rate). Deflate the balloon and increase the output to 5 mA. Slowly advance the catheter until ventricular capture occurs. Do not advance the catheter more than 10 cm beyond where the sensing indicator began to illuminate. If successful capture still has not occurred by this point, withdraw the catheter and rotate it 90 degrees. Readvance the catheter up to 10 cm. Continue to repeat the process until ventricular capture occurs and then decrease the ventricular rate to 70 or 80 beats/min. Unfortunately, even experienced clinicians occasionally fail despite multiple attempts with either technique, underscoring the benefits of fluoroscopic guidance.

Parameter Settings

Determine the pacing parameters, and record each when it is set.

1. *Rate:* If the patient shows no intrinsic heart rate, set the pacing rate at 70 to 80 beats/min to simulate the normal beating heart. If the patient is bradycardic, the same range can be used to raise the blood pressure and the heart rate. Record the rate chosen after setting the machine.

2. *Ventricular output:* The sensitivity is the voltage used (set the sensitivity between 1.5 and 3 mV), whereas the ventricular output is the current generated by the pacer, adjustable from 0.1 to 20 mA. Depending on technique, start with 1.5 to 5 mA and increase until capture is seen on the monitor. After reaching the level of output necessary to capture the ventricle, large spikes are seen (Fig. 232.7) followed by bundle branch block pattern complexes (wide QRS complexes, ST-segment elevation, and T-wave inversion, depending on the lead). The bundle branch block pattern occurs because the complex originates in the ventricle. A pulse should also be palpable, and it should generate a blood pressure. The ventricular output setting can then be reduced gradually, until capture is lost. The setting at which capture is lost is the pacing threshold, and this should be recorded. Resume pacing at 2 mA above this threshold. If capture occurs at less than 0.5 mA, the catheter may have become deeply embedded in the ventricular wall; be aware that withdrawal may cause perforation. If spikes are seen but no capture occurs, catheter manipulation is indicated. If levels of 5 to 6 mA or greater are required (which is common in fibrosis but is usually a result of poor electrode positioning), attempt to reposition the electrode. If spikes and bundle branch block pattern are seen with no pulse, the possibility of pulseless electrical activity (electromechanical dissociation) must be considered. With electromechanical dissociation, the proper ACLS management protocol should be followed and there may be benefit of an emergent echocardiogram (see Chapter 214, Emergency Department, Hospitalist, and Office Ultrasonography [Clinical Ultrasonography]).

Demand Pacing

If the patient's intrinsic rhythm is inadequate, a sensing threshold must be determined with the sensitivity knob. Occasionally a sensing threshold cannot be determined when the patient has a very slow rhythm.

Sensitivity is the control on the pacer that detects the amplitude of the patient's intrinsic R wave. The most sensitive setting is 1 mV, corresponding to full clockwise rotation of the knob. In the least sensitive setting, called *asynchronous pacing,* the pacer does not "care" if there is a rhythm and functions oblivious to the intrinsic rate. The asynchronous setting should be avoided when there is an intrinsic rhythm because the additional electric spikes generated by the pacer can cause an arrhythmia.

To determine sensing threshold, first set the rate about 10 beats/min below the patient's intrinsic rate. Gradually adjust the sensitivity control toward the highest sensitivity or entirely clockwise (to detect even the lowest-amplitude waves), which is known as the *full demand* setting. Pacer pulses should no longer be seen because all deflections are sensed and interpreted as QRS complexes. Every intrinsic or artifactual QRS complex should generate a flash of the sense indicator on the pacer. At this level the pacer senses almost all electrical activity and its firing is thus prevented. In fact, T waves, occasionally P waves (if the catheter is close to the atrium), chest muscle contractions, or even artifact may prevent the pacer from firing. This is called the *oversensing point.* This full demand setting is obviously too high for the pacer to function. The sensitivity control should then be turned counterclockwise, changing or decreasing the sensitivity toward higher numbers until ECG pacer spikes are seen that correspond to the patient's intrinsic rhythm, regardless of their capture. This level is the *sensing threshold* of the pacer. The pace indicator light (if the machine has one) should also flash. For *demand pacing* the sensing should be set at a level halfway between the oversensing point and the sensing threshold. This level should be recorded. Keep in mind that pacers can fail to sense when the sensitivity setting on the pacer is too low, when the lead is malpositioned, or when the intrinsic signal is of poor quality.

Once pacing is performing effectively, the length of wire that has been inserted transvenously should be recorded. Secure the electrode catheter to the skin with two sutures at two sites.

Confirmation of Lead Placement

1. A cross-table lateral and anteroposterior chest radiograph should be ordered. Pneumothorax should be ruled out. The tip of the catheter should be at the distal RV, in the apex, with no loops, kinks, or doublings. On the lateral view, the pacer should be to the left of the spine and slightly inferior and anterior, retrosternally.
2. A 12-lead ECG should demonstrate the expected left bundle branch block pattern because of the origination of electrical current in the RV (Fig. 232.8).
3. The pacer pulse generator should be secured to the bed, not the patient, for at least 24 hours. It should be covered to prevent inadvertent damage to the controls.

While a temporary pacer is in place, the patient's rhythm should be monitored and a hardwire or telemetry rhythm strip should be recorded frequently. Patients should be restricted to bed rest for at least 24 hours. Aseptic technique must be maintained when the catheter is handled, and appropriate skin care should be ordered. Sterile dressing changes should follow the intensive care unit's central venous line protocol. Unnecessary catheter manipulations should be avoided. Pacemaker function should be checked daily with a 12-lead ECG. A change in the morphology of the paced QRS on the 12-lead ECG may be the first sign of electrode displacement. Daily physical examination for friction rubs (a clue to perforation) or clicking noises (muscle stimulation) must be documented. Pacing threshold should also be determined daily and documented.

Troubleshooting: Failure to Pace

Failure to pace can occur for a variety of reasons, including—but not limited to—a faulty battery, dislodged or malpositioned leads,

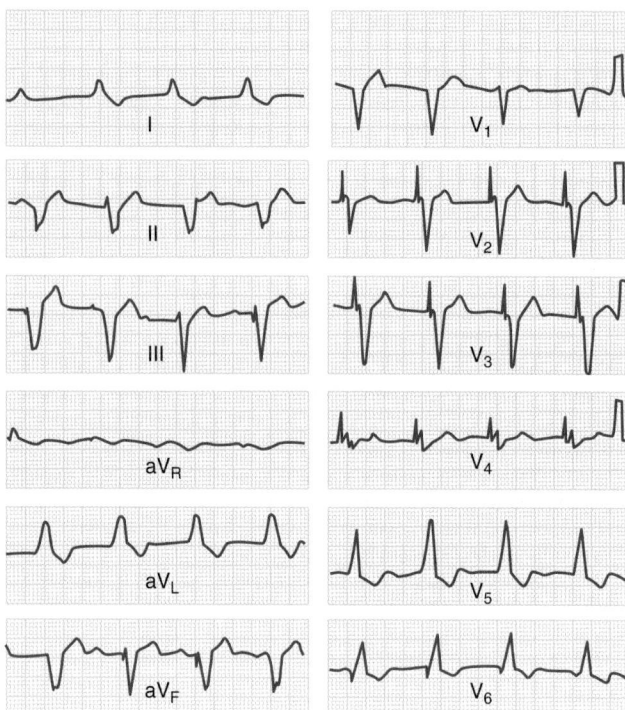

Fig. 232.8 Finished product: 12-lead electrocardiogram with pacer in place. (From Morelli RL, Goldschlager N. Temporary transvenous pacing: resolving postinsertion problems. *J Crit Illness.* 1987;2[3]:71.)

a loose connection, a damaged or fractured wire, electronic interference, or a faulty pacer. Some cardiac conditions cause very high pacing thresholds or preclude intrinsic pacing, including myocardial fibrosis or ischemia, drug toxicity from cardiac agents, myocardial perforation, and ventricular refractoriness from a low-grade, unsensed, intrinsic QRS complex.

If the pacer fails to work after it had been functioning previously, several questions should be considered: Has the catheter become dislodged? Are the wires loose or disconnected? Are the pacemaker settings correct? Has the battery failed? Is there electrical interference? Has the ventricle been perforated as a result of synchronous diaphragmatic or intracostal muscle contractions?

In an emergency situation, consider increasing the stimulation or pacing threshold to regain capture. Occasionally the area in the heart near the electrode has become fibrotic, requiring a higher stimulation. Also, the catheter tip could have become partially dislodged. If the problem is oversensing, that threshold should be reset.

If all else fails, another emergency maneuver is to switch the polarity of the pacer lead connections. Occasionally this technique will regain pacing, although it has not been well documented in the medical literature.

POSTPROCEDURE PATIENT EDUCATION

See the Postprocedure Patient Education section of Chapter 228, Central Venous Catheter Insertion. Also, if a patient will need a permanent pacemaker, see the Online Resources section of this chapter for patient education.

COMPLICATIONS

Most complications are infrequent and usually minor; life-threatening complications are rare. Complications are seen more frequently with emergent pacing, especially in a critically ill patient and when the operator is inexperienced.

- Pacing system dysfunction (18% to 43% of cases for transvenous), including failure to capture or sense the R wave properly. System malfunctions are usually due to problems with connections and lead placement or inappropriate setup of the device.
- Loss of pacing (failure of pacer, lead dislodgement, fracture of pacer wire).
- Failure to recognize that the pacer is not capturing or pacing.
- Pericardial friction rub, endocardial structural damage, myocardial damage, or infarction.
- Arrhythmia.
- Diaphragmatic stimulation; chest wall stimulation.

External (Transcutaneous)

- Failure to recognize the presence of underlying treatable ventricular fibrillation.
- Prolonged use is often associated with leads becoming dislodged; occasionally prolonged pacing is associated with a change in pacing threshold, requiring an increased pacing current.
- Third-degree burns have been reported in children, even when large electrodes were used. The risk of a burn increases if the electrodes are placed improperly or if prolonged pacing is necessary.

Internal (Transvenous)

Complications include the same as those for central venous line insertion; see Chapter 228, Central Venous Catheter Insertion.

- Infection, including bacteremia and septicemia (up to 20% of patients developed microbiologically confirmed septicemia when the pacing wire was left in place >48 hours, and this increases the risk of infection when a permanent pacemaker is placed).
- Interventricular septum or right ventricular perforation, with or without cardiac tamponade.
- Arterial or venous injury, including phlebitis and thrombosis (incidence is higher than expected).
- Pulmonary embolism.
- Air embolism.
- Electrical hazards (any extraneous currents, even microcurrents, can cause ventricular fibrillation if applied to a transvenous pacemaker catheter).

PATIENT EDUCATION GUIDES

See the sample patient education form available at www.expertconsult.com.

CPT/BILLING CODES

33210   Insertion or replacement of temporary transvenous single chamber cardiac electrode or pacemaker catheter
36556   Insertion of nontunneled centrally inserted central venous catheter, over age 5
92953   Temporary transcutaneous pacing

ICD-10-CM DIAGNOSTIC CODES

I21.09   ST elevation myocardial infarction other coronary artery of anterior wall

I21.19   ST elevation myocardial infarction other coronary artery of inferior wall

I21.29   ST elevation myocardial infarction involving other sites
I21.4   Non-ST elevation myocardial infarction
I44.2   Atrioventricular block, complete or third-degree heart block
I44.60   Left bundle branch hemiblock
I44.69   Left bundle branch block, complete
I45.10   Right bundle branch block
I44.0   First-degree atrioventricular block
I44.1   Mobitz type II block
I44.1   Other second-degree atrioventricular block, including Mobitz type I (Wenckebach's)
I45.2   Bifascicular or bilateral bundle branch block
I46.9   Cardiac arrest or asystole
I49.5   Sinoatrial node dysfunction or sinus bradycardia, persistent, severe, or sick sinus syndrome

Acknowledgment

The editors recognize the contributions of Len Scarpinato, DO, to this chapter in previous editions of this text.

SUPPLIERS

(See contact information available at www.expertconsult.com.)

See suppliers of pulmonary artery (Swan-Ganz) catheters, as well as the following:

Biosense Webster
Medtronic
St. Jude Medical

ONLINE RESOURCES

American Heart Association: www.heart.org (Information regarding temporary and permanent pacemakers)
Patient information: www.guidant.com (Guidant); www.medtronic.com (Medtronic); www.biotronik.com (Biotronic); www.sjm.com (St. Jude Medical)

RECOMMENDED READING

American Heart Association. *Advanced Cardiovascular Life Support Provider Manual.* Dallas: American Heart Association; 2015.
Dahlberg ST, Mooradd MG. Temporary cardiac pacing. In: Irwin RS, Cerra FB, Rippe JM, eds. *Irwin and Rippe's Intensive Care Medicine.* 7th ed. Philadelphia: Lippincott Williams & Wilkins; 2011.
Davis WR. Temporary cardiac pacemakers. In: Civetta JM, Taylor RW, Kirby RR, eds. *Critical Care.* 4th ed. Philadelphia: Lippincott Raven; 2009.
Larabee TM. Transcutaneous cardiac pacing. In: Reichman EF, ed. *Emergency Medicine Procedures.* 2nd ed. New York: McGraw-Hill; 2013:197–202.
Levine MD, Brown DFM. *Heart block, Third Degree;* 2009. www.emedicine.com/EMERG/topic235.htm.
Ferguson JD, Banning AP, Bashir Y. Randomised trial of temporary cardiac pacing with semirigid and balloon-flotation electrode catheters. *Lancet.* 1997;349:1883.
Francis GC, Williams SV, Achord JL, et al. Clinical competence in insertion of a temporary transvenous ventricular pacemaker: a statement for physicians from the ACP/ACC/AHA Task Force on Clinical Privileges in Cardiology. *Circulation.* 1994;89:1913.
Reichman EF, McClelland MC, Euerle B. Transvenous cardiac pacing. In: Reichman EF, ed. *Emergency Medicine Procedures.* 2nd ed. New York: McGraw-Hill; 2013:205–212.

CHAPTER 233

DRAWING BLOOD CULTURES

Theodore O'Connell

Bacteremia and septicemia are potentially life-threatening conditions caused by a variety of microorganisms. The successful isolation of microorganisms from blood requires an understanding of the intermittent nature of most bacteremias; the low order of magnitude of most bacteremias; the great variety of organisms capable of causing septicemia; inherent differences between aerobic, anaerobic, and fungal infections; and how to avoid contamination of the cultures obtained.

Consideration must first be given to the patient's clinical status. Indications for obtaining blood cultures are outlined later. Note that 25% of patients with documented bacteremia have periods without fever. In the elderly population, the proportion is even higher, with 50% of bacteremic patients older than 65 years of age being afebrile.

Because most bacteremias are intermittent, blood collections for culture ideally should be made intermittently during a 24-hour period. Two separate blood culture sets should be collected within a 24-hour period. However, if urgent administration of antibiotics is clinically indicated, two sets of cultures from two different sites should be obtained, separated by 20 to 30 minutes if possible. Cultures should also be obtained through any vascular access devices that have been in place at least 48 hours. Occasionally, three or four sets of blood cultures are indicated (Table 233.1). Increasing the number of sets improve not only sensitivity (an individual set is typically not more than 80% sensitive) but also specificity. Specificity is especially improved for microbes that can act as both a contaminant and a pathogen; microbes that appear in all sets are much more likely a pathogen, whereas microbes appearing in only some are more likely a contaminant. Each set of cultures should have two bottles—one aerobic and one anaerobic bottle.

Most bacteremias are of a very low magnitude, so an adequate volume of blood should be collected for each set of cultures. Small children usually have higher numbers (concentrations) of bacteria in the blood than adults, which means that smaller quantities of blood may be obtained from children. Appropriate volumes are noted in Table 233.2. At least 20 mL of blood should be obtained in adults; if short, use at least 10 mL for the aerobic bottle. In general, fungi are difficult to isolate in blood cultures, and it may take 4 to 6 weeks to obtain a positive result. If fungi are suspected, it is probably best to discuss which techniques to use with an infectious disease expert or the lab.

In the past, authorities argued that the primary source of contamination was in the laboratory processing of specimens; however, the current consensus is that the most common source is the process of phlebotomy and inoculation of blood culture bottles. This makes all the steps listed below vital to the process.

INDICATIONS

- Fever and unexplained alterations in mental status, functional status, or autonomic status in a previously healthy patient
- Fever and no source of infection, especially in a patient younger than 2 years of age or older than 65 years of age, or immunocompromised
- Fever of unknown origin
- All febrile infants younger than 2 months of age
- Persistent rigors, with or without fever
- Fever, or no fever in a patient with a toxic or "septic" appearance (including unexplained hypotension, altered mental status, or shock)
- Fever, or no fever and possible infectious endocarditis (hematuria and elevated sedimentation rate)
- Serious focal infections such as meningitis, septic arthritis, and osteomyelitis
- Patients with pneumonia or pyelonephritis and need for hospitalization or with signs of toxicity

NOTE: with widespread use of pneumococcal conjugate and *Haemophilus influenza* type B vaccines, the incidence of occult bacteremia in otherwise well-appearing febrile children is probably less than 1%. This may eventually change the recommended management of febrile children younger than 2 years old, perhaps decreasing the need for blood cultures. On the other hand, more regulatory agencies are mandating blood cultures in all patients being evaluated for pneumonia, which has dramatically increased the number of cultures obtained.

CONTRAINDICATIONS

There are essentially no contraindications to drawing blood cultures; however, blood should not be drawn through infected skin sites. When intravenous sampling is impossible, intraosseous sampling is acceptable (see Chapter 226, Intraosseous Vascular Access).

TABLE 233.1	Number of Blood Culture Sets to Be Obtained in Various Clinical Situations in Adults
Number of Sets	**Clinical Context**
Two sets	Pretest likelihood is low to moderate.
Three sets	Skin contaminants are a possible cause of the infectious process; the pretest probability of bacteremia is high or infectious endocarditis is a consideration but with a low to moderate pretest probability.
Four sets	Infectious endocarditis *and* either moderate to high pretest probability, or the patient has recently been taking antibiotics

TABLE 233.2	Optimal Specimen Volumes to Be Drawn per Blood Culture Set
Age Group	**Ideal Volume Per Set (mL)**
Neonates	1–2
Infants 5–10 kg	2–4
Children 7–20 kg	3–8
Children 20–40 kg	10
Children >40 kg	20–30
Adults	20–30

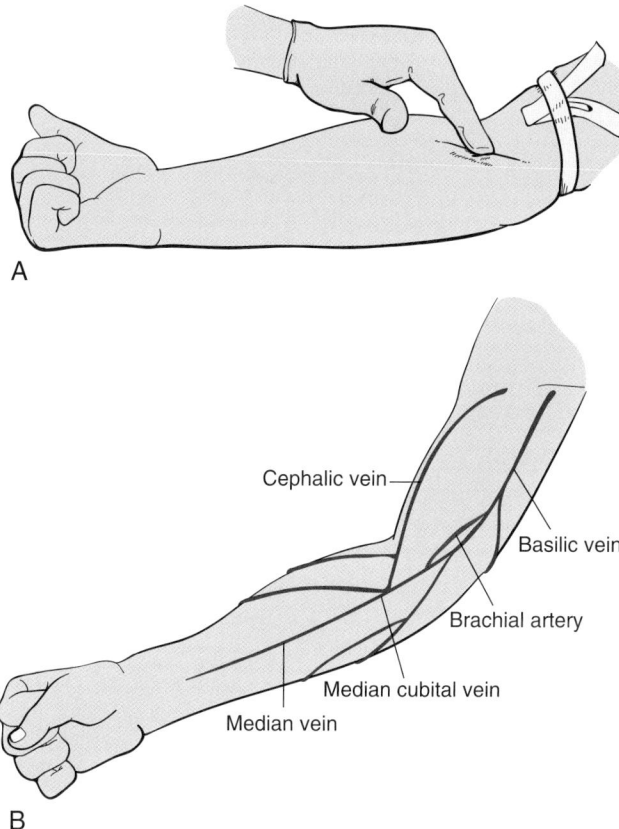

Fig. 233.1 Venipuncture. (A) After the tourniquet is applied, the vein is located. (B) Veins in arm.

EQUIPMENT

- Alcohol pads
- 2% tincture of iodine in 70% alcohol (alternatively, 2% iodine solution or 10% povidone-iodine [Betadine] may be used)
- Chlorhexidine (Hibiclens) for the iodine-allergic patient
- Tourniquet
- Gloves and any equipment needed to follow universal blood and body fluid precautions
- 21-gauge needle
- 30-mL syringe
- Set of blood culture bottles, aerobic and anaerobic, with labels

PREPROCEDURE PATIENT PREPARATION

Drawing blood for culture does not entail any more risk than drawing blood for any other purpose. Patients should be warned about the needlestick and the potential for bleeding, bruising, and infection. Written consent for this procedure is not necessary.

TECHNIQUE

1. Complete the laboratory order or request form and explain the procedure to the patient.
2. Apply the tourniquet and determine the location of the vein to be used for venipuncture (Fig. 233.1).
3. Cleanse the skin with alcohol swabs three times or until pads are free of surface dirt.
4. Allow the skin to dry.
5. Apply iodine three times in centrifugal circles from the anticipated site of venipuncture.

6. After the third swab, allow to dry at least 60 seconds.
7. Remove the protective cap and cleanse the top of the culture bottles with iodine, alcohol swabs, or both.
8. Wipe off dry iodine at the venipuncture site with alcohol swabs. Do not palpate the vein or the area where the needle will be inserted after disinfecting the site. Clinicians should follow universal blood and body fluid precautions.
9. Obtain the required volume of blood (see Table 233.1 for recommended blood volumes by patient size).
10. Immediately apply pressure to the puncture site (after removing the needle) with a clean cotton sponge.
11. Place up to 10 mL of blood in each culture bottle. (These two bottles constitute one blood culture set.)
12. Inoculate both bottles without changing needles.
13. Repeat at different sites or different times for the requisite number of blood culture sets.
14. Transport the blood cultures as soon as possible to start the incubating process.
15. Specimens need to be held for an extended duration when culturing blood for fungi or fastidious bacteria.

COMPLICATIONS

- Bleeding
- Bruising
- Infection
- False positive or negative results

INTERPRETATION OF RESULTS

In the case of a positive blood culture, the offending organism(s) are identified. If sensitivities have been ordered, the antibiotic susceptibility or resistance is reported.

One of the more challenging aspects of interpreting blood culture results is determining which positive blood cultures are actually false-positive results. Features of false-positive blood cultures are outlined as follows:

- Coagulase-negative staphylococci (*Staphylococcus epidermidis*) and *Streptococcus viridans* in a single bottle in patients not suspected of having infectious endocarditis and without chronic indwelling intravenous catheters are usually contaminants.
- *Corynebacterium, Propionibacterium acnes,* and *Bacillus* species are usually contaminants, but they can be pathogens in immunocompromised hosts.
- Multiple organisms growing from the same bottle suggests contamination.
- Species that grow out after a prolonged culture have a greater likelihood of being contaminants.
- The patient's symptoms have resolved or are inconsistent with sepsis. However, special consideration must be given to infectious endocarditis, which can have an indolent course.
- A primary infected source, such as urine, yields a different pathogenic isolate.

Another challenge with obtaining blood cultures is that anaerobic infections tend to occur in areas that are isolated from the bloodstream, such as poorly perfused tissue or locations that frequently evolve into abscesses. This phenomenon decreases the likelihood of detection by blood culture. Consequently, anaerobic cultures only account for 0.5% to 12% of positive blood cultures. For that reason, the clinician would not want to decrease the sensitivity of the aerobic culture if not enough blood is available; top priority should be placed on putting at least 10 mL in the aerobic culture bottle. In fact, some experts suggest that anaerobic cultures may not be needed unless the patient is at high risk of anaerobic bacteremia (Table 233.3).

TABLE 233.3	Clinical Settings at Higher Risk for Anaerobic Bacteremia
Number of Sets	**Clinical Context**
Infectious foci	Abdominal or pelvic infections
	Soft tissue or wound infections (e.g., myofasciitis)
	Sepsis with decubitus ulcers or necrotic tissue
	Aspiration pneumonia
	Odontogenic (dental) head and neck infections
Predisposing clinical features	Malignancy
	Immunosuppressive medications
	Recent abdominal or pelvic surgery
	Diabetes

CPT/Billing Codes

If cultures are grown in the office and organisms identified, laboratory codes are as follows:

87040	Culture, bacterial; blood, aerobic, with isolation and presumptive identification of isolates (includes anaerobic culture, if appropriate)
87103	Culture, fungi (mold or yeast) isolation, with presumptive identification of isolates, blood

There is no specific code for drawing blood. Add laboratory handling fee (99000) to office visit.

ICD-10-CM Diagnostic Codes

A40.9	Septicemia, streptococcal
A40.3	Septicemia, pneumococcal
A41.4	Septicemia, anaerobic
A41.9	Septicemia, unspecified
P36.8	Other bacterial sepsis of newborn
R78.81	Bacteremia

Suppliers

(See contact information available at www.expertconsult.com.)

BacT/Alert blood culture bottles
  Organon Teknika Biomerieux

Recommended Reading

Little JR, Murray PR, Traynor PS, Spitznagel E. A randomized trial of povidone-iodine compared with iodine tincture for venipuncture site disinfection: effects on rates of blood culture contamination. *Am J Med.* 1999;107:119–125.

Mandell GL, Bennett JE, Dolin R, eds. *Principles and Practice of Infectious Diseases.* 8th ed. New York: Churchill Livingstone; 2015.

Mimoz O, Karim A, Mercat A. Chlorhexidine compared with povidone-iodine as skin preparation before blood culture: a randomized, controlled trial. *Ann Intern Med.* 1999;131:834–837.

Roberts JR, Custalow CB, Thomsen TW, eds. *Roberts and Hedges' Clinical Procedures in Emergency Medicine.* 6th ed. Philadelphia: Elsevier; 2014.

CHAPTER 234

BLOOD PRODUCTS AND BLOOD BANKING

Graham V. Segal • M. Amer Wahed

Transfusion of blood and blood components is common in hospitals and emergency departments in the United States; 15 million blood donations take place per year and 14 million units of red blood cells are transfused. A working knowledge of what happens in the blood band and the necessary process for a transfusion is valuable for a primary care clinician working in an urgent care center, emergency department, or as a hospitalist. Knowledge of the different blood products available, their indications, as well as the possible complications from transfusions is also useful.

There are several blood bank tests that are routinely performed in a blood bank. These include ABO/Rh typing, antibody screen, and crossmatching. ABO typing is performed using two methods, and the conclusion of both methods should be the same. If not, additional testing will be required to resolve the discrepancy. An antibody screen is done to check for the presence of preformed antibodies against red blood cell (RBC) antigens. These antibodies of the patient may react with antigens of the transfused RBCs and cause hemolysis. If the antibody screen is positive, then additional tests will be performed to identify the antibody.

If the blood bank is a donor center, then several other tests are also performed on the donor's blood prior to it being released for general use. These tests are primarily to screen for transmissible infectious diseases. Donor blood is tested for hepatitis B, hepatitis C, HIV-1 and -2, HTLV-I and -II, *Treponema pallidum*, *Trypanosoma cruzi*, and West Nile virus. Since 1991, nucleic acid amplitude tests have been mandatory to screen for hepatitis C RNA; the American Association of Blood Bank (AABB) reports the risk of transmission is now less than 1 in a million transfusions. If the donor tests positive for any of these, the donor status is deferred and the blood is discarded. If test results are negative, the blood is released for further transfusion.

During transfusion, if there is evidence or suspicion of transfusion reaction (TR), then the transfusion is stopped and the clinical team initiates a TR workup. The blood component that was being transfused will be returned to the blood bank. The blood bank then conducts certain tests to address the issue.

To provide safe blood and avoid preventable risks associated with blood transfusions, all routine transfusion medicine services, starting with blood donation, testing, processing, and providing blood and blood products, and ending with administration and reporting adverse events are highly regulated by the Code of Federal Regulations and AABB Standards for Blood Banks and Transfusion Services.

SAMPLE COLLECTION

Since misidentification of the patient for blood products may have serious consequences, strict procedural steps must be followed. Blood sample collection should be performed directly by the phlebotomist/nurse after correct patient identification by full name and hospital identification number (attached wristband). The blood sample should be labeled at bedside. Tubes should not be prelabeled. Each patient has a red arm band with a unique blood bank identification number. This number should be included as part of the labeling of the tube. Acceptable tubes for blood bank testing are siliconized plain tubes (red top) with no additives or tubes with potassium ethylenediaminetetraacetic acid (K2EDTA) as an anticoagulant (purple top). Since purple top tubes are also used for a CBC, pink tubes with the same anticoagulant may be used for samples destined for the blood bank. Samples should be collected within less than 72 hours from a scheduled transfusion; otherwise complement dependent antibodies may be missed due to complement becoming unstable. New blood samples from recipients are needed for repeat pretransfusion testing every 72 hours if new transfusion orders are made. The age of the samples may be extended to up to a month in certain clinical settings, such as preoperative evaluation of elective surgery patients if they have a negative antibody screen and no RBC exposure via pregnancy or blood transfusions within the past 3 months. Blood samples may be rejected, and examples of reasons include improper labeling, inadequate amount, and hemolyzed sample. If both clerical check and samples are acceptable, the specimen is processed by immediate centrifugation and the RBCs and supernatant separated. Documentation of all steps from receipt of specimen to testing and result interpretation is performed manually or electronically, and records are kept confidential for a period of time in accordance with requirements of federal, state, and accrediting agencies.

ABO/RH(D) TYPING

Determination of the ABO blood group is performed in two steps: a forward and a reverse reaction. In the forward reaction, the presence of the A or/and B antigens is determined by mixing the RBCs to be tested with anti-A and anti-B reagents. If there is a reaction with only anti-A, then the patient has the A antigen on the red cells. His or her ABO blood group is A. If there is reaction with anti-B, then the patient has the B antigen. His or her blood group is B. If there is reaction with both anti-A and anti-B, then the patient has both AB antigens. His or her ABO blood group is AB. If there is no reaction, then the patient has neither A or B antigens. Thus his or her ABO blood group is O.

In the reverse reaction, the serum of the patient is mixed with reagent RBCs of A1 and B types to detect the presence of anti-A1 and anti-B antibodies. If there is reaction with A1 cells, then the patient has an anti-A1 antibody. If the patient has anti-A1 antibody, then he/she cannot have the A antigen. If there is reaction with B cells, then the patient has anti-B antibody. If the patient has anti-B antibody, then he/she cannot have the B antigen. Thus an individual with blood group A will have anti-B antibody. An individual with blood group B will have anti-A1 antibody. An individual with blood group AB will have none of the antibodies, and finally an individual with blood group O will have both the antibodies. If the forward and the reverse reaction lead to different conclusions regarding the ABO type, reaction strength is weaker than expected, and/or the historical blood type does not match the current one, the cause for the discrepancy must be fully investigated for a final interpretation of the ABO blood group type.

"Rh typing" is a misnomer because it does not involve phenotyping for all major antigens belonging to the Rh system, but only for the D antigen, the most immunogenic of all. The Rh or D type is determined in a similar was as the forward ABO typing, using anti-D reagent. Blood donors who type Rh-negative (D-negative) are further tested to detect the presence of so-called weak D antigen (Du) using more sensitive methods, such as the presence of antihuman globulin (AHG), which acts as an enhancer of the reaction between the D antigen and the anti-D reagent.

Determination of the weak D is required only for blood donors to establish the true D status and is performed by testing patient's RBCs IgG anti-D in AHG phase. If the weak D testing is positive, the Rh(D) type is interpreted as Rh(D)-positive, and if negative, the Rh(D) type is interpreted as a true negative. The weak D status is neither required nor routinely determined in recipients since Rh(D)-negative blood is safe to be transfused regardless of the true Rh(D) status of recipient. The presence of other antigens belonging to the Rh blood group is not determined for routine transfusions.

RED BLOOD CELL ANTIGENS AND ANTIBODIES

The Antibody Screen

There are more than 230 types of antigens present on the surface of RBCs, based on their chemical structures, and these can be grouped in two major categories: carbohydrates or polypeptides. The RBC antigens are encoded by specific genes and categorized into blood groups systems. Major blood group systems are ABO, Rh, Kell, Kidd, Duffy, Lutheran, and MNS.

Antigens belonging to the ABO, Lewis, I, and P blood system are carbohydrate in nature. Antibodies that are formed against these antigens do not require sensitization by prior RBC exposure. They are thus called naturally occurring antibodies. They are typically IgM in nature and are considered clinically insignificant, as they are not associated with hemolytic TRs or hemolytic disease of the newborn. A major exception to this is the antibodies formed against the antigens of the ABO blood group system. Antibodies to the ABO antigens are naturally occurring but clinically significant. In contrast, antigens belonging to the Rh, Kell, Kidd, Duffy, Lutheran, and MNS system are typically IgG in nature and are considered clinically significant, as they are associated with hemolytic TRs and hemolytic disease of the newborn. Antibody formation requires prior exposure to RBCs that possess these antigens. Prior exposure may be due to prior transfusion or pregnancy. An exception to this is anti-M and anti-N antibodies are typically clinically insignificant.

The antibody screen is performed by mixing the patient's plasma with three reagent RBCs with a known phenotype present in a commercially available kit containing a table of the antigenic profiles of RBC used, called *antigram*. For routine pretransfusion testing, the AABB requires that reagent RBC present in the antibody screen should contain at least one homozygous RBC positive for the following major RBC antigens: C, c, D, E, e, Fy^a, Fy^b, Jk^a, Jk^b, K, k, Le^a, Le^b, P_1, M, N, S, and s antigens. If the patient's plasma contains allo-antibodies against major RBC antigens, the antibody screen becomes positive and further testing by extended panel is required.

The antibody screen and panel are both indirect AHG tests performed with reagent RBCs prepared from donor of type O so that the naturally occurring anti-A or anti-B antibodies would not interfere with the testing. A positive antibody screen implies that recipient plasma might react with antigens present on the donor's red cell membrane. Additional tests will be required to determine the specificity of the antibody. A positive antibody screen can be seen if the patient has underlying alloantibodies or autoantibodies.

The blood bank needs to determine if the underlying antibody is an autoantibody or an alloantibody. If the antibody is an autoantibody, it needs to be determined whether the antibody is a warm autoantibody or a cold antibody. If the underlying antibody is an alloantibody, then the blood bank needs to determine the specificity of the antibody (i.e., the antigen against which the antibody is directed). If the alloantibody is a clinically significant one, then the blood bank must obtain blood from a donor which lacks that specific antigen to avoid hemolytic TRs.

Antibody Identification by Extended (Panel) Testing

Positive antibody screens require further testing by testing the patient's plasma against a panel of 10 to 12 RBCs (commercially available) of varying phenotypes. The identification of antibody specificity is done in two steps. In the first step, we identify RBCs that produce no reaction when tested with the patient's plasma. We may assume that if the patient's plasma had an antibody that is specific to the antigens present on these red cells, then there should have been a reaction. Since there is no reaction, then the patient's plasma does not have antibodies corresponding to the antigens present on these red cells. Thus several potential antibodies can be ruled out. In the next step, called "ruling in," the plasma reactivity pattern is compared with the profile of antigens across all cell lines. If at least three cell lines react with the patient's plasma, there is a 95% chance that the reactivity is due to an antibody corresponding to that antigen. Antibodies against major RBC antigens should be ruled out, and any additional reactivity should be explained, if possible. However, often, even if the major allo-antibodies are ruled out, an extra weak reactivity might still be present. The clinical significance of this weakly reactive nonspecific (WRNS) antibody is most likely limited if the patient does not have a history of prior RBC exposure, in which case crossmatch compatible RBC units are provided for the patient. However, if the patient had prior RBC sensitization via pregnancy or recent transfusion, the clinical significance of RBC is indeterminate, meaning that the developing allo-antibody with partial reactivity cannot be completely ruled out. In this case, additional testing, including determination of patient's RBC phenotype, may be indicated, and the safest blood to be provided for that patient would match the patient's profile.

Occasionally plasma reacts with all reagent RBCs tested (panreactivity), so if no negative reactions occur, the process of ruling out antibodies against major RBC antigens cannot be performed. The main differential diagnoses in such cases are autoantibodies, antibody against a high incidence antigen, and multiple antibodies. When plasma reacts with all reagent RBCs and the patient's own (positive autocontrol), an auto-antibody is suspected. Autoantibodies may be of warm type or cold type. With autoantibodies being present, it may not be possible to rule out underlying alloantibodies. In such situations, the patient's RBCs are phenotyped. This means the patient's RBC is tested for the presence of the major antigens. If we provide blood that is matched with the patient's RBC antigens, then even if the patient has any antibody, there should not be any corresponding antigen in the donor blood for it to react with. This is referred to as providing phenotypically matched blood.

Implications of Having Antibodies

Once an antibody is identified, a decision is made whether it belongs to a clinically significant class or not. If it belongs to a clinically significant class, then the patient must receive that particular antigen negative blood. Some antigens are quite prevalent in the donor population and some less so. Blood bank may require additional time to find blood that is negative for that particular antigen. This may be a significant problem if someone has multiple clinically significant antibodies.

TABLE 234.1	Blood Component Transfusion in a Bleeding Patient				
	PRBC	**FFP**	**Platelets**	**Cryoprecipitate**	
Threshold for transfusion	Hgb < 8–10 g/dL	INR > 1.5	<10,000 without bleeding; <50,000 with bleeding	Fibrinogen <100 mg/dL; uremic thrombocytopathia	
Dose (one)	One unit	Two single units or one jumbo FFP; 10–20 mL/kg	4–6 single units; one apheresis unit	10 units	
Expected rise post transfusion of one dose	Hgb by 1 g/dL or Hct by 3%	Unpredictable	30,000–60,000	Increase in fibrinogen by at least 50 mg/dL	

FFP, Fresh frozen plasma, *Hct*, hematocrit; *Hgb*, hemoglobin; *INR*, international normalized ratio; *PRBC*, packed red blood cells.

If a patient possesses a clinically insignificant antibody, such as a Lewis antibody, the blood bank will not try to find Lewis antigen negative blood. It will only provide crossmatch compatible blood.

CROSSMATCHING

There are two different types of crossmatch that can take place. One is the serologic crossmatch, which tests the blood compatibility between recipient and potential donor. It also serves to reconfirm the ABO type of the donor, and thus is a checkpoint for preventing ABO typing errors. There are two types of serologic crossmatch: major and minor. In the *major crossmatch*, the patient's plasma is tested against donor RBCs obtained from a segment of the blood product. The major crossmatch aims to detect whether the transfused RBCs will react with any antibody in the patient's blood and thus lead to hemolysis. The *minor crossmatch*, when the patient's RBCs are tested against donor's plasma to look for antibodies in the donor plasma that would react with patient's red cells, has been discontinued.

The method of performing the major crossmatch depends on the results of the antibody screen. If the antibody screen is negative and the patient does not have a history of clinically significant antibodies, the major crossmatch performed is only in immediate spin phase, so-called *incomplete crossmatch*. If the antibody screen is positive, the major crossmatch is performed in the AHG phase with selected antigen-negative RBC units.

The second method of crossmatch is the "computer crossmatch" or electronic crossmatch, wherein the ABO types of both donor and recipient are electronically confirmed and assessed for ABO compatibility by AABB-approved computer software, which is also acceptable when certain regulatory conditions are met.

BLOOD COMPONENTS

(See Table 234.1 for guidelines to transfuse various blood components in a bleeding patient, and Table 234.2 for when to transfuse blood components based on lab results.)

Whole Blood

Whole blood obtained from donors is typically separated into components; it is rarely used for transfusion directly. One reason is that the incidence of TRs following whole blood transfusion is approximately 2.5 times greater than with packed red blood cells (PRBCs). Whole blood also contains antigenic leukocytes and serum proteins that carry a higher risk for an allergic reaction (approximately 1%). However, some blood banks still stock units of whole blood for trauma cases. Warm whole blood has also recently seen an increase in popularity in military settings and others for massive transfusion protocols. Massive blood loss is typically defined as in the range of 30% to 40% or more of loss of blood volume. Whole blood is also used for exchange transfusion in neonates. However, in such situations, whole blood is made available by reconstitution by combining RBCs with FFP. Whole blood may also be used for autologous transfusions. If used, whole blood must be ABO identical to that of the patient. With storage, levels of labile coagulation factors diminish, as well as functional platelets.

TABLE 234.2	Use of Laboratory Evidence for Transfusion of Blood Components		
	CBC	**DIC Screen**	**TEG**
PRBCs	Low Hgb/Hct	NA	NA
FFP	NA	Prolonged PT/PTT. If TT is prolonged with normal fibrinogen levels, heparin may be an issue	TEG R value is prolonged. With heparinase, TEG R value does not decrease
Platelets	Low platelets	NA	TEG MA and angle alpha values are low
Cryoprecipitate	NA	Fibrinogen levels are low	TEG angle alpha value is low

CBC, Complete blood count; *DIC*, disseminated intravascular coagulation; *FFP*, fresh frozen plasma; *Hct*, hematocrit; *Hgb*, hemoglobin; *MA*, maximal amplitude; *NA*, not applicable; *PRBC*, packed red blood cells; *PT*, prothrombin time; *PTT*, partial thromboplastin time; *TEG*, thromboelastogram; *TT*, thromboplastin time.

Packed Red Blood Cells

PRBCs are the most commonly used blood component. PRBCs are prepared from whole blood by centrifugation or by apheresis collection and typically contain less sodium, potassium, ammonia, citrate, hydrogen ions, and antigenic protein than whole blood. This may be beneficial in patients with impaired renal, cardiovascular, or hepatic function. Typically one unit of PRBCs is approximately 350 mL in volume, of which RBC volume is 200 to 250 mL. The remaining volume is due to plasma (typically less than 50 mL), WBCs, platelets, and anticoagulants. The most commonly used anticoagulant is CPDA-1 (citrate, phosphate, dextrose, adenine), which allows for 35 days storage at 1° to 6°C. The hematocrit of such units is less than 80% (range 70% to 80%).

In the United States, most centers provide leukoreduced PRBCs. This is done by leukocyte reduction filters and done before storage. Residual leukocytes should not exceed 5 × 106 per unit. Leukocyte reduced units decrease alloimmunization and reduce chances of febrile nonhemolytic TRs. Leukocyte reduced units are also considered to be cytomegalovirus safe and can be given to cytomegalovirus-negative individuals.

In a nonemergency setting, PRBCs should be transfused at a rate of 1 to 2 mL/min for the first 15 minutes and then increased to 4 mL/min or as rapidly as the patient can tolerate. Transfusion should not exceed 4 hours. Potential life-threatening reactions most commonly occur within the first 15 minutes. In an emergency setting, PRBCs may be transfused at fast rates, and multiple units may need to be transfused. Massive RBC transfusions are defined as >10 units, but with such a transfusion, there is significant risk for metabolic and respiratory acidosis as well as hypocalcemia. Transfusion associated hypothermia and hyperkalemia are also recognized side effects of such a large transfusion.

Each unit of PRBC is expected to increase the hematocrit by 3% and hemoglobin level by 1g/dL. This effect can be measured 15 minutes after transfusion. In a bleeding patient, it must be kept in mind that transfusion of multiple units of PRBC will aggravate the coagulopathic state of the patient.

The unit of PRBC that is being transfused must be compatible with the recipient's plasma ABO antibodies. Thus if the recipient is blood group A, he/she has anti-B antibodies and cannot be transfused with B or AB units. If the recipient is B, he/she has anti-A antibodies and cannot be transfused with A or AB units. Both A and B patients can receive O units. If the recipient is AB, he/she has no anti-A or anti-B antibodies. Therefore, he/she can receive A, B, AB, or O units. If the recipient is O, he/she has anti-A and anti-B antibodies. He/she can receive only O units.

There are various types of PRBCs that may be made available in special circumstances:

PRBCs leukoreduced: In the United States, most centers provide PRBCs that are leukoreduced. This has decreased the incidence of febrile TRs. Leukoreduced products are also considered to be CMV safe. Leukoreduction also helps to prevent HLA alloimmunization.

PRBCs irradiated: Irradiated cellular products (RBCs and platelets) are used to prevent transfusion associated graft versus host disease (GVHD). Examples of indications for irradiation include transfusion to individuals who are immunodeficient, are on intensive chemotherapy, bone marrow transplant recipients, and Hodgkin disease patients. The maximum storage time after irradiation is 28 days post irradiation or the original expiration time, whichever comes first. Irradiation damages the red cell membranes, and there is increased leakiness of potassium. When irradiated RBCs are to be given to neonates, the unit needs to be washed to remove the excess potassium.

PRBCs washed: Washed PRBCs are generally requested when the patient has history of allergic reactions. Washing is performed with saline and removes plasma proteins and electrolytes. It further removes platelets and leukocytes. However, the unit must be transfused within 24 hours of washing. Washing of PRBCs (and also platelets) may also be done for transfusion to IgA deficient patients. Washing reduces the titers of anti-A and anti-B, thereby permitting safer transfusion of type O PRBCs into non-O recipients.

Frozen RBCs: Sometimes RBCs are frozen to preserve rare donor groups. They can be preserved for up to 10 years. Cryoprotective agents such as glycerol are used to prevent damage to red cells during freezing. When these frozen red cells are thawed for use, the cryoprotective agent (e.g., glycerol) must be removed. This is done by washing, and thus these units must be used within 24 hours.

Fresh Frozen Plasma

Fresh frozen plasma (FFP) is prepared from whole blood by separating and freezing the plasma within 8 hours of phlebotomy.

The approximate volume of 1 unit of FFP is 200 to 250 mL. FFP is stored at −18°C or lower for 1 year. Once thawed, it should be used within 24 hours. Thawed FFP should be stored at 1 to 6°C. One milliliter of FFP contains approximately one unit of coagulant factor activity. FFP is most often given to patients with elevated prothrombin time/international normalized ratio. It should be noted that FFP itself has an INR of approximately 1.3 to 1.4. Thus individuals with an INR of 1.5 or less do not typically need to be transfused with FFP. One conventional dose of FFP in a 70 kg individual is usually considered to be two units of FFP or one jumbo FFP (equivalent to two units of FFP). However, strictly speaking, one dose of FFP is 10 to 20 mL/kg, and this increases coagulation factors by 20%. One unit of FFP also contains about 400 mg of fibrinogen. Thus mild hypofibrinogenemia will improve with FFP transfusion. Since factor VII has a relatively short half-life (about 4 hours), the effect of FFP transfusion on INR values may be short-lived.

Indications for Fresh Frozen Plasma

- Bleeding patients with coagulopathy
- Bleeding patients requiring reversal of warfarin effect
- Correct coagulopathy in anticipation of surgery/invasive procedures

| TABLE 234.3 | Blood Type Compatibility for Fresh Frozen Plasma Transfusion |

	Donor Blood Group A; Donor Has Anti-B Antibody	Donor Blood Group B; Donor Has Anti-A Antibody	Donor Blood Group AB; Donor Has No Antibody	Donor Blood Group O; Donor Has Anti-A and Anti-B Antibody
Recipient blood group A	Safe to transfuse		Safe to transfuse	
Recipient blood group B		Safe to transfuse	Safe to transfuse	
Recipient blood group AB			Safe to transfuse	
Recipient blood group O	Safe to transfuse	Safe to transfuse	Safe to transfuse	Safe to transfuse

- Exchange fluid for therapeutic plasma exchange in certain situations (e.g., therapeutic plasma exchange for thrombotic thrombocytopenic purpura)
- Part of massive transfusion protocol (RBC:FFP should be 1:1)

Choice of FFP:
FFP has donor antibodies. These antibodies should be compatible with the recipient's red cells (Table 234.3).

Plasma Variants

FP24: This is plasma which has been frozen within 24 hours, rather than 8 hours. In this type of plasma factor VIII levels are approximately 20% to 25% less than that of conventional FFP.

Donor retested plasma: Donor retested plasma is a unit of donated FFP that has been held until the donor comes back a second time at least 112 days later. It has reduced infectivity for HIV-1 and 2, HCV, HBV, HTLV-1, and 2.

Solvent detergent–treated plasma: Solvent detergent–treated plasma is a pooled plasma product treated with a solvent and detergent to eliminate lipid-enveloped viruses such as HIV-1 and 2, HBV, HCV, and HTLV-1 and 2.

Cryo-poor plasma: This is the residual plasma that remains after cryoprecipitate has been removed. Cryo-poor fraction of FFP has been used in refractory cases of TTP.

Platelets

One unit of platelet may be derived from one unit of donated whole blood by centrifugation. Whole blood must be centrifuged twice to obtain platelets. The first centrifugation step yields RBCs and platelet rich plasma. The platelet rich plasma is spun again to produce platelets and plasma.

One unit of platelets has at least 5.5×10^{10} platelets, and the volume is 50 mL. This may be stored at 20 to 24°C, for a maximum of 5 days. Since one typical adult dose is six units, these individual units are frequently pooled. If pooled, then they should be used in 4 hours. Platelets may also be washed, just like RBCs, and if washed they should be used within 4 hours.

Platelets may also be obtained by apheresis. One apheresis procedure from one donor will yield at least one dose of platelets. This is equivalent to six units of platelets. The approximate volume is 250 mL to 300 mL. The number of platelets in one apheresis platelets is 3.0×10^{11}. The advantage of apheresis platelets is that the recipient is exposed to one donor for one dose of platelet transfusion, as opposed to six donors. It is possible to obtain more than one (two or three) doses from one donor by apheresis.

Platelets have platelet specific antigens, ABO and HLA antigens. The contaminating RBCs have Rh antigens. However, the amount of contaminating RBCs in one dose of platelets is less than 2 mL of RBCs. Thus crossmatch is not required for platelets.

That said, whenever possible, ABO compatible platelets should be used. With transfusion of ABO incompatible units, there arises two important issues. Firstly, the recipient's antibody against the A or B antigens may reduce platelet survival, as platelets also have ABO antigens. In reality in the majority of cases, this does not appear to be significant. In some individuals, this may be an issue. This is when the antigen expression on the platelets are high and the titers of antibodies in the recipients are also high. In such cases, post transfusion platelet count may be unsatisfactory. This should prompt a trial of group specific platelet transfusion. Secondly, platelets are suspended in plasma. The antibodies present from the donor may in theory react with the antigens on the recipient's red cells and cause hemolysis. This risk of hemolysis with apheresis platelets has been shown to be in the range of 1:3000 to 1:10,000. If this risk is to be minimized then when choosing ABO incompatible platelets, then think of the donor platelets as "plasma" and decide on the most suitable units for transfusion.

D negative individuals should ideally receive platelets from D negative donors. However, in men and postmenopausal women, this is not an issue. If an Rh negative premenopausal woman receives Rh-positive platelets, Rh Ig may be given.

Accumulation of cytokines in stored platelets may result in febrile reactions. For this and to prevent alloimmunization and for CMV negative units, leukocyte reduced platelets may be used.

Indications for Platelets

* Generally indicated for thrombocytopenia and thrombocytopathia

Contraindications for Platelets

* Not indicated for ITP, TTP, DIC
* Platelet transfusion may also be contraindicated in patients with heparin-induced thrombocytopenia

Dose: 1 unit/10 kg; conventionally six units or one apheresis dose. One dose of platelets usually increases the platelet count in a 70 kg person by 30,000 to 60,000/uL.

Threshold for platelet transfusion: For patients who are bleeding, the target platelet count is at least 50,000/uL, preferably closer to 100,000 u/L. This is especially true for intracerebral, ophthalmic, and pulmonary hemorrhage. For patients who are not bleeding, prophylactic platelet transfusion may be considered if count is less than 10,000 u/L. This may be raised to 20,000 u/L if the patient is coagulopathic, on heparin, or with an anatomic lesion likely to bleed.

Platelet refractoriness: When patients receive multiple platelet transfusions, there is a chance that there might occur a less than expected increase in platelet counts. Typically one dose of platelets should increase the platelet count by 30,000 to 60,000. Response to platelet transfusion can be determined by measuring platelet counts 10 minutes or 60 minutes post transfusion. Calculations are done to obtain a corrected count increment (CCI) value. It is considered that if the CCI is less 5000 after two consecutive transfusions, then there exists platelet refractoriness.

Platelet refractoriness is most often due to antibodies against HLA antigens. The recipient is exposed to donor HLA antigens from transfusion of cellular products (RBCs and platelets). This is why leukoreduced products reduce the incidence of HLA alloimmunization. Platelets possess HLA antigens. They possess class I but not class II antigens. Thus antibodies to HLA class I antigens will result in an inadequate rise in platelet count post transfusion. Other causes of platelet refractoriness include DIC, sepsis, fever, splenomegaly, or drugs. In the setting of platelet refractoriness due to HLA antibodies,

HLA-matched platelets may be transfused. HLA matched platelets need to be irradiated to prevent GVHD.

Most individuals have the HPA-1a antigen on the surface of their platelets. HPA-1a is also known as PlA1 antigen. If an individual who lacks this antigen receives platelets from a donor who has the antigen, then there is a chance of antibody formation against the antigen. This will also potentially cause platelet refractoriness to platelet transfusion. This mechanism as a cause of platelet refractoriness is quite rare. Rather, they are more often associated with neonatal alloimmune thrombocytopenia or posttransfusion purpura. The formula for CCI is as follows:

$$CCI = Posttransfusion\ platelet\ count - Pretransfusion\ platelet$$
$$count \times BSA \times 10^{11} / \left(platelets\ transfused \times 10^{11} \right)$$

Modified Platelet Products

Just like PRBCs, platelets can be leukoreduced, irradiated, or washed. If platelets are obtained from whole blood, then one donor of whole blood will provide one sixth of a dose of platelets. The six individual aliquots are sometimes pooled prior to transfusion.

Cryoprecipitate

Cryoprecipitate is obtained from thawing frozen plasma at 4°C followed by centrifugation. It is stored at −18°C or colder for 1 year. Once thawed, it has to be used within 6 hours or within 4 hours if pooled. Cryoprecipitate contains fibrinogen (150 mg/unit), Factor VIII (80 units/unit), Factor XIII (80 units/unit), von Willebrand factor, and fibronectin.

Indications for Cryoprecipitate

* Fibrinogen deficiency
* Factor XIII deficiency
* Uremia

The approximate volume of each unit of cryoprecipitate is 5 to 15 mL. Each unit raises fibrinogen level by 5 mg/dL. The minimum hemostatic level is at least 100 mg/dL. It is prudent for a bleeding patient to aim for 200 mg/dL. One conventional dose of cryoprecipitate is 10 units. Please note, thawed units or doses of cryo are not maintained in blood bank. Thus, once ordered, there is a delay of 20 to 30 minutes before the product can be made available.

Cryoprecipitate can also be used topically and is applied simultaneously with calcium and bovine thrombin to achieve hemostasis. This may, however, lead to formation of antibodies to thrombin and other procoagulant proteins in xenogenic products. This includes factor V. Virus inactivated fibrinogen concentrates are also available, reducing such uses of cryoprecipitate.

RELEASE OF BLOOD PRODUCTS

The process of releasing blood products is initiated when the blood bank receives a request for blood products. This is done by sending a form to blood bank, which contains all the pertinent information, such as patient information (which includes patient identifiers, red arm band number) and the type and number of blood products required. Blood products are selected from the blood bank inventory. The units are labeled with at least two independent patient identifiers, donor unit number, and compatibility test results. The blood components are placed in appropriate transport containers. PRBCs and plasma are placed in coolers, whereas platelets are placed in containers without ice packs. The containers are also labeled with patient information, and the containers are handed over or sent to the patient bedside.

On occasion, there is the necessity for emergency release of blood. In such situations, a physician must initiate the request, and a signed form needs to be sent to blood bank. O Rh negative blood will be sent from blood bank. Blood bank will continue with testing the patient's blood for ABO and RH typing, as well as the antibody screen. Once these are done, the patient can then be switched to the appropriate units.

AUTOLOGOUS BLOOD

Autologous blood may be collected from a patient prior to surgery, at the start of surgery, and during the intraoperative period. Use of autologous blood has the advantage of decreasing obvious risks of blood transfusion such as transmission of infectious diseases, transfusion-related acute lung injury (TRALI), and so on. Blood can be collected from a prospective patient, typically on a weekly schedule and then stored for transfusion during surgery. It is assumed that the patient's iron stores are adequate. If multiple donations are required, an erythropoietin injection may also be given.

Collection of blood just prior to start of surgery and then transfused at the end of surgery is known as acute normovolemic hemodilution. Blood that is lost during surgery can be collected under low vacuum pressure into a reservoir. RBCs in such cases are accompanied by activated clotting factors, platelets, and cellular debris. Anticoagulant is used to prevent the blood from clotting. When there is sufficient blood in the reservoir, it is pumped into a centrifuge bowl, where it is concentrated and washed with saline. From there, the blood is pumped to an infusion bag. Reinfusion should be within 4 hours after collection, to prevent bacterial growth. Typically, about one half of the blood lost may be salvaged. One typical unit of salvaged blood is 225 mL of saline suspended red cells, with a hematocrit of 50%. Intraoperative blood salvage instruments are referred to as cell savers.

Complications of Intraoperative Blood Salvage and Subsequent Reinfusion

- Fat and air embolism
- Coagulopathy
- DIC and acute respiratory distress syndrome due to activated platelets and white cells

TRANSFUSION REACTIONS

TRs are hazards of transfusion and are broadly divided into immunologic and nonimmunologic mechanisms. Immunologic TRs are:

- Febrile nonhemolytic
- Hemolytic: acute and delayed
- Allergic, anaphylactoid, and anaphylactic
- Post transfusion purpura
- TRALI
- GVHD

Nonimmunologic TRs are:

- Circulatory overload
- Bacterial contamination/sepsis
- Transmissible infections
- Air embolism
- Hypocalcemia
- Hyperkalemia
- Hypothermia

A common and important manifestation of TR is fever. Fever with or without chills are seen in

- Febrile nonhemolytic TR
- Hemolytic TR
- Bacterial contamination
- TRALI

Fever, in the setting of transfusion, is defined as a temperature elevation of 1°C or 2°F.

Febrile nonhemolytic TRs: These are due to cytokines from donor WBCs. WBCs are present in RBCs and platelets. With storage, cytokines accumulate in the bag, and when the unit is transfused, this may result in a febrile reaction. With the use of prestorage leukoreduction, the incidence of this particular type of reaction has significantly decreased. Premedication has no role in the prevention of febrile reactions. There is a 15% chance of recurrence of this type of reaction with future transfusions. If the unit is not a leukoreduced one, then the use of leukofilters at the time of transfusion will help.

Hemolytic TRs: Acute hemolytic TRs are rare and most often are due to clerical errors. Patient develops features of fever, flank pain, and hemoglobinuria are classical features. Hypotension may also be present and is a useful sign for anesthetized patients. Naturally, transfusion should be stopped and the patient should receive fluids and a potent diuretic started to maintain a significant urine output (e.g., 100 mL/hr or more). Causes of death in such a patient are acute tubular necrosis and DIC.

Delayed hemolytic TRs typically occur 2 to 10 days post transfusion. Alloantibodies to the Kidd and Duffy blood group system are typically implicated. The classical scenario is as follows: the patient lacks one of the antigens of the previously named blood group systems. The patient is transfused with red cells with that particular antigen. Patient then forms antibodies against that antigen. Levels of the antibody then decline to below detection levels. Prior to subsequent transfusion, the antibody screen is negative and crossmatching does not detect incompatibility. The patient again receives blood which has the same antigen. Antibody levels start to rise, and within a week there occurs hemolysis. The patient hemoglobin starts to drop. Serum haptoglobin declines. Bilirubin levels rise. The antibody is coating the surface of the transfused red cells. Thus a direct antibody test will be positive. Fortunately, this type of reaction and is not life threatening. Monitoring the patient and ensuring adequate hydration is effective in most situations.

Transfusion-related acute lung injury: TRALI is a clinical syndrome that takes place within 6 hours of transfusion and is characterized by shortness of breath due to noncardiogenic pulmonary edema, fever, and hypotension. TRALI can be seen with any blood products, but most often it is plasma or platelets that are implicated. In the United States, TRALI is now the leading cause of mortality due to transfusions. The mechanism of TRALI is not quite clear. However, antibodies in the donor product against HLA or neutrophils in the recipient are thought to play a role. Patients develop hypoxemia and may require intubation with mechanical ventilation. Treatment is supportive, and most patients improve within 2 to 4 days.

Transfusion related graft versus host disease: This is a rare but fatal complication and is due to concomitant transfusion of viable lymphocytes from cellular blood products. Normally the donor lymphocytes are destroyed by the host. However, if the immune system of the recipient is significantly compromised or there is HLA matching of the donor and the recipient, then the donor lymphocytes may not be destroyed. Thus in situations when transfusion-related graft versus host disease is a possibility, the donor products are irradiated to prevent the donor lymphocytes from having the ability to divide.

TRANSFUSION REACTION WORKUP

Whenever there is a suspicion of a TR, the transfusion should be stopped and an IV line kept open. This is in case medications and/or fluids need to be administered. A clinician needs to be notified who should assess the patient for TR. If a TR is considered, then a TR workup is initiated. The blood component is returned to the blood bank.

At the blood bank, a clerical check is performed. The relevant paperwork and the products with labels are checked for clerical errors. A sample of patient's blood is also provided, and a visual inspection for hemolysis is done. The patient's ABO group is rechecked on the posttransfusion sample. A DAT is performed and the results compared with a pretransfusion one, if available.

If there is a hemolytic TR, then visual inspection may reveal hemolysis. The posttransfusion sample DAT may be positive, and this is significant if the pretransfusion DAT is negative. Further testing for haptoglobin levels may be indicated. Haptoglobin levels fall with intravascular hemolysis. Subsequently serum bilirubin will rise and may also be tested for. At the conclusion of the TR workup, a report issued by the blood bank pathologist will be included in the patient's chart.

USE OF RhIG

RhIg is a high titered anti-D antibody (of human origin) preparation. It is used to prevent alloimmunization to the D antigen. In most instances, RhIg is given to Rh negative mothers when they are pregnant, if the father is Rh positive. They are also administered to Rh negative mothers after delivery if they give birth to an Rh-positive baby.

In cases of transfusion of red cells and platelets, for females who are Rh negative and who are of childbearing age, the blood bank will always try to provide products that are Rh negative. However, in certain situations, especially with platelet transfusions, this may not be possible. If Rh-positive red cells are given to an Rh negative individual, the use of RhIg is impractical. The patient needs to be tested for the development of anti-D antibody, and if it occurs, the patient must receive Rh negative blood. Platelets have a small amount of contaminating red cells. In apheresis donor units (which is one dose of platelets), this typically less than 2 mL. While platelets do not have Rh antigens, the contaminating red cells do. Thus if the platelet product is from an Rh-positive individual and the recipient is Rh negative, alloimmunization with formation of anti-D antibody is possible. To prevent the formation of anti-D antibody in these individuals, RhIg may be given. One dose of RhIg (300 µg) will be sufficient to suppress alloimmunization against 30 mL of whole blood or 15 mL of red cells. Thus one dose of RhIg is sufficient to prevent alloimmunization 6 to 8 doses (apheresis donor) of Rh-positive platelets.

RECOMMENDED READING

Kade CG, Thompson LR. In: Roberts JR, Custalow CB, Thomsen TW, eds. *Roberts and Hedges' Clinical Procedures in Emergency Medicine and Acute Care.* 7th ed. Philadelphia: Elsevier; 2019:500–522.
Kaushansky K, Lichtman MA, Prchal JT, Levi MM, Press OW, Burns LJ, et al. *Williams Hematology.* 9th ed. New York: McGraw Hill; 2016.

CHAPTER 235

PRINCIPLES OF X-RAY INTERPRETATION

W. MacMillan Rodney • J.R. MacMillan Rodney • K.M.R. Arnold

INTRODUCTION

Studies on imaging outcomes have documented quality of care for interpretation of radiographs by nonradiologists in family medicine and emergency medicine. This chapter provides a "how-to-do-it" guideline on the interpretation of the most common adult x-ray studies needed in primary care: common fractures of the long bones and the chest radiograph (posteroanterior [PA] and lateral). (For the treatment of fractures and further discussion, see Chapter 178, Fracture Care.) There will also be an overview of the purchase, maintenance, and staffing of equipment in the office. This includes the decision to have all or selected images interpreted by outside consultation. Published data suggest that consultation significantly changes management in less than 2% of cases if the physician has basic interpretation skills.

Who Reads the Film and Who Collects the Fee?

Practicing medicine in today's world entails medicolegal risk. It cannot be eliminated, but it can be lessened by timely application of procedural skills, such as the interpretation of radiologic images at the point of service. The advantages of bedside correlation and subsequent follow-up cannot be overemphasized.

Primary care residency training is adequate to train clinicians to interpret images or to seek consultation when needed. Levels of comfort vary from physician to physician. There is no legal requirement to have images interpreted by a radiologist. Physicians are entitled to reimbursement for the technical component and the professional component of the CPT-4 charges for the image if they own the equipment, and create the formal report for the medical record. Only the physician signing the final report is entitled to bill for the professional component of the fee.

Buying the Equipment

Digital radiography offers lower-cost and more reliable technology in the office. From a storage perspective, the space that developers, darkrooms, and films (both exposed and unexposed) occupy can be more efficiently used for patient care. Digital technology also promotes safety by eliminating developer chemicals that must be stored and disposed. Also, by decreasing the number of retakes, radiation to patients and office staff is reduced. Finally, images are easily stored and can be shared more quickly and efficiently, which prevents unnecessary repeated studies and minimizes expense and radiation exposure.

Computed radiography (CR) is less expensive and equally accurate as the picture archiving and communication systems purchased by hospitals. CR refers to the use of phosphor films that function in the cassettes of traditional x-ray equipment. The image is taken, the plate is transferred to a developer, and then the image is loaded digitally to the computer. Installation of a new digital CR system costs less than $60,000. Digital images can be inserted directly into most electronic medical record systems.

State Certification, Licensing Laws, and Insurances Vary

A lead-lined room is necessary to obtain state certification. This can be done for less than $10,000. Physicians do not require additional licensing to provide radiographs, but unlicensed staff must usually take a 6- to 10-day course and pass a state test for licensing. Hiring a dedicated radiology technician is an expensive option that may be beyond the budget of an office taking fewer than 25 images a day. Data suggest that offices order 3 to 8 radiographs per 100 patients per day. Geriatric and urgent care–open access practices have a higher demand.

Planning and cost–benefit analyses must be completed before the purchase of equipment and staff training (see Appendix L, Buying Major Office Equipment). Some HMO contracts forbid reimbursement to office-based physicians, but some emergency departments are charging more than $200 per chest film. An average Medicaid reimbursement may be less than $40 per image. Local reimbursement rates, insurance rules, governmental policies, and patient mix must be reviewed before purchasing an x-ray unit.

CHEST RADIOGRAPHY

One example of documentation that helps ensure that all aspects of the radiograph are reviewed is shown in Fig. 235.1. This documentation form helps maintain quality of care. Obtaining a second opinion (overreading by a second physician) is suggested until the reader becomes comfortable with the many variations of normal versus abnormal.

Interpretation Guidelines for the Adult Posteroanterior and Lateral Chest Radiograph

Clinical Context

The clinician who performs the history and bedside examination has a tremendous advantage compared with a radiologist remote in time and space. The immediacy of clinical data differentiates imaging as a diagnostic procedure for the patient in real time versus a radiologic consultation, which usually occurs after the patient has left the office. The bedside examination at the point of service minimizes errors of interpretation.

Validity

Images must be labeled and dated, and there must be a system in place to ensure this is done.

PA and *lateral* views are the standard views for the cooperative adult. "PA" simply means the beam travels in the direction from the back to the chest (posteroanterior; vs. AP [anteroposterior], from chest to back). The patient stands and takes a deep breath. Views are standardized as noted later. Cardiomegaly definitions are different on PA versus AP views, so it is important that radiographs be taken appropriately. Without a lateral view, lesions in the retrocardiac and

INTERPRETATION OF THE CHEST X-RAY

Please fill this form out completely.

I. CLINICAL CONTEXT

   Patient ID#/Name_____Age:_____   Sex:_____   Date: _____
   Are old films available for comparison?   Yes   No

   REVIEW OF SYSTEMS (circle those that apply)
      Cough   Dyspnea   Pleuritic Pain   Chest pain   Hemoptysis   HTN
      Other illnesses, signs, or symptoms _____
      DURATION OF PROBLEM in days, weeks, or months _____
      Circle the techniques used   PA   Lateral   AP   Portable Decubitus
      Is this film significantly rotated?   Yes   No
      Is there an adequate inspiration?   Yes   No
      Is the amount of penetration[exposure]within normal limits?   Yes   No

II. VALIDITY—Does the image need to be repeated?   Yes   No

III. Check the lateral—Are there abnormalities of the spine, diaphragms, anterior clear space or the posterior cardiac
      space?   Yes   No

IV. Bones and soft tissues. See any significant abnormalities?   Yes   No

V. Mediastinum. Is it normal?   Yes   No

VI. Cardiac silhouette. Is it normal?   Yes   No

VII. Diaphragms. Are there any significant abnormalities?   Yes   No

VIII. Lungs
      A. Are there any significant abnormalities on the left or right hilum?   Yes   No
      B. Any significant abnormalities to the lung parenchyma?   Yes   No
      C. Any significant abnormalities of the lung pleurae?   Yes   No

IX. My interpretation is[circle one]:
      A. Within normal limits.
      B. Normal, but I want to comment on some findings which are probably insignificant. Consultation not required.
      _____
      C. Questionable findings exist and consultation will be requested.
      D. Abnormal findings:
      _____

X. PLAN

XI. SIGNATURES
   Student/Resident:_____Attending Physician: _____CC:_____ Date:_____

Fig. 235.1   Interpretation of the chest x-ray report form.

poststernal (anterior clear space) space can be missed. Other potential views are not covered here.

"Perfect views" are not necessary to gain useful information, but a disclaimer describing any technique limitations must be inserted with every film. For chest films, the acronym RIP describes the characteristics of *rotation, inspiration, and penetration* (i.e., exposure). These validity checks must be addressed before any interpretation of findings.

POSTEROANTERIOR VIEW:

*   *Is this film rotated?* In the PA film, measure the distance from the spinous processes of the vertebral bodies to the medial heads of each of the clavicles. These are easily identifiable bony landmarks. Commonly, there is a 2- to 3-mm difference because of slight rotation, which does not invalidate the film, but in general, the distances on the right and the left should be approximately the same.
*   *Is there an adequate inspiration?* Inadequate inspiration is a cause of decreased specificity (increased opacity) for lung parenchyma. The "best" method for measuring inspiration is by counting *posterior* ribs as they join the spine. A minimally adequate inspiration uncovers nine ribs. Avoid counting anterior ribs, which are less predictable.

*   *Is the amount of penetration within normal limits?* Penetration describes the amount of radiation exposure applied to the tissue. A practical rule of thumb for evaluating overpenetration and underpenetration is the anatomic point at which the vertebral interspaces are no longer visible. An *overpenetrated* PA chest image will create a "spine film" with all elements of the vertebral bodies visible down into the abdomen. An *underpenetrated* film will be too "white." When penetration technique is ideal, intervertebral spaces disappear somewhere in the cardiac shadow and do not appear beneath the diaphragm.

Overexposure "burns out" the ability to see the lung parenchyma and vessels—that is, turns the lung fields black. The vessels normally start to disappear as they approach within 3 to 4 mm of the chest wall. Overexposure increases the probability of false-negative interpretation.

Physicians should comment on limitations of interpretation caused by suboptimal technique. The physician should request additional views or insert a disclaimer about technique if necessary. This includes the need for a lateral image in the ambulatory adult and older child.

These validity checks, and the following system for reviewing the film, establish guidelines for quality assurance.

Check the Lateral Image

Review the spine, diaphragms, anterior clear space, and the retrocardiac space. The majority of diagnoses will come from the PA view.

Does a Survey of the Bones and Soft Tissues Reveal Any Significant Abnormalities?

This area is of limited value when the radiograph has been ordered to investigate dyspnea, cough, hypertension, and other routine cardiovascular issues. However, a systematic sweep of the bones and soft tissues is mandatory.

Is the Appearance of the Mediastinum Within Normal Limits?

The physician cannot miss a shifted or widened mediastinum, which is associated with aortic dissections, pericardial tamponade, tumors of the thymus and thyroid, lymphoma, and germ cell teratomas. A quoted dimension for "wide" is 8 cm in the average adult. Another method measures the mediastinal width at the level of the carina. If it is more than 25% of the thoracic diameter, it is considered wide. A "thin" mediastinum has no significance. However, aortic dissections have occurred in mediastina measuring less than 8 cm. Normal children younger than 5 years frequently have a wide mediastinum and large cardiac silhouette.

Does a Review of the Cardiac Silhouette Reveal Any Significant Abnormalities on the Posteroanterior View?

Cardiomegaly exists if the transverse diameter of the heart on a PA view is greater than 50% of the transthoracic diameter measured at the same level. The thoracic diameter is measured from one side of the rib cage to the other at the level of the middle of the heart. An enlarged pulmonary artery segment can be seen as an extra hump on the left side of the PA heart. On the lateral, left ventricular enlargement can cause a shadow more than 2 cm posterior to the shadow of the inferior vena cava. Pneumopericardium creates a black line around the border of the heart. The thin heart of deep inspiration, such as in chronic obstructive pulmonary disease, is not indicative of cardiac disease.

Does a Review of the Diaphragms Reveal Any Significant Abnormalities (Posteroanterior View)?

Air beneath the diaphragms is a surgical emergency until proven otherwise (it documents a bowel perforation). Normally the right diaphragm is higher than the left by 2 to 20 mm. Abnormal elevation occurs from lung atelectasis, paralysis, effusion, lobectomy, and other causes.

Lungs

Now the lung tissue itself is evaluated.

1. *Are there any significant abnormalities on the left or right hilum?* In 70% of normal patients, the left hilum is higher than the right, and at equal elevations in 30%. The right hilum in not normally higher than the left. *Abnormal hilar adenopathy indicates serious infection, sarcoid, or malignancy in most cases.*
2. *Are there any significant abnormalities to the lung parenchyma?* A rapid visual "ping-pong" comparison of the left and right lung fields should detect flagrant asymmetries caused by pathologic processes such as hemothorax, metastatic nodules, sarcoid, primary tuberculosis, and pneumonias. Failure to detect an obvious abnormality in the face of a seriously ill patient may require consultation or hospitalization.

   Poor inspirations and AP views cause false-positive "fluffiness" similar to congestive heart failure (CHF) patterns. Normally on the PA film, the vascular markings stop short of the lung wall by 3 to 5 mm. Gravity causes subtle tapering of the vessels as they go toward the head (cephalad). "Cephalization of flow" is jargon for the phenomenon of enlarged lung vessels in the upper lung fields secondary to CHF.

   The *silhouette sign* helps the clinician to localize the lesion. In the chest, there are anatomic structures that exist in fixed air–soft tissue relationships. Given proper rotation and penetration, the heart borders, the ascending and descending aorta, the aortic knob, and the diaphragms are visible (Figs. 235.2 and 235.3). The silhouette sign describes the situation where parenchymal pathology masks the silhouette of a common anatomic landmark. The heart and diaphragm are most commonly affected. For example, when anterior left upper lobe pneumonia obscures the border of the left heart, it is called a silhouette sign. When pleural effusion obscures the contour of the diaphragm, it is a silhouette sign.

   Nodules are classified by their diameter of 5 to 30 mm. Above 30 mm, these lesions are classified as *masses*. Small lesions (2 to 10 mm) are common. Most of these are calcified granulomas, and vessels on end. They are small and innocent, and do not grow over time. They can be followed by serial radiographs and clinical history. Positron emission tomography scans can differentiate metabolically active lesions (malignant, infectious) from those that are metabolically quiescent (benign).
3. *Are there any significant abnormalities of the lung pleurae?* The absence of pulmonary vasculature extending out to the bony inner edge of the thorax indicates a pneumothorax until proven otherwise. The visceral pleura is the outer lining of the lung, and the parietal pleura is the inner lining of the chest cavity up against the bones and muscles. The area between the two, the pleural space, under

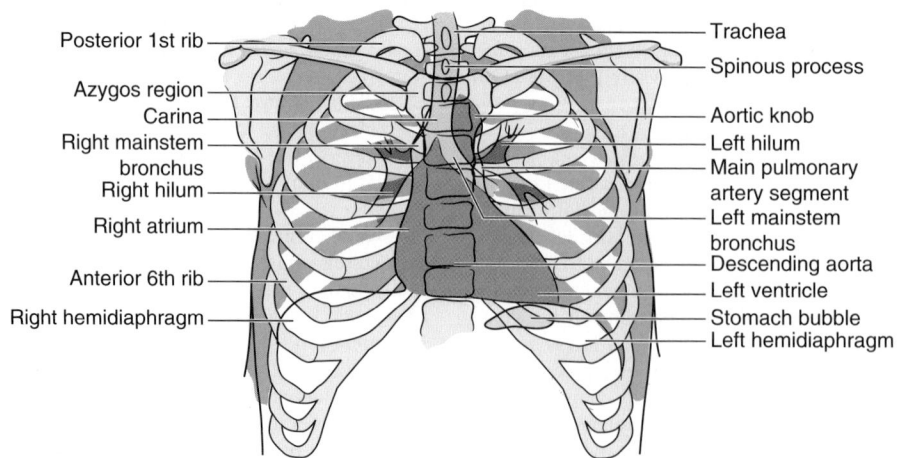

Fig. 235.2 Schematic anatomy of posteroanterior chest images.

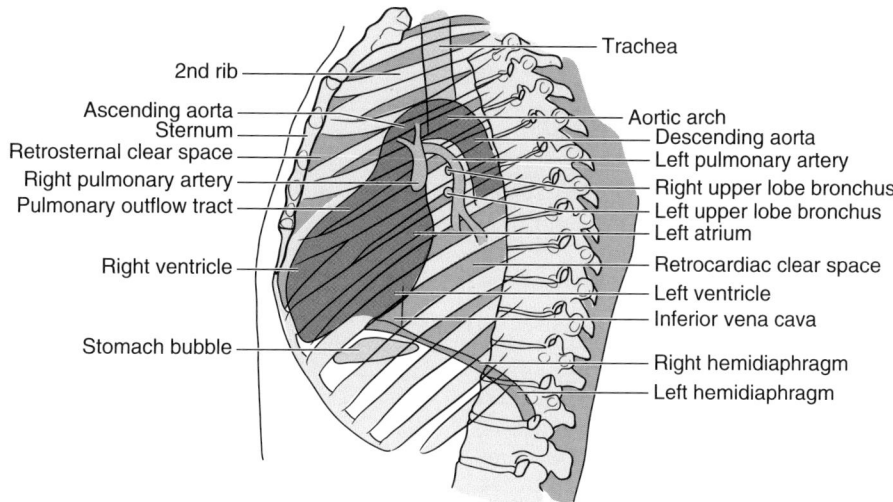

Fig. 235.3 Landmarks of the lateral chest film.

normal conditions, is a potential space. Pleural effusions are caused by primary disease processes such as infection, neoplasm, and inflammation. Specific diseases such as subphrenic abscess, hepatitis, and pancreatitis can cause effusions. Cardiac failure, renal failure, or any disease that alters the osmolar and hydrostatic equilibrium among the body compartments can cause effusions. Untreated chronic pleural effusions can cause loculations and adhesions.

Interpretation

1. Within normal limits.
2. Normal, but I want to comment on some findings which are probably insignificant. Consultation not required, but … (perhaps the penetration was not ideal or the entire right shoulder was not seen, etc.).
3. Questionable findings exist and consultation will be requested. This could include a computed tomography scan of the chest, which is the most commonly ordered test for ambiguous findings on the plain radiograph. Consultation reports can be ambiguous or wrong. CHF can appear to be pneumonia, and vice versa.
4. Abnormalities include the following: Naming the disease is not necessary. Stating that the entire right lung is "whited out," or that "multiple 2- to 3-cm nodules are present in both lungs," will lead to dramatic changes in management that will be mentioned in the plan.

Plan

By offering an interpretation or a preliminary interpretation in the office at the point of service, quality is improved. Clearly indicate in the report any intention of further diagnostic studies or follow-up, which can then be immediately explained to the patient. Poorly worded or ambiguous interpretations that arrive hours or days after the patient has left the office decrease the quality of care.

Consultant reports can be lost or misplaced. The beauty of imaging in the office is the high predictive value of a positive finding. Specificity is high when lesions are obvious, and delay of management pending formal interpretation is often not wise. The risk of a false-negative result (low sensitivity) is always present. Multiple studies have documented, however, that the rate of failure to diagnose a lesion of significance is less than 1% to 2%.

Top 10 "Normal" Tips

1. You are at the bedside. Integrate the history with the physical findings and be sure they correlate.
2. The clavicular heads are equidistant from the spinous processes.
3. There are at least nine ribs visible on a normal inspiratory PA view.

4. The intervertebral spaces should not be visible beneath the diaphragm.
5. Before 5 years of age, a normal thymus can make a large-appearing mediastinum.
6. In adults, the mediastinum should not measure more than 8 cm.
7. The left hilum is higher than the right hilum.
8. The right diaphragm is higher than the left.
9. The exact boundary distinguishing a granuloma from a nodule may not be as important as the clinical context, which includes a history for risk and the rate of growth. Lesions greater than 10 mm in diameter may benefit from a second opinion.
10. There is no exact formula for hilar enlargement and subtle parenchymal change. Chance favors the prepared mind. Read or perish.

Sample Chest Radiograph Presentations

Make copies of the report form (see Fig. 235.1) and fill it out for each of the following images. Check your findings against the information given in the figure legends.

Fig. 235.4: This is a 43-year-old African-American woman with a 3-month history of increasing fatigue and shortness of breath. Other than being overweight, her past medical history is noncontributory. Her lungs were clear to auscultation and vital signs were normal.

Fig. 235.5: A 59-year-old white man with a long history of chronic obstructive pulmonary disease reports a mild cough, a mild increase in dyspnea, and a fever last night. He has dropped out from care in the cardiology and pulmonary clinics. Many years ago he was told he needed a heart operation, but he has refused. He is demanding an antibiotic shot because his "pneumonias" start like this. His lungs are clear and his heart sounds are distant. His vital signs are normal, including a respiratory rate of 16 per minute.

Fig. 235.6: This patient complains of acute chest pain radiating to the back. A 33-year-old Latino man with an unremarkable past medical history walked away from a motor vehicle accident last night. He reports that he was hit in the chest very hard. He is in moderate distress, with a pulse of 110 beats/min and blood pressure of 100/70.

Fig. 235.7: A 23-year-old Latina woman presents with cough and fevers for 1 month. Past medical history is noncontributory.

Fig. 235.8: A 68-year-old white woman with a history of uncontrolled hypertension and dyspnea, worsening today. Vital signs are pulse 105, blood pressure 190/115 mm Hg, temperature 98°F, and respiratory rate 24 breaths/min. She is in mild distress.

Fig. 235.9: A 55-year-old smoker coughed up blood this morning and presents with cough, fever, and purulent sputum. Lateral view does not change management.

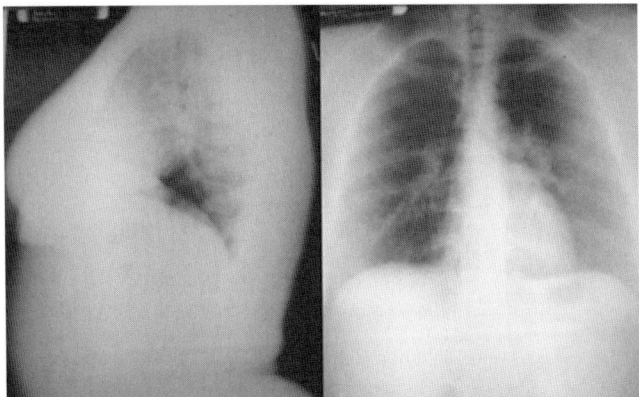

Fig. 235.4 On the posteroanterior (PA) film *(right)*, there is clinically insignificant rotation with an adequate inspiratory effort. The left costophrenic angle is partially cut off. Penetration (exposure) is somewhat strong but not clinically significant. The bones are normal, but soft tissue breast shadows are causing transparent opacity over the lower outer lung fields bilaterally. The mediastinum and cardiac shape are normal. The right hemidiaphragm is slightly higher than the left, and the left hilum is slightly higher than the right. Both hilar areas are enlarged and there is paratracheal node enlargement on the right in the area of the clavicle. There are parenchymal streaks extending down and outward from the hilar areas, but they do not constitute infiltrates. Although the lateral film *(left)* does not record an optimal inspiration, it does not change the findings on the PA film. Taken together, the films are adequate for an interpretation of "abnormal chest." Rather than repeating the films, the patient was sent for computed tomography of the chest. The differential diagnosis includes sarcoidosis, lymphoma, and tuberculosis, among others. This was biopsy-proven sarcoidosis.

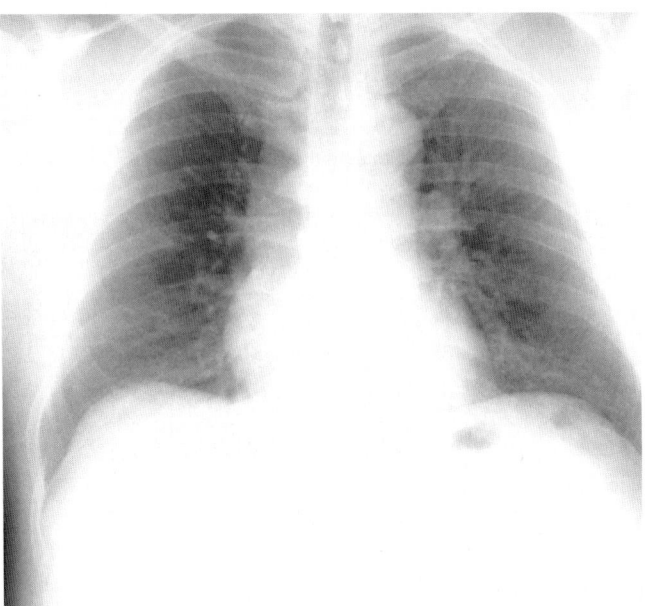

Fig. 235.6 The mediastinum is widened, and the diagnosis is traumatic aortic dissection. Overall, the film is insignificantly rotated with an adequate inspiration. Nine posterior ribs are showing, but the film is mildly underpenetrated–underexposed. Minor imperfections in technique are the rule, not the exception. The mediastinal findings are sufficient to send the patient to the hospital. The bones and soft tissues are inconsequential. The left hilum is higher than the right, and the right hemidiaphragm is higher than the left. The underexposure makes the parenchymal markings more prominent, but they do not represent infiltrates. As with all previous images, there is no air under the diaphragms.

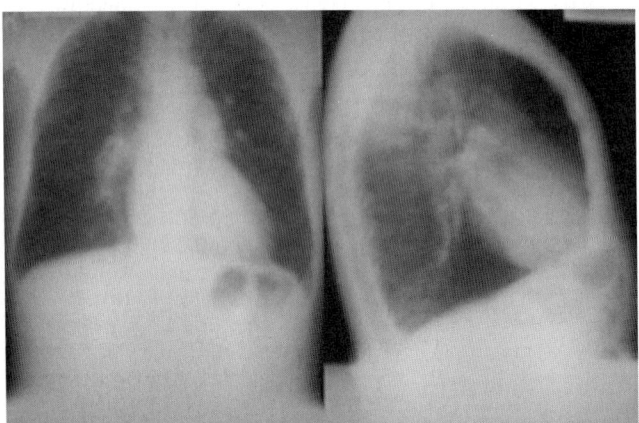

Fig. 235.5 The initial impression is overexposure with blackening of the lung fields, but the vertebral interspaces are not obvious. Clearly, there is an adequate inspiration without rotation. Bones and soft tissues are unremarkable, but the mediastinal and cardiac contours look abnormal. The diaphragms are flattened, as is common with patients with chronic obstructive pulmonary disease, suggesting a hyperaeration common with these patients. The opacities on the right do not constitute a mass or an infiltrate of significance. The lateral view *(right)* reveals flattened diaphragms and a barrel chest. This accentuates the anterior clear space in front of the heart and the retrocardiac space, which do not contain any abnormal findings. The extra hump on the left side of the heart is significant enlargement of the pulmonary artery segment, and it is likely that the patient has a compensated congenital heart defect.

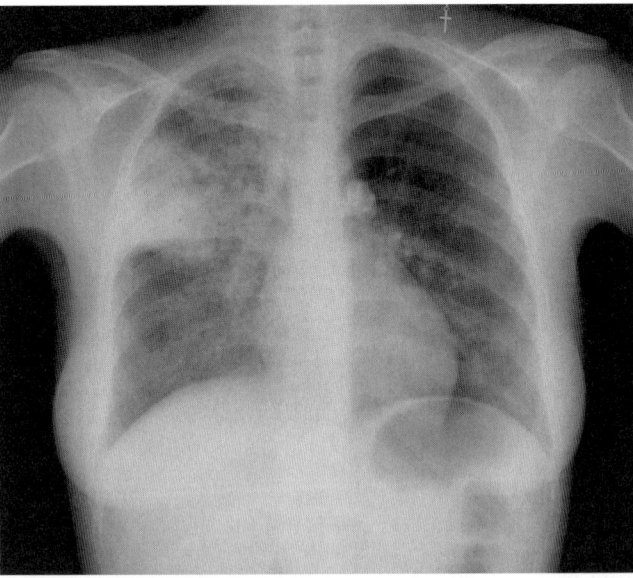

Fig. 235.7 Example of infiltrate on right, calcified hilar node on left, visible sequestration in minor fissure on left—and more. Lateral image did not add to the information seen here. The diagnosis is tuberculosis.

Fig. 235.10: This patient is a 27-year-old man with reported gunshot wounds to chest and pneumothorax. The patient is unable to stand and is tachycardic and clammy. The image was obtained using portable technique, AP view.

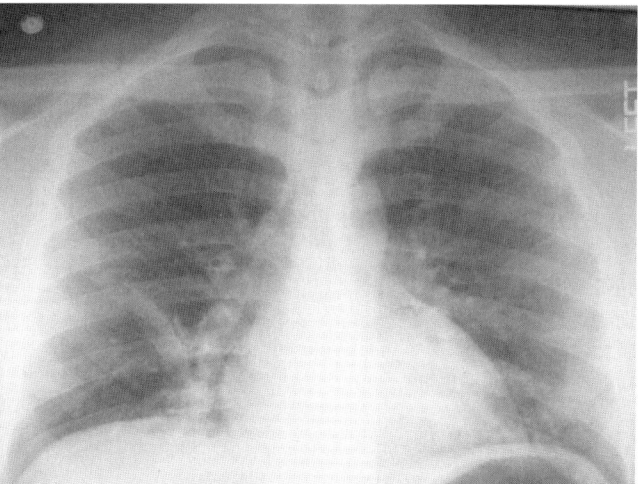

Fig. 235.8 Good example of cardiomegaly and "cephalization" of flow. Inspiration is adequate, with nine visible posterior ribs. The heart measures greater than 50% of the transthoracic distance. Blood vessels at a level superior to the tracheal bifurcation appear larger than those at the level of the mid-heart. This is the reverse of what would normally be seen. *Cephalization* is another term for the "reversal of flow" seen in congestive heart failure. This is a good view demonstrating the clavicular heads as equidistant from the spinous processes of the spinal column. In this case, the lateral image did not change the management.

LONG BONE FRACTURE RADIOGRAPHS

Tips for Reading Long Bone Fractures

- Study the terminology of fractures as given in Chapter 178, Fracture Care, and in a reprint of *Musculoskeletal Medicine/Office Orthopedics* by W. Rodney, MD (available at www.psot.com [see under rural family medicine, predoctoral section, ortho section, assigned reading]).
- Use comparison images of the injured with the noninjured bone in children with growth plates.
- Study the Salter system for fractures in children. Prognosis worsens as the Salter number increases. Salter 1 and 2 fractures can be managed conservatively.
- When any radiographic image is indicated, take the time to view each one in detail, looking at the bones too. This is what develops one's sense of "normal."

Finding fractures is guided by the location of the point tenderness. The clinician then requests two or three views to determine stability features such as displacement, angulation, and involvement of a joint. Positioning is an art, not a science. Make sure that you follow the cortex (edge of the bone) for any breaks in the line. These small defects are fractures, especially when they are associated with point tenderness.

Fracture detection is made more difficult by technique that is overpenetrated (too black). Nondigital films may be clarified by the use of a hot lamp technique in which the film is placed directly over a bright light. Digital films can be electronically corrected in several ways. Underpenetrated films (too white) may lead to false-negative findings. Without digital software, these images need to be retaken. Digital manipulations can correct some of the underpenetration errors in technique.

There are specific soft tissue clues that increase the probability of a fracture, even when one is not immediately visible. The best known is the *fat pad sign* associated with occult fractures of the bones surrounding the elbow. This sign is defined by a hypolucent (i.e., dark) space immediately adjacent to the injured bone. It usually represents blood released by the acute injury. A *posterior fat pad sign* is clearly abnormal, whereas an anterior fat pad may normally be visible for 1 to 2 mm. Larger than that is abnormal.

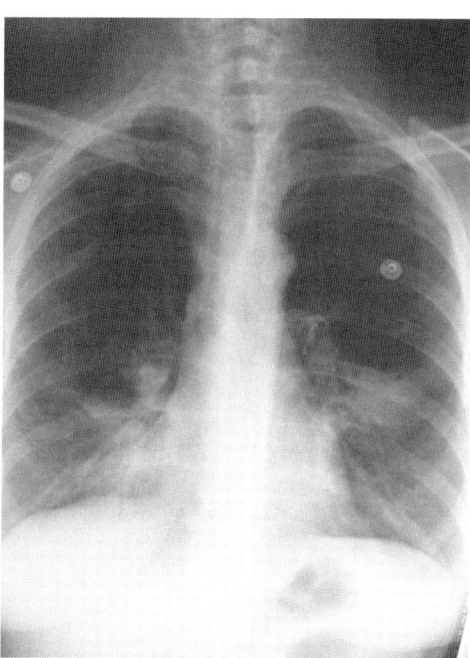

Fig. 235.9 Bilateral acute pneumonia. Note abnormalities of cardiac border on the left and right. This is a good example of the silhouette sign with the right heart border obscured by an inflammatory process. This man was sent for computed tomography, which led to tissue diagnosis of lung cancer.

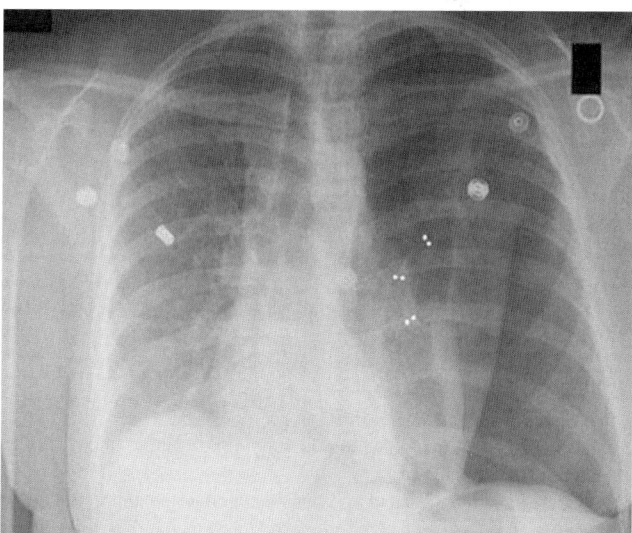

Fig. 235.10 Because the patient is unable to raise his arms, the scapulae are in the lung fields, but interpretation of the most significant event is reasonable. There is a bullet in the right side and buckshot in the left. The heart is shifted to the right and the radiograph confirms the need for chest tube insertion. The entire left lung is collapsed. Note the absence of vascular markings on the left. Although a lateral image would localize the depth of the bullet and buckshot, the emphasis should be on stabilizing these critical injuries.

Primary bone tumors are rare, but appear as hyperopaque (osteoblastic) or hypo-opaque (osteoclastic) lesions, with occasional detection by the spontaneous occurrence of pathologic fractures. Metastatic bone cancers, for example, from the prostate or breast, are more common. Fractures may be the first sign of an undiagnosed malignancy.

Those taking and reading their own radiographs should be reassured by the fact that most orthopedists depend on their own interpretations. The opportunity for clinical correlation is a tremendous help in achieving optimal management for the patient. The importance of examining the cortex with specific attention to the area of point tenderness cannot be overemphasized. Digital films allow magnification for subtle lesions. In the extremities, particularly in children, comparison views of the noninjured limb may lead to a more accurate diagnosis.

General Guidelines for Fracture Care

See Chapter 178, Fracture Care, for more detail.

- Even after the bones heal, many fractures have minor but residual discomfort and possible minor changes in function for up to 1 year later. Physical therapy will not remove this.
- Open (compound) fractures require immediate antibiotics.

- Stability governs prognosis, as well as the possible need for consultation.
- Fractures that are nondisplaced, nonangulated, transverse/oblique, and without involvement of the joint space are more stable.
- Fractures that are comminuted, spiral, and involving the joint space are less stable.
- Review the patient context and factor in comorbidity. For example, fractures in the elderly heal more slowly and are at higher risk of sustained discomfort. Patients with mental illness or sociopathic behavior require additional care.
- If providing care for a fracture, see the patient on days 2, 7, and 14 postinjury. If the pain is not resolving, consultation should be considered.
- Healing times and follow-up protocols vary. For nonoperative fractures, young people heal more rapidly than seniors.

Common Fractures

Make copies of the report form (Fig. 235.11) and fill it out for each of the following images. Check your findings against the information given in the figure legends.

X-RAYS FOR SPORTS, TRAUMA, AND WORKPLACE INJURIES

Medicos para la Familia; www.psot.com
Method of Wm. MacMillan Rodney, MD, FAAFP, FACEP
Original 1992; Updated June 3, 2008

Please fill this form out completely

I.   CLINICAL CONTEXT
     Patient Name/MRN #:_____Age:_____Sex:_____Date:_____

REVIEW OF SYSTEMS (briefly describe PMH, mechanism of injury, signs, and/or significant symptoms)
_____
_____

DURATION OF PROBLEM in days/wks/m/yrs_____
Old Films Available for Comparison?   Yes   No
II. LOCATION-ANATOMICAL AREA: Please circle areas of imaging interest
     Shoulder   Arm   Forearm   Wrist   Hand   Fingers
     Pelvis Thigh Knee Leg Ankle Foot Toes
     CSpine   Lspine   Sinus   Skull
III. VIEWS
     Views requested   AP/PA   Lateral   Oblique   Other-specify
     Number of views   1   2   other
IV. VALIDITY
     Is the amount of penetration acceptable to allow interpretation?   Yes   No
     Is the film labeled correctly   Yes   No
V.   FINDINGS
     A. Are there any significant abnormalities to the bones?   Yes   No
     B. Any significant abnormalities to the soft tissue?   Yes   No
     C. Any significant abnormalities to the joint?   Yes   No
VI. My interpretation is:
     A. Within normal limits.
     Normal, but I want to comment on some findings which are probably insignificant. Consultation not required.
     _____
     Questionable findings exist and consultation will be requested.
     Abnormalities include the following: _____
VII. PLAN: _____

VIII. SIGNATURES:
     Student/Resident: _____Attending MD/DO:_____Date:_____

Fig. 235.11 X-rays for sports, trauma, and workplace injuries report form.

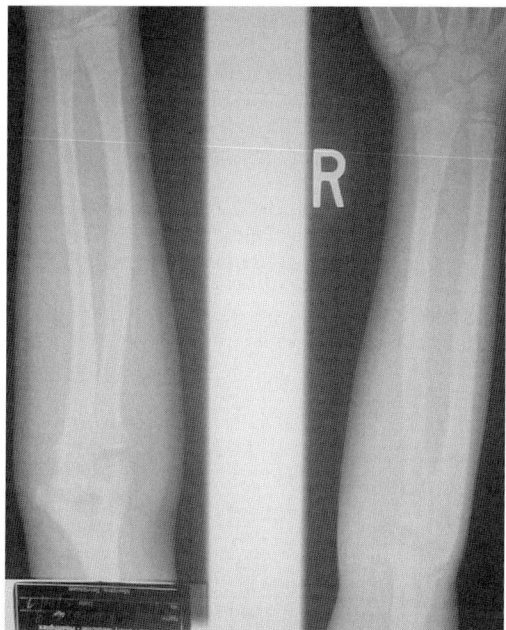

Fig. 235.12 A "bump" is visible on the radius proximal to normal epiphyses (growth plates). This is a torus fracture where the cortex of the bone has buckled. Although classified as a fracture, there is no displacement, angulation, joint involvement, or visible fracture line. Conservative management with simple protective devices will lead to a good result.

Fig. 235.12: A 10-year-old girl fell on her arm 2 hours ago while playing outside. There is point tenderness over the left distal radius, but otherwise she has no significant physical findings.

Fig. 235.13: A 19-year-old man "broke his arm 3 months ago and the cast was removed 4 weeks ago." He fell again today and wants to know if he refractured the forearm.

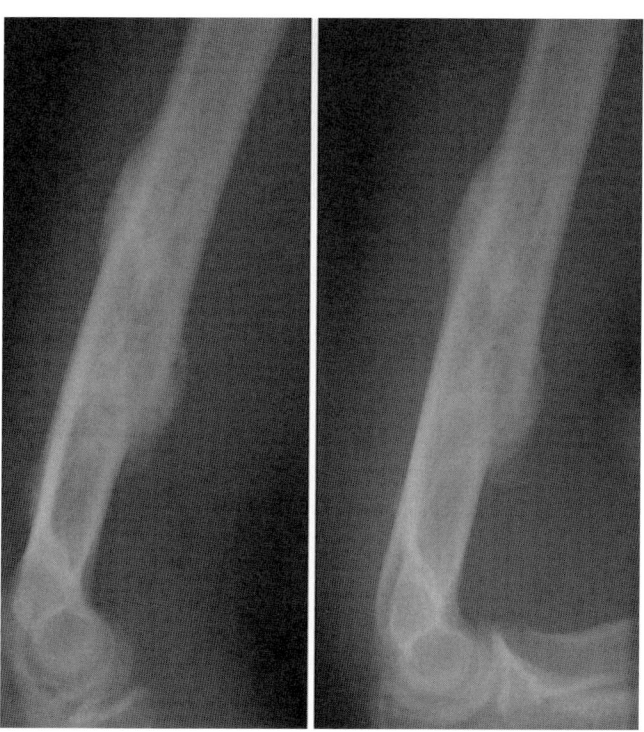

Fig. 235.13 Lateral views demonstrating normal callus formation with no evidence of a new fracture. Patient and family can be reassured. No additional casting is necessary.

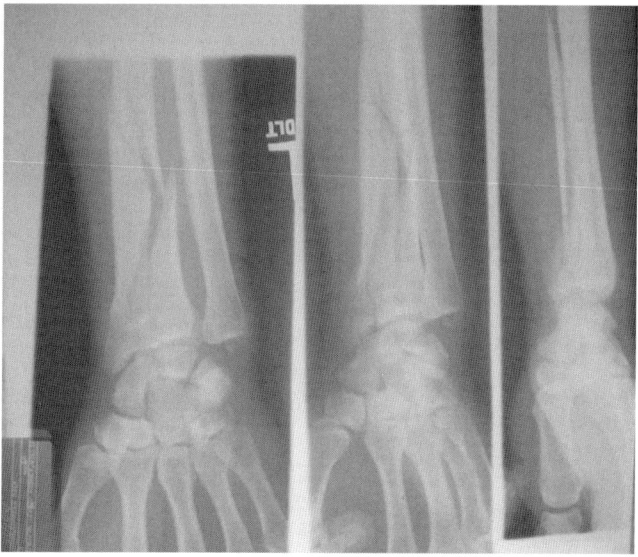

Fig. 235.14 Lateral, posteroanterior, and oblique views are the recommended views. Physicians should consider characteristics that affect fracture management. In this fracture, the joint space is involved, and this is associated with instability and a higher risk of subsequent arthritic pain. Instead of being transverse or oblique, this fracture has a spiral nature, but it is not distinctly comminuted (i.e., more than two pieces). It is a classic example of a complicated fracture destined for orthopedic surgery.

Fig. 235.14: A 27-year-old man fell on his arm yesterday, and he could not sleep last night. The arm is swollen and extremely painful to the touch. His neurovascular examination is negative, but there is limited range of motion secondary to pain.

Fig. 235.15: A 10-year-old boy experienced a collision on the soccer field this afternoon. He continued to play briefly, but states that he does not wish to move his arm.

Fig. 235.16: A 23-year-old man tripped playing touch football. He was unable to walk.

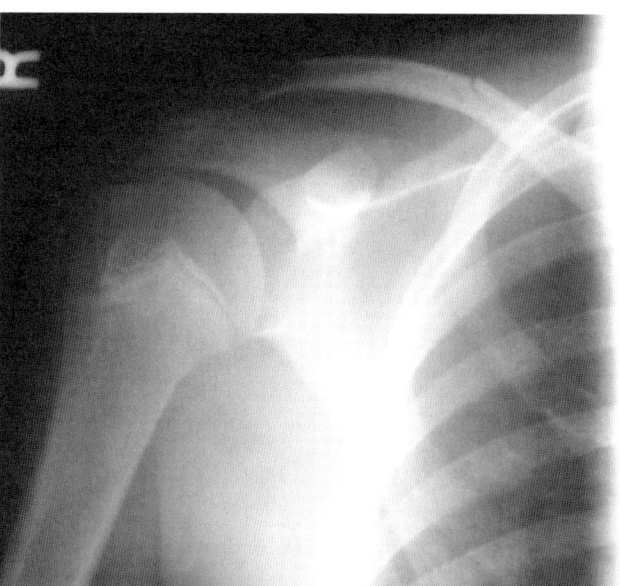

Fig. 235.15 The focal point of this image is the shoulder and its growth plate, which is normal. However, there is a nondisplaced, nonangulated fracture of the clavicle. We treated this with a sling and range-of-motion exercises three times a day.

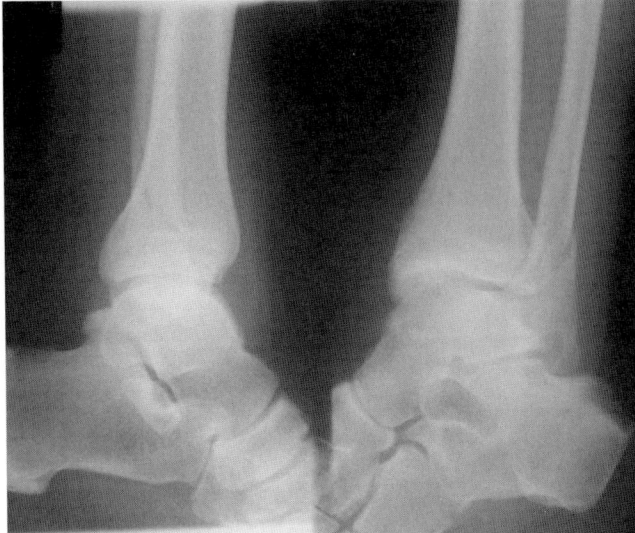

Fig. 235.16 Lateral *(left)* and oblique *(right)* views reveal a fracture of the distal fibula, which is simple, oblique, nonangulated, and nondisplaced, and does not involve an articular surface. It was immobilized with a cast for 6 weeks. No orthopedic consult was obtained.

Fig. 235.17: A 38-year-old jogger hit a pothole and inverted his ankle. There was an audible "pop," and exquisite pain was immediate. The neurovascular examination is negative.

Fig. 235.18: A 79-year-old farmer was brought by his daughter, who insisted that he be evaluated after a fall from a dumpster the preceding day. He is ambulating with a walker, and insisting that he "only needs a tetanus shot."

Fig. 235.19: A 23-year-old basketball fan hit the wall with his fist yesterday. The pain is great, and he would like an evaluation. His

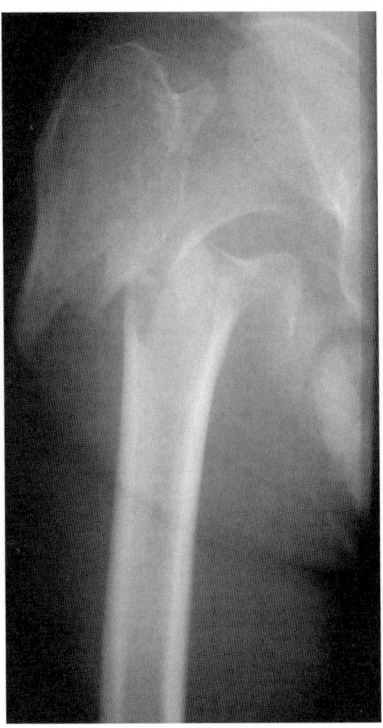

Fig. 235.18 This is a nonangulated but seriously displaced fracture of the proximal femur. It is probably intertrochanteric and transverse. It is not comminuted, but a request for surgical consultation should be noted in the medical record. The patient refused surgery and left with his walker. He died of pneumonia 9 months later (at home).

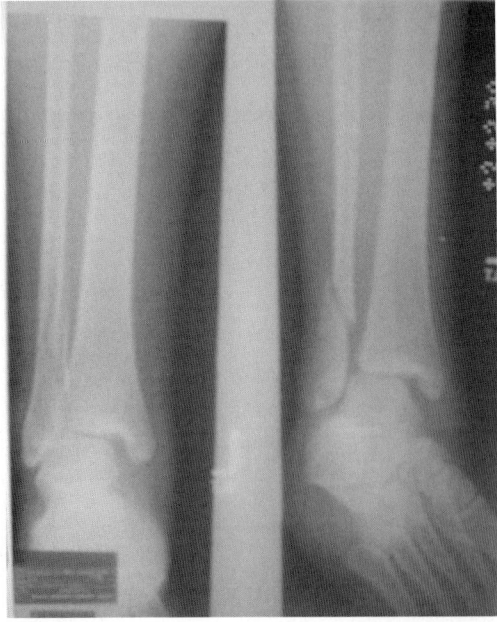

Fig. 235.17 This is a noncomminuted, nonangulated, nondisplaced, oblique fracture of the distal third of the fibula. There is no involvement of an articular surface. There is a spiral component to the fracture on the posteroanterior view *(left)*. Worse yet, there is displacement of the tibia on the talus. Note the abnormally large distance from the medial malleolus to the talus. This indicates separation of the interosseous membrane. This is a highly unstable fracture that received orthopedic surgery.

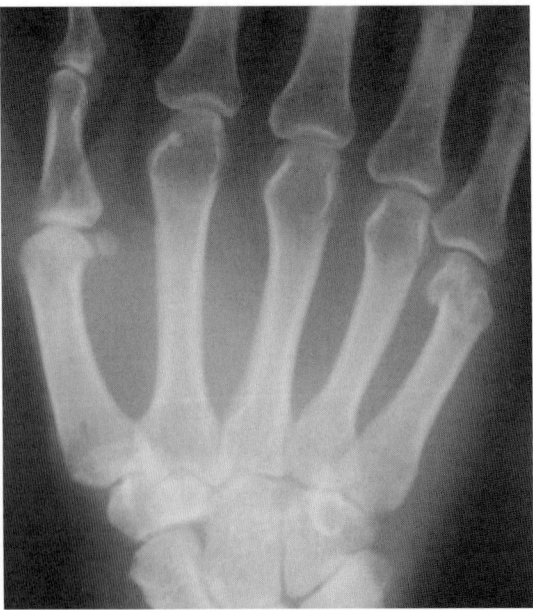

Fig. 235.19 In contrast to "compound" fractures, simple fractures are those in which the skin is unbroken and the bone is not "sticking out." This was the case here. There is a fracture at the distal fifth metacarpal bone, but it does not involve the articular surface of the joint. There is 45 degrees of angulation, but no displacement. This is the classic "boxer's fracture." Attempts at reduction are unlikely to affect the end result, which is good function and minor cosmetic deformity.

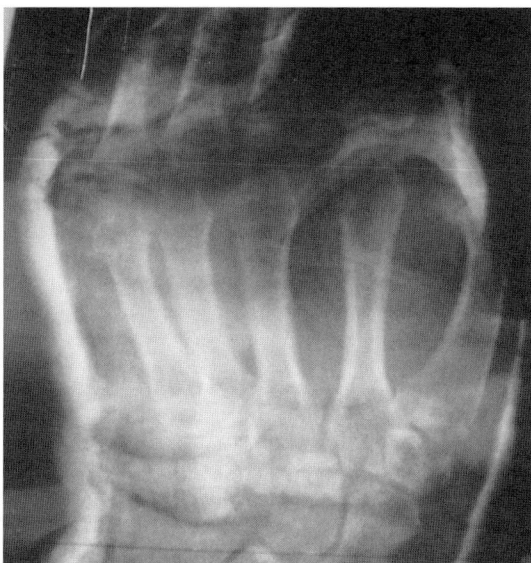

Fig. 235.20   A cast has been placed on the hand after a reduction maneuver. The radiograph has been taken with the cast on. It is tempting to deduce that the bone fragments are in better alignment, but at least two views would be necessary to make this judgment. Complete immobilization would require encasing the entire hand in concrete. This is not possible, and these fractures almost always return to their original position.

neurovascular examination is negative, but pain limits his ability to flex and extend the fourth and fifth digits.

Fig. 235.20: What has happened to the preceding case?

Fig. 235.21: A 14-year-old boy's hand was stepped on during his first football game. It is painful and swollen, but the worst pain occurs in the area of the third metacarpophalangeal joint. Is there a fracture?

Fig. 235.22: A 17-year-old female basketball player was trying to perform a dunk and landed on her outstretched hand with immediate

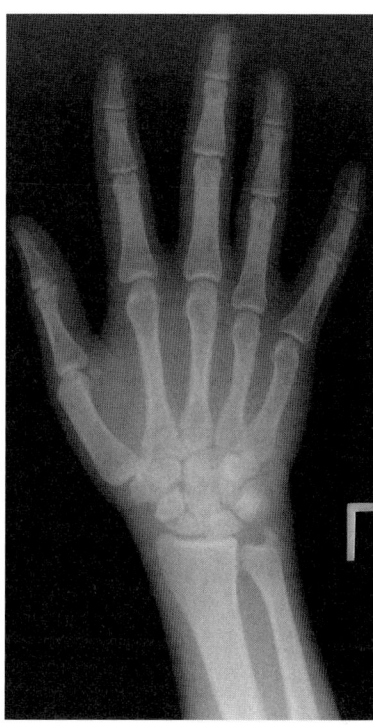

Fig. 235.22   This is a simple, noncomminuted, nondisplaced, nonangulated fracture of the scaphoid bone. A thumb spica cast should be applied for 6 to 8 weeks, and the patient should be warned about the possibility of nonunion.

pain, but little swelling. Neurovascular examination is negative, but there is a loss of range in motion at the wrist secondary to pain. Pain localizes to the area between the first metacarpal and distal radius.

ONLINE RESOURCES

LearningRadiology: www.learningradiology.com
Rodney W. Procedural Skills and Office Technology: www.psot.com.

RECOMMENDED READING

Ballinger PW, Frank EV, eds. *Merrill's Atlas of Radiographic Positions and Radiographic Procedures.* St. Louis: Mosby; 2003.
Black WS, Becker JA. Common forearm fractures in adults. *Am Fam Physician.* 200980:1107–1114.
Connolly JF. *Fractures and Dislocations: Closed Management.* Philadelphia: WB Saunders; 1995.
Griffin L, ed. *Essentials of Musculoskeletal Care.* 5th ed. Rosemont, IL: American Academy of Orthopaedic Surgeons; 2015.
Halvorsen JG, Kunian A, Gjerdingen D, et al. The interpretation of office radiographs by family physicians. *J Fam Pract.* 1989;28:426–432.
Hatch RL, Rosenbaum CI. Fracture care by family physicians: a review of 295 cases. *J Fam Pract.* 1994;38:238–244.
Muller NL, Silva CIS. *Imaging of the Chest.* Philadelphia: Saunders; 2008.
Simon HK, Khan NS, Nordenberg DF, Wright JA. Pediatric emergency physician interpretation of plain radiographs: is routine review by a radiologist necessary and cost-effective? *Ann Emerg Med.* 1996;27:295–298.
Smith P, Temte J, Beasley J, Mundt M. Radiographs in the office: is a second reading always needed? *J Am Board Fam Pract.* 2004;17:256–263.
Warren JS, Lara K, Hahn RG. Correlation of emergency department radiographs: results of a quality assurance review in an urban community hospital. *J Am Board Fam Pract.* 1993;6:255–259.

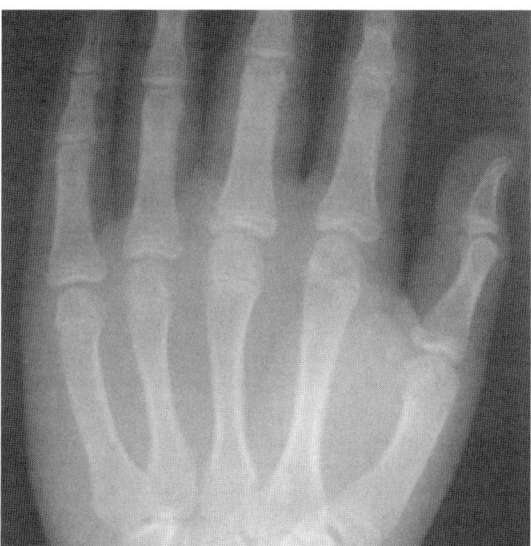

Fig. 235.21   A Canadian family physician, Robert Salter, created the Salter classification of pediatric fractures. This is a Salter 3 fracture with a fracture on the ulnar side of the epiphysis of the proximal third digit. It involves the joint space, but the size of the fracture is so small that it was treated conservatively.

APPENDIX A

COMMONLY USED INSTRUMENTS AND EQUIPMENT*

John L. Pfenninger

Listed here are the most commonly used instruments in a primary care clinician's office. This list provides a basic beginning for ordering equipment for the office. A clinician can alter the equipment depending on the procedures performed. Nonsterile gloves and equipment to follow universal blood and body fluid precautions should be available at all procedures.

Anoscope
- Every primary care office must have an anoscope to evaluate anal complaints. The Ives slotted anoscope is recommended, although others are acceptable (see Chapter 83, Anoscopy).
- Ives slotted (see Chapter 83, Anoscopy; Fig. 83.1D)
- Plastic, disposable
- Pediatric

Biopsy Instruments (Skin, Cervix, Endometrial, Colon, Breast)
- *Skin*: 2-, 3-, 4-, 5-mm disposable punches are inexpensive and stay sharp. They are preferable to the reusable Keyes punches (noted next). (See Chapter 26, Skin Biopsy.)
- *Skin*: A set of Keyes reusable punches is also an option for doing skin biopsies (Fig. A.1). However, they become dull quickly. Considering the time it takes to sterilize them and the sharpening costs, it may be advisable to consider the disposable punches.
- *Cervical*: Mini-Townsend, Baby Tischler, Kevorkian instruments are preferred (see Chapter 124, Colposcopic Examination; Fig. 124.9).
- *Endometrial*: Reusable Novak and disposable Endocell (Wallach), PipetCuret (Milex, CooperSurgical), and Pipelle (Unimar, CooperSurgical) instruments are useful (see Chapter 129, Endometrial Biopsy).
- *Colon/rectum*: For flexible sigmoidoscopy, colonoscopy, and esophagogastroduodenoscopy procedures, see Chapter 89, Flexible Sigmoidoscopy, Fig. 89.6. The small flexible biopsy forceps used for flexible sigmoidoscopy can be inserted through an anoscope to obtain adequate biopsies without causing excess bleeding. These can also be readily used for the high-resolution anoscopy procedure (see Chapter 84, High-Resolution Anoscopy).
- *Breast, Thyroid, Lymph Nodes*: Milex breast biopsy needle and Comeco syringe are optional (see Figs. 68.1 and 68.2).

Dermal Curettes
- Fox type (3-, 4-, 5-, 6-mm reusable (Fig. A.2); 2-, 3-, 4-, 5-mm disposable): Reusables work well for soft or necrotic tissue such as basal cell carcinomas. However, unless sharpened regularly, they perform poorly for more fibrotic tissue such as with warts. On the other hand, the disposables are so sharp

that they readily cut through any tissue, so if used for curetting out a basal cell, they may actually cut into normal tissue. It is advisable, then, to have both types of curettes. A disadvantage of using the disposables for larger very fibrotic lesions is that they bend. An excellent addition is the Curetteblade. The curette is disposable, so it stays sharp, and it fits on a scalpel handle. It is stronger and does not bend under pressure (see Chapter 26, Skin Biopsy, Fig. 26.1C).

Forceps
- Adson forceps with and without teeth, 4.5 inches (Fig. A.3)
- Splinter (Fig. A.4)
- Allis (Fig. A.5)
- Uterine packing (look like long, large hemostats)
- Ring (sponge)

Ring forceps can grasp tissue or clot during gynecologic procedures and are useful for holding gauze or cotton to apply solutions (such as antiseptics or acetic acid to the cervix during colposcopy) or to stop bleeding in the vagina or rectum (Fig. A.6).

Hemostats and Clamps
- Mosquito: 5-inch straight, 5-inch curved (for fine application) (Fig. A.7)
- Kelly: 5.5-inch straight, 5.5-inch curved (for larger application) (Fig. A.8)
- Towel clips (Fig. A.9)

Scissors
- Suture removal (Spencer 3.5-inch) (Fig. A.10)
- Suture cutting (William 4.5-inch) (Fig. A.11)
- Tissue
  - Mayo 6.75-inch (Fig. A.12)
  - Curved Metzenbaum 5-inch, 7-inch (Fig. A.13)
  - Fine tissue (iris) 4.125-inch (Fig. A.14)
- Bandage 5.5-inch (Fig. A.15)

Needle Driver 5-Inch (9-Inch for Vaginal/Uterine Procedures)
- Webster serrated jaws

NOTE: This is not the place to save a few pennies. Buy the best needle holders (Fig. A.16). They are often designated as the ones used for plastic surgery repairs. They are well worth it. Do not become frustrated by using the types provided in the disposable sets.

Minor Surgery Pack (Disposable Laceration Kit Is Similar)
- Scalpel handle with metric ruler inscribed on it (Fig. A.17)
- Fine hemostats (2), curved and straight
- 5-inch curved Metzenbaum scissors
- Pickups with teeth
- Pickups without teeth

---

*For a full list of supplier information, see Appendix D.

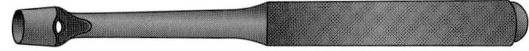

Fig. A.1 Keyes cutaneous punch, 4 mm.

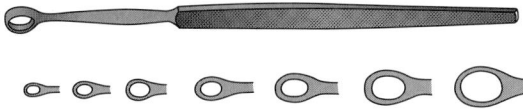

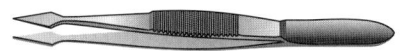

Fig. A.2 Fox dermal curette.

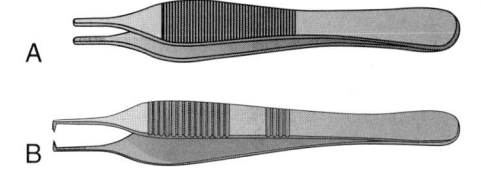

Fig. A.3 Adson forceps. (A) Serrated jaws. (B) With teeth.

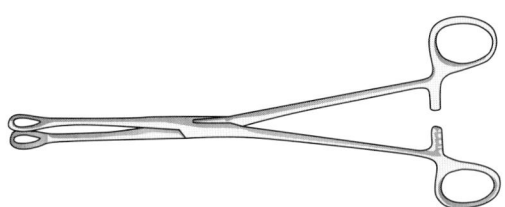

Fig. A.4 Carmalt splinter.

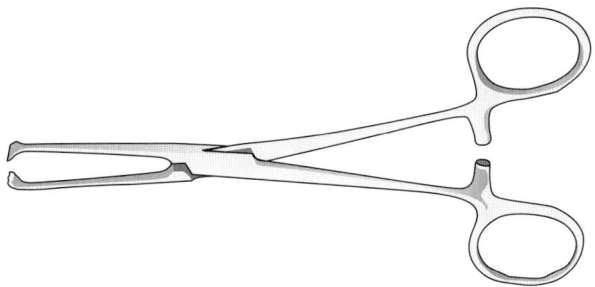

Fig. A.5 Allis tissue forceps.

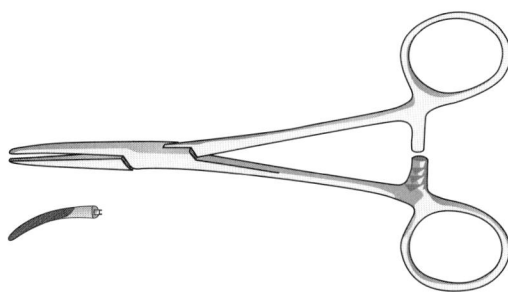

Fig. A.6 Foerster sponge/ring forceps.

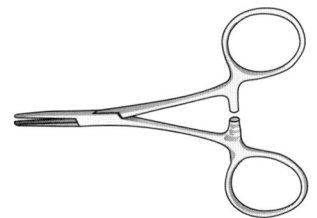

Fig. A.7 Pedifine Hartman mosquito hemostats.

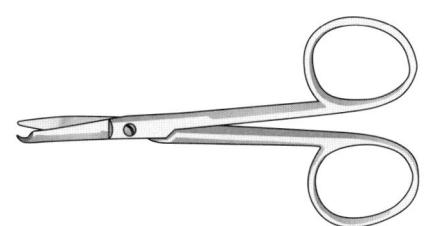

Fig. A.8 Kelly straight and curved (*inset*) hemostats.

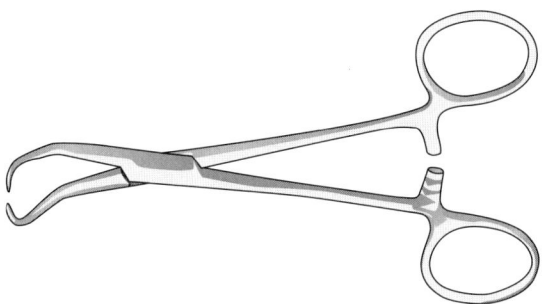

Fig. A.9 Backhaus towel clamps.

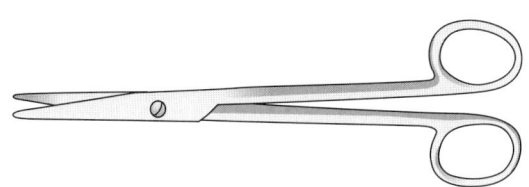

Fig. A.10 Spencer 3.5-inch suture removal scissors.

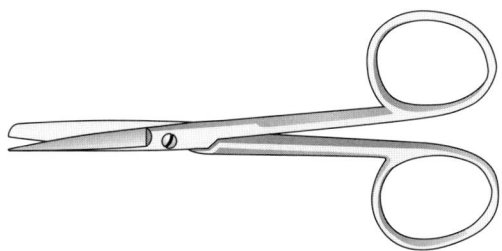

Fig. A.11 William 4.5-inch suture cutting scissors.

Fig. A.12 Mayo 6 ¾-inch operating scissors.

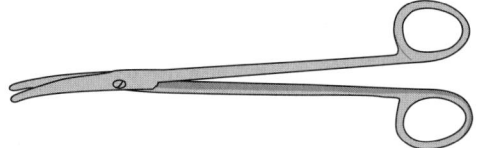

Fig. A.13 Curved Metzenbaum 5- and 7-inch operating scissors.

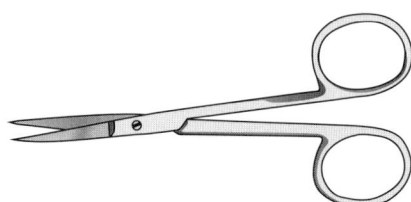

Fig. A.14 Fine tissue (iris) 4⅛-inch scissors.

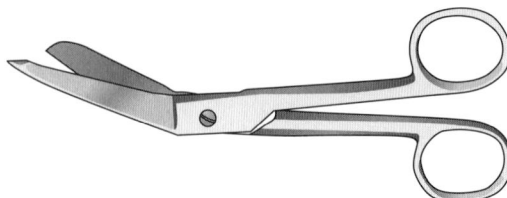

Fig. A.15 Bandage removal scissors.

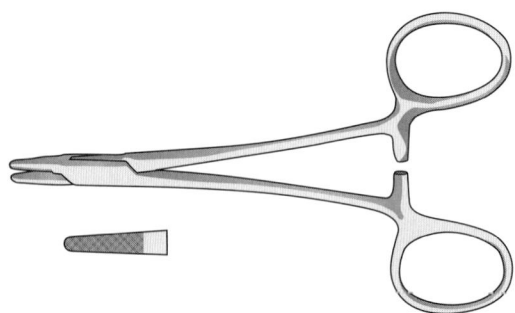

Fig. A.16 Webster serrated jaw needle holder.

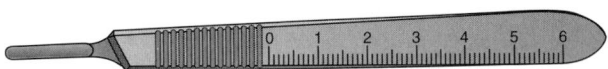

Fig. A.17 Scalpel handle with metric rule.

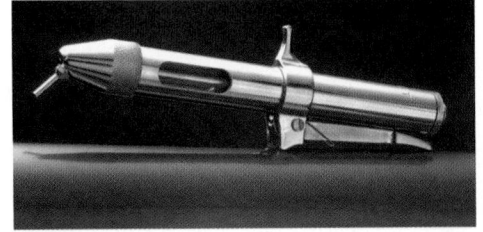

Fig. A.18 Madajet SL anesthetic injector. (Courtesy Mada Medical, Carlstadt, NJ.)

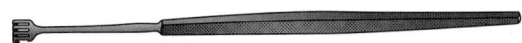

Fig. A.19 Seltzer skin hook.

- Suture scissors
- Stainless steel basin
- 4 × 4 gauze pads (8 to 10)
- Glass jar (or formalin-containing specimen bottle) for specimen
- Needle driver
- Also have available: sterile fenestrated drapes, appropriate suture, skin marking pens, alcohol wipes, betadine or chlorhexidine solution, dressings for the wound

Vasectomy Setup (No-Scalpel)
- Small curved hemostats (2 to 4)
- Hemoclip applicator (medium) and clips (or suture)
- Vas dissecting forceps
- Vas clamp (Wilson or Li)
- Sharp tissue scissors
- Battery-powered cautery unit
- Medicine cup
- 4 × 4 gauze pads, large pack
- For the no-needle method, will also need the Madajet anesthetic injector (urology version) (Fig. A.18) (see Chapter 111, Vasectomy).

Skin Hooks
- Useful for nontraumatic skin or wound edge retraction (Fig. A.19)

Staple Applicator
- See Chapter 196, Skin Stapling

Staple Remover
- Removes surgical stainless steel skin staples. Removers are sold as disposable, and many patients have staples, especially after being treated in the emergency room. Staple removers may be reused, however, with appropriate sterilization (Fig. A.20).

Syringes
- Clinicians need mostly 1-mL syringes for skin procedures (e.g., biopsies), as well as some 3-mL, a few 5-mL, and even fewer 10-mL (for excisions) syringes. Two 25-mL syringes may also come in handy for thoracenteses, knee aspirations, irrigations, and so forth.

Needles (for Injection)

NOTE: *The larger the number, the smaller the needle!* Clinicians need mostly 1.5-inch, 25-gauge and 0.5-inch, 30-gauge needles for skin local anesthesia. The larger 21-gauge and 18-gauge needles are used to aspirate viscous fluid (e.g., ganglions, 18G) or large amounts of fluid (e.g., knee aspiration). Eighteen-gauge needles are also used to draw up anesthetic; it goes much more quickly than with needles that are smaller.

5-Inch Needle Extender
- After twisting the extender on to a syringe, the practitioner then locks the needle to this "extender." It is reusable and can be used to reach deep areas like the cervix, posterior pharynx, anus, etc. (See Chapter 127, Loop Electrosurgical Excision Procedure for Treating Cervical Intraepithelial Neoplasia, Fig, 127.4.)

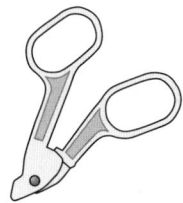

Fig. A.20 Davis & Geck staple remover.

Madajet

- A unique instrument for injecting solutions without a needle and with virtually no pain is the Madajet. Each application provides 0.1 mL of liquid for the intended site. It can be used to anesthetize for a simple skin biopsy or used in combination with steroids to treat hypertrophic and keloid scars. It is especially helpful in dense tissue where injecting with a needle is difficult. The instrument is cocked and then activated by pushing a button. This is the same basic unit that has been adapted for the no-needle vasectomy. (Be sure to order the correct device depending on whether it will be used for dermal applications or for vasectomies.) By using small volumes it also prevents distortion of tissue. Extenda Tips are available in varying lengths to reach tissue in the back of the mouth, the rectum, and other areas. It is easily cleaned between patients. Possible indications as listed by the manufacturer include anesthesia for digital block or prior to treating verrucae; steroids for keloids, lichen chronicus simplex, erythema nodosum, and lichen planus; injecting fasciitis, Morton's neuralgia, and more.

Suture

- Use cutting needles for the majority of patients:
  Skin: 3-0, 4-0, 5-0, and 6-0 nylon (for most interrupted skin closures)
  4-0 and 5-0 Prolene (for subcuticular procedures)
  Deep inverted: 3-0, 4-0, and 5-0 Vicryl
- See Chapter 19, Laceration and Incision Repair: Suture Selection.

Sterile Drapes, Fenestrated and Nonfenestrated

- Both polyurethane and paper drapes are available in solid and fenestrated versions. The area around the fenestration has an adhesive backing to keep it in place. The paper is cheaper but doesn't lie in place as well and can become soiled with blood.

Mayo Stand with Tray to Hold Instruments
Magnification Loupes

- Welch Allyn: 2.5× to 3×; has light with battery pack

Comedone Extractor

- Saalfeld or Unna types (Fig. A.21)

Ear Irrigation Setup

- A variety of units are available. One of the least expensive (approximately $40), most effective, and easiest to use is the Elephant Ear Wash System (Fig. A.22).

Ear Loop Curette

- For cerumen removal: Sklar #67-2513. These are available in both reusable metal and disposable, softer plastic. The latter are less traumatic and reduce the discomfort of removing cerumen.

For Ingrown Toenails

- Locke periosteal nail elevator (Fig. A.23)
- Nail splitter (Fig. A.24)

Chalazion Clamp (Small) with Curette (Figs. A.25 and A.26)
Vaginal Speculum

- Small, medium, large Graves'
- Nonconductive, vented for loop electrosurgical excision procedure
- Extra long (Snowman by CooperSurgical) for obese patients; very helpful for difficult cases

Endocervical Curette (Kevorkian, Without a Basket) (Disposable Available from Coopersurgical and Others)
Endocervical Speculum (Small, Large)

- For colposcopy and removal of cervical polyps (see Chapter 124, Colposcopic Examination)

Cervical Dilators (Including Silver Probe)

- For endometrial biopsy, cervical stenosis, and dilation and curettage (see appropriate chapters)

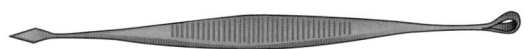

Fig. A.21 Saalfeld comedone extractor.

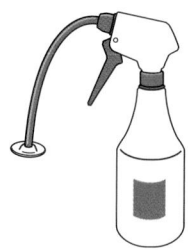

Fig. A.22 Elephant ear washer system.

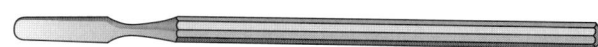

Fig. A.23 Locke elevator.

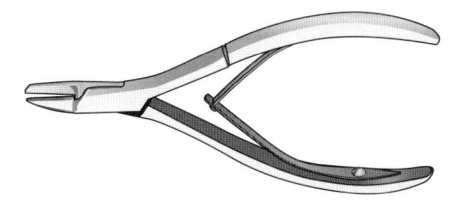

Fig. A.24 Nail splitter.

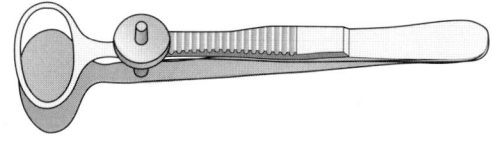

Fig. A.25 Desmarres chalazion clamp.

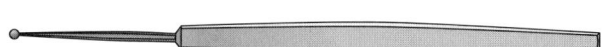

Fig. A.26 Skeele chalazion curette.

Dilateria (Thin, Medium Thick, Thick)

- For cervical stenosis
- Used to dilate a cervix atraumatically
- See Chapter 126, Cervical Stenosis and Cervical Dilation

Word Bartholin Cyst Catheter
Uterine Sound

- Malleable rod is used to determine the depth of the uterus (from external os to back wall). Such information decreases the likelihood of uterine perforation during procedures.

Vaginal Sidewall Retractors

- Used for cryotherapy of cervix, loop electrosurgical excision procedure (see Chapter 127, Loop Electrosurgical Excision Procedure for Treating Cervical Intraepithelial Neoplasia)

Single-Tooth Tenaculum for Cervix

- Used to stabilize the cervix for intrauterine device placement, endometrial biopsy, laminaria insertion, or dilation, or to perform colpocentesis (see Chapter 113, Pregnancy Termination: First-Trimester Suction Aspiration)

Intrauterine Device Remover
- See Chapter 135, Intrauterine Device Insertion and Removal

McGivney Hemorrhoid Ligator
- See Chapter 87, Office Treatment of Hemorrhoids; Fig. 87.4

Infrared Coagulator (Redfield)
- See Chapter 87, Office Treatment of Hemorrhoids; Fig. 87.7
- Used for hemorrhoids, warts, tattoos, nasal turbinates, and bleeders

Silver Probe
- This small malleable metal probe is basically a thickened wire with slightly bulbous ends. It is used to probe suspected fistulae around the anus and to probe for the cervical canal when the os is stenotic (see Chapter 85, Anal Fissure and, Lateral Sphincterotomy, and Anal Fistula).

Liquid Nitrogen Cryogun and Dewar (Brymill, Wallach) for Skin
- See Chapter 14, Cryosurgery

Casting Supplies
- See Chapter 175, Ankle and Foot Splinting, Casting, and Taping and Chapter 176, Cast Immobilization and Upper Extremity Splinting

Wall Blood Pressure Cuff with Stethoscope
Glucose Monitor
Oxygen Tank on Mobile Cart
Electrocardiography Machine
Pulse Oximeter and Vital Signs Monitor (Welch Allyn) (Consider Capnography if Performing Moderate Sedation)
Defibrillator
Banyan Emergency Kit
- See Chapter 212, Anaphylaxis

Electrosurgical Coagulation Unit
- See Chapter 25, Radiofrequency Surgery (Modern Electrosurgery) and Fig. 25.1
- Spend a little more and purchase a high-frequency unit for cutting (Ellman, Wallach, CooperSurgical)

Smoke Evacuator for Electrosurgical Application
- See Chapter 25, Radiofrequency Surgery, (Modern Electrosurgery) Fig. 25.17

Cart for Electrosurgical Coagulation Unit and Smoke Evacuator
- See Chapter 25, Radiofrequency Surgery (Modern Electrosurgery)

Otoscope and Ophthalmoscope
Sharps Containers
Safety Goggles

Examination Tables, Powered
- A matter of an inch or two makes a big difference. (Twenty-four inches is the ideal height when the table is as low as it can go. It cannot be higher.)

Examination Stools
Refrigerator for Medications
- Must be a separate unit from the one used to store lunches!

Autoclave
Portable DVD Player(S) or Online Access to Teaching Videos for Patient Education
Binocular Microscope

OPTIONAL EQUIPMENT TO CONSIDER

Air Purifier
Colonoscope
- See Chapter 90, Colonoscopy

Colposcope
- See Chapter 124, Colposcopic Examination, Fig. 124.8

Flexible Sigmoidoscope With Suction Pump and Light Source, Cart
- See Chapter 89, Flexible Sigmoidoscopy

Gastroscope
- See Chapter 91, Esophagogastroduodenoscopy
- Consider the new thin-diameter versions that do not require sedation.

Halogen Flexible Floor Light or Mobile High-Intensity Ceiling Surgical Light
Intravenous Pole
Nasopharyngoscope
- See Chapter 64, Nasolaryngoscopy

Nitrous Oxide Cryotherapy Unit
- See Chapter 125, Cryotherapy of the Cervix, Fig. 125.1
- Tips: 19- and 25-mm flat and slight conical for cervix
- Slanted end tips for skin
- Hemorrhoid tip (multifunctional for skin lesions; virtually never used for hemorrhoids!)

Stress Electrocardiography Unit
- See Chapter 74, Exercise (Stress) Testing

VE-11 Handzfree Anesthetic Bottle Holder
- See Chapter 5, Local Anesthesia, Fig. 5.1
- Saves time; holds multidose vials of anesthetic; inexpensive

INFORMED CONSENT

Patrick J. Haddad*

Before a clinician performs any procedure or offers other treatment, the patient and the clinician must discuss the reasons for it; the available alternatives; the possible material complications from the procedure or treatment, as well as those from forgoing it; and then the patient must consent. Consent is often considered to be simply a form which the patient needs to sign before a procedure or treatment begins, rather than being a process that results in the patient deciding, on an informed basis, whether to accept or reject treatment. Many clinicians mistakenly believe or hope that a signed consent form, by itself, will prevent a professional liability lawsuit. However, a consent form alone is not legally sufficient to protect a clinician from litigation or from liability if a suit is filed.

LEGAL CONSENT

A patient's consent to treatment is important to clinicians for various reasons, including liability exposure. *Clinicians have a legal liability exposure to claims for battery and the failure to obtain informed consent.* A clinician commits battery by treating a patient without consent. Battery is an intentional tort that does not require proof of negligence or of the intent to do harm. In general, a person commits battery by intentionally touching another individual without consent. The individual may be permitted to recover monetary damages absent bodily injury, although the damages awarded in such circumstances may be nominal. For medical care, consent may be express or implied by the patient seeking treatment or otherwise manifesting consent, or consent may be implied by law, such as in an emergency. If consent is given or implied, however, it is not limitless. A clinician remains exposed to liability for battery if the treatment furnished exceeds the boundaries of the consent given or implied.

A patient's consent may be sufficient for a clinician to successfully defend a battery claim. However, if the consent, or the patient's refusal of treatment, was not preceded by disclosure of the material benefits, risks, and alternatives, the clinician may continue to have a liability exposure, even if the procedure or treatment itself was furnished in a competent manner without technical error or if the procedure was declined. *For there to be liability for lack of informed consent, the patient generally must show that the clinician was negligent, the patient was injured and sustained damages, and the negligence was a proximate cause of the injury and damages.* Lack of informed consent is a claim based on professional negligence (i.e., malpractice). Unlike battery, which requires proof of an intentional touching without consent, a negligence claim requires proof of the applicable standard

of care and that the clinician failed to furnish care in conformity with that standard, in addition to proof of injury, damages, and causation. The standard of care, and whether the standard has been satisfied or breached, is typically established through the testimony of expert witnesses.

Across the United States, there are generally two alternative ways by which the standard of care is measured when lack of informed consent is alleged. One way is from *the perspective of clinicians—the reasonable clinician standard.* Under this standard, timely information must be given to the patient and in accordance with accepted standards of practice among clinicians with similar training and experience in the community, or nationally for care furnished by a specialist. This view is followed by a slight majority of jurisdictions in the United States. The alternative view, adopted by slightly less than one half of the jurisdictions in the United States, is from *the perspective of patients—the reasonable person standard,* under which the patient must be informed of the risks and alternatives that a reasonable person in the patient's position would consider material in deciding whether to accept or to reject the proposed treatment.

Both standards are measured objectively, rather than by the subjective intent of the clinician and the patient who are parties to a malpractice suit. Under either standard, risks that are not serious or are remote, or which are already known by the patient or which patients typically know, are generally not considered material.

Adults who do not have the capacity to make decisions about their own health may not give or withhold consent, or if they purport to do so, their consent will not be effective legally. Similarly, minor children typically may not consent to medical treatment, although some states have enacted exceptions by statute. For incompetent adults (adults lacking capacity) and minors, consent must be obtained from a legal guardian or parent. In emergencies, it is usually permissible to perform procedures or furnish treatment necessary to save the patient's life without consent when it cannot be obtained in a timely fashion.

Determining capacity is its own challenge; there is no definitive assessment tool to determine whether the patient understands what is being proposed and the consequences of their action or inaction. While there are multiple guidelines and standards for evaluating capacity, it is more generally a commonsense judgment made following the clinician's interaction with the patient. Simple questions such as the following (as quoted from Sabiston) may help with the assessment of capacity:

- What do you understand about what is going on with your health right now?
- What treatment (or diagnostic test or procedure) has been proposed to you?
- What are the benefits and risks?
- Why have you decided to _____?

Consider the following from the AMA Code of Medical Ethics: "When a patient lacks decision-making capacity, the clinician

* Mr. Haddad is a member of Kerr, Russell, and Weber, PLC, Detroit, Michigan. Mr. Haddad is cochair of the firm's health care law practice and is a member of the State Bar of Michigan Healthcare Law Section, the American Bar Association Health Law Section, and the American Health Lawyers Association. This chapter is presented for informational purposes only and does not constitute legal advice by Kerr, Russell, and Weber, PLC, or Mr. Haddad. Clinicians should consult with legal counsel knowledgeable in the laws of the jurisdictions in which they practice medicine.

has an ethical responsibility to identify an appropriate surrogate to make decisions on the patient's behalf. The could be the person the patient designated as surrogate through a durable power of attorney for healthcare or other mechanism or a family member or other intimate associate, in keeping with applicable law and policy if the patient has not previously designated a surrogate."

Some jurisdictions may excuse the obtaining of informed consent when the information might have a detrimental effect on the patient's physical or psychological well-being. The availability and scope of this so-called "therapeutic privilege" can vary among jurisdictions, and clinicians should use caution—and consult with legal counsel or with their liability carrier's risk management—before relying on it.

In addition, clinicians need to consider the ethical issues raised by postponing the disclosure of information to patients. Ethically, it may be appropriate in special circumstances to postpone or delay disclosure of certain information if early communication is clearly contraindicated. However, withholding medical information from patients without their knowledge is not ethically permissible. Although all information need not be communicated to the patient immediately or all at once, clinicians should assess the amount of information a patient is capable of receiving at a given time. Consult with the patient's family, professional colleagues, an ethics committee, or other institutional resource for help in assessing the risks and harms associated with delayed disclosure. Full disclosure should be offered to a patient when the patient is able to decide whether to receive the information. This should be done according to a definite plan so that disclosure is not permanently delayed.

Some states have codified by statute certain informed consent procedures. Texas, for example, has established panels of clinicians and lawyers who together write rules for informed consent for many surgical procedures, including the use of consent forms (Fig. B.1). Also, Michigan mandates that all women receive a state-approved booklet before mastectomy for breast cancer.

Clinicians should be aware of the law in their respective states, both legislative and judicial. Clinicians often have many resources available on consent issues, such as state and specialty medical societies. In addition, liability insurers will often furnish guidance to their insured clinicians on consent issues and may have available model consent forms.

In cases in which a legally mandated consent form is not required, a general consent form that identifies the patient, the procedure, the indications, and the risks can be used to document the clinician's disclosures and discussion with the patient, and the patient's consent (Fig. B.2). Some states may require a witness to sign the consent form. Many clinicians in office practice may ask nurses or other office staff to witness. Because of potential conflict-of-interest issues that may be raised in litigation, clinicians may consider having a family member or friend of the patient also witness the consent process, in addition to the clinician's staff, if possible.

MODELS OF MEDICAL DECISION MAKING

The courts have been criticized for setting standards that do not actually reflect medical practice and may interfere with the clinician-patient relationship. The problem may lie in the implementation, not in the actual concept. The ethical concept of informed consent includes the legal concept of consent, but it goes further: *the patient must be a partner in the decision-making process* (Box B.1). Just as the laws have evolved in clarifying informed consent, the transition toward involving the patient more in the process has also occurred.

There are essentially four models of medical decision making:

1. *Traditional model:* The clinician decides whether to perform a procedure and which procedure to perform; the patient's trust and confidence in the clinician replace the need for consent.
2. *Traditional informed consent:* The clinician decides whether to perform a procedure and which procedure to perform with the patient's informed consent.

3. *Collaboration:* The clinician and the patient work together to make a joint decision about the procedure.
4. *Patient choice:* The patient decides with the clinician's counsel.

If given a choice, some patients will choose the traditional model, and a few will choose the fourth model. Most patients and clinicians are more comfortable with either traditional informed consent or collaboration, and clinicians should learn how to use both models as well as how to determine which model to use for a specific patient.

Notwithstanding the model of medical decision making utilized, a clinician will be held, for liability purposes, to the standard of informed consent adopted by the jurisdiction in which he or she practices. This means that for liability purposes, the clinician must ensure that the necessary disclosures to the patient have been made and documented in the medical record and in any consent form used.

CONSENT IS A PROCESS

With the possible exception of treatment needed in emergencies, there is rarely an exception to the rule that all procedures or other treatment—whether office or facility based—should be preceded by disclosure of the material risks and benefits, and discussion that allows the patient to participate in and to decide whether to have the procedure or other treatment. In many instances, it may be permissible to obtain and to rely on the patient's oral consent, which should be documented explicitly by the clinician in the medical record summarizing all the essential points (risks, benefits, possible complications, alternatives, etc.). In other instances, particularly those involving surgical procedures, the patient should sign a consent form that documents the process utilized. Some states have laws that specify certain language on consent forms for certain procedures.

The process of discussing the procedure with the patient or guardian and providing education about the procedure itself, the possible complications, and aftercare responsibilities of the patient should all be considered part of the consent process. The relevant information provided should be appropriate to the patient's age and educational level. The consent form can be used as a patient education tool, with a copy containing the patient's signature to be given to the patient for reference. Patients can be educated during the consent process about the legal requirements for the signed form and the fact that results of medical procedures are not guaranteed. However, bringing the form out at the last minute for signature can produce some patient anxiety and suspicion. A better approach may be to start the process by giving the patient the consent form to read, then using the form to guide the discussion. For certain procedures, such as vasectomy, the form can be sent out before the consultation visit or given at the time of the consultation. The patient can read it, think about it, then return it before surgery. The consent form can include postprocedure instructions as well as instructions for contacting the clinician or an associate if complications occur after hours.

Many liability insurance companies advise that patients view videos discussing the proposed procedure. This ensures that the patient has an opportunity to consider all the pertinent information and serves as a record for defense of a lawsuit. However, a video is not a substitute for discussion between clinician and patient.

The process of informed consent can be summarized as follows:

1. Establish responsibility:
   * The clinician's role
   * The patient's role
2. Establish expected duration of responsibility.
3. Define the problem with the patient.
4. Set goals for treatment and establish whether cure is a reasonable expectation.
5. Select an approach to treatment; during this step the informed consent form is signed.
6. Perform extended treatment and follow-up.

State of Texas: 25 TAC §601.4(a)(1)

DISCLOSURE AND CONSENT
Medical and Surgical Procedures

TO THE PATIENT: You have the right, as a patient, to be informed about your condition and the recommended surgical, medical, or diagnostic procedure to be used so that you may make the decision whether or not to undergo the procedure after knowing the risks and hazards involved. This disclosure is not meant to scare or alarm you; it is simply an effort to make you better informed so you may give or withhold your consent to the procedure.

    I (we) voluntarily request Dr._____ as my physician, and such associates, technical assistants, and other health care providers as they may deem necessary, to treat my condition which has been explained to me (us) as:

_____

_____

_____ .

    I (we) understand that the following surgical, medical, and/or diagnostic procedures are planned for me and I (we) voluntarily consent and authorize these procedures:

_____

_____

_____ .

    I (we) understand that my physician may discover other or different conditions which require additional or different procedures than those planned. I (we) authorize my physician, and such associates, technical assistants, and other health care providers, to perform such other procedures which are advisable in their professional judgment.

    I (we) (do) (do not) consent to the use of blood and blood products as deemed necessary.

    I (we) understand that no warranty or guarantee has been made to me (us) as to result or cure.

    Just as there may be risks and hazards in continuing my present condition without treatment, there are also risks and hazards related to the performance of the surgical, medical, and/or diagnostic procedures planned for me. I (we) realize that common to surgical, medical, and/or diagnostic procedures is the potential for infection, blood clots in veins and lungs, hemorrhage, allergic reactions, and even death. I (we) also realize that the following risks and hazards may occur in connection with this particular procedure:

_____

_____

_____ .

    I (we) understand that anesthesia involves additional risks and hazards but I (we) request the use of anesthetics for the relief and protection from pain during the planned and additional procedures. I (we) realize the anesthesia may have to be changed, possibly without explanation to me (us).

    I (we) understand that certain complications may result from the use of any anesthetic including respiratory problems, drug reaction, paralysis, brain damage, or even death. Other risks and hazards which may result from the use of general anesthetics range from minor discomfort to injury to vocal cords, teeth, or eyes. I (we) understand that other risks and hazards resulting from spinal or epidural anesthetics include headache and chronic pain.

    I (we) have been given an opportunity to ask questions about my condition, alternative forms of anesthesia and treatment, risks of nontreatment, the procedures to be used, and the risks and hazards involved, and I (we) believe that I (we) have sufficient information to give this informed consent.

    I (we) certify this form has been fully explained to me (us), that I (we) have read it or have had it read to me (us), that the blank spaces have been filled in, and that I (we) understand its contents.

Fig. B.1   State of Texas disclosure and consent form for medical and surgical procedures. (Courtesy Texas Medical Board, http://www.tmb.state.tx.us/.)

PATIENT/OTHER LEGALLY RESPONSIBLE PERSON (signature required)

DATE:_____ TIME:_____ AM/PM

WITNESS:

Signature

Name (Print)

Address (Street or PO Box)

City, State, Zip Code

Fig. B.1, cont.

Patient Consent Form

I came to the office of Dr. _____ on _____ (date) for evaluation and treatment of the following condition:

_____
(description of diagnosis, etiology, and different diagnosis)

We discussed the different treatments possible, and discussed the risks of not treating the condition. Based on the advice given by Dr. _____ and my own judgment, I agree to undergo the following procedure:

_____
(description of anesthetic, procedure, and dressing)

We discussed the different outcomes that could occur, and most of the possible complications. I am aware that other complications could occur that we could not foresee. I agree to follow the instructions for self-care after the procedure, and to return for follow-up care on:_____. I will call the office or answering service if any problems arise before the scheduled follow-up visit.

_____   _____
Patient's signature   Date/time

_____   _____
Witness's signature   Clinician's signature

One copy for chart, one copy for patient.

Fig. B.2   Sample of patient consent form.

COMPLICATIONS HAPPEN AND THE CONSENT PROCESS WILL BE SCRUTINIZED

Surgical and other complications are at the core of many malpractice suits. Clinicians should not rely solely on a signed consent form for protection in a malpractice suit. Rather, they should rely on the process that resulted in the patient's consent, including the patient's participation in that process. In malpractice litigation, that process will be viewed through the lens of hindsight. A clinician who brings out a highly technical consent form to be signed by the patient at the last minute is not likely to be viewed favorably. By itself, such a form may not necessarily be evidence that the patient's consent was informed. A consent form is only one piece of evidence, and in lawsuits other evidence, such as the patient's testimony, is examined as well. *A consent form itself cannot—and is not intended to—substitute for a candid discussion* with the patient about the procedure and the inclusion of the patient in the decision-making process, or for

> **BOX B.1   Elements of Informed Consent**
>
> - Disclosure of information
> - Competency/capacity (the patient is not a minor, unconscious, intoxicated, or incapable of participating in the process)
> - Understanding
> - Voluntarism
> - Decision making
> - Patient participation

documentation in the medical record of the discussion before the patient signs the form. For some patients, particularly uninformed or anxious patients, knowledge of the risk may dissuade them from undergoing an otherwise needed procedure.

Many consent forms use language that is too technical; the forms are often too long to read and interpret during an office visit. Consent forms are often handed to patients during hospital registration by nonprofessional personnel, and some patients are unable to comprehend the procedure even after explanation. The consent form should be meaningful to the patient. *Likewise, to provide the additional type of documentation that is also useful in a court case, the clinician should include in the patient's chart a narrative of the discussion between clinician and patient during the decision-making process, in addition to the actual consent form.*

Clinicians should always *be careful not to "overpromise"* what a procedure can do. Honesty is best. "Never say never, and never say always!" There are always exceptions. If someone asks about a rare complication, the clinician should not say it *won't* happen! It could. An example should be given instead. If the patient plays the lotto, the clinician should ask if he or she is likely to win. The answer is usually "No." But could the patient win? Is it possible? The answer is usually "Yes." So it goes with complications. Will it happen? "Most likely not. But, in rare instances, it could."

It goes without saying that *no consent form will protect a clinician from true malpractice.* Competence and keeping up to date educationally are essential. Seeking expert advice and second opinions is encouraged, and knowing one's limits is essential. Especially in primary care, clinicians must be sure to inform the patient of their training and background; they should not pretend to be an orthopedist, or obstetrician, or gastroenterologist, or plastic surgeon. The patient should seek another opinion if he or she is at all uncomfortable.

As many have said before, the best way to minimize the risk of a lawsuit is to have an excellent clinician-patient relationship with both the patient and the family. Each patient is different. Some have a lot of questions that need to be addressed and answered.

Some have been let down by the medical system in the past and are fearful. Some have extreme anxiety, and no amount of reassurance helps them. Some want absolute assurances that are impossible.

Ultimately, it is the patient's decision whether to accept or reject treatment. As a matter of practicality, sometimes personalities just aren't compatible. When "the vibes are bad" between the patient and the caretaker, clinicians should learn to sense this and not try to "force" things. Providers should recognize that they can't always be all things to all people, and that referring a patient to "other experts" is often best for the relationship and to reduce liability exposure.

Complications occur, even though the clinician has furnished good quality care with technical perfection. Unfortunately, mistakes can and do happen. In the past, clinicians were typically advised by their hospitals, insurers, and legal counsel—and maybe ordered by their employers—to refrain from expressing sympathy or compassion to the patient or family in these circumstances. The reason is that such statements could have been construed as an admission of malpractice and used as evidence against the clinician in litigation. Expressions of sympathy were also seen as inviting malpractice suits. Nevertheless, most institutions have now enacted policies of transparency and accountability by admitting errors and volunteering fair settlements. The code of medical ethics of the AMA and the code of conduct of the American College of Surgeons states that adverse events and medical errors should be fully disclosed. As it turns out, it may not be as easy to sue a clinician who is also a person with human limitations as opposed to just a clinician. Originally anecdotal reports and now evidence suggest that this practice may reduce the number of malpractice suits, the dollar amount of settlements, and defense costs, although there is some debate as to whether the quantity of claims is affected. Most states have enacted laws—referred to as "I'm sorry" laws—that provide that expressions of sympathy and compassion by clinicians are inadmissible as an admission of liability in malpractice litigation. The scope of these laws varies among jurisdictions, but typically are narrowly drawn and normally will not shield statements that admit—or can be construed as admitting—fault. Consequently, clinicians, when caught up in the moment, could unwittingly express sympathy or compassion in such a way as to unfairly implicate himself or herself before a jury.

BILLING ISSUES

Evaluation and management codes are used to bill for surgical consultation, evaluation, and management services furnished by a clinician in the office. The informed consent process is included in the evaluation and management codes and is not a separately reimbursable service. The range of available evaluation and management codes varies according to the degree of the examination performed, the history taken, the complexity of the medical decision making, and the time spent with the patient and family. When extended counseling with the patient or family is necessary, the clinician should consult with his or her billing advisor to ensure that the appropriate evaluation and management codes are reimbursable and billed.

Acknowledgment

The editors recognize the contributions of Julie Graves Moy, MD, to this chapter in the previous edition of this text.

ONLINE RESOURCES

College of Registered Nurses of British Columbia statement on informed consent: http://www.crnbc.ca/downloads/359.pdf.
State of Texas Medical Board. http://www.tmb.state.tx.us/.

RECOMMENDED READING

American College of Surgeons Statements on Principals. *Code of Professional Conduct*; 2016. http://bulletin.facs.org/2016/09/american-college-surgeons-statements-principles/#code.

Informed consent and shared decision making. In: *American Medical Association. Code of Medical Ethics*. Chicago: American Medical Association; 2016:21–42.

American Medical Association, Code of Ethics Opinions 2.1.1 (http://www.tmb.state.tx.us/)(Informed Consent) and 2.1.3 (http://www.tmb.state.tx.us/) (Withholding Information from Patients).

Caterine JM, Miller B. Informed consent: procedure specific. *Iowa Med.* 1989;79:231.

Giordano J, Duffy J. Practical considerations for determining patient capacity and consent. *Am Fam Physician.* 2010;81(9):1090–1092.

Green JA. Minimizing malpractice risk by role clarification: the confusing transition from tort to contract. *Ann Intern Med.* 1988;109:234.

Hansson MO. Balancing the quality of consent. *J Med Ethics.* 1998;24:182.

Kaibara PD. 8 ways to improve the informed consent process. *J Fam Pract.* 2010;59:373.

King JS, Moulton BW. Rethinking conformed consent: the case for shared medical decision-making. *Am J Law Med.* 2006;32:429.

Lidz CW, Appelbaum PS, Meisel A. Two models of implementing informed consent. *Ann Intern Med.* 1988;148:1385.

Loewy EH. *Textbook of Healthcare Ethics.* New York: Plenum Press; 1996.

Mazur DJ. What should patients be told prior to a medical procedure? Ethical and legal perspectives on medical informed consent. *Am J Med.* 1986;81:1051.

Peters SK, Finberg J, Kroll JD. *The Law of Medical Practice in Michigan.* Ann Arbor, MI: Institute of Continuing Legal Education; 1981.

Savulescu J, Momeyer RW. Should informed consent be based on rational beliefs? *J Med Ethics.* 1997;23:282.

Sprung CL, Winick BJ. Informed consent in theory and practice: legal and medical perspectives on the informed consent doctrine and a proposed reconceptualization. *Crit Care Med.* 1989;17:1346.

Vaiani CE, Brody H. Ethics and professionalism in surgery. In: Townsend CM, Beauchamp RD, Evers BM, Mattox KL, eds. *Sabiston Textbook of Surgery.* 20th ed. Philadelphia: Elsevier; 2017:20–24.

Walter P. The doctrine of informed consent: a tale of two cultures and two legal traditions. *Issues Law Med.* 1999;14:357.

LATEX ALLERGY GUIDELINES

Sumana Reddy

Sensitivity to natural rubber latex (NRL) has gained increasing prominence over the last 3 decades. Current estimates of the prevalence of immediate hypersensitivity to latex in the general population is now 1%. Latex is now likely the second most important cause of intraoperative anaphylaxis, behind muscle relaxants. Although NRL has been in widespread use for over a century, multiple factors, including a dramatic increase in use and changes in production time and production quality, have led to now well-established reports of severe reactions. In 1997, the National Institute for Occupational Safety and Health (NIOSH) issued an advisory recommending that latex gloves be used only by those workers exposed to blood or body fluids, and not by food handlers, hobbyists, and those performing many housekeeping activities. NIOSH also recommends that if NRL gloves are to be used, they should be low protein and powder free. Increasingly, hospitals are making the decision to be latex-free in terms of glove purchases. It is a reasonable decision, given the prevalence of latex allergy, to do all procedures with nonlatex gloves. Although there are a variety of alternatives to latex, not all have the tensile strength, flexibility, and impermeability of NRL. The solution may be to use different glove materials for examination versus surgery and procedural use.

SYMPTOMS OF LATEX ALLERGY

Reactions to NRL are type I, immediate hypersensitivity reactions. They can cause local or systemic urticaria, symptoms of rhinoconjunctivitis or bronchospasm, and anaphylaxis. The proteins of NRL have been described as unique in that an unpredictable course may occur in the progression from no or mild symptoms to anaphylaxis. The sensitization begins and is perpetuated both as a contact allergen and as an inhalant. The greatest degree of sensitization occurs in areas where powdered latex gloves with a high NRL protein content are used. In these situations, the cornstarch powder particles appear to bind or adsorb latex to the surface. These latex-cornstarch powder particles have been demonstrated to aerosolize, especially when gloves are removed. Prolonged exposure through the lungs appears to cause high rates of sensitization. Those who are sensitized may crossreact to certain foods such as banana, kiwi, chestnut, or avocado. NRL gloves may also cause an irritant contact dermatitis from occlusion and frequent handwashing, or a delayed hypersensitivity reaction from chemicals used in processing. These are not reactions to latex itself (Box C.1).

RISK GROUPS

Those at greatest risk of sensitization are all those groups with cumulatively prolonged exposure to latex. The greatest prevalence appears to be in those who have undergone repeated surgeries, especially children with spina bifida or urogenital abnormalities. Others at risk include workers in the latex manufacturing industry and health care workers. Studies indicate 10% to 17% of health care workers have already become sensitized, and more than 2% have occupational asthma as a result of latex exposure. In addition, more than 50% of persons who are sensitive to latex have a history of atopic illness, or hay fever (Box C.2).

NONLATEX MATERIALS

The establishment of universal precautions in 1985 has led to an increased use of latex gloves through the spectrum of health services from phlebotomy to nursing home care. This use is now being reevaluated in light of growing understanding of the process of sensitization. As recommended by NIOSH, all health care providers should make purchasing decisions avoiding the use of powdered, high-protein latex gloves, and in favor of powder-free, low-protein gloves. Where possible, nonlatex gloves should be used. As mentioned, in the last decade this has become an increasingly popular solution. These measures have led to a probable drop in the incidence of latex allergy, and certainly a deceleration in the rate of newly sensitized individuals.

There is a range of surgical and nonsurgical gloves available in nonlatex materials. These have been American Society for Testing and Materials tested for barrier integrity and are expected to provide protection against viral particles such as the human immunodeficiency virus when used as recommended. Vinyl gloves are not as effective as other materials against viral penetration.

BOX C.1   Symptoms and Signs Associated With Latex Glove Use

Irritant Contact Dermatitis (Nonimmune)
Gradual onset, over days, caused by handwashing, occlusion, antiseptics, and glove chemicals
Redness
Cracks, fissures
Scaling

Allergic Contact Dermatitis, or Type IV (Delayed Hypersensitivity)
Onset 6–48 hr after contact, caused by chemicals
Erythema
Vesicles
Papules
Pruritus
Blisters
Crusting

Immediate Hypersensitivity, or Type I
Local and generalized urticaria onset within minutes, very rarely longer than 2 hr; caused by latex
Feeling of faintness
Feeling of impending doom
Angioedema
Nausea, vomiting, abdominal cramps
Rhinoconjunctivitis
Bronchospasm
Anaphylactic shock

Occupational latex exposure
  Health care workers
  Rubber industry workers
Medical patient exposure
  Spina bifida
  Urogenital abnormalities
  Other repeated or prolonged surgeries or mucous membrane
    exposure to latex devices, especially early in life
Atopic history or food allergy, especially bananas, avocados,
  kiwis, and chestnuts (cross-reacting protein epitopes)
Low risk: no identifiable risk factors

DIAGNOSIS

When performing procedures, there are issues with identifying the patient who may be latex allergic and with avoiding exposure through inadvertent use of a product containing latex. Use of a standardized questionnaire is recommended where any suspicion may exist (Box C.3). It is also important to prevent the development of latex sensitization in the health care workers performing and assisting in the procedure. The use of nonlatex gloves and supplies can streamline processes and has become more of an option as these gloves become competitively priced.

The diagnosis of latex sensitivity is not straightforward. It is made through a combination of thorough medical history and immunologic testing. Because symptoms can be generalized and nonspecific, the sensitized individual often remains unaware of the condition. While prick testing is available and is very effective (see Chapter 67, Allergy Testing and Immunotherapy), allergen extracts are not standardized in the United States. Therefore, such skin testing should be carried out only by centers with experience in preparing and managing extracts, which may cause a high incidence of anaphylaxis. Food and Drug Administration–approved and other in vitro tests to measure latex-specific IgE are available (e.g., Phadiatop, Thermo Fisher Scientific; ViraCor Eurofins Clinical Diagnostics; HYTEC, HYCOR Biomedical). The low specificity of these tests, with at least 20% false-negative results and unclear positive predictive value, gives them limitations. Negative serologic testing with a strongly positive history would suggest the value of skin prick testing in experienced hands to confirm the diagnosis. Because individuals with no risk factors or prior symptoms have had anaphylactic reactions, those who are asymptomatic with positive tests should be advised to exercise caution.

If in doubt at the time of performing a procedure, it is best to avoid use of latex-containing medical devices and products. Especially prone to cause reactions are gloves and urinary catheters placed in direct contact with mucosal surfaces (e.g., during pelvic examinations).

The task of identifying latex-containing medical devices has been simplified by Food and Drug Administration requirements indicating on packaging whether latex is contained in a product.

I. Allergies
* Have you had a history of hay fever, asthma, eczema, allergies, or problems with rashes?
* Are you allergic (rash, oral itching, swelling, or wheezing) to any foods, especially bananas, avocados, kiwi, or chestnuts?

II. Job-Related Symptoms
* Does your work involve any exposure to latex products, including latex gloves? Have you ever had allergic reactions to something in your work environment?
* If you have had a rash on your hands after wearing latex gloves, how long after putting on the gloves did the rash develop? What did it look like?

III. Hidden Reactions to Latex
* Have you ever had swelling, itching, hives, shortness of breath, cough, or other allergic symptoms during or after blowing up a balloon, undergoing a dental procedure, using condoms or diaphragms, or following a vaginal or rectal examination?
* Have you ever had an allergic reaction of unknown cause, especially during a medical or dental procedure?

IV. Surgical History
* Have you ever had surgery, and if so, what type?
* Do you have spina bifida or any urinary tract problem requiring surgery or catheterization?

Medical Devices With Potential Latex Content
Adhesive tape
Ambu-bags
Bandages
Bulb syringes
Dental devices
Electrode pads
Face masks
Gloves
Injection ports
Mattresses on stretchers
PCA syringes
Rubber syringe stoppers and medication vial stoppers
Stethoscope and BP cuff tubing
Tourniquets
Urinary catheters
Wound drains

Household Items With Potential Latex Content
Balloons
Buttons on electronic equipment
Carpet backing
Clothing, including elastic on underwear
Computer mouse pads
Condoms and diaphragms
Diapers
Erasers
Feeding nipples and pacifiers
Food handled with powdered latex gloves
Handles on racquets, tools
Many toys
Rubber bands
Sanitary and incontinence pads
Shoe soles
Sports equipment

BP, Blood pressure; *PCA*, patient-controlled analgesia.

A more detailed *and* periodically updated list of latex-containing products and nonlatex substitutes by brand name is available from the Spina Bifida Association of America (http://www.spinabifidaassociation.org).

BOX C.5 Latex Allergy Management Guidelines for the Hospital Setting

- Ask all patients about latex sensitivity, using a screening questionnaire if relevant.
- Place latex allergy identification bracelet on patient in admitting area.
- Label room as latex-safe and enter in all relevant areas of signage, notes, and databases.
- Disseminate latex allergy protocol and lists of nonlatex substitutes for latex-containing materials that may contact the patient.
- Remove all latex products that would contact the patient and remove all latex gloves. Use PVC tubing or wrap cotton gauze over the extremity if using latex cuffs and tubing or tourniquets.
- Ensure that adhesives and tapes, including ECG electrodes and dressing supplies, are checked for latex content.
- Have a latex-free crash cart available to follow the patient through his or her stay.
- Notify Pharmacy and Central Supply that the patient is latex-sensitive so that latex contact can be eliminated in preparation of materials or drugs for the patient.
- Notify Dietary of relevant food allergies and avoid handling food with powdered latex gloves (NIOSH recommended and mandated by many states).

ECG, Electrocardiogram; *NIOSH*, National Institute of Occupational Safety and Health; *PVC*, polyvinyl chloride.

Lists of latex-containing and latex-free devices may be obtained both directly from individual manufacturers and from the Spina Bifida Association of America. As Box C.4 shows, many medical and household items contain latex. To a sensitized person, all of these may be problematic. To an unsensitized person, the thin stretchy rubber of gloves, condoms, and balloons provides the greatest source of rubber particles leaching from the surface. Solid, molded rubber objects are less likely to leach proteins from their surfaces.

MANAGEMENT

A history of type 1 immediate hypersensitivity reactions necessitates a latex-safe environment. Patient records should be identified clearly for latex allergy, and at no time in treatment should latex gloves, tourniquets, catheters, or other materials come in direct contact with the patient. If blood pressure cuffs and tubing are made of latex, the patient's extremities should be wrapped to prevent contact. Although rubber medication vial and syringe stoppers are listed, to date there have been only rare reactions to medication in contact with latex. For the most part, then, extreme measures (e.g., only using medication from glass ampules or glass syringes) are not recommended. The hospital guidelines provided may be adapted as applicable for an outpatient setting (Box C.5).

Premedication with antihistamines or steroids is not helpful. It may only mask symptoms leading to anaphylaxis without preventing anaphylactic reactions. Persons with latex hypersensitivity should carry an epinephrine autoinjection kit and wear MedicAlert identification. In the medical office, it is always advisable to have available sterile nonlatex gloves for use.

SUPPLIERS

See Table C.1 for a list of suppliers of hypoallergenic nonlatex gloves.

CONCLUSION

For those who have been sensitized, avoidance is the cornerstone of management. In all settings where gloves are heavily used, avoiding sensitization through the purchase of powder-free gloves is recommended. Almost all hospitals have gone toward powder-free and low-protein gloves, and increasing numbers are opting to convert to entirely nonlatex products. This choice has already begun to have a positive impact on the patient with latex allergy and to prevent sensitization in the health care worker. Ironically, with this condition, it is the health care worker who is often the patient.

ICD-10-CM DIAGNOSTIC CODES

989.82   Latex allergy

TABLE C.1 Suppliers of Nonlatex Gloves*

Name of Glove	Material	Company
Dermaprene	Neoprene (polychloroprene polymer)	Ansell (800-321-9752), www.ansellpro.com
Sensicare	Polyisoprene	Medline (800-346-8849), www.medline.com
Elastyfree and Elastylite	Polyisoprene (no accelerators and nonchlorinated)	ECI Medical Technologies (800-668-5289), www.ecimedical.com
Neotech Biogel	Neoprene (polychloroprene polymer)	Regent Medical (800-843-8497)
True Advantage and Ultra Preserve	Butadiene-acrylonitrile (nitrile) and polychloroprene	Tillotson Dynarex (800-445-6830), www.thcnet.com
Elastylite and QualiTouch	Styrene butadiene co-polymer and butadiene-acrylonitrile (nitrile)	Smartpractice (800-522-0595)
Safeskin	Butadiene-acrylonitrile (nitrile), polyvinyl chloride	Kimberly Clark (800-524-3577), www.kchealthcare.com Ammex (800-274-7354), www.ammex.com
FreeForm, Supreno, NeoproEC	Nitrile† (butadiene co-polymer), polyvinyl chloride and polychloroprene	Microflex (800-876-6866), www.microflex.com
Nitrastretch, Synthatech	Nitrile† (butadiene co-polymer), polyvinyl chloride	Top Quality Manufacturing (800-483-8559), www.topqualitygloves.com
Allerderm	Polyvinyl chloride and nitrile	Allerderm (800-365-6868), www.allerderm.com
Duraprene and Esteem	Duraprene and polyisoprene	CardinalHealth (800-964-5227), www.cardinal.com
Allergard	Styrene butadiene block polymer	Allergard (800-255-2500)
N-DEX	Nitrile* (butadiene co-polymer)	Best Glove (800-241-0323)

*Kits containing everything needed for one latex-safe surgical procedure are obtainable from DeRoyal Surgical (800-251-9864), www.deroyal.com.
†Gloves made from nitrile are produced with the same accelerator (mercaptobenzathiazole) as some latex gloves. Those with suspected irritant or allergic contact dermatitis to latex gloves may also react to nitrile.

ONLINE RESOURCES

American Latex Allergy Association. www.latexallergyresources.org.
Latex allergy links. latexallergylinks.tripod.com/.
Spina Bifida Association of America. www.spinabifidaassociation.org.

RECOMMENDED READING

Ahmed S, Aw TC, Adisesh A. Toxicological and immunological aspects of occupational latex allergy. *Toxicol Rev.* 2004;23:123–134.

Arellano R, Bradley J, Sussman G. Prevalence of latex sensitization among hospital physicians occupationally exposed to latex gloves. *Anesthesiology.* 1992;77:905.

Adkinson NF, Bochner BS, Burks AW, Busse WW, Holgate ST, et al., eds. *Middleton's Allergy: Principles and Practice.* 8th ed. Philadelphia: Elsevier; 2014.

Beezhold DH, Beck WC. Surgical glove powders bind latex antigens. *Arch Surg.* 1992;127:1354.

Blumchen K, Bayer P, Buck D, et al. Effects of latex avoidance on latex sensitization, atopy and allergic diseases in patients with spina bifida. *Allergy.* 2010;65:1585–1593.

Condemi J. Allergic reactions to natural rubber latex at home, to rubber products and to cross-reacting foods. *J Allergy Clin Immunol.* 2002;110:2.

Epling C, Duncan J, Archibong E, Østbye T, Pompeii LA, Dement J. Latex allergy symptoms among health care workers: results from a university health and safety surveillance system. *Int J Occup Environ Health.* 2011;17:17–23.

Food and Drug Administration. Latex-containing devices: user labeling. *Fed Register.* 1996;61:32618–32620.

Kwittken PL, Becker J, Oyefara B, et al. Latex hypersensitivity reactions despite prophylaxis. *Allergy Proc.* 1992;13:123.

Lieberman P. Anaphylactic reactions during surgical and medical procedures. *J Allergy Clin Immunol.* 2002;110(suppl 2):S64–S69.

U.S. Department of Health and Human Services, Public Health Service, Centers for Disease Control and Prevention, National Institute for Occupational Safety and Health. *Preventing Allergic Reactions to Natural Rubber Latex in the Workplace.* Cincinnati: Government Printing Office; 1997. NIOSH Pub. No. 97-135.

U.S. Department of Health and Human Services, Public Health Service, Centers for Disease Control and Prevention, National Institute for Occupational Safety and Health. *High Impact: Preventing Occupational Latex Allergy in Health Care Workers.* Cincinnati: Government Printing Office; 2010. DHHS NIOSH publication 2011-118.

APPENDIX D

SUPPLIER INFORMATION

Accutome
263 Great Valley Pkwy.
Malvern, PA 19355
Phone: 800-979-2020
www.accutome.com

Accutron Inc.
Phone: 800-531-2221
www.accutron-inc.com

ACMI Circon Gyrus Olympus
136 Turnpike Rd.
Southborough, MA 01772-2104
Phone: 508-804-2600
www.olympusmedical.co.in/products/urology/
    cystoscopy/index.html

Acuderm
5370 NW 35 Terrace
Ft. Lauderdale, FL 33309
Phone: 800-327-0015
www.acuderm.com

Acuson (owned by Siemens)
1220 Charleston Rd.
P.O. Box 7393
Mountain View, CA 94039-7393
Phone: 800-422-8766
www.healthcare.siemens.com

**Advanced Meditech International Inc.
(AMI)**
86-38 53rd Ave.
Flushing, NY 11373
Phone: 800-635-2452
www.ameditech.com

Advanced Surgi-Pharm Inc.
850 Halpern Ave.
Dorval, QC
H9P 1G6 Canada
Phone: 800-661-5432
www.surgmed.com

Aesculap
3773 Corporate Pkwy.
Center Valley, PA 18034
Phone: 800-282-9000
www.aesculapusa.com

Agilent Technology (formerly Hewlett-
    Packard)
5301 Stevens Creek Blvd.
Santa Clara, CA 95051
Phone: 405-345-8886
www.agilent.com

**Aircast Inc. ([and DonJoy], now owned
    by DJO)**
1430 Decision St.
Vista, CA 92081
Phone: 800-336-6569
www.djoglobal.com

Air-Tite Products Company
565 Central Dr.
Virginia Beach, VA 23455
Phone: 800-231-7762
www.air-tite.shop.com

Akorn Pharmaceuticals
1925 W. Field Ct.
Suite 300
Lake Forest, IL 60045
Phone: 800-932-5676
www.akorn.com

Aldermna
17951 Sky Park Cir.
Suite G
Irvine, CA 92614
Phone: 949-250-8955 or 800-254-8505
Fax: 949-250-8821
www.aldermna.com

AliMed Inc.
297 High St.
Dedham, MA 02026
Phone: 800-225-2610
www.alimed.com

ALK Laboratory
1700 Royston Ln.
Round Rock, TX 78664
Phone: 800-252-9778
www.alk.net

Alkaline Corporation
Allergy Diagnostics Division
714 West Park Ave.
P.O. Box 306
Oakhurst, NJ 07755
Phone: 800-686-6483

Allegiance Healthcare Corp. (a Cardinal
    Health company)
7000 Cardinal Pl.
Dublin, OH 43017
Phone: 614-757-5000 or 800-234-8701
www.cardinal.com

Allergan Inc.
2525 Dupont Dr.
P.O. Box 19534
Irvine, CA 92623-9534
Phone: 800-433-8871 or 800-44BOTOX
www.allergan.com
www.botoxcosmetic.com (physician and
    consumer information)
www.aestheticenhance.org (CME accred-
    ited website; injection techniques)

Allergy Laboratories
P.O. Box 26492
Oklahoma City, OK 73126
Phone: 405-235-1451

Allermed Laboratories
7203 Convoy Ct.
San Diego, CA 92111
Phone: 800-221-2748
www.allermed.com

Allied Biomedical Corp.
3850 Ramada Dr., C-2
Paso Robles, CA 93446
Phone: 800-276-1322
www.alliedbiomedical.com

Allied Healthcare Products Inc.
1720 Sublette Ave.
St. Louis, MO 63110
Phone: 800-444-3940
www.alliedhpi.com

Alma Lasers
485 Half Day Rd.
#100
Buffalo Grove, IL 60089
Phone: 866-414-2562
Fax: 224-377-2050
www.almalasers.com

Aloka (now Hitachi-Aloka)
www.hitachi-aloka.com

Altair Instruments
321 Aviador St.
Suite 113
Camarillo, CA 93010
Phone: 805-388-8503
www.altairinstruments.com

American Medical Systems (now owned by
    Endo Pharmaceuticals)
10700 Bren Rd. West
Minnetonka, MN 55343
Phone: 800-328-3881
www.endo.com

American Sexual Health Association
P.O. Box 13827
Research Triangle Park, NC 27709
Phone: 919-361-8400
www.ashasexualhealth.org

American Society for Colposcopy and Cervical Pathology (ASCCP)
152 West Washington St.
Hagerstown, MD 21740
Phone: 800-787-7227 or 301-733-3640
www.asccp.org

American Society for Gastrointestinal Endoscopy
13 Elm St.
Manchester, MA 01944
Phone: 508-526-8330
www.asge.org

American Urological Association
1120 North Charles St.
Baltimore, MD 21201
Phone: 800-908-9414
www.auanet.com

Anatometal
411 Ingalls St.
Santa Cruz, CA 95060
Phone: 888-262-8663
www.anatometal.com

Angiodynamics
14 Plaza Dr.
Latham, NY 12110
Phone: 518-795-1400
Fax: 518-795-1401
www.angiodynamics.com

Antigen Laboratories Inc.
P.O. Box 123
Liberty, MO 64069
Phone: 800-821-7013
www.antigenlab.com

Arrow International Inc.
2400 Bernville Rd.
Reading, PA 19605
Phone: 800-523-8446
www.arrowintl.com

ArthroCare ENT
7500 Rialto Blvd.
Building 2
Suite 100
Austin, TX 78735
Phone: 800-797-6520
www.arthrocareent.com

American Association for Primary Care Endoscopy
11400 Tomahawk Creek Pkwy.
Leawood, KS 66211-2672
Phone: 913-906-6000, ext: 6706
Fax: 913-906-6092
www.aapce.org

Astra Tech Inc./Wellspect
Urology Division
21535 Hawthorne Blvd.
Suite 525
Torrence, CA 90503
Phone: 877-456-3742
www.wellspect.us

Atrium Medical Corp.
5 Wentworth Dr.
Hudson, NH 03051
Phone: 800-528-7486
www.atriummed.com

Augusta Medical Systems
1027 Broad St.
Augusta, GA 30903
Phone: 877-827-8382
www.augustams.com

B. Braun Medical Inc.
824 12th Ave.
Bethlehem, PA 18018
Phone: 800-523-9676
www.bbraunusa.com

B-Met Endoscopic Inc.
116 Saddle Ridge Dr.
Dallas, PA 18612
Phone: 570-255-1288

Banyan International Corp.
11629 49th Place West
Mukilteo, WA 98275
Phone: 888-STAT-KIT (782-8548)
customerservice@statkit.com
www.statkit.com

Bard Access Systems Inc.
605 North 5600 West
Salt Lake City, UT 84116
Phone: 801 522-5000
Fax: 801 522-4948 / 801 522-5415
medical.services@crbard.com
www.bardaccess.com

Bard Medical Division
8195 Industrial Blvd.
Covington, GA 30014
Phone: 770-784-6100
bardmedical.customerservice@crbard.com
www.bardmedical.com

Barr Pharmaceuticals Teva
Corporate Headquarters
5 Basel St.
Petach Tikva Israel, 49131
Phone: 972-3-9267267
Fax: 972-3-9234050
www.tevapharm.com

Bartor Pharmacal Co.
70 High St.
Rye, NY 10580
Phone: 914-967-4219

Bausch and Lomb
400 Somerset Corporate Blvd.
Bridgewater, NJ 08807
Phone: 800-828-9030
www.bausch.com

Baxter Healthcare Corp.
1 Baxter Pkwy.
Deerfield, IL 60015
Phone: 888-229-0001
www.baxter.com

Bayer Corp.
100 Bayer Rd.
Whippany, NJ 07981
Phone: 862-404-3000
www.bayer.us/

BD Diagnostics Tri Path
780 Plantation Dr.
Burlington, NC 27215
Phone: 336-222-9707 or 800-426-2176
Fax: 336-222-8819
www.bd.com

Becton, Dickinson and Co.
1 Becton Dr.
Franklin Lakes, NJ 07417
Phone: 888-237-2762
www.bd.com/en-us

Beiersdorf
P.O. Box 5529
Norwalk, CT 06856
Phone: 203-853-8008
www.beiersdorfusa.com
www.beiersdorf.org

Bella Products Inc.
27136 Burbank
Foothill Ranch, CA 92610
Phone: 877-550-5655
Fax: 949-855-0698
Email info@bellaproducts.com
www.bellaproducts.com

Belpro Medical Inc.
10450 Secant
Anjou
H1J 1S3 QC, Canada
Phone: 888-230-1010
Fax: 514-355-5554
e-mail: info@belpro.ca
www.belpro.ca

Benson Medical Instruments
310 Fourth Ave. South
Suite 5000
Minneapolis, MN 55415
Phone: 612-827-2222
Fax: 612-827-2277
sales@bensonmedical.com
www.bensonmedical.com

Bergen Brunswig Medical Corp. (Ameri-
SourceBergen)
1300 Morris Dr.
Chesterbrook, PA 19087
Phone: 610-727-7000
Fax: 800-640-5221
www.amerisourcebergen.com/abcnew/

Berkeley Medevices
1330 South 51st St.
Richmond, CA 94804-4628
Phone: 800-227-2388
Fax: 510-231-9880
E-Mail: contactmedevices@aol.com
www.berkeleymedevices.com

Beutlich LP Pharmaceuticals
7775 S. US Hwy 1, Suite H
Bunnell, FL 32110
Phone: 800-238-8542
www.beutlich.com

Bio-Therapeutic
2244 1st Ave. South
Seattle, WA 98134
Phone: 206-938-5800
info@bio-therapeutic.com
www.bio-therapeutic.com

Biodermis
1820 Whitney Mesa Dr.
Henderson, NV 89014
Phone: 800-322-3729
www.biodermis.com

Biodynamics Corp.
3809 Stone Way N #100
Seattle, WA 98103
Phone: 206-526-0205
www.biodyncorp.com

BioForm Medical
1875 South Grant St.
Suite 110
San Mateo, CA 94402
Phone: 650-286-4000
Fax: 650-286-4090
www.bioform.com

Biolitec
515 Shaker Rd.
East Longmeadow, MA 01028
Phone: 800-321-0790
Fax: 413-525-0611
www.biolitec.com

BioMedix
2025 Centre Point Blvd. Suite 200
St. Paul, MN 55120
Phone: 888-889-8997
www.biomedix.com

Bionix Corp.
5154 Enterprise Blvd.
Toledo, OH 43612
Phone: 800-551-7096
Fax: 800-455-5678
E-mail: sales@bionix.com
www.bionix.com

Biosense Webster
33 Technology Dr.
Irvine, CA 92618
Phone: 909-839-8500 or 800-729-9010
Fax: 909-468-2905
www.esaote.com/en-US/

BioSkin/Cropper Medical
240 E. Hersey St.
Suite 2
Ashland, OR 97520
Phone: 800-541-2455
Email: hello@bioskin.com
www.bioskin.com

Biosound Esaote Inc.
8000 Castleway Dr.
Indianapolis, IN 46250
Phone: 800-428-4374
www.esaote.com/en-US/

**BioTherapeutics, Education and Research
(BTER) Foundation**
36 Urey Ct.
Irvine, CA 92612
Phone: 949-679-3000
Fax: 949-509-7040
www.bterfoundation.org

Birtcher Medical Systems Conmed Corp.
310 Broad St.
Utica, NY 13501-1203
Phone: 714-753-9400

**Bivona Medical Technologies Smiths
Group**
6000 Nathan Ln. North
Plymouth, MN 55442
Phone: 763-383-3000

Bledsoe Breg Inc.
2885 Loker Ave. East
Carlsbad, CA 92010
Phone: 800-897-BREG (2734) and 800-
321-0607 (Customer Care)
www.bledsoebrace.com

Body Circle Designs
P.O. Box 68249
Seattle, WA 98168
Phone: 800-244-8430
www.bodycircle.com

Body Vision
1915 Mckinley Ave. Suite D
La Verne, CA 91750
Phone: 909-596-1802
www.bodyvision.net

Boston Medical Products
70 Chestnut St.
Shrewsbury, MA 01545
Phone: 508-898-9300
F: 508-898-2373
www.bosmed.com

Boston Scientific
300 Boston Scientific Way
Marlborough, MA 01752
Phone: 800-876-9960
www.bostonscientific.com

Bovie Medical Corporation
5115 Ulmerton Rd.
Clearwater, FL 33760-4004
Phone: 800-537-2790
www.boviemedical.com

Braintree Laboratories Inc.
60 Columbian St. West
P.O. Box 850929
Braintree, MA 02185
Phone: 800-874-6756
Email: webmaster@braintreelabs.com
www.braintreelabs.com

Breg Inc.
2885 Loker Ave. East
Carlsbad, CA 92010
Phone: 800-897-2734
www.breg.com

Briggs Corporation
4900 University Ave. West
Des Moines, IA 50266
Phone: 800-247-2343
www.briggshealthcare.com

Brymill Cryogenic Systems
105 Windmere Ave.
Ellington, CT 06029
Phone: 800-777-2796
www.brymill.com

BSN-Jobst USA
5825 Carnegie Blvd.
Charlotte, NC 28209
www.jobst.com
Phone: 800-537-1063

Burdick Quinton Mortara Welch Allyn
7865 N. 86th St.
Milwaukee, WI 53224
Phone: 888-667-8272
mor_tech.support@welchallyn.com
www.welchallyn.com/content/welchallyn/
   americas/en/about-us/Mortara-redirect-
   page.html

Burton Medical Products
2300 W Windsor Ct. Suite C
Addison, IL 60101
Phone: 800-444-9909
Fax: 800-765-1770
www.burtonmedical.com

Byron Medical Mentor
602 West Rillito
Tucson, AZ 85705
Phone: 800-777-3434
Fax: 520-746-1757
www.mentorcorp.com

Candela Syneron Apax Partners
530 Boston Post Rd.
Wayland, MA 01778
Phone: 800-733-8550
Fax: 508-358-5602
www.syneron-candela.com/na

Cardiac Science (formerly Burdick Quinton, now only sell AEDs)
N7 W22025 Johnson Dr.
Suite 100
Waukesha, WI 53186
Phone: 800-426-0337
www.cardiacscience.com

Cardinal Health
7000 Cardinal Pl.
Dublin, OH 43017
Phone: 800-964-5227
www.cardinal.com

CareFusion Becton Dickinson (BD)
1 Becton Dr.
Franklin Lakes, NJ 07417
Phone: 201-847-6800
www.carefusion.com
www.bd.com/en-us

Carl Zeiss Meditech Surgical Inc.
5160 Hacienda Dr.
Dublin, CA 94568
Phone: 925-557-4100
www.zeiss.com

Carolon Health Care Products
601 Forum Pkwy.
Rural Hall, NC 27045
Phone: 800-334-0414
info@carolon.com
www.carolon.com

Castle Group
Scarborough Business Park
Salter Rd.
Scarborough
North Yorkshire YO11 3UZ
United Kingdom
Phone: +44 (0)1723 584250
Fax: +44 (0)1723 583728
Contact: enquiries@castlegroup.co.uk
www.castlegroup.co.uk

Center Laboratories ALK-Abelló A/S
35 Channel Dr.
Port Washington, NY 11050-2216
Phone: 516-767-1800
www.alk.net/us/about-alk

Cetylite Industries Inc.
9051 River Rd.
Pennsauken, NJ 08110
Phone: 800-257-7740
www.cetylite.com

Dr. Charles Wilson
DrSnip—The Vasectomy Clinic
5402 47th Ave. NE
Seattle, WA 98105
Phone: 206-525-4090
www.drsnip.com/
www.thevasectomyclinic.com

Chattanooga Group Inc.
4717 Adams Rd.
Hixson, TN 37343
Phone: 800-592-7329
www.chattgroup.com

Cheshire Medical Specialties Inc.
P.O. Box 894
Cheshire, CT 06410
Phone: 800-243-3020 or 203-272-1364
Fax: 203-250-0557
Contact: chesmed@cheshire-medical.com
www.cheshire-medical.com

Claflin Medical Equipment
P.O. Box 6887
Warwick, RI 02887
Phone: 800-338-2372
www.cmecorp.com/
www.claflinequip.com

Clarion Medical
125 Fleming Dr.
Cambridge, Ontario
Canada N1T 2B8
Phone: 800-668-5236
www.clarionmedical.com

Clinical Innovations Inc.
747 W. 4170 South
Murray, UT 84123
Phone: 888-268-6222 (main) or 801-268-8200
clinicalinnovations.com

Colin Omron Colin Medical Corp.
5859 Farinon Dr.
San Antonio, TX 78249
Phone: 800-829-6427
www.omron.com/

College Pharmacy
3505 Austin Bluffs Pkwy. #101
Colorado Springs, CO 80907
Phone: 800-888-9358
www.collegepharmacy.com

Coloplast Corporation (formerly Mentor Corporation)
200 South 6th St.
Suite 900
Minneapolis, MN 55402
Phone: 800-533-0464
www.us.coloplast.com
www.coloplast.com

Commonwealth Medical Laboratories
4228 Aiken Dr.
Warrenton, VA 20187
Phone: 800-222-5775
www.allergytest.com

Conceptus Bayer (Essure discontinued 2018)
331 E. Evelyn Ave.
Mountain View, CA 94041
Phone: 877-ESSURE2 (877-377-8732)
www.essuremd.com

ConMed
525 French Rd.
Utica, NY 13402
Phone: 800-448-6505
www.conmed.com

Convatec Bristol-Myers Squibb
CenterPointe II
1160 Route 22 East
Bridgewater, NJ 08807
Phone: 800-422-8811
www.convatec.com

Cook Medical
750 Daniels Way
P.O. Box 489
Bloomington, IN 47402-0489
Phone: 800-457-4500
www.cookmedical.com/critical-care/ or
www.cookmedical.com

Cook Women's Health (mailing address for Cook Urological Inc.)
1100 West Morgan St.
P.O. Box 271
Spencer, IN 47460
Phone: 800-541-5591
Fax: 812-829-2022
www.cookmedical.com/urology/

Cooley and Cooley Temrex
8550 Westland West Blvd.
Houston, TX 77041
Phone: 800-215-4487
www.temrex.com

CooperSurgical
95 Corporate Dr.
Trumbull, CT 06611
Phone: 800-243-2974
www.coopersurgical.com

Corpak MedSystems Halyard Health
5405 Windward Pkwy.
Alpharetta, GA 30004
Phone: 844-HALYARD (1-844-425-9273)
www.halyardhealth.com

Corthel Inc.
440 Franklin St.
Building A
Bel Air, MD 21014
Phone 410-588-5484
www.corthel.com

Cosmetic R & D
4125 Pine Crest Ct.
Rocklin, CA 95677
Phone: 916-632-9134
www.dermasweep.com

Cosmos EuroPeel Plus
P.O. Box 27210
San Diego, CA 92198
www.cosmoseuropeel.com/files/EuroPeel_order_form2010.pdf
www.cosmoseuropeel.com

Covidien Medtronic
710 Medtronic Pkwy.
Minneapolis, MN 55432-5604
Phone: 800-962-9888
www.medtronic.com/covidien/en-us/
products.html

Creative Health Communications (Plainly
Creative Works Inc.)
4675 South Portsmouth Rd.
Bridgeport, MI 48722
Phone: 989-777-8485
www.plainlycreativeworks.com/

CryoPen LLC
800 North Shoreline
Suite 900
Corpus Christi, TX 78401
Phone: 888-246-3928
www.cryopen.com

CryoSurgery Inc.
5829 Old Harding Pike Rd.
Nashville, TN 37205
Phone: 800-729-1624
Fax: 615-354-0466
www.cryosurgeryinc.com

Curetteblade, Inc (S&A Tech)
10101 Stoltz Dr.
Rolla, MO 65401
Phone: 573-364-0122
Fax: 573-364-0123
www.stoeckertech.com/curetteblade

Custom Scripts Pharmacy
27732 Cashford Cir.
Wesley Chapel, FL 33544
Phone: 800-226-7094
rx@custom-rx.com; www.custom-rx.com

Cutera
3240 Bayshore Blvd.
Brisbane, CA 94005
Phone: 888-4-CUTERA or 415-657-5500
Fax: 415-330-2444
www.cutera.com

Cynosure Inc.
5 Carlisle Rd.
Westford, MA 01886
Phone: 978-256-4200
www.cynosure.com

CYTYC Hologic
250 Campus Dr.
Marlborough, MA 01752
Phone: 800-442-9892
Fax: 508-229-2860
www.hologic.com

Davol Bard Becton Dickinson
100 Crossings Blvd.
Warwick, RI 02886
Phone: 800-556-6275
Medical Services & Support: 800-562-0027
www.davol.com

Delasco Dermatologic Lab and Supply Co.
608 13th Ave.
Council Bluffs, IA 57501-6401
Phone: 800-831-6273
www.delasco.com

Dentsply Sirona
Susquehanna Commerce Center
221 W. Philadelphia St. Suite 60W
York, PA 17405
Phone: 800-877-0020
www.dentsplysirona.com/en-us

DermaMed Inc.
394 Parkmount Rd.
P.O. Box 198
Lenni, PA 19052-0198
Phone: 610-358-4447
dermamedsolutions.com/about/dermamed_
solutions_overview/
www.megapeel.com

Dermatology Lab & Supply Inc. (Delasco)
608 13th Ave.
Council Bluffs, IA 51501-6401
Phone: 800-831-6273 or 712-323-3269
Fax: 800-320-9612 or 712-323-1156
questions@delasco.com
www.delasco.com

Dey Mylan
1000 Mylan Blvd.
Canonsburg, PA 15317
Phone: 724-514-1800
www.epipen.com/

Diamond Medical Aesthetics
1 Madison St.
Bldg. C
East Rutherford, NJ 07073
Phone: 973-794-5343
bluediamondmd.com/

Diomed AngioDynamics
603 Queensbury Ave.
Queensbury, NY 12804
Phone: 800-772-6446
venacure-evlt.com

Don Joy DJO
1430 Decision St.
Vista, CA 92081
Phone: 800-321-9549
www.djoglobal.com/our-brands/donjoy
www.donjoy.com

Duramed Barr CooperSurgical
223 Quaker Rd.
Pomona, NY 10970
Phone: 800-222-0190
www.paragard.com

Dusa Sun Pharma
25 Upton Dr.
Wilmington, MA 01887
Phone: 877-533-DUSA (3872)
www.dusapharma.com

Dynatronics
7030 Park Centre Dr.
Salt Lake City, UT 84121
Phone: 800-874-6251
www.dynatronics.com

Eclipse, Ltd.
5916 Stone Creek Dr., Suite 120
The Colony, TX 75056
Phone: 972-380-2911 or 800-759-6876
Fax: 972-380-2953
sales@eclipsemed.com
www.eclipsemed.com

Edge Systems
2277 Redondo Ave.
Signal Hill, CA 90755
Phone: 800-603-4996

Edwards Life Sciences Corp
One Edwards Way
Irvine, CA 92614
Phone: 800-424-3278
www.edwards.com

Electro-Med Health Industries
500 6th Ave. NW
New Prague, MN 56071-1134
Phone: 952-758-9299
www.smartvest.com/about

Ellman Cynosure
400 Karin Ln.
Hicksville, NY 11801
Phone: 800-835-5355
www.ellman.com

EMPI DJO Global
599 Cardigan Rd.
St. Paul, MN 55126
Phone: 800-325-5663
www.djoglobal.com/our-brands/empi
www.empi.com

Endoscopy Support Services Inc.
3 Fallsview Ln.
Brewster, NY 10509
Phone: 800-349-3636
www.endoscopy.com

EngenderHealth
505 9th St. NW, Suite 601
Washington, DC 20004
Phone: 202-902-2000
www.engenderhealth.org

Emed Envy Medical Inc.
5150 E. Pacific Coast Hwy., Suite 720
Long Beach, CA 90804
Phone: 888-848-3633
www.silkpeel.com directed to envymedical.
com

ERBE USA Inc.
2225 Northwest Pkwy.
Marietta, GA 30067
Phone: 800-778-3723
us.erbe-med.com/us-en/

Ethicon Johnson & Johnson
Hwy. 22
P.O. Box 151
Somerville, NJ 08876-0151
Phone: 800-438-4426 or 908-218-0707
www.ethiconinc.com

Ethicon Endo-Surgery Johnson & Johnson
4545 Creek Rd.
Cincinnati, OH 45242
Phone: 800-USE-ENDO
www.jnj.com/media-center/press-releases/
    ethicon-endo-surgery-to-acquire-
    sterilmed
www.jnjgateway.com (video available)

Ethox Corp.
251 Seneca St.
Buffalo, NY 14204
Phone: 800-521-1022
www.ethoxcorp.com

Everything Birth Inc.
Chesterfield Township, MI
Phone: 586-648-4766
www.everythingbirth.com/

Feet Relief
1032 Irving St.
PMB 507
San Francisco, CA 94122-2200
Phone: 888-671-8027
www.feetrelief.com

Fem Cap
14058 Mira Montana Dr.
Del Mar, CA 92014
Phone: 858-922-7673
Fax: 858-792-2624
contact@femcap.com
www.femcap.com

Female Veru Healthcare
4400 Biscayne Blvd.
Suite 888
Miami, FL 33137
Phone: 305-509-6897
www.femalehealth.com or
www.fc2femalecondom.com

FLA BSN Orthopedics
5825 Carnegie Blvd.
Charlotte, NC 28209
Phone: 800-327-4110
www.flaorthopedics.com

Focus Medical LLC
23 Francis J. Clark Cir.
Bethel, CT 06801
Phone: 866-633-5273
www.focusmedical.com

Foot Smart
5250 Triangle Pkwy.
Suite 200
Norcross, GA 30092
Phone: 800-707-9928
www.footsmart.com

Fujinon Fujifilm Medical
10 High Point Dr.
Wayne, NJ 07470
Phone: 800-385-4666
www.fujifilmusa.com
www.fujinon.com

Futrex Inc.
6 Montgomery Village Ave.
#620
Gaithersburg, MD 20879
Phone: 800-255-4206
www.futrex.com

GC America Inc.
3737 West 127th
Alsip, IL 60803
Phone: 800-323-7063
www.gcamerica.com

GE Healthcare (Headquarters)
3000 North Grandview
Waukesha, WI 53188
Phone: 866-281-7545
www3.gehealthcare.com/en
www.gehealthcare.com/usen/cardiology/dia
    gnostic_ecg/products/amb_centerpg.html

General Electric Healthcare Bio-Sciences Corp
800 Centennial Ave.
P.O. Box 1327
Piscataway, NJ 08855-1327
Phone: 262-544-3011
www.gemedicalsystems.com or www3.gehea
    lthcare.com/en/global_gateway
www.gehealthcare.com

Genesis Biosystems
1500 Eagle Ct.
Lewisville, TX 75057
Phone: 888-577-7335
www.dermagenesis.com

Genzyme Biosurgery Vericel Sanofi
64 Sidney St.
Cambridge, MA 02142
Phone: 800-232-7546
vcel.com/

George Tiemann and Co.
25 Plant Ave.
Hauppauge, NY 11788-3804
Phone: 800-843-6266
www.georgetiemann.com

Gill Podiatry Supply and Equipment
22400 Ascoa Ct.
Strongsville, OH 44149
Phone: 800-432-9445
www.gillpodiatry.com

Gordon Stowe
3333 N Kennicott Ave.
Arlington Heights, IL 60004
Phone: 800-323-4371
www.gordonstowe.com

GPT Glendale Honeywell
Honeywell Safety Products USA
900 Douglas Pike
Smithfield, RI 02917
Phone: 800-430-5490

Graham-Field Inc.
400 Rabro Dr.
East Hauppauge, NY 11788
Phone: 516-582-5900
www.grahamfield.com

Grason-Stadler Inc.
10395 West 70th St.
Eden Prairie, MN 55344
Phone: 800-700 2282 (U.S.) or +1 952-278
    4402 (international)
Fax: +1 952-278 4401
Contact: info@grason-stadler.com
www.grasonstadler.com

Gulden Ophthalmics
225 Cadwalader Ave.
Elkins Park, PA 19027
Phone: 800-659-2250
www.guldenophthalmics.com

Gynecare Ethicon Johnson & Johnson
P.O. Box 151
Somerville, NJ 08876
Phone: 888-496-3227
www.ethicon.com/na/products/uterine-
    and-pelvic-surgery

Gyne-Tech Instrument Corp.
2819 Burton St.
Burbank, CA 91504
Phone: 323-849-5985
www.gynetech.com

Gynex
14603 NE 87th St.
Redmond, WA 98052
Phone: 888-486-4644 or 800-220-5988
Fax: 425-895-0115
www.gynexcorporation.com

Gyrus ACMI Olympus Surgical Technologies America
136 Turnpike Rd.
Southborough, MA 01772
Phone: 800-401-1086
medical.olympusamerica.com/

Haag-Streit
3535 Kings Mills Rd.
Mason, OH 45040
Phone: 866-417-3802
www.haag-streit-usa.com

Hardwood Puritan Medical Products Company
P.O. Box 149
Guilford, ME 04443
Phone: 888-289-3340 (U.S. & Canada)
www.hwppuritan.com or
www.hardwoodproductsco.com/

Hardy Diagnostics
1430 West McCoy Ln.
Santa Maria, CA 93455
Phone: 805-346-2766 or 800-266-2222
Fax: 805-346-2760
www.HardyDiagnostics.com

Heine USA
10 Innovation Way
Dover, NH 03820
Phone: 800-367-4872
www.heine.com

Hely & Weber
P.O. Box 832
Santa Paula, CA 93061-0832
Phone: 800-654-3241
www.hely-weber.com

HemCon Tricol Medical Technologies Inc.
720 SW Washington St., Suite 200
Portland, Oregon 97205
Phone: 503-245-0459
Fax: 503-245-1326
www.hemcon.com

Henry Schein Dental
135 Duryea Rd.
Melville, NY 11747
Phone: 631-843-5500 or 800-372-4346
www.henryschein.com/us-en/dental/Default.aspx?did=dental&stay=1 or
www.henryscheindental.com

Hitachi Medical Corp.
1959 Summit Commerce Park
Twinsburg, OH 44087
Phone: 800-800-3106
www.hitachi-aloka.com

Hollister-Stier Jubilant
3525 North Regal
Spokane, WA 99220-3145
www.jublhs.com

HOYA Conbio Cynosure
5 Carlisle Rd.
Westford, MA 01886
Phone: 800-886-2966
www.cynosure.com

HPSRx Enterprises Inc. (Ipas distributor)
3229 Brandon Ave.
Suite 2
Roanoke, VA 24018
Phone: 800-850-1657
Fax: 800-361-6984
www.hpsrx.com

Hull Anesthesia Inc.
7392 Vincent Cir.
Huntington Beach, CA 92648
Phone: 800-400-4484
Fax: 714-375-2658
www.hullanesthesia.com

Huot Instruments LLC (Wittenberg Visi-Punch and ElliptiPunch)
N50 W13740 Overview Dr.
Suite A
Menomonee Falls, WI 53051
Phone: 262-373-1700 or 866-212-8466
Fax: 262-373-1800
info@huotinstruments.com or Cust.Service@HuotInstruments.com
www.medicalmingle.com/huotinstruments

Hy-Tape International
P.O. Box 540
Patterson, NY 12563
Phone: 800-248-0101
www.hytape.com

ImageDerm
1600 N. San Fernando Rd.
2nd Floor
Los Angeles, CA 90065
Phone: 818-500-9034
imagederm.com

Industrial Strength
6115 Corte Del Cedro
Carlsbad, CA 92011
Phone: 760-438-8077
www.isbodyjewelry.com

Inhealth Industries
1110 Mark Ave.
Carpinteria, CA 93013-2918
Phone: 800-477-5968
www.inhealth.com

Innovative Med Inc. (KMI IMI Group)
4 Autry
Suite B
Irvine, CA 92618
Phone: 949-458-1897
www.kmiimigroup.com
www.imibeauty.com

Instromedix Card Guard Lifewatch
6779 Mesa Ridge Rd.
Suite 200
San Diego, CA 92121
800-633-3361
www.lifewatch.com

Instrument Specialists Inc.
32390 IH-10
Boerne, TX 78006-9214
Phone: 800-537-1945
www.isisurgery.com

Integra LifeSciences Corp.
311 Enterprise Dr.
Plainsboro, NJ 08538
Phone: 609-275-9004
www.integralife.com

Integrated Medical Systems Inc.
3316 2nd Ave. North
Birmingham, AL 35222
Phone: 800-783-9251
www.imsready.com

Interstitial Cystitis Association (ICA) National
7918 Jones Branch Dr.
Suite 300
McLean, VA 22102
Phone: 800-HELP-ICA (800-435-7422)
Fax: 301-610-5308
ICAmail@ichelp.org
www.ichelp.org

Interstitial Cystitis Network (ICN) National (A Division of J.H. Osborne Inc.)
P.O. Box 2159
Healdsburg, CA 95448
Phone: 800-928-7496
www.ic-network.com

IOMED DJO Global
1430 Decision St.
Vista, CA 92081
Phone: 760-727-1280
www.djoglobal.com

Ipas
P.O. Box 9990
Chapel Hill, NC 27515
Phone: 800-334-8446
customerservice@ipas.org
www.ipas.org

IQDr. Inc.
34 Sandra Ln.
Manitou Springs, CO 80829
Phone: 800-747-3184
www.iqdr.com

Iridex
1212 Terra Bella Ave.
Mountain View, CA 94043
Phone: 888-725-8115
Fax: 650-940-4710
www.iridex.com

Jobst/BSN Medical
5825 Carnegie Blvd.
Charlotte, NC 28209
Phone: 800-537-1063
www.jobst-usa.com
www.bsnmedical.com

Johnson & Johnson Professional Inc.
(extra-fast-setting casting splints available)
325 Paramount Dr.
Raynham, MA 02767-0350
Phone: 800-526-2459
https://www.jnj.com/healthcare-products

Juzo (Julius Zorn) Inc.
3690 Zorn Dr.
P.O. Box 1088
Cuyahoga Falls, OH 44223
Phone: 888-255-1300
www.juzousa.com

Karl Storz Endoscopy-America Inc.
600 Corporate Pointe
Culver City, CA 90230-7600
Phone: 800-421-0837
www.karlstorz.com

Kendall Cardinal Healthcare Products
15 Hampshire St.
Mansfield, MA 02048
Phone: 800-962-9888
www.kendallhq.com

Keystone Pharmacy (Compounding Pharmacy)
4021 Cascade Rd. SE
Grand Rapids, MI 49546
Phone: 616-974-9792
www.keystonerx.com

Kimberly-Clark/Ballard Halyard Medical
12050 Lone Peak Pkwy.
Draper, UT 84020
Phone: 800-528-5591
redirected to www.halyardhealth.com/

Krames Communications
1100 Grundy Ln.
San Bruno, CA 94066
Phone: 800-333-3032
www.krames.com

LabCorp
358 South Main St.
Burlington, NC 27215
Phone: 336-584-5171
www.labcorp.com

Laborie Medical Technologies
400 Ave. D
Suite 10
Williston, VT 05495
Phone: 800-522-6743
www.laborie.com

Langer Biomechanics (purchased Benefoot Inc.)
2905 Veterans Memorial Hwy
Ronkonkoma, NY 11779
Phone: 800-645-5520
www.langerbiomechanics.com

Lasering USA
220 Porter Dr., Suite 120
San Ramon, CA 94583
Phone: 866-471-0469
Contact: info@laseringusa.com
www.laseringusa.com

Levin, Salem (sump and feeding tubes; Bard Medical Division)
8195 Industrial Blvd.
Covington, GA 30014
Phone: 800-526-4455
www.bardmedical.com

Lhasa OMS Inc.
230 Libbey Pkwy.
Weymouth, MA 02189
Phone: 800-722-8775
www.lhasaoms.com

LifeCell Allergan Corporation
5 Giralda Farms
Madison, NJ 07940
Phone: 862-261-7000
www.lifecell.com or www.allergan.com/home

Lifesource Medical (A & D Medical)
1756 Automation Pkwy.
San Jose, CA 95131
Phone: 888-726-9966
www.lifesource.com or
medical.andonline.com/home

Life-Tech Thermo Fisher Scientific
4235 Greenbriar Dr.
Stafford, TX 77477-3995
Phone: 866-356-0354
www.thermofisher.com/us/en/home.html

Lincoln Diagnostics
P.O. Box 1128
Decatur, IL 62525
Phone: 800-537-1336
www.lincolndiagnostics.com

LPG
2966 NW 60 St.
Fort Lauderdale, FL 33309
Phone: 866-374-9401
www.endermologie.com/en-us/endermologie-lpg/

Lumenis ESC Medical Systems
2077 Gateway Place, Suite 300
San Jose, CA 95110
Phone: 877-Lumenis (877-586-3647)
www.lumenis.com

Lutronic
19 Fortune Dr.
Billerica, MA 01821
Phone: 888-588-7644
Fax: 609-275-3800
Contact: officeusa@lutronic.com
www.int.lutronic.com/intl/

Luxtec Integra LifeSciences
Integra LifeSciences
311 Enterprise Dr.
Plainsboro NJ, 08536
Phone: 609-275-0500
Fax: 609-750-4277
www.luxtec.com

MADA Medical Products
625 Washington Ave.
Carlstadt, NJ 07072
Phone: 800-526-6370
www.madamedical.com

Otometrics Natus
Natus Medical Incorporated
50 Commerce Dr. #180
Schaumburg, IL 60173
Phone: 855-283-7978
Contact: info@gnotometrics.dk
www.otometrics.natus.com or
www.otometrics.us

Maico Diagnostics
10393 West 70th St.
Eden Prairie, MN 55344
Phone: 888-941-4201 or 952-941-4200
www.maico-diagnostics.com

Mallinckrodt Pharmaceuticals
675 McDonnell Blvd.
Hazelwood, MO 63042
Phone: 314-654-2000
www.mallinckrodt.com/

Maquet Getinge Critical Care AB
45 Barbour Pond Dr.
Wayne, NJ 07470
Phone: 888-627-8383
www.maquet.com/us/specialities-and-therapies/critical-care/

Marina Medical
8190 West State Rd. 84
Davie, FL 33324
Phone: 954-924-4418 or 800-697-1119
Fax: 954-924-4419 or 800-748-2089
www.marinamedical.com

Matlock Endoscopic
830 Fesslers Pkwy., Suite 118
Nashville, TN 37210
Phone: 800-394-9822
www.matlockendo.com

Mattioli Engineering
1765 Greensboro Station Pl., Suite 900
McLean, VA 22102
Phone: 877-628-8364
www.mattioliengineering.com

McDavid Sports Medical Products
11488 Slater Ave.
Fountain Valley, CA 92708
Phone: 800-233-6956
www.mcdavidusa.com

Med-Aesthetic Solutions
2033 San Elijo Ave.
Suite 200
Cardiff-by-the-Sea, CA 92007
Phone: 877-733-7627
Redirected to www.yourmas.com

MedaSonics CooperSurgical
95 Corporate Dr.
Trumbull, CT 06611
Phone: 800-243-2974
www.coopersurgical.com/Our-Brands/MedaSonics

Medco Supply *Patterson Medical*
500 Fillmore Ave.
Tonawanda, NY 14150
Phone: 716-695-3244
www.medco-athletics.com

MedGyn Products Inc.
100 West Industrial Rd.
Addison, IL 60101
Phone: 630-627-4105
Toll-free: 800-451-9667
Fax: 630-627-0127
medgyn@medgyn.com
www.medgyn.com

Medical Graphics MGC Diagnostics Corporation
350 Oak Grove Pkwy.
St. Paul, MN 55127
Phone: 800-950-5597
www.medgraph.com

Medical Optics Inc.
10320 West McNab Rd.
Tamarac, FL 33321
Phone: 800-286-9542
www.medicaloptics.com

Medicis Valeant Bausch
7720 North Dobson Rd.
Scottsdale, AZ 85256
Phone: 866-222-1480
www.dysportusa.com

Medison Samsung
11075 Knott Ave.
Suite C
Cypress, CA 90630
Phone: 800-829-7666
www.samsungmedison.com

MediUSA
6481 Franz Warner Pkwy.
Whitsett, NC 27377
Phone: 800-633-6334
www.mediusa.com

MedSurge Advances Inc.
14850 Quorum Dr.
Suite 120
Dallas, TX 75254
Phone: 972-720-0425
www.medsurgeadvances.com ww5.medsurgeadvances.com

MedTech International
P.O. Box 162992
Altamonte Springs, FL 32716
Phone: 407-880-6904

Medtronic
710 Medtronic Pkwy. NE
Minneapolis, MN 55432-5604
Phone: 800-633-8766 or 800-505-4636 (bradyarrhythmia products)
www.medtronic.com/us-en/healthcare-professionals/products/cardiac-rhythm/pacemakers.html
www.medtronic.com

Medtronic Xomed Surgical Products Inc.
6743 Southpoint Dr. North
Jacksonville, FL 32216
Phone: 800-874-5797
www.medtronic.com/us-en/healthcare-professionals/products/advanced-surgical-technology.html or www.medtronic.com

Merz Pharmaceuticals
4215 Tudor Ln.
Greensboro, NC 27410
Phone: 888-925-8989
www.mederma.com or www.merzusa.com

Micro Audiometrics
655 Keller Rd.
Murphy, NC 28906
Phone: 386-888-7878
www.microaudiometrics.com

Micro Bio-Medics Henry Schein
846 Pelham Pkwy.
Pelham Manor, NY 10803
Phone: 800-431-2743
www.microbiomedics.com or https://www.henryschein.com/us-en/medical/default.aspx?did=medical&stay=1

Micro-Imaging Solutions Inc.
3134 Wyandot St.
Denver, CO 80211
Phone: 303-221-3677, ext. 2
www.micro-imaging.us

Microsulis AngioDynamics
603 Queensbury Ave.
Queensbury, NY 12804
Phone: 800-772-6446
www.angiodynamics.com

Miga Systems
3500 N. Holly Ln.
Suite 40
Plymouth, MN 55447
Phone: 800-913-6442
www.miga.com

Miles Bayer Pharmaceuticals
1127 Myrtle St.
Elkhart, IN 46514
Phone: 800-800-4793
www.pharma.bayer.com/

Milex Products Inc.
4311 N. Normandy
Chicago, IL 60634
Phone: 800-621-1278
Fax: 800-972-0696
www.milexproducts.com

Miltex Integra
700 Hicksville Rd.
Bethpage, NY 11714-3490
Phone: 800-645-8000
Fax: 866-854-8400
www.miltex.com or www.miltex.com/AboutUs.aspx

Mindray DP-6600 North America
800 MacArthur Blvd.
Mahwah, NJ 07430
Phone: 201-995-8000
Phone: 800-288-2121
www.mindraynorthamerica.com

Minogue Medical
180 Peel St., Suite 300
Montréal QC
H3C 2G7 Canada
Phone: 800-665-6466
www.minogue-med.com/

MJD Patient Communications
7910 Woodmont Ave.
Suite 1105
Bethesda, MD 20814
Phone: 301-657-8010
www.mjdpc.com

Mobile Instrument Service
333 Water Ave.
Bellefontaine, OH 43311
Phone: 800-722-3675
www.mobileinstrument.com

Mogen Circumcision Instrument Limited
437 Crown St.
Brooklyn, NY 11225
Phone: 718-604-8833

Monarch Labs
17875 Sky Park Cr.
Suite K
Irvine, CA 92614
Phone: 949-679-3000
Fax: 949-679-3001
www.monarchlabs.com

Moore Medical Corp
1690 New Britain Ave.
P.O. Box 4067
Farmington, CT 06032-4067
Phone: 800-234-1464
www.mooremedical.com

Mortara Welch Allyn Cardiology
7865 N. 86th St.
Milwaukee, WI 53224
Phone: 888-667-8272
mor_tech.support@welchallyn.com
www.welchallyn.com/content/welchallyn/americas/en/about-us/Mortara-redirect-page.html

M-Pact Jobst/BSN Medical
5825 Carnegie Blvd.
Charlotte, NC 28209
800-552-1157
www.m-pactmed.com or www.jobst.com

MRT Laboratories
50 Johnson Ave.
Hackensack, NJ 07601
Phone: 800-631-1379
www.mrtlabs.com

Myfootshop.com
1159 Cherry Valley Rd.
Newark, OH 43055
Phone: 888-859-8901
www.myfootshop.com

Nasostat Gottschalk
Los Angeles, CA 90049
Phone: 310-207-1445
www.nasostat.com

National Procedures Institute (NPI)
12012 Technology Blvd.
Suite 200
Austin, TX 78727
Phone: 866-NIP-CME1 or 512-870-8051
Fax: 512-329-0442
Contact: Info@npinstitute.com
www.npinstitute.com

Natus Medical Inc.
Corporate Headquarters
6701 Koll Center Pkwy. Suite 120
Pleasanton, CA 94566
Phone: 800-255-3901
www.natus.com

Nellcor Covidien Medtronic
6135 Gunbarrel Ave.
Boulder, CO 80301
Phone: 800-NELLCOR (635-5267)
respiratorysolutions.covidien.com or www.
    medtronic.com/covidien/en-us/index.html

NEUROMetrix Inc.
1000 Winter St.
Waltham, MA 02451
Phone (general assistance): 781-890-9989
Toll-free (customer service): 888-786-7287
www.neurometrix.com

Newport Cosmeceuticals Inc.
4695 MacArthur Ct.
Newport Beach, CA 92660
Phone: 949-825-5087
www.nciskincare.com

NG Strip Cardinal Health
7000 Cardinal Pl.
Dublin, OH 43017
Phone: 800-323-9088
www.cardinal.com

NightHawk Radiology Services
5944 Coral Ridge Dr.
Suite #276
Coral Springs, FL 33076
Phone: 866-379-0465
Fax: 954-866-5444
www.nighthawkradiology.com/

Norscan Medical, LLC.
13455 Ventura Blvd., Suite 237
Sherman Oaks, CA 91423
Phone: 818-735-0019
norscanmedical.com/laminaria-tents/

Northern Optotronics, Inc.
3 Progress Dr., Unit #1
Orillia, Ont L3V 0T7
Phone: 888-252-2219
Phone: 519-621-2666
www.noi.ca

Nuell Inc.
312 E. Van Buren St.
Leesburg, IN 46538
Phone: 800-829-7694
www.nuell.com

OBP Medical Inc.
360 Merrimack St., Bldg. 9
Lawrence, MA 01843
Phone: 978-291-6853
www.obpmedical.com

Olympic Natus Medical Corp
6701 Koll Center Pkwy., Suite 120
Pleasanton, CA 94566
Phone: 800-426-0353
www.natus.com

Olympus America Inc.
3500 Corporate Pkwy.
Center Valley, PA 11747
Phone: 800-401-1086
www.olympusamerica.com

OMS Llaso Medical Supplies (Oriental
    Medical Supplies)
Phone: 800-323-1839
OMS Medical Supplies/Lhaso OMS Inc.
230 Libbey Industrial Pkwy
Weymouth, MA 02189
www.lhasaoms.com/?SID=bf4b1566c9f175
    e2d1972307ec68e141

OraSure Technologies
220 E. First St.
Bethlehem, PA 18015
Phone: 800-ORASURE (800-672-7873)
www.orasure.com

Organon Teknika bioMérieux
100 Rodolphe St.
Durham, NC 27712
Phone: 800-682-2666
www.biomerieux-usa.com

**Ortho-McNeil Janssen Pharmaceuticals
    Johnson & Johnson**
Phone: 800-JANSSEN (526-7736)
www.janssenmd.com/
www.thepill.com (product of Janssen Phar-
    maceuticals)

Össur Americas
27051 Towne Centre Dr., Suite 100
Foothill Ranch, CA 92610
Phone: 800-233-6263
www.ossur.com

Otometrics Natus
50 Commerce Dr. #180
Schaumburg, IL, 60173
Phone: 855-283-7978
Phone: 800-289-2150
www.otometrics.us

Paddock Laboratories Perrigo
515 Eastern Ave.
Allegan, MI 49010
Phone: 269-673-8451
www.perrigo.com/

Padgett Integra LifeSciences
311 Enterprise Dr.
Plainsboro NJ, 08536
Phone: 800-654-2873
www.integralife.com/

Palomar Cynosure
5 Carlisle Rd.
Westford, MA 01886
Phone: 800-886-2966
www.cynosure.com/

Palumbo Orthopedics
8206 Leesburg Pike
Suite 402
Vienna, VA 22182
Phone: 800-292-7223
www.palumbobraces.com

Parks Medical Electronics
6000 S. Eastern Ave., Suite 10-B
Las Vegas, NV 89119
Phone: 888-557-2757
www.parksmed.com

Path Scientific LLC
P.O. Box 102
Carlisle, MA 01741
Fax: 978-369-7325
info@pathscientific.com
www.pathscientific.com

Pedicraft
4134 Saint Augustine Rd.
Jacksonville, FL 32247
Phone: 800-223-7649
www.pedicraft.com

Pentax Medical Company
102 Chestnut Ridge Rd.
Montvale, NJ 07645
Phone: 201-571-2300
www.pentaxmedical.com/pentax

Pharmacia Upjohn Pfizer
235 East 42nd St.
New York, NY 10017
Phone: 212-733-2323
www.pfizer.com

**Pharmacy Specialists Compounding Phar-
    macy** (Sam Pratt, RPh)
650 Maitland Ave.
Altamonte Springs, FL 32701
Phone: 800-224-7711
www.makerx.com/

Philips Medical Systems
22100 Bothell Everett Hwy.
Bothel, WA 98041
Phone: 800-263-3342
www.usa.philips.com/healthcare

pHion Nutrition
14201 North Hayden Rd.
Suite A4
Scottsdale, AZ 85260
Phone: 480-556-0210
Phone: 888-744-8589
www.phionbalance.com

Phlebology and Aesthetic Concepts
3725 South US Hwy.
Suite 1
Edgewater, FL 32141

Photo Therapeutics PhotoMedex Radiancy
147 Keystone Dr.
Montgomeryville, PA 18936
Phone: 215-619-3287

Precordial Stethoscopes (product)
Sedation Resource Inc.
Phone: 800-753-6376
www.sedationresource.com

Premier Medical Products
1710 Romano Dr.
P.O. Box 4500
Plymouth Meeting, PA 19462
Phone: 888-670-6100
www.premusa.com

Procter & Gamble Pharmaceuticals Warner Chilcott Actavis Allergen
5 Giralda Farms
Madison, NJ 07940
Phone: 862-261-7000
https://www.allergan.com/news/news/warner-chilcott-is-now-actavis

Pulpdent Corp.
80 Oakland St.
Watertown, MA 02471
Phone: 800-343-4342
www.pulpdent.com

Puritan Bennett Covidien Medtronic
6135 Gunbarrel Ave.
Boulder, CO 80301
Phone: 800-962-9888
http://www.medtronic.com/covidien/en-us/products/acute-care-ventilation.html

QIAGEN Inc.
27220 Turnberry Ln.
Valencia, CA 91355
Phone: 800-426-8157
www.thehpvtest.com and
www.qiagen.com/us/

QuickMedical
30200 SE 79th St., Suite 120
Issaquah, WA 98027
Phone: 888-345-4858
Fax: 425-222-6030
www.quickmedical.com

Raja Medical
801 South Olive Ave.
Suite 124
West Palm Beach, FL 33401
Phone: 877-880-4184
www.rajamedical.com

Redfield Corp.
336 West Passaic St.
Rochelle Park, NJ 07662
Phone: 800-678-4472
www.redfieldcorp.com

Redwing Book Company
202 Bendix Dr.
Taos, NM 87571
Phone: 800-873-3946
www.redwingbooks.com

Refine USA LLC
340 S. 3rd Ave. South, Suite C
Jacksonville Beach, FL 32250
Phone: 866-590-5533
www.refineusa.com

Reichert
3362 Walden Ave., Suite 100
Depew, NY 14043
Phone: 888-849-8955
www.reichert.com

Rejuveness LLC
28 Clinton St., Suite 3A
Saratoga Springs, NY 12866
Phone: 800-588-7455 or 518-584-5017
Fax: 518-584-3618
www.rejuveness.com

Reliant Technologies Thermage Bausch Health Companies
7031 Koll Center Pkwy. #260
Pleasanton, CA 94566
Phone: 877-782-2286
www.thermage.com

Richard Wolf Medical Instruments
353 Corporate Woods Pkwy.
Vernon Hills, IL 60061-3110
Phone: 800-323-WOLF (9653)
www.richardwolfusa.com/home.html

RS Medical
14001 SE 1st St.
Vancouver, WA 98684
Phone: 800-935-7763
www.rsmedical.com/

Rusch Teleflex
3015 Carrington Mill Blvd.
Morrisville, NC 27560
Phone: 866-246-6990
www.teleflex.com/usa/product-areas/urology/

Sam Wagner
P.O. Box 431
202 Dodd St.
Middlebourne, WV 26149
Phone: 304-758-2370
www.wagner-medical.com/

Sandstone Ellman
400 Karin Ln.
Hicksville, NY 11801
Phone: 800-835-5355
ellman.com/index.html

Saratoga Diagnostics Thomas Gerard Pallone
12619 Paseo Olivos
Saratoga, CA 95070
Phone: 800-998-1555
http://www.saratogaaesthetics.com/

Save-A-Tooth System Phoenix-Lazerus
2525 N Hayden Island Dr.
Portland, OR 97217 or
8 South Roland St.
Pottstown, PA 19464
Phone: 888-788-6684
www.saveatooth.com

ScarHeal Rejuvis Inc.
13191 Starkey Rd, Bldg. 11
Largo, FL 33773-1438
Phone: 888-722-7432 or 727-535-0022
www.scarheal.com

Schering-Plough Merck
2000 Galloping Hill Rd.
Kenilworth, NJ 07033
Phone: 908-740-4000
www.implanon-usa.com/en/consumer/index.xhtml

Sciton Inc.
925 Commercial St.
Palo Alto, CA 94303
Phone: 888-646-6999
Fax: 650-493-9146
www.sciton.com

The Scope Exchange Johnson & Johnson
5010 Cheshire Pkwy, Suite 2
Plymouth, MN 02360
Phone: 763-488-3400
www.sterilmed.com

Scripts Pharmacy
4059 Hollywood Rd.
St. Joseph, MI 49085
Phone: 269-428-2500
Fax: 269-428-2555

SDI Diagnostics Inc.
10 Hampden Dr.
Easton, MA 02375
Phone: 800-678-5782
www.sdidiagnostics.com

Seiler Precision Microscopes (Colposcopes)
3433 Tree Court Industrial Blvd.
St. Louis, MO 63122
Phone: 800-489-2282
www.seilermicro.com/products/medical-products/colposcopes/

Serolab
P.O. Box 400
Round Rock, TX 78680
Phone: 800-365-1700
serolab.us

Shippert Innovia Medical
6248 S. Troy Cir.
Suite A
Centennial, CO 80111
Phone: 800-888-8663
www.shippertmedical.com

Siemens/Acuson
40 Liberty Blvd.
Malvern, PA 19355
Phone: 888-826-9702
usa.healthcare.siemens.com/ultrasound

Sigvaris Inc.
1119 Hwy. 74 South
Peachtree City, GA 30269
Phone: 800-322-7744
www.sigvaris.com/usa/en-us

Silhouet-Tone USA
2043 NW 87th Ave.
Miami, FL 33172
Phone: 800-552-0418
www.silhouettone.com

Sims Portex Smiths Medical
10 Bowman Dr.
Keene, NH 03431
Phone: 800-258-5361
www.portexusa.com

Sirchie Fingerprint Laboratories Inc.
100 Hunter Pl.
Youngsville, NC 27596
Phone: 800-356-7311
www.sirchie.com/forensics/fingerprint-
taking.html

SkinMedica Allergan
5909 Sea Lion Pl.
Suite H
Carlsbad, CA 90210
Phone: 866-867-0110
www.SkinMedica.com

Slate Endo Pharmaceuticals
1400 Atwater Dr.
Malvern, PA 19355
Phone: 484-216-0000
Phone: 800-462-ENDO (3636)
www.testopel.com

Smart Practice
3400 E. McDowell Rd.
Phoenix, AZ 85008-7899
Phone: 800-522-0800
Fax: 800-522-8329
www.smartpractice.com

Smith & Nephew Inc.
150 Minuteman Rd.
Andover, MA 01810
Phone: 978-749-1000
www.smith-nephew.com/

**Smithers Bio-Medical Systems/Smithers-
Oasis Company**
P.O. Box 790
Kent, OH 44240
Phone: 800-321-8286
www.biofoamimpression.com

SmithKline Beecham Quest Diagnostics
Phone: 866-MYQUEST (866-697-8378)
www.questdiagnostics.com/home.html

Smiths Medical USA
5200 Upper Metro Pl., Suite 200
Dublin, OH 43017
Phone: 800-258-5361
www.smiths-medical.com

Solta Medical Inc.
7031 Koll Center Pkwy. #260
Pleasanton, CA 94566
Phone: 877-782-2286
Fax: 510-782-2287
www.solta.com or www.isolaz.com

Sonoscape USA
2730 North Berkeley Lake Rd., Suite
B-400
Duluth, GA 30096
Phone: 888-725-2959
www.sonoscapeusa.com/

SonoSite FUJIFILM
21919 30th Dr. SE
Bothell, WA 98021-3904
Phone: 888-482-9449
www.sonosite.com

SOS Medical
9259 Eton Ave.
Chatsworth, CA 91311
Phone: 800-863-1769
www.sosmedical.net/

SoundSkin Corp.
1703 South Prairie Ave.
Chicago. IL 60616
Phone: 630-554-5100
www.soundskin.com

SpaceLabs Healthcare OSI Systems
35301 SE Center St.
Snoqualmie, WA 98065
Phone: 800-522-7025
www.spacelabshealthcare.com

Stallergenes Greer Laboratories Inc.
P.O. Box 800
639 Nuway Cir.
Lenoir, NC 28645-0088
Phone: 800-438-0088
www.stallergenesgreer.com/

STD Pharmaceutical
Fields Yard, Plough Ln.
Hereford, UK HR4 0EL
Phone: +44-(0)1432-353684
www.stdpharm.co.uk

SterilMed Johnson & Johnson
5010 Cheshire Pkwy., Suite 2
Plymouth, MN
Phone: 763-488-3400
www.sterilmed.com/

St. Jude Medical Abbott
1 St. Jude Medical Dr.
St. Paul, MN 55117
Phone: 800-328-9634
www.sjm.com

Stoetling
620 Wheat Ln.
Wood Dale, IL 60191
Phone: 800-860-9775 or 630-860-9700
Fax: 630-860-9775
info@StoeltingCo.com
www.stoeltingco.com/

Storz (Bausch and Lomb)
180 Villa Verde Dr.
San Dimas, CA 91773
www.storzeye.com

Stryker Instruments
1410 Lakeside Pkwy.
Flower Mound, TX 75028
Phone: 866-726-3705 or 269-385-2600
www.stryker.com

SunTech Medical
507 Airport Blvd.
Suite 117
Morrisville, NC 27560
Phone: 800-421-8626
www.suntechmed.com

Surgical Optics LLC
7231 Garden Grove Blvd., Suite C
Garden Grove, CA 92841
Phone/Fax: 714-894-5400
cpmedscopes@yahoo.com
www.surgical-optics.com

Surgical Repair Technologies
325 Armour Ave.
St. Paul, MN 55075
Phone: 800-495-0297
srtrepair.com

Surgical Specialties Corporation
1100 Berkshire Blvd., Suite 308
Wyomissing, PA 19610
www.surgicalspecialties.com

Surgical Supply Service (Podiatric Supplies)
500 Fillmore Ave.
Tonawanda, NY 14150
Phone: 800-523-0706 (U.S.) or 716-743-
1529 (worldwide)
Fax (24-hour): 800-222-1934
customersupport@surgicalsupplyservice.com
www.surgicalsupplyservice.com

Swede-O Core Products International
808 Prospect Ave.
Osceola, WI 54020
Phone: 800-365-3047
www.coreproducts.com

Sybaritic
9220 S. James Ave.
Bloomington, MN 55431
Phone: 800-445-8418
www.sybaritic.com

Synectics Medical Medtronic Functional Diagnostics
3850 Victoria St. North
St. Paul, MN 55126-2907
Phone: 612-514-1700
www.medtronic.com

Syneron Inc.
3 Goodyear, Unit A
Irvine, CA 92618
Phone: 866-259-6661
www.syneron-candela.com/na
www.syneron.com

SYNOVA Healthcare Mayer Laboratories
P.O. Box 13323
Berkeley, CA 94712
Phone: 510-229-5300
www.todaysponge.com

Tao & Tao Technology Cook Medical
886 Sands Ln.
Camano Island, WA 98282
Phone: 800-457-4500
www.cookmedical.com/products/wh_dtca_
    webds/

Teleflex Medical
3015 Carrington Mill Blvd.
Morrisville, NC 27560
Phone: 866-246-6990
www.teleflex.com

TeraRecon
4000 East 3rd Ave.
Suite #200
Foster City, CA 94404
Phone: 877-996-0100
Contact: info@terarecon.com
www.terarecon.com

Terason Ultrasound Teratech
77 Terrace Hall Ave.
Burlington, MA 01803
Phone: 866-837-2766 (U.S. only) or 781-
    270-4143
Fax: 781-270-4145
www.terason.com

Terumo Medical Corp.
2101 Cottontail Ln.
Somerset, NJ 08873
Phone: 800-283-7866
www.terumotmp.com

Theraplex Company
6410 Poplar Ave., Suite 375
Memphis, TN 38119
Phone: 888-437-2753
www.theraplex.com

Thera-Tronics Everest
42 Broadway, 17th Floor
New York, NY 10004
Phone: 800-638-0308
www.theratronicsinc.com

Thermage Inc. (product of Solta Medical)
7031 Koll Center Pkwy. #260
Pleasanton, CA 94566
Phone: 877-782-2286
www.thermage.com

ThermoTek Inc.
1200 Lakeside Pkwy.
Suite 200 (Building 2)
Flower Mound, TX 75028
Phone: 972-874-4949 or 877-242-3232
Fax: 972-874-4945
Contact: info@thermotekusa.com
www.thermotekusa.com

Thomas Medical Inc.
6102 Victory Way
Indianapolis, IN 46278
Phone: 800-556-0349
www.thomasmedical.com

Three Dimensional Systems Inc. Abeo
Phone: 855-270-ABEO (2236)
www.abeofootwear.com/brand/3d3

3 Gen LLC
31521 Rancho Viejo Rd.
Suite 104
San Juan Capistrano, CA 92675
Phone: 949-481-6384
Fax: 949-240-7492
Contact: info@3GenLLC.com
www.dermlite.com/ (product)

3 M Health Information Systems
3 M Center
Bldg. 275-4E-01
St. Paul, MN 55144-1000
Phone: 800-228-3957
www.3m.com

TIMM Medical Technologies
2111 W. Wyatt Earp Blvd.
Dodge City, KS 67801
Phone: 800-438-8592
www.timmmedical.com

Topix Pharmaceuticals
174 Rte. 109
West Babylon, NY 11704
Phone: 800-445-2595
www.topixpharm.com

Toshiba Canon Medical Systems USA
2441 Michelle Dr.
Tustin, CA 92780
Phone: 800-421-1968 or 800-521-1968
www.us.medical.canon.com

Townsend Design
4615 Shepard St.
Bakersfield, CA 93313
Phone: 800-432-3466
www.townsenddesign.com

Travanti Pharma Inc. (formerly Birch
    Point Medical Inc.; for IontoPatch)
Phone: 866-467-2824
www.iontopatch.com

Ultradent Products Inc.
55 W. 10200 South (505)
South Jordan, UT 84095
Phone: 888-230-1420
www.ultradent.com

Unimax Supply Company
269 Canal St.
New York, NY 10013
Phone: 800-9-UNIMAX (864629)
store.unimaxshop.com/storefront.aspx

United Endoscopy
583 North Smith Ave., Suite B
Corona, CA 92880
Phone: 800-899-4847
www.endoscope.com

United Medical
832 Jury Ct.
San Jose CA, 95112
Phone: 408-278-9300 or 877-490-7036
Fax: 408-278-9797
www.umiultrasound.com

Universal Endoscopic Services
6861 SW 196th Ave.
Suite 402
Pembroke Pines, FL 33332
Phone: 800-266-1464
www.ues1.com

University Compounding Pharmacy
1875 Third Ave.
San Diego, CA 92101
Phone: 800-985-8065 or 619-683-2005
www.ucprx.com

**University of Washington Center for
    Health Sciences Interprofessional Edu-
    cation, Research & Practice**
1959 NE Pacific St.
Box 357266
Seattle, WA 98195
Phone: 206-685-1158
https://collaborate.uw.edu/

USSDG Sutures (now Syneture TYCO
    Healthcare)
195 McDermott Rd.
North Haven, CT 06473
Phone: 800-544-8772
www.tyco.com/markets/healthcare

Utah Medical Products Inc. (Europe)
Athlone Business and Research Park
Dublin Rd.
Athlone, County Westmeath
Republic of Ireland
Phone: 353-90-647-3932
www.utahmed.com

**Utah Medical Products Inc. (United
    States)**
7043 South 300 West
Midvale, UT 84047-1048
Phone: 866-754-9789 (main, toll-free) or
    800-533-4984 (customer support)

Valeant Bausch Pharmaceuticals
400 Somerset Corporate Blvd.
Bridgewater, NJ 08807
Phone: 800-556-1937

Valleylab Inc.
5920 Longbow Dr.
Boulder, CO 80301-3299
Phone: 800-255-8522
www.valleylab.com

VBM Medical Inc.
524 Herriman Ct.
Noblesville IN 46060
Phone: 317-776-1800
Phone: 800-580-7117
www.vbm-medical.com/products/

Venosan North America
300 Industrial Park Ave.
P.O. Box 1067
Asheboro, NC 27204-1067
Phone: 800-432-5347
www.venosanusa.com

Vidacare Teleflex
3015 Carrington Mill Blvd.
Morrisville, NC 27560
Phone: 866-246-6990
www.vidacare.com

Viora Inc.
213 West 35th St, Suite #500,
New York, NY 10001
Phone: l-888-415-1192
www.vioramed.com

Visual Changes Skin Care
4676 W. Jacquelyn Ave.
Fresno, CA 93722
Phone: 800-400-8901
customerservice@visualchanges.com
www.visualchanges.com

Vita Medical Technologies
5355 E. High St., #422
Phoenix, AZ 85054
Phone: 951-295-8087
www.vitamedtech.com

Vitalograph Inc.
13310 W. 99th St.
Lenexa, KS 66215
Phone: 800-255-6626
www.vitalograph.com

VNUS Medical Covidien
5799 Fontanoso Way
San Jose, CA 95138
Phone: 800-962-9888
Contact: info@vnus.com
www.vnus.com

WaisMed PerSys Medical
5310 Elm St.
Houston, TX 77081
Phone: 888-737-7978
ps-med.com

Wallach Surgical Devices Inc.
95 Corporate Dr.
Trumbull, CT 06611
Phone: 800-444-8456
www.wallachsurgical.com

Weck Closure Systems Teleflex Medical
3015 Carrington Mill Blvd.
Morrisville, NC 27560
Phone: 866-246-6990
www.teleflex.com/usa/product-areas/surgical/
    fascial-closure/weck-efx-fascial-closure-
    system/index?language_id=11

Welch Allyn Corporation
4341 State St. Rd.
P.O. Box 220
Skaneateles Falls, NY 13153-0220
Phone: 800-535-6663
www.welchallyn.com

Westone
2235 Executive Cr.
Colorado Springs, CO 80906
Telephone: 800-525-5071
www.westone.com

Wilson-Cook Medical Inc.
4900 Bethania Station Rd.
Winston-Salem, NC 27105
Phone: 336-744-0157
Fax: 336-744-1147

Wilson Ophthalmic Hilco
932 W. State Hwy. 152
Mustang, OK 73064
Phone: 405-376-9114
www.hilco.com

Xomed Medtronic
Medtronic ENT
6743 N. Southpoint Dr.
Jacksonville, FL 32216
Phone: 904-332-8319 or 800-874-5797
www.medtronic.com/us-en/healthcare-pro-
    fessionals/products/ear-nose-throat.html

Yama Inc.
650 Liberty Ave.
Union, NJ 07083
Phone: 800-699-8130
Fax: 908-206-8725

Z-Medica Corp.
4 Fairfield Blvd.
Wallingford, CT 06492
Phone: 877-750-0504
www.z-medica.com

Zeiss Carl Zeiss Meditec Inc.
5160 Hacienda Dr.
Dublin, CA 94568
Phone: 925-557-4100
www.meditec.zeiss.com/us

Zerowet
P.O. Box 4375
Palos Verdes Peninsula, CA 90274
Phone: 800-438-0938

Zimmer Biomet
345 East Main St.
Warsaw, IN 46580
Phone: 800-348-2759
www.zimmer.com

Zimmer Medizin Systems
3 Goodyear, Suite B
Irvine, CA 92618
Phone (office): 800-327-3576
Fax: 949-727-2154
info@zimmerusa.com
zimmerusa.com

APPENDIX E

RESOURCES FOR LEARNING AND TEACHING PROCEDURES

Stephen J. Wetmore • Steven E. Roskos

The well-rounded primary care clinician performs a variety of medical and surgical procedures in his or her practice. The skill in performing such procedures and resultant success will depend strongly on the training that one has received in performing those procedures. Advancing technology and changing practice patterns will likely lead primary care clinicians to add new procedures to their practices and to update their skills in procedures that they already perform. Regardless of whether the clinician is learning a procedure for the first time or wishing to update already existing skills, it is helpful to have a good understanding of the resources that are available to facilitate learning.

This appendix provides information about a variety of resources available for learning procedures and how these can be accessed. A new section in this appendix includes some tips for teaching and learning procedures in family medicine. This is also of considerable interest to teachers of procedural skills. It is not possible to include every resource, but each section will have examples and provide ideas about where to search for other similar resources.

POLICIES AND POSITION PAPERS ON VARIOUS PROCEDURES

The American Academy of Family Physicians (AAFP) has long provided policies and positions papers regarding various procedures. These are excellent references when considering obtaining privileges as well as when teaching students and residents about these procedures. They are all available online at www.aafp.org.

COURSES IN PROCEDURES FOR PRIMARY CARE CLINICIANS

In both Canada and the United States, national medical associations such as the College of Family Physicians of Canada and the AAFP provide opportunities to learn and update procedure skills. National and state or provincial meetings of these bodies often have seminars or workshops on common procedures in primary care. Seminars and workshops are excellent starting points for clinicians hoping to learn procedures because they include the pertinent background knowledge for each procedure, including indications, contraindications, technical details, typical pathology, and complications. Many of these workshops also include opportunities for hands-on experience, which allows clinicians to become familiar with equipment and techniques. These sessions are also suitable as updates for clinicians already familiar with the procedures; however, they often do not provide quite enough practical experience for new learners to commence performing them right away. They are, nevertheless, good starting points.

An example of an organization providing comprehensive, hands-on courses is The National Procedures Institute which was founded more than 30 years ago by the original senior editor of *Pfenninger and*

Fowler's Procedures for Primary Care, John (Jack) Pfenninger, MD. It is now wholly owned by the Texas Academy of Family Physicians. A variety of courses in procedure skills can be found on its website (www.npinstitute.com).

The following are examples of nationally recognized programs with standards and hands-on practical training that must be met to receive credit:

Advanced Cardiac Life Support
Advanced Life Support in Obstetrics
Advanced Trauma Life Support
American College of Sports Medicine (www.acsm.org)
Basic Life Support
Canadian Academy of Sports Medicine and Exercise Medicine (www.casm-acmse.org)
MOREOB program (http://moreob.com)
Neonatal Resuscitation Program
Newborn Advanced Life Support
Pediatric Advanced Life Support (www.americanheart.org)
Sideline Management Assessment Response Techniques

TEACHING PROCEDURES

Clinicians find themselves teaching procedures in various settings, both formal and informal. You may give a workshop to family medicine residents on a certain procedure. You may teach a procedure to a medical student spending time in your office. The principles of effective instruction remain the same, though their application to these different situations may vary.

Which procedures should be taught and learned? Each practice situation will require different procedural skills, so no list will be universal. Some good starting points include the core list of procedures for family physicians developed by the Working Group on Procedure Skills of the College of Family Physicians of Canada or the list of core procedures for family medicine developed by the Society of Teachers of Family Medicine Group on Hospital Medicine and Procedural Training.

Several other papers in the medical literature provide valuable information about procedure skills training in American and Canadian family medicine training programs. What should the content of teaching and learning procedures include? Although the first component that comes to mind is the technical skill, there is much more to learn about a medical procedure. The Working Group on the Certification Process of the College of Family Physicians of Canada has defined the key features that must be included for each procedure. These features are discussed in the following section.

EDITOR'S NOTE: Learning procedures and teaching procedures can be very different. It may take many years to really learn how to perform a certain procedure. While you may be competent performing the procedure much earlier, after many years, you may acquire additional tricks, such as how to be much more time-efficient. Over time, you may also learn more about your limitations and what to do no matter what type of patient, anatomy, body habitus, or complication comes along. But even after performing a procedure for many years, teaching a procedure can present unique challenges. After many years, you may know intuitively almost anything that can happen during a procedure, or what you might do, but you may not know what a particular learner will do. When teaching procedures for the first time, watch the learner very closely and carefully; only after many years of teaching procedures will you will also be able to anticipate almost anything any learner might do when performing the procedure.

KEY FEATURES OF PROCEDURAL SKILLS

1. When deciding whether to perform a procedure, consider the following:
   - Indications and contraindications to the procedure
   - Your own skills and readiness to do the procedure (e.g., your level of fatigue and any personal distracters)
   - Context of the procedure, including the patient involved, the complexity of the task, the time needed, the need for assistance, and location.
2. Before deciding to go ahead with the procedure, consider the following:
   - Discuss the procedure with the patient, including a description of the procedure and possible outcomes, both positive and negative, as part of obtaining consent.
   - Prepare for the procedure by ensuring appropriate equipment is ready.
   - Mentally rehearse the following:
     - The anatomic landmarks necessary to perform the procedure
     - The technical steps necessary in sequential fashion, including any preliminary examination
     - The potential complications and their management
3. During performance of the procedure
   - Keep the patient informed to reduce anxiety.
   - Ensure patient comfort and safety always.
4. When the procedure is not going as expected, stop, reevaluate the situation, and seek assistance as required.
5. Develop a plan with your patient for aftercare and follow-up after completion of a procedure.

A good working understanding of these key features is a prerequisite to performing any procedure and needs to be taught and learned in addition to the technical skill itself. The goal of teaching a procedure is that the learner will be able to perform the procedure in the real world on a real patient. When teaching medical procedures, it is best to treat them as a relatively "closed" skill—in other words, with specific steps that the learner should not deviate from. Once the procedure is mastered, variations can be introduced to address different anatomy or other variations in the clinical situation.

The OOMPA ED WASDM PF SIOMT acronym explained in the following sections can help you remember to incorporate all the steps to effective instruction.

Introduction

O: **O**bjective. To perform a given procedure on real patients in the real world.
O: **O**verview. Provide a quick summary of the steps involved.
M: **M**otivation. Why should the learner gain proficiency in this procedure? Provide information on how often this procedure is required, what the benefits are, and the consequences of not acquiring skill in this procedure.
P: **P**rerequisites. Before learning the technical skills required to perform a procedure, the learner needs to know the indications,

risks, anatomy, and so forth. This is a good opportunity to refer the learner to a chapter in this text. The best way to ensure that the learner knows the prerequisite information is to ask questions: "What are the indications for this procedure?" "What are the risks?" "What complications would you keep your eye out for?" Role playing works as well: "Pretend I am the patient and obtain informed consent for this procedure from me." Pictures and models are also very helpful in cementing this information in the learner's mind.
A: **A**genda. Describe what the learner can expect. If you are giving a formal lesson or workshop, describe what it will contain. If this is informal teaching in the office, explain that you will list and explain the steps, demonstrate them in some way, and ask the learner to demonstrate them as well.

Core Material

ED: **E**xplanation and **d**emonstration. This portion of the instruction is key. Even if the learner has performed this procedure several times, it is helpful to review the steps and then have the learner repeat them, and even have the learner demonstrate the procedure in some way before beginning the actual procedure on a patient.

The explanation and demonstration phase can be outlined by the WASDM acronym:

W: You **w**ill perform this procedure.
A: **A**ttend to these steps as I show you how to do them.
SD: **S**ay each step before **d**oing it.
M: Ask the learner to **m**emorize the steps and recall them before the practice.

Sometimes dividing the procedure into discrete steps can be difficult, and it is easy to leave a step out. Use this text as a starting point to list all the steps for a procedure. If the instruction is for a formal setting, ask others who are familiar with the procedure to review the steps. Then, ask someone who is unfamiliar with the procedure, perhaps someone who is nonmedical, to try to learn the procedure using this method. This person can often point out missing steps or incomplete instruction. If the situation is informal, add steps as you go if you realize that you have left some out. When teaching complex procedures, it may be best to divide them into segments and teach the segments separately, combining them later. For example, when teaching laceration repair, local anesthesia may be separated from suturing.

You may demonstrate a procedure in several ways. The best way is on a real patient. However, if you want the learner to perform a procedure on that patient, the patient probably doesn't need two procedures. On the other hand, if the patient needs both knees injected or two moles removed, this is the perfect opportunity to demonstrate and then have the learner perform the procedure, a classic case of "see one, do one." If several procedures are being performed in succession (e.g., several colonoscopies are scheduled in the endoscopy laboratory), you can demonstrate on the first one and let the learner try the second one. It is very important to follow the WASDM acronym when demonstrating so that the learner gains maximum benefit from the demonstration.

If a real patient is unavailable for demonstration, mock demonstration using capped needles or covered scalpels is useful. Video demonstration is an excellent alternative, and there are many resources available for video demonstration (see Table E.2).

PF: Following demonstration, **p**ractice with **f**eedback is very important. The learner can practice on a real or simulated patient. The learner should state the steps as they do them ("say, then **d**o"). It is important that the practice be in an environment that is encouraging and pleasant. If there really isn't time to teach the procedure, it is better to wait for another opportunity. A stressful and high-pressure setting is not conducive to learning and may discourage the learner from future attempts at learning a procedure.

Do your best to be encouraging and positive during the practice. If the learner is forgetting a step or not performing it properly, ask them to stop and think: "What step are you missing?" or "That's not quite right. How should you perform this step?" Specific feedback is very important. Rather than saying "good job," try pointing out specific things that were done well—for example, "you really kept that site sterile throughout the procedure" or "your conversation with the patient put him at ease."

Conclusion

Whether in a formal or informal instructional situation, it is important to review and summarize (SIOMT):

S: **S**ummary. Review the steps.
I: **I**ntegration. Explain how this procedure might fit in with other treatments for the same condition or other procedures that are related.
O: **O**bjective. Review the objective (to perform the procedure on a real patient in the real world).
M: **M**otivation. Review the motivation.
T: **T**est. If you need to assess competency, have the learner perform the procedure while you observe. The best situation is performing the procedure on a real patient. If this is not possible, then performing the procedure in some simulated fashion may suffice.

Teaching procedures is challenging and rewarding. Seeing a learner achieve competence and independence in performing procedures is one of the greatest rewards of the clinician–educator. Following these tips can help you do so effectively and efficiently.

GAINING PRACTICAL EXPERIENCE IN PROCEDURES

Although formal courses or workshops are suitable for learning information about procedures, equipment, and techniques, it may not be possible for the clinician to gain enough experience in this way to begin performing the procedure. Supervised practice is necessary to gain confidence in many procedures. In most cases, there is no consensus on how many supervised procedures are necessary to achieve competence. The number of supervised procedures necessary to achieve competence for any given procedure depends on the complexity of the procedure, and the confidence and physical dexterity of the operator, among other things. For example, a learner may need to perform 25 to 30 supervised flexible sigmoidoscopies to achieve competence but only 10 to 15 supervised no-scalpel vasectomies. Clinicians should consider performing procedures under the supervision of an experienced colleague until both are comfortable with the learner's competence. Even when everyone is comfortable, low-risk patients should be those chosen for quite some time for someone new at performing unsupervised procedures. Supportive colleagues can be a major resource for getting started in procedures and can provide backup and support when difficulties arise.

It should be noted that for the longest time, the AAFP refused to endorse a number of procedures needed to be performed to be considered competent for a particular procedure. And that was probably reasonable; we all know among our classmates there were some who could do a procedure five times and be competent. Meanwhile, other classmates would still not be competent after performing many, many more. Merely performing a certain number of procedures does not guarantee competence. That said, when the American College of Surgeons recommended that every surgery resident perform at least 50 colonoscopies during their training, the AAFP agreed with them. But these numbers are largely based on expert opinion. As it turns out, there are published studies regarding the learning curves of residents or practitioners in family medicine when obtaining competence in various procedures (e.g., gastroscopy, obstetric ultrasound, colonoscopy). It may be worthwhile for teachers of procedures to do some research regarding these learning curves. There are also guidelines for numbers of recommended procedures to obtain competence produced

by various other professional organizations. However, these are also predominantly based on expert opinion and not learning curves.

BOOKS ON PROCEDURES IN PRIMARY CARE

With the rise in technology and increasing use of CD-ROMs, DVDs, online videos, computer animations, and virtual reality, there is less emphasis on books for many of the things we do in practice. Nevertheless, textbooks remain a readily available source of practical information. One or two texts on procedural skills are an essential part of the primary care clinician's library. This book, *Pfenninger and Fowler's Procedures for Primary Care*, 4th ed., is one example of an ideal resource book because of its comprehensive nature, inclusion of background material, patient education, description of technique, helpful illustrations, company names and addresses for obtaining equipment, and billing and coding information. Many common primary care procedures are covered in *The Essential Guide to Primary Care Procedures*, 2nd ed., by E.J. Mayeaux Jr (2015), which has a companion website with patient education handouts and videos (Lippincott Williams & Wilkins). Another excellent resource for dermatology procedures is Habif's *Clinical Dermatology: A Color Guide to Diagnosis and Therapy*, 6th ed. (Elsevier, 2015), Usatine's text *Dermatologic and Cosmetic Procedures in Office Practice* (Elsevier, 2011) is a comprehensive review of dermatologic procedures.

The following are examples of other important texts; they are but a few of the must-have texts for any library:

Apgar's Principles and Practice of Colposcopy, 3rd ed. (Jaypee Brothers Medical Publishing, 2018)
Office Orthopedics for Primary Care: Treatment, by B.C. Anderson, 3rd ed. (Saunders, 2006)
Emergency Medicine Procedures, by E.F. Reichman, 3rd ed. (McGraw-Hill, 2018)
Essentials of Musculoskeletal Care, by A.D. Armstrong AD, M.C. Hubbard, 5th ed., with DVD (American Academy of Orthopedic Surgeons, 2015)
Essential Orthopedics, by M. Miller (Elsevier, 2009), comes with a DVD (videos on how to perform 29 joint injections, 7 common physical examinations, and 6 splinting and casting procedures) and full-text online access
Fracture Management for Primary Care, by M.P. Eiff, R.L. Hatch, 3rd ed. (Elsevier, 2017)
John Murtagh's Practice Tips, by J.M. Murtagh, 7th ed. (McGraw Hill, 2017)
Practical Guide to Joint and Soft Tissue Injections, by J.W. McNabb, 3rd ed. (Lippincott Williams & Wilkins, 2014)
Roberts and Hedges' Clinical Procedures in Emegency Medicine and Acute Care, by J. R. Roberts Jr, C.B. Custalow, and T.W. Thomsen, 7th ed. (Elsevier, 2019)
Surgery of the Skin, by J.K. Robinson, et al., 3rd ed. (Elsevier, 2014)

A more complete list of other available texts can be found in Table E.1.

RESOURCES FOR PROCEDURES IN PRIMARY CARE

These days, teaching videos for most procedures are available online with a simple search. The *New England Journal of Medicine* has a great library of such online videos. CD-ROMs and DVDs are also useful resources for purchase for learning procedures because the technology allows the integration of text with voice, pictures, computer animation, and video. These can be searched easily to focus on specific details of any given procedure. Like textbooks, CD-ROMs can provide all the relevant background information necessary to perform the procedure. Texts now often contain a DVD and online access (see Miller's *Essential Orthopedics*, cited previously). One strength of this technology is the capacity to incorporate video footage; the visual presentation of the technique is a powerful learning aid. CD-ROMs are portable and can be used in a variety of settings, including the office, clinic, or even the home. Access to such videos has often been expanded to online availability. As an example what started as a DVD, *Atlas of Essential* by Tuggy, and Garcia, is now available in print form and videos online. The original scripts for the videos were drafted from *Pfenninger and Fowler's Procedures for*

Primary Care, The quality of the videos and visualization of the techniques are excellent. This video and print package includes patient guides, voice or text instruction for each procedure, and access to CPT codes for each procedure. Many of the original videos from this project are now available on the website Procedures Consult, part of

TABLE E.I Procedures Books	
Book Title	**Authors and Publishing Data**
Atlas of Primary Care Procedures, for PDA	Thomas J. Zuber, EJ Mayeux Publisher: Lippincott Williams & Wilkins, 2004
Basic Soft-Tissue Surgery: An Illustrated Guide for the Family Physician	Thomas J. Zuber, Donald E. Dewitt Publisher: American Academy of Family Physicians, 2004
Blueprints Clinical Procedures	Laurie L. Marbas, Erin Case Publisher: Blackwell, 2004
Clinical Procedures for Medical Assistants	Kathy Bonewit-West, 9th ed. Publisher: Elsevier, 2014
Clinical Procedures for Ocular Examination	Nancy B. Carlson, Daniel Kurtz, 4th ed. Publisher: McGraw-Hill Medical Publishers, 2015
Clinical Procedures in Primary Eye Care	David B. Elliott Publisher: Butterworth-Heinemann, 2003
Clinical Skills for the Ophthalmic Examination: Basic Procedures	Lindy DuBois Publisher: SLACK Inc., 2006
Clinician's Pocket Reference	Leonard G. Gomella, Steven A. Haist, University of Kentucky College of Medicine, 11th ed. Publisher: McGraw-Hill, 2007
Current Procedures—Pediatrics	Denise M. Goodman, NetLibrary, Inc., et al. Publisher: McGraw-Hill, 2007
Emergency Medicine Procedures	Eric Reichman, 3rd ed. Publisher: McGraw-Hill Medical Publishing, 2018
Essential Clinical Procedures	Richard W. Dehn, David P. Asprey Publisher: Saunders Elsevier, 2013
Essential Emergency Procedures	Kaushal Shah, Chilembwe Mason Publisher: Wolters Kluwer Health/Lippincott Williams & Wilkins, 2008
The Essential Guide to Primary Care Procedures	EJ Mayeaux, 2nd ed. Publisher: Lippincott Williams & Wilkins, 2015
Medicine for the Outdoors: The Essential Guide to Emergency Medical Procedures and First Aid	Paul S. Auerbach Publisher: Lyons Press, 2003
Merrill's Atlas of Radiographic Positioning & Procedures	Bruce W. Long, Jeannean H Rollins, 13th ed. Publisher: Elsevier, 2015
Murtagh's Practice Tips	John Murtagh, 7th ed. Publisher: McGraw-Hill, 2017
Office Procedures	Robert S. Wigton, Thomas G. Tape Publisher: Mosby, 2004
Office Surgery	Gerald Amundsen, Brian Coleman, Kalyanakrishnan Ramakrishnan, Rhonda Sparks, American Academy of Family Physicians Publisher: American Academy of Family Physicians, 2003
On Call Procedures	Gregg A. Adams, Stephen D. Bresnick Publisher: Saunders, 2006
Ophthalmic Office Procedures: A Step-by-Step Approach	Kenneth C. Chern, Eliot Foley, Ashok Reddy Publisher: McGraw-Hill Medical Publishing (New York); McGraw-Hill (London), 2004
Orthopedics for Primary Care Physicians	Rene Cailliet Publisher: AMA Press, 2003
Pfenninger and Fowler's Procedures for Primary Care	John L. Pfenninger, Grant C. Fowler, 4th ed Publisher: Elsevier, 2019
Pfenninger and Fowler's Procedures for Primary Care, 4th ed. + Atlas of Essential Procedures Print and eBook with online videos	John L. Pfenninger, Michael Tuggy, Grant C. Fowler, Jorge Garcia Publisher: Elsevier, 2010
Pocket Guide to Orthopedic and Sports Medicine Procedures: 111 Commonly Performed Procedures for the Health Care Professional	J. Konin Publisher: SLACK, 2009
Primary Care Procedures in Women's Health	CB Heath, SM Sulik Publisher: Springer, 2009
Procedures for Primary Care Provider	Marilyn W. Edmunds, 3rd ed. Publisher: Elsevier, 2016
Roberts and Hedges, Clinical Procedures in Emergency Medicine and Acute Care	James R. Roberts, Catherine B. Custalow, Todd W. Thomsen Publisher: Elsevier, 2019
Roenigk's Dermatologic Surgery: Current Techniques in Procedural Dermatology	Randall K. Roenigk, John L. Ratz, Henry H. Roenigk Publisher: Informa Healthcare, 2007
Textbook of Pediatric Emergency Procedures	Christopher King, Fred M. Henretig, John Loiselle, Richard M. Ruddy Publisher: Wolters Kluwer Health/Lippincott Williams & Wilkins, 2008

Clinical Key, which is regularly updated, and video footage of additional procedures is also available and is described later. This works well for teaching many students and residents in a lecture format as well as small groups. Box E.1. lists many of the procedures found on Procedures Consult. An app for this book is also available from Usatine Media at www.usatinemedia.com.

Deutchman has produced two excellent DVDs: *Emergency and Trauma Ultrasound* and *Cesarean Delivery*. These products can be found at MedChallenger (www.challengercme.com). Descriptions and contents can be found in Box E.2.

The National Procedures Institute produces a series of learning DVDs that are listed in Box E.3.

MeisterMed recently launched its *Procedures: Hospital Collection* for iPhone and iPod touch (www.healthtap.com/apps/5655). It includes videos, images, and step-by-step details for 15 key inpatient procedures.

The American College of Physicians-American Society of Internal Medicine has two products: *Arthrocentesis and Joint Injection* (Alguire PC, Casey LM, eds., 1999) and *Common Skin Biopsy Techniques* (Alguire PC, Casey LM, eds., 1999) that include videotapes of the procedures.

WEBSITES

Elsevier has developed a subscription service called Clinical Key with an aim of integrating publications with other media to provide a source of clinical answers. Procedures Consult is available through Clinical Key and is an informative web-based resource that is constantly being updated. Many procedural topics are outlined, and each includes a short video clip of the procedure, as well the indications, contraindications, techniques, outcomes, and resources. Subscription is required but the value of the resource is worth it.

Another good resource for teaching is The Family Medicine Digital Resources Library, produced by the Society of Teachers in Family Medicine, available at resourcelibrary.stfm.org. This website contains user-posted conference presentations and handouts, and shared curricular materials such as PowerPoint lectures, learning modules, syllabi, digital images, video and audio recordings, and recommended websites. All the content has been peer reviewed, and anyone can search the database and download materials. Registration is required but free if you want to upload material to share with others. One example is a PowerPoint presentation entitled "Procedure World: A New Paradigm for Teaching Procedural Skills" by Ellen Johnson, which illustrates one teaching program for procedural skills.

BOX E.1 **Procedures Included on Clinical Key in Procedures Consult**

Abdominal paracentesis	Needle aspiration of breast cysts
Amniotomy	Neonatal circumcision
Anoscopy	No-scalpel vasectomy
Arthrocentesis—knee aspiration	Obstetric ultrasound
Banding of internal hemorrhoids	Optimal circumcision anesthesia
Barrier contraceptives (diaphragm)	Pap smear (and wet prep Pap smear with HPV sampling)
Bartholin gland—marsupialization	Paracervical block
Bartholin gland—Word catheter placement	Performing an instrument tie
Bladder catheterization—female	Pilonidal cyst excision
Bladder catheterization—male	Placing an Unna boot
Burn debridement	Punch biopsy
Cerumen impaction removal	Radiofrequency mole excision/shave biopsy
Cervical polyp removal	Radiofrequency spider vein ablation
Cervical sampling (wet smear with KOH preparation)	Removal of ingrown toenail
Cesarean section	Ring removal
Colposcopy	Scalp cyst excision
Complete nail removal	Shave biopsy
Curettage and cautery—basal cell carcinoma	Skin tag removal
Digital block	Subacromial shoulder injection
Endometrial biopsy	Subclavian line placement
Episiotomy—laceration repair	Subcuticular running stitches
Excisional skin biopsy	Suprapubic taps or aspirations
Flexible sigmoidoscopy	Thoracentesis
Ganglion injection/aspiration	Thyroid fine needle aspiration
Incision and drainage of abscesses	Tissue adhesives—use of tissue glues
Incision and drainage of thrombosed hemorrhoids	Topical anesthesia
Inverted subcuticular stitches	Topical hemostasis
IUD insertion	Trigger point injection
IUD removal	Tubal ligation
Joint injection—knee	Vaginal delivery
Joint injection—shoulder	Vulvar biopsy
Lipoma removal	V-Y flap closure
Lipoma removal by extrusion	Wart treatment (peripheral and plantar)
Local anesthesia	
Loop electrosurgical excision procedure (LEEP)	*HPV*, Human papillomavirus; *IUD*, intrauterine device; *KOH*, potassium hydroxide; *Pap*, Papanicolaou.
Lumbar puncture	From https://www.clinicalkey.com/#!/browse/procedures.Philadelphia: Elsevier,2019.
Mattress stitches	
Nasogastric intubation	
Nasopharyngoscopy	

BOX E.2 Contents of *Deutchman's Emergency and Trauma Ultrasound Examination and Cesarean Delivery* Course

Emergency and Trauma Ultrasound Examination

This course is designed to teach the basic technique of emergency ultrasound examination. The course contains a combination of still and video segments as well as diagrams, three-dimensional animation, and interactive multimedia that describe the key concepts of ultrasonography.

Chapters include the following:

Introduction
Physics and orientation
Trauma ultrasound examination
Cardiac examination
Right upper quadrant examination
Abdominal aorta examination
Renal examination
OB/GYN examination
Lower extremity venous examination (DVT)
Sonographic guidance of procedures

——————

http://www.challengercme.com

Cesarean Delivery

This course contains 50+ min of high-quality surgical video demonstrating all aspects and multiple variations of cesarean surgical technique and tubal ligation technique, as well as assisting at surgery. Although the procedure must ultimately be taught in the operating room, viewing high-quality video of the standard technique and its variation is helpful both to new learners and to more experienced clinicians interested in improving their skills.

These techniques are included:

Patient positioning and preparation
Abdominal incisions: vertical and transverse
Opening the uterus
Delivery of the infant from cephalic and breech presentations
Use of vacuum extractor
Delivery of the placenta
Closure of the uterus
Tubal ligation technique
Closure of the abdomen and skin

——————

http://www.challengercme.com
AMA, American Medical Association; *DVT*, deep vein thrombosis; *OB/GYN*, obstetrics/gynecology.
Courtesy Mark Deutchman, www.challengercme.com, Aurora, CO.

BOX E.3 DVDs Available from the National Procedures Institute

The Basics of Radiofrequency Surgery
Billing and Coding for Dermatologic Procedures
Cardiac Stress Testing for the Primary Care Physician
Common Office Dermatologic Procedures: Patient Cases
Excisions and Common Wound Repairs: Patient Cases
Hospitalist Procedures: Collection 1
Hospitalist Procedures: Collection 2
How to Perform Skin Biopsies
Joint Exam and Injections with an Introduction to Ultrasound
Learning No-Scalpel Vasectomy: A Guide for Clinicians—
    From Counseling Through Procedure
Learning to Work with Botox (Botulinum Toxin A): A Guide
    for Clinicians
No-Scalpel Vasectomy: 6 Patient Cases
Removal of Condyloma with Radiofrequency/Electrosurgery
Suturing and Excision Techniques: Exercises on Pigs' Feet
Working with Collagen and Newer Tissue Fillers: A Guide for
    Clinicians

The AAFP website now includes a self-study program on clinical procedures designed for clinicians to review and build confidence in procedural skills. Most of the programs (e.g., Joint Injection and Aspiration, No-Scalpel Vasectomy, and Soft Tissue Surgery) include a DVD and syllabus, which can be purchased online by both AAFP members and nonmembers. The website www.proceduresconsult.com is also paired with this text. Models are animated in three-dimensional (3-D) imagery.

Ethicon has several resources online. Not only is there a catalog of sutures, but a full 229-page comprehensive wound closure manual can be found at various sites online, such as http://web.mit.edu/2.75/resources/random/ethicon_wound_closure_manual.pdf.

More and more video clips of procedures and other resources are becoming available on the Internet. A more complete list is found in Table E.2.

ARTIFICIAL MODELS AND LEARNING PROCEDURES

Lack of opportunities for enough practice is a common obstacle to learning procedures in primary care. Models and simulations provide an opportunity to practice skills when patients requiring the procedure are not available. Many clinicians who have taken such courses as Advanced Cardiac Life Support, Advanced Trauma Life Support, Advanced Life Support in Obstetrics, Neonatal Advanced Life Support, the Neonatal Resuscitation Program, or the Sideline Management Assessment Response Techniques can appreciate the value of practicing and learning with models. Similar models are widely used in courses for teaching procedures. The National Procedures Institute relies on simulators for several courses, such as those for Hospitalist Medicine. Research has shown that artificial models can be effective for learning and retaining technical skills. They can also be helpful in the clinical setting to rehearse a procedure before performing it on a patient. Companies such as Medisim Corp. (www.medisim.ca), Sawbones (www.sawbones.com), 3-Dmed Surgical Training Aids (www.3-Dmed.com), the Chamberlain Group (www/thecgroup.com), Simulaids (www.simulaids.com), and Limbs & Things Ltd. (www.limbsandthings.com/us) offer highly realistic models for learning and practicing medical and surgical procedures. You will find a full listing of available models and costs at their websites.

Fig. E.1 shows a realistic pelvic model developed by Medisim Corp. in cooperation with Ontario College of Family Physicians as part of the Benign Uterine Conditions Project. The soft tissue component of this model was developed from a casting of a human model. Its highly realistic features allow for practicing pelvic examination, endometrial biopsy, intrauterine device insertion, and pessary fitting. This model has proved itself in teaching skills to family physicians and family medicine residents as part of the skills transfer workshop associated with the Benign Uterine Conditions Initiative (www.machealth.ca/programs/buc).

Fig. E.2 shows the artificial breast model developed by Medisim. The texture and feel of the skin and breast tissue are highly lifelike. With this model, a breast cyst can be palpated and aspirated. The cyst will actually disappear when aspirated properly in a very realistic simulation of a clinical situation.

TABLE E.2 Procedural Skills Videos on the Web

Title/Author	Address/Description
American Academy of Pediatrics Medical Procedures Videos	http://www.aap.org/en-us/professional-resources/ComPedMed/Pages/private/Common-Pediatric-Medical-Procedures.aspx 13 procedures including bladder catheterization, incision and drainage abscess, lumbar puncture, fracture splinting, reduction of simple dislocation, neonatal endotracheal intubation, umbilical catheterization, etc.
Atlas of Essential Procedures e-book and print: Expert Consult Online and Print. Tuggy M, Garcia J. Often sold as package deal with Pfenninger and Fowler's Procedures for Primary Care.	www.elsevier.com/books/atlas-of-essential-procedures/tuggy/978-1-4377-1499-9 ebook ISBN: 9781437735659 Hardcover ISBN: 9781437714999 Elsevier, 2010. $80
Canadian Family Physician Video Series	www.cfp.ca Search for each procedure. These procedures are offered as articles with photos. After clicking on the article, click on Figures & Data and the videos are available at the bottom as an HTML page attachment. Under this setting, the videos have mostly been migrated to YouTube. ~10 procedures including: cryotherapy, toenail resection, pilar cyst removal, skin tag removal, elliptical excision, punch biopsy, and more. Free.
Free podcasts on procedures, University of Ottawa Dept. of Emergency Medicine	http://www.freeemergencytalks.net/tag/procedures/ Search for tag for procedures where nearly 100 podcasts are available Free.
The Common Currency Project. Dalhousie University	http://virtualpatients.eu/resources/other-resources-2/videos-from-the-common-currency-project/ A project to develop general guidelines and concrete examples for the creation of a standard format, or "common currency," for shareable multimedia medical education materials. Free.
Google Video	http://video.google.com Type "medicine procedural skills" or name of specific skill. As with all resources, consider the source in evaluating usefulness.
NEJM Videos in Clinical Medicine	http://content.nejm.org/ Recent NEJM Video and More procedure videos (lower right panel) Free, registration required.
Papanicolaou Society of Cytopathology	http://www.papsociety.org/fna.html Fine Needle Aspiration video tutorials
PocketSnips Procedural Skills Project	Originally a crowd-sourcing project for teaching videos, the webpage is now defunct. But many procedure videos can be found on YouTube by searching the procedure and Pocketsnips. Free.
Procedures Consult. Elsevier	http://www.proceduresconsult.com/medical-procedures/ An online multimedia resource to with learning, performing, and testing of knowledge of the most frequent medical procedures. ~140 procedures. Annual subscription.
Root Atlas	http://www.rootatlas.com/ Ophthalmology videos showing how to use the slit lamp and manage foreign bodies. Free.
The Thorndale Lion's Medical Center	http://www.ingrowntoenails.ca/ Informational site on ingrown toenails, including speaking engagements
Vidéos sur la petite chirurgie La Fédération des médecins omnipraticiens du Québec (FMOQ)	http://www.fmoq.org/Accueil/Accueil/Index.aspx > Formation professionnelle > Outils de formation > Boîte à outils Free.
Webmed. University of Alberta	http://www.webmedtechnology.com/physician/video.html Procedures ranging from lumbar puncture to managing psychotic patients. ~15 procedures. Free.
YouTube	http://ca.youtube.com/ Type "medicine procedural skills" or name of specific skill. As with all resources, consider the source in evaluating usefulness.

Courtesy The Library Service of The College of Family Physicians of Canada, Room 106K, Natural Sciences Centre, UWO, London, Ontario, Canada N6A 5B7; clfm@uwo.ca or www.cpfc.ca/clfm, 2009.

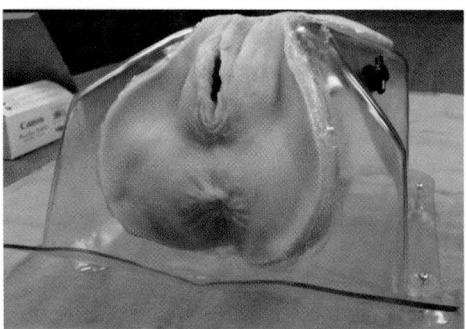

Fig. E.1 Artificial pelvis model. This model can be used to teach and learn pelvic examination, endometrial biopsy, intrauterine device insertion, and pessary fitting. (Courtesy Medisim Corp., Ontario, Canada.)

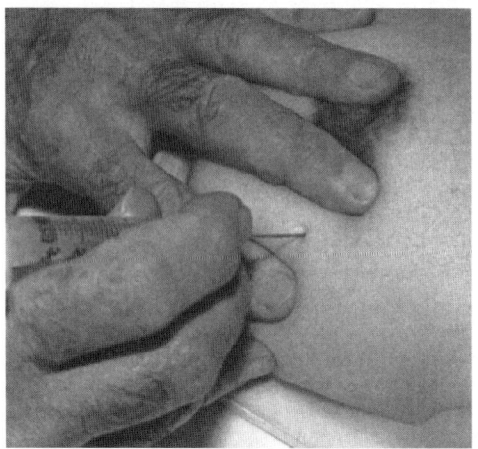

Fig. E.2 Artificial breast model. This lifelike model contains a cyst that can be aspirated as shown to simulate aspiration in a real clinical situation. (Courtesy Medisim Corp., Ontario, Canada.)

Fig. E.3 shows the simulated skin model produced by Limbs & Things Ltd. Once again, the skin is very lifelike when handled with instruments. Modifications of this model can be used to practice cyst or lipoma excision in a realistic fashion. The skin simulator can be adapted for different features, as is illustrated in Fig. E.4, which shows how the model can be used to simulate the excision of a sebaceous cyst.

Fig. E.5 shows the Face with Lesions produced by Limbs & Things Ltd. Some of these lesions can be excised, creating a realistic simulation of skin surgery of the face, where scar orientation, lines of tension, and similar issues must be considered.

Fig. E.6 shows the NPI Down's Cervical Model, which can be biopsied, frozen, and used for performing an endocervical curettage.

Fig. E.7 shows the very realistic NPI vasectomy model.

Fig. E.8 shows the use of an orange to practice shave biopsy.

3-Dmed Surgical Training Aids provides multiple models and simulators (www.3-Dmed.com). These items include portable endoscopic/laparoscopic trainers, open procedure surgical trainers (episiotomy repair, suturing pads, coordination models, etc.), computer interface equipment, and more.

The cost of commercially available models for practicing procedure skills can be considerable. There is always the possibility of using less expensive, less realistic models for learning procedures. In fact, many of these have been developed and described in various articles. Some of the models have been used in studies and shown success in improving a trainee's knowledge and confidence in procedure performance. In Table E.3, a variety of such models is listed. Some are quite traditional; some are very innovative. Nearly all are low cost, easily available, or reproducible. Appropriate references are provided in the table.

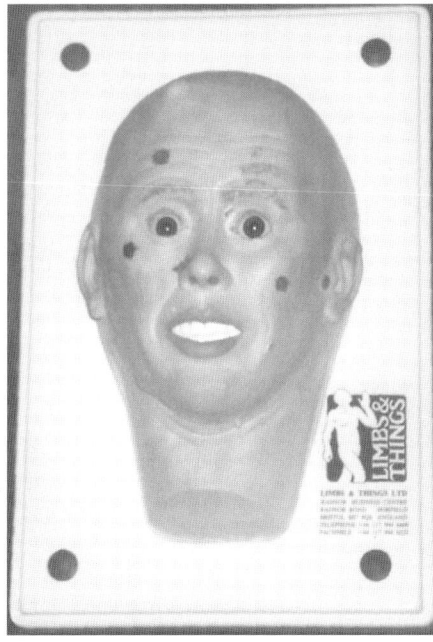

Fig. E.5 The Face with Lesions model has realistic skin lesions for diagnosis. Some lesions can be excised and the skin repaired to practice the fine surgical techniques necessary for the face. (Courtesy Limbs & Things Ltd., United Kingdom.)

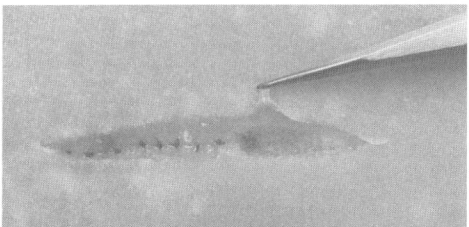

Fig. E.3 Skin simulator model. The artificial skin is very lifelike and feels realistic when using a scalpel or other instruments. It can be used to practice incisions and suture techniques. (Courtesy Limbs & Things Ltd., United Kingdom.)

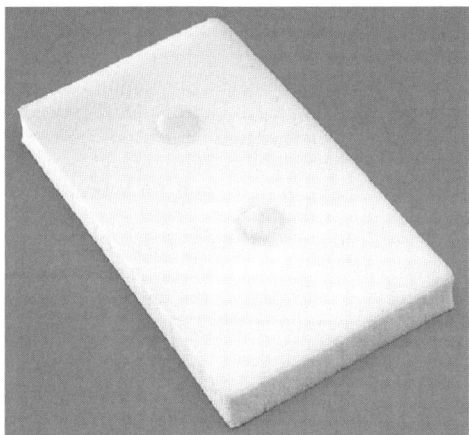

Fig. E.4 Adaptation of the skin simulator model, showing a sebaceous cyst that can be excised by the operator. The texture of the artificial skin and cyst is very lifelike and produces a realistic cyst excision procedure. (Courtesy Limbs & Things Ltd., United Kingdom.)

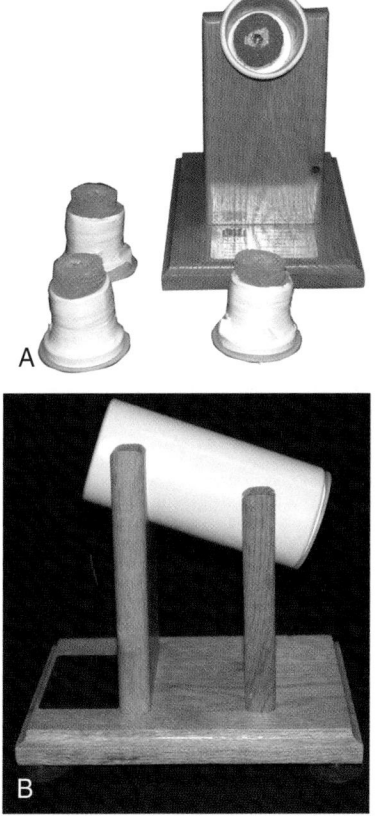

Fig. E.6 NPI Down's cervical model. This cervical model is unique because biopsies can be performed, endocervical curettage (ECC) can be practiced, and it can be frozen. (A) With replaceable inserts. (B) Side view. (Courtesy The National Procedures Institute, Midland, MI.)

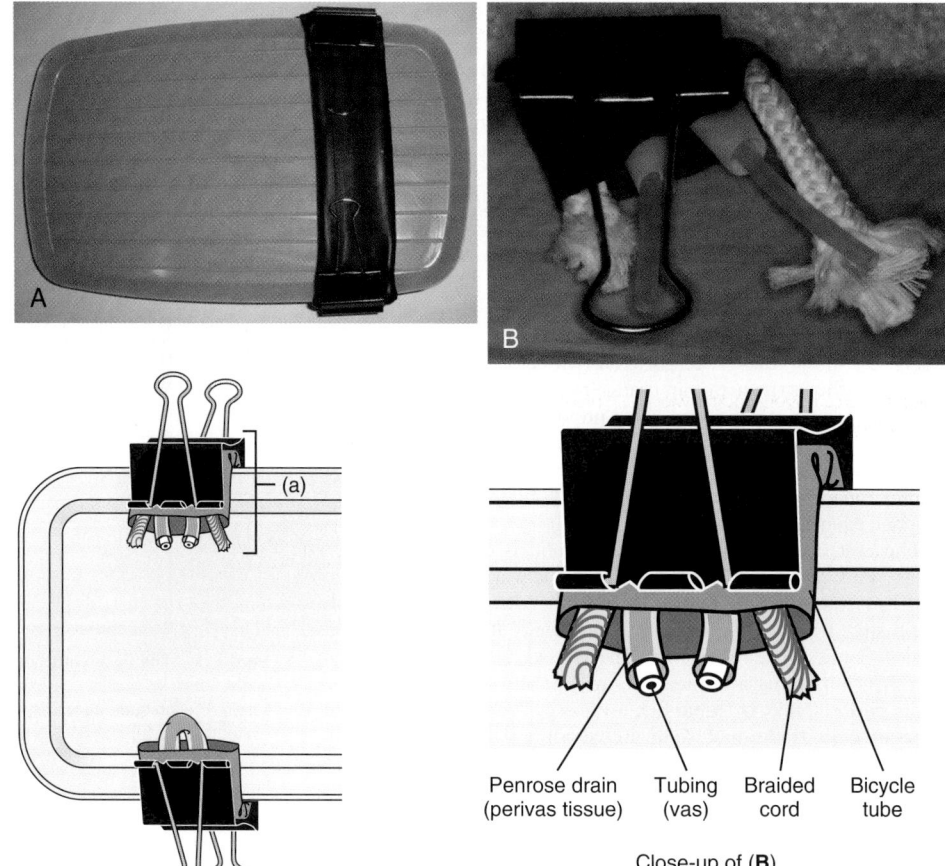

Fig. E.7 NPI vasectomy model. (A) Model. (B) An "underside view" of the components of the NPI vasectomy model. See diagram for explanation. (C) Illustration detailing the makeup of the model *(underside)* and what each material represents. The model is very realistic and provides a lifelike experience. (Courtesy The National Procedures Institute, Midland, MI.)

Penrose drain (perivas tissue)   Tubing (vas)   Braided cord   Bicycle tube

Close-up of (**B**)

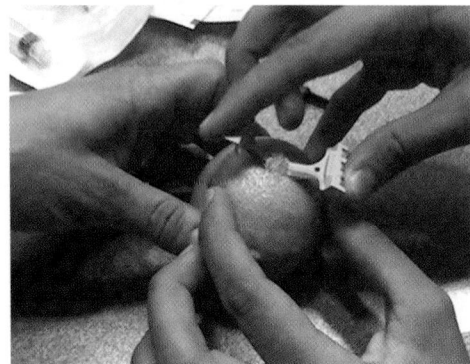

Fig. E.8 Using an orange to practice shave biopsy. (Courtesy of Linda Prine, MD.)

COMPUTER SIMULATION AND VIRTUAL REALITY IN LEARNING PROCEDURES

Simulation as a teaching technique has played a significant role in the training of pilots. The advent of virtual reality means that there is now the capability to combine 3-D visual imagery with the ability to interact. This can create very realistic simulations, which are useful for training surgeons. The use of simulation has been demonstrated for laparoscopic and neurosurgical procedures, and will be valuable for such techniques as sigmoidoscopy, colonoscopy, and hysteroscopy, among others. These simulations have proved very valuable for training in the various endoscopic techniques and ultrasound. While much of the attention has been given to

invasive or minimally invasive surgical procedures, such devices will be helpful for training in suturing, line placement, biopsy, lumbar puncture, and many other procedures in emergency medicine. It should be pointed out that a systematic review of simulation methods currently used for surgical training has not shown them to be any better than other forms of training; however, as there are such rapid advances in technology being made, there has to be continuous research in this area. In general, the more lifelike the simulations, the better the learning. Issenberg and associates have shown that high-fidelity medical simulations are educationally effective and complement usual medical training. Their value lies in the ability to receive feedback and experience repetitive practice. Application of such sophisticated training to the more common family medicine and emergency medicine procedures would be welcome. Although such virtual simulations are very expensive to develop, they can be reused indefinitely without deterioration and may be available, in part or in total, for long-distance learning over the Internet.

Many medical schools now have simulation centers, where models and computer simulations are used to train students and residents. You may wish to contact the nearest medical school to see if they have such a center and if it would be available to you for practice or teaching.

PROCEDURE-ORIENTED ASSOCIATIONS

In addition to the general societies, those interested should be made aware of the American Association for Primary Care Endoscopy (www.aapace.org), the American Institute of Ultrasound in Medicine (www.aium.org), and the American Society for Colposcopy and Cervical Pathology (www.asccp.org), which provide detailed learning in special interest areas. The Society of Teachers of Family

TABLE E.3   Models to Simulate and Practice Procedures

Model Type/Materials	Practice Use	Comments	Reference
Pig's feet	Suturing Minor skin surgery Laceration repair	Readily available from butchers and abattoirs	Snell GF. A method for teaching techniques of office surgery. *J Fam Pract.* 1978;7:987–990.
Pig abdominal skin	Suturing Minor skin surgery	Tough	
Chicken breast	Cryosurgery		
Beefsteak	Electrosurgery		
Chicken legs	Tendon repair		
Breast cyst aspiration model (balloons, flour, Vitamin E capsules, or bath beads for cysts)	Breast cyst aspiration	Easy to prepare Teaches importance of release of suction before withdrawal	Delva D, Tomatly L, Payne P. Practice tips: Fine needle aspiration of breast lumps. *Can Fam Phys.* 2002;48:1055–1056.
Neonatal circumcision (cocktail wiener and surgical glove)	Neonatal circumcision		Brill JR, Wallace B. Neonatal circumcision model and competency evaluation for family medicine residents. *Fam Med.* 2007;39:241–243.
Surgical towel/Face cloth model	Perineal laceration or episiotomy repair	Low cost Practice anywhere	Cain JJ, Shirar E. A new method for teaching the repair of perineal trauma of birth. *Fam Med.* 1996;2:107–110.
Sponge perineum	Fourth-degree perineal laceration repair	Low cost	Sparks RA, Beesley AD, Jones AD. The sponge perineum: An innovative method of teaching fourth-degree obstetrical perineal laceration repair to family medicine residents. *Fam Med.* 2006;38:542–544. (more info available at resourcelibrary.stfm.org)
Papaya fruit	Uterine aspiration		Paul M, Nobel K. Papaya: A simulation model for training in uterine aspiration. *Fam Med.* 2005;37:242–244.
Kiwi fruit	Endometrial aspiration, IUD insertion		

Bovine
    cervix Beefsteak
	Cervical
	    surgery Electrosurgical loop
	    excision
			Ferris DG, Waxman AG, Miller MD. Colposcopy and cervical biopsy educational training models. *Fam Med.* 1994;26:30.

Bovine colon	Sigmoidoscopy, colonoscopy		Sedlack RE, Baron TH, Downing SM, et al. Validation of a colonoscopy simulation for skills assessment. *Am J Gastroenterol.* 2007;102:64–74.
Hollowed-out fruit	Sigmoidoscopy	String fruit together	Empkie TM. Another exciting use for the cantaloupe. *Fam Med.* 1987;19:430.
Liver, beef or kidney (in surgical glove)	Fine needle aspiration of lumps		
Cow's eye	Corneal foreign body removal		
Peach	Musculoskeletal injections	Use a ripe peach and cut one side off flat for stability	
Sequential teaching model (surgical gloves and foam)	Perineal laceration repair		Montiel T. Rosenthal, MD Assistant Clinical Professor and Director of Maternity Services Department of Family Medicine University of Cincinnati The Christ Hospital/University of Cincinnati Family Medicine Residency Program 2123 Auburn Ave. Suite 340 Cincinnati, OH 45219 513-721-2221, ext. 12
Butternut pumpkin	Hysteroscopy		Kingston A, Abbott J, Lenart M, et al. Hysteroscopic training: The butternut pumpkin model. *J Am Assoc Gynecol Laparosc.* 2004;11:256–261.
Orange	Shave biopsy	See Fig. E.8	Photo courtesy Linda Prine, lindaprine@earthlink.net

Medicine Group on Hospital Medicine and Procedural Training is focused on all aspects of teaching procedural skills.

CONCLUSION

In conclusion, the resources available for learning procedures range from courses at medical association meetings, books, CD-ROMs,

DVDs, online videos, artificial models, and simulations, all the way to virtual reality.

Clinicians can learn the background for each procedure, indications, contraindications, complications, and techniques from books, CD-ROMs, DVDs and online videos. However, the ability to practice psychomotor skills is crucial to gaining confidence. Suitable practice can be achieved by using appropriate artificial models, biologic models, and other simulations. Such practice will facilitate learning in the clinical setting and skill maintenance.

Primary care clinicians should remember that their primary care colleagues and specialist consultants are valuable resources for learning procedures through their teaching, encouragement, and support during skill learning.

The listing of resources provided in this chapter should be helpful for teachers and learners in developing the skills and the support necessary to provide our patients with quality care in primary care procedures.

RECOMMENDED READING

Anastakis DJ, Regehr G, Reznick R, et al. Assessment of technical skills transfer from the bench training model to the human model. *Am J Surg.* 1999;177:167–170.

Harper MB, Mayeaux EJ, Pope JB, Goel R. Procedural training in family practice residencies: current status and impact on resident recruitment. *J Am Board Fam Pract.* 1995;8:189–194.

Issenberg SB, McGaghie WC, Petrusa ER, et al. Features and uses of high-fidelity medical simulations that lead to effective learning: a BEME systematic review. *Med Teach.* 2005;27:10–28.

Kelly BF, Sicilia JM, Forman S, et al. Advanced procedural training in family medicine: a group consensus statement. *Fam Med.* 2009;41:398–404.

Norris TE, Felmar E, Tolleson G. Which procedures should be taught in family practice residency programs? *Fam Med.* 1997;29:99–104.

Nothnagle M, Sicilia JM, Forman D, et al. Required procedural training in family medicine residency: a consensus statement. *Fam Med.* 2008;40:248–252.

Rodney WM, Hahn RC. Impact of the limited generalist (no hospital, no procedures) model on the viability of family practice training. *J Am Board Fam Pract.* 2002;15:191–200.

Sierpina VS, Volk RJ. Teaching outpatient procedures: most common settings, evaluation methods, and training barriers in family practice residencies. *Fam Med.* 1998;30:421–423.

Sutherland LM, Middleton PF, Anthony A, et al. Surgical simulation: a systematic review. *Ann Surg.* 2006;243:291–300.

Sweet RM, McDougall EM. Simulation and computer-assisted devices: the new minimally invasive skills training paradigm. *Urol Clin North Am.* 2008;35:519–531.

van der Goes T, Grzybowski SC, Thommasen H. Procedural skills training. Canadian family practice residency programs. *Can Fam Physician.* 1999;45:78–85.

Wetmore S, Allen T, Brailovsky C, et al. (The Working Group on the Certification Process, The College of Family Physicians of Canada): *The General Key Features of Procedure Skills (personal communication).*

Wetmore S, Rivet C, Tepper J, et al. (The Working Group on Procedure Skills): defining core procedure skills for Canadian family medicine training. *Can Fam Physician.* 2005;51:1364–1365.

Yelon S. *Powerful Principles of Instruction.* New York: Addison Wesley/Longman; 1996.

UNIVERSAL PRECAUTIONS

Madelyn Pollock

In discussion of universal precautions, it is important to understand the terminology used by the entities that promulgate the guidelines: primarily the Centers for Disease Control and Prevention (CDC) and the Occupational Safety and Health Administration (OSHA). Before 1983, the recommendations of public health agencies in handling blood and body fluids centered on special precautions taken with individuals known or suspected of being infected with bloodborne pathogens. These guidelines were known in the health care industry as "Blood and Body Fluid Precautions." With the increasing prevalence of human immunodeficiency virus (HIV) and hepatitis B virus (HBV) infections and the possibility that these diseases could be undiagnosed in patients, the CDC published "universal precautions" in 1983, recommending that blood and body fluids from *all patients* be considered potentially infectious and that rigorous infection control precautions be taken to minimize the risk of exposure to health care workers (HCWs).

In 1996, the CDC modified its recommendations for infection control in the hospital setting, introducing the terminology "standard precautions." To quote the CDC in *Guideline for Isolation Precautions in Hospitals*, "Standard Precautions synthesize the major features of Universal (Blood and Body Fluid) Precautions (designed to reduce the risk of transmission of bloodborne pathogens) and Body Substance Isolation (designed to reduce the risk of transmission of pathogens from moist body substances). Standard Precautions apply to (1) blood; (2) all body fluids, secretions, and excretions except sweat, regardless of whether or not they contain visible blood; (3) nonintact skin; and, (4) mucous membranes." These guidelines were updated in 2007.

In 1991, OSHA, a federal agency within the Department of Labor, issued a separate standard. OSHA's Bloodborne Pathogen Standards is based on the concept of universal precautions. It is intended to protect employees who might be exposed to blood or body fluids on the job. (See Online Resources for citation of the complete statute.)

A clinician or other administrator managing a health care facility must attend to both the practical matters of reducing risk to people as well as satisfying regulatory agencies through appropriate documentation and follow-through. This appendix focuses on the procedures, policies, and equipment recommended for reducing risk to HCWs and patients, as well as meeting statutory regulations, especially as they apply to office procedures. It also outlines the requirements of an "Exposure Control Plan" as required for all health care employers by OSHA. Be aware that OSHA focuses only on employee protection.

INFECTION PREVENTION STRATEGY: WORKERS

Recommended guidelines for prevention of infections in HCWs encompass four domains: (1) formulation and implementation of site-specific policies in infection control (an "Exposure Control Plan"), (2) HCW screening and education at time of employment, (3) HCW immunization at the time of entry into an employment situation with risk, and (4) HCW use of barrier protection at time of risk of exposure. *All aspects of the prevention strategy require regular reevaluation and updating*, as well as ongoing education of all workers.

The elements of an OSHA-compliant "Exposure Control Plan" are detailed in the statute and must be adapted to each individual site. Twenty-feight states have adopted their own OSHA-approved occupational safety guidelines and enforcement policies. They are usually identical to the federal guidelines, but you should check specifics for your state. In general, your plan must include common policies (Table F.1), as well as documentation of orientation and ongoing training of personnel. It must also delineate policies for record keeping (employee health screen information, records of training, records of any incidents or injuries, and so forth). The plan must be in written form and available to all employees. There should be evidence of periodic review of the plan for currency and accuracy. Proprietary agencies, including some medical supply marketers, sell "kits" for preparation of a site's "Exposure Control Plan" that include templates customizable to a site. Federal regulations require that all HCWs be evaluated initially with a health inventory. This should include determination of suitability for a position at risk for infectious exposure, as well as determination of the worker's immune status for vaccine-preventable illnesses (OSHA's only *required* immunization policy is for HBV vaccine). These health screens must be recorded in written form, and workers must be reevaluated periodically. Each employee in the facility should have a health record available and updated with the necessary information. This health record should be maintained separately from the employee's other employment record and must be maintained for 30 years by OSHA regulations. At this initial evaluation, a determination of the need for additional vaccination should be made. Current CDC recommendations are listed in Table F.2; those for workers with special conditions are listed in Table F.3.

After initial assessment, infection control in HCWs continues with education. Simple handwashing is the most important activity in reducing transmission of infections in the workplace. Education about policies such as sharps disposal, no recapping of needles, and prompt reporting of injury is crucial. Health care facilities should take steps to ensure initial orientation to infection control policies for all employees and periodic reinstruction of all established personnel. Policies should be written clearly and include supporting information so that employees can understand the rationale for the policies. Employees should be evaluated for the specific risk associated with their particular job and special education for risk reduction implemented and documented.

An often overlooked aspect of an infection control strategy is the immunization of HCWs who are at risk for vaccine-preventable diseases. Appropriate use of vaccines in susceptible individuals can not only help prevent nosocomial infections in HCWs but also reduce loss of workdays because of isolation following potential exposures. In addition, prevention of infection through optimal use of vaccinations and laboratory determination of immune status is much more cost effective than case management following an exposure in a nonimmunized HCW. Immune status of all health care facility personnel should be recorded at initiation of employment, and the hepatitis B vaccination series should be made available to all susceptible employees (OSHA Regulation, 2001). An employee who declines the vaccine should sign the Hepatitis B Vaccine Declination Form

TABLE F.1 Infection Control Policies for a Typical Health Care Provider's Office

Area	Specific Details to Include
Handwashing	Rules for areas with and without running water; handwashing before and after eating, drinking, smoking, applying cosmetics, handling contact lenses, or using the restroom as well as between patients
Contaminated sharps	Both disposable and reusable sharps; no recapping of needles or using one-handed recapping technique; disposal of filled sharps containers
Areas for eating, drinking, smoking, and applying cosmetics	Application of lip balm
Contaminated equipment	Manufacturers' guidelines for disinfection
Personal protection equipment	Use of gloves, gowns, masks, goggles, and impervious aprons
Cleaning/disposal of personal protection equipment	Method of documentation of cleaning
Contaminated spills	Choice of cleaning agent
Contaminated laundry	Bagging in room of use; use of closed bags for transport
Respiratory protection	FIT mask testing procedures
Employee hepatitis B virus vaccination	Hepatitis B vaccine declination form (OSHA Regulation, see Fig. F.1)
Postexposure evaluation and follow-up	Procedure to document details of injury; testing of both employee and source individual; document counseling; procedure for administration of antiretroviral agents
Employee training	Initial and ongoing training schedule
Specimen handling	Separation of food items and specimens; use of gloves when handling specimens
Triage of patients	Carefully screen patients for communicable diseases at check-in so that susceptible workers can avoid contact, and infectious patients can be removed promptly from contact with other waiting patients

TABLE F.2 Summary of Advisory Committee on Immunization Practices Recommendations for Health Care Workers

Vaccines	Recommendations in brief
Hepatitis B	If you don't have documented evidence of a complete hepatitis B vaccine series, or if you don't have an up-to-date blood test that shows you are immune to hepatitis B (i.e., no serologic evidence of immunity or prior vaccination) then you should • Get the 3-dose series (dose 1 now, dose 2 in 1 mo, dose 3 approximately 5 mo after dose 2). • Get anti-HBs serologic tested 1–2 mo after dose 3.
Influenza	Get 1 dose of influenza vaccine annually
MMR (Measles, Mumps and Rubella)	If you were born in 1957 or later and have not had the MMR vaccine, or if you don't have an up-to-date blood test that shows you are immune to measles or mumps (i.e., no serologic evidence of immunity or prior vaccination), get 2 doses of MMR (1 dose now and the second dose at least 28 days later). If you were born in 1957 or later and have not had the MMR vaccine, or if you don't have an up-to-date blood test that shows you are immune to rubella, only 1 dose of MMR is recommended. However, you may end up receiving 2 doses, because the rubella component is in the combination vaccine with measles and mumps. For HCWs born before 1957, see the ACIP vaccine recommendations for healthcare personnel in the reference below. Most of these individuals are probably immune, but if they lack laboratory evidence of immunity or laboratory confirmation of measles, mumps, or rubella, vaccination is recommended during an outbreak.
Varicella (Chickenpox)	If you have not had chickenpox (varicella), if you haven't had varicella vaccine, or if you don't have an up-to-date blood test that shows you are immune to varicella (i.e., no serologic evidence of immunity or prior vaccination), get 2 doses of varicella vaccine, 4 wk apart.
Tdap (Tetanus, Diphtheria and Pertussis)	Get a one-time dose of Tdap as soon as possible if you have not received Tdap previously (regardless of when previous dose of Td was received). Get Td boosters every 10 yr thereafter. Pregnant HCWs need to get a dose of Tdap during each pregnancy.
Meningococcal	Those who are routinely exposed to isolates of *N. meningitidis* should get one dose.

From Immunization of Health-Care Personnel. Recommendations of the Advisory Committee on Immunization Practices (ACIP). *MMWR* 2011;60(RR07):1–45. https://www.cdc.gov/mmwr/preview/mmwrhtml/rr6007a1.htm.

TABLE F.3 Summary of Advisory Committee on Immunization Practices Recommendations for Health Care Workers, Including Special Conditions

Worker Status	Hepatitis B Recombinant Vaccine	Influenza Vaccine	Measles/Mumps/Rubella Live-Virus Vaccine	Varicella Zoster Live-Virus Vaccine
Healthy, nonpregnant	R	R	R	R
Pregnant	R	R	C	C
HIV-positive	R	R	R*	C
Severe immunosuppression	R	R	C	C
Asplenia	R	R	R	R
Renal failure	R	R	R	R
Diabetes	R	R	R	R
Alcoholism and cirrhosis	R	R	R	R

*Contraindicated in persons with HIV infection and severe immunosuppression.
C, Contraindicated; *HIV*, human immunodeficiency virus; *R*, recommended.
Adapted from Centers for Disease Control and Prevention. Immunization of Health-Care Workers: Recommendations of the Advisory Committee on Immunization Practices (ACIP) and the Hospital Infection Control Practices Advisory Committee (HICPAC). *MMWR* 1997;46(No. RR-18):36. http://www.cdc.gov/mmwr/preview/mmwrhtml/00050577.htm.

Hepatitis B Vaccine Declination Form

I understand that due to my occupational exposure to blood or other potentially infectious materials I may be at risk of acquiring hepatitis B virus (HBV) infection. I have been given the opportunity to be vaccinated with hepatitis B vaccine, at no charge to myself. However, I decline hepatitis B vaccination at this time. I understand that by declining this vaccine, I continue to be at risk of acquiring hepatitis B, a serious disease. If in the future I continue to have occupational exposure to blood or other potentially infectious materials and I want to be vaccinated with hepatitis B vaccine, I can receive the vaccination series at no charge to me.

_____   _____
Signature of employee   Date

Fig. F.1 Hepatitis B Vaccine Declination (Mandatory) form. (From OSHA [Occupational Safety and Health Administration] Regulations [Standards, 29 CFR Part 1910.1030] [56 Fed. Reg. 64,004, Dec. 6, 1991, as amended at 57 Fed. Reg. 12,717, April 13, 1992; 57 Fed. Reg. 29,206, July 1, 1992; 61 Fed. Reg. 5507, Feb. 1996].)

(Fig. F.1). Barrier protection using personal protection equipment is the last line of prevention for HCW exposure to potentially infectious material. All HCWs must use appropriate personal protection equipment for the task at hand. In summary,

- Gloves should be worn when contact with any blood, body fluids, mucous membranes, or broken skin is anticipated or possible; this exposure includes contact with soiled items or surfaces and performing venipuncture.
- Masks and eye shields should be worn when splashes of blood or body fluids are possible or during procedures in which blood, body fluids, or tissue could be aerosolized.
- Gowns or impervious aprons should be worn in situations in which blood or body fluids could contaminate the HCW's clothing.
- Gowns, aprons, and gloves must be changed and discarded between patients.
- Mouth-to-mouth ventilation should be performed using a "mouth-to-mask" ventilation device with no direct contact between the patient's mouth and the HCW's.

See Table F.1 for an example of an office guideline, and consult the OSHA statute for a detailed discussion of the regulations.

ENVIRONMENTAL CONSIDERATIONS

Environmental considerations for prevention of infection from the HCW to the patient (or between patients) can be defined in three areas: (1) surface disinfection, (2) instrument sterilization/disinfection, and (3) policies regarding function of actively infected HCWs in the health care facility.

A full discussion of all the issues in the choice and use of agents for disinfection of surfaces and instruments is beyond of the scope of this appendix. The Association for Professionals in Infection Control and Epidemiology Inc. has published a comprehensive guideline that can serve as a reference for further details. In general, it is important to know some of the history of this area to understand some of the terminology. A classification developed in the 1960s by E.H. Spaulding is still used today to determine appropriate levels of decontamination of medical surfaces and equipment.

In general, Spaulding divided devices into three levels of decontamination. The first level is *critical*, meaning that the device enters sterile tissue or the vascular system. These devices must be *sterilized*—that is, devoid of microbial life, including spores. This can be

accomplished by heat, ethylene oxide gas, and a number of immersion techniques. For many physicians' offices, a small autoclave accomplishes the task of rendering reusable devices and instruments sterile between patients. For critical instruments that cannot be subjected to heat or for facilities in which use of heat or ethylene oxide sterilization is not available, several immersion fluids are available. Manufacturers' recommendations for use of these solutions, with special attention to treatment time, should be followed closely.

The second level is *semicritical* and applies to devices that touch mucous membranes. These instruments include endoscopes, endotracheal tubes, and laryngoscopes, as well as thermometers. These devices must be subjected to *high-level disinfection*. Because many of these instruments cannot be subjected to heat, special cleaning devices and fluids must be used for their disinfection. It is important to follow manufacturers' recommendations completely to avoid incomplete disinfection as well as damage to the instruments. Again, thorough cleaning of instruments prior to disinfection is important. Routine changing of fluids and cleaning tools is an important part of an effective routine.

The third level of decontamination according to Spaulding is *noncritical* and includes stethoscopes, examination room surfaces, and bedpans. These items should be cleansed appropriately with agents that are known to kill most surface microbes without significant corrosion of the items or without being excessively toxic to the HCW. Typical agents in this category include alcohols (ethyl and isopropyl), household bleach (5.2% sodium hypochlorite), phenols, iodophors, and quaternary ammonium compounds. These agents are commonly sold by medical supply companies for use on surfaces. Manufacturers' guidelines must be understood and followed. Be aware of the corrosive nature of some of these products on certain surfaces, and follow instructions for protection of HCWs from any potentially toxic fumes.

An important concept in the handling of reusable instruments is the direction of workflow. It is important that "clean" and "soiled" areas are separated and policies are established so that item flow does not risk contamination of "clean" items. There should be clearly defined areas for the receipt of contaminated items with physical barriers preventing accidental contamination. Policies for maintaining these processing standards should be clear to all workers.

Use and maintenance of autoclaves in an office should be governed by policies and routine, reflecting good infection control practices. The first step in sterilization of instruments is thorough cleaning (removal of surface debris) of all instruments to be sterilized. Biologic and chemical indicators for use in heat sterilizers should be used and checked consistently. Temperature and pressure and results of indicators should be recorded in a log form. Remember, biologic indicators require the use of a manufacturer-recommended incubator for proper use.

Regarding transmission of disease from the ill or potentially ill HCW to the patient, the health care facility's administration is responsible for development and implementation of policies to address this issue. At times, such policies may result in restriction of HCWs from patient contact; therefore, it is important that policies be designed to encourage reporting of exposures and illnesses protecting wages, benefits, and job status if possible. The policies should reflect exclusions resulting from both acute infection and known exposure. The policies should be clear regarding who in the facility is responsible for making isolation exclusions.

The decision making falls into two broad categories that require quite different management and follow-through. For chronic blood-borne communicable diseases such as HIV and HBV, the CDC recommends the HCW "...not perform exposure-prone, invasive procedures until counsel from an expert review panel has been sought, which will determine under what circumstances the worker may or may not perform exposure-prone, invasive procedures." Exposure-prone invasive procedures include those that involve manipulating a needle inside the body or placing the fingers and a needle or other sharp instrument in a poorly visualized or highly confined anatomic site. The CDC recommends no restrictions for workers with chronic hepatitis B if hepatitis B e antigen becomes negative and currently recommends no restriction regarding workers

TABLE F.4 Summary of Suggested Work Restrictions for Health Care Workers Exposed to or Infected With the Most Common Acute Communicable Diseases of Importance in the Ambulatory Setting

Disease/Problem	Work Restriction	Duration
Conjunctivitis	Restrict from patient contact and contact with the patient's environment	Until discharge ceases
CMV infection	No restriction	
Diarrheal Diseases		
Acute stage	Restrict from patient contact, contact with the patient's environment, and food handling	Until symptoms resolve
Convalescent stage (*Salmonella* spp.)	Restrict from care of high-risk patients	Until symptoms resolve; consult with local health agencies regarding need for negative cultures
Enteroviral infections	Restrict from care of infants, neonates, and immunocompromised patients and their environments	Until symptoms resolve
Hepatitis A	Restrict from patient contact, contact with the patient's environment, and food handling	Until 7 days after onset of jaundice
Herpes Simplex		
Genital	No restriction	
Hands (Whitlow)	Restrict from patient contact and contact with the patient's environment	Until lesions heal
Orofacial	Evaluate for need to restrict from care of high-risk patients	
Measles		
Active	Exclude from duty	Until 7 days after rash appears
Postexposure (susceptible)	Exclude from duty	From 5th day after first exposure through 21st day after last exposure or 4 days after rash appears
Meningococcal infection	Exclude from duty	Until 24 hr after start of effective therapy
Mumps		
Active	Exclude from duty	Until 9 days after onset of parotitis
Postexposure (susceptible)	Exclude from duty	From 12th day after first exposure through 26th day after last exposure or until 9 days after onset of parotitis
Pediculosis	Restrict from patient contact	Until treated and observed to be free of adult and immature lice
Rubella		
Active	Exclude from duty	Until 5 days after rash appears
Postexposure (susceptible)	Exclude from duty	From 7th day after first exposure through the 21st day after last exposure
Scabies	Restrict from patient contact	Until cleared by medical evaluation
***Staphylococcus aureus* infection**		
Active, still draining lesions	Restrict from patient contact, contact with patient's environment, and food handling	Until lesions have resolved
Carrier state	No restriction unless personnel are epidemiologically linked to transmission of the organisms	
Streptococcus, group A infection	Restrict from patient contact, contact with patient's environment, and food handling	Until 24 hr after adequate treatment started
Tuberculosis		
Active disease	Exclude from duty	Until proved noninfectious
PPD converter	No restriction	
Varicella		
Active	Exclude from duty	Until all lesions dry and crusted
Postexposure (susceptible)	Exclude from duty	From 10th day after first exposure through the 21st day (28th day if VZIG given) after last exposure
Zoster		
Localized in healthy person	Cover lesions, restrict from care of high-risk patients	Until all lesions dry and crusted
Generalized or localized in the immunocompromised person	Restrict from patient contact	Until all lesions dry and crusted
Postexposure (susceptible)	Restrict from patient contact	From 10th day after first exposure through the 21st day (28th day if VZIG given) after last exposure, or if varicella occurs, until all lesions dry and crusted
Viral URI, acute febrile	Consider excluding from the care of high-risk patients or contact with their environment during community outbreak of RSV and influenza	Until acute symptoms resolve

CMV, Cytomegalovirus; *PPD*, purified protein derivative; *RSV*, respiratory syncytial virus; *URI*, upper respiratory infection; *VZIG*, varicella zoster immunoglobulin.
From Current Postexposure Prophylaxis Recommendations. *MMWR Recomm Rep* 1998;47(RR-7):1. http://www.cdc.gov/ncidod/dhqp/gl_occupational.html.

with hepatitis C. Each facility should develop its own policy regarding HIV and hepatitis B– and C–infected workers.

For more acute disease entities, the CDC has developed guidelines that can be adapted for most facilities (Table F.4). The guidelines summarize recommended work restrictions, including duration. These guidelines apply to both exposure and infection with the disease. They should always be compared with any local or state guidelines that may apply in your area. Consideration of your facility's patient population and the worker's level of patient exposure is important. In jobs in which close contact with patients is unlikely, a worker might be able to remain on the job but could use certain precautions (such as wearing a mask) and still not jeopardize patients or coworkers.

Conclusion

It is important that the leadership of every health care facility, regardless of size, become familiar with the standards and regulations regarding infection control in the workplace. The facility must formulate and implement policies to protect HCWs as well as patients from communicable diseases. These policies should reflect current guidelines from the CDC and comply with regulations promulgated by OSHA. In addition to this appendix, the infection control officer of your local hospital should be considered as an ally and information source in the development or review of policies and procedures for your particular site.

General Resources

Association for Professionals in Infection Control and Epidemiology, Inc.
1275 K Street, NW, Suite 1000
Washington, DC 20005-4006
Phone: 202-789-1890
Website: www.apic.org

Centers for Disease Control and Prevention
1600 Clifton Road, NE
Atlanta, GA 30333

Phone: 404-639-3311
Division of AIDS/HIV Prevention: 800-843-6356
Website: www.cdc.gov

U.S. Department of Labor
Occupational Safety and Health Administration
200 Constitution Avenue, NW
Washington, DC 20210
Website: www.osha.gov

ONLINE RESOURCES

Centers for Disease Control and Prevention. "Workbook for Designing, Implementing, and Evaluating a Sharps Injury Prevention Program." For use in establishing a sharps policy. Available at: https://www.cdc.gov/sharpssafety/pdf/sharpsworkbook_2008.pdf. Accessed May 7, 2018.

Centers for Disease Control and Prevention. *Updated U.S. Public Health Service Guidelines for the Management of Occupational Exposures to HBV, HCV, and HIV and Recommendations for Postexposure Prophylaxis.* MMWR. 2001;50 (No. RR-11). Available at: http://www.cdc.gov/ncidod/dhqp/gl_occupational.html. Accessed May 7, 2018.

OSHA Regulation: Exposure Control Plan Occupational Safety and Health Administration, Department of Labor. 29 CFR Part 1910.1030, Occupational exposure to bloodborne pathogens; final rule. Revised 2001. Available at: http://www.osha.gov/SLTC/bloodbornepathogens/index.html. Accessed May 7, 2018.

The Guideline for Isolation Precautions. Preventing Transmission of Infectious Agents in Healthcare Settings 2007 Siegel JD, Rhinehart E, Jackson M, Chiarello L. *Am J Infect Control.* 2007;35(10 suppl 2):S65–164. Available at: https://www.cdc.gov/hai/pdfs/Isolation2007.pdf. Accessed May 7, 2018.

Updated US. Public Health Service guidelines for the management of occupational exposures to HIV and recommendations for postexposure prophylaxis. *Hospital Epidemiology.* 2013;34(9). Available at: https://stacks.cdc.gov/view/cdc/20711. Accessed May 7, 2018.

RECOMMENDED READING

Bolyard EA, Tablan OC, Williams WW, et al. The hospital infection control practices advisory committee: special article: guideline for infection control in healthcare personnel, 1998. *Am J Infect Control.* 1998;26:289.

NEOPLASMS OF THE SKIN: ICD-10 DIAGNOSTIC CODES

John L. Pfenninger

- For excision and repair CPT codes, see Chapter 19, Laceration and Incision Repair. Understand that "shave excisions" and "biopsies" have their own CPT codes.

- The following ICD-10 codes are only for neoplasms originating in the skin. Other, subcutaneous tumors have their own codes (see the section on Selected Tumor Codes).

	Malignant Primary	Malignant Secondary	Carcinoma in Situ	Benign	Uncertain Behavior	Unspecified Behavior
Neoplasm, neoplastic	C80.1	C79.9	D09.9	D36.9	D48.9	D49.9
—skin NOS	C44.90	C79.2	D04.9	D23.9	D48.5	D49.2
——abdominal wall	C44.509	C79.2	D04.5	D23.5	D48.5	D49.2
———basal cell carcinoma	C44.519	–	–	–	–	–
———specified type NEC	C44.599	–	–	–	–	–
———squamous cell carcinoma	C44.529	–	–	–	–	–
——ala nasi; see also Neoplasm, nose, skin	C44.301	C79.2	D04.39	D23.39	D48.5	D49.2
——ankle; see also Neoplasm, skin, limb, lower	C44.70	C79.2	D04.7	D23.7	D48.5	D49.2
——antecubital space; see also Neoplasm, skin, limb, upper	C44.60	C79.2	D04.6	D23.6	D48.5	D49.2
——anus	C44.500	C79.2	D04.5	D23.5	D48.5	D49.2
———basal cell carcinoma	C44.510	–	–	–	–	–
———specified type NEC	C44.590	–	–	–	–	–
———squamous cell carcinoma	C44.520	–	–	–	–	–
——arm; see also Neoplasm, skin, limb, upper	C44.60	C79.2	D04.6	D23.6	D48.5	D49.2
——auditory canal (external); see also Neoplasm, skin, ear	C44.20	C79.2	D04.2	D23.2	D48.5	D49.2
——auricle (ear); see also Neoplasm, skin, ear	C44.20	C79.2	D04.2	D23.2	D48.5	D49.2
——auricular canal (external); see also Neoplasm, skin, ear	C44.20	C79.2	D04.2	D23.2	D48.5	D49.2
——axilla, axillary fold; see also Neoplasm, skin, trunk	C44.509	C79.2	D04.5	D23.5	D48.5	D49.2
——back; see also Neoplasm, skin, trunk	C44.509	C79.2	D04.5	D23.5	D48.5	D49.2
——basal cell carcinoma	C44.91					
——breast	C44.501	C79.2	D04.5	D23.5	D48.5	D49.2
———basal cell carcinoma	C44.511					
———specified type NEC	C44.591					
———squamous cell carcinoma	C44.521					
——brow; see also Neoplasm, skin, face	C44.309	C79.2	D04.39	D23.39	D48.5	D49.2
——buttock; see also Neoplasm, skin, trunk	C44.509	C79.2	D04.5	D23.5	D48.5	D49.2
——calf; see also Neoplasm, skin, limb, lower	C44.70	C79.2	D04.7	D23.7	D48.5	D49.2
——canthus (eye) (inner) (outer)	C44.10	C79.2	D04.1	D23.1	D48.5	D49.2
———basal cell carcinoma	C44.11					
———sebaceous cell	C44.13					
———specified type NEC	C44.19					
———squamous cell carcinoma	C44.12					
——cervical region; see also Neoplasm, skin, neck	C44.40	C79.2	D04.4	D23.4	D48.5	D49.2
——cheek (external); see also Neoplasm, skin, face	C44.309	C79.2	D04.39	D23.39	D48.5	D49.2
——chest (wall); see also Neoplasm, skin, trunk	C44.509	C79.2	D04.5	D23.5	D48.5	D49.2
——chin; see also Neoplasm, skin, face	C44.309	C79.2	D04.39	D23.39	D48.5	D49.2
——clavicular area; see also Neoplasm, skin, trunk	C44.509	C79.2	D04.5	D23.5	D48.5	D49.2
——clitoris	C51.2	C79.82	D07.1	D28.0	D39.8	D49.59
——columnella; see also Neoplasm, skin, face	C44.309	C79.2	D04.39	D23.39	D48.5	D49.2
——concha; see also Neoplasm, skin, ear	C44.20	C79.2	D04.2	D23.2	D48.5	D49.2
——ear (external)	C44.20	C79.2	D04.2	D23.2	D48.5	D49.2
———basal cell carcinoma	C44.21					
———specified type NEC	C44.29					
———squamous cell carcinoma	C44.22					

	Malignant Primary	Malignant Secondary	Carcinoma in Situ	Benign	Uncertain Behavior	Unspecified Behavior
——elbow; see also Neoplasm, skin, limb, upper	C44.60	C79.2	D04.6	D23.6	D48.5	D49.2
——eyebrow; see also Neoplasm, skin, face	C44.309	C79.2	D04.39	D23.39	D48.5	D49.2
——eyelid	C44.10	C79.2	D04.1	D23.1	D48.5	D49.2
———basal cell carcinoma	C44.11					
———sebaceous cell	C44.13					
———specified type NEC	C44.19					
———squamous cell carcinoma	C44.12					
——face NOS	C44.300	C79.2	D04.30	D23.30	D48.5	D49.2
———basal cell carcinoma	C44.310					
———specified type NEC	C44.390					
———squamous cell carcinoma	C44.320					
——female genital organs (external)	C51.9	C79.82	D07.1	D28.0	D39.8	D49.59
———clitoris	C51.2	C79.82	D07.1	D28.0	D39.8	D49.59
———labium NEC	C51.9	C79.82	D07.1	D28.0	D39.8	D49.59
——— majus	C51.0	C79.82	D07.1	D28.0	D39.8	D49.59
——— minus	C51.1	C79.82	D07.1	D28.0	D39.8	D49.59
———pudendum	C51.9	C79.82	D07.1	D28.0	D39.8	D49.59
———vulva	C51.9	C79.82	D07.1	D28.0	D39.8	D49.59
——finger; see also Neoplasm, skin, limb, upper	C44.60	C79.2	D04.6	D23.6	D48.5	D49.2
——flank; see also Neoplasm, skin, trunk	C44.509	C79.2	D04.5	D23.5	D48.5	D49.2
——foot; see also Neoplasm, skin, limb, lower	C44.70	C79.2	D04.7	D23.7	D48.5	D49.2
——forearm; see also Neoplasm, skin, limb, upper	C44.60	C79.2	D04.6	D23.6	D48.5	D49.2
——forehead; see also Neoplasm, skin, face	C44.309	C79.2	D04.39	D23.39	D48.5	D49.2
——glabella; see also Neoplasm, skin, face	C44.309	C79.2	D04.39	D23.39	D48.5	D49.2
——gluteal region; see also Neoplasm, skin, trunk	C44.509	C79.2	D04.5	D23.5	D48.5	D49.2
——groin; see also Neoplasm, skin, trunk	C44.509	C79.2	D04.5	D23.5	D48.5	D49.2
——hand; see also Neoplasm, skin, limb, upper	C44.60	C79.2	D04.6	D23.6	D48.5	D49.2
——head NEC; see also Neoplasm, skin, scalp	C44.40	C79.2	D04.4	D23.4	D48.5	D49.2
——heel; see also Neoplasm, skin, limb, lower	C44.70	C79.2	D04.7	D23.7	D48.5	D49.2
——helix; see also Neoplasm, skin, ear	C44.20	C79.2	D04.2	D23.2	D48.5	D49.2
——hip; see also Neoplasm, skin, limb, lower	C44.70	C79.2	D04.7	D23.7	D48.5	D49.2
——infraclavicular region; see also Neoplasm, skin, trunk	C44.509	C79.2	D04.5	D23.5	D48.5	D49.2
——inguinal region; see also Neoplasm, skin, trunk	C44.509	C79.2	D04.5	D23.5	D48.5	D49.2
——jaw; see also Neoplasm, skin, face	C44.309	C79.2	D04.39	D23.39	D48.5	D49.2
——knee; see also Neoplasm, skin, limb, lower	C44.70	C79.2	D04.7	D23.7	D48.5	D49.2
———majora	C51.0	C79.82	D07.1	D28.0	D39.8	D49.59
———minora	C51.1	C79.82	D07.1	D28.0	D39.8	D49.59
——leg; see also Neoplasm, skin, limb, lower	C44.70	C79.2	D04.7	D23.7	D48.5	D49.2
——lid (lower) (upper)	C44.10	C79.2	D04.1	D23.1	D48.5	D49.2
———basal cell carcinoma	C44.11					
———sebaceous cell	C44.13					
———specified type NEC	C44.19					
———squamous cell carcinoma	C44.12					
——limb NEC	C44.90	C79.2	D04.9	D23.9	D48.5	D49.2
———basal cell carcinoma	C44.91					
———lower	C44.70	C79.2	D04.7	D23.7	D48.5	D49.2
——— basal cell carcinoma	C44.71					
——— specified type NEC	C44.79					
——— squamous cell carcinoma	C44.72					
———upper	C44.60	C79.2	D04.6	D23.6	D48.5	D49.2
——— basal cell carcinoma	C44.61					
——— specified type NEC	C44.69					
——— squamous cell carcinoma	C44.62					
——lip (lower) (upper)	C44.00	C79.2	D04.0	D23.0	D48.5	D49.2
———basal cell carcinoma	C44.01					
———specified type NEC	C44.09					
———squamous cell carcinoma	C44.02					
——male genital organs	C63.9	C79.82	D07.60	D29.9	D40.8	D49.59
———penis	C60.9	C79.82	D07.4	D29.0	D40.8	D49.59
———prepuce	C60.0	C79.82	D07.4	D29.0	D40.8	D49.59
———scrotum	C63.2	C79.82	D07.61	D29.4	D40.8	D49.59
——mastectomy site (skin); see also Neoplasm, skin, breast	C44.501	C79.2				

Continued

	Malignant Primary	Malignant Secondary	Carcinoma in Situ	Benign	Uncertain Behavior	Unspecified Behavior
——specified as breast tissue	C50.8	C79.81				
——meatus, acoustic (external); see also Neoplasm, skin, ear	C44.20	C79.2	D04.2	D23.2	D48.5	D49.2
——nates; see also Neoplasm, skin, trunk	C44.509	C79.2	D04.5	D23.5	D48.5	D49.2
——neck	C44.40	C79.2	D04.4	D23.4	D48.5	D49.2
———basal cell carcinoma	C44.41					
———specified type NEC	C44.49					
———squamous cell carcinoma	C44.42					
——nose (external); see also Neoplasm, nose, skin	C44.301	C79.2	D04.39	D23.39	D48.5	D49.2
——overlapping lesion	C44.80					
———basal cell carcinoma	C44.81					
———specified type NEC	C44.89					
———squamous cell carcinoma	C44.82					
——palm; see also Neoplasm, skin, limb, upper	C44.60	C79.2	D04.6	D23.6	D48.5	D49.2
——palpebra	C44.10	C79.2	D04.1	D23.1	D48.5	D49.2
———basal cell carcinoma	C44.11					
———sebaceous cell	C44.13					
———specified type NEC	C44.19					
———squamous cell carcinoma	C44.12					
——penis NEC	C60.9	C79.82	D07.4	D29.0	D40.8	D49.59
——perianal; see also Neoplasm, skin, anus	C44.500	C79.2	D04.5	D23.5	D48.5	D49.2
——perineum; see also Neoplasm, skin, anus	C44.500	C79.2	D04.5	D23.5	D48.5	D49.2
——pinna; see also Neoplasm, skin, ear	C44.20	C79.2	D04.2	D23.2	D48.5	D49.2
——plantar; see also Neoplasm, skin, limb, lower	C44.70	C79.2	D04.7	D23.7	D48.5	D49.2
——popliteal fossa or space; see also Neoplasm, skin, limb, lower	C44.70	C79.2	D04.7	D23.7	D48.5	D49.2
——prepuce	C60.0	C79.82	D07.4	D29.0	D40.8	D49.59
——pubes; see also Neoplasm, skin, trunk	C44.509	C79.2	D04.5	D23.5	D48.5	D49.2
——sacrococcygeal region; see also Neoplasm, skin, trunk	C44.509	C79.2	D04.5	D23.5	D48.5	D49.2
——scalp	C44.40	C79.2	D04.4	D23.4	D48.5	D49.2
———basal cell carcinoma	C44.41					
———specified type NEC	C44.49					
———squamous cell carcinoma	C44.42					
——scapular region; see also Neoplasm, skin, trunk	C44.509	C79.2	D04.5	D23.5	D48.5	D49.2
——scrotum	C63.2	C79.82	D07.61	D29.4	D40.8	D49.59
——shoulder; see also Neoplasm, skin, limb, upper	C44.60	C79.2	D04.6	D23.6	D48.5	D49.2
——sole (foot); see also Neoplasm, skin, limb, lower	C44.70	C79.2	D04.7	D23.7	D48.5	D49.2
——specified sites NEC	C44.80	C79.2	D04.8	D23.9	D48.5	D49.2
———basal cell carcinoma	C44.81					
———specified type NEC	C44.89					
———squamous cell carcinoma	C44.82					
——specified type NEC	C44.99					
——squamous cell carcinoma	C44.92					
——submammary fold; see also Neoplasm, skin, trunk	C44.509	C79.2	D04.5	D23.5	D48.5	D49.2
——supraclavicular region; see also Neoplasm, skin, neck	C44.40	C79.2	D04.4	D23.4	D48.5	D49.2
——temple; see also Neoplasm, skin, face	C44.309	C79.2	D04.39	D23.39	D48.5	D49.2
——thigh; see also Neoplasm, skin, limb, lower	C44.70	C79.2	D04.7	D23.7	D48.5	D49.2
——thoracic wall; see also Neoplasm, skin, trunk	C44.509	C79.2	D04.5	D23.5	D48.5	D49.2
——thumb; see also Neoplasm, skin, limb, upper	C44.60	C79.2	D04.6	D23.6	D48.5	D49.2
——toe; see also Neoplasm, skin, limb, lower	C44.70	C79.2	D04.7	D23.7	D48.5	D49.2
——tragus; see also Neoplasm, skin, ear	C44.20	C79.2	D04.2	D23.2	D48.5	D49.2
——trunk	C44.509	C79.2	D04.5	D23.5	D48.5	D49.2
———basal cell carcinoma	C44.519					
———specified type NEC	C44.599					
———squamous cell carcinoma	C44.529					
——umbilicus; see also Neoplasm, skin, trunk	C44.509	C79.2	D04.5	D23.5	D48.5	D49.2
——vulva	C51.9	C79.82	D07.1	D28.0	D39.8	D49.59
———overlapping lesion	C51.8					
——wrist; see also Neoplasm, skin, limb, upper	C44.60	C79.2	D04.6	D23.6	D48.0	D49.2

SELECTED TUMOR CODES

Lesions below the skin have their own ICD-9 diagnostic codes depending on the location. They are divided into similar categories including the following:

- Malignant
  - Primary
  - Secondary
- Benign
- Uncertain behavior
- Unspecified

Each lesion must be looked up individually. Some examples of benign tumors:

D21.0   Benign neoplasm connective and other soft tissue of head, face, and neck

D21.10 Benign neoplasm of connective and other soft tissue of unspecified limb, including shoulder

D21.6   Benign neoplasm of connective and other soft tissue of trunk, unspecified

Another way of coding some of these lesions would be more specific:

D17.0   Benign lipomatous neoplasm of skin and subcutaneous tissue of head, face, and neck

D17.1   Benign lipomatous neoplasm of skin and subcutaneous tissue of trunk

D17.30 Benign lipomatous neoplasm of skin and subcutaneous tissue of unspecified sites

D17.39 Benign lipomatous neoplasm of skin and subcutaneous tissue of other sites

Some examples of malignant tumors:

C49.0   Malignant neoplasm of connective and soft tissue of head, face, and neck

C49.10 Malignant neoplasm of connective and soft tissue of unspecified upper limb, including shoulder

C49.6   Malignant neoplasm of connective and soft tissue of trunk, unspecified

It is important to recognize that skin neoplasms are coded distinctly differently than tumors below the skin. For excision of these tumors, a separate set of CPT codes is used, based on the size (usually <3 cm or >3 cm) and whether they were subcutaneous or subfascial, or whether a radical removal/excision was required. See Chapter 19, Laceration and Incision Repair.

Using the "unspecified" codes for either skin neoplasms or for subcutaneous tumors is likely to generate rejections from insurance carriers or requests for further information.

PEARLS OF PRACTICE

John L. Pfenninger • Grant C. Fowler

> *I don't think I'm unique. Anybody can do quite a lot by refusing to give in to limitations.*
>
> Christopher Reeves

1. When repairing or removing scalp lesions, remember that patients do not like to have their hair shaved unless it is absolutely necessary. Shaving elsewhere does not decrease risk of infection; the scalp has a robust blood supply, and infections are rare. Remove minor lesions without shaving the hair. To keep the hair from continually falling into the operative field, use antibiotic ointment to flatten it down. Apply the ointment after performing the usual preparation.

2. The majority of skin lesion removals can be performed either with a shave technique or with curettement and cautery. Moist healing is the key to an excellent long-term outcome with minimal scarring. Eschars (scabs) impair the normal healing process. Healing tissue is much like a new lawn: It needs to be kept moist; but don't drown it. Unless under clothes, wounds should remain without a dressing, except for ointment, when possible. If under clothes, wounds will obviously need to be covered with an adhesive strip or other dressing. Likewise, facial areas will need to be covered at night. Basically, the patient just gently washes the area three to four times a day with mild soap and water and applies an ointment afterward. It does not necessarily have to be an antibacterial ointment; even petrolatum (Vaseline) will do. Avoid neomycin, hydrogen peroxide, or povidone-iodine (Betadine) because they may slow the healing process. For deeper shaves or curettements and for those who may experience slow healing (immune suppressed, diabetics, etc.), MediHoney works extremely well. The deeper the open wound, the longer it will be necessary to keep the area moist (generally 7 to 14 days). With sutured wounds, have the patient gently wash the area within 12 hours and apply antibiotic ointment three or four times a day (unless tissue glue or Steri-Strips have been applied). Cover with other dressings only as noted previously. An easier method for the patient that causes less inflammation is to use a moist healing occlusive dressing such as Tegaderm. It is transparent and allows the patient to see the wound. Should blood accumulate, it can be replaced either by the patient or the clinician. It is readily available at many stores. This is applied immediately after excision (or laceration repair) and left in place until the sutures are removed. The patient can also observe for signs of infection and return for evaluation if necessary. See the sample patient education handout online at www.expertconsult.com.

3. There is no need to stop warfarin (Coumadin), clopidogrel (Plavix), prasugrel (Effient) ticagrelor (Brilinta), dabigatran (Pradaxa), apixaban (Eliquis), rivaroxaban (Xarelto), or aspirin for routine dermatologic or dental procedures. Several articles have been published documenting that cardiovascular and embolic events occur during the period of stopping and restarting the medications. Instead, meticulous attention must be paid to hemostasis. Clotting parameters should be checked before significant excisional surgery. However, for shaves, curettements, and most excisions, it is unnecessary to stop any of these medications or to check laboratory results (see Alcalay, 2001; Schanbacher, 2000).

4. Bridge therapy is only necessary for certain high-risk patients on chronic anticoagulation who need elective invasive, high-risk surgery. It is defined as protected periprocedural discontinuation of warfarin (Coumadin) 3 to 4 days before performing procedures in patients at high risk for thromboembolism. The first step is initiation of low-molecular-weight heparin (LMWH) at full therapeutic dose on the day after warfarin is stopped (e.g., no warfarin Monday, begin LMWH on Tuesday morning). The patient receives the last dose of LMWH the morning of the day before the procedure. Then the invasive procedure or surgery occurs. Warfarin and LMWH are reintroduced later that day if deemed safe and hemostasis has been achieved. Subsequently, LMWH is discontinued after discharge once the international normalized ratio has been therapeutic for 3 or 4 days. Bridge therapy is used for patients with atrial fibrillation and a high risk of complications (i.e., recent cerebrovascular accident prosthetic valves, a recent [past 3 months] thromboembolic event, indications for prolonged warfarin therapy, or a history of a hypercoagulable state). This therapy avoids prolonged hospitalization, changing of anticoagulation while preparing for surgery, vitamin K administration, and a prolonged period without anticoagulation with the attendant risk for thromboembolism. The disadvantages are cost of LMWH, self-injection, and a relative lack of reversibility. (From James Lile, pharmacist, MidMichigan Medical Center, Midland, MI.) As a result of the BRIDGE study (Douketis, 2015), which showed a higher risk of bleeding and no decrease in thromboembolic events by bridging patients with atrial fibrillation (average CHADS2 score of 2.3) with Lovenox, many experts performing colonoscopy no longer use bridging therapy. Instead, they just stop the warfarin 5 days before the procedure. This higher risk of bleeding had also been seen in a meta-analysis of patients bridged with heparin (Siegel, 2012). On the other hand, other experts do not stop the anticoagulation for screening colonoscopy and just anticipate more bleeding and the use of more staples or clips with biopsy. As an in-between, although no guidelines have been written to support it, other experts use oral dabigatran (Pradaxa), apixaban (Eliquis), or rivaroxaban (Xarelto) for bridging therapy and withhold them 2 days prior to major surgery or 1 day for less significant surgery. Because apixaban is taken twice a day due to its shorter half-life, it would seem quicker to reverse by withholding it.

5. For those who want to diminish the pain of anesthetic injections, add a little bicarbonate to the anesthetic (1 part bicarbonate to 9 parts of anesthetic). Anesthetics sting with injection because of a low pH; this supposedly inhibits bacterial growth but at the same time is uncomfortable. The bicarbonate takes

the "sting" out of the injection. In addition, use a small needle (27 or 30 gauge), use warm solutions, and inject slowly. Injecting deeper into the dermis will cause less pain, but it takes longer for the anesthetic to work. Injecting more superficially will hurt a little more, but the anesthetic will work faster. Do not add sodium bicarbonate to bupivacaine (Marcaine), because it will precipitate in a neutral pH.

6. When injecting lidocaine into an area that needs to be palpable later (e.g., to feel a foreign body, find a vas during vasectomy), you can massage the lidocaine into the skin so that it does not obstruct your fine touch. Alternatively, perform a nerve block or a field block, thus eliminating any anesthetic in the area.

7. Melman (1999) has shown that it is perfectly okay to draw up anesthetic solutions in syringes up to 7 days before use. There is no increased bacterial contamination or growth, and the anesthetic still functions. We used to pull up our syringes at the beginning of the day and then discard them at the end of the day, but there is no need to do this. Currently, we fill numerous 1-mL syringes, date them, and continue to use them throughout the week. It is much more efficient for the nurse to pull up multiple syringes than to do just one at a time. It is inefficient for the clinician to spend time pulling up anesthetic! Many guidelines now prohibit use of multidose vials in hospital clinics, as well as predrawn syringes. This adds to the cost of medical care without really providing much benefit. At a minimum, the multidose vials have to be clearly labeled when they were first used and expiration date after first use.

8. Consider using the MadaJet for local injections. It is a small hand-held "gun" that "injects" medications without a needle. It is only for superficial injections but can be used to treat keloids and hypertrophic scars with steroids, etc. It has also been adapted for the no-needle vasectomy (Wilson, 2001). It is available from Delasco at 800-831-6273 (www.delasco.com) and Advanced Meditech International (AMI) (800-635-2452; www.ameditech.com).

9. When someone complains of an allergy to local anesthetics (including Novocain), he or she has usually received an ester. To date, there have been very few reported allergic reactions to the amides such as lidocaine (Xylocaine). Some patients still report that they have had a reaction to lidocaine or to "all local anesthetics." In these instances, they have usually had medication drawn from a multidose vial, which has preservatives (parabens) in it. If someone does complain of having a history of local anesthetic reaction, use single-dose vials of lidocaine, and he or she will be able to tolerate it without incident. It is inexpensive and helpful to have around. (Also see Pearl 43.)

10. AMI has designed a small anesthetic bottle holder that mounts on the wall (VE-11 Handzfree anesthetic bottle holder). The cost is only approximately $40, and in our office it is indispensable. It holds the anesthetic where it is readily available and makes filling syringes an easy task. It also allows the entire staff to see how much anesthetic is left in the bottle. There is nothing more frustrating than pulling out the drawer with the anesthetic solution and finding that the bottle is empty! Contact AMI at 800-635-2452 (www.ameditech.com).

11. Clinicians must maximize their time in the office. Inefficiency has to be eliminated. I (J.L.P.) literally tried to find 30 seconds to save on every patient. Having the syringes prefilled (see pearl 7) saves time! When I used to discuss this at our courses, initially there were chuckles about "the 30 seconds." Then I did the math. I was usually able to see 20 to 25 patients in a day. If I saved 30 seconds on each one, this was 10 to 12 minutes per day, which actually allows an extra office visit or procedure in a day. If you work 4 days a week, that is four extra visits a week. Working 45 weeks out of the year, this amounts to 180 visits. If you average $100 per visit, that is an extra $18,000 per year. At $150 per visit, that is an extra $27,000 a year—just for saving 30 seconds per patient! If you see more than 20 to 25 patients

per day, even more can be earned. Efficiency is essential. On the other hand, think of how much time is wasted by filling out forms that you are not compensated for! Look what you are losing!

12. OSHA has numerous requirements for a safe office practice. One of them is the use of fluid-resistant coats when performing procedures. My (J.L.P.'s) staff ordered these coats for me. They made an error and selected the coats with the knit cuff sleeves—how fortuitous! As residents rotate through the office, they frequently have the large sleeves that look like the old nuns' habits! The ends of the sleeves hang down 8 to 10 inches from the wrist. Subsequently when they reach for an instrument, the sleeve often drags across the sterile field. Knit cuffs help to protect a sterile field, and I highly recommend them. The fluid-resistant coats are also beneficial in that any fluid that gets on them is easily wiped off, and the coats last a long time. And remember, not using them could make you liable for a $25,000 OSHA fine! I change my white coat daily. If soiled with blood or pus, I change it during the day. I can't believe hospital guidelines that suggest not wearing neck ties but advise coats to be changed weekly!

13. I (J.L.P.) have found that a good way to explain the risk of complications to patients is to use the example of a lottery. In medicine, you "never say 'never' and never say 'always.'" And yet, the likelihood of some things happening is almost "never." So I ask the patients if they play the lotto. Most of them do, at least occasionally. I then ask them if they will ever win. Most of them say, "No." I then reply, "But you could, right?" and they say, "Yes." I then explain that many complications are just like that. It is not going to happen, but if you play "the lotto," it could. This example really helps them to understand the risk of complications. (So one day, a patient called up and said that he had won the lotto. A resident who was working with me got excited. I had to tell him that that wasn't good!)

14. I (J.L.P.) have always liked to explain to patients how the particular surgery or procedure went. I try to be very honest. I will often say, "Technically, things went well," or "Technically, this case was quite difficult and we had a few problems." Patients appreciate honesty. They know things cannot go perfectly all the time. I never tell patients that it was "an easy case"; should complications arise, they think you have done something wrong. However, if you tell them that the case was difficult, you are not looked on so negatively if complications do arise. In addition, if there are no complications with tough cases, they think you have done a better job. The point of this tip: Never overstate how well something went. Just say that technically things went well, but complications can still occur.

15. I (J.L.P.) have done perhaps 125 or 130 medicolegal cases as an expert witness. A brief tip to avoid litigation: When a patient comes in to the office, always review the last note to see what the complaint was. Ask the patient if the problem has resolved. Just jot a little note (e.g., "breast mass resolved" with the date, or "rectal bleeding gone" with the date, or perhaps "cough cleared"). Many times patients come into the office for a new complaint and the clinician forgets about a significant old complaint, but the patient thinks the clinician remembers. Just looking back at the record and asking that simple question could have cleared many clinicians from later malpractice suits. You would also be amazed how many problems persist that the patients don't complain about and clinicians subsequently overlook. And we are paid for following up on prior diagnoses, especially if they were complicated.

16. The height of your examination table is extremely important. When I (J.L.P.) opened a new office, I purchased a table that was only 2 inches higher than my current one. I found that older patients had a difficult time getting up on the table. The lowest height can be no more than 24 inches for these patients. A power table is essential if you are going to be doing procedures.

17. There are really few *medical emergencies* in a clinician's office. However, one of them can be *anaphylaxis* (see Chapter 212, Anaphylaxis). In addition to the Banyan kit ("a crash cart in a suitcase") that is mentioned there, I (J.L.P.) keep an EpiPen taped to one of our cupboard doors. Right beside it is a vial of atropine and some ammonia salts. I have only had occasion to use the EpiPen once after an injection with *Candida*. However, people were not rushing around looking for the proper dose of epinephrine, or the syringe, or even trying to find "the epi"! We just opened the cupboard door where it was taped and gave the injection. Consider having these three medications readily available in your office, especially if you perform a significant number of procedures or injections. The Banyan kit is the most cost-efficient, safe, and practical way to maintain resuscitation capabilities in your office.

18. I (J.L.P.) have developed a simple method for determining whether or not a patient is likely to faint during a procedure. I think vasovagal symptoms have occurred more with vasectomy than with any other procedure I do. Endometrial biopsy is probably the second most likely cause. As a result of having experienced these complications, prior to performing a procedure, I ask patients how well they tolerate pain. The options are "well," "okay," and "poorly." I also ask them if they have a tendency to faint or if they faint when they see blood. If the answer is that they tolerate pain well, I just use a local anesthetic. If they tolerate pain "okay," I'll offer them 10 mg of oral diazepam an hour before significant procedures (e.g., vasectomy). If they tolerate pain poorly or if they say they have a tendency to faint, in addition to the 10 mg of oral diazepam (if the procedure has been prescheduled), I'll give 0.5 of atropine intramuscularly on arrival to the office. (I'll often listen to the partner's answers, too, in addition to the man's response!) Since using this approach, I haven't had a single patient have a vasovagal episode while on the table during a vasectomy or any other procedure.

19. In the past it was believed that epinephrine should not be used in fingers, nose, penis, and toes. These are end-arterial, and it was thought that the vessels could go into spasm leading to necrosis. As with many past "teachings," this was an empirical one. Studies have not found this to be true, and "epi," in the doses used in local anesthetics, appears to be safe. By reducing blood flow, it may improve visualization of the anatomy and aid in closure. See the references in Chapter 5, Local Anesthesia. Interestingly, these very same areas (in addition to the anal and vulvar regions) are very sensitive. Warn patients that injections are very uncomfortable.

20. Now that I (J.L.P.) receive numerous referrals from primary care clinicians, I think the single largest error that I see involves anal complaints. Frequently, patients are sent to me for "hemorrhoids," and I have found fissures, fistulas, cancers, polyps, warts, and solitary anal ulcers. It seems that for both clinicians and patients, when there is any rectal bleeding, it is automatically assumed to be "hemorrhoids." My only plea would be to look. Many times just spreading the glutei will give you the diagnosis. If nothing else, perform a digital examination and a good anoscopy. In my opinion, the only anoscope to use is the Ive's slotted anoscope. The long cylindrical scopes just do not allow adequate visualization for anorectal complaints. If you as a clinician do not feel comfortable evaluating anorectal complaints, then don't treat them; but then don't make a diagnosis for the patient. Just send them to a clinician who is willing to evaluate them.

21. It always amazes me (J.L.P.) that when patients have anal complaints, one of the first things they are treated with is hydrocortisone cream for presumed hemorrhoids. I ask at many of my courses how many clinicians treat varicosities of the lower extremities with steroids. Not surprisingly, no one does. Then why does everyone treat "hemorrhoids," which are engorged veins, with steroids? It is an appropriate thing to do if the hemorrhoids are inflamed, but probably less than 10% of those with rectal bleeding truly have

inflammation. Again, the rule should be to examine the patient first before making the diagnosis of hemorrhoids and to use hydrocortisone preparations only if inflammation is present.

22. A study was performed that looked at absorbable versus nonabsorbable sutures after a punch biopsy. The study found that the cosmetic results 3 months later were equal.

23. When performing a punch biopsy of the skin, routinely use a 3-mm punch. The advantage is that it provides enough tissue for diagnosis but will not need suture closure. A 4-mm punch often requires a suture, and a 5-mm punch definitely does. However, when you close a circular lesion that is 5 mm with suture, you will end up with dog ears on each side. A 2-mm punch may not be adequate for diagnosis. The tissue is often macerated, and it is difficult to give the pathologist a good specimen. If a 3-mm punch defect is not closed, there will usually be no visible scar remaining. At the very worst, the patient may end up with a small acne pockmark-like lesion.

24. Performing a needle biopsy does not spread malignant cells in the needle track. It is safe even with nodes that contain metastatic melanoma. Similarly, shaving a nevus does not lead to malignant transformation. This may need to be explained to patients; urban myths exist which say otherwise. Rarely is a suture ever needed for biopsies 3 mm or less, unless in very cosmetic areas such as in young faces.

25. The work-up for abnormal uterine bleeding is currently generally managed with an endometrial biopsy (see Chapter 129, Endometrial Biopsy). In the past, fractional dilation and curettage (D&C) procedures were somewhat considered the standard. Endometrial biopsy has somewhat become the procedure of choice, with transvaginal ultrasound (TVUS) being an acceptable option in some women, especially those in whom endometrial biopsy was performed but the sample was insufficient for diagnosis. Many of us perform both. Although many of us have jumped to TVUS to evaluate abnormal uterine bleeding, there is an ethnic variance in normal endometrial lining thickness. Although the safe cut-off quoted is 5 mm of endometrial stripe, cancers have been found with only 3 mm of stripe in Japanese patients. Endometrial biopsy with ECC is still, in my (J.L.P.'s) estimation, the best way to evaluate abnormal uterine bleeding. That said, in 2009, ACOG stated when TVUS is performed for patients with postmenopausal bleeding and an endometrial thickness of less than or equal to 4 mm is found, endometrial sampling is not required. Regardless, the caveat is to be sure that the bleeding is "uterine" and that other potential causes are not overlooked.

26. Unless extensive stitching is to be done, sterile gloves are not needed for routine biopsies and most skin procedures. However, nonsterile gloves are recommended.

27. A potential pitfall in interpreting Papanicolaou (Pap) smear results is to confuse atypical squamous cells of undetermined significance (ASCUS) with atypical glandular cells (AGCs) and ASC-H (atypical squamous cells, high-grade lesion cannot be ruled out). Should a Pap smear come back with either AGCs or ASC-H, it is imperative that the patient undergo a complete work-up, beginning with colposcopy. A consensus of studies shows that approximately 10% of patients with AGC will have a cancer somewhere in the genital tract if indeed the cells are glandular and atypical. Another 10% to 15% will have high-grade dysplastic lesions. Be careful not to confuse atypical squamous cells with AGC.

28. I (J.L.P.) have found that using the medium titanium hemoclips for performing vasectomies for fascial occlusion has been a timesaver, reduces the amount of bleeding present during the procedure, and is cost effective. When introduced to the clips, I was resistant because I was going to have to incur another cost for the applicators. However, when suture material is used to perform the purse string around the fascia, the suture material also adds to the cost. In addition, bleeding often occurs with the insertion of the needle, and it takes more time. Currently, if there is bleeding

in the fascial tissues around the vas, the titanium clip will readily and quickly control it. Patients often ask if the clips set off metal detectors. Because they are nonmagnetic, they do not. After a vas there will often be a slight palpable nodule, but by 3 months, patients are unable to detect any sign of the clip. If the patient continues to be worried, I just tell him to think about all the men who have fought in various battles during wars and who have shrapnel remaining in their bodies that does not cause them problems. This example usually eases the patient's mind.

29. In regard to billing, consider billing a handling fee (99000) when any labs are sent out to the hospital or other laboratory. Although many health maintenance organizations, Medicare, and Medicaid may not reimburse it, a few private insurance companies do. This covers your costs for documenting that the labs were sent out, for receiving the labs back, and for calling the patient. Even if only a small percentage of these fees is paid, it is still worthwhile charging for them.

30. "Insurance only" statements on your bills may get you into trouble. If you write "insurance only," it negates the insurance company's obligation to pay you. Treating certain patients, such as clinicians and friends, for free is a medical tradition, but be careful. The changes in the law have made it a bad idea. The courts ruled in 1991 that clinicians cannot charge insurance companies if they make this statement! (Don't you just love how everyone else tells us what to do? My suggestion: Be creative, and be the clinician you want to be. You can figure out a way around this bureaucratic hassle.)

31. If you write off the patient portion of a Medicare bill, document well why it is a hardship case. Otherwise, Medicare can sue you and reclaim many of the fees they have paid you.

32. For Medicare, you cannot bill for treating your own family, which includes husband, wife, parents (even if you are adopted), children, siblings, step-relatives, grandparents, and domestic employees. It is okay for your partner to treat them, but not for insurance only. See Pearl 30.

33. For those of you who are audited and your current procedural terminology (CPT) coding is questioned, see King, 2000. He and colleagues found that giving the same procedure to various coding experts resulted in various methods of coding out the procedure. Their conclusion was that CPT coding is not objective. This finding may help you in court!

34. I (GCF) suggest that you spend some quality time on coding and that you buy a good book on coding. While writing the foreign body removal chapter, I found that "10120" is the routine code for general removal of a subcutaneous foreign body. However, if the foreign body is located in the area of the shoulder and is subcutaneous, the code is 23330 and the relative value units for this code are almost three times that for 10120! Knowing your coding and billing can markedly increase reimbursement.

35. It is difficult for us to know exactly what to charge for each procedure. I (J.L.P.) commonly refer to three books, which are updated annually: Yale Wasserman DMD Medical Publishers Ltd., Physicians' Fee Reference; The American Medical Association Current Procedural Terminology; and the Ingenix National Fee Analyzer. Certain experts have suggested setting fees at 110% of the best-paying PPO in town and understanding you will never receive your full charges. You should also review all fees at least twice a year. Otherwise, if a new PPO moves to town and is willing to pay you more, you will never receive it unless you charge for it.

36. Medicare did have a list of procedures in which they would reimburse a surgical tray. However, since 2003, a surgical tray fee is not allowed. They claim to have incorporated the cost of the tray into the reimbursement for the procedure (in other words, a nice way to cut reimbursement without admitting that they've done it!). However, a surgical tray can still be charged to other insurances with the procedures that require more medical supplies (e.g., loop electrosurgical excision procedure [LEEP]). A surgical tray should never be charged for routine laceration repair or lesion removal, because it is indeed incorporated into the usual reimbursement fee.

37. With coding and billing multiple procedures performed on the same day, always have the biller code out the highest reimbursed procedure first. The procedures listed second, third, fourth, and fifth may be reduced by as much as 50%. Those listed after that may be reduced to only 25% of the routine allowable charge. When seeing a new patient, it is essential to obtain a past medical history and evaluate the patient for other medical problems before performing the procedure. Proper coding and billing (CPT) allow for payment of an initial office visit along with the procedure that same day. If it has been less than 3 years but the patient is being seen for a different problem or procedure or another separate identifiable service has been provided (e.g., treatment for diabetes), a modifier 25 is used to receive reimbursement for both the procedure and the evaluation visit, even if performed on the same visit.

38. Some patients are sensitive to nonsteroidal antiinflammatory drugs and will have increased bleeding when using them. A simple way to check for this sensitivity is just to obtain a bleeding time on and off the drug. If the bleeding time is prolonged while on the drug, patients are indeed sensitive.

39. It is amazing to us that more clinicians are not incorporating ultrasound into the office practice. The newer units are cheaper and smaller and often can use a PC for the screen; apps can even be obtained for smart phones, and the definition has really been improved. Ultrasound is the modern stethoscope. If the stethoscope were developed today, we would call the health maintenance organization and get approval before we listen to someone's lungs to rule out pneumonia or congestive heart failure. Of course, approval for this procedure ("auscultation of the lungs") would probably cost $24.99! Clinicians should be embracing ultrasound technology as a means to enhance diagnostic capabilities, reduce delay in diagnosis, direct procedures, and actually bring down health care costs.

40. It concerns me (J.L.P.) that so many clinicians are jumping to the LEEP procedure to treat every dysplastic lesion on the cervix. Cryotherapy has worked for 30 years, and the documentation is excellent on efficacy and lack of complications. Cryotherapy fails only when there is a large extensive lesion or if the lesion goes into the os. It treats small CIN III lesions, as well as conization (whether it be by laser, cold knife, or the LEEP procedure). Appropriate treatment with cryotherapy removes approximately 3 to 4 mm of cervix. Treatment with LEEP not only costs four to six times more (don't forget about the pathology fee to interpret the sample) but removes a minimum of 8 mm of cervix and often 15 mm. Every study that has been done shows that in properly selected patients, cryotherapy of the cervix has the same cure rate as the LEEP procedure. (See, for example, Mitchell, 1998; Pfenninger, 1999.) Some OB/GYN residency programs do not even teach cryotherapy anymore! I have a difficult time understanding the lack of science in medicine. Studies have documented that 1 in 17 women who have had a LEEP will experience a complication of pregnancy. See Chapter 127 on the LEEP procedure and Appendix K for further information.

41. A fantastic buying resource for dermatologic equipment is Delasco (available at 800-831-6273 or www.delasco.com).

42. Now do you want to read something really interesting? See Harris, 1999, and Cha, 2001. When treating patients, always try to emphasize treating the whole patient. We need to include surgery, medicines, x-rays, faith, and the person himself or herself in the healing process. The second reference is fascinating. Women attending an infertility clinic in South Korea were placed in the study to evaluate the effects of prayer. Half of the group was prayed for in the United States; the other half was treated routinely. The average fertility rate for the clinic was 27% for the previous 2 years. For the control group, the average rate of pregnancy was 28%. For the group that was prayed for,

the average pregnancy rate was 56%! And the rest of the story: None of these patients or their clinicians even knew that they were enrolled in a study, let alone that they were being prayed for in the United States (while they were in South Korea)! I don't think we understand extrasensory perception, clairvoyance, or the power of prayer. But just because we don't understand it doesn't mean we shouldn't use it!

43. When injecting steroids into joints, many of the steroids will precipitate when mixed with multidose vials of anesthetic. (See Chapter 180, Joint and Soft Tissue Aspiration and Injection [Arthrocentesis].) When the steroids precipitate, small crystals are then injected into the joint space. Some have postulated that this may be one of the causes for the postinjection flare some people experience. To avoid this complication, use single-dose vials of the anesthetics that lack parabens, and the steroid will remain in solution. It is the reaction with the parabens that causes the precipitation. After reading about lidocaine being potentially toxic to bovine cartilage (Karpie, 2007), I (GCF) quit using it for intraarticular joint injections. Instead, I inject the straight steroid; this allows a higher dose of steroid to be injected. The undiluted steroid also seems to have an analgesic effect of its own.

44. For those who have to treat umbilical stump granulomas, an article by Lotan (2002) suggests using two ligatures rather than silver nitrate or other methods. The first ligature is tied to hold the stump and pull it up while a deeper ligature is placed to necrose the entire stump. It will fall off in 7 to 14 days and apparently has a better outcome than using silver nitrate.

45. Many people think that taking photographs of pathology (e.g., colposcopic findings) is beneficial and will help in a lawsuit situation. However, if you make a drawing to illustrate the findings, you are "the expert." In a photograph, a plaintiff's expert can contest what you identified. Drawing your findings may be more protective than photographing them.

46. Hypnotherapy can be a remarkable aid for controlling pain. Even if full hypnosis is not used, several relaxation techniques can be used. Use a low monotone voice during painful or uncomfortable procedures. Avoid noisy interruptions by the staff or too much noise in the hallways and around the room. Soft, soothing music helps. Engaging the patient to help relax is important.

47. Compounding pharmacists are currently readily available. They can make lollipops with lidocaine for anesthesia for oral procedures for children and with nicotine for those trying to stop smoking. "Rectal rockets" can make treatment of inflamed hemorrhoids easier. It is beneficial to learn what a compounding pharmacist can do.

48. Consider using a skin hook for vasectomies if you do not have the no-scalpel vasectomy instruments. It not only helps to stabilize the vas, it is also reassuring that the vas is isolated, because fascia will flatten out or tear with pressure or tension. The skin hook can also be used for the minimally invasive sebaceous cyst removal. It can fixate the cyst sac, making it easier to invert and remove the sac itself.

49. Aesthetic procedures have been really "hot" for some time. Not only do patients demand them, but the fees being charged are quite amazing! A 15- or 30-minute therapy may reimburse as much as 3 hours in the intensive care unit working on someone with diabetic ketoacidosis or cardiogenic shock. **Caution:** Much of the equipment being offered is very expensive. Be sure to do your homework and determine what the maintenance fees will be per year. They can often run to $10,000! Also, check on costs for supplies. Be cautious about the sales pitch that "everyone will be running to your office." Many of us have been caught with equipment that generates cash—not for the clinician, but for the salesperson and the manufacturer! See Appendix L on evaluating whether or not to purchase a piece of equipment.

50. The correct suture removal scissors can make a tough job much easier. Fine, tightly spaced sutures are often difficult to remove.

It is worth the money to obtain Shortbent Stitch Scissors (Sklar Surgical Instruments, or Miltex No. 9-101, Integra Miltex).

51. Good 2.5× to 3× optical magnification loops do help to evaluate lesions, treat telangiectasias, and remove foreign bodies and sutures. Consider the Welch Allyn LumiView, portable binocular microscope or flat surface magnifier (www.welchallyn.com) or Keeler Loupes (www.keeler.co.uk).

52. If you are having difficulty passing the sigmoidoscope or colonoscope at 25 cm, roll the patient all the way onto his or her back. This opens up the rectosigmoid junction and allows the scope to pass more easily (GCF). Sometimes even tilting the patients toward their back will have the same effect.

53. Pay critical attention to proper patient positioning for the slit-lamp examination, because this will greatly facilitate obtaining a good examination. Most ocular pathology can be visualized appropriately under low magnification. Use of high magnification causes many users to miss the forests for the trees (From Christopher J. Bigelow, Midland, MI).

54. The extensor tendons have a significant excursion over the metacarpophalangeal joints. When lacerations occur in this area, carefully explore the underlying joint capsule for penetration throughout the entire arc of motion. Unrecognized open joint injuries can lead to significant infection if not treated appropriately. Bites or tooth lacerations (usually resulting from fistfights) are especially bad. Use a low index of suspicion to start broad-spectrum antibiotics. A sizeable ganglion will typically transilluminate, thereby providing affirmation of the diagnosis (From David T. Bortel, Midland, MI).

55. Because fewer elective vaginal breech deliveries are being attempted, external cephalic version often provides the only option in attempting to avoid a cesarean section for breech presentation. If the initial attempt is unsuccessful, it is safe and cost effective to repeat the procedure in 1 week (From Andrew Coco, Hershey, PA).

56. Practice is the key to mastering laceration and incision repair. Begin with easy procedures and work up to larger excisions and skin flaps. Remember, it is okay to remove a suture that is made incorrectly and replace it (From William Jackson Epperson, Murrells Inlet, SC).

57. Consider event monitoring rather than Holter monitoring if the patient's symptoms are infrequent (From Dave Feller, Gainesville, FL).

58. Infarction Q waves can be normal in limb leads III, AVL, and precordial lead V1. ST segment elevation can be normal in healthy people but is ominous in the patient with chest pain (From Victor F. Froelicher, Stanford, CA).

59. The cesarean section is a lifesaving procedure that can be performed competently by family clinicians with adequate training. Hospital privileges should be granted on the basis of experience with the operation and expertise of the surgeon. The evaluation and selection of the patient for cesarean section is the most important step in the procedure. Knowledge of risk factors and indications for cesarean section is essential to proper patient care (From Rebecca H. Hart, Houston, TX).

60. Allergy screening with only 6 to 10 allergens can separate your allergic patient from nonallergic patients in a cost-effective way. Immunotherapy is the patient's only "cure" for allergic rhinitis (From Harold Hedges, Little Rock, AR).

61. Every spider vein, no matter how small, comes from venous incompetence that can be traced back to a perforator. Always try to inject the vein that is closest to the source of this incompetence. The longer postinjection compression (≤3 weeks) is used, the better the result (From Stanley A. Hirsch, Pittsburgh, PA).

62. Many paracentesis kits have a 16- or 18-gauge needle for the paracentesis. This size is generally too large. A smaller needle can limit the amount of "leakage" of ascitic fluid from the entry site after the procedure is completed (From Kenneth Hu, Santa Monica, CA).

63. Knee braces should be used only in conjunction with a rehabilitation program incorporating strength training, flexibility, activity modification, and technique refinement (From Scott A. Paluska, Seattle, WA).

64. A tissue diagnosis is required for any dominant breast mass, even if the mammogram and ultrasound are negative. Plan incisions carefully to achieve optimal cosmesis while preserving future surgical options if the lesion proves unexpectedly malignant (From Helen A. Pass, Royal Oak, MI).

65. Electrical cardioversion, unlike defibrillation, is the administration of DC current synchronized with the R wave of the QRS complex. Adequate anticoagulation of 3 weeks' duration and performance of an echocardiogram to evaluate left atrial diameter are generally considered necessary before cardioversion of atrial fibrillation of longer than 48 hours' duration (From David V. Power, Minneapolis, MN).

66. Send thoracocentesis fluid for protein, pH, and lactate dehydrogenase. Do not order other tests unless the fluid is an exudate (From Terry S. Ruhl, Altoona, PA).

67. When injecting a trigger point, inject directly into the area and then fan the needle to each side along the lines of the skin for best results. Trigger points are usually not round but are oblong and amenable to fanning (From Gary E. Ruoff, East Lansing, MI).

68. To best visualize the sides and top of the bladder, the cystoscope should be rotated around the long axis of the scope rather than levered from side to side. This minimizes patient discomfort (From Andrew C. Steele, Travis AFB, CA).

69. Endometrial ablation significantly improves PMS, moodiness, and dysmenorrhea. Postmenopausal bleeding resulting from hormone replacement therapy can be controlled completely by endometrial ablation (From Duane E. Townsend, Park City, UT).

70. When performing a punch biopsy, it is not necessary to obtain normal skin. The only time normal tissue is needed is with vesicular and bullous disease. For these entities, perform the biopsy on a new, fresh lesion right at the edge where it lifts up off the dermis. This location will afford the pathologist a better chance of making the correct diagnosis.

71. When using plastic endometrial aspirators for endometrial biopsy, it may be difficult to insert the unit into the os because of the flexibility of the tube. The aspirator can be "stiffened" by placing it in a freezer for a few minutes. When cold, it may easily enter the os. A full bladder often pushes the fundus posteriorly, opening the internal os if traction with a tenaculum has not succeeded in doing the same thing. Alternatively, a metal cervical dilator can be used.

72. The Centers for Disease Control and Prevention and other organizations have made the recommendation that, rather than frequent handwashing with soap and water, medical caretakers should use an antimicrobial hand gel. Various brands are available. In our office (J.L.P.), we use Prevacare (Johnson & Johnson). It is hypoallergenic and has moisturizers. Several of my staff have eczema, and frequent handwashing was really exacerbating symptoms. Using the new gels without any water improved their symptoms while producing a better compliance and efficacy rate than soap and water. We get the hand pump container and believe it's well worth the cost.

73. Some patients are allergic to iodine-containing substances, even those in topical preparations (e.g., Betadine). Consider Techni-Care surgical scrub (Care-Tech Laboratories, Inc., St. Louis, MO [phone: 1-800-325-9681]) with such cases. It is a broad-spectrum topical antiseptic microbicide with a 99.99% bacterial reduction in 30 seconds of contact. There is minimal to no dermal irritation. It is nonstinging and also safe on mucous membranes. The only difficulty is its tendency to foam up.

74. Children undergoing surgery develop more postsurgical scarring than adults. This is probably due to increased elasticity of the skin as well as an inability to get the children to limit activity. A report in the Family Practice News gives several pearls to limit the scarring:

- Use more subcutaneous sutures, and place them deeper. The Family Practice News report suggests that if you normally would use four sutures, then use eight for children! If the wound is fairly deep, consider using clear nylon for buried sutures, which will give permanent strength to the wound.
- Leave in nondissolving running subcuticular stitches. If not visible, they won't hurt anything. If the stitch begins to work out, remove it later.
- Place bulky dressings over the wound. This will inhibit some movement and help the child to remember that surgery has occurred.
- Immobilize the joints if there are any incisions over them.
- Provide written instructions, and emphasize the necessity of limiting activity.

RECOMMENDED READING

Alcalay J. Cutaneous surgery in patients receiving warfarin therapy. *Dermatol Surg.* 2001;27:756.

American College of Obstetricians and Gynecologists. The role of transvaginal ultrasonography in the evaluation of postmenopausal bleeding. Committee Opinion no. 426. *Obstet Gynecol.* 2009;113:462-464.

Cha KY, Wirth DP, Lobo RA. Does prayer influence the success of in vitro fertilization-embryo transfer? Report of a masked, randomized trial. *J Reprod Med.* 2001;46:9.

Douketis JD, Spyropoulos AC, Katz S, Becker RC, Caprini JA, The BRIDGE study group, et al. Perioperative bridging anticoagulation in atrial fibrillation. *N Engl J Med.* 2015;373:823–833.

Family Practice News. 2002;30.

Gabel EA, Jimenez GP, Eaglestein WH, et al. Performance comparison of nylon and an absorbable suture material (Polyglactin 910) in the closure of punch biopsy sites. *Dermatol Surg.* 2000;26:750.

Harris WS, Gowda M, Kolb JW, et al. A randomized, controlled trial of the effects of remote, intercessory prayer on outcomes in patients admitted to the coronary care unit. *Arch Intern Med.* 1999;159:2273.

Karpie J, Chi C. Lidocaine exhibits dose and time dependent cytotoxic effects on Bovine chondrocytes in vitro. *Am J Sports Med.* 2007;35:10.

King MS, Lipsky MS, Sharp L. Current procedural terminology coding: do the experts agree? *J Am Board Fam Pract.* 2000;13:144.

Lotan G, Klin B, Efrati Y. Double-ligature: a treatment for pedunculated umbilical granulomas in children. *Am Fam Physician.* 2002;65:2067.

Melman D, Siegel DM. *Dermatol Surg.* 1999;25:492.

Mitchell MF, Tortolero-Luna G, Cook E, et al. A randomized clinical trial of cryotherapy, laser vaporization, and loop electrosurgical excision for treatment of squamous intraepithelial lesions of the cervix. *Obstet Gynecol.* 1998;92:737.

Pfenninger JL. Good things still come in old packages: cryosurgery vs LEEP (Loop electrosurgical excision procedure). *J Am Board Fam Pract.* 1999;12:416.

Siegal D, Yudin J, Kaatz S, Douketis JD, Lim W, Spyropoulos AC. Periprocedural heparin bridging in patients receiving vitamin K antagonists: systematic review and meta-analysis of bleeding and thromboembolic rates. *Circulation.* 2012;126:1630–1639.

Schanbacher CF, Bennett RG. *Dermatol Surg.* 2000;26:785.

Wilson CL. No-needle anesthetic for no-scalpel vasectomy. *Am Fam Physician.* 2001;63:1295.

UNIVERSAL PROCEDURAL TRAINING IN FAMILY MEDICINE

Julie M. Sicilia • Stuart Forman

There has been a great deal of controversy over the fact that there are no universal standards defining which procedures are taught in family medicine residencies. In addition, there is a huge variance in regional and local areas. The inconsistent standardization of procedural training in family medicine residencies is the source of much consternation for patients, credentialing bodies, insurance companies, regulatory organizations, and other medical specialists, all of whom struggle to understand the scope of practice of family physicians, and which procedures family physicians are trained to perform.

The Society of Teachers of Family Medicine Group on Hospital Medicine and Procedural Training met as a Task Force in 2007 and again in 2008 to propose a standard procedural training curriculum. The group consisted of 17 family physician educators (15 faculty members, 2 in private practice) from rural, suburban, and urban areas. Ten states were represented. During the first Task Force meeting, multiple procedures were considered and classified into different categories based on the need to be included in the curriculum (Box I.1). A paper was published in *Family Medicine* that outlined the agreed-upon core procedures. Recommendations were sent to the American Academy of Family Physicians Commission on Education for potential consideration by the Residency Review Committee. The group met again in 2008 and revised and updated the core procedures, which are printed as Table I.1. Advanced procedures were also discussed (Table I.2), and a summary was published in 2009 in *Family Medicine*.

BOX I.1 Procedure Categories

A: All family medicine residency programs must provide training in each of these procedures.
- A0: Residents will have the ability to perform these basic procedures either upon graduation from medical school or through normal residency experience. These procedures do not require specific documentation of training or numbers performed.
- A1: All residents must be able to perform these procedures independently by graduation.
- A2: All residents must have exposure to these procedures and be given the opportunity to be trained to perform them independently by graduation.

B: These procedures are within the scope of family medicine and require focused training for residents to be able to perform independently by graduation.

C: These procedures are within the scope of family medicine and may require additional training beyond the usual 3 yr of training for family physicians to perform independently.

TABLE I.1 Core Procedures in Family Medicine

Area of Care	A0*	A1†	A2‡
		Category	
Skin	Remove corn/callous Drain subungual hematoma Skin staples Fungal studies (KOH) Laceration repair with tissue glues	Biopsies: punch, excisional, incisional Cryosurgery Remove warts, fingernail, toenail, foreign body Incision and drainage of abscess Simple laceration repair with sutures	Electrosurgery

Maternity care		Spontaneous vaginal delivery, including
		  Fetal monitoring
		  Fetal scalp electrode
		  IUPC and amnioinfusion
		  Amniotomy
		  Labor induction/augmentation
		  First- and second-degree laceration repair
		Vacuum-assisted vaginal delivery
			Third- and fourth-degree laceration repair
			Manual extraction of placenta

Women's health	Wet mount, KOH Diaphragm fitting	Pap smear Vulvar biopsy Bartholin cyst management Remove cervical polyp Endometrial biopsy IUD insertion/removal FNA of breast	Pessary fitting Paracervical block Cervical dilation Colposcopy Cervical cryotherapy Uterine aspiration/D&C

TABLE I.1 Core Procedures in Family Medicine—cont'd

Area of Care	Category		
	A0*	A1†	A2‡
Life support courses	Electrocardiography performance and interpretation	ACLS, NRP, PALS, ALSO, ATLS, or equivalent programs	

Musculoskeletal		Initial management of simple fractures
		  Closed reduction
		  Upper and lower extremity splints
		Injection/aspiration: large joint, bursa, ganglion cyst, trigger point
		Reduction of nursemaid's elbow
			Upper and lower extremity casts
			Reduction of shoulder dislocation

Pulmonary ultrasound	Hand-held spirometry		
Ultrasound		Basic OB ultrasound: AFI, fetal presentation, placental location U/S guidance for central vascular access, paracentesis, thoracentesis	Advanced OB ultrasound: dating, anatomic survey

Urgent care and hospital	Foreign body removal: ear, nose
	Ring removal
	Fish hook removal
	Phlebotomy
	Peripheral venous access
		Eye procedures
		  Fluorescein examination
		  Foreign body removal
		Anterior nasal packing for epistaxis
		Lumbar puncture
		FNA of mass or cyst
			Frenlotomy
			Slit lamp exam
			Endotracheal intubation
			Ventilator management
			Thoracentesis
			Paracentesis
			Arterial line
			Central venous catheter
			Venous cutdown
			Pediatric vascular access: peripheral, intraosseous, umbilical vein

Gastrointestinal and colorectal	Nasogastric tube, enteral feeding tube Fecal disimpaction Digital rectal exam	Anoscopy Excision of thrombosed hemorrhoid Incision and drainage of perirectal abscess Remove perianal skin tags	Flexible sigmoidoscopy or colonoscopy
Genitourinary	Urine microscopy Bladder catheterization	Newborn circumcision	Vasectomy Suprapubic tap
Anesthesia		Topical anesthesia Local anesthesia/field block Digital block	Peripheral nerve block Conscious sedation

ACLS, Advanced cardiac life support; *AFI,* amniotic fluid index; *ALSO,* advanced life support in obstetrics; *ATLS,* advanced trauma life support; *D&C,* dilation and curettage; *FNA,* fine needle aspiration; *IUD,* interuterine device; *IUPC,* intrauterine pressure catheterization; *KOH,* potassium hydroxide; *NRP,* neonatal resuscitation program; *OB,* obstetrics; *PALS,* pediatric advanced life support; *Pap,* Papanicolaou.
*All residents must be able to perform, but documentation not required.
†All residents must be able to perform independently by graduation.
‡All residents must be exposed to and have the opportunity to train to independent performance.

TABLE I.2 Advanced Procedures Within the Scope of Family Medicine

Area of Care	Category	
	B*	C†
Skin	Allergy testing Botulinum toxin injection Nonsurgical cosmetic aesthetics Skin flap advanced closures	
Maternity care	Amniocentesis Cesarean delivery Dilation and evacuation External cephalic version Forceps-assisted delivery	Cervical cerclage Vaginal twin delivery
Women's health	Contraceptive implant insertion and removal Loop electrosurgical excision procedure (LEEP) Non-FNA breast biopsy Tubal ligation	Hysteroscopy Laparoscopy
Musculoskeletal		Acupuncture

Continued

TABLE I.2   Advanced Procedures Within the Scope of Family Medicine—cont'd

Area of Care	Category B*	Category C†
Urgent care and hospital	Bone marrow biopsy Cardioversion Chest tube insertion, management, and removal Exercise stress test Nasorhinolaryngoscopy Peritonsillar abscess incision and drainage Swan-Ganz catheter insertion and management Tooth extraction	Bronchoscopy Myringotomy (PE) tubes Sleep study: perform and interpret Tonsillectomy
Gastrointestinal and colorectal	Endoscopic gastroduodenoscopy (EGD)	Appendectomy Anal fissure treatment including sphinctotomy and Botox injection
Genitourinary	Emergency dorsal slit procedure	Nonneonatal circumcision
Anesthesia	Intrathecal anesthesia	Epidural anesthesia

FNA, Fine needle aspiration.
*Require focused training in residency.
†May require additional training beyond residency or fellowship.

In 2018, the AAFP released Recommended Curriculum Guidelines for Family Medicine Residents in Point of Care Ultrasound. This will likely revolutionize not only diagnostic skills for future clinicians but also procedures. Many procedures can be facilitated or directed by ultrasound. (See Chapter 214, Emergency Department, Hospitalist, and Office Ultrasound [POCUS]).

This information is included here to provide a ready reference for those who need it. It is not meant to be all inclusive, or exclusive of any procedure. At some point, it is anticipated this list will be revised. However, at the time of this writing (late 2018), it had not been revised. In recent years, self-study courses for learning procedures in residency have been found to be effective (Deffenbacher, 2017); however, procedure workshops during residency did not (MacKenzie, 2010). Barriers to procedure training as well as methods to improve procedure training have been evaluated (Langner, 2016). There is interest by both residents and faculty to learn and teach more procedures during residency training (Newman, 2013).

RECOMMENDED READING

Deffenbacher B, Langner S, Khodaee M. Are self-study procedural teaching methods effective? A pilot study of a family medicine residency program. *Fam Med.* 2017;49(10):789–795.
Garcia-Rodriguez JA, Dickinson JA, Perez G, et al. Procedural knowledge and skills of residents entering Canadian family medicine programs in Alberta. *Fam Med.* 2018;50(1):10–21.

Harper MB, Mayeaux EJ, Pope JB, Goel R. Procedural training in family practice residencies: current status and impact on resident recruitment. *J Am Board Fam Pract.* 1995;8:189–194.
Kelly BF, Sicilia JM, Forman S, et al. Advanced procedural training in family medicine: a group consensus statement. *Fam Med.* 2009;41:398–404.
Langner S, Deffenbacher B, Nagle J, et al. Barriers and methods to improve office-based procedural training in a family medicine residency. *Int J Med Educ.* 2016;7:158–159.
MacKenzie MS, Berkowitz J. Do procedural skills workshops during family practice residency work? *Can Fam Physician.* 2010;56(8):e296–e301.
Newman RJ, Cummings DM, Lukosius E, Patel H, Carmon T. A survey of exercise stress test training in US family medicine residency programs. *Fam Med.* 2013;45(4):247–251.
Norris TE, Felmar E, Tolleson G. Which procedures should be taught in family practice residency programs? *Fam Med.* 1997;29:99–104.
Nothnagle M, Sicilia JM, Forman S, et al. Required procedural training in family medicine residency: a consensus statement. *Fam Med.* 2008;40:248–252.
Rodney WM, Hahn RC. Impact of the limited generalist (no hospital, no procedures) model on the viability of family practice training. *J Am Board Fam Pract.* 2002;15:191–200.
Tenore JL, Sharp LK, Lipsky MS. A national survey of procedural skill requirements in family practice residency programs. *Fam Med.* 2001;33:28–38.

OUTLINE FOR A COMPREHENSIVE OPERATIVE NOTE

John L. Pfenninger

Procedure(s) performed:
(1)
(2)
Surgeon:
Assistant:
Indications:
Preoperative diagnosis:
Postoperative diagnosis:
Findings:
Anesthesia:
Estimated blood loss:
Complications:
Pathology specimen sent?
Disposition:
>   Describe the patient's condition on the completion of the procedure and whether the patient was sent home, returned to the recovery room, and so on. If postoperative monitoring occurred, record that too.

Procedure:
>   Describe the surgical technique. Include the position of the patient; preparation; measurements; anesthetic administration; draping; details of the procedure itself, the findings, any specifics; any complications and what was done to manage; if tissue was removed, and if it was sent to the pathology department; methods of controlling bleeding, if applicable; closure (including types of sutures used, if applicable); dressing; and any other necessary pertinent information.

APPENDIX K

MANAGEMENT GUIDELINES FOR ABNORMAL CERVICAL CANCER SCREENING TESTS AND HISTOLOGIC FINDINGS

Gary R. Newkirk

In September 2012, a group of 47 experts representing 23 professional societies, national and international health organizations, and federal agencies met in Bethesda, Maryland, to revise the 2006 American Society for Colposcopy and Cervical Pathology Consensus Guidelines. The 2006 guidelines had replaced the original group of guidelines published in 2001. The group's goal in 2012 was to provide revised evidence-based guidelines for the management of women with abnormal cervical cancer screening tests, cervical intraepithelial neoplasia (CIN), and adenocarcinoma in situ. These guidelines followed in-turn adoption of cervical cancer screening guidelines incorporating longer screening intervals and co-testing. The process of revising these guidelines incorporated data from 1.4 million women in Kaiser Northern California Medical Care Plan, which provided evidence of risk following an abnormal test. This evidence was added to an updated literature review. Where data were available, guidelines prescribed similar management for women with similar risks for CIN 3, adenocarcinoma in situ, and cancer. Most prior guidelines were reaffirmed (Figs. K.1 through K.10).

Examples of updates include: human papillomavirus (HPV) negative atypical squamous cells of undetermined significance results are followed with co-testing at 3 years before return to routine screening and are not sufficient for exiting women from screening at age 65 years; women aged 21 to 24 years need less invasive management, especially for minor abnormalities; postcolposcopy management strategies incorporate co-testing; endocervical sampling reported as CIN 1 should be managed as CIN 1; unsatisfactory cytology should be repeated in most circumstances, even when HPV results from co-testing are known, while most cases of negative cytology with absent or insufficient endocervical cells or transformation zone component can be managed without intensive follow-up.

These guidelines are based on evidence whenever possible. However, for certain clinical situations, there is limited high-quality evidence, and in these situations the guidelines have, by necessity, been based on consensus expert opinion. The terms *recommended, preferred, acceptable, not recommended,* and *unacceptable* are used in these guidelines to describe various interventions. Table K.1 explains this terminology.

Several introductory caveats were provided with the 2006 guidelines, and they still apply: (1) clinical judgment should always be used when applying a guideline to an individual patient and (2) these guidelines should never substitute for clinical judgment.

The published algorithms for the 2012 Consensus Guidelines are presented as a valuable resource to clinicians who provide screening, diagnostic, and therapeutic management of cervical cancer precursors in women across the reproductive years and into the postmenopausal period. Appreciation is expressed to the ASCCP for granting inclusion of these guidelines. The complete guidelines are available at the ASCCP website and are cited in the references to this appendix.

Two high-risk HPV tests are now FDA-approved as the primary screening test in place of the Pap. As a result of these advancements and a better understanding of HPV screening, cervical cancer screening guidelines have been reconsidered. Interim Guidelines (Huh, et al., 2015) for Primary High-Risk HPV Screening were developed by representatives from the Society of Gynecologic Oncology, the American Society of Cytopathology, and the College of American Pathologists, in addition to American College of Obstetricians and Gynecologists and all groups authoring the 2012 Screening Guidelines. The Interim Guidelines state that because of equivalent or superior effectiveness, primary high-risk HPV screening can be used as an alternative to cytology. They did not recommend primary HPV screening in women younger than 25 years of age, and rescreening should not be repeated more frequently than every 3 years. In addition, although more research is necessary, the Interim Guidelines suggest that the best management of high-risk HPV-positive women is to triage positive tests with genotyping for 16/18 to colposcopy and to utilize reflex cytology for women positive for the 12 other high-risk genotypes.

The 2012 ASCCP and 2015 Interim Guidelines are cited throughout applicable areas of the text. Please see the following chapters:

- Chapter 120, Pap Smear and Related Techniques for Cervical Cancer Screening
- Chapter 121, Human Papillomavirus DNA Typing
- Chapter 124, Colposcopic Examination
- Chapter 125, Cryotherapy of the Cervix
- Chapter 127, Loop Electrosurgical Excision Procedure for Treating Cervical Intraepithelial Neoplasia
- Chapter 128, Cervical Conization

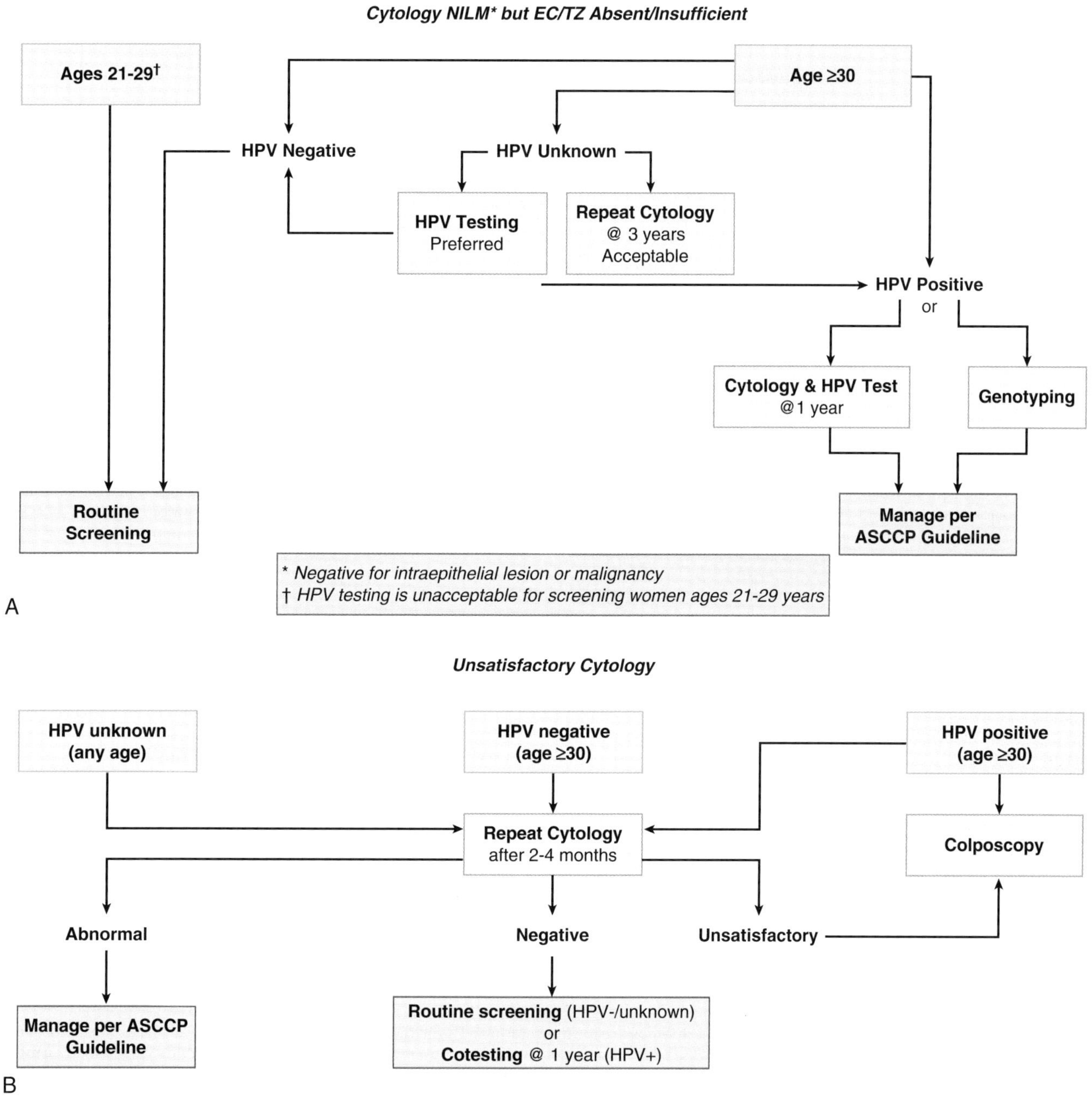

Fig. K.1 (A) Management of women with unsatisfactory cytology. (B) Management of women with negative cytology, but inadequate Pap smear (inadequate sample from endocervical cells or transformation zone). *ASCCP*, American Society for Colposcopy and Cervical Pathology; *EC/TZ*, endocervical/transformation zone; *HPV*, human papillomavirus. (Copyright 2013 American Society for Colposcopy and Cervical Pathology. http://www.asccp.org/asccp-guidelines.)

Management of Women ≥Age 30, who are Cytology Negative, but HPV Positive

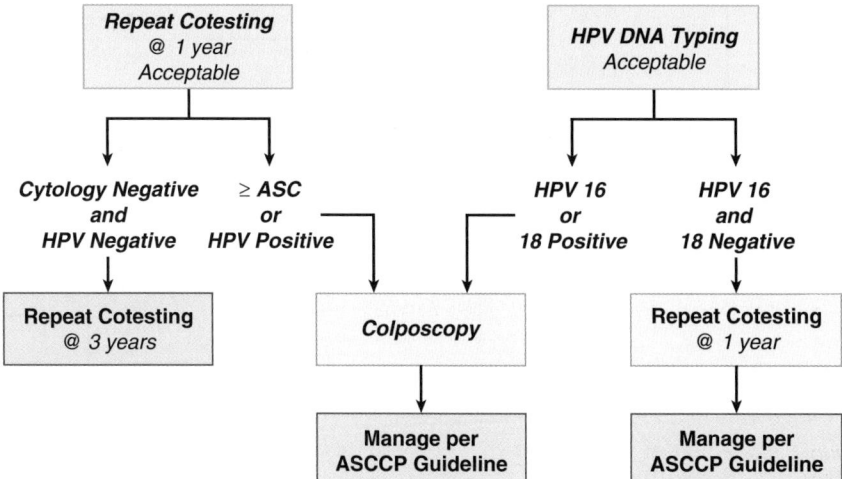

Fig. K.2   Management of women >age 30 years, cytology negative, human papillomavirus (HPV) positive. *ASC,* Atypical squamous cells; *ASCCP,* American Society for Colposcopy and Cervical Pathology. (Copyright 2013 American Society for Colposcopy and Cervical Pathology. http://www.asccp.org/asccp-guidelines.)

Management of Women with Atypical Squamous Cells of Undetermined Significance (ASC-US) on Cytology*

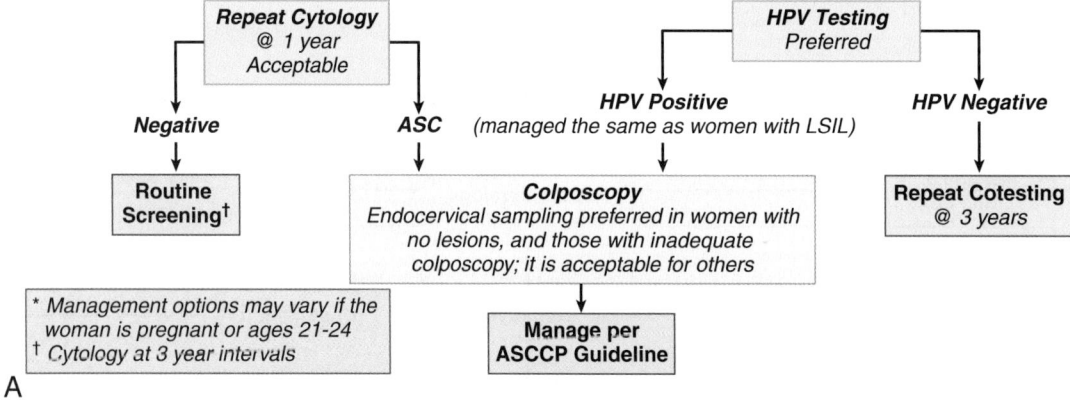

A

Fig. K.3   (A–D) Management of women with atypical squamous cells of undetermined significance (ASC-US) or with low-grade squamous intraepithelial lesion (LSIL) on cytology. *AGC,* Atypical glandular cells; *ASCCP,* American Society for Colposcopy and Cervical Pathology; *CIN,* cervical intraepithelial neoplasia; *HPV,* human papillomavirus. (Copyright 2013 American Society for Colposcopy and Cervical Pathology. All rights reserved. http://www.asccp.org/asccp-guidelines.)

Management of Women Ages 21-24 years with either Atypical Squamous Cells of Undetermined Significance (ASC-US) or Low-grade Squamous Intraepithelial Lesion (LSIL)

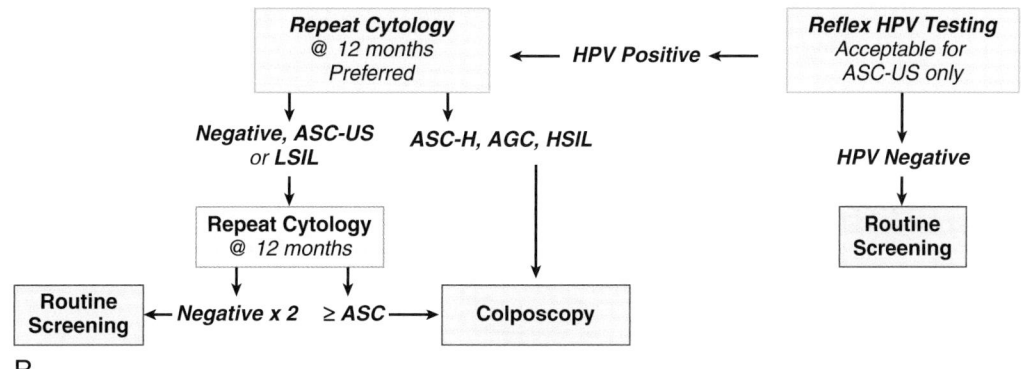

B

Management of Women with Low-grade Squamous Intraepithelial Lesions (LSIL) *†

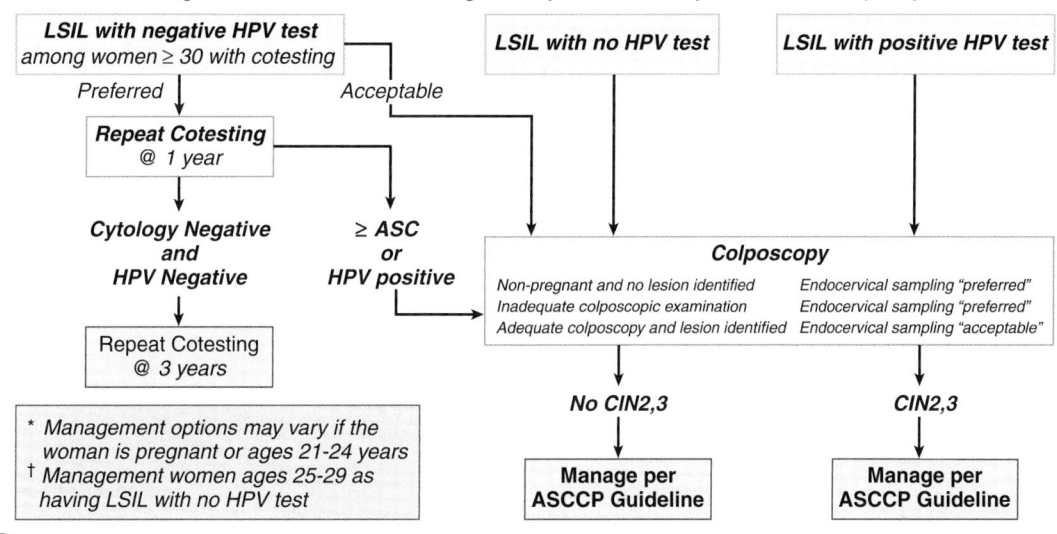

C

Management of Pregnant Women with Low-grade Squamous Intraepithelial Lesion (LSIL)

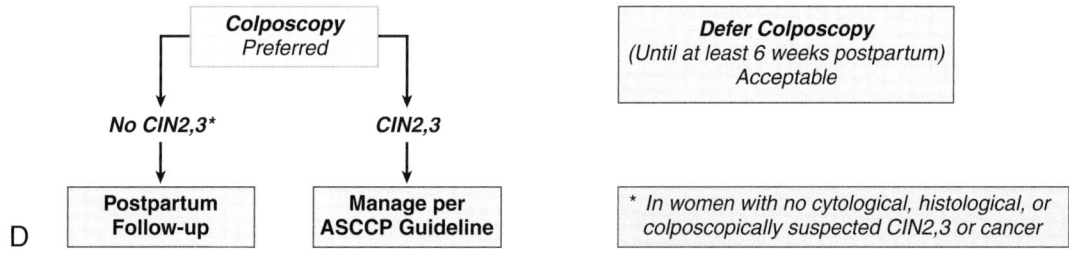

D

Fig. K.3, cont'd.

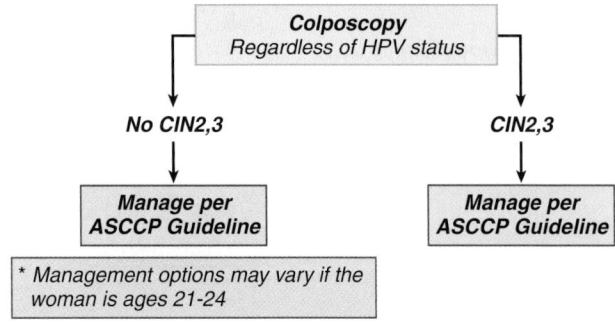

**Management of Women with Atypical Squamous Cells:
Cannot Exclude High-grade SIL (ASC-H)***

A

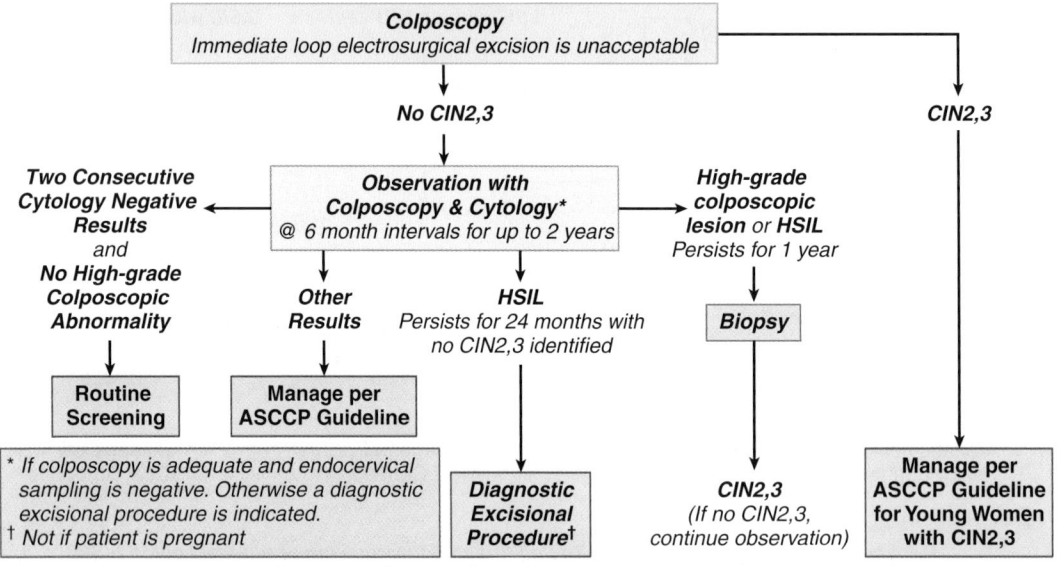

**Management of Women Ages 21-24 yrs with Atypical Squamous Cells, Cannot Rule Out
High Grade SIL (ASC-H) and High-grade Squamous Intraepithelial Lesion (HSIL)**

B

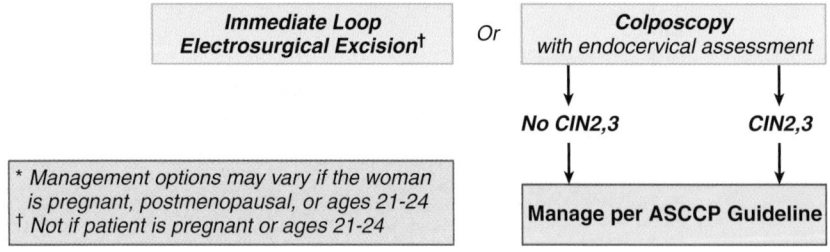

Management of Women with High-grade Squamous Intraepithelial Lesions (HSIL)*

C

Fig. K.4 (A–C) Management of women with atypical squamous cells: cannot exclude high-grade (ASC-H) squamous intraepithelial lesion (SIL) or with high-grade SIL (HSIL). (Copyright 2013 American Society for Colposcopy and Cervical Pathology. http://www.asccp.org/asccp-guidelines.)

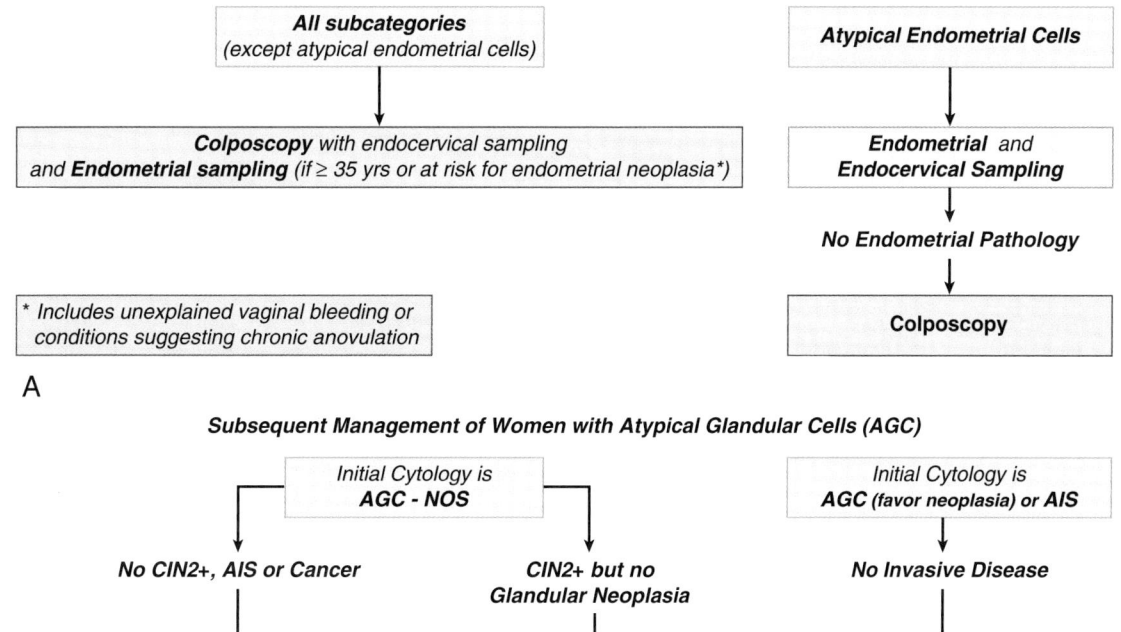

Fig. K.5 (A and B) Initial workup and management of women with atypical glandular cells (AGC) or adenocarcinoma in situ (AIS). *NOS,* Not otherwise specified. (Copyright 2013 American Society for Colposcopy and Cervical Pathology. http://www.asccp.org/asccp-guidelines.)

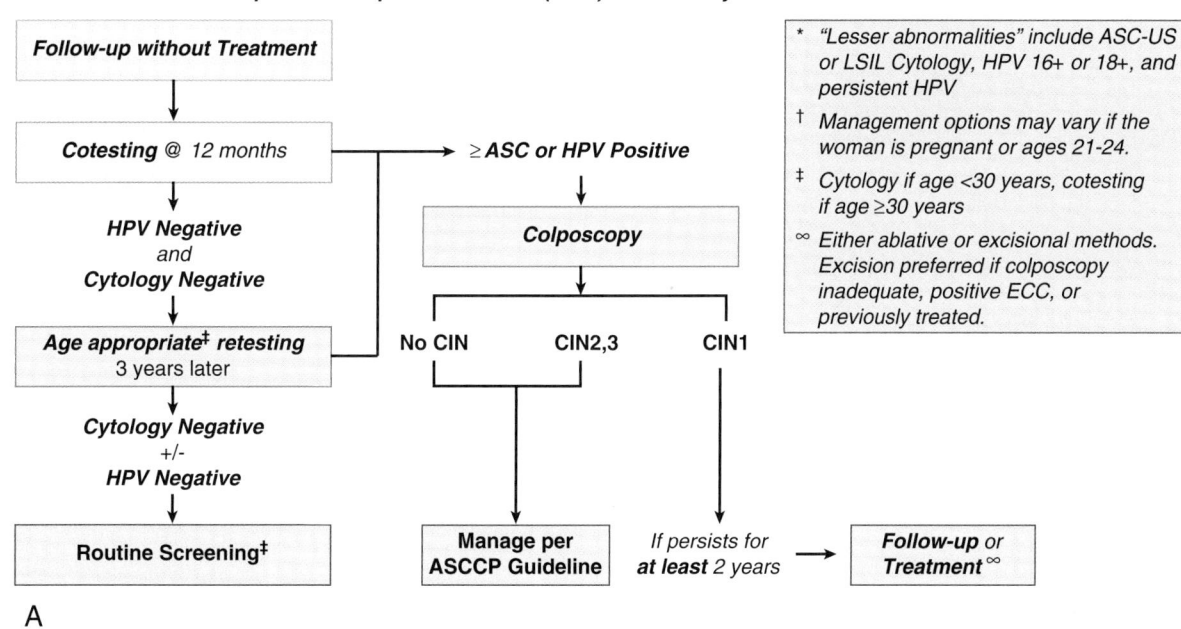

Fig. K.6 (A–C) Management of women with no lesion or biopsy-confirmed cervical intraepithelial neoplasia grade 1. (Copyright 2013 American Society for Colposcopy and Cervical Pathology. http://www.asccp.org/asccp-guidelines.)

(Continued)

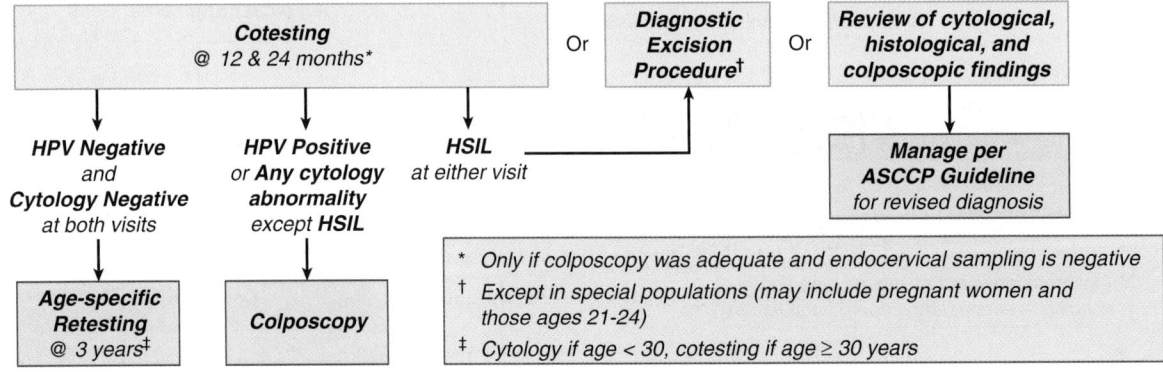

**Management of Women with No Lesion or Biopsy-confirmed Cervical
Intraepithelial Neoplasia – Grade 1 (CIN1) Preceded by ASC-H or HSIL Cytology**

B

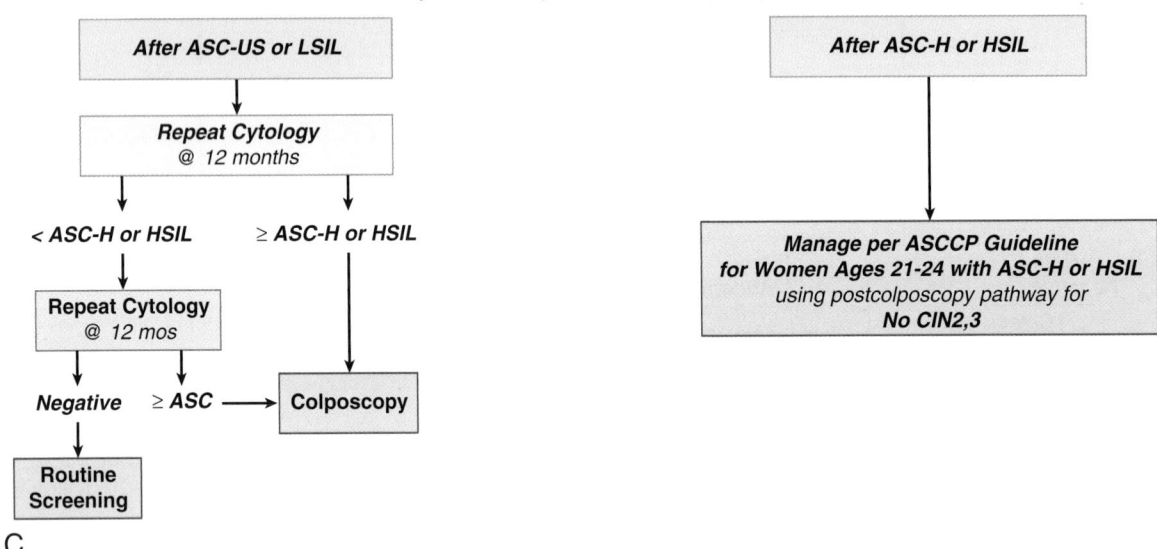

**Management of Women Ages 21-24 with No Lesion or Biopsy-confirmed Cervical
Intraepithelial Neoplasia – Grade 1 (CIN1)**

C

Fig. K.6, cont'd.

Management of Women with Biopsy-confirmed Cervical Intraepithelial Neoplasia – Grade 2 and 3 (CIN2,3)*

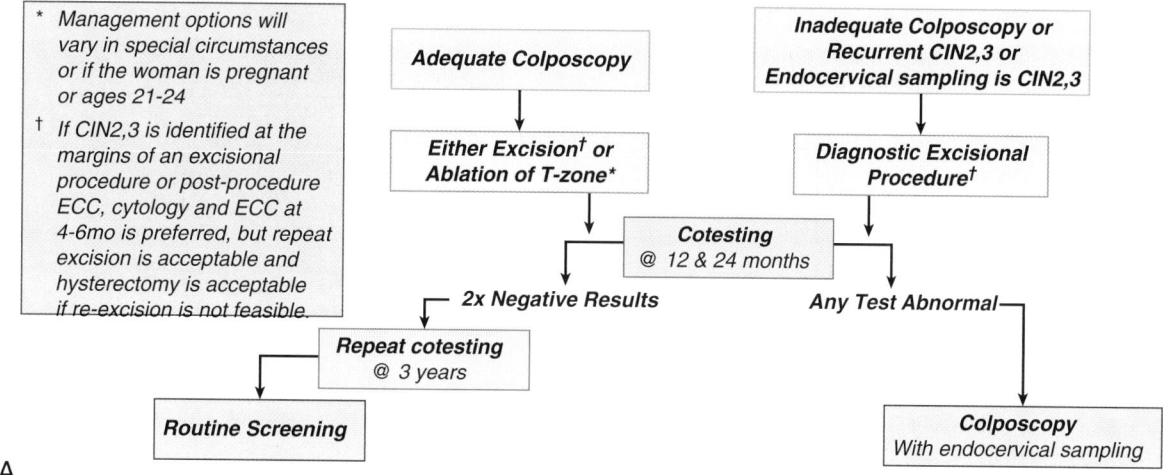

A

Management of Young Women with Biopsy-confirmed Cervical Intraepithelial Neoplasia – Grade 2,3 (CIN2,3) in Special Circumstances*

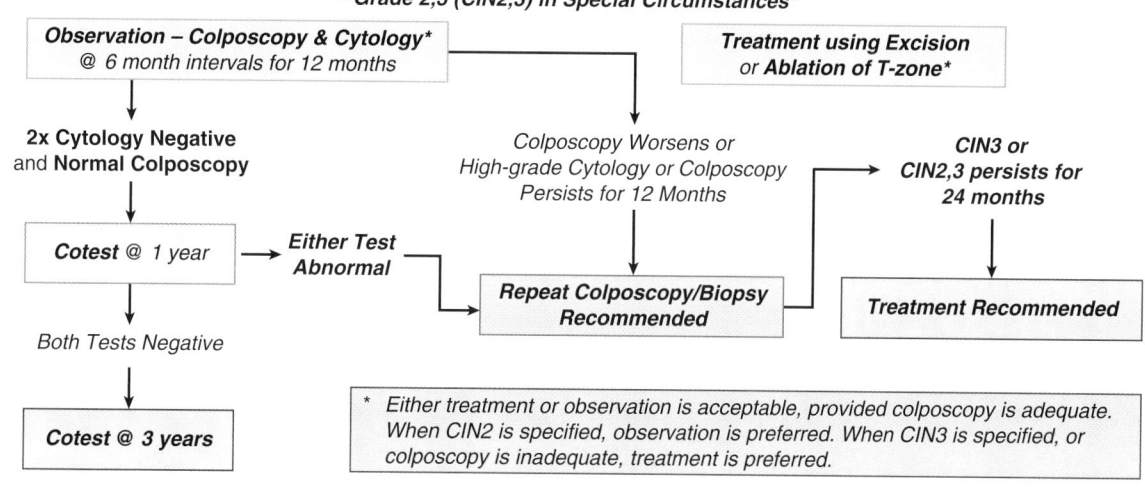

B

Fig. K.7   (A–B) Management of women with biopsy-confirmed cervical intraepithelial neoplasia grade 2 and 3 (CIN2,3). (Copyright 2013 American Society for Colposcopy and Cervical Pathology. http://www.asccp.org/asccp-guidelines.)

Management of Women Diagnosed with Adenocarcinoma in-situ (AIS) during a Diagnostic Excisional Procedure

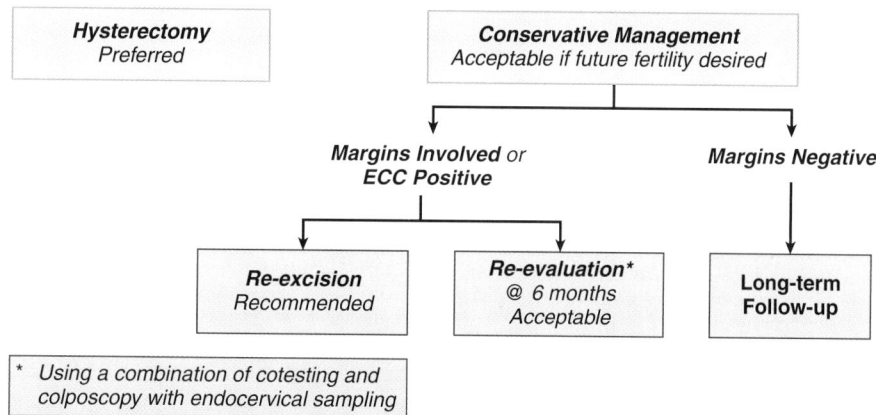

Fig. K.8   Management of women diagnosed with adenocarcinoma in situ (AIS) during a diagnostic excisional procedure. *ECC,* Endocervical curettage. (Copyright 2013 American Society for Colposcopy and Cervical Pathology. http://www.asccp.org/asccp-guidelines.)

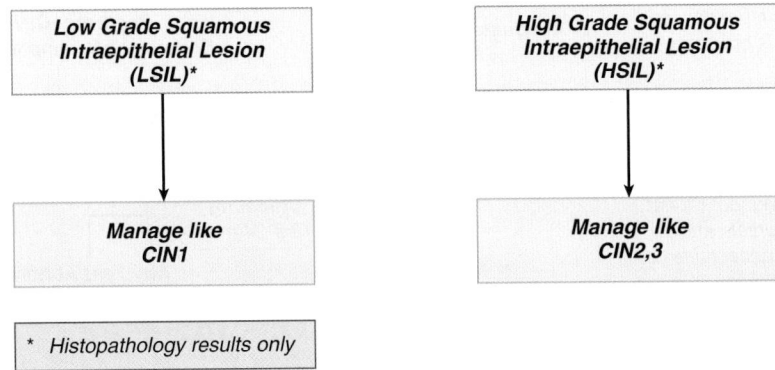

Interim Guidance for Managing Reports using the Lower Anogenital Squamous Terminology (LAST) Histopathology Diagnoses

Fig. K.9 Interim guidance for managing reports using the lower anogenital squamous terminology (LAST) histopathology diagnoses. (Copyright 2013 American Society for Colposcopy and Cervical Pathology. http://www.asccp.org/asccp-guidelines.)

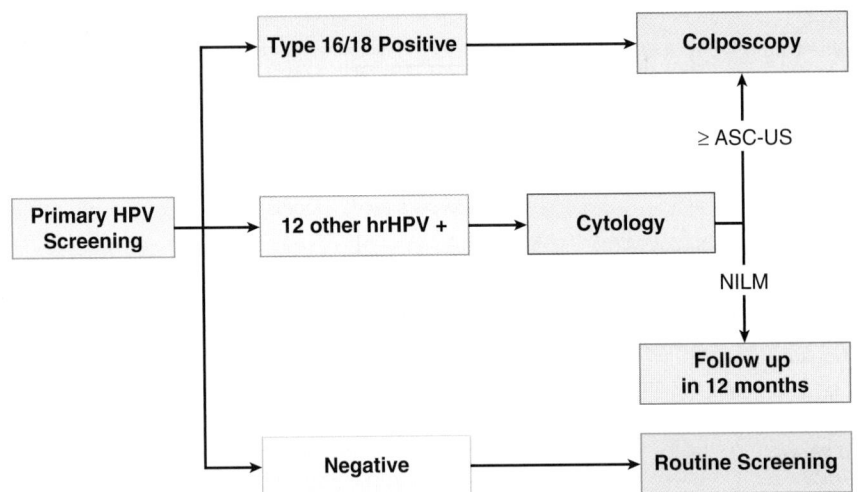

Fig. K.10 Interim Guidelines for Primary High-risk HPV Screening developed by representatives from the Society of Gynecologic Oncology, the American Society of Cytopathology, and the College of American Pathologists, in addition to American College of Obstetricians and Gynecologists and all groups authoring the 2012 Screening Guidelines. (From Huh WK, Ault KA, Chelmow D, Davey DD, Goulart RA, et al. Use of primary high-risk human papillomavirus testing for cervical cancer screening: interim clinical guidance. *Gynecol Oncol.* 2015;136(2):181.)

TABLE K.1	Terminology Used to Describe Interventions
Guideline Terminology	**Interpretation**
Recommended	Good data to support use when only one option is available
Preferred	Option is the best (or one of the best) when there are multiple options
Acceptable	One of multiple options when there is either
Not recommended	data indicating that another approach is
Unacceptable	superior or when there are no data to favor any single option
	Weak evidence against use and marginal risk for adverse consequences
	Good data against use

RECOMMENDED READING

American Society of Colposcopy and Cervical Pathology (ASCCP). www.asccp.org.

Huh WK, Ault KA, Chelmow D, Davey DD, Goulart RA, et al. Use of primary high-risk human papillomavirus testing for cervical cancer screening: interim clinical guidance. *Gynecol Oncol.* 2015;136(2):181.

Massad LS, Einstein MH, Huh WK, et al. 2012 ASCCP consensus guidelines conference: 2012 updated consensus guidelines for the management of abnormal cervical cancer screening tests and cancer precursors. *Obstet Gynecol.* 2013;121(4):829–846.

Wright TC, Massad LS, Dunton CJ, et al. 2006 consensus guidelines for the management of women with abnormal cervical cancer screening tests. *Am J Obstet Gynecol.* 2007;197:346–355.

Wright TC, Massad LS, Dunton CJ, et al. 2006 consensus guidelines for the management of women with cervical intraepithelial neoplasia or adenocarcinoma in situ. *Am J Obstet Gynecol.* 2007;197:340–345.

BUYING MAJOR OFFICE EQUIPMENT

Mark Needham • Bernard Katz

Throughout their careers, clinicians will be confronted with financial decisions that involve the investment of money with the hope for a profitable return. Buying a major piece of office equipment for a new diagnostic or therapeutic service is one example. Certain decisions, such as paying for office maintenance, are relatively straightforward. If the office is not maintained properly or the roof leaks, the practice obviously will do poorly. However, buying some office equipment is optional and requires investing money in a piece of equipment now with hopes of earning profit in the future. Certain financial tools, in particular the calculation of the net present value (NPV), can greatly increase the ability to determine whether to invest in the office equipment and how much to pay for it. This appendix explains how to estimate the value of a piece of office equipment over time so that you can make the right buying decisions.

If a clinician has a very strong desire to offer a certain procedure for personal or career goals, or for needs in the community, and is not strictly motivated by the financial result, the financial analysis that drives the purchase decision may be less important. However, for the most part, clinicians should base their decisions on sound financial principles. In so doing they should receive the best possible financial return for their investment.

Wise use of the tools of financial analysis increases the likelihood of making the correct decision so that the value of future dollars will exceed the value of the dollars invested today.

Presented here is a step-by-step approach that will increase the chances that the purchase will turn out to be financially successful. It is based on a simple Excel spreadsheet that includes all the financial information necessary for you to make an informed decision. To help understand how this is achieved, we will use an example of a practice that is considering whether to buy a bone densitometer (Fig. L.1). Make the following entries as shown in the sample in Fig. L.1.

ESTIMATE THE LIFETIME OF THE PROJECT

All equipment has a finite useful life. Equipment wears out; technology becomes obsolete; spare parts become unavailable; and so on. Estimate how long the equipment under consideration will last, and enter those years across the top of your spreadsheet. For the example of buying a bone densitometer (a DEXA unit), we have estimated a useful life of 10 years.

FORECAST THE ANNUAL REVENUE

Estimate the number of procedures that will be performed daily, and then scale that up to an annual number of procedures. Base your estimate on what you think will happen during the first year of operation. Later you will estimate what the growth rate in the number of procedures will be. Try to be conservative when you make an estimate. If your project exceeds your forecasts, you will only be pleased. But if your forecast is overly optimistic, the result may be a significant financial loss; time, money, and effort will have been expended on a losing project. In the example, it is estimated that during the first year 220 densitometry procedures will be performed.

FORECAST THE ANNUAL EXPENSE

Forecasting the annual expense is more complicated than forecasting revenue but equally important. Take a look at a recent income statement from your practice to ascertain all the categories of expense that need to be included and to assist with estimates in each category. There are generally two categories of expenses; those associated with startup and those that are recurring annual expenses. The recurrent expenses comprise both fixed and variable expenses. Fixed expenses will be incurred regardless of the number of procedures performed, and variable expenses will be dependent on the number of procedures done during the year.

Startup expenses include installation fees, delivery fees, remodeling or construction that may have to be done to ready the premises, licensing, staff training, and any other one-time expenses associated with getting the machine ready to go. Typical recurring annual expenses will include supplies and materials required to operate the machine, staff labor and benefit expense, repair and maintenance, marketing and advertising if required, travel for training, rent, telephone, data lines, insurance, and any other recurring expense associated with the annual operation of the machine.

CONSIDER THE OPPORTUNITY COST

It may not be easy to place a value on the opportunity cost, but it should be considered. In the example of the densitometry machine you need to know whether it is going to be placed into a vacant/unused area in the office, will displace some existing program, or requires new construction. Vacant and unused office space offers the best upside opportunity because the space is not currently generating any revenue for the practice. In that case the financial analysis simply compares the financial return from one project against the other. If a new piece of equipment is going to displace an existing program, then one must consider the revenue lost in displacing that program as part of the ongoing annual expense of the new project. It is important to factor in the lost revenue as an expense to the new project to properly decide if buying the new piece of equipment makes financial sense. If new office space has to be acquired or constructed to make room for the new equipment, then the cost of the new construction has to be included in the annual expense. But one can safely allocate that expense over a long time period and then apportion the expense per year. In the example of densitometry, the assumption is that the machine will be going into unused space in the office, so the opportunity cost is stated as zero dollars.

One must also factor in the opportunity cost of the clinician's time related to the equipment under consideration. Adding laser or colonoscopy equipment to the practice will ultimately require that the clinician spend time performing the procedure. That means when he or she is doing colonoscopy or laser procedures, the clinician cannot also be seeing patients in the office or otherwise generating revenue. For clinician-intense equipment, such as colonoscopes and lasers, you must factor in the clinician time expense into the

Example: Should I buy a DEXA machine?
Excel spreadsheet example

Name of project under consideration   Bone Densitometry

Estimated lifetime of project   10   years

Year of project	1	2	3	4	5	6	7	8	9	10
Estimated number of units of service per year	220	227	233	240	248	255	263	271	279	287
Estimated annual growth rate of units provided per year	3.00%									
Estimated revenue per unit of service	$ 110	$ 111	$ 112	$ 113	$ 114	$ 116	$ 117	$ 118	$ 119	$ 120
Estimated annual growth rate of revenue per unit	1%									
Forecasted annual revenue	$ 24,200	$ 25,175	$ 26,190	$ 27,245	$ 28,343	$ 29,485	$ 30,674	$ 31,910	$ 33,196	$ 34,534

Expense categories

One-time expenses
Installation	$ 1,000
Delivery	$ 300
Remodel/Construction	$ 5,000
License	$ -
Training	$ 2,500
Other One-time expense	$ -
Other One-time expense	$ -
Total One-time expense	$ 8,800

Recurrent expenses
Materials and supplies	$ 1,000
Labor	$ 10,000
Benefits	$ 1,000
Repair and maintenance	$ 1,800
Marketing and advertising	$ 500
Travel	$ -
Rent	$ -
Telephone	$ -
Utilities	$ 300
Insurance	$ 300
Taxes	$ 250
Opportunity cost/Expense	$ -
Clinician expense	$ -
Other recurring expense	$ -
Other recurring expense	$ -
Other recurring expense	$ -

Total recurring expense	$ 15,150	$ 15,908	$ 16,703	$ 17,538	$ 18,415	$ 19,336	$ 20,302	$ 21,318	$ 22,383	$ 23,503
Interest on loans	$ -	$ -	$ -	$ -	$ -	$ -	$ -	$ -	$ -	$ -
Total annual expenses	$ 23,950	$ 15,908	$ 16,703	$ 17,538	$ 18,415	$ 19,336	$ 20,302	$ 21,318	$ 22,383	$ 23,503

Estimated annual growth rate in recurring expenses   5.00%

Forecasted annual expense	$ 23,950	$ 15,908	$ 16,703	$ 17,538	$ 18,415	$ 19,336	$ 20,302	$ 21,318	$ 22,383	$ 23,503
Forecasted annual net income	$ 250	$ 9,268	$ 9,487	$ 9,707	$ 9,928	$ 10,150	$ 10,371	$ 10,592	$ 10,812	$ 11,031

Net present value (NPV) calculation

This estimates the present value of the future annual net income stream
Calculation is based on your selected discount rate

Selected discount rate   15.00%

Net present value $ 41,499

Initial cost of project $ 40,000
(price of equipment)

Sensitivity analysis

This shows the reduction in net present value if revenue forecasts fall short of the original estimate

90% of forecasted revenue
NPV $ 27,534

80% of forecasted revenue
NPV $ 13,569

70% of forecasted revenue
NPV $ (396)

Fig. L.1   Example of a spreadsheet that can help to determine if purchasing equipment makes fiscal sense for a practice.

annual expenses. Other office-based procedures, such as densitometry, are performed by a technician and require very little time for the clinician to interpret the results. Adding a procedure or service that does not require much time input from the clinician, although modest in revenue, may ultimately prove to be a better investment for the practice than adding a procedure that requires a lot of clinician labor, even though that procedure may produce more revenue. An exception might be a situation such as a laser procedure in which a technician administers the treatment under supervision of the clinician. Under those circumstances, clinician time must be considered at least for the initial consultation, and the technician cost must be included in the expenses.

It is a good exercise for any practice to determine what the average hourly net income is for each clinician in the practice. Once that number is determined you can estimate the average hourly net income for an examination room in the office. It is not a good idea to place machinery in an examination room that will ultimately produce net income less than that produced by usual patient care, unless the examination room is underutilized anyway. Similarly, it is not a good idea to have clinicians switch to doing procedures that result in an hourly net income that is lower than what they produce through usual patient care. Therefore certain strategic and career options may significantly affect this sort of decision. Just be aware that, because of limited resources, a decision to do one thing will typically result in an inability to do another thing.

FORECAST THE ANNUAL GROWTH RATE FOR REVENUE AND EXPENSE

Revenue growth depends on the expected increase in number of procedures performed and the change in reimbursement per procedure. In the densitometry example, it is forecasted that there will be a 3% annual growth rate in number of procedures performed and a 1% growth rate in revenue per procedure performed. If you do not think the growth will be a simple percentage annual increase, but instead might increase rapidly over the first few years and then taper off, then go ahead and manually enter the annual number of procedures forecast to be performed each year.

At the minimum, you should estimate that expenses will increase at a typical inflation rate, maybe 3% to 4%. However, for various reasons, medical expense growth seems to have outpaced inflation in recent years. For the densitometry example, we have forecasted an annual growth in expenses of 5%.

ESTIMATE THE TERMINAL VALUE

Most medical equipment wears out, becomes obsolete, or for some reason must be replaced after some finite period of time. You may be able to sell the equipment to a used machinery vendor or get some trade-in value if buying a replacement, but often the equipment has minimal value at the end of its useful life. It may be that you will be building some sort of business or revenue stream that might have value to a third party. If you can estimate what the resale value of the equipment or the sale value of the business would be at the end of the term under consideration, then you can add that value to the revenue received during the final year of the project. There are other ways to handle the so-called *terminal value*, but for our purposes this method will work well.

ESTIMATE THE RISK OF THE PROJECT

If you have gotten this far in your financial analysis then you should have a series of net annual income numbers along the bottom of your spreadsheet. That is what would be called the *annual cash flow for the project*. The Excel spreadsheet program has an extremely useful function called net present value (NPV) that indicates what the value of those cash flows is right now. When we compute the NPV of those cash flows we can then easily compare the value of the cash

flows over time, the NPV, with the cost or purchase price of the piece of equipment under consideration. If the NPV exceeds the purchase price, then the project is likely to be profitable. If the NPV does not meet the purchase price, then the project is a loser. When comparing two possible projects for likelihood of success, the project with the greatest NPV will likely be more financially successful. In calculating the value of the cash flows in today's dollars, the NPV calculation is easily able to compare projects of different duration, projects that may or may not have any residual value at the end of their expected lifetime, and projects with cash flows that vary over time.

To compute the NPV in Excel you will need the annual cash flows. To use Excel correctly, create and label a cell called NPV below your annual cash flow line. Next, insert the function called NPV. A dialogue box will appear that asks for "Rate," which will be described next, and "Value 1." Click on the "Value 1" box, and then drag the cursor across the annual cash flow line from the beginning to the end of the project. That will enter the annual cash flows into the formula. Ignore "Value 2."

You will also need to insert a number in your spreadsheet called the *discount rate*. When you open the dialogue box for the NPV function in Excel, it is called "Rate." The discount rate is a numeric estimate of the risk of the project. Think of the discount rate as the interest rate you would have to pay an outside investor to invest money in your project. If you were selling Treasury bonds backed by the US government, an investor would not require much of a premium beyond the bonds' interest rate to buy Treasury bonds from you because the payment of the interest and principle is virtually a sure thing. However, if you were buying a piece of office equipment to start a medical service in which you had little experience and there was a great deal of competition in your area providing the same service, then an outside investor might ask for a high interest rate, say 20%. This is because your chance of success and the investor's chance of being repaid is much less than if Treasury bills were the investment. The riskier the project, the higher the interest rate an investor will require because the failure rate increases and the risk of not being fully repaid increases. Investors require higher potential returns for assuming more risk.

Choosing a high discount rate, reflecting a high-risk venture, will cause the NPV of the future cash flows to be lower, whereas a low discount rate will increase the NPV. There is no ideal or perfect way to choose a discount rate. Using 15% is a reasonable discount rate to start with, adding 5% points if you think the project is high risk and reducing by 5% points if you think the project is rock solid. By varying the discount rate, you can see the rate at which the project breaks even (i.e., it returns over time the initial investment in the purchase or startup price of the project). If a discount rate less than 10% is required just to break even, you do not have much room for error on your project. Conversely, if a 30% discount rate still yields an NPV above your startup cost, then you have a project with a greater chance of profitability.

You can find the NPV function on the Excel spreadsheet by going to the menu across the top of the worksheet and finding "Insert." Pull down to "Function," and you will be given a list of possibilities. Choose NPV, or Net Present Value, and you will be shown a dialog box where you enter your chosen discount rate and your estimated annual cash flows. Enter the annual cash flows in the box called "Value 1," and enter your chosen discount rate in the box called "Rate." Percentage is entered as a decimal; for example, a chosen rate of 15% is entered in the "Rate" box as .15. Excel will then return the NPV for you to consider when you click "OK." You can ignore the box called "Value 2."

PERFORM A SENSITIVITY ANALYSIS

The next step is to challenge some of your forecasts. In performing a sensitivity analysis, you are going to make your forecasts for growth in annual revenue less optimistic and your forecasts for expense growth more pessimistic. In making these changes in your forecast, observe the effect the changes have on the NPV. The greater the amount that the NPV (i.e., the worth of the project over time) exceeds the cost of doing the project, the more likely that the project will be a financial success for you. Similarly, if the NPV exceeds the cost of doing the project, even when your sensitivity analysis subjects your revenue forecasts to only 60% or 70% of the originally forecasted net income, the more likely that your project will be a financial success. Conversely, if the NPV barely exceeds the cost of the project or the NPV actually drops below the cost of the project with minimal reduction in the net income forecasted, then it becomes more likely that the project will be a financial failure, especially when you factor in any "lost" opportunity cost.

It may be true that certain projects have "value" beyond the NPV. Adding a service line through purchase of new equipment may prevent a competitor from doing the same. By adding a procedure to your practice, you may learn a new skill that will allow you to do something else later that has financial benefits. The addition of a service line or procedure may simply make your practice more interesting and enjoyable. However, although these "intangibles" may have bearing on the final decision, just as the opportunity cost may, the most useful and reliable analytic tool that you can bring to the decision-making table is the NPV. Learning to make a forecast of cash flows for your project, estimating risk, calculating the NPV, and relying on this result to guide your decision to buy office equipment will greatly increase your chance of making the right decision.

Take a look at the densitometry example. The NPV of the cash flows over the 10 years of the project using a 15% discount rate is $41,499. That barely exceeds the asking price of the machine, which is $40,000. Effectively, that means that 10 years of densitometry will result in a profit of $1,499. That is a paltry return on a $40,000 investment. You'd be better off buying Treasury bonds and leaving that examination room empty or using it for storage until you find something better to do with it. However, let's say you went back to the salesperson and offered $28,000 for the machine and the offer was accepted. The expected profit would then increase to $13,499, which is approximately a 3% annual return on the $40,000, still not a great return but beginning to look more reasonable. You can see how knowing the NPV gives you a much firmer foundation to negotiate. A price of $40,000 would simply be unacceptable for the machine under these circumstances.

Establishing your demand price and walk-away price for purposes of negotiation is a great use of the NPV. You will be much less likely to overpay for equipment, office space, or any capital asset if you have a good sense of the current value (NPV) of your proposed project. The NPV is also useful when two or more potential projects might be competing in your mind for the same space, financial resources, or staff resources. If you use the same rigorous approach to developing the annual cash flows for each project, and appropriately assign a discount rate to each project based upon a fair estimate of the inherent risk of each project, then you will arrive at two NPVs that can be easily compared. Obviously, forecasts are subjective and subject to bias, but if you are even-handed in preparing your financial analysis and then subject each project to a sensitivity analysis, you can create a best case, expected case, and worst-case scenario for each project and then compare them side by side. This method requires less of a "gut" reaction or "seat of the pants" decision, but you will be far more competent at making financial decisions.

TALK TO YOUR ACCOUNTANT

After the numbers have been calculated, have a talk with your accountant. There may be some tax advantages or deductions available for capital expenditures, or methods of depreciation, especially if you own your practice.

CONCLUSION

Just as you might practice suturing on a pig's foot, you must practice NPV estimates by making a spreadsheet and "tinkering" around with the revenue forecasts, the expense forecasts, and the discount rate. In so doing, you will get a better understanding of what drives the value in a project, just as you might learn how different suture techniques affect the final appearance of a wound closure. Although your goal in a wound closure is an aesthetically appealing result for your patient, your goal in learning how to calculate the NPV is to win the negotiation with your vendor, your landlord, your banker, your broker, or anybody otherwise trying to take advantage of you in a sale. This may not be what you went to medical school for, but it is a handy skill if you want your practice to be more successful.

RECOMMENDED READING

Buford GA, House S. *Beauty and the Business*. Garden City, NY: Morgan James; 2010.

SPECIAL CONSIDERATIONS IN GERIATRIC PATIENTS

Lesca Hadley • Reena Mathews • Nnyekaa Collins • Christian Burton

Patients in the geriatric age group often have multiple chronic illnesses associated with functional decline of major organ systems. In addition, there are normal physiologic changes associated with aging that are universal to all. These diseases and changes, along with the medications used to treat them, may complicate outcomes of office procedures and influence clinician decisions regarding timing, technique, aftercare, and whether to perform the procedure at all.

Currently, people 65 years of age and older account for approximately 12% of the US population, a number expected to approach 20% by the year 2030. This group consumes approximately one-third of health care provided and a higher percentage of office surgical procedures. The clinician performing office procedures must understand the underlying physiologic changes associated with aging and approach them with caution to achieve the common goals of diagnostic accuracy, decreasing morbidity and mortality, and relief from symptoms, while maintaining functional independence, and improving quality of life.

The subclinical losses in organ function with advancing age, although rarely the cause of substantial illness or disability, impede optimal recovery and increase susceptibility to complications (Table M.1).

INFLUENCE OF COMORBIDITIES

The elderly are more likely to have poorly controlled chronic diseases such as coronary artery disease, diabetes mellitus, hypertension, peripheral vascular disease, or chronic obstructive pulmonary disease. In the absence of significant functional reserves, exposure to sustained physiologic stress may result in acute decompensation and organ failure.

Heart disease affects more than half the population 65 years of age and older. More than 70% of individuals have a greater than 50% lesion in a coronary artery by age 70. Orthopnea associated with congestive heart failure (CHF) influences patient positioning, frequently dictating the need to avoid Trendelenburg and flat supine positions, which may cause dyspnea. Electrolyte imbalance caused by diuretics may induce arrhythmias during procedures. Valvular heart lesions may dictate the need for endocarditis prophylaxis. In the presence of coronary artery disease, sublingual nitroglycerin should be available during surgery, and perioperative use of epinephrine should be minimized or avoided.

Hypertension is associated with perioperative bleeding and cardiovascular complications, as well as postoperative hematoma formation. Achieving normotension before even minor, elective surgery minimizes bleeding. Hypertensive responses to pain, hypoxia, hypercarbia, and hypothermia during surgery may be avoided through judicious use of analgesics, respiratory support, and maintaining ambient room temperature. Procedures may be performed while taking precautions to minimize stimuli elevating blood pressure and ensuring perioperative cardiovascular stability.

Patients with *diabetes mellitus* have defects in immune function, vasculopathy, and neuropathy, which increase risk for infection and poor healing. Efforts should be made to tighten blood sugar control before any significant procedure. Prophylactic antibiotics should be a strong consideration.

Hypoxemia and hypercapnia associated with *chronic obstructive pulmonary disease* can be associated with respiratory decompensation, as well as right-sided CHF, tissue edema, and impaired mental status. These patients may also be steroid dependent. Hypoxia, coexisting CHF, and steroid use delay wound healing. Once again, consider antibiotic prophylaxis for any surgical procedure. Oxygen, nebulized bronchodilators, and positioning options should be available for potential respiratory decompensation.

Peripheral vascular disease is chronic, progressive, and debilitating and adversely affects the patient's ability to perform daily activities. Ischemia and tissue hypoxemia associated with peripheral vascular disease delays wound healing. Postoperative infection may precipitate gangrene in areas already affected by critical ischemia. Prophylactic antibiotics may help to prevent this.

Bleeding diathesis due to anticoagulants or diseases such as myeloproliferative disorders may result in intraoperative bleeding and postoperative hematomas. These risks should be detected and corrected to minimize surgical complications.

Stroke victims more commonly have associated cardiac arrhythmias or coronary artery disease, so extra precaution needs to be taken in this population. In addition, commonly used antiplatelet agents or anticoagulants place this group at higher risk for wound hematoma and subsequent infection. Neurologic deficits may hinder recovery and postoperative care and may also present difficulties in obtaining informed consent.

Hypothyroidism may have protean manifestations (e.g., musculoskeletal or mobility disorders, depression and dementia, slowing of speech and thought processes, cerebellar dysfunction, neuropathy, and macrocytic anemia with or without pernicious anemia). Patients with mild to severe hypothyroidism may also have exaggerated responses to local anesthetics.

Neuropsychiatric manifestations of *vitamin B_{12} deficiency* may include fatigue, weakness, memory loss, and depression. Peripheral or sensory neuropathy may result in urinary or fecal incontinence, ataxia, spasticity, and abnormal gait. Hematologic features include pancytopenia and hepatic dysfunction. These manifestations may influence the informed consent process, as well as anesthetic and surgical techniques.

Hyperviscosity syndrome due to multiple myeloma, other plasma cell dyscrasias, leukemias, or polycythemia is generally not diagnosed until the seventh decade of life. Associated fatigue, weakness, skin and mucosal bleeding, and neurologic manifestations such as paresthesias and ataxia impede healing. Features of the illness and treatment measures (antimitotic agents and plasmapheresis) delay

TABLE M.I	Senescent Changes With Aging
Organ	**Changes and Effect**
Skin	Loss of subcutaneous fat, thinning of epidermis and dermis
	Decreased sensory perception
	Decrease in collagen, mast cells, fibroblasts, vascularity
	Greater susceptibility to injury, delay in wound healing, slowed reepithelization
Cardiovascular system	Thickening of LV, delayed LV relaxation, reduced LV filling
	Diminished cardiac output and vessel compliance
	Coronary atherosclerosis
	Decreased baroreceptor reflex sensitivity
	Cardiac decompensation and postural hypotension
Respiratory system	Weakness of pharyngeal muscles and diaphragm, intercostal muscle atrophy
	Diminished protective reflexes (cough, swallow), chest wall compliance
	Senile emphysema
	Diminished ventilatory response to congestive heart failure, chronic obstructive pulmonary disease, pneumonia
Central nervous system	Decrease in cognitive ability, increase in emotional lability
	Weakness, ataxia, instability
Kidney	Decreased glomerular filtration rate, renal blood flow, creatinine clearance,* impaired excretion of acid load, impaired concentrating/diluting capacity and ability to excrete/conserve elements
	Increased risk of renal failure in response to various stresses
	Reduced renal clearance of drugs; doses of medications need to be adjusted
Gastrointestinal tract	Delayed relaxation of lower esophageal sphincter and stomach emptying, diminished pepsin secretion, diminished strength and contractility of the colon, 90% with diverticulosis by age 90
Liver	Diminished hepatic metabolism
Immune system	Decrease in T cell–mediated immunity, decrease in delayed hypersensitivity
	Enhanced risk of infection
General	Loss in height and weight, increased fat to lean body mass, and increase in total body water
	Effect on drug distribution, binding

LV, Left ventricle.

*Serum creatinine is not an accurate reflection of creatinine clearance in the elderly.

wound healing, increase risk of infection, and influence the impact of any procedure.

Pedal edema not only can make lower extremity surgery more difficult, it also increases the likelihood of slow healing and infection. Whether the edema is from CHF, venous insufficiency, or other causes, any surgical intervention on the area should be accompanied by leg elevation, prophylactic antibiotics, and delayed removal of sutures.

Approximately 10% of elderly patients have some form of *cognitive impairment*, increasing to 47% among those institutionalized. Cognitive impairment may affect capacity and limit ability to give informed consent, follow instructions regarding aftercare, or comply with medication requirements. These patients are not excluded from office procedures, but there is an increased need to assess the level of functional independence and address the potential need to involve a surrogate caregiver. For those undergoing general anesthesia, any patient with known cognitive impairment and their caregiver should be counseled regarding increased risk of postoperative delirium and the potential for accelerated change in cognition afterwards.

PREOPERATIVE ASSESSMENT

It may be best to schedule the assessment weeks before the procedure so that a focused history, examination, and relevant tests can be carried out. This also allows for optimizing treatment of comorbidities, identification of barriers to obtaining informed consent, and mobilization of support systems. Most elderly patients depend on numerous family and social systems to maintain their independence, and these caregivers should be informed as to the treatment plan and details of postoperative care. Modifications to medications, antibiotic prophylaxis, and bowel preparation should also be addressed at the initial visit. In patients with multiple comorbidities, it may be beneficial to consult with other clinician colleagues to minimize risks and optimize outcomes.

The approach to the patient must be geriatric oriented. In addition to the history and physical, elements of functional assessment should be evaluated. The extent of assessment should be determined by the level and potential impact of the procedure on the patient. Psychosocial assessment should address cognitive, affective, functional, environmental, and economic issues.

Most, if not all, office procedures are "low risk," and there is insufficient evidence either to advocate routinely performing any given test on the basis of age or to clearly define preoperative tests that are of value. Morbidity after office procedures is not affected by commonly ordered preoperative tests, so laboratory tests should be ordered only when the history or an examination finding indicates a need. A chest radiograph and electrocardiogram do not reduce adverse postoperative outcomes and are not usually required.

Medication Issues

A detailed list of medications, including those available over the counter and herbal preparations, is important in assessing risks associated with office procedures. Medications can influence perioperative and postoperative outcomes by their effect on wound healing and hemostasis and through drug interactions. Classes of drugs affecting surgery include antiplatelet agents, anticoagulants, corticosteroids, nicotine, antineoplastic drugs, antihypertensives, antidepressants, and herbal medications. Most older Americans (80%) take at least one prescription medication and three over-the-counter drugs every day, and there is a linear relationship between the number of drugs taken and the potential for complications. Although it usually is unnecessary to alter or withhold medications, the risks and benefits of discontinuing medications must be carefully weighed with particular emphasis on potential complications, always with the goal of minimizing complications.

Aspirin, antiplatelet agents, selective serotonin reuptake inhibitors, and nonsteroidal antiinflammatory drugs (NSAIDs) may cause perioperative bleeding by inhibiting platelet aggregation. Traditionally, aspirin has been discontinued for 2 weeks and most NSAIDs 2 days before elective surgery. Nonaspirin, non-NSAID pain relievers are recommended postoperatively. Warfarin, a potent inhibitor of vitamin K–dependent factors, also increases bleeding risk. Recent publications have encouraged continuing both NSAIDs and other anticoagulants or aspirin during cutaneous or dental surgical procedures by demonstrating that complications are not reduced by their brief perioperative discontinuation. This is especially true if they have known cardiovascular disease. If it is necessary to stop oral anticoagulant therapy before performing the office procedure, warfarin can be replaced with bridge therapy using low-molecular-weight heparin (enoxaparin). Warfarin is usually stopped 5 days before the procedure and recommenced the day after. Enoxaparin is dosed at 1 mg/kg every 12 hours or 1.5 mg/kg daily in the interim. Both the low-molecular-weight heparin and warfarin are given for 2 to 3 days after the procedure to ensure anticoagulation while the warfarin takes effect. With any of these agents, meticulous hemostasis during office procedures must be ensured. Of note, the BRIDGE study showed no benefit to enoxaparin versus placebo in patients with atrial fibrillation regarding risk of stroke, systemic embolism, or transient ischemic attack. However, the risk of major bleeding in the placebo group was reduced by more than half.

TABLE M.2	Medications Interfering With Wound Healing
Agent	**Mechanism**
Aspirin, ticlopidine, dipyridamole, clopidogrel, prasugrel, ticagrelor, apixaban, rivaroxaban, dabigatran	Wound hematoma Disturbance of fibrin matrix
Corticosteroids	Decrease fibroblast and epidermal proliferation, formation of granulation tissue, protein and collagen production Decreased inflammatory response Increase wound infection rates
Nicotine	Vasoconstriction
Antineoplastic agents	Decreases immune response to infection, increased infection rates Interference with cell division
Colchicine, penicillamine, phenytoin	Interference with cellular turnover

Unwanted drug interactions are typically avoidable with careful preoperative assessment. Electrolyte levels should be monitored, if indicated based on comorbid illness or medication use, and imbalances corrected before surgery. The use of epinephrine in the presence of hypokalemia can induce cardiac arrhythmia. Propranolol, when used with epinephrine, has been known to cause malignant hypertension and reflex bradycardia. However, rebound hypertension and worsening angina may follow abrupt discontinuation of propranolol or other β-blockers. Abrupt withdrawal of benzodiazepines and antipsychotics may lead to significant hypertension and mental status changes; their use should therefore be continued. Monoamine oxidase inhibitors may interact with epinephrine, phenylephrine, and meperidine, leading to serotonin syndrome (hypertensive crises, mental status changes, fever, muscle cramps, seizures, and coma). Tricyclic antidepressants or selective serotonin reuptake inhibitors administered for chronic depression need not be discontinued before surgery because this may worsen anxiety, agitation, and depressed mood. It has been suggested that tricyclic antidepressants be stopped 1 to 2 weeks before surgery if use of epinephrine is anticipated, because of the potential arrhythmogenic effect; however, with the minimal doses used in the office setting, this is rarely, if ever, a significant factor. Potential complications of herbal supplements include coronary ischemia, stroke, bleeding, and interactions with anesthetic agents. Vitamin E, ginkgo biloba, ginseng, and garlic all inhibit platelet aggregation and increase risk of bleeding and hematoma.

Several agents commonly used in the elderly population delay wound healing (Table M.2).

Assistive Devices

Many older patients may have eyeglasses, hearing aids, and dentures that are essential to their independence, nutrition, and social interaction. Other assistive devices to be considered include pacemakers, prosthetic joints or extremities, and assistive mobility devices such as wheelchairs, canes, and walkers. Procedures should be modified to minimize intraoperative problems associated with these devices and minimally affect their postoperative use. In pacemaker-dependent patients, electrosurgery near the heart or pacemaker site should be avoided. If such surgery is contemplated, the indifferent (ground) electrode is placed far away from the pacemaker site and short bursts of current lasting less than 5 seconds should be used. The cutting currents have a higher likelihood of interfering with the pacer.

Competence, Capacity, and Informed Consent

Physical competence specifically refers to the patient's physical ability to participate in the preoperative, intraoperative, and postoperative phases of office procedures. Mental capacity, on the other hand, is defined as the patient's ability to understand the nature and risk

of the procedure, along with postoperative care instructions. The elements required to give informed consent include the ability to understand and remember treatment options, risks, and benefits and the capacity to make decisions consistent with personal values and goals. Sensory and cognitive impairment are associated with impaired understanding and difficulties in communication. Several effective methods have been used to improve understanding in these patients before obtaining consent, including simplified instructions, videos, instructions printed in large font, and use of health educators, patient quizzes, and multiple office visits to alleviate potential confusion. These strategies should be considered in designing materials, forms, policies, and procedures for obtaining informed consent. When the patient is deemed unable to fully understand the information and instructions, the next-of-kin or a legally appointed caregiver should participate in the process (see Appendix B, Informed Consent; included are some simple questions possibly helpful for assessing capacity).

ANTIBIOTIC PROPHYLAXIS

See Chapter 69, Antibiotic Prophylaxis, and Chapter 213, Prevention and Treatment of Wound Infections.

The goals of prophylactic antibiotics are (1) to prevent wound infection and (2) to avoid endocarditis. Antibiotics to prevent wound infection are probably indicated even in clean wounds in the oral cavity, axilla, and perineum or when there are minor breaks in aseptic technique, where the infection rate is less than 10%. Contaminated wounds (posttraumatic wounds, major breaks in sterile technique, wounds compounded by inflammation) have a 20% to 30% risk of infection and require antibiotics for 3 to 7 days. Wounds grossly contaminated with foreign bodies or with devitalized tissue have a 30% to 40% risk of infection and require more prolonged antibiotic treatment (7 to 14 days). There are no reliable studies confirming the effectiveness of this approach and the optimal duration of antibiotics in these classes of wounds.

In addition, for the office practice, wound prophylaxis should be strongly considered in the very old, those with suspected poor nutrition, those who are immunosuppressed for any reason or have diabetes, and for large wounds and for surgery on the lower extremities in the presence of edema or peripheral vascular disease.

Topical antibiotics facilitate wound healing by keeping the wound moist, increasing the removal of debris, and reducing the surface bacterial count. They may both promote and retard the rate of reepithelialization of wounds and may also cause allergic reactions. Sterile petrolatum is an inexpensive and effective alternative that is less likely to cause an allergic dermatitis or promote bacterial resistance. Although "moist healing" is the standard in the elderly, the moist environment may lead to maceration and skin breakdown. After the first few days, wounds may do better being left open to "dry" for a good portion of the day.

A significant proportion of reported cases of infective endocarditis have no known predisposing source, and most cases are not due to invasive procedures. Although antibiotic prophylaxis against endocarditis had been recommended in the past for dermatologic procedures in patients with valvular heart disease and prosthetic valves, more recent recommendations by the American Heart Association have not mandated this because of the low risk of endocarditis after these procedures. Office procedures associated with development of endocarditis include oral hygiene and dental procedures, especially in the presence of gum disease, nasal cautery for epistaxis, fiberoptic endoscopy of the gastrointestinal tract, barium enema, and genitourinary procedures such as urethral catheterization and prostate biopsy. Patients at high risk of development of endocarditis include those with cardiac prosthetic valves and those with previous episodes of endocarditis. Indwelling pacemakers pose a low risk of development of endocarditis. Most evaluations have also found routine prophylaxis for patients with prosthetic joints unnecessary.

AFTERCARE AND FOLLOW-UP

In the absence of any significant physical or cognitive limitations, most patients recover well after office procedures. Patients should be encouraged to resume activities of daily living as early as possible. Medication changes should be reviewed carefully. Written and verbal postprocedure instructions for wound care, pharmacotherapy, and follow-up should be given to the patient or caregiver.

If significant pain is anticipated after the procedure, analgesics should be continued, making allowances for temporary functional limitations they may impose. If narcotic analgesics are used, they should be accompanied by a gentle bowel stimulant such as Senna to prevent constipation and fecal impaction. Symptoms suggesting complications (e.g., wound infection, sepsis, deep venous thrombosis if immobilization is anticipated, bleeding and bowel perforation after endoscopy) should be explained to both patient and caregiver to maximize opportunities for early intervention. In cognitively impaired or homebound patients, a home health care agency or skilled nursing services may be useful in assisting with postprocedure monitoring and ensuring optimal recovery.

CONCLUSION

The 2 decades following the turn of the century have brought with them a large group of older people in need of health care and support. When contemplating office procedures, it is mandatory that clinicians familiarize themselves with the additional demands that aging, illness, polypharmacy, and the presence of assistive devices place on these patients.

ACKNOWLEDGMENTS

The editors recognize the contributions of Gerald A. Amundsen, MD, Kalyanakrishnan Ramakrishnan, MD, and Robert Salinas, MD, to this appendix in previous editions of this text.

RECOMMENDED READING

American Society of Health-System Pharmacists. *Snapshot of Medication Use in the U.S.* December: ASHP Research Report; 2000.

Dhesi JK, Partridge J. Surgery and anesthesia in the frail older patient. In: Fillit HM, Rockwood K, Young J, eds. *Brocklehurst's Textbook of Geriatric Medicine and Gerontology.* 8th ed. Philadelphia: Elsevier; 2018:232–240.

Douketis JD, Spyropoulos AC, Kaatz S, et al. BRIDGE investigators: perioperative bridging in patients with atrial fibrillation. *NEJM.* 2015;373:823–833.

Fleisher LA. Routine laboratory testing in the elderly: is it indicated? *Anesth Analg.* 2001;93:249–250.

Haas AF, Grekin RC. Antibiotic prophylaxis in dermatologic surgery. *J Am Acad Dermatol.* 1995;32:155–176.

Khazan M, Scheuering S, Adamson R, Mathis AS. Prescribing patterns and outcomes of enoxaparin for anticoagulation of atrial fibrillation. *Pharmacotherapy.* 2003;23:651–658.

O'Brien H, Mohan H, et al. Mind over matter? The hidden epidemic of cognitive dysfunction in the older surgical patient. *Ann Surg.* 2017;265(4):677–691.

Otley CC, Fewkes JL, Frank W, et al. Complications of cutaneous surgery in patients who are taking warfarin, aspirin, or non-steroidal anti-inflammatory drugs. *Arch Dermatol.* 1996;132:161–166.

Perron VD, Robinson BE. The aging process and functional assessment. *Arch Am Acad Orthop Surg.* 1998;2:1–8.

Smack DP, Harrington AC, Dunn C, et al. Infection and allergy incidence in ambulatory surgery patients using white petrolatum vs bacitracin ointment: a randomized controlled trial. *JAMA.* 1996;276:972–977.

Sprung J, Roberts RO, et al. Postoperative delirium in elderly patients is associated with subsequent cognitive impairment. *Br J Anaesth.* 2017;119(2):316–323.

Note: Page numbers followed by "f" indicate figures, "t" indicate tables, and "b" indicate boxes.

Unsatisfactory colposcopy, 843
Urethra
  in bladder catheterization, 684, 685f
  mucosa, biopsy of, 693
Urethroscopy, 692, 692f
Urinary incontinence, 707
  stress, pessaries for, 952, 953f
Urinary tract, fetal, 991–992
Urine, postvoid residual, 709
Urodynamic studies, bedside, 707–710
  complications of, 709
  contraindications to, 707
  cotton swab test in, 709, 709f
  cough/Valsalva stress test in, 708–709
  CPT/billing codes for, 710
  cystometry in, 708, 708f
  equipment for, 707–708, 708f
  ICD-10-CM diagnostic codes for, 710
  indications for, 707
  interpretations of results of, 709
  postprocedure patient education for, 709–710
  postvoid residual urine in, 709
  preprocedure patient preparation for, 708
  technique for, 708–709
  uroflowmetry in, 708
Uroflowmetry, simple, 708
Uropathy, obstructive, 1422–1424
Urticaria, 1402f
  in procedural sedation and analgesia, 5
US. see Ultrasonography
Uterine cavity septum, in hysteroscopy, 895
Uterine Explora, for endometrial biopsy, 881–882
Uterine fibroids, in first-trimester suction aspiration, 781
Uterine packing forceps, 1576
Uterine perforation, in first-trimester suction aspiration, 781
Uterine sound, 1579
Uterus. see also Endometrium
  adhesions of, 893f, 895
  anatomy of, 888
  bleeding of
    in endometrial biopsy, 884
    in hysteroscopy, 895
    intrauterine device and, 940
    Nexplanon and, 949–950
    in SIS, 925, 925f
    work-up for, 1626
  curettage of. see Dilation and curettage
  perforation of
    dilation and curettage and, 1096
    in endometrial biopsy, 884
    intrauterine device and, 940
  postdelivery inversion of, 1060
  septate, 930
Uveitis, 371

V
Vabra aspirator, in endometrial biopsy, 883
Vaccines, human papillomavirus, 960
Vacuum chamber, in vacuum devices, 745
Vacuum devices, for erectile dysfunction, 745–746
Vacuum dressings, 220, 221f
Vacuum erection devices, for erectile dysfunction, 741
Vacuum pump, in vacuum devices, 745
Vacuum-assisted delivery. see Delivery, vacuum-assisted
Vagina
  examination, colposcopic examination and, 851
  first-trimester bleeding from, 1418–1419
Vaginal approaches, in tubal ligation methods, 899b

Vaginal cream, after cryotherapy, 858
Vaginal delivery, 1053–1062. see also Delivery, vaginal
Vaginal discharge
  after colposcopic examination, 852
  pessaries and, 954
Vaginal mucosal injury, after cryotherapy, 858
Vaginal sidewall retractors, 1579
Vaginal speculum, 1579
Valsalva stress test, 708–709
Valves of Houston, 570, 615
Valvular heart disease, exercise ECG testing in, 479
Variable expenses, 1643
Varicose veins, 554
  light reflection rheography of, 537–538
  photoplethysmography of, 537–538
  physiology of, 534–535
  primary, 534–535
  secondary, 535
Vas deferens, 732, 755–756, 756f
Vasa deferentia, with vasectomy, 768
Vasal block technique, in no-scalpel vasectomy procedure, 760, 760f
Vascular access. see Venous cutdown
Vascular access, intraosseous. see Intraosseous vascular access
Vascular treadmill stress testing, 531–532
Vasectomy, 755–770
  anatomy for, 755–756, 756f
  artificial model of, 1612f
  bleeding with, 757, 764
  cautery instrument sterility in, 763, 767f
  closed-ended technique for, 759
  complications of, 764–768
  congestive epididymitis with, 765
  contraindications to, 756–757
  CPT/billing codes for, 769
  discomfort with, 764
  ecchymosis with, 764–765
  equipment for, 757–758, 757f
  hematoma with, 768, 768f
  hemospermia with, 765
  ICD-10-CM diagnostic codes for, 769
  indications for, 756
  laser, 755
  neuroma with, 765
  no-needle, 755
    anesthesia technique, 758–759, 758f
  no-scalpel, 755, 759–763, 760f, 762f–763f, 766f–767f
    anesthesia in, 760f, 765f
    operative report for, 764b
    traditional vasectomy vs., 759
  occlusion methods for, 759
  open-ended technique for, 759
  persistent sperm with, 765
  postoperative semen testing in, 768–769, 769f
  postprocedure patient care in, 763–764
  postvasectomy pain syndrome with, 765
  preprocedure patient preparation for, 756–757
  reversal, 769
  scrotal infection with, 768
  setup, 1578
  skin reaction in, 765
  sperm banking and, 753
  sperm granuloma with, 765
  superficial wound infection with, 765
  suture rejection with, 765
  swelling with, 764
  traditional, 759
Vas-fixing forceps, in vasectomy, 757
Vasospasm
  with endovenous chemical ablation, 554
  with umbilical artery catheterization, 1113

Vasovagal reactions
  after colposcopic examination, 852
  in first-trimester suction aspiration, 781
  intrauterine device and, 940
  to local anesthetics, 33–34
Vasovagal response, in endometrial biopsy, 884
VE-11 Handzfree anesthetic bottle holder, 1580
Vein(s), endovenous ablation of, 554–559
  chemical, 554
    catheter infusion technique for, 555, 555f
    complications of, 558
    direct needle injection technique for, 554, 555f
    foam sclerotherapy for, 554
    needle vs. catheter infusion for, 554–555
    Tessari technique for, 554, 555f
    vasospasm with, 554, 555f
  CPT/billing codes for, 558
  direct needle injection technique for, 554
  errors in, 558
  ICD-10-CM diagnostic codes for, 558
  laser ablation, 556, 556f
    complications of, 558
    contraindications to, 556
    equipment for, 556
    indications for, 556
    postprocedure patient care and education of, 558, 558f
    procedure of, 557–558, 557f
  radiofrequency, 556, 556f
    complications of, 558
    contraindications to, 556
    equipment for, 556, 556f
    indications for, 556
VelaShape, for cellulite treatment, 338f, 339
Vellus hairs, 246
Velocitometry, Doppler, for fetal monitoring, 1012
Velocity waveform analysis, 530, 531f
Venipuncture, 1556t
  contraindications to, 1556
  CPT/billing codes for, 1558
  equipment for, 1557
  ICD-10-CM diagnostic codes for, 1558
  indications for, 1556
  interpretation of, 1557, 1558t
  patient preparation for, 1557
  technique for, 1557, 1557f
Venous cutdown, 1515–1520
  basilic vein (antecubital fossa), 1517–1518
  cannulation in, 1518–1519, 1519f–1520f
  complications of, 1520
  contraindications to, 1515
  CPT/billing codes for, 1520
  distal saphenous vein (ankle), 1516–1517, 1517f–1518f
  equipment for, 1515–1516
  ICD-10-CM diagnostic codes for, 1520
  indications for, 1515
  minicutdown with angimocatheter or Seldinger wire, 1519–1520, 1520f
  patient preparation and general considerations for, 1516, 1516f
  proximal saphenous vein for, 1517, 1518f
Venous mini-cutdown, pediatric, 1106–1107
  complications of, 1107
  contraindications to, 1107
  CPT/billing codes for, 1107
  equipment and supplies for, 1107
  ICD-10-CM diagnostic codes for, 1108
  indications for, 1106
  postprocedure management of, 1107
  technique for, 1107, 1108f
Venous system, anatomy of, 534, 535f